PRINCIPLES OF ADDICTION MEDICINE

FOURTH EDITION

SENIOR EDITOR

Richard K. Ries, MD, FAPA, FASAM

Professor of Psychiatry
Director, Division of Addictions
Department of Psychiatry and Behavioral Sciences
University of Washington
Medical Director, Harborview Addictions and Rehabilitation Psychiatry Programs
Harborview Medical Center
Seattle, Washington

ASSOCIATE EDITORS

David A. Fiellin, MD

Associate Professor of Medicine and Investigative Medicine
Department of Internal Medicine
Yale University School of Medicine
New Haven, Connecticut

Shannon C. Miller, MD, FASAM, FAPA, CMRO

Associate Professor of Clinical Psychiatry
Associate Director for Education
Director, Addiction Psychiatry & Addiction Medicine Fellowships
Addiction Sciences Division
Department of Psychiatry
Cincinnati VAMC & University of Cincinnati
Cincinnati, Ohio

Richard Saitz, MD, MPH, FACP, FASAM

Professor of Medicine and Epidemiology
Director, Clinical Addiction Research and Education (CARE) Unit
Section of General Internal Medicine, Department of Medicine
Boston Medical Center/Boston University Schools of Medicine and Public Health
Boston, Massachusetts

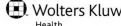

Lippincott Williams & Wilkins

Philadelphia • Baltimore • New York • London
Buenos Aires • Hong Kong • Sydney • Tokyo

AMERICAN SOCIETY OF ADDICTION MEDICINE FOUNDED 1954 ASAM

Acquisitions Editor: Charles W. Mitchell
Managing Editor: Sirkka E. Howes
Marketing Manager: Kimberly Schonberger
Project Manager: Jennifer Harper
Senior Manufacturing Manager: Benjamin Rivera
Design Coordinator: Stephen Druding
Production Services: Aptara, Inc.

530 Walnut Street
Philadelphia, PA 19106 USA
LWW.com

Printed in China

Library of Congress Cataloging-in-Publication Data

Principles of addiction medicine. — 4th ed. / senior editor, Richard K. Ries ; associate editors, David A. Fiellin, Shannon C. Miller, Richard Saitz.
p. ; cm.
Includes bibliographical references and index.
ISBN-13: 978-0-7817-7477-2 (alk. paper)
ISBN-10: 0-7817-7477-2 (alk. paper)
1. Substance abuse—Treatment. I. Ries, Richard.
[DNLM: 1. Substance-Related Disorders—therapy. 2. Substance-Related Disorders—complications. 3. Substance-Related Disorders—diagnosis. WM 270 P95656 2009]
RC564.P75 2009
616.86'06—dc22

2008051433

Care has been taken to confirm the accuracy of the information presented and to describe generally accepted practices. However, the authors, editors, and publisher are not responsible for errors or omissions or for any consequences from application of the information in this book and make no warranty, expressed or implied, with respect to the currency, completeness, or accuracy of the contents of the publication. Application of the information in a particular situation remains the professional responsibility of the practitioner.

The authors, editors, and publisher have exerted every effort to ensure that drug selection and dosage set forth in this text are in accordance with current recommendations and practice at the time of publication. However, in view of ongoing research, changes in government regulations, and the constant flow of information relating to drug therapy and drug reactions, the reader is urged to check the package insert for each drug for any change in indications and dosage and for added warnings and precautions. This is particularly important when the recommended agent is a new or infrequently employed drug.

Some drugs and medical devices presented in the publication have U.S. Food and Drug Administration (FDA) clearance for limited use in restricted research settings. It is the responsibility of the health care provider to ascertain the FDA status of each drug or device planned for use in their clinical practice.

To purchase additional copies of this book, call our customer service department at (800) 638-3030 or fax orders to (301) 223-2320. International customers should call (301) 223-2300.

Visit Lippincott Williams & Wilkins on the Internet: at LWW.com. Lippincott Williams & Wilkins customer service representatives are available from 8:30 am to 6 pm, EST.

10 9 8 7 6 5 4

CCS0211

Dedicated to all people whose lives
have been affected by

addiction and related conditions

and to those who care for them based on
respect and the best science available.

PREFACE

Welcome to the fourth edition of *Principles of Addiction Medicine*. Our goal, as with previous editions of *Principles*, is to provide a reference text that reflects the state of the art in the science and practice of addiction medicine. This goal is supported through the textbook's link to the American Society of Addiction Medicine (ASAM), the world's largest addiction medicine professional association, and through the involvement of the world's leading researchers and experts in our field. This edition of *Principles* is being released as ASAM certification has formed the basis of the new American Board of Addiction Medicine. With this and other developments, including legislation in the United States that promotes parity with other medical conditions in health insurance coverage, addiction medicine continues its movement towards improved integration into the mainstream of health care. We hope that this edition facilitates that movement.

The text is organized pyramidally under editor, coeditors, section editors, and authors. As in previous editions, new coeditors have joined the editorial team and include Richard Saitz, MD, and David Fiellin, MD, who strengthen our links to patient-oriented research, internal medicine and primary care, and Shannon Miller, MD, with his strengths in psychiatry and neuroscience and editorial links to ASAM's peer-reviewed medical journal, *Journal of Addiction Medicine* (JAM). Richard Ries, MD, is now senior editor, having worked on all of the previous editions of *Principles*, and brings his strengths in co-occurring psychiatric disorders and knowledge of how addiction treatment services function in community settings.

With this new edition of *Principles of Addiction Medicine*, ASAM inaugurates its publishing partnership with Lippincott Williams & Wilkins (LWW). This platform will enable *Principles* to reach a more global audience than ever before, with information for professionals about best practices and evidence-based principles relating to addiction medicine. The editors have been pleased to work with LWW in the development of this new edition, and have been joined in this task by managing editor Sirkka Howes.

Some particular issues of note for this edition:

The editors have updated, reorganized, deleted, and added chapters to provide more coherence and completeness to the text, with updates to all chapters and substantial revisions of most.

David Fiellin, MD, leads Section 1, "Basic Science and Core Concepts." The opening chapter, "Drug Addiction: The Neurobiology of Behavior Gone Awry," is written by Nora Volkow, MD, and T.K. Li, MD, directors of the National Institute on Drug Abuse (NIDA) and the National Institute on Alcohol Abuse and Alcoholism (NIAAA), respectively. Section 1 also includes a new chapter on the concept of behavioral addictions (Chapter 3).

Thomas Kosten, MD, leads Section 2 on pharmacology for this edition and has worked with his team to standardize the format for chapters, improve the content and illustrations, and better elucidate its clinical relevance to readers. Expansion into increasingly relevant topics such as dextromethorphan has been incorporated.

Section 3, led by Theodore Parran, Jr., MD, features an expanded chapter on screening and brief intervention (Chapter 18) and a new chapter on laboratory testing (Chapter 19).

Peter Friedmann, MD, leads Section 4 on Treatment. The section now includes chapters on historical and international perspectives on addiction treatment (Chapters 22 and 32, respectively) with contributions from individuals affiliated with the United Nations Office of Drug Control, the World Health Organization and the ASAM's international companion, the International Society of Addiction Medicine. In addition, NIAAA lends its expertise via Mark Willenbring, MD, to fully update the chapter on alcohol treatment.

In Section 5, "Special Issues in Addiction Medicine," new chapters have been developed around behavioral addictions, including gambling and sexual addictions (Chapters 38 and 39, respectively). Joan Zweben, PhD, and Peter Banys, MD, lead the section. We have also included new chapters on hot button issues such as prescription drug abuse (Chapter 33) and college drinking (Chapter 37), as well as a new chapter on cultural issues in addiction medicine (Chapter 36).

Adam Gordon, MD, and Andrew Saxon, MD, join us as the section editors of Sections 6 and 7, respectively. The management and pharmacologic treatment chapters in these sections have all been fully updated to include the most current information.

Richard Rosenthal, MD, leads Section 8 on behavioral therapies. The section incorporates the latest research in behavioral therapies and includes a new chapter on internet addiction (Chapter 64).

Marc Galanter, MD, now leads Section 9 on mutual help and twelve-step recovery programs and contributes a chapter on spirituality and recovery.

Section 10 is fully updated to include the latest research about medical disorders. J. Harry Isaacson, MD, is the section editor.

Section 11, led by Richard Ries, MD, includes a substantially revised chapter by Edward Nunes, MD, on co-occurring addiction and affective disorders (Chapter 84) as well as a new chapter on co-occurring addiction and posttraumatic stress disorder (PTSD) (Chapter 90).

Section 12 covers the increasingly relevant topic of pain and addiction and is led by Edward Covington, MD, Margaret

Kotz, DO, and Seddon Savage, MD, all of whom have also contributed chapters to the section.

Deborah Simkin, MD, John Knight, MD, and Ramon Solhkhah, MD, lead Section 13 on children and adolescents. The section has been greatly enhanced with new chapters on epidemiology (Chapter 97) and adolescent smoking (Chapter 101), as well as the addition of more dynamic attention to biological risk and protective factors in the developing human brain (Chapter 100).

Bonnie Wilford, MS and Robert DuPont, MD lead Section 14, "Ethical, Legal, and Liability Issues in Addiction Practice," which features an opening chapter by H. Westley Clark, MD, JD, Director of the Center for Substance Abuse Treatment under the Substance Abuse and Mental Health Services Administration (SAMHSA).

A NOTE ABOUT TERMINOLOGY

The editors of *Principles of Addiction Medicine* recognize that addiction is a medical condition with its own terminology used by not only clinicians and researchers but also patients, policy makers, the press, families, and other stakeholders. There are certain key terms that can have several meanings and, often unintended, effects. Most importantly, such terms can further the stigma about people and patients with addiction disorders. The terms *alcoholic* and *addict* are examples of such terms—they can be used by health care workers in a pejorative manner to label a problem medical patient, by family to label a member's violent and irresponsible behavior, by persons with substance dependence attending 12-step meetings as a positive label defining themselves as actively participating in recovery, by the general public to define anybody "who drinks too much" or "is a drug user," and by addiction professionals to indicate a patient's substance dependence. Pejorative terms can erode the motivation of people affected by these disorders to come forward for help from family, friends, or professionals. Inaccurate terms can cause confusion and lead to unclear research results, difficulty translating such results into practice, and inappropriate clinical care. Furthermore, inappropriate and imprecise terms can dehumanize patients as well as undermine and erode efforts toward scientifically informed and ethically appropriate public policy or legislation, including funding for research, treatment, or graduate medical education.

However, we must confess that consensus definitions of the many terms in addiction medicine have not yet been reached. As such, ASAM has commissioned The Descriptive and Diagnostic Terminology Action Group to begin to address these issues, hopefully finalizing an improved lexicon for the future. This group has identified a number of terms that have the potential to be inaccurate or even stigmatizing, and, therefore, we are attempting in this edition to avoid such terms—in particular those that can be stigmatizing.

Addiction medicine is shaped by constantly evolving science and practical clinical experience. It is our sincere hope that this book will embody the best of what both of these can offer to clinicians as we work to serve our patients and society.

ACKNOWLEDGMENTS

The editors wish to thank the American Society of Addiction Medicine (ASAM) for the opportunity to work on this textbook. Our section editors and authors generously lent their time and expertise. Robert Anthenelli, MD, B.J. Casey, PhD, and Monique Ernst, MD graciously reviewed chapters. Charley Mitchell and Sirkka Howes at Lippincott Williams & Wilkins helped bring the project to fruition. Finally, we wish to acknowledge the contributions of the editors of previous editions of *Principles of Addiction Medicine*.

SECTION EDITORS

Peter Banys, MD
Clinical Professor of Psychiatry
University of California, San Francisco
VA Medical Center
San Francisco, California

Edward C. Covington, MD
Director, Chronic Pain Rehabilitation Program
Cleveland Clinic
Cleveland, Ohio

John A. Dani, PhD
Professor of Neuroscience
Baylor College of Medicine
Houston, Texas

Robert L. DuPont, MD, FASAM
Clinical Professor of Psychiatry
Georgetown University
President, Institute for Behavior and Health
Rockville, Maryland

David A. Fiellin, MD
Associate Professor of Medicine and Investigative Medicine
Yale University School of Medicine
Department of Internal Medicine
New Haven, Connecticut

Peter D. Friedmann, MD, MPH
Professor, Departments of Medicine & Community Health
Alpert Medical School of Brown University
Director, Center on Systems, Outcomes & Quality in Chronic Disease & Rehabilitation
Providence Veterans Affairs Medical Center
Rhode Island Hospital
Providence, Rhode Island

Marc Galanter, MD, FASAM
Professor and Director, Division of Alcoholism and Drug Abuse
NYU School of Medicine
New York, New York

R. Jeffrey Goldsmith, MD
Professor of Clinical Psychiatry
College of Medicine, University of Cincinnati
Staff Psychiatrist
Mental Health Care Line
Cincinnati VA Medical Center
Cincinnati, Ohio

Adam J. Gordon, MD, MPH, FACP, FASAM
Assistant Professor of Medicine and Advisory Dean
University of Pittsburgh School of Medicine
Associate Clinical Director, Mental Illness Research & Education Center
Center for Health Equity Research and Promotion
VA Pittsburgh Healthcare System
Pittsburgh, Pennsylvania

David A. Gorelick, MD, PhD
Senior Investigator, Intramural Research Program
National Institute on Drug Abuse, National Institutes of Health
Adjunct Professor, Department of Psychiatry
University of Maryland School of Medicine
Baltimore, Maryland

J. Harry Isaacson, MD, FACP
Associate Professor of Internal Medicine
Cleveland Clinic Lerner College of Medicine
Vice Chairman, General Internal Medicine
Cleveland Clinic
Cleveland, Ohio

John R. Knight, MD
Associate Professor of Pediatrics
Harvard Medical School
Director, Center for Adolescent Substance Abuse Research
Children's Hospital Boston
Boston, Massachusetts

Thomas R. Kosten, MD
Professor of Psychiatry and Neuroscience
Baylor College of Medicine
Director and Vice Chair, Psychiatry, Addictions, and Neuroscience
Michael E. DeBakey Veterans Administration Medical Center
Houston, Texas

Margaret M. Kotz, DO
Associate Professor of Psychiatry
Case Medical Center
Director of Addiction Recovery Services
University Hospitals
Cleveland, Ohio

Theodore V. Parran, Jr., MD, FACP
Associate Clinical Professor, Department of Internal Medicine
Case Western Reserve University School of Medicine
Associate Medical Director, Rosary Hall Addiction Services
St. Vincent Charity Hospital
Cleveland, Ohio

Richard K. Ries, MD, FAPA, FASAM
Professor of Psychiatry
Director, Division of Addictions, Department of Psychiatry and Behavioral Sciences
University of Washington
Medical Director, Harborview Addictions and Rehabilitation Psychiatry Programs
Harborview Medical Center
Seattle, Washington

Richard N. Rosenthal, MD
Professor of Clinical Psychiatry
Columbia University College of Physicians & Surgeons
Chairman, Department of Psychiatry & Behavioral Health
St. Luke's-Roosevelt Hospital Center
New York, New York

Seddon R. Savage, MD, MS, FASAM
Director, Dartmouth Center on Addiction Recovery and Education (DCARE)
Pain Consultant, Manchester VA Medical Center
Associate Professor of Anesthesiology, Dartmouth Medical School, Adjunct Faculty
Hanover, New Hampshire

Andrew J. Saxon, MD
Professor of Psychiatry & Behavioral Sciences
University of Washington
Director, Addiction Patient Care Line, Mental Health Service
VA Puget Sound Health Care System
Seattle, Washington

Deborah R. Simkin, MD
Section Head, Division of Child and Adolescent Psychiatry
Residency Training Director, Adjunct Associate Professor
University of South Alabama Medical School
Mobile, Alabama

Ramon Solhkhah, MD
Director, The Child and Family Institute
Chief, Division of Child and Adolescent Psychiatry
St. Luke's-Roosevelt Hospital Center
Assistant Professor of Clinical Psychiatry
Columbia University College of Physicians and Surgeons
New York, New York

Bonnie B. Wilford, MS
Executive Director, Coalition on Physician Education in Substance Use Disorders (COPE)
Yale University School of Medicine
New Haven, Connecticut

Joan E. Zweben, PhD
Clinical Professor of Psychiatry
University of California, San Francisco
Executive Director
East Bay Community Recovery Project
Oakland, California

Daniel P. Alford, MD, MPH, FACP
Associate Professor of Medicine
Boston University
Attending Physician
Boston Medical Center
Boston, Massachusetts

Marie Armentano, MD
Psychiatrist
Belchertown, Massachusetts

Ashraf Attalla, MD
Clinical Assistant Professor of Psychiatry
Emory University School of Medicine
Director
Institute of Behavorial Medicine
Smyrna, Georgia

Sanford Auerbach, MD
Associate Professor of Neurology, Psychiatry and Behavioral Neurosciences
Boston University School of Medicine
Director, Sleep Disorders Center
Boston Medical Science
Boston, Massachusetts

Sudie E. Back, PhD
Assistant Professor, Department of Psychiatry
Clinical Neuroscience Division, Medical University of South Carolina
Charleston, South Carolina

Robert L. Balster, PhD
Butler Professor of Pharmacology and Toxicology
Director, Institute for Drug and Alcohol Studies
Virginia Commonwealth University
Richmond, Virginia

Kristen L. Barry, PhD
Research Associate Professor
Department of Psychiatry
University of Michigan
Department of Veterans Affairs
Serious Mental Illness Treatment Research and Evaluation Center (SMITREC)
Ann Arbor VAMC
Ann Arbor, Michigan

Andrea G. Barthwell, MD, FASAM
CEO, EMGlobal LLC
Arlington, Virginia

Robert Gordon Batey, MD, FRACP, FRCP (UK), FACHAM
Conjoint Professor of Medicine
University of Newcastle
Senior Staff Specialist, Addiction Medicine
Wyong Hospital
New South Wales, Australia

Neal L. Benowitz, MD
Professor of Medicine, Psychiatry, and Biopharmaceutical Sciences
University of California, San Francisco
Chief, Division of Clinical Pharmacology
San Francisco General Hospital
San Francisco, California

Nicolas Bertholet, MD, MSc
Clinical Epidemiology Center
Institute of Social and Preventive Medicine
Centre Hospitalier Universitaire Vaudois
Center for Alcohol Treatment
Department of Medicine and Public Health
Lausanne University, Switzerland

Aurelia N. Bizamcer, MD, PhD
Assistant Professor of Psychiatry
University of Massachusetts School of Medicine
Attending Psychiatrist
University of Massachusetts Medical Center
Worcester, Massachusetts

Anton C. Bizzell, MD
Vice President, Health and Clinical Services
DB Consulting Group, Inc.
Silver Spring, Maryland
Clinical Instructor, Community Health and Family Practice
Howard University Hospital
Washington, District of Columbia

Richard D. Blondell, MD
Professor of Family Medicine
University at Buffalo
Attending Physician
Erie County Medical Center
Buffalo, New York

Fred C. Blow, PhD
Department of Psychiatry
University of Michigan
Department of Veterans Affairs
Serious Mental Illness Treatment Research and Evaluation Center (SMITREC)
Ann Arbor, VAMC
Ann Arbor, Michigan

Lisa Borg, MD
Senior Research Associate, The Laboratory of the Biology of Addictive Diseases
The Rockefeller University
Associate Attending Physician
The Rockefeller University Hospital
New York, New York

Gilbert J. Botvin, PhD
Professor of Public Health and Psychiatry
Weill Cornell Medical Center
Attending Psychologist
Department of Psychiatry
The New York Presbyterian Hospital
New York, New York

Andria Botzet, MA
Research Program Coordinator
Department of Psychiatry
University of Minnesota
Minneapolis, Minnesota

Carol J. Boyd, PhD, MSN, RN, FAAN
Professor of Nursing
Director, Institute for Research on Women and Gender
University of Michigan
Ann Arbor, Michigan

Katharine A. Bradley, MD, MPH
Associate Professor of Medicine
University of Washington
General Internist
VA Primary and Medical Care Services, Division of General Internal Medicine
VA Puget Sound & University of Washington
Seattle, Washington

Kathleen T. Brady, MD, PhD
Professor of Psychiatry
Medical University of South Carolina
Charleston, South Carolina

Lawrence S. Brown, Jr., MD, MPH, FASAM
Clinical Associate Professor of Public Health
Weill Medical College, Cornell University
Executive Senior Vice President
Medical Services, Research & Information Technology
Addiction Research & Treatment Corporation
New York, New York

Richard A. Brown, PhD
Associate Professor, Department of Psychiatry and Human Behavior
Warren Alpert Medical School at Brown University
Director of Addictions Research
Butler Hospital
Providence, Rhode Island

John C. M. Brust, MD
Professor, Department of Neurology
Columbia University
Director of Neurology
Harlem Hospital Center
New York, New York

John S. Cacciola, PhD
Adjunct Associate Professor, Department of Psychiatry
University of Pennsylvania School of Medicine
Senior Scientist
The Treatment Research Institute (TRI)
Philadelphia, Pennsylvania

James W. Campbell, MD, MS
Professor of Family Medicine
Case Western Reserve University
Chairman, Family Medicine/Geriatrics
Metro Health
Cleveland, Ohio

Victor A. Capoccia, PhD
Senior Scientist
Center for Health Enhancement System Studies
Network for the Improvement of Addiction Treatment
University of Wisconsin
Madison, Wisconsin

Kathleen M. Carroll, PhD
Professor, Department of Psychiatry
Yale University School of Medicine
Director of Clinical Research
VA Connecticut Healthcare System
New Haven, Connecticut

Domenic A. Ciraulo, MD
Professor and Chairman, Department of Psychiatry
Boston University School of Medicine
Psychiatrist-in-Chief
Boston Medical Center
Boston, Massachusetts

H. Westley Clark, MD, JD, MPH, CAS, FASAM
Director, Center for Substance Abuse Treatment
Substance Abuse and Mental Health Services Administration
DHHS
Rockville, Maryland

Jeffrey S. Cluver, MD
Assistant Professor of Psychiatry
Medical University of South Carolina
Chief, Substance Abuse Treatment Clinic
Ralph H. Johnson VAMC
Charleston, South Carolina

Peggy Compton, RN, PhD, FAAN
Associate Professor, School of Nursing
University of California, Los Angeles
Los Angeles, California

Katherine Anne Comtois, PhD
Associate Professor, Department of Psychiatry and Behavioral Sciences
University of Washington
Clinical Director, Dialectical Behavior Therapy Program
Harborview Mental Health Services
Harborview Medical Center
Seattle, Washington

Edward C. Covington, MD
Director, Chronic Pain Rehabilitation Program
Cleveland Clinic Foundation
Cleveland, Ohio

Rosa M. Crum, MD, MHS
Professor
Department of Epidemiology, Psychiatry and Mental Health
Welch Center for Prevention, Epidemiology & Clinical Research
Johns Hopkins Medical Institutions
Baltimore, Maryland

Dennis C. Daley, PhD
Professor of Psychiatry
University of Pittsburgh
Chief, Addiction Medicine Services
Western Psychiatric Institute and Clinic
Pittsburgh, Pennsylvania

John A. Dani, PhD
Professor of Neuroscience
Baylor College of Medicine
Houston, Texas

Itai Danovitch, MD
Director, Addiction Psychiatry Clinical Services
Associate Director, Addiction Psychiatry Fellowship
Department of Psychiatry and Behavioral Neurosciences
Cedars-Sinai Medical Center
Los Angeles, California

Jose Carlos T. DaSilva, MD, MPH
Assistant Clinical Professor, Department of Medicine
Boston University School of Medicine
Staff Physician, Commonwealth Nephrology Association
Boston, Massachusetts

Linda C. Degutis, Dr.PH, MSN
Associate Professor, Emergency Medicine and Public Health
Department of Surgery
Yale University
New Haven, Connecticut

William E. Dickinson, DO, FASAM, FAAFP
Medical Director
Providence Behavioral Health Services
Everett, Washington

Linda A. Dimeff, PhD
Chief Scientific Officer
Behavioral Tech Research, Inc.
Seattle, Washington

Carson V. Dobrin, BS
Graduate Student
Neuroscience Program
Wake Forest University School of Medicine
Winston-Salem, North Carolina

Edward F. Domino, MD
Professor of Pharmacology
University of Michigan
Ann Arbor, Michigan

Gail D'Onofrio, MD, MS
Professor and Chief, Section of Emergency Medicine
Yale University
Chief, Department of Adult Emergency Services
Yale-New Haven Hospital
New Haven, Connecticut

Antoine Douaihy, MD
Assistant Professor of Psychiatry
University of Pittsburgh
Medical Director, Addiction Medicine Services
Western Psychiatric Institute and Clinic
Pittsburgh, Pennsylvania

Robert L. DuPont, MD, FASAM
Clinical Professor of Psychiatry
Georgetown University
President, Institute for Behavior and Health
Rockville, Maryland

Paul H. Earley, MD, FASAM
Medical Director
Talbott Recovery Campus
Atlanta, Georgia

Jon O. Ebbert, MD
Associate Professor, Department of Internal Medicine
Mayo Clinic
Rochester, Minnesota

Steven J. Eickelberg, MD, FASAM
President, Performax, P.C.
Sport Psychiatry
Addiction Psychiatry
Paradise Valley, Arizona

Nady el-Guebaly, MD
Professor and Head, Addiction Division
University of Calgary
Medical Director, Addictions Program
Calgary Health Region
Calgary, Alberta, Canada

Tamara Fahnhorst, MPH
Research Program Coordinator
Department of Psychiatry
University of Minnesota
Minneapolis, Minnesota

Kathleen J. Farkas, PhD, LISW-S, ACSW
Associate Professor
Mandel School of Applied Social Sciences
Case Western Reserve University
Cleveland, Ohio

Sergi Ferré, MD, PhD
Staff Scientist
Behavioral Neuroscience Branch
National Institute on Drug Abuse
Baltimore, Maryland

David A. Fiellin, MD
Associate Professor of Medicine and Investigative Medicine
Department of Internal Medicine
Yale University School of Medicine
New Haven, Connecticut

John W. Finney, PhD
Director, HSR&D Center for Health Care Evaluation
Department of Veterans Affairs
Stanford University School of Medicine
Menlo Park, California

Marc Fishman, MD
Assistant Professor of Psychiatry
Johns Hopkins University
Medical Director
Mountain Manor Treatment Center
Baltimore, Maryland

Michael F. Fleming, MD, MPH
Professor of Family Medicine
University of Wisconsin
Director, Addiction Medicine Programs
UW Hospital Clinics
Madison, Wisconsin

Keith Flower, MD
Scientist
Addiction Pharmacology Research Lab
California Pacific Medical Center Research Institute
St. Luke's Hospital
San Francisco, California

P. Joseph Frawley, MD
Co-Medical Director, Intensive Outpatient Program
Recovery Road Medical Center
Assistant Medical Director
Cottage Residential Treatment Center
Santa Barbara Cottage Hospital
Santa Barbara, California

Howard S. Friedman, MD
Clinical Professor of Cardiology
New York University School of Medicine
New York, New York

Peter D. Friedmann, MD, MPH
Professor, Departments of Medicine & Community Health
Alpert Medical School of Brown University
Director, Center on Systems, Outcomes & Quality in Chronic Disease & Rehabilitation
Providence Veterans Affairs Medical Center
Rhode Island Hospital
Providence, Rhode Island

Marc Galanter, MD, FASAM
Professor and Director
Division of Alcoholism & Drug Abuse
NYU School of Medicine
New York, New York

Rollin M. Gallagher, MD, MPH
Clinical Professor and Director for Pain Policy Research and Primary Care
Penn Pain Medicine
Departments of Psychiatry and Anesthesiology
University of Pennsylvania School of Medicine
Director of Pain Medicine
Philadelphia Veterans Affairs Medical Center
Philadelphia, Pennsylvania

Joseph E. Galligan, MA
Focal Therapist, Men's Treatment Team
Hazelden Springbrook
Newberg, Oregon

Gantt P. Galloway, PharmD
Scientist, Addiction Pharmacology Research Laboratory
California Pacific Medical Center Research Institute
San Francisco, California

Aaron M. Gilson, PhD, MS, MSSW
Director, Pain & Policy Studies Group
Madison, Wisconsin

Richard A. Glennon, PhD
Professor and Chair, Department of Medicinal Chemistry
Virginia Commonwealth University
Richmond, Virginia

Mark S. Gold, MD
Distinguished Professor and Chairman
Department of Psychiatry
University of Florida
Shands Hospital
Gainesville, Florida

Linn Goldberg, MD, FACSM
Professor and Head, Division of Health Promotion and Sports Medicine
Oregon Health & Science University
Portland, Oregon

Bruce A. Goldberger, PhD, DABFT
Professor and Director of Toxicology
Departments of Pathology, Immunology & Laboratory Medicine, and Psychiatry
University of Florida College of Medicine
Gainesville, Florida

R. Jeffrey Goldsmith, MD
Professor of Clinical Psychiatry
College of Medicine, University of Cincinnati
Staff Psychiatrist
Mental Health Care Line
Cincinnati VA Medical Center
Cincinnati, Ohio

David A. Gorelick, MD, PhD
Senior Investigator
Intramural Research Program
National Institute on Drug Abuse
National Institutes of Health
Adjunct Professor
Department of Psychiatry
University of Maryland School of Medicine
Baltimore, Maryland

Jon E. Grant, MD, JD, MPH
Associate Professor, Department of Psychiatry
University of Minnesota Medical School
Minneapolis, Minnesota

Kenneth W. Griffin, PhD, MPH
Associate Professor of Public Health
Weill Cornell Medical College
New York, New York

Roland R. Griffiths, PhD
Professor, Department of Psychiatry and Behavioral Sciences, Department of Neuroscience, Johns Hopkins University School of Medicine
Baltimore, Maryland

Paul J. Gruenewald, PhD
Senior Research Scientist
Prevention Research Center
Pacific Institute for Research and Evaluation
Berkeley, California

David H. Gustafson, PhD
Professor
Center for Health Enhancement Studies
University of Wisconsin
Madison, Wisconsin

Paul S. Haber, MD, FRACP, FAChAM
Head, Discipline of Addiction Medicine
University of Sydney
Medical Director, Drug Health Services
Royal Prince Alfred Hospital
Camperdown, New South Wales, Australia

Karen J. Hartwell, MD
Assistant Professor of Psychiatry
Medical University of South Carolina
Charleston, South Carolina

J. David Hawkins, PhD
Professor, School of Social Work
University of Washington
Seattle, Washington

J. Taylor Hays, MD
Associate Professor, Department of Internal Medicine
College of Medicine, Mayo Clinic
Chair, Division of General Internal Medicine
Mayo Clinic
Rochester, Minnesota

Derya Bora Hazar, MD
Assistant Clinical Professor of Medicine
Tufts University School of Medicine
Section Chief of Nephrology
Carney Hospital
Boston, Massachusetts

Stephen T. Higgins, PhD
Professor, Departments of Psychiatry and Psychology
University of Vermont
Burlington, Vermont

Harold D. Holder, PhD
Senior Scientist, Prevention Research Center
Pacific Institute for Research and Evaluation
Berkeley, California

Hon. Peggy Fulton Hora, JD (Ret)
Judge of the Superior Court of California (Retired)

Ryan Horvath, BA
Graduate Student in Pharmacology/Toxicology
Dartmouth Medical School
Hanover, New Hampshire

Matthew O. Howard, PhD
Frank A. Daniels Distinguished Professor, School of Social Work
University of North Carolina
Chapel Hill, North Carolina

Richard D. Hurt, MD, FASAM
Professor of Medicine
Director
Nicotine Dependence Center
Mayo Clinic
Rochester, Minnesota

Mark Hrymoc, MD
Clinical Instructor, Department of Psychiatry
Cedars-Sinai Medical Center
Los Angeles, California

Jerome H. Jaffe, MD
Clinical Professor, Department of Psychiatry
Division of Alcohol and Drug Abuse
University of Maryland
Baltimore, Maryland

Steven L. Jaffe, MD
Professor, Child & Adolescent Psychiatry
Emory University
Peachford Hospital
Atlanta, Georgia

Alain Joffe, MD, MPH
Associate Professor of Pediatrics
Johns Hopkins University School of Medicine
Johns Hopkins Hospital
Baltimore, Maryland

Laura M. Juliano, PhD
Assistant Professor, Department of Psychology
American University
Washington, DC

Christopher W. Kahler, PhD
Associate Professor (Research), Center for Alcohol and Addiction Studies
Brown University
Providence, Rhode Island

Lori D. Karan, MD, FACP, FASAM
Drug Dependence Research Laboratory
University of California, San Francisco
San Francisco, California

Jason R. Kilmer, PhD
Acting Assistant Professor, Department of Psychiatry and Behavioral Sciences
University of Washington
Seattle, Washington

Clifford M. Knapp, PhD
Associate Professor, Division of Psychiatry
Boston University School of Medicine
Boston, Massachusetts

John R. Knight, MD
Associate Professor of Pediatrics
Harvard Medical School
Director, Center for Adolescent Substance Abuse Research
Children's Hospital Boston
Boston, Massachusetts

Patricia K. Kokotailo, MD, MPH
Professor of Pediatrics
University of Wisconsin, School of Medicine and Public Health
University of Wisconsin Hospital and Clinics
Madison, Wisconsin

Thomas R. Kosten, MD
Professor of Psychiatry and Neuroscience
Baylor College of Medicine
Director and Vice Chair, Psychiatry, Addictions, and Neuroscience
Michael E. DeBakey Veterans Administration Medical Center
Houston, Texas

Margaret M. Kotz, DO
Associate Professor of Psychiatry
Case Western Reserve University School of Medicine
Director of Addiction Recovery Services
University Hospitals
Cleveland, Ohio

Henry R. Kranzler, MD
Professor of Psychiatry and General Clinical Research Center (GCRC) Program Director
University of Connecticut Health Center
Farmington, Connecticut

Igor Kravets, MD
Instructor of Clinical Investigation
Laboratory of Addictive Diseases
The Rockefeller University
Associate Attending Physician
The Rockefeller University Hospital
New York, New York

Mary Jeanne Kreek, MD
Professor and Head, Laboratory of the Biology of Addictive Diseases
The Rockefeller University; Senior Physician
Rockefeller University Hospital
New York, New York

Donald J. Kurth, MD, MBA, MPA, FASAM
Associate Professor, Departments of Psychiatry and Preventive Medicine
Loma Linda University
Chief of Addiction Medicine, Psychiatry Department
Loma Linda University Behavioral Medicine Center
Redlands, California

Maritza Lagos-Saez, MD
Assistant Professor, Department of Psychiatry
Michigan State University/Kalamazoo Center for Medical Studies
Attending Physician
Borgess Medical Center
Kalamazoo, Michigan

Bruce D. Lamb, JD, MA
Partner, Ruden McClusky
Tampa, Florida

Mary E. Larimer, PhD
Professor of Psychiatry and Behavioral Sciences
Clinical Psychologist
University of Washington
Seattle, Washington

David Y-W Lee, PhD
Associate Professor of Psychiatry
Harvard Medical School
Director, Bio-Organic and Natural Products Lab
McLean Hospital
Boston, Massachusetts

Elizabeth Mirabile Levens, MD
Waterbury Pulmonary Associates
Waterbury, Conneticut

Adam M. Leventhal, PhD
Postdoctoral Fellow
Center for Alcohol and Addiction Studies
Brown University
Providence, Rhode Island

Frances R. Levin, MD
Kennedy-Leavy Professor of Clinical Psychiatry
Columbia University
Research Psychiatrist
New York State Psychiatric Institute, Division on Substance Abuse
New York, New York

Sharon Levy, MD, MPH
Assistant Professor of Pediatrics
Harvard Medical School
Medical Director, Adolescent Substance Abuse Program
Children's Hospital Boston
Boston, Massachusetts

Ting-Kai Li, MD
Director
National Institute on Alcohol Abuse and Alcoholism
National Institutes of Health
Bethesda, Maryland

Michael R. Liepman, MD, FASAM, DFAPA
Clinical Professor and Director of Research
Department of Psychiatry
Michigan State University, College of Human Medicine
Kalamazoo Center for Medical Studies
Medical Director
Jim Gilmore Jr. Community Healing Center
Kalamazoo, Michigan

Marsha M. Linehan, PhD
Professor, Department of Psychology
Director, Behavioral Research & Therapy Clinics (BRTC)
University of Washington
Seattle, Washington

Scott E. Lukas, PhD
Professor of Psychiatry (Pharmacology)
Harvard Medical School
Boston, Massachusetts
Interim Director
Neuroimaging Center
McLean Hospital
Belmont, Massachusetts

Alan Ona Malabanan, MD, FACE
Assistant Professor of Medicine
Harvard Medical School
Attending Physician
Endocrinology, Diabetes and Metabolism
Beth Israel Deaconess Medical Center
Boston, Massachusetts

Issam A. Mardini, MD, PhD
Assistant Professor, Departments of Anesthesiology and Critical Care
University of Pennsylvania
Attending, Penn Pain Medicine Center and Department of Anesthesiology
University of Pennsylvania Health System
Philadelphia, Pennsylvania

John J. Mariani, MD
Assistant Professor of Clinical Psychiatry
Columbia University
Psychiatrist II
New York State Psychiatric Institute, Division on Substance Abuse
New York, New York

G. Alan Marlatt, PhD
Professor of Psychology
University of Washington
Seattle, Washington

Judith Martin, MD
Medical Director
BAART Turk Street Clinic
San Francisco, California

W. Alex Mason, PhD
Research Associate Professor
Social Development Research Group
School of Social Work
University of Washington
Seattle, Washington

Martha A. Maurer, MSW, MPH
Assistant Researcher
Pain & Policy Studies Group
University of Wisconsin
Madison, Wisconsin

Michael F. Mayo-Smith, MD, MPH
Chief Consultant, Primary Care
Patient Care Services
Department of Veterans Affairs
Washington, District of Columbia

Elinore F. McCance-Katz, MD, PhD
Professor of Psychiatry
University of California, San Francisco
San Francisco, California

Dennis McCarty, PhD
Professor
Department of Public Health & Preventive Medicine
Oregon Health & Science University
Portland, Oregon

Richard A. McCormick, PhD
Senior Scholar
Center for Health Care Research and Policy
Case Western Reserve University
Cleveland, Ohio

Barbara S. McCrady, PhD
Distinguished Professor of Psychology
Director, Center on Alcoholism, Substance Abuse and Addictions (CASAA)
University of New Mexico
Albuquerque, New Mexico

James R. McKay, PhD
Professor of Psychiatry
University of Pennsylvania
Director, Center of Excellence in Substance Abuse Treatment and Education
VA Medical Center
Philadelphia, Pennsylvania

Thomas McLellan, PhD
CEO, Treatment Research Institute
Professor in Psychiatry
University of Pennsylvania School of Medicine
Philadelphia, Pennsylvania

Mary G. McMasters, MD
Assistant Professor of Addiction Medicine and General Internal Medicine
University of Virginia
Co-Medical Director
Pantops Clinic (MMT)
Charlottesville, Virginia

David Mee-Lee, MD
Consultant
DML Training and Consulting
Davis, California

John Mendelson, MD
Senior Scientist, Addiction Pharmacology Research Laboratory
California Pacific Medical Center Research Institute
San Francisco, California

Delinda E. Mercer, PhD
Clinical Coordinator
Behavioral Health Unit
Regional West Medical Center
Scottsbluff, Nebraska

Lisa J. Merlo, PhD
Assistant Professor
Department of Psychiatry
Univesity of Florida
Gainesville, Florida

Shannon C. Miller, MD, FASAM, FAPA, CMRO
Associate Professor of Clinical Psychiatry
Associate Director for Education
Director, Addiction Psychiatry & Addiction Medicine Fellowships
Addiction Sciences Division
Department of Psychiatry
Cincinnati VAMC & University of Cincinnati
Cincinnati, Ohio

Rudolf H. Moos, PhD
Professor, Department of Psychiatry and Behavioral Sciences
Stanford University School of Medicine
Research Career Scientist, Research Service
Department of Veterans Affairs Health Care System
Palo Alto, California

Hugh Myrick, MD
Associate Professor of Psychiatry
Medical University of South Carolina
Director, Mental Health Service Line
Ralph H. Johnson VAMC
Charleston, South Carolina

Eric J. Nestler, MD, PhD
Nash Family Professor and Chair
Department of Neuroscience
Mount Sinai School of Medicine
New York, New York

Edward V. Nunes, MD
Professor of Clinical Psychiatry
Columbia University College of Physicians and Surgeons
New York State Psychiatric Institute
Associate Attending Psychiatrist
New York Presbyterian Hospital
New York, New York

Patrick G. O'Connor, MD MPH
Pofessor of Medicine
Yale University School of Medicine
Chief, Section of General Internal Medicine
Yale-New Haven Hospital
New Haven, Connecticut

Brian L. Odlaug, BA
Research Associate
Department of Psychiatry
University of Minnesota Medical School
Minneapolis, Minnesota

James A.D. Otis, MD
Associate Professor
Department of Neurology
Boston University School of Medicine
Director, Pain Management Group
Boston Medical Center
Boston, Massachusetts

Theodore V. Parran, Jr., MD, FACP
Associate Clinical Professor, Department of Internal Medicine
Case Western Reserve University School of Medicine
Associate Medical Director, Rosary Hall Addiction Services
St. Vincent Charity Hospital
Cleveland, Ohio

Rebecca A. Payne, MD
Resident, Department of Psychiatry and Behavioral Sciences
Clinical Neuroscience Division
Medical University of South Carolina
Charleston, South Carolina

J. Thomas Payte, MD
Medical Director
Drug Dependence Associates
San Antonio, Texas

Michael Perloff, MD
Resident, Department of Neurology
Boston University, Boston Medical Center
Boston, Massachusetts

Karran A. Phillips, MD, MSc
Staff Clinician
National Institutes of Health, National Institute on Drug Abuse
Intramural Research Program
Clinical Instructor
Division of General Internal Medicine
Johns Hopkins School of Medicine
Baltimore, Maryland

Marc N. Potenza, MD, PhD
Associate Professor
Department of Psychiatry and Child Study
Yale School of Medicine
New Haven, Connecticut

Vladimir Poznyak, MD, PhD
Coordinator, Management of Substance Abuse
Department of Mental Health and Substance Abuse
World Health Organization (WHO)
Geneva, Switzerland

James O. Prochaska, PhD
Professor and Director, Cancer Prevention Research Center
University of Rhode Island
Kingston, Rhode Island

Terri L. Randall, MD
Instructor, Department of Psychiatry and Human Behavior
Division of Child and Adolescent Psychiatry
Assistant Director, Child and Adolescent Psychiatry Fellowship Program
Thomas Jefferson University
Philadelphia, Pennsylvania

Lillian G. Remer, MA
Associate Research Scientist
Prevention Research Center
Pacific Institute for Research & Evaluation
Berkeley, California

Richard K. Ries, MD, FAPA, FASAM
Professor of Psychiatry
Director, Division of Addictions, Department of Psychiatry and Behavioral Sciences
University of Washington
Medical Director, Harborview Addictions and Rehabilitation Psychiatry Programs
Harborview Medical Center
Seattle, Washington

David C.S. Roberts, PhD
Professor
Department of Physiology and Pharmacology
Wake Forest University School of Medicine
Winston-Salem, North Carolina

Randall E. Rogers, PhD
Postdoctoral Fellow
University of Vermont Substance Abuse Treatment Center
University Health Center
Burlington, Vermont

Richard N. Rosenthal, MD
Professor of Clinical Psychiatry
Columbia University College of Physicians & Surgeons
Chairman, Department of Psychiatry & Behavioral Health
St. Luke's-Roosevelt Hospital Center
New York, New York

Bruce J. Rounsaville, MD
Professor of Psychiatry
Yale University School of Medicine
Director, New England Mental Illness Research and Education Center
VA Connecticut Healthcare
New Haven, Connecticut

Stanley Sacks, PhD
Director, Center for the Integration of Research & Practice
National Development & Research Institutes, Inc.
New York, New York

Richard Saitz, MD, MPH, FACP, FASAM
Professor of Medicine and Epidemiology
Boston University Schools of Medicine and Public Health
Director, Clinical Addiction Research and Education Unit
Department of Medicine
Boston Medical Center
Boston, Massachusetts

Michael E. Saladin, PhD
Associate Professor
Department of Health Sciences and Research and Department of Psychiatry and Behavioral Sciences
Clinical Neuroscience Division
Medical University of South Carolina
Charleston, South Carolina

Jeffrey H. Samet, MD, MA, MPH
Professor of Medicine
Boston University School of Medicine
Chief, General Internal Medicine
Boston Medical Center
Boston, Massachusetts

Jussi J. Saukkonen, MD
Assistant Professor of Medicine
Department of Pulmonary and Critical Care Medicine
Boston University School of Medicine
Boston, Massachusetts

Seddon R. Savage, MD, MS, FASAM
Director, Dartmouth Center on Addiction Recovery and Education (DCARE)
Pain Consultant, Manchestor VA Medical Center
Associate Professor of Anesthesiology, Dartmouth Medical School, Adjunct Faculty
Hanover, New Hampshire

Andrew J. Saxon, MD
Professor of Psychiatry and Behavioral Sciences
University of Washington
Director, Addiction Patient Care Line
Mantal Health Service
VA Puget Sound Health Care System
Seattle, Washington

William G. Schma, The Hon. (Ret)
Kalamazoo Circuit Court
Kalamazoo, Michigan

Jerome E. Schulz, MD, FASAM
Medical Director
Hazelden Center for Youth and Family
Plymouth, Minnesota

Neil Sharma, MD
Chief Resident Department of Internal Medicine
University of South Florida
Attending/Chief Resident
James A. Haley VA Hospital
Tampa, Florida

Steven J. Shoptaw, PhD
Professor, Department of Family Medicine
University of California, Los Angeles
Los Angeles, California

Gerald D. Shulman, MA, MAC, FACATA
President
Shulman & Associates, Training and Consulting in Behavioral Health
Jacksonville, Florida

Diana I. Simeonova, Dipl-Psych, MA
Associate Director
Institute for Behavioral Medicine
Smyrna, Georgia

Deborah R. Simkin, MD
Program Director, Psychiatry
Section Head, Division of Child and Adolescent Psychiatry
Residency Training Director
Adjunct Associate Professor
University of South Alabama Medical School
Mobile, Alabama

David A. Smelson, PsyD
Professor/Vice Chair of Clinical Research
Department of Psychiatry
University of Massachusetts Medical Center
Worcester, Massachusetts

Ramon Solhkhah, MD
Director, The Child & Family Institute
Chief, Division of Child and Adolescent Psychiatry
St. Luke's—Roosevelt Hospital Center
Assistant Professor of Clinical Psychiatry
Columbia University College of Physicians and Surgeons
New York, New York

Crystal R. Spotts, MEd
Senior Research Principal
Department of Psychiatry
University of Pittsburgh Medical Center
Western Psychiatric Institute and Clinic
Pittsburgh, Pennsylvania

Marc L. Steinberg, PhD
Assistant Professor of Psychiatry
Robert Wood Johnson Medical School
New Brunswick, New Jersey

Randy Stinchfield, PhD
Associate Director
Center for Adolescent Substance Abuse Research
Department of Psychiatry
University of Minnesota
Minneapolis, Minnesota

Susan M. Stine, MD, PhD
Associate Professor, Department of Psychiatry and Behavioral Neurosciences
Wayne State University School of Medicine
Director, Addiction Psychiatry Residency Program
Wayne State University School of Medicine and Detroit Medical Center
Detroit, Michigan

Amanda M. Stone, BS
Student
University of Florida
Gainesville, Florida

Carol A. Sulis, MD
Associate Professor of Medicine, Division of Infectious Diseases
Boston University School of Medicine
Hospital Epidemiologist
Attending Physician
Boston Medical Center
Boston, Massachusetts

Maria A. Sullivan, MD, PhD
Associate Professor of Clinical Psychiatry
Columbia University
Research Psychiatrist, Division on Substance Abuse
Columbia College of Physicians and Surgeons
New York State Psychiatric Institute
New York, New York

Zebulon Taintor, MD
Professor of Psychiatry
New York University School of Medicine
Consulting Attending Psychiatrist
Bellevue Hospital
New York, New York

Jeanette M. Tetrault, MD
Assistant Professor of Medicine
Department of Internal Medicine
Yale University School of Medicine
New Haven, Connecticut

Jennifer W. Tidey, PhD
Assistant Professor (Research), Center for Alcohol and Addiction Studies
Department of Psychiatry and Human Behavior
Warren Alpert Medical School of Brown University
Research Health Science Specialist
Providence Veterans Affairs Medical Center
Providence, Rhode Island

Juana Maria Tomás-Rosselló, MD, MPH
Drug Abuse Treatment Adviser
Global Challenges Section
United Nations Office on Drugs and Crime
Vienna, Austria

J. Scott Tonigan, PhD
Research Professor, Department of Psychology
Center on Alcoholism, Substance Abuse, and Addictions (CASAA)
University of New Mexico
Albuquerque, New Mexico

Andrew J. Treno, PhD.
Research Scientist
Prevention Research Center
Pacific Institute for Research and Evaluation
Berkeley, California

Himanshu P. Upadhyaya, MD, MBBS, MS
Associate Professor, Department of Psychiatry and Behavioral Sciences
Medical University of South Carolina
Charleston, South Carolina

Adrienne D. Vaiana, BS
Research Coordinator II
Department of Psychiatry
University of Massachusetts Medical School
Worcester, Massachusetts

Nora D. Volkow, MD
Director
National Institute on Drug Abuse
Chief
Laboratory of Neuroimaging
National Institute on Alcohol Abuse and Alcoholism
Bethesda, Maryland

Angela E. Waldrop, PhD
Assistant Professor
Department of Psychiatry and Behavioral Sciences
Medical University of South Carolina
Charleston, South Carolina

Hong Wang, MD, PhD
Instructor of Psychiatry
Havard Medical School
Bio-Organic and Natural Products Lab
McLean Hospital
Belmont, Massachusetts

Elizabeth A. Warner, MD
Associate Professor of Internal Medicine
University of South Florida College of Medicine
Medical Director, Ambulatory Services
Tampa General Hospital
Tampa, Florida

Michael F. Weaver, MD, FASAM
Associate Professor of Internal Medicine and Psychiatry
Virginia Commonwealth University
Medical Director, Substance Abuse Consult Service
Medical College of Virginia Hospital
Richmond, Virginia

Melissa Weddle, MD, MPH
Visiting Scholar
Department of Behavioral Neuroscience
Oregon Health and Science University
Portland, Oregon
Staff Physician
Department of Pediatrics Vancouver Clinic
Vancouver, Washington

Roger D. Weiss, MD
Professor of Psychiatry
Harvard Medical School
Boston, Massachusetts
Clinical Director, Alcohol and Drug Abuse Treatment Program
McLean Hospital
Belmont, Massachusetts

Sandra P. Welch, PhD
Professor
Department of Pharmacology and Toxicology
Virginia Commonwealth University
Richmond, Virginia

Joseph J. Westermeyer, MD, MPH, PhD
Professor of Psychiatry
University of Minnesota
Director, Mental Health Service
Minneapolis VAMC
Minneapolis, Minnesota

David B. Wexler, JD
Professor of Law
University of Puerto Rico
San Juan, Puerto Rico

William L. White, MA
Senior Research Consultant
Lighthouse Institute
Chestnut Health Systems
Bloomington, Illinois

Ursula Whiteside, MSD
NIAAA Postdoctoral Fellow
Department of Psychology
University of Washington
Seattle, Washington

Paula L. Wilbourne, PhD
Director, Addiction Treatment Service
VA Palo Alto Health Care System
Palo Alto, California

Bonnie B. Wilford, MS
Executive Director
Coalition on Physician Education in Substance Use Disorders (COPE)
Yale University School of Medicine
New Haven, Connecticut

Jeffery N. Wilkins, MD
Professor, Department of Psychiatry and Biobehavioral Sciences
David Geffen School of Medicine at UCLA
Vice Chair and Lincy/Moynihan-Heyward Chair in Addiction Medicine
Cedars-Sinai Medical Center
Los Angeles, California

Mark L. Willenbring, MD
Director, Division of Treatment and Recovery Research
National Institutes on Alcohol Abuse and Alcoholism
Bethesda, Maryland

Emily C. Williams, MPH
Doctoral Student, Health Services
University of Washington
Seattle, Washington

Vern Williams, MD
Medical Director
Hazelden Springbrook
Newberg, Oregon

Kevin C. Wilson, MD
Assistant Professor of Medicine
Boston University School of Medicine
Attending Physician, Pulmonary, Critical Care, and Allergy
Boston Medical Center
Boston, Massachusetts

Bruce J. Winick, JD
Professor of Law, School of Law
Professor of Psychiatry and Behavioral Sciences
University of Miami
Coral Gables, Florida

Ken C. Winters, PhD
Professor of Psychiatry
University of Minnesota Medical School
Minneapolis, Minnesota

Alex Wodak, MD, MB, BS, FRACP, FAChAM
Director, Alcohol and Drug Service
St. Vincent's Hospital
Sydney, Australia

John J. Woodward, PhD
Professor, Department of Neurosciences
Medical University of South Carolina
Charleston, South Carolina

Tara M. Wright, MD
Assistant Professor of Psychiatry
Medical University of South Carolina
Staff Psychiatrist, Medical Health Service Line
Ralph H. Johnson VAMC
Charleston, South Carolina

Martha J. Wunsch, MD, FAAP, FASAM
Associate Professor, Department of Behavioral Science
Center for Drug and Alcohol Research
University of Kentucky
Lexington, Kentucky

Stephen A. Wyatt, DO
Medical Director, Dual Day Treatment Program
Department of Psychiatry
Middlesex Hospital
Middletown, Connecticut

Sarah W. Yip, BA, MSc
Student, Department of Psychology
University College London
London, England

Christine Yuodelis-Flores, MD
Clinical Associate Professor of Psychiatry and Behavioral Sciences
University of Washington
Attending Psychiatrist
Harborview Medical Center
Seattle, Washington

Anne Zajicek, MD, PharmD
Pediatric Medical Officer, Associate Branch Chief
Obstetric and Pediatric Pharmacology Branch
Center for Research for Mothers and Children
Eunice Kennedy Shriver National Institute of Child Health and Human Development
National Institutes of Health
Bethesda, Maryland

Alexsandra Zgierska, MD, PhD
National Institute on Alcohol Abuse and Alcoholism (NIAAA)-funded Clinical Research Fellow
Department of Family Medicine
University of Wisconsin, School of Medicine and Public Health
Physician
NewStart Alcohol and Drug Treatment Program
Meriter Hospital
Madison, Wisconsin

Douglas M. Ziedonis, MD, MPH
Professor and Chairman, Department of Psychiatry
University of Massachusetts
Memorial Health Care and University of Massachusetts Medical School
Worcester, Massachusetts

Joan E. Zweben, PhD
Clinical Professor of Psychiatry
University of California, San Francisco
Executive Director
East Bay Community Recovery Project
Oakland, California

CONTENTS

SECTION 1

Basic Science and Core Concepts

CHAPTER 1

Nora D. Volkow, MD
Ting-Kai Li, MD

Drug Addiction: The Neurobiology of Behavior Gone Awry

Drug addiction manifests as a compulsive drive to take a drug despite serious adverse consequences. This aberrant behavior has traditionally been viewed as a bad "choice" that is made voluntarily by the addicted person. However, recent studies have shown that repeated drug use leads to long-lasting changes in the brain that undermine voluntary control. This, combined with new knowledge of how environmental, genetic, and developmental factors contribute to addiction, should bring about changes in our approach to the prevention and treatment of addiction.

Drugs, both legal (e.g., alcohol, nicotine) and illegal (i.e., cocaine, methamphetamine, heroin, marijuana) are misused for various reasons, including for pleasurable effects, altering mental state, improving performance and, in certain instances, self-medicating a mental disorder. Repeated drug use can result in addiction, which is manifested as an intense desire for the drug with an impaired ability to control the urges to take that drug, even at the expense of serious adverse consequences. To avoid confusion with physical dependence, the term *drug addiction* is used here instead of *drug dependence*, which is the clinical term favored by the *Diagnostic and Statistical Manual of Mental Disorders* (4th edition). Physical dependence results in withdrawal symptoms when drugs, such as alcohol and heroin, are discontinued, but the adaptations that are responsible for these effects are different from those that underlie addiction.

The aberrant behavioral manifestations that occur during addiction have been viewed by many as "choices" of the addicted individual, but recent imaging studies have revealed an underlying disruption to brain regions that are important for the normal processes of motivation, reward, and inhibitory control in addicted individuals (1,2). This provides the basis for a different view: that drug addiction is a disease of the brain and the associated abnormal behavior is the result of dysfunction of brain tissue, just as cardiac insufficiency is a disease of the heart and abnormal blood circulation is the result of dysfunction of myocardial tissue (3) (Fig. 1.1). Therefore, although initial drug experimentation and recreational use might be volitional, after addiction develops, control is markedly disrupted. Although imaging studies consistently show specific abnormalities in the brain function of addicted individuals, not all addicted individuals show these abnormalities. This highlights the need for further research to delineate other neurobiologic processes that are involved in addiction.

Chronic exposure to drugs of abuse is required for drug addiction, and its expression involves complex interactions between biologic and environmental factors. This might explain why some individuals become addicted and others do not, and why attempts to understand addiction as a purely biologic or a purely environmental disease have been largely unsuccessful. Recently, important discoveries have increased our knowledge of how drugs affect gene expression, protein products, and neuronal circuits (4), and how these biologic factors might affect human behavior. This sets the stage for a better understanding of how different environmental factors interact with biologic factors and contribute to patterns of behavior that lead to addiction.

Here, we summarize how new methodologies that allow us to study genes, molecular biology, and the human brain are providing us with a greater understanding of drug addiction, and the implications of these findings for the prevention and treatment of addiction.

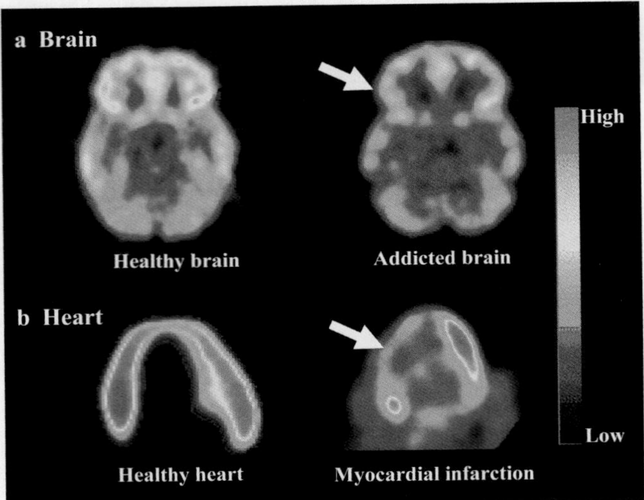

FIGURE 1.1. Drug addiction as a disease of the brain. Images of the brain **(A)** in a healthy control and in an individual addicted to a drug, and parallel images of the heart **(B)** in a healthy control and in an individual with a myocardial infarction. The images were obtained with positron emission tomography (PET) and [^{18}F]fluoro-2-deoxyglucose (FDG-PET) to measure glucose metabolism, which is a sensitive indicator of damage to the tissue in the brain and the heart. Note the decreased glucose metabolism in the orbitofrontal cortex (OFC, *arrow*) of the addicted person and the decreased metabolism in the myocardial tissue *(arrow)* in the person with a myocardial infarct. Damage to the OFC will result in improper inhibitory control and compulsive behavior, and damage to the myocardium will result in improper blood circulation. Although abnormalities in the OFC are some of the most consistent findings in imaging studies of addicted individuals (including alcoholics), they are not detected in all addicted individuals. This implies that disruption of this frontal region is not the only mechanism that underlies the addictive process. Heart images courtesy of H. Schelbert, University of California at Los Angeles.

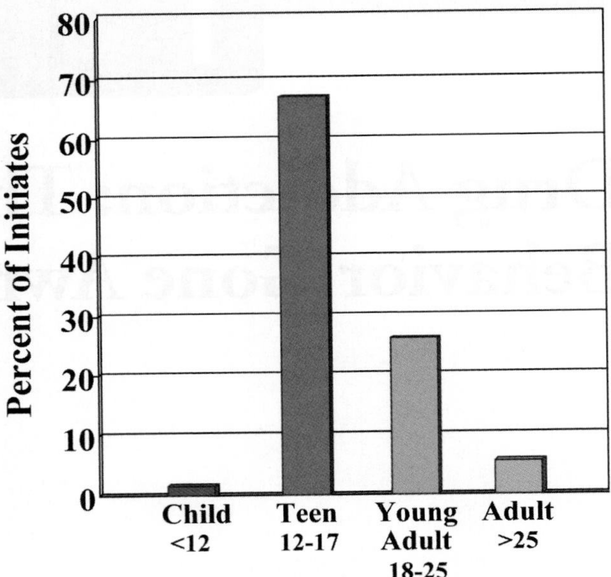

FIGURE 1.2. Age at which marijuana use is first initiated. Data from the National Survey of Drug Use and Health (64).

ADDICTION: A DEVELOPMENTAL DISORDER

Normal developmental processes might result in a higher risk of drug use at certain times in life than others. Experimentation often starts in adolescence, as does the process of addiction (5) (Fig. 1.2). Normal adolescent-specific behaviors (such as risk-taking, novelty-seeking, and response to peer pressure) increase the propensity to experiment with legal and illegal drugs (6), which might reflect incomplete development of brain regions (e.g., myelination of frontal lobe regions) (7) that are involved in the processes of executive control and motivation. In addition, studies indicate that drug exposure during adolescence might result in different neuroadaptations from those that occur during adulthood. For example, in rodents, exposure to nicotine during the period that corresponds to adolescence, but not during adulthood, led to significant changes in nicotine receptors and an increased reinforcement value for nicotine later in life (8). Future research might allow us to clarify whether this is the reason that adolescents seem to become addicted to nicotine after less nicotine exposure than adults (9). Similarly, further studies might enable us to determine whether the increased neuroadaptations to alcohol that occur during adolescence, compared with those that occur during adulthood (10) explain the greater vulnerability to alcoholism in individuals who start using alcohol early in life (11).

NEUROBIOLOGY OF DRUGS OF ABUSE

Many neurotransmitters, including GABA (γ-aminobutyric acid), glutamate, acetylcholine, dopamine, serotonin and endogenous opioid peptides, have been implicated in the effects of the various types of drugs of abuse. Of these, dopamine has been consistently associated with the reinforcing effects of most drugs of abuse. Drugs of abuse increase extracellular dopamine concentrations in limbic regions, including the nucleus accumbens (NAc) (12,13). Specifically, it seems that the reinforcing effects of drugs of abuse are due to their ability to surpass the magnitude and duration of the fast dopamine increases that occur in the NAc when triggered by natural reinforcers such as food and sex (14). Drugs such as cocaine, amphetamine, methamphetamine, and ecstasy increase dopamine by inhibiting dopamine reuptake or promoting dopamine release through their effects on dopamine transporters (15). Other drugs, such as nicotine, alcohol, opiates, and marijuana, work indirectly by stimulating neurons (GABA-mediated or glutamatergic) that modulate dopamine cell firing through their effects on nicotine, GABA, mu opiate, or cannabinoid CB1 receptors, respectively (16).

It seems that increases in dopamine are not directly related to reward per se, as was previously believed, but rather to the prediction of reward (17) and for salience (18). Salience refers to stimuli or environmental changes that are arousing or that elicit an attentional–behavioral switch (19). Salience, which, in addition to reward, applies to aversive, new, and unexpected stimuli, affects the motivation to seek the anticipated reward and facilitates conditioned learning (20,21). This provides a different perspective about drugs, because it implies that drug-induced increases in dopamine will inherently motivate further procurement of more drug (regardless of whether or not the effects of the drug are consciously perceived to be pleasurable). Indeed, some addicted individuals report that they seek the drug even though its effects are no longer pleasurable. Drug-induced increases in dopamine will also facilitate conditioned learning, so previously neutral stimuli that are associated with the drug become salient. These previously neutral stimuli then increase dopamine by themselves and elicit the desire for the drug (22). This explains why the addicted person is at risk of relapsing when exposed to an environment where he or she has previously taken the drug.

If natural reinforcers increase dopamine, why do they not lead to addiction? The difference might be due to qualitative and quantitative differences in the increases in dopamine induced by drugs, which are greater in magnitude (at least 5- to 10-fold) and duration than those induced by natural reinforcers (14). In addition, whereas the dopamine increases produced by natural reinforcers in the NAc undergo habituation, those induced by drugs of abuse do not (13). Nondecremental dopamine stimulation of the NAc from repeated drug use strengthens the motivational properties of the drug, which does not occur for natural reinforcers.

NEUROBIOLOGY OF DRUG ADDICTION

Addiction probably results from neurobiologic changes that are associated with chronic and intermittent supraphysiologic perturbations in the dopamine system, which occur in the same circuits that affect biologically important functions (1). We and others have postulated that adaptations in these dopaminergic circuits make the addicted individual more responsive to the supraphysiologic increases in dopamine that are produced by drugs of abuse and less sensitive to the physiologic increases in dopamine produced by natural reinforcers (23). Recent advances in both molecular biology and imaging have increased our insight into how these neural adaptations occur.

At a cellular level, drugs have been reported to alter the expression of certain transcription factors (nuclear proteins that bind to regulatory regions of genes, thereby regulating their transcription into mRNA), as well as a wide variety of proteins involved in neurotransmission in brain regions that are regulated by dopamine (18). The long-lasting changes that occur in the transcription factors δ FosB and cAMP-responsive element binding protein after chronic drug administration are of particular interest because they modulate the synthesis of proteins that are involved in synaptic plasticity (4). Indeed, chronic drug exposure alters the morphology of neurons in dopamine-regulated circuits. For example, in rodents, chronic cocaine or amphetamine administration increases neuronal dendritic branching and spine density in the NAc and prefrontal cortex—an adaptation that is thought to participate in the enhanced incentive motivational value of the drug (a process that results in increased "wanting" in contrast to just "liking" the drug) in the addicted person (24).

At the neurotransmitter level, addiction-related adaptations have been documented not only for dopamine, but also for glutamate, GABA, opiates, serotonin, and various neuropeptides. These changes contribute to the abnormal function of brain circuits. For example, in individuals who are addicted to cocaine, imaging studies have documented that disrupted dopamine activity in the brain (shown by reductions in dopamine D2 receptors) is associated with abnormal activity in the orbitofrontal cortex (OFC) and in the anterior cingulate gyrus—brain regions that are involved in salience attribution and inhibitory control (25) (Fig. 1.3). Abnormal function of these cortical regions has been particularly revealing in furthering our understanding of addiction, because their disruption is linked to compulsive behavior (OFC) and disinhibition (25) (cingulate gyrus). Therefore the abnormalities in these frontal regions could underlie the compulsive nature of drug administration in addicted individuals and their inability to control their urges to take the drug when they are exposed to it. In addition, animal studies have shown that drug-related adaptations in these frontal regions result in enhanced activity in the glutamatergic pathway that regulates dopamine release in the NAc (26). The adaptations in this pathway seem to be involved in the relapse that occurs after drug withdrawal in animals previously trained to self-administer a drug when they are again exposed to the drug, a drug stimulus, or stress (26).

At the circuit level, there is clear evidence that adaptations in the mesocortical circuit (including the OFC and cingulate gyrus) cause compulsive drug administration and poor inhibitory control, and they probably participate in relapse. However, adaptations also seem to occur in the mesolimbic circuit (including the NAc, amygdala, and hippocampus), which probably cause the enhanced saliency value of the drug and drug stimuli, and the decreased sensitivity to natural reinforcers (27). Furthermore, adaptations have also been reported in the nigrostriatal circuit (including the dorsal striatum), which might underlie habits that are linked to the rituals of drug consumption (28).

VULNERABILITY TO ADDICTION

Genetic Factors It is estimated that 40% to 60% of the vulnerability to addiction is attributable to genetic factors (29). In animal studies, several genes have been identified that are involved in drug responses, and their experimental modifications markedly affect drug self-administration (30). In humans, several chromosomal regions have been linked to drug abuse,

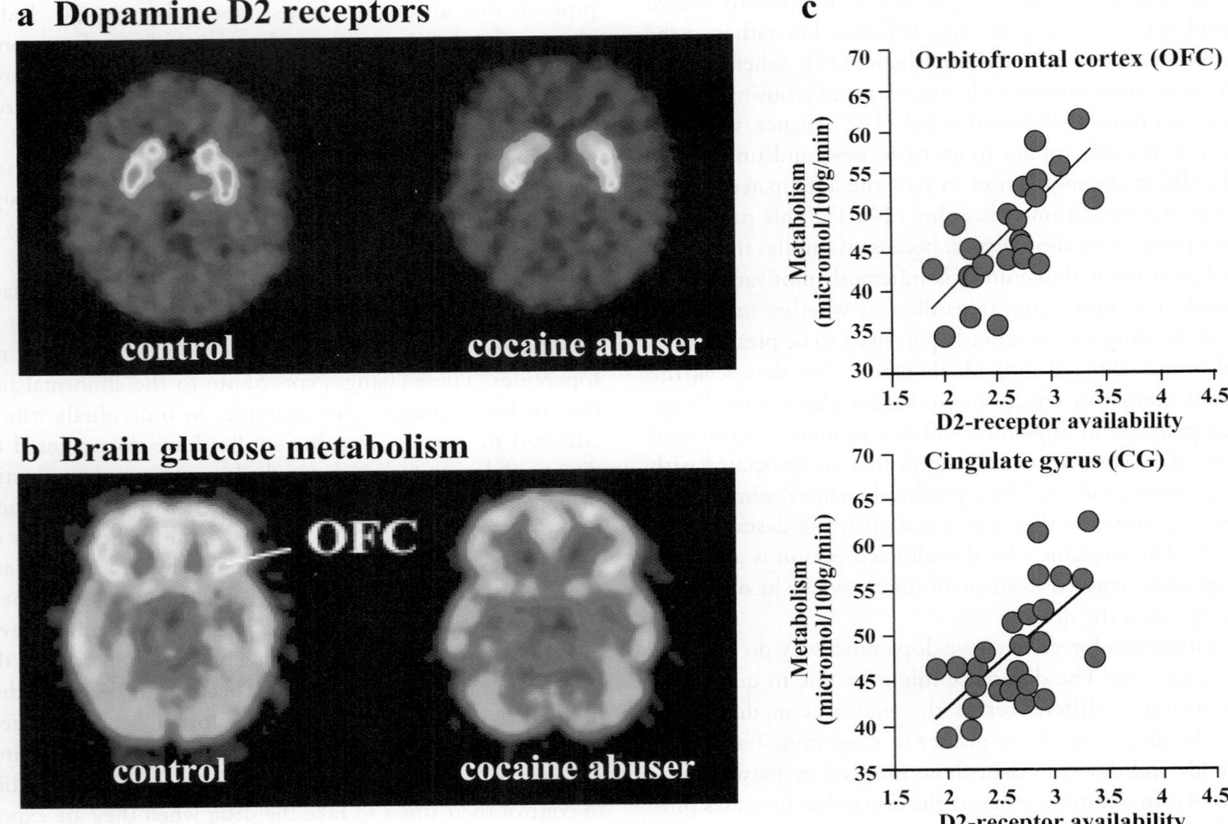

FIGURE 1.3. Dopamine D2 receptors and glucose metabolism in addiction. **A,B:** Positron emission tomography (PET) images showing dopamine D2 receptors and brain glucose metabolism in the OFC (orbitofrontal cortex) in controls and in individuals who abuse cocaine. Note that the individuals abusing cocaine have reductions in D2 receptors and in OFC metabolism. **C:** Correlation between measures of D2 receptors and brain glucose metabolism in the OFC and anterior cingulate gyrus (CG). The lower the D2-receptor expression, the lower the metabolism in the OFC and CG. Decreased activity in the OFC, a brain region that is implicated in salience attribution and whose disruption results in compulsive behavior, could underlie the compulsive drug administration that occurs in addiction. Decreased activity in the CG, a brain region that is involved in inhibitory control, could underlie the inability to restrain from taking the drug when the addicted person is exposed to it (2).

but only a few specific genes have been identified with polymorphisms (alleles) that either predispose to or protect from drug addiction (29). Some of these polymorphisms interfere with drug metabolism. For example, specific alleles for the genes that encode alcohol dehydrogenases ADH1B and ALDH2 (enzymes involved in the metabolism of alcohol) are reportedly protective against alcoholism (31). Similarly, polymorphisms in the gene that encodes cytochrome P-450 2A6 (an enzyme that is involved in nicotine metabolism) are reportedly protective against nicotine addiction (32). Furthermore, genetic polymorphisms in the cytochrome P-450 2D6 gene (an enzyme that is involved in conversion of codeine to morphine) seem to provide a degree of protection against codeine abuse (33).

Some polymorphisms in receptor genes that mediate drug effects have also been associated with a higher risk of addiction. For example, a number of convergent results support a CHRNA5/A3/B4 gene cluster association with nicotine dependence (34–37) and with the risk of such smoking-related diseases as lung cancer and peripheral arterial disease (38–40). An association has also been found between alcoholism and the genes for the GABA type A ($GABA_A$) receptors GABRG3 (41) and GABRA2 (42). D2-receptor polymorphisms have been linked to a higher vulnerability to drug addiction, although some studies have failed to replicate this finding (29). Replication of many of the genetic findings in substance abuse and addiction is still pending.

Environmental Factors Environmental factors that have been consistently associated with the propensity to self-administer drugs include low socioeconomic class, poor parental support, and drug availability. Stress might be a common feature in a wide variety of environmental factors that increase the risk for drug abuse. The mechanisms responsible for stress-induced increases in vulnerability to drug use and to relapse in people who are addicted are not yet well understood, but there is evidence that the stress-responsive neuropeptide corticotropin-releasing factor is involved through its effects in the amygdala and the pituitary–adrenal axis (43).

Imaging techniques now allow us to investigate how environmental factors affect the brain and how these, in turn, affect the behavioral responses to drugs of abuse. For example, in nonhuman primates, social status affects D2-receptor expression in the brain, which in turn affects the propensity for cocaine self-administration (44). Animals that achieve a dominant status in the group show increased numbers of D2 receptors and are reluctant to administer cocaine, whereas animals that are subordinate have lower D2-receptor numbers and readily administer cocaine. Because animal studies have shown that increasing D2 receptors in NAc markedly decreases drug consumption (which has been shown for alcohol) (45), this could provide a mechanism by which a social stressor could modify the propensity to self-administer drugs.

Comorbidity with Mental Illness The risk for substance abuse and addiction in individuals with mental illness is significantly higher than for the general population. The high comorbidity probably reflects, in part, overlapping environmental, genetic, and neurobiologic factors that influence drug abuse and mental illness (46).

It is likely that different neurobiological factors are involved in comorbidity depending on the temporal course of its development (that is, mental illness followed by drug abuse or vice versa). In some instances, the mental illness and addiction seem to co-occur independently (47), but in others there might be a sequential dependency. It has been proposed that comorbidity might be due to the use of the abused drugs to self-medicate the mental illness in cases in which the onset of mental illness is followed by abuse of some types of drug. But, when drug abuse is followed by mental illness, the chronic exposure could lead to neurobiologic changes, which might explain the increased risk of mental illness (46). For example, the high prevalence of smoking that is initiated after individuals experience depression could reflect, in part, the antidepressant effects of nicotine as well as the antidepressant effects of monoamine oxidase A and B inhibition by cigarette smoke (48). On the other hand, the reported risk for depression with early drug abuse (49) could reflect neuroadaptations in dopamine systems that might make individuals more vulnerable to depression.

The higher risk of drug abuse in individuals with mental illnesses highlights the relevance of the early evaluation and treatment of mental diseases as an effective strategy to prevent drug addiction that starts as self-medication.

STRATEGIES TO COMBAT ADDICTION

The knowledge of the neurobiology of drugs and the adaptive changes that occur with addiction is guiding new strategies for prevention and treatment, and identifying areas in which further research is required.

Preventing Addiction The greater vulnerability of adolescents to experimentation with drugs of abuse and to subsequent addiction underscores why prevention of early exposure is such an important strategy to combat drug addiction. Epidemiologic studies show that the prevalence of drug use in adolescents has changed significantly over the past 30 years, and some of the decreases seem to be related to education about the risks of drugs. For example, for marijuana, the prevalence rates of use in the United States in 1979 were as high as 50%, whereas in 1992 they were as low as 20% (50) (Fig. 1.4). This changing pattern of marijuana use seems to be related in part to the perception of the risks associated with the drug; when adolescents perceived the drug to be risky, the rate of use was low, whereas when they did not, the rate of use was high (Fig. 1.4). Similarly, the significant decreases in ecstasy use as well as cigarette smoking in adolescents seem to partly reflect effective educational campaigns (50). These results show that, despite the fact that adolescents are at a stage in their lives when they are more likely to take risks, interventions that educate them about the harmful effects of drugs with age-appropriate messages can decrease the rate of drug use (51,52). However, not all media campaigns and school-based educational programs have been successful (53). Tailored interventions that take into account socioeconomic, cultural, and age and gender characteristics of children and adolescents are more likely to improve the effectiveness of the interventions.

At present, prevention strategies include not only educational interventions based on comprehensive school-based programs and effective media campaigns and strategies that decrease access to drugs and alcohol, but also strategies that provide supportive community activities that engage adolescents in productive and creative ways. However, as we begin to understand the neurobiologic consequences that underlie the adverse environmental factors that increase the risks for drug use and for addiction, we will be able to develop interventions to counteract these changes. Similarly, in the future, as we gain knowledge of the genes and the proteins that they encode that make a person more or less vulnerable to taking drugs and to addiction, more targets will be available to tailor interventions for those at higher risk.

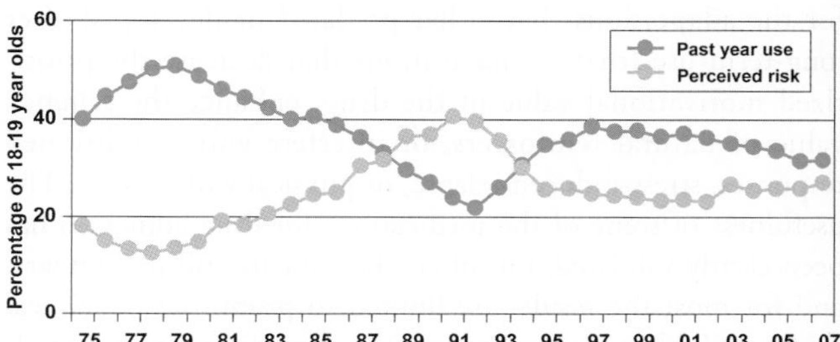

FIGURE 1.4. Use and risk perception of marijuana. The prevalence rate for marijuana use in the past 12 months and the perception of marijuana as a dangerous drug in 12th graders (18 to 19 years old) between 1975 and 2007 (50). When teenagers perceived marijuana as dangerous, the prevalence of drug use was low and vice versa.

Treating Addiction The adaptations in the brain that result from chronic drug exposure are long lasting; therefore, addiction must be viewed as a chronic disease. Long-term treatment will be required for most cases, just as for other chronic diseases (such as hypertension, diabetes, and asthma) (54). This perspective modifies our expectations of treatment and provides a new understanding of relapse. First, discontinuation of treatment, as for other chronic diseases, is likely to result in relapse. Also, as for other chronic medical conditions, relapse should not be interpreted as a failure of treatment (as is the view in most cases of addiction), but instead as a temporary setback because of lack of compliance or tolerance to an effective treatment (54). Indeed, the rates of relapse and recovery in the treatment of drug addiction are equivalent to those of other medical diseases (54).

The involvement of multiple brain circuits (reward, motivation, learning, inhibitory control, and executive function) and their associated disruption of behavior indicate the need for a multimodal approach in the treatment of the addicted individual. Therefore interventions should not be limited to inhibiting the rewarding effects of a drug, but should also include strategies to enhance the saliency value of natural reinforcers (including social support), strengthen inhibitory control, decrease conditioned responses, and improve mood if disrupted. The most obvious multimodal approach is the combination of pharmacologic and behavioral interventions, which might target different underlying factors and therefore have synergistic effects. For example, it might be predicted that addiction treatments that use behavioral interventions (such as 12-step programs [self-help support groups whose members attempt recovery from addiction, in part, by 'admitting' that they have a problem and by sharing experiences]) would be more effective if complemented with medications that could help the patient remain drug free.

Pharmacologic Intervention Pharmacologic interventions can be grouped into two classes. First, there are those that interfere with the reinforcing effects of drugs of abuse (that is, medications that interfere with the binding of the drug, drug-induced dopamine increase, postsynaptic responses, or with the drug's delivery to the brain, or medications that trigger aversive responses). Second, there are those that compensate for the adaptations that either predated or developed after long-term use (that is, medications that decrease the prioritized motivational value of the drug, enhance the saliency value of natural reinforcers, or interfere with conditioned responses, stress-induced relapse, or physical withdrawal). The usefulness of some of the medications for drug addiction has been clearly validated; for others the data are still preliminary, and for most the results are limited to promising preclinical findings. Table 1.1 summarizes proven medications and medications for which there are preliminary clinical data. Many of these promising new medications target different neurotransmitters (such as GABA, cannabinoids, or glutamate) from the older drugs, offering a wider range of therapeutic options.

Cognitive–behavioral Intervention In a similar fashion, behavioral interventions can be classified by their intended remedial function, such as to strengthen inhibitory control circuits, provide alternative reinforcers, and strengthen executive function. Traditionally, behavioral therapy has focused on symptom-based targets rather than underlying causes of addiction. However, for other brain disorders, new views of brain plasticity, which recognize the capacity of neurons in the adult brain to increase synaptic connections and in certain instances to regenerate (55), have resulted in more focused cognitive–behavioral interventions designed to increase the efficiency of dysfunctional brain circuits. This has been applied in attempts to improve reading in children with learning disabilities (56) and to facilitate motor and memory rehabilitation after brain injury (57), but has not yet been applied to the remediation of brain circuits altered by drug abuse. Dual approaches that pair cognitive–behavioral strategies with medications to compensate or counteract the neurobiologic changes induced by chronic drug exposure might, in the future, provide more robust and longer lasting treatments for addiction than either given in isolation.

Treating Comorbidities Abuse of multiple substances, such as alcohol and nicotine or alcohol and cocaine, should be considered in the proper management of the addicted individual. Similarly, comorbidities with mental illness will require treatment for the mental illness concurrent with treatment for drug abuse.

Because drugs of abuse adversely affect many organs in the body (Fig. 1.5), uncontrolled consumption contributes to the burden of many medical diseases, including cancer, cardiovascular and pulmonary diseases, HIV/AIDS, and hepatitis C, as well as to accidents and violence. Therefore substance-abuse treatment will help to prevent or improve the outcome for medical diseases. For example, drug abuse is a leading contributor

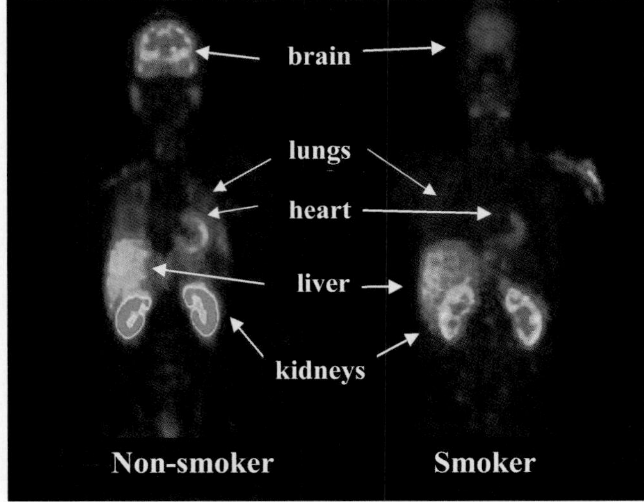

FIGURE 1.5. Monoamine oxidase B concentration and cigarette smoking. Positron emission tomography (PET) images of the concentration of the enzyme MAO-B (monoamine oxidase B) in the body of a healthy control and of a cigarette smoker. There are significant decreases in the concentration of the enzyme throughout the body of the smoker. Reproduced, with permission (66) © (2003) National Academy of Sciences, USA.

TABLE 1.1 Medications for Treating Drug and Alcohol Addiction*

Clinical target	Medication	Biological target
Alcoholism		
FDA approved (67)	Disulfiram (Antabuse; Wyeth-Ayerst) (67)	Aldehyde dehydrogenase (triggers aversive response)
	Naltrexone (67)	Mu opioid receptor (antagonist; interferes with reinforcement)
	Acamprosate (68, 69)	Glutamate related
	*Topiramate (Topamax; Ortho-McNeil) (70)	GABA/glutamate
Under investigation	*Valproate (71)	GABA/glutamate
	Ondansetron (72)	5-HT$_3$ receptor
	Nalmefene (73)	Mu opioid receptor (antagonist)
	Baclofen (Lioresal; Novartis) (74)	GABA$_B$ receptor (agonist)
	Pyrrolopyrimidine compound (Antalarmin; George Chrousos et al.) (75)	CRF1 receptor (inhibits stress-triggered responses)
	Rimonabant (Acomplia; Sanofi-Synthelabo) (76)	CB1 receptor (antagonist)
Smoking cessation		
FDA approved (77)	Nicotine replacement	Nicotinic receptor (substitution with different pharmacokinetics)
	Varenicline (78)	Nicotinic receptor (α4β2 partial agonist)
	Bupropion (77)	DA transporter blocker (amplifies DA signals)
Under investigation	Deprenyl (79)	MAO-B inhibitor (inhibits metabolism of DA)
	Rimonabant (Acomplia; Sanofi-Synthelabo) (76,80)	CB1 receptor (antagonist)
	Methoxsalen (81)	CYP2A6 (inhibits nicotine metabolism)
	Nicotine conjugate vaccine (NicVax; Nabi Biopharmaceuticals) (82)	Blocks entry into brain
	Naltrexone (83)	Mu opioid receptor (antagonist)
Heroin/opiate addiction		
FDA approved (84)	Naltrexone (85)	Mu opioid receptor (antagonist)
	Methadone (86)	Mu opioid receptor (substitution with different pharmacokinetics)
	Buprenorphine	Mu opioid receptor (substitution)
Cocaine addiction		
Under investigation	*Topiramate (Topamax; Ortho-McNeil) (87)	GABA agonist
	*γ-vinyl GABA (GVG) (Sabril; HoechstMarionRoussel) (88,89)	GABA transaminase (inhibits GABA metabolism)
	*Gabapentin (Neurontin; Parke-Davis) (90)	GABA/glutamate (synthesis)
	*Tiagabine (Gabitril; Abbott) (91)	GABA transporter (inhibitor)
	Baclofen (Lioresal; Novartis) (92)	GABA$_B$ receptor (agonist)
	Modafinil (93)	Glutamate (?)
	Disulfiram (Antabuse; Wyeth-Ayerst) (94)	Unknown for cocaine
	Cocaine vaccine (TA-CD; Xenova) (82,95)	Blocks entry into brain
	N-acetylcysteine (96)	Glutamate (?)

FDA, Food and Drug Administration; GABA, γ- aminobutyric acid; GABA$_B$, GABA type B; 5HT$_3$, 5-hydroxytryptamine (serotonin) receptor subtype 3; MAO-B, monoamine oxidase B.

Medications used for physical withdrawal are not included.

*Antiepileptic drugs that have been shown to decrease drug induced DA increases as well as conditioned response.

to the spread of HIV/AIDS, and treatment of addiction in some instances prevents its dissemination (58,59).

CHALLENGES FOR SOCIETY

In most cases, drug abuse and addiction alienate the individual from both family and community, increasing isolation, and interfering with treatment and recovery. Because both the family and the community provide integral aspects of effective treatment and recovery, this identifies an important challenge: to reduce the stigma of addiction that interferes with intervention and proper rehabilitation.

Effective treatment of drug addiction in many individuals requires consideration of social policy, such as the treatment of drug addiction in the criminal justice system, the role of unemployment in vulnerability to the use of drugs and family dysfunctions that contribute to stress and that might block the efficacy of otherwise effective interventions. For example, studies have shown that providing drug treatment to prisoners who were substance abusers and continuing the treatment after they left the prison dramatically reduced not only their rate of relapse to drugs, but also their rate of reincarceration (60,61). Similarly, drug courts in the United States, which incorporate drug treatment into the judicial system, have proved to be beneficial in decreasing drug use and arrests of offenders who are involved in drug-taking (62). However, despite these preliminary positive results, there are still many unanswered questions that future research should address. For example, what are the active ingredients in the treatment of the drug offender? How does the system deal with the fact that few offenders stay in treatment long enough to receive the minimally required services? What are the implications of these findings for pretrial diversion laws, post-prison reentry initiatives and so on?

The recognition of addiction as a disease that affects the brain might be essential for large-scale prevention and treatment programs that require the participation of the medical community. Engagement of pediatricians and family physicians (including the teaching of addiction medicine as part of medical students' training) might facilitate early detection of drug abuse in childhood and adolescence. Moreover, screening for drug use could help clinicians better manage medical diseases that are likely to be adversely affected by the concomitant use of drugs, such as cardiac and pulmonary diseases. Unfortunately, physicians, nurses, psychologists, and social workers receive little training in the management of addiction, despite it being one of the most common chronic disorders.

The participation of the medical community in many countries, including the United States, is further curtailed by the lack of reimbursement by most private medical insurance policies for the evaluation or treatment of drug abuse and addiction. This lack of reimbursement limits the treatment infrastructure and the choices that the addicted person has with respect to their treatment. It also sends a negative message to medical students who are interested in clinical practice, discouraging them from choosing a specialty for which the reimbursement of their services is limited by the lack of parity.

Another considerable obstacle in the treatment of addiction is the limited involvement of the pharmaceutical industry in the development of new medications. Issues such as stigma, lack of reimbursement for drug-abuse treatment, and the lack of a large market all contribute to the limited involvement of the pharmaceutical industry in the development of medications to treat drug addiction. The importance of this issue was identified by the Institute of Medicine of the United States, which recommended a program to provide incentives to the pharmaceutical industry as a way of helping to address this problem (63).

The translation of scientific findings in drug abuse into prevention and treatment initiatives clearly requires partnership with federal agencies such as the Substance Abuse and Mental Health Services Administration (which is responsible for U.S. programs to prevent and treat drug abuse) and the Office of National Drug Control Policy (which is responsible for U.S. programs to control availability and reduce demand for drugs of abuse). Furthermore, improved prevention and treatment programs could result from collaborations with other agencies and groups, such as the Department of Education (which can bring prevention interventions into the school environment), the Department of Justice (which can implement treatment strategies that will minimize the chances of recidivism and reincarceration of inmates with drug-abuse problems), and state and local agencies (which can bring evidence-based and science-based treatments into the communities).

As we learn more about the neurobiology of normal and pathologic human behavior, a challenge for society will be to use this knowledge to effectively guide public policy. For example, as we understand the neurobiologic substrates that underlie voluntary actions, how will society define the boundaries of personal responsibility in those individuals who have impairments in these brain circuits? This will have implications not only for the management of drug offenders, but also of other offenders with diagnoses such as antisocial personality disorder or conduct disorder. At present, critics of the medical model of addiction argue that this model removes the responsibility of the addicted individual from his or her behavior. However, the value of the medical model of addiction as a public policy guide is not to excuse the behavior of the addicted individual, but to provide a framework to understand it and to treat it more effectively.

SUMMARY

Remarkable scientific advances have been made in genetics, molecular biology, behavioral neuropharmacology, and brain imaging that offer new insights into how the human brain works and molds behavior. In the case of addiction, we can now investigate questions that were previously inaccessible, such as how environmental factors and genes affect the responses of the brain to drugs and produce neural adaptations that lead to the aberrant behavioral manifestations of addiction. This new knowledge is helping us to understand why drug addicts relapse even in the face of threats such as divorce, loss of child custody, and incarceration, even when, in some cases, the drug is no longer perceived as pleasurable, and is changing how we should approach prevention and treatment of addiction.

The field is at a crossroads where major advances in understanding the neurobiology of addiction have helped identify promising new medications, but where the translation of these findings into clinical practice is limited by several factors, including the limited involvement of the medical community in the treatment of addiction, the restricted involvement of the pharmaceutical industry, the lack of reimbursement by private insurance policies and the stigma associated with drug addiction. One of the main challenges for agencies like the National Institute on Drug Abuse and the National Institute on Alcohol Abuse and Alcoholism is to develop knowledge that will help to overcome these obstacles.

ACKNOWLEDGMENTS: *The authors thank T. Condon, M. Egli, J. Fowler, C. Kassed, R. Litten, A. Noronha, and J. Swanson* *for thoughtful comments and editorial assistance. This chapter is adapted from Volkow ND, Li TK. Drug addiction: the neurobiology of behaviour gone awry.* Nat Rev Neurosci *2004;5(12):963–970.*

REFERENCES

1. Volkow ND, Fowler JS, Wang G-J. The addicted human brain: insights from imaging studies. *J Clin Invest* 2003;111:1444–1451.
2. Volkow ND, Fowler JS, Wang G-J, et al. Dopamine in drug abuse and addiction: results of imaging studies and treatment implications. *Arch Neurol* 2007;64(11):1575–1579.
3. Leshner AI. Addiction is a brain disease, and it matters. *Science* 1997;278: 45–47.
4. Nestler EJ. Molecular basis of long-term plasticity underlying addiction. *Nat Rev Neurosci* 2001;2:119–128.
5. Wagner FA, Anthony JC. From first drug use to drug dependence: developmental periods of risk for dependence upon marijuana, cocaine, and alcohol. *Neuropsychopharmacology* 2002;26:479–488.
6. Spear LP. The adolescent brain and age-related behavioral manifestations. *Neurosci Biobehav Rev* 2000;24:417–463.
7. Sowell ER, Peterson BS, Thompson PM, et al. Mapping cortical change across the human life span. *Nat Neurosci* 2003;6:309–315.
8. Adriani W, Spijker S, Deroche-Gamonet V, et al. Evidence for enhanced neurobehavioral vulnerability to nicotine during periadolescence in rats. *J Neurosci* 2003;23:4712–4716.
9. Kandel DB, Chen K. Extent of smoking and nicotine dependence in the United States: 1991–1993. *Nicotine Tob Res* 2000;2:263–274.
10. Slawecki CJ, Roth J. Comparison of the onset of hypoactivity and anxiety-like behavior during alcohol withdrawal in adolescent and adult rats. *Alcohol Clin Exp Res* 2004;28:598–607.
11. Grant BF, Stinson FS, Harford TC. Age at onset of alcohol use and DSM-IV alcohol abuse and dependence: a 12-year follow-up. *J Subst Abuse* 2001;13:493–504.
12. Koob GF, Bloom FE. Cellular and molecular mechanisms of drug dependence. *Science* 1988;242:715–723.
13. Di Chiara, G. Nucleus accumbens shell and core dopamine: differential role in behavior and addiction. *Behav Brain Res* 2002;137:75–114.
14. Wise RA. Brain reward circuitry: insights from unsensed incentives. *Neuron* 2002;36:229–240.
15. Madras BK, Fahey MA, Bergman J, et al. Effects of cocaine and related drugs in nonhuman primates. I. [3H]cocaine binding sites in caudate-putamen. *J Pharmacol Exp Ther* 1989;251:131–141.
16. Kreek MJ, LaForge KS, Butelman E. Pharmacotherapy of addictions. *Nat Rev Drug Discov* 2002;1:710–726.
17. Schultz W, Tremblay L, Hollerman JR. Reward processing in primate orbitofrontal cortex and basal ganglia. *Cereb Cortex* 2000;10:272–284.
18. Lu L, Grimm JW, Shaham Y, et al. Molecular neuroadaptations in the accumbens and ventral tegmental area during the first 90 days of forced abstinence from cocaine self-administration in rats. *J Neurochem* 2003; 85:1604–1613.
19. Horvitz JC. Mesolimbocortical and nigrostriatal dopamine responses to salient non-reward events. *Neuroscience* 2000;96:651–656.
20. McClure SM, Daw ND, Montague PR. A computational substrate for incentive salience. *Trends Neurosci* 2003;26:423–428.
21. Schultz W. Reward signaling by dopamine neurons. *Neuroscientist* 2001;7:293–302.
22. Ito R, Dalley JW, Howes SR, et al. Dissociation in conditioned dopamine release in the nucleus accumbens core and shell in response to cocaine cues and during cocaine-seeking behavior in rats. *J Neurosci* 2000;20:7489–7495.
23. Volkow ND, Fowler JS, Wang GJ, et al. Dopamine in drug abuse and addiction: results from imaging studies and treatment implications. *Mol Psychiatry* 2004;9:557–569.
24. Robinson TE, Gorny G, Mitton E, et al. Cocaine self-administration alters the morphology of dendrites and dendritic spines in the nucleus accumbens and neocortex. *Synapse* 2001;39:257–266.
25. Volkow ND, Fowler JS. Addiction, a disease of compulsion and drive: involvement of the orbitofrontal cortex. *Cereb Cortex* 2000;10:318–325.
26. McFarland K, Davidge SB, Lapish CC, et al. Limbic and motor circuitry underlying footshock-induced reinstatement of cocaine-seeking behavior. *J Neurosci* 2004;24:1551–1560.
27. Martin-Soelch C, Chevalley A-F, Künig G, et al. Changes in reward-induced brain activation in opiate addicts. *Eur J Neurosci* 2001;14:1360–1368.
28. Porrino LJ, Lyons D, Smith HR, et al. Cocaine self-administration produces a progressive involvement of limbic, association, and sensorimotor striatal domains. *J Neurosci* 2004;24:3554–3562.
29. Uhl GR, Grow RW. The burden of complex genetics in brain disorders. *Arch Gen Psychiatry* 2004;61:223–229.
30. Laakso A, Mohn AR, Gainetdinov RR, et al. Experimental genetic approaches to addiction. *Neuron* 2002;36:213–228.
31. Chen CC, Lu R-B, Chen Y-C, et al. Interaction between the functional polymorphisms of the alcohol-metabolism genes in protection against alcoholism. *Am J Hum Genet* 1999;65:795–807.
32. Rao Y, Hoffmann E, Zia M, et al. Duplications and defects in the *CYP2A6* gene: identification, genotyping, and in vivo effects on smoking. *Mol Pharmacol* 2000;58:747–755.
33. Kathiramalainathan K, Kaplan HL, Romach MK, et al. Inhibition of cytochrome P450 2D6 modifies codeine abuse liability. *J Clin Psychopharmacol* 2000;20:435–444.
34. Bierut LJ, Madden PAF, Breslau N, et al. Novel genes identified in a high-density genome wide association study for nicotine dependence. *Hum Mol Genet* 2007;16(1):24–35.
35. Saccone SF, Hinrichs AL, Saccone NL, et al. Cholinergic nicotinic receptor genes implicated in a nicotine dependence association study targeting 348 candidate genes with 3713 SNPs. *Hum Mol Genet* 2007;16(1):36–49.
36. Berrettini W, Yuan X, Tozzi F, et al. α-5/α-3 Nicotinic receptor subunit alleles increase risk for heavy smoking. *Mol Psychiatry* 2008;13:368–373.
37. Schlaepfer IR, Hoft NR, Collins AC, et al. The CHRNA5/A3/B4 gene cluster variability as an important determinant of early alcohol and tobacco initiation in young adults. *Biol Psychiatry* 2008;63(11):1039–1046.
38. Thorgeirsson TE, Geller F, Sulem P, et al. Variant associated with nicotine dependence, lung cancer and peripheral arterial disease. *Nature* 2008;452(7187):638–642.
39. Amos CI, Wu X, Broderick P, et al. Genome-wide association scan of tag SNPs identifies a susceptibility locus for lung cancer at 15q25.1. *Nat Genet* 2008;40(5):616–622.
40. Hung RJ, McKay JD, Gaborieau V, et al. A susceptibility locus for lung cancer maps to nicotinic acetylcholine receptor subunit genes on 15q25. *Nature* 2008;452(7187):633–637.
41. Dick DM, Edenberg HJ, Xiaoling X, et al. Association of GABRG3 with alcohol dependence. *Alcohol Clin Exp Res* 2004;28:4–9.
42. Edenberg HJ, Dick DM, Xiaoling X, et al. Variations in *GABRA2*, encoding the α2 subunit of the $GABA_A$ receptor, are associated with alcohol dependence and with brain oscillations. *Am J Hum Genet* 2004;74:705–714.
43. Koob GF. Stress, corticotropin-releasing factor, and drug addiction. *Ann NY Acad Sci* 1999;897:27–45.
44. Morgan D, Grant KA, Gage HD, et al. Social dominance in monkeys: dopamine D2 receptors and cocaine self-administration. *Nat Neurosci* 2002;5:169–174.
45. Thanos PK, Volkow ND, Freimuth P, et al. Overexpression of dopamine D2 receptors reduces alcohol self-administration. *J Neurochem* 2001;78: 1094–1103.
46. Markou A, Kosten TR, Koob GF. Neurobiological similarities in depression and drug dependence: a self-medication hypothesis. *Neuropsychopharmacology* 1998;18:135–174.
47. Grant BF, Stinson FS, Dawson DA, et al. Prevalence and co-occurrence of substance use disorders and independent mood and anxiety disorders: results from the National Epidemiologic Survey on Alcohol and Related Conditions. *Arch Gen Psychiatry* 2004;61:807–816.
48. Fowler JS, Logan J, Wang GJ, et al. Monoamine oxidase and cigarette smoking. *Neurotoxicology* 2003;24:75–82.
49. Brook DW, Brook JS, Zhang C, et al. Drug use and the risk of major depressive disorder, alcohol dependence, and substance use disorders. *Arch Gen Psychiatry* 2002;59:1039–1044.

50. Johnston LD, O'Malley PM, Bachman JG, et al. Monitoring the future national survey results on drug use, 1975–2006: volume I, secondary school students. Bethesda, MD: National Institutes of Health Publication No. 07-6205, 2007.
51. Block LG, Morwitz VG, Putsis WP, et al. Assessing the impact of antidrug advertising on adolescent drug consumption: results from a behavioral economic model. *Am J Public Health* 2002;92:1346–1351.
52. Flynn BS, Worden JK, Secker-Walker RH, et al. Long-term responses of higher and lower risk youths to smoking prevention interventions. *Prev Med* 1997;26:389–394.
53. Gruber AJ, Pope HG, Jr. Marijuana use among adolescents. *Pediatr Clin North Am* 2002;49:389–413.
54. McLellan AT, Lewis DC, O'Brien CP, et al. Drug dependence, a chronic medical illness: implications for treatment, insurance, and outcomes evaluation. *JAMA* 2000;284:1689–1695.
55. Schaffer DV, Gage FH. Neurogenesis and neuroadaptation. *Neuromolecular Med* 2004;5:1–9.
56. Kujala T, Karma K, Ceponiene R, et al. Plastic neural changes and reading improvement caused by audiovisual training in reading-impaired children. *Proc Natl Acad Sci U S A* 2001;98:10509–10514.
57. Fraser C, Power M, Hamdy S, et al. Driving plasticity in human adult motor cortex is associated with improved motor function after brain injury. *Neuron* 2002;34:831–840.
58. Kelley MS, Chitwood DD. Effects of drug treatment for heroin sniffers: a protective factor against moving to injection? *Soc Sci Med* 2004;58: 2083–2092.
59. Treatment for cocaine use may have HIV benefits. Study shows how to achieve best results. *AIDS Alert* 2003;18:118–119.
60. Butzin CA, Martin SS, Inciardi JA. Evaluating component effects of a prison-based treatment continuum. *J Subst Abuse Treat* 2002;22:63–69.
61. Hiller ML, Knight K, Simpson DD. Prison-based substance abuse treatment, residential aftercare and recidivism. *Addiction* 1999;94:833–842.
62. Fielding JE, Tye G, Ogawa PL, et al. Los Angeles County drug court programs: initial results. *J Subst Abuse Treat* 2002;23:217–224.
63. Fulco CE, Liverman CT, Earley LE, eds. *Development of medications for the treatment of opiate and cocaine addictions: issues for the government and private sector* (Institute of Medicine). Washington DC: National Academy Press; 1995.
64. Gfroerer JC, Wu L-T, Penne MA. Initiation of marijuana use: trends, patterns and implications. SMA 02-3711. Analytic Series A-17. Rockville, MD: Substance Abuse and Mental Health Services Administration, Office of Applied Studies; 2002.
65. Goldstein RZ, Volkow ND. Drug addiction and its underlying neurobiological basis: neuroimaging evidence for the involvement of the frontal cortex. *Am J Psychiatry* 2002;159:1642–1652.
66. Fowler JS, Logan J, Wang G-J, et al. Low monoamine oxidase B in peripheral organs in smokers. *Proc Natl Acad Sci U S A* 2003;100: 11600–11605.
67. Anton RF. Pharmacologic approaches to the management of alcoholism. *J Clin Psychiatry* 2001;62(Suppl. 20):11–17.
68. Whitworth AB, Oberbauer H, Fleischhacker WW, et al. Comparison of acamprosate and placebo in long-term treatment of alcohol dependence. *Lancet* 1996;347(9013):1438–1442.
69. Anton RF, O'Malley SS, Ciraulo DA, et al. COMBINE Study Research Group. Combined pharmacotherapies and behavioral interventions for alcohol dependence: the COMBINE study; a randomized controlled trial. *JAMA* 2006;295(17):2003–2017.
70. Johnson BA, Ait-Daoud N, Bowden CL, et al. Oral topiramate for treatment of alcohol dependence: a randomised controlled trial. *Lancet* 2003;361:1677–1685.
71. Salloum IM, Cornelius JR, Daley DC, et al. Efficacy of valproate maintenance in bipolar alcoholics: a double blind placebo controlled study. *Arch Gen Psychiatry* 2005;62:37–45.
72. Johnson BA, Roache JD, Javors MA, et al. Ondansetron for reduction of drinking among biologically predisposed alcoholic patients: a randomized controlled trial. *JAMA* 2000;284:963–971.
73. Mason BJ, Salvato FR, Williams LD, et al. A double-blind, placebo-controlled study of oral nalmefene for alcohol dependence. *Arch Gen Psychiatry* 1999;56:719–724.
74. Addolorato G, Caputo F, Capristo E, et al. Baclofen efficacy in reducing alcohol craving and intake: a preliminary double-blind randomized controlled study. *Alcohol Alcohol* 2002;37:504–508.
75. Webster EL, Lewis DB, Torpy DJ, et al. In vivo and in vitro characterization of antalarmin, a nonpeptide corticotropin-releasing hormone (CRH) receptor antagonist: suppression of pituitary ACTH release and peripheral inflammation. *Endocrinology* 1996;137:5747–5750.
76. Fernandez JR, Allison DB. Rimonabant Sanofi-Synthelabo. *Curr Opin Investig Drugs* 2004;5:430–435.
77. George TP, O'Malley SS. Current pharmacological treatments for nicotine dependence. *Trends Pharmacol Sci* 2004;25:42–48.
78. Tonstad S, Tønnesen P, Hajek P, et al. Varenicline Phase 3 Study Group. Effect of maintenance therapy with varenicline on smoking cessation: a randomized controlled trial. *JAMA* 2006;296(1):64–71.
79. George TP, Vessicchio JC, Termine A, et al. A preliminary placebo-controlled trial of selegiline hydrochloride for smoking cessation. *Biol Psychiatry* 2003;53:136–143.
80. Maldonado R, Valverde O, Berrendero F. Involvement of the endocannabinoid system in drug addiction. *Trends Neurosci* 2006;29(4):225–232.
81. Sellers EM, Ramamoorthy Y, Zeman MV, et al. The effect of methoxsalen on nicotine and 4-(methylnitrosamino)-1-(3-pyridyl)-1-butanone (NNK) metabolism *in vivo*. *Nicotine Tob Res* 2003;5:891–899.
82. Kosten TR, Biegel D. Therapeutic vaccines for substance dependence. *Expert Rev Vaccines* 2002;1:363–371.
83. King A, de Wit H, Riley RC, et al. Efficacy of naltrexone in smoking cessation: a preliminary study and an examination of sex differences. *Nicotine Tob Res* 2006;8(5):671–682.
84. Krupitsky EM, Zvartau EE, Masalov DV, et al. Naltrexone for heroin dependence treatment in St. Petersburg, Russia. *J Subst Abuse Treat* 2004; 26:285–294.
85. Comer SD, Sullivan MA, Yu E, et al. Injectable, sustained-release naltrexone for the treatment of opioid dependence: a randomized, placebo-controlled trial. *Arch Gen Psychiatry* 2006;63(2):210–218.
86. Krantz MJ, Mehler PS. Treating opioid dependence: growing implications for primary care. *Arch Intern Med* 2004;164(3):277–288.
87. Kampman KM, Pettinati H, Lynch KG, et al. A pilot trial of topiramate for the treatment of cocaine dependence. *Drug Alcohol Depend* 2004;75: 233–240.
88. Brodie JD, Figueroa E, Dewey SL. Treating cocaine addiction: from preclinical to clinical trial experience with *v*-vinyl GABA. *Synapse* 2003;50:261–265.
89. Brodie JD, Figueroa E, Laska EM, et al. Safety and efficacy of gamma-vinyl GABA (GVG) for the treatment of methamphetamine and/or cocaine addiction. *Synapse* 2005;55(2):122–125.
90. Raby WN, Coomaraswamy S. Gabapentin reduces cocaine use among addicts from a community clinic sample. *J Clin Psychiatry* 2004;65:84–86.
91. Gonzalez G, Sevarino K, Sofuoglu M, et al. Tiagabine increases cocaine-free urines in cocaine-dependent methadone-treated patients: results of a randomized pilot study. *Addiction* 2003;98:1625–1632.
92. Shoptaw S, Yang X, Rotheram-Fuller EJ, et al. Randomized placebo-controlled trial of baclofen for cocaine dependence: preliminary effects for individuals with chronic patterns of cocaine use. *J Clin Psychiatry* 2003;64:1440–1448.
93. Dackis C, O'Brien C. Glutamatergic agents for cocaine dependence. *Ann N Y Acad Sc* 2003;1003:328–345.
94. Carroll KM, Fenton LR, Ball SA, et al. Efficacy of disulfiram and cognitive behavior therapy in cocaine-dependent outpatients: a randomized placebo-controlled trial. *Arch Gen Psychiatry* 2004;61:264–272.
95. Kosten T, Owens SM. Immunotherapy for the treatment of drug abuse. *Pharmacol Ther* 2005;108(1):76–85.
96. Mardikian PN, Larowe SD, Hedden S, et al. An open-label trial of N-acetylcysteine for the treatment of cocaine dependence: a pilot study. *Prog Neuropsychopharmacol Biol Psychiatry* 2007;31(2):389–394.

CHAPTER 2

Rosa M. Crum, MD, MHS

The Epidemiology of Substance Use Disorders

This chapter is organized to cover several areas. First, a few epidemiologic terms and types of epidemiologic studies are discussed. Second, some of the literature regarding prevalence and incidence of alcohol and drug use disorders is reviewed. The remainder of the chapter is devoted to discussing some of the correlates and risk factors associated with alcohol and drug use disorders.

SOME EPIDEMIOLOGIC PRINCIPLES

Epidemiology has been defined in many ways, but may be considered the study of how diseases are distributed in populations as well as the study of the determinants of disease and health (1–3). Some basic terms used in epidemiology deserve attention in this chapter, because they are important to understanding the literature and some of the studies reported here. *Prevalence* generally is taken to represent the ratio of the total number of cases of a particular disease, divided by the total number of individuals in a particular population at a specific time. *Incidence* refers to the occurrence of new cases of a disease, divided by the total number at risk for the disorder during a specified period (4). Prevalence takes into account both the incidence and duration of a disease, because it depends not only on the proportion of newly developed cases over time, but also on the length of time the disease exists in the population. In turn, the duration of the disorder is affected by the degree of recovery and death from the disease. Incidence generally is taken to represent the risk of disease, whereas prevalence is an indicator of the public health burden the disease imposes on the community (4).

The strength of association between a particular characteristic and the development of disease generally is represented by the *relative risk*, or the estimated relative risk (often called the odds ratio). The relative risk measures the incidence of disease among those with a particular characteristic (such as family history of alcohol addiction), divided by the incidence of disease among those without exposure to that characteristic. If there is no difference in the incidence among those with and without the characteristic, the ratio is equal to one. A relative risk greater than one indicates an increased risk of disease associated with a given characteristic. A relative risk less than one signifies a lower risk, which may indicate a protective effect associated with the characteristic.

Excellent detailed discussions of epidemiologic studies can be found elsewhere (1,2,4,5). For the purposes of this chapter, epidemiologic studies can be divided into two types: (i) observational or (ii) experimental. Observational studies may include cross-sectional, case-control, or cohort studies. In cross-sectional studies or surveys, individuals are assessed (by interview or physical examination, for example) at a particular point in time (4). Analytic studies usually are classified as case-control (retrospective) or cohort (longitudinal, prospective). Analytic studies generally test a hypothesis of a suspected association between a particular exposure (risk factor) and a disease or other outcome. In all observational studies, the investigator observes the study participants and gathers information for analysis (4). In contrast, experimental studies, such as randomized clinical trials, are designed by the investigator, study groups are selected, and often an intervention (such as a new type of treatment) is given to one group of participants. The study participants are followed and the outcomes of each group are measured and compared.

PREVALENCE OF ALCOHOL USE DISORDERS

A number of major surveys in the United States and internationally have assessed the prevalence of addiction. Comparison of these studies sometimes is difficult because they employ different definitions of addiction. Some surveys have used structured interviews according to criteria that have become universally recognized, such as the *Diagnostic and Statistical Manual of Mental Disorders* (6), now in a revised fourth edition (DSM-IV), and the *International Classification of Diseases*, now in its 10th revision (7). Throughout the text when we use the term *substance use disorder*, we are referring to substance abuse and/or dependence. The earliest survey to assess the epidemiology of psychiatric and substance use disorders in the United States using a structured psychiatric interview was the National Institute of Mental Health's Epidemiologic Catchment Area (ECA) study (8–10). Baseline interviews for this study were conducted between 1980 and 1984, when collaborators in the ECA assessed a probability sample of more than 20,000 adult participants in five metropolitan areas of the United States. Using the Diagnostic Interview Schedule (11), diagnoses of substance abuse and dependence were assessed according to criteria from the *Diagnostic and Statistical Manual of Mental Disorders, 3rd Edition* (DSM-III) (12). Overall occurrence of alcohol use disorders in the baseline ECA survey were 13.5% for lifetime prevalence, 4.8% for 6-month prevalence, and 2.8% for 1-month prevalence (13). More recent studies have identified alcohol use disorders according to the criteria of the revised third (DSM-III-R) and fourth (DSM-IV) editions of the DSM (14,15). Findings from the National Comorbidity Survey (NCS), completed between 1990 and 1992, which used DSM-III-R criteria for abuse and dependence and a modified version of the Composite International Diagnostic Interview, yielded higher lifetime and 12-month prevalence estimates than previously had been reported (16). Lifetime prevalence for alcohol abuse among males was found to be 12.5%, and among females was 6.4%. Lifetime prevalence of alcohol dependence was 20.1% for males and 8.2% for females. Twelve-month prevalence estimates from the National Comorbidity Survey also were higher for alcohol abuse (3.4% for males and 1.6% for females) and alcohol dependence (6.6% for males, and 2.2% for females) (16,17). Analyses of the NCS also have revealed that approximately one-third of adolescent drinkers will transition to alcohol abuse or dependence (18). Data from the 2001–2002 National Epidemiologic Survey on Alcohol and Related Conditions (NESARC), a nationally representative sample survey sponsored by the National Institute on Alcohol Abuse and Alcoholism, provides lifetime and 12-month estimates of alcohol use disorders based on DSM-IV criteria using the Alcohol Use Disorder and Associated Disabilities Interview Schedule (19–21). Twelve-month prevalence of alcohol abuse from the NESARC was found to be 6.9% among men and 2.6% among women. For alcohol dependence, the estimates were 5.4% for men and 2.3% for women. Overall lifetime prevalence of DSM-IV alcohol abuse and dependence was 17.8% and 12.5%, respectively (19). Most studies have found that the prevalence of alcohol use disorders is highest among young adults. For example, prevalence of 12-month alcohol use disorder is highest among the 18- to 29-year old age group in the NESARC baseline survey, and generally decreases among older age groups (19).

Differences in estimates across surveys may be due to variations in the diagnostic instrumentation, the version of the DSM that prevailed at the time the survey was completed, the size of the survey sample, and the locale of the survey participants (nationally representative samples vs. individual communities), as well as specific characteristics of the populations surveyed, including the age range of study participants. For example, the National Comorbidity Survey included a relatively younger population (persons ages 15 to 54 years) than some other surveys (17). In addition, specific methods used during data gathering (e.g., self-administered computerized vs. face-to-face interviews; use of identifiers for follow-up assessment vs. anonymity) may relate to differences in survey findings (22). Narrow and colleagues (23) have provided revised prevalence estimates, based on data from both the ECA and NCS, by focusing on clinical significance criteria among cases from both surveys that met diagnostic criteria. When the clinical significance criteria were used, disparities between the two surveys were attenuated. For example, the revised one-year prevalence of alcohol use disorders among adults aged 18 to 54 was estimated to be 6.5% once the clinical significance criteria were applied (as compared with 9.9% without the clinical significance criteria). A total of 1.7% of those age 18 and over had clinically significant drug abuse or dependence in the preceding year (23). Differences in survey findings also may occur from use of "gated" procedures (24). For example, to maximize efficiency, in some surveys only individuals who screen positive for abuse are assessed for dependence. This approach was recently assessed in several articles that reported relatively small differences in estimated prevalence for ascertainment of some types of substance dependence (i.e., cannabis, cocaine) when "gated" as compared with "ungated" protocols are in place (24,25), but more appreciable differences in other substance dependence assessment (i.e., alcohol) (26). As a consequence, some individuals with dependence may not be identified among population-based surveys when gated procedures are used (26,27). In some assessments, these cases appear to be less likely to have received treatment and therefore may be less likely to be clinically apparent cases, but may be more likely to occur among specific subgroups of the population, such as among women and racial-ethnic minorities (27,28).

INCIDENCE OF ALCOHOL USE DISORDERS

Data from the Swedish Lundby study provide one of the few estimates of incidence of alcohol abuse and dependence over a prolonged follow-up period (29). The Lundby community was interviewed for the first time in 1947, reinterviewed in 1957 (with 1% lost to follow-up), and then examined again in 1972 (29–31). Of the 2,550 participants in the original survey, 98%

of those still alive in 1972 were reinterviewed. The investigators found that, among males, the overall age-adjusted annual incidence of alcohol abuse or dependence was 0.3%. They further found a general decline in incidence with age, with a sharp drop in incidence of alcohol use disorders among men, beginning in their thirties (29). The highest annual incidence for an alcohol use disorder among men—0.67% annual incidence—was found among the youngest age group: those 10 to 19 years of age (29). Of the 925 women examined in the Lundby community in 1972, only 3 were identified as having an alcohol use disorder (30).

Fillmore examined longitudinal data from population-based U.S. samples and also found that incidence of drinking problems generally was lower for women than for men, and that incidence for both men and women declined with age (32,33). Drinking problems were identified using scales which included measures of binge drinking; drinking to cope; loss of control of alcohol use; belligerence; and drinking-related problems involving one's spouse, friends, job, finances, and the law. Fillmore's findings also indicated different patterns of drinking by gender. For example, women tended to develop problems associated with drinking later in life than men, and women were found to have higher rates of remission across all age groups than did men (33). Data from the 1-year follow-up of the ECA surveys are consistent with other studies (34). The estimated annual incidence of Diagnostic Interview Schedule–defined alcohol use disorders among men was highest for the youngest age group (those aged 18 to 29: 5.8 per 100 person years) and decreased with age, with an overall annual incidence of 3.7 per 100 person years for men. For women, incidence also decreased with age, with an overall incidence of 0.6 per 100 person years. The peak incidence in women also was among those 18 to 29 years of age (1.1 per 100 person years) (34). Analyses using the extended follow-up from the Baltimore site of the ECA, between 1981 and 1996, indicate similar trends for the development of alcohol dependence (35). The recent prospective data from the NESARC have provided annual incidence rates for DSM-IV alcohol abuse (1.0 per 100 person years), and alcohol dependence (1.7 per 100 person years), and also indicate that the greatest risk for alcohol use disorders occurs during young adulthood (36).

PREVALENCE OF DRUG USE DISORDERS

Although several major surveys estimate the prevalence of drug use in the United States (37,38), there are fewer population-based studies that have examined the prevalence and incidence of drug use disorders or drug addiction. Earlier analyses from the ECA surveys yield an overall lifetime prevalence of illicit drug abuse and dependence (including prescription drug use disorders) of 6.2% (39). As discussed with regard to alcohol disorders, men generally have a higher lifetime prevalence of drug use and drug use disorders (39,40). However, among drug users, lifetime prevalence differed little by gender (for male users, lifetime prevalence was 21%, whereas for female users, it was 19%) (39). More recent data on the prevalence of illicit drug use disorders have been provided by findings from the NCS (17). In that survey, the lifetime prevalence of DSM-III-R drug abuse without dependence was found to be 5.4% among males and 3.5% among females. The estimates for lifetime prevalence of drug dependence were 9.2% for males and 5.9% for females. The data showed that close to half of adolescent drug users developed drug abuse or dependence (18). The 2001–2002 NESARC survey has provided data on the prevalence of 12-month and lifetime DSM-IV drug abuse and drug dependence. Lifetime prevalence of drug abuse and dependence in this survey are 7.7% and 2.6%, respectively; and the corresponding estimates for 12-month prevalence are 1.4% and 0.6%, with prevalence being consistently higher for males (19). Since 2000, the National Survey on Drug Use and Health (NSDUH) has gathered information on substance use disorders within the prior year based on DSM-IV criteria. From the 2006 survey, prevalence of illicit drug use disorders in the year before the survey were reported to be 2.8% overall, with the largest prevalence among young adults ages 18 to 25 years (8.1%) (41). As indicated previously in the discussion on alcohol use disorders, differences in data collection methodology as well as diagnostic instrumentation may account for some of the variations found in prevalence estimates reported for these large national surveys (22).

Lifetime prevalence of nicotine dependence, estimated from the NCS, has been reported to be 24% (42). From the 2006 NSDUH, we know that 25% of the population is current tobacco cigarette smokers (38). Data from the 2001–2002 NESARC indicate that 12.8% of the population meets DSM-IV criteria for nicotine dependence in the year before the survey (43). A greater proportion of males (14.1%) than females (11.1%) have current nicotine dependence. The vast majority of the individuals with dependence use tobacco cigarettes (93.7%) (43).

INCIDENCE OF DRUG USE DISORDERS

There is a relative paucity of information regarding the incidence of drug use disorders as a group, with less information available for specific drugs. Early findings from the 1-year prospective ECA data showed that the incidence of illicit drug use disorders as a group is greater for men than for women across the entire lifespan (34). The estimated annual incidence was 1.09 per 100 person-years of risk (34). For men, the estimated annual incidence for drug abuse/dependence was 1.66 per 100 person-years of risk, whereas for women, the estimated annual incidence was 0.66 per 100 person-years of risk. As was the case for alcohol-related disorders, the highest incidence for both men and women was found in the 18- to 29-year-old age group; incidence dropped sharply after young adulthood. The incidence of drug use disorders was zero among those 65 years of age and older (34). Recent analyses of the 3-year prospective NESARC data have provided current data for annual incidence of drug use disorders (36). Annual incidence of drug abuse (0.28 per 100 person-years) and drug dependence (0.32 per 100 person-years) were similar. As discussed previously, variations in incidence may reflect a number of differences in methodology, survey design, and study population (36).

CORRELATES AND SUSPECTED RISK FACTORS

Several correlates and suspected risk factors for alcohol and drug use disorders have been examined. Some of these are discussed in this section for both alcohol and drugs, because the suspected risk factors are similar, and there are many findings in common. This section is restricted to a discussion of a selection of personal or individual characteristics that have been found to be associated with drug and alcohol addiction. The discussion is by no means exhaustive and reviews only a fraction of the investigations in this area.

Gender As discussed previously, alcohol disorders and alcohol-related problems are more common among men than among women. This consistent finding has been shown in a number of cross-sectional surveys (16,17,19–21,30,38,40,44,45), as well as in prospective studies (33,34,36). In the 2006 National Survey on Drug Use and Health (38), the occurrence of past-year alcohol dependence or abuse was twofold greater for males (10.3% and 5.1% for males and females, respectively). Women drinkers are less likely to transition to alcohol dependence or to have persistent dependence after it develops (20). Differences in prevalence and incidence between men and women have been attributed to a number of factors. Cultural norms, societal standards, and body size and differences in the metabolism of alcohol all may contribute to the finding that women appear to use less alcohol and to have lower rates of alcohol addiction. As reviewed by Greenfield (46), survey data over the past 20 years provide evidence that the prevalence of alcohol use disorders among women may be increasing, perhaps as the result of changes in drinking patterns. Some hypothesize that changes in patterns of drinking among women may be a result of deviations from traditional female social roles, or related to changes brought about by the increased number of women in the labor force, as well as the combined input of home and work environments (47,48). Many characteristics (e.g., marital status, full-time employment, ethnicity, age, occupation, educational level), as well as the occurrence of life events, and the presence of other psychopathology (such as depression), may play a role in gender variability with respect to alcohol consumption and the development of alcohol disorders (49,50). In addition, there may be gender differences in drinking as a response to stress and specific stressors (51). In their review, Wilsnack and Wilsnack (52) assessed drinking and problem drinking among women in the United States and found that certain subgroups of women were more likely to have heavy drinking patterns and adverse drinking consequences. These included younger women, those in nontraditional jobs, and unmarried women cohabiting with a partner. Assessments across cultural groups have reported on the impact of gender equity as well as social roles in explaining gender differences in drinking patterns (53,54). In some subpopulations, there may be a strong association between physical or sexual violence and alcohol use initiation (55) and the occurrence of problem drinking or alcohol use disorders (56). A history of childhood sexual abuse also has been found to be a potential predictor of women's risk for alcohol and drug use disorders (57). However, the relationship of childhood sexual abuse to alcohol disorders among women is complex, and may involve a number of other family characteristics (58). There also are gender differences with respect to illicit drug disorders. As discussed for alcohol, males (boys and men) generally are more likely to use illicit drugs (39,59) and may have a higher prevalence (39) and incidence (60) of drug use and disorders than females. However, gender differences will differ by the specific substance and the age of use. For example, in the 2006 Monitoring the Future survey (37), prevalence of cigarette and alcohol use was higher for female adolescents in some grades. The social or cultural restrictions that are possible explanations for the reduced prevalence of alcohol use among women also may apply to some types of illicit drug use. However, some (61) but not all data (62) show that among drug users, the proportion of males and females who develop dependence is similar. In more recent analyses, using data from the National Comorbidity Survey Replication, sex differences in the risk of progression from first use to dependence have been found for cannabis with relatively smaller differences found for other substances such as cocaine (63). In the 2006 NSDUH (38), the overall proportion of substance use disorder in the past year (abuse or dependence) among participants 12 years of age or older was approximately twice as large for males (12.3%) than females (6.3%). However, in the subgroup ages 12 to 17, the proportion with substance abuse or dependence was very similar (8.0% and 8.1% for boys and girls, respectively).

Age Prevalence of alcohol use disorders are generally lower among older adults (19,20,23,45,64). This may occur for a number of reasons. Because the measure of prevalence depends on the incidence as well as the duration of the disease (4,65), alcohol use disorders may be less prevalent among the elderly because (i) the incidence decreases over the lifespan, or (ii) the duration of the disorder is reduced, or (iii) some combination of the two factors is in effect. If the duration of the disorder is reduced, it may be a result of an increase in remission with age, or a reduction in survival. In other words, with age, prevalence may be reduced because fewer individuals develop the disease, because the addiction problems have resolved, or because addicted individuals die earlier. Explanations for a decreased prevalence with age also may include (i) a reduced tolerance to alcohol with age (66); (ii) poorer recall among older adults; or (iii) a cohort effect (45). Further, the means by which alcohol disorders are identified in young adults may not be relevant to the elderly (67), with the result that alcohol problems and disorders may be underrecognized in older adults (67,68). Surveys that include only household participants may miss many with alcohol disorders who reside in nursing homes; also, older community residents with alcohol disorders may be less willing to participate in household surveys. Although longitudinal analyses show declines in the proportion of older adults who consume alcohol (69), problems related to alcohol use among the elderly may occur at lower levels of consumption, and older adults with alcohol use disorders may be at greater risk for comorbid problems (70,71). Recent survey analyses do provide evidence that incidence of alcohol disorders generally decline with age (35,36). The hazard rate for alcohol abuse and dependence has been found to be highest at approximately age 19, with a steady reduction in hazard with increasing age (19).

The age of onset of alcohol use has been investigated as a predictor of subsequent alcohol abuse and dependence (72–74). In general, the earlier the age of first use, the greater the estimated risk associated with the subsequent development of an alcohol use disorder. In addition, early drinking onset is associated with elevated risk of alcohol-related injuries (75), motor vehicle accidents (76), physical violence after drinking (77), and the level of drinking in response to stressors (78). Moreover, early-onset drug use is associated with an increased risk for the development of drug use disorders, as well as alcohol dependence (79). Smoking at an early age has been identified as a predictor of drinking, increases the risk for transition to alcohol abuse and dependence, and is associated with greater severity of alcohol use disorders if they do develop (80).

As with alcohol disorders, age correlates with the occurrence of drug use disorders. The highest prevalence and incidence rates for illicit drug disorders are found among individuals in late adolescence and young adulthood (39). Although incidence is low among older adults, and survival may be decreased for individuals with drug disorders as they age, other factors also may be involved. Prevalence may be lower among older adults because of a cohort effect. Exposure and availability of illicit drugs differs by birth cohort. For example, the current cohort of older adults had no access to crack cocaine in their youth. When evaluating changes in the frequency of a disorder (in this case, drug and alcohol addiction), distinctions need to be made between changes that uniformly occur for all age groups during a particular historic period (period effect), changes that occur with age as the individual matures (age effect), and a cohort effect that reflects differences in disease rate for individuals born in different years (81,82). As with alcohol use disorders, incidence of drug abuse and dependence does decrease with age (34,36). Onset of drug use disorders is the highest at approximately age 19 years, with sharp declines thereafter, so that hazard rates after age 25 are relatively low (83). In addition, early onset of drug use is associated with elevated risk for subsequent substance abuse and dependence (73,79,84). Some analyses show that patterns of addiction have changed and show a greater prevalence of alcohol and illicit drug dependence among cohorts born since World War II (20,61,62). Similarly, the risk of nicotine dependence is greatest among smokers in the most recent birth cohorts (42). Evidence examining birth cohort associations with initiation of use for specific substances using data from the National Comorbidity Survey Replication also indicate that more recent birth cohorts have been more likely to initiate drug use in childhood and early adolescence, particularly for cannabis, cocaine, and other extramedical drugs (60).

Race and Ethnicity Information on the relationship between alcohol and illicit drug disorders and racial and ethnic background is complex and sometimes conflicting. Some of the inconsistent findings result from the relative paucity of data involving ethnic and racial subgroups, the classifications used to group ethnic minorities, variations in the social acceptability of drinking and drug use practices within groups, and the relationship of socioeconomic status and the availability of health care to ethnic minority populations.

Findings from some studies indicate that drinking patterns among African Americans differ from Whites (19,27,85). Among African Americans, the onset of heavy drinking appears to begin later, rates of consumption and prevalence of disorders tends to be lower, and abstention rates are higher (21,45,60, 86–91). Although the odds of alcohol dependence are lower for blacks compared with whites, after it develops, it is more likely to be chronic (20). In addition, frequent heavy drinking (defined in this study as drinking five or more drinks at one sitting at least weekly) has declined faster among whites (89,90). Analyses of the NESARC indicate that the proportion of alcohol dependence without abuse is higher among African Americans and Hispanics (27). Compared with whites, African Americans tend to suffer more medical consequences from drinking, including higher mortality and psychiatric comorbidity (92–95). This may relate to differences in socioeconomic status, health habits, access to health care, health service utilization, and differing social and cultural environments (87,92,96–102). For example, neighborhood poverty has a greater effect on alcohol problems among black relative to white or Hispanic men (103). When socioeconomic factors are taken into account, race is often not a risk factor for alcohol and other substance use (104–106).

Drinking patterns vary among Hispanic groups (107–111), and variations may reflect factors such as social and cultural environment, degree of acculturation, country of national origin, generational status, nativity, and time since immigration (110–123). Caetano found that Hispanic Americans (particularly Hispanic women) who were acculturated to U.S. society tended to drink more and were classified more frequently as heavy drinkers (110). Acculturation also relates to time of first alcohol use, and drinking level, and to characteristics which may relate to drinking such as suicide attempts, and self-reported health status (119,124,125). It is not clear if acculturation influences alcohol use patterns among those seeking treatment (126), or alters treatment response (127). Prevalence of alcohol abuse and dependence is lower for Hispanics relative to whites (19,128). Yet alcohol dependence among Hispanics may be more persistent after it develops (20). Furthermore, mortality from liver cirrhosis is higher for Hispanic populations (94,129).

Asian Americans generally have the lowest levels of alcohol consumption and lowest prevalence of alcohol use disorders (19,38,128). There is some evidence that this is the result of the discomfort that occurs with the physiologic effects of the flushing response present in many individuals of this ethnic background (130), because of variations in the aldehyde dehydrogenase gene (91,131–133). There also is evidence that genetic heterogeneity may explain differences in rates of alcoholism among certain subgroups (134). However, as with Hispanic Americans, the Asian American population is composed of many subgroups with different backgrounds and cultural drinking practices (135), and nativity and immigration status has been found to be associated with differential risk of some alcohol and drug use disorders (136). Native Americans historically have had the highest prevalence of alcohol use disorders in the United States (19,38,128,137), with high drinking-related death rates (138–140). However, it is not accurate to generalize to all Native American populations, as drinking practices are varied across tribal groups, and cultural factors as well as socioeconomic factors play a role (137,139,140).

Patterns of drug use and drug disorders also vary by racial-ethnic group (39,62). However, less information is available for drug addiction than for alcoholism among different ethnic populations, particularly for specific substances. Data from the NCS show that whites are more likely than African Americans or Hispanics to use drugs, but are less likely to have persistent dependence once the disorder develops (62). Data from the 2006 NSDUH show that as was found for alcohol use disorders, the occurrence of past year illicit drug abuse and dependence was highest among Native Americans (classified as American Indian or Alaskan Native in the NSDUH) and lowest for the Asian American subgroup (38). Similar relationships were documented in analyses of 12-month prevalence using the NESARC (128). However, there is limited evidence for differences in incidence of drug disorders by race-ethnicity as assessed with the prospective NESARC data (36). In assessments of specific nonmedical prescription drug use and disorders (sedative, tranquilizer, opioid, and amphetamine), relative to whites, black, Asian, and Hispanic subgroups were less likely and Native Americans more likely to report use and to have lifetime abuse or dependence (141). As with alcohol disorders, prevalence also varies by nativity, immigration status, country of origin, and degree of acculturation (122,136,142–144). It also has been shown that the relationship of some risk factors among adolescents (such as low family pride, depressed mood, and low self-esteem) differ by ethnic group (119). Comorbid patterns of substance use disorders (128,145) and consequences of drug use, such as risk of arrest, also vary by race-ethnicity (146). The evaluation of race and its association with addiction is complex. As stated in the discussion on alcohol disorders, when examining illicit drug use patterns among different ethnic groups, it is important to consider socioeconomic characteristics (100). One study found that, although national survey data indicated a higher prevalence of crack cocaine smoking among some ethnic minorities, when area of neighborhood residence was taken into account, differences in the prevalence of drug use between racial groups were attenuated (104).

Family History Alcohol disorders cluster in families (147–149). Twin studies (150–155), adoption and cross-fostering studies (156–159) have attempted to answer the question of whether such familial relationships are the result of genetic transmission or a shared environment. Linkage studies have provided evidence for specific genes that may be involved in alcohol dependence (160–162). Recent whole-genome association studies may provide evidence for possible novel genes related to alcoholism (163). There also have been a number of investigations of physiologic and biochemical markers associated with alcoholism (164–169). Studies examining familial patterns of alcoholism have indicated a possible genetic relationship. However, many individuals whose parents drink do not become alcoholic themselves (170,171), and many who develop alcohol disorders do not have a family history of alcoholism (147,172). Clearly, environmental influences also play a significant role (173,174). Studies to assess the relationship of genetic liability to drug use disorders have shown evidence for heritability involving nicotine (175,176), caffeine (177), cannabis (176), and illicit drugs such as cocaine, hallucinogens, stimulants, and opiates (178–183). Moreover, assessments of the liability for more than one substance use disorder (184–186) have found evidence indicating common genetic vulnerabilities among some diagnoses such as alcohol and nicotine dependence (184), and include recent genomewide association studies of dependence on a range of substances (187). Analyses also have examined the associations of genetic liability to drug disorders with personality traits such as antisocial traits (188), behavioral under control (189), and risk taking (190). Many of these studies have provided evidence for the importance of familial and potential genetic mechanisms in the development of drug disorders.

Employment Status and Occupation Employment, or working for pay, also is related to alcohol use and the occurrence of alcohol disorders (45). For example, McCord (191) found that individuals with alcoholism were more frequently unable to work on a regular basis than those without alcoholism. Similarly, study results from the ECA have reported that individuals who were unemployed 6 months or more in the preceding 5 years had higher prevalence rates of alcoholism (45) and greater risk for development of alcohol disorders (105). In the 2006 NSDUH, findings indicate that most individuals that binge or drink heavily are employed; however, the proportion of full-time employed individuals that binge (29.7%) or drink heavily (8.9%) is lower than the proportion among the unemployed (34.2% and 12.2%, respectively) (38). Early drinking behavior in youth may be associated with employment outcomes in adulthood (192). However, working relatively long work hours may increase alcohol and drug use among adolescents (193,194). In addition, the prevalence of alcohol use disorders differs by type of occupation (195). For example, higher prevalence of alcohol abuse and dependence and higher mortality from liver cirrhosis have been found among those in occupations typically associated with laborers, "blue collar" occupations, or those in lower socioeconomic levels (196,197). However, other studies find that employment in high occupational strata is associated with alcohol abuse and dependence (198). In addition, stressful working conditions may be associated with drinking level (199). There also is evidence that the relationship of employment status and occupation type with the frequency of alcohol-related health problems and drinking level is different for men than for women (200). Analyses of the ECA surveys also have provided evidence that the effect of alcohol abuse and dependence on income status may occur as a result of the indirect effects the disorders have on educational achievement and marriage (201).

In the 2006 NSDUH, a higher proportion of illicit drug use was reported among individuals who were unemployed (18.5%) or employed part-time (9.4%) than among full-time employees (8.8%) (38). However, there is a tendency for employed men with illicit drug disorders to have lower income (39). This was also found with recent analyses of the NESARC for drug use disorders overall (83), but not when examining some types of substance use disorders such as those related to nonmedical prescription drug use (141). Analyses of the NCS indicate that high occupational strata are associated with drug use disorders (198). Further, as with alcoholism, there appear to be differences in the prevalence of illicit drug disorders and cigarette smoking associated with specific occupations (202–204). Yet, with few exceptions (205,206), it is often difficult to know which developed first; that is, whether lack of employment led to heavy drinking or drug use, or whether alcohol or drug problems resulted in job loss, inability to obtain work, or selection into a particular type of occupation.

Marital Status Marital status also has been found to be related to the occurrence of alcohol disorders and drinking behavior, but understanding the temporal relationships may be difficult (207,208). Alcohol and drug addiction may predate the time that individuals make decisions about marriage, and problems associated with drinking and drug use may be the reason some individuals remain single, or become separated or divorced. Analyses of the NESARC indicate that individuals who never married or are separated, divorced, or widowed are less likely than married or cohabiting couples to have prevalent or incident alcohol use disorders (19,36). Persons in stable marriages or cohabiting had the lowest 12-month prevalence of alcohol use disorders (6.1%), as opposed to adults who had never married (15.9%) (19). However, depending on how marital status is categorized, findings may differ. For example, in earlier analyses of the ECA, cohabiting adults who never married had the highest prevalence of lifetime alcoholism (45). Furthermore, in longitudinal analyses, Wilsnack et al. (52) reported that cohabiting women may be at elevated risk for heavy drinking. Chilcoat and Breslau (209) found that the incidence of alcohol disorder symptoms was higher among single or divorced participants than in those who were married, similar to current analyses of the NESARC (36). There also is evidence that the risk of problem drinking is higher for women with spouses or partners who drink heavily (52), and that the quality of marital relationships varies as a function of the presence of current heavy drinking (210). Some prospective data (207,211) indicate that the time of transition to one's first marriage is associated with reduced drinking.

Lifetime prevalence rates of illicit drug disorders also have been found to vary by marital status. Anthony and Helzer found that, for both men and women and generally across all ages, individuals who lived with a partner but had never married had the highest lifetime prevalence of drug disorders. Cohabiting unmarried men had a 30.2% lifetime prevalence of an illicit drug disorder, compared with a 3.6% prevalence for married men. Cohabiting women had a lifetime prevalence of 19.9%, compared with 1.8% among women with a stable marital history (39). This contrasts to recent analyses of the NESARC, which find that individuals that never married (classified separately from those that are cohabiting) are the group with the highest prevalence of drug use disorders (83). Lack of marital stability and the periods of transition to and from marriage or divorce appear to influence substance use, treatment outcomes, and drug-related mortality (211–215). Moreover, the severity of alcohol and drug use effects marital functioning and is associated with risk of partner violence (216,217). However, as reviewed by Epstein and McCrady (218), couples treatment of alcohol and drug disorders may achieve improvements in marital functioning and substance use.

Educational Level Educational level often is included as part of broader socioeconomic or social class characteristics (96), and studies of the relationship between educational level and the development of alcohol abuse and dependence may yield conflicting results. Heavier consumption patterns have been found among those with lower educational levels (219). However, this may depend on how drinking is assessed. Recent analyses of the 2006 NSDUH show that when examining current drinking status, the proportion who reported drinking in the prior month increased with higher levels of education. Yet reports of binge and heavy alcohol use was lower for those who graduated from college than for those who had not completed college or had less schooling (38). Moreover, studies using prospective data have shown that dropping out of high school or leaving college early is associated with an increased risk of alcohol abuse and dependence in adulthood (105,220). Analyses of inner city school children also have provided evidence suggesting that poor educational achievement and some early school behaviors are associated with risk for alcohol use disorders (221). Academic competence has been reported to be important in studies of risk factors for problem drinking behavior among adolescents (222–224). Furthermore, the relationship between educational attainment and alcohol misuse may differ by race (225).

Lifetime prevalence of drug disorders also varies by educational level. Using data from the ECA surveys, Anthony and Helzer (39) showed that for men and women of all ages, lifetime prevalence of illicit drug disorders was highest for those who dropped out of high school, and for those who entered college but failed to earn a degree. Recent analyses of the 2006 NSDUH indicate that illicit drug use is lowest for individuals who had completed college (5.9%) than for those with less education (those with some college experience (9.1%), or who did or did not graduate from high school (8.6% and 9.2%, respectively)) (38). Furthermore, the proportion of those with substance abuse or dependence also is lowest for college graduates. Eggert and Herting (226) found that high-risk youth (defined as adolescents with a history of school problems and/or school dropout) had greater adverse consequences from drug use as well as greater access to drugs relative to students considered low-risk (those defined as typical high-school students). Performance on some achievement tests is different and lower for substance-abusing adolescents than for a comparison group of student controls (227). Moreover, in prospective analyses of high school seniors, there is evidence of an association between poor educational achievement and substance use after high school (228). In addition, early education indicators may be associated with increased risk for subsequent drug use disorders (229).

COMORBIDITY OF ALCOHOL AND DRUG USE DISORDERS

Many clinical studies and assessments from household survey samples document the comorbid occurrence of substance use disorders with psychopathology (13,83,123,230–236). Data from the NCS show that the majority of people with an alcohol use disorder had at least one psychiatric disorder (16). In addition, some types of comorbidity are more common among women (16,237,238), and may differ by race (92). Analyses of the NESARC found positive associations for mood, anxiety, and personality disorders with most substance use disorders (123,239). For example, Grant et al. (123) found that all the independent mood and anxiety disorders (those occurring independent from withdrawal and intoxication with the substances involved) including major depression, dysthymia, mania, hypomania, social and specific phobia, panic, and generalized anxiety disorders are associated with alcohol and drug dependence. Close to half of all individuals (47.7%) with a current drug use disorder also have at least one personality disorder (239). Compton et al. (83) found that antisocial personality disorder was strongly associated with drug dependence even after adjusting for sociodemographic factors and other psychiatric disorders. Furthermore, the prevalence of alcohol and other substance use disorder comorbidity is typically high. For example, the 12-month prevalence of alcohol abuse or dependence among those with a drug use disorder in the prior 12 months is more than 50% for most substances assessed in the NESARC (240). The prevalence of psychiatric disorders among individuals in alcohol and drug treatment programs, or drug use among mental health patients in clinical facilities also show high estimates, but with wide ranges of prevalence depending on the assessment methods, population characteristics, and type of treatment setting (241–246). Outcomes tend to be worse for individuals with co-occurring psychiatric and substance use disorders, than for those without the comorbid condition (e.g., poorer psychological adjustment, worse psychiatric symptoms, reduced treatment effectiveness, greater risk for relapse, homelessness, and rehospitalization) (247–259).

With respect to studies of the stages of drug use, patterns of progression have been described that begin with the use of tobacco or alcohol with progression to marijuana and the use of other illicit drugs (260,261). For example, among most cocaine and crack users, marijuana use is an antecedent. There are also gender differences with regard to the significant role of the early use of alcohol for young men and cigarettes for young women (262). Further, there may be differences by gender with respect to the pathways that lead to substance use disorders, as well as in the type and severity of comorbid psychopathologies (263).

Until recently, there were relatively few population-based studies that permitted a prospective examination of comorbid relationships. For example, prospective data provide evidence that the onset of alcohol abuse and dependence is elevated among individuals who have specific substance use and psychiatric diagnoses (36,220), and some conditions may have a bidirectional temporal relationship (36,264). Assessments of long-term outcomes highlight the impact that these types of co-occurring conditions can have on level of functioning and attainment in areas of educational achievement, occupation and social relationships (265). As more information becomes available from longitudinal studies, it will be possible to better assess these temporal relationships. In addition, future investigations into the progression of symptoms will provide valuable information for clinical treatment, as well as a better understanding of potential etiologic relationships.

CONCLUSIONS

This chapter has attempted to summarize a sampling of major findings in epidemiologic studies of alcohol and drug addiction. In contrast to clinical practice, or basic science and laboratory research, epidemiology is a study of populations. As discussed in detail by Kleinbaum et al. (82), it is through this study of populations that epidemiologic research aims to describe the health status and distribution of disease in populations, as well as to identify risk factors and potential etiologic agents of disease, which may enable us to better predict and prevent disease. The ultimate goals for the study of alcohol and drug use epidemiology are to improve our understanding of etiologic mechanisms, identify targets for intervention, and reduce the prevalence of addictive disorders.

ACKNOWLEDGMENTS: *This work was supported by a Scientist Development Award for Clinicians from the National Institute on Alcohol Abuse and Alcoholism (AA00168).*

REFERENCES

1. Gordis E. *Epidemiology,* 4th ed. Philadelphia: Saunders Elsevier, 2009.
2. Lilienfeld DE, Stolley PD. *Foundations of epidemiology,* 3rd ed. New York: Oxford University Press, 1994.
3. Last JM, ed. *A dictionary of epidemiology,* 4th ed. New York: Oxford University Press, 2001.

4. Mausner JS, Kramer S, eds. *Mausner and Bahn epidemiology: an introductory text.* Philadelphia: WB Saunders, 1985.
5. Rothman KJ, Greenland S, eds. *Modern epidemiology,* 2nd ed. Philadelphia: Lippincott-Raven, 1998.
6. American Psychiatric Association (APA). *Diagnostic and statistical manual of mental disorders,* 4th ed., text revision. Washington, D.C.: American Psychiatric Press, 2000.
7. World Health Organization. *The ICD-10 classification of mental and behavioural disorders.* Geneva, Switzerland: World Health Organization, 1992.
8. Eaton WW, Kessler LG. *Epidemiologic field methods in psychiatry; the NIMH Epidemiologic Catchment Area Program.* Orlando, FL: Academic Press, 1985.
9. Eaton WW, Kramer M, Anthony JE. Conceptual and methodological problems in estimation of the incidence of mental disorders from field survey data. In: Cooper B, Helgason T, eds. *Epidemiology and the prevention of mental disorders (World Psychiatric Association).* New York: Routledge, 1989:108–127.
10. Robins LN, Regier DA. *Psychiatric disorders in America: the Epidemiologic Catchment Area Study.* New York: The Free Press/MacMillan, Inc., 1991.
11. Robins LN, Healzer JE, Croughan J. National Institute of Mental Health diagnostic interview schedule: its history, characteristics, and validity. *Arch Gen Psychiatry* 1981;38:381–389.
12. American Psychiatric Association. *Diagnostic and statistical manual of mental disorders,* 3rd ed. Washington, DC: American Psychiatric Association, 1980.
13. Regier DA, Farmer ME, Rae DS, et al. Comorbidity of mental disorders with alcohol and other drug abuse: results from the Epidemiologic Catchment Area (ECA) Study. *JAMA* 1990;264(19):2511–2518.
14. American Psychiatric Association. *Diagnostic and statistical manual of mental disorders,* 3rd ed., revised. Washington, DC: American Psychiatric Association, 1987.
15. American Psychiatric Association. *Diagnostic and statistical manual of mental disorders,* 4th ed. Washington, DC: American Psychiatric Association, 1994.
16. Kessler RC, Crum RM, Warner LA, et al. Lifetime co-occurrence of DSM-III-R alcohol abuse and dependence with other psychiatric disorders in the National Comorbidity Survey. *Arch Gen Psychiatry* 1997;54: 313–321.
17. Kessler RC, McGonagle KA, Zhao S, et al. Lifetime and 12-month prevalence of DSM-III-R psychiatric disorders in the United States. *Arch Gen Psychiatry* 1994;51:8–19.
18. Warner LA, Canino G, Colon HM. Prevalence and correlates of substance use disorders among older adolescents in Puerto Rico and the United States: a cross-cultural comparison. *Drug Alcohol Depend* 2001;63(3):229–243.
19. Hasin DS, Stinson FS, Ogburn E, et al. Prevalence, correlates, disability, and comorbidity of DSM-IV alcohol abuse and dependence in the United States: results from the National Epidemiologic Survey on Alcohol and Related Conditions. *Arch Gen Psychiatry* 2007;64(7):830–842.
20. Grant BF. Prevalence and correlates of alcohol use and DSM-IV alcohol dependence in the United States: results of the National Longitudinal Alcohol Epidemiologic Survey. *J Stud Alcohol* 1997;58(5):464–473.
21. Grant BF, Harford TC, Dawson DA, et al. Prevalence of DSM-IV alcohol abuse and dependence. United States 1992. *Alcohol Health Res World* 1994;18(3):243–248.
22. Grucza RA, Abbacchi AM, Przybeck TR, et al. Discrepancies in estimates of prevalence and correlates of substance use and disorders between two national surveys. *Addiction* 2007;102(4):623–629.
23. Narrow WE, Rae DS, Robbins LN, et al. Revised prevalence estimates of mental disorders in the United States. *Arch Gen Psychiatry* 2002; 59(2):115–123.
24. Degenhardt L, Bohnert KM, Anthony JC. Assessment of cocaine and other drug dependence in the general population: "gated" versus "ungated" approaches. *Drug Alcohol Depend* 2008;93(3):227–232.
25. Degenhardt L, Cheng H, Anthony JC. Assessing cannabis dependence in community surveys: methodological issues. *Int J Methods Psychiatr Res* 2007;16(2):43–51.
26. Degenhardt L, Bohnert KM, Anthony JC. Case ascertainment of alcohol dependence in general population surveys: 'gated' versus 'ungated' approaches. *Int J Methods Psychiatr Res* 2007;16(3):111–123.
27. Hasin DS, Grant BF. The co-occurrence of DSM-IV alcohol abuse in DSM-IV alcohol dependence: results of the National Epidemiologic Survey on Alcohol and Related Conditions on heterogeneity that differ by population subgroup. *Arch Gen Psychiatry* 2004;61(9):891–896.
28. Hasin DS, Hatzenbueler M, Smith S, Grant BF. Co-occurring DSM-IV drug abuse in DSM-IV drug dependence: results from the National Epidemiologic Survey on Alcohol and Related Conditions. *Drug Alcohol Depend* 2005;80(1):117–123.
29. Ojesjo L, Hagnell O, Lanke J. Incidence of alcoholism among men in the Lundby community cohort Sweden, 1957–1972. Probabilistic baseline calculations. *J Stud Alcohol* 1982;43(11):1190–1198.
30. Ojesjo L. Prevalence of known and hidden alcoholism in the revisited Lundby population. *Soc Psychiatry* 1980;15:81–90.
31. Hagnell O. *A prospective study of the incidence of mental disorder.* Lund, Sweden: Svenska Bokforlaget, 1966.
32. Fillmore KM. Prevalence, incidence and chronicity of drinking patterns and problems among men as a function of age: a longitudinal and cohort analysis. *Br J Addict* 1987;82:77–83.
33. Fillmore KM. Women's drinking across the adult life course as compared to men's. *Br J Addict* 1987;82:801–811.
34. Eaton WW, Kramer M, Anthony JC, et al. The incidence of specific DIS/DSM-III mental disorders: data from the NIMH Epidemiologic Catchment Area Program. *Acta Psychiatr Scand* 1989;79:163–178.
35. Crum RM, Chan YF, Chen LS, et al. Incidence rates for alcohol dependence among adults: prospective data from the Baltimore Epidemiologic Catchment Area Follow-Up Survey, 1981–1996. *J Stud Alcohol* 2005;66(6):795–805.
36. Grant BF, Goldstein RB, Chou SP, et al. Sociodemographic and psychopathologic predictors of first incidence of DSM-IV substance use, mood and anxiety disorders: results from the Wave 2 National Epidemiologic Survey on Alcohol and Related Conditions. *Mol Psychiatry* 2008. Apr 22. [Epub ahead of print]
37. Johnston LD, O'Malley PM, Bachman JG, et al. *Monitoring the Future national results on adolescent drug use: overview of key findings, 2006.* NIH Publication No. 07-6202. Bethesda, MD: National Institute on Drug Abuse, 2007.
38. Substance Abuse and Mental Health Services Administration. Results from the 2006 National Survey on Drug Use and Health: National Findings. Office of Applied Studies, NSDUH Series H-32, DHHS Publication No. SMA 07-4293. Rockville, MD, SAMHSA, Office of Applied Studies, 2007.
39. Anthony JC, Helzer JE. Syndromes of drug abuse and dependence. In: Robins LN, Regier DA, eds. *Psychiatric disorders in America.* New York: The Free Press/Macmillan, 1991:116–154.
40. Robins LN, Helzer JE, Weissman MM, et al. Lifetime prevalence of specific psychiatric disorders in three sites. *Arch Gen Psychiatry* 1994;41:949–958.
41. Hughes A, Sathe N, Spagnola K. State estimates of substance use from the 2005–2006 National Surveys on Drug Use and Health. DHHS Publication No. SMA-08-4311, NSDUH Series H-33. Rockville, MD: Substance Abuse and Mental Health Services Administration, Office of Applied Studies, 2008.
42. Breslau N, Johnson EO, Hiripi E, et al. Nicotine dependence in the United States: prevalence, trends, and smoking persistence. *Arch Gen Psychiatry* 2001;58(9):810–816.
43. Grant BF, Hasin DS, Chou SP, et al. Nicotine dependence and psychiatric disorders in the United States: results from the national epidemiologic survey on alcohol and related conditions. *Arch Gen Psychiatry* 2004;61(11):1107–1115.
44. Caetano R, Tam TW. Prevalence and correlates of DSM-IV and ICD-10 alcohol dependence: 1990 U.S. National Alcohol Survey. *Alcohol Alcohol* 1995;39(2):177–186.
45. Helzer JE, Burnam A, McEvoy LT. Alcohol abuse and dependence. In: Robins LE, Regier DA, eds. *Psychiatric disorders in America.* New York: The Free Press, 1991:81–115.

46. Greenfield SF. Women and alcohol use disorders. *Harvard Rev Psychiatry* 2002;10(2):76–85.
47. Parker DA, Harford TC. Gender-role attitudes, job competition and alcohol consumption among women and men. *Alcohol Clin Exp Res* 1992;16(2):159–165.
48. Hall EM. Double exposure: the combined impact of the home and work environments on psychosomatic strain in Swedish women and men. *Int J Health Serv* 1992;22(2):239–260.
49. Gorman DM. Employment, stressful life events and the development of alcohol dependence. *Drug Alcohol Depend* 1988;22:151–159.
50. Wilsnack SC, Klassen AD, Schur BE, et al. Predicting onset and chronicity of women's problem drinking: A five-year longitudinal analysis. *Am J Public Health* 1991;81(3):305–318.
51. Dawson DA, Grant BF, Ruan WJ. The association between stress and drinking: modifying effects of gender and vulnerability. *Alcohol Alcohol* 2005;40(5):453–460.
52. Wilsnack SC, Wilsnack RW. Drinking and problem drinking in U.S. women. Patterns and recent trends. In: Galanter M, ed. *Recent developments in alcoholism.* New York: Plenum Press, 1995:29–60.
53. Bloomfield K, Gmel G, Wilsnack S. Introduction to special issue 'Gender, Culture and Alcohol Problems: a Multi-national Study'. *Alcohol Alcohol Suppl* 2006;41(1):i3–i7.
54. Wilsnack RW, Vogeltanz ND, Wilsnack SC, et al. Gender differences in alcohol consumption and adverse drinking consequences: cross-cultural patterns. *Addiction* 2000;95(2):251–265.
55. Hamburger ME, Leeb RT, Swahn MH. Childhood maltreatment and early alcohol use among high-risk adolescents. *J Stud Alcohol Drugs* 2008; 69(2):291–295.
56. Lown AE, Vega WA. Alcohol abuse or dependence among Mexican American women who report violence. *Alcohol Clin Exp Res* 2001;25(10): 1479–1486.
57. Wilsnack SC, Vogeltanz ND, Klassen AD, et al. Childhood sexual abuse and women's substance abuse: national survey findings. *J Stud Alcohol* 1997;58(3):264–271.
58. Fleming J, Mullen PE, Sibthorpe B, et al. The relationship between childhood sexual abuse and alcohol abuse in women—a case-control study. *Addiction* 1998;93(12):1787–1798.
59. Johnston LD, O'Malley PM, Bachman JG. Smoking, drinking, and illicit drug use among American secondary school students, college students, and young adults, 1975–1991; Vol. I, secondary school students. Rockville, MD: National Institute on Drug Abuse, 1992.
60. Degenhardt L, Chiu WT, Sampson N, et al. Epidemiological patterns of extra-medical drug use in the United States: evidence from the National Comorbidity Survey Replication, 2001–2003. *Drug Alcohol Depend* 2007;90:210–223.
61. Grant BF. Prevalence and correlates of drug use and DSM-IV drug dependence in the United States: results of the National Longitudinal Alcohol Epidemiologic Survey. *J Subst Abuse* 1996;8(2):195–210.
62. Warner LA, Kessler RC, Hughes M, et al. Prevalence and correlates of drug use and dependence in the United States. Results from the National Comorbidity Survey. *Arch Gen Psychiatry* 1995;52(3):219–229.
63. Wagner FA, Anthony JC. Male-female differences in the risk of progression from first use to dependence upon cannabis, cocaine, and alcohol. *Drug Alcohol Depend* 2007;86(2–3):191–198.
64. Kandel D, Chen K, Warner LA, et al. Prevalence and demographic correlates of symptoms of last year dependence on alcohol, nicotine, marijuana and cocaine in the U.S. population. *Drug Alcohol Depend* 1997;44(1):11–29.
65. Lilienfeld AM, Lilienfeld DE. *Foundations of epidemiology,* 2nd ed. New York: Oxford University Press, 1980.
66. Vestal R, McGuire EA, Tobin JD, et al. Aging and ethanol metabolism. *Clin Pharmacol Ther* 1977;21(3):343–354.
67. Graham K. Identifying and measuring alcohol abuse among the elderly: serious problems with existing instrumentation. *J Stud Alcohol* 1986; 47:322–326.
68. Blow FC. Treatment of older women with alcohol problems: meeting the challenge for a special population. *Alcohol Clin Exp Res* 2000;24 (8):1257–1266.
69. Adams WL, Garry PJ, Rhyne R, et al. Alcohol intake in the healthy elderly. Changes with age in a cross-sectional and longitudinal study. *J Am Geriatr Soc* 1990;28:211–216.
70. Dufour M, Fuller RK. Alcohol in the elderly. *Annu Rev Med* 1995;46: 123–132.
71. Liberto JG, Oslin DW, Ruskin PE. Alcoholism in older persons: a review of the literature. *Hosp Commun Psych* 1992;43(10):975–984.
72. DeWit DJ, Adlaf EM, Offord DR, et al. Age at First Alcohol Use: A risk factor for the development of alcohol disorders. *Am J Psychiatry* 2000; 157(5):745–750.
73. Grant BF, Dawson DA. Age at onset of alcohol use and its association with DSM-IV alcohol abuse and dependence: results from the National Longitudinal Alcohol Epidemiologic Survey. *J Subst Abuse* 1997;9:103–110.
74. Grant BF, Stinson FS, Harford TC. Age at onset of alcohol use DSM-IV alcohol abuse and dependence: a 12-year follow-up. *J Subst Abuse* 2001;13(4):494–504.
75. Hingson RW, Heeren T, Jamanka A, et al. Age of drinking onset and unintentional injury involvement after drinking. *JAMA* 2000;284(12): 1527–1533.
76. Hingson R, Heeren T, Levenson S, et al. Age of drinking onset, driving after drinking, and involvement in alcohol related motor-vehicle crashes. *Accid Anal Prev* 2002;34(1):85–92.
77. Hingson R, Heeren T, Zakocs R. Age of drinking onset and involvement in physical fights after drinking. *Pediatrics* 2001;108(4):872–877.
78. Dawson DA, Grant BF, Li TK. Impact of age at first drink on stress-reactive drinking. *Alcohol Clin Exp Res* 2007;31(1):69–77.
79. Grant BF, Dawson DA. Age of onset of drug use and its association with DSM-IV drug abuse and dependence: results from the National Longitudinal Alcohol Epidemiologic Survey. *J Subst Abuse* 1998;10(2):163–173.
80. Grant BF. Age at smoking onset and its association with alcohol consumption and DSM-IV alcohol abuse and dependence: results from the national longitudinal alcohol epidemiologic survey. *J Subst Abuse* 1998; 10(1):59–73.
81. O'Malley PM, Bachman JG, Johnston LD. Period, age, and cohort effects on substance use among young Americans: a decade of change, 1976–1986. *Am J Public Health* 1988;78(10):1315–1321.
82. Kleinbaum DG, Kupper LL, Morgenstern H. *Epidemiologic research.* New York: Van Nostrand Reinhold, 1982.
83. Compton WM, Thomas YF, Stinson FS, et al. Prevalence, correlates, disability, and comorbidity of DSM-IV drug abuse and dependence in the United States: results from the national epidemiologic survey on alcohol and related conditions. *Arch Gen Psychiatry* 2007;64(5):566–576.
84. McCabe SE, West BT, Morales M, et al. Does early onset of non-medical use of prescription drugs predict subsequent prescription drug abuse and dependence? Results from a national study. *Addiction* 2007;102(12): 1920–1930.
85. Lex BW. Review of alcohol problems in ethnic minority groups. *J Consult Clin Psychol* 1987;55(3):293–300.
86. Herd D. Rethinking Black drinking. *Br J Addict* 1987;82:219–223.
87. Otten MW, Teutsch SM, Williamson DF, et al. The effect of known risk factors on the excess mortality of black adults in the United States. *JAMA* 1990;263:845–850.
88. Caetano R, Clark CL. Trends in alcohol consumption patterns among whites, blacks and Hispanics: 1984 and 1995. *J Stud Alcohol* 1998;59(6): 659–668.
89. Caetano R, Kaskutas L. Changes in drinking patterns among Whites, Blacks, and Hispanics, 1984–1992. *J Stud Alcohol* 1995;56:558–565.
90. Jones-Webb R. Drinking patterns and problems among African Americans: Recent findings. *Alcohol Health Res World* 1998;22(4):260–264.
91. Higuchi S, Matsushita S, Murayama M, et al. Alcohol and aldehyde dehydrogenase polymorphisms and the risk for alcoholism. *Am J Psychiatry* 1995;152(8):1219–1221.
92. Hesselbrock MN, Hesselbrock VM, Segal B, et al. Ethnicity and psychiatric comorbidity among alcohol-dependent persons who receive inpatient treatment: African Americans, Alaska natives, Caucasians, and Hispanics. *Alcohol Clin Exp Res* 2003;27(8):1368–1373.
93. Polednak AP. Secular trend in U.S. black-white disparities in selected alcohol-related cancer incidence rates. *Alcohol Alcohol* 2007;42(2):125–130.

94. Stinson FS, Grant BF, Dufour MC. The critical dimension of ethnicity in liver cirrhosis mortality statistics. *Alcohol Clin Exp Res* 2001;25(8):1181–1187.
95. Caetano R. Alcohol-related health disparities and treatment-related epidemiological findings among whites, blacks, and Hispanics in the United States. *Alcohol Clin Exp Res* 2003;27(8):1337–1339.
96. Park P. Social-class factors in alcoholism. In: Kissin B, Begleiter H, eds. *The pathogenesis of alcoholism. Psychosocial factors.* New York: Plenum Press, 1983:365–404.
97. Jones-Webb RJ, Hsiao C-Y, Hannan P. Relationships between socioeconomic status and drinking problems among black and white men. *Alcohol Clin Exp Res* 1995;19(3):623–627.
98. Lillie-Blanton M, MacKenzie E, Anthony JC. Black-white differences in alcohol use by women: Baltimore survey findings. *Public Health Rep* 1991;106(2):124–133.
99. Herd D. Subgroup differences in drinking patterns among black and white men: results from a national survey. *J Stud Alcohol* 1990;51(3):221–232.
100. Herd D. Predicting drinking problems among black and white men: results from a national survey. *J Stud Alcohol* 1994;55(1):61–71.
101. Williams GD, Dufour M, Bertolucci D. Drinking levels, knowledge, and associated characteristics, 1985 NHIS findings. *Public Health Rep* 1986;101(6):593–598.
102. Schoenborn CA. Health habits of U.S. adults, 1985: the "Alameda 7" revisited. *Public Health Rep* 1986;101(6):571–580.
103. Jones-Webb R, Snowden L, Herd D, et al. Alcohol-related problems among black, Hispanic and white men: the contribution of neighborhood poverty. *J Stud Alcohol* 1997;58:539–545.
104. Lillie-Blanton M, Anthony JC, Schuster CR. Probing the meaning of racial/ethnic group comparisons in crack cocaine smoking. *JAMA* 1993;24:993–997.
105. Crum RM, Bucholz KK, Helzer JE, Anthony JC. The risk of alcohol abuse and dependence in adulthood: the association with educational level. *Am J Epidemiol* 1992;135(9):989–999.
106. Mensch BS, Kandel DB. Dropping out of high school and drug involvement. *Sociol Educ* 1988;61:95–113.
107. Nielsen AL. Examining drinking patterns and problems among Hispanic groups: results from a national survey. *J Stud Alcohol* 2000;61(2):301–310.
108. Dawson DA. Beyond black, white and Hispanic: race, ethnic origin and drinking patterns in the United States. *J Subst Abuse* 1998;10(4):321–339.
109. Lee DJ, Markides KS, Ray LA. Epidemiology of self-reported past heavy drinking in Hispanic adults. *Ethn Health* 1997;2(1–2):77–88.
110. Caetano R. Acculturation and drinking patterns among U.S. Hispanics. *Br J Addict* 1987;82:789–799.
111. Caetano R. Alcohol use among Hispanic groups in the United States. *Am J Drug Alcohol Abuse* 1988;14(3):293–308.
112. Strunin L, Edwards EM, Godette DC, et al. Country of origin, age of drinking onset, and drinking patterns among Mexican American young adults. *Drug Alcohol Depend* 2007;91(2–3):134–140.
113. Zayas LH, Rojas M, Malgady RG. Alcohol and drug use, and depression among Hispanic men in early adulthood. *Am J Community Psychol* 1998;26(3):425–438.
114. Ussher M, West R, Doshi R, et al. Acute effect of isometric exercise on desire to smoke and tobacco withdrawal symptoms. *Hum Psychopharmacol* 2006;21(1):39–46.
115. Polednak AP. Gender and acculturation in relation to alcohol use among Hispanic (Latino) adults in two areas of the northeastern United States. *Subst Use Misuse* 1997;32(11):1513–1524.
116. Caetano R, Raspberry K. Drinking and DSM-IV alcohol and drug dependence among white and Mexican-American DUI offenders. *J Stud Alcohol* 2000;61(3):420–426.
117. Zimmerman RS, Vega WA, Gil AG, et al. Who is Hispanic? Definitions and their consequences. *Am J Public Health* 1994;84(12):1985–1987.
118. Neff JA, Hoppe SK. Acculturation and drinking patterns among U.S. Anglos, blacks, and Mexican Americans. *Alcohol Alcohol* 1992;27(3):293–308.
119. Vega WA, Zimmerman RS, Warheit GJ, et al. Risk factors for early adolescent drug use in four ethnic and racial groups. *Am J Public Health* 1993;83(2):185–189.
120. Cervantes RC, Gilbert MJ, Salgado de Snyder N, et al. Psychosocial and cognitive correlates of alcohol use in younger adult immigrant and U.S.-born Hispanics. *Int J Addict* 1990;25(5A-6A):687–708.
121. Turner RJ, Gil AG. Psychiatric and substance use disorders in South Florida: racial/ethnic and gender contrasts in a young adult cohort. *Arch Gen Psychiatry* 2002;59(1):43–50.
122. Alegria M, Canino G, Stinson FS, et al. Nativity and DSM-IV psychiatric disorders among Puerto Ricans, Cuban Americans, and non-Latino Whites in the United States: results from the National Epidemiologic Survey on Alcohol and Related Conditions. *J Clin Psychiatry* 2006;67(1):56–65.
123. Grant BF, Stinson FS, Dawson DA, et al. Prevalence and co-occurrence of substance use disorders and independent mood and anxiety disorders: results from the National Epidemiologic Survey on Alcohol and Related Conditions. *Arch Gen Psychiatry* 2004;61(8):807–816.
124. Finch BK, Vega WA. Acculturation stress, social support, and self-rated health among Latinos in California. *J Immigr Health* 2003;5(3):109–117.
125. Finch BK, Hummer RA, Reindl M, et al. Validity of self-rated health among Latino(a)s. *Am J Epidemiol* 2002;155(8):755–759.
126. Arciniega LT, Arroyo JA, Miller WR, et al. Alcohol, drug use and consequences among Hispanics seeking treatment for alcohol-related problems. *J Stud Alcohol* 1996;57(6):613–618.
127. Arroyo JA, Miller WR, Tonigan JS. The influence of Hispanic ethnicity on long-term outcome in three alcohol-treatment modalities. J Stud Alcohol 2003;64(1):98–104.
128. Smith SM, Stinson FS, Dawson DA, et al. Race/ethnic differences in the prevalence and co-occurrence of substance use disorders and independent mood and anxiety disorders: results from the National Epidemiologic Survey on Alcohol and Related Conditions. *Psychol Med* 2006;36(7):987–998.
129. Bolen JC, Rhodes L, Powell-Griner EE, et al. State-specific prevalence of selected health behaviors, by race and ethnicity—Behavioral Risk Factor Surveillance System, 1997. *Mort Mortal Wkly Rep CDC Surveill Summ* 2000;49(2):1–60.
130. Suddendorf RF. Research on alcohol metabolism among Asians and its implications for understanding causes of alcoholism. *Public Health Rep* 1989;104(6):615–620.
131. Luczak SE, Elvine-Kreis B, Shea SH, et al. Genetic risk for alcoholism relates to level of response to alcohol in Asian-American men and women. *J Stud Alcohol* 2002;63(1):74–82.
132. Wall TL, Shea SH, Chan KK, et al. A genetic association with the development of alcohol and other substance use behavior in Asian Americans. *J Abnorm Psychol* 2001;110(1):173–178.
133. McCarthy DM, Wall TL, Brown SA, et al. Integrating biological and behavioral factors in alcohol use risk: the role of ALDH2 status and alcohol expectancies in a sample of Asian Americans. *Exp Clin Psychopharmacol* 2000;8(2):168–175.
134. Hsu Y-PP, Loh EW, Chen WJ, et al. Association of monoamine oxidase A alleles with alcoholism among male chinese in Taiwan. *Am J Psychiatry* 1996;153(9):1209–1211.
135. Nemoto T, Aoki B, Huang K, et al. Drug use behaviors among Asian drug users in San Francisco. *Addict Behav* 1999;24(6):823–838.
136. Breslau J, Chang DF. Psychiatric disorders among foreign-born and U.S.-born Asian-Americans in a U.S. national survey. *Soc Psychiatry Psychiatr Epidemiol* 2007;41(12):943–950.
137. Spicer P, Beals J, Croy CD, et al. The prevalence of DSM-III-R alcohol dependence in two American Indian populations. *Alcohol Clin Exp Res* 2003;27(11):1785–1797.
138. Gilliland FD, Becker TM, Samet JM, et al. Trends in alcohol-related mortality among New Mexico's American Indians, Hispanics, and non-Hispanic whites. *Alcohol Clin Exp Res* 1995;19(6):1572–1577.
139. Rhoades ER, Hammond J, Welty TK, et al. The Indian burden of illness and future health interventions. *Public Health Rep* 1987;102(4):361–368.
140. Christian CM, Dufour M, Bertolucci D. Differential alcohol-related mortality among American indian tribes in Oklahoma, 1968–1878. *Soc Sci Med* 1989;28(3):275–284.
141. Huang B, Dawson DA, Stinson FS, et al. Prevalence, correlates, and comorbidity of nonmedical prescription drug use and drug use disorders in

the United States: results of the National Epidemiologic Survey on Alcohol and Related Conditions. *J Clin Psychiatry* 2007;67(7):1062–1073.

142. Grant BF, Stinson FS, Hasin DS, et al. Immigration and lifetime prevalence of DSM-IV psychiatric disorders among Mexican Americans and non-Hispanic whites in the United States: results from the National Epidemiologic Survey on Alcohol and Related Conditions. *Arch Gen Psychiatry* 2004;61(12):1226–1233.
143. Burnam MA, Hough RL, Karno M, et al. Acculturation and lifetime prevalence of psychiatric disorders among Mexican Americans in Los Angeles. *J Health Soc Behav* 1987;28:89–102.
144. Gfroerer J, De La Rosa M. Protective and risk factors associated with drug use among Hispanic youth. *J Addict Dis* 1993;12(2):87–107.
145. Falk DE, Yi HY, Hiller-Sturmhofel S. An epidemiologic analysis of co-occurring alcohol and tobacco use and disorders: findings from the National Epidemiologic Survey on Alcohol and Related Conditions. *Alcohol Res Health* 2007;29(3):162–171.
146. Ramchand R, Pacula RL, Iguchi MY. Racial differences in marijuana-users' risk of arrest in the United States. *Drug Alcohol Depend* 2007; 84(3):264–272.
147. Cotton NS. The familial incidence of alcoholism. A Review. *J Stud Alcohol* 1979;40(1):89–116.
148. Dawson DA, Harford TC, Grant BF. Family history as a predictor of alcohol dependence. *Alcohol Clin Exp Res* 1992;16(3):572–575.
149. Dawson DA. The link between family history and early onset alcoholism: earlier initiation of drinking or more rapid development of dependence? *J Stud Alcohol* 2000;61(5):637–646.
150. Heath AC, Bucholz KK, Madden PA, et al. Genetic and environmental contributions to alcohol dependence risk in a national twin sample: consistency of findings in women and men. *Psychol Med* 1997;27(6):1381–1396.
151. Prescott CA, Kendler KS. Genetic and environmental contributions to alcohol abuse and dependence in a population-based sample of male twins. *Am J Psychiatry* 1999;156(1):34–40.
152. Kendler KS, Heath AC, Neale MC, et al. A population-based twin study of alcoholism in women. *JAMA* 1992;268(14):1877–1882.
153. Kendler KS, Neale MC, Heath AC, et al. A twin-family study of alcoholism in women. *Am J Psychiatry* 1994;151(5):707–715.
154. Hrubec Z, Omenn GS. Evidence of genetic predisposition to alcoholic cirrhosis and psychosis: twin concordances for alcoholism and its biological end points by Zygosity among male veterans. *Alcohol Clin Exp Res* 1981;5(2):207–215.
155. Kaprio J, Koskenvuo M, Langinvainio H, et al. Genetic influences on use and abuse of alcohol: A study of 5638 adult Finnish twin brothers. *Alcohol Clin Exp Res* 1987;11(4):349–356.
156. Cloninger Cr, Bohman M, Sigvardsson S. Inheritance of alcohol abuse. Cross-fostering analysis of adopted men. *Arch Gen Psychiatry* 1981;38: 861–868.
157. Goodwin DW, Schulsinger F, Hermansen L, et al. Alcohol problems in adoptees raised apart from alcoholic biological parents. *Arch Gen Psychiatry* 1973;28:238–243.
158. Sigvardsson S, Bohman M, Cloninger R. Replication of the Stockholm Adoption Study of alcoholism. Confirmatory cross-fostering analysis. *Arch Gen Psychiatry* 1996;53:681–687.
159. Yates WR, Cadoret RJ, Troughton E, Stewart MA. An adoption study of DSM-IIIR alcohol and drug dependence severity. *Drug Alcohol Depend* 1996;41(1):9–15.
160. Long CG, Williams M, Hollin CR. Treating alcohol problems: a study of programme effectiveness and cost effectiveness according to length and delivery of treatment. *Addiction* 1998;93(4):561–571.
161. Hill SY, Shen S, Zezza N, et al. A genome wide search for alcoholism susceptibility genes. *Am J Med Genet B Neuropsychiatr Genet* 2004;128B (1):102–113.
162. Prescott CA, Sullivan PF, Kuo PH, et al. Genomewide linkage study in the Irish affected sib pair study of alcohol dependence: evidence for a susceptibility region for symptoms of alcohol dependence on chromosome 4. *Mol Psychiatry* 2007;11(6):603–611.
163. Johnson C, Drgon T, Liu QR, et al. Pooled association genome scanning for alcohol dependence using 104,268 SNPs: validation and use to identify alcoholism vulnerability loci in unrelated individuals from the collaborative study on the genetics of alcoholism. *Am J Med Genet B Neuropsychiatr Genet* 2007;141(8):844–853.
164. Froehlich JC, Zink RW, Li TK, et al. Analysis of heritability of hormonal responses to alcohol in twins: beta-endorphin as a potential biomarker of genetic risk for alcoholism. *Alcohol Clin Exp Res* 2000;24(3):265–277.
165. Wall TL, Peterson CM, Peterson KP, et al. Alcohol metabolism in Asian-American men with genetic polymorphisms of aldehyde dehydrogenase. *Ann Intern Med* 1997;127(5):376–379.
166. Borras E, Coutelle C, Rosell A, et al. Genetic polymorphism of alcohol dehydrogenase in Europeans: the ADH2*2 allele decreases the risk for alcoholism and is associated with ADH3*1. *Hepatology* 2000;31(4): 984–989.
167. Begleiter H, Porjesz B. Potential biological markers in individuals at high risk for developing alcoholism. *Alcohol Clin Exp Res* 1988;12(4):488–493.
168. Rausch JL, Monteiro MG, Schuckit MA. Platelet serotonin uptake in men with family histories of alcoholism. *Neuropsychopharmacology* 1991;4(2):83–86.
169. Bailly D, Vignau J, Racadot N, et al. Platelet serotonin levels in alcoholic patients: changes related to physiological and pathological factors. *Psychiatry Res* 1993;47(1):57–88.
170. West MO, Prinz RJ. Parental alcoholism and childhood psychopathology. *Psychol Bull* 1987;102(2):204–218.
171. Ohannessian CM, Hesselbrock VM. The influence of perceived social support on the relationship between family history of alcoholism and drinking behaviors. *Addiction* 1993;88(12):1651–1658.
172. Schuckit MA. Alcoholic men with no alcoholic first-degree relatives. *Am J Psychiatry* 1983;140(4):439–443.
173. Kendler KS, Gardner CO, Prescott CA. Religion, psychopathology, and substance use and abuse; a multimeasure, genetic-epidemiologic study. *Am J Psychiatry* 1997;154(3):322–329.
174. Chilcoat HD, Dishion TJ, Anthony JC. Parent monitoring and the incidence of drug sampling in urban elementary school children. *Am J Epidemiol* 1995;141(1):25–31.
175. Kendler KS, Thornton LM, Pedersen NL. Tobacco consumption in Swedish twins reared apart and reared together. *Arch Gen Psychiatry* 2000;57(9):886–892.
176. Kendler KS, Neale MC, Thornton LM, et al. Cannabis use in the last year in a U.S. national sample of twin and sibling pairs. *Psychol Med* 2002;32(3):551–554.
177. Kendler KS, Prescott CA. Caffeine intake, tolerance, and withdrawal in women: a population-based twin study. *Am J Psychiatry* 1999;156(2): 223–228.
178. Tsuang MT, Lyons MJ, Eisen SA, et al. Genetic influences on DSM-III-R drug abuse and dependence: a study of 3,372 twin pairs. *Am J Med Genet* 1996;67(5):473–477.
179. van den Bree MB, Johnson EO, Neale MC, et al. Genetic and environmental influences on drug use and abuse/dependence in male and female twins. *Drug Alcohol Depend* 1998;52(3):231–241.
180. Kendler KS, Karkowski LM, Neale MC, et al. Illicit psychoactive substance use, heavy use, abuse, and dependence in a U.S. population-based sample of male twins. *Arch Gen Psychiatry* 2000;57(3):261–269.
181. Kendler KS, Prescott CA. Cocaine use, abuse and dependence in a population-based sample of female twins. *Br J Psychiatry* 1998;173: 345–350.
182. Pickens RW, Svikis DS. *Biological vulnerability to drug abuse.* NIDA Research Monograph 89. Rockville, MD: National Institute on Drug Abuse, 1988.
183. Cadoret RJ, Yates WR, Troughton E, et al. Adoption study demonstrating two genetic pathways to drug abuse. *Arch Gen Psychiatry* 1995;52: 42–52.
184. True WR, Xian H, Scherrer JF, et al. Common genetic vulnerability for nicotine and alcohol dependence in men. *Arch Gen Psychiatry* 1999;56(7): 655–661.
185. Hagnell O, Isberg PE, Lanke J, et al. Predictors of alcoholism in the Lundby Study. III. Social risk factors for alcoholism. *Eur Arch Psychiatry Neurol Sci* 1986;235(4):197–199.

186. Hettema JM, Corey LA, Kendler KS. A multivariate genetic analysis of the use of tobacco, alcohol, and caffeine in a population based sample of male and female twins. *Drug Alcohol Depend* 1999;57(1):69–78.
187. Uhl GR, Drgon T, Johnson C, et al. "Higher order" addiction molecular genetics: convergent data from genome-wide association in humans and mice. *Biochem Pharmacol* 2008;75(1):98–111.
188. Jang KL, Vernon PA, Livesley WJ. Personality disorder traits, family environment, and alcohol misuse: a multivariate behavioural genetic analysis. *Addiction* 2000;95(6):873–888.
189. Slutske WS, Heath AC, Madden PA, et al. Personality and the genetic risk for alcohol dependence. *J Abnorm Psychol* 2002;111(1):124–133.
190. Miles DR, van den Bree MB, Gupman AE, et al. A twin study on sensation seeking, risk taking behavior and marijuana use. *Drug Alcohol Depend* 2001;62(1):57–68.
191. McCord W, McCord J. A longitudinal study of the personality of alcoholics. In: Pittmen DJ, Snyder CR, eds. *Society, culture, and drinking patterns.* New York: John Wiley & Sons, Inc., 1962:413–430.
192. Mink M, Wang JY, Bennett KJ, et al. Early alcohol use, rural residence, and adult employment. *J Stud Alcohol Drugs* 2008;69(2):266–274.
193. McMorris BJ, Uggen C. Alcohol and employment in the transition to adulthood. *J Health Soc Behav* 2000;41(3):276–294.
194. Valois RF, Dunham AC, Jackson KL, et al. Association between employment and substance abuse behaviors among public high school adolescents. *J Adolescent Health* 1999;25(4):256–263.
195. Plant MA. Occupations, drinking patterns and alcohol-related problems: conclusions from a follow-up study. *Br J Addict Alcohol Other Drugs* 1979;74(3):267–273.
196. Olkinuora M. Alcoholism and occupation. *Scand J Work Environ Health* 1984;10:511–515.
197. Roberts RE, Lee ES. Occupation and the prevalence of major depression, alcohol, and drug abuse in the United States. *Environ Res* 1993; 61(2):266–278.
198. Diala CC, Muntaner C, Walrath C. Gender, occupational, and socioeconomic correlates of alcohol and drug abuse among U.S. rural, metropolitan, and urban residents. *Am J Drug Alcohol Abuse* 2004;30(2):409–428.
199. San Jose B, van de Mheen H, van Oers JA, et al. Adverse working conditions and alcohol use in men and women. *Alcohol Clin Exp Res* 2000; 24(8):1207–1213.
200. Lahelma E, Kangas R, Manderbacka K. Drinking and unemployment: contrasting patterns among men and women. *Drug Alcohol Depend* 1995;37(1):71–82.
201. Mullahy J, Sindelar JL. Alcoholism and income: the role of indirect effects. *Milbank Q* 1994;72(2):359–375.
202. Anthony JC, Eaton WW, Mandell W, et al. Psychoactive drug dependence and abuse: More common in some occupations than others? *J Employee Assist Res* 1992;1(1):148–186.
203. Mandell W, Eaton WW, Anthony JC, et al. Alcoholism and occupations: a review and analysis of 104 occupations [Review]. *Alcohol Clin Exp Res* 1992;16(4):734–746.
204. Bang KM, Kim JH. Prevalence of cigarette smoking by occupation and industry in the United States. *Am J Ind Med* 2001;40(3):233–239.
205. Claussen B. Alcohol disorders and re-employment in a 5-year follow-up of long-term unemployed. *Addiction* 1999;94(1):133–138.
206. Dooley D, Prause J. Effects of favorable employment change on alcohol abuse: one-and five-year follow-ups in the National Longitudinal Survey of Youth. *Am J Community Psychol* 1997;25(6):787–807.
207. Prescott CA, Kendler KS. Associations between marital status and alcohol consumption in a longitudinal study of female twins. *J Stud Alcohol* 2001;62(5):589–604.
208. Power C, Rodgers B, Hope S. Heavy alcohol consumption and marital status: disentangling the relationship in a national study of young adults. *Addiction* 1999;94(10):1477–1487.
209. Chilcoat HD, Breslau N. Alcohol disorders in young adulthood: effects of transitions into adult roles. *J Health Soc Behav* 1996;37(4):339–349.
210. McLeod JD. Spouse concordance for alcohol dependence and heavy drinking: evidence from a community sample. *Alcohol Clin Exp Res* 1993;17(6):1146–1155.
211. Curran PJ, Muthen BO, Harford TC. The influence of changes in marital status on developmental trajectories of alcohol use in young adults. *J Stud Alcohol* 1998;59(6):647–658.
212. Fu H, Goldman N. The association between health-related behaviours and the risk of divorce in the USA. *J Biosoc Sci* 2000;32(1):63–88.
213. Hartmann DJ, Sullivan WP, Wolk JL. A state-wide assessment: marital stability and client outcomes. *Drug Alcohol Depend* 1991;29:27–38.
214. Westhuis DJ, Gwaltney L, Hayashi R. Outpatient cocaine abuse treatment: predictors of success. *J Drug Educ* 2001;31(2):171–183.
215. Kallan JE. Drug abuse–related mortality in the United States: patterns and correlates. *Am J Drug Alcohol Abuse* 1998;24(1):103–117.
216. Chermack ST, Fuller BE, Blow FC. Predictors of expressed partner and non-partner violence among patients in substance abuse treatment. *Drug Alcohol Depend* 2000;58(1–2):43–54.
217. Mudar P, Leonard KE, Soltysinski K. Discrepant substance use and marital functioning in newlywed couples. *J Consult Clin Psychol* 2001;69(1): 130–134.
218. Epstein EE, McCrady BS. Behavioral couples treatment of alcohol and drug use disorders: current status and innovations. *Clin Psychol Rev* 1998;18(6):689–711.
219. Droomers M, Schrijvers CT, Stronks K, et al. Educational differences in excessive alcohol consumption: the role of psychosocial and material stressors. *Prev Med* 1999;29(1):1–10.
220. Crum RM, Helzer JE, Anthony JC. Level of education and alcohol abuse and dependence in adulthood: a further inquiry. *Am J Public Health* 1993;83(6):830–837.
221. Crum RM, Juon HS, Green KM, et al. Educational achievement and early school behavior as predictors of alcohol-use disorders: 35-year follow-up of the Woodlawn Study. *J Stud Alcohol* 2007;67(1):75–85.
222. Harrison PA, Luxenberg MG. Comparisons of alcohol and other drug problems among Minnesota adolescents in 1989 and 1992. *Arch Pediatr Adolesc Med* 1995;149(2):137–144.
223. Thomas BS. Drug use in a small midwestern community and relationships to selected characteristics. *J Drug Educ* 1993;23(3):247–258.
224. Thomas BS, Hsiu LT. The role of selected risk factors in predicting adolescent drug use and its adverse consequences. *Int J Addict* 1993;28(14): 1549–1563.
225. Paschall MJ, Flewelling RL, Faulkner DL. Alcohol misuse in young adulthood: effects of race, educational attainment, and social context. *Subst Use Misuse* 2000;35(11):1485–1506.
226. Eggert LL, Herting JR. Drug involvement among potential dropouts and "typical" youth. *J Drug Educ* 1993;23(1):31–55.
227. Braggio JT, Pishkin V, Gameros TA, et al. Academic achievement in substance-abusing and conduct-disordered adolescents. *J Clin Psychol* 1993;49(2):282–291.
228. Schulenberg J, Bachman JG, O'Malley PM, et al. High school educational success and subsequent substance use: a panel analysis following adolescents into young adulthood. *J Health Soc Behav* 1994;35: 45–62.
229. Fothergill KE, Ensminger ME, Green KM, et al. The impact of early school behavior and educational achievement on adult drug use disorders: a prospective study. *Drug Alcohol Depend* 2008;92(1–3):191–199.
230. Brown VB, Ridgely MS, Pepper B, et al. The dual crisis: mental illness and substance abuse. Present and future directions. *Am Psychol* 1989; 44(3):565–569.
231. Carey KB, Cocco KM, Simons JS. Concurrent validity of clinicians' ratings of substance abuse among psychiatric outpatients. *Psychiatr Serv* 1996;47(8):842–847.
232. Koegel P, Burnam MA, Farr RK. The prevalence of specific psychiatric disorders among homeless individuals in the inner city of Los Angeles. *Arch Gen Psychiatry* 1988;45(12):1085–1092.
233. Lambert MT, Griffith JM, Hendrickse W. Characteristics of patients with substance abuse diagnoses on a general psychiatry unit in a VA Medical Center. *Psychiatr Serv* 1996;47(10):1104–1107.
234. McHugo GJ, Drake RE, Burton HL, et al. A scale for assessing the stage of substance abuse treatment in persons with severe mental illness. *J Nerv Ment Dis* 1995;183:762–767.

235. Clark DB, Pollock N, Buckstein OG, et al. Gender and comorbid psychopathology in adolescent with alcohol dependence. *J Am Acad Child Adolesc* 1997;36(9):1195–1203.
236. Farell M, Howes S, Bebbington P, et al. Nicotine, alcohol and drug dependence and psychiatric comorbidity. Results of a national household survey. *Br J Addict* 2001;179:432–437.
237. Ross HE. DSM-III-R alcohol abuse and dependence and psychiatric comorbidity in Ontario: results from the Mental Health Supplement to the Ontario Health Survey. *Drug Alcohol Depend* 1995;39:111–128.
238. Husky MM, Mazure CM, Paliwal P, et al. Gender differences in the comorbidity of smoking behavior and major depression. *Drug Alcohol Depend* 2008;93(1–2):176–179.
239. Grant BF, Stinson FS, Dawson DA, et al. Co-occurrence of 12-month alcohol and drug use disorders and personality disorders in the United States: results from the National Epidemiologic Survey on Alcohol and Related Conditions. *Arch Gen Psychiatry* 2004;61(4):361–368.
240. Stinson FS, Grant BF, Dawson DA, et al. Comorbidity between DSM-IV alcohol and specific drug use disorders in the United States: results from the National Epidemiologic Survey on Alcohol and Related Conditions. *Drug Alcohol Depend* 2005;80(1):105–116.
241. Weaver T, Madden P, Charles V, et al. Comorbidity of substance misuse and mental illness in community mental health and substance misuse services. *Br J Psychiatry* 2003;183:304–313.
242. Caton CL, Drake RE, Hasin DS, et al. Differences between early-phase primary psychotic disorders with concurrent substance use and substance-induced psychoses. *Arch Gen Psychiatry* 2005;62(2):137–145.
243. Sakai JT, Hall SK, Mikulich-Gilbertson SK, et al. Inhalant use, abuse, and dependence among adolescent patients: commonly comorbid problems. *J Am Acad Child Adolesc Psychiatry* 2004;43(9):1080–1088.
244. Osher FC, Drake RE. Reversing a history of unmet needs: approaches to care for persons with co-occurring addictive and mental disorders. *Am J Orthopsychiatry* 1996;66(1):4–11.
245. Driessen M, Veltrup C, Wetterling T, et al. Axis I and Axis II comorbidity in alcohol dependence and the two types of alcoholism. *Alcohol Clin Exp Res* 1998;22(1):77–86.
246. Johnson ME, Brems C, Mills ME, et al. Psychiatric symptomatology among individuals in alcohol detoxification treatment. *Addict Behav* 2007;32(8):1745–1752.
247. Drake RE, Wallach MA. Substance abuse among the chronic mentally ill. *Hosp Comm Psych* 1989; 40(10):1041–1046.
248. Dixon L, McNary S, Lehman A. Substance abuse and family relationships of persons with severe mental illness. *Am J Psychiatry* 1995;152(3): 456–458.
249. Leon SC, Lyons JS, Christopher NJ, et al. Psychiatric hospital outcomes of dual diagnosis patients under managed care. *Am J Addict* 1998;7(1): 81–86.
250. Gupta S, Hendricks S, Kenkel AM, et al. Relapse in schizophrenia: is there a relationship to substance abuse? *Schizophr Res* 1996;20(1–2):153–156.
251. Swofford CD, Kasckow JW, Scheller-Gilkey G, et al. Substance use: a powerful predictor of relapse in schizophrenia. *Schizophr Res* 1996;20 (1–2):145–151.
252. Stanislav SW, Sommi RW, Watson WA. A longitudinal analysis of factors associated with morbidity in cocaine abusers with psychiatric illness. *Pharmacotherapy* 1992;12(2):114–118.
253. Owen RR, Fischer EP, Booth BM, et al. Medication noncompliance and substance abuse among patients with schizophrenia. *Psychiatr Serv* 1996;47(8):853–858.
254. Wolpe PR, Gorton G, Serota R, et al. Predicting compliance of dual diagnosis inpatients with aftercare treatment. *Hosp Comm Psych* 1993; 44(1):45–49.
255. Comtois KA, Ries R, Armstrong HE. Case manager ratings of the clinical status of dually diagnosed outpatients. *Hosp Community Psychiatry* 1994;45(6):568–573.
256. Willinger U, Lenzinger E, Hornik K, et al. Anxiety as a predictor of relapse in detoxified alcohol-dependent patients. *Alcohol Alcohol* 2002;37(6):609–612.
257. Upadhyaya HP, Deas D, Brady KT, et al. Cigarette smoking and psychiatric comorbidity in children and adolescents. *J Am Acad Child Adolesc Psychiatry* 2002;41(11):1294–1305.
258. Salloum IM, Cornelius JR, Douaihy A, et al. Patient characteristics and treatment implications of marijuana abuse among bipolar alcoholics: results from a double blind, placebo-controlled study. *Addict Behav* 2005;30(9):1702–1708.
259. Weisner C, Matzger H, Kaskutas LA. How important is treatment? One-year outcomes of treated and untreated alcohol-dependent individuals. *Addiction* 2003;98(7):901–911.
260. Kandel D. Stages in adolescent involvement in drug use. *Science* 1975; 28:912–914.
261. Donovan JE, Jessor R. Problem drinking and the dimension of involvement with drugs: a Guttman scalogram analysis of adolescent drug use. *Am J Public Health* 1983;73:543–552.
262. Kandel D, Yamaguchi K. From beer to crack: developmental patterns of drug involvement. *Am J Public Health* 1993;83(6):851–855.
263. Luthar SS, Cushing G, Rounsaville BJ. Gender differences among opioid abusers: pathways to disorder and profiles of psychopathology. *Drug Alcohol Depend* 1996;43(3):179–189.
264. Kushner MG, Sher KJ, Erickson DJ. Prospective analysis of the relation between DSM-III anxiety disorders and alcohol use disorders. *Am J Psychiatry* 1999;156:723–732.
265. Crawford TN, Cohen P, First MB, et al. Comorbid Axis I and Axis II disorders in early adolescence: outcomes 20 years later. *Arch Gen Psychiatry* 2008;65(6):641–648.

CHAPTER 3

Carson V. Dobrin, BS
David C.S. Roberts, PhD

The Anatomy of Addiction

Multiple brain structures are involved in the addiction process. Drug addiction involves increased and compulsive drug taking—often in the face of adverse consequences and at the expense of more socially or biologically important behaviors. Understanding the neurobiology of this phenomenon involves, at the most basic level, the identification of the neurotransmitter systems that mediate the reinforcing effects of specific drugs. However, to understand how the behavioral repertoire becomes subverted, it is necessary to consider the structures involved in decision making and in generating motivated behavior.

For the most part, the discussion of the anatomy of reinforcement and addiction maps onto structures associated with the limbic system and the basal ganglia. The first section of this chapter will offer a simplified overview—a primer—of the structures involved and their interconnections. The second section, entitled Neuroanatomy of Drug Reinforcement, will focus on the systems associated with the primary reinforcing effects of psychostimulants, opioids, and cannabinoids. To the extent that drug taking is a reinforced behavior, it is critical to understand the neural mechanisms that underlie drug reinforcement. We will focus on the concept of site of action, which defines the access points for a drug to influence a specific brain process. Another level of analysis is the study of how a reinforcing drug action influences other brain areas involved in the organization of the behavioral repertoire. This more broadly defined topic will be the subject of the third section entitled Neuroanatomy of Drug Addiction.

PRIMER ON NEUROANATOMY

The structures most often mentioned in the context of drug abuse are closely associated with the limbic system, lateral hypothalamus, basal ganglia, and frontal cortical regions. Here we present a brief description of each of these systems. Readers interested in a more complete description of the anatomy of these regions are referred to the following reviews (1–3).

Limbic System Research into the limbic system has a long and venerable history, but some scholars have suggested that the term may have outlived its usefulness. Nonetheless, a brief historic review of the term is a useful way of introducing some of the regions involved in drug addiction. The term *limbic* is derived from the Latin term *limbus*, meaning border, and was used to describe a ring of phylogenetically older cortex that separates the diencephalon and the neocortex. This limbic lobe consisted of the subcallosal area, cingulate, and parahippocampal gyri (Fig. 3.1). This purely anatomic distinction was expanded by MacLean (4) in 1952 to describe a functional unit that was proposed to be responsible for emotional expression. He made the distinction between the older, medial cortex and the more lateral neocortex which is involved in cognitive functions.

MacLean's concept was that most human behavior is the result of cooperation between three systems of the brain. The cerebral cortex is responsible for higher order reasoning and speech, whereas the limbic system was the source of emotions, aspects of personal identity, and fight or flight instincts. The third of MacLean's system is the reptilian brain. Early work with primates showed that when various parts of the limbic system were electrically stimulated a range of emotional responses was produced, such as rage, fear, and joy (5). This phylogenetically older brain is responsible for the organism avoiding things that are "disagreeable" and approaching those that are "agreeable"—reactions that MacLean saw as having survival value. It is now clear that structures associated with the limbic system (such as the hypothalamus, hippocampus, and

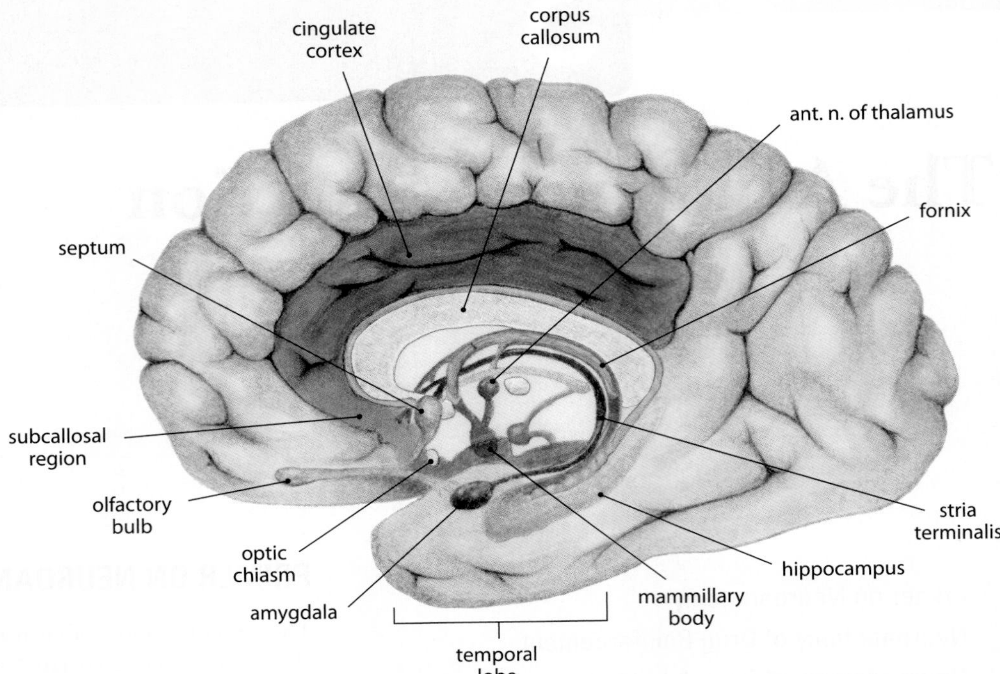

FIGURE 3.1. Regions of the human brain associated with the limbic system, which includes a loop of cortex extending from the subcallosal region through cingulate cortex to the parahippocampal gyrus. Also shown are the hippocampal formation, septum, amygdala, and mammillary bodies.

amygdala) are essential for not only learning and memory but also for the emotional context and the affective response to learned associations.

As will be detailed, many drugs of abuse have their sites of action within the limbic system and the neurochemistry within these structures is altered during the addiction process. This may help explain why decisions surrounding drug seeking and drug taking seem to be driven more by emotion and instinct rather than by logic.

From an anatomic perspective, MacLean defined the limbic system as the original limbic lobe along with other structures sharing direct connections with them. These include the olfactory cortex, hippocampal formation, amygdala, septum, hypothalamus, habenula, anterior thalamic nuclei, and parts of the basal ganglia. With further anatomic research, more and more areas were shown to share direct connections with these structures and some of these began to be included in the limbic system. The result was that the boundaries of the limbic system became overly broad. Brodal (6) observed that the term *limbic system* was becoming less useful and he argued that it should be discarded altogether; however, the concept of a phylogenetically older forebrain system responsible for emotional control is now firmly entrenched.

Swanson (7) has helped crystallize the anatomic definition by characterizing the limbic system as highly interconnected regions which appear to form the only major route for information transfer between the neocortex and the hypothalamus. Figure 3.1 illustrates these areas in the human brain.

Interface of the Limbic System and the Basal Ganglia The basal ganglia is traditionally thought of as a motor system; however, the idea that this system deals only with motor function while the limbic system deals with reinforcement and emotion is oversimplified and entirely misleading. As later sections will illustrate, there is reason to believe that parts of the basal ganglia are very much involved in memory formation and a variety of cognitive tasks. As more is learned about how the basal ganglia and limbic system communicate, it is becoming increasingly clear that the two systems are jointly involved in coordinating motivated behavior.

The largest mass associated with the basal ganglia is the striatum (caudate-putamen). The dorsal portion has long been considered part of the basal ganglia, whereas the ventral striatum is considered to be part of the limbic system (8). This dorsal/ventral distinction is clearly important; however, more recent debate has focused on the idea that gradations rather than sharp boundaries mark the transition from the dorsolateral to ventromedial striatum. Figure 3.2 shows the topographic organization of inputs to the striatum in the rat. Voorn et al. (9) makes the point, as Figure 3.2 illustrates, that no histologic or immunohistochemical border exists which can be used to define or divide the region. Note that although the dorsal-lateral parts receive primarily motor inputs and the ventromedial striatal areas receive primarily limbic projections, it is a gradual topographic transition.

The accumbens forms the ventral portion of the striatum, thus accumbens and ventral striatum are used synonymously in the addiction literature. Famously, in 1993, Mogenson et al. (10) described the ventral striatum as the crossroad of the limbic and motor systems and "the place where motivation is translated into action." Figure 3.2 also shows two regions identified as the nucleus accumbens (NAcc) core and shell. The involvement of these two regions in the behavioral and electrophysiologic responses to drug reinforcement has been

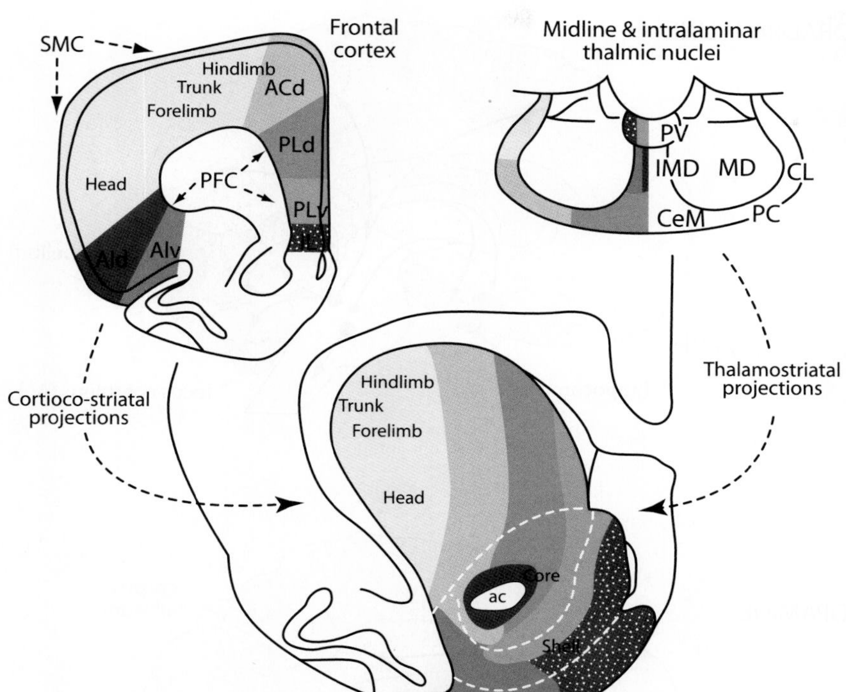

FIGURE 3.2. Connections of the dorsal and ventral striatum. Cortical and thalamic inputs to the striatum distribute in a dorsomedial-to-ventrolateral manner. To paraphrase Voorn et al. (9), afferents arising from the frontal cortex and projecting to the striatum are depicted. Sensorimotor projections innervate the dorsolateral striatum in a somatotopic fashion. Vicerolimbic inputs project to the ventromedial striatum. Areas in between dorsolateral and ventromedial striatum receive inputs from higher cortical association areas ac, anterior commissure; ACd, dorsal anterior cingulate cortex; AId, dorsal agranular insular cortex; AIv, ventral agranular insular cortex; IL, infralimbic cortex; PFC, prefrontal cortex; PLd, dorsal prelimbic cortex; PLv, ventral prelimbic cortex; SMC, sensorimotor cortex. Adapted from Voorn P, et al. *Trends Neurosci* 2004;27(8):468–474.

extensively studied and some debate has focused on which area is responsible for particular drug effects. Some of the core-shell debate might eventually give way to discussion of the function of subregions defined by projections.

Executive Function and Cortical Involvement

Executive function involves control over many aspects of behavior. Some of these include the ability to differentiate among conflicting thoughts, determine good and bad, better and best, same and different, future consequences of current activities, working toward a defined goal, expectation based on actions, behavioral inhibition, and social "control." The prefrontal cortex (PFC) is thought to be the "hub" of executive function in the brain.

The PFC in humans is subdivided into three main regions: (i) the orbitofrontal (OFC) and the ventromedial areas, which are thought to be involved in processing reward (11); (ii) the dorsolateral prefrontal cortex, more broadly involved in decision making (12); and (iii) the anterior and ventral cingulate cortex, which help to control whether or not a particular behavior will be performed, and to what intensity (13).

NEUROANATOMY OF DRUG REINFORCEMENT

"Site of action" is a pharmacologic concept that defines the access point for a drug to produce a specific response. If that response is defined behaviorally (e.g., anorexic, convulsant, antidepressant effect), then the site of action identifies the receptors and brain regions responsible for that particular behavioral response. It is one thing to describe all possible sites where a drug can affect the brain; it is a more difficult matter to narrow down the possibilities to a particular binding site in a circumscribed region. Research into the site of action for the reinforcing effects of psychostimulant drugs, such as cocaine and amphetamine, offer a good example of how this investigative process occurs.

In vitro experiments have shown that cocaine binds to dopamine, noradrenaline and serotonin (DA, NA, and 5-HT) transporters and blocks the reuptake of these neurotransmitters (14); amphetamine acts additionally as a releasing agent. Both of these actions result in an increased concentration of monoamine neurotransmitters in the synapse. Therefore psychostimulant drugs act as indirect agonists everywhere these transmitter are found.

An examination of the anatomic projections of the catecholamine systems shows that they have extensive and diffuse projections throughout the neural axis. The cell bodies of these transmitter systems are loosely organized in an anteroposterior fashion. Based on their histochemical mapping studies, Dahlstrom and Fuxe (15) proposed a nomenclature wherein cell clusters were numbered from posterior to anterior and given a letter prefix according to whether they were dopaminergic/noradrenergic (A) or serotoninergic (B). Figure 3.3A shows the distribution of NA fibers. The locus coeruleus (A6) is located in the dorsal brain stem and sends ascending projections to terminal regions of the cortex, hippocampus, and cerebellum. More caudal and ventral NA cells groups (A1–A5) innervate the hypothalamus and brain stem. Dopaminergic innervations are more circumscribed (Fig. 3.3B). DA cell groups within the ventral tegmental area (VTA) and substantia nigra (A8, A9 and A10) project in a topographic manner to the striatum. The more

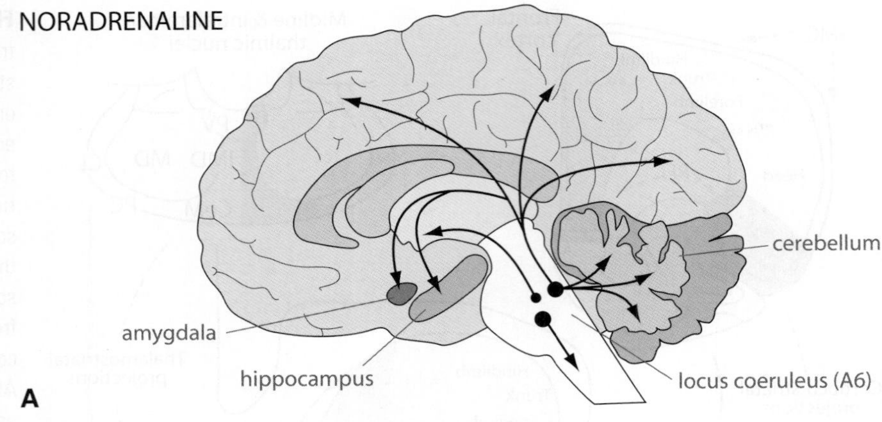

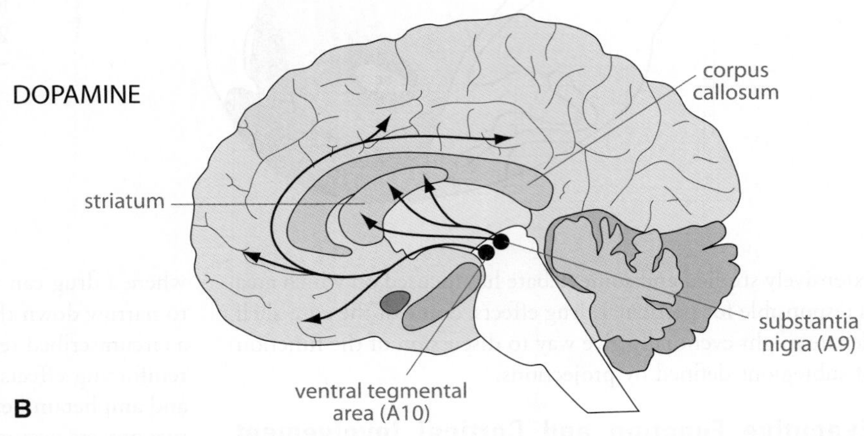

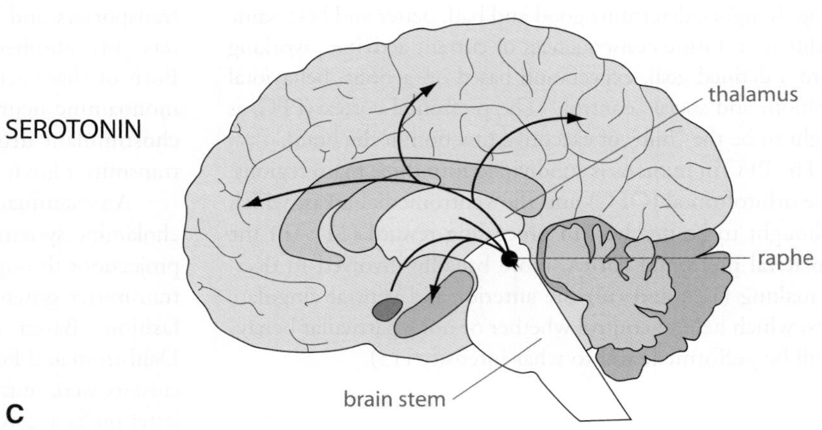

FIGURE 3.3. Schematic diagram illustrating the distribution of the main central neuronal pathways containing noradrenaline, **(A)**, dopamine **(B)**, and serotonin **(C)**. The location of cell bodies of origin is indicated by circles with the projections indicated by arrows.

medial group (A10) sends projections to the ventral striatum, whereas the more lateral groups form a nigrostriatal bundle that innervates the caudate-putamen. This latter projection is known to degenerate in Parkinson disease and is thus associated with motor function. An additional cluster of DA cells in the hypothalamus composes the tuberoinfundibular DA system, which innervates the external layer of the median eminence. Dahstrom and Fuxe (16) also described 5-HT cell groups (B1–B9), which lie near the midline of the pons and upper brain stem. Later studies showed clusters of cells also in the caudal locus coeruleus (LC), area postrema, and interpeduncular nucleus (14). Generally, the more caudal cell groups innervate the medulla and spinal cord, whereas the more anterior clusters project rostrally (Fig. 3.3C).

The main point to be taken from an examination of the areas innervated by DA, NA, and 5-HT is that there is hardly a region that is not innervated by at least two of the monoamines. Given that psychostimulants have an effect at the terminal regions of each of these systems, every area of the brain would be expected to be affected to some extent by an injection of cocaine or amphetamine. It has been a considerable challenge, therefore, sorting out what transmitter in which particular area produces toxic effects and adverse reactions on the one hand and pleasurable or positive reinforcing effects on the other.

Preclinical Studies of Drug Reinforcement Experiments with nonhuman primates and a variety of other laboratory animals have helped identify the important sites of action for drug reinforcement. It is important to note that, early on, there was considerable skepticism whether anything useful could be learned from laboratory animals regarding human drug taking. Given the premise that only humans abuse drugs, along with the observation that what distinguishes the human brain from other mammals is the development of the neocortex, the logical conclusion was that this region is responsible for drug addiction. This idea fit well with the idea that drugs were "mind expanding" and that the reasons why a person might take drugs has to do with their effects on consciousness. Interviews with drug users and introspective analysis of drug taking behavior suggested that some of the reasons that people take drugs is for "pleasure, curiosity, the desire to experiment, the sense of adventure, the search for self-knowledge . . . the relief of stress and tension, depression, the feeling of powerlessness and the lack of belief in the future" (17). Although these observations are entirely appropriate for discussion at one level, they also serve to perpetuate the idea that human consciousness and reasoning are the bases for drug reinforcement. The demonstration that nonhuman primates and rodents will voluntarily self-administer drugs such as cocaine and heroin has prompted a consideration of concepts other than human consciousness to account for drug abuse, forcing an examination of brain regions other than the cortex.

There is an extremely high correlation between the drugs that are abused by humans and drugs that are self-administered by other mammalian species such as rat, dog, cat, rabbit, and nonhuman primate (9,18). These data support the idea that drugs of abuse have their reinforcing actions on brain structures which have been relatively conserved through the course of human evolution—that is, limbic and brainstem areas. This being the case, the development of self-administration techniques, through intravenous (IV) (20–22), intracranial (23–25), and inhalation (26) routes, have provided a means to study brain structures responsible for drug reinforcement in animal models

Psychostimulants Pharmacologic experiments were the first to narrow down the range of possible sites of action for the reinforcing effects of psychostimulant drugs (27,28). In these studies, rats and monkeys were trained to self-administer cocaine and amphetamine until they showed a stable baseline level of responding (see sidebar). They were then pretreated with a variety of agonists or antagonists in an effort to identify the specific transmitter systems that modulate reinforcing efficacy. Importantly, it was shown that pretreatment with DA receptor antagonists caused the animals to self-administer cocaine and amphetamine more frequently (29–31). This is the same result one sees if the concentration of drug is diluted: the animals appear to compensate for the reduction in drug effect by increasing their intake. Note that pretreatment with NA or 5-HT antagonists did not have consistent effects on drug intake. These data prompted Wise (32,33) to champion the idea that stimulation of DA receptors must be essential for psychostimulant reinforcement.

Peripheral injections of DA antagonists narrowed the site of action to DA receptors, but it remained unclear which brain regions mediated this effect. Central manipulations were necessary to identify which brain regions were important. Neurotoxins specific to catecholamine and indolamine neurons provided a useful tool to examine whether the loss of a particular fiber

Sidebar

In self-administration studies, animals are implanted with permanent indwelling catheters and placed in an experimental chamber. The catheter is connected to a syringe pump through a fluid swivel that allows free movement throughout the chamber. A computer detects responses on a lever and controls the timing of drug delivery according to the schedule of reinforcement. For example, on a fixed ratio one schedule (FR1), every response on the lever results in an infusion of drug.

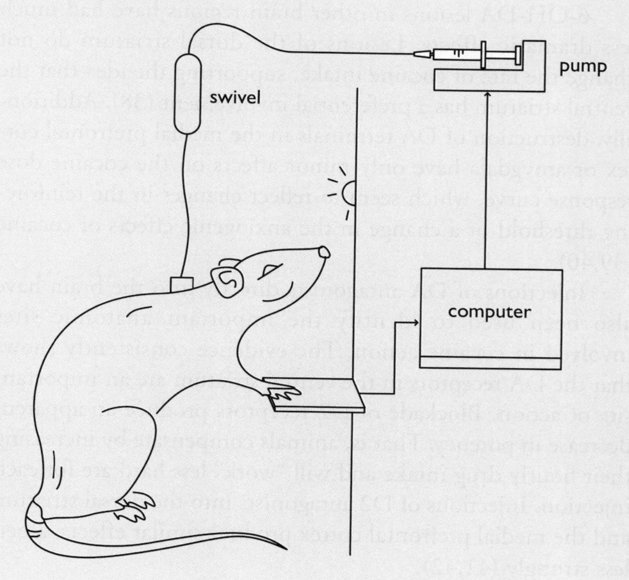

system would affect drug self-administration. A considerable literature developed around the neurotoxin 6-hydroxydopamine (6-OH-DA) that, depending on the site of injection and other parameters, could be used to completely deplete various brain regions of either DA or NA. Early experiments showed that removing the noradrenergic innervation of the entire forebrain had almost no effect on cocaine self-administration. By contrast, removal of the DA innervation of the NAcc resulted in a substantial reduction in cocaine's reinforcing effects (34–36). In fact, animals will no longer self-administer cocaine if DA levels in the NAcc are reduced by >80%. Destroying the DA neurons in the VTA also drastically reduced cocaine self-administration (37). These data were the first to draw attention to the NAcc (more recently referred to as ventral striatum) as a site for action for psychostimulant reinforcement.

6-OH-DA lesions in other brain regions have had much less dramatic effects. Lesions of the dorsal striatum do not change the rate of cocaine intake, supporting the idea that the ventral striatum has a preferential involvement (38). Additionally, destruction of DA terminals in the medial prefrontal cortex or amygdala have only minor affects on the cocaine dose response curve, which seem to reflect changes in the reinforcing threshold or a change in the anxiogenic effects of cocaine (39,40).

Injections of DA antagonists directly into the brain have also been used to identify the important anatomic sites involved in cocaine action. The evidence consistently shows that the DA receptors in the ventral striatum are an important site of action. Blockade of D2 receptors produce an apparent decrease in potency. That is, animals compensate by increasing their hourly drug intake and will "work" less hard are for each injection. Injections of D2 antagonists into the dorsal striatum and the medial prefrontal cortex produce similar effects, albeit less strongly (41,42).

In summary, the data presented are from a wide range of studies using neurotoxins and specific pharmacologic agents are consistent with the idea that the most important site of action for the reinforcing effects of cocaine and amphetamine is at DA terminals in the ventral striatum. It should be emphasized however that, although the ventral striatum is essential for the reinforcing effects of cocaine and amphetamine, other DA projection areas (such as the prefrontal cortex, amygdala, and dorsal striatum) also contribute to some extent.

The sight of action for the locomotor activating effects of psychostimulant drugs seem to largely overlap with the regions responsible for drug reinforcement. Experiments using either lesion or intracerebral injections of DA drugs have shown that stimulation of the DA receptors in the ventral striatum produces behavioral activating effects (locomotion); stimulation of DA receptors in the dorsal striatum produces stereotypy (43), which is characterized by repetitive sequences of movements, such as licking and grooming in rodents. 6-OH-DA–induced destruction of DA terminals in the ventral striatum almost completely abolishes the locomotor stimulant effects of cocaine while lesions of the dorsal striatum abolish psychostimulant stereotypy. Similarly, direct injections of DA agonists into the ventral striatum produce locomotion, whereas injections into the dorsal striatum produce stereotypy (44–46).

The stereotypic response elicited from the dorsal striatum may have relevance to addiction. In rats, stereotyped behavior is often measured on a categoric scale which includes licking chewing and gnawing. These high-frequency movements have the appearance of being "hard-wired" responses that are elicited by the drug. It should be emphasized, however, that almost any behavior can become stereotyped. In their influential article, Randrup and Munkvad (47) described how the precise forms of stereotyped behavior differ across species and offer the example of a man who repeatedly rebuilt his car engine. They suggested that inhibition of drug-induced stereotypy might be useful in screening antipsychotics. We know now that this is true because of the relationship between the importance of DA in stimulating stereotypy and the action of neuroleptic drugs. To re-emphasize, anything can become stereotyped.

Behaviors that occur with high frequency have a high likelihood of becoming stereotyped (i.e., they occur repetitively and ritualistically) if they occur in the presence of a drug (48). Lyon and Robbins (49) argue that stereotypy is a process in which there is an increase in frequency, in a diminishing number of response categories. The effect is that psychostimulant drugs narrow the behavioral repertoire such that only a few predominant behaviors remain. Put another way, the behavioral repertoire becomes focused around the things that occur most frequently. In the case of a person with addiction, the frequent behaviors associated with drug seeking and drug taking become repetitive and ritualistic.

In conclusion, strong evidence from studies using widely different strategies suggests that stimulation of DA receptors in the ventral striatum is associated with drug reinforcement. There is a wealth of evidence from a parallel literature showing that the mesolimbic DA system is also involved in reward from natural behaviors such as feeding (50–52), drinking (53,54), sexual behaviors (55,56), and intracranial self-stimulation (57–59). This enormous amount of literature has resulted in the mesolimbic DA system being called a *reward pathway*. Whether this term is accurate or biologically meaningful (we think it is not) lies outside the scope of this chapter. However, the immense interest in the mesolimbic DA pathway demands some discussions of its interconnections.

Data from electrophysiologic studies show that VTA-DA neurons respond to primary reinforcing stimuli (e.g., food) and to environmental cues which predict the presentation of rewards (60,61). It is therefore surprising that these neurons receive no direct input from visual, auditory, or somatosensory systems (62). It appears instead that the VTA is a part of, and receives inputs from, a widespread collection of neurons that belong to the "isodendritic core" (63). This system is a network of neurons stretching from brainstem to telencephalon. The neurons within the network have similar morphology, send out long projects, and are themselves the target of a great number of contacts from distant sources (64). It would appear that this network serves an integrative function and responses to changes in the environment that are biologically significant. At present, it remains unclear whether the VTA-DA neurons respond differentially than others in the network and whether they are specifically activated by reward or more generally by any other important stimulus.

Opioids Again, the process of identifying the site of action for the reinforcing effects of opioid begins with identifying all possible receptors sites. Opioid receptors are expressed throughout the brain, especially in limbic and limbic-related structures; they are found in the amygdala, insular cortex, caudate, anterior hypothalamus, cortex, parietal cortex, putamen, thalamus, and periaqueductal gray (65). There are three different types of G protein–coupled opioid receptors; μ, κ, and δ, which are acted on by both endogenous and exogenously applied opioids (66). Selective μ agonist drugs, such as morphine, heroin, and most clinically used opioid analgesics, produce analgesia, euphoria, respiratory depression, emesis, and antidiuretic effects. Selective κ agonist drugs, such as the experimental compounds ethylketazocine and bremazocine, produce analgesia, dysphoria, and diuretic effects, but no respiratory depression. There is less known about the direct role of δ receptors. Agonists at μ receptor are more likely to have abuse liability than κ agonists (67–69). Within the dorsal and ventral striatum there are areas of overlap between expression of opioid receptors; however, their expression patterns tend to differ. μ Receptors are expressed in patches, and κ and δ receptors being more diffusely distributed (70).

Almost all that is known about the neurobiology of opioid reinforcement is derived from animal models. Three approaches have been used to investigate the involvement of various brain regions in opioid reward: (i) intracerebral self-administration of opioid agonists, (ii) blockade of IV heroin self-administration by intracerebral injections of opioid antagonists, and (iii) disruption of IV heroin self-administration by lesions. Generally the focus has been on areas associated with the mesolimbic DA system (ventral striatum and VTA), although other regions have also been implicated.

Self-administration of drugs directly into various brain regions would seem to be the most straightforward test of their involvement in reinforcement processes; however, the procedures have a number of technical problems that limit their appeal. Issues involving diffusion, osmolarity and tissue damage demand thoughtful controls; see review (71). Nonetheless, several papers have provided evidence that opioid-like compounds are self-administered into discrete brain regions. The early work focused on the lateral hypothalamus (23,72,73) because this area was intensely studied for its ability to support intracranial electrical self-stimulation (74). Later, because of interest in the mesolimbic system, interest switched to the ventral striatum and the VTA. The role of the lateral hypothalamus has been challenged and it is possible that the early results were due to diffusion of drug to other areas (75). The ventral striatum appears to support intracranial self-administration of morphine (76) and methionine enkephalin (77). These data fit well with the demonstration that intra-NAcc opioids produce a conditioned place preference (78). Techniques have also been developed to study intracerebral self-injection in mice by using a Y-maze. Selection of one arm of the maze results in a morphine injection, whereas the other arm results in a saline injection. Using this method, mice have been shown to self-inject morphine into the lateral septum (79) and the ventral striatum but not the dorsal striatum (80).

By far the most sensitive site for intracerebral self-administration of opioids is the VTA. Both μ and δ opioids are self-administered into this region at doses that are not supported in other areas (25,81–83). The idea that opioids have a significant impact on reinforcement mechanisms through an action in the VTA is supported by other a variety of other techniques. For example, injections of opioid agonists into the VTA also produce a conditioned place preference (84), facilitate brain stimulation reward (85,86), and reinstate extinguished lever responding that was trained under IV heroin reward (87).

It should be noted that there are a few reports of reinforcing effects produced by intracerebral injections of opioids into the hippocampus (88) and periaqueductal gray. The doses used in these studies are relatively high and it remains unclear whether these are important but less sensitive sites or whether diffusion of the drug to other areas accounts for the data.

When self-administering IV heroin, animals respond to a decrease in the unit injection dose by taking injections more frequently. A similar phenomenon can be observed when animals are treated with a systemic injection of naloxone (a μ antagonist), suggesting that animals compensate for a reduced drug effect by increasing their intake (89). Several laboratories have used this compensatory response to evaluate the effects of opioid antagonists injected into various brain regions. Increases in IV heroin self-administration have been shown after injections of low doses of opioid antagonists into the NAcc (90–92), periaqueductal gray (91), stria terminalis (93), and lateral hypothalamus, but not the prefrontal cortex (94). Surprisingly, injections of an opioid antagonist into the VTA have relatively little effect (95). It remains unclear why many studies have shown that the VTA is one of the most sensitive brain sites for intracerebral self-administration of opioid agonists, whereas it is one of the least effective sites for disrupting IV heroin self-administration studies with an intracerebral injection of opioid antagonists.

Lesions offer a third method for identifying critical brain areas responsible for the reinforcing effects of opioids. Zito et al. (96) showed that the size of a kainic acid–induced lesion of the NAcc correlated with impaired heroin self-administration. This effect is site-specific because lesions of other areas, such as the lateral hypothalamus, do not necessarily affect heroin self-administration (97). More recent studies have attempted to define the relative contribution of subregions within the ventral striatum comparing acquisition of heroin self-administration after excitotoxic lesions of the NAcc core or shell. Rats with lesions of the NAcc core lesion group showed impairments in acquisition whereas the group with lesions of the NAcc shell was similar to controls. This effect was found either with acquisition of low dose heroin on a simple FR schedule (98) or with acquisition of a second order schedule with a high injection dose (99). These data suggest a relatively greater role for the NAcc core the acquisition of heroin-seeking behavior.

Martin et al. (100) examined regional differences in the ventral striatum by using beta-FNA. This drug is an irreversible antagonist at the μ-opioid receptor producing what amounts to a reversible lesion. Beta-FNA blocks the receptor rendering it unavailable for many days, until new receptor populations can be synthesized. Beta-FNA was found to produce site specific effects, attenuating heroin self-administration when injected into the caudal but not rostral NAcc.

The hypothesis that the mesolimbic DA systems mediate the reinforcing effects of opioids has been proposed. Certainly it is clear that psychostimulants and opioids have independent sites of action at the receptor level. DA antagonists potently affect cocaine but not heroin self-administration; conversely, opioid antagonists potently affect heroin but not cocaine self-administration (101,102). However, it has been shown that opioids indirectly affect DA cell firing through inhibition of GABA interneurons in the VTA (103). This disinhibition can result in enhanced DA release in the NAcc (104). Heroin self-administration increases DA in the accumbens, and this has been argued to be the mechanisms of action for heroin reinforcement (105).

Curiously, DA cells bodies in the VTA seem to be more important for heroin self-administration than the DA innervation of the ventral striatum. Bozarth and Wise (106) showed that 6-OHDA lesions of the VTA impair the acquisition of IV heroin self-administration. By contrast, 6-OHDA–induced depletion within of the NAcc having very little effect on heroin self-administration in spite of the fact that such lesions dramatically reduce or abolish cocaine self-administration (107,108). It appears that some, but not all, of the reinforcing effects of opioids are mediated through an action on DA mechanisms.

Cannabinoids The characterization of cannabinoid receptors in brain has been an important first step in identifying the site of action for the reinforcing effects of marijuana. Two cannabinoid receptors (CB1 and CB2) have been identified to date. Both are G protein–coupled receptors and function to inhibit adenylate cyclase. They are acted on by endogenous cannabinoids and exogenous activators such as marijuana. Figure 3.4 represents CB1 expression in the rat brain. As in humans, the CB1 receptor is highly expressed in the brain and found in the basal ganglia, hippocampus, cerebellum, cerebral cortex, and striatum (109). This expression may explain some of the behavioral effects of marijuana (motor, memory, or cognitive impairment (110). The CB2 receptor was once thought to be only expressed in peripheral immune cells, but has recently been identified in the brain at low levels (111).

Progress in identifying the brain mechanisms associated with the reinforcing effects of cannabinoids has been hampered until recently by the lack of a good animal model. Route of administration is a major influence on the reinforcing effects of drugs and smoking is the preferred route for marijuana use in humans. Smoking, of course, is not an option for studying cannabinoid use in rats, and there have been no reports of successfully training nonhuman primates to smoke marijuana. Instead, attempts have been made to demonstrate IV self-administration of Δ9-tetrahydrocannabinol, the active ingredient in marijuana, and other cannabinoid receptor agonists. Despite a good deal of effort, early studies provided little evidence that rats would self-administer Δ9-tetrahydrocannabinol (110), although self-administration of THC and anandamide analogs has been reported in squirrel monkeys (112,113). More success has been achieved with the synthetic CB1 receptor agonist WIN 55,212-2 which has shown to be self-administered by mice (114) and rats (115,116).

The neurobiologic investigation of cannabinoid self-administration is in the early stages although it appears that both opioid and DA mechanisms may interact with cannabinoid reinforcement (117–119).

NEUROANATOMY OF DRUG ADDICTION

The research questions that can be addressed by using animal models are necessarily different than those that can be asked with human subjects. Animal studies have a number of advantages and are well suited for the investigation of the site of action of drug reinforcement through the use of receptor agonists, antagonists, and lesion techniques. Animal self-administration

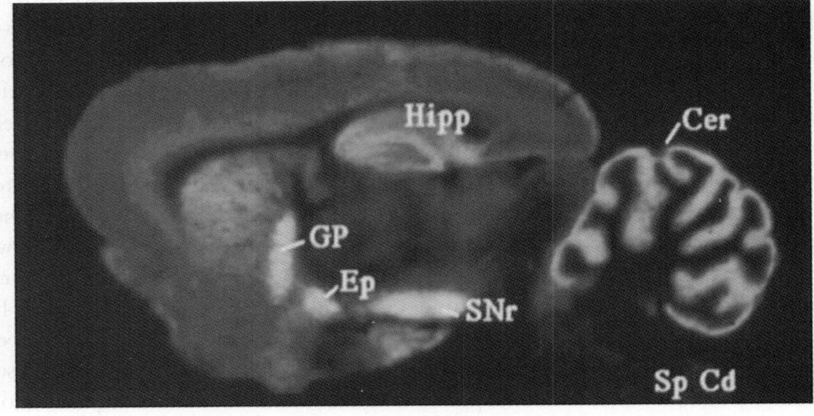

FIGURE 3.4. Cannabinoid receptor expression in the rat brain. Areas with brightest colors indicate a greater expression. Cannabinoid receptors are expressed in high numbers in the cerebellum (Cer), hippocampus (Hipp), globus pallidus (GP), external globus pallidus (Ep), and the substantia nigra pars reticulate (SNr). Spinal cord, Sp Cd. Image courtesy of Dr. Allyn Howlett.

studies allow tight control over many variables that could possibly affect the addiction process including genetics, frequency of access, dosage, route of administration, and drug history. Understandably this type of control is unattainable in the investigation of humans with addiction; however, human studies allow for the examination of aspects of addiction that are uniquely human. Addiction is a disease that lives in the real-world, and thus encompasses many different facets, such as poly drug use, comorbidity with other disorders, predisposition, drug use history, and environmental context. Thus the literature on human drug abuse offers quite different insights.

Imaging technology has been a key tool in the investigation of the neuroanatomy of addiction in human subjects. The two most widely used types of functional imaging are positron emission tomography (PET) and functional magnetic resonance imaging (fMRI). These technologies have very different temporal resolutions and lend themselves to assessing very different aspects of brain function. PET uses a radioisotope that is introduced into the body and binds to specific receptors, transporters, and enzymes. Specific ligands can be visualized, thereby offering insights into drug distribution and changes in receptor mechanism *in vivo*. fMRI offers much greater temporal resolution. Changes in the fMRI signal can be assessed on the order of seconds rather than minutes, making it possible to detect metabolic changes associated with transient cognitive demands or craving states.

Early imaging studies asked the questions, "Where does cocaine act in the brain, and how does it affect brain function?" One of the first imaging studies on cocaine-addicted individuals was conducted by Volkow et al. (120) in 1988. She found that chronic cocaine users have decreased relative cerebral blood flow (as measured by PET) in the prefrontal cortex. Volkow later showed changes in metabolic activity (as measured by fluorodeoxyglucose), which depended on the time since the last drug experience. An overall increase in metabolic activity was observed in frontal brain regions during the first week of withdrawal (121), whereas decreases in metabolic activity were found after several months (122). PET has also been used to map the binding sites of cocaine in the human brain. Fowler et al. (123) conducted the first of these studies showing high cocaine binding in the corpus striatum in nondrug using human subjects.

More recent work with PET has shown that striatal dopamine D2 receptor binding is reduced in cocaine (124), heroin (125), and methamphetamine abusers (126) and also in alcohol dependence (127). This area of work is in good concordance with nonhuman primate PET studies showing decreased D2 receptor availability in animals that are more susceptible to the reinforcing aspects of cocaine (128,129).

fMRI studies have been used to examine transient drug states, such as drug craving and the "rush" feeling associated with drug use. Much of the work in this area has been done by giving cocaine-dependent subjects (because of ethical limitations on giving drug-naive people cocaine) infusions of cocaine and other stimulants while in the fMRI scanner. Breiter (130) found that self-reports of craving for the upcoming infusion of cocaine corresponded to increases in activity in the NAcc and decreases in activity in the amygdala. He also observed increases in the ventral tegmentum (VTA and substantia nigra), pons, basal forebrain, caudate, and cingulate that correlated with self-reported feelings of rush. Further work into drug craving has shown that drug-dependent individuals have greater increases in brain activity in limbic areas and the prefrontal cortex following the presentation of drug associated cues (such as pictures of drugs and drug paraphernalia) when compared with nondrug users (131–133), and decreased responsiveness when presented with nondrug reinforcers (e.g., sexually evocative cues) (134).

Remarkably, drug-associated cues can produce limbic activation in cocaine users even when these stimuli are not consciously perceived. Childress et al. (135) presented stimuli for only 33 milliseconds. Although this short presentation was too brief for the image to be correctly identified, the drug-related stimuli nonetheless produced a strong increase in activity in the ventral pallidum and amygdala. The intensity of this response strongly predicted the magnitude of the subject's affective response when later shown visible versions of the same cues (135). These data suggest that drug cues can stimulate drug craving even before there is conscious awareness. Childress et al. (135) speculate that "by the time the motivational state is experienced and labeled as conscious desire, the ancient limbic reward circuitry already has a running start." The imaging field now provides concrete evidence of limbic involvement in drug craving that fits well with the wealth of evidence for animal studies.

REFERENCES

1. Zahm DS. The evolving theory of basal forebrain functional-anatomical 'macrosystems'. *Neurosci Biobehav Rev* 2006;30:148–172.
2. Gerfen CR. The neostriatal mosaic: multiple levels of compartmental organization in the basal ganglia. *Annu Rev Neurosci* 1992;15:285–320.
3. Squire LR, Stark CE, Clark RE. The medial temporal lobe. *Annu Rev Neurosci* 2004;27:279–306.
4. Maclean PD. Some psychiatric implications of physiological studies on frontotemporal portion of limbic system (visceral brain). *Electroencephalogr Clin Neurophysiol* 1952;4:407–418.
5. Hess WR, Akert K. Experimental data on role of hypothalamus in mechanism of emotional behavior. *AMA Arch Neurol Psychiatry* 1955;73:127–129.
6. Brodal A. *Neurological anatomy in relation to clinical medicine.* New York: Oxford University Press, 1969.
7. Swanson LW. Limbic system. In: Adelman G, Smith BH, eds. *Encyclopedia of neuroscience.* Amsterdam: Elsevier, 1987:1053–1055.
8. Heimer L, Switzer RC, van Hoesen GW. Ventral striatum and ventral pallidum: additional components of the motor system? *Trends Neurosci* 1982;5:83–87.
9. Voorn P, Vanderschuren LJ, Groenewegen HJ, et al. Putting a spin on the dorsal-ventral divide of the striatum. *Trends Neurosci* 2004;27: 468–474.
10. Mogenson GJ, Brudzynski SM, Wu M, et al. From motivation to action: a review of dopaminergic regulation of limbic → nucleus accumbens → ventral pallidum → pedunculopontine nucleus circuitries involved in limbic-motor integration. In: Kalivas PW, Barnes CD, eds. *Limbic motor circuits and neuropsychiatry.* Boca Raton: CRC Press, Inc, 1993: 93–236.

11. Wallis JD. Orbitofrontal cortex and its contribution to decision-making. *Annu Rev Neurosci* 2007;30:31–56.
12. Lee D, Seo H. Mechanisms of reinforcement learning and decision making in the primate dorsolateral prefrontal cortex. *Ann N Y Acad Sci* 2007;1104:108–122.
13. Kalivas PW, Volkow ND. The neural basis of addiction: a pathology of motivation and choice. *Am J Psychiatry* 2005;162:1403–1413.
14. Cooper JR, Bloom FE, Roth RH. *The biochemical basis of neuropharmacology.* 8th ed. Oxford University Press, 2003.
15. Dahlstrom A, Fuxe K. Evidence for the existence of monoamine-containing neurons in the central nervous system. I. Demonstration of monoamines in the cell bodies of brain stem neurons. *Acta Physiol Scand* 1965;62:1–55.
16. Dahlstrom A, Fuxe K. Evidence for the existence of monoamine neurons in the central nervous system. II. Experimentally induced changes in the intraneuronal amine levels of bulbospinal neuron systems. *Acta Physiol Scand* 1965;64:1–36.
17. LeDain G. *The report of the Canadian Government Commission of Inquiry into the non-medical use of drugs.* Ottawa, Canada: Information Canada, 1972.
18. Brady JV. Animal models for assessing drugs of abuse. *Neurosci Biobehav Rev* 1991;15:35–43.
19. Schuster CR, Johanson CE. An analysis of drug-seeking behavior in animals. *Neurosci Biobehav Rev* 1981;5:315–323.
20. Deneau G, Yanagita T, Seevers MH. Self-administration of psychoactive substances by the monkey. *Psychopharmacologia* 1969;16:30–48.
21. Thompson T, Schuster CR. Morphine self-administration, food-reinforced, and avoidance behaviors in rhesus monkeys. *Psychopharmacologia* 1964;5:87–94.
22. Weeks JR. Experimental morphine addiction: method for automatic intravenous injections in unrestrained rats. *Science* 1962;138:143–144.
23. Olds J, Yuwiler A, Olds ME, et al. Neurohumors in hypothalamic substrates of reward. *Am J Physiol* 1964;207:242–254.
24. Phillips AG, Rolls ET. Intracerebral self-administration of amphetamine by rhesus monkeys. *Neurosci Lett* 1981;24:81–86.
25. Bozarth MA, Wise RA. Intracranial self-administration of morphine into the ventral tegmental area in rats. *Life Sci* 1981;28:551–555.
26. Comer SD, Turner DM, Carroll ME. Effects of food deprivation on cocaine base smoking in rhesus monkeys. *Psychopharmacology (Berlin)* 1995;119:127–132.
27. Davis WM, Smith SG. Effect of haloperidol on (+)-amphetamine self-administration. *J Pharm Pharmacol* 1975;27:540–542.
28. Wilson MC, Schuster CR. The effects of chlorpromazine on psychomotor stimulant self-administration in the rhesus monkey. *Psychopharmacology* 1972;26:115–126.
29. Yokel RA, Wise RA. Increased lever pressing for amphetamine after pimozide in rats: implications for a dopamine theory of reward. *Science* 1975;187:547–549.
30. Yokel RA, Wise RA. Attenuation of intravenous amphetamine reinforcement by central dopamine blockade in rats. *Psychopharmacology* 1976;48:311–318.
31. De Wit H, Wise RA. Blockade of cocaine reinforcement in rats with the dopamine receptor blocker pimozide, but not with noradrenergic blockers phentolamine and phenoxybenzamine. *Can J Psych* 1977;31:195–203.
32. Wise RA. Catecholamine theories of reward: a critical review. *Brain Res.* 1978;152:215–247.
33. Wise RA. Brain substrates for reinforcement and drug self-administration. *Prog Neuropsychopharmacol* 1981;5:467–474.
34. Roberts DC, Mason ST, Fibiger HC. 6-OHDA lesion to the dorsal noradrenergic bundle alters morphine-induced locomotor activity and catalepsy. *Eur J Pharmacol* 1978;52:209–214.
35. Caine SB, Koob GF. Effects of mesolimbic dopamine depletion on responding maintained by cocaine and food. *J Exp Anal Behav* 1994;61: 213–221.
36. Lyness WH, Friedle NM, Moore KE. Destruction of dopaminergic nerve terminals in nucleus accumbens: effect on d-amphetamine self-administration. *Pharmacol Biochem Behav* 1979;11:553–556.
37. Roberts DCS, Koob GF, Klonoff P, et al. Extinction and recovery of cocaine self-administration following 6-hydroxydopamine lesions of the nucleus accumbens. *Pharmacol Biochem Behav* 1980;12:781–787.
38. Roberts DCS, Corcoran ME, Fibiger HC. Recovery of cocaine self-administration after 6-OHDA lesion of the N. accumbens correlates with residual dopamine levels. In: Usdin E, ed. *Catecholamines: basic and clinical frontiers.* Oxford: Pergamon Press, 1979:1774–1775.
39. McGregor A, Baker GB, Roberts DCS. Effect of 6-hydroxydopamine lesions of the amygdala on intravenous cocaine self-administration under a progressive ratio schedule of reinforcement. *Brain Res* 1994; 646:273–278.
40. McGregor A, Baker GB, Roberts DCS. Effect of 6-hydroxydopamine lesions of the medial prefrontal cortex on intravenous cocaine self-administration under a progressive ratio schedule of reinforcement. *Pharmacol Biochem Behav* 1996;53:5–9.
41. McGregor A, Roberts DCS. Dopaminergic antagonism within the nucleus accumbens or the amygdala produces differential effects on intravenous cocaine self-administration under fixed and progressive ratio schedules of reinforcement. *Brain Res* 1993;624:245–252.
42. McGregor A, Roberts DCS. Effect of medial prefrontal cortex injections of SCH 23390 on intravenous cocaine self-administration under both a fixed and progressive ratio schedule of reinforcement. *Behav Brain Res* 1995;67:75–80.
43. Kelly PH, Iversen SD. Selective 6OHDA-induced destruction of mesolimbic dopamine neurons: abolition of psychostimulant-induced locomotor activity in rats. *Eur J Pharmacol* 1976;40:45–56.
44. van Rossum JM. Mode of action of psychomotor stimulant drugs. *Int Rev Neurobiol* 1970;12:307–383.
45. Pijnenburg AJ, van Rossum JM. Stimulation of locomotor activity following injection of dopamine into the nucleus accumbens. *J Pharm Pharmacol* 1973;25:1003–1005.
46. Pijnenburg AJ, Honig WM, van Rossum JM. Inhibition of d-amphetamine-induced locomotor activity by injection of haloperidol into the nucleus accumbens of the rat. *Psychopharmacologia* 1975;41:87–95.
47. Randrup A, Munkvad I. Stereotyped behavior. *Pharmacol Ther [B]* 1975;1:757–768.
48. Ellinwood EH, Jr., Kilbey MM. Amphetamine stereotypy: the influence of environmental factors and prepotent behavioral patterns on its topography and development. *Biol Psychiatry* 1975;10:3–16.
49. Lyon M, Robbins TW. The action of central nervous system stimulant drugs: a general theory concerning amphetamine effects. *Curr Dev Psychopharmacol* 1975;2:81–163.
50. Ahn S, Phillips AG. Modulation by central and basolateral amygdalar nuclei of dopaminergic correlates of feeding to satiety in the rat nucleus accumbens and medial prefrontal cortex. *J Neurosci* 2002;22:10958–10965.
51. Ahn S, Phillips AG. Independent modulation of basal and feeding-evoked dopamine efflux in the nucleus accumbens and medial prefrontal cortex by the central and basolateral amygdalar nuclei in the rat. *Neuroscience* 2003;116:295–305.
52. Phillips AG, Ahn S, Howland JG. Amygdalar control of the mesocorticolimbic dopamine system: parallel pathways to motivated behavior. *Neurosci Biobehav Rev* 2003;27:543–554.
53. Agmo A, Galvan A, Talamantes B. Reward and reinforcement produced by drinking sucrose: two processes that may depend on different neurotransmitters. *Pharmacol Biochem Behav* 1995;52:403–414.
54. Agmo A, Federman I, Navarro V, et al. Reward and reinforcement produced by drinking water: role of opioids and dopamine receptor subtypes. *Pharmacol Biochem Behav* 1993;46:183–194.
55. Fibiger HC, Nomikos GG, Pfaus JG, et al. Sexual behavior, eating and mesolimbic dopamine. *Clin Neuropharmacol* 1992;15(Suppl 1, Pt A): 566A–567A.
56. Mitchell JB, Gratton A. Involvement of mesolimbic dopamine neurons in sexual behaviors: implications for the neurobiology of motivation. *Rev Neurosci* 1994;5:317–329.
57. Gratton A, Wise RA. Brain stimulation reward in the lateral hypothalamic medial forebrain bundle: mapping of boundaries and homogeneity. *Brain Res* 1983;274:25–30.

58. Tzschentke TM. The medial prefrontal cortex as a part of the brain reward system. *Amino Acids* 2000;19:211–219.
59. Wise RA. Brain reward circuitry: insights from unsensed incentives. *Neuron* 2002;36:229–240.
60. White FJ. Synaptic regulation of mesocorticolimbic dopamine neurons. *Annu Rev Neurosci* 1996;19:405–436.
61. Schultz W. Behavioral dopamine signals. *Trends Neurosci* 2007;30:203–210.
62. Phillipson OT. A Golgi study of the ventral tegmental area of Tsai and interfascicular nucleus in the rat. *J Comp Neurol* 1979;187:99–115.
63. Ramon-Moliner E, Nauta WJ. The isodendritic core of the brain stem. *J Comp Neurol* 1966;126:311–335.
64. Geisler S, Zahm DS. Afferents of the ventral tegmental area in the rat-anatomical substratum for integrative functions. *J Comp Neurol* 2005;490:270–294.
65. Martin M, Hurley RA, Taber KH. Is opiate addiction associated with longstanding neurobiological changes? *J Neuropsychiatry Clin Neurosci* 2007;19:242–248.
66. Dykstra LA, Preston KL, Bigelow GE. Discriminative stimulus and subjective effects of opioids with mu and kappa activity: data from laboratory animals and human subjects. *Psychopharmacology* 1997;130:14–27.
67. Koob GF, Vaccarino FJ, Amalric M, et al. Neurochemical substrates for opiate reinforcement. *NIDA Res Monogr* 1986;71:146–164.
68. Mucha RF, Herz A. Motivational properties of kappa and mu opioid receptor agonists studied with place and taste preference conditioning. *Psychopharmacology* 1985;86:274–280.
69. Tang AH, Collins RJ. Behavioral effects of a novel kappa opioid analgesic, U-50488, in rats and rhesus monkeys. *Psychopharmacology* 1985;85:309–314.
70. Mansour A, Khachaturian H, Lewis ME, et al. Autoradiographic differentiation of mu, delta, and kappa opioid receptors in the rat forebrain and midbrain. *J Neurosci* 1987;7:2445–2464.
71. Wise RA, Hoffman DC. Localization of drug reward mechanisms by intracranial injections. *Synapse* 1992;10:247–263.
72. Olds ME. Hypothalamic substrate for the positive reinforcing properties of morphine in the rat. *Brain Res* 1979;168:351–360.
73. Olds ME, Williams KN. Self-administration of D-Ala2-Met-enkephalinamide at hypothalamic self-stimulation sites. *Brain Res* 1980;194:155–170.
74. Olds J, Milner P. Positive reinforcement produced by electrical stimulation of septal area and other regions of rat brain. *J Comp Physiol Psychol* 1954;47:419–427.
75. Bozarth MA, Wise RA. Localization of the reward-relevant opiate receptors. *NIDA Res Monogr* 1982;41:158–164.
76. Olds ME. Reinforcing effects of morphine in the nucleus accumbens. *Brain Res* 1982;237:429–440.
77. Goeders NE, Lane JD, Smith JE. Self-administration of methionine enkephalin into the nucleus accumbens. *Pharmacol Biochem Behav* 1984;20:451–455.
78. van der Kooy D, Mucha RF, O'Shaughnessy M, et al. Reinforcing effects of brain microinjections of morphine revealed by conditioned place preference. *Brain Res* 1982;243:107–117.
79. Le Merrer J, Gavello-Baudy S, Galey D, et al. Morphine self-administration into the lateral septum depends on dopaminergic mechanisms: evidence from pharmacology and Fos neuroimaging. *Behav Brain Res* 2007;180:203–217.
80. David V, Cazala P. Anatomical and pharmacological specificity of the rewarding effect elicited by microinjections of morphine into the nucleus accumbens of mice. *Psychopharmacology* 2000;150:24–34.
81. David V, Durkin TP, Cazala P. Differential effects of the dopamine D2/D3 receptor antagonist sulpiride on self-administration of morphine into the ventral tegmental area or the nucleus accumbens. *Psychopharmacology* 2002;160:307–317.
82. Devine DP, Wise RA. Self-administration of morphine, DAMGO, and DPDPE into the ventral tegmental area of rats. *J Neurosci* 1994;14:1978–1984.
83. Welzl H, Kuhn G, Huston JP. Self-administration of small amounts of morphine through glass micropipettes into the ventral tegmental area of the rat. *Neuropharmacology* 1989;28:1017–1023.
84. Phillips AG, LePiane FG. Reinforcing effects of morphine microinjection into the ventral tegmental area. *Pharmacol Biochem Behav* 1980;12:965–968.
85. Jenck F, Gratton A, Wise RA. Opioid receptor subtypes associated with ventral tegmental facilitation of lateral hypothalamic brain stimulation reward. *Brain Res* 1987;423:34–38.
86. Broekkamp CL, Phillips AG. Facilitation of self-stimulation behavior following intracerebral microinjections of opioids into the ventral tegmental area. *Pharmacol Biochem Behav* 1979;11:289–295.
87. Stewart J. Reinstatement of heroin and cocaine self-administration behavior in the rat by intracerebral application of morphine in the ventral tegmental area. *Pharmacol Biochem Behav* 1984;20:917–923.
88. Corrigall WA, Linseman MA. Conditioned place preference produced by intra-hippocampal morphine. *Pharmacol Biochem Behav* 1988;30:787–789.
89. Koob GF, Pettit HO, Ettenberg A, et al. Effects of opiate antagonists and their quaternary derivatives on heroin self-administration in the rat. *J Pharmacol Exp Ther* 1984;229:481–486.
90. Britt MD, Wise RA. Ventral tegmental site of opiate reward: antagonism by a hydrophilic opiate receptor blocker. *Brain Res* 1983;258:105–108.
91. Corrigall WA, Vaccarino FJ. Antagonist treatment in nucleus accumbens or periaqueductal grey affects heroin self-administration. *Pharmacol Biochem Behav* 1988;30:443–450.
92. Vaccarino FJ, Bloom FE, Koob GF. Blockade of nucleus accumbens opiate receptors attenuates intravenous heroin reward in the rat. *Psychopharmacology* 1985;86:37–42.
93. Walker JR, Ahmed SH, Gracy KN, et al. Microinjections of an opiate receptor antagonist into the bed nucleus of the stria terminalis suppress heroin self-administration in dependent rats. *Brain Res* 2000;854:85–92.
94. Corrigall WA. Heroin self-administration: effects of antagonist treatment in lateral hypothalamus. *Pharmacol Biochem Behav* 1987;27:693–700.
95. Vaccarino FJ, Pettit HO, Bloom FE, et al. Effects of intracerebroventricular administration of methyl naloxonium chloride on heroin self-administration in the rat. *Pharmacol Biochem Behav* 1985;23:495–498.
96. Zito KA, Vickers G, Roberts DC. Disruption of cocaine and heroin self-administration following kainic acid lesions of the nucleus accumbens. *Pharmacol Biochem Behav* 1985;23:1029–1036.
97. Britt MD, Wise RA. Opiate rewarding action: independence of the cells of the lateral hypothalamus. *Brain Res* 1981;222:213–217.
98. Alderson HL, Parkinson JA, Robbins TW, et al. The effects of excitotoxic lesions of the nucleus accumbens core or shell regions on intravenous heroin self-administration in rats. *Psychopharmacology* 2001;153:455–463.
99. Hutcheson DM, Parkinson JA, Robbins TW, et al. The effects of nucleus accumbens core and shell lesions on intravenous heroin self-administration and the acquisition of drug-seeking behaviour under a second-order schedule of heroin reinforcement. *Psychopharmacology* 2001;153:464–472.
100. Martin TJ, Kim SA, Lyupina Y, et al. Differential involvement of mu-opioid receptors in the rostral versus caudal nucleus accumbens in the reinforcing effects of heroin in rats: evidence from focal injections of beta-funaltrexamine. *Psychopharmacology* 2002;161:152–159.
101. Ettenberg A, Pettit HO, Bloom FE, et al. Heroin and cocaine intravenous self-administration in rats: mediation by separate neural systems. *Psychopharmacology* 1982;78:204–209.
102. Gerber GJ, Wise RA. Pharmacological regulation of intravenous cocaine and heroin self-administration in rats: a variable dose paradigm. *Pharmacol Biochem Behav* 1989;32:527–531.
103. Johnson SW, North RA. Opioids excite dopamine neurons by hyperpolarization of local interneurons. *J Neurosci* 1992;12:483–488.

104. Hemby SE, Martin TJ, Co C, et al. The effects of intravenous heroin administration on extracellular nucleus accumbens dopamine concentrations as determined by in vivo microdialysis. *J Pharmacol Exp Ther* 1995;273:591–598.
105. Lecca D, Valentini V, Cacciapaglia F, et al. Reciprocal effects of response contingent and noncontingent intravenous heroin on in vivo nucleus accumbens shell versus core dopamine in the rat: a repeated sampling microdialysis study. *Psychopharmacology* 2007;194:103–116.
106. Bozarth MA, Wise RA. Involvement of the ventral tegmental dopamine system in opioid and psychomotor stimulant reinforcement. *NIDA Res Monogr* 1986;67:190–196.
107. Pettit HO, Ettenberg A, Bloom FE, et al. Destruction of dopamine in the nucleus accumbens selectively attenuates cocaine but not heroin self-administration in rats. *Psychopharmacology* 1984;84:167–173.
108. Gerrits MA, Van Ree JM. Effect of nucleus accumbens dopamine depletion on motivational aspects involved in initiation of cocaine and heroin self-administration in rats. *Brain Res* 1996;713:114–124.
109. Herkenham M, Lynn AB, Little MD, et al. Cannabinoid receptor localization in brain. *Proc Natl Acad Sci U S A* 1990;87:1932–1936.
110. Abood ME, Martin BR. Neurobiology of marijuana abuse. *Trends Pharmacol Sci* 1992;13:201–206.
111. Onaivi ES. Neuropsychobiological evidence for the functional presence and expression of cannabinoid CB2 receptors in the brain. *Neuropsychobiology* 2006;54:231–246.
112. Justinova Z, Tanda G, Redhi GH, et al. Self-administration of Δ9-tetrahydrocannabinol (THC) by drug naive squirrel monkeys. *Psychopharmacology* 2003;169:135–140.
113. Justinova Z, Solinas M, Tanda G, et al. The endogenous cannabinoid anandamide and its synthetic analog R(+)-methanandamide are intravenously self-administered by squirrel monkeys. *J Neurosci* 2005;25: 5645–5650.
114. Martellotta MC, Cossu G, Fattore L, et al. Self-administration of the cannabinoid receptor agonist WIN 55,212-2 in drug-naive mice. *Neuroscience* 1998;85:327–330.
115. Fattore L, Cossu G, Martellotta CM, et al. Intravenous self-administration of the cannabinoid CB1 receptor agonist WIN 55,212-2 in rats. *Psychopharmacology* 2001;156:410–416.
116. Fattore L, Spano MS, Altea S, et al. Cannabinoid self-administration in rats: sex differences and the influence of ovarian function. *Br J Pharmacol* 2007;152:795–804.
117. Justinova Z, Tanda G, Munzar P, et al. The opioid antagonist naltrexone reduces the reinforcing effects of Delta 9 tetrahydrocannabinol (THC) in squirrel monkeys. *Psychopharmacology* 2004;173:186–194.
118. Fadda P, Scherma M, Spano MS, et al. Cannabinoid self-administration increases dopamine release in the nucleus accumbens. *Neuroreport* 2006;17:1629–1632.
119. Lecca D, Cacciapaglia F, Valentini V, et al. Monitoring extracellular dopamine in the rat nucleus accumbens shell and core during acquisition and maintenance of intravenous WIN 55,212–2 self-administration. *Psychopharmacology* 2006;188:63–74.
120. Volkow ND, Mullani N, Gould KL, et al. Cerebral blood flow in chronic cocaine users: a study with positron emission tomography. *Br J Psychiatry* 1988;152:641–648.
121. Volkow ND, Fowler JS, Wolf AP, et al. Changes in brain glucose metabolism in cocaine dependence and withdrawal. *Am J Psychiatry* 1991; 148:621–626.
122. Volkow ND, Hitzemann R, Wang GJ, et al. Long-term frontal brain metabolic changes in cocaine abusers. *Synapse* 1992;11:184–190.
123. Fowler JS, Volkow ND, Wolf AP, et al. Mapping cocaine binding sites in human and baboon brain in vivo. *Synapse* 1989;4:371–377.
124. Volkow ND, Fowler JS, Wang GJ, et al. Decreased dopamine D2 receptor availability is associated with reduced frontal metabolism in cocaine abusers. *Synapse* 1993;14:169–177.
125. Wang GJ, Volkow ND, Fowler JS, et al. Dopamine D2 receptor availability in opiate-dependent subjects before and after naloxone-precipitated withdrawal. *Neuropsychopharmacology* 1997;16:174–182.
126. Volkow ND, Chang L, Wang GJ, et al. Low level of brain dopamine D2 receptors in methamphetamine abusers: association with metabolism in the orbitofrontal cortex. *Am J Psychiatry* 2001;158:2015–2021.
127. Volkow ND, Wang GJ, Fowler JS, et al. Decreases in dopamine receptors but not in dopamine transporters in alcoholics. *Alcohol Clin Exp Res* 1996;20:1594–1598.
128. Morgan D, Grant KA, Gage HD, et al. Social dominance in monkeys: dopamine D2 receptors and cocaine self-administration. *Nat Neurosci* 2002;5:169–174.
129. Nader MA, Morgan D, Gage HD, et al. PET imaging of dopamine D2 receptors during chronic cocaine self-administration in monkeys. *Nat Neurosci* 2006;9:1050–1056.
130. Breiter HC, Gollub RL, Weisskoff RM, et al. Acute effects of cocaine on human brain activity and emotion. *Neuron* 1997;19:591–611.
131. Garavan H, Pankiewicz J, Bloom A, et al. Cue-induced cocaine craving: neuroanatomical specificity for drug users and drug stimuli. *Am J Psychiatry* 2000;157:1789–1798.
132. Maas LC, Lukas SE, Kaufman MJ, et al. Functional magnetic resonance imaging of human brain activation during cue-induced cocaine craving. *Am J Psychiatry* 1998;155:124–126.
133. Wexler BE, Gottschalk CH, Fulbright RK, et al. Functional magnetic resonance imaging of cocaine craving. *Am J Psychiatry* 2001;158:86–95.
134. Garavan H, Pendergrass JC, Ross TJ, et al. Amygdala response to both positively and negatively valanced stimuli. *Neuroreport* 2001;12:2779–2783.
135. Childress AR, Ehrman RN, Wang Z, et al. Prelude to passion: limbic activation by "unseen" drug and sexual cues. *PLoS ONE* 2008;3:e1506.

CHAPTER 4

Eric J. Nestler, MD, PhD

From Neurobiology to Treatment: Progress Against Addiction

In terms of lost lives and productivity, drug addiction remains one of the most serious threats to our nation's public health. Addiction can be defined as the loss of control over drug use, or the compulsive seeking and taking of a drug regardless of the consequences. Available treatments for addiction remain inadequately effective for most individuals. Consequently, there is intense interest in better understanding the neurobiology of addiction in the hope that such knowledge will lead eventually to more effective treatments.

Diverse types of chemicals—drugs of abuse—cause addiction. Such drugs share no similarities in chemical structure, and yet they produce similar behavioral syndromes: addiction. Considerable progress has been made in understanding how drugs of abuse cause addiction. The initial protein targets for almost all drugs of abuse are known (Table 4.1) (1). Also, several circuits in the brain, containing these drug targets, are known to mediate the addicting actions of drugs of abuse (1–4). Most attention has been given to the nucleus accumbens (also called the ventral striatum) and its dopaminergic input from the ventral tegmental area of the midbrain as key substrates for these drug effects. Other brain regions interact with this circuit, including the amygdala, prefrontal and other limbic cortical regions, hippocampus, and hypothalamus, to name a few.

These brain structures represent reward pathways, which are very old from an evolutionary point of view and which presumably evolved to mediate an individual's response to natural rewards, such as food, sex, and social interaction. Drugs of abuse activate these reward pathways, in the absence of natural rewards, with a force and persistence not seen under normal conditions. Over time, repeated drug exposure causes adaptations in the brain's reward pathways, which seem to have two major consequences. First, during periods of active drug use or shortly after ceasing drug intake, the ability of natural rewards to activate the reward pathways is diminished, and the individual experiences depressed motivation and mood. Taking more drug is the quickest, easiest way for a person with addiction to feel "normal" again. Second, drug use causes long-lasting memories related to the drug experience, such that even after prolonged periods of withdrawal (months, years), stressful events or exposure to drug-associated cues can trigger intense craving, and in many cases relapse, in part by activating the brain's reward pathways. Roughly half the risk for addiction is genetic (5). A great deal of effort is aimed at identifying the specific genes involved and the mechanisms by which diverse nongenetic factors influence the development of an addictive disorder.

Addiction should be viewed as distinct from physical dependence, wherein individuals become physically sick when drug administration ceases (1,6). Physical dependence per se is neither necessary nor sufficient to cause addiction: some drugs of abuse do not cause appreciable physical dependence, and some medications used in general medicine cause physical dependence but are not addicting (e.g., β-adrenergic antagonists such as propranolol). Moreover, physical dependence and withdrawal syndromes are largely mediated to a great extent by different central nervous system regions than those important for addiction. Nevertheless, much of the clinical progress in the addiction field has come from improved methods of treating the physical dependence and severe withdrawal syndromes associated with opiates and alcohol (6). Knowledge of opiate action on opioid receptors at a cellular level led to the development of several medications now used to treat opiate withdrawal. Clonidine, an α_2-adrenergic agonist, produces cellular effects similar to opioid receptor activation, and was later shown to dampen many of the physical signs and symptoms of opiate withdrawal in humans (7,8). By combining clonidine with naltrexone, an opioid receptor antagonist, or with

TABLE 4.1 Acute Actions of Some Drugs of Abuse

Drug	Action	Receptor signaling mechanism
Opiates	Agonist at μ,δ and κ opioid receptors[a]	Gi
Cocaine	Indirect agonist at dopamine receptors by inhibiting dopamine transporters[b]	Gi and Gs[c]
Amphetamine	Indirect agonist at dopamine receptors by stimulating dopamine release[b]	Gi and Gs[c]
Ethanol	Facilitates $GABA_A$ receptor function and inhibits NMDA glutamate receptor function[d]	Ligand-gated channels
Nicotine	Agonist at nicotinic acetylcholine receptors	Ligand-gated channels
Cannabinoids	Agonist at CB_1 and CB_2 cannabinoid receptors[e]	Gi
Phencyclidine (PCP)	Antagonist at NMDA glutamate receptor channels	Ligand-gated
Hallucinogens	Partial agonist at $5HT_{2A}$ serotonin receptors	Gq
Inhalants	Unknown	

Data from Nestler EJ. Molecular basis of neural plasticity underlying addiction. *Nat Rev. Neurosci.* 2001;2:119–128.

[a]Activity at μ (and possibly) δ receptors mediates the reinforcing actions of opiates; κ receptors mediate aversive actions.

[b]Cocaine and amphetamine exert analogous actions on serotonergic and noradrenergic systems, which may also contribute to the reinforcing effects of these drugs.

[c]Gi couples D_2-like dopamine receptors, and Gs couples D_1-like dopamine receptors, both of which are important for dopamine's reinforcing effects.

[d]Ethanol affects several other ligand-gated channels, and at higher concentrations voltage-gated channels, as well. In addition, ethanol is reported to influence many other neurotransmitter systems, including serotonergic, opioidergic, and dopaminergic systems. It is not known whether these effects are direct or achieved indirectly via actions on various ligand-gated channels.

[e]Activity at CB_1 receptors mediates the reinforcing actions of cannabinoids; CB_2 receptors are expressed predominantly in the periphery. Endogenous ligands for the CB_1 receptor include the arachidonic acid metabolites, anandamide, and 2-arachidonylglycerol.

buprenorphine, an opioid receptor partial agonist, it is now possible to detoxify a patient from opiates over a few days with relatively minor distress (6). This is in striking contrast to the extremely painful "cold turkey" method that characterized opiate detoxification a generation ago. Similarly, based on the knowledge that benzodiazepines, such as alcohol, facilitate gamma-aminobutyric acid (GABA) receptor function, benzodiazepines are now used routinely to prevent the life-threatening sequelae of alcohol withdrawal.

The impact of these advances, however, is limited because treatment of physical dependence and withdrawal does not target the core clinical symptoms of addiction—namely, drug craving and relapse to drug use even after prolonged abstinence. Unfortunately, treatment of the core symptoms of addiction has proved much more difficult than treatment of physical withdrawal syndromes.

BLOCKADE OF DRUG TARGETS

Approaches pursued to date can be divided into several categories, including blockade of drug targets, mimicry of drug action, and blockade of the addiction process (Fig. 4.1). The most straightforward strategy is to block the drug from getting to its target. Such a treatment agent should have the additional requirement of not affecting that target on its own. The best example of this approach is naltrexone (6). In theory, naltrexone is inactive in the absence of an opiate, but blocks the ability of opiates to produce their many effects, including addiction. Indeed, naltrexone can be used to treat opiate addiction, but has its limitations. Naltrexone is not inactive in the absence of exogenous opiates. This is because the drug blocks the actions of the body's endogenous opioid peptides (enkephalin, dynorphin, endorphin); this can cause negative emotional effects (such as depressed mood), which reduce patient compliance (6). As a result, naltrexone is mostly effective for highly "motivated" addicts whose employment can be used to coerce compliance. Based on animal studies showing that alcohol's and nicotine's addicting actions are mediated in part via activation of endogenous opioidergic neurons (Fig. 4.1), naltrexone has been used to treat addiction to these drugs as well. Although some efficacy has been observed clinically, the effects of naltrexone are relatively small in magnitude (9).

A related approach with cocaine or other stimulants (amphetamine, methamphetamine) has not yet been effective. The most important mechanism of action of cocaine is inhibition of presynaptic dopamine transporters (Fig. 4.1). The goal for treatment would be to prevent cocaine's binding to the transporter without affecting the transporter's normal functioning. Despite intense effort, suitable molecules have not yet been developed and validated. An alternative to such a "cocaine antagonist" is the "cocaine vaccine," which would block cocaine's entry into the brain through immunologic approaches. By immunizing with cocaine coupled to a carrier, it has been possible to generate immunity in animals (10). When the animals are subsequently challenged with

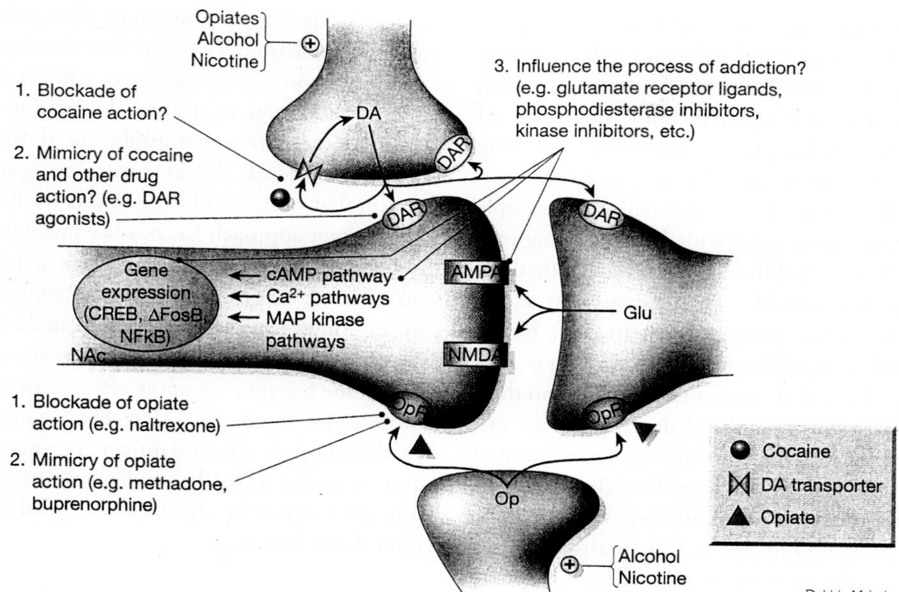

FIGURE 4.1. General Strategies Used to Treat Drug Addiction or Associated Physical Withdrawal Syndromes. A dendritic spine of a nucleus accumbens (NAc) neuron and its innervation by terminals of glutamatergic (Glu), dopaminergic (DA), and opioidergic (Op) neurons are shown. **1:** One approach is to block the ability of a drug to reach its initial protein target: for example, naltrexone's antagonism of opioid receptors (OR) or a hypothetical drug that interferes with cocaine's actions on the dopamine transporter. Not depicted is the use of immunologic methods (such as a cocaine or nicotine vaccine) to prevent a drug from entering the brain. **2:** A second approach is to mimic drug action: for example, sustained activation of OR by methadone, or activation of DA receptors (DAR) by various agonists or partial agonists. **3:** A third approach is to influence the process of addiction: for example, via perturbation of Glu receptors (AMPA, NMDA, metabotropic receptors) or a host of postreceptor signaling proteins (such as those involved in the cAMP, calcium, and MAP kinase pathways and in the regulation of gene expression—ΔFosB, CREB, or NFκB) that have been implicated in addiction (1,20).

cocaine, the drug's clearance is increased, its penetration into the brain is decreased, and its behavioral effects are attenuated. Cocaine vaccines are now in clinical development and could prove useful, but there are several potential drawbacks. First, cocaine already has a very short half-life. It is not clear whether increased clearance made possible by active immunity would have a functionally meaningful effect in humans. Second, a cocaine vaccine would not be active against other stimulants, and cocaine users could rapidly switch to another drug. The use of a cocaine vaccine also raises important ethical considerations, such as the potential loss of privacy (the presence of such antibodies would "mark" a person with addiction) and whether the vaccine should be voluntary (11). An alternative to such an active vaccine would be passive immunity, also under investigation, where a user would be injected at set intervals with anticocaine antibodies. Similar efforts are under way to generate a vaccine toward nicotine, which is in early clinical trials.

Cannabinoids, the active ingredients in marijuana, act through the stimulation of CB_1 receptors. Moreover, there is evidence that other drugs of abuse (e.g., opiates, alcohol) may produce part of their addicting effects via the activation of endogenous cannabinoids in the brain (Table 4.1) (12). This has led to the speculation that CB_1 antagonists may be of use in treating various addictions. Rimonabant is a CB_1 antagonist, approved in Europe for the treatment of obesity, but it is not yet known whether rimonabant is effective in treating drug addiction. However, an important cautionary note is that use of rimonabant is associated with the onset of depressive symptomatology in some patients, which may severely limit utility of this pharmacologic approach.

MIMICRY OF DRUG ACTION

Contrary to efforts to block drug effects, there has been considerable interest and progress in treating addiction by mimicking drug action. This approach is based on the notion that blocking drug targets, as mentioned previously, would leave the addicted person with an altered, addicted brain and the intense drug craving it produces. In contrast, by activating drug targets, it might be possible to partially alleviate this drug craving and allow the brain to slowly recover. A critical aspect of this approach, and presumably of brain recovery, is to use long-acting medications that would do more than simply mimic a drug of abuse; they would need to do so in a sustained manner, thereby avoiding the rapid on and off phases of repeated drug exposure. Although the effectiveness of drug mimicry has been documented clinically, it is poorly understood at the neurobiologic level. The best-established example of this approach is methadone, a particularly long-acting opioid receptor agonist. The only difference between methadone and other opiates is its long half-life, which means that, at the proper dose, opioid-dependent patients on methadone have a low level of sustained activation of opioid receptors. This enables patients to avoid the daily extremes of "highs" on drug administration and withdrawal as the drug effects wear off. This, in turn, enables the patients to return to a more normal life of steady work and social interactions. Decades of experience have documented the safety and efficacy of methadone and another long-acting opioid agonist, levo-alpha-acetylmethadol (LAAM), in the treatment of a subset of opiate addicts, although it is difficult to predict which individuals will respond (13,14). A variation in this theme is buprenorphine (15). As a high-affinity partial agonist, buprenorphine binds to opioid receptors and produces a mild agonist effect. Higher doses of the drug do not produce stronger effects because the ability of buprenorphine to activate the receptor is intrinsically low. However, buprenorphine, bound to the receptor at high affinity, can block the effects of opiate drugs of abuse, which limits the person with an addiction's attempts to obtain a drug "high" during treatment. Despite the clear utility of this general approach, and considerable success in many patients, there remains significant concern toward methadone and related treatments, because the addicted person is still being exposed to opiates and may be vulnerable to deleterious effects of these medications.

Another example of the mimicry approach is the use of nicotine patches or chewing gum to treat tobacco addiction. The resulting sustained release of low levels of nicotine can dampen craving for cigarettes in some patients long enough to help the individuals quit smoking (16). However, such approaches are not effective in most smokers, perhaps because of the very stable nicotine-induced changes in the brain that sustain the addiction. Perhaps agonists selective for particular nicotinic cholinergic receptors in the brain that mediate nicotine addiction would be more effective than low levels of nicotine itself. Indeed, one such nicotinic agonist, varenicline, has been approved recently for treatment of nicotine addiction, although much further clinical experience with the drug is needed to understand its effectiveness (17).

Mentioned briefly earlier is the important role of dopamine in drug addiction. Stimulation of dopaminergic transmission in the nucleus accumbens and elsewhere seems to be the most important mechanism of stimulant action and contributes to the actions of other drugs of abuse as well (Fig. 4.1) (3,4). Thus, activation of opioid, cholinergic, or cannabinoid receptors increases dopaminergic transmission in these brain regions. Based on this knowledge, there has been intense effort to use dopamine receptor antagonists and agonists in the treatment of addiction. The goal is to develop agents that regulate the general process of addiction, which might be equally effective for all drugs of abuse. Use of dopamine antagonists is based on the notion that inhibition of drug effects would limit drug use, whereas use of dopamine agonists is based on the notion that mimicry of drug effects would be more efficacious. The former approach has not been promising. Although dopamine receptor antagonists can block acute drug effects, there is no evidence that they limit drug craving or self-administration in the long term. They may even make animals and humans more sensitive to drugs of abuse via adaptive increases in dopamine receptor signaling efficacy. In contrast, there is some promise for the use of D1 receptor agonists and D2 receptor partial agonists, which dampen cocaine craving and relapse in animal models (18,19). Studies in humans are a high priority, but are limited by the lack of availability of suitable compounds for human use.

BLOCKADE OF THE ADDICTION PROCESS

A great deal has been learned over the past decade about the changes that drugs of abuse cause in the brain's reward pathways to produce addiction (1,20). Current research aims to exploit this information for the development of more effective treatments. However, efforts in this realm are almost entirely speculative and must be viewed with skepticism. It is clear, for example, that glutamatergic circuits are crucial for the normal activity of the nucleus accumbens and ventral tegmental area. Moreover, drugs of abuse alter levels or activity of glutamate receptors within these regions (2,21–24). This raises the possibility, untested to date in humans, that drugs aimed at any of several types of glutamate receptors might be of use in the treatment of addiction. Given the prominent role of glutamatergic mechanisms in learning and memory, and increasing evidence that important aspects of addiction can be viewed as a form of memory, it is possible that glutamatergic agents, given in conjunction with behavioral therapies, might be most efficacious at fundamentally altering addictive behavior. For example, we now know that extinction of a memory is not the passive process of undoing that memory, but rather the formation of an active new memory that supersedes the old one. Hence, a drug that enhances glutamatergic transmission, and, therefore, new memory formation, given in concert with behavioral extinction trials, might be a novel approach to treating addiction-related memories that are thought to underlie aspects of craving and relapse.

In a similar way, numerous other neurotransmitter, neuropeptide, and neurotrophic factor systems are altered by drugs of abuse and, in turn, modulate drug effects in laboratory animals: GABA, neuropeptide Y, corticotropin-releasing factor, serotonin, norepinephrine, melanocortins, and brain-derived neurotrophic factor, to name just a few. One example is gamma-vinyl GABA, a GABA transaminase inhibitor, which shows some promise toward cocaine and other stimulants in animal models and early clinical studies, although further work is needed to validate its true effectiveness (25). As these effects are better defined in animal models, and putative treatment agents suitable for human investigation are developed, these mechanisms can be tested in clinical populations.

Drug addiction also involves adaptations at postreceptor, intracellular signaling cascades, including alterations in gene expression (1,20). Moreover, modification of particular signaling proteins can have dramatic effects on an animal's responses to drugs of abuse. Examples include several proteins that regulate the function of G protein–coupled receptors: G proteins, G protein–receptor kinases, arrestins, and regulators of G protein signaling proteins (26–28). Because the acute targets of many drugs of abuse are G protein–coupled receptors, it is possible that agents affecting these modulatory proteins could exert interesting functional effects on the receptor systems so as to treat aspects of addiction. Similarly, given the evidence for an important role of the cyclic adenosine monophosphate (cAMP) pathway in addiction (1,29) and of the transcription factor ΔFosB (30), it is conceivable that novel agents directed against protein components of these pathways (such as phosphodiesterase inhibitors, which would enhance cAMP function) might warrant investigation as clinical treatments. Still another example is inhibitors of histone deacetylases (HDACs), enzymes that regulate gene expression by acetylating nearby histones. Recent evidence demonstrates that manipulation of specific histone deacetylases in the brain exerts a dramatic effect on drug-elicited behaviors (31). Drug discovery efforts should, of course, focus on subtypes of these intracellular signaling proteins that are highly enriched in the brain's reward pathways and would therefore represent potentially viable drug targets.

One of the central problems in approaching addiction is that truly effective treatments are not yet available. Thus, it is impossible to know what types of treatment are theoretically possible. For example, before the advent of antidepressant medications, there was considerable debate about the nature and magnitude of improvement possible with chemical treatments. By analogy, the drug abuse field now aims to identify medications that dampen drug craving or reward without interfering with motivation for natural rewards. Only as putative treatment agents are developed and tested in animals and humans will insight into the feasibility of this aim become available.

Perhaps an even greater obstacle in the development of new treatments for addiction is the relative lack of interest by the pharmaceutical industry. This problem has many factors, including the perceived stigma of dealing with addiction as well as the presumption that markets for addiction treatment agents might be too small. The latter would seem to represent a major miscalculation by the industry. Experience tells us that the size of many markets only becomes apparent when truly effective treatments are available. Antidepressants, now a worldwide market of more than $10 billion, are a case in point. By analogy, treatment agents that can correct compulsive behavior toward drug rewards, if they can be developed, would represent enormous successes, given their potential to treat not only drug addictions, but addictions to nondrug stimuli, such as gambling, food, and sex, which may be mediated by similar mechanisms. Such treatments could be highly successful and offer dramatic improvement in public health.

ACKNOWLEDGMENTS: *Preparation of this review was supported by grants from the National Institute on Drug Abuse. This chapter is adapted with permission of the publisher from Nestler EJ. From neurobiology to treatment: progress against addiction.* Nat Neurosci. *2002;5(Suppl):1076–1079. © 2002, Nature Neuroscience, New York, NY.*

REFERENCES

1. Nestler EJ. Molecular basis of neural plasticity underlying addiction. *Nat Rev. Neurosci* 2001;2:119–128.
2. Everitt BJ, Wolf ME. Psychomotor stimulant addiction: a neural systems perspective. *J Neurosci* 2002;22:3312–3320.
3. Koob GF, Le Moal M. Drug addiction, dysregulation of reward, and allostasis. *Neuropsychopharmacology* 2001;24:97–129.
4. Wise RA. Drug-activation of brain reward pathways. *Drug Alcohol Depend* 1998;51:13–22.
5. Kendler KS, Myers J, Prescott CA. Specificity of genetic and environmental risk factors for symptoms of cannabis, cocaine, alcohol, caffeine, and nicotine dependence. *Arch Gen Psychiatry* 2007;64:1313–1320.
6. Dackis C, O'Brien C. Neurobiology of addiction: treatment and public policy ramifications. *Nat Neurosci* 2005;8:1431–1436.
7. Aghajanian GK. Tolerance of locus coeruleus neurones to morphine and suppression of withdrawal response by clonidine. *Nature* 1978;276: 186–188.
8. Gold MS, Redmond DE Jr, Kleber HD. Clonidine blocks acute opiate-withdrawal symptoms. *Lancet* 1978;2:599–602.
9. Krystal JH, Cramer JA, Krol WE, et al. Veterans Affairs Naltrexone Cooperative Study 425 Group. Naltrexone in the treatment of alcohol dependence. *N Engl J Med* 2001;345:1734–1739.
10. Kantak KM, Collins SL, Bond J, et al. Time course of changes in cocaine self-administration behavior in rats during immunization with the cocaine vaccine IPC-1010. *Psychopharmacology* 2001;153:-334–340.
11. Cohen PJ. Immunization for prevention and treatment of cocaine abuse: legal and ethical implications. *Drug Alcohol Depend* 1997; 48:167–174.
12. Parolaro D, Vigano D, Rubino T. Endocannabinoids and drug dependence. *Curr Drug Targets CNS Neurol Disord* 2005;4:643–655.
13. National Consensus Development Panel on Effective Medical Treatment of Opiate Addiction. Effective medical treatment of opiate addiction. *JAMA* 1998;280:1936–1943.
14. Kreek MJ. Methadone-related opioid agonist pharmacotherapy for heroin addiction. History, recent molecular and neurochemical research and future in mainstream medicine. *Ann N Y Acad of Sci* 2000;909: 186–216.
15. Ling W, Smith D. Buprenorphine: blending practice and research. *J. Subst Abuse Treat* 2002;23:87–92.
16. Silagy C, Lancaster T, Stead L, et al. Nicotine replacement therapy for smoking cessation. *Cochr Database Syst Rev* 2001;3:CD000146.
17. Doggrell SA. Which is the best primary medication for long-term smoking cessation—nicotine replacement therapy, bupropion or varenicline. *Exp Opin Pharmacother* 2007;8:2903–2915.
18. Pulvirenti L, Koob GR. Dopamine receptor agonists, partial agonists and psychostimulant addiction. *Trends Pharmacol Sci* 1994;15:374–379.
19. Self DW, Barnhart WJ, Lehman DA, et al. (1996). Opposite modulation of cocaine-seeking behavior by D1-like and D2-like dopamine receptor agonists. *Science* 1996;271:1586–1589.

20. Hyman SE, Malenka RC, Nestler EJ. Neural mechanisms of addiction: the role of reward-related learning and memory. *Annu Rev Neurosci* 2006;29:565–598.
21. Carlezon WA Jr, Nestler EJ. Elevated levels of GluR1 in the midbrain: a trigger for sensitization to drugs of abuse? *Trends Neurosci* 2002;25: 610–615.
22. Kalivas PW. Glutamate systems in cocaine addiction. *Curr Opin Pharmacol* 2004;4:23–29.
23. Kauer JA, Malenka RC. Synaptic plasticity and addiction. *Nat Rev Neurosci* 2007;8:844–858.
24. Sutton MA, Schmidt EF, Choi KH, et al. Extinction-induced upregulation in AMPA receptors reduces cocaine-seeking behaviour. *Nature* 2003;421:70–75.
25. Brodie JD, Figueroa E, Laska EM, et al. Safety and efficacy of gamma-vinyl GABA (GVG) for the treatment of methamphetamine and/or cocaine addiction. *Synapse* 2005;55:122–125.
26. Bohn LM, Gainetdinov RR, Lin ET, et al. Mu-opioid receptor desensitization by beta-arrestin-2 determines morphine tolerance but not dependence. *Nature* 2000;408:720–723.
27. Rahman Z, Schwarz J, Zachariou V, et al. RGS9 modulated dopamine signaling in striatum. *Neuron* 2003;38:941–952.
28. Zachariou V, Georgescu D, Sanchez N, et al. Essential role for RGS9 in opiate action. *Proc Natl Acad Sci U S A* 2003;100:13656–13661.
29. Li S, Lee ML, Bruchas MR, et al. Calmodulin-stimulated adenylyl cyclase gene deletion affects morphine responses. *Mol Pharmacol* 2006;70: 1742–1749.
30. McClung CA, Ulery PG, Perrotti LI, et al. ΔFosB: a molecular switch for long-term adaptation in the brain. *Mol Brain Res* 2004;132: 146–154.
31. Renthal W, Maze I, Krishnan V, et al. Histone deacetylase 5 epigenetically controls behavioral adaptations to chronic emotional stimuli. *Neuron* 2007;56:517–529.

CHAPTER 5

Sarah W. Yip, BA, MSc
Marc N. Potenza, MD, PhD

Understanding "Behavioral Addictions": Insights from Research

The term *addiction* is derived from the Latin word *addicere*, meaning "bound to" or "enslaved by" (1). In its original formulation, the word was not linked to substance use behaviors. As of several hundred years ago, the word became associated first with excessive alcohol use and then with excessive drug use (2). By the time of the 1980s, the word was almost exclusively linked to excessive patterns of substance use, with experts involved in generating diagnostic criteria for drug dependence showing good agreement that the term applied to the condition of compulsive drug-taking (3). However, by the early part of the 2000s, a growing movement to consider nondrug behaviors-such as gambling, sex, and eating (although by strict definition this last category does involve a substance: food)-as addictive in nature was emerging (4). Aided by data from neurobiologic studies, this view is gaining momentum, leading to the consideration of changes in the Fifth edition of the *Diagnostic and Statistical Manual of Mental Disorders* (*DSM-V*) (5–8).

Addictions have been proposed to have several defining components: (i) continued engagement in a behavior despite adverse consequences; (ii) diminished self-control over engagement in the behavior; (iii) compulsive engagement in the behavior; and (iv) an appetitive urge or craving state before the engagement in the behavior (1,9). If these elements are considered the core features of addictions, then excessive patterns of gambling and other non–substance-related motivated behaviors might be considered addictions. Consistently, the term "behavioral addictions" has been used recently to describe these disorders. Particularly relevant to addictions are aspects of motivation, reward processing, and decision-making (10–12), and these features represent potential endophenotypes, or underlying constructs that may be more closely linked to biologic processes than are diagnoses, per se, that could be pursue in biologic investigations across a spectrum of substance- and non–substance-related addictive disorders.

Many disorders termed "behavioral addictions" are categorized as impulse control disorders (ICDs). The goals of this chapter will be to review similarities between ICDs and substance use disorders and to discuss the implications for treatment and theory. First, the category of ICDs in the *DSM-IV-TR* will be reviewed. Evidence from neurobiologic research, clinical reports, and pharmacotherapy studies regarding ICDs and their relationships with substance use disorders (SUDs) will be reviewed. In reviewing the individual ICDs, consideration will initially be given to disorders for which there have been arguably the most data supporting similarities with SUDs (e.g., in the areas of gambling and eating), with later portions focusing on ICDs for which there are arguably less data to support a categorization as a "behavioral addiction" (e.g., pathologic skin picking).

ICDs: "BEHAVIORAL ADDICTIONS"?

Many disorders that might be considered behavioral addictions are currently categorized in the *DSM* as "Impulse Control Disorders not Elsewhere Classified" (McElroy et al.,

ASAM 3rd edition 13). This title indicates that other disorders characterized by impaired impulse control, such as substance use disorders, attention deficit hyperactivity disorder (ADHD), bipolar disorder, cluster B personality disorders, among others, are categorized elsewhere in the manual. The ICDs within the "not elsewhere categorized" section include intermittent explosive disorder, kleptomania, pathologic gambling (PG), pyromania, trichotillomania, and impulse control disorder not otherwise specified. Additional ICDs currently under consideration for *DSM V* include ones related to excessive Internet or computer use, buying or shopping, sex, or skin-picking or nail-biting (14). In addition, research criteria for binge-eating disorder are currently in the manual (13), and a case for inclusion of obesity has been forwarded (5). Among issues being discussed within research workgroups are whether the ICDs might be best categorized separately, with substance use disorders as addictions, or with obsessive–compulsive disorder (OCD) as obsessive–compulsive spectrum disorders (5–8,14). Although the conceptualizations of ICDs as addictions or obsessive–compulsive spectrum disorders are not mutually exclusive and data exist to support each formulation, these frameworks have important clinical implications with respect to prevention and treatment strategies (15–17). In the following sections, we will review the ICDs, their main clinical features, and what is known regarding their biologies. A particular emphasis will be placed on PG because it is arguably the best studied of the ICDs to date. However, for a more detailed description of the clinical features of PG and its treatment we direct you to Chapter 39, "Pathologic Gambling: Clinical Characteristics and Treatment."

PG

PG has been considered a chronic, lifelong condition, although more recent data are challenging this notion (1,16,18). PG and SUDs share clinical characteristics and diagnostic criteria. Individuals with PG often experience withdrawal, craving, tolerance, and failed attempts to reduce or abate gambling behaviors—all common features of SUDs. The *DSM-IV*'s diagnostic criteria for PG reflect these similarities. A diagnosis of PG requires that the patient display five or more of the following: preoccupation with gambling; gambling with greater amounts of money to receive the same level of desired experience (tolerance); repeated, unsuccessful attempts to reduce or quit gambling; is restless/irritable when trying to stop gambling (withdrawal); gambles to escape from a dysphoric state; gambles to regain gambling-related losses ("chases" losses); lies in significant relationships about gambling; engages in illegal activity in order to fund gambling; has risked or lost a job or significant other because of gambling; and relies on others to fund gambling. Additionally an exclusionary criterion exists to specify that the gambling is not better accounted for by manic episodes.

A Nonsubstance Addiction? SUDs and PG share phenomenologic features. As with SUDs, PG often begins in adolescence and young adulthood, and prevalence estimates of PG tend to decrease across the lifespan (19). A common feature of SUDs and PG is "telescoping"—the phenomenon whereby the time between initiation and problematic engagement in the addictive behavior is shorter in females than in males (19). These commonalities suggest that there may be shared developmental vulnerabilities for both disorders. In particular, the high prevalence estimates in adolescents suggest common vulnerability factors (e.g., impaired impulse control) for both SUDs and PG. There additionally exist high comorbidity rates for PG and SUDs, with co-occurrence estimates as high as 39% for comorbid substance abuse in clinical populations (20) and elevated odds observed in community samples as well (21,22).

Neurocognition Neurocognitive measures provide insight into neurobiologic functioning. For example, neurocognitive research suggests a dysregulation of the ventromedial prefrontal cortex (vmPFC) and orbitofrontal cortex (OFC) in individuals with PG (23,24). Individuals with PG display impaired performance on the Iowa Gambling Task (IGT), a task involving risk/reward decision making (24,25). Other populations with impaired performance on the IGT include individuals with SUDs, schizophrenia, or vmPFC lesions. A recent cross-sectional study found that individuals meeting *DSM-IV-TR* criteria for PG and individuals with a history of alcohol dependence had impaired performance on neurocognitive tasks involving inhibition, time estimation, cognitive estimation, and planning tasks in comparison to normal controls and to individuals with Tourette's syndrome, who only had an impaired performance on inhibition tasks (24). These data highlight some of the clinical similarities between PG and SUDs and suggest similarities in underlying neurobiologic deficits. As such, neurocognitive research may be a useful tool in the identification of brain regions of interest warranting further investigation via more direct imaging-based modalities.

Delay Discounting Individuals with PG often make disadvantageous decisions, selecting small immediate rewards over larger delayed rewards. This rapid temporal discounting of rewards has been termed *delay discounting*, because rewards are more steeply discounted as a function of delay duration (26). This might reflect clinical situations in which delaying gratification is difficult for patients ("I'll go gambling now one last time").

Delay discounting has been studied in numerous different populations, including individuals with SUDs or PG. Illicit substance (i.e., cocaine and heroin) users perform worse on delay discounting measures (i.e., discount rewards more rapidly) than do non–substance-using individuals (26). A dose-dependent relationship has been found between level of alcohol use and patterns of delay discounting (26). Individuals with substance abuse discount rewards more rapidly than do healthy controls, and individuals with comorbid substance abuse and PG discount rewards more rapidly than do non-PG individuals with substance abuse problems (26,27). It is unclear whether comorbid substance abuse and PG promote delay discounting, or whether delay discounting is a vulnerability factor for comorbidity.

A similar additive effect has also been reported among heroin users in relation to needle-sharing: users who engaged in needle-sharing scored more highly than non–needle-sharing heroin users on delay discounting measures (26). Together, these data suggest that multiple risk factors may contribute to rates of delay discounting.

Although some data exist to suggest that abstinent substance users perform better (display less delay discounting) than do current substance users on delay discounting measures, other data suggest no significant differences (26). To our knowledge, delay discounting has not yet been studied in abstinent PG individuals. Further research into the effect of abstinence on delay discounting is needed.

Delay discounting involves aspects of reward evaluation, and multiple brain regions contribute to reward processing in humans. Amongst the most widely implicated brain regions in reward processing is the nucleus accumbens (NAcc), situated in the ventral striatum. A functional magnetic resonance imaging (fMRI) study of brain activation among healthy controls during a monetary incentive delay task found ventral striatal activation during anticipation of reward, whereas an increase in vmPFC activation was associated with the processing of actual reward outcomes (28). Recent preclinical research suggests that diminished serotonin (5-HT) activity in the forebrain may hypersensitize animals to delays, influencing patterns of delay discounting (29). Further research is needed to determine the relationship between 5-HT regulation, prefrontal cortical activation, and delay discounting behavior in humans (29).

The Neurobiology of PG The neurobiology of PG is incompletely understood, although several studies suggest that SUDs and PG may have similar pathophysiologies. Although PG was initially included in the *DSM* in 1980, relatively few investigations into the neurobiology have been performed (30).

Neurocircuitry Corticostriatal and forebrain neuromodualtory systems have been implicated in processing delayed and probabilistic rewards (29). Some research suggests that there is a dysregulation of the mesocorticolimbic dopamine (DA) system in PG. The mesocorticolimbic DA system, often referred to as the *reward pathway*, has long been implicated in SUDs (31). Given the phenomenologic (e.g., craving, tolerance) and neurocognitive (e.g., delay discounting) similarities between PG and alcohol and substance-use disorders, it is possible that these disorders may share similar neurobiologic abnormalities, and current investigations are examining this hypothesis.

There have been several fMRI studies of PG that suggest that specific brain regions contribute to the pathophysiology of PG. Potenza et al. (32) conducted echoplanar fMRI scans of 14 men with PG and 13 male controls during the presentation of videos depicting gambling and happy and sad scenarios. In response to gambling videos during the period before the subjective onset of emotional or motivational response, PG subjects displayed less activation of frontal cortex, basal ganglia, and thalamus activation than did controls. This finding is different from those observed in similar studies involving subjects with OCD in which relatively increased activation of these regions was observed in the patient group. When viewing the portion of the videotapes during which the most robust gambling stimuli (e.g., video clips of a gambling public service announcement involving slot reels or an advertisement for a casino in which table gambling is shown) were presented, individuals with PG displayed relatively less activation of the vmPFC. Diminished activation of the vmPFC in PG as compared with control subjects has also been observed in other studies. For example, during the performance of the Stroop color-word interference task (33) and during simulated gambling (31), PG as compared with control subjects displayed relatively less activation of the vmPFC. Similarly, individuals with cocaine dependence (either with or without PG) as compared with control subjects showed relatively diminished activation of the vmPFC during performance of the Iowa Gambling Task (34). Together, these data indicate an important role for the vmPFC in PG.

Reuter et al. (31) conducted an fMRI study of 12 pathological gamblers and 12 matched controls during a guessing task simulating gambling. They observed significantly less ventral striatal and vmPFC activation in the PG participants as compared with control subjects. Both right ventral striatal activation and vmpfc activation were inversely correlated with severity of gambling symptomatology in PG subjects, indicating that the less the activation of these brain regions, the greater the gambling pathology (31). Because DA is an important neurotransmitter for both vmPFC and ventral striatal functioning, Reuter et al. (31) proposed that these findings suggested a dysregulation of DA in PG. However, because DA levels were not measured in this study, further investigation into the relationship between DA and PG in relation to the reward pathways is needed to test this hypothesis.

Prepulse inhibition dysregularities have been reported in numerous different psychiatric populations, such as individuals with schizophrenia and individuals with OCD. Prepulse inhibition has been operationally defined as a measurement of DA activity in the PFC (35). Prepulse inhibition is a quantitative event-related potential measurement of the reduction of response amplitude to a given stimulus (S2) when stimulus presentation is immediately preceded by a brief tone or prepulse (S1) (35). It has been operationally defined as a measure of sensory motor gating, which is associated with the inhibition of neural processing of S2 to preserve processing of S1 (35). The PFC is associated with working memory, and dysregulated PFC function has been associated with an inability to use secondary inducers—regulated by working memory—in decision making on tasks such as the IGT (25). As such, sensory motor gating may be considered a measurement of PFC function, with the PFC representing an important region for decision making. Medial PFC lesions have been found to reduce the effects of DA agonists on PPI, implicating the mesocorticolimbic DA system in sensory motor gating (35).

Stonjanov et al. (35) recently investigated the role of endogenous DA in relation to sensory motor gating in a sample of individuals with PG. An increased startle response was observed in individuals with PG in comparison to controls, which is consistent with the notion of dysregulated DA neurotransmission in the PFC.

Neurochemistry

Serotonin (5-HT) Serotonin neurons project from the raphe nucleus of the brain stem to multiple brain regions including the hippocampus, amygdala, and prefrontal cortex. It has been hypothesized that dysregulated 5-HT functioning may mediate behavioral inhibition and impulsivity in PG (36,37). Data from studies of cerebrospinal fluid (CSF), pharmacologic challenge studies, and preclinical investigations together suggest a role for 5-HT in PG.

Low CSF levels of the 5-HT metabolite 5-hydroxyindoleacetic acid (5-HIAA) have been reported in individuals with PG (38). Low CSF levels of 5-HIAA in humans have been associated with violence, suicidality, and impulsive aggression (29), and observed in other psychiatric disorders including other impulse control disorders, and alcohol abuse/dependence. Preclinical research has also identified a correlation between risk-taking behaviors and lowered CSF levels of 5-HIAA in monkeys (29). Low levels of platelet monoamine oxidase (MAO) activity, considered a peripheral marker of 5-HT activity, have been reported in individuals with PG (36). Consistent with findings of 5-HIAA CSF levels, lowered levels of platelet MAO have additionally been reported in both suicidal and risk-taking individuals (36).

5-HT receptor sensitivity has been investigated via the administration of the 5-HT$_1$/5-HT$_2$ receptor partial agonist meta-chlorophenylpiperazine. Individuals with PG report a euphoric response to the meta-chlorophenylpiperazine, whereas control subjects report an unpleasant response (36). Phenomenologic accounts report a "high" subsequent to meta-chlorophenylpiperazine administration and an accompanying enhanced prolactin response among cocaine- and alcohol-dependent individuals (39). Cocaine-dependent individuals reported an abatement or reduction of cocaine cravings in relation to enhanced prolactin response, whereas alcohol-dependent individuals reported an increase in craving (39). A recent double-blind placebo-controlled investigation of prolactin response subsequent to meta-chlorophenylpiperazine administration found a significantly greater response among individuals with PG, in comparison to controls (39). This differential response was associated with severity of PG symptomatology, with higher scores on the Yale-Brown Obsessive-Compulsive Scale Modified for Pathological Gambling, a PG severity rating scale, significantly correlated with increased prolactin responses.

Other pharmacologic studies support the hypothesis that there is a dysregulation of the 5-HT system in PG. Serotonin reuptake inhibitors (SRIs), such as fluvoxamine and paroxetine, have been found to improve social functioning and reduce gambling behaviors and thoughts about gambling in PG. For example, a randomized double-blind study of fluvoxamine treatment for PG reported significant improvement on the PG Clinical Global Impression in response to fluvoxamine in comparison to placebo (40). However, another study did not observe a significant difference between active paroxetine and placebo with respect to measures of PG severity (41). As such, the precise role for SRIs in the treatment of PG remains an active area of investigation (42,43).

DA DA has been implicated in rewarding and reinforcing processes in drug addiction. Psychopharmacologic data suggest that the DA system may influence impulsive behavior, although the precise manner is not completely understood. Stimulants such as amphetamine increase DA release and prevent DA uptake within the synaptic cleft, and lead to improved impulse control in individuals with ADHD (29). However, amphetamine administration in PG has been associated with the priming of gambling motivations (44). Whereas dopamine agonists have been associated with PG and other impulse control disorders in the treatment of Parkinson disease (45), the dopamine D$_2$-like receptor antagonist haloperidol has been reported to enhance the rewarding and priming effects of gambling in PG (46). Investigations of CSF DA levels in PG have also yielded equivocal findings. Decreased CSF levels of DA and increased levels of the DA metabolites homovanillic acid and 3,4-dihydroxphenylacetic acid have been reported in PG (47). However, these findings were no longer present when correcting for CSF flow rate (38). A recent investigation reported increased levels of CSF homovanillic acid among individuals with PG (48). The authors additionally reported enhanced levels of 5-HIAA, a finding different from previous investigations of CSF 5-HT metabolite concentration levels (38). These data highlight the need for studies using larger carefully controlled samples, while accounting for mediating factors such as comorbid pathologies and CSF flow rate.

Norepinephrine and Arousal in PG Dysregulation of norepinephrine (NE)—a neurotransmitter implicated in arousal, attention, and sensation-seeking behavior—has been reported in individuals with PG. Individuals with PG have elevated urinary concentrations of NE, as well as elevated CSF levels of a metabolite of NE (metabolite 4-hydroxy-3-methoxyphenyl glycol) (49). Research has also shown abnormal NE regulation of the hypothalamic-pituitary-adrenal axis in PG. Meyer et al. (50) measured the neuroendocrine responses to real-life casino gambling in problem gamblers and found that problem gamblers had higher heart rates and elevated NE and DA levels in comparison to controls (50). Together, these data suggest that there may be an elevation of NE activity in PG that may be potentiated by gambling behaviors.

Opioids Pharmacologic challenge studies suggest a dysregulation of the opioid system in PG. Naltrexone and nalmefene, opioid receptor antagonists, have been found to reduce gambling-related thoughts and behaviors in individuals with PG (51).

Kim et al. (51) conducted a double-blind study of naltrexone in a sample of 89 individuals with PG, and found that naltrexone administration at a mean dosage of 188 mg/day reduced subjective craving reports, in comparison to placebo administration (51). Consistent with previous research demonstrating naltrexone's dose-dependent hepatotoxicity, approximately 20% of participants displayed liver function test abnormalities subsequent to naltrexone treatment (51,52). A recent randomized double-blind study of nalmefene, an opioid antagonist that has not been associated with hepatotoxicity (52), found significant improvement in PG symptoms subsequent to low-dose (25 mg/day) treatment in comparison to controls (52). Together, these data suggest an important role for opioid antagonists in the treatment of PG as there is in alcohol and opiate use disorders.

Population Genetics Family and twin-based studies of addiction indicate that genetic factors are important in the development of drug and alcohol abuse. Family studies of PG suggest a significant parental influence on the development of offspring gambling behaviors (53). Data from gene x environment studies suggest that the cross-generation transmission of drug addiction is a product of both environmental and genetic risk factors. Data derived from the Vietnam Twin Era Registry found that between 35% to 54% of the probability of meeting criteria for a *DSM-III-R* diagnosis of PG were attributable to inherited factors (54). Data from the same sample reported that 34% of the probability of developing drug dependence was attributable to inherited factors, suggesting similar degrees of heritability for PG and SUDs (55). Another study using the same population found that PG and alcohol dependence shared genetic and environmental contributions (56). Another study using the Vietnam Twin Era Registry population found substantial comorbid antisocial personality disorder, conduct disorder, and adult antisocial behavior among individuals with PG and found that these comorbidities were related to shared genetic and environmental influences (57).

Genetic Polymorphisms in PG Molecular genetic research has identified specific genetic alleles associated with PG. Genetic polymorphisms related to genes encoding for the DA-related moieties (*DRD1*Ddel, *DRD2* Taq I A, *DRD4* [exon III]) (58,59) and 5-HT (*5HTTLPR*) (60) and MAOA enzymes (*MAO-A* ([intron I], *MAO-A* [promoter], *MAO-B* [intron II]) have been reported with respect to PG (61). Similarities with respect to allelic distributions have been reported in PG and drug and alcohol dependence (e.g., variations in *DRD2* and *MAOA* genes have been linked to PG and alcohol abuse and dependence, and *DRD4* variants have been linked to PG and alcohol, cocaine and heroin abuse and dependence) (62). These and other molecular genetic studies of PG should be considered preliminary in nature given relatively small samples, incomplete subject characterization, and frequent absence of stratification by race/ethnicity (61), particularly as some early results have not replicated in studies using alternate designs (e.g., discordant sibling pairs) (63).

Conclusion Although the precise neurobiology of PG is incompletely understood, data from neurocognitive, neurochemical, neuroimaging, and genetic research suggest similarities with other disorders involving impaired impulse control, such as substance addictions. There are important treatment implications inherent in these similarities. For example, the biologic similarities between SUDs and PG could help to guide treatment development.

BINGE EATING

Introduction Changes in eating patterns are frequently observed in substance use and abuse (e.g., weight loss is associated with amphetamine and heroin use and weight gain is reported as a reason for smoking cessation failure). Conversely exogenous cannabinoids, such as tetrahydrocannabinol that is found in marijuana, increase food intake. Although specific drugs of abuse have different influences on eating behaviors, data suggest both substance use and eating behaviors may be modulated by the same motivational neurocircuitry.

The *DSM-IV-TR* category of eating disorders includes anorexia nervosa, bulimia nervosa, and eating disorder not otherwise specified. Anorexia nervosa, defined as "a refusal to maintain a minimally normal body weight" (13), is estimated to affect approximately 0.9% of women and approximately 0.3% of men (64). Bulimia nervosa, characterized by cycles of binge eating followed by purging, is thought to be slightly more prevalent, affecting up to 1.5% of women and 0.5% of men (64). Included for research purposes in the *DSM-IV-TR*, binge eating disorder (BED)—distinct from bulimia nervosa as it does not include compensatory behaviors such as purging—is associated with obesity and other negative sequelae. The recent rise in the prevalence of obesity within the population has led to more research on obesity and related disorders such as BED. Given that BED has an important of element of episodic behavioral dyscontrol similar to the formal impulse control disorders, this section will focus primarily on the neurobiology of this disorder. (For a review of anorexia nervosa and bulimia nervosa, see previous work) (64). Preclinical data relevant to BED and obesity will also be described.

Epidemiology Although not an official diagnostic category, the *DSM-IV-TR* contains provisional criteria and future research recommendations for BED. Features are similar to those of SUDs and impulse control disorders: recurrent episodes, impaired control, and marked distress in relation to binge eating. The *DSM-IV-TR* also notes that individuals may make repeated unsuccessful attempts to stop binge eating, and that they may report that their binge eating has detrimental social and occupational effects—two important criteria for substance dependence.

Obesity, a common consequence of binge eating, is an increasingly common phenomenon. Defined as "abnormal or excessive fat accumulation that may impair health" (65), it is estimated that up to 20.9% of the United States population meets the criteria for obesity (66). Globally, estimates from 2005 suggest that 1.6 billion adults are overweight, and that at least 400 million are obese (65). Associated medical conditions include type II diabetes, stroke, osteoarthritis, heart disease, and cancer (65,67). Psychiatric comorbidities include depression, anxiety, personality disorders, and lifetime SUDs.

Conceptualization and Treatment Along with the recent rise in the prevalence of obesity, there has been a concurrent rise in the number and diversity of treatment interventions. Such interventions range from preventive interventions, such as the incorporation of nutrition classes into school curriculums, to pharmaceutical interventions, such as the administration of appetite-suppressing drugs, to surgical innervations, such as gastric bypass surgery. Because some treatment interventions for obesity are highly invasive (e.g., gastric bypass, jaw-wiring), it is important to examine and assess not only efficacy, but also tolerability and impact on quality of life. It is also important to understand the pathophysiology underlying the disorder, particularly if individual differences contribute to selection of effective interventions.

The Biology of Eating Behaviors The hypothalamus is an important site for the maintenance of energy homeostasis. Lesions to the ventromedial hypothalamus result in hyperphagia and obesity, whereas lesions to the lateral hypothalamus result in hypophagia and weight loss. This finding led researchers to conceptualize the lateral hypothalamus as a "feeding center" and the ventromedial nucleus as a "satiety center." In this dual center model of eating behavior, the hypothalamus plays a central role, and hypothalamic function contributes significantly to homeostatic regulation within a larger motivational network (68).

Leptin Leptin, an adipose-derived hormone, is a chemical modulator involved in the maintenance of energy homeostasis and feeding behaviors (69). Leptin is also implicated in other reward-seeking behaviors (69,70). Leptin acts as a peripheral metabolic cue within the central nervous system to modulate neuronal activity in brain areas involved in appetite control, including the hypothalamus. Administration of exogenous leptin increases energy expenditure and reduces hyperphagia and obesity in genetically leptin-deficient mice and humans (*ob*/*ob*) (71). However, leptin deficiency syndrome is extremely rare in humans (69). Many obese rodents and humans have high plasma leptin concentrations, and both endogenous and exogenous leptin have reduced influence on energy intake in these individuals—a phenomenon referred to as leptin resistance (69).

The effects of exogenous leptin administration have been investigated in two adolescents with the rare disorder congenital leptin deficiency (72). An fMRI study presented visual food and non-food stimuli during a fasting state and a fed state, both before leptin treatment and after leptin treatment. Results yielded significant behavioral and neural response changes between conditions. When participants rated their level of preference for specific foods presented, leptin administration was associated with decreased preference ratings during the fed condition. Whereas activation in the nucleus accumbens and caudate nucleus of the striatum was positively correlated with preference ratings in both the fed and fasting conditions before leptin treatment, subsequent to leptin treatment striatal activation was only positively associated with preference ratings in the fasting condition. These data demonstrate extrahypothalamic action of exogenous leptin and suggest that leptin may help to encode palatability (72).

Leptin and DA-regulated Reward Processing Recent research suggests that mesolimbic reward pathways play an important role in eating behaviors. A recent fMRI study demonstrated an increase in activation of brain regions implicated in substance use and dependence—such as the OFC, insula, striatum, and midbrain—subsequent to the consumption of palatable food (73). Differential striatal activation in response to food has also been reported in obese individuals in comparison to healthy control subjects. An fMRI study of 13 obese females and 13 female controls visually exposed to food-related stimuli reported significantly increased activation of the dorsal striatum in response to images of high-calorie foods (74). In response to high-calorie food stimuli, body mass index (BMI) was also reported to be predictive of dorsal striatum, anterior insula, claustrum, posterior cingulate, and postcentral and lateral OFC activation (74). Based on previous reports of lowered DA levels in anorexia nervosa (75), one recent investigation compared the striatal responses of women who had recovered from anorexia to healthy controls during the performance of a monetary reward task, and found significant between-group differences in response to rewards and losses. Whereas unaffected control subjects displayed differential ventral striatal activation for rewards versus losses, recovered individuals showed no activation differences for wins and losses, suggesting a reduced experience of reward (76). A reduced availability of dopamine D2 receptors in the striatum has been reported in obese individuals, with receptor availability negatively correlated with BMI (77). Similar reductions in dopamine D2 receptor availability have been reported in individuals with SUDs. Preclinical research has demonstrated that genetically dopamine deficient mice display a failure to initiate feeding, though not an inability to feed (78). Together, these data suggest dysregulated striatal function in eating disorders that at least in part reflects dysregulated dopamine function.

Whereas leptin-modulated hypothalamic activity has been well-documented, research suggests that leptin acts directly on other brain regions, including the substantia nigra pars compacta and ventral tegmental area (VTA) of the midbrain. Dopamine neurons in the VTA and substantia nigra pars compacta project to the striatum and are implicated in reward, motivation, and addiction. Preclinical data from Figlewicz et al. (79) has demonstrated that dopamine neurons within the VTA express mRNA encoding for both leptin and insulin receptors. Exogenous leptin administration to the VTA results in a decrease in food consumption, and intravenous exogenous leptin administration reduces the firing of VTA dopamine neurons (80). The expression of mRNA encoding for the long form of the leptin receptor (ObRb) has additionally been reported in regions including the hippocampus, brain stem, cortex, thalamus, cerebellum, and substantia nigra (81). Leptin has additionally been reported to enhance synaptic plasticity in brain regions such as the hippocampus (82).

Preclinical research using self-administration of electrical brain stimulation of reward technology suggests that leptin influences drug-taking behaviors. An investigation by Fulton et al. (83) found increased brain-stimulation of reward in response to fasting conditions, which was attenuated by direct exogenous leptin administration. A different study found that leptin-deficient *ob/ob* mice have a lessened locomotor response to amphetamine administration, which is corrected by leptin administration (83). These data suggest that, in addition to its metabolic function, leptin may help to modulate mesolimbic reward circuits that may relate to both palatability and substance use.

Orexins Partially modulated by adipose-derived hormones such as leptin and ghrelin, the hypothalamic neuropeptides orexin A and orexin B—also referred to as hypocretin 1 and hypocretin 2—are important modulators of eating behavior and help to maintain energy homeostasis. The hypothalamus is the primary site of hypocretin-containing neurons, though these neurons project to other brain regions (84,85). Orexin administration has been demonstrated to increase feeding behaviors in preclinical populations (85). Orexin is also a crucial regulator of sleep and wakefulness, and orexin deficiency is implicated in narcolepsy (84).

Preclinical research has demonstrated that administration of orexin-A reinstates cocaine-seeking behaviors in a dose-dependent manner (86). Administration of orexin-A was also associated with increases in brain stimulation of reward, suggesting a negative regulation of reward circuits (86), consistent with orexin's role in opiate dependence and withdrawal (87). Similar research has demonstrated that the administration of an orexin receptor agonist abolishes reinstatement of cue-induced alcohol-seeking behaviors in rodents, further implicating orexin in substance-seeking behaviors (88).

Preclinical research conducted by Harris et al. (89) revealed a significant increase in hypothalamic orexin-containing neurons subsequent to preference conditioning for food, cocaine, or morphine, suggesting important similarities between the development of food and drug preferences. Whereas the number of orexin-containing neurons was positively correlated with increases in preference, no such correlations were found for any other type of hypothalamic neurons. This study additionally reported reinstatement of morphine preference subsequent to direct orexin administration to the VTA, one of the brain regions receiving projections from hypothalamic orexin neurons (89).

Orexin may directly influence dopamine neurons in the VTA. Direct administration of orexin A or B produced a locomotor-enhancing effect in mice that was prevented by prior administration of a dopamine receptor antagonist (90). The same study additionally demonstrated a lack of hyperlocomotion and a significantly lessened increase in dopamine in response to morphine (90). Increases in PFC dopamine subsequent to orexin A administration to the VTA have also been reported (91). Together, these data suggest that orexin may directly influence mesolimbic dopamine pathways implicated in reward and drug addiction.

Ghrelin Ghrelin is a gastrointestinal hormone that helps to maintain energy homeostasis. Unlike leptin and orexin, which are anorexigenic, ghrelin is orexigenic and increases food intake and body weight (92). Ghrelin may contribute importantly to the initiation of eating. One study measured ghrelin levels in the plasma of healthy controls during a 24-hour period and found significant increases in ghrelin levels before meal initiation followed by significant decreases after consumption (93). Reduced levels of circulating ghrelin have been reported in obese individuals, with an inverse correlation between BMI and ghrelin levels observed (94).

Although ghrelin is primarily synthesized in the stomach, recent research suggests that it may also mediate feeding behaviors via direct action on certain brain regions. Preclinical research has identified a ghrelin receptor, growth hormone secretagogue 1 receptor, in the hypothalamus and VTA. Ghrelin has been linked to increased synapse formation and dopamine turnover in the NAcc (95). Administration of exogenous ghrelin in the VTA prompted feeding behavior, and growth hormone secretagogue 1 receptor antagonist administration reduced feeding subsequent to food deprivation (95). These findings suggest that ghrelin may help to modulate the perceived reward of food. Further investigation is needed to determine the extent to which ghrelin is involved in other reward-seeking behaviors.

The NAcc: Opioid and Endocannabinoid Encoding of Palatability Research suggests that opioid receptors in the NAcc region of the ventral striatum may be particularly important for the encoding of food palatability. As with other regions of the striatum, dopamine is an important modulator of NAcc functioning. Preclinical research suggests that dopamine release in the NAcc modulates excitatory NAcc neuronal activity in response to previously learned reward-associated cues, thereby increasing the likelihood of cue responsiveness (e.g., performance of behaviors learned via operant conditioning) (96). Stimulation of NAcc opioid receptors has been found to increase food intake (97). Administration of opioid receptor antagonists, such as naloxone or naltrexone, extinguishes previously established preferences for sweetened versus unsweetened water in rats, whereas morphine has been demonstrated to enhance palatability and preference for sweet food (97,98). Importantly, such preclinical data demonstrates opioid involvement in the palatability—or reward value—encoding of food, that does not appear to directly effect caloric intake (97,98). This suggests that the opioid system is implicated in general reward processing, as opposed to specific appetitive control. These data nonetheless suggest shared neurobiological mechanisms in eating and substance use behaviors.

Preclinical research conducted by Taha and Fields (99) has identified two distinct populations of NAcc neurons responsive to food consumption: a group of neurons displaying primarily excitatory responses to increased palatability (i.e., increased sucrose), and a separate group of neurons displaying primarily inhibitory responses before initiation of feeding behaviors that does not appear to be related to palatability (99). This finding is consistent with other preclinical research demonstrating increases in nonappetitive food intake subsequent to NAcc inhibition (100). One possible interpretation of these data is that, in addition to neurons encoding for reward, a group of NAcc neurons may also be implicated in general habit formation or basic motor control of feeding behaviors, independent of palatability, although this hypothesis requires further testing. These data further support the hypothesis that the NAcc is an important brain region for the encoding of palatability as well as the initiation of feeding responses and highlight similarities between eating and substance use behaviors.

Human and animal studies also implicate the endocannabinoid system (composed of cannabinoid receptors, endocannabinoids, and associated enzymes) in eating behaviors (101,102). The endocannabinoid system is comprised of two endogenous ligands, anandamide (arachidonylethanolamide) and 2-arachidonoylglycerol, and two cannabinoid receptors, CB1 and CB2 (103). Cannabinoid receptors in the NAcc have been implicated in appetitive behavior.

Preclinical research suggests that CB1 receptors partially regulated by leptin (104) are involved in the presynaptic modulation of release of the neurotransmitters gamma-aminobutyric acid (GABA), glutamate, dopamine, noradrenaline, and serotonin (101,105), and has identified cannabinoid receptors (CB1/2) in the limbic forebrain, striatum, and NAcc (106). Colocalization of opioid and CB1 receptors in the striatum has also been reported (106). Preclinical investigations have additionally reported increases in feeding behaviors subsequent to administration of Δ^9-tetrahydrocannabinol and anandamide (an endogenous cannabinoid neurotransmitter) (106). Cannabinoids have long been associated with rewarding psychotropic effects and are additionally associated with increases in food intake. In addition to cannabinoid-induced increases in feeding behaviors, studies have implicated endogenous cannabinoids in the experience and encoding of food-associated reward. For example, direct anandamide administration to the NAcc shell has been found to significantly enhance "hedonic" reward and increase feeding behaviors in rats (106). Elevated anandamide blood levels have been reported in individuals with anorexia nervosa and individuals with BED, whereas no such elevation has been reported in individuals with bulimia nervosa (103). Despite evidence implicating the opioid system in eating behaviors, pharmaceutical challenge studies of opioid receptor antagonists such as naltrexone have yielded equivocal results in human populations and further research is needed to establish appropriate pharmacotherapies for the treatment of BED.

PFC Research from neuroimaging, neurocognitive, and lesion studies implicates prefrontal cortical modulation of eating behaviors. Frontotemporal dementia, a degenerative disorder involving atrophy of frontal, insular, and temporal cortical regions, is characterized by a variety of behavioral changes including changes in eating and sexual behaviors (107) as well as deficits in insight, empathy, and social interaction (107,108). Clinically reported changes in eating behaviors associated with frontotemporal dementia include increases in weight, food cravings/obsessions, and gluttony (108). Similarly, a recent study found that individuals with frontotemporal dementia meeting criteria for "gluttonous" overeating during "all-you-can-eat" 1-hour meal sessions had significantly increased atrophy of the OFC, right ventral insula, and striatum (109).

Evidence derived from positron emission tomography research additionally suggests a relationship between frontal lobe activity and eating behaviors. In a comparison of women classified as successful versus nonsuccessful dieters, successful dieters had significantly greater activation in dorsal prefrontal cortex, dorsal striatum, and anterior cerebellar lobe brain regions after meal consumption (110). Conversely, nonsuccessful dieters had significantly greater OFC activation after meal consumption (110). These data suggest differential modulation of eating behaviors by prefrontal regions. Further investigation is required to fully understand interactions between PFC regions in relation to eating behaviors.

Consistent with the finding that greater dietary restraint is negatively correlated with OFC activation and positively correlated with dorsal prefrontal cortex activation, one randomized double-blind parallel group study using repetitive transcranial magnetic stimulation found reduced self-reported craving sensations in response to exposure to craving-inducing foods subsequent to left DLPFC stimulation (111). DLPFC stimulation has also been reported to inhibit nicotine cravings and cigarette consumption in cigarette smokers, suggesting potentially similar neurobiological mechanisms for food and drug craving (111).

Neurocognitive research additionally implicates frontal lobe involvement in binge eating. Disadvantageous decision making—characterized by a disregard for future negative consequences in favor of immediate short-term gains—is associated with disorders characterized by impaired impulse control (e.g., SUDs, PG). Similar deficits have been reported in BED and obesity. In a sample of 41 healthy adult women, a tendency to overeat in response to stress and higher BMI both significantly predicted poorer IGT performance (112). Whereas IGT performance among nonobese/overweight women (BMI <25) improved over time, women classified as overweight or obese (BMI ≥ 25) showed no improvement in IGT performance (112).

Similar decision-making deficits have been reported in both anorexia nervosa and bulimia nervosa. Individuals with anorexia nervosa have been reported to perform significantly worse on the IGT in comparison to healthy controls and recovered anorexia nervosa patients (113). The same study additionally reported a significant reduction in skin conductance responses among individuals with anorexia nervosa in comparison to healthy controls and recovered anorexia nervosa individuals, consistent the hypothesis that somatic responses influence complex decision-making processes (113).

Similar deficits have been reported in bulimia nervosa, as measured by the Game of Dice Task (114). Similar to the IGT, the Game of Dice Task assesses decision making; however, unlike the IGT, it provides explicit information of reward-loss contingencies (115). In a comparison of 15 females with bulimia nervosa versus 15 matched control subjects, bulimia nervosa individuals performed significantly worse on the Game of Dice Task (114).

Serotonin (5-HT) Increases in both exogenous and endogenous serotonin (5-HT) are associated with a reduction of food intake and weight gain and an increase in energy expenditure (116). In relation to eating behaviors, research has focused on 5-HT and the hypothalamus. Serotonin neurons located in the dorsal raphe nucleus receive direct projections from hypothalamic orexin neurons and express orexin A and B receptors (117). Hypothalamic serotonin in part mediates the experience of satiety. Medial hypothalamic 5-HT is implicated in the temporal management of eating behavior, in particular with meal termination, as opposed to initiation. Preclinical research has demonstrated that d-fenfluramine—also known as Fen-Phen when combined with phentermine—an exogenous agent that increases 5-HT release while also blocking reuptake, may exert its anorexigenic effects via $5HT_{2C}$ receptor activation of pro-opiomelanocortin neurons in lateral hypothalamic regions (118). Further research is needed to establish the precise role of the central melanocortin system in the regulation of food intake; however, these data may help to develop alternative pharmacotherapies for BED and other eating disorders (118). 5-HT is also thought to be implicated in food preference. For example, preclinical studies have demonstrated that the injection of either exogenous 5-HT or drugs that increase 5-HT availability (such as fluoxetine) into the medial hypothalamus selectively inhibits carbohydrate intake, but has no significant effect on fat or protein intake. Conversely, elevated levels of tryptophan, a 5-HT amino acid precursor, and hypothalamic 5-HT, are associated with high-carbohydrate intake (116).

Sibutramine, a drug that blocks serotonin reuptake, is approved by the U.S. Food and Drug Administration for the treatment of obesity. In a 2-year follow-up of fluoxetine-treated individuals with BED, no significant improvements in BED symptoms were reported, despite significant improvements in depressive symptoms (119). In a recent randomized double-blind 12-week study of escitalopram versus placebo for the treatment of individuals with comorbid BED and obesity, individuals receiving high-dose escitalopram treatment had significantly greater reductions in weight, BMI, and total global illness severity (119). However, no significant between-group differences were found for the variables reduction of binge episodes, reduction of days with a binge episode, and reduction of obsessive–compulsive features of BED (119).

Conclusion Binge eating and comorbid obesity are increasingly common phenomena with wide-ranging public health implications. Recent neurobiologic findings, such as the involvement of the adipose-derived hormone leptin in the dopaminergic reward system, increasingly suggest that binge eating is a brain-based disorder that may share many of the same neurobiological features of SUD. Such findings have important treatment implications, and further investigation is required in order to provide the best possible treatment interventions.

COMPULSIVE SEXUAL BEHAVIOR

Compulsive sexual behavior (CSB) is an impulse control disorder characterized by excessive engagement in normative sexual behaviors. Not included in the current *DSM-IV*, CSB is often referred to as "sexual addiction".

Clinically relevant sexual behaviors may be divided into paraphilic and nonparaphilic behaviors. In paraphilic sexual behaviors, there is a disturbance in the object selection (e.g., an animal, unwilling person, inanimate object). In nonparaphilic sexual behaviors, the individual engages in socially normative sexual behaviors in an excessive, obsessive, or compulsive manner, without a disturbance of object choice. Paraphilic disorders are a distinct category of disorders, already included in the current *DSM-IV-TR*, and are outside the scope of this chapter.

Epidemiology There has been no systematic epidemiological study of compulsive sexual behavior, although estimates of 5% to 6% in the adult population have been reported (120,121). The majority of research on CSB has been conducted using predominantly male clinical populations. Co-occurring mood disorders (e.g., early-onset dysthymia), anxiety disorders, SUDs, ICDs, and ADHD have been reported in association with CSB (122,123).

Phenomenologic similarities between CSB and SUDs have been described. Individuals suffering from CSB often report feeling out of control. Estimates of comorbidity for SUDs and CSB range from 25% to 71% (122). Compulsive sexual behaviors are aimed at reward-seeking and anxiety-reduction. Individuals with compulsive sexual behaviors report feelings of regret and fear over losing loved ones or employment as a result of their behaviors (124).

Defining the Disorder Nonparaphilic impulsive or compulsive sexual disorders are not specifically listed in the *DSM-IV-TR*. CSB can be classified as either an impulse control disorder not otherwise specified (ICD-NOS) or a sexual disorder not otherwise specified. As with other impulse control disorders, CSB can be conceptualized along an impulsive compulsive spectrum (122). Coleman (125) has identified seven distinct CSB categories, all with their own unique constellation of symptoms: compulsive cruising and multiple partners, compulsive multiple love relationships, compulsive sexuality in a relationship, compulsive use of erotica, compulsive autoeroticism, compulsive use of the Internet, and compulsive fixation on an unattainable partner. When assessing sexual behaviors, Kinsey et al. (122) created the frequency measure of "total sexual outlet," defined as the number of orgasms per week. Kafka later redefined total sexual outlet as: # of orgasms / # of weeks (122). According to Kafka's criteria, a total sexual outlet score ≥7 is associated with both paraphilic and nonparaphilic (i.e., CSB) disorders. Other instruments, such as the Minnesota Impulsive Disorders Inventory, more closely resemble the diagnostic criteria for ICDs, such as PG: a preoccupation with sexual behaviors; repetitive sexual fantasies causing distress or associated with a loss of control; repetitive sexual urges causing distress or associated with a loss of control; repetitive engagement in sexual behaviors causing distress or associated with a loss of control (126). Similarly, Voon et al. (127) have proposed the following operational diagnostic criteria for hypersexuality (i.e., CSB): "1) maladaptive preoccupation with sexual thoughts; 2) inappropriately or excessively requesting sex from spouse or partner; 3) habitual promiscuity; 4) compulsive masturbation; 5) telephone sex lines or pornography; 6) paraphilias" (128).

Neurobiology of CSB Dopamine, serotonin, norepinephrine, and the opioid system contribute to human sexual behavior. However, no systematic studies of neurotransmitter systems involvement in CSB have been published to date. Lithium, tricyclic antidepressants, selective serotonin reuptake inhibitors (SSRIs), nefazodone, naltrexone, and atypical antipsychotics have all been used to treat CSB (129). However, the use of these medications has been typically open label and their efficacy in treating CSB has not been systematically examined. At present, most of the data on pharmacologic treatment for CSB is only from individual case reports, and further research is needed.

The neurotransmitter serotonin is implicated in sexual functioning and desire, and sexual dysfunctions, such as decreased libido, anorgasmia, and delayed ejaculation, are reported as adverse effects of SSRI treatment (120,130). There is mixed evidence to support the efficacy of SSRIs in treating CSB symptoms. In a randomized clinical trial, Wainberg et al. (131) tested the effect of citalopram versus placebo in a sample of 28 homosexual men with sexually compulsive behavior. As has been reported in relation to other ICDs, they observed a significant placebo effect; however, the patients taking citalopram reported a greater reduction of sexual desire, without a lessening in sexual satisfaction, than did controls (131). It is presently not clear whether the effectiveness of SSRI administration in reducing CSB symptoms can be attributed to an actual reduction of sexual thoughts or to the sexual side effects of the medication (120).

Pharmacologic tolerance to SSRI treatment has been reported in men with CSB, and comorbid ADHD is associated with CSB (132). Kafka and Hennen (132) examined the effect of psychostimulant augmentation during SSRI treatment in a sample of men with paraphilia or paraphilia-related (e.g., CSB) disorders. They found a significant reduction in paraphilias or paraphilia-related behaviors in response to SSRI treatment alone, and also reported a significant improvement subsequent to sustained-release methylphenidate. These preliminary data suggest an additive effect of methylphenidate administration in CSB populations that may help to counteract pharmacologic tolerance to SSRIs, and additionally implicate a dysregulation of the dopaminergic, serotonergic, and norepinephrine systems in CSB.

Nefazodone, a phenylpiperazine antidepressant that antagonizes 5-HT receptors and influences serotonin and norepinephrine reuptake, may be less frequently associated with sexual side effects than are SSRIs (120). A retrospective review of 14 individuals prescribed nefazodone for CSB found a significant reduction of sexual thoughts and an absence of substantial sexual side effects among individuals who received long-term nefazodone treatment (120). Because sexual side effects may deter patients from continuing SSRI treatment, nefazodone may be particularly beneficial in treating CSB. However, controlled trials are needed to examine their efficacy and tolerability.

Naltrexone, an opioid receptor antagonist, appears effective in treating both substance dependence and ICDs such as PG. Research suggests that the opioid system may mediate orgasm and arousal and that the endogenous opioid system is dysregulated in CSB (133). In a randomized, double-blind crossover design, Sathe et al. (133) administered either naltrexone (25 mg/day) or placebo to a sample of 20 sexually active men over a 3-day period. After 14 days, participants were administered either naltrexone or placebo (i.e., whichever they did not receive in the initial trial). As assessed via subject self-report, naltrexone administration was associated with increased sexual arousal, greater frequency of orgasms, and orgasm intensity in response to masturbatory behaviors.

Conversely, preliminary open-label studies of opioid receptor antagonists in CSB populations suggest possible efficacy. Beneficial response has typically been reported at high doses (134,135). Grant and Kim (136) administered naltrexone to a male patient with comorbid kleptomania and CSB who had previously not responded to SSRI or psychotherapy treatment. They reported a reduction in CSB symptoms during naltrexone treatment (150 mg/day), with reoccurring kleptomania and CSB symptoms after naltrexone discontinuation (136). Ryback (134) studied the efficacy of naltrexone treatment in a clinical population of male adolescent sex offenders. Patients were included in the study if they masturbated excessively, engaged in sexual fantasy for more than 30% of time awake, felt unable to control sexual arousal, or had sexual fantasies that interfered with treatment (134). Consistent with data obtained by Grant and Kim, this study suggests effective naltrexone-treatment of sexual symptoms only at high doses (e.g., 100 to 200 mg/day).

Together, these data suggest a complex relationship between endogenous opioids and CSB. In particular, the findings of increased sexual responsiveness subsequent to low-dose naltrexone administration in nonpsychiatric individuals, and decreased CSB-related behaviors in psychiatric individuals treated with high-dose naltrexone warrants further investigation. Other factors, including differences in patient populations and dosing durations also warrant consideration.

Topiramate, an anticonvulsant and mood-stabilizer, may help alleviate symptoms of CSB. Topiramate was reported to decrease anticipation before sexual behavior and to increase "sense of control," leading to cessation of sexual behaviors, in a patient who appeared nonresponsive to SSRI and combined SSRI-naltrexone therapy (129). The patient's CSB symptoms returned after topiramate discontinuation. The authors of this study propose that topiramate may help alleviate symptoms of CSB via the enhancement of inhibitory control (129).

Increased sexual desire and other impulse control behaviors have been observed in patients with Parkinson's disease or restless legs syndrome taking dopaminergic medications (137,128). Voon et al. (128) estimate that 2.4% of Parkinson's disease patients taking dopamine agonists meet the criteria for hypersexuality or pathologic sexual behavior. In a study of 70 restless legs syndrome patients without comorbid Parkinson's disease, 5% of respondents reported a high level of sexual desire and 4% reported that their desire had increased subsequent to taking dopaminergic medication (137). None of the patients with high levels of sexual desire had a personal or family history of CSB or sexual paraphilia. Further research is needed to examine the potential role of dopamine in the pathophysiology of CSB and other sexual behaviors in Parkinson's disease and restless legs syndrome.

Neuroanatomy of CSB To our knowledge, there have been no imaging studies of CSB performed. In human and preclinical populations, bilateral temporal lesions are associated with placidity, hyperorality, visual agnosia, and hypersexuality. Together, this constellation of symptoms has been termed Kluver-Bucy syndrome, and has also been observed in amygdalar lesioned patients (122). Extremely rare in humans, Kluver-Bucy syndrome's associated hypersexuality suggests an involvement of temporal lobe function in CSB and other paraphilia-related disorders. It is important to note that, in humans, individuals with this very rare disorder infrequently display hypersexual behaviors. In humans, Kluver-Bucy syndrome is most commonly associated with Alzheimer disease, herpes simplex encephalitis, ischemia/anoxia, and temporal lobectomies. Further research is needed to establish the relationship between temporal lobe and amygdalar function and CSB.

Conclusion CSB has been clinically acknowledged for years, but is not currently listed in the *DSM-IV*. As with other "behavioral addictions", CSB is negatively associated with distress and may interfere with personal and professional life.

PROBLEMATIC INTERNET USE

Introduction Not currently included in the DSM-IV, Internet or computer addiction is underresearched and very rarely addressed clinically. Internet or computer addictions have been defined as "non-chemical or behavioral addictions which involve human-machine interactions" (138). Internet use may have negative psychologic and social consequences (139). For example, face-to-face social activities may be substituted for Internet-based social interaction (139). As with compulsive shopping behavior, problematic Internet use involves excessive engagement in socially normative activities. As such, it may be hard to identify, and patients may be reticent to disclose excessive Internet behaviors, either from embarrassment or from a lack of awareness of the disorder.

Diagnostic Criteria There are no uniformly agreed on diagnostic criteria for problematic Internet use. Based on the *DSM-IV* definitions of SUDs, Young (140) proposed the following criteria for "Internet addiction:" withdrawal, tolerance, preoccupation with the Internet, longer than intended spent on the Internet, risk to significant other relationships or employment, lying about Internet use, and repeated, unsuccessful attempts to stop Internet use.

Co-occurring Disorders Greater frequencies of internet use have been associated with decreased social involvement and increased loneliness and depression (139). In an assessment of adults with problematic Internet use ($n = 20$), Shapira and colleagues (139) found significant social impairment, marked personal distress over Internet behaviors, vocational impairment, financial impairment, and legal problems. These results should be interpreted cautiously as all subjects met criteria for one or more Axis I disorders, primarily mood and anxiety disorders. Ten of the 20 participants had bipolar disorder and 12 had a substance use disorder.

As with SUDs, significant gender differences have been reported. In a Taiwanese study of adolescent internet behaviors ($n = 2,114$), higher levels of internet addiction were associated with higher rates of ADHD and depression across genders. However, higher rates of aggression were associated with increased severity of problematic internet use only among teenage males (142). Social phobia was also associated with Internet addiction, although not significantly after accounting for ADHD, depression, and hostility symptoms. These data suggest that ADHD, depression, and aggression may be vulnerability factors for problematic Internet use, and that social phobia may be a negative consequence of problematic Internet use (142). Further research is needed to identify the behavioral and neurobiologic correlates of problematic Internet use and to develop effective prevention and treatment strategies.

COMPULSIVE BUYING DISORDER

Classically referred to as "oniomania," compulsive shopping behavior has been clinically recognized for almost a century (143,144). Little is known about the pathophysiology of compulsive buying disorder (CBD). For example, there have been no imaging-based studies of CBD. Pharmacologic studies suggest certain similarities with SUDs, in particular with respect to the potential efficacy of naltrexone in CBD populations.

SSRIs A substantial placebo effect has been reported in pharmacologic treatment studies of SSRIs for CBD. A double-blind comparison of fluvoxamine (n = 12) versus placebo (n = 11) reported overall symptom improvement for all participants, and between-group differences in outcome were not observed despite the high doses of fluvoxamine (up to 300 mg/day) administered (145). A double-blind discontinuation trial of escitalopram among women with CBD (n = 26) (in which participants meeting criteria for responders after a 7-week open-label phase were randomized into placebo or continued escitalopram for a 9-week discontinuation phase) reported no significant differences between escitalopram versus placebo during the double-blind phase, suggesting that any initial improvements may have been due to placebo effects (146).

Opioid Antagonists There have been four case reports of successful naltrexone treatment in CBD (147,148). Kim (147) has reported successful CBD treatment with naltrexone (100 mg/day) in one individual with comorbid bulimia nervosa (which was also responsive to naltrexone treatment). Grant (148) reported three cases of successful high-dose naltrexone (100 to 200 mg/day) treatment for CBD. These open-label findings indicate the need for double-blind, placebo-controlled trials.

KLEPTOMANIA

Epidemiology Individuals with kleptomania suffer from a diminished ability to inhibit impulses to steal unnecessary or unwanted items, resulting in negative personal and professional consequences and experiences of regret and distress (149). *DSM-IV* diagnostic criteria for kleptomania reflect these aspects and include an increase in tension prior to theft followed by subjective pleasure/relief associated with theft (13).

Kleptomania generally begins in adolescence or early adulthood and appears more commonly in women than men (150). The natural history of kleptomania disorder may be chronic or acute (150). As with adolescent gambling, kleptomania is by definition illegal, and therefore poses specific negative consequences, such as incarceration, in addition to the more general negative consequences to personal and professional life. The necessarily illegal nature of these behaviors may increase both experiences of shame as well as reluctance to seek treatment. Although kleptomania has been reported to have a prevalence approaching 1% (151), the disorder has been omitted from major psychiatric epidemiological studies so its true prevalence is not precisely known.

Mood disorders, OCD, panic disorder, separation anxiety disorder, body dysmorphic disorder, and other ICDs have been associated with kleptomania (150). An association with first-degree relatives with alcohol and substance use problems suggests a shared genetic vulnerability between SUDs and kleptomania (151).

Neurobiology Neurocognitive and neuroimaging research suggest frontal lobe involvement in kleptomania. Using diffusion tensor imaging, one study reported reduced white matter integrity in inferior frontal regions in individuals with kleptomania versus controls (152). Performance deficits in neuropsychologic tasks associated with prefrontal regions (i.e., Wisconsin Card Sorting Test performance) have been found to correlate with kleptomania symptom severity (153).

Lesion-based studies also suggest frontal lobe involvement. Aizer and Lowengrub (154) have reported kleptomania subsequent to closed-head frontotemporal lobe blunt trauma in two male patients. A 43-year-old patient displayed behavioral changes (i.e., increased aggression), physical symptoms (i.e., headaches, insomnia, fatigue, and dizziness), and cognitive impairments (i.e., in memory and concentration) subsequent to trauma—in the absence of abnormal electroencephalogram, MRI, and computed tomography scans—followed by kleptomania behaviors. Combined citalopram and cognitive behavioral therapy effectively alleviated mood and kleptomania symptoms (154). In the second case, a 34-year-old patient began to display kleptomania and mood-disordered behaviors subsequent to trauma and a 3-day loss of consciousness. Pharmacotherapy (i.e., carbamazepine, valproic acid, paroxetine, combined venlafaxine and lithium, risperidone) was initially unable to alleviate symptoms (154). After a 3-month period of medication-abstinence, high-dose venlafaxine (150 mg/day) successfully remitted mood-related symptoms, and subsequent naltrexone augmentation (100 mg/day) 2 months later successfully treated kleptomania symptoms at a 1-year follow-up (154).

Nyfeller and Regard have reported one case of kleptomania-onset after frontolimbic damage during surgical removal of a craniopharyngioma in a 32-year-old male patient who displayed dysregular right hemispheric activity during postoperative electroencephalogram in the absence of any apparent neuropsychological changes (155). A few weeks subsequent to surgery, the patient began to develop a preoccupation with gambling and kleptomania and reported strong urges to steal objects of little to no value as well as subsequent guilt and regret, clinically similar to reports from non-lesioned individuals with kleptomania (155). Symptoms were unrelieved by SRI treatment (155). Kaplan (156) reported a case of comorbid left temporal lobe epilepsy and kleptomania onset in a 20-year-old female patient. Phenomenologically, the patient reported feeling tension before stealing, pleasure while stealing, and regret and shame subsequent to stealing. An MRI scan showed left mesial temporal sclerosis, and electroencephalogram revealed left temporal wave abnormalities. Symptoms were unrelieved by SRIs. Topiramate treatment (300 mg/day) successfully alleviated epileptic and kleptomania symptoms after 2 months (156).

Neurochemistry

SSRIs There have been several case reports of successful SSRI treatment for kleptomania (154). McElroy et al. (157) have reported successful fluoxetine treatment of kleptomania in four patients: two of the patients responded to fluoxetine treatment alone, whereas two other patients required augmented pharmacotherapy (either imipramine or lithium) (157). Burnstein (158) has also reported successful combined treatment of kleptomania with the combination of lithium and fluoxetine.

As has been reported in relation to OCD, the dosage targeted (80 mg/day) for efficacious fluoxetine treatment of kleptomania was higher than that typically used for treating depression (149,158). Kleptomania secondary to SSRI treatment for depression has been reported in three individuals (149). The equivocal efficacy of SSRIs in treating kleptomania, in conjunction with the report of SSRI-related kleptomania, suggests a potentially complex role for serotonin in kleptomania.

Opioid Antagonists There have been several case reports and one published open-label trial of effective naltrexone treatment in kleptomania. Kim (147) reported a reduction in urges to steal subsequent to naltrexone treatment in one individual with kleptomania and comorbid OCD. Grant and Kim (159) reported efficacious naltrexone treatment for kleptomania in an adolescent female. A recent open-label trial of naltrexone treatment for kleptomania found significant decreases in urge intensity and frequency subsequent to 12-week naltrexone administration (160).

Antiepileptics Topiramate, an antiepileptic drug used to treat partial and grand mal seizures, was reported in open-label fashion to effectively treat the symptoms of kleptomania in three published case reports (161). Research suggests that topiramate may also be efficacious in treating mood disorders, posttraumatic stress disorder, and binge-eating disorders. The interaction between neurobiologic mechanisms and topiramate is incompletely understood, and researchers have hypothesized that topiramate may partially inhibit GABAergic input into the NAcc in a similar manner to opioid antagonists such as naltrexone (161).

TRICHOTILLOMANIA

Hair twirling, lip and nail biting, skin picking, and other mildly uncomfortable or painful behaviors are common among the general population and are generally benign. Excessive engagement in such behaviors can have long-term medical consequences. Trichotillomania involves the pulling out of hair, most frequently from the scalp, although axillary, pubic, and perirectal regions may also be targeted.

Trichophagia (eating hair) may co-occur with trichotillomania. Resultant trichobezoars (hair balls) may cause gastrointestinal obstruction requiring surgical intervention (162). If untreated, trichobezoars may cause anemia, abdominal pain, hematemesis, nausea, vomiting, and bowel obstruction or perforation (162). However, the relationship between trichobezoars and trichotillomania has not yet been systematically assessed (162). Interpersonal consequences (i.e., negative effects to personal and professional life) (13) have additionally been reported.

Phenomenologic aspects of trichotillomania seem similar to those of SUDs. Hair-pulling is generally preceded by a sense of tension or experience of craving, and individuals report feeling unable to inhibit behaviors and experiencing of pleasure/relief during hair-pulling.

The duration of trichotillomania varies widely. Onset generally occurs in adolescence and may present as chronic and persistent across the lifespan or may abate without treatment (13). In addition to trichophagia, comorbid mood disorders, anxiety disorders, SUDs, OCD, eating disorders, personality disorders, and mental retardation have been reported in trichotillomania (13). Alopecia also commonly occurs with trichotillomania.

OCD and Trichotillomania Elevated levels of OCD have been reported in subjects with trichotillomania and their first degree relatives (163). Grant et al. (163) have suggested that differences in clinical presentations of trichotillomania may represent underlying differences in pathophysiology. For example, hair pulling, experienced as ego-dystonic in OCD, is experienced as ego-syntonic in trichotillomania, with 39% of individuals with trichotillomania reporting enjoyment in relation to hair-pulling behavior (163). This differential experience of hedonic enjoyment, which is typically not reported in OCD-related trichotillomania (and has been reported by some but not all trichotillomania patients) suggests that trichotillomania may have a different pathophysiology than OCD. Grant et al. (163) have suggested that two distinct pathophysiologies may underlie trichotillomania: one more resembling OCD and the other more similar to the pathophysiology of SUDs. This hypothesis is supported by pharmacological research demonstrating differential responses to SRIs in trichotillomania. Clinical findings suggest that there exist common features in SUDs and trichotillomania, such as craving, withdrawal, and tolerance.

Neuroimaging research has found differences in subjects with and without trichotillomania in parietal, frontal, and occipital cortical function (164). In comparison to healthy controls, neuroimaging studies have reported reduced left inferior frontal gyrus and left putamen volumes in trichotillomania (165,166). These abnormalities are distinct from those observed in OCD. In particular, reduced caudate volume, reported in OCD, has not been consistently found in trichotillomania. A single photon emission computed tomography analysis of female identical twins suggests that temporal pole abnormalities may be implicated in trichotillomania, with greater abnormalities associated with a more severe symptomatology (164).

Individuals with OCD display a blunted prolactin response to the serotonin agonist metachlorophenylpiperazine and have abnormal CSF levels of serotonin metabolites, whereas no such abnormalities have been found in trichotillomania (163). SRIs—an effective treatment for OCD—have been shown to alleviate some of the behaviors of trichotillomania; however, these findings are not consistent across individual patients, suggesting that there may be more than one pathophysiology in trichotillomania (163). Naltrexone, an opioid antagonist used to treat alcohol and opiate dependence, has been found to effectively treat trichotillomania symptoms (167). Naltrexone is not effective in treating OCD symptoms, suggesting a difference in the underlying biologies of the disorders.

Conclusion Trichotillomania is associated with negative psychiatric and medical features, including depression, social isolation, and alopecia. Although traditionally conceptualized as an impulse control disorder with strong similarities to OCD, clinical, phenomenologic, and neurobiologic research have identified important differences between trichotillomania and OCD that suggest different pathophysiologies. Similarities between trichotillomania and SUDs require further investigation, because they might carry important implications for patient care.

SKIN PICKING

Introduction Skin picking is currently listed in the *DSM-IV* under stereotypic movement disorder with self-injurious behavior. Stereotypic movement disorder is defined as repetitive, seemingly goal directed but nonfunctional motor behavior, resulting in self-inflicted injury or disruption to daily activities (13). Stereotypic movement disorder is most prevalent in individuals with mental retardation, and approximately 25% of adults institutionalized for mental retardation meet criteria (13).

Skin-picking behaviors, particularly in those individuals without mental retardation, share similarities with trichotillomania. Both skin picking and trichotillomania are generally done in isolation or only in the presence of close family members, thus discouraging socializing. We will use the term pathologic skin picking (PSP) — sometimes referred to as neurotic excoriation — to describe a pathological attention to, and duration of, skin-picking behavior that is impulsive, ritualistic, and repetitive (168). No single body area is uniquely associated with skin-picking behaviors, and any part of the body may be targeted. Individuals with this disorder may use a variety of implements to pick skin: tweezers, fingernails, pins, etc. As with other impulse control disorders, individuals who pick skin report spending up to 12 hours per day on picking. Clinical reports additionally suggest that suicidality is often a comorbid characteristic of individuals with PSP. Phenomenologically, trichotillomania and PSP appear similar. Bohne et al. (169) have proposed the term body-focused repetitive behaviors (BFRBs) based on such similarities.

Epidemiology As with trichotillomania, PSP most commonly occurs in females. There have been no widespread epidemiological studies of PSP, but data suggest that 3.8% of college students meet the criteria for neurotic excoriation, and that 2% of dermatology patients meet the criteria for skin picking (168). As in cases of other ICDs, individuals with PSP may feel ashamed of their behaviors and therefore be reluctant to seek psychologic or medical treatment. A recent study of ICD prevalence among adolescent psychiatric inpatients found that 11.8% met the criteria for skin picking (170).

Data derived from clinical populations estimate that 47.5% of treatment-seeking individuals had an onset of PSP before 10 years of age (171). PSP appears to be a chronic, often lifelong, condition that is associated with adverse medical and psychiatric outcomes. In trichotillomania, an early (childhood) age of onset is associated with a shorter disease course (often not continuing into adolescence), natural recovery, fewer co-occuring conditions and an equal prevalence in boys and girls, and is not associated with tension relief (172). Contrastingly, age of onset does not appear to have a substantial influence on PSP phenomenology or disease course (171). The finding that almost half of PSP sufferers experienced symptom onset before age 10 has important treatment implications, suggesting that the enhancement of public awareness of PSP may be especially important in the parents of young children.

OCD, ICD, and PSP A recent study conducted by Ferrão et al. (173) using the Structured Clinical Interview for DSM-IV (SCID-IV) assessed individuals with body-focused repetitive behaviors (i.e., PSP and trichotillomania) and individuals with OCD to assess any significant between-group differences in impulsive/compulsive characteristics. In comparison to individuals with OCD, individuals with BRFBs had the following statistically significant self-reported differences: (i) a more rapid impulse onset and a decreased ability to delay impulses; (ii) more immediate engagement in impulsive behaviors subsequent to impulses/desires and decreased time contemplating behaviors prior to initiation; (iii) an ego-syntonic or nonaversive/pleasurable experience during engagement in behaviors; (iv) a greater sensation of guilt subsequent to engaging in behaviors; (v) a lack of behavior-associated ritualistic behaviors; and (vi) fewer delusions of persecution (173).

Co-occurring Disorders PSP behaviors may be associated with different disorders including OCD, Prader-Willi syndrome, body dysmorphic disorder (BDD), and delusions (174). BDD is characterized by a distortion of body image resulting in a distressing and pathologic attention to body image (174). PSP has been found to co-occur with BDD (174–176). In PSP secondary to BDD, picking behaviors are aimed at improving the skin's appearance and mild or nonexistent imperfections are targeted (174,176). Grant et al. (174) studied the clinical characteristics and prevalence of PSP in a sample of 176 individuals with BDD: 44.9% of participants met criteria for lifetime PSP secondary to BDD and 36.9% met criteria for current PSP secondary to BDD.

Psychopharmacology Skin picking is categorized in *DSM-IV* as a stereotypic movement disorder (177). In an investigation of stereotypic movement disorder, Frecska et al. (177) compared opioid receptor sensitivity, as assessed via fentanyl-induced prolactin response, in individuals with trichotillomania in comparison to individuals with PSP. In comparison to individuals with trichotillomania or healthy controls, elevated prolactin level response was found for individuals with PSP (177). These findings suggest that dysregulation of the endogenous opioid system may play an important role in the pathophysiology of PSP. Researchers have hypothesized that PSP behaviors may be subjectively perceived as more self-injurious than is trichotillomania behaviors (177). As such, this finding is consistent with data suggesting an upregulation of opioid receptors in individuals with self-injurious behaviors.

As with trichotillomania, some, but not all, individuals with PSP may be successfully treated with SSRIs. Keuthen et al. (178) investigated the effects of escitalopram, an SSRI, in a sample of 29 individuals with PSP; however, only 19 individuals completed the 18-week open-label trial. Pre- and posttreatment data collected from the completers found a significant reduction in PSP symptoms: 11 (57.9%) individuals fully responded to treatment, 5 (26.3%) individuals partially responded, and 3 (15.8%) individuals experienced no abatement of PSP symptoms (i.e., were nonresponsive) (178). Given the potential for placebo responses, double-blind studies are needed to examine the efficacy of SRIs in the treatment of PSP.

There have been three published accounts of successful glutamatergic psychopharmacologic treatment in PSP. Grant et al. (179) tested the efficacy of lamotrigine, an anticonvulsant glutamatergic agent also used as a mood stabilizer, in treating PSP symptoms in a sample of 24 individuals and reported a subsequent improvement in 66% of participants. In a subject with PSP and co-occurring OCD, depression, and disordered eating behaviors (180), riluzole augmentation of fluoxetine was found to improve PSP behaviors in this patient whose PSP was previously nonresponsive to fluoxetine alone, combined fluoxetine and dextroamphetamine, and combined fluoxetine and lithium. *N*-acetyl cysteine was reported to successfully alleviate symptoms in a 52-year-old woman with PSP (181). The researchers also reported successful treatment with *N*-acetyl cysteine for two other individuals, one with trichotillomania, and the other with pathological nail biting (181). Together, these preliminary data suggest the need for more investigation of glutamate systems in the pathophysiology and treatment of PSP.

INTERMITTENT EXPLOSIVE DISORDER

Introduction Intermittent explosive disorder (IED) is characterized by a failure to inhibit aggressive impulses that are out of proportion to any precipitating stressor resulting in destruction of property or serious physical assault (13). Stressors may be internal (psychologic) or external (environmental). A diagnosis of IED is only given if the aggressive behavior cannot be explained by another mental disorder, such as a personality disorder or manic episode, or by substance use (13). Under earlier *DSM-III* criteria, a diagnosis of IED could not be given if the patient also met criteria for generalized aggression or impulsivity. As such, prevalence estimates based on older *DSM-III* criteria probably underestimate the prevalence of IED (182,183). Although arguably improved, the current *DSM-IV* criteria might benefit from further specification. At present, there is no time course or index of severity for disease onset/symptom presentation (182,184).

Based on data from the National Comorbidity Survey Replication, it has been estimated that as many as 7.3% of adults (approximately 11.5 to 16 million Americans) meet lifetime criteria for IED, and 3.9% meet criteria for 12-month IED (185). In a different community-based prevalence study assessing IED based on *DSM-IV* criteria, Coccaro et al. (186) estimated that up to 1.4 million Americans meet current IED criteria, and as many as 10 million may meet lifetime criteria (186).

Neurobiology The neuroanatomical literature on human aggressive behaviors has focused primarily on brain areas implicated in fear response such as the amygdala and the PFC, whereas neurochemical research has generally focused on corticotropin releasing factor, NE, and 5-HT. Current research suggests that neural circuitry connecting the OFC, vmPFC, DLPFC, anterior cingulate cortex, and amygdala may mediate emotion regulation and impulse control, with dysregulated function within this circuit associated with more impulsive aggressive behaviors and deficits in general emotion regulation (187).

Coccaro et al. (188) performed fMRI scans on 10 individuals with IED and 10 controls during a gender-decision task of emotional faces. There was no significant difference in fMRI gender-task performance accuracy or post-scan emotion-recognition task accuracy for IED versus control participants. Analyses of the fMRI data found a significant difference between the two groups for degree of amygdala and OFC activation. In response to angry faces, IED individuals displayed significantly greater amygdalar activation and significantly reduced OFC activation, and prior levels of aggressive behavior were associated with greater amygdalar activity. Whereas control subjects displayed an inverse relationship between the amygdala and OFC activations during presentation of emotional faces, as was consistent with previous research of fear processing, no such relationship was found for individuals with IED (188). These data suggest a dysregulation of inhibitory "top-down" OFC processes in individuals with IED.

Neurochemical research suggests that there is a dysregulation of the serotonin (5-HT) system in IED, and pharmacotherapy targeting the serotonin system has been found to reduce aggressive and impulsive behaviors (183). A reduced CSF concentration of 5-HIAA has been reported in individuals with IED, with lowered levels of 5-HIAA associated with more frequent or severe impulsive aggression (189). A study of aggressive behaviors is individuals with a personality disorder found an inverse relationship between platelet 5-HT concentration and a history of lifetime aggression (189). No significant relationship between platelet 5-HT concentration and impulsivity was reported (189).

CONCLUSION

ICDs share multiple features with SUDs and may be considered "behavioral addictions", although alternate conceptualizations also warrant consideration. Additional research is needed to determine how specific ICDs are related to one another and to specific SUDs, and how an improved understanding of the biologies of these disorders may be translated into improved prevention and treatment strategies.

REFERENCES

1. Potenza MN. Should addictive disorders include non-substance-related conditions? *Addiction* 2006;101:165–174.
2. Maddux JF, Desmond DP. Addiction or dependence? *Addiction* 2000; 95:661–665.
3. O'Brien CP, Volkow N, Li TK. What's in a word? Addiction versus dependence in DSM-V. *Am J Psychiatry* 2006;163:764–765.
4. Holden C. 'Behavioral' addictions: do they exist? *Science* 2001;294: 980–982.
5. Volkow ND, O'Brien CP. Issues for DSM-V: should obesity be included as a brain disorder? *Am J Psychiatry* 2007;164:708–710.
6. Potenza MN. Should addictive disorders include non-substance-related conditions? In Saunders JB, et al., eds. *Diagnostic issues in substance use disorders: refining the research agenda for DSM-V.* Washington, DC: American Psychiatric Press, Inc: 2007;251–268.
7. Petry NM. Should the scope of addictive behaviors be broadened to include pathological gambling. In: Saunders JB, Schuckit MA, Sirovatka PJ, et al., eds. *Diagnostic issues in substance use disorders: refining the research agenda for DSM-V.* Washington DC: American Psychiatric Press, Inc., 2007;269–283.
8. Potenza MN, Koran LM, Pallanti S. The relationship between obsessive-compulsive and impulse control disorders: a current understanding and future research directions. *Psychiatry Res.* In press.
9. Shaffer HJ. Strange bedfellows: a critical view of pathological gambling and addiction. *Addiction* 1999;94:1675–1678.
10. Redish AD, Jensen S, Johnson A. A unified framework for addiction: vulnerabilities in the decision process. *Behav Brain Sci* 2008;31(4):415–437.
11. Chambers R, Bickel WK, Potenza MN. A scale-free systems theory of motivation and addiction. *Neurosci Biobehav Rev* 2007;31:1017–1045.
12. Goldstein RZ, Alia-Klein N, Tomasi D, et al. Is decreased prefrontal cortical sensitivity to monetary reward associated with impaired motivation and self-control in cocaine addiction? *Am J Psychiatry* 2007;164:43–51.
13. Association AP. *Diagnostic and statistical manual of mental disorders.* Fourth edition–test revision. Washington, DC: American Psychiatric Press, Inc., 2000.
14. Hollander E, Kim S, Zohar J. OCSDs in the forthcoming DSM-V. *CNS Spectrums* 2007;12:320–323.
15. Potenza MN, Kosten TR, Rounsaville BJ. Pathological gambling. *JAMA* 2001;286:164–167.
16. Tamminga CA, Nestler EJ. Pathological gambling: focusing on the addiction, not the activity. *Am J Psychiatry* 2006;163:180–181.
17. Grant JE, Odlaug BL, Potenza MN. Addicted to hair-pulling? How an alternate model of trichotillomania may improve treatment outcome. *Harvard Rev Psychiatry* 2007;15:80–85.
18. Slutske WS. Natural recovery and treatment-seeking in pathological gambling: results of two national surveys. *Am J Psychiatry* 2006;163: 297–302.
19. Potenza MN, Steinberg MA, McLaughlin S, et al. Gender-related differences in the characteristics of problem gamblers using a gambling helpline. *Am J Psychiatry* 2001;181:1730–1735.
20. Comings DE, Gade-Andavolu R, Gonzalez N, et al. The additive effect of neurotransmitter genes in pathological gambling. *Clin Genet* 2001;60:107–116.
21. Desai R, Potenza M. Gender differences in the associations between problem gambling and psychiatric disorders. *Soc Psychiatry Psychiatr Epi* 2008;43:173–183.
22. Petry NM, Stinson FS, Grant BF. Co-morbidity of DSM-IV pathological gambling and other psychiatric disorders: results from the National Epidemiologic Survey on Alcohol and Related Conditions. *J Clin Psychiatry* 2005;66:564–574.
23. Goudriaan AE, Oosterlaan J, de Beurs E, et al. Psychophysiological determinants and concomitants of deficient decision making in pathological gamblers. *Drug Alcohol Depend* 2006;84:231–239.
24. Goudriaan AE, Oosterlaan J, de Beurs E, et al. Neurocognitive functions in pathological gambling: a comparison with alcohol dependence, Tourette syndrome and normal controls. *Addiction* 2006;101:534–547.
25. Bechara A. Risky business: emotion, decision-making, and addiction. *J Gambling Stud* 2003;19:23–51.
26. Reynolds B. A review of delay-discounting research with humans: relations to drug use and gambling. *Behav Pharmacol* 2006;17:651–667.
27. Petry NM. Pathological gamblers, with and without substance use disorders, discount delayed rewards at high rates. *Abnormal Psychol* 2001;110:482–487.
28. Knutson B, Fong GW, Bennett SM, et al. A region of mesial prefrontal cortex tracks monetarily rewarding outcomes: characterization with rapid event-related fMRI. *NeuroImage* 2003;18:263–272.
29. Cardinal RN. Neural systems implicated in delayed and probabilistic reinforcement. *Neural Netw* 2006;19:1277–1301.
30. Eber GB, Shaffer HJ. Trends in bio-behavioral gambling studies research: quantifying citations. *J Gambling Stud* 2000;16:461–467.
31. Reuter J, Raedler T, Rose M, et al. Pathological gambling is linked to reduced activation of the mesolimbic reward system. *Nat Neurosci* 2005;8:170–171.
32. Potenza MN, Steinberg MA, Skudlarski P, et al. Gambling urges in pathological gambling: a functional magnetic resonance imaging study. *Arch Gen Psychiatry* 2003;60:828–836.
33. Potenza MN, Leung HC, Blumberg HP, et al. An FMRI Stroop task study of ventromedial prefrontal cortical function in pathological gamblers. *Amer J Psychiatry* 2003;160:1990–1994.
34. Tanabe J, Thompson L, Claus E, et al. Prefrontal cortex activity is reduced in gambling and nongambling substance users during decision-making. *Hum Brain Mapp* 2007;28:1276–1286.
35. Stojanov W, Karayanidis F, Johnston P, et al. Disrupted sensory gating in pathological gambling. *Biol Psychiatry* 2003;54:474–484.
36. DeCaria CM, Begaz T, Hollander E. Serotonergic and noradrenergic function in pathological gambling. *CNS Spectrums* 1998;3:38–45.
37. Potenza MN. The neurobiology of pathological gambling. *Semin Clin Neuropsych* 2001;6:217–226.
38. Nordin C, Eklundh T. Altered CSF 5-HIAA disposition in pathological male gamblers. *CNS Spectrums* 1999;4:25–33.
39. Pallanti S, Bernardi S, Quercioli L, et al. Serotonin dysfunction in pathological gamblers: increased prolactin response to oral m-CPP versus placebo. *CNS Spectrums* 2006;11:956–964.
40. Hollander E, DeCaria CM, Finkell JN, et al. A randomized double-blind fluvoxamine/placebo crossover trial in pathological gambling. *Biol Psychiatry* 2000;47:813–817.
41. Grant JE, Kim SW, Potenza MN, et al. Paroxetine treatment of pathological gambling: a multi-centre randomized controlled trial. *Int Clin Psychopharmacol* 2003;18:243–249.
42. Brewer JA, Grant JE, Potenza MN. The treatment of pathological gambling. *Addict Disorders Treatment* 2008;7:1–13.
43. Brewer JA, Potenza, MN. The neurobiology and genetics of impulse control disorders: relationships to drug addictions. *Biochem Pharmacol* 2008;75:63–75.
44. Zack M, Poulos CX. Amphetamine primes motivation to gamble and gambling-related semantic networks in problem gamblers. *Neuropsyhcopharmacology* 2004;29:195–207.
45. Potenza MN, Voon V, Weintraub D. Drug insight: impulse control disorders and dopamine therapies in Parkinson's disease. *Nat Clin Practice Neurosci* 2007;3:664–672.
46. Zack M, Poulos CX. A D2 antagonist enhances the rewarding and priming effects of a gambling episode in pathological gamblers. *Neuropsychopharmacology* 2007;32:1678–1686.
47. Bergh C, Eklund T, Sodersten P, et al. Altered dopamine function in pathological gambling. *Psychol Med* 1997;27:473–475.
48. Nordin C, Sjödin I. CSF monoamine patterns in pathological gamblers and healthy controls. *J Psychiatric Res* 2006;40:454–459.
49. Roy A, Pickar D, De Jong J, et al. Norepinephrine and its metabolites in cerebrospinal fluid, plasma, and urine: relationship to hypothalamic-pituitary-adrenal axis function in depression. *Arch Gen Psychiatry* 1988;45:849–857.
50. Meyer G, Schwertfeger J, Exton M, et al. Neuroendocrine response to casino gambling in problem gamblers. *Psychoneuroendocrinology* 2004; 29:1272–1280.

51. Kim SW, Grant JE, Adson DE, et al. Double-blind naltrexone and placebo comparison study in the treatment of pathological gambling. *Biol Psychiatry* 2001;49:914–921.
52. Grant JE, Potenza MN, Hollander E, et al. Multicenter investigation of the opioid antagonist nalmefene in the treatment of pathological gambling. *Am J Psychiatry* 2006;163:303–312.
53. Gupta R, Derevensky J. Familial and social influences on juvenile gambling behavior. *J Gambling Stud* 1997;13:179–192.
54. Eisen SA, Lin N, Lyons MJ, et al. Familial influences on gambling behavior: an analysis of 3359 twin pairs. *Addiction* 1998;93:1375–1384.
55. Tsuang MT, Lyons MJ, Eisen SA, et al. Genetic influences on DSM-III-R drug abuse and dependence: a study of 3,372 twin pairs. *Amer J Med Genet* 1996;67:473–477.
56. Slutske WS, Eisen S, True WR, et al. Common genetic vulnerability for pathological gambling and alcohol dependence in men. *Arch Gen Psychiatry* 2000;57:666–673.
57. Slutske WS, Eisen S, True WR, et al. A twin study of the association between pathological gambling and antisocial personality disorder. *J Abnormal Psychol* 2001;110:297–308.
58. Comings DE, Gade R, Wu S, et al. Studies of the potential role of the dopamine D1 receptor gene in addictive behaviors. *Mol Psychiatry* 1997;2:44–56.
59. Comings DE, Rosenthal RJ, Lesieur HR, et al. A study of the dopamine D2 receptor gene in pathological gambling. *Pharmacogenetics* 1996;6: 223–234.
60. Perez de Castro I, Ibanez A, Saiz-Ruiz J, et al. Genetic contribution to pathological gambling: possible association between a functional DNA polymorphism at the serotonin transporter gene (5-HTT) and affected men. *Pharmacogenetics* 1999;9:397–400.
61. Ibanez A, Blanco C, de Castro IP, et al. Genetics of pathological gambling. *J Gambling Stud* 2003;19:11–22.
62. Kreek MJ, Nielsen DA, Butelman ER, et al. Genetic influences on impulsivity, risk taking, stress responsivity and vulnerability to drug abuse and addiction. *Nat Neurosci* 2005;8:1680–1687.
63. da Silva Lobo DS, Vallada HP, Knight J, et al. Dopamine genes and pathological gambling in discordant sib-pairs. *J Gambl Stud* 2007;23: 421–433.
64. Hudson JI, Hiripi E, Pope HG, Jr, et al. The prevalence and correlates of eating disorders in the National Comorbidity Survey Replication. *Biol Psychiatry* 2007;61:348–358.
65. Obesity and overweight. 2006. World Health Organization. Accessed 16 April 2008, from www.who.int/mediacentre/factsheets/fs311/en/.
66. Mokdad AH, Ford ES, Bowman BA, et al. Prevalence of obesity, diabetes, and obesity-related health risk factors, 2001. *JAMA* 2003;289: 76–79.
67. Joranby L, Pineda KF, Gold MS. Addiction to food and brain reward systems. *Sex Addict Compulsivity* 2005;12:201–217.
68. Swanson L. Cerebral hemisphere regulation of motivated behavior. *Brain Res* 2000;886:113–164.
69. Enriori P, Evans A, Sinnayah P, et al. Leptin resistance and obesity. *Obesity* 2006;14:254S–258S.
70. Trinko R, Sears RM, Guarnieri DJ, et al. Neural mechanisms underlying obesity and drug addiction. *Physiol Behav* 2007;91:499–505.
71. Halaas JL, Gajiwala KS, Maffei M, et al. Weight-reducing effects of the plasma protein encoded by the obese gene. *Science* 1995;269:543–546.
72. Farooqi SI, Bullmore E, Keogh J, et al. Leptin regulates striatal regions and human eating behavior. *Science* 2007;317:1355.
73. Small D, Zatorre R, Dagher A, et al. Changes in brain activity related to eating chocolate: from pleasure to aversion. *Brain* 2001;124:1720–1733.
74. Rothemund Y, Preuschhof C, Bohner G, et al. Differential activation of the dorsal striatum by high-calorie visual food stimuli in obese individuals. *NeuroImage* 2007;37:410–421.
75. Kaye WH, Guido KW, Frank GK, et al. Altered dopamine activity after recovery from restricting-type anorexia nervosa. *Neuropsychopharmacology* 1999;21:503–506.
76. Wagner A, Aizenstein H, Venkatraman VK, et al. Altered reward processing in women recovered from anorexia nervosa. *Amer J Psychiatry* 2007;164:1842–1849.
77. Wang G-J, Volkow ND, Logan J, et al. Brain dopamine and obesity. *Lancet* 2001;357:354–357.
78. Szczypka MS, Rainey MA, Kim DS, et al. Feeding behavior in dopamine-deficient mice. *Proc Natl Acad Sci* 1999;96:12138–12166.
79. Figlewicz DP, Evans SB, Murphy J, et al. Expression of receptors for insulin and leptin in the ventral tegmental area/substantia nigra (VTA/SN) of the rat. *Brain Res* 2003;964:107–115.
80. Hommel JD, Trinko R, Sears RM, et al. Leptin receptor signaling in midbrain dopamine neurons regulates feeding. *Neuron* 2006;51:801–810.
81. Elmquist, JK, Bjorbaek, C, Ahima, RS, et al. Distributions of leptin receptor mRNA isoforms in the rat brain. *J Comp Neurol* 1998; 395:535–547.
82. Shanley LJ, Irving AJ, Harvey J. Leptin enhances NMDA receptor function and modulates hippocampal synaptic plasticity. *J Neurosci* 2001; 21:186RC.
83. Fulton S, Woodside B, Shizgal P. Modulation of brain reward circuitry by leptin. *Science* 2000;287:125–128.
84. Chemelli, RM, Willie, JT, Sinton, CM, et al. Narcolepsy in *orexin* knockout mice: molecular genetics of sleep regulation. *Cell* 1999;98:409–412.
85. Sakurai T, Amemiya A, Ishii M, et al. Orexins and orexin receptors: a family of hypothalamic neuropeptides and G protein-coupled receptors that regulate feeding behavior. *Cell* 1998;92:573–585.
86. Boutrel B, Kenny PJ, Specio SE, et al. Role for hypocretin in mediating stress-induced reinstatement of cocaine-seeking behavior. *Proc Natl Acad Sci* 2005;102:19168–19173.
87. Georgescu D, Zachariou V, Barrot M, et al. Involvement of the lateral hypothalamic peptide orexin in morphine dependence and withdrawal. *J Neurosci* 2003;23:3106–3111.
88. Lawrence, JA, Cowen, MS, Yang, HJ, et al. The orexin system regulates alcohol-seeking in rats. *Br J Pharmacol* 2006;171:752–759.
89. Harris, GC, Wimmer, M, Aston-Jones, G. A role for lateral hypothalamic orexin neurons in reward seeking. *Nature*, 2005;437: 556–559.
90. Narita M, Nagumo Y, Hashimoto S, et al. Direct involvement of orexinergic systems in the activation of the mesolimbic dopamine pathway and related behaviors induced by morphine. *J Neurosci* 2006;26: 398–405.
91. Vittoz NM, Berridge CW. Hypocretin/orexin selectively increases dopamine efflux within the prefrontal cortex: involvement of the ventral tegmental area. *Neuropsychopharmacology* 2006;31:384–395.
92. Higgins SC, Gueorguiev M, Korbonits M. Ghrelin, the peripheral hunger hormone. *Ann Med* 2007;39:116–136.
93. Cummings DE, Purnell JQ, Frayo RS, et al. A preprandial rise in plasma ghrelin levels suggests a role in meal initiation in humans. *Diabetes* 2001;50:1714–1719.
94. Tschop M, Weyer C, Tataranni A, et al. Circulating ghrelin levels are decreased in human obesity. *Diabetes* 2001;50:707–709.
95. Abizaid A, Liu Z-W, Andrews Z, et al. Ghrelin modulates the activity and synaptic input organization of midbrain dopamine neurons while promoting appetite. *J Clin Invest* 2006;116:3229–3239.
96. Nicola SM, Taha SA, Kim SW, et al. Nucleus accumbens dopamine release is necessary and sufficient to promote the behavioral response to reward-predictive cues. *Neuroscience* 2005;135:1025–1033.
97. Kelley AE, Bakshi VP, Haber SN, et al. Opioid modulation of taste hedonics within the ventral striatum. *Physiol Behav* 2002;76:365–377.
98. Kelley AE, Bless EP, Swanson CJ. Investigation of the effects of opiate antagonists infused into the nucleus accumbens on feeding and sucrose drinking in rats. *J Pharmacol Exp Ther* 1996;278:1729–1737.
99. Taha SA, Fields HL. Encoding of palatability and appetitive behaviors by distinct neuronal populations in the nucleus accumbens. *J Neurosci* 2005;25:1193–1202.
100. Kelley AE, Baldo B, Pratt W, et al. Corticostriatal-hypothalamic circuitry and food motivation: integration of energy, action and reward. *Physiol Behav* 2005;86:773–795.
101. Cota D, Genghini S, Pasquali R, et al. Antagonizing the cannabinoid receptor type 1: a dual way to fight obesity. *J Endocrinol Invest* 2003;26:1041–1044.
102. Di Marzo V, Matias I. Endocannabinoid control of food intake and energy balance. *Nat Neurosci* 2005;8:585–589.

103. Monteleone P, Matias I, Martiadis V, et al. Blood levels of the endocannabinoid anandamide are increased in anorexia nervosa and in binge-eating disorder, but not in bulimia nervosa. *Neuropsychopharmacology* 2005;30:1216–1221.
104. Di Marzo V, Goparaju SK, Wang L, et al. Leptin-regulated endocannabinoids are involved in maintaining food intake. *Nature* 2001;410:822–825.
105. Schlicker E, Kathmann M. Modulation of transmitter release via presynaptic cannabinoid receptors. *Trends Pharmacol Sci* 2001;22:565–572.
106. Mahler SV, Smith KS, Berridge KC. Endocannabinoid hedonic hotspot for sensory pleasure: anandamide in nucleus accumbens shell enhances 'liking' of a sweet reward. *Neuropsychopharmacology* 2007;32:2267–2278.
107. Rosen HJ, Gorno-Tempini WP, Goldman RJ, et al. Patterns of brain atrophy in frontotemporal dementia and semantic dementia. *Neurol* 2002;58:198–208.
108. Mendez MF, Licht EA, Shapira JS. Changes in dietary or eating behavior in frontotemporal dementia versus Alzheimer's disease. *Amer J Alzheimers Dis Other Demen* 2008;23(3):280–285.
109. Woolley JD, Gorno-Tempini ML, Seeley WW, et al. Binge eating is associated with right orbitofrontal-insular-striatal atrophy in frontotemporal dementia. *Neurology* 2007;69:1654–1663.
110. Del Parigi A, Chen K, Salbe AD, et al. Successful dieters have increased neural activity in cortical areas involved in the control of behavior. *Int J Obes* 2007;31:440–448.
111. Uher R, Yoganathan D, Mogg A, et al. Effect of left prefrontal repetitive transcranial magnetic stimulation on food craving. *Biol Psychiatry* 2005;58:840–842.
112. Davis C, Levitan R, Muglia P, et al. Decision-making deficits and overeating: a risk model for obesity. *Obesity* 2004;12:929–935.
113. Tchanturia K, Liao P, Uher R, et al. An investigation of decision making in anorexia nervosa using the Iowa Gambling Task and Skin Conductance Measurements. *J Int Neuropsychol Soc* 2007;13:635–641.
114. Brand M, Kalbe E, Labudda K, et al. Decision-making impairments in patients with pathological gambling. *Psychiatry Res* 2005;133:91–99.
115. Brand M, Fujiwara E, Kalbe E, et al. Cognitive estimation and affective judgments in alcoholic Korsakoff patients. *J Clin Exp Neuropsychol* 2003;25:324–334.
116. Leibowitz SF, Alexander JT. Hypothalamic serotonin in control of eating behavior, meal size, and body weight. *Biol Psychiatry* 1998;44:851–864.
117. Halford JC, Harrold JA, Boyland EJ, et al. Serotonergic drugs: effects on appetite expression and use for the treatment of obesity. *Drugs* 2007;67:27.
118. Heisler LK, Cowley MA, Tecott LH, et al. Activation of central melanocortin pathways by fenfluramine. *Science* 2002;297:609–611.
119. Devlin MJ, Goldfein JA, Petkova E, et al. Cognitive behavioral therapy and fluoxetine for binge eating disorder: two-year follow-up. *Obesity* 2007;15:1702–1709.
120. Coleman E, Gratzer T, Nesvacil L, et al. Nefazodone and the treatment of nonparaphilic compulsive sexual behavior: a retrospective study. *J Clin Psychiatry* 2000;61:282–284.
121. Schaffer SD, Zimmerman ML. The sexual addict: a challenge for the primary care provider. *Nurse Pract* 1990;15:25–33.
122. Mick TM, Hollander E. Impulsive-compulsive sexual behavior. *CNS Spectrums* 2006;11:944–955.
123. Kafka MP, Prentky RA. Preliminary observations of DSM-III-R axis I comorbidity in men with paraphilias and paraphilia-related disorders. *J Clin Psychiatry* 1994;55:481–487.
124. Grant JE, Steinberg MA. Compulsive sexual behavior and pathological gambling. *Sex Addict Compulsivity* 2005;12:235–244.
125. Coleman E. Is your patient suffering from compulsive sexual behavior? *Psychiatric Ann* 1992;22:325.
126. Grant JE, Levine L, Kim D, et al. Impulse control disorders in adult psychiatric populations. *Amer J Psychiatry* 2005;162:2184–2188.
127. Voon V, Fox SH. Medication-related impulse control and repetitive behaviors in Parkinson disease. *Arch Neurol* 2007;64:1089–1096.
128. Voon V, Hassan K, Zurowski M, et al. Prevalence of repetitive and reward-seeking behaviors in Parkinson's disease. *Neurology* 2006;67: 1254–1257.
129. Fong TW, De La Garza R 2nd, Newton TF. A case report of topiramate in the treatment of nonparaphilic sexual addiction. *J Clin Psychopharmacol* 2005;25:512–514.
130. Hirschfeld RM. Long-term side effects of SSRI's: sexual dysfunction and weight gain. *J Clin Psychiatry*,2003;64:20–24.
131. Wainberg ML, Muench F, Morgenstern J, et al. A double-blind study of citalopram versus placebo in the treatment of compulsive sexual behaviors in gay and bisexual men. *J Clin Psychiatry* 2006;67:1968–1973.
132. Kafka MP, Hennen J. Psychostimulant augmentation during treatment with selective serotonin reuptake inhibitors in men with paraphilias and paraphilia-related disorders: a case series. *J Clin Psychiatry* 2000;61:664–670.
133. Sathe RS, Komisaruk BR, Ladas AK, et al. Naltrexone-induced augmentation of sexual response in men. *Arch Med Res* 2001;32:221–226.
134. Ryback RS. Naltrexone in the treatment of adolescent sexual offenders. *J Clin Psychiatry* 2004;65:982–986.
135. Grant JE, Kim SW. A case of kleptomania and compulsive sexual behavior treated with naltrexone. *Ann Clin Psychiatry* 2001;13:229–231.
136. Grant JE, Kim SW. A case of kleptomania and compulsive sexual behavior treated with naltrexone. *Ann Clin Psychiatry* 2001;13:229–231.
137. Driver-Dunckley ED, Noble BN, Hentz JG, et al. Gambling and increased sexual desire with dopaminergic medications in restless legs syndrome. *Clin Neuropharmacol* 2007;30:249–255.
138. Liu T, Potenza MN. Problematic Internet use: clinical implications. *CNS Spectrums* 2007;12:453–466.
139. Kraut R, Patterson M, Lundmark V, et al. Internet paradox: a social technology that reduces social involvement and psychological well-being? *Amer Psychol* 1998;53:1017–1031.
140. Young K. Psychology of computer use: XL. Addictive use of the Internet: a case that breaks the stereotype. *Psychol Rep* 1996;79:899–902.
141. Shapira N, Goldsmith T, Keck P, et al. Psychiatric features of individuals with problematic internet use. *J Affect Disord* 2000;57:267–272.
142. Yen J-Y, Ko C-H, Yen C-F, et al. The comorbid psychiatric symptoms of Internet addiction: attention deficit and hyperactivity disorder (ADHD), depression, social phobia, and hostility. *J Adolesc Health* 2007;41:93–98.
143. Kraepelin E. *Psychiatrie,* 8th ed. Leipzig: Verlag Von Johann Ambrosius Barth, 1915.
144. Lejoyeux M, Ades J, Tassain V, et al. Phenomenology and psychopathology of uncontrolled buying. *Amer J Psychiatry* 1996;176:1754–1759.
145. Black D, Gabel J, Hansen J, et al. A double-blind comparison of fluvoxamine versus placebo in the treatment of compulsive buying disorder. *Ann Clin Psychiatry* 2000;12:205–211.
146. Koran LM, Aboujaoude EN, Gamel NN. Escitalopram treatment of kleptomania: an open-label trial followed by double-blind discontinuation. *J Clin Psychiatry* 2007;68:422–427.
147. Kim SW. Opioid antagonists in the treatment of impulse-control disorders. *J Clin Psychiatry* 1998;59:159–164.
148. Grant JE. Three cases of compulsive buying treated with naltrexone. *International Journal of Psychiatry in Clinical Practice* 2003;7:223–225.
149. Durst R, Katz G, Teitelbaum A, et al. Kleptomania: diagnosis and treatment options. *CNS Drugs* 2001;15:185–195.
150. Presta S, Marazziti D, Dell'Osso L, et al. Kleptomania: clinical features and comorbidity in an Italian sample. *Compr Psychiatry* 2002;43:7–12.
151. Grant JE. Family history and psychiatric comorbidity in persons with kleptomania. *Compr Psychiatry* 2003;44:437–441.
152. Grant JE, Correia S, Brennan-Krohn T. White matter integrity in kleptomania: a pilot study. *Psychiatry Res* 2006;170:233–237.
153. Grant J, Odlaug B, Wozniak J. Neuropsychological functioning in kleptomania. *Behav Res Ther* 2007;45:1663–1670.
154. Aizer A, Lowengrub K, Dannon PN. Kleptomania after head trauma: two case reports and combination treatment strategies. *Clin Neuropharmacol* 2004;27:211–215.
155. Nyffeler T, Regard M. Kleptomania in a patient with a right frontolimbic lesion. *Neuropsychiatry Neuropsychol Behav Neurol* 2001;14: 73–76.
156. Kaplan Y. Epilepsy and kleptomania. *Epilepsy & behavior* 2007;11:474–475.
157. McElroy SL, Pope HG, Hudson JL. Kleptomania: a report of 20 cases. *Amer J Psychiatry* 1991;171:652–657.

158. Burstein A. Fluoxetine-lithium treatment for kleptomania. *J Clin Psychiatry* 1992;53:28–29.
159. Grant JE, Kim SW. Adolescent kleptomania treated with naltrexone: a case report. *Eur Child Adolesc Psychiatry* 2002;11:92–95.
160. Grant JE, Kim SW. An open-label study of naltrexone in the treatment of kleptomania. *J Clin Psychiatry* 2002;63:349–356.
161. Dannon PN. Topiramate for the treatment of kleptomania: a case series and review of the literature. *Clin Neuropharmacol* 2003;26:1–4.
162. Salaam K, Carr J, Grewal H, et al. Untreated trichotillomania and trichophagia: surgical emergency in a teenage girl. *Psychosomatics* 2005;46:362–366.
163. Grant JE, Odlaug BL, Potenza MN. Addicted to hair pulling? How an alternate model of trichotillomania may improve treatment outcome. *Harv Rev Psychiatry* 2007;15:80–85.
164. Vythilingum B, Warwick J, vanKradenburg J, et al. SPECT Scans in identical twins with trichotillomania. *J Neuropsychiatry Clin Neurosci* 2002;14:340–342.
165. Grachev ID. MRI-based morphometric topographic parcellation of human neocortex in trichotillomania. *Psychiatry Clin Neurosci* 1997; 51:315–321.
166. O'Sullivan R, Rauch S, Breiter H, et al. Reduced basal ganglia volumes in trichotillomania measured via morphometric magnetic resonance imaging. *Biol Psychiatry* 1997;42:39–45.
167. Carrion VG. Naltrexone for the treatment of trichotillomania: a case report. *J Clin Psychopharmacol* 1995;15:444–445.
168. Ferrão AY, Almeida V, Bedin ND, et al. Impulsivity and compulsivity in patients with trichotillomania or skin picking compared with patients with obsessive-compulsive disorder. *Compr Psychiatry* 2006;47:282–288.
169. Bohne A, Wilhelm S, Keuthen N, et al. Prevalence of body dysmorphic disorder in a German college student sample. *Psychiatry Res* 2002;109: 101–104.
170. Grant JE, Williams KA, Potenza MN. Impulse-control disorders in adolescent psychiatric inpatients: co-occurring disorders and sex differences. *J Clin Psychiatry* 2007;68:1814–1592.
171. Odlaug BL, Grant JE. Childhood-onset pathological skin picking: clinical characteristics and psychiatric comorbidity. *Compr Psychiatry* 2007;48:388–393.
172. Bohne A, Keuthen N, Wilhelm S. Pathologic hairpulling, skin picking, and nail biting. *Ann Clin Psychiatry* 2005;17:227–232.
173. Ferrao AY, Almeida V, Bedin N, et al. Impulsivity and compulsivity in patients with trichotillomania or skin picking compared with patients with obsessive-compulsive disorder. *Compr Psychiatry* 2006;47:282–288.
174. Grant JE, Menard W, Phillips KA. Pathological skin picking in individuals with body dysmorphic disorder. *Gen Hosp Psychiatry* 2006;28: 487–493.
175. Phillips KA, McElroy SL. Obsessive-compulsive disorder in relation to body dysmorphic disorder (letter). *Amer J Psychiatry* 1992;172:1284.
176. Phillips KA, Taub S. Skin picking as a symptom of body dysmorphic disorder. *Psychopharmacol Bull* 1995;31:279–288.
177. Frecska E, Arato M. Opiate sensitivity test in patients with stereotypic movement disorder and trichotillomania. *Progr Neuro-Psychopharmacol Biolo Psychiatry* 2002;26:909–912.
178. Keuthen NJ, Jameson M, Loh R, et al. Open-label escitalopram treatment for pathological skin picking. *Int Clin Psychopharmacol* 2007;22:268–274.
179. Grant JE, Odlaug BL, Kim SW. Lamotrigine treatment of pathologic skin picking: an open-label study. *J Clin Psychiatry* 2007;68:1384–1391.
180. Sasso DA, Kalanithi PS, Trueblood KV, et al. Beneficial effects of the glutamate-modulating agent riluzole on disordered eating and pathological skin-picking behaviors. *J Clin Psychopharmacol* 2006;26:685–687.
181. Odlaug BL, Grant JE. *N*-acetyl cysteine in the treatment of grooming disorders. *J Clin Psychopharmacol* 2007;27:227–229.
182. McCloskey MS, Berman ME, Noblett KL, et al. Intermittent explosive disorder-integrated research diagnostic criteria: convergent and discriminant validity. *J Psychiatric Res* 2006;40:231–242.
183. Coccaro EF, Kavoussi RJ, Berman ME, et al. Intermittent explosive disorder-revised: development, reliability, and validity of research criteria. *Compr Psychiatry* 1998;39:368–376.
184. Coccaro EF. Intermittent explosive disorder. In: Coccaro EF, ed. *Intermittent Explosive Disorder.* New York: Marcel Dekker Inc., 2003; 172–199.
185. Kessler RC, Coccaro EF, Fava M, et al. The prevalence and correlates of DSM-IV intermittent explosive disorder in the National Comorbidity Survey Replication. *Arch Gen Psychiatry* 2006;63:669–678.
186. Coccaro EF, Schmidt CA, Samuels JF, et al. Lifetime and 1-month prevalence rates of intermittent explosive disorder in a community sample. *J Clin Psychiatry* 2004;65:820–824.
187. Davidson R, Putnam K, Larson C. Dysfunction in the neural circuitry of emotion regulation—a possible prelude to violence. *Science* 2000;289:591–594.
188. Coccaro EF, McCloskey MS, Fitzgerald DA, et al. Amygdala and orbitofrontal reactivity to social threat in individuals with impulsive aggression. *Biol Psychiatry* 2007;62:168–178.
189. Goveas JS, Csernansky JG, Coccaro EF Platelet serotonin content correlates inversely with life history of aggression in personality-disordered subjects. *Psychiatry Res* 2004;126:23–32.

SECTION 2

Pharmacology

CHAPTER 6

Lori D. Karan, MD, FACP, FASAM
Elinore McCance-Katz, MD, PhD
Anne Zajicek, MD, PharmD

Pharmacokinetic and Pharmacodynamic Principles

Pharmacology is the study of drugs. Historically, drugs have been impure mixtures of components derived from plants and animals, whose composition was little understood. In contrast, today's drugs are highly formulated chemicals that are intended to specifically target pathogenesis as well as to maximize safety, convenience, and therapeutic efficacy. Illicit drugs are used for their mood-altering effects and often contain adulterants. Advances in pharmacology further our knowledge of both licit and illicit drugs.

Pharmacokinetics describes the movement of a drug within the body and especially how a drug's concentration in blood, body fluids, and tissues varies over time. A drug's concentration is determined by factors that influence its absorption, distribution, metabolism, elimination, and excretion. An understanding of pharmacokinetics is important because the magnitude of a drug's pharmacologic effect depends on the concentration of drug at its site of action.

The study of the biochemical and physiologic effects of drugs and their mechanisms of action is termed *pharmacodynamics*. Whereas pharmacokinetics can be explained as "what the body does to the drug," pharmacodynamics can be thought of as "what the drug does to the body."

As our knowledge of systems, circuits, receptors, and intracellular pathways advances, so does our ability to intervene pharmacotherapeutically. The chapters in this section summarize our advancing state of knowledge in these areas.

PHARMACOKINETICS

Absorption Psychoactive drugs can be inhaled (glue, solvents, amyl nitrate), smoked (nicotine, marijuana, freebase cocaine), sniffed intranasally (cocaine, heroin), taken orally (ethanol, caffeine, amphetamines, barbiturates, opiates), administered intravenously (heroin, cocaine, methamphetamine), or injected subcutaneously. Occasionally, such drugs are taken transdermally (fentanyl and nicotine patches), intramuscularly, sublingually, or rectally (Fig. 6.1).

The more rapidly a psychoactive drug is delivered to its site of action in the central nervous system, the greater is its reinforcing effect. Smoked and inhaled drugs bypass the venous system and thus have the most rapid rate of delivery. Absorption of inhaled drug depends on the physical characteristics of the drug, including its volatility, particle size, and lipid solubility (1). Drugs that reach the alveoli of the lungs have rapid access to the bloodstream through closely applied capillary alveolar surfaces. Because a large portion of the cardiac output passes through the pulmonary circulation, the delivery of drug from the alveoli to the brain is enhanced.

In contrast to inhaled drugs, different factors affect the rate of absorption for orally administered drugs. These factors include (i) the pharmaceutical properties of the oral dosage form, (ii) the pH of gastric contents (drugs can be destroyed by extreme acid or basic conditions), (iii) gastric emptying time (except dumping; faster gastric emptying time results in more rapid delivery to the small intestine, the site of absorption), (iv) intestinal transit time (for drugs absorbed in the small intestine, there is an increased rate of absorption with a faster intestinal transit time, unless saturation occurs), (v) integrity of intestinal epithelium, and (vi) the presence of food (which decreases the interaction time between the drug and the intestinal villi) (2).

With illicit drugs, dose often is difficult to determine because of the presence of adulterants in the preparations as well as imprecise measurement of the amount consumed (as compared to the quantity of active ingredients in prescription medications, which is known precisely).

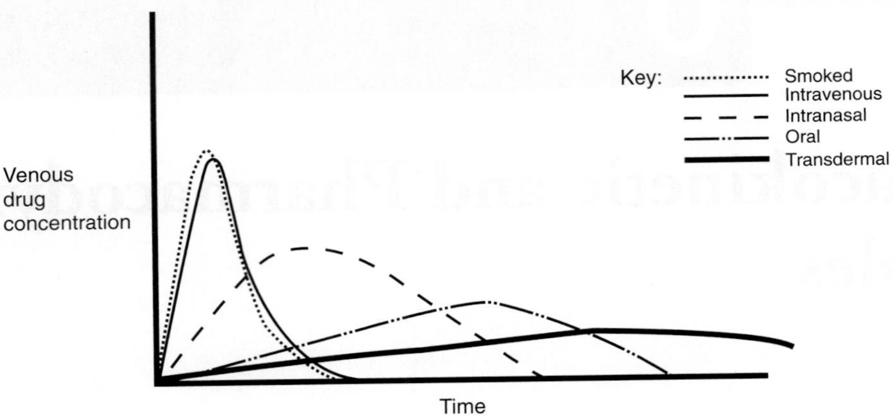

FIGURE 6.1. Venous drug concentrations after different routes of administration.

Bioavailability is defined as the fraction of unchanged drug that reaches the systemic circulation after administration by any route. The *bioavailability factor* (F) takes into account the portion of the administered dose that is able to enter the circulation unchanged. For intravenously administered drugs, F = 1.0 (100%). Bioavailability depends on a given drug's site-specific membrane permeability and its first-pass metabolism.

First-pass metabolism is the metabolism that occurs before a drug reaches the systemic circulation. Examples of drugs that show strong first-pass effects include morphine, methylphenidate, and desipramine. First-pass metabolism is particularly important for drugs administered by oral and deep rectal routes. After absorption across the gut wall, the portal blood delivers the drug to the liver before it enters into the systemic circulation. The liver can excrete the drug in the bile, and the drug can undergo enterohepatic recirculation. Metabolism by the gut and liver can significantly reduce a drug's bioavailable fraction.

First-pass metabolism is relatively unimportant for drugs administered through the intravenous, sublingual, intramuscular, subcutaneous, and transdermal routes. This is because drugs administered by these routes enter the general circulation directly.

Drugs must pass through biologic membranes to be absorbed. With passive diffusion, biologic membranes are more permeable to lipid soluble and uncharged molecules. Some drugs have diminished absorption because of a reverse transporter associated with p-glycoprotein. This reverse transporter actively pumps drug out of the gut wall cells back into the gut lumen. When p-glycoprotein is inhibited, increased drug absorption results.

Some food and drug interactions alter first-pass metabolism and absorption from the intestinal wall. For example, components of grapefruit juice and other foods that either inhibit or induce intestinal wall CYP3A4 or p-glycoprotein can lead to altered bioavailability of drugs that are substrates for this cytochrome (3). Also, the nonselective monoamine oxidase inhibitors (MAOIs) such as phenelzine and tranylcypromine—and, to a much lesser extent, the MAO B inhibitor selegiline and the reversible MAOI moclobemide—inhibit MAO A in the intestinal wall and liver. This inhibition diminishes the first-pass metabolism of tyramine, which is present in cheeses and various foods (4). When tyramine, an indirect-acting sympathomimetic amine, reaches the systemic circulation, it can produce increased release of norepinephrine from the sympathetic postganglionic neurons; this, in turn, can result in a severe pressor response and hypertensive crisis.

Upon absorption, when drug concentrations are graphed against time, a peak drug concentration (C_{max}) is reached at T_{max}. The trough concentration is C_{min}. The area under the concentration-time curve (AUC) is a measure of drug exposure that can be calculated (as the sum of trapezoids) and quantified.

Hastening gastric emptying can help to achieve a more rapid drug effect without altering bioavailability. Gastric emptying can be hastened by taking a drug on an empty stomach with at least 200 mL water and remaining in an upright position. Food, recumbency, heavy exercise, and drugs that slow gastric emptying (such as narcotics, anticholinergic drugs, and antacids) can result in later and lower peak concentrations of the index drug.

If the rate but not the extent of absorption is diminished, then the peak concentration decreases, the trough concentration increases, and the area under the curve is unchanged. The average steady-state concentration is unchanged, and there is no need to adjust the dose of a given drug to achieve therapeutic drug levels. In contrast, if the rate of absorption is unchanged but the extent of absorption is diminished, then both the peak and trough concentrations will be less. The area under the curve will decrease. Because the average steady-state concentration also will be diminished, a dose adjustment will be needed to achieve the therapeutic drug level. Therefore, when dosing prescribed drugs, a change in the rate of drug absorbed generally has less clinical significance than a change in the extent of drug absorbed.

Distribution Once absorbed, a drug is distributed to the various organs of the body. Distribution is influenced by how well each organ is perfused with blood, the organ's size, bind-

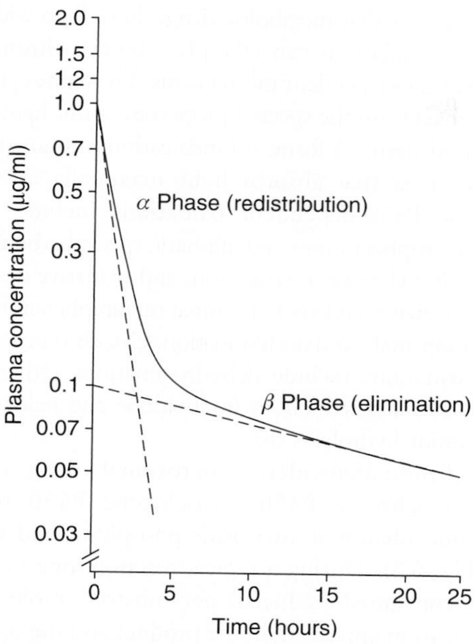

FIGURE 6.2. Plot of log concentration versus time for drug disposition characteristics consistent with an open two-compartment model.

ing of the drug within the blood and in the tissues, and the permeability of tissue membranes (5).

Distribution in the body can be understood by using a single "well-stirred" compartment, multiple compartments, or a model-independent approach. The single-compartment model assumes spontaneous equilibration of the drug between tissues and blood; it can be used when experimental data plotted on a logarithmic scale of drug concentration versus time yields a straight line with a declining slope.

In multicompartment models, spontaneous equilibration of the drug between the tissues and blood is not assumed, and the drug may be eliminated from one of several compartments. In a multicompartment model, the number of compartments required equals the number of exponential terms needed to describe the experimentally derived plasma concentration time curve (Fig. 6.2). Thus, a two-compartment model is best described by a bi-exponential equation, with constants used to describe the average transfer rate between compartments. For instance, a two-compartment model might include a central compartment and a tissue or peripheral compartment. Although drug distribution within a compartment is not homogenous and the concentrations of drug within and among such tissues may be quite variable, tissues of a compartment are grouped together because the time to achieve distribution equilibrium in such tissues is similar. Thus, the mathematically derived compartments may not be physiologically representative (5). Also, calculations involved in multicompartment models use differential equations and can become quite complex.

More recently, model-independent pharmacokinetic analysis has been developed as a simpler alternative to multicompartmental modeling. Noncompartmental pharmacokinetic analysis focuses on the average time drug molecules are in the body and uses calculations derived from a moment curve, which plots the product of concentration and time versus time alone.

When a drug distributes into all of the body compartments and tissues, it is said to distribute into an apparent *volume of distribution* (V_d). This volume has no direct physical equivalent because it describes the amount of serum, plasma, or blood that would be required to account for all drug in the body if the entire dose of that drug were spread uniformly throughout. V_d can be thought of as the amount of drug in the body (D = dose) divided by the concentration of drug (C) in the plasma, or

$$V_d = \frac{D}{C}$$

Drugs with a small V_d are confined primarily to the intravascular space of approximately 5 L. The drugs may be tightly bound to plasma proteins, or they may have a high molecular weight (large proteins, dextrans, and so forth). Drugs can have large V_d values up to 50,000 L if they are highly bound to tissue sites or are lipophilic.

Drugs with a large V_d thus partition into fat and bind to tissue. The volume of distribution and the fraction of unbound drug are terms that help quantify drug distribution. Acidic drugs commonly bind to albumin, the most abundant plasma protein. Drugs that bind primarily to albumin include barbiturates, benzodiazepines, and phenytoin. Basic drugs often bind to alpha$_1$-acid glycoprotein and to lipoproteins. Methadone is an example of a drug that primarily binds to alpha$_1$-acid glycoprotein, whereas amitriptyline and nortriptyline bind primarily to lipoproteins. Other binding proteins include gamma-globulin, transcortin, fibrinogen, and thyroid-binding globulin.

Several comparisons between albumin and alpha$_1$-acid glycoprotein can be made (6). Albumin, which is synthesized by the liver, can be decreased, especially with chronic illness and renal failure. Alpha$_1$-acid glycoprotein, which is an acute phase reactant produced by the liver, is relatively unaffected by chronic renal failure. Alpha$_1$-acid glycoprotein increases with chronic inflammatory disease, acute trauma, and stress. Alpha$_1$-acid glycoprotein levels vary relative to their total amount more than those of albumin. Also, alpha$_1$-acid glycoprotein (0.8 g/100 mL) is saturated much more readily than albumin (4.0 g/100 mL) because it is present in lower amounts.

The activity of a drug depends not on its total quantity but on the concentration of free drug at its site of action. This free concentration is clinically relevant for drugs such as phenytoin, warfarin, and thyroxine, which are more than 90% bound to plasma proteins.

The rate of blood flow delivered to specific organs and tissues is important. Well-perfused tissues can receive large quantities of drug, provided that the drug can cross the membranes or other barriers present between the plasma and tissue. In contrast, poorly perfused tissues, such as fat, receive drug at a slow rate. This action explains why the concentration of drug in fat can continue to increase long after the concentration in plasma has begun to decrease.

Most psychoactive drugs enter the brain because they are highly lipid soluble. The blood–brain barrier hinders the ability of non-lipid-soluble drugs to reach the brain tissue by diffusion (7). Unlike the fenestrated capillaries found throughout the body, which allow movement of molecules less than 25,000 daltons, the endothelial cells lining brain capillaries have tight junctions and do not permit these small molecules to pass through. Without fenestrations, drugs must cross the two membranes of the endothelial cell by passive diffusion in order to enter the brain. The blood–brain barrier limits the admittance of many drugs to the brain. However, for some compounds, specific active transport systems exist. These active transport systems enable glucose, amino acids, amines, purines, nucleosides, and organic acids to gain access to the brain. In contrast, p-glycoprotein is an efflux carrier present in the brain capillary endothelial cell, which bars the drug from translocating across the endothelial cell and actively exports the drug out of the brain.

It is important to note where the blood–brain barrier exists. The blood–brain barrier is found throughout the brain and spinal cord at all regions central to the arachnoid membrane, except for the floor of the hypothalamus and the area postrema, including the chemoreceptor trigger zone (where direct-acting chemicals can provoke vomiting).

Metabolism Metabolism is the process by which lipophilic drugs and foods are mostly transformed to more polar products that are more readily eliminated. Compared with the parent drug, drug metabolites usually have a diminished volume of distribution and diminished ability to penetrate cellular membranes. Not all metabolites are inactive or nontoxic; some biotransformation products have enhanced activity or toxic properties, including mutagenicity, teratogenicity, and carcinogenicity. Active metabolites need to be considered when assessing a drug's total activity. Also, scientists have made use of inherent drug-metabolizing enzymes to optimize drug delivery by designing pharmacologically inactive prodrugs that are converted in vivo to pharmacologically active molecules. One example of a prodrug is levodopa, which (after crossing the blood–brain barrier) is converted in the basal ganglia to dopamine.

Drugs can be metabolized by Phase I and/or Phase II reactions. Phase I reactions are nonsynthetic reactions in which the drug is chemically altered and oxidized. Phase II reactions are synthetic reactions in which the drug is conjugated with another moiety, such as glucuronide. Phase I reactions often provide the active site for Phase II reactions, but occasionally a Phase II conjugate becomes a substrate for a Phase I oxidation. Examples of nonsynthetic reactions include the oxidation of phenobarbital, amphetamine, meperidine, and codeine by microsomal enzymes. Examples of synthetic reactions include the glucuronidation of morphine and meprobamate, acetylation of clonazepam and mescaline, and methylation of dopamine and epinephrine. In each case, the drug is made more polar to facilitate elimination.

The enzymes that metabolize drugs do so for a wide variety of moieties. Oxidations can take place by cytochrome P450-dependent and independent mechanisms. The name cytochrome P450 is derived from the spectral properties of this hemoprotein. In its reduced (ferrous) form, it binds carbon monoxide to produce a complex that absorbs light maximally at 450 nm. Cytochrome P450-dependent oxidations include aromatic (phenytoin, amphetamine) and aliphatic (pentobarbital, meprobamate) hydroxylations, epoxidation, and oxidative dealkylation (morphine, caffeine, codeine), deamination (amphetamine), desulfuration (thiopental), and dechlorination. Cytochrome P450-independent oxidations include dehydrogenations (ethanol); azo, nitro, and carbonyl reductions (methadone and naloxone); and ester and amide hydrolyses (8).

Cytochrome-dependent microsomal drug oxidation requires cytochrome P450, cytochrome P450 reductase, nicotinamide adenine dinucleotide phosphate, and molecular oxygen (Fig. 6.3). During a typical reaction, one molecule of oxygen is consumed (reduced) per substrate molecule, with one oxygen atom appearing in the product and the other in the form of water. More than 50 individual CYPs have been identified in humans.

As a family of enzymes, CYPs are involved not only in the metabolism of dietary and environmental compounds and medications but in the degradation of bile acids from cholesterol, the metabolism of retinoic and fatty acids including prostaglandins and eicosanoids, and the synthesis of steroids. A large number of specialized CYPs with specific substrate preferences are involved in these latter endogenous functions in contrast to the relatively few numbers of CYPs that metabolize xenobiotics, which have wider ranging and overlapping capabilities. CYPs that metabolize medications not only have a tremendous capacity to oxidize a large number of structurally diverse compounds but can metabolize a single compound at different positions on that molecule (9). Drug metabolizing CYPs' large and fluid substrate binding sites contribute to their slow catalytic rates. In part, this explains why the half-lives of drugs are much longer than the half-lives of endogenous compounds.

Cloning and sequencing of CYP complementary DNAs, and more recently total genome sequencing, have revealed the existence of 57 putatively functional genes and 58 pseudogenes in humans (9). CYPs are named with the root CYP followed by a number designating the family, a letter denoting the subfamily, and another number designating the CYP form. Thus CYP2B6 is family 2, subfamily B, and gene number 6. Twelve CYPs (CYP1A1, 1A2, 1B1, 2A6, 2B6, 2C8, 2C9, 2C19, 2D6, 2E1, 3A4, and 3A5) are known to metabolize xenobiotics in humans (9,10). The CYP1A, CYP1B, CYP2A, CYP2B, and CYP2E subfamilies catalyze the metabolic activation of many protoxins and procarcinogens to their reactive metabolites, whereas CYP2C, CYP2D, and CYP3A subfamilies are more important for drug metabolism. CYP3A4 alone is responsible for metabolizing more than 50% of clinically prescribed drugs.

Genetic variability in drug metabolizing enzymes can influence drug response. Single nucleotide polymorphisms

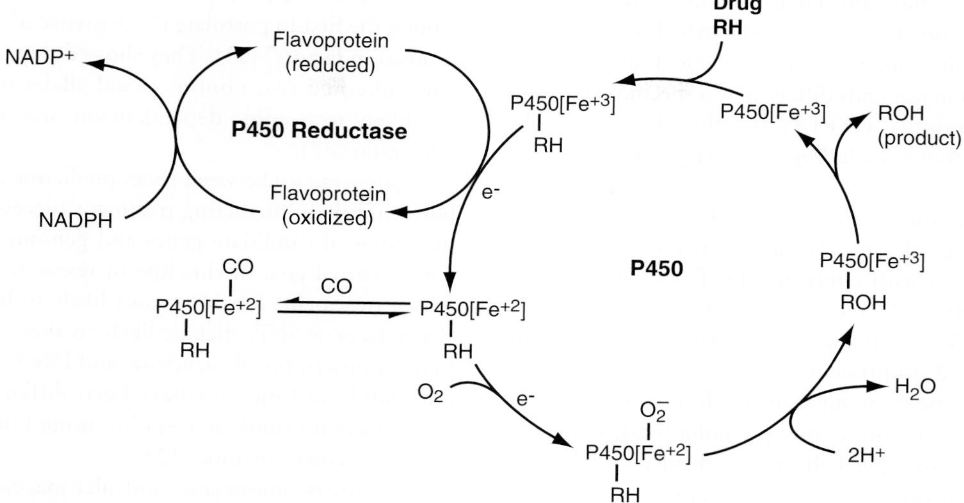

FIGURE 6.3. The potent oxidizing properties of this activated oxygen permit oxidation of a large number of substrates. Substrate specificity is very low for this enzyme complex. High lipid solubility is the only common structural feature of the wide variety of structurally unrelated drugs and chemicals that serve as substrates in this system. Cytochrome P450 cycle in drug oxidations. (RH, parent drug; ROH, oxidized metabolite; e$^-$, electron.) (From Katzung BG, *Basic & Clinical Pharmacology*, 10th ed. New York: McGraw-Hill; 2006, with permisson.) http://www.accessmedicine.com

(SNPs) may alter CYP activity (11). For example, for CYP2D6, the best studied of the drug metabolic enzymes, 48 mutations and 50 alleles have been identified. Genotype and enzyme activity are linked to ethnicity, which varies from no gene/no enzyme activity (6% of whites) to two copies of a fully active gene (33% of Ethiopians). Individuals can be genotyped for 2D6 enzyme function (with classification as poor, intermediate, extensive, and ultra-rapid metabolizers (12). CYP2D6 genotype is important to metabolism of numerous drugs that are substrates of the metabolic enzyme. For example, the metabolism of codeine to the potent analgesic, morphine, is determined by CYP2D6 genotype. Those with genotypes associated with an enzyme with reduced metabolic function can result in patients not obtaining effective analgesia with codeine administration.

CYP2B6 has been less well studied. However, important genotypic influences on enzyme function have been identified and examples of the importance of the variation in enzyme function on substrate metabolism follow. Several alleles have now been characterized as to enzyme amounts and activities, including CYP2B6 *1 (wild type), *2, *4, *5, *6, *9, and *18 (13). The *4 allele codes for an enzyme of higher function than the wild type. This allele has been associated, for example, with the toxicity of bupropion, an antidepressant medication and treatment for nicotine dependence. This toxicity is due to increased rates of conversion of bupropion to the active and longer-lasting metabolite, hydroxybupropion. Another substrate of CYP2B6 is the HIV medication, efavirenz. In a recent study of efavirenz metabolism, hydroxylation was noted to be significantly lower (relative to normal activity genotype CYP2B6*1/*1) in those with the CYP2B6*1/*6 and CYP2B6*6/*6 genotypes. Individuals with those genotypes were noted to have less enzyme present and lower enzyme activity as well. Genotypes CYP2B6*1/*5 and CYP2B6*5/*6 had lower amounts of protein present but no decrease in metabolic activity, likely owing to higher specific activity of the enzyme (14). The CYP2B6 allele *6 has also been found to be associated with diminished enzyme activity and can lead to toxicities related to increased plasma drug concentrations, which in the case of efavirenz was correlated with neuropsychologic toxicity (15).

CYP3A4 has also had numerous SNPs identified. However, thus far, none of 28 CYP3A4 SNPs identified in CYP3A4-phenotyped persons has been associated with low hepatic CYP3A4 protein expression or low CYP3A4 activity in vivo. Whites with low CYP3A4 activity have been screened for alleles and enzyme function. Allelic variants including CYP3A4*1B, CYP3A4*2, CYP3A4*4, CYP3A4*5, CYP3A4*6, CYP3A4*8, CYP3A4*11, CYP3A4*12, and CYP3A4*13 were examined, but none of these alleles correlated with reduced enzyme activity (10). Further, SNPs in human subjects who received one dose of midazolam, a CYP 3A4/5 substrate, and found up to an 11-fold difference in clearance and 18 SNPs. However, none of these SNPs correlated with enzyme activity. These results indicated that the genetic variants identified in the CYP3A4 and CYP3A5 genes have only a limited impact on CYP3A-mediated drug metabolism in vivo (16). Several opioids including methadone and buprenorphine are metabolized by CYP3A4. The role of genetic polymorphisms in metabolism of CYP3A4 substrates is unclear at this time and an area of active research.

Many drugs, foods, and environmental chemicals can induce and/or inhibit the activity of the cytochromes, speeding up or slowing down their own metabolism. Each cytochrome isozyme responds differently to specific exogenous chemicals. For example, CYP1A1 is induced by polycyclic aromatic hydrocarbons, including benzo[α]pyrene contained in cigarette smoke.

Drug interactions at the level of the cytochromes are often clinically significant. Methadone is metabolized primarily by CYP3A4, with contributions from CYP2B6 and to a lesser extent CYP2D6 and possibly CYP1A2 (17). Inhibitors of CYP3A4 including erythromycin, diltiazem, ketoconazole, and saquinavir, slow the metabolism of methadone and increase methadone levels. Inducers of CYP3A4 such as carbamazepine, phenobarbital, efavirenz, and Saint John's wort speed the metabolism of methadone and decrease methadone levels. Inhibitors tend to act more quickly than inducers. Awareness of potential interactions, clinical observation, and tailoring medication regimens and dosages are needed to optimize therapy and minimize potential toxicities.

Drug interactions also can cause altered *biotransformation*. When cocaine is used in conjunction with ethanol, the pharmacologic effect of cocaine is both prolonged and enhanced (18). A carboxylesterase catalyzes an ethyl transesterification of cocaine to cocaethylene, which is biologically active. In addition, ethanol inhibits cocaine metabolism. The increased levels of cocaine and cocaethylene can contribute to the prolonged and enhanced effects of cocaine.

Noninvasive markers are being developed to assess the activity of these cytochrome isozymes, including caffeine for CYP1A2, coumarin for CYP2A6, dextromethorphan for CYP2D6, and erythromycin for CYP3A4 (8,19). The new discipline of pharmacogenetics aims to elucidate cytochrome and other drug-metabolizing enzyme polymorphisms, the degrees of expression of these polymorphisms, and the functional significance of such expression. Understanding these polymorphisms can help to explain individual differences in drug response. For instance, slow metabolizers of a drug may have a relative deficiency of specific enzymes responsible for the drug's metabolism. Such poor metabolizers may experience increased side effects of specific drugs at lower drug doses.

Drug metabolism may influence risk of addiction, with relative protection for persons who experience adverse drug reactions at lower drug doses. Both the ADH1B2-His47Arg allele of alcohol dehydrogenase 1B and the ALDH-Glu487Lys allele of aldehyde dehydrogenase 2 alone or together can lead to flushing, nausea, and headache owing to the accumulation of acetaldehyde when alcohol is consumed. Each of these alleles leads to a reduction in the risk of alcoholism, with an additive protective effect when the same person carries both alleles. Persons of South Asian descent are likely to carry both alleles, whereas those with Jewish ancestry often carry the Arg47 allele. Heterozygous carriers of ALDH2 Lys487 have low levels of ALDH2 enzyme activity whereas ALDH2 Lys487/Lys487 homozygotes are nearly completely protected from alcoholism (20). Tyndale and colleagues were among the first to postulate the existence of "pharmacogenetic protection factors" (21). They showed that a sample of whites who inherited two nonfunctional alleles for CYP2D6 were less likely to become dependent on oral opiates (estimated odds ratio $>$7).

Convergence between genes predicting addiction vulnerability and those predicting treatment success are being sought in studies of candidate genes and genome-wide association. The eventual goal of this line of research is to develop and match treatments for those most likely to benefit from them. Recently, gene SNPs that are likely to alter cell adhesion, enzymatic, transcriptional, structural and DNA, RNA, and/or protein-handling functions have been differentially correlated with successful smoking cessation using bupropion and nicotine replacement methods (22).

Scientists, physicians, and pharmaceutical manufacturers also are interested in pharmacogenetics. Drug manufacturers would like to prevent adverse drug effects in consumers. One idea to help prevent adverse effects from drugs is to develop a registry that identifies persons lacking specific metabolic enzymes and cytochromes. Given a choice of medications, it would be better to choose a therapeutic regimen that does not require adjustment in dose due to pharmacologic predisposition or interaction with other medications (23).

Liver disease has many pharmacokinetic implications. The direction and quantity of these effects can change with the extent and course of illness. Reductions in liver blood flow, shunting of blood, alterations in plasma proteins and bile flow, and dysfunction of hepatocytes could be associated with the pathologic process. Drug bioavailability increases as first-pass metabolism decreases. The fraction of unbound drug could be altered. Modifications in the number and activity of metabolizing enzymes can take place, but these changes are not uniform among the liver enzyme classes (24,25).

Although drug metabolism occurs largely in the liver, most other tissues and organs, including the lungs, gastrointestinal tract, skin, and kidneys, carry out varying degrees of drug metabolism. Understanding brain metabolism can be especially important in understanding the activity of psychoactive drugs. Many P450 cytochromes have been shown to catalyze the metabolism of neurosteroids as well as psychoactive drugs such as neuroleptics and antidepressants. Alcohol produces a three- to fivefold increase in the level of brain P450 and induces CYP2C, CYP2E1, and CYP4A (26). Brain CYP2D6 can demethylate 3,4-methylenedioxy-N-methylamphetamine (MDMA or "ecstasy") forming a harmful metabolite, N-methyl-a-methyldopamine. Brain CYP2D6 can O-demethylate paramethoxyamphetamine (PMA), a synthetic psychostimulant and hallucinogen, into 4-hydroxyamphetamine, which is also toxic (27). CYP2B6 metabolizes cocaine, phencyclidine, and some amphetamines. Both CYP2B6 and CYP2D6 are inducible by nicotine (27). P450s in other brain areas are induced by different factors (e.g., levels of CYP2C and

CYP4A influence the activity of neurotransmitters such as dopamine, which use fatty acid metabolites as intracellular mediators).

Novel brain CYPs, such as 5α-androstane-3β, 17β-diol hydroxylase, CYP7B, and CYP2D4, continue to be discovered. Because the level of CYPs in the brain is approximately 0.5% to 2% of that in the liver and brain CYP isoenzymes are of different types than those found in the liver, brain CYPs appear to be locally active but contribute little to overall pharmacokinetics of drugs in the body (28). The regulation of cytochrome P450 isozyme expression in the brain and elsewhere is being studied.

Elimination and Excretion *Elimination* refers to disappearance of the parent and/or active molecule from the bloodstream or body, which can occur by metabolism and/or excretion. *Excretion* is the process of removing a compound from the body without chemically changing that compound. Drugs can be excreted through the urine or feces, exhaled through the lungs, or secreted through sweat or salivary glands.

The term *clearance* (Cl) represents the theoretical volume of blood or plasma that is completely cleared of drug in a given period of time (29). It is calculated as follows:

$$\frac{\text{Dose}}{\text{AUC}} = k_{el} \times V$$

Clearance is a *rate* whose units are volume over time. Because it is a rate, clearance is not an indicator of the amount of drug that is being removed.

The factors that determine hepatic clearance are hepatic blood flow (Q), the fraction of drug that is unbound (f_{ub}), and the drug's intrinsic clearance (Cl_{int}). The intrinsic clearance is a measure of the liver's ability to metabolize the drug. These terms are related by the following equation:

$$Cl_{hep} = \frac{Q\, f_{ub}\, Cl_{int}}{Q + f_{ub}\, Cl_{int}}$$

If the intrinsic clearance of an unbound drug is very small, the metabolic capacity of the liver, rather than hepatic blood flow, becomes the major determinant of hepatic clearance. If the intrinsic clearance of an unbound drug is very large, blood flow to the liver becomes rate-limiting.

The total clearance for a drug is the sum of its renal and nonrenal clearances. A convenient method to determine a given drug's renal clearance is to quantify the amount of drug excreted unchanged in the urine during a given time interval and to divide this value by the area under the plasma concentration versus time curve (AUC) for the same time interval (t_2-t_1). The equation for this determination is as follows:

$$Cl_R = \frac{C_{ur} \times V}{AUC_{t_2 - t_1}}$$

Here, C_{ur} is the drug concentration excreted in the urine collected during the time interval ($t_2 - t_1$), and V is the urine volume collected. Nonrenal clearance then is determined as the difference between the total and the renal clearances.

The *half-life* ($t_{1/2}$) of a drug is a measure of time required for a drug to arrive at or decay from steady state. This measure is such that 1 half-life represents a 50% change, and 2, 3, 4, and 5 half-lives represent 75%, 87.5%, 93.7%, and 96.8% changes, respectively.

Drugs that have dose-independent (first-order) disposition and elimination characteristics reach a steady-state concentration in 4 to 5 half-lives. In this case, the time to reach steady state depends on the duration of the half-life, whereas the amount of drug in the body at steady state will depend on the frequency of drug administration and its dose.

A drug's half-life ($t_{1/2}$) depends on its volume of distribution (V_d) and its clearance (Cl). This relationship can be written as follows:

$$t_{1/2} = \frac{0.693 \times V_d}{Cl}$$

The constant 0.693 in this equation is derived as an approximation of the natural logarithm of two [ln(2)]. Because drug elimination can be described by an exponential process, the time taken for a twofold decrease can be shown to be proportional to ln(2) (30).

Half-life is dependent on clearance and volume of distribution. For example, as clearance decreases because of aging or a disease process, half-life would be expected to increase. However with aging and disease, there may also be alterations in body water and lipid content influencing the volume of distribution. One cannot make assumptions about the volume of distribution or clearance of a drug based solely on knowledge of its half-life. If the half-life of a drug is lengthened, the clearance can be increased, decreased, or unchanged, depending on corresponding changes in the volume of distribution.

In addition, since $k_{el} = Cl/V_d$, the preceding equation can be written as $k_{el} = 0.693/t_{1/2}$, where k_{el} is a percentage of drug in the body that is eliminated per unit of time.

Most drugs display *first-order elimination* kinetics. When first-order kinetics are graphed, there is an exponential decay in the rate of elimination of the drug so that the concentration of drug in the body diminishes logarithmically over time. The *fraction* or *percentage* of the total amount of drug present in the body that is removed at any one time remains constant and is independent of dose. Given these relationships, a drug's plasma concentration can be calculated if its initial concentration, elimination half-life, and elapsed time are known:

$$C_t = C_o e^{-(k_{el} t)}$$

In contrast, drugs with *zero-order elimination* kinetics eliminate a constant amount of drug (rather than a constant fraction of drug). In most cases, the maximal rate of metabolism and/or elimination is due to the saturation of a key enzyme. Clearance then varies with the concentration of the drug, according to the Michaelis Menton equation. Because the half-life depends on the variable clearance, it too is not constant. Therefore, half-life is not particularly useful for drugs eliminated by zero-order kinetics. Ethanol, phenytoin, and salicylic

FIGURE 6.4. Extrapolating the decrease in blood alcohol concentration from two prior readings.

$$\text{Slope} = \frac{115\text{ mg/dl} - 75\text{ mg/dl}}{2\text{ hr}}$$

$$= \frac{40\text{ mg/dl}}{2\text{ hr}} = 20\,\frac{\text{mg/dl}}{\text{hr}}$$

expect at 4 hrs BAL to be 55 mg/dl
5 hrs BAL to be 35 mg/dl
6 hrs BAL to be 15 mg/dl
7 hrs BAL to have already reached 0.00 mg/dl

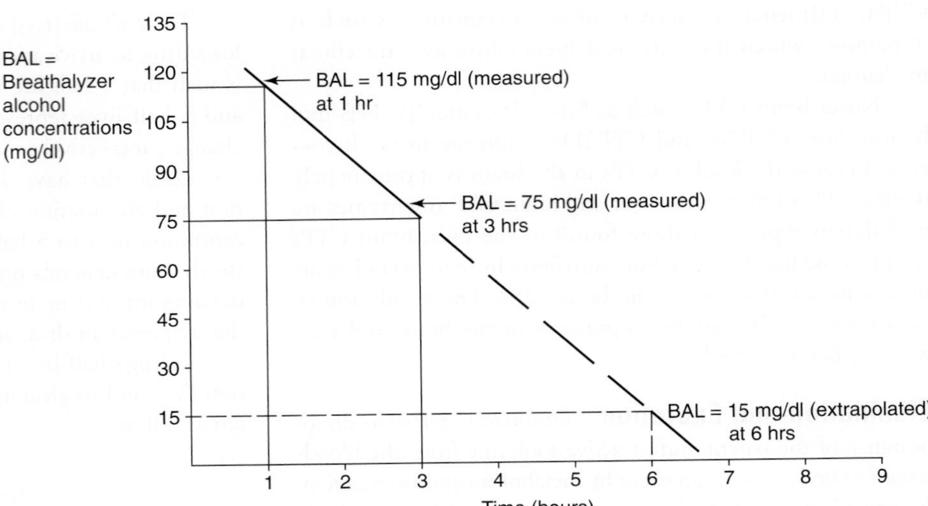

acid are prominent examples of drugs that display zero-order kinetics. Ethanol is eliminated at a constant rate no matter how much drug is in the system. With the use of regular graph paper, one can determine future alcohol concentrations at specific times by extrapolating a line from two data points, as shown in Figure 6.4.

According to multicompartmental modeling, a drug can have multiple half-lives rather than a single half-life. The terminal half-life is the most important, as it characterizes the elimination rate from the body. The other half-lives (alpha, beta, and so forth) can represent a combination of absorption, redistribution, and/or elimination.

Model-independent pharmacokinetics uses the concept of the mean residence time (MRT) to determine an elimination half-life without attention to the different phases. The MRT is the average amount of time a molecule resides in the body and is calculated as the area under the moment curve (AUMC) divided by the area under the concentration versus time curve (AUC), or:

$$\text{MRT} = \frac{\text{AUMC}}{\text{AUC}}$$

The area under the moment curve (AUMC) is derived from a plot of concentration multiplied by time ($c \times t$) on the y axis, versus time (t) on the x axis.

Therapeutics Based on Pharmacokinetic Calculations

Pharmacokinetics explores the relationship between drug dose and the time-varying concentration of drug at its site(s) of action. When pharmacokinetic equations are used to make therapeutic calculations, half-life can be used to determine the dosing interval, clearance to determine the dosing rate, the volume of distribution to determine the loading dose, and bioavailability to determine the dose adjustment.

A rational dosage regimen is based on the assumption that there is a target concentration that will produce a desired therapeutic effect. This target drug concentration falls within a therapeutic range whose lower bounds are a minimal therapeutic concentration and whose upper bounds are a minimum toxic concentration. Pharmacokinetic computations can be used to achieve such a dosage regimen.

First, a *maintenance dose* can be calculated as a product of the dosing rate and dosing interval, as follows:

$$\text{Maintenance dose} = \text{Dosing rate} \times \text{Dosing interval}$$

In a steady state, the dosing rate is primarily determined by the clearance of a drug. Because a *steady state* (^{ss}) is reached when the rate of drug acquisition into the body is equal to the rate of its elimination:

At steady-state, rate in = rate out:

$$\text{Bioavailability} \times \begin{matrix}\text{dosing}\\ \text{rate}\end{matrix} = \text{clearance} \times \begin{matrix}\text{desired}\\ \text{plasma}\\ \text{concentration}\end{matrix}$$

$$F \times \frac{\text{dose}}{\text{dosage interval}} = Cl \times Cp^{ss}$$

Rearranging the terms, the dosing rate can be calculated if the clearance, target concentration of the drug in plasma, and its bioavailability are known:

$$\begin{matrix}\text{Dosing}\\ \text{rate}\end{matrix} = \text{clearance} \times \frac{\begin{matrix}\text{desired steady}\\ \text{state plasma}\\ \text{concentration}\end{matrix}}{\text{bioavailability}} = \frac{Cl \times Cp^{ss}}{F}$$

The units (volume/time) should be consistent for the variables in the calculations.

TABLE 6.1 An Example Using Pharmacokinetic Calculations: Determination of a Loading Dose, the Expected Resulting Plasma Conceentration, an Infusion Rate, and an Ineremental Loading Dose

M.B. is a 4-year-old African American child, weighing 15 kg, who is to receive intravenous phenobarbital to treat his seizure disorder. The $t_{1/2}$ for phenobarbital is 48 hours. Given a V_d of 0.5 L/kg and a desired steady-state concentration (Cp^{SS}) between 15 and 40 mg/L, calculate an appropriate dosage regimen.

What loading dose would you recommend to achieve a concentration of 30 mg/L?

$C_{p\ desired} = 30$ mg/L

$V_d = 0.5$ L/kg $\times$ 15 kg $= 7.5$ L

Loading dose $= D = C_o \times V_d = 30$ mg/L $\times$ 7.5 L $= 225$ mg

If no further doses are given, what is the expected plasma concentration at 24 hours?

$K_{el} = 0.693/t_{1/2} = 0.693/48$ h $= 0.015$/h

$C_{24h} = C_o\, e^{-(kt)} = 30$ mg/l $[e^{-(.015/h)(24h)}] = 20.9$ mg/l

What is the infusion rate if M.B. were to be maintained at the 30 mg/L concentration level?

$Cl = k_{el} \times V_d = (0.015/h) \times (7.5\ L) = 0.113$ L/h

$$\text{Infustion rate} = K_o = \text{dosing rate} = \frac{Cl \times Cp^{ss}}{F}$$

$$= \frac{(0.113\,\frac{L}{H} \times 30\ mg/L)}{1} = 3.4\ mg/h$$

M.B. is not responding to a Cpss of 30 mg/L. You consider increasing his Cp^{ss} to 45 mg/L before adding another medication. To achieve this, what incremental loading dose would you now order?

$$\text{Incremental loading dose} = \frac{V_d \times Cp^{ss}}{F}$$

$$= \frac{V_d \times (C_{desired} - C_{current})}{F}$$

$$= \frac{7.5\ L(\frac{45\ mg}{L} - \frac{30\ mg}{L})}{1}$$

$$= 7.5\ L \times 15\ mg/L = 112.5\ mg$$

When it is essential to produce a therapeutic concentration of a drug quickly, a loading dose (D1) may be given:

$$\text{Loading dose} = \text{volume of distribution} \times \frac{\text{desired plasma concentration}}{\text{bioavailability}} = \frac{V_d \times Cp}{F}$$

A loading dose may be needed at the onset of therapy, especially if a drug's volume of distribution is large. Note that clearance does not enter into this calculation. If an incremental *loading dose* is needed, then the formula is as follows:

$$\text{Incremental loading dose} = \frac{V_d \times (C_{p\ desired} - C_{p\ initial})}{F}$$

Pharmacokinetic principles can be used to help practitioners attain target drug concentrations in their patients. A protocol designed by Holford in 2001 uses these calculations to individualize and adjust drug dosage. It has the following steps:

1. Choose the target concentration.
2. Predict V_d and Cl according to standard population values, with adjustments for factors such as weight and renal function.
3. Administer a loading dose or maintenance dose calculated by using target concentration, V_d, and Cl.
4. Measure the patient's response and drug concentration.
5. Revise V_d and/or Cl according to the measured concentration.
6. Repeat steps 3 to 5, adjusting the predicted dose to achieve the target concentration.

A clinical example applying these principles is illustrated in Table 6.1. In the preceding discussion, the estimates of dosing rate and average steady-state concentration (calculated by using clearance) are independent of any specific pharmacokinetic model. In contrast, the determination of the maximum and minimum steady-state concentrations require further pharmacokinetic assumptions. The accumulation factor assumes that the drug follows a one-compartment body model, and the peak concentration assumes that the absorption rate is more rapid than the elimination rate (30).

PHARMACODYNAMICS

The study of pharmacodynamics is the study of the biochemical and physiologic effects of drugs on the body. This study includes an understanding of the mechanisms of drug action, dose-response phenomena, and the body's regulatory response to this activity. A few drugs affect the body's physiologic functions by changing the environment of the cells rather than acting directly through cellular receptors. They include ammonium chloride, used to acidify the urine; antacids, used to neutralize gastric acidity; and sodium bicarbonate. Most drugs, however, act on specific endogenous targets, not to create new effects but rather to modulate the rate and extent of the body's endogenous functions. Receptors and their associated effector and transducer proteins coordinate signals from multiple ligands with the metabolic activities of the cell to act as integrators of this information.

The concept of the receptor dates to the turn of the 20th century. Paul Ehrlich introduced the term *receptor* as he

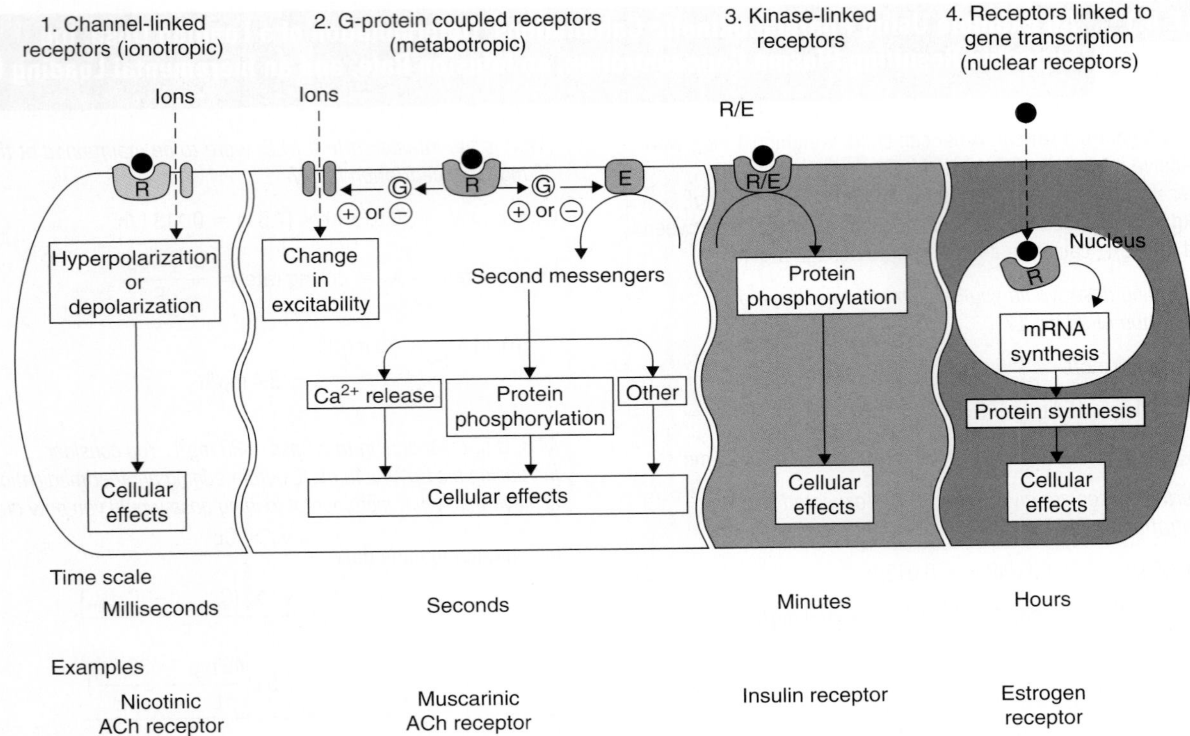

FIGURE 6.5. Types of receptor-effector linkage. (From Rang HP, Dale MM, Ritter JM, Moore PK, eds. *Pharmacology*, 5th ed. Philadelphia: Churchill Livingstone, 2003.)

described sites on what he believed to be a single very large molecule of cell protoplasm to which bacterial toxins (and later, drugs) bound to bring about changes in cellular metabolism. John Newport Langley investigated the actions of curare and nicotine on skeletal muscle and put forth the concept that drugs bind to specific binding sites or "receptive substance" to cause their effects. Alfred Joseph Clark then used a simple mathematical model to quantify the relationship between drug concentration and response. These discoveries laid the foundation for experimental pharmacology (31).

Originally, the term *receptor* was applied generically to all drug targets because there was no clear sense of how binding gave rise to a biologic effect. Some of these targets subsequently turned out to be structural proteins, enzymes of crucial metabolic or regulatory pathways, and proteins involved in transport processes of the cell. For example, some antibiotics work by disrupting bacterial cell membranes, and many chemotherapeutic agents alter intracellular DNA and/or RNA replication. This chapter focuses on the principles of pharmacology pertinent to psychoactive drugs. In this context, the term *receptor* will be used to designate controllers of regulatory processes, including transducers for neurotransmitters and hormones that produce endogenous biologic signals.

Receptor Physiology Receptors contain at least two functional domains: a ligand binding site and an effector or message propagation (i.e., signaling) area. Receptors can be grouped according to four common types. These are (i) ligand-gated ion channels, (ii) G protein–coupled receptor signaling, (iii) receptors with intrinsic enzymatic activity (guanylate cyclase, serine/threonine kinase, tyrosine kinase activity, tyrosine phosphatases), and (iv) receptors regulating nuclear transcription (Fig. 6.5). The relatively small number of mechanisms for cell signaling is fundamental to how target cells integrate signals from multiple receptors to produce sequential, additive, synergistic, or inhibitory responses.

Ligand-Gated Ion Channels These receptors selectively gate the flow of ions through channels into the cell. Each unit of these multisubunit proteins spans the plasma membrane several times. The association of the subunits allows the formation of a wall or pore. Binding to single or multiple subunits then enables these subunits to rapidly and cooperatively control channel opening and closing to alter cell membrane voltage potential. Excitatory neurotransmitters (e.g., acetylcholine and glutamate) result in a net inward current of cations such as Na^+, Ca^{+2}, and K^+, which depolarize the cell and increase the generation of action potentials. In contrast, inhibitory neurotransmitters (e.g., GABA and glycine) result in the inwards flux of anions such as Cl^-, which hyperpolarize the cell and decrease the generation of action potentials.

Ligand-gated channels enable rapid transformation of information across synapses. They are involved in synaptic plasticity required for learning and memory. Ligand-gated ion channels can be regulated by multiple mechanisms including endocytosis and phosphorylation.

G Proteins and Second Messengers "Serpentine" receptors coupled to G proteins have an extracellular amino (N) terminal and an intracellular carboxyl (C) terminal and commonly transverse the plasma membrane seven times. When agonists approach G protein receptors from the extracellular fluid, they bind to a site surrounded by the transmembrane regions. A change of confirmation occurs that is transmitted to the cytoplasmic loops of the receptor that in turn activates the appropriate G-protein. Several serpentine receptors exist as dimers or larger complexes. Dimerization may influence ligand preference and/or regulate the affinity and specificity of the complex for G protein and for other events important in the termination of action of the receptor (32). Examples of G protein receptors include muscarinic acetylcholinergic receptors, receptors for adrenergic amines, serotonin, and many peptide hormones.

G proteins modify the activity of regulatory proteins and/or ion channels, which in turn alter the activity of intracellular second messengers that enable signal transduction and amplification. Cells of different tissues may have different G protein–dependent responses to the same initial ligand (e.g., norepinephrine, acetylcholine, serotonin).

Among the well-established second messenger systems are cyclic adenosine monophosphate (cAMP) (by means of G_s and G_i), cyclic guanosine monophosphate (cGMP), and phosphoinositides (by means of G_q). β-Adrenergic amines, glucagon, histamine, serotonin, and numerous other hormones act on G_s to increase adenylyl cyclase and then increase the second messenger, cyclic adenosine monophosphate, whereas 2-adrenergic amines, muscarinic acetylcholine, opioids, serotonin, and others act on G_{i1}, G_{i2}, and G_{i3} to decrease adenylyl cyclase and then decrease cAMP. cAMP stimulates distinct cAMP-dependent protein kinases that are differentially expressed in varying tissues. When cAMP binds to the regulatory dimer (D) of the kinase, two catalytic (C) chains are released, which diffuse through the cytoplasm and nucleus, transferring phosphate from ATP to other specific enzymes and substrate proteins (Fig. 6.6a). When the hormonal stimulation stops, a diverse group of specific and nonspecific phosphatases quickly reverse the cAMP-induced phosphorylation of enzyme substrates, and cAMP is degraded to 5′AMP by several cyclic nucleotide phosphodiesterases. The cGMP-based signal transduction mechanism closely parallels the cAMP-mediated signaling mechanism, but its presence is limited to a few tissues including intestinal mucosa and vascular smooth muscle. Whereas methylxanthines (e.g., caffeine and theophylline) act by competitively inhibiting cAMP degradation, sildenafil produces vasodilation by inhibiting specific phosphodiesterases, which inhibit cGMP degradation.

Receptors for G_q including muscarinic acetylcholine, bombesin, serotonin (5-HT_{1C}), and others act through G proteins or tyrosine kinases to stimulate phospholipase C in the cell membrane that splits phosphatidylinositol-4,5-bisphosphate (PIP_2) into two second messengers, diacylglycerol (DAG) and inositol-1,4,5-triphosphate (IP_c or $InsP_3$) (Fig. 6.6b). Confined to the membrane, diacylglycerol activates a phospholipid- and

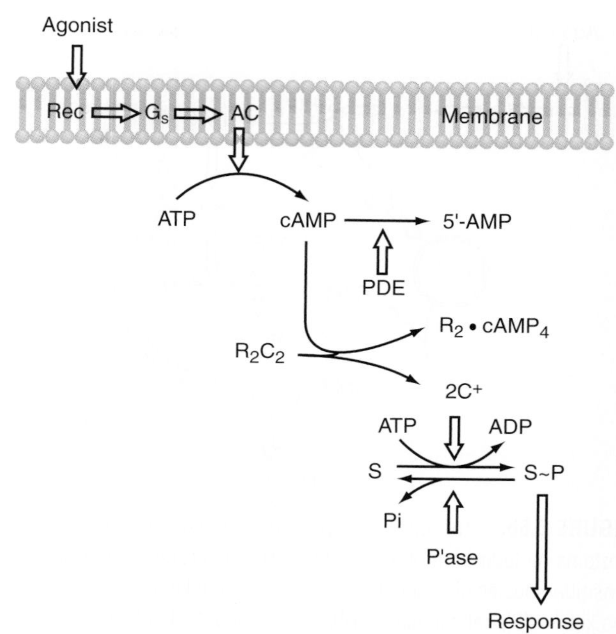

FIGURE 6.6a. The cAMP second messenger pathway. Key proteins include hormone receptors (Rec), a stimulatory G protein (G_s), catalytic adenylyl cyclase (AC), phosphodiesterases (PDE) that hydrolyze cAMP, cAMP-dependent kinases, with regulatory (R) and catalytic (C) subunits, protein substrates (S) of the kinases, and phosphatases (P'ase), which remove phosphates from substrate proteins. Open arrows denote regulatory effects. (From Katzung BG: *Basic & Clinical Pharmacology,* 10th ed. New York: McGraw-Hill; http://www.accessmedicine.com 2006, with permission.)

calcium-sensitive protein kinase C, whereas water-soluble IP_3 diffuses through the cytoplasm, enabling the release of Ca^{+2} from internal storage vesicles. Elevated cytoplasmic Ca^{+2} is bound to calmodulin, which regulates the activities of other enzymes, including calcium-dependent protein kinases. This signaling pathway is inactivated when IP_3 is dephosphorylated, and DAC is either phosphorylated to phosphatidic acid and converted back into phospholipids or deacylated to arachidonic acid, and Ca^{2+} is actively removed by calcium pumps from the cytoplasm. The phosphoinositide signaling pathway is more complex than the cAMP pathway owing to multiple second messengers and protein kinases. For instance, more than nine structurally distinct types of protein kinase C have been identified. In addition, protein kinases of different cell types may have general or specified substrate targets.

G protein receptors undergo pharmacodynamic tolerance. They acutely attenuate their response by reversible and rapid desensitization. When agonists induce conformational change of this receptor, it binds and activates a family of G protein–coupled receptor kinases (GRKs). The activated GRK then phosphorylates serine residues in the receptor's carboxy terminal tail, increasing the affinity for β-arrestin, which in turn diminishes the receptor's ability to interact with G_S, reducing the stimulation of adenylyl cyclase and the agonist response. Cellular

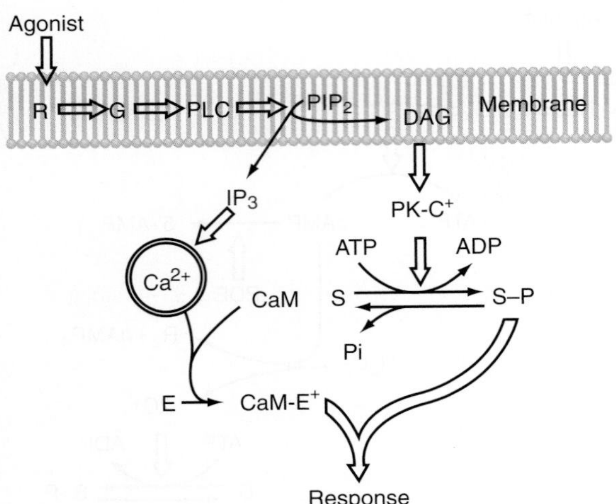

FIGURE 6.6b. The Ca^{2+}-phosphoinositide signaling pathway. Key proteins include hormone receptors (R), a G protein (G), a phosphoinositide-specific phospholipase C (PLC), protein kinase C substrates of the kinase (S), calmodulin (CaM), and calmodulin-binding enzymes (E), including kinases, phosphodiesterases, etc. (PIP_2, phosphatidylinositol-4,5-bisphosphate; DAG, diacylglycerol; IP_3, inositol trisphosphate. Asterisk denotes activitated state. Open arrows denote regulatory effects.) (From Katzung BG: *Basic & Clinical Pharmacology,* 10th ed. New York: McGraw-Hill; http://accessmedicine.com 2006, with permission.)

phosphatases can terminate GRK activation, facilitate removal of phosphate, and restore initial responsiveness to the agonist.

Desensitization may be homologous or heterologous. Homologous desensitization indicates feedback directed to the receptor molecule itself, whereas heterologous desensitization extends to the action of all receptors that share a common signaling pathway. Heterologous desensitization may involve inhibition of one or more downstream proteins that participate in signaling from other receptors as well.

Agonists can also induce endocytosis and membrane trafficking of receptors. β-Arrestin accelerates endocytosis of receptors from the plasma membrane by binding to endocytotic structures in the plasma membrane called *coated pits*. This endocytosis can either result in the receptor's recycling through the plasma membrane with continued cellular responsiveness or cause receptor trafficking to lysosomes such that degradation of the receptor causes down-regulation and attenuated cellular responsiveness. Recent work by Kim et al. showed (33) that increased endocytosis and recycling of opiate receptors in the plasma membrane (created by a knock-in mouse expressing mutant MOP-R) was associated with continued morphine analgesia but reduced tolerance and dependence.

Receptors with Intrinsic Enzyme Activity These polypeptide receptors typically consist of an extracellular growth factor or hormone-binding domain connected to a cytoplasmic enzyme domain by a hydrophobic segment that crosses the plasma membrane's lipid bilayer. The cytoplasmic enzyme domain may be a tyrosine kinase, a serine/threonine kinase, or a guanylate cyclase that, when activated, catalyses the activity of substrate proteins followed by additional downstream signaling proteins. For instance, when epidermal growth factor binds to its receptor, it converts the receptor from its inactive monomeric state to an active dimeric state of two noncovalently bound receptor polypeptides. The enzymatic cytoplasmic domains become activated and catalyze the phosphorylation of substrate proteins. Drugs may target the agonist binding site and/or the enzymatic activity of the receptor.

Some receptors including those for neurotrophic peptides and cytokines lack their own intracellular enzymatic domains. When responding to drug agonists, they bind or activate distinct protein kinases on the cytoplasmic face of the plasma membrane. For instance, cytokine receptors form dimers when activated. This dimerization results in separate activation of mobile Janus-kinase molecules that phosphorylate tyrosine residues on the receptor of signal transducers and activation of transcription molecules, which then travel to the nucleus to regulate transcription.

Signaling by insulin and atrial natriuretic peptide, as well as trophic hormones involved in growth and differentiation, begin their processes invoking enzymatic receptors. Once activated, enzymatic receptors may undergo endocytosis and down-regulation, as occurs with platelet-derived growth factor, or translocation in endocytic vesicles from the distal axon to the cell body, as occurs with nerve growth factor.

Receptors Regulating Nuclear Transcription Receptors that regulate nuclear transcription are soluble DNA-binding proteins that bypass the plasma membrane to reach their intracellular targets. They include (a) the steroid family of androgen, progesterone, glucocorticoid, and mineralocorticoid receptors, (b) the thyroid/retinoid family consisting of thyroid, vitamin D, and retinoic acid, and (c) the orphan receptor family, whose endogenous ligand, if any, remains unknown.

When inactive, these receptors are bound to proteins in the cytoplasm. They are then assembled as homodimers or heterodimers with ligand-binding, DNA-binding, and transcriptional regulation domains. The ligand-binding site confers a negative regulatory role. When hormone binds to the receptor, it relieves an inhibitory constraint, allowing the DNA-binding domain to bind to specific DNA sequences (called *response elements*) on the genome to activate or inhibit transcription of the nearby gene. For example, when cortisol binds to the glucocorticoid receptor, heat shock protein 90 is released. This allows the DNA-binding and transcription-activating domains of the receptor to fold into their functionally active conformations so that the activated receptor can initiate transcription of target genes.

As gene active hormones require time for synthesis of new proteins, they have a relatively slower onset and offset of action.

A Mechanistic Classification of Selected Drugs of Abuse

Abused drugs generally activate the mesolimbic system by (a) interacting with ion channel receptors, (b) binding to G_{io}-coupled receptors, or (c) interfering with monoamine

TABLE 6.2 The Mechanistic Classification of Drugs of Abuse

Name	Main molecular target	Pharmacology	Effect on dopamine (DA) neurons
Drugs that bind to ionotropic receptors and ion channels			
Nicotine	nAChR	Agonist	Disinhibition
Alcohol	$GABA_AR$, 5-HT_3R, nAChR, NMDAR, Kir3 channels	—	Disinhibition
Benzodiazepines	$GABA_AR$	Positive modulator	Disinhibition
Phencyclidine, ketamine	NMDAR	Antagonist	—
Drugs that activate G protein–coupled receptors			
Opioids	-OR (G_{io})	Agonist	Excitation, disinhibition (?)
Cannabinoids	CB1R (G_{io})	Agonist	Excitation, disinhibition (?)
γ-Hydroxybutyric acid (GHB)	$GABA_BR$ (G_{io})	Weak agonist	Disinhibition
LSD, mescaline, psilocybin	5-$HT_{2A}R$ (G_q)	Partial agonist	—
Drugs that bind to transporters of biogenic amines			
Cocaine	DAT, SERT, NET	Inhibitor	Blocks DA uptake
Amphetamine	DAT, NET, SERT, VMAT	Reverses transport	Blocks DA uptake, synaptic depletion
methylenedioxymethamphetamine (MDMA)	SERT > DAT, NET	Reverses transport	Blocks DA uptake, synaptic depletion

5-HTxR, serotonin receptor; CB1R, cannabinoid-1; DAT, dopamine transporter; GABA, - aminobutyric acid; Kir3 channels, G protein-coupled inwardly rectifying potassium channels; LSD, lysergic acid diethylamide; -OR, -opioid receptor; nAChR, nicotinic acetylcholine receptor; NET, norepinephrine transporter; NMDAR, *N*-methyl-D-aspartate receptor; SERT, serotonin transporter; VMAT, vesicular monoamine transporter;? indicates data not available.

Reprinted with permission from Katzung BG. *Basic & clinical pharmacology*, 10th ed. New York: McGraw-Hill Companies, Inc. http://www.accessmedicine.com (Katzung, Figure 32.1 reordered to match text).

transporters (34). Substances acting through the first two mechanisms tend to inhibit GABA inhibitory interneurons, resulting in a net release of dopamine. Drugs acting indirectly or directly upon ion channel receptors can additionally increase dopamine in the nucleus accumbens and ventral tegmental areas. Drugs that interfere with monoamine transporters block the reuptake or stimulate nonvesicular release of dopamine causing an accumulation of dopamine in target structures (Table 6.2).

Nicotine, benzodiazepines, phencyclidine, and ketamine work through ionotropic receptors. Nicotine activates the nicotinic acetylcholine receptor, and benzodiazepines are modulators of the $GABA_A$ receptor. Alcohol alters the function of several ionic receptors including $GABA_A$ receptors, K^+ inwardly rectifying or G protein activated inwardly rectifying K^+ channels (Kir3/GIRK), glycine receptors, *N*-methyl-D-aspartate (NMDA) receptors, and 5-HT_3 receptors. Alcohol also inhibits ENT1, the equilibrative nucleoside transporter for adenosine reuptake resulting in adenosine accumulation, stimulation of adenosine A_2 receptors, and enhanced cAMP response element-binding (CREB) signaling. Neither phencyclidine nor ketamine causes addiction or withdrawal, but both may lead to a long-lasting psychosis owing to noncompetitive antagonism of the NMDA receptor. Of the inhalants, nitric oxide acts on NMDA receptors whereas fuel additives enhance $GABA_A$ receptor function.

The opioids, cannabinoids, gamma-hydroxybutyric acid, and the hallucinogens all exert their action through G_{io}. Even though the mu, kappa, and delta opioid receptors all inhibit adenylyl cyclase, their selective neuronal expression results in different effects. For example, mu opioid agonists inhibit GABA inhibition of dopamine, causing a net release of mesolimbic dopamine, reinforcement, and euphoria. In contrast, kappa agonists inhibit dopamine neurons and induce dysphoria.

Cannabinoids cause presynaptic inhibition. The lipid soluble neurotransmitters 2-arachidonyl glycerol and anandamide bind to CB1 receptors to induce retrograde signaling from post- to presynaptic neurons, where they may inhibit the release of either glutamate or GABA.

The hallucinogens LSD, mescaline, and psilocybin neither stimulate dopamine release nor cause addiction. These drugs act through the 5-HT_{2A} receptor, which couples to G_q proteins and inositol triphosphate (IP_3) and leads to intracellular calcium release. Hallucinogens act by enhancing excitatory afferent input from the thalamus and increasing glutamate release in the cortex.

Cocaine, amphetamine, methamphetamine, and ecstasy bind to transporters of biogenic amines. Cocaine inhibits the dopamine transporter, decreasing dopamine clearance from the synaptic cleft and causing an increase in extracellular dopamine. Amphetamine competitively inhibits dopamine transport at the dopamine transporter and interferes with the vesicular monoamine transporter to lessen the storage of dopamine in the synaptic vesicles. As cytoplasmic dopamine increases, there is reversal of the dopamine transporter, increasing nonvesicular release of dopamine and further increasing extracellular dopamine. Ecstasy or methylenedioxymethamphetamine, like amphetamines, causes release of biogenic amines by reversing the serotonin and other transporters.

Allosteric Modulation of G Protein–Coupled Receptors: Activity Based Upon Conformational State It is now believed that G protein–coupled receptors can exist in multiple conformational states including ones that are active, inactive, partially active, and selectively active and those that produce nonproductive signaling though GTP-binding sites. If the conformational states of a receptor are in equilibrium and the inactive state predominates in the absence of drug, then the basal signal output from the downstream effector will be minimal or absent.

Drugs can bind to receptors at the same site or at a different site than the endogenous compound that physiologically activates that receptor. The relative affinity of the drug for various conformations of the receptor will determine the extent to which the equilibrium is shifted towards the active state. *Full agonists* have a higher affinity for the active conformation and drive the equilibrium toward the active state. *Partial agonists* bind to the receptor with only moderately more affinity for the active than for the inactive receptor. Even at saturating concentrations, partial agonists will not enable a full biologic response (Fig. 6.7).

Buprenorphine is an example of a highly potent mu opioid receptor partial agonist. The drug has a high affinity for mu receptors and displaces morphine, methadone, and other full opiate agonists from these receptors. In contrast to the full agonists, however, increases in buprenorphine dose may result in a longer duration of action but do not result in increased pharmacologic effects. Higher doses of buprenorphine can be given without respiratory depression. The partial agonist properties of buprenorphine may precipitate withdrawal in individuals who have a high level of physical dependence on opioids.

Antagonists have no effect upon response when used alone. They bind with equal affinity to the active and inactive conformations and prevent an agonist from inducing a response (35). Competitive antagonists may be reversed by adding excess agonist, but noncompetitive antagonists cannot be counteracted in this manner. With noncompetitive antagonists, there is a decrease in the agonist-induced E_{max} (maximal efficiency). The potency of some antagonists, particularly those that act by inhibiting the activity of an enzyme, often are expressed as an I_{50} value, which is the concentration of antagonist needed to elicit a 50% inhibition of enzyme activity.

Inverse agonists have preferential affinity for inactive receptor conformations when otherwise the equilibrium would be shifted towards an active receptor. In this case, inverse agonists produce an effect opposite to those of an agonist. However, if the basal equilibrium lies in the direction of the inactive receptor, then there will be little change in activity, and it will be difficult to distinguish inverse agonism from simple competitive antagonism (32).

Receptors can be constitutively in an active conformation or they can be activated by physiologic events even in the absence of an agonist. Pharmacologic agents that can induce or stabilize specific receptor conformations may be therapeutic. Inverse agonist drugs may be clinically useful if they can selectively prevent the pathologic aspects of receptor activation (36).

Agents that work at GABA-gated chloride ion channels illustrate this spectrum of drug activity. The endogenous agonist GABA acts at this receptor to produce inhibitory, hyperpolarizing postsynaptic potentials. Depending on variations in receptor structure and location in the central nervous system,

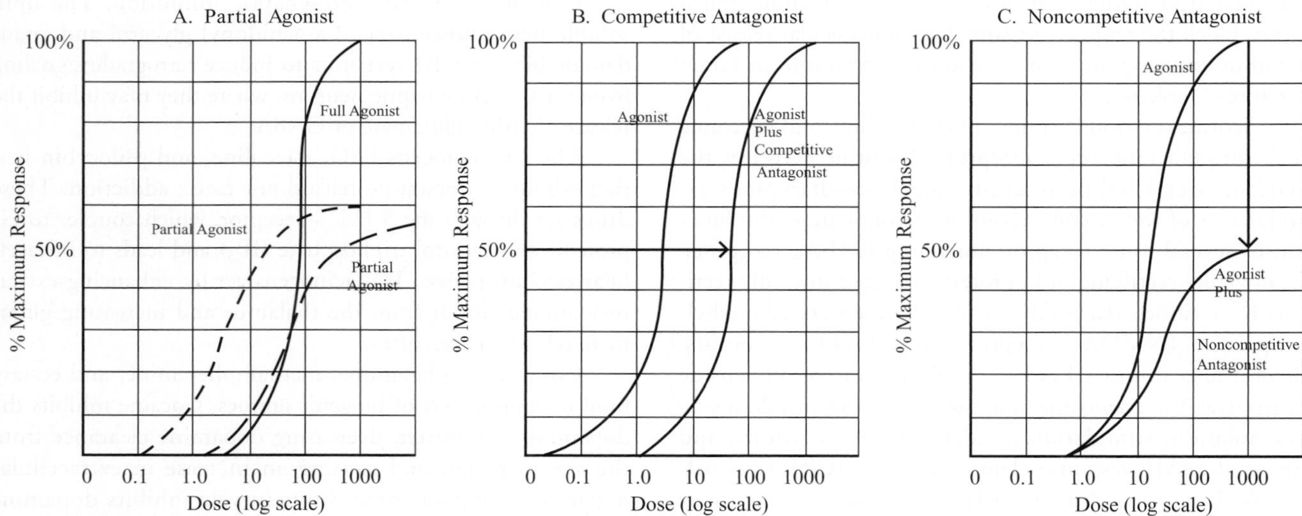

FIGURE 6.7. Full agonist, partial agonist, and competitive and noncompetitive antagonists. **A.** No matter how much the dose is increased, a partial agonist always will have a lower maximal efficiency (E_{max}). A partial agnoist may be more potent, less potent, or equally potent as the agonist. In this example, both partial agonists decrease E_{max}. However, one partial agonist is more potent, and the other partial agonist is equipotent, when compared to the full agonist. **B.** If there are no spare receptors, competitive agonists increase the EC_{50} but do not alter the other E_{max}. **C.** Non-competitive antagonists decrease the E_{max}. (Modified from Katzung BG & Masters SB (2002). Pharmacodynamics. In *Katzung & Trevor's Pharmacology Examination and Board Review.* New York, NY: Lange Medical Books/McGraw-Hill, 13.)

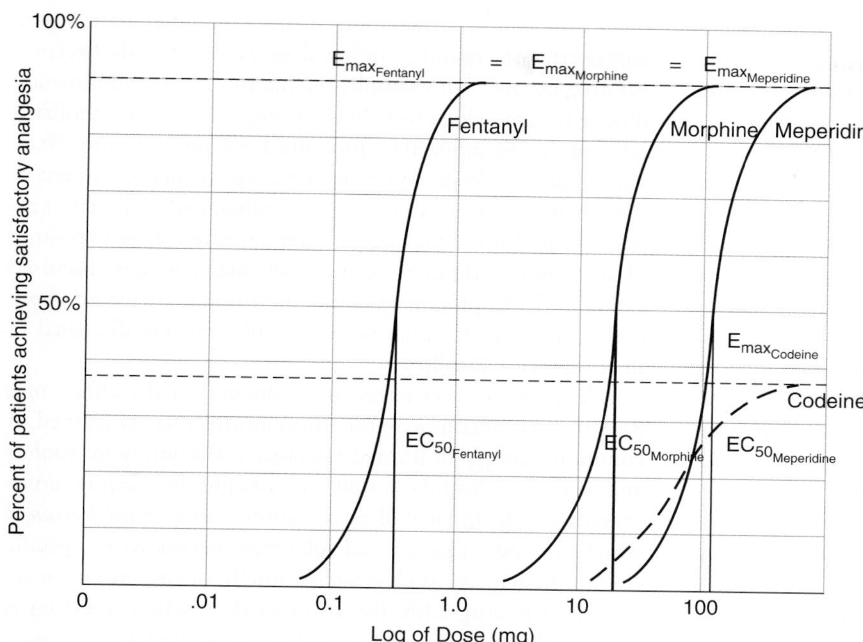

FIGURE 6.8. Dose response curves of some opioids. Fentanyl has a lower EC_{50} than morphine and is more potent than morphine. Both fentanyl and morphine have a higher Emax than codeine and are more efficacious than codeine. Meperidine is less potent than morphine but more efficacious than codeine.

this activity produces an assortment of sedative, anxiolytic, and anticonvulsant effects. Both barbiturates and benzodiazepines are pharmaceutical agonists that act at the GABA receptor. Binding of each of these drugs to the GABA receptor complex occurs at distinct sites and facilitates the activity of GABA to open the chloride-ion channel. Benzodiazepines increase the frequency of GABA-mediated chloride ion channel opening, whereas barbiturates increase the *duration* of this opening (37). Bicuculline, a competitive antagonist of GABA, binds selectively to the GABA site, interfering with GABA binding to that site. In contrast, picrotoxin, a noncompetitive antagonist of GABA, binds to the barbiturate site on the receptor, blocking the channel directly. Beta-carboline is an inverse agonist that reduces chloride ion conductance and increases excitability and irritability of the central nervous system; in fact, beta-carboline has no therapeutic use and can precipitate panic attacks. Flumazenil is an antagonist. Flumazenil lacks intrinsic activity but has therapeutic utility in treating benzodiazepine overdose. Flumazenil also blocks beta-carboline activity, although it does not antagonize the actions of ethanol or barbiturates.

Some drugs, depending on their concentrations, act as mixed agonists and antagonists. Mixed opioid agonist-antagonists have been developed in an attempt to produce analgesia with drugs that have less addictive potential and less respiratory depression. For example, nalbuphine and butorphanol are competitive mu receptor antagonists that exert their analgesic actions by acting as agonists at kappa receptors. Although each of these drugs has a place in the therapeutic armamentarium, unfortunately each is dependence-producing and associated with adverse effects, especially at higher doses.

Potency, Efficacy, and Dose Response When the response of a particular receptor-effector system is measured against increasing concentrations of drug, a graded dose-response graph is attained (Fig. 6.8). When drug dose is plotted on a logarithmic scale, a sigmoidal curve often results, permitting mathematical manipulation of the results. The *maximal efficacy* of a drug occurs at E_{max}, its maximal effect. Efficacy is the extent of functional change imparted to a receptor. Efficacy is determined mainly by the nature of the receptor and its associated effector system. In contrast, potency is primarily determined by the affinity of the receptor for the drug. *Potency* denotes the amount of drug needed to produce a given effect. The concentration of the drug needed to produce 50% maximal effect occurs at EC_{50}; the more potent the drug, the smaller the dose required to achieve maximal effect. In general, low potency is important only if the drug needs to be administered in undesirably large amounts. Because drug doses are readily adjusted, it is the maximal efficacy that is more often clinically relevant.

A similar sigmoidal curve is attained when the percentage of receptors that bind a drug is plotted against log drug concentration. Here, the concentration at which 50% of the receptors are bound is denoted K_d, and the maximum number of receptors bound are termed B_{max}. Both "dose response" and "dose-receptor bound" graphs have a linear or nearly linear middle segment, indicating a first-order process. As the concentration of drug increases, a constant proportion of the drug binds to the receptor, causing a proportionate drug effect.

A system is said to have spare receptors when the activation of fewer than 50% of the receptors achieves 50% of maximal effect. This determination is made by comparing the concentration for 50% of maximal effect, EC_{50}, with the concentration of 50% of maximal binding, K_d. If the EC_{50} is less than the K_d, spare receptors are said to be present. The presence of spare receptors does not alter the maximal biologic response, but it does increase the sensitivity to the drug ligand. This relationship occurs because drug-receptor interactions are more likely to appear when there are proportionately more available receptors.

When the log dose of a drug is plotted against the cumulative percentage of a population responding to a specified drug response, a quantal dose-response graph is achieved. The results of animal experiments can be plotted in this manner to discern the *median effective dose* (ED_{50}), *median toxic dose* (TD_{50}), and *median lethal dose* (LD_{50}). The *therapeutic index* is defined as the ratio of the TD_{50} to the ED_{50}. Because it is unethical to design experiments using a full range of drug doses to determine these indices in humans, the range of therapeutic drug concentrations and the margin of safety are estimated more broadly through extrapolation from animal studies, human drug trials, and clinical experience. In practice, both the risks and benefits of prescribing a medication are taken into account when making therapeutic decisions. Judgment about the clinically acceptable risk of toxicity often is influenced by the severity of the disease being treated.

Tolerance, Sensitization, and Physical Dependence Tolerance and sensitization reflect changes in the way the body responds to a drug *when it is used repeatedly*. Tolerance is the reduction in response to a drug after its repeated administration. Tolerance shifts the dose-response curve to the right, requiring higher doses than the initial doses to achieve the same effect. Sensitization indicates an increase in drug response after its repeated administration. Sensitization shifts the dose-response curve to the left, so that repeated doses cause a greater effect than that seen with the initial dose.

Tolerance and sensitization develop more readily to some drug effects than to other effects of the same drug. For example, tolerance to the euphoria produced by cocaine occurs much more rapidly than does tolerance to its cardiovascular effects. The discrepancy between tolerance to the "rush" experienced by drug users and tolerance to a drug's cardiovascular and respiratory effects can be an important cause of mortality in the user who overdoses. Also, chronic opiate users often have constipation and constricted pupils even though they no longer feel "high" after taking their drug. Differential toxicity can be explained by the dissimilar rates of drug tolerance that occur in diverse organ systems in individuals with unlike host characteristics.

Rodents experience sensitization, evidenced by an increase in locomotion, after being exposed to intermittent repeated doses of cocaine or amphetamine. In one study (38), this increase in behavioral activity was linked to an increase in dopamine levels in the extracellular fluid of the nucleus accumbens. Rats given repeated daily intraperitoneal cocaine injections (10 mg/kg) for 7 days had higher levels of dopamine detected by microdialysis on the seventh day than on the first day. Sensitization can be a phenomenon underlying chronic stimulant psychosis and/or alcohol withdrawal seizures.

There are several mechanisms by which tolerance can occur. *Pharmacokinetic tolerance* most often occurs as a consequence of increased metabolism of a drug after its repeated administration, resulting in less drug available at the receptor for drug activity. For example, the microsomal ethanol-metabolizing system, which usually is not important in metabolizing ethanol, can be induced by prolonged ethanol exposure. *Pharmacodynamic tolerance* refers to the adaptive changes in receptor density, efficiency of receptor coupling, and/or signal transduction pathways that occur after repeated drug exposure. Homologous and heterologous desensitization were discussed earlier under G protein receptors. Additional discussion about the mechanisms for pharmacologic tolerance are discussed in the chapters that follow.

Learned tolerance refers to a reduction in the effects of a drug because of compensatory mechanisms that are learned. A common example of learned tolerance is the ability for roofers and workers at heights to walk in a straight line despite motor impairment from alcohol intoxication. *Conditioned tolerance*, which is a subset of learned tolerance, occurs when specific environmental cues such as sights, smells, or circumstances are paired with drug administration so that, when the drug is taken in the presence of the specific environmental cue, a state of expectation occurs. With expectation, the drug effect may be experienced before the drug is taken—and an adaptive response may be learned (39). A powerful example of conditioned tolerance occurred in a study when rats died after being given a dose of opiates to which they previously had been tolerant. The deaths occurred when the rats were put in an unusual environment instead of the home cage where they were used to receiving the drug (40).

Cross-tolerance occurs when tolerance to the repeated use of a specific drug in a given category is generalized to other drugs in that same structural and mechanistic category. The cross-tolerance that occurs between alcohol, barbiturates, and benzodiazepines can be used to facilitate the smooth weaning of a patient from their drug of dependence during detoxification (see Section 6, "Management of Intoxication and Withdrawal").

Physical dependence is a state that develops as a result of the adaptation produced by resetting homeostatic mechanisms after repeated drug use. Withdrawal signs and symptoms can occur in a physically dependent person when drug administration is abruptly stopped. Withdrawal symptoms may reflect the interactions of numerous neurocircuits and organ systems. The molecular mechanisms of physical dependence caused by individual drugs are discussed in the chapters that follow.

Patients who take prescribed medications for appropriate medical indications can show tolerance, physical dependence, and withdrawal if the drug is stopped abruptly, even though they do not exhibit the compulsive drug use and negative consequences characteristic of drug addiction (39). The hypertensive rebound that occurs in patients when chronic administration of beta-adrenergic receptor blockers is abruptly discontinued is but one example of this phenomenon. Similarly, patients with pain may develop tolerance to opiates and require increased medication for pain relief. They may also develop physical withdrawal if chronically administered opiates are abruptly discontinued. Pain patients are not addicted to opiate medication unless they display compulsive behavior with adverse consequences despite being tolerant and/or physically dependent upon this medication (see Section 12, "Pain and Addiction").

CONCLUSIONS

This chapter gives an introduction to the pharmacologic principles that underlie the use of drugs for both therapeutic and nontherapeutic purposes. Pharmacokinetics, the study of how the concentration of a drug in the body varies over time, was discussed according to the processes of absorption, distribution, metabolism, elimination, and excretion. Pharmacodynamics, the study of the biochemical and physiologic effects of drugs and their mechanisms of action, was next covered. An introduction to receptor physiology of ligand-gated ion channels, G proteins and second messengers, receptors with intrinsic enzyme activity, and receptors regulating nuclear transcription built the foundation for discussing a mechanistic classification of selected drugs of abuse (41). Next, new concepts of allosteric modulation of G protein–coupled receptors formed the backdrop for a discussion of full and partial agonists as well as competitive and noncompetitive antagonists. The following chapters in this section elaborate on the pharmacology of individual mood and mind-altering chemicals and their drug classes, including further information about the topics of tolerance, sensitization, and physical dependence.

The conclusions in this paper represent the views of the authors and do not necessarily represent the views of NICHD or NIH.

REFERENCES

1. Meng Y, Lichtman AH, Bridgen DT, et al. Inhalation studies with drugs of abuse. In: Rapaka RS, Chiang N, Martin BR, eds. *Pharmacokinetics, metabolism, and pharmaceutics of drugs of abuse.* NIDA Research Monograph 173. Rockville, MD: National Institute on Drug Abuse, 1997:201–224.
2. Caviness MD, MacKichan J, Bottorff M, et al. *Therapeutic drug monitoring: a guide to clinical application.* Irving, TX: Abbott Laboratories, 1987. Diagnostics Division, 20.
3. Dresser GK, Spence JD, Bailey DG. Pharmacokinetic-pharmacodynamic consequences and clinical relevance of cytochrome P450 3A4 inhibition. *Clin Pharmacokinet* 2000;38(1):41–57.
4. Gardner DM, Shulman KI, Walker SE, et al. The making of a user friendly MAOI diet. *J. Clin Psychiatry* 1996;57(3):99–104.
5. Rowland M, Tozer TN. *Clinical pharmacokinetics: concepts and applications,* 3rd ed. Baltimore: Lippincott Williams & Wilkins, 1995.
6. Israili ZH, Dayton PG. Human alpha-1-glycoprotein and its interactions with drugs. *Drug Metab Rev* 2001;33(2):161–235.
7. Dziegielewska KM, Saunders NR. The ins and outs of brain barrier mechanisms. *Trends Neurosci* 2002;25(2):69–71.
8. Correia MA. Drug biotransformation. In: Katzung BG, ed. *Basic and clinical pharmacology,* 10th ed. Norwalk, CT: Appleton & Lange, 2007. http://www.accessmedicine.com.
9. Gonzalez FJ, Tukey RH. Drug metabolism. In: Brunton LL, Lazo JS, Parker KL eds. *Goodman & Gilman's the pharmacological basis of therapeutics,* 11th ed. New York: McGraw Hill Inc., 2005:71–91. Also in: http://www.accessmedicine.com.
10. Bertilsson L. Current status: pharmacogenetics/drug metabolism. In: Kalow W, Meyer UA, Tyndale RF, eds. *Pharmacogenomics.* New York: Marcel Dekker, Inc., 2001:33–50.
11. Flockhart DA, Bertilsson L. Clinical pharmacogenetics. In: Atkinson AJ, Abernathy DR, Daniels CE, et al., eds. *Principles of clinical pharmacology.* New York: Academic Press, 2007:179–195.
12. Daly, AK, Brockmoller J, Broly F, et al. Nomenclature for human CYP2D6 alleles. *Pharmacogenomics* 1996;6(3):193–201.
13. Zanger UM, Klein K, Saussele T, et al. Polymorphic CYP2B6: molecular mechanisms and emerging clinical significance. *Pharmacogenomics* 2007;8(7):743–759.
14. Desta Z, Saussele T, Ward B, et al. Impact of CYP2B6 polymorphism on hepatic efavirenz metabolism in vitro. *Pharmacogenomics* 2007;8(6):547–558.
15. Rotger M, Colombo S, Furrer H, et al. Swiss cohort study: influence of CYP2B6 polymorphism on plasma and intracellular concentrations and toxicity of efavirenz and nevirapine in HIV infected patients. *Pharmacogenet Genom* 2005;15(1):1–5.
16. He P, Court MH, Greenblatt DJ, et al. Genotype-phenotype associations of cytochrome P450 3A4 and 3A5 polymorphism with midazolam clearance in vivo. *Clin Pharmacol Ther* 2005;77(5):373–387.
17. Leavitt SB. Methadone-drug interactions. Pain treatment topics. [Special Report]. 2006b January. Available at: http://pain-topics.org/pdf/methadone-Drug_Intx_2006.pdf.
18. McCance-Katz EF, Kosten TR, Jatlow P. Concurrent use of cocaine and alcohol is more potent and potentially more toxic than use of either alone—a multiple-dose study. *Biol Psychiatry* 1998;44(4):250–259.
19. Zhu B, Ou-Yang DS, Chen XP, et al. Assessment of cytochrome P450 activity by a five-drug cocktail approach. *Clin Pharmacol Ther* 2001;70(5): 455–461.
20. Hejazi NS. Pharmacogenetic aspects of addictive behaviors. *Dialog Clin Neurosci* 2007;9(4):447–454.
21. Tyndale RF, Droll KP, Sellers EM. Genetically deficient CYP2D6 metabolism provides protection against oral opiate dependence. *Pharmacogenetics* 1997;7(5):375–379.
22. Uhl GR, Liu QR, Drgon T, et al. Molecular genetics of successful smoking cessation: convergent genome-wide association study results. *Arch Gen Psychiatry* 2008;65(6):683–693.
23. Wrighton SA, VandenBranden M, Ring BJ. The human drug metabolizing cytochromes P450. *J Pharmacokinet Biopharm* 1996;24(5):461–473.
24. Blaschke TF. Protein binding and kinetics of drugs in liver diseases. *Clin Pharmacokinet* 1977;2(1):32–44.
25. Blaschke TF. Effect of liver disease on dose optimization. *International Congress Series.* 2001;1220:247–258.
26. Warner M, Stromstedt M Wyss A, et al. Regulation of cytochrome P450 in the central nervous system. *J Steroid Biochem Mol Biol* 1993;47(1-6): 191–194.
27. Dutheil F, Beaune P, Loriot MA. Xenobiotic metabolizing enzymes in the central nervous system: contribution of cytrochrome P450 enzymes in normal and pathological human brain. *Biochimie* 2008;90(3):426–436.
28. Hedlund E, Gustafsson JA, Warner M. Cytochrome P450 in the brain: a review. *Curr Drug Metab* 2001;2(3):245–263.
29. Winter ME. *Basic clinical pharmacokinetics,* 2nd ed. Vancouver, WA: Applied Therapeutics, 1990.
30. Holford NGH. Pharmacokinetics and pharmacodynamics: rational dosing and the time course of drug action. In: Katzung BG, ed. *Basic and clinical pharmacology,* 8th ed. New York: Lange Medical Books/McGraw-Hill, 2001:35–50.
31. Flower R. Drug receptors: a long engagement. *Nature* 2002;415(6872):587.
32. Buxton, ILO. Pharmacokinetics and pharmacodynamics: the dynamics of drug absorption, distribution, action, and elimination. In: Brunton LL, Lazo JS, Parker KL, eds. *Goodman & Gilman's the pharmacological basis of therapeutics,* 11th ed. New York: McGraw Hill Inc., 2006:1–40. Also in: http://www.accessmedicine.com.

33. Kim JA, Bartlett S, He L, et al. Morphine induced receptor endocytosis in a novel knockin mouse reduces tolerance and dependence. *Curr Biol* 2008;18(2):129–135.
34. Luscher C. Drugs of abuse In: Katzung BG, ed. *Basic and clinical pharmacology*, 10th ed. New York: McGraw Hill Inc., 2007:511–526. Also in http://www.acessmedicine.com.
35. Gilchrist A. Modulating G protein-coupled receptors: from traditional pharmacology to allosterics. *Trends Pharmacol Sci* 2007;28(8): 431–437.
36. Buxton, ILO. Rethinking drug action in light of current models of receptor pharmacology. In: Brunton LL, Lazo JS, Parker KL, eds. *Goodman & Gilman's the pharmacological basis of therapeutics,* [Supplement to main textbook.] 11th ed. New York: McGraw Hill Inc., 2005: http://www.accessmedicine.com.
37. Trevor AJ, Way WL. Sedative-hypnotic drugs. In: Katzung BG, ed. *Basic and clinical pharmacology*, 8th ed. New York: Lange Medical Books/McGraw-Hill, 2001:364–381.
38. Kalivas PW, Duffy P. Effect of acute and daily cocaine treatment on extracellular dopamine in the nucleus accumbens. *Synapse* 1990;5(1): 48–58.
39. O'Brien CP. Drug addiction and drug abuse. In: Hardman JG, Limbird LE, Gilman AG, eds. *Goodman and Gilman's the pharmacologic basis of therapeutics*, 10th ed. New York: McGraw-Hill Inc., 2001: 621–642.
40. Siegel S, Hinson RE, Krank MD, et al. Heroin "overdose" death: the contribution of drug-associated environmental cues. *Science* 1982;216(4544):436–437.
41. Landry Y, Gies JP. Drugs and their molecular targets: an updated overview. *Fundam Clin Pharmacol* 2008;22(1):1–18.

CHAPTER 7

John J. Woodward, PhD

The Pharmacology of Alcohol

DEFINITION

Alcohol is a chemical name for a group of related compounds that contain a hydroxyl group (-OH) bound to a carbon atom. The form of alcohol that is voluntarily consumed by humans is ethyl alcohol or ethanol and consists of two carbons and a single hydroxyl group (written as C2H5OH or C2H6O). Unless otherwise noted, the term *alcohol* will be used throughout this chapter to mean ethanol.

SUBSTANCES INCLUDED IN THIS CLASS

In terms of human consumption, all commercially available alcoholic beverages contain ethyl alcohol, with concentrations depending upon the type of beverage. Beverages made by fermentation of sugar-containing fruits and grains include beer (3% to 8% ethanol by volume) and wines (11% to 13% ethanol by volume). Spirits are produced after distillation and generally contain at least 30% ethanol. Ethanol can be concentrated by simple distillation up to approximately 95%, whereas pure ethanol requires addition of benzene or related substances or dessication using glycerol. Denatured alcohol contains additives or toxins to prevent human consumption. Rubbing alcohol is prepared from denatured alcohol or isopropyl alcohol and is used for topical purposes.

FORMULATIONS AND METHODS OF USE

A bewildering array of alcoholic beverages is available for consumption, and these products contain a wide range of alcohol concentrations. In the United States, a standard alcoholic drink is defined as one that contains 0.6 fluid ounces of alcohol. Thus, this amount of alcohol is typically contained in 12 ounces of beer, 5 ounces of wine, or 1.5 ounces of distilled spirits (40% ethanol by volume), although this can vary depending on the specific type of beverage. Although most alcohol is consumed orally, there are isolated cases of individuals injecting ethanol intravenously (1). In addition, ethanol vapor can be inhaled, and machines called *AWOL* (alcohol without liquid; *www.awolmachine.com*) have been introduced into the United States as a novel means of self-administering alcohol. A number of U.S. states have since banned the sale or use of these devices.

CLINICAL USES

In addition to its use as a topical antiseptic, alcohol has several clinical indications including treatment of accidental or voluntary ingestion of methanol or ethylene glycol (2). Ethanol has a higher affinity for alcohol dehydrogenase than methanol and thus reduces the formation of methanol metabolites formaldehyde and formic acid. For both indications, hemodialysis is the recommended first line of treatment. Alcohol has also been used for treatment of various types of cysts (sclerotherapy) and was used historically for treatment of premature labor (2). Safer and more effective medications have largely replaced these uses. Alcohol combined with dextrose is used to increase caloric intake and for replenishing fluids. Alcohol, either given orally or IV, is sometimes used by physicians to treat withdrawal, particularly in a hospital setting. In a recent study, approximately one-half of inpatient hospital pharmacies surveyed reported having alcohol available for treatment of withdrawal, with surgical services requesting the majority of these uses (3).

BRIEF HISTORICAL FEATURES

Alcohol is one of the oldest used substances. Consumption of alcohol containing beverages predate recorded human history while written records of its use are found in Chinese and Middle Eastern texts as far back as 9,000 years ago. Alcoholic beverages have long been consumed as part of the daily diet and are also used for medicinal or symbolic effects. In modern times, alcohol is second only to caffeine in incidence of use, and its manufacture, distribution, and sale are of major economic importance across the world. Alcohol use worldwide is regulated by both societal and religious beliefs. In the United States, consumption of alcohol was legally restricted on the national level with passage of the Volstead Act and the Eighteenth Amendment to the U.S. Constitution in 1919 (4). Amid growing public outcry, prohibition was repealed in 1933 with the ratification of the Twenty-First Amendment that gave states the right to regulate the purchase and sale of alcohol. Today, sales and consumption of alcohol are under control of a wide variety of local and state laws.

EPIDEMIOLOGY

The lifetime exposure to alcohol is high, with nearly 88% of the U.S. population reporting using alcohol at least once in their lifetime (5). In 2006, current alcohol use (defined as use in the past 30 days) ranged from 3.9% among 12- to 13-year-olds to nearly 70% of 21- to 25-year-olds. Prevalence decreased among older groups although it was nearly 50% among 60- to 64-year-olds (5). Annual alcohol-related costs in terms of lost productivity and health care are estimated at $185 billion (6).

Clinical studies of alcohol abuse and alcoholism have led to the idea that there may be several types of alcohol use disorders, based on the appearance and severity of certain alcohol-related problems. Two particularly well-known examples of these classifications are the type I and type II forms proposed by Cloninger et al. and the Type A and B forms proposed by Babor (7). Cloninger's type I and Babor's type A share several similarities including (1) later onset of alcohol-related problems (younger than 25 years); (2) fewer childhood behavior problems; (3) relatively mild alcohol-related issues with fewer hospitalizations; and (4) lower degree of novelty seeking coupled with a preference toward harm avoidance. Type II and type B forms show essentially the opposite characteristics as type I and type A and include (1) familial alcoholism, (2) earlier onset of alcohol-related problems, (3) more incidents of alcohol-related problems or violence, and (4) higher preference for risk taking/novelty seeking. A recent analysis of the various proposed classifications of alcohol dependence suggests four general types of alcohol dependence: chronic/severe, depressed/anxious, mildly affected, and antisocial (8).

PHARMACOKINETICS

Alcohol is a small, water-soluble molecule that is rapidly and efficiently absorbed into the bloodstream from the stomach, small intestine, and colon. The rate of absorption depends on the gastric emptying time and can be delayed by the presence of food in the small intestine. Once in the bloodstream, alcohol is rapidly distributed throughout the body and gains access to all tissues, including the fetus in pregnant women. Although the relationship between alcohol intake and blood levels is body weight–dependent, gender is also important. When body weights are equivalent, women show a 20% to 25% higher blood alcohol level than men after ingestion of the same amount of alcohol. This appears to be due primarily to less gastric metabolism of alcohol in women as blood levels are not significantly different when alcohol is administered intravenously (9).

Alcohol is metabolized primarily by enzymatic pathways, and only small amounts of alcohol are excreted through the lungs as vapor. The odor of the breath is not a reliable indicator of alcohol consumption, because it is influenced by impurities in the alcoholic beverage. In the liver, alcohol is broken down by alcohol dehydrogenase (ADH) and mixed function oxidases such as P450IIE1 (CYP2E1). Levels of CYP2E1 may be increased in chronic drinkers. ADH converts alcohol to acetaldehyde, which subsequently can be converted to acetate by the actions of acetaldehyde dehydrogenase.

The rate of alcohol metabolism by ADH is relatively constant, as the enzyme is saturated at relatively low blood alcohol levels and thus exhibits zero order kinetics (constant amount oxidized per unit of time). Alcohol metabolism is proportional to body weight (and probably liver weight) and averages approximately 1 ounce of pure alcohol per 3 hours in adults. Thus, the time for an individual to become sober after even moderate intake of alcohol can be substantial. Although stimulants are often used to mask the depressant effects of alcohol, there do not appear to be any truly effective "alcohol antagonists" (amethystic agents) that can quickly reverse the intoxicating effects of alcohol. Naloxone (Narcan), the opiate antagonist, has been tested for its ability to reverse alcohol-induced coma but appears ineffective (10). Several $GABA_A$ receptor antagonists have also been examined, including flumazenil (Anexate), which is used to treat benzodiazepine overdose, and the experimental compound RO 15-4513. This compound, which is actually an inverse agonist, been reported to reverse some of the effects of low to moderate doses of alcohol in animals and may target a very specific subtype of $GABA_A$ receptor that shows sensitivity to very low concentration of ethanol (11). Although the clinical utility of an anti-alcohol medication for emergency medicine is undoubtedly high, moral, ethical, and medical concerns must be considered with respect to the development of such a drug as it would not be expected to alter the underlying deleterious effects of alcohol on organ systems.

PHARMACODYNAMICS

Central Nervous System Acutely, alcohol acts as a central nervous system (CNS) depressant. During the initial phase when blood alcohol levels are rising, a period of disinhibition often occurs, and signs of behavioral arousal are common. These include relief of anxiety, increased talkativeness, feelings of confidence and euphoria, and enhanced assertiveness. As drinking continues, there are impairments in judgment and reaction time, increased emotional outbursts, and ataxia. At higher blood levels, alcohol acts as a sedative and hypnotic, although the quality of sleep often is reduced after alcohol intake. In patients with sleep apnea, alcohol increases the frequency and severity of apneic episodes and the resulting hypoxia. Alcohol potentiates the sedative-hypnotic properties of both benzodiazepines and barbiturates, perhaps reflecting common mechanisms of action for these substances. Acute alcohol intoxication is not always associated with sedation or coma; indeed, some intoxicated individuals display violent behavior that requires administration of other sedative or antipsychotic agents. The use of these agents with a severely intoxicated individual must be approached cautiously to prevent respiratory failure. Chronic abuse of alcohol is associated with Wernicke's psychoses, and Korsakoff's, amnesia which are associated with deficiencies in nutrition and vitamin intake (particularly thiamine).

Other Organ Systems Acute alcohol ingestion usually produces a feeling of warmth as cutaneous blood flow is increased. This is accompanied by a reduction in core body temperature. Gastric secretions usually are increased, though the characteristics of these secretions depend on the concentration of alcohol ingested, with high concentrations (>20%) inhibiting secretions (12). Continual ingestion of high concentrations of alcohol can lead to a variety of pathologies associated with the gastrointestinal (GI) tract, including esophageal varices and bleeding, erosive gastritis, and diarrhea and malabsorption of nutrients and vitamins (12). Alcohol consumption is also associated with an increased risk of tumors in the GI system as well as in other tissues including lung and breast (13). Acute and chronic ingestion of alcohol generally decreases sexual performance in both men and women, although sexual behavior may be enhanced owing to loss of inhibitory control and judgment. The deleterious effect of alcohol on various organ systems is countered by protective effects of small amounts of alcohol on cardiovascular tissue (14). Low to moderate alcohol use is associated with a reduced risk of coronary disease. Although not completely understood, this may be related to alcohol-induced changes in plasma lipoproteins and alterations in cell protection pathways. Chronic alcohol ingestion is associated with increased fat accumulation in the liver that can progress to severe liver damage and cirrhosis. Alcohol-induced liver damage is due in part to the production of acetaldehyde that readily reacts with proteins, lipids and other compounds leading to impaired mitochondrial function.

DRUG–DRUG INTERACTIONS

Alcohol has depressant actions on the CNS that are similar to other centrally acting drugs such as such as barbiturates, benzodiazepines, general anesthetics, and anticonvulsants. Alcohol also enhances the sedative effects of antihistamines that are commonly used in the treatment of nasal congestion. Combining these medications with alcohol can result in significant CNS depression and reduced ability to safely carry out normal functions such as automobile driving. Alcohol can also enhance the hepatotoxic effects of acetaminophen (Tylenol) and the gastric irritating effects of nonsteroidal anti-inflammatory drugs, thus increasing the risk for development of gastritis and upper GI bleeding. Chronic alcohol use can interfere with the metabolism of certain drugs owing to enhanced levels of liver enzymes.

NEUROBIOLOGY (MECHANISMS OF ADDICTION)

A widely accepted tenet of addiction research is that addictive substances, by definition, produce pleasurable effects that engender actions promoting further drug seeking and drug taking. This concept suggests that drugs of abuse like alcohol must produce, at least initially, some form of positive reinforcement that provides incentive to reexperience the drug. As drug use proceeds, the degree of acute reinforcement or reward may be attenuated, leading to enhanced intake in an attempt to reach previous levels of reward. The repetitive nature of drug use also engages mechanisms of learning, leading to entrained behaviors that may become highly ritualistic and habit-like. These findings have led to the idea that drug and alcohol addiction is a form of dysfunctional, maladaptive learning that—once established—is difficult to reverse (15). In terms of brain systems that underlie the development of addiction, recent studies suggest an important interaction between dopamine-based reward systems and mechanisms of brain plasticity and learning that are mediated by the neurotransmitter glutamate.

As reviewed in various chapters in Section 1, all drugs of abuse, including alcohol, affect reward pathways by enhancing the release of dopamine from midbrain dopaminergic projections that regulate excitatory glutamatergic neurotransmission within mesolimbic and mesocortical areas of the forebrain (16). The DA neurons involved in this action originate in the midbrain ventral tegmental area (VTA) and project to discrete areas of the forebrain, including the nucleus accumbens, olfactory tubercle, frontal cortex, amygdala, and septal/hippocampal areas. These regions are thought to be involved in translating emotion and perception into action through the activation of motor pathways; thus, they may be important in initiating and sustaining drug-seeking behavior. Lesions of these discrete brain areas in experimental animals can reduce both the acquisition of drug-seeking as well as its reinstatement after long periods of abstinence (17).

The initial reinforcing actions of alcohol appear to involve excitation of VTA dopamine neurons. Acutely, alcohol enhances the firing rate of midbrain DA neurons, and animals will self-administer alcohol directly into the posterior but not anterior VTA (18,19). Chronic exposure to alcohol leads to a reduction in the excitability of these neurons in the absence of alcohol that may persist for significant periods of time (20,21). Electrophysiological studies have demonstrated enhanced efficiency of glutamatergic signaling in neurons following exposure to alcohol and other drugs of abuse (22,23). These findings suggest that enhanced firing of VTA DA neurons during exposure to alcohol facilitates glutamatergic transmission in mesolimbic and mesocortical areas, thus strengthening the association between behavioral action and outcome. Using in vivo microdialysis to monitor levels of dopamine in freely behaving rats, Weiss et al. (24) showed that rats self-administrating alcohol show significant dose-dependent increases in extracellular dopamine levels in the nucleus accumbens. Importantly, in rats that were genetically bred to consume large amounts of alcohol, significant increases in dopamine were also observed during the 15-minute waiting period that preceded alcohol self-administration. This finding suggests that the expected reward that the ingestion of alcohol may provide is sufficient to enhance activity in this pathway in the absence of alcohol. The subsequent pharmacologically induced elevation of dopamine that occurs during drinking may further strengthen the motivation to consume alcohol in future sessions. Genetic differences in the responsiveness of this pathway may contribute to the motivational factors that drive alcohol-seeking behavior in certain individuals.

Recent studies with human alcoholics have examined the neurobehavioral aspects of alcohol abuse, using drug discrimination procedures similar to those used in animal studies. In these studies, human alcoholics are asked to rate the effects produced by a variety of drugs in terms of their similarity to those produced by alcohol. For example, ketamine, a dissociative anesthetic that blocks the *N*-methyl-D-aspartate (NMDA) subtype of glutamate receptors, induces ethanol-like subjective effects in recently detoxified alcoholics (25). These effects were dose-dependent: At low doses, they mimicked the effects of one to two standard drinks of alcohol, whereas higher doses produced effects similar to those of eight to nine drinks. Interestingly, the effects of ketamine that were ethanol-like were associated with the descending phase of blood alcohol concentration that is associated with ethanol-induced sedation.

Other human clinical studies using selective pharmacological agents have implicated neurotransmitters such as γ-aminobutyric acid (GABA), serotonin, and the opiates in mediating the rewarding and craving aspects of alcohol action. Results from human imaging studies have begun to identify changes in brain activation during exposure to alcohol or alcohol-related cues between control and alcohol-dependent subjects (26). Such human studies are important in the context of understanding the underlying causes of alcohol abuse because alcohol, unlike most drugs of abuse, interacts with a wide variety of molecular and cellular processes to produce its pharmacologic, physiologic, and psychologic effects.

Molecular Sites of Alcohol Action Psychostimulants such as cocaine and amphetamine or opiates such as heroin and morphine all produce their primary effect by binding to specific protein receptors expressed on brain neurons. Alcohol, in contrast, is rather promiscuous and interacts with a wide variety of targets, including both lipids and proteins. Initial observations made by the German scientists Meyer and Overton more than 100 years ago led to a lipid disordering hypothesis of alcohol and anesthetic action owing to the correlation between lipid solubility and anesthetic potency. Support for this theory has waned in recent years because of several factors. For example, measurable changes in membrane fluidity require very high concentrations of alcohol, are relatively modest, and are less marked than the effects produced by small changes in temperature that are not associated with behavioral signs of intoxication (27). These findings and the demonstration of effects in lipid-free systems have led to the idea that alcohol's actions are likely due to effects on ion channel proteins that regulate the excitability of neurons (28). An important point to consider in these in vitro studies of alcohol action is whether the range of concentrations needed to cause significant effects are similar to those associated with the behavioral actions of alcohol. Blood alcohol concentrations in the of range 40 to 400 mg% are equivalent to 8 to 88 mM and are associated with the full spectrum of alcohol intoxication (described in more detail further). Thus, in vitro studies of alcohol's effect on ion channels are usually conducted at concentrations below 100 mM in order to better approximate levels found in the brain during drinking.

As shown in Table 7.1, many ligand-gated ion and voltage-activated ion channels that are expressed by neurons are sensitive to behaviorally relevant concentrations of alcohol. Alcohol's depressant action on neuronal excitability likely results from its ability to enhance the function of inhibitory ion channels while blocking the activity of excitatory receptors (Fig. 7.1).

γ-Aminobutyric acid$_A$ and Glycine Receptors As shown in Table 7.1, there are distinct families of subunits that make up $GABA_A$ and glycine receptors. Each class of subunits may have multiple members that differ slightly in their sequence and function. Different subunit combinations can give rise to a variety of $GABA_A$ and glycine receptors that show variable sensitivity to pharmacologic agents, including alcohol. Alcohol generally enhances $GABA_A$ and glycine receptor function, though $GABA_A$ ρ receptors are inhibited by alcohol. By using the oocyte

TABLE 7.1 Properties of Alcohol-Sensitive Ion Channels

Neurotransmitter agonist or activator	Channel name	Subunit families	Brain subtypes	Major permeant ions	Alcohol effect (acute)
GABA	$GABA_A$	α,β,γ,δ,ρ	α1/β1/γ2, α4(6)βxδ	Cl^-	Enhance
Glycine	Glycine	α,β	α1/β1	Cl^-	Enhance
Acetylcholine	nAchR	α,β	α4β2, α7–9, α6β2[a]	Na^+	Enhance/Inhibit (α7)
Serotonin	$5HT_3$	$5HT_{3a,b}$	$5HT_3$	Na^+	Enhance
ATP	$P2_X$	$P2X_{1-7}$	$P2X_3$, $P2X_4$	Na^+	Inhibit/Enhance
Glutamate	NMDA	NR1, NR2A–D	NR1/2A, NR1/2B	Ca^{++}/Na^+	Inhibit
Glutamate	Non-NMDA	GluR1–7	GluR1, GluR2/3	Na^+/Ca^{++}	Inhibit
Voltage-Gated	BK_{Ca}	α,β_{1-4}	α, α/β	K^+	Enhance
Voltage-Gated	L,N,P,Q,T	α (S,C,D) β,γ,δ	Multiple	Ca^{++}	Inhibit

Note: Ion channels are listed according to their natural agonist or mode of activation. Subunit families represent those found in the brain or spinal cord. Brain subtypes are examples of subunit combinations commonly expressed by neurons ([a] indicates other subunits likely required). Alcohol effect indicates change in ion channel function by alcohol acutely administered to recombinant or native receptor preparations.

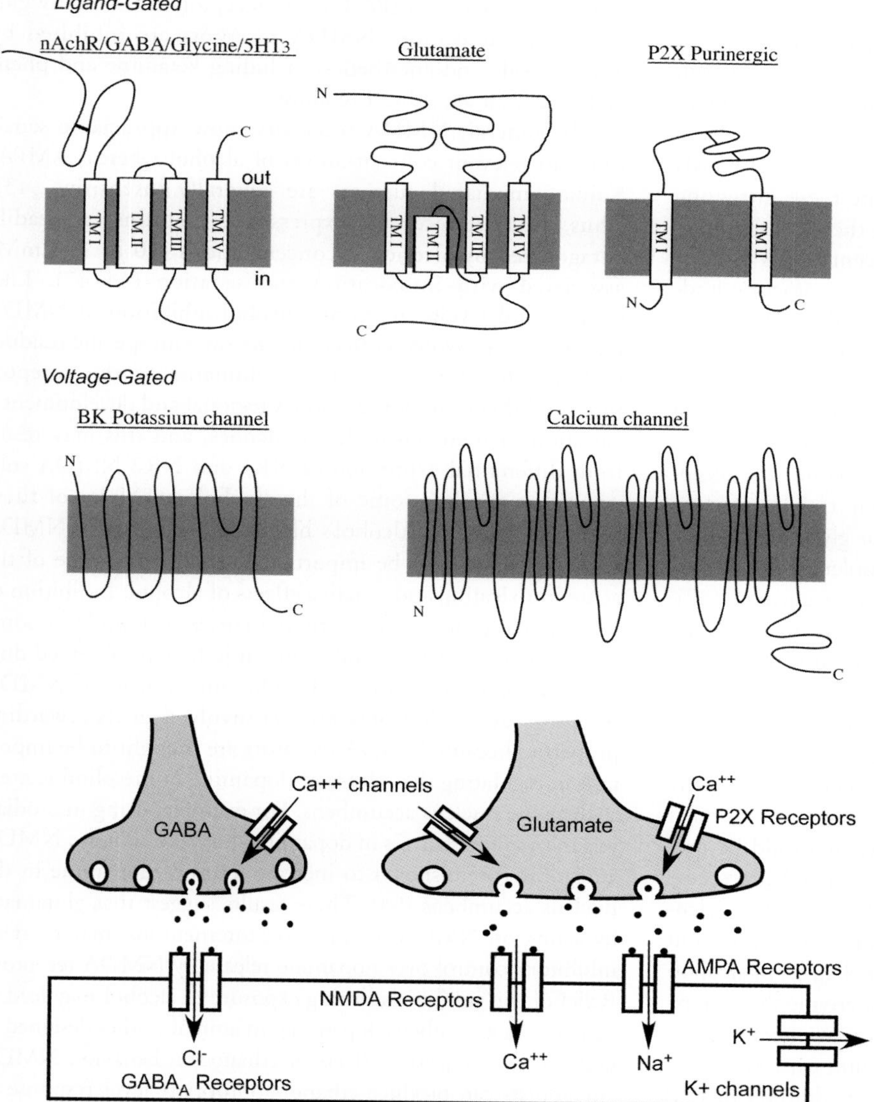

FIGURE 7.1. Structure and location of alcohol-sensitive ion channels in the neuronal synapse.

expression system, alcohol was shown to enhance the $GABA_A$ currents in receptors containing the γ2L variant of the GABA receptor, along with γ and γ subunits (29,30). This variant contains an additional eight amino acids that introduce a site for phosphorylation of the receptor by protein kinase C. Omission of the γ2L subunit or even substitution of other γ subunits (including the γ2 short variant) resulted in cells that did not show significant potentiation of the GABA-induced currents by alcohol. Despite these intriguing results, subsequent studies have shown that γ2L expression is not sufficient in itself to confer sensitivity to alcohol. In addition, knockout mice lacking this subunit show normal sensitivity to alcohol, though their responsiveness to benzodiazepines is enhanced (31,32). While these results appear to rule out a role for the γ2 subunit in mediating alcohol action of $GABA_A$ receptors, a recent study reported that the alcohol sensitivity of $GABA_A$ α1β2γ2 receptors is markedly enhanced when the kinase PKCε is inhibited (33). Mice lacking PKCε also show an enhanced response to ethanol suggesting that specific subtypes of $GABA_A$ receptors may show appreciable alcohol sensitivity under certain conditions (34).

In addition to γ-containing $GABA_A$ receptors, recent studies suggest that δ-containing GABA receptors possess high sensitivity to very low levels of alcohol. These receptors contain the α4(6), β and the δ subunit instead of the γ subunit and are affected by concentrations of ethanol (5 to 10 mM) achieved after only one drink (35). Despite these intriguing findings, not all studies have reported that these δ-containing $GABA_A$ receptors are sensitive to low concentrations of alcohol (36). While the reasons underlying these conflicting findings are not yet clear, they suggest the possibility that certain $GABA_A$ receptors may be especially important in mediating low-dose effects of alcohol.

A major approach that has revolutionized the study of alcohol action on ion channels is the use of mutagenesis to alter putative alcohol-sensitive amino acids within the receptor. These sites are often located within transmembrane domains of the receptor and in $GABA_A$ or glycine receptors, replacement of a conserved serine by an isoleucine abolished the potentiating effects of alcohol on receptor currents (37). Subsequent studies have shown that this site may also be involved in mediating the effects of some volatile anesthetics on $GABA_A$ and glycine receptor function (38). The identification of these alcohol-sensitive residues has allowed for detailed molecular modeling of these sites to better define the determinants for alcohol action and for the development of genetically modified animals that contain these mutations.

Based on results from in vitro studies, it would be predicted that animals lacking ethanol-sensitive $GABA_A$ receptors would show profound tolerance to some of the actions of alcohol. However, to date, results with $GABA_A$ receptor knock-out and knock-in mice have not revealed major changes in alcohol-induced behaviors (39,40). The reasons underlying these unexpected findings are not currently known but may involve powerful compensatory changes in GABA subunit expression that masks changes in alcohol sensitivity (41). In addition, there is now good evidence that some of the effects of alcohol on GABA receptor function arise from changes in the presynaptic release of GABA rather than a direct effect on the GABA receptor itself. Thus, in certain neurons of the amygdala, a brain structure highly involved in processing emotionally relevant stimuli, alcohol's potentiation of post-synaptic $GABA_A$ responses appears to be due to an increase in the release of GABA (42). The mechanism underlying the sensitivity of GABA release to alcohol is not currently known but could involve specific signaling pathways and proteins that normally regulate vesicle movement and fusion.

Glutamate Activated Ion Channels Glutamate is the major excitatory neurotransmitter in the brain and activates two major subtypes of ion channels called AMPA/Kainate and NMDA receptors. These channels mediate most of the fast excitatory synaptic transmission in the brain and are critical mediators of most forms of synaptic plasticity thought to underlie learning and memory. NMDA receptors are highly calcium-permeable and require both glutamate and glycine for activation whereas AMPA/Kainate receptors require only glutamate for activation. NMDA receptors are inhibited by nitrous oxide and anesthetics, including ketamine and phencyclidine, that are subject to abuse.

In general, NMDA receptors show appreciable sensitivity to relevant concentrations of alcohol whereas AMPA/Kainate–mediated currents are generally insensitive (43). Thus, NMDA receptors expressed in neurons are readily antagonized by alcohol at concentrations (10 to 100 mM) associated with intoxication and sedation (44–47). Like $GABA_A$ and glycine receptors, alcohol inhibition of NMDA receptors may involve a direct interaction with specific residues within defined transmembrane domains of the receptor (48,49). NMDA responses show a regional and developmental variation in their sensitivity to alcohol, and this may result from differential expression of NR1 and NR2 NMDA subunits that regulate some of the alcohol sensitivity of these receptors (50–52). Alcohol's blockade of excitatory NMDA signaling is likely to be important in mediating some of the acute intoxicating and sedative effects of alcohol. Inhibition of NMDA receptors in the prefrontal cortex may underlie some of the cognitive deficits and errors in judgment observed during alcohol intoxication (53). The antagonism of NMDA receptors by alcohol may also be involved in its rewarding properties because NMDA receptors are thought to be important in regulating the release of dopamine in mesolimbic areas such as the nucleus accumbens. For example, using microdialysis to monitor changes in dopamine in awake animals, NMDA antagonists were shown to increase levels of dopamine in the nucleus accumbens (54). These results suggest that glutamate, by acting on NMDA receptors on interneurons, may exert an inhibitory control over dopamine release by NMDA receptors. Relief of this inhibition during exposure to alcohol may lead to increases in accumbens dopamine. In animal studies designed to evaluate the subjective effects of ethanol on behavior, NMDA antagonists can produce ethanol-appropriate lever response in rats trained to discriminate ethanol from saline (55).

As NMDA receptor activity is a critical determinant of normal neuronal activity, it is perhaps not surprising that receptor function is also altered after chronic exposure to alcohol. In primary cultures of neurons, chronic exposure to alcohol increases the density and clustering of NMDA but not non-NMDA receptors (23,56). These changes take place specifically within the glutamatergic synapse as there is no change in NMDA receptors in nonsynaptic locations. These results suggest that NMDA receptors may serve as sensitive alcohol sensors and that neurons compensate for the inhibition of these receptors by moving more of them to the synapse where they can be activated by glutamate. One important outcome of this adaptive response is an increased susceptibility of animals and humans to seizures that develop during withdrawal from alcohol. Experiments with mice show that NMDA-induced seizure activity is elevated in mice made dependent on alcohol and that NMDA antagonists reduce or prevent seizures during withdrawal (57). More recent studies have suggested that the enhancement in NMDA receptor function after chronic alcohol may involve changes in the expression pattern of specific NMDA receptor subunits (58–60).

Other Ion Channel Subtypes

$5HT_3$ Receptors $5HT_3$ receptors are ligand-gated ion channels activated by serotonin. They are permeable primarily to monovalent cations, such as sodium and potassium. In cultured neurons and recombinant expression systems, low doses of alcohol appear to potentiate currents carried by $5HT_3$ receptor (61). In behavioral studies involving both rats and pigeons, $5HT_3$ receptor antagonists blocked the animal's ability to discriminate ethanol from saline, suggesting that alcohol's acute actions on $5HT_3$ receptors may underlie some of the subjective effects of alcohol (62). Human studies using the $5\text{-}HT_3$ antagonist ondansetron (Zofran) have generally found the drug reduces drinking though this effect appears more efficacious in early-onset alcoholics (63).

Acetylcholine Nicotinic Receptors Acetylcholine activates a variety of ligand-gated ion channels that are expressed in brain neurons and that are related to the nicotinic receptor expressed at the neuromuscular junction. Alcohol has been shown to either potentiate or inhibit acetylcholine receptors expressed in cultured neurons or oocytes (64,65). This biphasic effect appears to result from expression of different subtypes of nicotinic receptors by brain neurons that show a differential response to ethanol. Thus, heteromeric nicotinic receptors composed of $\alpha\beta$ subunits appear to be potentiated by ethanol, whereas homomeric receptors composed of just α subunits ($\alpha 7$, for example) are inhibited by ethanol (65). It is not yet clear how these different effects of ethanol on neuronal nicotinic receptors are manifested at the behavioral level. However, nicotinic receptors are expressed by neurons in the VTA, nucleus accumbens, and prefrontal cortex where they help shape the excitability of these neurons. Varenicline (Chantix), a newly approved medication for smoking cessation, is a partial agonist at the $\alpha 4\beta 2$ nicotinic receptor. Although not approved for the treatment of alcoholism, a recent preclinical study has reported that varenicline also reduces alcohol seeking in rodents without altering responding for sucrose (66).

Calcium and Potassium Selective Ion Channels Calcium-activated potassium channels (SK and BK channels) and those gated by G-proteins (GirK) channels are also affected either directly or indirectly by alcohol (67). These channels serve as a brake on excitatory glutamatergic transmission by hyperpolarizing the membrane and thus are critical regulators of neuronal activity. BK channel activity is acutely enhanced by alcohol, and this enhancement may contribute to the inhibition of vasopressin release from neurohypophysial terminals and the resulting diuresis that accompanies alcohol ingestion (67). Alcohol inhibits the function of native and some subtypes of recombinant ATP-gated purinergic receptors (68–70) and enhances currents through P2X3 receptors (71). Similarly, some types of voltage-gated calcium channels (L, N, and P/Q) are inhibited by alcohol, and L-type channels appear to be upregulated by chronic alcohol exposure (72).

Pharmacologic Studies Implicating Other Neurotransmitter Systems Much of the working knowledge of alcohol's effects on neuronal function comes from studies that have examined the ability of neurotransmitter specific agents to mediate alcohol drinking behavior. A brief review of this literature is presented here.

Adenosine Adenosine is a major inhibitory neurotransmitter in the brain and may serve as an endogenous anti-epileptic because of its ability to inhibit neuronal function. Alcohol has been shown to inhibit the function of a nucleoside transporter, leading to increased extracellular adenosine levels (73). This leads to activation of A2 adenosine receptors and increases cellular levels of cAMP that can activate PKA and stimulate cAMP-dependent changes in gene expression. A2 receptors show crosstalk with D2 dopamine receptors, and this interaction may be especially important in regulating the activity of medium spiny neurons in the nucleus accumbens. Block of this signaling pathway has been shown to reduce voluntary alcohol drinking in experimental animals (73).

Dopamine As mentioned earlier in this chapter, increases in mesolimbic and mesocortical dopamine are thought to be associated with the reinforcing effects of many drugs of abuse, including alcohol. Electrophysiologic studies have demonstrated that alcohol increases the firing of dopamine-containing neurons, located in the VTA leading to enhanced dopamine release in the nucleus accumbens and the prefrontal cortex (74). The mechanism underlying this effect of alcohol is not precisely known but may involve both a direct effect on a subtype of potassium channel that regulates the excitability of VTA neurons as well as indirectly via modulation of inputs into the VTA. Interestingly, the sensitivity of VTA neurons to alcohol-induced excitation is lower in mice that show a higher voluntary consumption of alcohol, suggesting that these animals may consume more alcohol to sufficiently activate a dopaminergic reward pathway (19,75).

The role of dopamine in alcohol addiction has also been explored by using pharmacologic agonists and antagonists that directly interact with dopamine receptors. The long-acting dopamine agonist bromocriptine (Parlodel), administered systemically, shift's a rat's preference from alcohol to water, especially in those strains of rats that show alcohol preference (76). Similar findings were demonstrated with another dopamine agonist, apomorphine. These results suggested that administration of direct dopamine agonists reduced the need for alcohol's dopamine-enhancing activity in these animals, such that the "reward state" was achieved at lower alcohol levels. Despite these promising results, human studies with these agents have not found significant effects on alcohol drinking or relapse (63).

Opioids and Other Neuropeptides The involvement of endogenous opioids (endorphins and enkephalins) and other neuropeptides in alcohol addiction is suggested by several lines of research. One of the first links between alcohol and opioids was suggested by the finding that acetaldehyde could undergo a metabolic reaction with monoamines to form compounds (tetrahydrisoquinolines or TIQs) that were structurally related to morphine (77). TIQs were shown to elicit alcohol-drinking behavior and alcohol preference even after cessation of TIQ administration (78). This hypothesis, although attractive, remains controversial because of the inability to replicate some of these findings and the demonstration that TIQ formation in vivo could be accounted by dietary factors rather than direct effects of alcohol (79). Alcohol does increase the release of certain opioid peptides (such as β-endorphin) from rat pituitary glands, and increases blood levels of β-endorphins in humans (80). If alcohol drinking is mediated in part by opioids, then selective opioid antagonists should inhibit alcohol-drinking behavior. Naloxone and naltrexone, two opioid receptor antagonists, reduce alcohol intake in both animals and humans, and various formulations of naltrexone (ReVia), including sustained-release and depot forms (Vivitrol, Naltrel, Depotrex), are now approved for treating alcoholism. These agents are thought to work by blocking alcohol induced increases in β–endorphin, thus reducing the acute rewarding effects of alcohol. A large number of laboratory studies and randomized, controlled trials have been conducted, and most of these report that naltrexone is better than placebo in reducing the risk of relapse (81). The results from these human studies are complemented by data obtained using mice genetically modified to lack the μ-opiate receptor. These animals do not self-administer alcohol or respond to the rewarding effects of opiates, nicotine, or cannanbinoids (82). Despite these dramatic effects in animal models and positive results in most human trials, the clinical efficacy of opiate antagonists in treating alcohol dependence is rather modest, suggesting that other factors may be important (63). As discussed in Chapter 47, "Pharmacologic Interventions for Alcoholism," the variability in response to opiate antagonists may be due to issues related to compliance as well as in differences in opiate receptor polymorphisms and other genetic changes among alcohol-dependent subjects that influence naltrexone efficacy (63).

Neuropeptides such as neuropeptide Y (NPY) and corticotropin-releasing factor (CRF) are involved in mediating stress and anxiety and have been shown to be important regulators of alcohol drinking. CRF is released after activation of the hypothalamic-pituitary-adrenal axis leading to elevated levels of cortisol that are indicative of a stress response. Alcohol also induces CRF release, and chronic alcohol use is associated with enhanced anxiogenesis that can be blocked by CRF antagonists (83). CRF antagonists appear to be especially effective in reducing the elevated drinking observed in alcohol-dependent rats without altering consumption in nondependent animals (84). Mice engineered to lack CRF1 receptors do not show enhanced drinking after the development of dependence, again suggesting an important link between stress and alcohol drinking (85). NPY is a neuropeptide associated with the general regulation of feeding behavior and anxiety. Injection of NPY reduces drinking in rodents while mice lacking NPY or the NPY Y1 receptor display enhanced ethanol intake (86). These effects may be related to anxiolytic effects of NPY.

Serotonin As mentioned, electrophysiologic studies have demonstrated that alcohol enhances cation conductance through $5HT_3$ receptors (61). Serotonin also interacts with a large number of non–ion channel G-protein linked receptors that are coupled to various signal transduction pathways. The direct effects of alcohol on these receptor systems are not as well characterized. However, there is a fairly large amount of literature describing the effects on alcohol-drinking behavior of various drugs that modulate serotonergic tone. 5HT and 5HT-metabolite levels are reduced in the cerebrospinal fluid of many alcohol abusers, suggesting that reduced 5HT levels or a reduction in 5HT-mediated neurotransmission may predispose certain people to uncontrollable drinking behavior (87).

It has been suggested that similar deficiencies in 5HT neurotransmission underlie the development of a variety of other disorders, including bulimia and obsessive-compulsive behavior, disorders that are characterized by a loss of behavioral control. Thus, pharmacologic agents that enhance 5HT neurotransmission (such as serotonin selective-uptake inhibitors) appear to be therapeutically effective in the treatment of these disorders. However, in terms of treating alcohol dependence, these agents (such as fluoxetine, Prozac and sertraline, Zoloft) appear to have limited efficacy (88,89). Of course, one drawback in using a transport inhibitor is the inability to selectively activate specific subtypes of 5-HT receptors. Interestingly, a variety of results from animals studies suggest that the 5-HT1b receptor may be especially involved in regulating alcohol intake, though the data are conflicting regarding whether receptor activity should be enhanced or blocked to produce these effects

(90–92). In addition, it is not completely clear whether these manipulations are selective for alcohol as 5-HT plays a central role in feeding and drinking behaviors.

Endocannabinoids The endogenous cannabinoid (EC) system has also been shown to be an important modulator of ethanol drinking. ECs are natural lipid-derived molecules that activate receptors (CB1, CB2) that also bind THC, the psychoactive constituent of marijuana. ECs are involved in regulating both GABAergic and glutamatergic synaptic transmission and are synthesized during periods of intense neuronal depolarization. Antagonists of the CB1 receptor (rimonabant, Acomplia) have been developed as weight loss drugs and though marketed in Europe, this drug has not yet been given FDA approval owing to concerns over psychiatric effects. However, CB1 antagonists reduce ethanol preference in wild-type mice and animals that lack CB1 receptors show reduced alcohol preference (93). In addition, the alcohol-induced increase in dopamine in the nucleus accumbens is prevented by a CB1 antagonist (94). This effect was also observed for cocaine and nicotine-induced increases in dopamine suggesting a link between the endogenous cannabinoid system and a variety of drugs of abuse that possess disparate acute mechanisms of action.

ADDICTION LIABILITY

Alcohol is an addictive substance although an individual's susceptibility to developing alcohol use disorders is influenced by a wide range of genetic and environmental factors. The 12-month prevalence for alcohol dependence for males is about 5.4% for men and 2.3% for women (95). Lifetime prevalence of alcohol dependence is approximately 13% and the risk of developing alcohol dependence shows a strong inverse correlation with the age at which heavy drinking begins (95). Chronic use of alcohol produces several neuroadaptive changes that may be important in the development of alcohol addiction.

Sensitization Sensitization is defined as an increase in the pharmacologic and physiologic response to a drug after repeated exposures. This phenomenon is best characterized by drugs of abuse such as cocaine or amphetamine, wherein it is associated with changes in glutamatergic signaling in the neurons of the VTA and nucleus accumbens (17). Sensitization to the locomotor effects of alcohol have been reported, but this effect is strain- and species-dependent. Another form of sensitization is characterized by an increase in the severity and intensity of withdrawal signs after multiple episodes of alcohol intoxication and withdrawal (96). This form of sensitization has been suggested to be similar to the kindling phenomena observed after repeated brain seizures and may involve some of the same mechanisms that underlie the adaptation of neurons to impaired neuronal signaling during chronic exposure to alcohol.

Tolerance and Dependence Tolerance is manifested as a reduced sensitivity to alcohol and is subdivided into several forms, depending on the specific action being measured and the time course over which it develops. For example, concentrations of alcohol required to produce sedation may increase in individuals or animals given alcohol chronically. In human alcoholics, tolerance to the sedative and even lethal effects of alcohol can be profound. For example, while the lethal dose of 50% (LD50) in non-tolerant humans is approximately 400 to 500 mg%, blood levels exceeding these values are often reported in individuals arrested for driving under the influence of alcohol (97). This form of tolerance is associated with changes in both the capacity to metabolize alcohol and in cellular adaptations that reduce sensitivity to alcohol. A form of short-term acute functional tolerance to alcohol (termed the *Mellanby effect*) is also demonstrated by differences in the degree of impairment produced by the same blood concentration of alcohol achieved during the rising phase of the blood alcohol curve as compared to the falling phase (98). Tolerance development has been extensively studied in rodent models, and the severity of the motor impairing effects of alcohol are strongly influenced by the context and environment in which they are measured (99). Dependence is defined by the occurrence of symptoms that appear after the cessation of alcohol drinking. These withdrawal symptoms include both physical (tremors, convulsions) and psychologic (negative emotions, craving) components. At the cellular level, tolerance and dependence also develop so that the acute effects of alcohol on ion channel or receptor function are diminished in animals chronically exposed to alcohol. As mentioned in the earlier section, this adaptation may involve changes in subunit expression or functional state of alcohol-sensitive ion channels as neurons adapt to the chronic presence of alcohol. Although reward mechanisms are undoubtedly important in the development of heavy alcohol use, processes and brain areas that underlie the development of dependence may be critical for maintaining continued drinking through negative reinforcement (anxiety, stress) generated during withdrawal. In support of this idea, a variety of studies now implicate activation of brain areas such as the amygdala and associated structures ("extended amygdala") with a relapse to drinking precipitated by alcohol specific cues or stress (100). These areas in combination with brain stress systems and areas involved in decision making (prefrontal cortex) may be critically important in driving continued drinking in alcohol dependent individuals (100).

A main feature of human alcoholism is the strong desire or craving for alcohol in subjects under treatment for alcohol abuse. Bouts of heavy drinking often follow periods of abstinence even when the symptoms of alcohol withdrawal have long subsided. This occurrence suggests that prolonged alcohol abuse may involve long-lasting or permanent changes in brain systems that alter a person's responsiveness to alcohol. Animal models of craving and relapse have been established and involve measuring consumption in alcohol-trained animals after various periods of deprivation (18,101). In most cases, animals display a robust increase in alcohol consumption after deprivation, and this effect is characterized by not only higher rates of drinking but increased preference for solutions containing higher alcohol concentrations. In addition, the alcohol deprivation effect in animals persists for very long periods of abstinence (up to 9 months; about one-third the lifespan of a rat), suggesting long-lasting or even irreversible changes in mechanisms regulating drinking behavior. Several studies have shown that drugs currently approved for treatment of alcoholism such as calcium N-acetylhomotaurine (acamprosate; Campral) and naltrexone (ReVia) can reduce or reverse the increase in ethanol intake produced by periods of forced deprivation (18). These results are important as they validate the utility and predictive value of animal models of craving and relapse and offer hope for the identification of better pharmacologic treatments to reduce or prevent relapse to drinking after withdrawal.

Toxicity States Alcohol produces a well-studied progression of behavioral symptoms that are highly correlated with blood alcohol levels. In nontolerant individuals, low levels (10 to 50 mg%) are anxiolytic and produce a feeling of well-being and increased sociabililty. As levels increase to 80 to 100 mg%, there is increased release from inhibitions and signs of impaired judgment and motor function. Higher levels (150 to 200 mg%) produce marked ataxia and reduced reaction time, and some individuals may experience blackouts, postintoxication periods wherein the individual cannot recall events that occurred during intoxication. As levels reach and exceed 300 mg%, an anesthetic level is approached, and individuals may show severe motor impairment and vomiting. As mentioned previously, lethal doses of alcohol in nontolerant individuals are on the order of 400 to 500 mg%, though this can vary widely. Alcohol is metabolized under zero order kinetics such that it is independent of dose and time and blood alcohol levels fall at a rate of about 20 mg/dl/hour.

Medical Complications Alcohol affects nearly all tissue and organ systems studied, and heavy drinkers show skeletal fragility and damage to tissues such as brain, liver, and heart and increased susceptibility to some cancers. Despite these negative effects, beneficial effects of moderate alcohol intake have been demonstrated; these include a reduced risk of coronary heart disease in individuals classified as light to moderate drinkers. Two factors that are important in determining whether alcohol drinking is associated with positive or negative effects are how an individual drinks and for how long. Most beneficial effects of alcohol are associated with light to moderate drinking, consisting of two or fewer drinks per day for men and one or fewer per day for women. These amounts are well below those experienced by alcohol abusers or alcoholics, who may consume more than 10 to 12 drinks per day. At higher levels, significant toxicity develops in most tissues, including the brain.

A variety of brain imaging techniques have been applied to the study of alcoholism and alcohol abuse. These techniques include computed tomography, magnetic resonance imaging (MRI), single-photon emission computed tomography (SPECT), and positron emission tomography (PET). Results from studies of human alcoholics has revealed increases in cortical cerebrospinal fluid in both gray and white matter that is distinct from that found in other neuropsychiatric disorders such as schizophrenia and Alzheimer disease (102,103). When corrected for age-related changes in these parameters, the frontal lobes and cerebellar gray matter are particularly sensitive to alcohol-induced damage. MRI studies have shown that volume deficits are found in anterior but not poster hippocampus and that these deficits were more severe in patients who displayed symptoms of memory loss and possible Korsakoff syndrome. Prenatal as well as adult exposure to alcohol was shown to disrupt and reduce the area of the corpus callosum. Functional imaging techniques such as magnetic resonance spectroscopy (MRS) or PET have been used to study alcohol-related changes in brain function (104,105). These techniques monitor the levels of certain metabolites (N-acetylaspartate and myo-inositol) or glucose metabolism that give useful information as to the integrity and functional status of the brain. These studies show reduced brain glucose metabolism in untreated alcoholics as compared with control subjects. Brain glucose metabolism has also been shown to increase 16 to 30 days after withdrawal, consistent with improvements in neuronal integrity measured by MRI. SPECT studies can detect changes in cerebral blood flow and have shown that alcoholics may have low perfusion of frontal lobe areas. Changes in blood flow coupled with structural damage to frontal brain areas may underlie the changes in cognitive and emotional behaviors observed in alcoholics.

Although a lifetime of heavy drinking long has been known to produce substantial changes in brain neuron density, recent data obtained in animal studies suggest that brief episodes of heavy drinking, or binges, also cause neuron loss (106). These findings are particularly relevant to alcohol use during adolescence and young adulthood, as these episodes of heavy binge drinking occur during critical periods of brain development (107).

The mechanisms underlying ethanol-induced neurotoxicity are not completely understood. There is a consensus that some forms of alcohol-induced damage may arise from overactivation of NMDA receptors during alcohol withdrawal. Thus, chronic exposure of neurons to ethanol induces an upregulation in the functional status of the NMDA receptor that is revealed during withdrawal (108). Enhanced receptor activation by glutamate may lead to above-normal production of cellular signals that contribute to cell death.

In other cases of ethanol-induced neurotoxicity, it appears that a non–NMDA-mediated mechanism is at work. In an acute binge model of alcohol intoxication, rats given large doses of alcohol over a 3- to 4-day period show pronounced loss of neurons in specific brain areas, including the entorhinal cortex and dentate gyrus. The toxic actions of ethanol were not blocked by NMDA antagonists but were attenuated by the diuretic furosemide (Lasix), suggesting other pathways for ethanol-induced brain damage (109).

Heavy alcohol use during pregnancy can lead to a variety of birth defects and alterations in normal growth and development of the newborn (110). Fetal alcohol spectrum disorder (FASD) consists of a variety of characteristic symptoms in newborns exposed to alcohol *in utero* and one in three infants born to alcoholic mothers displays symptoms of FASD. These include CNS dysfunction, such as low IQ and microcephaly, delayed growth, and facial abnormalities, among others. FASD generally is associated with heavy drinking, especially early in pregnancy, though it is not known whether there is any safe lower limit for alcohol consumption.

CONCLUSIONS/FUTURE RESEARCH

It is clear that, over the past 10 to 20 years, a great deal of progress has been made in understanding the sites and mechanisms of alcohol's effects on the brain. There is a growing appreciation that alcohol and other drugs of abuse initially target brain circuits involved in reward and learning and can induce long-lasting changes in the responsiveness of neurons within these areas. With regard to sites of action, a consensus has emerged that specific ligand-gated and voltage-gated ion channels represent a likely site for many of the acute effects of alcohol on neuronal function, though how alcohol actually produces its effect on these proteins is not yet clear. Compensatory mechanisms of neuroplasticity are likely engaged during repeated episodes of alcohol drinking as neurons and neuronal circuits attempt to adapted to the periodic presence of alcohol. These effects may involve changes in the expression and distribution of ion channel subunits and their downstream signaling processes that are normally involved in allowing an organism to learn and adapt to its environment. Chronic abuse of alcohol may usurp these mechanisms and result in a near permanent altered neuropsychologic state that promotes continued alcohol consumption. More work is needed with transgenic or knock-in animals that express proteins with altered alcohol sensitivity, so as to better understand the correlation between these targets and alcohol's behavioral effects. For example, if ion channels gated by glutamate, GABA, acetylcholine, and serotonin represent primary targets of alcohol action, how does perturbation of these channels lead to behaviors such as reward, craving, and reinforcement, that appear to involve complex neurocircuitry and multiple neurotransmitters, such as dopamine, opioids, and neuropeptides?

Other areas that need attention include elucidating the normal physiologic processes that operate in response to food and other natural reinforcers, as well as what genetic and environmental factors contribute to an individual's risk for developing an alcohol use disorder. Better use of brain imaging techniques in conjunction with electrophysiologic recording and network modeling would also improve our understanding of the neural regions that are involved in mediating the various behaviors associated with alcohol abuse and alcoholism.

ACKNOWLEDGMENTS: *Development of this chapter was supported by Grant RO1-AA09986 from the National Institute on Alcohol Abuse and Alcoholism.*

REFERENCES

1. Mahdi AS and McBride AJ. Intravenous injection of alcohol by drug injectors: Report of three cases. *Alcohol Alcohol* 1999;34:918–919.
2. Ethanol. In AltCareDex System [Internet database]. Updated periodically. Greenwood Village, CO: Thomson Healthcare.
3. Rosenbaum M, McCarty T. Alcohol prescription by surgeons in the prevention and treatment of delirium tremens: historic and current practice. *Gen Hosp Psychiatry* 2002;24:257–259.
4. Blocker JS Jr. Did prohibition really work? Alcohol prohibition as a public health innovation. *Am J Public Health* 2006;96:233–243.
5. Substance Abuse and Mental Health Services Administration. Results from the 2006 National Survey on Drug Use and Health: National Findings. Office of Applied Studies, NSDUH Series H-32, DHHS Publication No. SMA 07-4293. Rockville, MD: Author.
6. U.S. Department of Health and Human Services, Public Health Service, National Institutes of Health, National Institute on Alcohol Abuse and Alcoholism. Tenth special report to the U.S. Congress on alcohol and health. Washington, DC: Author, 2000.
7. Babor TF, Caetano R. Subtypes of substance dependence and abuse: implications for diagnostic classification and empirical research. *Addiction* 2006;101(Suppl 1):104–110.
8. Hesselbrock VM, Hesselbrock MN. Are there empirically supported and clinically useful subtypes of alcohol dependence? *Addiction* 2006;101(Suppl 1):97–103.
9. Baraona E, Abittan CS, Dohmen K, et al. Gender differences in pharmacokinetics of alcohol. *Alcohol Clin Exp Res* 2001;25:502–507.
10. Garces JM, de la Torre R, Gutierrez J, et al. Clinical effectiveness of naloxone in acute ethanol intoxication. *Revista Clin Espan* 1993;193:431–434.
11. Paul SM. Alcohol-sensitive GABA receptors and alcohol antagonists. *Proc Natl Acad Sci USA* 2006;103:8307–8308.
12. Bujanda L. The effects of alcohol consumption upon the gastrointestinal tract. *Am J Gastroenterol* 2000;95:3374–3382.
13. Boffetta P, Hashibe M. Alcohol and cancer. *Lancet Oncol* 2006;7: 149–156.
14. O'Keefe JH, Bybee KA, Lavie CJ. Alcohol and cardiovascular health: the razor-sharp double-edged sword. *J Am Coll Cardiol* 2007;50:1009–1014.
15. Berke JD, Hyman SE. Addiction, dopamine, and the molecular mechanisms of memory. *Neuron* 2000;25:515–532.
16. Koob GF, Roberts AJ, Schulteis G, et al. Neurocircuitry targets in ethanol reward and dependence. *Alcohol Clin Exp Res* 1998;22:3–9.
17. Kalivas PW. Glutamate systems in cocaine addiction. *Curr Opin Pharmacol* 2004;4:23–29.
18. Rodd ZA, Bell RL, Sable HJ, et al. Recent advances in animal models of alcohol craving and relapse. *Pharmacol Biochem Behav* 2004;79:439–450.
19. Brodie MS, Pesold C, Appel SB. Ethanol directly excites dopaminergic ventral tegmental area reward neurons. *Alcohol Clin Exp Res* 1999;23:1848–1852.
20. Okamoto T, Harnett MT, Morikawa H. Hyperpolarization-activated cation current Ih is an ethanol target in midbrain dopamine neurons of mice. *J Neurophysiol* 2006;95:619–626.
21. Hopf FW, Martin M, Chen BT, et al. Withdrawal from intermittent ethanol exposure increases probability of burst firing in VTA neurons in vitro. *J Neurophysiol* 2007;98:2297–2310.
22. Saal D, Dong Y, Bonci A, et al. Drugs of abuse and stress trigger a common synaptic adaptation in dopamine neurons. *Neuron* 2003;37:577–582.
23. Carpenter-Hyland EP, Woodward JJ, Chandler LJ. Chronic ethanol induces synaptic but not extrasynaptic targeting of NMDA receptors. *J Neurosci* 2004;24:7859–7868.
24. Weiss F, Hurd YL, Ungerstedt U, et al. Neurochemical correlates of cocaine and ethanol self-administration. *Ann N Y Acad Sci* 1992;654:220–241.
25. Krystal JH, Petrakis IL, Webb E, et al. Dose-related ethanol-like effects of the NMDA antagonist, ketamine, in recently detoxified alcoholics. *Arch Gen Psychiatry* 1998;55:354–360.
26. Sinha R, Li CS. Imaging stress- and cue-induced drug and alcohol craving: association with relapse and clinical implications. *Drug Alcohol Rev* 2007;26:25–31.

27. Forman SA, Miller KW. Molecular sites of anesthetic action in postsynaptic nicotinic membranes. *Trends Pharmacol Sci* 1989;10:447–452.
28. Franks NP, Lieb WR. Seeing the light: protein theories of general anesthesia. *Anesthesiology* 2004;101:235–237.
29. Wafford KA, Burnett DM, Leidenheimer NJ, et al. Ethanol sensitivity of the GABAA receptor expressed in xenopus oocytes requires 8 amino acids contained in the gamma2L subunit. *Neuron* 1991;7:27–33.
30. Wafford KA, Whiting PJ. Ethanol potentiation of $GABA_A$ receptors requires phosphorylation of the alternatively spliced variant of the gamma2 subunit. *FEBS Lett* 1992;313:113–117.
31. Homanics GE, Harrison NL, Quinlan JJ, et al. Normal electrophysiological and behavioral responses to ethanol in mice lacking the long splice variant of the gamma2 subunit of the gamma-aminobutyrate type A receptor. *Neuropharmacology* 1999;38:253–265.
32. Quinlan JJ, Firestone LL, Homanics GE. Mice lacking the long splice variant of the gamma2 subunit of the GABA(A.) receptor are more sensitive to benzodiazepines. *Pharmacol Biochem Behav* 2000;66:371–374.
33. Qi ZH, Song M, Wallace MJ, et al. Protein kinase C{epsilon} regulates {gamma}-aminobutyrate type a receptor sensitivity to ethanol and benzodiazepines through phosphorylation of {gamma}2 subunits. *J Biol Chem* 2007;282:33052–33063.
34. Hodge CW, Mehmert KK, Kelley SP, et al. Supersensitivity to allosteric GABA(A.) receptor modulators and alcohol in mice lacking PKCepsilon. *Nat Neurosci* 1999;2:997–1002.
35. Wallner M, Hanchar HJ, Olsen RW. Ethanol enhances alpha 4 beta 3 delta and alpha 6 beta 3 delta gamma-aminobutyric acid type A receptors at low concentrations known to affect humans. *Proc Natl Acad Sci USA* 2003;100:15218–15223.
36. Borghese CM, Storustovu S, Ebert B, et al. The delta subunit of gamma-aminobutyric acid type A receptors does not confer sensitivity to low concentrations of ethanol. *J Pharmacol Exp Ther* 2006;316:1360–1368.
37. Mihic SJ, Ye Q, Wick MJ, et al. Sites of alcohol and volatile anaesthetic action on GABAA and glycine receptors. *Nature* 1997;389:385–389.
38. Mascia MP, Mihic SJ, Valenzuela CF, et al. A single amino acid determines differences in ethanol actions on strychnine-sensitive glycine receptors. *Mol Pharmacol* 1996;50:402–406.
39. Werner DF, Blednov YA, Ariwodola OJ, et al. Knock-in mice with ethanol-insensitive alpha1-containing gamma-aminobutyric acid type A receptors display selective alterations in behavioral responses to ethanol. *J Pharmacol Exp Ther* 2006;319:219–227.
40. Mihalek RM, Bowers BJ, Wehner JM, et al. GABA(A.)-receptor delta subunit knockout mice have multiple defects in behavioral responses to ethanol. *Alcohol Clin Exp Res* 2001;25:1708–1718.
41. Woodward JJ. GABAA alpha 4 receptor subunits and ethanol: a knockout punch? *Alcohol Clin Exp Res* 2008;32:8–9.
42. Roberto M, Madamba SG, Moore SD, et al. Ethanol increases GABAergic transmission at both pre- and postsynaptic sites in rat central amygdala neurons. *Proc Natl Acad Sci USA* 2003;100:2053–2058.
43. Lovinger DM. Alcohols and neurotransmitter gated ion channels: past, present and future. *Naunyn-Schmiedeberg's Arch Pharmacol* 1997;356:267–282.
44. Lovinger DM, White G, Weight FF. Ethanol inhibits NMDA-activated ion current in hippocampal neurons. *Science* 1989;243:1721–1724.
45. Hoffman PL, Moses F, Tabakoff B. Selective inhibition by ethanol of glutamate-stimulated cyclic GMP production in primary cultures of cerebellar granule cells. *Neuropharmacology* 1989;28:1239–1243.
46. Woodward JJ, Gonzales RA. Ethanol inhibition of *N*-methyl-D-aspartate-stimulated endogenous dopamine release from rat striatal slices: reversal by glycine. *J Neurochem* 1990;54:712–715.
47. Gonzales RA, Woodward JJ. Ethanol inhibits *N*-methyl-D-aspartate-stimulated [3H]norepinephrine release from rat cortical slices. *J Pharmacol Exp Ther* 1990;252:1138–1144.
48. Ronald KM, Mirshahi T, Woodward JJ. Ethanol inhibition of *N*-methyl-D-aspartate receptors is reduced by site-directed mutagenesis of a transmembrane domain phenylalanine residue. *J Biol Chem* 2001;276:44729–44735.
49. Honse Y, Ren H, Lipsky RH, et al. Sites in the fourth membrane-associated domain regulate alcohol sensitivity of the NMDA receptor. *Neuropharmacology* 2004;46:647–654.
50. Woodward JJ. Ethanol and NMDA receptor signaling. *Crit Rev Neurobiol* 2000;14:69–89.
51. Ron D. Signaling cascades regulating NMDA receptor sensitivity to ethanol. *Neuroscientist* 2004;10:325–336.
52. Jin C, Woodward JJ. Effects of 8 different NR1 splice variants on the ethanol inhibition of recombinant NMDA receptors. *Alcohol Clin Exp Res* 2006;30:673–679.
53. Tu Y, Kroener S, Abernathy K, et al. Ethanol inhibits persistent activity in prefrontal cortical neurons. *J Neurosci* 2007;27:4765–4775.
54. Youngren KD, Daly DA, Moghaddam B. Distinct actions of endogenous excitatory amino acids on the outflow of dopamine in the nucleus accumbens. *J Pharmacol Exp Ther* 1993;264:289–293.
55. Colombo G, Grant KA. NMDA receptor complex antagonists have ethanol-like discriminative stimulus effects. *Ann N Y Acad Sci* 1992;654:421–423.
56. Iorio KR, Reinlib L, Tabakoff B, et al. Chronic exposure of cerebellar granule cells to ethanol results in increased *N*-methyl-D-aspartate receptor function. *Mol Pharmacol* 1992;41:1142–1148.
57. Grant KA, Valverius P, Hudspith M, et al. Ethanol withdrawal seizures and the NMDA receptor complex. *Eur J Pharmacol* 1990;176:289–296.
58. Blevins T, Mirshahi T, Woodward JJ. Increased agonist and antagonist sensitivity of *N*-methyl-D-aspartate stimulated calcium flux in cultured neurons following chronic ethanol exposure. *Neurosci Lett* 1995;200:214–218.
59. Follesa P, Ticku MK. Chronic ethanol treatment differentially regulates NMDA receptor subunit mRNA expression in rat brain. *Eur J Pharmacol* 1995;29:99–106.
60. Snell LD, Nunley KR, Lickteig RL, et al. Regional and subunit specific changes in NMDA receptor mRNA and immunoreactivity in mouse brain following chronic ethanol ingestion. *Mol Brain Res* 1996;40:71–78.
61. Lovinger DM, White G. Ethanol potentiation of 5-hydroxytryptamine3 receptor-mediated ion current in neuroblastoma cells and isolated adult mammalian neurons. *Mol Pharmacol* 1991;40:263–270.
62. Grant KA, Barrett JE. Blockade of the discriminative stimulus effects of ethanol with 5-HT3 receptor antagonists. *Psychopharmacology (Berl)* 1991;104:451–456.
63. Johnson BA. Update on neuropharmacological treatments for alcoholism: scientific basis and clinical findings. *Biochem Pharmacol* 2008;75:34–56.
64. Aistrup GL, Marszalec W, Narahashi T. Ethanol modulation of nicotinic acetylcholine receptor currents in cultured cortical neurons. *Mol Pharmacol* 1999;55:39–49.
65. Cardoso RA, Brozowski SJ, Chavez-Noriega LE, et al. Effects of ethanol on recombinant human neuronal nicotinic acetylcholine receptors expressed in Xenopus oocytes. *J Pharmacol Exp Ther* 1999;289:774–780.
66. Steensland P, Simms JA, Holgate J, et al. Varenicline, an alpha4beta2 nicotinic acetylcholine receptor partial agonist, selectively decreases ethanol consumption and seeking. *Proc Natl Acad Sci USA* 2007;104:12518–12523.
67. Brodie MS, Scholz A, Weiger TM, et al. Ethanol interactions with calcium-dependent potassium channels. *Alcohol Clin Exp Res* 2007;31:1625–1632.
68. Li C, Aguayo L, Peoples RW, et al. Ethanol inhibits a neuronal ATP-gated ion channel. *Mol Pharmacol* 1993;44:871–875.
69. Xiong K, Li C, Weight FF. Inhibition by ethanol of rat P2X4. receptors expressed in Xenopus oocytes. *British Journal of Pharmacology* 2000;130:1394-1398.
70. Koles L, Wirkner K, Furst S, et al. Trichloroethanol inhibits ATP-induced membrane currents in cultured HEK 293-hP2X3 cells. *Eur J Pharmacol* 2000;409:R3–R5.
71. Davies DL, Kochegarov AA, Kuo ST, et al. Ethanol differentially affects ATP-gated P2X(3.) and P2X(4.) receptor subtypes expressed in Xenopus oocytes. *Neuropharmacology* 2005;49:243–253.
72. Walter HJ, Messing RO. Regulation of neuronal voltage-gated calcium channels by ethanol. *Neurochem Int* 1999;35:95–101.
73. Mailliard WS, Diamond I. Recent advances in the neurobiology of alcoholism: the role of adenosine. *Pharmacol Ther* 2004;101:39–46.
74. Brodie MS, Shefner SA, Dunwiddie TV. Ethanol increases the firing rate of dopamine neurons of the rat ventral tegmental area in vitro. *Brain Res* 1990;508:65–69.

75. Brodie MS, Appel SB. Dopaminergic neurons in the ventral tegmental area of C57BL/6J and DBA/2J mice differ in sensitivity to ethanol excitation. *Alcohol Clin Exp Res* 2000;24:1120–1124.
76. Weiss F, Mitchiner M, Bloom FE, et al. Free-choice responding for ethanol versus water in alcohol preferring (P.) and unselected Wistar rats is differentially modified by naloxone, bromocriptine, and methysergide. *Psychopharmacology (Berlin)* 1990;101:178–186.
77. Davis VE, Walsh MJ. Alcohol, amines, and alkaloids: a possible biochemical basis for alcohol addiction. *Science* 1970;167:1005–1007.
78. Myers RD. Isoquinolines, beta-carbolines and alcohol drinking: involvement of opioid and dopaminergic mechanisms. *Experientia* 1989;45: 436–443.
79. Collins MA. Acetaldehyde and its condensation products as markers in alcoholism. *Recent Dev Alcohol* 1988;6:387–403.
80. Oswald LM, Wand GS. Opioids and alcoholism. *Physiol Behav* 2004;81: 339–358.
81. O'Brien CP. Anticraving medications for relapse prevention: a possible new class of psychoactive medications. *Am J Psychiatry* 2005;162:1423–1431.
82. Koob GF. The neurobiology of addiction: a neuroadaptational view relevant for diagnosis. *Addiction* 2006;101(Suppl 1):23–30.
83. Valdez GR, Roberts AJ, Chan K, et al. Increased ethanol self-administration and anxiety-like behavior during acute ethanol withdrawal and protracted abstinence: regulation by corticotropin-releasing factor. *Alcohol Clin Exp Res* 2002;26:1494–501.
84. Funk CK, Zorrilla EP, Lee MJ, et al. Corticotropin-releasing factor 1 antagonists selectively reduce ethanol self-administration in ethanol-dependent rats. *Biol Psychiatry* 2007;61:78–86.
85. Chu K, Koob GF, Cole M, et al. Dependence-induced increases in ethanol self-administration in mice are blocked by the CRF1 receptor antagonist antalarmin and by CRF1 receptor knockout. *Pharmacol Biochem Behav* 2007;86:813–821.
86. Thiele TE, Koh MT, Pedrazzini T. Voluntary alcohol consumption is controlled via the neuropeptide Y Y1 receptor. *J Neurosci* 2002;22:RC208.
87. Sellers EM, Higgins GA, Sobell MB. 5-HT and alcohol abuse. *Trends Pharmacol Sci* 1992;13:69–75.
88. Nunes EV, Levin FR. Treatment of depression in patients with alcohol or other drug dependence: a meta-analysis. *JAMA* 2004;291:1887–1896.
89. Kranzler HR, Mueller T, Cornelius J, et al. Sertraline treatment of co-occuring alcohol dependence and major depression. *J Clin Psychopharmacol* 2006;26:13–20.
90. Crabbe JC, Phillips TJ, Feller DJ, et al. Elevated alcohol consumption in null mutant mice lacking 5-HT1B serotonin receptors. *Nat Genet* 1996;14:98–101.
91. Yan QS, Zheng SZ, Feng MJ, et al. Involvement of 5-HT1B receptors within the ventral tegmental area in ethanol-induced increases in mesolimbic dopaminergic transmission. *Brain Res* 2005;1060:126–137.
92. Hoplight BJ, Sandygren NA, Neumaier JF. Increased expression of 5-HT1B receptors in rat nucleus accumbens via virally mediated gene transfer increases voluntary alcohol consumption. *Alcohol* 2006;38:73–79.
93. Wang L, Liu J, Harvey-White J, et al. Endocannabinoid signaling via cannabinoid receptor 1 is involved in ethanol preference and its age-dependent decline in mice. *Proc Natl Acad Sci USA* 2003;100:1393–1398.
94. Cheer JF, Wassum KM, Sombers LA, et al. Phasic dopamine release evoked by abused substances requires cannabinoid receptor activation. *J Neurosci* 2007;27:791–795.
95. Grant BF, Dawson DA, Stinson FS, et al. The 12-month prevalence and trends in DSM-IV alcohol abuse and dependence: United States, 1991–1992 and 2001–2002. *Drug Alcohol Depend* 2004;74:223–234.
96. Becker HC, Hale RL. Repeated episodes of ethanol withdrawal potentiate the severity of subsequent withdrawal seizures: an animal model of alcohol withdrawal "kindling." *Alcohol Clin Exp Res* 1993; 17:94–98.
97. Jones AW. The drunkest drinking driver in Sweden: blood alcohol concentration 0.545% w/v. *J Stud Alcohol* 1999;60:400–406.
98. Wu PH, Tabakoff B, Szabo G, et al. Chronic ethanol exposure results in increased acute functional tolerance in selected lines of HAFT and LAFT mice. *Psychopharmacology* 2001;155:405–412.
99. Kalant H. Research on tolerance: what can we learn from history? *Alcohol Clin Exp Res* 1998;22:67–76.
100. Koob G, Kreek MJ. Stress, dysregulation of drug reward pathways, and the transition to drug dependence. *Am J Psychiatry* 2007;164: 1149–1159.
101. Koob GF, Weiss F, Tiffany ST, et al. Animal models of craving: a round-table discussion. *Alcohol Res Health* 1999;23:233–236.
102. Sullivan EV, Pfefferbaum A. Neurocircuitry in alcoholism: a substrate of disruption and repair. *Psychopharmacology* 2005;180:583–594.
103. Harper C. The neurotoxicity of alcohol. *Hum Exp Toxicol* 2007;26: 251–257.
104. Martinez D, Kim JH, Krystal J, et al. Imaging the neurochemistry of alcohol and substance abuse. *Neuroimag Clin North Am* 2007;17: 539–555.
105. Volkow ND, Fowler JS, Wang GJ. The addicted human brain viewed in the light of imaging studies: brain circuits and treatment strategies. *Neuropharmacology* 2004;47(Suppl 1):3–13.
106. Obernier JA, White AM, Swartzwelder HS, et al. Cognitive deficits and CNS damage after a 4-day binge ethanol exposure in rats. *Pharmacol Biochem Behav* 2002;72:521–532.
107. Crews F, He J, Hodge C. Adolescent cortical development: a critical period of vulnerability for addiction. *Pharmacol Biochem Behav* 2007;86:189–199.
108. Chandler LJ, Newsom H, Sumners C, et al. Chronic ethanol exposure potentiates NMDA excitotoxicity in cerebral cortical neurons. *J Neurochem* 1993;60:1578–1581.
109. Collins MA, Zou JY, Neafsey EJ. Brain damage due to episodic alcohol exposure in vivo and in vitro: furosemide neuroprotection implicates edema-based mechanism. *FASEB J* 1998;12:221–230.
110. Spadoni AD, McGee CL, Fryer SL, et al. Neuroimaging and fetal alcohol spectrum disorders. *Neurosci Biobehav Rev* 2007;31:239–245.

CHAPTER 8

Domenic A. Ciraulo, MD
Clifford M. Knapp, PhD

The Pharmacology of Nonalcohol Sedative Hypnotics

Sedative hypnotic drugs represent a diverse group of chemical agents that suppress central nervous system (CNS) activity (1). They are used in medicine as anxiolytics, hypnotics, anticonvulsants, muscle relaxants, and anesthesia induction agents. Their calming effects are on a continuum with sleep-inducing effects, unconsciousness and, for some agents, coma and death. Substances discussed in this chapter include benzodiazepines, nonbenzodiazepine hypnotics, barbiturates, and miscellaneous related compounds.

FORMULATIONS AND CHEMICAL STRUCTURE

The basic structure of the benzodiazepines is the 1,4-benzodiazepine nucleus as shown in Figure 8.1 (2).

Various substitutions alter the efficacy, potency, and other properties of individual drugs (3). Variations on the benzodiazepine ring structure have produced (a) the triazole group: alprazolam, triazolam, estazolam; (b) the 2-keto group: diazepam, flurazepam, and clorazepate; (c) the 2-amino group: chlordiazepoxide; (d) the 3-hydroxy group: lorazepam, oxazepam, and temazepam; (e) the trifluoroethyl group: quazepam; (f) the imidazole group: midazolam, and (g) the 7-nitro group: nitrazepam and clonazepam.

More recently, four nonbenzodiazepine hypnotics have been introduced: (a) zopiclone, a cyclopyrolone; (b) eszopiclone, a stereoselective isomer of zopiclone; (c) zaleplon, a pyrazolopyrimidine; and (d) zolpidem, an imidazopyridine (4–6). Although these agents exert their hypnotic effects at the γ-aminobutyric acid ($GABA_A$) receptor, their actions are not identical to classic benzodiazepines (see "Pharmacodynamics" section). The clinically available formulations of benzodiazepines and related drugs are shown in Table 8.1.

Barbiturates have largely been replaced by benzodiazepines because the latter drugs have greater safety and less potential for abuse; however, barbiturates continue to be used in general anesthesia and for the treatment of seizures (3,7,8). In the practice of addiction medicine, phenobarbital is used to treat difficult cases of sedative hypnotic withdrawal; for example, in those cases unresponsive to benzodiazepines, detoxification from very high doses of sedative hypnotics, or when patients are abusing several different agents of this class. Specialists may also encounter patients who have been abusing analgesic preparations containing butalbital and require medically supervised detoxification. In these cases, heavy users may require phenobarbital withdrawal, whereas individuals taking ≤10 tablets per day of Fiorinal can usually be weaned off the medication gradually. Table 8.2 lists commonly used barbiturates (9).

There are a number of other sedative hypnotics that are rarely seen in clinical practice. These include paraldehyde, chloral hydrate, and ethchlorvynol. The clinician may occasionally see meprobamate, or more commonly the related drug carisoprodol, which is used as a muscle relaxant. All of these agents have abuse liability and produce a withdrawal syndrome

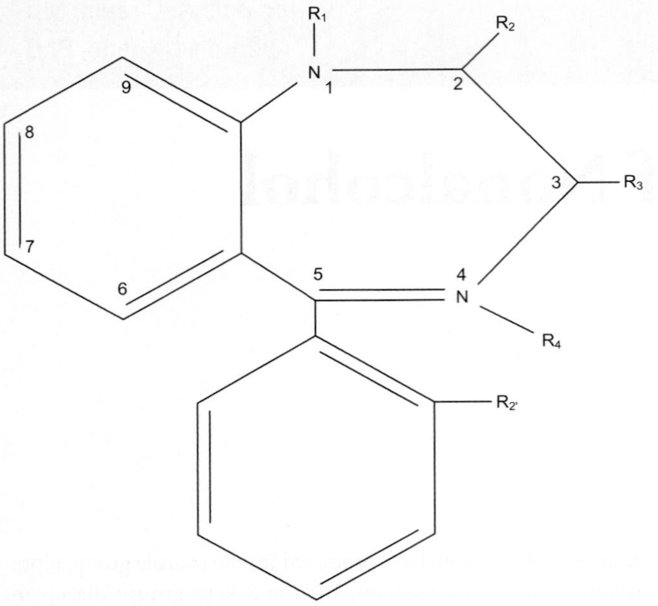

FIGURE 8.1. The 1,4-benzodiazepine nucleus.

upon abrupt discontinuation after chronic use. Phenobarbital withdrawal protocols are recommended for these drugs (10).

BRIEF HISTORICAL FEATURES

Barbituric acid was first prepared in 1864 by von Baeyer (7). Although not a central depressant itself, several of its derivatives have been used in medicine since the early 1900s. Barbital was introduced in 1903 and phenobarbital in 1912 (7). With respect to benzodiazepines, in the mid-1930s, Sternbach synthesized several heptoxdiazines, although it wasn't until 1955 when one of these quinazolines was treated with methylamine, that an active compound was developed (2). In 1957, the compound chlordiazepoxide was found to have hypnotic, sedative, and muscle-relaxing effects. The benzodiazepines provided advantages over the older barbiturates because they were less toxic in overdose and had fewer drug interactions. In addition, they had superior efficacy and safety compared to meprobamate, which was introduced as a tranquilizer in 1955 (2). Nonbenzodiazepine hypnotics have been the most recent addition and may offer some advantages of lower abuse liability, though clinical experience is insufficient to make definitive judgments.

EPIDEMIOLOGY

Estimates of the rates of abuse liability of benzodiazepines and related agents are made based on prescriptions issued, patterns of medical use, misuse by substance abusing patients, and national surveys. The American Psychiatric Association task force on benzodiazepine abuse reported that U.S. benzodiazepine prescriptions peaked at 87 million in 1973 (11). In 2007, there were 74 million prescriptions, and there is now a well-established pattern of higher sales among shorter-acting agents as compared to longer-acting ones. There has been a marked increase in U.S. zolpidem prescriptions, which have nearly doubled over the past 5 years.

In clinical populations, most patients take benzodiazepines for periods of <1 month. Between 7.4% and 17.6% of the U.S. population use a benzodiazepine for medical purposes at least once during a 1-year period, with about 1% using the medication for a year or longer (12). This is consistent with most studies in other countries, where 6 month use occurs in about 3% of the population, and 1-year use is about 1.7% (13), though the survey methodology used and the country studied can produce very different prevalence rates (13,14). Studies both in the United States and Europe indicate that long-term users are more likely to be older, women, and report high levels of chronic health problems and emotional difficulties. About 30% of psychiatric patients received benzodiazepines in one study, with the greatest use in patients with affective disorders, long duration of illness, and high users of psychiatric services (15). In general, the treatment of anxiety with medications has increased in recent years; however, the proportion of patients treated with antidepressants has grown while the percentage of those treated with anxiolytics has fallen slightly (16). In medical settings, most patients treated with benzodiazepines for anxiety do not increase their dose on their own. In fact, most patients tend to decrease the dose over time. Conversely, there are certain groups of high-risk patients where long-term use, misuse, and abuse are greater than in patients with anxiety disorders.

Benzodiazepine abuse is particularly high among alcoholics and methadone-treated patients (17–23). Approximately 15% to 20% of alcoholic patients presenting for treatment may be abusing benzodiazepines (1,24,25). In methadone clinics, rates of urines positive for benzodiazepines are common, with 30% to 90% reporting illicit use (26,27). Several groups report a positive mood enhancement from acute benzodiazepine doses, including moderate and heavy drinkers (28,29), abstinent alcoholics (30–32), and individuals who have strong family histories of alcoholism (33–35). Higher medical use of benzodiazepines has also been reported in the elderly, people with disabilities, and individuals with chronic pain (36–43).

The Treatment Episode Data Set, which maintains statistics on admissions to publicly funded U.S. treatment facilities, has consistently reported that admissions for primary "tranquilizer" use is rare, and most patients using benzodiazepines are also abusing alcohol, marijuana, and opioids other than heroin (44). The latest National Survey on Drug Use and Health found that 8% of the U.S. population 12 years old or older used tranquilizers for nonmedical purposes at some time in their life, with 0.7% having used them within the month prior to the survey (45). The Drug Abuse Warning Network reported that benzodiazepines were the most frequently reported psychotherapeutic drug mentioned in U.S. emergency department

TABLE 8.1 Formulations of Benzodiazepines and Nonbenzodiazepine Hypnotics

Benzodiazepines	Brand names	How supplied	Clinical doses
Alprazolam	Alprazolam Intensol Xanax Xanax XR Niravam	Oral solution: 1 mg/mL Tablets: 0.25 mg, 0.5 mg, 1 mg, 2 mg Extended-release tablets: 0.5 mg, 1 mg, 2 mg, 3 mg Orally disintegrating tablets: 0.25 mg, 0.5 mg, 1 mg, 2 mg	Initial dose: 0.25-0.5 mg 3 times daily, maximum dose 4 mg/day Initial dose: 0.5-1.0 mg daily, target dose 3-6 mg daily Initial dose: 0.25–0.5 mg 3 times daily, maximum dose 4 mg/day
Clonazepam	Klonopin Klonopin wafers	Tablets: 0.5 mg, 1 mg, 2 mg Tablets: 0.125 mg, 0.25 mg, 0.5 mg, 1 mg, 2 mg	Initial dose 0.25 mg 2 times daily, usual target dose 1–6 mg daily
Clorazepate	Tranxene T-Tab Tranxene-SD Tranxene-SD Half Strength	Tablets: 3.75 mg, 7.5 mg, 15 mg Tablets: 22.5 mg Tablets: 11.25 mg	15–60 mg daily Geriatric/Debilitated patients: 7.5–15 mg daily
Chlordiazepoxide	Librium	Capsules: 5 mg, 10 mg, 25 mg	Mild/Moderate: 5–10 mg, 3–4 times daily. Severe: 20–25 mg, 3–4 times daily. Geriatric patients: 5 mg, 2–4 times daily
Diazepam	Valium Diastat Diastat Acudial	Tablets: 2 mg, 5 mg, 10 mg Rectal delivery system: 2.5 mg Twin Pack Rectal delivery system: 10 or 20 mg delivery system	Depending on severity: 2–10 mg, 2–4 times daily Rectal gel: 0.2–0.5 mg/kg, depending on age
Estazolam	ProSom Estazolam	Tablets: 1 mg, 2 mg	Initial dosage: 1–2 mg before bedtime Geriatric patients: Initiate at 0.5 mg before bedtime
Flurazepam	Dalmane Flurazepam hydrochloride	Capsules: 15 mg, 30 mg Capsules: 15 mg, 30 mg	30 mg before bedtime Geriatric/Debilitated Patients: Initiate at 15 mg
Halazepam	Paxipam	(not available in the United States)	
Lorazepam	Ativan	Tablets: 0.5 mg, 1 mg, 2 mg	Usual range: 2–6 mg in divided doses
Midazolam	Versed Versed syrup (pediatric)	5 mg/mL, 10 mg/mL, 25 mg/mL, 50 mg/mL 2 mg of midazolam mL	Titrate to desired effect with multiple small doses Oral: 0.25–1.0 mg/kg; for pediatric patients, a maximum dose of 20 mg
Oxazepam	Serax	Capsules: 10 mg, 15 mg, 30 mg	10–15 mg, 3–4 times daily
Prazepam	Centrax	(not available in the United States)	
Quazepam	Doral	Tablets: 7.5 mg, 15 mg	Initiate at 15 mg, may be reduced to 7.5 mg before bedtime Geriatric patients: initiate at 7.5 mg before bedtime
Temazepam	Restoril Temazepam	Capsules: 7.5 mg, 15 mg, 22.5 mg, 30 mg Capsules: 7.5 mg, 15 mg, 22.5 mg, 30 mg	7.5–15 mg/day before bedtime Geriatric/Debilitated patients: 7.5 mg before bedtime
Triazolam	Halcion	Tablets: 0.125 mg, 0.25 mg	0.25 mg/day before bedtime Geriatric/Debilitated patients: 0.125–0.25 mg before bedtime
Nonbenzodiazepine hypnotics			
Eszopiclone	Lunesta	Tablets: 1 mg, 2 mg, 3 mg	2-3 mg before bedtime Geriatric/Debilitated patients: 1–2 mg before bedtime
Zaleplon	Sonata	Capsules: 5 mg, 10 mg	5–20 mg before bedtime Geriatric/Debilitated patients: 5–10 mg before bedtime
Zolpidem	Ambien Ambien CR	Tablets: 5 mg, 10 mg Tablets: 6.25 mg, 12.5 mg	10 mg before bedtime, Geriatric/Debilitated patients: 5 mg 12.5 mg before bedtime, Geriatric/Debilitated patients: 6.25 mg
Zopiclone	Imovane	(not available in the United States)	

TABLE 8.2 Barbiturates

Duration of action	Generic name	Therapeutic use
Ultra-short-acting (15 minutes to 3 hours)	Methohexital	General anesthetic
	Thiopental	General anesthetic, emergency treatment of seizures
Short-acting (3–6 hours)	Pentobarbital	Sedation, emergency treatment of seizures
	Secobarbital	Sedation, emergency treatment of seizures
Intermediate acting (6–12 hours)	Amobarbital	Hypnotic, sedation, emergency treatment of seizures
	Butabarbital	Hypnotic, sedative
	Butalbital	Combination with headache therapies
Long-acting (12–24 hours)	Phenobarbital	Sedation, seizures, many combination products
	Mephobarbital	Sedation, seizures

visits, comparable to the number of mentions for prescription opioids. Alprazolam was the benzodiazepine that was most frequently reported in emergency visits. Benzodiazepines were mentioned in 27% of suicide attempts (46).

PHARMACOKINETICS

Pathways that mediate the biotransformation of the benzodiazepines are presented in Figure 8.2.

Many benzodiazepines undergo hepatic metabolism involving oxidative reactions mediated by the cytochrome P450 (CYP450) enzymes (47–49). Oxidative metabolism reactions include N-dealkylation or aliphatic hydroxylation. The CYP enzymes involved in the metabolism of benzodiazepines are listed in Table 8.3. The CYP3A4 enzyme mediates the oxidative metabolism of many of the benzodiazepines and also plays a role in the biotransformation of the nonbenzodiazepine sedative-hypnotic agents, eszopicione, zaleplon, and zolpidem. Several of the benzodiazepines are converted into active metabolites such as desmethyldiazepam, which are very slowly cleared from the body. The final phase of metabolism for most benzodiazepines consists of conjugation of either the parent drug or their metabolites with glucuronide. Drugs or metabolites that undergo glucuronidation contain a hydroxyl group. Parent drugs, such as lorazepam and oxazepam, which undergo direct glucuronidation, are less subject to drug interactions or reduced clearance associated with impairment of hepatic function than are the other benzodiazepines.

The relationship between the pharmacokinetic profile of benzodiazepines and abuse liability is complex. It is generally believed that rapid onset of action is associated with euphoria (50). Onset of action after oral administration relies on the formulation of the drug, the intrinsic activity of the drug, lipid solubility, protein binding, and rate of entry into the brain. Some animal data suggest that greater lipid solubility increases the rate of brain uptake, with diazepam having more rapid brain uptake as compared to lorazepam (51). In clinical practice, pharmacokinetic factors do not always predict abuse liability. For example, clorazepate is rapidly decarboxylated in the stomach to desmethyldiazepam, which then reaches maximum plasma concentrations within 30 minutes or less (52), yet it is rarely cited as a benzodiazepine with high abuse potential. Subjective ratings by drug abusers of the "high" induced by clorazepate are lower than ratings of diazepam or lorazepam (53). Also, even though alprazolam and oxazepam differ only slightly in lipid solubility (54–56), intrinsic activity and rate of absorption are greater with alprazolam, which has higher abuse potential than oxazepam (30,31,57–60). Lower abuse potential is more consistently predicted with prodrugs that require hepatic metabolism to form the active moiety, such as the formation of desmethyldiazepam from halazepam, which appears to have lower abuse liability than diazepam (61). Therefore, the rate of absorption and entry into the brain may influence abuse liability, but other factors are also involved.

PHARMACODYNAMICS

Benzodiazepines exert their clinical effects through allosteric modulation of the $GABA_A$ receptor (62). As GABA is the major inhibitory neurotransmitter system in the brain, positive modulation of the receptor by benzodiazepines is responsible for sedative, anticonvulsant, hypnotic, and amnestic effects of the drug. The $GABA_A$ receptor is a pentameric protein structure surrounding a central chloride channel (63). These receptors may be activated directly by agonists such as muscimol, which opens the central channel leading to an influx of chloride ions, or indirectly by drugs such as benzodiazepines, which enhance the binding of GABA to the receptor and result in increased frequency of the opening of the central chloride channel (64). Both mechanisms lead to enhanced inhibitory effect by GABA neurons.

The five subunits that are linked to form the chloride ion channel are classified into several subtypes: alpha (α), beta (β),

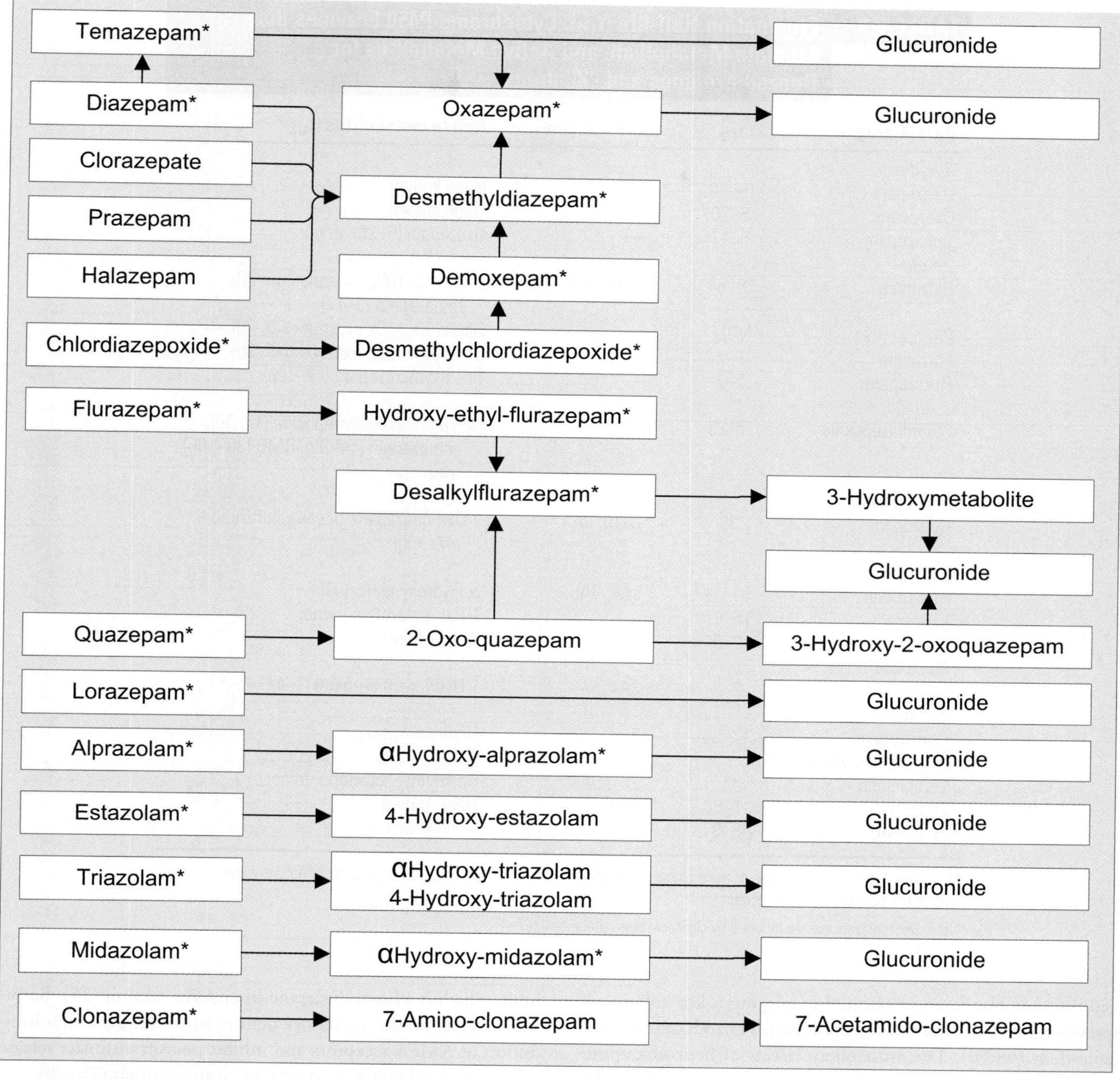

FIGURE 8.2. Biotransformation of benzodiazepines.

gamma (γ), delta (δ), epsilon (ϵ), rho (ρ), and pi (π), each of which has a unique sequence of amino acids (63). Minor alterations in amino acid sequences produce additional subtypes, which are designated by a number, and are relevant to the pharmacodynamic effects of drugs. Although the number of subunits, subtypes, and combinations may at first appear overwhelming, in reality only a relatively small number of combinations are of importance in humans. In the human brain, the most common structure of the $GABA_A$ receptor consists of two α, two β, and one γ subunit (63). Benzodiazepines bind at the interface of the γ2 and α subunits (62).

In humans, α 6 units have been identified and appear to be distributed in different regions of the brain, with the α1 unit located in the sensorimotor areas, cortex, globus pallidus, ventral thalamic complex, subthalamic nucleus, substantia nigra, and cerebellum in primates (65). $GABA_A$ receptors containing the α5 subunit are prominent in limbic areas (66). Receptors containing α1, α2, α3, and α5 subunits are sensitive to the effects of benzodiazepines. In contrast the presence of α4 or α6 subunits leads to a lack of sensitivity to benzodiazepines. $GABA_A$ receptors that contain α1 subunits appear to mediate the sedative-hypnotic effects of benzodiazepines (67–69). This

TABLE 8.3 Elimination Half-life ($t_{1/2}$), Cytochrome P450 Enzymes that Mediate Metabolism, and Active Metabolites for Benzodiazepines and "Z" drugs

Parent drug	$t_{1/2}$	CYP enzyme	Active metabolites ($t_{1/2}$)[a]
3-Hydroxy			
Lorazepam	10–20	—	None known
Oxazepam	5–20	—	None known
Temazepam	5–17	—	Oxazepam (5–20)–minor
2-Keto			
Diazepam	28–54	2C19, 3A4,	DMD (30–100), oxazepam (5–20), temazepam (5–17)
Clorazepate	ND/T	—	DMD (30–100); oxazepam (5–20)
Prazepam	1–2	—	DMD (30–100); oxazepam (5–20)
Flurazepam	2–3	—	Desalkylflurazepam (47–100)
2-Amino		—	
Chlordiazepoxide	7–25	—	Desmethylchlordiazepoxide (10–30), demoxepam (14–95), DMD (30–100), oxazepam (5–2)
Trifluoroethyl			
Quazepam	36	2C19, 3A4	2-Oxo-quazepam; desalkylflurazepam (47–100)
Triazole			
Alprazolam	10–14	3A4, 3A5	α-Hydroxy-alprazolam
Estazolam	15–17	—	1-Oxo-estazolam–minor
Triazolam	2–3	3A4	None known
Imidazole			
Midazolam	2–5	3A4, 3A5	1-Hydroxy-midazolam (1–4)
7-Nitro			
Clonazepam	17–56	3A4	None known
Non-benzodiazepines			
Eszopiclone	6	2E1, 3A4	Desmethyl-zopiclone–minor
Zaleplon	1–5	3A4	None known
Zolpidem	1.5–3	3A4, 1A2, 2D6	None known

*If known; ND/T, not detectable or trace amounts detected in plasma; DMD, desmethyldiazepam; minor, very low metabolite concentrations detected.

Note: Benzodiazepines are grouped by chemical class (italicized) (42–47).

subunit has also been implicated in playing a key role in the production of the ataxic effects of both benzodiazepines and zolpidem (68,70). The antianxiety effects of benzodiazepines may be mediated by receptors containing the α2, and possibly the α3 subunit (68,71). The α2 and α3 subunits also may be involved in the mediation of the muscle relaxant effects of benzodiazepines (72). The α5 unit is associated with sedation, learning, and memory in animal models (70,73).

Barbiturates share some pharmacodynamic properties with the benzodiazepines. At low concentrations, barbiturates act as positive modulators of the $GABA_A$ receptor via an allosteric mechanism (74). However, at higher concentrations, barbiturates act as direct $GABA_A$ receptor agonists by prolonging the duration of the opening of the chloride channel. $GABA_A$ receptors that contain the β2 or β3 subunit show greater sensitivity to the effects of pentobarbital than receptors with the β1 subunit (71). Pentobarbital shows the greatest efficacy as a GABA receptor agonist in receptor complexes that contain the α6 subunit, which is a benzodiazepine-insensitive subunit (75). Barbiturates may reduce excitatory neurotransmission through inhibition of AMPA receptors and inhibit neurotransmitter release by blockade of voltage-sensitive calcium channels (76–78).

Several nonbenzodiazepines compounds, which are commonly referred to as "the Z drugs," have been identified that act as positive modulators of the effects of GABA agonists on the $GABA_A$ receptor. These agents include the imidazopyridine, zolpidem; the pyrazolopyrimidine, zaleplon; and the cyclopyrrolone, zopiclone. (Zopiclone is marketed in the U.S. only as the more active S-enantiomer, eszopicione.) As would be expected, these drugs share many of the pharmacologic actions with the classic benzodiazepine agents including sedative-hypnotic, anxiolytic, myorelaxant, and anticonvulsant effects, although their selectivity for these actions differs. For example, animal studies suggest that zolpidem is more selective in its sedative effects as compared to its anticonvulsant actions than are quazepam, zaleplon, or zopiclone (79,80). Among the

Z drugs, eszopicione has the strongest antianxiety effect in animal models, which is produced at nonhypnotic doses (81,82). The Z drugs may differ from the classic benzodiazepines in that their amnestic effects may be less pronounced and tolerance is less likely to develop to their pharmacologic actions (4).

Electrophysiologic studies indicate that the Z drugs all act to enhance GABA-induced changes in chloride currents (5,6,83,84). This may occur through an allosteric mechanism that involves Z drug–induced increases in the affinity of GABA for the $GABA_A$ receptor. Evidence for this includes the finding that zaleplon enhances the binding of the $GABA_A$ receptor agonist muscimol to cerebellum tissue, as does diazepam (85).

Z drugs and benzodiazepines may act through overlapping binding sites on the interface between α and β subunits of the $GABA_A$ receptor. This is suggested by findings that the Z drugs inhibit the binding the benzodiazepine flunitrazepam to brain tissue (6,85,86). Also, the enhancement of muscimol binding produced by zaleplon is blocked by the administration of the benzodiazepine receptor antagonist flumazenil. Studies involving the selective replacement of the amino acids that comprise the $GABA_A$ receptor subunits indicate that zolpidem and zopiclone interact with amino acids located on specific sites on the α and β subunits that also interact with benzodiazepines (87–89). These studies have also demonstrated that zolpidem, however, binds to sites on these subunits that are not crucial for benzodiazepine activity.

Dissimilarities in the activity between individual Z drugs or between Z drugs and the classic benzodiazepines may arise, in part because of differences in the affinity of these drugs for the different subtypes of $GABA_A$ receptors. Benzodiazepines have roughly similar affinities for $GABA_A$ subtypes receptors that contain the α_1, α_2, α_3, and α_5 subunits. In contrast, zaleplon and zolpidem have more than 10-fold greater affinity for receptors with a $\alpha_1\beta_2\gamma_2$ composition than for those with a $\alpha_2\beta_2\gamma_2$ composition, whereas zopiclone has essentially equivalent affinity for these receptors (90). Zolpidem in contrast to the benzodiazepines and other Z drugs has little affinity for α_5-containing $GABA_A$ receptors, and the presence of the γ_3 subunit produces insensitivity to zolpidem (90).

Differences in binding affinities for the different $GABA_A$ receptor subtypes roughly correlate with the potency of the positive $GABA_A$ receptor modulators to enhance the GABA mediated currents (91). The full functional implications of differences in the affinities of Z drugs for the different $GABA_A$ receptor subtypes, however, remain far from being clear. A 10-fold difference in affinity for different receptor subtype may not be great enough to result in a distinct pharmacologic profile for a drug. There is some evidence, however, that zolpidem may have pharmacologic actions that are associated with a selective action on $GABA_A$ receptors that contain the α_1 subunit. In genetically altered mice that are missing the gene for the $GABA_A$ α_1 subunit, all of the high-affinity binding for zolpidem in the cortex is lost (92). In these mice, the hypnotic effects of zolpidem are greatly diminished whereas those of diazepam are increased, which is consistent with a selective action of zolpidem on the α_1 containing receptors (93).

DRUG–DRUG INTERACTIONS

The most serious drug–drug interactions occur when sedative hypnotics are combined with alcohol or other drugs that depress CNS activity. Benzodiazepines do not induce their own metabolism; however, those that are metabolized through CYP3A4 (Table 8.3) are subject to altered plasma levels by agents that inhibit this metabolic pathway. Common inhibitors are ketoconazole, itraconazole, macrolide antibiotics (erythromycin), fluoxetine, nefazodone, and cimetidine. Drugs that induce or inhibit CYP2C19 may also influence the metabolism of some benzodiazepines. For example, oral contraceptives containing estrogen and progesterone impair the metabolism of some substrates of CYP1A2, CYP3A4, and CYP2C19, although findings with benzodiazepines are inconsistent (94). One study found inhibition of alprazolam metabolism in women taking low-dose estrogen oral contraceptives (95), and another did not (96). Similarly, lorazepam metabolism was unaffected by oral contraceptives in one study (97), yet increased in another (95). The latter study also found enhanced elimination of temazepam. Oxazepam kinetics are not affected by oral contraceptives (97). The clearances of both chlordiazepoxide and diazepam are impaired in women taking oral contraceptives (98–100).

Barbiturates present a serious risk of CNS depression, coma, and death when taken in high doses or with ethanol or other sedative hypnotics. They induce their own metabolism (pharmacokinetic tolerance) and induce CYP2B6, CYP2C9, and CYP3A4, resulting in enhanced metabolism of drugs that are substrates of these cytochromes, reducing therapeutic effects. Patients taking phenobarbital may experience decreased effects of anticoagulants, oral contraceptives, corticosteroids, some antibiotics, and other drugs (101).

MECHANISM OF ADDICTION

Although the paths to sedative hypnotic addiction are complex and vary among individuals, it is helpful to consider three characteristics of the drug class that are related to misuse: (a) hedonic effects, (b) tolerance, and (c) the withdrawal syndrome. Use of benzodiazepines purely for the hedonic value, that is, to achieve a pleasurable or euphoric mood change, is rare unless they are used in combination with other drugs such as methadone, which results in a "boost." Benzodiazepines with a rapid onset of action, such as alprazolam or diazepam, probably present the greatest risk for this type of abuse.

Tolerance of clinical effects may lead some patients to escalate the dosage. The risk appears greatest when the drugs are used as hypnotics because tolerance of sedation occurs rapidly, though there is some evidence that temazepam (102) and eszopicione (103,104) have lower risk of tolerance than other agents. There is also evidence that tolerance does not develop to the anxiolytic action of benzodiazepines (105), and patients treated for panic disorder are more likely to decrease rather than increase their benzodiazepine dose; however, the issue of tolerance to the antianxiety effect remains controversial (106). There are also some reports of patients who have improvement in anxiety symptoms after discontinuation of long-term benzodiazepine treatment, suggesting that for some individuals, chronic treatment with these drugs actually exacerbates symptoms (107). Tolerance of the antiepileptic effects is well recognized and limits the use of these agents for long-term treatment of seizures, though the time to develop tolerance differs among drugs within the class (108). Partial tolerance develops to several other actions of the benzodiazepines, such as psychomotor and cognitive impairment (109–111), which may permit some patients to gradually escalate doses to supratherapeutic levels.

The withdrawal syndrome that appears upon decreasing dosage or abrupt discontinuation of treatment may produce uncomfortable mental and physical states that make it difficult for patients to terminate drug use. Rebound insomnia is a particular problem for patients who discontinue benzodiazepines. The withdrawal syndrome is discussed in greater detail later in this chapter.

Although the mechanism of therapeutic action is well known for benzodiazepines and barbiturates, the neurophysiologic basis of their reinforcing effects are not well understood. On the other hand, the pharmacodynamic mechanisms underlying the development of tolerance and withdrawal to sedative hypnotics are well studied. Tolerance, as evidenced by decreased responsiveness of $GABA_A$ receptors to benzodiazepines, has been demonstrated using measures of both electrophysiologic activity (112,113) and GABA-mediated chloride flux (114). The decreased ability of benzodiazepines to positively modulate $GABA_A$ receptors may result, in part, from the loss of interaction between benzodiazepine and GABA-binding sites within these receptors, referred to as "uncoupling" (115,116). Another possible mechanism of tolerance may involve benzodiazepine-induced internalization of surface $GABA_A$ receptors into intraneuronal sequestration sites (116). Alterations in sensitivities to the effects of benzodiazepines might also result from changes in the subunit composition of brain $GABA_A$ receptors. In vitro studies indicate that levels of the messenger RNAs (mRNAs) that are involved in the synthesis of the α_1 $GABA_A$ receptor subunit are reduced during prolonged exposure to benzodiazepines, whereas mRNAs for the benzodiazepine-insensitive α_4 subunit are increased soon after benzodiazepine withdrawal (117). In animals, tolerance to benzodiazepines has occurred in association with decreases in the density of binding sites for hippocampal $GABA_A$ receptors that contain the α_5 subunit (115). After withdrawal from the neurosteroid precursor, progesterone, α_4 subunit mRNAs and protein levels are increased in the brain, as may occur during withdrawal from benzodiazepines (118). These changes in α_4 subunit expression correlate with decreased sensitivity to the effects of benzodiazepines on GABA-mediated chloride currents (118). This loss of sensitivity can be prevented by blockade of the expression of α_4 subunits. These findings point to the possible role of increased α_4 subunit expression in early benzodiazepine withdrawal.

The glutamatergic system may play a major role in the benzodiazepine withdrawal syndrome. In animal models, anxiety associated with benzodiazepine withdrawal may involve upregulation of hippocampal AMPA receptors as evidenced by increased AMPA receptor GluR1 subunits and increased AMPA receptor binding (119–121). Other studies have confirmed increased AMPA receptor binding in the hippocampus and thalamus using different experimental paradigms of withdrawal but have not found corresponding alterations in levels of the GluR1 or GluR2 subunits in these brain regions (122).

ADDICTION LIABILITY

The benzodiazepines occupy an intermediate position of abuse liability, with barbiturates and older sedative hypnotics (e.g., methaqualone, ethchlorvynol) having greater risk of abuse, whereas anxiolytics and hypnotics that act via non-GABAergic mechanisms (e.g., buspirone, antidepressants, ramelteon) lack abuse potential. Many authorities believe that zolpidem, zopiclone, esopiclone, and zaleplon have lower potential for abuse than classic benzodiazepines; however, there are case reports of abuse and abstinence syndromes associated with abrupt discontinuation of high doses after prolonged use of these agents. More controversial is the issue of relative abuse liability among the benzodiazepines themselves. Using the sole criterion of a positive mood effect in humans, the benzodiazepines with the highest liability for abuse are flunitrazepam, diazepam, alprazolam, and possibly lorazepam. Those with the lowest positive reinforcing effects in humans are clonazepam, chlordiazepoxide, halazepam (61), prazepam (123), quazepam, and oxazepam. That said, individuals at risk for sedative-hypnotic abuse (e.g., alcoholics) may misuse any of the benzodiazepines, even those with relatively low potential for abuse. Benzodiazepines with the highest abuse potential produce a rapid onset of pleasant mood, well-being, relief of dysphoria, a sense of increased popularity, the belief that thoughts flow more easily, and a general state of contentment (124).

The relative abuse liability of the barbiturates and the Z drugs, compared to benzodiazepines, is a matter of some controversy. In human laboratory studies that assess abuse potential, these drugs produce euphoric effects at doses above their typical therapeutic ranges. For example, eszopicione, at doses of 6 mg and 12 mg, produced euphoric effects comparable to 20 mg of diazepam in previous sedative-hypnotic abusers. Studies examining the abuse liability of 25 mg, 50 mg, and 75 mg of zaleplon, in subjects with a history of sedative-hypnotic abuse, indicated abuse potential similar to benzodiazepines and benzodiazepine-like hypnotics. Zolpidem, 10 mg, produced effects similar to 0.25 mg of triazolam (125), but higher doses of triazolam (0.75 mg) were more often rated as similar to barbiturates than high doses of zolpidem (45 mg). Furthermore, postmarketing surveillance indicates a relatively low potential for abuse for zolpidem considering how often it is prescribed (126).

TOXICITY STATES AND THEIR MEDICAL MANAGEMENT

Toxicity must be considered whenever therapeutic agents are prescribed. With respect to sedative hypnotics, benzodiazepines provide a greater margin of safety than barbiturates and older agents. Despite the improved safety profile, prescription of benzodiazepines is associated with acute and chronic risks.

In the therapeutic context, acute toxicity of benzodiazepines includes sedation, psychomotor impairment, and memory problems. It is well established that acute doses of benzodiazepines produce anterograde amnesia, difficulty acquiring new learning (127), and sedation that may affect attention and concentration. Tolerance usually develops to most of the cognitive effects, but not in all patients. Those who use intermittent doses ("prn") of high-potency agents may not develop tolerance and continue to be at risk for impaired psychomotor and memory function, especially in the first few hours after taking a dose. Furthermore, studies (128) and clinical experience suggest that not all benzodiazepines produce the same type or severity of cognitive impairment. Although many studies have found no cognitive impairment associated with long-term benzodiazepine treatment (129,130), others have reported persistent problems in psychomotor function, learning, concentration, and visuospatial skills (21,131). In chronic high-dose users, greater impairment is seen in men, elderly, and individuals taking the highest doses (127). A meta-analysis suggested a pervasive cognitive impairment in chronic users, but the interpretation is complicated by comparing studies with different methods and populations (21). Even in patients with persistent cognitive impairment detected by neuropsychologic testing, there is substantial improvement when benzodiazepines are discontinued, though patients still perform worse than controls at 6 months after the medication is stopped (132). Most patients do not report persistent cognitive difficulties, either because they underestimate the impairment or because the neuropsychologic test findings have little relevance for everyday life.

Anterograde amnesia occurs with therapeutic doses of benzodiazepines, and the impairment in learning new information represents a major drawback of these medications. Some tolerance develops to the cognitive impairment, but it is not complete. Controlled studies that take into account alcohol use, psychiatric disorders, and age indicate that a mild cognitive disturbance may persist but that it does not interfere with the demands of everyday function.

An exception may be the elderly patient who is particularly vulnerable to falls and memory problems, though one study found the memory impairment in elderly taking benzodiazepines was rather small (133). Falls, conversely, present a serious problem for the elderly. Classic benzodiazepines, nonbenzodiazepine hypnotics, SSRI antidepressants, and antipsychotics have all been linked to falls and fractures in the elderly (134–136), making the treatment of insomnia in aged patients a challenge. Zolpidem also produces anterograde amnesia and has been associated with somnambulism and complex nocturnal behaviors, such as eating, shopping, and driving. Similar problems may be seen with zaleplon, especially at high doses. It is not known whether all hypnotics are capable of producing such effects; however, the U.S. Food and Drug Administration (FDA) issued a request for a label change requiring that benzodiazepine and nonbenzodiazepine hypnotics include a warning describing these complex sleep-related behaviors.

Several surveys in different countries have found that there is a higher incidence of motor vehicle accidents associated with benzodiazepines (137,138). It is not known whether this reflects acute psychomotor impairment, falling asleep at the wheel, or persistent visuospatial impairment.

The risks of benzodiazepines during pregnancy and lactation have been the subject of controversy. Data pooled from cohort studies have not demonstrated an increased risk of major malformations or cleft palate (139). Conversely, when data from case control studies were pooled in the same meta-analysis, a small but statistically significant association was found between exposure to benzodiazepines and oral cleft abnormalities or other major malformations. The rate of cleft palate in the general population is estimated at 0.06% (140), and case-control studies show that with benzodiazepines, the risk may be approximately doubled, still rather low at 0.12%. A review of older studies assessing the possible association of benzodiazepine use in the first trimester and cleft palate found that the use of different sampling schemes, different benzodiazepines at different doses for different durations, and failure of some studies to account for concurrent medications or illnesses contributed to the "confusion and controversy regarding the safety of benzodiazepine use during pregnancy" (141).

In a well-designed study of 873,879 infants whose mothers were registered in the Swedish Medical Birth Register, 1,979 infants were exposed to benzodiazepines or nonbenzodiazepine hypnotics (mainly zopiclone) but increased risk of orofacial clefts was not found (142). They did find an increased risk for low birth weight in infants that had both early and late exposure to benzodiazepines in utero, but it was most evident in women who also had been taking an antidepressant. They also found an unexpectedly high number of infants with pylorostenosis and alimentary tract atresia, although concomitant exposure to antidepressants and an anticonvulsant complicates the interpretation of the finding. Another study found that infants exposed in the first trimester to the combination of serotonin reuptake inhibitor antidepressants and benzodiazepines had increased risk of congenital anomalies and congenital heart disease compared to unexposed; however, when maternal illness was controlled, only the increased risk for congenital heart disease remained significant (143). Monotherapy with either class of drug was not associated with an increased risk. Most recent studies do not find an association of in utero benzodiazepine exposure alone with major congenital anomalies (144,145).

Although the major concern of clinicians has been congenital anomalies associated with benzodiazepines, two other clinically important problems may be encountered during pregnancy. Newborns who have been exposed to benzodiazepines in utero during the last trimester or during delivery may present with *floppy baby syndrome*, which is characterized by low Apgar scores, poor sucking, hypotonia, poor reflexes, and apnea (146). Neonatal withdrawal syndromes have also been reported (147).

Benzodiazepines administered to nursing mothers enter the breast milk but appear in such low concentrations that they do not usually cause adverse effects in infants (148–151). There are two important exceptions to this general rule: The risk to the infant is higher (a) if the benzodiazepine is given in high doses antepartum and continued postpartum and (b) if infants have impaired hepatic function, as evidenced by hyperbilirubinemia (150). Despite their relative safety, breastfed infants whose mothers are taking benzodiazepines should be monitored for lethargy, weight loss, and signs of an abstinence syndrome.

The use of anticonvulsants, including phenobarbital, by pregnant women with epilepsy has been associated with reports of harm to the fetus, although the findings are not consistent (152). The frequency of anticonvulsant embryopathy, defined as major malformations, growth retardation, and hypoplasia of the midface and fingers, is increased in infants exposed to phenobarbital alone or in combination with other anticonvulsants, compared to those whose mothers had a history of epilepsy but took no medications during pregnancy (153).

MEDICAL COMPLICATIONS

All sedative hypnotics produce effects on a continuum from sedation to obtundation. Barbiturates have a greater risk for respiratory depression than do benzodiazepines. In overdose situations, sedative hypnotics are often combined with ethanol or other CNS depressants. When high doses of benzodiazepines are ingested, either as a therapeutic intervention or overdose, initial signs of toxicity are ataxia and impaired gag reflex. Rarely sedative hypnotics produce disinhibition or paradoxical excitement.

A severe withdrawal syndrome after high-dose chronic administration of chlordiazepoxide or diazepam was demonstrated in the early 1960s (154,155) and, in its most severe form, can include grand mal seizures and psychosis. A characteristic abstinence syndrome may develop upon abrupt discontinuation of therapeutic doses of benzodiazepines that are administered for several weeks (11). When administered for short periods and at therapeutic doses, the withdrawal syndrome is usually mild, consisting of anxiety, headache, insomnia, dysphoria, tremor, and muscle twitching. After long-term treatment with therapeutic doses, the syndrome increases in severity and may include autonomic dysfunction, nausea, vomiting, depersonalization, derealization, delirium, hallucinations, illusions, agitation, and grand mal seizures. The time course of the abstinence syndrome is related to the half-life of the agent, with patients taking short-half-life agents (lorazepam, alprazolam, temazepam) developing symptoms within 24 hours of discontinuation, the severity of which peaks at 48 hours. With longer-half-life agents such as diazepam, symptoms may develop a week after drug discontinuation and last for several weeks. This timeline should be used as a general guideline, because some patients on long-acting agents will develop symptoms earlier than predicted by the pharmacokinetics of the drug. In addition, some clinicians believe that there is prolonged withdrawal syndrome that persists for several months, but it has not been clearly distinguished from return of original anxiety symptoms.

In general, longer treatment periods, higher doses, sudden drug discontinuation, and psychopathology increase the severity of the abstinence syndrome. Clinical experience has shown that there is great variability in the sensitivity of patients to discontinuation of benzodiazepines, and all patients who have been taking the drug for several weeks or longer should have the medication tapered.

The withdrawal syndrome from barbiturates was described by Wikler (156) using 0.8 to 2.2 g/day oral doses of secobarbital or pentobarbital for 6 weeks or longer. Upon abrupt discontinuation, apprehension, uneasiness, muscular weakness, coarse tremors, postural hypotension, anorexia, vomiting, and myoclonic jerks occurred within the first day and lasted up to 2 weeks. Grand mal seizure occurred within 2 to 3 days of discontinuation and lasted as long as 8 days. Delirium was most likely to develop 3 to 8 days after drug discontinuation and lasted up to 2 weeks. Strategies for management of the barbiturate withdrawal syndrome include transition to an equivalent dose of phenobarbital, determined either by a challenge dose or loading dose procedure (36).

CONCLUSION

Benzodiazepines are the most widely used and abused drugs of the sedative hypnotic class. In animal models and human laboratory studies, they occupy an intermediate position of abuse liability that is lower than barbiturates, but higher than anxiolytics such as buspirone (30) that do not act at the $GABA_A$ receptor complex. In patients with anxiety disorders, abuse is not common; however, certain subgroups of patients, such as individuals with alcohol dependence and those in methadone maintenance programs, are at high risk to misuse these agents. Compared to the general population, higher rates of benzodiazepine use are found in the elderly and patients with chronic pain; however, there is insufficient evidence to suggest these groups abuse benzodiazepines. The newer nonbenzodiazepine hypnotics, commonly referred to as the Z drugs, may have a lower potential for abuse, tolerance, and dependence, though they are not devoid of such risk. The identification of $GABA_A$ receptor subtypes and clarification of their function provide hope that drug development will lead to $GABA_A$ agonists and modulators that have fewer adverse effects, lower risk for dependence, and greater specificity of action (157).

REFERENCES

1. Ciraulo DA Sarid-Segal O. Sedative-, hypnotic-, or anxiolytic-related disorders. In: Sadock B, Sadock B, eds. *Comprehensive textbook of psychiatry.* New York: Lippincott Williams & Wilkins, 2004:1300–1318.
2. Greenblatt D Shader R. *Benzodiazepines in clinical practice.* New York: Raven Press, 1974.
3. Charney D, Mihic S, Harris R. Hypnotics and sedatives. In: Hardman J, Limbird L, Gilman A, eds. *The pharmacological basis of therapeutics.* New York: McGraw-Hill, Medical Publishing Edition, 2001.
4. Drover DR. Comparative pharmacokinetics and pharmacodynamics of short-acting hypnosedatives: zaleplon, zolpidem and zopiclone. *Clin Pharmacokinet* 2004;43(4):227–238.
5. Fleck MW. Molecular actions of (S)-desmethylzopiclone (SEP-174559), an anxiolytic metabolite of zopiclone. *J Pharmacol Exp Ther* 2002;302 (2):612–618.
6. Sanna E, Busonero F, Talani G, et al. Comparison of the effects of zaleplon, zolpidem, and triazolam at various GABA(A) receptor subtypes. *Eur J Pharmacoll* 2002;451(2):103–110.
7. Harvey D. Hypnotics and sedatives. In: Goodman L, Gilman A, eds. *The pharmacological basis of therapeutics.* New York: Macmillan Publishing Co., Inc., 1975:102–136.
8. Levy R, Mattson R, Meldrum B, et al., eds. *Antiepileptic drugs*, 5th ed. Philadelphia: Lippincott Williams & Wilkins, 2002.
9. Ciraulo DA, Shader RI, eds. *Clinical manual of chemical dependence.* Washington, DC: American Psychiatric Press, Inc., 1991:420.
10. Epstein S, Renner J, Ciraulo DA, et al. Opioids. In: Kranzler H Ciraulo DA, eds. *Clinical manual of addiction psychopharmacology.* Washington, DC: American Psychiatric Publishing, Inc., 2005:55–110.
11. American Psychiatric Association. *Benzodiazepine dependence, toxicity, and abuse.* Washington, DC: Author, 1990.
12. Piper A. Addiction to benzodiazepines—how common. *Arch Fam Med* 1995;4(11):964–970.
13. Zandstra S, Furer J, van de Lisdonk E, et al. Different study criteria affect the prevalence of benzodiazepine use. *Soc Psychiatry Psychiatr Epidemiol* 2002;37(3):139–144.
14. Lagnaoui R, Depont F, Fourrier A, et al. Patterns and correlates of benzodiazepine use in the French general population. *Eur J Clin Pharmacol* 2004;60(7):523–529.
15. Veronese A, Garatti M Cipriani A. et al. Benzodiazepine use in the real world of psychiatric practice: low-dose, long-term drug taking and low rates of treatment discontinuation. *Eur J Clin Pharmacol* 2007;63(9): 867–873.
16. Olfson M, Marcus S, Wan G, et al. National trends in the outpatient treatment of anxiety disorders. *J Clin Psychiatry* 2004;65(9):1166–1173.
17. Ciraulo DA, Nace EP. Benzodiazepine treatment of anxiety or insomnia in substance abuse patients. *Am J Addict* 2000;9(4):276–279; discussion, 280–284.
18. Darke S, Ross J, Teeson M, et al. Health service utilization and benzodiazepine use among heroin users: findings from the Australian treatment Outcome Study (ATOS). *Addiction* 2003;98(8):1129–1135.
19. Dinwiddie S, Cottler L, Compton W, et al. Psychopathology and HIV risk behaviors among injection drug users in and out of treatment. *Drug Alcohol Depend* 1996;43(1–2):1–11.
20. Ross J Darke S. The nature of benzodiazepine dependence among heroin users in Sydney, Australia. *Addiction* 2000;95(12):1785–1793.
21. Barker MJ, Greenwood KM, Jackson M, et al. Cognitive effects of long-term benzodiazepine use: a meta-analysis. *CNS Drugs* 2004;18(1):37–48.
22. Strain E, Brooner R, Bigelow G. Clustering of multiple substance use an dpsychiatric diagnosis in opiate addicts. *Drug Alcohol Depend* 1991;27(2):127–134.
23. Williams H, Oyefeso A, Ghodse A. Benzodiazepine misuse and dependence among opiate addicts in treatment. *Ir J Psychol Med* 1996;13:62–64.
24. Johansson B, Berglund M, Hanson M, et al. Dependence on legal psychotropic drugs among alcoholics. *Alcohol Alcohol* 2003;38(6):613–618.
25. Lejoyeux M, Solomon J, Ades J. Benzodiazepine treatment for alcohol-dependent patients. *Alcohol Alcohol* 1998;33(6):563–575.
26. Iguchi M, Handelsman L, Bickel W, et al. Benzodiazepine and sedative use/abuse by methadone maintenance. *Drug Alcohol Depend* 1993; 32(3):257–266.
27. Stitzer M, Griffiths R, McLellan A, et al. Diazepam use among methadone ainmtenance patients: patterns and dosages. *Drug Alcohol Depend* 1981;8(3):189–199.
28. deWitt H, McCarcken S, Uhlenhuth E, et al. Diazepine preference in subjects seeking treatment for anxiety. *NIDA Res Monogr* 1987;76:248–254.
29. deWitt H, Pierri J, Johanson C. Reinforcing and subjective effects of diazepam in nondrug-abusing volunteers. *Pharm Biochem Behav* 1991;33(1):205–213.
30. Ciraulo DA, Barnhill J, Ciraulo AM, et al. Alterations in pharmacodynamics of anxiolytics in abstinent alcoholic men: subjective responses, abuse liability, and electroencephalographic effects of alprazolam, diazepam, and buspirone. *J Clin Pharmacol* 1997;37(1):64–73.
31. Ciraulo DA, Barnhill J Greenblatt D, et al. Abuse liability and clinical pharmacokinetics of alprazolam in alcoholic men. *J Clin Psychiatry* 1988;49(9):333–337.
32. Ciraulo DA, Sands B Shader R. Critical review of liability for benzodiazepine abuse among alcoholics. *Am J Psychiatry* 1988;145(12):1501–1506.
33. Ciraulo DA, Sarid-Segal O, Knapp CM, et al. Liability to alprazolam abuse in daughters of alcoholics. *Am J Psychiatry* 1996;153(7):956–958.
34. Cowley DS, Roy-Byrne PP, Godon C, et al. Response to diazepam in sons of alcoholics. *Alcohol Clin Exp Res* 1992;16(6):1057–1063.
35. Ciraulo DA, Barnhill JG, Ciraulo AM, et al. Parental alcoholism as a risk factor in benzodiazepine abuse: a pilot study. *Am J Psychiatry* 1989; 146(10):1333–1335.
36. Kranzler H, Ciraulo DA. *Clinical manual of addiction psychopharmacology.* Washington, DC: American Psychiatric Publishing, Inc., 2005.
37. Gilson SF, Chilcoat HD, Stapleton JM. Illicit drug use by persons with disabilities: insights from the National Household Survey on Drug Abuse. *Am J Public Health* 1996;86(11):1613–1615.
38. Fishbain DA, Rosomoff HL, Rosomoff RS. Drug abuse, dependence, and addiction in chronic pain patients. *Clin J Pain* 1992;8(2):77–85.
39. Hardo PG, Kennedy TD. Night sedation and arthritic pain. *J R Soc Med* 1991;84(2):73–75.
40. Hendler N, Cimini C, Ma T, et al. A comparison of cognitive impairment due to benzodiazepines and to narcotics. *Am J Psychiatry* 1980; 137(7):828–830.
41. King SA, Strain JJ. Benzodiazepines and chronic pain. *Pain* 1990;41(1): 3–4.
42. King SA, Strain JJ. Benzodiazepine use by chronic pain patients. *Clin J Pain* 1990;6(2):143–147.
43. Kouyanou K, Pither CE, Wessely S. Medication misuse, abuse and dependence in chronic pain patients. *J Psychosom Res* 1997;43(5):497–504.
44. Substance Abuse and Mental Health Services Administration. *Treatment episode data set (TEDS) highlights.* Rockville, MD, Author: 2007.
45. Substance Abuse and Mental Health Services Administration, ed. *Results for the 2006 national survey on drug use and health: national findings.* Rockville, MD: Author, 2007.
46. Substance Abuse and Mental Health Services Administration. In: Drug Abuse Warning Network, ed. *National estimates of drug-related emergency department visits (DAWN).* Rockville, MD: Author, 2007.
47. Fukasawa T, Suzuki A, Otani K. Effects of genetic polymorphism of cytochrome P450 enzymes on the pharmacokinetics of benzodiazepines. *J Clin Pharm Ther* 2007;32(4):333–341.
48. Wang JS, DeVane CL. Pharmacokinetics and drug interactions of the sedative hypnotics. *Psychopharmacol Bull* 2003;37(1):10–29.
49. Chouinard G, Lefko-Singh K, Teboul E. Metabolism of anxiolytics and hypnotics: benzodiazepines, buspirone, zoplicone, and zolpidem. *Cell Mol Neurobiol* 1999;19(4):533–552.
50. Greenblatt DJ, Arendt RM, Shader RI. Pharmacodynamics of benzodiazepines after single oral doses: kinetic and physiochemical correlates. *Psychopharmacology Suppl* 1984;1:92–97.
51. Greenblatt DJ, Sethy VH. Benzodiazepine concentrations in brain directly reflect receptor occupancy: studies of diazepam, lorazepam, and oxazepam. *Psychopharmacology (Berl)* 1990;102(3):373–378.

52. Norman TR, Fulton A, Burrows GD, et al. Pharmacokinetics of N-desmethyldiazepam after a single oral dose of clorazepate: the effect of smoking. *Eur J Clin Pharmacol* 1981;21(3):229–233.
53. O'Brien CP. Benzodiazepine use, abuse, and dependence. *J Clin Psychiatry* 2005;66(Suppl 2):28–33.
54. Arendt RM, Greenblatt DJ, Liebisch DC, et al. Determinants of benzodiazepine brain uptake: lipophilicity versus binding affinity. *Psychopharmacology (Berl)* 1987;93(1):72–76.
55. Scavone JM, Friedman H, Greenblatt DJ, et al. Effect of age, body composition, and lipid solubility on benzodiazepine tissue distribution in rats. *Arzneimittelforschung* 1987;37(1):2–6.
56. Greenblatt DJ, Arendt RM, Abernethy DR, et al. In vitro quantitation of benzodiazepine lipophilicity: relation to in vivo distribution. *Br J Anaesth* 1983;55(10):985–989.
57. Griffiths RR, Bigelow G, Liebson I. Human drug self-administration: double-blind comparison of pentobarbital, diazepam, chlorpromazine and placebo. *J Pharmacol Exp Ther* 1979;210(2):301–310.
58. Griffiths RR, Bigelow GE, Liebson I, et al. Drug preference in humans: double-blind choice comparison of pentobarbital, diazepam, and placebo. *J Pharmacol Exp Ther* 1980;215(3):649–661.
59. Griffiths RR, McLeod DR, Bigelow GE, et al. Comparison of diazepam and oxazepam: preference, liking and extent of abuse. *J Pharmacol Exp Ther* 1984;229(2):501–508.
60. Griffiths RR, Wolf B. Relative abuse liability of different benzodiazepines in drug abusers. *J Clin Psychopharmacol* 1990;10(4):237–243.
61. Jaffe JH, Ciraulo DA, Nies A, et al. Abuse potential of halazepam and of diazepam in patients recently treated for acute alcohol withdrawal. *Clin Pharmacol Ther* 1983;34(5):623–630.
62. Jones-Davis DM, Song L, Gallagher MJ, et al. Structural determinants of benzodiazepine allosteric regulation of GABA(A) receptor currents. *J Neurosci* 2005;25(35):8056–8065.
63. Benarroch EE. GABAA receptor heterogeneity, function, and implications for epilepsy. *Neurology* 2007;68(8):612–614.
64. Korpi ER, Grunder G, Luddens H. Drug interactions at GABA(A) receptors. *Prog Neurobiol* 2002;67(2):113–159.
65. Dennis T, Dubois A, Benavides J, et al. Distribution of central omega 1 (benzodiazepine1) and omega 2 (benzodiazepine2) receptor subtypes in the monkey and human brain. An autoradiographic study with [3H]flunitrazepam and the omega 1 selective ligand [3H]zolpidem. *J Pharmacol Exp Ther* 1988;247(1):309–322.
66. Lingford-Hughes A, Hume SP, Feeney A, et al. Imaging the GABA-benzodiazepine receptor subtype containing the alpha5-subunit in vivo with [11C]Ro15 4513 positron emission tomography. *J Cereb Blood Flow Metab* 2002;22(7):878–889.
67. McKernan RM, Rosahl TW, Reynolds DS, et al. Sedative but not anxiolytic properties of benzodiazepines are mediated by the GABA(A) receptor alpha1 subtype. *Nat Neurosci* 2000;3(6):587–592.
68. Rowlett JK, Platt DM, Lelas S, et al. Different GABAA receptor subtypes mediate the anxiolytic, abuse-related, and motor effects of benzodiazepine-like drugs in primates. *Proc Natl Acad Sci U S A* 2005;102(3):915–920.
69. Rudolph U, Crestani F, Benke D, et al. Benzodiazepine actions mediated by specific gamma-aminobutyric acid(A) receptor subtypes. *Nature* 1999;401(6755):796–800.
70. Savic MM, Huang S, Furtmuller R, et al. Are GABAA receptors containing alpha5 subunits contributing to the sedative properties of benzodiazepine site agonists. *Neuropsychopharmacology* 2008;33(2):332–339.
71. Dias R, Sheppard WF, Fradley RL, et al. Evidence for a significant role of alpha 3-containing GABAA receptors in mediating the anxiolytic effects of benzodiazepines. *J Neurosci* 2005;25(46):10682–10688.
72. Crestani F, Low K, Keist R, et al. Molecular targets for the myorelaxant action of diazepam. *Mol Pharmacol* 2001;59(3):442–445.
73. Collinson N, Kuenzi FM, Jarolimek W, et al. Enhanced learning and memory and altered GABAergic synaptic transmission in mice lacking the alpha 5 subunit of the GABAA receptor. *J Neurosci* 2002;22(13):5572–5580.
74. Thompson SA, Whiting PJ, Wafford KA. Barbiturate interactions at the human GABAA receptor: dependence on receptor subunit combination. *Br J Pharmacol* 1996;117(3):521–527.
75. Drafts BC, Fisher JL. Identification of structures within GABAA receptor alpha subunits that regulate the agonist action of pentobarbital. *J Pharmacol Exp Ther* 2006;318(3):1094–1101.
76. Ko GY, Brown-Croyts LM, Teyler TJ. The effects of anticonvulsant drugs on NMDA-EPSP, AMPA-EPSP, and GABA-IPSP in the rat hippocampus. *Brain Res Bull* 1997;42(4):297–302.
77. Taverna FA, Cameron BR, Hampson DL, et al. Sensitivity of AMPA receptors to pentobarbital. *Eur J Pharmacoll* 1994;267(3):R3–R5.
78. Zhan RZ, Fujiwara N, Yamakura T, et al. Differential inhibitory effects of thiopental, thiamylal and phenobarbital on both voltage-gated calcium channels and NMDA receptors in rat hippocampal slices. *Br J Anaesth* 1998;81(6):932–939.
79. Sanger DJ. The pharmacology and mechanisms of action of new generation, non-benzodiazepine hypnotic agents. *CNS Drugs* 2004;18(Suppl 1):9–15; discussion, 41–45.
80. Sanger DJ, Morel E, Perrault G. Comparison of the pharmacological profiles of the hypnotic drugs, zaleplon and zolpidem. *Eur J Pharmacol* 1996;313(1–2):35–42.
81. Carlson JN, Haskew R, Wacker J, et al. Sedative and anxiolytic effects of zopiclone's enantiomers and metabolite. *Eur J Pharmacol* 2001;415(2-3):181–189.
82. Griebel G, Perrault G, Sanger DJ. Limited anxiolytic-like effects of non-benzodiazepine hypnotics in rodents. *J Psychopharmacol* 1998;12(4):356–365.
83. Im HK, Im WB, Hamilton BJ, et al. Potentiation of gamma-aminobutyric acid-induced chloride currents by various benzodiazepine site agonists with the alpha 1 gamma 2, beta 2 gamma 2 and alpha 1 beta 2 gamma 2 subtypes of cloned gamma-aminobutyric acid type A receptors. *Mol Pharmacol* 1993;44(4):866–870.
84. Mercik K, Piast M, Mozrzymas JW. Benzodiazepine receptor agonists affect both binding and gating of recombinant alpha1beta2gamma2 gamma-aminobutyric acid-A receptors. *Neuroreport* 2007;18(8):781–785.
85. Noguchi H, Kitazumi K, Mori M, et al. Binding and neuropharmacological profile of zaleplon, a novel nonbenzodiazepine sedative/hypnotic. *Eur J Pharmacol* 2002;434(1–2):21–28.
86. Doble A, Canton T, Dreisler S, et al. RP 59037 and RP 60503: anxiolytic cyclopyrrolone derivatives with low sedative potential. interaction with the gamma-aminobutyric acid A/benzodiazepine receptor complex and behavioral effects in the rodent. *J Pharmacol Exp Ther* 1993;266(3):1213–1226.
87. Davies M, Newell JG, Derry JM, et al. Characterization of the interaction of zopiclone with gamma-aminobutyric acid type A receptors. *Mol Pharmacol* 2000;58(4):756–762.
88. Hanson SM, Czajkowski C. Structural mechanisms underlying benzodiazepine modulation of the GABA(A) receptor. *J Neurosci* 2008;28(13):3490–3499.
89. Sancar F, Ericksen SS, Kucken AM, et al. Structural determinants for high-affinity zolpidem binding to GABA-A receptors. *Mol Pharmacol* 2007;71(1):38–46.
90. Damgen K, Luddens H. Zaleplon displays a selectivity to recombinant $GABA_A$ *Neuroscience Res Community* 1999;25:139–148.
91. Petroski RE, Pomeroy JE, Das R, et al. Indiplon is a high-affinity positive allosteric modulator with selectivity for alpha1 subunit-containing GABAA receptors. *J Pharmacol Exp Ther* 2006;317(1):369–377.
92. Kralic JE, Korpi ER, O'Buckley TK, et al. Molecular and pharmacological characterization of GABA(A) receptor alpha1 subunit knockout mice. *J Pharmacol Exp Ther* 2002;302(3):1037–1045.
93. Kralic JE, O'Buckley TK, Khisti RT, et al. GABA(A) receptor alpha-1 subunit deletion alters receptor subtype assembly, pharmacological and behavioral responses to benzodiazepines and zolpidem. *Neuropharmacology* 2002;43(4):685–694.
94. Granfors MT, Backman JT, Laitila J, et al. Oral contraceptives containing ethinyl estradiol and gestodene markedly increase plasma concentra-

tions and effects of tizanidine by inhibiting cytochrome P450 1A2. *Clin Pharmacol Ther* 2005;78(4):400–411.
95. Stoehr GP, Kroboth PD, Juhl RP, et al. Effect of oral contraceptives on triazolam, temazepam, alprazolam, and lorazepam kinetics. *Clin Pharmacol Ther* 1984;36(5):683–690.
96. Scavone JM, Greenblatt DJ, Locniskar A, et al. Alprazolam pharmacokinetics in women on low-dose oral contraceptives. *J Clin Pharmacol* 1988;28(5):454–457.
97. Abernethy D, Greenblatt D, Ochs H, et al. Lorazepam and oxazepam kinetics in women on low-dose oral contraceptives. *Clin Pharmacol Ther* 1983;33(5):628–632.
98. Abernethy D, Greenblatt D, Divoll M, et al. Impairment of diazepam metabolism by low-dose estrogen-containing oral-contraceptive steroids. *N Engl J Med* 1982;306(13):791–792.
99. Roberts RK, Desmond PV, Wilkinson GR, et al. Disposition of chlordiazepoxide: sex differences and effects of oral contraceptives. *Clin Pharmacol Ther* 1979;25(6):826–831.
100. Patwardhan RV, Mitchell MC, Johnson RF, et al. Differential effects of oral contraceptive steroids on the metabolism of benzodiazepines. *Hepatology* 1983;3(2):248–253.
101. Ciraulo DA, Shader RI, Greenblatt DJ, et al. *Drug interactions in psychiatry*. Baltimore: Williams & Wilkins, 1989:198–199.
102. van Steveninck AL, Wallnofer AE Schoemaker RC, et al. A study of the effects of long-term use on individual sensitivity to temazepam and lorazepam in a clinical population. *Br J Clin Pharmacol* 1997;44(3):267–275.
103. Krystal AD, Walsh JK, Laska E, et al. Sustained efficacy of eszopiclone over 6 months of nightly treatment: results of a randomized, double-blind, placebo-controlled study in adults with chronic insomnia. *Sleep* 2003;26(7):793–799.
104. Roth T, Walsh JK, Krystal A, et al. An evaluation of the efficacy and safety of eszopiclone over 12 months in patients with chronic primary insomnia. *Sleep Med* 2005;6(6):487–495.
105. Rickels K, Case WG, Downing RW, et al. Long-term diazepam therapy and clinical outcome. *JAMA* 1983;250(6):767–771.
106. Lader M, File S. The biological basis of benzodiazepine dependence. *Psychol Med* 1987;17(3):539–547.
107. Schweizer E, Rickels K, Case WG, et al. Long-term therapeutic use of benzodiazepines: II. Effects of gradual taper. *Arch Gen Psychiatry* 1990;47(10):908–915.
108. Riss J, Cloyd J, Gates J, et al. Benzodiazepines in epilepsy: pharmacology and pharmacokinetics. *Acta Neurol Scand* 2008;118(2):69–86.
109. File SE. Tolerance to the behavioral actions of benzodiazepines. *Neurosci Biobehav Rev* 1985;9(1):113–121.
110. Greenblatt DJ, Shader RI. Dependence, tolerance, and addiction to benzodiazepines: clinical and pharmacokinetic considerations. *Drug Metab Rev* 1978;8(1):13–28.
111. Rosenberg HC, Chiu TH. Time course for development of benzodiazepine tolerance and physical dependence. *Neurosci Biobehav Rev* 1985;9(1):123–131.
112. Zeng XJ, Tietz EI. Benzodiazepine tolerance at GABAergic synapses on hippocampal CA1 pyramidal cells. *Synapse* 1999;31(4):263–277.
113. Zeng XJ, Tietz EI. Role of bicarbonate ion in mediating decreased synaptic conductance in benzodiazepine tolerant hippocampal CA1 pyramidal neurons. *Brain Res* 2000;868(2):202–214.
114. Yu O, Chiu TH, Rosenberg HC. Modulation of GABA-gated chloride ion flux in rat brain by acute and chronic benzodiazepine administration. *J Pharmacol Exp Ther* 1988;246(1):107–113.
115. Li M, Szabo A, Rosenberg HC. Down-regulation of benzodiazepine binding to alpha 5 subunit-containing gamma-aminobutyric Acid(A) receptors in tolerant rat brain indicates particular involvement of the hippocampal CA1 region. *J Pharmacol Exp Ther* 2000;295(2):689–696.
116. Ali NJ, Olsen RW. Chronic benzodiazepine treatment of cells expressing recombinant GABA(A) receptors uncouples allosteric binding: studies on possible mechanisms. *J Neurochem* 2001;79(5):1100–1108.
117. Follesa P, Cagetti E, Mancuso L, et al. Increase in expression of the GABA(A) receptor alpha(4) subunit gene induced by withdrawal of, but not by long-term treatment with, benzodiazepine full or partial agonists. *Brain Res Mol Brain Res* 2001;92(1-2):138–148.
118. Smith SS, Gong QH, Hsu FC, et al. GABA(A) receptor alpha4 subunit suppression prevents withdrawal properties of an endogenous steroid. *Nature* 1998;392(6679):926–930.
119. Izzo E, Auta J, Impagnatiello F, et al. Glutamic acid decarboxylase and glutamate receptor changes during tolerance and dependence to benzodiazepines. *Proc Natl Acad Sci U S A* 2001;98(6):3483–3488.
120. Allison C, Pratt JA. Neuroadaptive processes in GABAergic and glutamatergic systems in benzodiazepine dependence. *Pharmacol Ther* 2003;98(2):171–195.
121. Van Sickle BJ, Xiang K, Tietz EI. Transient plasticity of hippocampal CA1 neuron glutamate receptors contributes to benzodiazepine withdrawal-anxiety. *Neuropsychopharmacology* 2004;29(11):1994–2006.
122. Allison C, Pratt JA. Differential effects of two chronic diazepam treatment regimes on withdrawal anxiety and AMPA receptor characteristics. *Neuropsychopharmacology* 2006;31(3):602–619.
123. Orzack MH, Cole JO, Ionescu-Pioggia M, et al. A comparison of some subjective effects of prazepam, diazepam, and placebo. *NIDA Res Monogr* 1982;41:309–317.
124. Ciraulo DA, Knapp CM, LoCastro J, et al. A benzodiazepine mood effect scale: reliability and validity determined for alcohol-dependent subjects and adults with a parental history of alcoholism. *Am J Drug Alcohol Abuse* 2001;27(2):339–347.
125. Jaffe JH, Bloor R, Crome I, et al. A postmarketing study of relative abuse liability of hypnotic sedative drugs. *Addiction* 2004;99(2):165–173.
126. Greenblatt DJ, Harmatz JS, von Moltke LL, et al. Comparative kinetics and response to the benzodiazepine agonists triazolam and zolpidem: evaluation of sex-dependent differences. *J Pharmacol Exp Ther* 2000; 293(2):435–443.
127. Stewart SA. The effects of benzodiazepines on cognition. *J Clin Psychiatry* 2005;66(Suppl 2):9–13.
128. Curran HV, Gorenstein C. Differential effects of lorazepam and oxazepam on priming. *Int Clin Psychopharmacol* 1993;8(1):37–42.
129. Lucki I, Rickels K, Geller AM. Chronic use of benzodiazepines and psychomotor and cognitive test performance. *Psychopharmacology (Berl)* 1986;88(4):426–433.
130. Buffett-Jerrott SE, Stewart SH. Cognitive and sedative effects of benzodiazepine use. *Curr Pharm Des* 2002;8(1):45–58.
131. Golombok S, Moodley P, Lader M. Cognitive impairment in long-term benzodiazepine users. *Psychol Med* 1988;18(2):365–374.
132. Barker MJ, Greenwood KM, Jackson M, et al. Persistence of cognitive effects after withdrawal from long-term benzodiazepine use: a meta-analysis. *Arch Clin Neuropsychol* 2004;19(3):437–454.
133. Bierman EJ, Comijs HC, Gundy CM, et al. The effect of chronic benzodiazepine use on cognitive functioning in older persons: good, bad or indifferent. *Int J Geriatr Psychiatry* 2007;22(12):1194–1200.
134. Vestergaard P, Rejnmark L, Mosekilde L. Anxiolytics, sedatives, antidepressants, neuroleptics and the risk of fracture. *Osteoporos Int* 2006; 17(6):807–816.
135. Hartikainen S, Lonnroos E, Louhivuori K. Medication as a risk factor for falls: critical systematic review. *J Gerontol Biol Sci Med Sci* 2007; 62(10):1172–1181.
136. Pariente A, Dartigues JF, Benichou J, et al. Benzodiazepines and injurious falls in community dwelling elders. *Drugs Aging* 2008;25(1):61–70.
137. Hebert C, Delaney JA, Hemmelgarn B, et al. Benzodiazepines and elderly drivers: a comparison of pharmacoepidemiological study designs. *Pharmacoepidemiol Drug Saf* 2007;16(8):845–849.
138. Engeland A, Skurtveit S, Morland J. Risk of road traffic accidents associated with the prescription of drugs: a registry-based cohort study. *Ann Epidemiol* 2007;17(8):597–602.
139. Dolovich LR, Addis A, Vaillancourt JM, et al. Benzodiazepine use in pregnancy and major malformations or oral cleft: meta-analysis of cohort and case-control studies. *BMJ* 1998;317(7162):839–843.
140. Addis A, Dolovich LR, Einarson TR, et al. Can we use anxiolytics during pregnancy without anxiety. *Can Fam Physician* 2000;46: 549–551.

141. Altshuler LL, Cohen L, Szuba MP, et al. Pharmacologic management of psychiatric illness during pregnancy: dilemmas and guidelines. *Am J Psychiatry* 1996;153(5):592–606.
142. Wikner BN, Stiller CO, Bergman U, et al. Use of benzodiazepines and benzodiazepine receptor agonists during pregnancy: neonatal outcome and congenital malformations. *Pharmacoepidemiol Drug Saf* 2007; 16(11):1203–1210.
143. Oberlander TF, Warburton W, Misri S, et al. Major congenital malformations following prenatal exposure to serotonin reuptake inhibitors and benzodiazepines using population-based health data. *Birth Defects Res B Dev Reprod Toxicol* 2008;83(1):68–76.
144. Czeizel AE, Rockenbauer M, Sorensen HT, et al. A population-based case-control study of oral chlordiazepoxide use during pregnancy and risk of congenital abnormalities. *Neurotoxicol Teratol* 2004;26(4):593–598.
145. Lin AE, Peller AJ, Westgate MN, et al. Clonazepam use in pregnancy and the risk of malformations. *Birth Defects Res Clin Mol Teratol* 2004;70(8):534–536.
146. Gillberg C. "Floppy infant syndrome" and maternal diazepam. *Lancet* 1977;2(8031): 244.
147. Iqbal MM, Sobhan T, Ryals T. Effects of commonly used benzodiazepines on the fetus, the neonate, and the nursing infant. *Psychiatr Serv* 2002;53(1):39–49.
148. Burt VK, Suri R, Altshuler L, et al. The use of psychotropic medications during breast-feeding. *Am J Psychiatry* 2001;158(7):1001–1009.
149. Menon SJ. Psychotropic medication during pregnancy and lactation. *Arch Gynecol Obstet* 2008;277(1):1–13.
150. Birnbaum CS, Cohen LS, Bailey JW, et al. Serum concentrations of antidepressants and benzodiazepines in nursing infants: a case series. *Pediatrics* 1999;104(1):e11.
151. McElhatton PR. The effects of benzodiazepine use during pregnancy and lactation. *Reprod Toxicol* 1994;8(6):461–475.
152. Bertollini R, Kallen B, Mastroiacovo P, et al. Anticonvulsant drugs in monotherapy. Effect on the fetus. *Eur J Epidemiol* 1987;3(2):164–171.
153. Holmes L, Harvey EA, Coull B, et al. The teratogenicity of anticonvulsant drugs. *N Engl J Med* 2001;344(15):1132–1138.
154. Hollister LE, Motzenbecker FP, Degan RO. Withdrawal reactions from chlordiazepoxide ("Librium"). *Psychopharmacologia* 1961;2:63–68.
155. Hollister LE, Bennett JL, Kimbell I, et al. Diazepam in newly admitted schizophrenics. *Dis Nerv Syst* 1963;24:746–750.
156. Wikler A. Diagnosis and treatment of drug dependence of the barbiturate type. *Am J Psychiatry* 1968;125(6):758–765.
157. Korpi ER, Sinkkonen ST. GABA(A) receptor subtypes as targets for neuropsychiatric drug development. *Pharmacol Ther* 2006;109(1–2): 12–32.

GHB

Keith Flower, MD, John Mendelson, MD, and Gantt P. Galloway, PharmD

Among the substances termed *club drugs* by the National Institute on Drug Abuse (NIDA) is γ-hydroxybutyrate (GHB). A sedative-hypnotic, it is a simple, four-carbon molecule synthesized in the early 1960s in a search for an orally active γ-aminobutyric acid (GABA) analog. It has been used as a general anesthetic and to induce absence seizures in animal models of epilepsy. More recently, it has been approved by the U.S. Food and Drug Administration (FDA) for the treatment of cataplexy in narcolepsy (marketed as Xyrem) and is used for treating alcohol and opiate dependence primarily in Italy and Sweden, where it is marketed as Alcover.

GHB abuse reports date to the early 1990s. Initially available as a dietary supplement in the United States, it was attractive to bodybuilders via reports that GHB raised levels of growth hormone. The substance is taken orally, with misusers reporting a euphoric "high" from the drug; the effects have been described anecdotally as comparable to both alcohol intoxication (with disinhibition, drowsiness, and loss of motor control) and MDMA/ecstasy use (enhanced sensuality, empathogenesis) (1). In the United States, GHB is a Schedule 1 controlled substance, except that the FDA-approved formulation (for narcolepsy) is classified as Schedule 3. Other countries maintain similar regulatory classifications.

GHB is inexpensive and readily available at some social events (notably "raves") or via kits and recipes for home manufacture found on the Internet. Other names for GHB include "G," "liquid ecstasy," "fantasy," "Grievous Bodily Harm," "cherry meth," "soap," "salty water," and "Georgia Home Boy" (2). GHB is usually sold in a salty-tasting, aqueous solution that may have a variable concentration, undoubtedly contributing to the high incidence of adverse effects. It is also sold as a white powder ready for dissolution. Legal restrictions on the purchase of GHB have led to increased abuse of two substances that convert to GHB in the body: γ-butyrolactone (GBL), whose street names include "lactone," "Renewtrient," "Blue Nitro," and "Verve," and 1,4-butanediol (BD), also known as "Pro-G," "Thunder," "Weight Belt Cleaner," and "Pine Needle Extract." Both substances are available as industrial solvents. GBL is a Drug Enforcement Administration (DEA) List 1 chemical in the United States, requiring justification for sales, and the FDA classifies BD as a Class I Health Hazard (i.e., a potentially life-threatening drug).

PHYSIOLOGY AND PHARMACOKINETICS

Found endogenously at very low concentrations in the brain, GHB is both a precursor and degradation product of GABA and is structurally similar to GABA. GHB interacts in a complex way with endogenous GABA (the primary inhibitory neurotransmitter in the brain) and with GABA receptors (3). Oral doses are rapidly absorbed, with maximum plasma concentrations reached in 30 to 50 minutes. Plasma elimination half-life is in the range of 20 to 30 minutes (4,5). GHB is metabolized to succinate and then to CO_2 and water via the citric acid cycle. GHB binds to and activates two receptors: the GABAb receptor, and a distinct GHB receptor. Human GHB receptors have recently been cloned and are pharmacologically distinct from GABA receptors; they are G-protein-coupled and do not bind GABA (6). GHB affects dopamine release biphasically: low GHB concentrations stimulate dopamine release (which may increase addiction liability by activating reward pathways), whereas higher concentrations inhibit dopamine release. GHB also influences serotonin turnover, and affects neurosteroid, acetylcholine, and growth hormone levels (3).

The pharmacologic profile of BD is similar to that of GHB (7), whereas GBL is more rapidly absorbed and has greater lipid solubility than GHB (8). GHB can be detected for approximately 5 hours in blood and oral fluid, and <12 hours in urine (9).

EPIDEMIOLOGY

Estimates vary on the frequency of GHB use. Overall, 0.05% of U.S. youths aged 16 to 23 in a 2002 survey reported lifetime use of GHB (10). Some researchers found a recent decline in GHB use among U.S. youth (11,12). Sizable minorities in some populations report higher use rates. 7% of young adults and adolescents in treatment for substance abuse reported lifetime use of GHB (13). A study of 450 "club" drug-using gay and bisexual men in New York City found that 29% recounted GHB use in the previous 4 months (14). There have been occasional reports of increased use in specific locales (15).

Intoxication Reasons given for GHB use include "to be sociable," to enhance sex, and to explore altered states of consciousness. Subjective effects of GHB include slurred speech, ease in socializing, feelings of increased sexual intimacy, drowsiness, and feelings of depression after the GHB "high" is past (16). GHB administered under controlled laboratory conditions produces sleepiness, sedation, fatigue, and feelings of being "easy going" or "mellow." Effects noted by observers of intoxicated subjects include decreased psychomotor performance and level of alertness

(*continued*)

GHB *(continued)*

and increased ratings of muscle relaxation and abnormal posture (17). In overdose, clinical characteristics include those expected from a CNS depressant—bradycardia, vomiting, somnolence, obtundation, stupor, and coma—but a literature review also identified agitation, combativeness, and self-injurious behavior as relatively common in persons using GHB alone and with cointoxicants (18). The frequent use of alcohol with GHB is thought to worsen GHB-induced sedation and may increase episodes of vomiting, hypotension, and respiratory depression (7).

Abuse Liability, Dependence, and Withdrawal Physical dependence and addiction have been reported with GHB, GBL, and BD (19,20), though knowledge of dependence on these drugs comes from a relatively small number of studies. One estimate places the likelihood for GHB abuse intermediate to triazolam and pentobarbital (17). Dependence may develop rapidly, usually with frequent (four or more times a day) dosing. Time course estimates for the development of physical dependence and severe withdrawal range from 7 days (21) to use over 2 months or more (20,22,23).

Though the withdrawal syndrome may be mild, with insomnia, agitation, anxiety, and limited sympathetic arousal, an analysis of reports of GHB withdrawal found that severe, potentially life-threatening withdrawal states may develop requiring vigorous inpatient clinical management. Signs and symptoms are similar to those seen in alcohol withdrawal: tremor, tachycardia, restlessness, and delirium, including hallucinations (24).

Adverse Effects Because the dose-response curve for GHB is steep and concentrations of GHB in illicitly purchased or homemade solutions are notoriously hard to predict, overdose is a hazard. Symptoms of CNS depression are dose-related, with reports of somnolence within 15 minutes at a dose of 30 mg/kg, and loss of consciousness and coma at doses exceeding 50 mg/kg (25). Overdose may lead to intubation and management in an ICU, although in one study the majority of overdose patients were discharged within 6 hours of presentation (26). Long-term sequelae of using GHB and congeners are not presently known.

GHB-associated deaths, both with and without cointoxicants, have been identified in the United States, Europe, and Australasia (27). GHB use is associated with risky behaviors such as coingestion of ethanol, driving under the influence of GHB (28), and risky sexual behaviors (29). GHB has been associated with drug-facilitated sexual assaults (30,31). Such use may be facilitated by GHB's properties of being colorless, odorless, sedating, purportedly causing amnesia, and detected poorly in urine after 12 hours.

TREATMENT

Treatment for GHB intoxication is largely supportive. McDonough, Kennedy, et al. conducted a retrospective analysis of treatment for GHB withdrawal and give recommendations for management. In their review, a tapering regimen of benzodiazepines was used in 91% of 38 cases, with a mean dose in diazepam equivalents of 335 mg (range 20 to 2,655 mg). Mean duration of withdrawal was 9 days. In 82% of the 38 cases, other drugs were used in combination with benzodiazepines: antipsychotics for psychosis and delirium, anticonvulsants, and non-benzodiazepine sedatives such as pentobarbital. They note that withdrawal delirium developed in more than one-half the cases wherein GHB use occurred every 8 hours or less, or with use of >30 g of GHB a day. They recommend inpatient management of withdrawal in these cases and note that though antipsychotics have been used for delirium and psychosis, they do not appear sufficient or necessary. Pentobarbital was effective where symptoms of withdrawal persisted despite high doses of benzodiazepines. They conclude by noting that management of GHB withdrawal requires more study (24).

REFERENCES

1. Galloway GP, Frederick-Osborne SL, Seymour R, et al. Abuse and therapeutic potential of gamma-hydroxybutyric acid. *Alcohol* 2000;20(3):263–269.
2. Maxwell JC. Party drugs: Properties, prevalence, patterns, and problems. *Subst Use Misuse* 2005;40(9–10):1203–1240.
3. Drasbek KR, Christensen J, Jensen K. Gamma-hydroxybutyrate—a drug of abuse. *Acta Neurol Scand* 2006;114(3):145–156.
4. Palatini P, Tedeschi L, Frison G, et al. Dose-dependent absorption and elimination of gamma-hydroxybutyric acid in healthy volunteers. *Eur J Clin Pharmacol* 1993;45(4):353–356.
5. Brenneisen R, Elsohly MA, Murphy TP, et al. Pharmacokinetics and excretion of gamma-hydroxybutyrate (GHB) in healthy subjects. *J Anal Toxicol* 2004;28(8):625–630.
6. Andriamampandry C, Taleb O, Kemmel V, et al. Cloning and functional characterization of a gamma-hydroxybutyrate receptor identified in the human brain. *FASEB J* 2007;21(3):885–895.
7. Thai D, Dyer JE, Jacob P, et al. Clinical pharmacology of 1,4-butanediol and gamma-hydroxybutyrate after oral 1,4-butanediol administration to healthy volunteers. *Clin Pharmacol Ther* 2007;81(2):178–184.
8. Kohrs FP, Porter WH. Gamma-hydroxybutyrate intoxication and overdose. *Ann Emerg Med* 1999;33(4):475–476.
9. Verstraete AG. Detection times of drugs of abuse in blood, urine, and oral fluid. *Ther Drug Monitor* 2004;26(2):200–205.
10. U.S. Department of Health and Human Services, Substance Abuse and Mental Health Services Administration, Office of Applied Studies. Results from the 2002 National Survey on Drug Use and Health: National Findings, 2003. *DHHS Publication No. SMA 03-2836. NSDUH Series H-22.* Accessed February 2008 at http://www.oas.samhsa.gov/nhsda/2k2nsduh/Results/2k2Results.htm.

GHB *(continued)*

11. Johnston LD, O'Malley PM, Bachman JG, et al. Monitoring the future: National results on adolescent drug use. National Institute on Drug Abuse, 2005. Accessed February 2008 at http://www.nida.nih.gov/PDF/overview2005.pdf.
12. Anderson IB, Kim SY, Dyer JE, et al. Trends in gamma-hydroxybutyrate (GHB) and related drug intoxication: 1999 to 2003. *Ann Emerg Med* 2006;47(2):177–183.
13. Hopfer C, Mendelson B, Van Leeuwen JM, et al. Club drug use among youths in treatment for substance abuse. *Am J Addict* 2006;15(1):94–99.
14. Halkitis PN, Palamar JJ. GHB use among gay and bisexual men. *Addict Behav* 2006;31(11):2135–2139.
15. Knudsen K, Greter J, Verdicchio M, et al. A severe outburst of GHB poisonings (gamma-hydroxybutyrate, gamma-hydroxybutyric acid) on the West Coast of Sweden. Mortality numbers ahead of heroin. *Clin Toxicol* 2006;44(5):637–638.
16. Sumnall HR, Woolfall K, Edwards S, et al. Use, function, and subjective experiences of gamma-hydroxybutyrate (GHB). *Drug Alcohol Depend* 2008;92:286–290.
17. Carter LP, Richards BD, Mintzer MZ, et al. Relative abuse liability of GHB in humans: a comparison of psychomotor, subjective, and cognitive effects of supratherapeutic doses of triazolam, pentobarbital, and GHB. *Neuropsychopharmacology* 2006;31(11):2537–2551.
18. Zvosec DL, Smith SW. Agitation is common in gamma-hydroxybutyrate toxicity. *Am J Emerg Med* 2005;23(3):316–320.
19. Galloway GP, Frederick SL, Staggers F Jr. Physical dependence on sodium oxybate. *Lancet* 1994;343(8888):57.
20. McDaniel CH, Miotto KA. Gamma hydroxybutyrate (GHB) and gamma butyrolactone (GBL) withdrawal: Five case studies. *J Psychoactive Drugs* 2001;33(2):143–149.
21. Perez E, Chu J, Bania T. Seven days of gamma-hydroxybutyrate (GHB) use produces severe withdrawal. *Ann Emerg Med* 2006;48(2):219–220.
22. Dyer J, Roth B, Hyma B. Gamma-hydroxybutyrate withdrawal syndrome. *Ann Emerg Med* 2001;37(2):147–153.
23. Miotto K, Darakjian J, Basch J, et al. Gamma-hydroxybutyric acid: patterns of use, effects and withdrawal. *Am J Addict* 2001;10(3):232–241.
24. McDonough M, Kennedy N, Glasper A, et al. Clinical features and management of gamma-hydroxybutyrate (GHB) withdrawal: a review. *Drug Alcohol Depend* 2004;75(1):3–9.
25. Okun MS, Boothby LA, Bartfield RB, et al. GHB: an important pharmacologic and clinical update. *J Pharm Sci* 2001;4(2):167–175.
26. Couper FJ, Thatcher JE, Logan BK. Suspected GHB overdoses in the emergency department. *J Anal Toxicol* 2004;28(6):481–484.
27. World Health Organization (WHO) 34th Expert Committee on Drug Dependence. Pre-review of gamma-hydroxybutyric acid (GHB). 2006. Accessed February 2008 at http://www.who.int/medicines/areas/quality_safety/5GHBPreReview.pdf.
28. Kim SY, Anderson IB, Dyer JE, et al. High-risk behaviors and hospitalizations among gamma hydroxybutyrate (GHB) users. *Am J Drug Alcohol Abuse* 2007;33(3):429–438.
29. Romanelli F, Smith KM, Pomeroy C. Use of club drugs by HIV-seropositive and HIV-seronegative gay and bisexual men. *Topics HIV Med* 2003;11(1):25–32.
30. Scott-Ham M, Burton FC. Toxicological findings in cases of alleged drug-facilitated sexual assault in the United Kingdom over a 3-year period. *J Clin Forensic Med* 2005;12(4):175–186.
31. Stillwell ME. Drug-facilitated sexual assault involving gamma-hydroxybutyric acid. *J Forensic Sci* 2002;47(5):1133–1134.

CHAPTER 9

Lisa Borg, MD
Igor Kravets, MD
Mary Jeanne Kreek, MD

The Pharmacology of Long-Acting as Contrasted with Short-Acting Opioids

DEFINITION OF DRUGS IN THE CLASS

Three distinct types of opioid receptors are found in the nervous system: mu, kappa, and delta. Opioids include the natural opiates (drugs derived from opium) and their manmade congeners, which are the agonist and antagonist drugs with mostly morphine-like activity (primarily at the mu-opioid receptor), as well as the other naturally occurring endogenous opioid peptides, products of three separate genes, which are also active at opioid receptors (1). The genes for each of these three receptors and each of these three classes of opioid peptides have been cloned from humans (2,3). These opioid receptors are members of the Gi-coupled, 7-transmembrane domain superfamily. The three main families of endogenous opioid peptides— beta-endorphin, enkephalins, and dynorphins—have a degree of selectivity for the three receptor types. For example, beta-endorphin and the met-enkephalins have relatively high affinity at mu- and delta-receptors, much lower at kappa. The dynorphins by contrast have relative selectivity for kappa-receptors over mu and delta. These receptors mediate a complex, partially overlapping, array of physiologic and neurobiologic functions (4). For the purposes of this chapter, we will concentrate on the mu-receptor as most of the clinically active opioids are active at this receptor. However, the endogenous opioid system plays an important role in responses to addictive opiates including morphine, codeine and heroin as well as to synthetic opioids (3). Dynorphin modulates mu opioid receptor responses through the kappa opioid receptor. Enkephalin peptides are derived from the processing of proenkephalin and function in the modulation of pain perception, affective state, and, possibly, reward and the addictions. Beta-endorphin is a breakdown product of proopiomelanocortin that is produced primarily in the anterior pituitary of humans. It is also produced in the central nervous system (CNS) and in the periphery. The three receptors mediate both the analgesic and rewarding effects of opioid compounds as well as their effects on many systems in the body, such as the hypothalamic-pituitary-adrenal (HPA) axis, immune, gastrointestinal (GI), and pulmonary function.

Opioids refer to all compounds, natural and synthetic, functionally related to opium derived from poppies, including the endogenous opioids. Opium is the naturally occurring drug mixture directly derived from the juice of the opium poppy, whereas opiates are drugs derived or synthesized from opium or from thebaine, another poppy product. Opiates are alkaloids, such as morphine and codeine. This chapter reviews the pharmacology of several exogenous opioids that are particularly significant in the area of opioid addiction and its treatment, i.e., heroin, morphine, oxycodone, codeine, meperidine, pentazocine, hydromorphone, and hydrocodone, as well as methadone, levo-alpha-acetylmethadol (LAAM), and buprenorphine.

SUBSTANCES INCLUDED IN THE CLASS

Heroin Diacetylmorphine was first synthesized in the 1870s by the Bayer company and marketed by Bayer under the name "heroin." Heroin is synthetically derived from the natural opioid morphine. Largely owing to its rapid onset of action and very short half-life, heroin is a popular drug of abuse. Heroin is classified in schedule I (i.e., not available for any therapeutic use in the United States), although it is available in a few countries as a pain medication for treatment of heroin addiction (5,6). Heroin is a prodrug, which is not itself active. It is most effective when used intravenously. Heroin increasingly is used intranasally and, sometimes, smoked in the free-base form (7), both to reduce the risk of human immunodeficiency virus (HIV-1) transmission from intravenous use and because of the wider availability of high-purity heroin in recent years. Heroin is rapidly deacetylated to 6-mono-acetylmorphine and morphine, both of which are active at the mu opioid receptor.

Morphine and Synthetic Compounds Morphine is a natural product of the seeds of the poppy plant, *Papaver somniferum*. Chemically, morphine is an alkaloid that belongs to the class of *phenanthrenes*. This class also includes codeine and thebaine. Modifications of the latter result in synthetic compounds discussed later (4). Morphine is prescribed primarily as a high-potency analgesic. Biotransformations or synthetic modifications of the chemical structure of the morphine molecule at the 3, 6, and 17 positions produce other compounds, including the mu-opioid receptor agonists such as morphine-6-glucuronide (M6G), a major pharmacologically active metabolite of morphine in humans. Synthetic compounds include hydrocodone (Vicodin), oxycodone (OxyContin), hydromorphone (Dilaudid) and heroin. Synthetic compounds also include antagonists such as naloxone (Narcan), naltrexone (Trexan or ReVia), and nalmefene (Revix), as well as partial agonists such as buprenorphine (Subutex) or, when combined with naloxone (Suboxone) (4).

Oxycodone Oxycodone has been used clinically since the early 1900s. It is combined with aspirin or acetaminophen for moderate pain and is available orally without coanalgesic for severe pain (8). It is a popular drug of abuse, especially in the controlled release formulation, which can be crushed for a potentially toxic, rapid "high" (9). Oxycodone is a semi-synthetic compound derived from thebaine, with agonist activity, primarily at mu receptors. Although structurally similar to codeine, it is pharmacodynamically comparable to morphine and has 1:2 equivalence with morphine (10).

Codeine Pierre-Jean Robiquet, a French pharmacist, first discovered several natural products including codeine (11). Codeine is methylmorphine, with methyl substitution on the phenolic hydroxyl group of morphine. It is more lipophilic than morphine and thus crosses the blood–brain barrier faster. It also has less first-pass metabolism in the liver, therefore, greater oral bioavailability than morphine, although it is less potent than morphine. A small part is metabolized to morphine via cytochrome 2D6 (4); however, morphine is twice as potent.

Meperidine Meperidine is a phenylpiperidine with a number of congeners. It is mostly effective in the CNS and bowel; however, it is no longer used for treatment of chronic pain owing to concerns regarding toxicity of its metabolite and should not be used for >48 hours or at doses >600 mg/day. It has serotonergic activity when combined with monoamine oxidase inhibitors (MAOIs), which can produce serotonin toxicity (clonus, hyper-reflexia, hyperthermia and agitation) (12).

Pentazocine Both parenteral and oral formulations of pentazocine were approved for marketing in the late 1960s. It is one of the initial "agonist-antagonist" medications, a weak antagonist or partial agonist (it has a "ceiling effect"; there is a plateau in maximal effect as contrasted with a full agonist wherein each increment in dose gives a greater effect) at the mu receptor and is also a kappa receptor partial agonist. In 1983, to block the effects of pentazocine if injected, it was manufactured in combination with naloxone (Talwin NX) as, if then injected, it would actually precipitate withdrawal in those with opioid dependence. Some data from the DAWN emergency room and medical examiner mentions indicated that abuse declined after this reformulation (13).

Hydromorphone Hydromorphone is a more potent opioid analgesic than morphine. It is used for the treatment of moderate to severe pain and is excreted along with its metabolites by the kidney. It can be given intravenously, by infusion, orally, and per rectum, with low oral bioavailability. On a milligram basis, it is five times more potent than morphine when given orally, and 8.5 times as potent when given intravenously (14). A minor pathway for the metabolism of morphine to hydromorphone has been identified (15).

Hydrocodone Hydrocodone is a prescription drug frequently prescribed for relatively minor (such as dental) pain. It is often used in combination with acetaminophen; thus there can be hepatotoxicity associated with its abuse (8).

Methadone Methadone is a synthetic long-acting full mu-opioid agonist given orally. It was first synthesized by Bayer as an analgesic in Germany in the late 1930s and first studied for human use in the 1950s in the United States. It has been used primarily as a maintenance treatment for heroin addiction since the first research done in 1964 (16), for which it was approved by the U.S. Food and Drug Administration (FDA) in 1972. It is also used and very effective in the treatment of chronic pain. The *l*(R)-methadone enantiomer has up to 50 times more analgesic activity and also the potential to produce more respiratory depression, than the *d*(S)-enantiomer. Both enantiomers have modest *N*-methyl-D-aspartate (NMDA) receptor antagonism. Methadone has a di-phenylheptylamine chemical structure and consists of a racemic mixture of *d(S)*- and *l(R)*-methadone. Again, the *l*(R)-enantiomer is responsible for the majority of opioid effects as it is up to 50 times more potent than the *d(S)*-enantiomer (17).

Levo-alpha-acetylmethadol LAAM is a synthetic, longer-acting (48-hour) congener of methadone that also is orally effective. LAAM was first studied in the 1970s for the treatment of heroin addiction (18) and approved in 1993 by the FDA (19) after a large multicenter safety trial. Postmarketing, after reports of prolonged QT_c intervals on electrocardiogram leading to *Torsade de Pointes* that may have been caused by LAAM, a black-box warning was added to the product label (20). This effect may have been the result of preexisting cardiac disease or undefined drug interactions (21), LAAM remains approved for humans in the United States. However, at this time, no company is manufacturing LAAM. As the new drug application for LAAM has not been withdrawn, LAAM could again be made available in the United States (22).

Buprenorphine Buprenorphine alone and in combination with naloxone was approved in 2002 by the FDA as an office-based sublingual treatment for heroin and opioid addiction (23–25) and, at the same time, buprenorphine was reclassified by the DEA from a Schedule V to a Schedule III drug (13). Buprenorphine or when combined with naloxone is a synthetic, primarily mu-opioid receptor-directed partial agonist and also a kappa partial agonist with a ceiling effect (i.e., there is a plateau in maximal effect versus that observed with the use of a high efficacy pure agonist where each increment in dose gives a greater effect). The chemical structure of buprenorphine is that of an oripavine with a C7 side chain, which contains a tert-butyl group. Norbuprenorphine is a major metabolite of buprenorphine in humans, with activity at the mu-opioid receptor as well (25).

EPIDEMIOLOGY OF OPIOID ABUSE AND ADDICTION

The pharmacology of opioids is of particular relevance to the treatment of addictive disorders, given reports of increases in the abuse of illicit opioids, as well as illicit use of prescribed opioid medications (26). It is estimated that more than 3.5 million Americans have used heroin, and more than 1 million people are addicted to heroin in the United States. More than 100,000 people aged 12 to 25 initiated use annually between 1995 and 2002 (3). According to the Office of National Drug Control Policy publication of January, 2008, more than 2.1 million teenagers in 2006 abused prescription drugs, and one third of new abusers of prescription drugs in 2006 were 12–17 year-olds. Among 12- to 13-year-olds, prescription drugs are the drug of choice (27). According to the Substance Abuse and Mental Health Services Administration (SAMHSA) Treatment Episode Data Set (TEDS), annual admissions to substance abuse treatment for primary heroin abuse increased from 228,000 in 1995 to 254,000 in 2005, with the percentage of primary heroin admissions remaining steady at about 14% to 15% of all substance abuse treatment admissions (7).

The majority of persons in treatment for heroin addiction are in methadone maintenance treatment. Also, currently, there are 8,911 U.S. physicians eligible to prescribe buprenorphine as office-based treatment to patients for treatment of opioid dependence (28). Eligibility requirements as established by the SAMHSA DATA 2000 (Drug Addiction Treatment Act 2000) for physicians to use buprenorphine in treatment of addiction are: completion of an 8-hour continuing medical education course; notification of the government of the intent to use buprenorphine for treatment of opioid-dependent patients; both having the capacity to provide or refer patients for ancillary services and, as of December 2006, and were in agreement to treat no more than 100 patients (increased from the original 30 maximum) at any one time in an individual or group practice (28,29).

Two cross-sectional studies conducted in New York City from 2000 to 2004 found that among new admissions to drug treatment who had stopped injecting heroin as of 6 months prior to the study, the most common reasons for cessation included concerns about health and preference for the intranasal route (30).

The recent and major problem of opioid abuse and addiction is the illicit (nonprescription) use of prescription opioids, obtained illicitly or frequently from family members or friends. As of 2007, eighth, tenth and 12th grade students nationwide continue to show a decline in the proportions reporting illicit drug use. Less than 1% of students in these grades report any use of heroin in 2007. However, the prevalence of other narcotic drug use reported for 12th graders was 9.2% (31). In an NIH-NIDA Research Report, published in 2001 and revised in 2005, it was reported that in addition to benzodiazepines, opioid pain relievers were the two most frequently reported prescription medications in drug abuse-related cases (32). In 2005, 30.1% of persons addicted to heroin sought treatment with methadone or buprenorphine maintenance, whereas only 19.9% of those addicted to prescription opioids illicitly used sought such pharmacotherapy (7).

PHARMACOKINETICS OF SPECIFIC DRUGS

It is beyond the scope of this chapter to provide a comprehensive table of dosing equivalents. There are a number of excellent reviews on this topic (4,8,33).

Heroin (Diacetylmorphine) Pharmacokinetics

Heroin is a very efficient lipid soluble pro-drug that is also more water-soluble and also more potent than morphine (34) but has no intrinsic opioid activity. It is synthesized from morphine by acetylation at both the 3 and 6 positions and metabolized in humans to active opioid compounds first by deacetylation to the active 6-mono-acetylmorphine (6-MAM) and then by further deacetylation to morphine (34). Well-designed studies of heroin pharmacokinetics in humans have been performed (35–38). Heroin given intramuscularly is about two times as potent as morphine for pain relief (36), with a faster onset of peak mood effect, however, it has less sustained effect (39). Heroin has an average half-life in blood of 3 minutes after intravenous administration; the half-life of 6-acetylmorphine in humans appears to be 30 minutes (35). Heroin given as an infusion to patients with chronic pain has an onset of pain relief after 15 to 45 minutes which occurs with the presence of 6-monoacetylmorphine in the blood, before the appearance of morphine (35). Oral heroin has complete first-pass metabolism (35,40) and, like morphine, has very limited systemic bioavailability when given orally, unlike methadone and LAAM. The blood clearance of heroin is greater than the upper range of hepatic blood flow in humans, indicating that organs other than the liver are likely involved in the metabolism of heroin, such as the GI wall and the kidney (35), as well as hepatic carboxylesterases such as butyrylcholinesterase (37). In comparing sublingual to oral absorption, the more lipid-soluble drugs (including methadone and heroin) are absorbed to the greatest degree, regardless of concentration of opioid, with increased absorption producing higher potential systemic bioavailability of the opioid (41).

The use of intranasal, intramuscular, and subcutaneous heroin all produce peak blood levels of heroin or 6-acetylmorphine within 5 minutes; however, intranasal use has about half the relative potency (36). Further research needs to be done on the role of 6-acetylmorphine (administered directly) in relation to the pharmacokinetics of parenteral heroin, particularly its onset of action and potency as compared with morphine. Most of the enzymes involved in the metabolism of opioids are part of the P450 microsomal enzyme system, though heroin and morphine are also biotransformed outside this system.

Morphine Pharmacokinetics Morphine is largely selective for the mu-opioid receptor at lower doses and is considered by most physicians in the United States the drug of choice for the treatment of cancer pain. Morphine is biotransformed mainly by hepatic glucuronidation to the major but inactive metabolite morphine-3-glucuronide (M3G) and the biologically active morphine 6-glucuronide (M6G) compound (42).

The pharmacokinetics of morphine and its metabolites vary, depending on the route of administration. Its favorable safety profile is due in large part to its pharmacokinetic profile. The oral bioavailability varies, from 35% to 75%, with a plasma half-life ranging from 2 to 3.5 hours. The half-life is less than the time course of analgesia, which is 4 to 6 hours, thus reducing accumulation. Morphine is metabolized mostly in the liver, with prolonged clearance because of enterohepatic cycling with oral dosing (43). In the setting of chronic liver disease, morphine oxidation is more affected than glucuronidation. Use of lower doses or longer dosing intervals is recommended to minimize the risk of accumulation of morphine when chronic liver disease is present, particularly with repeated dosing (41). Methadone is a better choice for chronic analgesia treatment in patients with chronic liver disease (see the "Methadone Pharmacokinetics" section).

At 24 hours, more than 90% of morphine has been excreted in urine. M6G elimination seems to be closely tied to renal function, so accumulation of metabolites can occur. With renal compromise, <10% of morphine and its metabolites are excreted in feces; therefore, morphine should be used with great caution in patients with renal disease (unlike methadone, which can be given relatively safely in these patients: see Methadone Pharmacokinetics) (41). The higher sensitivity of older adults to the analgesic properties of morphine may be related in part to altered pharmacokinetics (41).

Oxycodone Pharmacokinetics The onset of action begins after 1 hour, and in controlled-release form lasts for approximately 12 hours, with a plasma half-life of 3 to 4 hours for the immediate release. Stable plasma levels are achieved within 24 hours. Oral bioavailability ranges from 60% to 87%, with 45% protein-bound. Oxycodone is mostly metabolized in the liver, with the remainder as well as the metabolites metabolized in the kidneys. The two main metabolites are oxymorphone, which is also a potent analgesic, and the weaker analgesic noroxycodone, which is its major metabolite (10,44). In terms of protein binding and lipophilicity, oxycodone is similar to morphine, with slightly longer half-life and greater bioavailability. Unlike morphine, oxycodone is metabolized mostly by the cytochrome enzyme CYP2D6, while morphine in humans is primarily glucuronidated (45).

Codeine Pharmacokinetics Codeine is methyl morphine, with the methyl substitution on the phenolic hydroxyl group. Codeine has a high oral-parenteral effect, owing to low first-pass metabolism in the liver. Metabolites are mostly inactive and excreted in the urine, with about 10% demethylated to morphine via CYP2D6, which is mostly responsible for the analgesic effect of codeine, as it has very low affinity for opioid receptors. Genetic variations in this enzyme system may result in lower production of morphine-6-glucuronide. The allelic variants have different frequency in different ethnic groups and can affect the depth of analgesia. Repeated doses of codeine may result in the accumulation of the active metabolite M6G in patients with renal disease. Codeine is highly lipophilic and therefore is absorbed well transdermally (4).

Meperidine Pharmacokinetics Onset of analgesia begins with the oral route after 15 minutes, with peak in 1 to 2 hours, which is close to peak level in plasma, with duration of about 1.5 to 3 hours (4). It is absorbed by all routes, but intramuscular administration results in a less reliable peak plasma level after 45 minutes, with wide range of plasma concentrations. After oral administration, about 50% of the drug enters circulation without first-pass metabolism, with peak at 1 to 2 hours. Meperidine is mostly metabolized in the liver, with half-life of about 3 hours. Cirrhosis leads to increased bioavailability and half-life of both meperidine and normeperidine. Sixty percent of meperidine is protein-bound, and little is excreted unmetabolized (12).

Pentazocine Pharmacokinetics Pentazocine is a mixed agonist-antagonist that can be given intramuscularly or orally but is not currently available in the oral formulation. It can cause psychotomimetic effects, therefore has a very limited role in the treatment of chronic pain. Its duration of action is 3 to 6 hours. Its peak effect is at 0.5 to 1 hour when given intramuscularly and 1 to 2 hours when given orally (8). Sixty percent of the drug is bound to protein. Pentazocine is metabolized by the liver via oxidative and glucuronide conjugation with an extensive first-pass effect. When administered orally, the bioavailability of pentazocine is about 10%, except in patients with cirrhosis, which increases bioavailability to 60% to 70%. The drug half-life is 2 to 3 hours. Small amounts of unchanged pentazocine are excreted with urine (8).

Hydromorphone Pharmacokinetics Hydromorphone is shorter-acting than morphine. It is derived from morphine, although it may also be produced in the body in small amounts by N-demethylation of hydrocodone. It has an oral bioavailability of 30% to 40%, with an analgesic onset after 10 to 20 minutes, which peaks at about 30 to 60 minutes and persists for about 3 to 5 hours. The oral-parenteral ratio is about 5:1, with an equivalency of 1.5 mg of hydrocodone to 10 mg morphine (46).

Hydrocodone Pharmacokinetics Hydrocodone has a half-life of 2 to 4 hours, with a peak effect at 0.5 to 1 hour. Its duration of action is 3 to 4 hours (8). Codeine may show up as trace quantities of hydrocodone in urine testing as up to 11% of codeine is metabolized to hydrocodone (47), which could be misinterpreted as hydrocodone abuse.

Methadone Pharmacokinetics Methadone is a full mu-opioid receptor agonist. Methadone is a racemic compound; the *l*(R)-enantiomer is the active enantiomer and the other *d*(S)-enantiomer is the inactive enantiomer. Both enantiomers are weak NMDA receptor antagonists; therefore, racemic methadone, as used in human pharmacologic treatment, retards and attenuates the development of opioid tolerance (48). Methadone meets the two important criteria for a medication for the treatment of addiction: high systemic bioavailability (>90%) with oral administration and long apparent half-life with long-term administration in humans (49). The medical safety of long-term methadone maintenance treatment has been studied both prospectively and retrospectively (50).

Oral methadone has a rapid absorption but a delayed onset of action, with peak plasma levels achieved by 2 to 4 hours and sustained over a 24-hour dosing period (49,51–53). Moreover, the mean plasma apparent terminal half-life of racemic *d,l*-methadone in human subjects, as used for therapeutics in the United States, is around 24 hours (49). Further studies using stable isotopes have shown that the *l*-enantiomer has a half-life of 36 hours (54,55). Oral absorption is modestly affected by the drug's physical and chemical properties, gastric motility, gut perfusion, and pH (48,56). It has been shown that the biotransformation of methadone is accelerated in the third trimester; therefore, ideally the methadone dose should be increased in the final stages of pregnancy (57).

When taken on a chronic basis, methadone is stored and accumulated mostly in liver tissue (51,58). Methadone plasma levels are kept relatively constant because of the slow release of unmetabolized methadone into the blood, which extends the apparent terminal half-life. Methadone is more than 90% plasma protein bound both to albumin and all globulins (57,59). Methadone is relatively lipid soluble, with 34% to 75% absorption when given sublingually, depending on the pH (41). These properties help explain why methadone maintenance treatment is effective as a once-daily, orally administered pharmacotherapy for heroin addiction (16), unlike heroin and morphine, both of which have a relatively rapid onset and offset of the effect and short duration of action.

Owing to the long half-life of methadone, when beginning long-term methadone maintenance treatment (usually starting with a 20- to 40-mg daily dose), escalation of dose exceeding the rate of development of tolerance can result in accumulation, with sedation and even respiratory depression. Thus, dosages must be increased slowly, usually by 10 mg every 4 to 7 days. It is not yet fully understood why some patients in methadone maintenance treatment experience symptoms of opioid abstinence despite adequate dose (80 to 150 mg) and apparent therapeutic blood levels of 250 to 400 ng/mL (60). These symptoms may be due to pharmacodynamic factors not yet well understood or other factors such as concomitant illness or psychologic factors (e.g., depression) (59–61). Other cases, in which moderate to high doses of methadone do not result in apparent therapeutic levels of 250 to 400 ng/mL, may be due to "rapid metabolism" related to individual genetic differences of the cytochrome P450 or p-glycoprotein-related enzyme system (53,62,63). Methadone levels in the cerebrospinal fluid peak 3 to 8 hours after methadone dosing (64,65). Positron emission tomography studies found that mu-opioid receptor occupancy was lowered by only 19% to 32% in 14 former heroin addict volunteers who were maintained long-term (2 to 27 years) on daily doses of methadone, ranging from 30 to 90 mg/day, compared to 14 healthy control subjects (52).

Methadone is biotransformed in the liver by the cytochrome P450-related enzymes (primarily by the CYP3A4 and, to a lesser extent, the CYP2B6, CYP2D6, and CYP1A2 systems) to two N-demethylated biologically inactive metabolites, which undergo additional oxidative metabolism (17,48). Methadone and its metabolites are excreted in nearly equal amounts in urine and in feces (65–69). In patients with renal disease, methadone can be cleared almost entirely by the GI tract, unlike morphine and many other opiates, reducing potential toxicity by preventing accumulation (67–69). Less than 1% of unmetabolized methadone is removed in peritoneal dialysis, probably because of its extensive plasma protein binding and the small degree to which methadone is actually present in the blood (rather than stored in the liver) at any one point (69). Patients with severe long-standing liver disease have decreased methadone metabolism and thus slower metabolic clearance of methadone, yet lower than expected plasma methadone levels as a result of lower hepatic reservoirs of methadone because of reduced liver size. Methadone disposition is relatively normal in patients with mild to moderate liver impairment (65,70,71).

Other drugs can interact with methadone because of their effects on hepatic enzymes in the cytochrome P450-related enzyme system (59). The drug–drug interactions with methadone are complicated and in clinical practice may vary and must be considered on a case-by-case basis in individual patients (59). A number of studies are based upon hypothesized or measured pharmacokinetic changes with unclear clinical significance. The major categories of drugs potentially interacting with methadone include both inducers and inhibitors of CYP3A4, (as well as inhibitors of CYP2D6, such as paroxetine) (72). CYP3A4 inducers include rifampin (73), rifabutin (74), carbamazepine (75), phenytoin (76), and phenobarbital (46), some of which have been shown to have a documented effect, such as rifampin (73), carbamazepine (75), and phenytoin (76). Although CYP3A4 inhibitors, which include fluconazole (77), fluvoxamine (78), fluoxetine (79), paroxetine (72), and, possibly, erythromycin and ketoconazole have been hypothesized to result in significant drug interactions (17,48,59), very few of these medications have been shown to have a documented effect, either pharmacokinetic or pharmacodynamic, in humans at the doses used in methadone treatment, and some have been shown to have little or no effect, such as rifabutin (74) and fluoxetine (79).

A number of studies have examined specific antiretroviral medications used in the treatment of HIV-1 and their interaction with methadone. It has been shown that there are frequently pharmacokinetic interactions, usually through the 3A4 system, affecting either methadone or the antiretroviral medication, which sometimes have clinical manifestations (80,81).

Disulfiram, when used as a treatment for alcohol and cocaine dependence, has been shown to inhibit cytochrome P450-related enzymes (82). However, the metabolic interaction between methadone and disulfiram has been rigorously studied; there is no significant interaction between these two agents (17,82). Methadone levels are significantly affected by the regular consumption of more than four alcoholic drinks per day (83). Lowered methadone biotransformation secondary to hepatic enzyme competition occurs during excessive ethanol use, when blood measures of ethanol are very elevated (>150 mg/dL), with resultant increases in levels of methadone (84). When chronic use of alcohol is no longer present, the metabolism may be accelerated owing to the enhancement of the P450 enzymes (84), resulting in lower than expected plasma methadone levels.

St. John's wort (a dietary supplement sometimes self-administered by patients for depression) and grapefruit juice may affect the plasma concentration of methadone (85,86). Grapefruit juice may affect the pharmacokinetics of methadone probably via the CYP3A4 isoenzyme system and is not recommended during methadone maintenance treatment (86).

As methadone has slow onset of action owing to lipid solubility and slow offset of action owing to tissue reservoir coupled with long pharmacokinetic profile in humans, it has low primary abuse liability, with low rewarding effect. Abuse of methadone has been via the oral route, with a purpose of self-detoxification or self-maintenance, not for achieving a "high." This is sharply in contrast to short-acting narcotics.

Levo-alpha-acetylmethadol Pharmacokinetics

LAAM, a congener of methadone, shares with methadone the properties of long duration of effect (48 hours versus 24 hours for methadone, in part owing to its active metabolites norLAAM and dinorLaam, as well as its steady-state perfusion of mu opioid receptors), oral effectiveness (18), and function as a pure opioid agonist, active mostly at the mu opioid receptor. NorLAAM and dinorLAAM accumulate with chronic administration. In addition, LAAM and its metabolites bind to tissue proteins (18).

The clearance of norLAAM and LAAM is similar, whereas the clearance of dinorLAAM is more prolonged than that of its parent compound (18). The peak pharmacologic effect of LAAM as measured by amount of pupillary constriction occurred at 8 hours, then diminished at a rate most like that of norLAAM metabolism (18).

Because of the metabolism of LAAM by the cytochrome P450 3A4 system-related microsomal enzymes to norLAAM and dinorLAAM, drug interactions can occur (e.g., rifampin and long-term alcohol abuse tend to induce this enzyme system). In their presence, increased biotransformation of LAAM could accelerate the production of norLAAM and dinorLAAM. LAAM metabolism theoretically could be retarded if hepatic drug metabolism is diminished, as occurs in the presence of very large quantities of either ethanol or perhaps with large doses of benzodiazepines, or with intake of cimetidine (18).

Buprenorphine Pharmacokinetics Buprenorphine is metabolized to norbuprenorphine, which occurs by dealkylation in the cytochrome P450-related enzyme 3A4 system, of which buprenorphine itself is a weak inhibitor (87). Unlike methadone, buprenorphine undergoes extensive first pass in the liver, thus it is administered sublingually with 50% to 60% bioavailability. Despite the ceiling effect of buprenorphine as previously described, there have been a number of reported cases of deaths in Europe with concurrent benzodiazepine abuse (88). There have been many reports of the intravenous abuse of the sublingual preparation of buprenorphine in many countries in the world. A second formulation of sublingual buprenorphine, combined with naloxone, which was developed in 1984 and modeled after our early well-studied formulation of methadone/naloxone was developed and now is increasingly used in the United States and worldwide (50). In this formulation, naloxone will not precipitate withdrawal when taken sublingually because of its limited oral bioavailability; however, it may block the initial euphoric effects of buprenorphine if abused by the intravenous route, and may also then precipitate acute opioid withdrawal (89,90). The 4:1 ratio of buprenorphine to naloxone reduces any pleasurable effects of intravenous buprenorphine by blocking a small percentage of opioid receptors and may also produce modest withdrawal symptoms (90). However, naloxone apparently cannot effectively displace buprenorphine in overdose situations, particularly when benzodiazepines are present. With acute buprenorphine intoxication, there may be mild mental status changes, mild to minimal respiratory effects, small but not pinpoint pupils and essentially stable vital signs. In some situations, naloxone apparently can improve the respiratory depression but with limited effect on the other symptoms (91). Patients should be observed for 24 to 48 hours.

Initially developed as an analgesic, buprenorphine has been shown in most studies to be as effective as morphine in many situations. Buprenorphine has some modest kappa-opioid receptor activity, and recently it has been shown that the kappa activity of buprenorphine is that of a partial agonist (92). Owing to its ceiling effect, increasing doses in humans beyond 32 mg sublingually has no greater opioid agonist effect (93). Sixteen milligrams sublingual buprenorphine is the most commonly used dose in the treatment of opioid addiction, which is similar in efficacy to around 60 mg of methadone (94).

Buprenorphine has a long duration of action (24 to 48 hours) when administered on a chronic basis, not because of its pharmacokinetic profile but because of its very slow dissociation from mu-opioid receptors. Two important properties of buprenorphine are (1) its apparent lower severity of withdrawal signs and symptoms on cessation, compared with heroin, and, possibly, with methadone and LAAM and (2) its reduced potential to produce lethal overdose when used alone in opiate-naive or nontolerant persons because of its partial agonist properties. Given intravenously, buprenorphine has an apparent beta-terminal plasma half-life of about 3 to 5 hours. When given orally, it is relatively ineffective because of its first-pass metabolism (18), that is, rapid biotransformation, probably by the intestinal mucosa and, especially, by the liver. Sublingual preparations of buprenorphine can be liquid or tablet, both of which require about 120 minutes for time-to-peak. However, peak plasma concentrations of the sublingual tablet and mean area under the plasma concentration time curve are lower than that of the liquid at equivalent doses (93,95–97).

In two positron emission tomography studies of mu-opioid receptors using buprenorphine, studies initiated in 13 volunteers, who were treated with buprenorphine for up to 10 weeks maximum, and completed in 5 subjects, at dosages of 2 mg, 16 mg and 32 mg sublingually, it was found that buprenorphine induced dose-dependent reductions in mu-opioid receptor availability occupation far greater than that seen during moderate to high dose methadone maintenance treatment (52,98,99).

It was found that, at 2 mg, buprenorphine, sublingually, occupied about 37% to 47% of opiate receptors in different brain regions; at 16 mg, buprenorphine apparently occupied 85% to 92% of receptors, and at 32 mg, 85% to 98%. Both the 16-mg and 32-mg sublingual doses essentially completely blocked the effects of superimposed challenge with a single dose of hydrocodone. The mechanism by which buprenorphine blocks the effects of heroin or morphine are probably similar to those by which methadone, as used in maintenance treatment, blocks moderate to high doses of superimposed heroin or morphine, principally by tolerance and cross-tolerance (16).

PHARMACODYNAMICS

The pharmacodynamics of the clinically important mu-opioid receptor agonists are wide-ranging, with the most pronounced effects produced in the CNS and the GI tract.

The mechanism of action for all of the clinically relevant opioids described here is at the mu-opioid receptor, in which they act preferentially as agonists, except for buprenorphine, which is a partial mu-opioid agonist (99).

Morphine is the prototype for opioid analgesics. Both M6G and M3G cross the blood–brain barrier to a significant degree. With M3G, the major metabolite is essentially inactive but has excitatory effects in animals when injected directly into the CNS, suggesting that this metabolite may cause the neuroexcitatory effects that can be seen with large amounts of morphine given chronically. M6G is also an active metabolite which contributes to the analgesic effect of morphine. There is no evidence to suggest that any opioid has greater analgesic effect than morphine (42).

Opioids in general affect heat regulation mechanisms in the hypothalamus. Body temperature decreases slightly, except with chronic high doses temperature may be increased (4). Opioids also act in the hypothalamus to inhibit release of gonadotropin-releasing hormone and corticotropin-releasing hormone, producing a reduction in luteinizing hormone, follicle-stimulating hormone, adrenocorticotropin hormone (ACTH) and beta-endorphin (100). With decrease in these hormones, plasma concentrations of testosterone and cortisol are lowered. Mu agonists increase the amount of prolactin in plasma by decreasing dopaminergic inhibition. Given chronically, there is tolerance to the effects of morphine on the neuroendocrine system. Mu opioid agonists also tend to have antidiuretic effects (101–104).

Morphine also causes constriction of the pupil (4). Opioids can cause seizures at doses much higher than used for analgesia. Naloxone is less potent in antagonizing seizures with meperidine versus other opioids such as morphine or methadone, which may be owing to convulsant metabolites (normeperidine); therefore, meperidine is no longer used for chronic pain and is not to be used for >48 hours or >600 mg/day dose (12).

All opioids must be used cautiously in patients with impaired respiratory function. Also, opioids have the potential to elevate intracranial pressure (39) (e.g., in the setting of head injury it can produce an exaggerated respiratory depression, as well as mental status changes that can confuse the clinical picture). Typical side effects of all opioids include drowsiness, nausea, and constipation, while vomiting, pruritus, and dizziness are less common; however, all of these tend to lessen in intensity over time.

Codeine is commonly used to suppress cough at doses lower than used for analgesia (starting with 10 to 20 mg given orally) and can increase to higher doses for chronic (lower airway) cough. Codeine reduces cough via a central mechanism, with doses >65 mg not indicated owing to little increased effect with increasing side effects (4).

Pentazocine as a mixed agonist-antagonist drug has a "ceiling effect," like buprenorphine, which limits the degree of analgesia. It can lead to the development of severe psychotomimetic side-effects not reversible with naloxone; therefore, it may not be mediated through usual opioid receptors. Pentazocine has affinity for kappa receptors (105). Pentazocine can also produce withdrawal in opioid-tolerant patients due to its weak antagonist effects.

Methadone, like all mu opioid agonists, affects multiple organ systems, with tolerance developing at different rates to each effect. In the treatment of illicit opioid dependence or pain with prescribed opiates, proper dosing (titrated to the tolerance of the individual patient) is essential to avoid CNS depression. The precise neuronal and molecular mechanisms of physical tolerance have not been fully elucidated (102). However, it has been shown in studies of the *d*(R)-enantiomer of methadone (which is relatively inactive at the mu-opioid receptor) that this isomer has modest NMDA antagonist activity, which attenuates the development of morphine tolerance in rodents but does not affect physical dependence (106). Tolerance to the different effects of methadone occurs at different time points, with persistence (after at least 3 years of chronic treatment) of increased sweating and constipation (50) as well as a persistence of the pulsatile increase in prolactin entrained to the peak level of methadone, which occurs approximately 2 to 4 hours after daily administration (100,103,104).

With the use of oral methadone, analgesia occurs at 30 to 60 minutes. The analgesic effect of a single methadone dose given intramuscularly is equivalent to morphine, but its cumulative effects occur over time (8). Any euphoria produced by any opioid agonist, primarily short-acting opioids, apparently is mediated in part by the ventral tegmentum, where opioid agonist-mediated inhibition of GABAergic neurons results in disinhibition and thus activation of dopamine neurons extending to the nucleus accumbens. Norepinephrine-secreting cells in the locus ceruleus appear to play an important role in opioid withdrawal, whereas both serotonin and dopamine exert effects on dependence and craving (102,104).

Chronic administration of long-acting opioids (such as methadone) leads to the gradual development of tolerance to the effects on hypothalamic-releasing factors, with resumption of normal menses and return of plasma levels of testosterone to normal within 1 year as well as return to normal levels and activity of anterior pituitary-derived ACTH and beta-endorphin and normal ACTH stimulation in approximately 3 months (50,100). In humans, prolactin release is under tonic inhibition by tuberoinfundibular dopaminergic tone. With the use of short-acting opiates, there is a prompt increase in the release of prolactin because of an abrupt lowering of dopamine levels in the tuberoinfundibular dopaminergic system. With chronic methadone treatment, there is some tolerance to this response but not complete tolerance, because of the lowering of dopamine that is still present. Prolactin levels still rise after oral methadone dosing; however, both peak plasma levels of methadone and also prolactin are found at 2 to 4 hours after dosing; prolactin levels usually do not exceed the upper limit of normal (50,100,103,107,108).

The metyrapone test blocks 11-beta-hydroxylation of cortisol in the adrenal cortex. Heroin reduces the normal stress response to this test. However, a normal response is restored during chronic methadone maintenance treatment (50,100, 109,110). With heroin use, thyroid levels may be elevated because of raised thyroid-binding globulin; thus, there are increased measures without abnormal function (50,100). Hypothalamus and pituitary effects of opioids can produce antidiuretic effect by release of vasopressin and heat regulation changes (4,100).

Acutely, short-acting opiates can cause many effects. During chronic methadone maintenance treatment, many of these effects may diminish or present with a different time course. In the cardiovascular system, acute administration of opioids may cause peripheral vasodilatation, decreased peripheral resistance, reduced baroreceptor reflexes, histamine release, and decreased reflex vasoconstriction caused by raised PCO_2 (4). In the stomach, hydrochloric acid secretion may be inhibited, and somatostatin release from the pancreas may be elevated (4). Acetylcholine release from the GI tract is inhibited, and motility is slowed, as is absorption of drugs. The presence of increased feeding also has been noted. Biliary, pancreatic, and intestinal secretions may be reduced and digestion in the small intestine slowed. In the large intestine, there is reduced propulsion and higher tone (4,50,100,101). Tolerance develops to each of these effects. The short-acting opioids such as heroin or morphine, administered on an active or chronic basis, reduce rosettes formed by human T lymphocytes (100,101). Morphine reduces cytotoxic activity of natural killer cells and increases growth of implanted tumors (100,101). In contrast, with the chronic use of the long-acting opioid methadone, absolute numbers of T cells, T-cell subsets, B cells, and quantitative immunoglobulins are gradually restored to normal over 3 to 10 years, along with restoration of normal natural killer-cell activity (111). During the chronic use of short-acting narcotics, as here, these immunologic indices are abnormal with the use of heroin, possibly in part by mediation through the neuroendocrine system, since cortisol suppresses many parameters of immune function, and cortisol levels increase in opioid withdrawal. Thus, normalization of most of these immunologic indices may gradually occur with methadone maintenance treatment (50,100,101). During methadone maintenance treatment, no daily or multiple times per day withdrawal episodes occur.

TOLERANCE DEVELOPMENT

Tolerance may be defined as a loss of any effect after repeated use, leading to the need for higher doses to get the desired equivalent effect (102,112). Physical dependence is now known to be molecularly and clinically different from tolerance (102,112). All opiate and opioid medications lead to development of tolerance and physical dependence, though the rate of development of tolerance varies from one medication to another. Tolerance may develop at different rates for any side effects of any opioid medication and can occur over days, weeks, or years. Development of tolerance to opiates and opioids does not involve drug disposition and metabolism. There appears to be a complex interplay at both the single-cell and neuronal system levels (102).

Two unique characteristics distinguish methadone from almost all other therapeutic opiates and opioids. First, after binding to mu-opioid receptors, the methadone-opioid receptor complex undergoes rapid endocytosis, exactly like endogenous opioids (e.g., beta-endorphin or met-enkephalin) (102,112). Most opiates and opioids do not undergo endocytosis, or endocytosis is slow. The rapid endocytosis of the methadone-opioid receptor complex may contribute to the relatively slow rate of tolerance development. Second, it has been shown that both enantiomers of methadone, present in equal amounts in a racemic mixture, have modest NMDA-antagonist action, and that NMDA-antagonism attenuates or prevents tolerance to opiates and opioids (42,102). Thus, this modest NMDA-antagonist activity may contribute to the slow rate of development of tolerance to methadone (106).

Patients maintained on methadone rapidly develop partial or full tolerance to most of methadone's side effects (e.g., nausea and vomiting, miosis, sedation). However, tolerance develops at a slower rate to the neuroendocrine effects of the HPA and HPG (hypothalamic-pituitary-gonadal) axes. Tolerance develops even more slowly to the constipating effects of opioids, as has been shown in our prospective studies of chronic methadone maintenance patients (50). The only side effect to which tolerance does not develop is sweating (50), which is not excessive and does not interfere with extreme physical activities in heat or in sunlight; tolerance develops more rapidly to the "on-off" effects of short-acting narcotics (e.g., heroin, morphine, and even extended-release preparations of short-acting narcotics, such as oxycodone [OxyContin]). Therefore, the GI and neuroendocrine side effects of short-acting opioids tend to persist (49).

TOXICITY STATES AND THEIR MEDICAL MANAGEMENT

Acute opioid overdose is characterized by the triad of stupor or coma, respiratory depression, and "pinpoint" pupils. Needle marks may be noted.

Individualized dosing and reliance on regular clinical assessments are important, as diminished respiration occurs with opioids until tolerance develops. When any opioid is used beyond the degree of tolerance that is developed, reduced response to carbon dioxide centers in the pons and medulla can lead to CO_2 retention. Initially there is depressed cough (which is mediated by the medulla) as well as nausea and vomiting, which may be mediated by the area postrema of the medulla and which disappear rapidly with the development of tolerance. Constriction of the pupil is the result of parasympathetic nerve excitation. In opioid overdose, convulsions have been reported, probably because of inhibition of the release of GABA in the CNS (4).

Mydriasis or normal pupils may be observed in patients with an overdose of meperidine, propoxyphene, dextromethorphan, pentazocine, and diphenoxylate with atropine (i.e., Lomotil) (4,113,114).

A full opioid overdose can be effectively treated with an opioid antagonist; however, the pharmacokinetic profile of the opioid must be considered. Since naloxone has a half-life of only 30 minutes, more than one dose may be needed for management of any opioid overdose. When overdose occurs owing to excessive use of methadone in an opioid-naïve or weakly tolerant person, repeated intravenous doses or intravenous constant infusion of naloxone may be needed for up to 24 hours or longer. Most opioids have a half-life of 4 hours or longer; therefore, repeated naloxone administration is usually needed. Otherwise, the overdose may be only transiently reversed, and the patient may lapse back into the comatose overdose situation. Lack of full understanding of the pharmacokinetics of opioid antagonists, especially naloxone (Narcan), the most commonly used opioid antagonist, or the pharmacokinetics of various short-acting and long-acting opioids used in the treatment of addiction or pain, or used illicitly, have led to unnecessary deaths (83).

MEDICAL COMPLICATIONS OF OPIOIDS

Central Nervous System Effects of opioids on the CNS are minimal in therapeutic doses. The two main CNS effects of overdose of opioids are depression of the mental status and depression of respiratory activity. Depending on the dose ingested, mental status may vary from mild sedation to stupor and coma. Significant depression of mental status is accompanied by suppressed gag reflex predisposing the patient to aspiration of gastric contents into the lungs in the setting of centrally mediated nausea and vomiting. A few opioids may cause generalized seizures (e.g., high-dose meperidine). Respiratory depression manifests as low respiratory rate, hypoxia, hypercarbia; it is the most frequent cause of death owing to opioid overdose (4).

Pulmonary Effects of opioids on the pulmonary system are minimal in therapeutic doses. Besides centrally mediated respiratory depression, overdose of opioids may affect the respiratory system directly by causing non-cardiogenic pulmonary edema (NCPE) and bronchospasm. NCPE typically presents with frothy, pink bronchial secretions, cyanosis, and rales accompanying respiratory depression in a stuporous or comatose patient. NCPE is particularly associated with intravenous and inhalational use of heroin and occurs in 48% to 80% of patients hospitalized with heroin overdose. Heroin may also induce acute bronchospasm (4).

Cardiovascular Effects of opioids on the cardiovascular system are minimal in therapeutic doses. In overdose, the cardiovascular dysfunction occurs, mostly owing to hypoxia caused by respiratory depression. Opioids may cause a release of histamine leading to vasodilatation that, in turn, results in orthostatic hypotension. Morphine directly reduces peripheral vascular tone, an effect that is used therapeutically in pulmonary edema and myocardial infarction. The effect of opioids on heart rate is variable: Nausea and vomiting may stimulate vasovagal tone, leading to brachycardia; however, orthostatic hypotension may reflexively cause mild tachycardia. Overdose of propoxyphene may lead to direct myocardial toxicity. Cardiovascular problems associated with an intravenous route of opioid abuse include bacterial endocarditis, venous thrombosis, septic pulmonary emboli, emboli of cornstarch and talc to retina, lungs, kidney, liver, pseudoaneurysms, and mycotic aneurysms (114).

High (>300 mg/day) doses of methadone have been associated with prolongation of QT_c interval and with torsades de pointes (115). Many of these patients were receiving other medications as well, including some, such as antiretrovirals, that are known to prolong QT_c (116). Chlorobutanol, the preservative used in the only commercial formulation of parenteral methadone, potentiates methadone's ability to block ionic current through cardiac potassium channels, thus contributing to QT_c prolongation (117). A prospective cohort study (118) of methadone treatment showed a statistically significant (mean of 10.8 ms) prolongation of QT_c interval regardless of methadone dose, during the first 2 months of methadone treatment; however, this prolongation did not appear to be clinically significant. The mean QT_c value in this study was 428 ms; a QTc value of >500 ms is considered to be a potential risk for torsades de pointes (118). The degree of QT_c prolongation correlates with both the trough and peak serum methadone concentrations (119). In 2005, another study showed that methadone modestly increased both QT_c (by 14.1 ms) and QT_c dispersion (from 32.9 ± 12 ms to 42.4 ± 15 ms) after 6 months of therapy. The effect was not thought to be clinically significant (120). A 2006 cross-sectional study in Tel Aviv, Israel, showed that methadone maintenance therapy was safe, but QT_c interval must be measured before and during therapy with high doses (>120 mg/day) of methadone (121).

Gastrointestinal Besides nausea and vomiting, short-acting and also early maintenance treatment with long-acting opioids profoundly slows GI motility, leading to constipation and possible fecal impaction. This partially central and partially peripherally mediated effect may lead to changes in intestinal absorption. Morphine may cause spasm of the sphincter of Oddi; hence, it should not be used in biliary colic. However, clinical studies have not shown a significant difference between sphincter effects of morphine and meperidine, which is often recommended for biliary colic. Prospective studies determined that tolerance to the constipating effect of chronic methadone maintenance treatment develops within 3 years (50).

Renal Heroin, illicit methadone, and propoxyphene have been rarely associated with rhabdomyolysis, which may cause renal failure. However, there is considerable evidence that this is owing to admixtures of other chemicals with illicit drugs. Rhabdomyolysis has never been seen in methadone treatment. Heroin, morphine, and pentazocine may cause nephropathy when used intravenously, leading to glomerulonephritis (114).

Musculoskeletal Very high doses of opioids may induce centrally mediated muscle rigidity of the chest and abdominal wall. Intravenously abused opioids may cause osteomyelitis, septic arthritis, polymyositis, and fibrous myopathy (4).

Infectious Diseases Injection routes (intravenous, subcutaneous) of opioid abuse due to the use of shared unclean needles may lead to transmission of HIV-1 infection, hepatitis B, hepatitis C, as well as other bacteria causing cellulitis, skin and neck abscesses, endocarditis, and botulism (114).

CONCLUSIONS AND FUTURE RESEARCH DIRECTIONS

The specific neuronal and molecular basis of opioid tolerance and dependence has not been fully elucidated. Effects of opioids can be mediated by signal transduction, and exert their effect mostly through G-protein coupling (101). Neuroadaptation with sensitization as well as neurotoxicity do not occur with clinically used opioids in humans.

Morphine inhibits adenylyl cyclase, leading to inhibition of the cAMP-dependent cascade. With long-term morphine treatment, this initial inhibition results in a compensating increase of adenylyl cyclase and increase in the cAMP-dependent cascade (101). This compensation includes increases in protein kinase A, phosphorylated proteins, and cAMP-dependent response element binding protein. Chronic morphine treatment has been reported to produce an uncoupling of the mu-opioid receptor and its G-protein coupled inwardly rectifying potassium channels, which have been shown to cause reduced maximal outward current and reduced efficiency, with decreased opioid potency (101). Further research on the mechanisms and the differences in mechanisms among different opioids in eliciting each of these effects is needed.

Five single nucleotide polymorphisms have been identified in the coding region of the human muopioid receptor gene (122). Three of these five single-nucleotide polymorphisms lead to amino acid changes, and two (the A118G and the C17T variants) have high allelic frequencies: 2% to more than 40% in different cultural and ethnic groups. The C17T variant may have some association with opiate dependence, although significant associations have not been confirmed (122). Binding studies have shown that exogenous ligands, including methadone and morphine, bind similarly to the A118G variant and to the prototype receptor; however, the endogenous opioid beta-endorphin binds three times more tightly. Functional studies have shown that the endogenous opioid beta-endorphin produces three times more potent activation of one of the two major signal transduction systems when bound to the A118G variant (122). Genetic factors, such as the presence of this functional A118G variant, which regulate pharmacodynamics, may contribute to variability among patients with respect to intersubject response to opioids, or especially the opioid antagonists (122–124).

Atypical response to stress and stressors, as demonstrated by changes in hypothalamic-pituitary-adrenal (HPA) axis function, have been shown in heroin addicts with normalization of response after stabilization on a steady dose of methadone. During cycles of heroin addiction, there is a flattened circadian rhythm of levels of glucocorticoids, with increased levels during opiate withdrawal. With steady-state methadone treatment, both circadian rhythms and plasma levels of the HPA axis normalize, as do responses of the HPA axis to chemically-induced stress (109). With the use of heroin, the addicted individual may be seeking suppression of atypical (either endogenous or drug-induced) hyperresponsivity to stress and stressors, and the long-acting opioid methadone gradually produces normal responsivity of the stress-responsive systems. One imaging study using positron emission tomography showed only 19% to 32% greater occupancy of opiate receptors in specific brain areas related to pain and analgesia as well as addiction (caudate, putamen, amygdala, anterior cingulate cortex, and thalamus) during steady-dose methadone maintenance treatment compared with normal volunteers (52). The presence of these unoccupied receptors helps explain how physiologic systems dependent on mu-opioid receptor activation, which are disrupted during cycles of heroin abuse, can become normalized during methadone maintenance treatment.

The effects of another mu-opioid receptor partial agonist widely used in the treatment of opioid addiction, buprenorphine (or buprenorphine/naloxone), on specific indices of neuroendocrine function has not been extensively studied nor have any of the other aspects of physiology, such as known to be disrupted during cycles of opiate addiction and shown to be normalized during methadone treatment, such as effects on some immunological function. A very recent study from the group of Kakko et al. (125) in Sweden studied the effects of metyrapone in 20 buprenorphine-maintained former heroin addicts and 20 normal volunteers. They found that "response to metyrapone was subnormal in heroin addicts maintained on buprenorphine." This is precisely what we found in much earlier studies of heroin addicts and also during the first 1 or 2 months of methadone maintenance treatment (50,100). In medication-free, drug–free former heroin addicts, we found hyperresponsivity, as contrasted with subnormal responsivity in active heroin addicts (50,100). In repeated studies, in long-term (3 months or more) methadone-maintained treatment subjects, we have found normalization in response to metyrapone (50,100,109).

In the area of opioid agonist treatment pharmacology, more rigorous studies of complex drug interactions with methadone and other medications are needed, including studies of medications for patients with comorbid conditions, such as HIV-1, hepatitis C virus, and psychiatric illnesses. From a broader perspective, integration of basic science information at the molecular and animal level with clinical research and observation should be pursued (3). This research should include further elucidation of the differences in the stress-responsive HPA axis in persons maintained on other long-acting opioid agonist pharmacotherapy, such as buprenorphine, as with methadone, as compared with normal subjects, including areas such as possible gender differences.

Finally, studies conducted since the mid-1980s have demonstrated the effectiveness of "medical maintenance," which involves transferring patients already maintained at conventional methadone maintenance treatment programs to monthly office-based treatment with methadone.

In order to qualify in the early studies, methadone-maintained patients had to be abstinent from illicit substances for months to years, employed, and adhere to conventional treatment before they could be admitted to office-based methadone treatment (126–128).

However, the Federal Guidelines governing methadone maintenance treatment were rigorously reanalyzed by all three branches of the government, and the new interpretations of the guidelines published in the Federal Register, and were finally approved in early 2001 (21). Now, in accordance with Federal Guidelines, any patient may be transferred from a methadone maintenance clinic, constituted according to the old and new guidelines, to an individual physician's office-based practice at any time, based solely on the clinical assessment of the medical staff of the clinic and the physician who is accepting the patient. There is no constraint on length of time in a methadone clinic before moving to an office-based practice; there is no constraint on dose of methadone being used, nor length of time of abstinence from illicit use of substances (21). There are no further requirements other than the fact that the physicians offering office-based treatment will refer the patient back to the original methadone clinic or another methadone clinic with which a referral has been arranged if any significant problems ensue. However, individual states may impose more rigid regulations.

The guidelines governing entrance into methadone maintenance treatment remain very strict and far beyond establishment of a DSM-IV diagnosis of opiate addiction. Requirements include multiple daily self-administrations of heroin or any short-acting opiate for 1 year or more. To appropriately conduct a study of office-based induction to methadone maintenance treatment, the individual physicians involved each created a setting to adhere to the guidelines of a "methadone clinic," and one study reported outstanding success in office-based induction into methadone maintenance treatment (129).

To enter buprenorphine or buprenorphine/naloxone treatment, it is necessary only that a patient meet the DSM-IV criteria for "opioid dependence" (i.e., opioid addiction). Each physician administering buprenorphine (or buprenorphine/naloxone) maintenance treatment must take an 8-hour training course and should offer access to behavioral care. Office-based buprenorphine treatment has been found to be effective in many patients (130,131).

It has already been found that patients with high levels of tolerance to an opioid may not be able to be effectively treated with the partial agonist of buprenorphine or buprenorphine/naloxone, since the maximal effective dose of buprenorphine is around 24 or 32 mg sublingually, equal to 60 or 70 mg of methadone. Multiple studies performed over 44 years have documented that the majority of heroin addicts require 80 to 150 mg/day of methadone, as used in maintenance treatment (132). Fortunately, patients may be transferred with ease from buprenorphine to methadone maintenance treatment. The converse is not as simple, as the addition of buprenorphine will produce opioid withdrawal in patients who are being maintained on the usual doses of methadone. Thus, significant dose reduction of methadone to suboptimal treatment levels (e.g., 30 to 40 mg/day) must be used prior to starting buprenorphine treatment.

ACKNOWLEDGMENTS: *Support for this chapter has been provided by grants from the National Institutes of Health (NIH): National Institute of Drug Abuse (NIDA) Grant P60-DA05130 and the New York State Office of Alcoholism and Substance Abuse Services (OASAS). We also thank Eduardo Butelman, PhD; Ann Ho, PhD; Charles Inturrisi, PhD; Brenda Ray, NP; Elizabeth Ducat, NP; Jack Varon; and Meg West for assistance in preparation of the manuscript. We are especially grateful to Susan Russo, who helped in every stage of preparation of the manuscript.*

REFERENCES

1. Kreek MJ. Methadone-related opioid agonist pharmacotherapy for heroin addiction: history, recent molecular and neurochemical research and the future in mainstream medicine. *Ann N Y Acad Sci* 2000;909: 186–216.
2. LaForge KS, Yuferov V, Kreek MJ. Opioid receptor and peptide gene polymorphisms: potential implications for addictions. *Eur J Pharmacol* 2000:410:249–268.
3. Kreek M, Bart G, Lilly C, et al. Pharmacogenetics and human molecular genetics of opiate and cocaine addictions and their treatments. *Pharmacol Rev* 2005;57:1–26.
4. Gutstein HB, Akil H. Opioid analgesics In: Brunton L, Lazo JS, Parker KL, eds. *Goodman & Gilman's the pharmacological basis of therapeutics*, 11th ed. New York: McGraw-Hill, 2005:547–590.
5. Sell L, Zador D. Patients prescribed injectable heroin or methadone—their opinions and experiences of treatment. *Addiction* 2004;99: 442–449.
6. Blanken P, Hendriks V, Koeter M, et al. Matching of treatment-resistant heroin-dependent patients to medical prescription of heroin or oral methadone treatment: results from two randomized controlled trials. *Addiction* 2005;100:89–95.
7. Substance Abuse and Mental Health Services Administration Office of Applied Studies. *The DASIS Report: heroin—changes in how it is used: 1995–2005*. Rockville, MD: April 26, 2007.
8. Portenoy RK, Payne R, Passik SD. Acute and chronic pain. In: Lowinson JH, Ruiz P, Millman RB, et al., eds. *Substance abuse: a comprehensive textbook*. Baltimore: Williams & Wilkins, 1992:691–721.
9. Comer SD, Ashworth JB. The growth of prescription opioid abuse. In Smith HS, Passik SD, eds. *Pain and chemical dependency*. New York: Oxford University Press, 2008:19–23.
10. Ordonez Gallego A, Gonzalez Baron M, Espinosa Arranz E. Oxycodone: a pharmacological and clinical review. *Clin Translat Oncol* 2007;9: 298–307.
11. Warolin C, Robiquet P-J. *Rev Hist Pharm (Paris)* [Abstract]. 1999;47: 97.
12. Latta KS, Ginsberg B, Barkin RL. Meperidine: a critical review. *Am J Ther* 2002;9:53–68.
13. Fudala PJ, Johnson RE. Development of opioid formulations with limited diversion and abuse potential. *Drug Alcohol Depend* 2006;83S: S40–S47.
14. Sarhill N, Walsh D, Nelson KA. Hydromorphone: pharmacology and clinical applications in cancer patients. *Supp Care Cancer* 2001;9:84–96.
15. Cone E, Caplan Y, Moser F, et al. Evidence that morphine is metabolized to hydromorphone but not to oxymorphone. *J Anal Toxicol* 2008; 32:319–323.
16. Dole VP, Nyswander ME, Kreek MJ. Narcotic blockade. *Arch Intern Med* 1966;118:304–309.
17. Ferrari A, Coccia CP, Bertolini A, et al. Methadone—metabolism, pharmacokinetics and interactions. *Pharmacol Res* 2004;50:551–559.
18. Kreek MJ. Long-term pharmacotherapy for opiate (primarily heroin) addiction: Opiate agonists. In: Schuster C, Kuhar MK, eds. *Pharmacological aspects of drug dependence: toward an integrated neurobehavioral approach*. Berlin:Springer-Verlag, 1996:487–562.
19. Fudala PF, Vocci F, Montgomery A, et al. Levomethadyl acetate (LAAM) for the treatment of opioid dependence: a multisite, open label study of LAAM safety and an evaluation of the product labeling and treatment regulations. *J Maint Addict* 1997;1:9–39.
20. Kang J, Chen X-L, Wang H, et al. Interactions of the narcotic *l*-alpha-acetylmethadol with human cardiac K^+ channels. *Eur J Pharmacol* 2003; 458:25–29.
21. Kreek MJ, Vocci FJ. History and current status of opioid maintenance treatments: blending conference session. *J Subst Abuse Treat* 2002;23: 93–105.
22. Vocci F, Ling W. Medications development: successes and challenges. *Pharmacol Ther* 2005;108:94–108.
23. O'Connor PG, Oliveto AH, Shi JM, et al. A randomized trial of buprenorphine maintenance for heroin dependence in a primary care clinic for substance users versus a methadone clinic. *Am J Med* 1998; 105:100–105.
24. Casadonte P, Walsh R, Vocci F. Treatment of opioid dependence with buprenorphine naloxone in a solo private psychiatry practice. *Drug Alcohol Depend* 2001;63:92.
25. Huang P, Kehner GB, Cowan A, et al. Comparison of pharmacological activities of buprenorphine and norbuprenorphine: norbuprenorphine is a potent opioid agonist. *J Pharmacol Exp Ther*. 2001;297:688–695.
26. Compton WM, Volkow ND. Abuse of prescription drugs and the risk of addiction. *Drug Alcohol Depend* 2006;83S:S4–S7.
27. Office of National Drug Control Policy, Executive Office of the President. *Prescription for Danger*. Washington, DC: January, 2008.
28. Substance Abuse & Mental Health Services Administration. *Buprenorphine Physician and Treatment Program Locator*. Rockville, MD, 2008. http://buprenorphine.samhsa.gov/bwns_locator/aboutphysician.html.
29. Reckitt Benckiser Pharmaceuticals Inc. *Suboxone: Office-based treatment for opioid dependence*. Slough, UK, 2008. *http://*www.suboxone.com/officebasedtreatment.com.
30. Des Jarlais DC, Arasteh K, Perlis T, et al. The transition from injection to non-injection drug use: long-term outcomes among heroin and cocaine users in New York City. *Addiction* 2007;102:778–785.

31. Johnston L, O'Malley P, Bachman J, et al. *Overall, illicit drug use by American teens continues gradual decline in 2007.* Ann Arbor, MI [online] www.monitoringthefuture.org: University of Michigan News Service, 2007.
32. National Institute on Drug Abuse. *Prescription Drugs: abuse and addiction. NIDA Research Report Series,* NIH Publication Number 05-4881, Revised 2005. www.nida.gov/researchreports/prescription/prescription-drugs:abuseandaddiction, 2005.
33. Inturrisi CE. Opiates: clinical aspects. In Smith HS, Passik SD, eds. *Pain and chemical dependency.* New York: Oxford University Press, 2008:175–182.
34. Knapp CM, Ciraulo DA, Jaffe J. Opiates: clinical aspects. In: Lowinson JH, Ruiz P, Millman RB, et al., eds. *Substance abuse: a comprehensive textbook,* 4th ed. Philadelphia: Lippincott Williams & Wilkins, 2005: 180–195.
35. Inturrisi C, Max MB, Foley KM, et al. The pharmacokinetics of heroin in patients with chronic pain. *N Engl J Med* 1984;310:1213–1217.
36. Cone EJ, Holicky BA, Grant TM, et al. Pharmacokinetics and pharmacodynamics of intranasal "snorted" heroin. *J Anal Toxicol* 1993;17: 327–337.
37. Kamendulis LM, Brzezinski MR, Pindel EV, et al. Metabolism of cocaine and heroin is catalyzed by the same human liver carboxylesterases. *J Pharmacol Exp Ther* 1996;279:713–717.
38. Skopp G, Ganssmann B, Cone EJ, et al. Plasma concentrations of heroin and morphine-related metabolites after intranasal and intramuscular administration. *J Anal Toxicol* 1997;21:105–111.
39. Kaiko R, Wallenstein SL, Rogers AG, et al. Analgesic and mood effects of heroin and morphine in cancer patients with postoperative pain. *N Engl J Med* 1981;304:1501–1505.
40. Kraemer T, Paul LD. Bioanalytical procedures for determination of drugs of abuse in blood. *Anal Bioanal Chem* 2007;388:1415–1435.
41. Weinberg DS, Inturrisi CE, Reidenberg B, et al. Sublingual absorption of selected opioid analgesics. *Clin Pharmacol Ther* 1988;44:335–342.
42. Inturrisi CE. Clinical pharmacology of opioids for pain. *Clin J Pain* 2002;18:S3–S13.
43. Mazoit JX, Sandouk P, Scherrmann J-P, et al. Extrahepatic metabolism of morphine occurs in humans. *Clin Pharmacol Ther* 1990;4:613–618.
44. Lugo RA, Kern SE. The pharmacokinetics of oxycodone. *J Pain Palliat Care Pharmacother* 2004;18:17–30.
45. Davis MP, Varga J, Dickerson D, et al. Normal-release and controlled-release oxycodone: pharmacokinetics, pharmacodynamics, and controversy. *Supp Care Cancer* 2003;11:84–92.
46. Smith HS, Vanderah TW, McCleane G. Opioids for pain. In Smith HS, Passik SD, eds. *Pain and chemical dependency.* New York: Oxford University Press, 2008:183–202.
47. Oyler JM, Cone EJ, Joseph RE, et al. Identification of hydrocodone in human urine following codeine administration. *J Anal Toxicol* 2000;24:530–535.
48. Lugo RA, Satterfield KL, Kern SE. Pharmacokinetics of methadone. *J Pain Palliat Care Pharmacother* 2005;19:13–24.
49. Kreek MJ. Plasma and urine levels of methadone. *N Y State J Med* 1973;73:2773–2777.
50. Kreek MJ. Medical safety and side effects of methadone in tolerant individuals. *JAMA* 1973;223:665–668.
51. Dole V, Kreek MJ. Methadone plasma level: sustained by a reservoir of drug in tissue. *Proc Natl Acad Sci* 1973;70:10.
52. Kling MA, Carson RE, Borg L, et al. Opioid receptor imaging with positron emission tomography and [18F]cyclofoxy in long-term, methadone-treated former heroin addicts. *J Pharmacol Exp Ther* 2000;295:1070–1076.
53. Eap C, Buclin T, Baumann P. Interindividual variability of the clinical pharmacokinetics of methadone: implications for the treatment of opioid dependence. *Clin Pharmacokinet* 2002;41:1153–1193.
54. Hachey DL, Kreek MJ, Mattson DH. Quantitative analysis of methadone in biological fluids using deuterium-labelled methadone and GLC-chemical-ionization mass spectrometry *J Pharm Sci* 1977;66: 1579–1582.
55. Kreek MJ, Hachey DL, Klein PD. Stereoselective disposition of methadone in man. *Life Sci* 1979;24:925–932.
56. de Castro J, Aguirre C, Rodriguez-Sasiain JM, et al. The effect of changes in gastric pH induced by omeprazole on the absorption and respiratory depression of methadone. *Biopharmacol Drug Disp* 1996;17:551–563.
57. Pond SM, Kreek MJ, Tong TG, et al. Altered methadone pharmacokinetics in methadone-maintained pregnant women. *J Pharmacol Exp Ther* 1985;233:1–6.
58. Kreek MJ, Oratz M, Rothschild MA. Hepatic extraction of long and short-acting narcotics in the isolated perfused rabbit liver. *Gastroenterology* 1978;75:88–94.
59. Kreek MJ, Gutjahr CL, Garfield JW, et al. Drug interactions with methadone. *Ann N Y Acad Sci* 1976;281:350–371.
60. Borg L, Ho A, Peters JE,, et al. Availability of reliable serum methadone determination for management of symptomatic patients. *J Addict Dis* 1995;14:83–96.
61. Peles E, Schreiber S, Naumovsky Y, et al. Depression in methadone maintenance treatment patients: rate and risk factors. *J Affect Dis* 2007;99:213–220.
62. Eap CB, Broly F, Mino A, et al. Cytochrome P450 2D6 genotype and methadone steady-state concentrations. *J Clin Psychopharmacol* 2001; 21:229–234.
63. Levran O, O'Hara K, Peles E, et al. *ABCB1* (*MDR1*) genetic variants are associated with methadone doses required for effective treatment of heroin dependence. *Hum Mol Genet* 2008;17:2219–2227.
64. Rubenstein RB, Kreek MJ, Mbawa N, et al. Human spinal fluid methadone levels. *Drug Alcohol Depend* 1978;3:103–106.
65. Kreek MJ, Bencsath FA, Field FH. Effects of liver disease on urinary excretion of methadone and metabolites in maintenance patients: quantitation by direct probe chemical ionization mass spectrometry. *Biomed Mass Spectrom* 1980;7:385–395.
66. Kreek MJ, Bencsath FA, Fanizza A, et al. Effects of liver disease on fecal excretion of methadone and its unconjugated metabolites in maintenance patients: quantitation by direct probe chemical ionization mass spectrometry. *Biomed Mass Spectrom* 1983;10:544–549.
67. Bowen DV, Smit ALC, Kreek MJ. Fecal excretion of methadone and its metabolites in man: Application of GC-MS. In: Daily NR, ed. *Advances in mass spectrometry.* Philadelphia: Heyden & Son, 1978:7B, 1634–1639.
68. Kreek MJ, Kalisman M, Irwin M, et al. Biliary secretion of methadone and methadone metabolites in man. *Res Comm Chem Pathol Pharmacol* 1980;29:67–78.
69. Kreek MJ, Schecter AJ, Gutjahr CL, et al. Methadone use in patients with chronic renal disease. *Drug Alcohol Depend* 1980;5:197–205.
70. Novick DM, Kreek MJ, Fanizza AM, et al. Methadone disposition in patients with chronic liver disease. *Clin Pharmacol Ther* 1981;30: 353–362.
71. Novick DM, Kreek MJ, Arns PA, et al. Effect of severe alcoholic liver disease on the disposition of methadone in maintenance patients. *Alcohol Clin Exp Res* 1985;9:349–354.
72. Begre S, von Bardeleben U, Ledewig D, et al. Paroxetine increases steady-state concentrations of (R)-methadone in CYP2D6 extensive but not poor metabolizers. *J Clin Psychopharmacol* 2002;22:211–215.
73. Kreek MJ, Garfield JW, Gutjahr CL, et al. Rifampin-induced methadone withdrawal. *N Engl J Med* 1976;294:1104–1106.
74. Brown LS, Sawyer RC, Li R, et al. Lack of a pharmacologic interaction between rifabutin and methadone in HIV-infected former injecting drug users. *Drug Alcohol Depend* 1996;43:71–77.
75. Kuhn KL, Halikas JA, Kemp KD, et al. Carbamazepine treatment of cocaine dependence in methadone maintenance patients with dual opiate-cocaine addiction. *NIDA Res Monogr* 1989;95:316–317.
76. Tong TG, Pond SM, Kreek MJ, et al. Phenytoin-induced methadone withdrawal. *Ann Intern Med* 1981;94:349–351.
77. Cobb MN, Desai J, Brown LS, et al. The effect of fluconazole on the clinical pharmacokinetics of methadone. *Clin Pharmacol Ther* 1998;63:655–662.

78. Bertschy G, Baumann P, Eap CB, et al. Probable metabolic interaction between methadone and fluvoxamine in addict patients. *Ther Drug Monitor* 1994;16:42–45.
79. Bertschy G, Eap CB, Powell K, et al. Fluoxetine addition to methadone in addicts: pharmacokinetic aspects. *Ther Drug Monitor* 1996;18: 570–572.
80. McCance-Katz EF. Treatment of opioid dependence and coinfection with HIV and hepatitis C virus in opioid-dependent patients: the importance of drug interactions between opioids and antiretroviral agents. *Clin Infect Dis* 2005;41:S89–S95.
81. Bruce RD, Altice FL, Gourevitch MN, et al. Pharmacokinetic drug interactions between opioid agonist therapy and antiretroviral medications: implications and management for clinical practice. *J Acquir Immune Def Syndr* 2006;41:563–572.
82. Tong TG, Benowitz NL, Kreek MJ. Methadone-disulfiram interaction during methadone maintenance. *J Clin Pharmacol* 1980;20:506–513.
83. McHugh PF, Kreek MJ. The medical consequences of opiate abuse and addiction and methadone pharmacotherapy. In: Brick J, ed. *Handbook of the medical consequences of alcohol and drug abuse*, 2nd ed. New York: The Haworth Press, 2008:303–339.
84. Cushman P, Kreek M, Gordis E. Ethanol and methadone in man: a possible drug interaction. *Drug Alcohol Depend* 1978;3:35–42.
85. Markowitz JS, Donovan JL, DeVane CL, et al. Effect of St. John's wort on drug metabolism by induction of cytochrome P450 3A4 enzyme. *JAMA* 2003;290:1500–1504.
86. Benmebarek M, Devaud C, Gex-Febry M, et al. Effects of grapefruit juice on the pharmacokinetics of the enantiomers of methadone. *Clin Pharmacol Ther* 2004;76:55–63.
87. Kobayashi K, Yamamoto T, Chiba K, et al. Human buprenorphine N-dealkylation is catalyzed by cytochrome P450 3A4. *Drug Metab Disp* 1998;26:818–821.
88. Lintzeris N, Mitchell TB, Bond AJ, et al. Pharmacodynamics of diazepam co-administered with methadone or buprenorphine under high dose conditions in opioid dependent patients. *Drug Alcohol Depend* 2007;91:187–194.
89. Fudala PJ, Greenstein RA, O'Brien CP. Alternative pharmacotherapies for opioid addiction. In: Lowinson J, Ruiz JP, Millman RB, et al., eds. *Substance abuse: a comprehensive textbook*. Philadelphia: Lippincott Williams & Wilkins, 2008:641–653.
90. Mendelson J, Jones RT. Clinical and pharmacological evaluation of buprenorphine and naloxone combination: why the 4:1 ratio for treatment? *Drug Alcohol Depend* 2003;70:S29–S37.
91. Sporer KA. Buprenorphine: a primer for emergency physicians. *Ann Emerg Med* 2004;43:580–584.
92. Bidlack JM, Knapp BI. Buprenorphine and naltrexone are partial kappa agonists. Poster for the CPDD 70th Annual Scientific Meeting, San Juan, PR 2008.
93. Ciraulo DA, Hitzemann RJ, Somoza E, et al. Pharmacokinetics and pharmacodynamics of multiple sublingual buprenorphine tablets in dose-escalation trials. *J Clin Pharmacol* 2006;46:179–192.
94. Heit HA, Gourlay DL. Buprenorphine in pain and addiction. In: Smith HS, Passik SD, eds. *Pain and chemical dependency*. New York: Oxford University Press, 2008:303–307.
95. Schuh KJ, Johanson C-E. Pharmacokinetic comparison of the buprenorphine sublingual liquid and tablet. *Drug Alcohol Depend* 1999;56: 55–60.
96. Strain EC, Moody DE, Stoller KB, et al. Relative bioavailability of different buprenorphine formulations under chronic dosing conditions. *Drug Alcohol Depend* 2004;74:37–43.
97. Compton P, Ling W, Moody D, et al. Pharmacokinetics, bioavailability and opioid effects of liquid versus tablet buprenorphine. *Drug Alcohol Depend* 2006;82:25–31.
98. Zubieta J-K, Greenwald MK, Lombardi U, et al. Buprenorphine-induced changes in mu-opioid receptor availability in male heroin-dependent volunteers: a preliminary study *Neuropsychopharmacology* 2000;23:326–334.
99. Greenwald MK, Johanson C-E, Moody DE, et al. Effects of buprenorphine maintenance dose on μ-opioid receptor availability, plasma concentrations, and antagonist blockade in heroin-dependent volunteers. *Neuropsychopharmacology* 2003;28:2000–2009.
100. Kreek MJ. Medical complications in methadone patients. *Ann N Y Acad Sci* 1978;311:110–134.
101. Kreek MJ, LaForge KS, Butelman, E. Pharmacotherapy of addictions. *Nat Rev Drug Disc* 2002;1:710–726.
102. Kreek MJ. Molecular and cellular neurobiology and pathophysiology of opiate addiction. In: Davis KL, ed. *Neuropsychopharmacology: the fifth generation of progress*. Philadelphia: Lippincott Williams & Wilkins, 2002:1491–1506.
103. Cushman P, Kreek MJ. Methadone-maintained patients. Effects of methadone on plasma testosterone, FSH, LH and prolactin. *N Y State J Med* 1974;74:1970–1973.
104. Kreek MJ, Borg L, Zhou Y, et al. Relationships between endocrine functions and substance abuse syndromes: heroin and related short-acting opiates in addiction contrasted with methadone and other long-acting opioid agonists used in pharmacotherapy of addiction. In: Pfaff D, ed. *Hormones, brain and behavior*. San Diego: Academic Press, 2002: 781–830.
105. Bowdle TA. Adverse effects of opioid agonists and agonist-antagonists in anaesthesia. *Drug Safety* 1998;19:173–189.
106. Davis AM, Inturrisi CE. D-methadone blocks morphine tolerance and *N*-methyl-*D*-aspartate-induced hyperalgesia. *J Pharmacol Exp Ther* 1999;289:1048–1053.
107. Kreek MJ, Schluger J, Borg L, et al. Dynorphin A1-13 causes elevation of serum levels of prolactin through an opioid receptor mechanism in humans: gender differences and implications for modulations of dopaminergic tone in the treatment of addictions. *J Pharmacol Exp Ther* 1999;288:260–269.
108. Bart G, Borg L, Schluger JH, et al. Suppressed prolactin response to dynorphin A(1-13) in methadone maintained versus control subjects. *J Pharmacol Exp Ther* 2003;306:581–587.
109. Schluger JH, Borg L, Ho A, et al. Altered HPA axis responsivity to metyrapone testing in methadone maintained former heroin addicts with ongoing cocaine addiction. *Neuropsychopharmacology* 2001;24: 568–575.
110. Kreek MJ, Koob GF. Drug dependence: stress and dysregulation of brain reward pathways. *Drug Alcohol Depend* 1998;51:23–47.
111. Novick DM, Ochshorn M, Ghali V, et al. Natural killer cell activity and lymphocyte subsets in parenteral heroin abusers and long-term methadone maintenance patients. *J Pharmacol Exp Ther* 1989;250: 606–610.
112. Bailey CP, Connor M. Opioids: cellular mechanisms of tolerance and physical dependence. *Curr Opin Pharmacol* 2005;5:60–68.
113. White JM, Irvine RJ. Mechanisms of fatal opioid overdose. *Addiction* 1999;94:961–972.
114. Kleinschmidt KC, Wainscott M, Ford MD. Opioids. In: Ford MD, Delaney KA, Ling LJ, Erickson T, eds. *Ford: clinical toxicology*, 1st ed. Philadelphia: WB Saunders, 2001:627–639.
115. Krantz M, Lewkowiez L, Hays H, et al. Torsade de pointes associated with very-high-dose methadone. *Ann Intern Med* 2002;137:501–504.
116. Gil M, Sala M, Anguera I, et al. QT prolongation and Torsades de Pointes in patients with human immunodeficiency virus and treated with methadone. *Am J Cardiol* 2003;92:995–997.
117. Kornick C, Kilborn M, Santiago-Palma J, et al. QT_c interval prolongation associated with intravenous methadone. *Pain* 2003;105:499–506.
118. Martell B, Arnsten J, Ray B, et al. The impact of methadone induction on cardiac conduction in opiate users. *Ann Intern Med* 2003;139: 154–155.
119. Martell B, Arnsten J, Krantz M, Gourevitch MN. Impact of methadone treatment on cardiac repolarization and conduction in opioid users. *Am J Cardiol* 2005;95:915–918.
120. Krantz M, Lowery C, Martell B, et al. Effects of methadone on QT-interval dispersion. *Pharmacotherapy* 2005;25:1523–1529.

121. Peles E, Bodner G, Kreek MJ, et al. Corrected-QT intervals as related to methadone dose and serum level in methadone maintenance treatment (MMT) patients—a cross-sectional study. *Addiction* 2007;102: 289–300.
122. Bond C, La Forge KS, Tian M, et al. Single-nucleotide polymorphism in the human mu opioid receptor gene alters beta-endorphin binding and activity: possible implications for opiate addiction. *Proc Natl Acad Sci U S A* 1998;95:9608–9613.
123. Bart G, Heilig M, LaForge KS, et al. Substantial attributable risk related to a functional mu-opioid receptor gene polymorphism in association with heroin addiction in central Sweden. *Mol Psychiatry* 2004;9: 547–549.
124. Bart G, Kreek MJ, Ott J, et al. Increased attributable risk related to a functional mu-opioid receptor gene polymorphism in association with alcohol dependence in central Sweden. *Neuropsychopharmacology* 2005;30:417–422.
125. Kakko J, von Wachenfeldt J, Svanborg KD, et al. Mood and neuroendocrine response to a chemical stressor, metyrapone, in buprenorphine-maintained heroin dependence. *Biol Psychiatry* 2008;63:172–177.
126. Salsitz EA, Joseph H, Frank B, et al. Methadone medical maintenance (MMM): Treating chronic opioid dependence in private medical practice—a summary report (1983–1998). *Mount Sinai J Med* 2000;67: 388–397.
127. Novick DM, Joseph H, Salsitz EA, et al. Outcomes of treatment of socially rehabilitated methadone maintenance patients in physicians offices (medical maintenance). *J Gen Intern Med* 1994;33:127–130.
128. Schwartz RP, Brooner RK, Montoya ID, et al. A 12-year follow-up of a methadone medical maintenance program. *Am J Addict* 1999;8:293–299.
129. Fiellin DA, O'Connor PG, Chawarski M, et al. Methadone maintenance in primary care: a randomized controlled trial. *JAMA* 2001;286: 1724–1731.
130. Barry DT, Moore BA, Pantalon MV, et al. Patient satisfaction with primary care in office-based buprenorphine/naloxone treatment. *J Gen Intern Med* 2007;22:242–245.
131. Sullivan LE, Chawarski M, O'Connor PG, et al. The practice of office-based buprenorphine treatment of opioid dependence: is it associated with new patients entering into treatment? *Drug Alcohol Depend* 2005;79:113–116.
132. Schottenfeld RS. Opioid maintenance treatment. In: Galanter M, Kleber HD, eds. *The American Psychiatric Textbook of Substance Abuse Treatment.* Fourth Edition. Washington, DC: American Psychiatric Publishing, Inc., 2008:289–308.

CHAPTER 10

David A. Gorelick, MD, PhD

The Pharmacology of Cocaine, Amphetamines, and Other Stimulants

DEFINITION

Stimulants are a class of drugs that stimulate activity in the central and sympathetic peripheral nervous systems, chiefly by enhancing neurotransmitter activity at catecholaminergic synapses.

SUBSTANCES IN THE CLASS

Stimulants include both naturally occurring plant alkaloids, such as cocaine (Fig. 10.1) and ephedra, and more than a dozen synthetic compounds, such as the amphetamines and methylphenidate. Most of these are variants of the basic phenethylamine chemical structure, which is shared by the endogenous catecholamine neurotransmitters norepinephrine and dopamine (Fig. 10.2).

All stimulants share the same range of psychological and physiologic effects, while differing in potency and pharmacokinetic characteristics. Caffeine, the most widely used stimulant, is considered separately in Chapter 11, "Caffeine: Pharmacology and Clinical Effects." 3,4-Methylenedioxymethamphetamine (MDMA, "Ecstasy"), a structural analogue of methamphetamine with both stimulant and hallucinogenic characteristics, is considered separately in Chapter 14, "Hallucinogens and Mixed-Class Compounds."

HISTORY

Naturally occurring plant alkaloids have been used for their central nervous system (CNS) stimulant properties for thousands of years (1). Chinese medicine has used the herbal preparation ma-huang (ephedra) for at least 5,000 years. Chewing of coca leaves has been prevalent in the Andean regions of South America for at least 2,000 years (2). Coca leaves and pottery images of figures with bulging cheeks (presumably wads of coca leaf) have been found in 1,400-year-old Peruvian burial sites. The Spanish conquerors of South America found coca leaf chewing common in the Andean regions and noted its association with increased energy and decreased need for food and sleep. They did not discourage the practice, which continues to this day and is legal in Bolivia and Peru (3).

Coca received little attention in Europe until the second half of the 19th century. In 1860, a German graduate student, Albert Niemann, isolated cocaine as the active ingredient of coca leaf. This discovery helped generate the popularity of cocaine-containing products throughout Europe and North America. Cocaine-containing wines, such as Vin Mariani (containing 6 to 8 mg of cocaine per ounce), were widely advertised and endorsed by prominent political and cultural figures. A nonalcoholic beverage (containing 4.5 mg of cocaine per 6 ounces) was introduced in 1886 and quickly became one of the world's most popular soft drinks: Coca-Cola. A fluid extract of coca for medical use (containing 0.5 mg of cocaine per mL) appeared in the *U.S. Pharmacopeia* in 1882. The first specific use of cocaine in medicine came in 1884, when the German ophthalmologist Koller discovered its efficacy as a local anesthetic during surgery. In the same year, Sigmund Freud published his monograph, *Uber Coca*, describing the

FIGURE 10.1. Chemical structures of cocaine, mazindol, and methylphenidate.

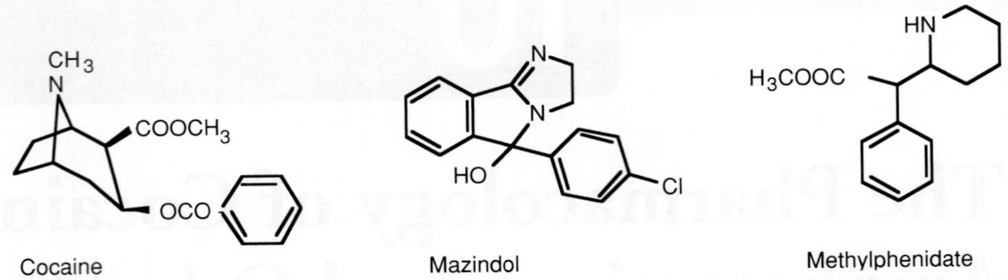

Cocaine Mazindol Methylphenidate

first systematic study of cocaine's psychological effects (albeit with a sample of one, himself) and suggesting its use as a treatment for morphine addiction.

With widespread use of cocaine came increasing reports of adverse effects. The first report of cocaine-associated cardiac arrest and stroke was published in 1886. By 1903, cocaine had been removed from Coca-Cola. In 1914, the Harrison Narcotic Act banned cocaine from over-the-counter (OTC) medications, beverages, and foods in the United States, restricting its use to prescription drugs. For the next 50 years, cocaine remained largely out of public view and medical attention, except for limited use as a local anesthetic.

Synthetic stimulants first appeared with the synthesis of amphetamine in 1887 (by Edeleau) and of methamphetamine in 1919. These attracted little attention until amphetamine became popular as an OTC bronchodilator (in the Benzedrine inhaler) in the early 1930s. By 1933, its CNS stimulant properties were recognized, leading to its use for weight

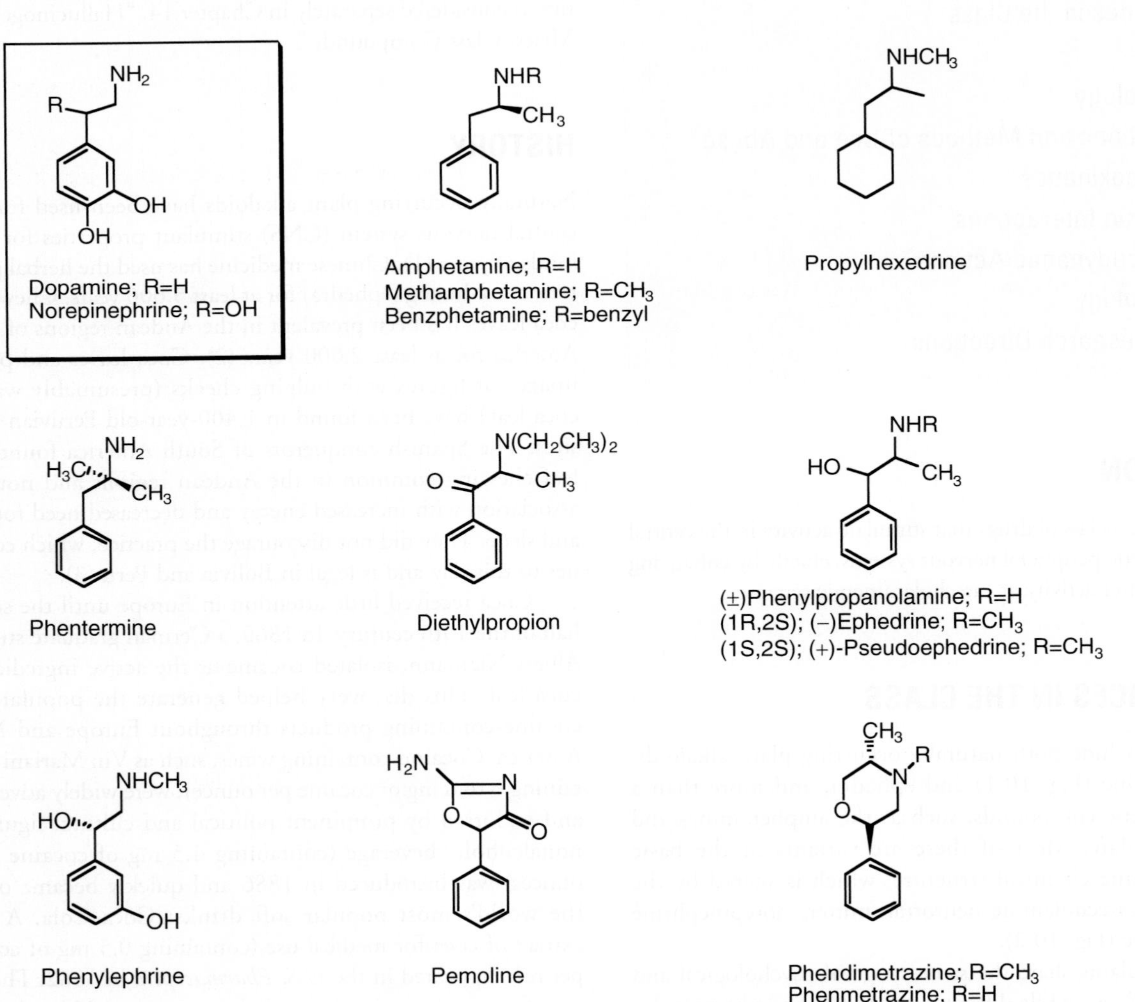

FIGURE 10.2. Chemical structures of endogenous catecholamine neurotransmitters (dopamine, norepinephrine) and phenethylamine stimulant drugs.

loss, narcolepsy, depression, and childhood hyperactivity. Amphetamine's advantages also were recognized by stimulant abusers. It largely replaced cocaine in illicit use because of its low cost, ready availability, and longer duration of action. This growing abuse pattern led to a switch in 1937 from OTC to prescription-only status. During World War II, amphetamine was widely used by the Allied and Axis countries to enhance the performance of troops and factory workers. After the war, widespread abuse in Japan and Sweden of large leftover stockpiles led to tight restrictions on amphetamine manufacture and dispensing. In response to increasing rates of intravenous abuse of amphetamine extracted from Benzedrine inhalers, the U.S. Food and Drug Administration (FDA) banned the inhalers in 1959. With passage of the Controlled Substances Act in 1970, cocaine, amphetamine, and methamphetamine were placed in Schedule II because they have high potential for abuse and accepted medical use only with severe restrictions. As recognition of their abuse potential grew, the number of prescription stimulants available in the United States declined from 65 (marketed by 40 different companies) in 1970 to eight (marketed by six companies) in 1995 (4).

EPIDEMIOLOGY

There are substantial geographic and sociodemographic differences in the epidemiology of stimulant use (5,6). In 2005, there were an estimated 14.3 million cocaine users worldwide, representing 0.3% of the 15- to 64-year-old population. Almost half (44%) were in North America (6.4 million; 2.2% prevalence), where use has remained stable over the past decade. Use has been increasing in Western and Central Europe (3.9 million; 1.2%), especially in Spain, United Kingdom, and Italy. Central and South America (including the Caribbean) had 2.2 million users (0.8%) and Oceania 0.2 million users (0.8%). There is very little cocaine use in Eastern Europe (0.1 million; 0.05%), Africa (although use in West Africa is increasing: 1 million; 0.2%), and Asia (0.3 million; 0.01%). In 2005, there were an estimated 24.8 million (0.6% prevalence) nonmedical users of other stimulants (primarily amphetamine and methamphetamine). Such misuse is most prevalent in Oceania (0.6 million; 2.9%), North America (3.8 million; 1.3%), Central and South America (1.9 million; 0.7%), Western and Central Europe (2.2 million; 0.7%), and Asia (13.7 million; 0.5%), especially East and Southeast Asia. There is relatively less use in Africa (2.1 million; 0.4%) and Eastern Europe (0.5 million; 0.2%). These patterns of stimulant use probably reflect availability and access, because the only source of cocaine is the Andean region of South America, whereas amphetamines can be readily synthesized anywhere.

Oral use of cocaine has a long cultural tradition and is legal in Bolivia and Peru. Surveys have found lifetime prevalence of coca leaf use up to 90% in Bolivia and 30% in Peru (3). Purified cocaine, suitable for intravenous, smoked, or intranasal administration, is illegal in all Andean countries. The lifetime prevalence of such cocaine use is similar to that reported in North America.

A detailed view of stimulant epidemiology in the United States comes from two annual national surveys conducted by the Substance Abuse and Mental Health Services Administration (SAMHSA). The National Survey on Drug Use and Health (NSDUH) surveys a representative sample of household residents 12 years and older that is sufficiently large (67,802 in 2006) to generate valid population estimates of drug use. NSDUH data may tend to underestimate overall drug use because the survey sample does not include some groups in which drug use is likely to be higher, such as persons in correctional settings, homeless persons, hospital patients, and residential college students. The NSDUH includes nonmedical use of prescription drugs but does not measure use of OTC medications or drugs considered dietary supplements, such as ephedra or caffeine (see Chapter 2, "The Epidemiology of Substance Use Disorders"). Information on adverse consequences of stimulant use comes from the Drug Abuse Warning Network (DAWN). DAWN is a nationwide survey of 355 general, nonfederal, short-stay hospitals with 24-hour emergency departments, selected to be representative of all U.S. hospitals. Data are collected on patient visits associated with the use of illegal drugs or nonmedical use of prescription and OTC medications. DAWN also surveys medical examiners/coroners in 35 metropolitan areas and six states for data on deaths (other than those due to homicide or acquired immunodeficiency syndrome) associated with medications or illegal drugs.

According to NSDUH data, cocaine is the second most widely used illegal drug in the United States, after marijuana. Cocaine use in the United States peaked during the mid-1980s. The 2006 NSDUH estimated that 35.3 million Americans (14.3% of the U.S. population 12 years old or older) had used cocaine at some time during their lifetimes (8.6 million [3.5%] by smoking "crack" cocaine); 6.1 million (2.5%) had used cocaine (1.5 million [0.6%] by smoking) within the preceding year; and 2.4 million (1.0%) had used cocaine (0.7 million [0.3%] by smoking) within the preceding month, considered current use (7). There were about 1 million new cocaine users in 2006 (0.25 million by smoking), with a mean age of 20.3 years. An estimated 1.7 million Americans met psychiatric diagnostic criteria (*DSM-IV*) (8) for cocaine abuse or dependence; about 928,000 people received specialty treatment for their cocaine use.

Cocaine use occurs in all segments of American society but is substantially more prevalent in certain population groups. Data from the 2001–2003 National Comorbidity Survey Replication (a representative, community-based sample of 5,692 adults) suggest that the most likely cocaine user is an unemployed, divorced/separated, non-Hispanic white male high school dropout or graduate in his 20s, living in a nonrural area in the Northeast or West, for whom religion is not important (9). These associations between cocaine use and age, gender, education level, and employment and marital status are generally found throughout the world (10).

Cocaine use is highly associated with legal substance use and with psychiatric syndromes. Cigarette smokers or heavy alcohol drinkers are each at least 10 times more likely to use cocaine than are nonsmokers or moderate (nonbinge) drinkers. Current cocaine users are twice as likely to have symptoms of depressive or anxiety disorders than are nonusers (11).

The 2006 NSDUH estimated that 20.1 million Americans (8.2% of the U.S. population aged 12 years or older) were nonmedical users of stimulants other than cocaine at some time during their lifetimes; 3.4 million (1.4%) had used such stimulants within the preceding year; and 1.2 million (0.5%) were current users. There were 845,000 new stimulant users in 2006, with a mean age of 23 years. An estimated 390,000 (0.2%) Americans met psychiatric diagnostic criteria (*DSM-IV*) for noncocaine stimulant abuse or dependence in 2006.

The most commonly misused stimulant is methamphetamine. The 2006 NSDUH estimated that 731,000 Americans (0.3% of population) were current users (7). Methamphetamine use is confined largely to the western two-thirds of the United States, with less use reported on the East Coast, even in cities with high rates of cocaine use (12).

Stimulant use often is associated with adverse consequences. In the 2005 DAWN survey, cocaine was the drug associated most often with visits to hospital emergency departments, with 448,481 visits (30.9% of all drug-related visits)—almost twice as often as the next most common drug, marijuana (16.7%) (13). Methamphetamine was associated with 108,905 visits (7.5%), amphetamines with 35,827 (2.5%), and methylphenidate with 3,212 (0.2%). Cocaine was the drug most often associated with deaths investigated by medical examiners in 2003, being reported in 39% of all drug misuse deaths (14). In about three-fourths of these cases, at least one other drug was also reported. Amphetamines or methamphetamine were among the 10 most commonly reported drugs in 16 of the 32 metropolitan areas. All but one of these was west of the Mississippi River, consistent with patterns of methamphetamine use and abuse.

Only a minority of stimulant users appear to seek drug abuse treatment. About one-quarter million persons who reported cocaine as their primary drug of abuse were admitted to publicly funded substance abuse treatment programs in 2005, of more than 1.8 million admissions overall (15). Almost three-fourths of patients smoked cocaine (as compared to about one-third cocaine smokers among the general population of cocaine users). Another 150,000 patients were admitted for primary methamphetamine use, 17,000 for use of other amphetamines and 981 for other stimulant use.

FORMULATIONS AND METHODS OF USE AND ABUSE

Plant-Derived Stimulants Several naturally occurring, plant-derived stimulants are widely available for traditional oral use in many areas of the world. These include cocaine (in South America), ephedra (in North America and East Asia), and khat (in East Africa and Arabia). Caffeine, the most widely used stimulant, is addressed in Chapter 11, "Caffeine: Pharmacology and Clinical Effects". Such use often is culturally sanctioned and may not be associated with abuse or dependence. Use of more potent formulations (e.g., the extracted active chemical) or more rapidly acting routes of administration has significant abuse potential and is illegal even where oral formulations are allowed.

Cocaine Cocaine is an alkaloid with a tropane ester chemical structure (Fig. 10.1) similar to that of scopolamine and other plant alkaloids. It occurs in leaves of the coca bush, *Erythroxylon coca*, which grows at altitudes of 1,500 to 6,000 feet in the Andean region of South America (chiefly Colombia, Peru, and Bolivia). The leaf contains cocaine (0.2% to 1%) and more than a dozen other tropane alkaloids (such as benzoylecgonine, methylecgonine, ecgonine, and cinnamoylcocaine), most of which are of unknown pharmacologic activity. Another *Erythroxylon* species, *E. novogranatense*, contains lesser amounts of cocaine and greater levels of other alkaloids (16). Cocaine exists as two stereoisomers: naturally occurring (−)-cocaine and (+)-cocaine, which has less affinity for the dopamine transporter and is relatively inactive in vivo because of its very rapid metabolism by butyrylcholinesterase (17).

About 157,000 hectares of coca were cultivated in Bolivia, Colombia, and Peru in 2006. This resulted in net production of about 984 metric tons of cocaine (6), most destined for export. Domestic use of oral cocaine is legal in these countries, usually as coca tea or by chewing the leaves. Coca leaves typically are chewed in conjunction with lime or plant ash, which alkalinizes the saliva and thus enhances absorption of the cocaine. Cocaine is legally available in the United States only as a 4% or 10% injectable solution (or powder for reconstitution) or viscous liquid for use as a local or topical anesthetic. Legal cocaine preparations rarely are diverted for misuse.

Illicit cocaine is smuggled into the United States specifically for abuse purposes from its countries of origin. An estimated 530 to 710 metric tons of cocaine entered the United States in 2006 (18). Based on samples seized by law enforcement agencies, the average wholesale (dealer) and retail (user) prices for cocaine in 2005 were $21 and $107 per gram, respectively, in the United States and $46 and $85 in Europe (6). In June, 2007, average U.S. wholesale and retail prices were $23 and $119, respectively, with a 10-fold range among various cities (19). U.S. federal law enforcement agencies seized 96,713 kg of cocaine in 2007.

Preparation of illicit cocaine begins with crushing the coca leaves and heating them in an organic solvent (often kerosene) to extract and partially purify the cocaine (20). After several more extraction and filtering steps, the coca paste (now 80% to 90% pure) is heated in an organic solvent (often ether or acetone) with concentrated acid to convert it to salt form. The salt is readily converted back to the base by heating it in an organic solvent at basic pH. This process is known as "freebasing," and was practiced by cocaine users during the 1980s, before cocaine base (or "freebase") was widely available on the retail street market. "Crack" as a street name for base cocaine reportedly derives from the crackling sound made during this process.

Cocaine is available for street use in two forms: base and salt (1,21). These have different physical properties, which favor different routes of administration. The base has a relatively low melting point (98°C) and vaporizes before substantial pyrolytic destruction has occurred. This allows cocaine base to be smoked, though the majority of the cocaine may be in the form of small particles (<5 microns) that reach the alveoli, rather than true cocaine vapor (22). Cocaine base is relatively insoluble in water (alcohol:water solubility ratio of 100:1), making it difficult to dissolve for injection purposes. In contrast, cocaine salt does not melt at <195°C, so heating it for smoking results in destruction of most of the cocaine. However, cocaine salt is highly water soluble (alcohol:water solubility ratio of 1:8), making it easy to dissolve for injection purposes and facilitating absorption across mucus membranes. Regardless of the chemical form or route of administration, the cocaine molecule exerts the same actions once it reaches the brain or other target organ (21).

The average purity of seized cocaine samples in the United States was 50% to 60% in 2007 (19). Diluents are added (that is, the cocaine is "cut") to enhance dealer profits. Diluents include both inert fillers that look like cocaine (such as dextrose, lactose, mannitol, or starch) and active chemicals that either mimic the local anesthetic effect of cocaine (such as benzocaine, lidocaine, or procaine) or provide some psychoactive effect (such as ephedrine, amphetamine, caffeine, or PCP) (20,23). Street cocaine also may contain contaminants from the preparation process (such as benzene, acetone, or sodium bicarbonate) (23).

Ephedra Ephedrine and pseudoephedrine are naturally occurring alkaloids with a phenethylamine chemical structure (Fig. 10.2) that are found in several *Ephedraceae* species (especially *Ephedra sinica, E. equisetina*, and *E. gerardiana*) (1,24). Ephedra is a preparation of dried young branches of *Ephedra* species, typically containing 1% to 3% ephedrine. This may be converted into a capsule, tincture, liquid extract, or tea. Ephedra products are widely used in East Asia and North America; they appear in the pharmacopoeias of China, Japan, and Germany.

Ephedra products often are advertised as legal versions of or alternatives to the more strictly regulated manufactured stimulants. They may appeal to consumers as safer than synthetic stimulants because they are "natural" or "herbal." Synthetic ephedrine and pseudoephedrine also are available as tablets or capsules (see subsequent text). Ephedra alkaloids have the same range of psychological and physiologic effects as do cocaine and amphetamines. There is limited evidence of their efficacy for weight loss in obese individuals (25). Ephedra use has been associated with severe cardiovascular and CNS effects, including death (26), leading to its banning from the U.S. market in 2006.

Khat *Khat* is the common term for preparations of the *Catha edulis* plant, which is native to East Africa (Sudan to Madagascar) and the southern Arabian peninsula (Yemen) (24,27,28). Fresh khat leaves contain at least two stimulant alkaloids with phenethylamine chemical structures: cathinone (present at 1% to 3%) and cathine (norpseudoephedrine).

Pure cathinone is a Schedule I controlled substance; cathine is in Schedule IV. The potent (Schedule I) cathinone congener methcathinone ("CAT"), known as ephedrone in Europe, is clandestinely synthesized from ephedrine or pseudoephedrine (20). Both cathinone and methcathinone inhibit the presynaptic neuronal dopamine and serotonin transporters with a potency similar to that of amphetamines (see further: Neurotransmitters) (29).

Khat use has been a widely accepted social custom for centuries, apparently predating the use of coffee (caffeine). The leaves are used in the same way as coca leaves in South America, that is, chewed and kept in the cheek for several hours. Less often, the leaves are brewed into tea or crushed with honey to make a paste. Moderate use reduces fatigue and appetite. Compulsive use may result in manic behavior or psychotic symptoms such as paranoia or hallucinations. The extent of abuse or dependence is unclear. Khat loses much of its potency within 2 days of harvesting, as cathinone is converted to the much less potent cathine. Some khat use is found among immigrant communities in Europe, but there appears to be negligible use of khat in the United States. Methcathinone is widely abused in Russia and the Baltic area.

Synthetic Stimulants More than a dozen synthetic stimulant medications are legally available in the United States, either by prescription (Table 10.1) or over the counter (Table 10.2). Most represent variations on the basic phenethylamine structure (Fig. 10.2). Common trade and street names, controlled substance scheduling, clinical uses (FDA-approved and otherwise), and typical doses are listed in Tables 10.1 and 10.2. All legal stimulants, other than cocaine, are sold for oral use in tablet, capsule, or liquid form.

Several stimulants are available in extended or sustained-release formulations (30,31). Methylphenidate is also available as a transdermal patch, which releases drug at a rate of 1.1–3.3 mg/hour, depending on patch size (32). Amphetamine is available as a prodrug, lisdexamfetamine, consisting of d-amphetamine coupled to the amino acid L-lysine (33,34). The active drug is formed as the inactive lysine is hydrolyzed off in the intestines and liver. All these formulations have two theoretical advantages over conventional immediate release formulations: improved patient compliance and effectiveness because of longer duration of action and reduced abuse liability because of slower onset of action and weaker peak subjective effects (35).

Some OTC stimulants also are available in aerosolized formulations for nasal inhalation (insufflation) for use as decongestants. Phenylephrine is available as a sterile solution for parenteral administration to treat hypotension.

Synthetic stimulants typically are abused by the oral or intravenous route. Amphetamines, especially highly pure crystallized methamphetamine ("ice"), may be used intranasally or smoked, as is cocaine. Some abused synthetic stimulants, such as methylphenidate, are diverted from legitimate sources and thus

TABLE 10.1 Stimulants Available by Prescription in the United States

Drug	Trade name	Street name	CSA schedule	Typical indications	Oral dose (mg/day)
Amphetamine (as d-isomer or racemic mixture)	Adderall, Dexedrine, Dextrostat, generic	Amp, bennies, dex, black beauties	II	ADHD, Narcolepsy, weight control, depression[a]	2.5–60
Lisdexamfetamine (L-lysine-d-amphetamine	Vyvanse		II	ADHD	30–70
Benzphetamine	Didrex	—	III	Weight control	25–150
Cocaine		Coke, crack, flake, snow	II	Local or topical anesthetic	—
Diethylpropion	Tenuate	—	IV	Weight control	75–100
Mazindol	Sanorex, Mazanor	—	IV	Weight control	1–3
Methamphetamine	Adipex, Desoxyn, Methedrine	Ice, meth, speed, crank, crystal	II	ADHD, Weight control	5–40 10–15
Methylphenidate (as d-isomer or racemic mixture)	Ritalin, Focalin, Concerta	Rits, Vitamin R	II	ADHD, narcolepsy	10–60 10–60
Phendimetrazine	Bontril, Plegine		III	Weight control	35–105
Phenmetrazine	Preludin		II	Weight control	25–75
Phentermine	Adipex-P, Fastin, Ionamin	—	IV	Weight control	15–90

ADHD, attention deficit/hyperactivity disorder; CSA, U.S. Controlled Substances Act.

[a]Not labeled for this indication by the U.S. Food and Drug Administration.

are of known content and purity. If oral administration is not intended, the original tablet or capsule may be crushed or opened to allow the drug to be taken intranasally or mixed with water for injection. In contrast, amphetamines, especially methamphetamine, usually are synthesized in clandestine laboratories directly for illicit use. This can be done with standard chemical reactions applied to legally available precursors. For example, methamphetamine (desoxyephedrine) can be made by reducing ephedrine or pseudoephedrine. For this reason, retail purchases in the United States of products containing ephedrine or pseudoephedrine are limited to 3.6 g/day and 9 g/month and require photographic identification. U.S. federal law enforcement agencies seized 1,086 kg of methamphetamine in 2007, the vast bulk in the western two-thirds of the United States (19).

Stimulants with a phenylisopropylamine structure (such as amphetamine, methamphetamine, ephedrine, pseudoephedrine, and phenylpropanolamine) have a chiral (stereoisomeric) center at the alpha-carbon atom (Fig. 10.2), and so exist in two (or more) stereoisomer forms that differ in pharmacodynamic and pharmacokinetic properties (36,37). The *d*- or S-(+) isomer generally has three to five times the CNS activity and about one-third the half-life of the *l*- or R-(−) isomer. The *l*-isomers have more peripheral alpha-adrenergic activity. For example, *d*-methamphetamine is a potent CNS stimulant, whereas *l*-methamphetamine (*l*-desoxyephedrine) has been used as a decongestant (as in the Vicks nasal inhaler) (38). Methylphenidate exists in four stereoisomeric forms, of which the *d*-threo enantiomer is the active one (39).

Clinical Uses Cocaine is used clinically only as a local or topical anesthetic, chiefly for eye, ear, nose, or throat surgery or procedures (40). Other prescription stimulants generally are

TABLE 10.2 Stimulants Available as Over-the-Counter Preparations in the United States

Drug	Trade name	Indications	Typical oral dose (mg/day)
Caffeine	(Various)	Weight control, alertness	50–250
Ephedrine	Marax, Quadrinal	Decongestant, bronchodilation	50–100
Phenylephrine	Comhist, Dristan, Neo-Synephrine	Decongestant	40–60
Pseudoephedrine	Sudafed, Sine-Aid	Decongestant	90–240
Propylhexedrine	Benzedrex, Dristan, Obesin	Decongestant, weight control	50–150

used for one of several FDA-approved indications: attention deficit/hyperactivity disorder (ADHD) in both children (41,42) and adults (43–45), narcolepsy and excessive daytime sleepiness (46,47), and appetite suppression to promote weight loss in exogenous obesity (48,49) (Table 10.1).

OTC stimulants generally are used for decongestion and bronchodilation in the treatment of asthma, upper respiratory infections, allergic rhinitis, sinusitis, or bronchitis, and for appetite suppression to promote weight loss in exogenous obesity (both of which are FDA-approved indications) (Table 10.2). Parenteral phenylephrine also is approved by the FDA as an adjunct to prolong the duration of spinal anesthesia, to terminate paroxysmal supraventricular tachycardia (probably indirectly by stimulation of arterial baroreceptors), and for immediate, short-term treatment of hypotension (especially when due to anesthesia, drugs, or hypersensitivity reactions).

In addition to their FDA-approved indications, oral stimulants have a long history of accepted clinical use for other indications (4,50). Amphetamines and methylphenidate are used as quick acting (2- to 3-day), short-term antidepressants in persons who are elderly, medically ill, HIV-infected, or those with neurologic conditions such as stroke or traumatic brain injury, especially those who cannot tolerate the side effects of standard antidepressants (4,51). Such patients may exhibit apathy, fatigue, and psychomotor retardation, rather than a full-blown classic depressive syndrome. Often, it is unclear whether the beneficial effect of stimulants in such patients is due to the drugs' activating effects or to true antidepressant actions (52). Stimulants also have been used to augment the response to standard antidepressants (53). Amphetamines have been used to improve recovery after stroke, but their efficacy is questionable (54). Amphetamines, methylphenidate, and mazindol have been used to potentiate opiate analgesia and to counteract opiate-induced sedation and respiratory suppression, thus allowing larger doses of opiates to be used (4,50). Cocaine has been used for this purpose as part of Brompton's cocktail (with alcohol and an opiate) in the treatment of cancer pain. Ephedrine and phenylephrine still are used parenterally to counteract hypotension associated with spinal anesthesia (especially in obstetrical and urologic surgery) (1). Most other clinical uses of stimulants for their pressor effect have been superceded by more selective agents.

There is no evidence that medical use of stimulants at therapeutic doses in appropriately diagnosed patients leads to stimulant abuse or increases the risk of serious adverse events, although there are little data from long-term, controlled trials (4,45,55). Prospective, longitudinal studies in children receiving stimulant treatment for ADHD found no increased risk of developing substance abuse (56).

Nonmedical Use, Abuse, and Dependence Oral stimulants (both prescription and OTC) have been widely used in work, school, military, and sports settings, often without medical supervision, for their alerting, antifatigue, sleep-suppressing, and performance-enhancing properties (57,58). Nonmedical use of prescription stimulants in the general U.S. population has increased substantially since the early 1990s (59), whereas use in the U.S. military has declined more than 80%, largely as the result of a comprehensive antidrug policy that includes mandatory urine drug testing. In 2005, 1.9% of U.S. military personnel had used cocaine, and 1.4% had used other stimulants within the preceding 12 months (60)—substantially less than among the general population of similar age and gender. Use by other occupational groups, such as long-distance truck drivers and night-shift workers, remains problematic.

The stimulants' antifatigue and sleep-suppression effects have been well demonstrated in laboratory and field studies. Enhancement of cognitive and psychomotor performance is more difficult to demonstrate in controlled studies and occurs more robustly in persons who already are fatigued or sleep-deprived. Stimulants are used by athletes to improve performance, especially in endurance sports such as cycling, which require anaerobic exercise, although there is little published evidence of their efficacy (61–63). Stimulants of all types (illicit, prescription, and OTC) are banned by the World Anti-Doping Agency and many other sports organizations (64).

All stimulants have a potential for misuse, abuse, and dependence, varying only in their potency. Cocaine, amphetamine, and methamphetamine have high abuse potential, as reflected in their placement in Schedule II. Community-based interview surveys suggest that up to one in six persons who use cocaine and one in nine who use prescription stimulants for other than medical purposes will become dependent (65). Even higher rates are found in treatment-seeking populations: up to four-fifths of those who have used cocaine several times and up to half of those who have used amphetamines become dependent (66). Heavier users and those who use the intravenous and smoked forms are more likely to become dependent than are lighter users or those who use the intranasal and oral forms (66–68). Even lower potency stimulants in Schedule IV, such as pemoline and phentermine, or OTC stimulants, such as ephedrine, pseudoephedrine, and phenylpropanolamine, have been misused and abused (69).

Studies of psychoactive drug use and abuse/dependence by pairs of fraternal (dizygotic) and identical (monozygotic) twins suggest that there is a genetic influence both on initiation and use of stimulants and on stimulant abuse and dependence (70,71). Findings are best explained by a single genetic factor influencing illegal drugs (as distinct from legal drugs such as alcohol, tobacco, and caffeine), which may account for about three-fourths of the variance in cocaine dependence and one-fourth of the variance in amphetamine dependence. There do not appear to be significant gender differences in genetic influence. Efforts to identify a specific gene or genes responsible for stimulant dependence have not been successful. Many candidates have been identified in genome-wide association studies, but none has been robustly replicated (72).

The greater abuse liability of intravenous and smoked (as opposed to oral and intranasal) routes of administration is considered owing to their faster rate of drug delivery to the brain (6 to 8 seconds, in the case of smoking), resulting in a faster onset of psychological effects (73,74). This faster onset is associated with a more intense pleasurable response and greater abuse liability (the so-called "rate hypothesis" of psychoactive drug action) (35).

Stimulants are used in a variety of patterns (75,76). "Binge" use involves short periods of heavy use (e.g., on weekends or after payday), separated by longer periods of little or no use. Others may use frequently for an extended period until their finances are exhausted or their access to drug is interrupted. A small number of users may use low doses daily without dose escalation over time. Some of these users may be self-medicating an underlying neuropsychiatric disorder such as ADHD or narcolepsy. Typical cocaine doses are 12 to 15 g orally (coca leaf chewing), 20 to 100 mg intranasally, 10 to 50 mg intravenously, and 50 to 200 mg smoked.

High rates of stimulant abuse have been documented in persons involved with the criminal justice system. A national survey of 6,982 local jail inmates in 2002 found that 20.7% reported using cocaine in the month before their offense; 10.6% had used cocaine at the time of their offense (77). The figures for use of other stimulants were 11.4% and 5.2%, respectively. These occurrence rates suggest an association between stimulant use and crime, violence, and aggression. There are several potential causal mechanisms for this association, including behaviors associated with the illegal manufacture, distribution, and marketing of drugs; behaviors associated with users obtaining drug (or the money to buy drug); or a direct pharmacologic effect of stimulants on behavior (78–80). The association also may reflect the co-occurrence of stimulant use and antisocial personality disorder (which is associated with high rates of criminal behavior).

Low doses of stimulants do increase aggressive behavior in human laboratory models of aggression (e.g., as evidenced by willingness to administer electric shock) (79). Numerous case reports document violent behavior due to stimulant-induced irritability, paranoia, or frank psychosis (81).

Unintended use of cocaine may occur in persons who swallow the drug in their possession to avoid arrest or prosecution ("body stuffers") or who swallow large quantities to transport it without detection by law enforcement authorities ("body packers," "mules") (82). The drug may be wrapped in plastic bags, balloons, condoms, paper, aluminum foil, or a combination. If the wrapper fails, the carrier may be exposed suddenly to large doses of cocaine in the gastrointestinal tract, resulting in severe acute cocaine intoxication.

Stimulants often are used in combination with other drugs, either concurrently or sequentially. Concurrent use of a stimulant and an opiate, sometimes in the same injecting syringe, is considered by many users to provide a qualitatively better subjective effect ("high") than either drug alone (83,84). Concurrent intravenous use of cocaine plus heroin is termed *speedballing*. Combined use of oral amphetamine plus an oral opiate (such as codeine) also is common. Human experimental studies suggest that the acute psychological effects of cocaine are somewhat enhanced with concurrent administration of cocaine and an opiate (85). Other drugs sometimes used concurrently with smoked cocaine include phencyclidine (PCP), marijuana, or tobacco (86). CNS depressant drugs, such as alcohol, benzodiazepines, opiates, and marijuana, often are used after cocaine use to temper unpleasant effects of cocaine intoxication (such as anxiety, paranoia, restlessness) and/or to relieve symptoms of cocaine withdrawal.

PHARMACOKINETICS

Absorption and Distribution Route of administration has a major effect on the pharmacokinetic characteristics of stimulants (87). Smoked stimulants (such as cocaine base or methamphetamine) are rapidly absorbed through the lungs and probably reach the brain in 6 to 8 seconds. Thus, the onset and peak effect occur within minutes of administration. As the stimulant redistributes from the brain, there is a rapid decline in effect. Intravenous administration produces peak brain uptake in 4 to 7 minutes, based on positron emission tomography (PET) studies with radiolabeled cocaine (88). Greatest cocaine uptake occurs in the striatum (caudate, putamen, and nucleus accumbens) and least uptake in the orbital cortex and cerebellum. Clearance to half-peak brain levels requires 17 to 30 minutes and is fastest in the orbital cortex, thalamus, and cerebellum and slowest in the striatum. The rapid offset after rapid onset often is experienced as a "crash" by users of smoked or intravenous stimulants. Heavy cocaine users have about 20% less brain cocaine uptake than do healthy nonusers (89). The mechanism of this difference is not known but could be related to differences in plasma protein binding or permeability of the blood–brain barrier.

Intranasal and oral stimulants have a slower absorption and onset of effect (30 to 45 minutes), a longer peak effect, and a more gradual decline from peak. The peak intensity of effect is weaker than with smoked or intravenous administration because less active drug reaches its site of action in the brain. Coca leaf chewing produces less than half the peak cocaine plasma concentrations of an equivalent dose of intranasal cocaine (90). However, even a single oral dose of cocaine (such as 2 mg in a cup of coca tea) may yield detectable urine concentrations of cocaine metabolites (91,92). Pharmacokinetic parameters for oral stimulants are given in Table 10.3.

Cocaine is well absorbed through mucus membranes and also is absorbed through intact skin or by passive inhalation of smoked cocaine or aerosolized particles (92–94). Passive exposure can result in adverse medical effects in infants (95,96) and detectable urine concentrations of cocaine metabolites in medical and laboratory personnel (94,97). In many cases, these concentrations are too low to trigger a positive result on routine urine drug testing.

Stimulants distribute into most tissues of the body. Cocaine is rapidly taken up into the heart, kidney, adrenal glands, and liver (17). In addition to blood and urine (98), cocaine and its hydrolytic metabolites, amphetamines, phentermine, and ephedrine and its analogues appear in hair (99–101), sweat (102), oral fluid (saliva) (103–105), nails (106), and breast milk (107), and cross the placenta to appear

TABLE 10.3 Pharmacokinetic Parameters of Oral Stimulants

Drug	T_{max} (h)	$T_{1/2}$ (h)	V_d (L/kg)	pK_a	F_b
Amphetamine	2–4	7–34[a]	3.2–5.6	9.9	0.16
Benzphetamine	—	—	—	6.6	—
Chlorphentermine	4	35–44	3.0	9.6	
Cocaine	1	0.75–1.5	1.6–2.7	8.6	0.92
Diethylpropion	—	2.5	—	—	—
Ephedrine	1	4–10	2.6–3.1	9.6	—
Mazindol	1	12–36	—	8.6	—
Methamphetamine	1–3	6–15[a]	3–7	9.9	0.1–0.2
Methylphenidate	1–3	1.4–4.2	11–33	8.8	0.15
Phendimetrazine	1	—	—	7.6	
Phenmetrazine	2	8	—	8.5	—
Phentermine	4	19–24	3–4	10.1	—
Phenylephrine	1	2–3	5	8.8	—
Propylhexedrine	—	—	—	10.4	—
Pseudoephedrine	2–3	3–16[a]	2–3	9.4	0.2

T_{max}, time of maximum plasma concentration (in hours); $T_{1/2}$, half-life (in hours); V_d, apparent volume of distribution (in liters per kg of body weight); pK_a, acid dissociation constant (= pH at which drug is 50% ionized); F_b, = fraction of bound drug.
[a]Urine pH-dependent: lower pH yields shorter half-life.
Source: Baselt, 2004 (36).

in umbilical cord blood, amniotic fluid, and meconium (106). Analysis of these tissues and fluids is used for drug detection in workplace, legal, and treatment settings (108). Stimulants can also be detected postmortem in body fluids and tissues (109).

Metabolism In humans (and other primates), 95% of cocaine is metabolized by hydrolysis of ester bonds to benzoylecgonine (the primary urinary metabolite) and ecgonine methylester by the action of carboxylesterases in the liver and butyrylcholinesterase in the liver, plasma, brain, lung, and other tissues (90,110–112). The remaining 5% of cocaine is N-demethylated to norcocaine by the CYP3A4 isozyme of the liver cytochrome P450 microsomal enzyme system. This is the predominant metabolic pathway in rodents.

Nococaine has some pharmacologic actions similar to those of cocaine and is hepatotoxic. This may account for the significant hepatotoxicity of cocaine in rodents, which is not found in primates. Cocaine's hydrolytic metabolites appear to be much less active pharmacologically, though this has not been well studied (113,114).

Amphetamines are metabolized in the liver via three different pathways: deamination to inactive metabolites, oxidation to norephedrine and other active metabolites, and parahydroxylation to active metabolites (115). Amphetamine itself is the initial metabolite of methamphetamine.

When cocaine is smoked, a pyrolysis product is formed (methylecgonidine or anhydroecgonine methylester), the presence of which allows identification of the smoked route of administration (87,90,112).

Elimination Stimulants and their metabolites are largely eliminated in the urine (36,90). Benzoylecgonine is the cocaine metabolite found in highest concentration in urine for several days after cocaine use. It is this substance, rather than the parent drug cocaine, that actually is measured in routine urine drug tests for cocaine. GI absorption and urinary elimination of amphetamines is highly pH-dependent (50). Because amphetamines are weak bases (pK_a around 9.9) (115), acidification of the GI tract or urine substantially decreases absorption and increases excretion, respectively (90). Conversely, alkalinization of the GI tract or urine can increase GI absorption and reduce excretion to negligible levels. This fact is exploited by drug users who take large doses of sodium bicarbonate to prolong the action of amphetamines and reduce the amount present in the urine for detection by drug tests (116).

DRUG–DRUG INTERACTIONS

The primary drug interaction of stimulants that is of clinical concern is with other stimulants or with other medications that also enhance catecholamine activity (4). Such interactions risk overstimulation of the sympathetic nervous system, with possible cardiac arrhythmia, hypertension, seizure, cardiovascular collapse, and death. The major potential for interaction is presented by monoamine oxidase inhibitors (MAOIs), which are used as antidepressants. MAOIs enhance catecholamine activity by inhibiting a major metabolic pathway for catecholamines. Potent prescription stimulants, such as amphetamine and methamphetamine, should not be used within 2 weeks of MAOI use. Stimulants should be used cautiously in conjunction with tricyclic antidepressants, many of which block presynaptic reuptake of catecholamines.

When cocaine is used in combination with alcohol, a new compound, cocaethylene, is formed by transesterification (117). Cocaethylene has pharmacologic actions similar to, but less potent than, those of cocaine, with a longer half-life. Formation of cocaethylene may contribute to more severe or longer-lasting toxic effects of cocaine when it is used along with alcohol. However, human laboratory studies of the cocaine/alcohol/cocaethylene interaction have given inconsistent results (118,119).

PHARMACODYNAMIC ACTIONS

Central Nervous System

Intoxication All stimulants produce a similar range of psychological, behavioral, and physiologic effects, with the intensity and duration depending on potency, dose, route of administration, and duration of use (see Section 6, Chapter 45, "Management of Stimulant, Hallucinogen, Marijuana, Phencyclidine, and Club Drug Intoxication and Withdrawal"). The initial effects—usually desired—include increased energy, alertness, and sociability; elation or euphoria; and decreased fatigue, need for sleep, and appetite (120). The intense pleasurable feeling has been described as a "total body orgasm" (121). These effects may occur after 5 to 20 mg of oral amphetamine, methamphetamine, or methylphenidate; 100 to 200 mg of oral cocaine; 40 to 100 mg of intranasal cocaine; or 15 to 25 mg of IV or smoked cocaine (121–123). Such single oral doses of stimulants improve cognitive and psychomotor performance in subjects whose performance has been impaired by fatigue, sleep deprivation, or alcohol, especially in tasks that require focused and sustained attention (vigilance) (122,124).

There is less consistent evidence that stimulants are of any benefit in subjects who are fully alert and attentive or engaged in tasks involving learning, memory, or problem solving. With increasing potency, dose, duration of use, or a more efficient route of administration, stimulant effects often progress to include dysphoric effects such as anxiety, irritability, panic attacks, interpersonal sensitivity, hypervigilance, suspiciousness, paranoia, grandiosity, impaired judgment, and psychotic symptoms such as delusions and hallucinations. Among non-treatment-seeking users, 10% to 40% may have sleep disturbance and weight loss (due to appetite suppression), and up to 25% may experience severe paranoia and/or hallucinations (125,126). In some case series, more than 50% of chronic cocaine and amphetamine users report psychotic symptoms (127–129), but this may reflect selection bias among users who come to medical or research attention.

Patients with stimulant psychosis may closely resemble those with acute schizophrenia (130,131)—perhaps not surprising, given that both conditions share the presumed pathophysiology of excessive brain dopamine activity (132). Cocaine-induced psychosis may differ from acute schizophrenic psychosis in being marked by less thought disorder and bizarre delusions and fewer negative symptoms such as alogia and inattention (129). Stimulant-induced hallucinations may be auditory, visual, or somatosensory (127,133). Tactile hallucinations are especially typical of stimulant psychosis and include the sensation of something (e.g., insects) crawling under the skin ("formication").

Parallel behavioral effects include restlessness, agitation, tremor, dyskinesia, and repetitive or stereotyped behaviors such as picking at the skin or foraging for drug ("punding," "hung-up activity") (134). Associated physiologic effects include tachycardia, pupil dilation, diaphoresis, and nausea, reflecting stimulation of the sympathetic nervous system. Criteria for the psychiatric diagnosis of stimulant intoxication are given in Appendix 4 (8). Treatment of acute stimulant intoxication is reviewed in Section 6, Chapter 45, "Management of Stimulant, Hallucinogen, Marijuana, Phencyclidine, and Club Drug Intoxication and Withdrawal." Cocaine and the more potent synthetic stimulants (such as amphetamines) produce these adverse effects at readily available doses by any route of administration. Less potent oral stimulants may require chronic, high-dose use or diversion to intravenous use to cause these effects. Even OTC stimulants have been associated with severe psychological effects, abuse, and dependence.

There is wide individual variability in the response to stimulants. The reasons are poorly understood but presumably are related to differences in genetics, psychological characteristics (including personality traits), previous drug experience, the setting in which the drug is taken, and the existence of psychiatric or medical comorbidities (121,135,136). Identical twins are highly concordant in their response to single doses of stimulants, suggesting an important genetic component. In animals, response to stimulants appears to be under polygenic control, with independent genetic influences on responses to cocaine or amphetamine (137). In rats, behavioral response to cocaine shows a negative correlation with baseline brain dopamine concentrations and a positive correlation with the increase in dopamine concentration elicited by a cocaine challenge (138).

Individual differences in tolerance and sensitization to stimulants (see later discussion: Neuroadaptations) may account for the poor correlation between stimulant plasma concentrations and toxic effects (121,139,140). Fatal cases of amphetamine or cocaine intoxication may present with 100-fold differences in plasma stimulant concentration (1).

Chronic Effects Chronic cocaine or amphetamine abuse is associated with cognitive impairment that may persist for at least several months of abstinence (141,142). Most affected are visuomotor performance, attention, inhibitory control, and verbal memory. Several studies have found abnormalities of behavioral regulation and risk-reward decision making. This type of impairment is associated with lesions of the frontal cortex, a brain area that shows decreased regional blood flow and metabolic activity in abstinent cocaine abusers.

Chronic cocaine use is associated with decreased gray and white matter volumes in the frontal cortex of the brain (143), enlarged basal ganglia, and lower concentrations of N-acetylaspartate (a magnetic resonance spectroscopy marker for normal neuronal function) and higher concentrations of creatine and myoinositol (markers of glial cell activity and inflammation) (144).

Chronic amphetamine or methamphetamine use (either oral or intravenous) can cause a psychotic syndrome (with paranoia and hallucinations) that may persist for years after the last drug use, even in persons with no personal or family history of psychiatric disorder (145,146). Methamphetamine psychosis may be associated with focal perfusion deficits in the frontal, parietal, and temporal lobes of the cerebral cortex (147). Psychotic flashbacks have been reported in methamphetamine abusers up to 2 years after their last drug use and often are precipitated by threatening experiences (146). A persisting psychosis after cocaine use has not been reported, except in patients with an underlying psychiatric disorder (such as schizophrenia or bipolar disorder) (148).

Withdrawal Cessation of stimulant use may result in a withdrawal syndrome that does not have prominent physiological features and is not life-threatening (149–151). Withdrawal symptoms generally are the opposite of those associated with stimulant intoxication and include depressed mood, anhedonia (inability to experience pleasure), fatigue, difficulty concentrating, increased total sleep and rapid eye movement sleep duration (but with poor sleep quality) (152), and increased appetite. Criteria for the psychiatric diagnosis of stimulant withdrawal are given in Appendix 4 (8). Treatment of stimulant withdrawal is reviewed in Section 6, Chapter 45, "Management of Stimulant, Hallucinogen, Marijuana, Phencyclidine, and Club Drug Intoxication and Withdrawal."

An early report of cocaine withdrawal among 30 outpatients described a complex triphasic syndrome lasting several months. This finding has not been replicated in subsequent inpatient or outpatient studies (149,151,153). Several studies of inpatients undergoing cocaine withdrawal found a monotonic decline in symptoms over 1 to 2 weeks.

Rodents undergoing cocaine or amphetamine withdrawal after a period of chronic drug exposure tend to show biphasic changes in the brain: initial increases in extracellular dopamine concentrations and expression of dopamine transporter and kappa and mu opiate receptors, followed by decreases in these variables (154,155). The few human studies on cocaine withdrawal do not find consistent changes in peripheral markers of dopamine activity, as in plasma concentrations of dopamine metabolites or of prolactin (a hormone under dopamine control) (156,157).

Human brain imaging studies suggest a modest increase in dopamine transporter binding during early cocaine withdrawal (using single-photon emission computed tomography [SPECT]) (158), followed by a decrease after 11 to 30 days of abstinence (using PET) (157). This pattern is consistent with most, but not all, postmortem studies of cocaine users (159).

Behavioral Pharmacology Cocaine, amphetamines, cathinone, ephedrine, and most other stimulants that have been tested in animals consistently produce increased motor activity, repetitive stereotyped behavior, drug discrimination, and evidence of reinforcing effects (such as drug self-administration and conditioned place preference) (160–162). Animals allowed free access to stimulants often self-administer in a "binge-abstinence" pattern: periods of high levels of drug intake (producing stereotyped behavior, hyperactivity, decreased eating, and little sleep), alternating with periods of abstinence, during which behavior returns to normal (138). Animals given unlimited access to stimulants may self-administer to the point of death during a binge period. The rewarding effect of stimulants in animals is influenced by the same factors as are other drug and natural reinforcers; for example, the dose of drug available, the schedule of reinforcement, the animal's past history of development and drug exposure, and the current environment and condition of the animal. Stimulant self-administration is reduced by increased work requirements, availability of an alternative potent reinforcer, or the concurrent presence of punishment (as by electric shock), and increased by food deprivation or stress (136,163).

Animals undergoing enforced abstinence after a period of stimulant self-administration initially increase their responding in an apparent attempt to obtain drug but eventually extinguish their drug-seeking behavior (138). However, they will promptly resume drug-seeking behavior if given a single "priming" dose of the drug or exposed to drug-associated stimuli or stress (such as electric foot shock) (164). This reinstatement of drug-seeking behavior has been considered an animal model of relapse to drug use after treatment.

Stimulants produce a distinctive set of subjective psychological effects (including euphoria, drug liking, increased energy, and increased alertness) in humans under controlled double-blind experimental conditions (161,165). *d*-Amphetamine, benzphetamine, cocaine, ephedrine, mazindol, methylphenidate, phenmetrazine, and phenylpropanolamine are readily distinguished from placebo or sedative drugs but often are not distinguished from each other when equipotent doses are given.

Other Central Nervous System Effects Acute stimulant administration is associated with transient increases in electroencephalographic (EEG) alpha, beta, and theta activity, which correlate with the acute psychological effects (166). Stimulant use by any route of administration is associated with seizures, even in persons without a pre-existing seizure disorder (167–169). These can occur with the first use and most often are single, generalized tonic-clonic seizures, although multiple seizures and status epilepticus can occur. Most cocaine-associated seizures occur within 90 minutes of drug use, during the time of peak plasma concentration.

Cocaine and amphetamine use are associated with cerebral vasoconstriction, cerebrovascular atherosclerosis, cerebrovascular disease, and stroke (170–172). In a study of more than 800,000 discharges from Texas hospitals in 2003, cocaine and amphetamine users had more than twice the risk of stroke than patients not using stimulants (173). Hemorrhagic stroke appears more common in intranasal or intravenous users, whereas ischemic stroke is more common in smokers. Neurologic symptoms usually appear within 3 hours of drug use, though a minority of patients may be asymptomatic for up to 24 hours. An underlying cerebrovascular abnormality (such as arterial aneurysm or arteriovenous malformation) probably increases the risk of cocaine-associated stroke, but the majority of such stroke patients do not have any cerebrovascular risk factors. The OTC stimulant phenylpropanolamine, marketed as a decongestant and appetite suppressant, was associated with a significant risk of hemorrhagic stroke in a recent case-control study, even in patients who used it at recommended doses (174). This finding led the FDA to remove phenylpropanolamine from the U.S. market in October 2000.

Stimulant use is associated with a variety of movement disorders, presumably as the result of increased dopamine activity in the basal ganglia and other brain areas that control movement (121,167,175). Such disorders include repetitive stereotyped behaviors (such as repeated dismantling of objects, cleaning, doodling, and searching for imaginary objects), acute dystonic reactions, choreoathetosis and akathisia (so-called "crack dancers"), buccolingual dyskinesias ("twisted mouth" or "boca torcida"), and exacerbation of Tourette's syndrome and tardive dyskinesia. Cocaine users are at increased risk of acute dystonic reactions to antipsychotic medications (176).

Cardiovascular System Stimulants act acutely on the cardiovascular system both directly (by increasing adrenergic activity at sympathetic nerve terminals) and via the CNS to increase heart rate, blood pressure, and systemic vascular resistance (170,177). Stimulant-induced increases in heart rate and blood pressure are significantly correlated with increases in plasma norepinephrine and epinephrine concentrations (178,179), suggesting mediation by increased activity of the sympathetic nervous system. The mechanism may be prolonged blockade of norepinephrine transporters in the heart, amplifying the action of endogenous norepinephrine.

Cocaine-induced tachycardia is blocked by beta-adrenergic receptor blockade (propranolol) but not by muscarinic receptor blockade (atropine) (180), further suggesting a sympathetic role. The resulting increase in myocardial oxygen demand, often accompanied by decreased coronary blood flow (from vasospasm and vasoconstriction), may cause acute myocardial infarction, even in young persons without atherosclerosis. This process may be promoted by cocaine-induced increases in circulating activated platelets, platelet aggregation, and thromboxane synthesis. Cocaine use is a factor in about one-fourth of nonfatal heart attacks in persons younger than 45 years (181). Frequent cocaine users are up to seven times more likely to have a nonfatal heart attack than are nonusers (181). Postmortem studies suggest that chronic cocaine use is associated with higher levels of coronary atherosclerosis (171).

Cocaine use is associated with cardiac arrhythmias (such as ventricular tachycardia or fibrillation) and sudden death (177,182). The mechanisms include blockade of myocyte sodium channels (resulting in impaired cardiac conduction and areas of localized conduction block) and increased concentration of plasma norepinephrine (which sensitizes the myocardium).

Chronic cocaine or amphetamine use is associated with cardiomyopathy and myocarditis (177,183,184). Case series of asymptomatic cocaine abusers have found up to half with echocardiographic abnormalities such as left ventricular hypertrophy and abnormal segmental wall motion. Cocaine-associated cases of dilated cardiomyopathy and myocardial fibrosis may be due to direct toxic effects of high concentrations of circulating norepinephrine. Cocaine-associated myocarditis (whose acute symptoms may mimic myocardial infarction) may be a direct toxic effect of cocaine or a hypersensitivity effect. Autopsy series of current cocaine users have found myocarditis in up to 20%.

Other Organ Systems No large surveys or prospective studies have comprehensively evaluated the natural history of stimulant use or the frequency of adverse effects. Existing knowledge derives largely from case reports or case series of persons who come to medical attention (185). In the absence of experimental data, it may be difficult to determine the extent to which an observed adverse effect is the result of a direct action on the affected organ or tissue, an indirect action, an effect of a street drug contaminant, or secondary to other factors that are part of a drug-using lifestyle, such as needle sharing, malnutrition, use of other substances, and the like. The most relevant indirect action of cocaine in producing adverse effects in many organs and tissues is ischemia and infarction. These result from several mechanisms, including vasoconstriction, vasospasm, damage to endothelium, and increased clotting as the result of increased number of circulating activated platelets, enhanced platelet aggregation, and increased thromboxane synthesis (167). These mechanisms often reinforce one another: for example, vasospasm may damage endothelium, endothelial damage increases thromboxane synthesis, and thromboxane causes platelet aggregation and vasoconstriction.

Adverse effects of stimulant use on particular organ systems often depend on the route of administration. For example, smoked stimulants produce lung toxicity not found with other routes, injection use is associated with infectious diseases such as human immunodeficiency virus and hepatitis C, and intranasal use is associated with damage to the nasal septum.

Pulmonary Smoked cocaine produces both acute and chronic pulmonary toxicity (186–189). Acute respiratory symptoms may develop in up to half of users within minutes to several hours after smoking. Symptoms include productive cough, shortness of breath, wheezing, chest pain, hemoptysis, and exacerbation of asthma. More severe, and rarer, acute effects include pulmonary edema, pulmonary hemorrhage, pneumothorax, pneumomediastinum, and thermal airway injury. Pulmonary edema also has been reported after intravenous cocaine use. Chronic cocaine smoking has been associated in case reports with pulmonary and peripheral eosinophilia, interstitial pneumonitis, and bronchiolitis obliterans. The pathophysiology of these adverse effects is not definitively understood but presumably involves a combination of direct damage by cocaine or inhaled microparticles to the alveolar-capillary membrane, vasoconstriction and damage to the pulmonary vascular bed, and/or interstitial disease.

The long-term effect of cocaine smoking on pulmonary function remains unclear (186). Standard pulmonary function tests (spirometry) have been normal in most studies. Some studies have found increased alveolar epithelial permeability and moderately decreased (up to 20%) pulmonary diffusion capacity among cocaine smokers without acute symptoms, although other studies have found normal function. The attribution of these abnormalities to cocaine use is confounded by the fact that the vast majority of cocaine-smoking subjects also were smokers of tobacco and/or marijuana.

Renal Stimulants have little direct toxic effect on the kidneys. Acute renal failure can occur as a result of renal ischemia or infarction, malignant hypertension, or rhabdomyolysis (see later discussion: Musculoskeletal (190–192). Release of myoglobin during rhabdomyolysis may cause renal tubular obstruction or direct myoglobin damage to renal tubules. Intrarenal arterial constriction with resulting renal medullary ischemia also may contribute to renal tubular damage.

Gastrointestinal Cocaine reduces gastric motility and delays gastric emptying, in part by affecting medullary centers that regulate these functions (167). The major gastrointestinal effects of cocaine use are due to vasoconstriction and ischemia: gastroduodenal ulceration and perforation, intestinal infarction and perforation, and ischemic colitis (167,185,193). The distribution of cocaine-associated ulcers is primarily in the greater curvature and prepyloric region of the stomach, pyloric canal, and first portion of the duodenum, whereas peptic ulcers occur primarily in the duodenal bulb. Concealing cocaine by swallowing large packets ("body packing") may result in severe acute toxicity if the wrapping deteriorates and allows cocaine into the gastrointestinal tract (175).

Liver Cocaine is hepatotoxic in rodents, presumably because of oxidative metabolism to norocaine by the cytochrome P450 microsomal enzyme system in the liver, with further transformation to reactive hepatotoxic compounds such as N-hydroxynorcocaine (175). This is a very minor metabolic pathway in humans (see previous discussion: Metabolism). There is no direct evidence that cocaine is hepatotoxic in humans. Liver abnormalities reported in case series of cocaine users can be accounted for by viral hepatitis from injection drug use, alcoholic liver disease, or other consequences of a drug-using lifestyle.

Pemoline has been associated with hepatocellular toxicity, sometimes resulting in fulminant liver failure and death (1,194). This led to pemoline's withdrawal from the U.S. market in 2005.

Endocrine Acute cocaine use activates the hypothalamic-pituitary-adrenal (HPA) axis, stimulating secretion of epinephrine, corticotropin-releasing hormone (CRH), ACTH, and cortisol (175,195,196). Acute cocaine use decreases plasma prolactin concentrations in cocaine-naive individuals, presumably because of increased dopamine activity (dopamine inhibits prolactin release from the pituitary). Chronic cocaine users may have increased, normal, or decreased prolactin levels and usually do not show changes in response to acute cocaine. Acute cocaine use increases plasma luteinizing hormone, but chronic cocaine users have normal levels of testosterone, cortisol, luteinizing hormone, and thyroid hormones. A blunted thyroid-stimulating hormone response to thyroid-releasing hormone stimulation has been reported in one study but has not been replicated. Cocaine use is associated with increased risk of diabetic keto-acidosis, either because of poor treatment adherence or acute stimulation of the HPA (197).

Musculoskeletal Stimulants may cause rhabdomyolysis by several different mechanisms: a direct toxic effect causing myofibrillar degeneration (probably rare except at very high doses), indirectly by vasoconstriction of intramuscular arteries resulting in ischemia, and secondary to stimulant-induced hyperthermia or seizures (167,198). Up to one-third of patients with rhabdomyolysis will develop acute renal failure, sometimes accompanied by disseminated intravascular coagulation and liver damage. This syndrome often is fatal.

Head and Neck Common head and neck complications of cocaine use depend on the route of administration (167,175). Intranasal cocaine use ("snorting") is associated with chronic rhinitis, perforated nasal septum and nasal collapse, oropharyngeal ulcers, and osteolytic sinusitis, presumably due to vasoconstriction and resulting ischemic necrosis (199). Changes in the sense of smell are rare, even in heavy users with intranasal damage (200). Oral cocaine use is associated with gingival ulceration and erosion of dental enamel (175). In South America, chronic coca leaf chewing has been associated with mild epithelial changes but no evidence of premalignant or malignant lesions (201). The observed changes may result from the alkaline ash usually chewed with the leaves to enhance cocaine extraction rather than from the cocaine itself. Smoked cocaine ("crack") may cause corneal ulcers (202). Cocaine use by any route of administration may reduce salivary secretions (xerostomia) and cause bruxism (203).

Immune System Cocaine use has been associated with a variety of vasculitic syndromes primarily affecting skin and muscle (204). These may mimic rheumatologic conditions such as Henoch Schönlein purpura, Steven-Johnson syndrome, or Raynaud phenomenon. Cocaine-associated midline destructive lesions may resemble Wegener's granulomatosis (205). In experimental studies, cocaine impairs innate immune mechanisms (e.g., the response of monocytes to bacterial lipopolysaccharide) (206).

Sexual Function Stimulants are commonly thought of as an aphrodisiac, but chronic use usually impairs sexual function (207,208). Men may experience erectile dysfunction or delayed or inhibited ejaculation. Priapism is rare. Women may develop irregular menses.

Cocaine has been applied to the penis or clitoris to use its local anesthetic effect to delay organism (208).

Reproductive, Fetal, and Neonatal Health Prescription stimulants, including cocaine and amphetamines, are classified by the FDA in pregnancy category C, meaning that risk cannot be ruled out because human studies are lacking. One exception is diethylpropion, which is category B (no evidence of risk in humans).

Prenatal (in utero) exposure to cocaine, amphetamines, or methylphenidate has been associated with vaginal bleeding, abruptio placenta, placenta previa, premature rupture of membranes, decreased head circumference, low birth weight, tremulousness, irritability, poor feeding, and autonomic instability (209–212). It is usually difficult in these studies to distinguish a direct effect of the stimulant from the effects of concomitant factors frequently present in drug users, such as other drug use (including alcohol, nicotine, and opiates), poor nutrition, and lack of prenatal care. The importance of concomitant factors is underscored by studies in which participation in prenatal care is associated with better outcomes even when stimulant use continues (213). Rodent and monkey studies, in which confounding factors can be excluded, show few direct adverse effects of prenatal exposure to cocaine (213).

The long-term effects of prenatal exposure to stimulants also are unclear (212). Well-controlled, prospective studies suggest that the mild cognitive deficits seen in the first 2 years of life largely resolve by the age of 4 years. However, subtler cognitive problems, as with habituation, have been noted in such children and require further study.

Cocaine, amphetamines, phentermine, ephedrine, and pseudoephedrine appear in breast milk (107). Cocaine and amphetamines may cause irritability, sleep disturbance, and tremors in the infant. Medical use by the mother of other prescription and OTC stimulants in appropriate doses usually does not have clinically significant adverse effects on nursing infants.

NEUROBIOLOGY

Mechanisms of Action

Neurotransmitters All stimulants act to enhance monoamine (dopamine, norepinephrine, and serotonin) activity in the central and peripheral nervous systems (Table 10.4). Potent stimulants, such as cocaine, amphetamines, mazindol, and methylphenidate, do this indirectly by acting on membrane reuptake pumps (transporters) for monoamines (214,215) (Fig. 10.3). These transporters at presynaptic nerve endings carry monoamine neurotransmitters from the synaptic cleft back into the nerve ending, thus ending their synaptic activity. Cocaine, mazindol, and methylphenidate block this transport, thus allowing more neurotransmitter to remain active in the synapse. Amphetamines and phentermine act as false substrates for the transporter. They are taken up into the presynaptic nerve ending in exchange for neurotransmitter released back into the synapse (hence, they are termed *releasers*). Once inside the nerve ending, amphetamines act as false substrates for the vesicular monoamine transporter 2 (VMAT2) located on the intracellular vesicles that store monoamine neurotransmitters within the presynaptic ending. As with the synaptic transporters, amphetamines are taken up into the vesicles in exchange for neurotransmitter released into the cytosol. This action makes more neurotransmitter available for release into the synapse. Less potent stimulants (e.g., OTC decongestants) act directly by binding to and activating norepinephrine receptors. Ephedrine, pseudoephedrine, phenylephrine, and phenylpropanolamine are more effective at alpha-adrenergic receptors, which mediate vasoconstriction (hence their use as decongestants and antihypotensive agents). Ephedrine also has some action at beta-adrenergic receptors, which mediate bronchodilation.

TABLE 10.4 Neuropharmacologic Actions of Selected Stimulants

	Catecholamines		Serotonin			
	Reuptake blockade	Presynaptic release	Reuptake blockade	Presynaptic release	MAO inhibition	Na channel blockade
Amphetamine	++	+++	+	+	+	0
Cocaine	+++	+	+++	+	0	+++
Ephedrine[a]	+	++	0	0	0	0
Mazindol	+++	0	+	0	0	0
Methamphetamine	++	+++	+	+++	+	0
Methylphenidate	+++	0	+	0	0	0
Phentermine	+	++	0	0	+	0

MAO, monoamine oxidase.

[a]Also direct agonist at adrenergic (norepinephrine) receptors.

Data from Rothman, Baumann, et al., 2001; (215) Howell and Kimmel, 2008 (246).

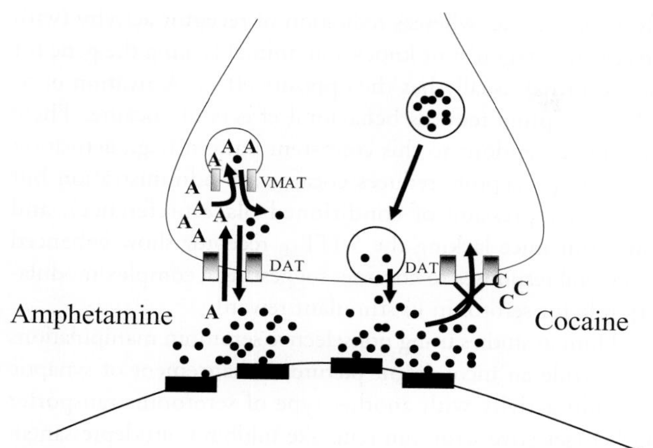

FIGURE 10.3. Mechanism of action of amphetamine and cocaine at dopamine synapse. Diagram of a dopamine synapse, showing the mechanism of action of amphetamine **(As)** left side and cocaine **(Cs)** right side. Amphetamine acts as a false substrate for the dopamine transporter (DAT) in the presynaptic nerve membrane, being taken up by the DAT from the synaptic cleft into the cytosol in exchange for release of dopamine (*black circles*) into the synaptic cleft. In addition, amphetamine, unlike cocaine, is a substrate for the intracellular vesicular monoamine transporter (VMAT), being taken up by the VMAT from the cytosol into the vesicle. This action results in release of dopamine from the vesicle into the cytosol, thus making more dopamine available for release from the presynaptic nerve cell into the synaptic cleft.

Cocaine blocks the uptake of dopamine by DAT from the synaptic cleft but is not itself transported.

These effects of amphetamine and cocaine result in more dopamine being available to cross the synaptic cleft and bind to postsynaptic dopamine receptors (*black bars*).

Cocaine and amphetamine have similar actions at presynaptic norepinephrine and serotonin transporters.

Dopamine Cocaine, amphetamines, and mazindol enhance synaptic dopamine activity by acting at presynaptic dopamine transporters, as described earlier (Table 10.4). The cocaine-binding site overlaps those for dopamine and amphetamine (216). Acute administration of cocaine or amphetamine transiently increases brain extracellular dopamine concentrations in animals and humans, especially in the striatum (which includes the nucleus accumbens) (217), and increases dopamine D_1 receptor density in the striatum. Repeated administration of cocaine or amphetamine increases D_1 receptor sensitivity in the nucleus accumbens but has variable effects on other dopamine receptor measures (218).

Postmortem studies of human brain suggest that cocaine abusers have decreased dopamine levels in the frontal cortex (219), normal levels of dopamine receptor binding (220), decreased VMAT transporter in striatum (221), and increased dopamine transporter binding in striatum (222), in conjunction with decreased transporter protein and messenger RNA levels (159,223,224). In vivo human studies using PET suggest that cocaine and methamphetamine users have decreased dopamine D_2 receptor binding in striatum and frontal cortex, which may persist for months of abstinence, and normal levels of dopamine transporter binding (217,225). In contrast, methamphetamine abusers have increased D_1 receptors in the nucleus accumbens (226) and decreased dopamine transporter density in nucleus accumbens, striatum, and prefrontal cortex (227).

Several lines of evidence from animal studies suggest that it is the increased synaptic dopamine activity in the mesocorticolimbic reward circuit that mediates the behavioral effects of stimulants (138,215). Fluctuations in extracellular dopamine concentrations and neuronal firing in the nucleus accumbens parallel cocaine self-administration (228). The potency of cocaine analogues and other stimulants for being self-administered or producing cocaine-like discriminative stimuli is highly correlated with their affinity for and speed of binding to the dopamine transporter (229) but not with their binding to other monoamine transporters or receptors (230). Conversely, lesions of dopamine neurons in the reward circuit (but not other brain regions) reduce cocaine self-administration (231), and mice genetically engineered with otherwise functional dopamine transporters that do not bind cocaine do not show reinforcing or other behavioral effects of cocaine (while still responding to amphetamine) (232–234). Mice lacking any dopamine transporters still find cocaine rewarding (235), but this is probably owing to cocaine's action on norepinephrine neurons, whose presynaptic norepinephrine transporters take up dopamine in place of the absent dopamine transporters (236).

Dopamine D_1 and D_2/D_3 receptors appear to play reciprocal roles in the behavioral effects of stimulants (218). Blockade of D_1 receptors in regions of the brain reward circuit (e.g., the shell of the nucleus accumbens or ventral tegmental area) reduces the rewarding effects of cocaine or amphetamine in the rat, as does stimulation of D_3 receptors (237–239). Knock-out mice that lack the D_1 receptor do not self-administer cocaine (240), whereas D_3 knock-out mice show enhanced responses to cocaine or amphetamine (241).

Evidence from human brain imaging studies using PET or SPECT is largely consistent with an important role for dopamine in the acute psychological effects of stimulants. The acute positive psychological response (euphoria or "high") to cocaine or methylphenidate correlates in time course and intensity with drug concentration in the brain, with dopamine transporter occupancy (in the case of cocaine) (230), and with extracellular dopamine release in the striatum (as measured by ligand displacement from dopamine receptors) (217,225). Exposure to cocaine-associated cues is also associated with dopamine release in the striatum; the degree of release is correlated with cocaine craving (217). Blockade of more than half the dopamine transporters is needed to reduce cocaine self-administration in animals (230) or reduce the subjective effects in humans.

Clinical evidence is not as supportive of an important role for dopamine activity in stimulant effects. Schizophrenic patients taking first-generation antipsychotics (which are potent dopamine D_2 receptor antagonists) at doses that well control their schizophrenic symptoms still experience the psychoactive effects of cocaine and frequently abuse it (242). Experimental attempts to block the acute psychological effects of cocaine or amphetamine with antipsychotic medication or by blocking dopamine and norepinephrine synthesis with the tyrosine hydroxylase inhibitor alpha-methyl-p-tyrosine have not been successful (243–245). These failures may have been due to the inability of subjects to tolerate sufficient doses of medication to influence cocaine's effects.

Norepinephrine Cocaine, amphetamines, mazindol, phentermine, and ephedrine enhance synaptic norepinephrine activity by acting at the presynaptic norepinephrine transporter, as described earlier (231) (Table 10.4). Consistent with this synaptic action, intravenous cocaine increases plasma norepinephrine and epinephrine concentrations within minutes of injection (178). There is a significant positive correlation between potency of norepinephrine release (measured in vitro) and the oral stimulant dose that produces stimulantlike subjective effects in humans, suggesting a role for norepinephrine in the psychological effects of stimulants (246). Chronic cocaine exposure increases norepinephrine transporter function in monkey and human brain (231,247). Knock-out mice lacking the norepinephrine transporter are supersensitive to the locomotor stimulation produced by cocaine or amphetamine and still find cocaine rewarding (235).

Ephedrine, pseudoephedrine, phenylephrine, and other direct-acting stimulants are agonists at alpha-adrenergic norepinephrine receptors. The effect of chronic administration of stimulants on adrenoreceptor subtypes has not been well studied.

Serotonin Cocaine, amphetamines, and mazindol enhance synaptic serotonin activity by acting at the presynaptic membrane serotonin transporter, as described (Table 10.4). Acute cocaine administration increases extracellular serotonin concentrations in the striatum and ventral tegmental area and reduces firing of serotonin neurons in the dorsal raphe (235). The latter action probably is mediated by negative feedback from stimulation of 5-HT_{1A} autoreceptors (248). Chronic cocaine exposure increases serotonergic terminal density and basal serotonin levels in the frontal cortex, probably by decreasing 5-HT_{1A} autoreceptor function in the median raphe nuclei (249). Human cocaine users have normal 5-HT_2 receptor availability in brain (250).

Serotonin's role in stimulant reward is unclear. Knock-out mice lacking the serotonin transporter still find cocaine rewarding (self-administration, conditioned place preference), whereas double knock-out mice lacking both the dopamine and serotonin transporters do not (235). Knock-out mice lacking both the norepinephrine and serotonin transporters show increased sensitivity to cocaine reward (235). These findings suggest a permissive, but not obligatory, role for the serotonin transporter in cocaine reward.

The various subtypes of serotonin receptors appear to play different roles in the behavioral effects of cocaine (235,251). Activation of 5-HT_{1A}, 5-HT_{1B}, 5-HT_{2A}, or 5-HT_3 receptors enhances both the locomotor hyperactivity and rewarding effects of cocaine, whereas reduction of receptor activity (with a receptor antagonist or knock-out animal lacking the gene for the receptors) usually has the opposite effect. Activation of 5-HT_{2C} receptors reduces behavioral effects of cocaine. There are some exceptions to this consistent pattern (e.g., activation of 5-HT_{1A} receptors reduces cocaine self-administration but enhances expression of conditioned place preference), and knock-out mice lacking the 5-HT_{1B} receptor show enhanced behavioral responses to cocaine, suggesting a complex modulatory role for serotonin in stimulant reward.

Human studies using nonselective serotonin manipulations also provide an inconsistent picture. Enhancement of synaptic serotonin activity with another type of serotonin transporter blocker (selective serotonin reuptake inhibitor antidepressants), activation of serotonin receptors with a partial agonist, or depletion of serotonin levels (via a tryptophan-free diet) all are reported to reduce the acute subjective effects ("high," craving) of cocaine (252,253). A postmortem study of human brain found higher serotonin levels in the frontal cortex among cocaine users than among matched controls (219). Clarification of the role of serotonin in stimulant reward must await the development for human use of selective agonists and antagonists at the more than dozen known serotonin receptor subtypes.

Endogenous Opiates Stimulants do not directly interact with opiate receptors but do influence endogenous opiate (endorphin, enkephalin) systems in the brain. In rats, single doses of cocaine or amphetamine increase extracellular endorphin levels in the nucleus accumbens and enkephalin and dynorphin mRNA levels in striatum (231). The mechanism is indirect, via other neurotransmitters, especially dopamine, that influence endogenous opiate release.

Repeated cocaine administration, especially in an intermittent binge pattern, increases brain mu and kappa opiate receptor binding in rodents, with no change in delta opiate receptors (254). Human cocaine users show increased mu opiate receptor binding in some brain regions with PET scanning, and this increased binding correlates with self-reported cocaine craving (255). Postmortem brains from fatal cocaine overdose victims show increased kappa opiate receptor binding in limbic areas (256).

Animal studies suggest that brain kappa opiate systems have an influence on cocaine effects. In general, activation of endogenous kappa opiate receptor systems (such as by administration of the endogenous ligand dynorphin) reduces behavioral and neuropharmacologic effects of stimulants (257).

Glutamate The acute administration of cocaine or amphetamine increases glutamate release in the ventral tegmental area, nucleus accumbens, dorsal striatum, ventral pallidum, septum, and cerebellum (258). Low doses of cocaine enhance glutamate-evoked neuronal firing and have variable effects on the different subtypes of glutamate receptors. Chronic cocaine exposure up-regulates some glutamate receptor subtypes, down-regulates others, and has bidirectional effects on others, depending on the brain region. Several glutamate receptor subtypes appear to play an important role in cocaine reinforcement. Blockade of *N*-methyl-D-aspartate receptors in the nucleus accumbens reduces cocaine reinforcement, as does reduction of mGluR5 receptor activity. Indirect reduction of glutamate activity by stimulating presynaptic mGluR2 receptors also reduces cocaine reinforcement, whereas reduction of mGluR2 activity enhances reinforcement.

A growing body of evidence suggests that glutamate plays an important role in relapse to cocaine or amphetamine abuse (258). Withdrawal from chronic cocaine or amphetamine exposure significantly alters brain glutamate receptor density in rodents. Readministration of the stimulant leads to a marked increase in extracellular glutamate levels and changes in glutamate receptor function in the nucleus accumbens that are absent after acute administration of the drug. A recent hypothesis proposes that the chronic administration of cocaine or amphetamine leads to the recruitment of cortical glutamatergic neurotransmission in the nucleus accumbens as a consequence of associations with the drug-taking environment. Thus, an environmental stimulus may evoke drug-seeking behavior through enhanced glutamate transmission.

Acetylcholine Cocaine and methamphetamine block neuronal nicotinic acetylcholine (ACh) receptors; cocaine also blocks muscarinic ACh receptors in the brain and on cardiac myocytes (259,260). Cocaine, amphetamine, and methamphetamine cause ACh release in several brain regions, including the striatum, nucleus accumbens, medial thalamus, and interpeduncular nucleus (260–262). Chronic cocaine exposure appears to cause down-regulation of brain cholinergic systems, reflected in decreased choline acetyltransferase activity and decreased nicotinic receptors. In contrast, chronic methamphetamine exposure appears to result in increased nicotinic receptor density (259).

Cholinergic receptors may play a role in cocaine reward. Rodents with reduced muscarinic receptor activity show decreased cocaine self-administration and conditioned place preference (263,264). Nicotinic receptor blockade has variable effects, depending on the receptor subtype and brain region (265). Enhancing cholinergic activity by inhibiting acetylcholinesterase (the enzyme that breaks down ACh) reduces the behavioral effects of cocaine but has no effect on those of methamphetamine (266,267).

Other Actions Some stimulants have additional neuropharmacologic actions (Table 10.4). Amphetamines and phentermine inhibit monoamine oxidase, which also would increase catecholamine activity. This action probably is not significant at the drug concentrations achieved with typical therapeutic or abused doses (268). Cocaine is unique in also blocking voltage-gated membrane sodium ion channels. This action accounts for its effect as a local anesthetic, and may contribute to cardiac arrhythmias.

Signal Transduction When monoamine neurotransmitters such as dopamine activate their membrane receptors on the nerve cell surface, they trigger a cascade of intracellular chemical events (269). The neurotransmitter receptors are coupled to G-proteins, which regulate adenylyl cyclase activity to alter levels of cyclic 3′,5′-adenosine monophosphate (cAMP), an intracellular "second messenger." Cyclic AMP, in turn, regulates the activity of protein kinases, phospholipases, and other intracellular enzymes. These enzymes regulate various intracellular processes, including the activity of transcription factors that regulate gene transcription by binding to specific DNA sequences in the regulatory regions of genes (see further: Gene Expression). Stimulants activate several signaling pathways in neurons of the brain reward circuit, including cAMP, extracellular signal-regulated kinase, mitogen-activated protein kinase, and phosphoinositide 3-kinase, as well as altering expression of proteins that regulate G-protein signaling. Direct manipulation of steps in these pathways can modify stimulant-induced behavior (270,271). Changes to these pathways from chronic exposure to stimulants may mediate tolerance and sensitization (see further: Neuroadaptation).

Gene Expression Acute administration of stimulants (such as cocaine, amphetamine, and methylphenidate) to rodents promptly activates (within 1 hour, without requiring protein synthesis) several "immediate early" genes in the brain, such as cAMP response element-binding protein (CREB), c-*fos*, *zif268*, and c-*jun*, probably via activation of dopamine receptors (272). The protein products of these genes are nuclear transcription factors that regulate gene expression. Repeated administration of stimulants results in a long-lasting blunting of the gene activation effect in many brain regions. Chronic stimulant administration leads to accumulation of some transcription factors, which may mediate the development of sensitization (see further: Neuroadaptation).

In animal studies, acute or chronic stimulant administration results in changes in expression of a variety of genes in many brain regions related to addiction, including genes involved in neuronal growth, cytoskeletal structure, synaptic plasticity, and receptors and signal transduction (273,274). Human postmortem studies of chronic cocaine users do not always find the same changes. Genes significantly up-regulated in human studies include cocaine- and amphetamine-related transcript, CREB, and several glutamate receptor subunits, whereas several myelin-related genes were down-regulated.

Neural Circuits and Systems Animal studies suggest that the rewarding effects of stimulants (and most other abused drugs) are mediated by a neural circuit involving connections among the ventral tegmental area (VTA) of the midbrain, the prefrontal cortex (PFC, including ventral orbitofrontal cortex and anterior cingulate), and the limbic regions of the basal forebrain sometimes called the *extended amygdala* (including the medial amygdala, medial ventral pallidum, and shell of the nucleus accumbens) (275). The VTA sends dopaminergic projections to the PFC, nucleus accumbens, and ventral pallidum. In return, it receives inhibitory GABAergic input from the ventral pallidum and nucleus accumbens, and excitatory glutamatergic input from the

PFC. The PFC also sends glutamatergic input to the nucleus accumbens, which in turn sends inhibitory GABAergic input to the ventral pallidum.

The nucleus accumbens and PFC appear to be the key sites for stimulant reward (138). In rodents, selective dopamine lesions or administration of dopamine receptor blockers in the nucleus accumbens, but not in other sites, abolish the rewarding effects of cocaine or amphetamine. Rodents will self-administer amphetamine directly into the nucleus accumbens or PFC and cocaine directly into the PFC but not into other brain sites. Cocaine administration into the PFC increases dopamine turnover in the nucleus accumbens. The relationship between cocaine self-administration and extracellular dopamine concentration in the nucleus accumbens also suggests a key role for this site (138). A period of cocaine self-administration increases tonic concentrations of extracellular dopamine, with each individual dose producing a time-locked phasic increase. The subsequent decline in dopamine concentration predicts the self-administration of the next dose. Overall, the animal appears to be titrating extracellular dopamine concentration in the nucleus accumbens to maintain an increase above baseline concentration.

The evidence for brain localization of stimulant effects in humans is very limited but somewhat consistent with the animal studies. Brain imaging studies using PET, SPECT, or functional magnetic resonance imaging have found stimulant-induced changes in blood flow or metabolic rate in a variety of brain regions, including frontal cortex, anterior cingulate, ventral striatum (which includes the nucleus accumbens), and amygdala (275). Chronic cocaine users have decreased dopamine release in response to amphetamine in many of these brain regions (225). Exposure to cocaine-associated stimuli that elicit cocaine craving has been associated with increased blood flow or metabolic activity in the prefrontal cortex, amygdala, and anterior cingulate gyrus.

Neuroadaptation Repeated exposure to stimulants results in two distinct neuroadaptations: sensitization (increased drug response) and tolerance (decreased drug response) (277,278). Sensitization tends to result from initial low-dose, intermittent exposure, and tolerance tends to result from more frequent, high-dose, or long-term exposure. The precise pharmacologic, neurobiologic, and behavioral factors that determine sensitization and tolerance are not well understood. There is growing evidence that the development of sensitization or tolerance depends on the balance of activity of gene transcription factors induced by the cAMP intracellular second messenger cascade (see previously: Signal Transduction and Gene Expression).

Sensitization Sensitization is the phenomenon whereby prior intermittent (rather than continuous) exposure to a drug results in an enhanced response to a later exposure. Sensitization is the opposite of tolerance and thus sometimes is termed *reverse tolerance*. Stimulants such as amphetamines or cocaine robustly produce sensitization in rodents, typically observed as a progressive increase in locomotor activity or stereotyped behavior with succeeding drug doses (279). Sensitization occurs not only to behavioral responses, but also to changes in EEG power spectrum (280) and HPA axis activation (281). Sensitization may occur after a single drug exposure (281) and last for months. There is cross-sensitization among stimulants so that previous exposure to amphetamine enhances the response to cocaine (282). However, there is some evidence of neuropharmacologic differences in the sensitization process induced by cocaine, amphetamine, and methylphenidate (283,284).

Behavioral sensitization has two temporally distinct phases: *initiation* or *induction* and *expression*. A combination of environmental and pharmacologic factors influence both phases (285,286). Sensitization may be influenced by circadian rhythm (287) and by the animal's prior drug experience in the environment in which the drug is administered (so-called "context-specific" or "conditioned" sensitization). Behavioral sensitization to stimulants is due, in part, to increased activity in glutamatergic pyramidal neurons in the medial prefrontal cortex, which project to the nucleus accumbens and ventral tegmental area (288). This increased excitatory input makes the dopaminergic neurons in these regions more responsive to stimulation.

Kindling is a process by which low-intensity, intermittent electrical or chemical stimulation of neurons results in a progressive increase in cellular response to subsequent stimulation. Kindling has been considered the neurophysiologic process mediating the sensitization that occurs after repeated stimulant administration and may play a role in cocaine-induced seizures (289).

Behavioral sensitization to stimulants has been suggested as a mechanism for drug craving and relapse (290) and for stimulant-induced psychosis (291). Neither has been directly demonstrated in humans. Several retrospective evaluations of patients presenting with stimulant-induced psychosis found that psychotic symptoms were more severe than during prior episodes of use or were elicited at lower doses that previously had not caused such symptoms (292). This pattern is consistent with sensitization (i.e., an enhanced response to the drug after prior exposure).

Attempts to demonstrate sensitization prospectively in humans have yielded inconsistent results (293). Studies using intravenous, intranasal, or oral cocaine in experienced cocaine users failed to show sensitization after one to several prior cocaine doses. However, one study using oral cocaine did find significant sensitization to cocaine's cardiovascular effects but not to its psychological effects (294). Studies using oral amphetamines in subjects with little or no prior stimulant exposure have shown sensitization to psychological and physiological (eye blink rate) responses after one to three prior oral amphetamine doses. This sensitized response was still present 1 year after the last amphetamine dose and included increased dopamine release in the ventral striatum (measured by PET scanning) (295). The failure to show sensitization in other studies may have been due to the substantial prior stimulant exposure of most subjects, resulting in sensitization already having occurred (i.e., a "ceiling" effect).

Tolerance Tolerance to the behavioral (including reinforcing and appetite-suppressing) effects of stimulants has been demonstrated in animals after high-dose, frequent, or continuous administration (121,278,296,297). Tolerance to cardiovascular, hyperthermic, and lethal effects occurs even more quickly, sometimes after just one or two exposures (121,298). Stimulant tolerance dissipates after 7 to 14 days of no exposure (296–298). There is significant cross-tolerance among various stimulants, but not between stimulants and other drug groups, such as opiates (299).

Stimulant tolerance is pharmacodynamic (i.e., due to adaptive changes in the brain) rather than pharmacokinetic; chronic stimulant exposure does not cause substantial changes in stimulant pharmacokinetics (296). Development of behavioral tolerance is associated with attenuation of the dopamine response to stimulants, decreased activation of immediate early genes, and increased activity of the signal transduction pathway involving protein kinase A and the gene transcription factor CREB (296,300).

In clinical use, tolerance to stimulants develops differentially to various effects. Patients typically become tolerant to the appetite-suppressing effects within several weeks of daily use, whereas the beneficial effects in narcolepsy or ADHD remain over months of treatment (121). In human laboratory studies, tolerance to psychological, cardiovascular, and neuroendocrine effects of cocaine and amphetamines may develop after several doses (301–303). There is some evidence that tolerance to cardiovascular effects develops more quickly and completely than does tolerance to psychological effects (303,304). Rapid tolerance to adverse effects presumably allows binge users to take large cumulative doses of stimulants (305).

Neurotoxicity In animal studies, cocaine and methylphenidate do not produce appreciable neurotoxicity of dopamine or serotonin neurons (29,306). In contrast, high doses of amphetamine or methamphetamine produce substantial dopamine and serotonin neurotoxicity, possibly through interference with monoamine transport and increased production of reactive oxygen species. Such neurotoxicity in human users has not been conclusively demonstrated. Chronic methamphetamine or methcathinone users have reduced density of dopamine transporters in the brain (measured by PET scanning) for at least 3 years after last use (307), but there is evidence of recovery after a year of abstinence (308). Thus, it is not clear whether the loss of transporters represents a reversible physiologic response (down-regulation) to chronic stimulant exposure or a true loss of dopamine nerve endings. Postmortem brain studies in methamphetamine abusers are more consistent with the former alternative. Their findings of decreased dopamine synthesis and dopamine transporter function, but intact vesicular transporter function, suggest that dopamine nerve terminals and the intracellular storage vesicles they contain remain intact (309).

Cocaine has caused DNA synthesis inhibition and cell death of brain neurons in rodents (310), but the clinical relevance of these findings is unknown.

FUTURE RESEARCH DIRECTIONS

Future research at both preclinical and clinical levels is needed to increase understanding of the mechanisms of stimulant addiction and to develop more effective prevention and treatment approaches. Productive areas for preclinical research include the neurochemical mechanisms that underlie stimulant sensitization and tolerance, the role of nondopamine neurotransmitter systems (e.g., glutamate, neuropeptides) in modulating the dopamine reward circuit, the intracellular signaling cascades triggered by stimulant attachment to membrane binding sites, and the role of various genes and gene transcription factors in stimulant action.

Productive areas for clinical research include the genetic, hormonal, psychological, and environmental factors that influence response to stimulants and the progression to stimulant addiction and the development of effective treatments for stimulant addiction and its medical consequences.

ACKNOWLEDGMENTS: *Dr. Gorelick is supported by the Intramural Research Program, National Institutes of Health, National Institute on Drug Abuse.*

REFERENCES

1. Karch SB. *The pathology of drug abuse*, 2nd ed. Boca Raton, FL: CRC Press, 1996.
2. Karch SB. *A brief history of cocaine*, 2nd ed. Boca Raton, FL: CRC Press, 2006.
3. Montoya ID, Chilcoat HD. Epidemiology of coca derivatives use in the Andean Region: A tale of five countries. *Subst Use Misuse* 1996;31(10):1227–1240.
4. Masand PS, Tesar GE. Use of stimulants in the medically ill. *Psychiatr Clin North Am* 1996;19(3):515–547.
5. Anthony JC, Helzer JE. Epidemiology of drug dependence. In: Tsuang MT, Tohen M, Zahner GEP, eds. *Textbook in psychiatric epidemiology*. New York: Wiley-Liss, 1995:361–406.
6. United Nations Office on Drugs and Crime. *2007 world drug report*. United Nations publication E.07.XI.5. Vienna, Austria: Author, 2007.
7. Substance Abuse and Mental Health Services Administration, Office of Applied Studies. *Results from the 2006 National Survey on Drug Use and Health: national findings*. NSDUH Series H-32, DHHS Publication No. SMA 07-4293. Rockville, MD: Office of Applied Studies, 2007.
8. American Psychiatric Association. *Diagnostic and statistical manual of mental disorders*, 4th ed. (text rev.). *(DSM-IV-TR)*. Washington, DC: American Psychiatric Press. 2000.
9. Degenhardt L, Chiu WT, Sampson N, et al. Epidemiological patterns of extra-medical drug use in the United States: evidence from the National Comorbidity Survey Replication, 2001-2003. *Drug Alcohol Depend* 2007;90:210–223.
10. Degenhardt L, Chiu WT, Sampson N, et al. Toward a global view of alcohol, tobacco, cannabis, and cocaine use: findings from the WHO World Mental Health Surveys. *PLoS Med* 2008;5:e141.
11. Kandel DB, Huang FY, Davies M. Comorbidity between patterns of substance use dependence and psychiatric syndromes. *Drug Alcohol Depend* 2001;64(2):233–241.
12. Maxwell JC, Rutkowski BA. The prevalence of methamphetamine and amphetamine abuse in North America: a review of the indicators, 1992–2007. *Drug Alcohol Rev* 2008;27:229–235.
13. Substance Abuse and Mental Health Services Administration, Office of Applied Studies. *Drug Abuse Warning Network, 2005: national estimates*

of drug-related emergency department visits. DAWN Series D-29, DHHS Publication No. SMA, 07-4256. Rockville, MD: Author, 2007.

14. Substance Abuse and Mental Health Services Administration, Office of Applied Studies. *Drug Abuse Warning Network, 2003: area profiles of drug-related mortality.* DAWN Series D-27, DHHS Publication No. SMA, 05-4023. Rockville, MD: Author, 2005.
15. Substance Abuse and Mental Health Services Administration, Office of Applied Studies. *Treatment Episode Data Set (TEDS): 2005. discharges from substance abuse treatment services,* DASIS Series: S-41, DHHS Publication No. SMA, 08-4314. Rockville, MD: Author, 2008.
16. Moore JM, Casale JF. In-depth chromatographic analyses of illicit cocaine and its precursor, coca leaves. *J Chromatogr* 1994;674:165–205.
17. Fowler JS, Volkow ND, Wang G-J, et al. [11]Cocaine: PET studies of cocaine pharmacokinetics, dopamine transporter availability and dopamine transporter occupancy. *Nucl Med Biol* 2001;28:561–572.
18. United States Office of National Drug Control Policy. *Cocaine smuggling in 2006.* Report ONDCP-01-07. Washington, DC: Author, 2007.
19. U.S. Drug Enforcement Administration. *Cocaine price/purity analysis of STRIDE data.* Washington, DC: Author, 2008.
20. Bono JP. Criminalistics—introduction to controlled substances. In: Karch SB, ed. *Drug abuse handbook.* Boca Raton, FL: CRC Press, 1998:1–75.
21. Hatsukami DK, Fischman MW. Crack cocaine and cocaine hydrochloride: are the differences myth or reality? *JAMA* 1996;276(19):1580–1588.
22. Snyder CA, Wood RW, Graefe JF, et al. "Crack smoke" is a respirable aerosol of cocaine base. *Pharmacol Biochem Behav* 1988;29(1):93–95.
23. Shesser R, Jotte R, Olshaker J. 1991). The contribution of impurities to the acute morbidity of illegal drug use. *Am J Emerg Med* 9:336–342.
24. Richardson WH III, Slone CM, Michels JE. Herbal drugs of abuse: an emerging problem. *Emerg Med Clin North Am* 2007;25:435–457.
25. Yanovski SZ, Yanovski JA. Drug therapy: obesity. *N Engl J Med* 2002; 346:591–602.
26. Haller CA, Benowitz NL. Adverse cardiovascular and central nervous system events associated with dietary supplements containing ephedra alkaloids. *N Engl J Med* 2000;343(25):1833–1838.
27. Al-Habori M. The potential adverse effects of habitual use of Catha edulis (khat). *Expert Opin Drug Saf* 2005;4:1145–1154.
28. Hassan NA, Gunaid AA, Murray-Lyon IM. Khat (Catha edulis): health aspects of khat chewing. *East Mediterr Health J* 2007;13:706–718.
29. Fleckenstein AE, Gibb JW, Hanson GR. Differential effects of stimulants on monoaminergic transporters: pharmacological consequences and implications for neurotoxicity. *Eur J Pharmacol* 2000;406:1–13.
30. Faraone SV. Stimulant therapy in the management of ADHD: mixed amphetamine salts (extended release). *Expert Opin Pharmacother* 2007;8:2127–2134.
31. Parasrampuria DA, Schoedel KA, Schuller R, et al. Assessment of pharmacokinetics and pharmacodynamic effects related to abuse potential of a unique oral osmotic-controlled extended-release methylphenidate formulation in humans. *J Clin Pharmacol* 2007;47:1476–1488.
32. Arnold LE, Lindsay RL, Lopez FA, et al. Treating attention-deficit/hyperactivity disorder with a stimulant transdermal patch: the clinical art. *Pediatrics* 2007;120:1100–1106.
33. Blick SK, Keating GM. Lisdexamfetamine. *Paediatr Drugs* 2007;9: 129–135.
34. Faraone SV. Lisdexamfetamine dimesylate: the first long-acting prodrug stimulant treatment for attention deficit/hyperactivity disorder. *Expert Opin Pharmacother* 2008;9:1565–1574.
35. Gorelick DA. The rate hypothesis and agonist substitution approaches to cocaine abuse treatment. *Adv Pharmacol* 1998;42:995–997.
36. Baselt RC. *Disposition of toxic drugs and chemicals in man,* 7th ed. Foster City, CA: Chemical Toxicology Institute, 2004.
37. Cho AK. Melega WP. Patterns of methamphetamine abuse and their consequences. *J Addict Dis* 2002;21:21–34.
38. Ellenhorn MJ, Schonwald S, Ordog G, et al. *Ellenhorn's medical toxicology: diagnosis and treatment of human poisoning,* 2nd ed. Baltimore: Williams & Wilkins, 1997.
39. Ding Y-S, Fowler JS, Volkow ND, et al. Chiral drugs: comparison of the pharmacokinetics of [11C]*d-threo* and *l-threo*-methylphenidate in the human and baboon brain. *Psychopharmacology* 1997;131:71–78.
40. Harper SJ, Jones NS. Cocaine: what role does it have in current ENT practice? A review of the current literature. *J Laryngol Otol* 2006;120: 808–811.
41. Pliszka S. Practice parameter for the assessment and treatment of children and adolescents with attention-deficit/hyperactivity disorder. *J Am Acad Child Adolesc Psychiatry* 2007;46:894–921.
42. Harpin VA. Medication options when treating children and adolescents with ADHD: interpreting the NICE guidance 2006. *Arch Dis Child Educ Pract Ed* 2008;93:58–65.
43. Nutt DJ, Fone K, Asherson P, et al. Evidence-based guidelines for management of attention-deficit/hyperactivity disorder in adolescents in transition to adult services and in adults: recommendations from the British Association for Psychopharmacology. *J Psychopharmacol* 2007;21: 10–41.
44. Tcheremissine OV, Salazar JO. Pharmacotherapy of adult attention deficit/hyperactivity disorder: review of evidence-based practices and future directions. *Expert Opin Pharmacother* 2008;9:1299–1310.
45. Peterson K, McDonagh MS, Fu R. Comparative benefits and harms of competing medications for adults with attention-deficit hyperactivity disorder: a systematic review and indirect comparison meta-analysis. *Psychopharmacology (Berl)* 2008;197:1–11.
46. Banerjee D, Vitiello MV, Grunstein RR. Pharmacotherapy for excessive daytime sleepiness. *Sleep Med Rev* 2004;8:339–354.
47. Morgenthaler TI, Kapur VK, Brown T, et al. Practice parameters for the treatment of narcolepsy and other hypersomnias of central origin. *Sleep* 2007;30:1705–1711.
48. Greenway FL, Caruso MK. Safety of obesity drugs. *Expert Opin Drug Saf* 2005;4:1083–1095.
49. Mancini MC, Halpern A. Pharmacological treatment of obesity. *Arq Bras Endocrinol Metabol* 2006;50:377–389.
50. Homsi J, Walsh D, Nelson KA. Psychostimulants in supportive care. *Support Care Cancer* 2000;8:385–397.
51. Candy M, Jones L, Williams R, et al. Psychostimulants for depression. *Cochrane Database Syst Rev* 2008;CD006722.
52. Glenn MB. Methylphenidate for cognitive and behavioral dysfunction after traumatic brain injury. *J Head Trauma Rehab* 1998;13(5):87–90.
53. DeBattista C. Augmentation and combination strategies for depression. *J Psychopharmacol* 2006;20:11–18.
54. Martinsson L, Hardemark H, Eksborg S. Amphetamines for improving recovery after stroke. *Cochrane Database Syst Rev* 2007;CD002090.
55. Winterstein AG, Gerhard T, Shuster J, et al. Cardiac safety of central nervous system stimulants in children and adolescents with attention-deficit/hyperactivity disorder. *Pediatrics* 2007;120:e1494–e1501.
56. Volkow ND, Swanson JM. Does childhood treatment of ADHD with stimulant medication affect substance abuse in adulthood? *Am J Psychiatry* 2008;165:553–555.
57. Svetlov SI, Kobeissy FH, Gold MS. Performance enhancing, non-prescription use of Ritalin: a comparison with amphetamines and cocaine. *J Addict Dis* 2007;26:1–6.
58. Wilens TE, Adler LA, Adams J, et al. Misuse and diversion of stimulants prescribed for ADHD: a systematic review of the literature. *J Am Acad Child Adolesc Psychiatry* 2008;47:21–31.
59. Blanco C, Alderson D, Ogburn E, et al. Changes in the prevalence of non-medical prescription drug use and drug use disorders in the United States: 1991–1992 and 2001–2002. *Drug Alcohol Depend* 2007;90: 252–260.
60. United States Department of Defense. *2005 Department of Defense survey of health related behaviors among active duty military personnel.* Arlington, VA: Author, 2006.
61. McDuff DR, Baron D. Substance use in athletics: a sports psychiatry perspective. *Clin Sports Med* 2005;24:885–888x.
62. Avois L, Robinson N, Saudan C, et al. Central nervous system stimulants and sport practice. *Br J Sports Med* 2006;40(Suppl 1):i16–i20.
63. Jones G. Caffeine and other sympathomimetic stimulants: modes of action and effects on sports performance. *Essays Biochem* 2008;44: 109–123.
64. Docherty JR. Pharmacology of stimulants prohibited by the World Anti-Doping Agency (WADA). *Br J Pharmacol* 2008;154:606–622.

65. Anthony JC, Warner LA, Kessler RC. Comparative epidemiology of dependence on tobacco, alcohol, controlled substances, and inhalants: basic findings from the National Comorbidity Survey. *Exp Clin Psychopharmacol* 1994;2:244–268.
66. Woody GE, Cottler LB, Cacciola J. Severity of dependence: data from the DSM-IV field trials. *Addiction* 1993;88:1573–1579.
67. Gorelick DA. Progression of dependence in male cocaine addicts. *Am J Drug Alcohol Abuse* 1992;18:13–19.
68. Gossop M, Griffiths P, Powis B, et al. Cocaine: Patterns of use, route of administration, and severity of dependence. *Br J Psychiatry* 1994;164: 660–664.
69. Tinsley JA, Watkins DD. Over-the-counter stimulants: abuse and addiction. *Mayo Clin Proc* 1998;73:977–982.
70. Kendler KS, Myers J, Prescott CA. Specificity of genetic and environmental risk factors for symptoms of cannabis, cocaine, alcohol, caffeine, and nicotine dependence. *Arch Gen Psychiatry* 2007;64: 1313–1320.
71. Agrawal A, Lynskey MT. Are there genetic influences on addiction: evidence from family, adoption and twin studies. *Addiction* 2008;103: 1069–1081.
72. Uhl GR, Drgon T, Johnson C, et al. "Higher order" addiction molecular genetics: convergent data from genome-wide association in humans and mice. *Biochem Pharmacol* 2008;75:98–111.
73. Volkow ND, Fowler JS, Wang G-J. Imaging studies on the role of dopamine in cocaine reinforcement and addiction in humans. *J Psychopharmacol* 1999;13:337–345.
74. Nelson RA, Boyd SJ, Ziegelstein RC, et al. Effect of rate of administration on subjective and physiological effects of intravenous cocaine in humans. *Drug Alcohol Depend* 2006;82:19–24.
75. Levin FR, Hess JM, Gorelick DA, et al. Patterns of cocaine use among cocaine-dependent outpatients. *Am J Addict* 1993;2(2):109–115.
76. Myers MG, Rohsenow DJ, Monti PM, et al. Patterns of cocaine use among individuals in substance abuse treatment. *Am J Drug Alcohol Abuse* 1995;21(2):223–231.
77. United States Bureau of Justice Statistics. *Substance dependence, abuse, and treatment of jail inmates, 2002.* Report NCJ 209588. Washington, DC: Author, 2005.
78. Giannini AJ, Miller NS, Loiselle RH, et al. Cocaine-associated violence and relationship to route of administration. *J Subst Abuse Treat* 1993;10: 67–69.
79. Licata A, Taylor S, Berman M, et al. Effects of cocaine on human aggression. *Pharmacol Biochem Behav* 1993;45:549–552.
80. Miller NS, Gold MS, Mahler JC. Violent behaviors associated with cocaine use: possible pharmacological mechanisms. *Int J Addict* 1991;26(10):1077–1088.
81. Fukushima A. Criminal responsibility in amphetamine psychosis. *Jpn J Psychiatry Neurol* 1994;48(Suppl):1–4.
82. Sporer KA, Firestone J. Clinical course of crack cocaine body stuffers. *Ann Emerg Med* 1997;29:596–601.
83. Grella CE, Anglin MD, Wugalter SE. Patterns and predictors of cocaine and crack use by clients in standard and enhanced methadone maintenance treatment. *Am J Drug Alcohol Abuse* 1997;23:15–42.
84. Kreek MJ. Opiate and cocaine addictions: challenge for pharmacotherapies. *Pharmacol Biochem Behav* 1997;57:551–569.
85. Foltin RW, Fischman MW. Effects of methadone or buprenorphine maintenance on the subjective and reinforcing effects of intravenous cocaine in humans. *J Pharmacol Exp Ther* 1996;278:1153–1164.
86. Gorelick DA, Simmons MS, Carriero N, et al. Characteristics of smoked drug use among cocaine smokers. *Am J Addict* 1997;6:237–245.
87. Cone EJ, Tsadik A, Oyler J, et al. Cocaine metabolism and urinary excretion after different routes of administration. *Ther Drug Monit* 1998;20:556–560.
88. Telang FW, Volkow ND, Levy A, et al. Distribution of tracer levels of cocaine in the human brain as assessed with averaged [11C]cocaine images. *Synapse* 1999;31:290–296.
89. Volkow ND, Wang G-J, Fowler JS, et al. Cocaine uptake is decreased in the brain of detoxified cocaine abusers. *Neuropsychopharmacology* 1996;14(3):159–168.
90. Jenkins AJ, Cone EJ. Pharmacokinetics: drug absorption, distribution, and elimination. In: Karch SB, ed. *Drug abuse handbook.* Boca Raton, FL: CRC Press, 1998:151–201.
91. Jackson GF, Saady JJ, Poklis A. Urinary excretion of benzoylecgonine following ingestion of health Inca tea. *Forens Sci Int* 1991;49:57–64.
92. Kavanagh KT, Maijub AG, Brown JR. Passive exposure to cocaine in medical personnel and its effect on urine drug screening tests. *Otolaryngol Head Neck Surg* 1992;107:363–366.
93. Cone EJ, Yousefnejad D, Hillsgrove MJ, et al. Passive inhalation of cocaine. *J Anal Toxicol* 1995;19:399–411.
94. Le SD, Taylor RW, Vidal D, et al. Occupational exposure to cocaine involving crime lab personnel. *J Forens Sci* 1992;37(4):959–968.
95. Mott SH, Packer RJ, Soldin SJ. Neurologic manifestations of cocaine exposure in childhood. *Pediatrics* 1994;93(4):557–560.
96. Mirchandani HG, Mirchandani IH, Hellman F, et al. Passive inhalation of free-base cocaine ('crack') smoke by infants. *Arch Pathol Lab Med* 1991;115:494–498.
97. Bruns AD, Zieske LA, Jacobs AJ. Analysis of the cocaine metabolite in the urine of patients and physicians during clinical use. *Otolaryngol Head Neck Surg* 1994;111(6):722–726.
98. Verstraete AG. Detection times of drugs of abuse in blood, urine, and oral fluid. *Ther Drug Monit* 2004;26:200–205.
99. Musshoff F, Driever F, Lachenmeier K, et al. Results of hair analyses for drugs of abuse and comparison with self-reports and urine tests. *Foren Sci Int* 2006;156:118–123.
100. Boumba VA, Ziavrou KS, Vougiouklakis T. Hair as a biological indicator of drug use, drug abuse or chronic exposure to environmental toxicants. *Int J Toxicol* 2006;25:143–163.
101. Moore C, Coulter C, Crompton K. Determination of cocaine, benzoylecgonine, cocaethylene and norcocaine in human hair using solid-phase extraction and liquid chromatography with tandem mass spectrometric detection. *J Chromatogr B Analyt Technol Biomed Life Sci* 2007;859:208–212.
102. Follador MJ, Yonamine M, de Moraes Moreau RL, Silva OA. Detection of cocaine and cocaethylene in sweat by solid-phase microextraction and gas chromatography/mass spectrometry. *J Chromatogr B Analyt Technol Biomed Life Sci* 2004;811:37–40.
103. Pil K, Verstraete A. Current developments in drug testing in oral fluid. *Ther Drug Monit* 2008;30:196–202.
104. Cone EJ, Huestis MA. Interpretation of oral fluid tests for drugs of abuse. *Ann N Y Acad Sci* 2007;1098:51–103.
105. Samyn N, Laloup M, De BG. Bioanalytical procedures for determination of drugs of abuse in oral fluid. *Anal Bioanal Chem* 2007;388: 1437–1453.
106. Gray T, Huestis M. Bioanalytical procedures for monitoring in utero drug exposure. *Anal Bioanal Chem* 2007;388:1455–1465.
107. American Academy of Pediatrics, Committee on Drugs. The transfer of drugs and other chemicals into human milk. *Pediatrics* 2001;108(3): 776–789.
108. Caplan YH, Goldberger BA. Alternative specimens for workplace drug testing. *J Anal Toxicol* 2001;25(5):396–399.
109. Drummer OH. Postmortem toxicology of drugs of abuse. *Forens Sci Int* 2004;142:101–113.
110. Cone EJ. Pharmacokinetics and pharmacodynamics of cocaine. *J Anal Toxicol* 1995;19:459–478.
111. Warner A, Norman AB. Mechanisms of cocaine hydrolysis and metabolism in vitro and in vivo: a clarification. *Ther Drug Monit* 2000;22:266–270.
112. Maurer HH, Sauer C, Theobald DS. Toxicokinetics of drugs of abuse: current knowledge of the isozymes involved in the human metabolism of tetrahydrocannabinol, cocaine, heroin, morphine, and codeine. *Ther Drug Monit* 2006;28:447–453.
113. Wang J, Carpentier RG. Electrophysiologic in-vitro effects of cocaine and its metabolites. *Int J Cardiol* 1994;46:235–242.
114. Gorelick DA. Pharmacokinetic approaches to treatment of drug addiction. *Expert Rev Clin Pharmacol* 2008;1(2):277–290.
115. de la Torre R, Farre M, Navarro M, et al. Clinical pharmacokinetics of amfetamine and related substances: monitoring in conventional and non-conventional matrices. *Clin Pharmacokinet* 2004;43:157–185.

116. Braithwaite RA, Jarvie DR, Minty PSB, et al. Screening for drugs of abuse: I. Opiates, amphetamines and cocaine. *Ann Clin Biochem* 1995;32:123–153.
117. Pennings EJ, Leccese AP, Wolff FA. Effects of concurrent use of alcohol and cocaine. *Addiction* 2002;97:773–783.
118. Baker J, Jatlow P, Pade P, et al. Acute cocaine responses following cocaethylene infusion. *Am J Drug Alcohol Abuse* 2007;33:619–625.
119. Harris DS, Everhart ET, Mendelson J, Jones RT. The pharmacology of cocaethylene in humans following cocaine and ethanol administration. *Drug Alcohol Depend* 2003;72:169–182.
120. Romanelli F, Smith KM. Clinical effects and management of methamphetamine abuse. *Pharmacotherapy* 2006;26:1148–1156.
121. Angrist B. Clinical effects of central nervous system stimulants: a selective update. In: Engel J, Oreland L, Ingvar DH, et al., eds. *Brain reward systems and abuse.* New York: Raven Press, 1987:109–127.
122. Baselt RC. *Drug effects on psychomotor performance.* Foster City, CA: Biomedical Publications, 2001.
123. Fischman MW, Foltin RW. Cocaine self-administration research: Implications for rational pharmacotherapy. In: Higgins ST, Katz JL, eds. *Cocaine abuse: behavior, pharmacology, and clinical applications.* San Diego: Academic Press, 1998:181–207.
124. Heishman SJ. Effects of abused drugs on human performance: laboratory assessment. In: Karch SB, ed. *Drug abuse handbook.* Boca Raton, FL: CRC Press, 1998:206–235.
125. Hando J, Topp L, Hall W. Amphetamine-related harms and treatment preferences of regular amphetamine users in Sydney, Australia. *Drug Alcohol Depend* 1997;46:105–113.
126. Williamson S, Gossop M, Powis B, et al. Adverse effects of stimulant drugs in a community sample of drug users. *Drug Alcohol Depend* 1997;44:87–94.
127. Cubells JF, McCance-Katz EF, Grieg T, et al. Phenotypic assessment of cocaine-induced paranoia and psychotic symptoms (CIPPS). *Biol Psychiatry* 2000;47(Suppl):167S–168S.
128. Hall W, Hando J, Darke S, et al. Psychological morbidity and route of administration among amphetamine users in Sydney, Australia. *Addiction* 1996;91(1):81–87.
129. Serper MR, Chou JC, Allen MH, et al. Symptomatic overlap of cocaine intoxication and acute schizophrenia at emergency presentation. *Schizophr Bull* 1999;25(2):387–394.
130. Harris D, Batki SL. Stimulant psychosis: symptom profile and acute clinical course. *Am J Addict* 2000;9(1):28–37.
131. Thirthalli J, Benegal V. Psychosis among substance users. *Curr Opin Psychiatry* 2006;19:239–245.
132. Featherstone RE, Kapur S, Fletcher PJ. The amphetamine-induced sensitized state as a model of schizophrenia. *Prog Neuropsychopharmacol Biol Psychiatry* 2007;31:1556–1571.
133. Mahoney JJ III, Kalechstein AD, De La GR, Newton TF. Presence and persistence of psychotic symptoms in cocaine- versus methamphetamine-dependent participants. *Am J Addict* 2008;17:83–98.
134. Fasano A, Barra A, Nicosia P, et al. Cocaine addiction: from habits to stereotypical-repetitive behaviors and punding. *Drug Alcohol Depend* 2008;96:178–182.
135. Laviola G, Adriani W, Terranova ML, et al. Psychobiological risk factors for vulnerability to psychostimulants in human adolescents and animal models. *Neurosci Biobehav Rev* 1999;23:993–1010.
136. LeSage MG, Stafford D, Glowa JR. Preclinical research on cocaine self-administration: environmental determinants and their interaction with pharmacological treatment. *Neurosci Biobehavl Rev* 1999;23:717–741.
137. Elmer GI, Miner LL, Pickens RW. The contribution of genetic factors in cocaine and other drug abuse. In: Higgins ST, Katz JL, eds. *Cocaine abuse: behavior, pharmacology, and clinical applications.* San Diego: Academic Press, 1998:289–311.
138. O'Brien CP, Gardner EL. Critical assessment of how to study addiction and its treatment: human and non-human animal models. *Pharmacol Ther* 2005;108:18–58.
139. Blaho K, Logan B, Winbery S, et al. Blood cocaine and metabolite concentrations, clinical findings, and outcome of patients presenting to an ED. *Am J Emerg Med* 2000;18(5):593–598.
140. Stephens BG, Jentzen JM, Karch S, et al. Criteria for the interpretation of cocaine levels in human biological samples and their relation to the cause of death. *Am J Forensic Med Pathol* 2004;25:1–10.
141. Rogers RD, Robbins TW. Investigating the neurocognitive deficits associated with chronic drug misuse. *Curr Opin Neurobiol* 2001;11: 250–257.
142. Yucel M, Lubman DI, Solowij N, Brewer WJ. Understanding drug addiction: a neuropsychological perspective. *Aust N Z J Psychiatry* 2007;41:957–968.
143. Lim KO, Wozniak JR, Mueller BA, et al. Brain macrostructural and microstructural abnormalities in cocaine dependence. *Drug Alcohol Depend* 2008;92:164–172.
144. Magalhaes AC. Functional magnetic resonance and spectroscopy in drug and substance abuse. *Top Magn Reson Imaging* 2005;16:247–251.
145. Flaum M, Schultz SK. When does amphetamine-induced psychosis become schizophrenia? *Am J Psychiatry* 1996;153(6):812–815.
146. Yui K, Ishiguro T, Goto K. et al. Factors affecting the development of spontaneous recurrence of methamphetamine psychosis. *Acta Psychiatr Scand* 1998;97:220–227.
147. Buffenstein A, Heaster J, Ko P. Chronic psychotic illness from methamphetamine. *Am J Psychiatry* 1999;156(4):662.
148. Satel SL, Seibyl JP, Charney DS. Prolonged cocaine psychosis implies underlying major psychopathology. *J Clin Psychiatry* 1991;52(8): 349–350.
149. Coffey SF, Dansky BS, Carrigan MH. et al. Acute and protracted cocaine abstinence in an outpatient population: a prospective study of mood, sleep and withdrawal symptoms. *Drug Alcohol Depend* 2000;59:277–286.
150. Cottler LB, Shillington AM, Compton WM III, et al. Subjective reports of withdrawal among cocaine users: Recommendations for *DSM-IV. Drug Alcohol Depend* 1993;33:97–104.
151. Lago JA, Kosten TR. Stimulant withdrawal. *Addiction* 1994;89:1477–1481.
152. Morgan PT, Malison RT. Cocaine and sleep: early abstinence. *Sci World J* 2007;7:223–230.
153. Satel SL, Price LH, Palumbo JM, et al. Clinical phenomenology and neurobiology of cocaine abstinence: a prospective inpatient study. *Am J Psychiatry* 1991;148:1712–1716.
154. Pilotte NS. Neurochemistry of cocaine withdrawal. *Curr Opin Neurol* 1997;10:534–538.
155. Sharpe LG, Pilotte NS, Shippenberg TS, et al. Autoradiographic evidence that prolonged withdrawal from intermittent cocaine reduces mu-opioid receptor expression in limbic regions of the rat brain. *Synapse* 2000;37:292–297.
156. Kuhar MJ, Pilotte NS. Neurochemical changes in cocaine withdrawal. *Trends Pharmacol Sci* 1996;17:260–264.
157. Wu JC, Bell K, Najafi A, et al. Decreasing striatal 6-FDOPA uptake with increasing duration of cocaine withdrawal. *Neuropsychopharmacology* 1997;17:402–409.
158. Malison RT, Best SE, van Dyck CH, et al. Elevated striatal dopamine transporters during acute cocaine abstinence as measured by [$^{123}\beta$]beta-CIT SPECT. *Am J Psychiatry* 1998;155:832–834.
159. Little KY, McLaughlin DP, Zhang L, et al. Brain dopamine transporter messenger RNA and binding sites in cocaine users. *Arch Gen Psychiatry* 1998;55:793–799.
160. Glennon RA. Arylalkylamine drugs of abuse: an overview of drug discrimination studies. *Pharmacol Biochem Behav* 1999;64(2):251–256.
161. Kollins SH, MacDonald EK, Rush CR. Assessing the abuse potential of methylphenidate in nonhuman and human subjects. A review. *Pharmacol Biochem Behav* 2001;68:611–627.
162. Preston KL, Walsh SL. Evaluating abuse liability: methods and predictive value. In: Karch SB, ed. *Drug abuse handbook.* Boca Raton, FL: CRC Press, 1998:276–306.
163. Bergman J, Katz JL. Behavioral pharmacology of cocaine and the determinants of abuse liability. In: Higgins ST, Katz JL, eds. *Cocaine abuse: behavior, pharmacology, and clinical applications.* San Diego, CA: Academic Press, 1998:51–79.
164. Bossert JM, Ghitza UE, Lu L, et al. Neurobiology of relapse to heroin and cocaine seeking: an update and clinical implications. *Eur J Pharmacol* 2005;526:36–50.

165. Heishman SJ, Henningfield JE. Discriminative stimulus effects of *d*-amphetamine, methylphenidate, and diazepam in humans. *Psychopharmacology* 1991;103:436–442.
166. Reid MS, Flammino F, Howard B, et al. Topographic imaging of quantitative EEG in response to smoked cocaine self-administration in humans. *Neuropsychopharmacology* 2006;31:872–884.
167. Boghdadi MS, Henning RJ. Cocaine: pathophysiology and clinical toxicology. *Heart Lung* 1997;26:466–483.
168. Brust JCM. Acute neurologic complications of drug and alcohol abuse. *Neurol Clin North Am* 1998;16(2):503–519.
169. Neiman J, Haapaniemi HM, Hillbom M. Neurological complications of drug abuse: pathophysiological mechanisms. *Eur J Neurol* 2000;7:595–606.
170. O'Connor AD, Rusyniak DE, Bruno A. Cerebrovascular and cardiovascular complications of alcohol and sympathomimetic drug abuse. *Med Clin North Am* 2005;89:1343–1358.
171. Darke S, Kaye S, Duflou J. Comparative cardiac pathology among deaths due to cocaine toxicity, opioid toxicity and non-drug-related causes. *Addiction* 2006;101:1771–1777.
172. Treadwell SD, Robinson TG. Cocaine use and stroke. *Postgrad Med J* 2007;83:389–394.
173. Westover AN, McBride S, Haley RW. Stroke in young adults who abuse amphetamines or cocaine: a population-based study of hospitalized patients. *Arch Gen Psychiatry* 2007;64:495–502.
174. Kernan WN, Viscoli CM, Brass LM. et al. Phenylpropanolamine and the risk of hemorrhagic stroke. *N Engl J Med* 2000;343(25): 1826–1832.
175. Warner EA. Cocaine abuse. *Ann Intern Med* 1993;119:226–235.
176. van Harten PN, van Trier JCAM, Horwitz EH, et al. Cocaine as a risk factor for neuroleptic-induced acute dystonia. *J Clin Psychiatry* 1998;59: 128–130.
177. Afonso L, Mohammad T, Thatai D. Crack whips the heart: a review of the cardiovascular toxicity of cocaine. *Am J Cardiol* 2007;100: 1040–1043.
178. Sofuoglu M, Nelson D, Babb DA, et al. Intravenous cocaine increases plasma epinephrine and norepinephrine in humans. *Pharmacol Biochem Behav* 2001;68:455–459.
179. Volkow ND, Wang GJ, Fowler JS, et al. Cardiovascular effects of methylphenidate in humans are associated with increases of dopamine in brain and of epinephrine in plasma. *Psychopharmacology (Berl)* 2003;166:264–270.
180. Vongpatanasin W, Mansour Y, Chavoshan B, et al. Cocaine stimulates the human cardiovascular system via a central mechanism of action. *Circulation* 1999;100:497–502.
181. Qureshi AI, Suri FK, Guterman LR, et al. Cocaine use and the likelihood of nonfatal myocardial infarction and stroke. *Circulation* 2001;103:502–506.
182. Lange RA, Hillis LD. Cardiovascular complications of cocaine use. *N Engl J Med* 2001;345(5):351–358.
183. Ghuran A, Nolan J. Recreational drug misuse: issues for the cardiologist. *Heart* 2000;83:627–633.
184. Yeo KK, Wijetunga M, Ito H, et al. The association of methamphetamine use and cardiomyopathy in young patients. *Am J Med* 2007;120: 165–171.
185. Glauser J, Queen JR. An overview of non-cardiac cocaine toxicity. *J Emerg Med* 2007;32:181–186.
186. Tashkin DP. Airway effects of marijuana, cocaine, and other inhaled illicit agents. *Curr Opin Pulm Med* 2001;7:43–61.
187. Wolff AJ, O'Donnell AE. Pulmonary effects of illicit drug use. *Clin Chest Med* 2004;25:203–216.
188. Restrepo CS, Carrillo JA, Martinez S, et al. Pulmonary complications from cocaine and cocaine-based substances: imaging manifestations. *Radiographics* 2007;27:941–956.
189. Wilson KC, Saukkonen JJ. Acute respiratory failure from abused substances. *J Intensive Care Med* 2004;19:183–193.
190. Gitman MD, Singhal PC. Cocaine-induced renal disease. *Expert Opin Drug Saf* 2004;3:441–448.
191. Bemanian S, Motallebi M, Nosrati SM. Cocaine-induced renal infarction: report of a case and review of the literature. *BMC Nephrol* 2005;6:10.
192. Jaffe JA, Kimmel PL. Chronic nephropathies of cocaine and heroin abuse: a critical review. *Clin J Am Soc Nephrol* 2006;1:655–667.
193. Hagan IG, Burney K. Radiology of recreational drug abuse. *Radiographics* 2007;27:919–940.
194. Marotta PJ, Roberts EA. Pemoline hepatotoxicity in children. *J Pediatr* 1998;132:894–897.
195. Mello NK, Mendelson JH. Cocaine's effects on neuroendocrine systems: clinical and preclinical studies. *Pharmacol Biochem Behav* 1997; 57(3):571–599.
196. Warner EA, Greene GS, Buchsbaum MS, et al. Diabetic ketoacidosis associated with cocaine use. *Arch Intern Med* 1998;158:1799–1802.
197. Nyenwe EA, Loganathan RS, Blum S, et al. Active use of cocaine: an independent risk factor for recurrent diabetic ketoacidosis in a city hospital. *Endocr Pract* 2007;13:22–29.
198. Doctora JS, Williams CW, Bennett CR, Howlett BK. Rhabdomyolysis in the acutely cocaine-intoxicated patient sustaining maxillofacial trauma: report of a case and review of the literature. *J Oral Maxillofac Surg* 2003;61:964–967.
199. Goodger NM, Wang J, Pogrel MA. Palatal and nasal necrosis resulting from cocaine misuse. *Br Dent J* 2005;198:333–334.
200. Gordon AS, Moran DT, Jafek BW, et al. The effect of chronic cocaine abuse on human olfaction. *Arch Otolaryngol Head Neck Surg* 1990;116: 1415–1418.
201. Hamner JE 3rd, Villegas OL. The effect of coca leaf chewing on the buccal mucosa of Aymara and Quechua Indians in Bolivia. *Oral Surg Oral Med Oral Pathol* 1969;28:287–295.
202. Ghosheh FR, Ehlers JP, Ayres BD, et al. Corneal ulcers associated with aerosolized crack cocaine use. *Cornea* 2007;26:966–969.
203. Pallasch TJ, Joseph CE. Oral manifestations of drug abuse. *J Psychoactive Drugs* 1987;19(4):375–377.
204. Bhinder SK, Majithia V. Cocaine use and its rheumatic manifestations: a case report and discussion. *Clin Rheumatol* 2007;26:1192–1194.
205. Peikert T, Finkielman JD, Hummel AM, et al. Functional characterization of antineutrophil cytoplasmic antibodies in patients with cocaine-induced midline destructive lesions. *Arthritis Rheum* 2008;58: 1546–1551.
206. Irwin MR, Olmos L, Wang M, et al. Cocaine dependence and acute cocaine induce decreases of monocyte proinflammatory cytokine expression across the diurnal period: autonomic mechanisms. *J Pharmacol Exp Ther* 2007;320:507–515.
207. Carey JC. Pharmacological effects on sexual function. *Obstet Gynecol Clin North Am* 2006;33:599–620.
208. Palha AP, Esteves M. Drugs of abuse and sexual functioning. *Adv Psychosom Med* 2008;29:131–149.
209. Chiriboga CA. Fetal alcohol and drug effects. *Neurologist* 2003;9: 267–279.
210. Kuczkowski KM. The effects of drug abuse on pregnancy. *Curr Opin Obstet Gynecol* 2007;19:578–585.
211. Phupong V, Darojn D. Amphetamine abuse in pregnancy: the impact on obstetric outcome. *Arch Gynecol Obstet* 2007;276:167–170.
212. Williams JH, Ross L. Consequences of prenatal toxin exposure for mental health in children and adolescents: a systematic review. *Eur Child Adolesc Psychiatry* 2007;16:243–253.
213. Schama KF, Howell LL, Byrd LD. Prenatal exposure to cocaine. In: Higgins ST. Katz JL, eds. *Cocaine abuse: behavior, pharmacology, and clinical applications.* San Diego: Academic Press, 1998:159–179.
214. Fleckenstein AE, Volz TJ, Riddle EL, et al. New insights into the mechanism of action of amphetamines. *Annu Rev Pharmacol Toxicol* 2007;47: 681–698.
215. Howell LL, Kimmel HL. Monoamine transporters and psychostimulant addiction. *Biochem Pharmacol* 2008;75:196–217.
216. Beuming T, Kniazeff J, Bergmann ML, et al. The binding sites for cocaine and dopamine in the dopamine transporter overlap. *Nat Neurosci* 2008;11:780–789.
217. Volkow ND, Fowler JS, Wang GJ, et al. Imaging dopamine's role in drug abuse and addiction. *Neuropharmacology* 2008. In press.
218. Goodman A. Neurobiology of addiction. An integrative review. *Biochem Pharmacol* 2008;75:266–322.

219. Little KY, Patel UN, Clark TB, et al. Alteration of brain dopamine and serotonin levels in cocaine users: A preliminary report. *Am J Psychiatry* 1996;153(9):1216–1218.
220. Meador-Woodruff JH, Little KY, Damask SP, et al. Effects of cocaine on D3 and D4 expression in the human striatum. *Biol Psychiatry* 1995;38:263–266.
221. Little KY, Krolewski DM, Zhang L, Cassin BJ. Loss of striatal vesicular monoamine transporter protein (VMAT2) in human cocaine users. *Am J Psychiatry* 2003;160:47–55.
222. Qin Y, Ouyang Q, Pablo J, Mash DC. Cocaine abuse elevates alpha-synuclein and dopamine transporter levels in the human striatum. *Neureport* 2005;16:1489–1493.
223. Letchworth SR, Nader MA, Smith HR, et al. Progression of changes in dopamine transporter binding site density as a result of cocaine self-administration in rhesus monkeys. *J Neurosci* 2001;21:2799–2807.
224. Wilson JM, Levey AI, Bergeron C, et al. Striatal dopamine, dopamine transporter, and vesicular monoamine transporter in chronic cocaine users. *Ann Neurol* 1996;40:428–439.
225. Martinez D, Kim JH, Krystal J, bi-Dargham A. Imaging the neurochemistry of alcohol and substance abuse. *Neuroimag Clin North Am* 2007;17:539–555.
226. Worsley JN, Moszczynska A, Falardeau P, et al. Dopamine D_1 receptor protein is elevated in nucleus accumbens of human, chronic methamphetamine users. *Mol Psychiatry* 2000;5:664–672.
227. Sekine Y, Iyo M, Ouchi Y, et al. Methamphetamine-related psychiatric symptoms and reduced brain dopamine transporters studied with PET. *Am J Psychiatry* 2001;158(8):1206–1214.
228. Anderson SM, Pierce RC. Cocaine-induced alterations in dopamine receptor signaling: implications for reinforcement and reinstatement. *Pharmacol Ther* 2005;106:389–403.
229. Wee S, Carroll FI, Woolverton WL. A reduced rate of in vivo dopamine transporter binding is associated with lower relative reinforcing efficacy of stimulants. *Neuropsychopharmacology* 2006;31:351–362.
230. Kimmel HL, O'Connor JA, Carroll FI, Howell LL. Faster onset and dopamine transporter selectivity predict stimulant and reinforcing effects of cocaine analogs in squirrel monkeys. *Pharmacol Biochem Behav* 2007;86:45–54.
231. Weinshenker D, Schroeder JP. There and back again: a tale of norepinephrine and drug addiction. *Neuropsychopharmacology* 2007;32:1433–1451.
232. Chen R, Tilley MR, Wei H, et al. Abolished cocaine reward in mice with a cocaine-insensitive dopamine transporter. *Proc Natl Acad Sci U S A* 2006;103:9333–9338.
233. Tilley MR, Cagniard B, Zhuang X, et al. Cocaine reward and locomotion stimulation in mice with reduced dopamine transporter expression. *BMC Neurosci* 2007;8:42.
234. Tilley MR, Gu HH. Dopamine transporter inhibition is required for cocaine-induced stereotypy. *Neuroreport* 2008;19:1137–1140.
235. Filip M, Frankowska M, Zaniewska M, et al. The serotonergic system and its role in cocaine addiction. *Pharmacol Rep* 2005;57:685–700.
236. Carboni E, Silvagni A. Dopamine reuptake by norepinephrine neurons: exception or rule? *Crit Rev Neurobiol* 2004;16:121–128.
237. Koob GF. The role of the striatopallidal and extended amygdala systems in drug addiction. *Ann N Y Acad Sci* 1999;877:445–460.
238. Pierre PJ, Vezina P. D_1 dopamine receptor blockade prevents the facilitation of amphetamine self-administration induced by prior exposure to the drug. *Psychopharmacology* 1998;138:159–166.
239. Ranaldi R, Wise RA. Blockade of D1 dopamine receptors in the ventral tegmental area decreases cocaine reward: possible role for dendritically released dopamine. *J Neurosci* 2001;21(15):5841–5846.
240. Caine SB, Thomsen M, Gabriel KI, et al. Lack of self-administration of cocaine in dopamine D1 receptor knock-out mice. *J Neurosci* 2007;27:13140–13150.
241. Zhang J, Xu M. Toward a molecular understanding of psychostimulant actions using genetically engineered dopamine receptor knockout mice as model systems. *J Adict Dis* 2001;20:7–18.
242. Buckley PF. Substance abuse in schizophrenia: a review. *J Clin Psychiatry* 1998;59:26–30.
243. Brauer LH, de Wit H. High dose pimozide does not block amphetamine-induced euphoria in normal volunteers. *Pharmacol Biochem Behav* 1997;56:265–272.
244. Kuhar MJ, Ritz MC, Boja JW. The dopamine hypothesis of the reinforcing properties of cocaine. *Trends Neurosci* 1991;14:299–302.
245. Stine SM, Krystal JH, Petrakis IL, et al. Effect of alpha-methylpara-tyrosine on response to cocaine challenge. *Biol Psychiatry* 1997;42:181–190.
246. Rothman RB, Baumann MH, Dersch CM, et al. Amphetamine-type central nervous system stimulants release norepinephrine more potently than they release dopamine and serotonin. *Synapse* 2001;39:32–41.
247. Mash DC, Ouyang Q, Qin Y, Pablo J. Norepinephrine transporter immunoblotting and radioligand binding in cocaine abusers. *J Neurosci Methods* 2005;143:79–85.
248. Muller CP, Carey RJ, Huston JP, et al. Serotonin and psychostimulant addiction: focus on 5-HT_{1A}-receptors. *Prog Neurobiol* 2007;81:133–178.
249. Horne MK, Lee J, Chen F, et al. Long term administration of cocaine or serotonin reuptake inhibitors results in anatomical and neurochemical changes in noradrenergic, dopaminergic and serotonin pathways. *J Neurochem* 2008;106:1731–1734.
250. Wang G-J, Volkow ND, Logan J, et al. Serotonin 5-HT_2 receptor availability in chronic cocaine abusers. *Life Sci* 1995;56:PL299–PL303.
251. Muller CP, Huston JP. Determining the region-specific contributions of 5-HT receptors to the psychostimulant effects of cocaine. *Trends Pharmacol Sci* 2006;27:105–112.
252. Buydens-Branchey L, Branchey M, Fergeson P, et al. Craving for cocaine in addicted users: Role of serotonergic mechanisms. *Am J Addict* 1997;6:65–73.
253. Walsh SL, Cunningham KA. Serotonergic mechanisms involved in the discriminative stimulus, reinforcing and subjective effects of cocaine. *Psychopharmacology* 1997;130:41–58.
254. Unterwald EM. Regulation of opioid receptors by cocaine. *Ann N Y Acad Sci* 2001;937:74–92.
255. Gorelick DA, Kim YK, Bencherif B, et al. Imaging brain mu-opioid receptors in abstinent cocaine users: time course and relation to cocaine craving. *Biol Psychiatry* 2005;57:1573–1582.
256. Staley JK, Rothman RB, Rice KC, et al. κ_2 Opioid receptors in limbic areas of the human brain are upregulated by cocaine in fatal overdose victims. *J Neurosci* 1997;17:8225–8233.
257. Shippenberg TS, Zapata A, Chefer VI. Dynorphin and the pathophysiology of drug addiction. *Pharmacol Ther* 2007;116: 306–321.
258. Gass JT, Olive MF. Glutamatergic substrates of drug addiction and alcoholism. *Biochem Pharmacol* 2008;75:218–265.
259. Garcia-Rates S, Camarasa J, Escubedo E, Pubill D. Methamphetamine and 3,4-methylenedioxymethamphetamine interact with central nicotinic receptors and induce their up-regulation. *Toxicol Appl Pharmacol* 2007;223:195–205.
260. Williams MJ, Adinoff B. The role of acetylcholine in cocaine addiction. *Neuropsychopharmacology* 2008;33:1779–1797.
261. Hussain RJ, Taraschenko OD, Glick SD. Effects of nicotine, methamphetamine and cocaine on extracellular levels of acetylcholine in the interpeduncular nucleus of rats. *Neurosci Lett* 2008;440:270–274.
262. Rada P, Hernandez L, Hoebel BG. Feeding and systemic D-amphetamine increase extracellular acetylcholine in the medial thalamus: a possible reward enabling function. *Neurosci Lett* 2007;416:184–187.
263. Carrigan KA, Dykstra LA. Behavioral effects of morphine and cocaine in M1 muscarinic acetylcholine receptor-deficient mice. *Psychopharmacology (Berl)* 2007;191:985–993.
264. Mark GP, Kinney AE, Grubb MC, et al. Injection of oxotremorine in nucleus accumbens shell reduces cocaine but not food self-administration in rats. *Brain Res* 2006;1123:51–59.
265. Zanetti L, Picciotto MR, Zoli M. Differential effects of nicotinic antagonists perfused into the nucleus accumbens or the ventral tegmental area on cocaine-induced dopamine release in the nucleus accumbens of mice. *Psychopharmacology (Berl)* 2007;190:189–199.

266. Takamatsu Y, Yamanishi Y, Hagino Y, et al. Differential effects of donepezil on methamphetamine and cocaine dependencies. *Ann N Y Acad Sci* 2006;1074:418–426.
267. Grasing K, He S, Yang Y. Dose-related effects of the acetylcholinesterase inhibitor tacrine on cocaine and food self-administration in rats. *Psychopharmacology (Berl)* 2008;196:133–142.
268. Rothman RB, Baumann MH. Neurochemical mechanisms of phentermine and fenfluramine: therapeutic and adverse effects. *Drug Dev Res* 2000;51:52–65.
269. McGinty JF, Shi XD, Schwendt M, et al. Regulation of psychostimulant-induced signaling and gene expression in the striatum. *J Neurochem* 2008;104:1440–1449.
270. Lu L, Koya E, Zhai H, et al. Role of ERK in cocaine addiction. *Trends Neurosci* 2006;29:695–703.
271. Stipanovich A, Valjent E, Matamales M, et al. A phosphatase cascade by which rewarding stimuli control nucleosomal response. *Nature* 2008;453:879–884.
272. Yano M, Steiner H. Methylphenidate and cocaine: the same effects on gene regulation? *Trends Pharmacol Sci* 2007;28:588–596.
273. Yuferov V, Nielsen D, Butelman E, Kreek MJ. Microarray studies of psychostimulant-induced changes in gene expression. *Addict Biol* 2005;10:101–118.
274. Hemby SE. Assessment of genome and proteome profiles in cocaine abuse. *Prog Brain Res* 2006;158:173–195.
275. Kalivas PW. Neurobiology of cocaine addiction: implications for new pharmacotherapy. *Am J Addict* 2007;16:71–78.
276. Lingford-Hughes A. Human brain imaging and substance abuse. *Curr Opin Pharmacol* 2005;5:42–46.
277. Koob GF. Drug addiction: the yin and yang of hedonic homeostasis. *Neuron* 1996;16:893–896.
278. Schenk S, Partridge B. Sensitization and tolerance in psychostimulant self-administration. *Pharmacol Biochem Behav* 1997;57(3):543–550.
279. Robinson TE, Berridge KC. The psychology and neurobiology of addiction: an incentive-sensitization view. *Addiction* 2000;95:S91–S117.
280. Ferger B, Stahl D, Kuschinsky K. Effects of cocaine on the EEG power spectrum of rats are significantly altered after its repeated administration: do they reflect sensitization phenomena? *Naunyn Schmiedebergs Arch Pharmacol* 1996;353:545–551.
281. Vanderschuren LJMJ, Schmidt ED, De Vries TJ, et al. A single exposure to amphetamine is sufficient to induce long-term behavioral, neuroendocrine, and neurochemical sensitization in rats. *J Neurosci* 1999;19(21): 9579–9586.
282. Bonate PL, Swann A, Silverman PB. Context-dependent cross-sensitization between cocaine and amphetamine. *Life Sci* 1997;60(1):PL1–PL7.
283. Gaytan O, Yang P, Swann A, et al. Diurnal differences in sensitization to methylphenidate. *Brain Res* 2000;864:24–39.
284. Vanderschuren LJMJ, Kalivas PW. Alterations in dopaminergic and glutamatergic transmission in the induction and expression of behavioral sensitization: a critical review of preclinical studies. *Psychopharmacology* 2000;151:99–120.
285. Ohmori T, Abekawa T, Ito K, et al. Context determines the type of sensitized behaviour: a brief review and a hypothesis on the role of environment in behavioural sensitization. *Behav Pharmacol* 2000;11(3-4):211–221.
286. Robinson TE, Browman KE, Crombag HS, et al. Modulation of the induction or expression of psychostimulant sensitization by the circumstances surrounding drug administration. *Neurosci Biobehav Rev* 1998;22(2):347–354.
287. Gaytan O, Lewis C, Swann A, et al. Diurnal differences in amphetamine sensitization. *Eur J Pharmacol* 1999;374:1–9.
288. Steketee JD. Cortical mechanisms of cocaine sensitization. *Crit Rev Neurobiol* 2005;17:69–86.
289. Witkin JM, Levant B, Zapata A, et al. The dopamineD3/D2 Agonist R-(+)-trans-3,4a,10b-tetrahydro-4-propyl-2H,5H-[1]benzopyrano[4,3-b]-1,4-oxazin-9 -ol [(+)-PD-128,907] protects against acute and cocaine-kindled seizures in mice: further evidence for the involvement of D3 receptors. *J Pharmacol Exp Ther* 2008;326:930–938.
290. Kalivas PW, Pierce RC, Cornish J, et al. A role for sensitization in craving and relapse in cocaine addiction. *J Psychopharmacol* 1998;12(1): 49–53.
291. Post RM, Weiss SRB. Stimulant-induced behavioral sensitization: a model for neuroleptic nonresponsiveness. In: Simon P, Soubrie P, Wildlocer D, eds. *Animal models of psychiatric disorders*. Basel, Switzerland: S Karger, 1988:52–60.
292. Ujike H, Sato M. Clinical features of sensitization to methamphetamine observed in patients with methamphetamine dependence and psychosis. *Ann N Y Acad Sci* 2004;1025:279–287.
293. Leyton M. Conditioned and sensitized responses to stimulant drugs in humans. *Prog Neuropsychopharmacol Biol Psychiatry* 2007;31: 1601–1613.
294. Kollins SH, Rush CR. Sensitization to the cardiovascular but not subject-rated effects of oral cocaine in humans. *Biol Psychiatry* 2002; 51(2):143–150.
295. Boileau I, Dagher A, Leyton M, et al. Modeling sensitization to stimulants in humans: an [^{11}C]raclopride/positron emission tomography study in healthy men. *Arch Gen Psychiatry* 2006;63:1386–1395.
296. Hammer RP Jr, Egilmez Y, Emmett-Oglesby MW. Neural mechanisms of tolerance to the effects of cocaine. *Behav Brain Res* 1997;84: 225–239.
297. King GR, Xiong Z, Ellinwood EH Jr. Withdrawal from continuous cocaine administration: time dependent changes in accumbens 5-HT_3 receptor function and behavioral tolerance. *Psychopharmacology* 1999;142:352–359.
298. Tella SR, Schindler CW, Goldberg SR. Cardiovascular responses to cocaine self-administration: acute and chronic tolerance. *Eur J Pharmacol* 1999;383:57–68.
299. Woolverton WL, Weiss SRB. Tolerance and sensitization to cocaine: an integrated view. In: Higgins ST, Katz JL, eds. *Cocaine abuse: behavior, pharmacology, and clinical applications*. San Diego: Academic Press, 1998:107–134.
300. Nestler EJ. Molecular neurobiology of addiction. *Am J Addict* 2001;10:201–217.
301. Comer SD, Hart CL, Ward AS, et al. Effects of repeated oral methamphetamine administration in humans. *Psychopharmacology* 2001;155: 397–404.
302. Mendelson JH, Sholar M, Mello NK, et al. Cocaine tolerance: behavioral, cardiovascular, and neuroendocrine function in men. *Neuropsychopharmacology* 1998;18:263–271.
303. Ward AS, Haney M, Fischman MW, et al. Binge cocaine self-administration in humans: Intravenous cocaine. *Psychopharmacology* 1997;132: 375–381.
304. Perez-Reyes M, White WR, McDonald SA, et al. Clinical effects of daily methamphetamine administration. *Clin Neuropharmacol* 1991;14(4): 352–358.
305. Cho AK, Melega WP, Kuczenski R, et al. Relevance of pharmacokinetic parameters in animal models of methamphetamine abuse. *Synapse* 2001;39:161–166.
306. Yuan J, McCann U, Ricaurte G. Methylphenidate and brain dopamine neurotoxicity. *Brain Res* 1997;767:172–175.
307. McCann UD, Wong DF, Yokoi F, et al. Reduced striatal dopamine transporter density in abstinent methamphetamine and methcathinone users: evidence from positron emission tomography studies with [11C]WIN-35,428. *J Neurosci* 1998;18(20):8417–8422.
308. Volkow ND, Chang L, Wang G-J, et al. Loss of dopamine transporters in methamphetamine abusers recovers with protracted abstinence. *J Neurosci* 2001;21(23):9414–9418.
309. Cho AK, Melega WP. Patterns of methamphetamine abuse and their consequences. *J Addict Dis* 2002;21:21–34.
310. Li J-H, Lin L-F. Genetic toxicology of abused drugs: a brief review. *Mutagenesis* 1998;13(6):557–565.

CHAPTER 11

Laura M. Juliano, PhD
Sergi Ferré, MD, PhD
Roland R. Griffiths, PhD

The Pharmacology of Caffeine

Caffeine is the most widely used mood altering drug in the world. In the United States, 87% of children and adults regularly consume foods and beverages containing caffeine (1). As a nonselective A_1 and A_{2A} adenosine receptor antagonist and mild central nervous system stimulant, caffeine produces various physiologic and psychologic effects. Caffeine is not highly associated with any life-threatening illnesses, and typical daily dietary doses can be consumed under many circumstances without incident. However, caffeine is not completely innocuous. It has the potential to produce clinically significant negative physiologic and psychologic effects, tolerance and withdrawal, discrete psychiatric symptoms and disorders (e.g., caffeine-induced anxiety disorder), and features of a substance dependence syndrome. Furthermore, its coadministration with some commonly used psychotherapeutic and recreational drugs may have important clinical implications. The ubiquitous and passive use of caffeine and its integration in daily customs and routines (e.g., coffee break) can result in a lack of appreciation for the role that caffeine plays in one's daily subjective experiences; thus making the recognition and treatment of caffeine-associated problems particularly challenging.

DRUGS IN THE CLASS

Caffeine is the common name for 1,3,7-trimethylxanthine (Fig. 11.1). More than 60 types of caffeine containing plants have been identified, including coffee, tea, cola, cacao, guarana, and yerba maté. Caffeine is a member of the methylxanthine class of alkaloids, which includes the structurally related dimethylxanthines, theophylline, and theobromine. Caffeine in its free base form is a bitter white powder that is moderately soluble in water (21.7 mg/mL) (2). Pharmaceutical preparations of caffeine include caffeine anhydrous, caffeine sodium benzoate, and citrated caffeine.

Common Sources of Caffeine As shown in Table 11.1, sources of caffeine include beverages, foods, dietary supplements, and over-the-counter and prescription medications. A significant problem in estimating caffeine exposure occurs because of the wide variety of caffeinated products, large differences in common serving sizes, and a wide range of caffeine content in products even of the same type. For example, a 12-oz cup of coffee may contain anywhere from 107 to 420 mg of caffeine, whereas an energy drink, which can vary in size from 8 to 24 oz, can contain between 50 and 505 mg of caffeine.

History Cultivation of tea in China, coffee in Ethiopia, and cacao pod in South America date back to time immemorial

FIGURE 11.1. The chemical structure of caffeine. The chemical structure of caffeine (1,3,7-trimethylxanthine) and adenosine. Adenosine is an endogenous neuromodulator that has structural similarities to caffeine. Most of the physiologic effects of caffeine, including the central nervous system stimulant effects, are likely mediated through adenosine receptor antagonism.

CAFFEINE
(an adenosine receptor antagonist)

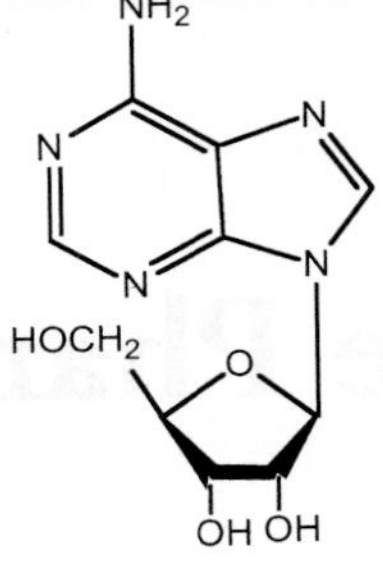

ADENOSINE
(an endogenous neuromodulator)

(3). Records of caffeine use date back at least 2,000 years for tea in China. With the development of worldwide trade in the 17th and 18th centuries, caffeinated foods and beverages rapidly spread from their original constrained geographic origins. Numerous failed attempts to eliminate or suppress the use of caffeine-containing foods on the basis of political, religious, economic, or medical grounds have been documented worldwide (including Arabia, Turkey, England, France, and Prussia) (3,4). In America, the protest of a British tax on tea became a symbolic focal point for revolution, resulting in the famous "Boston tea party" in 1773. After the Continental Congress passed a resolution against tea consumption, America was transformed from a predominately tea drinking land to one in which coffee was the caffeinated drink of choice (4). Presently, coffee is a major agricultural import of the United States, second only after oil in total value of all imports. The last century has seen the development and growing use of caffeinated soft drinks and energy drinks. The U.S. Food and Drug Administration limits the amount of caffeine in soft drinks to 0.02% (or 71.5 mg per 12 oz serving). In recent years, caffeine has been added to an increasingly wide variety of foods (e.g., candy, potato chips) and beverages (e.g., beer, energy drinks). It is notable that energy drinks, which typically contain much higher concentrations of caffeine than soft drinks, have been growing in popularity in the United States over the past decade and represent a multibillion dollar industry. Some countries ban the sale of energy drinks or strictly regulate their caffeine content because of concerns about negative health effects.

Therapeutic Uses As a mild central nervous system stimulant, caffeine is widely used to increase energy. Because of its putative analgesic-enhancing effects, caffeine is found in the formulations of a wide range of over-the-counter and prescription analgesic products that are frequently used to treat various types of pain, including migraine (5). Not surprisingly, caffeine alone is the most effective treatment for caffeine withdrawal headache, with prophylactic caffeine administration recognized as an effective way to prevent postsurgical headaches in caffeine consumers (6,7). As a respiratory stimulant, caffeine is used to treat apnea in neonates and infants (8). Intravenous caffeine has also been administered before electroconvulsive therapy to lengthen seizure duration; however, its therapeutic merits are unclear (9). Caffeine has been used to treat postprandial hypotension, although its effectiveness has been questioned (10). Because of its lipolytic and thermogenic effects, caffeine is commonly used in weight loss preparations and nutritional supplements. Caffeine is also used to facilitate athletic performance because of its ergogenic effects, although meaningful enhancements may be limited to well-conditioned athletes (11).

Epidemiology More than 85% of children and adults in the United States consume caffeine on a regular basis (1). Mean daily intake of caffeine for adult caffeine consumers has been estimated to be about 280 mg in the United States, with higher intakes estimated for consumers in the United Kingdom and Denmark (12). A recent epidemiologic survey found the highest caffeine consumption to be among males ages 35 to 54 years (i.e., 336 mg/day) (1).

PHARMACOKINETICS

Absorption and Distribution Caffeine is rapidly and completely absorbed after oral administration, with peak levels reached in 30 to 45 minutes (13). Caffeine is readily distributed throughout the body, with concentrations in blood correlating with those in saliva, breast milk, amniotic fluid, fetal tissue, semen, and the brain (14). Binding to plasma proteins is estimated to range between 10% and 35% (15). Saliva caffeine concentrations, which often exceed 75% of plasma concentrations, are used as a noninvasive alternative to serum monitoring.

Metabolism Caffeine metabolism is complex, with more than 25 metabolites identified in humans (16). The primary metabolic pathways involve the cytochrome P-450 liver enzyme system, which is responsible for the demethylation of caffeine to three biologically active dimethylxanthines: paraxanthine, theobromine, and theophylline, accounting for 80%, 10%, and 4% of caffeine metabolism, respectively (15). The large amounts of paraxanthine, coupled with the demonstration of similar sympathomimetic effects of paraxanthine and caffeine, suggest that paraxanthine needs to be considered in understanding the clinical pharmacology of caffeine (17).

TABLE 11.1 Caffeine Content of Common Foods and Medications

Product	Serving size (volume or weight)	Typical caffeine content (mg)	Range (mg)
Beverages			
Coffee			
Brewed/drip	12 oz	200	107–420
Instant	12 oz	140	40–260
Espresso	1 oz	70	60–95
Decaffeinated	12 oz	8	0–20
Starbucks drip	12 oz	260	
Starbucks bottled frappuccino	9.5 oz	85	
Tea			
Brewed	6 oz	40	30–90
Instant	6 oz	30	10–35
Canned or bottled	12 oz	20	8–32
Chocolate milk	6 oz	4	2–7
Cocoa/hot chocolate	6 oz	7	2–10
Soft drinks			
Typical amount	12 oz	40	22–69
Coca-cola Blak	12 oz	69	
Mountain Dew/ Diet Mountain Dew	12 oz	55	
Coke classic/Diet Coke	12 oz	47/35	
Sunkist/Diet Sunkist	12 oz	41/42	
Dr. Pepper/ Diet Dr. Pepper	12 oz	41	
Pepsi-Cola/Diet Pepsi	12 oz	38/36	
A&W cream soda/ diet cream soda	12 oz	29/22	
Barq's root beer/ diet root beer	12 oz	23	
Energy drinks			
Typical amount	varies	varies	50–505
Wired-X-505	23.5oz	505	
FIXX	20 oz	500	
Spike Shooter	8.4 oz	300	
Cocaine	8.2 oz	280	
Jolt	23.5 oz	278	
Rockstar	16 oz	160	
Monster	16 oz	160	
Full Throttle	16 oz	144	
Tab	10.5 oz	95	
Red Bull	8.3 oz	80	
Sobe Adrenaline Rush	8.3 oz	78	
Airforce Nutrisoda	8.4 oz	50	
Caffeinated water			
Buzzwater	16.9 oz	100 or 200	
Water Joe	16.9 oz	60	
Alcohol beverages			
Typical	varies	varies	
Bud Extra Beer	16 oz	80	
Tilt malt beverage	16 oz	71	
Moonshot Beer	12 oz	69	
Sparks malt beverage	16 oz	15	
Foods			
Chocolate			
Snickers Charged	1.83 oz	60	

(continued)

TABLE 11.1 Caffeine Content of Common Foods and Medications (Continued)

Product	Serving size (volume or weight)	Typical caffeine content (mg)	Range (mg)
Hershey's unsweetened baking chocolate	1.0 oz	30	
Hershey's special dark	1.45 oz	18	
Hershey's chocolate bar	1.55 oz	9	
Hershey's chocolate syrup	2 Tbsp	7	
Snickers bar	2.07 oz	2	
Miscellaneous foods			
Stay-Alert caffeinated gum	1 stick	100	
Extreme Sport Beans jelly beans	1 oz	50	
Jolt caffeinated gum	1 stick	33	
Dannon coffee yogurt	6 oz	30	
Starbucks classic coffee ice cream	4 oz	30	
Penguin peppermints	1 mint	7	
Over-the-counter medications			
Stimulants			
Typical	1 tablet	100 or 200	100–200
Vivarin	1 tablet	200	
Ultra Pep-Back	1 tablet	200	
No-Doz/No-Doz maximum strength	1 tablet	100/200	
Analgesics			
Excedrin extra strength	2 tablets	130	
Anacin Advanced Headache	2 tablets	130	
BC Fast Pain Relief	1 powder packet	33.3	
Goody's headache powder	1 powder packet	32.5	
Menstrual pain relief/diuretics			
Pamprin Max	2 caplets	130	
Midol Menstrual Complete	2 caplets	120	
Diurex Water Pills	2 tablets	100	
Dietary supplements/weight loss products			
Typical	1 or 2 tablets	Varies	50–300
Swarm Extreme Energizer	1 capsule	300	
Stacker 3	1 capsule	254	
Leptopril	2 capsules	220	
Twinlab Ripped Fuel	2 capsules	220	
Hydroxycut weight loss formula	2 caplets	200	
Metabolife Ultra	2 caplets	150	
Dexatrim Max	1 caplet	50	
Prescription Medications			
Headache/migraine/pain			
Cafergot	2 tablets	200	
Fiorinal	2 capsules	80	
Fioricet/Esgic/Many others	2 tablets	80	
Norgesic	2 tablets	60	

Sources: Barone JJ, Roberts HR. Caffeine consumption. *Food Chem Toxicol* 1996;34:119–129. McCusker RR, Fuehrlein B, Goldberger BA, et al. Caffeine content of decaffeinated coffee. *J Anal Toxicol* 2006;30:611–613. McCusker RR, Goldberger BA, Cone EJ. Caffeine content of specialty coffees. *J Anal Toxicol* 2003;27:520–522.

Caffeine values for all brand name products were obtained directly from product labels, the manufacturer's Web site, or customer service department.

Elimination On average, caffeine half-life is 4 to 6 hours; however, there are wide individual differences in rates of caffeine elimination, with half-lives varying more than a 10-fold range in healthy adults (15). An important implication of the central role of cytochrome P-450 liver enzymes in metabolizing caffeine is that drugs or conditions that affect this metabolic system significantly alter caffeine elimination. Caffeine's half-life is prolonged with liver disease (15), presumably because of lower CYP1A2 activity (18). Although caffeine half-life does not differ between younger and older adults (19), caffeine half-life is markedly increased in premature and full-term newborns (half-life of 80 to 100 hours) whose liver enzyme capacity is not completely developed until about 6 months of age (20). Cigarette smoking, which induces liver enzymes, decreases caffeine half-life by as much as 50% (21). Numerous compounds have been shown to inhibit caffeine metabolism, including high doses of caffeine itself, oral contraceptive steroids, cimetidine, some quinoline antibiotics, fluvoxamine, and mexiletine (16,22). Caffeine half-life increases markedly during the end of pregnancy (23). Caffeine elimination may vary over the course of the menstrual cycle, with reduced clearance during the luteal phase relative to the follicular phase (24).

MECHANISMS OF ACTION

The primary cellular site of action of caffeine is the adenosine receptor. Adenosine is an endogenous purine nucleoside found throughout the brain. It is formed from the breakdown of adenosine triphosphate (ATP) and modulates a variety of central and peripheral nervous system effects. Caffeine is structurally similar to adenosine (Fig. 11.1). As a competitive A_1 and A_{2A} adenosine receptor antagonist, caffeine produces a variety of effects that are opposite to the effects of adenosine (e.g., central nervous stimulation, vasoconstriction).

More specifically, caffeine produces its motor and reinforcing effects by releasing the pre- and postsynaptic brakes that adenosine imposes on striatal dopaminergic neurotransmission. At the presynaptic level, caffeine induces dopamine release by a glutamate-independent mechanism, by targeting adenosine A_1 receptors localized in striatal dopaminergic terminals. Furthermore, caffeine induces dopamine release by a glutamate-dependent mechanism, by targeting A_1 receptors that form heteromers with adenosine A_{2A} receptors in striatal glutamatergic terminals. These presynaptic effects of caffeine are potentiated by postsynaptic effects, which depend on the existence of strong antagonistic adenosine-dopamine receptor-receptor interactions. These interactions depend on the ability of A_1 and A_{2A} receptors to form heteromers with dopamine D_1 and D_2 receptors, respectively. The effects of caffeine on sleep do not seem to be dopamine-dependent and are related to the ability of adenosine to act as an endogenous sleep-promoting substance by acting on A_1 and A_{2A} receptors localized in the brainstem, basal forebrain and hypothalamic areas. These effects are discussed in greater detail in the following sections.

Adenosine A_1 and A_{2A} Receptor Antagonism

Among the four cloned adenosine receptors (A_1, A_{2A}, A_{2B}, and A_3 receptors), A_1 and A_{2A} receptors are the ones predominantly expressed in the brain. Caffeine is a nonselective adenosine receptor antagonist, with similar in vitro affinities for A_1, A_{2A}, and A_{2B} receptors and with much lower affinity for A_3 receptors (25,26). A_1 and A_{2A} receptors are the preferential targets for caffeine in the brain, because physiologic extracellular levels of adenosine are sufficient to occupy and, therefore, stimulate A_1 and A_{2A} receptors. On the other hand, A_{2B} receptors have a lower affinity for adenosine and they are only activated by high pathologic extracellular levels of adenosine (25). A_1 receptors are widely expressed in the brain, including the striatum, whereas A_{2A} receptors are highly concentrated in the striatum (25,27). The striatal localization of both receptors seems to underlie the motor-activating and reinforcing effects of caffeine (see the following section). On the other hand, A_1 receptors localized in the brainstem and basal forebrain and A_{2A} receptors localized in the hypothalamus have been suggested to be involved in caffeine effects on sleep regulation.

There has been a long debate about the preferential involvement of A_1 and A_{2A} receptors in the psychostimulant effects of caffeine (28,29). By comparing both quantitative and qualitative aspects of the motor activity induced by caffeine and selective A_1 and A_{2A} receptor antagonists, recent studies have clearly shown that caffeine, when administered acutely, shows a profile of a nonselective adenosine receptor antagonist with preferential A_1 receptor antagonism (30,31). Also, recent drug discrimination experiments support a key role of A_1 receptors in the psychostimulant effects of acutely administered caffeine (26). Importantly, chronic exposure to caffeine differentially modifies its motor effects dependent on A_1 and A_{2A} receptor blockade. Thus chronic exposure to caffeine in the drinking water in rats results in partial tolerance to the motor effects of an additional acute administration of caffeine and total cross-tolerance to the motor effects of an A_1 but not an A_{2A} receptor antagonist (31). This indicates that tolerance to the effects of A_1 receptor blockade is mostly responsible for the tolerance to the motor-activating effects of caffeine and that the residual motor-activating effects of caffeine in tolerant individuals might be mostly because of A_{2A} receptor blockade.

An important amount of experimental evidence supports a key role of dopamine in the psychostimulant effects of caffeine in animals and humans. For instance, dopamine depletion or blockade of dopamine receptors significantly impairs the motor and discriminative stimulus effects of caffeine (32,33). Most probably, the same basic dopamine-mediated mechanisms are involved in the motor-activating and reinforcing effects of caffeine, as happens with classical psychostimulants (34,35). The key to understanding these mechanisms of action is to appreciate how adenosine modulates dopaminergic neurotransmission in the brain.

The effects of caffeine on sleep regulation do not seem to be dopamine-dependent and they are related to its ability to antagonize the sleep-promoting effects of adenosine (36–39). Although previous results suggested that A_1 receptors are involved in sleep regulation by inhibiting ascending cholinergic neurons of the basal forebrain (36,39), more recent studies, which include experiments with A_{2A} and A_1 receptor knockout mice, indicate that A_{2A} receptors play a crucial role in the sleep-promoting effects of adenosine and the arousal-enhancing effects of caffeine (37,38). Those A_{2A} receptors are localized in the ventrolateral preoptic area of the hypothalamus and their stimulation promotes sleep by inducing gamma-aminobutyric acid (GABA) release in the histaminergic tuberomammillary nucleus, thereby inhibiting the histaminergic arousal system (37,38).

Adenosine is a key modulator of dopaminergic and glutamatergic neurotransmission in the striatum (40). Recent studies suggest that astroglia plays a fundamental role in the formation of extracellular adenosine, which can influence synaptic transmission. Astrocytes express glutamate receptors (mostly metabotropic) and ATP receptors that, when activated, induce astrocytes to release glutamate and ATP (41,42). Astroglial-released ATP is then converted to adenosine in the extracellular space by means of ectonucleotidases (43). Finally, there is an increasing amount of data suggesting the existence of a neurotransmitter-like formation of adenosine, a synaptic pool of adenosine. Adenosine can be produced from ATP coreleased with glutamate, which is also metabolized to adenosine by means of ectonucleotidases (27,40). GABAergic enkephalinergic and dynorphinergic medium sized spiny neurons constitute more than 90% of the striatal neuronal population (44). In the striatum, A_{2A} receptors are localized postsynaptically in the dendritic spines of enkephalinergic medium spiny neurons, colocalized with D_2 receptors and presynaptically in glutamatergic terminals, colocalized with A_1 receptors (27,40,45,46). In addition to the glutamatergic terminals, A_1 receptors are localized in a fraction of dopaminergic nerve terminals (47) and, postsynaptically, in the dendritic spines of dynorphinergic medium spiny neurons, colocalized with D_1 receptors (46). Antagonistic interactions between A_{2A} and D_2 receptors modulate the function of the enkephalinergic medium spiny neuron and antagonistic interactions between A_1 and D_1 receptors modulate the function of the dynorphinergic medium spiny neuron (48,49). This gives the explanation at the neuronal level of an important number of pharmacologic findings indicating a selective modulation of A_1 and A_{2A} receptor ligands on D_1 and D_2 receptor–mediated behavioral effects, respectively (32,46,50).

Postsynaptic Mechanisms: Adenosine-dopamine Receptor Interactions The molecular mechanisms responsible for the selective antagonistic A_1-D_1 and A_{2A}-D_2 receptor interactions have been found to involve "intramembrane receptor-receptor interactions," a common property of neurotransmitter receptor heteromers (45,51). There is compelling evidence for the existence of A_1-D_1 and A_{2A}-D_2 receptor heteromers in artificial cell systems and in the striatum (45,51). In the A_{2A}-D_2 heteromer, the stimulation of the A_{2A} receptor decreases the binding of dopamine to the D_2 receptor (52). This intramembrane interaction controls neuronal excitability and, consequently, neuronal firing and neurotransmitter (GABA) release by the GABAergic enkephalinergic neuron (27,48,53,54). Furthermore, there is a reciprocal antagonistic A_{2A}-D_2 receptor interaction by which D_2 receptor stimulation counteracts the effects induced by A_{2A} receptor stimulation at the level of adenylyl cyclase and, consequently, at the level of protein phosphorylation and gene expression (55–57).

The A_{2A}-D_2 intramembrane receptor-receptor interaction seems to play a key role in the motor-activating effects of caffeine. In fact, this A_{2A}-D_2 receptor interaction has been given a lot of attention in the literature, more recently with the application of A_{2A} receptor antagonists as an adjuvant therapy for levodopa in Parkinson's disease (58). But, as mentioned previously, A_1-D_1 receptor interactions are also of significant functional and pharmacologic importance. Thus A_1 receptor antagonists selectively potentiate the motor activating effects of D_1 receptor–mediated motor activation in different animal models (49,59). Similar to what happens with the A_{2A}-D_2 receptor heteromers, A_1 and D_1 receptors antagonistically interact both at intramembrane level and at the adenylyl cyclase level. However, in this case, the interactions are not reciprocal, and stimulation of A_1 receptors inhibits both the binding of dopamine to the D_1 receptor (60,61) and the D_1 receptor-mediated activation of cAMP-PKA signaling pathway and the expression of genes, such as *c-fos* and *preprodynorphin* (61,62).

Presynaptic Mechanisms: Modulation of Glutamate and Dopamine Release Different studies have repeatedly shown that A_1 and A_{2A} receptors exert opposite modulatory roles on extracellular levels of glutamate and dopamine in the striatum, with activation of A_1 receptors inhibiting and activation of A_{2A} receptors stimulating glutamate and dopamine release (28,29). More recently, it has been shown that systemic or striatal administration of caffeine or an A_1, but not an A_{2A}, receptor antagonist produces a significant increase in the extracellular concentrations of glutamate and dopamine in the ventral striatum, particularly in the most medial part, the medial shell of the nucleus accumbens (63,64). It was hypothesized that dopamine release mostly depended on glutamate release induced by blockade of A_1 receptors localized in glutamatergic terminals and on stimulation of ionotropic glutamate receptors localized in dopaminergic terminals (64,65). Importantly, chronic administration of caffeine in the rat's drinking water completely counteracted the effects of caffeine or an A_1 receptor antagonist on dopamine and glutamate, whereas the effect of an A_{2A} receptor antagonist was not modified (63). Thus these biochemical changes are consistent with the studies on motor activity described previously (31), strongly suggesting an involvement of presynaptic mechanisms in the psychostimulant effects of caffeine. The ability of caffeine to release dopamine in the nucleus accumbens was questioned by another research group (66), but a recent study demonstrated the existence of subregional differences in the effect of A_1 receptor blockade in different parts of the nucleus accumbens and other striatal areas, most probably related to subregional differences in the level of tonic activation by endogenous adenosine (47). Furthermore, glutamate-independent mechanisms were also found to be involved in A_1 receptor blockade-mediated striatal dopamine release, which depended on A_1 receptors localized in dopaminergic nerve terminals (47).

Dopamine release in the very medial striatal compartments seems to be involved in both motor-activating and reinforcing effects of psychostimulants (34). Therefore the motor and reinforcing effects of caffeine most probably depend on the pre- and postsynaptic dopaminergic mechanisms mentioned previously (striatal dopamine release and adenosine-dopamine receptor-receptor interactions) taking place in the medial striatal compartments. At least two factors related to the dopamine-releasing effects of caffeine could explain its weaker reinforcing effects as compared with other psychostimulants: its specific subregional effects (47) and the development of tolerance (63).

Under chronic caffeine exposure, different factors might contribute to the predominant tolerance of the effects of A_1 receptor blockade. Upregulation of A_1 receptors has been repeatedly demonstrated (31,68–70), but its significance as a mechanism involved in caffeine tolerance has been seriously questioned (71). Modifications in the function of A_1-A_{2A} receptor heteromers might play a key role in the development of caffeine tolerance. Thus radioligand binding experiments have shown that chronic treatment with caffeine causes an increase in the potency of A_{2A} receptor agonist–mediated inhibition of A_1 receptor agonist binding and a significant reduction in the affinity of the striatal A_{2A} receptor for caffeine (67). An additional factor that might play a significant role in caffeine tolerance is the significant increase in plasma and extracellular concentrations of adenosine with chronic caffeine exposure (72). The higher adenosine levels and lower affinity of the A_{2A} receptor for caffeine could allow endogenous adenosine to stimulate A_{2A} receptors even in the presence of caffeine, which would not reach enough concentration to compete with adenosine for binding A_{2A} receptors. Under these conditions, A_1 receptor signaling in the A_1-A_{2A} receptor heteromer would be expected to be chronically turned down, because of its continuous blockade by caffeine and because of the strong A_{2A} receptor–mediated inhibition of A_1 receptor agonist binding. On the other hand, an additional administration of caffeine would be expected to produce a blockade of the residual A_{2A} receptor signaling.

PHYSIOLOGIC EFFECTS

Cardiovascular At moderate dietary dose levels, caffeine produces increases in blood pressure (73). Caffeine tends to have no effect (74) or to reduce heart rate in humans (75).

Gastrointestinal Caffeine stimulates gastric acid secretions and is a colonic stimulant, with caffeinated coffee producing colonic motor activity similar to that produced by a meal (76).

Renal and Urinary Caffeine is a diuretic, increasing urine volume 30% or more for several hours after caffeine ingestion (77). Caffeine also increases detrusor pressure on the bladder of patients with complaints of urinary urgency and confirmed detrusor instability (78).

Respiratory Caffeine is a respiratory stimulant (79) and a bronchodilator at high doses (80).

Skeletal Muscle Caffeine is ergogenic across a variety of exercise situations, and in particular during prolonged exercise (81), with activity potentially mediated via multiple mechanisms, including effects on muscle contractility (82).

Hormonal Caffeine increases plasma epinephrine, norepinephrine, renin, and free fatty acids, particularly in nontolerant individuals (17,83,84). It also increases adrenocorticotropic hormone and cortisol (85–87). Caffeine increases insulin levels in healthy subjects (88) and increases postprandial glucose and insulin responses among patients with type 2 diabetes who are habitual coffee drinkers (88,89). Heavy caffeine use (>300 mg per day) is associated with shorter menses and shorter menstrual cycles (90).

EFFECTS ON PHYSICAL HEALTH

The body of research on the health effects of caffeine is vast and has been the focus of several scholarly books and reviews (91–93). Although caffeine is not associated with any life-threatening illnesses, there are some medical conditions that may be adversely affected by caffeine or coffee consumption. Epidemiologic research has also provided evidence that caffeine or coffee consumption may have some protective effects against specific diseases.

Adverse Health Effects Caffeine can increase blood pressure by 5 to 15 mm Hg systolic and 5 to 10 mm Hg diastolic for several hours in healthy adults (93). It has been argued that such effects are clinically significant and represent an important cardiovascular risk factor (94), although this has been debated (93). Caffeine can influence heart rate variability and increase arterial stiffness (95), but the implications of these findings are unclear (96). Both caffeinated and decaffeinated coffees contain lipids that raise total and low-density lipoprotein cholesterol with higher levels obtained from unfiltered brewing methods (e.g., French press, boiled) (97).

Although some early case control studies reported positive associations between caffeine consumption and certain types of cancer including pancreatic, bladder, and ovarian cancer, more recent and carefully controlled studies have not provided convincing evidence that caffeine consumption increases the risk of cancer development (91,92).

Coffee has been shown to exacerbate gastroesophageal reflux (98), however it is not clear if it is due to caffeine or other coffee constituents (99,100). There is no clear association between caffeine use and peptic or duodenal ulcers (14,101).

Caffeine is a general risk factor for urinary incontinence (102) and contributes to urinary incontinence in psychogeriatric patients (103). Likewise, caffeine reduction can decrease urinary incontinence (104).

Caffeine increases urinary calcium excretion. Thus it has been suggested that caffeine may negatively affect overall calcium balance and increase the risk of osteoporosis; however, the clinical significance of the calcium loss is debated (93). Associations between high caffeine consumption and bone fractures have been observed in some epidemiologic studies, particularly among women with low calcium intake (105); however, a direct effect of caffeine on the increased likelihood of fractures has not been confirmed.

Caffeine readily crosses the placenta barrier and is distributed to all fetal tissues including the central nervous system (23). Furthermore, caffeine elimination decreases substantially over the course of pregnancy (23). Some recent large scale studies and a meta-analysis of previous studies suggest that maternal caffeine use increases the rate of spontaneous abortion in a roughly dose-dependent fashion (106,107). Caffeine use is also associated with decreased fecundity and reduced fetal growth, although methodologic differences across studies prohibit definitive conclusions (93). It has been suggested that polymorphisms in the CYP1A2 gene may interact with caffeine dose and increase the risk of pregnancy loss and other negative pregnancy outcomes (108,109). A review of research on caffeine and pregnancy concluded that reproductive aged women should consume no more than 300 mg caffeine per day (93).

Health Protective Effects Case control and epidemiologic studies have elucidated a relationship between caffeine consumption and reduced risk of Parkinson's disease (110–113). Epidemiologic studies have also reported an association between coffee drinking and reduced incidence of chronic liver disease (114), although the potential mechanisms are unclear (115) and may be unrelated to caffeine. Additionally, epidemiologic studies have reported a protective effect of coffee drinking for risk of developing type 2 diabetes (116,117), with the effects attributed to coffee constituents other than caffeine (118).

EFFECTS ON HUMAN PERFORMANCE

A large number of studies have examined the effects of caffeine on human performance. The most consistent generality to emerge is that caffeine reliably increases performance on task performance that has been degraded by fatigue (e.g., under conditions of sleep deprivation or prolonged vigilance) (14,119,120). Although the results are variable (14,121), and observed effects are often small (121), compared with placebo, caffeine at normal dietary doses may improve tapping speed, reaction time, sustained attention (or vigilance), and perhaps focused attention (121). The effect of caffeine on various memory tasks has also been investigated, but is inconclusive (121). A growing literature on the effects of caffeine on exercise performance suggests that, relative to placebo, caffeine can enhance performance during long-term (30 to 60 minutes) aerobic exercise (11,81), can reduce ratings of perceived exhaustion (122), and can improve speed or power output in simulated race conditions (11,123). Some studies have also demonstrated caffeine induced enhancement during short-term, high-intensity exercise (123,124), but these effects are generally more difficult to demonstrate (11). A problem in interpreting the effects of caffeine on performance is that most studies have compared the effects of caffeine and placebo on the performance of habitual caffeine users who have been required to abstain from caffeine, usually overnight. Thus improvements in performance after caffeine relative to placebo may simply reflect a relief of withdrawal symptoms or restoration to baseline performance (125,126). Studies have shown caffeine-related performance enhancements among light non-dependent caffeine consumers and nonconsumers (127,128), although it has been argued that population differences or self-selection of groups in such studies are important confounds (129). Based on the preclinical literature, which clearly documents the behavioral stimulant effects of caffeine, it seems quite likely that caffeine enhances human performance on some types of tasks (e.g., vigilance), especially among nontolerant individuals. Among high-dose habitual caffeine consumers, performance enhancements above and beyond withdrawal reversal effects are likely to be modest at best (129).

SUBJECTIVE EFFECTS

Human laboratory studies demonstrate that single low to moderate doses of caffeine typically produce a profile of positive subjective effects, including increased well-being, happiness, energy, arousal, alertness, and sociability (130). Positive effects are more likely to be observed in studies that require participants abstain from caffeine before testing and that administer a caffeine dose in the range of typical dietary consumption (e.g., 20 to 200 mg) (131). Physical dependence also increases the positive mood effects of caffeine, likely through suppression of low-grade withdrawal symptoms (129,132). However, positive mood effects occur among nonhabitual users and those maintained on a caffeine-free diet, as well as under conditions of minimal caffeine deprivation (125,127,133–136).

In general, acute doses of caffeine >200 mg are more likely to produce negative subjective effects, such as increased anxiety, nervousness, jitteriness, tense negative mood, upset stomach, and "bad effects" (130). Individual differences in sensitivity and tolerance seem to play an important role in the likelihood and severity of negative subjective effects. Individuals with panic disorder and generalized anxiety disorder, as well as nonclinical populations with higher anxiety sensitivity, tend to be particularly sensitive to the anxiogenic effects of caffeine

(137–140). Although high-dose subjective effects of caffeine show some overlap with the subjective effects of *d*-amphetamine, caffeine produces greater negative effects (e.g., anxiety) and fewer positive effects (e.g., positive mood) (127,141,142). In most cases, the negative subjective effects of caffeine are relatively mild and short-lived. However, acute and/or chronic use of caffeine, especially in very high doses, can cause distress and discrete psychopathology, as discussed in subsequent sections.

DISCRIMINATIVE STIMULUS EFFECTS

Carefully controlled double-blind studies show that the majority of individuals (>80%) can learn to reliably discriminate caffeine from placebo (143), using initial caffeine doses ranging from 100 to 320 mg. Studies that have explicitly trained discrimination of progressively lower caffeine doses show that caffeine doses as low as 1.8 to 10 mg can be reliably discriminated by some participants (134,135,144). These studies documenting that caffeine can produce reliable discriminative effects at very low doses are consistent with studies showing that low doses of caffeine (e.g., 9–12.5 mg) can produce improvements in behavioral performance (145,146). Drug discrimination studies in humans and animals have demonstrated both similarities and differences between caffeine and other stimulant drugs (e.g., cocaine, *d*-amphetamine, methylphenidate) (130).

REINFORCING EFFECTS

The circumstantial evidence for caffeine functioning as a reinforcer is compelling. Caffeine is the most widely self-administered mood-altering drug in the world and, historically, repeated efforts to restrict or eliminate consumption of caffeinated foods have been completely unsuccessful. Several carefully controlled research studies over the past 20 years provide unequivocal evidence for the reinforcing effects of caffeine (130). Caffeine reinforcement has been demonstrated with various participant populations, using a variety of methodological approaches (e.g., choice procedures, ad libitum self administration), and across different caffeine vehicles (e.g., coffee, soft drinks, capsules). The average incidence of caffeine reinforcement across studies in normal caffeine users is approximately 40%, with higher rates observed (i.e., 82% to 100%) among certain subsamples such as high caffeine consumers, those with histories of drug or alcohol abuse, in studies involving repeated exposure to caffeine and placebo test conditions before reinforcement testing (130,147), and in the context of having to perform a vigilance task after drug administration (136). Doses as low as 25 mg per cup of coffee and 33 mg per serving of soft drink function as reinforcers (148–150). Doses >50 or 100 mg tend to decrease choice or self-administration, with relatively high doses of caffeine (e.g., 400 or 600 mg) sometimes producing significant caffeine avoidance (151). The subjective effects of caffeine covary with caffeine reinforcement (131). Positive subjective effects of caffeine predict the subsequent choice of caffeine relative to placebo, and negative subjective effects predict the subsequent choice of placebo relative to caffeine. Furthermore, caffeine users who report negative effects of placebo (i.e., withdrawal symptoms) also tend to choose caffeine over placebo (152). Avoidance of caffeine withdrawal symptoms clearly plays a central role in the reinforcing effects of caffeine among regular caffeine consumers. For example, in studies that prospectively manipulated caffeine physical dependence, subjects chose caffeine more than twice as often when they were physically dependent than when they were not physically dependent (153,154).

A series of studies has used a conditioned flavor preference paradigm to provide suggestive evidence of caffeine reinforcement. These studies have shown that abstinent caffeine consumers who are repeatedly given a novel flavored drink paired with either caffeine (e.g., 70 mg) or placebo, rate the caffeine-paired drink as more pleasant or preferred, and the placebo-paired drink as less so (155,156). The ability of caffeine to produce changes in flavor liking appears to be primarily driven by the alleviation of withdrawal symptoms among habitual caffeine consumers (i.e., negative reinforcement) (157). In the natural environment, the development of such conditioned flavor preferences over many days of self-administration likely play an important role in engendering strong consumer preferences for specific types and brands of caffeine-containing beverages.

Caffeine reinforcement has also been investigated in animals using self-injection or conditioned place preference paradigms. Animals will self-inject caffeine, sometimes showing patterns of irregular intake (e.g., high rates of intake alternating irregularly with periods of low intake) (130). Somewhat consistent with self-injection studies of nicotine, caffeine does not reliably maintain self-administration across animals and studies to the extent that is observed in studies of classic abused stimulants (e.g., cocaine, *d*-amphetamine). Low doses of caffeine produce conditioned place preference in rats, whereas higher doses produce clear place avoidance (130). Similar to the self-injection data, a direct comparison of place preference between caffeine and cocaine suggested that cocaine has greater reinforcing effects (158).

CAFFEINE TOLERANCE

The degree of tolerance development to caffeine can be expected to depend on the caffeine dose, the dose frequency, the number of doses, and the individual's elimination rate (159). Tolerance has been clearly demonstrated in both animals and humans; however, quantitative parametric information is quite fragmentary. Complete tolerance does not occur at low daily dietary doses. Very high doses of caffeine (750 to 1,200 mg/day spread throughout the day) administered daily, produce "complete" tolerance (i.e., caffeine effects are no longer different from baseline or placebo) to some but not all effects. For example, in one study, differences in ratings of mood and other subjective effects were observed between participants given 300 mg of caffeine three times daily and those given placebo three times daily only during the first 4 days of an 18-day study, clearly suggesting tolerance development (152). Tolerance develops to the sleep-disrupting effects of caffeine (160,161) and to physiologic effects including diuresis, parotid gland salivation, increased metabolic rate (oxygen consumption), increased plasma norepinephrine and epinephrine, and increased plasma renin activity (143). Tolerance also develops to blood pressure increases caused by caffeine ingestion; however, controlled research has shown that tolerance to such pressor effects is incomplete (94,162,163).

Studies in animals have demonstrated complete, insurmountable tolerance to high doses of caffeine. Caffeine tolerance occurs across different animal species (e.g., mice, rats, monkeys) and a wide range of experimental measures (e.g., locomotor activity, schedule-controlled responding, reinforcement thresholds for electrical brain stimulation, caffeine-induced seizure thresholds, discriminative responding in caffeine-trained animals) (130).

CAFFEINE INTOXICATION

The potential for caffeine intoxication to cause clinically significant distress is reflected by the inclusion of caffeine intoxication as a diagnosis in DSM-IV-TR (*Diagnostic and statistical manual of mental disorders*, 4th ed., text revision) (164) and in the ICD-10 (International Statistical Classification of Diseases and Related Health Problems). Reports of caffeine intoxication can be found in the medical literature dating back to the 1800s (165). "Caffeinism" is an older term that has been used to describe negative or toxic consequences of caffeine resulting from acute or chronic use (166). Unlike many other drugs of dependence, but similar to nicotine, the high-dose intoxicating effects of caffeine are not usually sought out by users.

Diagnostic Criteria for Intoxication Caffeine intoxication is defined by a number of symptoms and clinical features that emerge in response to recent consumption of caffeine. As listed in Table 11.2, common features of caffeine intoxication include restlessness, nervousness (anxiety), insomnia, gastrointestinal disturbance, tremors, tachycardia, and psychomotor agitation. In addition, there have been reports of patients with caffeine intoxication having fever, irritability, sensory disturbances, tachypnea, and headaches (165). Although DSM-IV diagnostic guidelines suggest that diagnosis be dependent on the recent daily consumption of at least 250 mg of caffeine, the equivalent of just two and a half cups of brewed coffee, intoxication is typically observed at much higher doses of caffeine (i.e., >500 mg). However, individual sensitivity (e.g., metabolic differences) and tolerance are likely to influence the dose effects. A person with high sensitivity and little tolerance might show signs and symptoms of caffeine intoxication in response to doses of caffeine much lower than a regular user. However, it should be noted that caffeine intoxication can occur in a person who has been using caffeine for many years with no apparent problems (167).

TABLE 11.2 Diagnostic Criteria for Caffeine Intoxication (DSM-IV-TR)

A. Recent consumption of caffeine, usually in excess of 250 mg (e.g., more than 2 to 3 cups of brewed coffee).

B. Five (or more) of the following signs, developing during, or shortly after, caffeine use:
1. Restlessness
2. Nervousness
3. Excitement
4. Insomnia
5. Flushed face
6. Diuresis
7. Gastrointestinal disturbance
8. Muscle twitching
9. Rambling flow of thought and speech
10. Tachycardia or cardiac arrhythmia
11. Periods of inexhaustibility
12. Psychomotor agitation

C. The symptoms in Criterion B cause clinically significant distress or impairment in social, occupational, or other important areas of functioning.

D. The symptoms are not due to a general medical condition and are not better accounted for by another mental disorder (e.g., an anxiety disorder).

Epidemiology There have been very few studies examining the incidence and prevalence of caffeine intoxication in the general population. Although many may experience the negative effects of caffeine on occasion, caffeine intoxication serious enough to come to clinical attention is considered relatively rare. One random-digit telephone survey found that 7% of current caffeine users met DSM-IV criteria for caffeine intoxication by reporting use of more than 250 mg, five or more symptoms (Table 11.2), and that symptoms interfered with their functioning at work, school, or home (168). Prior studies that have used ambiguous criteria and have focused on special populations (e.g., psychiatric patients, college students) have reported caffeine intoxication rates ranging from 2% to 19%. There have also been case reports of caffeine intoxication occurring in patients with eating disorders and athletes. A recent large-scale twin study found that 29% reported having felt ill or shaky or jittery after consuming caffeinated beverages (169). Caffeine was implicated in 4,656 reports to poison control centers in the United States in 2005, with half warranting treatment in a health care facility (170). Another recent study evaluated 265 cases of caffeine intoxication that were reported to a local area poison center between 2001 and 2004 after ingestion of caffeinated products other than coffee or tea (171). They found that caffeine was in the form of a medication in 77% of the cases, a caffeine enhanced beverage in 16% of cases, and a dietary supplement in 14% of cases. Patients were typically young (21 years old on average), half were female, and 12% required hospitalization. It has been suggested that the emergence of highly caffeinated energy drinks that seem to have particular appeal to young and perhaps nontolerant users, could increase rates of caffeine intoxication. For example, a recent series of case reports based on poison control center data found that a particular energy drink containing 250 mg of caffeine was repeatedly implicated in caffeine intoxication reports. The most common symptoms reported were hypertension, jitteriness, agitation, tremors, nausea, vomiting, and dizziness (172).

Identification and Management of Intoxication

Because of the many features of caffeine intoxication that overlap with other medical and psychiatric disorders, identifying recent ingestion of caffeine is critical in diagnosing caffeine intoxication. Serum or saliva assays of caffeine can be used to verify caffeine use. Caffeine intoxication should be considered as a differential diagnosis when assessing possible intoxication and withdrawal from other drugs, medication side effects (e.g., akathisia), other psychiatric disorders (e.g., anxiety disorders, mania, sleep disturbances), and somatic disorders (e.g., arrhythmia, hyperthyroidism). Caffeine intoxication resolves rapidly (consistent with caffeine's half-life of 4 to 6 hours) and usually appears to have no long-lasting consequences. When significant caffeine overdose occurs, patients should receive close monitoring, symptomatic treatment (e.g., for tachycardia), stomach aspiration, and assessment of serum caffeine level. Caffeine can be lethal after ingestion of very high doses (i.e., about 5 to 10 g) and there is documentation of accidental overdose and suicide by caffeine ingestion, usually in the form of pills (130).

ANXIETY AND CAFFEINE

There is abundant evidence that caffeine is anxiogenic. Acute doses of caffeine generally >200 mg can increase anxiety ratings in both individuals with anxiety disorders (138,139,173) and nonclinical samples (174–176), with higher doses sometimes producing unequivocal panic attacks (174,177,178). Individuals with anxiety disorders appear to be particularly sensitive to the effects of caffeine. Individuals with anxiety disorders tend to report greater anxiety after consuming caffeine than control subjects (137–139,173,179). Genetic factors may underlie individual sensitivity to the anxiogenic effects of caffeine. Genetic polymorphisms in the A_{2A} receptor gene (ADORA2A) were shown in two studies to predict an anxiogenic response to 150 mg dose of caffeine among low caffeine consumers (180,181). Furthermore, first-degree relatives of patients with panic disorder also show heightened anxiogenic responses to high doses of caffeine (182).

It has been suggested that individuals with anxiety disorders may find the stimulus effects of caffeine aversive and therefore may naturally limit their caffeine intake. Indeed the choice to consume caffeine in double-blind choice procedures has been shown to be associated with lower prestudy anxiety levels (151,152). It has been observed in some studies that patients with anxiety disorders, such as panic disorder, report lower levels of caffeine than healthy controls (178,179,183,184). However, some studies have failed to show a relationship between anxiety disorders or greater anxiety levels and caffeine use (139,185,186). Finally, other studies have shown a positive relationship between self-reported caffeine use and anxiety levels (187). In light of these disparate data, it seems reasonable to conclude that some but not all individuals with high anxiety levels will naturally avoid caffeine, and it is possible that some individuals may fail to recognize the role that caffeine plays in their anxiety symptoms.

Caffeine-induced Anxiety Disorder Caffeine-induced anxiety disorder is a diagnosis included in DSM-IV-TR. There is no research specifically examining this disorder, although clinical features of caffeine-induced anxiety have been described (188). Caffeine cessation has been shown to produce improvements in anxiety in some patients, with some requiring no additional treatment (189). Clinicians should consider advising anxiety patients to eliminate caffeine to rule out an etiological role of caffeine in anxiety symptoms.

SLEEP AND CAFFEINE

It is widely accepted that caffeine affects sleep. Caffeine increases wakefulness and reduces decrements in performance under conditions of sleep deprivation. Because of its ability to cause insomnia, sleep researchers use caffeine as a challenge agent to study insomnia in healthy volunteers (190). Caffeine's effects on sleep appear to be determined by a variety of factors including dose, the time between caffeine ingestion and attempted sleep, and individual differences in sensitivity or tolerance to caffeine (191). Caffeine administered immediately before bedtime or throughout the day has been shown to delay sleep onset, reduce total sleep time, alter the normal stages of sleep, and decrease the reported quality of sleep (191–193). There is also some evidence that caffeine taken early in the day can disrupt nighttime sleep (194). Genetic factors may underlie individual sensitivity in the sleep disruptive effects of caffeine. In one study, certain polymorphisms in the adenosine A_{2A} receptor gene were shown to be associated with differential responses to caffeine's effects on electroencephalogram beta activity in non-REM sleep and self-reported caffeine sensitivity (195). In another, genetic variations of adenosine deaminase and the adenosine A_{2A} receptor gene were related to intensity and sleep architecture (196).

Caffeine-induced Sleep Disorder Caffeine-induced sleep disorder is a diagnosis included in DSM-IV-TR (164). Caffeine-induced sleep disorder is characterized by a prominent disturbance of sleep etiologically related to caffeine use. Caffeine use is most often associated with insomnia; however, excessive sleepiness after caffeine consumption has been documented as well (197). There is little information about the incidence or prevalence of caffeine-induced sleep disorder. Patients who complain of sleep problems should be advised to eliminate caffeine as a first line of treatment.

TABLE 11.3 Empirically Validated Signs and Symptoms Resulting from Caffeine Abstinence

Headache
Tiredness/fatigue
Drowsiness/sleepiness
Decreased energy/activeness
Decreased alertness/attentiveness
Decreased contentedness/well-being
Irritability
Depressed mood
Difficulty concentrating
Muggy/foggy/not clearheaded
Flulike symptoms
Nausea/vomiting
Muscle pain/stiffness

Source: Juliano LM, Griffiths RR. A critical review of caffeine withdrawal: empirical validation of symptoms and signs, incidence, severity, and associated features. *Psychopharmacology (Berlin)* 2004;176:1–29.

CAFFEINE WITHDRAWAL

The caffeine withdrawal syndrome has been well-characterized. A recently published review of 57 experimental studies and 9 survey studies of caffeine withdrawal identified symptoms of caffeine withdrawal and pharmacologic and psychologic parameters affecting withdrawal (132). The authors identified 13 symptoms of caffeine withdrawal judged to be reliable across carefully controlled studies (Table 11.3). Symptoms with a strong empirical basis were conceptually clustered into five categories: headache; fatigue or drowsiness; dysphoric mood, depressed mood, or irritability; difficulty concentrating; and flulike somatic symptoms nausea, vomiting, and muscle pain/stiffness. The review found that, for 13% of individuals, the withdrawal symptoms produced clinically significant distress and/or functional impairment (e.g., unable to care for children, missed work) (198).

Time Course of Withdrawal The caffeine withdrawal syndrome follows an orderly time course. Onset usually occurs 12 to 24 hours after terminating caffeine intake, although onset as early as 6 hours and as late as 43 hours has been documented (132). Peak withdrawal intensity occurs in the range of 20 to 51 hours after abstinence (132). The duration of withdrawal appears to range from 2 to 9 days (132), although some have suggested that caffeine withdrawal headache may last for up to 3 weeks (199).

Dosing Parameters Although there is wide variability across individuals, the incidence and severity of caffeine withdrawal appears to be roughly an increasing function of daily caffeine dose (200). However, caffeine withdrawal occurs after abstinence from a dose as low as 100 mg/day (200,201). Caffeine withdrawal also occurs after relatively short-term exposure to daily caffeine, such that significant withdrawal can occur after only 3 consecutive days of 300 mg/day caffeine, with somewhat greater severity shown after 7 and 14 consecutive days of exposure (200). Another study showed that caffeine withdrawal headache occurred in three individuals who normally abstained from caffeinated beverages but were given 600 to 750 mg/day caffeine for 6 or 7 days (202). The spacing of caffeine dose throughout the day (i.e., 300 mg once daily versus 100 mg three times daily) does not appear to influence the range or severity of caffeine withdrawal symptoms (200). Low doses of caffeine are capable of suppressing caffeine withdrawal. For example, when individuals were maintained on 300 mg caffeine/day and tested with a range of lower doses (200, 100, 50, 25, and 0 mg/day), a substantial reduction in caffeine dose (to $<$100 mg/day) was necessary for the manifestation of caffeine withdrawal. Interestingly, just 25 mg/day was sufficient to suppress significant caffeine withdrawal headache (200).

Individual Differences There are substantial differences within and across individuals with regard to incidence or severity of caffeine withdrawal. For example, only about 50% of regular caffeine consumers report headache after any single episode of caffeine abstinence. One study that evaluated repeated abstinence trials showed that at least 36% of subjects who showed statistically significant elevations in headache failed to report this effect consistently across repeated trials (203).

Caffeine Withdrawal (ICD-10 Diagnosis and DSM-IV Proposed Criteria) The potential for caffeine withdrawal to cause clinically significant distress and/or impairment in functioning is reflected by the inclusion of caffeine withdrawal as an official diagnosis in ICD-10 and as a proposed diagnosis in DSM-IV-TR (164). Carefully controlled research on caffeine withdrawal has more than doubled since the DSM-IV was published in 1994, now providing a sound empirical basis for a diagnosis of caffeine withdrawal (132). The proposed criteria for a DSM-IV-TR research diagnosis of caffeine withdrawal require the presence of headache and one or more of the following: marked fatigue or drowsiness, marked anxiety or depression, nausea or vomiting (164). Anxiety is a proposed symptom in the DSM-IV-TR, although it does not appear to be a valid symptom of caffeine withdrawal (132). Furthermore, the suggested criteria fail to include other valid symptoms of caffeine withdrawal (Table 11.3). The only epidemiological study to evaluate the incidence of caffeine withdrawal using the criteria for the DSM-IV research diagnosis was a random-digit telephone survey (168). In this study, 44% of caffeine users reported having stopped or reduced caffeine use for at least 24 hours in the past year. Of those, 41% reported that they experienced one or more DSM-IV–defined caffeine withdrawal symptoms. Among individuals who attempted to permanently stop using caffeine, at least 71% reported experiencing DSM-IV–defined symptoms, and 24% reported having headache plus other symptoms that interfered with performance.

Caffeine withdrawal symptoms overlap with various psychologic and physical complaints. Caffeine withdrawal should be considered in the differential diagnosis in individuals presenting with headaches, fatigue, mood disturbances, impaired concentration, and flulike symptoms. It should also be noted that caffeine withdrawal has been observed in neonates as a result of in utero exposure to caffeine (204,205).

Short-term Caffeine Abstinence for Medical Procedures Patients are often asked to stop food and fluids before certain blood tests, surgery, or procedures such as endoscopies, colonoscopies, and cardiac catherizations. Whether patients scheduled to undergo these procedures could be allowed caffeine supplements to avoid symptoms of withdrawal should be considered. Caffeine withdrawal has been identified as a significant cause of postoperative headaches, the risk of which can be reduced if regular caffeine users are given caffeine on the day of the surgical procedure (206,207).

Caffeine Withdrawal in Animals Of the dozen or so reports of caffeine withdrawal in laboratory animals (mice, rats, cats, monkeys), most have documented substantial behavioral disruptions after cessation of chronic caffeine dosing (e.g., 50% to 80% reductions in spontaneous locomotor activity; 20% to 50% reductions in operant responding) (143,208). Similar to human studies, the severity of withdrawal in laboratory animals is an increasing function of the caffeine maintenance dose, with maximal withdrawal effects occurring on the first or second day of caffeine withdrawal (209,210). It has been speculated and there is some evidence supporting that increased functional tissue sensitivity to endogenous adenosine is the mechanism underlying some caffeine withdrawal effects (211–213).

CAFFEINE DEPENDENCE

The diagnosis of substance dependence is based on several features of problematic drug use including but not limited to withdrawal, tolerance, difficulty controlling use, using more than intended, and use despite harm. The ICD-10 recognizes a diagnosis of substance dependence due to caffeine (214,215), whereas the DSM-IV-TR does not, despite the two having very similar criteria. The rationale for excluding caffeine dependence from DSM-IV-TR was that although caffeine withdrawal had been documented, there was no available database pertaining to other important features of substance dependence such as inability to stop use and use despite harm (216,217).

More recently, five studies have identified adults and adolescents who report problematic caffeine consumption and fulfill DSM-IV-TR criteria for substance dependence on caffeine (168,198,218–221). Individuals meeting criteria for caffeine dependence have shown a wide range of daily caffeine intake (e.g., 129 to 2,548 mg/day in one study) and have been consumers of various types of caffeinated products (e.g., coffee, soft drinks, tea, medications). A diagnosis of caffeine dependence has been shown to prospectively predict a greater incidence of caffeine reinforcement (150) and more severe withdrawal (198). Furthermore, among a sample of pregnant women advised by their physician to eliminate all caffeine throughout pregnancy, a caffeine dependence diagnosis predicted greater use of caffeine during pregnancy and a history of daily cigarette smoking (221). In this study, those with a caffeine dependence diagnosis and a family history of alcoholism used potentially problematic amounts of caffeine during pregnancy (i.e., 50% used >300 mg/day). Caffeine dependence has also been shown to be associated with a history of alcohol abuse or dependence (198). The one study to examine the prevalence of caffeine dependence in the general population found that 30% of caffeine consumers fulfilled DSM-III-R diagnostic criteria for caffeine dependence (168). The most commonly endorsed symptom was desire or unsuccessful efforts to cut down or control use (56%). Additional research is needed to more fully characterize the prevalence of substance dependence on caffeine, its clinical significance and prognosis, its relationship with other drug dependencies, and effective treatment strategies. Table 11.4 lists some guidelines for assisting patients to reduce or eliminate caffeine.

TABLE 11.4 Practical Guidelines for Assisting Patients to Eliminate or Reduce Caffeine Use

1. Educate the patient about all sources of caffeine. For example, some individuals might not be aware that caffeine is present in noncola soft drinks or analgesics. It is also important to inform the patient of the wide variability in caffeine content within and across product types (see Table 11.1).
2. Determine usual caffeine consumption via a self-monitoring period using a food diary or via patient self-report of caffeine consumption over the past week.
3. Identify all sources of caffeine and calculate the total daily caffeine consumption in milligrams.
4. Choose a caffeine reduction or cessation goal depending on the needs of the patient. Patients who would like to avoid physical dependence on caffeine should be advised to consume no more than 50 mg of caffeine daily or to only use caffeine on an occasional basis. Present caffeine cessation as a temporary trial for patients who are resistant to treatment, or who appear to have a caffeine-related disorder but do not believe that caffeine is the cause of their complaints.
5. Generate a graded reduction (i.e., fading) schedule with the patient. A reasonable decrease would be 10% to 25% of the usual dose every few days or so.
6. Have the patient identify a noncaffeinated substitute for his or her usual caffeine-containing beverage. If the patient is a coffee drinker, he or she can start by mixing decaffeinated and caffeinated coffee and then progressively increase the percentage of decaffeinated until the desired level is achieved. If he or she consumes soft drinks, caffeinated and caffeine-free soft drinks can be alternated or mixed until the caffeinated soft drink is reduced or eliminated.
7. Discuss the possibility of relapse with the patient. Discuss triggers (i.e., antecedent conditions) for caffeine use and offer suggestions for coping with situations that pose a high risk of relapse (e.g., stress, withdrawal symptoms).
8. Suggest that the patient continue to self-monitor his or her caffeine consumption and encourage the patient to reward him or herself for successful behavior change.

HERITABILITY OF CAFFEINE USE

Genetic factors account for some of the individual variability in the use and effects of caffeine. Genetic variability in the adenosine A_{2A} receptor gene has been shown to be associated with levels of caffeine consumption (222) as well as differential effects of caffeine on measures of sleep and anxiety (180,181, 195,196). Large-scale twin studies have shown that relative to dizygotic twins, monozygotic twins have higher concordance rates for total caffeine consumption, heavy caffeine consumption, coffee and tea intake, caffeine tolerance, caffeine withdrawal, and caffeine intoxication with heritabilities ranging between 34% and 77% (169,198,223–225). Interestingly, three twin studies using multivariate structural equation modeling of caffeine, cigarette, and alcohol use concluded that a common genetic factor (polysubstance use) underlies the use of these three substances, with 28% to 41% of the heritable effects of caffeine use (or heavy use) shared with alcohol and smoking (224–226). A recent study of monozygotic and dizygotic male and female twin pairs found that caffeine and nicotine dependence were substantially influenced by genetic factors unique to these licit drugs and distinct from genetic factors found to be common among illicit drugs (227). As a whole, these genetic data underscore the fact that caffeine use and associated problems have an underlying biologic basis, part of which is shared with other commonly abused substances.

ASSOCIATIONS BETWEEN CAFFEINE AND OTHER DRUGS

Nicotine and Cigarette Smoking Cigarette smokers consume more caffeine than nonsmokers (228), and twin and cooccurrence studies suggest links between caffeine use and smoking (224–226,229). In a recent study, pregnant women were nine times more likely to report a history of daily cigarette smoking if they met criteria for substance dependence on caffeine (221). These finding are partially explained by the observation that cigarette smoking increases the rate of caffeine metabolism (21). Coffee drinking and cigarette smoking tend to temporally covary (230). Human and animal studies demonstrate that caffeine can increase the reinforcing and discriminative stimulus effects of intravenous nicotine (231–234). However, caffeine administration has not been shown to reliably increase cigarette or nicotine self-administration, or alter the effects of nicotine (141,235,236), suggesting that the coffee smoking interaction is not controlled by the pharmacologic effects of caffeine alone. However, studies have shown that caffeine can increase the analgesic effects of cigarette smoking (237) and moderate decreases in arousal after cigarette smoking (238). Several studies have shown that cigarette smoking abstinence can produce substantial increases in caffeine blood levels among heavy caffeine consumers, presumably because of the reversal of cigarette smoking-induced caffeine metabolism (239,240); however, the clinical significance during smoking cessation attempts has not been demonstrated (228,241,242).

Alcohol Heavy use and clinical dependence on alcohol is associated with heavy use and clinical dependence on caffeine (229,241,243). One study reported substantial increases in caffeine consumption after alcohol detoxification in alcoholics (244). A study of individuals fulfilling DSM-IV diagnostic criteria for substance dependence on caffeine found that almost 60% had a past diagnosis of alcohol abuse or dependence (198). It is common lore that caffeine reverses the impairing effects of alcohol; however, controlled research suggests that such effects are generally incomplete and highly inconsistent across different types of behavioral and subjective measures (245). Some recent studies have shown that individuals consuming caffeine along with alcohol underestimate their levels of intoxication and impairment (245,246) and may be more prone to injury (247). The growing trend of combining energy drinks and alcohol, presumably to offset the sedative effects of alcohol, and the growing market of caffeinated beers, malt beverages, and liquors suggests there is a need for more research in this area.

Other Drug Interactions Animal studies show that caffeine increases acquisition of cocaine self-administration, reinstates self-administration behavior previously maintained by cocaine, and potentiates the stimulant and discriminative stimulus effects of cocaine (32). In human experimental studies, oral caffeine increases drug-appropriate responding in individuals trained to discriminate cocaine (248). Caffeine and ephedrine have been shown to mutually potentiate each other's stimulus effects (249). There is preclinical evidence to suggest that caffeine may increase the toxic effects of other stimulant drugs such as d-amphetamine, cocaine, and MDMA (250–252).

Both animal and human studies suggest a mutually antagonistic relationship between caffeine and benzodiazepines (253). Although it is possible that this interaction occurs at the benzodiazepine receptor, the lack of uniform antagonism across measures suggests that the effect is functional in nature (253–255).

There is some evidence that caffeine inhibits the metabolism of the antipsychotic clozapine to an extent that might be clinically significant (256). Because caffeine and theophylline mutually inhibit each others metabolism, caffeine consumption during theophylline therapy should be monitored. Lithium toxicity may occur after caffeine withdrawal because of decreased renal clearance of lithium (16).

ACKNOWLEDGMENTS: *Preparation of this review was supported, in part, by U.S. Public Health Service grant R01 DA03890 from the National Institute on Drug Abuse and by intramural funds of the National Institute on Drug Abuse.*

REFERENCES

1. Frary CD, Johnson RK, Wang MQ. Food sources and intakes of caffeine in the diets of persons in the United States. *J Am Diet Assoc* 2005;105: 110–113.

2. Budavari S, O'Neil M, Smith A, et al., eds. *The Merck index*. Whitehouse Station, NJ: Merck Research Laboratories, 1996.
3. Weinburg BA, Bealer BK. *The world of caffeine: the science and culture of the world's most popular drug*. New York: Routledge, 2001.
4. Pendergrast M. *Uncommon grounds: the history of coffee and how it transformed our world*. New York: Basic Books, 1999.
5. Sawynok J, Yaksh TL. Caffeine as an analgesic adjuvant: a review of pharmacology and mechanisms of action. *Pharmacol Rev* 1993;45:43–85.
6. Fennelly M, Galletly DC, Purdie GI. Is caffeine withdrawal the mechanism of postoperative headache? *Anesth Analg* 1991;72:449–453.
7. Hampl KF, Schneider MC, Ruttimann U, et al. Perioperative administration of caffeine tablets for prevention of postoperative headaches. *Can J Anaesth* 1995;42:789–792.
8. Schmidt B, Roberts RS, Davis P, et al. Long-term effects of caffeine therapy for apnea of prematurity. *N Engl J Med* 2007;357:1893–1902.
9. Rosenquist PB, McCall WV, Farah A, et al. Effects of caffeine pretreatment on measures of seizure impact. *Convuls Ther* 1994;10:181–185.
10. Jansen RW, Lipsitz LA. Postprandial hypotension: epidemiology, pathophysiology, and clinical management. *Ann Intern Med* 1995;122: 286–295.
11. Graham TE. Caffeine and exercise: metabolism, endurance and performance. *Sports Med* 2001;31:785–807.
12. Barone JJ, Roberts HR. Caffeine consumption. *Food Chem Toxicol* 1996;34:119–129.
13. Mumford GK, Benowitz NL, Evans SM, et al. Absorption rate of methylxanthines following capsules, cola and chocolate. *Eur J Clin Pharmacol* 1996;51:319–325.
14. James JE. *Understanding caffeine*.Thousand Oaks, CA: Sage Publications, Inc., 1997.
15. Denaro CP, Benowitz NL. Caffeine metabolism: Disposition in liver disease and hepatic-function testing. In: *Drug and alcohol abuse reviews, vol. 2: liver pathology and alcohol*. Watson, RR, ed. Totowa, NJ: The Human Press, Inc., 1991;513–539.
16. Carrillo JA, Benitez J. Clinically significant pharmacokinetic interactions between dietary caffeine and medications. *Clin Pharmacokinet* 2000;39:127–153.
17. Benowitz NL, Jacob P, Mayan H, et al. Sympathomimetic effects of paraxanthine and caffeine in humans. *Clin Pharmacol Ther* 1995;58: 684–691.
18. Frye RF, Zgheib NK, Matzke GR, et al. Liver disease selectively modulates cytochrome P450–mediated metabolism. *Clin Pharmacol Ther* 2006;80:235–245.
19. Blanchard J, Sawers SJ. Comparative pharmacokinetics of caffeine in young and elderly men. *J Pharmacokinet Biopharm* 1983;11:109–126.
20. Parsons WD, Neims AH. Prolonged half-life of caffeine in healthy term newborn infants. *J Pediatr* 1981;98:640–641.
21. Parsons WD, Neims AH. Effect of smoking on caffeine clearance. *Clin Pharmacol Ther* 1978;24:40–45.
22. Denaro CP, Brown CR, Wilson M, et al. Dose-dependency of caffeine metabolism with repeated dosing. *Clin Pharmacol Ther* 1990;48: 277–285.
23. Aldridge A, Bailey J, Neims AH. The disposition of caffeine during and after pregnancy. *Semin Perinatol* 1981;5:310–314.
24. Vo HT, Smith BD, Elmi S. Menstrual endocrinology and pathology: caffeine, physiology, and PMS. In: Smith BD, Gupta U, Gupta BS, eds. *Caffeine activation theory: effects on health and behavior*. Boca Raton, FL: Taylor & Francis Group, 2007:181–197.
25. Fredholm BB, Irenius E, Kull B, et al. Comparison of the potency of adenosine as an agonist at human adenosine receptors expressed in Chinese hamster ovary cells. *Biochem Pharmacol* 2001;61:443–448.
26. Solinas M, Ferré S, Antoniou K, et al. Involvement of adenosine A1 receptors in the discriminative-stimulus effects of caffeine in rats. *Psychopharmacology (Berlin)* 2005;179:576–586.
27. Schiffmann SN, Fisone G, Moresco R, et al. Adenosine A_{2A} receptors and basal ganglia physiology. *Prog Neurobiol* 2007;83:277–292.
28. Ferré S, Ciruela F, Borycz J, et al. Adenosine A_1-A_{2A} receptor heteromers: new targets for caffeine in the brain. *Front Biosci* 2008;13:2391–2399.
29. Ferré S. An update on the mechanisms of the psychostimulant effects of caffeine. *J Neurochem*, 2008;105:1067–1079.
30. Antoniou K, Papadopoulou-Daifoti Z, Hyphantis T, et al. A detailed behavioral analysis of the acute motor effects of caffeine in the rat: involvement of adenosine A_1 and A_{2A} receptors. *Psychopharmacology (Berlin)* 2005;183:154–162.
31. Karcz-Kubicha M, Antoniou K, Terasmaa A, et al. Involvement of adenosine A_1 and A_{2A} receptors in the motor effects of caffeine after its acute and chronic administration. *Neuropsychopharmacology* 2003;28: 1281–1291.
32. Ferré S, Fuxe K, von Euler G, et al. Adenosine-dopamine interactions in the brain. *Neuroscience* 1992;51:501–512.
33. Garrett BE, Griffiths RR. The role of dopamine in the behavioral effects of caffeine in animals and humans. *Pharmacol Biochem Behav* 1997;57: 533–541.
34. Ikemoto S. Dopamine reward circuitry: two projection systems from the ventral midbrain to the nucleus accumbens-olfactory tubercle complex. *Brain Res Rev* 2007;56:27–78.
35. Wise, RA. Dopamine, learning and motivation. *Nat Neurosci Rev* 2004; 5:483–494.
36. Basheer R, Strecker RE, Thakkar MM, et al. Adenosine and sleep-wake regulation. *Prog Neurobiol* 2004;73:379–396.
37. Ferré S, Diamond I, Goldberg SR, et al. Adenosine A_{2A} receptors in ventral striatum, hypothalamus and nociceptive circuitry implications for drug addiction, sleep and pain. *Prog Neurobiol* 2007;83:332–347.
38. Huang ZL, Urade Y, Hayaishi O. Prostaglandins and adenosine in the regulation of sleep and wakefulness. *Curr Opin Pharmacol* 2007;7: 33–38.
39. Porkka-Heiskanen T, Strecker RE, McCarley RW. Brain site-specificity of extracellular adenosine concentration changes during sleep deprivation and spontaneous sleep: an in vivo microdialysis study. *Neuroscience* 2000;99:507–517.
40. Ferré S, Agnati LF, Ciruela F, et al. Neurotransmitter receptor heteromers and their integrative role in 'local modules': the striatal spine module. *Brain Res Rev* 2007;55:55–67.
41. Hertz L, Zielke HR. Astrocytic control of glutamatergic activity: astrocytes as stars of the show. *Trends Neurosci* 2004;27:735–743.
42. Newman EA. New roles for astrocytes: regulation of synaptic transmission. *Trends Neurosci* 2003;26:536–542.
43. Pascual O, Casper KB, Kubera C, et al. Astrocytic purinergic signaling coordinates synaptic networks. *Science* 2005;310:113–116.
44. Gerfen CR. Basal Ganglia. In: Paxinos, G, ed. *The rat nervous system*. Amsterdam: Elsevier Academic Press, 2004:445–508.
45. Agnati LF, Ferré S, Lluis C, et al. Molecular mechanisms and therapeutical implications of intramembrane receptor/receptor interactions among heptahelical receptors with examples from the striatopallidal GABA neurons. *Pharmacol Rev* 2003;55:509–550.
46. Ferré S, Fredholm BB, Morelli M, et al. Adenosine-dopamine receptor-receptor interactions as an integrative mechanism in the basal ganglia. *Trends Neurosci* 1997;20:482–487.
47. Borycz J, Pereira MF, Melani A, et al. Differential glutamate-dependent and glutamate-independent adenosine A_1 receptor-mediated modulation of dopamine release in different striatal compartments. *J Neurochem* 2007;101:355–363.
48. Ferré S, O'Connor WT, Fuxe K, et al. The striopallidal neuron: a main locus for adenosine-dopamine interactions in the brain. *J Neurosci* 1993;13:5402–5406.
49. Ferré S, O'Connor WT, Svenningsson P, et al. Dopamine D_1 receptor-mediated facilitation of GABAergic neurotransmission in the rat strioentopenduncular pathway and its modulation by adenosine A_1 receptor-mediated mechanisms. *Eur J Neurosci* 1996;8:1545–1553.
50. Ferré S, Popoli P, Gimenez-Llort L, et al. Adenosine/dopamine interaction: implications for the treatment of Parkinson's disease. *Parkinsonism Relat Disord* 2001;7:235–241.
51. Ferré S, Ciruela F, Woods AS, et al. Functional relevance of neurotransmitter receptor heteromers in the central nervous system. *Trends Neurosci* 2007;30:440–446.

52. Ferré S, von Euler G, Johansson B, et al. Stimulation of high-affinity adenosine A_2 receptors decreases the affinity of dopamine D_2 receptors in rat striatal membranes. *Proc Natl Acad Sci U S A* 1991;88:7238–7241.
53. Azdad K, Gall D, Woods AS, et al. Antagonistic modulatory role of adenosine A_{2A} receptor on dopamine D_2 receptor regulation of down- to up-state transitions in striatopallidal neurons: Involvement of A_{2A}-D_2 receptor heteromerization. *Neuropsychopharmacology*, in press.
54. Stromberg I, Popoli P, Muller CE, et al. Electrophysiological and behavioural evidence for an antagonistic modulatory role of adenosine A_{2A} receptors in dopamine D_2 receptor regulation in the rat dopamine-denervated striatum. *Eur J Neurosci* 2000;12:4033–4037.
55. Svenningsson P, Lindskog M, Ledent C, et al. Regulation of the phosphorylation of the dopamine- and cAMP-regulated phosphoprotein of 32 kDa in vivo by dopamine D_1, dopamine D_2, and adenosine A_{2A} receptors. *Proc Natl Acad Sci U S A* 2000;97:1856–1860.
56. Hakansson K, Galdi S, Hendrick J, et al. Regulation of phosphorylation of the GluR1 AMPA receptor by dopamine D_2 receptors. *J Neurochem* 2006;96:482–488.
57. Lindskog M, Svenningsson P, Pozzi L, et al. Involvement of DARPP-32 phosphorylation in the stimulant action of caffeine. *Nature* 2002;418: 774–778.
58. Muller CE, Ferré S. Blocking striatal adenosine A_{2A} receptors: a new strategy for basal ganglia disorders. *Recent Patents CNS Drug Discov* 2007;2:1–21.
59. Popoli P, Gimenez-Llort L, Pezzola A, et al. Adenosine A_1 receptor blockade selectively potentiates the motor effects induced by dopamine D_1 receptor stimulation in rodents. *Neurosci Lett* 1996;218:209–213.
60. Ferré S, Popoli P, Gimenez-Llort L, et al. Postsynaptic antagonistic interaction between adenosine A_1 and dopamine D_1 receptors. *Neuroreport* 1994;6:73–76.
61. Ferré S, Torvinen M, Antoniou' K, et al. Adenosine A_1 receptor-mediated modulation of dopamine D_1 receptors in stably cotransfected fibroblast cells. *J Biol Chem* 1998;273:4718–4724.
62. Ferré S, Rimondini R, Popoli P, et al. Stimulation of adenosine A_1 receptors attenuates dopamine D_1 receptor-mediated increase of NGFI-A, c-fos and jun-B mRNA levels in the dopamine-denervated striatum and dopamine D_1 receptor-mediated turning behaviour. *Eur J Neurosci* 1999;11:3884–3892.
63. Quarta D, Ferré S, Solinas M, et al. Opposite modulatory roles for adenosine A_1 and A_{2A} receptors on glutamate and dopamine release in the shell of the nucleus accumbens. Effects of chronic caffeine exposure. *J Neurochem* 2004;88:1151–1158.
64. Solinas M, Ferré S, You ZB, et al. Caffeine induces dopamine and glutamate release in the shell of the nucleus accumbens. *J Neurosci* 2002;22:6321–6324.
65. Quarta D, Borycz J, Solinas M, et al. Adenosine receptor-mediated modulation of dopamine release in the nucleus accumbens depends on glutamate neurotransmission and *N*-methyl-D-aspartate receptor stimulation. *J Neurochem* 2004;91:873–880.
66. De Luca MA, Bassareo V, Bauer A, et al. Caffeine and accumbens shell dopamine. *J Neurochem* 2007;103:157–163.
67. Ciruela F, Casado V, Rodrigues RJ, et al. Presynaptic control of striatal glutamatergic neurotransmission by adenosine A_1-A_{2A} receptor heteromers. *J Neurosci* 2006;26:2080–2087.
68. Boulenger J-P, Patel J, Post RM, et al. Chronic caffeine consumption increases the number of brain adenosine receptors. *Life Sci* 1983; 32:135–142.
69. Hawkins M, Dugich MM, Porter N, et al. Effects of chronic administration of caffeine on adenosine A_1 and A_2 receptors in the brain. *Brain Res Bull* 1988;21:479–482.
70. Jacobson KA, von Lubitz DK, Daly JW, et al. Adenosine receptor ligands: differences with acute versus chronic treatment. *Trends Pharmacol Sci* 1996;17:108–113.
71. Holtzman SG, Mante S, Minneman KP. Role of adenosine receptors in caffeine tolerance. *J Pharmacol Exp Ther* 1991;256:62–68.
72. Conlay LA, Conant JA, deBros F, et al. Caffeine alters plasma adenosine levels. *Nature* 1997;389:136.
73. James JE. Critical review of dietary caffeine and blood pressure: a relationship that should be taken more seriously. *Psychosom Med* 2004; 66:63–71.
74. Sudano I, Spieker L, Binggeli C, et al. Coffee blunts mental stress-induced blood pressure increase in habitual but not in nonhabitual coffee drinkers. *Hypertension* 2005;46:521–526.
75. Quinlan PT, Lane J, Moore KL, et al. The acute physiological and mood effects of tea and coffee: the role of caffeine level. *Pharmacol Biochem Behav* 2000;66:19–28.
76. Rao SS, Welcher K, Zimmerman B, et al. Is coffee a colonic stimulant? *Eur J Gastroenterol Hepatol* 1998;10:113–118.
77. Wemple RD, Lamb DR, McKeever KH. Caffeine vs. caffeine-free sports drinks: effects on urine production at rest and during prolonged exercise. *Int J Sports Med* 1997;18:40–46.
78. Creighton SM, Stanton SL. Caffeine: does it affect your bladder? *Br J Urol* 1990;66:613–614.
79. Pianosi P, Grondin D, Desmond K, et al. Effect of caffeine on the ventilatory response to inhaled carbon dioxide. *Respir Physiol* 1994;95:311–320.
80. Becker AB, Simons KJ, Gillespie CA, et al. The bronchodilator effects and pharmacokinetics of caffeine in asthma. *N Engl J Med* 1984; 310:743–746.
81. Doherty M, Smith PM. Effects of caffeine ingestion on exercise testing: a meta-analysis. *Int J Sport Nutr Exerc Metab* 2004;14:626–646.
82. Tarnopolsky M, Cupido C. Caffeine potentiates low frequency skeletal muscle force in habitual and nonhabitual caffeine consumers. *J Appl Physiol* 2000;89:1719–1724.
83. Patwardhan RV, Desmond PV, Johnson RF, et al. Effects of caffeine on plasma free fatty acids, urinary catecholamines, and drug binding. *Clin Pharmacol Ther* 1980; 28:398–403.
84. Robertson D, Wade D, Workman R, et al. Tolerance to the humoral and hemodynamic effects of caffeine in man. *J Clin Invest* 1981;67: 1111–1117.
85. al'Absi M, Lovallo WR, McKey B, et al. Hypothalamic-pituitary-adrenocortical responses to psychological stress and caffeine in men at high and low risk for hypertension. *Psychosom Med* 1998;60:521–527.
86. Lin AS, Uhde TW, Slate SO, et al. Effects of intravenous caffeine administered to healthy males during sleep. *Depress Anxiety* 1997;5:21–28.
87. Lovallo WR, Farag NH, Vincent AS, et al. Cortisol responses to mental stress, exercise, and meals following caffeine intake in men and women. *Pharmacol Biochem Behav* 2006;83:441–447.
88. MacKenzie T, Comi R, Sluss P, et al. Metabolic and hormonal effects of caffeine: randomized, double-blind, placebo-controlled crossover trial. *Metabolism* 2007;56:1694–1698.
89. Lane JD, Feinglos MN, Surwit RS. Caffeine increases ambulatory glucose and postprandial responses in coffee drinkers with type 2 diabetes. *Diabetes Care* 2008;31:221–222.
90. Fenster L, Quale C, Waller K, et al. Caffeine consumption and menstrual function. *Am J Epidemiol* 1999;149:550–557.
91. Higdon JV, Frei B. Coffee and health: a review of recent human research. *Crit Rev Food Sci Nutr* 2006;46:101–123.
92. James JE. *Caffeine and health*. San Diego, CA: Academic Press, Inc., 1991.
93. Nawrot P, Jordan S, Eastwood J, et al. Effects of caffeine on human health. *Food Addit Contam* 2003;20:1–30.
94. James JE. Blood pressure effects of dietary caffeine are a risk for cardiovascular disease. In: Smith BD, Gupta U, Gupta BS, eds. *Caffeine and activation theory: effects on health and behavior*. Boca Raton, FL: Taylor & Francis Group, 2007:133–153.
95. Vlachopoulos C, Hirata K, Stefanadis C, et al. Caffeine increases aortic stiffness in hypertensive patients. *Am J Hypertens* 2003;16:63–66.
96. Smith BD, Aldridge K. Acute cardiovascular effects of caffeine: hemodynamics and heart function. In: Smith BD, Gupta U, Gupta BS, eds. *Caffeine and activation theory: effects on health and behavior*. Boca Raton, FL: Taylor & Francis Group, 2007:81–91.
97. Wei M, Schwertner HA. Effects of coffee and caffeine consumption on serum lipids and lipoproteins. In: Smith BD, Gupta U, Gupta BS, eds. *Caffeine and activation theory: effects on health and behavior*. Boca Raton, FL: Taylor & Francis Group, 2007:155–178.

98. Boekema PJ, Samsom M, van Berge Henegouwen GP, et al. Coffee and gastrointestinal function: facts and fiction. A review. *Scand J Gastroenterol Suppl* 1999;230:35–39.
99. Pehl C, Pfeiffer A, Wendl B, et al. The effect of decaffeination of coffee on gastro-oesophageal reflux in patients with reflux disease. *Aliment Pharmacol Ther* 1997;11:483–486.
100. Wendl B, Pfeiffer A, Pehl C, et al. Effect of decaffeination of coffee or tea on gastro-oesophageal reflux. *Aliment Pharmacol Ther* 1994;8:283–287.
101. Aldoori WH, Giovannucci EL, Stampfer MJ, et al. A prospective study of alcohol, smoking, caffeine, and the risk of duodenal ulcer in men. *Epidemiology* 1997;8:420–424.
102. Holroyd-Leduc JM,Straus SE. Management of urinary incontinence in women: scientific review. *JAMA* 2004;291:986–995.
103. James JE, Sawczuk D,Merrett S. The effect of chronic caffeine consumption on urinary incontinence in psychogeriatric inpatients. *Psychol Health* 1989;3:297–305.
104. Bryant CM, Dowell CJ, Fairbrother G. Caffeine reduction education to improve urinary symptoms. *Br J Nurs* 2002;11:560–565.
105. Hallstrom H, Wolk A, Glynn A, et al. Coffee, tea and caffeine consumption in relation to osteoporotic fracture risk in a cohort of Swedish women. *Osteoporos Int* 2006;17:1055–1064.
106. Fernandes O, Sabharwal M, Smiley T, et al. Moderate to heavy caffeine consumption during pregnancy and relationship to spontaneous abortion and abnormal fetal growth: a meta-analysis. *Reprod Toxicol* 1998;12:435–444.
107. Weng X, Odouli R, Li DK. Maternal caffeine consumption during pregnancy and the risk of miscarriage: a prospective cohort study. *Am J Obstet Gynecol* 2008;198:279, e1–e8.
108. Grosso LM, Bracken MB. Caffeine metabolism, genetics, and perinatal outcomes: a review of exposure assessment considerations during pregnancy. *Ann Epidemiol* 2005;15:460–466.
109. Sata F, Yamada H, Suzuki K, et al. Caffeine intake, CYP1A2 polymorphism and the risk of recurrent pregnancy loss. *Mol Hum Reprod* 2005;11:357–360.
110. Tan EK, Tan C, Fook-Chong SM, et al. Dose-dependent protective effect of coffee, tea, and smoking in Parkinson's disease: a study in ethnic Chinese. *J Neurol Sci* 2003;216:163–167.
111. Paganini-Hill A. Risk factors for Parkinson's disease: the leisure world cohort study. *Neuroepidemiology* 2001;20:118–124.
112. Ascherio A, Zhang SM, Hernan MA, et al. Prospective study of caffeine consumption and risk of Parkinson's disease in men and women. *Ann Neurol* 2001;50:56–63.
113. Ross GW, Abbott RD, Petrovitch H, et al. Association of coffee and caffeine intake with the risk of Parkinson disease. *JAMA* 2000;283: 2674–2679.
114. Ruhl CE, Everhart JE. Coffee and tea consumption are associated with a lower incidence of chronic liver disease in the United States. *Gastroenterology* 2005;129:1928–1936.
115. Cadden IS, Partovi N, Yoshida EM. Review article: possible beneficial effects of coffee on liver disease and function. *Aliment Pharmacol Ther* 2007;26:1–8.
116. Pereira MA, Parker ED, Folsom AR. Coffee consumption and risk of type 2 diabetes mellitus: an 11-year prospective study of 28,812 postmenopausal women. *Arch Intern Med* 2006;166:1311–1316.
117. van Dam RM, Hu FB. Coffee consumption and risk of type 2 diabetes: a systematic review. *JAMA* 2005;294:97–104.
118. van Dam RM. Coffee and type 2 diabetes: from beans to beta-cells. *Nutr Metab Cardiovasc Dis* 2006;16:69–77.
119. McLellan TM, Kamimori GH, Voss DM, et al. Caffeine effects on physical and cognitive performance during sustained operations. *Aviat Space Environ Med* 2007;78:871–877.
120. van der Stelt O, Snel J. Caffeine and human performance. In: Snel J, Lorist MM, eds. *Nicotine, caffeine, and social drinking*. Amsterdam, Netherlands: Harwood Academic Publishers, 1998:167–183.
121. Stafford LD, Rusted J, Yeomans MR. Caffeine, mood, and performance: a selective review. In: Smith BD, Gupta U, Gupta BS, eds. *Caffeine and activation theory: effects on health and behavior*. Boca Raton, FL: Taylor & Francis Group, 2007:283–309.
122. Doherty M, Smith PM. Effects of caffeine ingestion on rating of perceived exertion during and after exercise: a meta-analysis. *Scand J Med Sci Sports* 2005;15:69–78.
123. Wiles JD, Coleman D, Tegerdine M, et al. The effects of caffeine ingestion on performance time, speed and power during a laboratory-based 1 km cycling time-trial. *J Sports Sci* 2006;24:1165–1171.
124. Doherty M, Smith P, Hughes M, et al. Caffeine lowers perceptual response and increases power output during high-intensity cycling. *J Sports Sci* 2004;22:637–643.
125. James JE. Acute and chronic effects of caffeine on performance, mood, headache, and sleep. *Neuropsychobiology* 1998;38:32–41.
126. Rogers PJ, Heatherley SV, Hayward RC, et al. Effects of caffeine and caffeine withdrawal on mood and cognitive performance degraded by sleep restriction. *Psychopharmacology (Berlin)* 2005;179:742–752.
127. Childs E, de Wit H. Subjective, behavioral, and physiological effects of acute caffeine in light, nondependent caffeine users. *Psychopharmacology (Berlin)* 2006;185:514–523.
128. Haskell CF, Kennedy DO, Wesnes KA, et al. Cognitive and mood improvements of caffeine in habitual consumers and habitual non-consumers of caffeine. *Psychopharmacology (Berlin)* 2005;179:813–825.
129. James JE, Rogers PJ. Effects of caffeine on performance and mood: withdrawal reversal is the most plausible explanation. *Psychopharmacology (Berlin)* 2005;182:1–8.
130. Griffiths RR, Juliano LM, Chausmer AL. Caffeine pharmacology and clinical effects. In: Graham AW, Schultz TK, Mayo-Smith M. et al., eds. *Principles of addiction medicine,* 3rd ed. Chevy Chase, MD: American Society of Addiction Medicine, 2003;193–224.
131. Griffiths RR, Mumford GK. Caffeine-A drug of abuse? In: Bloom FE, Kupfer DJ, eds. *Psychopharmacology: the fourth generation of progress*. New York: Raven Press, Ltd., 1995;1699–1713.
132. Juliano LM, Griffiths RR. A critical review of caffeine withdrawal: empirical validation of symptoms and signs, incidence, severity, and associated features. *Psychopharmacology (Berlin)* 2004;176:1–29.
133. Christopher G, Sutherland D, Smith A. Effects of caffeine in non-withdrawn volunteers. *Hum Psychopharmacol* 2005;20:47–53.
134. Mumford GK, Evans SM, Kaminski BJ, et al. Discriminative stimulus and subjective effects of theobromine and caffeine in humans. *Psychopharmacology (Berlin)* 1994;115:1–8.
135. Silverman K, Griffiths RR. Low-dose caffeine discrimination and self-reported mood effects in normal volunteers. *J Exp Anal Behav* 1992;57: 91–107.
136. Silverman K, Mumford GK, Griffiths RR. Enhancing caffeine reinforcement by behavioral requirements following drug ingestion. *Psychopharmacology (Berlin)* 1994;114:424–432.
137. Boulenger JP, Uhde TW, Wolff EA, 3rd, et al. Increased sensitivity to caffeine in patients with panic disorders. Preliminary evidence. *Arch Gen Psychiatry* 1984;41:1067–1071.
138. Bruce M, Scott N, Shine P, et al. Anxiogenic effects of caffeine in patients with anxiety disorders. *Arch Gen Psychiatry* 1992;49: 867–869.
139. Charney DS, Heninger GR, Jatlow PI. Increased anxiogenic effects of caffeine in panic disorders. *Arch Gen Psychiatry* 1985;42:233–243.
140. Telch MJ, Silverman A, Schmidt NB. Effects of anxiety sensitivity and perceived control on emotional responding to caffeine challenge. *J Anxiety Dis* 1996;10:21–35.
141. Chait LD, Griffiths RR. Effects of caffeine on cigarette smoking and subjective response. *Clin Pharmacol Ther* 1983;34:612–622.
142. Chait LD, Johanson CE. Discriminative stimulus effects of caffeine and benzphetamine in amphetamine-trained volunteers. *Psychopharmacology (Berlin)* 1988;96:302–308.
143. Griffiths RR, Mumford GK. Caffeine reinforcement, discrimination, tolerance, and physical dependence in laboratory animals and humans. In: Schuster CR, Kuhars MJ, eds. *Pharmacological aspects of drug dependence: toward an integrated neurobehavioral approach*. Heidelberg: Springer-Verlag, 1996:315–341.
144. Griffiths RR, Evans SM, Heishman SJ, et al. Low-dose caffeine discrimination in humans. *J Pharmacol Exp Ther* 1990;252:970–978.

145. Smit HJ, Blackburn RJ. Reinforcing effects of caffeine and theobromine as found in chocolate. *Psychopharmacology (Berlin)* 2005;181:101–106.
146. Haskell CF, Kennedy DO, Milne AL, et al. Caffeine at levels found in decaffeinated beverages is behaviourally active. *Appetite* 2008;50:559.
147. Evans SM, Critchfield TS, Griffiths RR. Caffeine reinforcement demonstrated in a majority of moderate caffeine users. *Behav Pharmacol* 1994;5:231–238.
148. Hughes JR, Hunt WK, Higgins ST, et al. Effect of dose on the ability of caffeine to serve as a reinforcer in humans. *Behav Pharmacol* 1992;3: 211–218.
149. Hughes JR, Oliveto AH, Bickel WK, et al. The ability of low doses of caffeine to serve as reinforcers in humans: a replication. *Exp Clinl Psychopharmacol* 1995;3:358–363.
150. Liguori A, Hughes JR. Caffeine self-administration in humans: 2. A within-subjects comparison of coffee and cola vehicles. *Exp Clin Psychopharmacol* 1997;5:295–303.
151. Griffiths RR, Woodson PP. Reinforcing effects of caffeine in humans. *J Pharmacol Exp Ther* 1988;246:21–29.
152. Evans SM, Griffiths RR. Caffeine tolerance and choice in humans. *Psychopharmacology (Berlin)* 1992;108:51–59.
153. Garrett BE, Griffiths RR. Physical dependence increases the relative reinforcing effects of caffeine versus placebo. *Psychopharmacology (Berlin)* 1998;139:195–202.
154. Griffiths RR, Bigelow GE, Liebson IA. Human coffee drinking: reinforcing and physical dependence producing effects of caffeine. *J Pharmacol Exp Ther* 1986;239:416–425.
155. Rogers PJ, Richardson NJ, Elliman NA. Overnight caffeine abstinence and negative reinforcement of preference for caffeine-containing drinks. *Psychopharmacology (Berlin)* 1995;120:457–462.
156. Yeomans MR, Jackson A, Lee MD, et al. Expression of flavour preferences conditioned by caffeine is dependent on caffeine deprivation state. *Psychopharmacology (Berlin)* 2000;150:208–215.
157. Tinley EM, Yeomans MR, Durlach PJ. Caffeine reinforces flavour preference in caffeine-dependent, but not long-term withdrawn, caffeine consumers. *Psychopharmacology (Berlin)* 2003;166:416–423.
158. Patkina NA, Zvartau EE. Caffeine place conditioning in rats: comparison with cocaine and ethanol. *Eur Neuropsychopharmacol* 1998;8:287–291.
159. Shi J, Benowitz NL, Denaro CP, et al. Pharmacokinetic-pharmacodynamic modeling of caffeine: tolerance to pressor effects. *Clin Pharmacol Ther* 1993;53:6–14.
160. Bonnet MH, Arand DL. Caffeine use as a model of acute and chronic insomnia. *Sleep* 1992;15:526–536.
161. Zwyghuizen-Doorenbos A, Roehrs TA, Lipschutz L, et al. Effects of caffeine on alertness. *Psychopharmacology (Berlin)* 1990;100:36–39.
162. Farag NH, Vincent AS, McKey BS, et al. Hemodynamic mechanisms underlying the incomplete tolerance to caffeine's pressor effects. *Am J Cardiol* 2005;95:1389–1392.
163. Farag NH, Vincent AS, Sung BH, et al. Caffeine tolerance is incomplete: persistent blood pressure responses in the ambulatory setting. *Am J Hypertens* 2005;18:714–719.
164. American Psychiatric Association. *Diagnostic and statistical manual of mental disorders, 4th ed. text revision*. Washington, DC: American Psychiatric Press, 2000.
165. Griffiths RR, Reissig CJ. Substance abuse: caffeine use disorders. In: Tasman A, Kay J, Lieberman HR et al., eds. *Psychiatry*, 3rd ed. Chichester, UK: John Wiley & Sons, 2008:1019–1040.
166. American Psychiatric Association. *Diagnostic and statistical manual of mental disorders, 3rd ed. revised*. Washington, DC: American Psychiatric Press, 1987.
167. Greden JF, Pomerleau OF. Caffeine-related disorders and nicotine-related disorders. In: Kaplan HI, Sadock BJ, eds. *Comprehensive textbook of psychiatry IV*. Baltimore, MD: Williams & Wilkins, 1995:799–810.
168. Hughes JR, Oliveto AH, Liguori A, et al. Endorsement of DSM-IV dependence criteria among caffeine users. *Drug Alcohol Depend* 1998; 52:99–107.
169. Kendler KS, Myers J, Gardner, CO. Caffeine intake, toxicity and dependence and lifetime risk for psychiatric and substance use disorders: an epidemiologic and co-twin control analysis. *Psychol Med* 2006;36: 1717–1725.
170. Lai MW, Klein-Scwartz W, Rodgers GC, et al. 2005 annual report of the American Association of Poison Control Centers' National Poisoning and Exposure Databases. *Clin Toxicol* 2006;44:803–932.
171. McCarthy D, Mycyk M, DesLauriers C. Hospitalization for caffeine abuse is associated with concomitant abuse of other pharmaceutical products. *Ann Emerg Med* 2006;48:101.
172. Walsh MJ, Marquardt KA, Albertson TE. Adverse effects from the ingestion of redline energy drinks. *Clin Toxicol* 2006;44:642.
173. Beck JG, Berisford MA. The effects of caffeine on panic patients: response components of anxiety. *Behav Ther* 1992;23:405–422.
174. Nickell PV, Uhde TW. Dose-response effects of intravenous caffeine in normal volunteers. *Anxiety* 1994;1:161–168.
175. Stern KN, Chait LD, Johanson CE. Reinforcing and subjective effects of caffeine in normal human volunteers. *Psychopharmacology (Berlin)* 1989;98:81–88.
176. Botella P, Parra A. Coffee increases state anxiety in males but not in females. *Hum Psychopharmacol* 2003;18:141–143.
177. Nardi AE, Valenca AM, Lopes FL, et al. Caffeine and 35% carbon dioxide challenge tests in panic disorder. *Hum Psychopharmacol* 2007;22:231–240.
178. Uhde TW. Caffeine provocation of panic: a focus on biological mechanisms. In: Ballenger, JC, ed. *Neurobiology of panic disorder*. New York: Alan R. Liss, Inc., 1990:219–242.
179. Lee MA, Cameron OG, Greden JF. Anxiety and caffeine consumption in people with anxiety disorders. *Psychiatry Res* 1985;15:211–217.
180. Alsene K, Deckert J, Sand P, et al. Association between A_{2a} receptor gene polymorphisms and caffeine-induced anxiety. *Neuropsychopharmacology* 2003;28:1694–1702.
181. Childs E, Hohoff C, Deckert J, et al. Association between ADORA2a and DRD2 polymorphisms and caffeine-induced anxiety. *Neuropsychopharmacology* 2008 Feb 27. Epub ahead of print.
182. Nardi AE, Valenca AM, Nascimento I, et al. A caffeine challenge test in panic disorder patients, their healthy first-degree relatives, and healthy controls. *Depress Anxiety* 2007 Sept 6. Epub ahead of print.
183. Lee MA, Flegel P, Greden JF, et al. Anxiogenic effects of caffeine on panic and depressed patients. *Am J Psychiatry* 1988;145:632–635.
184. Rihs M, Muller C, Baumann P. Caffeine consumption in hospitalized psychiatric patients. *Eur Arch Psychiatry Clin Neurosci* 1996;246:83–92.
185. Hewlett P, Smith A. Correlates of daily caffeine consumption. *Appetite* 2006;46:97–99.
186. Holle C, Heimberg RG, Sweet RA, et al. Alcohol and caffeine use by social phobics: an initial inquiry into drinking patterns and behavior. *Behav Res Ther* 1995;33:561–566.
187. Winstead DK. Coffee consumption among psychiatric inpatients. *Am J Psychiatry* 1976;133:1447–1450.
188. Greden JF. Anxiety or caffeinism: a diagnostic dilemma. *Am J Psychiatry* 1974;131:1089–1092.
189. Bruce MS, Lader M. Caffeine abstention in the management of anxiety disorders. *Psychol Med* 1989;19:211–214.
190. Paterson LM, Wilson SJ, Nutt DJ, et al. A translational, caffeine-induced model of onset insomnia in rats and healthy volunteers. *Psychopharmacology (Berlin)* 2007;191:943–950.
191. Snel J. Coffee and caffeine: sleep and wakefulness. In: Garattini S, ed. *Caffeine, coffee, and health*. New York: Raven Press, Ltd., 1993:255–290.
192. Alford C, Bhatti J, Leigh T, et al. Caffeine-induced sleep disruption: effects of waking the following day and its reversal with a hypnotic. *Hum Psychopharmacol* 1996;11:185–198.
193. Hindmarch I, Rigney U, Stanley N, et al. A naturalistic investigation of the effects of day-long consumption of tea, coffee and water on alertness, sleep onset and sleep quality. *Psychopharmacology (Berlin)* 2000;149: 203–216.
194. Landolt HP, Werth E, Borbely AA, et al. Caffeine intake (200 mg) in the morning affects human sleep and EEG power spectra at night. *Brain Res* 1995;675:67–74.
195. Retey JV, Adam M, Khatami R, et al. A genetic variation in the adenosine A_{2A} receptor gene (ADORA2A) contributes to individual

sensitivity to caffeine effects on sleep. *Clin Pharmacol Ther* 2007;81: 692–698.
196. Retey JV, Adam M, Honegger E, et al. A functional genetic variation of adenosine deaminase affects the duration and intensity of deep sleep in humans. *Proc Natl Acad Sci U S A* 2005;102:15676–15681.
197. Regestein QR. Pathologic sleepiness induced by caffeine. *Am J Med* 1989;87:586–588.
198. Strain EC, Mumford G, Silverman K, et al. Caffeine dependence syndrome: evidence from case histories and experimental evaluations. *JAMA* 1994;272:1043–1048.
199. Richardson NJ, Rogers PJ, Elliman NA, et al. Mood and performance effects of caffeine in relation to acute and chronic caffeine deprivation. *Pharmacol Biochem Behav* 1995;52:313–320.
200. Evans SM, Griffiths RR. Caffeine withdrawal: a parametric analysis of caffeine dosing conditions. *J Pharmacol Exp Ther* 1999;289: 285–294.
201. Griffiths RR, Evans SM, Heishman SJ, et al. Low-dose caffeine physical dependence in humans. *J Pharmacol Exp Ther* 1990;255:1123–1132.
202. Driesbach RH, Pfeiffer C. Caffeine-withdrawal headache. *J Lab Clin Med* 1943;28:1212–1219.
203. Hughes JR, Oliveto AH, Bickel WK, et al. Caffeine self-administration and withdrawal: incidence, individual differences and interrelationships. *Drug Alcohol Depend* 1993;32:239–246.
204. Martin I, Lopez-Vilchez MA, Mur A, et al. Neonatal withdrawal syndrome after chronic maternal drinking of mate. *Ther Drug Monit* 2007; 29:127–129.
205. McGowan JD, Altman RE,Kanto WP, Jr. Neonatal withdrawal symptoms after chronic maternal ingestion of caffeine. *South Med J* 1988;81: 1092–1094.
206. Galletly DC, Fennelly M, Whitwam JG. Does caffeine withdrawal contribute to postanaesthetic morbidity? *Lancet* 1989;1:1335.
207. Weber JG, Klindworth JT, Arnold JJ, et al. Prophylactic intravenous administration of caffeine and recovery after ambulatory surgical procedures. *Mayo Clin Proc* 1997;72:621–626.
208. Fredholm BB, Battig K, Holmen J, et al. Actions of caffeine in the brain with special reference to factors that contribute to its widespread use. *Pharmacol Rev* 1999;51:83–133.
209. Finn IB, Holtzman SG. Tolerance to caffeine-induced stimulation of locomotor activity in rats. *J Pharmacol Exp Ther* 1986; 238:542–546.
210. Holtzman SG. Complete, reversible, drug-specific tolerance to stimulation of locomotor activity by caffeine. *Life Sci* 1983;33:779–787.
211. Ahlijanian MK, Takemori AE. Cross-tolerance studies between caffeine and (−)-N6-(phenylisopropyl)-adenosine (PIA) in mice. *Life Sci* 1986; 38:577–588.
212. Hirsh K. Central nervous system pharmacology of the dietary methylxanthines. *Prog Clin Biol Res* 1984;158:235–301.
213. von Borstel RW, Wurtman RJ, Conlay LA. Chronic caffeine consumption potentiates the hypotensive action of circulating adenosine. *Life Sci* 1983;32:1151–1158.
214. World Health Organization. *The ICD-10 classification of mental and behavioural disorders: clinical descriptions and diagnostic guidelines.* Geneva, Switzerland: World Health Organization, 1992.
215. World Health Organization. *International statistical classification of diseases and related health problems,* 10th rev. Vol. 1. Geneva, Switzerland: World Health Organization, 1992.
216. Hughes JR. Caffeine withdrawal, dependence, and abuse. In: *American Psychiatric Association: Diagnostic and Statistical Manual of Mental Disorders,* 4th edition. Washington, DC: American Psychiatric Association, 1994:129–134.
217. Hughes JR, Oliveto AH, Helzer JE, et al. Should caffeine abuse, dependence, or withdrawal be added to DSM-IV and ICD-10? *Am J Psychiatry* 1992;149:33–40.
218. Bernstein GA, Carroll ME, Thuras PD, et al. Caffeine dependence in teenagers. *Drug Alcohol Depend* 2002;66:1–6.
219. Jones HA, Lejuez CW. Personality correlates of caffeine dependence: the role of sensation seeking, impulsivity, and risk taking. *Exp Clin Psychopharmacol* 2005;13:259–266.
220. Oberstar JV, Bernstein GA,Thuras PD. Caffeine use and dependence in adolescents: one-year follow-up. *J Child Adolesc Psychopharmacol* 2002; 12:127–135.
221. Svikis DS, Berger N, Haug NA, et al. Caffeine dependence in combination with a family history of alcoholism as a predictor of continued use of caffeine during pregnancy. *Am J Psychiatry* 2005;162:2344–2351.
222. Cornelis MC, El-Sohemy A, Campos H. Genetic polymorphism of the adenosine A_{2A} receptor is associated with habitual caffeine consumption. *Am J Clin Nutr* 2007;86:240–244.
223. Kendler KS, Prescott CA. Caffeine intake, tolerance, and withdrawal in women: a population-based twin study. *Am J Psychiatry* 1999;156: 223–228.
224. Swan GE, Carmelli D, Cardon LR. The consumption of tobacco, alcohol, and coffee in Caucasian male twins: a multivariate genetic analysis. *J Subst Abuse* 1996;8:19–31.
225. Swan GE, Carmelli D, Cardon LR. Heavy consumption of cigarettes, alcohol and coffee in male twins. *J Stud Alcohol* 1997;58:182–190.
226. Hettema JM, Corey LA, Kendler KS. A multivariate genetic analysis of the use of tobacco, alcohol, and caffeine in a population based sample of male and female twins. *Drug Alcohol Depend* 1999;57:69–78.
227. Kendler KS, Myers J,Prescott CA. Specificity of genetic and environmental risk factors for symptoms of cannabis, cocaine, alcohol, caffeine, and nicotine dependence. *Arch Gen Psychiatry* 2007;64:1313–1320.
228. Swanson JA, Lee JW, Hopp JW. Caffeine and nicotine: a review of their joint use and possible interactive effects in tobacco withdrawal. *Addict Behav* 1994;19:229–256.
229. Kozlowski LT, Henningfield JE, Keenan RM, et al. Patterns of alcohol, cigarette, and caffeine and other drug use in two drug abusing populations. *J Subst Abuse Treat* 1993;10:171–179.
230. Emurian HH, Nellis MJ, Brady JV, et al. Event time-series relationship between cigarette smoking and coffee drinking. *Addict Behav* 1982;7: 441–444.
231. Gasior M, Jaszyna M, Munzar P, et al. Caffeine potentiates the discriminative-stimulus effects of nicotine in rats. *Psychopharmacology (Berlin)* 2002;162:385–395.
232. Jones HE, Griffiths RR. Oral caffeine maintenance potentiates the reinforcing and stimulant subjective effects of intravenous nicotine in cigarette smokers. *Psychopharmacology (Berlin)* 2003;165:280–290.
233. Shoaib M, Swanner LS, Yasar S, et al. Chronic caffeine exposure potentiates nicotine self-administration in rats. *Psychopharmacology (Berlin)* 1999;142:327–333.
234. Tanda G, Goldberg SR. Alteration of the behavioral effects of nicotine by chronic caffeine exposure. *Pharmacol Biochem Behav* 2000;66:47–64.
235. Blank MD, Kleykamp BA, Jennings JM, et al. Caffeine's influence on nicotine's effects in nonsmokers. *Am J Health Behav* 2007;31:473–483.
236. Perkins KA, Fonte C, Stolinski A, et al. The influence of caffeine on nicotine's discriminative stimulus, subjective, and reinforcing effects. *Exp Clin Psychopharmacol* 2005;13:275–281.
237. Nastase A, Ioan S, Braga RI, et al. Coffee drinking enhances the analgesic effect of cigarette smoking. *Neuroreport* 2007;18:921–924.
238. Rose JE, Behm FM. Psychophysiological interactions between caffeine and nicotine. *Pharmacol Biochem Behav* 1991;38:333–337.
239. Benowitz NL, Hall SM, Modin G. Persistent increase in caffeine concentrations in people who stop smoking. *BMJ* 1989;298:1075–1076.
240. Brown CR, Jacob P, 3rd, Wilson M, et al. Changes in rate and pattern of caffeine metabolism after cigarette abstinence. *Clin Pharmacol Ther* 1988;43:488–491.
241. Hughes JR, Oliveto AH. Coffee and alcohol intake as predictors of smoking cessation and tobacco withdrawal. *J Subst Abuse* 1993;5: 305–310.
242. Oliveto AH, Hughes JR, Terry SY, et al. Effects of caffeine on tobacco withdrawal. *Clin Pharmacol Ther* 1991;50:157–164.
243. Istvan J, Matarazzo JD. Tobacco, alcohol, and caffeine use: a review of their interrelationships. *Psychol Bull* 1984;95:301–326.
244. Aubin HJ, Laureaux C, Tilikete S, et al. Changes in cigarette smoking and coffee drinking after alcohol detoxification in alcoholics. *Addiction* 1999;94:411–416.

245. Marczinski CA, Fillmore MT. Clubgoers and their trendy cocktails: implications of mixing caffeine into alcohol on information processing and subjective reports of intoxication. *Exp Clin Psychopharmacol* 2006; 14:450–458.
246. Ferreira SE, de Mello MT, Pompeia S, et al. Effects of energy drink ingestion on alcohol intoxication. *Alcohol Clin Exp Res* 2006;30: 598–605.
247. Oteri A, Salvo F, Caputi AP, et al. Intake of energy drinks in association with alcoholic beverages in a cohort of students of the School of Medicine of the University of Messina. *Alcohol Clin Exp Res* 2007;31:1677–1680.
248. Oliveto AH, McCance-Katz E, Singha A, et al. Effects of d-amphetamine and caffeine in humans under a cocaine discrimination procedure. *Behav Pharmacol* 1998;9:207–217.
249. Young R, Gabryszuk M, Glennon RA. (−)Ephedrine and caffeine mutually potentiate one another's amphetamine-like stimulus effects. *Pharmacol Biochem Behav* 1998;61:169–173.
250. Derlet RW, Tseng JC, Albertson TE. Potentiation of cocaine and d-amphetamine toxicity with caffeine. *Am J Emerg Med* 1992;10:211–216.
251. McNamara R, Kerans A, O'Neill B, et al. Caffeine promotes hyperthermia and serotonergic loss following co-administration of the substituted amphetamines, MDMA ("Ecstasy") and MDA ("Love"). *Neuropharmacology* 2006;50:69–80.
252. McNamara R, Maginn M, Harkin A. Caffeine induces a profound and persistent tachycardia in response to MDMA ("Ecstasy") administration. *Eur J Pharmacol* 2007;555:194–198.
253. White JM. Behavioral effects of caffeine coadministered with nicotine, benzodiazepines and alcohol. *Pharmacopsychoecologia* 1994;7:119–126.
254. Oliveto AH, Bickel WK, Hughes JR, et al. Functional antagonism of the caffeine-discriminative stimulus by triazolam in humans. *Behav Pharmacol* 1997;8:124–138.
255. Roache JD, Griffiths RR. Interactions of diazepam and caffeine: behavioral and subjective dose effects in humans. *Pharmacol Biochem Behav* 1987;26:801–812.
256. Hagg S, Spigset O, Mjorndal T, et al. Effect of caffeine on clozapine pharmacokinetics in healthy volunteers. *Br J Clin Pharmacol* 2000;49: 59–63.

CHAPTER 12

John A. Dani, PhD
Thomas R. Kosten, MD
Neal L. Benowitz, MD

The Pharmacology of Nicotine and Tobacco

Tobacco use is the leading cause of death in the United States, and it is projected to be responsible for 10% of all deaths globally by 2015 (1–3). Its use causes approximately 440,000 deaths each year in the United States and produces more than $75 billion in direct medical costs annually. This chapter examines the pharmacology of nicotine, which is the main addictive component of tobacco. Understanding the pharmacology of nicotine is important in devising effective interventions for smoking cessation and in developing nicotine as a therapeutic agent.

DRUGS IN THE CLASS

Nicotine is a naturally occurring alkaloid that serves as an insecticide in many plants. Nicotine is a tertiary amine that consists of a pyridine and a pyrrolidine ring (Fig. 12.1). There are two stereoisomers of nicotine. The (S)-nicotine form is the active isomer that binds to nicotinic acetylcholine receptors (nAChRs) and is found in tobacco. The (R)-nicotine form is a weak agonist at cholinergic receptors. During smoking, some racemization takes place, and small quantities of (R)-nicotine are found in cigarette smoke. In humans, nicotine is a psychostimulant and mood modulator (1,3).

METHODS OF ABUSE

Nicotine and the reinforcing sensory stimulation associated with tobacco use are responsible for the compulsive use of tobacco in the form of cigarettes, bidis, cigars, pipes, snuff, and chewing tobacco (1,3–5). Nicotine replacement medications, which are used to facilitate smoking cessation, include nicotine polacrilex gum, transdermal patches, nasal spray, inhalers, buccal lozenges, and oral nicotine solutions. Nicotine and its analogues are also being investigated as potential therapeutic agents for ulcerative colitis, Parkinson's disease, Alzheimer's disease, attention deficit/hyperactivity disorder (ADHD), schizophrenia, anxiety, depression, obesity, sleep apnea, and Tourette syndrome.

HISTORICAL FEATURES

Native American tribes cultivated and used tobacco for many different purposes for thousands of years before the arrival of Europeans. Tobacco was first commercially grown for the European market at the first permanent English settlement in America, Jamestown, which was founded in 1607. Tobacco became an important economic influence in the British American colonies and the early United States (6). The World Health Organization estimates that one third of the global adult population smokes, and because tobacco use is on the rise in developing countries, it is one of the few causes of death that is increasing (2).

PHARMACOKINETICS

Absorption, Distribution, Metabolism, and Elimination The absorption of nicotine depends on its pH. Below pH 6, smoke contains <1% unprotonated (free) nicotine. As the pH rises, so does the proportion of unprotonated nicotine. At pH 7.26, 15% of the nicotine is unprotonated,

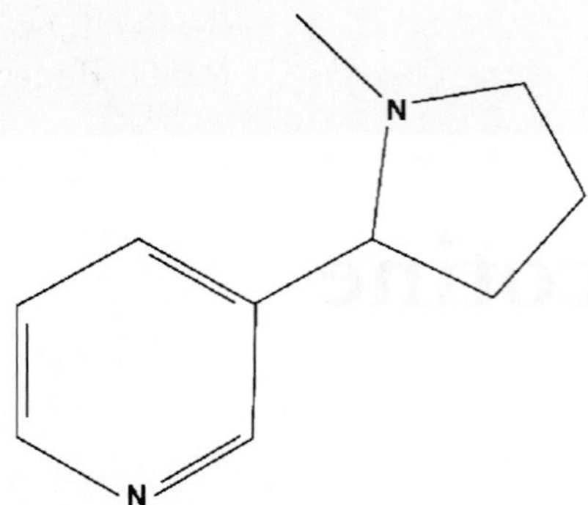

FIGURE 12.1. The chemical structure of nicotine. The chemical IUPAC name is 3-(1-methylpyrrolidin-2-yl)pyridine and the chemical formula is $C_{10}H_{14}N_2$.

increasing to 50% at pH 8. Unprotonated nicotine is present mainly in the vapor phase of the smoke, whereas protonated nicotine is contained primarily within particles in the smoke aerosol (7). Unprotonated nicotine is absorbed through the mucous membranes of the oral and nasal cavities (8,9). Tobacco products such as cigars, many pipe tobaccos, snuffs, and chewing tobaccos present nicotine either as a unionized (unprotonated), vaporized component of smoke or as an alkaline solution of nicotine. Tobacco smoke with pH levels above 6.2 contains increasing amounts of free ammonia, nitrates that are partially reduced to ammonia during smoking, and other volatile basic components (10).

Because alkaline smoke is irritating to the pharynx, it is harsh and difficult to inhale. Therefore smoke from cigarettes and from some pipe tobaccos has an acidic pH. The ionized nicotine in such smoke is largely dissolved in the aerosol droplets. After small droplets of tar-containing nicotine are inhaled and deposited in small airways and alveoli, the protonated nicotine is buffered to a physiologic pH and absorbed. Inhaled nicotine avoids first-pass metabolism. It is quickly delivered from the large surface area of the alveoli and circulation in the lung to the arterial bloodstream and then to the tissues and the nicotinic receptors in the brain.

Nicotine begins to reach the brain in approximately 20 seconds after inhalation, but then it gradually increases occupancy of nAChRs over many minutes. Smoking of a cigarette leads to high occupancy of the high-affinity $\alpha 4\beta 2$ nAChRs for >3 hours (11). The brain is exposed to high peak levels of nicotine, so that the arterial levels of nicotine after cigarette smoking exceed venous levels by two- to six-fold (12,13). Although levels of nicotine bound to nicotinic cholinergic receptors in the brain continue to rise slowly and are maintained for hours (11), the initial rapid arrival of nicotine is believed to contribute to the enhanced capacity of cigarettes to cause addiction. Environmental and sensory cues, such as smoke odor and sensation in the throat and airways, also contribute to the overall addictive drive (4,5,14).

The rapid delivery of nicotine to the brain in the smoking process allows precise dose titration so that the smoker can obtain the desired effects. Smokers can control nicotine intake by altering their puff volume, the number of puffs they take from a cigarette, the intensity of puffing, and the depth to which they inhale. Smokers also can increase smoke intake by blocking the ventilation holes of the filter with their fingers or their lips. Because of the complexity of smoking, the exact dose of nicotine cannot be accurately predicted from the nicotine content of the tobacco or a cigarette's machine-rated yield (15). Individuals smoke to obtain desired levels of nicotine from cigarettes in ways that largely compensate for the engineering features that reduce the amount of nicotine deposited on a filter pad in standard smoking machine tests.

Nicotine is poorly absorbed from the stomach because of the acidity of the gastric fluid, but it is well absorbed in the small intestine, which has an alkaline pH as well as a large surface area. When nicotine is administered in capsules, peak concentrations are reached in just over an hour. Nicotine undergoes first-pass metabolism; its oral bioavailability is approximately 45% (16).

After it is absorbed, nicotine enters the bloodstream. Nicotine has a volume of distribution of about 180 L, with <5% binding to plasma proteins. Nicotine crosses the placenta freely and has been found in the amniotic fluid and in the umbilical cord blood of neonates. Nicotine also is found in breast milk at concentrations approximately twice those found in blood.

Nicotine obtained from tobacco reaches high initial concentrations in the arterial blood, lung, and brain; subsequently, it is distributed to storage adipose and muscle tissue. The average steady-state concentration of nicotine in the body tissues is 2.6 times the average steady-state concentration of nicotine in the blood (16). The initial rate of rise of nicotine at brain targets, which meaningfully occurs in minutes (11), is likely to be the determinant for nicotine's immediate impact on the central nervous system (CNS).

Based on a half-life of 2 hours or more, nicotine accumulates over 6 to 8 hours (3 to 4 half-lives) of regular smoking and persists for 6 to 8 hours after smoking ceases. Steady-state plasma nicotine levels, which plateau in the early afternoon, typically range between 10 and 50 ng/mL. The increment in blood nicotine concentration after smoking a single cigarette ranges from 5 to 30 ng/mL, depending on how the cigarette is smoked (16). Peak blood concentrations of nicotine are similar for cigar smokers, users of snuff, chewers of tobacco, and those who smoke cigarettes, although the rate of rise of nicotine concentrations is slower for the nonsmoking methods of tobacco use. Individual smokers seem to manipulate their nicotine intake to maintain a consistent level of nicotine from day to day (15). Based on positron emission tomography imaging, the distribution of nicotine onto nAChRs is slower than the rise in the bloodstream (11).

Smoking represents a multiple-dosing situation, with considerable accumulation of nicotine in the body tissues (including the brain) while smoking. Nicotine persists in the body around the clock. Peaks and troughs in blood nicotine concentrations follow each cigarette, but those variations are smoothed

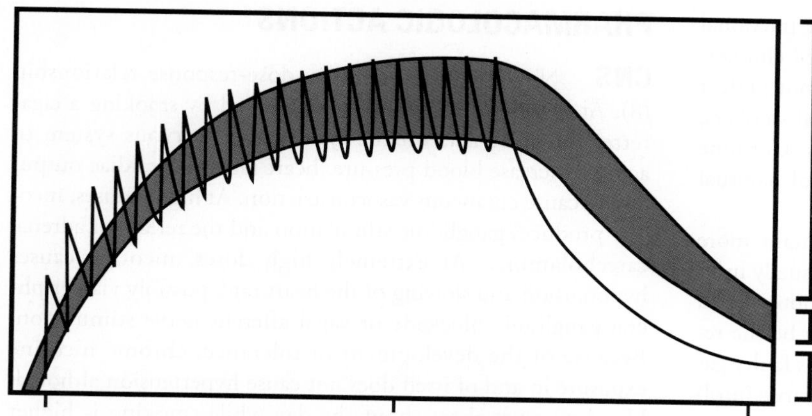

FIGURE 12.2. A simulation of the plasma nicotine concentration throughout the day in relation to psychoactive effect.

out within the brain. As the day progresses for the regular smoker, the overall level of nicotine rises and the potential influence of each dose becomes less important. Tolerance occurs, so that the effects of individual cigarettes tend to lessen throughout the day. Overnight abstinence allows considerable, but not complete resensitization of nicotinic receptors to nondesensitized states (Fig. 12.2). The populations of nAChR subtypes will begin to change as other molecular mechanisms involving neuroadaptations come into play after days and weeks of tobacco use (1,17,18).

Nicotine is extensively metabolized, primarily in the liver and to a lesser extent in the lung and in the brain (16). On average, 80% of nicotine is metabolized to cotinine, with a smaller fraction (4%) metabolized to nicotine-N-oxide. Cotinine is further metabolized to trans 3′ hydroxycotinine, the major nicotine metabolite found in the urine, as well as cotinine methonium ion, 5′ hydroxycotinine, and cotinine-N-oxide. About 17% of cotinine is excreted unchanged in the urine (16). CYP 2A6 is primarily responsible for both the C-oxidation of nicotine to cotinine and for the oxidation of cotinine to trans 3′ hydroxycotinine. Nicotine, cotinine, and trans 3′ hydroxycotinine are further metabolized by glucuronidation.

Renal clearance accounts for about 10% (range 2% to 35%) of total nicotine clearance. The renal clearance of unchanged nicotine increases in acidic urine and decreases in alkaline urine. Cotinine excretion is influenced less by urinary pH than nicotine because it occurs primarily in the unionized form within physiologic pH.

Sex and race influence nicotine metabolism. Women metabolize nicotine faster than men, and women who take estrogen-containing oral contraceptives metabolize nicotine faster than women who do not (19). The metabolism of nicotine during pregnancy is even faster, consistent with a dose effect of estrogen on CYP2A6 activity (20). African Americans obtain on average 30% more nicotine per cigarette, and they clear nicotine and cotinine more slowly than do Caucasians (21). The slower nicotine clearance is due to the less rapid oxidative metabolism of nicotine to cotinine, related at least in part to a higher prevalence of CYP2A6 gene variants associated with reduced activity in African Americans (22). African Americans also exhibit population polymorphism in the rate of nicotine N-glucuronidation, with a subpopulation of slow metabolizers, not found in Caucasians (23). Black men also have a higher incidence of mortality from lung cancer than do white men (24). Chinese Americans have both a lower nicotine intake per cigarette and smoke fewer cigarettes per day than do Caucasians (23). Chinese Americans also metabolized nicotine and cotinine more slowly than do Caucasians or Hispanic Americans. Slower metabolism in Chinese Americans is consistent with the higher prevalence of CYP2A6 alleles associated with slow metabolism among Asians (25). Because nicotine intake per cigarette is a marker for tobacco smoke exposure per cigarette, these findings suggest why Chinese American smokers have lower rates of lung cancer than either African Americans or Caucasians (24). Ethnic variations in nicotine intake per cigarette, the number of cigarettes smoked, and the metabolism of nicotine may form the basis for population-based differences in the incidence and prevalence of progression from nicotine use to addiction, as well as the associated risk of tobacco-related disease.

Biochemical Assessment of Exposure to Nicotine and Tobacco Blood, salivary, and plasma cotinine are most commonly used as biochemical markers of nicotine intake (26). Other measures of smoking include expired carbon monoxide concentrations, blood carboxyhemoglobin concentrations, and plasma or salivary thiocyanate concentrations. Measurement of the minor tobacco alkaloids anabasine and anatabine in urine can be used as a biomarker of tobacco use in individuals who are using nicotine medications (27).

The 16-hour half-life of cotinine makes it useful as a plasma and salivary marker of nicotine intake. Salivary cotinine concentrations correlate well with blood cotinine concentrations ($r = 0.82–0.90$) (28). The cotinine level produced by a single cigarette is 8 to 10 ng/mL. It takes several hours for the cotinine to peak after a cigarette is smoked. A cotinine value >14 ng/mL typically is taken to indicate smoking (29). A smoker with a plasma cotinine concentration of 100 ng/mL would have an estimated intake of 8 mg nicotine per day, which corresponds to smoking approximately a half pack of cigarettes per day (26). Cotinine blood levels average about 250 to 300 ng/mL in regular smokers, but range from 10 to

900 ng/mL. Because of individual variability in the fractional conversion of nicotine to cotinine and in the rate of elimination of cotinine itself, blood levels of cotinine are not perfect quantitative markers of nicotine intake in individual smokers, but are useful in studying populations of smokers. Cotinine levels may persist for up to 7 days after cessation of habitual smoking.

Breath measurements of expired air that contain more than 10 parts per million carbon monoxide (CO) usually indicate tobacco smoking within the past 8 to 12 hours (29). Elevated CO levels in the absence of smoking may be the result of exposure to environmental pollutants, such as faulty gas boilers, car exhausts, and smog. Persons who are lactose intolerant exhale hydrogen after ingesting milk. Several monitors misinterpret this exhaled hydrogen as CO (30).

Hydrogen cyanide is inhaled as a combustion product of nitrogen-containing compounds. It is metabolized in the body from thiosulfate to thiocyanate, which can be detected in the blood and saliva (31). Thiocyanate levels also may be affected by consumption of common foods (such as almonds, tapioca, cabbage, broccoli, and cauliflower). Assays of thiocyanate are insensitive to low amounts of smoking, and thiocyanate levels can remain elevated for weeks after smoking has ceased. CO and cotinine levels generally are preferred to thiocyanate levels in the assessment of smoking.

Drug Interactions with Nicotine and Tobacco

Smoking accelerates the metabolism of many drugs, particularly those metabolized by CYP1A2 (32). Polycyclic aromatic hydrocarbons are believed to account for the enzyme-inducing effects of smoking although other smoke components may play a role. Nicotine does not induce most enzymes, but may increase CYP2E1 and inhibit CYP2A6 enzymatic activity. Cigarette smoking induces the metabolism of theophylline, propranolol, flecainide, tacrine, caffeine, olanzapine, clozapine, imipramine, haloperidol, pentazocine, estradiol, and other drugs. When smokers stop smoking, as often occurs during hospitalization for an acute illness, the doses of these medications may need to be lowered to avoid toxicity.

Several pharmacodynamic interactions arise between cigarette smoking and other drugs. Cigarette smoking results in faster clearance of heparin, possibly because of smoking-related activation of thrombosis, with enhanced heparin binding to antithrombin III. Cigarette smoking and oral contraceptives interact synergistically to increase the risk of stroke and premature myocardial infarction in women. Cigarettes appear to enhance the procoagulant effect of estrogens. For this reason, oral contraceptives are relatively contraindicated in women who smoke cigarettes. The stimulant actions of nicotine inhibit reductions in blood pressure and heart rate from beta-adrenergic blockers. Smoking results in less sedation from benzodiazepines and less analgesia from some opioids. Smoking also impairs the therapeutic effects of histamine H2-receptor antagonists using in treating peptic ulcers. Cutaneous vasoconstriction by nicotine can slow the rate of absorption of subcutaneously administered insulin.

PHARMACOLOGIC ACTIONS

CNS Nicotine has a complex dose-response relationship (8). At low doses (such as those achieved by smoking a cigarette), nicotine acts on the sympathetic nervous system to acutely increase blood pressure, heart rate, and cardiac output and to cause cutaneous vasoconstriction. At higher doses, nicotine produces ganglionic stimulation and the release of adrenal catecholamines. At extremely high doses, nicotine causes hypotension and slowing of the heart rate, possibly via peripheral ganglionic blockade or vagal afferent nerve stimulation. Because of the development of tolerance, chronic nicotine exposure in and of itself does not cause hypertension although blood pressure throughout the day while smoking is higher compared with when that person is not smoking (33). Nicotine also causes muscle relaxation by stimulating discharge of the Renshaw cells or pulmonary afferent nerves while inhibiting the activity of motor neurons.

Psychoactive Effects The primary CNS effects of nicotine in smokers are arousal, relaxation (particularly in stressful situations), and enhancement of mood, attention, and reaction time, with improvement in performance of some behavioral tasks. Some of this improvement results from the relief of withdrawal symptoms in addicted smokers, rather than as a direct enhancing effect (34–36). Smoking may mainly reverse the effects of abstinence, rather than directly relieving stress and improving cognition. In a comparison of self-rated feelings of stress, arousal, pleasure, and evaluations of cognitive function in 25 cigarette smokers, 25 temporarily abstaining smokers, and 25 nonsmokers, the abstaining smokers reported significantly worse psychologic states on every assessment measure than did the nonsmokers and nondeprived smokers, who did not differ from each other (37). Smokers may need regular doses of nicotine to feel normal rather than to enhance their capabilities.

The psychoactive effects of nicotine and tobacco are determined not only by the route and speed of drug administration and the pharmacokinetic parameters that determine the concentration at receptor sites over time, but also by a variety of host and environmental factors. The magnitude of nicotine's subjective effects may depend on the predrug subjective state, level of activity, genetic predisposition, history or current intake of other drugs, expectancy of the individual, and other situational factors (4,5,38–40).

Nicotine's effects are baseline dependent. Low-activity rats become more active on exposure to nicotine, whereas the reverse occurs in high-activity rats (41). Similarly, nicotine has stimulant like effects on human electroencephalograms during quiet conditions, but minimal effects during high-noise conditions (42).

Nicotine's ability to cause stimulation when smoked at a low level of arousal (such as fatigue) and to affect relaxation when smoked at a high level of arousal (such as anxiety) underlies its reinforcing effects under a range of conditions (43). Smokers increase their smoking under both low- and high-arousal conditions (44). Subtle stimulation or relaxation effects may be thought beneficial by users who would like to fine tune their disposition at a given time. The subtle modulatory effects preferred by tobacco users are in contrast to the flagrant intoxicating effects desired by some users of alcohol and other psychoactive substances.

Gender differences appear to affect nicotine responsiveness. Women have less sensitivity to changes in nicotine dose during nicotine discrimination experiments, and they may not benefit as much as men from nicotine replacement therapy during smoking cessation (45). Women may be influenced more by nonnicotine stimuli, such as the olfactory and taste attributes of cigarette smoke, indicating greater conditioned reinforcement (46).

Genetic Predisposition Monozygotic twins are more similar than dizygotic twins with respect to smoking behavior (38). Data from large twin registries suggest that about half of the total variance (range 28%–84%) in smoking behavior can be attributed to genetic effects (39,47). Twin studies also demonstrate a genetic influence on nicotine withdrawal symptoms (36).

Animal studies show that genetics mediate differences in sensitivity to nicotine (48). Different mice strains react differently to nicotine, self-administer nicotine to different extents (49), differ in the ability to develop tolerance, and have different numbers of nicotine receptor-binding sites (50).

Family linkage studies and candidate gene association studies suggest a number of loci or particular genes that are associated with smoking behavior, although smoking phenotypes vary considerably from study to study (38). Candidate genes coding for nicotine receptor subtypes, dopamine receptors or transporter, GABA receptors, and others have been identified in various studies as being associated with different aspects of smoking behavior (51). However, subsequent research has not replicated many of these earlier findings.

Recent genome-wide association studies point to several genes that are promising signals for genetic determinants of nicotine dependence, including the alpha5, alpha3, and beta3 nicotinic receptor genes, neurexin 1, VPS13A (vacuolar sorting protein), KCNJ6 (a potassium channel), and the GABA A4 receptor genes (52,53). Some of these genes, such as the neurexin 1 gene, are related to cell communication. Other genome-wide association studies have identified a number of genes affecting cell adhesion and extracellular matrix molecules that are common among various addictions, consistent with the idea that neural plasticity and learning are key determinants of individual differences in vulnerability to nicotine as well as other drug addictions (54).

Psychiatric Comorbidity Tobacco use is most highly prevalent and more intense among psychiatric patients and among those who abuse other drugs (1). Individuals with schizophrenia, depression, and ADHD have a higher prevalence of cigarette smoking than the population as a whole. These groups of patients have more difficulty in quitting compared with smokers without mental illness, often experiencing greater depression after stopping smoking than others.

Among patients with schizophrenia, 70% to 88% are smokers (55). Schizophrenic patients have diminished sensory gating to repeated stimuli, an abnormality reversed by nicotine and clozapine, but not haloperidol (56). Nicotine also reverses some haloperidol dose-related impairments on a variety of cognitive tasks (57) and relieves some of the negative symptoms (such as blunted affect, emotional withdrawal, and lack of spontaneity and flow of conversation) that occur with schizophrenia. Genetic linkage in schizophrenic families supports a role for the α7 nicotinic receptor subunit, with potential linkage at the α7 locus on chromosome 15 (58). These data suggest there may be a shared underlying neurobiology for both cigarette smoking and schizophrenia. Smokers experience fewer side effects from antipsychotic drugs, presumably from the stimulating effects of nicotine, which also may contribute to a higher prevalence of smoking among schizophrenics.

Rates of nicotine dependence are substantially higher among adults with ADHD (40%) than in the general population (26%) (59). Among adult smokers, the presence of ADHD is associated with early initiation of regular cigarette smoking, even after controlling for confounding variables such as socioeconomic status, IQ, and psychiatric comorbidity (60). Nicotine administered through transdermal patches improves the attentional symptoms of ADHD (61).

Population-based epidemiologic Catchment Area studies (62) found a lifetime prevalence of depression of 59% among subjects who had ever smoked, compared with 17% in the general population. Other reports confirm that the prevalence of smoking in individuals with major depression is twice that observed in the general population. A history of major depression may speed the progression from nicotine use to dependence. Twin studies support a model with common risk factors for both depression and cigarette smoking (63).

Depression sensitizes smokers to the influences of stress (1,64), making the individual more susceptible to drug reward. Depression and anxiety often accompany nicotine withdrawal, particularly for abstinent smokers with psychiatric illness. Relief from specific aspects of those symptoms motivates relapse. Thus smokers become conditioned to expect nicotine to provide partial relief from stress and depression as it does from the symptoms of withdrawal (64). Smokers with a history of depression who stop smoking are at risk of developing more severe withdrawal symptoms, have poorer outcomes, and are more likely to experience a depressive episode, especially during the first 3 months after stopping smoking (1,64).

Nicotine also has been studied as a potential treatment for Tourette syndrome (65), and may be protective against the development of Parkinson disease (66).

Discrimination and Self-Administration Squirrel monkeys and rodents are able to distinguish the subjective effects of nicotine and nicotine analogues from drugs of other classes. This effect is attenuated by pretreatment with mecamylamine, a centrally acting nicotinic receptor antagonist, but not with hexamethonium, a peripheral antagonist that does not enter the brain. Animals will self-administer nicotine, but the environment, dose, and timing of the reinforcement schedule are more critical with nicotine than with cocaine.

Human volunteers will self-administer intravenous nicotine (62). They describe the experience as pleasurable and similar to that evoked by cocaine. Human smokers regulate the nicotine levels that they self-administer. For example, they block the ventilation holes on the cigarette filter, puff harder, inhale more deeply, and smoke more frequently when smoking "light" cigarettes (15). Smokers pretreated with mecamylamine smoke more to overcome the blocking effects of this antagonist (34).

Human smokers get "secondary reinforcement" from the irritant effects of nicotine on the tissues of the mouth and throat. Experienced smokers can use the tissue irritant effects to assess how much nicotine they are receiving when smoking (4). A short-term reduction in cigarette craving is seen when the sensory input from tobacco smoke is simulated with ascorbic acid or black pepper extract. Products that replicate the taste, flavor, throat, and chest sensations of cigarette smoking or the sensorimotor handling of a cigarette may reduce craving and some of the symptoms of nicotine withdrawal. Some of these products are being developed as smoking cessation aids.

Dependence, Tolerance, and Withdrawal Nicotine obtained through chewing tobacco and cigarettes often precedes the use of other drugs (67). The earlier the age at which use begins, the more difficult it is for the user to quit. Many persons have been exposed to nicotine in utero as a result of smoking by their mothers (68). Nicotine exposure alters nicotine receptor numbers and influences their function. In smokers who progress to chronic use, tolerance develops rapidly to the headache, dizziness, nausea, and dysphoria associated with the first cigarette. However, tolerance is incomplete; the ingestion of as little as 50% more than the usual dose can result in symptoms of toxicity. Chronic use is associated with the regular ingestion of quantities far larger than those used initially, even though consumption levels typically remain steady for many years after addiction has been established.

Conditioned cues (drug-associated memories) become established during the fine-tuned dosing of nicotine. Desiring a cigarette becomes associated with everyday events such as driving a car, finishing a meal, talking on the telephone, waking from sleep, and taking a break. Tobacco users link the need to modulate their moods with smoking. The imagery promoted by cigarette advertising adds to this expectation. Thus a person who begins smoking a pack of cigarettes per day at age 17 would experience thousands of finely tuned doses of nicotine-conditioned internal emotional states and external cues by their mid-20s. The quantity and power of this conditioning is unique to cigarette smoking, and it is one of the reasons that smokers find cigarette smoking so difficult to quit.

The regular use of tobacco commonly leads to its compulsive use. There have been attempts to correlate the severity of nicotine addiction with factors such as the duration of smoking, potency of cigarettes, puff frequency, puff duration, and inhalation volume. However, these variables only weakly correlate with biochemical measures, and they do not predict the intensity and extent of withdrawal symptoms. The Fagerström Test of Nicotine Dependence is one of the most widely accepted measures of the severity of nicotine dependence. Many studies show a relationship between the Fagerström Test of Nicotine Dependence and the ability to achieve tobacco cessation.

There is a high rate of relapse among individuals who try to quit smoking (1). Population surveys consistently find that up to 75% of adults who smoke want to stop. About one-third actually try to stop each year, but <3% succeed (69). Among persons who experience myocardial infarctions, laryngectomies, chronic obstructive pulmonary disease, and other medical sequelae of smoking, ≥50% revert to cigarette use within days or weeks after leaving the hospital.

Withdrawal Tobacco use is sustained, in part, by the need to prevent the symptoms of nicotine withdrawal (1,34,35). These symptoms vary, but include craving for nicotine, irritability and frustration or anger, anxiety, depression, difficulty concentrating, restlessness, and increased appetite. Performance measures such as reaction time and attention are impaired during withdrawal. Although these symptoms often are distressing and can be disruptive to interpersonal functioning, they are not in themselves life-threatening. Most acute withdrawal symptoms reach maximum intensity at 24 to 48 hours after cessation and then gradually diminish over a few weeks. Some (including dysphoria, mild depression, and anhedonia) may persist for months. The extinction of tobacco-associated conditioned cues requires months to years. That nicotine itself is responsible for the withdrawal symptoms is supported by the appearance of similar symptoms with the sudden withdrawal from the use of chewing tobacco, snuff, or nicotine gum, and relief of those symptoms provided by nicotine replacement. Another motivating factor for some abstinent smokers is an average weight gain of 3 to 4 kg during the first year after smoking cessation.

There is evidence that the activation of the extrahypothalamic corticotropin-releasing factor (CRF)-CRF1 receptor system contributes to negative affect during nicotine withdrawal. During precipitated nicotine withdrawal in rats, which is associated with anxiety-like behavior, CRF is released in the central nucleus of the amygdala (70). CRF activation produces anxiety behavior, and pharmacologic blockade of CRF1 receptors inhibits the anxiogenic effects of nicotine withdrawal. Withdrawal from other drugs of abuse such as alcohol, cocaine, opiates, and cannabinoids is also associated with activation of the extrahypothalamic CRF system, suggesting that this is a common mechanism of affective manifestations of drug withdrawal. Both the hypoactivity of the dopaminergic system and the activation of the CRF system appear to mediate nicotine withdrawal symptoms that often precipitate relapse to smoking.

NEUROBIOLOGIC MECHANISMS OF ACTION

nAChRs Nicotinic acetylcholine receptors belong to a superfamily of ligand-gated ion channels that includes gamma-aminobutyric acid, glycine, and 5-hydroxytryptamine serotonin receptors. The most basic conformational states of a nAChR channel are the closed state at rest, the open state, and the desensitized state (71). Acetylcholine (ACh), the endogenous agonist, and nicotine, the exogenous agonist, both stabilize the open conformation of the nAChR channel. After binding ACh or nicotine, the nAChR ion channel is stabilized in the open conformation for several milliseconds. Then the open pore of the receptor/channel complex returns to a resting state or closes to a desensitized state that is unresponsive to ACh or other agonists for many milliseconds or longer. While open, nAChRs conduct cations that cause a local depolarization of the membrane and produce an intracellular ionic signal. Although sodium and potassium ions carry most of the current through nAChR channels, calcium also can make a small but significant contribution.

The nicotinic receptor-channel complex consists of five polypeptide subunits assembled like staves of a barrel around a central water-filled core (71). Various subunit combinations produce many different nAChR types. Three functional classes of nAChRs are recognized: muscle nAChRs (not discussed here), neuronal nAChRs formed from alpha-beta combinations ($\alpha 2$ to $\alpha 6$ and $\beta 2$ to $\beta 4$), and neuronal nAChRs formed only of alpha subunits ($\alpha 7$ to $\alpha 9$ or $\alpha 10$ with $\alpha 9$). Among the types, only homomeric $\alpha 7$ is widely distributed in the mammalian CNS. Some evidence suggests that subunits of the separate classes are capable of combining to form nAChRs, but such combinations may be rare.

Genetic studies in mice indicate a primary role for the alpha4 beta2 containing ($\alpha 4\beta 2^*$) nAChRs in mediating nicotine dependence. In $\beta 2$-subunit knockout mice, nicotine is less able to release dopamine in the brain, and these animals do not self-administer nicotine (40). Genetic manipulation of the $\alpha 4$ subunit alters the sensitivity to the effects of nicotine (72).

The Cholinergic Systems Cholinergic neurons project throughout the CNS, providing diffuse, sparse innervation to practically all of the brain (71). Despite its relatively sparse innervation in the CNS, cholinergic activity influences a wide variety of behaviors. By acting initially on nAChRs, nicotine or nicotinic cholinergic innervation can increase arousal, heighten attention, influence stages of sleep, produce states of euphoria, decrease fatigue, decrease anxiety, act centrally as an analgesic, and influence cognitive function. It is thought that cholinergic systems affect discriminatory processes by increasing the signal-to-noise ratio and helping to evaluate the significance and relevance of stimuli.

Nicotinic Mechanisms in the CNS The most widely observed synaptic role of nAChRs in the mammalian CNS is to influence neurotransmitter release (71). Presynaptic nAChRs are thought to initiate a direct and indirect calcium signal that boosts the release of neurotransmitters. Exogenous application of nicotinic agonists can enhance, and nicotinic antagonists often can diminish, the release of ACh, dopamine, norepinephrine, serotonin, GABA, and glutamate. In many cases, the $\alpha 7^*$ nAChRs, which are highly calcium permeable, mediate the increased release of neurotransmitter, but in other cases different nAChR types are involved.

Nicotinic AChRs also have roles in neuronal development and plasticity (73). The density of nAChRs varies during the course of development, and nAChRs can contribute to activity-dependent calcium signals. Nicotinic regulatory, plasticity, and developmental influences may be important in the etiology of disease. Biologic changes that inappropriately alter nicotinic mechanisms could immediately influence the release of many neurotransmitters and alter circuit excitability. Moreover, nicotinic dysfunction could have long-term developmental consequences that are expressed later in life.

The tremendous diversity of nAChRs provides the flexibility necessary for them to play multiple, varied roles. Broad, sparse cholinergic projections ensure that nicotinic mechanisms modulate the neuronal excitability of relatively wide circuits. Although fast nicotinic transmission is not the predominant driving force, it can contribute excitatory input to many synapses at one time. Presynaptic and preterminal nAChRs modulate the release of many neurotransmitters. As a result of volume ACh transmission, nAChRs also can influence circuit excitability at locations outside the synapse (71).

Nicotine's Influence on Dopaminergic Neurons

Much evidence supports the theory that nicotine is the major addictive component of tobacco (1,74–76). Under controlled laboratory conditions, nicotine reinforces intravenous self-administration and elicits conditioned place preference by animals and humans. In addition, nicotine cessation produces a withdrawal syndrome with both somatic and affective symptoms, which are relieved by nicotine replacement.

Addiction research has focused on dopamine's complex participation in the processes associated with reinforcing behaviors that lead to reward. Although many areas of the brain participate, the mesocorticolimbic dopamine (DA) system serves a vital role in the acquisition of behaviors that are inappropriately reinforced by addictive drugs. An important dopaminergic pathway originates in the ventral tegmental area of the midbrain and projects to the prefrontal cortex, as well as the limbic and striatal structures, including the nucleus accumbens. A role for the mesocorticolimbic DA system in nicotine addiction is supported by a number of findings (1,74–76). For example, blocking DA release in the nucleus accumbens with antagonists or lesions reduces nicotine self-administration in rodents (77).

Nicotine Activates and Desensitizes nAChRs on Mesocorticolimbic Neurons In rat brain slices, nicotine, at concentrations obtained from tobacco, can activate and desensitize nAChRs on ventral tegmental area DA neurons and thereby potently modulate the firing of ventral tegmental area neurons (1,76).

Nicotine that arrives in the brain reaches nAChRs at every location, including those at presynaptic, postsynaptic, and nonsynaptic (including somal) locations. On the DA neuron's cell bodies and postsynaptically, most of the nAChRs contain $\alpha4\beta2$ subunits (often in combination with $\alpha5$ or $\alpha6$) that have a high affinity for nicotine. The $\alpha4\beta2$-containing ($\alpha4\beta2^*$) nAChRs also predominate on inhibitory GABAergic neurons innervating this area. However, mainly $\alpha7^*$ nAChRs, which have a low affinity for nicotine, are located on the presynaptic terminals of excitatory glutamatergic afferents into this midbrain area (in rodent studies). This arrangement of the nAChRs is hypothesized to underlie their enhancement of excitatory synaptic potentiation (1,76).

When nicotine first arrives in the midbrain DA area, it excites nAChRs, particularly the high-affinity $\alpha4\beta2^*$ nAChRs and, to a lesser degree, the $\alpha7^*$ nAChRs. Activation of the presynaptic nAChRs enhances the release of glutamate. At this time, the postsynaptic (and somal) $\alpha4\beta2^*$ nAChRs contribute to the depolarization of the DA neurons, helping NMDA receptors to participate in glutamatergic synaptic potentiation. After the initial exposure to nicotine and potentiation of glutamatergic afferents, there is significant desensitization of the high-affinity $\alpha4\beta2^*$ receptors. Consequently, the inhibitory GABA transmission decreases because the $\alpha4\beta2^*$ nAChRs desensitize, and the GABAergic inhibition of the DA neurons is decreased because any afferent cholinergic activity that normally boosted GABA release no longer can act on the $\alpha4\beta2^*$ receptors.

Glutamatergic excitation of the DA neurons remains elevated because the synaptic potentiation that was initiated by the transient $\alpha4\beta2^*$ nAChR activity persists for longer time periods. In addition, the presynaptic $\alpha7^*$ nAChRs on the glutamatergic afferents are much less desensitized by the low concentrations of nicotine that are present. Therefore, $\alpha7^*$ nAChRs continue to enhance glutamate release, particularly at the potentiated synapses that provide ongoing excitation of the DA neurons (1,71,76).

Hypotheses to Extrapolate the Cellular Results to Smokers On the basis of the cellular studies of nAChR activation and desensitization, it is possible to infer some of the effects of smoking cigarettes, which delivers about 50 to 500 nM nicotine to the brain (11,78). Initially, the brain is free of nicotine and the nAChRs should be responding normally to cholinergic synaptic activity. When nicotine first arrives, nAChRs are activated, causing the neurons to depolarize and fire action potentials. This process occurs throughout the brain, with multiple consequences (79) (Fig. 12.3). DA neurons are activated, contributing to the increase in DA that has been detected in the nucleus accumbens. Present theories hold that these neuronal events reinforce the behaviors that produce the DA release (1,74–76,80). Thus, smoking and associated behaviors, whether incidental or meaningful, are reinforced (in a type of learning process). As the nicotine from the cigarette lingers, desensitization of nAChRs begins. This process decreases the effect obtained by smoking more than a few cigarettes in a row. However, the desensitization process is not complete and, in fact, there is considerable variability in desensitization of the various nAChR subtypes.

Nicotinic receptor desensitization has other effects (1,71,76). When nicotine obtained from tobacco is present, the high-affinity nicotine sites (including $\alpha4\beta2^*$ nAChRs) are more likely to desensitize. At cholinergic synapses, nAChRs experience repeated exposures to synaptic ACh and are exposed to nicotine from the cigarette. The combination of agonist exposures increases the probability that nAChRs at active cholinergic synapses (or experiencing ongoing cholinergic activity) will enter desensitization. Thus, smoking will turn down the gain for information arriving via nicotinic cholinergic synapses because fewer nAChRs will be able to respond to the released ACh. In summary, nicotine not only sends inappropriate information through the mesocorticolimbic DA system, but it also decreases the amplitude for normal nicotinic cholinergic information processing.

Long-term nicotine exposure increases the number of nAChRs in brains of humans, rats, and mice (81). After long periods (months or years) of exposure to smoking, nAChRs enter the desensitized state more often, eventually leading to an overall increase in number as a homeostatic reaction of decreased sensitivity (i.e., desensitization).

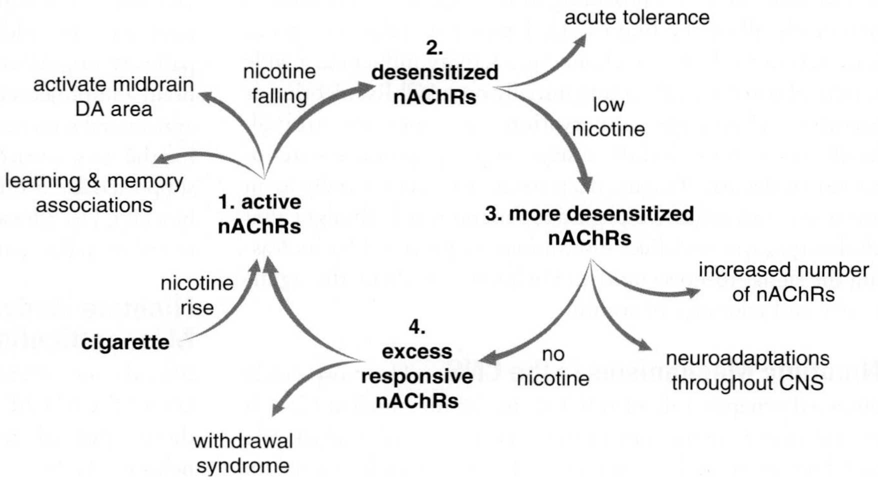

FIGURE 12.3. A simplified cycle for continued tobacco use, based on nicotine's cellular actions. The nicotinic acetylcholine receptors (nAChRs) are initially and transiently activated when nicotine first arrives. The desensitization of the receptors follows as the concentration of nicotine slowly decreases. The increased number of nAChRs and the neuroadaptations are hypothesized to develop after chronic use of nicotine. The learned associations occur over the course of tobacco use as nicotine causes reinforcements via the midbrain dopaminergic systems (79).

When nicotine is removed from the brain, some of the excess nAChRs recover from desensitization, resulting in an excess excitability of the nicotinic cholinergic systems of smokers. This hyperexcitability, where nAChRs have been up-regulated, could contribute to the unrest and agitation that contribute to the smoker's motivation for the next cigarette, which "medicates" the smoker by desensitizing the excess number of nAChRs back toward a more normal level.

These receptor changes may underlie the most common pattern of cigarette smoking. Most smokers report that the first cigarette of the day is the most pleasurable. After a night of abstinence, nicotine concentrations in the brain are at their lowest level. Thus, smoking the first cigarette most strongly activates nAChRs, possibly causing the largest activity of the midbrain DA areas and contributing to the most reinforcing effects (Fig. 12.3, Step 1). After a few cigarettes, there is significant (albeit incomplete) desensitization, causing some acute tolerance and less effect from additional cigarettes (Fig. 12.3, Step 2). The process of activation and desensitization affects different nAChR types differently and influences synaptic plasticity, contributing to the long-term changes associated with addiction. When smoking continues for long periods, the nicotinic system undergoes neuroadaptations, including an increase in the number of high-affinity nAChRs (Fig. 12.3, Step 3). Cigarettes are smoked throughout the day, in part driven by smaller, variable rewards and by the agitation arising, in part, from the excess nAChRs and hyperexcitability at cholinergic synapses experienced during abstinence (Fig. 12.3, Step 4).

Episodes of cigarette smoking are often separated by hours of abstinence. During that time, nicotine levels drop and some nAChRs recover from desensitization. Smokers often report that cigarettes smoked during the day help them to focus and relax so that they can work more efficiently. As an individual smokes several times during the course of a day, the background level of nicotine slowly increases. Therefore, a smoker experiences some exposure to nicotine throughout the day, ensuring that some types of nAChRs visit states of desensitization. These episodes of nAChR desensitization ensure that the number of nAChRs becomes and remains elevated. If nicotine is avoided for a few weeks, the number of nAChRs begins to return to the lower value seen in nonsmokers. Although this readjustment suggests the "quitting" process is under way, the nicotine-associated learning and memory is not lost. Thus, smoking-associated conditioned cues can continue to motivate tobacco use for long periods beyond this stage.

Most attempts to quit fail. Over years of smoking, long-term synaptic changes result in learned associations, including associations with the events, people, and context in which smoking takes place. Because these behaviors are reinforced by repeated variable reinforcements from cigarettes, associations become conditioned cues that motivate tobacco usage such that the desire for cigarettes extinguishes slowly and sometimes incompletely. Desires for cigarettes may be experienced even years after having quit, cued by learned associations (1,34,35,80).

Monoamine Oxidase and Tobacco Dependence

Cigarette smoking is associated with reduced activity of the enzymes monoamine oxidase A (MAO A) and monoamine oxidase B (MAO B), as demonstrated by positron emission tomography scanning of the brain using MAO substrates (82,83). Inhibition of MAO is produced not by nicotine, but by condensation products of acetaldehyde with biogenic amines, such as benzoquinones, 2-naphylamine, Harmon, and other chemicals. A main function of MAO is to metabolize catecholamines, including dopamine. Inhibition of MAO would be expected to result in higher brain levels of dopamine after exposure to nicotine. Studies in rats show that pretreatment with drugs that inhibit MAO make nicotine more rewarding and increase the likelihood and rate of acquisition of nicotine self-administration (84). Therefore MAO inhibition may contribute to the addictiveness of smoking. In addition, given that medications that inhibit MAO have antidepressant action, smoking-induced inhibition of monoamine oxidase might contribute to the perceived benefit of smoking by some depressed patients.

SYSTEMIC TOXICITY

Particulate and Gaseous Components of Tobacco Smoke Tobacco smoke is composed of volatile (gaseous) and particulate phases that contain substances other than nicotine that are primarily responsible for human morbidity and mortality. The volatile phase contains more than 500 gaseous compounds, including nitrogen, CO, carbon dioxide, ammonia, hydrogen cyanide, and benzene. There are about 3,500 different compounds in the particulate phase, including the pharmacologically active alkaloids nornicotine, anabasine, anatabine, myosmene, nicotyrine, and nicotine. Assays for some of these alkaloids are used as biomarkers of tobacco use (27). The "tar" in a cigarette is composed of the particulate matter minus its alkaloid and water content. Tar contains many carcinogens, including polynuclear aromatic hydrocarbons, N-nitrosamines, and aromatic amines.

Cardiovascular, Pulmonary, and Oncologic Toxicities Smokers are exposed to about 4,000 different chemicals, including at least 50 known carcinogens. The increased risk of cardiovascular disease among cigarette smokers likely is related to exposure to oxidant chemicals and CO, as well as hydrogen cyanide, carbon disulfide, cadmium, and zinc (85). Although CO reduces oxygen delivery to the heart, oxidant chemicals are primarily responsible for endothelial dysfunction, platelet activation, thrombosis, and coronary vasoconstriction.

Cigarette smoking has significant detrimental effects on both the structure and function of the lung. Cigarette smoking causes an imbalance between proteolytic and antiproteolytic forces in the lung and heightens airway responsiveness. Chronic obstructive lung diseases are linked with exposure to tar, nitrogen oxides, hydrogen cyanide, and volatile aldehydes, enhanced by inducers of superoxide and H_2O_2.

The agents contributing most significantly to lung cancer are expected to be the carcinogenic polynuclear aromatic hydrocarbons and the tobacco-specific N-nitrosamines, followed by polonium-210 and volatile aldehydes. Catechol, the weakly acidic agents, volatile aldehydes, and nitrogen oxides that can serve as precursors in the exogenous and endogenous formation of N-nitrosamines enhance tobacco smoke-induced tumorigenesis (86). Active smokers with elevated levels of DNA damage from polynuclear aromatic hydrocarbons in their white blood cells (DNA adducts) are three times more likely to be diagnosed with lung cancer 1 to 13 years later than are smokers with lower adduct concentrations (odds ratio, 2.98; 95% confidence interval, 1.05–8.42; $p = 0.04$) (87). As with other tobacco-related diseases, the risk of cancer of the mouth, larynx, esophagus, lung, stomach, pancreas, kidney, urinary bladder, and uterine cervix as well as leukemia is directly related to the intensity and duration of exposure to cigarette smoke.

Other Physiologic Effects and Toxicities Cigarette smoking is associated with skin changes, including yellow staining of fingers, vasospasm and obliteration of small skin vessels, precancerous and squamous cell carcinomas on the lips and oral mucosa, and enhanced facial skin wrinkling. Tobacco smoke and exposure to ultraviolet A radiation each cause wrinkle formation. When excessive sun exposure (>2 hours/day) and heavy smoking (>35 pack years) occur together, the risk of developing wrinkles is 11.4 times higher than that of nonsmokers and those with less sun exposure at the same age (88). The induction of matrix metalloproteinase-1, mediated by reactive oxygen species (especially in people with low glutathione content fibroblasts), is thought to be an important mechanism underlying premature skin aging caused by cigarette smoking and exposure to ultraviolet A radiation.

Current smokers of 20 or more cigarettes per day have statistically significant increases in nuclear sclerosis and posterior subcapsular cataracts compared with individuals who never smoked. After adjusting for age and average number of cigarettes smoked per day, former smokers who had quit smoking 25 or more years previously have a 20% lower risk of cataracts, but still higher than among subjects who never smoked (89). Current smokers of more than 20 cigarettes per day also have an increased risk of age-related macular degeneration (90).

Cigarette smoking in women is associated with lower levels of estrogen, earlier menopause, and increased risk of osteoporosis (91). The alkaloids in tobacco smoke diminish estrogen formation by inhibiting an aromatase enzyme in granulosa cells or placental tissue.

In men, smoking may impair penile erection, primarily in people with underlying vascular disease, through the impairment of endothelium-dependent smooth muscle relaxation (92). Smoking doubles the likelihood of moderate or complete erectile dysfunction associated with other risk factors, such as coronary artery disease and hypertension. Because the prevalence of erectile dysfunction in former smokers is no different from that in individuals who never smoked, erectile dysfunction is believed to improve with smoking cessation (92).

Nicotine causes both appetite suppression and an increase in metabolic rate (93). Smokers weigh an average 2.7 to 4.5 kg (6 to 10 lb) less than nonsmokers. With smoking cessation, individuals typically crave sweets. Individuals who stop smoking typically gain weight to approximately the levels of never smokers in the 6 to 12 months after smoking cessation.

Through release of catecholamines, nicotine increases lipolysis and releases free fatty acids, which are taken up by the liver (94). This could contribute to the increase in very low-density lipoprotein and low-density lipoprotein and the decrease in high-density lipoprotein seen in smokers.

Cigarette smoking is associated with the occurrence and delayed healing of peptic ulcers. Mechanisms include decreases in the mucous bicarbonate barrier in the stomach, reduction in the production of endogenous prostaglandins in the gastric mucosa, and increased proliferation of *Helicobacter pylori* (95).

Tobacco and Pregnancy Smoking during pregnancy nearly doubles the relative risk of having a low birthweight infant; the relative risks of spontaneous abortion and perinatal and neonatal mortality are increased by about one-third (96). The components of tobacco smoke responsible for obstetric and fetal problems have not been definitively identified. CO clearly is detrimental, because it markedly reduces the oxygen-carrying capacity of fetal hemoglobin (97).

The effect of smoking in lowering birthweight interacts with the metabolic genes CYP1A1 and GSTT1 (96). Infants born to smoking mothers who had genetic variants associated with reduced CYP1A1 activity—Aa and aa (heterozygous and homozygous variant types)—and reduced or absent GSTT1 activity had greater reductions in birthweight than did infants born to smoking mothers who had the normal metabolic activity genes CYP1A1 AA (homozygous wild type) or GSTT1 genotype. The CYP1A1 and GSTT1 enzymes have roles metabolizing and excreting some toxic chemicals in cigarette smoke.

In the developing fetus, nicotine can arrest neuronal replication and differentiation and can contribute to sudden infant death syndrome (98). Nicotine prematurely activates nicotinic cholinergic receptors in the fetal brain, resulting in abnormalities of cell proliferation and differentiation that lead to shortfalls in cell numbers and eventually to altered synaptic activity. Comparable alterations occur in peripheral autonomic pathways and are hypothesized to lead to increased susceptibility to hypoxia-induced brain damage, perinatal mortality, and sudden infant death (16,96,98).

Secondhand Smoke Secondhand smoke (SHS) is the complex mixture formed by the escaping smoke of a burning tobacco product, as well as smoke that is exhaled by a smoker. Sidestream smoke contains higher concentrations of some toxins than mainstream smoke. As SHS combines with other constituents in the ambient air and ages, its characteristics may change (99). Exposure to SHS is causally associated with acute and chronic coronary heart disease, lung cancer, nasal sinus cancer, and eye and nasal irritation in adults. SHS is causally associated with asthma, chronic respiratory symptoms, and acute lower respiratory tract infections such as bronchitis and pneumonia in children. SHS also is causally associated with low birthweight and sudden infant death syndrome in infants. Young children's exposure to tobacco smoke comes mainly from smokers in the home, especially parents. Maternal smoking has the greatest effect on children's measured cotinine levels. Additional contributors include paternal smoking, smoking by other household members, and smoking by child care personnel.

An average salivary cotinine level of 0.4 ng/mL corresponds to an increased lifetime mortality risk of 1/1,000 for lung cancer and 1/100 for heart disease (100). Assuming a prevalence of 28% for unrestricted smoking in the workplace, passive smoking would yield 4,000 heart disease deaths and 400 lung cancer deaths annually in the United States. More than 95% of SHS-exposed office workers exceeded the significant risk level for heart disease mortality and more than 60% exceeded the significant risk level for lung cancer mortality established by the Occupational Safety and Health Administration (100).

Morbidity and Mortality The cumulative result of these health effects is that each pack of cigarettes sold in the United States costs the nation an estimated $7.18 in medical care expenditures and lost productivity (101). Smoking is a leading cause of preventable death in the United States, accounting for an estimated 402,374 premature deaths annually between 1995 and 1999. This includes 148,605 deaths (36.9%) from cardiovascular causes, 155,761 deaths (38.7%) from cancer, and 98,008 deaths (24.3%) from nonmalignant pulmonary disease (101). Cigarette smoking also increases the risk of developing and increases the severity of respiratory tract infections, including influenza, pneumococcal pneumonia, and tuberculosis (102). On average, adult men and women smokers lost 13.2 and 14.5 years of life, respectively. In contrast, the annual mortality attributable to passive smoking between 1995 and 1999 was estimated at 39,060 deaths, including 35,053 from cardiovascular diseases, 3,000 from lung cancer, and 1,007 from perinatal conditions (101).

Tobacco and Other Addictions There is a strong correlation between smoking and alcohol abuse (1). More severely dependent drinkers smoke more and are less likely to quit. Tobacco also synergizes with alcohol in causing a number of medical complications. Smoking and heavy drinking, in combination, are associated with substantially increased rates of oral and esophageal cancers (103). Because lit cigarettes smolder when they fall onto upholstered furniture, alcohol use combines with smoking to cause household fires that claim more than 1,000 deaths per year among children and adults (104). Persons recovering from other substance use disorders often die from tobacco-related illnesses. In a landmark population-based retrospective cohort study, death certificates were examined for 214 of 854 persons who were admitted between 1972 and 1983 to an inpatient program for the treatment of alcoholism and other nonnicotine drugs of dependence (105). Of the deaths reported, 50.9% were caused by tobacco use, whereas 34.1% were attributable to alcohol use. The cumulative 20-year mortality was 48.1% versus an expected 18.5% for a demographically matched control population ($p < 0.001$).

Benefits of Cessation The good news is that smoking cessation has benefits for smokers of all ages. The immediately decreased risk of cardiovascular death in those who stop smoking may reflect a decrease in blood coagulability, improved tissue oxygenation, and reduced predisposition to cardiac arrhythmias. Among former smokers, the reduced risk of death compared with continuing smokers begins shortly after quitting and continues for at least 10 to 15 years. After 10 to 15 years' abstinence, the risk of all-cause mortality returns nearly to that of persons who never smoked (106).

REFERENCES

1. Dani JA, Harris RA. Nicotine addiction and comorbidity with alcohol abuse and mental illness. *Nat Neurosci* 2005;8:1465–1470.
2. Mathers CD, Loncar D. Projections of global mortality and burden of disease from 2002 to 2030. *PLoS Med* 2006;3:e442.
3. Benowitz NL. Clinical pharmacology of nicotine: implications for understanding, preventing, and treating tobacco addiction. *Clin Pharmacol Ther* 2008;83:531–541.
4. Rose JE. Nicotine and nonnicotine factors in cigarette addiction. *Psychopharmacology (Berlin)* 2006;184:274–285.
5. Palmatier MI, Liu X, Matteson GL, et al. Conditioned reinforcement in rats established with self-administered nicotine and enhanced by noncontingent nicotine. *Psychopharmacology (Berlin)* 2007;195:235–243.
6. Gately I. Tobacco: A cultural history of how an exotic plant seduced civilization. Grove Press, New York, New York. 2002.
7. Pankow JF, Tavakoli AD, Luo W, et al. Percent free base nicotine in the tobacco smoke particulate matter of selected commercial and reference cigarettes. *Chem Res Toxicol* 2003;16:1014–1018.
8. Benowitz NL. Pharmacologic aspects of cigarette smoking and nicotine addiction. *N Engl J Med* 1988;319:1318–1330.
9. Henningfield JE, Radzius A, Cooper TM, et al. Drinking coffee and carbonated beverages blocks absorption of nicotine from nicotine polacrilex gum. *JAMA* 1990;264:1560–1564.
10. Hoffmann D, Hoffmann I. The changing cigarette, 1950–1995. *J Toxicol Environ Health* 1997;50:307–364.
11. Brody AL, Mandelkern MA, London ED, et al. Cigarette smoking saturates brain alpha 4 beta 2 nicotinic acetylcholine receptors. *Arch Gen Psychiatry* 2006;63:907–915.
12. Henningfield JE, Stapleton JM, Benowitz NL, et al. Higher levels of nicotine in arterial than in venous blood after cigarette smoking. *Drug Alcohol Depend* 1993;33:23–29.
13. Gourlay SG, Benowitz NL. Arteriovenous differences in plasma concentration of nicotine and catecholamines and related cardiovascular effects after smoking, nicotine nasal spray, and intravenous nicotine. *Clin Pharmacol Ther* 1997;62:453–463.
14. Megerdichian CL, Rees VW, Wayne GF, et al. Internal tobacco industry research on olfactory and trigeminal nerve response to nicotine and other smoke components. *Nicotine Tob Res* 2007;9:1119–1129.
15. Benowitz NL, Shopland DR, Burns DM, et al. Compensatory smoking of low yield cigarettes. In: *Yields of tar and nicotine.* Bethesda, MD: NIH Publication No. 02-5074, 2001:39–64.
16. Hukkanen J, Jacob P 3rd, Benowitz NL. Metabolism and disposition kinetics of nicotine. *Pharmacol Rev* 2005;57:79–115.

17. Mathieu-Kia AM, Kellogg SH, Butelman ER, et al. Nicotine addiction: insights from recent animal studies. *Psychopharmacology (Berlin)* 2002;162:102–118.
18. Corringer PJ, Sallette J, Changeux JP. Nicotine enhances intracellular nicotinic receptor maturation: a novel mechanism of neural plasticity? *J Physiol Paris* 2006;99:162–171.
19. Benowitz NL, Lessov-Schlaggar CN, Swan GE, et al. Female sex and oral contraceptive use accelerate nicotine metabolism. *Clin Pharmacol Ther* 2006;79:480–488.
20. Dempsey D, Jacob P, 3rd, Benowitz NL. Accelerated metabolism of nicotine and cotinine in pregnant smokers. *J Pharmacol Exp Ther* 2002; 301:594–598.
21. Perez-Stable EJ, Herrera B, Jacob P 3rd, et al. Nicotine metabolism and intake in black and white smokers. *JAMA* 1998;280:152–156.
22. Mwenifumbo JC, Sellers EM, Tyndale RF. Nicotine metabolism and CYP2A6 activity in a population of black African descent: impact of gender and light smoking. *Drug Alcohol Depend* 2007;89:24–33.
23. Benowitz NL, Perez-Stable EJ, Fong I, et al. Ethnic differences in N-glucuronidation of nicotine and cotinine. *J Pharmacol Exp Ther* 1999;291:1196–1203.
24. Haiman CA, Stram DO, Wilkens LR, et al. Ethnic and racial differences in the smoking-related risk of lung cancer. *N Engl J Med* 2006;354:333–342.
25. Malaiyandi V, Sellers EM, Tyndale RF. Implications of CYP2A6 genetic variation for smoking behaviors and nicotine dependence. *Clin Pharmacol Ther* 2005;77:145–158.
26. Benowitz NL. Cotinine as a biomarker of environmental tobacco smoke exposure. *Epidemiol Rev* 1996;18:188–204.
27. Jacob P 3rd, Hatsukami D, Severson H, et al. Anabasine and anatabine as biomarkers for tobacco use during nicotine replacement therapy. *Cancer Epidemiol Biomarkers Prev* 2002;11:1668–1673.
28. Jarvis M, Tunstall-Pedoe H, Feyerabend C, et al. Biochemical markers of smoke absorption and self reported exposure to passive smoking. *J Epidemiol Community Health* 1984;38:335–339.
29. Benowitz NL, Jacob P 3rd, Ahijevych K, et al. Biochemical verification of tobacco use and cessation. *Nicotine Tob Res* 2002;4:149–159.
30. McNeill AD, Owen LA, Belcher M, et al. Abstinence from smoking and expired-air carbon monoxide levels: lactose intolerance as a possible source of error. *Am J Public Health* 1990;80:1114–1115.
31. Tsuge K, Katoaoka M, Seto Y. Cyanide and thiocyanate levels in blood and saliva of healthy adult volunteers. *J Health Sci* 2000;46:343–350.
32. Zevin S, Benowitz NL. Drug interactions with tobacco smoking. An update. *Clin Pharmacokinet* 1999;36:425–438.
33. Benowitz NL, Hansson A, Jacob P 3rd. Cardiovascular effects of nasal and transdermal nicotine and cigarette smoking. *Hypertension* 2002;39: 1107–1112.
34. Rose JE, Behm FM, Westman EC. Acute effects of nicotine and mecamylamine on tobacco withdrawal symptoms, cigarette reward and ad lib smoking. *Pharmacol Biochem Behav* 2001;68:187–197.
35. Kenny PJ, Markou A. Conditioned nicotine withdrawal profoundly decreases the activity of brain reward systems. *J Neurosci* 2005;25: 6208–6212.
36. Xian H, Scherrer JF, Madden PA, et al. Latent class typology of nicotine withdrawal: genetic contributions and association with failed smoking cessation and psychiatric disorders. *Psychol Med* 2005;35: 409–419.
37. Parrott AC, Kaye FJ. Daily uplifts, hassles, stresses and cognitive failures: in cigarette smokers, abstaining smokers, and non-smokers. *Behav Pharmacol* 1999;10:639–646.
38. Lessov-Schlaggar CN, Pergadia ML, Khroyan TV, et al. Genetics of nicotine dependence and pharmacotherapy. *Biochem Pharmacol* 2008;75:178–195.
39. Schnoll RA, Johnson TA, Lerman C. Genetics and smoking behavior. *Curr Psychiatry Rep* 2007;9:349–357.
40. Mineur YS, Picciotto MR. Genetics of nicotinic acetylcholine receptors: relevance to nicotine addiction. *Biochem Pharmacol* 2008;75: 323–333.
41. Rosecrans JA. The psychopharmacological basis of nicotine's differential effects on behavior: individual subject variability in the rat. *Behav Genet* 1995;25:187–196.
42. Gilbert DG, Estes SL, Welser R. Does noise stress modulate effects of smoking/nicotine? Mood, vigilance, and EEG responses. *Psychopharmacology (Berlin)* 1997;129:382–389.
43. Grobe JE, Perkins KA. Behavioral factors influencing the effects of nicotine. In: Piasecki M, Newhause P (eds). *Nicotine: neurotropic and neurotoxic effects*. American Psychiatric Press, Washington, D.C. 2000.
44. Parrott AC. Nesbitt's Paradox resolved? Stress and arousal modulation during cigarette smoking. *Addiction* 1998;93:27–39.
45. Perkins KA. Nicotine discrimination in men and women. *Pharmacol Biochem Behav* 1999;64:295–299.
46. Perkins KA, Gerlach D, Vender J, et al. Sex differences in the subjective and reinforcing effects of visual and olfactory cigarette smoke stimuli. *Nicotine Tob Res* 2001;3:141–150.
47. Carmelli D, Swan GE, Robinette D, et al. Heritability of substance use in the NAS-NRC Twin Registry. *Acta Genet Med Gemellol (Roma)* 1990;39:91–98.
48. Mohammed AH. Genetic dissection of nicotine-related behaviour: a review of animal studies. *Behav Brain Res* 2000;113:35–41.
49. Robinson SF, Marks MJ, Collins AC. Inbred mouse strains vary in oral self-selection of nicotine. *Psychopharmacology (Berlin)* 1996;124:332–339.
50. Tritto T, Stitzel JA, Marks MJ, et al. Variability in response to nicotine in the LSxSS RI strains: potential role of polymorphisms in alpha4 and alpha6 nicotinic receptor genes. *Pharmacogenetics* 2002;12:197–208.
51. Ho MK, Tyndale RF. Overview of the pharmacogenomics of cigarette smoking. *Pharmacogenomics J* 2007;7:81–98.
52. Bierut LJ, Madden PA, Breslau N, et al. Novel genes identified in a high-density genome wide association study for nicotine dependence. *Hum Mol Genet* 2007;16:24–35.
53. Saccone SF, Hinrichs AL, Saccone NL, et al. Cholinergic nicotinic receptor genes implicated in a nicotine dependence association study targeting 348 candidate genes with 3713 SNPs. *Hum Mol Genet* 2007;16:36–49.
54. Uhl GR, Liu QR, Drgon T, et al. Molecular genetics of nicotine dependence and abstinence: whole genome association using 520,000 SNPs. *BMC Genet* 2007;8:10.
55. Dalack GW, Healy DJ, Meador-Woodruff JH. Nicotine dependence in schizophrenia: clinical phenomena and laboratory findings. *Am J Psychiatry* 1998;155:1490–1501.
56. Martin LF, Freedman R. Schizophrenia and the alpha7 nicotinic acetylcholine receptor. *Int Rev Neurobiol* 2007;78:225–246.
57. Levin ED, Wilson W, Rose JE, et al. Nicotine-haloperidol interactions and cognitive performance in schizophrenics. *Neuropsychopharmacology* 1996;15:429–436.
58. Leonard S, Adler LE, Benhammou K, et al. Smoking and mental illness. *Pharmacol Biochem Behav* 2001;70:561–570.
59. Sullivan MA, Rudnik-Levin F. Attention deficit/hyperactivity disorder and substance abuse. Diagnostic and therapeutic considerations. *Ann N Y Acad Sci* 2001;931:251–270.
60. Milberger S, Biederman J, Faraone SV, et al. ADHD is associated with early initiation of cigarette smoking in children and adolescents. *J Am Acad Child Adolesc Psychiatry* 1997;36:37–44.
61. Levin ED, Conners CK, Sparrow E, et al. Nicotine effects on adults with attention-deficit/hyperactivity disorder. *Psychopharmacology (Berlin)* 1996;123:55–63.
62. Lasser K, Boyd J W, Woolhandler S, et al. Smoking and mental illness: a population-based prevalence study. *JAMA* 2000;284:2606–2610.
63. Kendler KS, Neale MC, MacLean CJ, et al. Smoking and major depression. A causal analysis. *Arch Gen Psychiatry* 1993;50:36–43.
64. Balfour DJ, Ridley DL. The effects of nicotine on neural pathways implicated in depression: a factor in nicotine addiction? *Pharmacol Biochem Behav* 2000;66:79–85.
65. Shytle RD, Baker M, Silver AA, et al. Smoking nicotine and movement disorders. In: Piasecki M, Newhause P (eds). Nicotine: neurotropic and neurotoxic effects. Washington DC: American Psychiatric Press, 2000.

66. Newhouse PA, Whitehouse PJ. Nicotinic cholinergic aystems in Alzheimer's and Parkinson's diseases. In: *Nicotine: neurotropic and neurotoxic effects*. Washington DC: American Psychiatric Press, 2000.
67. Haddock CK, Weg MV, DeBon M, et al. Evidence that smokeless tobacco use is a gateway for smoking initiation in young adult males. *Prev Med* 2001;32:262–267.
68. Weissman MM, Warner V, Wickramaratne PJ, et al. Maternal smoking during pregnancy and psychopathology in offspring followed to adulthood. *J Am Acad Child Adolesc Psychiatry* 1999;38:892–899.
69. MMWR. State-specific prevalence of cigarette smoking and quitting among adults—United States. 2005;54:1124–1127.
70. George O, Ghozland S, Azar MR, et al. CRF-CRF1 system activation mediates withdrawal-induced increases in nicotine self-administration in nicotine-dependent rats. *Proc Natl Acad Sci U S A* 2007;104: 17198–17203.
71. Dani JA, Bertrand D. Nicotinic acetylcholine receptors and nicotinic cholinergic mechanisms of the central nervous system. *Annu Rev Pharmacol Toxicol* 2007;47:699–729.
72. Tapper AR, McKinney SL, Nashmi R, et al. Nicotine activation of alpha4* receptors: sufficient for reward, tolerance, and sensitization. *Science* 2004;306:1029–1032.
73. Broide RS, Leslie FM. The alpha7 nicotinic acetylcholine receptor in neuronal plasticity. *Mol Neurobiol* 1999;20:1–16.
74. Balfour DJ, Wright AE, Benwell ME, et al. The putative role of extrasynaptic mesolimbic dopamine in the neurobiology of nicotine dependence. *Behav Brain Res* 2000;113:73–83.
75. Di Chiara G. Role of dopamine in the behavioural actions of nicotine related to addiction. *Eur J Pharmacol* 2000;393:295–314.
76. Mansvelder H D, McGehee D S. Cellular and synaptic mechanisms of nicotine addiction. *J Neurobiol* 2002;53:606–617.
77. Corringer PJ, Bertrand S, Galzi JL, et al. Mutational analysis of the charge selectivity filter of the alpha7 nicotinic acetylcholine receptor. *Neuron* 1999;22:831–843.
78. Rose JE, Behm FM, Westman EC, et al. Arterial nicotine kinetics during cigarette smoking and intravenous nicotine administration: implications for addiction. *Drug Alcohol Depend* 1999;56:99–107.
79. Dani JA, Heinemann S. Molecular and cellular aspects of nicotine abuse. *Neuron* 1996;16:905–908.
80. Dani JA, Montague PR. Disrupting addiction through the loss of drug-associated internal states. *Nat Neurosci*, 2007;10:403–404.
81. Buisson B, Bertrand D. Chronic exposure to nicotine upregulates the human (alpha)4(beta)2 nicotinic acetylcholine receptor function. *J Neurosci* 2001;21:1819–1829.
82. Fowler JS, Logan J, Wang GJ, et al. Monoamine oxidase and cigarette smoking. *Neurotoxicology* 2003;24:75–82.
83. Lewis A, Miller JH, Lea RA. Monoamine oxidase and tobacco dependence. *Neurotoxicology* 2007;28:182–195.
84. Guillem K, Vouillac C, Azar MR, et al. Monoamine oxidase inhibition dramatically increases the motivation to self-administer nicotine in rats. *J Neurosci* 2005;25:8593–8600.
85. Benowitz NL. Basic cardiovascular research and its implications for the medicinal use of nicotine. *J Am Coll Cardiol* 2003;41:497–498.
86. Hecht SS. Human urinary carcinogen metabolites: biomarkers for investigating tobacco and cancer. *Carcinogenesis* 2002;23: 907–922.
87. Tang D, Phillips DH, Stampfer M, et al. Association between carcinogen-DNA adducts in white blood cells and lung cancer risk in the physicians health study. *Cancer Res* 2001;61:6708–6712.
88. Yin L, Morita A, Tsuji T. Skin aging induced by ultraviolet exposure and tobacco smoking: evidence from epidemiological and molecular studies. *Photodermatol Photoimmunol Photomed* 2001;17:178–183.
89. Weintraub JM, Willett WC, Rosner B, et al. Smoking cessation and risk of cataract extraction among U.S. women and men. *Am J Epidemiol* 2002;155:72–79.
90. Jager RD, Mieler WF, Miller JW. Age-related macular degeneration. *N Engl J Med* 2008;358:2606–2617.
91. Department of Health and Human Services. Women and smoking. A Report of the Surgeon General. U.S. Department of Health and Human Services Washington, D.C. 2001.
92. McVary KT, Carrier S, Wessells H. Smoking and erectile dysfunction: evidence based analysis. *J Urol* 2001;166:1624–1632.
93. Chiolero A, Faeh D, Paccaud F, et al. Consequences of smoking for body weight, body fat distribution, and insulin resistance. *Am J Clin Nutr* 2008;87:801–809.
94. Campbell SC, Moffatt RJ, Stamford BA. Smoking and smoking cessation—the relationship between cardiovascular disease and lipoprotein metabolism: a review. *Atherosclerosis* 2008; May 13. Epub ahead of print.
95. Rhodes J, Green J, Thomas G. Nicotine and the gastrointestinal tract. In: Benowitz NL (ed). *Nicotine safety and toxicity.* New York: Oxford University Press, 1998:161–166.
96. Wang X, Zuckerman B, Pearson C, et al. Maternal cigarette smoking, metabolic gene polymorphism, and infant birth weight. *JAMA* 2002; 287:195–202.
97. Dempsey DA, Benowitz NL. Risks and benefits of nicotine to aid smoking cessation in pregnancy. *Drug Saf* 2001;24:277–322.
98. Slotkin TA. Fetal nicotine or cocaine exposure: which one is worse? *J Pharmacol Exp Ther* 1998;285:931–945.
99. DHHS. The health consequences of involuntary exposure to tobacco smoke. A Report of the Surgeon General. U.S. Department of Health and Human Services Washington, D.C. 2006.
100. Repace JL, Jinot J, Bayard S, et al. Air, nicotine, and saliva cotinine as indicators of workplace passive smoking exposure and risk. *Risk Anal* 1997;18(1):71–83.
101. Centers for Disease Control and Prevention (CDC). Annual smoking-attributable mortality, years of potential life lost, and economic costs—United States, 1995–1999. *MMWR Morb Mortal Wkly Rep* 2002;51: 300–303.
102. Arcavi L, Benowitz NL. Cigarette smoking and infection. *Arch Intern Med* 2004;164:2206–2216.
103. DHHS. The health consequences of smoking. A Report of the Surgeon General. U.S. Department of Health and Human Services Washington, D.C. 2004.
104. Leistikow BN, Martin DC, Milano CE. Fire injuries, disasters, and costs from cigarettes and cigarette lights: a global overview. *Prev Med* 2000;31:91–99.
105. Hurt RD, Offord KP, Croghan IT, et al. Mortality following inpatient addictions treatment: role of tobacco use in a community-based cohort. *JAMA* 1996;275:1097–1103.
106. NCI. Changes in cigarette-related disease risks and their implication for prevention and control. U.S. National Institutes of Health, National Cancer Institute Bethesda, MD. 2001:39–64.

CHAPTER 13

Sandra P. Welch, PhD

The Pharmacology of Cannabinoids

Cannabis sativa, obtained from hemp plants, historically is one of the oldest and most widely used drugs in the world (1). An elegant review summarizes the chemistry and uses of the hemp plant throughout history (2).

DRUGS IN THE CLASS

Δ^9-Tetrahydrocannabinol (THC), the major psychoactive ingredient in marijuana, first was isolated and purified in 1965 (3). This important discovery was the first step in elucidating the site and mechanism of action of the cannabinoids—the term for all compounds that are structurally related to THC. More than 400 chemicals are synthesized by the hemp plant, approximately 60 of which are cannabinoids. Four decades of the investigation of the complex pharmacologic properties of THC culminated in the discovery of neuronal cannabinoid receptors, which in turn stimulated the search for endogenous ligands for cannabinoid receptors (4–7). Natural ligands, which bind to cannabinoid receptors, include arachidonoylethanolamide (anandamide (8), 2-arachidonoylglycerol (2-AG) (9), noladin ether (10), virodhamin (11), and N-arachidonoyldopamine (12)). These lipid signaling molecules are referred to as endocannabinoids. There are two known cannabinoid receptor subtypes, CB_1 (13) and CB_2 (14). The discovery of the receptors has led to the development of numerous receptor agonists and antagonists, some of which have been shown to have medicinal benefit. A CB_1 cannabinoid antagonist, SR141716A (rimonabant), has been described (15), as has the cannabinoid CB_2 receptor antagonist, SR144528 (16). Sativex (a 1:1 mixture of THC and cannabidiol) has been approved by Health Cananda. A mixed-ratio of THC and cannabidiol in capsular formulation produced by Cannador (Cannador, European Institute for Oncology and Immunological Research, Germany) is also available. In addition, synthetic Δ^9-tetrahydrocannabinol (dronabinol, Marinol) is available, as is nabilone, a synthetic cannabinoid with therapeutic use as an antiemetic, appetite stimulant, and as an adjunct analgesic for neuropathic pain. Nabilone is a synthetic cannabinoid, which mimics the main ingredient of marijuana (THC), but produces minimal euphoria. Nabilone is not derived from the cannabis plant, as is dronabinol. In Canada, the United States, the United Kingdom, and Mexico, nabilone is marketed as Cesamet. Both dronabinol and nabilone are marketed as Schedule III preparations.

HISTORY

The use of cannabis dates back over 12,000 years (17). Cannabis use is believed to have started in central Asia and continued to flourish in Southeast Asia and India. Its uses include that of making clothes and rope from hemp by the ancient Chinese and Greeks. It is believed that cannabis was introduced into the Americas in the 1600s by the English settlers and Spanish conquistadors. Cannabis was cultivated early in American history for its fiber. Medicinally, it has long been used in China, India, the Middle East, South America, and South Africa. The earliest references to its medicinal uses date back to 2700 BC (18). Uses in ancient China included treatment for constipation, malaria, rheumatic pains, and female disorders. The euphoric properties were discovered in India around 2000 BC, and cannabis was recommended for reducing fevers, producing sleep, stimulating the appetite, relieving headaches, and curing venereal diseases (19). The medicinal uses of cannabis in Azerbaijan are described in medieval texts from as early as the ninth century AD; uses for the drug in modern medicine, some based on folkloric uses, have been proposed as reviewed elsewhere (2). In 1842, O'Shaughnessy, a British army physician in India, published a review on the use of cannabis in the treatment of various medical conditions (20). Interestingly, several of these early references to the medical uses of marijuana include disease states on which research continues today (21,22). Recreational use of cannabis began to surge in the 1930s during the Prohibition Era. Although cannabis was recognized as an official drug and was listed in the U.S. Pharmacopoeia from 1850 until 1942, its medical use in the United States was essentially abolished in 1937 when the Marijuana Tax Act was enacted. In addition, cannabis was placed in Schedule 1 of the Controlled Substances Act in 1970. A dramatic increase in cannabis use was observed during the 1960s, which led to extensive research in the field of cannabinoid pharmacology.

EPIDEMIOLOGY

Marijuana remains the nation's most commonly used illicit drug. The National Survey on Drug Use and Health 2006 report (23) including data from all 50 states indicates that 44% of males and 35% of all females studied have used marajuana at least once in their life time. Based on the National Survey on Drug Use and Health (23,24), 6.8% (1.7 million) youth ages 12 to 17 used marijuana in the past month and 3.5% (891,000) smoked "blunts" (cigars with marijuana in them) in the past month. An estimated 39.2% of daily marijuana users were dependent on or abused marijuana compared with 13.5% of less-than-daily marijuana users. In 2004, marijuana was used by 76.4% of illicit drug users. An estimated 56.8% of current illicit drug users used only marijuana, 19.7% used marijuana and another illicit drug, and the remaining 23.6% used only an illicit drug other than marijuana in the past month (24).

According to the Drug Abuse Warning Network, marijuana reports were the second most frequently recorded major substance of abuse (excluding alcohol). The prevalence was highest in patients ages 18 to 24. The prevalence of male admissions was more than triple that for females in all areas. In addition, it was reported the combination of marijuana with alcohol contributes to nearly 10% of the admissions and nearly 14% of admissions for detoxification (25). Thus, the use of marijuana remains high throughout the country. The most widely abused substance is cannabis (used at least once per year by more than 150 million people). There is increasing consumption in South America, and expanding markets in Western and Eastern Europe, as well as in Africa. Production of cannabis declined in 2005. This decline follows several years of sustained growth. The demand for treatment of cannabis addiction has increased globally for the last 10 years (26).

THERAPEUTIC USE

A minimum of 21 therapeutic potentials for cannabinoids are under investigation, including nonpsychoactive cannabinoids such as cannabidiol (27). The problems associated with such uses have also been reviewed (28,29). In addition, the development of modulators of the endocannabinoid systems provides a increasingly large number of potential therapeutic uses. Controlled clinical trials of using cannabis have only recently been conducted (30) and indicate that smoked cannabis significantly decreases neuropathic pain in those individuals that are HIV-positive. Several side effects of the cannabis were noted, but were not serious life-threatening events. Cannabis is not a U.S. Food and Drug Administration (FDA)-approved preparation. However, two novel cannabis-derived preparations are either in testing or approved in countries other than the United States. The most promsing is a standardized oromucosal spray from GW Pharmaceuticals called Sativex. Sativex (a 1:1 mixture of THC and cannabidiol) has been approved by Health Cananda, shows promise in treatment of numerous types of neurologic pain in the United Kingdom and is in more than 15 current clinical trials in the United States and Europe (31). The indicated use for Sativex at present is as an adjuct for neuropathic pain in multiple sclerosis patients and intractable pain in cancer patients. The second cannabis derived product is a mixed ratio of THC and cannabidiol in capsular formulation produced by Cannador (Cannador, European Institute for Oncology and Immunological Research, Germany). The efficacy of this preparation for neuropathic pain from multiple sclerosis was not demonstrated and the study was discontinued, although studies with Cannador continue.

Therapeutic Indications and Proposed Indications Therapeutic uses for cannabis have been anecdotally reported for thousands of years. Only recently have several uses described in folk medicine been formally evaluated. The most intense interest has been directed toward the prevention of weight loss in AIDS patients, management of pain, prevention of emesis, control of glaucoma, and control of movement disorders. The use of smoked cannabis remains both politically and scientifically controversial although some studies of smoked cannabis are under way in the United States, as discussed previously. The availability of synthetic THC in capsule form provides a potential alternative to the smoked plant material as do a variety of novel delivery systems, including vaporizors. The potential for development of alternative methods of drug delivery using either pure THC or one of the newer THC derivatives may obviate the problems and the controversial nature of the use of the smoked plant material. In addition, more data describing the role or roles of the endocannabinoid system in the etiology of disease states, coupled with the pharmacologic activity of the endocannabinoids administered exogenously, have opened a new and exciting area for the development of potential therapeutic agents.

Antiemetic Effect Two oral formulations described previously, dronabinol (synthetic THC) (Marinol) and nabilone (Cesamet), are approved by the FDA for use in emesis refractory to conventional antiemetic therapy and as an appetite stimulant in patients with AIDS-wasting or cancer. In a recent review of antiemetics (32), cannabinoids were shown to be slightly more efficacious than the conventional antiemetics used such as metoclopromide, phenothiazines, and haloperidol at doses of 5 to 10 mg every 4 hours for dronabinol and 1 to 2 mg twice per day for nabilone. However, side effects such as dizziness and dysphoria limit the use of such drugs. There is some evidence that the combination of a dopamine antagonist and cannabinoid is superior to either alone and is particularly effective in preventing nausea (33). In addition, cannabidiol not only ameliorates vomiting, but also decreases the anticipatory effects of the onset of nausea and vomiting, an effect likely related to effects on learning (34).

Appetite Stimulation and Cachexia The cannabinoid effect most commonly discussed is the effect on appetite. Smoked cannabis is well known to stimulate appetite. AIDS patients have lobbied to make cannabis available to those suffering from cachexia, the body wasting resulting from HIV infection. Clinical trials indicate some improvement in appetite, slight increases in caloric intake, and weight gain (35). Although dronabinol (Marinol) use was associated with declining health in patients undergoing antiretroviral therapies, all clinical indicators of pancreatitis improved in the patients who used the dronabinol (36). In AIDS patients with the lowest CD4+ counts, utilization of dronabinol was not harmful and the long-term, safe use of THC for anorexia associated with weight loss in patients with AIDS was reported (37). One placebo-controlled, within-subjects study in individuals with HIV-induced cachexia evaluated marijuana and dronabinol across a range of behaviors including eating (38). As compared with placebo, marijuana and dronabinol dose-dependently increased daily caloric intake and body weight in HIV-positive marijuana smokers. However, at the doses used, cannabis produced significant intoxication and the low-dose dronabinol (5 mg) formulation did not.

The onset of the "munchies" after THC use led to the development of the cannabinoid antagonist, SR141716A (rimonabant), as an agent for weight reduction (39). Several trade names of the drug are used worldwide (Acomplia, Riobant, Slimona, Rimoslim, and Zimulti). Riobant, Slimona, and Rimoslim are generic forms available in India. If approved in the United States, it is intended to be marketed under the name Zimulti. At of the end of 2007, the drug was approved for marketing in more than 50 countries, but not in the United States. In June 2007, the FDA's Endocrine and Metabolic Drugs Advisory Committee voted against recommending rimonabant for approval (for review of clinical trials and summary of the results see FDA Briefing Document) (40). However, the effects of rimonabant on weight reduction have opened an expanding new area of research as to the regulation of appetite and metabolic processes by the cannabinoids and endocannabinoids.

The detailed biochemical effects of cannabinoids on increased food uptake have been recently reviewed (39,41). From the time of birth, the endocannabinoid system may be a factor in our food intake. Newborn mice given the cannabinoid antagonist, SR141716A, fail to suckle, lose weight, and die if not rescued with administrations of THC or endocannabinoids such as 2-AG. Endocannabinoids regulate energy balance and food intake in newborns and suckling behaviors at both central and peripheral sites (42). Central control appears to be via the limbic system (site of the desire or "craving" for food), as well as the hypothalamus and hindbrain. Peripheral intestinal control and endocannabinoid effects on adipose tissue are additional players in the control of appetite. The endocannabinoid system interacts with a number of better known molecules involved in appetite and weight regulation, including leptin, ghrelin, and the melanocortins (43). It has been shown that CB_1 receptor knockout mice eat less than their wild-type littermates and endocannabinoids in the hypothalamus tonically activate CB_1 receptors to maintain food intake. The mechanism by which endocannabinoids appear to regulate food intake includes modulation of leptin, the major signaling peptide through which the hypothalamus senses satiety. Defects in the leptin/endocannabinoid interplay have been proposed to underly obesity in genetically obese rats and may underly obesity in humans (41). Endocannabinoids appear to increase leptin production from adipocytes, because CB_1 receptor–deficient mice contain less circulating leptin than wild-type mice. Conversely, ghrelin, released during food deprivation, signals the hypothalamus the need for energy intake. Ghrelin upregulates hypothalamic endocannabinoid levels. Thus, two key hormones controlling food intake, leptin and ghrelin, are not only regulated by endocannabinoids, but also regulate endocannabinoid levels in seemingly opposing ways, an effect under control of CB_1 receptors. Data from both animal studies and clinical trials with rimonabant indicate that these and other regulatory effects occur also in peripheral tissues, particularly in adipocytes, and that the endocannabinoid system may play an important role not only in energy intake but also in lipid metabolism and accumulation, in both animals and humans. The important new insights as to the role of endocannabinoids in eating has provided novel new therapeutic possibilities for the treatment of a variety of eating disorders via the use of drugs designed to alter perpheral, but not central cannabinoid receptors (44).

Anticonvulsant Effect Cannabis's therapeutic potential as an anticonvulsant was shown in the 1940s when children, poorly controlled on conventional anticonvulsant medication, were improved after the use of cannabis (45). Recently, cannabidiol has been shown to have anticonvulsant effect in children who are refractory to other therapies (46). Cannabidiol, a natural component of cannabis with practically no THC-like psychoactivity, has some moderate anticonvulsant activity in animals (47). There is interest in cannabidiol because the recent observation that CB_1-receptor knockout mice are prone to seizures (48). The role of the endocannabinoid system in the regulation of neuronal firing, action potential modulation, and excitotoxicity has led to numerous new studies as to the role of CB_1 receptors in epilepiform activity (49). In addition, in animal studies, it has been shown that the CB_1 receptor when activated by exogenous or endogenous cannabinoids produces an anticonvulsant effect (50), whereas the development of status epilepticus in rats results in a redistribution of the CB_1 receptor that persists and results in altered coupling of the receptor to G-proteins (51). Such data indicate that the CB_1 receptor plays a critical role in neuronal firing and as such could be the target of therapeutic approaches to the treatment of epilepsy and other diseases resultng in convulsant behaviors, such as in those with head trauma.

Neurologic and Movement Disorders There are numerous anecdotal reports that smoked cannabis is effective in relieving spasticity arising from multiple sclerosis and spinal cord injury. However, there have been few controlled studies comparing the effectiveness of either cannabis or THC with other therapies. A recent review indicated that the endocannabinoid system is subject to plasticity changes of various durations in pathologic conditions such as in neurologic, neuropsychiatric, and movement disorders (52). In addition, endocannabinoid tone appears to play a critical role in the modulation of basal ganglia mediation of the spasticity in Parkinson's disease. In multiple sclerosis patients, a nearly fourfold increase in anandamide levels is observed along with an increase in the CB_2 receptor. The importance of such changes is yet to be determined. Clearly, the endocannabinoid tone plays a critical role in numerous neurologic disorders and imbalance in the system may underlie such disorders. Such recent work opens up a new area for increased research involving the role of the endocannabinoids in neuromuscular and neurodegenerative diseases resulting in movement disorders. There have been several clinical trials that have yielded data indicating that cannabinoids can ameliorate spasticity and pain and improve quality of sleep in multiple sclerosis patients (53). In questionnaires sent to multiple sclerosis patients, >90% reported improvement after taking cannabis. Preclinical evidence in animal models of demyelination indicates that cannabinoid receptor agonists can decrease motor dysfunction in a manner similar to the effects in humans.

Analgesia A variety of pharmacologic, anatomic, and electrophysiologic investigations indicate the CB_1 receptor system plays a fundamental role in regulating pain behavior (54–57). CB_1 receptors are expressed at high levels in a variety of peripheral (58) and central (59) neurons that participate in pain perception. CB_1 agonists produce analgesia by acting at several sites along pathways for pain transmission peripherally (60,61), spinally (62–65), and supraspinally (66,67). Natural ligands, which bind to cannabinoid receptors such as the endocannabinoids previously described in this chapter, have become the targets of the majority of studies of the CB_1 and CB_2 receptors in the modulation of pain. In addition, modulators of the synthesis, transport, and degradation of the endocannabinoids have become increasingly important therapeutic targets.

Multiple enzymes are involved in the biosynthesis and degradation endocannabinoids (68). A specific phospholipase D (NAPE-PLD) has been proposed to hydrolyze N-acyl-phosohatidylethanolamine to anandamide (69). The highest concentrations of this enzyme are found in brain, kidney, and testis of the mouse. Two sn-1–specific diacylglycerol lipases ($DAGL_a$ and $DAGL_b$) have been identified that can hydrolyze diacylglycerol to 2-arachidonoylglycerol (70). Degradative enzymes include fatty acid amide hydrolase (FAAH) as the enzyme primarily responsible for anandamide catabolism (71) and the serine lipase monoacylglycerol lipase responsible for 2-AG degradation (72).

Anandamide (AEA) (73) and 2-AG (74) produce antinociception when administered to animals. The short half-lives of the endocannabinoids (75) present a significant challenge in investigating their function. However, the identification of fatty acid amide hydrolase (FAAH) as the enzyme primarily responsible for anandamide catabolism and the serine lipase monoacylglycerol lipase responsible for 2-AG degradation (72) have provided valuable targets to increase endogenous levels of each of these respective endocannabinoids, by using genetically engineered mice devoid of FAAH as well as pharmacologic inhibitors of each of these enzymes. As expected, $FAAH^{(-/-)}$ mice have an impaired ability to metabolize anandamide, as well as noncannabinoid fatty acid amides. Consequently, they possess highly elevated endogenous levels of these compounds in the central nervous system (CNS) and periphery (71). $FAAH^{(-/-)}$ mice display phenotypic hypoalgesia in the tail immersion, hot plate, and formalin tests, which are completely normalized by rimonabant (71,76). $FAAH^{(-/-)}$ mice also exhibit decreased inflammatory responses in the formalin (76) and carrageenan paw edema.

Both irreversible (e.g., URB597) and reversible (e.g., OL-135) inhibitors of FAAH produce similar pharmacologic effects as those observed in $FAAH^{(-/-)}$ mice, including increased brain anandamide levels, increased sensitivity to the pharmacologic effects of injected anandamide, and a CB_1-mediated decrease in pain sensitivity in the tail immersion, hot plate, and formalin tests (76,77). Thus FAAH inhibitors such as URB-597 as well as MAGL inhibitors (6) produce antinociception. In addition, the endogenous cannabinoid system appears to be an active component of chronic pain, in that the CB_1 antagonist, SR141716A (rimonabant), has been shown to produce hyperalgesia in rats (64,78) and mice (60).

Other research has demonstrated that pain can lead to functional adaptations within the endocannabinoid system. For example, spinal nerve ligation in the rat has been found to upregulate CB_1 receptors in the thalamus (79) and spinal cord

(65). In an analogous study, anandamide levels in the periaqueductal grey region (PAG) were increased by an injection of formalin into a hind paw (80). Moreover, electrical stimulation of the dorsal PAG led to the release of anandamide in this brain region along with a CB_1 receptor–mediated analgesia (80).

Anandamide is synthesized and released postsynaptically to act in a retrograde manner on presynaptic CB_1 cannabinoid receptors. However, the ultimate fate of anandamide in the synaptic cleft is unclear. There is evidence of a specific transporter that might participate in reuptake of anandamide, a subject surrounded by considerable controversy (81,82). In a recent report, inhibitors of the putative anandamide reuptake transporter did not produce antinociceptive effects when administered alone, but were able to potentiate the effects of exogenously administered anandamide (83). It remains to be established whether these agents will prove to be clinically useful as analgesic agents.

There is increasing evidence that the CB_2 receptor is a critical component of inflammatory pain (84), in addition to having multiple effects on imflammation, autoimmune responses and bone density, all potential players in the etiology of such pain. However, CB_2 receptors were recently identified in brainstem neurons which could be a possible site of action (85). In addition, sciatic nerve section or spinal nerve ligation causes an upregulation of CB_2 receptors in the dorsal horn of the spinal cord (86). It is reasonable to speculate that the analgesic and anti-inflammatory effects of CB_2 selective agonists result from a combination of actions at both neuronal and immune sites. Several CB_2 selective analogues have been developed that are effective in acute pain and inflammatory models at doses that do not produce behavioral effects ascribed to the CB_1 receptor (87).

The use of THC as an adjunct to the opioids for pain control, prevention of opioid tolerance, and dependence, has become an area of increasing interest. Early experiments to evaluate the analgesic effects of the cannabinoids dealt mainly with an examination of the effects of THC, the principal active ingredient in cannabis. Studies in human subjects indicate that, at oral doses of 10 and 20 mg/kg, THC is no more effective than codeine as an analgesic, while producing a significant degree of dysphoric side effects (88). When tested after intravenous administration to human dental patients, THC produced antinociception that was accompanied by dysphoria and anxiety (89). Thus it appears that THC analgesia could be elicited only at doses producing other behavioral side effects. In addition, THC appears to be no more potent than the more commonly used opioid analgesics. Cannabinoids are active as analgesic drugs when administered to laboratory animals by several routes of administration. Early studies by Sofia and colleagues (90) and Moss and Johnson (91) established that oral THC is effective in the rat paw pressure test. Similarly, it has been shown that the synthetic cannabinoid, WINN 55,212-2 alleviates the pain associated with sciatic nerve constriction in rats (92) and capsaicin-induced hyperalgesia in rats (93) and in rhesus monkeys (94).

Considerable evidence for the interactions of the cannabinoids with opioid systems in the modulation of nociception exists (95–97). Anatomic studies have reported a similar distribution of CB_1 cannabinoid and the opioid receptors in the dorsal horn of the spinal cord (54,98) and in several brain structures associated with nociceptive transmission (99). The kappa opioid receptor (KOR) antagonist, nor-binaltorphimine, and dynorphin antisera block THC-induced antinociception, but do not block catalepsy, hypothermia, or hypoactivity (100,101). This is an exciting finding in that it is the first time that the behavioral effects of the cannabinoids have been separated. These findings suggest the possibility of enhancing antinociception by opioid/THC interactions without enhancing other effects of THC. In addition, the discovery of the bidirectional cross-tolerance of THC to KOR agonists in the tail-flick test (100) indicates that cannabinoids release endogenous kappa opioids. THC releases dynorphin A (1–17), as well as leucine enkephalin, in the spinal cord (102,103). The attenuation of the antinociceptive effects of THC by antisense to the KOR (104), by nor-binaltorphimine, and by dynorphin antibodies implicates dynorphins in the spinal mechanism of action of the cannabinoids (105). In addition, as animals are rendered tolerant to THC, dynorphin A release is only elicited by very high doses of THC, suggesting that tolerance to THC involves a decrease in the release of dynorphin A (103). Thus, the acute antinociceptive effects of THC appear to be due at least in part to dynorphin release.

It is unlikely that either THC-induced antinociception or tolerance is totally due to dynorphin release. The events that precede and follow dynorphin release, and which are likely to modulate dynorphin release, have not yet been characterized. Cannabinoid-induced release of dynorphin most likely is a modulator of other downstream systems (possibly decreasing Substance P release or calcitonin gene-related peptide (CGRP) release), which culminate in antinociception on administration of cannabinoids. Cannabinoid receptors colocalize with Substance P receptors in the striatum (106), providing additional evidence for the interactions of the two systems. Recently, it was demonstrated that in CB_1 knockout mice, brain levels of Substance P, dynorphin, and enkephalin are significantly increased. Thus, it is likely that the CB_1 receptor plays a role in the tonic regulation of these peptides (107). In summary, THC-induced release of endogenous KOR-interating peptides plays a role in the production of THC-induced antinociception.

THC and morphine synergize in the production of antinociception in mice (108) and in normal and arthritic rats (109). The release of leucine enkephalin by THC is a critical factor in THC/morphine analgesia enhancement spinally in the rat. Recent work with dynorphin, enkephalin, and mu opioid receptor (MOR) knockout mice suggests that the antinociceptive effects of THC are attenuated (110). Increases in prodynorphin and proenkephalin mRNA (precursors of dynorphins and enkephalins) after exposure to THC have been shown (111). Prevention of the metabolism of dynorphin A (1-17) to dynorphin (1-8) or to leucine enkephalin prevents the enhancement of morphine-induced antinociception by THC (105). The functional coupling of the mu/delta and mu/kappa receptors may lead to enhanced antinociceptive effects of opioids by the cannabinoids. Consistent with that hypothesis, it has been demonstrated that the heterodimerization of mu/delta complexes increases the affinity of morphine for binding to the receptor complex (112). Miaskowski et al. (113) and others further suggest that all three types of opioid receptors may interact to produce antinociceptive synergy (114). Thus, THC-induced release of an endogenous opioid (leucine enkephalin) with interactions at the delta opioid receptor (DOR) likely enhances morphine in a similar manner. For example, transgenic knockout studies show that not only DOR, but also MORs, are required for DOR ligand-mediated antinociception. Others have also suggested that formation of mu/delta heterodimers may explain the enhancement of MOR-mediated analgesia by DOR-specific ligands (115). Recently, it has been shown that cannabinoid and opioid receptors form dimers that alter the affinity of both receptors (116). Thus, the enhancement of morphine antinociception by THC could be occurring not only through the release of endogenous opioids that might interact with proximal receptors, but also through a direct stimulation of receptor coupling or dimerization.

Tolerance does not develop to a low-dose combination of subactive doses of morphine and THC and a low dose of THC will prevent the development of tolerance to morphine (117,118). Thus, an important potential clinical ramification of these studies is the understanding that combination cannabinoid/opioid treatment produces effective antinociception with reduced development of tolerance and, most likely, dependence. In summary, cannabinoids produce antinociception by interfacing with the opioid system in the control of pain. The mechanisms that underlie such an interaction between the two systems are not known but clearly involve the release of endogenous opioids by cannabinoids, particularly dynorphins. The clinical implications of the interplay of the cannabinoid and opioid systems may lead investigators to an increased therapeutic potential for the drugs used in combination. A review addresses several animal models to evaluate the complex cannabinoid/opioid interactions and the neurochemical substrates involved in such interactions (119). Several additional elegant reviews have discussed parallel pathways by which the endocannabinoids and endogenous opioids control pain (12,120). The endogenous cannabinoid system appears to play a role in the suppression of chronic pain. It has been shown that in chronic neuropathic pain, an endocannabinoid analogue retains the ability to modulate nociception whereas opioids lose the ability to reduce nociception (121). Thus, the endocannabinoid system does not appear to require the opioid system for antinociception in a chronic pain state. Similar results using THC and morphine in chronic intractable pain have led to the conclusion that cannabinoid and opioid pathways are independent in such types of pain and further, that the cannabinoid system may be superior to the opioid system in terms of pain relief (120).

Glaucoma Although there is some variability among studies, most reveal that smoking cannabis lowers intraocular pressure to a significant degree. The synthetic cannabinoid, nabilone, is marketed in Europe for the treatment of glaucoma (122). However, evidence is lacking that cannabis is capable of lowering intraocular pressure sufficiently to prevent optic nerve damage. The necessity of smoking cannabis or the systemic administration of synthetic cannabinoids for beneficial effects has tempered enthusiasm for their use in managing glaucoma.

One of the major drawbacks of cannabis is that it has to be smoked at relatively short intervals to depress intraocular pressure. There is one report of a topical preparation of cannabis that is effective for glaucoma and is marketed as Canasol in Jamaica (123). However, there is no evidence that cannabis or THC is more effective than other agents in controlling glaucoma or that it is effective in patients refractory to current therapies. Development of a cannabinoid derivative that is effectively topically could be beneficial in that it would most likely exert its effects through a mechanism distinct from that of current medications.

In summary, multiple lines of evidence suggest that endocannabinoids and cannabinoid receptors, in particular CB_1, play an important role in the regulation of intraocular pressure, although the mechanism underlying such effects is not known. Topically applied endocannabinoids or their modulators and cannabinoid ligands may be of significant benefit in the treatment of glaucoma. A recent review also includes the potential for the endocannabinoid tone to play a role of potential therapeutic use in the treatment of glaucoma (124).

ABSORPTION AND METABOLISM

Preparations The concentration of THC varies among the three most common forms of cannabis: marijuana, hashish, and hash oil. Marijuana is prepared from the dried flowering tops and leaves of the harvested plant. However, potency decreases through the upper leaves, lower leaves, stems, and seeds. THC concentrations in marijuana containing mostly leaves and stems ranges from 0.5% to 5%. On the other hand the "sinsemilla," the flowering tops from unfertilized female plants, may have THC concentrations of 7% to 14%. Hashish, dried cannabis resin and compressed flowers, has a 2% to 8% THC content. Hash oil obtained by extracting THC from hashish (or marijuana) with an organic solvent, is a highly potent substance with between 15% and 50% THC concentration. The "fiber-type" cannabis has low THC content (typically <0.4%) coupled with high cannabidiol content.

Kinetics The most common route of administration is smoking marijuana as a hand-rolled "joint," the size of a cigarette or larger, often with tobacco added to assist burning. A typical joint contains between 0.5 and 1.0 g of cannabis varying in THC content between 5 and 150 mg (i.e., typically between 1% and 15%). The actual amount of THC delivered in the smoke has been estimated at 20% to 70%. Only a small amount of smoked cannabis (e.g., 2 to 3 mg of available THC) is required to produce a brief, pleasurable "high" for the occasional user. A water pipe known as a "bong" is a popular implement for all cannabis preparations because the water cools the hot smoke and loss of the drug through side stream smoke is decreased. Smokers generally inhale and hold their breath, which increases absorption of THC by the lungs in which the blood supply is extensive. Thus, inhalation produces the most rapid onset and intense "high" of the major routes of administration in humans.

Marijuana and hashish may also be taken orally via food products. However, the onset of the psychoactive effects is slow (about an hour) and absorption is irratic. The kinetics of oral absorbtion leads to a slower onset, but also a slower offset of action. The "high" is of lesser intensity but longer in duration. THC is insoluble in water, and so little or no drug is actually present in certain THC extracts, which have been known to be injected intravenously. Human studies have used THC doses of 10, 20, and 25 mg oraly as low, medium, and high doses (125).

The synthetic chemistry of THC and its metabolism has been extensively reviewed (126). THC is metabolized to the active metabolite, 11-OH-THC, which is unlikely to contribute significantly to THC's pharmacologic effects because it is rapidly converted to conjugated 11-*nor*-9-carboxy-THC, which is inactive but serves as the primary urinary marker for detecting cannabis use. THC can be deposited in fatty tissues for long periods after use. However, there is no evidence that THC exerts a deleterious effect when slowly released from fat tissues. The relationship between blood levels of THC and pharmacologic effects is not initially linear with a slight delay between the rapid appearance in plasma of THC and the onset of behavioral effects, which makes the impairment produced by THC difficult to predict based soley on plasma concentrations. However, after THC is distributed completely to all body compartments, the behavioral effects of THC are proportional to the plasma concentrations (127). Lack of correlation of blood concentrations and pharmacologic effects is a confound to the interpretation of impairment after THC use (128). However, complex mathemathic models (129) allow for the estimation of time elapsed since marijuana usage based on THC/metabolite ratios, a topic of importance in criminal cases in which libility is to be assessed due to drug use. Study of human volunteers led to the development and validation of two equations, Model I based on THC concentration (which predicts time since usage best in infrequent users) and Model II based on 11-*nor*-9-carboxy-THC/THC ratio (predicting time since useage in all users, frequent and infrequent, as well as oral administration). Both models were evaluated and found valid for forensic use with 95% confidence intervals of detection.

PHARMACOLOGIC ACTIONS

Psychomotor effects Marijuana modifies object distance and outlines leading to distortion, as are the ability to discriminate shapes and to make rapid critical judgments after smoked cannabis use (130,131). In addition, slowed reaction time and information processing; impaired perceptual-motor coordination and motor performance; impaired short-term memory, attention, signal detection, tracking behavior; and slowed time perception are observed (132). There is an additive effect of marijuana and alcohol on performance tasks such as driving. However, studies of the effects of cannabis on on-road driving performance have found at most minor impairments (133,134). Eye-tracking performance is disrupted by THC smoking in human subjects, but the residual effects of a single marijuana cigarette on eye-tracking performance are minimal 24 hours later (135). The effects of cannabis on psychomotor tasks is generally dose-related (132). The effects are generally larger, more consistent, and of increased persistence in difficult tasks that involve sustained attention (136,137).

Behavioral Effects Cannabis use has been associated with reports of an "amotivational syndrome." However, such a syndrome has little scientific evidence to support its existence in a recent human study (138). Studies have been narrow in scope and small in number (139–141). An increased risk of quitting high school and increased job turnover in young adults has been shown, but such studies fail to account for the initial aspirations and goal orientation of the study participants. Numerous behavioral end points have been examined in recent studies. The use of properly controlled longitudinal studies have been shown to provide the most cogent interpretations of the data on neurocognitive function following cannabis use. In one such study, control values for various behavioral functions were determined before the initiation of marihuana smoking: light (5 joints per week) and heavy (15 joints per week). It was concluded that residual marijuana effects are evident beyond the acute intoxication period in current heavy users but similar deficits are no longer apparent 3 months after cessation of regular use, even among former heavy using young adults (142). A recent review delineates many confounds associated with such studies (143). There are marked patterns of individual variability of substance use (e.g. duration, frequency, dosage, type) and, with the exception of a few studies, most researchers have not been able to definitively isolate the effects of a specific drug because of a history of polysubstance use. It remains to be seen if concurrent use of different substances (e.g., cannabis and alcohol) may potentiate the long-term adverse effects of each drug.

Cognitive Effects Marijuana use is associated with decreased cognition and memory that is subtle in nature via alterations in memory, attention, and integration of complex information. A recent review indicates that cannabis impairs cognitive processes, that cannabis users show persistent deficits in specific cognitive functions beyond the period of acute intoxication and that neurobiologic studies indicate involvement of the endogenous cannabinoid system after repeated exposure to cannabis (144). In humans, all stages of memory including encoding, consolidation, and retrieval are altered (145). Long-term potentiation and long-term depression and the inhibition of neurotransmitter release of gamma-aminobutyric acid, glutamate, acetylcholine, and dopamine release lead to amnestic effects of cannabinoids. Other behaviors altered are time and space perception, and sense of self ("depersonalization") (146). Pope and Todd-Yurgelun (147) found heavy marijuana use (subjects had smoked marijuana a median of 29 days in the last 30 days and who also displayed cannabinoids in their urine) associated with residual effects on memory and learning, thus implicating even short-term heavy use with persistent neuronal changes. The longer that cannabis is used, the more pronounced is the cognitive impairment (144). However, there is no evidence that marijuana use produces cognitive impairments like those found in chronic heavy alcohol drinkers. Studies examining the acute effects of THC in humans using positron emission tomography methods indicate that administration of THC leads to increased activation in frontal and paralimbic regions and the cerebellum consistent with the behavioral effects of the drug. There is only equivocal evidence that chronic cannabis use results in structural brain changes, functional magnetic resonance imaging studies in chronic users indicate neuroadaptations of brain networks responsible for higher cognitive functions that may not be reversible with abstinence (148).

Recent evidence in animals indicates that the endocannabinoid system is a selective and rapid modulator of hippocampal synapse function via effects on neurotransmitter release (149). CB_1 receptors located in the hippocampus are a crucial element of this influence. In general, exogenous administration of cannabinoids inhibits neurotransmitter release in hippocampus. In vivo studies in which memory duration is enhanced in rimonabant-treated mice and CB_1 knockout mice are consistent with the notion that endocannabinoids are tonically active to dampen memory. However, whether endocannabinoids, such as anandamide and 2-AG, tonically modulate the neural pathways that underlie cognition, remains unclear. CB_1 receptor-mediated signaling centrally is involved in the facilitation of behavioral adaptation after the acquisition of aversive memories. The cannabinoid analogue, WINN 55212-2, as well as THC and AEA, block the formation of new synapses in rat hippocampal cells in culture (150). The changes in the plasticity of the hippocampal system may explain the memory deficits observed in THC users and abusers. Several human psychiatric disorders such as generalized anxiety disorders, and posttraumatic stress disorder appear to involve failure to "forget" aversive memories. Thus, modulation of the endocannabinoid system might be a valuable therapeutic target for the treatment of these disorders.

A review by Kalant (151) decribes several case studes of long-term users of marijuana. Compared with matched controls who had used marijuana the heavy users had significantly lower educational achievement, lower income, and a subjective self-assessment of impaired cognitive function, social life, and health. Very similar findings were reported in a study in New Zealand in which a significant correlation between the level of cannabis use during adolescence and young adulthood and the failure to complete school or university programs were correlated. However, such studies are confounded by the social surroundings of the subjects.

Acute cognitive impairments after use of cannabis include loss of concentration and short-term memory and goal-directed activities (152). Other reported effects of THC include disturbances of fine motor control and coordination and problems in visual perception. Complex reaction time, perception, reading, arithmetic performance, recall, and memory were affected in all studies. THC also may have more pronounced effects on cognition if a person is using other drugs simultaneously. It has been shown that the effects of THC on cogitive behavior is decreased profoundly and in a synergistic manner if the human is also using the stimulant MDMA, also known as "ecstasy" (153). Given the polypharmacy that accompanies much THC use, it is possible that other drugs of abuse would have a similar effect in combination with THC.

MECHANISMS OF ACTION

The effects of THC are due to both peripheral and CNS activity. Behavioral effects are characterized at low doses as a mixture of depression and stimulation and, at higher doses, as predominantly CNS depression (154), leading to hyperreflexia. Cannabinoids generally cause a reduction in spontaneous locomotor activity and a decrease in response rates. In addition to hypoactivity, other effects that have been shown in the mouse include hypothermia (155), immobility (catalepsy), and antinociception. These comprise the "tetrad" of tests for cannabinoid activity (156). The mechanisms that underlie the other effects of the cannabinoids as tested in the tetrad have been shown to be sensitive to pertussis toxin (66) and thus probably are mediated by G-protein activation.

Neurobiology: Cannabinoid Receptors Δ^9-THC is the prototypical cannabinoid and major psychoactive component in marijuana. Δ^9-THC is a noncrystalline, waxy-liquid substance at room temperature. The pharmacologic activity of Δ^9-THC is stereoselective, with the (−)-trans isomer having 6 to 100 times more potency than the (+)-trans isomer, depending on the pharmacologic test (157). It was initially thought that because of the lipophilic nature of Δ^9-THC and the central depressant effects, cannabinoids mediated their actions through the disruption of membrane ordering. In vitro studies revealed a distinct relationship between cannabinoid interaction with attenuation of G protein–mediated cAMP production and behavioral effects (158,159). The enantioselectivity of Δ^9-THC reinforced the hypothesis that cannabinoid effects are receptor-mediated (160). Definitive evidence for a specific cannabinoid receptor became apparent when the receptors were cloned (13,14) and had homology with other receptors that interacted with G proteins in the cell membrane. The mRNA distribution of the receptor clone paralleled that of the cannabinoid receptor. Confirmation of the identity of the clone occurred when adenylyl cyclase was inhibited on exposure to THC in cells transfected with the clone. The human cannabinoid receptor was subsequently cloned and found to have almost identical homology to the rat receptor (161). The cannabinoid CB_1 receptor, a saturable binding site for which cannabinoids possess high affinity, has been identified primarily in tissues of central nervous system origin (13). A splice variant of the cannabinoid CB_1 receptor, the cannabinoid CB_{1A} receptor, has also been characterized (162). However, no pharmacologic relevance has been attributed to this splice variant. A cannabinoid antagonist for the CB_1 receptor, SR141716A (rimonabant), has been described (15) and appears to selectively attenuate cannabinoid CB_1 receptor–mediated activity in vivo and in vitro (53,163).

The CB_2 receptor was first identified on splenic macrophages (14). It has been found in both peripheral an central (brain) sites (164,165). A specific antagonist for the CB_2 receptor has also been discovered, SR144528 (16). The physiologic role of the CB_2 receptors in the spleen and at other peripheral sites remains elusive. Even though the CB_1 and CB_2 receptors share only 40% homology, Δ^9-THC has similar binding affinity for both receptor subtypes. The use of CB_1 receptor knockout mice demonstrated that the main pharmacologic responses to Δ^9-THC, as well as the addictive properties of cannabinoids, are almost completely mediated by the CB_1 receptor (166). The cannabinoid CB_1 receptor has been shown to be the major player in the behavioral effects of cannabis and THC across a range of species. A recent review discusses the role of the CB_1 receptor in the maintenance of chronic marijuana smoking in humans, as well as providing an excellent review of human and animal studies of reward, subjective effects, and the development of dependence and withdrawal (167). The CB_1 receptor when activated chronically by THC is required for the development of tolerance and physical dependence to THC. The clinical relevance of such studies to the treatment modalities possible through the use of cannabinoid antagonists to treat dependence on cannabis is an area of considerable research.

Endocannabinoids The behavioral effects of the first endocannabinoid discovered, anandamide (8), are comparable to those of other psychoactive cannabinoids and cross-tolerance with other cannabinoids has been demonstrated (168–171). AEA is one of a family of arachidonic acid derivatives that have cannabinoid effects (2,57). Another major endocannabinoid is 2-AG, discovered by Mechoulam et al. (9) in canine gut. In addition, a variety of endogenous substances known as "entourage proteins" have been shown to be released with and protect the degradation of 2-AG (172). 2-AG levels are higher in the brain than are those of AEA. The nature of such a distinct difference in concentrations is yet to be determined but have been the subject of several recent reviews (29,52).

After the initial discovery of the endocannabinoids, several synthetic pathways for the AEA and 2-AG were proposed. The hydrolysis by phospholipase D of arachidonylethanolamide from a precursor N-acylphosphatidylethanolamine has been conclusively shown (57). It has been shown that AEA and 2-AG are synthesized "on demand" and then released after cell depolarization or the mobilization of intracellular calcium stores. The process requires activation G_q/G_{11} protein–coupled receptors. N-arachidonoylphosphatidylethanolamine is the precursor of anandamide produced by transferring of arachidonic acid to phosphatidylethanolamine, via a mechanism that has not been discovered. The enzyme termed NAPE-selective phospholipase D is enzymatically distinct from other phospholipase D enzymes. Several redundant systems for the synthesis of anandamide have recently been discovered (57). Thus, the PLD system is but one of several mechanism for the generation of this endocannabinnoid.

2-AG has higher selectivity and efficacy for CB_1 and CB_2 receptors than AEA and the regulatory process for 2-AG are different than for AEA. 2-Arachidonate–containing DAG can be generated either from phosphoinositides by a specific phospholipase C or from phosphatidic acid phosphohydrolase (163). DAGs are then converted into 2-AG by selective DAG lipases, $DAGL_a$ (most abundant in adult brain), and $DAGL_b$ (most abundant in the developing brain).

AEA is taken up into cells via a putative AEA transporter which also transports 2-AG into cells (173) and is thought to be the first step in the termination of activity of both endocannabinoids. An AEA transporter inhibitor, AM404, has been synthesized (174), but no transporter protein has been cloned and remains the subject of intense interest. A fatty acid amide hydrolase, FAAH, was found in membrane fractions from brain (175–177) and later cloned (178). FAAH has been shown to degrade intracellular AEA (Fig. 13.1). FAAH also hydrolyses 2-AG, but the reaction proceeds to completion at least four times faster than with AEA (179). An alternative metabolic pathway for AEA, which has been less studied, involves cytochrome P450s and results in epoxides or hydroxylated eicosanoids (180). The function of such prostanoids is not known. A number of FAAH inhibitors have been synthesized and the structure-activity relationships for the endocannabinoid interactions with both the transporter and with FAAH have been reviewed (181). Recent work indicates that the FAAH-induced regulation of AEA may be the key regulator of AEA levels and thus AEA signaling pathways. In FAAH knockout mice, pain sensation is significantly reduced, an effect correlated with increased AEA levels. Thus, FAAH may be the target for increased research and pharmaceutical interventions into the functions of the endocannabinoid system and its tonic control of pain perception (71).

Monoacylglycerol lipase (MAGL) inactivates 2-AG. MAGL has been cloned from human, mouse and rat. A second MAGL has also been discovered (182) It is distributed in the CNS in the same brain regions as CB_1 receptors and, unlike FAAH, is a presynaptic enzyme in agreement with the role of 2-AG as a retrograde signal to be discussed in the next section.

Intracellular Mechanisms of Action It is now well recognized that THC and other cannabinoids produce their psychoactive effects through their binding to CB_1 receptors. Investigations using CB_1 knockout mice have provided evidence that the activation of CB_1 receptors is necessary for the elicitation of antinociception, decreased spontaneous activity,

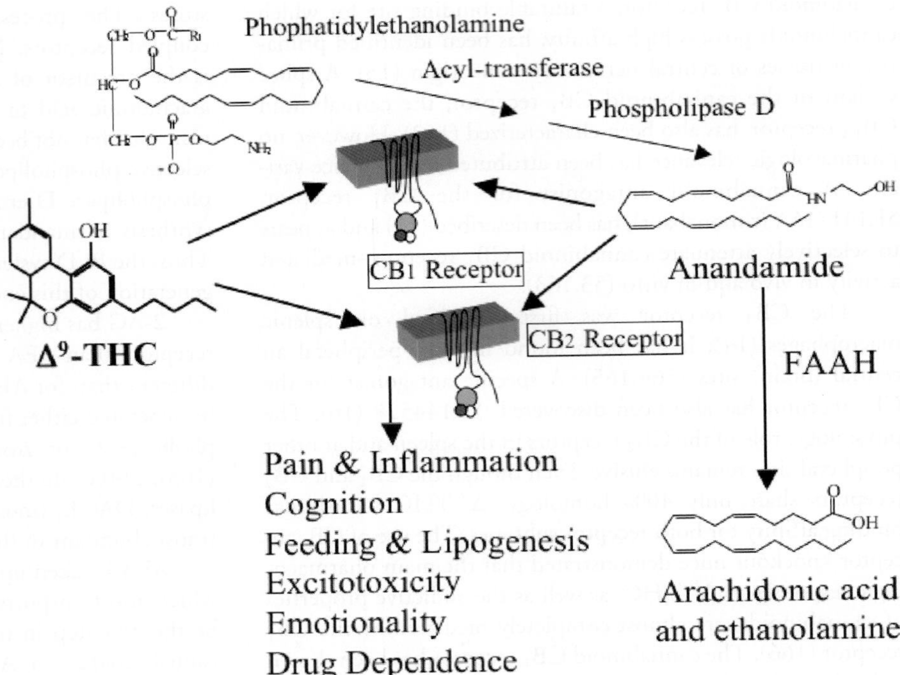

FIGURE 13.1. Endocannabinoid system.

and other psychopharmacologic effects (107,166) There is considerable evidence that indicates that CB_1 receptors are coupled to G proteins, some of which are Gi/Go and others, which are Gs. Activation of the Gi/Go proteins leads to an inhibition of adenylate cyclase, whereas activation of the Gs proteins by psychoactive cannabinoids leads to an activation of adenylate cyclase (183). These results may explain the bidirectional aspects of many of the CNS effects of the cannabinoids but this still remains to be proven. One example of these bidirectional effects is the ability of THC, synthetic cannabinoids and the endocannabinoids to either stimulate or inhibit nitrous oxide formation.

The functional activity of G protein–coupled receptors can be measured directly using receptor-stimulated binding of the hydrolysis-resistant GTP analogue, $[^{35}S]GTP\gamma S$, in membranes and tissue sections (184). These studies have shown cannabinoid receptor-stimulated G proteins in brain regions that contain cannabinoid receptors (184,185). Previous studies using agonist-stimulated $[^{35}S]GTP\gamma S$ binding have demonstrated cannabinoid receptor-activated G proteins in membrane homogenates and sections of brains from mouse (186), rat (187), and guinea pig (188). The receptor specificity of agonist-stimulated $[^{35}S]GTP\gamma S$ binding has been confirmed by demonstrating 1) specific anatomic localization corresponding to appropriate receptor distribution, 2) antagonist reversibility of the response, and 3) concentration-dependent and saturable nature of stimulation (184). In addition, agonist-stimulated $[^{35}S]GTP\gamma S$ binding has allowed the investigation of desensitization of cannabinoid (185,189) receptors after chronic agonist treatment; receptor efficiency (defined as the ratio of activated G protein to receptor B_{max}) (185) and agonist efficacy (maximal stimulation) (185,188).

Protein phosphorylation plays an important role in the development of tolerance and dependence to opioids and cannabinoids. The intracellular modulation of enzymes by both cannabinoids and endocannaboids has recently been reviewed (163). Mitogen-activated protein kinase (MAPK), which is modulated by CB_1 receptor activation, catalyses protein phosphorylation (190), and this effect coupled with the inhibition of cAMP-dependent protein kinase A (PKA), is the basis of a number of cannabinoid actions. MAPK activation by cannabinoids may occur independently from inhibition of PKA or be due at least in part to inhibition of cAMP formation. The stimulation of CB_1 receptors may regulate MAPK activity indirectly through its effects on cAMP accumulation. A decrease in cAMP levels and consequently in PKA activity, may participate in the stimulatory effects of CB_1 receptor activation on the MAP kinase pathway. It also has been proposed that the inhibition of adenylate cyclase and PKA may be involved in the CB_1-induced activation of focal adhesion kinases in hippocampal slices, an effect suggested to lead to modulation by cannabinoids of synaptic plasticity and learning processes. These effects of cannabinoids on multiple families of kinases suggest the importance of alterations in protein phosphorylation in the mechanism of action of cannabinoids. Other systems of cannabinoid receptor signal transduction pathways have been shown (163). There are two signal transduction pathway proposed for the activation of MAPK by the CB_1 receptor. The first involves the activation of PI3K/PKB, which in turn mediates tyrosine phosphorylation and activation of Raf. The second pathway is initiated by sphingomyelin hydrolysis, release of the lipid second messenger ceramide, and the subsequent activation of the Raf MAPK cascade.

Studies show that cannabinoids activate the inositol phospholipid pathway. This pathway involves the receptor activation of a G protein that in turn activates phospholipase C. Phospholipase C cleaves phosphatidylinositol-bisphosphate into inositol-triphosophate and DAG. DAG activates protein kinase C (PKC), and inositol-triphosophate triggers calcium release from intracellular stores (191). It has been shown that cannabinoids increase the activity of brain PKC in vitro (192). Phosphorylating the CB_1 receptor with PKC attenuates N- and P/Q-type calcium currents and the inwardly rectifying potassium currents after cannabinoid receptor activation (193). Therefore, cannabinoid-induced acivation of PKC decreases neuronal excitability and synaptic activity. It has been shown electrophysiologically that cannabinoids inhibit an omega conotoxin sensitive, high voltage–activated N-type calcium channel (29). Cannabinoids also have been reported to enhance the low-voltage A-type potassium channels (194).

The CB_2 receptor also is coupled to the G_i protein and inhibits adenylate cyclase (195). CB_2 receptors also produce the activation of MAPK. The pathway proposed is by activation of PI3K/PKB, which in turn induces translocation of Raf-1 to the membrane and phosphorylation of p42/p44 MAPK (84,163). There is also evidence that the CB_2 receptor induces the expression of genes through a PKC-dependent activation of MAPK. However, evidence exists that the CB_2 receptor is not coupled to phospholipase C or phospholipase D signal transduction pathways, mobilization of intracellular Ca^{2+} stores and does not inhibit voltage-gated Ca currents or activate inwardly rectifying potassium channels (195). There is also intriguing evidence that the CB_2 receptor is inducible in various pain states (84).

The endocannabinoids bind both CB_1 and CB_2 receptors and produce effects on transduction pathways similar to those of the cannabinoids (29,57,163,196). The endocannabinoids have been shown to be released postsynaptically to have "retrograde messenger" activity resulting in the regulation of the synaptic release of neurotransmitters from the presynaptic neuron. CB_1 receptors inhibit presynaptic voltage-gated calcium channels via activation of the postsynaptic cell, either by depolarization or activation of $Gq/_{11}$-linked receptors. The diffusion in a retrograde fashion of the endocannabinoids activates presynaptic the CB_1 receptors inhibiting presynaptic calcium channels leading to decreased neurotransmitter release. Depolarization-induced suppression of inhibition is induced when inhibitory transmission is attenuated. Conversely, depolarization-induced suppression of stimulation is induced when excitatory transmission is inhibited). Additional forms of inhibition of metabotropic glutamate receptors have also been shown as well as a long-term inhibition of neurotransmitter release. The net effect of the endocannabinoid system is to function as a regulator or "rheostatic" mechanism on neuronal excitability.

Olvanil, an endocannabinoid, has been shown to interact with the vanilloid receptor. The vanilloid receptor, TRPV1, is widely distributed in brain and spinal cord, is heat activated and activated by the application of capsaicin, an ingredient in hot chili peppers. TRPV1 activation gates calcium entry to cells, in particular sensory neurons. AEA activation of TRPV1-mediated cardiovascular processes has also been shown (197). Thus, the interactions with TRPV1 appear to be unique to the endocannabinoids versus the exogenous or synthetic cannabinoids, and may indicate a role for endocannabinoids in the modulation of pain and cardiovascular responses independent of CB receptor activation.

Other non-CB1/non-CB2–mediated effects of endocannabinoids have recently been reported such as the presence of AEA-induced antinociception in CB_1 knockout mice (mice devoid of the CB_1 receptor) and the lack of blockade of the effects of AEA and certain other endocannabinoids by SR141716A (189).

Given the wide array of effects produced by cannabinoids, in addition to effects of the drugs that appear CB-independent, it is becoming apparent that another cannabinoid receptor may exist. A recent review of two novel cannabinoid-like receptors GPR55 and GPR119 (198) summarizes numerous non-CB_1/non-CB_2 effects mediated by both orphan G protein–coupled receptors. Given the plethora of effects of the cannabinoids and endocannabinoids, it is unlikely that such effects are mediated by two receptors. The mechanisms associated with these and other novel receptors will provide researchers with multiple preclinical targets for potential clinical therapies.

ADDICTION LIABILITY

In animal studies, marijuana is self-administered and acts via reward neuroanatomy similar to those of other drugs of abuse (199). Although it is difficult to establish self-administration paradigms for THC, rats have been observed to readily self-administer the THC analogue, WINN 55,212-2 (200). In addition, self-administratin in rhesus monkeys followed by withdrawal signs on cessation of the drug indicate that dependence can be produced in the monkeys (201). The self-administration of THC and WINN 55,212-2 can be abolished by the administration of the CB_1 antagonist SR141716A. Thus, as with many other pharmacologic effects of THC (107), the abuse potential appears at this point to be mediated by CB_1 receptor activation.

Interactions with Other Drugs of Abuse Cannabis use typically preceeds involvement with other drugs such as stimulants (202,203). There is no scientific evidence of neurobiologic basis for such a "gateway" effect of cannabis smoking (204,205). Such an effect may be due to the increased opportunity of cannabis users to associate with users of other types of drugs or the group peer pressure to use other drugs (206,207). A combination of THC and alcohol in humans may result in increased levels of THC because of ethanol-induced increases in THC absorption resulting in enhanced subjective effects on mood. It is proposed that the effects of alcohol on THC may enhance the abuse of the drugs in combination. In addition, the chronic administration of THC produces sensitization to the effects of amphetamine and heroin in rats. Interestingly, the rats most profoundly affected by the THC sensitization were those "high responding" rats subject to high intrinsic levels of drug-seeking behavior. Alhough the data are preliminary, they could indicate a propensity of THC to increase drug seeking in those individuals particularly sensitive or vulnerable to addictive behaviors (208). The acute euphoric effects of THC in human studies appear to be due to CB_1 receptor activation and blocked by the CB_1 antagonist, SR141716A (128,209).

Tolerance Tolerance develops to the pharmacologic effects of cannabinoids in a variety of animal species, including pigeons, rodents, dogs, monkeys, and rabbits (210). Tolerance has occurred to antinociception (156), anticonvulsant activity and catalepsy (211), depression of locomotor activity (212), hypothermia (213), hypotension (214), corticosteroid release (215), ataxia in dogs (216), and schedule-controlled behavior (217). In mice, tolerance has been shown to occur to most THC-induced behaviors (218). The precise mechanism of the development of tolerance is unknown. Most of the research efforts to date have been directed toward receptor regulation by evaluation of receptor inactivation or desensitization, or on decreased receptor number (downregulation). In addition, tertiary signalling processes and plasticity of other neurotransmitter/neuromodulatory systems have been evaluated, such as those described previously for the endogenous opioid system. Desensitization can involve a conformation change in the receptor, internalization of the receptor, uncoupling or the receptor from G proteins, or a combination of such processes. The process of downregulation includes loss of receptors from the membrane as evidenced by a decrease in receptor number in binding assays or changes in mRNA and protein levels for such receptors. There is little evidence that chronic administration of cannabinoids alters disposition or metabolism of cannabinoids in the brain or periphery (219), suggesting that tolerance is pharmacodynamic in nature rather than a consequence of reduced bioavailability.

Autoradiographic studies have shown that downregulation of the CB_1 receptor occurs in all CB_1 receptor–containing brain regions. Downregulation occurs more rapidly and with greater magnitude in the hippocampus and cerebellum compared with the basal ganglia. These regional differences in adaptation suggest that CB_1 receptor regulation of signaling proteins can also vary by brain region. The cannabinoid receptor is rapidly internalized after binding of an agonist. The internalization appears to occur through clathrin coated pits and is reversible after short treatment ($<$15 minutes), but not after long treatment ($>$90 minutes). Internalization is not blocked by pretreatment with pertussis toxin or cholera toxin, suggesting activation of G proteins is not required for internalization. This pathway appears similar to that of the beta2-adrenergic receptor (29).

Receptor internalization is highly dependent on kinase-induced phosphorylation. The decreased responsiveness of the β-AR after stimulation with a near saturating concentration of ligand appears to be caused by rapid cyclic AMP-dependent protein kinase (PKA) and G protein–coupled protein kinase (GRK) phosphorylation. GRK phosphorylation in turn promotes b-arrestin binding and receptor internalization (220). There is indirect evidence that a variety of kinases, not just PKA and GRK, could be involved in the development of tolerance to cannabinoids.

In nontolerant animals, acute administration of THC or anandamide decreases cAMP formation by inhibiting adenylyl cyclase. This reduction in cAMP formation also decreases the likelihood that cAMP-dependent protein kinase (PKA) will be activated. The injection of the PKA inhibitor KT-5720 did not affect the antinociceptive potency of THC (221). These results suggest that adenylyl cyclase is not constitutively active in sites mediating antinociception in nontolerant animals. Homologous desensitization to the inhibition of cAMP accumulation occurs during chronic cannabinoid exposure (222). In rats, chronic exposure enhances the adenylyl cyclase pathway, as shown by the significant increase in cAMP levels and PKA activity in the same areas that CB_1 receptor downregulation is observed (i.e., cerebellum, striatum and cortex) (223). Thus, during tolerance, CB_1 receptors lose the ability to inhibit adenylyl cyclase, either through desensitization or switching to G-protein stimulation. Thus, the adenylyl cyclase cascade appears to become constitutively active during tolerance. In support of this, KT-5720 completely reversed THC-induced tolerance (221).

Under conditions of acute cannabinoid exposure, CB_1 and CB_2 receptors are G protein–coupled to $G_{i/o}$ proteins that, when activated by phosphorylation, inhibit the activity of adenylyl cyclase as previously discussed (224). However, on agonist binding, the $\beta\gamma$ subunit disassociates from the a subunit of the G protein (225). The $\beta\gamma$ subunit has been linked to stimulation of other cellular events such as the activation of Src tyrosine kinase, one of numerous types of tyrosine kinases. G protein–coupled receptors interact with tyrosine kinases in intracellular signaling subsequently involving MAPK. Src tyrosine kinase has been shown to activate the factor, Ras, which can activate MAPK. It has been clearly demonstrated that CB_1 receptor activation stimulates MAPK (16,190). The Src tyrosine kinase inhibitor PP1 (226) has been tested in mice (221). In nontolerant mice, PP1 had no effect on the antinociceptive potency of THC. However, PP1 completely reversed THC tolerance (221).

Anandamide and THC increase the activity of brain PKC in vitro (192). Anandamide appears to act by increasing phosphatidylserine-induced PKC activation, as well as acting at the diacylglycerol site on PKC. Because PKC plays a part in activating MAPK, it is possible that PKC activators (phorbol esters) and PKC inhibitors modulate the antinociceptive effects of THC and the endocannabinoids. PKC appears to directly affect CB_1 receptors. Phosphorylation of the CB_1 receptor with PKC suppresses the modulation of calcium channels by cannabinoids (193). However, application of neurotransmitters that stimulate the PI cascade and activate PKC restore the neuronal excitability and synaptic activity inhibited by cannabinoids.

In summary, desensitization has been shown to occur after repeated administration of cannabinoids. The process of desensitization appears to mimic that of the beta-adrenergic receptor, involves several kinase phosphorylation steps, and possibly the constituitive activation of several of the kinases. Downregulation of cannabinoid receptors after tolerance to cannabinoids is an area of research in which several inconsistencies exist. Abood et al. (227) found no alterations in cannabinoid receptor mRNA or protein levels in mouse whole brain homogenates after a chronic injection paradigm sufficient to induce 27-fold tolerance in a behavioral assay. However, the possibility remains that in distinct brain regions receptor mRNA and protein levels are altered, and by measuring whole-brain homogenates these changes would not be apparent. Conversely, Oviedo et al. (219) observed dose-dependent alterations in the cannabinoid receptor number and affinity in rat brain regions using autoradiography and a decrease in mRNA for the CB1 receptor was noted in the caudate. Downregulation of receptors after chronic THC in rat was likewise observed in striatum and nigrostriatal and mesolimbic areas in another study (228). Conversely, tolerance to THC in the vas deferens model did not involve an alteration in the number of cannabinoid receptors (229).

There is a bidirectional cross-tolerance noted between the kappa opioids and THC, which implies a common mechanism of tolerance may underlie both classes of drugs (104). KOR antisense administration blocks the antinociceptive effects of THC. Another mechanism of tolerance that must not be discounted is the role of the G protein subunit, G_{i2T}, which appears to be involved in opioid-induced tolerance. Antisense specific for the G_{i2T} subunit blocks morphine-induced antinociception and to different degrees also blocks the effects of different mu agonists. Therefore, alterations in G proteins, or an uncoupling at the receptor, could account for cannabinoid-induced tolerance via the interaction of the cannabinoids with kappa-opioids (104).

In summary, marijuana use is still considered by many to be a "safe" drug (25). Marijuana has all of the properties consistent with a drug that is reinforcing including a fast onset after inhalation, and rapid entry to brain and spinal cord sites. The long half-life combined with euphoric activity enhance the potential for physical dependence. As previously discussed, the newer forms of cannabis have higher levels of THC that make the drug effects increasingly rewarding. In addition, the majority of the chemical entities present in the cannabis, as well as the pyrolysis (burning) products, have not been evaluated for either psychoactive or toxicologic properties. Thus the effects of prolonged drug use are difficult to predict, although clearly neurochemical changes are observed on tolerance and dependence to THC as discussed.

Dependence Animals develop dependence to the effects of THC on repeated exposure (118,210). Both the DSM-IV-TR and the World Health Organization recognize cannabis dependence (151). Clinical and epidemiologic evidence indicates that a cannabis dependence syndrome occurs in heavy, chronic users of cannabis as exhibited by a lack of control of their cannabis use, and continued use of the drug despite adverse personal consequences (230–232). The risk of lifetime cannabis users becoming dependent on cannabis is approximately 9% (233). However, recent surveys indicate a slight increase in cannabis use. It is not known if this will translate into an increase in the occurrence of dependence (234).

Withdrawal Marijuana abstinence has been observed in human experimental studies (230,235–238) and includes effects that are typically the opposite of those produced by the drug, such as insomnia, anorexia, anxiety, irritability, depression, and tremor. The characteristics of cannabis withdrawal are characteristic of a true drug withdrawal syndrome although the predominant symptoms are behavioral and affective symptoms (238). Human chronic heavy cannabis users develop tolerance to its subjective and cardiovascular effects; users experience withdrawal symptoms on the abrupt cessation of cannabis use (230). The cannabis withdrawal syndrome has been compared to that of tobacco. Based on the withdrawal severity associated with cannabis alone and tobacco alone, the drugs were similar in intensity of withdrawal. However, simultaneous cessation of both substances was more severe than for each substance alone (239). Relapse rates following cannabis withdrawal are higher than for many other drugs of abuse (240). Withdrawal symptoms can serve as a negative reinforcement for further use (241). One study reviewed indicated that 27% of the cannabis users reported the use of cannabis to relieve or avoid withdrawal. The amount of cannabis consumed and the duration of use are critical components of the intensity of the withdrawal syndrome and duration of the withdrawal signs (241). In addition, oral THC administration has been shown in placebo-controlled studies to decrease many of the abstinence-associated unpleasant effects and also decrease the craving for cannabis (242).

In animal studies, a few reports have noted that abrupt cessation of chronic cannabinoid administration produces certain behavioral changes that include increased grooming and motor activity (243), aggression (201), and susceptibility to electroshock-induced convulsions (47). The development of a specific cannabinoid antagonist, rimonabant (15), led to the demonstration that a withdrawal syndrome could be elicited in many species of animals treated chronically with THC (149). Studies in rats and mice chronically injected or infused with THC and then challenged with rimonabant elicited behavioral signs such as head shakes, facial tremors, tongue rolling, biting, wet-dog shakes, eyelid ptosis, facial rubbing, paw treading, retropulsion, immobility, ear twitch, chewing, licking, stretching, and arched back (244,245). Administration of clonidine, an alpha-2 receptor antagonist, decreased withdrawal signs (149). Subsequently, Aceto et al. (246) observed spontaneous withdrawal after abrupt cessation of chronic treatment with the synthetic cannabinoid, WIN WINN 55,212-2. These studies provide convincing evidence that cannabinoids can produce dependence in animals. In additon, several studies have linked withdrawal from cannabinoids with the opioids system. It appears that the opioid/endogenous opioid system may play a modulatory role in the severity of cannabinoid withdrawal signs (247) because cannabinoid withdrawal is lessened in MOR knockout mice (149) and proenkephalin knockout mice (247). Conversely, in CB_1 knockout mice, the withdrawal effects from morphine are reduced (166). However, the relationship between these animal models and the abuse pattern of cannabinoids in humans remains to be understood in terms of the neuronal systems that subserve the cannabis withdrawal syndrome. Manipulation of these systems may provide a means for treating individuals who seek assistance in terminating their marijuana use.

TOXICITY/ADVERSE EFFECTS

Intoxication Marijuana users frequently report euphoria, hunger, and relaxation and less often, panic, anxiety, nausea, and dizziness. In rare instances marijuana can increase paranoia and panic attacks at doses of 20 mg or higher (248). These effects are most often reported by naive users or patients receiving THC therapeutically who are unfamiliar with the drug's effects. Discussions of potential effects can reduce the intensity of such experiences. Experienced users rarely report these effects.

Psychopathology Given the data previously discussed concerning the effects of the cannabinoid antagonist rimonabant in clinical trials that have prevented FDA approval of the drug in the United States, and the clinical studies indicating higher levels of endocannabinoids in the cerebrospinal fluid of patients with schizophrenia (249), there has been increased interest in the role of the cannabinoid receptor and the use of cannabis in mental illness and various psychopathologies. Numerous large prospective, longitudinal studies in humans suggests that the use of cannabis increases the risk for schizophenia, worsens symptoms, and is associated with a poorer prognosis, effects related to the dose of drug smoked and other risk factors (250,251). In addition, the data suggest that those persons with genetic vulnerability to psychoses, or having had previous psychotic episodes, as well as those who initiate cannabis use in early adolescence, are particulary prone to to the development of schizophrenia. It is unclear as to the causal relationship between cannabis use and schizophrenia. Given the number of environmental factors that are likely interacting with genetic factors in the development of the disease state, cannabis appears to at least be a risk factor. The use of cannabis has been shown to produce a nearly threefold increased risk of psychotic illnesses (250). In an extensive review of the extant studies of cannabis use on psychoses, as well as depression, suicidal ideations and other affective disorders, cannabis use increased the risk of psychosis. The correlation between depression and cannabis use is less significant because of a lack of studies and additional confounds such as polydrug use (251). Human studies of suicidal ideations and affective disorders in cannabis users remain unclear as to the risk of cannabis use (251). Some reviews warn that cannabis use may result in "amotivational symptoms" (23), whereas others find no differences in motivation in cannabis users, but do report a significant effect on general health and wellbeing proposed to account for the motivational effects observed (252).

Preclinical studies indicate that the endocannabinoid system is altered in neurological disorders (52,124,173) with a significant amount of change in the synthesis and degradation of the endocannabinoids on chronic administration of THC to rodents. Such changes and the duration of the alterations have been proposed to indicate that chronic THC exposure has the potential to produce neuronal plasticity changes of therapeutic and clinical significance in numerous disease states.

Effects on Major Organ Systems

Respiratory The major adverse health effect associated with marijuana smoking is damage to the respiratory system. Many of the same mutagens and carcinogens in nicotine cigarettes are found in marijuana smoke (253). Marijuana smoking has been shown to increase airway resistance and decrease pulmonary function, produce chronic cough, airway inflammation, and abnormal cell growth that may indicate the onset of cancer (254). However, clinical and epidemiologic evidence linking marijuana smoking to chronic obstructive pulmonary disease or respiratory cancer is equivocal. It has been shown that chronic use of marijuana impairs alveolar macrophages increasing the chance for pulmonary infection. The concurrent use of tobacco by marijuana smokers increases the risk of lung cancers or lung injury (255). Both cross-sectional and longitudinal studies of lung function showed significantly poorer functioning and significantly greater abnormalities in small airways among tobacco smokers (regardless of concomitant cannabis use), whereas marijuana smokers showed poorer large airways functioning than nonmarijuana smokers (regardless of concomitant tobacco use) (256). Many such effects are not reversed on abstinence (257). However, the International Agency for Research on Cancer found the epidemiologic data inconclusive as to the increased risk of cancer from cannabis use versus that of tobacco smokers (258).

Immunologic The existence of the CB_2 receptor that is expressed on cells of the immune system, bone, and in the CNS has led to the hypothesis that the cannabinoid system plays a significant role not only in immune modulation, but also in numerous additional pathologic states (84,164). The effects of CB_2 receptor activation extend beyond the initial effects observed on the macrophage to include effects on most modulatory systems involved in neuropathic pain and autoimmune disorders (165). The role of both agonists and antagonists of the CB_2 receptor is likely to become one of the major new therapeutic "fronts" for drug development, especially because the CB_2 agonists do not appear to have the psychoactive effects associated with the CB_1 receptor. Immunomodulatory effects of THC on macrophage function are abolished in CB_2 knockout mice shown to be devoid of CB_2 receptors (84). In addition, it has been shown that modulation of the cAMP/PKA pathway by the CB_2 receptor is critical for the gene regulation of immune cells possibly via the decreased production of various chemokines such as interleukin-1 (259) leading to immune suppression.

Immune suppression by THC results in protective effects on pancreatic beta cells in an experimental model of autoimmune diabetes (41). However, such work is confounded by other data indicating a potential stimulation of immune responses via lymphocyte activation (260). Thus, cannabinoid use to decrease inflammation (261) could also be accompanied by an increase in viral infections (262,263). Overall, it is apparent that THC will decrease macrophage function (264) and decrease natural killer cell activity. It has also been reported that THC increases HIV-1 host infection in cell lines (265). Thus, the effects of cannabinoid activation or endocannabinoid activation of the immune system are complex, but numerous studies are in agreement that host resistance is impaired by THC administration (266,267). The preclinical and clinical evidence for increased rates of infectious disease after THC administration or cannabis use have been reviewed. The increase in mortality after THC administration to animals is highly dependent upon the infectious agent. Of importance in humans was an observed increase in mortality of HIV-positive cannabis users (268).

Cardiovascular Marijuana increases heart rate and produces orthostatic hypotension, which is blocked by rimonabant (124). However, both CB_1 and CB_2 receptors have been implicated in a number of cardiovascular processes, including vasodilation, cardiac protection, modulation of the baroreceptor reflex in the control of systolic blood pressure, and inhibition of endothelial inflammation and the progress of atherosclerosis making cannabinoid drugs potential targets for therapeutic use in a number of cardiovascular disease states (269). Endocannabinoids may regulate platelet function and possibly lead to thrombogenesis (270), and may also influence haematopoiesis, which can worsen cardiac conditions and increase hypertension. The endogenous cannabinoid system has also been implicated in the mechanism of hypotension associated with hemorrhagic, endotoxic, and cardiogenic shock. A protective role of endocannabinoids in myocardial ischemia has also been documented. Recent studies also indicate the existence of a novel endothelial and cardiac receptor that mediates certain endocannabinoid-induced cardiovascular effects. Furthermore, cannabinoids have been considered as novel antihypertensive agents (124). Direct stimulation of the cardiac pacemaker by marijuana leads to an increase in heart rate, making the drug less safe in cardiac patients (257). In healthy young users, these cardiovascular effects are unlikely to be of clinical significance. Similar studies have indicated that THC and its analogues have profound hypotensive and bradycardic effects in rats which are mediated by the CB_1 receptor (124). The critical therapeutic role of reversing the endocannabinoid effects in such states as endotoxic and haemorrhagic shock may provide alternative therapies for such conditions.

Liver Considerable experimental evidence indicates that cannabinoid receptors play a crucial role in the pathogenesis of a variety of conditions related to liver diseases (271). In mice, activation of CB_1 receptors contributes to alcohol-induced steatosis, an increase in liver fibrous tissue with a reduced rate of viral elimination. Daily cannabis use is a predictor of fibrosis progression via a steatogenic effect. Thus, daily cannabis use in patients with liver disease can have deleterious effects. The predominant effects of cannabis in the liver of healthy human cannabis users is an effect on liver microsomes resulting in cannabis-induced prolongation the action of barbiturates because of inhibition of liver microsomes by THC and cannabidiol (272). Cannabis users metabolize and activate or inactivate drugs more slowly than normal (273). In preclinical studies, hashish induces carcinogen-metabolizing enzymes potentiating the deleterious effects of N-nitrosamines and aromatic hydrocarbons (e.g., benzo(a)pyrene in the liver) (274).

Kidney Renal complications are rare following cannabis use, with only one case of renal infarction documented in a recent review (275). An additional case report of nephropathy associated with marijuana smoking has recently been reported (276).

Endocrine THC has been shown to alter pituitary hormones (277). Virtually no hormonal system remains unaffected by activation of cannabinoid receptors, although the effects are more often observed in preclinical than clinical studies. Effects of cannabinoids include inhibitory effects on pituitary lutenizing hormone, prolactin, and growth hormone and with little effect on the secretion of follicle-stimulating hormone (278). Cannabinoids have been shown to inhibit growth hormone secretion because of stimulation of somatostatin release (277). Recent work indicates that the cannabinoid analogue WINN 55,212-2–induced modulation of pituitary hormones occurs via the CB_1 receptor, particular in the anterior lobe of the pituitary, site of release of growth hormone and prolactin (inhibited by the WINN 55,212-2) in normal and hyperactive pituitary states (279). Cannabinoids also affect thyroid function via a reduction of iodine accumulation and reduction of levels of thyroxine and thyroid-stimulating hormones in animals. However, there are no data regarding the effect of cannabinoids on thyroid function in humans (277). Basal and stress-induced plasma levels of adrenocorticotropin (ACTH) and corticosterone are higher in CB_1-receptor knockout mice versus wild-type controls. Thus the role of the CB_1 receptor activation in stress responses, release of ACTH and production of cortisol has been shown (280). THC-induced increases in ACTH and corticosterone require cannabinoid and opioid receptors (281). It is hypothesized that human neuropsychiatric disorders, including anxiety and posttraumatic stress disorders, involve abnormal responses to stress, an effect likely resulting from altered activation of the ACTH/cortisol pathway. Activation of the CB_1 receptor by endocannabinoids has been shown in rodent models to be involved in responses of the animals to acute, repeated and variable stress, an effect enhanced by prior stress of the animals. Thus, modulation of the hypothalamic-pituitary-adrenal axis via cannabinoids may have therapeutic potential in such disease states (282). In addition, the role of cannabinoid receptors in bone and the subsequent effects on the development of osteoporosis has been reviewed. Mice lacking the CB_1 receptor have lower bone density than their wild-type controls, leading to the hypothesis that cannabinoid agonists may improve bone density (124).

Reproductive Marijuana can disrupt the female reproductive system and induce galactorrhea (283). Animal studies using CB_1 and CB_2 knockout mice indicate that the endocannabinoid system is plays a role in the development and implantation of the embryo by synchronizing the developmental stage of the embryo to the receptive stage for implantation in the uterus. Such studies indicate that far more research is needed to determine the role of the endocannabinoid system in reproduction and potential adverse effects of THC use on pregnancy (284,285). Studies of smoking marijuana during pregnancy are unclear as to effects on the fetus because of "polypharmacy" (use of several drugs in combination) that is often observed with marijuana smokers. However, women who smoke marijuana during pregnancy often have children with low birth weights possibly from a shorter gestation (286). The lipid solubility of THC allows for rapid transit to the fats in breast milk, where it has been shown to accumulate and be passed to the newborn (287). In male animals, chronic administration of high doses of THC disrupts reproductive function in animals, reducing the secretion of testosterone, and sperm production, motility, and viability, but effects in human males are not conclusive (288). Thus, overall, the effects of THC on reproduction and fetal development are areas of research wrought with difficulties from the polypharmacy of most cannabis users and the large number of confounding variables, such as diet and age, which have not been controlled in many studies.

FUTURE RESEARCH DIRECTIONS

Cannabinoids are an ancient class of compounds with a rich history of anecdotal uses for both recreational and therapeutic purposes. It has only been within the recent decade that the mechanisms underlying cannabinoid actions have been ascertained aided by the discovery of receptors, antagonists for those receptors, and new transgenic technology in which the receptors are genetically "removed" from an animal. Despite all the advances into the pharmacology of the cannabinoids, considerable controversies remain as to the potential uses of the cannabinoids for a variety of disease states, as well as the route of administration of the active ingredient, THC, and other cannabinoid compounds.

As was evident from the ancient sources, cannabinoids appear to have a variety of potentially useful therapeutic effects. The problem that will need to be addressed by research is how to develop a cannabinoid agent devoid of undesirable side effects. The hypotheses that the CB_1 and CB_2 receptors may not be the only cannabinoid receptors is supported by several lines of research indicating non-CB_1, non-CB_2 effects of the drugs. If such novel cannabinoid receptors exist, they certainly will become therapeutic targets by which the multiplicity of the cannabinoid effects may be separated. In addition, the increasing knowledge of the endocannabinoid system's role in tonic regulation of analgesia, cognition, food intake, and cardiovascular tone indicate that possible analogues of the endocannabinoids, or modulators of endocannabinoid pathways, may become targets for drug development. The goal of novel therapeutic interventions will clearly be to decrease the potential for tolerance and dependence to the cannabinoid drugs.

In summary, the cannabinoids are a class of drugs with a diverse profile of pharmacologic activities. The endocannabinoids and cannabinoid receptors are highly conserved phylogenically. For the researcher today remains the task of determining the reasons for the preservation of the cannabinoid system through both invertebrate and vertebrate evolution, and the roles such receptors, known and yet to be found, play in diseases, including addictive behaviors.

REFERENCES

1. Harris LS, Dewey WL, Rasdan RK. Cannabis: its chemistry, pharmacology and toxicology. In: WR Martin, ed. *Handbook of experimental pharmacology*. New York: Springer-verlag, 1977:371–429.
2. Mechoulam R, Hanus L. A historical overview of chemical research on cannabinoids. *Chem Phys Lipids* 2000;108:1–13.
3. Mechoulam R, Gaoni Y. A total synthesis of dl-D1-tetrahydrocannabinol, the active constituent of hashish. *J Amer Chem Soc* 1965;87:3273–3275.
4. Cravatt BF, Lichtman AH. The endogenous cannabinoid system and its role in nociceptive behavior. *Jf Neurobiol* 2004;61(1):149–160.
5. De Petrocellis L, Bisogno T, Di MarzoV. Neuromodulatory actions of endocannabinoids in pain and sedation. *Adv Exp Med Biol* 2003;523: 215–225. [Review]
6. Fowler CJ, Tiger G, Ligresti A, et al. Selective inhibition of anandamide cellular uptake versus enzymatic hydrolysis—a difficult issue to handle. *Eur J Pharmacol* 2004;492(1):1–11.
7. Di Marzo V, De Petrocellis L, Bisogno T. The biosynthesis, fate and pharmacological properties of endocannabinoids. *Handbook Exp Pharmacol* 2005;168:147–185.
8. Devane WA, Hanus L, Breuer A, et al. Isolation and structure of a brain constituent that binds to the cannabinoid receptor. *Science* 1992; 258(5090):1946–1949.
9. Mechoulam R, Ben-Shabat S, Hanus L, et al. Identification of an endogenous 2-monoglyceride, present in canine gut, that binds to cannabinoid receptors. *Biochem Pharmacol* 1995;50:83–90.
10. Hanus L, Abu-Lafi S, Fride E, et al. 2-arachidonyl glyceryl ether, an endogenous agonist of the cannabinoid CB1 receptor. *Proc Natl Acad Sci U S A* 2001;98(7):3662–3665.
11. Porter AC, Sauer JM, Knierman MD, et al. Characterization of a novel endocannabinoid, virodhamine, with antagonist activity at the CB1 receptor. *J Pharmacol Exp Ther* 2002;301(3):1020–1024.
12. Walker JM, Huang SM. Endocannabinoids in pain modulation. *Prostagland Leuk Essen Fatty Acids* 2002;66(2–3):235–242.
13. Matsuda LA, Lolait SJ, Brownstein MJ, et al. Structure of a cannabinoid receptor and functional expression of the cloned cDNA. *Nature* 1990;346:561–564.
14. Munro S, Thomas KL, Abu-Shaar M. Molecular characterization of a peripheral receptor for cannabinoids. *Nature* 1993;365:61–65.
15. Rinaldi-Carmona M, Barth F, Heaulme M, et al. SR141716A, a potent and selective antagonist of the cannabinoid receptor. *FEBS Lett* 1994;350:240–244.

16. Rinaldi-Carmona M, Barth F, Millan J, et al. SR 144528, the first potent and selective antagonist of the CB2 cannabinoid receptor. *J Pharmacol Exp Ther* 1998;284:644–650.
17. Abel EL. *A comprehensive guide to the cannabis literature.* Westport, CT: Greenwood Press, 1979.
18. Grinspoon L, Bakalar JB. *Marihuana: the forbidden medicine.* New Haven, CT: Yale University Press, 1993.
19. Mechoulam R, Feigenbaum JJ. Towards cannabinoid drugs. *Progr Med Chem* 1987;24:159–207.
20. O'Shaughnessy WB. On the preparation of Indian hemp or gunjah. *Transcr Med Phys Soc Bombay* 1842;8:421–461.
21. Hollister LE. An approach to the medical marijuana controversy. *Drug Alcohol Depend* 2000;58(1–2):3–7.
22. Russo E. Cannabinoids in pain management. Study was bound to conclude that cannabinoids had limited efficacy. *Br Med J* 2001;323(7323): 1249–1251.
23. U.S. Department of Health and Human Services, Substance Abuse and Mental Health Services Administration, Office of Applied Studies. *National survey on drug use and health 2006.* Research Triangle Park, NC: Research Triangle Institute, and Ann Arbor, MI: Inter-university Consortium for Political and Social Research, 2008.
24. Substance Abuse and Mental Health Services Administration. *Results from the 2004 National Survey on Drug Use and Health: national findings.* Rockville, MD: Office of Applied Studies, NSDUH Series H-28, DHHS Publication No. SMA 05-4062, 2005.
25. Substance Abuse and Mental Health Services Administration, Office of Applied Studies. *Drug Abuse Warning Network, 2005: national estimates of drug-related emergency department visits.* Rockville, MD: DAWN Series D-29, DHHS Publication No. (SMA) 07-4256, 2007.
26. United Nations World Drug Report, *United Nations Office of Drugs and Crime,* 2007:95–121.
27. Mechoulam R, Peters M, Murillo-Rodriguez E, et al. Cannabidiol—recent advances. *Chem Biodivers* 2007;4(8):1678–1692. Review.
28. McCarberg BH, Barkin RL. The future of cannabinoids as analgesic agents: a pharmacologic, pharmacokinetic, and pharmacodynamic overview. *Amer J Ther* 2007;14:475–483.
29. Mackie, K. From active ingredients to the discovery of the targets: the cannabinoid receptors. *Chem Biodivers* 2007;4(8):1693–1706. Review.
30. Abrams DI, Vizoso HP, Shade SB, et al. Vaporization as a smokeless cannabis delivery system: a pilot study. *Clin Pharmacol Ther* 2007; 82(5):572–578.
31. Rog D, Nurmikko T, Young C. Oromucosal delta-9-tetrahydrocannabinol/cannabidiol for neuropathic pain associated with multiple sclerosis: an uncontrolled, open-label, 2-year extension trial. *Clin Ther* 2007;29(9):2068–2079.
32. Jordan K, Schmol HJ, Aapro MS. Comparative activity of antiemetic drugs. *Crit Rev Oncol Hematol* 2007;61:162–175.
33. Slatkin NE. Cannabinoids in the treatment of chemotherapy-induced nausea and vomiting: beyond prevention of acute emesis. *J Support Oncol* 2007;5(5 Suppl 3):1–9.
34. Parker LA, Burton P, Sorge RE, et al. Effect of low doses of delta9-tetrahydrocannabinol and cannabidiol on the extinction of cocaine-induced and amphetamine-induced conditioned place preference learning in rats. *Psychopharmacology (Berlin)* 2004;175(3):360–366.
35. Plasse TF, Gorter RW, Krasnow SH, et al. Recent clinical experience with dronabinol. *Pharmacol Biochem Behav* 1991;40:695–700.
36. Whitfield RM, Bechtel LM, Starich GH. The impact of ethanol and Marinol/marijuana usage on HIV+/AIDS patients undergoing azidothymidine, azidothymidine/dideoxycytidine, or dideoxyinosine therapy. *Alcohol Clin Exp Res* 1997;21(1):122–127.
37. Beal JE, Olson R, Lefkowitz L, et al. Long-term efficacy and safety of dronabinol for acquired immunodeficiency syndrome-associated anorexia. *J Pain Symp Manage* 1997;14(1):7–14.
38. Haney M, Gunderson EW, Rabkin J, et al. Dronabinol and marijuana in HIV-positive marijuana smokers. Caloric intake, mood, and sleep. *J Acq Immune Defic Syndr* 2007;45(5):545–554.
39. Nissen SE, Nicholls SJ, Wolski K, et al.; STRADIVARIUS Investigators. Effect of rimonabant on progression of atherosclerosis in patients with abdominal obesity and coronary artery disease: the STRADIVARIUS randomized controlled trial. *JAMA* 2008;299(13):1547–1560.
40. Sanofi Aventis, Advisory Committee. Zimulti (rimonabant) tablets, 20 mg. *FDA Briefing Document,* NDA 21-888, 2007.
41. Matias I, Gonthier MP, Orlando P, et al. Regulation, function, and dysregulation of endocannabinoids in models of adipose and beta-pancreatic cells and in obesity and hyperglycemia. *J Clin Endocrinol Metab* 2006;91(8):3171–3180.
42. Fride E, Ginzburg Y, Breuer A, et al. Critical role of the endogenous cannabinoid system in mouse pup suckling and growth. *Eur J Pharmacol* 2001;419(2–3):207–214.
43. Fride E, Bregman T, Kirkham TC. Endocannabinoids and food intake: newborn sucking and appetite regulation in adulthood. *Exp Biol Med (Maywood, N.J.)* 2005;230(4):225–234.
44. Horvath TL. The unfolding cannabinoid story on energy homeostatis: central or peripheral site of action? *Int J Obes (Lond)*, 2006;30(Suppl 1): S30–S32.
45. Davis JP, Ramsey HH. Antiepileptic action of marijuana-active substances. *Feder Proc* 1949;8:284–285.
46. Cortesi M, Fusar-Poli P. Potential therapeutical effects of cannabidiol in children with pharmacoresistant epilepsy. *Med Hypoth* 2007;68(4): 920–921.
47. Karler R, Turkanis SA. The cannabinoids as potential antiepileptics. *J Clin Pharmacol* 1981;21(8–9 Suppl):437S–448S.
48. Steiner H, Bonner TI, Zimmer AM, et al. Altered gene expression in striatal projection neurons in CB1 cannabinoid receptor knockout mice. *Proc Natl Acad Sci U S A* 1999;96(10):5786–5790.
49. Alger BE. Endocannabinoids and their implications for epilepsy. *Epilepsy Curr* 2004;4(5):169–173.
50. Wallace MJ, Martin BR, DeLorenzo RJ. Evidence for a physiological role of endocannabinoids in the modulation of seizure threshold and severity. *Eur J Pharmacol* 2002;452(3):295–301.
51. Falenski KW, Blair RE, Sim-Selley LJ, et al. Status epilepticus causes a long-lasting redistribution of hippocampal cannabinoid type 1 receptor expression and function in the rat pilocarpine model of acquired epilepsy. *Neuroscience*,2007;146(3):1232–1244.
52. Bisogno T, Di Marzo V. Short- and long-term plasticity of the endocannabinoid system in neuropsychiatric and neurological disorders. *Pharmacol Res* 2007;56(5):428–442.
53. Pertwee RG. Cannabinoids and multiple sclerosis. *Mol Neurobiol* 2007;36(1):45–59.
54. Hohmann AG. Spinal and peripheral mechanisms of cannabinoid antinociception: behavioral, neurophysiological and neuroanatomical perspectives. *Chem Phys Lipids* 2002;121(1–2):173–190.
55. Goya P, Jagerovic N, Hemandez-Folgado L. Cannabinoids and neuropathic pain. *Mini Revi Med Chem* 2003;3(7):765–772.
56. Hohmann AG, Suplita RL 2nd. Endocannabinoid mechanisms of pain modulation. *AAPS J* 2006;8(4):E693–E708.
57. Di Marzo V, Petrosino S. Endocannabinoids and the regulation of their levels in health and disease. *Curr Opin Lipidol* 2007;18(2):129–140.
58. Sañudo-Peña MC, Tsou K, Walker JM. Motor actions of cannabinoids in the basal ganglia output nuclei. *Life Sci* 1999;65(6–7):703–713.
59. Tsou K, Brown S, Sañudo-Peña MC, et al. Immunohistochemical distribution of cannabinoid CB1 receptors in the rat central nervous system. *Neuroscience* 1998;83(2):393–411.
60. Richardson J, Aanonsen L, Hargreaves KM. SR141716A, a cannabinoid receptor antagonist, produces hyperalgesia in untreated mice. *Eur J Pharmacol* 1997;319:3R–5R.
61. Calignano A, La Rana G, Giuffrida A, et al. Control of pain initiation by endogenous cannabinoids. *Nature* 1998;394(6690):277–281.
62. Yaksh TL. The antinociceptive effects of the intrathecally administered levonantradol and desacetyllevonantradol in the rat. *J Clin Pharmacol* 1981;21:334S–340S.
63. Lichtman AH, Martin BR. Spinal and supraspinal mechanisms of cannabinoid-induced antinociception. *JfPharmacol Exp Ther* 1991;258:517–523.

64. Martin WJ, Loo CM, Basbaum AI. Spinal cannabinoids are antiallodynic in rats with persistent inflammation. *Pain* 1999;82(2):199–205.
65. Lim G, Sung B, Ji, RR, et al. Upregulation of spinal cannabinoid-1 receptors following nerve injury enhances the effects of win 55,212-2 on neuropathic pain behaviors in rats. *Pain* 2003;105(1–2):275–283.
66. Lichtman AH, Meng Y, Martin BR. Inhalation exposure to volatilized opioids produces antinociception in mice. *J Pharmacol Exp Ther* 1996; 279:69–76.
67. Monhemius R, Azam, IJ, Green DL, et al. CB1 receptor mediated analgesia from the nucleus reticularis gigantocellularis pars alpha is activated in an animal model of neuropathic pain. *Brain Res* 2001; 908(1):67–74.
68. Ueda, N. Endocannabinoid hydrolases. *Prostagland Other Lipid Mediat* 2002;68–69:521–534.
69. Okamoto Y, Morishita J, Tsuboi K, et al. Molecular characterization of a phospholipase d generating anandamide and its congeners. *J Biol Chem* 2004;279(7):5298–5305.
70. Bisogno T, Howell F, Williams G, et al. Cloning of the first sn1-dag lipases points to the spatial and temporal regulation of endocannabinoid signaling in the brain. *J Cell Biol* 2003;163(3):463–468.
71. Cravatt BF, Demarest K, Patricelli MP, et al. Supersensitivity to anandamide and enhanced endogenous cannabinoid signaling in mice lacking fatty acid amide hydrolase. *Proc Nat Acad Sci* 2001;98(16): 9371–9376.
72. Dinh TP, Carpenter D, Leslie FM, et al. Brain monoglyceride lipase participating in endocannabinoid inactivation. *Proc Nat Acad Sci U S A* 2002;99(16):10819–10824.
73. Fride E, Mechoulam R. Pharmacological activity of the cannabinoid receptor agonist, anandamide, a brain constituent. *Eur J Pharm* 1993; 231:313–314.
74. Kogan NM, Mechoulam R. The chemistry of endocannabinoids. *J Endocrin Invest* 2006;29:3–14. Review.
75. Willoughby KA, Moore SF, Martin BR, et al. The biodisposition and metabolism of anandamide in mice. *J Pharm Exp Ther* 1997;282: 243–247.
76. Lichtman AH, Leung D, Shelton CC, et al. Reversible inhibitors of fatty acid amide hydrolase that promote analgesia: evidence for an unprecedented combination of potency and selectivity. *J Pharm Exp Ther* 2004a;311(2):441–448.
77. Kathuria S, Gaetani S, Fegley D, et al. Modulation of anxiety through blockade of anandamide hydrolysis. *Nat Med* 2003;9(1):76–81.
78. Strangman NM, Patrick SL, Hohmann AG, et al. Evidence for a role of endogenous cannabinoids in the modulation of acute and tonic pain sensitivity. *Brain Res* 1998;813(2):323–328.
79. Siegling A, Hofmann HA, Denzer D, et al. Cannabinoid CB(1) receptor upregulation in a rat model of chronic neuropathic pain. *Eur J Pharm* 2001;415(1):R5–R7.
80. Walker JM, Hohmann AG, Martin WJ, et al. The neurobiology of cannabinoid analgesia. *Life Sci* 1999;65(6–7):665–673.
81. Fegley D, Kathuria S, Mercier R, et al. (2004). Anandamide transport is independent of fatty-acid amide hydrolase activity and is blocked by the hydrolysis-resistant inhibitor am1172. *Proc Nat Acad Sci U S A* 2004;101(23):8756–8761.
82. Hillard C J, Jarrahian, A. Accumulation of anandamide: evidence for cellular diversity. *Neuropharmacology* 2005;48(8):1072–1078.
83. Ligresti A, Cascio MG, Pryce G, et al. New potent and selective inhibitors of anandamide reuptake with antispastic activity in a mouse model of multiple sclerosis. *Br J Pharmacol* 2006;147(1):83–89.
84. Buckley NE. The peripheral cannabinoid receptor knockout mice: an update. *Br J Pharmacol* 2008;153(2):309–318.
85. Van Sickle MD, Duncan M, Kingsley PJ, et al. Identification and functional characterization of brainstem cannabinoid CB2 receptors. *Science* 2005;310(5746):329–332.
86. Wotherspoon G, Fox A, McIntyre P, et al. Peripheral nerve injury induces cannabinoid receptor 2 protein expression in rat sensory neurons. *Neurosci* 2005;135(1):235–245.
87. Valenzano KJ, Tafesse L, Lee G, et al. Pharmacological and pharmacokinetic characterization of the cannabinoid receptor 2 agonist, gw405833, utilizing rodent models of acute and chronic pain, anxiety, ataxia and catalepsy. *Neuropharmacology* 2005;48(5):658–672.
88. Noyes R Jr,, Brunk SF, Avery DA, et al. The analgesic properties of delta-9-tetrahydrocannabinol and codeine. *Clin Pharmacol Ther* 1975;18:84–89.
89. Raft D, Gregg J, Ghia J, et al. Effects of intravenous tetrahydrocannabinol on experimental and surgical pain. Psychological correlates of the analgesic response. *Clin Pharmacol Ther* 1977;21(1):26–33.
90. Sofia RD, Nalepa SD, Harakal JJ, et al. Anti-edema and analgesic properties of delta-9-tetrahydrocannabinol (THC). *J Pharmacol Exp Ther* 1973;186:646–655.
91. Moss DE, Johnson RL. Tonic analgesic effects of delta9 tetrahydrocannabinol as measured with the formalin test. *Eur J Pharmacol* 1980; 61(3):313–315.
92. Herzberg U, Eliav E, Bennett GJ, et al. The analgesic effects of R(+)-WIN 55,212-2 mesylate, a high affinity cannabinoid agonist, in a rat model of neuropathic pain. *Neurosci Lett* 1997;221:157–160.
93. Li J, Daughters RS, Bullis C, et al. The cannabinoid receptor agonist WIN 55,212–2 mesylate blocks the development of hyperalgesia produced by capsaicin in rats. *Pain* 1999;81(1–2):25–33.
94. Ko MC, Woods JH. Local administration of delta-9-tetrahydrocannabinol attenuates capsaicin-induced thermal nociception in rhesus monkeys: a peripheral cannabinoid action. *Psychopharmacology* 1999; 143:322–326.
95. Cichewicz DL. Synergistic interactions between cannabinoid and opioid analgesics. *Life Sci* 2004;74(11):1317–1324.
96. Manzanares J, Corchero J, Romero J, et al. Pharmacological and biochemical interactions between opioids and cannabinoids. *Trends Pharmacol Sci* 1999;20:287–294.
97. Viganò D, Rubino T, Parolaro D. Molecular and cellular basis of cannabinoid and opioid interactions. *Pharmacol Biochem Behav* 2005;81(2):360–368.
98. Salio C, Fischer J, Franzoni MF, et al. CB1-cannabinoid and mu-opioid receptor co-localization on postsynaptic target in the rat dorsal horn. *Neuroreport* 2001;12(17):3689–3692.
99. Yaksh TL, Al-Rodhan NR, Jensen TS. Sites of action of opiates in production of analgesia. *Progr Brain Res* 1988;77:371–394.
100. Smith PB, Welch SP, Martin BR. Interactions between delta9-tetrahydrocannabinol and kappa opioids in mice. *J Pharmacol Exp Ther* 1994; 268:1382–1387.
101. Pugh GJ, Abood ME, Welch SP. Antisense oligonucleotides to the kappa-1 receptor block the antinociceptive effects of delta-9-THC in the spinal cord. *Brain Res* 1995;689:157–158.
102. Mason DL, Welch SP. A diminution of 9-tetrahydrocannabinol modulation of dynorphin A-(1–17) in conjunction with tolerance development. *Eur J Pharmacol* 1999a;381:105–111.
103. Mason DJ, Welch SP. Cannabinoid modulation of dynorphin A: correlation to cannabinoid-induced antinociception. *Eur J Pharmacol* 1999b;378:237–248.
104. Rowen DW, Embrey JP, Moore CH, et al. Antisense oligodeoxynucleotides to the kappa1 receptor enhance delta9-THC-induced antinociceptive tolerance. *Pharmacol Biochem Behav* 1998;59(2): 399–404.
105. Pugh GJ, Smith PB, Dombrowski DS, et al. The role of endogenous opioids in enhancing the antinociception produced by the combination of delta-9-THC and morphine in the spinal cord. *J Pharmacol Exp Ther* 1996;279:608–616.
106. Mailleux P, Vanderhaeghen JJ. Localization of cannabinoid receptor in the human developing and adult basal ganglia. Higher levels in the striatonigral neurons. *Neurosci Lett* 1992;148(1–2):173–176.
107. Zimmer A, Zimmer AM, Hohmann AG, et al. Increased mortality, hypoactivity, and hypoalgesia in cannabinoid CB1 receptor knockout mice. *Proc Nat Acad Sci* 1999;96(10):5780–5785.
108. Cichewicz DL, McCarthy EA. Antinociceptive synergy between Δ9-tetrahydrocannabinol and opioids after oral administration. *J Pharmacol Exp Ther* 2003;304:1010–1015.

109. Cox ML, Welch SP. The antinociceptive effect of delta9-tetrahydrocannabinol in the arthritic rat. *Eur J Pharmacol* 2004;493(1–3):65–74.
110. Zimmer A, Valjent E, Konig M, et al. Absence of delta-9-tetrahydrocannabinol dysphoric effects in dynorphin-deficient mice. *J Neurosci* 2001;21(23):9499–9505.
111. Corchero J, Avila MA, Fuentes JA, et al. Delta-9-tetrahydrocannabinol increases prodynorphin and proenkephalin gene expression in the spinal cord of the rat. *Life Sci* 1997;61:PL39–PL43.
112. Gomes I, Filipovska J, Jordan BA, et al. Oligomerization of opioid receptors. *Methods* 2002;27(4):358–365.
113. Miaskowski C, Sutters KA, Taiwo YO, et al. Antinociceptive and motor effects of delta/mu and kappa/mu combinations of intrathecal opioid agonists. *Pain* 1992;49(1):137–144.
114. Sutters KA, Miaskowski C, Taiwo YO, Levme, et al. Analgesic synergy and improved motor function produced by combinations of mu-delta- and mu-kappa-opioids. *Brain Res* 1990;530(2):290–294.
115. Traynor JR, Elliott J. Delta-opioid receptor subtypes and cross-talk with mu-receptors. *Trends Pharmacol Sci* 1993;14(3):84–86. Review.
116. Rios C, Gomes I, Devi LA. Opioid and CB1 cannabinoid receptor interactions: reciprocal inhibition of receptor signaling and neuritogenesis. *Br J Pharmacol* 2006;148:387–395.
117. Cichewicz DL, Haller VL, Welch SP. Changes in opioid and cannabinoid receptor protein following short-term combination treatment with delta(9)-tetrahydrocannabinol and morphine. *J Pharmacol Exp Ther* 2001;297(1):121–127.
118. Smith PA, Selley DE, Sim-Selley LJ, et al. Low dose combination of morphine and delta9-tetrahydroncannabinol circumvents antinociceptive tolerance and apparent desensitization of receptors. *Eur Jf Pharmacol* 2007;571(2–3):129–137.
119. Tanda G, Goldberg SR. Cannabinoids: reward, dependence, and underlying neurochemical mechanisms—a review of recent preclinical data. *Psychopharmacology (Berlin)* 2003;169(2):115–134.
120. Mao J, Price DD, Lu J, et al. Two distinctive antinociceptive systems in rats with pathological pain. *Neurosci Lett* 2000;280(1):13–16.
121. Kawasaki Y, Kohno T, Ji RR. Different effects of opioid and cannabinoid receptor agonists on C-fiber-induced extracellular signal-regulated kinase activation in dorsal horn neurons in normal and spinal nerve-ligated rats. *J Pharmacol Exp Ther* 2006;316(2):601–607.
122. Puccio M, Nathanson L.The cancer cachexia syndrome. *Semin Oncol* 1997;24(3):277–287.
123. Noyes R Jr, Baram DA. Cannabis analgesia. *Compr Psychiatry* 1974; 15(6):531–535.
124. Pacher P, Bákai S, Kunos G. The endocannabinoid system as an emerging target of pharmacotherapy. *Pharmacol Rev* 2006;58(3):389–462.
125. Perez-Reyes M, Di Guiseppi S, Davis KH, et al. Comparison of effects of marihuana cigarettes to three different potencies. *Clin Pharmacol Ther* 1982;31(5):617–624.
126. Martin BR, Cone EJ. Chemistry and pharmacology of cannabis. In: Kalant H, Corrigall W, Hall W, eds. *The health effects of cannabis*. Centre for Addiction and Mental Health, Addiction Research Foundation, Toronto, Ontario, Canada 1999:21–68.
127. Cone EJ, Heustis MA, Relating blood concentrations of tetrahydrocannabinol and metabolites to pharmacologic effects and time of marijuana usage. *Ther Drug Monitor* 1993;15:527–532.
128. Huestis MA, Henningfield JE, Cone EJ. Blood cannabinoids. II. Models for the prediction of time of marijuana exposure from plasma concentrations of delta9-tetrahydrocannabinol (THC) and 11-nor-9-carboxy-delta9-tetrahydrocannabinol (THCCOOH). *J Anal Toxicol* 1992;16(5):283–290.
129. Huestis MA, Elsohly M, Nebro W, et al. Estimating time of last oral ingestion of cannabis from plasma THC and THCCOOH concentrations. *Ther Drug Monitor* 2006;28(4):540–544.
130. Isbell H, Gorodetzsky CW, Jasinski DR. Effects of (-) transtetrahydrocannabinol in man. *Psychopharmacologia* 1967;11:184–188.
131. Adams IB, Ryan W, Singer M. Evaluation of the cannabinoid receptor binding and the in vivo activities for the anandamide analog. *J Pharmacol Exp Ther* 1995;273:1172–1182.
132. Chait LD, Pierri J. Effects of smoked marijuana on human performance: a critical review. In L Murphy, A Bartke, eds. *Marijuana/cannabinoids neurobiology and neurophysiology*. Boca Raton, FL: CRC, 1992;387–424.
133. Klonoff H. Marijuana and driving in real-life situations. *Science* 1974; 317–324.
134. Sharma S, Moskowitz H. Effect of marihuana on the visual autokinetic phenomenon. *Perceptual and Motor Skills* 1972;35:891–894.
135. Fant RV, Heishman SJ, Bunker EB, et al. Acute and residual effects of marijuana in humans. *Pharmacol Biochem Behav* 1998;60(4):777–784.
136. Hansteen RW, Miller RD, Lonero L, et al. Effects of cannabis and alcohol on automobile driving and psychomotor tracking. *Ann N Y Acad Sci* 1976;282:240–256.
137. Smiley A, Moskowitz H. Effects of long-term administration of buspirone and diazepam on driver steering control. *Am J Med* 1986; 31:80(3B):22–29.
138. Barnwell SS, Earleywine M, Wilcox R. Cannabis, motivation, and life satisfaction in an internet sample. *Subst Abuse Treat Prev Policy* 2006;1(1):2.
139. Hollister LE. Health aspects of cannabis. *Pharmacol Rev* 1986;38:1–20.
140. Dornbush RL. Marijuana and memory: effects of smoking on storage. *Ann N Y Acad Sci* 1974;36(1):94–100.
141. Negrete JC. Effect of cannabis use on health. *Acta Psiq Psico Am Latina* 1983;29(4):267–276.
142. Fried PA, Watkinson, B, Gray, R. Neurocognitive consequences of marihuana—a comparison with pre-drug performance. *Neurotoxicol Teratol* 2005;27:231–239.
143. Yücel M, Lubman D I, Solowij N, et al. Understanding drug addiction: a neuropsychological perspective. *Aust N Z J Psychiatry* 2007;41: 957–968.
144. Solowij N, Michie PT. Cannabis and cognitive dysfunction: parallels with endophenotypes of schizophrenia? *J Psychiatry Neurosci* 2007;32(1):30–52.
145. Ranganathan M, D'Souza DC. The acute effects of cannabinoids on memory in humans: a review. *Psychopharmacology (Berlin)* 2006;188(4): 425–444.
146. Mathew RJ, Wilson WH, Humphreys D, et al. Depersonalization after marijuana smoking. *Biol Psychiatry* 1993;33:431–441.
147. Pope HG, Todd-Yurgelun D. The residual cognitive effects of heavy marijuana use in college students. *JAMA* 1996;275:521–527.
148. Chang L, Chronicle EP. Functional imaging studies in cannabis users. *Neuroscientist* 2007;13(5):422–432.
149. Lichtman AH, Varvel SA, Martin BR. Endocannabinoids in cognition and dependence. *Prostagland Leukot Essent Fatty Acids* 2002;66(2–3): 269–285.
150. Kim DJ, Thayer SA.Activation of CB1 cannabinoid receptors inhibits neurotransmitter release from identified synaptic sites in rat hippocampal cultures. *Brain Res* 2000;852(2):398–405.
151. Kalant H. Adverse effects of cannabis on health: an update of the literature since 1996. *Prog Neuropsychopharmacol Biol Psychiatry* 2004; 28(5):849–863.
152. Grotenhermen F. The toxicology of cannabis and cannabis prohibition. *Chem Biodivers* 2007;4(8):1744–1769.
153. Croft RJ, Mackay AJ, Mills AT, et al. The relative contributions of ecstasy and cannabis to cognitive impairment. *Psychopharmacology (Berlin)* 2001;153(3):373–379.
154. Dewey WL. Cannabinoid pharmacology. *Pharmacol Rev* 1986;38: 151–175.
155. Compton DR, Rice KC, De Costa BR, et al. Cannabinoid structure-activity relationships: Correlation of receptor bonding and in-vivo activities. *J Pharmacol Exp Ther* 1993;265:218–226.
156. Martin BR. Characterization of the antinociceptive activity of intravenously administered delta-9-tetrahydrocannabinol in mice. In: DJ Harvey, ed. *Marihuana '84, proceedings of the Oxford symposium on cannabis*. Oxford, England: IRL Press, 1985:685–692.
157. Dewey WL, Martin BR, May EL. Cannabinoid stereoisomers: pharmacological effects. In: DF Smith, ed. *CRC handbook of stereoisomers: drugs in psychopharmacology*. Boca Raton, FL: CRC Press, 1984:317–326.

158. Howlett AC, Johnson MR, Melvin LS, et al. Nonclassical cannabinoid analgetics inhibit adenylate cyclase: development of a cannabinoid receptor model. *Mol Pharmacol* 1988;33:297–302.
159. Howlett AC, Evans DM, Houston DB. The cannabinoid receptor. In: L Murphy, A Bartke, eds. *Marijuana/cannabinoids: neurobiology and neurophysiology.* Boca Raton, FL: CRC Press, 1992:35–72.
160. Mechoulam R, Feigenbaum JJ, Lander N, et al. Enantiomeric cannabinoids: stereospecificity of psychotropic activity. *Experientia* 1988;44: 762–764.
161. Gerard CM, Mollerearu C, Vasart G, et al. Molecular cloning of a human cannabinoid receptor which is also expressed in testis. *Biochem J* 1991;279:129–134.
162. Shire D, Carillon C, Kaghad M, et al. An amino-terminal variant of the central cannabinoid receptor resulting from alternative splicing. *J Biol Chem* 1995;270:3726–3731.
163. Gomez-Ruiz M, Hernández M, de Miguel R, et al. An overview on the biochemistry of the cannabinoid system. *Mol Neurobiol* 2007;36:3–14.
164. Onaivi ES, Ishiguro H, Gong JP, et al. Discovery of the presence and functional expression of cannabinoid CB2 receptors in brain. *Ann N Y Acad Sci* 2006;1074:514–536.
165. Guindon J, Hohmann AG. Cannabinoid CB2 receptors: a therapeutic target for the treatment of inflammatory and neuropathic pain. *Br J Pharmacol* 2008;153(2):319–334.
166. Ledent C, Valverde O, Cossu G, et al. Unresponsiveness to cannabinoids and reduced addictive effects of opiates in CB1 receptor knockout mice. *Science* 1999;283:401–404.
167. Cooper ZD, Haney M. Cannabis reinforcement and dependence: role of the cannabinoid CB1 receptor. *Addict Biol* 2008;13(2):188–195.
168. Pertwee RG, Stevenson LA, Griffin G. Cross-tolerance between delta-9-THC and the cannabimimetic agents, CP 55,940, WIN 55,212- 2 and anandamide. *Br J Pharmacol* 1993;110:1483–1490.
169. Welch SP, Dunlow LD, Patrick GS. Characterization of anandamide- and fluoroanandamide-induced antinociception and cross-tolerance to delta-9-THC following intrathecal administration to mice: blockade of delta-9-THC-induced antinociception. *J Pharmacol Exp Ther* 1995; 273:1235–1244.
170. Vogel Z, Barg J, Levy R, et al. Anandamide, a brain endogenous compound, interacts specifically with cannabinoid receptors and inhibits adenylate cyclase. *J Neurochem* 1993;61:352–355.
171. Felder CC, Briley EM, Axelrod J, et al. Anandamide, an endogenous cannabimimetic eicosanoid, binds to the cloned human cannabinoids receptor and stimulates receptor-mediated signal transduction. *Cell Biol* 1993;90:7656–7660.
172. Ben-Shabat S, Fride E, Sheskin T, et al. An entourage effect: inactive endogenous fatty acid glycerol esters enhance 2-arachidonoyl-glycerol cannabinoid activity. *Eur J Pharmacol* 1998;353(1):23–31.
173. Mangieri RA, Piomelli D. Enhancement of endocannabinoid signaling and the pharmacotherapy of depression. *Pharmacol Res* 2007;56(5):360–366.
174. Beltramo M, Stella N, Calignano A, et al. Functional role of high affinity anandamide transport, as revealed by selective inhibition. *Science* 1997;277(5329):1094–1097.
175. Desarnaud F, Cadas H, Piomelli D. Anandamide amidohydrolase activity in rat brain microsomes: Identification and partial characterization. *J Biol Chem* 1995;270:6030–6035.
176. Hillard C J, Wilkison DM, Edgemond WS, et al. Characterization of the kinetics and distribution of N-arachidonylethanolamine (anandamide) hydrolysis by rat brain. *Biochim Biophys Acta* 1995;1257: 249–256.
177. Ueda N, Kurahashi Y, Yamamoto S, et al. Partial purification and characterization of the porcine brain enzyme hydrolyzing and synthesizing anandamide. *J Biol Chem* 1995;270:23823–23827.
178. Cravatt BF, Giang DK, Mayfield SP, et al. Molecular characterization of an enzyme that degrades neuromodulatory fatty-acid amides. *Nature* 1996;384(6604):83–87.
179. Goparaju SK, Ueda N, Yamaguchi H, et al. Anandamide amidohydrolase reacting with 2-arachidonoylglycerol, another cannabinoid receptor ligand. *FEBS Lett* 1998;422(1):69–73.
180. Bornheim LM, Kim KY, Chen B, et al. Microsomal cytochrome P450-mediated liver and brain anandamide metabolism. *Biochem Pharmacol* 1995;50:677–686.
181. Reggio PH, Traore H. Conformational requirements for endocannabinoid interaction with the cannabinoid receptors, the anandamide transporter and fatty acid amidohydrolase. *Chem Phys Lipids* 2000;108(1–2):15–35.
182. Marrs W, Stella N. 2-AG + 2 new players = forecast for therapeutic advances. *Chem Biol* 2007;14(12):1309–1311.
183. Howlett AC. Pharmacology of cannabinoid receptors. *Annu Rev Pharmacol Toxicol* 1995;35:607–634.
184. Sim LJ, Selley DE, Childers SR. In vitro autoradiography of receptor-activated G-proteins in rat brain by agonist-stimulated guanylyl 5'-[gamma-[35S]thio]-triphosphate binding. *Proc Natl Acad Sci* 1995;92: 7242–7246.
185. Sim LJ, Selley DE, Xiao R, et al. Differences in G-protein activation by mu and delta opioid, and cannabinoid, receptors in rat striatum. *Eur J Pharmacol* 1996;307:95–107.
186. Selley DE, Rorrer WK, Breivogel CS, et al. Agonist efficacy and receptor efficiency in heterozygous CB1 knockout mice: Relationship of reduced CB1 receptor density to G-protein activation. *J Neurochem* 2001;77(4):1048–1057.
187. Sim-Selley LJ, Brunk LK, Selley DE. Inhibitory effects of SR141716A on G-protein activation in rat brain. *European Journal of Pharmacology* 2001;414(2–3):135–143.
188. Sim LJ, Childers SR. Anatomical distribution of mu, delta, and kappa opioid- and nocioception/orphanin FQ-stimulated [35S]guanylyl-5'-O-(gamma-thio)-triphosphate binding in guinea pig brain. *J Comp Neurol* 1997;386(4):562–572.
189. Breivogel CS, Griffin G, Di Marzo V, et al. Evidence for a new G protein-coupled cannabinoid receptor in mouse brain. *Molec Pharmacol* 2001;60(1):155–163.
190. Bouaboula M, Poinot-Chzel C, Bourrie B, et al. Activation of mitogen-activated protein kinases by stimulation of the central cannabinoid receptor CB1. *Biochem J* 1995;312:637–641.
191. Chaudry A, Thompson RH, Rubin RP, et al. Relationship between delta-9-tetrahydrocannabinol-induced arachidonic acid release and secretagogue-evoked phosphoinositide breakdown and Ca2+ mobilization of exocrine pancreas. *Mol Pharmacol* 1988;34:543–548.
192. Hillard CJ, Auchampach A. In vitro activation of brain protein kinase C by the cannabinoids. *Biochim Biophys Acta* 1994;1220:163–170.
193. Garcia DE, Brown S, Hille B, et al. (1998). Protein kinase C disrupts cannabinoid actions by phosphorylation of the CB1 cannabinoid receptor. *J Neurosci* 1998;18(8):2834–2841.
194. Deadwyler SA, Hampson RE, Bennett BA, et al. Cannabinoids modulate potassium current in cultured hippocampal neurons. *Receptors Channels* 1993;1:121–134.
195. Felder CC, Joyce KE, Briley EM, et al. Comparison of the pharmacology and signal transduction of the human cannabinoid CB1 and CB2 receptors. *Mol Pharmacol* 1995;48(3):443–450.
196. Lovinger DM. Endocannabinoid liberation from neurons in transsynaptic signaling. *J Mol Neurosci* 2007;33:87–93.
197. Zygmunt PM, Petersson J, Andersson DA, et al. Vanilloid receptors on sensory nerves mediate the vasodilator action of anandamide. *Nature* 1999;400(6743):452–457.
198. Brown AJ. Novel cannabinoid receptors. *Br J Pharmacol* 2007;152: 567–575.
199. Gardner EL, Lowinson JH. Marijuana's interaction with brain reward systems: update 1991. *Pharmacol Biochem Behav* 1991;40:571–580.
200. Fattore L, Cossu G, Martellotta CM, et al. Intravenous self-administration of the cannabinoid CB1 receptor agonist WIN 55,212–2 in rats. *Psychopharmacology (Berlin)* 2001;156(4):410–416.
201. Beardsley PM, Balster RL, Harris LS. Dependence on tetrahydrocannabinol in rhesus monkeys. *J Pharmacol Exp Ther* 1986;239(2): 311–319.
202. Donovan JE, Jessor R. Problem drinking and the dimension of involvement with drugs: a Guttman scalogram analysis of adolescent drug use. *Am J Public Health* 1983;73(5):543–552.

203. Yamaguchi K, Kandel DB. Patterns of drug use from adolescence to young adulthood: II. Sequences of progression. *Am J Public Health* 1984;74(7):668–672.
204. Kandel DB. Does marijuana use cause the use of other drugs? *JAMA* 2003;289(4):482.
205. Kandel DB, Yamaguchi K, Klein LC. Testing the gateway hypothesis. *Addiction* 2006;101(4):470–472.
206. Baumrind D. Specious causal attributions in the social sciences: the reformulated stepping-stone theory of heroin use as exemplar. *J Personal So Psychol* 1983;45(6):1289–1298.
207. Goode E. The criminogenics of marijuana. *Addict Dis* 1974;1(3): 297–322.
208. Lamarque S, Taghzouti K, Simon H. Chronic treatment with delta-9-tetrahydrocannabinol enhances the locomotor response to amphetamine and heroin. Implications for vulnerability to drug addiction. *Neuropharmacology* 2001;41(1):118–129.
209. Huestis MA, Gorelick DA, Heishman SJ, et al. Blockade of effects of smoked marijuana by the CB1-selective cannabinoid receptor antagonist SR141716. *Arch Gen Psychiatry* 2001;58(4):322–328.
210. Martin BR, Sim-Selley LJ, Selley DE. Signaling pathways involved in the development of cannabinoid tolerance. *Trends Pharmacol Sci* 2004;25(6):325–330.
211. Pertwee RG. Tolerance to the effect of delta1-tetrahydrocannabinol on corticosterone levels in mouse plasma produced by repeated administration of cannabis extract or delta1-tetrahydrocannabinol. *Br J Pharmacol* 1974;51(3):391–397.
212. Karler R, Calder LD, Turkanis SA. Changes in CNS sensitivity to cannabinoids with repeated treatment: tolerance and auxoesthesia. *NIDA Res Monogr* 1984;54:312–322.
213. Thompson GR, Fleischman RW, Rosenkrantz H, et al. Oral and intravenous toxicity of delta9-tetrahydrocannabinol in rhesus monkeys. *Toxicol Appl Pharmacol* 1974;27(3):648–665.
214. Birmingham MK. Reduction by 9-tetrahydrocannabinol in the blood pressure of hypertensive rats bearing regenerated adrenal glands. *Br J Pharmacol* 1973;48(1):169–171.
215. Miczek KA, Dixit BN. Behavioral and biochemical effects of chronic delta9-tetrahydrocannabinol in rats. *Psychpharmacology (Berlin)* 1980; 67(2):195–202.
216. Martin BR, Dewey WL, Harris LS, et al. 3H-delta9-tetrahydrocannabinol tissue and subcellular distribution in the central nervous system and tissue distribution in peripheral organs of tolerant and nontolerant dogs. *J Pharmacol Exp Ther* 1976;196(1):128–144.
217. McMillan DE, Harris LS, Frankenheim JM, et al. I-Dgr9-trans-tetrahydrocannabinol in pigeons: tolerance to the behavioral effects. *Science* 1970;196(3944):501–503.
218. Compton DR, Aceto MD, Lowe J, et al. In vivo characterization of a specific cannabinoid receptor antagonist (SR141716a): inhibition of delta9 tetrahydrocannabinol-induced responses and apparent agonist activity. *J Pharmacol Exp Ther* 1996;277(2):586–594.
219. Oviedo A, Glowa J, Herkenham M. Chronic cannabinoid administration alters cannabinoid receptor binding in rat brain: a quantitative autoradiographic study. *Brain Res* 1993;616(1–2):293–302.
220. Seibold A, January BG, Friedman J, et al. Desensitization of beta2- adrenergic receptors with mutations of the proposed G proteincoupled receptor kinase phosphorylation sites. *J Biol Chem* 1998;273(13):7637–7642.
221. Lee MC, Smith FL, Stevens DL, et al. The role of several kinases in mice tolerant to delta9-tetrahydrocannabinol. *J Pharmacol Exp Ther* 2003; 305(2):593–599.
222. Dill JA, Howlett AC. Regulation of adenylate cyclase by chronic exposure to cannabimimetic drugs. *J Pharmacol Exp Ther* 1988;244(3):1157–1163.
223. Rubino T, Vigano D, Massi P, et al. Chronic delta-9-tetrahydrocannabinol treatment increases cAMP levels and cAMP-dependent protein kinase activity in some rat brain regions. *Neuropharmacology* 2000;39(7):1331–1336.
224. Howlett AC, Fleming RM. Cannabinoid inhibition of adenylate cyclase. Pharmacology of the response in neuroblastoma cell membranes. *Mol Pharmacol* 1984;26(3):532–538.
225. Childers SR, Deadwyler SA. Role of cyclic AMP in the actions of cannabinoid receptors. *Biochem Pharmacol* 1996;52(6):819–827.
226. Daub H, Wallasch C, Lankenau A, et al. Signal characteristics of G protein-transactivated EGF receptor. *EMBO J* 1997;16(23): 7032–7044.
227. Abood ME, Sauss C, Fan F, et al. Development of behavioral tolerance to delta9-THC without alteration of cannabinoid receptor binding or mRNA levels in whole brain. *Pharmacol Biochem Behav* 1993;46(3):575–579.
228. Rodriguez de Fonseca F, Gorriti MA, Fernandez-Ruiz JJ, et al. Downregulation of rat brain cannabinoid binding sites after chronic delta9-tetrahydrocannabinol treatment. *Pharmacol Biochem Behav* 1994;47(1): 33–40.
229. Pertwee RG, Griffin G. A preliminary investigation of the mechanisms underlying cannabinoid tolerance in the mouse vas deferens. *Eur J Pharmacol* 1995;272(1):67–72.
230. Budney AJ, Hughes JR, Moore BA, et al. Review of the validity and significance of cannabis withdrawal syndrome. *Am J Psychiatry* 2004; 161(11):1967–1977.
231. Hasin D, Hatzenbuehler ML, Keyes K, et al. Substance use disorders. Diagnostic and Statistical Manual of Mental Disorders, fourth edition (DSM-IV) and International Classification of Disease, tenth edition (ICD-10). *Addiction* 2006;101(Suppl 1):59–75.
232. Budney AJ. Are specific dependence criteria necessary for different substances: how can research on cannabis inform this issue? *Addiction* 2006;101(Suppl. 1):125–133.
233. Anthony JC, Warner LA, Kessler RC. Comparative epidemiology of dependence on tobacco, alcohol, controlled substances, and inhalants: basic findings from the National Comorbidity Study. *Clin Exp Psychopharmacol* 1994;2:244–268.
234. Degenhardt L, Chiu WT, Sampson N, et al. Epidemiological patterns of extra-medical drug use in the United States: evidence from the National Comorbidity Survey Replication, 2001–2003. *Drug Alcohol Depend* 2007;90:210–223.
235. Mendelson JH, Meyer RE, Rossi AM. Behavioral and biological concomitants of chronic marihuana smoking by heavy and casual users. In: *Marijuana: a signal of misunderstanding (technical papers, vol. 1)*. Rockville, MD: National Institute on Drug Abuse, 1972:68–246.
236. Mendelson JH, Mello NK, Lex BW. Marijuana withdrawal syndrome in a woman. *Am J Psychiatry* 1984;141:1289–1290.
237. Jones RT. Drug of abuse: cannabis. *Clin Chem* 1987;33(11 Suppl): 72B–81B.
238. Budney AJ, Hughes JR. The cannabis withdrawal syndrome. *Curr Opin Psychiatry* 2006;19(3):233–238.
239. Vandrey RG, Budney AJ, Hughes JR, et al. A within-subject comparison of withdrawal symptoms during abstinence from cannabis, tobacco, and both substances. *Drug Alcohol Depend* 2008;92:48–54.
240. Copeland J, Swift W, Roffman R, et al. A randomized controlled trial of brief cognitive-behavioral interventions for cannabis use disorder. *J Subst Abuse Treatment* 2001;21(2):55–64; discussion 65–66.
241. Copersino ML, Boyd SJ, Tashkin DP, et al. Cannabis withdrawal among non-treatment-seeking adult cannabis users. *Am J Addict* 2006;15(1):8–14.
242. Haney M, Hart CL, Vosburg SK, et al. Marijuana withdrawal in humans: effects of oral THC or divalproex. *Neuropsychopharmacology* 2004;29(1):158–170.
243. Kaymakcalan S, Ayhan IH, Tulunay FC. Naloxone-induced or postwithdrawal abstinence signs in delta9-tetrahydrocannabinol-tolerant rats. *Psychopharmacology (Berlin)* 1977;55(3):243–249.
244. Tsou K, Patrick SL, Walker JM. Physical withdrawal in rats tolerant to delta9-tetrahydrocannabinol precipitated by a cannabinoid receptor antagonist. *Eur J Pharmacol* 1995;280(3):R13–R15.
245. Aceto MD, Scates SM, Lowe JA, et al. Cannabinoid precipitated withdrawal by the selective cannabinoid receptor antagonist, SR 141716A. *Eur J Pharmacol* 1995;282(1–3):R1–R2.
246. Aceto MD, Scates SM, Martin BB. Spontaneous and precipitated withdrawal with a synthetic cannabinoid, WIN 55212-2. *Eur J Pharmacol* 2001;416(1–2):75–81.

247. Valverde O, Maldonado R, Valjent E, et al. Cannabinoid withdrawal syndrome is reduced in pre-proenkephalin knock-out mice. *J Neurosci* 2000;20(24):9284–9289.
248. Grotenhermen F, Leson G, Berghaus G, et al. Developing limits for driving under cannabis. *Addiction* 2007;102:1910–1917.
249. Leweke FM, Giuffrida A, Wurster U, et al. Elevated endogenous cannabinoids in schizophrenia. *Neuroreport* 1999;10:1665–1669.
250. Semple DM, McIntosh AM, Lawrie SM. Cannabis as a risk factor for psychosis: systematic review. *J Psychopharmacol* 2005;19(2):187–194.
251. Moore TH, Zammit S, Lingford-Hughes A, et al. Cannabis use and risk of psychotic or affective mental health outcomes: a systematic review. *Lancet* 2007;370(9584):319–328.
252. Barnwell SS, Earleywine M, Wilcox R. Cannabis, motivation, and life satisfaction in an internet sample. *Subst Abuse Treat Preven Pol* 2006; 1(1):2.
253. Sherman MP, Aberland EE, Wong VZ, et al. Effects of smoking marijuana, tobacco or cocaine alone or in combination on DNA damage in human alveolar macrophages. *Life Sci* 1997;56:2301–2307.
254. Tashkin DP. Smoked marijuana as a cause of lung injury. *Monaldi Arch Chest Dis* 2005;63(2):93–100.
255. Gil E, Kelp E, Webber M, et al. Acute and chronic effects of marijuana smoking on pulmonary alveolar permeability. *Life Sci* 1995;56:2193–2199.
256. Tashkin DP. Pulmonary complications of smoked substance abuse. *West J Med* 1990;152(5):525–530.
257. Tashkin DP, Shapiro BJ, Lee EY, et al. Subacute effects of heavy marijuana smoking pulmonary function in healthy young mates. *N Engl J Med* 1976;294:125–129.
258. Hashibe M, Straif K, Tashkin DP, et al. Epidemiologic review of marijuana use and cancer risk. *Alcohol* 2005;35(3):265–275.
259. Condie R, Herring A, Koh WS, et al. Cannabinoid inhibition of adenylate cyclase-mediated signal transduction and interleukin 2 (IL-2) expression in the murine T-cell line, EL4.IL-2. *J Biol Chem* 1996; 271(22):13175–13183.
260. Kaminski NE, Koh WS, Yang KH, et al. Suppression of the humoral immune response by cannabinoids is partially mediated through inhibition of adenylate cyclase by a pertussis toxin-sensitive G-protein coupled mechanism. *Biochem Pharmacol* 1994;48(10):1899–1908.
261. Mechoulam R. The pharmacohistory of Cannabis sativa. In: R Mechoulam, ed. *Cannabinoids as therapeutic agents.* Boca Raton, FL: CRC Press, 1986:1–9.
262. Klein TW, Newton C, Friedman H. Cannabinoid receptors and the cytokine network. *Adv Exp Med Biol* 1998;437:215–222.
263. Klein TW, Newton C, Friedman H. Cannabinoid receptors and immunity. *Immunol Today* 1998;19(8):373–381.
264. McCoy KL, Matveyeva M, Carlisle SJ, et al. Cannabinoid inhibition of the processing of intact lysozyme by macrophages: evidence for CB2 receptor participation. *J Pharmacol Exp Ther* 1999;289(3):1620–1625.
265. Noe SN, Newton C, Widen R, et al. Modulation of CB1 mRNA upon activation of murine splenocytes. *Adv Exp Med Biol* 2001;493:215–221.
266. Klein TW, Newton C, Larsen K, et al. The cannabinoid system and immune modulation. *J Leuk Biol* 2003;74(4):486–496.
267. Massi P, Vaccani A, Parolaro D. Cannabinoids, immune system and cytokine network. *Curr Pharma Design* 2006;12(24):3135–3146.
268. Friedman H, Newton C, Klein TW. Microbial infections, immunomodulation, and drugs of abuse. *Clin Microbiol Rev* 2003;16(2):209–219.
269. Ashton JC, Smith PF. Cannabinoids and cardiovascular disease: the outlook for clinical treatments. *Curr Vasc Pharmacol* 2007;5(3):175–185.
270. Randall MD. Endocannabinoids and the haematological system. *Br J Pharmacol* 2007;152(5):557–558.
271. Hézode C, Zafrani ES, Roudot-Thoraval F, et al. Daily cannabis use: a novel risk factor of steatosis severity in patients with chronic hepatitis C. *Gastroenterology* 2008;134(2):432–439.
272. Paton WDM, Pertwee RG. Effect of cannabis and certain of its constituents on pentobarbitone sleeping time and phenazone metabolism. *Br J Pharmacol* 1972;44:250–261.
273. Paton WD. Cannabis and its problems. *Proc Roy Soc Med* 1973;66(7): 718–721.
274. Sheweita SA. Narcotic drugs change the expression of cytochrome P450 2E1 and 2C6 and other activities of carcinogen-metabolizing enzymes in the liver of male mice. *Toxicology* 2003;191(2–3):133–142.
275. Crowe AV, Howse M, Bell GM, et al. Substance abuse and the kidney. *QJM Int J Med* 2000;93(3):147–152.
276. Bohatyrewicz M, Urasinska E, Rozanski J, et al. Membranous glomerulonephritis may be associated with heavy marijuana abuse. *Transpl Proc* 2007;39(10):3054–3056.
277. Brown TT, Dobs AS. Endocrine effects of marijuana. *J Clin Pharmacol* 2002;42(11 Suppl):90S–96S.
278. Wenger T, Toth BE, Martin BR. Effects of anandamide (endogenous cannabinoid) on the anterior pituitary hormone secretion in adult ovariectomized rats. *Life Sci* 1995;56:2057–2063.
279. Pagotto U, Marsicano G, Fezza F, et al. Normal human pituitary gland and pituitary adenomas express cannabinoid receptor type 1 and synthesize endogenous cannabinoids: first evidence for a direct role of cannabinoids on hormone modulation at the human pituitary level. *J Clin Endocrinol Metab* 2001;86(6):2687–2696.
280. Barna I, Zelena D, Arszovszki AC, et al. The role of endogenous cannabinoids in the hypothalamo-pituitary-adrenal axis regulation: in vivo and in vitro studies in CB1 receptor knockout mice. *Life Sci* 2004;75(24):2959–2970.
281. Manzanares J, Corchero J, Fuentes JA. Opioid and cannabinoid receptor-mediated regulation of the increase in adrenocorticotropin hormone and corticosterone plasma concentrations induced by central administration of delta(9)-tetrahydrocannabinol in rats. *Brain Res* 1999; 839(1):173–179.
282. Carrier EJ, Patel S, Hillard CJ. Endocannabinoids in neuroimmunology and stress. *Curr Drug Targets CNS Neurolog Disord* 2005;6:657–665.
283. Cohen S. Marijuana and reproductive functions. *Drug Abuse Alcohol News* 1985;13:1.
284. Paria BC, Song H, Dey SK. Implantation: molecular basis of embryouterine dialogue. *Int J Dev Biol* 2001;45(3 Spec No):597–605.
285. Fride E. The endocannabinoid-CB receptor system: Importance for development and in pediatric disease. *Neuro Endocrinol Lett* 2004; 25(1–2):24–30.
286. Tennes K. Effect of marijuana on pregnancy and fetal development in the human. In: MC Braude, JP Ludford, eds. *Marijuana effects on the endocrine and reproductive systems (NIDA research monograph 44).* Rockville, MD: National Institute on Drug Abuse, 1984:115–123.
287. Fehr KO, Kalant H. Addiction Research Foundation/World Health Organization Meeting on Adverse Health and Behavioral Consequences of Cannabis Use. Toronto, Ontario. *Addict Res* 1983:257–354.
288. Mendelson JH, Mello NK. Effects of marijuana on neuroendocrine hormones in human males and females. In: *Effect of marijuana on pregnancy and fetal development in the human (NIDA research monograph 44).* Rockville, MD: National Institute on Drug Abuse, 1984:97–114.

CHAPTER 14

Richard A. Glennon, PhD

The Pharmacology of Classical Hallucinogens and Related Designer Drugs

Hallucinogens are agents that, typically on ingestion of a single dose, consistently produce alterations in thought, mood, and perception; produce minimal autonomic side effects and craving; and fail to produce excessive stupor or central stimulation (1). This broad classification encompasses agents with varied chemical structures that can elicit varied pharmacologic effects. The *classical hallucinogens*, a subclass of the larger family of hallucinogens, are divided into indolealkylamine and phenylalkylamine hallucinogens (2).

Classical hallucinogens represent the single largest category of abusable drugs (3). Because these agents act as agonists at serotonin receptors, they sometimes are referred to as *serotonergic hallucinogens*. Structural modification of these agents can result in so-called "designer drugs" that retain hallucinogenic properties, display diminished hallucinogenic character, or display a novel action with or without hallucinogenic character.

HISTORICAL

Evidence suggests use of mescaline-containing plants >5,000 years ago (4), and mescaline was probably the first (classical) hallucinogen to be studied in depth because of its early identification and synthesis at the beginning of the 20th century (5). It was not until the 1940s that LSD (lysergic acid diethylamide) was accidentally discovered by Albert Hofmann, and its incredible potency realized. Interestingly, these two agents represent extremes in potency with LSD being >1,000 times more potent than mescaline. Initial excitement during the 1950s centered on the possibility that LSD-induced effects might represent a model psychosis and lead to a better understanding of schizophrenia (6). Because of structural similarities between LSD and the tryptamine neurotransmitter serotonin (5-hydroxytryptamine; 5-HT), first synthesized in the early 1950s, as well at the ability of LSD to either antagonize or mimic certain actions of 5-HT, interest in examining related 5-HT-like substances was heightened. Certain hallucinogenic tryptamines and "cyclic tryptamines" or beta-carbolines were isolated from Central and South American plant sources (7). During the late 1950s and into the 1960s, animal and human studies were conducted with these agents. It was also during this period that new structural analogues were synthesized and pharmacologic investigations performed. Certain ring-substituted analogues of the phenylisopropylamine central stimulant amphetamine were found to lack stimulant character but, rather, behaved as hallucinogens. Popular interest in exploring these "mind-altering" substances or psychedelics for religious, artistic, and recreational purposes rose during the 1960s. Subsequently, clinical studies with hallucinogens became unpopular, and the Controlled Substances Act (1970) placed restrictions and prohibitions on human investigations with such substances. For approximately 40 years, few new human studies were sanctioned whereas, at the same time, the list of agents was growing exponentially. Throughout this period, attempts were made to develop animal models of hallucinogen action, but none was found reliable (8); this is likely because the agents termed *hallucinogens* or *psychotomimetics*, as defined by Hollister (1) represented a pharmacologically diverse and heterogeneous group of substances. Later, using drug discrimination techniques with animals, it was possible to better define and classify these agents as belonging to different categories (8). One of the categories of hallucinogens was defined the classical hallucinogens (2) as represented by LSD, mescaline, 1-(2,5-dimethoxy-4-methylphenyl)-2-aminopropane (DOM), and other agents described in this chapter. Drug discrimination studies were also employed to investigate the mechanisms of actions of these agents. In the mid 1990s, human evaluation of hallucinogens was allowed once again and the first agents examined were the tryptamine hallucinogens N,N-dimethyltryptamine (DMT) and psilocybin (9,10). Other studies have been reported more recently (see the following section) and additional studies are ongoing (11).

By the late 1970s, it had been shown, for those phenylisopropylamine hallucinogens examined in animal or human subjects, that their R(−)-isomers were more effective/potent than their S(+)-enantiomers; however, for the N-methyl analogue of 1-(3,4-methylenedioxyphenyl)-2-aminopropane (MDA), MDMA, the S(+)-isomer was more potent/effective than its R(−)-isomer (12). This seeming exception led to additional studies with MDMA and related agents. MDMA was found to lack hallucinogenic action and behaved more like a central stimulant than a hallucinogen. But, it also displayed empathogenic character (i.e., increased empathy and sociability, as well as enhanced feelings of well-being). MDMA was legally available for a number of years leading to a rise in its popularity. MDMA, despite now being a controlled substance, is one of today's most popular recreational drugs. MDMA came along at a time when human studies were not sanctioned; hence, nearly all the early literature on MDMA derives from animal studies. Mechanism of action was investigated and additional analogues were synthesized and examined. Today, human investigation with MDMA has resumed.

The agents in this chapter are all structurally related. However, it should be appreciated that subtle structural modification of these molecules can result in dramatic alterations in potency or action. Now that human evaluations are once again being conducted, it is anticipated that the gap between the extensive amount of currently available animal data and the paucity of human studies will be bridged.

DRUGS IN THE CLASS

Classical hallucinogens are agents that possess an arylalkylamine skeleton of the indolealkylamine or phenylalkylamine type, although not all arylalkylamines are hallucinogenic. Most of these agents have not been thoroughly investigated in humans, but many have seen at least some human evaluation (13–15). Agents from this class do not necessarily produce identical effects. However, all have been shown to bind at 5-HT_2 serotonin receptors and, where they have been investigated, all (except certain beta-carboline derivatives) have been demonstrated to behave as 5-HT_2 receptor agonists or partial agonists. Nearly all examples of classical hallucinogens described herein have been examined in tests of stimulus generalization using animals trained to discriminate DOM from vehicle. And a significant correlation exists between stimulus generalization potency and human hallucinogenic potency (for those agents where human data are available) (2). Classical hallucinogens, the indolealkylamines and the phenylalkylamines, are collectively referred to as arylalkylamines (Fig. 14.1). The indolealkylamines are further divided into tryptamines (amine-substituted or N-alkyltryptamines and alpha-alkyltryptamines), ergolines (or lysergamides), and, possibly, beta-carbolines. The phenylalkylamines consist of phenylethylamines and phenylisopropylamines. Common drugs in the arylalkylamine class include LSD, mescaline (a constituent of the peyote cactus), DOM, psilocybin (the active ingredient in various mushroom species), and harmaline (a hallucinogen used primarily in some South American countries, but with increasing popularity in the United States); but, many others are known. Certain, so-called designer drugs or controlled substance analogues, are structurally related to these agents and one in particular, MDMA, is related to 1-(3,4-methylenedioxyphenyl)-2-aminopropane (MDA).

Idolealkylamines

N-Alkyltryptamines (such as DMT, Psilocin, Psilocybin, and constituents of "shrooms") One of the best investigated classical hallucinogens is DMT (Table 14.1) (Fig. 14.1), which is considered the prototype of this subclass of agents (1,16). DMT is a naturally occurring substance, but is readily synthesized in the laboratory. Its actions are characterized by a rapid onset (typically <5 minutes) and short duration of action (about 30 minutes) depending on route of administration. DMT-like agents possess a characteristically unpleasant odor, particularly when free-based or smoked. DMT, like some other members of this family, is not orally active, but generally is administered by inhalation, by smoking, and—less frequently—by injection (16). It should be noted that DMT might be orally active when given as an admixture such as in *ayahuasca* (see the following section)—a decoction recently approved for religious use in the United States (17). The corresponding secondary amine (N-monomethyltryptamine) and primary amine (tryptamine) are not known to be hallucinogenic, most likely because they lack sufficient lipophilicity to readily penetrate the blood–brain barrier, and because what little gets into the brain is quickly metabolized by monoamine oxidase. Other tertiary amine DMT-related agents, such as N-ethyl-N-methyltryptamine, N,N-diethyltryptamine, N,N-di-*n*-propyltryptamine, and some secondary amines, also are hallucinogenic in humans (15). If the N-alkyl or N,N-dialkyl substituents are sufficiently bulky and lipophilic, these tryptamines can be orally active (Table 14.1).

Relatively few aryl-substituted tryptamine analogues have been systematically examined, but substitution in the benzenoid ring can enhance or diminish potency depending on the specific nature and location of the substituents. Some of the more frequently encountered derivatives of DMT, their common names, and their approximate human potency are shown in Table 14.1. N,N-Dimethylserotonin (bufotenine, 5-OH DMT) might be a weak hallucinogen, but the results of human studies are controversial. Because of its polar hydroxyl group, bufotenine does not readily penetrate the blood–brain barrier but produces considerable peripheral effects (facial

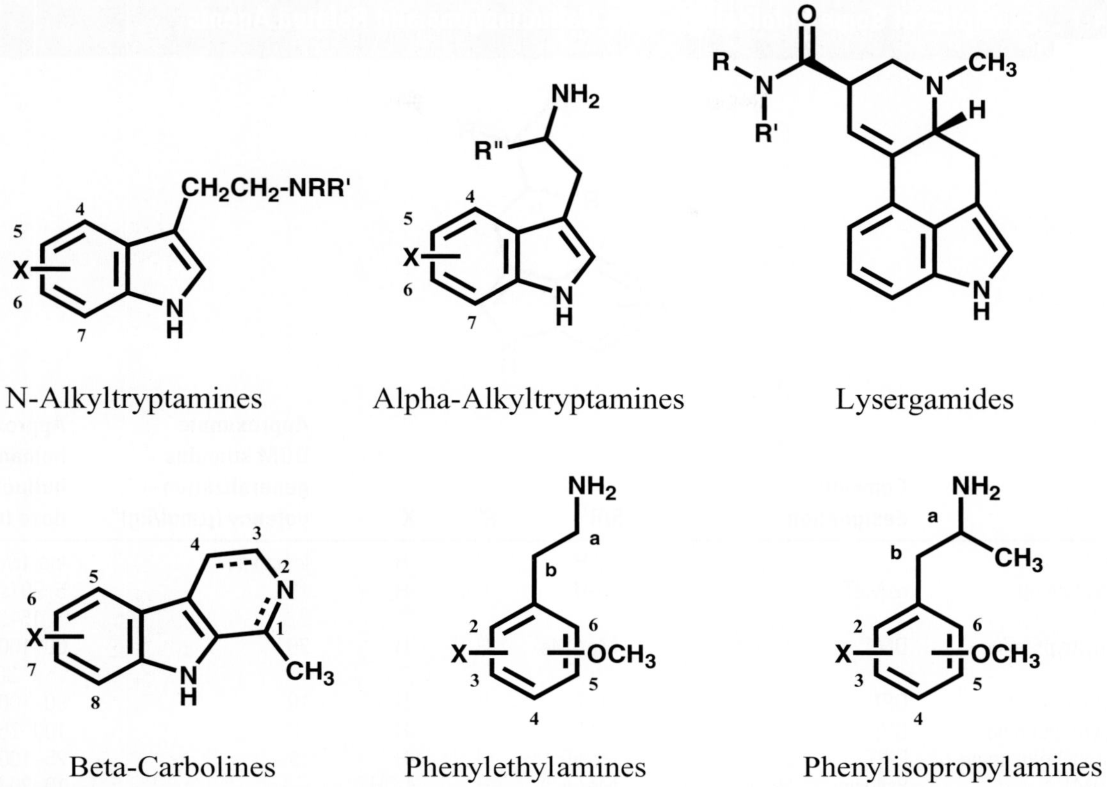

N-Alkyltryptamines Alpha-Alkyltryptamines Lysergamides

Beta-Carbolines Phenylethylamines Phenylisopropylamines

FIGURE 14.1. General structures of classical arylalkylamine hallucinogens. The structural subcategories include indolealkylamine hallucinogens such as the N-alkyltryptamines, alpha-alkyltryptamines, lysergamides, and (perhaps) the beta-carbolines, and the phenylalkylamine hallucinogens including phenylethylamines and phenylisopropylamines.

flushing, cardiovascular actions) that have prevented evaluation of an extended dose range in humans. O-Methylation of bufotenine decreases its polarity and results in 5-OMe DMT. 5-OMe DMT, a naturally occurring substance found as a constituent of a number of plants and grasses, is one of the more potent N-alkylated tryptamines. Bufotenine and 5-OMe DMT are found in the skin of certain frogs and might be responsible for the anecdotal phenomenon known as "toad licking." Psilocin is 4-hydroxy DMT; with a polar hydroxyl group like bufotenine, psilocin might not have been expected to enter the brain. Yet, psilocin is hallucinogenic. Although there is no documented support for the concept, it is speculated that the 4-hydroxyl group forms a hydrogen bond with the terminal amine to reduce polarity just enough so that psilocin penetrates the blood–brain barrier. Psilocin and its phosphate ester, psilocybin, are widely found in certain species of mushrooms and have given rise to the terms *shrooms* and *shrooming*. There are no reports that 6-methoxy DMT or 7-methoxy DMT is hallucinogenic. Of late, use of 5-methoxy-N,N-diisopropyltryptamine ("Foxy Methoxy") has seen an increase in popularity. It is quite difficult to make strict human potency comparisons within this series because of the varied routes of administration employed (Table 14.1). In drug discrimination studies using DOM-trained animals (Table 14.1), generalization potency follows the order of 5-OMe DMT > 4-OMe DMT > DMT; 6- and 7-OMe DMT failed to substitute for DOM (2).

Alpha-Alkyltryptamines Hallucinogenic alpha-alkyltryptamines typically possess an alpha-methyl group (R″ = Me; Fig. 14.1) and *X* is either a hydrogen atom or a methoxy group at the four- or five-position (2). Two optical isomers are possible for alpha-alkyltryptamines. Tryptamine is not hallucinogenic, but introduction of an alpha-methyl group seems to enhance lipophilicity and protect against metabolic degradation with the result being that alpha-methyltryptamine (Table 14.1) is at least twice as potent as DMT, and is orally active (18). In general, alpha-methyltryptamines, where they have been investigated, are somewhat more potent than their corresponding DMT counterparts. Otherwise, their structure-activity relationships (SARs) are similar to those of DMT analogues. For example, in animal studies, racemic 5-methoxy-alpha-methyltryptamine (5-OMe αMeT) is about twice as potent as 5-OMe DMT (Table 14.1). Where they have been investigated, the *S*(+)-isomers of alpha-methyltryptamines are more potent than their *R*(−)-enantiomers (2). Homologation of the alpha-methyl group to an alpha-ethyl group affords alpha-ethyltryptamines; these will be discussed in the section on designer drugs.

TABLE 14.1 Examples of Some Indolealkylamine Hallucinogens and Related Agents

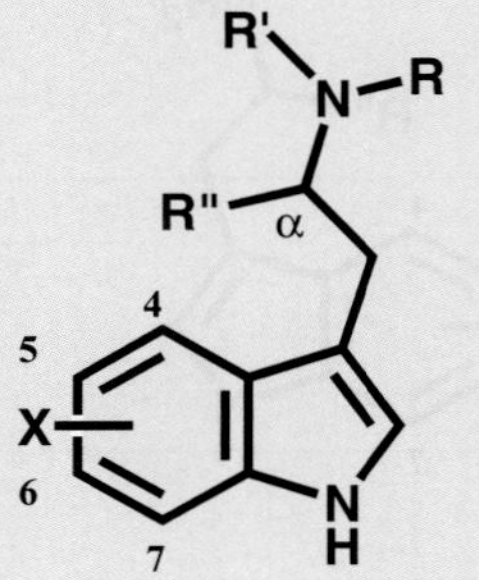

Agent	Common designation	R/R′	R″	X	Approximate DOM stimulus generalization potency (μmol/kg)[a]	Approximate human hallucinogenic dose (mg)[b]
Tryptamine		-H/-H	-H	-H	Inactive	Inactive
α-Methyltryptamine	α-MeT	-H/-H	-Me	-H	15	5–20 (s) 15–30 (po)
N,N-Dimethyltryptamine	DMT	-Me/-Me	-H	-H	26	60–100 (s) 4–30 (iv)
N,N-Diethyltryptamine	DET	-Et/-Et	-H	-H	10	50–100 (po)
N,N-Dipropyltryptamine	DPT	-Pr/-Pr	-H	-H	8	100–250 (po)
N,N-Diisopropyltryptamine	DIPT	-iPr/-iPr	-H	-H	9	25–100 (po)
4-Hydroxy DMT	Psilocin	-Me/-Me	-H	4-OH	—	10–20 (po)
4-Methoxy DMT	4-OMe DMT	-Me/-Me	-H	4-OMe	12	Unknown
5-Hydroxytryptamine	Serotonin	-H/-H	-H	5-OH	Inactive	Inactive
5-Hydroxy DMT	Bufotenine	-Me/-Me	-H	5-OH	Inactive	Unknown
5-Methoxy DMT	5-OMe DMT	-Me/-Me	-H	5-OMe	4	6–20 (s); 2–3 (iv)
5-Methoxy-N, N-di-isopropyltryptamine	Foxy Methoxy	-iPr/iPr	-H	5-OMe	3	6–12 (po)
(±)5-Methoxy α-MeT	5-OMe α-MeT	-H/-H	-Me	5-OMe	2	2.5–4.5 (po)

s, smoked; po, oral; iv, intravenous.

[a]Drug discrimination data, transformed to approximate μmol/kg dose, from Glennon (34,35).

[b]Data from Shulgin and coworkers (13,15).

Ergolines or Lysergamides (LSD, "Acid," "Blotter") (+)LSD (Fig. 14.1; R = R′ = Et) is perhaps the best known, and one of the most potent, of the classical hallucinogens. Although LSD itself is not naturally occurring, many related ergolines and synthetic precursors are found in nature. In terms of potency, LSD is active at total human doses of ≤0.1 to 0.2 mg (100–200 micrograms). Although numerous derivatives of LSD are possible, relatively few have been investigated in humans. Some work has been reported on the SAR of LSD (6,19). No hallucinogen has been as extensively studied in animals or humans as LSD (reviewed in 1,6,20). Its actions in humans can be divided into three major categories: perceptual (altered shapes and colors, heightened sense of hearing), psychic (depersonalization, visual hallucinations, alterations in mood and sense of time), and somatic (nausea, blurred vision, dizziness) (6). In terms of overall principal effects, there seem to be few qualitative differences between those produced by LSD, psilocybin, and mescaline. Although LSD has been sold on the clandestine market in tablet form, it is not uncommon to find this material available on "blotter paper" because of its extreme potency (21). Blotter paper is a sheet of porous paper impregnated with a solution of LSD, and the dried sheet later is cut to afford the desired dose.

Beta-carbolines (Harmaline, Harmine) The beta-carbolines (Fig. 14.1) represent an interesting and controversial class of agents, that are referred to as "harmala alkaloids." Several are naturally occurring in South American plants; for example, beta-carbolines are found in certain vines and lianas (e.g., *Banisteriopsis caapi*). In the Old World, beta-carbolines are found as constituents of Syrian Rue (*Pegnum harmala*). Naturally occurring harmala alkaloids can have a double-bond at the C1-N2 position or at both the C1-N2 and C3-C4 positions; *X* generally is a hydrogen atom or a 7-methoxy group. South American Indians use beta-carboline–containing plants to prepare a variety of concoctions and snuffs—the most notable of which is ayahuasca—for their hallucinogenic and visionary healing properties. Based on the number of reports that have appeared, there is little question that such concoctions are psychoactive; however, the plant preparations usually consist of admixtures in which indolealkylamines such as DMT or 5-OMe DMT sometimes have been identified (17). Some beta-carbolines possess activity as monoamine oxidase (MAO) inhibitors, and it has been suggested that the MAO inhibitory effect of the beta-carbolines simply potentiates the effect of any indolealkylamine hallucinogen present in the admixture by interfering with its metabolism. There have been very few studies with individual beta-carbolines, especially under carefully controlled clinical settings. The most commonly occurring beta-carbolines are harmine, harmaline, and tetrahydroharmine. Evidence suggests that harmine and harmaline are hallucinogenic in humans (with potencies not greater than that of DMT) (7,22). Harmaline has seen some limited experimental application as an adjunct to psychotherapy (22). As with other classical hallucinogens, certain beta-carbolines bind at 5-HT_{2A} receptors (23) and, in animal studies, DOM-stimulus generalization occurs to harmaline (24). However, none of the examined beta-carbolines produced the type of 5-HT_{2A} agonist effects (phosphoinositol hydrolysis) common to other classical hallucinogens (23); hence, they cannot yet be formally classified as classical hallucinogens. Moreover, an ibogaine stimulus, but not an LSD stimulus, generalized to certain of these beta-carbolines (25,26). In any event, over the past decade or so, beta-carbolines have begun to make an appearance on the clandestine market. They have been referred to as *fantasy-enhancing agents* (7) and have the potential to serve as templates for the development of novel designer drugs. Because relatively little is known about these agents, there is increased interest in their investigation. This may be particularly true now that ayahuasca has been legalized for religious use in the United States.

Phenylalkylamines

Phenylethylamines (Mescaline, Peyote) Phenylethylamines and phenylisopropylamines (Fig. 14.1), collectively referred to as phenylalkylamines, represent the largest group of classical hallucinogens (2,14). The phenylethylamines are the alpha-*des*methyl counterparts of the phenylisopropylamines. As with the indolealkylamines, the presence of the alpha-methyl group increases an agent's lipid solubility and reduces its susceptibility to metabolism. Phenylethylamine hallucinogens typically produce behavioral effects that are similar to those of their corresponding phenylisopropylamines, but usually are several-fold less potent; phenylethylamine counterparts of weak phenylisopropylamines might even be inactive. Although there is a temptation to view phenylethylamines simply as abbreviated versions of phenylisopropylamines (which, structurally, they are), evidence suggests that the presence or absence of the alpha-methyl group might play a greater role than previously appreciated in differences in receptor binding, receptor selectivity, efficacy, and the "functional selectivity" of the two series (27–32).

A large number of phenylalkylamines has been examined in human and animal studies (14). Certain hallucinogenic phenylisopropylamines are described as possessing some stimulant character, which can be minimized or altogether absent in the corresponding phenylethylamines. At the alpha-position, the phenylisopropylamines (Fig. 14.1) possess a chiral center that is absent in the phenylethylamines. Otherwise, the behavioral SARs of the two groups of agents are relatively similar. Consequently, the phenylethylamines will not be discussed here in detail; see Shulgin and Shulgin (14) for an extended discussion of phenylethylamine hallucinogens. One of the best recognized phenylethylamine hallucinogens is mescaline. A constituent of the peyote (and other) cactus, mescaline is a relatively weak hallucinogenic agent. Because it is one of the oldest investigated hallucinogens, mescaline often serves as a standard and the potencies of other agents are compared with it (e.g., in terms of MU or mescaline units). As with many of the hallucinogens, mescaline is a Schedule I substance under the federal Controlled Substances Act; however, the use of peyote in certain Native American religious practices is legally sanctioned.

Phenylisopropylamines (DOM, DOB, DMA, MDA)

Structural modification of mescaline and related substances by introduction of an alpha-methyl group and by deletion or rearrangement of the position of its methoxy groups results in a series of agents known as the phenylisopropylamine hallucinogens (Fig. 14.1; Table 14.2). Numerous names and terminologies have been used to describe these phenylisopropylamine hallucinogens (14), but one of the more common and readily applied nomenclatures is that associated with the number and location of methoxy groups in the molecule. Analogues with two methoxy groups are called DMAs (i.e., dimethoxy analogues), whereas analogues with three methoxy groups are called trimethoxy analogues, or TMAs. For example, introduction of an alpha-methyl group to mescaline results in 3,4,5-TMA (Table 14.2). There are three possible mono-methoxyphenylisopropylamines: the *ortho*-methoxy analogue OMA, the *meta*-methoxy analogue MMA, and the *para*-methoxy analogue PMA (Table 14.2). Although PMA is classified as a Schedule I substance, none of the three monomethoxy analogues has been demonstrated to be hallucinogenic in humans. PMA possesses weak central stimulant actions, acts as a 5-HT–releasing agent, and has been found on the clandestine market; several deaths have been attributed to PMA overdose (e.g., 33). (PMA is discussed in the section on designer drugs.) There are six isomeric DMA analogues. These analogues have not been extensively investigated in humans, and few produce DOM-like stimulus effects in animals (Table 14.2). None is more potent than DOM. One of the more potent positional isomers, and one that has been evaluated in humans, is 1-(2,5-dimethoxyphenyl)-2-aminopropane or 2,5-DMA (sometimes referred to simply as DMA). There are six different TMA analogues (Table 14.2). Most show some activity, but the 2,4,5-

TABLE 14.2 Examples of Some Psychoactive Phenylisopropylamines and Related Agents

Agent	X_2	X_3	X_4	X_5	X_6	DOM-stimulus generalization potency (μmol/kg)[a]	Approximate human hallucinogenic dose (mg)[b]
Amphetamine	-H	-H	-H	-H	-H	NSG	NH
OMA	-OMe	-H	-H	-H	-H	NSG	NH
MMA	-H	-OMe	-H	-H	-H	NSG	NH
PMA	-H	-H	-OMe	-H	-H	NSG	NH
2,3-DMA	-OMe	-OMe	-H	-H	-H	NSG	(?)
2,4-DMA	-OMe	-H	-OMe	-H	-H	21.0	>60 (?)
2,5-DMA	-OMe	-H	-H	-OMe	-H	23.8	120 (80–160)
2,5-DMA, *R*(−)-	-OMe	-H	-H	-OMe	-H	14.0	(?)
2,6-DMA	-OMe	-H	-H	-H	-OMe	NSG	(?)
3,4-DMA	-H	-OMe	-OMe	-H	-H	NSG	>500 (?)
3,5-DMA	-H	-OMe	-H	-OMe	-H	NSG	(?)
2,3,4-TMA	-OMe	-OMe	-OMe	-H	-H	29.8	>100 (?)
2,3,5-TMA	-OMe	-OMe	-H	-OMe	-H	63.0	>80 (?)
2,3,6-TMA	-OMe	-OMe	-H	-H	-OMe	—	>30 (?)
2,4,5-TMA	-OMe	-H	-OMe	-OMe	-H	13.7	30 (20–40)
2,4,6-TMA	-OMe	-H	-OMe	-H	-OMe	13.9	38 (25–50)
3,4,5-TMA	-H	-OMe	-OMe	-OMe	-H	24.2	175 (100–250)
MEM	-OMe	-H	$-OC_2H_5$	-OMe	-H	22.9	35 (20–50)
DOM	-OMe	-H	$-CH_3$	-OMe	-H	1.8	7 (3–10)
DOM, *R*(−)-	-OMe	-H	$-CH_3$	-OMe	-H	0.9	(?)
DOM, *S*(+)-	-OMe	-H	$-CH_3$	-OMe	-H	6.9	(?)
DOET	-OMe	-H	$-C_2H_5$	-OMe	-H	0.9	4 (2–6)
DOPR	-OMe	-H	$-nC_3H_7$	-OMe	-H	0.6	4 (2.5–5)
DOBU	-OMe	-H	$-nC_4H_9$	-OMe	-H	3.2	(?)
DOAM	-OMe	-H	$-nC_5H_{11}$	-OMe	-H	NSG	(?)
DON	-OMe	-H	$-NO_2$	-OMe	-H	2.7	4 (3–4.5)
DOC	-OMe	-H	-Cl	-OMe	-H	1.2	2.5 (1.5–3)
DOB	-OMe	-H	-Br	-OMe	-H	0.6	2 (1–3)
DOB, R(−)-	-OMe	-H	-Br	-OMe	-H	0.3	1.0–1.5 (?)
DOI	-OMe	-H	-I	-OMe	-H	1.2	2.5 (1.5–3)
DOOC	-OMe	-H	-COOH	-OMe	-H	NSG	(?)
DOOH	-OMe	-H	-OH	-OMe	-H	NSG	(?)

NH, material has not been reported to be hallucinogenic; NSG, no stimulus generalization (i.e., the agent did not produce DOM-like stimulus effects); (?), the material has not been well investigated or that its actions or potency are essentially unknown; DOM, 1-(2,5-dimethoxy-4-methylphenyl)-2-aminopropane.

[a]Drug discrimination data represent ED_{50} values and are from Glennon (2,34,35).

[b]Data are primarily from Shulgin and coworkers (13,14). Where a dose range was reported in the original literature, the arithmetic mean is also provided here to facilitate comparison and the original range is given in parenthesis; the values should not be taken as a measure of precision. In fact, doses are approximate and no implication is made that the different agents produce an identical effect.

timethoxy analogue 2,4,5-TMA is the most potent of the series. Most of the trimethoxy analogues are recognized by DOM-trained animals, but none is more potent than DOM itself (2,34,35). The presence of the 2,5-methoxy substitution pattern in 2,5-DMA and 2,4,5-TMA might be noted. Replacement of the 4-methoxy group of 2,4,5-TMA with a methyl group results in DOM or 1-(2,5-dimethoxy-4-methylphenyl)-2-aminopropane. DOM represents the prototype member of this family of agents. Increasing the length of this 4-methyl group to an ethyl or *n*-propyl group (that is, DOET and DOPR, respectively) results in enhanced potency on a molar basis. Further extension of the alkyl chain results in decreased potency or loss of action. Active agents such as DOB (Table 14.2) and DOI result from substituting hydrophobic, electron-withdrawing groups at the four-position. DOB is quite potent and has been misrepresented on the clandestine market as LSD both in tablet and "blotter" form.

Where optical isomers of phenylisopropylamines have been examined, activity resides primarily with the *R*(−)isomer; the *S*(+)isomers typically are less potent, inactive, or have received little study (2). For example, although not well investigated, it appears that *R*(−)DOM and *R*(−)DOB show activity at total human doses of about 4 mg and 1 mg, respectively. Animal (drug discrimination) studies show that, for all of the phenylisopropylamine hallucinogens investigated, the R(−)isomers are more potent than their S(+)isomers by several-fold. N-Monomethylation reduces potency or abolishes activity; for example, the N-monomethyl analogues of DOM and DOB are about one-tenth as potent as their primary amine counterparts. SARs for the DOM-like actions of phenylisopropylamine hallucinogens have been summarized (2,36). The phenylisopropylamine MDA is structurally distinct from many of the other hallucinogenic phenylisopropylamines by virtue of lacking methoxy groups and possessing a methylenedioxy group instead. MDA has been reported to produce effects in humans akin to a combination of cocaine and LSD. MDA produces both amphetamine-like and DOM-like stimulus effects in animals; furthermore, animals trained to discriminate MDA recognize central stimulants (such as amphetamine and cocaine) as well as classical hallucinogens (such as LSD, mescaline, and DOM) (37). The hallucinogenic qualities of MDA reside primarily with its R(−)isomer, whereas the S(+)isomer seems primarily responsible for its stimulant character. Table 14.2 provides a comparison of the approximate human doses of various phenylisopropylamines when administered by the oral route. These agents represent a mere sampling of the agents that have been examined (14). Using only those functional groups shown in Table 14.2, it can be imagined how many different analogues are possible on the basis of structural rearrangement. There is no reason to suspect that each of these agents produces identical effects. In fact, the actions of some of these agents have been reported to be quite unique and range from hallucinations and closed-eye imagery to intellectual and sensory enhancement to erotic arousal (14).

Designer Drugs Clandestine chemists have developed designer drugs, or *controlled substance analogues* by making designed SAR changes in existing hallucinogens. To illustrate, DOB is a potent hallucinogen; removal of the alpha-methyl group of DOB should, according to established SAR, result in a phenylethylamine analogue that retains—although with several-fold reduced potency—the actions of DOB. Its effects in humans might not be identical with those of DOB, but significant similarities should exist. Even though alpha-*des*methyl DOB was known earlier in the scientific literature, it made an appearance on the clandestine market as "Nexus" or "2-CB." As expected, the agent is hallucinogenic and is somewhat less potent than DOB.

Aryl-unsubstituted phenylisopropylamine is amphetamine (Fig. 14.2); that is, removal of the 4-methyl group and the two methoxy groups of DOM results not in a hallucinogenic agent but in a central stimulant (see Chapter 5). Amphetamine is rather unusual in that few phenylisopropylamines retain its central stimulant character and very few analogues retain a level of potency similar to that of amphetamine. One of the best known examples of a phenylisopropylamine analogue that retains potent stimulant properties is the N-monomethyl counterpart of amphetamine, or methamphetamine (Fig. 14.2). Nevertheless, structural variation of amphetamine can result in controlled substance analogues. For example, cathinone is the beta-keto analogue of amphetamine; cathinone is a naturally occurring substance (a constituent of the shrub *Catha edulis* or *khat*) that retains central stimulant character (see Chapter 5). Cathinone can be transformed through N-monomethylation into methcathinone or ephedrone ("CAT"; Fig. 14.2)—a potent stimulant and drug of abuse. Structurally, methcathinone is to cathinone what methamphetamine is to amphetamine. In this manner, designer drugs have appeared that are structurally related to either the hallucinogens or stimulants. In many instances, their actions are what might have been expected on the basis of published SARs.

Not all designer drugs result in actions that are entirely predictable. One of the most popular designer drugs is MDMA (Fig. 14.2) (also called methylenedioxymethamphetamine, Ecstasy, XTC, Adam, X, or e). On the basis of established SAR, it might have been expected that N-monomethylation of a phenylisopropylamine stimulant would enhance the amphetamine-like stimulant actions of MDA, whereas the same structural modification would diminish its hallucinogenic or DOM-like action. Although this appears to be the case, what emerged was an agent that, in addition to its stimulant character, also produces an empathogenic effect. MDMA was explored for several years as an adjunct to psychotherapy and then as a legal recreational drug before its emergency scheduling under the federal Controlled Substances Act as a Schedule I substance. This agent has been extensively investigated; while studies have shown that both optical isomers are active, the *S*(+)isomer is the more active of the two (12). A structurally related, but less popular, agent is its N-ethyl homolog MDE ("Eve"). The consensus today is that MDMA probably is an empathogen with amphetamine-like stimulant side effects. Homologation of the alpha-methyl group of phenylisopropylamine stimulants and hallucinogens

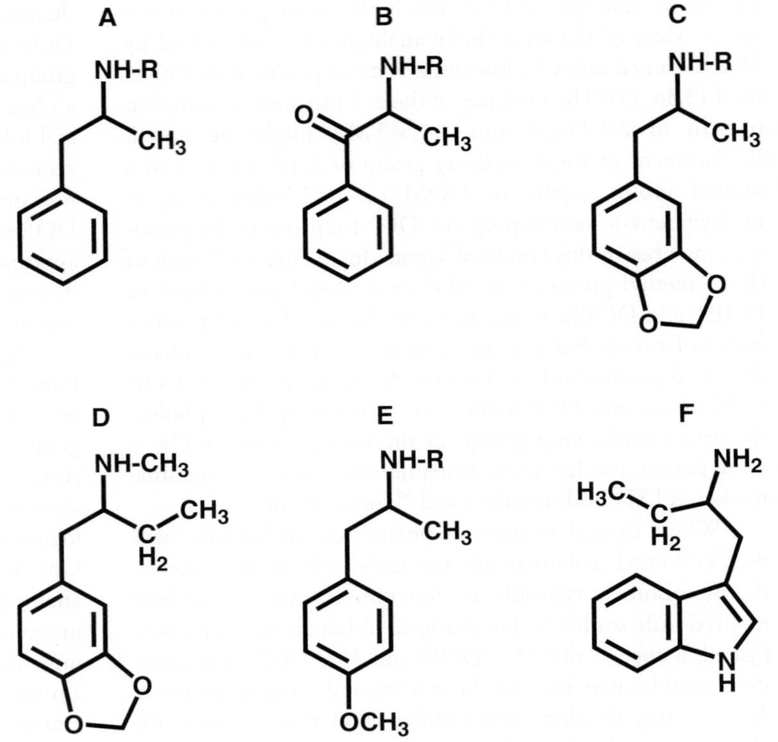

FIGURE 14.2. Chemical structures of **(A)** amphetamine and methamphetamine (R = -H and $-CH_3$, respectively), **(B)** cathinone and methcathinone (R = -H and $-CH_3$, respectively), **(C)** 1-(3,4-methylenedioxyphenyl)-2-aminopropane (MDA) and 3,4-methylenedioxymethamphetamine (MDMA) (R = -H and $-CH_3$, respectively), **(D)** MBDB, **(E)** PMA and PMMA (R = -H and $-CH_3$, respectively), and **(F)** α-ethyltryptamine.

typically diminishes their potency or abolishes their activity; however, the alpha-ethyl homolog of MDMA, MBDB or N-methyl-1-(3,4-methylenedioxyphenyl)-2-aminobutane (Fig. 14.2), retains MDMA-like actions, but apparently lacks amphetamine-like central stimulant character (38,39).

In recent times, agents such as MDA, PMA, PMMA (see the following section), and others have been represented and sold as MDMA on the illicit drug market. Possibly because of the adverse cardiovascular effects associated with PMA or its potential neurotoxicity (40), there is concern among MDMA users about the authenticity of the drugs they use. Test kits and assays have been developed so that users can, at least to some extent, validate the authenticity of the substances they are using. An agent closely related in structure to MDMA is PMMA or N-methyl-1-(4-methoxyphenyl)-2-aminopropane (Fig. 14.2). PMMA is a hybrid structure of two phenylisopropylamine stimulants: PMA and methamphetamine. Surprisingly, in contradiction to established stimulant SAR, PMMA lacks significant central stimulant actions. Unlike PMA and methamphetamine, PMMA is not recognized by (+)amphetamine-trained animals. PMMA has seen little controlled human evaluation (14). Because PMMA is structurally related to metabolites of MDMA, it was examined in MDMA-trained animals in tests of stimulus generalization; PMMA substituted for and was several-fold more potent than MDMA. PMMA has been suggested to be the structural parent of MDMA-like agents. As with MDMA, PMMA has been reported to produce neurotoxic effects in animals (40). Animals have been trained to discriminate PMMA from vehicle, and PMMA stimulus generalization occurs to racemic MDMA, *S*(+)MDMA, *S*(+)MBDB, *R*(−)MBDB, *S*(+)3,4-DMA, and *R*(−)3,4-DMA, but not to DOM, (+)amphetamine, *R*(−)MDMA, or *R*(−)PMMA (41,42). These results, coupled with the earlier discussion of MDMA, suggest that some phenylisopropylamines might not be best described as being merely central stimulants or hallucinogens, but as possessing yet a third action that needs to be accounted for. This third type of effect, shared by PMMA and MBDB in animal studies, is one that requires further clinical investigation. On the basis of drug discrimination studies, it has been proposed that phenylalkylamines with abuse potential can produce one or more of at least three distinct stimulus effects in animals: a hallucinogenic or DOM-like effect (*D*), a central stimulant or (+)amphetamine-like effect (*A*), and a PMMA-like effect (*P*) (Fig. 14.3). Compounds such as DOM fall into the *D* category of the Venn diagram, whereas (+)amphetamine serves as the prototype of the *A* agents. The *P* category is typified by PMMA and MBDB. MDMA produces both PMMA-like and amphetamine-like effects and would fall into the *A*/*P* intersect. MDA has been shown to possess MDMA-like actions in addition to the hallucinogenic and stimulant actions described earlier. Hence, R(−)MDA falls into the *D*/*P* intersect, and S(+)MDA falls into the *A*/*P* intersect. Racemic MDA (that is, an equal combination of MDA optical isomers commonly encountered on the clandestine market) actually falls into the common intersect (shaded area of Fig. 14.3) because it produces all three types of stimulus effects (43). Other agents recently demonstrated to produce a PMMA-like stimulus effect include PMA ("chicken powder," "white Mitsubishi," "death"), and 4-MTA or 1-(4-methylthio)phenylisoprop-

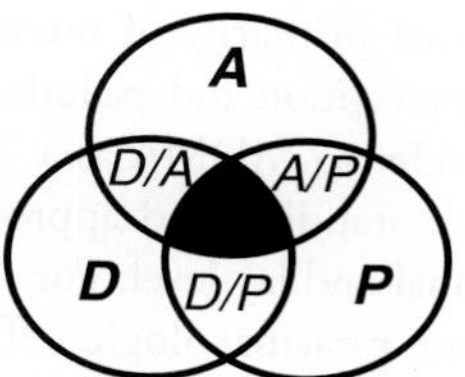

FIGURE 14.3. Venn diagram showing a relationship between the stimulus properties of 1-(2,5-dimethoxy-4-methylphenyl)-2-aminopropane (DOM)-like hallucinogens (D), amphetamine-like stimulants (A) and PMMA-like agents (P) (adapted from Glennon et al. [41]). Some agents produce only one of the three possible effects, whereas other agents can produce effects, such as stimulant and PMMA-like effects, that are best represented by the A/P intersect. See text for additional discussion. Racemic 3,4-methylenedioxy amphetamine (MDA) produces all three stimulus effects and is best represented by the common (i.e., shaded) intersect.

ylamine ("flatliners," "golden eagles") (44). It must be emphasized that this proposal was developed on the basis of animal studies; although it appears to reflect the human actions of the agents, additional work, particularly in a clinical setting, is obviously required to further substantiate the model. Nevertheless, the classification scheme suggests that there will be at least three different SARs and three different mechanisms of action. Certain agents, because they fall into more than one category, represent mechanistic and structure-activity composites. The same can be said of indolealkylamine designer drugs; indeed, it may be the particular "mix" of actions that makes certain designer drugs attractive as drugs of abuse. Recent evidence suggests that alpha-ethyltryptamine (alpha-ET, alpha-EtT, AET, "ET"; Fig. 14.2) represents a novel agent of abuse that possesses several kinds of actions. alpha-ET was briefly marketed in the early 1960s as an antidepressant, but was withdrawn shortly after its introduction. alpha-ET acts as a MAO inhibitor, but it has been shown that alpha-ET is hallucinogenic in humans and also behaves as a central stimulant (16,18,20). It was more recently shown that *S*(+)alpha-ET produces both DOM- and PMMA-like effects but not (+)amphetamine-like effects, whereas *R*(−)alpha-ET produces (+)amphetamine- and PMMA-like effects but not DOM-like effects; both optical isomers of alpha-ET produce MDMA-like actions (45). The last is consistent with the mention of alpha-ET being sold as a substitute for MDMA (46). In the classification scheme shown in Figure 14.3 *S*(+)alpha-ET might best be described as falling into the *D/P* intersect, whereas *R*(−)alpha-ET falls into the *A/P* intersect. Certain designer drugs, then, behave like classical hallucinogens and, hence, involve a serotonergic mechanism. Others might produce more than one effect; that is, certain agents (for example, MDA) possess hallucinogenic character but also produce other effects. Evidence exists for the involvement of other serotonin receptor subpopulations in the actions of designer drugs. For example, as discussed in the following section, the 5-HT_{1A} agonist 8-OH DPAT seems to potentiate the effect of DOM. In addition, 8-OH DPAT and both its optical isomers substitute for MDMA in animals trained to discriminate MDMA from vehicle (47). As a consequence, because MDMA and classical hallucinogens sometimes are used in combination at "raves" for a heightened drug effect (a process known as "flipping" or "candy-flipping"), it has been suggested that this phenomenon may, at least in part, involve both a 5-HT_2 and a 5-HT_{1A} receptor mechanism.

ABSORPTION AND METABOLISM

Few detailed studies have been conducted on the human metabolism of hallucinogenic agents. Simple indolealkylamines such as DMT and 5-OMe DMT undergo multiple routes of metabolism, including N-demethylation, cyclization to tetrahydro-beta-carbolines, and N-oxidation; however, their major route of metabolism is via oxidative deamination by MAO (48). Ring-substituted derivatives such as psilocybin are hydrolyzed to psilocin, whereas certain methoxy derivatives might also be O-demethylated. Most metabolic studies on LSD were conducted some time ago, when analytic techniques were not as refined as they are today. This fact, coupled with the small drug doses necessary to produce behavioral effects, has created some controversy about the exact structures of LSD metabolites formed after administration of pharmacologically relevant LSD doses (6). Detailed investigations of the metabolism of phenylalkylamine hallucinogens also are scant, but most phenylalkylamines are believed to be substrates for MAO and cytochrome P450. DOM is one of the better investigated hallucinogens. The *S*(+)-isomer of DOM is metabolized more rapidly than its *R*(−)-enantiomer, and the aromatic methyl group is oxidized to the corresponding hydroxymethyl and subsequently oxidized to a carboxylate. DOM also is O-demethylated by rabbit liver homogenates to afford its 2-O-demethylated, 5-O-demethylated, and 2,5-di-O-demethylated products (49). It has been suggested that the latter metabolite might undergo oxidation to a quinone and behave as a neurotoxin in vivo (49). Both individual O-*des*methyl metabolites of DOM are pharmacologically active, but neither is as potent as the parent agent (50). DOB (51,52) and DOI (53) also undergo metabolism via O-demethylation.

Various hallucinogenic and nonhallucinogenic phenylisopropylamines are substrates or inhibitors of human cytochrome P450; methylenedioxy analogues, such as MDA and MDMA, display particularly high affinity for the enzyme (54). Recent interest in MDMA has led to extensive investigations of its metabolism. One of the major metabolites of MDMA is its N-desmethyl analogue, MDA. The methylenedioxy rings both of MDMA and MDA are attacked by cytochrome P450 to give ring-opened products: HHMA (N-methyl-3,4-dihydroxyamphetamine) and HHA (3,4-dihydroxyamphetamine), respectively. These dihydroxy compounds are O-methylated, primarily to HMMA (N-methyl-4-hydroxy-3-methoxyamphetamine) and HMA (4-hydroxy-3-methoxyamphetamine). For a detailed description of the metabolism of MDA, MDMA, and the MDMA homologs MDE and MBDB, as well as the specific cytochrome P450 isozymes involved in their metabolism, see review (55). The major human urinary MDMA metabolite is HHMA (56).

PHARMACOLOGIC ACTIONS

The effects of various indolalkylamine hallucinogens are not necessarily identical, but they generally produce alterations in thought, mood, or perception (1,9). Intravenous administration of 0.3 mg/kg DMT to human subjects produces a (nearly immediate) spectrum of "psychedelic" effects, including an abstract, rapidly moving, intensely colored, kaleidoscopic display of visual effects, transient anxiety, elation, and euphoria. On the other hand, cognition was relatively unimpaired, and there was a heightening of evaluative processes (57). Similar doses of DMT also produced (n = 13) increased heart rate (by up to >30%) and blood pressure (by up to 15%) within 5 minutes, elevated prolactin (variable) and cortisol (by 30% at 60 minutes) levels, and hyperthermia (56 and references therein). Psilocybin (0.25 mg/kg, orally) produced a psychotic syndrome that included disturbances of emotion and sensory perception, difficulty in thinking and reality appraisal, and loss of ego boundaries. Symptoms appeared 20 to 30 minutes after administration, peaked after another 30 to 40 minutes, and completely subsided after 5 or 6 hours. During the peak period, perceptual alterations included auditory and visual hallucinations ranging from illusions to complex scenery hallucinations (9,58). Because of the rapid hydrolysis of psilocybin to psilocin in humans (59), it is quite likely that the effects observed after administration of the former are due to psilocin (60–67).

Mescaline, one of the oldest known phenylalkylamine hallucinogens (4), is active at total oral doses of 200 to 400 mg/kg, has a slow onset (1 to 3 hours) and long duration of action (approximately 8 to 10 hours) (5). Although >1,000-fold less potent than LSD, the two agents were found to produce similar effects including visual changes and changes in body image (5,68,69). In a series of comparative studies, the same subjects were administered oral doses of LSD, psilocybin, and mescaline; although the mescaline experience was found most intense (68,69), the clinical effects of the three agents were comparable in "kind and degree" (68). This led to speculation that all three agents might be working through a common mechanism (68). Mescaline is naturally occurring in certain cacti (e.g., peyote, *Lophophora williamsii*), and peyote is used as a religious sacrament by members of the Native American Church. A recent study found no evidence of psychologic or cognitive deficits among American Indians using peyote regularly in a religious setting (70).

Somewhat distinct from these effects are the actions of the designer drug MDMA. Indeed, the designer drugs do not represent a homogeneous class of agents; that is, certain designer drugs are hallucinogens, some are stimulants, others are empathogens, and yet others can be of mixed action. Few designer drugs have been investigated in detail. However, several clinical investigations of MDMA have been reported; in them, MDMA has been found to produce a rather unique spectrum of effects that would not be considered "hallucinogenic" in nature. For example, the acute effects of MDMA include extroversion, heightened mood (heightened sense of confidence and well-being), dry mouth and increased thirst, difficulty in concentrating, impaired balance, dizziness, jaw clenching, lack of appetite, and restlessness (71). Perceptual changes induced by MDMA are modest and consist primarily of intensification of tactile, visual, and acoustic perception and exclude frank hallucinations (71–73). In fact, to refer to MDMA as a "hallucinogen" might only confuse an understanding and appreciation of its actions both at the professional and lay level. For detailed discussion of the biochemical and pharmacologic effects of MDMA in rodents and humans, the interested reader is referred to a comprehensive review by Green and coworkers (74).

MECHANISMS OF ACTION

An argument can be made that human subjects provide the most reliable assessment of the actions and potency of hallucinogenic agents. Unfortunately, extensive human data, particularly data from well-controlled clinical studies with large subject populations, are available for only a very few agents (i.e., LSD, DMT, psilocybin, and mescaline). Information about most agents, where human data are available, is from studies that involved limited subject populations or from studies that investigated only few drug doses, with or without proper controls. Some of what is known, and often cited, comes from anecdotal reports, from which even the identity or purity of the test material might not have been authenticated. Today, for example, an enormous amount of anecdotal information on the human effects of hallucinogenic agents can be found on the Internet (75), but such information (although it should not be ignored) must be considered in the proper context.

Many attempts have been made to develop animal models of hallucinogenic activity but, to date, no single animal model accounts for the actions of these agents as a class (reviewed in 8). In contrast, one animal procedure that has found considerable application in the classification of hallucinogenic agents is the drug discrimination paradigm (reviewed in 76). In this procedure, which typically uses operant conditioning, animals are trained to recognize or discriminate the stimulus effects of a specific training drug from vehicle. After animals have reliably learned the stimulus, tests of *substitution* or *stimulus generalization* can be conducted. That is, novel agents can be administered to the trained animals to determine if they produce stimulus effects similar to those of the training drug. The results are quantitative as well as qualitative and, where substitution occurs, an estimation of potency (an ED_{50} value) can be calculated. This procedure does not represent a general model of hallucinogenic activity. In fact, the drug discrimination paradigm has seen broad application in the investigation of a wide variety of centrally acting agents and drugs of abuse (76,77). With this procedure, large numbers of animals can be used, numerous drugs and drug doses can be evaluated, testing parameters can be widely manipulated and mechanistic studies can be conducted.

Many types of hallucinogens and psychoactive agents have been used as training drugs, and the results of such studies have contributed to the categorization of these agents. It is presumed that animals can distinguish drug effects much in the same way that humans do. Animals trained to discriminate LSD, for example, do not recognize (substitute for, generalize to) phencyclidine (PCP), just as animals trained to discriminate PCP do not recognize LSD. Neither LSD nor PCP-trained animals recognize tetrahydrocannabinol. LSD-trained animals, however, recognize mescaline, DOM, and certain other hallucinogens. LSD and DOM have seen the most extensive application as training drugs for investigations of mechanism of action, classification, and SARs of hallucinogenic agents (35,45,78). Through use of the drug discrimination technique, it has been possible to identify what are termed the classical hallucinogens—agents that share common (although not necessarily identical) stimulus character and that probably act by a shared mechanism of action (45). Drug discrimination data have been shown to be significantly correlated with human hallucinogenic potency (2). It has been further demonstrated that the classical hallucinogens bind at 5-HT_2 receptors and behave as agonists (2,79). In the mid-1980s, it was shown that the 5-HT_2 serotonin receptor affinities of classical hallucinogens are significantly correlated both with their DOM-stimulus generalization potencies and their human hallucinogenic potencies (79). Today, the classical hallucinogens are thought to produce their effect by acting as agonists at 5-HT_2 receptors in the brain—the "5-HT_2 hypothesis of classical hallucinogen action"—and, hence, derivation of the term *serotonergic hallucinogens* (reviewed in 2). Radiolabeled analogues of DOB and its iodinated counterpart DOI (for example, [^{3}H]DOB, [^{125}I]DOI) are available for the investigation of 5-HT_2 receptor pharmacology. Later, it was demonstrated that 5-HT_2 receptors represent a family of 5-HT receptors consisting of 5-HT_{2A}, 5-HT_{2B}, and 5-HT_{2C} receptor subpopulations. Relatively few arylalkylamines have been compared, but it appears that they show little selectivity for one subpopulation over the others (80). Studies with 5-HT_{2A} receptor antagonists suggest that 5-HT_{2A} receptors play a predominant role in the discriminative stimulus actions of these agents (81–83).

Although activation of 5-HT_{2A} receptors seems to be responsible for the actions that the classical hallucinogens have in common, other neurochemical mechanisms might account for their differences. For example, LSD is a very promiscuous agent that binds with high affinity at many receptor populations for which most other classical hallucinogens show little to no affinity. Also, many indolalkylamine hallucinogens bind with high affinity at multiple populations of 5-HT receptors, and some display comparable or higher affinity at these receptors (for example, 5-HT_{1A}, h5-HT_{1D}, 5-HT_6) than they do at 5-HT_{2A} receptors. In contrast, the phenylalkylamine hallucinogens are quite selective for 5-HT_2 receptors. Some beta-carbolines, although they bind at 5-HT_2 receptors (23), possess activity as MAO inhibitors (20); α-ET also is an inhibitor of MAO (20). Thus these mechanistic complexities might account for the somewhat dissimilar (i.e., nonidentical) actions of these agents. Other neurotransmitter mechanisms also might contribute to the actions of the hallucinogens. For example, although DOM does not bind at 5-HT_{1A} receptors, the 5-HT_{1A} receptor agonist 8-hydroxy-2-(N,N-di-*n*-propylamino)tetralin (8-OH DPAT) enhances the stimulus potency of DOM (2). Hence certain indolalkylamine hallucinogens might be more potent than expected because they activate both 5-HT_{2A} and 5-HT_{1A} receptors. In similar fashion, PCP, which does not bind at 5-HT_{2A} receptors, potentiates the actions of DOM (84). Interaction of hallucinogens with 5-HT_{2A} receptors might be too simplistic an explanation to account for all the actions of the classical hallucinogens. However, the one feature that all these hallucinogens have in common is that they bind at 5-HT_{2A} receptors (the "common component hypothesis") (2). Although the 5-HT_2 hypothesis of classical hallucinogen action was first proposed in 1984 (79), it was not for another 15 years that clinical results to support the hypothesis would become available. In 1998 Volenweider and colleagues (60) showed that the 5-HT_2 antagonist ketanserin dose-dependently antagonized the psychotomimetic effects of psilocybin in healthy human volunteers.

It has been nearly 25 years since the "5-HT_2 hypothesis of classical hallucinogen action" was first described (79). Yet there are issues that remain to be resolved. For example, why is it that some 5-HT_{2A} agonists lack hallucinogenic character, and why is it that phenylethylamines, although they possess 5-HT_{2A} receptor affinities similar to that of their phenylisopropylamine counterparts, are less active even though they are equi-effective as 5-HT_{2A} agonists (i.e., is it simply a matter of lipid solubility and blood-brain barrier penetrability, or the effect of metabolic rate)? Also, where in the brain do hallucinogens produce their effects? These issues remain unanswered, but progress is being made.

5-HT_2 receptors, members of the G-protein coupled receptor superfamily, are associated primarily with the $G_{\alpha q}$ class of G proteins resulting in activation of phospholipase C and mobilization of intracellular calcium (85,86). Using $G_{\alpha q}$ knockout mice, certain, but not all, DOI-induced behaviors were shown to be eliminated, leading to speculation that other effector systems must be involved in the actions of these agents (87). More specifically, 5-HT_{2A} and 5-HT_{2C} receptors are coupled to $G_{q/11}$ and $G_{12/13}$ proteins and influence both phospholipase C and phospholipase A_2 (31,88). That is, 5-HT_2 agonists increase phospholipase C–mediated inositol phosphate production and phospholipase A_2–mediated release of arachidonic acid. According to traditional receptor theory, the effector activity of an agonist is a generally thought to be a function of the receptor stimulus produced by an agonist and is independent of the effector pathway to which it is coupled. However, there is evidence of differential effector activation by agonists and this has been difficult to explain. To account for this, Kenakin (89) postulated that an agonist might preferentially induce or stabilize one of several (or, at least, more than one) active conformational states over another ("agonist-induced trafficking of a receptor stimulus"). That is, a receptor, R, might be capable of existing in more than one active conformation (R*, R**) and, in this manner, might be able to preferentially activate one effector system over another. This implies that it is not only the affinity for a particular receptor subtype that is important for selectivity, but that selective activation (via receptor conformational stabilization or induction) of one effector mechanism over another—through the same receptor type—can give rise to *functionally selective agonists*. In support of the concept, the potency rank-order for a small series of agonists was found to differ for 5-HT_{2A} receptor–mediated inositol phosphate accumulation versus arachidonic acid release (88). Comparing several hallucinogens and nonhallucinogens, differential activation of phospholipase C or phospholipase A_2 signaling was not observed; however, most of the agents displayed greater potency for activating the phospholipase A_2 pathway (90). In another study, the actions of the hallucinogenic 5-HT_{2A} agonist LSD and the nonhallucinogenic 5-HT_{2A} agonist lisuride were explained on the basis of receptor trafficking (91). There also is evidence that the absence or presence of an alpha-methyl group (i.e., comparing phenylethylamines with phenylisopropylamines) might selectively activate one postsynaptic effector system over another (28,30,32,90,92,93).

MDMA increases central monoamine levels by releasing serotonin, norepinephrine, and, to a lesser extent, dopamine (74). The ability of MDMA, MDA, and their optical isomers to release these three transmitters has been compared (94). MDMA is not usually considered to produce hallucinogenic effects. However, MDMA is metabolized, at least in part, to MDA, and MDA is a weak hallucinogenic agent. Consistent with this concept, MDMA has been reported to produce "slight hallucinogen-like effects," consisting of increased vividness of perception, including an intensification of colors and tactile awareness (71). These MDMA-induced perceptual alterations, as well as the hyperthermic actions of MDMA—hyperthermia also being a consequence of 5-HT_2 agonism (8)—were attenuated by pretreatment of human volunteers with ketanserin (71).

ADDICTION LIABILITY

Although relatively few studies have been conducted, classical hallucinogens are not generally considered to possess amphetamine-like or cocaine-like reinforcing properties on the basis of self-administration studies. There are a few exceptions, notably MDMA and MDA. MDMA is self-administered by nonhuman primates (95,96) and produces conditioned place preference in rats (97,98). MDA is self-administered by baboons (99) and rats (100), but is about 20 to 30 times less potent than (+)amphetamine (99). Perhaps these agents stand apart from most classical hallucinogens because MDMA is metabolized, at least to some extent, to MDA, and both MDMA and MDA have been demonstrated to possess amphetamine-like character. Referring to Figure 14.3, agents classified as hallucinogens (that is, those falling into the "D" category) likely lack reinforcing properties, whereas those classified as "A" (for example, amphetamine and methamphetamine, as well as cocaine) are reinforcing. The "A/P"-type agents like MDA and MDMA are less reinforcing than amphetamine, but preexposure to MDMA facilitates acquisition of cocaine self-administration in rats, suggesting that MDMA users might be at risk for developing psychomotor stimulant abuse (101). Finally, although hallucinogens have shown no addiction liability in animal models, a small percentage (2% to 3%) of users appears to develop a "hallucinogen dependence syndrome" (102).

Toxicity/Adverse Effects The most widely investigated agent with respect to adverse effects is MDMA; and even here, data are relatively scant. Furthermore, environmental factors have been shown to have an effect on the actions of MDMA, and some self-reporting studies (e.g., by use of questionnaires) have indicated the uncertainty of the drug involved (see the following section). The literature has been reviewed regarding the acute effects of MDMA on executive, attention, visual, motor, and auditory function, subjective experiences, and various physiologic measures in healthy volunteers (103). Another review concluded that adult females are more susceptible than males to the acute and subacute psychologic and physical adverse effects of MDMA, whereas males appear more sensitive to the acute physiologic effects (104).

MDMA was one of the first phenylalkylamines shown to produce neurotoxic effects in animals. The neurotoxicity of MDMA and other phenylalkylamines has been reviewed (98,105–109). High-dose MDMA users, in particular, run a significant risk of persistent cognitive impairment and disturbances of affect and personality (108). The possibility cannot be overlooked that these sequelae might be a result of the neurotoxic actions of MDMA. MDMA has been shown to destroy brain serotonin neurons in animals by creating long-lasting decrements in the number of axon terminals, decreasing the major metabolite of serotonin—5-hydroxyindoleacetic acid, and interfering with the rate-limiting 5-HT biosynthetic enzyme tryptophan hydroxylase and the 5-HT reuptake transporter. Studies with humans also indicate that some MDMA users may have selective decrements in cerebrospinal 5-hydroxyindoleacetic acid and 5-HT reuptake transporter levels and that humans with a history of MDMA use show lasting decrements in global brain transporter binding (110). It has been suggested that reactive metabolites (111) of MDA and MDMA, such as HHMA (56), or free radicals derived from MDMA, might play important roles in producing the neurotoxic effect. But, it seems that 5-HT deficits are not always synonymous with axonal death (112). Other MDMA-associated adverse effects (e.g., cardiovascular and hyperthermic effects) also appear to involve noradrenergic and dopaminergic mechanisms, respectively (112). In addition to the possible neurotoxic effects associated with MDMA (see previous section) and PMMA (40), PMA and PMMA are not infrequently sold as substitutes for MDMA. The increasing number of deaths involving PMA or PMMA abuse is raising concern about these agents (33). Furthermore, abuse of MDMA has been associated with the production of "serotonin syndrome"; because certain antidepressants (particularly MAO inhibitors) can add to this risk, it has been suggested that screening for MDMA use be considered when prescribing certain antidepressants (113). However, it is appropriate to put this information in perspective: it has been stated that there are about 12 to 15 MDMA-associated deaths per year in the United Kingdom when it is estimated that 500,000 persons consume the drug every week (114).

Another problem associated with MDMA use is its possible adverse cardiovascular actions. MDMA has been shown to induce fenfluramine-like proliferative actions on human cardiac valvular interstitial cells in vitro by activation of 5-HT_{2B} receptors (94). A new study involving MDMA users now has provided the first evidence that MDMA use might lead to mild to moderate valvular heart disease (115).

It should be noted that the previous discussion focused primarily on MDMA, an agent that is not a classical hallucinogen. In general, classical hallucinogens seem to be free of toxicity—but it is not known if this is the case, or whether this is simply because these agents have not been investigated for such. For example, various phenylisopropylamines are 5-HT_{2B} receptor agonists, but their cardiotoxicity has yet to be investigated.

SUMMARY

Classical or serotonergic hallucinogens consist of a very large class of agents (numbering in the hundreds) that possess an arylalkylamine (i.e., indolalkylamine or phenylalkylamine) structure. Not all arylalkylamines are hallucinogenic; some are devoid of this action, some are CNS stimulants, and yet others (depending on pendant substituents) are empathogens—with or without hallucinogenic character. The classical hallucinogens may or may not produce identical effects, but have in common the ability to bind at and (nearly all, with the exception of the harmala derivatives) activate 5-HT_{2A} serotonin receptors (79). Whereas phenylalkylamine hallucinogens are fairly selective in their affinity for 5-HT_{2A} receptors, indolalkylamine hallucinogens (due, perhaps, to their structural similarity to the endogenous neurotransmitter serotonin), bind at multiple populations of 5-HT receptors—particularly 5-HT_{1A} receptors. It might be the lack of 5-HT_2 selectivity of the latter that accounts for differences in the action of indolalkylamine versus phenylalkylamine hallucinogens. Moreover, certain hallucinogens (particularly the harmala derivatives and alpha-ET) also act as inhibitors of MAO. Structural modification of the arylalkylamines results in designer drugs that (again, depending on pendant substituents) possess or lack hallucinogenic character. A classification scheme (Fig. 14.3) has been proposed to account for the actions of these agents. Structural modification of arylalkylamines has resulted in the appearance of a variety of designer drugs on the clandestine market, and many, many more are theoretically possible. The most popular of the so-called designer drugs is MDMA. MDMA has been called an "empathogen" with some CNS stimulant properties. Although neither considered a classical hallucinogen nor a CNS stimulant, MDMA produces a number of central effects including mild central stimulation and mild euphoria, and its actions seem to involve the neurotransmitters serotonin, norepinephrine, and dopamine. (97,113, and subsequent articles). Certain actions of MDMA might be a result of its metabolic conversion to MDA. Substantial effort is required to further understand the actions of the arylalkylamines. Classical hallucinogens appear to act by activation of 5-HT_{2A} serotonin receptors (79) and although this hypothesis is nearly 25 years old, recent evidence suggests that it might be the functional selectivity of these agents for one effector system over others that accounts for their various actions.

ACKNOWLEDGMENT: *Work from the author's laboratory was supported by U.S. Public Health Service grant DA 01642.*

REFERENCES

1. Hollister LE. *Chemical psychoses.* Springfield, IL: Charles C Thomas, 1968.
2. Glennon RA. Classical hallucinogens. In: Schuster CR, Kuhar MJ, eds. *Pharmacological aspects of drug dependence.* Berlin, Germany: Springer, 1996:343–371.
3. Glennon RA. Pharmacology of hallucinogens. In: Tarter RE, Ammerman RA, and Ott PJ, eds. *Handbook of substance abuse. neurobehavioral pharmacology.* New York: Plenum Press, 1988:217–227.
4. Bruhn JG, De Smet PAGM, El-Seedi HR, et al. Mescaline use for 5,700 years. *Lancet* 2002;359:1866.
5. Hoffer A, Osmond H. *The hallucinogens.* New York: Academic Press, 1967:1–81.
6. Siva Sankar DV, ed. *LSD—a total study.* Westbury, NY: PJD Press, 1975.
7. Naranjo C. Psychotropic properties of harmala alkaloids. In Efron DK, Holmstedt B, and Kline NS, eds. *Ethnopharmacologic search for psychoactive drugs.* Washington DC: U.S. Government Printing Office, 1967:385–391.
8. Glennon RA. Animal models for assessing hallucinogenic agents. In Boulton AA, Baker GB, Wu PH, eds. *Animal models of drug addiction.* Totowa, NJ: Humana Press, 1992:345–381.
9. Strassman RJ. Human psychopharmacology of N,N-dimethyltryptamine. *Behav Brain Res* 1996;73(1–2):121–124.
10. Strassman R. *DMT: the spirit molecule.* Rochester, VT: Park Street Press, 2001.
11. Morris K Research on psychedelics moves into the mainstream. *Lancet* 2008;371:1491–1492.
12. Nichols DE, Oberlender R. Structure-activity relationships of MDMA-like substances. In Ashgar K, De Souza E, eds. *Pharmacology and toxicology of amphetamine and related designer drugs (NIDA research monograph 94).* Rockville, MD: National Institute on Drug Abuse, 1989:1–29.
13. Jacob P III, Shulgin AT. Structure-activity relationships of classical hallucinogens and their analogs. In: Lin LC, Glennon RA, eds. *Hallucinogens: an update (NIDA research monograph 146).* Rockville, MD: National Institute on Drug Abuse, 1994:74–91.
14. Shulgin AT, Shulgin A. *Pihkal.* Berkeley, CA: Transform Press, 1991.
15. Shulgin AT, Shulgin A. *Tihkal.* Berkeley, CA: Transform Press, 1997.
16. Brimblecombe RW, Pinder RM. *Hallucinogenic agents.* Bristol, UK: Wright-Scientechnica, 1975.
17. Gable RS. Risk assessment of ritual use of oral dimethyltryptamine (DMT) and harmala alkaloids. *Addiction* 2007;192:24–34.
18. Murphree HB, Dippy RH, Jenney EH, et al. Effects in normal man of alpha-methyltryptamine and alpha-ethyltryptamine. *Clin Pharmacol Therapeu* 1961;2:722–726.
19. Pfaff RC, Huang X, Marona-Lewicka D, et al. Lysergamides revisited. In Lin JC, Glennon RA, eds. *Hallucinogens: an update (NIDA research monograph 146).* Rockville, MD: National Institute on Drug Abuse, 1994:52–73.
20. Hoffer A, Osmond H. *The hallucinogens.* New York: Academic Press, 1967.
21. Pellerin C. *Trips.* New York: Seven Stories Press, 1998.
22. Naranjo C. *The healing journey.* New York: Pantheon Books, 1973.
23. Glennon RA, Dukat M, Grella B, et al. Binding of beta-carbolines and related agents at serotonin (5-HT_2 and 5-HT_{1A}), dopamine (D_2) and benzodiazepine receptors. *Drug Alcohol Depend* 2000;60:121–132.
24. Grella B, Dukat M, Young R, et al. Investigation of hallucinogenic and related beta-carbolines. *Drug Alcohol Depend* 1998;50:99–107.

25. Helsley S, Fiorella D, Rabin RA, et al. A comparison of N,Ndimethyltryptamine, harmaline, and selected congeners in rats trained with LSD as a discriminative stimulus. *Progr Neuropsychopharmacol Biol Psychiatry* 1998;22(4):649–663.
26. Helsley S, Rabin RA, Winter JC. The effects of beta-carbolines in rats trained with ibogaine as discriminative stimulus. *Eur J Pharmacol* 1998;345(2):139–143.
27. Nichols DE, Frescas S, Marona-Lewicka D, et al. 1-(2,5-Dimethoxy-4-(trifluoromethyl)phenyl)-2-aminopropane: a potent 5-$HT_{2A/2C}$ agonist. *J Med Chem* 1994;37:4346–4351.
28. Acuna-Castillo C, Villalobos C, Moya PR, et al. Differences in potency and efficacy of a series of phenylisopropylamine/penylethylamine pairs at 5-HT_{2A} and 5-HT_{2C} receptors. *Br J Pharmacol* 2002;136:510–519.
29. Nichols DE. Hallucinogens. *Pharmacol Therap* 2004;101:131–181.
30. Parrish JC, Braden MR, Gundy E, et al. Differential phospholipase C activation by phenylalkylamine serotonin 5-HT_{2A} receptor agonists. *J Neurochem* 2005;95:1575–1584.
31. McLean TH, Parrish JC, Braden MR, et al. 1-Aminomethylbenzocycloalkanes: conformationally restricted hallucinogenic phenethylamine analogues as functionally selective 5-HT_{2A} receptor agonists. *J Med Chem* 2006;49:5794–5803.
32. Moya PR, Berg KA, Gutierrez-Hernandez MA, et al. Functional selectivity of hallucinogenic phenethylamine and phylisopropylamine derivatives at human 5-hydroxytryptamine $(5\text{-HT})_{2A}$ and 5-HT_{2C} receptors. *J Pharmacol Exp Thera* 2007;321:1054–1061.
33. Lin DL, Liu HC, Yin HL. Recent paramethoxymethamphetamine (PMMA) deaths in Taiwan. *J Anal Toxicol* 2007;31:109–113.
34. Glennon RA. Synthesis and evaluation of amphetamine analogs. In Klein M, Sapienza F, McClain H, et al., eds. *Clandestinely produced drugs, analogues, and precursors.* Washington DC: U.S. Department of Justice, Drug Enforcement Administration, 1989:39–65.
35. Glennon RA. Discriminative stimulus properties of hallucinogens and related designer drugs. In Glennon RA, Jarbe TUC, and Frankenheim J, eds. *Drug discrimination: applications to drug abuse research (NIDA research monograph 116).* Rockville, MD: National Institute on Drug Abuse, 1991:25–44.
36. Nichols DE, Glennon RA (1984). Medicinal chemistry and structure activity relationships of hallucinogens. In Jacobs BL, ed. *Hallucinogens: neurochemical, behavioral, and clinical perspectives.* New York: Raven Press, 1984:95–142.
37. Young R, Glennon RA. A three-lever operant procedure differentiates the stimulus effects of R(−)-MDA from S(+)-MDA. *J Pharmacol Exp Therap* 1996;276:594–601.
38. Nichols DE. Differences between the mechanism of action of MDMA, MBDB, and the classical hallucinogens: identification of a new therapeutic class: entactogens. *J Psychoact Drugs* 1986;18:305–313.
39. Oberlender R, Nichols DE. (+)N-Methyl-1-(1,3-benzodioxol-5-yl)-2-butanamine as a discriminative stimulus in studies of 3,4-methylenedioxyamphetamine-like behavioral activity. *J Pharmacol Exp Therap* 1990;255:1098–1106.
40. Steele TD, Katz JL, Ricaurte GA. Evaluation of the neurotoxicity of N-methyl-1-(4-methoxyphenyl)-2-aminopropane (para-methoxymethamphetamine, PMMA). *Brain Res* 1992;589(2):349–352.
41. Glennon RA, Young R, Dukat M, et al. Initial characterization of PMMA as a discriminative stimulus. *Pharmacol Biochem Behav* 1997;57:151–158.
42. Rangisetty JB, Bondarev ML, Chang-Fong J, et al. PMMA-stimulus generalization to the optical isomers of MBDB and 3,4-DMA. *Pharmacol Biochem Behav* 2001;69:261–267.
43. Glennon RA, Young R. Effect of 1-(3,4-methylenedioxyphenyl)-2-aminopropane and its optical isomers in PMMA-trained rats. *Pharmacol Biochem Behav* 2002;72:379–387.
44. Dukat M, Young R, Glennon RA. Effect of PMA optical isomers and 4-MTA in PMMA-trained rats. *Pharmacol Biochem Behav* 2002;72:299–305.
45. Glennon RA. Arylalkylamine drugs of abuse: an overview of drug discrimination studies. *Pharmacol Biochem Behav* 1999;64:251–256.
46. Martinez DL, Geyer MA. Characterization of the disruptions of prepulse inhibition and habituation of startle induced by alphaethyltryptamine. *Neuropsychopharmacology* 1997;16:246–255.
47. Glennon RA, Young R. MDMA stimulus generalization to the 5-HT_{1A} serotonin agonist 8-hydroxy-2-(di-*n*-propylamino)tetralin. *Pharmacol Biochem Behav* 2000;66(3):483–488.
48. Barker SA, Littlefield-Chabaud MA, David C. Distribution of the hallucinogens N,N-dimethyltryptamine and 5-methoxy-N,N-dimethyltryptamine in rat brain following intraperitoneal injection: application of a new solid-phase extraction LC-APcI-MS-MS-isotope dilution method. *J Chromatogr B Biomed Scient Appl* 2001;751(1):37–47.
49. Zweig JS, Castagnoli N. In vitro O-demethylation of the psychotomimetic amine 1-(2,5-dimethoxy-4-methylphenyl)-2-aminopropane. *J Med Chem* 1977;20:414–419.
50. Eckler JR, Chang-Fong J, Rabin RA, et al. Behavioral characterization of 2-O-desmethyl and 5-O-desmethyl metabolites of the phenylethylamine hallucinogen DOM. *Pharmacol Biochem Behav* 2003;75(4):845–852.
51. Ewald AH, Fritschi G, Bork WR, et al. Designer drugs 2,5-dimethoxy-4-bromo-amphetamine (DOB) and 2,5-dimethoxy-4-bromo-methamphetamine (MDOB): studies on their metabolism and toxicological detection in rat urine using gas chromatographic/mass spectrometric techniques. *J Mass Spectrom* 2006;41(4):487–498.
52. Beránková K, Szkutová M, Balíková M. Distribution profile of 2,5-dimethoxy-4-bromoamphetamine (DOB) in rats after oral and subcutaneous doses. *Forensic Sci Int* 2007;170(2–3):94–99.
53. Ewald AH, Fritschi G, Maurer HH. Metabolism and toxicological detection of the designer drug 4-iodo-2,5-dimethoxy-amphetamine (DOI) in rat urine using gas chromatography-mass spectrometry. *J Chrom B Analyt Tech Biomed Life Sci* 2007;857(1):170–174.
54. Wu D, Otton V, Inaba T, et al. Interactions of amphetamine analogs with human liver CYP2D6. *Biochem Pharmacol* 1997;53:1605–1612.
55. Maurer HH, Bickeboeller-Friedrich J, Kraemer T, et al. Toxicokinetics and analytical toxicology of amphetamine-derived designer drugs ('Ecstasy'). *Toxicol Letts* 2000;112–113:133–142.
56. Segura M, Ortuno J, Farre M, et al. 3,4-Dihydroxymethamphetamine (HHMA). A major in vivo 3,4-methylenedioxymethamphetamine (MDMA) metabolite in humans. *Chem Res Toxicol* 2001;14:1203–1208.
57. Strassman RJ, Qualls CR, Berg LM. Differential tolerance to biological and subjective effects of four closely spaced doses of N,N-dimethyltryptamine in humans. *Biol Psychiatry* 1996;39(9):784–795.
58. Vollenweider FX, Vontobel P, Hell D, et al. 5-HT modulation of dopamine release in basal ganglia in psilocybin-induced psychosis in man—A PET study with $[^{11}C]$raclopride. *Neuropsychopharmacology* 1999;20:425–433.
59. Hasler P, Bourquin D, Brenneisen R, et al. Determination of psilocin and 4-hydroxyindole-3-acetic acid in plasma by HPLC-ECD and pharmacokinetic profiles or oral and intravenous psilocybin in man. *Pharma Acta Helv* 1997;72:175–184.
60. Vollenweider FX, Vollenweider-Scherpenhuyzen MF, Babler A, et al. Psylocybin induces schizophrenia-like psychosis in humans via a serotonin-2 agonist action. *Neuroreport* 1998 9:3897–3902.
61. Gouzoulis-Mayfrank E, Thelen B, Habermeyer E, et al. Psychopathological, neuroendocrine and autonomic effects of 3,4-methylenedioxyethylamphetamine (MDE), psilocybin and d-methamphetamine in healthy volunteers. Results of an experimental double-blind placebo-controlled study. *Psychopharmacology (Berlin)* 1999;142(1):41–50.
62. Gouzoulis-Mayfrank E, Schreckenberger M, Sabri O, et al. Neurometabolic effects of psilocybin, 3,4-methylenedioxyethylamphetamine (MDE) and d-methamphetamine in healthy volunteers. A double-blind, placebo-controlled PET study with [18F]FDG. *Neuropsychopharmacology* 1999;20(6):565–581.
63. Gouzoulis-Mayfrank E, Thelen B, Maier S, et al. Effects of the hallucinogen psilocybin on covert orienting of visual attention in humans. *Neuropsychobiology* 2002;45(4):205–212.
64. Hasler F, Grimberg U, Benz MA, et al. Acute psychological and physiological effects of psilocybin in healthy humans: a double-blind, placebo-controlled dose-effect study. *Psychopharmacology (Berlin)* 2004;172(2):145–156.

65. Carter OL, Pettigrew JD, Hasler F, et al. Modulating the rate and rhythmicity of perceptual rivalry alternations with the mixed 5-HT_{2A} and 5-HT_{1A} agonist psilocybin. *Neuropsychopharmacology* 2005;30(6): 1154–1162.
66. Griffiths RR, Richards WA, McCann U, et al. Psilocybin can occasion mystical-type experiences having substantial and sustained personal meaning and spiritual significance. *Psychopharmacology (Berlin)* 2006;187(3):268–283.
67. Wittmann M, Carter O, Hasler F, et al. Effects of psilocybin on time perception and temporal control of behaviour in humans. *J Psychopharmacol* 2007;21(1):50–64.
68. Hollister LE, Hartman AM. Mescaline, lysergic acid diethylamide and psilocybin: comparison of clinical syndromes, effects on color perception and biochemical measures. *Comp Psychiatry* 1962;3:235–241.
69. Hollister LE, Sjoberg BM Clinical syndromes and biochemical alterations following mescaline, lysergic acid diethylamide and psilocybin. *Comp Psychiatry* 1964;5:170–178.
70. Halpern JH, Sherwood AR, Hudson JI, et al. Psychological and cognitive effects of long-term peyote use among native Americans. *Biol Psychiatry* 2005;58:624–631.
71. Liechti ME, Saur MR, Gamma A, et al. Psychological and physiological effects of MDMA ("Ecstasy") after pretreatment with the 5-HT_2 antagonist ketanserin in healthy humans. *Neuropsychopharmacology* 2000;23: 396–404.
72. Vollenweider, FX, Gamma A, Liechti M, et al. Psychological and cardiovascular effects and short-term sequelae of MDMA ("Ecstasy") in MDMA-naïve healthy volunteers. *Neuropsychopharmacology* 1998;19: 241–251.
73. Cami J, Farre M, Mas M, et al. Human pharmacology of 3,4-methylenedioxymethamphetamine ("ecstasy") psychomotor performance and subjective effects. *Clin Psychopharmacol* 2000;20(4):455–466.
74. Green RA, Mechan OA, Elliott JM, et al. The pharmacology and clinical pharmacology of 3,4-methylenedioxymethamphetamine (MDMA, "Ecstasy"). *Pharmacol Rev* 2003;55:463–508.
75. Halpern JH, Pope HG Jr. Hallucinogens on the internet: a vast new source of underground drug information. *Am J Psychiatry* 2001;158(3): 481–483.
76. Glennon RA, Jarbe TUC, Frankenheim J, eds. *Drug discrimination: applications to drug abuse research (NIDA research monograph 116).* Rockville, MD: National Institute on Drug Abuse, 1991.
77. Colpaert FC, Slangen JL, eds. *Drug discrimination: applications in CNS pharmacology.* Amsterdam, The Netherlands: Elsevier, 1982.
78. Appel JB, White FJ, Holohean AM. Analyzing mechanism(s) of hallucinogenic drug action with drug discrimination procedures. *Neurosci Biobehav Rev* 1982 6(4):529–536.
79. Glennon RA, Titeler M, McKenney JD. Evidence for 5-HT_2 involvement in the mechanism of action of hallucinogenic agents. *Life Sci* 1984;35:2505–2511.
80. Nelson DL, Lucaites VL, Wainscot DB, et al. Comparisons of hallucinogenic phenylisopropylamine binding affinities at cloned human 5-HT_{2A}, 5-HT_{2B}, and 5-HT_{2C} receptors. *Naunyn Schmiedebergs Arch Pharmacol* 1999;359:1–6.
81. Ismaiel AM, De Los Angeles J, Teitler M, et al. Antagonism of 1-(2,5-dimethoxy-4-methylphenyl)-2-aminopropane stimulus with a newly identified 5-HT_2- versus 5-HT_{1C}-selective antagonist. *J Med Chem* 1993;36:2519–2525.
82. Schreiber R, Brocco M, Millan MJ. Blockade of the discriminative stimulus effects of DOI by MDL 100,907 and the "atypical" antipsychotics, clozapine and risperidone. *Eur J Pharmacol* 1994;264(1): 99–102.
83. Fiorella D, Rabin RA, Winter JC. The role of the 5-HT_{2A} and 5-HT_{2C} receptors in the stimulus effects of hallucinogenic drugs. I: antagonist correlation analysis. *Psychopharmacology (Berlin)* 1995;121(3):347–356.
84. Rabin RA, Doat M, Winter JC. Role of serotonergic 5-HT_{2A} receptors in the psychotomimetic actions of phencyclidine. *Int J Neuropsychopharmacol* 2000; 3:333–338.
85. Free RB, Hazelwood LA, Namkung Y, et al. Synaptic transmission: Intracellular signaling. In: Sibley DR, Hanin I, Kuhar M, et al., eds. *Handbook of contemporary neuropharmacology.* John Wiley & Sons, Hoboken, NJ 2007:59–106.
86. Roth BL, Berry SA, Kroeze WK, et al. Serotonin 5-HT_{2A} receptors: molecular biology and mechanism of regulation. *Crit Rev Neurobiol* 1998;12:319–338.
87. Garcia EE, Smith RL, Sabders-Bush E. Role of G_q protein in the behavioral effects of the hallucinogenic drug 1-(2,5-dimethoxy-4-iodophenyl)-2-aminopropane. *Neuropharmacology* 2007;52:1671– 1677.
88. Berg KA, Maayani S, Goldfarb J, et al. Effector pathway-dependent relative efficacy at serotonin type 2A and 2C receptors: Evidence for agonist-directed trafficking of receptor stimulus. *Mol Pharmacol* 1998;54: 94–104.
89. Kenakin T. Agonist-receptor efficacy II: agonist trafficking of receptor signals. *Trends Pharmacol Sci* 1995;16:232–238.
90. Kurrasch-Orbaugh DM, Watts VJ, Barker EL, et al. Serotonin 5-hydroxytryptamine$_{2A}$ receptor-coupled phospholipase C and phospholipase A2 signaling pathways have different receptor reserves. *J Pharmacol Exp Therap* 2003;304:229–237.
91. Gonzalez-Maeso J, Weisstaub NV, Zhou M, et al. Hallucinogens recruit specific cortical 5-HT_{2A} receptor-mediated signaling pathways to affect behavior. *Neuron* 2007;53:439–452.
92. Shi J, Damjanoska J, Singh RK, et al. Agonist induced-phosphorylation of $G_{\alpha 11}$ protein reduces coupling to 5-HT_{2A} receptors. *J Pharmacol Exp Therap* 2007;322:248–256.
93. McClean TH, Parrish JC, Braden MR, et al. 1-Aminomethylbenzocycloalkanes: conformationally restricted hallucinogenic phenethylamine analogues as functionally selective 5-HT_{2A} receptor agonists. *J Med Chem* 2006;46:5794–5803.
94. Setola V, Hufeisen SJ, Grande-Allen KJ, et al. 3,4-methylenedioxymethamphetamine (MDMA, "Ecstasy") induces fenfluramine-like proliferative actions on human cardiac valvular interstitial cells in vitro. *Mol Pharmacol* 2003;63(6):1223–1229.
95. Beardsley PM, Balster RL, Harris LS. Self-administration of methylenedioxymethamphetamine (MDMA) by rhesus monkeys. *Drug Alcohol Depend* 1986;18:149–157.
96. Lamb R, Griffiths RR. Self-injections of d-3,4-methylenedioxymethamphetamine (MDMA) in the baboon. *Psychopharmacology* 1987; 91:268–272.
97. Marona-Lewicka D, Rhee GS, Sprague JE, et al. Reinforcing effects of serotonin-releasing amphetamine derivatives. *Pharmacol Biochem Behav* 1996;53:99–105.
98. De La Garza R, Miczek KA. Editorial: a contemporary view of MDMA. *Psychopharmacology* 2007;189:403–405. (Plus subsequent articles in this special issue [volume 189, issue 4) devoted to MDMA, including its self-administration and neurotoxicity.)
99. Griffiths RR, Winger G, Brady JV, et al. Comparison of behavior maintained by infusions of eight phenylethylamines in baboons. *Psychopharmacologia* 1976;24:251–258.
100. Markert LE, Roberts DCS. 3,4-Methylenedioxy amphetamine (MDA) self-administration and neurotoxicity. *Pharmacol Biochem Behav* 1991; 39:569–574.
101. Fletcher PJ, Robinson SR, Slippoy DL. Pre-exposure to 3,4- methylenedioxymethamphetamine (MDMA) facilitates acquisition of intravenous cocaine self-administration in rats. *Neuropsychopharmacology* 2001;25: 195–203.
102. Slone AL, O'Btien MS, De La Torre A, et al. Who is becoming hallucinogen dependent soon after hallucinogen use starts? *Drug Alcohol Depend* 2007;87:153–163.
103. Dumont GJ, Verkes RJ A review of the acute effects of 3,4-methylenedioxymethamphetamine in healthy volunteers. *J Psychopharmacol* 2006;20(2):176–187.
104. Allott K, Redman J. Are there sex differences associated with the effects of ecstasy/3,4-methylenedioxymethamphetamine (MDMA)? *Neurosci Biobehav Rev* 2007;31(3):327–347.
105. Curran HV. Is MDMA ('Ecstasy') neurotoxic in humans? An overview of evidence and of methodological problems in research. *Neuropsychobiology* 2000;42:34–41.
106. Gibb JW, Johnson M, Elayan I, et al. Neurotoxicity of amphetamines and their metabolites. In: Rapaka RS, Chiang N, Martin BR, eds.

Pharmacokinetics, metabolism, and pharmaceutics of drugs of abuse (NIDA research monograph 173). Rockville, MD: National Institute on Drug Abuse, 1997:128–145.

107. Kalant H. The pharmacology and toxicology of "ecstasy" (MDMA) and related drugs. *Can Med Assoc J* 2001;165:917–928.
108. Morgan MJ. Ecstasy (MDMA): a review of its possible persistent psychological effects. *Psychopharmacology* 2000;152:230–248.
109. Seiden LS, Sabol KE. Methamphetamine and methylenedioxymethamphetamine: possible mechanisms of cell destruction. In: Majewska, MD, ed. *Neuropathology and neurotoxicity associated with cocaine/stimulant abuse (NIDA research monograph 163)*. Rockville, MD: National Institute on Drug Abuse, 1996:251–276.
110. Ricaurte GA, McCann UD, Szabo Z, et al. Toxicodynamics and long-term toxicity of the recreational drug, 3,4-methylenedioxymethamphetamine (MDMA, "Ecstasy"). *Toxicol Lett* 2000;112–113:143–146.
111. Bai F, Jones DC, Lau SS, et al. Serotonergic neurotoxicity of 3,4-methylenedioxyamphetamine and 3,4-methylendioxymethamphetamine (ecstasy) is potentiated by inhibition of gamma-glutamyl transpeptidase. *Chem Res Toxicol* 2001;14(7):863–870.
112. Baumann MH, Wang X, Rothman RB. 3,4-Methylenedioxymethamphetamine (MDMA) neurotoxicity in rats: a reappraisal of past and present findings. *Psychopharmacology* 2007;189:407–424.
113. Silins A, Copeland I, Dillon P. Qualitative review of serotonin syndrome, ecstasy (MDMA) and the use of other serotonergic substances: hierarchy of risk. *Aust N Z J Psychiatry* 2007;41(8):649–655.
114. Green RA. MDMA: fact and fallacy, and the need to increase knowledge in both the scientific and popular press. *Psychopharmacology* 2004;173:231–233.
115. Droogmans S, Cosyns B, D'haenen H, et al. Possible association between 3,4-methylenedioxymethamphetamine abuse and valvular heart disease. *Am J Cardiol* 2007;100:1442–1445.

CHAPTER 15

Edward F. Domino, MD
Shannon C. Miller, MD
FASAM, FAPA, CMRO

The Pharmacology of Dissociatives

DEFINITION (DRUGS IN THIS CLASS)

Several heterogeneous chemicals are antagonists of the N-methyl-D-aspartate (NMDA) receptor subtype of the major excitatory neurotransmitter, glutamic acid, in the brain. Termed *dissociatives*, these substances can be distinguished pharmacologically and clinically from true hallucinogens (see Chapter 14). A simplified view suggests that dissociatives and hallucinogens share common features; however, hallucinogens affect primarily the 5HT2a receptor instead of the NMDA receptor, and hallucinogens are associated with a somewhat different clinical syndrome of intoxication (whereby dissociation or impaired reality testing is less typically involved, and visual hallucinations are more commonly involved). Dissociatives include various arylcyclohexylamines (of which phencyclidine and ketamine are best known), dizocilpine (MK-80l), dextromethorphan, and, perhaps surprisingly, the gaseous anesthetic, nitrous oxide. Ketamine and nitrous oxide are used clinically in animals and humans as general anesthetics, usually in combination with other agents. Dextromethorphan is used clinically as an antitussive in more than 100 over-the-counter cough preparations.

Most of the known NMDA antagonists are drugs of abuse when used in subanesthetic doses/concentrations. Subanesthetic doses of phencyclidine and ketamine induce a psychotomimetic state, which resembles many but not all of the signs and symptoms of schizophrenia (1). Dextromethorphan (DXM) in large doses is readily metabolized to dextrorphan (DXO), a significant NMDA-antagonist pharmacodynamically akin to phencyclidine and ketamine. An emerging drug of abuse, DXM was reviewed in detail in 2005 (2). Nitrous oxide or "laughing gas" has not yet been classified as a psychotomimetic. Its euphoric and dysphoric properties have been known for more than 200 years, but have not been well studied.

This chapter reviews the known pharmacology of these diverse substances, which have multiple mechanisms of action, primarily including NMDA receptor antagonism. The pharmacology of hallucinogens and other drugs capable of producing psychoses is discussed in greater detail in their respective chapters in this section. The specific treatment of dissociative intoxication and withdrawal states is discussed in Section 6 of this book.

SUBSTANCES INCLUDED IN THIS CLASS

The chemical structures of abused arylcyclohexylamines are shown in Figure 15.1. Phencyclidine (PCP) and ketamine are the principal abused illicit compounds. DXM is the principal abused over-the-counter compound. Ketamine is a racemic mixture of its D- and L-isomers. The (S)-isomer is more potent and is claimed to have less clinical dysphoric effects. Other members of this class that are less commonly abused include cyclohexamine (N-ethyl-1-phenylcyclohexylamine, CI, 400), 1-(1-2-thienylcyclohexyl) piperidine, 1-(1-phenylcyclohexyl) pyrrolidine, and 4-methyl pip PCP (1-(phenylcyclohexyl)-4-methylpiperidine). Dextromethorphan (DM, DXM, D-3-methoxy-N-methylmorphinan) is the D-isomer of a codeine analogue, methorphan. In contrast to the L-isomer, which is an opioid analgesic, dextromethorphan is not.

FIGURE 15.1. Chemical structures of major abused drugs of this class.

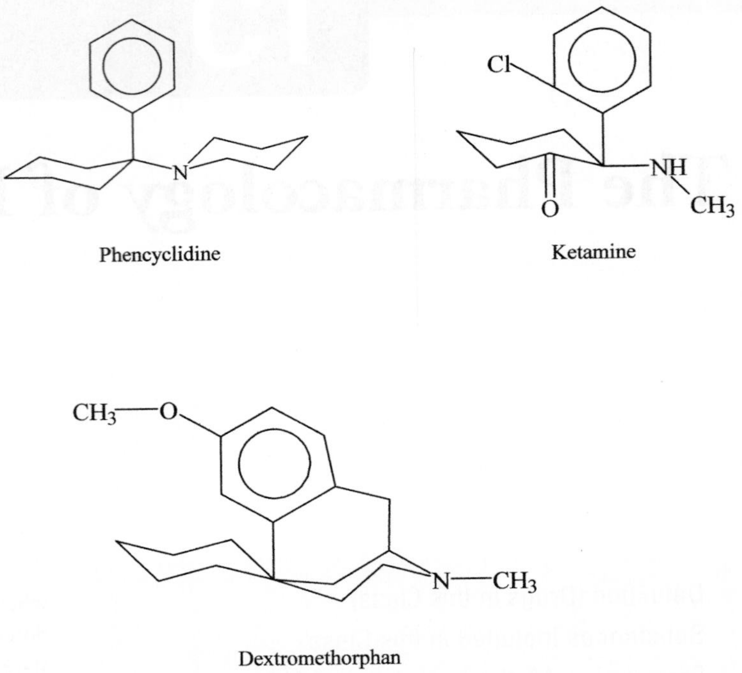

Phencyclidine

Ketamine

Dextromethorphan

FORMULATION, METHODS OF USE AND ABUSE

U.S. Food and Drug Administration–approved Formulations Ketamine is available as a sterile solution in 10-mL bottles for use in general anesthesia in both animals and humans as a Schedule III substance. It has also been used for prehospital analgesia and anesthesia (3) and conscious sedation (4). It is used most often in children, who appear less susceptible than adults to emergent delirium (5). In medical settings, it is injected intravenously or intramuscularly in doses of 0.1 to 1.0 mg/kg, depending on its clinical use. However, it is also effective when insufflated, smoked, or taken orally. It is abused by various routes in different doses. Doses of ketamine as large as 900 to 1,000 mg given intravenously or intramuscularly are lethal.

PCP is no longer available as a medical commercial preparation approved by the U.S. Food and Drug Administration (FDA). It is available in many illicit preparations in various forms and is used in a wide range of doses. It has many of the pharmacologic effects of ketamine, but is more potent, longer acting, and more likely to produce seizures. Doses of only 120 mg of PCP may cause death. It has been used as a general anesthetic in animals. It is prepared illegally in various forms: powder, tablets, and liquid (salt in water, base in ether). The latter are typically sprayed onto plant leaves such as ginger, marijuana, mint, oregano, or parsley and then smoked. PCP and some of its congeners are Schedule I substances.

Legal DXM preparations are administered orally. They are usually available as dextromethorphan hydrobromide and less as dextromethorphan polistirex. Capsules, tablets, lozenges, or solutions of dextromethorphan hydrobromide are available alone or in combination with many other substances as cough, cold, and flu relief preparations. The usual antitussive dosage for adults is 10 to 20 mg every 4 hours or 30 mg every 6 to 8 hours, not to exceed 120 mg daily. Extended release forms are given as 60 mg twice daily. Larger doses of DXM are abused for their mental effects. Fortunately, dextromethorphan has a low toxicity. Death is usually unlikely in doses much greater than therapeutic doses. However, deaths have been reported. Moreover, the additional ingredients in over-the-counter preparations make for additional hazards: decongestant/pseudoephedrine (causing cardiac toxicity), antihistamine/chlorpheniramine (antihistamine toxicity), pain/acetaminophen (liver toxicity), and bromides (bromide toxicity). Serotonin syndrome has also been reported (2). Lastly, death from behavioral impairment has been reported—such as drowning while intoxicated and dissociating (6).

HISTORICAL FEATURES

The discovery of phencyclidine, or PCP, has been well documented by those involved with its therapeutic development (7). The drug was developed as an intravenous anesthetic. The unique anesthesia it produced was complicated by a prolonged emergence delirium; this quickly led to its demise as a clinically useful agent. PCP is associated with symptoms that model both the positive (delusions, hallucinations) and negative (blunted affect, ambivalence, asociality, autistic-like effects) symptoms of schizophrenia, making for perhaps one of the more useful pharmacologic models of schizophrenia (8). Its trade name was Sernyl or Semylan. Years later, PCP was rediscovered by the drug abuse community in the form of "PCP," "angel dust," "hog," and "crystal" (9). It is now also known as "Chuck Norris," "Hulk Hogan," and "riding the imaginary leprechaun," among others.

The desirable anesthetic properties of Sernyl were retained in the short-acting arylcyclohexylamine derivative ketamine (Ketalar, Ketanest, and Ketaset), which produced a much briefer emergence delirium. The term *dissociative anesthetic* was coined to emphasize that the anesthetized patient was psychologically "disconnected" from his or her environment. Ketamine subsequently was discovered by the drug abuse community, where it is known as "K," "super K," "special K," and "cat Valium," among others. Ketamine also has the perception among users as being medically safe to use because it is made and packaged by pharmaceutical companies, most often for veterinary use (10).

Arylcyclohexylamine abuse occurs primarily in large metropolitan areas. Because the drugs are easy to synthesize, they are relatively inexpensive substitutes for many street drugs. The user may not realize that he or she has used an arylcyclohexylamine, because the drugs frequently are misrepresented as LSD, amphetamine, or synthetic marijuana. Moreover, they may be added to marijuana by the user to enhance marijuana's desired effects.

In contrast to the arylcyclohexylamines, MK-801 (dizocilpine) was developed as an anticonvulsant (11) and subsequently was used as a brain protective agent; however, it was discarded because of its PCP-like effects (12). Clinical trials of MK-801 have been extremely limited, and the results are not publicly available. Very little is known of its properties in humans.

The history of DXM begins with the synthesis of racemethorphan (deoxydihydrothebaiodine) or methorphan, and its patent to Hoffmann-LaRoche in 1954 as an opioid analgesic. After the D- and L-isomers were isolated, it was discovered that the D-isomer was antitussive and had less analgesic and narcotic-like properties. Compared with codeine as an antitussive, DXM was nearly equal. However, unlike codeine, DXM is fairly devoid of other opioid effects such as analgesia, central nervous system depression, and respiratory suppression. Although it is metabolized to DXO, an NMDA receptor antagonist, its binding sites in the brain are distributed beyond the NMDA receptor. DXM's mechanism in low doses as an antitussive is unknown. In doses of typically 300 to 1,800 mg (20 to 120 times the recommended dose), DXM produces PCP-like mental effects (13,14). However, larger doses (237 times the recommended dose) have been reported as regularly abused (15). DXM abuse has been a concern since at least the 1960s. The over-the-counter tablet form of DXM, Romilar, was replaced by a cough syrup to attempt to reduce its recreational use in 1973. In 1990, the FDA Drug Abuse Advisory Committee assessed DXM use by teenagers and recommended against placing the drug on the Controlled Drug Schedule, but desired more study of the problem (16). Although abuse of DXM began originally with abuse of liquid cough syrup (known to hamper the abuse of large doses of DXM because of the distasteful nature of cough syrup), more convenient consumer products have been developed to include both high-dose (30 mg) tablets as well as high-dose gel capsules—eventually being found as preferable to those whom abuse DXM. Moreover, a free-base extraction technique has since been developed by users of the cough syrup (17). DXM has recently become popular, particularly in children and adolescents, owing to this population incorrectly perceiving DXM as a "SMART" choice of drugs to abuse, because they perceive DXM abuse as without *stigma*, not costing much *money* to procure, having easy *access* at local stores, being devoid of medical *risks*, and not included in routine employment or home-based drug *testing* (18). The FDA has continued to express its concern over the abuse of DXM, in particular the purified powder form purchased via the Internet (19). Slang terms of the cough medicine preparations are "dex," "robo," "skittles" (owing to some tablets appearance being akin to red Skittles candies), "tussin," and "triple Cs." Recreational use of DXM can be described as "dexing," "roboing," and "robotripping" (referring to the popular DXM cough syrup Robitussin).

Nitrous oxide has been known for more than 226 years. It is widely used today in anesthesia. In addition, its recreational use as "laughing gas" has been well described since it first was discovered. Ketamine and nitrous oxide still are medically used in humans as anesthetic agents. Ketamine is used in circumstances in which other anesthetic agents are relatively contraindicated. In contrast, nitrous oxide is widely used today as part of the mixture of anesthetics used to achieve "balanced anesthesia."

The desirable "brain protective" properties of NMDA antagonists, including DXM, have been pursued slightly by the pharmaceutical industry in developing relatively weak derivatives of amantadine, and other so-called sigma agonists and antagonists. For example, amantadine is an antiviral agent used in the prophylaxis and therapy of influenza A and to treat parkinsonism. Patients with Parkinson's disease who took amantadine reported that it improved their motor symptoms. The mechanism of action of amantadine is unclear, but may include dopamine release or blockade of its reuptake and possible muscarinic anticholinergic action. Amantadine and a related compound, memantadine, have been shown to be NMDA receptor antagonists (20), but are relatively weak and do not appear to be abused.

EPIDEMIOLOGY

PCP abuse appears to be more of a problem in large cities such as Houston, Los Angeles, Philadelphia, and Washington, DC, compared with the rest of the United States (21). Five percent of emergency department major drug abuse reports in the city of Houston between January and June 2006 were related to PCP abuse. Relative to other drugs of abuse, PCP does not appear to be a major problem in any of the Community Epidemiology Working Group (CEWG) areas. According to Drug Abuse Warning Network data, since 1999, PCP-related emergency room visits have increased 109% (from 3,663 to 7,648) with increases from 2000 to 2002 of 42% (from 5,404). Long-term Drug Abuse Warning Network trends show that PCP visits began increasing in 1999 at about the same time that LSD visits began a sharp decline. Among the 21 metropolitan areas represented in Drug Abuse Warning Network; Washington, DC, and Philadelphia had the highest rates of PCP-related emergency room visits. Nationally, patients in PCP-related emergency department visits were more likely to be male than female (22), which is also supported in the National Survey on Drug Use and Health (23).

Ketamine has often been considered as typically used with other drugs (24); however, sole use of ketamine has been reported (10). Although ketamine has often been self-administered by insufflation, other data suggest an emerging problem in youth of injecting ketamine. Importantly, such youth may be more likely to engage in multiple injections, shared bottles of ketamine, and use of syringes obtained from secondary sources—practices that increase risk for hepatitis C, HIV, and other infectious diseases (25).

DXM is considered one of the most commonly abused over-the-counter medications in the United States. The proportion of U.S. students who reported having used DXM during the prior year for the expressed purpose of "getting high" was 4%, 5%, and 7% in grades 8, 10, and 12, respectively (26). There is an increasing trend of DXM abuse in older adults (27,28), and particularly in adolescents (29). Cases of DXM abuse reported to the California Poison Control System increased 10-fold in all age groups and 15-fold in adolescents between 1999 and 2004. The average effect was an almost 50% increase in the frequency of reported cases each year. Similar trends were seen in national databases. Approximately 75% of California cases were ages 9 to 17 years old. The highest frequency of abuse was in 15 to 16 year olds. The most commonly abused DXM product was Coricidin HBP Cough & Cold Tablets. The extent of DXM abuse is likely far greater than what has been reported, because only the most severe cases are reported into the poison control databases, and nearly all routine drug screening kits do not screen or test for DXM or DXO. Studies of DXM in blood samples of suspected impaired drivers in the state of Wisconsin between 1999 and 2005 support an increasing prevalence of DXM-positive drivers, with a mean concentration of 207 ng/mL—compared with an expected therapeutic concentration range of 0.5 to 5.9 ng/mL (with the highest concentrations being in males ages 16 to 20 years) (30).

PHARMACOKINETICS

The pharmacokinetics of PCP in humans have never been well studied with psychoactive doses using modern methods (31). Blood PCP concentrations from 7 ng/mL to 240 ng/mL (mean, 75) were found in arrested persons intoxicated in public or driving under its influence. The blood/plasma concentration ratio is 1. The plasma half-life ($t_{1/2}$) of PCP has been reported to vary from 7 to 46 hours, suggesting that dose or the alpha and beta $t_{1/2}$s are involved. Terminal gamma $t_{1/2}$s of 1 to 4 days have been reported in cases of severe phencyclidine poisoning. PCP is biotransformed in the liver to several metabolites and excreted in the urine as both free and glucuronide conjugates. Acidification of the urine increases its renal clearance because PCP is a base; however, the clinical utility of this is no longer recommended because of the risk of increasing urinary myoglobin precipitation (32).

Ketamine exists as the (S)- and (R)-enantiomers in combination, which is how it usually is available in the United States. (S)-Ketamine in vitro has a lower inhibition constant for the NMDA receptor and a higher one for the sigma-binding site than does (R)-ketamine. (S)-Ketamine is available as the preferred intravenous anesthetic, especially in Germany, and there is some evidence of its superior analgesic potency. From a practical clinical point of view, the separate enantiomers have properties that are grossly similar to those of the racemic mixture. Thus the pharmacology of ketamine is that of the mixture. The fact that ketamine is more lipophilic than phencyclidine accounts for its rapid onset, short anesthetic duration of action, and shorter period of emergence delirium. Plasma concentrations of ketamine vary widely depending on the dose, route, and time elapsed since administration. Anesthetic doses produce plasma or serum concentrations of 1 mg/mL to 6.3 ng/mL.

Nonanesthetic psychoactive blood concentrations of ketamine are in the low nanogram per milliliter range. Ketamine has at least two plasma $t_{1/2}$s when it is given intravenously: a beta $t_{1/2}$ of 3 to 4 hours has been reported, but it has a much shorter alpha $t_{1/2}$ of about 7 minutes because of rapid redistribution. As used in general anesthesia, an intravenous dose of 2.0 mg/kg produces rapid induction. This dose produces an onset in 30 seconds, with the coma lasting for 8 to 10 minutes. The intramuscular injection of ketamine has a latency of 3 to 5 minutes and a duration of 10 to 20 minutes or more, depending on the dose administered.

DXM is readily absorbed from the gut. Peak serum levels are reached at 2 to 3 hours for immediate release, 6 hours for sustained release preparations. DXO levels peak at 1.6 to 7 hours (33). Humans have a genetic polymorphism for the biotransformation of DXM (31). Rapid metabolizers have a plasma elimination $t_{1/2}$ of about 3.4 hours and slow metabolizers may have $t_{1/2}$'s exceeding 24 hours. Slow metabolizers of DXM represent about 10% to 15% of the population. Both O- and N-demethylation to DXO occur. The latter is also an antitussive. Subsequent biotransformation results in various, less active compounds, both free and conjugated. Phenotypic "slow" metabolizers of DXM report fewer intoxication effects than normal subjects (34). Thus clinically slow metabolizers might be at higher risk for developing DXM dependence/addiction (2).

PHARMACODYNAMICS

Depending on the dose and specific arylcyclohexylamine ingested, patients who have taken PCP or ketamine present with widely different neurologic and psychiatric signs and symptoms. These signs and symptoms can be generally subdivided into three major clinical pictures, including confusion,

TABLE 15.1 Dose-Related Effects of Phencyclidine in Normal Subjects

Total dose by intravenous infusion mg/kg:	**1 mg** 0.014	**2 mg** 0.03	**7 mg** 0.10	**7–10 mg** 0.20	**14 mg** 0.20	**17.5 mg** 0.25	**35 mg** 0.50	**70 mg** 1.0
Acute effects								
Subjective effects	+	+						
Nystagmus			+					
Gait ataxia			+					
Increased blood pressure			+					
Confusional state				+				
Theta slowing (electroencephalogram)			−	±	+	+	+	+
Anesthesia-analgesia (loss of consciousness, no response to painful or auditory stimuli)					−			
Amnesia						+	+	+
Purposeless movements (state of agitation)							+	
Muscle rigidity and extensor posturing (severe rigidity and catatonia)								+
Seizure activity								+
Respiration depression								−

Data summarized by Burns & Lerner in Domino EF, ed. *Phencyclidine: historical and current perspectives.* Ann Arbor, MI: NPP Books, 1981:450.

delirium, and psychosis; semicoma and coma; and coma with seizures. One can observe patients becoming progressively more obtunded and eventually comatose—or the reverse when the patient is emerging from coma and showing emergence delirium. Table 15.1 lists the various clinical correlates of PCP signs and symptoms at different blood levels. Figure 15.2 further correlates the molecular target sites with doses, concentrations, and clinical effects (35). Most PCP abusers do not grossly overdose themselves to the point of semicoma and coma. Hence most patients intoxicated with PCP show a clinical picture of confusion, delirium, and psychosis. Rats show marked behavioral sensitization to both PCP and MK-801 with asymmetric cross-sensitization (36–38). However, the significance of this phenomenon for humans is unknown. Whether individuals who abuse PCP or ketamine show enhanced psychotomimetic effects over time is unknown. Tolerance occurs with PCP, and to a greater degree with continuous dosing (39). Animal models show severe withdrawal with PCP exposure: vocalizations, bruxism, oculomotor hyperactivity, diarrhea, piloerection, somnolence, tremor, and seizures (40).

When ketamine first was developed as a general anesthetic, the early clinical trials found that about a third of patients experienced an obvious emergence delirium. Why two-thirds did not remains unexplained, but suggests the importance of preoperative and postoperative medications, dosage, environmental, and psychologic or genetic factors. Schizophrenic patients appear to be much more susceptible to a prolonged psychotic episode related to PCP than do other individuals. In addition, environmental and genetic factors influence PCP biotransformation in animals and humans. After the initial induction dose, an intravenous drip of 15 to 30 mcg/kilogram/minute (or about 1 to 2 mcg/kg/hour) provides adequate amnesia and analgesia, in combination with $N_20:0_2$

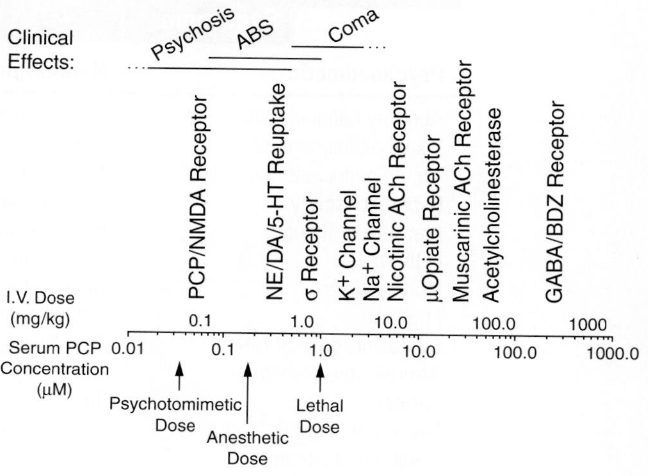

FIGURE 15.2. PCP doses, serum concentrations, molecular target sites, and clinical effects.

and a skeletal muscle relaxant. Muscle relaxants are necessary for intubation and for maintenance, because ketamine causes no relaxation of the jaw and other skeletal musculature; rather, it increases muscle tone. Abnormal jerky muscle movements of the extremities can occur during anesthesia or coma. Diazepam 0.3 to 0.5 mg/kg given intravenously reduces the occurrence of jerky muscle movements. Both agents should be given only when persons are competent to maintain an airway.

During and after slow intravenous administration of 2.0 mg/kg ketamine, the following sequence of eye signs is observed: blinking, staring, closure of lids, nystagmus, strabismus, and loss of lid reflex. Initially, when the patient falls into a dissociative or cataleptic state, the eyelids are widely open, and horizontal or vertical nystagmus is seen. Later, the eyeballs become centrally fixed in a gaze. During this stage, both somatosensory and visual stimulation elicit evoked potentials in the cortex. This finding supports the contention that the patient's brain cannot interpret the afferent impulses because of the disruption of the normal connections of sensory cortex with association areas. Such eye signs are differentiated from those caused by other intravenous and inhalational anesthetics or coma-producing substances by the fact that the eyes remain open during the course of anesthesia (after a transient closure immediately after induction), despite coma and adequate analgesia. The difficulty of relying on the eye signs of anesthesia to determine anesthetic or coma depth is one of the major disadvantages of ketamine as an anesthetic agent.

Ketamine induces coma in a dose-dependent manner. A minimum of 0.5 mg/kg intravenously is necessary to induce coma for approximately 1.5 minutes. A dose of 1.0 mg/kg induces coma for approximately 5.8 minutes, whereas a dose of 2.0 mg/kg induces coma for approximately 10 minutes. Persons who abuse ketamine may use a variety of routes of administration. The objective of their use is the low-dose mental state that is considered reinforcing by substance abusers. One exception is the giving of large doses surreptitiously to an unsuspecting person as one of the "date rape" drugs.

The clinical effects of ketamine are akin to PCP and can include analgesia, dissociation, hallucinations, and anesthesia, in addition to lessened agitation and cardiovascular and respiratory stimulation effects when compared with PCP. Violence and accidents may also result (41). Long-term chronic effects may include dysphoria, reduced memory and cognition, apathy, and irritability (42). Although evidence supports the potential for tolerance and physical dependence with ketamine (reference), further research is needed.

DXM has significant serotonergic properties, including increasing the synthesis and release of serotonin, as well as inhibiting the reuptake of serotonin from the synaptic cleft. DXM in clinical therapeutic doses produces relatively few side effects. These may include body rash, itching, nausea, and vomiting when combined with the other ingredients in cough preparations. Depending on dose, the drug can cause drowsiness, dizziness, altered vision, cardiovascular, and significant central nervous system effects that may resemble PCP intoxication. Euphoria and hallucinosis can occur within 15 to 30 minutes of ingestion of intoxicating doses, with peak effects experienced in roughly 2.5 hours. Clinical effects of DXM are summarized in Table 15.2 (2). The intoxication state can persist in varying degrees for about 3 to 6 hours (called a "plateau"). DXO is a weaker sigma opioid agonist and a stronger NMDA antagonist than DXM. DXO is relatively inactive at mu, kappa, and delta opioid receptor sites; thus, it is essentially devoid of the more conventional opiate properties; although respiratory depression has been reported with massive ingestion (43).

TABLE 15.2 Characteristics of the Dextromethorphan (DXM) Intoxication Syndrome

Psychomimetic	Neurologic	General
Auditory hallucinations	Slurred speech	Nausea
Visual hallucinations	Ataxia	Vomiting
Tactile hallucinations	Mydriasis	Diaphoresis
Hyperexcitability	Blurry vision	Hypertension
Pressure of thought	Bidirectional nystagmus	Respiratory suppression[a]
Lethargy	Hypertonia	Coma[a]
Nervousness	Choreoathetoid movements	Fatality[a]
Euphoria	Dystonic movements	
Confusion/disorientation	Dyskinesia	
Altered time perception	Restlessness	
Paranoia	Tremor	
Feeling of "floating"	Hyperreflexia	
Heightened perceptual awareness	Seizures[a]	

[a]Condition occurs only rarely.

Reprinted with permission from Bobo WV, Miller SC, Martin BD. The abuse liability of dextromethorphan among adolescents: a review. *J Child Adolesc Subst Abuse* 2005;14(4):55–75. http://www.informaworld.com.

DRUG–DRUG INTERACTIONS

Many centrally acting drugs can produce an algebraic summation of effects with all of the agents described herein. Therapeutic combinations of ketamine, with benzodiazepines reduce its emergence delirium depending on the pharmacokinetics of the drug involved. Clonidine and related alpha-adrenergic agonists such as dexmedetomidine have been given clinically with ketamine with beneficial effects.

DXM can induce a serotonin syndrome when taken with monoamine oxide inhibitors, selective serotonin reuptake inhibitors, or other serotonergically active substances. Genetic polymorphism in the biotransformation of DXM via CYP2D6 may enhance the toxicity of the former by inhibitors of the latter. These include many drugs such as chlorpromazine, delavirdine, fluoxetine, miconazole, paroxetine, pergolide, quinidine, quinine, ritonavir, and ropindole, as well as acute alcohol abuse.

NEUROBIOLOGY

The action of arylcyclohexylamines on NMDA receptors of glutamic acid first was described by Lodge and colleagues (44). Other investigators suggested different mechanisms of action involving biogenic amines and sigma-binding sites (45–47). However, noncompetitive blockade of NMDA receptors is a primary mechanism of action of low concentrations of these agents (1). This important conclusion stimulated interest in the role of glutamic acid in the disorder of schizophrenias (48–50). Krystal and colleagues (51–55) have been especially active in studying ketamine and possible antagonists in human volunteers. Moreover, understanding the role of glycine and other agonists in modulating NMDA-receptor function has led to possible novel therapeutic approaches to schizophrenia.

Recent imaging data have shown that ketamine-induced antagonism of the NMDA receptor is directly correlated with the Brief Psychiatric Rating Scale negative subscale, suggesting that dissociatives may induce negative symptoms via NMDA antagonism (56).

It has also been hypothesized that dissociatives induce positive symptoms via enhancing glutamate release. As discussed by Deakin et al. (57), Olney and Farber (58) have previously suggested that NMDA antagonists block excitation of gamma-aminobutyric acid interneurons (59) resulting in removal of gamma-aminobutyric acid restraint of cholinergic, serotonergic, and glutamatergic afferents to posterior cingulate cortex; suggesting a mechanism for triple excitoxicity and subsequent posterior cingulate pyramidal cell neurodegeneration observed after PCP administration. Subsequent studies using in vivo microdialysis have confirmed that the administration of NMDA antagonists causes increased glutamate release in the frontal cortex. Alternatively, mGluR2 (metabotropic glutamate 2/3 receptor) agonists, acting presynaptically to decrease the release of glutamate, have been shown in rats to reverse the behavioral effects of PCP (60).

Ketamine administration has been shown to induce a rapid, focal decrease in ventromedial frontal cortex regional blood oxygenation level-dependent signals that strongly predicted its dissociative effects and to cause significantly increased blood oxygenation level-dependent activity in midposterior cingulate, thalamus, and temporal cortical regions—increases that were correlated with Brief Psychiatric Rating Scale psychosis scores. Importantly, when pretreated with lamotrigine (a sodium channel blocker that decreases glutamate release), lamotrigine prevented many of the blood oxygenation level-dependent changes and Brief Psychiatric Rating Scale psychosis scores. Thus dissociatives may induce positive symptoms via enhancing glutamate release (57). Of course, there may be other mechanisms at play that relate to the association of positive and negative symptomatology with dissociative exposure.

A coincidental finding that has important clinical implications is that two patients with complex regional pain syndrome given a low-dose infusion of ketamine recovered from their associated depression (61). A follow-up study of 18 subjects with treatment-resistant depression given a single dose of ketamine showed rapid improvement in depression symptoms for up to 1 week (62). The mechanism for the rapid mood-elevating properties of ketamine is a recent area of research (63).

The fact that nitrous oxide is an NMDA antagonist has been another major advance in our knowledge, and has stimulated much new thinking (64–66) that may have clinical applications. N_2O is thought to stimulate the neuronal release of endogenous opioid peptide or dynorphins; the molecular aspects of how N_2O initiates this process are as yet unknown (67). Moreover, nitrous oxide may have an excitatory role on neurons via gamma-aminobutyric acid A receptor-mediated disinhibition (68).

Addiction Liability Why substances such as PCP, and now ketamine, are reinforcing is difficult to understand except in the context of individuals who wish to experience the feelings of floating in space, dissociation, sensory isolation, mental distortions, and so forth that dissociatives provide. It is known that dissociatives are self-administered. Rhesus monkeys self-administer PCP, and social stimulation among monkeys in adjoining cages leads to enhanced reinforcing strength of PCP (69). Changes in dopaminergic or cAMP signal cascades induced by repeated PCP treatment in mice likely play an important role in the development of PCP-induced rewarding effects (70). Rodent and primate animal studies of DXM support reinforcement by DXO, akin to PCP. Stimulus discrimination to DXO and stimulus generalization to PCP have been reported for DXM. Moreover, DXM has been shown to be strongly self-administered (71).

Toxicity/Adverse Effects Since the 1970s, when Olney described its neurotoxic effects, glutamic acid excess has been a target for finding brain-protective agents. NMDA antagonists have remarkable effects on brain neurons (72), including toxicity (73), which can be reduced or prevented (74). These agents induce significant vesicular changes (termed

Olney lesions) in rat brain posterior cingulate retrosplenial neurons. Not all species of animals evidence these changes. The relationship of such neurotoxicity to humans who use or abuse NMDA antagonists is as yet unclear. That such neurotoxic changes can be reduced by pretreatments with benzodiazepines is noteworthy; further supporting the mechanism outlined above of NMDA antagonists blocking gamma-aminobutyric acid interneuron activity, resulting in disinhibition of cholinergic, serotonergic, and glutamatergic afferents—resulting in excitotoxicity. Such vesicular Olney lesions have not been reported as much in DXM toxicity in rats (75). However, repeated high-dose administration of DXM during adolescence in rats may induce permanent deficits in cognitive function, and increased expression of NMDA receptor AR 1 subunits in the prefrontal cortex and hippocampus may play a role in these DXM-induced memory deficits (76). This has concerning implications in the setting of the increasing prevalence of DXM abuse in adolescents coincident with a remarkable period of brain growth during this age range.

Intoxication and Overdose Intoxication is discussed in greater detail in Section 6 of this book. Although a preliminary diagnosis of arylcyclohexylamine intoxication can be made on the basis of history, clinical signs, and symptoms, only a drug-positive blood or urine specimen will unequivocally establish it. Most clinical screening panels include PCP, but not the other agents discussed herein; thus, special requests may be required for specialized testing from a lab. A large variety of different chemical assays is available, but gas chromatography-mass spectrometry is often still ideal for confirmation. The brain wave changes induced by arylcyclohexylamines are unusual, and an electroencephalogram can be helpful if the patient is cooperative or comatose. Serum skeletal creatinine phosphokinase levels are increased, and the urine can contain myoglobin because of rhabdomyolysis. End-organ kidney damage may result.

The first step in the differential diagnosis of arylcyclohexylamine intoxication must be on the basis of whether the patient is in coma with or without seizures, emerging from coma, descending into coma, or in a psychotic state. The patient in coma—with or without seizures—has a differential diagnosis that includes all other causes of coma and seizures. The history and laboratory analysis are crucial. This is further discussed in Section 6 of this book.

Psychotic manifestations of arylcyclohexylamine poisoning can be confused with catatonic schizophrenia, an acute toxic psychosis induced with other hallucinogens, and various acute organic brain syndromes. Arylcyclohexylamine intoxication readily induces nystagmus, an organic brain syndrome, as well as cardiovascular and renal complications that are seldom, if ever, seen with other psychiatric syndromes. Body image loss (especially numbness of the entire body), feelings of being in outer space, and relatively rare visual hallucinations suggest arylcyclohexylamine abuse as opposed to use of hallucinogens such as LSD or related agents. DXM can be associated with psychosis at doses >300 to 600 mg or in fast metabolizers of DXO (15). Psychosis may occur at lower doses when DXM is combined with other drugs or alcohol. Folate deficiency may also be associated with DXM abuse (77). DXM abuse may also result in brain damage, seizure, loss of consciousness, and irregular heart beat (19). Respiratory depression from DXM has been reported to be reversed with naloxone (78). The National Guideline Clearinghouse (*www.guideline.gov*) provides detailed guidelines for management of DXM poisoning. An evidence-based consensus guideline for out-of-hospital management of DXM toxicity has recently been published (79). Use of medications to reduce relapse risk on DXM is virtually unexplored (80).

CONCLUSIONS AND FUTURE RESEARCH

Dissociatives include an array of compounds sharing activity at the NMDA receptor (among other actions on the human brain) and resulting in a clinical syndrome involving dissociation or disconnection of the brain from its external and internal environments. Such a disconnection is described by users as the desired end-state when abusing these compounds; however, it is not uncommon for users to exceed the dosing required for these effects, resulting in untoward psychiatric and medical effects. It is often only then that such patients present for medical assistance. Researchers are confronted with several key foci toward better understanding of drugs of this class. Antidotes do not as yet exist for these compounds, making for supportive care the underlying treatment modality. The issue of addiction liability of these drugs requires further exploration. The exploration of this drug class for its neuroprotective qualities may prove increasingly fruitful as the American population increases in average lifespan and need for such agents increases as well. Rapid antidepressant qualities relating to ketamine infusion is a recent discovery already resulting in increased research (81). Finally, the apparent trend of increasing prevalence and significance of DXM abuse is alarming, particularly for its concentrated involvement of young people who appear unaware of its potential toxicities warrants closer attention. Early data suggest neuronal toxicity and resultant neuropsychologic impairment may result from DXM abuse, particularly in the adolescent, developing brain. As such, public policy may be increasingly directed towards the controlled access of DXM versus its current over-the-counter (or behind the counter) availability.

REFERENCES

1. Krystal JH, Perry EB Jr, Gueorguieva R, et al. Comparative and interactive human psychopharmacologic effects of ketamine and amphetamine: implications for glutamatergic and dopaminergic model psychoses and cognitive function. *Arch Gen Psychiatry* 2005;62:985–994.
2. Bobo WV, Miller SC, Martin BD. The abuse liability of dextromethorphan among adolescents: a review. *J Child and Adolescent Substance Abuse* 2005 Summer;14(4):55–75.
3. Svenson JE, Abernathy MK. Ketamine for prehospital use: new look at an old drug. *Am J Emerg Med* 2007;25(8):977–980.

4. Mikhael MS, Wray S, Robb ND. Intravenous conscious sedation in children for outpatient dentistry. *Br Dent J* 2007;203(6):323–331.
5. Bhutta AT. Ketamine: a controversial drug for neonates. *Semin Perinatol* 2007;31(5):303–308.
6. Miller, SC, unpublished forensic data, 1999.
7. Domino EF, ed. *Phencyclidine: historical and current perspectives.* Ann Arbor, MI: NPP Books, 1981.
8. Javitt DC. Glutamate and schizophrenia: phencyclidine, N-Methyl-d-Aspartate receptors, and dopamine-glutamate interactions. *Int Rev Neurobiol* 2007;78:69–108.
9. Domino EF. From Sernyl to angel dust: the return of PCP. *Univ Mich Med Center J* 1981;XLVII:1–5. (Available from the author.)
10. Bobo WV, Miller SC. Ketamine as a preferred substance of abuse. *Am J Addictions* 2002;11(4):332–334.
11. Troupin AS, Mendius JR, Cheng F, et al. MK-801. In: Meldrum BS, Porter RJ, eds. *Epilepsy.* London, England: John Libbey & Co., 1986:191–201.
12. Piercey MF, Hoffman WE, Kaczkofsky P. Functional evidence for PCP-like effects of the anti-stroke candidate MK-801. *Psychopharmacology* 1988;96:561–562.
13. McFee RB, Mofenson HC, Caraccio TR. Dextromethorphan: another ecstasy? *Arch Family Med* 2000;9:123.
14. Nordt SP. DXM: a new drug of abuse? *Ann Emerg Med* 1998;31:794–795.
15. Miller SC. Dextromethorphan psychosis, dependence, and physical withdrawal. *Addiction Biol* 2005;10(4):325–327.
16. U.S. Food and Drug Administration. Drug Abuse Advisory Committee, Open Session, Vol. 1. Washington, DC: Public Health Service, 1990.
17. Hendrickson RG, Cloutier RL. "Crystal dex": free-base dextromethorphan. *J Emerg Med* 2007;32(4):393–396.
18. Miller SC. Coricidin HBP Cough and Cold Addiction. *J Am Acad Child Adolesc Psychiatry* 2005;44(6):509–510.
19. FDA Talk Paper. FDA warns against abuse of dextromethorphan (DXM), 2005. Accessed November 10, 2007, from http://www.fda.gov/bbs/topics/ANSWERS/2005/ANS01360.html.
20. Stoof JC, Booij J, Drukarch B. Amantadine as N-methyl-D-aspartic acid receptor antagonist: new possibilities for therapeutic application? *Clin Neurol Neurosurg* 1992;94:S4–S6.
21. Proceedings of the Community Epidemiology Working Group, National Institute on Drug Abuse. Epidemiologic trends in drug abuse: highlights and executive summary. National Bethesda, MD: Institutes of Health, 2007. Accessed August 2008, from http://www.drugabuse.gov/PDF/CEWG/Vol1_607.pdf.
22. Office of Applied Studies, SAMHSA, Drug Abuse Warning Network, 2002 (03/2003 update). Accessed August 2008, from http://dawninfo.samhsa.gov/old_DAWN/pubs_94_02/shortreports/files/TDR_PCPa.pdf.
23. Office of Applied Studies, SAMHSA, National Survey on Drug Use and Health, 2004. Accessed August 2008, from http://www.oas.samhsa.gov/2k7/hallucinogen/hallucinogen.htm.
24. Lankenau SE, Clatts MC. Patterns of polydrug use among ketamine injectors in New York City. *Subst Use Misuse* 2005;40(9–10):1381–1397.
25. Lankenau SE, Clatts MC. Ketamine injection among high-risk youth: preliminary findings from New York City. *J Drug Issues* 2002;32(3):893–905.
26. Johnston LD, O'Malley PM, Bachman JG, et al. Teen drug use continues down in 2006, particularly among older teens; but use of prescription-type drugs remains high. University of Michigan News and Information Services: Ann Arbor, MI. Accessed December 5, 2007, from http://www.monitoringthefuture.org/pressreleases/06drugpr.pdf.
27. Bobo WV, Miller SC, Smith CJ. Possible physiologic dependence on dextromethorphan. *West J Med* 2002;176(5):(available from Dr. Miller).
28. Desai S, Aldea D, Daneels E, et al. Chronic addiction to dextromethorphan cough syrup: a case report. *JABFM* 2006;19:320–323.
29. Bryner JK, Wang UK, Hui JW, et al. Dextromethorphan abuse in adolescence: an increasing trend: 1999–2004. *Arch Pediatr Adolesc Med* 2006;160:1217–1222.
30. Cochems A, Harding P, Liddicoat L. Dextromethorphan in Wisconsin drivers. *J Anal Toxicol* 2007;31:227–232.
31. Baselt RC. *Disposition of toxic drugs and chemicals in man.* Foster City, CA: Chemical Toxicology Institute, 2000:456–458, 676–679.
32. Stone CK, Humphries RL, eds. *Current diagnoses and treatment: Emergency medicine,* 6th ed. New York: McGraw Hill, 2008.
33. Silvasti M, Karttunen P, Tukiainen H, et al. Pharmacokinetics of dextromethorphan and dextrorphan: a single dose comparison of three preparations in human volunteers. *Int J Clin Pharmacol Therap Toxicol* 1987;9,493–497.
34. Zawertailo LA, Kaplan HL, Busto UE, et al. Psychotropic effects of dextromethorphan are altered by CYP2D6 polymorphism: a pilot study. *J Clin Psychopharmacol* 1998;18:332–337.
35. Javitt DC, Zukin SR. Recent advances in the phencyclidine model of schizophrenia. *Am J Psychiatry* 1991;148:1301–1308.
36. Xu X, Domino EF. Phencyclidine induced behavioral sensitization. *Pharmacol Biochem Behav* 1994;47:603–608.
37. Xu X, Domino EF. Asymmetric cross-sensitization to the locomotor stimulant effects of phencyclidine and MK-801. *Neurochem Int* 1994;25:155–159.
38. Xu X, Domino EF. A further study on asymmetric cross-sensitization between MK-801 and phencyclidine-induced ambulatory activity. *Pharmacol Biochem Behav* 1999;63:413–416.
39. Balster RL. Clinical implications of behavioral pharmacology research on phencyclidine. *NIDA Res Monogr Serv* 1986;64:148–161.
40. Balster RL, Woolverton WL. Continuous access phencyclidine self-administration by rhesus monkeys leading to physical dependence. *Psychopharmacology (Berlin)* 1980;70:5–10.
41. White JM, Ryan CF. Pharmacological properties of ketamine. *Drug Alcohol Rev* 1996;15(2):145–155.
42. Soyka M, Krupinski G, Volki G. Phenomenology of ketamine-induced psychosis. *Sucht [Germ J Addiction Res Pract]* 1993;5:327–331.
43. Paterson JW, Lulich KM. Antiallergic drugs and antitussives. In: Aronson JK, Dittman S, Dukes MNG, eds. *Meyler's side effects of drugs.* Amsterdam, The Netherlands: Elsevier Science B.V., 1996.
44. Anis NA, Berry SC, Burton NR, et al. The dissociative anesthetics, ketamine and phencyclidine selectively reduce excitation of central mammalian neurons by N-methyl-D-aspartate. *Br J Pharmacol* 1983;79:565–575.
45. Tadimeti S, Rao HS, Kim JL, et al. Differential effects of phencyclidine (PCP) and ketamine on mesocortical and mesostriatal dopamine release in vivo. *Life Sci* 1989;45:1065–1072.
46. Rao TS, Kim HS, Lehmann J, et al. Interactions of phencyclidine receptor agonist MK-801 with dopaminergic system: regional studies in the rat. *J Neurochem* 1990;54:1157–1162.
47. Rabin RA, Doat M, Winter JC. Role of serotonergic 5-HT_{2A} receptors in the psychotomimetic actions of phencyclidine. *Int J Neuropsychopharmacol* 2000;3:333–338.
48. Abi-Saab WM, D'Souza DC, Moghaddam B, et al. The NMDA antagonist model for schizophrenia: promise and pitfalls. *Pharmacopsychiatry* 1998;31(Suppl 2):104–109.
49. Loh M, Rolls ET, Deco G. A dynamical systems hypothesis of schizophrenia. *PLoS Comput Biol* 2007;311):e228. [Epub ahead of print.]
50. Javitt, DC. Glycine transport inhibitors and the treatment of schizophrenia. *Biol Psychiatry* 2008;63(1):6–8.
51. Krystal JH, Karper LP, Seibyl JP, et al. Subanesthetic effects of the noncompetitive NMDA antagonist, ketamine, in humans. Psychotomimetic, perceptual, cognitive, and neuroendocrine responses. *Arch Gen Psychiatry* 1994;51(3):199–214.
52. Krystal JH, Karper LP, Bennett A, et al. Interactive effects of subanesthetic ketamine and subhypnotic lorazepam in humans. *Psychopharmacology* 1998;135(3):213–229.
53. Krystal JH, Petrakis IL, Webb E, et al. Dose-related ethanol-like effects of the NMDA antagonist, ketamine, in recently detoxified alcoholics. *Arch Gen Psychiatry* 1998;55(4):354–360.
54. Krystal JH, D'Souza DC, Karper LP, et al. Interactive effects of subanesthetic ketamine and haloperidol in healthy humans. *Psychopharmacology* 1999;145(2):193–204.
55. Krystal JH, Bennet A, Abi-Saab D, et al. Dissociation of ketamine effects on rule acquisition and rule implementation: possible relevance to

NMDA receptor contribution to executive cognitive function. *Biol Psychiatry* 2000;47(2):137–143.
56. Stone JM, Erlandsson K, Arstad E, et al. Relationship between ketamine-induced psychotic symptoms and NMDA receptor occupancy—a [123I]CNS-1261 SPET study. *Psychopharmacology* 2008;197: 401–408.
57. Deakin JFW, Lees J, McKie S, et al. Glutamate and the neural basis of the subjective effects of ketamine: a pharmaco-magnetic resonance imaging study. *Arch Gen Psychiatry* 2008;65(2):154–164.
58. Olney JW, Farber N. Glutamate receptor dysfunction and schizophrenia. *Arch Gen Psychiatry* 1995;52(12):998–1007.
59. Drejer J, Honore T. Phencyclidine analogues inhibit NMDA stimulated [3H]GABA release from cultured cortex neurons. *Eur J Pharmacol* 1987;143:287–290.
60. Moghaddam B, Adams BW. Reversal of phencyclidine effects by a group II metabotropic glutamate receptor agonist in rats. *Science* 1998;281 (5381):1349–1352.
61. Correll GE, Futter GE. Two cases of patients with major depression disorder given low-dose (subanesthetic) ketamine infusions. *Pain Med* 2006;7(1):92–95.
62. Zarate CA Jr, Singh JB, Carlson PJ, et al. A randomized trial of an N-methyl-D-aspartate antagonist in treatment-resistant major depression. *Arch Gen Psychiatry* 2006;63(8):856–864.
63. Witkin JM, Marek GJ, Johnson BG, et al. Metabotropic glutamate receptors in the control of mood disorders. *CNS Neurol Disord Drug Targets* 2007;6(2):87–100.
64. de Lima J, Hatch D, Torsney C. Nitrous oxide analgesia-A 'sting in the tail'. *Anaesthesia* 2000;55(9):932–933.
65. Franks NP, Lieb WR. A serious target for laughing gas. *Nat Med* 1998;4(4):383–384.
66. Maze M, Fujinaga M. Recent advances in understanding the actions and toxicity of nitrous oxide [editorial]. *Anaesthesia* 2000;55: 311–314.
67. Emmanouil DE, Quock RM. Advances in understanding the actions of nitrous oxide. *Anesth Prog* 2007;54(1):9–18.
68. Nagashima K, Zorumski CF, Izumi Y. Nitrous oxide (laughing gas) facilitates excitability in rat hippocampal slices through gamma-aminobutyric acid A receptor-mediated disinhibition. *Anesthesiology* 2005;102(1): 230–234.
69. Newman JL, Perry JL, Carroll ME. Social stimuli enhance phencyclidine (PCP) self-administration in rhesus monkeys. *Pharmacol Biochem Behav* 2007;87(2):280–288.
70. Noda Y, Nabeshima T. Involvement of signal transduction cascade via dopamine-D1 receptors in phencyclidine dependence. *Ann N Y Acad Sci* 2004;1025:62–68.
71. Nicholson KL, Hayes BA, Balster RL. Evaluation of the reinforcing properties and phencyclidine-like discriminative stimulus effects of dextromethorphan and dextrorphan in rats and rhesus monkeys. *Psychopharmacology* 1999;46:49–59.
72. Johanson CE, Balster RL. A summary of results of a drug self-administration study using substitution procedures in rhesus monkeys. *Bull Narc* 1978;30:43.
73. Allen HL, Iversen LL, Olney JW, et al. Phencyclidine, dizocilpine, and cerebrocortical neurons. *Science* 1990;247:221.
74. Olney JW, Labruyere J, Wang G, et al. NMDA antagonists neurotoxicity: mechanism and prevention. *Science* 1991;254:1515–1518.
75. Carliss RD, Radovsky A, Chengelis CP, et al. Oral administration of dextromethorphan does not produce neural vacuolation in the rat brain. *Neurotoxicology* 2007;28(4):813–818.
76. Zhang TY, Cho HJ, Lee S, et al. Impairments in water maze learning of aged rats that received dextromethorphan repeatedly during adolescent period. *Psychopharmacology* 2007;191(1):171–179.
77. Au WY, Tsang J, Cheng TS, et al. Cough mixture abuse as a novel case of megaloblastic anemia and peripheral neuropathy. *Br J Haematol* 2003;123:956–958.
78. Schneider SM, Michelson EA, Boucek CD. Dextromethorphan narcosis reversed by naloxone. *Vet Hum Tox* 1986;31:376.
79. Chyka PA, Erdman AR, Manoguerra AS, et al.; American Association of Poison Control Centers. Dextromethorphan poisoning: an evidence-based consensus guideline for out-of-hospital management. *Clin Toxicol (Phil)* 2007;45(6):662–677.
80. Miller SC. Treatment of dextromethorphan dependence with naltrexone. *Addictive Disord Treatment* 2005;4(4):145–148.
81. Mathew SJ, Manji HK, Charney DS. Novel drugs and therapeutic targets for severe mood disorders. *Neuropsychopharmacology.* 2008 August; 33(9):2080–2092. Epub 2008 January 2. Review. Erratum in: *Neuropsychopharmacology.* 2008 August; 33(9):2300.

CHAPTER 16

Robert L. Balster, PhD

The Pharmacology of Inhalants

DEFINITION

There is good consensus on what constitutes inhalant abuse. Typically, abused inhalants are breathable chemicals that can be self-administered as gases or vapors. The products can be gases, liquids, aerosols, or, in some cases, solids, but products that begin as liquids or solids are vaporized and inhaled. There are historical examples of liquids that are both inhaled and consumed orally (e.g., ether) and there is a recent appearance of devices for alcohol inhalation, but the overwhelming majority of abused inhalants, by definition, are inhaled. Drugs such as crack cocaine, which is aerosolized, and cannabis, which is smoked, are consumed by inhalation but are not generally, or usefully, classified as inhalants.

DRUGS IN THE CLASS

With other drugs of abuse, it has proved most useful for addiction medicine to classify the substances primarily on the basis of shared pharmacologic and behavioral effects rather than by structure, source, or form. It would be desirable if the same could be done for inhalants (1). The problem is that there is not sufficient knowledge of the effects of inhalants to make very fine distinctions among them. In addition, the toxicologic effects of these compounds differ, and these differences do not necessarily follow classifications based on acute abuse-related pharmacologic and behavioral effects. Nonetheless, three subdivisions of abused inhalants are useful, as shown in Table 16.1. The rationale for this subclassification has been presented elsewhere (1), and is summarized in this chapter.

Volatile Alkyl Nitrites The prototypic alkyl nitrite is amyl nitrite, used medically as a vasodilator for treatment of angina. Amyl nitrite is available as a volatile liquid in ampules that are broken open and the vapor inhaled. At one time, the ampules were available over the counter and abusers would "pop" them open—hence the street name "poppers." When amyl nitrite was brought under prescription control by the U.S. Food and Drug Administration, retailers made room for odorizer products from other alkyl nitrites with names such as "locker room" (nitrites smell like a locker room), "rush," "hardware," and "climax." The latter connote their use in the context of sexual activity. As of this writing, cyclohexyl nitrite appears to be the most easily obtained volatile nitrite, for reasons described in the following sections. Very little is known about the safety of these products.

Relatively little research has been done to determine the mechanisms of action for the abuse-related effects of volatile nitrites. It is clear from animal studies that they do not produce acute intoxications similar to those of abused solvents such as toluene and trichloroethane. It seems likely that they are abused because of their ability to produce syncope secondary to venous pooling in the periphery and because of their effects on tumescence and smooth muscles, making them popular as aids to sexual activity. The attractiveness of syncope as a drug effect might be questioned until one recalls that even children like to hold their breath or twirl around until dizzy. It also may be that during dancing, for example, the pounding in the head one might experience from anoxia could enhance a user's appreciation of the situation. More research is needed on this point.

Nitrous Oxide Nitrous oxide is somewhat distinct in that it is a gas at room temperature and pressure. It is popular to

TABLE 16.1 Pharmacologic Classification of Abused Inhalants

Class	Examples	Sources
Volatile alkyl nitrites	Amyl nitrite	Antianginal medication ampules
	Butyl nitrite	Room odorizers
Nitrous oxide		Whipped creme chargers, cylinders for anesthesia, racing fuels, dairy industry foaming agent
Solvents, fuels, and anesthetics	Toluene	Adhesives, paint removers and thinners (toluol), inks, nail polish and remover, industrial solvents and degreasers
	Xylene	Adhesives and printing inks, paints and varnishes, pesticides
	Trichloroethane	A solvent in water repellants, automotive cleaners, paints, adhesives and silicone lubricants, correction fluids, spray paints and paint removers, spot removers and other cleaning products
	Trichloroethylene	Correction fluids, stains and varnishes, paint removers
	Methylene chloride	A solvent in water repellants, automotive cleaners, primers and paints, adhesives and silicone lubricants, correction fluids, spray paints and paint removers, rust and spot removers and other cleaning products
	Tetrachloroethylene	A solvent in water repellants, brake and carburetor cleaners, paints, adhesives and silicone lubricants, correction fluids, paint removers
	Diflouroethane, tetrafluroethane, dichlorodifluromethane	Compressed gas dusters for computers and other uses
	Butane, isopropane	Cigarette lighter fuel, aerosol propellant, bottled gas
	Ether, isoflurane	Anesthetics
	Ketones (MBK, MEK)	Solvents, adhesives

divert anesthetic nitrous oxide for illegitimate use. The tanks can be used to fill balloons for ready sale at concerts, "raves," or parties. The acute pharmacologic and behavioral effects of subanesthetic concentrations of nitrous oxide are poorly understood. Certainly, it can produce euphoria ("laughing gas") and feelings of intoxication (2,3), but the qualitative nature of this intoxication appears to be different from that produced by anesthetic vapors such as isofluorane and sevofluorane or by other drugs of abuse (2,4). It should be remembered that nitrous oxide is very impotent as an anesthetic, requiring concentrations of about 15% to 20% to produce intoxication. In fact, many users breathe almost 100% nitrous oxide (e.g., from a balloon). This action, of course, can lead to some anoxia and, as with nitrite-produced syncope, has acute psychologic effects as well.

Another interesting aspect to nitrous oxide pharmacology is that, unlike vaporous anesthetics, it can produce good analgesia, as seen in animal models, and there is some evidence for opiate receptor involvement in the analgesic effects (5), although opiate antagonists do not appear to reverse either anesthesia or subanesthetic intoxication with nitrous oxide (2). Gamma-aminobutyric acid (GABA)-ergic effects may be responsible for the anesthetic and other depressant effects of nitrous oxide (5).

Volatile Solvents, Fuels, and Anesthetics This category includes a large collection of chemicals which further research probably will reveal to have different profiles of acute effects as well, but the state of the science is insufficient at this point to propose a further subclassification. Among the prototypic chemicals for this class are 1,1,1-trichloroethane (TCE) and other halogenated hydrocarbons; toluene and other alkyl benzenes; butane and other alkanes; and various ketones, alcohols, and ethers (Table 16.1). It has been hypothesized that many of these commercial chemicals share profiles of acute effects with subanesthetic concentrations of volatile anesthetics such as halothane, sevoflurane, and isoflurane (6,7). These anesthetics offer a safer alternative to the study of toluene and similar chemicals in humans, and they have been directly compared in many animal studies (8,9). As a point of comparison, it is useful to recall that beverage alcohol (ethanol) also is a solvent and produces a type of anesthesia at very high blood levels. Ethanol actually is much less potent than the other solvents for acute central nervous system (CNS) effects, discouraging use by inhalation. Alcohol shares pharmacologic and behavioral effects with depressant drugs such as the barbiturates, nonbarbiturate sedatives, and benzodiazepines, and perhaps abuse of these solvents and anesthetics could be viewed clinically as special instances of abuse of depressant drugs (6). To be sure, the acute depressantlike intoxication and presentation of overdose can be the same among all these compounds.

History The abuse of inhalants has a long history. Perhaps the best known instances are the use of anesthetics for purposes of intoxication that began with their discovery more than 200 years ago. The euphoriant effects of nitrous oxide were noted by Sir Humphrey Davy, who synthesized the substance in 1798 and began calling it "laughing gas." Laughing gas subsequently was used as part of comedic traveling shows at the beginning of the 19th century. The early vapor anesthetics, including ether and chloroform, were used recreationally and as "nerve tonics," both by inhalation and drinking. It may seem odd to drink an anesthetic, but one must remember that alcohol is a highly volatile liquid with irritant properties, yet its oral consumption surprises no one.

Today, abused inhalants differ widely in their availability. Some, such as nitrous oxide and amyl nitrite, are under control of the U.S. Food and Drug Administration as prescription medications, although forms of nitrous oxide are available commercially (e.g., as "whippets"). Commercial sales of volatile alkyl nitrites are regulated in the United States by the Consumer Product Safety Commission, a step that has greatly reduced the availability and abuse of most of these substances. However, many are still advertised for sale on Internet sites. Many other types of abused inhalants can be found in homes or workplaces or are readily purchased at retail establishments. Gasoline, a very complex mixture of volatile compounds, is available everywhere, and butane lighter fluid is not very difficult to obtain. There have been discussions of strategies to prevent access to abused inhalants, to change their labeling, or to reformulate products to limit their abuse potential. Each of these strategies needs to be viewed on a case-by-case basis to be certain that it will achieve the desired effect and not result in abusers seeking potentially more toxic products that almost certainly cannot be restricted (e.g., gasoline). Harwood (10) has undertaken a policy analysis of the inhalant abuse problem in the United States, including the roles of treatment and prevention.

Epidemiology Results of national surveys suggest that the prevalence of inhalant use is greatest among 12 to 17 year olds compared with other age groups. For example, the school-based Monitoring the Future national survey in the United States of 8th, 10th, and 12th graders (11) estimated that inhalant use in 2007 was somewhat less than its peak in the mid 1990s, yet it still remains high (Fig. 16.1). One important difference from other dugs of abuse is that the prevalence of inhalant use actually decreases from 8th to 12th grade. Except for alcohol and tobacco, the prevalence of inhalant use among youth is second only to marihuana in this age range. The 2006 U.S. National Survey on Drug Use and Health estimated lifetime, past year, and past month prevalence for marijuana, inhalants, and cocaine in the United States (12). About 1 in 10 youths used inhalants sometime in their life and 4.4% used them in the past year (Fig. 16.2). Among older youth and adults, the prevalence of inhalant use falls considerably below that of marijuana, cocaine, and heroin, but current users remain a significant minority of substance abusers. Use of inhalants in the United States is common among both sexes but disproportionately involves non-Hispanic white youths compared with other age and ethnic groups (13). Although many inhalant users quit as they reach young adulthood, it is incorrect to characterize this problem as a passing fad in youth. For about half of current users, duration of use exceeds 1 to 2 years, with about 10% using inhalants for 6 years or more (13). Abuse of inhalants is an even more significant problem in other parts of the world, particularly in developing countries (14,15).

Inhalant users often develop substance use disorders. In one study (16), 8% of past-year inhalant users 18 years and older met *Diagnostic and statistical manual of mental disorders* criteria for inhalant abuse or dependence within that period. Inhalant use is also associated with other substance use disorders and may be an even stronger predictor of subsequent drug abuse problems than marijuana use. Several studies have shown a clear progression from early inhalant use to later use of drugs such as cocaine and heroin. In one such study, researchers found that youth who had used inhalants by age 16 had more than a ninefold greater likelihood of using heroin by age 32 than did youth who had not used inhalants, even when controlling for other risk factors associated with inhalant abuse (17). In another study, a history of inhalant use independently increased the odds of becoming an injection drug user by more than fivefold (18). In the latter study, the magnitude of the increased risk associated with inhalant use exceeded that for

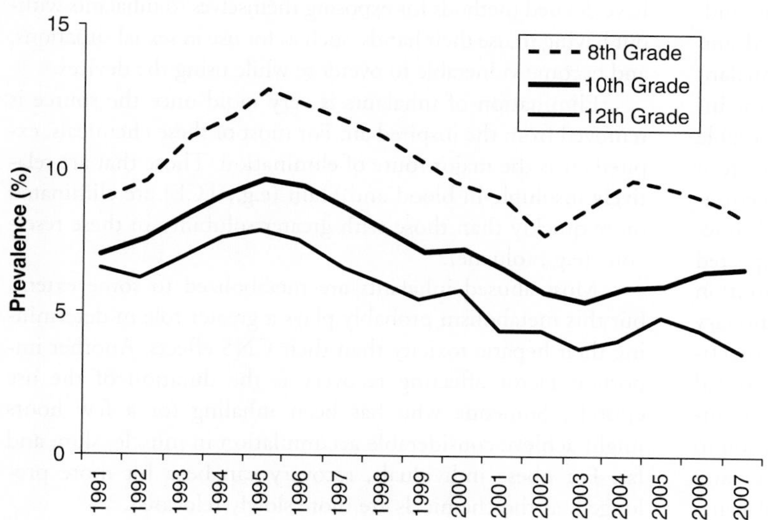

FIGURE 16.1. Trends in the annual prevalence of the use of inhalants for 8th, 10th, and 12th graders in the United States. Shown is estimated use in the past year during each of the reporting years between 2001 and 2007. Data are from the Monitoring the Future school-based study (Johnston, O'Malley et al., 2007).

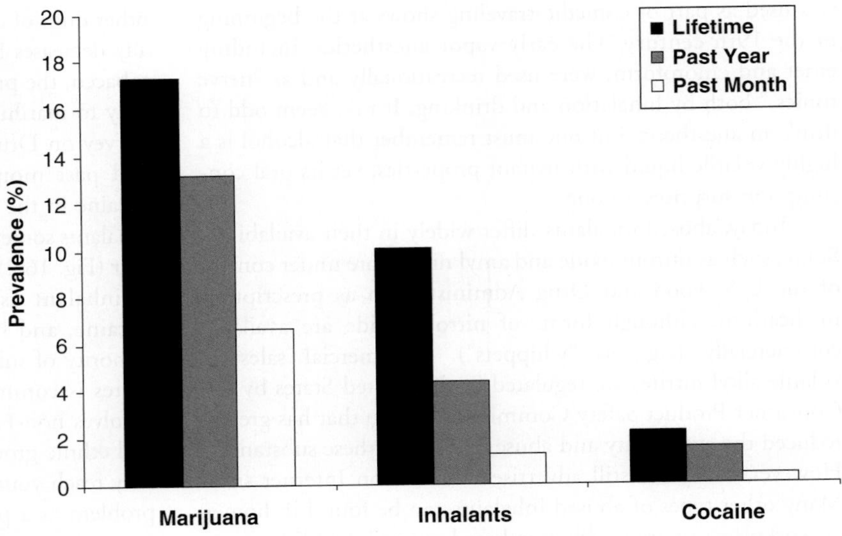

FIGURE 16.2. Lifetime, past-year, and past-month prevalence estimates for marijuana, inhalant, and cocaine use in 2006 for youth ages 12 to 17 in the United States. Data are from the National Household Survey on Drug Use and Health (Substance Abuse and Mental Health Services Administration, 2007).

marijuana use. There is also evidence that users of both inhalants and marijuana are at especially greater risk. For example, among adolescents who had used both (19), 35 % had a 1-year prevalence of alcohol abuse or dependence and 39% had a drug abuse disorder.

ABSORPTION AND METABOLISM

The abused inhalants include compounds that are self-administered as gases, vapors, and aerosols. These three forms of inhalants have somewhat different absorption characteristics and require different methods of use (e.g., balloons for gases and bags or rags for volatile liquids). In the case of abused aerosol products such as spray paint, the likely "active ingredient" for abusers is the propellant (e.g., butane) that exists in the aerosol can under pressure; however, the other materials in the cans (e.g, pigments) also can be absorbed.

A useful way to think about the bioavailability of abused inhalants is to apply knowledge of inhalation anesthesia. Gases and vapors rapidly penetrate deep into the lung and, because of their high lipophilicity, are rapidly absorbed and distributed into arterial blood. What distinguishes inhalant abuse from anesthetic use is that the partial pressure of the inhalant vapor inhaled generally is very high and quite variable over time, as users intermittently sniff from balloons or from rags or bags saturated with liquid. With these high concentrations in the inspired air, effects on the brain are almost immediate. As with anesthetics, key factors that would be expected to affect brain concentrations of inhalants are concentration in the inspired air, pulmonary ventilation rate, pulmonary blood flow, and the amount of body fat; however, the practical significance of these variables outside of a well-controlled anesthesia situation is uncertain. Because physical activity increases cardiac out put, it is likely that inhalant distribution to the brain in someone who is active will be markedly greater than in someone at rest. Inhalants easily cross the placenta and expose the fetus, with consequences that will be discussed later.

The situation with aerosols is somewhat different. Aerosol propellants typically are gases or vapors. Some of the constituents of aerosol products actually are droplets (that is, aerosols) when inhaled and, for these, the rapidity and efficiency of absorption are determined by particle size (median aerodynamic diameter). For all practical purposes, even aerosols have an almost immediate onset of action. Thus, it is common for inhalant users to breathe the gas or vapor and instantly stumble or fall down, posing a risk to themselves and others.

It is likely that, for many use situations with inhalants, the concentrations in inspired air exceed concentrations that would be lethal if the user were to be exposed continuously. Lethal concentrations could occur, for example, if a user became unconscious while still exposed to the inhalant. This situation is probably the most common form of acute overdose. It happens when someone using a rag or a bag laden with solvent falls in such a way as to maintain contact with the solvent. Also, some users have devised methods for exposing themselves to inhalants without having to use their hands, such as for use in sexual situations, and become vulnerable to overdose while using the devices.

Elimination of inhalants is very rapid once the source is removed from the inspired air. For most of these chemicals, expired air is the major route of elimination. Those that are relatively insoluble in blood and brain (e.g., TCE) are eliminated more quickly than those with greater solubility in these reservoirs (e.g., toluene).

Most abused inhalants are metabolized to some extent, but this metabolism probably plays a greater role in determining their hepatic toxicity than their CNS effects. Another important factor affecting recovery is the duration of the use episode. Someone who has been inhaling for a few hours might achieve considerable accumulation in muscle, skin, and fat. For obese individuals, recovery can be a bit more prolonged, as the chemicals are more slowly relocated.

The nature of postintoxication effects after an episode of inhalant abuse is poorly understood. It is reasonable to assume they might produce a "hangover" and headaches sometimes are reported. Whether the aversiveness of postintoxication motivates continued use is completely unknown. Nevertheless, intoxication with inhalants is of shorter duration than with other drugs of abuse, with the result that many health care providers, as well as friends and family of users, rarely see an inhalant abuser who is grossly intoxicated. Unless comatose, such users typically are not brought to emergency departments because they will have recovered before they get there. Law enforcement personnel occasionally encounter intoxicated users if they come upon them during a use episode, but there is little they can do, even in cases of driving under the influence, because of the rapid recovery time. Perhaps it is this lack of direct experience with intoxicated inhalant users and the difficulty of obtaining confirming clinical chemistry that has contributed to an under appreciation of the adverse public health effects of this form of substance abuse.

MECHANISMS OF ACTION

The neuropharmacologic mechanisms by which inhalant intoxication occurs are poorly understood. After they are inhaled, solvents rapidly enter the brain and distribute to lipid-containing membranes within the CNS, placing them in proximity to key functional components. Although it is presumed that the inhalants disrupt normal neural function, it is not clear which systems are most affected and the mechanism by which such disruption occurs. Even the question of whether specific receptors are affected by these agents remains unresolved.

Because of the properties that solvents share with alcohol, it is logical to turn to new discoveries about the mechanisms for the abuse-related effects of ethanol for hypotheses about how abused solvents might act in the brain. Evidence is accumulating that ethanol and solvents can have effects at certain ligand-gated and other ion channel receptors, including those for $GABA_A$, glutamate, and acetylcholine (20). The best current evidence is that acute solvent intoxication is probably associated with enhancement of $GABA_A$ and antagonism at N-methyl-D-aspartate receptors (21–23). Of particular interest is the discovery that these effects can be very selective for different structural subtypes of these heteromeric proteins, with different chemicals having somewhat different profiles of selectivity. Also important is the finding that vaporous chemicals that do not have depressantlike acute behavioral effects (e.g., flurothyl, a convulsant vapor) do not act like the abused chemicals in these in vitro procedures (21,24). Nevertheless, definitive knowledge about the cellular mechanisms for the abuse of inhalants lags far behind our knowledge of most other classes of abused drugs.

Although scientific evidence would support the view that most of the chemicals in this class of inhalants produces alcohol- and depressant druglike effects, published descriptions include a much wider array of potential subjective and pharmacologic effects, including hallucinations, tremor, and seizures. Certainly vapors can have excitatory effects in animals (such as flurothyl); and animal studies provide some evidence that even aromatic hydrocarbons such as benzene or the isoparaffins can produce a different profile of acute effects than the prototypic depressant solvents such as toluene (25,26). Considering how many commercial products containing very complex mixtures are inhaled, it should not be surprising that users experience a diverse array of acute effects, depending on the product used.

ADDICTION LIABILITY

All of the vapors that have been tested produce clear, reversible, druglike behavioral effects in animal studies (6). In addition, self-administration studies in rodents (27), primates (28), and humans (4) have shown toluene, chloroform, and nitrous oxide to have reinforcing properties. Toluene also produces a conditioned place preference in rats and mice (29,30). When given repeatedly to animals, many drugs of abuse produce sensitization to their locomotor stimulant effects, a phenomenon thought to reflect engagement of addictive processes in the brain. Trichloroethane has been shown to produce locomotor sensitization in mice (31), and repeated toluene exposure in rats produces cross-sensitization to cocaine and increased cocaine-produced dopamine release (32). Indeed, toluene itself has been shown to enhance dopaminergic function in various portions of the brain reward system (33,34), suggesting that there may be a common neural basis for abuse of inhalants and other well-studied drugs of abuse.

Tolerance and Dependence Little is known about the development of tolerance to and dependence on inhalants, but in general they do not appear to be prominent features. It may be useful first to describe what has been learned from carefully controlled animal studies of tolerance and dependence, in which exposure conditions are easily manipulated. Under conditions in which many drugs of abuse show considerable tolerance development when given repeatedly, abused inhalants do not readily produce a significant degree of tolerance to their behavioral effects (35). It has also been difficult to demonstrate cross-tolerance with other depressant drugs of abuse. This fact is somewhat surprising because animal models for tolerance to ethanol are readily established. However, with continuous exposure (such as that achieved with mice in inhalation exposure chambers), a mild withdrawal syndrome can be observed with TCE (36); other vapors have not been systematically studied. The withdrawal effects appear within hours after discontinuation of exposure and can be considered excitatory in nature. Ethanol and barbiturates can suppress these withdrawal signs, suggesting a cross-dependence within the depressant class.

Inhalant abuse typically is episodic in nature and thus generally would not occur with sufficient frequency and intensity to maintain a constant exposure throughout a day, much less the weeks or months it might take for physical dependence to develop. Thus, it is not surprising that physical dependence on inhalants is not seen often, if at all, in clinical settings. Signs and symptoms occurring a day or so after discontinuation of use (37) obviously would not correspond to the elimination of these chemicals from the body and may not represent a true abstinence syndrome so much as a manifestation of toxicity. There is little evidence of use of inhalants to avoid a withdrawal syndrome and a characteristic withdrawal syndrome is not included in the *Diagnostic and statistical manual of mental disorders*-IV Inhalant Dependence Disorder criteria set. However, regular users of inhalants clearly can develop a pattern of uncontrolled use, marked by a devotion of considerable time and efforts to obtaining and using inhalants that is characteristic of all the substance abuse problems.

Clinical Chemistry Although few, if any, clinical facilities will routinely conduct tests for the presence of abused inhalants, such tests can be ordered through special services provided by commercial laboratories. Typically, these tests are performed on blood or urine and appear to be available mainly for the abused solvents such as toluene, TCE, and methyl ethyl ketone. Because inhalants are eliminated so rapidly after acute exposure, such tests would be expected to have a high probability of producing false negatives. Nevertheless, technologic advances can be expected in this area. Problems associated with postmortem detection of abused volatile solvents have also been described (38).

TOXICITY/ADVERSE EFFECTS

It is difficult to summarize what is known and not known about the adverse consequences of inhalant abuse. The discussion that follows focuses almost exclusively on the subclass of inhaled solvents, fuels, and anesthetics. Their toxicity differs depending on which of this broad array of chemicals and chemical mixtures is being abused. The toxicology of commonly used solvents is reviewed in reference texts (39), which can be consulted for specific information on compounds of interest. A brief overview of the information is provided here. Nitrous oxide will be mentioned when appropriate, but the situation with alkyl nitrites is probably very different. The known side effects of organic nitrites used for smooth muscle relaxation would be relevant to abuse of these compounds, but a systematic study of the health consequences in nitrite abusers has not been done. The health effects of nitrite abuse have been reviewed (40).

Acute Effects Deaths related to the acute effects of inhalants are well documented (41–43). There are two primary sources: behavioral toxicity and overdose. Because the solvent class of inhalants can produce profound intoxication and even anestheticlike effects at high concentrations, it would not be surprising for accidents and injuries related to behavioral toxicity to occur. Vulnerability to these events probably is enhanced by the rapid onset of intoxication. Additive effects would be expected when these inhalants are used in combination with alcohol or other CNS depressant drugs. Overdose occurs when users lose consciousness while being continually exposed, allowing lethal concentrations to accumulate in the brain. As with anesthetic vapors, the concentration-effect curves for inhalants are very steep, with toxic exposures achieved easily under the poorly regulated exposure conditions of actual use.

It appears that the proximate cause of most overdose deaths is CNS depression, leading to respiratory problems or suffocation. Treatment of overdose rarely occurs in emergency departments because overdose victims usually are either dead or recovered by the time they arrive. In addition to these overdose situations, at least some of the inhalants appear capable of producing acute cardiotoxicity, even in otherwise healthy young users. The mechanism may be increased sensitivity of the myocardium to circulating catecholamines, which may occur when an intoxicated individual engages in some strenuous activity. This phenomenon has been termed "sudden sniffing death" (41) and has been associated particularly with the abuse of aerosols containing chlorofluorocarbon and butane propellants and refrigerants that contain them. The contribution of hypoxia to the acute toxicity of inhalants should be considered, especially with the use of nitrous oxide, in which even 100% concentrations are not lethal except for the loss of oxygen.

Chronic Toxicity Because of the diverse array of chemicals subject to inhalant abuse, it is difficult to summarize their chronic toxicity. The situation is made even more complicated by the fact that few chronic users confine themselves to a single product or a single chemical agent. Add to this the fact that many abused commercial products are complex mixtures, and it becomes difficult for a toxicologist to ascertain the specific etiology of any adverse health effects seen in inhalant users. Some adverse effects may be secondary to inhalant abuse and reflect lifestyles seen in solvent abusers. These may include such known predictors of poor health as homelessness, inadequate diet, and other substance abuse. Thus, data from case reports in inhalant abusers always should be viewed cautiously. Careful epidemiologic work that controls for key covariants in this population has yet to be done.

In animal studies, it is easier to study individual chemicals, but research in this area typically has been done to simulate the long duration and low concentration exposures that might be experienced in the home or workplace. Few studies attempt to model the repeated high concentration and intermittent exposure most typical of inhalant abusers. Many chronic inhalant abusers manifest adverse health effects, some of which can be used in diagnosing the problem. Common target organs are the nose and mouth area, lungs, brain, liver, and kidney. There also are physical dangers in using highly inflammable and explosive chemicals.

Neurotoxicity Many, if not all, abused inhalants can be neurotoxic and some components of abused products are well-characterized neurotoxicants. Among these are hexane and methyl-n-butyl-ketone, which produce axonopathies. The lead in leaded gasoline (still used in many countries throughout the world) produces classic demyelination. Other commonly abused chemicals (such as toluene, TCE, and propane) have less well described chronic effects on the brain and behavior. Human neural imaging studies and clinical observations suggest that they can produce neurotoxic effects at high exposures, but systematic studies with proper controls are lacking. Most of the information on neurotoxicity of inhalants comes from case reports or small series of patients. It is not known what percentage of abusers have detectable brain damage nor whether the inhalants alone were responsible for the observed effects. Brain scanning, neurologic, and neuropsychologic assessment or autopsy reports of inhalant abusers show many types of neuropathologies, including loss of white matter, brain atrophy, and damage to specific neural pathways (44–46). Of particular concern are the effects of abused inhalants on the developing nervous system where animal studies have revealed evidence for developmental delays (47,48).

Psychiatric Disorders The association of early inhalant abuse with increased risk of many substance use disorders has been described. For example, Wu and Howard (49) recently reported a very high rate of psychiatric disorders among inhalant abusers in the general U.S. population. For example, 70% of inhalant users in this sample met criteria for at least one lifetime mood, anxiety, or personality disorder and 38% experienced a mood or anxiety disorder in the past year. Females were more likely than males to have multiple comorbid psychiatric illness. Conduct disorder, mood disorders, and suicidality are common among adolescent inhalant abusers (50,51).

Effects on Major Organ Systems Many chronic solvent users develop irritation of the eyes, nose, and mouth and exhibit rhinitis, nose bleeding, conjunctivitis, and a localized skin rash. When these signs are accompanied by the odor of solvents on the breath or in clothing; by paint, adhesive, or other similar stains on clothing, or by possession of abusable products in unusual circumstances or amounts, inhalant abuse should be considered. With chronic use, inflammation of the lungs can result in coughing and may compromise respiration and bone mass toxicity has been reported.

The liver is an important target in chronic exposure to many solvents, particularly those that undergo some metabolism. Of particular concern are some of the halogenated hydrocarbons, such as carbon tetrachloride. It could be speculated that persons with other types of liver disease, such as hepatitis or alcoholism, would be particularly vulnerable. Kidney damage also has been reported, in the form of glomerulonephritis, kidney stones, and renal tubular acidosis. Benzene and vinyl chloride are known carcinogens. Nitrites and methylene chloride can produce methemoglobinemia.

Fetal Solvent Syndrome It has been estimated that as many as 12,000 women use inhalants while pregnant in the United States alone. The research on inhalant abuse and pregnancy (47) suggests that decreased fertility and spontaneous abortions in some women may be related to inhalant abuse. Clinical reports of adverse effects in the offspring of solvent abusers include low birth weight, facial and other physical abnormalities, microcephaly, and delayed neurologic and physical maturation. Because certain features seen in these children resemble the fetal alcohol syndrome, a "fetal solvent syndrome" has been proposed. Whether these features result from direct teratologic effects of the abused chemicals or some lifestyle covariants associated with solvent abuse is unknown at this time. Nevertheless, confirmation of adverse effects of prenatal solvent exposure has been obtained in animal studies (47,48). Thus, clinicians should be alert to this possibility in patients who abuse inhalants during pregnancy.

FUTURE RESEARCH DIRECTIONS

Inhalant abuse is one of the least understood substance abuse problems. This is primarily related to the fact that there has been little research in this area (52), generally because of mistaken beliefs about inhalant abuse that even exist within the scientific community. These beliefs include the ideas that (i) inhalant abuse is a transient phenomenon of adolescence that has relatively little associated morbidity and mortality, (ii) abused inhalants have "nonspecific effects" on the brain and behavior that do not lend themselves to study with modern technologies in behavioral and molecular neurobiology, (iii) laboratory studies of vapors and gases are very difficult to perform, and (iv) there are too many chemicals to successfully sort out the similarities and differences in terms of their abuse potential and toxicity.

Our understanding should improve with the increasing information available from animal models (48). However, there are some unique problems inherent in the study of inhalant abuse. The most significant is that it will be difficult to conduct laboratory-based human exposure studies of many of these compounds at behaviorally active concentrations. Such studies have been very important with other drugs of abuse. One approach to overcoming this problem may be to draw lessons about the effects of chemicals of this type by studying general anesthetics. This approach has been used successfully by Zacny and colleagues (2–4). It is particularly useful in studying nitrous oxide. Animal studies of abused inhalants will be especially important because there are fewer limitations on the exposure conditions.

Epidemiologic studies are made difficult by the numerous types of products and chemicals subject to inhalant abuse and by the fact that subclassifications have differed from study to study. There has been an increased appreciation that alkyl nitrite abuse differs from the rest, and this difference is reflected in separate analyses of prevalence data in many reports. The U.S. National Survey on Drug Use and Health now contains a breakdown of specific subtypes of abused inhalant products, which should be useful for analyses, although it may complicate comparing prevalence figures from one survey to another. Such progress should lead to a better understanding of inhalant abuse and improved treatment and prevention strategies.

Although it seems clear that inhalants can cause damage to the brain and other organs, much more information is needed about the patterns of use that produce such effects and whether the chemicals themselves cause the damage or whether inhalant abuse interacts with other factors to produced the observed effects in some users. Considering the very large number of persons who have experimented with inhalants it seems certain that only a fraction of these experience organ damage. Much more data are needed on the etiologic factors in observed cases of organ toxicity in inhalant abusers and more general population studies with appropriate control groups are needed to assess the incidence of these effects.

ACKNOWLEDGMENT: *The preparation of this chapter was supported by NIDA grant DA-01442.*

REFERENCES

1. Balster RL. Neural basis of inhalant abuse. *Drug Alcohol Depend* 1998;51:207–214.
2. Zacny JP, Coalson DW, Lichtor JL, et al. Effects of naloxone on the subjective and psychomotor effects of nitrous oxide in humans. *Pharmacol Biochem Behav* 1994;49:573–578.
3. Zacny JP, Klafta JM, Coalson DW, et al. The reinforcing effects of brief exposures to nitrous oxide in healthy volunteers. *Drug Alcohol Depend* 1996;42:197–200.
4. Zacny JP, Janiszewski D, Sadeghi P, et al. Reinforcing, subjective, and psychomotor effects of sevoflurane and nitrous oxide in moderate-drinking health volunteers. *Addiction* 1999;94:1817–1828.
5. Emmanouil DE, Quock RM. Advances in understanding the actions of nitrous oxide. *Anesthes Progr* 2007;54:9–18.
6. Evans EB. Balster RL. CNS depressant effects of volatile organic solvents. *Neurosci Biobehav Rev* 1991;15:233–241.
7. Bowen SE, Batis JC, Paez-Martinez N, et al. The last decade of solvent research in animal models of abuse: mechanistic and behavioral studies. *Neurotoxicol Teratol* 2006;28:636–647.
8. Moser VC, Balster RL. Effects of toluene, halothane and ethanol vapor on fixed-ratio performance in mice. *Pharmacol Biochem Behav* 1985;22: 797–802.
9. Bowen SE, Balster RL. Desflurane, isoflurane and ether produce ethanol-like discriminative stimulus effects in mice. *Pharmacol Biochem Behav* 1997;57:191–198.
10. Harwood HJ. Inhalants: a policy analysis of the problem in the United States. In: Kozel N, Sloboda Z, De La Rosa M, eds. *Epidemiology of inhalant abuse: an international perspective (NIDA research monograph 148).* Rockville, MD: National Institute on Drug Abuse, 1995:274–303.
11. Johnston LD, O'Malley PM, Bachman JG, et al. *Monitoring the future national survey results on drug use, 1975–2006. Volume I: secondary school students* (NIH Publication No. 07-6205). Bethesda, MD: National Institute on Drug Abuse, 2007.
12. Substance Abuse and Mental Health Services Administration. Results from the National Survey on Drug Use and Health: National Findings, 2007. Office of Applied Statistics. Accessed January 10, 2008, from http://oas.samhsa.gov/nsduh/2k6nsduh/2k6Results.cfm#TOC.
13. Neumark YD, Delva J, Anthony JC. The epidemiology of adolescent inhalant drug involvement. *Arch Pediatr Adolesc Med* 1998;152:781–786.
14. Kozel N, Sloboda Z, De La Rosa M, eds. *Epidemiology of inhalant abuse: an international perspective (NIDA research monograph 148).* Rockville, MD: National Institute on Drug Abuse, 1995.
15. Medina-Mora ME, Real T. Epidemiology of inhalant use. *Curr Opin Psychiatry* 2008;21(3):247–251.
16. Wu L-T, Ringwalt CL. Inhalant use and disorders in the United States. *Drug Alcohol Depend* 2006;85:1–11.
17. Johnson EO, Schütz CG, Anthony JC, et al. Inhalants to heroin: a prospective analysis from adolescence to adulthood. *Drug Alcohol Depend* 1995;40:159–164.
18. Schütz CG, Chilcoat HD, Anthony JC. The association between sniffing inhalants and injecting drugs. *Compr Psychiatry* 1994;35:99–105.
19. Wu L-T, Pilowsky, DJ, Schlenger WE. High prevalence of substance use disorders among adolescents who use marijuana and inhalants. *Drug Alcohol Depend* 2005;78:23–32.
20. Bowen SE, Batis JC, Paez-Martinez N, et al. The last decade of solvent research in animal models of abuse: Mechanistic and behavioral studies. *Neurotoxicol Teratol* 2006;28:636–647.
21. Cruz SL, Balster RL, Woodward JJ. Effects of volatile solvents on recombinant N-methyl-D-aspartate receptors expressed in Xenopus oocytes. *Br J Pharmacol* 2000;131:1303–1308.
22. Cruz SL, Mirshahi T, Thomas B, et al. Effects of the abused solvent toluene on recombinant NMDA and non-NMDA receptors expressed in Xenopus oocytes. *J Pharmacol Exp Therap* 1998;286:334–340.
23. Mihic SJ, Ye Q, Wock MJ, et al. Sites of alcohol and volatile anaesthetic action on $GABA_a$ and glycine receptors. *Nature* 1997;389:385–389.
24. Bowen SE, Wiley JL, Evans EB, et al. Functional observational battery comparing the effects of ethanol, 1,1,1-trichloroethane, ether and flurothyl. *Neurotoxicol Teratol* 1996;18:557–585.
25. Tegeris JS, Balster RL. A comparison of the acute behavioral effects of alkylbenzenes using a functional observational battery in mice. *Fundam Appl Toxicol* 1994;22:240–250.
26. Balster RL, Bowen SE, Evans EB, et al. Evaluation of the acute behavioral effects and abuse potential of a C8-C9 isoparaffin solvent. *Drug Alcohol Depend* 1997;46:125–135.
27. Blokhina EA, Dravolina OA, Bespalov AY, et al. Intravenous self-administration of abused solvents and anesthetics in mice. *Eur J Pharmacol* 2004;485:211–218.
28. Wood RW. Stimulus properties of inhaled substances. An update. In: Mitchell CD, ed. *Nervous system toxicology.* New York: Raven Press, 1982:199–212.
29. Funada M, Sato M, Makino Y, et al. Evaluation of the rewarding effect of toluene by the conditioned place preference procedure in mice. *Brain Res Protocols* 2002;10:47–54.
30. Gerasimov MR, Collier L, Ferrieri A, et al. Toluene inhalation produces a conditioned place preference in rats. *Eur J Pharmacol* 2004;477:45–52.
31. Bowen SE, Jones HE, Balster RL. Repeated exposure to 1,1,1-trichloroethane produces both tolerance and sensitization to effects on mouse behavior. *Fundam Appl Toxicol Toxicol* 1997;36(Suppl):62.
32. Beyer SE, Stafford D, LeSage MG, et al. Repeated exposure to inhaled toluene induces behavioral and neurochemical cross-sensitization to cocaine in rats. *Psychopharmacology* 2001;154:198–204.
33. Riegel AC, Zapata A, Shippenberg TS, et al. The abused inhalant toluene increases dopamine release in the nucleus accumbens by directly stimulating ventral tegmental area neurons. *Neuropsychopharmacology* 2007;32: 1558–1569.
34. Gerasimov MR, Schiffer WK, Marstellar D, et al. Toluene inhalation produces regionally specific changes in extracellular dopamine. *Drug Alcohol Depend* 2002;65:243–251.
35. Moser VC, Scimeca JA, Balster RL. Minimal tolerance to the effects of 1,1,1-trichloroethane on fixed-ratio responding in mice. *Neurotoxicology* 1985;6:35–42.
36. Evans EB, Balster RL. Inhaled 1,1,1-trichloroethane produced physical dependence in mice: effects of drugs and vapors on withdrawal. *J Pharmacol Exp Therap* 1993;264:726–733.
37. Evans AC, Raistrick D. Phenomenology of intoxication with toluene-based adhesives and butane gas. *Br J Psychiatry* 1987;150:769–773.
38. Willie SMR, Lambert WEE. Volatile substance abuse—post-mortem diagnosis. *Forensic Sci Int* 2004;142:135–156.
39. Snyder R. *Ethel Browning's toxicity and metabolism of industrial solvents,* 2nd ed., vol. 1. Hydrocarbons. Amsterdam, The Netherlands: Elsevier, 1987.
40. Haverkos HW, Dougherty JA, eds. *Health hazards of nitrite inhalants (NIDA research monograph 83).* Rockville, MD: National Institute on Drug Abuse, 1988.
41. Bass M. Sudden sniffing death. *JAMA* 1970;212:2075–2079.

42. Garriott J, Petty CS. Death from inhalant abuse: toxicological and pathological evaluation. *Clin Toxicol* 1980;16:305–315.
43. Bowen SE, Daniel J, Balster RL. Deaths associated with inhalant abuse in Virginia from 1987 to 1996. *Drug Alcohol Depend* 1999;53:239–245.
44. Aydin K, Sencer S, Demir T, et al. Cranial MR findings in chronic toluene abusers. *Am J Neuroradiol* 2002;23:1173–1179.
45. Filley CM, Halliday W, Kleineschmidt-DeMasters BK. The effects of toluene on the central nervous system. *J Neuropathol Exp Neurol* 2004;63:1–12.
46. Borne J, Riascos R, Cueller H, et al. Neuroimaging in drug and substance abuse part II: opioids and solvents. *Top Magnet Res Imaging* 2005;16: 239–245.
47. Jones HE, Balster RL. Inhalant abuse in pregnancy. *Obstet Gynecol Clin N Am* 1998;25:153–167.
48. Bowen SE, Batis JC, Mohammadi MH, et al. Abuse pattern of gestational toluene exposure and early postnatal development. *Neurotoxicol Teratol* 2005;27:105–116.
49. Wu L-T, Howard MO. Psychiatric disorders in inhalant users: results from the National Epidemiologic Survey on Alcohol and Related Conditions. *Drug Alcohol Depend* 2007;88:146–155.
50. Sakai JT, Hall SK, Mikulich-Gilbertson SK, et al. Inhalant use, abuse and dependence among adolescent patients: commonly comorbid problems. *J Am Acad Child Adolesc Psychiatry* 2004;43:1080–1088.
51. Sakai JT, Mikulich-Gilbertson SK, Crowley TJ. Adolescent inhalant use among male patients in treatment for substance and behavior problems. *Am J Drug Alcohol Abuse* 2006;32:29–40.
52. Balster RL. Inhalant abuse: A forgotten drug abuse problem. In: Harris LS, ed. *Problems of drug dependence 1996: proceedings of the 58th annual scientific meeting (NIDA Research Monograph 174).* Rockville, MD: National Institute on Drug Abuse, 1997:3–8.

SUGGESTED READINGS

Balster RL. Abuse potential evaluation of inhalants. *Drug Alcohol Depend* 1987;19:7–15.

Dinwiddie SH. In: Tarter RE, Ammerman RT, Ott PJ, eds. *Handbook of substance abuse: neurobehavioral pharmacology*. New York: Plenum Press, 1988:269–279.

Edwards RW, Oetting ER. Inhalant abuse in the United States. In: Kozel N, Sloboda Z, De La Rosa M, eds. *Epidemiology of inhalant abuse: an international perspective (NIDA research monograph 148).* Rockville, MD: National Institute on Drug Abuse, 1995:8–28.

CHAPTER 17

Scott E. Lukas, PhD

The Pharmacology of Anabolic Androgenic Steroids

Drugs in the Class
Therapeutic Use and Misuse
Adverse Effects
Addiction Liability
Absorption and Metabolism
Mechanisms of Action
Future Vistas

Within the addiction field, the term *steroids* has come to define those compounds that possess anabolic or tissue-building effects, but because most also have some androgenic properties, they are more appropriately called anabolic-androgenic steroids (AAS). This profile of effects distinguishes them from the corticosteroids and the female gonadotrophic hormones, neither of which are subject to abuse. There is a rather long list of anabolic-androgenic steroids that have been produced for both human and veterinary use; the major source of abused steroids is diversion from licit manufacture and distribution, as clandestine laboratory synthesis of these products is very rare. The major distinction between use and abuse is that abusers employ supraphysiologic dose compounds to increase muscle growth and performance. It is the consequence of these extremely high doses that results in rather dangerous, but often reversible, organ toxicity.

DRUGS IN THE CLASS

The prototypic hormone, testosterone, is the standard to which all of the synthetic products are compared and it is one of four structurally distinct groups of anabolic-androgenic steroids. The other three groups are: 17α-alkylated derivatives of testosterone, 17β-esterified derivatives of testosterone, and modified ring structure analogues (1). The history of how testosterone and its effects on male sexual development and tissue building were discovered is well detailed by Kochakian (2). Although hormonal involvement in male sexual development was known in 1849, it was not until 1930 when androsterone (a metabolite of testosterone) was isolated from human urine. In the 1940s, after chemists had succeeded in synthesizing testosterone, their efforts were directed toward separating its anabolic from its androgenic effects and to make a formulation that could be taken orally. The androgenic component of these synthetics has never been completely separated from the anabolic effects; only the relative percentage of the two has been manipulated. Commercially prepared products were used briefly during World War II to promote wound healing. In 1939, Boje postulated that anabolic-androgenic steroids might not only increase muscle mass, but improve physical performance as well (3). Hartgens and Kuipers provide a comprehensive review of the pharmacology and toxicity of AAS in athletes (4).

The introduction of anabolic-androgenic steroids to the United States has been traced to the 1954 World Weightlifting Championships in Vienna, when the Soviet Union's coach informed the U.S. coach that his team members were taking testosterone (5). In the ensuing years, use of anabolic-androgenic steroids by elite weight lifters, power lifters, and bodybuilders increased. Over the years, their use spread to many professional sports, especially those in which strength and body weight were important for success (e.g., football). Testosterone was the drug of choice in the 1950s, which was replaced by more elegant synthetic compounds over the next three decades, primarily because of their slightly higher percent of anabolic versus androgenic effects and their relative resistance to detection by current laboratory tests. Use spread to collegiate and amateur athletes as evidenced by the 50% positive tests obtained by the International Olympic committee during unannounced urine screens in 1984 and 1985 (6). The 1990s saw a return to the use of testosterone, which is thought to be due to improved gas chromatographic methods of detecting the synthetic compounds and the continued difficulty of accurately detecting exogenously administered testosterone (7). However, another trend toward using other types of performance-enhancing aids has evolved in the wake of pure anabolic-androgenic steroid abuse.

It often is difficult to determine whether the attraction of the drugs is related to any beneficial effect on the individual's performance, because the drugs rarely are taken in the absence of a training program that includes exercise and sound nutrition (8). This concept punctuates the second aspect of anabolic-androgenic steroid abuse among athletes—it usually occurs during training periods, which typically can begin weeks and even months before a competitive event or season. The need for these drugs by most athletes decreases during actual competition, and so the active use can decline. However, with the advent of mandatory urine testing at major athletic events, the risk of being caught also curtails use. Positive urine screens that are collected during the actual competitive event are usually due to the high sensitivity of the analytic methods to detect small amounts of metabolites that have persisted long since use of the anabolic-androgenic steroid has ceased. The fact that a hair gas chromatographic test has been validated may have a greater impact on detecting AAS among athletes (9). Despite the enhanced methods of detecting these complex compounds, controversial use of AAS has tainted a large number of sporting events including Major League Baseball, track and field, and professional cycling—some of these have led to congressional investigations and elite athletes continue to be stripped of accolades because of discovered abuse.

New-Generation "Performance Enhancers" With the advent of more sophisticated urine testing procedures, the likelihood that an athlete can avoid being caught using AAS is decreasing somewhat. This situation has yielded to the increased popularity of an entirely new generation of performance enhancing drugs and nutritional supplements that are not currently illegal or banned substances. Moreover, some of these agents have been extremely difficult to detect using standard laboratory procedures, not because the technology is limited but because these substances are found naturally in the body (10) and so carbon isotope mass spectrometry is needed (11). These include other hormones such as human growth hormone (somatotropin), dehydroepiandrosterone, erythropoietin, and thyroxine. Cadaver pituitary growth hormone has been replaced by recombinant human growth hormone and the latter has been found to increase strength, peak power output, and fat-free mass index decreased after only a short course of the recombinant hormone (12).

Other drugs that may enhance performance include the mixed agonist/antagonist opioids such as butorphanol and nalbuphine; the beta adrenergic agonist clenbuterol; "hormone helpers" such as gamma hydroxybutyrate, clonidine and human chorionic gonadotropin; and testosterone stimulants such as clomiphene and human chorionic gonadotropin. In addition, a variety of diuretics (acetazolamide, furosemide, spironolactone, and triamterene) are used to help clear the anabolic-androgenic steroids and their metabolites from the urine before drug testing. Knowledge of these drugs, where to get them, doses to use and even recipes for adding them to training programs can be found in a number of "underground" guides as well as from a variety of Web sites.

At-risk Populations It is now well established that athletes are not the only individuals to use and abuse AAS. Abuse has now appeared in adult nonathletes and even in young boys who may be using them to simply improve their appearance (13). Women are also using these drugs, but all estimates indicate that the percentage is lower than in males. These factors encouraged the U.S. Congress to enact the Anabolic Steroids Control Act, which effectively placed all of these compounds, including testosterone and its many analogues, in Schedule III of the federal Controlled Substances Act (states, of course, have the option of scheduling these drugs even more restrictively under state law). Schedule III includes opioids such as nalorphine, stimulants such as benzphetamine, and depressants such as butabarbital and thiopental.

The 1990s were rife with a number of surveys demonstrating that the incidence of AAS use and abuse by adults and adolescents was lower than that of other drugs of abuse (14,15). The data suggested that AAS were used by <2% of the adolescents surveyed and <1% for older respondents. However, in the past 5 to 6 years, new data have revealed some concerning trends in AAS abuse, particularly among the youth. Use among boys in general is now reported to be >3% (16) and in certain populations of 15- to 19-year-old boys, nearly 10% reported using AAS (17). In a recent cross-sectional assessment using the 2003 Centers for Disease Control and Prevention National School–based Youth Risk Behavior Survey database (18), Elliot et al. (19) reported that 5.3% of the 7,544 females in grades 9 to 12 used AAS. In addition, these young women also engaged in a number of other unhealthy life choices including using tobacco, marijuana, diet pills, carrying weapons, and having sexual relations before the age of 13. These authors also noted that AAS using females were *less* likely to participate in team sports; this fuels the belief that children and adolescents have poor body image (20). This rate of AAS use among females punctuates the twofold to fourfold increase in AAS use that was reported by Yesalis et al. (21) in the 1990s. However, steroid use appears to decline with age, and desire to weigh more was a strong predictor of AAS use by males, but female AAS users were more likely to have higher body mass indices and a poorer knowledge of nutrition (22). Another complicating factor in obtaining accurate information about AAS use in teenage girls is that surveys may contain imprecise language so that the term *steroid* is misinterpreted (23), leading to an inflated estimate of AAS use. The clinician may need to weigh the impact of the media, peer pressure, and teasing/comments from parents as factors that predict or at least facilitate AAS use among young boys. Smolak and Stein reported that the media as well as endorsements about male physical characteristics were strong correlates of a desire to attain a more muscular body (24). Indeed, in a Web-based survey of 500 AAS users, 78% were noncompetitive bodybuilders and not otherwise engaged in athletic events (25).

However, the use of nutritional supplements has increased dramatically and in particular, testosterone precursors such as androstenedione, dehydroepiandrosterone, and androstenediol, have been used by adolescent athletes (26–29). The use of these supplements continues in spite of repeated evidence that small to moderate doses resulted in transient and modest increases in testosterone and as such had no discernible effect on body composition or performance (30–36). This dissociation between real efficacy and perceived effects is thought to be due to a lack of knowledge about supplements so that a comprehensive educational program might be useful in curtailing the use of these supplements (37).

In the Syrian hamster animal model, there is compelling evidence that adolescents are far more sensitive to the effects of AAS than their adult counterparts (38). The AAS-treated adolescent males had significantly higher sexual and aggressive behavior, whereas similarly treated adults had significantly lower levels of sexual and aggressive behavior. This model relates to the clinical condition as it is suspected that the neural "rewiring" that occurs in males during puberty sets the tone for future aggressive and violent tendencies (39) and that exposure to AAS during this critical time can increase the likelihood that aggressive acts result in violent behavior. The link between testosterone and aggressive behavior was further made by van Bokhoven et al. who reported that 16-year-old boys who had criminal records had elevated testosterone levels than their peers and concluded that there was a positive relationship between testosterone and proactive and reactive aggression and self-reported delinquent behavior (40).

Figure 17.1 depicts some of the more commonly identified effects and side effects of AAS use in adolescents. High-dose AAS use during adolescence has the potential of causing significantly more problems when adulthood is reached (41). Some of the effects are easier to identify than others, so the challenge to the clinician in detecting AAS use in his or her patients is to know the risk factors and ask the correct questions when exploring use patterns (42). But more importantly, the clinician must be well informed and be able to present themselves as a credible source of information.

THERAPEUTIC USE AND MISUSE

Therapeutic Use Although one might think that the therapeutic uses of anabolic-androgenic steroids is of less concern to the addiction medicine specialist, in reality, most physicians are asked to give prescriptions for these drugs far more often than they are asked to help treat someone who is dependent on the drugs. Thus, knowledge of these medical situations might help in discussions with a potential abuser because these individuals are likely to be aware of the medical reasons for their prescription and may use such information in their initial attempts to obtain legal medications to support their training or alter their appearance.

Males may receive anabolic-androgenic steroids for replacement therapy when the testicles fail to function, either because of congenital or traumatic factors, or when puberty is delayed and short stature would result. The doses that are prescribed, however, are much lower than those used by bodybuilders. The equivalent of 75 to 100 mg per week of testosterone suffices as replacement, but weight lifters and bodybuilders have reportedly used weekly doses of 1,000 to 2,100 mg of methandienone (43,44). Women are occasionally treated with androgens when metastatic breast cancer has spread to bone. Methyltestosterone is combined with estrogen (Premarin) to help alleviate some of the signs and symptoms of menopause. Very recently, nandrolone has been used in combination with exercise to increase lean body mass in patients who are on dialysis (45).

Both males and females might receive the more anabolic agents during treatment of a rare form of hereditary angioedema.

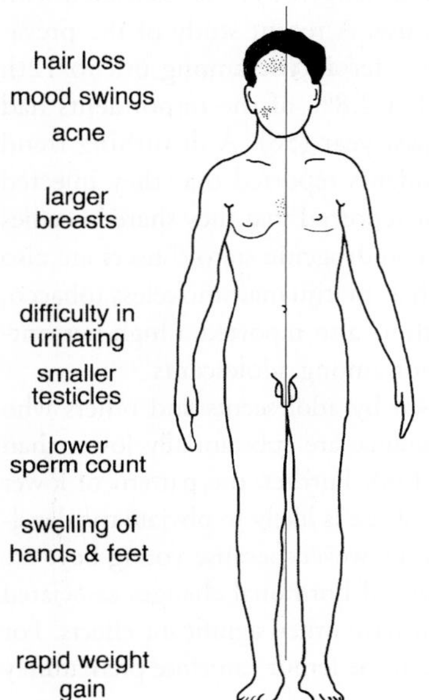

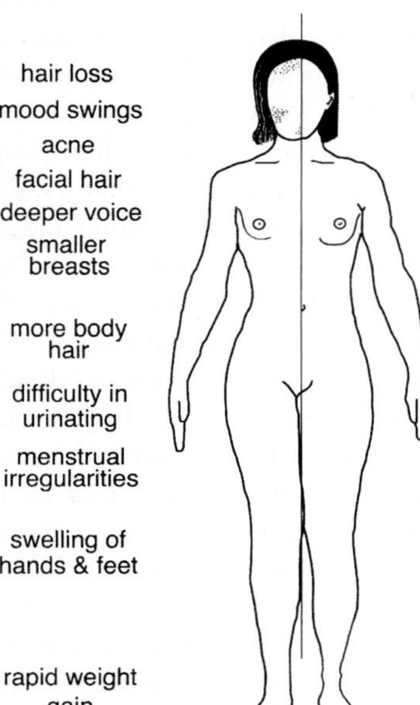

FIGURE 17.1. Side effects of anabolic-androgenic steroids.

Acquired aplastic anemia and myelofibrosis both result in deficiencies of red blood cell production, which is combated with drugs that have equal amounts of anabolic and androgenic effects. Sometimes these drugs can be useful in treating the trauma associated with burns and AIDS. Finally, just as was done in post–World War II, steroids with more anabolic activity are useful in treating muscle wasting that is secondary to starvation.

Misuse Anabolic-androgenic steroids are abused by three distinct populations: (i) athletes who use them to improve performance; (ii) aesthetes who use them solely to improve appearance and perhaps gain some weight; and (iii) the fighting elite who use them to enhance aggression and fighting skills (46). Identifying to which of these three populations a patient belongs is the first step to understanding the pattern of use and determining the best treatment plan to follow.

Athletes Athletes use anabolic-androgenic steroids for one reason: to improve their performance. Perhaps one of the greatest mistakes a clinician makes in dealing with an athlete is attempting to dissuade their use on the grounds that the drugs cannot improve performance. In fact, this is not true. The older research studies that purported to show that the effects of anabolic-androgenic steroids were no different than placebo suffered from a number of methodologic problems, did not control for motivation, and failed to document the amount of physical training. In addition, ethical considerations prevented the investigators from administering extremely high doses, which are considered necessary to achieve the muscle-building effect. Negative findings also have been attributed to the use of only one drug at a time in the research studies, whereas athletes in training typically use multiple drugs in combination. The continued use of these drugs is based on the belief that they increase muscle capacity, reduce body fat, increase strength and endurance, and hasten recovery from injury (47). Many athletes also believe that anabolic-androgenic steroid-assisted training allows the user to increase both the frequency and the intensity of workouts—factors that contribute to any direct benefits of the drugs (48). A recent Web-based survey revealed that bodybuilders and weightlifters use on average 3.1 agents, engage in cycles that last 5 to 10 weeks in length and use doses that are 5 to 29 times greater than physiologic replacement doses (49). Rates of use among individuals in fitness centers is also much higher (approximately 12.5%) than the general population (50).

In the world of professional weightlifting and body building, anabolic-androgenic steroids are used in three basic patterns: "stacking," "pyramiding," and "cycling." *Stacking* is the practice of using multiple products at the same time. Users believe that the beneficial effects of one drug will complement those of another, and that they will only achieve real benefits through a specific combination. There are now animal data to support the notion that stacking AAS can result in an altered pharmacologic response. Wesson and McGinnis administered a number of combinations of testosterone, stanozolol, and nandrolone to adolescent male rats and found that behavioral and endocrine effects were altered. Furthermore, this simulated "stacking" procedure revealed that the level of androgen receptor occupation did not directly correlate with the effects of the combined agents (51).

A *pyramid* plan involves starting with a low dose and then gradually increasing the dose until peak levels are achieved a number of weeks before competition. The individual then slowly decreases or tapers the drug dose down and, because the beneficial effects of anabolic-androgenic steroids persist long after their use has been discontinued, the athlete will be primed for the competitive event.

Cycling refers to the practice of using different combinations over a period to avoid the development of tolerance or loss of effectiveness. Thus different combinations of drugs are used over a 6- to 12-week period, after which another drug or combination is substituted.

When prescriptions for AAS cannot be obtained, individuals may sometimes turn to veterinary products. It is an interesting paradox when young bodybuilders profess to be on strict diets and use only the purest of vitamin and dietary supplements, yet they will self-administer drugs for which use in humans has not been approved. Products that are not approved for use in the United States typically are obtained by mail order from abroad. Because the testing of these products in some other countries is not as stringent as that in the United States, patients should be cautioned about using such products. Finally, there is an extensive black market of anabolic-androgenic steroids that supports a rather large percentage of inactive products that are falsely advertised as containing anabolic steroids.

Aesthetes Another group of users is composed of young boys and girls who use these drugs primarily to increase their weight or to improve their physical appearance (52–55). This desire for weight gain among a group of adolescent boys who are not yet taking anabolic-androgenic steroids may place them at risk for initiating use (54). This trend is disturbing because these authors noted that a significant number of the boys were unaware of the most dangerous risks associated with anabolic-androgenic steroid use. A recent study of the prevalence of anabolic-androgenic steroid use among 6th to 12th grade Canadians revealed that 2.8% of the respondents had used these drugs over the past year (56). A disturbing trend was that 29.4% of these students reported that they injected the drugs and 29.2% of these reported that they shared needles with friends. Young anabolic-androgenic steroid users are also likely to use other drugs such as marijuana, smokeless tobacco, and cocaine (57). These authors also reported a high percentage of needle-sharing behavior among adolescents.

In general, the doses used by adolescents and others who want to improve their appearance are substantially lower than those used by adult athletes (58). Further, the pattern of lower doses and intermittent cycles of use is likely to obviate the development of major side effects. However, because young boys are often still in transition because of hormonal changes associated with puberty, these drugs can have other significant effects. For example, the epiphyseal plate of the femur can close prematurely and actually stunt a boy's growth (59), which is contrary to what a significant number of adolescents believe. More importantly, these young users may be particularly sensitive to the increased aggressive effects resulting from their use (58).

Apparently, a substantial proportion of these adolescents are also unaware of the side effects of anabolic-androgenic steroids. Although educational programs have been slow to incorporate these drugs in the lesson plans, the real reason that the public is so unaware of the risks is that these drugs are probably not a severe health hazard when taken intermittently and in low to moderate doses (58). Because programs that simply emphasize the negative aspects of drugs of abuse are ineffectual at curtailing use (60), the health professional should balance the discussion about anabolic-androgenic steroid abuse with the straight facts and not try to overstate the degree of harm. Such actions will only alienate the patient. Unfortunately, these young people know that only a small percentage of users actually experience very serious and deadly outcomes and that it will not happen to them. For the others, the side effects (except for some effects in women) are largely reversible.

Fighting Elite Very little is known about this population of anabolic-androgenic steroid users. This profile was originally described by Brower and includes individuals who seek to increase their strength in order to perform their job (46). Another desired effect is the increase in aggressiveness that may also help them with their jobs. Thus, bouncers at bars, security personnel, and even law enforcement officers (61,62) have been reported to take these drugs.

Personality Profiles A study of the personalities of anabolic-androgenic steroid abusers by Cooper and colleagues identified a high rate of abnormal personality traits in a sample of 12 bodybuilders who used anabolic-androgenic steroids compared with a matched group who did not (63). Along with being heavier than the controls, the users were more likely to score higher on measures of paranoia, schizoid, antisocial, borderline, histrionic, narcissistic, and passive-aggressive personality profiles. Further, the incidence of abnormal personality traits before anabolic-androgenic steroid use began was not different from the control group, suggesting that such disturbances are secondary to their use. Users also reported that they believe that anabolic-androgenic steroids not only enhance physical strength and athletic ability, but increase confidence, assertiveness, feelings of sexuality, and optimism (64). There appears to be both a pathologic perception of body image and a very narrow (stereotypic) view of what a male body should look like among AAS users (65). The term *reverse anorexia nervosa* has been coined by this group to describe symptoms association with muscle dysmorphia or a pathological preoccupation with muscularity (e.g., not willing to let their bodies be seen in public). This particular form of body dysmorphic disorder may be associated with psychopathology as evidenced by a greater incidence of suicide attempts, higher frequency of substance abuse, and poorer quality of life (66).

ADVERSE EFFECTS

A great deal is known about the side effect and toxic profile of these drugs. Side effects are generally reversible, but more serious medical consequences and even toxic reactions appear to involve primarily blood chemistry, endocrine function, liver, the cardiovascular system, and the nervous system. Reports that excessive amounts of these drugs leads to certain types of malignant cancers have not been substantiated. Overall, even the more serious side effects have disappeared within 3 months of discontinuing their use, yet benefits such as increases in lean body mass and increased diameter of muscle fibers remain (67). Although the side effect profile of AAS has been well documented in adults, less is known about how chronic use of high doses of AAS will affect adolescent users.

Administration of the 17-alkylated androgens can cause a dramatic reduction in high-density lipoprotein (HDL) cholesterol, but because there is a nearly equal increase in low-density lipoprotein (LDL) cholesterol, there is no net change in total cholesterol levels (68). Other agents such as nandrolone and testosterone esters fail to produce this profile (68,69). Although the long-term detrimental effects of altered HDL/LDL ratios are known to predispose humans to atherosclerosis, documented morbidity and mortality as a result of anabolic-androgenic steroid use has been rare (70,71). The lack of direct correlations may also be due to the fact that different steroids have varied effects on lipid dynamics (69). Thus, although users stack different drugs to improve the beneficial effects, this practice may actually afford some protection against these side effects. Further, the relative paucity of coronary vascular disease in athletes who use these drugs may also be due to the fact that other risk factors (e.g., diet, exercise, low body fat) compensate for any negative contribution afforded by the HDL/LDL profile. Such protection, however, may not be present in individuals who use anabolic-androgenic steroids just to improve their appearance and do not engage in athletic activity. Platelet aggregation (72) and increased red blood cell production and slight increases in systolic blood pressure have been suggested to be important factors that increases an individual's risk for thromboembolic disorders (1,73).

Because testosterone exerts an inhibitory action on the hypothalamic-pituitary axis, administration of natural or synthetic analogues of testosterone decreases testicular size and sperm count (74,75). Residual amounts of active metabolites may keep the levels of follicle-stimulating hormone and luteinizing hormone low and coupled with the relatively long cycle to produce sperm, the recovery is likely to be slow, but often is complete. Aromatization is the process by which steroid hormones are interconverted. For example, testosterone is converted to estradiol and estrone and high-dose male anabolic-androgenic steroid users can have circulating estrogen levels of normally cycling women (1). These circulating estrogens exert the usual feminizing effects, such as gynecomastia. Compounds that resist aromatization (e.g., fluoxymesterolone, mesterolone, stanozolol) may not result in the feminizing effects (76).

Although a wide variety of medical disorders (and even exercise) can increase the amount of liver enzymes in the blood, this response is primarily limited to the use of oral, 17-alkylated anabolic-androgenic steroids. The relationship between these drugs and elevated enzyme levels exists because: these orally effective drugs are metabolized by the liver, the first-pass effect delivers an exceptionally large percentage of the dose to the liver, and abusers typically take excessive doses that further stress liver function. This profile often results in cholecystic jaundice (77), but because inflammation and necrosis are not present, the symptoms are limited to an accumulation of bile, which spills over into the blood. Interestingly, many bodybuilders use this side effect as a metric of their dosing regimen and titrate themselves to levels that just precipitate jaundice (78).

Peliosis hepatitis is a disorder characterized by blood-filled cysts scattered throughout the liver; a detailed description of the history of this disorder and its relationship to anabolic-androgenic steroid abuse is presented elsewhere (79). It has been associated with the 17-alkylated androgens, rarely results in symptoms and likely resolves with discontinuation (80).

The evidence linking 17-alkylated androgens with hepatic tumors is well established. Except for the fact that the androgen-related adenomas are typically larger, the profile resembles that of women who take birth control pills. The risk for developing hepatocellular adenomas ranges from 1% to 3% of users (68), and as with peliosis hepatitis, these adenomas rarely result in symptoms and are often not documented until a routine autopsy is performed.

Anabolic-androgenic steroids affect the cardiovascular system via their effects on HDL/LDL ratios and other blood products. However, there are reports that these drugs can directly affect myocardial tissue. The bulk of the evidence comes from animals studies in which high doses of methandrostenolone result in myocyte necrosis, cellular edema, and mitochondrial swelling (81,82). Because these changes cannot be duplicated by exercise alone, it is likely that these effects were responsible for the clinical case report of an anabolic-androgenic steroid user who suddenly died of cardiac arrest (83).

An adverse effect of anabolic-androgenic steroid use during high-intensity training periods that is not well documented is the incidence of injury that may occur as a direct result of their use. A recent case of bilateral quadriceps rupture profiles the risks involved (84). Although it might seem that the fact that users can train with the drugs beyond what they would be able to tolerate without the drugs is responsible for injuries of this type, it is possible that the growth of muscle mass is not paralleled by an increase in ligament support.

Controversy remains over the degree and extent of the severity of anabolic-androgenic steroid-induced extreme psychiatric effects often referred to as "roid rage." These eruptions of frenzied violent behavior during a cycle of high-dose anabolic-androgenic steroids have been described in a few case reports, but no laboratory studies verifying such reactions have been published. More frequently, cases in which psychiatric effects appear associated with drug use have been reported (85–89). The constellation of symptoms appears to most closely resemble those of hypomania or mania. The energized user of anabolic-androgenic steroids talks faster, has more energy, sleeps less, and is be more impulsive, even to the extent of purchasing expensive cars (88). At the far end of the spectrum, mania may lead to delusions and even hallucinations. Interestingly, many individuals with body dysmorphic disorder present with delusions as well (90). Two studies (91,92) have attempted to standardize the collection of these data and found that using structured interviews, the incidence of a full affective syndrome was present in 22% of a population of 41 bodybuilders (92). Another 12% displayed psychotic symptoms that clearly emerged during anabolic-androgenic steroid use. The cohort of 20 weight lifters who used anabolic-androgenic steroids experienced more somatic, depressive, anxious, hostile, and paranoid complaints than those who did not use these drugs (91).

Empirical evidence of drug effects on aggressive behavior has been obtained using the Karolinska Scale of Personality (93) and a human laboratory model of aggression, the Point Subtraction Aggression Paradigm (94). More recently, psychiatric side effects after supraphysiologic doses of combinations of AAS were reported to correlate with severity of abuse (95). Results from the personality scale indicate that a cohort of anabolic-androgenic steroid users exhibit significantly more verbal aggression, impulsiveness, and indirect aggression. Yates et al. (96) reported that three measures of the Buss-Durkee Hostility Inventory (97), assault, indirect aggression, and verbal aggression were elevated in a group of current or recent anabolic-androgenic steroid users. The Point Subtraction Aggression Paradigm directly measures the amount of provoked aggressive behavior in the laboratory by ostensibly taking away points (that are worth money) from an individual who believes he is playing against another person. In reality, the subject plays against a computer program and the rate of provocation is controlled by the experimenter. Both aggressive and nonaggressive behavior is recorded, so the effects of various drugs on responding per se can be viewed independent from aggressive responding. Using this model, moderately high doses of testosterone cypionate (600 mg, intramuscularly, once per week) can increase aggressive responding in individuals who had not used steroids before (98). Interestingly, animal models have confirmed that anabolic-androgenic steroid administration increases aggressive behavior (99). As weight lifters and bodybuilders have reportedly used weekly doses that exceed three times that used in research studies, it is reasonable to suspect that aggressive behavior can result from these training programs.

Collectively, it appears that anabolic-androgenic steroid use can result in hypomania and even psychotic symptoms, whereas depression may ensue during withdrawal. The lack of well-controlled prospective studies has prevented a more definitive association between anabolic-androgenic steroid use and psychiatric disorders. It is unlikely that such data will become available in the near future because ethical constraints will preclude the conduct of any double-blind assessments of supraphysiologic doses of these drugs.

ADDICTION LIABILITY

Anabolic-androgenic steroid abuse includes a variety of social and psychologic components that are not easy to imitate in either animal models or in currently validated methods of assessing abuse liability in human volunteers. The concepts of perception, motivation, and expectation play a more pivotal role in the initial use and subsequent abuse of these compounds. Because the anabolic effects of AAS can be profound, but slow to develop, it has been difficult to separate these "desired" muscle building effects from direct reinforcement. Demonstrating tolerance and physical dependence on these agents has also proved to be elusive because there are limitations in the doses that can be given to human subjects.

Reward Although the anabolic steroid addiction hypothesis was proposed nearly 20 years ago (100), few empirical studies have been conducted to actually test it. In the last 8 years, animal models of conditioned place preference and self-administration have been employed and evidence is mounting that AAS may possess some weak reinforcing effects that are not related to athletic performance. In the one study by Su et al., healthy non-AAS users described feeling euphoric, full of energy, and having increased sexual arousal after an acute dose of methyltestosterone (101). Although the magnitude of the response was modest, the results were consistent, but have not been replicated.

Perhaps the most important concept to understand about anabolic-androgenic steroid abuse is that these agents are not used in the typical patterns that are observed with traditional drugs of abuse such as cocaine, heroin, alcohol, nicotine, and marijuana. Indeed, AAS are often taken or injected once per week as part of an exercise program. It is well known that if the subjective effects of a psychoactive drug are sufficiently delayed after self-administration, then the drug's reinforcing efficacy decreases and drug-seeking behavior is reduced (102). Although there are a few scattered anecdotal reports that high-doses of anabolic-androgenic steroids can elevate mood, no controlled studies have demonstrated that these drugs produce immediate positive mood effects or euphoria. Anabolic-androgenic steroids can act within minutes to hours on cell membrane receptor sites, but the real beneficial effects of such action (e.g., protein synthesis) takes more time. So, because of the difficulties of conducting such studies with humans, animal models have proven to be most valuable in discerning the nature of the reinforcing effects of these compounds.

Testosterone was shown to be self-administered as hamsters preferred aqueous solutions of the steroid over water (103). The rewarding effects of testosterone using conditioned place preference were described (104), but appeared to be dependent on the environmental cues as conditioned stimuli. A recent study in male rats demonstrated that these drugs may alter the sensitivity of brain reward systems (105). In that study, a 2-week treatment with methandrostenolone alone had no effect on brain reward systems, but a 15-week treatment with a cocktail of three different anabolic-androgenic steroids resulted in a shift in the response patterns to brain electrical reward and amphetamine. In a related study, dopamine receptor density in nucleus accumbens was altered by supraphysiologic doses of testosterone in male rats, suggesting that dopamine levels are increased after AAS (106). This action was verified using positron emission tomography and found that chronic AAS treatment caused an upregulation of the binding potential of dopamine in rat striatum (107).

Another potential link to drugs of abuse is that AAS share brain sites of action and neurotransmitter systems with opioids. In humans, AAS abuse is often associated with prescription opioid use and in animals, AAS overdose produces symptoms resembling opioid overdose (108). This study also demonstrated that AAS modifies the activity of the endogenous opioid system.

The pharmacologic profile of the AAS is thought to be due to androgen binding to intracellular androgen receptors. This process takes about 30 minutes and ultimately alters gene expression, but it is now believed that AAS possess a nongenomic action that can be mobilized in seconds or minutes (109). There have been some recent advances in the understanding of how testosterone metabolites interact with the $GABA_A$/benzodiazepine receptor complex or dopaminergic neurons in nucleus accumbens to mediate testosterone's hedonic effects (110).

The absence of a well-defined pattern of self-administration in animals is confirmed by the finding that humans cannot tell whether they have been given an active anabolic-androgenic steroid or placebo (111). Marginal discriminations were made in two studies, but only after a period of extended testing had been employed (44,112). However, it is likely that it was the side effects of these drugs that were detected, rather than any positive reinforcing effects. Because the latter are thought to regulate drug-taking behavior in both humans and animals, the question that remains is "why do humans use and abuse anabolic-androgenic steroids?"

Collectively, these data from animal models suggest that AAS may very well be reinforcing, but the magnitude and strength of the direct rewarding effects of these agents is modest at best and does not appear to approach that of the more classic drugs of abuse such as heroin, cocaine, or nicotine. Because of testosterone's role in a number of socially labile situations, it may be that it intensifies the rewarding aspects of these other behaviors and that is what contributes to the persistent use by a small fraction of the population.

Tolerance The evidence supporting tolerance development is not strong, although there is a belief among users that cycling is a necessary practice to avoid its development. Twenty percent of a sample of weight lifters believes that tolerance develops, but more than 80% believe that dependence develops. Nevertheless, such concerns over lost efficacy with time appear to be without hard empirical evidence. As such, it must be assumed that the escalating doses that elite athletes use are not taken because tolerance develops to their effects, but to increase the magnitude of the desired effects. The doses are increased slowly to minimize the side effects or to allow time to acclimate to them. When presented with this fact, some users are likely to confuse their behavior with tolerance.

Dependence Although evidence of physical dependence on anabolic-androgenic steroids have not been widespread, there are a few detailed reports of clear signs of withdrawal when their use was abruptly stopped (113–115). In a study of 49 male weight lifters (115), 84% reported experiencing withdrawal effects and the most frequently reported symptoms were: craving for more steroids (52%), fatigue (43%), depressed mood state (41%), restlessness (29%), anorexia (24%), insomnia (20%), decreased libido (20%), and headaches (20%). Interestingly, 42% of these subjects were dissatisfied with their body image during withdrawal as well. Those who reported being dependent on anabolic-androgenic steroids generally took higher doses, completed more cycles of use and reported more aggressive symptoms than those who did not report being dependent. However, the extent of dependence on anabolic-androgenic steroids in the larger population of users may be considerably smaller as there have been no reported cases of withdrawal effects in female athletes or among patients who have been prescribed high doses for legitimate medical purposes.

Anabolic-androgenic steroids in fact can increase muscle mass and body weight, especially when used along with a regular training program. However, many of the "black market" anabolic-androgenic steroid preparations sold during the late 1980s actually were devoid of any active ingredients, including anabolic-androgenic steroids. In spite of the spread of these counterfeit drugs, users claimed to have experienced improvements in their performance. Herein lies the real difficulty in assessing the abuse liability of these compounds. They are not expected to have immediate beneficial effects and so the delay in any improvement does not raise suspicion that the preparation may be inert. Nevertheless, whether these drugs actually increase muscle mass, improve performance, or increase endurance is really not the question that confronts the addiction medicine specialist. The fact that anabolic-androgenic steroid-seeking behavior exists and that extremely high doses are used over relatively long periods suggests that there is a problem and should trigger further inquiry and subsequent treatment.

Physical dependence on AAS may be more insidious than with other drugs. It is quite likely that the initial involvement with AAS is related to the anticipated increased physical strength and body mass. Brower proposed a two-stage model of AAS dependence that incorporated the anabolic benefits early on, but that physical dependence ensues after prolonged use of extremely high doses (116).

Thus, although physical dependence on anabolic-androgenic steroids may be more rare than dependence on other drugs of abuse, the prudent clinician will be ever-vigilant to identify the constellation of signs and symptoms that may signify dependence. Attempts to label the withdrawal signs and symptoms as opiate-like or ethanol-like may complicate the issue only because such an effort may conceal a real dependence on these other drugs. Thus, when obvious signs of distress are observed during periods of forced abstinence, it is worthwhile to consider the possibility that the individual may, in fact, be dependent on other drugs. There have been a few reports of opioid dependence in bodybuilders (117,118), and these individuals clearly met criteria for dependence on both drug classes. Thus, the possibility of polydrug abuse should always be considered when dealing with anabolic-androgenic steroid abusers. Interestingly, according to the American Psychiatric Association's *Diagnostic and Statistical Manual of Mental Disorders, 4th Edition* (DSM-IV; 119), the diagnosis of polysubstance dependence cannot be made if the individual meets criteria for dependence on one of the substances; the criteria for polydrug abuse appear to be geared toward identifying individuals who experiment with a number of different drugs.

Diagnostic Classifications It is apparent from the historical literature that anabolic-androgenic steroid users have met formal criteria for dependence in the American Psychiatric Association's *DSM,* 3rd ed., revised (DSM-IIIR; 120) by having three or more of the following: (a) use continues over longer periods than desired; (b) attempts to stop are unsuccessful; (c) substantial time is spent obtaining, using or recovering from their use; (d) use continues despite knowledge of their harmful effects; (e) physical signs of withdrawal appear upon cessation of use; and (f) they are taken to relieve the withdrawal symptoms (100). The criteria for the DSM-IV are similar, except that a seventh factor of tolerance development, as defined by a need to increase the dose to achieve the desired effect or that a markedly diminished effect occurred with continued use of the same dose, was added.

There is another factor that must be considered when attempting to diagnosis anabolic-androgenic steroid abuse. In a study of 108 bodybuilders, Pope and colleagues noted a rather high percentage of anorexia nervosa and uncovered a body image disorder that they labeled *reverse anorexia* (121). This condition shares many signs and symptoms of body dysmorphic syndrome (122). The profile of the former is that they view themselves as being too small and weak, when they are quite large and strong. The incidence of this disorder was 8% among anabolic-androgenic steroid users and was not observed in any of the non users. The authors postulate that these body image disorders may have some influence on an individual's decision to use anabolic-androgen steroids. Because the perceived size, shape, and attractiveness of one's body is likely tied to self-esteem (123), and, in general, men want to be three pounds heavier, taller, and have wider shoulders (124), anabolic-androgenic steroid use may be viewed as a way of speeding up the process to attain physical attractiveness. This similarity in profiles between body image disorders and drug use might suggest that anabolic-androgenic steroid abusers who present with a profile of body image disturbance may respond to the same treatments that have been used for body dysmorphic syndrome. Serotonin reuptake blockers have been marginally successful in treating body dysmorphic disorder (125), and although there have been no published studies to this effect with anabolic-androgenic steroid users, fluoxetine has been marginally successful in a small sample of bodybuilders who presented with depression during withdrawal from anabolic-androgenic steroid use (126).

ABSORPTION AND METABOLISM

Anabolic-androgenic steroids are taken either orally or injected deep into the muscle; there is no intravenous formulation, nor is there a smokable product. By far the greatest influence on subsequent development of toxic side effects is the route of administration. About half of an oral dose of testosterone is metabolized via the first-pass effect, so very large doses are needed. Some 17α-alkylated analogues of testosterone such as methyltestosterone resist such metabolism and so can be given orally in smaller doses. The oral route gives rise to a number of 17-alkylated metabolites, which are formed in the liver. This overload, not only of the metabolizing enzymes, but also because the doses taken are so high, causes significant stress on this organ.

Testosterone is metabolized to 5α-dihydrotestosterone in certain tissues such as prostate gland, seminal vesicles, and pubic skin. Because 5α-dihydrotestosterone has two to three times the affinity for the androgen receptor as the parent hormone, the effects of testosterone are enhanced in these tissues. One of the more interesting aspects of testosterone's metabolic pathway is that it is converted to estradiol in tissues that contain an aromatase enzyme (127). The biologic significance of circulating estrogens in males is unknown, but they may be involved with sex hormone–binding globulin and lipoproteins. Further, the estrogen that results from this metabolic process may interact with estrogen receptors to produce an anabolic effect (99,128). The 17α-alkylated analogues discussed above are not metabolized to either 5α-dihydrotestosterone or estrogen. Instead, they interact with the androgen receptor (1,129). Thus, the overall profile of relative anabolic to androgenic effects is not only due to the parent compound, but to the profile of metabolites that result. With the advent of widespread use of these drugs during athletic competition, a number of analytic laboratories have been set up to detect either the parent drug or its metabolites (130,131). In addition to providing quantitative analyses of the various synthetic analogues, most labs attempt to measure the testosterone/epitestosterone ratio as a metric of exogenous testosterone administration.

MECHANISMS OF ACTION

About 95% of the testosterone in males is synthesized in the testes, whereas the remaining 5% comes from the adrenals. The cholesterol used in the synthetic pathway comes from acetate that is stored in the testes, and not from circulating blood levels. Anabolic-androgenic steroids have long been thought to exert their effects in the periphery, primarily by increasing the rate of RNA transcription (7,132). About half of the circulating testosterone is tightly bound to sex hormone–binding globulin, and the other half is lightly bound to albumin, from which it freely dissociates and from whence it can diffuse passively into target cells. After attaching to a steroid receptor in the cytoplasm, the hormone-receptor complex moves into the nucleus where it binds to sites on the chromatin, resulting in new mRNA. If the target tissue is skeletal muscle, then new myofilaments are formed which causes myofibrils to divide (1,133). Because it is not completely understood whether this activity occurs at the supraphysiologic doses typically taken by anabolic-androgenic steroid abusers, another mechanism was sought. It has been suggested that high doses of anabolic-androgenic steroids cross-react with glucocorticoid receptors that control the catabolic rates of protein (1,134,135). The significance of the anticatabolic effect of these drugs is often ignored in lieu of the more direct effect of these steroids on protein synthesis. It is also possible that the stress of strenuous workouts is not felt by athletes taking these compounds because the stress-induced increase in cortisol is somehow blocked. This action would also permit the workouts to be longer and more vigorous, further improving performance.

It is possible that the physical changes attributed to a direct effect of anabolic-androgenic steroids on protein synthesis may actually be mediated via a direct effect on the central nervous system. Such effects might result in increased motivation and intensity of training to a degree that performance is improved. Increased aggressive behavior may also play a role in the training process. It is likely that the use of supraphysiologic doses of these drugs can have both a direct effect on muscle tissue and an indirect effect by altering emotions such as motivation and drive such that the training periods are longer and more productive, resulting in improved performance.

The pharmacologic profile of the AAS is thought to be due to androgen binding to intracellular androgen receptors. This process takes about 30 minutes and ultimately alters gene expression, but it is now believed that AAS possess a non genomic action that can be mobilized in seconds or minutes (109). There have been some recent advances in the understanding of how testosterone metabolites interact with the $GABA_A$/benzodiazepine receptor complex or dopaminergic neurons in nucleus accumbens to mediate testosterone's hedonic effects (110). The concept that AAS interact directly with peripheral benzodiazepine receptors in rat brain was explored over a decade ago (136). These receptors are mitochondrial proteins that are involved with regulating steroid synthesis and transport, so it seems plausible that their activation via exogenous anabolic-androgenic steroids could have an impact on behavior that is mediated by these receptors.

The increase in body weight, especially during the first weeks of use, is almost certainly attributed to the stimulation of mineralocorticoid receptors, resulting in sodium and, ultimately, water retention as well as increasing amounts of circulating estrogen that has been aromatized from testosterone. This effect gives the muscles, particularly the deltoid, a "puffy" appearance. The increase in red blood cell production is probably the major reason that long-distance runners may use these drugs because endurance, rather than bulk muscle mass, is an asset in this sport. Blood volume probably increases as a result of erythropoietin synthesis. This effect is due to direct action on bone marrow and easily leads to a rise in hematocrit (137).

FUTURE VISTAS

Although AAS are not specifically mentioned in the Healthy People 2010 initiative, the federal government has set a national goal to increase the "proportion of adolescents not using alcohol or any illicit drugs during the past 30 days" (138). These drugs continue to be used and abused by individuals for a wide range of reasons. Further, as former heavy users of anabolic androgenic steroids enter middle age, it remains to be seen whether there are psychiatric of other medical consequences of this form of drug abuse (139). The addiction liability of AAS may have a central nervous system mechanism that complements the anabolic effects. As quantitative methods for detecting AAS have become more sophisticated and specific, individuals have switched to using nutritional supplements, endogenous peptides such as growth hormone and epoetin. Although the anabolic effects of many of these supplements are not well documented, side effects can still occur and remain a concern. Because these novel peptides can now be detected, the way has been paved for an emerging biotechnique that implements recombinant DNA such that manipulated genes can be inserted into mammalian cells. This practice, called gene doping or performance-enhancing genetics, has been defined by the World Anti-Doping Agency or as "the non-therapeutic use of genes, genetic elements and/or cells that have the capacity to enhance athletic performance" (140). This commission is unique in that human gene doping has not yet occurred, but World Anti-Doping Agency has taken the initiative to set standards for future events. Conceptually, gene doping would involve using scientific techniques to manipulate DNA in a manner that would improve athletic performance (141,142).

ACKNOWLEDGMENTS: *This manuscript was supported by Research Scientist Award K05 DA00343 from the National Institute on Drug Abuse.*

REFERENCES

1. Wilson JD. Androgen abuse by athletes. *Endocr Rev* 1988;9:181–199.
2. Kochakian CD. History of anabolic-androgenic steroids. In: Lin GC, Erinoff L, eds. *Anabolic steroid abuse (NIDA research monograph 102).* Rockville, MD: National Institute on Drug Abuse, 1990:29–59.
3. Boje O. Doping. *Bull Health Org League Nations* 1939;8:439–469.
4. Hartgens F, Kuipers H. Effects of androgenic-anabolic steroids in athletes. *Sports Med* 2004;34:513–554.
5. Todd T. Anabolic steroids: the gremlins of sport. *J Sports Hist* 1987; 14:87–107.
6. Yesalis C, Anderson W, Buckley W, et al. (Incidence of the nonmedical use of anabolic-androgenic steroids. In: *Anabolic steroid abuse.* Rockville, MD: National Institute on Drug Abuse, 1990.
7. Lukas SE. Current perspectives on anabolic-androgenic steroid abuse. *Trends Pharmacol Sci* 1993;14:61–68.
8. Bahrke MS, Yesalis III CE. Weight training: a potential confounding factor in examining the psychological and behavioural effects of anabolic-androgenic steroids. *Sports Med* 1994;18(5):309–318.
9. Gambelunghe C, Sommavilla M, Ferranti C, et al. Analysis of anabolic steroids in hair by GC/MS/MS. *Biomed Chromatogr* 2007;21(4): 369–375.
10. McHugh CM, Park RT, Sönksen PH, et al. Challenges in detecting the abuse of growth hormone in sport. *Clin Chem* 2005;51:1587–1593.
11. Graham MR, Davies B, Grace FM, et al. Anabolic steroid use: patterns of use and detection of doping. *Sports Med* 2008;38:505–525.
12. Graham MR, Baker JS, Evans P, et al. Physical effects of short-term recombinant human growth hormone administration in abstinent steroid dependency. *Horm Res* 2008;69:343–354.
13. Yesalis CE, Kennedy NJ, Kopstein AN, et al. Anabolic-androgenic steroid use in the United States. *JAMA* 1993;270(10):1217–1221.
14. Substance Abuse and Mental Health Services Administration. *National household survey on drug abuse: main findings 1994.* Washington, DC: U.S. Government Printing Office (DHHS Publication No. [SMA] 96-3085), 1996.
15. National Institute on Drug Abuse. *National survey results on drug use from the Monitoring The Future Study, 1975–1994, vol. II.* Bethesda, MD: National Institutes of Health (NIH Publication No. 96-4139), 1996.
16. Irving LM, Wall M, Neumark-Sztainer D, et al. Steroid use among adolescents: findings from Project EAT. *J Adolesc Health* 2002;4: 243–52.
17. Cafri G, Thompson JK, Ricciardelli L. Pursuit of the muscular ideal: physical and psychological consequences and putative risk factors. *Clin Psychol Rev* 2005;25:215–239.
18. National Center for Chronic Disease Prevention and Health Promotion. Youth Risk Behavior Surveillance System. Healthy Youth! National data files & documentation: 1991–2005. Accessed June 16, 2008, from http://www.cdc.gov/HealthyYouth/yrbs/index.htm.
19. Elliot DL, Cheong J, Moe EL, et al. Cross-sectional study of female students reporting anabolic steroid use. *Arch Ped Adolesc Med* 2007; 161(6):572–577.
20. Smolak L. Body image in children and adolescents: where do we go from here? *Body Image* 2004;1:15–28.
21. Yesalis CE, Barsukiewicz CK, Koopstein AN, et al. Trends in anabolic-androgenic steroid use among adolescents. *Arch Pediatr Adolesc Med* 1997;151:1197–1206.
22. vandenBerg P, Neumark-Sztainer D, Cafri G, et al. Steroid use among adolescents: longitudinal findings from Project EAT. *Pediatrics* 2007; 119:476–486.
23. Kanayama G, Boynes M, Hudson JI, et al. Anabolic steroid abuse among teenage girls: an illusory problem? *Drug Alcohol Depend* 2007; 88:156–162.
24. Smolak L, Stein JA. The relationship of drive for muscularity to sociocultural factors, self-esteem, physical attributes gender role, and social comparison in middle school boys. *Body Image* 2006;3:121–129.
25. Parkinson AB, Evans NA. Anabolic androgenic steroids: a survey of 500 users. *Med Sci Sports Exerc* 2006;38:644–651.
26. Laos C, Metzl JD. *Adolesc Med Clin* 2006;17(3):719–731.
27. Castillo EM, Comstock RD. Prevalence of use of performance-enhancing substances among United States adolescents. *Pediatr Clin North Am* 2007;54:663–675.
28. Smurawa TM, Congeni JA. Testosterone precursors: use and abuse in pediatric athletes. *Pediatr Clin North Am* 2007;54:787–796.
29. Hoffman JR, Faigenbaum AD, Ratamess NA, et al. Nutritional supplementation and anabolic steroid use in adolescents. *Med Sci Sports Exerc* 2008;40:15–24.
30. Wells S, Jozefowicz R, Statt M. Failure of dehydroepiandrosterone to influence energy and protein metabolism in humans. *J Clin Endocrinol Metab* 1990;71:1259–1264.
31. Broeder CE, Quindry J, Brittingham K, et al. The andro project: physiological and hormonal influences of androstenedione supplementation in men 35 to 65 years old participating in a high-intensity resistance training program. *Arch Intern Med* 2000;160:3093–3104.

32. Brown GA, Vukovich MD, Sharp RL, et al. Effect of oral DHEA on serum testosterone and adaptations to resistance training in young men. *J Appl Physiol* 1999;87:2274–2283.
33. Brown GA, Vukovich MD, Reifenrath TA, et al. Effects of anabolic precursors on serum testosterone concentrations and adaptations to resistance training in young men. *Int J Sport Nutr Exerc Metab* 2000; 10:340–359.
34. Ziegenfuss TN, Berardi JM, Lowrey LM. Effects of prohormone supplementation in humans: a review. *Can J Appl Physiol* 2002;27:628–645.
35. Foster ZJ, Housner JA. Anabolic-androgenic steroids and testosterone precursors: ergogenic aids and sport. *Curr Sports Med Rep* 2004;3:234–241.
36. Bahrke MS, Yesalis CE. Abuse of anabolic androgenic steroids and related substances in sport and exercise. *Curr Opin Pharmacol* 2004; 4:614–620.
37. Petróczi A, Naughton DP, Mazanov J, et al. Performance enhancement with supplements: incongruence between rationale and practice. *J Int Soc Sports Nutr* 2007;12:19–28.
38. Salas-Ramirez KY, Montalto PR, Sisk CL. Anabolic androgenic steroids differentially affect social behaviors in adolescent and adult male Syrian hamsters. *Horm Behav* 2008;53:378–385.
39. McGinnis MY. Anabolic androgenic steroids and aggression: studies using animal models. In: Devine J, Gilligan J, Miczek KA, et al., eds. Youth violence: scientific approaches to prevention. New York: New York Academy of Sciences, 2004:399–409.
40. van Bokhoven I, van Goozen SH, van Engeland H, et al. Salivary testosterone and aggression, delinquency, and social dominance in a population-based longitudinal study of adolescent males. *Horm Behav* 2006;50: 118–125.
41. Sato SM, Schulz KM, Sisk CL, et al. Adolescents and androgens, receptors and rewards. *Horm Behav* 2008;53:647–658.
42. Holland-Hall C). Performance-enhancing substances: is your adolescent patient using? *Pediatr Clin North Am* 2007;54:651–662.
43. Yesalis CE, Herrick RT, Buckley WE, et al. Self-reported use of anabolic androgenic steroids by elite powerlifters. *Physiol Sportsmed* 1988; 16:91–100.
44. Freed DLJ, Banks AJ, Longson D, et al. Anabolic steroids in athletics: crossover double-blind trial on weightlifters. *Br Med J* 1975;2:471–473.
45. Johansen KL, Painter PL, Sakkas GK, et al. Effects of resistance training and nandrolone deconoate on body composition and muscle function among patients who receive hemodialysis: a randomized, controlled trial. *J Am Soc Nephrol* 2006;17:2307–2314.
46. Brower KJ. Rehabilitation for anabolic-androgenic steroid dependence. *Clin Sports Med* 1989;1:171–181.
47. Haupt HA, Rovere GB. Anabolic steroids: a review of the literature. *Am J Sports Med* 1984;12:469–484.
48. Anderson W, McKeag B. *The substance use and abuse habits of college student athletes. Research paper no. 2.* Mission, KS: National Collegiate Athletic Association, 1985.
49. Perry PJ, Lund BC, Deninger MJ, et al. Anabolic steroid use in weightlifters and bodybuilders: an internet survey of drug utilization. *Clin J Sports Med* 2005;15:326–330.
50. Perikles S, Striegel H, Aust F, et al. Doping in fitness sports: estimated number of unreported cases and individual probability of doping. *Addiction* 2006;101:1640–1644.
51. Wesson DW, McGinnis MY. Stacking anabolic androgenic steroids (AAS) during puberty in rats: a neuroendocrine and behavioral assessment. *Pharmacol Biochem Behav* 2006;83:410–419.
52. Buckley WE, Yesalis CE, Friedl KE, et al. Estimated prevalence of anabolic steroid use among male high school seniors. *JAMA* 1988; 260:3441–3445.
53. Yesalis CE, Streit AL, Vicary JR, et al. Anabolic steroid use: indications of habituation among adolescents. *J Drug Ed* 1989;19:103–116.
54. Wang MQ, Fitzhugh EC, Yesalis CE, et al. Desire for weight gain and potential risk of adolescent males using anabolic steroids. *Percept Motor Skills* 1994;78:267–274.
55. Tanner SM, Miller DW, Alongi C. Anabolic steroid use by adolescents: Prevalence, motives, and knowledge of risks. *Clin J Sports Med* 1995;5:108–115.
56. Melia P, Pipe A, Greenberg L. The use of anabolic-androgenic steroids by Canadian students. *Clin J Sports Med* 1996;6(1):9–14.
57. Durant RH, Rickert VI, Ashworth CS, et al. Use of multiple drugs among adolescents who use anabolic steroids. *N Engl J Med* 1993; 328:922–926.
58. Rogol AD, Yesalis CE 3d. Anabolic-androgenic steroids and the adolescent. *Pediatr Ann* 1992;21(3):175–188.
59. Moore WB. Anabolic steroid use in adolescents. *JAMA* 1988;260: 3484–3486.
60. Goldberg L, Bents R, Bosworth E, et al. Anabolic steroid education and adolescents: Do scare tactics work? *Pediatrics* 1991;87:283–286.
61. Dart R. Drugs in the workplace: anabolic steroid abuse among law enforcement officers. *Police Chief* 1991;58(7):18.
62. Swanson C, Gaines L, Gore B. Abuse of anabolic Steroids. *FBI Law Enforce Bull* 1991;60(8):19–23.
63. Cooper CJ, Noakes TD, Dunne T, et al. A high prevalence of abnormal personality traits in chronic users of anabolic-androgenic steroids. *Br J Sports Med* 1996;30(3):246–250.
64. Schwerin MJ, Corcoran KJ. Beliefs about steroids: user vs. non-user comparisons. *Drug Alcohol Depend* 1996;40(3):221–225.
65. Kanayama G, Barry S, Hudson JI, et al. Body image and attitudes toward male roles in anabolic-androgenic steroid users. *Am J Psychiatry* 2006;163:697–703.
66. Pope CG, Pope HG, Menard W, et al. Clinical features of muscle dysmorphia among males with body dysmorphic disorder. *Body Image* 2005;2:395–400.
67. Hartgens F, Kuipers H, Wijnen JAG, et al. Body composition, cardiovascular risk factors and liver function in long term androgenic-anabolic steroids using body builders three months after drug withdrawal. *Int J Sports Med* 1996;17:429–433.
68. Friedl KE. Reappraisal of the health risks associated with high doses of oral and injectable androgenic steroids. In: Lin GC, Erinoff L, eds. *Anabolic steroid abuse (NIDA research monograph 102).* Rockville, MD: National Institute on Drug Abuse, 1990:142–177.
69. Thompson PB, Curinane AN, Sady SP, et al. Contrasting effects of testosterone and stanozolol on serum lipoprotein levels. *JAMA* 1989;261:1165–1168.
70. McNutt RA, Ferenchick GF, Kirlin PC, et al. Acute myocardial infarction in a 22 year old, world-class weightlifter using anabolic steroids. *Am J Cardiol* 1988;62:164.
71. Bowman S. Anabolic steroids and infarction. *Br Med J* 1990;300:750.
72. Ferenchick BS. Are androgenic steroids thrombogenic? *N Engl J Med* 1990;322:476.
73. Lenders JWM, Demacker PN, Vos JA, et al. Deleterious effects of anabolic steroids on serum lipoproteins, blood pressure and liver function in amateur bodybuilders. *Int J Sports Med* 1988;9:19–23.
74. Palacios A, McClure RB, Campfield A, et al. Effect of testosterone enanthate on testis size. *J Urol* 1981;26:46–48.
75. Allen M, Suominen J. Effect of androgenic and anabolic steroids on spermatogenesis in power athletes. *Int J Sports Med* 1984;5 (Suppl):189.
76. Kashkin KB. Anabolic steroids. In: Lowinson JH, Ruiz P, Millman RB, et al., eds. *Substance abuse: a comprehensive textbook,* 2nd ed. Baltimore, MD: Williams & Wilkins, 1992:380–395.
77. Pecking A, Lejolly JM, Najean Y. Hepatic toxicity of androgen therapy in aplastic anemia. *Nouvelle Revue Francaise D Hematologie* 1980;22:257–265.
78. Lukas SE. *Steroids.* Hillside, NJ: Enslow Publishers, 1994.
79. Karch SB. Anabolic steroids. Karch's pathology of drug abuse. 3E Boca Raton FL: CRC Press, 2002:481–499.
80. Westaby B, Ogle SJ, Paridians FJ, et al. Liver damage from long-term methyltestosterone. *Lancet* 1977;1(8032):261–263.
81. Appell H, Heller-Umpfenbach B, Feraudi M, et al. Ultra-structural and morphometric investigations on the effects of training and administration of anabolic steroids on the myocardium of guinea pigs. *Int J Sports Med* 1983;4:268–274.
82. Behrendt H, Boffin H. Myocardial cell lesions caused by an anabolic hormone. *Cell Tissue Res* 1977;181:423–426.

83. Luke J, Farb A, Virmani R, et al. Sudden cardiac death during exercise in a weight lifter using anabolic androgenic steroids: pathological and toxicological findings. *J Forensic Sci* 1991;35(6):1441–1447.
84. David HG, Green JT, Grant AJ, et al. Simultaneous bilateral quadriceps rupture: A complication of anabolic steroid abuse. *J Bone Jt Surg (Brit)* 1995;77(1):159–160.
85. Annitto WR, Layman WA. Anabolic steroids and acute schizophrenic episode. *J Clin Psychiatry* 1980;41:143–144.
86. Freinhar JP, Alvarez W. Androgen-induced hypomania. *J Clin Psychiatry* 1985;46:354–355.
87. Conacher GN, Workman DG. Violent crime possibly associated with anabolic steroid use. *Am J Psychiatry* 1989;146:679.
88. Pope HG Jr, Katz DL. Body-builder's psychosis. *Lancet* 1987;1:863.
89. Wilson IC, Prange AJ Jr, Lara PP. Methyltestosterone with imipramine in men: Conversion of depression to paranoid reaction. *Am J Psychiatry* 1974;131:21–24.
90. Phillips KA, McElroy SL, Keck PE Jr, et al. A comparison of delusional and nondelusional body dysmorphic disorder in 100 cases. *Psychopharmacol Bull* 1994;30(2):179–186.
91. Perry PJ, Yates WR, Anderson KH. Psychiatric effects of anabolic steroids: A controlled retrospective study. *Ann Clin Psychiatry* 1990;2:11–17.
92. Pope HG Jr, Katz DL. Affective and psychotic symptoms associated with anabolic steroid use. *Am J Psychiatry* 1988;45(4):487–490.
93. Galligani N, Renck A, Hansen S. Personality profile of men using anabolic androgenic steroids. *Horm Behav* 1996;30(2):170–175.
94. Cherek DR. Effects of smoking different doses of nicotine on human aggressive behavior. *Psychopharmacology* 1981;75:339–345.
95. Pagonis TA, Angelopoulos NV, Koukoulis GN, et al. Psychiatric side effects induced by supraphysiological doses of combinations of anabolic steroids correlate to the severity of abuse. *Eur Psychiatry* 2006;21:551–62.
96. Yates WR, Perry P & Murray S. Aggression and hostility in anabolic steroid users. *Biological Psychiatry* 1992;31:1232–1234.
97. Buss AH, Durkee A. An inventory for assessing different kinds of hostility. *J Consult Psychol* 1957;21:343–349.
98. Kouri EM, Lukas SE, Pope HG Jr, et al. Increased aggressive responding in male volunteers following the administration of gradually increasing doses of testosterone cypionate. *Drug Alcohol Depend* 1995;40:73–79.
99. Svare BB. Anabolic steroids and behavior: a preclinical research prospectus. In: Lin GC, Erinoff L, eds. *Anabolic steroid abuse (NIDA research monograph 102).* Rockville, MD: National Institute on Drug Abuse, 1990:224–241.
100. Kashkin KB, Kleber HD. Hooked on hormones? An anabolic steroid addiction hypothesis. *JAMA* 1989;262(22):3166–3170.
101. Su TP, Pagliaro M, Schmidt PJ, et al. Neuropsychiatric effects of anabolic steroids in male normal volunteers. *JAMA* 1993;269:2760–2764.
102. Balster RL, Schuster CR. Fixed-interval schedule of cocaine reinforcement: effect of dose and infusion duration. *J Exp Anal Behav* 1973;20(1):119–129.
103. Johnson LR, Wood RI. Oral testosterone self-administration in male hamsters. *Neuroendocrinology* 2001;73:285–292.
104. Arnedo MT, Salvador A, Martinez-Sanchis S, et al. Rewarding properties of testosterone in intact male mice: a pilot study. *Pharmacol Biochem Behav* 2000;65:327–332.
105. Clark AS, Lindenfeld RC, Gibbons CH. Anabolic-androgenic steroids and brain reward. *Pharmacol Biochem Behav* 1996;53(3):741–745.
106. Kindlundh AM, Lindblom J, Bergström L, et al. The anabolic-androgenic steroid nandrolone decanoate affects the density of dopamine receptors in the male rat brain. *Eur J Neurosci* 2001;13: 291–296.
107. Kindlundh AM, Bergström M, Monazzam A, et al. Dopaminergic effects after chronic treatment with nandrolone visualized in rat brain by positron emission tomography. *Prog Neuropsychopharmacol Biol Psychiatry* 2002;26:1303–1308.
108. Peters KD, Wood RI. Androgen dependence in hamsters: overdose, tolerance, and potential opioidergic mechanisms. *Neuroscience* 2005;130: 971–981.
109. Michels G, Hoppe UC. Rapid action of androgens. Front *Neuroendocrinol* 2008;29:182–198.
110. Frye CA. Some rewarding effects of androgens may be mediated by actions of its 5alpha-reduced metabolite 3alpha-androstanediol. Pharmacol Biochem Behav 2007;86:354–367.
111. Ariel G, Saville W. The physiological effects of placebos. *Med Sci Sports* 1972;4:124.
112. Crist DM, Stackpole PJ, Peake GT. Effects of androgenic-anabolic steroids on neuromuscular power and body composition. *J Appl Physiol* 1983;54:366–370.
113. Brower KJ, Eliopulos GA, Blow FC, et al. Evidence for physical and psychological dependence on anabolic-androgenic steroids in eight weightlifters. *Am J Psychiatry* 1990;147:510–512.
114. Brower KJ. Anabolic steroids: addictive, psychiatric, and medical consequences. *Am J Addictions* 1992;1(2):100–114.
115. Brower KJ, Blow FC, Young JP, et al. Symptoms and correlates of anabolic-androgenic steroid dependence. *Br J Addiction* 1991;86:759–768.
116. Brower KJ. Anabolic steroid abuse and dependence. *Curr Psychiatry Rep* 2002;4:377–387.
117. vans WS, Bowen JN, Giordano FL, et al. A case of Stadol dependence (letter). *JAMA* 1985;253(15):2191–2192.
118. McBride AJ, Williamson K, Petersen T. Three cases of nalbuphine hydrochloride dependence associated with anabolic steroid use. *Br J Sports Med* 1996;30(1):69–70.
119. American Psychiatric Association (1994). *Diagnostic and statistical manual of mental disorders, 4th ed.* Washington DC: American Psychiatric Association.
120. American Psychiatric Association (1987). *Diagnostic and statistical manual of mental disorders, 3rd ed., revised.* Washington DC: American Psychiatric Association.
121. Pope HG Jr, Katz DL, Hudson JI. Anorexia nervosa and "reverse anorexia" among 108 male bodybuilders. *Comp Psychiatry* 1993;34(6):406–409.
122. Phillips KA. Body dysmorphic disorder: diagnosis and treatment of imagined ugliness. *J Clin Psychiatry* 1996;57(Suppl 8):61–65.
123. Lombardo JA. Anabolic-androgenic steroids. In: Lin GC, Erinoff L, eds. *Anabolic steroid abuse (NIDA research monograph 102).* Rockville, MD: National Institute on Drug Abuse, 1992:60–73.
124. Wroblewski AM. Androgenic-anabolic steroids and body dysmorphia in young men. *J Psychosom Res* 1997;42(3):225–234.
125. Hollander E, Liebowitz MR, Winchel R, et al. Treatment of body-dysmorphic disorder with serotonin reuptake blockers. *Am J Psychiatry* 1989;146(6):768–770.
126. Malone DA Jr, Dimeff RJ. The use of fluoxetine in depression associated with anabolic steroid withdrawal: a case series. *J Clin Psychiatry* 1992;53(4):130–132.
127. Martini L. The 5-alpha-reduction of testosterone in the neuroendocrine structures: biochemical and physiological implications. *Endocr Rev* 1982;3:1–25.
128. Bardin CW, Catterall JF, Janne OA. The androgen-induced phenotype. In: Lin GC, Erinoff L, eds. *Anabolic steroid abuse (NIDA research monograph 102).* Rockville, MD: National Institute on Drug Abuse, 1990: 131–141.
129. Winters SJ. Androgens: endocrine physiology and pharmacology. In: Lin GC, Erinoff L, eds. *Anabolic steroid abuse (NIDA research monograph 102).* Rockville, MD: National Institute on Drug Abuse, 1990:113–130.
130. Schanzer W. Metabolism of anabolic androgenic steroids. *Clin Chem* 1996;42(7):1001–1020.
131. Catlin DH. Detection of drug use by athletes. In: Strauss RH, ed. *Drugs and performance in sports.* Philadelphia, PA: WB Saunders, 1987: 103–120.
132. Lukas SE. CNS effects and abuse liability of anabolic-androgenic steroids. *Annu Rev Pharmacol Toxicol* 1996;36:333–357.
133. Rogivkin BA. The role of low molecular weight compounds in the regulation of skeletal muscle genome activity during exercise. *Med Sci Sports* 1976;8:104.
134. Mayer M, Rosen F. Interaction of glucocorticoids and androgens with skeletal muscle. *Metabolism* 1977;27:937–962.
135. Raaka BM, Finnerty M, Samuels HH. The glucocorticoid antagonist 17 alpha-methyltestosterone binds to the 10S glucocorticoid receptor and

blocks agonist-mediated disassociation of the 10S oligomer to the 4S deoxyribonucleic acid-binding subunit. *Mol Endocrinol* 1989;3: 322–341.

136. Masonis AE, McCarthy MP. Direct interactions of androgenic/anabolic steroids with the peripheral benzodiazepine receptor in rat brain: implications for the psychological and physiological manifestations of androgenic/anabolic steroid abuse. *J Steroid Biochem Mol Biol* 1996;58(56): 551–555.
137. Narducci WA, Wagner JC, Hendrickson TP, et al. Anabolic steroids—a review of the clinical toxicology and diagnostic screening. *Clin Toxicol* 1990;28(3):287–310.
138. DHHS. US Department of Health and Human Services. Healthy People 2010. Washington, DC: Goal 26-10, 2000. Accessed June 16, 2008, from http://www.healthypeople.gov/Document/tableofcontents.htm# Volume2.
139. Kanayama G, Hudson JI, Pope HG. Long-term psychiatric and medical consequences of anabolic-androgenic steroid abuse: A looming public health concern? *Drug Alcohol Depend* 2008;98:1–12.
140. World Anti-Doping Agency. The 2007 prohibited list: international standard. Montreal (Canada): WADA; 2006.
141. Unal M, Unal DO. Gene doping in sports. *Sports Med* 2004;34:357–362.
142. Azzazy HME, Mansour MMH, Christenson RH. Doping in the recombinant era: strategies and counterstrategies. *Clin Biochem* 2005;38: 959–965.

SUGGESTED READINGS

Cowart VS. Some predict increased steroid use in sports despite drug testing, crackdown on supplies. *JAMA* 1987;257:3025–3029.

Elliott D, Goldberg L. Intervention and prevention of steroid use in adolescents. *Am J Sports Med* 1996;24(6):5–46, 1996.

Johnson MD, Jay MS, Shoup B, et al. Anabolic steroid use by male adolescents. *Pediatrics* 1989;83(6):921–924.

Karila T, Laaksonen R, Jokelainen K, et al. The effects of anabolic androgenic steroids on serum ubiquinone and dolichol levels among steroid abusers. *Metabolism* 1996;45(7):844–847.

Kouri EM, Pope HG Jr, Katz DL, et al. Fat-free mass index in users and nonusers of anabolic-androgenic steroids. *Clin J Sports Med* 1995;5(4): 223–228.

National Institute on Drug Abuse. *National survey results on drug use from the monitoring the future study, 1975–1995, vol. I.* Bethesda, MD: National Institutes of Health (NIH Publication No. 96-4027), 1996.

O'Connor JS, Baldini FD, Skinner JS, et al. Blood chemistry of current and previous anabolic steroid users. *Mil Med* 1990;155(2):72–75.

Substance Abuse and Mental Health Services Administration. *Results from the 2006 National Survey on Drug Use and Health: National Findings* (Office of Applied Studies, NSDUH Series H-32, DHHS Publication No. SMA 07-4293). Rockville, MD, 2007.

Substance Abuse and Mental Health Services Administration. *Proceedings of the National Consensus Meeting on the Use, Abuse and Sequelae of Abuse of Methamphetamine with Implications for Prevention, Treatment and Research.* Washington, DC: U.S. Government Printing Office (DHHS Publication Number [SMA] 96-8013), 1996.

VanItallie TB, Yang MU, Heymsfield SB, et al. Height-normalized indices of the body's fat-free mass and fat mass: Potentially useful indicators of nutritional status. *Am J Clin Nutrition* 1990;52:953–959.

Wood RI. Reinforcing aspects of androgens. *Physiol Behav* 2004;83: 279–89.

Yesalis CE, Vicary JR, Buckley WE, et al. Indications of psychological dependence among anabolic-androgenic steroid abusers. In: GC Lin GC, Erinoff L, eds. *Anabolic steroid abuse (NIDA research monograph 102).* Rockville, MD: National Institute on Drug Abuse, 1990: 196–214.

SECTION 3

Diagnosis, Assessment and Early Intervention

CHAPTER 18

Aleksandra Zgierska MD, PhD
Michael F. Fleming, MD, MPH

Screening and Brief Intervention

Alcohol use disorders occur in 10% to 20% of patients presenting to the offices of primary care physicians and admitted to a hospital. The frequency varies by age, culture and comorbid medical and mental health problems. These rates are higher in trauma patients and those presenting to emergency departments and approach 50% in some high-risk settings. Rates of illicit and prescription drug use disorders in primary care and hospital settings vary from 5% to 10% with considerable overlap with alcohol use disorders. Prescription opioid abuse is becoming an increasing problem. Substance misuse and use disorders are an enormous burden to the health care system with no easy solution.

What is a doctor to do when every fifth patient coming into the office has an alcohol and/or drug use disorder? Every day, a primary care physician will provide medical care to three to five patients with addictive disorders. How should hospital-based physicians care for the one in five admissions directly related to substance abuse? What is the appropriate response for health care systems, payors, hospitals? How do physicians manage the complex comorbidity with which alcohol and drug use are closely associated with, and are sometimes the etiologic agents responsible for the patient's disease? A number of serious medical problems, including tobacco dependence, liver failure, hypertension, obesity, glucose intolerance, memory loss, and a variety of other medical and mental health conditions are directly related to problematic alcohol use. One promising solution is screening and brief intervention (SBI), and—when appropriate—a referral to a specialty, addiction treatment program (SBIRT).

Brief intervention (BI) is one of many treatment methods available to help patients with excessive alcohol use and alcohol and drug use disorders. BI is a time-limited, client-centered counseling session designed to reduce substance use. It is generally delivered by a health care professional in the context of routine clinical care. The average duration of a BI can range from 5 to 20 minutes. Studies suggest that multiple BI sessions are more effective than a single contact. Having an established relationship with a patient seems to increase the likelihood of success. BI does not seem to be linked to a patient's stated "readiness to change" and can work in precontemplators as well as persons who are ready to change.

One of the primary differences between BI and other types of therapy ranging from behavioral and pharmacologic professional treatments to self-help meetings such as Alcoholic Anonymous (AA) is the treatment goal. BI is based on a harm reduction paradigm that emphasizes reduction in use rather than abstinence in order to reduce the risk of negative, drinking-related consequences (e.g., trauma, depression, hypertension or violence). There is a clear dose-response relationship between the level of alcohol consumption and the risk for alcohol related harms. For example, patients who drink four or more drinks per day have a two- to three-fold increase in the risk of a fatal accident and the development of liver failure, cancer, or ischemic heart disease; if the patient can reduce alcohol use to one to two drinks per day and never drinks more than three to four drinks on an occasion, the risk of harm will be substantially reduced.

SBI has been studied and used in clinical practice for a long time. Although most physicians have received limited formal training in brief "talk therapy" or brief counseling, it is one of the essential elements of being a physician. SBI technique is one of the most popular clinical "tools" utilized by primary care providers who employ the SBI basics with nearly every patient to change a variety of the patient's harmful behaviors including smoking, overeating, poor medication compliance, or sedentary life style. SBI can be viewed as a part of the provider's responsibilities, in addition to ordering tests, performing surgical procedures, prescribing medications, and filling out medical records.

NATIONAL RECOMMENDATIONS ON THE IMPLEMENTATION OF SUBSTANCE ABUSE SCREENING AND TREATMENT IN MEDICAL CARE SETTINGS

Over the past four decades, research has demonstrated the feasibility and benefits of SBI as a behavioral therapy for substance use in a variety of public health and clinical care settings. Based on this evidence, recent years have witnessed structured efforts to disseminate SBI into clinical practice.

The U.S. Preventive Services Task Force (USPSTF) recommends routine SBI to reduce alcohol "misuse" by adults, including pregnant women and in primary care settings and strongly recommends that clinicians screen all adults, including pregnant women, for tobacco use and provide tobacco cessation interventions for tobacco users. The USPSTF concludes that the evidence is insufficient to formally recommend for or against routine SBI to prevent or reduce alcohol misuse or tobacco use among children and adolescents. The USPTF does not recommend universal SBI for illicit drug use because of the insufficient evidence for efficacy of this specific practice (1).

Many health care organizations such as the American Medical Association (AMA), the American Academy of Child and Adolescent Psychiatry, the American Academy of Family Physicians, the American Academy of Pediatrics (AAP), the American College of Obstetricians and Gynecologists, and the American College of Surgeons (ACS) have adopted policies calling on their members to be knowledgeable, trained, and involved in all phases of prevention and SBI for alcohol, tobacco, and other drug problems. The ACS Committee on Trauma requires screening of all level I and level II trauma patients for alcohol misuse as well as providing BI for those patients who screen positive in level 1 trauma centers (2). Recommendations to implement SBI in general and mental health care settings have been endorsed by the National Institute on Alcohol Abuse and Alcoholism (NIAAA), National Institute on Drug Abuse (NIDA), Substance Abuse and Mental Health Services Administration (SAMHSA) and the National Quality Forum (NQF), a voluntary consensus evidence-based standard-setting organization. The NQF recommends that all patients 10 years of age or older should be screened for alcohol misuse and any tobacco use during new-patient encounters, and at least annually (2a). Those who screen positive should receive a more detailed assessment, and, when appropriate, treatment including BI.

Adoption of the new codes for structured screening and BI by the AMA (Level I Current Procedural Terminology, CPT codes: 99408 for 15 to 30 minutes, and 99409 for more than 30 minutes of SBI for substance use disorders other than tobacco-related) and by the Centers for Medicare and Medicaid Services (HCPCS H codes: H0049 for screening, and H0050 for 15 minutes of BI) represent a major step toward dissemination of SBI in clinical settings.

CLINICAL GUIDELINES

"If you aren't already doing so, we encourage you to incorporate alcohol screening and intervention into your practice. You're in a prime position to make a difference."

These first lines of the booklet "Helping Patients Who Drink Too Much: A Clinician's Guide" summarize the current NIAAA guidelines on SBI for primary care and mental health providers (2b). This guide recommends the following approach for the assessment and management of alcohol use disorders in nonaddiction health care settings.

Screening for At-Risk Drinking, Alcohol Abuse, and Alcohol Dependence One can start with a *prescreening question* about *any* alcohol use ("Do you sometimes drink beer, wine, or other alcoholic beverages?"); this can help "ease" the patient into the more detailed questions about alcohol consumption. *Screening* can be achieved with a *single* question about the frequency of heavy drinking, defined as at least five drinks per day for men up to age 65, and at least four drinks per day for men older than 65 years and for women. (*How many times in the past year have you had . . . 5 or more* drinks in a day? *(for men) 4 or more* drinks in a day? *(for women).*

Additional questions include asking about the usual frequency and quantity of alcohol consumed in the previous 30 days, followed with the CAGE or the Alcohol Use Disorders Identification Test (AUDIT) surveys to assess the severity of the drinking problem. The CAGE questions are: Have you ever felt you should *cut* down on your drinking? Have people *annoyed* you by criticizing your drinking? Have you ever felt bad or *guilty* about your drinking? Have you ever had a drink first thing in the morning to steady your nerves or get rid of a hangover (*eye*-opener)? The 10 AUDIT questions are available in the Guide (2b).

During screening, it can be helpful to present the patient with a chart describing what constitutes a "standard drink." One standard drink is equivalent to 12 ounces of beer, 5 ounces of wine, or 1.5 ounces of 80-proof spirits. Negative answers about heavy drinking *and* a negative AUDIT score (no more than 7 for men up to age 65 and no more than 3 for men older than 65 years and for women) indicate a *negative screen* that should be followed with individually tailored advice to maintain alcohol consumption below the "at-risk drinking" limits (see below), or reduce use or abstain from alcohol, if medically indicated.

Positive screen results mandate determining the patient's average weekly alcohol consumption by asking two questions: "On average, how many days a week do you have an alcoholic drink?" and "On a typical drinking day, how many drinks do you have?", and determining the presence or absence of alcohol abuse or dependence. If the "safe" drinking limits are exceeded (at least 5 drinks per day and/or more than 14 drinks per week for men up to age 65, and at least 4 drinks per day and/or more than 7 drinks per week for men older than age 65 and for women), and the criteria for abuse and/or dependence are not met, then the patient is diagnosed with "at-risk drinking," which is a risk factor for the development of alcohol abuse or dependence in the future.

Brief Intervention ("Advise and Assist") for At-Risk Drinking and Persons Who Meet Criteria for Alcohol Abuse or Dependence A patient should be provided, in an empathic and nonconfrontational manner, with an *assessment* of his or her drinking and its consequences as well as clear *recommendations.*

"You're drinking more than is medically safe, I strongly recommend that you cut down." "I believe that you have a serious alcohol problem and strongly recommend that you quit drinking." "As your physician I am willing to help you reduce or quit drinking."

The next step is to assess the patient's *readiness to change* drinking and negotiate a *drinking goal.* The goal should be patient-specific. For some patients, cutting down from daily drinking to 3 days a week may be appropriate. For college students, cutting down from 12 to 15 drinks to 5 to 6 drinks on a weekend night may reduce the risk for significant harm and convince the student to begin the process of cutting back even further to low-risk levels. For patients who meet criteria for alcohol dependence and those with specific comorbid medical or psychiatric problems, abstinence should be advised as a primary treatment goal.

For otherwise "healthy" people who drink at-risk amounts or those who should, but are not willing, to abstain, cutting down may be a reasonable choice. Abstinence has been associated with better treatment outcomes than reduced drinking in people with abuse or dependence; however, drinking reduction may be more acceptable to some patients as a treatment goal than abstinence and has been related to a decrease in alcohol-related harms. If the patient is willing to change, the clinician should discuss a *treatment plan* to achieve the patient's drinking goals. This plan should involve setting specific steps the patient will take to reduce/quit drinking (e.g., how to prevent and manage high-risk situations, establish a support network, track the amount of consumed alcohol).

Alcohol-dependent patients should be *referred* and encouraged to see an addiction specialist and attend a mutual self-help group such as AA. In addition, they should be assessed for the need for medically managed *treatment,* such as detoxification and pharmacotherapy, and for mental health disorders. All patients should be provided with educational materials and scheduled follow-up appointments.

If the patient is not willing to change his or her drinking, the clinician should restate the drinking-related health concerns, reaffirm a willingness to help when the patient is ready, and encourage the patient to reflect about perceived "benefits" of continued drinking versus decreasing or stopping drinking, and barriers to change.

Follow-Up Sessions With patients who adhere to goals to decrease use, the clinician should reinforce and support continued adherence, renegotiate drinking goals, if indicated, and encourage follow-up. At follow-up, patient progress should be documented ("Was the patient able to meet and sustain his drinking goals?"). Former "at-risk drinkers" should be rescreened annually. Patients who are alcohol-dependent need careful monitoring for follow-through with an alcohol treatment program and self-help groups, coordination of care with addiction specialists, and treatment of coexisting medical (e.g., hypertension, hyperglycemia) and mental health conditions (e.g., mood disorders, insomnia, nicotine and other drug use disorders).

Patients who do not meet their treatment goals should be additionally supported; the provider should acknowledge that change is difficult, reemphasize his willingness to help, readdress the impact of continued drinking, re-evaluate the diagnosis, treatment goals, and plan, consider engaging significant others, and schedule close follow-up.

CURRENT EVIDENCE ON SCREENING AND BRIEF INTERVENTIONS: A BRIEF SUMMARY

Screening and Brief Intervention for Unhealthy Alcohol Use (At-Risk Use through Dependence)

Brief intervention for alcohol problems is one of the most clinically effective and cost-effective preventive services from among services recommended by the USPSTF, with economic savings similar to screening for colorectal cancer, hypertension or visual acuity (adults older than 64), and to influenza or pneumococcal immunization (3).

In contrast to those other services, screening and counseling for unhealthy alcohol use are currently delivered at much lower rates, with only 8.7% of problem drinkers in a national survey reporting having been asked and counseled about their alcohol use in the last 12 months (4).

Cost-benefit studies have demonstrated savings of $30,000 to 40,000 for each $10,000 invested in the health care system for SBI (5). In a primary care setting, SBI can reduce alcohol use and at-risk drinking by 10% to 30% during a 12-month follow-up (6,7), with one study reporting maintenance of improved drinking patterns for 48 months (5,7a). All adults in primary care should be screened for alcohol misuse (1).

In trauma settings, SBI seems to reduce drinking, drinking-related harms, and recurrence of injuries requiring emergency department care or hospital admissions among injured at-risk drinkers (2,8–11). However, the overall evidence is not as strong as for a primary care setting. Level I and II trauma centers are required to provide screening, and level I trauma centers to deliver BI to those who screened positive (2).

In emergency department (ED) settings, limited and conflicting research suggests that SBI can reduce drinking and result in fewer subsequent ED visits among at-risk drinkers (11a,12,13). Emergency medical professionals are encouraged to incorporate SBIRT into clinical ED practice (13,14) though some high-methodologic-quality studies in ED settings have yielded negative results (15,16).

In general inpatient settings, evidence on the effectiveness of opportunistic alcohol SBI is inconclusive and suggests that SBI may be beneficial but does not work as well as for primary care, trauma, or ED patients (17,18). One of the key issues in this setting is that the vast majority of general medical inpatients, identified as "positive" by screening, have alcohol dependence. BIs have less proven success for decreasing drinking or linking alcohol-dependent patients with addiction-specific treatment after hospital discharge.

Limited evidence suggests that SBI can reduce morbidity and mortality in the population of problem drinkers. SBI appears to work in adults (5,18a,19,20), including young adults ages 18 to 25 (21) and older adults ages 65 and older (22,23), college students (24–26), pregnant women and women of child-bearing age (7a,60), though in the latter the evidence is mixed.

There is insufficient evidence on SBI efficacy in adolescents and in different cultural groups; however, the early evidence is encouraging (28,29). A single, short 5- to 15-minute intervention can be effective; however, a multiple-contact BI, usually including one to three booster sessions, seems to be more effective and is recommended (1,6,7).

The BI studies with the largest effect sizes utilized primary care clinicians to deliver the intervention (5,19,30–32). The counseling style of effective BIs is based on motivational interviewing and commonly includes elements such as empathy, feedback, advice with an emphasis on patient responsibility and self-efficacy, and a treatment plan with a menu of options (28,33).

There has been a growing support for different ways of SBI delivery (e.g., via mail, phone, or web-based, rather than in person) (26,34,35). The optimal interval for SBI is unknown. Patients with past alcohol-related problems, young adults, and other high-risk groups (e.g., smokers) may benefit from frequent screening and BI, if indicated (1). A recent expert panel advised screening all patients 10 years or older during new-patient encounters and at least annually for established patients (36). Alcohol screening and/or assessment alone has been associated with drinking reduction in clinical research settings (16,37).

Screening and Brief Intervention for Illicit Drug Use Current evidence is insufficient to assess the balance of benefits and harms of screening adolescents, adults and pregnant women for illicit drug use (38). Although standardized questionnaires to screen adolescents and adults for drug use have been shown to be valid and reliable, there is insufficient evidence to assess the clinical utility of these instruments when applied widely in primary care settings (38). One such screening tool that could be used is the Drug Abuse Screening Test (see Chapter 20, "Assessement") SAMHSA has suggested use of a single question ("Have you used street drugs more than 5 times in your life?"). A single item has recently been validated in primary care (as yet unpublished; personal communication Dr. Richard Saitz, October 13, 2008): "How many times in the past year have you used an illegal durg or used a prescription medication for non-medical reasons?" One or more is a positive screening test result.

Limited research has evaluated the efficacy of SBI for illicit drug use and disorders. The strongest evidence exists for cannabis use and dependence (39). There is also some indication that SBI may be beneficial for cocaine and heroin use and amphetamine use (39a,40), and may reduce risk of human immunodeficiency virus (HIV) transmission. The evidence for the SBI efficacy is very limited for people identified by screening in comparison to those who seek help.

Overall there is little evidence of harm reduction associated with either screening for illicit drug use or behavioral interventions used in treatment for abuse or dependence (38). There is fair evidence that people who reduce or stop drug use have a lower risk of negative health outcomes (38).

Screening and Brief Intervention for Prescription Opioid Misuse Research designed to develop screening methods for the detection of prescription opioid abuse or dependence has been growing. Most studies have focused on survey-based screening for aberrant, drug-related behaviors, and toxicology screens. A recent study found that four aberrant behaviors were strongly associated with opioid dependence (41). There is limited information on the sensitivity and specificity of routine toxicology drug screening in opioid-treated chronic pain patients in primary care settings.

There is no current literature on the efficacy of SBI for prescription opioid-related abuse or dependence. Although not considered traditional BI, treatment contracts for prescription opioids often incorporate many of the basic BI principles including a client-centered agreement to minimize or stop alcohol and illicit drug use and obtaining these medications from other physicians.

SYSTEMATIC REVIEWS AND META-ANALYSES OF SCREENING AND BRIEF INTERVENTIONS FOR UNHEALTHY ALCOHOL USE

The following papers were used to support the summary statements in the previous sections. What follows is a brief overview of SBI-related research for unhealthy alcohol use and illicit drug use/disorders.

Solberg et al. conducted a meta-analysis of primary care studies and evaluated the clinically preventable burden (CPB) and cost-effectiveness of SBI implementation and compared these values across other (1) recommended preventive services (3). The CPB was calculated as the product of effectiveness times the alcohol-attributable fraction of both mortality and morbidity (measured in quality-adjusted life years, or QALYs). Cost-effectiveness from both the societal perspective and the health-system perspective was estimated. Randomized controlled trials (RCTs; $n = 10$) and cost-effectiveness studies were included. The mean percentage of SBI effectiveness for both heavy drinking and hazardous drinking in primary care was found to be 17.4% (range, 9.8% to 30.1%), reflecting behavior change at 6 months to 2 years after intervention. The calculated CPB was 176,000 QALYs saved over the lifetime of a birth cohort of 4,000,000 people. From both the societal and health-system perspectives, SBI is cost-effective and may be cost-saving. This meta-analysis suggests SBI as one of the highest-ranking preventive services among the 25 effective services evaluated using standardized methods. As current levels of delivery are the lowest of comparably ranked services, SBI deserves special attention by clinicians and care delivery systems for improvement. A meta-analysis was conducted by the Cochrane Group, led by Kaner (7), to evaluate the effectiveness of SBI to reduce alcohol consumption among nontreatment-seeking patients in primary care settings, including EDs. The meta-analysis included 21 RCTs ($n = 7{,}286$ participants), showing robust results that participants receiving SBI significantly reduced their alcohol consumption as compared to the control group (mean difference, −41 g/per week or 4 to 5 units), with substantial heterogeneity noted between trials. The percentage of heavy drinkers and binge drinkers was significantly reduced in the SBI as compared to the control group. The analysis confirmed the benefit of SBI in men (significant mean difference, −57 g/per week studied was relatively small (nonsignificant mean difference, -10 g/per week; $n = 499$ women). When compared with brief BI, extended BI was associated with an insignificantly greater reduction in alcohol consumption (mean difference = −28 g/per week), and with a trend to an increased reduction in alcohol use of 1.1 g/per week and for each extra minute of treatment exposure ($p = 0.06$). Reduction of drinking was also observed in some control groups. Mean loss-to-follow-up was 27%, with more subjects lost in the SBI than control group (significant 3% difference). The results of efficacy trials were comparable to those in the effectiveness trials. The results of this meta-analysis are broadly similar to previous work focused on primary care samples (42–44) and showed that SBI consistently produced reductions in alcohol consumption. The effect was clear in men at one year of follow-up but unproven in women.

The systematic review and meta-analysis by Bertholet et al. evaluated the efficacy of SBI aimed at reducing long-term alcohol use and related harms in the nontreatment-seeking individuals in primary care settings (44). Nineteen RCTs ($n = 5{,}639$ subjects) were analyzed. The BIs in the studies ranged from 5 to 45 minutes per session (mostly 5 to 15 minutes), and the majority included booster sessions. The control groups received either brief advice (up to 5 minutes) or "usual care" or no intervention. The adjusted, intention-to-treat analysis showed a significant mean pooled difference of −38 g/wk of ethanol (approximately 4 standard drinks) in favor of the SBI group. Most of the effective interventions lasted 5 to 15 minutes and included written handouts. Reduction in alcohol consumption at 6 months was comparable to that at 12 months, and comparable between men and women. Intervention modality (type of provider, session duration, use of the motivational interviewing technique, presence of booster sessions) did not play a significant role. No negative effects of SBI were reported. Evidence of efficacy for other outcome measures was inconclusive. Based on this meta-analysis, SBI appears effective in reducing alcohol consumption at 6 and 12 months among nontreatment-seeking primary care patients, regardless of gender.

A systematic review by Whitlock et al. (6), prepared as a summary of evidence for the USPSTF, focused on the efficacy of SBI to reduce at-risk and harmful alcohol consumption among adults in primary care settings. The review included 12 controlled trials. At 6 to 12 month follow-up, brief, multicontact BIs (up to 15 minutes of initial contact and at least one booster session) resulted in drinking reduction by 2.9 to 8.7 drinks per week (13% to 34% net reductions, respectively) more than in controls, and the proportion of participants drinking at moderate or safe levels was 10% to 19% greater as compared to controls. One study reported the maintenance of an improved drinking pattern for 48 months (5). Very brief (<5 minutes) or brief (up to 15 minutes) single-contact interventions were less effective or ineffective in reducing at-risk or harmful drinking but were better than no intervention. No adverse effects of SBI were noted. The review concluded that brief multicontact BI can provide an effective component of a public health approach to reducing at-risk or harmful alcohol use among adult primary care patients.

The meta-analysis by Ballesteros et al. assessed gender-specific effects of alcohol BI in primary care settings (43). Seven studies ($n = 2{,}981$ subjects) with a follow-up of 6 to 12 months were included. The effect sizes of BI for the reduction of alcohol consumption were statistically significant and similar for men (0.25) and women (0.26). The odds ratios (OR) for drinking below hazardous levels at 6 to 12 months were also similar (OR = 2.3 for both men and women; $p < 0.05$). This analysis supports the similarity of outcomes among men and women achieved by BI for hazardous drinking in primary care settings.

A systematic review and meta-analysis by Beich et al. evaluated the effectiveness of screening, as a part of a SBI program, for excessive alcohol use in general practice (45). The 8 included studies used health questionnaires for screening, and the BIs included feedback, information, and advice. In 1,000 screened patients, 90 screened positive and required further assessment, after which 25 qualified for BI. After 1 year, 2.6 reported they drank less than the maximum recommended level. Although SBI can reduce excessive drinking, screening in general practice may be inefficient as a precursor to BIs targeting excessive alcohol use. This meta-analysis raised questions about the feasibility of screening in general practice for excessive alcohol use. Although the authors reported efficacy of the BI data, the findings should be interpreted with caution, as this study was not designed primarily to evaluate the efficacy of BI but rather to assess potential effectiveness of the screening process.

A meta-analysis by Poikolainen (42) evaluated the effectiveness of BIs to reduce drinking in primary care settings. It included 14 RCTs with follow-up time at 6 to 12 months. Significant heterogeneity was observed when data on very brief BIs among men and women were pooled (which is consistent with the findings of the meta-analysis of Bertholet et al. (44). For brief BIs (5 to 20 minutes), the change in alcohol consumption was not significant among men or women. For extended BIs (several visits), the pooled effect estimate of change in alcohol intake was –51 g of alcohol per week among women. Among men, the estimate was of similar magnitude, but lack of homogeneity was noted. In sum, extended BIs were effective among women but not men. Other BIs seemed to be effective sometimes but not always, and the average effect could not be reliably estimated.

A meta-analysis by Wilk et al. assessed the effectiveness of BIs in primary care heavy or problem drinkers (46). Twelve RCTs (n = 3,948) were included. The BI sessions lasted for up to 1 hour and incorporated simple techniques of motivational interviewing. The pooled OR (1.9; $p < 0.05$) was in favor of BIs over no intervention, and was consistent across gender and the intensity of intervention. Compared to no-intervention controls, heavy drinkers who received a BI were almost twice as likely to moderate their drinking at 6 to 12 months.

A systematic review and meta-analysis by Rubak et al. evaluated the effectiveness of motivational interviewing in different conditions, including alcohol consumption, and the factors potentially influencing treatment outcomes (47). Seventy-two RCTs were included. When using motivational interviewing in brief encounters of 15 minutes, 64% of the studies showed an effect. More than one encounter with the patient increased the effectiveness of motivational interviewing. Meta-analysis showed a significant effect of motivational interviewing for standard ethanol content (N = 648 subjects) and blood alcohol concentration (N = 278 subjects). This report indicates that motivational interviewing-based BIs can reduce alcohol consumption as evaluated by standard ethanol content and blood alcohol concentration.

The meta-analysis by Cuijpers et al. evaluated effects of BIs on mortality in problem drinkers (18a). Among the included 32 studies (n = 7,521 subjects), 6 reported unverified deaths, and 4 reported verified mortality status. The total number of deaths was relatively low. The pooled relative risk (RR) of dying was approximately 0.5 ($p < 0.05$). The prevented fraction of deaths was about 0.3, indicating that about one in every three deaths can be prevented by the intervention. The number needed to treat (NNT) ranged from 154 to 317. In the studies with verified mortality status, the NNT was 282, indicating that 282 subjects have to be treated in order to prevent one death. Based on the limited evidence, BIs appear to reduce mortality by about 23% to 36% in the population of problem drinkers.

A meta-analysis by Moyer assessed efficacy of BI for alcohol problems in the treatment-seeking and nontreatment-seeking ("opportunistic") samples (48). Fifty-six studies were included. Most studies of the treatment-seeking samples compared BI to extended treatments (n = 20); most studies of the opportunistic samples compared BI to a control condition (n = 34). In the nontreatment-seeking samples, BI tended to be briefer and delivered by general health care professionals, whereas BI in the treatment-seeking samples were usually more intensive and delivered by therapists or counselors. In the treatment-seeking samples, no substantial differences were found between the efficacy of brief compared to extended BIs. In the opportunistic samples, compared to controls, small to medium aggregate effect sizes in favor of BI emerged across different follow-up points; the most pronounced effect size for alcohol consumption (0.67) and all drinking-related outcomes (0.3) was noted at the earliest follow-up (no more than 3 months), and the least pronounced and statistically nonsignificant effect size (0.12 to 0.20) was found at follow-up longer than 12 months, suggesting dissipation of the BI effects over time. Larger effect of BI compared to a control condition was also noted when individuals with more severe alcohol problems were excluded. In a small number of studies reporting outcomes by gender, BI efficacy did not differ between men and women. This meta-analysis indicates that BI is efficacious for drinking reduction; however, its effects may fade over time. The BI efficacy was increased when dependent drinkers were excluded. Brief and extended BIs show similar efficacy.

A systematic review by the Cochrane Group, led by Dinh-Zarr, assessed the effect of interventions intended to reduce alcohol consumption or prevent injuries or their antecedents among "problem drinkers" in diverse settings (49). Seventeen RCTs were included. Among those, seven evaluated BIs in the clinical setting. BIs were associated with a significant reduction of injury-related deaths (RR=0.65) and showed beneficial effects on diverse nonfatal injury–related outcomes. Interventions, including BIs, for problem drinking appear to reduce injuries and their antecedents.

INDIVIDUAL STUDIES OF SCREENING AND BRIEF INTERVENTION FOR UNHEALTHY ALCOHOL USE

Primary Care Settings SBI is efficacious for alcohol misuse and recommended in primary care settings. Implementation of SBI in primary care settings can allow for a better integration of medical care and substance abuse treatment. Such an integrated approach may benefit individuals with substance abuse-related medical conditions and be cost-effective compared to a "treatment-as-usual model," in which primary care and substance abuse treatment are provided separately (50).

Project TrEAT and Project Health are examples of the positive SBI trials in primary care. Project TrEAT was the first U.S. study to evaluate long-term efficacy and cost-benefit of SBI among 774 at-risk drinkers in primary care (5,19,20). After two short BI sessions delivered by a clinician, each followed by a phone call, at-risk adult drinkers who received BI significantly decreased alcohol use, health resource utilization, and alcohol-related costs compared to controls. These effects were observed at 6 months and maintained during a 48-month follow-up.

In Project Health, after a very short BI, delivered by a clinician as a part of a routine primary care visit, participants significantly reduced drinking and were less likely to relapse to at-risk drinking than controls at 6 and 12 months (31,32). Only one study evaluated efficacy of SBI over a period >4 years (51). After up to three sessions of BI, delivered over a 6-month period, 554 at-risk and harmful drinkers in the BI group significantly reduced their drinking at 9 months compared to "no-treatment" controls. The differences between the groups dissipated at 10-year follow-up; however, at 10 years, both the BI and control groups tended to drink less than at baseline or at 9 months, which suggests "assessment effects" or a favorable natural history of risky alcohol use.

Emergency Department Settings In the emergency department (ED) setting, as many as 24% to 31% of "general" patients and 50% of severely injured trauma patients screen positively for problematic alcohol use (13); however, <10% of ED patients in need of treatment actually receives it (51a). Although research is limited, it suggests SBI feasibility and efficacy in the ED setting, for both injured patients (9,10,10a) and general adult ED patients (11a,12,13). Alcohol SBI may also be beneficial for adolescents (29) and young adults (52) presenting to the ED for alcohol-related injury. In spite of many positive studies, it is important to note there have been a number of high-quality negative trials. Combined with existing evidence on SBI efficacy in primary care along with high prevalence of at-risk and problematic drinking among ED patients, evidence is sufficient to recommend incorporating SBI into clinical ED practice.

A review by D'Onofrio and Degutis (10) identified only four relevant RCTs evaluating efficacy of SBI for injured ED patients with alcohol misuse. Three of these studies were conducted in the ED setting exclusively (9,29,52a) and one in a trauma center (8). The authors concluded that SBI is feasible and effective in the ED setting.

A systematic review by D'Onofrio et al. was conducted to determine the strength of the recommendation for alcohol SBI in the ED setting (13). Thirty RCTs and nine cohort studies, including individuals 12 to 70 years old, were reviewed; four studies were conducted exclusively in the ED setting, and two included ED subsamples. The BIs were of varied intensity (initial session of 5 to 60 minutes' duration, followed by 0 to 6 booster sessions) and most commonly based on motivational interviewing principles. Among the reviewed studies, 82% demonstrated a positive effect of the BI; 90% showed reduction in alcohol consumption; 38% found decreased mortality and morbidity secondary to alcohol-related illness/injuries; and 13% showed fewer ED/hospital admissions or outpatient visits, decrease in social consequences, or increase in treatment referrals.

Longabaugh et al., in a 3-arm RCT, compared the efficacy of a single-session or a two-session BI to "usual ED trauma care" in 539 injured ED patients who were identified as misusing alcohol (9). The BI session was 40 to 60 minutes long and was delivered by a trained researcher. At 12 months, all three groups significantly reduced drinking and the number of injuries compared to baseline; however, only the two-session BI group, but not the single-BI group, significantly reduced alcohol-related negative consequences and injuries compared to controls, indicating that SBI, especially multisession, can be helpful to injured ED patients with at-risk drinking.

The Academic ED SBIRT Research Collaborative study was a quasi-experimental (not randomized) study that evaluated the efficacy of a single 10-minute BI session accompanied by a handout in the general ED setting among 1,132 patients, heavy or harmful drinkers (12). A part of efforts to evaluate implementation of SBI in ED settings, this study demonstrated that BI, delivered by a diverse ED staff, can result in a significant drinking reduction among heavy or harmful drinkers at a 3-month follow-up.

Not all studies confirm efficacy of ED-delivered SBI for injured at-risk drinkers. Two recent studies with a 12-month follow-up failed to show benefit of SBI compared to controls (15,16). Daeppen (16) compared effects of a single brief SBI to two control groups who received either brief screening with an assessment, or screening only, in a sample of 947 injured, at-risk drinkers treated in the ED. Compared to controls, BI-treated subjects did not decrease alcohol use or health resource utilization. Interestingly, all three groups decreased drinking at 12 months, suggesting that even screening for alcohol misuse may have positive effects or that the natural history of the condition is favorable, as this trajectory is observed in most SBI studies across settings.

D'Onofrio et al. evaluated the efficacy of brief BI (<10 minutes long), delivered by the ED practitioner, compared to routine discharge instructions containing advice to reduce drinking, in a sample of 494 hazardous or harmful drinkers treated in the ED ("Project ED Health") (15). Although both BI and control groups decreased the number of drinks per week and the number of binge drinking bouts at 12 months compared to baseline, the changes were comparable between the groups. In this patient population, brief BI was not more efficacious for the reduction of drinking and related harms than brief advice provided in discharge instructions.

Hungerford found that alcohol SBI can be feasible and highly accepted by young ED patients (53). Approximately 90% of age-appropriate patients consented to participate, and 90% of eligible patients were counseled. Median times for obtaining consent, screening, and intervention were 4, 4, and 14 minutes, respectively.

Inpatient Settings Evidence for the effectiveness of opportunistic SBI in inpatient settings is inconclusive, especially for general hospital patients. Results of limited research on SBI efficacy in inpatient trauma settings are more encouraging.

A systematic review by Emmen evaluated the effectiveness of SBI for problem drinking among general nontreatment-seeking inpatients (17). Eight controlled trials (n = 1,597 subjects, 2- to 18-month follow-up), most with methodologic weaknesses, were included. Six studies were based in the inpatient setting (medical and surgical) and two in specialist outpatient setting. Only one study, conducted in an outpatient hypertension clinic, using a relatively intensive BI and a short, 2-month follow-up period, showed a significant reduction in alcohol consumption in the BI group compared to controls. Evidence for the effectiveness of opportunistic SBI for problem drinkers in a general hospital setting is inconclusive.

A recent study by Saitz et al. of 341 adult medical inpatients produced results consistent with the conclusions drawn by the above review (18). Saitz et al. compared the effects of a single BI session, delivered by a trained counselor during a patient's hospitalization and followed up by a letter, to informed consent alone for inpatients identified with unhealthy alcohol use (18). At 12 months, both groups significantly decreased drinking, but no significant differences between the groups were found, indicating lack of SBI efficacy. Several factors could have contributed to such findings. First, 77% of patients identified by screening in this setting met criteria for alcohol dependence. Selecting nondependent inpatients could improve SBI efficacy (33). Second, at 12 months, only 37% of the BI-treated subjects recalled having a BI session, and 28% of the control group claimed having it. This recall (unassessed in most studies) may suggest that hospitalized medical patients may be less receptive to counseling than outpatient individuals. However, significant drinking reduction in both groups, and the fact that almost a half of alcohol dependent individuals sought treatment for alcohol use disorders after hospital discharge, can be viewed as encouraging findings, at least regarding the natural history of the condition, and suggesting a need for further research in this setting.

Gentilello, after a single BI session, delivered by a psychologist and followed up by a letter, noted a significant, nearly 50% drinking reduction in the BI, but not in the "no-treatment" control group, at 12 months (8). In addition, compared to controls, the BI group non-significantly reduced number of injuries requiring ED, trauma center, or hospital admission during the 12- to 36-month follow-up. Despite the substantial loss to follow-up, this study, based on 762 at-risk drinkers and drinkers with alcohol use disorders admitted to a trauma center, created a foundation for the recommendation on screening and BIs for alcohol misuse in level I and level II trauma centers (2).

An RCT by Schermer et al. evaluated effects of BI on the risk of Driving Under the Influence (DUI) arrest among 126 at-risk or harmful drinkers admitted to a trauma center after motor vehicle collisions (54). Although limited by the relatively small sample size, the results of this study suggested that patients who receive BI during a trauma center admission they are less likely to be arrested for DUI within 3 years of discharge.

Another trauma-based inpatient study, conducted by Soderstrom et al., compared a single 15- to 20-minute BI session, followed up by a letter and two booster phone calls, to a "brief advice" group (n = 497 subjects) (11). This study did not include a "no-treatment" control condition. Both interventions resulted in a significant reduction of drinking and related consequences at 6 and 12 months. Sommers et al. compared the efficacy of two types of BIs for alcohol consumption and drinking-related harms among 187 patients admitted to a level I trauma center for alcohol-related vehicular injury (55). No significant differences in the main treatment outcomes were found between the groups at 12 months.

Adolescents and Young Adults Research on alcohol SBI efficacy for adolescent drinking is limited. The USPSTF evaluated it as insufficient to recommend for or against universal screening of adolescents in primary care. However, other professional organizations, such as the AMA, the AAP and the NQF, advise such a screening based on promising early evidence on SBI efficacy in this vulnerable population. Data indicate that rates of adolescent alcohol use range from 5% among general ED admissions to nearly 50% among trauma admissions, and alcohol use by adolescents is associated with increases in severity of injury and cost of medical treatment (56).

A review by Tevyaw and Monti presented the use and efficacy of motivational enhancement and other brief interventions for substance use, particularly drinking, in adolescents and young adults (28). This review found that positive results demonstrated in clinical trials using motivational enhancement interventions with adolescents and college students primarily stem from reductions in alcohol-related problems and, to a lesser extent, from reductions in drinking. Although most young people do mature out of hazardous drinking patterns, motivational enhancement-based interventions may help accelerate that maturation process in high-risk individuals. The review concluded that motivational enhancement-based BIs can decrease alcohol-related negative consequences, reduce alcohol use, and increase treatment engagement among adolescents and young adults.

Spirito et al. evaluated outcomes of a single BI session in the ED setting among 152 adolescents admitted for an alcohol-related injury (29). The BI was delivered by a researcher, included a personalized feedback and a handout, and was compared to a control condition, consisting of brief advice and a handout. Over 12 months, both groups significantly reduced number of drinks per occasion. Those with problematic alcohol use (almost 50% of the sample) significantly more reduced frequency of drinking and high-volume drinking if they received BI, indicating that BIs had some efficacy, particularly for those adolescents who engage in the most risky drinking behavior.

Grossberg (21), as a part of Project TrEAT (19), examined 226 primary care at-risk drinkers aged 18 to 30 years. Young adults who received the BI significantly reduced drinking, had fewer ED visits, motor vehicle crashes and events, and fewer arrests for controlled substance or liquor violation over the 4-year follow-up. SBIs seem feasible and accepted by young adults (53).

Older Adults SBIs seem effective for older adults. Project GOAL, conducted in parallel to Project TrEAT (19) and based on similar methodology, showed that SBI can decrease alcohol use among older primary care at-risk drinkers during the 2-year follow-up (22,23).

College Students About 40% of college students report binge drinking in the prior 2 weeks (56a); a third meet criteria for alcohol abuse and 6% for alcohol dependence in the prior year (57). SBIs seem effective for reducing at-risk drinking in college students in general (24,25), in mandated college students, and in students admitted to the ED (56b,57a). College students seem receptive to alcohol SBIs (24,25).

A review by Larimer et al. summarized the results of 16 studies evaluating effects of alcohol SBIs in college settings and concluded that research provides strong support for the efficacy of SBIs (26). The strongest evidence exists for interventions in the form of brief, personalized, individual, motivational feedback based interviews. There also is emerging support for the efficacy of mailed or computerized feedback alone in producing at least short-term reductions in students' alcohol consumption. A systematic review by Zisserson et al. (34) reviewed evidence for the utility of SBIs delivered without direct, real-time contact to college students engaging in at-risk drinking. The results suggest that "no-contact" interventions (e.g., printed materials or computer-based modalities), are feasible, and may have efficacy in this population. The "noncontact" interventions may be helpful with broader dissemination of SBIs to college students.

A study described by Mariatt (24) and Baer (25) included 461 college freshmen, identified as at-risk drinkers or a "normative control" group during their final high-school year. At-risk drinkers were randomized into the "no treatment" control arm or the BI arm, which received one to two BI sessions, delivered by psychologists, with a personalized feedback letter. Over 4 years, at-risk students, in both intervention and control groups, significantly reduced drinking and related harmful consequences, with changes significantly favoring the BI group. These long-term benefits occurred even in the context of maturational, natural trends, observed in the "normative control" group.

Pregnant Women and Women of Child-Bearing Age

Approximately 6.7 million women of child-bearing age in the United States, including 13% of nonpregnant and 2% of pregnant women, engaged in binge drinking during the period of 2001 and 2003 (57b). As there does not appear to be a "zero-risk level" of alcohol consumption during pregnancy, pregnant women and women contemplating pregnancy should abstain from drinking to avoid the potential harmful alcohol effects on the fetus (58). Limited studies provide encouraging evidence on the benefits of SBI in pregnancy (7a,59,60), but more research on the efficacy of primary care screening and behavioral intervention for alcohol misuse among pregnant women is needed (1).

A review by Chang presented evidence on perinatal effects of SBI (59). Selected reviewed studies documented positive effects of SBI on alcohol-related maternal and fetal outcomes during current and subsequent pregnancies among subgroups of pregnant drinking women and women of child-bearing age who were risky drinkers, though benefits were not observed in overall samples. SBI can help eliminate or at least reduce women's prenatal alcohol use, minimize fetal risk, and maximize pregnancy outcome.

A study by Manwell et al. provided the first direct evidence that SBI is associated with sustained reductions in alcohol consumption by women of child-bearing age, especially those who are pregnant. Recent studies corroborated these findings (7a,27,60).

Project CHOICES, conducted jointly with the Centers for Disease Control and Prevention (CDC) (27), included 830 nonpregnant women of child-bearing age engaging in risky drinking and other risky behaviors, and compared the efficacy of an extended, five-session BI, delivered over 14 weeks, to a brochure-only control condition, in reducing risk of an alcohol-exposed pregnancy. At 9 months, the odds ratio of being at reduced risk for alcohol-exposed pregnancy was twofold greater in the BI group as compared to controls. The BI group was significantly more likely to reduce alcohol consumption to below risk level and to use effective contraception compared to controls.

O'Connor and Whaley assessed efficacy of SBI for reducing alcohol-related perinatal harm among 255 pregnant drinkers, enrolled on average at 18 weeks of gestational age (60). The group that received a short SBI, delivered during each prenatal visit, as needed, by nonmedical professionals in a community setting, compared to controls, was more likely to report abstinence by the third trimester. Newborns whose mothers received the BI had higher birth weights and birth lengths and lower fetal mortality rates compared with newborns in the control group.

INDIVIDUAL STUDIES OF SCREENING AND BRIEF INTERVENTION FOR ILLICIT DRUG USE AND DISORDERS

Evidence on SBI efficacy for illicit drug use or disorders is limited and inconsistent, nonetheless encouraging. Best evidence on potential benefits of SBI exists for cannabis use and disorders in adults (60a,61,62), adolescents and young adults (63,64). However, these studies were not done in patients identified by universal screening, in whom results would be expected to be less favorable. Some promising effects of SBI on substance use have been reported in cocaine and heroin users identified by screening (39a), amphetamine users (40), and in methadone clinic patients (65). Marsden reported lack of efficacy of BI for increasing abstinence among young, 16- to 22-year-old ecstasy and cocaine users (64a).

A systematic review by the Cochrane group, led by Denis, evaluated the efficacy of psychosocial interventions for cannabis abuse or dependence—the first published systematic review in this area. Six RCTs (n = 1,297 subjects) were included (39). Studies were not pooled in meta-analysis because of heterogeneity. The studies suggested that counseling approaches might have beneficial effects for the treatment of cannabis dependence. Extended therapy had better results than BI. However, both had positive effects (61,62). Abstinence rates were relatively small. The included studies were too heterogenous and could not allow drawing clear conclusions. The low abstinence rate indicated that cannabis dependence is not easily treated by psychotherapies in outpatient settings. Finally, subjects studied were not identified by screening.

A review by Ritter and Cameron assessed the efficacy and effectiveness of harm reduction interventions to reduce substance use (66). More than 650 articles, providing evaluation data (before, after, or control group comparisons), were included. The evidence was limited in its support for the efficacy and effectiveness of BIs for illicit drug use.

A systematic review by the Cochrane Group, led by Gates, evaluated the effectiveness of interventions for the prevention of drug use by young people (under age 25) delivered in nonschool settings (67). Seventeen RCTs, evaluating four different types of interventions, including BI, were found; they were too dissimilar and too few to combine using meta-analysis and to draw firm conclusions. There is a lack of evidence for the BI effectiveness for the prevention of drug use by young people in nonschool settings.

A systematic review by Tait and Hulse evaluated the effectiveness of BIs in adolescents (mean age, younger than 20 years) in reducing alcohol, tobacco, or other drug use (68). Eleven studies (n = 3,734 adolescents) were included. Follow-up ranged from 6 weeks to 24 months. Motivational interviewing was the predominant approach (n = 8 studies); the remaining studies provided personalized health information. Seven papers reported outcomes for alcohol interventions, and four involved other substances (including one with separate alcohol outcomes). The effect size from the eight alcohol interventions (n = 1,075) was significant but "small" (d = 0.28). The two interventions with tobacco involved a substantial sample (n = 2,626) but had a very small effect (d = 0.04). Although the two interventions addressing multiple substances involved few participants (n = 110), they had a medium-to-large effect (d = 0.78).

A systematic review by Dunn examined the effectiveness of brief BI across four behavioral domains: substance abuse, smoking, HIV risk, and diet/exercise (69). Twenty-nine RCTs were included in the review. There was substantial evidence that motivational interviewing–based interventions are effective for substance abuse when used by nonspecialist clinicians, particularly when enhancing entry to and engagement in more intensive substance abuse treatment. No significant association was found between the length of follow-up time and the magnitude of effect sizes across the studies.

Bernstein et al. examined the efficacy of a single BI session, delivered by a "peer-educator," and augmented by a follow-up phone call, compared to a handout-only control condition (39a). Among 1,175 adult cocaine and/or heroin users, recruited from urgent care and other outpatient settings, those in the BI group were 1.5 times more likely to be abstinent from cocaine, heroin, or both drugs and report greater improvements on the drug and medical subscales than controls at 6 months. Corresponding effect sizes were small.

Baker focused on efficacy of BI in 214 adult amphetamine users from diverse clinical and community settings (40). Participants in the BI arm received two or four BI sessions delivered by a psychologist or a social worker and accompanied by a self-help booklet, whereas controls were given a booklet only. At 6 months, all groups significantly reduced their daily amphetamine use, with those attending BI sessions being more likely to report abstinence than controls.

The Marijuana Treatment Project Research Group study of 450 adult cannabis-dependent smokers showed significant reduction of marijuana use and associated consequences at 4 months, and maintained at 15 months, after a two-session BI, delivered by therapists over 5 weeks, compared to controls (62).

SUMMARY

Like so much in medicine, it takes one to two generations of physicians to implement and disseminate new clinical interventions. The test of time is also a critical factor as many therapies come and go once there is sufficient evidence to support or disprove the therapy. There are many examples, including the decline of angioplasty and other surgical therapies, owing to lack of evidence, dozens of medications that did more harm than good such as the use of estrogen to reduce cardiovascular risk, decreased use of inpatient treatment for alcoholism, and traditional "insight" psychotherapy for mental illness. SBI has survived the test of time and is now on the forefront of our efforts to reduce alcohol-related harms and the suffering alcohol use disorders inflict on individuals, their families, and society. The implementation of SBI in all clinical settings has become a high priority for federal and foundation funding initiatives and health care systems.

From an evidence and research perspective, much work needs to be done. Implementation science, especially for substance use disorder–related therapy, remains in its infancy with a limited number of scientists working in this area. Electronic medical record systems offer a good opportunity to move SBI into point of care and routine clinical practice.

The evidence for the use of SBI for adolescents in general clinical settings remains weak. Identification and treatment of illicit drug misuse and prescription drug abuse in primary care and specialized clinical settings is a relatively new area of work and the utility of SBI for these problems is unclear. More research is needed on the use of SBI for hospitalized patients, a large proportion of whom is alcohol-dependent, and on the impact of SBI on morbidity and mortality. The use of SBI in psychiatric or dual diagnosis settings remains an understudied area, with no studies reported in the literature.

Even with the foregoing areas that need further study, SBI has come a long way since the first large study reported by Wallace in 1988 (30) demonstrated strong evidence for SBI efficacy in many populations.

REFERENCES

1. U.S. Preventive Services Task Force. *Guide to clinical preventive services, 2007: recommendations.* Retrieved January 23, 2008, from http://www.ahrq.gov/clinic/pocketgd07/.
2. Committee on Trauma, American College of Surgeons. *Resources for optimal care of the injured patient: 2006.* Chicago; American College of Surgeons, 2006.
2a. National Quality Forum. *National voluntary consensus standards for the treatment of substance use conditions: evidence-based treatment practices; a*

consensus report. (Item No.: NQFCR-19–07). Washington DC: Author, 2007. Retrieved January 23, 2008, from http://www.qualityforum.org/publications/reports/sud-2007.asp.

2b. National Institutes on Alcohol Abuse and Alcoholism. *Helping patients who drink too much: a clinician's guide* [Updated 2005 edition]. NIH Publication No. 07–3769. Washington, DC: Author, 2007 (revised). Retrieved February 1, 2008, from www.niaaa.nih.gov/guide.

3. Solberg LI, Maciosek MV, Edwards NM. Primary care intervention to reduce alcohol misuse ranking its health impact and cost effectiveness. *Am J Prev Med* 2008;34(2):143–152.

4. D'Amico EJ, Paddock SM, Burnam A, et al. Identification of and guidance for problem drinking by general medical providers: results from a national survey. *Med Care* 2005;43:229–236.

5. Fleming MF. Brief physician advice for problem drinkers: long-term efficacy and benefit-cost analysis. *Alcohol Clin Exp Res* 2002;26(1): 36–43.

6. Whitlock EP, Polen MR, Green CA, et al. U.S. Preventive Services Task Force. Behavioral counseling interventions in primary care to reduce risky/harmful alcohol use by adults: a summary of the evidence for the U.S. Preventive Services Task Force. *Ann Intern Med* 2004;140: 557–568.

7. Kaner EF. Effectiveness of brief alcohol interventions in primary care populations. *Cochrane Database Syst Rev* 2007;18(2):CD004148.

7a. Manwell LB, Fleming MF, Mundt MP, et al. Treatment of problem alcohol use in women of childbearing age: results of a brief intervention trial. *Alcohol Clin Exp Res* 2000;24(10):1517–1524.

8. Gentilello LM. Alcohol interventions in a trauma center as a means of reducing the risk of injury recurrence. *Ann Surg* 1999;230(4):473–80.

9. Longabaugh R. Evaluating the effects of a brief motivational intervention for injured drinkers in the emergency department. *J Stud Alcohol* 2001;62(6):806–816.

10. D'Onofrio G, Degutis LC. Screening and brief intervention in the emergency department. *Alcohol Res Health* 2004/2005;28(2):63–72.

10a. Blow FC, Barry KL, Walton MA, et al. The efficacy of two brief intervention strategies among injured, at-risk drinkers in the emergency department: impact of tailored messaging and brief advice. *J Stud Alcohol* 2006;67(4):568–578.

11. Soderstrom CA, DiClemente CC, Dischinger PC, et al. A controlled trial of brief intervention versus brief advice for at-risk drinking trauma center patients. *J Trauma* 2007;62(5):1102–1111; discussion 1111–1112.

11a. Crawford MJ, Patton R, Touquet R, et al. Screening and referral for brief intervention of alcohol-misusing patients in an emergency department: a pragmatic randomised controlled trial. *Lancet* 2004;364(9442):1334–1339.

12. Academic ED SBIRT Research Collaborative. The impact of screening, brief intervention, and referral for treatment on emergency department patients' alcohol use. *Ann Emerg Med* 2007;50(6):699–710.

13. D'Onofrio G. Preventive care in the emergency department: screening and brief intervention for alcohol problems in the emergency department: a systematic review. *Acad Emerg Med* 2002;9(6):627–638.

14. Jouriles NJ, Chaney WC, Jones CA, et al., eds. *Advancing emergency care: policy compendium.* Dallas: American College of Emergency Physicians, 2007. Retrieved February 2, 2008, from http://www.acep.org/workarea/showcontent.aspx?id=9104,.

15. D'Onofrio G, Pantalon MV, Degutis LC, et al. Brief intervention for hazardous and harmful drinkers in the emergency department. *Ann Emerg Med* 2008;51:742–750.

16. Daeppen JB. Brief alcohol intervention and alcohol assessment do not influence alcohol use in injured patients treated in the emergency department: a randomized controlled clinical trial. *Addiction* 2007;102(8): 1224–1233.

17. Emmen MJ. Effectiveness of opportunistic brief interventions for problem drinking in a general hospital setting: systematic review. *BMJ* 2004;328(7435):318. Epub 2004 January 16, 2004.

18. Saitz R, Palfai TP, Cheng DM, et al. Brief intervention for medical inpatients with unhealthy alcohol use: a randomized, controlled trial. *Ann Intern Med* 2007;146(3):167–176.

18a. Cuijpers P, Riper H, Lemmers L. The effects on mortality of brief interventions for problem drinking: a meta-analysis. *Addiction* 2004;99(7):839– 845.

19. Fleming MF. Brief physician advice for problem alcohol drinkers. A randomized controlled trial in community-based primary care practices. *JAMA* 1997;277(13):1039–1045.

20. Fleming MF. Benefit-cost analysis of brief physician advice with problem drinkers in primary care settings. *Med Care* 2000;38(1):7–18.

21. Grossberg PM. Brief physician advice for high-risk drinking among young adults. *Ann Fam Med* 2004;2(5):474–480.

22. Fleming MF. Brief physician advice for alcohol problems in older adults: a randomized community-based trial. *J Fam Pract* 1999;48(5):378–384.

23. Mundt MP, French MT, Roebuck MC, et al. Brief physician advice for problem drinking among older adults: an economic analysis of costs and benefits. *J Stud Alcohol* 2005;66(3):389–394.

24. Marlatt GA. Screening and brief intervention for high-risk college student drinkers: results from a 2-year follow-up assessment. *J Consult Clin Psychol* 1998;66(4):604–615.

25. Baer JS. Brief intervention for heavy-drinking college students: 4-year follow-up and natural history. *Am J Public Health* 2001;91(8):1310–1316.

26. Larimer ME, Cronce JM, Lee CM, et al. Brief intervention in college settings. *Alcohol Res Health* 2004/2005;28(2):94–104.

27. Floyd RL, Project CHOICES Efficacy Study Group. Preventing alcohol-exposed pregnancies: a randomized controlled trial. *Am J Prev Med* 2007;32(1):1–10.

28. Tevyaw TO, Monti PM. Motivational enhancement and other brief interventions for adolescent substance abuse: foundations, applications, and evaluations. *Addiction* 2004;99(Suppl 2):63–75.

29. Spirito A, Monti PM, Barnett NP, et al. A randomized clinical trial of a brief motivational intervention for alcohol-positive adolescents treated in an emergency department. *J Pediatr* 2004;145(3):396–402.

30. Wallace P, Cutler S, Haines A. Randomised controlled trial of general practitioner intervention in patients with excessive alcohol consumption. *BMJ* 1988;297(6649):663–668.

31. Ockene JK, Adams A, Hurley TG, et al. Brief physician- and nurse practitioner-delivered counseling for high-risk drinkers: does it work. *Arch Intern Med* 1999;159(18):2198–2205.

32. Reiff-Hekking S, Ockene JK, Hurley TG, et al. Brief physician and nurse practitioner-delivered counseling for high-risk drinking. Results at 12-month follow-up. *J Gen Intern Med* 2005;20(1):7–13.

33. Vasilaki EI, Hosier SG, Cox WM. The efficacy of motivational interviewing as a brief intervention for excessive drinking: a meta-analytic review. *Alcohol Alcohol* 2006;41(3):328–335.

34. Zisserson RN, Palfai T, Saitz R. 'No-contact' interventions for unhealthy college drinking: efficacy of alternatives to person-delivered intervention approaches. *Subst Abuse* 2007;28(4):119–131.

35. Brown RL. Randomized-controlled trial of a telephone and mail intervention for alcohol use disorders: three-month drinking outcomes. *Alcohol Clin Exp Res* 2007;31(8):1372–1379.

36. National Quality Forum. *National voluntary consensus standards for the treatment of substance use conditions: evidence-based treatment practices; a consensus report.* (Item No.: NQFCR-19–07). Washington DC: Author, 2007. Retrieved January 23, 2008, from http://www.qualityforum.org/publications/reports/sud-2007.asp.

37. Nordqvist C, Wilhelm E, Lindqvist K, et al. Can screening and simple written advice reduce excessive alcohol consumption among emergency care patients. *Alcohol Alcohol* 2005;40(5):401–408.

38. U.S. Preventive Services Task Force. *Screening for illicit drug use, topic page.* Rockville, MD: Agency for Healthcare Research and Quality, January 2008. Retrieved February 1, 2008, from http://www.ahrq.gov/clinic/uspstf/uspsdrug.htm.

39. Denis C. Psychotherapeutic interventions for cannabis abuse and/or dependence in outpatient settings. *Cochrane Database Syst Rev* 2006;3: CD005336.

39a. Bernstein J, Bernstein E, Tassiopoulos K, et al. Brief motivational intervention at a clinic visit reduces cocaine and heroin use. *Drug Alcohol Depend* 2005;77(1):49–59.

40. Baker A. Brief cognitive behavioural interventions for regular amphetamine users: a step in the right direction. *Addiction* 2005;100(3):367–378.

41. Fleming MF. Substance use disorders in a primary care sample receiving daily opioid therapy. *J Pain* 2007;8(7):573–582.

42. Poikolainen K. Effectiveness of brief interventions to reduce alcohol intake in primary health care populations: a meta-analysis. *Prev Med* 1999; 28(5):503–509.
43. Ballesteros J. Brief interventions for hazardous drinkers delivered in primary care are equally effective in men and women. *Addiction* 2004;99(1): 103–108.
44. Bertholet N. Reduction of alcohol consumption by brief alcohol intervention in primary care: systematic review and meta-analysis. *Arch Intern Med* 2005;165(9):986–995.
45. Beich A. Screening in brief intervention trials targeting excessive drinkers in general practice: systematic review and meta-analysis. *BMJ* 2003; 327(7414):536–542.
46. Wilk AI, Jensen NM, Havighurst TC. Meta-analysis of randomized control trials addressing brief interventions in heavy alcohol drinkers. *J Gen Intern Med* 1997;12(5):274–283.
47. Rubak S, Sandbaek A, Lauritzen T, et al. Motivational interviewing: a systematic review and meta-analysis. *Br J Gen Pract* 2005;55(513):305–312.
48. Moyer A. Brief interventions for alcohol problems: a meta-analytic review of controlled investigations in treatment-seeking and non-treatment-seeking populations. *Addiction* 2002;97(3):279–292.
49. Dinh-Zarr T, Goss C, Heitman E, et al. Interventions for preventing injuries in problem drinkers. *Cochrane Database Syst Rev* 2004;(3):CD001857.
50. Weisner C, Mertens J, Parthasarathy S, et al. Integrating primary medical care with addiction treatment: a randomized controlled trial. *JAMA* 2001;286(14):1715–1723.
51. Wutzke SE, Conigrave KM, Saunders JB, et al. The long-term effectiveness of brief interventions for unsafe alcohol consumption: a 10-year follow-up. *Addiction* 2002;97(6):665–675.
51a. Rockett IR, Putnam SL, Jia H, et al. Assessing substance abuse treatment need: a statewide hospital emergency department study. *Ann Emerg Med* 2003;41(6):802–813.
52. Monti PM. Motivational interviewing versus feedback only in emergency care for young adult problem drinking. *Addiction.* 2007;102(8):1234–1243.
52a. Monti PM, Colby SM, Barnett NP, et al. Brief intervention for harm reduction with alcohol-positive older adolescents in a hospital emergency department. *J Consult Clin Psychol* 1999;67(6):989–994.
53. Hungerford DW. Feasibility of screening and intervention for alcohol problems among young adults in the ED. *Am J Emerg Med* 2003;21(1):14–22.
54. Schermer CR, Moyers TB, Miller WR, et al. Trauma center brief interventions for alcohol disorders decrease subsequent driving under the influence arrests. *J Trauma* 2006;60(1):29–34.
55. Sommers MS, Dyehouse JM, et al. Effectiveness of brief interventions after alcohol-related vehicular injury: a randomized controlled trial. *J Trauma* 2006;61:523–533.
56. Sindelar HA, Barnett NP, Spirito A. Adolescent alcohol use and injury. A summary and critical review of the literature. *Minerva Pediatr* 2004; 56(3):291–309.
56a. Johnston LD, O'Malley PM, Bachman JG, et al. *Monitoring the future: national survey results on drug use, 1975–2003. Volume II: College Students and Adults Ages 19—45.* NIH Pub. No. 04–5508. Bethesda, MD: National Institute on Drug Abuse, 2004.
56b. White HR, Young Mun E, Pugh L, et al. Long-Term Effects of Brief Substance Use Interventions for Mandated College Students: Sleeper Effects of an In-Person Personal Feedback Intervention. *Alcohol Clin Exp Res* 2007;31(8):1380–1391.
57. Knight JR, Wechsler H, Kuo M, et al. Alcohol abuse and dependence among U.S. college students. *J Stud Alcohol* 2002;63(3):263–270.
57a. Helmkamp JC, Hungerford DW, Williams JM, et al. Screening and brief intervention for alcohol problems among college students treated in a university hospital emergency department. *J Am Coll Health* 2003; 52(1):7– 16.
58. American College of Obstetricians and Gynecologists. At-risk drinking and illicit drug use: ethical issues in obstetric and gynecologic practice. *Obstet Gynecol* 2004;103(51):1021–1031.
59. Chang G. Screening and brief intervention in prenatal care settings. *Alcohol Res Health* 2004l2005;28(2):80–84.
60. O'Connor MJ, Whaley SE. Brief intervention for alcohol use by pregnant women. *Am J Public Health* 2007;97(2):252–258.
60a. Stephens RS, Roffman RA, Curtin L. Comparison of extended versus brief treatments for marijuana use. *J Consult Clin Psychol* 2000; 68(5):898–908.
61. Copeland J, Swift W, Roffman R, et al. A randomized controlled trial of brief cognitive-behavioral interventions for cannabis use disorder. *J Subst Abuse Treat* 2001;21(2):55–64; discussion 65–66.
62. Marijuana Treatment Project Research Group. Brief treatments for cannabis dependence: findings from a randomized multisite trial. *J Consult Clin Psychol* 2004;72(3):455–466.
63. Martin G. The adolescent cannabis check-up: randomized trial of a brief intervention for young cannabis users. *J Subst Abuse Treat* 2007. [Epub ahead of print]
64. McCambridge J. The efficacy of single-session motivational interviewing in reducing drug consumption and perceptions of drug-related risk and harm among young people: results from a multi-site cluster randomized trial. *Addiction* 2004;99(1):39–52.
64a. Marsden J. An evaluation of a brief motivational intervention among young ecstasy and cocaine users: no effect on substance and alcohol use outcomes. *Addiction* 2006;101(7):1014–1026.
65. Saunders B, Wilkinson C, Phillips M. The impact of a brief motivational intervention with opiate users attending a methadone programme. *Addiction* 1995;90(3):415–424.
66. Ritter A, Cameron J. A review of the efficacy and effectiveness of harm reduction strategies for alcohol, tobacco and illicit drugs. *Drug Alcohol Rev* 2006;25(6):611–624.
67. Gates S, McCambridge J, Smith LA, et al. Interventions for prevention of drug use by young people delivered in non-school settings. *Cochrane Database Syst Rev* 200625;(1):CD005030.
68. Tait RJ, Hulse GK. A systematic review of the effectiveness of brief interventions with substance using adolescents by type of drug. *Drug Alcohol Rev* 2003;22(3):337–346.
69. Dunn C. The use of brief interventions adapted from motivational interviewing across behavioral domains: a systematic review. *Addiction* 2001;96(12):1725–1742.

Screening and Brief Intervention for Pregnant Women

Nicolas Bertholet, MD, MSc, and Richard Saitz, MD, MPH, FACP, FASAM

ALCOHOL

Introduction Alcohol has a harmful effect on the fetus that is completely preventable (by not drinking), and can be responsible for lifelong consequences such as the fetal alcohol syndrome (FAS; see Chapter 81, "Alcohol and Other Drug Use During Pregnancy: Management of the Mother and Child") (1,2). In addition, the consumption of 7 to 14 standard drinks per week is associated with developmental problems such as moderate intellectual and behavioral deficits. These "fetal alcohol effects" are similar to FAS but less severe and much more common (3–5). Alcohol exposure during the first trimester of pregnancy is associated with low birth weight, decreased birth length and head circumference, minor physical abnormalities, and alcohol-related neurodevelopmental disorders (6). Second- and third-trimester exposure can lead to developmental delay (3). Though minimal alcohol consumption (e.g., one drink every 10 days or less) might be very low risk during pregnancy, no definitive threshold level of safe alcohol consumption has been identified, mostly because of differences in fetal vulnerability to the toxic effects of alcohol (7). The U.S. Surgeon General states that no level of alcohol consumption by pregnant women can be considered safe and that pregnant women and women who may be or are considering pregnancy should abstain from alcohol (8). Effective prevention of alcohol use by pregnant women is an important public health measure with direct impact on infant outcomes.

Screening The goal of screening is to identify pregnant women and women who are considering or planning pregnancy and are using any alcohol and to advise them to abstain (and to advise those who are abstinent to remain so). The evaluation of prenatal alcohol use is challenging: many women will reduce their alcohol use as soon as they are aware of their pregnancy (9). Assessing alcohol use during the pregnancy will therefore not be an accurate evaluation of what the alcohol consumption was at the time of conception. Day et al. have demonstrated that asking women about their alcohol consumption before pregnancy was a more accurate measure of drinking during the first trimester (10).

Because of fear and stigma associated with alcohol use during pregnancy, pregnant women may underreport their alcohol consumption (11). In addition, despite the widespread effort to inform women about the harmful effects of alcohol use on the fetus (e.g., via warning labels on containers), many women believe that the consumption of small amounts will not have harmful consequences.

Screening instruments developed for general populations may perform less well in women and in women of childbearing age (7). Consequently, instruments have been developed specifically to ascertain drinking among pregnant women. The T-ACE, based on the "CAGE" (12) (each letter stands for one key word in each of the items), is a four-question instrument (13). T-ACE stands for T (*Tolerance)*: How many drinks does it take to make you feel high? A: Have people *annoyed* you by criticizing your drinking? C: Have you ever felt you ought to *cut down* on your drinking? E *(Eye-opener)*: Have you ever had a drink first thing in the morning to steady your nerves or get rid of a hangover? Affirmative answers to questions A, C, or E are 1 point each. Reporting tolerance to more than two drinks (T question) is scored 2 points. A score of 2 or more is considered positive. The TWEAK, also derived from the CAGE, is a five-question instrument (14). TWEAK stands for T *(Tolerance)*: How many drinks can you hold? (positive if $\geq$6 drinks) *Or* How many drinks does it take before you begin to feel the first effects of alcohol? (positive if $\geq$3 drinks) W: Have close friends or relatives *worried* or complained about your drinking in the past year? E *(Eye-opener)*: Do you sometimes take a drink in the morning when you first get up? A *(Amnesia)*: Has a friend or a family member ever told you about things you said or did while you were drinking that you could not remember? K: Do you sometimes feel the need to *cut down* on your drinking? Affirmative answers to question E, A, K are 1 point each. Affirmative answers to question W and T are 2 points each. The cut-off score is 2. The NET is a three-question instrument. It shares two questions with the T-ACE (Eye opener and Tolerance) and one with the Michigan Alcohol Screening Test (MAST) (Do you feel you are a normal drinker?). The tolerance question scores 2 points, the two other questions score 1 point each, and $\geq$2 is considered positive.

Tested in routine assessment in gynecology and obstetrics services, the T-ACE questionnaire showed better sensitivity compared to the Alcohol Use Disorders Identification Test (AUDIT) and the Short MAST (SMAST) for a lifetime diagnosis of an alcohol use disorder, risky drinking, and current alcohol use in pregnant women (13,15). It outperformed obstetrics staff assessment of any alcohol use (15), and its brevity makes it useful for routine practice (16). Russell et al. demonstrated that the TWEAK and the T-ACE were sensitive for periconceptional risky drinking (17) and outperformed the CAGE and the MAST. At a

(*continued*)

Screening and Brief Intervention for Pregnant Women *(continued)*

cutoff of 2, the NET appears to be less sensitive than the T-ACE, the TWEAK, and the MAST (14). In conclusion, the T-ACE and the TWEAK are two brief questionnaires with satisfactory performance among pregnant women (and those in the periconception stage). The National Institute on Alcohol Abuse and Alcoholism (NIAAA) single screening question has not been tested specifically among pregnant women.

Brief Intervention Various studies of brief intervention included but did not specifically report on women of childbearing age. One of the largest studies to date conducted in primary care, a randomized controlled trial (Trial for Early Alcohol Treatment, project TrEAT) (18), reported results of a subgroup analysis of 205 women aged 18 to 40. Brief intervention decreased the number of drinks consumed in the past 7 days and the number of heavy drinking episodes in the past month by about 20% to 25% (19). This study included women who drank more than 11 drinks per week, more than four standard drinks per occasion, or had positive CAGE screening tests (2+) but excluded women with alcohol dependence. The brief intervention consisted of two 15-minute visits with a physician, 1 month apart, and supportive phone calls by a nurse 2 weeks after each clinician visit. These results support the hypothesis that brief interventions conducted in primary care among women of childbearing age with unhealthy alcohol use are effective in reducing alcohol consumption and heavy drinking episodes.

Few studies focusing on pregnant women have been published. Chang et al. randomly assigned 250 pregnant women identified using the T-ACE questionnaire (score ≥2) as they attended prenatal care (20). Women with gestational age >28 weeks and women without alcohol consumption in the 6 months preceding study participation were excluded. Women were randomly assigned to a comprehensive assessment only or to a comprehensive assessment and a 45-minute brief intervention. Brief intervention included review of the subject's health and pregnancy, review of lifestyle changes made since pregnancy, articulation of drinking goals while pregnant and reasons for these goals, recommendation of abstinence as the most prudent drinking goal, and identification of high-risk situations for drinking and alternatives to drinking. There was a similar decrease in alcohol consumption during pregnancy in the control and intervention groups (0.4 vs. 0.3 drinks per drinking day, respectively). The groups did not differ on the number of drinking episodes either (1.0 vs. 0.7 episodes, respectively). There was an effect of brief intervention on the subgroup of women who were abstinent at study entry, with significantly more maintenance of abstinence in the intervention group (86% vs. control group 72%).

In 2005, Chang et al. published a randomized controlled trial of a 25-minute brief intervention that could involve a partner among pregnant women (21). The partner could be a spouse, father of the child, or any other supportive adult and was chosen by the pregnant woman. Women were enrolled as they initiated prenatal care in obstetric practices and included if they scored 2 or more on the T-ACE, reported any alcohol consumption while pregnant, reported consumption of at least one drink per day in the 6 months before study enrollment, or drank during a previous pregnancy. Women were excluded if they were receiving treatment for a substance use disorder, had physical dependence to alcohol requiring medically supervised detoxification, or used cocaine, opiates, or other illicit drugs. The brief intervention included knowledge assessment with feedback on drinking and pregnancy, goal setting, and behavioral modification (identification of high-risk situations, alternative behaviors, support from the partner). Both intervention and control groups showed similar reductions in alcohol consumption. Brief intervention was, however, effective in reducing drinking among women drinking more heavily. In another subgroup analysis, authors reported a significant impact of brief intervention when a partner participated.

In 2007, Connor and Whaley published the results of a randomized controlled trial of brief intervention versus advice to stop drinking only, among 345 pregnant currently drinking women (22). Brief interventions were delivered by trained nutritionists as part of an individual nutrition education program and included education, feedback, goal setting, cognitive-behavioral procedures, and a contract. There was a substantial decrease in alcohol use in both groups, and authors reported a significant effect of the intervention on abstinence by the third trimester: Women in the intervention group were five times more likely to abstain than were women in the control group. Brief intervention also improved birth weight and reduced fetal death (from 2.9% to 0.9%).

Several other studies are noteworthy. Handmaker et al. published findings of a pilot randomized study of a 1-hour motivational interviewing intervention with 42 pregnant women that showed an impact of the intervention on women with the highest drinking levels at study enrollment (23). In another study, 300 women drinking more than three drinks per week during conception were randomly assigned postpartum to receive or not receive a brief intervention aimed at reducing prenatal alcohol use during the next pregnancy. The intervention decreased alcohol use and improved infant out-

(continued)

Screening and Brief Intervention for Pregnant Women *(continued)*

comes (low birth weight, fewer premature deliveries) (24). Floyd et al. randomly assigned 830 nonpregnant women aged 18 to 44 years and currently at risk for alcohol exposed pregnancies (drinking more than five drinks any day or more than eight drinks per week and having unprotected sex) to receive information or information and a brief motivational alcohol intervention (four sessions) and one contraception consultation (25). For up to 9 months, women in the intervention group were significantly less likely to be at risk for an alcohol-exposed pregnancy (either by drinking risky amounts or by not using effective contraception), confirming results from a previous report (26).

OTHER DRUGS

Introduction Drug use is associated with medical complications in pregnant women (e.g., placental abruption, chorioamnionitis, placental insufficiency, spontaneous abortion, postpartum hemorrhage, and preeclampsia) (27). In addition, evidence of impact of drug use on the fetus is growing, especially for the combined use of illicit drugs and alcohol (see Chapter 82) (28).

Screening Unlike those for testing alcohol usage, drug use screening tools to address use during pregnancy have not been extensively studied. Chasnoff et al. reported using three questions (have you ever drank alcohol, how much alcohol did you drink in the month before your pregnancy, how many cigarettes did you smoke in the month before your pregnancy) to identify and refer women for a full drug and alcohol assessment in the context of prenatal exam (29). In a later study, Chasnoff et al. demonstrated that the 4Ps Plus, a five-item instrument derived from the three questions cited earlier, was a reliable measure with good sensitivity and specificity for substance use (alcohol, marijuana, heroin, cocaine, and methamphetamines) during pregnancy (30). The questionnaire (positive if questions about use during or before pregnancy are affirmative) asks about *P*ast substance use, use during *P*regnancy, and use by *P*arents and *P*artners. The questions are:

- Did either of your parents ever have a problem with alcohol or drugs?
- Does your partner have a problem with alcohol or drugs?
- Have you ever drunk beer, wine, or liquor?
- In the month before you knew you were pregnant, how many cigarettes did you smoke?
- In the month before you knew you were pregnant, how many beers/how much wine/how much liquor did you drink?

Brief Intervention According to the 2008 recommendation of the U.S. Preventive Services Task Force, there is insufficient evidence to determine the benefits and harms of screening for illicit drug use among pregnant women. The Committee on Ethics of the American College of Obstetricians and Gynecologists (ACOG), based on an ethical rationale, recommends screening and brief intervention for illicit drug use (31). Screening and brief interventions are usually delivered with protection of confidentiality, notably to enhance accuracy of screening and establish trust in the clinician–patient relationship. This confidentiality may be challenged in states where the law requires physicians to report illicit drug use by pregnant women, and where laws define this use as criminal behavior (see Section 14). Physicians should also be aware of their state's law regarding the reporting of substance use during pregnancy.

CONCLUSION AND RECOMMENDATIONS

Alcohol Alcohol has toxic effects on the fetus, and there is currently no safe threshold identified for its consumption during pregnancy. The current recommendation for pregnant women, women who might be pregnant, and women who are trying to conceive is to abstain from alcohol. Physicians should inform patients of this recommendation. For breastfeeding mothers, recommendations are to avoid consumption of alcohol or at least not to nurse for at least 2 hours per drink after drinking (that is, if the mother takes two drinks, at least 4 hours should elapse after the last drink) (32), as alcohol is concentrated in breast milk, and its use can inhibit milk production, decrease milk intake by the child, and cause delayed motor development (33).

Women of childbearing age, including pregnant women, should be screened using validated tools. Brief, validated instruments are available for screening pregnant women and those considering pregnancy (T-ACE, TWEAK) and should be used in routine practice. Women positive by screening should then receive a brief intervention.

Pregnancy itself, or assessment of alcohol use, may lead women to decrease or stop drinking. In addition to that effect, brief intervention can decrease risky use in young women (pregnant or not), and although not extensively confirmed in the literature to date, can decrease drinking during pregnancy and the risk of alcohol-exposed pregnancy, may increase abstinence, and may improve fetal outcomes. Some studies suggest that brief intervention effects are limited to women who drink the largest amounts. But even if brief interventions are effective predominantly in

(continued)

Screening and Brief Intervention for Pregnant Women *(continued)*

the highest risk drinkers, screening, advice to abstain from alcohol during pregnancy and before a planned pregnancy, and at least feedback on consequences of alcohol use on the fetus should be included in routine practice, as preventing alcohol use is the only way to prevent FAS and other alcohol-related effects on infants. Depending on resources available, the intervention can be repeated over a few sessions and/or include the partner, as partner involvement may have beneficial effects. Brief interventions conducted among pregnant women should include specific feedback on consequences of drinking on the fetus and infant as well as medical complications related to alcohol use during pregnancy and identification of risky situations (and potential coping strategies). Parents should be informed of potential legal consequences of reporting their alcohol use if applicable (e.g., loss of parental rights).

Other Drugs Use of illicit drugs during pregnancy has a negative impact on the course of pregnancy and on the fetus (27). There is currently insufficient evidence to determine the benefits and harms of screening for illicit drug use among pregnant women. Nevertheless, given its potential preventive benefits, it seems reasonable, if not ethically required, for physicians to give at least feedback on consequences of use as well as advice to abstain. Even in the absence of scientific data on screening and brief intervention efficacy among pregnant women, one would ask about medications, illicit drug use, and alcohol and tobacco use as part of a prenatal exam. If drug abuse or dependence is suspected, women should be referred for a comprehensive assessment, in order to address substance use severity and associated psychosocial issues (27). For that purpose, one instrument, the 4 Ps Plus, has been validated among pregnant women. As for alcohol, information on illicit drug use and tobacco use consequences on the fetus should also be provided to women of childbearing age. It should be noted that the specific context of pregnancy and the potential legal consequences will impact the accuracy of the screening and necessary ingredients of brief intervention, and clinicians will face ethical challenges, having to balance principles of beneficence and respect for autonomy as they apply to both women and their children.

REFERENCES

1. Jones KL, Smith DW, Ulleland CN, Streissguth P. Pattern of malformation in offspring of chronic alcoholic mothers. *Lancet* 1973;1: 1267–1271.
2. Jones KL, Smith DW. Recognition of the fetal alcohol syndrome in early infancy. *Lancet* 1973;2:999–1001.
3. Jacobson JL, Jacobson SW. Drinking moderately and pregnancy: effects on child development. *Alcohol Res Health* 1999;23:25–30.
4. O'Connor MJ, Kasari C. Prenatal alcohol exposure and depressive features in children. *Alcohol Clin Exp Res* 2000;24:1084–1092.
5. Manning MA, Hoyme HE. Fetal alcohol spectrum disorders: a practical clinical approach to diagnosis. *Neurosci Biobehav Rev* 2007;31:230–238.
6. Day NL, Jasperse D, Richardson G, et al. Prenatal exposure to alcohol: effect on infant growth and morphologic characteristics. *Pediatrics* 1989;84:536–541.
7. Bradley KA, Boyd-Wickizer J, Powell SH, Burman ML. Alcohol screening questionnaires in women: a critical review. *JAMA* 1998; 280:166–171.
8. U.S. Surgeon General. News Release. Accessed May 9, 2008, from www.hhs.gov/surgeongeneral/pressrelease/sg02222005.html.
9. Smith IE, Lancaster JS, Moss-Wells S, et al. Identifying high-risk pregnant drinkers: biological and behavioral correlates of continuous heavy drinking during pregnancy. *J Stud Alcohol* 1987; 48:304–309.
10. Day NL, Cottreau CM, Richardson GA. The epidemiology of alcohol, marijuana, and cocaine use among women of childbearing age and pregnant women. *Clin Obstet Gynecol* 1993;36:232–245.
11. Jacobson SW, Chiodo LM, Sokol RJ, Jacobson JL. Validity of maternal report of prenatal alcohol, cocaine, and smoking in relation to neurobehavioral outcome. *Pediatrics* 2002;109:815–825.
12. Mayfield D, McLeod G, Hall P. The CAGE questionnaire: validation of a new alcoholism screening instrument. *Am J Psychiatry* 1974;131: 1121–1123.
13. Sokol RJ, Martier SS, Ager JW. The T-ACE questions: practical prenatal detection of risk-drinking. *Am J Obstet Gynecol* 1989;160: 863–868; discussion 868–870.
14. Russell M, Martier SS, Sokol RJ, et al. Screening for pregnancy risk-drinking. *Alcohol Clin Exp Res* 1994;18:1156–1161.
15. Chang G, Wilkins-Haug L, Berman S, et al. Alcohol use and pregnancy: improving identification. *Obstet Gynecol* 1998;91: 892–898.
16. Fabbri CE, Furtado EF, Laprega MR. Alcohol consumption in pregnancy: performance of the Brazilian version of the questionnaire T-ACE. *Rev Saude Publica* 2007;41:979–884.
17. Russell M, Martier SS, Sokol RJ, et al. Detecting risk drinking during pregnancy: a comparison of four screening questionnaires. *Am J Public Health* 1996;86:1435–1439.
18. Fleming MF, Barry KL, Manwell LB, et al. Brief physician advice for problem alcohol drinkers. A randomized controlled trial in community-based primary care practices. *JAMA* 1997;277:1039–1045.
19. Manwell LB, Fleming MF, Mundt MP, et al. Treatment of problem alcohol use in women of childbearing age: results of a brief intervention trial. *Alcohol Clin Exp Res* 2000;24:1517–1524.
20. Chang G, Wilkins-Haug L, Berman S, Goetz MA. Brief intervention for alcohol use in pregnancy: a randomized trial. *Addiction* 1999;94: 1499–1508.
21. Chang G, McNamara TK, Orav EJ, et al. Brief intervention for prenatal alcohol use: a randomized trial. *Obstet Gynecol* 2005;105:991–998.
22. O'Connor MJ, Whaley SE. Brief intervention for alcohol use by pregnant women. *Am J Public Health* 2007;97:252–258.
23. Handmaker NS, Miller WR, Manicke M. Findings of a pilot study of motivational interviewing with pregnant drinkers. *J Stud Alcohol* 1999;60:285–287.
24. Hankin JR. Fetal alcohol syndrome prevention research. *Alcohol Res Health* 2002;26:58–65.
25. Floyd RL, Sobell M, Velasquez MM, et al. Preventing alcohol-exposed pregnancies: a randomized controlled trial. *Am J Prev Med* 2007; 32:1–10.

(continued)

Screening and Brief Intervention for Pregnant Women *(continued)*

26. Ingersoll K, Floyd L, Sobell M, Velasquez MM. Reducing the risk of alcohol-exposed pregnancies: a study of a motivational intervention in community settings. *Pediatrics* 2003;111:1131–1135.
27. Helmbrecht GD, Thiagarajah S. Management of addiction disorders in pregnancy. *J Addict Med* 2008;2:1–16.
28. Rivkin MJ, Davis PE, Lemaster JL, et al. Volumetric MRI study of brain in children with intrauterine exposure to cocaine, alcohol, tobacco, and marijuana. *Pediatrics* 2008;121:741–750.
29. Chasnoff IJ, Neuman K, Thornton C, Callaghan MA. Screening for substance use in pregnancy: a practical approach for the primary care physician. *Am J Obstet Gynecol* 2001;184:752–758.
30. Chasnoff IJ, Wells AM, McGourty RF, Bailey LK. Validation of the 4P's Plus screen for substance use in pregnancy validation of the 4P's Plus. *J Perinatol* 2007;27:744–748.
31. The American College of Obstetricians and Gynecologists, Committee on Ethics. At-risk drinking and illicit drug use: ethical issues in obstetric and gynecology practice. In: the American College of Obstetricians and Gynecologists (eds.). *Gynecologists*. Washington, DC: ACOG Committee Opinion, 2004.
32. American Academy of Pediatrics. Breastfeeding and the use of human milk. *Pediatrics* 2005(4);496–506.
33. Anderson PO. Alcohol and breastfeeding. *J Hum Lact* 1995;11:321–323.

Trauma Centers, Hospitals, Emergency Departments

Richard D. Blondell, MD

Compared to those in the general population, individuals with substance use disorders are overrepresented among patients presenting to emergency departments (1,2) and among those hospitalized for general medical conditions (3,4) or for traumatic injuries (5,6). Alcohol is the major risk factor for virtually all categories of fatal and nonfatal injury, including traffic accidents, burns and fires, drowning, air traffic injuries, occupational injuries, homicides, suicides, and domestic violence (7). The prevalence of substance use disorders among hospitalized patients varies with the population studied and has been observed to be as low as 7.4% of all general hospital admissions (8) to up to 70% of those with life-threatening injuries (9). Trauma centers, hospitals, and emergency departments are ideal places for clinicians to use the "teachable moment" generated by the hospital visit to implement screening, brief intervention, and referral to treatment for substance use disorders. In the United States, a "Level I Trauma Center" provides the highest level of surgical care to victims of traumatic injury, and these centers must have the capability to provide an intervention for patients identified as problem drinkers (10).

CASE FINDING AND SCREENING

Routine clinical information alone will identify many patients with alcohol and drug problems. Some patients may freely admit that their hospitalization was related to substance abuse (e.g., "I had too much to drink and fell down the stairs"). At other times, the illness may be obviously related to an alcohol use disorder (e.g., delirium tremens) or drug use (e.g., a gunshot wound sustained in a "crack house") or there may be a well-documented history of a substance use disorder in the medical record. In these instances, no additional "screening questions" are required. However, clinical "case finding" has its limitations as clinicians can even fail to recognize patients who are acutely intoxicated (11).

There is no shortage of screening instruments that could be used to detect subclinical substance use disorders among hospitalized patients. Examples include the four "CAGE" questions (12), the 10-item "Brief MAST" (Brief Michigan Alcoholism Screening Test) (13), or the 10-item "AUDIT" (Alcohol Use Disorders Identification Test) (14). These instruments can be modified to screen for drug use disorders. It can be an administrative challenge to incorporate these screening questionnaires into a busy clinical service that is focused on treatment of acute problems. Some authorities suggest a practical way to put screening into actual practice: Start with a single question, such as, "When was the last time you had more than 5 drinks (4 drinks for women) in one day?" Additional questions could then be asked of those who admit to exceeding these limits within the past 3 months (15).

A number of biochemical markers may suggest the presence of an alcohol use disorder (e.g., elevations of liver enzymes or the mean corpuscular volume); however, none have sufficient sensitivity or specificity for routine screening. Other biochemical markers have been investigated as screening tests for alcohol use disorders among trauma patients, such as carbohydrate-deficient transferrin (16), but these have not been incorporated into routine practice. There are no biochemical markers that are useful as screening tests for drug abuse.

Mandatory toxicology testing can be an important first-line screening test used to detect substance use disorders among acutely ill patients (17,18). In some states, however, health insurance regulations may serve as a barrier to toxicology testing (19). The sensitivity, specificity, and predictive value of toxicology as a marker for alcohol or drug use disorders among inpatients has not been well studied. Toxicology results can be difficult to interpret because they often detect only recent use, and it is not always easy to distinguish between licit and illicit drug use, and there are limitations of the tests. For example, many opioids do not cross-react with the urine "opiate" test, which is usually standardized to morphine.

Obtaining patient prescription records directly from pharmacies or statewide electronic databases can provide important information about the types and dosages of medications dispensed to the patient (20). Excessive prescriptions, dosages, and visits to multiple physicians for controlled substances can suggest a licit drug use disorder.

CLINICAL ASSESSMENT

If clinical information or the results of screening techniques suggest a diagnosis of a substance use disorder, additional information is required to determine patient "willingness to change" and the severity of disease. Some patients can be surprisingly honest about their situation, (e.g., "Doc, I know I have a problem with these drugs"), whereas others will maintain a strong denial of a problem. Likewise, the severity of disease can vary from "problem use" to "abuse" or "dependence." Therefore, the appropriate clinical intervention might vary from a brief counseling session designed to increase patient willingness to change a pattern of problem

(*continued*)

Trauma Centers, Hospitals, Emergency Departments *(continued)*

drinking to a referral for treatment of an advanced addiction disorder.

A clinical assessment that suggests alcohol or drug dependence is of immediate clinical importance, as treatment to prevent or manage a withdrawal syndrome may be indicated. Patients with the most severe alcohol problems are at the greatest risk for the development of alcohol withdrawal syndrome (AWS) and delirium tremens (21). Those patients with a history of heavy drinking (i.e., eight or more drinks per day) who have withdrawal symptoms early in the course of hospitalization, or who have a high admission blood alcohol concentration (>150 mg/dL), and those who also have a concurrent acute medical illness may be at particularly high risk for severe AWS (22–25). A history of licit or illicit use of sedatives should place the physician on the alert for a sedative withdrawal syndrome which can also be life-threatening.

INITIAL MANAGEMENT OF WITHDRAWAL SYNDROMES

Parenteral thiamine should always be administered as a priority to alcohol-dependent patients in the emergency department before glucose-containing intravenous fluids are given to prevent the development of Wernicke's encephalopathy.

Based on reviews of available data, long-acting benzodiazepines are the drugs of choice to prevent and treat AWS (26,27). The management of drug withdrawal among hospitalized patients is largely anecdotal and based mostly on expert opinion and uncontrolled studies. Withdrawal from short-acting benzodiazepines, such as alprazolam, may begin within the first 24 hours after hospital admission, whereas withdrawal from long-acting benzodiazepines or barbiturates may be delayed for several days. Although opioid withdrawal is not necessarily life-threatening, it can complicate the initial assessment and treatment of inpatients as well as preoperative, intraoperative, and postoperative patient care and should therefore be treated (e.g. with long-acting opioids such as methadone).

INTERVENTION AND DISCHARGE PLANNING

Hospitalized patients with substance use disorders are good candidates for an intervention to prevent future problems because they are in a controlled environment under the direction of health care professionals. An acute illness usually captures the attention of the patient and the patient's family. An acute medical problem or the pain from a traumatic injury can diminish the usual patient denial of problem drinking or illicit drug use. If approached at the right time, hospitalized patients can be surprisingly receptive toward an intervention designed to address an alcohol or drug problem.

Although most physicians are capable of addressing alcohol and drug problems among their patients prior to hospital discharge if given proper training, they are often appropriately focused on providing acute medical or surgical care. Therefore, it is usually necessary for other members of the hospital team (e.g., social workers, nurses, psychologists, lay volunteers) to discuss a substance use disorder treatment plan with the patient prior to hospital discharge. For example, when victims of alcohol-related traumatic injuries were given a single motivational interview by a "psychologist trained in the use of brief interventions," these patients consumed fewer drinks per week over the 12 months after their hospital discharge as compared to a control group who did not receive the brief intervention (28). However, this effect was observed primarily for patients who were considered to be "problem drinkers" and less so for alcohol-dependent patients. Patients who are in denial about their alcohol problems or who are highly dependent on alcohol may respond to an intensive counseling session (29). Many large hospitals have a "substance abuse consult service" that can be called upon to intervene with patients with alcohol or drug problems (30). Nurses can be trained to deliver structured interventions that are effective with hospitalized medical patients (31). Peers who are in recovery could also be asked to visit hospitalized patients (32). In emergency departments, lay people who are trained as "Health Promotion Advocates" have been used to increase patient access to substance abuse treatment services after discharge (33).

The authors of one systematic review found that the evidence for the effectiveness of opportunistic brief interventions in general hospitals for problem drinkers is inconclusive (34). There are conflicting reports about the effectiveness of brief interventions in emergency department settings, with some reports suggesting a positive benefit (35,36), whereas others suggest a lack of any benefit (37). It may be that the effectiveness of brief interventions varies with setting of the study, the population included in the study, the severity of the substance use disorder studied, the type of intervention that was used, and outcome measured. One well-designed randomized trial of brief interventions in a trauma center demonstrated a reduction in drinking among problem drinkers and a trend toward the reduction of future injuries (28). Payment for professional services related to screening, brief interventions, referral, and

(continued)

Trauma Centers, Hospitals, Emergency Departments *(continued)*

treatment can be a problem. In the majority of the states, an insurer is permitted to withhold payments to the hospital and the treating physicians if there is information that indicated that the patient was intoxicated at the time of an injury (38).

Even when the patient admits to having a serious alcohol or drug problem and is willing to comply with a clinical recommendation, it is not always easy to coordinate a treatment referral. Treatment centers may require a significant amount of data regarding patient demographics, insurance information, medical clearance, or even a written treatment referral signed by the attending physician. A referral to a treatment program may also involve a lengthy and complicated health insurance company "preauthorization" process. Despite this, the conventional wisdom is that doing something that addresses an underlying substance use disorder produces better outcomes than simply treating the primary medical or surgical problem alone.

Acknowledgments: *This work was supported, in part, by grant (K23-AA015616) from the National Institute on Alcohol Abuse and Alcoholism.*

REFERENCES

1. Rockett IR, Putnam SL, Jia H, Smith GS. Declared and undeclared substance use among emergency department patients: a population-based study. *Addiction* 2006;101:706–712.
2. D'Onofrio G, Becker B, Woolard RH. The impact of alcohol, tobacco, and other drug use and abuse in the emergency department. *Emerg Med Clin North Am* 2006;24:925–967.
3. Fach M, Bischof G, Schmidt C, Rumpf HJ. Prevalence of dependence on prescription drugs and associated mental disorders in a representative sample of general hospital patients. *Gen Hosp Psychiatry* 2007;29:257–263.
4. Brown RL, Leonard T, Saunders LA, Papasouliotis O. The prevalence and detection of substance use disorders among inpatients ages 18-49: an opportunity for prevention. *Prev Med* 1998;27:101–110.
5. Rivara FP, Mueller BA, Fligner CL, et al. Drug use in trauma victims. *J Trauma* 1989;29:462–470.
6. Soderstrom CA, Dischinger PC, Smith GS, et al. Psychoactive substance dependence among trauma center patients. *JAMA* 1992;267: 2756–2759.
7. Lunetta P, Smith GS. The role of alcohol in injury deaths. In: preedy VR, Watson RR, eds. Comprehensive handbook of alcohol related pathology, vol 1. London: elsevier, 2005:147–164.
8. Smothers BA, Yahr HT, Ruhl CE. Detection of alcohol use disorders in general hospital admissions in the United States. *Arch Intern Med* 2004;164:749–756.
9. Madan AK, Yu K, Beech DJ. Alcohol and drug use in victims of life-threatening trauma. *J Trauma* 1999;47:568–571.
10. American College of Surgeons, Committee on Trauma. Alcohol screening and brief intervention (SBI) for trauma patients. Accessed April 25, 2008, from www.facs.org/trauma/publications/sbirtguide.pdf.
11. Gentilello LM, Villaveces A, Ries RR, et al. Detection of acute alcohol intoxication and chronic alcohol dependence by trauma center staff. *J Trauma* 1999;47:1131–1135; discussion 1135–1139.
12. Ewing JA. Detecting alcoholism. The CAGE questionnaire. *JAMA* 1984;252:1905–1907.
13. Pokorny AD, Miller BA, Kaplan HB. The brief MAST: a shortened version of the Michigan Alcoholism Screening Test. *Am J Psychiatry* 1972;129:342–345.
14. Babor TF. From clinical research to secondary prevention: international collaboration in the development of the Alcohol Use Disorders Identification Test (AUDIT). *Alcohol Health Res World* 1989;13: 371–374.
15. Canagasaby A, Vinson DC. Screening for hazardous or harmful drinking using one or two quantity-frequency questions. *Alcohol Alcohol* 2005;40:208–213.
16. Spies CD, Emadi A, Neumann T, et al. Relevance of carbohydrate-deficient transferrin as a predictor of alcoholism in intensive care patients following trauma. *J Trauma* 1995;39:742–748.
17. Parran TV Jr, Weber E, Tasse J, et al. Mandatory toxicology testing and chemical dependence consultation follow-up in a level-one trauma center. *J Trauma* 1995;38:278–280.
18. Carrigan TD, Field H, Illingworth RN, et al. Toxicological screening in trauma. *J Accid Emerg Med* 2000;17:33–37.
19. Rivara FP, Tollefson S, Tesh E, Gentilello LM. Screening trauma patients for alcohol problems: are insurance companies barriers? *J Trauma* 2000;48(1):115–118.
20. Blondell RD, Dodds HN, Blondell MN, Droz DC. Is the Kentucky prescription reporting system useful in the care of hospitalized patients? *J Ky Med Assoc* 2004;102:15–19.
21. Spies CD, Rommelspacher H. Alcohol withdrawal in the surgical patient: prevention and treatment. *Anesth Analg* 1999;88: 946–954.
22. Vinson DC, Menezes M. Admission alcohol level: a predictor of the course of alcohol withdrawal. *J Fam Pract* 1991;33:161–167.
23. Ferguson JA, Suelzer CJ, Eckert GJ, Zhou XH, Dittus RS. Risk factors for delirium tremens development. *J Gen Intern Med* 1996;11: 410–414.
24. Wojnar M, Bizon Z, Wasilewski D. The role of somatic disorders and physical injury in the development and course of alcohol withdrawal delirium. *Alcohol Clin Exp Res* 1999;23:209–213.
25. Glickman L, Herbsman H. Delirium tremens in surgical patients. *Surgery* 1968;64:882–890.
26. Mayo-Smith MF. Pharmacological management of alcohol withdrawal. A meta-analysis and evidence-based practice guideline. American Society of Addiction Medicine Working Group on Pharmacological Management of Alcohol Withdrawal. *JAMA* 1997;278: 144–151.
27. Holbrook AM, Crowther R, Lotter A, et al. Meta-analysis of benzodiazepine use in the treatment of acute alcohol withdrawal. *CMAJ* 1999;160:649–655.
28. Gentilello LM, Rivara FP, Donovan DM, et al. Alcohol interventions in a trauma center as a means of reducing the risk of injury recurrence. *Ann Surg* 1999;230:473–480; discussion 480–473.
29. Dunn CW, Donovan DM, Gentilello LM. Practical guidelines for performing alcohol interventions in trauma centers. *J Trauma* 1997;42:299–304.
30. Fleming MF, Wilk A, Kruger J, et al. Hospital-based alcohol and drug specialty consultation service: does it work? *South Med J* 1995;88: 275–282.

(*continued*)

Trauma Centers, Hospitals, Emergency Departments *(continued)*

31. Chick J, Lloyd G, Crombie E. Counselling problem drinkers in medical wards: a controlled study. *Br Med J (Clin Res Ed)* 1985; 290(6473):965–967.
32. Blondell RD, Looney SW, Northington AP, et al. Can recovering alcoholics help hospitalized patients with alcohol problems? *J Fam Pract* 2001;50:447.
33. Bernstein E, Bernstein J, Levenson S. Project ASSERT: an ED-based intervention to increase access to primary care, preventive services, and the substance abuse treatment system. *Ann Emerg Med* 1997;30: 181–189.
34. Emmen MJ, Schippers GM, Bleijenberg G, Wollersheim H. Effectiveness of opportunistic brief interventions for problem drinking in a general hospital setting: systematic review. *BMJ* 2004;328(7435): 318.
35. Monti PM, Barnett NP, Colby SM, et al. Motivational interviewing versus feedback only in emergency care for young adult problem drinking. *Addiction* 2007;102:1234–1243.
36. Academic ED SBIRT Research Collaborative. The impact of screening, brief intervention, and referral for treatment on emergency department patients' alcohol use. *Ann Emerg Med* 2007;50:699–710, e691–e696.
37. Daeppen JB, Gaume J, Bady P, et al. Brief alcohol intervention and alcohol assessment do not influence alcohol use in injured patients treated in the emergency department: a randomized controlled clinical trial. *Addiction* 2007;102:1224–1233. Errata 2007;102:1995.
38. American College of Surgeons. Statement on insurance, alcohol-related injuries, and trauma centers. *Bull Am Coll Surg* 2006;91(9)ST-55. Accessed April 25, 2008, from www.facs.org/fellows_info/statements/st-55.html.

Implementation of Screening and Brief Intervention in Clinical Settings Using Quality Improvement Principles

Katharine A. Bradley, MD, MPH, and Emily C. Williams, MPH

Despite evidence-based recommendations that alcohol screening and brief intervention (SBI) be routinely implemented in primary care settings, widespread efforts by researchers to implement SBI have been disappointing. Some research efforts to implement SBI have succeeded (1–6), but none has resulted in sustained SBI after research ended. Even studies that were designed based on established models for implementing evidence-based care (7) have met with marginal success in the degree of implementation (8). A review of implementation studies concluded that research trials to date have been too heterogeneous and in need of longer follow-up times to provide conclusive information regarding the circumstances under which SBI is likely to be successfully implemented in health care settings (9). Therefore, clinical managers or clinicians who wish to implement SBI in their health care systems currently have little research on successful implementation to guide them.

However, some integrated health care systems are making progress toward implementation of SBI. One such example is the Veterans Affairs (VA) health care system. Implementation of SBI offers unique challenges owing to the complexity of measures taken to implement SBI in randomized trials: alcohol screening, clinician training, comprehensive assessments of severity, systems to ensure receipt of interventions, and follow-up visits. Therefore, the VA started by focusing on implementing alcohol screening as a first step and later has followed with efforts to implement brief intervention. Following is a retrospective analysis of this implementation process based on a model developed by Greenhalgh and colleagues to explain the spread and sustainability of health care innovations (10).

The Greenhalgh and colleagues model (figure), which is based on a thorough literature review, outlines the importance not only of the nature of an **Innovation** but of characteristics of the **User System** and **Innovators,** and the **Linkage** between the two. Innovations are more likely to be successfully implemented if they are simple, relevant to the user, easily transferable, and can be tried by users without any commitment to continued use. Further, successful innovations consist of a "core" of essential elements, but they also typically have more flexible or modifiable "peripheral" elements that allow users to adapt the innovations to their own circumstances. Important components of **User Systems** that help determine the success of innovations include system antecedents, system readiness for a specific innovation, characteristics of adopters, the implementation process, and evaluating and addressing consequences of implementation. *System antecedents* that foster innovation include structural features (e.g., large size, differentiation, decentralization, availability of dedicated time and resources), a capacity for sharing new knowledge; and

Adaptation of Greenhalgh Model of Diffusion of Innovations in Service Organizations

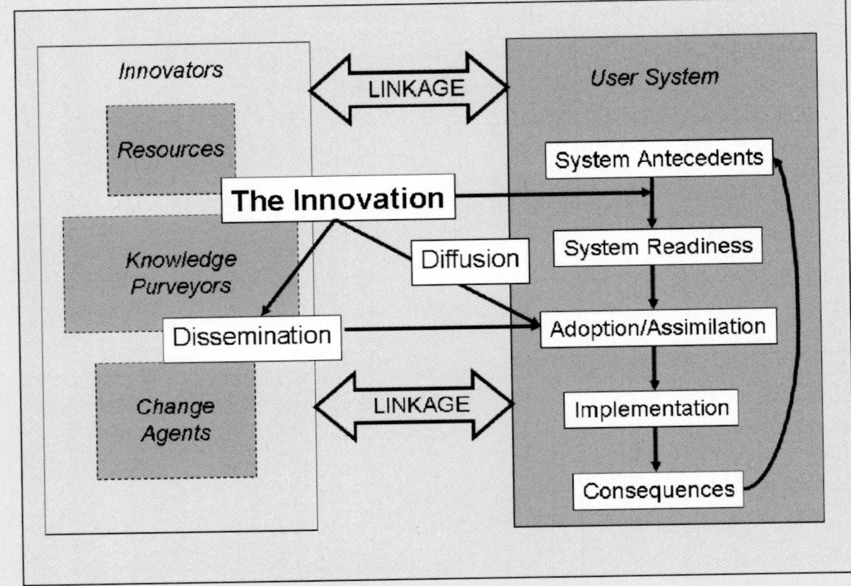

Factors That influence the success of implementation. (Adapted from Greenhalgh T. *Milbank Quart* 2004;82:581–692, with permission.)

(*continued*)

Implementation of Screening and Brief Intervention in Clinical Settings Using Quality Improvement Principles *(continued)*

receptivity to change (e.g., leadership with clear goals and vision and a willingness to take risks, systems to measure and respond to results of implementation efforts). *System readiness for a particular innovation* is affected by institutional pressures for and against change, innovation-system fit, balance of power between supporters and opponents of change, dedication of time and resources to implementation of the innovation, and the capacity for monitoring and feedback. *Adopters'* needs, motivation, values, goals, and learning styles and adopter social networks also affect the success of an implementation. Innovations based on a "shared meaning" between innovators and adopters are more likely to be successfully implemented. Important components of the *implementation process* include ongoing support from leadership, availability and timeliness of support materials to staff, and effective communication across departmental boundaries. Timely evaluation to identify intended and unintended *consequences* of implementation, and the extent to which those consequences are considered when implementing further innovations are the final components of the User System. The outcome of efforts to implement health care innovations also depends on the **Innovators,** who typically consist of "teams" of experts ("knowledge purveyors") and leaders able to actualize change ("change agents") with access to resources required to implement an innovation. These teams might be formal or informal, with some emerging transiently to implement an innovation. Depending on the communication and influence of the Innovators and characteristics of an innovation, successful implementation efforts range from spontaneous passive diffusion, when innovations are readily adopted with little active support, to active dissemination with formal, planned marketing often facilitated by champions, "boundary spanners," and change agents. Finally, efforts to implement service innovations are most successful when there is **Linkage** between the innovators and the user system, both during the development of an innovation and throughout the implementation process.

ESSENTIAL VA SYSTEM ANTECEDENTS TO SBI

The VA health care system has many of the system antecedents required for successful innovation, which provided an essential foundation for SBI implementation efforts. Starting in 1995, the VA underwent a complete redesign of health care delivery (11–13) in line with quality improvement principles (14). Improvements have included implementation of a nationwide electronic medical record (EMR) with a system of clinical reminders, a system of evolving nationwide performance measures to encourage evidence-based practices (15), financial incentives for network leaders linked to annual performance measures, and systems of measuring performance on a monthly and quarterly basis using medical record review and patient satisfaction surveys. EMR clinical reminders can be developed and edited locally but can also be transferred to other VA facilities. A system of national monthly educational video conferences for quality managers and a national VA employee educational system were also established. In 1998, the VA also launched the Quality Enhancement Research Initiative (QUERI) to conduct implementation research on specific conditions common among VA patients, including one QUERI center focused on substance use disorders (SUD QUERI). Each QUERI center has a research coordinator, a clinical coordinator, and an implementation coordinator (i.e., a team of "boundary-spanning" experts), and a small core budget. The QUERI centers were asked to develop research programs to identify important gaps in the quality of VA care, to evaluate interventions to address the identified gaps, and to develop and evaluate strategies for implementation (16,17).

VA READINESS FOR SBI

Several important developments led to VA system readiness for SBI. First, beginning in 1998 as part of the VA's initial wave of performance measures for preventive care based on recommendations of the U.S. Preventive Service Task Force, alcohol screening with a valid instrument was required annually. Most sites initially chose to use the CAGE questionnaire, a validated screen for alcohol use disorders.

At the same time, clinician researchers from the SUD QUERI had identified the need to screen for "unhealthy" drinking (the spectrum from drinking above recommended limits to meeting diagnostic criteria for alcohol use disorders) (18,19) in order to identify patients who benefit from brief intervention. These researchers validated the AUDIT-C, the first three questions of the WHO's 10-item Alcohol Use Disorders Identification Test, as an effective brief screen for identifying BI's target population. Clinician researchers from the QUERI educated local leaders and a national mental health leader in informatics about the limitations of the CAGE in the late 1990s. As a result, the AUDIT-C was implemented at one site, and a self-scoring AUDIT-C was

(*continued*)

Implementation of Screening and Brief Intervention in Clinical Settings Using Quality Improvement Principles *(continued)*

programmed into the electronic medical record, which laid the foundation for national use. SUD QUERI researchers also integrated a clinician informatics expert with detailed knowledge of the VA's EMR into the research team and began exploring ways to use the VA's EMR to prompt providers to offer brief intervention to patients who screened positive for alcohol misuse.

In addition, the VA conducted the Large Health Study of Veterans, which found that among the 4% of patients who reported drinking more than four drinks daily, 83% indicated they were not getting the help with their drinking that they needed from the VA (18). This report created pressure for VA leadership to do more for the recognition and treatment of unhealthy alcohol use (18) and led analysts in the Office of Quality and Performance to evaluate rates of follow-up among patients who screened positive on the CAGE.

Linkage of the "User System" and Innovators The national VA Office of Quality and Performance contacted QUERI researchers for assistance in planning next steps. Once the communication between quality managers (change agents) and QUERI researchers (knowledge purveyors) was established, researchers shared unpublished analyses consistent with findings of the Large Health Survey (20–22). Researchers also educated national quality leaders about evidence for the efficacy of brief intervention, the target population for brief interventions (patients with unhealthy alcohol use), and the fact that many patients who screened positive on the CAGE no longer drank alcohol (23). QUERI experts were then invited to present two educational seminars via teleconferences for quality managers nationwide (one on screening and one on brief intervention) and then to recommend options for performance improvement to the national VA group that set performance measures. This presentation led to a new performance measure that required the full AUDIT or the three-item AUDIT-C for annual alcohol screening beginning in fiscal year 2004. Plans were also made to add relevant measures to data systems already in place (medical record review and patient satisfaction surveys) to evaluate performance on alcohol screening.

Implementation of Alcohol Screening After announcement of the new performance measure for screening for unhealthy alcohol use, the Office of Quality and Performance convened a group consisting of QUERI researchers (alcohol experts) and a VA clinician widely regarded as the national expert in clinical reminder development (informatics expert) to design a clinical reminder in the EMR that incorporated the self-scoring AUDIT-C. This clinical reminder was made available to VA sites by the informatics expert, which resulted in rapid diffusion of the clinical reminder nationwide. Although the "core" of the innovation was alcohol screening with the AUDIT-C, sites could tailor the innovation as they wished. The clinical reminder was available and could be edited or combined with other clinical reminders (e.g., for smoking) and could be activated for nurses and/or for primary care providers. Finally, sites could have patients provide the answers on paper, in interviews, or on a computer terminal.

Adopters At the time the performance measure was announced, no attention had been paid to educating clinicians nationwide about the rationale for the change. The relative neglect of provider education at the time of dissemination of the clinical reminder led to a lack of shared meaning between innovators and individual adopters within the user system. Quality managers at some individual VA sites asked national quality managers what should happen after patients screened positive. Others initially planned to refer all patients with a positive screen to addictions treatment, not understanding that the new goal of screening was to identify patients with the spectrum of unhealthy alcohol use, many of whom would benefit from brief interventions and not be appropriate for specialty treatment. In addition, e-mails forwarded to QUERI researchers from national quality leaders indicated that the inconsistency between a patient's responses to individual AUDIT-C questions (which underestimate drinking) and the results of screening based on the AUDIT-C total *score* undermined acceptance of the screening performance measure. QUERI worked to meet the educational need by creating a Frequently Asked Questions document, making the slides from the national teleconferences available to sites and developing a VA intranet web site with clinician resources. In addition, a clinical reminder for brief alcohol counseling, which had been developed with the support of two research career grants, was shared with sites that requested it and was rapidly disseminated at one eight-site facility where clinicians routinely used clinical reminders (24).

Evaluation of Consequences of Implementing Alcohol Screening High rates of alcohol screening were achieved relatively rapidly (25), and the systems in place to monitor performance offered an important opportunity to identify

(continued)

Implementation of Screening and Brief Intervention in Clinical Settings Using Quality Improvement Principles *(continued)*

consequences of the implementation effort. In particular, drawing on the pre-existing collaboration with the Office of Quality and Performance, QUERI was able to compare medical record review data with patient report data from surveys. These analyses revealed that many patients who reported drinking on patient surveys were identified in medical records as "nondrinkers" (26). In addition, a higher proportion of patients screened positive on the AUDIT-C via mailed survey than had screened positive based on clinical screening documented in the medical record (33% vs. 25%) (26). As a result, changes were made to the screening performance measure and alcohol screening clinical reminder to encourage asking screening questions verbatim. Finally, patient surveys suggested that rates of alcohol-related advice remained relatively low (25). New medical record measures were piloted to monitor documented follow-up of positive alcohol screening tests. In 2007, QUERI investigators collaborated with national clinical leaders in primary care and mental health as well as quality improvement leaders to develop a performance measure for appropriate follow-up on positive alcohol screens that was implemented in 2008.

FLEXIBLE RESOURCES FOR IMPLEMENTATION OF INNOVATIONS

As is clear from this discussion, the implementation of SBI in VA involved the collaboration of researchers with expertise in alcohol screening and brief intervention but was driven by quality managers, clinical leaders in mental health and primary care, informatics experts, and feedback based on performance monitoring. Initial work, including validation of the AUDIT-C and development of clinical reminders for both alcohol screening and follow-up brief intervention, was funded via project grants from the VA and the University of Washington's Alcohol and Drug Abuse Institute, two 4- to 5-year career grants from National Institute on Alcohol Abuse and Alcoholism and the Robert Wood Johnson Foundation, and funding from VA Centers of Excellence for Health Services Research and Substance Abuse Treatment and Education. During the implementation phase, however, the extensive resources required for implementation and monitoring of SBI came from the VA's national Office of Quality and Performance, and individual sites supported alcohol screening by dedicating clinical staff time to screening and monitoring performance. Recent stages of implementation have been supported and made possible by ongoing support from national primary care and mental health leaders, who have launched a nationwide effort to integrate mental health care into primary care settings. Ongoing dedicated resources have been paramount to any success in implementation of SBI in the VA.

SUMMARY

The application of the Greenhalgh model to the VA's experience in implementing SBI, as outlined earlier, demonstrates important lessons for other health care systems wishing to implement SBI. First, a quality improvement infrastructure as well as an EMR created an essential institutional foundation for SBI. Other essential system antecedents included the availability of data systems for monitoring, feedback and performance measurement. Second, data on patients' unmet needs, the QUERI infrastructure, and other informal linkage between alcohol and informatics experts and quality improvement leaders led to the VA's readiness for SBI. The implementation process was flexible but included performance measures to motivate leaders and providers nationwide, which, in turn, led to the commitment of necessary resources. Ongoing attention to adopters' educational needs and feedback to adopters regarding performance have been essential, so that intended consequences could be improved upon and unintended consequences could be addressed. Finally, after initial funding of innovations by research, the implementation of SBI has been supported by ongoing clinical and quality improvement resources.

REFERENCES

1. Babor T, Higgins-Biddle JC. Cutting back (R): managed care screening and brief intervention for risky drinking. March 2004; 1–13. Accessed August 8, 2005, from http://www.rwjf.org/reports/npreports/cuttingback.htm.
2. Seale JP, Shellenberger S, Boltri JM, Okosun IS, Barton B. Effects of screening and brief intervention training on resident and faculty alcohol intervention behaviours: a pre- post-intervention assessment. *BMC Fam Pract* Nov 4 2005;6:46.
3. Seale JP, Shellenberger S, Tillery WK, et al. Implementing alcohol screening and intervention in a family medicine residency clinic. *Subst Abuse* 2005;26(1):23–31.
4. Kaner EF, Lock CA, McAvoy BR, Heather N, Gilvarry E. A RCT of three training and support strategies to encourage implementation of screening and brief alcohol intervention by general practitioners. *Br J Gen Pract* 1999;49(446):699–703.
5. Lock CA, Kaner EF. Implementation of brief alcohol interventions by nurses in primary care: do non-clinical factors influence practice? *Fam Pract* 2004;21(3):270–275.

(*continued*)

Implementation of Screening and Brief Intervention in Clinical Settings Using Quality Improvement Principles *(continued)*

6. Ockene J, Adams A, Hurley T, et al. Brief physician- and nurse practitioner-delivered counseling for high-risk drinkers: does it work? *Arch Intern Med* 1999;159(18):2198–2205.
7. Fixsen DL, Naoom SF, Blase KA, Friedman RM, Wallace F. Implementation research: a synthesis of the literature. Tampa, FL: university of South Florida, 2005.
8. Rodriguez-Martos A, Castellano Y, Salmeron JM, Domingo G. Simple advice for injured hazardous drinkers: an implementation study. *Alcohol Alcohol* 2007;42(5):430–435.
9. Nilsen P, Aalto M, Bendtsen P, Seppa K. Effectiveness of strategies to implement brief alcohol intervention in primary healthcare. a systematic review. *Scand J Prim Health Care* 2006;24(1):5–15.
10. Greenhalgh T, Robert G, Macfarlane F, et al. Diffusion of innovations in service organizations: systematic review and recommendations. *Milbank Q* 2004;82(4):581–629.
11. Kizer KW. The "new VA": a national laboratory for health care quality management. *Am J Med Qual* 1999;14(1):3–20.
12. Kizer KW, Demakis JG, Feussner JR. Reinventing VA health care: systematizing quality improvement and quality innovation. *Med Care* 2000;38(6 Suppl 1):I7–16.
13. Oliver A. Public-sector health-care reforms that work? A case study of the U.S. Veterans Health Administration. *Lancet* 2008;371:1211–1213.
14. Institute of Medicine. Crossing the quality chasm: a new system for the 21st Century. Washington, DC: National Academy Press, 2001.
15. Kerr EA, Fleming B. Making performance indicators work: experiences of U.S. Veterans Health Administration. *BMJ* 2007;335(7627): 971–973.
16. Demakis JG, McQueen L, Kizer KW, Feussner JR. Quality Enhancement Research Initiative (QUERI): a collaboration between research and clinical practice. *Med Care* 2000;38(6 Suppl 1):I17–125.
17. McQueen L, Mittman BS, Demakis JG. Overview of the Veterans Health Administration (VHA) Quality Enhancement Research Initiative (QUERI). *J Am Med Inform Assoc* 2004;11(5):339–343.
18. Kalman D, Miller DR, Ren XS, et al. Health behaviors of veterans in the VHA: alcohol consumption and services. A Report of the 1999 Large Health Survey. Washington DC and Bedford, MA: department of Veterans Affairs Office of Quality and Performance and Center for Health Quality, Outcomes, and Economic Research, 1999.
19. Saitz R. Clinical practice. Unhealthy alcohol use. *N Engl J Med* 2005; 352(6):596–607.
20. McCormick KA, Cochran NE, Back AL, et al. How primary care providers talk to patients about alcohol: a qualitative study. *J Gen Intern Med* 2006;21:966–972.
21. Burman ML, Kivlahan DR, Buchbinder MB, et al. Alcohol-related advice for VA primary care patients: who gets it, who gives it? *J Stud Alcohol* 2004;65(5):621–630.
22. Williams EC, Kivlahan DR, Saitz R, et al. Readiness to change in primary care patients who screened positive for alcohol misuse. *Ann Fam Med* 2006;4(3):213–220.
23. Bradley KA, Maynard C, Kivlahan DR, et al. The relationship between alcohol screening questionnaires and mortality among male veteran outpatients. *J Stud Alcohol* 2001;62(6):826–833.
24. Bradley KA, Williams EC, Achtmeyer C, et al. Measuring performance for brief alcohol counseling in medical settings: a review of the options and lessons learned from the Veterans Affairs health care system. *Subst Abuse* 2007;28:4.
25. Bradley KA, Williams EC, Achtmeyer CE, et al. DR. Implementation of evidence-based alcohol screening in the Veterans Health Administration. *Am J Manag Care* 2006;12(10):597–606.
26. Hawkins E, Kivlahan DR, Williams EC, Wright S, Craig T, Bradley KA. Examining quality issues in alcohol misuse screening. *Subst Abuse* 2007;28(3):53–65.

Screening for Alcoholism and Other Drug Abuse in the Elderly

James W. Campbell, MD, MS

EPIDEMIOLOGY

The population of elders in the United States is growing dramatically. The 2000 census reported 33 million Americans over the age of 65. Current projections are that by 2030, one in five Americans will be elderly and that the older population will reach 50 million by 2019 (1). Alcoholism is present in 6% to 11% of older persons admitted to hospitals (2). A common misconception—that older individuals have less alcoholism—partially stems from the change in nonproblematic drinking, as 60% of men and 30% of women report a decline in alcohol use after age 65. Alcoholism is estimated to be the third most common psychiatric disorder among elderly persons. Rates have been estimated to be approximately twice as common in men as in women (3). Clearly, detection rates are suboptimal in elders and especially in elderly women. Estimates are as many as three-fourths of older alcoholics admitted to hospitals are not diagnosed. Table 1 summarizes rates in specific clinical arenas.

Definitions are confounded in this population, and screening tools have to be appropriate for the biopsychosocial reality of elderly persons. Older alcoholics are classified as late onset if they present beyond the age of 65. It is estimated that one-third of older alcoholics are late onset, or approximately 700,000 individuals. Care must be taken in labeling a person as late onset, as many older individuals may have had undetected symptomatology in their remote past. The older cohort is especially adverse to the label of *alcoholic* and is more amenable to accepting that their alcohol intake is negatively impacting their health. Elders are more likely to be widowed, retired, and socially isolated, all contributing to poor alcoholism detection rates.

PATHOPHYSIOLOGY

Elders have altered pharmacokinetics that impact on the metabolism of alcohol. They have proportionally more body fat and less water than younger individuals, and therefore achieve higher blood alcohol concentrations with ingestion of lower quantities of alcohol. They also have significant use of pharmacologic agents, many of which have narrow therapeutic windows and concentrations significantly altered by alcohol.

Older individuals are less likely to be screened and are more likely to have their symptoms attributed to aging or to diseases common in elders than suspected as an alcohol problem. Table 2 summarizes factors leading to low detection rates. An older person's alcoholism has a great diversity of clinical presentations. In addition, alcohol's impact on etiology or exacerbation of common diseases is likely to be overlooked in older persons. Many older alcoholics present as a new medical diagnosis or an exacerbation of a chronic medical condition. Table 3 reviews diseases common in elders, wherein alcohol is a possible etiologic factor or a significant contributor to worsening disease.

Screening instruments that exist are specific to the geriatric population and standard tools that are age-adjusted for

TABLE 1 Rates of Alcoholism in Elderly Clinical Settings

10% of cases in geriatric mental health outreach program
11% of older male admissions to psychiatric facilities
15% of older patients presenting to a psychiatrist
18% of general medical/surgical hospitalized elderly
30% of all calls for alcohol information from persons aged 55
40%–60% in a Midwestern United States nursing home

TABLE 2 Age-Related Factors Affecting Rate and Impact of Alcoholism

Underdiagnosis by health care providers
Less socialization, less awareness by peers of drinking behaviors
Family unwillingness to report
Institutionalized persons not in community surveys
Less job or legal pressure to initiate treatment
Patient unaccepting of diagnosis

TABLE 3 Clues Attributed to Coexisting Diseases with High Prevalence in Older Persons

Depression
Delirium
Chronic fatigue
Seizures
Repeated infections
Hypertension
Malnutrition
Peripheral neuropathy
Sexual dysfunction
Cardiomyopathy

(*continued*)

Screening for Alcoholism and Other Drug Abuse in the Elderly *(continued)*

TABLE 4 Test Sensitivity and Specificity when Used on Older Individuals (4,5)

Tool	Sensitivity	Specificity
MAST	1.0	0.83
UMAST	0.96	0.86
GMAST short version	0.94	0.78
Cyr/Wartman	0.52	0.76
CAGE (1 of 4 considered positive screen)	0.91	0.48
ARPS short version	0.92	0.51

Data from Buchsbaum DG, Buchanan BA, Welsh MA, et al. Screening for drinking in the elderly using the CAGE questionnaire. *J Am Geriatr Soc* 1992;40:662; Widlitz M, Marin DB. Substance abuse in older adults: an overview. *Geriatrics* 2002;57:29.

number of responses that indicate a positive screen. Table 4 summarizes a few of the more common tools.

Use of lab tests to aid in the diagnosis is of limited utility. Tests such as mean corpuscular volume (MCV) and gamma GT already nonspecific in younger persons have even worse specificity in older individuals.

Impact of Alcoholism on Health In elders, the negative consequences of alcohol abuse are even more severe than in younger populations. Neurocognitive impairment already common in this population is worsened by alcoholism. It is estimated that as many as 10% of patients with diagnosed Alzheimer's disease may have an alcoholic dementia or a dementia presentation worsened by alcoholism (6). Many health and sensory realities of aging also make alcohol abuse manifestations more severe. A classic example, hip fracture, is associated with alcoholism through not only an increase in falls but a direct effect by exacerbating osteoporosis (7).

Intervention Mechanisms to guide a patient into treatment are similar to other age groups, and brief office or urgent care/emergency department (ED) intervention is effective (8). Modification to the approach is valuable as previously stated, and the nonlabeling approach is more readily accepted by this cohort. In addition, the realistic benefits are different. As opposed to job and legal issues, older folks are more concerned with health, disability, and—particularly—the ability to live independently. The value of an elderly specific treatment milieu or group is debated. Although logical, no evidence exists to support differential benefit of an elderly specific treatment.

SUMMARY

In summary, the age wave is upon us, and rates of alcoholism and other drug abuse—especially prescription drug abuse—in elders approach the rates in younger populations. The diagnosis is often missed as a result of poor screening techniques, cohort underreporting, age bias, and misattribution of alcohol-related health issues to either aging or diseases common in elders. Appropriate screening tools do exist and are useful, though markedly underused. In addition, brief intervention and standard treatment strategies, including AA, are effective. The health yield of sobriety is tremendous as alcoholism is even more dangerous when it occurs in older persons. Finally, alcohol recovery rates are at least as favorable in elders as in younger populations.

REFERENCES

1. Hetzel L, Smith A. The 65 years and older population: 2000. Oct. 2001. Retrieved July 11, 2008, from http://www.census.gov/prod/2001pubs/c2kbr01-10.pdf.
2. National Institute on Alcohol Abuse and Alcoholism. Alcohol Alert No. 40: alcohol and aging. Bethesda, MD: Author, 1998.
3. Blow FC. Treatment of older women with alcohol problems: meeting the challenge for a special population. *Alcohol Clin Exp Res* 2000; 24(8):1257.
4. Buchsbaum DG, Buchanan BA, Welsh MA, et al. Screening for drinking in the elderly using the CAGE questionnaire. *J Am Geriatr Soc* 1992;40:662.
5. Widlitz M, Marin DB. Substance abuse in older adults: an overview. *Geriatrics* 2002;57:29.
6. Meldon S, Ma J, Woolard R, eds. *Geriatric emergency medicine.* New York: McGraw-Hill Publishers, 2003:553.
7. Berg KM, Kunins HV, et al. Association between alcohol consumption and both Osteoporotic fracture and bone density. *Am J Med* 2008;121(5):406.
8. Arndt S, Schultz SK, Turvey C, et al. Screening for alcoholism in the primary care setting: are we talking to the right people? *J Fam Pract* 2002;51(1):41.

CHAPTER 19

Elizabeth A. Warner, MD
Neil Sharma, MD

Laboratory Diagnosis

Laboratory testing can play a key role in the diagnosis and evaluation of substance abuse and dependence. Testing can include direct identification and measurement of suspected drugs of abuse in body fluids or tissues or can indirectly measure consequences of substance use. The accurate interpretation of laboratory findings requires knowledge of the type of test performed, the limits of detection, and the recognition of the possibility of false-positive and false-negative tests (1). Clinicians need to understand that laboratory tests ordered to screen for substance abuse and dependence are intended for clinical care and are not intended to be used in legal proceedings.

Testing for substances of abuse is often performed in clinical settings. When suggested by clinical findings, laboratory testing can assist in the initial diagnosis of a substance use disorder and can identify substances associated with overdoses or trauma (2). Laboratory tests also are used both to monitor abstinence in patients in drug treatment programs and to monitor treatment adherence (e.g., in methadone treatment programs).

APPROACH TO DRUG TESTING

Interpretation of Test Results Although tests for drugs of abuse are widely available and reasonably simple to perform, skill is required in the interpretation of the resulting data. Laboratory results should be interpreted in the clinical context. The clinician should know which drugs are detected by the tests ordered and how long the drug is detectable after use. Knowledge of which substances can give either false-positive or false-negative results is also important. Many laboratories use commercially available kits for drug testing. The manufacturers of these tests publish package inserts that report the concentration at which drugs are detected. The inserts also list drugs that cross-react with the assay and thus cause false-positive tests. The inserts are available from the laboratory, and many are available online.

Body Fluids for Testing Virtually any body fluid or tissue can be assayed for drugs of abuse but, for practical purposes, such testing is limited to specimens that can be obtained in a reasonably noninvasive manner. Sources commonly used for clinical drug testing include urine and blood. Other sources are oral fluid, sweat, hair, and meconium, which can be used to screen for prenatal exposure to drugs in the neonate (3).

Urine Urine is the most common source for testing for drugs of abuse because it can be collected easily and noninvasively. A large quantity is available, and drugs are often present in high concentrations. However, clinicians must be aware that (even when observed) urine specimens are easily adulterated or substituted (4). Commonly used parameters for measuring to ensure a valid specimen include temperature, pH, specific gravity, and creatinine.

Blood Blood testing is more helpful than urine testing for quantitating recent ingestion. In addition, blood is less likely to be adulterated or substituted than is urine. However, alcohol and other drugs are generally present in the blood for much shorter periods than in the urine. Also, venipuncture requires training, is invasive, and poses a higher risk of infection to the personnel obtaining the specimen. Many injection drug users have poor venous access from prior venous thrombosis, so obtaining specimens may be difficult.

Oral Fluid Oral fluid, which is a mixture of saliva, fluid from gingival crevices, and food remnants, can be used to screen for drugs of abuse (5). Oral fluid collection is noninvasive, and directly observed collection does not have the same issues as with urine collection. Adulteration during sample collection is less likely with oral fluid than with urine. Measurements of drug concentrations in oral fluid can closely estimate circulating concentrations in the plasma and can be used to assess for recent drug use. On the other hand, drugs are present in oral fluid for a shorter period of time than in urine. Differences in collection technique can affect drug concentrations in oral fluid. Contamination of oral fluid from recently smoked or ingested drugs can affect measurements in oral fluid (6).

Sweat Drugs are secreted into sweat, and sweat can be used to monitor substance abuse. Patches can be applied to the skin to absorb sweat. Such tests can identify drug excretion over an extended period of time. However, sweat can be collected in only relatively small amounts, and quantification of drug levels in sweat is difficult because it is usually not possible to measure total amount of sweat secreted (7).

Hair Hair testing has been used to test for drugs of abuse and is probably more applicable to forensic or research study testing than to clinical or workplace testing. Hair can be collected easily and noninvasively, and adulteration and substitution are less likely than with urine. Substances are deposited from the blood into the hair during keratinization, diffused into the hair shaft from the surrounding skin tissues, or incorporated from the external environment, and remain in the hair shaft in a fixed position indefinitely (8). Deposition into the hair is related to melanin content; pigmented hair has higher concentration of basic drugs than nonpigmented hair. Cosmetic treatments and ultraviolet light exposure can lead to decreasing concentrations of the drug in hair over time.

Environmental contamination makes hair analysis more difficult to interpret. The only unambiguous proof of systemic administration would be the detection of endogenous metabolites in hair (8). Hair testing involves a more labor-intensive preparation than urine testing, requiring extraction of the drug into a solvent or enzymatic digestion of the hair. Concentrations of drugs in hair are low, requiring sensitive assays. Currently, most hair testing is done with gas chromatography/mass spectroscopy.

If hair is assumed to grow approximately 1 cm per month, segmented analysis can give a qualitative account of the history of ingestion. However, hair testing is not helpful in assessing acute intoxication, because significant amounts of drug are not found in hair until 1 to 2 weeks after use (9). Theoretically, hair analysis can provide a history of the pattern of substance use over a longer time span than other studies, complementing the information obtained from short-term measures such as urine testing.

Collection Procedures Proper collection and processing of specimens are essential for accurate results. Universal handling precautions are recommended for all specimens. The timing of the collection should be noted, so results can be interpreted in the context of the time of ingestion. The identity of the person supplying the specimen needs to be confirmed, and the specimen needs to be properly labeled. Chain-of-custody regulations in forensic or workplace testing have been developed to prevent specimen misidentification, especially when the testing has legal implications. However, when testing is done for clinical purposes, chain-of-custody regulations are not routinely followed. This fact should be considered when interpreting testing results in clinical settings.

Specimen Validity Testing Testing for urine specimen validity is required in federal workplace testing (10). In clinical settings, validity testing is not required, and practices vary. For federal workplace testing, extensive guidelines mandate that all specimens be tested for creatinine concentration and pH to ensure that the specimens are within the range of normal human urine. For specimens with creatinine concentrations <20 ng/mL, measurement of specific gravity is required. The temperature of recently collected urine specimens should approximate body temperature. An acceptable temperature range is 90°F to 100°F within 4 minutes of collection. A lab may refuse a urine specimen that is not within this temperature range. Regulations for federal workplace testing define a dilute urine as having a creatinine concentration ≥2 mg/dL and <20 mg/dL *and* a specific gravity greater than 1.0010 but less than 1.0030. A substituted urine, which is not consistent with normal or dilute human urine, is defined as having a creatinine <2 mg/dL *and* a specific gravity of not more than 1.0010 or at least 1.0200.

Testing for potential adulteration is required in federal workplace testing. Potential adulterants include in vivo adulterants, which are pills, capsules, or "tea" that is ingested before giving a urine specimen. Many of these products require increased fluid intake; in order not to dilute the urine excessively, they may also contain creatine or creatinine. In vitro adulterants include common household products, such as bleach, vinegar, liquid detergent, table salt, and baking soda, as well as commercially available kits, such as "Urine Luck," which can be added to urine to interfere with the urine test (11). Active ingredients in current commercial in vitro adulterants include glutaraldehyde, sodium or potassium nitrite, pyridinium chlorochromate, and peroxide/peroxidase (4). Federal workplace testing mandates testing every urine specimen with one or more validity tests for oxidizing adulterants. A number of commercially available urine specimen validity dipsticks are available for testing in clinical or nonregulated settings (12).

Laboratory Methods The initial procedure for drug testing usually is a screening urine immunoassay (1). Immunoassays are inexpensive, easily automated, and yield rapid results. In these tests, an antibody reacts to a portion of the drug or its metabolite. A major limitation of immunoassays is cross-reactivity. The antibody can interact with antigens other than the one used to produce the antibody, yielding a false positive result (Table 19.1) (13). Commercial immunoassays from different manufacturers use various antibodies, and not all assays share the same cross-reactivities. With the development of more specific antibodies, many currently available immunoassays no longer have cross-reactivities with substances previously reported to give false-positive results. The package insert of the immunoassay lists which compounds the manufacturers have found to cross-react with the assay. Such cross-reactivity information usually is listed for the parent drug

TABLE 19.1 Compounds that May Cause False-Positive Results in Urine Immunoassays

Amphetamine/methamphetamine	Marijuana
Benzphetamine (Didrex)	Efavirenz
Bupropion	Pantoprozole
Chloroquine	Quinaprine
Chlorpromazine	Methadone
Ephedrine	Quetiapine
Fenfluramine	Opiates
Labetalol	Gatifloxacin
Mexiletine	Levofloxacin
N-acetyl procainamide	Ofloxacin
Phentermine	Papaverine
Phenylephrine	Rifampicin
Phenylpropanolamine	Poppy seeds
Propranolol	Phencyclidine
Pseudoephedrine	Dextromethorphan
Quinacrine	Diphenhydramine
Ranitidine	Thioridazine
Selegiline	Venlafaxine
Trazodone	Propoxyphene
Tyramine	Cyclobenzaprine
Vick's inhaler	Diphenylhydramine
Barbiturate	Doxylamine
Phenytoin	Imipramine
Benzodiazepines	Methadone
Oxaprozin	
Sertraline	
LSD	
Amitriptyline	
Chlorpromazine	
Doxepin	
Fluoxetine	
Haloperidol	
Metoclopramide	
Risperidone	
Sertraline	
Thioridazine	
Verapamil	

and does not include cross-reactivity information on endogenous metabolites (13). Therefore, this information should be interpreted with caution, recognizing that metabolites of a compound may have cross-reactivity, even though the parent compound does not.

Because of the serious consequences that may ensue after a positive urine screen, positive tests on immunoassay can be confirmed with a second analytic procedure to verify the results. The second procedure should be independent of the initial test and should use a different technique and chemical principle from that of the initial test in order to insure reliability and accuracy. Although confirmatory testing is required for workplace or forensic testing, it is not required for clinical testing. The College of American Pathologists recommends that clinical toxicology results for tests that have not been confirmed should be reported as "presumptively positive," and there should be a statement that the results are intended for diagnostic use only (14). Confirmatory testing is often not available on-site in hospital laboratories. Because of the delay in obtaining results when sent out to a reference laboratory, results of confirmatory studies would not likely be available for clinical decision making in urgent clinical settings. When a precise identification of the drug is needed or when there are anticipated medicolegal issues, the clinician can request confirmatory studies.

Chromatography is most commonly used as a confirmatory test. Gas chromatography with mass spectroscopy (GC/MS) couples the powerful separation potential of gas chromatography with the precise detection and identification capability of mass spectroscopy. This technique can identify and quantify extremely small amounts of drugs or metabolites, rendering GC/MS the "gold standard" for confirming positive immunoassays. For workplace or forensic testing, confirming a positive immunoassay by GC/MS is required before reporting the test positive (similar to performing a Western blot test to confirm a positive enzyme-linked immunosorbent assay test when testing for human immunodeficiency virus [HIV]).

Cutoff A cutoff is a defined concentration of an analyte in a specimen at or above which the test result is reported as positive and below which it is reported negative. The factors that are considered in establishing a cutoff include the goals of testing, the sensitivity of the assay, the desired duration of detection of drug use, and data from pharmacologic studies. If a drug is detected in a specimen in concentrations lower than the defined cutoff, the test result will be reported as negative, even though the drug was in fact detected. For screening tests, if a test result is reported as negative, generally no further testing is done. If a specimen is reported as positive, a confirmatory test may be ordered.

Knowledge of the cutoff level for a particular test is helpful in estimating the length of time after drug ingestion that a test result will be positive. Lower cutoff levels are associated with a higher sensitivity and with longer detection times. Table 19.2 lists approximate duration of detection time from the time of last use, using commonly used cutoffs.

On-Site Testing Point-of-care or on-site testing refers to tests that are performed outside of the laboratory. Commercially available immunoassay kits are available to test urine or oral fluid for commonly abused drugs. These tests are performed at the time of specimen collection. The assays are rapid and easy to perform and require little training. However, the interpretation of these tests is somewhat subjective. Cutoffs are not standardized and may be different than those suggested by the Substance Abuse and Mental Health Services Administration (SAMHSA; Table 19.3) (15). Recent studies evaluating oral point-of-collection devices find improved sensitivity and performance from previous studies (16). Point-of-care tests are more expensive than tests performed in large numbers by laboratories, although commercially available point-of-care 10-drug urine tests can be purchased for approximately $10. Such tests clearly are designed for use as screening tests, and many manufacturers recommend that any positive results be

TABLE 19.2 Approximate Detection Time Using Screening Urine Immunoassays (with Commonly Used "Cut-Offs")

Drug	Duration of detection[a] (approximate)
Amphetamine	1–3 days
Methamphetamine	3 days
Barbiturate	
Short-acting	1–4 days
Long-acting	Several weeks
Cocaine	3 days
Marijuana	
Single joint (using 50 ng/mL cutoff)	2 days
Heavy use (using 20 ng/mL cutoff)	Up to 27 days
Opioids	
Heroin, codeine, morphine	1–2 days
Methadone (using a specific assay for methadone)	2–3 days
PCP	7 days

[a]The duration of detection is variable and depends on dose, route of administration, pattern of use, laboratory cutoff, and individual metabolism.

confirmed by more specific laboratory methods. Nevertheless, many of these tests have been accepted for use in clinical and nonregulated workplace testing.

Federal Regulations The SAMHSA, an operational division of the U.S. Department of Health and Human Services, oversees drug testing of federal workers (10). The U.S. Department of Transportation (DOT) requires drug and alcohol testing of safety-sensitive transportation employees in aviation, trucking, mass transit, railroad, pipelines, and other transportation industries (17). Both agencies have developed extensive guidelines for specimen collection, chain-of-custody procedures, and specimen validation. Initial screening tests are performed by immunoassay, followed by confirmation of all positive screening test results by GC/MS. The federal guidelines for federal workplace and DOT drug testing limit drug testing to five substances (amphetamines, cannabinoids, cocaine, opiates, PCP) and establish cutoff values for screening and confirmatory testing of these substances. DOT and federal workplace testing must be done in laboratories certified by the National Laboratory Certification Program.

Clinical Laboratories Clinical laboratories perform drug and alcohol testing for diagnostic purposes. Since clinical laboratories can select which substances to include in their drug screens, the assays may vary among laboratories. Specimens obtained for clinical use, however, are not subject to the same collection and testing requirements used in federal workplace testing. Although clinical laboratories are not required to use the cutoffs chosen for workplace testing for federal workers, many clinical laboratories use the same cutoffs.

DRUG-SPECIFIC TESTS

Alcohol Tests that are widely used to monitor recent alcohol ingestion include gamma-glutamyl-transferase (GGT), aspartate amino transferase (AST), and erythrocyte mean cell volume (MCV). Of these tests, the GGT is the most sensitive marker of alcohol abuse (18). GGT levels are elevated in approximately 75% of persons with diagnosed alcohol

TABLE 19.3 Cutoffs for Urine Drug Screening Tests

Drug	SAMHSA cutoff[a]	SAMHSA confirmation[a]	Commonly used in clinical laboratories
Amphetamines	1,000 ng/mL	Amphetamine 500 ng/mL Methamphetamine 500 ng/mL (must also have presence of amphetamine 200 ng/mL)	1,000 ng/mL
Cannabinoids (THC-COOH)	50 ng/mL	15 ng/mL	50 or 100 ng/mL
Cocaine (benzoylecgonine)	300 ng/mL	150 ng/mL	300 ng/mL
Opiates	2,000 ng/mL	Morphine 2,000 ng/mL Codeine 2,000 ng/mL 6-monoacetylmorphine 10 ng/mL (must be tested if morphine >2,000 ng/mL)	300 ng/mL
Phencyclidine (PCP)	25 ng/mL	25 ng/mL	25 ng/mL
Barbiturates[b]	—	—	200 or 300 ng/mL
Benzodiazepines[b]	—	—	200 or 300 ng/mL
LSD[b]	—	—	0.5 ng/mL
Methadone[b]	—	—	150 or 300 ng/mL

[a]U.S. Department of Health and Human Services, 2004.

[b]Not included in federal workplace drug testing programs.

dependence, approximately 50% of patients hospitalized for alcohol-related problems, and approximately 30% of people who drink heavy amounts and have related problems. It is important to note that the GGT is not specific for alcohol use disorders and is also elevated in patients with fatty liver and obstructive liver disease and in those using certain medications, including anticonvulsants. As such, the GGT is not generally useful for universal screening. The exact amount of alcohol consumption required to raise a patient's GGT is variable and likely is a function of the patient's weight, gender, and individual hepatic function. An estimate is that five drinks a day for approximately 2 weeks will yield an elevation in GGT in most individuals (19). GGT levels generally are reduced by half with approximately 2 weeks of abstinence and can return to normal over 6 to 8 weeks. One study examined the use of monitoring GGT to detect relapse in abstinent subjects. Using a 30% increase in baseline GGT values to detect relapse, the sensitivity was 32% and 29% and the specificity was 92% and 89% in men and women, respectively (20).

With abstinence, the MCV will fall, but because the life span of the red blood cell (RBC) is 120 days, it may take approximately 3 months to see improvement in the MCV after abstinence. Non–alcohol-related conditions that increase the MCV include chronic liver disease, hypothyroidism, folate deficiency, and megaloblastic disorders. Because the MCV takes longer to decline than the GGT, it is less helpful in following up patients in the weeks after they enter alcohol abuse treatment (21). Furthermore, the MCV is not very sensitive for detecting heavy drinking.

A less commonly used marker for heavy alcohol use is the carbohydrate-deficient transferrin (CDT). In the setting of heavy alcohol ingestion, the glycosylation process of transferrin is impaired, rendering the transferrin missing some carbohydrate terminal chains, termed carbohydrate-deficient transferrin (22). Drinking four to seven standard drinks (or about 50 to 80 g of alcohol) per day for a week is required to elevate CDT levels. The half-life of CDT is approximately 15 days. Other etiologies of elevated CDT include advanced liver disease and genetic variations of transferrin.

In one study that examined simultaneous measurements of CDT, GGT, and MCV in patients seen in an emergency department or primary care center, the sensitivity and specificity of the tests as markers of alcohol consumption of >60 g a day were 0.58 and 0.82 for CDT, 0.69 and 0.65 for GGT, and 0.27 and 0.91 for MCV, respectively (23). Using the combination of CDT and GGT increases sensitivity by 20% above either marker alone, without compromising specificity (24).

Serum aminotransferases, particularly aspartate amino transferase (AST) and alanine amino transferase (ALT), may be elevated in patients with alcohol use disorders. However, these tests are not as sensitive as markers for alcohol abuse as the GGT. The AST is usually more elevated than the ALT in patients with alcohol-related liver disease. When the aminotransferases are elevated and ALT is more elevated than the AST, alcohol is less likely to be the cause of the liver disease. Although elevations of the aminotransferases may suggest alcohol-related liver disease, none of the abnormal liver enzymes can predict alcohol dependence or intoxication.

A number of promising markers for alcohol abuse have been proposed, including hexosaminidase, 5-hydroxytryptophol, sialic acid, fatty acid ethyl esters (FAEE), whole blood–associated acetaldehyde (WBAA), and acetaldehyde adducts. Although WBAA, FAEE, and hexosaminidase all appear to have increased sensitivity and specificity, routine clinical use is limited by short half-lives, technical difficulties, and cost. Also, the bulk of the data comes from chronic and heavy alcohol use; limited data support use in patients outside of these categories (25).

It is important to note that despite the increasing sensitivity and specificity of even the newer biomarkers, there are a number of potential pitfalls to their clinical use, which must be kept in mind. First, as with many other clinical tests, their sensitivity and specificity directly relates to pretest probability when being used as a general screening tool. Thus patients with a low pretest probability are more likely to have false-positive results. Dose-response relationships are not well established, making it difficult to use these tests as a direct quantifier for alcohol consumption (26). None of the currently available biomarkers are sufficiently sensitive and specific to be used as generalized "screening tests" for alcohol use disorders.

Acute Alcohol Intoxication Laboratory testing to confirm alcohol ingestion relies on measurement of ethanol from body fluids. These measurements can confirm recent alcohol intake but do not necessarily determine impairment, because some individuals develop tolerance to the effects of alcohol. Both blood and breath tests can estimate a person's alcohol ingestion.

Blood alcohol concentration detects alcohol use within the preceding few hours. Testing for alcohol levels in blood can be done using enzymatic analysis or gas chromatography of the headspace. Specimens for venipuncture should be drawn using an alcohol-free antiseptic. The enzymatic analysis measures the amount of nicotinamide adenine dinucleotide (NADH) formed during oxidation of ethanol; this may produce falsely elevated readings in the presence of isopropanol, methanol, and ethylene glycol. High levels of acetone, such as found in diabetic ketoacidosis (DKA) or starvation, can be metabolized to isopropanol, giving falsely elevated ethanol levels by the enzymatic analysis (27).

In the headspace analysis, a specimen is obtained in a vacutainer tube that is not completely filled. Ethanol equilibrates between the blood and the air space (headspace) above the liquid. A portion of the vapor from the tube is injected onto a chromatographic column and then quantitated (28). Although gas chromatography is considered the gold standard for measuring ethanol in forensic laboratories, many clinical laboratories use enzymatic methods.

Most states define intoxication based on whole blood alcohol levels; the most commonly used are 80 or 100 mg/dL. Clinical laboratories, however, measure ethanol in serum or plasma. Because the water content of serum is higher than that of whole blood, the same specimen will show a higher level of ethanol in serum than in whole blood (29). An estimate of the ratio of serum to whole blood is 1.14/1.00. If a clinical specimen of serum or plasma is used to estimate whole blood levels, the appropriate correction needs to be calculated.

Less invasive means of detecting the blood alcohol concentration include analysis of alcohol in the exhaled air. Breath alcohol testing is usually done in traffic law enforcement and DOT testing. The ratio of blood to breath concentration of alcohol is approximately 2100:1, though this probably underestimates venous levels by about 10% (30). In the United States, breath alcohol concentration is usually reported in grams per 210 liters, so that a breath level of 0.1 g/210 liters is equivalent to a whole blood alcohol level of 0.10 g/dL.

In order to allow clearance of any ethanol that may be in the mouth, a 15-minute waiting period is required before a breath test is performed. The alveolar concentration of ethanol is most accurately measured when the subject takes a deep breath, with the measurement taken in the last third of the breath. Failure to obtain a deep breath specimen can lead to an underestimate of blood alcohol level (30). In a study with patients with documented gastroesophageal reflux, breath alcohol analysis was not affected by the presence of such reflux (31).

Oral fluid can also be used to estimate serum ethanol concentration. The concentration of ethanol in saliva theoretically is similar to that in serum, although salivary alcohol levels do not correlate as well with breath tests in measuring blood alcohol levels (32). Patients with chronic alcohol ingestion may have difficulty producing adequate oral fluid samples. This may be explained by some degree of parotid dysfunction related to chronic alcohol use. The U.S. DOT has approved on-site oral fluid tests for alcohol screening of safety-sensitive employees in the transportation industry.

Urine testing for alcohol provides a qualitative marker of recent alcohol ingestion. The presence of alcohol in the urine suggests alcohol intake within the preceding 8 hours. However, urine concentrations are variable compared to blood levels and are related to the length of time the urine has been in the bladder, so quantitative measures of alcohol levels in the urine are difficult to interpret. Ethanol glucuronide (Etg), a metabolite of alcohol, can be detected in the urine for 22 to 31 hours after drinking (33) and has been used as a marker to monitor abstinence. Etg testing is highly sensitive, but the effect of incidental alcohol exposure (such as from commercial products including mouthwashes) has not been well-defined. Because of lack of proven specificity, the SAMHSA advises that the use of Etg testing is inappropriate for monitoring abstinence when legal or disciplinary actions can result from a positive test result (19).

Amphetamines Amphetamines are a group of stimulants that include amphetamine, methamphetamine, "Ecstasy," which is MDMA (3,4-methylenedioxymethamphetamine) or MDA (3,4-methylenedioxyamphetamine), and "Eve," which is MDEA (3,4-methylenedioxy-N-ethylamphetamine). Amphetamine and methamphetamine have d- and l-isomers. As the d-isomers of amphetamine and methamphetamine have stronger central nervous system effects, they are associated with more abuse potential than the l-isomers. Screening tests for amphetamines can be selective for detecting d-amphetamine and d-methamphetamine, or they can be less selective, also targeting MDMA or MDA. Therefore, one should not routinely assume that MDMA would be detected on an amphetamine immunoassay. The package insert for the assay can be reviewed to determine the concentration of MDMA required to produce a positive result. Routine GC/MS amphetamine assays can distinguish methamphetamine from amphetamine but cannot distinguish the d-isomers from the l-isomers. Specialized GC/MS testing, chiral analysis, can differentiate l-isomers from d-isomers (34).

Of the frequently tested drugs of abuse, amphetamines have the most false-positive screening tests. Many sympathomimetic amines with structures similar to amphetamines have cross-reactivity with the immunoassays, causing false-positive results (35). Examples of compounds that have been reported to cause positive results include the decongestants phenylpropanolamine, pseudoephedrine, and l-methamphetamine (found in the nasal decongestant used in Vick's nasal inhaler) and appetite suppressants containing ephedrine and phentermine. Other prescription drugs, such as selegiline or benzphetamine, are metabolized either to amphetamine or methamphetamine and can also cause positive results. Amphetamine is a metabolite of methamphetamine and is detected in the urine after the use of methamphetamine.

Since a significant amount of amphetamine and methamphetamine are excreted unchanged in the urine, most urinary detection methods are targeted for these compounds rather than their metabolites. Urine pH influences the excretion of amphetamines. At high pH levels, there is a marked reduction in amphetamine and methamphetamine excretion. Individuals have been known to ingest large quantities of bicarbonate to reduce the amount of amphetamines excreted in the urine. The duration of detection of amphetamine in the urine by immunoassay is variable but generally accepted to be 1 to 3 days (36). With repeating daily use of methamphetamine, detection was up to 3 days in urine and 1 day in oral fluid after last use (37).

Barbiturates Barbiturates, which are central nervous system depressants, are divided into three categories, depending on their duration of action. Thiopental is an ultra-short-acting barbiturate used in anesthesia. The short-acting barbiturates, which include pentobarbital (Nembutal), secobarbital (Seconal), and amobarbital (Amytal), are the most widely abused. The long-acting barbiturates, such as phenobarbital, are used therapeutically as anticonvulsants and have low abuse potential. With the exception of phenobarbital, only a small portion of the parent drug is found in the urine. However, most urine immunoassays are directed toward the parent compound secobarbital, using a cutoff concentration of either 200 or 300 ng/mL. The amount of cross-reactivity with other compounds varies with each assay.

The duration of detection after barbiturate use is variable and depends on dose. In general, short-acting barbiturates such as butalbital, pentobarbital, and secobarbital, can be detected from 1 to 4 days after use, while long-acting barbiturates such as phenobarbital can be detected for several weeks after use (38). Testing for therapeutic levels of phenobarbital involves a separate assay; it is not an appropriate use of urine drug screens.

Benzodiazepines The interpretation of urine immunoassays for benzodiazepines is complicated by the multiple drugs available, their variable potencies (allowing a large dose range), and their diverse metabolites, which may show poor cross-reactivity with commonly used immunoassays. Chlorazepate, chlordiazepoxide, diazepam, and temazepam are metabolized to oxazepam, which in turn is conjugated into an inactive glucuronide metabolite. The nitrobenzodiazepines, which include clonazepam, are metabolized to the 7-amino benzodiazepine (39). Alprazolam, lorazepam, and triazolam are excreted as glucuronide conjugates, distinct from oxazepam glucuronide. Urine specimens usually contain little of the parent benzodiazepine (40). Many of the benzodiazepine immunoassays are designed to detect unconjugated oxazepam (41). An immunoassay that is targeted to detect oxazepam is less likely to detect clonazepam, lorazepam, or triazolam, unless they are present in high doses (40). Reviewing the package insert can identify the sensitivity of the particular assay for different benzodiazepines.

The cutoff for benzodiazepines immunoassays usually is either 200 or 300 ng/mL, which can detect high doses but may not detect a therapeutic dose. The high-potency benzodiazepines, such as triazolam, are more difficult to detect in immunoassays because they are prescribed in low doses (42). The benzodiazepine antagonist, flumazenil, is not detected on a benzodiazepine immunoassay.

Substances reported to give false positive results on immunoassay include oxaprozin, sertraline, and tolmetin (43,44). Because there is considerable variation in the half-life of benzodiazepines, it is difficult to estimate the time of use based on screening tests.

Cocaine Cocaine hydrochloride is the powdered form of cocaine. It is water-soluble and can be snorted or mixed with water and injected. The alkaloid form of cocaine, "crack" or freebase, is not water-soluble but vaporizes when heated and can be smoked (45). Screening urine immunoassays measure benzoylecgonine, the major urinary cocaine metabolite, commonly using a cutoff of 300 ng/mL. The detection of cocaine in the urine is variable and depends on the amount of drug ingested. The usual detection time after cocaine use is 2 to 3 days, though there are reports of positive urine assays up to 22 days after high-dose binges (46).

Immunoassays for benzoylecgonine are quite specific and have not been reported to have false positives with other drugs. Immunoassays and GC/MS do not differentiate cocaine hydrochloride from crack cocaine.

Lysergic Acid Diethylamide The hallucinogen LSD (lysergic acid diethylamide) is synthesized from lysergic acid and is structurally similar to the ergot alkaloids. LSD is extensively metabolized so that <1% appears unchanged in the urine. The major human metabolite is nor-LSD (N-desmethyl-LSD). At a cutoff of 0.5 ng/mL, urine immunoassays detect LSD for 2 to 5 days after use (47). Confirmatory testing can be done by chromatography.

One study found a 4% false-positive testing on immunoassay in patients and found in vivo false positives with multiple drugs, including amitriptyline, chlorpromazine, doxepin, fluoxetine, haloperidol, metoclopramide, risperidone, sertraline, thioridazine, and verapamil (48). Because of the high number of false positives, caution must be exercised in interpreting these tests (49).

Marijuana The primary psychoactive component of the marijuana plant is tetrahydrocannabinol (THC). When smoked, THC is absorbed quickly into the circulation, with an elimination half-life estimated to be between 20 and 30 hours. THC has a highly lipophilic nature and is stored in fat tissues, where it is slowly released back into the circulation. Most laboratories measure the inactive metabolite 11-nor-Δ9-THC-9-carboxylic acid (THC-COOH).

Urine screening tests for marijuana typically use cutoffs of 20, 50 or 100 ng/mL. The current federally mandated cutoff for workplace testing is 50 ng/mL. The detection time for marijuana is variable and depends on the amount ingested, whether the person is a chronic or an occasional user, and the sensitivity of the assay. In the 1980s, when assays were less specific for TCH-COOH, studies reported detection of marijuana in urine for weeks or months after use. Current research suggests that the detection time is shorter than previously described (50). The mean detection time of a single marijuana cigarette is <2 days using a 50 ng/mL cutoff immunoassay (51) and is 3 to 4 days using a 15 ng/mL cutoff on GC/MS (52). In frequent users, urine specimens were found positive for THC-COOH up to 27 days after last use using an immunoassay with a cutoff of 20 ng/mL (53).

A positive test is helpful in identifying past marijuana use, but it does not correlate with level of impairment. Oral ingestion of hemp seed oil or dronabinol (Marinol), a synthetic THC used for treatment of chemotherapy-associated nausea and HIV-related anorexia, can result in positive urine test results for marijuana (54). In the past, immunoassays gave false-positive results with nonsteroidal antiinflammatory drugs such as ibuprofen and naproxen sodium. Current assays have been modified to eliminate this cross-reactivity. Confirmation by GC/MS of a positive screening immunoassay can be done when there are legal implications.

There has been some debate about the degree to which passive exposure to marijuana smoke influences drug screens. In experimental studies using extreme conditions, urine specimens of individuals passively exposed to high concentrations of marijuana smoke did test positive with immunoassays (55). However, on quantitative GC/MS, the concentrations of THC-COOH during more realistic exposure generally are <10 ng/mL, below the cutoffs used in federal workplace or clinical testing (56).

Opiates and Opioids Opiates are drugs derived from opium, the extract of the seeds of the opium poppy, and include morphine, codeine, and heroin. The term *opioid* is more comprehensive and includes all agonists and antagonists with morphine-like activity, including natural opiates, semisynthetic drugs such as hydrocodone and hydromorphone, and synthetic drugs, such as oxycodone, methadone, buprenorphine, and fentanyl. The evaluation of opiate drug screens can be confusing. Many physicians assume the immunoassays for "opiates" are a reliable screen for all opioids. However, currently available opiate immunoassays are targeted to detect morphine and have little or no cross-reactivity with synthetic opioids such as fentanyl, propoxyphene, buprenorphine, or methadone and variable cross-reactivity with hydrocodone, hydromorphone, and oxycodone. This differs from past practice, when the opiate immunoassays were even less sensitive to oxycodone. To determine which opioids show significant cross-reactivity with opiate immunoassays, one should review the package insert, where the concentrations of drugs that produce positive tests are listed. There are currently available immunoassays specific for oxycodone (57) or buprenorphine that are distinct from the opiate assays. Dextromethorphan and the opioid antagonists nalmefene, naltrexone, and naloxone do not cross-react with immunoassays for opiates (58–60). The opioids meperidine, fentanyl, and pentazocine also are not detected in routine urine opiate drug screens.

Both heroin and codeine are metabolized to morphine. In the process of heroin metabolism, 6-monoacetylmorphine (6-MAM) is produced, which then is hydrolyzed to morphine. Poppy seeds contain small quantities of codeine and morphine, and ingestion of them can result in positive urine opiate screens for 48 hours at a cutoff of 300 ng/mL (61). Morphine can be detected in the urine after ingestion of heroin, codeine, morphine, or poppy seeds. The only finding in the urine that unequivocally proves heroin use is the detection of 6-monoacetylmorphine. This metabolite is the specific byproduct of heroin metabolism and not a metabolite of morphine, codeine, poppy seeds, or other synthetic opioids (62). However, 6-MAM is rapidly eliminated and usually detected in the urine for <8 hours after heroin use (63). Although regulations for federal workplace programs require testing for 6-MAM when opiate immunoassay results are positive, most clinical laboratories do not routinely check for 6-MAM. In 1997, the federal government raised the screening cutoff for opioid testing in workplace programs from 300 ng/mL to 2,000 ng/mL to reduce the number of false-positive results, although many clinical laboratories still use a cutoff value of 300 ng/mL.

Methadone Most drug testing for methadone is done to assess compliance with methadone therapy. Methadone is not detected in the standard opiate drug screens and requires a specific test. Screening immunoassays for methadone have little cross-reactivity with other opioids. Using a cutoff of 300 ng/mL, screening immunoassays detect methadone in the urine for about 2 or 3 days after use. If there is concern that an individual may be spiking a urine specimen with methadone, further testing can be done to detect the presence of the major metabolite, 2-ethylidene-1,5-dimethyl-3,3-diphenylpyrrolidine (64).

Phencyclidine Phencyclidine (PCP) in powdered form ("angel dust") can be snorted or smoked, or PCP can be ingested in tablet form. The federal government requires PCP testing in drug screening programs for federal employees. Laboratories that are not federally regulated may include PCP in the drug screen, depending on the prevalence of PCP use in a given community.

Using a cutoff value of 25 ng/dL, urine immunoassay results are positive for approximately 7 days after a single dose and for up to 21 days after chronic use. Saliva tests are promising because saliva levels of PCP are higher than blood levels, and PCP may be more stable in saliva than urine (47).

Club Drugs Standard urine drug screens do not detect many of the new "designer" drugs. At one time, MDMA and MDA were not detected by amphetamine immunoassays; however, newer-generation tests have improved cross-reactivity to these compounds. The drugs ketamine and gamma-hydroxybutyrate are not detected by routine urine drug tests and require specialized testing (65).

Ethical Considerations Though there are extensive guidelines for drug testing in the workplace, very few guidelines on the use of such tests for clinical purposes have been developed. The American Medical Association and the U.S. Preventive Services Task Force (USPSTF) recommend asking about alcohol use (and about drug use when there is a clinical indication) when obtaining a patient history, but neither recommend routine laboratory screening for alcohol or drugs in asymptomatic adults. The American College of Emergency Physicians found that urine drug screens in alert, awake, and cooperative patients with a psychiatric complaint did not affect emergency department management and were not required (66). In clinical practice, drug testing is commonly ordered under the general "consent to treatment" without specific informed consent, as a diagnostic test to guide treatment. However, because of concerns about the technical limitations of drug testing in the clinical setting, patient autonomy, and the implications of a positive drug test, some favor obtaining informed consent before ordering urine drug screens (67). The USPSTF endorses drug testing in clinical situations in which "there is reasonable suspicion of substance abuse" and recommends obtaining informed consent prior to performing such tests (68). The American Academy of Pediatrics (AAP) recommends that physicians approach drug testing in the same manner as other diagnostic tests: as an aid in diagnosis and in formulating treatment recommendations. The AAP recommends that adolescents should not be tested without informed consent (69,70).

The actual benefit of urine drug testing has been examined in several clinical situations. The immediate management was affected by the results of urine drug screening in fewer than 5% of emergency department patients with suspected drug overdoses (71). Urine drug testing, however, can help identify cocaine use in patients with ischemic chest pain and guide decisions on appropriate pharmacotherapy. Urine drug testing is also helpful in the management of patients on chronic opioid therapy; both to assess, adherence with prescribed therapy and to detect drug abuse.

CONCLUSIONS

Laboratory testing in the evaluation of patients with known or suspected substance use disorders, when performed in an appropriate clinical setting, can assist in making an accurate diagnosis. However, the physician must understand the limitations of any test used. For alcohol, breath and blood testing can quantitate recent ingestion, but none of the markers for chronic alcohol abuse are ideal screening tests. For other drugs, urine testing can identify drug use, usually within the preceding few days, but does not confirm drug dependence.

An important consideration is that laboratory testing in the clinical setting is intended to guide diagnosis and treatment planning and does not follow the stringent requirements of workplace or forensic testing. The clinician must combine the findings from the history and physical exam with that of the laboratory testing for accurate interpretation and management.

REFERENCES

1. Wolff K, Farrell M, Marsden J, et al. A review of biological indicators of illicit drug use, practical considerations and clinical usefulness. *Addiction* 1999;94:1279–1298.
2. Wu AH, McKay C, Broussard LA, et al. National Academy of Clinical Biochemistry Laboratory Medicine practice guidelines: recommendations for the use of laboratory tests to support poisoned patients who present to the emergency department. *Clin Chem* 2003;49:357–379.
3. Gareri J, Klein J, Koren G. Drug of abuse testing in meconium. *Clin Chim Acta* 2006;366:101–111.
4. Jaffee WB, Trucco E, Levy S, et al. Is this urine really negative? A systematic review of tampering methods in urine drug screening and testing. *J Subst Abuse* Treat 2007;33:33–42.
5. Cone EJ, Huestis MA. Interpretation of oral fluid tests for drugs of abuse. *Ann N Y Acad Sci* 2007;1998:51–103.
6. Crouch DJ. Oral fluid collection: the neglected variable in oral fluid testing. *Forensic Sci Int* 2005;150:165–173.
7. Kidwell DA, Holland JC, Athanaselis S. Testing for drugs of abuse in saliva and sweat. *J Chromatogr B Biomed Sci Appl* 1998;713:111–135.
8. Pragst F, Balikova MA. State of the art in hair analysis for detection of drug and alcohol abuse. *Clin Chim Acta* 2006;370:17–49.
9. Spiehler V. Hair analysis by immunological methods from the beginning to 2000. *Forensic Sci Int* 2000;107:249–259.
10. Substance Abuse and Mental Health Services Administration. Mandatory guidelines for federal workplace drug testing programs. *Federal Register* 2004;69(19644-19673):249–259.
11. Wu, AH, Bristol, B, Sexton, K, et al. Adulteration of urine by "Urine Luck." *Clin Chem* 1999;45:1051–1057.
12. Dasgupta A. The effects of adulterants and selected ingested compounds on drugs-of-abuse testing in urine. *Am J Clin Pathol* 2007;128:491–503.
13. Colbert DL. Drug abuse screening with immunoassays: unexpected cross-reactivities and other pitfalls. *Br J Biomed Sci* 1994;51:136–146.
14. Caplan YH, Kwong TC. Evaluation of toxicology test results. Accessed on January 8, 2008, from www.cap.org/apps/docs/disciplines/toxicology/toxeval.pdf.
15. George S, Braithwaite RA. Use of on-site testing for drugs of abuse. *Clin Chem* 2002;48:1639–1649.
16. Walsh JM, Crouch DJ, Danaceau JP, et al. Evaluation of ten oral fluid point-of-collection drug- testing devices. *J Anal Toxicol* 2007;31:44–54.
17. U.S. Department of Transportation. 49 CFR Part 40. Procedures for transportation workplace drug and alcohol testing programs. Accessed March 31, 2008, from http://ecfr.gpoaccess.gov/cgi/t/text/text-idx?c=ecfr&tpl=/ecfrbrowse/Title49/49cfr40_main_02.tpl.
18. Conigrave KM, Saunders JB, Whitfield JB. Diagnostic tests for alcohol consumption. *Alcohol Alcohol* 1995;30:13–26.
19. U.S Department of Health and Human Services, Substance Abuse and Mental Health Services Administration. Substance abuse treatment advisory. 2006; 5:4. Accessed June 24, 2008, from http://kap. samhsa.gov/products/manuals/advisory /pdfs/0609_biomarkers.pdf.
20. Anton RF, Lieber C, Tabakoff B, CDTect Study Group. Carbohydrate-deficient transferrin and gamma-glutamyltransferase for the detection and monitoring of alcohol use: results from a multisite study. *Alcohol Clin Exp Res* 2002;26:1215–1222.
21. Sillanaukee P. Laboratory markers of alcohol abuse. *Alcohol Alcohol* 1996;31:613–616.
22. Litten RZ, Allen JP, Fertig JB. Gamma-glutamyltranspeptidase and carbohydrate deficient transferrin: alternative measures of excessive alcohol consumption. *Alcohol Clin Exp* Res 1995;19:1541–1546.
23. Yersin B, Nicolet J, DeCrey H, et al. Screening for excessive alcohol drinking. *Arch Intern Med* 1995;155:1907–1911.
24. Hietala J, Koivisto H, Anttila P, et al. Comparison of the combined marker GGT-CDT and the conventional laboratory markers of alcohol abuse in heavy drinkers, moderate drinkers and abstainers. *Alcohol Alcohol* 2006;41:528–533.
25. Hannuksela ML, Liisanantti MK, Nissinen AE, et al. Biochemical markers of alcoholism. *Clin Chem Lab Med* 2007;45:953–956.
26. Allen JP, Sillanaukee P, Strid N, et al. Biomarkers of heavy drinking. National Institute of Alcohol Abuse and Alcoholism, 2004. Accessed January 13, 2008, from http://pubs.niaaa.nih.gov/publications/Assesing%20Alcohol/biomarkers.htm1.
27. Jones AW, Pounder DJ. Measuring blood-alcohol concentration for clinical and forensic purposes. In: Karch SB, ed. *Drug abuse handbook*. Boca Raton, FL: CRC Press, 1998:327–355.
28. Porter W. Clinical toxicology. In: Burtis C, Ashwood E, eds. *Tietz textbook of clinical chemistry*. Philadelphia: WB Saunders Co., 1999: 906–981.
29. Frajola WJ. Blood alcohol testing in the laboratory: problems and suggested remedies. *Clin Chem* 1993;39:377–399.
30. Mason MF, Dubowski KM. Breath-alcohol analysis: uses, methods, and some forensic problems–review and opinion. *J Forensic Sci* 1976; 21: 9–41.
31. Kechagias S, Jonsson KA, Franzen T, et al. Reliability of breath-alcohol analysis in individuals with gastroesophageal reflux disease. *J Forensic Sci* 1999;44:814–818.
32. Bendtsen P, Hultberg J, Carlsson M, et al. Monitoring ethanol exposure in a clinical setting by analysis of blood, breath, saliva, and urine. *Alcohol Clin Exp Res* 1999;23:1446–1451.
33. Dahl H, Stephanson N, Beck O, et al. Comparison of urinary excretion characteristics of ethanol and ethyl glucuronide. *J Anal Toxicol* 2002;26: 201–204.
34. Swotinsky RB, Smith DR. Pharmacology, metabolism, and interpretation of alcohol and specific drugs. In: *The medical review officer's manual*. Beverly Farms, MA: OEM Press, 2006:205–251.
35. Kraemer T, Maurer HH. Determination of amphetamine, methamphetamine and amphetamine-derived designer drugs or medicaments in blood and urine. *J Chromatogr B Biomed Sci Appl* 1998;713:163–187.
36. Verstraete AG. Detection times of drugs of abuse in blood, urine, and oral fluid. *Ther Drug Monit* 2004;26:200–205.
37. Huestis MA, Cone EJ. Methamphetamine disposition in oral fluid, plasma, and urine. *Ann N Y Acad Sci*2007;1098:104–121.
38. Simpson D, Braithwaite RA, Jarvie DR, et al. Screening for drugs of abuse (II): cannabinoids, lysergic acid diethylamide, buprenorphine, methadone, barbiturates, benzodiazepines and other drugs. *Ann Clin Biochem* 1997;34(5): 460–510.
39. Drummer OH. Methods for the measurement of benzodiazepines in biological samples. *J Chromatogr B Biomed Sci Appl* 1998;713:201–225.

40. Fitzgerald RL, Rexin DA, Herold DA. Detecting benzodiazepines: immunoassays compared with negative chemical ionization gas chromatography/mass spectrometry. *Clin Chem* 1994;40:373–380.
41. Nishikawa T, Ohtani H, Herold DA, et al. Comparison of assay methods for benzodiazepines in urine. A receptor assay, two immunoassays, and gas chromatography-mass spectrometry. *Am J Clin Pathol* 1997;107: 345–352.
42. Becker J, Correll A, Koepf W, et al. Comparative studies on the detection of benzodiazepines in serum by means of immunoassays (FPIA). *J Anal Toxicol* 1993;17:103–108.
43. Camara PD, Audette L, Velletri K, et al. False-positive immunoassay results for urine benzodiazepine in patients receiving oxaprozin (Daypro). *Clin Chem* 1995;41:115–116.
44. Joseph R, Dickerson S, Willis R, et al. Interference by nonsteroidal anti-inflammatory drugs in EMIT and TDx assays for drugs of abuse. *J Anal Toxicol* 1995;19:13–17.
45. Warner EA. Cocaine abuse. *Ann Intern Med* 1993;119:226–235.
46. Weiss RD, Gawin FH. Protracted elimination of cocaine metabolites in long-term, high-dose cocaine abusers. *Am J Med* 1988;85:879–880.
47. Schneider S, Kuffer P, Wennig R. Determination of lysergide (LSD) and phencyclidine in biosamples. *J Chromatogr B Biomed Sci Appl* 1998;713: 189–200.
48. Ritter D, Cortese CM, Edwards LC, et al. Interference with testing for lysergic acid diethylamide. *Clin Chem* 1997;43:635–637.
49. Wu AH, Feng YJ, Pajor A, et al. Detection and interpretation of lysergic acid diethylamide results by immunoassay screening of urine in various testing groups. *J Anal Toxicol* 1997;21:181–184.
50. Fraser AD, Collins L, Worth D. Drug and chemical metabolites in clinical toxicology investigations: the importance of ethylene glycol, methanol and cannabinoid metabolite analyses. *Clin Biochem* 2002;35: 501–511.
51. Huestis MA, Mitchell JM, Cone EJ. Detection times of marijuana metabolites in urine by immunoassay and GC-MS. *J Anal Toxicol* 1995;19:443–449.
52. Huestis MA, Mitchell JM, Cone EJ. Urinary excretion profiles of 11-nor-9-carboxy-delta-9-tetrahydrocannabinol in humans after single smoked doses of marijuana. *J Anal Toxicol* 1996;20:441–452.
53. Smith-Kielland A, Skuterud B, Morland J. Urinary excretion of 11-nor-9-carboxy-delta9-tetrahydrocannabinol and cannabinoids in frequent and infrequent drug users. *J Anal Toxicol* 1999;23:323–332.
54. Gustafson RA, Levine B, Stout PR, et al. Urinary cannabinoid detection times after controlled oral administration of Δ^9-tetrahydrocannabinol to humans. *Clin Chem* 2003;49:1114–1124.
55. Cone EJ, Johnson RE, Darwin WD, et al. Passive inhalation of marijuana smoke: urinalysis and room air levels of delta-9-tetrahydrocannabinol. *J Anal Toxicol* 1987;11:89–96.
56. Mule, SJ, Lomax, P, Gross, SJ. Active and realistic passive marijuana exposure tested by three immunoassays and GC/MS in urine. *J Anal Toxicol* 1988;12:113–116.
57. Abadie JM, Allison KH, Black DA, et al. Can an immunoassay become a standard technique in detecting oxycodone and its metabolites? *J Anal Toxicol* 2005;29:825–829.
58. Storrow AB, Wians FH Jr, Mikkelsen SL, et al. Does naloxone cause a positive urine opiate screen? *Ann Emerg Med* 1994;1151–153.
59. Storrow AB, Magoon MR, Norton J. The dextromethorphan defense: dextromethorphan and the opioid screen. *Acad Emerg Med* 1995;2: 791–794.
60. Storrow AB, Hernandez AV, Norton JA. Nalmefene and the urine opiate screen. *Clin Chem* 1998;44:346–348.
61. Hayes LW, Krasselt WG, Mueggler PA. Concentrations of morphine and codeine in serum and urine after ingestion of poppy seeds. *Clin Chem* 1987;33:806–808.
62. Mule SJ, Casella GA. Rendering the "poppy-seed defense" defenseless: identification of 6-monoacetylmorphine in urine by gas chromatography/mass spectroscopy. *Clin Chem* 1998;34:1427–1430.
63. Cone EJ, Dickerson S, Paul BD, et al. Forensic drug testing for opiates: V. Urine testing for heroin, morphine, and codeine with commercial opiate immunoassays. *J Anal Toxicol* 1993;7:156–164.
64. George S, Parmar S, Meadway C, et al. Application and validation of a urinary methadone metabolite (EDDP) immunoassay to monitor methadone compliance. *Ann Clin Biochem* 2000;37(3):350–354.
65. Kankaanpaa A, Liukkonen R, Ariniemi K. Determination of gamma-hydroxybutyrate (GHB) and its precursors in blood and urine samples: a salting-out approach. *Forensic Sci Int* 2007;170:133–138.
66. Lukens TW, Wolf SJ, Edlow JA, et al. Clinical policy: critical issues in the diagnosis and management of the adult psychiatric patient in the emergency department. *Ann Emerg Med* 2006;47:79–99.
67. Warner EA, Walker RM, Friedmann PD. Should informed consent be required for laboratory testing for drugs of abuse in medical settings? *Am J Med* 2003;115:54–58.
68. U.S. Preventive Services Task Force Screening for drug abuse. *Guide to clinical preventive services*. Baltimore: Williams and Wilkins, 1996:583–594.
69. American Academy of Pediatrics Committee on Substance Abuse [anonymous]. Testing for drugs of abuse in children and adolescents. *Pediatrics* 1996:98(2):305–307.
70. Knight JR, Mears CJ, Committee on Substance Abuse, American Academy of Pediatrics, Council on School Health. Testing for drugs of abuse in children and adolescents: addendum—testing in schools and at home. *Pediatrics* 2007;119:627–630.
71. Kellermann AL, Fihn SD, LoGerfo JP, Copass MK. Impact of drug screening in suspected overdose. *Ann Emerg Med* 1987;16:1206–1216.

CHAPTER 20

Theodore V. Parran, Jr., MD, FACP
Richard A. McCormick, PhD
John S. Cacciola, PhD

Assessment

ASSESSMENT IN MANAGING PATIENTS WITH SUBSTANCE USE DISORDERS

Individualized patient assessment is a basic clinical skill and one of the foundations of quality patient care. As such, it is introduced in the earliest levels of health professional training, and the development of assessment skills is critically evaluated by health educators. Patient assessment can also be an extremely complex and sophisticated clinical or research evaluation involving a multidisciplinary team and multiple forms of patient testing. The importance of assessment in patient evaluation, treatment planning and evolution of the treatment plan, patient safety, and provision of optimal patient care cannot be overstated. Quality assessment bridges the gap between patient diagnosis and the initiation of treatment, ensuring the accuracy of the initial diagnosis and identifying the most effective and efficient care. Patient assessment is as important when dealing with substance use disorders as it is for other medical or psychiatric illness.

Addictive disease is a brain disease that when active affects the behavioral control areas. As a consequence, signs and symptoms of active addictive disease are primarily behavioral. Contrary to most other diseases, when dealing with addictions the morbidity of this disease moves from the intrapersonal sense of self (self-image, self-respect, self-concept, sense of self-efficacy, and even psychiatric symptomatology are often the earliest evidence of disease), to interpersonal relationships (first family and close friends and then social relationships suffer), to avocations and hobbies, to financial status, to legal standing, to employment or school performance, and finally to physical or end-organ damage. Addictive disease typically affects all of these varied domains of life and is affected in turn by many domains, including legal and licensure status, insurance eligibility, comorbid medical and psychiatric conditions, and family relationships (CSAT TIP #27) (1). This is why the assessment process is such a critical aspect of the approach to addictive disease.

NEEDS OF DIFFERENT ASSESSORS

Different clinicians have different clinical decision-making needs when it comes to the initial assessment of substance use disorders, and these different clinicians can be generally divided into four groups; primary care clinicians, addiction medicine or psychiatry specialists, substance use disorders treatment programs, and substance use disorder researchers.

The primary care provider needs to perform a reasonably brief patient assessment to quickly verify the diagnosis, stage the severity of the disease from the perspective of psychosocial morbidity/end-organ damage/physical dependence, stage the patient's readiness for behavior change, and screen for immediately important medical or psychiatric comorbidities (Table 20.1). This needs to be done in parts of one or more office visits thorough patient interview, questionnaire and, if possible, corroboration in person or by phone from collateral sources (family, friends, other health care providers). The primary care practice should utilize a structured approach to this assessment as much as possible to try to ensure an appropriately careful and through evaluation.

The addiction medicine or psychiatry specialist might approach the assessment from a different perspective. Certainly assessing the severity of the addictive disease and stage of readiness for behavior change, as well as expert evaluation for

TABLE 20.1 Assessing Addictive Disease Using Screening Tool Data

Domains levels	Physical dependence	Organ system damage	Psychosocial morbidity
Mild	One or more of the following: • Inability to stop • Insomnia • Irritability • Anxiety • AUDIT (Questions 1-3) Combined score >5: • Frequency (20) • Average # of drinks (22) • Six or more drinks (23)	One of the following: • High normal GGT • Memory loss • Physical injury • Bloodshot eyes • Depression • Sexual dysfunction • High blood pressure • Gastritis/ulcers • Headaches • Osteoporosis	One of the following: CAGE: • Cut down (C) • Annoyed (A) • Guilty (G) AUDIT: • Failed expectations (13) • Remorse (10) • Memory loss (24) • Injured self or others (5) • Concern expressed by others (31)
Moderate	Any of the above mild symptoms with one or more of the following: • Hand tremor • "Eye opener" • Diaphoresis • Blood alcohol level ≥100 • Positive urine toxicology	Two or three of the following: • Elevated aspartate aminotransferase • Memory loss • Injury/broken bones • Elevated MCV • Elevated liver enzyme • Depression • Sexual dysfunction • High blood pressure • Gastritis/ulcers • Headaches • Osteoporosis	Two of the following: CAGE: • Cut down (C) • Annoyed (A) • Guilty (G) AUDIT: • Failed expectations (13) • Remorse (10) • Memory loss (24) • Injured self or others (5) • Concern expressed by others (31)
Severe	Any of the above mild or moderate symptoms with one or more of the following: • Hallucinations • Seizures • DTs • BAL >200 • Prolonged positive toxicology	Four or more of the following: • Elevated aspartate aminotransferase • Memory loss • Injury/broken bones • Elevated MCV • Elevated liver enzymes • Depression • Sexual dysfunction • High blood pressure • Gastritis/ulcers • Headaches • Osteoporosis • Hepatomegaly • Elevated prothrombin time	Positive on three or more of the following: CAGE: • Cut down (C) • Annoyed (A) • Guilty (G) AUDIT: • Failed expectations (13) • Remorse (10) • Memory loss (24) • Injured self or others (5) • Concern expressed by others (31)

medical withdrawal or detoxification needs, must be accomplished. Further evaluation for co-occurring psychiatric disorders, a more thorough family assessment, careful evaluation of prior attempts at treatment, patterns of substantial remissions and relapses, and the potential role for pharmacotherapy should all be part of this specialist assessment process.

The substance use disorders treatment program must spend less time on evaluating patient readiness for behavior change and more emphasis on prior treatment experiences, identification and management of co-occurring medical and psychiatric conditions, family issues and the therapeutic milieu of the living environment, and past relapse patterns (see Chapter 27).

The substance use disorder research organization has a very different goal when it comes to assessment. The focus tends to be on quantitative evaluation of the degree of accumulated morbidity in the patient's life, patient-entered research into treatment matching efforts, identification and exploration of patient characteristics that predict response to treatment, and the elucidation of different types and sub-types of addictive disorders.

TASKS OF THE ASSESSMENT PROCESS

Assessment of substance use disorders within the context of the rest of the patient's life circumstances is a process that should be utilized when evaluating every patient. The nature of the assessment process is influenced not only by patient factors but by clinician and organizational factors. Therefore, the tools

TABLE 20.2 Major Areas for Addiction Assessment

1. Diagnostic criteria
2. Presence and level of intoxication
3. Suicidal or homicidal ideation
4. Physiologic dependence and withdrawal potential
5. Level of addiction-associated morbidity
6. Medical comorbidities
7. Psychiatric comorbidities
8. Legal issues
9. Readiness for behavior change
10. Prior treatment successes and relapse patterns

used in an assessment may change depending upon the clinical situation, the skills and resources available to the clinician, and the specific characteristics of patient presentation, but the basic areas to be assessed remain fairly constant as indicated in Table 20.2.

Generally speaking, assessment of a substance use disorder is utilized for one or more of the following tasks: diagnostic verification, assessing for physiologic dependence, staging disease severity, identifying the domains of life affected by the disease, evaluating for additional medical or psychiatric diagnosis, quantifying the disease-associated morbidity, identifying characteristics of the disease that are important from a prognostic or a treatment-matching perspective, quantifying the impact of treatment on disease-associated morbidity, or attempting to determine subtypes of addictive disease.

The assessment process can also be thought about from the perspective of timing. Since 1990, the addiction treatment field has been challenged to improve the *pretreatment* assessment of alcoholism and other addictions in order to provide better treatment decisions (Institute of Medicine). More recently, the concept of *intratreatment* and even *posttreatment assessment* has gained favor, urging formal on-going assessment performed at transition points in the treatment process. This permits the continued adaptation of the treatment plan, a key criterion for most treatment program accreditation reviews (26). *Pretreatment* assessments are focused on identifying the treatment needs of the patient, identifying positive and negative predictive factors for treatment retention, quantifying the pretreatment level of morbidity and impairment of functioning from the addictive disease, and screening for urgent comorbid medical psychiatric and psychosocial issues. *Intratreatment* assessment updates should be performed at periodic intervals during the formal treatment and aftercare phase, especially at times of treatment transition or whenever substantial additional or new clinical information becomes available. This intratreatment assessment update should focus on organizing the accumulating data from the treatment experience in such a way as to inform the ongoing treatment planning and patient diagnostic process. *Posttreatment* assessment can be performed during the final aspect of treatment to summarize the treatment experience, inform after-care and follow-up monitoring, focus on relapse prevention, reorder the problem list, and focus attention on additional, new, or previously deferred problems. In addition, posttreatment assessment can be used to quantify the patient's posttreatment or post-posttreatment level of morbidity and impairment of functioning from addictive disease. The difference between pretreatment and post-posttreatment assessment can, therefore, quantify and characterize the difference in patient morbidity, and thus measure the impact of addiction treatment.

SOURCES OF ASSESSMENT INFORMATION

As domains of patient life affected by addictive disease include such varied areas as intrapersonal, interpersonal, avocations and hobbies, financial status, legal issues, employment or school performance, and physical or end-organ damage, it becomes incumbent on the assessment process to gather information from many different—and at times atypical—sources. This is in contrast to the assessment of most medical or surgical conditions wherein the usual and adequate sources for assessment and management are provided by an initial history and physical followed by laboratory and diagnostic study review.

Sources that commonly are utilized in assessing addictive disease include patient history, physical exam, and laboratory results; toxicology testing; family interview; use of pharmacology (licit and illicit) with special emphasis on the controlled drug use history; medical-legal history questioning, educational; and occupational interview; and readiness for behavior change evaluation. These areas of questioning and examination are even more important than during routine medical care. Substance use disorders are some of the most highly stigmatized disorders in our society. As a result, issues of the reliability of patient self-report are even more suspect than with other health problems faced by clinicians. It is important to interview patients in ways that avoid defensiveness about the behaviors resulting from their addictive disease. Just as in the area of screening and brief intervention, patient self-report reliability can be improved by using a consistent series of questions that progress from general and open-ended to specific information sought in a more closed-ended question form and by utilizing the family or significant other interview whenever possible.

Owing to high rates of psychiatric symptomatology, a psychiatric screening interview and specific screening for suicidal or homicidal ideation are required. Rates of interpersonal violence are quite high in patients with chemical dependence, either as a child or as an adult or both, so assessing for abuse history is necessary. Even the cultural background, spiritual inclination, and belief system that the patient holds regarding substance use disorders can be essential areas of assessment. As a consequence, assessment entails extensive patient interview, family interview, checking pharmacy profiles, documenting legal issues and the actual causes of legal issues, and careful review of prior treatment and relapse experiences. Thus, the assessment process typically is extended in time and multidisciplinary in nature.

ASSESSMENT TOOLS

A thorough assessment should evaluate each area of patient function that is necessary for the needs of the clinician performing or requesting the assessment. In addition, the assessment tool used should be reliable, reproducible, and verifiable. Diagnostic and assessment strategies are often evaluated based upon their convergent validity (consistency with an established best practice of "gold standard") and ability to predict different outcomes (predictive validity). A quality assessment tool should also have face-validity (seem to be clear, logical, and make sense), as well as retest and interrater reliability (reoffering the assessment to the same patient by the same or different staff member should produce a consistent result).

This section suggests tools to assist the clinician in key assessments. The clinician often begins by assessing the severity of the patient's substance use problem. There are a number of options that vary in the effort required and the range of use they span. The instruments highlighted have been shown to be reliable and valid for the purposes suggested. Some of the tools (AUDIT and AUDIT-C, DAST, CAGE) are primarily *screening tools*, but the assessment process is a clear and direct extension of the screening and diagnosis process. As a consequence, extending the use of a screening tool by asking straightforward follow-up questions for each positive screening response can result in a substantial assessment without needing to use additional clinical tools. Table 20.3 demonstrates this process of extending a screening tool for use in assessment. Further information on many of these tools, and other assessment options, can be found on-line at *niaaa.nih.gov/publications, drugabuse.gov,* or *samsha.gov.*

Often the first step in conducting an addiction assessment is to establish degree of risk associated with the current level of acute intoxication or withdrawal. The CIWA-Ar (1a) is a brief 10-item scale that can be administered in less than 5 minutes. It quantifies the severity of the alcohol withdrawal syndrome by rating 10 common alcohol withdrawal symptoms and can be clinically useful in monitoring progress over time.

The Alcohol Use Disorders Identification Test (AUDIT) (2,3) was developed by the World Health Organization to identify hazardous use, harmful use, and dependence on alcohol in primary care. The 10-item Core questionnaire includes three questions on consumption (the AUDIT-C) and seven on the impact of alcohol use. The AUDIT has been shown to have good sensitivity and specificity in medical and general populations and has recently been shown to be useful for screening patients with major psychiatric disorders and as an assessment instrument for patients seeking alcohol treatment (4,5). The consumption items (AUDIT-C) provide an efficient standardized method for assessing the quantity and frequency of alcohol use and have been demonstrated to account for much of the discriminative power of the test in medical populations (6). The AUDIT can serve as a key first step in developing and implementing brief interventions for alcohol misuse or early abuse, which have been shown to have significant positive impact. Similar instruments, such as the Drug Abuse Screening Test (DAST) (7), a widely used 20-item questionnaire, screen for abuse of drugs other than alcohol.

The Psychoactive Substance Use Disorders module of the Structured Clinical Interview for DSM-IV (SCID) (8,9) is a semistructured diagnostic interview that establishes DSM-IV Axis I diagnoses for substance use disorders. It is widely used and considered the "gold standard" for establishing reliable diagnoses in research applications. Questions paralleling the DSM-IV diagnostic criteria establish lifetime and current abuse and dependence diagnoses for alcohol and each psychoactive substance included in DSM-IV. Age of onset and an estimate of current severity are also obtained. The expectation is that the interviewer will be trained to an acceptable level of reliability on the instrument. Depending on the complexity of the substance use history, the interview should take from 30 to 60 minutes to administer.

The Addiction Severity Index (ASI) Drug/Alcohol Use section provides a reliable measure of lifetime use and use within the past 30 days for a full range of commonly used substances (27). The ASI has been widely used in both clinical and research applications. It was designed to be administered by a trained interviewer as a semistructured interview. It yields both a composite score, which is mathematically calculated based on selected quantifiable items, and a rater-generated severity score. A self-administered computerized version is also available.

As noted, substance use disorders, including hazardous or harmful use, have broad impact on the physical and psychosocial functioning of the patient. The full ASI assesses additional key dimensions of functioning: medical status; vocational; legal; family, including history, and social; and psychiatric status. Composite scores and severity ratings are determined for each dimension based on the structured interviews, which take approximately 1 hour to administer. The ASI sections can be readministered to assess progress over time. More recently, modifications of the ASI have been introduced tailored to the needs of women (10) and teenagers (11).

Self-report instruments that are available also provide a *broadened assessment of the consequences of use.* The Drinker Inventory of Consequences (DrInc) (12) measures the adverse consequences of alcohol abuse in five domains: physical, social, impulsive, interpersonal, and intrapersonal. The 50-item test takes only about 10 minutes, yielding lifetime and last 3-month scores for each domain and an overall score. The DrInc has been used widely in clinical trials, including in a repeated measure design. A companion instrument, the Inventory of Drug Use Consequences (InDUC) (30) provides similar information for a broader population of patients abusing drugs or drugs and alcohol.

As highlighted earlier, patients with substance use disorders often present with *psychiatric co-morbidities* that require concomitant or sequential treatment. The full SCID has modules for each of the other major syndrome groups: anxiety disorders, affective disorders, and psychotic disorders, as well as other comorbidities that are common in substance abuse, most notably the other disorders of impulse control, such as eating disorders and pathologic gambling, and the personality disorders. Each module may stand alone for the assessment of a particular diagnostic syndrome. Administration of the full SCID can take 2 hours or more depending on the complexity of the patient's presenting problems.

Short self-report instruments are available to measure some of the most common comorbidities. For example, the Beck Depression Inventory (13) and the Beck Anxiety Inventory are both relatively short (21-item) instruments that take about 10 minutes to administer and can be readministered over time to monitor progress. Special versions for children (ages 7 to 14) are also available. One of the most common concomitant disorders of impulse control, pathologic or problem gambling has been effectively screened for and assessed using the South Oaks Gambling Screen (SOGS) (14), a short self-report instrument that has been demonstrated to reliably identify substance abusers with problem or pathological gambling.

It is important to assess the *motivational level* of the patient for engaging in treatment. Self-report instruments are available, including the Stages of Change Readiness and Treatment Eagerness Scale (SOCRATES) (15). The 19-item short form of the self-report instrument assesses motivation to change drinking behavior. A personal drug use version is also available. Based on the trans-theoretical model of change, it assesses the patient's level of recognition of a problem, ambivalence or uncertainty about changing, and whether the patient is taking steps to change. It has been employed to monitor motivational level and predict compliance with and outcome of treatment. A similar instrument, the University of Rhode Island Change Assessment (URICA) (16) is slightly longer (32 items) and can readily be modified to assess motivation for change across a range of behaviors, including alcohol, other drugs, or concomitant unhealthy behaviors. Both instruments are easy to administer and have been used successfully with a wide range of patients, including the dually diagnosed severely mentally ill (17).

When a more comprehensive assessment of *resistance to treatment* is needed, most often in the context of a specialized treatment program, the Recovery Attitude and Treatment Evaluator (RAATE) (18) provides both a 35 item semistructured clinical interview option (RAATE-CE) (19) and a 94-item self-report version (RAATE-QI) (19). They both measure five constructs: resistance to initial treatment, resistance to continuing care, severity of biomedical problems, severity of psychiatric/psychologic problems, and social/environmental support for recovery. The RAATE-CE is designed for administration by someone with adequate substance abuse expertise to make the ratings required. The QI version provides a more direct patient perspective on the constructs. Both take approximately 30 minutes to complete.

Assessment instruments can be valuable aids in constructing a *relapse prevention* plan: the patient's knowledge of the situations that trigger the use of substances. This is an important element in a relapse prevention plan. The Inventory of Drinking Situations (20) is a 100-item self-report instrument that allows a patient to assess his or her tendency to drink in a variety of situations that can be categorized as: urges and temptations; personal control; unpleasant emotions; pleasant emotions; conflict; social pressure; physical discomfort; and pleasant times with others.

In helping the patient prepare a relapse prevention plan, it is also useful to understand the *coping skills* that the patient possesses. A number of instruments are available to assess coping repertoire. The Coping Response Inventory (CRI) (21) is a relatively short (48-item) self-report instrument that assesses four types of avoidant coping (emotional discharge, cognitive avoidance, seeking alternative rewards, resigned acceptance) and four types of approach coping (logical analysis, problem solving, seeking guidance and support, positive reappraisal). A youth version is also available.

Although there is ample evidence that treatment can work, *adherence to treatment* remains a major impediment to recovery. Self-efficacy and expectations about the effect of alcohol and drugs have been demonstrated to be related to adherence across a broad range of disorders. Self-efficacy for alcohol-related situations can be measured using the Situational Confidence Questionnaire (SCQ) (22), a 39-item self-report instrument that asks patients to imagine themselves in a variety of situations and rate their confidence that they can resist the urge to drink in these situations. It takes approximately 15 minutes to complete. A companion instrument, the Drug Taking Confidence Questionnaire (23) assesses self-efficacy for drug-related situations. Expectations about the effect of alcohol or drugs can also influence adherence. Specific instruments exist to measure expectations (e.g., the Adult Alcohol Expectancy Questionnaire (24)).

SELECTING THE RIGHT ASSESSMENT TOOL

Assessment is a necessary part of the evaluation of patients with addictive disease and is a critical bridge between screening and diagnosis and treatment planning. There are many tools available to assist in the assessment process. Choosing the right tool for the clinical needs of the patient and the capability of the treatment program can be difficult. The level of staff training and the availability of time and assessment resources (e.g., computerized data base access, etc.) can all impact on the selection of assessment tools. Some suggestions follow.

Primary Care Office Setting The assessment resources available to the primary care practitioner are limited but quite adequate to perform an addiction assessment. Following up on the results of typically used *screening tools* like the CAGE, AUDIT, DAST, and s-MAST provide assessment information about patterns of use, adverse consequences of use, possible physiologic dependence, and quantity/frequency data (Table 20.3). This helps with assessing psychosocial morbidity, risk of withdrawal, and need for detoxification. In addition, the

TABLE 20.3 Moving from Screening Tools to Patient Assessment

The following are simple follow-up questions that can be asked after encountering a positive response to the CAGE screening questions. The goal of the follow-up interview is to establish whether the positive responses were "true" or "false" positives, helping to establish the diagnosis and begin the assessment process.

1) Cut down
   a. When did you cut down?
   b. How did you cut down?
   c. How was it cutting down: easy, hard, etc.?
   d. Why did you cut down?
   e. Why weren't you able to stay cut down?
2) Annoyed by comments
   a. Who has made the comments?
   b. Anyone else?
   c. What is your relationship like?
   d. What comments did they make?
   e. Why did it sort of get under your skin?
   f. Why do you think they made comments?
3) Embarrassed, bashful, or guilty
   a. What happened?
   b. What else has happened?
   c. Why do you think it happened?
   d. Why did it make you feel bad afterward?
   e. What did you do as a result of it happening?
4) Eye-openers
   a. Why do you use in the morning?
   b. What would happen if you did not?
   c. Do you use even when you try not to?

primary care physician would want to inquire about prior success or failure with abstinence, prior treatment experience, and affiliation with the 12-step or self-help community. Brief depression screening is always important, as well as laboratory evaluation including a urine drug screen, complete blood count, and liver profile. One strategy for utilizing these office-based resources to assess the addictive disease (stage the disease severity) from the perspectives of psychosocial morbidity, physiologic dependence, and end-organ damage is outlined in Table 20.1.

Addiction Physician Setting The addiction medicine or psychiatry physician needs when approaching the assessment process require much more in-depth evaluation and typically necessitate the use of more formal tools for staging the addictive disease.

The use of the aforementioned screening tools and a more extensive diagnostic interview is required. In addition, formal depression and anxiety screening with tools, such as the Beck Depression Inventory and the Hamilton Anxiety Scale, are often performed. Thorough review of prior treatments, length and characteristics of remissions, patterns and triggers for relapse, and current supports and resources available for treatment is essential. Assessment of the readiness for behavior change, level of commitment to a recovery program, and possibilities for pharmacotherapy are necessary. Careful evaluation for acute, subacute and post-acute withdrawal issues is necessary.

Addiction Treatment Program Setting The addiction treatment program must use a formalized addiction assessment process for quality control and accreditation reasons. A full medical history and physical exam are mandatory focusing on the aforementioned areas but also a structured interview such as the ASI or even the SCID should be used. Programs that deal with a high prevalence of psychiatric dual diagnosis will utilize the more extensive SCID or at least will need to use specific anxiety and depression screens (Beck or Hamilton, etc.). Assessing treatment readiness and treatment resistance, as well as relapse patterns and coping skills, are all typically a part of the addiction treatment program assessment process.

SUMMARY

Quality assessment bridges the gap between patient screening and diagnosis and the initiation of treatment, ensuring the accuracy of the initial diagnosis and identifying patient treatment needs from the perspective of effectiveness and efficiency. Quality assessment permits the development of a comprehensive problem list and a thorough treatment plan. Assessment of all of the various domains of life affected by addictive disease as well as medical and psychiatric comorbidities, detoxification needs, prior treatment, relapse patterns, readiness for change, and treatment resistance are all critical areas of focus. Finally, some assessment tools can quantify the impact of addictive disease on patient's lives and measure the level of morbidity and the residual level of functioning. Repeating the use of these quantitative tools can measure improved functioning and decreased morbidity as well as help to continue to inform the ongoing process of treatment planning (25–30).

REFERENCES

1. Center for Substance Abuse Treatment. Treatment Improvement Protocol #27. Comprehensive Case Management for Substance Abuse Treatment. SAMSHA. DHHS Publication No. (SMA) 98-3222. Washington, DC: 1998.

1a. Sullivan JT, Sykora K, Schneiderman J, et al. Assessment of alcohol withdrawal: the revised Clinical Institute Withdrawal Assessment for Alcohol scale (CIWA-AR). *Br J Addict* 1989;84:1353–1357.

2. Babor TF, Higgins-Biddle JC, Saunders JB, Monteiro MG. AUDIT: the Alcohol Use Disorders Identification Test. Guidelines for Use in Primary Care. Geneva: World Health Organization, 2001.

3. Bohn MJ, Babor TF, Kranzler HR. The Alcohol Use Identification Test (AUDIT): validation of a screening instrument for use in medical settings. *J Stud Alcohol* 1995;56:423–432.

4. Donovan DM, Kivlahan DR, Doyle SR, et al. Concurrent validity of the Alcohol Use Disorders Test (AUDIT) and AUDIT zones in defining levels of severity among outpatients with alcohol dependence in the COMBINE study. *Addiction* 2006;101:1696–1704.

5. Cassidy CM, Schmitz N, Malla A. Validation of the Alcohol Use Disorders Identification Test and the Drug Abuse Screening Test in first episode psychosis. *Can J Psychiatry* 2008;53:26–33.
6. Rodriguez-Martos A, Santamarina E. Does the short form of the Alcohol Use Disorders Test (AUDIT-C) work at a trauma emergency department? *Subst Use Misuse* 2007;42:923–932.
7. Skinner HA. The Drug Abuse Screening Test. *Addict Behav* 1982;7: 363–371.
8. Spitzer RL, Williams JB, Gibbon M, et al. The Structured Clinical Interview for DSM-III-R (SCID). I: History, rationale, and description. *Arch Gen Psychiatry* 1992:49(8):624–629.
9. First MB, Spitzer RL, Gibbon ML, et al. *Structured Clinical Interview for DSM-IV-TR Axis I Disorders, Research Version, Patient Version (SCID I/P).* New York: New York State Psychiatric Institute, Biometrics Research Department, 2001.
10. Brown E, Frank D, Friedman A. *Supplementary Administration Manual for the Expanded Female Version of the Addiction Severity Index (ASI) Instrument. The ASI-F.* Herndon, VA: Head & Co., Inc., 1995.
11. Kaminer Y, Wagner E, Plumer B, Seifer R. Validation of the teen addiction severity index (T-ASI): preliminary findings. *Am J Addict* 1993;*2*(3): 250–254.
12. Miller WR, Tonigan JS, Longabaugh R. *The Drinker Inventory of Consequences (DrInC): an Instrument for assessing adverse consequences of alcohol abuse.* Project MATCH Monograph Series, Vol. 4, DHHS Publication No. 95-3911. Rockville, MD: National Institute on Alcohol Abuse and Alcoholism, 1995.
13. Beck AT, Ward CH, Mendelson M, et al. An inventory for measuring depression. *Arch Gen Psychiatry* 1961;4:561–571.
14. Lesieur HR, Blume SB. The South Oaks Gambling Screen (SOGS): a new instrument for the identification of pathological gamblers. *Am J Psychiatry* 1987;144:1184–1188.
15. Miller W, Tonigan JS. Assessing drinker's motivations for change: the Stages of Change Readiness and Treatment Eagerness Scale (SOCRATES). *Psychol Addict Behav* (1996);10(2):81–89.
16. DiClemente CC, Hughes SO. Stages of change profiles in alcoholism treatment. *J Subst Abuse* 1990;2:217–235.
17. Zhang AY, Harmon JA, Werkner J, McCormick RA. Impacts of motivation for change on the severity of alcohol use by patients with severe and persistent mental illness. *J Stud* Alcohol 2004;65:392–397.
18. Mee-Lee D. An instrument for treatment progress and matching: the Recovery Attitude and Treatment Evaluator (RAATE). *J Subst Abuse Treat* 1988;*5*:183–186.
19. Smith MB, Hoffmann NG, Nederhoed R. The development and reliability of the RAATE-CE. *J Subst Abuse* 1992;4:355–363.
20. Annis HM, Graham JM, Davis CS. *Inventory of drinking situations (IDS): user's guide.* Toronto: Addiction Research Foundation, 1987.
21. Moos R. *Coping Response Inventory Manual.* Palo Alto, CA: Center for Health Care Evaluation, Department of Veterans Affairs and Stanford University Medical Center, 1992.
22. Annis HM, Graham JM. Situational Confidence Questionnaire (SCQ-39): user's guide. Toronto: Addiction Research Foundation, 1988.
23. Annis HM, Skylar Turner NE. *The Drug Taking Confidence Questionnaire: user's guide.* Toronto: Addiction Research Foundation, 1997.
24. Brown SA, Christiansen BA, Goldman MS. The Alcohol Expectancy Questionnaire: an instrument for the assessment of adolescent and adult alcohol expectancies. *J Stud Alcohol* 1987;48:483–491.
25. Institute of Medicine. *Broadening the base of treatment for alcohol problems: a report of a study by a committee of the Institute of Medicine, Division of Mental Health and Behavioral Medicine.* Washington, DC: National Academy Press, 1990.
26. The Joint Commission. A Practical Guide to Documentation in Behavioral Health. 2008; ISBN: 978-1-59940-186-7, The Joint Commission, Oak Brook Terrace, IL.
27. McLellan AT, Kushner H, Metzger D. The fifth edition of the Addiction Severity Index. *J Subst Abuse Treat* 1992;9:199–213.
28. Moos RH. *Coping Responses Inventory—Adult Form Professional Manual.* Odessa, FL: Psychological Assessment Resources, 1993.
29. Smith MB, Hoffman NG, Nederhoed R. Development and reliability of the Recovery Attitude and Treatment Evaluator-Questionnaire I (RAATE-QI). *Int J Addict* 1995;30(2):147–160.
30. Tonigan JS, Miller WR. The Inventory of Drug Use Consequences (InDUC): test-retest stability and sensitivity to change. *Psychol Addict Behav* 2002;16(2):165–168.

CHAPTER 21

Andrew J. Treno, PhD
Paul J. Gruenewald, PhD
Harold D. Holder, PhD
Lillian G. Remer, MA

Environmental Approaches to Prevention

Alcohol-involved problems are a serious public health issue. The prevention of these problems is a major need in contemporary America and has been a continual source of public concern. Total annual alcohol-related deaths in the United States for 2001 have been estimated at 75,000 or more, representing roughly 2.3 million years of potential life lost (1,2). Estimates of the extent of alcohol involvement in trauma include 39% of traffic-crash fatalities (3), 47% of homicides, 29% of suicides (4), 30% to 40% for fatal recreational injuries (5), and 10% to 25% for home injuries (6,7). Alcohol is involved in a substantial percentage of injuries caused by falls, drowning, and burns (8,9). More than 5% of all hospital discharges other then childbirth include at least one alcohol-related diagnosis (10).

Though medical care costs resulting from the physiologic damage caused by excessive drinking are substantial ($26.3 billion per year) (11), injuries and deaths related to alcohol use and their associated social costs are broadly experienced throughout the United States by drinkers and nondrinkers alike. The economic and social costs due to alcohol use accrue, owing to accidents and injuries and the interpersonal violence associated with drinking among adults and young people. In addition to the estimated 17,000 persons who die each year in alcohol-related traffic crashes (3), some 2.7 million violent victimization events involving alcohol occur each year (12), many of which result from violence between partners (13). Alcohol involvement in violence-related injuries has been estimated as 28% to 43% (14). Much of the violence associated with drinking takes place among young people between the ages of 15 and 20. This sadly includes high rates of both interpersonal violence (15) and suicide (16). Alcohol consumption is also a major problem in the U.S. work force, linked to increased medical costs, worker's compensation claims, sick leave/absenteeism, accidents, early retirement, and loss of productivity (17,18). Crime and injuries related to drinking account for some $32.2 billion per year. Lost productivity related to drinking accounts for some $87.6 billion per year (11).

Treatment alone has seldom been an adequate response to any major public health problem, and alcohol-related problems are no different. Treatment of individuals hurt by alcohol-involved trauma or drinking problems is the most expensive response. Prevention and reduction of alcohol-related problems can have immediate short-term, as well as long-term, value. In the past, however, many prevention efforts have shown limited success (19,20). Limiting factors have included incomplete conceptual models or theory, poor program or policy design, and inadequate research and evaluation (21–23). It is now clear that alcoholics do not account for all alcohol problems and that alcohol problems are widely dispersed in society (11) and are linked to a broader system of relationships between persons, places, and drinking patterns (24). Today, prevention researchers recognize that alcohol-related problems result from the interaction between individuals and their larger environment, which encompasses social, cultural, economic, and political factors (25–27). Fortunately, some of the larger features of the alcohol environment can be easily, and sometimes inexpensively, changed. This chapter is divided into three sections. The first section provides a brief summary of the environmental perspective on the reduction of alcohol and other drug problems. The second section describes several examples of major demonstration projects developed in keeping with this perspective. The third section discusses how environmentally based studies provide the core scientific research needed to develop adequate theoretical models of the ecologies of drinking and related problems and how these ecologies will lead to more effective environmental prevention programs.

ENVIRONMENTAL STRATEGIES

Prior to the development of the environmental perspective, most prevention programs relied heavily upon various methods to persuade individuals to avoid use by providing them with messages or strategies to prevent initiation, encourage desistance or reduce use, and change the social influences that surround young people (28–32). As a complement to these approaches, environmental strategies were developed and shaped into programs that communities could implement to reduce alcohol and drug problems but did not require direct intervention with specific individuals (33–36). Though differing somewhat in details, these programs shared a common heritage of policy, regulatory, and enforcement interventions that attempted to reduce problems related to substance abuse by changing the economic, physical, or social environment in which alcohol or drugs are obtained or used (23,37–39).

Environmental approaches to the reduction of alcohol and drug problems share a number of important characteristics and contrast sharply to more traditional approaches that focused on individuals and abstinence or treatment. First, environmental approaches seek to change "community systems" that are related to substance use and the occurrence of related problems. Such efforts often include changing formal institutions (e.g., reducing hours and days of sale of alcohol) but also may include attempts to change informal systems (e.g., breaking up markets for illegal drugs) (25). The second way in which the two approaches differ is in their use of the media. Traditional approaches target individuals whereas environmental approaches typically target policymakers or gatekeepers such as state legislators, law enforcement agencies, or even parents within families. Changes in community systems cannot be accomplished without the support of relevant gatekeepers to systems that enable prevention efforts. Thus, media efforts in environmental prevention programs often are intended to motivate gatekeepers to pursue activities that are extensions of their normal efforts. Environmental interventions can also use media to increase public awareness or to influence social norms. The community is viewed as a resource to mobilize for structural and system change with a subsequent focus on policy interventions.

A third important distinction between environmental and traditional approaches to prevention is their orientation toward persons at risk. Rather than targeting individuals at risk directly, the environmental approach targets the broader alcohol and drug environment. Thus, a workplace-based environmental intervention may be aimed at altering workplace policies toward alcohol, but these policies will affect everyone at the workplace, not just those who abuse alcohol (40). The primary consequences of this broad focus are the secondary effects of environmental prevention on persons indirectly at risk. Research shows that nonabusers suffer collateral damage from alcohol and drug abuse (41,42), and awareness of their risk may lead them to support the implementation of environmental prevention programs. Fourth, as a final distinction, traditional approaches attempt to reduce the individual demand for drugs, whereas environmental approaches seek to reduce supply of a substance or the risks associated with its use. Environmental efforts may include enforcement actions to reduce youth purchases of alcohol (43), drug interdiction (44), efforts to target risks specifically related to sales (e.g., responsible beverage service programs) (45), safe needle programs (37), and efforts to change drug distribution to ameliorate problem "hot spots" (46).

Though alcohol and drug use can lead to both "acute" and "chronic" problem outcomes, environmental prevention programs generally target acute problems such as motor vehicle crashes, injuries, and violence, rather than chronic medical conditions, such as alcohol dependence or liver cirrhosis. Similarly, in the case of illegal drugs, environmental efforts generally target reductions in drug-related crime (47). Though it is clear that environmental approaches to prevention may lead to reductions in alcohol or drug use, reductions in use are not a precondition to alcohol- or drug-related harm reduction. In fact, environmental prevention efforts rarely focus on reduced use; rather, they attempt to reduce the harm resulting from use. Thus, prevention programs that are oriented toward regulating problem outcomes related to alcohol use, such as responsible beverage service (45), may reduce one harmful outcome related to alcohol use (motor vehicle crashes). It follows that environmental prevention programs may reduce proximal acute harms related to alcohol and drug abuse (such as motor vehicle crashes and AIDS transmission through needle-sharing among injection drug users) without changing the chronic problems that result from prolonged use (such as heart and liver disease).

The importance of the focus on acute problems is illustrated by the social costs of alcohol and drug abuse in terms of years of life lost owing to acute harm (48). For example, the total economic costs attributed to alcohol-related motor vehicle crashes, violence, and premature death ($218 billion) accounts for a very substantial portion of the $246 billion total costs of alcohol abuse (49). When all acute harms related to drug and alcohol use are considered (including all injuries and violent crimes related to illegal drug use), the costs are estimated at $305 billion per year. The immediate short-term burden that acute alcohol and drug problems place on the health care and enforcement systems thus renders them more costly to society than many other major health problems. Acute problems are so costly because they are distributed so widely in the population of drinkers and drug users. Thus, one often hears reference to the "prevention paradox" (50), which is the observation that while high-risk individuals produce more problems on an individual basis, lower-risk individuals produce more problems on an aggregate basis. From a public health perspective of reducing aggregate alcohol and drug problems in the community, a focus on high- and low-risk individuals makes sense. Environmental strategies have the advantage of affecting all drinkers and drug users, regardless of their levels of use and, highly important, affect all individuals at risk.

DOMAINS OF ENVIRONMENTAL PREVENTION

Environmental prevention programs act in three domains: the physical, the social, and the economic. Prevention programs may alter physical access by affecting proximity to sources of alcohol, drugs, and tobacco. College dormitories may prohibit alcohol in dorm rooms, college administrators may eliminate the sale of tobacco through vending machines, and public markets for illegal drugs may be disrupted by matrix enforcement programs (37). Environmental prevention programs may alter social access by affecting the social networks that encourage and enable distribution of these substances. They may alter social access to alcohol by restricting social activities at which alcohol is freely served (as during on-campus celebrations), reduce social access to tobacco through increased counter-advertising, and moderate social access to illegal drugs by establishing and enforcing drug-free zones in a community. Prevention programs may alter economic access by increasing the real costs of alcohol, drugs, and tobacco and changing the economic geography of availability.

The three domains of environmental influence interact in producing alcohol and drug problems. For example, physical, social, and economic availability of alcohol (represented by outlets, use by others, and beverage prices) intersect at places wherein alcohol problems occur. The presence of other drinkers at outlets exposes the patron of a bar both to social influences for drinking and much greater risks of violence (51). Prices for alcoholic beverages at bars are much greater than at off-premise establishments, changing both the nature of drinking at bars and its relationship to problem outcomes, such as driving while intoxicated and alcohol-related crashes (52). The purchasing patterns of others at these establishments naturally influence the behaviors of drinking groups, as by encouraging much greater levels of intoxication (53). Naturally, parallel arguments can be constructed for illegal drugs. Concentrated use of illegal drugs (for example, in and around crack houses) is associated with substantial degrees of crime and elevated rates of disease (37,47). Prices of illegal drugs may be influenced by drug interdiction efforts (modestly) but certainly affect the distribution of drug purchases (54). Favored drugs for abuse change as social access is restructured by enforcement efforts or other changes in informal social systems that support drug distribution.

STRUCTURE OF ENVIRONMENTAL PREVENTION

Environmental prevention programs are part of the natural ecology of local communities—the psychologic, social, and economic geographies of people, places, and things with which everyone interacts in daily life. Nothing in environmental prevention takes place in a vacuum, and everything is contingent on something else. Thus, in environmental prevention, the relationships between physical, social, and economic contexts of human behavior become very important. These relations are not naively additive, contributing to the balance sheet of risk and protective factors (26) but represent ecologic contexts that interact with the relationships between individual predispositions to problem outcomes and their realization in different settings (46,55,56).

Individual use of drugs and alcohol produces problems. Drinking may lead to drinking and driving, or illegal drug use may lead to crime. The alcohol environment is not simply producing problems or influencing personal activities. Instead, the environment creates a stage on which human activities play themselves out to produce problems. With this in mind, there are four ways in which the alcohol environment can affect problems related to drinking and drug use:

1. The alcohol environment may directly affect use (as when reduced availability leads to reduced use).
2. The alcohol environment may indirectly affect problems through its effect on use (as when reduced availability leads to reduced use and, hence, fewer problems related to use).
3. The alcohol environment may directly affect outcomes (as when increased safety belt use leads to reductions in alcohol-involved fatal crashes, independent of rates of alcohol use).
4. The alcohol environment may moderate the relationship between substance use and problem outcomes (as when densities of bars and restaurants moderate the relationship between traffic flow patterns and automobile crashes).

In the third and fourth arenas, the effects of the environment are most compelling, as environmental changes can accelerate or decelerate the rates of alcohol and drug problems (46).

Direct Effects on Substance Use The most obvious way in which environmental prevention activities reduce problems related to alcohol and drugs is to alter the behaviors of drinkers and drug users. Behavioral change was, in fact, the primary goal of prevention studies through much of the latter half of the 20th century. Environmental prevention research has demonstrated that demographic, economic, and physical restrictions on availability can reduce use and problems. For example, increasing the minimum legal drinking age to 21 has been linked to a 13% reduction in the number of high school seniors reporting drinking, as well as lower drinking levels across demographic groups (57).

Price increases are clearly associated with declines in alcohol consumption (58); heavy drinkers and youthful drinkers are particularly sensitive to price changes (59). Estimates from these studies suggest that if beer prices had been indexed to inflation over the past decades, youth drinking could be reduced by 9% and youth heavy drinking by 20% (60). Increases and decreases in the physical availability of alcohol have been linked to increases and decreases in alcohol sales (61), suggesting that a 10% reduction in outlet densities would be associated with a 3% reduction in alcohol sales. Thus, in large aggregate studies across the United States, reductions in the demographic, economic, and physical availability of alcohol appear to be related to reductions in use.

Additional mechanisms also have been found through which the environment may directly affect drinking behaviors. For example, reductions have been achieved through the introduction of responsible beverage service programs, which are linked to lower levels of intoxication (62), or local enforcement of underage sales laws, which can reduce underage alcohol sales in off-premise establishments by half (43). Conversely, increases in alcohol use have been related to the privatization of alcohol monopolies, which yield lower prices, greater numbers of outlets, and increased sales (63).

Environmental efforts to reduce underage access to alcohol have proved particularly effective. The implementation of community-based alcohol policies to reduce youth access have led to reduced sales to youth in on-premise outlets by 24% and off-premise outlets by 8%, with a concomitant 7% reduction in past 30-day drinking (64).

Indirect Effects on Problems Empirical studies have clearly demonstrated the potential impact of environmental change on problem outcomes such as traffic crashes. For example, raising the legal drinking age to 21 has been linked to a 20% reduction in single-vehicle nighttime crashes (the commonly used surrogate for alcohol-involved crashes) among youthful drivers (57,64). Similarly, reflecting the potential impact of changes in the economic availability of alcohol, higher alcohol prices have been linked to lower rates of traffic deaths and cirrhosis mortality (65). Mandated server-training policies have been linked to reductions in alcohol-involved crashes (66). Conversely, increased availability of spirits at bars and restaurants has been linked to substantial increases in alcohol-involved crashes (67). At the local level of neighborhoods within communities, lower densities of alcohol outlets have been linked to decreases in alcohol-involved crashes (42,68,69) pedestrian injury collisions (70,71), and violence (72–76).

Direct Effects on Problems As suggested in the previous section, environmental conditions that support drinking or drug use can indirectly affect problems. Changes in one can produce reductions in the other through a simple causal chain. Environmental prevention efforts also can directly affect problem outcomes and provide alternative paths to prevention. Aspects of the psychologic, social, economic, and physical environments apparently unrelated to alcohol and drug use can confound research efforts to evaluate any prevention activity, but they also can become an important part of environmental prevention. As a confound or "nuisance," these aspects of the environment disrupt simple cause-and-effect relationships between environmental prevention activities (such as reduced availability) and prevention outcomes (e.g., reduced motor vehicle crashes). Any attempt to evaluate the effects of reduced alcohol availability on drinking and driving traffic crashes must isolate the unique effects of this policy from such factors as vehicle miles traveled by drivers, characteristics of urban and rural traffic flow, other safety measures on roadway systems (such as stoplights) and within automobiles (such as safety belts), and sources of distraction (such as cell phones). Thus, differences in traffic flow rates and patterns can be substantive predictors of traffic crashes and pedestrian collisions in general and alcohol-related motor vehicle crashes and pedestrian injuries in particular (42,71). Sociodemographic characteristics of resident populations around retail centers (such as poverty) are related to violence independent of the number of alcohol outlets (75). The availability of alcohol in different venues (such as taverns and grocery stores) may mitigate the effects of a price increase (46). However, the same "nuisance" factors also can become part of environmental prevention efforts. Thus, low rates of driving after drinking in urban settings where public transportation is widely available points to a natural environmental strategy for the reduction of alcohol-related crashes: safe-ride programs. The former confounding variable now becomes a potential intervention. Changing rates of safety belt use may confound an evaluation of the direct effects of a liquor tax increase on alcohol-related fatal crashes but become part of an effective strategy to reduce this particular alcohol-related harm. Thus, most environmental prevention studies recognize that multiple environmental supports must be incorporated in the prevention of problem outcomes. As an example, Hingson et al. (77) showed that a combination of media campaigns, enforcement of speed and DUI limits, and community awareness reduced fatal motor vehicle crashes by as much as 25%. Holder et al. (39) demonstrated that environmental prevention programs oriented toward alcohol-related problems (such as alcohol-related crashes, violence, drownings, burns, and falls), rather than alcohol use can be effective in reducing problems and changing patterns of use.

Effects on Relationships Between Substance Use and Problem Outcomes The social, economic, and physical environments determine the nature of problems experienced by individuals. No violence occurs in the absence of social interaction, no motor vehicle crashes without cars or trucks, no falls occur without the opportunity for falling. Thus, participation in the routine activities of daily life condition the occurrence of problem outcomes (78). The environment may encourage or discourage alcohol and drug use, but it certainly moderates the relationship between use and problems related to specific drinking events. The moderating effects of environmental variables on the relationship between substance use and problem outcomes have been investigated in only a few studies to date. In each case, however, researchers found strong indications that environmental contexts focus problems in ways that can be taken advantage of in future preventive intervention programs. In the case of alcohol-related traffic crashes, as shown by Gruenewald and Treno (46), local patterns of traffic flow are directly related to rates of motor vehicle crashes, but this relationship is significantly moderated by the presence of on-premise alcohol outlets (bars and restaurants). The location of alcohol outlets along different types of roadways affects drinking, driving, and crashing. Within low traffic flow areas of communities, greater numbers of alcohol outlets do not lead to significantly greater numbers of alcohol-related crashes. Within high traffic flow areas of communities, conversely, greater numbers of alcohol outlets lead to substantively greater numbers of alcohol-related crashes.

The differences in these contexts suggest that 10% greater densities of alcohol outlets will be related, systematically, to no change in crash rates within downtown areas with low traffic flow, to 20% greater crash rates within areas with greater traffic flow (particularly along highway systems). Clearly, regulations governing outlet densities and locations within community areas should be developed to be sensitive to these local characteristics.

Similar observations are beginning to emerge in studies of violence related to alcohol outlets and problems related to illegal drug markets. The frequently observed relationship between densities of alcohol outlets (particularly bars) and rates of violence (72,73) must be supplemented with two other pieces of contextual information. First, rates of violence are not simply a function of the number of outlets and populations characteristics of a local area but are a function of population characteristics of people living in nearby areas (75). Second, densities of alcohol outlets do not appear to be a direct source of violence in geographic areas but rather a moderator of the rates at which populations produce violence (76). Rates of assault are greater in neighborhoods with specific population characteristics (e.g., more poverty, disorganization, immigration, and residential mobility). They are accelerated in neighborhoods with more taverns and off-premises alcohol establishments (79). A similar pattern is found with regard to illegal drug markets: Disrupting the geographic link between location of sales and location of users leads to reduced drug sales and problems (80).

ENVIRONMENTAL STRATEGIES AND ALCOHOL POLICY

"Policy" usually refers to structural change, as through a regulation, law, or enforcement priority. As suggested by this chapter, communities have begun to go beyond policy to affect the drinking environment itself as an approach to reducing alcohol-involved problems. Local policymakers can establish the priorities for community action to reduce risky behavior involving drinking, which, in turn, can reduce the number of alcohol-involved problems. For example, local alcohol policies can make it a priority to enforce laws against drinking and driving, violence, or sales of alcohol to youth; to mandate server training for bars, pubs, and restaurants; or to promote written policies and training for responsible alcoholic beverage service by licensed retail establishments. Existing national and state or provincial laws provide the legal basis for many local policies and can enable local communities to prioritize uses of existing resources within legal frameworks to achieve specific objectives. In short, national as well as state, regional, or provincial laws often establish the base for local policies, including legal drinking ages, regulation of alcohol outlets, the legal blood alcohol level for driving after drinking, advertising restrictions, and service to obviously intoxicated persons and underage persons. Local policies often address the implementation and enforcement of these existing laws. In sum, environmental prevention strategies appear to have a critical role in reducing alcohol problems. Such strategies have demonstrated effectiveness in terms of population-level outcome measures (e.g., reductions in alcohol-involved motor vehicle crashes) and drinking among both heavy and moderate users and have been characterized by maintained effects extending beyond the initial implementation periods. Environmental interventions are politically feasible because they do not target specific subgroups in a discriminatory manner. In general, they are cost-effective because they do not require case finding, service provision, or cost maintenance. Moreover, environmental prevention strategies provide a number of levers for change, including tax codes, alcohol beverage control laws, laws regulating drinking and driving and minimum drinking ages, administrative regulation of outlets, planning and zoning regulations and conditional use permits, and law enforcement policies. A number of issues do, however, remain unresolved.

Table 21.1 presents an overall evaluation of what is known in terms of specific policy interventions in terms of the underlying implied mechanisms demonstrated effects, and overall strengths and weaknesses. In general, it would appear as if there are three basic policy strategies used to reduce alcohol related problems.

The first class of interventions reduces alcohol availability by limiting the times and days that alcohol outlets may sell or serve alcohol (i.e., control of days and hours of legal sales) or by reducing the number of outlets that provide opportunities for such purchases (i.e., outlet density restrictions or state-controlled monopoly). It may be argued here that these are strong approaches in that they seek to influence the alcohol environment directly and that they have generally been proven effective while being relatively inexpensive to implement. On the downside, they tend to generate political opposition and may take long periods to implement. It is not surprising to find that such approaches are often opposed by the manufacturers, distributors, and even the consumers of alcoholic beverages as they conflict with their interests.

A second group of interventions operate through the application of specific penalties to either consumers or providers either by establishing liability for second parties for serving alcohol to persons of specific statuses (minimum legal drinking age) or to levels of intoxication (dram shop liability), or by punishing persons for consuming alcohol in specific amounts conjoint to specific activities (DUI enforcement). It may be argued here that these are somewhat weaker approaches in that they seek to influence the alcohol environment through the application of specific penalties to either consumers or providers. The strengths here are less clear, particularly in the case of establishing second-party

TABLE 21.1 Policy Interventions

Intervention	Mechanism	Strengths	Weaknesses	Effects	Studies
Reducing availability					
Control of hours and days of sales	Increased inconvenience in obtaining sales and service.	Low enforcement costs	Very difficult to enact required legislation. Political opposition from owners and managers.	Reductions in drunkenness, domestic and public violence, drunk driving, and ED admissions.	Chikritzhs & Stockwell, 2002 (99); Ragnarsdottir and Daviosdottir, 2002 (100); Duailibi, Ponicki, Grube, et al., 2007 (101); Norstrom and Skog, 2005 (102); Baker, Johnson, Voas, and Lange, 2000 (103)
Outlet density restrictions	Increased difficulty in obtaining alcohol in terms of required travel costs and reductions in pressures to lower prices.	High system impact	Very difficult to enact required legislation. Changes in densities take a long time to occur. Political opposition from owners and managers.	Reductions in overall consumption, heavy drinking and a host of social problems including child abuse, crashes and assaults.	Gruenewald, Freisthler, Remer, et al., 2006 (79); Lipton and Gruenewald, 2002 (104); Parker and Rebhun, 1995 (105); Scribner, Mackinnon and Dwyer, 1995 (73); Zhu, Gorman and Horel, 2004 (106); Norstrom, 2000 (107).
Monopoly regulatory system	Increased difficulty in obtaining alcohol in terms of required travel costs and reductions in pressures to lower prices.	High system impact	Very difficult to enact required legislation.	General reductions in consumption.	Wagenaar and Holder, 1995 (108); Trolldal, 2005 (109).
Minimum-age drinking laws	Deterrent effect based on perceived severity of penalties for servers and sellers with resulting reduction in availability to youth.	High system impact	Continued enforcement costs.	Reductions of use, crashes, suicides, homicides, and vandalism among youth.	24 major studies reviewed in Wagenaar and Toomey, 2002 (110).
Penalties					
Server liability laws	Deterrent effect based on perceived severity of penalties for servers and sellers.	Shifts responsibility from drinker to the outlet requiring little voluntarism on the part of the drinker	Difficulties in determining liability and difficulty in enactment of necessary legislation. Political opposition from owners and managers.	Some effects in reduced crashes.	Mosher, 1984 (111); Holder et al., 1993 (112); Sloan et al., 2000 (113).
Increased DUI enforcement	Increased real and perceived risk of arrest and punishment.	Generally effective	High implementation costs. Questionable legality in some jurisdictions.	Demonstrated reductions in crashes.	McKnight and Voas, 2001 (114), Voas, Holder, and Gruenewald, 1997 (96), Voas, Lange, and Treno, 1997 (115).
Drinking environment					
Server training.	Change of server behavior.	Moderate implementation costs	Low system impact due to high server turnover. Most effective when embedded in larger multi-component strategies.	Mixed results with some small changes in server behavior.	Major studies reviewed in Haines and Graham, 2005 (116); Homel 1997 (51); Maguire et al., 2003 (117); Wallin et al., 2003 (93).

liability wherein issues of "fairness" may arise. An additional weakness involves costs associated with case finding.

A third approach focuses on altering the alcohol environment though training of providers (server training). While having the advantage of being the least politically controversial, it would seem the least effective largely owing to high turnover rates in the hospitality industry, low levels of monitoring of servers, and competitive economic pressures to overserve patrons and to sell to minors. Server training and written establishment policies may suffer from excessive "voluntarism" whereas the potentially most effective and cost-efficient interventions are those likely to raise the most political opposition. Still, when contrasted with more traditional approaches (treatment, brief interventions, and school-based education) environmental strategies can be more cost-effective relative to system impact.

EFFICACY TRIALS

Based upon the promising results found from basic policy studies, several important community-based environmental preventive intervention studies were undertaken. Each involved at least one aspect of the alcohol environment, and each employed a clearly environmental approach to prevention. These projects went beyond the scientific evidence to test whether environmental prevention efforts could be effective at the community level in preventing three harmful outcomes related to alcohol: drinking and driving, underage access and use, and violence related to alcohol.

The Saving Lives Project The Saving Lives Project, conducted in six communities in Massachusetts, was designed to reduce alcohol-impaired driving and related problems such as speeding (77). Programs were designed locally and involved a host of activities, including media campaigns, business information programs, speeding and drunk driving awareness days, speed watch telephone hotlines, police training, high school peer-led education, Students Against Drunk Driving chapters, and college prevention programs. The program evaluation involved a quasi-experimental design and five communities as controls. Though the control communities were slightly more affluent than the experimental sites, they had similar demographic characteristics, rates of traffic citations, and fatal crashes. The outcome evaluation of the project included measures of fatal and injury crashes, safety belt use, telephone surveys, and traffic citations. The study found that Saving Lives cities experienced a 25% decline in fatal crashes when compared to the rest of Massachusetts (that is, from 178 crashes to 120), a 42% reduction in fatal motor vehicle crashes within the experimental communities, a 47% reduction in the number of fatally injured drivers who tested positive for alcohol, and an 8% decline in crash injuries among 15- to 25-year-olds. In addition, there was a decline in self-reported driving after drinking (specifically among youth). The greatest fatal and injury crash reductions occurred in the 15- to 25-year-old age group.

The Communities Mobilizing for Change on Alcohol Project The Communities Mobilizing for Change on Alcohol (CMCA) project was designed to reduce access to alcohol among youth under the legal drinking age of 21 (64). The project was composed of five core components intended to influence (1) community policies, (2) community practices, (3) youth alcohol access, (4) youth alcohol consumption, and subsequently (5) youth alcohol problems. Though the project clearly was communitywide in terms of the institutions involved, it was focused on youth younger than 21 years. The CMCA project recruited 15 communities in Minnesota and western Wisconsin, matched them on size, state, proximity to a college or university, and baseline data from an alcohol purchase survey, then randomly assigned members of each pair to intervention or control groups (81). The CMCA project hired from within each community a part-time local organizer who was responsible for community organizing activities that activated the community members, who would, in turn, select interventions designed to influence underage access to alcohol. The interventions that could be selected included a broad array of programs that affect youth access: decoy operations with alcohol outlets, citizen monitoring of outlets selling to youth, keg registration, sponsorship of alcohol-free events for youth, policy action to shorten hours of sale for alcohol, implementation of responsible beverage service training programs, and development of educational programs for youth and adults. The experimental sites were free to shape these interventions to fit their own ends. Evaluation data were collected at baseline and at about 30 months after the interventions began. Results showed that merchants increased the frequency of checks for age identification, reduced sales to minors, and reported more care in controlling sales to youth (82). A telephone survey of 18- to 20-year-olds showed reductions in attempts to purchase alcohol, reduced levels of alcohol use, and reduced propensity to provide alcohol to other teens (64). In addition, the project found a statistically significant net decline in drinking and driving arrests among 18- to 20-year-olds and disorderly conduct violations among 15- to 17-year-olds in the CMCA cities as compared to the controls (64).

The Community Trials Project The Community Trials (CT) project was a five-component community-level intervention conducted in three experimental communities matched to three controls (83). The goals of the project were to reduce alcohol-related harm among all persons in the three experimental communities. The outcomes of the project reflected the primary sources of acute injury and harm related to alcohol: injuries and fatalities related to drinking and driving or to violence, drownings, burns, and falls (84). Each environmental prevention component was based on prior scientific evidence (34), but this mix of components had not been tested for mutually supportive or synergistic effects (83). The project design recognized the complex systems environment in which environmental preventive interventions take place (25). Community Trials fielded five intervention components: (1) a "Media and Mobilization" component to develop community organization and support for the goals and strategies of the project; (2) a "Responsible Beverage Service" (RBS) component to reduce service to intoxicated patrons at bars and restaurants; (3) a "Sales to Youth" component to reduce underage access; (4) a "Drinking and Driving" component to increase enforcement activities related to driving while intoxicated (DWI) offenses; and (5) an "Access" component to reduce the availability of alcohol. The final evaluation of the project covered key problem areas through data collected in a large population survey and from archival sources and emergency departments (85). Comparison of the effects of the interventions on relative risks of injury outcomes between matched communities showed significant reductions in nighttime injury crashes (10%) and in crashes in which the driver was found by police to "have been drinking" (6%). Assault injuries observed in emergency departments declined by 43%, and all hospitalized assault injuries declined by 2%. Analyses of survey data showed a 49% decline in episodes of driving after "having had too much to drink" and 51% in self-reports of driving when "over the legal limit." Surprisingly, though the drinking population increased slightly in the experimental sites over the course of the study, there was a significant reduction in problematic alcohol use: The average number of drinks per occasion declined by 6%, and the variance in drinking patterns (an indirect measure of heavy drinking) declined by 21% (39).

The Sacramento Neighborhood Alcohol Prevention Project The primary goal of the Sacramento Neighborhood Alcohol Prevention Project (SNAPP) was to implement and evaluate neighborhood-level interventions intended to reduce youth and young-adult access to alcohol, risky drinking, and associated problems, particularly in low-income ethnically diverse neighborhoods (86). SNAPP represented an extension of the CT project in that it posed three basic questions. First, could an environmental approach be tailored to the unique needs of economically and ethnically diverse populations? Second, could environmental strategies address the problem of intentional injuries (i.e., assaultive violence) in the context of more economically and ethnically diverse settings? Finally, could these more specifically tailored interventions be implemented at the neighborhood level? To address these questions, SNAPP set as its goal the reduction of alcohol access, drinking, and related problems in two low-income, predominantly ethnic minority neighborhoods, focusing on individuals between ages 15 and 29.

SNAPP implemented five project interventions: a mobilization component, a community awareness component, a responsible beverage service component, an underage-access law enforcement component, and an intoxicated-patron law enforcement component. These were phased in one area of the city early in the project, then fielded in another similar area about 2 years later. To mobilize the neighborhoods in support of the overall project goals and interventions, project lead agencies worked with collaborative advisory committees composed of members drawn from each of the two geographic areas and that worked to ensure intervention implementation and fidelity to project design. The Community Awareness Component intended to increase awareness of the problems associated with youth and young-adult drinking to catalyze support for community mobilization efforts. Activities included neighborhood presentations of research findings and local statistics related to underage and problematic drinking to parents and other community groups, distribution of informational flyers and brochures, and youth participation as volunteers in data collection activities related to neighborhood alcohol availability. The RBS Component was designed to help retailers develop policies and train staff to reduce alcohol sales to minors and intoxicated persons. This component increased compliance with existing alcohol policies by obtaining sponsorship and support from local and state hospitality organizations, providing manager and server training for all on- and off-premise licensed alcohol outlets in the selected neighborhoods using a standard curriculum, developing a process to increase enforcement of existing laws regarding service to intoxicated customers, and obtaining endorsement of RBS from neighborhood bodies and organizations. The Underage-Access Enforcement Component focused on increasing actual and perceived enforcement of laws prohibiting alcohol sales to minors and was accomplished by working with neighborhood police to increase the number of off-premise sting operations. These efforts were designed to parallel those of the off-premise intervention. Letters from the local police were sent to all premises in and around the study sites informing them that stepped-up enforcement of laws regarding sales to intoxicated patrons and minors would become a regular police activity, that undercover police would visit all establishments at least once during the following year, and that minors might be used to determine whether sales were made to underage persons.

Overall, the project found significant reductions in assaults as reported by police, aggregate emergency medical services (EMS) outcomes, EMS assaults, and EMS motor vehicle accidents. Specifically, it found an estimated reduction of 3.9% in police calls involving assaults and reductions of 33.4% in EMS calls involving motor vehicle accidents in the South. Similarly, the project found an estimated reduction of 36.5% in police calls involving assaults and an estimated reduction of 37.4% in EMS calls involving assaults in the North.

International Contexts In addition to these successful U.S. environmental prevention programs, several other important efforts were fielded at the same time throughout the world. In Australia, the Surfers' Paradise Safety Action Project (51,87), and its later replications (88,89), featured three primary strategies focused on alcohol outlets, communities, and enforcement leaders. One component focused on the development and implementation of risk assessments, model house policies, and a code of practice by night club managers that addressed security and safety inside and outside of venues (supported by staff education and training, incident reporting, and other measures), staff responsibility, responsible use of alcohol, quality service and entertainment, and honest and accurate advertising. A second component involved a community forum and community-based task groups that used monitoring and risk assessments to regulate managers. The third component, an effort to strengthen external regulation of licensed premises by police and liquor licensing authorities—with an emphasis on preventive rather than reactive strategies—was largely unsuccessful. As a whole, the program showed a marked initial impact of the project on establishment practices (e.g., reductions in binge-drinking incentives; improvements in security practices and entertainment) (87). The intervention was also associated with substantial declines in physical and verbal aggression inside and outside of drinking establishments. Though, as Graham et al. (90,91) point out, the absence of a comparison community makes interpretations regarding the causal role of the intervention difficult, the convergence of evidence across several dependent variables (e.g., unobtrusive observations of the frequency of aggression in licensed premises; police statistics and security company reports of assaults, serious assaults, and disorderly conduct), and subsequent successful replications (88,89) support the interpretation that reductions in violence were related to changes in the drinking environment. Despite its initial success, within 2 to 3 years after the intensive intervention, violence levels in Surfers Paradise increased nearly to the pre-intervention rates (87).

The STAD project in Stockholm, Sweden is another multi-component intervention designed to reduce interpersonal violence in and around licensed premises (92,93). This 10-year community alcohol prevention program has been conducted since 1996 in the northern part of central Stockholm, with a control area in the southern part of central Stockholm. The project's main components include RBS training of servers, community mobilization, and stricter enforcement of existing alcohol laws. The outcome measure—police-reported violence—included assaults, illegal threats and harassment, and violence and threats targeted at officials (including policemen and doormen). Time series analyses using Autoregressive Integrated Moving Average (ARIMA) modeling indicated that during the project period violent crimes decreased significantly by 29% in the project area while they increased slightly in the control area. In addition, to these two examples, notable environmental strategies have been implemented and tested in many countries throughout the world, including Brazil, Sweden, Finland, Denmark, Italy, Israel, Australia, New Zealand, and Canada. See Table 21.1 for a summary of these projects.

EMERGENCE OF ECOLOGIC RESEARCH

One of the serendipitous, but by no means unintended, side benefits of the CT, CMCA, Saving Lives, and SNAPP projects has been the development of a set of core research findings suggestive of directions in which environmentally based prevention science might be directed. These projects were, indeed, efficacy trials for environmental preventive interventions but efficacy trials "with a twist," so-to-speak. Each manipulated with some success different components of complex community systems related to drinking and the emergence of drinking problems (25). Each produced fundamental research findings on the mechanisms of success and failure and unintended consequences that environmental preventive interventions can have in community settings. Each has guided the field toward more direct ecologic studies of alcohol-related problems. Still, further ecologic studies are needed to develop a deeper understanding of how community systems work. Through a better understanding of the processes and relationships that generate alcohol and other drug-related problems, improved intervention strategies can be developed.

Despite the demonstrated effectiveness of environmentally based preventive interventions, much empirical research and efficacy testing remains to be done. To date, most approaches that study relationships between alcohol environments and alcohol problems rely upon statistical evaluations of empirical correlations (e.g., between measures of outlet density and rates of child abuse and neglect) (94) to elucidate plausible person-environment interactions. In this sense, we are in the prestage of truly ecologic studies. We have moved from demonstrating that environmental interventions are effective to considering which are the most effective. Yet the mechanisms that make them work are not understood. The causal status of arguments based on correlational data can be strengthened by longitudinal analyses that identify the same associations over time. However, without a convincing theoretical statement of plausible mechanisms that relate observed environmental measures to outcomes (i.e., a stated mechanism by which greater outlet densities lead to more neglect and abuse) and without accompanying empirical tests of these mechanisms, the causal processes that support these correlations remain unknown. Tests of unique predictions from social ecologic models (e.g., that the time heavy drinking parents spend either intoxicated or drinking outside the home reduces parental monitoring and leads to child neglect) are required. Moreover, it is clear that such studies would need to incorporate individual-level data (e.g., surveys) into analyses that have typically relied on aggregate level data. The ultimate goal here is to state and test strong social ecologic theories about alcohol-related problems such as drinking and drunken driving, intimate partner violence and alcohol, parental alcohol use and child abuse and neglect, and the relationships of community policy and enforcement activities to underage drinking.

To summarize, a number of important points should be noted. First, almost all of the interventions reviewed earlier have to do with regulating availability, punishing "bad" drinkers, or punishing purveyors of alcohol. This rather primitive view, though consistent with overall effects, ignores those situations where such approaches are likely to fail (e.g., people die in alcohol-involved crashes before they get stopped). Second, by maintaining an individual focus, traditional approaches ignore the broader economic and community structures that support alcohol problems. Specifically, the social and commercial distribution of alcohol in communities may distort social systems in specific ways that may lead to great harm. In developing and developed countries, where commercialization of distribution and sales is championed by myopic interests, these distortions can be quite excessive, leading to much harm (and the institutionalization of systems that produce and maintain harm). Third, careful consideration should be given to the roles outlets play in producing problems. Here, at least three theories present themselves, each with different implications for prevention policy. First, outlets may cause problems through their effect on consumption levels. In this case, the target of policy interventions is appropriately to be found in the regulation of the alcohol that flows through them. Second, outlets may serve as places where problems "congregate" as a result of the concentration of drinkers into drinking cultures and environments with generally permissive norms regarding the expression of aggression (95). In this case, alcohol would appear to be somewhat secondary, and attention would need to be focused on more general policing of establishments and the development of policies designed to thwart the development of such "subcultures of violence." Finally, outlets might simply be markers of social pathology. Outlets may simply concentrate in low-income areas where political opposition to their development is absent or ineffectual. Unfortunately, given our current state of knowledge, we are only beginning to put together a suitable ecologic explanatory framework.

ENVIRONMENTAL STRATEGIES AND DRUG POLICY

Environmental strategies for the reduction of harm related to the use of illicit drugs are in their infancy when compared to alcohol prevention programs. As Caulkins (37) points out, much of what is conceived as "environmental" is instead only "enforcement" when considering illegal substances. That the enforcement activities of police take place in the drug-selling and drug-using environment does make this sort of activity a form of environmental intervention, but whether it is prevention or selective incapacitation (the removal of drug users and sellers from activity on the streets) is another question. Ideally, the equivalent action with regard to alcohol (arrests for drunken driving) are intended to reduce this illegal activity by deterring driving after drinking, as described in specific and general deterrence theories (96). Arrests make enforcement an environmental prevention activity (that is, an action that may, in the future, discourage an apprehended, drunk driver from driving after drinking). In the arena of illegal drug sales, it is difficult to ascribe such preventive benefits to enforcement outside of the greater costs incurred by users through the disruption of drug supply networks (80). In a similar manner, greater costs for drugs may arise through the "War on Drugs" and other interdiction activities. However, the effectiveness of such strategies has been shown to be very limited (54).

Other prevention strategies with regard to illegal drug use are oriented to individuals or families, not the environment of drug use. The majority of these efforts are programs to educate young people to resist use, to help moderate the dire consequences of disrupted families on youth use, and more general media campaigns to encourage users to stop and discourage nonusers from beginning to use drugs (97). Strikingly, though there is extensive research literature discussing the many environments in which drug use and related crime take place, there is little literature on environmental prevention per se (37,98). Were one to modify community environments, what would be the consequences to illegal drug sales and use? What aspects of the community environment are most likely to enable reductions of sales and use? These questions remain largely unanswered (99–117).

ACKNOWLEDGMENTS: *This work was supported by NIAAA grant P60-AA06282 (Environmental Approaches to Prevention).*

REFERENCES

1. Midanik LT, Chaloupka FJ, Saitz R, et al. Alcohol-attributable deaths and years of potential life lost due to excessive alcohol use, United States, 2001. *JAMA* 2004;292:2831–2832.
2. National Institute for Alcohol Abuse and Alcoholism. *Report to the Extramural Advisory Board, August 16–17, 2006: Division of Epidemiology & Prevention Research Strategic Planning Document.* Washington, DC: US DHHS, 2006.
3. National Highway Traffic Safety Administration. *Traffic Safety Facts 2004 Data: Alcohol.* Washington DC: Department of Transportation, 2005. Retrieved http://www-nrd.nhtsa.dot.gov/pdf/nrd-30/NCSA/TSF2004/809905.pdf.
4. Smith G, Brannings KC, Miller T. Fatal non-traffic injuries involving alcohol. *Ann Emerg Med* 1999;33:699–702.
5. Mayhew DR, Donelson AC, Beirness DJ, et al. Youth, alcohol and the relative risk of crash involvement. *Accid Anal Prev* 1986;18: 273–288.
6. Center for Disease Control. Alcohol as a risk factor for injuries—U.S. *MMWR* 1983;32:61–62.
7. Fell J, Nash C. The nature of the alcohol problem in U.S. fatal crashes, *Health Ed Q* 1989;16:335–343.
8. Howland J, Hingson R. Alcohol as a risk factor for drownings: a review of the literature (1950–1985). *Accid Anal Prev* 1988;20:19–25.
9. Hingson R, Howland J. Alcohol as a risk factor for injury or death resulting from accidental falls: a review of the literature, *J Stud Alcohol* 1987;48:212–219.
10. Chen CA, Yi HY, Hilton ME. *Trends in alcohol-related morbidity among short-stay community hospital discharges, U.S., 1979–2003.* NIAAA Surveillance Report #72. Bethesda, MD: National Institute on Alcohol Abuse and Alcoholism, 2005.
11. Harwood H. *Updating estimates of the economic cost of alcohol abuse: estimates, updating methods, and data.* Bethesda, MD: National Institute on Alcohol Abuse and Alcoholism, 2000.
12. Greenfield L. *Alcohol and crime: an analysis of national data on the prevalence of alcohol involvement in crime.* Washington DC; U.S. Department of Justice, 1998.
13. Cunradi CB, Caetano R, Clark CL, et al. Alcohol-related problems and intimate partner violence among white, black, and Hispanic couples in the U.S. *Alcohol Clin Exp Res* 1999;23:1492–1501.
14. Cherpitel CJ, Yu Y, Bond J. Attributable risk of injury assoc with alcohol use *American J Public Health* 2005;95:266–272.
15. Department of Health and Human Services. *Youth violence: a report of the Surgeon General.* Washington DC: U.S. Government Printing Office, 2001.
16. Cohen Y, Spirito A, Brown LK. Suicide and suicidal behavior. In: DiClemente RJ, Hansen WB, Ponton LE, eds. *Handbook of adolescent health risk behavior.* New York: Plenum, 1996:193–224.
17. Wrich JT. *The impact of substance abuse at the workplace.* New York: The Conference Board, 1986.

18. Hingson RW, Lederman RI, Walsh DC. Employee drinking patterns and accidental injury: a study of four New England states. *J Stud Alcohol* 1985;46:298–303.
19. Gorman DM. Do school-based social skills training programs prevent alcohol use among young people? *Addict Res* 1996;4:191–210.
20. Gorman DM. The failure of drug education. *Public Interest* 1997;129: 50–60.
21. Blane HT. Education and prevention of alcoholism. In: Kissin B, Begleiter H, eds., *Social aspects of alcoholism*. New York: Plenum, 1976:519–578.
22. Gorman DM. The irrelevance of evidence in the development of school-based drug prevention policy, 1986–1996, *Eval Rev* 1998;22:118–146.
23. Holder HD, Flay B, Howard J, et al. Phases of alcohol problem prevention research. *Alcohol Clin Exp Res* 1999;23(1):183–194.
24. Mubayi A, Greenwood P, Castillo-Chávez C, et al. Heavy drinking is increased by equally divided residence time in low- and high-risk environments. *Socio-economic planning sciences* 2008 (in press).
25. Holder HD. *Alcohol and the community: a systems approach to prevention*. Cambridge: Cambridge University Press, 1998.
26. Hawkins JD, Catalano RF, Miller JY. Risk and protective factors for alcohol and other drug problems in adolescence and early adulthood: implications for substance abuse prevention. *Psychol Bull* 1992;112(1):64–105.
27. Ammerman RT, Ott PJ, Tarter RE. *Prevention and societal impact of drug and alcohol abuse*. Mahwah, NJ: Lawrence Erlbaum, 1999.
28. Botvin GJ, Schinke SP, Orlandi MA. Psychosocial approaches to substance abuse prevention: theoretical foundations and empirical findings. *Crisis J Crisis Interv Suicide Prev* 1989;10:62–77.
29. Hansen WB. Prevention of alcohol use and abuse. *Prev Med* 1994;23: 683–687.
30. Perry CL, Kelder SH. Models for effective prevention. *J Adolesc Health* 1992;13:355–363.
31. Flay BR, Sobel JL. The role of mass media in preventing adolescent substance abuse. In: Glynn TJ, Leukefeld CG, Ludford JP, eds. *Preventing adolescent drug abuse: intervention strategies*. Rockville MD: National Institute on Drug Abuse, 1983:5–35.
32. Kumpfer KI. Prevention of alcohol and drug abuse: a critical review of risk factors and prevention strategies. In: D Shaffler, I Philips & N Enzer, eds. *Prevention of mental disorders, alcohol, and other drug use in children and adolescents*. Rockville, MD: Office of Substance Abuse Prevention, 1989:309–371.
33. Howard J. Community organizing, public policy and the prevention of alcohol problems. *Alcohol Clin Exp Res* 1996;20(Suppl 8):265A–269A.
34. Holder HD, Grube JW, Gruenewald PJ, et al. Community approaches to prevention of alcohol-related accidents. In: Watson RR, ed. *Drug and alcohol abuse reviews*, vol. 7: *Alcohol, cocaine, and accidents*. Totowa, NJ: Humana Press, Inc., 1995:175–194.
35. Pentz MA. Institutionalizing community-based prevention through policy change. *J Commun Psychol* 2000:28.
36. Wagenaar AC, Perry CL. Community strategies for the reduction of youth drinking: theory and application. *J Res Adolesc* 1994;4:319–345.
37. Caulkins JP. Measurement and analysis of drug problems and drug control efforts. In: D Duffee, ed. *Measurement and analysis of crime and justice*, vol. 4: *Criminal justice 2000*. Washington, DC: National Institute of Justice, 2000:391–449.
38. Hingson R, Howland J. Alcohol, injury, and legal controls: some complex interactions. *Law Med Health Care* 1989;17:58–68.
39. Holder HD, Gruenewald PJ, Ponicki WR, et al. Effect of community-based interventions on high risk drinking and alcohol-related injuries. *JAMA* 2000;284:2341–2347.
40. McCrady BS, Zucker RA, Brooke SG, et al. Social environmental influences on the development and resolution of alcohol problems. *Alcohol Clin Exp Res* 2006;30:688–699.
41. Wechsler H, Moeykens B, Davenport A, et al. The adverse impact of heavy episodic drinkers on other college students. *J Stud Alcohol* 1995;56:628–634.
42. Gruenewald PJ, Millar AB, Treno AJ, et al. The geography of availability and driving after drinking. *Addiction* 1996;91:967–983.
43. Grube JW. Preventing sales of alcohol to minors: results from a community trial. *Addiction* 1997;92:S251–S260.
44. Reuter P. Quantity illusions and paradoxes of drug interdiction: federal intervention into vice policy. *Law Contemp Probl* 1988;51:233–252.
45. Saltz RF, Stanghetta P. A community-wide responsible beverage service program in three communities: early findings. *Addiction* 1997;92:S237–S249.
46. Gruenewald PJ, Treno AJ. Local and global alcohol supply: economic and geographic models of community systems. *Addiction* 2000;95:S537–S545.
47. White HR, Gorman DM. Dynamics of the drug-crime relationship. In: LaFree G, ed. *Criminal justice 2000*, Vol. 1: *The nature of crime: continuity and change*. 2000:151–218. NIJ http://www.NCJRS.ORG/CRIMINAL_JUSTICE2000/vol_1/02D.pdf
48. Single E, Robson L, Xie X, et al. *The costs of substance abuse in Canada*. Ottawa, Canada: CCSA, 1996.
49. Harwood H, Fountain D, Livermore G. *The economic costs of alcohol and drug abuse in the United States, 1992*. Washington, DC: U.S. Government Printing Office, 1998.
50. Kreitman N. Alcohol consumption and the preventive paradox. *Br J Addict* 1986;81:353–363.
51. Homel R. *Policing for prevention: reducing crime, public intoxication and injury*. New York, NY: Criminal Justice Press, 1997.
52. Gruenewald PJ, Johnson FW, Millar A, et al. Drinking and driving: explaining beverage specific risks. *J Stud Alcohol* 2000;61:515–523.
53. Hennessy M, Saltz RF. Modeling social influences on public drinking. *J Stud Alcohol* 1993;54:139–145.
54. Reuter P, Caulkins JP. Redefining the goals of drug policy: report of a working group. *Am J Public Health* 1995;85:1059–1063.
55. Gruenewald PJ, Millar AB, Treno AJ. Alcohol availability and the ecology of drinking behavior. *Alcohol Health Res World* 1993;17: 39–45.
56. Stockwell T, Gruenewald PJ. Controls on the physical availability of alcohol. In: Heather N, Peters TJ. Stockwell T, eds. *International handbook of alcohol dependence and problems*. New York: John Wiley & Sons, Ltd., 2001:699–719.
57. O'Malley PM, Wagenaar AC. Effects of minimum drinking age laws on alcohol use, related behaviors and traffic crash involvement among American youth: 1976–1987. *J Stud Alcohol* 1991;52:478–491.
58. Kenkel D, Manning W. Perspectives on alcohol taxation. *Alcohol Health Res World* 1996;20:230–238.
59. Coate D, Grossman M. Effects of alcoholic beverage prices and legal drinking ages on youth alcohol use. *J Law Econ* 1988;31:145–171.
60. Laixuthai AF, Chaloupka FJ. Youth alcohol use and public policy. *Contemp Policy Issues* 1993;11:70–81.
61. Gruenewald PJ, Ponicki WR, Holder HD. The relationship of outlet densities to alcohol consumption: a time series cross-sectional analysis. *Alcohol Clin Exp Res* 1993;17:38–47.
62. Hennessy M, Saltz RF. The situational riskiness of alcoholic beverages. *J Stud Alcohol* 1990;51:422–427.
63. Wagenaar AC, Holder HD. The scientific process works: seven replications now show significant wine sales increases after privatization. *J Stud Alcohol* 1996;57:575–576.
64. Wagenaar AC, Murray DM, Gehan JP, et al. Communities mobilizing for change on alcohol: outcomes from a randomized community trial. *J Stud Alcohol* 2000;61:85–94.
65. Cook PJ, Tauchen G. Effect of liquor taxes on heavy drinking. *Bell J Econ* 1982;13:379–390.
66. Holder HD, Wagenaar AC. Mandated server training and reduced alcohol-involved traffic crashes: a time series analysis of the Oregon experience. *Accid Anal Prev* 1994;26:89–97.
67. Holder HD, Blose JO. Impact of changes in distilled spirits availability on apparent consumption: A time series analysis of liquor-by-the-drink. *Br J Addict* 1987;82:623–631.
68. Scribner RA, MacKinnon DP, Dwyer JH. Alcohol outlet density and motor vehicle crashes in Los Angeles County cities. *J Stud Alcohol* 1994;5:447–453.
69. Jewell RT, Brown RW. Alcohol availability and alcohol-related motor vehicle accidents. *Appl Econ* 1995;27:759–765.
70. LaScala EA, Gerber D, Gruenewald PJ. Demographic and environmental correlates of pedestrian injury collisions: a spatial analysis. *Accid Anal Prev* 2000;32:651–658.

71. LaScala EA, Johnson F, Gruenewald PJ. Neighborhood characteristics of alcohol-related pedestrian injury collisions: a geostatistical analysis. *Prev Sci* 2001;2:123–134.
72. Roncek DW, Maier PA. Bars, blocks, and crimes revisited: linking the theory of routine activities to the empiricism of "hot spots." *Criminology* 1991;29:725–753.
73. Scribner RA, MacKinnon DP, Dwyer JH. The risk of assaultive violence and alcohol availability in Los Angeles County. *Am J Public Health* 1995;85:335–340.
74. Stevenson RJ, Lind B, Weatherburn D. The relationship between alcohol sales and assault in New South Wales, Australia. *Addiction* 1999;94: 397–410.
75. Gorman D, Speer PW, Gruenewald PJ, et al. Spatial dynamics of alcohol availability, neighborhood structure and violent crime. *J Stud Alcohol* 2001;62:628–636.
76. Gruenewald PJ, Remer LG. Changes in outlet densities affect violence rates. *Alcohol Clin Exp Res* 2006;30:1184–1193.
77. Hingson R, McGovern T, Howland J, et al. Reducing alcohol impaired driving in Massachusetts: the Saving Lives program. *Am J Public Health* 1996;86:791–797.
78. Felson M. Routine activities and crime prevention in the developing metropolis. *Criminology* 1987;25:911–931.
79. Gruenewald PJ, Freisthler B, Remer LG, et al. Ecological models of alcohol outlets and violent assaults: Crime potentials and geospatial analysis. *Addiction* 2006;101(5):666–677.
80. Moore MH. Supply reduction and drug law enforcement. In: Tonry M, Wilson JQ, eds. *Drugs and crime,* Vol. 13: *Crime and justice: a review of research*. Chicago: University of Chicago Press, 1990.
81. Murray D. *Design and analysis of group-randomized trials*. New York: Oxford University Press, 1998.
82. Wagenaar AC, Toomey TL, Murray DM, et al. Sources of alcohol for underage drinkers. *J Stud Alcohol* 1996;57:325–333.
83. Holder HD, Saltz RF, Grube JW, et al. A community prevention trial to reduce alcohol-involved accidental injury and death: Overview. *Addiction*, 1997;92(Suppl 2):S155–S171.
84. Holder HD, Howard J, eds. *Community prevention trials for alcohol problems: methodological issues*. Westport, CT: Praeger Publishers, 1992.
85. Gruenewald PJ. Analysis approaches to community evaluation. *Eval Rev* 1997;21:209–230.
86. Treno AJ, Gruenewald PJ, Lee JP, et al. The Sacramento Neighborhood Alcohol Prevention Project: outcomes from a community prevention trial, *J Stud Alcohol Drugs* 2007;68(2):197–207.
87. Homel R, McIlwain G, Carvolth R. Creating safer drinking environments. In: Heather N, Peters TJ, Stockwell T, eds. *International handbook of alcohol dependence and problems*. Chichester, UK: John Wiley and Sons, 2001:721–740.
88. Hauritz M, Homel R, McIlwain G, et al. Reducing alcohol-related harm through local government safety action projects: the Queensland experience. *Contemp Drug Prob* 1998;25:511–551.
89. Hauritz M, Homel R, McIlwain G, et al. Reducing violence in licensed venues: community safety action projects. *Trends Issues Crime Justice* 1998;101:1–6.
90. Graham K, Homel R. Creating safer bars. In: Plant M, Single E, Stockwell T, eds. *Alcohol: minimising the harm*. London: Free Association Press, 1997:171–192.
91. Graham K, Jelley J, Purcell J. Training bar staff in preventing and managing aggression in licensed premises. *J Subst Use* 2005;10:48–61.
92. Wallin E, Gripenberg J, Andreasson S. Overserving at licensed premises in Stockholm: effects of a community action program. *J Stud Alcohol* 2005;66:806–815.
93. Wallin E, Norstrom T, Andreasson S. Alcohol prevention targeting licensed premises: a study of effects on violence. *J Stud Alcohol* 2003;64(2):270–277.
94. Freisthler B, Midanik LT, Gruenewald PJ. Alcohol outlets and child physical abuse and neglect: applying routine activities theory to the study of child maltreatment. *J Stud Alcohol* 2004;65:586–592.
95. Gruenewald PG. The spatial ecology of alcohol problems: niche theory and assortative drinking. *Addiction* 2007;102:870–878.
96. Voas RB, Holder HD, Gruenewald PJ. The effect of drinking and driving interventions on alcohol-involved traffic crashes within a comprehensive community trial. *Addiction* 1997;92:S221–S236.
97. Advisory Council on the Misuse of Drugs. *Drug use and the environment*. London: Her Majesty's Stationery Office, 1998.
98. Harrison LD, Backenheimer M. Research careers in unraveling the drug-crime nexus in the United States. *Subst Use Misuse* 1998;33: 1763–2003.
99. Chikritzhs T, Stockwell TR. The impact of later trading hours for Australian public houses (hotels) on levels of violence. *J Stud Alcohol* 2002;63:591–599.
100. Ragnarsdottir P, Kjartansdottir A, Davidsdottir S. Effect of extended alcohol serving hours in Reykyavik, Iceland. In: Room R, ed. *Effect of Nordic alcohol policies: what happens to drinking and harm when alcohol controls change?* Helsinki, Finland: Nordic Council for Alcohol and Drug research, 2002.
101. Duailibi S, Ponicki W, Grube J, et al. The effect of restricting opening hours on alcohol-related violence. *Am J Public Health* 2007;97: 2276–2280.
102. Norström T, Skog OJ. Saturday opening of alcohol retail shops in Sweden: an experiment in two phases. *Addiction* 2005;100:767–776.
103. Baker TK, Johnson MB, Voas RB, et al. To reduce youthful binge drinking: call an election in Mexico. *J Safety Res* 2000;31:61–69.
104. Lipton R, Gruenewald PJ. The spatial dynamics of violence and alcohol outlets. *J Stud Alcohol* 2002;63:187–195.
105. Parker RN, Rebhun LA. *Alcohol and homicide: a deadly combination of two American traditions*. Albany: State University of New York Press, 1995.
106. Zhu L, Gorman DM, Horel S. Alcohol outlet density and violence: a geospatial analysis, *Alcohol Alcohol* 2004;39:369–375.
107. Norström T. Outlet density and criminal violence in Norway, 1960–1995. *J Stud Alcohol* 2000;61:907–911.
108. Wagenaar A, Holder HD. Changes in alcohol consumption resulting from elimination of retail wine monopolies: results from five U.S. states, *J Stud Alcohol* 1995;56:566–572.
109. Trolldal B. *Availability and sales of alcohol: experiences from Canada and the U.S. Centre for Social Research on Alcohol and Drugs,* Dissertation Series #2. Stockholm: Almqvist & Wiksell International, 2005.
110. Wagenaar AC, Toomey TL. Effects of minimum drinking age laws: review and analyses of the literature from 1960–2000. *J Stud Alcohol* 2002;(Suppl)14:206–225.
111. Mosher JF. The impact of legal provisions on barroom behavior: toward an alcohol-problems prevention policy. *Alcohol Int Biomed J* 1984;1: 205–211.
112. Holder HD, Janes K, Mosher J, et al. Alcoholic beverage server liability and the reduction of alcohol-involved problems. *J Stud Alcohol* 1993;54:23–36.
113. Sloan FA, Stout EM, Whetten-Goldstein K, et al. *Drinkers, drivers, and bartenders: balancing private choices and public accountability*. Chicago: University of Chicago Press, 2000.
114. McKnight AJ, Voas RB. Prevention of alcohol-related road crashes. In: Heather N, Peters TJ, Stockwell T, eds. *International handbook of alcohol dependence and problems*. Chichester, UK: John Wiley and Sons, 2001: 741–770.
115. Voas RB, Lange J, Treno AJ. Documenting community-level outcomes: lessons from drinking and driving, *Eval Rev* 1997;21:191–208.
116. Haines B, Graham K. Violence prevention in licensed premises. In: Stockwell T, Gruenewald PJ, Toumbourou J, et al., eds. *Preventing harmful substance use: the evidence base for policy and practice*. New York: Wiley, 2005:163–176.
117. Maguire M, Nettleton H. *Reducing alcohol-related violence and disorder: an evaluation of the TASC project*. Home Office Research Study No. 265. London: Home Office, 2003.

SECTION 4

Overview of Addiction Treatment

CHAPTER 22

William L. White, MA

Addiction Medicine in America: Its Birth and Early History (1750–1935) with a Modern Postscript

The Birth of Addiction Medicine

The recent recognition of addiction medicine as a medical specialty obscures the fact that American physicians have been involved in the treatment of severe and persistent alcohol- and other drug-related problems for more than two centuries. This chapter describes the birth of addiction medicine in the late 18th century, the professionalization of addiction medicine in the second half of the 19th century, and the virtual collapse of addiction medicine as an organized specialty in the opening decades of the 20th century. The review includes early pioneers of addiction medicine, conceptual and clinical breakthroughs, the evolving settings in which addiction medicine was practiced, the larger currents in American medicine, and the evolving social policies that influenced the early practice of addiction medicine.

THE BIRTH OF ADDICTION MEDICINE

The roots of addiction medicine began not in a young America but in the ancient civilizations of Africa and Europe. Special methods to care for those addicted to alcohol were developed in ancient Egypt, and references to chronic drunkenness as a sickness that enslaved body and soul date to Heroditus (5th century BC), Aristotle (384–322 BC), and Seneca (4 BC–65 AD). St. John Chrysostom (1st century AD) provided one of the earliest comparisons of chronic alcohol inebriety to other diseases (1). These earliest intimations of the concept of addiction and its treatment reflect the fleeting observations of individuals rather than an organized cultural response to alcohol and other drug problems.

The earliest American medical responses to alcoholism emerged within the systems of medicine practiced by Native-American tribes. Alcohol-related problems rose dramatically in Native America as alcohol became increasingly used as a tool of economic, political, and sexual exploitation in the 18th and early 19th centuries (2,3). Native tribes actively resisted these problems through political/legal advocacy, organizing sobriety-based cultural revitalization movements and through the medical treatment of those affected. Native-American healers used botanical agents to suppress cravings for alcohol (hop tea), to induce an aversion to alcohol (the root of the trumpet vine), and to facilitate personal transformation within sobriety-based cultural and religious revitalization movements (4).

In colonial America, there was pervasive consumption of alcoholic beverages but no recognition of excessive drinking as a distinct medical problem (5). This changed in response to increased alcohol consumption (a near tripling of annual per capita alcohol consumption between 1780 and 1830), a shift in preference from fermented to more potent forms of distilled alcohol, and the emergence of a pattern of socially disruptive "frontier drinking" (6,7). It was in this changing context that several prominent Americans "discovered" the phenomenon of addiction (8).

In 1774, the philanthropist and social reformer Anthony Benezet published a treatise, *Mighty Destroyer Displayed*, that recast alcohol from its status as a gift from God to that of a "bewitching poison." He noted the presence of "unhappy dram-drinkers bound in slavery" and observed that drunkenness had a tendency to self-accelerate: "Drops beget drams, and drams beget more drams, till they become to be without weight or measure" (9).

Benezet's warning was followed by a series of publications by Dr. Benjamin Rush (1746–1813). Rush's work is particularly important given his prominence in colonial society and his role in the history of American medicine and psychiatry. Rush's 1784 pamphlet, *Inquiry into the Effects of Ardent Spirits on the Human Mind and Body*, was the first American treatise on alcoholism, and it almost single-handedly launched the American temperance movement. In this pamphlet, Rush catalogued the symptoms of acute and chronic drunkenness, described the progressiveness of these symptoms, and suggested that chronic drunkenness was a "disease induced by a vice" (10). Rush was the first prominent physician to claim that many confirmed drunkards could be restored to full health and responsible citizenship through proper medical treatment and to call for the creation of a special facility (a "Sober House") to care for the drunkard (11).

Rush's writings were mirrored in the work of physicians in other countries, most notably the Edinburgh physician, Dr. Thomas Trotter, whose 1788 publication, *Essay, Medical Philosophical, and Chemical, on Drunkenness and its Effects on the Human Body,* shared many of Rush's ideas (12). Another contribution that influenced the subsequent development of addiction medicine in America was the work of Christopher Wilhelm Hufeland, who in 1819 described a clinical condition characterized by uncontrollable cravings for alcoholic spirits that triggered periodic "drink storms." Hufeland labeled this condition *dipsomania*. During the same decade, Lettsom, Armstrong, and Pearson described the condition that Thomas Sutton subsequently christened *delirium tremens* (13).

By the late 1820s, the subject of chronic drunkenness was taken up in a number of medical dissertations. Most notable among these were the works of Drs. Daniel Drake and William Sweetser. Drake speculated on the causes of "habitual drinking," elaborated on Rush's list of systems of the body effected by alcohol, and hinted at what would later become the concepts of *inability to abstain* and *loss of control* ("the habit being once established, he will not, I almost say cannot, refrain") (14). In 1828, Sweetser provided a detailed account of the pathophysiology of chronic alcohol intoxication, including depictions of the addictiveness of alcohol and the potential role of heredity in chronic drunkenness. He concluded that intemperance created a "morbid alteration" in nearly all the major structures and functions of the human body. Cycles of compulsive drinking were viewed by Sweetser as the product of a devastating paradox: The poison (alcohol) was itself its only antidote (15).

The 1827 publication of the Reverend Lyman Beecher's *Six Sermons on the Nature, Occasion, Signs, and Remedy of Intemperance* exerted their own influence on the emerging concept of addiction. Bridging the gap between moral and medical models, Beecher described the intemperate as being "addicted to the sin" and suffering from an "insatiable desire for drink." Beecher provided two other contributions to this developing concept. First, he described the early warning signs of addiction, linking these to the later signs that Rush, Drake, Sweetser, and others had catalogued. Second, he challenged these very physicians who, in the case of Rush, had tried to get their patients to moderate their drinking by switching from distilled alcohol to fermented drinks such as wine or beer. Beecher's declaration, "There is no remedy for intemperance but the cessation of it" marked the call for complete abstinence as a personal and social strategy for the resolution of alcohol problems (16).

Between 1774 and 1829, America "discovered" addiction through the collective observations of her physicians, clergy, and social activists. There was an emerging view that chronic drunkenness was a problem with biologic roots and consequences and thus the province of the physician. These earliest pioneers declared that chronic intoxication was a diseased state, and they articulated the major elements of an addiction disease concept: biologic predisposition, drug toxicity, pharmacologic tolerance, disease progression, morbid appetite (craving), loss of volitional control of alcohol/drug intake, and the pathophysiologic consequences of sustained alcohol and opiate ingestion. Though their treatments could involve such "heroic" methods as purging, blistering, bleeding, and the use of highly toxic medicines, they also used surprisingly modern strategies (e.g., aversive conditioning) and recognized many pathways to the initiation of sobriety (e.g., from religious conversion to witnessing an alcohol-related death). The writings of this period portray addiction recovery not as an enduring process but as a climactic decision. This view focused the attention of the emerging temperance movement on the pledge of lifetime abstinence (from distilled alcohol) as a central strategy in their early attempts at rescue work with confirmed drunkards.

Addiction medicine emerged in the shift from treating medical consequences of alcohol addiction to treating the addiction itself. The earliest practice of addiction medicine predated institutional treatment and was practiced out of the private offices of individual physicians. Alcohol was not the only drug of concern to these physicians. During the 16th and 17th centuries, physicians in Germany, Holland, Portugal, and England had begun to conceptualize opium as "a kind of poison" that required regular and increasing use that, when stopped, created a unique sickness that drove people to return to the drug (17). In 1701, the English physician, John Jones, provided an exceptionally detailed account of opiate withdrawal in his book, *The Mysteries of the Opium Reveal'd* (18). Three events between the early and mid-19th century profoundly altered the future of narcotic addiction in America: the isolation of morphine from opium, the introduction of the hypodermic syringe, and the emergence of a patent drug industry. These events produced drugs of greater potency, created a more efficient and euphorigenic method of drug ingestion, and increased the availability and promotion of powerful psychoactive drugs (19,20).

Early Professionalization and Medical Advancements (1830–1900) In 1828, Dr. Eli Todd, superintendent of the Hartford Retreat for the Insane, called for the creation of a physician-directed inebriate asylum. Under his influence, the Connecticut State Medical Society passed a resolution supporting this idea in 1830 (21). A year later, Dr. Samuel Woodward, superintendent at the Hospital for the Insane at Worcester, Massachusetts, wrote a series of influential essays echoing the Connecticut recommendations. He declared:

> *A large proportion of the intemperate in a well-conducted institution would be radically cured, and would again go into society with health reestablished, diseased appetites removed, with principles of temperance well grounded and thoroughly understood, so that they would be afterwards safe and sober men* (22).

Woodward argued that intemperance was a physical disease requiring medical remedies and, breaking with Rush, declared that "the grand secret of the cure for intemperance is total abstinence from alcohol in all its forms" (22). This total abstinence position was given greater weight in light of the failed efforts to cure drunkards through the use of public pledges to refrain only from distilled alcohol. The number of drunkards who continued their debauchery through fermented alcoholic drinks contributed to the temperance movement's shift from the partial pledge to the T-total pledge (23).

What followed in the 1830s and 1840s was a series of clinical contributions to the understanding of chronic drunkenness that exerted considerable influence on the emerging field of addiction medicine (24). First, there were new experiments and clinical observations on the pathophysiology of alcohol, such as those of Prout, Beaumont, and Percy on the effects of alcohol on the stomach and the blood (25). Dr. Robert Macnish's *Anatomy of Drunkenness* (1835) offered one of the earliest typologies of alcohol addiction, noting seven clinical subtypes (26). Macnish also referenced a subject that continued as a medical controversy for much of the 19th century: the claimed spontaneous combustion of alcohol inebriates (27,28).

In 1838, France's leading expert on drunkenness, Dr. Esquirol, argued that the disease of intemperance was a "monomania"—a "mental illness whose principle character is an irresistible tendency toward fermented beverages" (29). This was followed in 1840 by Dr. R.B. Grinrod's text, *Bacchus*, in which he declared, "I am more than ever convinced that drunkenness is a disease, physical as well as moral, and consequently requires physical as well as moral remedies" (30–32).

One of the most significant milestones in the history of addiction medicine was the 1849 publication of Magnus Huss's text, *Chronic Alcoholism*. After an extensive review of the chronic effects of intoxication, Huss declared:

> *These symptoms are formed in such a particular way that they form a disease group in themselves and thus merit being designated and described as a definite disease . . . It is this group of symptoms which I wish to designate by the name Alcoholismus chronicus* (33,34).

Huss's text stands as the landmark addiction medicine text of the mid-19th century. It contributed a clinical term—*alcoholism*—that came into increasing medical and public popularity in the transition between the 19th and 20th centuries.

The Washingtonian Revival of the 1840s and the fraternal temperance societies and reform clubs that followed brought the issue of recovery from alcoholism onto center cultural stage. Local Washingtonian groups encountering "hard cases" needing more than an occasional sobriety support meeting began organizing lodging houses that evolved into America's first addiction treatment institutions. A multibranched treatment field emerged in the mid-19th century. Inebriate homes emerged out of alcoholic mutual aid societies that viewed addiction recovery as a process of moral reformation (35). There were medically-directed inebriate asylums, the first of which was the New York State Inebriate Asylum, chartered in 1857 and opened in 1864, under the leadership of Dr. Joseph Turner (36,37). There were also privately franchised, for-profit addiction cure institutions such as the Keeley, Neal, Gatlin, and Oppenheimer Institutes. These institutions generated considerable controversy over their claim to have medicinal specifics that could cure addiction (38) and their practice of hiring physicians who were in recovery from addiction (39,40). Inebriate homes and asylums and the private addiction cure institutes competed with bottled patent medicine addiction cures (most containing alcohol, opium, morphine, or cocaine), some of which were promulgated by physicians, and religiously sponsored inebriate colonies and rescue missions (21). By the late 1870s, large urban hospitals, such as Bellevue Hospital in New York City, had also started opening inebriate wards (41). Annual alcoholic admissions at Bellevue rose to 4,190 by 1895—a number that continued to climb to more than 11,300 per year in the opening decade of the 20th century (21).

In 1870, Dr. Joseph Parrish led the creation of the American Association for the Cure of Inebriety (AACI), which brought together the heads of America's most prominent inebriate homes and asylums. The AACI by-laws posited that

> *1. Intemperance is a disease. 2. It is curable in the same sense that other diseases are. 3. Its primary cause is a constitutional susceptibility to the alcoholic impression. 4. This constitutional tendency may be either inherited or acquired* (42).

The AACI held regular meetings to exchange ideas and published the first specialized medical journal on addiction—the Journal of Inebriety. The Journal, edited by Dr. T. D. Crothers during its entire publication life (1876–1914), was filled with essays by addiction medicine specialists and with advertisements promoting various treatment institutions (43,44). A similar inebriety treatment movement was under way in Europe during the last decades of the 19th century, and the first international meetings of addiction medicine specialists were held during this period (45).

American physicians specializing in addiction began releasing texts on the nature of addiction and their treatment methods in the 1860s: Dr. Albert Day's *Methomania: A Treatise on Alcoholic Poisoning and Dr. W. Marcet's On Chronic Alcoholic Intoxication.* The production of such literature virtually exploded in the 1880s and 1890s. Among the most prominent texts either written in America or that exerted a significant influence on the practice of addiction medicine in America during this period were Dr. H. H. Kane's *Drugs That Enslave: The Opium, Morphine, Chloral and Hashish Habits;* Dr. Fred Hubbard's *The Opium Habit and Alcoholism;* Dr. Joseph Parrish's *Alcoholic Inebriety: From a Medical Standpoint with Cases from Clinical Records;* Dr. Asa Meyerlet's *Notes on the Opium Habit;* Dr. T. L. Wright's *Inebriism;* Franklin Clum's *Inebriety: Its Causes, Its Results, Its Remedy;* Dr. T. D. Crothers' *The Disease of Inebriety from Alcohol, Opium and Other Narcotic Drugs;* Dr. Norman Kerr's *Inebriety or Narcomania: Its Etiology, Pathology, Treatment and Jurisprudence;* and Dr. Charles Palmer's *Inebriety: Its Source, Prevention, and Cure* (21).

The central organizing concept of 19th-century addiction medicine specialists was that of *inebriety*. Inebriety was viewed as a disease that manifested itself in numerous varieties. These varieties were meticulously detailed by clinical subpopulation and drug choice. Addiction medicine texts were often organized under such headings as *alcoholic inebriety, opium inebriety, cocaine inebriety*, and *ether inebriety*. Inebriety was viewed as a disease that sprang from multiple etiologic pathways, unfolded in many diverse patterns, and had a variable course and outcome. Inebriety specialists talked eloquently about the need to individualize treatment and, by the 1880s, had begun to recognize and study the problem of posttreatment relapse (46).

The treatment methods of the two physician-directed branches of the inebriety movement (the inebriate asylums and the private addiction cure institutes) were quite different, and the conflicts between these branches reflected allopathic and homeopathic approaches to medicine in this period. The inebriate asylum physicians advocated a sustained (1 to 3 years), legally enforced course of treatment that consisted of drug-assisted detoxification, collateral medical treatments, and a sustained period of institutional convalescence. The addiction cure institute physicians boasted medicinal specifics (daily hypodermic injections and liquid tonics) that could "unpoison" the addict's cells, destroy the craving and compulsion to use alcohol, opiates, and cocaine—all in 4 short weeks—cash in advance. Drug treatments within both branches included such substances as cannabis, cocaine, chloral hydrate, paraldehyde, strychnine, atropine, hyoscine, and apomorphine. Although some addiction medicine specialists used cocaine as a tonic during detoxification, most warned of the addictive properties of the drug (21).

Most inebriate asylums and addiction cure institutes treated all drug addictions, whereas others, such as Dr. Jansen Mattison's Brooklyn Home for Habitues (opened in 1891), specialized in the treatment of opiate and cocaine addiction (47). The inebriety literature of this period is filled with debates over whether medically supervised opiate withdrawal should be abrupt, rapid (over days), or sustained (over weeks and months). One also finds discussions of such contemporary issues as the addictiveness and psychologic toxicity of cocaine, problems of drug substitution, and the management of the relapsed patient (45).

Understanding of the potential physiologic foundations and consequences of addiction increased during the last two decades of the 19th century. Carl Wernicke's 1881 discovery of a psychosis with polyneuritis that resulted from chronic alcoholism and Sergei Korsakoff's 1887 description of an alcoholism-induced psychosis characterized by confusion, memory impairment, confabulation, hallucinations, and stereotyped and superficial speech both underscored the potential organic basis of alcoholic behavior. There was considerable discussion about the potential hereditary transmission of inebriety, as there is today. Between 1899 and 1903, there were also antibody theories of alcoholism that led to experiments with an alcoholism vaccine called *equizine* (48).

A new addiction-related medical society was founded in 1891. The American Medical Temperance Association (AMTA) was formed in Washington, D.C. at the annual meeting of the American Medical Association (AMA). Dr. N. S. Davis of Chicago was its founder and first president. The AMTA published the *Bulletin of the American Medical Temperance Association* under the editorship of Dr. J. H. Kellogg, director of the Battle Creek Sanatarium. (49).

In summary, the field of addiction medicine experienced professionalization and specialization between 1830 and 1900. There were many addiction medicine pioneers who founded medically directed treatment institutions, men such as Turner, Parrish, Crothers, Day, and later, Dr. Agnes Sparks, one of the first female physicians specializing in addiction medicine. The practice of addiction medicine shifted from the private physician's practice to the institutional setting. Within this institutional practice, there was a growing understanding of the physiologic consequences of chronic alcoholism and an extension of the concept of inebriety to embrace dependence upon opium, morphine, cocaine, chloral hydrate, chloroform, and ether. There was a well-articulated addiction disease concept with elaborate protocol for detoxification and rehabilitation, though there was considerable conflict between allopathic and homeopathic approaches to addiction treatment.

The growing field of addiction medicine was infused with optimism in the early 1890s. Dr. T. D. Crothers proclaimed, "The future looks promising, and it is believed that the public will support inebriate asylums with increasing generosity" (50). There were reasons for Crothers' optimism. There was a well-articulated disease concept of inebriety and two addiction-related medical organizations that embraced a field that had grown from a handful of specialized treatment institutions in 1870 to several hundred by the turn of the century. But forces outside the medical profession that were stirring would drive a wedge between the physician and those addicted to alcohol and other drugs.

Demedicalization and the Collapse of Addiction Treatment (1900–1935) There was a further profusion of addiction medicine texts in the first decade of the 20th century: J. B. Mattison's *The Mattison Method in Morphinism: A Modern and Human Treatment of the Morphine Disease*; T. D. Crothers's *The Drug Habits and their Treatment*; T. D. Crothers's *Morphinism*; and George Cutten's *The Psychology of Alcoholism*. The proliferation of addiction literature couldn't hide the fact that America's response to alcohol and other drug problems was shifting. Between 1900 and 1920, addiction treatment institutions closed in great numbers in the wake of a weakened infrastructure of the field, rising therapeutic pessimism, economic austerity triggered by unexpected depressions, and a major shift in national policy. The country turned its gaze to state and national prohibition laws as the solution to alcohol and other drug-related problems.

As inebriate homes and asylums and the private addiction cure institutes closed in tandem with the spread of local and state prohibition laws, alcoholics were relegated to other institutions. These included the "foul wards" of large city hospitals, the back wards of aging state psychiatric asylums, and the local psychopathic hospital, all of which did everything possible to discourage the admission of alcoholics. Wealthy alcoholics/addicts sought discrete detoxification in a new genre of private hospital or sanitarium established for this purpose. These latter institutions were known as "dip shops" (derived from the term *dipsomania*), "jitter joints," or "jag-farms" (21). There were also efforts to integrate medicine, religion, and psychology in the treatment of alcoholism, most notably within the Emmanuel Clinics in New England (51). For all but the most affluent, the management of the alcoholic shifted from a strategy of treatment to a strategy of control and punishment via inebriate penal colonies. The large public hospitals also bore much of the responsibility for the medical care of the chronic alcoholic (52).

The shift from viewing the alcoholic as a diseased person in need of help to a person of weak character was reflected in the medical literature of the early 20th century. Kurtz and Kraepelin coined the term *alcohol addiction* to depict those whose will was "not strong enough to abandon the use of alcohol even if drinking causes them serious economic, social and somatic changes" (34). Addiction medicine organizations struggled in this shifting cultural climate. The AMTA and the American Association for the Study and Cure of Inebriety merged in 1904 to create the American Medical Society for the Study of Alcohol and Other Narcotics. In 1906, the Scientific Temperance Federation was founded by Dr. T. D. Crothers and Frances Stoddard. The Federation published the *Scientific Temperance Journal.* A year later, the *Journal of Inebriety* merged with *The Archives of Physiological Therapy.* This marked the progressive demise of both the *Journal of Inebriety* and its parent organization. The last issue of the *Journal of Inebriety* was published in 1914, and the American Association for the Study and Cure of Inebriety collapsed in the early 1920s after passage of the Volstead Act and the subsequent sharp decline in demand for treatment. Alcohol-related problems decreased dramatically in the early 1920s but rose to pre-prohibition levels by the late 1920s (21). The 18th Amendment to the U.S. Constitution transferred cultural ownership of alcohol problems from physicians to law enforcement authorities. A similar process was underway with drugs other than alcohol, but it took two decades for this shift in approach to fully emerge.

Early 20th-century addiction texts by physicians such as George Pettey and Ernest Bishop boldly proclaimed that narcotic addiction was a disease, and Dr. Foster Kennedy declared that morphinism was "a disease, in the majority of cases, initiated, sustained and left uncured by members of the medical profession" (53–55). Physicians such as Dr. Charles Terry and Dr. Willis Butler had already begun operationalizing this addiction disease concept by advocating and offering clinic-directed detoxification and maintenance of incurable narcotic addicts (56–59). The medical treatment of narcotic addicts was dramatically altered by passage of the Harrison Anti-Narcotic Act of 1914. This federal act designated physicians and pharmacists as the gatekeepers for the distribution of opiates and cocaine. Although this law was not presented as a prohibition law, a series of Supreme Court interpretations of the Harrison Act (particularly the 1919 *Webb vs. the United States* case) declared that for a physician to maintain an addict on his or her customary dose is not in "good faith" medical practice under the Harrison Act and therefore an indictable offense (19).

There was one brief opportunity to alter the subsequent history of narcotic control policy and the history of addiction. It came in the form of the France Bill, which was introduced in Congress in 1919. This proposed legislation would have provided federal support for physician-directed, community-based treatment of narcotic addicts. The Bill did not have enough support to come to a vote. Despite this lack of federal leadership, physicians in 44 communities operated morphine maintenance clinics between 1919 and 1924. These clinics, which were sponsored by local health departments and even local police departments, all eventually closed under threat of federal indictment (19,21). The Harrison Act, in effect if not intent, transferred responsibility for the care of addicts from physicians to criminal syndicates and the criminal justice system by threatening physicians with both loss of license and incarceration if they provided maintenance rather than rapid detoxification of addicts (60).

Physician culpability in the problem of narcotic addiction made it difficult for the AMA to oppose this government infringement in medical practice. In 1919, the AMA passed a resolution opposing ambulatory treatment, in effect opposing narcotic maintenance as treatment. There were, however, many physicians who became harsh critics of the Harrison Act and this new era of criminalization. Such criticism was reflected in the new addiction medicine texts that emerged in the 1920s, such as Dr. Ernest Bishop's *The Narcotic Drug Problem* and Dr. E. H. Williams's *Opiate Addiction: Its Handling and Treatment* (61–63).

The influence of psychiatry on the characterization and treatment of addiction increased in tandem with the decline of a specialized field of addiction medicine. Karl Abraham's 1908 essay, *The Psychological Relations between Sexuality and Alcoholism*, marked the shift from seeing alcoholism as a primary medical disorder to seeing the condition as a symptom of underlying psychiatric disturbance (64). Abraham's essay marked a long series of psychoanalytic writings that viewed alcoholism as a manifestation of latent homosexuality. In the mid-1920s, Public Health Service psychiatrist, Dr. Lawrence Kolb, published a series of articles challenging earlier physiologic explanations of narcotic addiction. Kolb portrayed addiction as a product of defects in personality—a characterization that reflected the growing portrayal of addicts as psychopathic and constitutionally inferior (65). The first American Standard Classified Nomenclature of Disease (1933) included the diagnoses of "alcohol addiction," "alcoholism without psychosis," and "drug addiction" and classified these conditions as personality disorders (66).

Few institutional resources existed for the treatment of alcoholism and narcotic addiction during the 1920s and early 1930s, but the growing visibility of these problems began to generate new proposals for their management. The opening of the California Narcotics Hospital at Spadra in 1928 marked the beginning of state support for addiction treatment (67). Physicians working within the federal prison system were writing about the problems posed by a growing population of incarcerated addicts and advocating more specialized treatment of the addict (68).

There were important addiction-related research studies in the 1920s. Drs. Arthur B. Light and Edward G. Torrance conducted research on opiate addicts at the Philadelphia General Hospital under the auspices of the Philadelphia Committee for Clinical Study of Opium Addiction Research. They demonstrated that withdrawal from opiates is not life threatening and usually not dangerous—a finding that was misused by policy makers to withhold medical care for addicts (69). In 1928, the Bureau of Social Hygiene published Charles Terry and Mildred Pellens' work, *The Opium Problem* (70). In this important report, Terry and Pellens made a strong argument in favor of addiction maintenance as the most appropriate treatment for addicts who are not able to sustain abstinence. Their views were viciously attacked, and it would only be years later that *The Opium Problem* would be recognized as one of the best treatises on opiate addiction ever written (58).

Medical treatments for narcotic addiction in the first 3 decades of the 20th century continued to focus on managing the mechanics of narcotic withdrawal. Heroin was briefly used in the detoxification of morphine addicts, and its subsequent emergence as the drug of preference among addicts bred caution in the choice of any narcotic as a withdrawal agent. This fear of exposing patients to other addicting agents led to experimentation with a wide variety of nonnarcotic withdrawal procedures. These procedures included various belladonna treatments (scopolamine and hyoscine) that were known to induce hallucinations; peptization treatments (sodium thiocyanate) that could induce long-lasting psychosis; sleep treatments (sodium bromide) that had a 20% mortality rate; injected Narcosan—a lipoid treatment thought to eliminate toxins and stimulate new blood formation but which actually worsened withdrawal; insulin treatments that had no effect on the withdrawal process; and serum and blood therapies in which either previously drawn blood or serum (the latter drawn from induced blisters) was reinjected as a purported aid to detoxification (71–73).

The first decades of the 20th century were marked by a profound therapeutic pessimism regarding treatment of alcoholism and narcotic addiction. Biological views of addiction fell out of favor and were replaced by psychiatric and criminal models that placed the source of addiction within the addict's character and argued for the control and sequestration of the addict.

The Rebirth of Addiction Treatment (1935–1970)

After the early 20th-century collapse of systems of care for those addicted to alcohol and other drugs, addiction medicine was revived within the larger context of two movements.

The "modern alcoholism movement" was ignited by the founding of Alcoholics Anonymous (1935), a new scientific approach to alcohol problems in post-Repeal America led by the Research Council on Problems of Alcohol (1937) and the Yale Center of Alcohol Studies (1943) and by a national recovery advocacy effort led by the National Committee for Education on Alcoholism (1944). Two goals of this movement were to encourage local hospitals to detoxify alcoholics and to encourage local communities to establish post-hospitalization alcoholism rehabilitation centers (74). This movement spawned new institutional resources for the treatment of alcoholism from the mid-1940s through the 1960s, including "AA wards" in local hospitals, model outpatient alcoholism clinics developed in Connecticut and Georgia, and a model community-based residential model pioneered by three alcoholism programs in Minnesota: Pioneer House (1948), Hazelden (1949), and Willmar State Hospital (1950). Dr. Nelson Bradley, who led the developments at Willmar, later adapted the Minnesota Model for delivery within a community hospital. That adapted model was franchised throughout the United States in the 1980s via Parkside Medical Services and was replicated by innumerable hospital-based treatment programs.

The spread of these models nationally was aided by efforts to legitimize the work of physicians in the treatment of alcoholism. Early milestones in this movement included landmark resolutions on alcoholism passed by the AMA (1952, 1956, 1967) and the American Hospital Association (1944, 1951, 1957) that paved the way for hospital-based treatment of alcoholism. The former were championed by Dr. Marvin Block, chairman of the AMA's first Committee on Alcoholism. Mid-century alcoholism treatments included nutritional therapies, brief experiments with chemical and electroconvulsive therapies, psychosurgery and new drug therapies, including the use of disulfiram (Antabuse), stimulants, sedatives, tranquilizers, and LSD (21).

A mid-20th-century reform movement advocating medical rather than penal treatment of the opiate addict also helped spawn the rebirth of addiction medicine. This began with the founding of state-sponsored addiction treatment hospitals (e.g., Spadra Hospital in California) and led to the creation of two U.S. Public Health Hospitals within the Bureau of Prisons—one in Lexington, Kentucky (1935), the other in Fort Worth, Texas (1938). Many of the pioneers of modern addiction medicine and addiction research—Drs. Marie Nyswander, Jerry Jaffe, George Vaillant, Patrick Hughes—received their initial training at these facilities. The documentation of relapse rates after community reentry from Lexington and Forth Worth confirmed the need for community-based treatment. Three replicable models of treatment emerged: ex-addict directed therapeutic communities, methadone maintenance pioneered by Drs. Vincent Dole and Marie Nyswander, and outpatient drug-free counseling (21).

State and federal funding for alcoholism and addiction treatment slowly increased from the late 1940s through the 1960s and was followed by landmark legislation in the early 1970s that created the NIAAA and the National Institute on Drug Abuse (NIDA)—the beginning of the federal, state, and local community partnership that has been the foundation of modern addiction treatment. Parallel efforts were under way to provide insurance coverage for the treatment of alcoholism and other drug dependencies. The expansion of such insurance coverage in the 1960s and 1970s and the establishment of accreditation standards for addiction treatment programs by the Joint Commission on Accreditation of Hospitals set the stage for the dramatic growth of hospital-based and free-standing, private addiction treatment programs in the 1980s. NIAAA and NIDA also made heavy investments in research that led to dramatic breakthroughs in understanding the neurobiology of addiction that encouraged more medicalized approaches to severe alcohol and other drug problems (75).

The growing sophistication of addiction science was aided by other key organizations. The College of Problems of Drug Dependence, which dates from the Committee on Problems of Drug Dependence established in 1929, hosts an annual scientific meeting and publishes the journal *Drug & Alcohol Dependence*. The Research Society on Alcoholism, founded in 1976, also holds an annual scientific conference and publishes the journal *Alcoholism: Clinical and Experimental Research*.

Addiction Medicine Comes of Age (1970–2008)

The reemergence of addiction medicine as a clinical specialty of medical practice has been significantly advanced by two professional associations: the American Society of Addiction Medicine (ASAM) and the American Academy of Addiction Psychiatry (AAAP).

The ASAM can trace its roots to the establishment of the creation of a New York City Medical Committee on Alcoholism in 1951 by the National Council on Alcoholism, the 1954 founding of the New York State Medical Society on Alcoholism under the leadership of Dr. Ruth Fox, and the movement of this group in 1967 to establish itself as a national organization—the American Medical Society on Alcoholism (AMSA). AMSA was later evolved into the American Medical Society on Alcoholism and Other Drug Dependencies and then into the ASAM.

ASAM's achievements include the following:

- advocating the AMA's addition of addiction medicine to its list of designated specialties (achieved in June 1990)
- offering a certification and recertification process for addiction medicine specialists based on the early work of the California Society of Addiction Medicine
- hosting its annual addiction medicine conference
- publishing its widely utilized patient placement criteria
- development of the *Principles of Addiction Medicine*
- publishing first the *Journal of Addictive Diseases* and presently the *Journal of Addiction Medicine*

ASAM has been very influential in establishing addiction medicine as a legitimate medical specialty. There are currently more than 4,000 ASAM-certified physicians.

The AAAP (formerly the American Academy of Psychiatrists in Alcoholism and the Addictions) was established in 1985 with the goal of elevating the quality of clinical practice in addiction psychiatry. The AAAP's contributions include successfully advocating that the American Board of Psychiatry and Neurology grant addiction medicine a subspecialty status (1991), administering an addiction psychiatry certification and recertification process, hosting an annual conference on addiction psychiatry, publishing the *American Journal on Addictions*, and promoting fellowships in addiction psychiatry (76).

Several additional initiatives have advanced addiction-related medical education. The NIAAA and the NIDA created the Career Teacher Program (1971–1981) that develop addiction-related curricula for the training of physicians in 59 U.S. medical schools. In 1976, Career Teachers and others involved in addiction-related medical education and research established the Association of Medical Education and Research in Substance Abuse (AMERSA). AMERSA draws its members primarily from American medical school faculty, hosts an annual meeting, and publishes the journal *Substance Abuse*. In 1980, the Consortium for Medical Fellowships in Alcoholism and Drug Abuse was established to promote addiction-focused research and teaching specialists.

Today (2008), there are more than 14,400 physicians working within a network of 13,200 specialized addiction treatment programs in the United States who help care for the more than 1.9 million individuals and families admitted for treatment each year (77). As this history has reviewed, addiction medicine rose in the United States in the mid-19th century, collapsed in the opening decades of the 20th century, but reemerged and became increasingly professionalized in the late 20th and early 21st centuries.

REFERENCES

1. Crothers TD. *The disease of inebriety from alcohol, opium and other narcotic drugs: Its etiology, pathology, treatment and medico-legal relations*. New York: E. B. Treat, Publisher, 1893.
2. Mancall P. *Deadly medicine: Indians and alcohol in early America*. Ithica, New York: Cornell University Press, 1995.
3. Unrau W. *White man's wicked water: The alcohol trade and prohibition in Indian country, 1802–1892*. Lawrence: University Press of Kansas, 1996.
4. Coyhis D, White W. *Alcohol problems in native America: The untold story of resistance and recovery*. Colorado Springs, CO: White Bison, Inc., 2006.
5. Lender M, Martin J. *Drinking in America*. New York: The Free Press, 1982.
6. Rorabaugh W. *The alcoholic republic: An American tradition*. Oxford: Oxford University Press, 1979.
7. Winkler AM. Drinking on the American frontier. *Q J Stud Alcohol* 1968; 29:413–445.
8. Levine H. The discovery of addiction: Changing conceptions of habitual drunkenness in America. *J Stud Alcohol* 1978;39(2):143–174.
9. Benezet A. *A lover of mankind. Mighty destroyer displayed in some account, of the dreadful havock made by the mistaken use as well as abuse of distilled spirituous liquors*. Philadelphia: Joseph Crukshank, 1774.
10. Rush B. *An inquiry into the effect of ardent spirits upon the human body and mind, with an account of the means of preventing and of the remedies for curing them*, 8th rev. ed. Brookfield, MA: E. Merriam & Co., 1814.
11. Rush B. Plan for an asylum for drunkards to be called the Sober House. Reprinted in: Corner G (ed.). *The autobiography of Benjamin Rush*. Princeton: Princeton University Press, 1948.
12. Trotter T. *Essay, medical philosophical, and chemical aspects of drunkenness: Thesis*. Edinburgh: University of Edinburgh, 1788.
13. Romano J. Early contributions to the study of delirium tremens. *Ann Med Hist* 1941;3:128–139.
14. Drake D. A discourse on intemperance. In: Grob G (ed.). *Nineteenth century medical attitudes toward alcohol addiction*. New York: Arno Press, 1981:54.

15. Sweetser W. A dissertation on intemperance. In: Grob G (ed.). *Nineteenth century medical attitudes toward alcohol addiction.* New York: Arno Press, 1981.
16. Beecher L. *Six sermons on the nature, occasions, signs, evils and remedy of intemperance,* 3rd ed. Boston: T. R. Martin, 1828.
17. Sonnedecker G. Emergence of the concept of opiate addiction. *J Mondial Pharm* 1962;3:275–290.
18. Jones J. *The mysteries of the opium reveal'd.* London: Printed for Richard Smith, 1701.
19. Musto D. *The American disease: Origins of narcotic controls.* New Haven: Yale University Press, 1973.
20. Howard-Jones N. A critical study of the origins and early development of hypodermic medication. *J Hist Med* 1947;Spring:201–249.
21. White W. *Slaying the dragon: The history of addiction treatment and recovery in America.* Bloomington, IL: Chestnut Health Systems, 1998.
22. Woodward, SB. Essays on asylums for inebriates (1836). In: Grog, G. (ed.). *Nineteenth-century medical attitudes toward alcohol addiction.* New York: Arno Press, 1981.
23. Blair H. *The temperance movement.* Boston: William E. Smythe Company, 1888.
24. Bynum W. Chronic alcoholism in the first half of the 19th century. *Bull Hist Med* 1968;42:160–185.
25. Wilkerson A. *A history of the concept of alcoholism as a disease* [DSW dissertation]. University of Pennsylvania, Philadelphia, PA:1966.
26. MacNish R. *Anatomy of drunkenness.* New York: William Pearson & Co., 1835.
27. Oliver J. Spontaneous combustion. *Bull Med Hist* 1936;4:559–572.
28. Jellinek EM. Scientific views on the spontaneous combustion of alcoholics. *Q J Stud Alcohol* 1942;2:804–805.
29. Paredes A. The history of the concept of alcoholism. In: Tarter R, Sugerman A (eds.). *Alcoholism: Interdisciplinary approaches to an enduring problem,* 3rd ed. Reading, MA: Addison-Wesley, 1976:9–52.
30. Grindrod R. *Bacchus: An essay on the nature, causes, effects and cure of intemperance.* Columbus, OH: J & H Miller, Publisher, 1840.
31. Grindrod R. *Bacchus: An essay on the nature, causes, effects and cure of intemperance.* Columbus, OH: J & H Miller, Publisher, 1886.
32. Hargreaves W. *Alcohol and science.* New York: National Temperance Society and Publication House, 1884.
33. Huss M. *Alcoholismus chronicus: Chronisk alcoholisjudkom: Ett bidrag till dyskrasiarnas känndom.* Stockholm: Bonner/Norstedt, 1849.
34. Marconi J. The concept of alcoholism. *Q J Stud Alcohol* 1959;20(2): 216–235.
35. Baumohl J, Room R. Inebriety, doctors, and the state: alcoholism treatment institutions before 1940. In: Galanter M (ed.). *Recent developments in alcoholism,* vol. 5. New York: Plenum Publishing, 1987:135–174.
36. Turner J. *History of the first inebriate asylum in the world.* New York: Privately printed, 1888.
37. Crowley J, White W. *Drunkard's refuge: The lessons of the New York inebriate asylum.* Amherst: University of Massachusetts Press, 2004.
38. Inside the history of the Keeley cure. *JAMA* 1907;49:1861–1864, 1941–1951.
39. Crothers TD. Reformed men as asylum managers. *J Inebriety* 1897; 19:79, 897.
40. White WL. The role of recovering physicians in 19th century addiction medicine: An organizational case study. *J Addict Dis* 1999;19(2):1–10.
41. Dana C. A study of alcoholism as it occurs in the Belleville Hospital Cells. *N Y Med J* 1890;51:564–647.
42. *Proceedings of the 1870–1875 American Association for the Cure of Inebriates.* New York: Arno Press, 1981.
43. Crothers TD. A review of the history and literature of inebriety, the first journal and its work to present. *J Inebriety* 1912;33:139–151.
44. Weiner B, White W. The journal of inebriety (1876–1914): history, topical analysis and photographic images. *Addiction* 2007;102:15–23.
45. Crothers TD. Inebriate asylums. In: Stearns JN (ed.). *Temperance in all nations.* New York: National Temperance Society and Publication House, 1893.
46. Parrish J. *Alcoholic inebriety: From a medical standpoint with cases from clinical records.* Philadelphia: P. Blakiston, Son & Co., 1883.
47. Brooklyn Home for Habitues. *Q J Inebriety* 1891;July:271–272.
48. Jellinek EM (ed.). *Alcohol addiction and chronic alcoholism.* New Haven: Yale University Press, 1942.
49. Weiner B, White W. The history of addiction/recovery-related periodicals in America: literature as cultural/professional artifact. *Contemp Drug Probl* 2002;28:531–557.
50. Crothers TD. Inebriate asylums. In: *Cyclopaedia of temperance and prohibition.* New York: Funk and Wagnall's, 1891:247–248.
51. Worcester E, McComb S, Coriat I. *Religion and medicine.* New York: Funk & Wagnall's, 1908.
52. Moore M, Gray M. The problem of alcoholism at the Boston City Hospital. *N Engl J Med* 1937;217:381–388.
53. Pettey G. *Narcotic drug diseases and allied ailments.* Philadelphia: F. A. Davis Co., 1913.
54. Bishop E. *The narcotic drug problem.* New York: The Macmillan Company, 1920.
55. Kennedy F. The effects of narcotic drug addiction. *N Y Med J* 1914; 22:20–22.
56. Terry C. Some recent experiments in narcotic control. *Am J Public Health* 1921;11:35.
57. Butler W. How one American city is meeting the public health problems of narcotic addiction. *Am Med* 1922;28:154–162.
58. Courtwright D. Charles Terry: The opium problem and American narcotic policy. *J Drug Issues* 1986;16:422–425.
59. Courtwright D. Willis Butler and the Shreveport narcotic clinic. *Social Pharmacol* 1987;1:13–24.
60. King R. The Narcotics Bureau and the Harrison Act: jailing the healers and the sick. *Yale Law Review* 1953;62:736–749.
61. Bishop E. Morphinism and its treatment. *JAMA* 1912;58:1499–1504.
62. Williams EH. *Opiate addiction.* New York: Arno Press, 1922.
63. Williams H. *Drug addicts are human beings.* Washington, DC: Shaw Publishing Company, 1938.
64. Abraham K. The psychological relations between sexuality and alcoholism. *Int J Psycho-Anal* 1926;7:2–10.
65. Kolb L. Clinical contributions to drug addiction: The struggle for care and the conscious reasons for relapse. *J Nerv Ment Dis* 1927;66:22–43.
66. Schuckit M, Nathan PE, Helzer JE, et al. Evolution of the DSM diagnostic criteria for alcoholism. *Alcohol Health Res World* 1991;15:278–283.
67. Joyce T. California State Narcotic Hospital. *Calif West Med* 1929; 31:190–192.
68. Bennett C. Hospitalization of narcotic addicts, U.S. Penitentiary, Leavenworth, KS. *J Kansas Med Soc* 1929;30:341–345.
69. Acker C. *Creating the American junkie: Addiction research in the classical era of narcotic control.* Baltimore: The Johns Hopkins University Press, 2002.
70. Terry C, Pellens M. *The opium problem.* Montclair, NJ: Patterson Smith, 1928.
71. Reddish W. The treatment of morphine addiction by blister fluid injection. *Ky Med J* 1931;29:504.
72. Kolb L, Himmelsbach C. Clinical studies of drug addiction: a critical review of the withdrawal treatment with method of evaluating abstinence syndromes. *Am J Psychiatry* 1938;94:759–797.
73. Kleber H, Riordan C. The treatment of narcotic withdrawal: a historical review. *J Clin Psychiatry* 1982;43(6):30–34.
74. Mann, M. Formation of a National Committee for Education on Alcoholism. *Q J Stud Alcohol* 1944;5(2):354.
75. Nature Neuroscience (multiple authors). Focus on neurobiology of addiction [Special issue]. *Nat Neurosci* 2005;8(11).
76. Galanter, M, Frances, R. Addiction psychiatry: Challenges for a new psychiatric subspecialty. *Hosp Commun Psychiatry* 1992;43(11):1067–1070.
77. Substance Abuse and Mental Health Services Administration. *Alcohol and drug services study (ADSS): The National Substance Abuse Treatment System: Facilities, Clients, Services, and Staffing.* Office of Applied Studies. Rockville, MD, Author, 2003.

CHAPTER 23

Mark L. Willenbring, MD

Treatment of Heavy Drinking and Alcohol Use Disorders

Attempts to change the course and consequences of heavy drinking undoubtedly started soon after the discovery that fermenting grain or fruit yielded a drink that changed the way humans felt and behaved, because some of them behaved badly. Throughout most of history, personal, moral, social, and legal methods have composed the tools available for this task. Other than purely custodial care, professional treatment for alcohol use disorders (AUD) is a relatively recent addition, beginning with the promulgation of professional treatment programs in the latter part of the 20th century. Research concerning the nature and course of AUD and the efficacy of various treatments has grown considerably since then, providing a growing evidence base for clinicians. Consequently, the evidence base upon which addiction medicine rests is considerable, as good as or better than that for many other common complex disorders. At the same time, recent research advances have led to a reconsideration of some basic assumptions upon which treatment and research have been based. New research inspired by this reconsideration will likely lead to development of new and innovative approaches for treating AUD. It is likely that the number and effectiveness of treatments available for treating AUD will increase significantly in the next decade.

This enthusiasm is tempered by limitations of the infrastructure for providing treatment and implementing new treatments when they become available. Treatments are only effective if they are accessible and acceptable to those with the disorder. Very few people, only about one in eight who develop alcohol dependence ever seek or receive treatment in an addiction treatment center (1,2). (Throughout this chapter, I distinguish between treatment, which is delivered by trained professionals for a fee, and mutual support obtained through groups such as Alcoholics Anonymous [AA].) In addition, most treatment offered lasts a few weeks for a disorder that often lasts years. This limits the population level impact of treatment, and means that many people suffer needlessly. A related but independent challenge is lack of implementation of new research findings and treatments in clinical settings. The addiction treatment system is not configured to facilitate implementation of new treatments (3) and the quality of care for heavy drinking and AUD in general medical settings is among the worst in health care (4). Although not the focus of this chapter, these limitations are so important that any discussion about treatment must consider them, and how to overcome them. Unless these barriers are addressed, treatment for AUD will have a small impact on the overall problems of heavy drinking and AUD in our society.

This chapter provides an overview of current research on treatment for heavy drinking and AUD. The various behavioral and pharmacologic treatments are addressed in detail in other chapters; therefore, the goal of this overview is to provide a context to help guide interpretation of the research and guidelines provided in other chapters. There are four parts. Part 1 briefly reviews recent historic trends in research on change in drinking behavior, including a discussion of different ways to assess outcome. Part 2 presents a framework for conceptualizing heavy drinking and alcohol use disorders along a spectrum, proposes a continuum of care that corresponds to the spectrum of disorder, and raises the question of how to define a goal of treatment for different stages of the disorder. The third part briefly discusses overall treatment effectiveness and addresses the question of what causes change in drinking behavior. Part 4 examines the challenge of applying research findings to individual patients; that is, the art of evidence-based medicine.

DEVELOPMENT OF MODERN APPROACHES TO TREATMENT

Compared with other areas of medicine, professional treatment for AUD that is supported by a base of basic and clinical research is a relatively new field. For most of history, custodial treatment was all that was available. Modern behavioral treatment approaches grew initially out of the success of AA on the one hand and the growth of academic psychiatry and psychology after World War II on the other. AA was established in 1935, and its Big Book was published in 1939 and it spread rapidly (5). The Minnesota Model of treatment was initially conceived by a psychologist and a physician working at Willmar State Hospital in Minnesota in the 1950s. They collaborated with two early recovery centers run by recovering AA members, Pioneer House and Hazelden, to create a treatment model that combined counseling and education and the Twelve Steps of AA. Dan Anderson, a cocreator of the model, moved to the Hazelden Foundation in 1961, an organization that has been influential in its popularization (6). The Johnson Institute, another Minnesota organization, was established in 1966 to help spread the Minnesota Model; it also developed the procedure known as an intervention, where people close to an alcohol dependent person come together to share their concern (and usually shuttle the soon-to-be patient off to treatment). Subsequently, the Minnesota model has been adopted internationally, and it is the most prevalent form of treatment available in the United States (3,6).

Key features of the Minnesota Model of treatment are the use of both professional staff and staff who are recovering from alcohol dependence, patient and family education, strong linkage to AA—a requirement of abstinence from all addictive substances other than tobacco and caffeine—and belief that alcoholism is a primary, progressive disease that cannot be cured, although it can be arrested through abstinence and AA. It was initially provided only in 28-day programs in hospitals or residential facilities, but is now provided in outpatient settings as well. The primary modalities used in most programs are group counseling and education (7). Twelve-step facilitation is a manualized version of the Minnesota Model that has been adapted for an individual outpatient approach (8).

At about the same time, the fields of psychology and psychiatry were undergoing substantial development and expansion, primarily because the Veterans Administration rapidly expanded mental health services after World War II (9,10). Pavlov discovered classic conditioning in the 1920s (11) and B. F. Skinner first published on operant conditioning in 1935 (12). The concepts of group therapy and therapeutic community were first proposed in the mid-1940s, with subsequent development and spread in the 1950s and 1960s (13). Albert Ellis developed the first type of cognitive-behavior therapy, Rational-Emotive Therapy, in the mid-1950s (14), and Aaron Beck developed cognitive therapy for depression in the 1960s (15). Specific therapies for alcohol dependence based on these earlier psychologic theories include therapeutic communities, aversion therapy, cognitive-behavior therapy, skills training, community reinforcement, and contingency management. More recently, William Miller and colleagues developed an approach based on stages of change and motivation (16).

Over the same period, pharmacotherapy for alcohol dependence was attempted with many new psychiatric medications as they were discovered or developed. Examples include lithium carbonate, anxiolytics, tricyclic antidepressants, antipsychotics, and phenytoin. Although initial studies reported efficacy in open-label studies, subsequent research for all except disulfiram failed to substantiate early claims. Disulfiram was approved for use as a deterrent or aversive agent in 1949. It took 46 years for the next medication, naltrexone, to be approved for treatment of alcohol dependence in 1995. More recently, acamprosate and topiramate have been shown to be effective (17,18). Multiple pharmacotherapy agents are now under investigation, and it is very likely that there will be additional medications available in the future.

Research on the nature, causes, consequences, course, and treatment of AUD developed in parallel during this time. Major advances have been made in identifying genetic, developmental, and environmental risk factors for AUD, describing its natural history and treatment response, as well as social and biomedical consequences of heavy drinking and AUD. Excellent animal models now exist for studying the neurobiology of the disorder as well as identifying potential treatment approaches. The methodology for clinical studies has advanced as well, resulting in refinement of methods and widespread agreement on use of various instruments for determining outcome. Manualization and sophisticated monitoring of the application of behavioral techniques has allowed true comparisons of efficacy with a high degree of confidence in the validity of the trials.

It is obvious that considerable progress towards enlightened, humane, and effective treatment has been made in a relatively short time. Nevertheless, the historic development of modern treatment also created some unique obstacles that must be overcome for progress to continue. In more than 90% of community programs (not including the Veterans Affairs health care system), group counseling and referral to AA provided by counselors with minimal education are the only modalities offered (3). In most cases, there is no physician involvement in treatment other than treating withdrawal. Furthermore, treatment is time-limited, focused on inducing and maintaining remission, and offers little except repetition for patients who do not respond. Because of the lack of integration of addiction treatment programs with medical and psychiatric treatment, few programs are able to identify and treat coexisting mental and physical disorders in their patients, even though these are very common in a treatment-seeking population. The quality of counseling in community programs is poor, often consisting of casual talk unrelated to therapy (19), and supervision is minimal. Very few community treatment programs offer currently available pharmacotherapy or even educate their patients about it (3). In sum, although progress has been made, much remains to be done.

How Should Treatment Outcome be Determined?

An additional legacy of the unique history of treatment for alcohol dependence is controversy about what the goal of treatment should be, and how outcome should be measured. Until relatively recently, total, continuous, permanent abstinence was considered by most to be the only goal of treatment and the only measure of outcome. Reasons for this are complex, but include the strongly held belief of AA members and Minnesota Model treatment providers that anything less than a commitment to total lifetime abstinence would result in failure. Additionally, abstinence was easier for researchers to measure and verify. Also, certain strains of American Protestantism have held the view that any consumption of alcohol is sinful and dangerous (20,21). Thus, for a habitual drunkard, becoming abstinent is equated with moral redemption. AA grew out of early members' experience with the Oxford Group, which was grounded in Christian evangelism and incorporated sharing of one's sins to others in a group that included others who had already experience a spiritual transformation. In fact, Bill Wilson, one of the founders of AA, experienced a sudden transformative experience he called his "hot flash" (5). To this day, a spiritual awakening is considered to be at the heart of the path of AA (22).

On the other hand, some researchers believed that drinking (including heavy drinking) was a learned behavior, and that it might therefore be possible for patients to learn new ways of (moderate) drinking. Treatment methods based on this idea were developed and eventually compared to abstinence-based approaches, which generated considerable controversy and outright animosity (23). Whether abstinence or reduced drinking should be the goal remains a matter of contention. Reduced drinking as a goal has been labeled as *harm reduction*, an unfortunate term that describes a pragmatic public drug policy most interested in results, as opposed to a more idealistic one focused more on intention. In the case of clinical care, the term is used to describe a pragmatic approach when abstinence cannot be obtained, either because the individual is unwilling to endorse a goal of abstinence or because treatment is unable to help the patient achieve and maintain abstinence.

A more recent twist on this debate is whether abstinence or nonabstinent remission is equivalent to "recovery." One prominent 12-step–oriented treatment facility convened a consensus panel to define recovery (24). The panel concluded that recovery required sobriety (in this case abstinence from alcohol and all other nonprescribed drugs) as a necessary but not sufficient condition for recovery. In their view, in addition to sobriety, recovery required personal health (improved quality of life, physical, mental, and spiritual health) and citizenship (social health, contributing and interacting with the community at large). A study of recovering volunteers from the community (25) found that most considered total abstinence necessary for recovery. However, recovery entailed additional goals, such as well-being, a new life, or a second change, suggesting not only wellness as a goal but also regaining what was lost through addiction. Subjects also believed that recovery was an ongoing process or way of life rather than something that is achieved at a specific point in time. This emphasis on recovery coincides with a similar focus on recovery from mental illnesses recovery (26), and an overall increase in attention to patient-rated outcomes in health care (27). More research on recovery processes and trajectories is needed.

The research community has developed increasingly sophisticated ways to measure outcome, although they are far from perfect. There are three broad categories of outcome: drinking behavior, symptoms or diagnostic criteria of dependence, and functioning in multiple life areas such as occupational achievement, social function, and psychologic and physical health. Depending on the method used, these functional areas may or may not be explicitly linked to drinking behavior. That is, some instruments or studies attempt to quantify adverse life consequences of drinking, whereas others simply measure functioning without reference to drinking.

Drinking behavior is most often determined by taking the individual through a structured process of retrospective reconstruction; the most commonly used instrument for this is the Timeline Follow-Back (28).

Retrospective self-report is still the standard approach in treatment trials, and most research supports its validity and reliability (29). Recent research using interactive voice response and personal digital assistants offer one alternative that may eliminate memory errors (30,31), but daily monitoring of drinking may itself lead to drinking reductions, thus complicating interpretation (32,33). Eventual development of biosensors that can measure blood alcohol concentration continuously will likely supplant self-report measures, but they may also cause drinking reductions themselves.

Another way to measure outcome is whether or not the disorder, as determined by diagnostic criteria, is still present after treatment. Although different studies use slightly different approaches, a reasonable approach for clinicians mirrors that used for other disorders. For the outcome of treatment of dependence, and using the Diagnostic and Statistical Manual of the American Psychiatry Association, Fourth Edition (DSM-IV) criteria (34), recovery is defined as no longer meeting any of the seven criteria of dependence (full remission), irrespective of drinking. Partial remission means meeting one or two dependence criteria, but not enough to qualify for the dependence diagnosis, and nonremission is continuing to meet three or more criteria. (Although the definitions in DSM-IV are clear, the clinical utility and predictive validity of these categories is not fully established.) In some studies meeting one or more abuse criteria, but not three or more dependence criteria, is also considered partial remission (recurrence of symptoms but not syndrome). Importantly, since drinking quantity and frequency are not included in the diagnosis, they are not considered in DSM-IV. A recent epidemiologic study divided outcomes into these categories: abstinent recovery, nonabstinent recovery (meeting no diagnostic criteria for abuse or dependence and not exceeding maximum drinking recommendations from the National Institute on Alcohol Abuse and Alcoholism), risk drinking (meeting no criteria for dependence, but exceeding maximum drinking recommendations), symptomatic but not dependent (meeting one or two dependence criteria or one or more abuse criteria), and dependent (meeting three or more criteria) (35).

In the earliest studies of outcome, this type of categorical or dichotomous measures (abstinent or drinking, relapse or not) was used. Over time, use of simple categories was largely supplanted by variable-based approaches, where average values of a continuous drinking variable were compared among groups using increasingly sophisticated statistical techniques. Percent days abstinent and percent days heavy drinking are common examples. This variable-centered approach has advantages, such as using more data and allowing use of parametric statistics, thus increasing statistical power. This approach also allows for a wider range of outcomes rather than a few predetermined categories. However, variable-based approaches also hide complexity. For example, in medication trials especially, it seems likely that with any one medication, only a portion of the study population will demonstrate a response, whereas the majority may not respond at all. Consequently, a robust response in a minority of individuals may only move the mean a small distance, suggesting that the treatment is only minimally effective overall (which is true for the entire study population). Variable-centered analysis may miss such an effect entirely. For example, in a reanalysis of two studies of naltrexone, both of which were negative with the a priori variable-based analysis, trajectory analysis found that naltrexone recipients were significantly more likely to be in an abstinent trajectory (36). Trajectory analysis also yields results that are more clinically intuitive. For example, one such analysis examined three different trajectories through the follow-up period: stable remission, stable non-remission, and unstable (37). Comparing the likelihood of being in various trajectories for different treatments is easier for most people to grasp, compared with a change in a continuous variable such as mean percent days abstinent. Consequently, trajectory analysis is likely to be used more often. Rapid development in pharmacogenomics suggests the possibility of being able to identify likely responders to different medications before treatment starts. However, at this time, no genetic marker which reliably predicts response has been identified.

In some other medical disorders such as cardiovascular disease, outcomes are often measured in terms of reduction in disease-related adverse consequences. For example, the value of therapies for hypertension or hyperlipidemia is determined by how well they reduce the risk for adverse consequences such as stroke, myocardial infarction, and death. Similarly, heavy drinking is the third leading preventable cause of death in the United States, after smoking and obesity/lack of exercise (38). According to one estimate (39), 54% of premature deaths due to alcohol consumption are due to acute conditions and 46% to chronic conditions. Because acute deaths due primarily to trauma differentially affect young people, the years of life lost is higher for acute (65%) compared with chronic (35%) conditions. In middle age, chronic dependence is associated with a host of physical disorders such as liver fibrosis and cirrhosis, cancer, and cardiovascular disease (40); social consequences such as unemployment and divorce; and mental illness such as depression and suicide. The relationship between these outcomes and alcohol consumption is complex, however, mediated by genetic vulnerability, other lifestyle factors such as smoking, social factors, and possibly choice of beverage (41).

Further complicating matters, alcohol consumption carries not only risks but potential benefits. Moderate alcohol consumption in middle age adults is associated with decreased incidence of cardiovascular disease and death, diabetes, Alzheimer disease, and stroke, although heavy drinking increases risk for these disorders in some studies (42,43). Thus one must subtract potential beneficial effects of drinking from potential risk for adverse events when developing risk estimates. Most mortality data on people with AUDs have been obtained with samples of people seeking or receiving treatment for alcohol dependence. These studies have found that annual mortality is 1.4 to 4.7 times that of matched controls, depending on the sample studied (44–47). Because treatment-seekers have more severe dependence, a higher prevalence of comorbid conditions and less social capital than nontreatment seekers, information obtained by studying treatment populations applies only to the 20% or less of people with AUDs with the most severe and recurring form of dependence (48–50).

Social consequences are mediated by comorbid mental disorders, especially antisocial personality disorder (51), and are also highly context dependent. For example, whether one is arrested for driving while intoxicated depends on the laws of the particular jurisdiction in which driving occurs and how they are enforced, as well as whether an individual has a coexisting antisocial personality disorder. Societies vary markedly in their tolerance for various forms of social behavior associated with intoxication or dependence. At the same time, there remains a strong association between overall physical, mental, occupational and social function, and presence and degree of dependence. In a recent large community sample, as the number of diagnostic criteria met increased, function decreased, and functional impairment for severe dependence (6–7 criteria met) was similar to that for anxiety disorders and depression (52). Similarly, in a treatment sample, problems associated with drinking were strongly (but imperfectly) correlated with drinking outcomes (37). In a longitudinal study of help-seeking older adults with alcohol dependence, long-term abstinence was strongly associated with improved functional outcomes (53).

In sum, measures of drinking behavior are the easiest to measure reliably across studies and can be used as either categorical or continuous variables. Quantity and frequency alone are sufficient to determine whether a patient's drinking constitutes a risk factor for future problems. However, drinking becomes an alcohol use disorder when it causes clinically significant distress or impairment, and these variables are more difficult to measure. Similarly, the relationship between social and occupational function is complex and bidirectional. Because abstinence or low-risk drinking without symptoms of an alcohol use disorder (remission) are most robustly predictive of continued recovery as well as function, yet are easier to measure, they may serve as the best single outcome measure. Categoric approaches, such as full remission, partial remission or risk drinking, and non-remission, offer an attractive and clinically intuitive way to measure outcome, and analysis of groups with different trajectories may prove to be more sensitive to detecting meaningful treatment effects in some studies.

THE SPECTRUM OF HEAVY DRINKING AND ALCOHOL USE DISORDERS

New research has provided a new and more complete view of the range of drinking, alcohol use disorders and alcohol-related harms. However, some definitions are needed to describe drinking behavior and relate it to adverse events. In the United States, a single alcohol serving is defined as the amount of ethanol in 1.5 oz (45 mL) of 80 proof spirits, 12 oz of beer, or 5 oz of table wine, each containing about 14 g of absolute ethanol (Table 23.1). Because actual alcohol levels in beer and wine vary, these amounts are meant to be approximate. The National Institute of Alcohol Abuse and Alcoholism of the National Institutes of Health recommends that men drink no more than 4 alcohol servings per day and 14 servings per week and that women drink no more than 3 servings per day and 7 servings per week (Table 23.2). Drinking within these limits is considered "low-risk" drinking. Lower limits or abstinence may be indicated in the presence of coexisting medical or psychiatric disorders, in older people, or when medication interactions are a concern. Women who are pregnant or at risk of becoming pregnant are advised to abstain. In this chapter, a day on which the limit is exceeded is considered a "heavy drinking day," and "heavy drinking" is defined as drinking in excess of the maximum limits on a regular basis, such as exceeding the daily limits weekly or more often. "At-risk drinking" is heavy drinking in the absence of meeting any criteria for an alcohol use disorder, whereas heavy drinking includes both at-risk drinking and symptomatic drinking (alcohol use disorders).

TABLE 23.1 Typical Beverages and Drink Sizes and the Approximate Number of U.S. Standard Drinks in Each

Beverage	Percent ethanol	Serving size	Number of drinks
Beer	5	12 oz	1
Malt liquor	7	12 oz	1.5
		40 oz	4.5
Wine	12	5 oz	1
		750 mL bottle	5
Fortified wine	24	2.5 oz	1
80 proof spirits	40	1.5 oz	1
		1 L bottle	22

The continuum of drinking in U.S. adults is shown in Figure 23.1 About 70% of the U.S. adult population report either being abstinent or engaging in low-risk drinking in any given year, about 21% are at-risk drinkers and 9% have an alcohol use disorder (5% abuse and 4% alcohol dependence) (52). At-risk drinking places an individual at higher risk for developing alcohol-related problems, such as an alcohol use disorder, liver disease, or a mental disorder. As a health risk factor, at-risk drinking

TABLE 23.2 Characteristics of Individuals in Each Category of Drinking Behavior

	Drinking pattern (example)	Alcohol use disorder criteria	Disability	Treatment
Abstinent/low risk	Less than NIAAA limits	None	None	Health promotion/ primary prevention
At-risk drinking	Above NIAAA daily limits 1–7 days per week	0–2 dependence only	None	Brief counseling Facilitated self-change
Harmful drinking	Episodic to daily	0–2 dependence 0–1 abuse	Limited	Brief counseling Facilitated self-change Addiction focused behavioral therapy Pharmacotherapy
Dependent drinking	Daily or near daily 5–10 drinks per day	3–5 dependence 0–1 abuse	Mild to moderate	Behavioral and pharmacologic treatment
Chronic dependence	Daily or near daily 10+ drinks per day	6–7 dependence 2–4 abuse	Moderate to severe	Behavioral and pharmacologic treatment Long-term care management

NIAAA, National Institute on Alcohol Abuse and Alcoholism.

Alcohol Use Disorder criteria refer to all 11 DSM-IV criteria for abuse and dependence treated as a single dimensional disorder. NIAAA maximum recommended drinking limits are: women: 3 drinks per day and 7 per week; men: 4 drinks per day and 14 per week. Information in all cells is provided for illustrative purposes only, and is not meant to imply formal definitions.

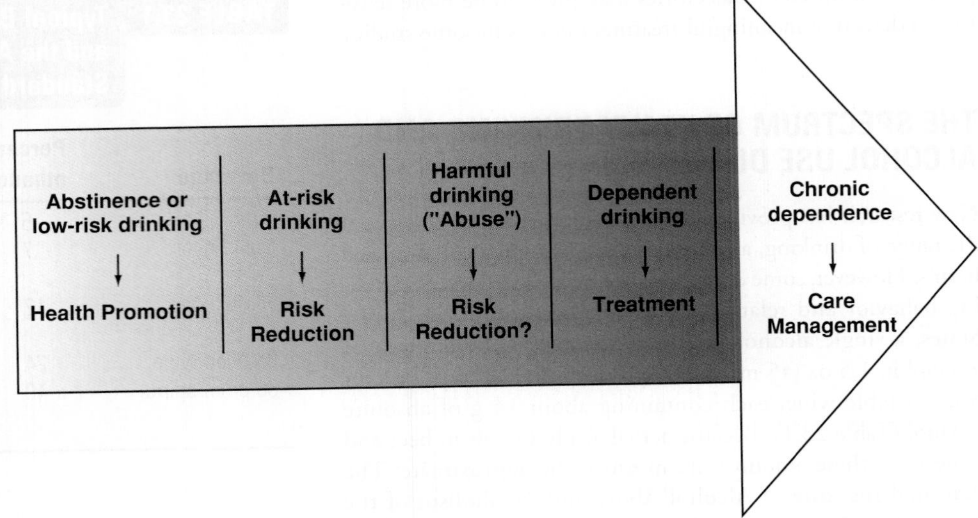

FIGURE 23.1 Spectrum of drinking and alcohol use disorders at any given time. A conceptualized continuum of care is projected upon the spectrum. See Table 23.2 for more details about each category.

is analogous to high blood pressure or hyperlipidemia before end-organ damage. Also, alcohol addiction from dysregulation of the brain systems involved with motivation and reward can be thought of as end organ damage to the brain caused by heavy drinking (54). Most heavy drinking occurs between the ages of 18 and 25, which is also when the prevalence of alcohol use disorders peaks (55). Not all heavy drinkers develop alcohol-related problems, and which type of problem a heavy drinker develops varies. Importantly, more than 40% of daily or near daily heavy drinkers do not meet any criteria for alcohol use disorder (1). Similarly, only 20 to 40% of people with alcoholic liver cirrhosis also have alcohol dependence (56,57). Finally, not all alcohol-related harms occur in people who have alcohol use disorders, in part because there are twice as many at-risk drinkers as there are people with alcohol use disorders. Trauma, in particular, may occur because of a single occasion of heavy drinking, or in someone who only drinks to excess occasionally.

In this scheme, harmful drinking is a category that includes DSM-IV abuse but not dependence, and includes drinking which has resulted in complications of coexisting medical or psychiatric illnesses, or to end-organ damage such as liver fibrosis. Under DSM-IV, recurrent drinking despite psychologic or physical symptoms because of or exacerbated by drinking (such as hangover) is categorized under dependence. Only drinking despite recurrent social, legal, or interpersonal problems or recurrent use that is physically hazardous such as drunk driving is considered abuse. The category of harmful drinking is included in the ICD-10 diagnostic scheme, which is defined as use that is harmful to physical or mental health. In contrast to dependence, which usually involves drinking on a regular basis, often daily or near-daily, even episodic or sporadic intoxication can cause serious harm. Examples include drunk driving and motor vehicle crashes, trauma from assaults, falls, drowning, sexual assault, and suicide. On the other hand, daily or near-daily heavy drinking can result in liver fibrosis or heart failure in the absence of symptoms of dependence (56,57). Harmful drinking is meant here to include both.

Diagnostic criteria for alcohol dependence can be grouped as: (1) impaired control (going over limits, failed attempts to quit or cut down, continued drinking despite adverse psychologic or physical effects), (2) increased salience (spending much time anticipating, drinking and recovering, and reduced involvement in non-drinking activities, and (3) physiologic adaptation (increased tolerance and withdrawal) (34). Drinking must also be causing clinically significant impairment or distress. Thus heavy drinking itself is not considered an alcohol use disorder, even if it results in physical harm. Drinking quantity and frequency patterns vary considerably among people who meet minimum criteria for alcohol dependence, but most often involve drinking 4 to 7 days per week. Note, however, that many heavy daily drinkers do not meet criteria for an alcohol use disorder. People with alcohol dependence vary in many other ways as well, suggesting that the clinical diagnosis is actually comprised of an unknown number of subgroups. This heterogeneity presents a serious problem for treatment research, because treatment of a depressed, anxious 38-year-old married woman drinking six drinks per day would presumably differ from that for a 22-year-old antisocial male with cannabis dependence who drinks a liter of vodka twice weekly. However, although there are exceptions, most studies of treatment have included all people meeting criteria for dependence. Similarly, most treatment programs essentially provide the same treatment to everyone entering the program. Attempts to subtype dependence according to clinical and demographic characteristics have not been productive in terms of predicting differential response to treatment. Therefore there is a pressing need to identify more robust subtypes of heavy drinkers, in particular subtypes that predict treatment response. Until that occurs, the individual physician must attempt to assimilate the latest information from randomized controlled trials and skillfully apply that information to an individual patient's situation.

The Spectrum of Drinking, Disorders, and Treatment The goal of treatment depends on the nature, extent, and severity of the disorder. In place of the "one size fits all" approach initially developed for people with severe, relapsing dependence, an individualized approach that takes patient preferences into account is required. Coexisting conditions or circumstances are also important determinants of the therapeutic approach and methods used. The continuum of drinking presented in Figure 23.1 serves as a template on which to project a continuum of care (Table 23.2).

Abstainers and low-risk drinkers require health promotion, such as education about the recommended maximum limits adjusted for that person's individual situation. Health promotion is especially important for adolescents and women who are pregnant or at risk of becoming pregnant. High-risk groups, such as youth with a primary relative with alcohol dependence, or who have conduct disorder, may require modification of advice and possibly more intensive interventions to prevent the development of heavy drinking and alcohol use disorders. The goal for at-risk drinkers is to reduce consumption, preferably below recommended maximum limits, to reduce risk of future harm. At-risk drinkers (and possibly those with mild dependence) respond well to facilitated self-change (58) and brief counseling by physicians in primary care, with about a 25% overall reduction in drinking 1 year later, and a greater decrease in heavy drinking (59). Evidence is accumulating that college students respond to Internet-based individualized feedback as well as to brief counseling (60). Whether brief counseling is effective in emergency care settings is unclear, with some studies showing an effect and others not (61). For individuals with more than minimal levels of dependence, however, more intensive forms of treatment are needed. Brief counseling alone is not effective with dependent drinkers in general (59) or hospitalized heavy drinkers (because most are dependent) (62).

Treatment of abuse without dependence or of frequent heavy drinking resulting in end-organ damage when alcohol use disorder criteria are not met is not well developed. Most patients presenting to addiction treatment programs have dependence, and may meet several criteria for abuse as well. In studies of screening and brief intervention in primary care, participants with abuse were combined with heavy drinkers not meeting any criteria for alcohol use disorder, and this combined group was differentiated from dependence, which was an exclusionary condition. Diagnostic confusion contributes to a lack of studies focused on DSM-IV abuse alone. This is unfortunate, because abuse may persist for decades without progressing to dependence (63,64). Recent epidemiologic studies have found that in persons who have abuse but do not qualify for dependence, about 90% qualify for abuse because of physically hazardous use, mostly drunk driving (65). Other abuse criteria (role failure, interpersonal problems, and legal problems) are typically met only in individuals who also meet criteria for dependence, and are associated with greater severity of alcohol use disorder than drink-driving (66,67). More research is needed on abuse-only identification and treatment.

Most studies of treatment of dependence have been done on middle-aged, treatment-seeking adults, especially white males and veterans. Because the average age of onset of alcohol dependence is 21 years (52) and the average age in most treatment studies is about 40, this means that most study subjects have chronic, relapsing, severe alcohol dependence, and have been ill for a decade or more. This chronically ill group, which also has considerable comorbidity, represents a minority of people who develop dependence at some point in their lives. The extensive study of this subgroup (and lack of study of others) has created a picture of alcohol dependence as an inevitably severe, chronic disorder resistant to treatment. In fact, new research has demonstrated that 72% of U.S. adults with a lifetime diagnosis of dependence have a single episode, lasting on average 3 to 4 years (52). Those with more than one average five episodes of decreasing length, suggesting that failure to achieve permanent remission after the first episode predicts a more chronic course (52).

At the same time, treatment study recruitment has shifted over time from patients in treatment programs to volunteers solicited through newspaper ads. Research volunteers recruited from community settings differ systematically from volunteers recruited from treatment programs; they are more functional, more likely to be employed, have less severe alcohol dependence, and are less likely to have coexisting other substance, mental or physical disorders (68). Furthermore, efficacy studies typically exclude people with significant comorbidities, homelessness, or lack of transportation. Consequently, generalizing from such studies to clinical populations where these co-occurring conditions are common is not straightforward. There is a gap in research knowledge on the effectiveness of treatments in more natural settings with a broader population, especially for studies of specific behavioral or pharmacotherapy treatments. That overall outcomes from miller treatment studies do not differ substantially from those in efficacy trials is reassuring (69,70), but more effectiveness research is needed, particularly in different settings such as primary care and general psychiatry.

Another pressing need to is develop and test treatment approaches for people with mild to moderate dependence and relatively few comorbidities. Such patients are unlikely to seek treatment in addiction treatment programs (50). In this type of patient, treatment with oral naltrexone plus brief behavioral support by health care clinicians is at least as effective as state-of-the-art outpatient addiction therapy (71,72). These findings suggest that pharmacotherapy with medical management may be an effective approach for patients with similar characteristics. If so, making such treatment available in primary care and general psychiatry would substantially increase access to effective care.

About two thirds of individuals who develop dependence do so in adolescence or young adulthood. However, only about half of them go on to a chronic course (52). Those who do are more likely to have a family history of alcohol dependence and antisocial personality traits and to have started drinking in early adolescence (50). A pressing need is more research on early intervention in the course of illness for those at high risk for chronicity. Another third of dependent persons have midlife onset of moderate severity dependence, and those who do are more likely to have coexisting psychopathology (50).

This suggests that primary care and general psychiatry may be ideal settings in which to identify and treat this group.

For those who do not respond to self-change efforts and non-intensive or brief treatment, referral to specialty addiction treatment is needed. This type of stepped care approach is implied in the Patient Placement Criteria, Second Edition by the American Society of Addiction Medicine (73). However, although the stepped care approach makes sense intuitively, its effectiveness has not been adequately examined. Stepped care or adaptive treatment designs are methodologically complex and require sophisticated design and analysis as well as large numbers of subjects. Adaptive study design is an emerging area of interest, however, and recent advances in statistical techniques make it more feasible. Such research can help answer questions about the best ways to structure the treatment system and to most effectively match patient needs and services offered. Attempts to improve outcomes by matching patient characteristics to treatment type have not yet yielded information of much use to clinicians, but such a body of knowledge is likely to develop over time.

At the most severe end of the spectrum are those unfortunate individuals with severe and persistent or recurrent alcohol dependence. In this group, coexisting substance, mental and physical disorders, and social disabilities are common, including antisocial personality, as is a family history of alcohol dependence and very early onset. Not surprisingly, they are the most likely to seek and receive treatment, often because of overt coercion (50). Even though most of this group has a chronic or recurrent course, addiction treatment programs typically offer treatment for only a few weeks or months. Furthermore, few programs are staffed to address the serious comorbidities present, so they are ignored or dealt with through referral (3). The effectiveness of treatment programs for this group is difficult to evaluate because there are many factors present that may be driving change. For example, serious physical illness, legal mandates, homelessness, unemployment and poverty and family pressure frequently cause or contribute to a decision to seek treatment. Many of these factors are quite powerful and could account for much or all of whatever change occurs. More research is needed on the mechanisms of behavior change among heavy drinkers including those with severe disorders.

Research on long-term care management strategies similar to those used for other chronic disorders is promising, especially for people with alcohol dependence and serious mental or physical disorders. For example, studies of heavy drinkers with severe medical complications such as liver cirrhosis suggest that addressing drinking using a care management approach in the context of general medical care is effective at reducing drinking and inducing abstinence (74). In two studies of this approach, 2-year mortality was about half of that in comparison groups receiving usual medical care (75,76). Integrating substance use interventions into community support programs for severely mentally ill people also has some support. These studies suggest that for harmful drinkers with serious medical or psychiatric illnesses, addressing drinking directly in the context of medical or psychiatric treatment is preferable to referral to a standard addiction treatment program, which are not staffed so as to be able to address serious medical or psychiatric illnesses. At this time there are no treatment approaches shown to be effective with severe and persistent alcohol dependence in the absence of comorbidities that cause serious dysfunction. Because people with severe dependence are frequently heavy consumers of health care and social and criminal justice services, development of more effective treatments is a priority. It may be that external motivating factors, such as skillful application of legal coercion or contingency management may be effective with this group, especially when combined with "wrap-around" services that integrate addiction, psychiatric and medical care as well as social services and sober housing. What is clear is that treatment for these individuals needs to be structured with the goal of providing services intermittently or continuously for years to decades rather than weeks or months.

To summarize, recent research has shown that drinking and associated symptoms and problems occur along a continuum ranging from none to mild, moderate, and severe. A large majority of U.S. adults abstains or drinks at low-risk levels. Most heavy drinkers are without current symptoms or problems, but are at increased risk for physical, mental, and substance use disorders developing over time. Most heavy drinkers with an abuse-only diagnosis do so by virtue of drinking and driving. In contrast to popular belief, most people who meet dependence criteria do not have a chronic course and most recover without professional treatment or even attendance at mutual help groups. It appears that most people, on recognizing a problem attempt to change alone or with informal help, and the majority are eventually successful, albeit after several years of active dependence. Seeking help from mutual help groups or non-addiction professionals (about 25%) or professional treatment programs (13%) occurs when informal attempts to change fail (or because of an external contingency such as a driving while intoxicated charge). A significant proportion of help-seekers respond with improvement or remission, leaving a small but important group with severe and persistent dependence. This continuum of drinking and associated symptoms and problems suggests a corresponding continuum of care (Table 23.2).

Unfortunately, most of this continuum of care is not yet implemented or available. The quality of care for heavy drinking and alcohol use disorders in primary care is the lowest among 30 chronic conditions (4), and attempts to increase screening and brief intervention for at risk drinking have met with little success in spite of a robust evidence base for their efficacy (59). Large numbers of Americans lack health insurance, and private insurance companies have disinvested in addiction treatment, so that most treatment provided today is publicly funded (77). Treatment programs suffer from insufficient funds, resulting in poorly trained and underpaid staff and excessive turnover (3). The proportion of people with current dependence receiving treatment actually declined between 1991 and 1992 and 2001 and 2002 (52), and there is no evidence that the prevalence or public health burden of heavy drinking or alcohol dependence has decreased, with the important exception of a reduction in premature deaths among adolescents because of stricter drink-driving laws (78). Thus much remains to be done and many challenges lie ahead. Nevertheless, this fuller understanding of the spectrum of drinking, disorders, and treatment approaches provides one possible conceptual framework for advancing investment and development of the continuum of care.

A major public health challenge is to provide earlier identification and appropriate treatment to a much broader spectrum of individuals who drink heavily or who have alcohol dependence than is currently the case. There is a pressing need to identify early intervention strategies for youth who begin drinking in early adolescence and who are at high risk for later development of severe chronic dependence. Early identification and treatment of heavy drinking and dependence in primary care and general mental health care would provide access for millions of people who otherwise will not receive treatment. Needed also is a better understanding of the factors driving change in heavy drinkers and how to facilitate that change both in addiction treatment and in other settings. Finally, effective and cost-effective care management strategies for managing chronic severe dependence need to be implemented. To provide this type of comprehensive care, the specialty addiction treatment sector will require substantial development so that addiction, psychiatric, medical, and social services can be provided in an integrated way and over longer periods.

TYPES OF TREATMENT AND TREATMENT EFFECTIVENESS

Multiple treatment modalities have been shown to be effective in the treatment of alcohol dependence. However, the best way to match the type and intensity of treatment to the individual needs of a patient with alcohol dependence remains unclear. For example, no systematic outcome advantage has been demonstrated for residential or intensive day program treatment compared with once or twice weekly outpatient treatment (79). Similarly, no behavioral treatment has been shown to be better than others that are conceptually distinct and use different behavioral techniques (80). Attempts to match specific behavioral therapies with clinical characteristics of patients have yielded little (80). Several medications are efficacious in reducing relapse or heavy drinking during early recovery, but none are clearly better than others, and there is not yet a way to predict how likely a patient is to respond to one rather than another. Achieving the goal of "personalized" medicine through the use of biomarkers and pharmacogenomics is the focus of extensive research across medicine (81). Finally, approximately 10% of people with alcohol dependence have a severe chronic form of the disorder, yet most treatment programs offer a few weeks or months of treatment, and information on management of alcohol dependence as a chronic illness is limited. In sum, current recommendations and practice regarding the selection and sequencing of treatments are based upon clinical experience and expert consensus and not randomized controlled trials. In practical terms, the addiction treatment offered or available likely depends on patient preference, availability, access, coercion, urgent needs such as imminent withdrawal or suicide risk, and clinician orientation rather than on scientific evidence. One of the key research challenges ahead is to develop methods to compare the effectiveness of different stepwise or adaptive strategies for deploying treatment modalities with demonstrated efficacy.

The outcome of treatment varies according to the diagnosis, or stage of illness. At-risk drinkers (and possibly those with abuse-only diagnoses) who are identified and offered education and brief motivational counseling on average reduce drinking about 25% over the following year (59). Treatment outcome for dependence is remarkably similar across studies and treatment modalities, both behavioral and pharmacologic (70). In a typical treatment study, about one third of subjects will be in full abstinent or nonabstinent remission for the following year, 30 to 40% will show substantial improvement but will have at least some episodes of heavy drinking, and 20% to 30% will not show an effect (37,70,79). However, over the course of the ensuing 5 to 10 years, most will suffer at least some relapse (64). Detailed information about each different behavioral and pharmacologic modality is provided in the appropriate chapters of this text. However, no particular treatment or technique has proved to be overall more effective than others, thus raising the question of what the mechanisms of change really are. In fact, many people start reducing their drinking prior to treatment entry, and both study protocols and treatment programs may require that a patient be abstinent at treatment entry, whether or not they required medical support for withdrawal. For that matter, there are no clear criteria for distinguishing "still drinking" from "abstinent," because treatment cannot take place if an individual is intoxicated. In other words, it is often arbitrary how long abstinence is required in order to qualify as "abstinent." In another randomized controlled trial of two behavioral treatments for alcohol dependence that failed to detect a difference between brief motivational counseling versus a more extensive multimodal program of care, Orford and colleagues (82) qualitatively examined the process leading to help-seeking in study subjects. They identified a "catalyst system" consisting of increasing problems and distress related to drinking, pressure from others, and a trigger event, which in turn led to the realization "I can't do this on my own." Factors outside the treatment context continued to be important throughout the recovery process, especially after the discontinuation of treatment services. In another study of 15 community treatment programs, 5-year outcomes of patients who dropped out of treatment early did not differ from program completers (83). These findings suggest that the process of deciding to seek help is itself part of the change process, and is arguably the most important, although it is not well understood. In the next section, we will examine the question of what causes change.

What Causes and Maintains Change in Drinking Behavior? Help-seeking is strongly associated with increased odds of achieving recovery, but help-seekers differ systematically from non–help-seekers. Help-seekers on average are older, have more severe dependence and more coexisting mental and physical disorders as well as less social support (1,84), and are more likely to have the relapsing form of the illness (52). For those who do seek help, both professional treatment and 12-step participation are associated with increased likelihood of recovery, especially abstinent recovery (1). For individuals older than 35 years, abstinence is much more stable an outcome than even light drinking without problems (83,85), whereas in younger persons light drinking without problems (non-abstinent remission) is similar to abstinence in predicting continued remission 3 years later (85). In people who have been treated for alcohol dependence, recovery is in turn strongly associated with improved mortality (46). Thus full remission, whether abstinent or non-abstinent, should be the goal of treatment for dependence, tempered with the recognition that full recovery cannot always be achieved.

Unfortunately, such studies are not able to establish causality. Although help-seeking and participation in treatment and 12-step groups are associated with improved outcomes and decreased mortality, it cannot be ruled out that people who have decided to change will seek treatment, whereas those who do not want to change do not, or that people who respond to treatment early develop more hope and motivation to continue. That is, treatment participation or continuation may be a result of change rather than the converse. There may be other unmeasured differences between the groups as well. At the same time, it is clear that people who achieve full remission of drinking have much better overall functional and medical outcomes that those with partial or no response. Furthermore, it appears that treatment followed by 12-step participation is a frequent and effective (but not the only) path to recovery for many people. Recently, Rudolf Moos has emphasized the importance of the interaction of personal and social resources instrumental in promoting remission (86). Specific theories and treatment components he identifies include social control theory (support, goal direction, and structure), behavioral economics and behavioral choice theory (an emphasis on rewards that compete with substance use), social learning theory (focus on abstinence-oriented norms and models), and stress and coping theory (attempts to develop self-efficacy and coping skills). Conceptualizations such as these provide guidance for both research and clinical practice, and are particularly helpful to approach the relationship of factors at different levels of analysis (neurobiologic, personal, and social). This type of integrative thinking and research will become increasingly important as the question of determinants of change is further explored. As an indication of this trend, the U.S. National Institute on Alcohol Abuse and Alcoholism has undertaken a major research initiative to promote interdisciplinary research into mechanisms of behavior change related to initiation of positive change among heavy drinkers (87), and the National Institutes of Health recently approved a similar initiative to understand health behavior change across a wide variety of disorders.

Integrating the Evidence and Personalizing Practice Given the proliferation of new research, published in an ever expanding number of professional journals, it is a challenge to understand and incorporate new findings into practice. Unfortunately, although studies of the efficacy of various treatments may help determine how one treatment compares with another treatment or to no treatment, there are few studies that address directly questions of central importance to clinicians. For example, should one recommend a few sessions of motivational enhancement therapy or an intensive day program for the treatment of dependence? If an at-risk drinker does not respond to brief motivational counseling, what is the appropriate next step? Is the stepped care strategy, where the least restrictive and expensive option for a particular patient's situation is offered first, the best approach? How much evidence is required before recommending a new treatment? How much evidence is required before failure to offer or recommend a treatment based on personal taste or ideology is ethically indefensible?

Although it is not possible at this time to provide definitive or even approximate answers for many such questions, certain conclusions emerge from the current body of evidence. First, although differences among different behavioral techniques tend to be minor, the quality of behavioral treatment is important. Specifically, empathic and skillful therapy is more effective than confrontation and education. Furthermore, it is more important to engage someone with alcohol dependence in treatment than which particular treatment is used, as long as the treatment has been shown to be effective and it is delivered skillfully. Therefore it makes sense to offer a variety of treatment options, because patients are likely to vary in their preferences. The same holds true for the setting of treatment. Unless someone is unable to abstain from living in the community, there is no systematic advantage of residential versus outpatient treatment. Second, available medications offer small but clinically important benefit in early recovery and therefore patients should routinely be offered the opportunity to use them. As with behavioral treatments, however, there is no consensus that any one medication is better than another, or that there is a specific sequence in which they should be used. There is no evidence at this time that combining medications is more beneficial than monotherapy. For appropriate patients (moderate levels of dependence, little or no coexisting psychopathology, socially stable and motivated to change drinking), medication with medical care management and encouragement to abstain, adhere to treatment, and attend mutual help groups is as effective as specialized alcohol counseling. Third, a social network supportive of abstinence is at least as important as whatever treatment occurs in determining outcome (88). Except for referral to mutual help groups, this aspect of treatment tends to be neglected, to the detriment of our patients. Behavioral marital therapy, for example, has a strong evidence base (89). Finally, for any given diagnosis (e.g., at-risk drinking versus dependence), there is not yet a way to identify patient characteristics that reliably predict differential response to different treatments, although research in this area is promising.

SUMMARY AND CONCLUSIONS

From humble beginnings in recovery houses staffed by volunteer members of AA, the treatment for alcohol use disorders has evolved in remarkable ways. Much has been learned about the genetics, neurobiology, psychology, social manifestations, epidemiology, and natural history of heavy drinking and alcohol dependence. Animal models available to study alcohol dependence are among the best available for any disease (90). With dedicated funding from the National Institutes of Health, a formidable research community has developed, providing a substantial body of sophisticated genetic and genomic, behavioral, neurobiologic, and pharmacotherapy research on which to base treatment decisions and development of new treatments. The focus of current research has evolved from whether treatment works to questions of how it works, for whom, how to individualize treatment, and how to increase access to affordable and appealing treatment. Unfortunately, the clinical infrastructure has not developed in concert with growth in scientific understanding, thus making implementation of new findings difficult. Changing this situation will first require changing how drinking and its attendant risks and adverse effects are conceptualized. The public health model described in this chapter provides a framework for understanding drinking, risk, and disorders as existing along a continuum, which in turn suggests a corresponding comprehensive continuum of care. This model may be helpful in formulating new directions for research and policy. It also provides a framework for integrating information about different types of prevention and treatment activities for the purposes of treatment planning. It has important implications about what treatment is, where and to whom should be offered, and who should provide it.

More than conceptual change will be required, however. Fully implementing a continuum of care for heavy drinking and alcohol use disorders requires the continued development of new treatments, especially medications, and new ways to provide behavioral support for change to large numbers of people. Physicians, in particular, must play a central role in helping to design systems that can provide care to people in existing primary care and psychiatric practices. A reinvestment into the specialty treatment sector is also required, but with a new focus: providing true comprehensive specialty care over longer periods. A reinvigorated addiction medicine specialty approach must integrate treatment for addiction with treatment of physical and mental disorders as well as social services such as housing and vocational services. Changes in how services are funded, where they occur, and how they are staffed will be necessary, so the configuration of funding streams must change as well, because funding mechanisms tend to reflect and therefore support the current configuration of services.

At the same time, in the next decade, we are likely to witness major advances in the understanding of and treatments available for heavy drinking and related disorders. Development of more effective pharmaceuticals and identification of indicators predicting response in individual patients will be central features. Having more effective, cost-effective and appealing treatments may then drive system changes to facilitate their implementation.

ACKNOWLEDGMENT: *The opinions expressed in this article are those of the author and do not necessarily reflect the views of the National Institute on Alcohol Abuse and Alcoholism or any other government agency.*

REFERENCES

1. Dawson DA, Grant BF, Li TK. Quantifying the risks associated with exceeding recommended drinking limits. *Alcohol Clin Exp Res* 2005;29(5):902–908.
2. Dawson DA, Grant BF, Stinson FS, et al. Estimating the effect of help-seeking on achieving recovery from alcohol dependence. *Addiction* 2006;101(6):824.
3. McLellan AT, Meyers K. Contemporary addiction treatment: a review of systems problems for adults and adolescents. *Biol Psychiatry* 2004; 56(10):764.
4. McGlynn EA, Asch SM, Adams J, et al. The quality of health care delivered to adults in the United States. *N Engl J Med* 2003;348(26): 2635–2645.
5. Pittman B. *AA: the way it began.* Seattle, WA: Glen Abbey Books, 1988.
6. White WL. *Slaying the dragon: the history of addiction treatment and recovery in America.* Bloomington, IN: Chestnut Health Systems, 1998.
7. Anderson DJ, McGovern JP, DuPont RL. The origins of the Minnesota Model of addictions treatment—a first person account. *J Addict Dis* 1999;18:107–114.
8. Nowinski J, Baker S, et al. *Twelve step facilitation therapy manual: a clinical research guide for therapists treating individuals with alcohol abuse and dependence*, vol. 1. Project MATCH Monograph Series. Rockville, MD: National Institute on Alcohol Abuse and Alcoholism, 1992.
9. Menninger R, Nemiah J. *American psychiatry after World War II: 1944–1994.* Washington, DC: American Psychiatric Press, 2000.
10. Compas B, Gotlib I. *Introduction to clinical psychology.* New York: McGraw-Hill Higher Education, 2002.
11. Pavlov IP. *Conditioned reflexes; an investigation of the physiological activity of the cerebral cortex.* London: Oxford University Press, Humphrey Milford, 1927.
12. Skinner BF. Two types of conditioned reflex and a pseudo type. *J Gen Psychol* 1935:66–77.
13. Pines M. Forgotten pioneers: the unwritten history of the therapeutic community movement. *Therap Comm* 1999;20:23–42.
14. Ellis A. *Reason and emotion in psychotherapy.* Secaucus, NJ: Citadel, 1962.
15. Beck AT. Cognitive therapy and the emotional disorders. *Int. Univ. Press,* New York:1976.
16. Miller WR, Rollnick S. *Motivational interviewing: preparing people to change addictive behavior.* New York: The Guilford Press, 1991.
17. Bouza C, Angeles M, Munoz A, et al. Efficacy and safety of naltrexone and acamprosate in the treatment of alcohol dependence: a systematic review. *Addiction* 2004;99(7):811–828.
18. Johnson BA, Rosenthal N, Capece JA, et al. Topiramate for treating alcohol dependence: a randomized controlled trial. *JAMA* 2007;298(14): 1641–1651.

19. Carroll KM, Farentinos C, Ball SA, et al. MET meets the real world: design issues and clinical strategies in the Clinical Trials Network. *J Subst Abuse Treat* 2002;23(2):73–80.
20. United Methodist Church Book of Discipline 2004 English Red. Abingdon Press, Nashville, TN:2003.
21. Land R, Duke B. (2008, 2006/07/25/). On alcohol use. Accessed March 31, 2008, from http://erlc.com/article/on-alcohol-use.
22. Alcoholics Anonymous. *The big book,* 3rd ed. New York: Alcoholics Anonymous World Services, 1976.
23. Sobell MB, Sobell LC. The aftermath of heresy: a response to Pendery et al.'s (1982) critique of 'individualized behavior therapy for alcoholics'. *Behav Res Ther* 1984;22(4):413–440.
24. What is recovery? A working definition from the Betty Ford Institute. *J Subst Abuse Treat* 2007;33(3):221–228.
25. Laudet AB. What does recovery mean to you? Lessons from the recovery experience for research and practice. *J Subst Abuse Treat* 2007;33(3):243.
26. National Consensus Statement on Mental Health Recovery, 2004. Retrieved August 8, 2008, from http://mentalhealth.samhsa.gov/ publications/allpubs/sma05-4129/.
27. Cella D, Yount S, Rothrock N, et al. The Patient-Reported Outcomes Measurement Information System (PROMIS): progress of an NIH roadmap cooperative group during its first two years. *Med Care* 2007;45(5 Suppl. 1):S3–S11.
28. Sobell LC, Sobell MB. *Timeline followback user's guide: a calendar method for assessing alcohol and drug use.* Toronto, Ontario, Canada, The Addiction Research Foundation, 1996.
29. Del Boca FK, Darkes J. The validity of self-reports of alcohol consumption: state of the science and challenges for research. *Addiction* 2003;98(s2):1–12.
30. Searles JS, Helzer JE, Rose GL, et al. Concurrent and retrospective reports of alcohol consumption across 30, 90, and 366 days: interactive voice response compared with the timeline follow back. *J Stud Alcohol* 2002;63(3):352.
31. Toll BA, Cooney NL, et al. Correspondence between Interactive Voice Response (IVR) and Timeline Followback (TLFB) reports of drinking behavior. *Addict Behav* 2006;31(4):726–731.
32. Helzer JE, Badger GJ, et al. Decline in alcohol consumption during two years of daily reporting. *J Stud Alcohol* 2002;63(5):551.
33. Ball SA, Todd M, Tennen H, et al. Brief motivational enhancement and coping skills interventions for heavy drinking. *Addict Behav* 2007; 32(6):1105.
34. American Psychiatric Association. *Diagnostic and statistical manual,* 4th ed., revised—text revision. Washington, DC: American Psychiatric Press, 2000.
35. Dawson DA, Grant BF, et al. Recovery from DSM-IV alcohol dependence: United States, 2001–2002. *Addiction* 2005;100(3): 281–292.
36. Gueorguieva R, Wu R, et al. New insights into the efficacy of naltrexone based on trajectory-based reanalyses of two negative clinical trials. *Biol Psychiatry* 2007;61(11):1290–1295.
37. Cisler RA, Kowalchuk RK, Saunders SM, et al. Applying clinical significance methodology to alcoholism treatment trials: determining recovery outcome status with individual- and population-based measures. *Alcohol Clin Exp Res* 2005;29(11):1991–2000.
38. Mokdad AH, Marks JS, Stroup DF, et al. Actual causes of death in the United States, 2000. *JAMA* 2004;291(10):1238–1245.
39. Chikritzhs TN, Jonas HA, Stockwell TR, et al. Mortality and life-years lost due to alcohol: a comparison of acute and chronic causes. *Med J Aust* 2001;174(6):281–284.
40. Chase V, Neild R, Sadler CW, et al. The medical complications of alcohol use: understanding mechanisms to improve management. *Drug Alcohol Rev* 2005;24(3):253–265.
41. Satre DD, Gordon NP, Weisner C. Alcohol consumption, medical conditions, and health behavior in older adults. *Am J Health Behav* 2007; 31(3):238–248.
42. Dawson DA. Alcohol consumption, alcohol dependence, and all-cause mortality. *Alcohol Clin Exp Res* 2000;24(1):72–81.
43. Ellison RC. Balancing the risks and benefits of moderate drinking. *Ann N Y Acad Sci* 2002;957:1.
44. Johnson JE, Finney JW, Moos RH. Predictors of 5-year mortality following inpatient/residential group treatment for substance use disorders. *Addict Behav* 2005;30(7):1300–1316.
45. Costello RM. Long-term mortality from alcoholism: a descriptive analysis. *J Stud Alcohol* 2006;67(5):694–699.
46. Timko C, DeBenedetti A, et al. Predictors of 16-year mortality among individuals initiating help-seeking for an alcoholic use disorder. *Alcohol Clin Exp Res* 2006;30(10):1711.
47. Saitz R, Gaeta J, Cheng DM, et al. Risk of mortality during four years after substance detoxification in urban adults. *J Urban Health* 2007; 84(2):272–282.
48. Bischof G, Rumpf H, et al. Types of natural recovery from alcohol dependence: a cluster analytic approach. *Addiction* 2003;98(12): 1737–1746.
49. Fein G, Landman B. Treated and treatment-naive alcoholics come from different populations. *Alcohol* 2005;35(1):19–26.
50. Moss HB, Chen CM, et al. Subtypes of alcohol dependence in a nationally representative sample. *Drug Alcohol Depend* 2007;91(2–3):149–158.
51. Young R, Sweeting H, West P. A longitudinal study of alcohol use and antisocial behaviour in young people. *Alcohol Alcohol* 2008;43(2): 204–214.
52. Hasin DS, Stinson FS, Ogburn E, et al. Prevalence, correlates, disability, and comorbidity of DSM-IV alcohol abuse and dependence in the United States: results from the national epidemiologic survey on alcohol and related conditions. *Arch Gen Psychiatry* 2007;64(7):830–842.
53. Moos RH, Moos BS. Long-term influence of duration and frequency of participation in Alcoholics Anonymous on individuals with alcohol use disorders. *J Consult Clin Psychol* 2004;72(1):81–90.
54. Koob GF. The neurobiology of addiction: a neuroadaptational view relevant for diagnosis. *Addiction* 2006;101(s1):23–30.
55. Grant BF, Stinson FS, Dawson DA, et al. Prevalence and co-occurrence of substance use disorders and independent mood and anxiety disorders: results from the National Epidemiologic Survey on Alcohol and Related Conditions. *Arch Gen Psychiatry* 2004;61(8):807–816.
56. Wodak AD, Saunders JB, Ewusi-Mensah I, et al. Severity of alcohol dependence in patients with alcoholic liver disease. *Br Med J* 1983; 287(6403):1420.
57. Smith S, White J, Nelson C, et al. Severe alcohol-induced liver disease and the alcohol dependence syndrome. *Alcohol Alcohol* 2006; 41(3): 274–277.
58. Sobell MB, Sobell LC. Guided self-change model of treatment for substance use disorders. *J Cogn Psychother* 2005;19(3):199–210.
59. Whitlock EP, Polen MR, Green CA, et al. Behavioral counseling interventions in primary care to reduce risky/harmful alcohol use by adults: a summary of the evidence for the U.S. Preventive Services Task Force. *Ann Intern Med* 2004;140(7):557–568.
60. Zisserson RN, Palfai T, Saitz R. "No-contact" interventions for unhealthy college drinking: efficacy of alternatives to person-delivered intervention approaches. *Subst Abuse* 2007;28(4):119.
61. Nilsen P, Baird J, Mello MJ, et al. A systematic review of emergency care brief alcohol interventions for injury patients. *J Subst Abuse Treat* 2008; 35(2):184–201.
62. Saitz R, Palfai TP, Cheng DM, et al. Brief intervention for medical inpatients with unhealthy alcohol use: a randomized, controlled trial. *Ann Intern Med* 2007;146(3):167–176.
63. Schuckit MA, Smith TL, Danko GP, et al. Five-year clinical course associated with DSM-IV alcohol abuse or dependence in a large group of men and women. *Am J Psychiatry* 2001;158(7):1084–1090.
64. Vaillant GE. A 60-year follow-up of alcoholic men. *Addiction* 2003; 98(8):1043.
65. Grant BF, Dawson DA, Stinson FS, et al. The 12-month prevalence and trends in DSM-IV alcohol abuse and dependence: United States, 1991–1992 and 2001–2002. *Drug Alcohol Depend* 2004;74(3):223–234.
66. Saha TD, Chou SP, Grant BF. Toward an alcohol use disorder continuum using item response theory: results from the National Epidemiologic Survey on Alcohol and Related Conditions. *Psychol Med* 2006; 36(7):931–941.
67. Saha TD, Stinson FS, Grant BF. The role of alcohol consumption in future classifications of alcohol use disorders. *Drug Alcohol Depend* 2007;89(1):82–92.

68. Humphreys K, Weingardt KR, Horst D, et al. Prevalence and predictors of research participant eligibility criteria in alcohol treatment outcome studies, 1970–98. *Addiction* 2005;100(9):1249–1257.
69. Moos RH, Finney JW, Ouimette PC, et al. A comparative evaluation of substance abuse treatment: I. Treatment orientation, amount of care, and 1-year outcomes. *Alcohol Clin Exp Res* 1999;23(3):529–536.
70. Miller WR, Walters ST, Bennett ME. How effective is alcoholism treatment in the United States? *J Stud Alcohol* 2001;62(2):211–220.
71. O'Malley SS, Rounsaville BJ, Farren C, et al. Initial and maintenance naltrexone treatment for alcohol dependence using primary care vs. specialty care: a nested sequence of 3 randomized trials. *Arch Intern Med* 2003;163(14):1695–1704.
72. Anton RF, O'Malley SS, Ciraulo DA, et al. Combined pharmacotherapies and behavioral interventions for alcohol dependence: the COMBINE study: a randomized controlled trial. *JAMA* 2006;295(17):2003–2017.
73. American Society of Addiction. *ASAM patient placement criteria for the treatment of substance-related disorders,* 2nd ed.—rev. Annapolis Junction, MD: ASAM Publications Distribution, 2001.
74. Lieber CS, Weiss DG, Grozsmann R, et al. I. Veterans Affairs Cooperative Study of polyenylphosphatidylcholine in alcoholic liver disease: effects on drinking behavior by nurse/physician teams. *Alcohol Clin Exp Res* 2003;27(11):1757–1764.
75. Willenbring ML, Olson DH, Bielinski J. Integrated outpatient treatment for medically ill alcoholic men: results from a quasi-experimental study. *J Stud Alcohol* 1995;56(3):337–343.
76. Willenbring ML, Olson DH. A randomized trial of integrated outpatient treatment for medically ill alcoholic men. *Arch Intern Med* 1999; 159(16):1946–1952.
77. Mark TL, Levit KR, Buck JA, et al. Mental health treatment expenditure trends, 1986–2003. *Psychiatric Serv* 2007;58(8):1041.
78. Hingson R, McGovern T, Howland J, et al. Reducing alcohol-impaired driving in Massachusetts: the saving lives program. *Am J Public Health* 1996;86(6):791.
79. Finney JW, Hahn AC, Moos RH. The effectiveness of inpatient and outpatient treatment for alcohol abuse: the need to focus on mediators and moderators of setting effects. *Addiction* 1996;91(12):1773–1796.
80. Matching alcoholism treatments to client heterogeneity: Project MATCH posttreatment drinking outcomes. *J Stud Alcohol* 1997;58(1): 7–29.
81. Lee C, Morton CC. Structural genomic variation and personalized medicine. *N Engl J Med* 2008;358(7):740–741.
82. Orford J. Effectiveness of treatment for alcohol problems: findings of the randomised UK alcohol treatment trial (UKATT). *Br Med J* 2005; 331(7516):541–544.
83. McKellar JD, Harris AH, Moos RH. Predictors of outcome for patients with substance-use disorders five years after treatment dropout. *J Stud Alcohol* 2006;67(5):685–693.
84. Timko C, Billow R, DeBenedetti A. Determinants of 12-step group affiliation and moderators of the affiliation-abstinence relationship. *Drug Alcohol Depend* 2006;83(2):111–121.
85. Dawson DA, Goldstein RB, Grant BF. Rates and correlates of relapse among individuals in remission from DSM-IV alcohol dependence: a 3-year follow-up. *Alcohol Clin Exp Res* 2007;31(12):2036.
86. Moos RH. Theory-based processes that promote the remission of substance use disorders. *Clin Psychol Rev* 2007;27(5):537–551.
87. Willenbring ML. A broader view of change in drinking behavior. *Alcohol Clin Exp Res* 2007;31(s3):84s–86s.
88. Zywiak WH. Decomposing the relationships between pretreatment social network characteristics and alcohol treatment outcome. *J Stud Alcohol* 2002;63(1):114–121.
89. Powers MB, Vedel E, Emmelkamp PM. Behavioral couples therapy (BCT) for alcohol and drug use disorders: a meta-analysis. *Clin Psychol Rev* 2008;28(6):952–962.
90. Heilig M, Egli M. Pharmacological treatment of alcohol dependence: target symptoms and target mechanisms. *Pharmacol Therap* 2006;111(3): 855–876.

CHAPTER 24

Andrea G. Barthwell, MD, FASAM
Lawrence S. Brown, Jr., MD, MPH, FASAM

The Treatment of Drug Addiction: An Overview

Drug addiction is a complex illness. Compulsive (at times uncontrollable) drug craving, seeking, and use, which persist even in the face of extremely negative consequences, characterize the disorder. For many patients, drug addiction is a chronic disease, with relapses possible even after long periods of abstinence. Patients with substance use disorders are heterogeneous in a number of clinically important features and domains. Because addiction has so many dimensions and disrupts so many aspects of an individual's life, treatment for this illness never is simple; generally, a multimodal approach to treatment is required. Drug treatment must help the individual stop using drugs and maintain a drug-free lifestyle while achieving productive functioning in the family, at work, and in society. After repeated failures of appropriately matched treatment, some individuals are deemed unable to stop using drugs. In this instance, it is appropriate to work to achieve intermediate outcomes that include a reduction in the use and effects of substances, reduction in frequency and severity of relapse to substance use, and improvement in psychologic and social functioning. Physicians are cautioned that the latter is hard to achieve with continued drug use.

Effective treatment programs typically incorporate many components, each directed to a particular aspect of the illness and its consequences. In practice, specific pharmacologic and psychosocial treatments are often combined because combined treatments lead to better treatment retention and outcomes (1). Three decades of scientific research and clinical practice have yielded a variety of approaches to addiction treatment; the most effective match the patient's assessed needs to services that research suggests might have the most impact. Evidence suggests that substance-dependent individuals who achieve sustained abstinence from the abused substance have the best long-term outcomes (2,3). Extensive data show that such treatment is as effective as treatment for most other chronic medical conditions (4). Of course, not all drug treatment is equally effective or applied in a standardized way. To overcome inconsistency and to improve fidelity to conceptualized models, the National Institute on Drug Abuse has manualized therapies. Research also has revealed a set of overarching principles that characterize the most effective drug addiction treatments and their implementation (Table 24.1).

GOALS OF DRUG ADDICTION TREATMENT

Drug addiction is a complex disorder that can involve virtually every aspect of an individual's functioning—in the family, at work, and in the community. Because of addiction's complexity and pervasive consequences, addiction treatment typically must involve many components. Some of those components focus directly on the individual's drug use, whereas others, such as employment training, focus on restoring the addicted individual to productive membership in the family and society (Table 24.2). Treatment of drug abuse and addiction is delivered in many different settings, using a variety of behavioral and pharmacologic approaches. In the United States, more than 11,000 specialized drug treatment facilities provide rehabilitation, counseling, behavioral therapy, medication, case management, and other types of services to persons with drug use disorders.

Care of individuals with substance use disorders includes assessing needs, providing treatment for intoxication and withdrawal, and developing, with appropriate support, the treatment

TABLE 24.1	Principles of Effective Treatment	
1.	No single treatment is appropriate for all individuals.	Matching treatment settings, interventions, and services to each individual's particular problems and needs is critical to his or her ultimate success in returning to productive functioning in the family, workplace, and society.
2.	Treatment needs to be readily available.	Because individuals who are addicted to drugs may be uncertain about entering treatment, taking advantage of opportunities when they are ready for treatment is crucial. Potential treatment applicants can be lost if treatment is not immediately available or is not readily accessible.
3.	Effective treatment attends to multiple needs of the individual.	To be effective, treatment must address the individual's drug use and any associated medical, psychologic, social, vocational, and legal problems.
4.	An individual's treatment and services plan must be assessed continually and modified as necessary to ensure that the plan meets the person's changing needs.	A patient may require varying combinations of services and treatment components during the course of treatment and recovery. In addition to counseling or psychotherapy, a patient at times may require medication, other medical services, family therapy, parenting instruction, vocational rehabilitation, and social and legal services. It is critical that the treatment approach be appropriate to the individual's age, gender, race/ethnicity, and culture.
5.	Remaining in treatment for an adequate period is critical for treatment effectiveness.	The appropriate duration for an individual depends on his or her problems and needs. Research indicates that, for most patients, the threshold of significant improvement is reached at about 3 months in treatment. After this threshold is reached, additional treatment can produce further progress toward recovery. Because people often leave treatment prematurely, programs should include strategies to engage and keep patients in treatment.
6.	Counseling (individual and group) and other behavioral therapies are critical components of effective treatment.	In therapy, patients address issues of motivation, build skills to resist drug use, replace drug-using activities with constructive and rewarding nondrug-using activities, and improve their problem-solving abilities. Behavioral therapy also facilitates interpersonal relationships and the individual's ability to function in the family and community.
7.	Medications are an important element of treatment for many patients, especially when combined with counseling and other behavioral therapies.	Methadone and levo-alpha-acetylmethadol are very effective in helping individuals addicted to heroin and other opiates stabilize their lives and reduce their illicit drug use. Naltrexone is an effective medication for some opiate dependent patients and some patients with co-occurring alcohol dependence. For persons addicted to nicotine, a nicotine replacement product (such as patches or gum) or an oral medication (such as bupropion) can be an effective component of treatment. For patients with co-occurring mental disorders, both behavioral treatments and medications can be critically important.
8.	Addicted or drug-abusing individuals with cooccurring mental disorders should have both disorders treated in an integrated way.	Because addictive disorders and mental disorders often occur in the same individual, patients presenting for either condition should be assessed and treated for the co-occurrence of the other type of disorder.
9.	Medical detoxification is only the first stage of addiction treatment and by itself does little to change long-term drug use.	Medical detoxification safely manages the acute physical symptoms of withdrawal associated with stopping drug use. Although detoxification alone is rarely sufficient to help addicts achieve long-term abstinence, for some individuals it is a strongly indicated precursor to effective addiction treatment.
10.	Treatment does not need to be voluntary to be effective.	Strong motivation can facilitate the treatment process. Sanctions or enticements in the family, employment setting, or criminal justice system can increase significantly both entry into treatment and retention in treatment, as well as the success of treatment interventions.
11.	Possible drug use during treatment must be monitored continuously.	Lapses to drug use can occur during treatment. The objective monitoring of a patient's drug and alcohol use during treatment, as through urinalysis or other tests, can help the patient withstand urges to use drugs. Such monitoring also can provide early evidence of drug use so that the individual's treatment plan can be adjusted. Feedback to patients who test positive for illicit drug use is an important element of monitoring.
12.	Treatment programs should provide assessment for HIV/AIDS, hepatitis B and C, tuberculosis, and other infectious diseases, and counseling to help patients modify or change behaviors that place themselves or others at risk for infection.	Counseling can help patients avoid high-risk behaviors. Counseling also can help those who are already infected manage their illnesses.
13.	Recovery from drug addiction can be a long-term process and frequently requires multiple episodes of treatment. As with other chronic illnesses, relapses to drug use can occur during or after successful treatment episodes.	Addicted individuals may require prolonged treatment and multiple episodes of treatment to achieve long-term abstinence and fully restore functioning. Participation in self-help support programs during and following treatment often is helpful in maintaining abstinence.

From National Institute on Drug Abuse (1999). *Principles of drug addiction treatment: a research-based guide*. Rockville, MD: NIDA (NIH Publication No. 99-4180), 1999:1–3.

TABLE 24.2 Components of Comprehensive Addiction Treatment

The best treatment programs provide a combination of therapies and other services to meet the needs of the individual patient.

Core components of addiction treatment	Intake processing/assessment Treatment planning Clinical and case management Substance use monitoring Behavioral therapy and counseling Pharmacotherapies Self-help/peer support groups Continuing care
Ancillary services include	Mental health services Medical services HIV/AIDS services Educational services Vocational services Legal services Financial services Housing/transportation services Family services Child care services

From National Institute on Drug Abuse (1999). *Principles of drug addiction treatment: a research-based guide.* Rockville, MD: NIDA (NIH Publication No. 99-4180), 1999:14.

plan that may consist of referrals to psychosocial care. The treatment plan should address how the patient will achieve abstinence without medical compromise; achieve and maintain abstinence after withdrawal; and gain improvement in functioning in the medical, social, and psychologic domains.

TREATMENT SETTINGS

The addiction treatment delivery system is a specialty care delivery system, often separate from the medical/surgical delivery system. Funding for care in the system is usually separate, and the professionals in the system are different. Treatment settings vary widely with regard to services and medical support available and the milieu or philosophy. For physicians, assessment for treatment matching and knowledge of referral and funding options in the community are important, as every community is different. Hospital social work departments generally know the local resources, and health maintenance organization case managers can assist with locating specialty providers of addiction medicine. Mental health carve-outs make accessing care complicated for the patient, and physicians may not be allowed to refer to preferred providers who are out of the network of care. Underinsurance for addiction care is common, and benefit limits (any coverage) or lifetime caps (remaining coverage) may preclude care for patients relapsing following prior treatment.

Decisions regarding the site of care should be based on the patient's ability to cooperate with and benefit from the treatment offered, refrain from illicit use of substances, and avoid high-risk behaviors, as well as the patient's need for structure and support or particular treatments that may be available only in certain settings. Patients move from one level of care to another based on these factors and an assessment of their ability to benefit from a different level of care. Delivery system discontinuities occur when coverage is available for a limited number of levels of care, but not the one indicated based on the assessment carried out using a standardized system such as the American Society of Addiction Medicine (ASAM) Patient Placement Criteria (PPC). ASAM PPC describes four levels of care: (1) general outpatient; (2) intensive outpatient or day hospital; (3) medically monitored inpatient residential care; and (4) medically managed inpatient care. An in-hospital consultant or a member of the medical staff who is knowledgeable and interested in patients with addictive disorders can make criteria-based placement. Sometimes the payer will insist that external case managers employed by the payer make criteria-based decisions. In some instances, placement decisions are not criteria-based.

Hospital-based physicians may find their management of addiction limited to detoxification and referral. It is uncommon to refer outside of the hospital, either because the payer requires referral to a contracted provider, or the patient lacks coverage and needs referral to the public system of care. Hospital-based physicians can create an inpatient Addiction Medicine Consultation Service with specialty-trained clinicians and nonphysician clinicians who assess addiction severity and withdrawal potential, manage withdrawal, and refer to posthospital addiction care when the patient no longer requires care in the hospital setting.

Detoxification According to ASAM PPC-2R, detoxification refers not only to the attenuation of the physiologic and psychologic features of withdrawal syndromes, but also to the process of interrupting the momentum of compulsive use in persons diagnosed with substance dependence (5). This phase of treatment frequently requires a great intensity of treatment to establish treatment engagement and patient role induction. It can be delivered in ambulatory settings with and without extended onsite monitoring. In residential or inpatient settings, it is delivered under clinically managed, medically monitored, or medically managed conditions. There is increasing intensity of services and involvement of nursing and medical personnel across the latter continuum. A full description of services available in each setting can be found in Chapter 26.

Hospital Settings Hospitalization is appropriate for patients whose assessed need cannot be treated safely in an outpatient or emergency department setting because of (1) acute intoxication, (2) severe or medically complicated withdrawal potential, (3) co-occurring medical or psychiatric conditions that complicate detoxification or impair treatment engagement and response, (4) failure of engagement in treatment at a lower level of care, (5) life- or limb-threatening medical conditions that would require hospitalization, (6) psychiatric disorders that make the patient an imminent threat to self or others, and (7) failure to respond to care at any level such that the patient endangers others or poses a self-threat. Aside from detoxification and management of overdose or intoxication, most patients are receiving services incident to a medical-surgical need to manage a biomedical condition or complication or a psychiatric need to manage an emotional or behavioral condition in a primary psychiatric setting. The physician must evaluate the timing and intensity of addiction medicine services in the context of other concerns.

Partial Hospital Programs and Intensive Outpatient Partial hospitalization is considered for patients who require intensive care but have a reasonable chance of making progress on treatment goals in the intertreatment interval, including maintenance of abstinence. It is often provided to individuals whose treatment is hospital or residential initiated and who still require frequent and concentrated contact with treatment professionals to monitor their behavior and manage their risk of relapse. These patients often have a history of relapse after completion of treatment or are returning to a high-risk environment and have a need to develop support for their recovery-focused efforts beyond the treatment system. Lack of motivation to continue to build on the gains made in treatment, allowing the treatment effect to erode, is often cause to continue the patient in this highly intensive and structured setting. The difference between partial hospital programs and intensive outpatient is seen in intensity, number of hours per day, setting of the program, and structure of the program. Patients who are not successful in intensive outpatient may have clinical contact increased by transfer to partial hospital programs.

Outpatient Programs This treatment varies in the types and intensity of services offered. It costs less than residential or inpatient treatment and often is more suitable for individuals whose ASAM PPC shows insight into his or her disease, a high degree of predicted compliance, low symptomatology, high resource availability and use, and a supportive structure in his or her home environment. Low-intensity programs may offer little more than drug education and admonition; however, as in the other treatment settings, a comprehensive approach is optimal, using—where indicated—a variety of psychotherapeutic and pharmacologic interventions along with behavioral monitoring. High rates of attrition can be problematic, particularly in the early phase. Because outcomes are highly correlated with time in treatment, retention should be one focus of treatment, along with self-efficacy regarding adherence to the abstinence plan. Self-help participation is useful (7).

Other outpatient models, such as intensive day treatment, can be comparable to residential programs (see below) in services and effectiveness, depending on the individual patient's characteristics and needs. In many outpatient programs, as in much of treatment in general, group counseling is emphasized. Some outpatient programs are designed to treat patients who have medical or mental health problems in addition to their drug disorder (8).

Most alcohol abuse and dependence is treated outside of the hospital after medical complications associated with detoxification are addressed (9,10). Similarly, cocaine abuse and dependence (11), nicotine dependence (12), and marijuana abuse and dependence are treated on an outpatient basis as long as the focus on reduced substance use can be maintained and there are no other reasons for hospitalization (13,14).

RESIDENTIAL PROGRAMS, INCLUDING THERAPEUTIC COMMUNITY

Residential programs provide care 24 hours a day, generally in non-hospital settings. Residential care is generally provided to patients who do not meet the clinical criteria for hospitalization but whose lives are transformed by and focused on substance use. These individuals are unlikely to maintain abstinence in the absence of continued application of a variety of therapeutic techniques in a highly structured and supportive environment. Short-term programs provide intensive but relatively brief residential treatment based on a modified 12-step approach and may or may not include elements of therapeutic communities (TCs) (see the following paragraph). The duration of residential treatment should be determined by the clinical response to therapy and the length of time necessary for the patient to meet specific criteria predictive of success in a lower level of care according to ASAM PPC. In general, longer programs provide better outcomes (15). These programs originally were designed to treat alcohol problems, but during the cocaine epidemic of the mid-1980s, many began to treat illicit drug abuse and addiction. The original residential treatment model consisted of a 3- to 6-week hospital-based inpatient treatment phase, followed by extended outpatient therapy and participation in a self-help group such as Alcoholics Anonymous. Reduced health care coverage for addiction treatment has resulted in a diminished number of these programs, and the average length of stay under managed care review is much shorter than in early programs.

One residential treatment model is the TC, but residential treatment programs also employ other models, such as cognitive behavioral therapy. TCs are residential programs with planned lengths of stay from 6 to 12 months. TCs focus on the "resocialization" of the individual and use the program's entire "community"—including other residents, staff, and the social context—as active components of treatment. Addiction is viewed in the context of an individual's social and psychologic deficits, so treatment focuses on developing personal accountability and responsibility and socially productive lives. Treatment is highly structured and can at times be confrontational, with activities designed to help residents examine damaging beliefs, self-concepts, and patterns of behavior, and to adopt new, more harmonious and constructive ways to interact with others. Many TCs are quite comprehensive and include employment training and other support services onsite or through formal linkage agreements. Compared with patients in other forms of drug treatment, the typical TC resident has more chronicity and criminal involvement. Research shows that TCs can be modified to treat individuals with special needs, including adolescents, women (16,17), those with severe mental disorders (18), and individuals in the criminal justice system. Recently, with pressure from reimbursement sources, the elements of TCs have been incorporated into shorter term residential programs and institutional criminal justice settings.

Heroin addiction has been effectively treated in the TC; however, return to use rates after TC treatment are higher than 80% in most long-term follow-up studies, indicating a need for selectivity in application of this modality over medication-assisted clinical settings (19). Data regarding the effectiveness of traditional long-term TC are limited by the low completion rates of 15% to 25%, with most attrition occurring during the first 3 months (20). Retention lengths predict outcomes on abstinence with abstinence success rates of 90% for graduates of 2-year programs and 25% for dropouts of the same programs completing less than 1 year (21). Retention rates differ with program sites (22).

Community Residential Rehabilitation Community residential rehabilitation facilities include "halfway houses" or "sober living facilities," with the former providing more structure and supervision. Individuals referred to these settings are generally deemed to be at risk for relapse without such support. Often this setting is offered to the individual whose environmental risk is great or those needing a number of services after primary treatment to address deficits in vocation, employment, and social supports. These services have been shown to significantly improve substance use outcomes for both sexes, but are variable in their impact on young people (24–26).

Case Management Case management is a collaborative process that assesses, plans, implements, coordinates, monitors, and evaluates the options and services to meet an individual's health needs (27). It uses communication and available resources to promote quality, cost-effective outcomes.

Case management, although difficult to assess for effectiveness in a rigorous fashion, has been shown to be an effective adjunctive treatment for patients with alcohol use disorders, patients with substance use disorders co-occurring with psychiatric disorders (27), and adolescents (28). Case management is provided to individuals whose social situation and complex needs would impair their ability to adhere to a prescribed treatment plan and follow-up care. Basic needs are often met as part of the service array, which includes as psychoeducation and assistance in comprehension of the extent and nature of the disease for which treatment is provided and advocated (29,30).

Aftercare Programs Aftercare generally follows an episode of care and is focused on maintenance of gains made in treatment over a prescribed period with less frequent contact than the primary episode of care (e.g., once weekly monitoring and group therapy after a 6-week intensive outpatient program in which the patient is seen nightly for 3 hours). The patient's affiliation with a 12-step program is encouraged and the transition to self-efficacy is monitored.

Treatment in the Physician's Office, Including Screening and Brief Interventions The addiction treatment enterprise has traditionally been separate and distinct from addiction medicine, with addiction medicine provided in the context of addiction treatment in sometimes limited ways. Public policies, practices, and laws have worked against the provision of care by physicians for the addicted. For example, The Harrison Narcotics Tax Act was a U.S. federal law that regulated and taxed the production, importation, and distribution of opiates. The courts interpreted this to mean that physicians could prescribe narcotics to patients in the course of normal treatment but not for the treatment of addiction. Despite longstanding barriers to care and the risk of prosecution, physicians have recognized a need to provide care to addicted individuals. Early identification through screening for addictive disorders and brief interventions or referral to treatment is a federal initiative supported by demonstration grants from the Center for Substance Abuse Treatment of the U.S. Department of Health and Human Services.

Brief interventions for alcohol use disorders had been studied before being adopted and expanded for substance use disorders (31). Interventions were intended to facilitate treatment of alcohol abuse in settings other than those in the addiction treatment enterprise (e.g., mental health clinics, physician's offices) (32,33).

Brief interventions include assessment, feedback, responsibility for change, advice, and menu of options provided using empathic listening and encouraged self-efficacy (34). Chapter 20 of this textbook provides a more extensive review of this area. The most critical take-home message is that this clinical approach can be used by primary care providers for their patients with harmful substance use because only a small portion of these patients warrant a clinical diagnosis of substance abuse or substance dependence.

Criminal Justice Settings for Mandated Treatment, Including Drug Courts Research has shown that combining criminal justice sanctions with drug treatment can be effective in decreasing drug use and related crime. Individuals under legal coercion tend to stay in treatment for a longer period and do as well as or better than others not under legal pressure (35). Often, drug-addicted persons encounter the criminal justice system earlier than other health or social systems, and intervention by the criminal justice system to engage the individual in treatment may help to interrupt and shorten a career of drug use (36). Addiction treatment may be delivered before, during, after, or in lieu of incarceration.

Prison-based Treatment Programs Offenders with drug disorders may encounter a number of treatment options while incarcerated, including didactic drug education classes, self-help programs, and treatment based on TC or residential milieu therapy models. The TC model has been studied extensively and found to be quite effective in reducing drug use and recidivism to criminal behavior (37). Those in treatment are generally segregated from the general prison population, so that the "prison culture" does not overwhelm progress toward recovery. As might be expected, treatment gains can be lost if inmates are returned to the general prison population after treatment. Research shows that relapse to drug use and recidivism to crime are significantly lower if the drug offender continues treatment after returning to the community (38,39).

Community-based Treatment for Criminal Justice Populations Several criminal justice alternatives to incarceration have been tried with offenders who have drug disorders, including limited diversion programs, pretrial release conditional on entry into treatment, and conditional probation with sanctions. The drug court is a promising approach. Drug courts mandate and arrange for drug addiction treatment, actively monitor progress in treatment, and arrange other services for drug-involved offenders. Federal support for planning, implementation, and enhancement of drug courts is provided under the U.S. Department of Justice Drug Courts Program Office. As a well-studied example, the Treatment Accountability and Safer Communities program provides an alternative to incarceration by addressing the multiple needs of drug-addicted offenders in a community-based setting (35). Treatment Accountability and Safer Communities programs typically include counseling, medical care, parenting instruction, family counseling, school and job training, and legal and employment services. The key features of Treatment Accountability and Safer Communities include coordination of criminal justice and drug treatment; early identification, assessment, and referral of drug-involved offenders; monitoring offenders through drug testing; and use of legal sanctions as inducements to remain in treatment.

TREATMENT SERVICES

This section presents several examples of evidence-based treatment approaches and components that have been developed and tested through research supported by the National Institute on Drug Abuse. Each approach is designed to address certain aspects of drug addiction and their consequences for the individual, family, and society. These approaches are best used to enhance and standardize the quality of best practices in existing treatment programs. This section is not a complete list of empirically supported treatment approaches. Additional approaches are under development as part of National Institute on Drug Abuse's continuing support of treatment research and are reviewed in this section, as well as in Chapters 6, 7, and 8 of this textbook.

Somatic services are defined as those used to manage intoxication, withdrawal syndromes, and pathophysiologic effects and other clinical manifestations of the substance used. Medications are seen as adjunctive to behavioral therapies and self-help involvement and are viewed as best used on a platform of talk therapy. Behavioral therapies and medications are provided in a number of settings, including hospitals and by hospitalists and other primary care specialists in office-based settings. These services are based on scientific advances in the behavioral sciences and neurobiology for a wide range of drugs, alcohol, tobacco, and other psychoactive substances. These services are discussed in more detail in Sections 7 and 8 of this textbook.

Clinical Monitoring As with the treatment of other medical disorders and irrespective of the therapeutic approach chosen, clinical monitoring is extremely important in achieving successful clinical options. Although many studies have underscored the limitations of relying solely on a patient's self-report (40), this type of information is most useful in the context of a nonconfrontational, nonjudgmental, patient-provider relationship based on openness, understanding, and empathy. It should also be explicitly recognized that patients receiving care for other chronic disorders also underreport unhealthy behaviors to their caregivers, and, because substance use is stigmatized and often illegal, underreporting is understandable as is the expectation that reports be objectively verified.

Because of the limitations of self-report in the initial assessment and during clinical monitoring, clinical drug testing represents an important tool for addiction medicine specialists (42,43) but is underused and often misunderstood by primary care providers (44,45). When used in concert with a good history, physical examination, and biologic markers, clinical drug testing facilitates screening, assessment, diagnosis, and clinical monitoring of a substance use disorder in the hands of an experienced practitioner. Drug testing provides useful information about a patient's potential for achieving desirable clinical outcomes with co-occurring medical or psychiatric disorders.

Managing Intoxication and Withdrawal Similar to the treatment of other clinical disorders, patients with substance use disorders exhibit varied clinical presentations, from acute and subacute to chronic manifestations. Some manifestations, such as intoxication and withdrawal, can be life-threatening without appropriate, if not emergent intervention. The therapeutic response is contingent on the substance used, the presence or absence of evidence of a compromised cardiopulmonary system, and the underlying health status of the patient. Pharmacotherapy is the cornerstone for patients suffering from either intoxication or withdrawal, although effective treatment for intoxication requires a hospital setting, whereas withdrawal can be treated in either an inpatient or outpatient setting.

Detoxification is a commonly used approach in responding to patients with clinical signs of intoxication or withdrawal. It is a process in which, under the care of a physician, individuals are systematically withdrawn from addicting drugs in an inpatient or outpatient setting. Detoxification is intended to reduce or eliminate the medical consequences of withdrawal, the pain of withdrawal, or the acute increase in craving experienced by the patient. Detoxification is a precursor to treatment because it addresses the acute physiologic effects of stopping drug use. Medications are available for detoxification from opiates, nicotine, benzodiazepines, alcohol, barbiturates, and other sedatives. Detoxification is not designed to address the psychologic, social, and behavioral problems associated with addiction; therefore, this clinical approach does not typically produce the type of lasting behavior changes necessary for recovery. Detoxification is most useful when it incorporates formal processes of assessment and referral to subsequent addiction treatment (45).

Behavioral Therapy Numerous studies have demonstrated that behavioral counseling is effective treatment for substance use disorders. Although these services are a part of most treatment modalities in most settings, they are particularly important for the treatment of substance use disorders for which pharmacologic treatments are inefficacious. These therapies attempt to arrest compulsive substance use through modification of behaviors, feelings, social functioning, and thoughts. They address a set of common tasks and attempt to increase motivation, expand the coping repertoire, change reinforcement contingencies to increase the frequency of positive behaviors, improve mood, and enhance interpersonal connection and the number of social supports. Because no form of psychotherapy has proven superior to another for all patients, successful referral to services is more important than physician determination of the most useful approach. In other words, a lack of knowledge regarding how to match patients to the various techniques should not be an excuse to avoid this task. In fact, failure to refer to adjunctive psychotherapy is associated with reduced efficacy of known effective pharmacotherapy because medications frequently address only part of the substance dependence syndrome (47–49).

Cognitive-Behavioral Therapy Cognitive-behavioral therapy is based on the theory that learning processes play a critical role in the development of maladaptive patterns of behavior. Cognitive-behavioral therapy targets two processes, dysfunctional thoughts and maladaptive behaviors. Thought-based interventions focus on increasing the patient's resolve not to use—based on negative and positive consequences of use—and confronting thoughts about use. Relapse prevention is an example of cognitive-behavioral therapy with which physicians might be familiar. Relapse prevention was developed for the treatment of problem drinking and later adapted to other substance use disorders. Relapse prevention encompasses several cognitive-behavioral strategies that facilitate abstinence as well as provide help for persons who experience relapse. The goal of relapse prevention is to help addicted individuals learn to identify and correct problematic behaviors. For example, the relapse prevention approach to the treatment of cocaine addiction consists of a collection of strategies intended to enhance self-control (50). Specific techniques include exploring the positive and negative consequences of continued use, self-monitoring to recognize drug cravings early on and to identify situations that pose high risk of use, and developing strategies for coping with and avoiding high-risk situations and the desire to use. A central element of this treatment is anticipating the problems patients are likely to meet and helping them develop effective coping strategies. Research indicates that the skills individuals learn through relapse prevention therapy remain after the completion of treatment (51). In one study, most persons receiving this cognitive-behavioral approach maintained the gains they made in treatment throughout the year after discharge (52–57).

Motivational Enhancement Therapy Motivational enhancement therapy is a patient-centered counseling approach that attempts to initiate behavior change by helping patients resolve their ambivalence about engaging in treatment and stopping drug use. This approach employs strategies to evoke rapid and internally motivated change in the client, rather than guiding the client stepwise through the recovery process. The therapy provides feedback generated from an initial assessment to stimulate discussion regarding personal substance use and to elicit self-motivational statements. Motivational interviewing principles are used to strengthen motivation and build a plan for change. Coping strategies for high-risk situations are suggested and discussed with the client. Over time, the therapist monitors change, reviews cessation strategies being used, and continues to encourage commitment to change or to sustained abstinence. Clients sometimes are encouraged to bring a significant other to sessions. This approach has been used successfully with alcohol- and cannabis-dependent individuals (53–55).

Community Reinforcement Approach Plus Vouchers Community reinforcement approach is an intensive outpatient therapy for the treatment of cocaine addiction. The treatment has dual goals: to achieve cocaine abstinence long enough for patients to learn new life skills that will help sustain abstinence and to reduce alcohol consumption for patients, whose drinking is associated with cocaine use. Patients attend one or two individual counseling sessions per week, where they focus on improving family relations, learning a variety of skills to minimize drug use, receiving vocational counseling, and developing new recreational activities and social networks. Those who also abuse alcohol receive clinic-monitored disulfiram (Antabuse) therapy. Patients submit urine samples two or three times per week and receive vouchers for cocaine-negative samples. The value of the vouchers increases with consecutive clean samples. Patients may exchange their vouchers for retail goods that are consistent with a cocaine-free lifestyle. This approach facilitates patients' engagement in treatment and systematically aids them in gaining substantial periods of cocaine abstinence. The approach has been tested in urban and rural areas and used successfully in outpatient detoxification of opiate-addicted adults and with inner-city methadone maintenance patients who have high rates of intravenous cocaine abuse (56,57).

Voucher-based Reinforcement Therapy in Methadone Maintenance Treatment Voucher-based reinforcement therapy helps patients achieve and maintain abstinence from illegal drugs by providing them with a voucher each time they provide a drug-free urine sample. The voucher has monetary value and can be exchanged for goods and services consistent with the goals of treatment. Initially, the voucher values are low, but their value increases with the number of consecutive drug-free urine specimens the individual provides. Cocaine- or heroin-positive urine specimens reset the value of the vouchers to the initial low value. The contingency of escalating incentives is designed specifically to reinforce periods of sustained drug abstinence. Studies show that patients receiving vouchers for drug-free urine samples achieved significantly more weeks of abstinence and significantly more weeks of sustained abstinence than patients who were given vouchers independent of urine toxicology results. In another study, urine toxicology positive for heroin decreased significantly when the voucher program was started and increased significantly when the program was stopped (58).

Day Treatment with Abstinence Contingencies and Vouchers This approach was developed to treat crack addiction among homeless persons (59). For the first 2 months, participants were required to spend 5.5 hours daily in the program, which provided lunch and transportation to and from shelters. Interventions included individual assessment and goal setting, individual and group counseling, multiple psychoeducational groups (for example, didactic groups on community resources, housing, cocaine, and HIV/AIDS prevention; establishment and review of personal rehabilitation goals; relapse prevention; and weekend planning), and patient-governed community meetings, in which patients reviewed contract goals and provided support and encouragement to each other. Individual counseling occurs once per week, and group therapy sessions are held three times per week. After 2 months of day treatment and at least 2 weeks of abstinence, participants graduate to a 4-month work component that pays wages, which can be used to rent inexpensive, drug-free housing. A voucher system also rewards drug-free social and recreational activities (60). This innovative day treatment was compared with treatment consisting of twice-weekly individual counseling and 12-step groups, medical examinations and treatment, and referral to community resources for housing and vocational services. Innovative day treatment followed by work and housing (dependent on drug abstinence) had a more positive effect on alcohol use, cocaine use, and days of homelessness (65,66).

Psychodynamic Therapy/Interpersonal Therapy Individualized counseling focuses directly on reducing or stopping the patient's illicit drug use. It also addresses related areas of impaired functioning—such as employment status, illegal activity, and family/social relations—as well as the content and structure of the patient's recovery program. Through its emphasis on short-term behavioral goals, individualized drug counseling helps the patient develop coping strategies and tools for abstaining from drug use and then maintaining abstinence. The addiction counselor, social worker, or psychologist encourage 12-step program participation and makes referrals for needed supplemental medical, psychiatric, employment, and other services. Individuals are encouraged to attend sessions one or two times per week. In a study that compared opiate dependent patients receiving methadone alone with those receiving methadone coupled with counseling, individuals who received methadone alone showed minimal improvement in reducing opiate use (61). The addition of counseling produced significantly more improvement. The addition of onsite medical, psychiatric, employment, and family services further improved outcomes. In another study with cocaine dependent patients, individualized drug counseling, together with group counseling, was quite effective in reducing cocaine use (62). Thus it appears that this approach has great utility in outpatient treatment for both heroin and cocaine addiction.

Supportive expressive psychotherapy is a time-limited, focused psychotherapy that has been adapted for heroin- and cocaine-addicted individuals (63). The therapy has two main components: supportive techniques to help patients feel comfortable in discussing their personal experiences and expressive techniques to help patients identify and work through interpersonal relationship issues. Special attention is paid to the role of drugs in relation to problem feelings and behaviors and how problems may be solved without recourse to drugs. The efficacy of individual supportive-expressive psychotherapy has been tested with patients in methadone maintenance treatment who had co-occurring psychiatric disorders (64). In a comparison with patients receiving drug counseling only, both groups fared similarly with regard to opiate use, but the supportive-expressive psychotherapy group had lower cocaine use and required less methadone. In addition, the patients who received supportive-expressive psychotherapy maintained many of the gains they had made. In an earlier study, supportive-expressive psychotherapy, when added to drug counseling, improved outcomes for opiate dependent patients in methadone treatment with moderately severe psychiatric problems (65,66).

Treatment of the Adolescent with Multidimensional Family Therapy Multidimensional family therapy is an outpatient, family-based, drug treatment approach for adolescents. It approaches adolescent drug use in terms of a network of influences (individual, family, peer, and community) and suggests that reducing unwanted behavior and increasing desirable behavior occur in multiple ways in different settings. Treatment includes individual and family sessions held in the clinic, in the home, or with family members at the family court, school, or other community locations. During individual sessions, the therapist and adolescent work on important developmental tasks, such as decision-making, negotiation, and problem-solving skills. Teens acquire skills in communicating their thoughts and feelings to deal better with life stressors and vocational skills. Parallel sessions are held with family members. Parents examine their particular parenting styles, learn to distinguish influence from control, and learn how to have a positive and developmentally appropriate influence on their child (67,68).

Multisystemic Therapy Multisystemic therapy addresses the factors associated with serious antisocial behavior in children and adolescents who use drugs. These factors include characteristics of the adolescent (for example, favorable attitudes toward drug use), the family (poor discipline, family conflict, or parental drug abuse), peers (positive attitudes toward drug use), school (dropout, poor performance), and neighborhood (criminal subculture) (69). By participating in intense treatment in natural environments (homes, schools, and neighborhood settings), most youths and families complete a full course of treatment. Multisystemic therapy significantly reduces adolescent drug use during treatment and for at least 6 months after treatment. Reduced numbers of incarcerations and out-of-home placements of juveniles (70) offset the cost of providing this intensive service and maintaining the clinicians' low caseloads (71). For more information on treatment of adolescents, see Section 13 of this textbook.

PHARMACOLOGIC THERAPIES

Opioid Agonist Treatment Also referred to as agonist or maintenance treatment for opiate-dependent patients, opioid agonist treatment usually is conducted in outpatient treatment settings, such as methadone treatment programs or the physician's office. These programs use a long-acting synthetic opiate medication, usually methadone or buprenorphine, administered orally for a sustained period at a dose sufficient to prevent opiate withdrawal, block the effects of illicit opiate use, and decrease opiate craving. Patients stabilized on adequate, sustained doses of methadone or buprenorphine can function normally. They can hold jobs, avoid the crime and violence of the drug culture, and reduce their exposure to HIV by stopping or decreasing injection drug use and drug-related high-risk sexual behaviors (72–76). Indeed, the infection reducing benefit of substance abuse treatment programs is most robust in those programs providing opiate agonist therapies (77,78). Patients stabilized on opiate agonists can engage more readily in counseling and other behavioral interventions that are essential to recovery and rehabilitation. The most effective opiate agonist maintenance programs include individual or group counseling, as well as provision of, or referral to, other needed medical, psychologic, and social services. Criteria for management in the physician's office have been described and physicians are advised to engage with local providers of substance abuse care to provide services that may be beyond the scope or ability of the office-based practice.

Narcotic Antagonist Treatment Using Naltrexone Antagonist therapies are used to block or counteract the physiologic or subjective reinforcing effects of substances. Treatment of opiate dependent patients with naltrexone usually is conducted in outpatient settings, although initiation of the medication often begins after medical detoxification in a residential setting. Naltrexone is a long-acting synthetic opiate antagonist with few side effects that is taken orally, either daily or three times per week, for a sustained period. Candidates for therapy with naltrexone must be medically detoxified and opiate-free for several days before the drug can be given, to avoid precipitating the opiate abstinence syndrome. When naltrexone is used in this fashion, it completely blocks the effects of self-administered opiates, including euphoria. The theory behind this treatment is that the repeated lack of the desired opiate effects, as well as the perceived futility of using the opiate, will gradually extinguish the habit of opiate addiction. Naltrexone itself has no subjective effects or potential for abuse and is not addicting. Patient noncompliance is a common problem; therefore, a favorable treatment outcome requires that there also be a positive therapeutic relationship, effective counseling or therapy, and careful monitoring of medication compliance (79). Many experienced clinicians have found naltrexone most useful for highly motivated, recently detoxified patients who desire total abstinence because of external circumstances, including impaired professionals, parolees (80), probationers, and prisoners in work-release status. Patients stabilized on naltrexone can function normally. They can hold jobs, avoid the crime and violence of the street culture, and reduce their exposure to HIV by stopping injection drug use and drug related high-risk sexual behaviors. Compared with naloxone, naltrexone has a good oral bioavailability and a relatively long half-life. Its availability as a long-acting injectable preparation may improve treatment adherence (81,82).

CONCLUSION

Although this chapter has not been exhaustive in its coverage of all the behavioral or medication-assisted therapies in use; at the writing of this chapter, many other pharmacotherapies are in various stages of development. Similarly, variants of current behavioral therapies and combinations of pharmacotherapies and behavioral therapies are also under investigation, focused on expanding the array of options to treat substance use disorders associated with the most prevalent psychoactive substances. Even so, dissemination remains a challenge that requires the highest priorities if patients with substance use disorders in various clinical settings are to benefit from the advances in the past 30 years and those in the future.

REFERENCES

1. Siqueland L, Crits-Christoph P. Current developments in psychosocial treatments of alcohol and substance abuse. *Curr Psychiatry Rep* 1999;1:179–184.

2. Vaillant GE. A long-term follow-up of male alcohol abuse. *Arch Gen Psychiatry* 1996;53:243–249.
3. Vaillant GE. A 60-year follow-up of alcoholic men. *Addiction* 2003;98: 1043–1051.
4. McLellan AT, O'Brien CP, Lewis DL, et al. Drug addiction as a chronic medical illness: implications for treatment, insurance, and evaluation. *JAMA* 2000;284:1689–1695.
5. ASAM PPC-2R. Mee-Lee D, ed. *ASAM patient placement criteria for the treatment of substance-related disorders, 2nd edition–revised.* Chevy Chase, MD: American Society of Addiction Medicine, 2001.
6. Paist S. Teaching MDs the ABCs of addiction. *Behav Health Manage* 2005;1 May.
7. Klamen DL. Education and training in addictive diseases. *Psychiatric Clin N Am* 1999;22(2).
8. Kleber H, Slobetz F. Outpatient drug-free treatment. In: DuPont RL, Goldstein A, O'Donnell J, eds. *Handbook on drug abuse.* Rockville, MD: National Institute on Drug Abuse, 1979:31–38.
9. Institute of Medicine. *Treating drug problems.* Washington, DC: National Academy Press, 1990.
10. McLellan AT, Grisson G, Durell J, et al. Substance abuse treatment in the private setting: are some programs more effective than others? *J Subst Abuse Treatment* 1993;10:243–254.
11. Simpson DD, Joe GW, Brown BS. Treatment retention and follow-up outcomes in the Drug Abuse Treatment Outcome Study. *Psychol Addict Behav* 1997;11:294–307.
12. Higgins ST, Budney AJ, Bickel WK, et al. Incentives improve outcome in outpatient behavioral treatment of cocaine dependence. *Arch Gen Psychiatry* 1994;51:568–576.
13. Fiore MC, Smith SS, Jorenby DE, et al. The effectiveness of the nicotine patch for smoking cessation: a meta-analysis. *JAMA* 1994;271:1940–1947.
14. Miller WR, Wilbourne PL, Hettema JE. What works? A summary of alcohol treatment outcome research. In: Hester RK, Miller WR, eds. *Handbook of alcoholism treatment approaches: effective alternatives,* 3rd ed. Needham Heights, MA: Allyn & Bacon, 2003:13–63.
15. Leukefeld C, Pickens R, Schuster CR. Improving drug abuse treatment: recommendations for research and practice. In: Pickens RW, Luekefeld CG, Schuster CR, eds. *Improving drug abuse treatment (NIDA research monograph series).* Rockville, MD: National Institute on Drug Abuse, 1991.
16. Lewis BF, McCusker J, Hindin R, et al. Four residential drug treatment programs: project IMPACT. In: Inciardi JA, Tims FM, Fletcher BM, eds. *Innovative approaches in the treatment of drug abuse.* Westport, CT: Greenwood Press, 45-60:1993.
17. Stevens S, Arbiter N, Glider P. Women residents: expanding their role to increase treatment effectiveness in substance abuse programs. *Int J Addictions* 1989;24(5):425–434.
18. Stevens SJ, Glider PJ. Therapeutic communities: substance abuse treatment for women. In: Tims FM, De Leon G, Jainchill N, eds. *Therapeutic community: advances in research and application (NIDA research monograph 144).* Rockville, MD: National Institute on Drug Abuse, 1994;162–180.
19. Sacks S, Sacks J, DeLeon G, et al. Modified therapeutic community for mentally ill chemical abusers: background; influences; program description; preliminary findings. *Subst Use Misuse* 1998;32(9):1217–1259.
20. Simpson DD, Sells S, eds. *Opioid addiction and treatment: a 12-year follow-up.* Melbourne, FL: Robert E. Krieger, 1990.
21. De Leon G, Schwartz S. Therapeutic communities: what are the retention rates? *Am J Drug Alcohol Abuse* 1984;10:267–284.
22. De Leon G. *The therapeutic community: study of effectiveness.* Rockville, MD: National Institute on Drug Abuse, 1984.
23. Simpson DD, Joe GW, Brown BS. Treatment retention and follow-up outcomes in the Drug Abuse Treatment Outcome Study (DATOS). *Psychol Addict Behav* 1997;11:294–307.
24. Friedmann PD, Hendrickson JC, Gerstein DR, et al. The effect of matching comprehensive services to patients' needs on drug use improvement in addiction treatment. *Addiction* 2004;99:962–972.
25. Lemke S, Moos RH. Treatment and outcomes of older patients with alcohol use disorders in community residential programs. *J Stud Alcohol* 2003;64:219–226.
26. Jason LA, Davis MI, Ferrari JR, et al. Oxford House: a review of research and implications for substance abuse recovery and community research. *J rug Educ* 2001;31:1–27.
27. National Case Management Task Forces. *CCM certification guide.* Rolling Meadows, IL: CIRSC/Certified Case Manager, 1993.
28. Weiner DA, Abraham ME, Lyons J. Clinical characteristics of youths with substance use problems and implications for residential treatment. *Psychiatr Serv* 2001;52:793–799.
29. Drake RE, Mercer-McFadden C, Mueser KT, et al. Review of integrated mental health and substance abuse treatment for patients with dual disorders. *Schizophr Bull* 1998;24:589–608.
30. Godley MD, Godley SH, Dennis ML, et al. Preliminary outcomes from the assertive continuing care experiment for adolescents discharged from residential treatment. *J Subst Abuse Treat* 2002;23:21–32.
31. Graham K, Timney CB. Case management in addictions treatment. *J Subst Abuse Treat* 1990;7:181–188.
32. McNeese-Smith DK. Case management within substance abuse treatment programs in Los Angeles County. *Care Manage J* 1999;1:10–18.
33. Miller WR, Rollnick S. *Motivational interviewing: preparing people for change,* 2nd ed. New York: Guilford, 2002.
34. Edwards G, Orford J, Egert S, et al. Alcoholism: a controlled trial of "treatment" and "advice." *J Stud Alcohol* 1977;38:1004–1031.
35. Bien TH, Miller WR, Tonigan JS. Brief interventions for alcohol problems: a review. *Addiction* 1993;88:315–335.
36. Baker A, Lewin T, Reichler H, et al. Evaluation of a motivational interview for substance use within psychiatric in-patient services. *Addiction* 2002;97:1329–1337.
37. Anglin MD, Hser Y. Treatment of drug abuse. In: Tonry M, Wilson JQ, eds. *Drugs and crime.* Chicago, IL: University of Chicago Press, 1990;393–460.
38. Hiller ML, Knight K, Broome KM, et al. Compulsory community based substance abuse treatment and the mentally ill criminal offender. *Prison J* 1996;76(2):180–191.
39. Inciardi JA, Martin SS, Butzin CA, et al. An effective model of prison-based treatment for drug-involved offenders. *J Drug Issues* 1997;27(2): 261–278.
40. Wexler HK. Therapeutic communities in American prisons. In: Cullen E, Jones L, Woodward R, eds. *Therapeutic communities in American prisons.* New York: Wiley & Sons, 1997.
41. Wexler HK, Falkin GP, Lipton DS. Outcome evaluation of a prison therapeutic community for substance abuse treatment. *Crim Just Behav* 1990;17(1):71–92.
42. Chen JT, Fang CC, Shyu RS, et al. Underreporting of illicit drug use by patients at emergency departments as revealed by two-tiered urinalysis. *Addictive Behav* 2006;31:2304–2308.
43. Brown RL. Identification and office management of alcohol and drug disorders. In: Fleming MF, Barry KL, eds. *Addictive disorders.* Baltimore, MD: Mosby Yearbook, 1992.
44. Cone EJ. New developments in biological measures of drug prevalence. In Harrison L, Hughes A, eds. *The validity of self-reported drug use: improving the accuracy of survey estimates (NIDA research monograph 167).* Bethesda, MD: National Institute on Drug Abuse, 1997.
45. Warner EA, Friedmann, PD. Laboratory testing for drug abuse. *Arch Pediatr Adolesc Med* 2006;160:854–864.
46. Levy S, Harris SK, Sherritt L, et al. Drug testing of adolescents in ambulatory medicine: physician practices and knowledge. *Arch Pediatr Adolesc Med* 2006;160:146–150.
47. Reisfield GM, Bertholf R, Barkin RL, et al. Urine drug test interpretation: what do physicians know? *J Opioid Manage* 2007;3:80–86.
48. Kleber HD. Outpatient detoxification from opiates. *Prim Psychiatry* 1996;1:42–52.
49. Carroll KM, Sinha R, Nich C, et al. Contingency management to enhance naltrexone treatment of opioid dependence: a randomized clinical trial of reinforcement magnitude. *Exp Clin Psychopharmacol* 2002;10: 54–63.
50. Fuller RK, Branchey L, Brightwell DR, et al. Disulfiram treatment of alcoholism: a Veterans Administration cooperative study. *JAMA* 1986; 256:1449–1455.

51. Rounsaville BJ, Carroll KM, Back S. Individual psychotherapy. In: Lowinson JH, Ruiz P, Millman RB, et al., eds. *Substance abuse: a comprehensive textbook,* 4th ed. Baltimore, MD: Lippincott, Williams & Wilkins, 2004:653–670.
52. Carroll K, Rounsaville B, Keller D. Relapse prevention strategies for the treatment of cocaine abuse. *Am J Drug Alcohol Abuse* 1991;17(3):249–265.
53. Carroll K, Rounsaville B, Nich C, et al. One-year follow-up of psychotherapy and pharmacotherapy for cocaine dependence: delayed emergence of psychotherapy effects. *Arch Gen Psychiatry* 1994;51: 989–997.
54. Marlatt G, Gordon JR, eds. *Relapse prevention: maintenance strategies in the treatment of addictive behaviors.* New York: Guilford Press, 1985.
55. Budney AJ, Kandel DB, Cherek DR, et al. College on problems of drug dependence meeting, Puerto Rico (June 1996). Marijuana use and dependence. *Drug Alcohol Depend* 1997;45:1–11.
56. Miller WR. Motivational interviewing: research, practice and puzzles. *Addictive Behav* 1996;61(6):835–842.
57. Stephens RS, Roffman RA, Simpson EE. Treating adult marijuana dependence: a test of the relapse prevention model. *J Consult Clin Psychol* 1994;62:92–99.
58. Higgins ST, Budney AJ, Bickel WK, et al. Incentives improve outcome in outpatient behavioral treatment of cocaine dependence. *Arch Gen Psychiatry* 1994;51:568–576.
59. Higgins ST, Budney AJ, Bickel WK, et al. Outpatient behavioral treatment for cocaine dependence: one-year outcome. *Exp Clin Psychopharmacol* 1995;3(2):205–212.
60. Silverman K, Higgins ST, Brooner RK, et al. Sustained cocaine abstinence in methadone maintenance patients through voucher-based reinforcement therapy. *Arch Gen Psychiatry* 1996;53:409–415.
61. Silverman K, Wong C, Higgins S, et al. Increasing opiate abstinence through voucher-based reinforcement therapy. *Drug Alcohol Depend* 1996;41:157–165.
62. Milby JB, Schumacher JE, McNamara C, et al. *Abstinence contingent housing enhances day treatment for homeless cocaine abusers. (NIDA research monograph series 174).* Rockville, MD: National Institute on Drug Abuse, 1996.
63. Milby JB, Schumacher JE, Raczynski JM, et al. Sufficient conditions for effective treatment of substance abusing homeless. *Drug Alcohol Depend* 1996;43:39–47.
64. McLellan AT, Arndt I, Metzger DS, et al. The effects of psychosocial services in substance abuse treatment. *JAMA* 1993;269(15):1953–1959.
65. McLellan AT, Woody GE, Luborsky L, et al. Is the counselor an "active ingredient" in substance abuse treatment? *J Nerv Mental Dis* 1988;176:423–430.
66. Woody GE, Luborsky L, McLellan AT, et al. Psychotherapy for opiate addicts: does it help? *Arch Gen Psychiatry* 1983;40:639–645.
67. Luborsky L. *Principles of psychoanalytic psychotherapy: a manual for supportive-expressive (SE) treatment.* New York: Basic Books, 1984.
68. Woody GE, McLellan AT, Luborsky L, et al. Twelve month followup of psychotherapy for opiate dependence. *Am J Psychiatry* 1987;144: 590–596.
69. Woody GE, McLellan AT, Luborsky L, et al. Psychotherapy in community methadone programs: a validation study. *Am J Psychiatry* 1995; 152(9):1302–1308.
70. Diamond GS, Liddle HA. Resolving a therapeutic impasse between parents and adolescents in multidimensional family therapy. *J Consult Clin Psychol* 1996;64(3):481–488.
71. Schmidt SE, Liddle HA, Dakof GA. Effects of multidimensional family therapy: relationship of changes in parenting practices to symptom reduction in adolescent substance abuse. *J Family Psychol* 1996; 10(1):1–16.
72. Dole VP, Nyswander M, Kreek MJ Narcotic blockade. *Arch Intern Med* 1996;118:304–309.
73. Lowinson JH, Payte JT, Joseph H, et al. Methadone maintenance. In: Lowinson JH, Ruiz P, Millman RB, et al., eds. *Substance abuse: a comprehensive textbook.* Baltimore, MD: Lippincott, Williams & Wilkins, 405–414:1996.
74. Simpson DD. Treatment for drug abuse: follow-up outcomes and length of time spent. *Arch Gen Psychiatry* 1981;38(8):875–880.
75. Simpson DD, Joe GW, Bracy SA. Six-year follow-up of opioid addicts after admission to treatment. *Arch Gen Psychiatry* 1982;39(11): 1318–1323.
76. Novick DM, Joseph J, Croxson TS, et al. Absence of antibody to human immunodeficiency virus in long-term, socially rehabilitated methadone maintenance patients. *Arch Intern Med* 1990;150(1):97–99.
77. Brown LS, Kritz SA, Goldsmith RJ, et al. Health services for HIV/AIDS, hepatitis C virus, and sexually transmitted infections in substance abuse treatment programs. *Public Health Rep* 2007:122:441–451.
78. Brown LS, Kritz SA, Goldsmith JR, et al. Characteristics of substance abuse treatment programs providing services for HIV/AIDS, hepatitis C virus infection, and sexually transmitted infections: the National Clinical Trials Network. *J Substance Abuse Treatment* 2006:30: 315–321.
79. Cornish JW, Metzger D, Woody GE, et al. Naltrexone pharmacotherapy for opioid dependent federal probationers. *J Substance Abuse Treatment* 1997;14(6):529–534.
80. Greenstein RA, Arndt IC, McLellan AT, et al. Naltrexone: a clinical perspective. *J Clin Psychiatry* 1984;45(9 Part 2):25–28.
81. Resnick RB, Schuyten-Resnick E, Washton AM. Narcotic antagonists in the treatment of opioid dependence: review and commentary. *Compr Psychiatry* 1979;20(2):116–125.
82. Resnick RB, Washton AM. Clinical outcome with naltrexone: predictor variables and followup status in detoxified heroin addicts. *Ann N Y Acad Sci* 1978;11:241–246.

CHAPTER 25

A. Thomas McLellan, PhD
James R. McKay, PhD

Integrating Evidence-Based Components into a Functional Continuum of Addiction Care

INTRODUCTION

Problems in Delivery of Effective Addiction Treatment Addictive disorders—here defined as any substance use disorder meeting DSM-IVR criteria for abuse or dependence—occur in approximately 10% to 15% of the adult population (1) and result in dramatic costs to society such as lost productivity, social disorder, and excessive health care utilization (2–4). It is disturbing and potentially dangerous to public health and safety that less than 15% of those who meet diagnostic criteria for a substance use disorder receive any kind of addiction treatment (1). Many studies of emergency rooms, general medical care settings, and psychiatric clinics document high rates of easily detected signs of abuse or dependence, yet there has been no meaningful increase in the rates of screening, early intervention, or referral to specialty care for addictive disorders among the general medical community (1). Indeed, only the welfare and especially the criminal justice systems have made a concerted effort to screen for substance use disorders intervene with those clients and refer them to specialty care (5). But the problems go beyond simply getting care to those who need it. Among those who do enter treatment, more than 80% receive outpatient care, usually in a nonprofit (69%) community-based specialty treatment program that is not affiliated with any part of the larger health care system (6). Perhaps for these reasons, studies of state treatment systems indicate that the modal duration of outpatient treatment is only one to three visits; less than 30% remain actively engaged in outpatient care by 60 days (7).

Although research over the past several decades has documented effective medications, behavioral therapies, and other interventions that can be used during treatment (8), the great majority of outpatient addiction treatment programs provide only group counseling and referral to Alcoholics Anonymous (AA) (6). Note here that this type of counseling is typically generic problem sharing in a group format and is typically not the type of focused "therapy" that has been studied and shown to be effective in individual and group settings. One reason for this is that many studies of addiction counselors—the major care providers within the system—show that their training, licensure, and certification does not require proficiency or even understanding of most of the contemporary therapies, medications, or biologic discoveries in addiction (9). Moreover, counselor turnover rates have ranged from 35% to 50% each year, making it impractical from a business standpoint to invest training resources into this group (10). Of course, it is true many other sectors within the health care field also fail to deliver the kind of evidence-based treatments that work; studies have shown that the quality of addiction treatment is frequently worse than quality of general health care (11). Thus individuals with addictive disorders simply cannot count on receiving attractive, individualized, effective, or, sometimes, even adequate care.

This serious situation sets the background and drives the focus of the present chapter. Given these contemporary infrastructure issues that so profoundly affect the delivery of care within the addiction treatment system, the usual listing of evidence-based medications, therapies, and other clinical interventions might reasonably be considered irrelevant. Health services and policy research studies over the past 10 years have suggested that conceptual, organizational, and operational issues at the national and state systems level set real limits on the potential clinical benefits that may be derived from even the best combination of evidence-based clinical interventions. Thus, this chapter is written in three parts. Part 1 describes research over the past 5 to 7 years investigating these conceptual, political, organizational, and operational factors that we refer to as the treatment infrastructure. This part of the chapter ends with a rather bleak picture of the decline in organizational infrastructure of the addiction treatment system. In contrast, Part 2 describes some of the conceptual and organizational changes that have occurred over the past two decades within the primary care system in the management of other chronic illnesses. The staged approach, use of treatment teams, inclusion of patients and families in the development, and maintenance of their care and the systematic use of clinical information systems to monitor and support patient change are discussed as a model for what a staged continuum of care might look like in addiction treatment. With this as background, Part 3 of the chapter then discusses contemporary evidence-based clinical practices—the components of care—in the context of the described stages of the addiction treatment continuum.

PART 1—THE CONCEPTUAL, ORGANIZATIONAL, AND FINANCIAL INFRASTRUCTURE OF CONTEMPORARY ADDICTION TREATMENT

Conceptual Issues Addiction to alcohol and other drugs has variously been conceptualized as a sin, a sign of weak character, a bad habit, or some type of disease (12). This conceptualization has had significant implications for whether this condition should be dealt with through confrontation, reeducation, and peer modeling, as one might with a bad habit, or through medications and therapies, as one might with a disease.

Over the past decade, work originally done by Anglin and later by many other researchers (13) suggested that, at least for many of the more serious cases of addiction, the "condition" might be best considered as a chronic illness, similar in terms of onset, course, management, and outcome to chronic illnesses such as hypertension, diabetes, and asthma (14).

Although the concept of addiction as a chronic illness has been attractive in research and even clinical circles, this conceptual shift has so far not led to much change in the way addictions have been treated, insured, or evaluated. In brief, when a condition is considered to be a *medical illness*, at-risk individuals are screened by physicians or other health care providers to identify and treat incipient cases; more advanced cases are provided medications, interventions, and therapies by well-trained, primary health care professionals. Cases that require specialized services are transferred to specialty care that is linked to the primary care system.

By extension, when an illness is considered to be a *chronic illness,* it is expected that no time-limited intervention is likely to cure the illness, and the best strategy will be disease management and monitoring for a significant period of time (15). Indeed, *chronic care teams* involving a multidisciplinary treatment staff negotiate a long-term treatment plan with the patient and his or her family; and this plan typically includes long-term support and monitoring by the primary care team, to maintain patient function and prevent relapses and expensive reutilization of emergency room or hospital beds (15,16).

It also follows that the process of outcome evaluation in the management of chronic illnesses—as with the care itself—should be an ongoing clinical process. Standard measures of symptom severity and patient function are an integral part of most health care clinical information systems (17). Clinicians are expected to evaluate individual patients during regularly scheduled appointments. These evaluations measure important elements such as symptom number and severity, side effects of any treatments, and patient function. Importantly, these clinical evaluations serve the dual purposes of measuring patient improvement and also providing decision support for judgments on whether to change the treatment. This is critical because without ongoing care, management, and evaluation, time-limited forms of treatment can be expected to result in relapse, reoccurrence of serious symptoms, and significant expense.

Organization, Management, and Financing Issues

Given this conceptual background, it should not be surprising that the administration, regulation, and financing of the addiction treatment system has occurred outside the mainstream health care system, or that addiction treatment has been organized and financed as an acute care system. Specialty addiction treatment in the United States is historically one of the youngest treatment systems in operation. As detailed by Musto (18) and White (12), the contemporary system was designed during the early 1970s after the emergence of a drug culture among the college-aged baby boomers during the 1960s and particularly after the return of Viet Nam veterans suffering from opioid dependence. The existing health care systems of the day were neither trained for accepting, nor particularly eager to accept, patients with addictive disorders and so a new system was designed and financed separately. Originally, these state systems were well funded and organizationally placed at the highest levels of government bureaucracy, reflecting the political importance of the issue at the time. The treatments that emerged were conceptualized in various ways and in turn, a very wide range of care providers (e.g., clergy, counselors) became part of addiction treatment teams (3,12). With the exception of the methadone maintenance programs, most addiction care was time-limited. However, patients treated in therapeutic community settings (approximately 30% of patients) received 6 to 12 months of care (3).

Over the ensuing decades, there was no emergent cure for alcohol or other drug use disorders. Health care spending became an increasingly important issue within the private sector.

Employers became disenchanted with Employee Assistance Program efforts to control workplace substance use problems and took special efforts to reduce employee health care benefits for addiction treatment through managed care organizations. Meanwhile, in the public sector, the political position of most state drug agencies became reduced in visibility, budget, and organizational power (19). By 2000, most addiction treatment was purchased with government funding (primarily state block grant and Medicaid dollars), and private insurance accounted for less than 12% of all care episodes (3). One important but seldom acknowledged implication of this is that, in the rest of health care, pharmaceutical benefits from private insurance packages fostered development of new medications with the promise of cheaper and more effective treatments. In the addiction field, care was already very inexpensive, there was little physician involvement, and no provision for pharmacy benefits through insurance. Because addiction was not accepted as an illness, medications were considered inappropriate by some providers, unnecessary by many state Medicaid systems, and clearly not profitable by most pharmaceutical companies. Consequently, until the 1990s, there were very few medications available to treat addiction and little active research to develop new ones (20).

As is evident from this short description, contemporary addiction treatment as an industry is in significant trouble. Conceptual confusion regarding the nature of addiction has confused the content of treatment interventions, insurance benefits, provider credentialing, and outcome evaluation methods. Organizational devolution of state addiction offices, "carving out" of addiction from most private insurance plans, and the lack of access to pharmaceutical insurance benefits have left physicians with few new medications and thus little incentive to make a career in this field. At this writing, drug counselors are the most prevalent professional group in the addiction field and group counseling is by far the most prevalent component of care—just as it was in the 1960s.

PART 2—WHAT MIGHT AN APPROPRIATE CONTINUUM OF ADDICTION CARE LOOK LIKE?

Development of a Continuum of Care in Mainstream Health Although the past two decades have been a period of decline for the addiction specialty care system, they have been a period of significant advance for the treatment of other chronic illnesses in the primary care system. Because chronic illnesses are by far the most prevalent and expensive forms of illness facing contemporary health care, there are now well-developed efforts to screen and intervene early with patients having genetic or behavioral indication of incipient illness. Among patients with disease progression, the emerging standard of primary care includes individualized treatment planning and involvement of the family to foster long-term behavioral change (e.g., training in food preparation for families of patients with diabetes and hypertension). Patients who have reduced the severity of their symptoms and adopted lifestyle changes toward the goal of self-management of their illness are nonetheless followed by the care team, albeit through less invasive means such as telephone, Internet, and home visits. At this stage of treatment, the goal is to maintain the gains from prior, more intensive stages of care, and to prevent clinically damaging and costly relapses. These stages of treatment and management are referred to as the *continuum of care*. Care management throughout this continuum is considered a team responsibility, using a shared clinical information system (patient registry) to monitor and adapt components of care to changes in the symptoms and function of the patient (15,16). Because most chronic illnesses have broad effects on patient and family function and because these effects may compound the course (and potential expense) of the illness, medical insurance now covers a broad array of treatment components (e.g., medications, behavioral therapies, family interventions).

With this as a general model, it is reasonable to ask what an appropriately conceptualized and organized continuum of care for addiction treatment might look like and how such a system might make contact with the rest of mainstream health care. Taking other chronic illnesses as a model, it also seems reasonable to think of clinical stages linked conceptually and organizationally toward the overall goal of promoting patient self-management of their addiction. Each stage of care within the continuum would have specific clinical goals, but achieving the goals of the early stages would prepare the patient for advancement to succeeding stages of care. Within each stage of care, various treatment components (medications, behavioral therapies, other interventions) would be evaluated with regard to their ability to affect the symptom and function goals appropriate to the particular stage of care of the patient. Because these stages and their clinical goals are conceptually linked, it is reasonable to think that many of the currently available treatment components might have a role at multiple stages of patient care, but to address different problems and goals. One implication of this type of model is that it would no longer be useful to ask the following typical research question "Is cognitive behavioral therapy effective in the treatment of alcohol dependence?" A much more relevant and useful question would be "Is cognitive behavioral therapy effective in reducing cocaine craving among patients in residential care, who have been stabilized through detoxification?" Or similarly, "Is cognitive behavioral therapy effective in reducing situational anxiety among recovering alcohol dependent patients in outpatient treatment?"

Toward a More Developed Continuum of Addiction Care Given that much of the chapter to this point has been rather negative about the condition of the addiction treatment system, it is important to note that there has been substantial development in the continuum of care over the past 30 years, and there is now at least the potential for many more options in many more venues than in the past. To illustrate this, we have represented the stages and major clinical components of the continuum of addiction care during the 1970s in

FIGURE 25.1. Continuum of addiction care, circa 1970–1980.

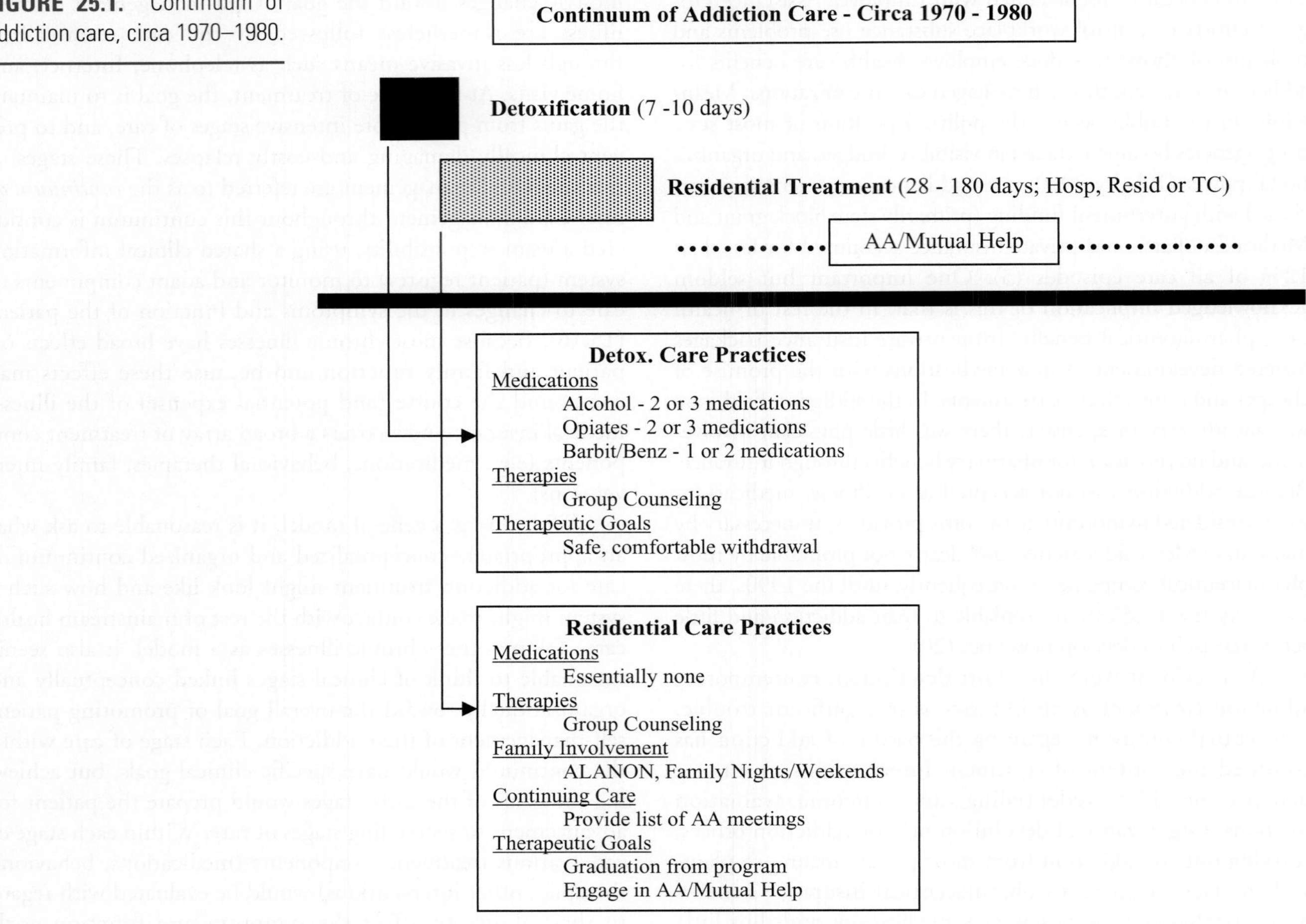

Figure 25.1. During this era, there were rarely more than two stages of abstinence-oriented care (we have not included methadone maintenance), detoxification, and residential treatment. Within each of these stages, there were very few therapeutic components. Note particularly that there were essentially no treatment options for addiction treatment outside of the specialty care system; that apart from detoxification, there were few medications or medical procedures to engage physicians; and that although the rehabilitation stage of care was much longer, it was still time limited with no continuing care options available other than referral to AA.

Figure 25.2 provides a depiction of what a contemporary continuum of care *could* look like given the previously described changes in conceptual approach to addiction and the many clinical discoveries brought about by the past two decades of National Institutes of Health–funded research. The most obvious difference between the two figures is the number of stages. In addition, there would be many more venues in which patients may access one or more stages addiction care. These changes in number and placement of care access points have provided the opportunity to detect and address early substance use disorders and provide continuing care for the more severe and chronic cases. This is the subject of Part 3 of this chapter.

PART 3—EVIDENCE-BASED CLINICAL PRACTICES WITHIN AND ACROSS THE CONTINUUM OF ADDICTION TREATMENT

Screening, Brief Interventions, and Brief Treatments Though work on screening and brief interventions has been under way for more than 20 years (21), the past 5 to 7 years has seen several parts of the mainstream medical establishment embrace it. The now large and still growing research in this area is well represented by Fleming and colleagues' (22,23) studies of screening and brief interventions within primary care practices in Wisconsin. His study screened for and found alcohol use problems in 723 newly admitted patients in 17 primary care practices. Half of those who screened positive (randomly selected) then received a 10- to 15-minute intervention delivered by those primary care physicians. His findings showed that there were significant reductions from baseline to 12 months in 7-day alcohol use (19 to 11 for the experimental group versus 19 to 15 for controls). In addition, monthly episodes of binge drinking decreased from baseline to 12 months for the experimental group (6 to 3) versus controls (5 to 4).

There are similar studies showing significant prevalence of alcohol and other substance use disorders in emergency room

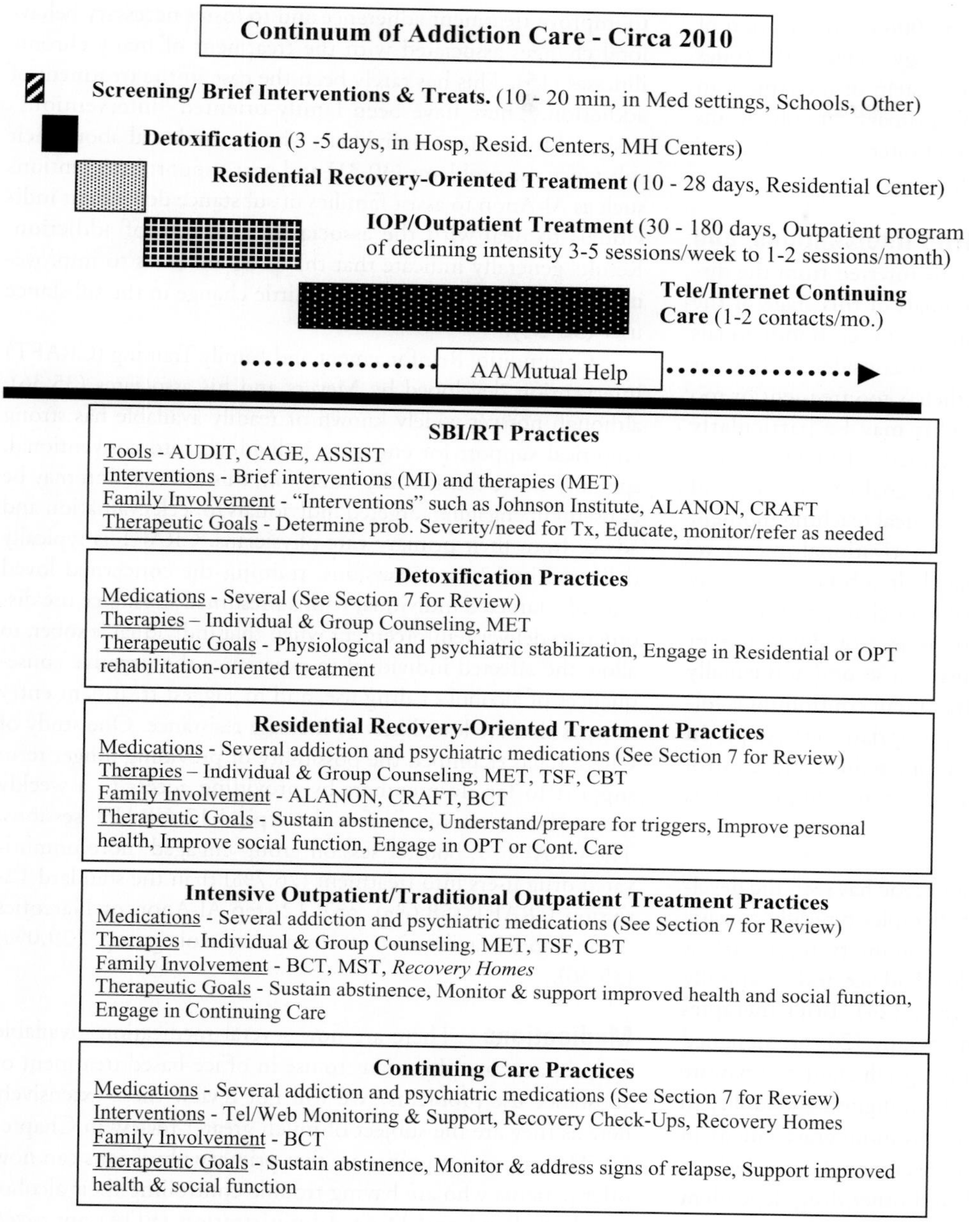

Continuum of Addiction Care - Circa 2010

Screening/ Brief Interventions & Treats. (10 - 20 min, in Med settings, Schools, Other)

Detoxification (3 -5 days, in Hosp, Resid. Centers, MH Centers)

Residential Recovery-Oriented Treatment (10 - 28 days, Residential Center)

IOP/Outpatient Treatment (30 - 180 days, Outpatient program of declining intensity 3-5 sessions/week to 1-2 sessions/month)

Tele/Internet Continuing Care (1-2 contacts/mo.)

AA/Mutual Help

SBI/RT Practices
Tools - AUDIT, CAGE, ASSIST
Interventions - Brief interventions (MI) and therapies (MET)
Family Involvement - "Interventions" such as Johnson Institute, ALANON, CRAFT
Therapeutic Goals - Determine prob. Severity/need for Tx, Educate, monitor/refer as needed

Detoxification Practices
Medications - Several (See Section 7 for Review)
Therapies – Individual & Group Counseling, MET
Therapeutic Goals - Physiological and psychiatric stabilization, Engage in Residential or OPT rehabilitation-oriented treatment

Residential Recovery-Oriented Treatment Practices
Medications - Several addiction and psychiatric medications (See Section 7 for Review)
Therapies – Individual & Group Counseling, MET, TSF, CBT
Family Involvement - ALANON, CRAFT, BCT
Therapeutic Goals - Sustain abstinence, Understand/prepare for triggers, Improve personal health, Improve social function, Engage in OPT or Cont. Care

Intensive Outpatient/Traditional Outpatient Treatment Practices
Medications - Several addiction and psychiatric medications (See Section 7 for Review)
Therapies – Individual & Group Counseling, MET, TSF, CBT
Family Involvement - BCT, MST, *Recovery Homes*
Therapeutic Goals - Sustain abstinence, Monitor & support improved health and social function, Engage in Continuing Care

Continuing Care Practices
Medications - Several addiction and psychiatric medications (See Section 7 for Review)
Interventions - Tel/Web Monitoring & Support, Recovery Check-Ups, Recovery Homes
Family Involvement - BCT
Therapeutic Goals - Sustain abstinence, Monitor & address signs of relapse, Support improved health & social function

FIGURE 25.2. Continuum of addiction care, circa 2010.

populations, trauma centers, primary mental health centers, and school health settings (22). Brief intervention (i.e., educational and motivational interventions lasting less than 10 minutes) and brief treatment (similar interventions of two to five sessions) studies within these populations have generally shown significant reductions in substance use, lasting at least 6 to 12 months. The content of brief intervention settings varies depending on the severity of an individual's problems. It includes several common elements known by their acronym FRAMES: feedback, responsibility, advice, menu of strategies, empathy, and self-efficacy (24).

Beyond the fact that identifying and addressing early-stage substance use disorders is an important public health problem in itself, there is also evidence that primary care physicians can often improve the outcomes and reduce the substantial costs of treating common, chronic illnesses such as diabetes, hypertension, asthma, several types of cancer, and sleep—simply by identifying and managing their cooccurring substance use problems (25). One central source of this evidence is the Program of Research to Integrate Substance Use Information into Mainstream Healthcare project, which commissioned 13 systematic reviews regarding the role of alcohol and other substance use problems in the course, complications, outcomes, and costs of treating prevalent chronic illnesses. These reviews, written by physician specialists in the target disease and all published in mainstream medical journals, showed that even subdiagnostic levels of heavy drinking or other substance use can significantly impair the diagnosis, complicate the treatment and elevate the costs of most chronic illnesses. These data, combined with the results of two decades of screening and brief intervention research, led in 2008 to the creation of Medicaid Current Procedural Terminology codes (CPT codes 99408 and 99409, a numeric coding system of the American Medical Association) that now enable primary care physicians to be reimbursed for screening and brief interventions directed toward alcohol and smoking problems.

Goals within the Screening, Brief Interventions, and Brief Treatments Stage As may be inferred from the discussion in the previous section, the goals of this stage of the substance abuse treatment continuum are to reach individuals whose substance use may be below that considered abuse or dependence, but whose use is nonetheless too frequent or too serious for their medical health. This may be particularly important for those with diagnosed medical or psychiatric conditions. Once identified, a linked goal of this stage of treatment is to use the power of the medical teaching moment as well as clinical techniques such as motivational interviewing to help patients understand that their substance use may be a problem and that they are capable of changing their substance use. Because these interventions are not always potent enough to produce the desired changes, a second and equally important goal of this stage of the treatment continuum is follow-up monitoring to determine appropriate next steps. In those cases in which the patient cannot reduce and control substance use, referral to a specialty care treatment program is warranted.

Behavioral Therapies The last decade has seen the development and testing of several brief therapies typically consisting of two to twelve sessions. One session intervention such as motivational interviewing is considered advice and is typically administered within medical contexts (24). Brief therapies such as motivational enhancement therapy (26) are designed to promote problem recognition among reluctant or unaware substance abusers, to foster a sense of willingness and ability to address the problem, and, often, to promote engagement in treatment. These brief therapies have been tested extensively in more than 100 trials with alcohol- and other drug-dependent individuals usually as a strategy for encouraging, nontreatment-seeking individuals to enter into formal treatment, but also as a treatment intervention (27,28). Studies of nontreatment-seeking individuals typically show small to medium effect sizes compared against no intervention at all, with the best effects seen for individuals with less severe forms of addiction (28). Studies of brief interventions as a treatment intervention have shown posttreatment outcomes that are not different from those seen among individuals with more extensive treatments (26,28,29). Because of their brevity they have been particularly attractive to primary care physicians dealing with alcohol-dependent individuals in family medicine or emergency medical settings (29).

Family Involvement Mainstream health care has long acknowledged the benefits of engaging family and social supports to improve treatment adherence and to foster necessary behavioral changes associated with the treatment of many chronic illnesses (15). This has rarely been the case in the treatment of addiction. There have been family-oriented "interventions" designed to confront individuals who are in denial about their substance use problems (30,31) and peer support interventions such as Al-Anon to assist families of substance dependent individuals to deal with the associated problems of addiction. Results generally indicate that this program leads to improvements in family functioning, but little change in the substance user (32–35).

Community Reinforcement and Family Training (CRAFT) intervention developed by Meyers and his associates (35,36), although not yet widely known or readily available has strong empirical support for engaging individuals into conventional, specialty care treatment. By extension, this intervention may be as useful in engaging targeted individuals to seek evaluation and advice from their primary care physicians. CRAFT is typically delivered in 12 to 14 sessions, training the concerned loved ones of a targeted individual with a presumed substance use disorder, to deliver reinforcement when that individual is sober, to allow the affected individual to experience the negative consequences of alcohol or drug use, and to suggest treatment entry in ways that are least likely to increase resistance. One study of CRAFT has examined the possibility of providing longer term support to family members by providing access to a weekly group "booster session" after the typical 12 CRAFT sessions. The CRAFT + booster session group engaged more unmotivated drug users into treatment (76.7%) than the standard 12-session CRAFT (58.6%), or a 12-step Al-Anon or Narcotics Anonymous facilitation training control group (29.0%) (35,36).

Medications There are now several medications available for primary care physicians to use in office-based treatment of substance use problems. We will not review these extensively here as they are the subject of much greater review in Chapter 50. The important points are that primary physicians can now offer patients who are having trouble controlling their alcohol use, U.S. Food and Drug Administration (FDA)-approved medications such as acamprosate (Campral), disulfiram (Antabuse), or naltrexone (Revia, Vivitrol). Naltrexone for example blocks alcohol-mediated stimulation of endogenous opioids, thus blunting some of alcohol's pleasurable effects. At this writing, there have been more than 20 field studies of the medication with a variety of clinical samples (8,37). Overall, these studies have shown a statistically and clinically significant response compared with placebo or with standard outpatient treatment involving no medication. O'Malley has found that the best candidates for naltrexone include those with high levels of alcohol dependence, a familial history of alcohol dependence, significant cravings for alcohol and lower educational levels (38). In early 2006, a sustained-release, injectable form of naltrexone (Vivitrol) was FDA approved for use. This preparation provides clinically effective blood levels of the medication for at least 30 days. Early findings with this formulation indicated that more than 85% of those given the initial injection returned for five additional monthly injections, that side effects were modest, and that the effectiveness was substantially greater than placebo injections (39).

Finally, for patients whose use of opiates is not able to come under control, there are two medications available for primary care physicians. Although the opiate agonist methadone is clearly the most reliable and well studied of all medications for opiate dependence, federal and state restrictions prevent its use outside of licensed methadone maintenance programs (40). However, a partial agonist, buprenorphine, was approved in 2002 by the FDA for treatment of opioid dependence in general practice settings. Buprenorphine is administered sublingually and is also effective in reducing opiate craving for 24 to 36 hours. The partial agonist actions of buprenorphine has some advantages over methadone, such as few or no withdrawal symptoms after discontinuation and lower risk of overdose even if combined with other opiates (40). The fears of diversion that accompanied the release of the medication for office-based practice have not been borne out, likely because of three policy efforts that were put into place to minimize these risks. Only "certified" physicians who complete an instructional course are able to prescribe the medication. Second, physician caseloads were restricted to 30 patients until late 2006 when demand for the medication combined with the safety record to that point led to a change to a 100-patient caseload. Finally, the manufacturer of the medication agreed to develop a combined formulation (Suboxone) that included naloxone with the buprenorphine to prevent injection use of the medication. At this writing, the use of this medication has increased steadily in response to its acceptance by patients, its efficacy in reducing withdrawal symptoms and preventing new opioid use, and the low level of individual and community side effects.

Detoxification Stage of Treatment The first specialty treatment stage within the proposed substance use care continuum is also the most specialized stage of care.

Goals of Detoxification Detoxification is a relatively brief, explicitly medical procedure, usually provided in a hospital setting and designed to stabilize the physical and emotional effects of recent termination of heavy alcohol or drug use. This stage of treatment is designed for people who experience frank withdrawal symptoms or significant physiologic or emotional instability after a period of prolonged abuse of drugs. Significant physiologic withdrawal is not present in all cases—even those with the more serious forms of addiction. However, alcohol, opioid, and sedative/tranquilizer dependence may produce a characteristic rebound physiologic withdrawal syndrome 8 to 30 hours after the last dose of the drug (depending on the drug, dose, and period of use). Users of amphetamine, cocaine, and even marijuana can also experience substantial emotional and physiologic symptoms and often require a period of stabilizing treatment.

The purpose of the detoxification stage of treatment is not to produce cure or lasting sobriety, but rather to prepare an unstable patient to do well in the subsequent rehabilitation phase of treatment. The major components of this phase of care include medications to relieve physiologic and emotional symptoms and to reduce craving for the abused substances. These medications are typically accompanied by rest and motivational forms of therapy, usually in the context of a residential or hospital setting.

Continuing care in an appropriate specialty treatment setting is considered an important clinical goal of this stage of treatment because on its own, detoxification is rarely effective in helping patients achieve lasting recovery, particularly patients with more severe or protracted histories of substance dependence. Thus this stage of treatment is best considered preparation for continued rehabilitation.

Medications There have been significant advances in the use of medications to reduce the dangers and alleviate the suffering associated with the withdrawal and stabilization of physiologic and emotional problems attendant to the cessation of heavy substance use. This area of addiction medicine is quite specialized and well beyond the scope of this chapter (see Section 7 for more detailed discussion).

Behavioral Therapies Because detoxification is a typically short (3 to 5 days) medical procedure and because patients' attention and concentration may be compromised for much of this period, extended therapies within this context are not typically possible. However, the same brief interventions and brief therapies described in the Screening and Brief Interventions stage of care are also possible and sensible in this context. In this context, the goal of these forms of behavioral therapy should generally be to have the patient understand that they have a significant substance use problem and that their ability to gain control over that problem will benefit from continued participation in a rehabilitation form of treatment (residential or outpatient).

Residential Recovery–Oriented Stage of Treatment Residential rehabilitation or "recovery"-oriented treatment is appropriate for patients who are no longer suffering from the acute physiologic or emotional effects of recent substance abuse. Recovery-oriented treatments are provided in outpatient and methadone maintenance settings as well as residential settings. Indeed, outpatient programs account for about 80% of all treatment programs. However, residential treatment is qualitatively different in that it offers protected and secluded care to enable patients to regain personal health and social functioning as well as control over their substance use urges. As with detoxification, residential recovery-oriented care may be best considered preparation for continuing recovery-oriented treatment in a less protected outpatient environment (see the following section).

"Recovery" and Rehabilitation Both here and in prior publications (41–43), the authors have argued for a rather broad set of rehabilitation treatment goals that go well beyond just the reduction of alcohol and drug use to capture a number of other important behavioral changes. This formulation is quite similar to the concept of "recovery" used by the large number of formerly addicted individuals to describe their new sober, responsible, spiritual lives since gaining control over their addictions. In this regard, a recent consensus conference comprised researchers, policy makers, clinicians, and others put forward an initial operational definition of "recovery" as "a voluntarily maintained lifestyle comprised of sobriety, personal health and citizenship" (44).

At this writing, this definition has not yet been broadly adopted, and the suggested measures of each domain from the World Health Organization Quality of Life instrument (45) have not yet been broadly used. Thus there has been very little research on the extent to which this definition of recovery can be an expectable outcome from rehabilitation-oriented care. Moreover, many of those now "in recovery" never received any type of formal treatment to achieve their changed lifestyle. However, we do see this recent definition as evidence of conceptual convergence in outcome expectations among patients, payers, providers, and researchers. One point in particular bears emphasis. Although continuation of abstinence from alcohol and other drugs of abuse is widely considered *necessary* for achieving recovery, abstinence by itself is not *sufficient* to assure the equally desirable qualities of improved personal health and independent social function. This is important in understanding the varied clinical practices that have been employed in this stage of addiction treatment.

Goals of Recovery-Oriented Treatments Patients suitable for residential rehabilitation treatments usually also have significant problems in medical and mental health, family and social relationships, and sometimes legal and employment problems that may have resulted from or led to their substance use problems (43). Regardless of the etiology of these associated problems, patients will typically require substantial therapeutic effort to address and manage these associated problems if the substance use is expected to remain under control. Thus residential recovery oriented treatments for addiction have the following goals.

- Maintain physiologic and emotional improvements initiated during detoxification; enhance and sustain reductions in alcohol and drug use (virtually all residential programs suggest a goal of complete abstinence).
- Teach, model, and support behaviors that lead to improved personal health, family and social function, and reduced threats to public health and public safety.
- Motivate behavioral and lifestyle changes that are incompatible with substance use.

These are significant and challenging goals requiring broad and sustained changes in patients' behaviors and their social structures. It is clear that, especially for those with more serious and protracted forms of addiction, these goals will require not just appropriate medications, therapies, and interventions, but also a period of protected living. It is equally clear that a period of 20 to 30 days of residential recovery-oriented living will only initiate this recovery process. Engagement in continuing outpatient, recovery-oriented treatment, or at least informal continuing care (discussed in the next sections) will be necessary for continuing the recovery process and achieving these clinical goals.

Medications As described earlier in this chapter, there are now three FDA-approved medications for the treatment of alcohol dependence (disulfiram/Antabuse, acamprosate/Campral, and naltrexone/Revia and Vivitrol); and two FDA-approved medications for the treatment of opiate dependence (beyond methadone) (naltrexone/Trexan and buprenorphine/Suboxone). There are also some promising medications for the treatment of cocaine dependence (modafinil, topiramate/Topamax). These were summarized in that section of the chapter and are more thoroughly reviewed in other chapters (see Section 7) and are not discussed further here.

Again, in the context of the broad goals of this stage of the continuum of substance abuse treatment, other medications, beyond those designed to control alcohol and other substance use, may also be helpful in effecting recovery goals. For example, there is a large and important literature sample that examines the use of medications to reduce psychiatric problems among addicted individuals (46–48). This is an important area for physician involvement. Psychiatric disorders such as depression, anxiety, phobia, and others are prominent among nicotine-, alcohol-, opiate-, cocaine-, and benzodiazepine-dependent individuals. There is abundant evidence that addicted individuals with concurrent psychiatric problems are more likely to drop out of standard drug dependence treatments, more likely to perform poorly during those treatments, and more likely to relapse early after those treatments (49–51). Finally, there is increasing evidence that the prescription of *appropriate* psychotropic medications can alter that prognosis (46–48).

Behavioral Therapies Significant research has taken place in the past two decades to develop behavioral interventions not only to help patients control their urges to use and to remain abstinent, but also to help them deal with the emotional and relationship problems that so often accompany substance dependence. Most of these therapies have been primarily applied in outpatient settings and thus are reviewed below under that stage of the care continuum. Several of the behavioral therapies and interventions discussed in the next section may also be appropriate for use in residential settings, but have rarely been studied in that context. Two that seem particularly pertinent to the goals of residential care are described here and also in the section that follows.

12-Step Facilitation Therapy Twelve-step facilitation (TSF) therapy was originally developed as a practical control condition, to be implemented by counselors, and compared against theoretically derived therapies implemented by trained therapists in a controlled trial with alcohol-dependent patients in an outpatient setting of care (26). It is described here because it is designed to assist in one of the main goals of this stage of care: engaging patients into accepting their inability to control their substance use; acknowledging the effects of their substance use on their lives and the lives of their loved ones; and ultimately taking steps to deal with the problems through the 12 steps and 12 traditions of AA (52). TSF is typically delivered as a time-limited (12- to 15-session) intervention, either as an individual treatment or in groups (53). In either format, TSF is a highly structured intervention whose sessions begin with a review of the patient's recovery week, including any 12-step meetings attended, episodes of substance, and urges to drink or use drugs. Each session concludes with assignments to recovery-oriented tasks such as readings from the AA literature and attending AA meetings that the patient agrees to undertake between sessions. One aspect of TSF that clearly separates it from other therapies is its active promotion of spirituality as a key to lasting recovery. In this context, spirituality is considered a force that provides direction and meaning to one's life.

The evidence for effectiveness of TSF was first shown in the large, multisite National Institute on Alcohol Abuse and Alcoholism Project MATCH study of alcohol-dependent patients (26). There were no overall differences among the three therapies tested in that study over the 3-year period, but, as designed, the TSF group was more successful in getting patients involved with AA and, in turn, more effective in getting patients to be abstinent from alcohol than either of the other two groups (54).

Individual Drug Counseling Similar in several ways to TSF, the drug-dependence field has employed a structured form of individual counseling employing many of the same practical elements, but not a formal spiritual component (55,56). Individual counseling, delivered in a structured manner to foster abstinence and general adjustment in 12 to 24 sessions, has been extensively studied. It has typically been studied in outpatient settings and in almost all studies patients who have received this form of counseling (even those who initially did not want it) had better during and posttreatment outcomes (57,58), with those who attended a greater frequency of sessions typically showing the best results (59–61). Individual counseling is discussed here briefly because it is widely used within recovery-oriented residential settings and because it has shown benefits in helping patients to adjust and improve during that stage of care. This component is discussed in more detail in the Outpatient section that follows.

Linking Patients to AA or Other Mutual-Help Groups Virtually all alcohol-dependence rehabilitation programs and most cocaine-dependence rehabilitation programs refer patients to AA with instructions to get a sponsor, "share and chair" at meetings, and to attend 90 meetings in 90 days as a continued commitment to sobriety. Note that although there are also many Cocaine Anonymous and Narcotics Anonymous groups, these are typically less prevalent, and most AA groups now accept individuals with a range of addiction problems. For these reasons, we discuss mutual-help organizations generically under the rubric of AA. Research studies done to date have generally found that only about 25% to 35% of those who attend one meeting of AA go on to active participation (e.g., attend 90 meetings, acquire a sponsor). However, for those who do attend, there is every indication that this peer support component of rehabilitation is valuable for maintaining rehabilitation (62,63). There are now many controlled trials and field studies of AA showing that participation in posttreatment self-help groups is related to better outcome among cocaine- or alcohol-dependent individuals (48,64,65).

Intensive/Traditional Outpatient Stage of Treatment Outpatient treatment is the final stage of the formal substance abuse treatment process and is appropriate for patients who have initiated the major goals of rehabilitation, particularly behavioral control over their urges to use substances. Thus outpatient treatment is designed to provide continuing support for the behavioral changes achieved during detoxification or residential treatment and to support personal changes in health and social function while monitoring early threats to relapse. Many of the more intensive forms of outpatient treatment (e.g., intensive outpatient and day hospital) begin with full or half-day sessions three to five times per week for approximately 1 month. As the rehabilitation progresses, the intensity of the treatment reduces to shorter sessions of 1 to 2 hours delivered one to three times per week and then tapering gradually to once per month, typically in association with parallel involvement in AA.

Goals of Intensive/Outpatient Treatments Outpatient treatments share many of the goals and therapeutic components of more intensive, residential recovery oriented treatment. In general, the medications, therapies, and services that have been applied and studied in the rehabilitation/recovery phase of treatment can also be applied in the outpatient phase of treatment. Outpatient treatment is a formal part of the specialty care treatment system and the programs that deliver it are licensed and accredited in much the same way as the more intensive programs. Specifically, outpatient treatments for addiction have the following three goals:

- maintain physiologic and emotional improvements initiated during detoxification or residential treatments;
- maintain abstinence from alcohol and other drugs; and
- motivate and support behavioral and lifestyle changes that are incompatible with substance use.

Once again, even this duration and intensity of treatment may not be adequate to sustain the gains made in earlier treatment stages or to forestall relapse. Thus a final goal of this stage of treatment is engagement in continuing recovery-oriented care (discussed in the next sections). Here we review those interventions that have been typically provided and studied in outpatient settings.

Medications All antiaddiction medications previously described earlier in this part of the chapter, are also useful—and may be particularly important—in this stage of the addiction continuum. In addition, because at least half of substance dependent patients in treatment suffer from cooccurring problems of depression, anxiety, or phobia, standard psychotropic medications can be important in the achievement and maintenance of improved mental health. This an important goal in the overall recovery effort, but in addition, patients with concurrent psychiatric problems are more likely to perform poorly during outpatient treatment and most likely to drop out prematurely (8,37,40).

It is important to note that psychotropic and antiaddiction medications may not control the targeted substance use or mental health problems when used in the context of a primary care setting. Nonetheless, these same medications may be very helpful within the context of a recovery-oriented outpatient treatment program because the added benefits of the peer support, intensified therapeutic setting, and additional social services and family involvement may enhance the actions of these same medications (66). The inverse is also true; more severely dependent patients or those with more psychiatric problems may do poorly in outpatient treatment without medications for their symptoms. The assistance of these medications may provide pharmacologic support for the benefits of traditional behavioral and social interventions.

Behavioral Therapies With the exceptions of individual drug counseling and linkage to AA, most evidence-based behavioral therapies are not widely used during this stage of the addiction continuum (see Part 1). Interventions designed to engage family and to change previous peer relationships may be particularly important at this stage of the continuum as the patient attempts to develop and sustain a new recovery-oriented lifestyle within the home setting.

Cognitive Behavioral Therapy Cognitive behavioral therapy (CBT) in the treatment of addictions, emphasizes the role of thinking and behavior in determining both craving for drugs and the ensuing drug seeking and use. Put simply, the therapy is based on the findings that biased or inaccurate thoughts and beliefs, coupled with poor coping skills, lead to a greater risk for relapse. Therefore CBT treatments involve techniques to modify biased or inaccurate beliefs and expectancies and to improve behavioral coping skills. There are several approaches to, or variations on CBT, including rational emotive behavior therapy, rational behavior therapy, rational living therapy, cognitive therapy, and dialectic behavior therapy. In the addiction field, most of the versions studied have been adapted from Marlatt and Gordon's relapse prevention treatment for problem drinking (67). As studied in most research trials, the therapy is usually individual (but also group) delivered in 8 to 16 weekly sessions. Change in thinking about and reactions to relapse-provoking situations and improvements in coping abilities require practice and time. Thus one of the hallmarks of CBT is homework assignments to provide practice in the cognitive and behavioral techniques learned during the formal sessions. CBT may be the most studied of all the therapies in addiction due perhaps to the very carefully developed manuals developed to train and guide the provision of the therapy (68,69). Studies of CBT with cocaine-dependent patients have shown general acceptance by patients (attendance at more than 50% of planned sessions) and better posttreatment rates of abstinence than patients given no therapy or group counseling alone (70,71). Similarly, CBT has also been associated with generally good engagement and posttreatment outcomes among alcohol-dependent patients (72). Although the evidence for the effectiveness of this therapy is quite consistent across studies, the effects have been generally modest in clinical impact, and CBT has generally not proved to be superior to other well-delivered treatments of similar intensity and duration (73–76).

12-Step Facilitation Therapy TSF therapy was described previously in the residential stage of care. However, it was developed and is most widely used in outpatient treatment. In either stage, one aspect of TSF that clearly separates it from other therapies is its active promotion of spirituality as a key to lasting recovery. In this context, spirituality is considered a force that provides direction and meaning to one's life.

As described previously, many studies have confirmed the effectiveness of this therapy versus usual care. For example, Thevos et al. studied female alcoholics who received TSF over 12 weeks in a random assignment comparison with motivational counseling. Women who received CBT or TSF had better outcomes than women who received the control condition (77). It should be noted that most treatment provided in addictions specialty care programs has elements of TSF, but the actual TSF intervention developed for Project MATCH and implemented in other research studies is not widely available in such programs.

Timko and colleagues conducted a study to determine whether more intensive referral to self-help groups during outpatient treatment would promote higher and more sustained rates of participation and better outcomes than standard clinic practices (78). The intervention consisted of detailed lists of local self-help meetings that had been favored by prior patients, directions to the meetings, and material that described self-help meetings and addressed common questions and typical concerns about the program. The counselor also arranged a meeting between the patient and a participating member of a self-help group and provided the patient with a journal to record attendance at meetings and reactions to the meetings. Attendance at self-help meetings was monitored over the next two outpatient sessions. For patients who had attended a self-help meeting, attempts were made to link the patient with a sponsor. For those who had not attended a meeting, the process of linking the patients with a self-help volunteer was repeated.

Results indicated that patients in the intensive referral condition had higher rates of overall involvement in self-help programs at 6 months than those in the standard referral condition. These patients were more likely to be doing service work at meetings, to have reported having a "spiritual awakening," to have a sponsor, and to have worked on more of the steps in the 12-step program. In addition, in those patients who had relatively little prior experience with self-help programs, the intensive referral intervention produced higher rates of attendance at self-help meetings than standard referral. With regard to substance use outcomes, the intensive referral condition produced better alcohol and drug use outcomes at 6 months, as assessed by Addiction Severity Index (ASI) composite scores, and higher rates of total abstinence from drugs than the standard referral condition (78).

Individual Drug Counseling Individual counseling, delivered in structured sessions (12 to 24) to foster abstinence and general adjustment, has been extensively studied in outpatient settings. In almost all studies, patients who have received this form of counseling had better during and posttreatment outcomes (57,58), with those who attended a greater frequency of sessions typically showing the best results (59–61). Importantly, there are very few studies that have shown positive effects from *group* drug counseling. Indeed, in one large trial among cocaine-dependent patients, it was only individual counseling and not group counseling that was associated with improved outcomes (76). This is important in that *group* drug counseling is by far the most prevalent component of treatment in the national treatment system (7).

A meta-analysis of studies examining the effects of counseling in agonist maintenance showed a clinically modest and not statistically significant effect of counseling when added to methadone treatment. One study that did find a significant effect of adding counseling in methadone was done within the Veterans Administration methadone program in Philadelphia (66). In that study, all participants were treated with methadone within the same treatment program and received the same methadone dose. These individuals were randomly assigned to receive counseling or no counseling in addition to the methadone (66). Results showed that 68% of patients assigned to the no counseling condition failed to reduce their drug use (confirmed by urinalysis) and 34% of those patients required at least one episode of emergency medical care. In contrast, no patient in the counseling group required emergency medical care, 63% showed sustained elimination of opiate use, and 41% showed sustained elimination of cocaine use over the 6 months of the trial.

A study by Fiorentine and Anglin (57) also demonstrated the contribution of counseling to drug rehabilitation. In that study, group counseling was the most common modality (averaging 9.5 sessions per month), followed by 12-step meetings (7.5 times per month) and individual counseling (4.7 times per month). Greater frequency of both group and individual counseling sessions was shown to reduce the likelihood of relapse over the subsequent 6 months. These findings obtained even among those who had approximately the same length of stay in the programs. Thus it may be that beyond the simple effects of attending a program, greater involvement in counseling activities is important for improved outcomes.

Other Interventions and Services Though medications and behavioral therapies have been the most extensively studied components of care, there are additional types of interventions and services that have also been shown to be effective in initiating and sustaining abstinence from alcohol and other substances.

Voucher-Based Reinforcement of Abstinence Higgins and colleagues (79–81) brought laboratory principles of behavioral change to the treatment of cocaine dependence. In a now-classic set of studies in a clinical laboratory setting, cocaine-dependent patients seeking outpatient treatment were randomly assigned to receive either standard drug counseling and referral to AA or a multicomponent behavioral treatment in which vouchers for desirable goods and services, provided by community shops and stores were provided contingent on drug-negative urine tests. Voucher-based reinforcement of abstinence retained more patients in treatment, produced more abstinent patients, longer periods of abstinence, and greater improvements in personal function than the standard counseling approach. In the decade since the publication of these early studies, the technique of providing positive reinforcement contingent on drug-free urines has been replicated and extended in alcohol-, cocaine-, opiate-, and methamphetamine-dependent patients, all with similarly positive findings (80). Moreover, because voucher-based reinforcements have been criticized for their expense and administrative problems, investigators have tested partial reinforcement schedules using a lottery system where drug-free urine tests afford patients an opportunity to draw for a range of small to large valued prizes (82). This procedure has reduced costs in real-world settings and appears to provide an enjoyable and treatment-compatible means of delivering the reinforcers. A very promising extension of the voucher-based reinforcement procedure has been developed and studied by Silverman and colleagues (83,84). These investigators operate a data entry center where recovering patients may learn data entry skills and to earn wages for data entry, contingent upon their providing a drug-free urine sample (83). This procedure appears to be practical and potentially useful as a means of extending the principles of contingency management practices into real world settings (82).

Clinical Case Management and Wraparound Services The majority of patients admitted to substance abuse treatment have significant problems in one or more other areas of life function such as medical status, employment, family relations, or psychiatric function. Studies have documented that "wraparound services"—such as primary medical care, housing, employment training, psychiatric care and parenting assistance for these addiction-related problems can be effective adjuncts to standard addiction-focused care in either residential or outpatient settings and in either the rehabilitative or continuing care stages of treatment.

As indicated in Part 1 of this chapter, most specialty care treatment programs do not have access to many of the types of wraparound services that would be useful to their clients; for this reason, most field studies have employed clinical case managers to link patients to available services in the community and to encourage follow-through by those patients (85). Studies of case management with alcohol- and drug-addicted patients show mixed results. Although there are many studies that have found improved patient function with the addition of case management to standard addiction services, the effectiveness of this form of care management seems to be more related to the availability and attractiveness of the services that are being managed than to the theoretical or methodological aspects of the case management process itself (85). For these reasons, this review treats special services as the active ingredients and case management as the vehicle for linking those services to the patient.

A study by Milby and colleagues (86) illustrates the importance of providing supplemental social support services to homeless, substance (typically cocaine and alcohol)-dependent individuals who sought health care services (not explicitly drug abuse treatment) from the Birmingham Health Care for the Homeless Coalition. In that study, 176 subjects were recruited and randomized into usual care (primarily 12-step group counseling) and enhanced (addition of employment, housing and psychiatric services to usual care) conditions, conducted in separate facilities. Enhanced care patients attended therapy more regularly and at 6-month follow up were two times more likely to be employed and four times less likely to be homeless than the usual care patients. It appears that the supplemental services were associated with significant and broad improvements.

Not all studies of wraparound services have required clinical case management. Similar findings have been seen from adding wraparound services to standard addiction treatment through special computer systems or special training of counselors. Better outcomes have been seen when the services were "matched" to the problems presented by the patients and when those services were requested by the patients. For example, Friedmann et al. (87) conducted a large-scale study of services-to-needs matching, with a sample of more than 3,100 addiction treatment patients. The study focused on the degree to which reported needs in five domains—medical, mental health, family, vocational, and housing—were addressed with services, and whether better matching produced better substance use outcomes. Overall, higher rates of services-to-problems matching predicted better substance use outcomes. The effect was concentrated in patients who reported problems in more areas (e.g., at least four of the five domains), and was strongest among patients in long-term residential facilities. Matching of vocational and housing services was particularly important.

Family Involvement As discussed earlier in this part of the chapter, the idea of involving family in the ongoing support, monitoring, and management of loved ones entering the recovery process is a relatively new one. As described earlier, interventions such as Al-Anon have been widely applied to assist families of substance-dependent individuals. There has not been much support for the effectiveness of this approach though the literature is still limited. Results generally indicate that Al-Anon leads to improvements in family functioning, but little change in the substance user (32–35,89,90).

Marital, Family, and Couples Therapies Over the past 15 years, there have been more than 60 studies in which marital, family, or couples therapies have been provided to reduce substance abuse, or substance abuse–related problems such as violence. In a recent review of controlled studies of this type with alcohol-dependent patients, marital and family therapy, and particularly behavioral couples therapy, was significantly more effective than individual treatments at inducing and sustaining abstinence, improving relationship functioning, and reducing domestic violence and emotional problems of children (90). Similar reductions in substance use and partner violence have also been seen in controlled trials of marital, family, or couples therapy with opiate- and cocaine-dependent patients (81,91,92).

Behavioral Couples Therapy Behavioral couples therapy treats the substance-abusing patient with his or her spouse to arrange a daily "sobriety contract" in which the patient states his or her intent not to drink or use drugs, and the spouse expresses support for the patient's efforts to stay abstinent. Behavioral couples therapy also teaches communication and nonsubstance-associated positive activities for couples. Findings show that behavioral couples therapy produces more abstinence and better relationship function than typical individual-based treatment and also reduces social costs and domestic violence (90,93,94).

CRAFT CRAFT is based on a combination of standard functional analysis of behavior combined with principles of reinforcement. The therapy was developed to teach and promote the practice of these principles by members of a household. Specifically, families who learn the CRAFT intervention are taught skills for modifying a loved one's alcohol or drug-using behavior and for enhancing treatment engagement (95). The intervention has been generally well accepted by families and several studies have shown that CRAFT produces greater likelihood of entry and engagement of substance abusing family members and greater likelihood of post treatment abstinence than standard treatments (34,35). In addition, families of the substance abusers in these studies show significantly less depression, anxiety, anger, and physical abuse than families of patients who received standard treatment (35,95).

The Continuing Care Stage of Treatment The term *continuing care* has been used to indicate the stage of treatment that follows an initial episode of more intensive care, usually inpatient/residential or intensive outpatient. At one point, this phase of care was referred to as "aftercare," but the more common term is now continuing care, which better conveys the idea that active treatment continues in this phase. Continuing care is provided in a variety of formats and modalities, including group counseling, individual therapy, telephone counseling, brief checkups, and self-help meetings. These interventions are usually 3 months or longer in duration, with some interventions lasting as long as 2 years. The results of recent reviews indicate that continuing care interventions were more likely to produce positive treatment effects when they had a longer planned duration (e.g., 12 months or more), made more active efforts to deliver treatment to patients (e.g., active outreach, counseling via telephone, home visits), or provided incentives to clients or practitioners for continued participation (96).

Historically, formal continuing care interventions were often not included as part of standard treatment. However, with the change in approach toward addiction as a chronic condition, substantial research showing the value of participation in AA, and the emerging research on the value of simply contacting, supporting, and monitoring the condition of previously treated patients has shown its importance. For these reasons, there is an increasing number of formal treatment settings that offer continuing care, and some states have begun to reimburse for this stage of the continuum. Nonetheless, at this writing, most continuing care is still AA or another mutual help group and most insurance programs and public substance abuse benefit designs do not reimburse care at this stage. As discussed in Part 2 of this chapter, the major venue for continuing care in the rest of medicine is the primary care setting. As should be clear from the early parts of this chapter, primary care physicians have clear reason and an increasing number of tools to manage substance use disorders. Again, these disorders are being regarded as medical conditions in their own right (14) and "unhealthy substance use" is now widely associated with increased complications, management problems, poor outcomes, and significant expense in the treatment of other chronic illnesses (25).

From a cost-effectiveness perspective, the types of care available and the therapeutic components within the continuing care stage are among the least costly, but may provide the most value for sustaining the patient recovery that may have been initiated in one of the earlier stages. Put differently, substance-dependent patients who complete detoxification, residential, and/or outpatient treatment stages *without* engaging into continuing care are at great risk of relapse and return to the more intensive, expensive stages of care if they do not adequately participate in the continuing care stage of the continuum.

Goals of Continuing Care Continuing care shares many of the goals and therapeutic components of outpatient treatment. Indeed, low-frequency outpatient visits have been considered continuing care in some treatment systems. However, care at this stage of the continuum is generally less formalized, involves less contact in specialty care settings (i.e., treatment may also be provided by phone or home visit), and is more dedicated to monitoring for early signs of relapse while simultaneously supporting engagement in AA and any parts of a lifestyle that provide insurance against relapse. Continuing care has the following goals.

- Maintain physiologic and emotional improvements initiated during residential or outpatient treatments.
- Monitor progress in recovery and possible relapse and intervene where appropriate on signs of relapse.
- Continue to teach and foster more effective coping behaviors and self-care.
- Support healthy relationships and behaviors that are incompatible with substance use and promote recovery.

Medications All antiaddiction medications previously described earlier are also useful in this stage of the addiction continuum. As noted earlier, cooccurring problems of depression, anxiety, or phobia are prevalent and may reoccur when the patient returns to their former environments and relationships. Thus psychotropic medications can be important in the achievement and maintenance of improved mental health. The assistance of these medications may provide pharmacologic support for the benefits of traditional behavioral and social interventions.

Behavioral Therapies All the behavioral therapies discussed under the residential and outpatient stages of the continuum are as likely to be useful in this stage of treatment. Interventions designed to engage family supports and to change previous peer relationships may be particularly valuable as the recovering patient attempts to integrate a new recovering lifestyle into the historical environment and relationships. In this section, we review effective continuing care strategies that have not been covered in the section on outpatient treatment.

Types or Modalities of Continuing Care Participation in AA/Narcotics Anonymous/Cocaine Anonymous AA remains the most prevalent form of continuing care for individuals who are actively participating in outpatient treatment; or who have completed residential treatment. Because of the anonymous quality of AA, not much research was done to evaluate this important part of rehabilitation until recently (26,78,97–99). This research has shown that treated patients who have participated in AA have much better continuing abstinence records than patients who have received rehabilitation treatments but have not continued in AA. There is now little question that individuals who frequently attend AA and other self-help programs usually do better than those who do not (51,54).

McKay and colleagues (49,100) found that participation in posttreatment self-help groups also predicted better outcomes among a group of cocaine- or alcohol-dependent veterans in a day-hospital rehabilitation program. Timko et al. (50) found that more AA attendance was associated with better 1-year outcomes among previously untreated problem drinkers, regardless of whether they received inpatient, outpatient, or no other treatment. Moos and Moos (98) also found that faster affiliation with AA and longer participation predicted better 1-, 8-, and 16-year alcohol-related outcomes. Individuals who attended AA at least five times per week for the first year had almost a 90% likelihood of abstinence at 1 year, and participation in AA had a positive effect on alcohol related outcomes over and above the effects of formal treatment (98,101). McKay et al. (102) examined whether measures of motivation, coping and mood, social support, comorbid problem severity, treatment attendance, employment, and self-help participation assessed at 6-month intervals predicted subsequent cocaine use over a 2-year follow-up, In multivariate analyses, degree of self-help participation emerged as the strongest and most consistent predictor of cocaine use.

Office-Based Therapy We have chosen to include office-based therapy in the continuing care stage of the continuum, though we recognize there are arguments for placing it in other stages. Although office-based therapy is formal treatment and is reimbursed under many insurance plans, this type of care is not part of the specialty addiction treatment spectrum. Also, it is our impression that the majority of care delivered in this modality is not focused on the symptoms of substance use per se, but perhaps more appropriately directed at problems of relationships, mood, and adjustment—the types of problems that are so often confronted by those seeking to change their lives to cope with recovery from an addictive disorder. This is an area that is clearly in need of research to inform the addiction field.

An examination of a city phone directory under "addiction treatment" reveals far more "addiction therapists" than addiction programs. More individuals receive treatment for substance use disorders from these private therapists than from treatment "programs." However, it is very difficult to characterize the nature of this treatment in even the most basic terms. Most states do not require a license to treat addictive disorders and many to most of the patients who receive care in these offices do not use their insurance to pay for it. Consequently, there are few records to describe who these therapists are or who their patients are. Many of the articles in the "trade magazines" devoted to counseling and case management suggest that individuals with a very wide range of background training are providing addiction treatment. This includes psychiatrists, psychologists, nurses, social workers, and counselors as well as clergy and many others. It is also not clear how frequently or for what duration treatment occurs in this setting or what kinds of activities are provided (e.g., urine screening, family counseling, case management). This is an area in need of fundamental descriptive and qualitative research.

Telephone Continuing Care Clinical researchers have been studying methods for extending the positive effects of outpatient rehabilitative care. Consistent with a "disease management" perspective, several groups have shown that extended therapeutic contact provided via the telephone can have positive effects (103). For example, McKay and colleagues have been studying various continuing care interventions for alcohol and cocaine-dependent patients after their participation in intensive outpatient programs (IOP). The continuing care services in these studies have been provided by experienced addictions counselors. One study compared telephone-based continuing care with two clinic-based continuing care treatments, standard group counseling and CBT relapse prevention (104,105). The continuing care interventions were provided for 12 weeks after graduation from IOP, and participants were followed up for 2 years from intake into continuing care. Results indicated that the telephone condition produced better abstinence outcomes than standard group counseling, and better outcomes than relapse prevention on several outcomes (e.g., cocaine urine toxicology, liver function measures indicative of heavy drinking). Further analyses showed that the telephone continuing care intervention was superior to the two clinic-based interventions for patients who made reasonable progress toward achieving the goals of IOP when they were in that phase of treatment, which was 80% of the study sample (101,105).

McKay and colleagues are currently evaluating a longer term, telephone-based adaptive alcoholism treatment package (102). In this study, patients who achieved initial engagement and stabilization in the first 2 weeks of IOP were randomized to standard care only, standard care plus 18 months of monitoring and feedback via brief telephone contacts (5 to 10 minutes), or standard care plus 18 months of telephone monitoring and counseling (20- to 30-minute calls), along with a stepped care protocol that provided additional telephone contacts or more intensive, face-to-face treatment, as needed. Preliminary analyses indicated that the more comprehensive telephone intervention produced more days of abstinence than standard care during months 6 through 12 of the follow-up and more days of abstinence than the brief telephone monitoring condition during months 3 through 9. At the 12-month follow-up, 73% of those in more comprehensive telephone condition reported no alcohol or cocaine use in the prior month, compared with 65% in the telephone monitoring condition and 45% in standard care (106).

Recovery Management Check-ups Another approach to the long-term management of substance use disorders is to provide brief "checkups" on a regular basis, with referral to treatment if necessary. Scott, Dennis, and colleagues from Chestnut Health Systems have developed such a protocol, which they refer to as "Recovery Management Checkups" (RMC) (107). In this protocol, substance abusers who have entered treatment are followed and interviewed every 3 months. For those individuals who are not currently in treatment or in a controlled environment such as jail, need for further treatment is determined through a relatively brief assessment. Individuals who met criteria for need for treatment are transferred to a linkage manager, who uses motivational interviewing techniques to help the participant recognize and acknowledge the problem and need for treatment, addresses any existing barriers to reentering treatment, and arranges scheduling and transportation to treatment.

The RMC protocol was evaluated in a study in which 448 adults presenting at a central intake unit were randomized to RMC or quarterly research follow-ups and followed for 24 months (108). The results of the study indicated that the RMC intervention led to better management of the patients over time. First, patients in RMC were more likely to be readmitted to treatment, were readmitted sooner, and received more treatment during the 2-year follow-up than those in the control condition. Second, patients in RMC had better substance use outcomes over the course of the follow-up than those in the control condition. Specifically, RMC patients were less likely to meet criteria for needing treatment in five or more quarters than patients in the control condition (23% vs. 32%). In recent work, the effectiveness of the RMC protocol has been improved via the addition of urine drug testing to assess need for treatment, better transportation assistance, and practices to increase retention in individuals who are referred to treatment following their checkup.

Extended Medical Monitoring There is accumulating evidence that continuing care for substance use disorders and cooccurring medical problems can be provided through primary care practices. For example, Willenbring and Olson (109) tested whether a treatment model that provided extended integrated medical and addiction treatment for alcohol with severe medical problems would yield better outcomes than standard treatment. The integrated care model, referred to as "Integrated Outpatient Care" or IOT, provided monthly clinic visits with a nurse practitioner or physician. Motivational interviewing techniques were used in the sessions, and family members were included when possible to support change and reduce behaviors on the part of family members that may have enabled drinking. Outreach attempts were made to reengage patients who missed sessions. Patients in the control condition received standard care, which consisted of referral to traditional specialty addictions treatment and advice from medical staff to abstain from alcohol.

The results indicated that the integrated care model produced much higher rates of extended participation in both medical and addiction treatment over the 2-year follow-up than standard care. For example, patients in IOT had an average of 42 treatment visits over 2 years versus 17 visits in standard care. IOT also produced better substance use outcomes. At the end of the 2-year follow-up, 74% of IOT patients were abstinent versus only 47% of those in standard care. More patients in standard care died during the 2-year follow-up compared with IOT (30% vs. 18%).

SUMMARY AND CONCLUSIONS

We began this chapter with a review of the concepts under which addiction has been treated. Based on that mixed and sometimes confused conceptual formulation about the "condition" of addiction we described how the current specialty care addiction system was organized, funded, and regulated independent from the rest of mainstream health care. Although this organization was likely necessary in the early 1970s, we argue that this segregated system is finding it increasingly difficult to meet the needs of its patients or to deliver evidence-based quality care.

We then turned our attention to an examination of how mainstream health care has developed new models of treating chronic illness in a staged approach by employing team treatment management through a "continuum of care." We argued that this "disease management" approach might serve as a model for what a functional continuum of care in addiction treatment might be. In this regard, scientific advances during the past two decades have provided many evidence-based medications, behavioral therapies, and other interventions—the components of care—that could form the basis for a functional continuum of addiction treatment. Thus in the last part of the chapter, we reviewed these evidence-based components of care within the context of a proposed five-stage continuum of addiction care.

Although these stages of the proposed continuum have distinct goals, they are conceptually linked with the earlier, more intensive stages designed to prepare patients for later, less intensive, self-management–oriented stages. Importantly, the medications, behavioral therapies, and other interventions discussed in this part of the chapter were seen as having multiple roles at different stages of the continuum, hopefully leading to a more nuanced series of research studies designed to elucidate those roles. The conclusions possible from this part of the chapter are very optimistic. There is an increasing range of evidence-based treatment components. There are adequate medications and a medical basis for treatment, as well as compensation to attract and provide a meaningful role for physicians in the treatment of addiction. There are also individual- and family oriented behavioral therapies that sophisticated therapists from various backgrounds can use to change the substance use and its associated personal and family pathologies. Moreover, work in these important areas is continuing with new progress made each month. The possibilities for improved treatment are significant.

The limiting factors in this otherwise optimistic future are the conceptual, organizational, and financial foundations of the contemporary specialty care addiction treatment system. Without an informed conceptualization of addiction as a chronic illness, the health care system simply will not train primary care physicians, develop disease management protocols, build information systems with standard measures of illness progression and patient improvement, or develop adaptive care management practices. Further, without a commitment to related changes in the way addiction treatment is organized, financed, and managed, addiction treatment is not likely to improve, regardless of the advances in specialty care medications or therapies. Although there will always be a continuing need for new and more sophisticated treatment interventions and components, there is a pressing need for financial and organizational development to permit the treatment system to provide the kind of quality care that is possible.

ACKNOWLEDGMENTS: *Preparation was supported by grants from the Center for Substance Abuse Treatment, the National Institute on Drug Abuse, the National Institute on Alcoholism and Alcohol Abuse and The Robert Wood Johnson Foundation.*

REFERENCES

1. National Household Survey on Drug Use and Health (NHSDUH): results from the 2006 survey. SAMHSA. Accessed August 11, 2008, from http://www.oas.samhsa.gov/nsduh/2k6nsduh/2k6Results.pdf.
2. Institute of Medicine (IOM). *Managing managed care: quality improvement in behavioral health.* Washington, DC: National Academy Press, 1997.
3. Institute of Medicine (IOM). *Crossing the quality chasm for mental and substance use disorders.* Washington, DC: National Academy Press, 2006.
4. Harwood HJ, Fountain D, Livermore G. *The economic costs of alcohol and drug abuse in the United States.* Rockville, MD: National Institute on Drug Abuse, 1998.
5. Morgenstern J, McCrady BS, Blanchard K, et al. Barriers to employability among substance dependent and nonsubstance-affected women on federal welfare: implications for program design. *J Studies Alcohol* 2003;64:24–38.
6. National Survey of Substance Abuse Treatment Services (NSSATS), 2006. Accessed August 11, 2008, from http://wwwdasis.samhsa.gov/webt/state_data/US06.pdf.
7. Treatment Episode Dataset (TEDS), 2006. SAMHSA. Accessed August 11, 2008, from http://wwwdasis.samhsa.gov/webt/quicklink/US06.htm.
8. Willenbring ML. Medications to treat alcohol dependence: adding to the continuum of care. *JAMA* 2007;298(14):1691–1692.
9. Kerwin ML, Walker-Smith M, Kirby K. Comparative analysis of state requirements for the training of substance abuse and mental health counselors *J. Substance Abuse Treatment* 2006;30(3):173–181.
10. Meyers K, McLellan AT. The American Treatment System for Adolescent Substance Abuse: formidable challenges, fundamental revisions and mechanisms for improvements. In: Seligman MEP, Evans DL, eds. *Current issues in adolescent health.* Oxford, UK: Oxford University Press, 2004:210–244.
11. McGlynn E, Asch J, Adams J, et al. The quality of health care delivered to adults in the United States. *N Engl J Med* 2003;348:2635–2645.
12. White W. *Slaying the dragon: the history of addiction treatment and recovery in America.* Bloomington, IL: Chestnut Health Systems, 1998.
13. Anglin MD, Hser Y, Grella CE. Drug addiction and treatment careers among clients in the Drug Abuse Treatment Outcomes Study (DATOS). *Psychol Addictive Behav* 1997;11(4):308–323.
14. McLellan AT, O'Brien CP, Lewis D, et al. Drug addiction as a chronic medical illness: implications for treatment, insurance and evaluation. *JAMA* 2000;84:1689–1695.
15. Bodenheimer T, Wagner E, Grumbach K. Improving primary care for patients with chronic illness. *JAMA* 2002;288(14):1775–1779.
16. Wagner E, Austin BT, Von Korff M. Organizing care for patients with chronic illness. *Milbank Q* 1996;74(4):511–544.
17. McLellan AT, McKay JR, Forman R, et al. Reconsidering the evaluation of addiction treatment: from retrospective follow-up to concurrent recovery monitoring. *Addiction* 2005;100:447–458.
18. Musto DF. *The American disease: the origins of narcotic control.* New Haven, CT: Yale University Press, 1973.
19. Gelber S. Funding and financing of california's alcohol/drug treatment system: issues for system efficiency, access, management, coordination and improvement. Testimony before the California Little Hoover Commission. Sacramento CA, 2002.
20. Vocci FJ, Elkashef A. Pharmacotherapy and other treatments for cocaine abuse and dependence. *Curr Opin Psychiatry* 2005;18:3:265–270.
21. Babor TF, Higgins-Biddle JC, Higgins PS, et al. Training medical providers to conduct alcohol screening and brief interventions. *Subst Abuse* 2004;25(1):17–26.
22. Bertholet J, Daeppen J, Wietlisbach V, et al. 2005; Reduction of alcohol consumption by brief alcohol intervention in primary care. *Arch Intern Med* 2005;165:986–995.
23. Fleming MF, Barry KL, Manwell LB, et al. Brief physician advice for problem alcohol drinkers: a randomized controlled trial in community-based primary care practices. *JAMA* 1997;277:1039–1045.
24. Miller RW, Rollnick S. *Motivational interviewing: preparing people for change,* 2nd ed. New York: Guilford, 2002.
25. Program of Research to Integrate Substance Use Information into Mainstream healthcare (PRISM) 2008. Accessed August 11, 2008, from http://www.tresearch.org/add_health/about_prism.htm.
26. Project MATCH Research Group. Matching alcoholism treatments to client heterogeneity: project MATCH post treatment drinking outcomes. *J Studies Alcohol* 1997;58:7–29.
27. Bien T, Miller WR, Tonigan JS. Brief interventions for alcohol problems: a review. *Addiction* 1993;88(3):315–336.
28. Moyer A, Finney JW, Swearingen CE, et al. Brief interventions for alcohol problems: a meta-analytic review of controlled investigations in treatment-seeking and non-treatment-seeking populations. *Addiction* 2002;97(3):279–292.
29. Saitz R, Horton N, Larson MJ, et al. Primary medical care and reductions in addiction severity: a prospective cohort study. *Addiction* 2005; 100(1):70–78.
30. Copello A, Velleman R, Templeton L. Family interventions in the treatment of alcohol and drug problems. *Drug Alcohol Rev* 2005;24(4): 369–385.
31. Johnson V. How to help someone who doesn't want help. Minneapolis, MN: Johnson Institute Books, 1986.
32. Barber JG, Gilbertson R. An experimental study on brief unilateral intervention for the partners of heavy drinkers. *Res Soc Work Pract* 1996;6(2):325–336.
33. Dittrich JE, Trapold MA. A treatment program for wives of alcoholics: an evaluation. *Bull Soc Psychol Addict Behav* 1984;3(2):91–102.
34. Kirby KC, Marlowe DB, Festinger DS, et al. Community reinforcement training for family and significant others of drug abusers: a unilateral intervention to increase treatment entry of drug users. *Drug Alcohol Depend* 1999;56(1):85–96.
35. Meyers RJ, Miller WR, Smith JE, et al. A randomized trial of two methods for engaging treatment-refusing drug users through concerned significant others. *J Consult Clin Psychol* 2002;70(5):1182–1185.
36. Meyers RJ, Miller WR, Smith JE. Community reinforcement and family training (CRAFT). In: Meyers RJ, Miller WR, eds. *A community reinforcement approach to addiction treatment.* New York: Cambridge University Press, 2001:147–160.
37. O'Brien CP. Anti-craving medications for relapse prevention: a possible new class of psychoactive medications. *Am J Psychiat* 2005;162(8): 1423–1431.
38. O'Malley S, Jaffe A, Chang G, et al. Six-month follow-up of naltrexone and psychotherapy for alcohol dependence. *Arch Gen Psychiatry* 1996;53:217–224.
39. Garbutt JC, Kranzler HR, O'Malley SS, et al. Efficacy and tolerability of long-acting injectable naltrexone for alcohol dependence: a randomized controlled trial. *JAMA* 2005;293:1617–1625.
40. O'Brien CP, McKay JR. Psychopharmacological treatments of substance use disorders. In: Nathan PE, Gorman JM, eds. *Effective treatments for DSM-IV disorders,* 2nd ed. New York: Oxford University Press, 2002: 125–156.
41. McLellan AT, McKay J. Components of successful addiction treatment: what does research say? In: Graham AW, Schultz T, eds. Principles of addiction medicine, 4th ed. Chicago: University of Chicago Press, 2005:34–45.
42. McLellan AT, Alterman AI, Woody GE, et al. Great expectations: a review of the concepts and empirical findings regarding substance abuse

treatment. In: *Alcohol and substance dependence.* London, UK: Royal Task Force on Substance Dependence, 1994.
43. McLellan AT, Weisner C. Achieving the public health potential of substance abuse treatment: implications for patient referral, treatment "matching" and outcome evaluation. In: Bickel W, DeGrandpre R, eds. *Drug policy and human nature.* Philadelphia: Williams & Wilkins, 1996.
44. Betty Ford Institute Consensus Panel. What is recovery? A working definition from the Betty Ford Institute. *J. Subst Abuse Treatment* 2007; 33(2):39–47.
45. WHO Quality of Life Group. The World Health Organization Quality of Life assessment (WHOQL): development and general psychometric properties. *Soc Sci Med* 1998;46:569–1585.
46. Simpson DD. Effectiveness of drug abuse treatment: review of research from field settings. In: Egertson JA, Fox DM, Leshner AI, eds. *Treating drug abusers effectively.* Cambridge, MA: Blackwell, 1997.
47. Simpson DD, Joe GW, Brown BS. Treatment retention and follow-up outcomes in the Drug Abuse Treatment Outcome Study (DATOS). *Psychol Addictive Behav* 1997;11(4):294–301.
48. McLatchie BH, Lomp KG. Alcoholics Anonymous affiliation and treatment outcome among a clinical sample of problem drinkers. *Am J Drug Alcohol Abuse* 1988;14:309–324.
49. McKay JR, Alterman AI, Cacciola JS, et al. Group counseling vs. individualized relapse prevention aftercare following intensive outpatient treatment for cocaine dependence: initial results. *J Consult Clin Psychol* 1997;65:778–788.
50. Timko C, Moos RH, Finney JW, et al. Outcome of treatment for alcohol abuse and involvement in Alcoholics Anonymous among previously untreated problem drinkers. *J Mental Health Admin* 1994;21:145–160.
51. Tonigan JS, Toscova R, Miller WR. Meta-analysis of the literature on Alcoholics Anonymous: sample and study characteristics moderate findings. *J Studies Alcohol* 1996;57:65–72.
52. Nowinski J, Baker S, Carroll K. *The twelve-step facilitation manual: a clinical research guide for therapists treating individuals with alcohol abuse and dependence.* Project MATCH Monograph Series, Vol. 1. Rockville, MD: National Institute on Alcohol Abuse and Alcoholism, 1995.
53. Maude Griffin P, Hohenstein J, Humfleet G, et al. Superior efficacy of cognitive-behavioral therapy for urban crack cocaine abusers: main and matching effects. *J Consult Clin Psychol* 1998;66(5):832–837.
54. Tonigan JS, Connors GJ, Miller WR. Participation and involvement in Alcoholics Anonymous. In: Babor T, DelBoca F, eds. *Treatment matching in alcoholism.* New York: Hollis Press, 2000.
55. Woody GE, McLellan AT, Luborsky L, et al. Psychotherapy and counseling for methadone-maintained opiate addicts: results of research studies. *NIDA Res Monogr* 1990;104:9–23.
56. Woody GE, McLellan AT, Luborsky L, et al. Psychotherapy in community methadone programs: a validation study. *Am J Psychiatry* 1995; 152(9):1302–1308.
57. Fiorentine R, Anglin DM. More is better: counseling participation and the effectiveness of outpatient drug treatment. *J Subst Abuse Treatment* 1996;13(4):232–240.
58. McLellan AT, Woody GE, Luborsky L, et al. Is the counselor an "active ingredient" in substance abuse rehabilitation? *J Nerv Mental Dis* 1988; 176:423–430.
59. Simpson DD. A conceptual framework for drug treatment process and outcomes. *J Substance Abuse Treatment* 2004;27:99–121.
60. Moos RH. Addictive disorders in context: principles and puzzles of effective treatment and recovery. *Psychol Addictive Behav* 2003;17(1):3–14.
61. McLellan AT. The outcomes movement in substance abuse treatment: comments, concerns, and criticisms. In: Sorenson J, et al., eds. *Drug abuse treatment through collaboration: practice and research partnerships that work.* Washington, DC: American Psychological Association Press, 2002:58–63.
62. Humphreys K. *Circles of recovery: self-help organizations for addictions.* Cambridge, England: Cambridge University Press, 2003.
63. Humphreys K, Wing S, McCarty B, et al. Self-help organizations for alcohol and drug problems: toward evidence-based practice and policy. *J Subst Abuse Treatment* 2004;26(3):151–158.
64. Moos RH, Finney JW, Cronkite RC. *Alcoholism treatment: context, process, and outcome.* New York: Oxford University Press, 1990.
65. Morgenstern J, Labouvie E, McCrady B, et al. Affiliation with Alcoholics Anonymous following treatment: a study of its therapeutic effects and mechanisms of action. *J Consult Clin Psychol* 1997;65:768–778.
66. McLellan AT, Arndt IO, Woody GE, et al. Psychosocial services in substance abuse treatment? A dose-ranging study of psychosocial services. *JAMA* 1993;269(15):1953–1959.
67. Marlatt GA, Gordon JR, eds. *Relapse prevention: maintenance strategies in the treatment of addictive behaviors.* New York: Guilford Press, 1985.
68. National Institute on Drug Abuse (NIDA). *Therapy manual for drug addiction: manual 1, a cognitive-behavioral approach: treating cocaine addiction.* DHHS, NIH Publ. No. 98-4308. Washington, DC: U.S. Government Printing Office, 1998.
69. Kadden R, et al., eds. *Cognitive-behavioral coping skills therapy manual: a clinical research guide for therapists.* NIAAA, Project MATCH Series, Vol 3. DHHS., NIH Pub. No. 98-2620. Washington, DC: U.S. Government Printing Office, 1997.
70. Morgenstern J, Blanchard, KA, Morgan TJ, et al. Testing the effectiveness of cognitive-behavioral treatment for substance abuse in a community setting: within treatment and post-treatment findings. *J Consult Clin Psychol* 2001;69(6):1007–1017.
71. Carroll KM, Onken L. Behavioral therapies for drug abuse. *Am J Psychiat* 2005;162:1452–1460.
72. Balldin J, Berglund M, Borg S, et al. A 6-month controlled naltrexone study: combined effect with cognitive behavioral therapy in outpatient treatment of alcohol dependence. *Alcoholism Clin Exp Res* 2003;27(7):1142–1149.
73. Ouimette PC, Finney JW, Moos R. Twelve step and cognitive behavioral treatment for substance abuse: a comparison of treatment effectiveness. *J Consult Clin Psychol* 1997;65(2):230–240.
74. Morgenstern J, Longabaugh R. Cognitive-behavioral treatment for alcohol dependence: a review of evidence for its hypothesized mechanisms of action. *Addiction* 2000;95:1475–1490.
75. Leichsenring F, Leibing E. The effectiveness of psychodynamic therapy and cognitive behavior therapy in the treatment of personality disorders: a meta-analysis. *Am J Psychiatry* 2003;60:1223–1232.
76. Crits Christoph P, Siqueland L, Blaine J, et al. Psychosocial treatments for cocaine dependence: National Institute on Drug Abuse Collaborative Cocaine Treatment Study. *Arch Gen Psychiatry* 1999;56:493–502.
77. Thevos A, Thomas S, Randall C. Social support in alcohol dependence and social phobia: treatment comparison. *Res So Work Pract* 2001; 11(4):458–472.
78. Timko C, DeBenedetti A, Billow R. Intensive referral to 12-step self-help groups and 6-month substance use disorder outcomes. *Addiction* 2006;101:678–688.
79. Higgins ST, Budney AJ, Bickel WK, et al. Achieving cocaine abstinence with a behavioral approach. *Am J Psychiatry* 1993;150:763–769.
80. Higgins ST, Budney AJ, Bickel WK, et al. Incentives improve outcome in outpatient behavioral treatment of cocaine dependence. *Arch Gen Psychiatry* 1994;51:568–576.
81. Higgins S, Budney A, Bickel W, et al. Participation of significant others in outpatient behavioral treatment predicts greater cocaine abstinence. *J Drug Alcohol Abuse* 1994;20:38–45.
82. Petry NM. A comprehensive guide to the application of contingency management procedures in clinical settings. *Drug Alcohol Depend* 2000;58:9–26.
83. Silverman K, Higgins ST, Brooner RK, et al. Sustained cocaine abstinence in methadone maintenance patients through voucher-based reinforcement therapy. *Arch Gen Psychiatry* 1996;53:409–415.
84. Silverman K, Wong CJ, Umbricht Schneiter A, et al. Broad beneficial effects of reinforcement of cocaine abstinence in methadone patients. *J Consult Clin Psychol* 1998;66:811–824.
85. McLellan AT, Hagan TA, Meyers K, et al. Supplemental social services improve outcomes in public addiction treatment. *Addiction* 1998; 93(10):1489–1499.
86. Milby JB, Schumacher JE, Raczynski JM, et al. Sufficient conditions for effective treatment of substance abusing homeless persons. *Drug Alcohol Depend* 1996;43:39–47.

87. Friedmann PD, Hendrickson JC, Gerstein DR, et al. The effect of matching comprehensive services to patients' needs on drug use improvement in addiction treatment. *Addiction* 2004;99:962–972.
88. Miller WR, Meyers RJ, Tonigan JS. Engaging the unmotivated in treatment for alcohol problems: a comparison of three strategies for intervention through family members. *J Consult Clin Psychol* 1999;67(5):688–697.
89. Sisson R, Azrin N. Family-member involvement to initiate and promote treatment of problem drinkers. *J Behav Ther Exp Psychiatry* 1986; 17(1):15–21.
90. O'Farrell T, Fals Stewart W. Behavioral couples and family therapy for substance abusers. *Curr Psychiatry Rep* 2002;4:371–376.
91. Fals-Stewart W, O'Farrell T, Birchler B. Behavioral couples therapy for male methadone maintenance patients: effects on drug using behavior and relationship adjustment. *Behav Ther* 2001;32(2):391–411.
92. Fals-Stewart W. Behavioral couples therapy for drug-abusing patients: effects on partner violence. *J. Substance Abuse Treatment* 2002;22(2): 87–96.
93. McCrady B, Epstein E, Hirsch B. Maintaining change after conjoint behavioral alcohol treatment for men: outcomes at 6 months. *Addiction* 1999;94(9):1381–1396.
94. Winters J, Fals Stewart W, O'Farrell TJ, et al. Behavioral couples therapy for female substance-abusing patients: effects on substance use and relationship adjustment. *J Consult Clin Psychol* 2002;70:344–355.
95. Smith JE, Meyers RJ. Motivating substance abusers by treating their loved ones: the CRAFT Program. New York: Guilford Press, 2008.
96. McKay JR, Kivlahan D, Lash S, et al. Continuing care research: what we've learned and where we're going. *J Subst Abuse Treatment* 2009;36(1): 113–131.
97. McCrady BS, Miller WR. *Research on Alcoholics Anonymous: opportunities and alternatives.* New Brunswick, NJ: Rutgers Center of Alcohol Studies, 1993.
98. Moos R, Moos B. Participation in treatment and Alcoholics Anonymous: a 16-year follow-up of initially untreated individuals. *J Clin Psychol* 2006;62:735–750.
99. Weisner CM, Matzger H, Kaskutas L. How important is treatment? One-year outcomes of treated and untreated alcohol-dependent individuals. *Addiction* 2003;98(7):901–911.
100. McKay JR, Alterman AI, McLellan AT. et al. Treatment goals, continuity of care, and outcome in a day hospital substance abuse rehabilitation program. *Am J Psychiatry* 1994;151:254–259.
101. McKay JR, Lynch KG, Shepard DS, et al. Do patient characteristics and initial progress in treatment moderate the effectiveness of telephone-based continuing care for substance use disorders? *Addiction* 2005;100: 216–226.
102. McKay JR. The role of continuing care in outpatient alcohol treatment programs. In: Galanter M, ed. *Recent developments in alcoholism, vol. XV: services research in the era of managed care.* New York: Kluwer, 2001: 357–372.
103. McKay JR. Is there a case for extended interventions for alcohol and drug use disorders? *Addiction* 2005;100:1594–1610.
104. McKay JR, Lynch KG, Shepard DS, et al. The effectiveness of telephone-based continuing care in the clinical management of alcohol and cocaine use disorders: 12 month outcomes. *J Consult Clin Psychol* 2004;72:967–979.
105. McKay JR, Lynch KG, Shepard DS, et al. The effectiveness of telephone based continuing care for alcohol and cocaine dependence: 24 month outcomes. *Arch Gen Psychiatry* 2005;62:199–207.
106. McKay JR, Lynch KG, Van Horn D, et al. Effectiveness of extended telephone continuing care. Presented at the Research Society on Alcoholism, Washington DC, 2008.
107. Dennis M, Titus JC, Diamond G, et al. The Cannabis Youth Treatment (CYT) experiment: rationale, study design and analysis plans. *Addiction* 2002;97(Suppl 1):16–34.
108. Dennis ML, Scott CK, Funk R. An experimental evaluation of recovery management checkups (RMC) for people with chronic substance use disorders. *Eval Progr Plan* 2003;26:339–352.
109. Willenbring ML, Olson DH. A randomized trial of integrated outpatient treatment for medically ill alcoholic men. *Arch Intern Med* 1999;159:1946–1952.
110. Amato, Davoli M, Perucci C, et al. An overview of systematic reviews of the effectiveness of opiate maintenance therapies: available evidence to inform clinical practice and research. *J Substance Abuse Treatment* 2005;28(4):321–329.

SUGGESTED READINGS

Inciardi JA, Martin SS, Butzin CA, et al. An effective model of prison-based treatment for drug-involved offenders. *J Drug Issues* 1997;27(2): 261–278.

McKay JR. Adaptive continuing care and the management of drug use disorders. Washington, DC: American Psychological Association Press, 2009.

McKay JR, Alterman AI, Cacciola JS, et al. Continuing care for cocaine dependence: comprehensive 2-year outcomes. *J Consult Clin Psychol* 1999;67:420–427.

McKay JR, Longabaugh R, Beattie MC, et al. Does adding conjoint therapy to individually-focused alcoholism treatment lead to better family functioning? *J Subst Abuse* 1993;5:45–60.

McKay JR, McLellan AT, Alterman AI. An evaluation of the Cleveland Criteria for Inpatient Treatment of Substance Abuse. *Am J Psychiatry* 1992;149:1212–1218.

McKay J, McLellan AT, Alterman A, et al. Predictors of participation in aftercare sessions and self-help groups following completion of intensive outpatient treatment for substance abuse. *J Stud Alcohol* 1998;43: 345–361.

McLellan AT, Cacciola J, Kushner H, et al. The Fifth Edition of the Addiction Severity Index: cautions, additions and normative data. *J Subst Abuse Treat* 1992;9(5):461–480.

McLellan AT, Grissom G, Brill P. Improved outcomes from treatment service "matching" in substance abuse patients: a controlled study. *Arch Gen Psychiatry* 1997;54:730–735.

McLellan AT, Woody GE, Metzger D, et al. Evaluating the effectiveness of treatments for substance use disorders: reasonable expectations, appropriate comparisons. *Milbank Q* 1996;74(1):51–85.

Miller WR, Benefield RG, Tonigan JS. Enhancing motivation for change in problem drinking: A controlled comparison of two therapist styles. *J Consult Clin Psychol* 1993;61:455–461.

Miller WR, Hester RK. Inpatient alcoholism treatment: who benefits? *Am Psychol* 1986;41:794–805.

Morgenstern J, Blanchard KA, McCrady BS, et al. Effectiveness of intensive case management for substance-dependent women receiving temporary assistance for needy families. *Am J Public Health* 2006;96:2016–2023.

National Institutes of Health. Presentation at the Consensus Conference on the Treatment of Opiate Addiction. Bethesda, MD; NIH, 1997.

O'Brien CP. A range of research-based pharmacotherapies for addiction. *Science* 1997;278:66–70.

Smith JE, Meyers RJ. Motivating substance abusers by treating their loved ones: The CRAFT Program. New York: Guilford Press, 2008.

CHAPTER 26

John W. Finney, PhD
Rudolf H. Moos, PhD
Paula L. Wilbourne, PhD

Effects of Treatment Setting, Duration and Amount on Patient Outcomes

Treatment Settings
Duration and Amount of Treatment
Implications for Policymakers and Service Providers

This chapter examines research evidence on the effects of substance use disorder (SUD) treatment settings, duration, and amount, drawing heavily on research syntheses. Most of the research focuses on treatment for alcohol use disorders, but research on treatment of other drug use disorders also is considered. We argue that research findings (e.g., those on the relative effects of inpatient/residential versus outpatient treatment) have been extrapolated to populations beyond those involved in the studies (e.g., patients with serious comorbid psychiatric conditions) and that key issues remain unaddressed. Those issues include determining the specific types of persons who benefit more from initial treatment in inpatient/residential than in outpatient settings, whether certain types of individuals benefit from longer or more intensive treatment, and whether treatment should be spread out over longer periods for some patients.

TREATMENT SETTINGS

Although inpatient treatment is more prevalent in some other countries (e.g., in Germany), only about 10% of SUD patients in the United States receive residential treatment and only 1% receive inpatient treatment where presumably medical or psychiatric care also is readily available (1). Considerable research has focused on whether inpatient/residential or outpatient treatment is more effective overall, but the more pressing issue is whether certain types of patients benefit more from an initial phase of inpatient/residential treatment before continuing outpatient care than from outpatient treatment alone.

Rationales for Inpatient/Residential and Outpatient Treatment At least five rationales have been put forward for the superiority of an initial phase of treatment in inpatient/residential SUD treatment settings (2). One is that such settings provide a respite for patients, removing them from unstructured and unsupportive environments that perpetuate their addiction, thereby allowing their efforts toward abstinence to be consolidated (see Chapter 28). Second, inpatient/residential settings may allow patients to receive more treatment because treatment is more intensive and patients may be less likely to drop out of treatment (3). A third rationale is that inpatient/residential settings provide medical/psychiatric care (inpatient settings) and other comprehensive services to patients who otherwise would not have access to such care or support. Such services are seen as crucial to achieving optimal substance use outcomes (4). Fourth, inpatient/residential treatment prepares a patient better to engage in continuing outpatient treatment (e.g., by stressing the need for continuing care) (5). Finally, some proponents argue that inpatient/residential treatment suggests to patients that their problems are more severe and that resolving them is more paramount than would be the case if treatment were offered in an outpatient setting (6).

Arguments in favor of outpatient treatment also have focused on the patient's usual life situation, but stress the advantages of leaving the patient in, rather than removing him or her from that context (7,8). Proponents have suggested that outpatient treatment provides an opportunity for more accurate assessments of the antecedents of substance use and for testing coping skills in real-life situations while the patient remains in a supportive therapeutic relationship. Accordingly, greater generalization of learning should take place than would be the case in the atypical environment of an inpatient/residential treatment program (9). In addition, outpatient treatment might mobilize help in the patient's natural environment (e.g., from a family physician or self-help groups), to a greater extent than does inpatient or residential treatment. Finally, proponents have argued that outpatient treatment results in a more successful transition to continuing care when, for example, a patient begins to attend self-help group meetings near his or her home while still in treatment.

Relevant Research Several early research reviews examined the relative effectiveness of alcohol treatment in inpatient and outpatient settings and concluded inpatient/residential treatment was no more effective than outpatient treatment (9–11). A later review by Finney et al. (2) found that 7 of 14 relevant studies had significant setting effects on one or more drinking-related outcome variables at one or more follow-up points. In five studies, the outcome difference favored inpatient/residential (sometimes followed by continuing outpatient treatment) over outpatient treatment; in the other two, the outcome difference favored day hospital over inpatient treatment. Patients in the "superior" setting usually received more treatment.

This "box-score" approach to synthesizing the research literature has serious limitations. Nonsignificant differences between treatment groups may simply reflect lack of statistical power; significant findings may emerge by chance when multiple tests for treatment effects are conducted and not adjusted for "experiment wise" error. Indeed, Finney et al. (2) found that the seven studies yielding significant setting effects had greater statistical power and conducted more treatment contrasts, on average, than the studies with no difference in outcome. The shortcomings of box-score reviews prompted the development of meta-analytic techniques (12) that use an "effect size" to gauge treatment efficacy. A common effect size in this context is the difference in the average posttreatment functioning of two groups divided by the pooled standard deviation of outcome scores for the two groups. A between-group, standardized effect size allows one to determine by how many standard deviation units, or by what proportion of a standard deviation unit, the functioning of one group is superior to that of another. When Finney and Moos (13) calculated average, cross-study effect sizes on drinking-related outcome variables, only the effect size of 0.22 at 3-month follow-ups was significant and favored inpatient/residential over outpatient treatment (the effect sizes at 6- and 12- to 14-month follow-ups were not significant).

Although some recent studies of mixed SUD treatment have found small or scattered effects on a few of many outcome variables that favored inpatient or residential treatment (5,14–20), others focusing on treatment for alcohol use disorders (21–23) and cocaine abuse (24) have not. Likewise, reviews of the relevant research on outpatient methadone maintenance by Anglin and Hser (25) and outpatient drug-free treatment by Crits-Christoph and Siqueland (26) reported few differences in outcomes in comparison with residential therapeutic community programs.

Extracting appropriate policy implications from this research literature requires consideration of the representativeness and types of patients who have been included in the studies. In some studies, relatively low percentages of patients in treatment have actually participated in the research. For example, 6 of the 14 studies reviewed by Finney et al. (2) noted the percentage of patients in treatment that participated in the research; in 4 of those studies, the percentage was 25% or lower. Most studies, especially randomized trials, have examined a restricted set of patients. Ethical concerns have prevented random assignment to outpatient treatment of highly impaired patients who on clinical grounds were candidates for inpatient/residential treatment. Accordingly, studies often have excluded patients with major medical or psychiatric disorders, or insufficient resources, such as an inability to commute to treatment, homelessness, or a lack of a telephone. Thus the findings may not generalize well to more impaired individuals or those with fewer social resources for whom inpatient/residential treatment might provide the most benefit. It perhaps is no coincidence that many of the investigations indicating superiority of inpatient/residential treatment have come from naturalistic studies of more impaired patients receiving treatment in publicly funded programs (5,19).

Who Benefits from Inpatient/Residential Treatment? Even though some degree of patient homogeneity resulting from ethical concerns in randomized trials or from admission criteria for public and private programs operates against its emergence, considerable evidence suggests that more impaired patients benefit more from an initial episode of inpatient or residential treatment than from outpatient treatment alone. In other words, patient impairment has been found to interact with treatment setting in affecting patient outcomes.

A diagnosis of a serious psychiatric disorder often has been an exclusion criterion in studies of inpatient versus outpatient alcohol treatment (2), precluding its broad examination as a matching variable. Nevertheless, Ritson (27) found that patients in outpatient treatment who had personality disorders tended to have poor outcomes, though no relationship was found between personality disorders and outcome among inpatients. Likewise, research by Moos et al. (28) found that, for patients with psychiatric disorders, an episode of inpatient treatment before transfer to a community residential facility was associated with better outcomes than direct placement in a community residential facility. With respect to social resources, Kissin et al. (29) reported that more socially stable alcoholic patients experienced better outcomes in outpatient treatment, whereas socially unstable patients had better outcomes after inpatient treatment. Among both alcohol and drug use disorder patients with middle-level psychiatric severity (defined by scores from one standard deviation above to one standard deviation below the mean Addiction Severity Index psychiatric severity rating), McLellan et al. (30) observed that those who had more serious family, legal, or employment problems experienced poorer outcomes after receiving outpatient versus inpatient treatment.

At least six studies (5,22,31–34) have found that patients with greater alcohol or drug use severity at treatment intake who receive an initial episode of inpatient or residential treatment experience better outcomes than those receiving only outpatient treatment (cf 35). On the other hand, Rychtarik et al.'s (22) study yielded no support for the hypothesis that patients who come from environments that promote heavy drinking benefit more from a residential stay than they do from outpatient treatment.

The evidence summarized here provides general support for matching patients to different treatment settings. However, the strength of the interactions, which statistically indicate how strongly different treatment settings are linked to different outcomes for different types of patients, is usually difficult to determine from research reports. In one study providing this information (34), the two interaction effects found, although significant, were weak, each accounting for less than 1% of the outcome variance after main effects had been taken into account. The highly impaired sample from Veterans Administration facilities may have been constrained the strength of these interactions, because stronger interactions are more likely to emerge with greater variability among the patients studied. Likewise, we know little about the precise levels of severity at which more impaired patients do better in inpatient/residential versus outpatient treatment. In the study by Tiet et al. (34), only patients who had very extreme scores on Addiction Severity Index alcohol and drug composites did better when they had an initial episode of inpatient/residential treatment versus only outpatient treatment.

Overall, the general concept of the American Society of Addiction Medicine's (ASAM) Patient Placement Criteria (36) is supported by the research reviewed here (see also Chapter 27, "The ASAM Placement Criteria and Matching Patients to Treatment"). The criteria attempt to match patients to five levels of care: (1) early intervention; (2) outpatient treatment; (3) intensive outpatient/partial hospitalization treatment; (4) residential/inpatient treatment; and (5) medically managed intensive inpatient treatment. Placement decisions are based on a patient's standing on six dimensions: (1) acute intoxication or withdrawal potential; (2) biomedical conditions and complications; (3) emotional/behavioral conditions or complications; (4) treatment acceptance/resistance; (5) relapse/continued use potential; and (6) recovery/living environment. However, research is needed to validate the specific placement assessments and algorithms used in the ASAM system (37,38). We do not have precise, empirically supported guidelines for allocating patients to different levels of care. Magura et al. (39) voiced the concern that "[w]ithout well-validated placement criteria that justify intensive treatments on the basis of their greater effectiveness, the pressures of managed care to reduce costs will continue to threaten addiction treatment quality" (39).

A more fundamental issue not addressed in existing studies is the relative *attractiveness* of treatment in the two types of settings; that is, their ability to induce certain types of individuals to seek and enter treatment. In randomized trials, patients already have opted for treatment and are usually preselected for their willingness to accept either inpatient/residential or outpatient treatment. Under normal conditions of treatment delivery, inpatient/residential programs may be more effective than outpatient programs in attracting individuals who have significant barriers to receiving treatment in other settings (e.g., homeless individuals and persons who lack transportation or who live some distance from a treatment facility) (40). Milby et al.'s (19) findings support the beneficial effects of providing homeless individuals a place to stay, especially abstinence-oriented housing, while receiving SUD treatment. More broadly, if inpatient/residential programs are not available, administrators may be able to point to "reduced treatment demand" as evidence to support cutbacks in SUD treatment services.

DURATION AND AMOUNT OF TREATMENT

Although the chronic, relapsing nature of many individuals' substance use disorders would suggest the need for treatment extended over a long period, the tendency in the United States has been toward shorter episodes of treatment, given reduced insurance coverage for SUD care (41). This section reviews evidence on the effectiveness longer versus shorter stays in inpatient/residential treatment, and the effects of participation in continuing outpatient care.

Because Chapter 18 reviews the evidence on screening and brief interventions, we only note here the need for more research to determine who is as likely to benefit from a brief intervention as from more extensive care. However, at present, low to moderate alcohol severity patients with positive life contexts and without severe skills deficits appear to be the best candidates for brief interventions. In this vein, Edwards et al. (42) noted that the patients in their classic study of brief advice versus treatment were socially stable and suggested that "patients with a lesser degree of social support might . . . be less able to respond to the advice regimen—extrapolation to a population of homeless men would be risky" (42). Also, Ashton (43) pointed to evidence suggesting that brief motivational interventions are best directed toward persons who are ambivalent about changing the substance use behavior. Persons already committed to reducing or eliminating their substance use may be "set back" by consideration of positive aspects of substance use that is a component of some brief interventions using motivational interviewing principles.

Length of Stay in Inpatient/Residential Treatment

Mattick and Jarvis (10) and Miller and Hester (11) reviewed several randomized trials comparing different lengths of inpatient or residential treatment for alcohol abuse. The consistent finding was no difference in outcome. Several more recent randomized trials also have found no, or only isolated (i.e., on a few outcomes) beneficial effects for longer inpatient/residential alcohol or substance abuse treatment (15,16,44–48). These findings suggest it is not useful to assign unselected clients to longer stays in residential or inpatient treatment. In contrast, many naturalistic studies of substance abuse treatment have found longer stays in treatment to be associated with better outcomes, even a reduction in premature mortality (49). For example, longer episodes of inpatient and residential care (50–52), extended care (28), community residential care (53–56), and care in therapeutic communities (57) have been associated with better substance use outcomes and psychosocial functioning, as well as lower readmission rates for subsequent inpatient care, including among SUD patients with cooccurring psychiatric disorders (58).

It may be that beneficial effects of longer stays in inpatient/residential treatment apply only to more impaired patients with fewer social resources. For example, Welte et al. (50) found no relationship between length of stay and outcome of alcoholism treatment for higher social stability patients; in contrast, for patients with lower social stability, those with longer stays had better outcomes (60,61). That individuals in naturalistic studies have better outcomes with longer treatment than clients who stay in treatment for shorter periods suggests that many clients may be able to determine whether or not they will benefit from longer treatment. Thus having longer courses of treatment available can be important for clients who seek them.

Continuing Outpatient Care Most SUD treatment providers recommend additional outpatient treatment (i.e., continuing care or aftercare) to maintain or enhance the therapeutic gains achieved during inpatient/residential or intensive or initial outpatient (e.g., day hospital) treatment. Considerable correlational evidence (26,62–66) is consistent with this recommendation. Do controlled trials also provide empirical support for continuing care? McKay (67) reviewed 11 controlled studies that compared some form of continuing care to minimal or no treatment; 7 (64%) had findings supporting the efficacy of continuing care. Importantly, when McKay compared the studies with positive and negative results, he found that an active approach to engaging patients in continuing care (e.g., "taking the intervention to the patient") and a longer duration of prescribed continuing care characterized the positive studies.

Research by Schaefer et al. (68) highlights some active methods for engaging SUD patients in continuing care. They focused on the continuity of care practices of staff at the point of discharge from residential or intensive outpatient treatment. Although staff practices were not linked to continuing care among residential patients, such practices as coordinating care among providers, connecting patients to community resources, maintaining contact with patients over time, and ensuring continuity in providers were associated with a longer period of continuing care for individuals receiving initial intensive outpatient treatment. Subsequent analyses (60) indicated that engagement in continuing care mediated a relationship between continuity of care practices and abstinence for the individuals receiving initial intensive outpatient treatment.

Lash and colleagues (70) used a "contracting, prompting, and reinforcement" intervention to foster ongoing engagement in continuing care. Patients signed a behavioral contract that expressed their commitment to attend an aftercare group weekly, Alcoholics Anonymous/Narcotics Anonymous weekly, and an individual therapy session monthly for at least 8 weeks (they also were informed they would be recontacted after 8 weeks to commit to remaining in continuing care for 1 year). Prompts consisted of a letter from the therapist before the first continuing care session, mailed appointment cards for all continuing care sessions and Alcoholics Anonymous/Narcotics Anonymous meetings, automated telephone reminders of appointments, and a letter and telephone call from the therapist after missed appointments. Social reinforcement included a letter from the therapist congratulating the patient on attending the first session, an encouraging letter accompanying the appointment card following the third group session, a "90 Days of Treatment" certificate for attending at least six group sessions and two individual sessions, and a medallion for attending eight group and three individual sessions in the first 3 months. Participants were reinforced for maintaining long-term participation in continuing care with a 1-year certificate and a medallion. A randomized trial demonstrated greater effectiveness for "contracting, prompting, and reinforcement" than standard treatment on engaging patients in continuing care and patient abstinence.

With respect to effective durations of continuing care, all three studies reviewed by McKay (67) that provided continuing care for a minimum of 12 months yielded significant results supporting continuing care. Of course, the two features distinguishing effective forms of continuing care are connected: active means of engaging patients help maintain their engagement in continuing care over longer periods.

Naturalistic studies have shown a "dose-response" relationship between the amount of outpatient mental health care and psychiatric patients' outcomes (71–73). Similarly, naturalistic studies have provided evidence for the effectiveness of a longer duration of care for patients with substance use disorders. In a nationwide sample of SUD patients in an index episode of care, patients who received specialty outpatient mental health care experienced better risk-adjusted substance use and psychiatric symptom outcomes than did patients who did not receive such care (74). Patients who had longer index episodes of mental health care improved more than did those who had shorter episodes. There was some evidence that the duration of care contributed more to better outcomes among patients with only substance use disorders, whereas the intensity of care was more important for patients with both substance use and psychiatric disorders.

A long-term study by Moos and Moos (75) focused on the duration of participation in professional treatment for previously untreated individuals with alcohol use disorders. Compared with individuals who remained untreated, individuals who obtained a longer duration of treatment in the first year after seeking help were more likely to be abstinent and had fewer drinking problems at 8-year and 16-year follow-ups. These finding suggest that more emphasis should be placed on ensuring that patients enter specialty care and on keeping them in treatment.

Telephone care is a cost-effective means to extend care over time (76). McKay et al. (77,78) found that 12 weeks of telephone monitoring and counseling, along with weekly group counseling in the first 4 weeks, was as effective at a 1-year follow-up for alcohol- and cocaine-dependent patients on most outcomes compared with 12 weeks of relapse prevention or standard 12-step group counseling. For individuals with only alcohol dependence, the telephone condition had better 1-year alcohol use outcomes than the 12-step condition. At 24 months, individuals in the telephone group were more likely to be abstinent and had similar percentages of days abstinent and number of consequences of substance use to those in the other two conditions. However, individuals who had not made much progress during their initial intensive outpatient treatment did better with the twice weekly face-to-face group therapy than with telephone care (79).

Taken together, these studies and reviews of treatment intensity, length of stay, and outpatient care suggest that an effective strategy may be to provide lower intensity addiction treatment over a longer duration—that is, treatment spread out at a lower rate over a longer period (64,76). The effectiveness of spreading substance abuse treatment over a longer period is suggested by the positive findings for outpatient care after inpatient treatment (e.g., 64) and for interventions that incorporate somewhat extended (e.g., 12 weeks), but relatively few (e.g., 4) contacts with patients (e.g., 80). More extended treatment may improve patient outcomes because it provides patients with ongoing support and the potential to discuss and resolve problems before the occurrence of a full-blown relapse. In this vein, brief interventions may be most effective for relatively healthy patients who have intact community support systems. Patients who have severe substance dependence, concomitant psychiatric disorders, or insufficient social resources appear to be appropriate candidates for longer treatment and intensive monitoring (26,81) to address their multiple co-occurring problems and the chronic, relapsing nature of their substance use disorders.

IMPLICATIONS FOR POLICYMAKERS AND SERVICE PROVIDERS

Studies on substance use disorder treatment settings, amount, and duration, along with reviews of this research, have had a positive impact on health care policy: They appropriately called into question the blanket application of expensive forms of treatment. For example, in the United States, in the early 1980s, insurance coverage for alcohol treatment was such that if a socially stable individual wanted covered treatment, inpatient treatment was the only option. The advent of managed care in the United States in the 1990s brought an increasing emphasis on outpatient treatment so that in 2005, 89% of the individuals in treatment for alcohol and other drug use disorders were seen in less expensive outpatient settings (1). In recent years, findings for selected samples in some studies have been used to justify denial of inpatient/residential treatment and more intensive treatment to persons who may need such treatment. Thus the pendulum may have swung too far in the opposite direction.

An important agenda over the next decade will be to validate specific placement criteria for allocating individuals to different settings of care and to determine appropriate durations and intensities of care for different types of individuals. In the meantime, we believe that the best approaches for treatment providers today are those recommended in previous reviews and largely embodied in the ASAM Patient Placement Criteria (36; see Chapter 27): (1) provide outpatient treatment for those individuals who have sufficient social resources and no serious medical/psychiatric impairment; (2) use less costly intensive outpatient treatment options for patients who have failed with brief interventions or for whom a more intensive intervention seems warranted, but who do not need the structured environment of a residential setting; (3) retain residential options for those with few social resources or a living environment that is a serious impediment to recovery; (4) reserve inpatient treatment options for individuals with serious medical/psychiatric conditions; (5) have longer term treatment options available for clients who desire them; and (6) use active methods of engagement at the start of treatment (e.g., motivational interventions) and when clients transition to continuing care (e.g., "contracting, prompting, and reinforcement").

With respect to treatment duration and amount, brief interventions in medical and settings other than specialty SUD treatment can be effective, especially for individuals with moderate alcohol misuse. For individuals with more severe alcohol or drug use disorders, existing research indicates that uncomplicated patients should be provided less intensive treatment; patients with substance use disorders complicated by co-occurring psychiatric disorders, medical problems, or social barriers to treatment should receive more intensive treatment. For many patients with alcohol or drug dependence, outpatient treatment, in some cases following an initial episode of residential care, should be provided over an extended period. Care also can be extended by linking (not just referring) patients with self- or mutual-help groups, such as Alcoholics Anonymous (82) or, for those with cooccurring psychiatric conditions, to such groups as Double Trouble in Recovery (83) or Dual Recovery Anonymous.

As suggested by Humphreys and Tucker (84), "stepped care" (85,86) can be an "organizing principle" for efficiently providing treatment for SUD. Individuals for whom a less intensive (and less costly) initial approach is not successful can be "stepped up" to a more intensive form of treatment. In this regard, brief motivational interventions have been shown to enhance the effectiveness of more intensive treatments that follow them (87). Individuals who function well over for a period of time can be "stepped down" to a less intensive form of care (e.g., continuing outpatient care after a period of intensive outpatient treatment). Later, care intensity can be reduced even further, to consist only of monitoring the individual's functioning. As McKay (88) notes, "newer models of continuing care in the addictions are designed to improve the long-term management of substance use disorders by engaging patients into flexible, or 'adaptive,' treatment algorithms that change in focus and intensity as symptoms wax and wane over time" (88).

Such a model is embodied in the Recovery Management Checkup (RMC) developed by Dennis et al. (89). The RMC tracks individuals quarterly over time; assesses for early indications of relapse or problems; uses motivational techniques to maintain or reinitiate desired behavioral changes; stresses the need for early reengagement in treatment, as indicated; and assists with treatment reengagement. Compared with patients randomized to an attention condition (quarterly follow-up assessments over 2 years; referral to treatment only in emergency situations), RMC patients were more likely to reenter treatment, to do so sooner, and to receive more days of treatment, but to be less likely to need further treatment at the end of the 2 years (as determined by current substance use and negative consequences). Although these results are promising, two-thirds of the patients in need of treatment in the RMC condition did not obtain it. Of those reentering treatment, only one in four remained engaged in treatment for 90 days. The investigators conclude there is room for improvement in the RMC protocol, such as having a staff member who would focus on retaining people in treatment once they reentered.

For communities and health care organizations, an ideal management system would encompass the full continuum of care with respect to treatment settings, duration, and amount. In addition, coordinated comprehensive services, such as social, housing, legal and medical services, would be available (4; also see Chapter 28, "Linking Addiction Treatment with Other Medical and Psychiatric Treatment Systems"). To maximize the impact of the system's resources, not only would there be easy access to them, but they would be coordinated, for example by case managers (90), so that rather than merely having services available and referring individuals to them, the system would track and monitor individuals with substance misuse and disorders, and actively reach out to them in periods of poor functioning to engage and reengage them in treatment.

ACKNOWLEDGMENTS: *Preparation of this revised chapter was supported by the U.S. Department of Veterans Affairs, Veterans Health Administration, Health Services Research and Development Service, and NIAAA Grant AA15685. The views expressed are those of the authors and do not necessarily reflect the views of the Department of Veterans Affairs.*

REFERENCES

1. Substance Abuse and Mental Health Services Administration, Office of Applied Studies *National Survey of Substance Abuse Treatment (NSSAT): 2005. Data on Substance Abuse Treatment Facilities* (Vol. DHHS Publication No. SMA 06-4206). Rockville, MD, 2006.
2. Finney JW, Hahn AC, Moos RH. The effectiveness of inpatient and outpatient treatment for alcohol abuse: the need to focus on mediators and moderators of setting effects. *Addiction* 1996;91:1773–1796.
3. Alterman AI, O'Brien CP, McLellan AT, et al. Comparative effectiveness and costs of inpatient and day hospital cocaine rehabilitation treatment. *J Nerv Ment Dis* 1994;182:157–163.
4. Friedmann PD, Hendrickson JC, Gerstein DR, et al. The effect of matching comprehensive services to patients' needs on drug use improvement in addiction treatment. *Addiction* 2004;99:962–972.
5. McKay JR, Donovan DM, McLellan AT, et al. Evaluation of full vs. partial continuum of care in the treatment of publicly funded substance abusers in Washington State. *Am J Drug Alcohol Abuse* 2002;28:307–338.
6. Panepinto W, Galanter M, Bender SH, et al. Alcoholics' transition from ward to clinic: group orientation improves retention. *J Stud Alcohol* 1980;41:940–945.
7. McLachlan JFC, Stein RL. Evaluation of a day clinic for alcoholics. *J Stud Alcohol* 1982;43:261–272.
8. McCrady B, Longabaugh R, Fink E, et al. Cost effectiveness of alcoholism treatment in partial hospital versus inpatient settings after brief inpatient treatment: 12-month outcomes. *J Consult Clin Psychol* 1986;54:708–713.
9. Annis HM Is inpatient rehabilitation cost effective? Con position. *Adv Alcohol Substance Abuse* 1986;5:175–190.
10. Mattick RP, Jarvis T. In-patient setting and long duration for the treatment of alcohol dependence? Out-patient care is as good. *Drug Alcohol Rev* 1994;13:127–135.
11. Miller MR, Hester RK Inpatient alcoholism treatment: who benefits? *Am Psychol* 1986;41:794–805.
12. Cooper H, Hedges LV, eds. *The handbook of research synthesis.* New York: Russell Sage Foundation, 1994.
13. Finney JW, Moos RH Effectiveness of inpatient and outpatient treatment for alcohol abuse: Effect sizes, research design issues, and explanatory mechanisms [response to commentaries]. *Addiction* 1996;91:1813–1820.
14. Budde D, Rounsaville F, Bryant K. Inpatient and outpatient cocaine abusers: clinical comparisons at intake and one-year follow-up. *J Subst Abuse Treatment* 1992;9:337–343.
15. Guydish J, Werdegard D, Sorensen JL, et al. Drug abuse day treatment: a randomized clinical trial comparing day and residential treatment programs. *J Consult Clin Psychol* 1998;66:280–289.
16. Guydish J, Sorensen JL, Chan M, et al. A randomized trial comparing day and residential drug abuse treatment: 18-month outcomes. *J Consult Clin Psychol* 1999;67:428–434.
17. Greenwood GL, Woods WJ, Guydish J, et al. Relapse outcomes in a randomized trial of residential and day drug abuse treatment. *J Substance Abuse Treatment* 2001;20:15–23.
18. McNeese-Smith D, Nyamathi A, Longshore D, et al. Processes and outcomes of substance abuse treatment between two programs for clients insured under managed care. *Am J Drug Alcohol Abuse* 2007;33:439–446.
19. Milby JB, Schumacher JE, Wallace D, et al. To house or not to house: the effects of providing housing to homeless substance abusers in treatment. *Am J Public Health* 2005;95:1259–1265.
20. Witbrodt J, Bond J, Kaskutas LA, et al. Day hospital and residential addiction treatment: randomized and nonrandomized managed care clients. *J Consult Clin Psychol* 2007;75:947–959.
21. Magura S, Fong C, Staines GL, et al. The combined effects of treatment intensity, self-help groups and patient attributes on drinking outcomes. *J Psychoactive Drugs* 2005;37:85–92.
22. Rychtarik RG, Connors GJ, Wirtz PW, et al. Treatment settings for persons with alcoholism: evidence for matching clients to inpatient versus outpatient care. *J Consult Clin Psychol* 2000;68:277–289.
23. Weithmann G, Hoffmann M. A randomised clinical trial of in-patient versus combined day hospital treatment of alcoholism: primary and secondary outcome measures. *Eur Addiction Res* 2005;11:197–203.
24. McKay JR, Alterman AI., McLellan AT, et al. Random versus nonrandom assignment in the evaluation of treatment for cocaine abusers. *J Consult Clin Psychol* 1998;66:697–701.
25. Anglin MD, Hser Y-I. Treatment of drug abuse. In: Tonry M, Wilson JQ, eds. *Drugs and crime (vol. 13).* Chicago, IL: University of Chicago Press, 1990.
26. Crits-Christoph P, Siqueland L. Psychosocial treatment for drug abuse: selected review and recommendations for national health care. *Arch Gen Psychiatry* 1996;53:749–756.
27. Ritson B. The prognosis of alcohol addicts treated by a specialised unit. *Br J Psychiatry* 1968;114:1019–1029.
28. Moos RH, King M, Patterson M. Outcomes of residential treatment of substance abuse in hospital- versus community-based programs. *Psychiatric Serv* 1996;47:68–74.

29. Kissin B, Platz A, Su WH. Social and psychological factors in the treatment of chronic alcoholism. *J Psychiatric Res* 1970;8:13–27.
30. McLellan AT, Luborsky L, Woody GE, et al. Predicting response to alcohol and drug abuse treatments: role of psychiatric severity. *Arch Gen Psychiatry* 1983;40:620–625.
31. Harrison PA, Asche SE. Comparison of substance abuse treatment outcomes for inpatients and outpatients. *J Substance Abuse Treatment* 1999; 17:207–220.
32. Pettinati HM, Meyers K, Evans BD, et al. Inpatient alcohol treatment in a private healthcare setting: which patients benefit and at what cost? *Am J Addictions* 1999;8:220–233.
33. Simpson DD, Joe GW, Fletcher BW, et al. A national evaluation of treatment outcomes for cocaine dependence. *Arch Gen Psychiatry* 1999; 56:507–514.
34. Tiet QQ, Ilgen MA., Byrnes HL, et al. Treatment setting and baseline substance use severity interact to predict patients' outcomes. *Addiction* 2007;102:432–440.
35. Burdon WM, Dang J, Prendergast ML, et al. Differential effectiveness of residential versus outpatient aftercare for parolees from prison-based therapeutic community treatment programs. *Substance Abuse Treatment Prevent Policy* 2007;2:16.
36. Mee-Lee D, Shulman G, Fishman M, et al. *Patient placement criteria for the treatment of substance-related disorders, 2nd edition-revised.* Chevy Chase, MD: American Society of Addiction Medicine, 2001.
37. Gastfriend DR, Lu S-H, Sharon E. Placement matching: Challenges and technical progress. *Substance Use Misuse* 2000;35:2191–2213.
38. McKay JR, Cacciola JS, McLellan AT, et al. An initial evaluation of the psychosocial dimensions of the American Society of Addiction Medicine criteria for inpatient versus intensive outpatient substance abuse rehabilitation. *J Studies Alcohol* 1997;58:239–252.
39. Magura S, Staines G, Kosanke N, et al. Predictive validity of the ASAM patient placement criteria for naturalistically matched vs. mismatched alcohol dependent patients. *Am J Addictions* 2003;12:386–397.
40. Beardsley K, Wish ED, Fitzelle DB, et al. Distance traveled to outpatient drug treatment and client retention. *J Substance Abuse Treatment* 2003;25:279–285.
41. McKay JR. Is there a case for extended interventions for alcohol and drug use disorders? *Addiction* 2005;100:1594–1610.
42. Edwards G, Orford J, Egert S, et al. Alcoholism: a controlled trial of "treatment" and "advice." *J Studies Alcohol* 1977;38:1004–1031.
43. Ashton M. The motivational hallo. *Drug Alcohol Findings* 2005;13:23–30.
44. Kamara SG, Van der Hyde VA. Outcomes of regular vs. extended alcohol/drug outpatient treatment. I. Relapse, aftercare, and treatment re-entry. *Med Law* 1997;16:607–620.
45. Kamara SG, Van der Hyde VA. Employment outcomes of regular versus extended outpatient alcohol and drug treatment. *Med Law* 1998;17: 625–632.
46. Kamara SG, Van der Hyde VA. Outcomes of regular versus extended outpatient alcohol/drug treatment. Part II. Medical, psychiatric, legal and social problems. *Med Law* 1998;17:131–142.
47. Nemes S, Wish E, Messina N. Comparing the impact of standard and abbreviated treatment in a therapeutic community: findings from the District of Columbia Treatment Initiative Experiment. *J Substance Abuse Treatment* 1999;17:339–347.
48. Trent LK. Evaluation of a four- versus six-week length of stay in the Navy's alcohol treatment program. *J Studies Alcohol* 1998;59:270–279.
49. Bunn JY, Booth BM, Cook CA, et al. The relationship between mortality and intensity of inpatient alcoholism treatment. *Am J Public Health* 1994;84:211–214.
50. Darke S, Ross J, Teesson M, et al. Factors associated with 12 months continuous heroin abstinence: findings from the Australian Treatment Outcome Study (ATOS). *J Substance Abuse Treatment* 2005;28:255–263.
51. Peterson K, Swindle R, Phibbs C, et al. Determinants of readmission following inpatient substance abuse treatment: a national study of VA programs. *Med Care* 1994;32:535–550.
52. Timko C, Finney JW, Moos RH. Short-term treatment careers and outcomes of previously untreated alcoholics. *J Substance Abuse* 1995;7:43–59.
53. Jason LA, Davis MI, Ferrari JR. The need for substance abuse aftercare: longitudinal analysis of Oxford House. *Addict Behav* 2007;32: 803–818.
54. Moos RH, Pettit E, Gruber V. Longer episodes of community residential care reduce substance abuse patients' readmission rates. *J Studies Alcohol* 1995;56:433–443.
55. Rosenheck R, Frisman L, Gallup P. Effectiveness and cost of specific treatment elements in a program for homeless mentally ill veterans. *Psychiatric Serv* 1995;46:1131–1139.
56. Simpson DD. Treatment for drug abuse: follow-up outcomes and length of time spent. *Arch Gen Psychiatry* 1981;38:875–880.
57. Condelli WS, Hubbard RL. Relationship between time spent in treatment and client outcomes from therapeutic communities. *J Substance Abuse Treatment* 1994;11:25–33.
58. Brunette MF, Drake RE., Woods M, et al. A comparison of long-term and short-term residential treatment for dual diagnosis patients. *Psychiatric Serv* 2001;52:526–528.
59. Welte J, Hynes G, Sokolow L, et al. Effect of length of stay in inpatient alcoholism treatment on outcome. *J Studies Alcohol* 1981;42: 483–491.
60. Gottheil E, McLellan AT, Druley KA. Length of stay, patient severity and treatment outcome: sample data from the field of alcoholism. *J Studies Alcoholism* 1992;53:69–75.
61. Messina NP, Wish ED, Nemes S. Therapeutic community treatment for substance abusers with antisocial personality disorder. *J Substance Abuse Treatment* 1999;17:121–128.
62. Donovan DM. Continuing care: promoting the maintenance of change. In: Miller WR, Heather N, eds. *Treating addictive behaviors*, 2nd ed. New York: Plenum, 1998:317–336.
63. Ito J, Donovan DM. Predicting drinking outcome: demography, chronicity, coping, and aftercare. *Addictive Behav* 1990;15:553–559.
64. Moos RH, Finney JW, Ouimette PC, et al. A comparative evaluation of substance abuse treatment: I. Treatment orientation, amount of care, and 1-year outcomes. *Alcohol Clin Exp Res* 1999;23:529–536.
65. Onken LS, Blaine JD, Boren JJ. *Beyond the therapeutic alliance: keeping the drug-dependent individual in treatment (NIDA research monograph 165)* (NIH Publication No. 97-4142). Rockville, MD: National Institute on Drug Abuse, 1997.
66. Greenberg GA, Rosenheck RA, Seibyl CL. Continuity of care and clinical effectiveness: outcomes following residential treatment for severe substance abuse. *Med Care* 2002;40:246–259.
67. McKay JR. Continuing care research: what we've learned and where we're going. *J Subst Abuse Treat* in press.
68. Schaefer JA, Ingudomnukul E, Harris AHS, et al. Continuity of care practices and substance use disorder patients' engagement in continuing care. *Med Care* 2005;43:1234–1241.
69. Schaefer JA, Harris AHS, Cronkite RC, et al. Continuity of care practices, engagement in continuing care, and patients' abstinence outcomes following intensive outpatient substance use disorder treatment. *J Studies Alcohol Drugs* 2008;69:747–756.
70. Lash SJ, Stephens RS, Burden JL, et al. Contracting, prompting, and reinforcing substance use disorder continuing care: a randomized clinical trial. *Psychol Addictive Behav* 2007;21:387–397.
71. Howard KI, Kopta SM, Krause MJ, et al. The dose-effect relationship in psychotherapy. *Am Psychologist* 1986;41:159–164.
72. Steenbarger BN. Duration and outcome in psychotherapy: an integrative review. *Prof Psychol Res Pract* 1994;25:111–119.
73. Svartberg M, Stiles TC. Comparative effects of short-term psychodynamic psychotherapy: a meta-analysis. *J Consult Clin Psychol* 1991;59: 704–714.
74. Moos R, Finney JW, Federman B, et al. Specialty mental health care improves patients' outcomes: findings from a nationwide program to monitor the quality of care for patients with substance use disorders. *J Studies Alcohol* 2000;61:704–713.
75. Moos R, Moos B. Participation in treatment and Alcoholics Anonymous: a 16-year follow-up of initially untreated individuals. *J Clin Psychol* 2006;62:735–750.

76. Stout RL, Rubin A, Zwick W, et al. Optimizing the cost-effectiveness of alcohol treatment: a rationale for extended case monitoring. *Addictive Behav* 1999;24:17–35.
77. McKay JR, Lynch KG, Shepard DS, et al. The effectiveness of telephone-based continuing care in the clinical management of alcohol and cocaine use disorders: 12-month outcomes. *J Consult Clin Psychol* 2004;72:967–979.
78. McKay JR, Lynch KG, Shepard DS, et al. The effectiveness of telephone-based continuing care for alcohol and cocaine dependence: 24-month outcomes. *Arch Gen Psychiatry* 2005;62:199–207.
79. McKay JR, Lynch KG, Shepard DS, et al. Do patient characteristics and initial progress in treatment moderate the effectiveness of telephone-based continuing care for substance use disorders? *Addiction* 2005;100:216–226.
80. Project Match Research Group. Matching alcoholism treatments to client heterogeneity: Project MATCH posttreatment drinking outcomes. *J Studies Alcohol* 1997;58:7–29.
81. Higgins ST, Budney AJ, Bickel WK, et al. Achieving cocaine abstinence with a behavioral approach. *Am J Psychiatry* 1993;150:763–769.
82. Timko C, DeBenedetti A. A randomized controlled trial of intensive referral to 12-step self-help groups: one-year outcomes. *Drug Alcohol Depend* 2007;90:270–279.
83. Laudet AB, Cleland CM, Magura S, et al. Social support mediates the effects of dual-focus mutual aid groups on abstinence from substance use. *Am J Commun Psychol* 2004;34:175–185.
84. Humphreys K, Tucker J. Toward more responsive and effective intervention systems for alcohol-related problems. *Addiction* 2002;97:126–132.
85. Breslin F, Sobell MB, Sobell LC, et al. Problem drinkers: evaluation of stepped-care approach. *J Substance Abuse* 1998;10:217–232.
86. Sobell MB, Sobell LC. Stepped care as a heuristic approach to the treatment of alcohol problems. *J Consult Clin Psychol* 2000;68:573–579.
87. Hettema J, Steele, J, Miller WR. Motivational interviewing. *Annu Rev Clin Psychol* 2005;1:91–111.
88. McKay JR. Continuing care in the treatment of addictive disorders. *Curr Psychiatry Rep* 2006;8:355–362.
89. Dennis ML, Scott CK, Funk R. An experimental evaluation of recovery management checkups (RMC) for people with chronic substance use disorders. *Eval Progr Plan* 2003;26:339–352.
90. McLellan AT, Hagan TA, Levine M, et al. Does clinical case management improve outpatient addiction treatment? *Drug Alcohol Depend* 1999; 55:91–103.

CHAPTER 27

David Mee-Lee, MD
Gerald D. Shulman, MA, MAC, FACATA

The ASAM Placement Criteria and Matching Patients to Treatment

The Patient Placement Criteria for the Treatment of Substance-Related Disorders of the American Society of Addiction Medicine (ASAM PPC) have their roots in the mid 1980s, even before managed behavioral health care began to significantly impact addiction treatment. Multidisciplinary groups worked to develop one national set of consensus criteria to promote a common language and placement guidelines for the treatment of addiction disorders. The ASAM PPC was designed to help clinicians and payers use and fund levels of care in a rational and individualized, cost-effective, and therapeutic manner. This moved the addiction treatment field away from fixed length programs to an assessment-based, clinically driven, and outcomes-oriented continuum of care. The continuing development and refinement of the criteria represent a shift from:

- Unidimensional to multidimensional assessment.
- Program-driven to clinically driven treatment.
- Fixed length of service to variable length of service.
- A limited number of discrete levels of care to a continuum of care.

The ASAM PPC describes six assessment dimensions that are used to differentiate client needs for services across levels of care. The first edition, *Patient Placement Criteria for the Treatment of Psychoactive Substance Use Disorders*, was published by ASAM in 1991 (1). A second edition was developed in 1996, *ASAM PPC-2* (2) and in 2001, a revision of PPC-2 was published, *ASAM PPC-2R* (3).

There are separate criteria sets for adults and adolescents. About 30 states require the use of the ASAM criteria to varying degrees. The Department of Defense's addiction treatment programs mandate the PPC around the world; and there are about 50 million lives under managed care companies that indicate they use the ASAM PPC for decisions on authorizing addiction treatment.

SELECTING AN APPROPRIATE TREATMENT

Evolving Approaches to Treatment Matching The process of matching patients to treatment services has evolved through at least four approaches, each with a fundamentally different philosophy (4,5).

Complications-driven treatment gives only cursory attention to the diagnosis of a substance use disorder. In this approach, rather than actively treating the primary alcohol or other drug disorder that is causing the patient's symptoms, only secondary complications or sequelae are addressed. For example, the gastritis or bleeding esophageal varices are controlled, the depression is medicated, fractures are splinted or pinned, but care for the addiction disorder is superficial or nonexistent.

In contrast, *diagnosis, program-driven treatment* recognizes the primacy of the substance use disorder, but the diagnosis alone drives the treatment plan, rather than the assessed needs of the individual patient. For example, by policy, a diagnosis of substance abuse may assign the patient to outpatient treatment, whereas a substance dependence diagnosis sends the patient to inpatient treatment without regard to the patient's service needs. Patients are assigned to fixed lengths of stay in programs with static approaches, often in response to a mandated referral, policy guidelines, or available funding or benefit structures.

Individualized, assessment-driven treatment emphasizes multidimensional assessment. Problems are identified and prioritized in the context of the patient's severity of illness, interference with treatment or recovery and level of function. Treatment services are matched to the patient's needs over a continuum of care (6). Ongoing assessment of progress and treatment response influence future treatment recommendations and length of treatment. This cycle—assessment, treatment matching, level of care placement, and progress evaluation through assessment—represents an ideal approach to care toward which much of the addiction treatment field strives (7).

Outcomes-driven treatment, the most recent approach, adds the element of measurement of outcomes in real time, so that progress and treatment response is more explicit. The focus on "during-treatment" feedback of outcomes, patient engagement, and therapeutic alliance allows real-time modification of the treatment plan. Here, tracking the most salient outcomes and measures of alliance and patient engagement inform decisions about which problems are prioritized and what changes are made in strategies and level of care (Fig. 27.1).

Uses of Placement Criteria Placement criteria are irrelevant to the first two approaches to patient placement (complications-driven and program-driven treatment). In the latter two approaches, the ASAM criteria play an integral role by providing a multidimensional assessment structure, initially to generate a service plan that leads to appropriate placement and then a formal treatment plan that meets the patient's assessed needs and improves the prospects for a positive outcome once in treatment. The ASAM criteria also provide a nomenclature and guidelines to describe an expanded set of treatment options and promote the use of a wider continuum of services. The ASAM criteria thus are intended to enhance the efficient use of limited resources, increase patient retention in treatment, improve outcome, and prevent relapse. Thus the ASAM criteria advocate for individualized, assessment-driven treatment and the flexible use of a broad continuum of care.

Increasingly, however, treatment must be driven not only by the assessment, but more importantly by the outcome of treatment measured in real time. No single treatment is appropriate for all individuals at all times (8). Therefore matching treatment settings, interventions, and services to each individual's particular problems and needs is critical to his or her ultimate success in returning to productive functioning in the family, workplace, and society. Measurement during treatment that tracks real-time outcomes and the quality of the patient's engagement and therapeutic alliance allows for modification of the strategies and level of care depending on patient progress or lack of it (9,10).

The Concept of "Unbundling" At present, most addiction treatment services are "bundled," meaning that several different services are packaged together and paid for as a unit. Similarly, the first edition of the ASAM criteria "bundled" clinical services with environmental supports in fixed levels of care. Today, however, there is increasing recognition that clinical services can be and often are provided separately from environmental supports. Indeed, many managed care companies and public treatment systems are suggesting that treatment modality and intensity be "unbundled" from the treatment setting (11,12).

Unbundling is a practice that allows any type of clinical service (such as psychiatric consultation) to be delivered in any setting (such as a therapeutic community); or for example, partial hospitalization or intensive outpatient level of service combined with supportive living (e.g., sober house) instead of residential care for those patients who are not in imminent danger. With unbundling, the type and intensity of treatment are based on the patient's needs and not on limitations imposed by the treatment setting. The unbundling concept

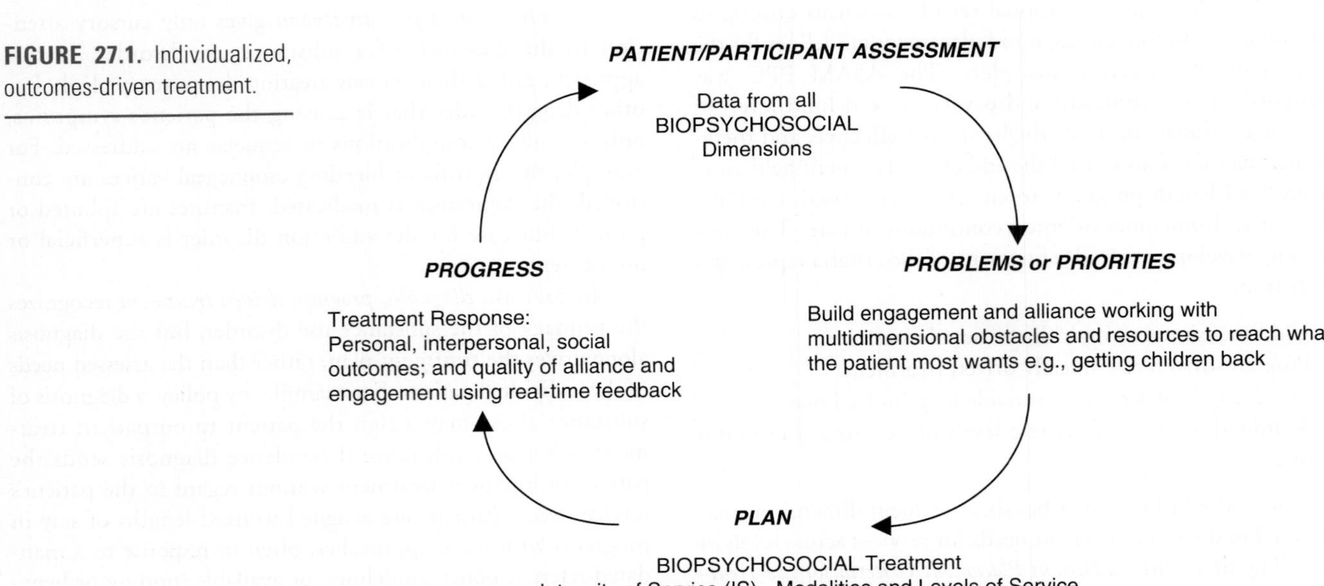
PATIENT/PARTICIPANT ASSESSMENT
Data from all BIOPSYCHOSOCIAL Dimensions
PROBLEMS or PRIORITIES
Build engagement and alliance working with multidimensional obstacles and resources to reach what the patient most wants e.g., getting children back
PLAN
BIOPSYCHOSOCIAL Treatment
Intensity of Service (IS) - Modalities and Levels of Service
(Clinical and Wrap-around services)
PROGRESS
Treatment Response:
Personal, interpersonal, social outcomes; and quality of alliance and engagement using real-time feedback

FIGURE 27.1. Individualized, outcomes-driven treatment.

thus is designed to maximize individualized care and to encourage the delivery of necessary treatment in any clinically feasible setting.

A transition to unbundled treatment would require systemic changes in state program licensure and public funding and insurance reimbursement. In terms of treatment, there would no longer be "programs," but rather a constellation of services to meet the needs of each patient. The systems in use for program licensure or accreditation, billing, reimbursement, and funding would not support unbundled treatment. However, the ASAM criteria encourage exploration of unbundling by suggesting ways to match risk and severity of needs with specific services and intensity of treatment. To assist clinicians and programs to advance this approach, the revised second edition of the ASAM criteria (3) proposed a future directions matrix. Although it requires empirical validation, the *Matrix for Matching Multidimensional Risk with Type and Intensity of Services* found in Appendix A for adults (3, pp. 281–312) and Appendix B for adolescents (3, pp. 313–339) is designed to assist the user to determine the level of risk using a five-point risk rating scale in each dimension, the needed services, and the appropriate level of care.

UNDERSTANDING THE ASAM PATIENT PLACEMENT CRITERIA

Four features characterize the ASAM Patient Placement Criteria: (1) comprehensive, individualized treatment planning, (2) ready access to services, (3) attention to multiple treatment needs, and (4) ongoing reassessment and modification of the plan.

Functionally, the criteria are used to match treatment settings, interventions, and services to each individual's particular problems and (often-changing) treatment needs. The ASAM criteria advocate for individualized, assessment-driven treatment and the flexible use of services across a broad continuum of care.

The criteria also advocate for a system in which treatment is readily available, because patients may be lost when the treatment they need is not readily accessible (13). By expanding the criteria to incorporate more use of outpatient care, especially for those in early stages of readiness to change, the ASAM criteria have helped to reduce waiting lists for residential treatment and thus have improved access to care (14).

The criteria are based on a philosophy that effective treatment attends to multiple needs of each individual, not just his or her alcohol or drug use (8). To be effective, treatment must address any associated medical, psychologic, social, vocational, legal problem, and environmental problems. Through its six assessment dimensions, the ASAM criteria underscore the importance of multidimensional assessment and treatment. To engage the patient in a collaborative therapeutic alliance, the assessment is in the service of what the patient wants (e.g., "Get my children back"). It serves to identify obstacles and resources; liabilities and strengths within each of the assessment dimensions (Fig. 27.2)

Objectivity The criteria are as objective, measurable, and quantifiable as possible. Certain aspects of the criteria require subjective interpretation. In this regard, the assessment and treatment of substance-related disorders are no different from biomedical or psychiatric conditions in which diagnosis or assessment and treatment are a mix of objectively measured criteria and clinical judgment.

Principles Guiding the Criteria Several important principles have guided development of the ASAM criteria.

Goals of Treatment The goals of intervention and treatment (including safe and comfortable detoxification, motivational enhancement to accept the need for recovery, the attainment of skills to maintain abstinence, and the like) determine the methods, intensity, frequency, and types of services provided. The health care professional's decision to prescribe a type of service and subsequent discharge of a patient from a level of care are based on how that treatment and its duration will influence the resolution of the dysfunction and improve the patient's prognosis.

Thus, in addiction treatment, the treatment may extend beyond simple resolution of observable symptoms to the achievement of overall healthier functioning, the difference between abstinence alone and recovery. The patient demonstrates a response to treatment through new insights, attitudes, and behaviors. Addiction treatment programs have as their goal not simply stabilizing the patient's condition but altering the course of the patient's substance use disorder and their overall functioning.

Individualized Treatment Plan Treatment should be tailored to the needs of the individual and guided by an individualized treatment plan that is developed in collaboration with the patient. Such a plan should be based on the patient's goals for treatment, a comprehensive biopsychosocial assessment of the patient, and, when possible, a comprehensive evaluation of the family (8–10).

Organizations that survey the quality of care such as the Joint Commission on Accreditation of Healthcare Organizations and the Commission on Accreditation of Rehabilitation Facilities publish consensus quality standards about treatment planning. These standards indicate that the treatment plan should list problems prioritized by obstacles to treatment and risks and arranged according to severity (such as obstacles to recovery, knowledge or skill deficits, dysfunction, or loss), strengths (such as readiness to change, a positive social support system, and a strong connection to a source of spiritual support), goals (a statement to guide realistic, achievable, short-term resolution, or reduction of the problems), methods or strategies (the treatment services to be provided, the site of those services, the staff responsible for delivering treatment), and a timetable for follow-through with the treatment plan that promotes accountability.

The plan should be written to facilitate measurement of progress. As with other disease processes, length of service should be linked directly to the patient's response to treatment

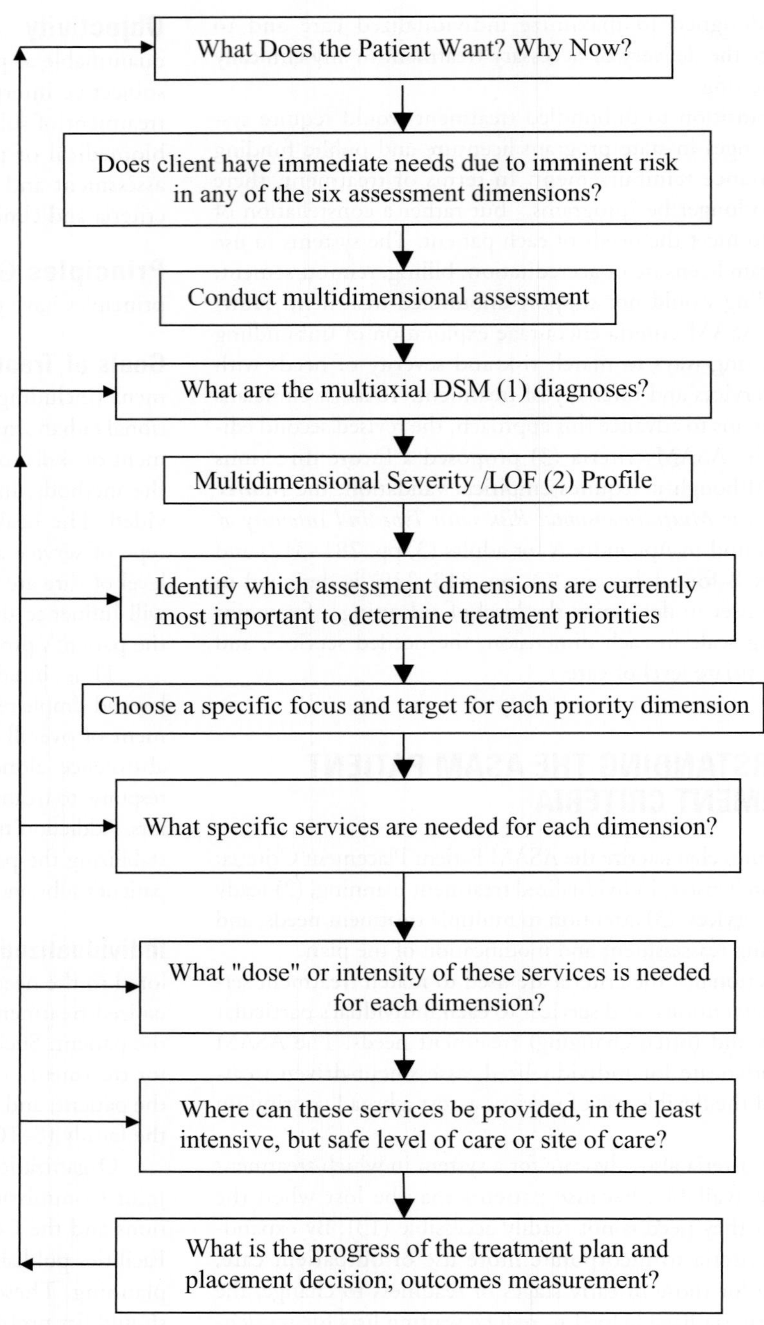
What Does the Patient Want? Why Now?
Does client have immediate needs due to imminent risk in any of the six assessment dimensions?
Conduct multidimensional assessment
What are the multiaxial DSM (1) diagnoses?
Multidimensional Severity /LOF (2) Profile
Identify which assessment dimensions are currently most important to determine treatment priorities
Choose a specific focus and target for each priority dimension
What specific services are needed for each dimension?
What "dose" or intensity of these services is needed for each dimension?
Where can these services be provided, in the least intensive, but safe level of care or site of care?
What is the progress of the treatment plan and placement decision; outcomes measurement?
(1) = Diagnostic and Statistical Manual of Mental Disorders, American Psychiatric Association
(2) = Level of Function

FIGURE 27.2. Decision tree to match assessment and treatment/ placement assignment.

(e.g., attainment of the treatment goals and degree of resolution of the identified clinical problems) rather than a predetermined time frame based on the length of the treatment program or the reimbursement.

Choice of Treatment Levels The goal that underlies the criteria is the placement of the patient in the most appropriate level of care. Referral to a specific level of care must be based on a careful assessment of the patient. For both clinical and financial reasons, the preferred level of care is the least intensive level that meets treatment objectives, while providing safety and security for the patient. Moreover, although the levels of care are presented as discrete levels, in reality they represent benchmarks or points along a continuum of treatment services through which the patient might progress in a variety of ways, depending on a his or her needs and response. For example, a patient could begin at a more intensive level and move to a more or less intensive level of care, depending on individual needs.

For patients who have been previously treated and have relapsed, the choice of the current level of care should be based on an assessment of the patient's history and current functioning, not automatic placement in a more intensive level of care (15). Such placement by policy assumes that relapse after treatment indicates that the previous level of care was of insufficient intensity. In fact, poorly matched services may have been the problem (e.g., "recovery"), relapse prevention services for a patient at an early stage of change who needs "discovery" motivational enhancement services.

Continuum of Care To provide the most clinically appropriate and cost-effective treatment system, a continuum of care must be available. Such a continuum may be offered by a single provider or multiple providers. For the continuum to promote continuity of care and improve patient retention, it is best distinguished by at least three characteristics: (1) seamless transfer between levels of care which links the patient to the next level of care rather than merely referring the patient to another agency or level of care, (2) philosophical congruence among the various providers of care, and (3) timely arrival of the patient's clinical record at the next provider (16). It is most helpful if providers envision admitting the patient into the continuum *through* their program rather than admitting the patient *to* their program.

Many providers of treatment services offer only one of the many levels of care described. In such situations, movement between levels might mean referring the patient out of the provider's own network of care. Although lack of reimbursement for some levels of care, or lack of availability of other levels of care may render this ideal unattainable at present, one goal of these criteria is to stimulate the development of an accessible, efficient, and effective system of comprehensive care for people with the spectrum of substance use disorders and cooccurring service needs.

Progress through the Levels of Care As a patient moves through treatment in any level of care, his or her progress in all six dimensions should be continually assessed to ensure that treatment is addressing the patient's changing needs (8,16). Such multidimensional assessment ensures comprehensive treatment. In the process of patient assessment, certain problems and priorities are identified as justifying admission to a particular level of care. The resolution of those problems and priorities determines when a patient can be treated at a different level of care or discharged from treatment. The appearance of new problems may require services that can be effectively provided at the same level of care, or that require a more or less intensive level of care.

Each time the patient's response to treatment is assessed, new priorities for recovery are identified. The intensity of the strategies incorporated in the treatment plan helps to determine the most efficient and effective level of care that can safely provide the care articulated in the individualized treatment plan. Patients may, however, worsen or fail to improve in a given level of care or with a given type of program. When this happens, changes in the level of care or program should be based on a reassessment of the treatment plan, with modifications to achieve a better therapeutic response (8–10).

Should a patient drink or use drugs during treatment, the immediate response should be to revise the treatment plan rather than automatically change the level of care or administratively discharge the patient. Additionally, some benefit managers require that a patient be "motivated for sobriety" as a requirement for admission to a program. Given the characteristic symptoms of denial and lack of readiness to change of addiction disorders, the only requirement should be that the patient is willing to enter treatment. Clinicians then facilitate the patient's self change process along the stages of change.

Length of Stay The patient's progress toward achieving his or her treatment plan goals and objectives determines length of stay or service level. Fixed length of stay or program-driven treatment is not individualized and does not respond to the particular problems of a given patient. Although fixed length of stay programs are more convenient and predictable for the provider, they may be less effective for individuals (17,18).

Clinical versus Reimbursement Considerations The ASAM criteria describe a wide range of levels and types of care. Not all of these services are available in all locations, nor are they covered by all payers. Clinicians who make placement decisions are expected to supplement the criteria with their own clinical judgment, their knowledge of the patient, and their knowledge of the available resources. The ASAM criteria are not intended as a reimbursement guideline, but rather as a clinical guideline for making the most appropriate placement recommendation for an individual patient with a specific set of symptoms and behaviors. If the criteria only covered the levels of care commonly reimbursable by private insurance carriers, they would not address many of the resources of the public sector and, thus, would tacitly endorse limitations on a complete continuum of care.

Treatment Failure Two incorrect assumptions are associated with the concept of "treatment failure." The first is that the disorder is acute rather than chronic, so that the only criterion for success is total and complete cure and elimination of the problem. Such expectations are recognized as inappropriate in the treatment of other chronic disorders, such as diabetes or hypertension. No one expects that simply because a patient has been treated on one occasion for his or her hypertension, there will never be another episode. The same recognition of chronicity should be applied to the treatment of addiction disorders, for which appropriate criteria would involve reductions in the intensity or severity of symptoms, the duration of symptoms, and the frequency of symptoms.

The second assumption is that responsibility for treatment "failure" always rests with the patient (as in, "The patient was not ready"). However, poor treatment outcomes also may be related to a provider's failure to provide services tailored to the patient's needs.

Finally, there is a concern that some benefit managers require that a patient "fail" at one level of care as a prerequisite for approving admission to a more intensive level of care (for example, "failure" in outpatient treatment as a prerequisite for admission to inpatient treatment). In fact, such a requirement is no more rational than treating every patient in an inpatient program or using a fixed length of stay for all; or requiring all breast cancer patients to first have a lumpectomy as a requirement for a mastectomy. Such a strategy potentially puts the patient at risk because it delays care at a more appropriate level of treatment, and potentially increases health care costs if restricting the appropriate level of treatment allows the addiction disorder to progress.

The ASAM Criteria and State Licensure or Certification The ASAM criteria contain descriptions of treatment programs at each level of care, including the setting, staffing, support systems, therapies, assessments, documentation, and treatment plan reviews typically found at that level. This information should be useful to providers who are preparing to serve a particular group of patients, as well as to clinicians who are making placement decisions. Nevertheless, the descriptions are not requirements and are not intended to replace or supersede the relevant statutes, licensure, or certification requirements of any state.

ASSESSMENT DIMENSIONS

The ASAM criteria identify six assessment areas (dimensions) as the most important in formulating an individualized treatment plan and in making subsequent patient placement decisions. Table 27.1 outlines the six dimensions and the assessment and treatment planning focus of each dimension.

There is an increased focus on recovery and strength-based, person-centered assessments and services. A strength-based multidimensional assessment addresses not only a patient's needs, obstacles, and liabilities; but also his or her strengths, assets, resources, and supports to promote recovery. For example, in assessing a person's relapse, continued use, or continued problem potential (Dimension 5), the focus should not restrict inquiry to cravings, peer refusal skill problems, relapse triggers, or other impulses; but also identification of any periods of sobriety or mental health wellness. Even if these were for relatively short periods, assessment of how the patient changed attitudes, knowledge, skills, or behavior to achieve success identifies strategies that can be included in the individualized service plan.

Similarly, if a person has been suicidal before, but has never needed hospitalization or medical care for serious cutting or overdose behavior, this may suggest a level of impulse control that can be harnessed in the emotional, behavioral, or cognitive (Dimension 3) part of the treatment plan. Or if a patient is homeless, but has one family member who is still invested in the person's well-being, that is a recovery support (Dimension 6) that should be engaged early in treatment.

TABLE 27.1 ASAM Criteria Assessment Dimensions

Assessment dimensions	Assessment and treatment planning focus
1. Acute intoxication and/or withdrawal potential	Assessment for intoxication or withdrawal management. Detoxificationin a variety of levels of care and preparation for continued addiction services.
2. Biomedical conditions and complications	Assess and treat cooccurring physical health conditions or complications. Treatment provided within the level of care or through coordination of physical health services.
3. Emotional, behavioral, or cognitive conditions and complications	Assess and treat cooccurring diagnostic or subdiagnostic mental health conditions or complications. Treatment provided within the level of care or through coordination of mental health services.
4. Readiness to change	Assess stage of readiness to change. If not ready to commit to full recovery, engage into treatment using motivational enhancement strategies. If ready for recovery, consolidate and expand action for change.
5. Relapse, continued use, or continued problem potential	Assess readiness for relapse prevention services and teach where appropriate. Identify previous periods of sobriety or wellness and what worked to achieve this. If still at early stages of change, focus on raising consciousness of consequences of continued use or continued problems as part of motivational enhancement strategies.
6. Recovery environment	Assess need for specific individualized family or significant other, housing, financial, vocational, educational, legal, transportation, childcare services. Identify any supports and assets in any or all of the areas.

Interactions across Dimensions in Assessing for Level of Care The ASAM criteria promotes a holistic, biopsychosocial approach to patient care. Thus a patient's needs are not discretely confined to one assessment dimension independent from other dimensions. To ensure that the whole person's needs and strengths are assessed each dimension is considered independently but also in terms of the interaction across dimensions. For example, when assessing an individual for severity, a history of moderate or severe withdrawal *without* any current intoxication or withdrawal, or current intoxication without a history of significant withdrawal problems should generate a lesser level of concern than a combination of a history of moderate or severe withdrawal *with* current symptoms of intoxication or withdrawal.

In reality, there is considerable interaction across dimensions. For example, significant problems with readiness to change (Dimension 4), coupled with a poor recovery environment (Dimension 6) may increase the risk of relapse (Dimension 5). Another commonly seen combination involves problems in Dimension 2 (such as chronic pain that distracts the patient from the recovery process) coupled with problems in Dimensions 4, 5, or 6.

The converse also is true. For example, problems with relapse potential (Dimension 5) may be offset by a high degree of readiness to change (Dimension 4) or a very supportive recovery environment (Dimension 6). The interaction of these factors may result in a lower level of severity than is seen in any dimension alone.

The lesson here is that assessments are most accurate when they take into account all of the factors (dimensions) that affect each individual's receptivity and ability to engage in treatment at a particular point in time.

Continued Service and Discharge Criteria In a departure from earlier editions, the current edition of the criteria (*ASAM Patient Placement Criteria for the Treatment of Substance-Related Disorders, Second Edition-Revised* [*ASAM PPC-2R*]) (3), contains only admission criteria, leaving the decisions about continued service, transfer, or discharge to general guidelines and the judgment of the treatment professional. This change was made in recognition of the fact that, in the process of patient assessment, certain problems and priorities are identified as justifying admission to a particular level of care. It is the resolution of those problems and priorities that determines when a patient can be treated at a different level of care or discharged. The appearance of new problems may require services that can be provided effectively at the same level of care or transfer of the patient to a more or less intensive level of care.

The assessment process for continued service or discharge/transfer is the same as for admission, with the reassessment of multidimensional severity determining the treatment priorities, intensity of needed services, and the decision about ongoing level of care. Decisions concerning continued service, transfer, or discharge involve review of the treatment plan and assessment of the patient's progress. That is, they require the same type of multidimensional assessment process that led to admission to the current level of care.

LEVELS OF CARE

The ASAM criteria conceptualize treatment as a continuum marked by five basic levels of care, which are numbered in numerals from Level 0.5 through Level IV. Thus the ASAM criteria provide the addiction field with a nomenclature for describing the continuum of addiction services, as follows:

Level 0.5: Early intervention
Level I: Outpatient services
Level II: Intensive outpatient/partial hospitalization services
Level III: Residential/inpatient services
Level IV: Medically managed intensive inpatient services

Within each level, a decimal number (ranging from 0.1 to 0.9) expresses gradations of intensity within the existing levels of care. This structure allows improved precision of description and better "interrater" reliability by focusing on five broad levels of care. Thus the ASAM criteria describe gradations within each level of care. For example, a II.1 level of care provides a benchmark for intensity at the minimum description of Level II care (also see the Rapid Reference section of this text for a summary crosswalk of the levels of care). For more detail on each of the levels of care within the broad levels of care, see Table 27.2.

PLACEMENT DILEMMAS

Even those using the ASAM criteria regularly encounter "real-world" dilemmas surrounding access, reimbursement, funding, resource allocation, and availability of services, particularly for patients with cooccurring medical or psychiatric disorders.

Cooccurring Disorders When the first edition of the ASAM criteria was published in 1991, the criteria were designed for programs that offered only addiction treatment services. However, even that early edition also acknowledged that some patients come to treatment with medical (Dimension 2) and psychiatric (Dimension 3) disorders that coexist with their substance-related problems. Clinical reality suggests that programs and practitioners who are committed to meeting the total needs of the patients they serve must be able to meet the needs of people with cooccurring disorders, either directly or through referral or consultation. This concept is particularly relevant today, as the range of patient needs and clinical variability continues to broaden.

Factors contributing to this clinical reality include the expansion of substance use and substance-related disorders in younger populations; greater sensitivity to substance use problems in the mental health, methadone maintenance, welfare, and criminal justice populations; and increased commitment to earlier intervention in substance use disorders in preference to fragmented services and incarceration. A major factor has been the growing body of scientific evidence pointing to addiction disorders as diseases of the brain; another is the development of pharmacotherapies for addiction. Greater understanding of the uses and effects of psychosocial and cognitive-behavioral strategies also has heightened awareness of a broadened range of modalities to meet individual needs.

TABLE 27.2 ASAM Criteria Levels of Care

ASAM PPC-2R level of detoxification service for adults	Level	(Note: There are no separate detoxification services for adolescents)
Ambulatory detoxification without extended onsite monitoring	I-D	Mild withdrawal with daily or less than daily outpatient supervision; likely to complete detoxification and to continue treatment or recovery.
Ambulatory detoxification with extended onsite monitoring	II-D	Moderate withdrawal with all-day detoxification support and supervision; at night, has supportive family or living situation; likely to complete detoxification.
Clinically managed residential detoxification	III.2-D	Minimal to moderate withdrawal, but needs 24-h support to complete detoxification and increase likelihood of continuing treatment or recovery.
Medically monitored inpatient detoxification	III.7-D	Severe withdrawal and needs 24-h nursing care and physician visits as necessary; unlikely to complete detoxification without medical, nursing monitoring.
Medically managed inpatient detoxification	IV-D	Severe, unstable withdrawal and needs 24-h nursing care and daily physician visits to modify detoxification regimen and manage medical instability.
ASAM PPC-2R Levels of Care	Level	Same Levels of Care for Adolescents except Level III.3
Early intervention	0.5	Assessment and education for at risk individuals who do not meet diagnostic criteria for substance-related disorder.
Outpatient services	I	Less than 9 h of service/week (adults); less than 6 h/week (adolesecents) for recovery or motivational enhancement therapies/strategies
Intensive outpatient	II.1	9 or more hours of service/week (adults); 6 or more h/week (adolesecents) in a structured program to treat multidimensional instability.
Partial hospitalization	II.5	20 or more hours of service/week in a structured program for multidimensional instabilty not requiring 24-h care.
Clinically managed low-intensity residential	III.1	24-h structure with available trained personnel with emphasis on reentry to the community; at least 5 h of clinical service/week.
Clinically managed medium-intensity residential	III.3	24-h care with trained counselors to stablize multidimensional imminent danger. Less intense milieu and group treatment for those with cognitive or other impairments unable to use full active milieu or therapeutic community.
Clinically managed high-intensity residential	III.5	24-h care with trained counselors to stabilize multidimensional imminent danger and prepare for outpatient treatment. Able to tolerate and use full active milieu or therapeutic community.
Medically monitored intensive inpatient	III.7	24-h nursing care with physician availablity for significant problems in Dimensions 1, 2, or 3. 16 h/day counselor ability.
Medically managed intensive inpatient	IV	24-h nursing care and daily physician care for severe, unstable problems in Dimensions 1, 2, or 3. Counseling available to engage patient in treatment.
Opioid maintenance therapy	OMT	Daily or several times weekly opioid medication and counseling available to maintain multidimensional stability for those with opioid dependence.

ASAM, American Society of Addiction Medicine; PPC, Patient Placement Criteria.

The *ASAM PPC-2R* thus incorporates criteria that address the large subset of individuals who present for treatment with cooccurring Axis I substance-related disorders and cooccurring Axis I/Axis II mental disorders. Table 27.3 summarizes what kinds of patients with cooccurring mental and substance-related disorders are best treated in three kinds of programs: Addiction Only Services; Dual Diagnosis Capable; and Dual Diagnosis Enhanced. Because cooccurring disorders are so prevalent, the ASAM criteria encourage all programs to be at least Dual Diagnosis Capable (Table 27.4).

Assessment of Imminent Danger Residential treatment has often been used for patients with chronic relapse problems; those with poor recovery environments or homeless; and to "break through denial." In the ASAM PPC, residential treatment is reserved for stabilization of those in imminent danger. Such patients need a residential program that offers clinical staff and services 24 hours per day to respond to the patient's issues that pose the imminent danger (i.e., that there is a strong probability certain behaviors such as continued drug or alcohol use will occur, and that such behaviors will present a significant risk of adverse consequences to the

TABLE 27.3 Matching Patients with Co-occurring Disorders to Services

Characteristics of cooccurring disorders	
Patients	**Services**
Addiction-only patients: Individuals who exhibit substance abuse or dependence problems without co-occurring mental health problems or diagnosable Axis I or II disorders	Addiction-only services: Services directed toward the amelioration of substance-related disorders without services for the treatment of cooccurring mental health problems or diagnosable disorders. Such services are clinically inappropriate for dually diagnosed individuals.
Patients with cooccurring MH problems of mild to moderate severity: Individuals who exhibit (1) subthreshold diagnostic (i.e., traits, symptoms) Axis I or II disorders or (2) diagnosable but stable Axis I or II disorders (i.e., bipolar disorder but compliant with and stable on lithium).	Dual-diagnosis capable: Primary focus on substance use disorders but capable of treating patients with subthreshold or diagnosable but stable Axis I or II disorders. Psychiatric services available onsite or by consultation; at least some staff members are competent to understand and identify signs and symptoms of acute psychiatric conditions.
Patients with co-occurring mental health problems of moderate to high severity: Individuals who exhibit moderate to severe diagnosable Axis I or II disorders, who are not stable and require mental health as well as addiction treatment.	Dual-diagnosis enhanced: Psychiatric services available onsite or closely coordinated; all staff cross-trained in addiction and mental health and are competent to understand and identify signs and symptoms of acute psychiatric conditions and treat mental health problems along with the substance use disorders. Treatment for both mental health and substance abuse disorders is integrated. This service is most similar to a traditional "dual-diagnosis" program.

individual or others; and that such adverse events will occur in the very near future) (3, p. 12).

Mandated Level of Care or Length of Service In some cases, an individual is referred for treatment at a specific level of care or for a specific length of service (for example, an offender in the criminal justice system may be given a choice of a prison term or a fixed length of stay in a treatment center). Such mandated or court-ordered referrals may not be based on clinical considerations and thus may be inconsistent with a placement decision arrived at through the ASAM criteria. In such a case, the provider should make reasonable attempts to have the order amended to reflect the assessed clinical level or length of service.

If the court order or other mandate cannot be amended, the individual may be continuing treatment at a level of care or for a length of stay greater than is clinically indicated. The resident's readiness for discharge or transfer and the staff's attempts to implement a clinically appropriate placement should be noted in the clinical record, and the treatment plan should be updated in a manner that provides the resident with the opportunity to continue the recovery process at the same level of care even though it could be continued at a less intensive level of care.

Logistical Impediments Logistic problems can arise anywhere, but present major challenges in rural and frontier areas because of large distances and few treatment resources or personnel. Underserved inner-city areas with lower socioeconomic and disadvantaged people may lack the resources for people to easily access services. When logistic considerations are an impediment to the indicated services (for example, lack of available transportation is a barrier to a patient's access to an indicated outpatient program), an outpatient service combined with unsupervised/minimally supervised housing may be an appropriate treatment intervention. In cities or towns, such a domiciliary option might be found in a group living situation (such as a Salvation Army program, motel accommodations, YMCA/YWCA, or mission). In rural and other underserved areas, options could include the creation of a supervised housing situation by using unused treatment beds, assertive community treatment models in which the treatment is brought to rural areas (such as Native American settlements) and provided in weekend intensive models at sites such as community centers and churches, vans that are sent out to pick up patients and bring them to a treatment site, and using a van or motor home as an office or group therapy room.

Need for a Safe Environment When a patient lives in a recovery environment that is so toxic as to preclude recovery efforts (as through victimization or exposure to an active addict) and a Level I or II outpatient service is indicated, the patient may need referral to a safe place to live while in treatment, as well as to treatment itself. One example might be combining a women's shelter with a Level II.1 or II.5 treatment program.

Assuring Individualized Treatment Many programs claim to provide individualized care, but how can quality auditors know that such care actually is provided? There are at least three efficient ways to determine whether a program is providing truly individualized treatment.

1. Take 10 closed clinical case records and compare the treatment plans. If the reviewer cannot clearly distinguish patients by their treatment plans, the treatment is not individualized.

TABLE 27.4 Application of the ASAM Criteria to Clinical Presentations

Use of the *ASAM Patient Placement Criteria* in treatment planning involves much more than simply a decision about level of care. The assessment dimensions and the broad continuum of care surveyed by the ASAM dimensions provide an opportunity to focus treatment, consistent with a disease management approach. The following vignettes, which represent segments of comprehensive assessments, are designed to illustrate some of the more common problems encountered in determining severity of illness, developing treatment plans, and making placement decisions. Each vignette illustrates an initial response, a discussion, and a revised response.

Case 1: Mr. A

Mr. A is a 58-year-old male who meets diagnostic criteria (19) (DSM-IV-TR) for "Alcohol Dependence with Physiological Dependence." In terms of Dimension 1, he is currently in mild withdrawal from alcohol (Clinical Institute Withdrawal Assessment of Alcohol Scale, Revised, CIWA-Ar, score of 7) with a history of no more than moderate severity withdrawal. However, he stopped drinking only 2 hours ago. Mr. A is hypertensive by history, not well-controlled with medication even when sober, and current blood pressure is 140/100. Severity in Dimensions 3 through 6 is low.

Initial Response

Based on only mild withdrawal severity in Dimensions 1, Mr. A is referred for Level I-D detoxification, ambulatory detoxification without extended on-site monitoring. For his Dimension 2 problem, he is referred back to his primary care physician for review of his hypertension.

Discussion

Given that Mr. A is withdrawing from alcohol, a sedative drug, the resultant autonomic arousal will create an increase in blood pressure. His current blood pressure reading is only 2 hours since his last drink and insufficient time has elapsed for the full withdrawal syndrome to have developed. It can be assumed that the autonomic arousal could markedly increase his blood pressure and because his baseline blood pressure is already elevated, the interaction between Dimension 1 and 2 increases his overall severity.

Revised Response

Because of the high severity resulting from the interaction between Dimensions 1 and 2, Arthur should be treated in Level III.7-D medically monitored inpatient detoxification service. An alternative might be referral to a Level II-D ambulatory detoxification with extended onsite monitoring if the patient enters treatment early in the week and could be observed for a number of days; or if the II-D service operates 7 days per week.

Case 2: Ms. P

A 16-year-old woman is brought to the emergency department of an acute care hospital with a report that, in the course of an argument with her parents, she has thrown a chair. Her parents suspect drug intoxication is the cause and report that she has been staying out unusually late at night and mixing with "the wrong crowd." They report a great deal of family discord, anger, and frustration, particularly directed by the young woman toward her father. Ms. P has no history of psychiatric or addiction treatment.

The parents both are present in the emergency department, although Ms. P was brought in by the police after her mother called for help. An emergency physician and a nurse from the psychiatric unit jointly evaluate Ms. P; they agree that she needs to be hospitalized in view of the animosity at home, her violent behavior, and the possibility that she is using an unknown drug.

Following the ASAM assessment dimensions, they organize the clinical information as follows:

Dimension 1: acute intoxication and/or withdrawal potential: Although she was intoxicated at the time of the chair-throwing incident, Ms. P is no longer intoxicated and has not been using alcohol or other drugs in sufficient quantities or for a long enough period to suggest the possibility of a withdrawal syndrome.

Dimension 2: biomedical conditions and complications: Ms. P is not taking any medications, is physically healthy, and has no current complaints.

Dimension 3: emotional, behavioral, or cognitive conditions and complications: Ms. P has complex problems with anger management, as evidenced by the chair-throwing incident, but is not impulsive at present if separated from her parents, especially her father.

Dimension 4: readiness to change: Ms. P is willing to talk to a therapist, blames her parents for being overbearing and not trusting her, and agrees to come into treatment, but does not want to be at home with her father.

Dimension 5: relapse, continued use, or continued problem potential: The team concludes that Ms. P is likely to engage in drug use if released. They believe that, if she returns home immediately, there may be a reoccurrence of the fighting and, possibly, violence.

Dimension 6: recovery environment: Ms. P's parents are frustrated and angry as well. They are mistrustful of their daughter and want her hospitalized to provide a break in the family fighting.

Initial Response

Based on Ms. P's recent history of violent acting out, the emergency physician and the psychiatric nurse recommend that she be admitted to the hospital's psychiatric unit, at least for the night.

Discussion

Ms. P's acting out occurred when she was intoxicated, which she no longer is. The major conflict appears to be a family issue, particularly between Ms. P and her father. There is no indication of a severe or imminently dangerous biomedical, emotional, behavioral, or cognitive problem that requires the resources of a medically managed intensive inpatient setting.

Revised Response

The initial goal is to separate Ms. P from her father, which might be done by arranging for Ms. P to stay with a relative or family friend overnight, or by having Ms. P and her mother stay at a motel for the night. Based on the available information, Ms. P's behavior and conflict with her parents may reflect normal adolescent struggles rather than psychopathology. To address this, outpatient family counseling should be considered. Given the information available, there is also nothing indicating that Ms. P suffers from a diagnosable substance use disorder.

In crisis or mandated treatment situations, clinicians often come under pressure from family or referral agencies to provide a certain level of care. However, when the essential information is organized according to the ASAM dimensions, the patient's real severity and needs are more easily identified. This leads to a more appropriate clinical plan and avoids wasteful use of resources by focusing on the services needed to meet the patient's individual needs.

ASAM, American Society of Addiction Medicine.

2. Review the progress notes and determine whether they relate back to the objectives or strategies in the treatment plan.
3. For programs that receive reimbursement from multiple payers, compare lengths of service by sources of payment. If the lengths of stay correspond to payer type, then the program is payment-driven rather than offering individualized treatment.

Fidelity to the Spirit and Content of the ASAM PPC

The following implementation issues suggest that clinicians and programs still struggle with understanding the full intent of the ASAM criteria.

1. Programs that describe their services as a fixed length of stay program as evidenced by description of the program as a "30-Day Inpatient Program" or "27-session IOP." Or, if the program claims no fixed length of stay, check what clients say if you ask: "How long do you have to be here?" An answer involving fixed numbers of sessions or weeks reveals regression to a program driven model.
2. Language used: "extended residential"—length of stay should be determined by severity, function, and progress, not a priori that the patient needs extended length of stay in a residential setting; "graduate" and "complete the program" reveal a focus on a fixed plan and program rather than on functional improvement as the determinant of level of care.
3. Waiting lists for residential when admission criteria require "imminent danger."
4. States and counties that fund only a few levels of care, which discourages a seamless continuum of care; licensure and contractual arrangements that keep levels of care in fixed programs that discourages flexible overlapping of levels (e.g., a state may contract only for Level III.7D that forces the program to staff for and document on every patient as if they are continually a III.7D severity, when that may change in 2 days).
5. Levels of detoxification available are often only IV-D or III.7-D, which drives up cost and allows only brief length of stay in high intensity settings. This leads to rapid relapse when the patient is not fully detoxified. An ambulatory level might be both more clinically appropriate and less costly. Use of the five levels of detoxification would allow longer length of stay for the same or less resources.

Exceptions to the Patient Placement Criteria In making treatment placement decisions, three important factors override the patient-treatment match with regard to levels of care.

1. Lack of availability of appropriate, criteria-selected care.
2. Failure of a patient to progress at a given level of care, so as to warrant a reassessment of the treatment plan with a view to modifying the treatment approach. Such situations may require transfer to a specialized program at the same level of care or to a more intensive or less intensive level of care to achieve a better therapeutic response.
3. State laws regulating the practice of medicine or licensure of a facility that require the use of different criteria.

Unique clinical presentations or extenuating circumstances require some flexibility in application of the criteria to ensure the safety and welfare of the patient.

Gathering Data to Improve Systems of Care There are no ideal continuums of care that have seamless levels of care; and where all policy, licensure and funding obstacles have been removed. Clinicians should resist the impulse to immediately place a patient in what is locally available and pragmatic. If sufficient multidimensional assessment reveals that an appropriately matched level of care is not available, this provides an opportunity to gather data to assist in systems change. It would take 30 seconds to note on a form the date; patient's name and case number; and fill in the level of care or service clinically indicated; the level of care or service actually received; and then to note the particular reasons for the difference in your region. These data can identify the greatest gaps in services and prioritize where resources need to be concentrated to improve the system of care (Table 27.5).

TABLE 27.5 Data Gathering on Discrepancy between Needed and Available Services

Placement Summary
Level of care/service indicated: Insert the level of care and/or type of service that offers the most appropriate level of care/service that can provide the service intensity needed to address the client's current functioning/severity.
Level of care/service received: If the most appropriate level/service is not able to be used, insert the most appropriate placement/service available and circle the reason for the difference between indicated and received level/service.
Reason for difference: Circle only one number. 1: level of care or service not available; 2: provider judgment; 3: patient preference; 4: patient is on waiting list for appropriate level/service; 5: level of care or service available, but no payment source; 6: geographic inaccessibility; 7: family responsibility problems (e.g., no childcare); 8: language; 9: not applicable; 10: not listed.

Research on the ASAM Criteria The ASAM criteria are the most intensively studied set of addiction placement criteria. A considerable body of work exists on the ASAM PPC including at least nine evaluations involving a total of 3641 subjects. Federal agencies—including the National Institute on Drug Abuse, the National Institute on Alcohol Abuse and Alcoholism, and the Center for Substance Abuse Treatment—have invested more than $7 million in this research (20). Several controlled studies have found that treatment based on the ASAM PPC are associated with less morbidity, better client functioning, and more efficient service utilization than mismatched treatment (21).

A prospective, naturalistic study examined the validity and impact of the PPC, comparing the placement of 287 adults within Washington State versus 240 adults within Oregon, where a statewide PPC training model was fully implemented. Results showed that the use of standardized criteria such as the PPC showed good potential for changing treatment planning behavior, increasing individualization, and improving utilization of new levels of care (14).

Given the complexity of the PPC multidimensional branching logic, researchers at the Massachusetts General Hospital Addiction Research Program implemented the ASAM criteria as a comprehensive computerized interview (22). It consists of a sequence of questions and scoring options for real-time use by the counselor or research assistant. This real-time, computerized method yielded good interrater reliability for the level-of-care assignment (intraclass correlation coefficient = 0.77; $P < 0.01$) (23).

To date, three prospective studies have tested this method in three different samples (public system Medicaid and uninsured patients, insured patients, and Veterans Administration) using three different outcomes (acute no-show to treatment, 90-day drinking rates, and long-term hospital utilization)—but all three trials used the same computerized algorithm to implement the PPC-1 in a standardized fashion (22). The first prospective study, a multisite trial in Massachusetts, is the only randomized, controlled trial of placement criteria to be conducted to date. In this project, 700 subjects were randomized to Level II or Level III treatment, either matched or mismatched according to the recommendation of the PPC-1 algorithm. Results showed good concurrent validity (22) and evidence for predictive validity, because higher acute no-show rates occurred in patients who were mismatched to a lower level of care than was recommended overall and in subsamples with high-frequency cocaine use (24) and in the subset of patients with comorbid symptomatology—which also had *higher no-show rates* when mismatched to higher level of care than recommended (25).

These results support the predictive validity of the use of PPC. They also indicate that the PPC have valid clinical decision-making guidelines, good feasibility and reliability through standardized computer assessment instruments, and good concurrent validity in treating patients throughout the multidimensional assessments (26). The ultimate goal of this ongoing research work is revision of the PPC that will emerge not simply from the current expert consensus process but also through the findings from multiple national and international research studies.

CONCLUSIONS

Four important missions underlie the ASAM criteria: to (1) enable patients to receive the most appropriate and highest quality treatment services; (2) encourage the development of a continuum of comprehensive care; (3) promote the effective, efficient use of care resources; and (4) help protect access to and funding for care. The use of placement criteria in treatment planning thus represents far more than a narrow utilization review or case management process. Correctly applied and implemented, the ASAM criteria can assist patients in accessing a much broader continuum of care and menu of services than is typically available (4).

Effective implementation of the ASAM criteria will require a shift in thinking toward outcomes-driven case planning. A variety of agencies will need to make this shift, including regulatory agencies, clinical and medical staff, and referral sources, such as courts, probation officers, child protective services, employers, and employee assistance professionals (27).

The ASAM criteria offer a system for improving patient-centered, comprehensive care through the use of multidimensional assessment and treatment planning that permits more objective evaluation of patient outcomes. With improved outcome analysis driving treatment decisions, the problems of access to care and funding of treatment can be championed more effectively.

REFERENCES

1. Hoffmann NG, Halikas JA, Mee-Lee D, et al. *Patient placement criteria for the treatment of psychoactive substance use disorders (PPC-1)*. Washington, DC: American Society of Addiction Medicine, 1991.
2. Mee-Lee D, Shulman GD, Gartner L. *ASAM patient placement criteria for the treatment of substance-related disorders, 2nd ed. (ASAM PPC-2)*. Chevy Chase, MD: American Society of Addiction Medicine, 1996.
3. Mee-Lee D, Shulman GD, Fishman M, et al. *ASAM patient placement criteria for the treatment of substance-related disorders, 2nd ed.-revised (ASAM PPC-2R)*. Chevy Chase, MD: American Society of Addiction Medicine, 2001.
4. Mee-Lee D. Persons with addiction disorders, system failures, and managed care. In: Ross EC, ed. *Managed behavioral health care handbook*. Gaithersburg, MD: Aspen Publishers, Inc., 2001:225–266.
5. Mee-Lee D, Shulman GD. The ASAM patient placement criteria and matching patients to treatment. In: Graham AW, Schultz TK, Mayo-Smith MF, eds. *Principles of addiction medicine*, 3rd ed. Chevy Chase, MD: American Society of Addiction Medicine, 2003.
6. Shulman GD. Continued treatment for substance abuse: an effective system for referral *Cont Care* 1994:13:27–33.
7. Mee-Lee D. Use of patient placement criteria in the selection of treatment. In Graham AW, Schultz TK, eds. *Principles of addiction medicine,* 2nd ed. Chevy Chase, MD: American Society of Addiction Medicine, 1998.
8. National Institute on Drug Abuse (NIDA). *Principles of drug addiction treatment: a research-based guide* (NIH Publication No. 00-4180). Rockville, MD: National Institute on Drug Abuse, 1999.

9. McLellan AT, McKay JR, Forman R, et al. Reconsidering the evaluation of addiction treatment—from retrospective follow-up to concurrent recovery monitoring. *Addiction* 2005;100:447–458.
10. Miller SD, Mee-Lee D, Plum B, et al. Making treatment count: client-directed, outcome informed clinical work with problem drinkers. In: Lebow J, ed. *Handbook of clinical family therapy*. New York: Wiley, 2005.
11. The role and current status of patient placement criteria in the treatment of substance use disorders: the recommendations of a consensus panel. Co-Chairs: Lee Gartner and David Mee-Lee. Treatment improvement protocol No. 13. The Center for Substance Abuse Treatment, Rockville, MD, 1995.
12. McGee MD, Mee-Lee D. Rethinking patient placement: the human services matrix model for matching services to needs. *J Substance Abuse Treatment* 1997;14(2):141–148.
13. McCarty D, Gustafson DH, Wisdom JP, et al. The Network for the Improvement of Addiction Treatment (NIATx): enhancing access and retention. *Drug Alcohol Depend* 2007;11;88(2-3):138–145.
14. Deck D, Gabriel R, Knudsen J, et al. Impact of patient placement criteria on substance abuse treatment under the Oregon Health Plan. *J Addict Dis* 2003;22(Suppl 1):27–44.
15. Gastfriend DR, Rubin A, Sharon E, et al. New constructs and assessments for relapse and continued use potential in the ASAM patient placement criteria. Addition treatment matching—research foundations of the American Society of Addiction Medicine (ASAM) criteria. *J Addictive Dis* 2003;22(Suppl 1):2.
16. Berry LL, Seiders K, Wilder SS. Innovations in access to care: a patient-centered approach. *Ann Intern Med* 2003;139:568–574.
17. Miller WR, Hester RK. Inpatient alcoholism treatment: who benefits? *Am Psychologist* 1986;41(7):794–805.
18. Institute of Medicine. *Broadening the base of treatment for alcohol problems.* Washington, DC: National Academy Press, 1990.
19. American Psychiatric Association. *Diagnostic and statistical manual of mental disorders, 4th edition, text revision (DSM-IV-TR).* Washington, DC: American Psychiatric Association, 2000.
20. Gastfriend DR, ed. Addition treatment matching—research foundations of the American Society of Addiction Medicine (ASAM) criteria. *J Addictive Dis* 2003:22(Suppl 1):2.
21. Gastfriend DR, Mee-Lee D. The ASAM patient placement criteria: context, concepts, and continuing development. Addition treatment matching—research foundations of the American Society of Addiction Medicine (ASAM) criteria. *J Addictive Dis* 2003;22(Suppl 1):2.
22. Turner WM, Turner KH, Reif S, et al. Feasibility of multidimensional substance abuse treatment matching: automating the ASAM patient placement criteria. *Drug Alcohol Depend* 1999;55:35–43.
23. Baker SL, Gastfriend DR. Reliability of multidimensional substance abuse treatment matching: implementing the ASAM patient placement criteria. *J Addictive Dis* 2003;22(Suppl 1):45–60.
24. Kang SK, Sharon S, Pirard S, et al. Predictors for residential rehabilitation and treatment no-show in high frequency cocaine users: validation of the American Society of Addiction Medicine (ASAM) criteria. Paper presented at the annual meeting and symposium of the American Academy of Addiction Psychiatrists, Las Vegas, NV, December 15, 2002.
25. Angarita GA, Reif S, Pirard S, et al. No-show for treatment in substance abuse patients with comorbid symptomatology: validity results from a controlled trial of the ASAM patient placement criteria. *J Addict Med* 2007;1:79–87.
26. Mee-Lee D. Development and implementation of patient placement criteria. New developments in addiction treatment. Academic highlights. *J Clin Psychiatry* 2006;67:11:1805–1807.
27. Heatherton B. Implementing the ASAM criteria in community treatment centers in Illinois: opportunities and challenges. *J Addictive Dis* 2000; 19(2):109–116.

CHAPTER 28

Peter D. Friedmann, MD, MPH
Karran A. Phillips, MD, MSc
Richard Saitz, MD, MPH, FACP, FASAM
Jeffrey H. Samet, MD, MA, MPH

Linking Addiction Treatment with Other Medical and Psychiatric Treatment Systems

Persons with substance use problems are at substantial risk for coexisting medical and mental health problems (see Section 10, "Medical Disorders and Complications of Addiction," and Section 11, "Co-Occurring Addictions and Psychiatric Disorders"), so it comes as little surprise that they present in significant numbers to medical and mental health settings. Similarly, patients in addictive disorder treatment commonly experience medical and psychiatric problems, which can distract from recovery and increase relapse risk (1–3). In both medical and addictive disorder treatment settings, the provision of comprehensive care for individuals with alcohol and other drug use disorders presents challenges to clinicians, who traditionally have been concerned only with issues reflecting their own training and perspectives. For example, medical practitioners typically address the toxic effects of a particular substance, such as seizures or cirrhosis, or the health consequences of a high-risk lifestyle, such as viral hepatitis or HIV. Psychiatrists and other mental health professionals focus on the mental health issues so prevalent among substance-using patients. Meanwhile, addiction medicine specialists typically focus on the individual's destructive preoccupation with obtaining and consuming a psychoactive chemical substance and the negative consequences of such actions. For the patient, these problems are inseparable, yet the providers operate in distinct systems of care, each with its own—often exclusive—focus. For example, the medical literature contains instances of medical practitioners not attending to the addictive disorders of their patients by failing to screen, intervene, or refer (4–6). Similarly, patients in addictive disorder treatment programs report unmet psychologic and medical needs (7). It is as if substance-using patients with psychiatric or medical illnesses sometimes are bounced between systems—told that they must be abstinent before they can receive treatment for their psychiatric and medical problems or that they are too sick (medically or psychiatrically) to get into an addiction treatment program—resulting in a clinical "Catch-22."

Patients who present with complex, interrelated, comorbid problems make apparent the disconnect between these parallel yet typically separate systems of care. The growth of addiction medicine will help to close these gaps. However, for most systems that lack access to a certified addiction medicine physician (8), linkages across the separate medical, mental health, and addictive disorder disciplines will be needed to improve the quality of care delivered to patients with addictive disorders. This chapter briefly reviews the benefits to linkages between primary medical care, mental health, and addictive disorder services; identifies the potential barriers to such linkages; outlines recommendations for coordination of care by advisory bodies; and describes published linkage models."

BENEFITS OF LINKED SERVICES

Effective linkage may benefit individuals with substance use problems in the following common scenarios: when issues related to addictive disorders are not addressed in primary care and mental health settings, when medical and mental health issues are not addressed in addictive disorder treatment, and when the patient is seen in two or more of these settings but no effective communication between or within the systems occurs.

From a patient's perspective, the potential for improved overall care is the motivating force for linkage of systems (Table 28.1). For example a patient on methadone maintenance who receives efavirenz, which can decrease methadone blood levels, without coordination of care might experience

TABLE 28.1 Benefits of Linking Addiction Treatment with Other Medical and Psychiatric Services

From the patient's perspective
- Structured format
- Improves overall quality of care
- Facilitates access to addictive disorders treatment for patients in medical care settings
- Enhances access to primary medical care for patients receiving addictive disorder treatment
- Improves patient well-being in terms of addictive disorder severity and medical problems
- Provides care that may be easier to access
- Increases the patient's satisfaction with his or her health care

From the primary care provider's perspective
- Promotes screening of all patients for alcohol problems
- Facilitates inclusion of alcohol and drug causes when considering a differential diagnosis
- Allows more achievable access to the addictive disorder treatment system
- Supports the prevention of relapse to alcohol and drug abuse
- Encourages other mental health services for primary care patients
- Enhances adherence with appointments and medical regimens
- Provides addictive disorder training opportunities for personnel

From the addiction treatment provider's perspective
- Improves addictive disorder treatment outcomes
- Reduces stigma about addictive disorder issues among medical providers
- Provides training opportunities about addictive disorder–related medical problems
- Promotes healthier behaviors
- Enhances medical providers' appreciation of the value of addictive disorder treatment
- Creates support for reimbursement parity for addictive disorder services
- Develops ongoing quality improvement efforts within addictive disorder programs

From a societal perspective
- Reduces costs of healthcare, criminal justice, and loss of productivity
- Reduces duplication of services and administrative costs
- Improves health outcomes of specific populations

withdrawal symptoms, toxicity, provider unease about possible methadone diversion, or relapse. Other examples of improved quality of care from such linkages include the potential for improved pain control in a patient receiving substance abuse treatment services, proper attribution of side effects of medications (versus substance use or withdrawal), and better access to detoxification and treatment for patients in the medical system. A profound benefit of linked systems is the improved well-being of individual patients in terms of addictive disorder severity, medical and psychiatric problems, and overall quality of life (9). A pragmatic patient benefit is the provision of convenient, comprehensive, and coordinated care. As this would likely result in increased service utilization, as noted in the broader spectrum of patients presenting to primary care–based buprenorphine treatment programs (10), careful assessment of its appropriateness would be necessary. Finally, linking services also may decrease stigma, as all providers would acknowledge and support the patient's recovery efforts, and all medical and psychiatric conditions may be addressed in the same location.

From the perspective of the primary care provider and the mental health clinician, possible benefits of linkage include early identification of and relapse prevention for substance use disorders (11), increased consideration of alcohol and drug problems in the formulation of differential diagnoses, better access to addictive disorder treatment services, enhanced patient adherence to appointments and medications, and improved addictive disorder training and experience for personnel. From an addiction treatment provider's perspective, stronger linkages could yield improved outcomes of addictive disorder treatment, similar to that demonstrated with the addition of needed psychosocial services (12,13). Ready availability of needed medical and mental health services also would allow addictive disorder professionals to do what they do best: focus on the core substance use issues. Exposure to examples of successful treatment could reduce stigma on the part of medical and mental health professionals toward addictive disorders and enhance their appreciation of the value of addictive disorder treatment. Bringing addictive disorder treatment closer to mainstream medical care and exposing its similarities to the care of other chronic illnesses could support the effort to achieve reimbursement parity for addictive disorders. Addictive disorder providers could learn about the medical and mental health complications of addictions and enhance their appreciation of clients' conditions, health care needs, and prevention approaches. Conceivably, the linkage of services could provide an opportunity to affect other behavior-related issues, such as sexually transmitted diseases (including human immunodeficiency virus) and smoking. Finally, linkage of services could enhance quality improvement efforts within addictive disorder treatment systems—as articulated in a relatively recent accreditation requirement from the Joint Commission on Accreditation of Healthcare Organizations (*http://www.jointcommission.org/AccreditationPrograms/BehavioralHealthCare/*) and by the focus of a recent Institute of Medicine report (14) —by taking lessons from medical settings that have grappled with these issues as part of the restructuring of medical care systems.

From a societal perspective, stronger linkages might lower long-term costs, including savings from reduced HIV incidence and other health-related sequelae of averted substance use, reduced incarceration and other criminal justice expenditures, and increased productivity (15,16). Other benefits include reduced duplication of services across these systems. Finally, a potential public health achievement would be improved health outcomes for specific populations burdened with the substantial morbidity associated with alcohol or drug use disorders.

BARRIERS TO OPTIMAL LINKAGE

Many barriers impede better linkage of services. One well-documented problem has been the perspective of many medical practitioners that addressing alcohol and drug abuse issues is not providing medical care and thus is outside his or her purview (17). This viewpoint is slowly changing within the profession. Medical education about substance dependence has been sorely deficient in past years (18). In the mid-1980s, medical students' suboptimal knowledge, perceived responsibility for caring for patients with alcoholism, and confidence in clinical skills was related to reported screening and referral practices; resident physicians perceived even less of a responsibility for care, had less confidence in their skills, and had more negative attitudes (19). These reports suggested that curricula needed improvement and that education, though necessary, may not be sufficient to maintain appropriate attitudes and practices on the part of physicians. Efforts to rectify that situation have been under way, most notably in the past decade, with development of appropriate standards, curricula, and effective addictive disorder educators within many disciplines, including most recently an effort by the Health Resources and Services Administration and the Center for Substance Abuse Treatment to have addiction educators in place in every health professional school in the United States (20–25). Nevertheless, progress requires time, dedicated resources, attention to continuing medical education, and maintenance of high-quality care.

Medical clinicians in practice generally report having received minimal training in substance use disorders, and they screen inadequately for preclinical cases (23,26). Because they neither find patients with less severe addictive disorders nor follow up those who have had success in treatment, most physicians have experienced few successes. This latter product of poor linkages biases the spectrum of medical providers' clinical experience and further discourages physician involvement. In effect, only patients who do poorly and develop severe medical and psychosocial problems are "visible" (27). In such an environment, it is difficult to convince even well-meaning providers that the diagnosis and management of these disorders are worthwhile; however, training can help overcome these barriers (28–30).

Payment and Service Linkage Issues In our current health care system, payment for addiction treatment and mental health care has been limited, compared with payments for other medical services (31,32). Though there have been efforts to achieve parity for health care benefits, parity has not been the norm.

In 1950, the Uniform Accident and Sickness Policy Provision Law (UPPL) stating insurers are not liable for any loss sustained or contracted while the insured is intoxicated or under the influence of any narcotics was passed. The refusal of reimbursement serves as a disincentive for physicians to screen and document alcohol use and the opportunity for intervention is missed despite an estimated health savings of 3.81 U.S. dollars for every 1.00 U.S. dollar spent on screening and intervention (33). As of January 1, 2007, this law was enacted in all but nine states (CO, CT, IA, MD, NV, NC, RI, SD, WA).

Moreover, many managed behavioral health plans have "carved out" addictive disorder benefits, separating the financing of care for mental and addictive disorders from that for the rest of the patient's ailments (34–37). Such plans have reduced the utilization of services for addictive disorders, and the effect they have had on clinical outcomes, quality of care, integration of care, and physician attitudes remains unclear. Separate systems could foster the continuation of episodic, poorly coordinated care for substance-abusing patients.

However, in March 2008, the House of Representatives passed the Paul Wellstone Mental Health and Addiction Equity Act of 2007 (HR 1424) sponsored jointly by Congressman Patrick J. Kennedy (D-RI) and congressman Jim Ramstad (R-MN), which seeks to improve health for all Americans by granting greater access to mental health and addiction treatment and prohibiting health insurers from placing discriminatory restrictions on treatment. HR 1424 goes beyond the 1996 Mental Health Parity Act, which required equality only for annual and lifetime limits by requiring equality across the terms of the health plan. President Bush signed this bill into law on October 3, 2008 as part of the Emergency Economic Stabilization Act of 2008.

Current systems of payment often do not cover addictive disorder services provided by primary care physicians. Financial reimbursements to medical and behavioral health clinicians generally are taken from separate budgets, and the financial benefits of averted medical complications occur late. Consequently, the cost of treatment for an addictive disorder that prevents subsequent HIV infection may be appreciated as a treatment expense, rather than as a savings of future medical care costs. Another financial disincentive to linked services is the perception that costs of such care may be limitless. The fear of the cost of appropriate addictive disorder services persists, despite analyses that document the limited effect even a worst case scenario would have on health care expenditures (38). In January 2001, the Office of Personnel Management required parity of mental health and substance abuse coverage for all federal employees. A 2006 study comparing seven Federal Employee Health Benefit Plans with a matched set of plans that did not have parity of mental health and substance abuse benefits found that implementation of parity was associated with an increase in service utilization in one of the seven federal plans (+0.78%; $p < 0.05$), decrease utilization in one of the seven plans (−0.96%; < 0.05), and no significant difference in the five other plans (range, −0.38% to +0.23%; $p > 0.05$ for each comparison). Additionally, they found that there was a statistically significant decrease in spending attributable to parity in three plans (range, −\$201.99 to −\$68.97; $p < 0.05$ for each comparison) and no significant change in spending attributable to the implementation of parity in the remaining four plans (range, −$42.13 to +$27.11; $p > 0.05$ for each comparison). The authors concluded that implementation of parity in insurance benefits for mental health and substance dependence coupled with management of care can improve insurance protection without increasing total costs (39).

In October 2007, the White House Office of National Drug Control Policy (ONDCP) announced new health care codes for substance abuse SBI. The American Medical Association's new Level I Current Procedural terminology (CPT) codes (99408 and 99409) went into effect on January 1, 2008, and allow health care providers to report and be reimbursed for structured screening and brief intervention (*http://www.whitehousedrugpolicy.gov/news/press07/101107.html*).

Concerns About Confidentiality and Stigma Well-meaning concerns about patient confidentiality can be barriers to effectively linked medical, mental health, and addictions care. Practical difficulties interfere with obtaining timely two-way written releases of information. Substance dependence programs are required to comply with both the federal confidentiality regulations (42 CFR Part 2 or Part 2) and with the "Standards for Privacy of Individually Identifiable Health Information" final rule (Privacy Rule), pursuant to the Administrative Simplification provisions of the Health Insurance Portability and Accountability Act of 1996 (HIPAA), 45 CFR Parts 160 and 164, Subparts A and E (*http://www.hipaa.samhsa.gov/download2/SAMHSA'sPart2-HIPAAComparison-ClearedWordVersion.doc*). Addictive disorder information must be specified in information releases to be shared and is often kept separate from the standard medical record. Though the protection of patient confidentiality is noble, in some cases it can impede integrated care.

Stigma remains a fundamental barrier in the treatment of any patient with alcohol or drug abuse. In addition to effects on patient behavior, such as limiting recognition of needs and readiness to accept services, stigma might result in medical clinicians' disinclination toward spending time addressing drug and alcohol issues or a perception of diminished stature of substance abuse treatment providers. Both outgrowths of stigma impede overall progress.

Medical and mental health providers often inadequately appreciate the efficacy of treatment for addictive disorders despite an overwhelmingly supportive body of research. For example, physicians do not appreciate the comparable therapeutic value of treatment for alcohol or heroin dependence relative to standard treatment for other chronic disorders, such as diabetes mellitus or asthma (40–42).

In summary, the barriers to an integrated system of care for patients with substance use disorders are manifold. Barriers include issues of professional responsibility, education among providers, financial disincentives, concerns about confidentiality, and stigma, among others. Though the barriers can appear to be extensive, they are not insurmountable. At the "macro" level, addressing systems linkages would go a long way toward improving integrated care. Examples of systems approaches include implementation of the following: linkage models of care, payment systems that encourage linkage, and quality measures that value coordinated care. Parity of health care benefits for mental health, addictive disorders, and medical problems (as part of legislative efforts in Connecticut and Minnesota) can help to reduce stigma and improve care coordination, but impediments to the care of addictive disorders in primary care settings exist even in states where parity legislation has been enacted. These impediments include the arbitrary health insurance practice of discounting or denying primary care reimbursement for visits in which the provider indicates a mental or addictive disorder as the primary diagnosis (43).

Confidentiality issues can be addressed at the systems level by having all care occur under the umbrella of one health system facilitating records availability and at an individual patient-clinician level by having office systems that prompt clinicians and staff to obtain patient information releases to allow health care providers to communicate. Recently published and future studies demonstrating the feasibility and effectiveness of these models should help to convince payers and practitioners of the need to move in this direction.

The advent of office-based opioid agonist treatment has enhanced communication between some primary medical care providers and opioid treatment staff members and provides models for the opportunity of integrated medical and/or psychiatric care with addiction treatment. At the clinician level, various approaches can be taken simultaneously to help overcome the barriers to integration. Physician attitudes, skills, and practices can be changed by active learning educational programs (28,29). Convincing theoretical and empirically proven benefits of linked services also will lead clinicians to favor better-integrated care (44,45).

MODELS OF LINKED SERVICES

Alcohol and drug-abusing patients use services in "inefficient" ways (e.g., emergency department presentations rather than outpatient clinic visits), and they do not receive care in the continuous, longitudinal, and comprehensive manner that is often essential for the high-quality management of any chronic disease (46–48). Two basic models have been proposed to bring the system of care for patients with substance use disorders closer to a primary care or chronic disease management model (Table 28.2). One model uses a centralized approach in which treatment of addictive disorders, primary medical care, and mental health services are co-located at a single site. A second model uses a distributive approach to facilitate effective patient referrals to services at different sites. This section describes these models of linked primary medical, mental health, and addictive disorder services and reviews the available evidence of their success in facilitating the multidisciplinary care of addicted patients.

Centralized Models Centralized or on-site models bring primary care, mental health, and/or addictive disorder services

TABLE 28.2 Features of Centralized and Distributive Integrated Service Models

Centralized models

- Addiction treatment and pharmacotherapy in primary medical care and mental health services sites
- Addiction providers located in group HMOs, private practices, or clinics
- Behavioral medicine and primary medical provider offices co-located in shared space
- Addiction treatment delivered at public health clinics (e.g., sexually transmitted infections, HIV or tuberculosis care)
- Addiction treatment delivered in a general hospital with proximate medical and mental health clinics
- Addiction treatment and primary care services co-located in a community mental health setting
- Addiction-trained nurse practitioner or physician available in a primary care practice to prescribe and monitor naltrexone, to prescribe and monitor buprenorphine, and to initiate and manage detoxification
- Addiction and mental health specialty teams present in medical care sites (e.g., consult teams in emergency departments or hospitals)
- Smoking cessation counseling and pharmacotherapy delivered as part of primary care
- Brief interventions and advice for unhealthy substance use in doctor's offices, emergency departments, and hospitals
- Primary medical care and mental health services delivered at addiction treatment sites
- Medical and mental health providers or clinic located at a methadone treatment program
- Co-located primary care and addiction care
- An integrated alcohol and medical clinic
- An addiction medicine physician with medical and psychiatric skills
- A multiservice community agency with a central location

Distributive

- Health maintenance organizations or preferred provider organizations with defined, yet decentralized referral networks
- Addiction triage and referral, or central intake and assessment centers that perform medical and mental health assessments and referral for multiple addiction treatment programs
- Community-based case management
- Evaluation at addiction treatment sites with external referral for ongoing medical and mental health care
- Defined networks of providers with facilitated communication and financial/contractual links and systems
- Informal links between clinicians or agencies facilitated by releases of information, transportation, and case management
- A multiservice community agency with a single owner but several locations

together at a single site. This fully integrated, "one-stop-shopping" model has been best described in primary care medical clinics and in addictive disorder treatment programs. In addition to overcoming the substantial political, bureaucratic, attitudinal, and financial barriers that separate addicted persons from needed services (49,50), centralized delivery overcomes the problems of geographic separation, patient disorganization, and poor motivation that inhibit patients with addictive disorders from keeping outside appointments (50,51).

Willenbring and Olson (1999) reported favorable results for a model of integrated alcohol treatment in a primary care clinic for poorly motivated, medically ill alcoholics." Their model included at least monthly visits (28), outreach to patients who missed appointments (20), clinic notes that cued the primary care provider to monitor alcohol intake at each visit (52), provider-delivered brief advice that emphasized reducing the harm from alcohol use and cutting down rather than strict abstinence (53), verbal and graphic feedback of improvement and deterioration in biologic markers such as gamma-glutamyl transferase (GGT) (54), and on-site mental health services as needed (55,56). In a randomized design, medically ill alcoholic patients in the integrated clinic were compared with similar patients referred to traditional alcohol dependence treatment and ambulatory medical care." During 2 years of follow-up, patients in the integrated clinic had improved alcohol treatment outcomes (including greater abstinence), improved outpatient visit adherence, and lower mortality. Though this model may prove too elaborate for many primary care settings, it serves as a starting point for a disease management system for substance use disorders similar to those used for asthma, diabetes mellitus, and congestive heart failure (46,57). With further study, this model may prove cost-effective for recalcitrant alcohol-dependent patients or for other poorly motivated or complicated substance-abusing patients. Less resource-intensive intervention models developed for problem drinkers in primary care also have proved feasible. The cost analysis of Project TrEAT, a randomized study of physician-delivered brief interventions, showed substantial improvements in drinking outcomes and substantial savings for society and health systems (58). A primary care study from the University of Massachusetts reported that 2.5 hours of primary care provider training in patient-centered alcohol brief intervention was feasible (28) and reduced alcohol consumption among problem drinkers (59). An early study suggested that simple feedback about changes in biologic markers, such as GGT in alcoholic patients, can itself reduce sick days, hospital days, and mortality (60). Saitz et al. (58) demonstrated that a systems intervention (physician prompting with suggested courses of action) can improve counseling for alcohol problems and reduce drinking (61). In another model of alcohol treatment in primary care, O'Connor reported the successful treatment of a series of alcohol dependent patients with naltrexone (62). Other models have successfully incorporated behavioral health personnel into primary care practices (63,64). However, if these efforts are to be generalized to primary care settings as they exist today, substantial training of clinicians will be required as physicians often estimate their competence in alcohol-related behavior change lower than in other health-related behavior change such as smoking cessation, stress, exercise, and weight management (65).

Prior to the Drug Addiction Treatment Act of 2000, few American studies had integrated treatment of illicit drug dependence into primary care. Though general practitioners have frequently participated in the management of these disorders elsewhere in the world, this has only recently occurred in the United States with the enactment of legislation permitting office-based treatment of opioid dependence with Schedule III, IV, or V pharmacologic agents approved by the U.S. Food and Drug Administration (FDA). Sublingual buprenorphine and a combination of buprenorphine and naloxone have been used for this purpose in the United States since 2003. Several studies have found that buprenorphine works as well as methadone for patients with opiate addiction of mild to moderate severity. In a 12-week randomized trial of 46 opiate-dependent patients treated with buprenorphine maintenance, there was higher retention in the primary care setting than in a drug treatment program (78% vs. 52%; $p = 0.06$), and lower rates of opioid use based on urine toxicology (63% vs. 85%; $p < 0.01$) (66). In addition to achieving positive treatment outcomes, office-based buprenorphine has been well received by patients. Barry (67) surveyed 142 opioid-dependent patients receiving primary care–based buprenorphine/naloxone. Their mean overall satisfaction with treatment was 4.4 (of 5). Patients were most satisfied with the medication and ancillary services; and they indicated a strong willingness to refer a substance-abusing friend for the same treatment. With the development and dissemination of new pharmacologic therapies for alcohol and other drug use disorders, the impetus for addictive disorder services in the primary care setting will only increase.

Though methadone is an effective treatment for opioid dependence, its use is heavily regulated. Few experimental programs have looked at the use of medical methadone maintenance involving stabilized methadone patients in a medical setting. In a recent study by Merrill et al. (68) regulatory exemptions were granted to establish a methadone medical maintenance program. Of the 30 enrolled stable methadone patients transferred to a medical office for care, 28 remained after 1 year and only two patients had opioid–positive urine tests. In addition to good substance dependence treatment outcomes, previously unmet medical needs were attended to as demonstrated by an improvement in the medical composite score of the Addiction Severity Index ($p = 0.02$) and patient and physician satisfaction were high with an improved attitude of physicians towards methadone maintenance ($p = 0.007$).

Centralizing primary medical care, substance dependence treatment, and psychiatric services has also proven an effective way to manage concomitant medical conditions such as hepatitis C and tuberculosis. Substance dependence treatment physicians often perform initial hepatitis C management including screening for hepatitis C virus antibodies, recommending hepatitis A and B vaccines, and referring patients to subspecialists for hepatitis C treatment (69). In a 2007 study by Sylvestre and Clements (70), methadone maintenance patients received hepatitis C treatment in a community-based nonprofit clinic providing on-site medical and psychiatric treatment. Adherence to hepatitis C treatment (defined as taking at least 80% of prescribed interferon and ribavirin) occurred in 68%, and those who were adherent were more likely to achieve a sustained hepatitis C virologic response (42% vs. 4% in nonadherent patients; $p = 0.001$). Furthermore, pegylated interferon does not appear to precipitate opioid withdrawal in HCV and HIV co-infected methadone maintenance patients (71). Less is known about tuberculosis management within a centralized medical care and substance dependence setting. However, O'Connor et al. (72) demonstrated that by utilizing an admixture of isoniazid and methadone, 72% of methadone maintenance patients eligible for tuberculosis chemoprophylaxis completed therapy.

Centralized models of primary medical and mental health care in addiction treatment settings may also improve addicted patients' access to these services (73). Umbricht-Schneiter et al. (50) found that 92% of patients randomly assigned to a centralized model in a methadone treatment program received medical services, compared with only 35% of patients referred to a local clinic. A recent trial of veterans found that primary care onsite in an addiction treatment program increased attendance at primary care (adjusted odds ratio [OR] = 2.20; 95% confidence interval [CI] = 1.53 to 3.15) and engagement in addiction treatment at 3 months (adjusted OR = 1.36; 1.00 to 1.84) but showed no effect on overall health status or costs (74). Among patients with substance abuse–related medical conditions, integrated care models compared to independent care models have shown significant decreases in hospitalization rates ($p = 0.04$), inpatient days ($p = 0.05$), and emergency room use ($p = 0.02$) (75). Similarly, Friedmann et al. (73) found that on-site delivery of primary care to methadone maintenance patients and long-term residential patients reduced subsequent ED and hospital use (15). Other work suggests that integration of addictive disorder treatment and community mental health services reduces relapse and improves social stability for patients dually diagnosed with addictive disorders and mental illness (55,76,77).

In general, patients with nicotine dependence, at-risk drinking, and low-severity illicit drug use can be managed in primary care settings without subspecialty addiction medicine consultation. Conversely, patients with addictive disorders or substance dependence generally should be cared for in collaboration with addiction specialists and/or treatment counselors (whether integrated in a primary care office or located elsewhere). Recent advances support and encourage a major role for primary care physicians and office-based psychiatrists in the pharmacologic management of patients with opioid or alcohol dependence while at the same time recognizing the need for substantial collaboration and coordination with addiction treatment providers. For example, with the availability of the highly effective and safe option of office-based buprenorphine/naloxone, the primary care physician or general psychiatrist can prescribe medication for opioid dependence while counseling is delivered by either the physician, a health behavior expert in the practice, or by referral. Similarly, though not specifically tested in primary care, medications for alcohol dependence can have efficacy when given along with low-intensity medication management counseling that addresses adherence, side effects, and alcohol use (53); such counseling can be done in medical settings because it is similar to adherence counseling for medications for other chronic conditions such as hypertension and diabetes mellitus. Medications for alcohol dependence can be as effective when delivered with medication management counseling as with more specialized behavioral counseling.

All patients should have primary and preventive health care—again, where this care is delivered will depend on the system of care. An ideal centralized model of care can provide addiction, mental health, and medical care at a single site. Whether specialty addiction medicine or addiction psychiatry services are delivered at an addiction specialty treatment site or within the primary care setting, the key is that systems be integrated to deliver the most appropriate and efficient care.

Distributive Models In light of the lack of parity in reimbursement for the treatment of substance use disorders and the absence of unified budgets for medical and behavioral health services (78), most providers lack resources to provide comprehensive, centralized services for addicted patients (73). Moreover, patients (especially those in long-term recovery) may object to long-term primary care in settings primarily identified as addiction treatment programs. Therefore, the development and dissemination of effective decentralized or distributive models is an important step toward service integration in the current health care environment.

Successful referral is the central task of the distributive model. Anecdote and limited data suggest that simple referral alone cannot integrate the care of addicted patients in primary care settings. For example, among 1,440 patients who were in addiction treatment with a primary care physician, 45% reported that the physician who cared for them was unaware of their addictive disorder (6). A study of one community in California similarly noted that 45% of drug users had contact with the mainstream health care system in a given year, but medical or mental health providers were major client referral sources or destinations for fewer than 10% of addictive disorder programs (79). Thus, the substantial interorganizational distance between addiction treatment programs and mainstream health care presents great barriers to successful referral. Because substance-abusing populations can have disorganized lifestyles and poor motivation, contemporary distributive models typically use case management to facilitate referrals. Community-based case management can effectively link substance-dependent patients to needed services (54,80).

In addiction treatment programs, distributive arrangements are commonly used to link patients to medical and mental health services (81–83). Distributive arrangements range, for example, from an addictive disorder treatment unit that contracts with a local group practice to provide physical examinations and routine medical care to its patients to one that makes ad hoc referrals to a local community mental health center. The advantage of this model is that it makes use of existing health care systems. For example, patients in an inpatient detoxification unit who received a facilitated referral to primary care in the local community from a multidisciplinary team (physician, nurse, and social worker) were more likely to link with primary medical care (84). This model requires no rearrangement of existing health care delivery systems; however, it does require efforts (and therefore costs) to assure that linkage is facilitated.

Case management or transportation assistance can facilitate these referrals (81,85,86). A study of public addiction treatment programs found that contracted referral with case management increased medical services utilization two- to threefold over ad hoc referrals (87). More recent work has emphasized the importance of transportation assistance to increase the delivery of needed services (85).

Disease Management Model Chronic disease management (CDM) is a care delivery approach based on the chronic care model described by Wagner that links, integrates, and coordinates primary and specialty care (88,89). The key components are an informed and motivated patient, a proactive team, and an established delivery system resulting in maximized chronic disease management and outcomes. Such an approach has been successfully applied to many chronic diseases but not yet to substance dependence. Saitz et al. have proposed that the implementation of CDM focused on substance dependence should include attention to (1) systems of care, (2) addressing medical, psychiatric, and social problems, and (3) addiction-specific treatments (Saitz et al., unpublished). The systems component addresses the fragmentation of care through on-site longitudinal service delivery, referral agreements, multidisciplinary teams, coordination of an explicit care plan, patient reminders, electronic medical records, and collaboration of addiction, medical and psychiatric physicians. Medical, psychiatric, and social components include assessment, management, and coordination of care with specialty referral. Addiction-specific components include all treatments with evidence for efficacy such as motivational interviewing, relapse prevention counseling, ambulatory detoxification, and appropriate referral. It is hypothesized that strong CDM linkages within and between systems of care and integrated case management will increase access and receipt of, and retention in, effective substance dependence and medical treatment that in turn will improve utilization and health outcomes.

Vulnerable Populations Integrated models may be most germane and show the most benefit to vulnerable populations including HIV-infected, homeless, and incarcerated individuals. They have been found to promote delivery of HIV-related care, medication adherence, and outpatient medical services (82,85,90,91). An analysis of data gathered from New York State Medicaid claims found that regular drug abuse and medical care reduced hospitalizations by approximately 25% among HIV-positive and HIV-negative patients with drug abuse diagnoses (92). Basu et al. (93) outlined four possible models for the integration of addiction disorder treatment with buprenorphine into the primary HIV care setting: (1) the HIV primary care model wherein the HIV primary care physician provides buprenorphine maintenance services; (2) the on-site specialist model wherin an addiction specialist provides buprenorphine maintenance therapy at an HIV primary care clinic; (3) the hybrid model wherein buprenorphine induction is performed by a specialist and maintenance by the HIV care provider; and (4) the drug treatment model wherein buprenorphine maintenance is provided through a substance abuse clinic with HIV care services. Further research is needed to determine which of these models will be most feasible and effective and whether they can be applied to other addiction disorder treatments in addition to buprenorphine. A randomized trial of integrated primary care in an addiction treatment program concluded that integrated care may be cost-effective for patients with addictive disorder-related medical conditions (75,94).

With the increasing prevalence of substance abuse/dependence and polysubstance use among urban homeless persons, these individuals have unique needs that will require tailored interventions (95). Homeless individuals have high rates of social instability, comorbidity, and chronic drug use, which make them ideally suited for systems of integrated care. Alford et al. (52) conducted a retrospective medical record review of 44 homeless and 41 housed patients enrolled in office-based opioid treatment over 12 months and found that homeless patients receiving buprenorphine/naloxone fared comparably to housed. Treatment failure for the homeless (21%) and housed (22%) did not differ (p = .94). Both groups had similar proportions with illicit opioid use (odds ratio [OR], 0.9; 95% CI, 0.5 to 1.7 p = .8), utilization of counseling (homeless, 46%; housed, 49%; p = .95), and participation in mutual-help groups (homeless, 25%; housed, 29%; p = .96) at 12 months.

Substance dependence is common in incarcerated individuals with a recent systematic review finding drug abuse or dependence in male prisoners ranging from 10% to 48% and in female prisoners from 30% to 60% (96). Despite the high prevalence of substance use disorders in correctional settings, a survey of the medical directors of all 50 states and the federal prison system demonstrated that among respondents who had jurisdiction over 88% of U.S. prisoners, 48% used methadone, predominantly for short-term detoxification and pregnant inmates, and only 8% referred opiate-dependent inmates to methadone programs upon release (97). The high prevalence of substance use disorders in incarcerated individuals and the limited treatment options create a gap in services. Efforts to close that gap should include improved treatment matching and linkage of services both during and after incarceration (98).

In summary, several effective models of centralized and distributive linkage in primary care and specialty addiction treatment settings have been developed. Addiction interventions in medical settings are appropriate for a spectrum of patients: at-risk drinkers and substance use disorders of mild-to-moderate severity; medically ill substance-dependent patients who refuse formal treatment referral; and substance-dependent patients who receive rehabilitative counseling elsewhere yet would benefit from substance-related pharmacotherapy and management of their medical problems. With adequate support, primary care physicians also can have a productive role in outpatient detoxification (99). Minimally motivated patients who will accept only harm-reduction interventions can benefit from management in the primary care setting as well. For patients in formal addiction treatment, linkage to needed medical and psychologic services can improve access to health care, improve physical and mental health, and reduce relapse. Both centralized and distributive models show promise for integrating care across these systems. The distributive model predominates in the United States (81). Though it can be less effective than the centralized model in linking substance-abusing patients to needed services (50,85), its relatively low cost, flexibility, and adaptability (especially to integration of secondary and tertiary care services), suggest that the distributive model, with further refinements, is likely to remain the method of coordinated services in the near future.

PROSPECTS FOR IMPROVED LINKAGE

Despite the enormity of the challenge, the time is right for a transformation in the configuration of addictive disorder treatment and health care services. A number of signs suggest that a window of opportunity exists for innovation. The staggering burden of medical and mental health problems affecting substance-abusing patients is now well documented, from HIV, hepatitis C, and drug overdose to depression, anxiety, and victimization (100–103). The enormous economic burden that substance use problems place on our society, through costs related to health care, criminality/incarceration, and loss of productivity, is increasingly recognized and forces policymakers to consider alternative approaches to the management and care of this population (104). Moreover, advances in the diagnosis and treatment of substance-related disorders, including pharmacologic and behavioral approaches applicable in the primary care setting, promise to change the approach to clinical management of these prevalent disorders. The perspective that the 21st century is an opportune time to advance the linkage of substance use treatment with mental health and medical care was fully endorsed in report from the Institute of Medicine, "Improving the quality of healthcare for mental and substance-use conditions: The quality chasm" series (14). An underlying theme in the book is that only by addressing substance use and mental health problems can one achieve optimal benefit for patients engaged in medical care. One of the most important recommendations of the IOM report pertains to the delivery of coordinated care among primary care, mental health, and substance-use treatment providers. The basis of this recommendation lies in the *Crossing the Quality Chasm* "Rules" that endorse "shared knowledge and the free flow of information" and "cooperation among clinicians."

Primary care and disease management systems are not achievable if only adopted by physicians but rather require a multidisciplinary team. Thus, the reported sense of overburdening of physicians should not preclude the development of linkage systems but rather influence its development so that its implementation does not solely rely on physicians' functions (105). The ability to treat addictive disorders in less intensive settings will promote cost savings and cost-effectiveness. Increased attention to the improvement of quality in health care systems also presents opportunities to address linkage to addictive disorder treatment as a quality issue. Finally, the current era has seen rapid reorganization of health care services. Despite the difficulties associated with such periods, they challenge policymakers to rethink inadequate systems and can create a climate of innovation toward the delivery of high-quality, comprehensive, and coordinated care for patients with substance use disorders (14,106–109).

REFERENCES

1. Friedmann PD. Effect of primary medical care on addiction and medical severity in substance abuse treatment programs. *J Gen Intern Med* 2003;18(1):1–8.
2. Bradizza CM. Qualitative analysis of high-risk drug and alcohol use situations among severely mentally ill substance abusers. *Addict Behav* 2003;28(1):157–169.
3. Saxon AJ, Wells EA, Fleming C, et al. Pre-treatment characteristics, program philosophy and level of ancillary services as predictors of methadone maintenance treatment outcome. *Addiction* 1996;91(8): 1197–1209.
4. Friedman LS. Evaluation of substance-abusing adolescents by primary care physicians. *J Adolesc Health Care* 1990;11(3):227–230.
5. Moore RD, Bone LR, Geller G, et al. Prevalence, detection, and treatment of alcoholism in hospitalized patients. *JAMA* 1989;261:403–407.
6. Saitz R, Mulvey KP, Plough A, et al. Physician unawareness of serious substance abuse. *Am J Drug Alcohol Abuse* 1997a;23:343–354.
7. Etheridge RM, Craddock SG, Dunteman GH, et al. Client services in two national studies of community-based drug abuse treatment programs. *J Subst Abuse* 1995;7:9–26.
8. Laine C, Newschaffer C, Zhang D, et al. Models of care in New York State Medicaid substance abuse clinics. Range of services and linkages to medical care. *J Subst Abuse Treat* 2000;12:271–285.
9. D'Aunno TA. Linking substance abuse treatment and primary health care. In: Egertson JA, Fox DM, Leshner AI, eds. *Treating drug abusers effectively*. Malden, MA: Blackwell Publishers, 1997:311–351.
10. Sullivan LE, Chawarski M, O'Connor PG, et al. The practice of office-based buprenorphine treatment of opioid dependence: is it associated with new patients entering into treatment? *Drug Alcohol Depend* 2005;79(1):113–116.
11. Friedmann PD, Saitz R. Management of adults recovering from alcohol or other drug problems: relapse prevention in primary care. *JAMA* 1998;279:1227–1231.
12. McLellan AT, Arndt IO, Metzger DS, et al. The effects of psychosocial services in substance abuse treatment. *JAMA* 1993;269:1953–1959.
13. McLellan AT, Hagan TA, Levine M, et al. Supplemental social services improve outcomes in public addiction treatment. *Addiction* 1998;93: 1489–1499.
14. Institute of Medicine. *Improving the quality of healthcare for mental and substance-use conditions: the quality chasm series.* Washington, DC: The National Academies Press, 2005.
15. Friedmann PD, Hendrickson JC, Gerstein DR, et al. Do mechanisms that link addiction treatment patients to primary care influence subsequent utilization of emergency and hospital care. *Med Care* 2006; 44(1):8–15.
16. Schermer CR, Moyers TB, Miller WR, Bloomfield LA. Trauma center brief interventions for alcohol disorders decrease subsequent driving under the influence arrests. *J Trauma* 2006;60(1):29–34.
17. Chappel JN, Schnoll SH. Physician attitudes: effect on the treatment of chemically dependent patients. *JAMA* 1977;237:2318–2319.
18. Lewis DC, Niven RG, Czechowicz D. A review of medical education in alcohol and other drug abuse. *JAMA* 1987;257:2945–2948.
19. Geller G, Levine DM, Mamon JA, et al. Knowledge, attitudes, and reported practices of medical students and house staff regarding the diagnosis and treatment of alcoholism. *JAMA* 1989;261:3115–3120.
20. Adger H, Macdonald DI, Wenger S. Core competencies for involvement of health care providers in the care of children and adolescents in families affected by substance abuse. *Pediatrics* 1999;103:1083–1084.
21. Brown RL, Marcus M, Amodeo M, et al. The HRSA-AMERSA interdisciplinary faculty development fellowship program in substance abuse [abstract]. *Subst Abuse* 2001;22:127.
22. Fiellin DA, Butler R, D'Onofrio G, et al. The physician's role in caring for patients with substance use disorders: implications for medical education and training. *Subst Abuse* 2002;23(3 suppl):207–212.
23. Isaacson JH, Fleming M, Kraus M, et al. A national survey of training in substance use disorders in residency programs. *J Stud Alcohol* 2000;61: 912–915.
24. Sirica C, ed. *Training about alcohol and substance abuse for all primary care physicians* [conference proceedings, October 2–5, 1994]. New York: Josiah Macy Jr. Foundation, 1995.
25. Haack MR, Adger H. Strategic plan for interdisciplinary faculty development. Arming the nation's health professional workforce for a new approach to substance use disorders. *Subst Abuse* 2002;23(Suppl 3).
26. Friedmann PD, McCullough D, Chin MH, et al. Screening and intervention for alcohol problems. A national survey of primary care physicians and psychiatrists. *J Gen Intern Med* 2000;15:84–91.
27. Cohen P, Cohen J. The clinician's illusion. *Arch Gen Psychiatry* 1984;41:1178–1182.
28. Adams A, Ockene JK Wheeler EV, et al. Alcohol counseling: physicians will do it. *J Gen Intern Med* 1998;13:692–698.
29. Saitz R, Sullivan LM, Samet JH. Training community-based clinicians in screening and brief intervention for substance abuse problems: translating evidence into practice. *Subst Abuse* 2000;21:21–32.
30. D'Onofrio G, Nadel ES, Degutis LC, et al. Improving emergency medicine residents' approach to patients with alcohol problems: a controlled educational trial. *Ann Emerg Med* 2002;40:50–62.
31. Goldman W, McCulloch J, Sturm R. Costs and use of mental health services before and after managed care. *Health Affairs* 1998;17: 40–52.
32. Schoenbaum M, Zhang W, Sturm R. Costs and utilization of substance abuse care in a privately insured population under managed care. *Psychiatr Serv* 1998;49:1573–1578.
33. Gentilello LM, Ebel BE, Wickizer TM, et al. Alcohol interventions for trauma patients treated in emergency departments and hospitals: a cost benefit analysis. *Ann Surg* 2005;241(4):541–550.
34. Larson MJ, Samet JH, McCarty D. Managed care of substance abuse disorders. Implications for generalist physicians. *Med Clin North Am* 1997;81:1053–1069.
35. Stein B, Reardon E, Sturm R. Substance abuse service utilization under managed care: HMOs versus carve-out plans. *J Behav Health Serv Res* 1999;26:451–456.
36. Sturm R. Tracking changes in behavioral health services: how have carve-outs changed care? *J Behav Health Serv Res* 1999;26:360–371.
37. Sturm R, McCulloch J. Mental health and substance abuse benefits in carve-out plans and the Mental Health Parity Act of 1996. *J Health Care Fin* 1998;24:82–92.
38. Sturm R, Zhang W, Schoenbaum M. How expensive are unlimited substance abuse benefits under managed care? *J Behav Health Serv Res* 1999; 26:203–210.
39. Goldman HH, Frank RG, Burnam MA, et al. Behavioral health insurance parity for federal employees. *N Engl J Med.* 2006;354(13): 1378–1386.

40. McLellan AT, Woody GE, Metzger D, et al. Evaluating the effectiveness of addiction treatments: reasonable expectations, appropriate comparisons. *Milbank Q* 1996;74:51–85.
41. McLellan AT, Lewis DC, O'Brien CP, et al. Drug dependence, a chronic medical illness: implications for treatment, insurance, and outcomes evaluation. *JAMA* 2000;284:1689–1695.
42. O'Brien CP, McLellan AT. Myths about the treatment of addiction. *Lancet* 1996;347:237–240.
43. Bosl RH. The illusion of parity [letter]. *Intern Med News* 2001;8.
44. Gourevitch MN, Chatterji P, Deb N, et al. On-site medical care in methadone maintenance: associations with health care use and expenditures. *J Subst Abuse Treat* 2007;32(2):143–151.
45. Saitz R, Horton NJ, Larson MJ, Winter M. Primary medical care and reductions in addiction severity: a prospective cohort study. *Addiction* 2005;100:70–78.
46. Bodenheimer T. Disease management in the American market. *Br Med J* 2000;320:563–566.
47. Kimball HR, Young PR. Statement on the generalist physician from the American Boards of Family Practice and Internal Medicine. *JAMA* 1994;271:315-316.
48. Saitz R, Mulvey KP, Samet JH. The substance abusing patient and primary care: linkage via the addiction treatment system? *Subst Abuse* 1997b;18:187–195.
49. Center for Substance Abuse Treatment. *State methadone maintenance treatment guidelines*. Rockville, MD: CSAT, Substance Abuse and Mental Health Services Administration, 1993. DHHS Publication No. SMA 93-1991.
50. Umbricht-Schneiter A, Ginn DH, Pabst KM, et al. Providing medical care to methadone clinic patients: referral vs. on-site. *Am J Public Health* 1994;84:207–210.
51. Teitelbaum M, Walker A, Gabay M, et al. *Analysis of barriers to the delivery of integrated primary care services and substance abuse treatment: case studies of nine linkage program projects*. Rockville, MD: Health Resources and Services Administration and Abt Associates, Inc., 1992.
52. Alford DP, LaBelle C, Richardson JM, et al. Treating homeless opioid dependent patients with buprenorphine in an office-based setting. *J Gen Intern Med* 2007;22:171–176.
53. Anton RF, O'Malley SS. Combined pharmacotherapies and behavioral interventions for alcohol dependence: the COMBINE study: a randomized controlled trial. *JAMA* 2006;295:2003–2017.
54. Ashery RS, ed. *Progress and issues in case management* (NIH publication no. ADM 92-1946). Rockville, MD: National Institute on Drug Abuse, 1992.
55. Bach-Beisel J, Scott J, Dixon L. Co-occurring severe mental illness and substance use disorders: a review of recent research. *Psychiatr Serv* 1999;50:1427–1434.
56. Willenbring ML, Olson DH, Bielinski J, et al. Treatment of medically ill alcoholics in the primary-care setting. In: Beresford T, Gomberg E, eds. *Alcohol and aging*. New York: Oxford University Press, 1995: 249–259.
57. Finney JW, Willenbring ML, Moos RH. Improving the quality of VA care for patients with substance-use disorders: the Quality Enhancement Research Initiative (QUERI) substance abuse module. *Med Care* 2000; 38:I105–I113.
58. Fleming MF, Mundt MP, French MT, et al. Benefit-cost analysis of brief physician advice with problem drinkers in primary care settings. *Med Care* 2000;38:7–18.
59. Ockene JK, Adams A, Hurley TG, et al. Brief physician and nurse practitioner-delivered counseling for high-risk drinkers: Does it work. *Arch Intern Med* 1999;159:2198–2205.
60. Kristenson H, Ohlin H, Hulten-Nosslin MB, et al. Identification and intervention of heavy drinking in middle-aged men: results and follow-up of 24-60 months of long-term study with randomized controls. *Alcohol Clin Exp Res* 1983;7:203–209.
61. Saitz R, Horton NJ, Sullivan LM, et al. Addressing alcohol problems in primary care: a cluster randomized, controlled trial of a systems intervention. The screening and intervention in primary care (SIP) study. *An Intern Med* 2003;138(5):372–382.
62. O'Connor PG, Farren CK, Rounsaville BJ, et al. A preliminary investigation of the management of alcohol dependence with naltrexone by primary care providers. *Am J Med* 1997;103:477–482.
63. Bray JH, Rogers JC. The linkages project: training behavioral health professionals for collaborative practice with primary care physicians. *Fam Syst Health* 1997;15:55–61.
64. Kunnes R, Niven R, Gustafson T. Financing and payment reform for primary health care and substance abuse treatment. *J Addict Dis* 1993; 12:23–42.
65. Geirsson M, Bendtsen P, Spak F. Attitudes of Swedish general practitioners and nurses to working with lifestyle change, with special reference to alcohol consumption. *Alcohol Alcohol* 2005;40(5):388–393.
66. O'Connor PG, Oliveto AH, Shi JM. A randomized trial of buprenorphine maintenance for heroin dependence in a primary care clinic for substance users versus a methadone clinic. *Am J Med* 1998;105: 100–105.
67. Barry DT. Patient satisfaction with primary care office-based buprenorphine/naloxone treatment. *J Gen Intern Med* 2007;22(2):242–245.
68. Merrill JO, Jackson TR, Schulman BA, et al. Methadone medical maintenance in primary care. An implementation evaluation. *J Gen Intern Med* 2005;20(4):344–349.
69. Litwin AH, Kunins HV, Berg KM, et al. Hepatitis C management by addiction medicine physicians: results from a national survey. *J Subst Abuse Treat* 2007;33(1):99–105.
70. Sylvestre DL, Clements BJ. Adherence to hepatitis C treatment in recovering heroin users maintained on methadone. *Eur J Gastroenterol Hepatol* 2007;19(9):741–747.
71. Berk SI, Litwin AH. Effects of pegylated interferon alfa-2b on the pharmacokinetic and pharmacodynamic properties of methadone: a prospective, nonrandomized, crossover study in patients coinfected with hepatitis C and HIV receiving methadone maintenance treatment. *Clin Ther* 2007;29(1):131–138.
72. O'Connor PG, Shi JM, Henry S, et al. Tuberculosis chemoprophylaxis using a liquid isoniazid-methadone admixture for drug users in methadone maintenance. *Addiction* 1999;94(7):1071–1075.
73. Friedmann PD, Alexander JA, Jin L, et al. On-site primary care and mental health services in outpatient drug abuse treatment units. *J Behav Health Serv Res* 1999;26:80–94.
74. Saxon AJ, Malte CA, Sloan KL, et al. Randomized Trial of Onsite Versus Referral Primary Medical Care for Veterans in Addictions Treatment. *Med Care* 2006;44(4):334–342.
75. Parthasarathy S, Mertens J, Moore C, et al. Utilization and cost impact of integrating substance abuse treatment and primary care. *Med Care* 2003;41(3):357–367.
76. Baker F. *Coordination of alcohol, drug abuse, and mental health services*. Rockville, MD: Center for Substance Abuse Treatment; 1991. (Publication no. SMA 00-3360, Technical Assistance Publication Series, No. 4.)
77. Crits-Christoph P, Siqueland L. Psychosocial treatment for drug abuse: selected review and recommendations for national health care. *Arch Gen Psychiatry* 1996;53:749–756.
78. Mechanic D. Integrating mental health into a general health care system. *Hosp Community Psychiatry* 1999;45:893–897.
79. Weisner C, Schmidt LA. Expanding the frame of health services research in the drug abuse field. *Hosp Serv Res* 1995;30:707–726.
80. Brindis CD, Pfeffer R, Wolfe A. A case management program for chemically dependent clients with multiple needs. *J Case Manage* 1995;4: 22–28.
81. Friedmann PD, D'Aunno TA, Jin L, et al. Medical and psychosocial services in drug abuse treatment: do stronger linkages promote client utilization. *Hosp Serv Res* 2000;35:443–465.
82. Samet JH, Saitz R, Larson MJ. A case for enhanced linkage of substance abusers to primary medical care. *Subst Abuse* 1996;17:181–199.
83. Peter D, Hart Research Associates. *The road to recovery a landmark national study on public perceptions of alcoholism and barriers to treatment*. New York: The Recovery Institute, 1999.
84. Samet JH, Larson MJ, Horton NJ, et al. Linking alcohol and drug dependent adults to primary medical care: a randomized controlled trial

of a multidisciplinary health evaluation in a detoxification unit (the Health Evaluation and Linkage to Primary Care [HELP] Study). *Addiction* 2003;98:509-516.

85. Friedmann PD, Lemon SC, Stein MD, et al. Linkage to medical services in the Drug Abuse Treatment Outcome Study. *Med Care* 2001;39:284–295.
86. Schwartz M, Baker G, Mulvey KP, et al. Improving publicly funded substance abuse treatment: the value of case management. *Am J Public Health* 1997;87:1659–1664.
87. McLellan AT, Hagan TA, Levine M, et al. Does clinical case management improve outpatient addiction treatment. *Drug Alcohol Depend* 1999;55:91-103.
88. Wagner EH. The role of patient care teams in chronic disease management. *Br Med J* 2000;320:569–572.
89. Wagner EH, Austin BT, Von Korff M. Organizing care for patients with chronic illness. *Milbank Q* 1996;74:511–544.
90. Newschaffer CJ, Laine C, Hauck WW, et al. Clinic characteristics associated with reduced hospitalization of drug users with AIDS. *J Urban Health* 1998;75:153–169.
91. Selwyn PA, Budner NW, Wasserman WC, et al. Utilization of onsite primary care services by HIV-seropositive and seronegative drug users in a methadone maintenance program. *Public Health Rep* 1993;108:492–500.
92. Laine C, Hauck WW, Gourevitch MN, et al. Regular outpatient medical and drug abuse care and subsequent hospitalization of persons who use illicit drugs. *JAMA* 2001;285:2355–2362.
93. Basu S, Smith-Rohrberg D, Bruce RD, et al. Models for integrating buprenorphine therapy into the primary HIV care setting. *Clin Infect Dis* 2006;42(5):716–721.
94. Weisner C, Mertens J, Parthasarathy S, et al. Improved effectiveness from integrating primary medical care with addiction treatment. A randomized controlled trial. *JAMA* 2001;286:1715–1723.
95. O'Toole TP. Substance-abusing urban homeless in the late 1990s: how do they differ from non-substance-abusing homeless persons. *J Urban Health* 2004;81(4):606–617.
96. Fazel S, Bains P, Doll H. Substance abuse and dependence in prisoners: a systematic review. *Addiction* 2006;101:181–191.
97. Rich JD, Boutwell AE, Shield DC, et al. Attitudes and practices regarding the use of methadone in U.S. state and federal prisons. *J Urban Health* 2005;82(3):411–419.
98. Belenko S, Peugh J. Estimating drug treatment needs among state prison inmates. *Drug Alcohol Depend* 2005;77:269–281.
99. O'Connor PG, Waugh ME, Carroll K, et al. Primary care-based ambulatory opioid detoxification: the results of a clinical trial. *J Gen Intern Med* 1995;10:255–260.
100. Liebschutz JM, Mulvey KP. Victimization among substance-abusing women. Worse health outcomes. *Arch Intern Med* 1997;157:1093–1097.
101. O'Connor PG, Selwyn PA, Schottenfeld RS. Medical care for injection-drug users with human immunodeficiency virus infection. *N Engl J Med* 1994;331:450–459.
102. Schiff ER. Hepatitis C and alcohol. *Hepatology* 1997;26:39S–42S.
103. Sporer KA. Acute heroin overdose. *Ann Intern Med* 1999;130:584–590.
104. National Institute on Drug Abuse & National Institute on Alcohol Abuse and Alcoholism. In: Harwood HJ, Fountain D, Livermore D, eds. *The economic costs of alcohol and drug abuse in the United States—1992.* Washington, DC: Author, 1998. Retrieved June 25, 2001, from http://www.nida.nih.gov/economiccosts/index.html.
105. St. Peter RF, Reed MC, Kemper P, et al. Changes in the scope of care provided by primary care physicians. *N Engl J Med* 1999;341:1980–1985.
106. Saitz R, Horton NJ, Sullivan LM, et al. Addressing alcohol problems in primary care: a cluster randomized, controlled trial of a systems intervention (the Screening and Intervention in Primary Care [SIP] Study). *Ann Intern Med* 2003 Mar 4; 138(5):372–382.
107. Saitz R, Larson M, LaBelle C, et al. The case for chronic disease management for addiction *J Addict Med* 2008;2(2):55–65.
108. Samet JA, Stein MD. Models of medical care for HIV-infected drug users. *Subst Abuse* 1995;16:131–139.
109. Willenbring ML, Olson DH. A randomized trial of integrated outpatient treatment for medically ill alcoholic men. *Arch Intern Med* 1999;159:1946–1952.

CHAPTER 29

David Y-W Lee, PhD
Hong Wang, MD, PhD

Alternative Therapies for Alcohol and Drug Addiction

Addiction is a complex process with physiologic, behavioral, psychologic, and social components, so treatment is usually multifaceted. There are two fundamental approaches: prevention of the onset of compulsive use and prevention of relapse and the craving that leads to relapse. In the past, much medical attention has been directed at the symptoms of acute abstinence (detoxification), and these symptoms can be treated with available therapies and medications. However, relapse, which is often precipitated by withdrawal and/or intense craving even after prolonged abstinence, poses the most serious therapeutic challenge. In view of the complexity of drug dependence and a limited number of effective treatments, it is conceivable that certain selected alternative pharmacotherapies may have important clinical significance. This chapter reviews traditional herbal medicines and therapies for the prevention of drug and alcohol relapse.

HERBAL REMEDIES WITH ANTI-ADDICTIVE POTENTIALS

Poppy has been known in China for 12 centuries and its medicinal use for 9 centuries. Opiates, alkaloids derived from poppy, effectively activate the endogenous opioid system in the body. This activation produces many cardiovascular, endocrine, immune, and neuropsychologic effects including euphoria, analgesia, and addiction. It has been clear that the effects of opiate drugs are mediated through interaction with opioid receptors. Moreover, studies of the binding of various related opioid compounds in the brain indicate the existence of a multitude of opioid-receptor types and subtypes such as μ-, κ-, and δ (1). Since the rewarding effects of opiates are mediated through action at μ-opioid receptors, interference with actions at these receptors presents a rational strategy for developing medications for opiate addiction (2,3). Specifically, medications that block activation of μ-opioid receptors (e.g., naltrexone) might reduce drug-seeking behavior (1,3,4).

It was not until the middle of the 19th century that smoking opium for recreational purposes was practiced throughout China. The quantity of opium imported into China rose from 5,000 chests in 1820 to 16,000 in 1830, 20,000 in 1838, and 70,000 in 1858. After more than a century of steady demoralization, with half the Chinese population (nearly that of the U.S. population today) addicted, China finally determined to give up opium, which ultimately led to the "Opium Wars." During this period, Chinese herbal remedies were developed for treating addiction or relieving the withdrawal syndrome.

The Chinese remedies developed during the Opium Wars era were combinations of more than a dozen herbs, thus a mixture of herbs may well represent a multitargeted approach acting on opioid receptors that would have the benefits of improved overall efficacy with reduced toxicity. However, it is necessary to isolate and characterize the bioactive compounds as well as elucidate the mechanism of actions for further development of safe and complementary natural medications for drug abuse. Few original remedies have been investigated scientifically. One, YGT (NPI-025), consists of five herbs (Qiang Huo, Gou Teng, Chun Xiong, Fu Zi, and Yan Hu Suo) most frequently used for substance abuse treatment in China. Yang et al. (5) studied YGT among 300 individuals with addiction

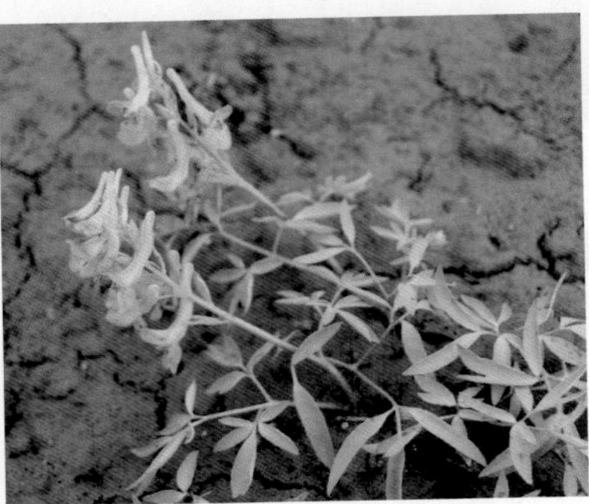

FIGURE 29.1. *Corydalis yanhusuo.*

over a 10-year period and reported that NPI-025 significantly reduced withdrawal symptoms (−48%) compared to addicts without treatment. Follow-up visits of many "cured" patients 1 to 3 years after treatment revealed that NPI-025 was helpful in overcoming craving for drugs.

After the cloning of the mouse κ-opioid receptor (6,7), μ, δ, and κ-receptors of several species were cloned (for reviews, see 8,9). These cloned opioid receptors provide excellent tools for pharmacologic screening of traditional remedies for drug abuse. For instance, YGT (NPI-025), used clinically in Hong Kong (5,10), was subjected to bioactivity-guided fractionation and showed potent opioid receptor-binding activities (11). These studies provide important evidence for further development of such natural products.

Corydalis yanhusuo *Corydalis yanhusuo* (Fig. 29.1) is one of the five Chinese medicinal plants in NPI-025. Chemical fractionation resulted in the isolation and characterization of *d,l*-tetrahydropalmatine *d,l*-THP; Fig. 29.2) as one of the bioactive components. Optical resolution or chemical synthesis resulted in pure *l*-THP, which is the active compound with significant binding activities to D1 and D5 dopamine receptors (Fig. 29.2).

Dopamine Receptors and Pharmacologic Actions of *l*-THP Despite extensive research for new approaches, there is currently no effective pharmacotherapy for cocaine or methamphetamine addiction (12–14) The effects of *l*-THP on cocaine and methamphetamine self-administration have been demonstrated (15,16) Cocaine binds differentially to the dopamine-, serotonin-, and norepinephrine-transporter proteins and directly prevents the reuptake of dopamine, serotonin, and norepinephrine into presynaptic neurons (17–19). Inhibition of reuptake subsequently elevates the synaptic concentrations of each of these neurotransmitters, thus reduces craving for cocaine and methamphetamine.

Two types of dopamine receptors, D1 class and D2 class, mediate dopamine neurotransmission. The D1 class includes both D1 and D5 receptors, while the D2 class includes D2, D3, and D4 receptors (20). There is a high-density distribution of D1 and D2 receptors in the striatum, which is relevant to the pharmacology of cocaine. Recent preclinical studies suggest that drugs that are selective for D1 or D2 receptors may effectively reduce some aspects of cocaine self-stimulation (21,22) or ethanol self-administration (23). Though both selective D1 and D2 receptor agonists can reduce cocaine self-administration, these agents can also mimic the discriminative stimulus produced by cocaine and stimulate locomotor activity (24–26); therefore, there is a risk that these drugs may also have abuse potential and would not be ideal for cocaine treatment.

Though selective D1 receptor agonists or D2 receptor antagonists might modulate cocaine-induced behavior (27), they have side effects that prevent them from becoming useful therapeutic agents. Indeed, preliminary clinical studies have not provided promising results (28,29). Because of the limited success of these selective compounds, interest has turned to drugs that may have dual actions. In particular, a drug that stimulates D1 receptors and blocks D2 receptors may have the right profile to become a promising treatment for cocaine or drug abuse. A recent study of one such compound, an ergoline derivative (LEK-8829) with D1 agonistic and D2 antagonist characteristics attenuated reinstatement of cocaine seeking induced by cocaine priming injections and diminished cocaine intake in cocaine self-administration sessions (30). Thus, it has a better profile than selective D1 receptor agonists alone for inhibiting cocaine self-administration. Furthermore, LEK-8829 reduced cocaine reinstatement behavior but did not induce reinstatement of cocaine. The combined results suggest that the strategy of using compounds with dual D1 receptor agonist/D2 receptor antagonist properties to treat drug addiction is worth pursuing.

Similar to LEK-8829, plant-derived *l*-THP has both D1 receptor agonist and D2 receptor antagonist actions. Its effects on cocaine and methamphetamine addiction have been demonstrated (15,16) *l*-THP could suppress the expression of stimulant-induced conditioned place preference (CPP). *L*-THP could also block the discrimination behavior for methamphetamine and the reestablishment after its distinction. Interestingly, it has been reported that *l*-THP suppresses

FIGURE 29.2. Structure of dopamine, isocorypalmine, and *l*-tetrahydropalmatine (THP).

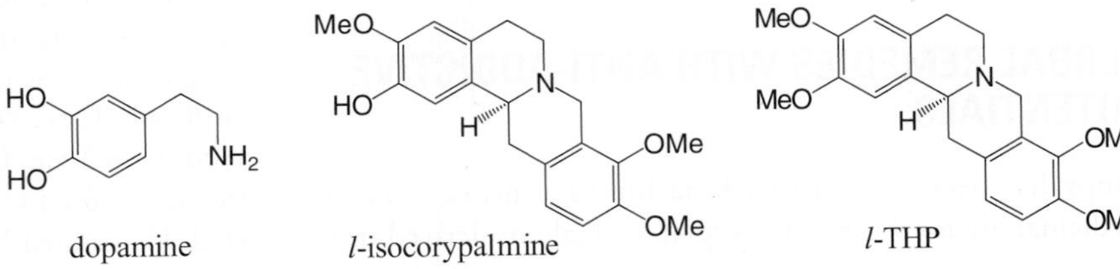

dopamine

l-isocorypalmine

l-THP

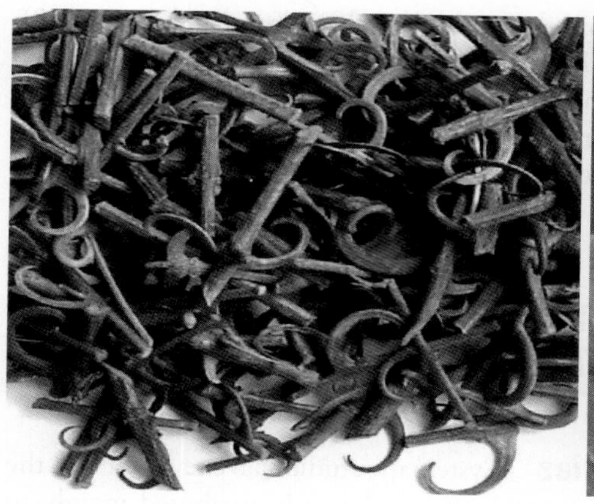

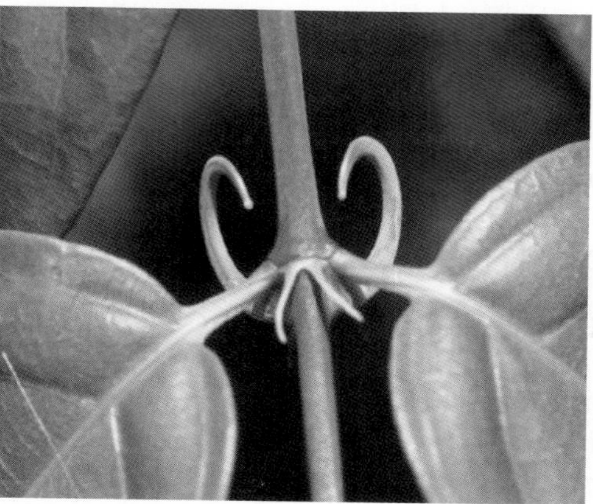

FIGURE 29.3. Uncaria rhynchophylla.

the craving/relapse for cocaine in addiction. Thus, these findings strongly suggest that *l*-THP could be a novel natural medication for inhibiting the craving/relapse of the psychostimulants addiction including cocaine and methamphetamine.

In summary, *l*-THP and isocorypalmine, a demethylated analog of *l*-THP, are two interesting compounds isolated from *Corydalis yanhusuo*. In vitro binding study showed that both *l*-THP and *l*-isocorypalmine have affinity toward D1 and D5 receptors. In the functional assay, *d,l*-isocorypalmine is more potent than *l*-THP as D1 and D5 partial agonists. It is interesting to note that the partial skeleton of both *l*-THP and isocorypalmine resembles the dopamine molecule (Fig. 29.2) with different number of methoxy-group attached. These bioactive compounds derived from fractionation and in vitro screening may provide a better understanding of the mechanism of action of NPI-025 as a whole.

Uncaria rhynchophylla *Uncaria rhynchophylla* (Fig. 29.3) is an important traditional Chinese medicine used in the treatment of pain, infantile convulsions, headaches, dizziness, hypertension, and rheumatoid arthritis. *U. rhynchophylla* is another ingredient in NPI-025 (5). In order to clarify the mechanism of action, 12 compounds have been isolated by solvent extraction, followed by silica gel fractionation and Toyopearl HW-40, MCI gel column chromatography. Two major alkaloids, rhynchophylline and isorhynchophylline (Fig. 29.4), have been identified as the anti-addictive components with moderate binding activity for dopamine receptors [^{3}H]DIP rMOR and [^{3}H]DIP mDOR.

TRANSCUTANEOUS ELECTRICAL ACUPUNCTURE STIMULATION AS A NONINVASIVE ALTERNATIVE THERAPY FOR ALCOHOL AND DRUG ABUSE

In a serendipitous observation in 1972, Dr. H. L. Wen in Hong Kong noted that electroacupuncture relieved a patient's withdrawal from opium (31). Dr. Wen and Dr. Cheung at the Kwong Wah Hospital (31) subsequently reported that, in a study of 40 individuals addicted to heroin and/or opium, acupuncture combined with electrical stimulation was effective in relieving withdrawal. This method was later adopted in

Rhynchophylline

Isorhynchophylline

3,4-dihydroxytoluene

2,5-dihydroxypyranone

Chlorogenic acid

FIGURE 29.4. Structures of rhynchophylline and isorhynchophylline.

many clinical settings in Western countries, including the Lincoln Hospital in New York. However, the body acupuncture points originally used by Wen and Cheung on the arm and hand were gradually omitted, with only auricular acupuncture being used (32), and electrical stimulation also was omitted, leaving only needles staying in situ. Whether these two omissions will affect therapeutic efficacy deserves further investigation.

The discovery of morphine-like substances (endorphins) in the mammalian brain (33) had a great impact on acupuncture research. It was soon made clear that acupuncture-induced analgesia (manual needling) can be blocked by the narcotic antagonist naloxone, suggesting the involvement of endogenous opioid substances (34). In animal experiments, manual acupuncture or acupuncture combined with electrical stimulation (electroacupuncture, or EA) was shown to accelerate the production and release of endorphins that can interact with different kinds of opioid receptors to ease pain (35). It was further clarified that endorphins are, in fact, a group of neuropeptides possessing different characteristics. Among these neuropeptides, β-endorphin and enkephalin are primarily agonists at μ- and δ-opioid receptors, whereas dynorphin is an agonist at κ-receptors (36). Interestingly, electrical stimulation of different frequencies can induce the release of different kinds of endorphins. For example, low-frequency (2 to 4 Hz) EA accelerates the release of enkephalins to interact with μ- and δ-receptors, whereas high-frequency (100 Hz) EA accelerates the release of dynorphin to interact with κ-receptors (37). These findings strengthen the scientific basis of this ancient healing art and point the way to its use in areas beyond pain control.

It is natural to hypothesize that, if acupuncture can release endogenous opioids in the brain to ease pain, it might relieve withdrawal symptoms. In fact, the first observation made by Dr. Wen in 1972 was that he attempted to use acupuncture for reducing surgical pain and incidentally found that it ameliorated the opiate withdrawal syndrome. This hypothesis was tested in morphine-dependent rats. Withdrawal signs were significantly reduced by high-frequency (100 Hz) EA administered on the hind limb acupoints St 36 and Sp 6 (38). This effect was much greater than that induced by low-frequency (2 Hz) stimulation. On the basis of these results, EA was applied to heroin addicts and obtained very promising results. However, it was inconvenient for patients to go to the clinic for treatment several times a day. As a result, they missed sessions, thus affecting the therapeutic outcome. One possible solution was to have patients treat themselves by using acupoints stimulation without a needle but still under the control of a physician. To overcome this problem, Han et al. developed a constant current electrical stimulator: Han's Acupoint Nerve Stimulator (HANS).

Experiments in the rat using HANS showed that electrical stimulation applied at the surface of the skin over acupoints can produce an analgesic effect similar to that produced by EA (39). Satisfactory results were obtained using this transcutaneous electrical acupoint stimulation (TEAS) by HANS for the treatment of heroin withdrawal syndrome in humans (40). Later, the method was shown to suppress CPP, an animal model of craving for drugs of abuse for morphine in rats (41). Subsequent human studies revealed that this form of stimulation could indeed suppress craving in heroin-dependent patients.

OPIATE DETOXIFICATION WITH TRANSCUTANEOUS ELECTRICAL ACUPUNCTURE STIMULATION

Animal Studies Systematic studies have revealed that the mechanism of acupuncture analgesia is attributed mainly to the increased release of endogenous opioid peptides in the central nervous system (CNS) (35). A rational extrapolation would be that the activation of the endogenous opioid system by acupuncture should ease opiate withdrawal symptoms.

Transauricular electrostimulation was reported to suppress the naloxone-induced morphine withdrawal syndrome in mice (42) and rats (43). Auriacombe et al. (44) demonstrated that Transcutaneous Electro-Nerve Stimulation (TENS) with an intermittent high-frequency current effectively attenuated signs in the rat after abrupt cessation of morphine; the mechanism remains obscure. Based on the findings that low-frequency EA (2 Hz) accelerated the release of β-endorphin and enkephalin in the CNS, whereas high-frequency EA (100 Hz) accelerated the release of dynorphin (37,45) in the spinal cord, the effect of EA was tested in naloxone-precipitated morphine withdrawal in the rat. Because the effect of 2 Hz EA is to accelerate the release of the morphine-like opioid peptides enkephalin and endorphin, it was predicted that 2 Hz would be more effective than 100 Hz in replacing morphine and ameliorating the abstinence syndrome. However, 2 Hz was only marginally effective in reducing two of five withdrawal signs, whereas 100 Hz suppressed all five signs (38).

Human Studies To observe the effect of TEAS on the withdrawal syndrome in heroin-dependent patients, the method was applied for 30 minutes once a day for 10 days in an addiction treatment center (40). In addition to a standard questionnaire, two objective parameters were measured-heart rate and body weight.

Single Treatment To observe the immediate effect on heart rate, the two pairs of output leads were placed on four acupoints in the upper extremities: one pair at *Hegu* (LI4) on the dorsum of the hand and on the palmar aspect of the hand opposite to LI4 *Laogon*, P-8) to complete the circuit, the other pair at *Neiguan* (PC6) on the palmar side of the forearm 2 inches above the palmar groove between the two tendons, and *Waiguan* (TE5) on the opposite side of PC6. A dense-and-disperse (DD) mode of stimulation was administered, with 2 Hz alternating automatically with 100 Hz, each lasting 3 seconds. This mode was shown to release four of the opioid peptides in the CNS (37), thus producing maximal

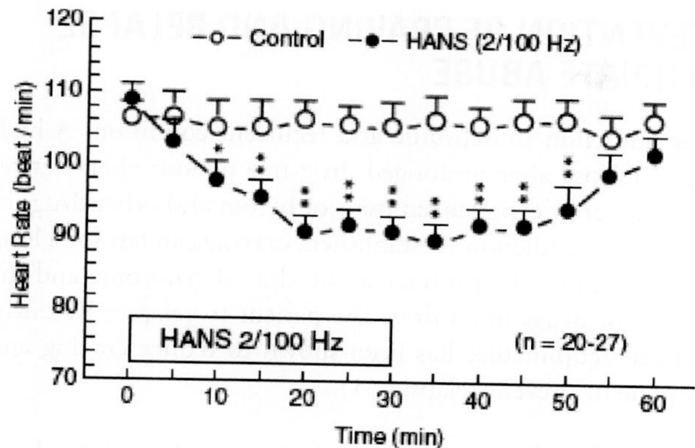

FIGURE 29.5. Effects of 2/100 Hz electric stimulation (HANS) on the heart rate of heroin addicts during episodes of withdrawal. *,** represent $p < 0.05$ and p , 0.01, respectively, compared with control groups. (Reprinted with permission from Han JS, Trachtenberg AI, Lowinson JH. Acupuncture. In: Lowinson JH, et al., eds. *Substance abuse: a comprehensive textbook.* Philadelphia: Lippincott Williams & Wilkins, 2004:743–782.)

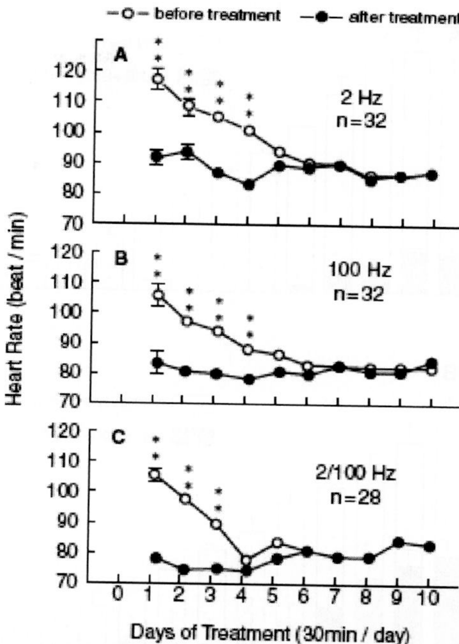

FIGURE 29.6. Changes of heart rate before and after treatment by TEAS administered every day: A normalization of the heart rate was obtained by day 4 **(C)** or day 5 **(A and B)**. ** $p < 0.01$ compared with after treatment (ANOVA). (Reprinted with permission from Han JS, Trachtenberg AI, Lowinson JH. Acupuncture. In: Lowinson JH, et al., eds. *Substance abuse: a comprehensive textbook.* Philadelphia: Lippincott Williams & Wilkins, 2004:743–782.)

therapeutic effect. The control group received the same placement of electrodes, which were disconnected from the circuitry. The average heart rate of the abstinent addicts was 109 beats per minute before treatment. DD stimulation for 30 minutes reduced the heart rate significantly, as shown in Figure 29.5. Reduction occurred within the first 5 to 10 minutes, continued for 20 minutes, and plateaued at 90 per minute in the last 10 minutes. The after-effect remained for 20 minutes, after which the heart rate began to return to the original level (46).

Multiple Treatment To observe the cumulative effect of multiple daily treatments with TEAS, 117 heroin addicts were divided randomly into four groups. Three groups received TEAS of 2 Hz (constant frequency), 100 Hz (constant frequency), or 2/100 Hz (2 Hz alternating with 100 Hz, DD mode). The control group received mock stimulation, where the skin electrodes were placed on the points and connected to the stimulator with blinking signals but with the electric circuitry disconnected. The treatment was applied for 30 minutes a day over 10 consecutive days. Heart rate was measured with an electrocardiogram before and immediately after the TEAS stimulation. Figure 29.6 shows the results. In the 2-Hz group, for example, on the first day of observation, the heart rate averaged 110, which dropped to 90 immediately after the TEAS treatment $p < 0.01$). On the second day, the heart rate averaged 102, then fell to 91 after TEAS $p < 0.01$). This trend continued for days 3 and 4. On day 5, there was no significant difference before and after the treatment (91 vs. 89), suggesting that the rate had returned to "normal" (40). In the three TEAS groups, 100 Hz produced a slightly better result than 2 Hz. In the 2/100 Hz group, the after-TEAS rate reached an even lower level (72 beats). Also, the 2/100 Hz returned to "normal" in day 4, 1 day earlier than the fixed frequency groups (day 5). In the control group (n = 30) receiving mock TEAS, the rate did not come down to 100 until the eighth day of treatment. These results suggest that repeated daily EA treatment is effective in reducing tachycardia in heroin addicts, with an order of DD > 100 Hz > 2 Hz (Fig. 29.5). Body weight was also affected. The patients ages ranged from 17 to 35, and their average weight was only 49 to 51 kg. In the control group receiving mock TEAS, weight declined by 1 kg at the end of the first week, probably owing to the presence of withdrawal distress. In the TEAS groups, weight had increased significantly after 4 days of treatment and continued to increase thereafter. By day 10, the TEAS groups weighed 5 kg more than the control group. This 10% increase was apparently due to reduced withdrawal symptoms and increased food and water intake. Though the DD mode was significantly better than the fixed frequency mode in reducing tachycardia, weight change did not differ among the three TEAS groups, suggesting that the mechanisms modulating heart rate and body weight may not be identical (40).

In clinical practice, opiate withdrawal symptoms could be reduced but not abolished by the TEAS treatment, especially in those cases with a history of heroin abuse for more

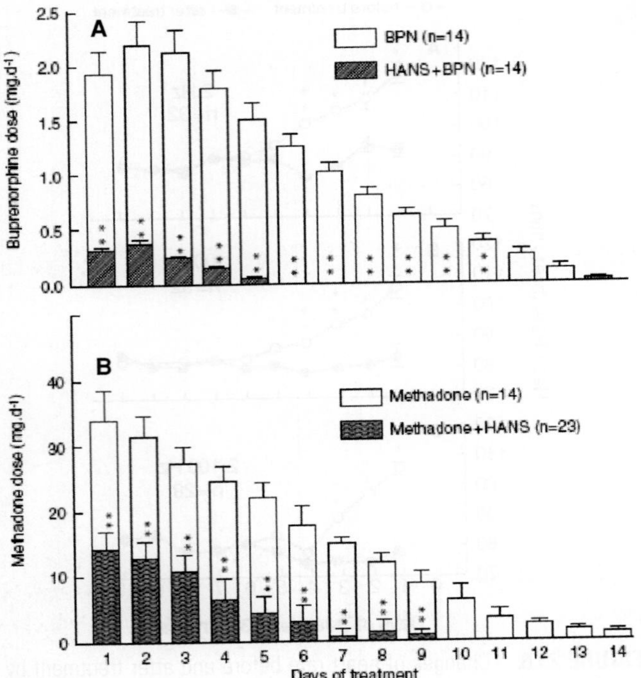

FIGURE 29.7. Influence of 2/100 Hz electric simulation (HANS) on the requirement of buprenorphine (BPN) (**A**) or methadone (**B**) for heroin detoxification. ** $p < 0.01$ compared with the corresponding control group. (Reprinted with permission from Han JS, Trachtenberg AI, Lowinson JH. Acupuncture. In: Lowinson JH, et al., eds. *Substance abuse: a comprehensive textbook.* Philadelphia: Lippincott Williams & Wilkins, 2004:743–782.)

than 5 years. To obtain a quantitative estimate of the efficacy of TEAS (47): (a) TEAS was applied on the acupoints *Hegu/Laogong, Neiguan/Waiguang* and *Xingjian/Sanyinjiao*). Buprenorphine (BPN, i.m.) was used as a supplement to TEAS when the patient experienced a specified degree of withdrawal distress and was given immediately upon request. The purpose of this arrangement was to maintain a comfortable detoxification procedure without any withdrawal syndrome. In this study, 28 heroin addicts were randomly divided into BPN only and TEAS+BPN groups. Figure 29.7A shows the results. The group receiving TEAS required only 8% of the BPN required by the group not receiving TEAS. This can be taken as a quantitative estimate of the effect of TEAS for opiate detoxification. The sharp difference observed between the mild and short-lasting therapeutic effect on day 1 (Fig. 29.5) and the large effect by day 14 (Fig. 29.7) suggests an accumulation of efficacy produced by repetitive treatments. A similar reduction occurred in another group of heroin addicts with a methadone-reduction protocol for the control group and "a TEAS (2/100 Hz) plus methadone" experimental group with a reduction of 75% methadone use for the TEAS + methadone group (48).

PREVENTION OF CRAVING AND RELAPSE TO OPIATE ABUSE

Drug addiction is a chronic and recurrent condition. A high rate of relapse after prolonged drug-free periods characterizes the behavior of experienced users of heroin and other drugs of abuse. Once addiction is established, craving can last for a long period of time. The protracted withdrawal syndrome and the craving for drugs often drive the patient to relapse. Recently, electrical acupuncture has been shown to reduce craving and postpone or prevent relapse (41).

Animal Studies Several animal procedures have been proposed to model craving (49). CPP has been frequently used (50). The drug (unconditioned stimulus) is given in one chamber of a two- or three-chamber apparatus, thereby becoming associated with the environmental stimuli unique to that chamber (color, floor texture, etc.). After repeated pairings, the rat will spend more time in the chamber associated with drug. The ratio between the times spent in drug-associated and vehicle-associated areas is assumed to reflect the degree of craving. CPP has been regarded as a relatively pure measure of psychic dependence in that the preference for the drug-associated chamber can be demonstrated when the rat is in the undrugged condition and free of withdrawal symptoms. Experiments were done to determine whether acupuncture could suppress the expression of CPP.

Wang et al. (41) were among the first to explore the effect of EA on morphine CPP in the rat. They found that 2 Hz and 2/100 Hz significantly suppressed CPP but that 100 Hz did not (Fig. 29.8A). Since the effect of EA can be reversed by a dose of the opioid receptor antagonist naloxone (Fig. 29.8B) that is sufficient to block μ- and δ- but not κ-receptors, it was concluded that the effect of EA is mediated by endogenously released μ- and δ-opioid agonists, most likely endorphins and enkephalins, to ease craving for exogenous opiate (in this case, morphine). Another issue deserving attention is that the effect of EA was demonstrable 12 hours after application. Acupuncture-induced analgesia usually disappears within 1 hour. Thus, EA might sensitize endogenous opioid circuits to produce a continuous release of opioid peptides, resulting in a long-lasting effect.

In the everyday life of the drug addicts, craving and relapse can be triggered by stress or by a very small dose of opioid. This phenomenon can be reproduced in the rat CPP model. Wang et al. (41) reported that morphine-induced CPP disappeared after a 9-day extinction period and was reinstated by foot shock stress or by a small dose of morphine or amphetamine. Reinstated CPP could be reversed by 2 Hz or 2/100 Hz EA, an effect easily reversed and by naloxone (51). However, the mechanisms of EA suppression of morphine CPP may involve different neural pathways.

Human Study of Cravings To obtain a quantitative estimate of suppression of craving in response to acupuncture or related techniques, a visual analogue scale (VAS) in heroin

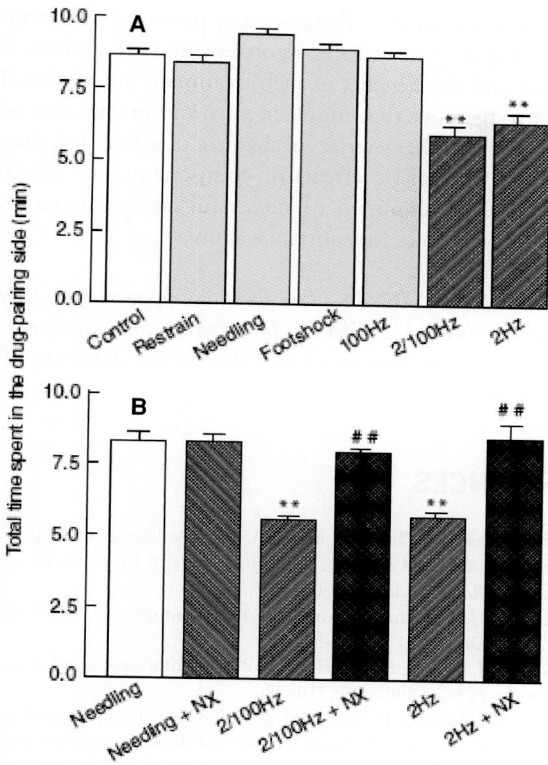

FIGURE 29.8. **A:** Effects of electroacupuncture on 4 mg/kg morphine-induced CPP (n = 11–12). ** $p < 0.01$, compared with four control groups as well as the group treated with 100 Hz stimulation. **B:** Naloxone blockade of the inhibitory effect of electroacupuncture on morphine-induced CPP (n = 9–0). ** $p < 0.01$, compared with needling control group. ## $p < 0.01$, compared with their corresponding naloxone treated group. (Reprinted with permission from Han JS, Trachtenberg AI, Lowinson JH. Acupuncture. In: Lowinson JH, et al., eds. *Substance abuse: a comprehensive textbook.* Philadelphia: Lippincott Williams & Wilkins, 2004:743–782.)

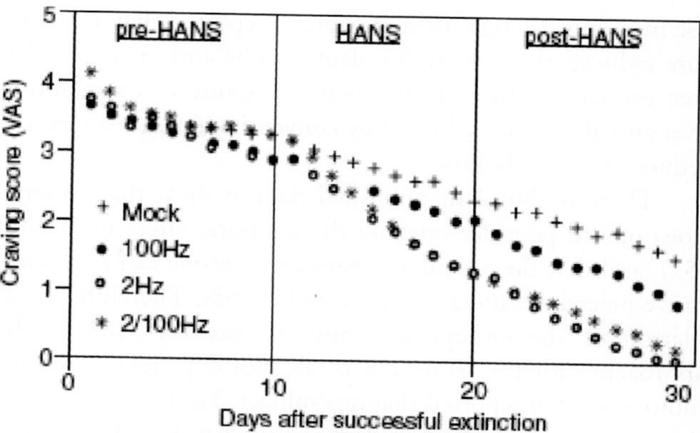

FIGURE 29.9. Effects of HANS on craving scores in heroin addicts (n = 29–30 in each group). HANS of 2 Hz and 2/100 Hz accelerated the decay of craving scores during the 10-day treatment period. (Reprinted with permission from Han JS, Trachtenberg AI, Lowinson JH. Acupuncture. In: Lowinson JH, et al., eds. *Substance abuse: a comprehensive textbook.* Philadelphia: Lippincott Williams & Wilkins, 2004:743–782.)

addicts at least 1 month after detoxification was used. The scale is 100 mm long; 0 = no craving, 100 = the most severe craving imaginable. One hundred seventeen subjects were assigned randomly into four groups. Three groups received TEAS at 2 Hz, 100 Hz, or 2/100 Hz. Self-adhesive skin electrodes were placed on four acupoints: *Hegu* and *Laogong* (palmar side of the *Hegu* point) on the left (or right) hand to complete the circuit, and *Neiguan* and *Weiguan* on the right (or left) arm to complete the circuit. The intensity was increased from threshold on the first day to two or three times threshold on the following days. The mock TEAS control group was processed like the other groups except that the intensity was minimal (at threshold stimulation for 3 minutes, followed by 1 mA thereafter). The results, shown in Figure 29.9 indicate a slow decline of the VAS in the mock TEAS group and a parallel slow decline in 100 Hz group, in contrast with a dramatic decline in the 2 Hz and 2/100 Hz groups. In summary, the results in humans coincided with the results in rats, that low frequency is more effective than high frequency in reducing craving for opiates (51).

On the basis of the experimental effects of TEAS described earlier, the subjects were encouraged to take with them a portable TEAS unit when they were discharged from the detoxification center. The purpose was to ameliorate the protracted withdrawal syndrome and to suppress the craving induced by environmental cues. At least one 30-minute session before going to bed was recommended to facilitate sleep, as was use whenever they encountered a cue. It was found that the anti-craving effect usually appears within 20 minutes.

ACUPUNCTURE AND ALCOHOL ABUSE

Acupuncture was considered promising for the treatment of alcohol addiction in the 1980s. The orthodox ear points suggested by National Institute on Drug Abuse were used, with points 3 to 5 mm apart as a nonspecific control. Two papers provided positive results (52,53). However, these results could not be replicated in the United States (54) or Sweden (55). A recent randomized placebo-controlled clinical trial of auricular acupuncture (56) (N = 503) was unique in that, aside from the "specific" ear acupuncture group, "nonspecific" ear acupuncture group, and conventional treatment group, there was a symptom-based acupuncture group for which the acupuncturists were not constrained to the four ear points stipulated for the other acupuncture groups, and the point prescription could be changed from day to day according to the patients' discomfort. Six treatments per week were given for as long as 3 weeks to maximize the effect. All four groups showed significant improvement, with few differences associated with treatment assignment and no treatment difference on alcohol use measures, though 49% of subjects reported that acupuncture reduced their desire for alcohol. The authors concluded that ear acupuncture did not make a significant contribution over and above that achieved by conventional treatment in the reduction of alcohol use.

There is abundant published data to show that endogenous opioid peptides mediate the euphoric effect of alcohol (57), and that the opioid antagonist naltrexone can assist cognitive behavioral therapy for alcoholics (58). Therefore, modulation of the endogenous opioid system is one of the approaches for the treatment of alcohol dependence. Yoshimoto et al. (59) reported that rats subjected to repeated restriction stress consumed more alcohol than controls. EA at hind limb points *Zusanli* (ST 36) significantly reduced alcohol seeking, but EA at the lumbar point *Shenshu* (BL-23) did not. EA at ST36 was accompanied by a higher dopamine level in the striatum than was EA at BL23. These findings provide intriguing information for understanding alcohol-drinking behavior and for treating alcoholics.

CONCLUSION

The continued rise in the use of opiates, stimulants, and alcohol has led to the search for alternative therapies. Traditional Chinese medicines have been used for treatment of human disease for more than 2,000 years. It is estimated that roughly one-half of current pharmaceuticals originally were procured from plants (60). Examples include foxglove leaf (digitalis), belladonna tops (atropine), poppy herb (morphine), white willow tree bark (salicin), and cinchona bark (quinine). Modern drugs developed from plant products include warfarin from coumarin anticoagulants found in sweet clover silage, ergotamine from ergot alkaloids of a fungus that infects rye grass, antineoplastic vincristine from the vinca alkaloid fractions of the rosy periwinkle, the anti-cancer drug taxol from pacific yew tree, and anti-malaria artemisin from Qingao (61). It is therefore reasonable that medications development for drug and alcohol abuse should seek active isolates from traditional herbal remedies.

That said, many believe that a combination of medicinal plants with synergistic effects is a better approach. Though it is difficult to prove the synergism of multi-component herbal remedies, the concept of a multitargeted approach is familiar to Western medicine as the basis of chemotherapy for most cancers and highly active retroviral therapy for HIV disease. It is also conceivable that a multitargeted approach would improve the overall efficacy and reduce toxicity. For example, Chung et. al. (62), reported the in vitro receptor-binding affinities of natural products used successfully to treat psychotic illness in Korean traditional medicine.

Though acupuncture and related acupoint therapies are most commonly recognized for analgesic effect, their medical applications extend beyond pain treatment. Based on our and other studies, TEAS represents a promising, noninvasive, and safe physical method for the prevention of alcohol and drug relapse.

Though alternative therapies may provide new treatments for existing drug treatments, rigorous studies to evaluate both the risks and the benefits of such treatments are needed. Biologic investigations that couple in vitro and in vivo pharmacologic models to characterize mechanism of action and the possibility of synergistic effects of components are crucial to further the development of successful complementary and alternative therapies for substance abuse.

ACKNOWLEDGMENTS: *The work is supported by a grant funded by NCCAM/NIAAA for Center for Excellence for Research on Complementary and Alternative Medicine (P01-AT002038).*

REFERENCES

1. Shippenberg TS, Chefer VI, Zapata A, et al. Modulation of the behavioral and neurochemical effects of psychostimulants by kappa-opioid receptor systems. *Ann N Y Acad Sci* 2001;937:50–73.
2. Kreek MJ. Cocaine, dopamine and the endogenous opioid system. *J Addict Dis* 1996;15(4):73–96.
3. Kreek MJ, LaForge KS, Butelman E. Pharmacotherapy of addictions. *Nat Rev Drug Discov* 2002;1(9):710–726.
4. Schenk S, Partridge B, Shippenberg TS. U69593, a kappa-opioid agonist, decreases cocaine self-administration and decreases cocaine-produced drug-seeking. *Psychopharmacology (Berl)* 1999;144(4):339–346.
5. Yang MMP, Yeun RCF, Kwok JSL. *Effect of certain Chinese herbs on drug addiction.* In: *Advances in Chinese medicinal materials research.* In: Chang HM, et al., ed. Singapore: World Scientific Publishing, 1985:147–158.
6. Kieffer BL, Befort K, Gaveriaux-Ruff C, et al. The delta-opioid receptor: isolation of a cDNA by expression cloning and pharmacological characterization. *Proc Natl Acad Sci U S A* 199289(24):12048–12052.
7. Evans CJ, Keith DE Jr, Morrison H, et al. Cloning of a delta opioid receptor by functional expression. *Science* 1992;258(5090):1952–1955.
8. Kieffer BL. Recent advances in molecular recognition and signal transduction of active peptides: receptors for opioid peptides. *Cell Mol Neurobiol* 1995;15(6):615–635.
9. Knapp RJ, Malatynska E, Collins N, et al. Molecular biology and pharmacology of cloned opioid receptors. *Faseb J* 1995;9(7):516–525.
10. Yang MMP, Yuen RCF, Kok SH. Experimental studies on the effects of certain Chinese herbs on morphine withdrawal syndrome in rats. *J Am Coll Trad Chinese Med* 1983;2:3–24.
11. Ma Z, Xu W, Liu-Chen LY, et al. Novel coumarin glycoside and phenethyl vanillate from Notopterygium forbesii and their binding affinities for opioid and dopamine receptors. *Bioorg Med Chem* 2008;16:3231–3236.
12. Gottschalk PC, Jacobsen LK, Kosten TR. Current concepts in pharmacotherapy of substance abuse. *Curr Psychiatry Rep* 1999;1(2): 172–178.
13. de Lima MS, de Oliveira Soares BG, Reisser AA, et al. Pharmacological treatment of cocaine dependence: a systematic review. *Addiction* 2002;97(8):931–949.
14. Majewska MD. Cocaine addiction as a neurological disorder: implications for treatment. *NIDA Res Monogr* 1996;163:1–26.
15. Luo J, Ren Y, Zhu R, et al. The effect of l-tetrahydropalmitine on cocaine-induced conditioned place preference. *Chin J Drug Depend* 2003;12(3):177–179.
16. Ren Y, Zhang K. Effect of L-tetrahydrapalmitine on discrimination of methamphetamine in rats. *Chin J Drug Depend* 2002;9(2):108–110.
17. Heikkila RE, Orlansky H, Cohen G. Studies on the distinction between uptake inhibition and release of (3H)dopamine in rat brain tissue slices. *Biochem Pharmacol* 1975;24(8):847–852.
18. Reith ME, Meisler BE, Sershen H, et al. Structural requirements for cocaine congeners to interact with dopamine and serotonin uptake sites

in mouse brain and to induce stereotyped behavior. *Biochem Pharmacol* 1986;35(7):1123–1129.

19. Ritz MC, Lamb RJ, Goldberg SR, et al. Cocaine receptors on dopamine transporters are related to self-administration of cocaine. *Science* 1987;237(4819):1219–1223.
20. Sibley DR, Monsma FJ Jr. Molecular biology of dopamine receptors. *Trends Pharmacol Sci* 1992;13(2):61–69.
21. Koob GF. Animal models of craving for ethanol. *Addiction* 2000;95(Suppl 2):S73–S81.
22. Everitt BJ, Dickinson A, Robbins TW. The neuropsychological basis of addictive behaviour. *Brain Res Brain Res Rev* 2001;36(2–3):129–138.
23. Silvestre JS, O'Neill MF, Fernandez AG, et al. Effects of a range of dopamine receptor agonists and antagonists on ethanol intake in the rat. *Eur J Pharmacol* 1996;318(23):257–265.
24. Callahan PM, Appel JB, Cunningham KA. Dopamine D1 and D2 mediation of the discriminative stimulus properties of d-amphetamine and cocaine. *Psychopharmacology (Berl)* 1991;103(1):50–55.
25. Caine SB, Negus SS, Mello NK, et al. Effects of dopamine D(1-like) and D(2-like) agonists in rats that self-administer cocaine. *J Pharmacol Exp Ther* 1999;291(1):353–360.
26. Self DW, Barnhart WJ, Lehman DA, et al. Opposite modulation of cocaine-seeking behavior by D1- and D2-like dopamine receptor agonists. *Science* 1996;271(5255):1586–1589.
27. Platt DM, Rowlett JK, Spealman RD. Behavioral effects of cocaine and dopaminergic strategies for preclinical medication development. *Psychopharmacology (Berl)* 2002;163(3–4):265–282.
28. Haney M, Collins ED, Ward AS, et al. Effect of a selective dopamine D1 agonist (ABT–431) on smoked cocaine self-administration in humans. *Psychopharmacology (Berl)* 1999;143(1):102–110.
29. Berger SP, Hall S, Mickalian JD, et al. Haloperidol antagonism of cue-elicited cocaine craving. *Lancet* 19961347(9000):504–508.
30. Milivojevic N, Krisch I, Sket D, et al. The dopamine D1 receptor agonist and D2 receptor antagonist LEK-8829 attenuates reinstatement of cocaine-seeking in rats. *Naunyn Schmiedebergs Arch Pharmacol* 2004; 369(6):576–582.
31. Wen HL, Cheung SYC. Treatment of drug addiction by acupuncture and electrical stimulation. *Asian J Med* 1973;9:138–141.
32. McLellan AT, Grossman DS, Blaine JD, et al. Acupuncture treatment for drug abuse: a technical review. *J Subst Abuse Treat* 1993;10(6):569–576.
33. Hughes J, Smith TW, Kosterlitz HW, et al. Identification of two related pentapeptides from the brain with potent opiate agonist activity. *Nature* 1975;258(5536):577–580.
34. Mayer DJ, Price DD, Rafii A. Antagonism of acupuncture analgesia in man by the narcotic antagonist naloxone. *Brain Res* 1977;121(2):368–372.
35. Han JS, Terenius L. Neurochemical basis of acupuncture analgesia. *Annu Rev Pharmacol Toxicol* 1982;22:193–220.
36. Herz A, ed. *Handbook of experimental pharmacology*, vol. 104/I. Berlin: Springer-Verlag, 1993.
37. Han JS, Wang Q, Mobilization of specific neuropeptides by peripheral stimulation of different frequencies. *News Physiol Sci* 1992;7:176–180.
38. Han JS, Zhang RL, Suppression of morphine abstinence syndrome by body electroacupuncture of different frequencies in rats. *Drug Alcohol Depend* 1993;31(2):169–175.
39. Wang JQ, Mao L, Han JS. Comparison of the antinociceptive effects induced by electroacupuncture and transcutaneous electrical nerve stimulation in the rat. *Int J Neurosci* 1992;65(1–4):117–129.
40. Wu LZ, Cui CL, Han JS. Han's acupoint nerve stimulator for the treatment of opiate withdrawal syndrome. *Chin J Pain Med* 1995;1:30–35.
41. Wang B, Luo F, Xia YQ, et al. Peripheral electric stimulation inhibits morphine-induced place preference in rats. *Neuroreport* 2000;11(5):1017–1020.
42. Choy YM, Tso WW, Fung KP, et al. Suppression of narcotic withdrawals and plasma ACTH by auricular electroacupunture. *Biochem Biophys Res Commun* 1978;82(1):305–309.
43. Ng LK, Douthitt TC, Thoa NB, et al. Modification of morphine-withdrawal syndrome in rats following transauricular electrostimulation: an experimental paradigm for auricular electroacupuncture. *Biol Psychiatry* 1975;10(5):575–580.
44. Auriacombe M, Tignol J, Le Moal M, et al. Transcutaneous electrical stimulation with Limoge current potentiates morphine analgesia and attenuates opiate abstinence syndrome. *Biol Psychiatry* 1990;28(8): 650–656.
45. Han JS, Chen XH, Sun SL, et al. Effect of low- and high-frequency TENS on Met-enkephalin-Arg-Phe and dynorphin A immunoreactivity in human lumbar CSF. *Pain* 1991;47(3):295–298.
46. Wu LZ, Cui CL, Han JS. Effect of Han's acupoint nerve stimulator (HANS) on the heart rate of 75 inpatients during heroin withdrawal. *Chin J Pain Med* 1996;2:98–102.
47. Wu LZ, Cui CL, Han JS. Treatment on heroin addicts by 4 channel Han's Acupoint Nerve Stimulator (HANS). *J Beijing Med Univ* 1999;31:239–242.
48. Wu LZ, Cui CL, Han JS. Reduction of methadone dosage and relief of depression and anxiety by 2/100 Hz TENS for heroin detoxification. *Chin J Drug Depend* 2001;10:124–126.
49. Markou A, Weiss F, Gold LH, et al. Animal models of drug craving. *Psychopharmacology (Berl)* 1993;112(2–3):163–182.
50. Bardo MT, Bevins RA, Conditioned place preference: what does it add to our preclinical understanding of drug reward? *Psychopharmacology (Berl)* 2000;153(1):31–43.
51. Wang B, Zhang B, Ge X, et al. Inhibition by peripheral electric stimulation of the reinstatement of morphine-induced place preference in rats and drug-craving in heroin addicts. *Beijing Da Xue Xue Bao*, 2003;35(3):241–247.
52. Bullock ML, Umen AJ, Culliton PD, et al. Acupuncture treatment of alcoholic recidivism: a pilot study. *Alcohol Clin Exp Res* 1987;11(3):292–295.
53. Bullock ML, Culliton PD, Olander RT. Controlled trial of acupuncture for severe recidivist alcoholism. *Lancet* 1989;1(8652):1435–1439.
54. Worner TM, Zeller B, Schwarz H, et al. Acupuncture fails to improve treatment outcome in alcoholics. *Drug Alcohol Depend* 1992;30(2): 169–173.
55. Sapir-Weise R, Berglund M, Frank A, et al. Acupuncture in alcoholism treatment: a randomized out-patient study. *Alcohol Alcohol* 1999;34(4): 629–635.
56. Bullock ML, Kiresuk TJ, Sherman RE, et al. A large randomized placebo controlled study of auricular acupuncture for alcohol dependence. *J Subst Abuse Treat* 2002;22(2):71–77.
57. Olive MF, Koenig HN, Nannini MA, et al. Stimulation of endorphin neurotransmission in the nucleus accumbens by ethanol, cocaine, and amphetamine. *J Neurosci* 2001;21(23):RC184.
58. Anton RF, Moak DH, Waid LR, et al. Naltrexone and cognitive behavioral therapy for the treatment of outpatient alcoholics: results of a placebo-controlled trial. *Am J Psychiatry* 1999;156(11):1758–1764.
59. Yoshimoto K, Kato B, Sakai K, et al. Electroacupuncture stimulation suppresses the increase in alcohol-drinking behavior in restricted rats. *Alcohol Clin Exp Res* 2001;25(Suppl 6):63S–68S.
60. Fugh-Berman A. Clinical trials of herbs. *Prim Care* 1997;24(4):889–903.
61. Clark AM, Natural products as a resource for new drugs. *Pharm Res* 1996;13(8):1133–1144.
62. Chung IW, Kim YS, Ahn JS, et al. Pharmacologic profile of natural products used to treat psychotic illnesses. *Psychopharmacol Bull* 1995;31(1):139–145.

CHAPTER 30

Alex Wodak, MD, MB BS, FRACP, FAChAM

The Harm Reduction Approach to Prevention and Treatment

Harm reduction policies and programs, spanning prevention and treatment, aim to decrease the adverse health, social, and economic consequences of legal and illegal psychoactive drugs *without necessarily* diminishing drug consumption (1). This approach continues to gain increasing support while more conventional policy approaches focusing on reducing consumption are increasingly regarded as ineffective, expensive and counter-productive (2–4).

WHAT IS HARM REDUCTION?

Defining Harm Reduction The term *harm reduction*, sometimes also known as *harm minimization*, is used with a bewildering variety of interpretations (5). The ambiguity of the term adds to the confusion of an area already complicated by emotional fervor and lack of terminologic clarity. The alcohol and drug field is also often characterized by attempts to force dichotomous categorizations even though most phenomena in the discipline are distributed on a continuum. Harm reduction is better considered as a difference in emphasis rather than a radical departure from conventional responses. The essence of harm reduction is a paramount focus on pragmatically reducing adverse consequences of drug use whereas any impact on drug consumption is regarded as a lower priority. In contrast, supply control–dominated approaches regard a reduction of consumption as the primary objective, with any reduction of adverse consequences considered a bonus.

The notion that the best should never be allowed to be the enemy of the good is the essence of harm reduction, and is important throughout public health and many other areas of public policy. Adopting and then ensuring delivery of achievable but suboptimal objectives is far more effective in public policy than aiming for utopian objectives and then failing to achieve them. The risk-compensation hypothesis in psychology and the concept of moral hazard in economics and finance resemble the concept of harm reduction. The common thread in these approaches is the concern that individuals insulated from risk may behave less prudently than they would if still exposed to risk.

Harm reduction objectives are often ranked in a hierarchy with the most feasible but still acceptable options preferred over unachievable but more desirable options. For example, the least-worst option from an human immunodeficiency virus (HIV) prevention perspective for injecting drug users unable or unwilling to abstain from injecting drugs is ensuring the use of sterile injecting equipment on every drug-injecting occasion. In contrast, the sharing of needles and syringes is the worst option. Opponents of harm reduction consider that the only objective worth achieving is enduring abstinence and that anything less than that is not worth considering.

In its simplest form, harm reduction refers to "policies, programs and projects which aim primarily to reduce the health, social and economic harms associated with the use of psychoactive substances" (6). Harm reduction embodies the recognition that "many people throughout the world use psychoactive substances, and that society is unlikely to ever be drug-, drink-, or nicotine-free. Harm reduction does not exclude abstinence as a goal for individuals who are dependent but, rather, provides people with more pragmatic choices. . . ." (6). Beneficiaries of harm reduction include people who use drugs, their families, and their communities.

A more expanded view of harm reduction emphasizes the maximization of the potential benefits of psychoactive substances as an aim additional to minimizing potential harms. Accordingly, emphasis is given to more judicious use of dependence-producing medications. For example, the common practice of suboptimal prescription of opioids in the management of cancer and chronic nonmalignant pain often results in considerable distress from inadequate pain relief. Excessive fear of inducing drug dependence despite a cancer patient's limited life expectancy is often a significant factor in the decision to prescribe subtherapeutic doses of analgesics. Similarly, the evidence that medicinal use of cannabis is relatively safe and has many worthwhile benefits is growing. Benefits include amelioration of distressing symptoms of cancer chemotherapy and AIDS sometimes unrelieved by conventional medications. Evidence of efficacy and safety is now accepted by many as compelling (7,8). Yet availability of medicinal cannabis is still limited. This concerns many harm reduction supporters who favor policy based on the same kind of rigorous evaluation of costs and benefits as in other medical attempts to prolong life or alleviate suffering.

Though harm reduction approaches are not intended primarily to reduce consumption of drugs, this is often an unintended long-term result. For example, random breath testing of car drivers was introduced to reduce the incidence of alcohol-related road crash deaths and serious injuries by deterring intoxicated citizens from driving. Random breath testing had the unanticipated benefit of encouraging many car drivers, who form the majority of the adult population in developed countries to consume less alcohol. Similarly, many drug users who have attended needle syringe programs for some time canvass the idea of achieving abstinence and request referral to drug treatment (9,10). Though harm reduction grew largely out of concerns to protect public health, respect for human rights has become an increasingly important consideration.

History of Harm Reduction Though harm reduction is often misrepresented as a recent development in the alcohol and drug field, it has a long history. In ancient China, authorities attempted unsuccessfully to limit alcohol consumption as a means of preventing inebriated citizens falling into wintry canals and freezing to death. Though it was not possible to eliminate public intoxication, the simple installation of barriers around the canals was found to effectively prevent such deaths. Compulsory car safety belt legislation was introduced in the 1960s in a number of countries when authorities became alarmed by increasing numbers of alcohol-related road crash deaths. Efforts at that time to reduce per capita alcohol consumption were singularly unsuccessful. Though attempts to ensure that car drivers wore safety belts while driving had no discernible effect on alcohol consumption or drunk driving, alcohol-related road crash deaths and serious injuries were dramatically reduced. Fears that safety belts would result in an increase in speeding or reckless driving as compensation for increased safety proved groundless. Alcohol policy researchers in the 1970s spoke of the need to "make the world safe for drunks." Support for harm reduction policies and programs increased dramatically in the mid-1980s after recognition of the HIV pandemic and the realization that uncontrolled epidemics involving injecting drug users threatened immense health, social, and economic costs for the whole community.

Misconceptions about Harm Reduction The commonest misconception regarding harm reduction is that this approach and efforts to promote abstinence from psychoactive drugs are mutually exclusive options. In some ways, abstinence from drugs is the most complete form of harm minimization. However, it is undeniable that relapse is not only a very common phenomenon but extremely dangerous. Also, some drug users are unable or unwilling to consider abstinence. Harm reduction reminds clinicians of the supreme importance of keeping drug users alive and preferably also avoiding irreversible damage. Perhaps at some time in the future, some of the people who have hitherto been unable or unwilling to abstain will aim for abstinence and remain abstinent from drugs indefinitely?

Harm reduction is also often misconstrued as rejecting the role of drug law enforcement. On the contrary; harm reduction usually involves a far closer partnership between law enforcement and health. Police in many countries have become convinced of the importance of allowing needle syringe and methadone programs to function without undue law enforcement interference in order to ensure that the significant community benefits of these programs are not jeopardized. Health workers accepting harm reduction have also slowly come to better understand the considerable difficulties of illicit drug law enforcement and the importance of collaborating with police in certain areas, such as reducing alcohol-related violence or deaths from drug overdose. Strong partnerships among health, law enforcement, injecting drug users, clinicians, researchers, and government officials increase the effectiveness of harm reduction. In many countries where harm reduction has been well accepted for some years, police have begun to reverse earlier opposition to methadone programs and supported their expansion, recognizing the ability of these programs to substantially reduce crime (11). Some senior police also recognize that harm reduction may reduce official corruption that so often accompanies largely unsuccessful attempts to control the supply of drugs through reliance on drug law enforcement. Providing ready availability of methadone treatment in Zurich, Switzerland reduced the estimated number of new heroin users from 850 in 1990 to 150 in 2002 while also reducing the number of new HIV infections, deaths from drug overdose, crime and, judging by the decreasing quantity of heroin seizures, the size of the drug market (12).

Though sometimes misrepresented as a radical threat to conventional policies, harm reduction has received support from prestigious international health authorities.

> *"A concern often expressed about harm reduction strategies is their potential for communicating a message condoning drug use. Such concerns have been expressed, for instance, concerning mass media programs that encourage drinking groups to nominate a nondrinking 'designated driver,' as this message might seem to condone drunkenness in the other group members, and concerning those that provide information about methods for solvent inhalation that reduce the risk of fatalities and other harm. Often these concerns could be alleviated by targeting the message to those already*

involved in hazardous drug use. In considering such strategies, it should be kept in mind that the public health sector has always been in favour of reducing the immediate drug-related harm, even if this involves some risk of a more distant hazard or can be seen as condoning drug use" (13).

For some trenchant critics, harm reduction is still simply the thin edge of an ugly wedge of drug legalization. For others in hostile political environments, achieving even minimal harm reduction in a situation where HIV is spreading at alarming rates among injecting drug users is a major accomplishment. In these settings, any consideration of drug policy reform is a luxurious distraction. A third situation is where the major and self-evident benefits derived from harm reduction justifies taking reform further, including rigorously evaluating some form of regulation of currently illicit drugs (14). It is hard to deny in some countries that a drug policy heavily reliant on law enforcement causes more harm than good. Accordingly, harm reduction in these countries often attempts to reduce the harm resulting from drug law enforcement. A study carried out in 89 large cities in the United States (15) compared the number of injecting drug users per capita and their HIV seroprevalence with per capita drug arrests, police employees, and corrections expenditures. Drug arrests, police employees, and corrections expenditures did not correlate with the numbers of injecting drug users per capita, but the greater these legal measures were in a particular city, the higher the HIV prevalence among injecting drug users.

It is undeniable that in some countries, harm reduction opened up drug policy reform as an issue. However, this is not in itself sufficient reason to permanently suppress all consideration of harm reduction policies and programs. Some modest degree of drug policy reform is required to maintain HIV control among injecting drug users. It is important that no country that has started harm reduction has ever regretted doing so and then terminated their harm reduction programs.

Examples of Harm Reduction Approaches It has been known since at least the early 1990s that HIV among injecting drug users can be easily controlled by the early and vigorous implementation of a comprehensive "harm reduction package" (16). This package consists of education, needle syringe programs, drug treatment, and community development of drug users. Needle syringe programs and opiate substitution treatment with methadone or buprenorphine are often considered the epitome of harm reduction. The evidence that both these interventions are effective, safe, and cost-effective is now very compelling (17,18) and very widely accepted.

As with any medical treatment for any condition, harm reduction services must attract, retain, and benefit large numbers of individuals to have an impact at the population level. They need to be effective in reducing the harms associated with drug use including HIV, but just as important, they must also be attractive and considered useful by the populations who need to attend them. The advantage of providing a coordinated package of services is that it offers many entry points for drug users to obtain access to health treatment from "low threshold-low intensity" contacts to "high threshold-high intensity" treatment and everything in between. *Threshold* here refers to the ease of gaining access to an intervention while the intensity of the intervention refers to the degree of commitment required by drug users and the extent of service provision.

Needle syringe programs increase the use of sterile injecting equipment and decrease the use of used injecting equipment, thereby decreasing the circulation time of used needles and syringes. In some countries, sterile injecting equipment can now be purchased from pharmacies and supermarkets. Vending machines have been installed in some areas with high populations of injecting drug users with considerable benefit (19). Though most programs emphasize an exchange of new equipment for old, some simply provide sterile injecting equipment as needed. Laws restricting the availability of injecting equipment undermine efforts to control HIV. Needle syringe programs usually provide a great deal of practical education and also serve as important entry points for drug treatment and provision of other basic services.

Education of injecting drug users about the HIV risks of sharing injecting equipment are most effective if they are simple, explicit, peer-based, and factual. Basic information is required about behaviors associated with the risk of HIV transmission and practical ways of reducing that risk.

Drug treatment is a critical part of the package, especially opiate substitution treatments. Methadone and buprenorphine maintenance treatment have been shown convincingly to reduce HIV spread and result in many other benefits. Substitution treatment also ensures that antiretroviral treatment achieves similar results for injecting drug users as it does for other groups at high risk of HIV. What makes methadone and buprenorphine treatments examples of harm reduction is the prescription of drugs of dependence to drug-dependant persons to reduce the high health, social, and economic costs of injecting street heroin. The lack of an effective pharmacotherapy for stimulant (amphetamine, cocaine) injectors is a major problem in the many countries where stimulants are the most commonly injected drug.

Opiate substitution treatment is the most frequently evaluated intervention in all of medicine. Abundant, consistent, and compelling evidence supports the effectiveness of methadone maintenance treatment in reducing HIV among injecting drug users and the achievement of multiple other important benefits including substantially reducing drug overdose deaths, crime, and illicit drug use (20). Social functioning is also improved during substitution treatment. The ratio of economic benefits to costs is estimated to be about four to one (21). In 2004, the United Nations Drug Office on Drugs and Crime, the UNAIDS, and the World Health Organization (WHO) endorsed opiate substitution treatment (22), and the WHO included methadone and buprenorphine in the List of Essential Medicines (23).

In harm reduction settings, patients undergoing drug treatment often are encouraged to negotiate treatment goals and parameters with clinicians. Cycles of remission and relapse are regarded as part of the natural history of drug dependence rather than as a reflection of poor motivation or defective character. Harm reduction treatments are generally based on evidence rather than moral, religious, or spiritual considerations. Retention in treatment is stressed and correlated with favorable outcomes. Harm reduction treatments often favor minimal improvements for many rather than heroic gains for the few. Drug treatment in a harm reduction framework is regarded as similar to the management of many relapsing and remitting chronic medical conditions rather than as an offshoot of law enforcement.

Not all drug users accept or benefit from pharmacotherapies, so nonpharmacologic treatments should generally also be provided (even though evidence of their effectiveness is weak). Counseling can be useful for many drug users, including those undergoing pharmacologic treatments. Though the emphasis of drug treatment from an HIV control perspective is always appropriately focused on injecting drug users, it is also important to offer assistance to people who consume drugs without injecting (such as those who smoke or snort drugs). This includes responding effectively to factors that increase the likelihood of drug users undertaking a transition to injecting. Some who take drugs without injecting may switch to injecting if street drug prices increase or purity declines. Lack of assistance for people who consume drugs without injecting but have developed problems provides a perverse incentive for these people to begin injecting in order to get help.

From a public health perspective of HIV control, some "bridge populations" require particular attention. These groups include men who have sex with men and also inject drugs and sex workers who also inject drugs. Other populations of great public health interest include injecting drug users with severe mental illness, prison inmates, and those from indigenous and other minority backgrounds.

Medically supervised injecting centers are particularly effective at attracting severely disadvantaged injecting drug users in proximity to major drug markets. These centers provide many worthwhile benefits including reducing fatal and non-fatal overdoses and improving neighborhood amenity without producing significant unintended consequences such as increasing crime (24). In practice, these facilities have proved very difficult to evaluate, often because their opponents have ensured that the excessively stringent operational conditions unduly constrain clinical activities (25).

The often disappointing results from education programmers aimed at reducing drug use among young people have stimulated greater interest in broader approaches. Greater success may be achieved by identifying and, where possible, reducing risk factors such as individual characteristics, family factors, and peer relationships, along with structural determinants such as poor education, housing, health services, and limited employment opportunities (26,27).

Understanding and responding to the needs of drug users from disadvantaged groups improves service design and use. Community development of injecting drug users helps to ensure that this population becomes part of the solution rather than constituting the crux of the problem. Involving injecting drug users in the design and implementation of HIV prevention strategies increases their effectiveness. To this end, government funded organizations of injecting drug users have been established in many countries. The low status of injecting drug users means they have few opportunities to participate in societal decision making. The inclusive nature of organizations of drug users reduces the marginalization of this population. Specific evidence on the effectiveness of drug user organization is difficult to gather. However, research with other consumer groups, such as those with a mental illness, shows that training outcomes are improved and service effectiveness increased when consumers of services are employed in their development and delivery (28).

Harm reduction should also include efforts to improve the basic social conditions of injecting drug users including their general health, housing, welfare and employment. Harm reduction should mean more than simply reducing the harms of drug use (29).

Harm reduction is needed not only in community settings but in so-called "closed settings" such as detention centers, jails, and prisons. Reliance on drug law enforcement to control illicit drugs inevitably means that many injecting drug users spend long periods of their drug injecting careers in correctional institutions. However, with so little to lose, high-risk drug injecting often continues in closed settings. Once behind bars, the risk of acquiring HIV infection is further increased by multiple factors including the large number of injecting equipment–sharing partners, the severely degraded condition of needles and syringes, the lack of HIV prevention strategies found in community settings, and the mixing of diverse demographic and geographic groups in prison.

Applications of harm reduction to alcohol in licensed premises are diverse and include the replacement of glasses with shatterproof drinking containers and the provision of heavy furniture bolted to the floor. Fortification of flour with thiamine virtually eliminates the Wernicke-Korsakoff syndrome, a form of brain damage strongly associated with severe alcohol dependence. The application of harm reduction to tobacco is more controversial, but nicotine replacement therapy to help smokers quit is analogous to the use of methadone to help heroin users quit.

Official Responses to Harm Reduction Harm reduction has been explicitly accepted as the national drug policy in a number of developed countries, including Australia, Canada, and France. A national meeting in Australia of the then–prime minister and the then–governors of each state declared in 1985 that "the aim [of drug policy] is to minimize the harmful effects of drugs on Australian society" (30).

There is strong and growing support for harm reduction at the national level. Needle syringe programs and opioid substitution programs are now provided in more than 60 countries (31). Numerous countries report substantial unmet demand for methadone treatment. Unfortunately, despite abundant and high-quality evidence and extensive international experience, the United States has maintained a ban on federal government funding for needle syringe programs. This ban has been immensely influential in many other countries. All 25 members of the European Union now provide needle syringe programs and methadone or buprenorphine maintenance treatment. In eastern and central Europe and Central Asia, needle syringe programs is becoming more common though coverage is still poor. Several populous countries in Asia are now implementing harm reduction programs. China set a target in 2005 to have 300,000 patients on methadone maintenance treatment by the end of 2008. India is rapidly expanding its buprenorphine programs and commencing methadone maintenance treatment. The National Assembly of Vietnam passed legislation supporting harm reduction. Malaysia and Indonesia have started needle syringe programs and methadone maintenance treatment. Indonesia became the first country in Asia to provide methadone maintenance treatment to some prison inmates. Taiwan and then Malaysia soon followed. Iran has become a world leader in implementation and expansion of harm reduction to control HIV among injecting drug users. However, the coverage of harm reduction programs in prisons worldwide remains very poor.

Support for harm reduction is now also strong at the international level. The United Nations Office on Drugs and Crime (UNODC), which is responsible for coordinating international illicit drug law enforcement and global supply control initiatives within the United Nations system, increasingly (though still somewhat ambivalently) supports harm reduction. The largest section of the UNODC is now harm reduction. The UNODC now employs more staff providing harm reduction than any other organization in the world—around 30% of the organization's 2005 expenditure was allocated to harm reduction activities (32). Harm reduction is now supported by virtually all of the United Nations organizations with responsibility for illicit drugs including WHO, UNAIDS, UNICEF, and the World Bank. Many international organizations now support harm reduction including the International Red Cross and the Global Fund for AIDS, TB, and Malaria. The International Narcotics Control Board, a quasi-UN organization with responsibility for monitoring implementation of the international drug treaties, is the last organization within the United Nations system to still oppose harm reduction.

Support for harm reduction within the United Nations system has been growing for some time. A document drawn up by an Expert Committee of the WHO used the term *harm reduction* in the sense of preventing adverse consequences of drug use without setting out primarily to reduce drug consumption (13). This interpretation of harm reduction has existed comfortably and apparently without controversy in an organization that carefully positions itself in the middle ground of the family of nations. Examples of harm reduction referred to included needle syringe programs to control the spread of HIV among injecting drug users, nicotine patches for tobacco users, and attempts to reduce physical injuries associated with alcohol intoxication by making environments in which people drink less dangerous. The committee commented that "in the harm minimization approach attention is directed to the careful scrutiny of all prevention and treatment strategies in terms of their intended and unintended effects on levels of drug-related harm" (13).

The Expansion of Harm Reduction The dissemination of information about harm reduction is improving through the establishment of organizations, conferences, and publications. A series of international conferences on the Reduction of Drug-Related Harm have been held annually after an initial conference in Liverpool, United Kingdom, in 1990. In 1996, an International Harm Reduction Association and an Asian Harm Reduction Network were established. The establishment of other regional harm reduction networks then followed. These include the Eurasian Harm Reduction Network (initially called the Central and Eastern European Harm Reduction Network) in 1997; the Latin American Harm Reduction Network in 1998; and the Middle East and North Africa Network on Harm Reduction in 2007. The International Harm Reduction Association holds an annual conference, publishes a journal, and disseminates information and materials through its impressive Web site. In 2008, about 1,500 delegates from about 90 countries attended the International Harm Reduction Conference. The first National Harm Reduction Conference in the United States was held in Oakland, CA, in September 1996. The National Harm Reduction Coalition is a United States–based group established in 1993.

The International Harm Reduction Development Program was established in 1995 as part of the Open Society Institute. It focused initially on eastern Europe and Russia and has always strongly emphasized human rights (33,34). Both organizations assist training of harm reduction workers, especially in developing and transitional countries. The availability of manuals, guidelines, and training in harm reduction continues to expand (35). Material is increasingly available in languages other than English. The growing use of the internet and e-mail has made it a great deal easier and less expensive to disseminate information and materials.

A comprehensive and up-to-date survey of harm reduction implementation was published in 2008 (36). The growing international acceptance of methadone was confirmed in a survey carried out by the Health Department of Canada (37). Long-term methadone maintenance was accepted in 16 countries by 1995: Australia, Canada, Denmark, Finland, France, Germany, Hong Kong, Hungary, Israel, Italy, Mexico, The Netherlands, New Zealand, Spain, Switzerland, and the United States. Three countries (Belgium, England, and Sweden) regarded methadone with eventual withdrawal as the only acceptable form of treatment. Controls and regulations differed considerably. Switzerland had the highest number of patients per million (2,000) followed by Hong Kong (1,818), Belgium (1,000), Australia (964), Netherlands (732), Denmark (542), New Zealand (495), Spain (459), and the United States (441). In 2008, methadone or buprenorphine maintenance treatment was available in 63 countries, 77 countries providing some form of needle syringe program and 82 countries supporting harm reduction (36). Methadone programs for inmates were operating in correctional systems in 33 countries with needle syringe programs for prison inmates operating in at least eight countries in 2008.

When methadone maintenance is provided in countries that are sympathetic to harm reduction, adequate doses (80 to 120 mg/day) are generally provided for a duration that is largely determined by the patient and may extend for several years. These characteristics of treatment have been demonstrated repeatedly to maximize benefits (38). In most countries, methadone may also be provided under supervision of a family doctor who has completed a brief training course, but this is not considered acceptable in the United States, where office-based buprenorphine for a maximum of 30 patients (later increased to 100 patients) was first approved in 2000. In virtually all countries providing opioid substitution treatment, demand considerably outstrips demand.

Outcomes of Harm Reduction Approaches Reviews of the evidence for needle syringe programs have concluded that these programs are effective in reducing HIV infections and unaccompanied by serious unintended negative consequences (including inadvertently increasing illicit drug use). These include reviews commissioned by or conducted by agencies of the United States government (9,39,40–44) and an international review commissioned by the WHO (17).

As more data have become available over time, confidence in the findings of these major studies has increased immeasurably (45). The evidence that needle syringe schemes reduce HIV spread among injecting drug users is strong. Comparisons of needle syringe attendees with non-attendees have generally shown a reduction in risk behavior among the former. A reduction of at least one-third in the incidence of HIV among injecting drug users who attended needle syringe programs was estimated using a mathematical model. A study commissioned by the Commonwealth Department of Health in Australia (46) estimated that by 2000, needle syringe programs cost Australia's governments $A122 million ($US 113 million) but prevented 25,000 HIV and 21,000 hepatitis C infections and, by 2010, will have prevented 4,500 AIDS deaths and 90 deaths from hepatitis C. Needle syringe programs saved Australian governments at least $A2.4 billion ($US 2.2 billion) allowing for a 5% annual discount for future benefits (as is conventional in government accounting). If this discount is not deducted, the savings were estimated to be as much as $A7.7 billion ($US 7.2 billion). This major evaluation was based on a study of data from 103 cities around the world. Cities with needle syringe programs had an average annual 18.6% decrease in HIV, compared with an average annual 8.1% increase in HIV in cities without such programs. The mean annual increase in seroprevalence, weighted according to the number of subjects sampled, was 3.6% in cities without and 0.2% in cities with needle syringe programs. Though a standard methodology for measurement of HIV seroprevalence between and within cities was not used, it is difficult to envisage any systematic design flaw capable of producing these results.

Virtually all court challenges mounted in the United States against needle syringe programs have been dismissed. Public support for needle syringe programs in opinion surveys was demonstrated in Australia and the United States. Cost-effectiveness analyses estimated that needle syringe programs in the United States can generally prevent an HIV infection for between $4,000 and $12,000 (47). Using conservative assumptions drawn from published studies, it was estimated (48) that between 4,000 and 10,000 HIV infections could have been prevented in the United States had needle syringe programs been implemented at the same rate as in Australia. These infections will ultimately cost up to half a billion U.S. dollars in HIV/AIDS treatment costs.

Compelling evidence supporting the effectiveness of methadone treatment against a range of important outcomes is drawn from a large literature, including randomized controlled trials and a vast number of observational studies (38). Methadone treatment has been demonstrated to reduce deaths from drug overdose, total mortality, morbidity, HIV risk behavior, HIV seroprevalence, HIV seroincidence, unemployment rates, and crime. The magnitude and consistency of these findings is extremely impressive. Improved outcomes are seen with higher doses of methadone, strengthening the confidence in these findings. Cost-benefit studies have shown much larger benefits than costs. Methadone treatment costs much less than other treatment modalities, incarceration, or no treatment. Methadone programs also are far more successful than other treatment modalities in attracting, retaining, and benefiting large numbers of drug users. In general, retention in drug treatment is closely linked to satisfactory outcomes. Early implementation of harm reduction policies and programs has been associated with persistently low HIV seroprevalence rates in a number of cities around the world (49) and impressive claims have been made for an averted HIV epidemic in Britain based on harm reduction programs (50).

Comparison of the HIV epidemics in Australia and the United States are illuminating (45). It was estimated that 14% of the 1.5 million injecting drug users in the 96 metropolitan areas of the United States with a population exceeding 500,000 are infected with HIV (52). More needles and syringes are dispensed each year in Australia (32 million) than in the United States (25 million) even though the population of the United States is more than 15 times greater. The proportion of annual AIDS cases in the United States attributed to injecting drug use increased from 12% in 1981 to 28% in 1993 (43). The United States epidemic is even more dominated by injecting drug users than AIDS data suggest. Fifty percent of incident HIV infections are estimated to occur among injecting drug users, excluding infections from injecting drug users to sex partners and children (52). Yet the prevalence of HIV infection is consistently low (less than 2%) among injecting drug users in Australia who do not report male-to-male sexual contact (53). Annual surveys of attendees at needle syringe programs in all states have been carried in Australia since 1995, and these have consistently found that many fewer than 2% of attendees with no history of male-to-male sexual contact were HIV-positive (54).

Alternatives to Harm Reduction Societal responses to illicit drug use were conventionally divided into law enforcement, education, and treatment. A more contemporary division refers to supply reduction, demand reduction, and harm reduction.

Demand Reduction Demand reduction typically involves a broad range of educational measures including mass and school campaigns and programs directed at established drug users and high-risk groups. Treatment of drug users is also classified as a form of demand reduction.

Some measures intended to reduce demand also reduce supply and vice versa. For example, methadone treatment might be regarded as simply reducing demand for street drugs in a small number of heroin-dependent individuals. However, those seeking entry to methadone maintenance programs are usually severely dependent and probably include many of the heaviest consumers in the community. Removing these individuals from the heroin market could have a significant effect on demand. As many of these users also are likely to traffic in drugs, their entry into treatment may temporarily disrupt the heroin supply system. A study conducted in Zurich, Switzerland supports this notion (12).

Supply Reduction Also sometimes referred to as *use reduction*, supply reduction forms the core of traditional international drug policy. The paramount aim of supply reduction is to decrease consumption of (usually illicit) mood-altering substances with any reduction in harm regarded as a bonus. Supply reduction involves attempts to reduce crop production, drug production, transport from countries of origin to countries of destination (interdiction), entry to the country of destination (customs), distribution (police) at wholesale and retail levels, and financial surveillance. Supply reduction usually receives the overwhelming majority of government expenditure in response to illicit drugs.

Use reduction is based implicitly on the premise that adverse consequences of drug use are closely correlated with consumption. This relationship is valid in the case of legal drugs such as alcohol and tobacco. Both drugs have significant intrinsic toxicity, and adverse health consequences correlate closely with individual or societal consumption. Consumption of alcohol and tobacco correlates closely with changes in price or availability. Decreases in price or increases in availability of alcohol and tobacco generally result in increased consumption and worse health outcomes. The converse is also true. Above a threshold, alcohol toxicity increases, linearly for some conditions, exponentially for others, and in a J-curve relationship for other conditions (54). Tobacco toxicity is generally linear. There seems to be no threshold below which smokers can consume tobacco with impunity.

Among developed countries, one of the strongest supporters of use reduction is the United States government. The Anti-Drug Abuse Act passed by Congress in 1988 stated in 5252-B that "it is the declared policy of the United States to create a Drug-Free America by 1995." Members of Congress who supported the Anti-Drug Abuse Act did so notwithstanding the fact that this lofty policy goal clearly was not achievable within the specified 7-year time frame and is probably never achievable. Whether drug consumption or drug-related harm should be considered the more appropriate target of U.S. government policy was answered clearly in an official policy statement that declared "we must come to terms with the drug problem in its essence: use itself. Worthy efforts to alleviate the symptoms of epidemic drug abuse-crime and disease for example-must continue unabated. But a largely ad-hoc attack on the holes in the dike can have only an indirect and minimal effect on the flood itself" (55).

Contrasts between Harm Reduction and Alternative Approaches The public health tradition accepts that incremental improvements often are all that can be achieved in areas of great complexity and difficulty. Aggregate results from the combination of multiple interventions are often very rewarding, though each intervention on its own produces relatively minor benefit. An elderly and somewhat decrepit Groucho Marx responded to the question, "What do you think of old age?" by noting that it was better than the alternative. This remark encapsulates the spirit of harm reduction, choosing between realistic options while recognizing that often all options are far from perfect. Harm reduction programs do not pretend to be a panacea, always producing complete success for all, but they do have a strong case to be regarded as more effective than alternative approaches.

Outcomes of Alternative Approaches A review of the global illicit drug situation by a body charged with responsibility for international supply reduction concluded that "countries that are not suffering from the harmful consequences of drug abuse are the exception rather than the rule" (56). This deterioration in the global illicit drug situation has occurred despite progressive strengthening of illicit drug law enforcement over several decades.

Illicit drug use was a problem in only a few developed countries a generation ago. During the 1960s, illicit drug use spread to most developed countries. During the 1980s, illicit drug use began to spread to developing countries. By the early 1990s, it was estimated that there were more than 5 million drug injectors (57) spread over more than 120 countries (58). In 2004, the number of injecting drug users in the world was estimated to be 13.2 million (59). The estimated global turnover of the illicit drug trade was recently estimated to be $US 322 billion (60). Global production of opium increased 102% from 4,346 tons in 1990 to 8,880 tons in 2007 while global cocaine production increased 20% from 825 tons in 1990 to 994 tons in 2007. The UNODC describes the current situation as "containment." These changes reflected a steady growth in global cultivation and production of illicit drugs. Technologic changes in transport, communications, and computers made movement of contraband substances and profits around the globe much easier for drug traffickers while control of illicit drug trafficking became much more difficult for law enforcement authorities.

This inexorable deterioration of the global illicit drug situation was accompanied by increasingly serious consequences of illicit drug use. Soon after the AIDS epidemic was first recognized in the early 1980s, it was evident that HIV had spread alarmingly among and from populations of injecting drug users in several developed countries, including the United States. HIV has irrevocably changed the nature of injecting drug use and has had an equally dramatic influence on the way injecting drug use is now perceived. Hepatitis C is now recognized to be globally more prevalent among injecting drug users than HIV, including those countries where HIV prevalence has reached alarming levels (61). Though there is still some uncertainty about the natural history of hepatitis C, it is apparent that this infection results in considerable morbidity but only modest mortality. Multi-drug-resistant TB has appeared as a significant health problem in some countries and is now recognized to be closely associated with uncontrolled HIV epidemics in injecting drug users.

Demand Reduction Approaches. There is a large literature evaluating the effectiveness of efforts to reduce demand for illicit substances using educational programs. There is little evidence of significant and sustained reduction in demand from mass audience, school-based, or specially targeted educational campaigns (62). Some educational programs have demonstrated improvements in knowledge, others in attitudes, some in both. However, evidence of reduced consumption or—more significantly—a reduction in drug-related problems is scant.

Demand for illicit substances appears to be greater in populations with high levels of youth unemployment, poor housing, limited educational opportunities, poor health services, and neglected, crime-ridden neighborhoods. It is difficult to assess the role of these factors in stimulating demand for drugs. Lack of data for the influence of these factors on demand should not be taken as evidence that they are unimportant.

Supply Reduction Approaches A substantial literature, including empirical (63) and theoretical (64–66) studies document the relative ineffectiveness of supply reduction and predict continuing failure. An impressive study commissioned by the United States Army and carried out by the RAND Corporation evaluated the return on a $1 investment in a variety of measures designed to reduce the societal cost of cocaine. The return was 15 cents for crop reduction and eradication in South America, 32 cents for interdicting transport of cocaine between South America and the United States, 52 cents for U.S. customs and police, and $7.46 for drug treatment of cocaine users (67). The ineffectiveness of supply reduction and likelihood of continuing failure prompted a review body to despair that

> *"over the past two decades in Australia we have devoted increased resources to drug law enforcement, we have increased the penalties of drug trafficking and we have accepted increasing inroads on our civil liberties as part of battle to curb the drug trade. All the evidence shows, however, not only that our law enforcement agencies have not succeeded in preventing the supply of illicit drugs to Australian markets but that it is unrealistic to expect them to do so. If the present policy of prohibition is not working then it is time to give serious consideration to the alternatives, however radical they may seem" (68).*

Consideration of alternatives (69) is now beginning in a number of countries and has even been undertaken by the research arm of the Congress (70).

The experience of most countries and the international experience has been that global drug production has for decades increased almost every year apart from occasional reductions in production caused by bad weather in growing areas. Illicit drug use is spreading to more and more countries around the world. The range of drugs used has increased. Many countries have experienced an exponential growth in drug-related crime and other adverse outcomes, including drug-related deaths. The response to this national and global deterioration of the illicit drug situation has been an ever-increasing emphasis on attempts to restrict the supply of illicit drugs. International collaboration has increased. More funds have been allocated to attempts to reduce drug cultivation and production. Penalties for drug trafficking or drug use have been increased. Drug squads have been expanded. The number of prison inmates serving sentences for drug related offences has increased. Financial surveillance has been intensified.

Strengthening supply reduction has required ever-increasing funding at a time of growing scarcity of public resources. Greater inroads have been made into civil liberties, and corruption of the criminal justice system also has increased. Few attempts to eliminate harm have been successful whereas harm reduction has rarely failed. To many, harm reduction has been a way of curbing the excesses of a drug policy that has unrealistically emphasized supply reduction. Though many countries have now adopted harm reduction, no country has yet established and then closed harm reduction programs.

Estimates of the allocation of government expenditure in response to illicit drugs have shown consistently that drug law enforcement is very generously funded while health and social interventions are generally funded parsimoniously.

The alarming possibility exists that supply reduction may have inadvertently exacerbated health problems. Emphasis on supply reduction and public health goals may be inimical. Anti-opium policies adopted in Hong Kong (1945), Thailand (1959), and Laos (1972) were followed by the disappearance of opium smoking—which was replaced by heroin injecting (71), setting the scene for a later epidemic of HIV infection beginning among injecting drug users in Thailand in 1988, which then seeded uncontrolled epidemics involving the general populations of Thailand, Burma, Malaysia, Vietnam, China, and India.

CONCLUSIONS

Harm reduction, with a paramount concern for a reduction in the adverse health, social, and economic consequences of legal and illegal drug use, has now become the mainstream global drug policy. It has gained acceptance from most developed and many developing countries and virtually all United Nations organizations with responsibility for drug policy. Harm reduction is now accepted as a legitimate component of a contemporary response to legal and illegal psychoactive drugs alongside measures to reduce supply and demand. The United States is the most important nation still opposed to harm reduction and is now supported by only a dwindling number of other countries. A more effective global and national response to the problems of illicit drugs requires a better balance of supply, demand, and harm reduction rather than an almost exclusive reliance on supply reduction. Recognition of the substantial health, social, and economic costs of uncontrolled spread of HIV among and from injecting drug users prompted many countries in recent decades to accept harm reduction. The scientific debate about the effectiveness and safety of major harm reduction interventions (such as needle syringe programs and methadone and buprenorphine maintenance treatment) is now over. However implementation of these measures in most countries in the world is still very poor. The major obstacle to greater acceptance of harm reduction comes from entrenched advocates of supply control. Harm reduction increasingly emphasizes the importance of protecting the human rights of drug users. Other important aspects of harm reduction include basing policy, programs, and practice on evidence; valuing the importance of incremental gains for the many rather than requiring heroic gains for a select few; cost-effectiveness; and involvement of affected populations including, especially injecting drug users but also other major stakeholders.

REFERENCES

1. Wodak A., Saunders W. Harm reduction means what I choose it to mean [editorial]. *Drug Alcohol Rev* 1995;14:269–271.
2. Birt L. Prime Minister's Strategy Unit. *Strategy Unit drugs project. Phase 1 report: understanding the issues project report.* London: UK Cabinet Office, 2003.
3. RSA Drugs Commission. *The report of the RSA Commission on illegal drugs, communities and public policy. Drugs—facing facts.* London: The Royal Society for the Encouragement of Arts, Manufactures & Commerce, 2007.
4. Nadelmann E. Drug prohibition in the United States: costs, consequences, and alternatives. *Science* 1989;245(4921):939–947.
5. Strang J. Drug use and harm reduction: responding to the challenge. In: Heather N, Wodak A, Nadelmann E, O'Hare P, eds. *Psychoactive drugs and harm-reduction: from faith to science.* London: Whurr Publishers, 1993:3–20.
6. International Harm Reduction Association. Organisation Web site, 2006. Retrieved July 10, 2008, from http:// www.ihra.net/ Whatisharm reduction.
7. Select Committee on Science and Technology, House of Lords. *Cannabis: the scientific and medical evidence (report to the United Kingdom Parliament).* London: The Stationery Office, 1998.
8. Joy JE, Watson SJ, Benson JA. *Marijuana and medicine: assessing the science base.* Washington DC: National Academy of Sciences, Institute of Medicine, 1999.
9. Lurie P, Reingold AL, Bowser B, et al. *The public health impact of needle exchange programs in the United States and abroad,* vol. I. San Francisco: University of California, 1993.
10. Heimer R. Can syringe exchange serve as a conduit to substance abuse treatment? *J Subst Abuse Treat* 1998;15:183–191.
11. National Consensus Development Panel on Effective Medical Treatment of Opiate Addiction. *Journal of the American Medical Association* 1998;280(22):1936–1943.
12. Nordt C, Stohler R. Incidence of heroin use in Zurich, Switzerland: a treatment case register analysis. *Lancet* 2006;367:1830–1834.
13. World Health Organization Expert Committee on Drug Dependence. *WHO Technical Report Series* (Twenty-eighth Report). Geneva, Switzerland: World Health Organization, 1993.
14. King County Bar Association, Drug Policy Project. *Effective drug control: toward a new legal framework.* Seattle: King County Bar Association 2005.
15. Friedman SR, Cooper HLF, Tempalski B, et al. Relationships of deterrence and law enforcement to drug-related harms among drug injectors in U.S. metropolitan areas. *AIDS* 2006;20:93–99.
16. United Nations Office on Drugs and Crime. *Reducing the adverse health and social consequences of drug abuse: a comprehensive approach.* Vienna: Author, 2008.
17. Wodak A., Cooney A. Do needle syringe programs reduce HIV infection among injecting drug users: a comprehensive review of the international evidence. *Subst Use Misuse* 2006;41(6–7):777–816.
18. National Institute for Health and Clinical Excellence. Methadone and buprenorphine for the management of opioid dependence. London: Author, 2007. Retrieved August 4, 2008, from http://www.guideline.gov/summary/summary.aspx?ss=15&doc_id=10483&nbr=5506.
19. Islam MM, Wodak A, Conigrave KM. The effectiveness and safety of syringe vending machines as a component of needle syringe programmes in community settings. *Int J Drug Policy* 2007:31. [Epub ahead of print]
20. Farrell M, Gowing L, Marsden J, et al. Effectiveness of drug dependence treatment in HIV prevention. *Int J Drug Policy* 2005;16:67–75.
21. National Institute on Drug Abuse International Program. *Methadone research Web guide.* Bethesda: U.S. National Institutes of Health, 2006. Accessed May 1, 2008, from http://international.drugabuse.gov/ methadone/methadone_web_guide/part_b/partb_question15.html#harwood.
22. World Health Organization, United Nations Office on Drugs and Crime & UNAIDS. *Substitution maintenance therapy in the management of opioid dependence and HIV/AIDS prevention: position paper.* Geneva: WHO, 2004.
23. Kerr T, Wodak A, Elliot R, et al. Opioid substitution and HIV/AIDS treatment and prevention. *Lancet* 2004;364:1918–1919.
24. Wood E, Tyndall MW, Montaner JS, Kerr T. Summary of findings from the evaluation of a pilot medically supervised safer injecting facility. *CMAJ* 2006;175:1399–1404.
25. Hall W, Kimber J. Being realistic about benefits of supervised injecting facilities. *Lancet* 2005;366:271–272.
26. Spooner C, Hall W. Preventing drug misuse by young people: we need to do more than "just say no." *Addiction* 2002;97(5):478–481.
27. Spooner C, Hall W, Lynskey M. *Structural determinants of youth drug use.* Woden: Australian National Council on Drugs, 2001.
28. Cook JA, Jonikas JA, Razzano L. A randomized evaluation of consumer versus nonconsumer training of state mental health service providers *Community Ment Health J* 1999;31(3):229–238
29. Pauly B. Harm reduction through a social justice lens. *Int J Drug Policy* 2008;19(2):4–10.
30. Department of Health. *National campaign against drug abuse.* Canberra, Australia: Australian Government Publishing Service, 1985:2.
31. International Harm Reduction Development. *Harm reduction* development 2005: Countries with injection-driven HIV epidemics. New York: Open Society Institute. 2006.
32. United Nations Office on Drugs and Crime. UNODC 2005 Annual Report. Geneva: Author, 2005.
33. Coffin P. Marketing harm reduction: a historical narrative of the International Harm Reduction Development Program. *Int J Drug Policy* 2002;13(3):213–220.
34. Open Society Institute and SOROS Foundation. *International Harm Reduction Development Program Official Web site,* 2008. Retrieved May 1, 2008, from http://www.soros.org/initiatives/ health/focus/ihrd.
35. Centre for Harm Reduction, Macfarlane Burnet Centre for Medical Research, Asian Harm Reduction Network. *Manual for reducing drug-related harm in Asia.* Melbourne: Author, 2003.

36. International Harm Reduction Association. *Global state of harm reduction 2008. Mapping the response to drug-related HIV and hepatitis C epidemics*. London: International Harm Reduction Association. 2008. Accessed on December 18, 2008, http://www.ihra.net/Assets/582/i/GSHRFull Report.pdf.
37. Ruel J-M. *International survey of the use of methadone in the treatment of narcotic addiction*. Ottawa, Canada: Health, Canada, 1996.
38. Ward J, Mattick R, Hall W. *Methadone maintenance treatment and other opioid replacement therapies*. Amsterdam, The Netherlands: Harwood Academic Publishers, 1998.
39. National Commission on Acquired Immune Deficiency Syndrome. *The twin epidemics of substance use and HIV*. Washington, DC: National Commission on Acquired Immune Deficiency Syndrome, 1991.
40. United States General Accounting Office. *Needle exchange programs: research suggests promise as an AIDS prevention strategy*. Report No. GAO/HRD93-60. Washington, DC: U.S. Government Printing Office, 1993.
41. Satcher D. *Note to Jo Ivey Boufford*. Washington, DC: Drug Policy Foundation, 1995.
42. National Research Council and Institute of Medicine. *Preventing HIV transmission. The role of sterile needles and bleach*. Washington, DC: National Academy Press, 1995.
43. Office of Technology Assessment. *The effectiveness of AIDS prevention efforts*. Washington, DC: Author, 1995.
44. Committee on the Prevention of HIV Infection among Injecting Drug Users in High Risk Countries. *Preventing HIV infection among injecting drug users in high risk countries: an assessment of the evidence*. Washington: National Academies Press, 2006.
45. Wodak A, Lurie P. A tale of two countries: attempts to control HIV among injecting drug users in Australia and the United States. *J Drug Issues* 1997; 27(1):117–134.
46. Law MG, Batey RG. Injecting drug use in Australia: needle/syringe programs prove their worth, but hepatitis C still on the increase. *MJA* 2003;178(5):197–198.
47. Kahn JG. Are NEPs cost-effective in preventing HIV infection? In: Lurie P, Reingold AL, Bowser B, et al., eds. *The public health impact of needle exchange programs in the United States and abroad*, vol I. San Francisco: University of California, 1993.
48. Lurie P, Drucker E. *An Opportunity Lost: Estimating the Number of HIV Associated with the U.S. Government Opposition to Needle Exchange* Programs. Presented at XI International Conference on AIDS, Vancouver, British Columbia, July 1996.
49. Des Jarlais DC, Hagan H, Friedman SR, et al. Maintaining low HIV seroprevalence in populations of injecting drug users. *JAMA* 1995;274: 1226–1231.
50. Stimson GV. Has the United Kingdom averted an epidemic of HIV-l infection amongst drug injectors? [editorial]. *Addiction* 1996;91(8):1085–1088.
51. Holmberg SD. The estimated prevalence and incidence of HIV in 96 large U.S. metropolitan areas. *Am J Public Health* 1996;86:642–654.
52. Kaldor J, Elford J, Wodak A, et al. HIV prevalence among IDUs in Australia: a methodological review. *Drug Alcohol Rev* 1993;12:175–184.
53. National Centre in HIV Epidemiology and Clinical Research. *Australian NSP Survey. National Data Report. 2003–2007. Prevalence of HIV, HCV and injecting and sexual behaviour among IDUs at needle syringe programs*. Sydney: Author, 2008.
54. Edwards G, Anderson P, Babor TF, et al. Alcohol policy and the public good: a good public debate. *Addiction* 1996:91(4):477–81.
55. White House. *Drug Control Strategy*. Washington, DC: Government Printing Office, 1989:11.
56. International Narcotics Control Board (INCB). *Report of the International Narcotics Control Board for Medicine* 1993. Vienna: INCB, 1993.
57. Mann JM, Tarantola DJM, Netter TW. *AIDS in the World. The Global AIDS Policy Coalition*. Cambridge, MA: Harvard University Press, 1992:406–411.
58. Stimson GV, Choopanya K. Global perspectives on drug injecting. In: Stimson GV, des Jarlais DC, Ball A, eds. *Drug injecting and HIV infection: Global dimensions and local responses*. Geneva: World Health Organization, 1998.
59. Aceijas C, Stimson GV, Hickman M, Rhodes T. United Nations reference group on HIV/AIDS prevention and care among IDU in developing and transitional countries. *AIDS* 2004;18(17):2295–2303. Retrieved August 4, 2008, from http://www.ncbi.nlm.nih.gov/pubmed/15577542.
60. United Nations Office on Drugs and Crime. World Drug Report. Vienna, 2007.
61. Garfein RS, Vlahov D, Galai N, et al. Viral infections in short-term injection drug users: the prevalence of the hepatitis C, B, human immunodeficiency and human T-lymphotropic viruses. *Am J Public Health* 1996;86: 655–661.
62. Cohen J. Achieving a reduction in drug-related harm through education. In: Heather N, Wodak A, Nadelmann E, O'Hare P, eds. *Psychoactive drugs and harm-reduction: from faith to science*. Londonand: Whurr Publishers, 1993:65–76.
63. Commission on Narcotic Drugs. *Economic and social consequences of drug abuse and illicit trafficking: an interim report*. Vienna, Austria: United Nations Economic and Social Council, 1995.
64. Wisotsky S. *Breaking the impasse in the war on drugs*. Westport, CT: Greenwood Press, 1986.
65. Thornton M. *The economics of prohibition*. Salt Lake City: University of Utah Press, 1991.
66. Center for Strategic and International Studies. *The transnational drug challenge and the new world order: new threats and opportunities*. Washington, DC: Author, 1993.
67. Rydell CP, Everingham SS. *Controlling cocaine. supply versus demand programs*. Santa Monica, CA: RAND Drug Policy Research Center, 1994.
68. Parliamentary Joint Committee on the National Crime Service. Canberra. Parliament of the Commonwealth of Australia. 1989.
69. Nadelmann E. Thinking seriously about alternatives to drug prohibition. *Daedalus* 1992;121:85–132.
70. United States General Accounting Office. *Confronting the drug problem: debate persists on enforcement and alternative approaches*. Report No. GAOl GGD-93-82. Washington, DC: U.S. Government Printing Office, 1993.
71. Westermeyer J. The pro-heroin effects of anti-opium laws in Asia. *Arch Gen Psychiatry* 1976;33:1135–1139.

CHAPTER 31

Dennis McCarty, PhD
Victor A. Capoccia, PhD
David H. Gustafson, PhD

Quality Improvement for Addiction Treatment

Outcomes from addiction treatment services compare favorably with treatments for other chronic conditions such as hypertension, diabetes and asthma (1). Policy makers, purchasers, families, and practitioners, nonetheless, are not satisfied and challenge the field to enhance treatment outcomes and improve the quality of care.

Dissatisfaction with the outcomes of addiction treatment may reflect broader and more visible social impacts (e.g., family integrity, crime, employment); the impacts from other chronic illness such as diabetes may be less visible. Effective treatment interventions for hypertension, diabetes, and asthma, moreover, have been in use for longer periods while more recent and emerging research guides evidence-based treatments for addiction. A consequence of the discrepancies between substance use disorders and other chronic illnesses is a persistent expectation that patients with diagnosed drug and alcohol disorders remain symptom-free (i.e. without substance use) after their treatment ends. A contemporary understanding of addiction as a treatable health condition includes a recognition that withdrawal of treatment or related supports may promote a reemergence of symptoms; continuing care including active self-management and recovery supports is essential to sustaining positive outcomes associated with treatment (2,3).

Efforts to improve the consistency and quality of addiction treatment and enhance treatment effectiveness generally fall into four categories:

1. building the science and knowledge of addiction and treatment interventions (continue to gain understanding of the condition and what works to treat the condition)
2. defining and measuring the results of treatment (measure the results of treatment)
3. accrediting and licensing programs that deliver treatment
4. building delivery-system capacity to deliver effective treatments consistently (improve the capacity to deliver what we know works)

This chapter examines efforts to measure and track results, efforts to accredit programs that deliver treatment, and the efforts to improve quality and capacity to deliver effective treatments consistently. First, current interest in improved outcomes is placed within the broad context of reports and expectations from the Institute of Medicine. The chapter goes on to review research on measuring treatment and outcomes, outlines accreditation activities, and discusses opportunities for the development of systems and improving processes that support delivery of treatments that work.

INSTITUTE OF MEDICINE REPORTS

The Institute of Medicine (IOM) within the National Academy of Sciences advises federal policy makers about health concerns and public health policy issues. In a series of reports, the Institute identified needs for better health care and outlined strategies to improve the quality of health care in America. *To Err is Human: Building a Safer Health System* (4) found that medical error was a major source of morbidity and mortality in the U.S. health care system and challenged health care systems to track and eliminate error through implementation of performance standards that emphasize patient safety. *Crossing the Quality Chasm: A New Health System for the 21st Century* (5) was the follow-up report providing guidance on redesigning systems of health care to better address chronic care, make greater use of information and technology, coordinate care, incorporate process and outcome measures into systems of care, and continually improve the effectiveness of service providers. Six dimensions of quality were specified: Care should be safe, effective, patient-centered, timely, efficient, and equitable. The most recent report, *Improving the Quality of Health Care for Mental Health and Substance Use Conditions* (6), asserts that the *Crossing the Quality Chasm* framework can be extended to treatments for alcohol, drug, and mental health disorders. The report notes that proven science-based treatments are not used routinely and that substandard care leads to greater expense and suffering. The report, sponsored by the Substance Abuse and Mental Health Services Administration, explicitly recommends that alcohol, drug, and mental health treatment systems emphasize the six dimensions of quality of care and that public agencies and other payers promote the development of process and outcome measures that track quality of care (6).

Over the next decade, drug and alcohol treatment services can anticipate mandates for evidence-based, patient-centered care delivered in ways that are safe, timely, efficient and equitable. One important common theme that carried across all three IOM reports on quality is that system design, reimbursement processes, and service delivery have more impact on treatment results (patient outcomes) than variation in individual practitioner knowledge or behavior. In other words, improved outcomes will come more readily from improved systems than from additional training. Though human resource development is important, better system design trumps improvement of skills as a leverage point for improving outcomes for populations.

DEFINING AND MEASURING QUALITY TREATMENT AND OUTCOMES

Public expectations, demands for accountability from payers and policy makers, and a strong desire from within the field of addiction medicine to improve performance drive efforts to define and measure effective treatments and treatment outcomes. Measurement is a key to improvement. Measures of performance before and after the introduction of changes enable managers to verify desired impacts and to monitor, track and maintain performance over time. Payers, including the U.S. Department of Health and Human Services, Substance Abuse and Mental Health Services Administration (SAMHSA) and its Center for Substance Abuse Treatment (CSAT), and state and county governments are collaborating with researchers, treatment providers, and professional trade groups to construct robust measurement systems and to promote quality improvements. Their efforts to define and measure the quality of addiction treatment include measures that track system performance (i.e., National Outcome Measures, Washington Circle Measures) and catalogues that identify and promote the use of proven treatments (i.e., National Quality Forum Consensus Standards).

National Outcome Measures and the State Outcomes Measurement and Management System

SAMHSA is implementing a national system to monitor state performance related to treatment and prevention of alcohol, drug, and mental health disorders: the State Outcome Measurement and Management System (SOMMS). For treatment of alcohol and drug disorders, states must report 10 measures at client admission and discharge that contribute to six National Outcome Measures (NOMs):

- abstinence from alcohol and other drugs
- employment/education
- crime and criminal justice
- stability in housing
- access capacity
- retention

Measures are under development for three additional dimensions:

- social support/social connectedness
- perception of care
- use of evidence-based practices

States will also provide data for estimates of cost effectiveness.

The NOMs measures represent a combination of patient outcome, system performance, and process measures. Data collected through the state's admission and discharge datasets and reported to SAMHSA as part of the Treatment Episode Data Set provide the raw material for NOMs. The reports are required as a condition of federal funding through the Substance Abuse Prevention and Treatment Performance Partnership Block Grant. The measures are designed to increase the accountability of state systems and participating treatment services. See the SAMHSA Web pages (*http://nationaloutcomemeasures.samhsa.gov/./welcome.asp*) for detail (accessed October 28, 2007).

Washington Circle Measures CSAT supports the Washington Circle process to develop and test measures that monitor the performance of health plans and public treatment systems. Three measures are in current use:

1. identification of alcohol and drug disorders among members (percent with an alcohol or drug disorder diagnosis)
2. treatment initiation (percent of individuals who entered inpatient or outpatient care and completed another treatment session within 14 days
3. treatment engagement (percent of individuals who initiated care and completed at least two additional treatment visits within 30 days) (7).

The initiation and engagement measures are included in the Health Plan Employer Data and Information Set (HEDIS) measures that health plans submit annually to the National

Commission for Quality Improvement. HEDIS reports suggest that health plan performance on these measures varies by type of plan: commercial (initiation = 45%; engagement = 14%), Medicare (initiation = 51%; engagement = 5%), and Medicaid (initiation = 41%; engagement = 10%) (8). Moreover, the rates seem disappointingly low; only 40% to 50% of the individuals with a diagnosed alcohol or drug disorder initiate care, and only 5% to 15% complete a minimum two additional visits within 30 days. Furthermore, these rates have declined over the relatively brief period during which health plans have been reporting the data (8).

The impact of these measures on treatment outcomes is unclear. An analysis of administrative data from Oklahoma found that individuals who initiated and engaged in treatment for alcohol and drug disorders were less likely to be arrested or incarcerated (9). The proximal process measures seem to anticipate improvements on distal outcome measures. A study of addiction treatment centers within the VA examined relationships between center performance on Washington Circle measures and improvements in scores on the Addiction Severity Index (ASI) alcohol and drug domains and found no significant influence: Better rates of identification, initiation, and engagement were not related to more improvement on the ASI measures (10).

National Quality Forum The National Quality Forum (NQF) is a Congressionally chartered membership organization charged with using empirically based consensus process to define and disseminate standards and measures for the health care system. The federal Office of Management and Budget (OMB) directs Federal agencies (e.g., The Center for Medicare and Medicaid Service [CMS]) to use voluntary consensus standards in lieu of government-unique standards in procurement and regulatory matters. A recent NQF report, *National Voluntary Consensus Standards for the Treatment of Substance Use Conditions*, identifies 11 treatment practices, organized into four domains and subdomains, as evidence-based treatments for alcohol, tobacco, and drug use disorders (11). Table 31.1 summarizes the domains and subdomains.

The endorsement of these practices by NQF's members (more than 365 organizations, including health care providers, consumer groups, professional associations, purchasers, federal and state agencies, research and quality improvement organizations, and suppliers) is the first formal consensus on evidence-based practices for treatment of substance use conditions. Follow-up work continues to define, test and disseminate operational measures for the NQF sanctioned practices.

ACCREDITATION FOR TREATMENT PROGRAMS

Performance measures are often examined in accreditation reviews. Accreditation is recognition by peers that an organization meets standards of performance that represent safe and competent treatment. Three bodies—the Joint Commission on Accreditation of Health Care Organizations (JCAHO), the Commission on Accreditation of Rehabilitation Facilities (CARF), and the Council on Accreditation for Children and Family Services (COA)—are the primary entities that provide peer-reviewed accreditation for alcohol and drug treatment programs (12). The 2006 National Survey of Substance Abuse Treatment Services (N-SSATS) notes that less than half of the facilities reported accreditation from JCAHO (22%), CARF (18%), or COA (4%) (13).

Accreditation Process Accreditation requires an organization to conduct an extensive internal analysis of its performance. Accreditation standards focus on broad domains, including governance, consumer rights and privacy, human resource development, use of treatment and or clinical interventions, methods to continually improve quality, maintenance and use of records, business systems, and facilities. The standards are aimed at minimum at promoting patient safety and optimally at improving patient outcomes. The organizational self-analysis is followed by a site visit by peers, or accreditation surveyors, who independently verify the existence and performance of components noted in the self-assessment. Surveyors identify strengths and the need for improvement and then present a recommendation to the accrediting body for multi-year, limited, conditional, or denial of accreditation.

Accreditation for Opioid Treatment Programs An exception to the limited accreditation of treatment programs are outpatient opioid treatment programs. As a result of a transfer of authority from the U.S. Food and Drug Administration (FDA) to SAMHSA in 2001, Federal regulations (42 CFR Part 8) require that opioid treatment programs receive certification from a national accreditation organization or state agency documenting that the treatment program meets regulatory standards and will comply with the standards. Accreditation was expected to promote more consistent use of individualized treatment plans based on current best practice guidelines for medical and clinical care and facilitate evaluation of clinical outcomes (14). The CARF and The Joint Commission are approved to provide national accreditation. They review opioid treatment programs to confirm that the services comply with federal standards, including the elements found in regular accreditation reviews and some specific to opioid treatment services: specialized services for pregnant patients, HIV counseling and education, and procedures to dispense medications in compliance with federal rules (14).

To assess the feasibility of using accreditation to monitor regulatory compliance, CSAT sponsored a pilot assessment. Most programs (90 of 110: 82%) achieved accreditation (15). Programs had the most difficulty meeting the standards for organizational administration, performance improvement, and screening and assessment (15). The challenge in complying with expectations for continuous quality improvement suggests the addiction treatment field needs to develop its capacity for continuous improvement.

TABLE 31.1 Summary of National Quality Forum Consensus Standards for the Treatment of Substance Use Conditions

Domain #1: Identification of Substance Use Conditions

Screening and Case Finding

During new patient encounters and at least annually, patients in general and mental health care settings should be screened for at-risk drinking, alcohol use problems and illnesses, and any tobacco use.

To identify patients who use drugs, health care providers should employ a systematic method that considers epidemiologic and community factors and the potential health consequences of drug use for their specific population.

Diagnosis and Assessment

Patients who have a positive screen for—or an indication of—a substance use problem or illness should receive further assessment to confirm that a problem exists and determine a diagnosis. Patients with a diagnosed substance use illness should receive a multidimensional, biopsychosocial assessment to guide patient-centered treatment planning for substance use illness and any coexisting conditions.

Domain #2: Initiation and Engagement in Treatment

Brief Intervention

All patients identified with alcohol use in excess of National Institute on Alcohol Abuse and Alcoholism guidelines and/or any tobacco use should receive a brief motivational counseling intervention by a health care worker trained in this technique.

Promoting Engagement in Treatment for Substance Use Illness

Health care providers should systematically promote patient initiation of care and engagement in ongoing treatment for substance use illness. Patients with substance use illness should receive supportive services to facilitate their participation in ongoing treatment.

Withdrawal Management

Supportive pharmacotherapy should be available and provided to manage the symptoms and adverse consequences of withdrawal, based on a systematic assessment of the symptoms and risk of serious adverse consequences related to the withdrawal process. Withdrawal management alone does not constitute treatment for dependence and should be linked with ongoing treatment for substance use illness.

Domain #3: Therapeutic Interventions to Treat Substance Use Illness **Psychosocial Interventions**

Empirically validated psychosocial treatment interventions should be initiated for all patients with substance use illnesses.

Pharmacotherapy

Pharmacotherapy should be recommended and available to all adult patients with diagnosed opioid dependence and without medical contraindications. Pharmacotherapy, if prescribed, should be provided in addition to and directly linked with psychosocial treatment/support.

Pharmacotherapy should be offered and available to all adult patients with diagnosed alcohol dependence and without medical contraindications. Pharmacotherapy, if prescribed, should be provided in addition to and directly linked with psychosocial treatment/support.

Pharmacotherapy should be recommended and available to all adult patients with diagnosed nicotine dependence (including those with other substance use conditions) and without medical contraindications. Pharmacotherapy, if prescribed, should be provided in addition to and directly linked with brief motivational counseling.

Domain #4: Continuing Care Management of Substance Use

Patients with substance use illness should be offered long-term, coordinated management of their care for substance use illness and any co-existing conditions, and this care management should be adapted based on ongoing monitoring of their progress.

BUILDING SYSTEM CAPACITY TO DELIVER EFFECTIVE TREATMENTS

Since 2001, a number of national-level efforts have focused on improving the quality of treatment offered, particularly among the more than 13,000 publicly supported programs that deliver the 70% of care paid for by public sources of support. According to Roman and associates in their 15 year follow-up of more than 400 programs, fewer than 10% offered medication-assisted treatment, and fewer than half offered psychosocially based interventions supported by empirical research (16–18). McLellan and colleagues noted that weak infrastructure in the form of high turnover, low use of technology, and minimal presence of medical expertise, may make it difficult to make substantive improvements in treatment effectiveness (19). An analysis of admission and retention rates of adults and adolescents in residential treatment for drug disorders noted that the design of systems accounted for more barriers to admission and detachment form treatment than did "client resistance" or need for additional staff training (20).

Contemporary quality improvement strategies begin with recognition that insufficient quality often reflects poor system and process design. Process improvement strategies, therefore, strive to construct processes that minimize variability and eliminate error to improve efficiency and enhance customer satisfaction with the product or service. Shewhart (21,22) and his students Deming (23) and Juran (24) were pioneers in the application of these techniques to manufacturing. Over time, the concepts have been extended to health care and to services (25,26).

Network for the Improvement of Addiction Treatment The Network for the Improvement of Addiction Treatment (NIATx) applies process improvement strategies to the programs that treat alcohol and drug disorders. NIATx members learn to use process improvement to reduce time to admission, decrease no-shows, enhance retention in care, and increase admissions (27,28). Participating programs form a learning community that shares problems and solutions and uses a simplified set of five key process-improvement principles to facilitate organizational changes that enhance the quality of addiction treatment services: understand the customer, fix key problems, pick a powerful change leader, seek outside ideas and encouragement, and use rapid PDSA (Plan-Do-Study-Act) cycles (29). Together, these principles have the potential to influence organizational culture and reflect an orientation to continuous improvement.

Understand the Customer Process improvement stresses the need to understand and involve customers in identifying and fixing problems. Focus groups and interviews with clients can help increase understanding of treatment experiences. Another useful tool is the walk-through. Change leaders use walk-throughs to gain insight into problems in treatment processes. Observers simulate the patient experience and walk through processes that are required for patients. NIATx participants typically start with the admission process. A senior manager develops a patient script (description of the patient and the presenting problems), calls the treatment center for an appointment, completes the admission process, and notes positive and negative findings. Typically, the walk-through scenario includes a "family member" (e.g., sister, spouse, or parent) who shares the experience and makes additional observations. The walk-throughs create stories with impact and illuminate problematic facets of the process.

A review of walk-through reports from 327 applicants to NIATx revealed conflicting and incorrect information to applicants, redundant and burdensome intake forms, unanswered telephone lines, and unreturned voice mail (30). There were also challenges addressing complex patient needs and weaknesses in agency infrastructure (30). Change teams use the results of walk-through to identify process problems that can be corrected and improved.

Fix Key Problems Agency change requires active support from the highest levels of the organization. The chief executive will be most supportive if the change team addresses problems that are central to the organization's success. Issues that affect organizational efficiency and productivity often impact revenues generated and costs of service delivery and get attention and support from organizational leadership. Missed appointments, for example, reduce counselor productivity, and anticipated revenue is lost. Strategies to reduce no-show rates, therefore, can lead to increased revenues and improved counselor productivity.

A number of treatment services participating in the NIATx report improved business cases as a result of the work on NIATx. Acadia Hospital in Bangor, Maine, for example, completed a walk-through; they found that their admission process included 4 days between the first contact with a potential patient and the beginning of intensive outpatient services; required multiple phone calls between the patient and program staff; and that only 25% of the initial contacts led to an admission (27). To reduce the delays and eliminate multiple calls, the program implemented a next-day admission policy: Potential clients were told to be at the clinic at 7:30 the next morning. Intake assessments were completed and clients began care later in the morning. As a result of the change, the days to admission declined to 1 day, and 65% of the first contact telephone calls led to a treatment admission. Over the next 2 years, program revenues increased 56% (27).

Pick a Powerful Change Leader Serving as a change leader (the individual who leads a team in creating and implementing organizational change) can be an excellent career development opportunity. Not every counselor or employee, however, has the skill to lead change, and many do not seek the responsibility of leading change. It is important, therefore, to choose individuals who can effect change. Change leaders should have the respect of their peers and of staff and leaders throughout the organization. They must also have access to agency management. Over time, a well-developed organization will use the opportunity to lead change teams as a strategy for grooming future managers and leaders within the corporation.

Seek Outside Ideas and Encouragement NIATx members get ideas for service improvements from other NIATx participants and from other industries. The vice-president of quality improvement at the Ritz Carlton spoke at a NIATx Summit and shared his perspectives on serving hotel guests and the hotel's expectations for customer orientation among all employees: "Ladies and Gentlemen Serving Ladies and Gentlemen." Though the Ritz typically serves a clientele different from that found in most publicly funded drug abuse treatment services, its emphasis on treating guests and staff as ladies and gentlemen can be applied in any business, including addiction treatment.

A second aspect of the principle is that it is important to get encouragement as well as ideas from other organizations. Making organizational change can be a lonely experience. Internal pressures encourage attention to more immediate and pressing needs. NIATx participation includes regularly scheduled learning sessions wherein programs report on projects and set targets for gains; the public process creates pressure to meet expectations and continue to improve. The NIATx also provides "interest circle" telephone calls whereby change leaders working on similar processes discuss their experiences and share ideas for success. The outside support encourages organizations to continue to improve and to benefit from the group norms and experiences.

Use Rapid PDSA Cycles PDSA (Plan, Do, Study Act) cycles are a central component of process improvement. Change teams need to plan (plan). Planning includes specification of the problem that will be fixed, collection of data to assess the extent of the problem, and development of a change that will implemented. Process improvement is about action. Change teams test the proposed change—(do). A key facet is that the test is for a limited time and limited number of patients. Initially, it is a feasibility test. Can we make the change and does the change reduce the problem rate? A few simple measures are collected and analyzed (study): Did a change occur in the frequency or extent of the problem? Based on the planning, doing, and studying, the change team decides what to do next (act). The change can be abandoned if it does not work. It may be modified to enhance the effect. Hopefully, it expands to include more patients and more counselors and eventually can be institutionalized. PDSA cycles are rapid. One to two weeks (and sometimes much less time) is usually sufficient to learn whether the change is viable and if additional time and resources should be invested.

The first cohort of NIATx participants reported organizational changes that led to a 43% reduction in days to treatment and 25% improvements in early retention (28). Analysis of admissions data over a 15-month reporting period, moreover, found a 37% decline in days to treatment, from about 20 days in October 2003 to 12 days in December 2004 (28). Significant improvements were also observed in retention in care. In October 2003, about 72% of the patients who completed one unit of care returned for a second unit of care; by December 2004, 85% of the admissions received at least two units of care (28). Although gains may appear to be modest, the impact of process improvement seemed to increase over time, and preliminary analyses suggest that programs can sustain the improvements in access and retention. Additional analysis of NIATx data suggests that reduction in days to treatment enhances retention in care (31). Finally, a qualitative analysis of NIATx implementation found that some treatment programs struggled with the development change measures and use of process data (32).

NIATx evaluation results are suggestive. Before-and-after analyses suggest that programs can make changes to reduce days to admission and to enhance retention in care. These analyses, however, have been unable to disaggregate the influence of different NIATx strategies: It is not feasible to determine which changes are more responsible for the observed effects. A more systematic trial of the NIATx is required to identify the most influential facets of the process improvement strategy and, thus, the next variation in the NIATx—NIATx 200.

NIATx 200 With support from the National Institute on Drug Abuse, nearly 200 treatment programs in Massachusetts, Michigan, New York, Oregon, and Washington State were recruited to participate in the NIATx 200. The programs were randomly assigned to four levels of support for the implementation of process improvement: (i) interest circle telephone calls plus access to the NIATx Web site, (ii) coaching plus access to the NIATx Web site, (iii) learning sessions plus access to the NIATx Web site, and (iv) interest circle telephone calls, coaching, learning sessions plus access to the NIATx Web site. Analyses will assess the influence of each study condition on change in days to treatment and retention in care. A calculation of the benefit/cost ratios will assess the relative value of the more expensive (learning sessions) and less expensive (interest circle telephone calls) interventions.

Scaling up the NIATx for the NIATx 200 requires more systemization of the NIATx components. Walk-through procedures and reports are standardized. Coaches work within more structured guidelines, and interest circle calls are more scripted. Data collection relies on state data systems to minimize burden on the participating treatment programs. Successful implementation of the NIATx 200 will be a big step in developing process improvement technology that can be spread throughout the treatment systems for alcohol, drug and mental health disorders.

Strengthening Treatment Access and Retention—State Implementation: the NIATx State Initiative

Launched in 2006, the 3-year Strengthening Treatment Access and Retention—State Implementation (STAR-SI) program promotes widespread dissemination of quality improvement in state addiction treatment systems. CSAT supports work in Florida, Illinois, Iowa, Maine, Ohio, South Carolina, and Wisconsin. The Robert Wood Johnson Foundation funds awards to New York and Oklahoma. Finally, Montana is supporting its own participation. Although the NIATx offered a methodology to improve performance at the organizational level, policy makers wondered whether "spread" could be achieved faster by focusing on state-level purchasing and regulating agencies to improve performance at the delivery level. Thus, in the STAR-SI, the participating state agencies create incentives and provide support mechanisms to promote statewide adoption of NIATx principles and results. The State Initiative encourages states to involve larger numbers of treatment programs in process improvement and to review and improve their own systems and processes.

Advancing Recovery The most recent facet of the NIATx process improvement strategy is to invite states and providers to collaborate and facilitate the implementation of evidence-based practices for the treatment of alcohol and drug disorders. Advancing Recovery is sponsored by the Robert Wood Johnson Foundation and designed to promote implementation of the National Quality Forum's five sets of evidence-based practices: (i) use of medications, (ii) screening and brief interventions in primary care settings, (iii) seven psychosocial interventions (motivational interviewing, moti-

TABLE 31.2 Advancing Recovery Model for Spreading and Sustaining System Change

Drivers of change
- Clear and measurable project aims
- A few simple measures of progress and success
- A business case for spreading and sustaining the change
- A financing plan to spread and sustain the change
- A purchasing plan to spread and sustain the change
- A cyclical change model built with rapid testing, modification and retesting

Relationships to support change
- Select changes that organizational leadership will commit to for implementation, spreading, and sustaining.
- Participate in a learning community for support to stimulate thinking and to encourage continued action.
- Select changes that meet an important customer need.

Contextual supports for change
- Select changes that help key stakeholders address strategically important issues.
- Identify and address key barriers to spreading and sustaining change.
- Identify and build key organizational relationships to spread and sustain change.

vational enhancement therapy, cognitive behavioral therapy, structured family therapy, contingency management, community reinforcement, and 12-step facilitation), (iv) posttreatment aftercare, and (v) case management, wraparound, and supportive services. Participating states (Alabama, Arkansas, Colorado, Delaware, Florida, Kentucky, Maine, Missouri, Rhode Island, and West Virginia) and cities (Baltimore and Dallas) seek to make changes in systems to support and encourage the use of these categories of treatment services. Maine, for example, added buprenorphine and naltrexone to the Medicaid formulary, requested and received funding in their state appropriation to support medications for uninsured patients, modified regulations, and worked with treatment programs to support the adoption and use of medications. Similarly, Missouri and Florida are working to promote the adoption of medications for treatment of alcohol use disorders. Rhode Island developed a new reimbursement code to facilitate the use of continuing care and a new process that no longer requires cases to be closed when patients move from acute treatment to continuing care. A model of change is emerging from the Advancing Recovery experience to guide the change efforts and provide structure for state and provider initiatives. The model summarized in Table 31.2 articulates drivers, relationships, and contextual variables that promote spreading and sustaining system change.

Advancing Recovery extends the NIATx model to the use of evidence based practices. The initiative also recognizes the critical role that state agencies play in building and sustaining system change.

CONCLUSIONS

Quality improvement efforts are affecting the organization and delivery of treatment for alcohol and drug disorders. Strategies to define, measure, and improve quality of addiction treatment services influence standards of care and the ways in which quality is evaluated. The NOM system increases attention to both proximal and distal treatment outcomes. Other quality improvement strategies emphasize system change. Quality interventions that build on the foundation of the NIATx may be especially promising.

Treatment programs participating in the NIATx gain encouragement and ideas from participation in learning communities and support the application of process improvement to systems of care for alcohol and drug disorders. Outcome studies suggest that process changes can lead to reductions in days to admission and to improvements in retention in care. NIATx change initiatives have many advantages and the key resources needed to widely spread and sustain changes.

The NIATx also attempts to promote a spread of process improvements across statewide treatment systems. The STAR-SI model uses the state treatment and prevention authority as a key player to create an environment wherein it is clearly in the providers' best interest to make certain changes. In doing so, states often provide incentives to providers to promote the implementation, sustaining, and spreading of change. The state authority can model organizational improvements and improve its regulatory and contracting processes. These changes often stimulate provider change so that they can take advantage of the modified processes. The provider sees changes in paperwork requirements or rules and regulations that influence the ease with which a patient are admitted.

Advancing Recovery is another effort to spread system change. There is an explicit focus on changes in state regulations and financing to sustain and spread process improvements and evidence based practices. The key NIATx principles of change work for individual organizations and are also applicable to multiorganizational system changes to facilitate adoption of evidence based practices. Additional principles, however, also need to be considered when addressing statewide adaptations/changes not only at the provider and SSA level but within other state agencies such as Medicaid and Youth and Families. Formal working relationships, for example, need to be stabled between organizations when large-scale systems change are planned.

All of these strategies are being evaluated, but probably the most thorough evaluation will be of the first type of improvement: individual organizational change built within a learning collaborative framework. A randomized clinical trial funded by the NIDA will be assessing the relative contribution of the different components of the NIATx strategy.

One area not addressed in this chapter is innovation. As in any field, resources need to be allocated to leaps forward rather than incremental change. The addiction treatment field is well positioned to benefit from innovation. It is a labor-intensive field with poorly paid staff and high turnover. There are customers that are not touched at all by addiction treatment services, not only people with addictions but family members, many of whom could be very effective resources to partner with treatment agencies if they had a modest set of supports. Certainly the work that is being conducted to find cost-effective medications is crucial. However, there are many other initiatives that might be considered in the areas of automation: computer-based screening and brief interventions; computer-based relapse prevention programs; computer-based programs to assist the parents and partners of women and men struggling with alcohol and drug disorders. The point is that investment in innovation needs to share space with investment in improvement.

REFERENCES

1. McLellan AT, Lewis DC, Obrien CP, Kleber HD. Drug dependence a chronic medical illness: Implications for treatment, insurance and outcomes evaluation. *JAMA* 2000;284:1689–1695.
2. White WL. Addiction recovery: Its definition and conceptual boundaries. *J Subst Abuse Treat* 2007;33:229–241.
3. The Betty Ford Institute Consensus Panel. What is recovery? A working definition from the Betty Ford Institute. *J Subst Abuse Treat* 2007;33: 221–228.
4. Institute of Medicine. *To err is human: Building a safer health system.* Washington, DC: National Academy Press, 2000.
5. Institute of Medicine. *Crossing the quality chasm: a new health system for the 21st century.* Washington, DC: National Academy Press, 2001.
6. Institute of Medicine. *Improving the quality of health care for mental and substance-use disorders: Quality Chasm Series.* Washington, DC: National Academy Press, 2006.
7. Garnick DW, Lee MT, Chalk M, et al. Establishing the feasibility of performance measures for alcohol and other drugs. *J Subst Abuse Treat* 2002;23(4):375–385.
8. National Committee for Quality Assurance. *The state of health care quality: Industry trends and analysis.* Washington, DC: Author, 2006.
9. Garnick D, Horgan C, Lee MT, et al. Are Washington Circle performance measures associated with decreased criminal activity following treatment. *J Subst Abuse Treat* 2007. In press.
10. Harris A, Humphreys KN, Finney JW. Is medical centers' performance on Washington Circle indicators associated with the case-mix adjusted effectiveness of their substance abuse treatment services? *J Subst Abuse Treat* 2007. In press.
11. National Quality Forum. *National voluntary consensus standards for the treatment of substance use conditions: Evidence-based treatment practices.* Washington, DC: Author, 2007.
12. Institute of Medicine. *Managing managed care: Quality improvement in behavioral health.* Washington, DC: National Academy Press, 1997.
13. Substance Abuse and Mental Health Services Administration. *National Survey of Substance Abuse Treatment Services (N-SSATS): 2006. Data on Substance Abuse Treatment Facilities.* Rockville, MD: Substance Abuse and Mental Health Services Administration, 2007.
14. Substance Abuse and Mental Health Services Administration. Opioid drugs in maintenance and detoxification treatment of opiate addiction: Final rule. *Federal Register* 2001;66(11):4076–4102.
15. Wechsberg WM, Kasten JJ. *Methadone maintenance treatment in the U.S.: a practical question and answer guide.* New York: Springer Publishing Company, 2007.
16. Ducharme LJ, Knudsen HK, Roman PM, Johnson JA. Innovation adoption in substance abuse treatment: Exposure, trialability and the Clinical Trials Network. *J Subst Abuse Treat* 2007;32:321–329.
17. Knudsen HK, Ducharme LJ, Roman PM. The adoption of medications in substance abuse treatment: Associations with organizational characteristics and technology clusters. *Drug Alcohol Depend* 2007; in press.
18. Roman PM, Johnson JA. Adoption and implementation of new technologies in substance abuse treatment. *J Subst Abuse Treat* 2002;22: 211–218.
19. McLellan AT, Carise D, Kleber HD. Can the national addiction treatment infrastructure support the public's demand for quality care? *J Subst Abuse Treat* 2003;25:117–121.
20. Ebener P, Kilmer B. *Barriers to treatment entry: Case studies of applicants approved for admission.* Santa Monica, CA: Drug Policy Research Center, Rand; 2003. Report No. DRU-2949-PH.
21. Shewhart WA. *Economic control of quality of manufactured product.* New York: D. Norstrand Co., Inc., 1931.
22. Shewhart WA. *Statistical method from the viewpoint of quality control.* Lancaster, PA: Lancaster Press, 1939.
23. Deming WE. *Out of the crisis.* Cambridge, MA: MIT-CAES, 1986.
24. Juran JM. *Juran's quality control handbook.* New York: McGraw-Hill Publishing Company, 1988.
25. Barney M, McCarty T. *The new six sigma: A leader's guide to achieving rapid business improvement and sustainable results.* Upper Saddle River, NJ: Prentice Hall, 2003.
26. Berwick D. Escape fire: Designs for the future of health care. San Francisco: Jossey Bass, 2005.
27. Capoccia VA, Cotter F, Gustafson DH, et al. Making "stone soup": How process improvement is changing the addiction treatment field. *Joint Commission Journal on Quality and Patient Safety* 2007;33:95–103.
28. McCarty D, Gustafson DH, Wisdom JP, et al. The Network for the Improvement of Addiction Treatment (NIATx): enhancing access and retention. *Drug Alcohol Depend* 2007;88:138–145.
29. Gustafson DH, Hundt SA. Findings of innovation research applied to quality management principles for health care. *Health Educ Q* 1995;20(2):16–33.
30. Ford J, Green CA, Hoffman KA, et al. Process improvement needs in substance abuse treatment: admissions walkthrough results. *J Subst Abuse Treat* 2007;33:379–389.
31. Hoffman KA, Ford JH, Choi D, et al. Replication and sustainability of improved access and retention within the Network for the Improvement of Addiction Treatment. *Drug and Alcohol Dependence* 2008; 98:63–69.
32. Wisdom JP, Ford J, Hayes RA, et al. Addiction treatment agencies' use of data: A qualitative assessment. *J Behav Health Serv Res* 2006;33(4): 394–407.

CHAPTER 32

Nady el-Guebaly, MD
Vladimir Poznyak, MD, PhD
Juana Maria Tomás-Rosselló, MD, MPH

International Perspectives on Addiction Management

Historically, international efforts to control use of psychoactive substances have focused on reducing the worldwide supply. International efforts to decrease the demand for drugs are more recent and are gaining momentum. This chapter will focus on major international endeavors: The first two sections will describe the relevant activities under the umbrella of the United Nations: the World Health Organization (WHO) and the United Nations Office of Drug Control (UNODC). The third part describes the mostly volunteer efforts of physicians to develop international networks to address the public health aspects of the use of drugs. These collaborations have resulted in a number of international medical organizations committed to demand reduction, including the World Medical Association, the World Psychiatric Association and the International Society of Addiction Medicine.

Disclaimer: The views expressed herein are those of the authors, Drs. V. Poznyak, J. Tomas, and N. el-Guebaly, and do not necessarily reflect the positions, decisions, or stated policies of the World Health Organization, United Nations Office on Drugs and Crime, the World Psychiatric Association, or the International Society of Addiction Medicine.

WORLDWIDE PREVALENCE OF PSYCHOACTIVE SUBSTANCE USE

Worldwide psychoactive substance use is highly prevalent, and large segments of the world population are exposed to the effects of dependence-producing substances. Alcohol is the most widely used psychoactive substance worldwide, and about 2 billion people use alcohol beverages around the world (1). Currently there are more than 1 billion people in the world who smoke tobacco (2) and around 200 million people using illicit drugs (3). Significant proportions of populations repeatedly exposed to such dependence-producing substances as alcohol, tobacco, or drugs develop substance use disorders. According to WHO estimates, in 2000, the number of people with alcohol dependence or harmful use of alcohol worldwide reached 76.4 million, and number of people with drug use disorders was 15.3 million (4).

The UNODC's World Drug Report 2007 estimates the total number of drug users at 200 million people, equivalent to about 5% of the global population aged 15 to 64. Cannabis (162 million) represents the first, and amphetamine-type stimulants, or ATS (35 million) the second most widely used substances, followed by opiates (16 million) and cocaine (13 million). UNODC estimates indicate that 25 million people, equivalent to 0.6% of the world population aged 15 to 64, are drug-dependent (3) (Fig. 32.1).

The reports to the Commission on Narcotic Drugs (CND) on the world situation with regard to drug abuse (5) are based on the opinion of national experts as reported by the member states in the Annual Reports Questionnaire (ARQ) (6). The 2008 report provides an overview of trends in consumption of the main types of illicit drugs from 1998 to 2006 and contributes to the global evaluation of progress towards the achievement of the United Nations General Assembly Special Session (UNGASS) goals set in 1998 (5). The available information suggests that the consumption of opioids and cocaine is stabilizing or decreasing particularly in high-consumption countries (cocaine in North America and heroin in Western and Central Europe, in particular), and the prevalence

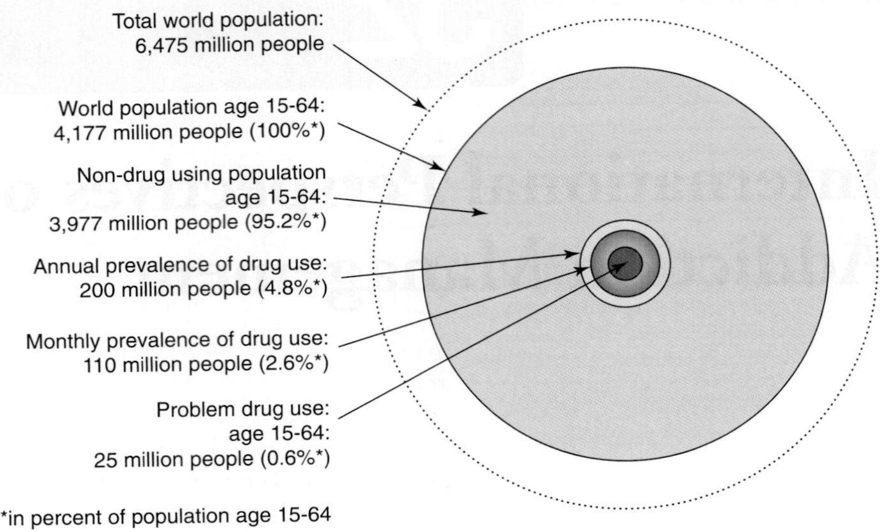

FIGURE 32.1. Illegal drug use at the global level (2005/2006). (Reprinted from World Drug Report, UNODC, 2007.)

of heroin injection remains highest in Central Asian and Eastern European countries. Increases in use of ATS are reported to be tapering off as consumption tends to stabilize or even decrease in Western and Central Europe, East and South-East Asia, North America, and Oceania. In contrast, cannabis consumption remains globally widespread, as experimentation among youth continues to increase.

In the last 25 years, one of the most visible negative consequences of drug dependence has been human immunodeficiency virus and acquired immunodeficiency syndrome (HIV/AIDS), and it is estimated that more than 10% of all HIV infections worldwide are due to the use of contaminated drug injecting equipment. If sub-Saharan Africa and the Caribbean are excluded, this rate of injecting drug users rises even to 30% to 40% among those with HIV infection. Data on the size of the injection drug user (IDU) population from 130 countries indicates that there are 13.1 million IDUs worldwide. It also indicates that sharing of contaminated injection equipment is a major route of HIV transmission in many regions, including Eastern Europe, Central, South, and South East Asia, and some countries in Latin America (7).

HISTORICAL SYNOPSIS OF INTERNATIONAL DRUG TREATIES

International drug treaties concluded between 1912 and 1988 provide the legal basis for the present international drug control system aimed at reducing the supply of and demand for illicit narcotic drugs and psychotropic substances. The three major international drug control treaties are complementary and aim at ensuring the availability of narcotic and psychotropic substances for medical and scientific purposes while preventing their diversion into illicit channels, with a view to reducing human suffering and protecting the public health and welfare (8–10).

Particularly relevant to addiction medicine, the Conventions specify that signatory countries take all practicable measures for the prevention of abuse of drugs and for the early identification, treatment, education, after-care, rehabilitation, and social reintegration of the persons involved, including interventions to counteract the social and health consequences of drug abuse. They also require parties to promote the training of personnel involved in delivering such interventions and to facilitate an understanding of the problems of drug abuse among professionals and the general public.

Further clarifying such provisions in the Conventions, the International Narcotics Control Board (INCB), in its 2003 report, noted that "Governments needed to adopt measures that may decrease the sharing of hypodermic needles among injecting drug abusers in order to limit the spread of HIV/AIDS." At the same time, the INCB stressed that such measures should not promote and/or facilitate drug abuse. The same report also observes that "many Governments have opted in favour of drug substitution and maintenance treatment" and that "the implementation of this treatment does not constitute any breach of treaty provisions, whatever substance may be used for such treatment in line with established national sound medical practice" (6).

The Conventions further state that when drug abusers have committed drug offences, countries may provide drug treatment, education, after-care, rehabilitation, and social reintegration either as an alternative or an addition to conviction or punishment. Such bridges between the criminal justice system and the treatment system may be established at different stages of the criminal process, including the prosecution stage or at the stage of enforcement of a prison sentence.

In June 1998, the United Nations General Assembly's 20th special session (UNGASS) was convened as the largest multilateral gathering ever held on combating illegal drug trafficking and abuse. Member States agreed on a Political Declaration (11) that set out a number of drug control targets to be achieved by 2008 and recognized the strategic significance of the human rights dimension in both supply and demand reduction activities. The adoption of a Declaration on the Guiding Principles of Drug Demand Reduction (12) established a new equilibrium, recognizing demand reduction as one of the pillars of the new global strategy. The Declaration emphasized that demand reduction programs should cover all areas of prevention, from discouraging initial use to reducing the negative health and social consequences of drug abuse for the individual and society as a whole.

The Declaration called for demand reduction policies built on knowledge acquired from research and evaluation of past programs and on systematic and periodic situation assessments. It advocated a community-wide participatory and partnership approach integrated into broader health and social welfare programs; highlighted the importance of appropriate training of policy makers, program planners, and practitioners; and reinforced the Conventions' agreements that social integration of drug-abusing offenders should be pursued, either as an alternative or in addition to punishment, through education, treatment, and rehabilitation services.

As the 10-year period closes in 2008, the international community is assessing the progress made in reaching the UNGASS goals and targets set in 1998. At the 51st session of the CND in March 2008, Member States agreed to establish five intergovernmental expert working groups to review progress and propose future action on the topics outlined in 1998 in preparation of a new Political Declaration to be discussed and adopted by a high-level segment at the 52nd session of the CND in March 2009 (13). The international NGO community is also preparing for this assessment through "Beyond 2008," an international initiative led by the Vienna NGO Committee on Narcotic Drugs in partnership with the UNODC.

SELECTED ACTIVITIES OF THE UNITED NATIONS OFFICE ON DRUGS AND CRIME

The United Nations has had drug control functions since its inception, having inherited them from the League of Nations to provide leadership for international drug control efforts. In response to the various mandates reflected under the three major international drug control treaties, work on demand reduction is an integral part of the activities of the UNODC. This important area of work was given further impetus by the special United Nations session in 1998 and thereafter through the adoption of the Political Declaration, the Declaration on the Guiding Principles of Demand Reduction, and the Action Plan for its implementation, which provide focus for the UNODC's work in providing assistance to Member States towards the goal of achieving significant and measurable results in the field of demand reduction by the year 2008. The UNODC's program of work aims specifically at improving national and global information systems for reporting on activities for the reduction of demand for illicit drugs, sharing of information on best practices, and supporting Member States seeking expertise in developing their own strategies and activities for the reduction of demand for illicit drugs (14).

Progress Toward Reaching a Balance Between Supply and Demand Reduction As reported by Member States to the UNODC through the Biennial Reports Questionnaire, despite the size of the problem and the enormous costs related to drug abuse, in many countries specialized services are not available or, if present, are not accessible. Although treatment and rehabilitation interventions are being expanded, they are still well below the amount and quality that is needed. For instance, opioid dependence detoxification remains the most common reported approach despite evidence of its lack of effectiveness as a stand-alone intervention, while the intervention with the most solid evidence base—pharmacologic maintenance—remains rather infrequently used in most regions. Interventions for reducing the negative health and social consequences of drug abuse have registered a strong increase at the global level and have overtaken treatment and rehabilitation interventions in terms of reported coverage of activities. In some regions, this trend appears to be associated with efforts to prevent the spread of HIV and other infections among IDUs.

UNODC advocates a comprehensive approach including prevention, treatment, and prevention of health and social consequences in line with the evidence base and has recently released a paper highlighting the complementarities of all those measures and calling for a continuum of care in services for drug users (15). In such a continuum, steps are taken to reach out to and engage drug users in prevention, treatment, and care strategies that protect them, their partners, and families from infectious disease, other health problems, and negative social consequences. Within this model, a wide range of community-based services offer easy access to different target groups, responding to diverse age, gender, and other needs, and encourage entry to social and health care, and substance dependence treatment, and rehabilitation. The UNODC-WHO discussion paper on principles of drug dependence treatment (16) notes that interventions and investments in treatment within such a model would be guided by human rights and evidence-based good practice, and the high-quality standards that are required to approve pharmacologic or psychosocial interventions in all the other medical disciplines. Community and prison-based treatment and rehabilitation programs can form part of the same overall treatment system and guarantee the same level of quality. In an international context, such interventions and strategies need to be adapted to the diverse regional, national, and local circumstances, taking into account cultural and economic factors.

Unfortunately, underutilization of such approaches represents a longstanding problem for the field, and those who would most benefit from research advances (community treatment agencies and the clients they serve) have historically been the least likely to be exposed to innovative evidence-based methods. Training of prevention and treatment professionals from early on in their careers and evaluation and feedback on service performance are essential to improve knowledge and disseminate evidence-based methodologies worldwide.

Key Initiatives and Tools: Youthnet and Treatnet—Knowledge Transfer Initiatives With the aim of supporting countries in achieving significant results in reducing demand for drugs by 2008, the UNODC supports the Global Youth Network (*www.unodc.org/youthnet*) for the prevention of drug abuse. Regional networks reach with information, resources, and training more than 500 youth groups around the world and provide grants to some 125 organizations to implement comprehensive drug abuse prevention activities. Unfortunately, many prevention programs around the world, while well intentioned, implement activities that do not have the backing of scientific evidence (e.g., life skills education and family skills training programs) (17–20).

The UNODC aims at positioning drug dependence treatment as a key public health and development intervention. Its work, therefore, will increasingly focus on raising awareness about addiction as a treatable, multifactorial disease and about the need to improve the quality and coverage of drug treatment services around the world. Treatnet, the "International Network of Drug Dependence Treatment and Rehabilitation Resource Centres" *(www.unodc.org/treatnet)* aims to improve the provision of diversified and effective drug treatment and rehabilitation services, including the support to HIV/AIDS prevention and care, in all regions. The Network's members included, in its first stage from 2005 to 2007, 20 drug dependence treatment and rehabilitation resource centers, a training consortium led by UCLA/ISAP, and other partners. In its second phase, starting in 2008, it will evolve into regional networks and involve in addition to treatment centers universities and governmental institutions in charge of treatment and rehabilitation. The work of the network has focused on and developed good-practice documents on four key topics: community-based treatment (21), treatment in prison settings (22), treatment and HIV/AIDS prevention and care (23), and sustained recovery management (24). Through Treatnet, the UNODC has developed a comprehensive training package on treatment and rehabilitation (25) and training of trainers in 14 countries who in turn have trained more than 1,000 physicians, psychologists, counselors, social workers, nurses, and other professionals. The trainers have assessed very positively the comprehensive training package and, in many cases, have continued to disseminate the training well beyond the UNODC's supported program.

The UNODC's Global Assessment Programme (GAP) on Drug Abuse aims at improving the local and global knowledge of the drug abuse situation and at building the capacity to design and implement effective responses to the drug abuse problem through establishing drug epidemiologic surveillance and monitoring and evaluation systems for drug demand reduction. The GAP has been operational since 2000 in several regions of the world and is currently providing training and technical assistance in the Russian Federation, Central Asia, West and Central Africa, and the Middle East and North Africa.

The UNODC is a cosponsor of the Joint United Nations Programme on HIV/AIDS (UNAIDS) and the lead agency for HIV/AIDS prevention and care among IDUs and in prison settings. The UNODC is also responsible for assisting countries in implementing large-scale and wide-ranging interventions to prevent HIV infections and providing care and support to people living with HIV/AIDS. The UNODC advocates that evidence-informed, comprehensive and large-scale interventions for IDUs be an integral part of national HIV/AIDS frameworks.

SELECTED ACTIVITIES OF THE WORLD HEALTH ORGANIZATION RELATED TO ADDICTION MEDICINE

The WHO, as the UN specialized agency on health, is concerned with all psychoactive substances irrespective of their legal status in the international treaties and advocates for a public health approach to problems related to tobacco, alcohol, illicit drugs, and other psychoactive substance use.

Global Burden of Disease Attributable to Psychoactive Substance Use Better understanding of the impact of psychoactive substance use on the population health resulted from the influential Global Burden of Disease (GBD) study, a groundbreaking international effort to quantify the disease burden of different diseases and health conditions using mortality estimates and the estimates of disease burden expressed in Disability Adjusted Life Years (DALYs) lost (26). In 2000, the WHO published its World Health Report with figures of comparative contribution of different risk factors to the disease burden in different parts of the world (27). Tobacco, alcohol, and illicit drug use were among the top leading preventable risk factors to health, responsible for 8.9% of the total disease burden if taken together (28).

The public health impact of psychoactive substance use is not limited to substance use disorders, and significant harm comes from acute intoxication, risks associated with the form of administration, or toxic effects of a substance (28). The proportion of the burden attributable to substance use disorders in the overall burden attributable to psychoactive substances is at least moderate. For example, according to the WHO estimates for 2002, alcohol use disorders are responsible for 1.4% of the total global disease burden, whereas drug use disorders account for 0.5%, compared to a much higher contribution of alcohol and drug use as risk factors to the global disease burden (illustrated in Table 32.1). At the same time, alcohol and drug use disorders (harmful use/abuse and dependence) are the second largest contributor—after unipolar depressive disorders—to the global disease burden among "neuropsychiatric disorders," which are responsible for 13% of the total global disease burden in 2002 (29). These data have important policy implications: From a public health perspective, effective reduction of the disease burden attributable to psychoactive substance use cannot be achieved just by treatment of substance dependence and implies a broader spectrum of effective policies. These include reducing exposure to psychoactive substances, limiting

TABLE 32.1 Percentage of Total Global Mortality and DALYs Attributable to Tobacco, Alcohol, and Illicit Drugs, 2000

Risk factor	High mortality developing countries		Low mortality developing countries		Developed countries		Worldwide
	Males	Females	Males	Females	Males	Females	
Mortality							
Tobacco	7.5	1.5	12.2	2.9	26.3	9.3	8.8
Alcohol	2.6	0.6	8.5	1.6	8.0	−0.3	3.2
Illicit drugs	0.5	0.1	0.6	0.1	0.6	0.3	0.4
DALYs							
Tobacco	3.4	0.6	6.2	1.3	17.1	6.2	4.1
Alcohol	2.6	0.5	9.8	2.0	14.0	3.3	4.0
Illicit drugs	0.8	0.2	1.2	0.3	2.3	1.2	0.8

Source: Neuroscience of psychoactive substance use and dependence. Geneva: World Health Organization, 2004.

their availability in populations, and specific targeted interventions aimed at reducing the harm associated with continued use of psychoactive substances.

Prevention and Treatment of Substance Use Disorders

Tobacco WHO work on tobacco is an example of a comprehensive public health approach to problems caused by psychoactive substances. Reducing tobacco use is one of the key objectives of the current WHO work on the global tobacco epidemic supported by the WHO Framework Convention on Tobacco Control—a multilateral international treaty aimed at preventing tobacco-related diseases and promoting health (30). The WHO advocates for the six most effective tobacco control policies: raising taxes and prices; banning advertising, promotion, and sponsorship; protecting people from secondhand smoke; warning everyone about the dangers of tobacco; offering help to people who want to quit; and carefully monitoring the epidemic and prevention policies (2). Tobacco dependence treatment is one of the key effective measures in controlling tobacco-related harm, but a full range of treatment for tobacco dependence and at least partial financial support is available to only 5% of the world's population in developed countries in spite of the fact that tobacco use and dependence has the largest impact on health in populations of less-resourced countries and that, by 2030, more than 80% of deaths attributable to tobacco will occur in low- and middle-income countries (31). Significant impact on public health can be achieved provided that coverage of effective interventions is sufficient and population-based measures are included in a comprehensive societal response and are properly implemented. This is equally applicable to prevention and treatment interventions.

Alcohol and Other Drugs The WHO for many years advocated for the promotion of screening and brief interventions procedures for hazardous and harmful use of alcohol in health care and other settings, which have strong evidence base for their effectiveness and cost-effectiveness (32). The WHO sponsored the Project on Identification and Management of Alcohol-Related Problems in numerous countries with the objective of adoption of screening and brief interventions in national or regional health care systems to achieve the impact on population's health (33). Applying the principles of AUDIT-based screening and brief interventions for alcohol problems, the WHO initiated and supported the development of a screening instrument for hazardous and harmful use of any psychoactive substance, from tobacco to heroin and cocaine, which resulted in the development and testing of the WHO instrument called ASSIST (Alcohol Screening and Substance Involvement Screening Test) (34). The WHO sponsored the randomized controlled trial of screening and brief interventions for drug use implemented in the framework of the WHO ASSIST project in several countries, including Australia, Brazil, India, and the United States. Results of the study proved the effectiveness of brief interventions in reducing cannabis, opioid, and stimulant use among clients of health care settings (35).

One of the conclusions in the WHO report "Neuroscience of psychoactive substance use and dependence" was that substance dependence "is not a failure of will or of strength of character but a medical disorder that could affect any human being" and "a complex disorder with biological mechanisms affecting the brain and its capacity to control substance use" (28). Pharmacologic interventions for some substance use disorders proved their effectiveness and became an important component of public health interventions in many parts of the world. Reflecting the growing public health importance of pharmacologic interventions for substance use disorders, a new section, "Medicines used in substance dependence programmes," was introduced in the WHO Model List of Essential Medicines, and methadone and buprenorphine were the first medications included in the complementary list of essential medicines recommended by WHO under this section

(36). The public health relevance and importance of drug dependence treatment, including opioid agonist pharmacotherapy, is increasingly recognized worldwide in connection with HIV epidemics among injecting drug users, and this is reflected in several WHO policy documents (37,38).

Treatment Systems for Substance Use Disorders

Development of a treatment system for substance use disorders should be an integral part of the overall response to health and social problems (39). In many countries, substance use disorders are being addressed in the framework of existing mental health care services. The World Health Report 2001 addressed priority areas for actions for countries with different levels of resources for developing mental health care, which are directly relevant to developing treatment systems for substance use disorders. These priority areas include the following: provision of treatment in primary health care; making psychotropic drugs available; providing care in the community; educating the public; involving communities, families, and consumers; establishing national policies, programs, and legislation; developing human resources; linking with other sectors; monitoring community mental health; and supporting more research (40). New opportunities for supporting improvement of treatment systems emerge with evolving methodology of their structured assessment developed by the WHO for mental health care services (41) and in the process of development for prevention and treatment systems for substance use disorders.

THE EVOLVING ROLE OF INTERNATIONAL MEDICAL ASSOCIATIONS

The founding of medical associations created opportunities for addressing issues of global concern by medical professionals. The World Medical Association has several position statements in relation to the use of substances (*http://www.wma.net/e/policy/a8.htm*) (42). After World War II, the World Medical Association modernized the Hippocrates Oath in 1948 to what became known as the "Declaration of Geneva" enshrining an International Code of Medical Ethics. Spurred by similar ethical concerns in relation to the treatment of mental disorders, the World Psychiatric Association (WPA) was founded in 1950. It currently includes a Section of Addiction Psychiatry that organizes educational activities about substance and behavioral addictions at meetings of the WPA and provides an addiction perspective on international strategies such as the development of a physician health and wellness international network or the optimal psychiatric response to comorbidities. It also contributes to the WPA role as a watchdog against the occurrence or recurrence of abuses of those suffering from mental illness and addictions.

To address the international aspects of Addiction Medicine, the need for an international society was recognized by international attendants at a number of meetings of the American Society of Addiction Medicine in the mid-1980s. On April 26, 1998, 25 physicians representing 11 countries from four continents met in New Orleans and decided to formalize their international collaboration. In 1999, at a founding meeting at the Betty Ford Center in Palm Springs, the International Society of Addiction Medicine (ISAM) came into being. The ISAM committed itself to advance the knowledge about addiction seen as a treatable disease, advocate for the major role physicians worldwide have to play in its management as well as enhance the credibility of their role and, last, develop educational activities including consensus guidelines.

Nine years later, the ISAM has a membership spanning 98 countries from all continents. It has added to the initial membership-based organization a network of national societies. It has a special affiliation agreement with the Austrian, Canadian, Dutch, Egyptian, Finnish, Icelandic, and Indian Addiction Medicine Societies, and a number of other agreements with national societies are in the works. We welcome associate memberships from allied health disciplines as well; the only activity restricted to physicians is board membership. Differential dues based on their economic potential follow the four World Bank categories of countries.

The Advocacy Role The same objectives guiding the advocacy of the American Society of Addiction Medicine (ASAM) are at play in various countries of the world. Embarking on a career in addiction medicine means battling the public stigma attached to the disease that rubs off on the care providers. By and large, the general attitudes of the medical profession mirror those of the public. As the national organizations are involved in similar struggles within different resource constraints, an umbrella international organization can provide the external validation required to strengthen national advocacy. For example, several national medical insurance schemes, such as Canada's, successfully provide parity coverage for the treatment of addiction disorders, thus contributing to the experimental validation required by the U.S. struggle for such a parity.

International medical associations help bolster the perception of addiction as a treatable disease by disseminating information about empirically based treatment practices arising from various parts of the globe while respectful of the local culture. This often involves a local needs assessment gathered by local medical opinion leaders and a culturally sensitive stepwise approach to remedial action. The ISAM has supported the research surrounding the experimental application of the ASAM's Patient Placement Criteria in diverse systems of care (43).

International Dissemination of Information From the onset, a major goal for the ISAM was to hold an annual meeting in different parts of the world to overcome the barriers of distance and travel costs and network with practitioners worldwide. The ISAM have so far held or cosponsored meetings in Palm Springs, Cairo, Tel Aviv, Trieste, Ljubjana, Reykjavik, Amsterdam, Helsinki, St. Petersburg, Oporto, Buenos Aires, and Mar del Plata. Travel fellowships supported by the WHO for members from developing countries and the

National Institute on Drug Abuse (NIDA) for young scientists help reduce the burden of cost. For members of the ISAM, the world becomes a much smaller place, connections with colleagues from across the globe are established, their programs and practices are directly observed, and the impact of their national drug strategies is compared. At each meeting, the local organizing committee strives to display their country's reservoir of hospitality and ensure optimal safety. In most ISAM meetings, about 40% of the scientific presentations originate from North America, anchored by presentations from the NIDA and the National Institute of Alcohol Abuse and Alcoholism (NIAAA), a third originate from Europe and Australasia, and one-fourth from the rest of the world. The presentations are in English, but a half-day track may be allotted to presentations in the local language. The meetings are a forum for the exchange of cutting-edge research as well as local and international clinical experience. The meetings bring visibility to the field locally and raise public awareness through media reports. International and local opinion leaders enhance one anothers' credibility in comparing empirically based practices.

A number of complementary educational activities have also been developed, including an information Web site (*www.isamweb.org*), a newsletter, and several position papers. The ISAM members are also playing key roles in the previously described UNODC TreatNet and the UNGASS feedback.

International Accreditation of Specialists The development of a field with specialized expertise must be accompanied by an accreditation process. Since 2005, an International Certification in Addiction Medicine with an international editorial board has been held with applicants from six countries and 40 certificants so far (*www.isamweb.org*) (44). Based on the ASAM's pioneering efforts, the International Certification strives to provide affordable, valid, and comparable international credentialing. It is mainly a test of knowledge with several clinical judgment questions. It is not meant to compete with national qualifications but rather to be a main resource for countries that do not have such a validation instrument and eventually establish an internationally standardized core test of knowledge in addiction medicine. National legislation and/or cultural requirements as well as observation of clinical skills could be easily tagged along the core knowledge test. The criteria of eligibility of physicians for writing the exam are meant to be inclusive. The certification test also helps point "new knowledge" frontiers to be promoted in the educational activities. Currently, knowledge about behavioral addictions as well as the management of pain and addiction constitute two such frontiers. Another challenge is for the exam to be as "culturally neutral" as possible.

Reaching out to Colleagues from Developing Countries Resource constraints are a major impediment to our colleagues in many areas of the world. Aside from a differential fee structure, organizing meetings in different continents, and maximizing our electronic outreach, the ISAM has collaborated with the WHO and NIDA in providing fellowships to colleagues from developing nations and young investigators (44).

Impact of Culture on Medical Practice Policies addressing the use of various drugs including alcohol and tobacco vary from country to country. The management of opioid dependence may, arguably, arouse the most polarizing divide among national drug policies and, more specifically, the support or denial of the need for opioid maintenance therapy. Unfortunately, in areas of the world where the use of opioids creates the heaviest burden of morbidity, cultural and structural factors have impeded the dissemination of opioid maintenance treatment. The International Medical Associations are striving to promote empirically based practices that account for the local culture and economic resources. In many Islamic countries, for example, a thriving network of therapeutic communities with religious underpinning is the main resource for the management of opioid dependence. More recently, however, countries such as Iran and China are incorporating methadone maintenance and/or buprenorphine as part of their strategic panoply to combat opioid dependence (45).

Many countries limit their efforts to opioid detoxification. This preference has spurred the development of controversial practices such as Rapid Antagonist Induction Under General Anesthesia. Despite modifications and improvement (46), the potential serious morbidity and mortality of this procedure along with its relatively high cost has led to charges of exploitation of the patient's desire for a "pain-free" detoxification. The long-term effect of the procedure is not supported by evidence (47) (see Sidebar, "Ultra Rapid Opiate Detoxification," in Chapter 44).

CONCLUSIONS

Though demand reduction has gained international momentum in recent decades, increased, political support and financial commitment are needed to develop further effective and ethical policies and programs for prevention and treatment of substance use disorders. Development of adequate international responses to problems related to psychoactive substance use requires concerted action. Synergy is emerging among the main international bodies involved in the management of legal and illegal drug problems, such as the WHO and the UNODC, research institutes such as the NIDA and the NIAAA in the United States, and the medical associations, such as the ISAM, concerned with the related problems. However, each organization has the need for resources to facilitate the necessary collaborations.

Prevention and treatment approaches delivered within the community and as a continuum of care can maximize coverage and response to needs as well as help reduce stigma and discrimination. International mechanisms for knowledge transfer such as communities of knowledge, networks, and partnership schemes are key to disseminating evidence-based practices and ultimately improving the quality and effectiveness of interventions. Health professionals, and particularly specialists in addiction medicine, have an important role in development, shaping, and implementation of international responses. The medical associations have a major peer-led educational role either through their meetings and fellowships or in collaboration with other organizations' activities. The associations promote culturally sensitive, empirically based medical practices at the local level and may credential local medical practitioners.

To achieve public health goals and impact on population health, it is imperative to go beyond individual-level interventions and promote and support effective problem- and population-based preventive strategies and measures on an international basis.

REFERENCES

1. World Health Organization. *Global Status Report on Alcohol 2004.* Geneva: WHO, 2004.
2. World Health Organization. *WHO Report on the Global Tobacco Epidemic, 2008: The MPOWER package.* Geneva: WHO, 2008.
3. UNODC. *World Drug Report 2007.* Vienna:UNODC, 2007. Retrieved November 11, 2008 from http://www.unodc.org/pdf/research/wdr07/WDR_2007.pdf.
4. Mathers CD, Stein C, Fat DM, et al. *Global burden of disease 2000: version 2 methods and results.* GPE Discussion paper 50. Geneva: WHO, 2001.
5. Commission on Narcotic Drugs. *World situation with regard to drug abuse.* Report of the Secretariat, Commission on Narcotic Drugs. Vienna, 2008—E/CN. Retrieved July 7, 2008, from. http://documents-dds-ny.un.org/doc/UNDOC/GEN/V08/501/18/pdf/V0850118.pdf?OpenElement.
6. International Narcotics Control Board Report of the International Narcotics Control board for 2003 (E/INCB/2003/1). Retrieved November 11, 2008 from http://www.incb.org/incb/annual_report_2003.htm.
7. Mathers B. Degenhardt I., Phillips B. Wiessing I., Hickman M. Strathdec S, Wodak A, Panda S, Tyndall M, Toufik A, Muttick RP and the Reference Group to the United Nations on HIV and injecting drug use. The global epidemiology of injecting drug use and HIV among people who inject drugs: a systematic review. *Lancet* 2008; 372 published online, 24 September 2008.
8. Single Convention on Narcotic Drugs, 1961 (amended by the Protocol of 25 March 1972), United Nations. Retrieved November 11, 2008 from http://www.unodc.org/pdf/convention_1961_en.pdf.
9. Convention on Psychotropic Substances, 1971, United Nations. Retrieved November 11, 2008 from http://www.unodc.org/pdf/convention_1971_en.pdf.
10. Convention against the Illicit Traffic in Narcotic Drugs and Psychotropic Substances, 1988, United Nations. Retrieved November 11, 2008 from http://www.unodc.org/pdf/convention_1988_en.pdf.
11. Political Declaration on the World Drug Problem, 1998 — General Assembly Resolution S-20/2, Annex. Retrieved November 11, 2008 from http://www.un.org/ga/20special/polecia.html.
12. Declaration on the Guiding Principles of Drug Demand Reduction, General Assembly Special Session, 1998. Retrieved November 11, 2008 from http://www.unodc.org/pdf/report_1999-01_1.pdf.
13. Report on the Fifty-first Session, Commission on Narcotic Drugs — Resolution 51/4 — E/CM.7/2008/15 — United Nations, New York 2008 (Advanced Unedited Version) – Retrieved November 11, 2008 from http://www.unodc.org/documents/commissions/CND-Session51/E200828CVn-AUE.pdf.
14. UNODC Annual Report 2008. Retrieved November 11, 2008 from http://www.unodc.org/documents/about-unodc/AR08_web.pdf.
15. Reducing the adverse health and social consequences of drug abuse: A comprehensive approach, UNODC, 2008. Retrieved November 11, 2008 from http://www.unodc.org/docs/treatment/reducing-adverse-consequences-drug-abuse%5B1%5D.pdf
16. Principles of Drug Dependence Treatment. Discussion paper. UNODC, WHO, 2008. Retrieved November 11, 2008 from http://www.unodc.org/documents/drug-treatment/UNODC-WHO-Principles-of-Drug-Dependence-Treatment-March08.pdf.
17. Foxcroft DR, Ireland D, Lister-Sharp DJ, et al. Longer-term primary prevention for alcohol misuse in young people: a systematic review. *Addiction* 2003;98:397–411.
18. Foxcroft DR, Ireland D, Lowe G, Breen R. Primary prevention for alcohol misuse in young people. *Cochrane Database System Rev* 2002;3: CD003024.
19. Foxcroft DR. *Alcohol misuse prevention for young people: a rapid review of recent evidence.* WHO Technical Report. Geneva: World Health Organization, 2006.
20. Faggiano F, Vigna-Taglianti FD, Versino E, et al. School-based prevention for illicit drugs' use. *Cochrane Database System Rev* 2005;2:CD003020.
21. United Nations Office of Drug Control. *Treatnet good practice document—drug dependence treatment: community based treatment.* Geneva: UNODC, 2008.
22. United Nations Office of Drug Control. *Treatnet good practice document—drug dependence treatment in prison settings.* Geneva: UNODC, 2008.
23. United Nations Office of Drug Control. *Treatnet good practice document—drug dependence treatment—its role in HIV/AIDS prevention and care.* Geneva: UNODC, 2008.
24. United Nations Office of Drug Control. *Treatnet good practice document—drug dependence treatment—sustained recovery management.* UNODC, 2008.
25. United Nations Office of Drug Control. *Treatnet drug dependence treatment training package.* UNODC, 2008.
26. Murray CJL, Lopez AD, eds. *The global burden of disease: a comprehensive assessment of mortality and disability from diseases, injuries and risk factors in 1990 and projected to 2020.* Cambridge, MA: Harvard University Press, 1996.
27. World Health Organization. *The World Health Report 2002. Reducing risks, promoting healthy life.* Geneva: World Health Organization, 2002.
28. World Health Organization. *Neuroscience of psychoactive substance use and dependence.* Geneva: World Health Organization, 2004.
29. World Health Organization. *The World Health Report 2004: changing history.* Geneva: World Health Organization, 2004.
30. World Health Organization. *WHO framework convention on tobacco control.* WHO 2003 [updated reprint 2004, 2005]. Geneva: WHO.
31. Mathers CD, Loncar D. Projections of global mortality and burden of disease from 2002 to 2030. *PLoS Med* 2006;3(11):442.
32. Whitlock EP, et al. Behavioral counseling interventions in primary care to reduce risky/harmful use by adults: a summary of the evidence for the U.S. Preventive Services Task Force. *Ann Intern Med* 2004;140:557–568.
33. Heather N, ed. *WHO Project on identification and management of alcohol-related problems: report on phase IV.* Geneva: WHO, 2006. Retrieved November 11, 2008 from http://www.who.int/substance_abuse/publications/identification_management_alchoholproblems_phaseiv.pdf.
34. WHO ASSIST Working Group. The alcohol, smoking and substance involvement screening test (ASSIST): development, reliability and feasibility. *Addiction* 2002;97:1183–1194.
35. The effectiveness of a brief intervention for illicit drugs linked to the alcohol, smoking and substance involvement screening test (ASSIST) in primary health care settings: a technical report of phase III findings of the WHO ASSIST randomized controlled trial. Retrieved November 11, 2008 from http://www.who.int/substance_abuse/ activities/assist_technicalreport_phase3_final.pdf
36. WHO Expert Committee on the Selection and Use of Essential Medicines. *14th report (including the 14th model list of essential medicines).* Geneva: World Health Organization, 2005.

37. World Health Organization. *Substitution maintenance therapy in the management of opioid dependence and HIV/AIDS prevention: position paper.* Geneva: WHO, UNODC, UNAIDS, 2004.
38. World Health Organization. *Basic principles for treatment and psychosocial support of drug dependent people living with HIV/AIDS.* Geneva: World Health Organization, 2006.
39. World Health Organization, WHO Expert Committee on Drug Dependence. *30th report.* Geneva: World Health Organization, 1998.
40. World Health Organization. *The World Health Report 2001: mental health: new understanding, new hope.* Geneva: World Health Organization, 2001.
41. World Health Organization. *Assessment instrument for mental health systems,* Version 2.2. Geneva: WHO, 2005.
42. World Medical Association: World Medical Association Statement on the Prescription of Substitute Drugs in the Outpatient Treatment of Addicts to Opiate Drugs. Adopted by the 47th General Assembly Bali, Indonesia, September 1995 and rescinded at the WMA General Assembly, Pilanesberg, South Africa, 2006. Retrieved 11/11/2008 from http://www.wma.net/e/policy/a8.htm.
43. Gastfriend DR ed. *Addiction treatment matching. Research foundations of the American Society of Addiction Medicine Criteria.* Binghamton, NY: Haworth Medical Press, 2003.
44. International Society of Addiction Medicine. ISAM Web page. Retrieved November 11, 2008 from www.isamweb.org.
45. Lu L, Zhao D, Bao-Y-P, Shi J. Methadone maintenance treatment of heroin abuse in China. *Am J Drug Alcohol Abuse* 2008;34:127–131.
46. Brewer C. Ultra-rapid, antagonist-precipitated opioid detoxification under general anesthesia or sedation. *Addict Biol* 1997;2:291–302.
47. Collins ED, Kleber HD, Whittington RA, et al. Anaesthesia-assisted vs. buprenorphine- or clonidine-assisted heroin detoxification and naltrexone inductions. A randomized trial. *JAMA* 2005;294:903–913.

SECTION 5

Special Issues in Addiction Medicine

CHAPTER 33

Martha J. Wunsch, MD, FAAP, FASAM
Carol Boyd PhD, MSN, RN, FAAN
Mary G. McMasters, MD

Nonmedical Use of Prescription Medications

The rapid growth of inappropriate use of scheduled prescription medications presents serious public health concerns and unique medical and policy issues when compared with the abuse of illegal drugs such as heroin or cocaine. Scheduled medications are socially sanctioned to relieve pain, anxiety, depression, insomnia, narcolepsy, and attention deficit disorders. Yet, these medications have pharmacologic properties that may lead to misuse, abuse, addiction, diversion, and doctor shopping. Such nonmedical use presents a unique challenge to the provision of medical and nursing care (1–3). There has been a remarkable increase in the number of persons who report they are new abusers of scheduled prescription medications over the past several decades. This trend has been most notable over the past 5 years (Fig. 33.1) (4,5). The four scheduled drug classes most often involved are stimulants, sedative-hypnotics, sedative-anxiolytics, and opioid analgesic medications. Nonmedical use occurs for many reasons among all age groups (5,6,7), and often escapes medical attention in primary care offices (8), pain clinics (9,10), and addiction treatment programs (11,12). Physicians, dentists, and other prescribers are understandably concerned about their role in the misuse, abuse, and diversion of controlled prescriptions.

This chapter will present an overview of what is known about the new phenomenon of nonmedical use of prescription medications, including discussion of serious consequences such as poisoning and overdose deaths (13). In many fatalities, multiple prescription medications are involved and identified on toxicology. Finally, we introduce some strategies for prevention when prescribing these medications and the identification and management of the individuals who are using prescription medications in medically unintended ways.

DEFINITIONS

There are no commonly accepted definitions of abuse, addiction, problematic use, or nonmedical use of prescription medications (NUPM), among the scientific, clinical, or research community. The National Institute on Drug Abuse defines abuse of prescription drugs as "any intentional use of a medication with intoxicating properties outside of a physician's prescription for a bona fide medical condition, excluding accidental misuse" (4). According to the National Institute on Drug Abuse, prescription drug abuse includes taking a medication prescribed for someone else, even if it is taken for an appropriate medical condition. The federal Drug Enforcement Administration defines *abuse* as the use of Schedule I through V medications in a manner or amount that is inconsistent with the medical or social pattern of a culture (14). The Drug Enforcement Administration also notes that abuse involves the use of prescription medications outside "the scope of sound medical practice" (14). This definition emphasizes social deviance. Both the American Society of Addiction Medicine and the American Psychiatric Association use DSM-IV TR criteria to define abuse and addiction, emphasizing physical and psychosocial consequences but not specifically addressing problematic use or nonmedical use of prescription medications (15).

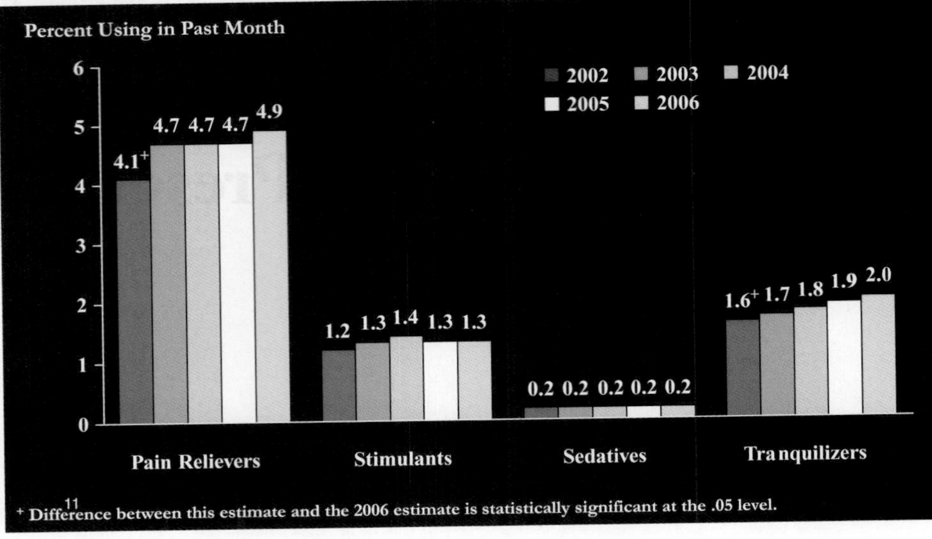

FIGURE 33.1. Past month nonmedical use of prescription drugs among adults (18–25 years). Trend from 2002–2006 (5).

Nonmedical Use of Prescription Medications

Boyd and McCabe (16) argue that nonmedical use of scheduled prescription medications involves a variety of subtypes that are not adequately or consistently distinguished in the current literature. Additionally, they suggest that careful attention is needed to refine both the measurement and definition of such use. For the purpose of this chapter, the term *NUPM* will be used as an overarching term to refer to the use of a scheduled, prescription medication without the prescribing clinician's knowledge. For example, patients may share or sell a prescription written for them, obviously without the physician's permission or awareness. Thus NUPM encompasses misuse, abuse, and addiction and can occur both among patients with prescriptions and among those without. NUPM also includes behaviors such as patients increasing their dose without a physician's knowledge, nonpatients using a diverted medication from a friend or family member, patients snorting or injecting their medications to achieve euphoria (rather than the intended purpose), or the procurement of scheduled medications via theft, duplicitous doctor shopping or illegal drug dealing.

In addition to confusion about nomenclature among professionals, the definition of NUPM is not clearly understood by our patients either. In a review by Hubbard (17) of the National Household Survey on Drug Abuse, 70% of respondents who said they were not engaging in NUPM admitted to either taking their medications more often, taking in greater amounts than prescribed, or taking medication that was borrowed or bought without a prescription. Few endorsed taking a drug for kicks, to get "high," to feel good, or for curiosity. These findings were reported over a decade ago; however, they indicate that, for the general public, NUPM only includes behavior such as seeking euphoria or an altered state. Self-treatment with someone else's medication is not seen as a problem. Prescribers would be wise to educate their patients about appropriate use of medications because sharing medication, taking more or more often, as well as combining prescription medications, can lead to serious consequences including overdose death.

Misuse versus Abuse The term *misuse* is equally fraught with confusion. According to Compton and Volkow, misuse of scheduled prescription medications differs from abuse because it does not include motivation to achieve euphoria. Furthermore, they note that misuse is associated with a specific pattern of social, familial, and individual predictors (4). For this chapter, the misuse of a scheduled prescription medication, as distinguished from abuse, refers to the incorrect use of a medication by *patients with legal prescriptions.* For misuse to occur, the patient must engage in the misuse for the purpose of self-treating a perceived medical condition and further, at least one of the following three intentional behaviors must be present: the medication is taken more often than prescribed, the medication is taken for a longer period than prescribed, or too much medication is taken at one time (18). Misuse can lead to abuse and addiction, but not necessarily.

Finally, our review of the literature revealed many different conceptual approaches to describing nonmedical use of prescription medications across research studies. We caution the reader that varying definitions of misuse, abuse, addiction, and dependence are employed across studies and authors do not always clearly specify definitions. Whenever possible, we have employed the terms used by authors in reporting their work.

PREVALENCE

All national studies over the past 15 years have shown an increase in reports of the nonmedical use of prescription medications. One such epidemiologic survey is the annual National Survey on Drug Use and Health (NSDUH) (5), formerly the National Household Survey on Drug Abuse. NSDUH uses a computer assisted survey method to ask respondents "Have you ever, even once, used *[insert the name of a specific medication]* that was not prescribed for you or that you took only for the experience or feeling it caused?"; the NSDUH uses pill cards with pictures to assist the respondent in identification of medications that were used in this manner. According to the 2006 NSDUH 7 million persons aged 12 or older used psychotherapeutics nonmedically (any prescription type pain relievers, tranquilizers, stimulants, or sedatives) in the past month. Prescription pain medication is the drug class most often used nonmedically among the general population (5). However, it is conceivable that individuals with very different sources and motivations for use may answer the questions in the affirmative, affecting interpretation of NSDUH. For instance, a teen who is given one of a parent's prescribed hydrocodone pills while awaiting evaluation for a sports injury would answer this query in the same manner as a teen who has snorted hydrocodone seeking euphoria.

Nonmedical Use of Prescription Medication: Prescription Opioids The reported prevalence of nonmedical use of prescription medication (NUPM), in the case of opioids, varies from almost none to nearly half of patients studied. There are several significant problems with the validity of such reports. A lack of agreement in the definition of misuse, abuse, addiction, or problematic behavior confounds the results and variation in the criteria used to define opioid abuse or addiction, from loosely defined behavioral criteria to results of urine toxicology tests or DSM-III and DSM-IV criteria, make interpretation difficult. In some cases, addiction to prescription opioids is reported alone; others also report addiction to benzodiazepines, barbiturates, and prescription stimulants. The populations studied may include patients with cancer, patients with nonmalignant pain only, patients in treatment for addiction, or patients in primary care settings. In some studies patients with known addiction are excluded.

Among primary care patients, NUPM is reported to occur in one quarter to one third of patients while among patients coming to addiction treatment opioid addiction is reported to occur more often among women, individuals from rural areas, and among patients prescribed opioids for the treatment of chronic pain (8,9,11,12). In an exhaustive review of 25 studies in which opioids were prescribed for the treatment of chronic nonmalignant pain, Hojsted and Sjögren found the rates of addiction, dependence, aberrant drug taking, abuse, misuse, and problematic opioid use varied widely, between 0 and 49.7% (19). Given the range of prevalence, the reader is referred to this work for further description of the complex issue of NUPM among patients with chronic pain.

The Researched Abuse, Diversion, and Addiction-Related Surveillance (RADARS) was a system designed specifically to monitor the abuse of oxycodone (OxyContin) by reporting information from drug abuse experts, law enforcement, and poison control centers (20). RADARS reported an increase in prescription opioid abuse of all opioids in the United States; however, extended-release and immediate-release oxycodone and hydrocodone were the most widely abused drugs in the country. These investigators and others report that there are pockets regionally where there is more abuse of opioid medications. Individuals who abused prescription opioids were more likely to live in rural, suburban, and small- to medium-sized urban areas, although these demographic factors may be changing.

NUPM: Benzodiazepine Medications Less is known about the prevalence and incidence of NUPM of the tranquilizers and sedative-hypnotics. In an analysis of NSDUH participants, 2.3% of individuals reported nonmedical use of these medications and among those 9.8% met criteria for abuse or dependence. Of note, these individuals also had anxiety symptoms, and serious mental illness, and were more likely than nonmedical users to be engaged in illicit drug use, to have initiated drug use at a younger age, and to have used intravenous drugs. From this information and clinical experience, physicians should be aware that individuals use sedative hypnotics and tranquilizers for a variety of reasons and are at higher risk for other forms of substance abuse as well. Nonmedical use of benzodiazepines can be missed when clinicians do not have an appropriate index of suspicion for such behaviors (21,22).

NONMEDICAL USE AMONG ADOLESCENT AND YOUNG ADULTS

Nonmedical use of prescription medications is of particular concern among youth, especially given the understanding that earlier onset of alcohol, tobacco, and marijuana substance use is associated with development of abuse and dependence in adulthood (23,24). A similar picture is emerging for early nonmedical use of prescription opioids (25,26). In an analysis of data from the 2001–2002 National Epidemiologic Survey on Alcohol and Related Conditions, researchers (24) found that if respondents reported using a scheduled prescription medication nonmedically before age 13 they were significantly more likely than those who began nonmedical use at 21 years (or older) to have a diagnosis of prescription medication abuse or dependence at the time of the National Epidemiologic Survey on Alcohol and Related Conditions interview. In a school-based sample of adolescents, this same research team found that NUPM was associated with other drug use, including alcohol, tobacco, marijuana, and other illicit drugs as well as reports of drug abuse problems (26).

Prevalence According to the NSDUH, the nonmedical use of prescription medications remains a concern, with 7 million Americans engaging in NUPM in the previous month (Fig. 33.2). Young adults have the highest prevalence rates for NUPM, with an estimated 5% reporting the nonmedical use of a scheduled pain medication in the past month (5). The NSDUH 2006 reported prescription opioid analgesics

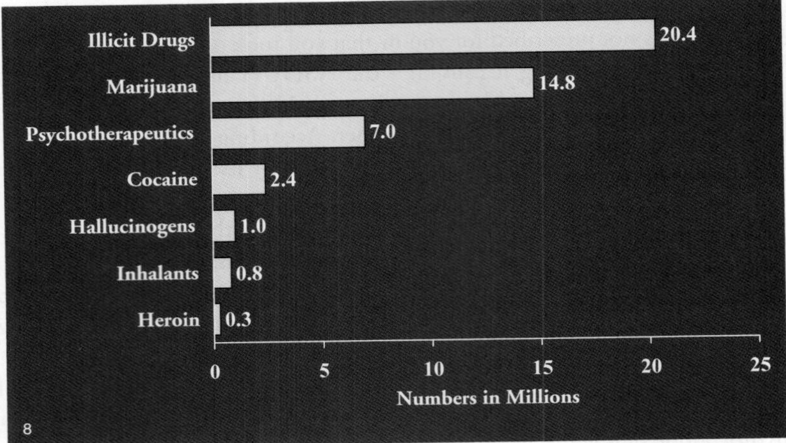

FIGURE 33.2. Past month use of specific illicit drugs among persons aged 12 or older: 2006 (5).

surpassing marijuana as the most commonly used drug for new initiates each year. (Fig. 33.3).

The nonmedical use of stimulants appears to be most prevalent after high school, among young adults aged 18 to 25. Although the primary motivation for prescription stimulant misuse (dextroamphetamine, Adderall, methylphenidate) is often to increase attention or improve concentration (27), to party, to reducing hyperactivity, and to study, nonmedical use often occurs with alcohol and other substances (with males more likely than females to engage in polydrug abuse [28]).

Motivation for Adolescent/Young Adult Misuse

Boyd and colleagues found that adolescents and young adults who engaged in NUPM frequently endorsed self treatment as a reason for use, suggesting a distinctive rationale associated with this misuse. In one Web-based survey of Midwestern 10- to 18-year olds, adolescents were asked to endorse reasons for their nonmedical use of prescription medications (29,30). Respondents most often endorsed treatment of symptoms for which a medication is often prescribed, including using stimulants to study, focus, and lose weight; pain medication to relieve pain; and tranquilizers and sedative hypnotics for anxiety or as sleep aids. In addition, some respondents also endorsed experimentation, "to get high" and "because I'm addicted" as reasons for use. Clearly, the motivations for nonmedical use may vary from "self-treatment," to experimentation, to partying in a "club drug scene". Those who endorsed reasons other than self-treatment for nonmedical use were significantly more likely to have substance abuse problems as indicated by high scores on the Drug Abuse Screening Test-10 (29,30,31).

Sources of Prescription Medications (Fig. 33.4)

Controlled prescription medications used non medically are most often obtained from friends and family, although other sources include doctor shopping, theft from pharmacies, online purchases, and stealing from friends or family members who have them legally prescribed (29,32–34). The NSDUH data indicate that, among respondents age 12 or older, the most common source of opioid and stimulant medications was "from a friend or relative for free" (59.8%) whereas 16.8% obtained medication from one doctor, and <1% bought on the Internet (5). Purchase from street sources was less common, with only 4.3% buying pain relievers from a drug dealer

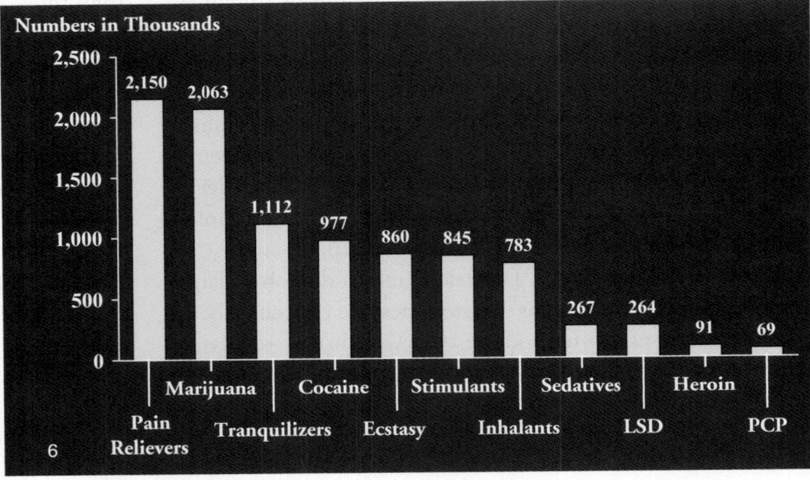

FIGURE 33.3. Past year initiates for specific illicit drugs among persons age 12 or older: 2006 (5).

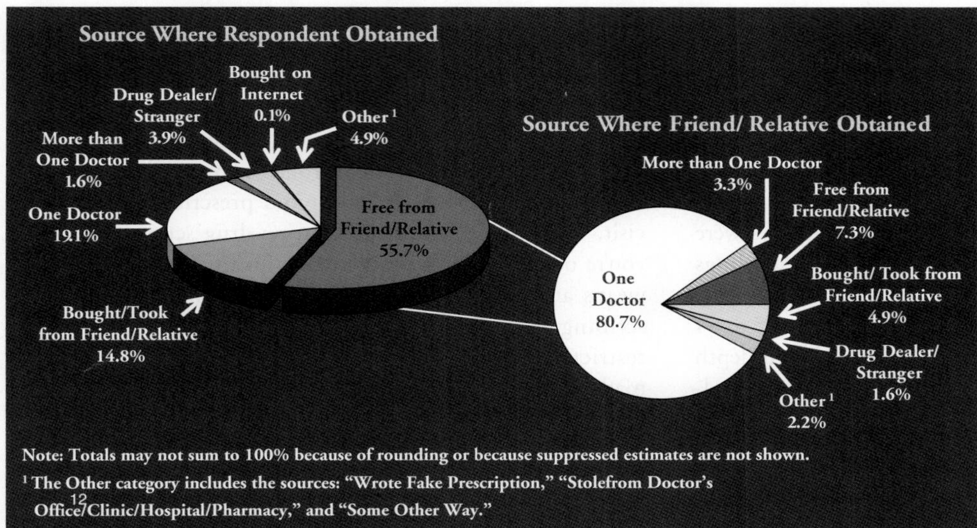

FIGURE 33.4. Source where pain relievers were obtained for most recent nonmedical use among past year users age 12 or older: 2006 (5).

or other stranger; however, in the case of stimulant medications, 6.5% bought the drug from a drug dealer or other stranger, and 7.2% bought on the Internet. Although most surveys report relatively little use of the Internet as a source for NUPM, there is a proliferation of "new prescription Web sites" that sell and ship primarily prescription Schedule IV and III scheduled medications (35,36,37). The sources of benzodiazepines are not well described in the literature; however, it is likely that they are commonly obtained, as other prescription medications, from friends and family.

Methods of obtaining medication may vary by age and gender (37). Younger students in middle and high school are more likely to get medication from family or friends (38). Male college students are more likely to obtain diverted medications from peers, but family members remain the source of sedative hypnotic, sleeping, and pain medications for women (39). In the case of nonmedical use of stimulants, high school and college students are often approached at school to divert their own legitimately prescribed medications (38,39,40).

Adolescents may take bottles of medications from their parents' medicine cabinets to parties to distribute for recreational use, a practice described as "pharming" (41). When prescription medications are used by teenagers and young adults in such a setting, they are often used in combination with over-the-counter medications, including dextromethorphan and pseudoephedrine (42). Other medications used opportunistically and intermittently in this social setting include benzodiazepines (alprazolam, diazepam), opioids (hydrocodone, oxycodone), and stimulants (methylphenidate, amphetamine). Club drug users who abuse prescription benzodiazepines and opioids will often do so in an intermittent or chronic pattern of high doses. As in adults, chronic use can result in a withdrawal syndrome that may require detoxification with cross-tolerant medication (clonazepam or phenobarbital for benzodiazepine withdrawal; methadone or buprenorphine for opioid withdrawal). For older adolescents with opioid dependence, medication-assisted treatment with buprenorphine or methadone may be indicated to stabilize symptoms, thus facilitating engagement in the psychosocial and counseling aspects of treatment.

SOCIAL, LEGAL, AND MEDICAL CONSEQUENCES

Legal consequences of NUPM and diversion may include arrest for prescription forgery, theft, and trafficking of these medications for illegal purposes. In one study of 233 arrestees administered a modified Addiction Severity Index in rural southwestern Virginia, those abusing prescription medications were more likely to abuse alcohol, illicit drugs, and to have engaged in criminal behavior than arrestees primarily abusing alcohol (43). Additionally, a study of subjects abusing and addicted to oxycodone in the same region revealed psychiatric comorbidity, associated criminal activity, and psychosocial problems such as those of any person with addiction to illicit opioids (44).

The increase in nonmedical use of prescription medications has been accompanied by an increased number of deaths from overdose where these medications are identified on toxicology (45,46). Poisoning, which include overdoses involving illicit drugs, alcohol, and medications, is the leading cause of injury death for individuals' ages 35 to 44 years old and prescription opioid-related overdose deaths have increased at an alarming rate in portions of the United States (46,47). At the same time that heroin poisonings increased by 12.4% from 1999 to 2002, the number of opioid analgesic poisonings in the United States increased by 91.2% (48). Medical examiners report increased opioid-related drug deaths in Maine, New Hampshire, Vermont, Maryland, Utah, and New Mexico involving predominantly the prescription medications oxycodone, hydrocodone, and methadone (49).

In an analysis of 893 medical examiner prescription medication, accidental overdose deaths from rural southwestern Virginia prescription medications were found more often than illicit drugs, polydrug overdose cases predominated (57.9%); and medications found on toxicology included prescription opioids (74.0%), antidepressants (49.0%), and benzodiazepines (39.3%) (50).

As would be expected from the national epidemiologic reports of drug abuse and addiction, the majority of the deaths were male. However, contrary to epidemiologic reports of NUPM, in five of the six states, the highest death rates were among adults ages 35 to 54 years old (47). Similar findings emerged in the review of medical examiner cases in rural Virginia where 60% of the decedents were older adults (35 to 54 years old). In contrast to epidemiologic reports, this in-depth review reported that 37% of the decedents were female, a finding replicated in other reviews of prescription fatalities (46–49).

Methadone prescribed as an analgesic (tablet form) accounts for more inadvertent deaths than methadone prescribed for agonist maintenance (liquid form). Because methadone is prescribed in the treatment of addiction, identification of the cause of death helps address public concern, thus preserving access to medication assisted treatment with methadone (51). In medical examiner decedent cases investigations in North Carolina, Texas, New Hampshire, and Hennepin County, Minnesota, where methadone is identified on toxicology, this medication was more likely to have been diverted illegally from physician prescription than diverted from an opioid treatment program (52–56). In Texas, there was a threefold increase in methadone-associated mortality between 1999 and 2002, but deaths of patients in opioid treatment programs declined (41). In New Hampshire, prescription opioid deaths doubled between 2000 and 2003 at a time when prescriptions of methadone for analgesia had increased by 563% (57).

Medical examiners and forensic toxicologists have access to a wealth of information about the circumstances in deaths where prescription medications are identified on toxicology. In such decedent cases, often multiple prescription medications (opiates, benzodiazepines, antidepressants), illicit drugs, and alcohol are found on toxicology, making precise determination of the cause of death difficult (52,53). Attribution to suicide or unintentional death may also be difficult to ascertain. Furthermore, it may be unknown if the concentration of the medication was lethal or pharmacologic and physiologic interactions were at work (58,59).

In the case of prescription medication overdose, whether the nature of death involves suicide or accidental and decedent cases involve one prescription medication or a combination along with other psychoactive substances, the increase in overdose deaths is a public health problem.

STRATEGIES FOR IDENTIFICATION OF NONMEDICAL USE OF PRESCRIPTION MEDICATIONS

Physicians prescribing any prescription medication with potential for euphoria, abuse, and addiction, including opioids, benzodiazepines, and prescription stimulants, are charged with the treatment of disease while minimizing abuse, misuse, diversion, and preventing addiction. The lack of guidelines in doing so may result in differing responses by providers. In a survey of practitioners, Bhamb identified "best guess" responses from physicians concerned about medication diversion, which included "no controlled substance prescribing," "no opioid prescribing," "no opioid prescribing on the first visit," "one strike (unexpected urine drug screen result) and you're out," "no high dosage narcotics (mandatory cutoffs or weans at preset dosages)," "no high potency narcotics prescribing (no fentanyl, morphine, methadone)," "practice restricted to lower potency narcotics (hydrocodone, tramadol)," and "urine drug screen on suspicion only"(60). The variety of these responses reflects the legal liability concerns and clinical uncertainties of many physicians in addressing NUPM.

Patients who are using prescription medications nonmedically and have a diagnosis of addiction are not easily identified (61–64). Prescribers can rarely differentiate between the medication compliant patient and those seeking medications to abuse or divert. Although many screening tools have been developed for evaluation of NUPM in chronic pain patients prescribed opioids (60), there are no accepted and validated screening assessments for use in the case of NUPM with nonopioid medications. Nonetheless, some of the strategies in use to assess for problematic opioid use may be helpful in evaluation for misuse, abuse, diversion of, and addiction to other scheduled medications.

For example, Savage (65) proposed schemata for identifying addiction in the chronic pain patient. Although this approach was developed specifically for use in the chronic pain patient, this model may be useful when applied to NUPM of any scheduled medications. The "4 Cs" could be applied to the diagnosis of attention deficit hyperactivity disorder in the case of stimulants, or anxiety disorders when prescribing benzodiazepines (Table 33.1). In this scenario, the patient prescribed benzodiazepines or stimulants therapeutically will have stable or improving activity, mood, sleep, and relationships. Furthermore, there will be few medication incidents, and a pill count, requested and performed shortly after a prescription is dispensed, will indicate appropriate use of medications. When pill counts are used, they should be performed randomly and at differing intervals after prescriptions are given. Abstinence from alcohol and illicit drug use, by report of support network and family and of negative urine drug screens, can validate that the patient is using medications appropriately and not combining prescription medication with other substances, illicit, legal, and prescribed. When monitoring a patient prescribed controlled medications, urine drugs screens should be requested to assay for both prescribed and nonprescribed psychoactive substances. In the case of opiates, prescribers must look for both illicit and prescribed opioids, and for synthetic opioids including buprenorphine to identify the patient using heroin as well as those ingesting nonprescribed opioids. Assays for stimulants must differentiate

TABLE 33.1 Assessment for Addiction During Opioid Therapy of Pain (looking for the four "Cs")

Pattern may suggest addiction	Pattern suggests therapeutic use
Adverse consequences/harm from use	Favorable therapeutic response to use
Intoxicated/somnolent/sedated	No significantly altered consciousness
Declining activity	Stable or improving activity
Irritable/anxious/labile mood	Stable or improved mood
Increasing sleep disturbance	Stable or improved sleep
Increasing pain complaints	Stable or improving pain
Increasing relationship dysfunction	Improving relationships
Impaired control over use/compulsive use	Able to use as prescribed
Reports lost or stolen prescriptions or medications	Rare or no medication incidents
Frequent early renewal requests	Uses medications as prescribed
Urgent calls or unscheduled visits	Doses discussed at clinical visits
Abusing other drugs or alcohol	No alcohol or drug abuse
Cannot produce medications on request	Has expected amount of medication left
Withdrawal noted at clinic visits	No withdrawal signs
Observers report overuse or sporadic use	Observers report appropriate use
Preoccupation with use because of craving	Seeking pain relief not opioid reward
Frequently misses appointments unless opioid renewal expected	Makes most appointments
Does not try nonopioid treatments	Shows up for recommended evaluations
Cannot tolerate most medications	Gives reasonable treatment recommendations a fair trial
Requests medications with high reward	Medication sensitivities and favorable responses not predictable by medication abuse liability
No relief with anything except opioids	Adopts self management strategies (can demonstrate/discuss techniques)

Reprinted with permission from Savage SR. Assessment for addiction in pain-treatment settings. *Clin J Pain* 2002;18:S28–S38.

among those prescribed and the illicit stimulants. When prescribing benzodiazepines, urine drug screens must include testing for the specific medications, thus identifying any benzodiazepines being abused but not prescribed. In summary, urine drug screens should identify specific medications, thus differentiating the prescribed from nonprescribed and helping the physician identify NUPM.

Universal precautions, as described by Heit and Gourlay, although not empirically validated for use other than with the patient prescribed opioids, might also be used by physicians to identify and minimize NUPM (Table 33.2) (66,67). Before prescribing a controlled substance, the physician should require documentation of the diagnosis with an appropriate differential, a psychologic assessment including risk of addictive disorders, and patient-centered urine drug testing for the presence of illicit and nonprescribed licit medications. Informed consent should outline proposed treatment plans, including the risk of addiction for medications with euphoric effects. Equally important is a clear description of behavioral expectations, including the consequences of aberrant behavior. After medication is prescribed, the clinician should request random pill counts to assure that a patient is not undertaking or overtaking a medication. Furthermore, a family member, if there is a diagnosis of addiction, or a 12-Step sponsor may need to be identified to help in management of medications. Throughout treatment a regular review of response to medication, as well as the status of comorbid conditions is helpful. Finally, clear and concise documentation is indicated in these cases.

Prescription Monitoring Programs In response to concerns about misuse, abuse, and diversion, and in an effort to assure continued access for patients to medications, state and federal governments have implemented systems to monitor the prescription and distribution of controlled substances. Additionally, some state medical boards have released controlled substance abuse guidelines derived from a model document from the Federation of State Medical Boards to assist practitioners in the treatment of pain (63–66).

Prescription Monitoring Programs (PMP), both computerized and noncomputerized, monitor prescribing practices of controlled substances in an attempt to decrease diversion of prescription medications. Ideally, use of the PMPs by practitioners allow appropriate medication for chronic pain, anxiety and depression, and attention deficit disorders while providing the assurance that a patient is not procuring controlled substances from multiple physicians. There are few studies evaluating the efficacy of specific state PMPs in decreasing NUPM. (68,69)

Designed and directed by state agencies, the most common goals of these programs are education, delivery of information, execution of public health initiatives, early intervention and prevention of diversion, investigation and

TABLE 33.2 Ten Steps of Pain Management

1. Make a Diagnosis with Appropriate Differential
   Identify any treatable causes for pain, where they exist, and direct therapy to the pain generator
   Address any comorbid conditions, including substance use disorders and other psychiatric illness.
2. Psychologic Assessment Including Risk of Addictive Disorders
   Inquire about personal and family history of substance misuse
   Discuss patient-centered urine drug testing (UDT) with all patients regardless of what medications they are currently taking
   Assess patients using illicit or unprescribed licit drugs and offer or refer for further assessment for possible substance use disorders
3. Informed Consent
   Discuss with and answer any questions the patient may have about the proposed treatment plan including anticipated benefits and foreseeable risks
   Explore specific issues of addiction, physical dependence, and tolerance at the patient's level of understanding
4. Treatment Agreement
   Clarify expectations and obligations of both the patient and the treating practitioner either verbally or in writing
5. Pre- and Postintervention Assessment of Pain Level and Function
   Conduct an ongoing assessment after initiation of treatment and document success in meeting clinical goals to support the continuation of any mode of therapy
6. Appropriate Trial of Opioid Therapy ± Adjunctive Medication
   Assure that pharmacologic regimens are individualized and based on subjective, as well as objective, clinical findings
7. Reassessment of Pain Score and Level of Function
   Assess the patient and use corroborative support from family or other knowledgeable third parties to help document continued therapy
8. Regularly Assess the "Four As" of Pain Medicine
   Document how analgesia, activity, adverse effects, and aberrant behavior and affect to support pharmacologic options
9. Periodically Review Pain Diagnosis and Comorbid Conditions, including Addictive Disorders
   Assess for evolution of underlying illnesses evolve and shift treatment focus as needed
10. Documentation
    Carefully and completely record initial and follow-up evaluations to support the best interest of all parties

Created from Gourlay DL, Heit HA, Almahrezi A. Universal precautions in pain medicine: a rational approach to the treatment of chronic pain. *Pain Med* 2005;6(2):107–112.

enforcement of abuse, and protection of confidentiality (70,71). Nineteen states have legislative mandates for prescription monitoring program, each differing in specific details, including the need for patient consent to access information, the means by which physicians garner information, those classes of medications tracked, and the timeliness of reporting by pharmacies.

In many states, the system requires informed consent from the patient; however, this should not be a barrier to accessing the system. The use of computer technology allows prescribing physicians access the database immediately, sometimes while a patient is undergoing evaluation in the practitioner's office. The PMP is one mechanism the physician can use to decrease diversion by determining when a patient is receiving multiple prescriptions from multiple providers for a controlled substance. More importantly, the use of computerized data bases for PMP decrease stigmatization while giving physicians and other providers access to data to affirm appropriate use of medication by patients.

ADDICTION TREATMENT: PRESCRIPTION MEDICATIONS

There are many circumstances under which concern arises about misuse, abuse of, or addiction to prescription medications, and the addiction clinician must parse them to design an effective intervention or treatment plan. In some cases, medications were not prescribed and euphoria was the primary goal of use. In other cases, the patient may be diverting his or her own prescribed medication by selling on the street or altering a prescription. Alternatively, some patients in treatment for chronic pain, anxiety, or attention deficit hyperactivity disorder may use alcohol, marijuana, or other illicit drugs along with medications. In this scenario, prescription of medication may be discontinued because of a urine drug test positive for illicit drugs or evidence of intoxication. In the case of prescription misuse, unlike the case where a drug of abuse is illegal, a patient may be overtaking prescribed medication or combining medications. This patient may be at risk for medical complications, such as overdose. Diversion may be occurring without patient awareness when the pill count is incorrect because a family member is diverting. Although the diagnosis of dependence is not met, such behavior is still a problem and prescribing may be jeopardized.

A patient may lose access to medications despite the fact that, in the patient's opinion, this nonmedical use was justified for adequate treatment of his or her pain, anxiety, depression, or attention deficit hyperactivity disorder. They may not agree that use of alcohol or illicit drugs, in addition to their medications, is a problem. Because these medications were prescribed for them, patients may feel entitled to medication and disagree with the diagnosis of abuse or addiction. Some may obtain prescription medications illicitly because they no longer have a "legitimate prescription." With the loss of access to prescribed medications, patients may engage in doctor shopping. Some patients may attempt to secure prescriptions or pills from emergency rooms or from other physicians or community clinics. Others will buy medications "on the street" or borrow or steal from family members or friends. As in every area of medicine, every patient and every history will require a tailored response.

A careful history, including information from family members and others who support the patient, should be combined with urine drug screen to formulate a diagnosis. Sometimes a pattern emerges over several months; still, the physician must watch closely for behavior that may jeopardize patient or public safety or indicate diversion. In some cases, the physician may discontinue prescribing the controlled substances while still caring for the patient. In other cases, prescription of smaller amounts of medication, more frequent patient visits, more pill counts, and attention to patient behavior is indicated. A good review of this topic and clinical management, again with a focus on chronic pain, is presented by Weaver (72,73).

When there is an untreated diagnosis of addiction to either prescription or illicit drugs, it is difficult to effectively treat chronic pain with opioids, an anxiety disorder with benzodiazepines, and an attention disorder with stimulants. Stabilization of the addiction diagnosis is essential, in some cases including the treatment of withdrawal.

There is no evidence in the literature that patients addicted to or abusing prescription medications have less severity in their diagnosis of addiction, although their drug of abuse is a manufactured pharmaceutical. As with other addiction, they require treatment of comorbid psychiatric and medical diagnosis. Treatment for patients abusing or addicted to prescription medications varies little from treatment for each corresponding drug class. Medication-assisted treatment with the prescription of methadone or buprenorphine may be indicated in those cases of opioid dependence, stabilization with a cross-tolerant long acting-medication, such as phenobarbital or a long-acting benzodiazepine such as diazepam, may be needed for benzodiazepine addiction. Those patients addicted to stimulants will benefit from strategies used in the treatment of the cocaine- or methamphetamine-addicted patient, including contingency management and intensive counseling. As is common in addiction, the diagnoses of depression and anxiety often require concurrent treatment. In short, the treatment modalities employed for any patient with addiction should be employed in the patient abusing and addicted to prescription medication tailored to the primary substance of abuse. Treatment for comorbid psychiatric diagnosis, ongoing psychologic evaluation and support, individual counseling, and therapeutic group treatment should be prescribed as required. Education about and encouragement to use community-supported 12-step programs are helpful.

After addiction problems and psychiatric comorbid conditions are stabilized, these patients will require collaborative treatment with medical providers for the treatment of chronic pain, anxiety, depression, or attention disorders. Ideally, the clinical setting for treatment is one in which there is multidisciplinary collaboration between addiction medicine and other clinicians, all aware of the potential for misuse, abuse, and diversion of controlled substances, a model well described in the pain literature (71–73). For further discussion of the treatment of pain with co-morbid addition the reader is referred to the case discussion by Weaver (73) and Section 7 in this textbook. In the case of benzodiazepines, O'Brien reminds us that it is important to distinguish between addiction to and normal physical dependence (74). As he notes, those intentionally abusing benzodiazepines usually have concurrent substance abuse problems and use these medications secondarily to augment the high of another drug or treat withdrawal symptoms. Normal physiologic dependence is distinguished from addiction, and is best treated with appropriate dose tapering, medication switching, or medication augmentation.

SUMMARY

In summary, misuse, abuse, diversion, and addiction to prescription medications is increasing in the United States. Prevention and treatment of the problem is complicated by the absence of an accepted definition and the complex interaction between access to medications for patients and nonmedical use of prescription medications. Prescribers should use a consistent and nondiscriminatory approach with patients prescribed medications with potential for abuse with the understanding that identification of patients at risk can be difficult. Use of precautions, clear documentation, and utilization of state prescription monitoring programs, although not yet a strategy studied for evidence of efficacy, may be helpful to the clinician. When concern about misuse, abuse, and addiction occur, physicians must determine the circumstances that have led to problematic use of a prescribed medication. The patient diagnosed with abuse and addiction presents an opportunity for intervention to prevent morbidity and overdose, as with the case of addiction to any substance.

When indicated, treatment of NUPM should balance medical considerations of comorbid conditions as well as abuse and addiction. Patients abusing prescription medication will need treatment for withdrawal, stabilization, treatment of addiction, and reassessment of the contributing medical conditions that necessitated prescription of controlled medications. Treatment of this population differs only in the path to addiction, not the opportunity for intervention and treatment and potential for recovery.

REFERENCES

1. Boyd CJ. The nonmedical use of prescription medications: what nurses should know. *J Addict Nurs* 2007;18:113–118.
2. Manchikanti L. National Drug Control Policy and Prescription Drug Abuse: facts and fallacies. *Pain Phys* 2007;10:399–424.
3. Zacny J, Bigelow G, Compton P, et al. College on Problems of Drug Dependence taskforce on prescription opioid non-medical use and abuse: position statement. *Drug Alcohol Depend* 2003;69:215–232.
4. Compton WM, Volkow ND. Abuse of prescription drugs and the risk of addiction. *Drug Alcohol Depend* 2006;83S:S4–S7.
5. Substance Abuse and Mental Health Services Administration, Office of Applied Studies. Results from the 2006 National Survey on Drug Use and Health: (NSDUH) 2007. www.oas.samhsa.gov/nsduh/2kbnsduh/slides.ppt.
6. Boyd CJ, McCabe SE, Teter CJ. Medical and nonmedical use of prescription pain medication by youth in a Detroit-area public school district. *Drug Alcohol Depend* 2006;81(1):37–45.
7. McCabe SE, Cranford JA, Boyd CJ. Motives, diversion and routes of administration associated with nonmedical use of prescription opioids. *Addict Behav* 2007;32:562–575.
8. Reid MC, Engles-Horton LL, Weber MB, et al. Use of opioid medications for chronic non cancer pain syndromes in primary care. *J Gen Intern Med* 2002;17:173–179.
9. Compton P, Darakjian J, Miotto K. Screening for addiction in patients with chronic pain and "problematic" substance use: evaluation of a pilot assessment tool. *J Pain Symptom Manage* 1998;16:355–363.
10. Cowan DT, Wilson-Barnett J, Griffiths P, et al. A survey of chronic noncancer pain patients prescribed opioid analgesics. *Pain Med* 2003;4:340–351.
11. Brands B, Blake J, Sproule B, et al. Prescription opioid abuse in patients presenting for methadone maintenance treatment. *Drug Alcohol Depend* 2004;73:199–207.
12. Miller NS, Greenfeld A. Patient characteristics and risk factors for development of dependence on hydrocodone and oxycodone. *Am J Therap* 2004;11:26–32.
13. Centers for Disease Control and Prevention. Unintentional and undetermined poisoning deaths-11 states, 1990–2001. *MMWR Wkly* 2004;53(11):233–238.
14. Drug Enforcement Administration (DEA), U.S. Department of Justice (2002). Information available at www.usdoj.gov/dea/concern/drugclassesp.html.
15. American Psychiatric Association. Diagnostic and Statistical Manual of Mental Disorders. 4th ed., text revision. Washington, DC: American Psychiatric Association, 2000.
16. Boyd CJ, McCabe SE. Coming to terms with the nonmedical use of prescription medications (Commentary). *Substance Abuse Treat Prevent Policy.*
17. Hubbard ML, Pantula J, Lessler JT. Effects of decomposition of complex concepts. In: Turner CF, Lessler JT, Gfroerer JC, eds. *Survey measurement of drug use: methodological studies.* DHHS publication no. (ADM) 92-1929. Washington, DC: Government Printing Office, 1992.
18. Boyd CJ. Adolescents' nonmedical use of prescription opioid analgesics. Pain, opioids, and addiction: an urgent problem for doctors and patients. Washington, DC: National Institute on Drug Abuse and American Heart Association, March 5–6, 2007.
19. Hojsted J, Sjogren P. Addiction to opioids in chronic pain patients: a literature review. *Eur J Pain* 2007;11(5):490–518.
20. Cicero TJ, Dart RC, Inciardi JA, et al. The development of a comprehensive risk-management program for prescription opioid analgesics: Researched Abuse, Diversion and Addition-Related *Surveillance* (RADARS). *Pain Med* 2007:8(2):157–170.
21. Miller NS, Gold MS. Benzodiazepines: a major problem. *Subst Abuse Treatment* 1991;8(1-2):3–7.
22. Miller NS, Gold MS. Benzodiazepines: tolerance, dependence, abuse, and addiction. *J Psychoactive Drugs* 1990;22(1):23–33.
23. Lubman DI, Hides L, Yücel M, et al. Intervening early to reduce developmentally harmful substance use among youth populations. *Med J Aust* 2007;187(7 Suppl):S22–S25.
24. Anthony JC, Petronis KR. Early-onset drug use and risk of later drug problems. *Drug and Alc Dep* 1995;40:9–15.
25. McCabe SE, West BT, Morales M, et al. Does early onset of non-medical use predict prescription drug abuse and dependence? Results from a national study. *Addiction* 2007;102(12):1920–1930. Epub 2007 Oct 4.
26. McCabe SE, Boyd CJ, Young AM. Medical and Nonmedical use of prescription drugs among secondary school students. *J Adolesc Health* 2007;40:76–83.
27. Barrett SP, Darredeau C, Bordy LE, et al. Characteristics of methylphenidate misuse in a university student sample. *Can J Psychiatry* 2005;50(8):457–461.
28. White BP, Becker-Blease KA, Grace-Bishop K. Stimulant medication use, misuse, and abuse in an undergraduate and graduate student sample. *J Am Coll Health* 2006;54(5):261–268.
29. McCabe SE, Boyd CJ. Sources of prescription drugs for illicit use. *Addict Behav* 2005;30:1342–1350.
30. Boyd CJ, McCabe SE, Cranford JA, et al. Adolescents' motivations to abuse prescription medications. *Pediatrics* 2006;118:2472–2480.
31. McCabe SE, Boyd CJ, Cranford JA, et al. A modified version of the drug abuse screening test among undergraduate students. *J Subst Abuse Treatment* 2006;31:297–303.
32. Goldsworthy RC, Schwartz NC, Mayhorn CB. Beyond abuse and exposure: framing the impact of prescription-medication sharing. *Am J of Pub Health* 2008;98(6):1115–1121.
33. Novak SP, Kroutil LA, Williams RL. et al. The nonmedical use of prescription ADHD medications: results from a national internet panel. *Sub Ab Treat, Prev & Policy* 2007; 2(32):13–17.
34. Quintero G, Peterson J, Young B. An explaratory study of socio-cultural factors contributing to prescription drug misuse among college students. *J of Drug Issues* 2005;35(4):903–932.
35. Forman RF, Woody GE, McLellan T, et al. The availability of web sites offering to sell opioid medications without prescriptions. *Am J Psychiatry* 2006;163(7):1233–1238.
36. Forman RF, Marlowe DB, McLellan AT. The Internet as a source of drugs of abuse. *Curr Psychiatry Rep* 2006;8(5):377–382.
37. Haydon E, Rehm J, Fischer B, et al. Prescription drug abuse in Canada and the diversion of prescription drugs into the illicit drug market. *Can J Public Health* 2005;96(6):459–461.
38. Boyd CJ, McCabe SE, Cranford JA, et al. Gender differences in prescription drug abuse and diversion among adolescents in a southeast Michigan school-district. *Arch Adolesc Pediatr Med* 2007;161:276–281.
39. McCabe SE, Teter CJ, Boyd CJ. Medical use, illicit use and diversion of abusable prescription drugs. *J Am Coll Health* 2006;54(5):269–278.
40. Musser CJ, Ahmann PA, Theye FW, et al. Stimulant use and the potential for abuse in Wisconsin as reported by school administrators and longitudinally followed children. *J Develop Behav Pediatr* 1998;19:187–192.
41. Levine DA. "Pharming": the abuse of prescription and over-the-counter drugs in teens *Curr Opin Pediatr* 2007;19(3):270–274.
42. Weaver MF, Schnoll SH. Hallucinogens and club drugs. In: Galanter M, Klebert HD, eds. *Textbook of substance abuse treatment,* 4th ed. Washington, DC: American Psychiatric Press, 2008.

43. Wunsch MJ, Nakamoto K, Goswami A, et al. Prescription Drug abuse among prisoners in rural southwestern Virginia. *J Addict Dis* 2007;26(4): 15–22.
44. Wunsch MJ, Cropsey KL, Campbell ED, et al. OxyContin use and misuse in three populations: substance abuse patients, pain patients, and criminal justice participants. *J Opioid Manage* 2008;4(2):73–80.
45. Centers for Disease Control and Prevention. Unintentional and undetermined poisoning deaths-II states, 1990–2001. *MMWR Weekly* 2004; 53(11):233–238.
46. Substance Abuse and Mental Health Services Administration, Office of Applied Studies. Drug Abuse Warning Network, 2003: area profiles of drug-related mortality. DAWN Series D-27, DHHS Publication No. (SMA) 05-4023. Rockville, MD, 2005.
47. Substance Abuse Mental Health Services Administration, Office of Applied Studies. (19:2006). The DAWN Report: opiate-related drug misuse deaths in six states: 2003. Rockville, MD.
48. Paulozzi LJ, Budnitz DS, Youngli X. Increasing deaths from opioid analgesics in the United States. *Pharmacoepidemiology and Drug Safety* 2006;15:618–627.
49. Substance Abuse Mental Health Services Administration, Office of Applied Studies. (July 2004). The DAWN Report: Oxycodone, hydrocodone, and Polydrug use, 2002. Rockville, MD.
50. Wunsch MJ, Nakamonto K, Behonick G. et al. Opioid deaths in rural Virginia: A description of the high prevalence of accidental fatalities involving prescribed medications. *Am J on Addictions* 18:1. In Press.
51. Center for Substance Abuse Treatment. *Methadone-associated mortality: report of a national assessment.* DHHS Publication No. (SMA) 04-3904. Rockville, MD: Center for Substance Abuse, 2004.
52. Sanford C. Deaths from unintentional drug overdoses in North Carolina, 1997–2001: a DHHS investigation into unintentional poisoning related deaths. North Carolina Department of Health and Human Services, 2002.
53. Sorg MH, Greenwald M. Maine drug-related mortality patterns: 1997–2002. Augusta, ME: Office of the Maine Attorney General, 2002.
54. Ballesteros MF, Budnitz DS, Sanford CP, et al. Increase in deaths due to methadone in North Carolina. *JAMA* 2003;290:40.
55. Barret DH, Luk AJ, Parrish RG, et al. An investigation of medical examiner cases in which methadone was detected, Harris County, Texas, 1987–1992. *J Forensic Sci* 1996;41(3):442–448.
56. Gagajeewski A, Apple FS. Methadone-related deaths in Hennepin County, Minnesota: 1992–2002. *J Forensic Sci* 2003;48(3):668–671.
57. Andrew TA, Daval JV. *Impact of methadone on drug-related mortality in New Hampshire.* Office of the Chief Medical Examiner, State of New Hampshire 2004. Program and Abstracts, Joint Meeting of SOFT and TIAFT, 2004.
58. Landen MG, Castle S, Nolte KB, et al. Methodological issues in the surveillance of poisoning, illicit drug overdose, and heroin overdose deaths in New Mexico. *Am J Epidemiol* 2003;157:273–278.
59. Cone E, Rant RV, Rohal JM, et al. Oxycodone involvement in drug abuse deaths: a DAWN-based classification scheme applied to an oxycodone postmortem database containing over 1,000 cases. *J Anal Toxicol* 2003; 27:57–67.
60. Bhamb B, Brown D, Hariharan J, et al. Survey of select practice behaviors by primary care physicians on the use of opioids for chronic pain. *Curr Med Res Opin* 2006;22(9):1859–1865.
61. Manchikanti L, Giordano J, Boswell MV, et al. Psychological factors as predictors of opioid abuse and illicit drug use in chronic pain patients. *J Opioid Manage* 2007;3(2):89–100.
62. Ballantyne JC, LaForge KS. Opioid dependence and addiction during opioid treatment of chronic pain. *Pain* 2007;129(3):235–255.
63. Ives TJ, Chelminski PR, Hammett-Stabler CA, et al. Predictors of opioid misuse in patients with chronic pain: a prospective cohort study. *BMC Health Serv Res* 2006;6:46.C.
64. Chabal C, Erjavec MK, Jacobson L, et al. Prescription opiate abuse in chronic pain patients: clinical criteria, incidence and predictors. *Clin J Pain* 1997;13:150–155.
65. Savage SR. Assessment for addiction in pain-treatment settings. *Clin J Pain* 2002;18:S28–S38.
66. Heit HA. Addiction, physical dependence, and tolerance: precise definitions to help clinicians evaluate and treat chronic pain patients. *J Pain Palliat Care Pharmacother* 2003;17(1):15–29.
67. Gourlay DL, Heit HA, Almahrezi A. Universal precautions in pain medicine: a rational approach to the treatment of chronic pain. *Pain Med* 2005;6(2):107–112.
68. Kasprak J. State programs for electronic monitoring of controlled substance prescriptions. Hartford, CT: Connecticut General Assembly OLR Research Report, 2003.
69. Alliance of States with Prescription Monitoring Programs. The goals of prescription monitoring. Quincy, MA: National Association of State Controlled Substances Authorities, 1999. http://www.nascsa.org/alliance/Goals.PDF.
70. Fishman SM, Papazian JS, Gonzalez S, et al. Regulating Opioid prescribing through prescription monitoring programs: balancing drug diversion and treatment of pain. *Pain Med* 2004;5(3):309–324.
71. Joranson DE, Carrow GM, Ryan KM, et al. Pain management and prescription monitoring. *J Pain Symptom Manage* 2002;23:231–238.
72. Weaver M, Schnoll S. Addiction issues in prescribing opioids for chronic non-malignant pain. *J Addiction Medicine* 2007;1(1):2–10.
73. Weaver M, Heit H, Savage S, et al. Clinical case discussion: chronic pain management. *J Addiction Medicine* 2007;1(1):11–14.
74. O'Brien CP. Benzodiazepine use, abuse, and dependence. *J Clin Psychiatry* 2005;66(Suppl 2):28–33.

SUGGESTED READINGS

Wilford BB. Legislative digest. American Medical Association, Chicago, IL, 1998.

Joranson DE, Cleeland CS, Weissman DE, et al. Opioids for chronic cancer and noncancer pain—a survey of state medical board members. *Fed Bull* 1992:15–49.

CHAPTER 34

Joan E. Zweben, PhD

Special Issues in Treatment: Women

Within the past decade, treatment providers have devoted increasing attention to defining and addressing the unique needs of women. Gender disparities were largely ignored until the 1970s, when interest grew in the biomedical and psychosocial aspects of women's use of alcohol and other drugs. Prompted by the women's movement, the federal government initiated efforts to focus scientific and public attention on women's issues (1,2). This focus has generated new research, services specifically tailored to women's needs, new materials for clinicians in the field, and reconsideration of public policy. However, there still are many ways in which the needs of women in alcohol and drug treatment remain unmet. According to Substance Abuse and Mental Health Services Administration's facility locator, based on 2006 data, only 24% of the 11,000 programs listed offered specific services for women (3). This chapter will discuss treatment issues specific to women, including the relationship of drug and alcohol use problems to psychiatric and medical conditions, and review new findings on gender-specific treatment.

EPIDEMIOLOGY

Gender Differences in Alcohol and Other Drug Use Several large-scale epidemiologic studies document gender differences in the use of alcohol and almost all other drugs, with higher rates found in men (4,5). The Epidemiological Catchment Area study, with data collected in the 1980s, reported that men had five times greater 1-month prevalence rates for alcohol and three times greater 1-month prevalence for other drugs (5). The more recent National Comorbidity Study (4) documented similar differences, but the gap appears to be diminishing. A subsequent National Household Survey on Drug Abuse (6) study, conducted in 1998, showed smaller gender differences for all age groups except adolescents ages 12 to 17 years. For this group, the gap virtually disappeared for alcohol, marijuana, cocaine, and cigarettes. Thus, gender patterns are evolving according to changing social conditions, with reported rates of use becoming more similar for men and women (7). Nonmedical use of prescription drugs in general and opioids in particular has been identified as a significant emergent problem since the late 1990s. Among use, such use of opioids is also associated with first use of illicit drug use at age 24 or older, serious mental illness, and cigarette smoking (8). A subgroup of women (and men) who are opioid dependent report that the energy they get from opioids is very reinforcing and the drug seems to relieve depression. This phenomenon warrants further study.

Stimulants such as cocaine and methamphetamine have a particular appeal for women. Their use is associated with loss of appetite and desirable weight loss, and the stimulating effects are often initially perceived as alerting and beneficial in a world of undone work and household chores.

Common Psychiatric Disorders in Women with Addictive Disorders Most men and women in treatment for addictive disorders have at least one coexisting mental disorder, but the pattern differs for women. The higher the intensity of care, the greater the likelihood of dual disorders. Both the Epidemiologic Catchment Area Study (5) and the National Comorbidity Study (4) found that women were more likely to have an affective disorder than men (with the exception of mania, for which rates were the same). Women were significantly more likely than men to have experienced a major depressive episode. Data from the National Comorbidity

Study showed a lifetime prevalence of 21.3% and a 12-month prevalence of 12.9% for women, compared with 12.7% and 7.7% for men. Dysthymia also was more common in women, with a lifetime prevalence of 8% and a 12-month prevalence of 3% compared with 4.8% and 2.1% for men. Women also had a higher lifetime and 12-month prevalence of three or more disorders.

In addition, women who have experienced childhood sexual abuse are at greatly increased risk of developing a wide range of psychopathology, particularly bulimia, alcoholism, and other drug dependence (9). In a carefully done twin study, the researchers concluded that their results could not be explained by pre-existing familial-environmental factors.

MEDICAL CONSIDERATIONS

Alcohol The influence of alcohol on women's health has been much more carefully studied than other drugs. Although women are less likely than men to drink heavily or even moderately (10), when they do so, they are more vulnerable to alcohol-related liver damage, cardiovascular disease, and brain damage (11). A large prospective study that followed 13,000 adults for 12 years found that women developed alcohol-related liver disease at approximately half the consumption levels of men (12). For women, the risk of alcohol-induced liver disease and alcohol-related cirrhosis rose once consumption levels exceeded 7 to 13 drinks (84 to 156 g of alcohol) per week. Alcohol increased women's susceptibility to myopathy and cardiomyopathy, and studies suggest that female alcoholics suffer from a generalized skeletal fragility that increases the risks from falls (11). Negative consequences occur at lower levels of consumption and after much shorter periods of drinking. This is referred to as the "telescoped course" in women. In a recent review, Blume and Zilberman (13) note that there is growing evidence that women develop many of the pathologic effects of alcohol more rapidly than men. Their examples include fatty liver, hypertension, anemia, malnutrition, gastrointestinal hemorrhage, and peptic ulcer requiring surgery.

Mumenthaler and colleagues reviewed studies of alcohol absorption, distribution, elimination, and impairment, and they explored the mechanisms by which women achieve higher blood alcohol concentrations than men after drinking equivalent amounts of alcohol, even when doses are adjusted for body weight (14). Women tend to have lower levels of alcohol dehydrogenase and lower volumes of distribution, leading to an increased effect of alcohol from an equivalent exposure in a man. Their review also noted women's relatively greater susceptibility to alcohol's effects on cognitive functions, such as divided attention and impaired memory. They concluded that the menstrual cycle is not likely to affect alcohol pharmacokinetics and is not a significant influence on alcohol's effects on performance. The relationship between drinking and breast cancer risk has been also studied since the 1980s. Alcohol consumption raises breast cancer risk even after adjustment for age, family history, and other known dietary and reproductive risk factors (11). The increased risk appears to be modest and dose-related, and the form of alcohol appears to be irrelevant.

It is important that clinicians make use of opportunities to educate women about their greater risks, even those who are highly educated and articulate (15). There is still widespread public naivete about what constitutes moderate or low-risk drinking. For example, many interpret their increased tolerance or the absence of short-term negative consequences to mean they are drinking moderately. In this recent study, none of the 150 respondents discussed gender differences in their in-depth interview, indicating a surprising lack of awareness given how long the information on differential impact has been available.

Prenatal Alcohol Exposure Drinking during pregnancy remains a serious concern, with physicians in a key position to reinforce social norms that encourage the elimination of drinking during this time. Fetal alcohol syndrome (FAS) is a set of birth defects considered the single leading nonhereditary cause of mental retardation. The growth deficiency and characteristic set of facial traits tend to become more normal over time, but the alcohol-induced damage to the developing brain is enduring. These mental impairments include deficits in general intellectual functioning and specific difficulties with learning, memory, attention, and problem solving, in addition to manifestations in psychosocial arenas. The impairments are dose-related and may be evident in children without the distinguishing physical features of FAS (11). Several terms have been developed to describe alcohol-related conditions. The term *alcohol-related birth defects* refers to alcohol-related physical abnormalities of the skeleton and certain organ systems (for example, heart and kidney) that occur in the absence of the characteristic growth deficiency and facial characteristics of FAS. The term *alcohol-related neurodevelopmental disorder* refers to the mental impairments in the absence of FAS. The introduction of a new diagnostic system for categorizing fetal alcohol effects has facilitated more systematic research. Neuroimaging studies provide insight into the structural damage to the brain, and specific patterns of behavioral impairment have been more carefully delineated. Heavy prenatal exposure to alcohol leads to neurobehavioral impairment, but the effects of lower levels of exposure are less clear, although documented in some studies (11). Simply stated, there is no demonstrated safe level of alcohol consumption during pregnancy.

Compounding these defects are the caregiving deficits in the child's immediate family when one or both parents are drinking heavily. These deficits include inconsistent nurturance; lack of parental support, monitoring, and communication; high levels of conflict; and physical and sexual abuse (16). Comprehensive treatment of the substance-abusing woman needs to address these wide-ranging needs, as described later in this chapter.

Drugs Although evidence of gender differences in the effects of drug use is not extensive at this time, there are indications that gender may be a factor for understanding the pharmacokinetic effects of some drugs. A study of treatment-seeking female cocaine users concluded that some women may have greater vulnerability to the effects of cocaine relative to men, resulting in more rapid progression of pathology (17). Biomedical research also suggests that women may be more sensitive to some behavioral effects of cocaine. Mechanisms suggested include female steroid hormones (18), estrogen (19), and differences in receptor function (20). Investigations of the influence of menstrual cycle phase have yielded contradictory results (21–23). Unfortunately, there is scant literature examining differing effects of other drugs such as heroin on men and women. However, it is well known that a woman's substance use is heavily influenced by her male partner (24–26) and that she can underestimate her level of harm if her main reference point is her partner's behavior.

Stereotypes about methadone being "just another addiction" can have prejudicial influence on medical decisions. Methadone is considered the gold standard maintenance treatment for opioid-dependent pregnant women. It is important that the dose be adequate. Contrary to common expectations, higher doses are not associated with increased risks of neonatal abstinence (27). Despite the fact that some of the women were on relatively high doses of methadone (ranging from 25 to 180 mg/day), levels in breast milk were small and no adverse events were detected. Women should not be discouraged from breastfeeding if they are not using illicit drugs and do not have specific contraindications (28).

Buprenorphine is not currently approved by the U.S. Food and Drug Administration for use in pregnancy, and it, along with methadone, is category C in pregnancy. This allows a risk-benefit clinical decision to start or continue to maintain pregnant patients on sublingual buprenorphine/naloxone when methadone treatment is not an option or is not acceptable to the patient. A large-scale, multisite study is under way to evaluate its safety and efficacy of buprenorphine in pregnancy (29). The Maternal Opioid Treatment: Human Experimental Research project is a double-blind, double-dummy, flexible-dosing, parallel-group clinical trial involving eight clinical sites. Inasmuch as women on buprenorphine may become pregnant, or may prefer buprenorphine to methadone, the Maternal Opioid Treatment: Human Experimental Research project seeks to develop guidelines based on risk-benefit ratios. It is important to use buprenorphine alone rather than the buprenorphine/naloxone combination to avoid prenatal exposure to naloxone. Transferring a methadone patient to buprenorphine is challenging and there is no medication transition procedure that avoids the risk of withdrawal, which carries the risks of fetal distress, miscarriage, and stillbirth. In research studies, this transition has been accomplished using intravenous morphine in a hospital (30), but this is not a practical option for community treatment providers. Buprenorphine may pose complications for pain management during labor and delivery. The same features that produce an enhanced safety profile for buprenorphine may mean that pain medications fail to reach the target receptors. Buprenorphine in pregnancy is covered in more detail in Chapter 81.

In summary, although methadone is the treatment of choice for opioid-dependent pregnant women, the emergence of buprenorphine as an option is an important development with potential to expand treatment access in rural areas and in other circumstances.

It is especially important to reduce early treatment dropout in pregnant women, because participation in treatment is associated with better maternal and neonatal outcomes. Drug craving and withdrawal were important precipitants of relapse, especially for heroin users who did not receive methadone maintenance (31).

Domestic Violence In 1994, a Bureau of Justice report indicated that more than half a million women were treated in hospital emergency departments for violence-related injuries, usually inflicted by an intimate partner (32). At least 4.4 million women in the United States each year suffer from related health problems. Women who have been battered report that their general health is fair or poor, that they have had sexually transmitted diseases and other gynecologic problems, and that they have needed medical care that they have not received. Chronic headaches, as well as hearing, vision, and concentration problems, can reflect neurologic damage. A variety of stress-related symptoms, such as irritable bowel syndrome, also can manifest (33). For these reasons, psychosocial treatment efforts must integrate good medical care to be fully comprehensive. It is especially important that residential and outpatient programs without such care on site develop effective case management. Addiction medicine specialists can help such programs develop protocols and procedures to ensure that the counseling staff members are aware of the woman's medical status and are clear in their role to facilitate adherence to treatment recommendations. Larger programs have found that a "medical coordinator" who functions as a medical case manager can provide more systematic attention to medical concerns.

HIV/AIDS Women account for a steadily increasing proportion of AIDS cases. In 1985, <5% of new AIDS cases in the United States were among girls older than 13 years of age and adult women. By 2005, it was nearly 27%, with women of color heavily impacted. HIV/AIDS is the leading cause of death for African American women ages 25 to 34 (34). Having sex with a man with HIV is the most common mode of transmission, followed by sharing injection drug works used by someone with HIV (35). Similar patterns of increase, particularly among women of color, also are beginning to be apparent in the distribution of reported hepatitis C cases. Socially sanctioned imbalance of power plays a major role in influencing risk reduction behavior in women. Inasmuch as the condom remains the major method to reduce sexual transmission of HIV, women are at a disadvantage for determining their exposure. Women must either gain the cooperation of their male partners in using a condom or must decide not to have sexual relations if the man refuses (36,37). Many women lack the self-esteem and communication skills to negotiate condom use. Young women in particular often lack the fortitude to insist if their partners balk at the prospect. Addicted women are at an additional disadvantage in attempting to practice safer sex. Many women fear emotional or physical abuse if they do so. Indeed, a woman's greatest risk of assault is from her male partner (38). The development of an effective protective method that is under the woman's control and can be used without the knowledge of her sexual partner is a key element in reducing women's risk.

For the HIV-infected women, managing caretaking responsibilities often is an issue added to the physical and psychiatric burdens of the disease. They worry about transmission of the virus to family members and must be both well informed and reassured. They struggle with how to address their health issues and their possible death with their children. Women who have given birth to HIV-positive children have an added layer of anxiety and guilt. Initially, they must choose whether to carry the child to term. After delivery, women in these circumstances are often socially isolated and welcome the opportunity to share with other women in a support group, which can help to bypass their shame and express their feelings more openly, with less fear of rejection (39).

PSYCHIATRIC DISORDERS

The need for treatment interventions that are sensitive to gender differences has brought increasing attention to co-occurring disorders and their effect on addicted women. It is preferable to address multiple disorders with an integrated approach. Although the addiction treatment field has made great progress in addressing co-occurring disorders in the past decade, advances in understanding and practice vary greatly in their degree of dissemination. Physicians can expect wide variation in sophistication and responsiveness among community providers and should attempt to refer or place the patient according to specific conditions and behaviors that indicate the need for particular services or levels of care. These conditions and behaviors are described in the recent revision of the American Society of Addiction Medicine's Patient Placement Criteria (40), in which community service levels are described in terms of "addiction treatment only," programs that focus primarily if not exclusively on addiction; programs that are "dual diagnosis capable," for those whose psychiatric disorders have been stabilized; and those that are "dual diagnosis enhanced," for those who are unstable or disabled to the extent of needing specific psychiatric support, monitoring, and accommodation. Many community providers describe themselves as offering treatment for co-occurring psychiatric disorders without having the resources to handle the full range of problems (41,42). A clear picture of the strengths and limits of programs available in the community can lead to more appropriate referrals, as well as help in guiding the development of services needed to fill the gaps.

It has become more widely accepted in the addiction treatment community that psychotropic medications are compatible with recovery, especially when prescribed by physicians knowledgeable about addiction. Indeed, appropriately prescribed medications enhance the effects of psychosocial interventions. Effective pharmacotherapy requires careful education and a clear treatment contract (43): "The essential principles are that pharmacotherapy targets specific symptoms, is time limited, is modified only one change at a time, is monitored for compliance, and is provided only in the context of a comprehensive psychosocial treatment plan" (p. 1002). The physician's role as a member of a multidisciplinary team is crucial to achieving these objectives. Counseling staff members typically are responsible for implementing major elements of the plan, and good communication and a structure for coordination improve patient cooperation with physician recommendations.

In this section, we will review the most common psychiatric disorders found in women with substance abuse problems: anxiety disorders (especially posttraumatic stress disorder [PTSD]), mood disorders, eating disorders, and borderline personality disorder.

Anxiety Disorders As a group, anxiety disorders constitute the most common psychiatric disorders among women, with a total lifetime prevalence of 30.5% and a 12-month prevalence of 22.6% (4). The experience of anxiety is characterized by sensations of nervousness, tension, apprehension, and fear that arise from the anticipation of internal or external danger. These feelings constitute important survival signals, so the task is to distinguish what is normal and appropriate from states that require intervention. Certainly, women in early recovery will experience heightened distress as they try to cope with situations in which they previously relied on alcohol and other drugs, and also as they more clearly see the impact of their self-destructive behaviors. However, overwhelming anxiety is debilitating, interferes with new learning, and contributes to relapse. Psychosocial strategies are beneficial for the management of anxiety regardless of whether it is normal or excessive. The task for the woman and the clinician is to determine when the level is high enough to impair daily function and to justify medication. Fortunately, the first-line medications for anxiety and panic disorders are no longer the benzodiazepines, but the selective serotonin reuptake inhibitors, historically misunderstood as antidepressants only.

It can be easy to underestimate her level of distress when a woman's description is viewed as "dramatic"; in earlier eras, women reporting the same symptoms as men often were labeled "hysterics." Both depression and anxiety can occur in the context of a wide variety of other disorders, and it may be difficult to disentangle the interacting elements and identify the predominant disorders. When anxiety symptoms do not resolve with abstinence, a variety of psychosocial interventions can be used, selected to address the tasks specific to the woman's stage of recovery. In early recovery, calming reassurance, reality-oriented support, exercise, meditation, breathing management, and other relaxation techniques can be helpful when added to group activities designed to encourage exchange of experiences and transmission of skills. In the later stages of treatment, a variety of supportive, cognitive, and psychodynamic therapies can be used, but anxiety-arousing explorations should be avoided in early recovery. Insight-oriented therapy should be used in the context of a firm recovery support system (including regular self-help group attendance) by a therapist familiar with recovery issues. Familiarity with relapse hazards, warning signs, and prevention strategies are important. Severe or chronic anxiety can be a significant relapse hazard, so it is important to develop a medication stance that does not make a virtue out of excessive suffering. However, the patient must develop new ways of coping with everyday distress, and it is undesirable to seek to eliminate most of the unpleasant feeling states that are inevitable in recovery.

Benzodiazepines, commonly prescribed for anxiety disorders, can be problematic for those with a personal or family history of addiction. They are best avoided when possible or used in circumscribed situations (44). Nonreinforcing alternatives, such as sedating antidepressants or buspirone (BuSpar) for anxiety or trazodone (Desyrel) for insomnia, are recommended. Anticonvulsants, antihypertensives, or the newer atypical neuroleptic medications can also be used. When reasonable alternatives have failed, benzodiazepines can be used with careful monitoring. This includes consideration of abstinence from substances, adherence to prescribed medication regimens, and participation in recovery efforts (44).

Of all the anxiety disorders, PTSD is arguably the most difficult and complex to manage. In the National Comorbidity Study, the estimated lifetime prevalence of PTSD was 7.8%, with a striking gender difference—a prevalence of 10.4% in women as compared with 5.0% in men. (45). This finding is consistent with several studies by Breslau and colleagues (46–48). Wasserman and colleagues (49) concluded that the relationship between female gender and PTSD is robust across patient populations. Rape and sexual molestation were the most frequently reported "most upsetting event(s)," with childhood parental neglect and childhood physical abuse reported more frequently by women. Female victims were more than twice as likely as male victims to develop PTSD (20% compared with 8.2%). A lifetime history of at least one other disorder was present in 79% of women with PTSD, and more than one third of the women with PTSD failed to recover from their PTSD, even after many years and even if they received professional treatment.

Participants in addiction treatment have much higher rates of traumatic experiences and PTSD than the general population. Studies of both residential and outpatient treatment programs that serve both middle class insured and indigent populations show high levels of childhood abuse and adult trauma (49–55). These findings require treatment providers to equip themselves to meet complex needs. As Brown and colleagues (56) demonstrated, such a high "level of burden" promotes early dropout, increases the difficulty of treatment in a variety of ways, and makes it more difficult to obtain a positive outcome.

Childhood experiences set the stage for later manifestation of a wide range of disorders and enhance the likelihood of dysfunctional coping responses in adulthood (57). Studies differ in terms of the types of trauma they consider and how they measure it, making it difficult to compare across studies. Russell and Wilsnack (58) discuss the methodologic problems in comparing the studies that started to emerge in the 1990s. They examined available studies using a conservative definition of childhood sexual abuse that and included both intrafamilial and extrafamilial sexual abuse, but excluded noncontact experiences, before the age of 18. By these criteria, in community samples, more than one third of female children experienced sexual abuse by age 18. This included incest, defined as sexual abuse by a relative before the age of 18.

Newer studies and reviewers support these findings. In a population-based study of female twins, Kendler and colleagues (9) found that 30.4% reported childhood sexual abuse of a variety of kinds (sexual invitation, sexual kissing, fondling, exposing, sexual touching), and 8.4% reported intercourse. They analyzed their data to examine the relationship of childhood sexual abuse and common psychiatric disorders and substance abuse, controlling for background familial factors. They concluded that women with childhood sexual abuse are at high risk for developing a wide range of psychopathology. In their National Comorbidity study, Kessler and colleagues (45) came to similar conclusions regarding the relationship between sexual trauma, PTSD, and other psychiatric disorders in women.

Women in substance abuse treatment show higher rates than the general population (59,60). Addictive disorder is only one of many sequelae. Others include low self-esteem, depression, suicide, anxiety, difficulties in interpersonal relationships, sexual dysfunction, and a tendency toward revictimization (49). These girls are at nearly a fourfold increased risk of any psychiatric disorder and a threefold risk of addictive disorder (61).

It appears that among adult stressors, rape is the most consistently severe in its effect (46) and is associated with a range of psychiatric symptoms (62). Koss and Burkart (63) noted that almost half of the victims of rape seek some type of professional psychotherapy, often years after the assault. One study indicated that nearly 20% of the women who reported rapes in 1984 had attempted suicide and as many as 80% to 97% developed symptoms of PTSD (64). Newer studies support this finding (65). Intimate partner violence is especially associated with suicidal ideation and other psychiatric symptoms (66).

Mood Disorders In assessing for depression, it is important to rule out the direct effects of alcohol, illicit drugs, or medications, as well as general medical conditions, such as hypothyroidism, that can lower mood. Agencies should have protocols for assessing suicide risk and protective factors. These risks are often but not exclusively attendant to mood disorders.

Pregnant patients with mood disorders fared worse on drug use outcomes than those with an anxiety disorder or no cooccurring disorder (67), highlighting the importance of rapid identification and intervention during pregnancy.

For diagnostic purposes, negative mood states that are the direct result of alcohol or illicit drugs generally clear within 2 to 3 weeks, with symptoms of longer duration suggesting an independent mood disorder (68,69). Distress, which is not the same as depression, can persist for a long period. It is important to inquire carefully, because women in recovery often use the term *depressed* to describe brooding anxiety, misery, obsessive guilt, apprehension, and other forms of wretchedness that are not synonymous with clinical depression. There is a substantial literature on known pregnancy risk profiles of common antidepressants (70,71).

It also is important to remember that a sad or depressed mood is only one of many signs and symptoms of a clinically significant depression and may not be the most prominent feature. Other indications include disturbances in emotional, cognitive, behavioral, or somatic regulation. The mood disturbance itself can include apathy, anxiety, or irritability along with, or instead of, sadness. Not all clinically depressed patients feel sad, and many who feel sad are not clinically depressed. Clinicians need to have good skills for drawing patients out and helping them describe their feelings. Women in subcultures that place a high value on functioning can mask depressive symptoms. Those in leadership or caregiver roles can initially manifest depression in more disguised forms, especially if they have a high investment in performance or in continuing to function despite distress. Some depressed women do not describe a low mood, but their interest in or capacity for pleasure or enjoyment may be markedly reduced, making it difficult for them to experience rewards in recovery or to invest in new social relationships with others who do not drink or use drugs.

Eating Disorders Despite the recognition that eating disorders are relatively common in substance-abusing women, careful assessment is not routine and integrated treatment is rare. Eating disorders are more prevalent among substance-abusing women than in the general population, and substance-abusing women report more disordered eating behavior than women in the general population. A review of the comorbidity of eating disorders and addictive disorder (72) indicated that bulimia is more common than anorexia. It appears that women with bulimia and alcohol dependence are more likely to have major depression, drug dependence, tobacco dependence, and obsessive compulsive disorder than women with either disorder alone (73). Krahn and colleagues (74,75) studied eating abnormalities and substance use (including alcoholism) and suggested that levels of symptoms below the threshold required to meet criteria for eating disorders are important for the clinician to address. They caution that dieting-related attitudes and behaviors in young women may be related to increased susceptibility to alcohol and other drug use. Stimulants and over-the-counter diet preparations are particularly appealing to women seeking to lose or control weight.

Among alcohol- and drug-using women, there are many possible relationships between substance use and eating disorders. The eating disorder may present before the onset of alcohol and drug problems. Eating disorders can coexist with substance use in a variety of ways. Some patients report that heroin is appealing because it facilitates vomiting. Drinking alcohol can provide the feeling of release also gained from vomiting. Stimulants are attractive because they make women feel capable, energetic, and suppress the appetite. Alcohol can be used to suppress the panic associated with bingeing and vomiting or to quash the shame that follows an episode. Eating disorders also can be part of a pattern of symptom substitution in abstinent substance users. For example, women concerned about weight gain once abstinent from stimulants may begin to vomit or purge to cope with their anxiety about body image.

It is important for programs serving women to develop proficiency in addressing eating disorders and obesity, especially given the demise of many specialized eating disorder programs. Because secrecy is a feature of both disorders, careful inquiry is important during the initial assessment, and observation by staff members is necessary throughout treatment. A woman in treatment may gain or lose 20 pounds without a disorder being addressed by her individual counselor or in her groups. Eating disorder specialists agree that treatment of these conditions requires specialized training. A thorough medical evaluation should assess possible problems and be part of a plan for nutritional stabilization, including strategies to stop aberrant eating behaviors, as well as medication planning and discharge planning that actively addresses both disorders (76). Selective serotonin reuptake inhibitors have been shown to be beneficial in treating bulimia, but not restrictive anorexia. Addiction specialists should avoid the temptation to apply a variant of the 12-step model as the sole treatment for eating disorders and should be selective about which elements are applied. Cognitive-behavioral approaches to eating disorders, which are well-supported by empirical evidence, are designed to reduce dietary restraint (in contrast with promoting abstinence from particular foods), address abnormal attitudes about body weight and shape, and alter thinking about eating and personal control. Psychotherapy to address related personal issues is encouraged much earlier in the recovery process (77) than is the case with addictive disorders.

Borderline Personality Disorder When receiving a patient with a borderline diagnosis, it is important to review the diagnosis for accuracy. Misdiagnosis of borderline personality disorder unfortunately is quite common, because of confusion of borderline characteristics with the behaviors exhibited during active alcohol and drug use and early recovery. Although the DSM-IV (78) introduced clear criteria for differential diagnosis, patients diagnosed before that time or from settings in which diagnostic rigor is not the norm may be improperly classified. Thus, it is advisable to reconsider the diagnosis. This reconsideration is especially important because borderline patients are viewed in many settings as difficult and unrewarding to treat. Clinicians treating addictive disorder are accustomed to seeing women present with behaviors consistent with borderline personality disorder, who settle down markedly and look far less pathologic with a year or so of sobriety and a good recovery program.

Enduring characteristics of borderline personality disorder include unstable mood and self-image; unstable, intense, interpersonal relationships; extremes of overidealization and devaluation; and marked shifts from baseline to impulsive outbursts, anxiety states, or other extreme moods. Prevalence of borderline personality disorder is estimated to be about 2% of the general population, 10% of those seen in outpatient mental health clinics, and 20% of psychiatric inpatients. Women constitute about 75% of those with the diagnosis (79). Initial formulations and discussion of borderline personality disorder emerged from the psychoanalytic tradition and downplayed the possibility that abuse experiences were real, in favor of the view that fantasy distortion, strong impulses in a weak ego structure, maternal conflicts, and separation and loss experiences were decisive. The possibility that fearfulness, anger, and suspicion of the borderline patient might have its roots in real childhood trauma was minimized (80). Cultural denial of childhood abuse was pervasive until the attention to PTSD created a knowledge base that revised earlier notions about abuse as mere fantasy (81,82). Herman, van der Kolk, and others have explored the possibility that actual traumatic experiences play a key role in the etiology of borderline pathology. Subsequently, a literature has emerged that described a relationship between borderline pathology and childhood physical and sexual abuse. Although childhood trauma does not always predict borderline personality disorder, it can be a significant contributing factor (83–86). A history of childhood sexual abuse and a family history of substance use disorder is associated with longer time to remission of borderline personality disorder (87).

In summary, the prevalence of co-occurring disorders in women underlines the importance of offering psychiatric services, although funding may be more difficult to obtain except for those with severe mental illness. In addition to education about addiction, programs should include material on co-occurring mental disorders and how they can influence relapse and recovery. This education should have many of the same components as alcohol and other drug use (AOD) topics: (1) nature of the disorders commonly found in women; their usual course and prognosis; (2) important factors such as genetics, environmental stressors, and traumatic experiences; (3) misunderstandings about medication; (4) relapse warning signs; and (5) how to maximize recovery potential. Patients benefit from clarification of what constitutes effective teamwork with the physician (e.g., log of symptoms, notes about physician recommendations, when to call and when to wait).

According to the large National Epidemiologic Survey on Alcohol and Related Conditions, women are also at greater risk of avoidant, dependent, and paranoid personality disorders (88). Although this increases the risk of greater global impairment, treatment dropout, and relapse, there has been little focus on specific treatment interventions for this group of women.

SPECIAL POPULATIONS

Variations in cultural subgroups and sexual orientation also play an important role in treatment. Gender roles vary greatly, especially among immigrant groups, in which the degree of acculturation determines many of the constraints on the woman's role. Use of alcohol and other drugs may be taboo for women, so recognition of their use, or seeking treatment for problems related to use, may be impossible. Those from patriarchal cultures can face strong taboos about disclosing family secrets, especially around interpersonal violence. Women can fear abandonment if they violate cultural norms. Those disclosing sexual violations can risk severe devaluation within or expulsion from their community, and they can lack the hope for improvement that could propel them past this barrier. Many fear institutions such as the police, social services, and mental health agencies that might provide alternative resources (89,90). Culturally sensitive and specific education and prevention messages have begun to be developed for women in some subgroups, but much more work in this area remains to be done.

Another subgroup of women, lesbians, is at particular risk because of the extensive use of alcohol and drugs as part of the culture (91). Socializing patterns built around bars and drug-sharing increase the risk of addiction but do not necessarily lead to recognition of the attendant problems. These women generally are more dependent on lesbian friendship networks than on families or marital bonds, and their adaptive system of mutual reliance may be inappropriately pathologized as codependence. Historically, lesbian bars were seen as gathering places and safe arenas for self-expression and, in many areas, they still are the only place where such behavior can occur. Even when problems are recognized, they can avoid treatment agencies if they fear discrimination or lack of understanding about their specific needs (92).

ADDITIONAL TREATMENT ISSUES

In a recent review of 280 articles published between 1975 and 2005, Greenfield and colleagues examined substance abuse treatment entry, retention, and outcomes in women (93). Although the gender ratio is variable in different studies, it is lower than the gender ratio of prevalence of alcohol and drug use disorders in the population. This may be in part because of women's tendency to seek help in medical or mental health settings (94,95). Barriers vary, but include lack of pregnancy services, lack of child care, fears of loss of custody or of prosecution, and inadequate services for women with cooccurring disorders. With respect to treatment retention, Greenfield and colleagues conclude that larger studies suggest gender is not a significant predictor overall, but specific treatment elements improve outcomes for various subgroups. For example, inclusion of children enhances engagement and retention for women seeking residential treatment. Some of these key issues are explored further in the following sections.

Management and Retention Issues The epidemiologic finding that women have high rates of three or more disorders has consequences for treatment. New work on readiness to change shows promise for improving women's treatment. Brown and colleagues (96) noted that candidates for addiction treatment can vary in their commitment to make changes in a variety of areas that will affect their prospects. They have developed a Steps of Change Model that covers four areas in which changes may be relevant: (i) domestic violence, (ii) risky sexual behaviors, (iii) addictive disorder behaviors, and (iv) emotional problems. Their work supports the hypothesis that the most immediate or threatening problems will be what a woman focuses on first, and she selects her treatment modality accordingly. Women with addictive disorders who are in domestic violence situations are relatively resistant to addressing their alcohol and drug use. They are preoccupied with achieving greater safety and see their alcohol and other drug problems as secondary. By contrast, women with other mental health problems are more receptive to treatment for their addictive disorders. Treatment providers need to be willing to start by addressing those problems the woman is most ready to change while cultivating readiness in other areas identified by the clinician as important for long-term success.

The number and severity of problems experienced by women clients can be translated into a measure of level of burden. In studies of high-burden clients, such women tend to be at greatest risk of early termination and poor outcomes even when they do remain in treatment for longer periods (56). Integrated treatment for multiple disorders thus is especially important in designing or selecting a treatment program to meet women's needs. It generally is agreed by providers that women-only programs or activities are an important aspect of effective treatment, and although research on this question supports this view, much remains to be covered. An examination of the services offered in women-only programs compared with mixed-gender programs in southern California found that the most consistent difference was the provision of services specific to women's needs, particularly those associated with pregnancy and parenting (97). These services included parenting classes; children's activities; and pediatric, prenatal, and postpartum services. Women-only programs also were more likely to assist with housing, transportation, job training, and practical skills training. Thus, even though programs can present themselves as doing individualized treatment planning, women-only programs appear to be better equipped to meet women's needs. These programs also were more likely to be funded through the Medicaid system instead of fees or private insurance, reflecting the lower socioeconomic status of their client population.

A prospective longitudinal study examining service needs, utilization and outcomes in women-only and mixed-gender programs found that those in women-only programs had greater problem severity but better outcomes in the areas of drug use and legal problems (98). This study had a large, ethnically diverse sample of women in community based treatment in eight different programs in California. The 189 women in women-only programs tended to be in residential treatment, whereas the 871 women in mixed-gender programs were in outpatient treatment. Those in women-only programs had greater Addiction Severity Index (ASI) scores in the areas of alcohol, drug, family, medical, and psychiatric domains.

It appears that gender-specific treatment is also associated with higher rates of continuing care. In a quasi-experimental retrospective study of women and children in residential treatment, those in specialized, women-only programs who completed the residential phase were more likely to continue appropriate care than those in mixed-gender programs (99).

Aside from the different needs and characteristics of male and female substance abusers, there is reason to think that women-only groups tend to foster greater interaction, emotional and behavioral expression, and more variability in style than mixed-gender groups. Women in mixed groups tend to engage in a more restricted type of behavior, whereas the behavior of the men shows a wider variability (100).

It is not known whether these differences are most influenced by the overall characteristics of the women-only treatment setting, or by specific services provided by these programs. As McLellan and colleagues have shown, the tightness of fit between the individual's problem profile and the actual services received are more relevant than the specific treatment setting (101,102). It is also possible that women-only programs create a distinctive type of synergy that makes it difficult to disentangle the active ingredients.

Physical and Sexual Abuse and Domestic Violence Although more than a third of women with PTSD fail to recover after many years, even with professional treatment, the average duration of symptoms was shorter among women in treatment (45), suggesting that existing treatments did confer some benefit. Co-occurring psychopathology typically is associated with less favorable addiction treatment outcomes. However, in a study by Gil-Rivas et al. (52), abused clients were more likely than their nonabused counterparts to participate in counseling and just as likely to complete treatment and remain drug-free during and up to 6 months after treatment.

Trauma-related difficulties can impair parenting in a variety of ways (103). Women with histories of childhood trauma can have attachment problems that impact their own parenting, particularly their ability to nurture. They often lack appropriate role models, leading to reliance on physical punishment, difficulties setting appropriate boundaries, and neglect. They may be unable to integrate protective discipline and affection. Women with sexual abuse histories may be deeply mistrustful of men but at the same time miss danger signs that their children are at risk. Obviously, current alcohol and other drug use will exacerbate these vulnerabilities. It is important to keep in mind that not all women with histories of abuse will abuse their children. Clinicians should be observant but avoid conveying a pessimistic attitude towards a woman's prospects for being a good parent.

Efforts are under way to modify service systems to meet the needs of clients with histories of abuse and violence. At minimum, these systems need to be *trauma informed*, or knowledgeable about and sensitive to trauma-related issues present in survivors. Most importantly, these services will be delivered in a way that avoids retraumatization and encourages consumer participation in treatment. *Trauma-specific services* include appropriate assessment methods and specific interventions to address trauma issues (104). Parenting classes offered to women should be trauma-informed.

Seeking Safety (105,106) is a well accepted and widely disseminated trauma-specific treatment intervention for those with substance abuse and a trauma history. It is an early-stage intervention designed to stabilize the patient (create safety) with respect to both substance abuse and PTSD, integrated within a manualized but flexible treatment approach. It has been unusually well accepted by clinical staff and clients alike. (For more information, go to *www.seekingsafety.org*.)

It has been noted that children with battered mothers experience posttraumatic stress reactions themselves. These children often are subjected to ongoing marital conflict, family dysfunction, dislocations, and relocations of home, lack of parental care, economic and social disadvantage, and interactions with the police and court. Preschool children are more vulnerable to the effects of domestic violence (33) than older children.

The extensive variety and complexity of children's reactions to domestic violence argues for routine assessment and case management for these families. Partnerships between substance abuse treatment programs and organizations focused on children can be excellent ways of bringing specialized services to augment what can be provided in-house. Children can develop a variety of other problems in response to traumatic events, including thought suppression, sleep problems, exaggerated startle responses, developmental regressions, deliberate avoidances, panic, irritability, psychophysiologic disturbances, hypervigilance, and fear of recurrence. Children can engage in repetitive play in which the trauma is reenacted, cope by psychic numbing and withdrawal, show uncharacteristic behavior patterns, and/or become fearful of mundane things (33). Cognitive and emotional problems include a preoccupation with physical aggression, withdrawal and suicidal ideation, anxiety, depression, and social withdrawal. Behavioral problems include conduct problems, hyperactivity, diminished social competence, school problems, bullying, truancy, clinging behaviors, and speech disorders. Physical symptoms include bed-wetting, sleep disturbances, headaches, gastrointestinal problems, and failure to thrive (33).

Treatment Culture Women clients and treatment providers have noted that the male-dominated treatment culture characteristic of some programs (particularly many therapeutic communities and veterans' programs) is not conducive to meeting women's needs (107). They stress the importance of a more supportive and less confrontational approach to treatment. In addition to the gender imbalance in the client population, reliance on aggressive confrontation contributed to premature dropout and a treatment environment that can be experienced as disrespectful at best and frankly abusive at worst. An emphasis on harsh confrontation is particularly problematic in populations with a high frequency of traumatic experiences. Treatment methods that exacerbate a woman's sense of powerlessness discourage her from revealing and exploring key issues. In addition, women with severe psychiatric disorders can decompensate and leave treatment if confrontation is too intense. Reducing the emphasis on confrontation and broadening the skill base of clinicians has proved a difficult task in some treatment modalities, particularly those that rely primarily on staff members without advanced professional training. Although these practitioners may have extensive training and many have acquired addiction credentials, the style of intervention they learned first is difficult to change, particularly if it involves charismatic or dogmatic personal role models of recovery.

Both the National Institute on Drug Abuse and the Center for Substance Abuse Treatment have funded specialized research and treatment demonstration programs focused on women, and these programs have enhanced the development of provider groups committed to improving women's treatment. Additional resources made available through Center for Substance Abuse Treatment's Addiction Technology Transfer Centers, launched in the mid-1990s, made it easier to broaden the skill base of frontline practitioners working with an indigent population. There appears to be less coordinated activity focused on women in treatment facilities that serve the insured population. Provider groups serving women also emphasize the importance of female leadership at all levels of the organization to serve as role models and to avoid perpetuating the view that major decision-making influence is reserved for men. Some programs hire only female staff members to facilitate the task of dealing with sensitive issues such as incest, rape, and battering. Male staff members in a residential program are in a difficult position and must have clear boundaries and a supervision structure that protects them and the patients from potential boundary violations. This situation also is an issue for female staff members, particularly in areas with a large lesbian population, because boundary violations among women usually are more taboo to reveal.

Women and the Criminal Justice System Women constitute the fastest growing segment of the criminal justice population nationally and yet have the fewest appropriate social services available to them (108). Women today are more likely than men to serve time in prison for drug offenses (109). Between 1982 and 1991, the number of women arrested for drug offenses increased 89% (108). Since 1991, increasing numbers of women have been incarcerated for crimes committed in the service of drug use. Half the women reported committing their crimes while under the influence of drugs or alcohol, and about 40% reported using drugs daily before arrest. Fifty-three percent of the women in federal prison were unemployed at the time of arrest (109).

Typically, incarcerated women report that they started using drugs at an early age. These women commonly were confronted with obstacles such as absent parents, educational setbacks, parenthood, poverty, drug accessibility (109), and minimal social resources (108). Most came from communities in which crime was rampant. Additionally, most were victims of childhood sexual or physical abuse, as well as traumatic experiences as adults. Consequently, they had high rates of depressive and other psychiatric disorders (110). They often suffered from low self-esteem, depression, addiction, and shame, and frequently attempted to self-medicate their struggle with illicit drugs.

Insufficient job skills as a result of poor education undermine self-esteem in incarcerated women. Low income or poverty results in desperation, thus making illegal activities more acceptable, especially in the service of drug use. Major child-rearing responsibilities with inadequate social support systems contribute to the development of psychiatric disorders in mothers and behavior problems in children (110). Thirty-four percent of the women in U.S. prisons report being sexually abused, and another 34% report being physically abused (109). Women's social status and gender roles affect sexual risk behaviors and the ability to take steps to reduce the risk of HIV infection (36), contributing to the high incidence of HIV in drug-using and incarcerated women. A subsequent study of 3,315 subjects found rates of 7.5% in incarcerated women, several times higher than found in community samples (111).

Intergenerational and familial transmission of drug use and associated criminality makes the obstacles confronting these women more debilitating. National data on women in prison show that 40% of the women reported that an immediate family member also was in jail (109). In California, 59% of inmate women reported that family members were currently incarcerated (112). One third of the inmates reported that a parent or guardian had abused drugs or alcohol. For these and other complex and interwoven factors, it is necessary to intervene decisively in prison prerelease programs to break the cycle of drug use and criminality and to include family members in the treatment experience whenever possible. Various states have invested in treatment in-custody and postrelease, but many challenges remain to be surmounted (such as a trained workforce of adequate size) and the data currently supports only modest benefits.

Prison-based treatment is growing rapidly, and specialized programs for women are included in this development. Both research and clinical experience indicate that community-based services after treatment in prison significantly increases the percentage of offenders who remain drug-free 18 months after release. Thus, programs in large states such as California emphasize the importance of a seamless transition to services in the community and provide substantial funding to accomplish these goals. Although the implementation remains imperfect, segments of the criminal justice system are increasing their understanding of what it takes to achieve and maintain positive outcomes. Drug courts and diversion initiatives such as California's Proposition 36 have also shown success in reducing recidivism, likely in proportion to their access to psychiatric and social services.

CONCLUSIONS

Although gender differences have been well-studied in specific areas, there are many gaps in our understanding. Biomedical effects are far better understood for alcohol than for the illicit drugs. Research and treatment funding incentives over the past 20 years have provided a much better understanding of women's treatment needs and preferences. Removing obvious barriers, such as transportation and child care, increases women's participation in treatment. Treatment for women must be comprehensive, including their spouses, partners, and children. Research is needed to determine how best to intervene with children to reduce the negative effects of their parents' addictive disorders. Programs need to be capable of addressing co-occurring mood and anxiety disorders, particularly PTSD and eating disorders. When queried, women report that women-only groups and other activities and role models at all levels of decision-making in the organization are important to them. Advocacy is still needed for research to clarify which gender-specific treatment components are most influential in improving outcomes.

REFERENCES

1. Blume S. Alcohol and other drug problems in women. In: Lowinson JH, Ruiz P, Millman RB, et al., eds. *Substance abuse: a comprehensive textbook.* Baltimore, MD: Williams and Wilkins, 1992:794–807.
2. Blume SB. Understanding addictive disorders in women. In: Graham AW, Schultz TK, eds. *Principles of addiction medicine,* 2nd ed. Chevy Chase, MD: American Society of Addiction Medicine, 1998.
3. Substance Abuse and Mental Health Services Administration. Facilities offering special programs or groups for women (2006). Rockville, MD. Accessed May 26, 2008 from: http://findtreatment.samhsa.gov/ufds/listsearch_00.process_query.
4. Kessler RC, McGonagle KA, Zhao, S, et al. Lifetime and 12 month prevalence of DSM-IIIR psychiatric disorders in the United States. *Arch Gen Psychiatry* 1994;51:8–19.
5. Regier DA, Farmer ME, Rae DS, et al. Comorbidity of mental disorders with alcohol and other drug abuse. *JAMA* 1990;264(19):2511–2518.
6. Greene JM, Marsden ME, Sanchez RP, et al. National household survey on drug abuse: main findings 1998. Rockville, MD: Department of Health and Human Services, Office of Applied Studies, 2000.
7. Kuczkowski KM. The effects of drug abuse on pregnancy. *Curr Opin Obstet Gynecol* 2007;19(6):578–585.
8. Tetrault JM, Desai RA, Becker WC, et al. Gender and non-medical use of prescription opioids: results from a national US survey. *Addiction* 2008;103(2):258–268.
9. Kendler KS, Bulik CM, Silberg J, et al. Childhood sexual abuse and adult psychiatric and substance use disorders in women. *Arch Gen Psychiatry* 2000;57:953–959.
10. Dawson D, Archer L. Gender differences in alcohol consumption: effects of measurement. *Br J Addiction* 1992;87(1):119–123.

11. National Institute on Alcohol Abuse and Alcoholism (NIAAA). 10th Special Report to the U.S. Congress on Alcohol and Health. Rockville, MD: U.S. Department of Health and Human Services, 2000.
12. Becker U, Deis A, Sorensen TI, et al. Prediction of risk of liver disease by alcohol intake, sex and age: a prospective population study. *Hepatology* 1996;23(5):1025–1029.
13. Blume SB, Zilberman ML. Alcohol and women. In: Lowinson JH, Ruiz P, Millman RB, Langrod JG eds. *Substance abuse: a comprehensive textbook* (4th ed) Philadelphia, PA: Lippincott Williams & Wilkins, 2005;1049–1064.
14. Mumenthaler MS, Taylor JL, O'Hara R, et al. Gender differences in moderate drinking effects. *Alcohol Res Health* 1999;23(1):55–64.
15. Green CA, Polen MR, Janoff SL, et al. "Not getting tanked": definitions of moderate drinking and their health implications. *Drug Alcohol Depend* 2007;86:265–273.
16. Young NK. Effects of alcohol and other drugs on children. *J Psychoactive Drugs* 1997;29(1):23–42.
17. McCance-Katz EF, Carroll KM, Rounsaville BJ. Gender differences in treatment-seeking cocaine abusers-Implications for treatment and prognosis. *Am J Addictions* 1999;8:300–311.
18. Woolfolk DR, McCreary AC, Cunningham KA. An electrophysiologic study of ventral tegmental area dopamine neurons in male vs. female rats. In: Harris LS, ed. *Problems in drug dependence, 1998* (NIDA Research Monograph 179). Rockville, MD: National Institute on Drug Abuse, 1999:148.
19. Sell, SL, Scalzitti JM, Thomas ML, Cunningham KA. The influence of ovaria hormones on the acute locomotor response to cocaine in female rats. In: Harris (ed). *Problems of drug dependence* Bethesda, MD: U.S. Department of Human Services. NIDA Monograph, 1998;179:148.
20. Carmona GN, Tella SR, Greig NH, et al. The gender-specified psychomotor stimulatory effects of cocaine may not be due to hepatic mechanisms. In: Harris LS, ed. *Problems in drug dependence, 1998* (NIDA Research Monograph 179). Bethesda, MD: National Institute on Drug Abuse, 1999:149.
21. Mendelson JH, Sholar MB, Mello NK, et al. Cocaine pharmacokinetics in men and in women during two phases of the menstrual cycle. In: Harris LS, ed. *Problems in drug dependence, 1998* (NIDA Research Monograph 179). Rockville, MD: National Institute on Drug Abuse, 1999:149.
22. Sholar MB, Mendelson JH, Mello NK, et al. Gender differences in ACTH and cortisol response to I.V. cocaine administration. In: Harris LS, ed. *Problems in drug dependence, 1998* (NIDA Research Monograph 179). Rockville, MD: National Institute on Drug Abuse, 1999:150.
23. Sofuoglu M, Dudish-Poulsen S, Nelson D, et al. Subjective effects of cocaine are altered by gender and menstrual phase in humans. In: Harris LS, ed. *Problems in drug dependence, 1998* (NIDA Research Monograph 179). Rockville, MD: National Institute on Drug Abuse, 1999:150.
24. Amaro H, Zuckerman B, Cabral H. Drug use among adolescent mothers: a profile of risk. *Pediatrics* 1989;84:144–151.
25. Anglin MD, Hser YI, McGothlin W. Sex differences in addict careers II: becoming addicted. *Am J Drug Alcohol Abuse* 1987;13(1–2):59–71.
26. Hser YI, Anglin MD, McGlothlin W. Sex differences in addict career, I: initiation of use. *Am J Drug Alcohol Abuse* 1987;13(1–2):33–57.
27. McCarthy JJ, Leamon MH, Parr MS, et al. High-dose methadone maintenance in pregnancy: maternal and neonatal outcomes. *Am J Obstet Gynecol* 2005;193(3 Pt 1):606–610.
28. McCarthy JJ, Posey BL. Methadone levels in human milk. *J Hum Lact* 2000;16(2):115–120.
29. Jones HE, Martin PR, Heil SH, et al. Treatment of opioid-dependent pregnant women: clinical and research issues. *J Subst Abuse Treat* 2008; Jan 11. [Epub ahead of print.]
30. Jones HE, Suess P, Jasanski JR, et al. Transferring methadone-stabilized pregnant patients to buprenorphine using an immediate release morphine transition: an open-label exploratory study. *Am J Addict* 2006; 15(1):61–70.
31. Kissin WB, Svikis DS, Moylan P, et al. Identifying pregnant women at risk for early attrition from substance abuse treatment. *J Subst Abuse Treat* 2004;27(1):31–38.
32. Rand MR, Strom K. *Violence-related injuries treated in hospital emergency departments* (Bureau of Justice Statistics special report NCJ-156921). Washington, DC: Bureau of Justice, 1997.
33. Campbell JC, Lewandowski LA. Mental and physical health effects of intimate partner violence on women and children. *Psychiatry Clin N Am* 1997;20(2):353–374.
34. National Women's Health Information Center and Office of Women's Health. *Women & HIV/AIDS*. Rockville, MD: U.S. Department of Health and Human Services, 2008.
35. Centers for Disease Control and Prevention. *HIV/AIDS and women*. Rockville, MD: U.S. Department of Health and Human Services, 2008.
36. Amaro H. Love, sex and power. Considering women's realities in HIV prevention. *Am Psychol* 1995;50(6):437–447.
37. Amaro H, Hardy-Fanta C. Gender relations in addiction and recovery. *J Psychoactive Drugs* 1995;27(4):325–356.
38. Koss MP, Goodman LA, Browne A, et al. *No safe heaven: male violence against women at home, at work, and in the community.* Washington DC: American Psychological Association, 1994.
39. Chung JY, Magraw MM. A group approach to psychosocial issues faced by HIV-positive women. *Hosp Comm Psychiatry* 1992;43(9):981–894.
40. Mee-Lee D, Shulman G, Fishman M, et al. *ASAM patient placement criteria for the treatment of substance-related disorders,* 2nd ed., rev. (ASAM PPC-2R). Chevy Chase, MD: American Society of Addiction Medicine, 2001.
41. McLellan AT, Meyers K. Contemporary addiction treatment: a review of systems problems for adults and adolescents. *Biol Psychiatry* 2004; 56(10):764–770.
42. McGovern MP, Xie H, Segal SR, et al. Addiction treatment services and co-occurring disorders: prevalence estimates, treatment practices, and barriers. *J Subst Abuse Treat* 2006;31(3):267–275.
43. Gastfriend DR, Lillard P. Anxiety disorders. In: Graham AW, Schultz TK, eds. *Principles of addiction medicine,* 2nd ed. Chevy Chase, MD: American Society of Addiction Medicine, 1998:993–1006.
44. Nitenson N, Gastfriend DR. Co-occurring addictive and anxiety disorders. In: Graham AW, Schultz TK, Mayo-Smith MR, et al., eds. *Principles of addiction medicine*. Chevy Chase, MD: American Society of Addiction Medicine, 2003:1287–1296.
45. Kessler RC, Sonnega A, Bromet E, et al. Posttraumatic stress disorder in the National Comorbidity Survey. *Arch Gen Psychiatry* 1995;52(12): 1048–1060.
46. Breslau N, Davis GC, Andreski P, et al. Traumatic events and posttraumatic stress disorder in an urban population of young adults. *Arch Gen Psychiatry* 1991;48:216–222.
47. Breslau N, Davis GC, Andreski P, et al. Sex differences in posttraumatic stress disorder. *Arch Gen Psychiatry* 1997;54(11):1044–1048.
48. Breslau N, Davis GC, Peterson EL, et al. Psychiatric sequelae of posttraumatic stress disorder in women. *Arch Gen Psychiatry* 1997;54(1): 81–87.
49. Wasserman DA, Havassy BE, Boles SM. Traumatic events and posttraumatic stress disorder in cocaine users entering private treatment. *Drug Alcohol Depend* 1997;46(1–2):1–8.
50. Boyd CJ, Blow F, Orgain LS). Gender differences among African-Americans. *J Psychoactive Drugs* 1993;25(4):301–305.
51. Dansky BS, Brady KT, Saladin ME, et al. (1996). Victimization and PTSD in individuals with substance use disorders: gender and racial differences. *Am J Drug Alcohol Abuse* 1996;22(1):75–93.
52. Gil-Rivas V, Fiorentine R, Anglin MD, et al. Sexual and physical abuse: do they compromise drug treatment outcomes? *J Subst Abuse Treat* 1997;14(4):351–358.
53. Janikowski TP, Glover NM. Incest and substance abuse: implications for treatment professionals. *J Subst Abuse Treat* 1994;11(3):177–183.
54. Teets JM. The incidence and experience of rape among chemically dependent women. *J Psychoactive Drugs* 1997;29(4):331–336.
55. Yandow V. Alcoholism in women. *Psychiatric Ann* 1989;19:243–247.

56. Brown VB, Huba GJ, Melchior LA. Level of burden: women with more than one co-occurring disorder. *J Psychoactive Drugs* 1995;27(4): 321–325.
57. Zweben JE, Clark HW, Smith DE. Traumatic experiences and substance abuse: mapping the territory. *J Psychoactive Drug* 1994;26(4):327–345.
58. Russell SA, Wilsnack S. Adults survivors of childhood sexual abuse: substance abuse and other consequences. In: Roth P, ed. *Alcohol and drugs are women's issues,* vol. I. Netuchen, NJ: Women's Action Alliance and The Scarecrow Press, 1991.
59. Najavits LM, Weiss RD, et al. The link between substance abuse and posttraumatic stress disorder in women. A research review. *Am J Addict* 1997;6(4):273–283.
60. Wilsnack SC, Wonderlich SA, et al. Self-reports of forgetting and remembering childhood sexual abuse in a nationally representative sample of U.S. women. *Child Abuse Negl* 2002;26(2):139–147.
61. Finkelhor D, Dziuba-Leatherman D. Victimization of children. *Am Psychol* 1994;49(3):173–183.
62. Faravelli C, Giugni A, Salvatori S, et al. Psychopathology after rape. *Am J Psychiatry* 2004;161(8):1483–1485.
63. Koss MP, Burkhart BR. A conceptual analysis of rape victimization. *Psychol Women Q* 1989;13:27–40.
64. Green BL. Psychosocial research in traumatic stress: an update. *J Traum Stress* 1994;7:341–362.
65. Ullman SE, Brecklin LR. Sexual assault history and suicidal behavior in a national sample of women. *Suicide Life Threat Behav* 2002;32(2): 117–130.
66. Weaver TL, Allen JA, et al. Mediators of suicidal ideation within a sheltered sample of raped and battered women. *Health Care Women Int* 2007;28(5):478–489.
67. Fitzsimons HE, Tuten M, Vaidya V, et al. Mood disorders affect drug treatment success of drug-dependent pregnant women. *J Subst Abuse Treat* 2007;32(1):19–25.
68. Brown S, Schuckit M. Changes in depression among abstinent alcoholics. *J Studies Alcohol* 1988;49(5):412–417.
69. Brown SS, Inaba RK, Gillin JC, et al. Alcoholism and affective disorder; clinical course of depressive symptoms. *Am J Psychiatry* 1995;152(1): 45–51.
70. Misri S, Kendrick K. Treatment of perinatal mood and anxiety disorders: a review. *Can J Psychiatry* 2007;52(8):489–498.
71. ACOG. ACOG Practice Bulletin: Clinical management guidelines for obstetrician-gynecologists number 92, April 2008 (replaces practice bulletin number 87, November 2007). Use of psychiatric medications during pregnancy and lactation. *Obstet Gynecol* 2008;111(4): 1001–1020.
72. Holderness CC, Brooks-Gunn J, Warren MP. Co-morbidity of eating disorders and substance abuse review of the literature. *Int J Eating Disord* 1994;16(1):1–34.
73. Duncan AE, Neuman RJ, Kramer JR, et al. Lifetime psychiatric comorbidity of alcohol dependence and bulimia nervosa in women. *Drug Alcohol Depend* 2006;84(1):122–132.
74. Krahn D, Kurth C, Demitrack M, et al. The relationship of dieting severity and bulimic behaviors to alcohol and other drug use in young women. *J Subst Abuse* 1992;4(4):341–353.
75. Krahn DD. The relationship of eating disorders and substance abuse. *J Subst Abuse* 1991;3(2):239–253.
76. Marcus RN, Katz JL. Inpatient care of the substance-abusing patient with a concomitant eating disorder. *Hosp Comm Psychiatry* 1990; 41(1):59–63.
77. Wilson GT. Eating disorders and addictive disorders. In: Brownell KD, Fairburn CG, eds. *Eating disorders and obesity: a comprehensive handbook.* New York: Guilford Press, 1997.
78. American Psychiatric Association. *Diagnostic and statistical manual of mental disorders,* 4th ed. (DSM-IV). Washington, DC: American Psychiatric Press, 1994.
79. American Psychiatric Association. *Diagnostic and statistical manual of mental disorders,* 4th ed., text revision (DSM-IV-TR). Washington, DC: American Psychiatric Press, 2000.
80. van der Kolk B. The body keeps score: memory and the evolving psychobiology of posttraumatic stress. *Harvard Rev Psychiatry* 1994;1(5): 253–265.
81. Herman J. Complex PTSD: a syndrome in survivors of prolonged and repeated trauma. *J Traum Stress* 1992;5:377–391.
82. Herman J. *Trauma and recovery.* New York: Basic Books, 1992.
83. Golier JA, Yehuda R, Bierer LM, et al. The relationship of borderline personality disorder to posttraumatic stress disorder and traumatic events. *Am J Psychiatry* 2003;160(11):2018–2024.
84. Bandelow B, Krause J, Wedekind D, et al. Early traumatic life events, parental attitudes, family history, and birth risk factors in patients with borderline personality disorder and healthy controls. *Psychiatry Res* 2005;134(2):169–179.
85. Bradley R, Jenei J, Westen D. Etiology of borderline personality disorder: disentangling the contributions of intercorrelated antecedents. *J Nerv Ment Dis* 2005;193(1):24–31.
86. Grover KE, Carpenter LL, Price LH, et al. The relationship between childhood abuse and adult personality disorder symptoms. *J Personal Disord* 2007;21(4):442–447.
87. Zanarini MC, Frankenburg FR, Hennen J, et al. Prediction of the 10-year course of borderline personality disorder. *Am J Psychiatry* 2006;163(5):827–832.
88. Grant BF, Hasin DS, Ogburn E, et al. Prevalence, correlates, co-morbidity, and comparative disability of DSM-IV generalized anxiety disorder in the USA: results from the National Epidemiologic Survey on Alcohol and Related Conditions. *Psychol Med* 2005;35(12): 1747–1759.
89. Brainin-Rodriguez JE. Traumatic experiences in substance abusing women. Paper presented at the Traumatic Experiences in Substance Abusing Women: Implications for Recovery, San Francisco, CA; January 29, 1998.
90. Comas-Dias L, Greene B, eds. *Women of color: integrating ethnic and gender identities in psychotherapy.* New York: Guilford Press, 1994.
91. Wilsnack SC, Hughes TL, et al. Drinking and drinking-related problems among heterosexual and sexual minority women. *J Stud Alcohol Drugs* 2008;69(1):129–139.
92. Hall JM. Lesbians and alcohol: patterns and paradoxes in medical notions and lesbians' beliefs. *J Psychoactive Drugs* 1993;25(2): 109–119.
93. Greenfield SF, Brooks AJ, Gordon SM, et al. Substance abuse treatment entry, retention, and outcome in women: a review of the literature. *Drug Alcohol Depend* 2007;86(1):1–21.
94. Weisner C, Schmidt L. Gender disparities in treatment for alcohol problems. *JAMA* 1992;268(14):1872–1876.
95. Weisner C. Toward an alcohol treatment entry model: a comparison of problem drinkers in the general population and in treatment. *Alcohol Clin Exp Res* 1993;17(4):746–752.
96. Brown VB, Melchior LA, Panter AT, et al. Women's steps of change and entry into drug abuse treatment. A multidimensional stages of change model. *J Subst Abuse Treat* 2000;18(3):231–240.
97. Grella CE, Polinsky ML, Hser YI, et al. Characteristics of women only and mixed-gender drug abuse treatment programs. *J Subst Abuse Treat* 1999;17(1–2):37–44.
98. Niv N, Hser YI. Women-only and mixed-gender drug abuse treatment programs: service needs, utilization and outcomes. *Drug Alcohol Depend* 2007;87(2–3):194–201.
99. Claus RE, Orwin RG, Kissin W, et al. (Does gender-specific substance abuse treatment for women promote continuity of care?) *J Subst Abuse Treat* 2007;32(1):27–39.
100. Hodgins DC, el-Guebaly N, et al. Treatment of substance abusers: single or mixed gender programs? *Addiction* 1997;92(7):805–812.
101. McLellan AT, Grisson GR, Zanis D, et al. Problem-service matching in addiction treatment. *Arch Gen Psychiatry* 1997;54:730–735.
102. McLellan AT, Hagan TA, Levine M, et al. Supplemental social services improve outcomes in public addiction treatment. *Addiction* 1998; 93(10):1489–1499.
103. Hien D, Litt LC, Cohen LR, et al. *Reclaiming Pandora: integrating trauma services for women in substance abuse programs.* Trauma Services

for Women in Substance Abuse Treatment: An Integrated Approach. Washington DC: APA Books. 2008.
104. Jennings A. *Models for developing trauma-informed behavioral health systems and trauma specific services.* Rockville, MD: U.S. Department of Health and Human Services, 2004.
105. Najavits LM, Weiss RD, Shaw SR, et al. "Seeking safety": outcome of a new cognitive-behavioral psychotherapy for women with posttraumatic stress disorder and substance dependence. *J Trauma Stress* 1998; 11(3):437–456.
106. Najavits LM. *Seeking safety: a treatment manual for PTSD and substance abuse.* New York: Guilford, 2002.
107. Brown V, Sanchez S, Zweben JE, et al. Challenges in moving from a traditional therapeutic community to a women and children's TC model. *J Psychoactive Drugs* 1996;28(1):39–46.
108. Wellisch J, Anglin MD, Prendergast ML. Numbers and characteristics of drug-using women in the criminal justice system: implications for treatment. *J Drug Issues* 1993;23:7–30.
109. Bureau of Justice Statistics. *Women in prison.* Washington, DC: U.S. Department of Justice, 1994.
110. Jordan KB, Schlenger WE, Fairbank JA, et al. Prevalence of psychiatric disorders in incarcerated women. II. Convicted felons entering prison. *Arch Gen Psychiatry* 1996;53:513–519.
111. Altice FL, Marinovich A, et al. Correlates of HIV infection among incarcerated women: implications for improving detection of HIV infection. *J Urban Health* 2005;82(2):312–326.
112. Arnaudy M, Lee S, Relojo E. *Report on the health care status of incarcerated women.* San Francisco, CA: Department of Public Health, 1996.

CHAPTER 35

Fred C. Blow, PhD
Kristen L. Barry , PhD

Treatment of Older Adults

The increase in medical conditions in later life can lead to higher utilization of health care among older adults (1–4). Many of the medical and psychiatric disorders experienced in aging are influenced by lifestyle choices and behaviors such as the consumption of alcohol and use/misuse of medications/drugs. Older adults are more vulnerable to the effects of alcohol and medications and, combined with their increased risk of comorbid diseases, may seek health care for a variety of conditions that are not immediately associated with increased alcohol consumption and medication use/misuse. These include greater risk for harmful drug interactions, injury, depression, memory problems, liver disease, cardiovascular disease, cognitive changes, and sleep problems (5–7). Therefore, systematic screening, brief interventions, and referral to appropriate treatments for problems related to alcohol and prescription drug use are particularly relevant to providing high-quality health care to this population. Older adults with alcohol problems are a special and vulnerable population who require elder-specific screening and intervention procedures focused on the unique issues associated with alcohol and prescription drug misuse in later life. At-risk and problem drinking are the largest classes of substance use problems seen in older adults. However, with the aging of the "Baby Boom" generation, it is anticipated that clinicians will see a greater use of illicit drugs (8,9). Recent results from the National Epidemiologic Survey on Alcohol and Related Conditions (10) showed that lifetime rates of nonmedical prescription drug use disorders for the oldest age group (65+) were relatively low (<1% with odds ratios of 1) and that the younger age groups were most likely to abuse sedatives, tranquilizers, opioids, or amphetamines. Of note is the 45 to 64 year age group who had somewhat higher rates of nonmedical prescription drug abuse than today's elderly (sedatives: 1.3%; OR = 19.4; tranquilizers: 1.0%; OR = 7.9; opioids: 1.3%; OR = 8.6; amphetamines: 2.1%; OR = 19.0). Illicit drug use and dependence are more common in cohorts born after World War II (11,12). These finding indicate that the Baby Boom cohort, with the leading edge at age 62, more need more intervention and treatment options than have been available for the current elderly.

SCOPE OF THE PROBLEM IN OLDER ADULTHOOD

Despite significant advances over the last two decades in the understanding of the aging process with its attendant health problems and in the understanding of alcohol problems and alcoholism, little attention has been paid to the intersection of the fields of gerontology/geriatrics and alcohol studies. In recent years, however, there has been an increased interest in alcohol problems among the elderly. Although studies in this area are limited, prevalence estimates and typical characteristics of older problem drinkers now are being reported (13–15). Specific treatment and intervention strategies for older adults who are alcohol dependent or hazardous drinkers are only beginning to be disseminated.

In community surveys over the years, the prevalence estimates of problem drinking in older adults have ranged from 1% to 15% (13–15). These rates vary widely because of differing definitions and sample methodologies. Among clinical populations, however, estimates of alcohol abuse/dependence are substantially higher because problem drinkers of all ages are more likely to present in health care settings (16).

Older adults are at higher risk for inappropriate use of medications than younger groups. Older persons regularly consume on average between two and six prescription medications and between one to three over-the-counter (OTC) medications (17). Combined difficulties with alcohol and medication misuse may affect up to 19% of older Americans (18–21). In contrast to younger substance abusers who most often abuse illicit drugs, substance abuse problems among elderly individuals more typically occur from misuse of OTC and prescription drugs. Drug misuse can result from the overuse, underuse, or irregular uses of either prescription or OTC drugs. For some older adults, misuse may become drug abuse and dependence (22,23). Factors such as previous or coexisting drug, alcohol, or mental health problems, old age, and being female also increase vulnerability for misusing prescribed medications (24–28).

Despite the high prevalence of alcohol problems, most elderly patients with alcohol problems go unidentified by health care personnel. Signs and symptoms of potential problems related to alcohol use in older adults are shown in Table 35.1; these signs and symptoms can be applied to other age groups but, because of the lack of recognition in health care settings, they are described here with a focus on older adults. Moreover, few elderly patients with alcohol problems seek help in specialized addiction treatment settings. Given the high utilization of general medical services by the elderly, physicians and other health care professionals can be crucial in identifying those in need of treatment and providing appropriate interventions based on clinical need (29).

Most research conducted on substance use and misuse in older adults has focused on drinking and alcohol abuse. The rates of illegal drug abuse in the current elderly cohort are poorly documented but are thought to be very low (6). The potential for abuse of psychoactive drugs is a growing concern with midlife and older adults. Simoni-Wastila et al. (30) found that an estimated 11% of older women (age 50+ in their review) misuse prescription drugs and they estimated that nonmedical use of prescription drugs will increase for this age group to 2.7 million by 2020. Being female, social isolation, a history of substance abuse or mental health disorders, and medical exposure to prescription drugs with abuse potential were associated with psychoactive drug misuse/abuse. Nicotine dependence remains prevalent across age groups including older adults. In an analysis of the 2006 National Health Survey, the Centers for Disease Control and Prevention estimated the percentages of current smokers by age group (31). Approximately 24% of adults age 18 to 44 smoke, whereas 10.2% of those age 65+ are current smokers. Although nicotine dependence is common among older adults and interventions to reduce smoking have tremendous benefits, issues related to treatment of smoking are not unique to older adults and will not be a focus of this report. With the exception of psychoactive drugs, most prescription misuse can be addressed without formal treatment.

Substance Abuse/Dependence Diagnostic Classification for Older Adults Clinicians often rely on the criteria published in the American Psychiatric Association's Diagnostic and Statistical Manual of Mental Disorders, Fourth Edition (DSM-IV), for classifying alcohol-related problems (32). There are concerns that these criteria may not apply to older adults with substance use problems because older adults may not experience some of the legal, social, or psychologic consequences specified in the criteria and often seen in younger adults with abuse/dependence. "A failure to fulfill major role obligations at work, home, or school" may be not be as applicable to individuals who are retired and have fewer familial and work obligations (6). Additionally, a lack of "tolerance" may not indicate that an older adult is without problems related to alcohol use. DSM criteria for tolerance is mostly based on increased consumption over time and does not take into account the physiologic changes of aging that can mean increased tolerance with less alcohol consumption. (See Table 35.2 for the relationship between current DSM-IV criteria for substance abuse/dependence and issues of older adulthood.) The criteria related to physical and emotional consequences of alcohol use may be especially important.

TABLE 35.1 Signs and Symptoms of Potential Alcohol Problems in Older Adults: Time to Ask Questions

Mental/cognitive/relationship changes	Physical health	Alcohol and medication
Anxiety	Poor hygiene	Increased alcohol tolerance
Depression	Falls, bruises	Unusual medication response
Social isolation	Poor nutrition	
Excessive mood swings	Incontinence	
Disorientation	Sleep problems	
Memory loss		
New decision-making problems		
Idiopathic seizures		

Adapted from Barry KL, Oslin D, Blow FC. *Alcohol problems in older adults: prevention and management.* New York: Springer Publishing, 2001.

TABLE 35.2 Substance Abuse/Dependence Criteria Considerations in Diagnosing Older Adults

1. Tolerance: older adults may have problems with even low levels of intake because of their increased sensitivity to alcohol and higher blood alcohol levels.
2. Withdrawal: many adults with late-onset alcohol use disorders do not develop symptoms of physiologic dependence.
3. Taking larger amounts or over a longer period: self-monitoring is more difficult with increased cognitive impairment and that can interfere with an individual's ability to recall if he or she is drinking more than was intended.
4. Unsuccessful efforts to cut down or control use: this issue is similar for individuals across the lifespan.
5. Spending much time to obtain and use alcohol: because the negative consequences of alcohol can occur at relatively low levels, older adults may not report this behavior.
6. Giving up activities because of use: older adult may decrease their activity level for a variety of reasons making detection of problems by others more difficult.
7. Continuing use despite physical or psychologic problems: some older adults may not know or understand that some of the problems they are experiencing can be related to their use of alcohol or drugs/medications.

Modified from Barry KL, Oslin D, Blow FC. *Alcohol problems in older adults: prevention and management.* New York: Springer Publishing, 2001; Blow FC. *Substance abuse among older adults.* Rockville, MD: U.S. Department of Health and Human Services, Public Health Service, Substance Abuse and Mental Health Services Administration, Center for Substance Abuse Treatment; Treatment Improvement Protocol (TIP) Series, 1998.

Issues Unique to Older Adults Older individuals may have unique drinking patterns and alcohol-related consequences, social issues, and treatment needs (33). In addressing alcohol problems or prescription medication misuse in later life, the use of nonjudgmental, motivational approaches can be a key to successfully engaging these patients in care. Older adults also present challenges in applying brief intervention strategies for reducing alcohol consumption. Because of historical and cultural factors that lead to stigma, older adults who drink at risk levels can find it particularly difficult to identify their own risky drinking. In addition, chronic medical conditions may make it more difficult for clinicians to recognize the role of alcohol in decreased functioning and quality of life. These issues present barriers for both clinicians and their older adult patients in identifying the need for changes in use patterns. In working with patients who do not recognize that their level of alcohol consumption can lead to problems, brief education regarding changes in metabolism with aging related to alcohol use, the interactions between alcohol and specific medications (e.g., sedatives), the potential for falls, and the relationship between alcohol and some medical problems (e.g., hypertension), can be helpful.

Cooccurring Disorders in Older Adulthood Psychiatric comorbidities complicate treatment and relapse prevention. Studies of older adults with substance use disorders indicate the common presence of cooccurring psychiatric illnesses. Rates of psychiatric illness in older adults with substance use disorders range from 21% to 66% (34–38). Depression and co-occurring risk drinking in older adults are associated with increased suicidality and greater inpatient and outpatient service utilization (39–44). In addition, illnesses, bereavement, job loss, and retirement can all be issues that can affect depressed feelings and alcohol use in this age group.

Depression and alcohol use are the most commonly cited co-occurring disorders in older adults. For example, nearly half of community dwelling older adults with a history of alcohol abuse have co-occurring depressive symptoms (36). Approximately 29% of older veterans receiving treatment for alcohol use disorders have a co-occurring psychiatric disorder (45), most commonly an affective disorder (46). Among an at-risk population of older adults receiving in-home services, 9.6% had an alcohol abuse problem and two thirds of those individuals (6% of the overall sample) had a comorbid psychiatric illness such as depression or dementia (37). Among older adults with a recognized substance abuse disorder attending an alcohol dependence rehabilitation treatment program, 23% had dementia and 12% had affective disorders (38). Finally, psychiatric comorbidity was prevalent among older persons (age 65+) hospitalized for prescription drug dependence, with indications that 32% had a mood disorder and 12% had an anxiety disorder (24).

The nature of substance misuse among older adults complicates the relationship between psychiatric illness and substance abuse. Most older adults who are experiencing problems related to their alcohol consumption do not meet DSM-IV criteria for alcohol abuse or dependence (6,47). However, drinking even small amounts of alcohol can increase risks for developing problems in older adults, particularly when coupled with the use of some OTC or prescription medications. The combination of some psychoactive medications, particularly sedatives, with alcohol use increases the risk of many unfavorable reactions (48,49).

Research has indicated how alcohol consumption, as well as at-risk and problem drinking can aggravate affective disorders, such as depression, among elders (50–53). Low and moderate levels of drinking among older adults with psychiatric problems may also influence treatment outcomes for a variety of diagnoses. There is a small body of literature addressing comorbid alcohol abuse/dependence and affective disorders in older adults. Research has shown a strong association between depression and alcohol use disorders across age cohorts; this linkage continues in later life. In a national study of persons age 65 and older, 13.3% of those with major lifetime depression also met criteria for a lifetime alcohol use disorder, whereas only 4.5% had a lifetime alcohol use disorder without a history of depression (54).

Studies of clinical populations have demonstrated the prevalence of comorbid affective disorders and alcohol abuse among older adults. Blixen et al. (55) found 38% of older adults admitted to a freestanding psychiatric hospital had both a substance abuse disorder and another psychiatric disorder, primarily depression. Blow et al. (34) found major depression among 8% to 12% of older alcohol dependent patients in treatment and dysthymic disorder among 5% to 8% of the same population.

At-risk and problem drinking among the elderly is likely to exacerbate existing depressive disorders (51,56). Associations have been shown between current alcohol consumption and depression scores on the Center for Epidemiological Studies-Depression scale in persons age 65 and older (53) and past alcohol consumption and current depressive disorders in older men (50).

Subsyndromal depression may be aggravated by drinking leading to a major depressive disorder. This is exemplified in grief-associated depressive symptoms or late life adjustment disorders with depressed mood (51) that may increase to levels indicative of a major depressive disorder. For example, a recently widowed person may be depressed and use alcohol in an attempt to mitigate these feelings. The reinforcing positive feelings associated with the drinking can then lead to continued alcohol use, which may increase depressive symptoms—both those associated with loss of the partner as well as those brought on by alcohol misuse (e.g., health-related difficulties, rejection by others from drinking, financial strain). Further drinking episodes can be used to attempt to assuage increasing depressed feelings, and the resultant cycle of alcohol use and depressed feelings can lead to a major depression episode.

Comorbid depressive symptoms are not only common in late life but are also an important factor in the course and prognosis of psychiatric disorders. Depressed alcohol dependent patients have been shown to have a more complicated clinical course of depression with an increased risk of suicide and more social dysfunction than nondepressed alcoholics (39,40). Moreover, they were shown to seek treatment more often. Relapse rates for those who were alcohol dependent, however, did not appear to be influenced by the presence of depression. Alcohol use before late-life has also been shown to influence treatment of late-life depression. Cook et al. found that a prior history of alcohol abuse predicted a more severe and chronic course for depression (40). The co-occurrence of alcohol use disorders and depression heightens late-life suicide risk, as does at-risk and problem drinking among elders (57).

Alcohol Use Guidelines for Older Adults The National Institute on Alcohol Abuse and Alcoholism (NIAAA) and the CSAT Treatment Improvement Protocol on older adults recommend that persons, male or female, age 65 and older consume no more than one standard drink/day or seven standard drinks/week (21,58). In addition, older adults should consume no more than four standard drinks on any drinking day. These drinking limit recommendations are consistent with data regarding the relationship between heavy consumption and alcohol-related problems within this age group (6). These recommendations are also consistent with the current evidence for a beneficial health effect of low-risk drinking (59,60). Drinking guidelines also highlight an important distinction between problem drinking or at-risk drinking and alcohol dependence. Clarification of terms is essential in a discussion of alcohol problems (see the following section for levels of risk) among older adults.

- At-risk use: Use that increases the chances that an individual will develop problems and complications is *at-risk use.* Persons older than age 65 who drink more than seven drinks/week—one per day—are in the at-risk use category. Although they may not currently have a health, social, or emotional problem caused by alcohol, they may experience family and social problems and, if this drinking pattern continues over time, health problems could be exacerbated.
- Problem use: Older adults engaging in *problem use* are drinking at a level that has already resulted in adverse medical, psychologic, or social consequences (61). Potential consequences can include injuries, medication interaction problems, and family problems, among others. Some older adults who drink even small amounts of alcohol can experience alcohol-related problems.
- Abuse/dependence: The terms alcohol *abuse* or *dependence* are used as defined in the DSM-IV (32).

Screening and Detection of Alcohol Problems in Older Adults To practice prevention and early intervention with older adults, clinicians need to screen for alcohol use (frequency and quantity), drinking consequences, and alcohol/medication interaction problems. Screening can be done as part of routine mental and physical health care and updated annually, before the older adult begins taking any new medications, or in response to problems that may be alcohol- or medication-related. Clinicians can obtain more accurate histories by asking questions about the recent past; embedding the alcohol use questions in the context of other health behaviors (i.e., exercise, weight, smoking, alcohol use), and asking straightforward questions in a nonjudgmental manner. The "brown bag approach"—where the clinician asks the patient to bring all of his or her medications, OTC preparations, and herbs in a brown paper bag to the next clinical visit—is often recommended to determine medication use. Additionally, many states allow physicians or pharmacists to query a state database of triplicate prescriptions without a patient's prior consent. This can reveal multiple prescribers for controlled substances, such as opiate analgesics, and can also be helpful in determining potential problematic use. This provides an opportunity for the provider to determine what the patient is taking and what, if any, interaction effect these medications, herbs, and so on may have with each other and with alcohol.

OTC use often remains unevaluated in clinical settings and the use of some OTC preparations can be problematic with alcohol or prescription medications.

Screening questions can be asked by verbal interview, by paper-and-pencil questionnaire, or by computerized questionnaire. All three methods are reliable and valid (61,62). Any positive responses can lead to further questions about consequences. To successfully incorporate alcohol (and other drug) screening into clinical practice with older adults, it should be simple and consistent with other screening procedures already in place (63).

Before asking any screening questions, the following conditions are helpful: the interviewer needs to be empathetic and nonthreatening; the purpose of the questions should be clearly related to health status; the information must be confidential; and the questions need to be easy to understand. In some settings (such as waiting rooms), screening instruments are given as self-report questionnaires with instructions for patients to discuss the meaning of the results with their health care providers.

The following interview guidelines can be used. For patients requiring emergency treatment or for those who are temporarily impaired, it is best to wait until their condition has stabilized, if possible. However, assessing the current condition of the patient can be done at any point. Signs of alcohol or drug intoxication should be noted. Patients who have alcohol on their breath or appear intoxicated may give incomplete responses, so consideration should be given to following up the initial interview when the level of intoxication is not a factor. If the alcohol questions are embedded in a longer health interview, a transitional statement is needed to move into the alcohol-related questions. The best way to introduce alcohol questions is to give the patient a general idea of the content of the questions, their purpose, and the need for accurate answers (61). This statement should be followed by a description of the types of alcoholic beverages typically consumed. If necessary, clinicians may include a description of beverages that may not be considered alcoholic (e.g., cider, low alcohol beer). Determinations of consumption are based on "standard drinks." A standard drink is a 12-ounce bottle of beer, a 4-ounce glass of wine, or 1.5 ounces (a shot) of liquor (e.g., vodka, gin, whiskey).

Screening for alcohol-related problems is not always standardized and not all standardized instruments have good reliability and validity with older adults. The following section is focused on four widely used screening instruments. In addition to quantity/frequency questions to ascertain use, the Michigan Alcoholism Screening Test–Geriatric version (MAST-G) and the shortened version, the SMAST-G, the CAGE, and the Alcohol Use Disorders Identification Test (AUDIT) are often used with older adults. Of these, the MAST-G and SMAST-G were developed specifically for older adults.

It is important to note that clinicians under strict time constraints may have time to ask a patient only one screening question about his or her alcohol consumption. One study (64) has shown that a positive response to the question "On any single occasion during the past 3 months, have you had more than 5 drinks containing alcohol?" accurately identifies patients who meet either NIAAA's criteria for at-risk drinking or the criteria for alcohol abuse or dependence specified in the *Diagnostic and Statistical Manual of Mental Disorders, Fourth Edition* (DSM-IV) (32). Although this has not been validated with older adults and the number of drinks considered binge drinking may be less (generally 4 drinks/occasion), this question could provide a quick screener for problems.

The Michigan Alcoholism Screening Instrument—Geriatric Version (MAST-G) (Table 35.3) was developed at the University of Michigan (Blow, et al, 1992) as an elderly alcoholism screening instrument for use in a variety of settings. Psychometric properties of this instrument are superior to other screening tests for the identification of elderly persons with alcohol abuse/dependence. The MAST-G was the first major elderly-specific alcoholism screening measure to be developed with items unique to older problem drinkers. It is a 24-item scale with good sensitivity and specificity in older adults (see Table 35.4). Similar values were found after excluding those subjects who did not currently drink. The Short Michigan Alcoholism Screening Test-Geriatric version (SMAST-G) is a validated shortened form of the MAST-G containing 10 items.

The CAGE questionnaire (65) has been the most widely used alcohol screening test in clinical practice over the last three decades. It contains four items regarding alcohol use: felt they should Cut down, felt Annoyed that people criticized their drinking, felt Guilty about their drinking, and had a drink upon awakening in the morning to get rid of a hangover—an Eye-opener. Two positive responses are considered a positive screen and indicate that further assessment is warranted. CAGE alcohol items can be asked alone but are sometimes embedded along with CAGE-like items about exercise, smoking, and weight (66). Like most of the screening instruments reviewed, the sensitivity and specificity of the CAGE varies from 60% to 95% and 40% to 95%, respectively, (61,67) depending on sample characteristics. This measure had less sensitivity with older adults (Table 35.4).

The CAGE has not been well-validated with at-risk drinkers, women, older adults and non-Caucasian ethnic groups. Older adults may not screen positive on the CAGE while still having problems with alcohol use. For example, they may not have been annoyed by others who spoke to them about their drinking because their family may not know and they may not have close contact with friends. In addition, very few older adults need a drink upon rising, an "eye-opener." They may consume alcohol at a level they used when younger and not believe they need to cut down. On the other hand, older women have been more likely to say they feel guilty while using very little alcohol. Follow-up questions are always needed for positive screens on these questions to determine what prompted each positive response.

TABLE 35.3 Short Michigan Alcoholism Screening Test—Geriatric Version (SMAST-G)

	YES (1)	NO (0)
1. When talking with others, do you ever underestimate how much you actually drink?	____	____
2. After a few drinks, have you sometimes not eaten or been able to skip a meal because you didn't feel hungry?	____	____
3. Does having a few drinks help decrease your shakiness or tremors?	____	____
4. Does alcohol sometimes make it hard for you to remember parts of the day or night?	____	____
5. Do you usually take a drink to relax or calm your nerves?	____	____
6. Do you drink to take your mind off your problems?	____	____
7. Have you ever increased your drinking after experiencing a loss in your life?	____	____
8. Has a doctor or nurse ever said they were worried or concerned about your drinking?	____	____
9. Have you ever made rules to manage your drinking?	____	____
10. When you feel lonely, does having a drink help?	____	____
TOTAL S-MAST-G SCORE (0–10)	____	

Scoring: 2 or more "yes" responses indicative of alcohol problem.

For further information, contact Frederic C. Blow, PhD, at the University of Michigan Department of Psychiatry, 4250 Plymouth Road, Box 5765, Ann Arbor, MI 48109; (734) 761–2210.

The Alcohol Use Disorders Identification Test (AUDIT) is well-validated in adults under 65 in primary care settings (68–70) and has had initial validation in a study of older adults (71). The AUDIT comprises two sections: a 10-item scale with alcohol-related information for the previous year only, and a "clinical screening procedure" which includes a trauma history and a clinical examination. The questionnaire is introduced by a section explaining to the respondent that questions about alcohol use in the previous year only are included. The questionnaire is often used as a screener without the clinical examination. The recommended cutoff score for the AUDIT has been 8, but Blow et al. (71) found a Cronbach's alpha reliability of 0.95, with good sensitivity and specificity in a sample of older adults with a cutoff score of 7 (Table 35.4). A copy of this tool can be found at: *http://www.niaaa.nih.gov/NR/rdonlyres/287137A9–62BF-4EDE-A752–4A351C57A0B8/0/Audit.pdf.* The AUDIT-C (the first three questions: quantity, frequency, binge) had psychometric properties similar to the full AUDIT (Table 35.5).

TABLE 35.4 Screening Instruments: Sensitivity and Specificity with Older Adults

	Sensitivity (%)	Specificity (%)
Michigan Alcoholism Screening Test–geriatric version	95	78
Cut down, Annoyed, Guilty, Eye-opener (CAGE)	65	40
Alcohol Use Disorders Identification Test	83	91

BROAD-BASED ASSESSMENT OF SUBSTANCE USE PROBLEMS

Clinicians can follow-up the brief questions about consumption and consequences such as those in the MAST-G, AUDIT, and the CAGE with a few more in-depth questions about consequences, health risks, and social/family issues.

To assess dependence, questions should be asked about alcohol- or drug-related problems, a history of failed attempts to stop or cut back, or withdrawal symptoms such as tremors. Clinicians should refer any patient thought to be dependent for a diagnostic evaluation and possible specialized elder alcohol treatment. Medication assessments include questions about prescriptions, particularly antidepressants, benzodiazepines, opioid pain medications, OTC medications, and herbal remedies. If there is evidence of prescription drug dependence, the patient should also be referred to a specialist for treatment.

For older adults with positive screens, assessments are needed to confirm the problem, to characterize the dimensions of the problem, and to develop individualized treatment plans. For insurance reimbursement purposes, the assessment should follow criteria in the DSM-IV (32) or other relevant criteria, keeping in mind that these criteria may not apply directly to planning older adults' treatment. The application of the DSM criteria can be difficult in older adult populations because the

TABLE 35.5 Alcohol Use Disorders Identification Test-C Alcohol Screening

1. How often did you have a drink containing alcohol in the past year?	
• Never	(0 points)
If you answered never score questions 2 and 3 as zero.	
• Monthly or less	(1 point)
• Two to four times per month	(2 points)
• Two to three times per week	(3 points)
• Four or more times a week	(4 points)
How many drinks did you have on a typical day when you were drinking in the past year?	
• 1 or 2	(0 points)
• 3 or 4	(1 point)
• 5 or 6	(2 points)
• 7 to 9	(3 points)
• 10 or more	(4 points)
How often did you have six or more drinks on one occasion in the past year?	
• Never	(0 points)
• Less than monthly	(1 point)
• Monthly	(2 points)
• Weekly	(3 points)
• Daily or almost daily	(4 points)

The Alcohol Use Disorders Identification Test-C is scored on a scale of 0–12 (scores of 0 reflect no alcohol use). A score of 3 or more in older adults is considered positive and suggests the need for further evaluation. Generally, the higher the AUDIT-C score, the more likely it is that the patient's drinking is affecting his/her health and safety Dawson DA, BF, Grant F, Stinson S, et al. Effectiveness of the derived Alcohol Use Disorders Identification Test (AUDIT-C) in screening for alcohol use disorders and risk drinking in the U.S. general population. *Alcohol Clin Exp Res* 2005;29(5):844–854.

symptoms of other medical diseases and psychiatric disorders overlap to a considerable extent with substance use-related disorders.

Substance Abuse Assessment Instruments The use of validated substance abuse assessment instruments can be of great help to clinicians by providing a structured approach to the assessment process as well as a checklist of items that should be evaluated with each older adult receiving a substance abuse assessment. Specialized assessments are generally conducted by substance abuse treatment program personnel or trained mental and physical health care providers. Structured assessment interviews "possess (at least potentially) the desired qualities of quantifiability, reliability, validity, standardization, and recordability" (72).

Despite problems with criteria used to assess older adults for substance use disorders, two structured assessment instruments have been developed: the Structured Clinical Interview for DSM-III-R (SCID) (73) and the Diagnostic Interview Schedule (DIS) for DSM-IV (74) are available. The SCID is a multimodule assessment that covers disorders of: substance use, psychosis, mood, anxiety, somatoform, eating, adjustment, and personality. It takes a trained clinician approximately 30 minutes to administer the 35 SCID questions that probe for alcohol abuse or dependence. The DIS was originally developed by Robins et al. (74) with DSM-III criteria and has been updated as DSM criteria have evolved. The DIS is a highly structured interview that does not require clinical judgment and can be used by nonclinicians. The DIS assesses both current and past symptoms and is available in a computerized version. It has been translated into a number of languages. Because of the time required for administration, these measures are generally used for research rather than for clinical administration.

BRIEF ALCOHOL INTERVENTIONS WITH OLDER ADULTS

Low-intensity, brief interventions have been suggested as being cost-effective and practical techniques that can be used as an initial approach to at-risk and problem drinkers in primary care settings. Over the last two decades, there have been a number of controlled clinical trials to evaluate the effectiveness of early identification and secondary prevention using brief intervention strategies for treating problem drinkers, especially those with relatively mild to moderate alcohol problems who are potentially at-risk for developing more severe problems. The majority of clinical trials have shown the efficacy of brief alcohol interventions in these settings (29,50,75–78). Brief interventions are characterized by few sessions (five or fewer; often one or two) of relatively brief duration (a few minutes to an hour) (79). Research has shown the efficacy and effectiveness of a variety of brief interventions across treatment settings including primary care and emergency settings, populations, and providers (80,81). Often used to reduce alcohol consumption among individuals with at-risk or hazardous drinking, brief interventions can often also motivate patients to seek and engage in additional treatment as needed. Brief interventions can provide immediate attention to individuals at risk and help facilitate the level of care needed to address substance use problems and prevent or minimize potential consequences. Brief interventions are also attractive as a cost-effective, efficient way to prevent and treat substance use problems (82,83).

In general, the results of brief intervention studies to support the recommendations of the expert committee report (79) and the NIAAA (21) that early identification/screening and brief interventions are effective should be a matter of routine practice in primary and other health care settings to detect patients with hazardous or harmful patterns of alcohol use. Early identification and secondary prevention of alcohol problems directed in straightforward, nontechnical terms at an audience likely to be motivated to change could have broad positive public health implications. The NIAAA has developed a guide for clinicians to aid in working with patients around issues of alcohol use. "Helping Patients Who Drink Too Much: A Clinician's Guide" is available online at *http://pubs.niaaa.nih.gov/ publications/Practitioner/CliniciansGuide2005/clinicians_guide.htm.*

This is an excellent guide including screening with the AUDIT (see Table 35.5 for the AUDIT-C), assessment materials, brief intervention support materials, and frequently asked questions.

Effectiveness of Brief Alcohol Interventions with Older At-Risk Drinkers There had been little attention given to brief intervention research in older adults until recently. The spectrum of alcohol interventions for older adults range from prevention/education for persons who are abstinent or low-risk drinkers to minimal advice or brief structured interventions for at-risk or problem drinkers, and formalized alcoholism treatment for drinkers who meet criteria for abuse or dependence. Formalized treatment is generally used with persons who meet criteria for alcohol abuse or dependence and cannot discontinue drinking with a brief intervention protocol. Nonetheless, preintervention strategies are also appropriate for this high-problem population.

To date, there have been two brief alcohol intervention trials with older adults. Fleming et al. (29) and Blow and Barry (85) have conducted randomized clinical brief intervention trials to reduce hazardous drinking in older adults using advice protocols in primary care settings. These studies have shown that older adults can be engaged in brief intervention protocols, the protocols are acceptable in this population, and there is a substantial reduction in drinking among the at-risk drinkers receiving the interventions compared with a control group.

The first, Project GOAL: Guiding Older Adult Lifestyles withdrawal (7a) was a randomized, controlled clinical trial conducted in Wisconsin with 24 community-based primary care practices (43 practitioners) located in 10 counties. Of the 6,073 patients screened for problem drinking, 105 males and 53 females met study inclusion criteria (N = 158) and were randomized into a control (n = 71) or intervention group (n = 87). One hundred forty-six subjects participated in the 12-month follow-up procedures. The intervention consisted of two, 10- to 15-minute, physician-delivered counseling visits that included advice, education, and contracting using a scripted workbook. No significant differences were found between groups at baseline on alcohol use, age, socioeconomic status, smoking status, rates of depression or anxiety, frequency of conduct disorders, lifetime drug use, or health care utilization. At baseline, both groups consumed an average of 15 to 16 drinks/week. At 12-month follow-up, the intervention group drank significantly less than the control group $p < .001$).

The second elder-specific intervention study, the Health Profile Project (84,85), contained both brief advice/discussion by either a psychologist or a social worker, as used in the World Health Organization studies, and motivational interviewing techniques including feedback. A total of 452 subjects were randomized in this trial, with more than 26% being African American. Follow-up rates of 92% were obtained at the 12-month follow-up. They found results similar to those of Fleming et al. (29) in terms of 7-day alcohol use and binge drinking over the course of the study. These randomized, controlled clinical trials extend the potential of brief interventions from younger at-risk drinkers to even more vulnerable populations of older adults.

BRIEF INTERVENTION CONTENT AND STEPS

Following identification of older adults who are at-risk or problem drinkers through screening techniques, a semistructured brief intervention can be conducted. Workbooks can be used for guiding the intervention. With or without the use of workbooks, the important aspects of brief interventions include screening, feedback on behavior, motivation to change, strategies for change, a behavioral agreement, and follow-up to determine if more intensive steps are needed.

The following steps are often included in a brief intervention for older adults.

1. Identifying future goals is important for many older adults. Discuss how the older person would like his or her life to improve and be different in the future (e.g., "What are some of your goals for the next 3 months to a year regarding your physical and emotional health, activities and hobbies, relationships and social life, and your financial situation and other parts of your life?"). This helps to set the context for the brief intervention and generally provides increased motivation for the individual to change.
2. Customized feedback in the form of a health profile on screening questions relating to drinking patterns and other health habits (may also include smoking, nutrition, tobacco use) (e.g., "You indicated that, on average, you drink alcohol almost every day and drink two drinks at a time").
3. Introduce the concept of standard drinks, that the alcohol content of various beverages is roughly equivalent for a

12-ounce beer, 1.5 ounces of distilled spirits, 5 ounces of wine, or 4 ounces of sherry or liqueur. This concept provides the context for a discussion of sensible drinking limits.

4. Discuss the types of drinkers in the United States and where the patient's drinking pattern fits into the population norms for their age group (e.g., "National guidelines recommend that men your age drink no more than [seven drinks/week: no more than one/day]. Your pattern of alcohol use fits into the at-risk drinking category").
5. Reasons for drinking, weighing the pros and cons of drinking, and reasons to cut down or quit drinking. The intervenor needs to understand both the positive and negative role of alcohol in the context of the older patient's life, including coping with loss and loneliness (e.g., "We've spent some time talking before about your sleep problems, your blood pressure problems, the fall you took in the bathroom, and your loneliness since your wife died"). Some older patients may experience problems in physical, psychologic, or social functioning even though they are drinking below cutoff levels (e.g., "Even though your drinking is close to the limit for people your age and you drank at this level for years, I am concerned about some of the health problems you've had and your loneliness"). Maintaining independence, physical health, and mental capacity can be key motivators in this age group (e.g., "I am concerned that the amount you are drinking could be making some of these problems worse. Our goal is for you to remain as independent as possible and have a good quality of life").
6. Considering changing quitting or cutting down on drinking. Discussion of how changing drinking levels could have important benefits for the individual.
7. Sensible drinking limits and strategies for cutting down or quitting. *Note:* Strategies that are useful in this age group include developing social opportunities that do not involve alcohol, getting reacquainted with hobbies and interests from earlier in life, and pursuing volunteer activities, if possible.
8. Drinking agreement. Negotiated drinking limits that are signed by the patient and the intervenor are particularly effective in changing drinking patterns.
9. Coping with risky situations. Social isolation, boredom, and negative family interactions can present special problems in this age group. *Note:* Work with the patient to develop strategies to deal with such issues as social isolation and negative family interactions.
10. Summary of the session. The summary should include the drinking limits, encouragement, discussion of drinking diary cards (calendar) to be completed for the next month, and the recommendation to refer back to the workbook materials given to the individual during the intervention session.

Brief interventions generally include some educational information on the adverse effects of alcohol in older adults and the warning signs of alcohol problems and alcohol impairment. Clear limits can be established to minimize the adverse effects of alcohol use.

Summary Brief motivational interventions have been used successfully in a variety of treatment settings. There is a large body of research indicating that brief interventions and brief advice are effective across a variety of clinical settings. To summarize the results of brief intervention research, the 12 studies that met review criteria for U.S. Preventive Services Task Force (English-language; multicontact behavioral intervention; primary care–based; 6- to 12-month follow-up; nondependent drinkers) (80), participants reduced average number of drinks/week by 13% to 34% compared with controls. The proportion of participants in intervention condition drinking at moderate or safe levels was 10% to 19% greater than controls after 12 months.

SBIRT Model Out of all of the research on alcohol and drug screening and brief interventions, a comprehensive model for addressing alcohol and drug use in medical settings, SBIRT, (Screening, Brief Intervention, Referral to Treatment) has been developed. SBIRT includes screening, brief intervention, and referral to treatment. Screening quickly assesses the severity of substance use and identifies the appropriate level of intervention/treatment. Brief intervention focuses on increasing insight and awareness regarding substance use and motivation for behavioral change. Referral to treatment provides those identified as needing more extensive treatment with access to specialized care, where appropriate (86). Referral to treatment can take place at any point in this continuum and is based on severity.

The SBIRT model with screening, brief interventions, and referral to treatment for substance use employs the results of randomized clinical trials and best evidence-based practices to provide a framework for early detection, focused motivational enhancement, and targeted encouragement to seek needed substance abuse treatment. This model can be applied to both younger and older adults, and can enhance engagement in treatment for those individuals who are experiencing problems that cannot be addressed by brief interventions and brief motivational treatments. The model has been tested and incorporated most often into emergency care settings but has been expanded to primary care. The entire SBIRT model is the subject of a number of current research initiatives.

FORMAL SUBSTANCE ABUSE TREATMENT IN OLDER ADULTHOOD

Although alcoholism is a significant and growing health problem in the United States (87), there have been few systematic studies of formal alcoholism treatment outcome for older adults (33). Because traditional residential alcoholism treatment programs provide services to very few older individuals, sample sizes for treatment outcome studies have often been inadequate. The study of treatment outcomes for older adults has become a critical issue. Because traditional residential alcoholism treatment programs generally provide services to few older adults, sample size issues have been a barrier to studying treatment outcomes for elderly alcoholics in most settings.

Pharmacologic treatments are seldom used in the long-term treatment of older alcohol dependent adults and, therefore, they have not been adequately studied in this population. Until recently, disulfiram was the only medication approved by the U.S. Food and Drug Administration for treating alcohol dependence and it was seldom used for older adults because of concerns regarding potential side effects. Naltrexone, an opioid antagonist, has demonstrated efficacy in large samples that have included older adults and in studies of older adults exclusively (88–92). Krystal et al. (93), however, in multicenter, double-blind, placebo-controlled evaluation of veterans (mean age 49), found no significant differences in percentage of days drinking and drinks/day at 52-week follow-up. One of the few studies testing naltrexone (50 mg/day) in older adults was conducted by Oslin et al. (91), who enrolled 44 veterans older than age 50 in a 12-week double-blind placebo-control efficacy trial. There were no significant differences between the groups in abstinence, but half as many subjects in the treatment group lapsed into significant drinking compared to the control group. Naltrexone was well-tolerated by older adults and had efficacy in preventing relapse.

Acamprosate has also been studied as a promising agent in the treatment of alcohol dependence (94,95). There is clinical evidence for the use of acamprosate. There are, however, no studies to date of the efficacy or safety of acamprosate with older patients. It can be anticipated that future research will answer these questions.

Psychosocial Interventions with Older Adults

Because traditional residential alcohol treatment programs generally provide services to few older adults, there have been few studies with large enough populations of older adults to determine the efficacy of residential programming in this age group. There are a few naturalistic studies suggesting that older adults who do engage in treatment have better outcomes compared with younger adults (88,96–99). Older adults also seem to do best in programs that offer age appropriate care with providers who are knowledgeable about aging issues (98).

One of the few randomized controlled trials of treatment outcomes for older adults is a study of 137 male veterans (age 45 to 59 years, n = 64; age 60 to 69 years, n = 62; age 70 years and older, n = 11) with alcohol problems who were randomly assigned after detoxification to age-specific treatment or standard mixed-age treatment (100). Outcome data showed that those in the age-specific treatment programs were 2.1 times more likely at 1 year to report abstinence compared with patients in mixed-age groups. Because baseline alcohol consumption and alcohol severity data were not collected as part of the study, baseline data could not be compared for those variables.

Most of the treatment outcome research on older adults with substance use disorders has focused on *compliance* with treatment program expectations, in particular the patient's fulfillment of prescribed treatment activities and goals, including drinking behavior (33). Results from compliance studies have shown that age-specific programming improved treatment completion and resulted in higher rates of attendance at group meetings compared to mixed age treatment (101). In addition, older adults with substance use disorders were significantly more likely to complete treatment than younger patients. Atkinson et al. (96) also found that the proportion of older male alcoholics completing treatment was twice that of younger men.

Age of onset of alcohol problems has been a major focus of research for elderly treatment compliance studies in the elderly. In one of the few early studies in this area (102) using a matched-pairs, post hoc design, rates of completion of 6-month day treatment for 23 older male and female alcoholics (age 55 and older) whose problem drinking began before age 50 (early onset) were compared with 23 who began problem drinking after age 50 (late onset). Those classified as late onset problem drinkers were significantly more likely to complete treatment. In another study of 132 male alcoholic veterans 60 years of age and older, the sample was divided into the following subgroups: early onset (age 40 and younger, n = 50), mid-life onset (41–59, n = 62), and late onset (age 60 and older, n = 20) (103). Age of onset was related to program completion and to weekly meeting attendance, with the late onset subgroup showing the best compliance. However, a subsequent analysis of 128 men, age 55 and older, in alcoholism treatment found that drinking relapses during treatment were unrelated to age of onset (96). Furthermore, onset age did not contribute significantly to variance in program completion, but was related to meeting attendance rate.

In a study of treatment matching, Rice et al. (104) compared drinking outcomes for randomly assigned male and female alcoholics 3 months after beginning one of three age-mixed outpatient treatment protocols scheduled to last for 4 months. The sample included 42 individuals, age 50 years and older; with 134 patients, 30 to 49 years old; and 53 patients, 18 to 29 years old. There were no main effects of age or treatment condition on treatment compliance. There were, however, significant age by group effects by treatment protocol effects. For older patients, the number of days abstinent was greatest and the number of heavy drinking days fewest among those treated in an individual-focused rather than in a group condition. This study suggested that elderly alcoholics may respond better to individual-focused interventions, rather than traditional mixed-age, group-oriented treatment.

Studies on the effect of age of onset on treatment compliance have yielded mixed results. Major limitations remain in the treatment compliance literature, including a lack of drinking outcome data, failure to report on treatment dropouts, and variations in definitions of treatment completion. In addition, there have been fewer recent studies that have focused on older adults in treatment settings than were conducted in the 1990s. Few carefully controlled, prospective treatment outcome studies including sufficiently large numbers of older subjects who meet criteria for alcohol dependence have been conducted to address the methodologic limitations of prior work.

Limitations of Treatment Outcome Research

Although the examination of factors related to completion of programming is important for the identification of patient characteristics for those who will remain in treatment, existing studies have an inherent selectivity bias and provide no information on treatment dropouts or on short- or long-term treatment outcomes. Other issues with sampling may also limit the generalizability of previous studies. For example, the majority of reports on alcoholism treatment outcome for older adults have included only male subjects. Furthermore, age cutoffs for inclusion in studies have varied widely, and have included nonelderly individuals in the "older" category. In addition to these issues, the majority of studies have used relatively unstructured techniques for assessing alcohol-related symptoms and consequences of drinking behavior. Finally, the manner in which outcomes have been assessed has been narrow in focus. Most studies have dichotomized treatment outcome (abstention versus relapse) based solely on drinking behavior. Given evidence that heavy or binge drinking is more strongly related to alcohol consequences than is average alcohol consumption (e.g., 105), it is possible that there are important differences in outcome for nonabstinent individuals, depending on whether their reuse of alcohol after treatment involves binge drinking. Furthermore, most studies have not addressed other relevant domains that may be positively affected by treatment, such as physical and mental health status, and psychologic distress.

Relapse Prevention Older adults have age-related risks with relapse that need to be considered. Barrick and Connors reviewed the literature regarding relapse prevention among older adults with alcohol use disorders (88) and highlighted how psychosocial factors such as social isolation, loneliness, loss and grief, and depression can become antecedents to alcohol use for older adults, and how older drinkers tend to report using alcohol to alleviate negative emotional states (88,102,106). Comorbid medical conditions also put older adults at higher risk for relapse. For example, Brennan et al. (107) studied the relationship of alcohol use and pain among older adults. They found that more pain was related to increased use of alcohol to manage pain and that this relationship was stronger for older adults with drinking problems than for those who did not have problems with alcohol use.

Relapse prevention with older adults requires planning for the potential psychosocial and physical health factors that place them at risk for relapse. Barrick and Connors (88) provide a summary of the types of relapse prevention treatment approaches such as cognitive-behavioral therapy, group and family therapies, self-help groups, and pharmacologic adjuncts that provides useful information for the development of appropriate clinical relapse prevention models.

A Group Treatment Approach to Substance Abuse Relapse Prevention The Substance Abuse and Mental Health Services Administration recently published a manual entitled *Substance Abuse Relapse Prevention for Older Adults: A Group Treatment Approach* (108) developed by Schonfeld and Dupree. This manual details a relapse prevention method using cognitive-behavioral and self-management treatment techniques adapted specifically for use with older adults in a counselor-led group treatment setting. The approach, which was designed for use in outpatient group settings, can be adapted for use in other treatment settings such as inpatient, outpatient or intensive outpatient settings. The goals of this cognitive-behavioral/self-management relapse prevention approach with older adults are: to engage and support clients as they receive skill training and to analyze, understand, and control the day-to-day factors that have led clients to abuse substances.

This innovative model of care for older adults uses nonjudgmental, classroom-oriented approaches that are empowering to participants and report positive outcomes.

CONCLUSION

The results of research on screening, brief interventions, brief treatments and formal treatment for older adults indicate that a nonconfrontational, respectful approach as that used in brief interventions and elder-specific treatment is the most acceptable and generally effective with older adults who are experiencing physical or mental health difficulties related alcohol or medications. There are research questions that remain regarding the "active ingredients" that are needed in across clinical settings and the appropriate length and complexity of the intervention needed for this population.

It is clear studies are developing a spectrum of potential effective approaches to address alcohol and medication use/misuse/abuse in older adults. Real-world implementation strategies to address time, logistical barriers will be the key to more widespread use. The use of appropriate screening, brief interventions, brief therapies, referral to substance abuse treatment, and nonconfrontational elder-specific treatments, where appropriate, will provide state-of-the-art targeted choices for use by providers and other health care treatment staff for this vulnerable population to improve outcomes and manage costs.

REFERENCES

1. Waldo DR, Sonnefeld ST, McKusick DR, et al. Health expenditures by age group: 1977 and 1987. *Health Care Financ Rev* 1989;10(4): 111–120.
2. Schneider EL, Guralnik J. The aging of America: impact on health care costs. *JAMA* 1990;263(17):2335–2340.
3. Fuchs V. Health care for the elderly: how much? Who will pay for it? *Health Aff (Millwood)* 1999;18:11–21.
4. Krop JS, Powe NR, Weller WE, et al. Patterns of expenditures and use of services among older adults with diabetes: implications for the transition to capitated managed care. *Diabetes Care* 1998;21(5):747–752.

5. Barry KL. *Alcohol and drug abuse. Fundamentals of clinical practice: a textbook on the patient, doctor, and society.* New York: Plenum Medical Book Company, 1997.
6. Blow FC, Gillespie BW, Barry KL, et al. Brief screening for alcohol problems in an elderly population using the Short Michigan Alcoholism Screening Test-Geriatric version (SMAST-G). Research Society on Alcoholism, June 20–24, 1998.
7. Gambert SR, Katsoyannis KK. Alcohol-related medical disorders of older heavy drinkers. In: Alcohol and Aging, Beresford T, Gomberg E., eds. New York: Oxford University Press, 70–81;1995.

7a. Fleming MF, Manwell LB, Barry KL, et al. Brief physician advice for alcohol problems in older adults: A randomized community-based trial. *Journal of Family Practice,* 1999;48(5):378–384.

8. Blow FC, Barry KL, Fuller B, et al. Analysis of the National Health and Nutrition Examination Survey (NHANES): longitudinal analysis of drinking over the lifespan. In: Korper SP, Council CL, eds. *Substance use by older adults: estimates of future impact on the treatment system.* Rockville, MD: Substance Abuse and Mental Health Services Administration, Office of Applied Studies. (DHHS Publication No. SMA 03-3763, Analytic Series A-21), 2002:125–141.
9. Blow FC, Barry KL, Welsh D, et al. National Longitudinal Alcohol Epidemiologic Survey (NLAES): alcohol and drug use across age groups. In: Korper SP, Council CL, eds. *Substance use by older adults: estimates of future impact on the treatment system.* Rockville, MD: Substance Abuse and Mental Health Services Administration, Office of Applied Studies. (DHHS Publication No. SMA 03–3763, Analytic Series A-21), 2002:105–122.
10. Huang B, Dawson DA, Stinson FS, et al. Prevalence, correlates, and comorbidity of nonmedical prescription drug use and drug use disorders in the United States: results of the national epidemiologic survey on alcohol and related conditions. *J Clin Psychiatry* 2006;67: 1062–1073.
11. Grant BF. Prevalence and correlates of drug use and DSM-IV drug dependence in the United States; results of the national longitudinal alcohol epidemiologic survey. *J Subst Abuse* 1996;8(2):195–210.
12. Compton WM, Thomas YF, Stinson FS, et al. Prevalence, correlates, disability and comorbidity of DSM-IV drug abuse and dependence in the United States. *Arch Gen Psychiatry* 2007;64:566–576.
13. Adams WL, Barry KL, Fleming MF. Screening for problem drinking in older primary care patients. *JAMA* 1996;276(24):1964–1967.
14. Robins LN, Helzer JE, Weissman MM, et al. Lifetime prevalence of specific psychiatric disorders in three sites. *Arch Gen Med* 1984;41(10): 949–958.
15. Gurland BJ, Cross PS. Epidemiology of psychopathology in old age: some implications for clinical services. *Psychiatr Clin North Am* 1982; 5(1):11–26.
16. Institute of Medicine. Who provides treatment? Committee of the Institute of Medicine (Division of Mental Health and Behavioral Medicine). *Broadening the base of treatment for alcoholism.* Washington, DC: National Academy Press, 1990:8–141.
17. Larsen P, Martin J. Polypharmacy and elderly patients. *AORN Journal,* 1999;70(3),619–627.
18. Bucholz KK, Hesselbrock VM, Shayka JJ, et al. Reliability of individual diagnostic criterion items for psychoactive substance dependence and the impact on diagnosis. *J Stud Alcohol* 1995;56(5):500–505.
19. D'Archangelo E. Substance abuse in later life. *Can Fam Phys* 1993;39: 1986–1993.
20. National Institute on Alcohol Abuse and Alcoholism. Drinking in the United States: main findings from the 1992 National Longitudinal Alcohol Epidemiologic Survey (NLAES). NIH Publication No. 99-3519, 1998.
21. NIAAA *Helping patients who drink too much: a clinician's guide, updated edition.* Accessed http://pubs.niaaa.nih.gov/publications/Practitioner/CliniciansGuide2005/cliniciansguide.htm, 2005.
22. Patterson TL, Jeste DV. The potential impact of the baby-boom generation on substance abuse among elderly persons. *Psychiatr Serv* 1999;50(9):1184–1188.
23. Ellor JR, Kurz DJ. Misuse and abuse of prescription and nonprescription drugs by the elderly. *Nurs Clin North Am* 1982;17(2):319–330.
24. Finlayson RE, Davis LJ, Jr. Prescription drug dependence in the elderly population: demographic and clinical features of 100 inpatients. *Mayo Clin Proc* 1994;69(12):1137–1145.
25. Finlayson RE. Comorbidity in elderly alcoholics. In: Beresford T, Gomberg ESL, eds. *Alcohol and aging.* New York: Oxford University Press, 1995:56–69.
26. Finlayson RE. Misuse of prescription drugs. *Int J Addict* 1995;30(13-14):1871–1901.
27. Cooperstock R, Parnell P. Research on psychotropic drug use. A review of findings and methods. *Soc Sci Med* 1982;16(12):1179–1196.
28. Sheahan SL. Drug misuse among the elderly: a covert problem. *Health Values* 1989;13(3):22–29.
29. Fleming MF, Manwell LB, Barry KL, et al. Brief physician advice for alcohol problems in older adults: a randomized community-based trial. *J Fam Pract* 1999;48(5):378–384.
30. Simoni-Wastila L, Yang HK. Psychoactive drug abuse in older adults. *Am J Geriatr Pharmacother* 2006;4:380–394.
31. Centers for Disease Control and Prevention. Cigarette smoking among adults—United States, 2006. *MMWR Weekly* 2007;56(44):1157–1161.
32. American Psychiatric Association. *Diagnostic and statistical manual of mental disorders,* 4th ed. Washington, DC: American Psychiatric Association, 1994.
33. Atkinson RM. Treatment programs for aging alcoholics. In: Beresford TP, Gomberg ESL, eds. *Alcohol and aging.* New York: Oxford University Press, 1995:186–210.
34. Blow FC, Cook CA, Booth BM, et al. Age-related psychiatric comorbidities and level of functioning in alcoholic veterans seeking outpatient treatment. *Hosp Comm Psychiatry* 1992;43:990–995.
35. Brennan PL, Schutte KK, Moos RH. Pain and use of alcohol to manage pain: prevalence and 3-year outcomes among older problem and non-problem drinkers. *Addiction* 2005;100(6):777–786.
36. Blazer D, Williams CD. Epidemiology of dysphoria and depression in an elderly population. *Am J Psychiatry* 1980;137:439–444.
37. Jinks MJ, Raschko RR. A profile of alcohol and prescription drug abuse in a high-risk community-based elderly population. *Ann Pharmacother* 1990;24(10):971–975.
38. Finlayson RE, Hurt RD, Davis LJ Jr, et al. Alcoholism in elderly persons: a study of the psychiatric and psychosocial features of 216 inpatients. *Mayo Clin Proc* 1988;63:761–768.
39. Conwell Y. Suicide in elderly patients. Diagnosis and treatment of depression in late life. (pp. 397–418). Washington, DC: American Psychiatric Press, 1991.
40. Cook BL, Winokur G, Garvey MJ, et al. Depression and previous alcoholism in the elderly. *The British Journal of Psychiatry* 1991;158:72–75.
41. Bartels SJ, Oxman TE, Constantino G, et al. Suicidal and death ideation in older primary care patients with depression, anxiety, and at-risk alcohol use. *Am J Geriatr Psychiatry,* 2002;10(4), 417–427.
42. Brennan PL, Kagay C, Geppert JJ, et al. Predictors and Outcomes of Outpatient Mental Health Care: A 4-Year Prospective Study of Elderly Medicare Patients With Substance Use Disorders. *Medical Care,* 2001;39(1):39–49.
43. Wu LT, Ringwalt CL, Williams CE. Use of substance abuse treatment services by persons with mental health and substance use problems. *Psychiatr Serv* 2003;54(3):363–369.
44. Hoff RA, Rosenheck RA. Long-term patterns of service use and cost among patients with both psychiatric and substance abuse disorders. *Med Care* 1998;36(6):835–843.
45. Brennan PL, Nichols KA, Moos RH. Long-term use of VA mental health services by older patients with substance use disorders. Psychiatr Serv, 2002;53(7):836–41.
46. Blow FC, Brower KJ, Schulenberg JE, et al. The Michigan Alcoholism Screening Test—geriatric version (MAST-G): a new elderly-specific screening instrument. *Alcohol Clin Exp Res* 1992;16:372.
47. Barry KL, Oslin D, Blow FC. *Alcohol problems in older adults: prevention and management.* New York: Springer Publishing, 2001.
48. Substance Abuse and Mental Health Administration. Substance Abuse Among Older Adults (Treatment Improvement Protocol (TIP) Series.

Rockville, MD: U.S. Department of Health and Human Services, 1998.

49. Korrapati VR. Alcohol and medications in the elderly: complex interactions. In: Gomberg E, ed. *Alcohol and aging*. New York: Oxford; 1995: 42–55.
50. Saunders PA, Copeland JR, Dewey ME, et al. Heavy drinking as a risk factor for depression and dementia in elderly men. *Br J Psychiatry* 1991; 159:213–216.
51. Atkinson RL. Depression, alcoholism and ageing: a brief review. *Int J Geriatr Psychiatry* 1999;14:905–910.
52. Coyne J, Katz IR. Improving the primary care treatment of late life depression: progress and opportunities. *Med Care* 2001;39(8):756–759.
53. Graham K, Schmidt G. Alcohol use and psychosocial well-being among older adults. *J Stud Alcohol* 1999;60:345–351.
54. Grant BF, Harford TC. Comorbidity between DSM-IV alcohol use disorders and major depression: results of a national survey. *Drug Alcohol Depend* 1995;39:197–206.
55. Blixen CE, McDougall GJ, Suen L. Dual diagnosis in elders discharged from a psychiatric hospital. *Int J Geriatr Psychiatry* 1997;12:307–313.
56. Coyne JC, Schwenk TL. The relationship of distress to mood disturbance in primary care and psychiatric populations. *J Consult Clin Psychol* 1997;65:161–168.
57. Blow FC, Brockmann LM, Barry KL. Role of alcohol in late-life suicide. *Alcohol Clin Exp Res* 2004;28(5 Suppl):48S–56S.
58. U.S. Department of Health and Human Services; U.S. Department of Agriculture. Dietary Guidelines for American: Finding Your Way to a Healthier You. *http://www.health.gov/dietaryguidelines/dga2005/document/html/brochure.htm,* 1995.
59. Chermack ST, Blow FC, Hill EM, et al. The relationship between alcohol symptoms and consumption among older drinkers. *Alcohol Clin Exp Res* 1996;20:1153–1158.
60. Klatsky A L, Armstrong MA. Alcoholic beverage choice and risk of coronary artery disease mortality: do red wine drinkers fare best? *Am J Cardiol,* 1993;71(5): 467–469.
61. Barry KL, Fleming MF. Computerized administration of alcoholism screening tests in a primary care setting. *J Am Board Fam Pract* 1990;3:93–98.
62. Greist JH, Klein MH, Erdman HP, et al. Comparison of computer- and interviewer-administered versions of the Diagnostic Interview Schedule. *Hosp Community Psychiatry* 1987;8(12):1304–1311.
63. Barry KL, Blow FC. Screening and assessment of alcohol problems in older adults. Lichtenberg P, ed. *Handbook of assessment in clinical gerontology.* New York: Wiley, 2000.
64. Taj N Devera-Sales A, Vinson DC. Screening for problem drinking: does a single question work? *J Fam Practice* 1998;46(4):328–335.
65. Mayfield D, McLeod G, Hall P. The CAGE questionnaire: validation of a new alcoholism screening instrument. *Am J Psychiatry* 1974;131(10): 1121–1123.
66. Fleming MF, Barry KL, MacDonald R. The Alcohol Use Disorders Identification Test (AUDIT) in a college sample. *Int J Addict* 1991;26: 1173–1185.
67. Beresford TP, Blow FC, Hill E, et al. Comparison of CAGE questionnaire and computer-assisted laboratory profiles in screening for covert alcoholism. *Lancet* 1990;336:482–485.
68. Babor TF, Kranzler HR, Lauerman RJ. Early detection of harmful alcohol consumption: comparison of clinical, laboratory, and self-report screening procedures. *Addict Behav* 1989;14(2):139–157.
69. Fleming MF, Barry KL. A three-sample test of a masked alcohol screening questionnaire. *Alcohol Alcohol* 1991;26:81–91.
70. Schmidt A, Barry KL, Fleming MF. Detection of problem drinkers: the Alcohol Use Disorders Identification Test (AUDIT). *South Med J* 1995;88(1):52–59.
71. Blow FC. *Substance abuse among older adults.* Rockville, MD: U.S. Department of Health and Human Services, Public Health Service, Substance Abuse and Mental Health Services Administration, Center for Substance Abuse Treatment; Treatment Improvement Protocol (TIP) Series, 1998.
72. Oslin DW, Cary MS. Alcohol-related dementia: validation of diagnostic criteria. *Am J Geriatr Psychiatry* 2003;11(4):441–447.
73. Spitzer RL, Williams JBW, Skodol AE. DSM III: the major achievements and an overview. *Am J Psychiatry* 1980;137(2):151–164.
74. Robins LN, Helzer JE, Croughan J, et al. National Institute of Mental Health Diagnostic Intervniew Schedule. Its history, characteristics, and validity. Archives of General Psychiatry. 1981:38(4):381–389.
75. Wallace P, Cutler S, Haines A. Randomised controlled trial of general practitioner intervention in patients with excessive alcohol consumption. *Br Med J* 1988;297(6649):663–668.
76. Chick J, Lloyd G, Crombie E. Counseling problem drinkers in medical wards: a controlled study. *Br Med J* 1985;290:965–967.
77. Fleming MF, Barry KL, Manwell LB, et al. Brief physician advice for problem drinkers: a randomized controlled trial in community-based primary care practices. *Alcohol Alcohol* 1997;277:1039–1045.
78. Blow FC, Barry KL, Walton MA, et al. The efficacy of brief tailored alcohol messages among injured at risk drinkers in the emergency department. *J Stud Alcohol* 2006;67(4):568–578.
79. Barry KL. *Brief interventions and brief therapies for substance abuse.* Rockville, MD: U.S. Department of Health and Human Services, Public Health Service, Substance Abuse and Mental Health Services Administration, Center for Substance Abuse Treatment, 1999.
80. Whitlock EP, Polen MR, Green CA, et al.; U.S. Preventive Services Task Force. Behavioral counseling interventions in primary care to reduce risky/harmful alcohol use by adults: a summary of the evidence for the U.S. Preventive Services Task Force. *Am Coll Phys Clin Guidelines* 2004; 140:554–556.
81. Harvard A, Shakesshaft A, Sanson-Fisher R. Systematic review and meta-analyses of strategies targeting alcohol problems in emergency departments: interventions reduce alcohol-related injuries. *Addiction* 2008;103:368–376.
82. Fleming MF, Mundt MP, French MT, et al. Benefit-cost analysis of brief physician advice with problem drinkers in primary care settings. *Med Care* 2000;38(1):7–18.
83. Mundt MP, French MT, Roebuck MC, et al. Brief Physician advice for problem drinking among older adults: an economic analysis of costs and benefits. *J Stud Alcohol* 2005;66(3):389–394.
84. Blow FC, Barry KL, Walton MA, et al. The efficacy of brief interventions with older primary care patients, (manuscript in process), 2008.
85. Blow FC, Barry KL. Older patients with at-risk and problem drinking patterns: new developments in brief interventions. *J Geriatr Psychol Neurol* 2000;13(3):115–123.
86. Substance Abuse and Mental Health Services Administration Center for Substance Abuse Treatment (CSAT). Screening, Brief Intervention, and Referral to Treatment: What is SBIRT? *http://sbirt.samhsa.gov/,* 2008.
87. AMA Council on Scientific Affairs. Alcoholism in the elderly. *JAMA* 1996;275:797–801.
88. Barrick C, Connors GJ. Relapse prevention and maintaining abstinence in older adults with alcohol-use disorders. *Drugs Aging,* 2002;19(8): 583–594.
89. O'Malley S. *Naltrexone and alcoholism treatment.* Rockville, MD: U.S. Department of Health and Human Services, Public Health Service, Substance Abuse and Mental Health Services Administration, Center for Substance Abuse Treatment; Treatment Improvement Protocol (TIP) Series #28, 1998.
90. O'Malley SS, Jaffe AJ, Chang G, et al. Naltrexone and coping skills therapy for alcohol dependence: a controlled study. *Arch Gen Psychiatry* 1992;49(11):881–887.
91. Oslin D, Liberto JG, O'Brien J, et al. Naltrexone as an adjunctive treatment for older patients with alcohol dependence. *Am J Geriatr Psychiatry* 1997;5(4):324–332.
92. Volpicelli JR, Alterman AI, Hayashida M, et al. Naltrexone in the treatment of alcohol dependence. *Arch Gen Psychiatry* 1992;49(11): 876–880.
93. Krystal JH, Cramer JA, Krol WF, et al., for the Veterans Affairs Naltrexone Cooperative Study 425 Group. Naltrexone in the treatment of alcohol dependence. *N Engl J Med* 2001;345(24):1734–1739.

94. Sass H, Soyka M, Mann K, et al. Relapse prevention by acamprosate. Results from a placebo controlled study in alcohol dependence. *Arch Gen Psychiatry* 1996;53(8):673–680. [erratum: *Arch Gen Psychiatry* 1996;53(12):1097).
95. Pelc I, Verbanck P, Le Bon O, et al. Efficacy and safety of acamprosate in the treatment of detoxified alcohol-dependent patients. A 90-day placebo-controlled dose-finding study. *Br J Psychiatry* 1997;171:73–77.
96. Atkinson RM, Tolson RL, Turner JA. Factors affecting outpatient treatment compliance of older male problem drinkers. *J Stud Alcohol* 1993;54(1):102–106.
97. Lemke S, Moos RH. Treatment and outcomes of older patients with alcohol use disorders in community residential programs. *J Stud Alcohol* 2003;64(2):219–226.
98. Oslin DW, Pettinati H, Volpicelli JR. Alcoholism treatment adherence: older age predicts better adherence and drinking outcomes. *Am J Geriatr Psychiatry* 2002;10(6):740–747.
99. Satre DD, Mertens J R, Arean PA, et al. Five-year alcohol and drug treatment outcomes of older adults versus middle-aged and younger adults in a managed care program. *Addiction* 2004;99(10),1286–1297.
100. Kashner TM, Rodell DE, Ogden SR, et al. Outcomes and costs of two VA inpatient treatment programs for older alcoholic patients. *Hosp Community Psychiatry* 1992;43(10):985–989.
101. Wiens AN, Menustik CE, Miller SI, et al. Medical-behavioral treatment of the older alcoholic patient. *Am J Drug Alcohol Abuse* 1982;9(4):461–475.
102. Schonfeld L, Dupree LW. Antecedents of drinking for early- and late-onset elderly alcohol abusers. *J Stud Alcohol* 1991;52(6):587–592.
103. Atkinson RM. Aging and alcohol use disorders: diagnostic issues in the elderly. *Int Psychogeriatrics* 1990;2(1):55–72.
104. Rice C, Longabaugh R, Beattie M, et al. Age group differences in response to treatment for problematic alcohol use. *Addiction* 1993;88:1369–1375.
105. Chermack S, Blow FC, Hill EM, et al. The relationship between alcohol symptoms and consumption among older drinkers. Alcoholism: Clinical and Experimental Research, 1996;20(7):1153–1158.
106. Brown S A, Goldman MS, Inn A, et al. Expectations of reinforcement from alcohol: their domain and relation to drinking patterns. *J Consult Clin Psychol,* 1980;48(4):419–420.
107. Brennan P L, Schutte KK, Moos RH. Pain and use of alcohol to manage pain: prevalence and 3-year outcomes among older problem and non-problem drinkers. *Addiction,* 2005;100(6):777–786.
108. Center for Substance Abuse Treatment. *Substance abuse relapse prevention for older adults: a group treatment approach* (Report No. DHHS Publication No. (SMA) 05-4053). Rockville, MD: Substance Abuse and Mental Health Services Administration, 2005.

Not Cited:

Bush B, Shaw S, Cleary P, et al. Screening for alcohol abuse using the CAGE questionnaire. *Am J Med* 1987;82:231–235.

Dawson DA, BF, Grant F, Stinson S, et al. Effectiveness of the derived Alcohol Use Disorders Identification Test (AUDIT-C) in screening for alcohol use disorders and risk drinking in the U.S. general population. *Alcohol Clin Exp Res* 2005;29(5):844–854. (cited in Table 4)

Gilman SE, Abraham HD. A longitudinal study of the order of onset of alcohol dependence and major depression. *Drug Alcohol Depend* 2001;63: 277–286.

Harris KB, Miller WR. Behavioral self-control training for problem drinkers. *Psychol Addict Behav* 1990;4(2):82–90.

Heather N, Tebutt J. Definitions of non-abstinent and abstinent categories in alcoholism treatment outcome classifications: a review and proposal. *Drug Alcohol Depend* 1989;24(2):83–93.

Kofoed LL, Tolson RL, Atkinson R, et al. Treatment compliance of older alcoholics: an elder-specific approach is superior to "mainstreaming." *J Stud Alcohol* 1987;48(1):47–51.

Oslin DW. Evidence-based treatment of geriatric substance abuse. *Psychiatr Clin N Am* 2005;28:897–911.

Wetle T. Living longer, aging better: aging research comes of age. *JAMA* 1997;278(16):1376–1377.

CHAPTER 36

Joseph J. Westermeyer, MD, MPH, PhD

Cultural Issues in Addiction Medicine

Addictive disorders vary widely across nations and cultural groups. For example, unusually high rates of alcohol abuse and dependence occur among some countries of Eastern Europe (1) and some aboriginal peoples of Australia (2) and North America (3). Likewise, some ethnic groups in Asia have unusually high rates of opium dependence (4). Social disruption can lead to widespread addiction (5). Some nationalities and groups have also demonstrated the ability to notably reduce the prevalence of addiction. An example was the decline of opium use in China during the latter half of the 20th century (6).

Clinicians may need to appreciate the interaction of culture and addiction in hopes of enhancing their clinical effectiveness. Cultural factors can increase the risk of addiction and undermine patients' and clinicians' efforts at recovery (7). Similarly, an appreciation of cultural factors influencing patients and their social networks can enhance treatment outcomes (8). Basic to assessing cultural factors is the ability to take a culture-ethnicity history and to assess the patient's current cultural and ethnic affiliations.

DEFINITIONS RELATED TO SUBSTANCE USE AND ABUSE

Several concepts related to culture are helpful in guiding the addiction specialist in understanding the role of culture in contributing to, as well as alleviating addictive disorders (Table 36.1 for a list of these terms). *Cultures* typically have laws or traditions regarding substance production, distribution, and consumption. Within a culture, however, *ethnic groups* can differ greatly in their use of alcohol and other psychoactive substances, even when they live in the same community. Their attitudes, values, or practices may resemble or differ from those of the culture at large (9). Groups of people with substance use disorder can comprise *subcultures*, such as a drug subculture or a drinking subculture tied to a particular location where use occurs (e.g., neighborhood tavern, cocktail lounge, crack house) (10).

Cultural competence in this chapter includes the individual's ability to use psychoactive substances as prescribed by a group without abusing the substance or becoming addicted to it. Failure to become culturally competent may increase the risk to addiction, and addiction can impede the development of cultural competence among adolescents (11). *Clinical cultural competence* applies to a clinician's ability to provide care for people whose culture, ethnicity, or subculture differs from that of the clinician.

Alcohol and drug use are subject to cultural norms (12). An *ideal norm* may require use of a substance under certain circumstances, such as alcohol drinking during Jewish Passover or consumption of peyote in the Native American Church. Or the norm may demand abstinence, such as abstention from alcohol by many Moslem sects or tobacco by Seventh Day Adventists. Laws may forbid teenagers to consume alcohol on their own recognizance, but some teenagers in the culture may choose to ignore this stricture and some adults may support them—a norm gap or dissonance between the ideal and behavioral norms. Addicted people may possess their own unique

TABLE 36.1 Definition of Culture-related Terms with Utility in Understanding, Assessing, and Treating Substance Use Disorders

Term	Definition
Culture	The sum total of a people's way of life, including their geography, topography, climate, work and recreation, technology and economic production, political organization, law and law enforcement, family organization and function, child raising and education, life cycle patterns and age-sex roles, language and communication, clothing, beliefs and norms, customs and ceremonies, recreation and "time out" from social roles, and diet and health care.
Ethnicity	Groups within a culture who share their own unique cultural attributes, which may include national origin, language, shared ancestors, religion, traditions, clothing, and/or beliefs or norms.
Subculture	Groups within a culture that share major sociocultural characteristics, such as occupation, identity, or values. Examples include professional groups, guilds or unions, political parties, recovery organizations, commercial groups, or recreational associations. Subcultures depend on the majority culture for their existence; they are not freestanding and cannot sustain themselves.
Cultural competence	The ability to function effectively within a culture. Such competence depends on the ability to communicate with others, earn a living, function within family and community groups, avoid interpersonal or legal problems insofar as possible, and develop an identity consistent with cultural expectations.
Clinical cultural competence	The ability of a clinician to interact effectively with people from cultures different from that of the clinician; this ability is fostered by (1) awareness of one's own cultural world view, (2) positive attitudes toward cultural differences, (3) knowledge regarding the range of cultural practices and world views, and (4) skill in evaluating and treating patients from cultures different from the clinician's own culture.
Norm	Behaviors within a culture that possess positive or negative valance; norms typically exist with any behavior that is viewed in a judgmental way or has moral overtones.
Ideal norm	These norms describe the manner in which a person should behave.
Behavior norm	These norms describe the manner in which the people in a group actually do behave, regardless of the expressed ideal norm.
Identity	An individual's view of himself or herself based on group affiliations.
Enculturation	Training of children to become culturally competent—a process sometimes also termed "ensocialization" (50).
Acculturation	A process by which two adjacent cultural groups adapt certain aspects of one another's culture; also applied to migrants into a new culture, who must acquire attitudes, knowledge, and skill of the new culture to function as an adult (18).

behavioral norms, even though they may share the ideal norms of their ethnic group or the norms of the culture at large (13). For example, they may express commitment to their own substance use while believing that others (such as their children) should never use substances as they do.

Exploring the individual's identity can lead to valuable insights that can guide interventions, such as motivational interviewing. For example, asked about his identity, one patient replied, "I'm what you might call a common drunk, doc, but I'm not an alcoholic." This response led to a useful conversation regarding the patient's criteria for these categories and why he was willing, even anxious, to accept one identity while vehemently rejecting the other. Entrenched negative identities (such as being a "common drunk" or a "pot head") can serve as a justification for continued addiction and avoidance of recovery (14).

CULTURE AND PATTERNS OF SUBSTANCE USE AND ABUSE

Cultures prescribe or proscribe the use of various psychoactive substances. For example, cultures and ethnic groups associated with Judaism or Roman Catholicism require the use of alcoholic beverage at specific ceremonies (e.g., Passover dinner, Catholic mass). On the other hand, cultures and ethnic groups associated with Islam and certain fundamentalist Christian sects forbid alcohol drinking. Among groups in which ideal norms and behavioral norms are identical, substance abuse is infrequent, if not nonexistent. On the other hand, groups that proscribe use and yet permit use manifest a gap between the ideal norm and the behavioral norm with regard to substance use. Such norm gaps are associated with substance abuse in the culture or ethnic group. Table 36.2

TABLE 36.2 Consequences of Substance Use Depending on Presence vs. Absence of Norm Gap

Characteristic	Norm gap present	Norm gap absent
Enculturation source	Peers	Parents, extended family
Enculturation context	Surreptitious, hidden	Open, acknowledged
Context of use	Secular, drinking is primary activity	Religious or communal, eating or celebration occurs
Locus of control	The individual controls frequency and amount of use	The family, extended family, or entire community determines frequency and amount of use
Psychological correlates	Shame, guilt, denial	Satisfaction, group cohesion, enhanced identity
Risk for substance abuse	Risk of abuse/dependence is high	Risk of abuse/dependence is low
Legal aspects	Use may be illegal or socially unacceptable	Use is legal and socially acceptable
Cost of substance	High cost because of heavy taxes (to discourage use) or from illegal import or production	Low or moderate cost from legal production and distribution

shows the consequences of substance use in a society with presence-versus-absence of norm gaps with regard to psychoactive substance use (15). Resolution of the underlying ambivalence that gives rise to norm gaps may be helpful in ameliorating substance abuse (12).

Some authors have attempted to describe individual ethnic patterns of substance use and abuse in the United States (16). A review of these general trends may be informative to the beginning clinician who is unfamiliar with general trends outside of his or her own community or ethnic group. However, relying on such general overviews (or stereotypes) of several major racial-ethnic groups can be misleading, for the following reasons.

- Within any major group, there are considerable differences among subgroups. For example, Korean Americans tend to have higher rates of substance abuse than other Asian-American groups (17).
- Rates of substance abuse may change with the generations since immigration. For example, Mexican American women have extremely low rates in the first generation after immigration, but rates comparable to other American women in the second and subsequent generations (11,18).
- Sociocultural changes within ethnic groups can affect the pattern of substance use and abuse over time. For example, many Hispanic Americans have abandoned Roman Catholicism for abstinent-oriented Protestantism in an effort to resolve alcohol abuse (19). A new Asian American immigrant group, the Hmong, formerly had no norm gap with regard to alcohol use and virtually no alcohol abuse. However, widespread conversation to abstinent-oriented Protestantism has resulted in the recent appearance of a norm gap regarding drinking and the appearance of alcohol abuse (20).
- Clinicians must conduct individual assessments for each new patient, while avoiding stereotyping. Failure to do so will result in both missed diagnosis (in patients from groups with low rates of substance abuse) and erroneous overdiagnosis (in patients from groups with high rates of substance abuse).

CULTURAL ASPECTS OF CLINICAL ASSESSMENT

General History The first step in conducting a cultural history consists of asking the patient about the ethnic origins of his or her parents and grandparents (21). This would include their place of birth, national origin, language learned at home, migrations, roles and affiliations in the ethnic community and in the community-at-large, educational experiences, and marital history. For example, did family ancestors receive all of their education in ethnic or specific religious settings? Over the last few generations, have family ancestors married within the same religious or ethnic group or into other groups? Have family ancestors achieved roles or status within the ethnic community, the community-at-large, or both communities?

The second step consists of assessing the parent's overall enculturation of the patient in his or her ethnic groups-of-origin. Was one or more of the parenting adults actively abusing substances during the patient's childhood? Parental substance abuse can disrupt a health identity formation and undermine cultural competence.

Migration may occur within a country or across countries. Adoption or foster home placement can affect ethnic affiliation and identity, especially if the new parents differ in their ethnic origins from the biologic parents (22). The developing child's enculturation, which may involve integrating distinctly different cultural norms and values, can affect the use of psychoactive substances. During late adolescence or early adulthood, the patient may have chosen to relocate away from the family/community-of-origin and into a more mainstream community, such as college, the military, or a cross-ethnic marriage (23). Learning to live in another culture can involve stressors that may precipitate excessive substance use (24).

SUBSTANCE-SPECIFIC HISTORY

Cultural groups prescribe or proscribe particular socialization experiences in relation to psychoactive substance use. These developmental events fall into several categories.

- *Observations of role models*: What substances did the parenting adults use in the home or outside of the home? Was the use excessive or associated with problems or disruptions in the home?
- *Socialization into psychoactive substance use*: Who first taught or guided the patient's use of psychoactive substances? Did this occur in the home and family, or outside with peer groups? Who were these mentors and what substances or instruction did they provide? How old was the patient at the time?
- *Early experience with substance use*: Who determined the substances, occasions for use, dose, and patterns of use? Was it the patient, family, family friends, or peers? Were these teachers substance abusers themselves? How did early use assist coping in the family, in school, or while dating?
- *Linkage with other developmental tasks*: Was the patient learning other developmental tasks at the same time? These other developmental tasks might include recreation, courting, acquisition of social skills, early sexual experiences, or coping with illness or anxiety.

ADDICTION AND PATIENTS' CULTURAL FUNCTION

The relationship between psychoactive substances and social performance is a complex one. Psychoactive substance use may foster social coping, at least initially. For example, use of stimulants may initially help with a variety of tasks, such as acquiring new memory, performing athletic feats, producing on a factory assembly line, or coping with lack of sleep while in combat or driving an over-the-road truck (25). Nonproblematic use of psychoactive substances can be a manifestation of successful enculturation or acculturation; an example in the United States could be the nonproblematic use of alcohol in social settings. Likewise, abusive or addictive use of a psychoactive substance provides evidence for lack of cultural competence in psychoactive use. Over time, addiction generally undermines cultural performance.

Psychoactive substances can aid young people in acquiring social competence, or at least the appearance of social competence. An example in the 19th century was the use of the herbal anticholinergic drug *belladonna* or "beautiful woman" to produce rosy cheeks: young women seeking male courtiers at balls or seasonal celebrations used belladonna to project an image of health and vigor. Alcohol use may relieve social anxiety or alleviate performance anxiety. Symptom-relieving use may escalate if the original anxiety persists and competence fails to appear, as in the following case.

Case Example

A college freshman found that one drink before appearing at a sorority party alleviated her severe anxiety at meeting and socializing with new people. By her third year, however, she required several drinks to achieve the same effect as formerly achieved with one or two drinks. Consequently, she was showing up intoxicated at social events. This led to an intervention by her peers, who had become alarmed at her drunken behavior. She sought professional opinion regarding her use, complied with treatment recommendations, and was successfully treated for social phobia. Abstinence was recommended, and she joined an abstinence-oriented recovery group composed of college students.

Loss of social coping during the course of substance use disorder is a common feature of addiction in all cultures (26). Indeed, the achievement of a certain social stature in a community followed by gradual loss of status is a common presenting feature in addictive disorders. Examples of competence loss include the following:

1. Marital status: divorce, repeated failed marriages of ever-shorter duration.
2. Employment status: jobs of brief duration at a status below one's level of training or education, longer periods of unemployment, inability to obtain a job, losing jobs because of positive alcohol or drug screening tests.
3. Housing: living with friends who abuse substances, living in institutional settings (e.g., halfway house), homelessness.
4. Community participation: alienation and isolation from non-substance-related groups, events, and activities.
5. Friends: most friends use substances heavily.
6. Legal: breaking laws related to driving under the influence of alcohol or drugs, drug possession or sale, property law offenses.
7. Financial: inability to pay bills, selling property to buy alcohol or drugs, bankruptcy.

The addiction subculture may comprise a welcome identity group to a person who is estranged from family and other groups. Drug subcultures do not impose hurdles of the kind that distinguish career advancement, achievement on the sports field, or investment of time or effort in family and community activities. The norms and values of the drug subgroup are congenial to the addicted person, unlike norms and values of community associations or religious organizations. Thus the young person who has failed to achieve social competence may drift toward the identity proffered by a drug subculture (12,27).

CULTURE, TREATMENT, AND RECOVERY

Addiction and the Intimate Social Network The normal social network consists of 20 to 30 people, typically organized into four or five groups (28) (Table 36.3). Typical groups include the face-to-face living group, relatives, friends, coworkers, and perhaps another group or two (e.g., neighbors,

TABLE 36.3 Characteristics of the Intimate Social Network in Relation to Clinical Characteristics

Category	Number of people	Number of groups	Reciprocity	Connectedness*	Other
Normal	20–30	4–5	Symmetric	80%	Stable, long lasting
Dysfunction, outpatient, self-help group	10–19	2–3	Symmetric	60%	Unstable, may include pets, caregivers, deceased
Disabled, inpatient, day or residential program	0–9	1	Asymmetric	100%	Stable, alienation can lead to no network

*Likelihood that any one person in the network knows anyone else in the network.

association members, church or recreational group members). The chance that any one person knows another in the proband's (the identified individual) social network (the network "connectedness") is about 80%. The group tends to be stable: even if a proband dyad (i.e., the proband and another member) becomes alienated for a time, the group tends to override antipathy and foster rapprochement. Thus social networks foster the settling of inevitable interpersonal problems, thereby enhancing maturation and interpersonal intimacy over time. Such groups are reciprocal: that is, each individual exchanges work, time, or resources with other members of group—a major factor in the limitation of such groups to around 20 to 30 people (and rarely into the 40s or more). Favazza observed that middle class, middle-age, married, employed alcohol-dependent patients coming to treatment had "normal" social networks by the criteria enumerated here (29). However, they lost about half of their social network members during early abstinence, because these heavy drinkers met in places and organized their lives around activities focused on drinking.

The "neurotic" or "addictive" social network usually involves around 10 to 19 people, with two or three groups (often family and relatives) and then some one-to-one relationships. The "connectedness" of the network tends to be less, about 60%, and some of the one-to-one relationships are recent rather than long lasting. Although the element of reciprocity persists, the proband is often a client of other people in the network. The latter consist of drug dealers, bar tenders, hair stylists, clergy, social workers, and health and mental health professionals. These patients sometimes report network members not ordinarily reported in "normal" groups. Examples include caregivers, deceased persons, pet animals, or people who were friends years ago but rarely seen in recent years (30).

"Disabled" social networks consist of less than 10 people, all of who tend to know one another. Their common connection involves nonreciprocal relationships with the proband, who cannot return time, resources, or instrumental support. For example, a parent, a social worker, a homeless shelter manager, and a law enforcement officer may all know another through their common efforts to help the proband. Eventually, the alienated proband may not have a social network containing even a single person (31).

Social network reconstruction can compose a potent means of intervening in the addiction process and then providing support during recovery (32). A key element involves elimination of active substance abusers from the network, with retention of those committed to the patient's ultimate recovery (8). This approach has proven useful even in cases possessing limited family or economic resources (33).

Case Example

A surgeon referred a Native American veteran who reported that the preoperative sedative provided him with the first full night of sleep that he had experienced in years. The patient, in for surgical repairs related to shrapnel injuries, had been seriously wounded in combat, with polytrauma and probable traumatic brain injury from a nearby blast injury. Despite these injuries, he completed post-college professional training. After his return from combat, he would go to his basement once or twice a month to drink a quart of whiskey alone and think about his experiences and deceased comrades-in-arms. Aside from his spouse (a second marriage) and two children, he had minimal social contacts or commitments outside of his professional work. Raised on a reservation by his grandparents, and exposed to English and majority society only when he began grade school, he had achieved notable success in the military, in his educational pursuits, and in his professional role. Evaluation revealed chronic posttraumatic stress disorder in addition to alcohol abuse. After the patient had a 3-month period of sobriety and good relief from his posttraumatic stress disorder and insomnia, we began to work on social network reconstruction. He chose first to expand his affiliation with and support of his former combat unit, providing him with opportunities to obtain support from those with similar experiences and, eventually, to provide support to others (similar to the role of sponsors in Alcoholics Anonymous). Two years later, he became active with the alumni group where he received his professional training, providing him with opportunities to "pay back" that institution as well as provide a role model (and support) for Native American students at that school. Mostly recently, he has begun efforts to help others in his extended family, as well as the people on his reservation. This began humbly, with his first attending social events, but has led to his assuming more substantive roles as a clan patriarch and community resource on his reservation.

This case demonstrates several principles of social network reconstruction. First, the patient had a period of sobriety and psychologic recovery from his posttraumatic stress disorder before initiating a process that can be stressful and produce rejection or loss. Second, he chose a sequence of groups that he discerned would accept him without putting demands on him. Whereas the clinician might have chosen the extended family or reservation first, he chose his veteran comrades first. He recognized (and rightly, as it turned out) that his veteran group would accept him whatever his circumstances, given his combat experience and injuries. Third, he began by merely attending social gatherings, whether these were veterans' meetings, extended family events (weddings, funerals), or reservation ceremonies (pow-wows, historical remembrances). Fourth, as opportunities to help others or assume leadership positions occurred, he considered their impact on his family, his work, and his available time and energy.

Cultural Recovery in Addictive Disorders Reconstruction of the intimate social network poses a serious challenge for several reasons. First, most other people have a full complement of people with whom they have reciprocal relationships. Thus they do not readily take on another person, especially someone who comes as an individual rather than a group. Nonetheless, a number of strategies have proven useful in social network reconstruction during recovery.

- Joining a recovery group whose members are also looking for new associates (e.g., Alcoholics Anonymous) (34).
- Joining a group who share similar interests, such as a community action group, church or parish, a sports club, an avocational group, a professional work group or guild, or a political party (35).
- Joining a charitable organization, or a social group with a charitable purpose (36,37).
- Volunteering at a health care facility, a school, a nursing home, or similar facility (38).
- Returning to a group or organization from the past, such as an ethnic association or church group (39).
- Going back to school or taking a job (part time or full time), which leads to new contacts (40).

These strategies will lead to affiliation with new people and groups, affording the recovering person a new lease on life. They replace the groups associated with psychoactive substance use in the person's previous life (41).

Often, a more difficult task lies in building bridges back to relatives and family members. These people have probably been hurt or alienated by the addiction-related behaviors of the past. Frequently, they have come to distrust the recovering person. Consequently, the recovering person should not expect to be immediately welcomed back and lauded for the Herculean efforts required in recovery. On the contrary, the recovering person should expect a long period of rebuilding trust. This takes at least a year and often longer. Relatives will want to know if the recovering person can follow through on appointments and commitments, engage in reciprocal acts of mutual support, and adapt a predictable life style (28). For all of these reasons, it may be wise to delay rebuilding these family relationships until a modicum of sobriety has been established, say 6 months or even a year. If the recovering person undergoes a series of slips or recurrences—common in the early months or recovery—this can reaffirm the family's worse fears (9). Awash with renewed negative expectations, after an initial spurt of hope and optimism, family members may become ever more entrenched in their opposition to accepting the addicted member back into the family fold (42). Fortunately for those involved in Twelve Step work, several of the steps prepare the recovering person for making amends to family members and former friends who have suffered from the consequences of addiction (26).

Resumption of former cultural competence and affiliation can give rise to emotionally warm and spiritually uplifting experiences. Such a social or cultural "rebirth" can feel like a second chance, a turning back the clock, a visit back to familiar places and habits. This experience can elicit feelings of acceptance, belonging, and positive identify. By the same token, these journeys back can be suffused with pain and regret. In general, most patients have more of the former rather than the latter response. A few patients will experience such negative feelings that they may seek other social groups. These new affiliations may include adoption of a new religion, a new ethnic affiliation, or marriage to someone from another ethnic group.

Culture-Specific Treatment Therapies specific to particular cultures, ethnic groups, nationalities, and religions can contribute to recovery from substance use disorders. Participation can aid the recovering person in several ways: provision of a stable and sober environment, engagement in meaningful and productive work, availability of emotional support from other members, and establishing a new social identity as a "recovering person."

Some of these interventions are ceremonial in nature, such as a healing ceremony, pow-wow, or religious ritual (43). Entry into a new sober environment may occur in religion-oriented residential facilities, halfway houses, and working farms or ranches with a rehabilitation emphasis. Active participation in ethnic-specific religious groups has benefited numerous people afflicted with addictive disorders (44,45). Community-wide endeavors to reduce widespread and excessive drinking or drug use have proven useful (46).

Pharmacotherapies can also play pharmacocultural roles during rehabilitation. For example, clinicians can provide disulfiram to recovering alcohol-dependent patients who will inevitably be exposed to alcohol use in their home communities. Taking disulfiram can be an acceptable excuse for not participating in a group binge, when such a refusal may be viewed as a hostile rejection of a friendly invitation (47). Likewise, prescribing naltrexone may assist recovering opioid-dependent patients who find themselves in a situation where refusal to use an opioid compound may be interpreted as an unfriendly act (48).

Referral to treatment that undermines the patient's cultural or ethnic values, or that introduces unacceptable beliefs, can be counterproductive. For example, some people may dislike the concept of a "higher power" emphasis in Alcoholic Anonymous. In such cases, clinicians might refer the patient to Rational Recovery. Some culture-related groups may not specifically address addiction, but can nonetheless support recovery. For example, some Buddhist communal experiences can be extremely useful in selected cases (49).

Folk modalities can be either risky or helpful, depending on timing. For example, sweat baths can pose a risk if the patient in still in withdrawal or has secondary cardiovascular problems. On the other hand, many Native Americans, Asians, and Northern Europeans find group sweats relaxing and supportive.

CONCLUSIONS

Substance use is much too important in most cultures to be left to individual judgments and decisions. Across history, cultural groups have fostered specific norms with regard to substance use. Disparity between ideal and behavioral norms, or "norm gap," results in substance abuse that is costly to many individuals as well as the society or culture at large. In addition, cultural groups with widespread addiction have developed approaches for intervening in addiction.

Clinicians can increase their effectiveness by understanding the cultural elements that the patient brings to the clinic. This task begins with understanding the patient's enculturation from childhood to young adulthood and possible subsequent acculturation experiences. Current and past cultural affiliations can be helpful in devising a successful recovery plan. Assessing the patient's intimate social network is a critical first step in this plan. Although cultural factors have contributed to the onset of substance abuse in all substance-abusing patients, likewise cultural resources and traditions can serve clinicians and patients in the challenging process of recovery.

REFERENCES

1. Partanen J. Failures in alcohol policy: lessons from Russia, Kenya, Truk, and history. *Addiction* 1993;88(supplement):129S–134S.
2. Eastwell HD. Petrol-inhalation in Aboriginal towns. *Med J Aust* 1979; 2:221–224.
3. Walker RD, Lambert MD, Walker PS, et al. Alcohol abuse in urban Indian adolescents and women: a longitudinal study for assessment and risk evaluation. *Am Indian Alsk Native Ment Health Res* 1996;7(1):1–47.
4. Westermeyer J, Lyfoung T, Westermeyer M, et al. Opium addiction among Indochinese refugees in the U.S.: characteristics of addicts and their opium use. *Am J Drug Alcohol Abuse* 1991;17:267–277.
5. Goodhand J. From holy war to opium war? A case study of the opium economy in North-Eastern Afghanistan. *Disasters* 2000;4:87–102.
6. Westermeyer J. The sociocultural environment in the genesis and amelioration of opium dependence. In: Pogge J, ed. *Anthropological research: process and application.* New York: State University of New York Press, 1992:115–132.
7. Westermeyer J. The role of cultural and social factors in the cause of addictive disorders. *Psychiatric Clin N Am* 1999;22(2):253–273.
8. Galanter M. *Network therapy for alcohol and drug abuse.* New York: Basic Books, 1993.
9. Catalano RF, Morrison DM, Wells EA, et al. Ethnic differences in family factors related to early drug initiation. *J Stud Alcohol* 1992;53(3): 208–217.
10. Dumont M. Tavern culture: the sustenance of homeless men. *Am J Orthopsychiatry* 1967;37:938–945.
11. Caetano R. Acculturation and drinking patterns among U.S. Hispanics. *Br J Addict* 1987;82:789–799.
12. Kulis S, Napoli M, Marsiglia EF. Ethnic pride, biculturalism, and drug use norms in urban American Indian adolescents. *Social Work Res* 2002; 26(2):101–112.
13. Miller JS, Sensenig J, Stocker RB, et al. Value patterns of drug addicts as a function of race and sex. *Int J Addict* 1973;8:589–598.
14. Westermeyer J. Ethnic identity problems among 10 Indian psychiatric patients. *Int J Soc Psychiatry* 1979;25:188–197.
15. Arif A, Westermeyer J, eds. *A manual for drug and alcohol abuse: guidelines for teaching.* New York: Plenum, 1988.
16. Gaw A. *Culture and ethnicity.* New York: Praeger Press, 1993.
17. Chi I, Lubben J, Kitano H. Differences in drinking behavior among three Asian American groups. *J Stud Alcohol* 1989;50(1):15–23.
18. Markides KS. Acculturation and alcohol consumption among Mexican Americans: a three-generation study. *Am J Public Health* 1988;78(9): 1178–1181.
19. Porter E. Protestant faiths appeal to Hispanics and win many over. *Wall Street J* 2002:1–6.
20. Bennett LA, Ames GM, eds. *The American experience with alcohol: contrasting cultural perspectives.* New York: Plenum, 1985.
21. Westermeyer J. Cultural aspects of substance abuse and alcoholism: assessment and management. *Psychiatric Clin N Am* 1995;18(3):589–605.
22. Westermeyer J. Cross-racial foster home placement among Native American psychiatric patients. *J Natl Med Assoc* 1977;69(4):231–236.
23. Silverman I, Lief VF, Shah RK. Migration and alcohol use: a careers analysis. *Int J Addict* 1971;6:195–213.
24. Berry JW, Kim V, Minde T, et al. Comparative studies of acculturative stress. *Int Migration Rev* 1987;21:491–511.
25. Tamura M. Japan: stimulant epidemics past and present. *UN Bull Narcotics* 1989;41:81–93.
26. Westermeyer J. *A clinical guide to alcohol and drug problems.* New York: Praeger, 1986:325.
27. Kleinfeld J. Getting it together at adolescence: case studies of positive socializing environments for Eskimo youth. In: Manson SM, ed. *New directions in prevention among American Indian and Alaska Native communities.* Portland, OR: University of Oregon, 1982:341–365.
28. Speck RV, Attneave CL. *Family networks.* New York: Pantheon, 1973.
29. Favazza A, Thompson JJ. Social networks of alcoholics: some early findings. *Alcohol Clin Exp Res* 1984;8:9–15.
30. Westermeyer J, Pattison EM. Social networks and mental illness in a peasant society. *Schiz Bull* 1981;7(1):125–134.
31. Kroll J, Carey K, Hagedorn D, et al. A survey of homeless adults in urban emergency shelters. *Hosp Comm Psychiatry* 1986;37(3):283–286.
32. Pattison EM. Clinical social systems interventions. *Psychiatry Dig* 1977;38:25–33.
33. Red Horse Y. A cultural network model: perspectives for adolescent services and para-professional training. In: Manson S, ed. *New directions in prevention among American Indian and Alaska Native communities.* Portland, OR: University of Oregon, 1982:173–185.
34. Lieberman MA, Borman LD. Self-help groups. *J Appl Behav Sci* 1976; 12:261–303.
35. Willie E. The story of Alkalai Lake: anomaly of community recovery or national trend in Indian country? *Alcohol Treatment Q* 1989;6(3/4):167–174.
36. Kearny M. Drunkenness and religious conversion in a Mexican village. *Q J Stud Alcohol* 1970;31:248–249.

37. Galanter M, Westermeyer J. Charismatic religious experience and large-group psychology. *Am J Psychiatry* 1980;137(12):1550–1552.
38. Koski-Jannes A. The role of children in the recovery of alcoholic clients. *Contemp Drug Problems* 1991;18(4):629–643.
39. White WL. Addiction recovery mutual aid groups: an enduring international phenomenon. *Addiction.* 2004;99(5):535–538.
40. Bell M, Greig T, Gill P, et al. Work rehabilitation and patterns of substance use among persons with schizophrenia. *Psychiatric Serv* 2002;53(1):63–69.
41. Pattison EM. Social system psychotherapy. *Am J Psychother* 1973;27:396–409.
42. Birchwood M, Cochrane R, Macmillan F, et al. The influence of ethnicity and family structure on relapse in first-episode schizophrenia. *Br J Psychiatry* 1992;161:783–790.
43. Jilek WG. Indian healing power: indigenous therapeutic practices in the Pacific Northwest. *Psychiatric Ann* 1974;4:13–21.
44. Bergman RL. Navaho peyote use: its apparent safety. *Am J Psychiatry* 1971;128:695–699.
45. Brady M. Giving away the grog: an ethnography of Aboriginal drinkers who quit without help. *Drug Alcohol Rev* 1993;12:401–411.
46. Chelsea P, Chelsea A. *Honour of all: the people of Alkalai lake.* British Columbia, Canada: Alkalai Lake Tribal Council, 1985.
47. Savard RJ. Effects of disulfiram therapy in relationships within the Navaho drinking group. *Q J Stud Alcohol* 1968;29:909–916.
48. Westermeyer J. *Poppies, pipes and people: opium and its use in Laos.* Berkeley, CA: University California Press, 1982.
49. Johnson DR, Westermeyer J. Psychiatric therapies influenced by religious movements. In: Boehnlein J, ed. *Psychiatry and religion: the convergence of mind and spirit.* Washington, DC: American Psychiatric Press, Inc., 2000:87–108.
50. LittleSoldier L. To soar with the eagles: enculturation and acculturation of Indian children. *Childhood Ed* 1995;61(3):185–191.

CHAPTER 37

Mary E. Larimer, PhD
Jason R. Kilmer, PhD
Ursula Whiteside, MSD

College Student Drinking

PREVALENCE AND CONSEQUENCES

Heavy drinking and significant alcohol-related problems are commonly reported by college students nationwide (1). Peak lifetime alcohol use generally occurs in an individual's late teens and early twenties. The prevalence of heavy episodic (or binge) drinking (currently defined by the National Institutes on Alcohol Abuse and Alcoholism (NIAAA) as reaching a blood alcohol level of .08 or higher, usually by consuming five or more drinks for men, four or more for women, in a 2-hour period) (1), and the detrimental consequences resulting from this type of drinking have led the U.S. Department of Health and Human Services and the Surgeon General to classify college student binge drinking as a major public health problem. Though extensive research and administrative efforts have been aimed at decreasing college student binge drinking, research suggests binge drinking, driving under the influence, and unintentional student deaths related to alcohol are on the rise (2). What follows is a review of the research on college student drinking, including prevalence rates and consequences, a review of risk factors, as well as the empirically supported interventions and treatment practices.

Drinking Rates and Disorders among College Students Approximately 85% of college students have consumed alcohol, and 73% have been drunk at least once in their lives (3). In the past month, nearly half (48%) report having been drunk, and 5% report drinking daily, while 40% have engaged in heavy episodic drinking (five or more drinks in a row) in the past 2 weeks (3). These rates are comparable to nonncollege students, with the exception that college students are more likely to engage in heavy episodic drinking. Estimated prevalence of alcohol abuse and dependence varies across studies (4); however, approximately 18% of college students met criteria for an alcohol use disorder (12% abuse, 6% dependence) (5). Of students diagnosed during early college with alcohol abuse or dependence, an estimated 43% continue to meet criteria after college (6).

Alcohol-Related Problems and Consequences

An estimated 1,700 unintentional college student deaths per year involve alcohol (2). College-specific, drinking-related consequences range from the more extreme (death, injury, assault, sexual abuse, unsafe sex, health problems and suicide, drunk driving) to the less problematic but still life-interfering (academic problems, vandalism, property damage, police involvement). The NIAAA Task Force on College Drinking (7) categorized college student drinking consequences as damage to self, others, or the institution (as well as the overlapping categories of drinking and driving, high-risk sexual behavior, and physical and sexual aggression).

Damage to Self Nausea, vomiting, and hangovers are among the most common negative effects produced by alcohol (7). Higher levels of drinking are associated with poorer academic records, as indicated by grade point averages (8). Additionally, alcohol-related health problems (e.g., accidental overdose, memory problems) are reported by 2% of students (2). College students are increasingly likely to put themselves at risk for arrest (31% report driving while under the influence in the past year), to be involved with local or campus police because of drinking (5%) (9), or to be arrested for an alcohol related offense (2%) (2).

Damage to Others In addition to direct harm to self, there are numerous secondary effects or problems resulting from peer drinking. These include being affected by alcohol-related automobile accidents, vandalism and litter, noise, fighting, public urination, vomiting, and encounters with people who are intoxicated. For example, among students who live on campus (e.g., dormitories, fraternities, or sororities) and drink lightly or not at all, 60% experienced interrupted study or sleep, 48% took care of a drunk student, almost 20% had a serious argument or experienced an unwanted sexual overture (for females) (9). It is estimated that approximately half a million college students annually are unintentionally injured because of drinking and almost 700,000 experience assault by another drunken student—of these, approximately 97,000 experience alcohol-related sexual assault or date rape (2).

Damage to Institution College administrators, staff, and campus police often have to deal with the consequences of students' alcohol use, and resulting problems such as violence, vandalism, and property damage are relatively common. More than one fourth of colleges with low rates of drinking, and more than half of those with high rates of drinking, have moderate to major problems with alcohol-related vandalism and property damage (10). Approximately 11% of students have damaged property while under the influence (9), and sporadic binge drinkers and frequent binge drinkers were 4 and 10 times more likely, respectively, to report having damaged property than were nonbingers (11). Roark (12) estimated that somewhere between 50% and 80% of violence occurring on campuses is alcohol-related.

Risk Factors Related to College Student Drinking

Certain factors put some college students at particularly high risk for heavy drinking and related problems. Identified risk factors include demographic and environmental influences, cognitive and motivational factors (e.g., perceptions of the normative nature of drinking, expectations of positive outcomes from drinking), and affective factors (mood or anxiety problems, a desire to avoid negative emotions or enhance positive ones) among others (13).

Demographics

Sex and Ethnicity On average, college men drink more often, consume larger quantities of alcohol, and are more likely to engage in binge drinking than are college women (3,14). College males are also more likely to meet criteria for an alcohol use disorder and experience more alcohol-related problems (15–17). However, it has been hypothesized that current measures of alcohol-related problems assess primarily externalizing behavior problems owing to alcohol and do not assess internalizing problems (e.g., drinking related to the management of anxiety and depression), which may be more inclusive of females (18).

Research on both the national and local levels has found that white college students are most likely to engage in heavy episodic drinking and, similar to Native American/Alaskan Native students, experience more problems related to drinking (10,19). In contrast, African American students are least likely to engage in heavy drinking and, along with Asian American students, are less likely to experience alcohol-related problems (19). Based on a review of national studies of adolescents and young adults, O'Malley and Johnston (19) estimated that 40% to 50% of white students engage in binge drinking, in comparison to 30% to 40% of Hispanic/Latino and 10% to 20% of African American students (19). Compared to Hispanic/Latino and white gender differences, African American female college students drink proportionally less than do African American male students.

Athletics For both males and females, involvement in athletics at the high school or college level is related to more frequent drinking, including binge drinking and other risk behaviors (20). Team captains and leaders are particularly vulnerable to these behaviors, and the level of participation in sports from nonparticipation to team captain is positively associated with binge drinking (20). One need not be a team member to be considered high risk—across 140 colleges, students (team and nonteam members) who rated athletics as important have higher rates of heavy drinking (10).

Membership in the Fraternity/Sorority (Greek) System Fraternity and sorority organizations are environments in which heavy drinking is considered normative, and is considered a sexuality, friendship, and socialization enhancer (21,22). Members of the Greek system consume alcohol at greater frequencies and quantities than their non-Greek peers (10,22). Cashin et al. (22) surveyed more than 25,000 students across 61 colleges and found that Greek organization members also experienced greater alcohol-related problems than non-Greek members. Greek membership (for males) was also found to be the highest risk factor (of 17 others) for heavy episodic drinking (10). Even when accounting for individuals' expectations for drinking, high school drinking rates, and family history of drinking, living in a fraternity was related to greater alcohol-related problems and more frequent drinking than were students living elsewhere (23). However, there can be a great deal of variability in drinking rates within a fraternity or sorority, and not all Greek organization members drink heavily (24).

Drinking Expectancies Alcohol expectancies are the set of beliefs, positive and negative, one carries about the effects of alcohol consumption. Drinking expectancies begin to form as early as the third grade (25). Positive expectancies, or the anticipated or valued effects of alcohol consumption, are stronger predictors of drinking than negative expectancies (26). Positive expectancies have been shown to predict drinking (27) as well as differentiate between problem and nonproblem college student drinking (26). Positive expectancies have been found to explain a large degree of variance in the relationship between early experiences with alcohol (e.g., parental, peer, and media modeling) and subsequent problem drinking in adolescence (25). Among adolescents, positive alcohol expectancies have been found to be a more successful predictor of problem drinking than family history of alcohol problems (28).

Drinking Motives Overlapping the drinking expectancies literature is the alcohol motives literature. Drinking motives, or reasons for drinking, not surprisingly predict alcohol use behaviors (29,30). Conformity, enhancement, social, and coping reasons are the most cited drinking motives (29). Of these motives, social and enhancement motives are most commonly endorsed by students, followed by coping motives (31,32).

Drinking for emotional enhancement reasons (including for social reasons) and drinking to cope with feelings of depression or anxiety (29) are two types of emotion-regulatory processes that are phenomenologically different from each other. A study of adolescent and adult alcohol use found support for two types of adolescent drinkers. The first group drinks to cope and has greater depression problems, whereas the second group's drinking is related to sensation seeking. Though the second group consumes more alcohol, they experience fewer drinking related problems than the first (33).

Social Norms and Misperceptions Research in social psychology has provided some insight into the social factors that put college students at risk for heavy drinking. Perceptions of what is "normal behavior" for a group of individuals, or social norms, are known to influence behavior. One of the major forms of human learning is facilitated by the process of modeling—whereby one individual or group, consciously or unconsciously, displays a behavior that others imitate. The college student drinking literature has examined how attitudes toward and drinking behavior of students' social groups (e.g., peers, family, close friends, other social affiliations) impact their own drinking behaviors. One consistent finding is that college students overestimate the rates at which other college students drink (34), the amount other college students drink (35), and the extent to which other students support heavy drinking (18). The degree to which students overestimate other students' drinking predicts their own increased consumption (36), and this overestimation was recently found to be the strongest predictor of college student drinking when controlling for a variety of other individual risk factors (37).

Environmental Risk and Protective Factors Environmental factors can also impact alcohol consumption. Presley et al. (14) note that the cost of alcohol in and surrounding the campus environment can be related to alcohol use and that increases in total cost can reduce consumption. This has significant implications for colleges surrounded by bars frequently offering drink specials or "happy hour" promotions in which the cost of a drink is dramatically reduced for a limited amount of time (which could also impact a student's rate of consumption). The authors also note the impact of the density of sites where drinking can take place (both outlets for sale of alcohol and party venues), finding that when multiple drinking venues exist, long-term and short-term drinking problems also increase. Clapp and Shillington (38) learned that, among other predictors, students who were in a setting where many people were intoxicated were almost 13 times more likely to report consumption of five or more drinks than peers not present in such a setting.

Rates of college student drinking are also impacted by high-risk specific events associated with increased consumption of alcohol, suggesting that annual celebrations should be included in a consideration of risk factors. Events associated with higher rates of drinking are generally well known (e.g., New Year's Eve, St. Patrick's Day, spring break, Halloween, and high-profile sporting events) or may be personal events, including 21st birthdays, graduations, or major accomplishments (39). A phenomenon associated with the way in which college students consume alcohol involves the playing of "drinking games," such as "beer pong" prior to a primary drinking event or, in fact, as the event itself. Drinking games can be as simple as having everyone drink when a word or phrase is uttered during a movie, can be time-focused (e.g., one sip per minute), can be team sport–focused such that losers of a game must drink, or could be quite complicated with a range of rules surround gambling, card games, motor skills, or verbal skills (40). Drinking games have been identified as a risk factor for "problematic" drinking (13) and have been associated with heavy drinking episodes (38). In some places, the birthday tradition of downing one shot of hard liquor for every year of age increases risks for frank alcohol poisoning and/or aspiration of vomitus.

Involvement in athletics is associated with risk for higher rates of drinking and for consequences associated with alcohol consumption (13,41). Yet the culture surrounding collegiate sporting events seems to also influence and be influenced by alcohol, with many students and alumni participating in "tailgating," significant sporting events being associated with increased drinking, the frequency of alcohol advertising aired during televised sports, and the association of alcohol with celebration (39,41,42).

However, environmental variables can also serve as protective factors against high-risk drinking. Many colleges have seen the emergence of designated substance-free housing options and 12-step recovery groups on campus. Although students may self-select into various living options, including Greek systems, residence halls, and substance-free housing, it has been suggested that living in a designated substance-free housing environment, even for those who drink, is a protective factor for negative consequences, including heavy episodic or binge drinking, and is associated with increased use of preventative behaviors (including less drinking-game involvement and increasing use of a number of strategies for altering one's approach to drinking) (43). Clapp and Shillington (38) found that the only protective variable associated with lower risk of heavy episodic drinking was whether the event in which drinking occurred was a date. In attempting to explain this finding, the authors speculate that students who are dating may be less likely to use alcohol as a "social lubricant" and suggest additional research is needed to further examine this apparent protective factor.

College Drinking Prevention Strategies Given the high prevalence of college student alcohol use and related harm, considerable research has focused on development of prevention and intervention approaches for this population. The NIAAA has taken a major leadership role in compiling, disseminating, and stimulating research to address the serious public health problem of college student drinking. The NIAAA's influential report of the Task Force on College Drinking (44) represented the joint efforts of researchers and college presidents to address the harms of and solutions to college drinking. Based on comprehensive reviews of the literature on college drinking prevention, the Task Force report designated four tiers of prevention strategies. Tier I involved interventions with documented, replicated evidence of efficacy in college populations. Tier II involved interventions with documented evidence of efficacy in general populations that could be adapted for college students. Tier III involved interventions with logical and theoretical promise in need of more research, and tier IV involved interventions with evidence of ineffectiveness. The Task Force report was accompanied by increased college drinking prevention research supported by NIAAA and was supported by other organizations including the Department of Education and The Substance Abuse and Mental Health Services Administration. In addition, several comprehensive reviews of the prevention literature have been conducted in support of the Task Force Report (45–52). Thus, over the past decade, there has been considerable progress and growing consensus in determining what works in college drinking prevention. The following sections briefly review the evidence regarding the efficacy of interventions designated as tier I, II, or III approaches in the Task Force report.

Cognitive-Behavioral Skills-Based Interventions

Cognitive-behavioral skills-based interventions have received considerable support in the college drinking prevention literature, and two skills-based approaches were designated as tier I interventions in the NIAAA Task Force Report (44). The first of these encompassed multicomponent skills-based interventions. These interventions typically combine cognitive-behavioral skills training (such as identifying and planning for or avoiding risky situations, using protective behavioral strategies such as drink spacing, counting drinks, and limit setting to reduce intoxication during drinking events, discussing myths about alcohol's effects, and communicating assertively about drinking decisions) with norms clarification (correcting misperceptions about drinking norms, exploring assumptions that everybody drinks), using a motivational interviewing (53) style to reduce resistance and promote change. Larimer and Cronce (47,48) reviewed 18 studies including a multicomponent skills intervention and found 11 of 18 produced statistically significant reductions in alcohol use, harmful consequences, or both. Methodologically stronger studies (i.e., larger samples, longer follow-up, appropriate control groups) were more likely to report statistically significant effects of the multicomponent skills approach.

A second cognitive-behavioral intervention designated as tier I in the Task Force report (44) was expectancy challenge interventions (see "Drinking Expectancies" in preceding section). Expectancy challenge interventions, aimed at changing students' positive expectations for alcohol intoxication, are delivered by two methods. The first method is experiential—the alcohol placebo effect is directly applied to demonstrate how one's expectations about drinking influence his or her experience. Typically, students told they are drinking alcohol but actually receive a nonalcoholic drink (i.e., a placebo) still show the social or interpersonal effects associated with drinking for them (i.e., they become more social, talkative). Alternatively, students told they are not drinking alcohol when their beverage is actually alcoholic do not exhibit these social effects; instead, they feel some of the physical effects of drinking (e.g., feel sleepy, flushed) but attribute these feelings to factors other than alcohol. The second method is didactic, wherein students are educated about this phenomena (e.g., discussion of alcohol myths, such as "I can't be outgoing at a party without alcohol" and placebo effects). Initial reviews (47) suggested demonstrations of the placebo effect (54) but not education about this effect were associated with reduced alcohol use at short-term follow-up for college males. A more recent review (48) found two of seven studies supported demonstrations of the placebo effect in producing short-term reductions in alcohol use, with results again more positive in males. One study (55) suggested education about the placebo effect may have iatrogenic effects for women, whereas a more recent study (56) found demonstrating the placebo effect was associated with reductions in alcohol use for both men and women at 1-month follow-up, but these effects did not maintain at the 6-month follow-up. Thus, results regarding efficacy of expectancy challenge interventions are mixed, and practical issues regarding the demonstration of the placebo effect (i.e., administering alcohol to college students as part of the intervention) currently limit wider application of this approach.

Interestingly, an even simpler behavioral approach has shown efficacy in several recent studies of college drinking prevention. Specifically, Larimer and Cronce (47,48) reviewed four studies of self-monitoring or self-assessment of alcohol use and/or consequences in the absence of other intervention strategies, and all four reported significant reductions in alcohol use and/or consequences relative to minimal assessment. For example, Carey et al. (57) found addition of a Timeline Followback interview (a method for assessing drinking in detail on a daily basis over the past 3 months) to standard assessment (58) resulted in reductions in peak and typical quantity as well as frequency of heavy consumption at 1-month follow-up, perhaps owing to increased awareness of harmful drinking patterns. This beneficial effect of recalling and reporting one's drinking levels to others may contribute to overall efficacy of approaches utilizing screening and brief intervention methods (49,59).

Brief Motivational Interventions There is growing consensus that brief motivational interventions (typically incorporating assessment and personalized feedback regarding alcohol use, norms, and consequences) are efficacious in reducing and preventing excessive alcohol use and related harm in college populations. Motivational interviewing is based on the work of Miller and Rollnick (53) and Marlatt et al (60,61), who developed and published a manual for the BASICS intervention (Brief Alcohol Screening and Intervention for College Students). Brief, in-person motivational feedback interventions for college drinking have amassed the strongest evidence to date in support of efficacy (46–48,52). BASICS (61) includes a comprehensive assessment followed by a 1-hour personalized feedback interview. The interview is delivered in motivational interviewing style, designed to elicit personally relevant reasons for change and the adoption of cognitive-behavioral strategies to implement the desired changes, through use of specific strategies including open questions, reflective listening, summarizing key observations or points, and supporting and affirming the client. The interview is structured around a review of graphic feedback generated from the assessment. Larimer and Cronce (47,48) reviewed 22 brief motivational interventions for college drinking, most involving BASICS or similar interventions, and found 18 of 22 were associated with reductions in alcohol use, consequences, or both, across follow-up periods up to 4 years. A recent meta-analysis (46) found effect sizes for these interventions were generally in the small-to-medium range, with effects on alcohol use emerging within 1 month and effects on consequences emerging 6 months or more after intervention. Effects generally weakened or decayed by 12-month follow-up, which may be a function of the natural trajectory of alcohol use in college to be a reduction in use over time even among the control group (46,60). Thus, these interventions may work to hasten the natural developmental process out of high-risk drinking, reducing harmful consequences during this risky period. Studies have successfully employed brief motivational intervention approaches in both group (62) and individual formats (56,63), with men (63), women (62), and both genders (56), and with high-risk volunteers (60) as well as mandated or judicially referred students (64). Further, this strategy has been successfully implemented in a variety of settings, including campus health clinics (65) and fraternity social organizations (63). Thus, this type of intervention appears to be flexible and robust, reliably producing drinking reductions in a wide segment of the campus population.

Feedback-Only Interventions Though BASICS and related motivational interventions have substantial evidence of efficacy and have been successfully utilized in a variety of settings, there are barriers to the more widespread utilization of this approach. Specifically, the approach requires the availability of trained providers and the resources and time to meet individually or in small groups with students. Some of these barriers can be diminished through use of trained peers to provide the intervention (63,66) rather than professional providers and/or the integration of brief interventions into health or mental health settings through training of existing providers (65). Nonetheless, the majority of campuses do not have the resources to extend in-person BASICS to all students who would benefit from intervention (nor do all students who would benefit wish to voluntarily attend an in-person session), and typically this approach is reserved for the highest-risk students. As a result, researchers and practitioners have begun to evaluate more cost-effective methods for reaching a broader audience of students, using minimal intervention strategies such as provision of written, mailed, or Internet motivational feedback. In addition, studies have evaluated the extent to which in-person intervention improves efficacy in comparison to feedback alone. Results of this research are encouraging. Specifically, Larimer and Cronce (47,48) reviewed 11 interventions involving assessment and mailed, computerized, or written motivational feedback alone and found 10 of 11 were associated with reductions in alcohol use after intervention. A recent mailed feedback and tips intervention was found to both prevent initiation of drinking among abstainers and reduce likelihood of heavy drinking at 1-year follow-up (67). Two studies (64,68) found no differences between in-person and mailed or written feedback, though neither study included an assessment-only control condition. In their recent meta-analysis, Carey et al. (46) found effect sizes were largest for in-person, individual motivational feedback interventions as compared to mailed/computerized interventions, but feedback alone was nonetheless associated with significant reductions in drinking. In addition, Larimer and Cronce (48) identified four studies that evaluated computerized normative feedback alone in reducing drinking. These interventions provide simple information comparing the participant's own use to his or her perceptions of the typical college student's drinking pattern, and the actual norm for college students (e.g., 69). All four studies found reductions in alcohol use and/or consequences over follow-up periods ranging from 1 to 6 months. Some evidence suggests gender specific information (i.e., comparison to typical female college student) improves outcomes for women as compared to gender neutral information (70). Taken together, these findings suggest minimal interventions involving mailed or computerized feedback may be an important addition to the overall college drinking prevention toolbox.

Environmental Interventions With data clearly supporting the use of brief intervention with high-risk or at-risk college students, there is reason for optimism surrounding efforts to decrease harm and risk among college students who choose to drink alcohol. Although less empirical evidence support prevention efforts that target the college environment, such efforts are emerging as important components of an overall prevention strategy. DeJong and Langford (71) propose a prevention typology that identifies environmental change as one of four areas of intervention. Utilizing this framework, they suggest that there are five subcategories of strategic interventions within the environmental change category: (i) promoting alcohol-free options (e.g., creating or promoting alcohol-free events, publicizing volunteer opportunities, expanding hours for alcohol-free settings, promoting consumption of nonalcoholic beverages at events); (ii) creating an environment that supports health-promoting norms (e.g., modifying the academic schedule, offering substance-free residence halls, increasing faculty-student contact, creating programs to correct student misperceptions of drinking norms); (iii) limiting alcohol availability on- and off-campus (e.g., banning or restricting use of alcohol on campus, instituting responsible server-training programs, limiting number and concentration of alcohol outlets near campus); (iv) restricting alcohol promotion and marketing on- and off-campus (e.g., banning or restricting alcohol advertising on campus, banning alcohol promotions with special appeal to underage drinkers, instituting cooperative agreements to limit special drink promotions); and (v) developing and enforcing policies and laws surrounding alcohol consumption (e.g., revising campus policy as needed, increase checks of identification at on-campus functions, increasing disciplinary sanctions for violation of campus policies).

In their discussion of high-risk specific events, Neighbors et al. (39) provide a number of recommendations involving environmental change for spring break, one particular high-risk period. These recommendations include inviting parents to visit campus during spring break, providing alternative activities (including community service trips), advertising available activities early before students plan spring break trips, and encouraging faculty to schedule major papers or exams the week after spring break. When considering prevention of risky drinking games, Borsari (40) also noted the importance of providing social alternatives to drinking games and taking steps to ensure students are aware of nondrinking related activities as part of an environmental strategy.

Issues surrounding enforcement of policy are also of great importance, and steps can be taken to promote an environment that may increase the effectiveness of minimum drinking age laws (72). Keeling (73) highlighted the finding that more laws restricting underage drinking and governing the volume of sales are associated with lower levels of drinking and that student support for "cracking down" on underage drinking differs by their own alcohol consumption (77% of underage students who do not engage in binge drinking support more enforcement, compared to 29% of their binge drinking peers). Because of some findings that suggest inconsistent or ineffective enforcement of drinking laws, Kypri et al. (74) stress the importance of effective communication surrounding laws, including clear definitions of key terms (e.g., no clear definition of *intoxication* in laws in which more clarity could aid in enforcement).

When the community and college or university campus both stand to benefit from efforts aiming to reduce consumption or related consequences, use of a campus-community coalition has been encouraged (71). A campus-community coalition typically assembles key stakeholders from both settings who can collaborate together in efforts to reduce problems on campus and in the surrounding area. Stakeholders generally include faculty, student leaders, administrators, staff (residence life, counseling center, health center, etc.), police, bar or restaurant owners, or landlords near campus. Clapp and Stanger (75) detail four examples in which a coalition (the Collegiate-Community Alcohol Prevention Partnership) successfully worked with bars frequented by students to provide responsible beverage service training and to take steps toward modifying advertising practices, took steps to halt a bus provided by a bar in a Mexican border town that was unsafely transporting students, provided students with tips on hosting a safe party, and worked to remove paraphernalia associated with the promotion of heavy drinking from campus stores.

CONCLUSIONS AND FUTURE DIRECTIONS

Alcohol use on college campuses is an important health, safety, liability, and risk management issue, and advances have been made in identifying effective strategies to reduce alcohol consumption and associated consequences. Increasingly, colleges and universities are recognizing the need for a strategic plan with multiple components, targets, and delivery strategies as they seek to reduce the harm associated with college student drinking.

It is important to recognize that alcohol use does not occur in a vacuum, and attention should be paid to the context of college student alcohol use. Research suggests that 34% of college students also report use of an illicit drug in the past year, with 30% of students reporting past-year use of marijuana and 18% of students reporting past-year use of any illicit drug other than marijuana (3). Efforts to prevent or intervene with alcohol will necessarily need to consider these related behaviors. Future studies will need to measure the impact on other drug use when alcohol is targeted through prevention or intervention efforts and will need to identify effective strategies for working with polysubstance using college students.

Also related to the context of student alcohol use are co-occurring mental health problems. In a national survey of counseling center directors, 92% of directors felt that psychologic problems were becoming more severe (76). Schwartz (77) documented a more than fivefold increase in students prescribed psychotropic medication on college campuses over a recent 10-year period. A number of explanations have been suggested for the perceived increase in the severity of mental health disorders on college campuses, including increased management of depression and anxiety with psychotropic medications (allowing attendance of more severely ill students that otherwise would not have attended college), students using alcohol and drugs while on medication (resulting in an accentuation of depressant effects), or students stopping use of medication when entering college because, among other possible reasons, they want to use alcohol or other drugs instead (78). Given success with brief interventions targeting depression (79) and targeting alcohol (48), future research must consider strategies to address the overlap of mental health issues and substance use.

Research to date indicates that brief motivational interventions utilizing assessment and in-person feedback are consistently efficacious in reducing alcohol use in a number of college student settings. In addition, cognitive-behavioral skills-based interventions have clear evidence of efficacy. Given the difficulties with encouraging participation in in-person interventions on college campuses, integration of these resources into existing points of contact (including academic courses, residence halls, Greek social organizations, student services, and campus health and mental health settings) holds promise for reaching students in need of services. Although it may seem intuitive to screen for alcohol problems in a campus health setting, the data do not suggest that this is a widespread practice. Although approximately one third of health centers at 4-year colleges or universities routinely screen for alcohol problems, only 17% of these used standardized instruments as part of their screening (80). Thus, in addition to integrating services into points of contact, reliable and valid screening strategies should be used (68).

There is also reason for promise as various delivery strategies are considered. Given the recent success of mailed and computerized feedback (69,70,81), the widespread implementation of a program of screening and brief feedback intervention is now feasible on many college campuses. Research on commercially available computerized products is emerging, and more research through randomized controlled trials evaluating the efficacy of such approaches is needed.

There are documented barriers to dissemination, adoption, implementation, and maintenance of empirically tested approaches; fortunately, these are surmountable (82). College student alcohol use and associated consequences are not unique problems on any one campus. Instead, there are shared challenges across campuses and, increasingly, shared successes. As colleges and universities move toward developing campus-community coalitions and getting involved in statewide coalitions, efforts to impact college student health become more than the responsibility of the individual campus. With an ever-changing and ever-growing population, it is possible that the strategies used to reduce use and consequences will need to change accordingly.

REFERENCES

1. National Institute on Alcohol Abuse and Alcoholism. *What colleges need to know: an update on college drinking research.* Bethesda, MD: U.S. Department of Health and Human Services, Public Health Service, National Institutes of Health, 2007.
2. Hingson R, Heeren T, Winter M, et al. Magnitude of alcohol-related mortality and morbidity among U.S. college students ages 18–24: changes from 1998 to 2001. *Annu Rev Public Health* 2005;26:259–279.
3. Johnston LD, O'Malley PM, Bachman JG, et al. *Monitoring the future national survey results on drug use, 1975–2006:* vol II, *College students and adults ages 19–45.* Bethesda, MD: National Institute on Drug Abuse, 2007.
4. American Psychiatric Association. *Diagnostic and statistical manual of mental disorders,* 4th ed. Washington, DC: Author, 1994.
5. Slutske WS. Alcohol use disorders among U.S. college students and their non-college-attending peers. *Arch Gen Psychiatry* 2005;62:321–327.
6. Sher KJ, Gotham HJ. Pathological alcohol involvement: a developmental disorder of young adulthood. *Dev Psychopathol* 1999;11:933–956.
7. National Institute on Alcohol Abuse and Alcoholism. *High-risk drinking in college: what we know and what we need to learn: final report of the panel on contexts and consequences: epidemiology of alcohol use among college students.* Bethesda, MD: U.S Department of Health and Human Services, Public Health Service, National Institutes of Health, 2002.
8. Singleton RA. Collegiate alcohol consumption and academic performance. *J Stud Alcohol Drugs* 2007;68:548–555.
9. Wechsler H, Lee JE, Kuo M, et al. Trends in college binge drinking during a period of increased prevention efforts: findings from 4 Harvard School of Public Health College Alcohol Study surveys: 1993–2001. *J Am Coll Health* 2002;50:203–217.
10. Wechsler H, Dowdall GW, Davenport A, et al. Correlates of college student binge drinking. *Am J Public Health* 1995;85:921–926.
11. Wechsler H, Lee JE, Kuo M, et al. College binge drinking in the 1990s: a continuing problem. Results of the Harvard School of Public Health 1999 College Alcohol Study. *J Am Coll Health* 2000;48:199–210.
12. Roark ML. Conceptualizing campus violence: definitions, underlying factors, and effects. *J Coll Student Psychother* 1993;8:1–27.
13. Ham LS, Hope DA. College students and problematic drinking: a review of the literature. *Clin Psychol Rev* 2003;23:719–759.
14. Presley CA, Meilman PW, Leichliter, JS. College factors that influence drinking. *J Stud Alcohol* 2002;(Suppl 14):82–90.
15. Clements R. Prevalence of alcohol-use disorders and alcohol-related problems in a college student sample. *J Am Coll Health* 1999;48:111–118.
16. Hill EM, Chow K. Life-history theory and risky drinking. *Addiction* 2002;97:401–413.
17. Read JP, Wood MD, Davidoff OJ, et al. Making the transition from high school to college: the role of alcohol-related social influence factors in students' drinking. *Subst Abuse* 2002;23:53–65.
18. Perkins HW. Surveying the damage: a review of research on consequences of alcohol misuse in college populations. *J Stud Alcohol* 2002;(Suppl): 14:91–100.
19. O'Malley PM, Johnston LD. Epidemiology of alcohol and other drug use among American college students. *J Stud Alcohol* 2002(Suppl)14:23–39.
20. Leichliter JS, Meilman PW, Presley CA, et al. Alcohol use and related consequences among students with varying levels of involvement in college athletics. *J Am Coll Health* 1998;46:257–262.
21. Baer JS. Effects of college residence on perceived norms for alcohol consumption: an examination of the first year in college. *Psychol Addict Behav* 1994;8:43–50.
22. Cashin JR, Presley CA, Meilman PW. Alcohol use in the Greek system: follow the leader? *J Stud Alcohol* 1998;59:63–70.
23. Larimer ME, Anderson BK, Baer JS, et al. An individual in context: predictors of alcohol use and drinking problems among Greek and residence hall students. *J Subst Abuse* 2000;11:53–68.
24. Harrington N, Brigham NL, Clayton RR. Differences in alcohol use and alcohol-related problems among fraternity and sorority members. *Drug Alcohol Depend* 1997;47:237–246.
25. Dunn ME, Goldman MS. Age and drinking-related differences in the memory organization of alcohol expectancies in 3rd-, 6th-, 9th-, and 12th-grade children. *J Consult Clin Psychol* 1998;66:579–585.
26. Young RM, Connor JP, Ricciardelli LA, et al. The role of alcohol expectancy and drinking refusal self-efficacy beliefs in university student drinking. *Alcohol Alcohol* 2006;41:70–75.
27. Greenbaum PE, Del Boca FK, Darkes J, et al. Variation in the drinking trajectories of freshmen college students. *J Consult Clin Psychol* 2005;73: 229–238.
28. Smith GT, Goldman MS. Alcohol expectancy theory and the identification of high-risk adolescents. *J Res Adolesc* 1994;4:229–248.
29. Cooper ML. Motivations for alcohol use among adolescents: development and validation of a four-factor model. *Psychol Assess* 1994;6:117–128.
30. Cooper ML, Russell M, Skinner JB, et al. Stress and alcohol use: moderating effects of gender, coping, and alcohol expectancies. *J Abnorm Psychol* 1992;101:139–152.
31. Brennan AF, Walfish S, AuBuchon P. Alcohol use and abuse in college students: I. A review of individual and personality correlates. *Int J Addict* 1986;21:449–474.
32. Neighbors C, Larimer ME, Geisner IM, et al. Feeling controlled and drinking motives among college students: contingent self-esteem as a mediator. *Self Identity* 2004;3:207–224.
33. Cooper ML, Frone MR, Russell M, et al. Drinking to regulate positive and negative emotions: a motivational model of alcohol use. *J Person Soc Psychol* 1995;69:990–1005.
34. Borsari B, Carey KB. Descriptive and injunctive norms in college drinking: a meta-analytic integration. *J Stud Alcohol* 2003;64:331–341
35. Baer JS, Stacy A, Larimer M. Biases in the perception of drinking norms among college students. *J Stud Alcohol* 1991;52:580–586.
36. Clapp JD, McDonnell AL. The relationship of perceptions of alcohol promotion and peer drinking norms to alcohol problems reported by college students. *J Coll Stud Dev* 2002;41:19–26.
37. Neighbors C, Lee CM, Lewis MA, et al. Are social norms the best predictor of outcomes among heavy-drinking college students? *J Stud Alcohol Drugs* 2007;68:556–565.

38. Clapp JD, Shillington AM. Environmental predictors of heavy episodic drinking. *Am J Drug Alcohol Abuse* 2001;27:301–313.
39. Neighbors C, Walters ST, Lee CM, et al. Event-specific prevention: addressing college student drinking during known windows of risk. *Addict Behav* 2007;32:2667–2680.
40. Borsari B. Drinking games in the college environment: a review. *J Alcohol Drug Ed* 2004;48:29–51.
41. Martens MP, Dams-O'Connor K, Beck NC. A systematic review of college student-athlete drinking: prevalence rates, sport-related factors, and interventions. *J Subst Abuse Treat* 2006;31:305–316.
42. Neal DJ, Fromme K. Hook 'em horns and heavy drinking: alcohol use and collegiate sports. *Addict Behav* 2007;32:2681–2693.
43. Boyd CJ., McCabe SE, d'Arcy H. Collegiate living environments: a predictor of binge drinking, negative consequences, and risk-reducing behaviors. *J Addict Nurs* 2004;15:111–118.
44. National Institute on Alcohol Abuse and Alcoholism. *A call to action: changing the culture of drinking at U.S. colleges.* Bethesda, MD: U.S. Department of Health and Human Services, Public Health Service, National Institutes of Health, 2002.
45. Barnett NP, Read JP. Mandatory alcohol intervention for alcohol-abusing college students: a systematic review. *J Subst Abuse Treat* 2005;29: 147–158.
46. Carey KB, Scott-Sheldon LA, Carey MP, et al. Individual-level interventions to reduce college student drinking: a meta-analytic review. *Addict Behav* 2007;32:2469–2494.
47. Larimer ME, Cronce JM. Identification, prevention and treatment: a review of individual-focused strategies to reduce problematic alcohol consumption by college students. *J Stud Alcohol* 2002;(Suppl)14:148–163.
48. Larimer ME, Cronce JM. Identification, prevention, and treatment revisited: individual-focused college drinking prevention strategies 1999–2006. *Addict Behav* 2007;32:2439–2468.
49. Larimer ME, Cronce JM, Lee CM, et al. Brief interventions in college settings. *Alcohol Res Health* 2005;28:94–104.
50. Walters ST, Miller E, Chiauzzi E. Wired for wellness: e-interventions for addressing college drinking. *J Subst Abuse Treat* 2005;29:139–145.
51. Walters ST, Neighbors C. Feedback interventions for college alcohol misuse: what, why and for whom? *Addict Behav* 2005;30:1168–1182.
52. White HR. Reduction of alcohol-related harm on United States college campuses: the use of personal feedback interventions. *Int J Drug Policy* 2006;17:310–319.
53. Miller WR, Rollnick S. *Motivational interviewing*, 2nd ed. New York: Guilford Press, 2002.
54. Darkes J, Goldman MS. Expectancy challenge and drinking reduction: experimental evidence for a mediational process. *J Consult Clin Psychol* 1993;61:344–353.
55. Corbin WR, McNair LD, Carter JA. Evaluation of a treatment-appropriate cognitive intervention for challenging alcohol outcome expectancies. *Addict Behav* 2001;26:475–488.
56. Wood MD, Capone C, Laforge R, et al. Brief motivational intervention and alcohol expectancy challenge with heavy drinking college students: a randomized factorial study. *Addict Behav* 2007;32:2509–2528.
57. Carey KB, Carey MP, Maisto SA, et al. Brief motivational interventions for heavy college drinkers: a randomized controlled trial. *J Consult Clin Psychol* 2006;74:943–954.
58. Sobell LC, Sobell MB. *Timeline followback user's guide: a calendar method for assessing alcohol and drug use.* Toronto, Ontario, Canada: Addiction Research Foundation, 1996.
59. Kypri K, Saunders JB, Gallagher SJ. Acceptability of various brief intervention approaches for hazardous drinking among university students. *Alcohol Alcohol* 2003;38:626–628.
60. Marlatt GA, Baer JS, Kivlahan DR, et al. Screening and brief intervention for high-risk college student drinkers: results from a 2-year follow-up assessment. *J Consult Clin Psychol* 1998;66:604–615.
61. Dimeff LA, Baer JS, Kivlahan DR, et al. *Brief alcohol screening and intervention for college students (BASICS).* New York: The Guilford Press, 1999.
62. LaBrie JW, Thompson AD, Huchting K, et al. A group motivational interviewing intervention reduces drinking and alcohol-related negative consequences in adjudicated college women. *Addict Behav* 2007;32: 2549–2562.
63. Larimer ME, Turner AP, Anderson BK, et al. Evaluating a brief alcohol intervention with fraternities. *J Stud Alcohol* 2001;62:370–380.
64. White HR, Morgan TJ, Pugh LA, et al. Evaluating two brief substance-use interventions for mandated college students. *J Stud Alcohol* 2006;67: 309–317.
65. Martens MP, Cimini MD, Barr AR, et al. Implementing a screening and brief intervention for high-risk drinking in university-based health and mental health care settings: reductions in alcohol use and correlates of success. *Addict Behav* 2007;32:2563–2572.
66. Fromme K, Corbin W. Prevention of heavy drinking and associated negative consequences among mandated and voluntary college students. *J Consult Clin Psychol* 2004;72:1038–1049.
67. Larimer ME, Lee CM, Kilmer JR, et al. Personalized mailed feedback for college drinking prevention: a randomized clinical trial. *J Consult Clin Psychol* 2007;75:285–293.
68. Murphy JG, Benson TA, Vuchinich RE, et al. A comparison of personalized feedback for college student drinkers delivered with and without a motivational interview. *J Stud Alcohol* 2004;65:200–203.
69. Neighbors C, Larimer ME, Lewis MA. Targeting misperceptions of descriptive drinking norms: efficacy of a computer-delivered personalized normative feedback intervention. *J Consult Clin Psychol* 2004;72: 434–447.
70. Lewis MA, Neighbors C. Who is the typical college student? Implications for personalized normative feedback interventions. *Addict Behav* 2006;31:2120–2126.
71. DeJong W, Langford LM. A typology for campus-based alcohol prevention: moving toward environmental management strategies. *J Stud Alcohol* 2002;(Suppl)14:140–147.
72. Toomey TL, Wagenaar AC. Environmental policies to reduce college drinking: options and research findings. *J Stud Alcohol* 2002;(Suppl)14: 193–205.
73. Keeling RP. Binge drinking and the college environment. *J Am Coll Health* 2002;50:197–201.
74. Kypri K, Paschall MJ, Maclennan B, et al. Intoxication by drinking location: a web-based diary study in a New Zealand university community. *Addict Behav* 2007;32:2586–2596.
75. Clapp JD, Stanger L. Changing the college AOD environment for primary prevention. *J Prim Prev* 2003;23:515–523.
76. Gallagher RP. *National survey of counseling center directors.* Monograph Series Number 8Q. Pittsburgh: The International Association of Counseling Services, Inc., 2007.
77. Schwartz AJ. Are college students more disturbed today? Stability in the acuity and qualitative character of psychopathology of college counseling center clients: 1992–1993 through 2001–2002. *J Am Coll Health* 2006; 54:327–337.
78. The National Center on Addiction and Substance Abuse at Columbia University. *Depression, substance abuse and college student engagement: a review of the literature.* New York: Author, 2003.
79. Geisner IM, Neighbors C, Larimer ME. A randomized clinical trial of a brief, mailed intervention for symptoms of depression. *J Consult Clin Psychol* 2006;74:393–399.
80. Foote J, Wilkens C, Vavagiakis P. A national survey of alcohol screening and referral in college health centers. *J Am Coll Health* 2004;52:149–157.
81. Kypri K, Saunders JB, Williams SM, et al. Web-based screening and brief intervention for hazardous drinking: a double-blind randomized controlled trial. *Addiction* 2004;99:1410–1417.
82. Larimer ME, Kilmer JR, Lee CM. College student drug prevention: a review of individually oriented prevention strategies. *J Drug Issues* 2005;35:431–456.

CHAPTER 38

Jon E. Grant, MD, JD, MPH
Brian L Odlaug, BA
Marc N. Potenza, MD, PhD

Pathologic Gambling: Clinical Characteristics and Treatment

Pathologic gambling is a psychiatric disorder characterized by persistent and recurrent maladaptive patterns of gambling behavior, which is associated with impaired functioning, reduced quality of life, and high rates of bankruptcy, divorce, and incarceration (1). Excessive gambling behaviors have been reported for millennia across cultures and have been discussed in the medical literature since the early 1800s (2). Pathologic gambling, however, was recognized by the American Psychiatric Association only in 1980 in their third edition of the Diagnostic and Statistical Manual (DSM-III) (3).

Currently classified in DSM-IV-TR as an "impulse control disorder not elsewhere classified," the diagnosis of pathologic gambling requires that a person meet five of the possible 10 criteria listed for the disorder (Table 38.1). The term *problem gambling* has been used to describe forms of disordered gambling, sometimes inclusive and at other times exclusive of pathologic gambling. Problem gambling, like problem drinking, is not an officially recognized disorder by the American Psychiatric Association.

There remains controversy about whether pathologic gambling is better understood as a compulsive disorder or an addictive disorder. This is probably so because pathologic gambling is often resistant to treatment, and it remains unclear whether the treatment technologies of traditional addiction treatment (group, twelve-step participation, relapse prevention, motivational enhancement, etc.) are superior, inferior, equivalent, or need to be combined with those of psychiatric treatments (medication, cognitive behavioral therapy [CBT], psychotherapy). Nonetheless, evidence supports significant phenomenologic, clinical, epidemiologic, and biologic links with substance use disorders. These data support the conceptualization of pathologic gambling as a "behavioral"—as opposed to a chemical—addiction. As such, it seems increasingly important that individuals involved in the prevention and treatment of substance use disorders have a current understanding of pathologic gambling and the potential for future research findings to guide prevention and treatment efforts for addictions in general.

EPIDEMIOLOGY

A range of prevalence estimates have been reported for pathologic gambling depending upon the time frame of the study and the instruments used to diagnose the disorder. Only four national studies and one meta-analysis of state and regional surveys have examined prevalence estimates of pathologic gambling in the general population. The first national study in 1976 noted that 0.8% of 1,749 adults contacted via telephone survey had a significant gambling problem (4). Twenty years later, the National Opinion Research Center at the University of Chicago conducted a national telephone survey (requested by the National Gambling Impact Study Commission) of 2,417 adults and found a lifetime prevalence estimate of 0.8% of pathologic gambling and an additional 1.3% of problem gambling (5). Another national telephone survey of 2,628 adults found that 1.3% had current pathologic gambling measured by the Diagnostic Interview Schedule and 1.9% when measured by the South Oaks Gambling Screen, and an additional 2.8% to 7.5% had problem gambling (6). A recent study, the National Epidemiologic Survey on Alcohol and Related Conditions (NESARC), however, found that only 0.42% of adults in a community sample met current criteria for pathologic gambling (7). A meta-analysis of 120 prevalence estimate surveys completed in North America from the late 1970s to the late 1990s found that the lifetime estimate of pathologic gambling was 1.6% and of problem gambling was 3.85%, for a combined rate of 5.45% for some kind of disordered gambling (8).

The incidence of pathologic gambling appears higher in clinical samples. In subjects seeking treatment for substance use disorders, lifetime estimates of pathologic gambling range

TABLE 38.1 Diagnostic Criteria for Pathologic Gambling

A. Persistent and recurrent maladaptive gambling behavior as indicated by five (or more) of the following:
   (1) Is preoccupied with gambling (e.g., preoccupied with reliving past gambling experiences, handicapping or planning the next venture, or thinking of ways to get money with which to gamble)
   (2) Needs to gamble with increasing amounts of money in order to achieve the desired excitement
   (3) Has repeated unsuccessful efforts to control, cut back, or stop gambling
   (4) Is restless or irritable when attempting to cut down or stop gambling
   (5) Gambles as a way of escaping from problems or of relieving a dysphoric mood (e.g., feelings of helplessness, guilt, anxiety, depression)
   (6) After losing money gambling, often returns another day to get even ("chasing" one's losses)
   (7) Lies to family members, therapist, or others to conceal the extend of involvement with gambling
   (8) Has committed illegal acts such as forgery, fraud, theft, or embezzlement to finance gambling
   (9) Has jeopardized or lost a significant relationship, job, or educational or career opportunity because of gambling
   (10) Relies on other to provide money to relieve a desperate financial situation caused by gambling

B. The gambling behavior is not better accounted for by a Manic Episode.

Note: Reprinted with permission from the Diagnostic and Statistical Manual of Mental Disorders, 4th edition [Text revision]. American Psychiatric Association. 2000: Washington, DC: Permission has been obtained.

from 5% (9) to 33% (10). In studies of psychiatric inpatients estimates of lifetime pathologic gambling have ranged from 4.9% in adolescents to 6.9% in adults (11,12).

There has been an accelerated proliferation of gambling venues during the past decade, particularly with Native American casinos and riverboat gambling (13,14). With increased opportunity to gamble, some research suggests that we can expect greater rates of pathologic gambling in the future (8,15,16). Physicians, therefore, will likely be seeing more individuals struggling with pathologic gambling and need to be skilled in assessing and treating this disorder.

Clinical Characteristics A Pathologic gambling often begins in adolescence or early adulthood, with males tending to start at earlier ages (8,17). Although prospective studies are largely lacking, pathologic gambling appears to follow a trajectory similar to that of substance dependence, with high rates in adolescent and young adult groups, lower rates in older adults, and periods of abstinence and relapse (18). Pathologic gambling is a serious psychiatric disorder, but there is recent evidence that approximately one-third of individuals with pathologic gambling experience natural recovery (i.e., without formal treatment or attendance at Gamblers Anonymous) (19). The research on natural recovery, however, is based on retrospective reports, and there is no data regarding whether these individuals who are symptom-free for 1 year remain free of symptoms beyond that time or whether they switch to some other addictive behavior.

Significant clinical differences have been observed in men and women with pathologic gambling. Men with pathologic gambling are more likely to be single and living alone as compared to women with the disorder (20). Male pathologic gamblers are also more likely to have sought treatment for substance abuse (21), have higher rates of antisocial personality traits (17), and have marital consequences related to their gambling (17). Though men seem to start gambling at earlier ages and have higher rates of pathologic gambling, women, who constitute approximately 32% of pathologic gamblers in the United States, seem to progress more quickly to a pathologic state than do men (22,23).

The types of gambling preferred by men tend to be different from those preferred by women. Men with pathologic gambling have higher rates of "strategic" forms of gambling, including sports betting, video poker, and blackjack. Women, on the other hand, have higher rates of "nonstrategic" gambling, such as slot machines or bingo (23). In regard to gambling triggers, though both men and women report that advertisements trigger their urges to gamble, men tend to report gambling for reasons unrelated to their emotional state whereas women report gambling to escape from stress or owing to depressive states (21,23,24). Higher rates of sensation-seeking or "action"-seeking behavior in men have been suggested as a possible reason for this difference in gambling preference (23,25).

Functional Impairment, Quality of Life, and Legal Difficulties Individuals with pathologic gambling suffer significant impairment in their ability to function socially and occupationally. Many individuals report intrusive thoughts and urges related to gambling that interfere with their ability to concentrate at home and work (24). Work-related problems such as absenteeism, poor performance and job loss are common (22). The inability to control behavior about which a person has mixed feelings may lead to feelings of shame and guilt (24). Pathologic gambling is also frequently associated with marital problems (24) and diminished intimacy and trust within the family (26). Financial difficulties (44% of pathologic gamblers report loss of savings or retirement funds and 22% report losing homes or automobiles or pawning valuables owing to gambling) often exacerbate personal and family problems (24).

With the functional impairment that individuals with pathologic gambling experience, it is not surprising that they also report poor quality of life. In two studies systematically evaluating quality of life, individuals with pathologic gambling reported significantly poorer life satisfaction compared to general, nonclinical adult samples (27,28).

Pathologic gambling is also associated with greater health problems (for example, cardiac problems, liver disease) and increased use of medical services (29,30). Possible reasons for the association of pathologic gambling with health problems might be the sedentary nature of gambling, reduced leisure and exercise time, reduced sleep, increased stress, and increased nicotine and alcohol consumption.

Many individuals with pathologic gambling report the need for psychiatric hospitalization owing to the depression, and rarer, suicidality, they feel was brought on by their gambling losses (24). Research on individuals in gambling treatment centers has found that 48% of individuals report having had gambling-related suicidal ideation at some time (31). Pathologic gambling may also contribute to attempted or completed suicide. A study of Gamblers Anonymous participants (recruited through a gambling telephone hotline) found that 17% to 24% reported having attempted suicide owing to gambling (32).

In addition to the emotional impact of problem and pathologic gambling, many individuals with pathologic gambling have faced legal difficulties related to their gambling. One study found that 27.3% of pathologic gamblers had committed at least one gambling-related illegal act (33). Problem or pathologic gambling may lead people to engage in illegal behavior including embezzlement, stealing, and writing bad checks in order to either finance the gambling behavior or to compensate for past losses related to the excessive gambling (32). One study found high percentages of pathologic gamblers endorsing prior acts of embezzlement (31%) and robbery (14%) (34).

Although pathologic gambling is associated with multiple legal and functional difficulties, one caveat is that the research is based on relatively small numbers of individuals with pathologic gambling and the studies may reflect the more severe cases when individuals may be more likely to come for treatment.

Comorbidity Psychiatric comorbidity is common in individuals with pathologic gambling. Frequent co-occurrence has been reported between substance use disorders (including nicotine dependence) and pathologic gambling, with the highest odds ratios generally observed between gambling and alcohol use disorders (6,35). A Canadian epidemiologic survey estimated that the relative risk for an alcohol use disorder is increased 3.8-fold when disordered gambling is present (36).

Among clinical samples, 52% of Gambler's Anonymous participants reported either alcohol or drug abuse (37) and 35% to 63% of individuals seeking treatment for pathologic gambling also screened positive for a lifetime substance use disorder (1), rates notably higher than that found in the general population (26.6%) (38).

Other studies examining co-occurring disorders in pathologic gamblers have also noted high estimates of mood disorders (34% to 78%) (24,39–41). In 1984, McCormick et al. (39) studied 38 cases of treatment-seeking pathologic gamblers with major depressive disorder and found that, in 86% of cases, the gambling problem preceded the onset of depression. This raises the question of whether co-occurring mood disorders may be secondary to pathologic gambling. However, the finding of shared genetic contributions to pathologic gambling and major depression in men (42) suggests a possible shared biological predisposition to the co-occurrence of the disorders.

High prevalence estimates of co-occurring anxiety disorders (28% to 40%) also exist in pathologic gamblers (37,40), but not all anxiety disorders are seen with equal frequency. Recent research suggests that estimates of co-occurring generalized anxiety disorder range as high as 40% among pathologic gamblers (35), whereas those of obsessive-compulsive disorder may be as low as 1% (1). The relationship of obsessive compulsive disorder to pathologic gambling, however, has produced a mixed picture, with some studies reporting high estimates (17% to 20%) (36,37) and other investigations generating low estimates (1%) (35). The rates of co-occurring disorders often have wide ranges, and this may be owing to lack of structured clinical interviews used in assessing comorbidity, the small sample sizes of gamblers assessed, and the possible heterogeneity of pathologic gambling.

Significantly fewer data are available regarding the frequencies of Axis II personality disorders in pathologic gamblers. Studies have shown that estimates of any personality disorder in pathologic gamblers range from 25% to 93% (40,43,44). Borderline (3% to 70%), narcissistic (5% to 57%), avoidant (5% to 50%), and obsessive-compulsive (5% to 59%) personality disorders are most commonly reported (40,43,44). One of the best-studied personality disorders in pathologic gambling, antisocial personality disorder has been found in 15% to 40% of pathologic gamblers, a frequency higher than the 0.6% to 3% estimates reported for the general population (45,46). Although multiple reasons may explain the elevated rates of comorbid antisocial personality disorder in pathologic gambling, recent evidence suggests a possible shared genetic vulnerability between pathologic gambling and antisocial personality disorder (47).

Family History High frequencies of psychiatric disorders are seen in the first-degree relatives of those with pathologic gambling. Commonly reported conditions include mood, anxiety, substance use, and antisocial personality disorders (27,48,49). In two studies of first-degree relatives of pathologic gamblers, 17% to 33% had a mood disorder, and 18% to 24% reported an alcohol use disorder (37,48). In another study of 51 pathologic gamblers, 50% had a parent with an alcohol use disorder (49).

Studies have also found that 20% of the first-degree relatives of pathologic gamblers also have pathologic gambling (50). Gambino et al. (51) found that problem gamblers at a Veteran's hospital were up to eight times more likely to have a parent with a gambling problem than were non-problem gamblers. In one of the few studies to use a psychometrically sound instrument (Family History Research Diagnostic Criteria) to collect family history data, the researchers found that 31% of first-degree relatives of pathologic gamblers had a lifetime alcohol use disorder and 19% had lifetime major depressive disorder (27).

In one of the few studies to use a control group to examine familial aggregation of psychiatric disorders among pathologic gamblers, Black et al. (52) examined 31 pathologic gambler probands and 31 control probands. Lifetime estimates of pathologic gambling were significantly higher in family members of pathologic gamblers (8.3%) compared to control subjects (2.1%) (odds ratio of 4.49; $p = .018$). Similarly elevated estimates were observed for substance use disorders (odds ratio of 4.21) and antisocial personality disorder (odds ratio of 7.73) (52).

TREATMENT

Psychotherapy Although there is a long literature of case reports using psychodynamic psychotherapy and psychodynamic psychotherapy is often incorporated into multimodal, eclectic, and integrated approaches to PG, there are no randomized controlled trials supporting its use (53). Similarly, although some evidence exists that Gamblers Anonymous (54–57) and self-exclusion contracts (58) may be beneficial for pathologic gamblers, no controlled study for these interventions has been published.

A variety of psychosocial treatments have been examined in controlled studies for the treatment of pathologic gambling. Cognitive strategies have traditionally included cognitive restructuring, psychoeducation, and irrational cognition awareness training. Behavioral approaches focus on developing alternate activities to compete with reinforcers specific to pathologic gambling as well as the identification of gambling triggers.

Cognitive Therapy To date, 15 randomized clinical trials using CBT have been conducted for pathologic gambling. There have been three controlled studies examining the effect of cognitive restructuring in pathologic gambling. One study used a combination of individual cognitive therapy and relapse prevention strategies in 40 subjects (59). When subjects were assessed at 12-months, the treatment group showed significant reductions in both gambling frequency and the subjects' perceived self-control over their gambling behavior. The study did not, however, include data from the 11 subjects who withdrew from the study. The same techniques of cognitive therapy with relapse prevention were utilized in a group of 88 pathologic gambling subjects over a period of 3 months compared to a wait-list control. Although 41% of the subjects dropped out of treatment, those in the group who completed treatment experienced gambling symptom improvement at 3 months (reduced urges to gamble, reduced gambling behavior), and 71% of the completers maintained that improvement at a 12-month follow-up (60).

Group cognitive therapy was tested against a wait-list control condition in 71 subjects with pathologic gambling (61). Groups met weekly for 10 weeks, and each session lasted 2 hours; 74% completed all sessions. After 10 sessions, 65% of those in group cognitive behavior therapy (CBT) who completed it no longer met criteria for pathologic gambling, compared to 20% in the wait-list condition. At 24-month follow-up, 68% of those who completed the 24-month follow-up (33% of the original sample) did not meet criteria for pathologic gambling.

Behavioral Therapy Behavioral approaches have also been examined in three controlled studies. In the first study, researchers reported significant reductions in gambling behaviors in a comparison of imaginal desensitization (i.e. subjects were taught relaxation and then instructed to imagine experiencing and resisting triggers to gambling) to traditional aversion therapy in the randomized treatment of 20 compulsive gamblers (62). Both therapies had positive outcomes, but at 1-year follow-up, 70% of the group assigned to imaginal desensitization were still maintaining reductions in gambling urges and behavior compared to 30% of those assigned to aversion therapy.

In another study, 20 inpatient subjects were randomly assigned to receive either imaginal desensitization or imaginal relaxation in 14 sessions over a 1-week period. Both groups improved after treatment; however, therapeutic gains were not maintained by either group at a 12-month follow-up (63).

McConaghy et al. (64) examined long-term outcomes in a larger study of 120 subjects randomly assigned to aversion therapy, imaginal desensitization, in vivo desensitization, or imaginal relaxation; 53% of subjects were available for assessment 2 to 9 years later, and 79% of subjects assigned to imaginal desensitization had decreased or ceased gambling as compared to 33% in the other groups. No difference ws reported among treatment groups, however, in rates of abstinence.

Cognitive Behavioral Therapy Echeburua et al. (65) conducted a randomized study of cognitive behavioral therapy (CBT) in slot machine-playing pathologic gamblers with subjects assigned to one of four groups: (1) individual stimulus control and in vivo exposure with response prevention, (2) group cognitive restructuring, (3) a combination of 1 and 2, and (4) a wait-list control. At 12 months, rates of abstinence or minimal gambling (defined as no more than one or two gambling episodes with the total amount spent gambling being no greater than a week's worth of gambling at baseline) were higher in the individual treatment (69%) compared with group cognitive restructuring (38%) and the combined treatment (38%). The same investigators further assessed individual and group relapse prevention for completers of a 6-week individual treatment program. At 12 months, 86% of those receiving individual relapse prevention and 78% of those in group relapse prevention had not relapsed, compared to 52% with no follow-up (66).

Milton et al. (67) compared CBT to CBT combined with interventions designed to improve treatment compliance (interventions included positive reinforcement, identifying barriers to change, and applying problem-solving skills) in 40 subjects using eight sessions of manualized, individual therapy. Of these, 65% of the CBT-plus-interventions group completed treatment while only 35% of the CBT-alone group did so. At 9-month follow-up, there was no difference in outcome between treatments, though both produced clinically significant change in the amount of money spent gambling.

Melville et al. (68) described two studies that used a three-topic mapping system (targeting understanding randomness, problem solving, and relapse prevention) to improve outcome. In the first study, 13 subjects were assigned to either 8 weeks of group CBT, group CBT with the mapping-enhanced treatment, or wait-list. In the second study, 19 subjects were assigned to a mapping group or a wait-list group for 8 weeks. For those subjects who were in the CBT-with-mapping group, significant improvement was maintained both after treatment and at a 6-month follow-up.

Petry et al. (55) examined an eight-session manualized form of CBT. In this study, 231 subjects were referred to Gamblers Anonymous and randomly assigned to weekly CBT sessions with an individual counselor, to self-directed use of the CBT manual, or to no additional treatment. Though all groups reduced their gambling, those subjects assigned to individual therapy or the self-help workbook reduced gambling behaviors to a greater degree than did those only with a referral to Gamblers Anonymous. Only some effects were maintained throughout follow-up. Attendance at Gamblers Anonymous and number of therapy sessions or workbook exercises completed were associated with gambling abstinence.

In a study examining cognitive-motivational behavior therapy (CMBT), a method that combines gambling-specific CBT with motivational interviewing techniques to aid in resolving treatment ambivalence and subsequently improve retention rates, nine subjects received manualized treatment as compared to a control group of 12 who received treatment as usual (TAU). All nine subjects (100%) in the CMBT group completed treatment versus eight (66.7%) in the TAU group. Significant improvements were observed through a 12-month follow-up for the CMBT group (69).

Brief Interventions and Motivational Interviewing In one study of brief interventions, Dickerson et al. (70) randomly assigned 29 subjects to either workbook or to workbook plus a single in-depth interview. The workbook included CBT and motivational enhancement techniques. Both groups reported significant reductions in gambling at 6 months.

Another study assigned 102 gamblers to a CBT workbook, a workbook plus a telephone motivational enhancement intervention, or a wait-list. Rates of abstinence at 6 months did not differ between groups, though the frequency of gambling and money lost in gambling were lower in the motivational intervention group (71). Compared to the workbook alone, those gamblers assigned to the motivational intervention and workbook reduced gambling throughout a 2-year follow-up period; however, 77% of the entire follow-up sample was still rated as improved at the 24-month assessment (72).

A recent study used relapse prevention–based pamphlets in 169 subjects who had recently quit gambling. Subjects were randomly assigned to receive either a summary booklet that detailed all relapse prevention information available (single-mailing group) or the same booklet and seven additional informational booklets mailed over the course of the next 12 months (repeated-mailing group). At the 12-month assessment, groups did not differ in frequency of gambling or extent of gambling losses (73).

Assessment of Psychosocial Therapies Although cognitive behavioral therapy appears promising for the treatment of pathologic gambling, several limitations exist in the psychologic treatment studies performed and published to date. First, though some psychologic treatment studies approximate well-powered, rigorous studies, the studies have generally lacked a large enough sample for adequate statistical power. One exception is the study by Petry et al. (55) that was adequately powered at the time of enrollment (N = 231). CBT has shown efficacy for PG, but no manualized CBT treatment has been examined in a confirmatory study by another independent investigator. In addition, manualized treatments of psychosocial therapies for pathologic gambling, with the exception of the Hodgins et al. study, have generally lacked published therapist adherence and competence measures. Third, no study has examined whether certain individuals with pathologic gambling would benefit differentially from specific behavioral treatments.

CBT studies have shown that both brief interventions and longer-term therapy are potentially effective, but no study has yet examined the optimal duration of treatment. Predictors of a positive response to CBT have largely yet to be identified, and there are limited data concerning the effectiveness of psychosocial therapies for pathologic gambling with co-occurring psychiatric conditions.

Pharmacotherapy No medication is currently approved by the U.S. Food and Drug Administration for treating pathologic gambling. Thirteen randomized, placebo-controlled trials of pharmacotherapy treatment in pathologic gambling have been conducted, and these studies suggest that medications may be beneficial in treating pathologic gambling.

Opioid Antagonists Given their ability to modulate dopaminergic transmission in the mesolimbic pathway and to block mu opioid receptors, opioid receptor antagonists have been investigated in the treatment of pathologic gambling. An initial double-blind study suggested the efficacy of naltrexone (ReVia), an FDA-approved treatment for alcohol dependence, in reducing the intensity of urges to gamble, gambling thoughts, and gambling behavior (74). In an 11-week, double-blind, placebo-controlled study of 45 pathologic gambling subjects, significant improvement was seen in 75% of naltrexone subjects (mean end-of-study dose of 188 mg/day) compared to 24% of placebo subjects (74). Individuals reporting higher-intensity gambling urges at treatment onset responded preferentially to active treatment (74), and this supports the theory that targeting cravings via opiate blockade/dopamine modulation reduces the endpoint target of cravings.

Findings from the initial study were recently replicated in a larger, longer study of 77 subjects randomly assigned to either naltrexone or placebo over an 18-week period. Subjects assigned to naltrexone had significantly greater reductions in gambling urges and gambling behavior compared to subjects on placebo. Subjects assigned to naltrexone also had greater improvement in psychosocial functioning. By study endpoint, 39.7% of those on naltrexone were able to abstain from all gambling for at least 1 month, whereas only 10.5% on placebo attained complete abstinence for the same time period (75).

Another opioid antagonist, nalmefene, has shown promise in the treatment of pathologic gambling. In a large, multicenter trial using a double-blind, placebo-controlled, parallel-arm design, 207 subjects were assigned to receive either nalmefene at varying doses or placebo. At the end of the 16-week study, 59% of those assigned to nalmefene showed significant reductions in gambling urges, thoughts, and behavior compared to 34% on placebo (76).

Although these studies of opioid antagonists are of relatively short duration (11 to 18 weeks) and the sample sizes in two of them are small to moderate (45 and 77 subjects), the fact that three double-blind studies have demonstrated significant benefit of these medications compared to placebo offers clinicians and patients a promising treatment option.

"Antidepressants"—Serotonin Reuptake Inhibitors and Bupropion Antidepressant medications have been examined for pathologic gambling based on the proposed neurobiology of pathologic gambling. Low levels of the serotonin metabolite 5-hydroxyindole acetic acid (5-HIAA) and blunted serotonergic response within the ventromedial prefrontal cortex (vmPFC) have been associated with impulsive behaviors (77,78). As compared to control comparison subjects, individuals with pathologic gambling demonstrate diminished activation of the vmPFC when viewing gambling-related videotapes or during prepotent response inhibition when performing the Stroop color-word interference task (79). Individuals with pathologic gambling also show relatively diminished activation of the vmPFC during a simulated gambling task, and severity of gambling problem correlated inversely with signal intensity within this brain region (80). Together, the findings suggest that decreased serotonin function within vmPFC may engender disinhibition and contribute to pathologic gambling. Thus, drugs targeting serotonin neurotransmission have been examined.

Two studies examining paroxetine (Paxil) have been conducted, and the results have been mixed. The first 8-week study of 53 pathologic gamblers demonstrated significantly greater improvement for those pathologic gamblers assigned to paroxetine compared to placebo (61% of subjects on paroxetine showed improvement versus only 23% on placebo) (81). A 16-week, multi-center study of paroxetine in 76 pathologic gamblers, however, did not find a statistically significant difference between active drug and placebo, perhaps in part owing to the high placebo response rate (48% to placebo, 59% to active drug) (82).

Fluvoxamine (Luvox) has also demonstrated mixed results in two placebo-controlled, double-blind studies, with one 16-week, crossover study (N = 15) supporting its efficacy at an average dose of 207 mg/day (83), and a second 6-month parallel-arm study (N = 32) with high rates of drop-out finding no significant difference in response to active or placebo drug (84).

In a double-blind, 6-month, placebo-controlled trial using sertraline (Zoloft), a mean dosage of 95 mg/day demonstrated no statistical advantage over placebo in a group of 60 pathologic gamblers (85).

Escitalopram (Lexapro) was used in a 12-week, open-label trial with an 8-week double-blind discontinuation phase for responders in 13 subjects with co-occurring pathologic gambling and anxiety disorders (86). At the end of the open-label phase (mean dose, 25.4 mg/day), six subjects were considered responders with respect to gambling and anxiety symptomatology. Improvement was maintained for those randomly assigned to continue receiving escitalopram while assignment to placebo was associated with a return of gambling and anxiety symptoms.

In the only controlled study of a non-SRI antidepressant, Black et al. (87) examined the efficacy of bupropion (Wellbutrin), a dopaminergic and noradrenergic antidepressant, in a 12-week, double-blind, placebo-controlled study of 39 subjects with pathologic gambling. Although bupropion alone among antidepressants has been shown efficacious in smoking cessation, it was not significantly more efficacious than placebo for pathologic gambling. When subjects with at least one post-randomization visit were assessed, nearly 36% of bupropion subjects and 47% of placebo subjects were classified as responders. However, high treatment discontinuation rates of nearly 44% were observed in this study, making definitive statements regarding the efficacy of bupropion in PG difficult.

The antidepressant trials for pathologic gambling have produced mixed results, with some studies reporting significant improvement over placebo and others not. These findings may be owing to the fact that serotonergic dysfunction is merely a peripheral aspect of pathologic gambling, the small sample sizes of the studies, or the heterogeneity of pathologic gambling. Antidepressant medications may be helpful for co-occurring conditions in pathologic gamblers (i.e., depression or anxiety) but cannot be recommended for targeting the core symptoms of pathologic gambling based on current studies.

Mood Stabilizers Mood stabilizers have been examined in pathologic gambling with the hypothesis that they are beneficial in reducing impulsivity and hypermotoric activation. Sustained-release lithium carbonate was used in a 10-week, double-blind, placebo-controlled study of 40 subjects with bipolar spectrum disorders and pathologic gambling. Lithium (mean level, 0.87 meq/liter) reduced the thoughts and urges associated with pathologic gambling. However, no significant difference was found in the episodes of gambling per week, time spent per gambling episode, or the amount of money lost (88).

Based on only one double-blind study that resulted in moderate benefits, no recommendation can be made at this time for the use of mood stabilizers in pathologic gambling.

Glutamatergic Agents Because improving glutamatergic tone in the nucleus accumbens has been implicated in reducing the reward-seeking behavior of animals (89), N-acetyl cysteine (NAC), a glutamate-modulating agent that is available through health food stores without a prescription, was administered to 27 pathologic gambling subjects over an 8-week period with responders randomly assigned to receive an additional 6-week double-blind trial of NAC or placebo. Of those subjects, 59% in the open-label phase experienced significant reductions in pathologic gambling symptoms and were classified as responders. At the end of the double-blind phase (N = 13), 83% of those assigned to receive NAC were still classified as responders compared to only 28.6% of those assigned to placebo (90).

Assessment of Pharmacotherapies Several conclusions as well as limitations can be made regarding the pharmacologic literature. First, given three double-blind studies of opioid antagonists and a confirmatory study of naltrexone, naltrexone should be considered a first-line treatment for pathologic gambling. Though different classes of medication have shown some benefit in small studies, no comparison studies of medications have been performed in a randomized, placebo-controlled design. In addition, no study has examined whether certain individuals with pathologic gambling would benefit differentially from specific pharmacotherapies. With one exception, there have been no systematic dose-response studies for medication. The exception showed that 25 mg/day and 50 mg/day, but not 100 mg/day, of nalmefene was more effective than placebo (76). Furthermore, the long-term effects of medication for pathologic gambling remain largely untested. Only two studies have examined pharmacologic effects for 6 months, but these studies experienced dropout rates of 59% (84) and 44% (85). No study has examined pharmacologic treatment effects for longer than 6 months or whether the effects of acute treatment last beyond the 8 to 18 weeks. With regard to predictors of a positive response to pharmacotherapy, preliminary findings suggest that PG subjects with more intense gambling urges respond better to naltrexone (74) and males and younger PG subjects respond better to fluvoxamine (84). There are limited data concerning the effectiveness of pharmacotherapy for pathologic gamblers with co-occurring psychiatric conditions. Preliminary data suggest that individuals with pathologic gambling and bipolar symptoms may respond to lithium (88) and those with pathologic gambling and anxiety respond to escitalopram (86).

Treatment Recommendations Pathologic gambling is a common, disabling psychiatric disorder that is associated with high rates of co-occurring disorders, particularly substance use disorders, and high rates of illegal activities. Psychotherapy and pharmacotherapy have shown promise in the treatment of pathologic gambling. Based on the treatment literature, the off-label use of naltrexone would appear the most promising pharmacologic option. An SSRI antidepressant used off-label may also be beneficial particularly when the individual has comorbid depression or anxiety. In terms of psychosocial treatments, cognitive behavior therapy appears promising. One manualized form of this therapy is that developed by Petry et al. (91). Although the stronger evidence suggests eight sessions of CBT should be considered (55), some data suggest that even fewer sessions may be effective. With a manualized treatment, counselors with a background in Alcoholics Anonymous should be able to deliver the treatment with minimal training.

Even knowing the evidence for various treatment options for pathologic gambling, other factors may influence which treatment option is chosen for a particular patient. First, many clinicians are simply unaware of pathologic gambling. Therefore, if a clinician is referring a patient for either medication management or psychotherapy, it may simply be difficult to find people who know how to treat the behavior. This problem can be minimized by having a list of providers who know about pathologic gambling and can provide treatment. For example, if no one is available to do CBT for pathologic gambling, then perhaps medication management should be maximized. Second, there are no clear recommendations of treatment for the clinician to follow. For example, it is unclear exactly how many sessions of CBT are most helpful for pathologic gambling. The exact dose of medication or duration of medication trial for optimal treatment is also unknown. These gaps in knowledge make it difficult to inform patients about what their care may entail and what expectations they may have. Third, individuals with pathologic gambling exhibit high rates of placebo response in treatment studies. Clinicians need to understand that for many patients with pathologic gambling, simply talking about their problem will help substantially at first. This initial robust response, however, may cause the clinician to believe that his or her treatment approach is successful. Clinicians should carefully monitor the patient for several months and not assume they will continue to do well. Fourth, impulsive patients do not often follow recommendations or follow-up with treatment. The treatment data show that drop-out rates are high for pathologic gambling. This may be owing to two factors: One, patients often believe they are doing better than in fact they are and therefore they see treatment as unnecessary, and two, they do not have an instantaneous response and therefore do not stay with treatment. Both of these concerns can be minimized by providing psychoeducation about the illness, detailing the expectations of treatment, and the expressing the need to stay in treatment.

ACKNOWLEDGMENTS: *This research was supported in part by a Career Development Award (JEG - K23 MH069754-01A1)*

REFERENCES

1. Argo TR, Black DW. Clinical characteristics. In: Grant JE, Potenza MN, eds. *Pathological gambling: a clinical guide to treatment.* Washington, DC: American Psychiatric Publishing, 2004:39–54.
2. Petry NM, ed. *Pathological gambling: etiology, comorbidity, and treatment.* Washington, DC: American Psychological Association, 2005.
3. American Psychiatric Association. *Diagnostic and statistical manual of mental disorders,* 3rd ed. (DSM-III). Washington, DC: American Psychiatric Publishing, 1980.
4. Kallick MD, Suits T, Deilman T, et al. *A survey of American gambling attitudes and behavior.* Research report series Survey Research Center, Institute for Social Research, Ann Arbor, MI: University of Michigan Press, 1979.
5. Gerstein D, Murphy S, Toce M, et al. *Gambling impact and behavior study: final report to the National Gambling Impact Study Commission.* Chicago: National Opinion Research Center, 1999.
6. Welte J, Barnes G, Wieczorek W. Alcohol and gambling pathology among U.S. adults: prevalence, demographic patterns and comorbidity. *J Stud Alcohol* 2001;62(5):706–712.
7. Petry NM, Stinson FS, Grant BF. Comorbidity of DSM-IV pathological gambling and other psychiatric disorders: results from the National Epidemiologic Survey on Alcohol and Related Conditions. *J Clin Psychiatry* 2005;66(5):564–574.
8. Shaffer HJ, Hall MN, Vander Bilt J. Estimating the prevalence of disordered gambling behavior in the United States and Canada: a research synthesis. *Am J Public Health* 1999;89(9):1369–1376.
9. Lesieur HR, Blume SB, Zoppa RM. Alcoholism, drug abuse, and gambling. *Alcohol Clin Exp Res* 1986;10(1):33–38.
10. Daghestani AN, Elenz E, Crayton JW. Pathological gambling in hospitalized substance abusing veterans. *J Clin Psychiatry* 1996;57:360–363.
11. Grant JE, Levine L, Kim D, et al. Impulse control disorders in adult psychiatric inpatients. *Am J Psychiatry* 2005;162(11):2184–2188.
12. Grant JE, Williams KA, Potenza MN. Impulse-control disorders in adolescent psychiatric inpatients: co-occurring disorders and sex differences. *J Clin Psychiatry* 2007;68(10):1584–1592.
13. National Research Council. *Pathological gambling: a critical review.* Washington, DC: National Academy Press, 1999.
14. Dickson-Gillespie L, Rugle L, Rosenthal R, et al. Preventing the incidence and harm of gambling problems. *J Prim Prev* 2008;Mar 29 [Epub ahead of print].
15. Volberg RA. *Gambling and problem gambling in Iowa: a replication survey.* Report to the Iowa Department of Human Services, 1995.
16. Grant Stitt B, Nichols M, Giacopassi D. Perceptions of the extent of problem gambling within new casino communities. *J Gambl Stud* 2000;16(4):433–451.
17. Ibáñez A, Blanco C, Moreryra P, et al. Gender differences in pathological gambling. *J Clin Psychiatry* 2003;64(3):295–301.
18. Grant JE, Potenza MN. Impulse control disorders: clinical characteristics and pharmacological management. *Ann Clin Psychiatry* 2004;16(1): 27–34.
19. Slutske WS. Natural recovery and treatment-seeking in pathological gambling: results of two U.S. national surveys. *Am J Psychiatry* 2006; 163(2):297–302.
20. Crisp BR, Thomas SA, Jackson AC, et al. Not the same: a comparison of female and male clients seeking treatment from problem gambling counseling services. *J Gambl Stud* 2004;20(3):283–299.
21. Ladd GT, Petry NM. Gender differences among pathological gamblers seeking treatment. *Exp Clin Psychopharmacol* 2002;10:501–507.
22. Grant JE, Kim SW. Gender differences in pathological gamblers seeking medication treatment. *Comp Psychiatry* 2002;43(1):56–62.
23. Potenza MN, Steinberg MA, McLaughlin SD, et al. Gender-related differences in the characteristics of problem gamblers using a gambling helpline. *Am J Psychiatry* 2001;158(9):1500–1505.
24. Grant JE, Kim SW. Demographic and clinical characteristics of 131 adult pathological gamblers. *J Clin Psychiatry* 2001;62(12):957–962.
25. Vitaro F, Arseneault L, Tremblay RE. Dispositional predictors of problem gambling in male adolescents. *Am J Psychiatry* 1997;154:1769–1770.
26. Pallanti S, Baldini Rossi N, Hollander E. Pathological gambling. In: Stein DJ, Hollander E, eds. *Clinical manual of impulse control disorders.* Washington, DC: American Psychiatric Publishing, 2006:251–289.
27. Black DW, Moyer T, Schlosser S. Quality of life and family history in pathological gambling. *J Nerv Ment Disord* 2003;191:124–126.
28. Grant JE, Kim SW. Quality of life in kleptomania and pathological gambling. *Comp Psychiatry* 2005;46(1):34–37.
29. Morasco BJ, Vom Eigen KA, Petry NM. Severity of gambling is associated with physical and emotional health in urban primary care patients. *Gen Hosp Psychiatry* 2006;28(2):94–100.
30. Morasco BJ, Petry NM. Gambling problems and health functioning in individuals receiving disability. *Disabil Rehabil* 2006;28(10):619–623.
31. Ledgerwood DM, Petry NM. Gambling and suicidality in treatment-seeking pathological gamblers. *J Nerv Ment Disord* 2004;192(10): 711–714.
32. Potenza MN, Steinberg MA, McLaughlin SD, et al. Illegal behaviors in problem gambling: an analysis of data from a gambling helpline. *J Am Acad Psychiatry Law* 2000;28:389–403.
33. Ledgerwood DM, Weinstock J, Morasco BJ, et al. Clinical features and treatment prognosis of pathological gamblers with and without recent gambling-related illegal behavior. *J Am Acad Psychiatry Law* 2007;35(3): 294–301.
34. Blaszczynski A, Silove D. Pathological gambling: forensic issues. *Aust N Z J Psychiatry* 1996;30:358–369.
35. Cunningham-Williams RM, Cottler LB, Compton WM 3rd, et al. Taking chances: problem gamblers and mental health disorders—results from the St. Louis Epidemiologic Catchment Area Study. *Am J Public Health* 1998;88(7):1093–1096.
36. Bland RC, Newman SC, Orn H, et al. Epidemiology of pathological gambling in Edmonton. *Can J Psychiatry* 1993;38(2):108–112.
37. Linden RD, Pope HG, Jonas JM. Pathological gambling and major affective disorders: preliminary findings. *J Clin Psychiatry* 1986;47:201–203.
38. Kessler RC, McGonagle KA, Zhao S, et al. Lifetime and 12-month prevalence of DSM-III-R psychiatric disorders in the United States. Results from the National Comorbidity Survey. *Arch Gen Psychiatry* 1994;51(1): 8–19.
39. McCormick RA, Russo AM, Rameriz LF, et al. Affective disorders among pathological gamblers seeking treatment. *Am J Psychiatry* 1984;141: 215–218.
40. Black DW, Moyer T. Clinical features and psychiatric comorbidity of subjects with pathological gambling behavior. *Psychiatr Serv* 1998;49: 1434–1439.
41. Specker SM, Carlson GA, Christenson GA, et al. Impulse control disorders and attention deficit disorder in pathological gamblers. *Ann Clin Psychiatry* 1995;7(4):175–179.
42. Potenza MN, Xian H, Shah K, et al. Shared genetic contributions to pathologicalgambling and major depression in men. *Arch Gen Psychiatry* 2005;62(9):1015–1021.
43. Specker S, Carlson G, Edmonson K, et al. Psychopathology in pathological gamblers seeking treatment. *J Gambl Stud* 1996;12:67–81.
44. Blaszczynski A, Steel Z. Personality disorders among pathological gamblers. *J Gambl Stud* 1998;14:51–71.
45. Compton WM, Conway KP, Stinson FS. Prevalence, correlates, and comorbidity of DSM-IV antisocial personality syndromes and alcohol and specific drug use disorders in the United States: results from the national epidemiologic survey on alcohol and related conditions. *J Clin Psychiatry* 2005;66(6):677–685.
46. Lenzenweger MF, Lane MC, Loranger AW, et al. DSM-IV personality disorders in the National Comorbidity Survey Replication. *Biol Psychiatry* 2007;62(6):553–564.
47. Slutske WS, Eisen S, Xian H, et al. A twin study of the association between pathological gambling and antisocial personality disorder. *J Abnorm Psychol* 2001;110(2):297–308.
48. Roy A, Adinoff B, Roehrich L, et al. Pathological gambling: a psychobiological study. *Arch Gen Psychiatry* 1988;45:369–373.
49. Ramirez LF, McCormack RA, Russo AM, et al. Patterns of substance abuse in pathological gamblers undergoing treatment. *Addict Behav* 1983;8:425–428.

50. Ibáñez A, Blanco C, Sáiz-Ruiz J. Neurobiology and genetics of pathological gambling. *Psychiatr Ann* 2002;32:181–185.
51. Gambino B, Fitzgerald R, Shaffer HJ, et al. Perceived family history of problem gambling and scores on the SOGS. *J Gambl Stud* 1993;9:169–184.
52. Black DW, Monahan PO, Temkit M, et al. A family study of pathologic gambling. *Psychiatry Res* 2006;141(3):295–303.
53. Rosenthal RJ. Psychodynamic psychotherapy and the treatment of pathological gambling. *Brazil J Psychiatry* 2008 [Epub ahead of print].
54. Hodgins DC, Peden N, Cassidy E. The association between comorbidity and outcome inpathological gambling: a prospective follow-up of recent quitters. *J Gambl Stud* 2005;21(3):255–271.
55. Petry NM, Ammerman Y, Bohl J, et al. Cognitive-behavioral therapy for pathological gamblers. *J Consult Clin Psychol* 2006;74(3):555–567.
56. Stewart RM, Brown RI. An outcome study of gamblers anonymous. *Br J Psychiatry* 1988;152:284–288.
57. Taber JI, McCormick RA, Ramirez LF. The prevalence and impact of major life stressors among pathological gamblers. *Int J Addict* 1987;22(1):71–79.
58. Ladouceur R, Jacques C, Giroux I, et al. Analysis of a casino's self-exclusion program. *J Gambl Stud* 2000;16(4):453–460.
59. Sylvain C, Ladouceur R, Boisvert JM. Cognitive and behavioral treatment of pathological gambling: A controlled study. *J Couns Clin Psychol* 1997;65(5):727–732.
60. Ladouceur R, Sylvain C, Boutin C, et al. Cognitive treatment of pathological gambling. *J Nerv Ment Dis* 2001;189(11):774–780.
61. Ladouceur R, Sylvain C, Boutin C, et al. Group therapy for pathological gamblers: a cognitive approach. *Behav Res Ther* 2003;41(5):587–596.
62. McConaghy N, Armstrong MS, Blaszczynski A, et al. Controlled comparison of aversive therapy and imaginal desensitization in compulsive gambling. *Br J Psychiatry* 1983;142:366–372.
63. McConaghy N, Armstrong MS, Blaszczynski A, et al. Behavior completion versus stimulus control in compulsive gambling. Implications for behavioral assessment. *Behav Mod* 1988;12(3):371–384.
64. McConaghy N, Blaszczynski A, Frankova A. Comparison of imaginal desensitisation with other behavioural treatments of pathological gambling: a two- to nine-year follow-up. *Br J Psychiatry* 1991;159:390–393.
65. Echeburúa E, Baez C, Fernández-Montalvo J. Comparative effectiveness of three therapeutic modalities in psychological treatment of pathological gambling: long term outcome. *Behav Cogn Psychother* 1996;24:51–72.
66. Echeburúa E, Fernández-Montalvo J, Baez C. Predictors of therapeutic failure in slot-machine pathological gamblers following behavioural treatment. *Behav Cogn Psychother* 2001;29:379–383.
67. Milton S, Crino R, Hunt C, et al. The effect of compliance-improving interventions on the cognitive-behavioural treatment of pathological gambling. *J Gambl Stud* 2002;18(2):207–229.
68. Melville CL, Davis CS, Matzenbacher DL, et al. Node-link-mapping-enhanced group treatment for pathological gambling. *Addict Behav* 2004;29:73–87.
69. Wulfert E, Blanchard EB, Freidenberg BM. Retaining pathological gamblers in cognitive behavior therapy through motivational enhancement. *Behav Mod* 2006;30(3):315–340.
70. Dickerson M, Hinchy, J, England SL. Minimal treatments and problem gamblers: a preliminary investigation. *J Gambl Stud* 1990;6(1):87–102.
71. Hodgins DC, Currie S, el-Guebaly N. Motivational enhancement and self-help treatments for problem gambling. *J Couns Clin Psychol* 2001;69(1):50–57.
72. Hodgins DC, Currie S, el-Guebaly N, et al. Brief motivational treatment for problem gambling: a 24-month follow-up. *Psychol Addict Behav* 2004;18(3):293–296.
73. Hodgins DC, Holub A. Treatment of problem gambling. In: Smith G, Hodgins DC, Williams RJ, eds. *Research and measurement issues in gambling studies*. Burlington, MA: Elsevier, 2007:371–397.
74. Kim SW, Grant JE, Adson DE, et al. Double-blind naltrexone and placebo comparison study in the treatment of pathological gambling. *Biol Psychiatry* 2001;49(11):914–921.
75. Grant JE, Kim SW, Hartman, BK. A double-blind, placebo-controlled study of the opiate antagonist, naltrexone, in the treatment of pathological gambling urges. *J Clin Psychiatry* 2008;69(5):783–789.
76. Grant JE, Potenza MN, Hollander E, et al. Multicenter investigation of the opioid antagonist nalmefene in the treatment of pathological gambling. *Am J Psychiatry* 2006;163(2):303–312.
77. Linnoila M, Virkkunen M, George T, et al. Impulse control disorders. *Int Clin Psychopharmacol* 1993;8(Suppl 1):53–56.
78. Virkkunen M, Goldman D, Nielsen DA, et al. Low brain serotonin turnover rate (low CSF 5-HIAA) and impulsive violence. *J Psychiatry Neurosci* 1995;20(4):271–275.
79. Potenza MN, Leung HC, Blumberg HP, et al. An FMRI Stroop task study of ventromedial prefrontal cortical function in pathological gamblers. *Am J Psychiatry* 2003;160(11):1990–1994.
80. Reuter J, Raedler T, Rose M, et al. Pathological gambling is linked to reduced activation of the mesolimbic reward system. *Nat Neurosci* 2005;8(2):147–148.
81. Kim SW, Grant JE, Adson DE, et al. A double-blind placebo-controlled study of the efficacy and safety of paroxetine in the treatment of pathological gambling. *J Clin Psychiatry* 2002;63(6):501–507.
82. Grant JE, Kim SW, Potenza MN, et al. Paroxetine treatment of pathological gambling: a multi-centre randomized controlled trial. *Int Clin Psychopharmacol* 2003;18(4):243–249.
83. Hollander E, DeCaria CM, Finkell JN, et al. A randomized double-blind fluvoxamine/placebo crossover trial in pathologic gambling. *Biol Psychiatry* 2000;47(9):813–817.
84. Blanco C, Petkova E, Ibáñez A, et al. A pilot placebo-controlled study of fluvoxamine for pathological gambling. *Ann Clin Psychiatry* 2002;14(1):9–15.
85. Sáiz-Ruiz J, Blanco C, Ibáñez A, et al. Sertraline treatment of pathological gambling: a pilot study. *J Clin Psychiatry* 2005;66(1):28–33.
86. Grant JE, Potenza MN. Escitalopram treatment of pathological gambling with co-occurring anxiety: an open-label pilot study with double-blind discontinuation. *Int Clin Psychopharmacol* 2006;21(4):203–209.
87. Black DW, Arndt S, Coryell WH, et al. Bupropion in the treatment of pathological gambling: a randomized, double-blind, placebo-controlled, flexible-dose study. *J Clin Psychopharmacol* 2007;27(2):143–150.
88. Hollander E, Pallanti S, Allen, A., et al. Does sustained-release lithium reduce impulsive gambling and affective instability versus placebo in pathological gamblers with bipolar spectrum disorders? *Am J Psychiatry* 2005;162(1):137–145.
89. Kalivas PW, Peters J, Knackstedt L. Animal models and brain circuits in drug addiction. *Mol Interv* 2006;6(6):339–344.
90. Grant JE, Kim SW, Odlaug BL. N-acetyl cysteine, a glutamate-modulating agent, in the treatment of pathological gambling: a pilot study. *Biol Psychiatry* 2007;62(6):652–657.
91. Petry NM. *Pathological gambling: etiology, comorbidity, and treatment.* Washington, DC: American Psychological Association, 2005.

CHAPTER 39

Steven J. Shoptaw, PhD

Sexual Addiction

The notion that individuals can become addicted to a behavior as fundamental as sex carries controversy, in both the professional and the lay communities (1). Yet, individuals affected by such a behavior disorder commonly express symptoms that parallel dependence to nicotine, alcohol, and illicit drugs (2). The parallels are striking, including repetitive, compulsive behaviors that impact on neurobiology, social environments, and the health of the individual and the public during the development, maintenance, and treatment of the disorder. The concept of sexual addiction shares other defining features with substance dependence, including clinically significant distress due to negative consequences of compulsive and impulsive sexual behaviors.

The Task Force on the Fifth Edition of the Diagnostic and Statistical Manual of Mental Disorders adopted the charge of considering a formal definition for sexual addiction. This effort would classify the disorder as a variant of obsessive-compulsive disorder, more precisely as "compulsive-impulsive sexual behavior" (3). As implied by the name, the diagnostic category reflects the central feature of compulsive sexual behaviors due to impaired impulse inhibition. This chapter reviews the scientific evidence regarding the concept of sexual addiction, discusses the known epidemiology of the disorder, recognizes the comorbidities with sexual addiction, provides evaluation of measures used to assess sexual addiction, and discusses the evidence for different approaches to treatment.

DEFINITIONS

Sixty years after Kinsey's groundbreaking reports on male (4) and female (5) sexuality, there is still a wide range of opinion on what defines abnormal or pathologic sexual behaviors. Two current boundaries that define pathologic (and illegal) sexual behavior involve inclusion of sexual partners who are children and sexual partners who are subjected to aggression, physically or emotionally. Among clinicians who treat individuals seeking relief from sexual addiction, whether for pathologic/illegal sexual behaviors or for behaviors that are legal but carry distress to the individual and family, the notion that sexual behavior can manifest as an addiction conforms well to the presentation of addictions to chemicals (2,6). Still, outside legal sanctions against behaviors that involve pedophilia, violence, or abuse, there are no agreed upon cut points that distinguish "normal" from "out-of-control" sexual behaviors (7,8). Formal definitions of human sexual urges as abnormal or excessive remain as culturally defined and historically influenced (9). Earlier reviews consider these and other issues related to definitions of normal and abnormal human sexual behaviors (10).

Understandably, research and clinical reports on sexual addiction have yet to arrive at an agreed-upon title for the concept. A variety of definitional terms have been used to refer to the phenomenon, including *sexual addiction* (6,11), *compulsive sexual behavior* (12,14,15), *pathologic sexual behavior*, *erotomania*, *hypersexuality* (16,17), *paraphilias* and *paraphilia-related disorders* (18), and *sexual impulsivity* (19). As currently referenced in the DSM-IV-Text Revision, disorders consistent with sexual addiction are defined as paraphilias and paraphilia-related disorders that involve "recurrent, intense sexually arousing fantasies, urges or behaviors involving (1) nonhuman objects, (2) the suffering or humiliation of oneself or one's partner, or (3) children or other non-consenting persons" (20).

Throughout this chapter, the term *sexual addiction* is used except when describing outcomes in which authors reference a different term.

Sexual addiction shares many of the elements and problems of other behavioral disorders defined by excessive consumption and that cause clinical distress. While many professionals and affected individuals agree that sexual addiction is defined by repetitive, frequent, and compulsive sexual behaviors, there are few evidence-based, quantitative definitions of sexual addiction that are based on amount of sexual behaviors. Moreover, existing quantitative definitions are not adopted consistently across the field (21). The etiology of sexual addition is articulated primarily based on retrospective clinical reports. As with many other behavioral disorders, there are no pathogens recognized as causal and only initial suggestions that brain dysfunction might be identified to account for the distress caused by compulsive sexual behaviors. Complicating efforts at nosology, behaviors consistent with the concept of sexual addiction are common features of major psychiatric diagnoses, especially those indicating impaired impulse inhibition (e.g., bipolar disorder, schizophrenia, stimulant dependence, and antisocial personality disorder).

Although there may be utility in a diagnostic category that defines the disorder of sexual addiction, the DSM-IV-Text Revision (22) does not formally classify sexual addiction as an addictive behavior. Instead, clinicians code the behavior under diagnostic entities that either feature impaired impulse control (e.g., Impulse-Control Disorders Not Otherwise Specified) or as a variant of the paraphilia disorders (Paraphilic Sexual Disorder, Non-paraphilic Sexual Disorder) (23). Recommendations by the Task Force guiding revisions to the DSM-V on a diagnostic category defining compulsive-impulsive sexual behavior using behavioral criteria sets will undoubtedly help to clarify defining elements of the clinical phenomenon and to improve quality of research on incidence, prevalence, etiology and treatment.

Although repetitive, compulsive sex, obsessive thoughts about sex, and the consequences of these are central defining features, sexual addiction can vary greatly in presentation in different groups of individuals. Among heterosexual men, the issue of sexual conquest of many female partners (i.e., "the hunt") can play a central role, and the focus can center on physical sexual gratification (23,24). Women as well can express insatiable desires for sexual intercourse linked to conquest issues (25) but can also present with "dependency needs" that are relieved with frequent sexual activity with multiple male partners (26). Women also can focus on the romantic or emotional aspects of sexuality (24). Across both genders, excessive masturbation is common in sexual addiction.

The presentation of sexual addiction among gay and bisexual men, however, varies somewhat for important reasons. In general, gay and bisexual men have more sexual partners than heterosexual men (27), even when comparing stimulant-dependent gay and bisexual men with stimulant-dependent heterosexual men (28). This may be owing to easier access to sexual partners willing to sexually liaise approached at sexual venues and the Internet. As well, anxiety and conflicts about ones' homosexual orientation, including societal homophobia, may contribute to obsessive thinking and sexual compulsivity (2,27). There are no published reports of behaviors consistent with sexual addiction in lesbians. Indeed, it appears that lesbian women report lower numbers of sexual episodes compared to heterosexual women (29).

Specific sexual behaviors engaged in by individuals and society's sanctions against the behaviors vary systematically across groups, as well. For example, heterosexual men and gay and bisexual men with sexual addictions differ significantly in that men who meet criteria for nonparaphilia-related disorders (i.e., persistent and disinhibited forms of socially tolerated sexual behaviors) are significantly more likely to be gay or bisexual than heterosexual. By contrast, men with paraphilias (repetitive, socially deviant, and sanctioned expressions of intensified sexual arousal and associated behaviors, including exhibitionism, voyeurism, pedophilia, sexual masochism and sadism, fetishism, transvestic fetishism, frotteurism, and telephone scatologia) are significantly more likely to be heterosexual and less likely to be gay or bisexual (30).

DIAGNOSIS

The group of individuals easiest to diagnose with a form of sexual addiction are those (primarily men) who meet criteria for paraphilia disorders (18). The societal and legal sanctions on many of these sexual behaviors frequently require individuals with paraphilias to submit to the justice system for remedy and to the medical establishment for treatment (including chemical castration). Outside the paraphilias, however, sexual addiction typically presents with specific behaviors that are not socially sanctioned but that often cause significant clinical distress and that may be concomitant with other problems, such as substance abuse or mental disorders (2,6).

One of the behavioral complaints common to individuals who seek treatment for sexual addiction involves the large amounts of time they take from their days to plan or engage in sexual behaviors, either alone or with partners. These behaviors include hours spent on the Internet seeking their next sexual connections (in chat rooms or sex sites), seeking out sex venues, engaging in public sex, and masturbating to pornography (31). As well, individuals complain of sexual behaviors that are repetitive, persistent, compulsive, and out-of-control and, when not engaged in the behaviors, individuals report obsessive thoughts about their sexual behaviors (13). The characteristic of obsessive sexual thoughts in such individuals contributed to development of a model defining the disorder as a variant of obsessive-compulsive disorder (3). Negative self-evaluations or feelings are also part of the definition of sexual addiction and that result from their sexual behaviors, including feeling abnormal or sick; feeling degraded, guilty, or shamed; feeling regret, depression, or discomfort; or feeling numb, hollow, or empty (32).

The presentation of sexual addiction conforms well to application of diagnostic criteria for substance abuse disorders (2). Consistent with substance abuse disorders, individuals with sexual addiction engage in sexually compulsive behaviors repeatedly despite knowledge of adverse medical, legal, and/or interpersonal consequences. Obsessive sexual thoughts can serve as a coping mechanism during periods of stress or interpersonal conflict, contributing to large amounts of time planning, engaging in, or recovering from the behavior (6). Some note the need for increased sexual activities and describe experiences consistent with the concept of tolerance (i.e., that more of the behavior is needed to get the feelings one got when she or he first started the behavior) and extreme mood changes that are related to sexual activity (euphoria) or its abstinence (depression) (2). Finally, many with sexual addiction will engage in the behavior at the neglect of social-recreational activities and role responsibilities (6).

One notable attempt to quantify sexually compulsive behavior and to distinguish between socially conforming sexual behaviors and behaviors that are nonsocially conforming defines "hypersexual desire" in men as persistence of seven or more orgasms per week for a minimum duration of 6 months or more after age 15 (33). This definition characterizes between 3% and 8% of responses in nationally representative surveys of male sexual behavior in the United States (33,34) and Sweden (35). The definition also shows particular relevance to men with paraphilia or paraphilia related disorders: Some 72% met the threshold for "hypersexual desire" as indicated by spending 1 to 2 hours per day engaged in their compulsive sexual behaviors (33). The definition, however, may not extend as well to females, as fewer women in the population engage in high rates of sexual behavior. In one national telephone survey of 987 white or black women, 24.1% reported sexual intercourse several times per week but only 1.1% daily, with far fewer reporting masturbation several times per week (4.5%) and only 1.6% reporting daily masturbation (36).

There are no evidence-based estimates of the prevalence of sexual addiction. In one online survey,17% of 9,265 respondents reported symptoms consistent with sexual compulsivity using Kalichman's Sexual Compulsivity Scale (37). Yet, this percentage is high when compared to probability-based surveys of sexual behaviors showing a very low percentage of younger American males and females (aged 15 to 44) who report three or more sexual partners in any year (38), which would indicate that a much smaller minority of Americans might meet the criteria for this disorder than convenience samples might indicate. Finally, there are no reports on the incidence of such a disorder; however, retrospective self-reports of individuals seeking treatment for sexual addiction suggest the condition typically begins in the late teens or early twenties and is chronic or intermittent (12).

ETIOLOGY

The quality of evidence supporting the etiology of a sexual addiction is poor, with much of the literature describing etiology being based on theory. In one comprehensive report (20), several theories are reviewed that may be the basis for the development of paraphilias and hypersexual disorders. These include endocrine dysfunctions, the monoamine hypothesis, incomplete developmental processes (including an "imprinting hypothesis"—particular sentinel experiences during adolescence becoming the model of compulsive sexual behaviors in adulthood), and a courtship disorder (i.e., an adolescent who fails to successfully negotiate one of the stages to establish an intimate relationship may associate with the type of compulsive sexual behavior in adulthood), social learning theory, and psychodynamic theories (10). Each of these theories, however, is descriptive and provides no data.

From a developmental perspective, human sexual behavior typically initiates in early to mid-adolescence, with most individuals initiating sexual behaviors by early adulthood. From this developmental stance, acquisition of sexual behavior during adolescence is a period of life marked by exploration, particularly regarding sex (39). Thus, engaging in one or a few episodes of uncommon sexual behaviors while an adolescent would not seem especially pathognomonic, but repetitiously engaging multiple sexual partners, not using condoms consistently, and combining alcohol/substance use with sex could indicate sexual behavior problems in youth (40). Still, there are no indications that the concept of sexual addiction extends down to adolescents or that the behaviors noted in retrospective studies significantly predict those individuals who go on to develop sexual addiction in adulthood (32).

There are, however, better data documenting trauma in the histories of individuals who develop sexual addiction. Developmental traumatic experiences commonly recognized among individuals with sexual addiction include childhood sexual abuse (2,6,24,26), early substance use, impulse inhibition problems, and peer and family influences (32,40). In a retrospective report of a large survey on the sexual health of adults in Sweden, both men and women who scored above 90% on measures consistent with hypersexual behaviors (i.e., times masturbated [past month]; times viewed pornography [past month]; number sexual partners [past year]; more than one current sexual partner; prefer casual sex; and had group sex) reported significant correlations with separation from parents during childhood, earlier age of first sexual experience, and more varied sexual behaviors while young (35). As well, these respondents reported significantly greater likelihood of being current cigarette smokers, being substantially drunk in the past month, ever having used illegal drugs, and ever having gambled (35). Finally, one report indicates a high co-occurrence of individuals with sexual addiction and the experience of having family members with sexual or other types of addiction (41).

The foregoing reports are associational in nature and provide little guidance about the types of trauma that might discriminate youth who develop sexual addiction in adulthood from those who do not. Specifically, many more youth experience childhood sexual abuse, early substance use, attention deficit hyperactivity disorder (ADHD) and impoverished social and family backgrounds and do not develop sexual addiction than those who have these experiences and go on to develop sexual addiction. One notable exception, however, are some unique data that distinguish men who develop pedophilia from those who develop sexual addictions that do not focus on children as erotic targets. Specifically, there is an interesting correlation between number of head injuries experienced prior to age 13 and preference of children as erotic stimuli. In a forensic sample of men (N = 685) tested using penile tumescence measures and detailed sexual histories to determine whether the men adjudicated for sexual offenses preferred children or adults in erotic stimuli, men who reported a history of three or more head traumas before age 13 were significantly more likely to have pedophilia (become aroused by children in erotic stimuli) than were men with fewer than three head traumas before age 13 (42). Additional significant correlates for the group of men with more than three injuries prior to age 13 included childhood ADHD. Men who preferred erotic stimuli with adults older than 17 reported fewer than three head traumas before age 13 but were significantly more likely to report substance abuse histories. Though this is only a single report correlating tumescence and sexual history data, findings provide a suggestion that the development of pedophilia may be unique and emphasize repeated early head trauma, especially in comparison to the development of sexual compulsive behaviors that have adults as the erotic focus.

Sexual Addiction and Gay Men Although sexual addiction may be expressed differently in gay and bisexual men than in heterosexual men, studies provide strong evidence that the concept of sexual addiction appears to differentiate a group of gay and bisexual men whose sexual behaviors are more compulsive, more repetitive, and more distressing than for gay and bisexual men in general. Using the Sexual Compulsivity Scale (14) to select a sample that scored one standard deviation or higher above the mean, qualitative interview data for 146 gay and bisexual men indicated there are five intrinsic explanations for sexually compulsive behaviors: negative affect, low self-esteem, needs for validation and affection, stress release, and having a high sex drive (27). Explanations that were external to the men that were offered for explaining their sexually compulsive behaviors include relationship issues, the easy availability of gay sex, childhood sexual abuse, and parental conflicts/deficiencies. Findings are consistent with a large venue-based sample of gay and bisexual men who reported sex in the past 3 months with a casual partner, although findings from this latter sample emphasized associations showing higher expectations for engaging in unprotected sex when alcohol or drugs are used before or during sex (43).

Several studies in gay and bisexual men correlate Sexual Compulsivity Scale scores and various indices of sexual behaviors. In two studies of gay and bisexual men positive for human immunodeficiency virus (HIV), high scores on the Sexual Compulsivity Scale (implicating sexually compulsive behaviors) corresponded with remarkably similar behavioral and psychologic outcomes. In the most recent (N = 217), higher scores on the Sexual Compulsivity Scale associated significantly with older age, using methamphetamine before or during sex, going to sex venues or street corners for sex partners, low self-efficacy for condom use, low levels of self-esteem, higher disinhibition, and a higher number of HIV-negative or status-unknown sexual partners (44). An earlier report (45) (N = 112) found higher Sexual Compulsivity Scale scores associated significantly with more frequent unprotected sexual acts with more partners, greater use of cocaine during sex, enjoyment of high-risk sex, and low self-esteem. In an online survey of 513 gay and bisexual men recruited in a gay chat room, Sexual Compulsivity Scale scores correlated significantly with ratings of internalized homophobia and numbers of male sexual partners met online (46). Venue-based questionnaire results collected for 687 gay and bisexual men who attended large gay community events in New York City and who reported having more than one sexual partner found that 82 (12%) of respondents indicated they self-identified as a "barebacker" — engages in unprotected anal sex (47). Factors significantly associated with identity as a engaging in unprotected anal sex were use of methamphetamine during sex in the past 3 months and higher peer norms for unprotected sexual behaviors. Findings reported are drawn from venue based and convenience samples, which does not support estimates of prevalence of sexual addiction in gay and bisexual men. It does appear, however, that the concept of sexual addiction can be observed in gay and bisexual men similar as in heterosexual groups, albeit with somewhat different defining criteria. Across these studies, there are remarkably strong associations between reported substance use, particularly stimulant use, and sexual behaviors consistent with sexual addiction.

Neurobiology of Sexual Addiction There exists a small literature on the neurobiology of healthy male sexual behavior. One report described regional cerebral blood flow as being diminished throughout brain during orgasm in eight healthy males undergoing single-photon emission computed tomography excepting regions in the right temporal lobe (48). An alternate approach to imaging studies experimentally manipulates presentation of erotic and neutral stimuli among young adult male heterosexual subjects under positron emission tomography (49,50,51). Findings indicate that erotic visual stimuli activate brain regions that include the right insula and claustrum (somatosensory processing and recognition of erection), the hypothalamus and striatum (areas of dopamine neurotransmission), the anterior cingulate gyrus (shifting attention, repetitive behavior, endocrine and gonadal secretions), in addition to activation in the occipital cortex (visual processing) (49,50). It is possible that studies of neurobiology of individuals with sexual addiction will one day articulate dysfunction in brain regions that may advise development of medication and/or behavioral approaches to treatment. For example, in one study, men with pedophilia (N = 65) completed T-$_1$ weighted functional magnetic resonance imaging scans and voxel-based morphometry, which were compared to 62 men who were nonsexual offenders. Findings showed significant reductions in white matter volume in the fiber bundles of the superior fronto-occipital fasciculus and the right arcuate in the pedophilia group. No such associations were observed in scans from the 62 men who were nonsexual offenders included as a control condition (52). These differences are observed in fibers that connect areas of the brain that respond to sexual cues, suggesting that pedophilia may result from disruption of the networks of brain regions connected by these fibers.

Observational evidence describes neurobiologic events and neurotransmission factors that can support development of sexual compulsivity later in the lifespan that can give some indications of mechanisms (35,53). Patients with brain injury in the right temporal areas develop sexual compulsivity, which is very consistent with positron emission tomography studies indicating these areas are associated with male heterosexual response (49,50,51). Patients with stroke and with multiple sclerosis also experience high rates of sexual behaviors that develop later in life and after occurrence of these conditions (35).

Dopamine neurotransmission is also strongly implicated in the expression of sexual addiction. Among 300 patients with Parkinson disease, 58 (19.3%) self-reported they developed behavioral compulsions. Of those who reported compulsive behaviors, 25 (43.1%) reported sexual compulsivity, and the remainder reported gambling compulsion. Of interest, all of those who developed sexual compulsivity were male, and all were on stable dopamine agonist therapy (54). Preexisting histories of an impulse control disorder (e.g., substance abuse) increased the odds of developing compulsive sexual disorder under dopamine agonist treatment, leaving some to believe that patients and their families should be warned of this potential serious adverse event before starting such care (55). Multiple case reports noted development of different forms of compulsive sexual behaviors when patients with Parkinson's disease engage in long-term treatment using dopamine agonists (56) such as selegiline and pergolide (57,58).

PSYCHIATRIC COMORBIDITY

Reports consistently implicate impulsivity, obsessions, and compulsivity as central issues in the expression of sexual addiction. Several psychiatric conditions share one or more of these features. Impulsivity is a core feature of ADHD, bipolar disorders, and substance abuse and dependence. In the original work describing experiences with 932 individuals with sexual addiction (6), 28% of individuals with sexual addiction reported working compulsively, 26% reported spending compulsively, 38% reported disordered eating, and 42% reported substance dependence. A more recent report is consistent with this initial finding (41). About one-third of psychiatric inpatients had comorbid impulse control disorders in one sample, with 4.4% of these having current and 4.9% lifetime prevalence of comorbid sexual compulsive behaviors (59). Though the study did not include formal assessment of sexual compulsive behaviors in 403 adolescents seen in primary care settings, those rated as having three or more symptoms of Axis II diagnoses reported higher numbers of sexual partners than those with symptoms of two or fewer Axis II diagnoses. The association was stronger in females than in males (60).

In samples of men with paraphilia and paraphilia-related disorders, psychiatric comorbidity is highly prevalent. In one sample of clinic-referred males diagnosed with paraphilias (N = 88), 60 of whom who were sex offenders, and paraphilia-related disorders (n = 32), 86% met criteria for any mood disorder, 46% met criteria for any anxiety disorder, and 49% met criteria for any psychoactive substance abuse (61). Men with paraphilias reported a broader range of problems with impaired impulse inhibition than those with paraphilia related disorders; specifically, significantly higher rates of lifetime cocaine abuse (18.1% vs. 3.1%), ADHD (42.0% vs. 18.7%), and conduct disorder (22.7% vs. 0%).

High prevalence of psychiatric comorbidities is also observed in community samples of individuals who defined their behavior as sexually compulsive. In one (N = 36), 39% met criteria for lifetime mood disorders, 50% for lifetime anxiety disorders, and 64% for lifetime substance abuse disorders (12). In another (N = 24, including two females), all subjects met lifetime criteria for any Axis I disorder (mood disorders, 71%; anxiety disorders, 96%). Fully 88% met criteria for any current Axis I disorders (mood disorders, 33%; anxiety disorders, 42%), with 29% and 71% who met criteria for any substance use disorder current and lifetime, respectively, and the most frequent diagnosis involving alcohol. On Axis II, 46% met criteria for any disorder, predominantly cluster C disorders (31). In a retrospective chart review of 85 patients treated for compulsive sexual behavior and psychiatric diagnoses, few symptoms of borderline personality disorder were observed, and only one patient was diagnosed with the disorder (62).

Depression Among individuals with substance abuse and dependence, there is a high rate of psychiatric comorbidities, particularly depression (63). As noted, in small samples recruited from the community, depressive disorders correspond significantly with sexual compulsivity (12,31). In a report of 220 male participants recruited via an online newsletter, high scores on the sexual addiction screening test (SAST) correlated significantly and positively with scores on the Beck depression inventory (BDI). Though no information about prevalence of either of these disorders can be inferred from this report (as neither the SAST nor the BDI scores are sufficient for inferring clinical diagnoses), findings do provide an indication of the high co-occurrence of depressive symptoms in men who self-report behaviors consistent with sexual addiction.

Anxiety The prevalence of current and lifetime anxiety disorders are reported earlier. Presence of anxiety symptoms appears to be somewhat higher in individuals with behaviors consistent with sexual addiction as compared to controls. In an early study, participants recruited from 12-step self-help venues were classified into three groups based on their behavioral presentations: sexual addiction (n = 32), pathologic gamblers (n = 38), and nonaddict controls (64). Comparison of scores for the symptom checklist-90-R along depression, anxiety, interpersonal sensitivity, and obsessive compulsive subscales showed significantly higher scores for individuals in the sexual addiction group than for controls.

Attention Deficit Hyperactivity Disorder Some retrospective reports suggest associations between ADHD during childhood and presence of sexual addiction (65). Seventy-two individuals seeking treatment for sexual addiction completed a variety of scales to assess symptoms of sexual compulsivity; 34% scored in the range of probable ADHD diagnosis. As noted, data collected from a forensic setting (42) showed presence of ADHD and more than three head traumas before age 13 corresponded with hypersexuality in the form of pedophilia in adult men. Similar findings are reported in a much smaller sample of individuals diagnosed with paraphilias (n = 42) and paraphilia-related disorders (n = 18). This report indicated the only significant variable discriminating between the two groups of men was symptoms consistent with ADHD during childhood as measured using the Wender Utah Retrospective Scale and paraphilia (66). Though retrospective reports indicate significant correlation of ADHD in samples of men with behaviors consistent with sexual addiction, it is possible that childhood ADHD is a correlate of sexual behaviors in adult men that are sanctioned.

ASSESSMENT

Individuals who present to a clinician for treatment or to a researcher for evaluation need careful evaluation to define the presenting problem, as would occur in any clinical or research setting involving those experiencing pathology and/or distress. Standard areas to review include current presentation and history of the sexual addiction: Did something precipitate the visit? Exactly what is the patient doing, at what frequency, and under what circumstances to define compulsive sexual behaviors? What is the gender and age of the partners involved with the individual? What is the development of the behavior—from childhood to present? What is the individual's experience with sexual abuse, physical abuse, and head or other physical trauma as a child? When were symptoms or distress the worst? What has helped reduce the severity of symptoms or distress in the past?

In addition, careful review of ways in which the sexual addiction impacted areas of functioning is crucial. This starts with thorough review of medical history (especially regarding treatments for sexually transmitted infections), employment background and pattern, involvement with alcohol and drugs (including nicotine and marijuana) that may be used before, during, and after sexually compulsive behaviors, detailed history of legal problems (whether formal charges were or were not recorded), quality of relationships with family, friends, and intimates (if any), and mental health functioning, including both diagnosable psychiatric conditions and subthreshold mood, affect, and cognitive disturbances. This ancillary information provides strong indications as to whether the behaviors indicating sexual addiction are localized or are more generalized across most domains of functioning for the individual.

Over the past 15 years or so, several measures have been developed, and psychometric properties are established for their use, in arriving at valid and reliable assays of sexually compulsive behaviors. These include the Total Sexual Outlet Inventory, the Compulsive Sexual Scale, the Compulsive Sexual Behavior Inventory, and the Sexual Arousal and Desire Inventory. A female-specific measure used in gynecologic practice and research—the Female Sexual Function Index (67,68,69)—is frequently used to assess sexual dysfunction in women, but there are few reports of the scale used to measure women with sexual addiction, and the scale is not reviewed. As well, some investigators and clinicians have developed measures used in specific clinical or research projects, but they are not reviewed owing to their limited use and limited descriptions of their psychometrics. A notable example of this is the Compulsive Sexual Behavior Consequences Scale, which was used in a small randomized, placebo-controlled trial of citalopram for compulsive sexual behavior (70).

Sexual Addiction Screening Test The SAST (71), is a 25-item test in which respondents answer questions with yes or no regarding various aspects of their sexual behaviors. The test is very popular and can easily be found on various Web sites that provide services to individuals considering intervention for sexually compulsive behaviors. A simple sum is computed of all items answered affirmatively, with scores >10 interpreted to suggest need for consultation for treatment of sexual addiction and scores >13 as indicating immediate need for treatment. In the original sample of 191 men with sexual addiction and 67 controls, alphas were reported as .92 and .85, respectively, which are similar to that reported in a recent report of 629 veterans receiving treatment for addiction problems who also completed the SAST (72). More recent reports, however, in a sample of 125 college students who completed the male version of the SAST (G-SAST) had alpha of .66 (73). Although the psychometrics may vary somewhat, perhaps with greater internal consistency as age increases, the SAST test remains the most popularly available assessment used to define sexual addiction.

Sexual Outlet Inventory The Sexual Outlet Inventory is a clinician-administered rating scale that quantifies sexual fantasies, urges, and behaviors to distinguish unconventional (paraphilic) from conventional (not paraphilic) sexual behavior. Total Sexual Outlet measures the number of orgasms achieved in a week. Men who have a Total Sexual Outlet score of seven or more orgasms per week for a minimum duration of 6 months with onset after age 15 are defined as having "*hypersexual desire*" (18). This criterion reflects only 3% to 8% of males in nationally representative samples of sexual behavior who report a Total Sexual Outlet greater than this level and 72% of men diagnosed with paraphilia or paraphilia-related disorders who report a Total Sexual Outlet greater than this level (18). The Total Sexual Outlet score has been used in several of Kafka's studies on the monoamine hypothesis among men with paraphilia- and nonparaphilia-related disorders, including a treatment study on sertraline (74).

Sexual Compulsivity Scale The scale most frequently used in reports of sexual addiction is Kalichman's Sexual Compulsivity Scale (SCS). The SCS was originally developed on two samples (296 gay and bisexual men and 158 inner-city men and women) to measure sexual behaviors that corresponded to engaging risk behaviors involved in HIV transmission (14). The scale is composed of 32 items that are answered on a Likert scale ranging from 1 (not at all like me) to 4 (very much like me). Scores are calculated as means for the total items and for three subscales. Reliability for the gay male and low income heterosexual samples (respectively) were sexual sensation seeking (11 items; $\alpha = .82, .79$), nonsexual sensation seeking (11 items; $\alpha = .81, .79$), and sexual compulsivity scales (10 items; $\alpha = .86, .87$). Psychometric properties of the SCS in 876 heterosexual college students showed similar high reliability for the overall totals ($\alpha = .82$), and with male ($\alpha = .77$) and female subgroups ($\alpha = .81$); (75). High scores on the SCS also correlated significantly with higher numbers of sexual partners, more episodes of masturbation, and reports of public sex experiences.

The scale also has strong content validity. HIV-negative men who have sex with other men, who report recent commission of one or more acts of unprotected anal intercourse with other than a main partner, and who score in the highest quartile of the SCS also reported significantly more sexual partners and that they met more partners in Internet sites than men with lower SCS scores (76). There is published information indicating the SCS performs well in ethnic groups. In a sample of primarily African American males receiving treatment at a clinic for sexually transmitted infections, subjects who scored one standard deviation above the mean for the Sexual Compulsivity Scale ($\geq$80% or a total score of $\geq$24) had significantly more sexual partners, had significantly more recent diagnoses of sexually transmitted infections, and had higher rates of sexual risk behaviors with casual or one-time sexual partners (77). High scores on the SCS are not sufficient to diagnose individuals with sexual compulsivity or sexual addiction. Instead, the scores provide one marker of impaired impulse inhibition in the domain of sexual behavior. As noted, diagnoses of sexual compulsivity or addiction should be arrived at using multiple and consistent sources of information. As well, SCS scores provide no indication of an individual's readiness to engage in treatment for their sexual compulsivity, as there are no significant associations between SCS scores and scores indicating readiness to change as measured using the Stages of Change scale (78). Instead it appears that many individuals seeking intervention are highly ambivalent and likely to discontinue treatment early, regardless of SCS score (79).

Compulsive Sexual Behavior Inventory The Compulsive Sexual Behavior Inventory (CSBI) was originally developed to measure factors of control (over sexual behaviors), abuse (sexual and physical), and violence (current and historical) (80). Though developed on small samples of men with nonparaphilic compulsive sexual behaviors (n = 15), pedophiles (n = 35), and controls (n = 42), the total score for the scale correctly discriminated 92% of subjects with compulsive sexual behaviors from control subjects. In a much larger sample, 1,026 Latino men recruited via the Internet completed the scale (81), and a two-factor solution (control and violence) emerged, generally replicating the original findings. Men with higher CSBI scores also reported behaviors consistent with aspects of compulsive sexual behavior problems, including being high/drunk, feeling depressed, and feeling lonely. Scores above the median CSBI also correlated with higher numbers of sexual partners. In addition to demonstrating psychometric abilities when used in ethnic samples, an equivalent version of the scale is available in Spanish language.

TREATMENT APPROACHES

Behavior Therapies Treatment approaches for sexual addictions involve behavioral and/or pharmacologic approaches. Reflecting the nascent state of the treatment field, behavioral models for treating sexual addiction are largely descriptive and draw upon existing models for treating substance abuse (e.g., cognitive behavioral therapy, motivational interviewing). All reports on behavioral therapies are either reports of open trials or case reports, which provide descriptive feasibility information but no information about efficacy.

One early open trial of outpatient psychotherapy for compulsive sexual behavior in gay and bisexual men (82) indicated that the 15 subjects who were able to retain in treatment of the 30 subjects followed, the men reported significant reductions in numbers of sexual partners, in public sex and in combining drugs and alcohol with sex. Another open trial commented on the experiences of individuals who completed five consecutive 8-day treatment programs in a 1-year period (38 completers of 53 who initiated treatment, or 71.7%), reported generally favorable reductions in psychologic distress and some indices of sexually compulsive behaviors (83). Literature documenting outcomes for residential treatment is also poorly developed, with one report indicating that 71% of 202 individuals followed up over a 4-year period relapsed to compulsive sexual behaviors, yet that most reported positive outcomes associated with retention in treatment (84). Outcomes from these open trial reports of various types of psychotherapy for sexual addiction are generally unimpressive and confirm the bromide familiar to all psychotherapy researchers: "treatment works for who it works for." There is little direction from this literature that might identify groups of subjects for whom treatment works well or what might be considered for the larger group of patients who terminate early or who show only partial or wholly inadequate responses to treatment. Not one published randomized controlled trial exists to document outcomes of behavioral treatments for sexual addiction that might provide evidence to guide the decisions of clinicians working with this pathology group.

In a comprehensive review of family therapies for sexual addiction, two papers include data to describe experiences of family members of sexual addicts who are undergoing family therapy (85). In one, a description of 94 participants is provided, indicating sexual problems in the couple and describing problems when disclosing information about the sexual addiction to children (86). In the other, qualitative reports of 39 wives of sexual addicts were compared to 36 wives of men who were not sexual addicts and showed wives of sexual addicts were more likely to report early histories of chaotic families of origin (e.g., abuse, abandonment) than wives of men without sexual addiction (87). The review references a few psychodynamic family therapy reports, but these are limited to descriptions of models or processes. As earlier, there are no controlled trials to document the value of family therapy for treating sexual addiction.

An issue important to any form of treatment for sexual addiction is how to address the topic of sexual addiction within the family. In one clinical report, female spouses/partners of male sexual addicts are presented as having a central role in maintaining the dysfunction of the compulsive sexual behaviors of the male (88,89). Some data describe outcomes when disclosing sexual addiction in families. Individuals in treatment for sexual addiction typically prefer not to disclose information to their spouses and/or children. When female spouses (N = 63) learned of their husbands' sexual addiction, 75% did so from their discovery; few found out via planned disclosures by the husband (90). Once the disclosure is made, however, the impact on the women was traumatic regardless of whether finding out accidentally or from a planned disclosure. Disclosures by parents with sexual addiction (N = 57) to children, whether made in anger or in unplanned or forced disclosures (i.e., someone threatened to tell), predictably caused upset in the children. By contrast, planned disclosures allowed for forethought about what information to tell the children and allowed the discloser to emphasize the amount of disturbance he has caused the family rather than provide accounts of his behaviors (91).

Cognitive Behavioral Therapy Cognitive behavioral therapy (CBT) is a general approach to treating addictive behavioral disorders that teach patients skills to instill abstinence and to return to abstinence upon relapse. The approach is highly didactic and involves the counselor adopting the role of a coach to the patient. The approach is based largely in social learning theory (92) and conceptualizes compulsive sexual behaviors as being maintained both by experiences that initiated and sustained the behaviors and by a lack of noncompulsive sexual behavior experiences that might be engaged in lieu of the behaviors. One generic cognitive behavioral therapy strategy involves identification of "triggers" (i.e., persons, places, things, or internal experiences) that are specific to sexually compulsive behavior (93).There are no randomized controlled trials of cognitive behavioral therapy for sexual addiction. There is, however, one randomized controlled trial of cognitive behavioral therapy-based HIV-prevention interventions for men who have sex with men. In men who completed baseline measures of sexual compulsivity along with measures of sexual risk behaviors, no differences were observed between the condition that received an HIV prevention approach that used cognitive behavioral therapy procedures and a standard condition (76). Post hoc analyses of these data showed that subjects in the lowest and highest quartiles of the SCS reported engaging in unprotected sex with status-unknown or presumed-positive men at significantly higher rates than those in the interim quartiles (76). These correlational data underscore both the clinical challenge to the therapist in successfully teaching individuals to reduce high-risk sexual behaviors who engage in sexually compulsive behaviors and the need to develop and evaluate treatments that specifically address these behaviors.

Though not specifically addressing sexual addiction, there is a growing body of work illustrating that reduction in drug use by providing evidence-based, cognitive behavioral treatments for drug dependence corresponds with reductions in high-risk sexual behaviors. One controlled clinical trial found that among gay and bisexual male methamphetamine abusers, treatment-associated reductions in high-risk sexual behaviors are observed to 1 year after treatment entry (94), a finding that was recently replicated (95). A qualitative report on the experiences of the men in the initial research project indicated that the participants noted the primary mechanism driving reductions in their high-risk sexual behaviors, both in numbers of partners and in episodes of unprotected anal sex, was treatment-associated reductions in methamphetamine use. The manual developed and validated for these research projects is available for download at *www.uclaisap.org*.

12-Step and Self-Help Groups There are no controlled studies of the efficacy of 12-step self-help groups in the reduction of behaviors consistent with sexual addiction. Still, the primary advantage to 12-step group attendance for those with sexual addiction is that the groups are convenient and are available both in urban and rural contexts. The social process of recovery that involves selection of a "sponsor" to provide around the clock assistance in managing sexual obsessions and compulsive urges also assists affected individuals who can comply with the procedures of a 12-step program of recovery. Moreover, as even the most efficacious program of psychotherapy or of medication taken for the treatment of sexual addiction eventually ends, involvement with a 12-step program for sexual addiction can continue for many years. There are four adapted versions of Alcoholics Anonymous and/or using a 12-Step approach to assist individuals in recovering from sexual addiction: Sexaholics Anonymous, *www.sa.org;* Sex Addicts Anonymous, *www.saa-recovery.org;* Sex and Love Addicts Anonymous, *www.slaafws.org;* and Sexual Compulsives Anonymous, *www.sca-recovery.org;* (96). The Web sites listed can assist individuals seeking support additional to ongoing psychotherapy and/or medical procedures for sexual addiction.

PHARMACOTHERAPY STRATEGIES

Antidepressants One strategy to pharmacotherapy of sexual addiction involves treatment of dysphoric mood symptoms commonly experienced during initial (and perhaps sustained) abstinence. If antidepressant medications diminish dysphoric mood symptoms, patients may be able to sustain their sexual behavior goals. Owing to involvement of serotonin in sex addiction, this class of antidepressants is considered separately in the section that follows. There are no randomized, placebo-controlled trials of sexual behavior outcomes for patients treated with antidepressants other than selective serotonin reuptake inhibitors (SSRIs). In one open-label trial of nefazodone (200 mg/day) in 14 subjects with nonparaphilic sexual disorders, of 11 subjects who adhered to the medication, 6 reported "good control" of sexual obsessions and compulsions; 5 reported complete remission of their paraphilic behaviors (97). One case report described use of clomipramine and valproic acid with a 21-year-old woman with sexual addiction (98).

Selective Serotonin Reuptake Inhibitors Use of SSRI as treatment for sexual addiction is based largely on the theorized mechanism of serotonergic dysfunction that may underlie the condition (18). Preclinical data show clearly that serotonin depletion in the presence of testosterone greatly potentiates sexual behavior in laboratory animals (99). Conversely, common side effects to treatment for depression using SSRIs frequently include reduction in sexual libido, particularly for males but also for females (68). The potential mechanism explaining sexual addiction (i.e., serotonin depletion in the presence of testosterone) provides strong rationale for using SSRIs in treatment.

Recent randomized placebo-controlled evidence indicates that in healthy adult males, 4 weeks of treatment with citalopram significantly increases time to orgasm compared to men in a placebo condition, with men assigned to fluoxetine showing similar but nonstatistically significant delays to orgasm as compared to placebo (100). Neither medication, however, significantly dampened sexual desire or penile tumescence measurements, which suggests SSRIs may have differential effects on dampening libido and sexual function in men who are not depressed or who do not have compulsive sexual behavior disorders. Evidence for this suggestion comes from the only randomized, placebo-controlled trial of an SSRI for the treatment of sexual addiction/sexual compulsivity. Gay and bisexual male subjects who were randomly assigned to 12 weeks of citalopram (20 to 60 mg/day) as a potential treatment for compulsive sexual behaviors reported significant reductions in sexual drive, in frequency of masturbation, and in viewing of pornography compared to placebo (70). There were, however, no significant effects on sexual behaviors involving partners.

Reports from open-label trials with SSRIs cannot address efficacy owing to inherent design weaknesses and, as such, do not provide the highest level of evidence upon which to guide decisions on clinical practice. Such reports, however, can provide useful descriptions of the feasibility of a particular medication approach. In one, 17 of 24 men with paraphilias and nonparaphilia-related disorders treated with SSRIs showed sustained reductions in total sexual occasions that lasted a minimum of 4 weeks (18). In another open-label trial, generally positive outcomes for 13 patients who presented for treatment of sexual addictions were reported with specifically poorer outcomes for men with diagnosed paraphilias as compared to men diagnosed with nonparaphilia-related disorders (101). There are also several case reports describing experiences with unique patients and should only be interpreted as an outline of SSRIs that have been used with patients, particularly as no case studies describe a treatment that failed for sexual addiction. Case reports of using SSRIs, either alone or in combination with psychotropic medication for other psychiatric disorders, describe experiences with lamotrigine and fluoxetine (102) and citalopram (103).

On balance, there is some initial controlled evidence supporting use of the SSRI citalopram for sexual addiction, particularly with gay and bisexual men. This also supports the rationale emphasizing the role of serotonin dysregulation in sexually compulsive behaviors and the suggestion that medications that increase serotonin availability may help patients achieve their sexual behavior goals in treatment. There exists, however, no evidence to support use of other types of antidepressants to target reduction in mood dysphoria as a strategy for treating sexual addiction.

Opioid Antagonists

Naltrexone Naltrexone is an opioid antagonist approved for use in treating alcoholism and opioid dependence. The mechanism of action for considering naltrexone treatment for sexual abuse involves opioid antagonist effects in dampening dopamine release, thereby reducing the euphorigenic properties of fantasizing and tension buildup that are usually the initial steps in compulsive sexual behaviors (104). Especially for nonparaphilia-related disorders, naltrexone may be a reasonable candidate for evaluation in clinical trials. Unfortunately, there are no randomized, placebo-controlled trials of opioid antagonists for sexual addiction. In one open-label trial, high doses of naltrexone were used with 22 adolescent (ages 13 to 17) sexual offenders, with doses between 150 mg and 200 mg/day (divided doses) reduced frequency of masturbation, sexual fantasies, and nocturnal emissions. The trial used an escalating dose strategy against symptoms of masturbation, sexual fantasy and, nocturnal emissions until they slowed to acceptable levels. Although this open-label trial cannot address efficacy, symptoms did not remit for patients at naltrexone doses of <100 mg/day (105). Three case reports describe experiences in using high-dose naltrexone with patients with different types of compulsive sexual behaviors (47,104,106).

Hormone Therapies The strategy of administering hormone therapies to men with sexual addiction is based on eliminating sexual compulsivity and obsessions using medications that chemically stop production of testosterone, such as luteinizing hormone-releasing hormone agents. Because this approach is often referred to as *chemical castration*, the strategy is usually reserved for treating men with paraphilias that involve sexual offenses involving children or violence against adults. Similar to other pharmacologic approaches to treatment of sexual addiction, there are no placebo-controlled clinical trials that might guide use of any medications. A review of multiple open-label trials is consistent with case reports describing remission of paraphilia behaviors when patients take hormone medications (107,108), yet these descriptions provide only weak evidence to advise expected outcomes using hormone therapies, especially in patients with nonparaphilia-related behaviors. There are several case studies with hormone therapy, including one showing serious bone loss when using triptorelin therapy (109). There are no reports or evidence that might describe the utility of these drugs in women with paraphilia.

CONCLUSIONS

The concept of sexual addiction carries a great deal of controversy as it is defined primarily by abrogation of social, historical, and sometimes legal constructs of what is acceptable human sexual behavior. Much of the research on the concept over the past 15 to 20 years has focused on the defining features of sexual addiction. It appears probable that the DSM-V will include a diagnostic category intended to describe the behavior. One of the complications to defining the category is its frequent comorbidity with psychiatric disorders, particularly bipolar disorder, stimulant dependence, and cluster C personality disorders. There are no data to describe the prevalence or incidence of sexual addiction. Similarly, there are few randomized controlled trials to guide treatment approaches to sexual addiction, though there is one initial placebo-controlled randomized trial indicating subjects receiving citalopram demonstrated significant reductions in pornography viewing and masturbation compared to subjects assigned to placebo. Hormone therapies are frequently used in treating men with paraphilias, particularly pedophilia, as an approach to chemical castration. A variety of psychotherapy models are described in the treatment of sexual addiction but only in the absence of a comparison condition. Even when conducting open-label trials of behavioral therapies for sexual addiction, outcomes are modest and relapse is common. There are four 12-step self-help organizations that provide resources to individuals seeking recovery from sexual addiction and represent an important component to a coordinated treatment approach, especially for those individuals who can comply with the requirements of a 12-step approach (65,79,110–116).

REFERENCES

1. Holden C. 'Behavioral' addictions: do they exist? *Science* 2001;294:980–982.
2. Schneider JP, Irons RR. Assessment and treatment of addictive sexual disorders: relevance for chemical dependency relapse. *Subst Use Misuse* 2001;36:1795–1820.
3. Dell'Osso B, Altamura AC, Allen A, Marazziti D. Epidemiologic and clinical updates on impulse control disorders: a critical review. *European Arch Psychiatry Clin Neurosci* 2006;256:464–475.
4. Kinsey AC, Pomeroy WB, Martin CE. *Sexual behavior in the human male*. Philadelphia: W.B. Saunders, 1948.
5. Kinsey AC, Pomeroy WB, Martin CE, Gebhard PH. *Sexual behavior in the human female*. Philadelphia: W.B. Saunders, 1953.
6. Carnes P. *Don't call it love: recovery from sexual addiction*. New York: Bantam, 1991.
7. Orford J. Hypersexuality: Implications for a theory of dependence. *Br J Addict* 1978;73:299–310.
8. Levine MP, Troiden RR. The myth of sexual compulsivity. *J Sex Res* 1988;25:347–363.
9. Kinsey AC, Pomeroy WB, Martin CE, Gebhard PH. Concepts of normality and abnormality in sexual behavior. In: Hoch PH, Zubin J, eds. *Psychosexual development in health and disease*. New York: Grune and Stratton, 1949:11–32.
10. Goodman A. What's in a name? Terminology for designating a syndrome of driven sexual behavior. *Sex Addict Compulsiv* 2001;8:191–213.
11. Goodman A. Diagnosis and treatment of sexual addiction. *J Sex Marital Ther* 1993;19:225–251.
12. Black DW, Kehrberg LLD, Flumerfelt DL, Schlosser SS. Characteristics of 36 subjects reporting compulsive sexual behavior. *Am J Psychiatry* 1997;154:243–249.
13. Coleman E. The obsessive-compulsive model for describing compulsive sexual behavior. *Am J Prev Psychiatry Neurol* 1990;1:9–14.
14. Kalichman SC, Rompa D. Sexual sensation seeking and compulsivity scales: reliability, validity and predicting HIV risk behavior. *J Person Assess* 1995;65:385–397.
15. Quadland MC. Compulsive sexual behavior: definition of a problem and an approach to treatment. *J Sex Marital Ther* 1985;11:121–132.
16. Montaldi DF. Understanding hypersexuality with an Axis II model. *J Psychol Hum Sex* 2002;14:1–23.
17. Rinehart NJ, McCabe MP. Hypersexuality: psychopathology or normal variant in sexuality. *Sex Marital Ther* 1997;12:45–60.
18. Kafka MP. Sertraline pharmacotherapy for paraphilias and paraphilia-related disorders: An open trial. *Ann Clin Psychiatry* 1994;6:189–195.
19. Barth RJ, Kinder BN. The mislabeling of sexual impulsivity. *J Sex Marital Ther* 1987;13:15–23.
20. Krueger RB, Kaplan MS. The paraphilic and hypersexual disorders: an overview. *J Psychiatr Pract.* 2001;7(6):391–403.
21. Gold SN, Heffner CL. Sexual addiction: many conceptions, minimal data. *Clin Psychol Rev* 1998;18:367–381.
22. American Psychiatric Association. *Diagnostic and statistical manual,* 4th ed. (text rev). Washington DC: American Psychiatric Association, 2004.

23. Kaplan BJ, Sadock VA. *Kaplan & Sadock's synopsis of psychiatry: behavioral sciences/clinical psychiatry,* 10th ed. Lippincott Williams & Wilkins: New York, 2007:715.
24. Black DW. The epidemiology and phenomenology of compulsive sexual behavior. *CNS Spectr* 2000;5:26–72.
25. Kasl CD. *Women, sex and addiction: a search for love and power.* New York: Ticknor & Fields, 1986.
26. Roller CG. Sexually compulsive/addictive behaviors in women: a women's healthcare issue. *J Midwif Women's Health* 2004;52:486–491.
27. Parsons JT, Kelly BC, Bimbi DS, et al. Explanations for the origins of sexual compulsivity among gay and bisexual men. *Arch Sex Behav* 2008;37:817–826.
28. Twitchell G, Huber A, Reback C, Shoptaw S. Comparison of general and detailed HIV risk assessments among methamphetamine abusers. *AIDS Behav* 2002;6:153–162.
29. Laumann EO. *The social organization of sexuality: sexual practices in the United States.* Chicago: University of Chicago Press, 1994.
30. Kafka MP, Hennen J. A DSM-IV Axis I comorbidity study of males (n = 120) with paraphilias and paraphilia related disorders. *Sex Abuse* 2002;14: 349–366.
31. Raymond NC, Coleman E, Miner MH. Psychiatric comorbidity and compulsive/impulsive traits in compulsive behavior. *Compr Psychiatry* 2003;44:370–380.
32. Sussman S. Sexual addiction among teens: a review. *Sex Addict Compulsiv* 2007;14:257–278.
33. Kafka MP. Hypersexual desire in males: an operational definition and clinical implications for males with paraphilias and paraphilia-related disorders. *Arch Sex Behav* 1997;26:505–526.
34. Kafka MP, Hennen J. Hypersexual desire in males: are males with paraphilias different from males with paraphilia-related disorders. *Sex Abuse* 2003;15:307–321.
35. Langstrom N, Hanson RK. High rates of sexual behavior in the general population: correlates and predictors. *Arch Sex Behav* 2006;35:37–52.
36. Bancroft J, Loftus J, Long JS. Distress about sex: a national survey of women in heterosexual relationships. *Arch Sex Behav* 2003;32:193–208.
37. Cooper A, Delmonico DL, & Burg R. Cybersex users, abusers, and compulsives: New findings and implications. *Sex Addict Compulsiv* 2000;7:5–29.
38. Mosher WD, Chandra A, Jones J. Sexual behavior and selected health measures: men and women 15–44 years of age, United States, 2002. *Adv Data* 2005;362:1–55.
39. Seegers JA. The prevalence of sexual addiction symptoms on the college campus. *Sex Addict Compulsiv* 2003;10:247–258.
40. Sussman S. The relations of cigarette smoking with risky sexual behavior among teens. *Sex Addict Compulsiv* 2005;12:181–199.
41. Carnes PJ, Murray RE, Charpentier L. Bargains with chaos: sex addicts and addiction interaction disorder. *Sex Addict Compulsiv* 2005;12: 79–120.
42. Blanchard R, Kuban ME, Klassen P, et al. Self-reported head injuries before and after age 13 in pedophilic and nonpedophilic men referred for clinical assessment. *Arch Sex Behav* 2003;32:573–581.
43. Bimbi DS, Nanin JE, Parsons JT, et al. Assessing gay and bisexual men's outcome expectancies for sexual risk under the influence of alcohol and drugs. *Subst Use Misuse* 2006;41:643–652.
44. Semple SJ, Zians J, Grant I, Patterson TL. Sexual compulsivity in a sample of HIV-positive methamphetamine-using gay and bisexual men. *AIDS Behav* 2006;10:587–598.
45. Benotsch EG, Kalichman SC, Kelly JA. Sexual compulsivity and substance use in HIV-seropositive men who have sex with men: prevalence and predictors of high-risk behaviors. *Addict Behav* 1999;24:857–868.
46. Dew BJ, Chaney MP. The relationship among sexual compulsivity, internalized homophobia, and HIV at-risk sexual behavior in gay and bisexual male users of Internet chat rooms. *Sex Addict Compulsiv* 2005;12: 259–273.
47. Parsons JT, Bimbi DS. Intentional unprotected anal intercourse among men who have sex with men: barebacking—from behavior to identity. *AIDS Behav* 2007;11:277–287.
48. Tiihonen J, Kuikka J, Kupila J, et al. Increase in cerebral blood flow of right prefrontal cortex in man during orgasm. *Neurosci Lett* 1994;170: 241–243.
49. Arnow BA, Desmond JE, Banner LL, et al. Brain activation and sexual arousal in healthy, heterosexual adult males. *Brain* 2002;125: 1014–1023.
50. Redouté J, Stoléru S, Grégoire MC, et al. Brain processing of visual sexual stimuli in human males. *Hum Brain Map* 2000;11:162–177.
51. Stoléru S, Grégoire MC, Gérard D, et al. Neuroanatomical correlates of visually evoked sexual arousal in human males. *Arch Sex Behav* 1999;28:1–21.
52. Cantor JM, Kabani N, Christensen BK, et al. Cerebral white matter deficiencies in pedophilic men. *J Psychiatr Res* 2008;42:167–183.
53. Bancroft J, Vukadinovic Z. Sexual addiction, sexual compulsivity, sexual impulsivity, or what? Toward a theoretical model. *J Sex Res* 2004;41: 225–234.
54. Singh A, Kandimala G, Dewey RB, O'Suilleabhain P. Risk factors for pathologic gambling and other compulsions among Parkinson's disease patients taking dopamine agonists. *J Clin Neurosci* 2007;14:1178–1181.
55. Weintraub D, Siderowf AD, Potenza MN, et al. Association of dopamine agonist use with impulse control disorders in Parkinson disease. *Arch Neurol* 2006;63:969–673.
56. Ivanco LS, Bohnen NI. Effects of donepezil on compulsive hypersexual behavior in Parkinson disease: a single case study. *Am J Ther* 2005;12(5): 467–468.
57. Shapiro MA, Chang YL, Munson SK, et al. Hypersexuality and paraphilia induced by selegiline in Parkinson's disease: report of 2 cases. *Parkinsonism Relat Disord* 2006;12:392–395.
58. Cannas A, Solla P. Hypersexual behaviour, frotteurism and delusional jealousy in a young parkinsonian patient during dopaminergic therapy with pergolide: a rare case of iatrogenic paraphilia. *Prog Neuropsychopharmacol Biol Psychiatry* 2006;30:1539–541.
59. Grant J, Luxford Y, Darbyshire P. Culture, communication and child health. *Contemp Nurse* 2005;20:134–142.
60. Lavan H, Johnson JG. The association between axis I and II psychiatric symptoms and high-risk sexual behavior during adolescence. *J Personal Disord* 2002;16:73–94.
61. Kafka MP, Hennen J. A DSM-IV Axis I comorbidity study of males (n =120) with paraphilias and paraphilia-related disorders. *Sex Abuse* 2002;14:349–366.
62. Lloyd M, Raymond NC, Miner MH, Coleman E. Borderline personality traits in individuals with compulsive sexual behavior. *Sex Addict Compulsiv* 2007;14:187–206.
63. Weiss D. The prevalence of depression in male sex addicts residing in the United States. *Sex Addict Compulsiv* 2004;11:57–69.
64. Raviv M. Personality characteristics of sexual addicts and pathological gamblers. *J Gambl Stud* 1993;9:17–30.
65. Blankenship R, Laaser M. Sexual addiction and ADHD: is there a connection. *Sex Addict Compulsiv* 2008;11:7–20.
66. Kafka MP, Prentky R. Fluoxetine treatment of nonparaphilic sexual addictions and paraphilias in men. *J Clin Psychiatry* 1992;53:351–358.
67. Meston CM. Validation of the Female Sexual Function Index (FSFI) in women with female orgasmic disorder and in women with hypoactive sexual desire disorder. *J Sex Marital Ther* 2003;29:39–46.
68. Rosen RC, Lane RM, Menza M. Effects of SSRIs on sexual function: a critical review. *J Clin Psychopharmacol* 1999;19:67–85.
69. Wiegel M, Meston C, Rosen R. The female sexual function index (FSFI): cross-validation and development of clinical cutoff scores. *J Sex Marital Ther* 2005;31:1–20.
70. Wainberg ML, Muench F, Morgenstern J, et al. A double-blind study of citalopram versus placebo in the treatment of compulsive sexual behaviors in gay and bisexual men. *J Clin Psychiatry* 2006;67:1968–1973.
71. Carnes P. *Contrary to love.* Center City, MN: Hazeldon, 1989.
72. Nelson KG, Oehlert ME. Evaluation of a Shortened South Oaks Gambling Screen in veterans with addictions. *Psychol Addict Behav* 2008; 22:309–312.
73. Abell JW, Steenbergh TA, Boivin MJ. Cyberporn use in the context of religiosity. *J Psychol Theol* 2006;34:165–171.

74. Kafka MP, Prentky R. Fluoxetine treatment of nonparaphilic sexual addictions and paraphilias in men. *J Clin Psychiatry* 1992;53:351–358.
75. Dodge B, Reece M, Cole SL, Sandfort TGM. Sexual compulsivity among heterosexual college students. *J Sex Res* 2004;41:343–350.
76. Dilley JW, Loeb L, Marson K, et al. Sexual compulsiveness and change in unprotected anal intercourse: unexpected results from a randomized controlled HIV counseling intervention study. *J Acquir Immune Defic Syndr* 2008;48:113–114.
77. Kalichman SC, Cain D. The relationship between indicators of sexual compulsivity and high risk sexual practices among men and women receiving services from a sexually transmitted infection clinic. *J Sex Res* 2004;41:235–241.
78. McConnaughy EA, Prochaska JO, Velicer WF. Stages of change in psychotherapy: Measurement and sample profiles. *Psychother Theory Res Pract* 1983;20:368–375.
79. Reid RC. Assessing readiness to change for clients seeking help for hypersexual behavior. *Sex Addict Compulsiv* 2007;14:167–186.
80. Coleman E, Miner M, Ohlerking F, Raymond N. Compulsive sexual behavior inventory: a preliminary study of reliability and validity. *J Sex Marital Ther* 2001;27:325–332.
81. Miner MH, Coleman E, Center BA, et al. The compulsive sexual behavior inventory: psychometric properties. *Arch Sex Behav* 2007;36: 579–587.
82. Quadland MC. Compulsive sexual behavior: definition of a problem and an approach to treatment. *J Sex Marital Ther* 1985;11:121–132.
83. Klontz B. The effectiveness of brief multimodal experiential therapy in the treatment of sexual addiction. *Sex Addict Compulsiv* 2005;12: 275–294.
84. Wan M, Finlayson R, Rowles A. Sexual dependence treatment outcome study. *Sex Addict Compulsiv* 2000;7:177–196.
85. Phillips LA. Literature review of research in family systems treatment of sexual addictions. *Sex Addict Compulsiv* 2006;15:241–246.
86. Schneider JP. Compulsive and addictive sexual disorders and the family. *CNS Spectr* 2000;5:53–62.
87. Wildmon-White ML, Young JS. Family of origin characteristics among women married to sexually addicted men. *Sex Addict Compulsiv* 2002;9: 265–273.
88. Schneider JP. Compulsive and addictive sexual disorders and the family. *CNS Spectr* 2000;5:53–62.
89. Schneider JP. Effects of cybersex addiction on the family: results of a survey. *Sex Addict Compulsiv* 2000b;7:31–58.
90. Steffens BA, Rennie RL. The traumatic nature of disclosure for wives of sexual addicts. *Sex Addict Compulsiv* 2006;13:247–267.
91. Corley MD, Schneider JP. Sex addiction disclosure to children: the parents' perspective. *Sex Addict Compulsiv* 2003;10:291–324.
92. Marlatt GA, Gordon JR. Relapse prevention: maintenance strategies in the treatment of addictive behaviors. The Gulford Press.
93. Parsons JT, Kelly BC, Bimbi DS, et al. Accounting for the social triggers of sexual compulsivity. *J Addict Dis.* 2007;26:5–16.
94. Shoptaw S, Reback CJ, Peck JA, et al. Behavioral treatment approaches for methamphetamine dependence and HIV-related sexual risk behaviors among urban gay and bisexual men. *Drug Alcohol Depend* 2005;78: 125–134.
95. Shoptaw S, Reback CJ, Larkins S, et al. Outcomes using two tailored behavioral treatments for substance abuse in urban gay and bisexual men. *J Subst Abuse Treat* 2008;Mar 6. Epub ahead of print.
96. Manley G. Treatment and recovery for sexual addicts. *Nurse Pract* 1990;15:34–41.
97. Coleman E, Gratzer T, Nesvacil L, Raymond NC. Nefazodone and the treatment of nonparaphilic compulsive sexual behavior: a retrospective study. *J Clin Psychiatry* 2000;61(4):282–284.
98. Gulsun M, Gulcat Z, Aydin H. Treatment of compulsive sexual behaviour with clomipramine and valproic acid. *Clin Drug Investing* 2007; 27:219–223.
99. Gessa GL. Essential role of testosterone in the sexual stimulation induced by p-chlorophenylalanine in male animals. *Nature* 1970;227:616–617.
100. Madeo B. The effects of citalopram and fluoxetine on sexual behavior in healthy men: evidence of delayed ejaculation and unaffected sexual desire. a randomized, placebo-controlled, double-blind, double-dummy, parallel group study. *J Sex Med* 2008. Epub ahead of print.
101. Stein DJ, Hollander E, Anthony DT, et al. Serotonergic medications for sexual obsessions, sexual addictions, and paraphilias. *J Clin Psychiatry* 1992;53:267–271.
102. Schupak C. Case report: lamotrigine/fluoxetine combination in the treatment of compulsive sexual behavior. *Prog Neuropsychopharmacol Biol Psychiatry* 2007;31:1337–1338.
103. Malladi SS. Hypersexuality and its response to citalopram in a patient with hypothalamic hamartoma and precocious puberty. *Int J Neuropsychopharmacolol* 2005;8:635–636.
104. Bostwick JM, Bucci JA. Internet sex addiction treated with naltrexone. *Mayo Clin Proc* 2008;83:226–230.
105. Ryback RS. Naltrexone in the treatment of adolescent sexual offenders. *J Clin Psychiatry* 2004;65:982–986.
106. Grant JE, Kim SW. A case of kleptomania and compulsive sexual behavior treated with naltrexone. *Ann Clin Psychaitry* 2001;13:229–231.
107. Briken P, Hill A, Berner W. Pharmacotherapy of paraphilias with long-acting agonists of luteinizing hormone-releasing hormone: a systematic review. *J Clin Psychiatry* 2003;64:890–897.
108. Schober JM, Kuhn PJ, Kovacs PG, et al. Leuprolide acetate suppresses pedophilic urges and arousability. *Arch Sex Behav* 2005;34:691–705.
109. Hoogeveen J, Van Der Veer E. Side effects of pharmacotherapy on bone with long-acting gonadorelin agonist triptorelin for paraphilia. *J Sex Med* 2008;5:626–630.
110. Carnes P. *Contrary to love*. Center City, MN: Hazeldon, 1989.
111. Cooper A, Delmonico DL, Burg R. Cybersex users, abusers, and compulsives: new findings and implications. *Sex Addict Compulsiv* 2000;7:5–29.
112. Gulsun M, Gulcat Z, Aydin H. Treatment of compulsive sexual behaviour with clomipramine and valproic acid. *Clin Drug Invest* 2007;27:219–223.
113. Larkins S, Reback CJ, Shoptaw S. HIV risk behaviors among gay male methamphetamine users: before and after treatment. *J Gay Lesbian Psychother* 2006;10:123–129.
114. Munech F, Morgenstern J, Hollander E, et al. The consequences of compulsive sexual behavior: the preliminary reliability and validity of the Compulsive Behavior Consequences Scale. *Sex Addict Compulsiv* 2007; 14:207–220.
115. Raymond NC, Grant JE, Kim SW, Coleman E. Treatment of compulsive sexual behavior with naltrexone and serotonin reuptake inhibitors: two case studies. *Int Clin Psychopharmacol* 2002;17:201–205.
116. Schneider J, Sealy J, Montgomery J, Irons R. Ritualization and reinforcement: keys to understanding mixed addiction involving sex and drugs. *Sex Addict Compulsiv* 2005;12:121–148.

CHAPTER 40

Paul H. Earley, MD, FASAM

Physician Health Programs and Addiction among Physicians

The available research about addiction in physicians and physician health programs (PHPs) is extensive and has been well documented; several excellent overviews provide a comprehensive analysis of the topic (1–5). Bissell and Haberman (6), Angres et al. (7), Nace (8), and Coombs (9) have written complete texts dedicated to the issues of addiction in physicians and other health professionals. Physicians are a convenient population to study; they are accessible both prior to and after treatment and are articulate about their disease. Research on physician addiction elucidates the natural course of addiction in a highly regulated and monitored population. At the same time, physicians differ from the general population in terms of education, income, and regulatory oversight. Thus, though informative, conclusions made from physician studies about the efficacy of treatment should be viewed as atypical compared to the population at large.

PREVALENCE

We have 20 years of debate about the actual and changing prevalence of addiction in physicians (10). Kessler et al. (11) reported that 3.8% of the general population at any given time has any substance disorder, 1.3% meet criteria for alcohol dependence and 0.4% for drug dependence. Lifetime prevalence has been estimated at between 8% and 13% for alcohol and drug dependence in the general population. Studies that attempt to determine the prevalence of addiction in physicians are based upon anonymous questionnaires (10,12–19). Hughes et al. (17) reported a lifetime prevalence of alcohol abuse or dependence and drug abuse or dependence in physicians at 7.9%, somewhat less than the percentage reported in the general population by Kessler (11). However methodologic differences may account for this difference. The Hughes study surveyed 9,600 physicians by mail with a lower response rate (59%) and relied on honest and denial-free reports by the physicians; the Kessler study utilized face-to-face interviews with trained interviewers.

In 1970, Vaillant et al. (20) reported on the types of substances physicians use. At that time, he noted that physicians were just as likely to smoke cigarettes and drink alcohol as the general population but more likely to take tranquilizers and sedatives. In a more comprehensive study 29 years later, Hughes et al. (15) noted that physicians were *less* likely to smoke cigarettes than nonphysicians and more likely to consume benzodiazepines and opiates. The change in cigarette use was presumably due to increasing medical data about the health risks of tobacco. The recent decrease in smoking was reiterated by Mangus et al. in 1998 (21). Hughes et al. (17) stated that physicians drink more alcohol than the general population; the authors attributed this in part to their higher socioeconomic status. They also noted that 11.4% of physicians had used unsupervised benzodiazepines and 17.6% reported the unsupervised use of opioids. Vaillant (22), in his commentary on the Hughes study, rang an alarm bell by stating "physicians are five times as likely [than the general population] to take sedatives and minor tranquilizers without medical supervision." The use of opioids and minor tranquilizers commonly begins prior to or in medical school, since medical students use more of these drugs than age-matched cohorts (23). Clark examined substance abuse in medical students using a 4 year longitudinal study (24). Eighteen percent met the study research criteria for alcohol abuse in the first 2 years of medical school. They reported that a family history of alcoholism was associated with alcohol abuse in the medical student.

Another view of physician drug abuse can be derived from complaints heard by state medical boards. Morrison and Wickersham (25) noted that 14% of board disciplinary actions were alcohol- or drug-related, and another 11% were due to inappropriate prescribing practices—many of which are also addiction-related. In 2003, Clay and Conatser (26) reported similar disciplinary rates, with 21% due to alcohol and drug issues and 10% due to inappropriate prescribing or drug possession. Alcohol- and drug-related work impairment was the primary impetus for the formation of state physician health programs (PHPs) in the United States and continues to account for the majority of physician impairment cases seen by most PHPs today (2). Ethnic variation in substance abuse in the general population is described in the National Epidemiological Survey on Alcohol and Related Conditions; whites, Native Americans, and Hispanics have a higher prevalence of dependence than Asians; but no published data about physician addiction have been reported to date using ethnicity as an independent variable.

In summary, though the prevalence of addiction to all chemicals appears to be about the same as in the general population, currently physicians consume less tobacco and more opioids and sedatives. Research data do suggest that physicians consume more alcohol than the general population.

CHARACTERISTICS OF ADDICTED PHYSICIANS

Age Berry (27) has suggested a bimodal distribution of age at first presentation for treatment; physicians in training and early practice comprise the first wave, and physicians in mid- to late career comprise the second. Talbott et al. (28) reported a decrease in the age of presentation in treatment from 51 years to 44 years between 1975 and 1985. In a 2008 analysis of more than 1,400 medical students, residents, and physicians at the same southeastern treatment program, Earley and Weaver (29) noted an age range from 25.3 to 83.7 years, with a median age of 45.8, the ages disbursed in a bell curve (Fig. 40.1). Despite the earlier report that physicians are arriving earlier in the course of their addictive disease, the age at presentation in treatment in more recent years increased from 42.5 in 1998 to 48.2 in 2007 (Fig. 40.2). Of possible correlation, heavy drinking decreases with age in the general population but increases with age in physicians (10).

Gender Males account for the majority of physician addiction cases, with reported ratios varying between 7 to 1 (30) and 10 to 1 (29), male to female. This contrasts with the 3-to-1 male-to-female ratio in the physician population at large (31). Although fewer females than males have drinking problems, female physicians are more likely to report problematic drinking by the end of medical school (5) and are more likely to have alcohol problems later in life than their nonmedical counterparts (32). At intake into one of four PHP programs, female physicians were more likely to be younger and to have medical and psychiatric comorbidity (33). Female physicians were more likely to have past or current suicidal ideation and were more likely to have attempted suicide regardless of whether they were under the influence at the time. Wunsch et al. (33) report that female physicians are more likely to abuse sedative/hypnotics than men. Interestingly, women physicians are the subject of more severe sanctions by medical boards than their male counterparts (25).

Specialty Bissell and Jones (32), writing in 1976, were among the first to systematically study addiction in physicians. Using a follow-up questionnaire of physicians in Alcoholics

FIGURE 40.1. Distribution of physician age at presentation to treatment.

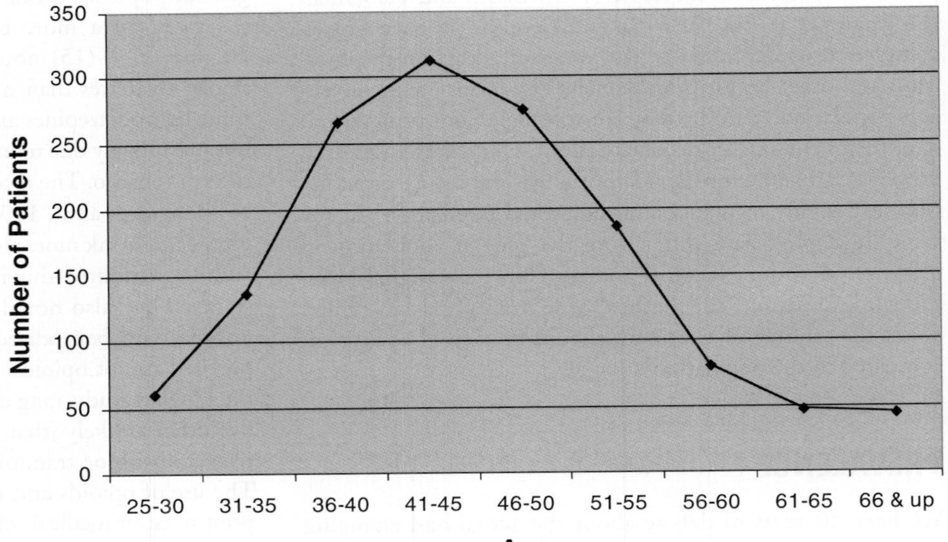

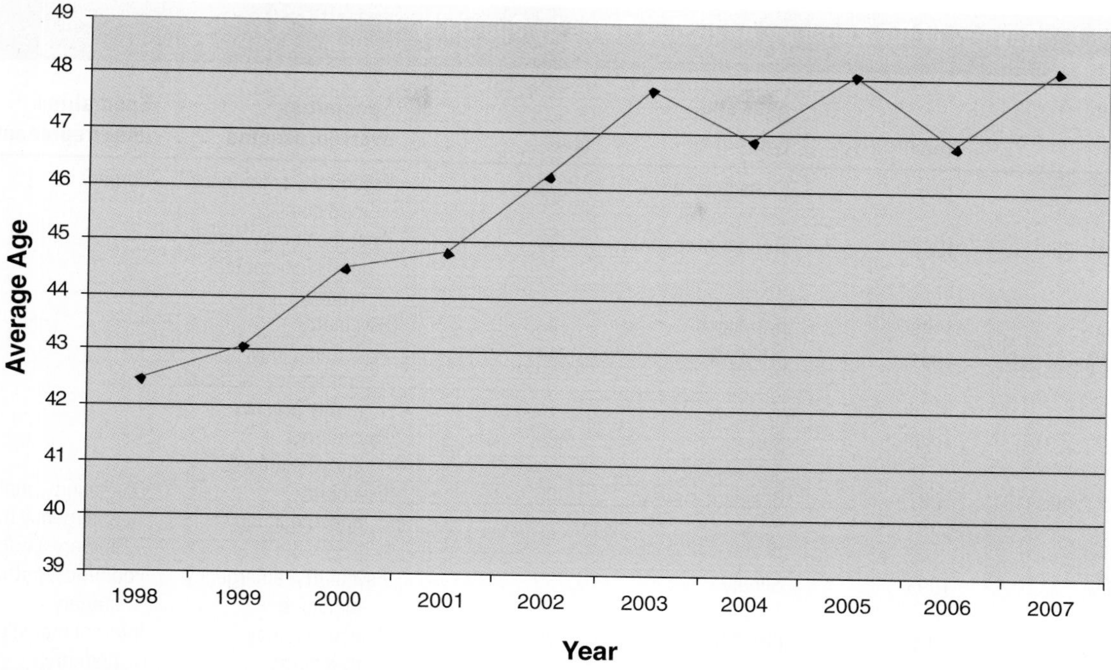

FIGURE 40.2. Increasing age of physician entry into treatment over time.

Anonymous, she noted that psychiatrists and emergency medicine physicians were overrepresented in Alcoholics Anonymous (overrepresentation was defined as the percentage of a cohort higher than predicted by the percentage of that cohort in the population of physicians at large). Hughes et al. (15) surveyed physician use by an anonymous survey. Reported substance use was highest in psychiatrists and emergency medicine physicians and lowest in surgeons and pediatricians.

A synopsis of the literature on addiction rates by specialty appears in Table 40.1. This table covers multiple authors and modes of analysis. Sufficient information was not available to allow meta-analysis. However, the combined literature looks at the breakdown by specialty from multiple angles; it consistently suggests that psychiatry and emergency medicine physicians have higher substance problems. Table 40.1 also suggests that family practice physicians might be overrepresented, and pediatricians and pathologists appear to be at lower risk for addiction.

The problem of addiction in anesthesiologists continues to attract research and debate. Lutsky et al. (14) noted anesthesiologists were heavier users of marijuana and psychedelics when compared with medicine and surgery physicians but suggested caution in the interpretation of these data owing to age differences between the medicine and surgery cohort and the anesthesiology cohort. Talbott et al. (28) and Earley and Weaver (29) note that anesthesiologists account for 5% of all physicians, yet they account for 13% (Talbott) to 15% (Earley) of all physician patients in residential treatment. In contrast, Hughes et al. (16) noted a low overall rate of substance use in anesthesiology, both in residency and after completing training (15). Lutsky et al. (14) noted that the use of fentanyl (and its relatives) occurred only in anesthesiologists in their study. Hughes et al. (15) noted a trend toward more frequent use of the major opioids, such as fentanyl, in anesthesiologists, but the statistical analysis did not support significance.

Gold et al. (41) and McAuliffe et al. (42) have recently hypothesized that anesthesiologists may be sensitized to opioids and propofol (an anesthesia induction agent) through the inhalation of picograms of these potent agents in the operating room air. Assays of operating room air, especially when taken near the expiration point of the anesthetized patient, detected these agents. This hypothesis rests on an uncertain foundation (the notion that sensitization directly contributes to the etiology of addiction, the assumption the quantities are sufficient to produce sensitization, etc.) but does introduce additional avenues of research.

With one significant exception in the data (15), the anesthesiologist appears be a more frequent user of highly potent opioids and is strikingly overrepresented in treatment settings. Access to large quantities of these high-potency opioids (and other drugs) in the day-to-day practice of anesthesia is the most likely culprit for the prevalence of anesthesia personnel in treatment settings.

DRUGS ABUSED

Alcohol Two types of studies are used to assess the types of drugs abused by physicians: anonymous questionnaires (10,13–19) and self-reports of drugs of choice of physicians as

TABLE 40.1 Review of Research on Addiction Rates by Specialty

Research	Year	Research type	No.	Specialties overrepresented	Specialties underrepresented
Bissell (32)	1976	Closed survey	98	Psychiatry, emergency medicine	Surgery
Talbott et al. (28)	1987	Treatment records	1,000	Anesthesiology, family medicine/general practice	—
Shore (100)	1987	PHP/MB	34	Psychiatry	—
Pelton and Ikeda (99)	1991	PHP/MB	247	Anesthesiology, emergency medicine, family practice	—
McAullife et al. (13)	1986	Survey	489	Psychiatry, anesthesiology	—
Myers and Weiss (101)	1987	Resident survey	1,805	Psychiatry, anesthesiology	Community health, emergency medicine, surgery, pediatrics
Hughes (15)	1999	Survey	1,785	Psychiatry, emergency medicine	Pediatrics, pathology, surgery
Morrison and Wickersham (25)	1998	PHP/MB	375	Anesthesiology, psychiatry	Internal medicine, pediatrics
Knight (94)	2007	PHP/MB	120	Anesthesiology, emergency medicine	Pediatrics
Earley and Weaver (29)	2008	Treatment records	618	Anesthesiology, emergency medicine	Pathology, pediatrics, radiology

PHP/MB, Physicians Health Program or Medical Board record study.

they appear in treatment or monitoring programs (28,29). Both types of research underscore that alcohol is, as expected, the most frequent primary drug of abuse by physicians, just as in the general population.

Nicotine Tobacco dependence has been suggested as a risk factor for alcohol and other drug dependence in physicians (34) as in the general population (35). Tobacco use in physicians has decreased over time (20,21). Emergency medicine and surgery physicians are twice as likely to smoke as are other physicians (15).

Opioids Opioids are the second most frequently abused substance by physicians arriving in treatment (29,36). This finding has been remarkably stable over time, but the type of opioids used continues to change. Hughes et al. (15) differentiates opioid use into the major opioids (morphine, meperidine, fentanyl, and other injectable narcotics) and the minor opioids (hydrocodone, oxycodone, codeine, and other oral drugs). Distinguishing in this manner, they reported that family practice and obstetrics and gynecology specialists have a higher probability of abusing minor opioids. This study goes on to report that anesthesiologists were less likely than other physicians to use minor opioids, with a trend toward increased use of major opioids. If one assumes that use of major opioids results in a more aggressive manifestation and progression of addiction, this would partly account for the overrepresentation of anesthesiologists over other specialties in physician treatment programs (28,29). Several authors (15,17,37) posit that exposure to drugs of abuse in the workplace leads to higher abuse of those workplace drugs. This postulate is supported by the data on major opioid use by anesthesiologists and the use of minor opioids by family physicians.

Cocaine In one study, professions that use cocaine medicinally (ophthalmology, head and neck surgery, plastic surgery, and otolaryngology) had a (nonstatistically significant) trend to higher cocaine use (15). Hyde and Wolfe (38) noted that when cocaine is abused by surgery residents, it often comes from hospital sources.

Benzodiazepines One hypothesis of substance misuse among physicians suggests that drugs that are seen as helpful in a physician's line of work might be more commonly abused by the physicians themselves. Survey-based studies report that psychiatrists have a greater misuse of benzodiazepines; 26.3% report using unsupervised benzodiazepines in the past year, in comparison with 11.4% in other physician groups (15). This high rate of benzodiazepine misuse is reflected in the overrepresentation of psychiatrists in treatment. Family medicine and obstetrics and gynecology physicians are frequent prescribers and use more minor opioids than other specialties (15).

Illicit Drugs The most common street drug of abuse among medical residents is marijuana (16). Many kinds of specialists abuse marijuana, with emergency medicine, anesthesiology, family practice, and psychiatry physicians displaying elevated odds of marijuana abuse over physicians as a whole (15). Cocaine use is more common in emergency medicine physicians, presumably from street sources. Several authors (37,39,40) have postulated that the personality style of these specialties attract them to these drugs of abuse.

Other Drugs Physicians are also found to abuse drugs that are not generally available or not recognized as abusable by the general public. Skipper (43) reported an ominous increase in the abuse of and dependence upon tramadol (Ultram, Ultracet). Propofol (Diprivan) abuse has occurred in 18% of anesthesia training programs (44). The prevalence of propofol abuse in the past decade has increased fivefold in comparison with the previous decade. In this study by Wischmeyer et al. (44), 25 personnel were identified, and seven died as a result of propofol abuse. This study showed a positive correlation between availability (as defined by the lack of control over drug access) and the prevalence of abuse in a given training program. It is unclear whether this propofol abuse pattern is limited to physicians in training. Finally, Moore and Bostwick (45) described two cases of ketamine abuse in anesthesiologists; most professionals' treatment programs see several ketamine dependent physicians per year.

RISK FACTORS

The risk for addiction in physicians is an area with many speculators and limited research. Issues related to workplace stress and family-of-origin are covered in the natural history section.

Genetics The strongest predictor of alcohol or drug problems in physicians is the same as in the general population: a family history of alcoholism or drug dependence (5). Of note is the work of Moore (34) who observed that cigarette use of one pack or more per day was highly correlated with alcohol abuse in physicians.

Personality All physician specialties are burdened with common stereotypes, and it has long been tempting to speculate about causal personality factors in the development of physician addiction. At the outset, it must be noted that in the general population, decades of research have failed to discern an "addictive personality." As in all etiologic studies, physician-related personality dynamics may be an epiphenomenon to the true etiology of the addictive process. With the preceding caveats, it is interesting to review published speculations about physician personality types and addiction. Although personality issues may or may not be causative in addiction, they do play a central role in the progression and treatment of addiction disorders, and are covered below.

McAullife et al. (46) noted "sensation seeking" as a personality factor that is correlated with recreational drug use in physicians in training. These authors speculate that such individuals gravitate to specialties such as emergency medicine. Emergency medicine physicians may self-select high-risk or illicit drugs owing to the same personality characteristics that draws them to their specialty. Emergency medicine physicians, as reported by Hughes et al. (15) were twice as likely to use marijuana as other specialties. Their data also suggested cocaine use was higher in this cohort. This hypothesis is contradicted by data from other similar specialties that attract sensation-seeking individuals, such as surgery, which are not overrepresented in treatment settings.

Bissell and Jones (32) suggest perfectionist behavior and high ranking in class are risk factors for addiction. This is supported by Higgins Roche (47), who noted that addicted anesthesiologists are often in the top 10% to 20% of their class. Udel (48) notes that compulsive personality disorder (or traits) is the most common personality diagnosis of physicians presenting for treatment. No data differentiating the occurrence of compulsive traits in addicted or nonaddicted physicians is available, and one might think that compulsive traits are beneficial in physician training and work. Zeldow (37) and Yufit (39) speculate that the introverted and introspective qualities as well as a drive for an internal locus of control are partially responsible for the drug of choice selection in this population.

Drug Access O'Connor and Spickard described a subset of physicians who began abusing benzodiazepines and opioids only after receiving prescribing privileges (1). Shifting drug use has occurred over time, especially within the opioid class. Green et al. in 1976 (49) and Talbott et al. (28) in 1987 reported the predominant opioid abused by physicians at the time was meperidine (Demerol). A more recent (2004) review of the Michigan and Alabama Physicians Health Programs reports hydrocodone as the number-one opioid abused (40% of all opioid cases), meperidine dropping to 10% of cases. Skipper (43) reported an alarming increase in the abuse of tramadol (nearly 10% of all of studied opioid addiction cases) between 1994 and 2002. The tramadol addiction rate in physicians is worrisome; it may be a harbinger for an increase in tramadol abuse by the general population. The most likely hypothesis for shifts in the drug of choice by physicians over time is the changing prescribing patterns and shifting availability of these drugs to the physician.

Biologic Effect of the Drug of Choice The physical effects of the drugs used by an addict color the characteristics of the addiction disorder itself. Drug-of-choice characteristics may result in a skew in the physician-patients seen in treatment programs. For example, all opioids produce intense tolerance, resulting in abuse at escalating doses. If a physician diverts opioid drugs from a work setting and escalates the dose, he increases the probability of detection. This could explain why treatment-seeking or treatment-mandated physicians tend to present disproportionately with opioid abuse histories.

Major anesthetic opioids (such as fentanyl) when consumed parenterally produce a rapid downhill course owing to the development of a remarkable level of tolerance. The accelerated course of addiction when using the most potent opioids can be postulated as contributing to rapid demise and resultant high percentage of anesthesiologists seen in physician treatment programs. In addition, rapid onset (and the resolution of tolerance with brief periods of abstinence) and/or low therapeutic ratio may account for the high mortality rate in fentanyl-, sufentanil-, and alfentanil- and remifentanil-abusing anesthesiologists, as suggested by Collins (3). Increased awareness along with checks and balances to account for the remaindered volumes of fentanyl used in hospitals may detect diversion more rapidly and save lives of anesthesia personnel (14).

ADDICTION COMORBIDITY

Thought and Mood Disorders Physicians suffer from a spectrum of emotional and psychiatric problems similar to the general population. However, addicted physicians rarely have comorbid primary schizophrenia and related thought disorders. Although it is unclear whether physicians have higher or lower rates of unipolar depression, physicians who successfully complete suicide are more likely to have a drug abuse problem in their lives; self-prescribed psychoactive substances; a recent alcohol-related problem; a history of emotional problems prior to 18 years of age; and/or a family history of alcohol abuse and/or mental illness (50). Substance dependence, self-criticism, and dependant personality characteristics are predictors of depression in physicians (51). Bipolar disorder, both types I and II, may contribute to the intensity of addictive disease in physicians, particularly for drinking during manic intervals (52).

Pain PHPs are working with an increasing number of physicians with pain and chronic opioid use, many of whom have become physiologically dependent; in turn, a percentage of those go on to become addicted. Eventual addiction is thought to be more common in patients with pain disorders (53) and, when combined with the 25% of physicians who self-prescribe (13), a perfect storm of high-risk factors emerges. Physicians who have significant pain *and* addiction disorders pose diagnostic, treatment, and management difficulties for assessors, treatment providers, and the PHPs. Regulatory issues cloud the treatment of addicted physicians with pain: Should a formerly addicted physician on opioid drugs be allowed to practice? Is it logical for state boards to prohibit methadone or buprenorphine maintenance for addiction treatment but permit potent opioids for pain management? These are complex questions that wind up being responded to in terms of ideology rather than data. Scientific data on the safety of allowing physicians to practice on opioids, whether addicted or not, is absent.

Posttraumatic Stress Disorder Posttraumatic stress disorder (PTSD) and alcoholism are closely intertwined (54), and PTSD increases the probability of addiction relapse in PTSD-related contexts (55). However, no studies about the prevalence of PTSD in physicians have been published. Physicians, like anyone else, are not immune from prior trauma histories. Several physician specialties, including emergency medicine, trauma surgeons, and military psychiatrists, treat the immediate and chronic consequences of trauma. Although combat exposure is known to increase the statistical risks of addiction in veterans, no data exist to indicate whether such trauma increases the likelihood of substance abuse disorders in military physicians. Treating trauma can be, in itself, traumatizing to the caregiver.

THEORIES OF ADDICTION IN PHYSICIANS

The natural history of addiction is, on the surface, similar in physicians to that of any other addicted or alcohol-dependent person. McAuliffe (40) reports that 27% of medical students and 22% of physicians had family histories of alcohol dependence. And, the genetic research literature now supports inherited genetic vulnerabilities for all major classes of addictive drugs.

Clark (19) reported that excessive alcohol consumption in medical students was positively associated with better grades in the first year and a strong tendency toward better scores on Part One of the National Board of Medical Examiners test. Alcohol abuse was found to have no discernable impact on clinical rotations in years 3 and 4 of medical school in this study. This led Clark to speculate that hard-drinking students may be prone to discount warnings and feel invulnerable to the effects of alcohol; their own internal experience does not match cautionary information provided to them during their medical education. This may exacerbate an emerging "us" (doctors) and "them" (patients) view of the world.

Stress is often cited by the physician-patient as the primary agent that drives self-medication. Stress is an elusive concept; its exact correlation with substance use and addiction is unclear. Physicians report similar levels of stress as other health professionals (60). Physicians in treatment for chemical dependency report that the stress of medical training, when combined with social isolation, provides a fertile soil for the growth of drug consumption (3). Jex (61) suggests that the physician's unhealthy *response* to stress is a more important determinant of addiction than the ubiquitous *presence* of stress itself.

No evidence supports a specific professional personality type as being determinant in addiction. Personality dynamics specific to physicians do play a role in the course of the illness and its treatment, however. Vaillant (58) has suggested that physicians commonly experience an emotionally barren childhood. This postulate is echoed by Johnson and Connelly (59), who identified 72% of a 50-physician sample hospitalized for addiction as experiencing parental deprivation in their childhood. Khantzian (63) eloquently depicts the physician's efforts at caring for others as a partially successful transformation of the conflict about being cared for themselves and an attempt to correct the barren nature of their parental nurturance. When this transformation fails, the addiction-prone physician turns to or increases his or her substance use.

Physicians in the act of saving human life develop a varying degree of omnipotence (4). This omnipotence, when combined with knowledge of the drugs they prescribe, produces a feeling of invulnerability regarding drug or alcohol use. Vaillant (22) has speculated that self-prescribing (related to physician self-sufficiency and false omnipotence) plays a permissive role in the development of addiction in physicians. Physicians' illusion of mastery over pharmaceuticals keeps them from distinguishing their lack of control over chemical use, opening the door to a progressive demise into substance abuse.

Genetic vulnerability and the priming effects of the drug itself are the best-understood etiologic agents for addiction. The childhood experiences, medical school training about pharmaceuticals, and the life-and-death nature of a physician's work modify the quality and progression of a nascent addiction disorder. Physicians are taught in medical school and residency (and often in their childhood) to appear self-sufficient and in control. An evolving addiction disorder wages against this external façade of competence. Such a physician is at baseline more secretive and duplicitous and, once abusing drugs or alcohol, his or her secretive nature further fuels chemical use. Emotional regression and dysregulation is produced by the illicit and secretive qualities of addiction and their resultant stressors.

The physician's behavior deteriorates first at home, then with friends, and finally surfaces at the workplace. By the time the physician exhibits problems at work, significant familial discord (marital strife, divorce, difficulties with acting out in children) commonly exists. Rarely does the family "turn in" an addicted spouse or other family member (64). Often hospital staff or a colleague becomes publically worried about the physician. The physician is then confronted at work when an undeniable incident occurs or a series of smaller incidents push colleagues and the hospital medical staff to confront the doctor. An active PHP, especially one that is supportive and confidential, can be very beneficial in reducing the threshold for reporting to punitive agencies and thus, can promote early detection. Most physicians arrive in treatment with thin scraps of their façade remaining. They exhibit a demeanor of superiority and knowledge, deny any loss of control, and have a need to appear competent, in stark contrast to their crumbling lives.

IDENTIFICATION, INTERVENTION, AND ASSESSMENT

Identification Physicians come to light with a broad spectrum of symptom severity, from a physician self-identifying his alcoholism while in couples' therapy, all the way to an apneic and asystolic physician on the floor of the operating room bathroom. In the past, denial, shame, and fear of reprisal tended to keep the physician from seeking proper help until significant external consequences coalesced (2). In more recent years, the emergence of clinically oriented, supportive, and confidential PHPs has stimulated earlier reporting, either by self or colleagues. Physician-patients have often had years of familial and social discord while struggling to maintain acceptable work performance, until this last refuge, too, collapses. Thus, disturbances of social or familial functioning may be more sensitive early indicators of substance dependence in the physician. Unfortunately the family often protects the alcoholic or drug-addicted "bread winner" physician.

A variety of work-related behaviors can be clues to substance use. O'Conner and Spickard (1) describe conditions and warning signs that can help detect addiction, including genetic history, drug access, domestic problems, appearance of being drunk at social functions, intoxication or the odor of alcohol on the breath at work, highly irregular hours for rounds, self-prescribing, neglect of responsibilities, anger outbursts, frequent medical complaints without a reasonable diagnosis, staff concerns about physician behavior, depression or weight change, and citations for driving while under the influence (DUI or DWI). Talbott and Wright (64) have independently reported a similar list of behavioral signs of addiction in the physician.

If problems are not addressed early, the doctor's work quality and attendance often suffers. In contrast, if a physician obtains drugs at work (e.g., samples from a drug closet or drugs diverted from the OR or ICU), he or she displays the opposite behavior—volunteering for additional shifts, arriving early for work, and signing up for more complex (i.e., easier drug access) cases.

Modes of Intervention Several comprehensive guides to intervention have been published (2,65). In recent years, PHPs have become very skilled at directing the physician-patient into treatment. The formal "Johnson Model Intervention" is seldom used today. Tension involved in the intervention process can be reduced by directing the physician suspected of addictive disease to undergo an evaluation rather than insisting that addiction exists and treatment is indicated. The physician in question is told about the concerns (often without divulging the source of information) and the importance of resolving said concerns by undergoing a thorough and authoritative evaluation. Ultimately, the goal of intervention is early detection of whatever problem is causing concerns. The immediate goal is to get the physician in question into a "safe harbor," to undergo appropriate evaluation.

If handled with tact, as is common with experienced PHPs, physicians can usually be "gently coerced" into an evaluation, given the alternative of possible Medical Board referral, evaluation, and possible legal action. However, some physicians, especially those who have felt assaulted by a legal process or have undergone previous interventions, require additional external pressure to begin the evaluation and/or treatment process. Regardless of the level of encouragement needed to get physician-patients into evaluation, they often arrive with a thinly fabricated story depicting their entry into evaluation or treatment as self-motivated.

Most states have reporting laws ("snitch laws") that require hospitals and colleagues to report to the state PHP or their state medical board a physician who is suspected of being impaired by alcohol or drugs. Treating physicians must have knowledge of the laws in their state before embarking down the road of caring for physician patients. In 2001, the Joint Commission pressured hospital organizations to address the wellness of their medical staff (67). This Joint Commission standard has helped formalize a physician health process in most hospitals and formalize the support and intervention network in hospitals. In most states, the PHP is willing to take on or assist the hospital in meeting this standard (68). Hospital physician health committees or officers can be effective in early identification and referral of addicted physicians if the process maintains a balance of compassion with a firm directive hand.

Impairment commonly occurs in physicians as addiction progresses. In a study of impairment of all types (and clearly not focused solely on substance-induced impairment), Igartua (69) reported that 7% of residents in her survey reported working with an impaired physician supervisor. Impaired supervisory physicians are no longer protected and enabled by their juniors. Reuben and Noble (70) reported that 72% of house officers would report an impaired attending physician.

Assessment Physicians vary on their need for assessment. Some are quickly identified and agree to cooperate with their treatment needs or at least with an outpatient evaluation. Physicians who are more entrenched in their addiction, have more complex presentations, or are frankly resistant need formal assessment. In these cases, timely and proper diagnosis is often best made by a multidisciplinary evaluation using the guidelines established by the Federation of State Physician Health Programs. Assessment can be completed at the least intensive level of care that results in a comprehensive view of the patient and his or her family and social system. The examination process must prevent the assessed physician from hiding continued drug use, withdrawal, and addiction-related interpersonal behaviors. Because of the complexity and comprehensive nature of these evaluations, most evaluators conduct them in a residential or partial hospitalization setting where the physician can be observed continuously. Such evaluations have come to be called a "Ninety-six Hour Evaluation," a moniker derived from the time usually taken to complete this process. A comprehensive evaluation is best performed by removing the doctor from his or her work role to a center with expertise and willingness to take on the sometimes laborious and difficult task of physician evaluation. Most PHPs have established criteria and maintain a list of competent evaluators. Allowing physicians to self-select an evaluator often results in their selecting a friend or colleague or someone not equipped with proper expertise for the nuances of a physician addiction evaluation. This results in an inadequate and partial evaluation and thus a missed chance at early diagnosis. The evaluation should include information from, but should not be carried out by, a current or past therapist, psychiatrist, or other caregiver (8). Among the criteria listed by PHPs for competent evaluation are that the evaluation be performed by a multidisciplinary team composed of an addiction medicine physician and an addiction psychiatrist; include psychologic and neuropsychologic testing, family assessment, review of previous medical records, and the collection of collateral information from coworkers, hospital employees, friends, and PHPs themselves; and/or any other important source of information needed to thoroughly assess the physician. The purpose of each component of a comprehensive addiction evaluation for physicians is outlined in Table 40.2.

The team involved in a multidisciplinary evaluation meets repeatedly during the course of the evaluation and once again when all data has been collected. Final diagnoses and recommendations are best produced by discussion (often *lively* discussion) by the evaluation team. The patient then meets with one or all members of the evaluation team to review the diagnosis and recommendations. The patient may elect to involve a family member. The evaluation team is best served by including the PHP or other referral source in the summation session; this action decreases confusion and splitting regarding the outcome. A comprehensive, integrated report is commonly sent to both the evaluatee and other relevant parties.

TREATMENT

Approximately a dozen programs in the United States have experience and special expertise in the treatment of addicted physicians and other health professionals; some programs have more than 30 years of experience and have treated thousands of addicted physicians. However, some states are trending towards increased law enforcement actions against addicted physicians, as opposed to treatment. California, for example, has decided to "sunset" the Physician Diversion Program in 2009, and it is far from clear what kind of structures will replace it. Strong political voices are heard to say that addicted physicians deserve no "strikes," that they are, in essence disposable in a competitive medical economy.

Clinical Considerations with Addicted Physicians as Patients It has been alleged that physicians "make the worst patients" (72). Physicians often deny symptoms of any disease, seek substandard care, and put off appropriate care for serious symptoms (74). As in any other medical situation, the physician-patient in addiction treatment has difficulty giving up the provider role and assuming the obligations of the sick role (73). In treatment settings with an admixture of physician and nonphysician patients, the treatment program must set firm limits prohibiting the physician from providing medical advice to other patients. If a patient is the only physician in a given treatment setting, that patient will likely remain or lapse into his or her physician's role the first moment another patient asks for medical advice or for stories from the physician's career. This is a recipe for treatment failure. By contrast, when

TABLE 40.2 Components of a Suggested Comprehensive Physician Addiction Assessment

Required components	Purpose[a]
Addiction medicine evaluation	Determine the existence and extent of any type of addictive disorder.
Addiction psychiatry evaluation	Determine comorbid Axis I and II disorders that interact with the addictive disease and impede treatment. Can be combined with the above assessment.
History and physical and review of medical records	Determine the existence and extent of medical consequences of substance use. Evaluate comorbid medical conditions (chronic pain, etc.).
Psychological testing	Correlate with psychiatric evaluation; determine interaction of personality and treatment.
Neuropsychologic testing	Determine if cognitive deficits exist and ultimately, the physician's ability to practice from a cognitive standpoint.
Family assessment	Determine how the evaluatee's family of origin and current nuclear family contributes to psychological, psychiatric, and addiction problems and suggest methods of correcting them.
Collection of collateral information	Evaluate effects of addiction on the workplace, family and social life. Catalog behavioral observations that correlate with addiction-related behaviors, personality problems, and stressors.
Hair and body fluid drug testing	Correlate with addiction history from multiple sources. Determine honesty of self disclosures.
Spiritual history	Assess past involvement with spiritual and religious pursuits. Determine potential pitfalls with twelve-step programs.
Optional components	
Forensic interview with or without polygraphic exam	Determine the level of honesty on a broad base of issues related to chemical use and attendant behaviors.
Pain evaluation	Determine the interaction between an acute or chronic pain disorder and the addiction. Distinguish between pseudo-addiction and addiction.
Milieu interaction	Evaluate physician for social difficulties and personality issues. Assist the physician in entering the patient role.
Sexual issues evaluation	Evaluate need for sexual compulsivity treatment, predator treatment, or special sexual issues therapy.

[a]All components of the evaluation contribute to determining whether an addictive disease exists, the level of care needed, and treatment planning for eventual care, if any.

a physician falls into self-diagnosis, it is best to use this as grist for the therapeutic mill.

Physicians will attempt to fit the treatment into what they know: school and testing. Physician-patients have little trouble learning the didactic parts of treatment. Physicians early in treatment may arrive at a group therapy session with pen and paper in hand, hoping to glean one piece of information that will rocket them into recovery, or at least accelerate their discharge. The change required of all patients in addiction treatment is an emotional, interpersonal, and spiritual shift. Physicians have little experience in this area. They often become stuck trying to obtain an "A" in treatment and, in this way, miss the necessary emotional, experiential, interpersonal, and spiritual changes that are needed to truly recover. When staff attempt to correct the physician's approach to treatment, they risk becoming ensnared in the physician's tendency toward excess perfectionism. The resultant projection of this hostility produces negative transference and poorly veiled contempt for "less educated" treaters (73).

Physicians work and interact in an environment filled with physical and emotional pain. In order to succeed, they must at times distance themselves from the strife around them. When combined with an achievement-oriented childhood, the physician-patient defaults to intellectualization of his emotional experience or, on occasion, frank alexithymia (without-word-for-feelings) (75). Treatment will necessarily reacquaint the physician with the subtle nuances of feeling states. One particularly difficult emotional state is shame. Most addicts view their addiction and their lives through a lens of shame, and physicians seem to have a surfeit of shame. Fayne and Silvan (73) note that a key task in recovery is an honest appraisal of how the physician's addiction has interfered with his ability to function as a physician. This requires a vigilant therapeutic group that models self-disclosure and self-examination. The physician, owing to childhood and training-induced drives for accomplishment and perfection, risks turning the task of self-examination into self-loathing. Treatment of such individuals mandates that the treatment staff and community encourage fearless self-examination without inadvertently pulling the hair trigger of the physician's self-loathing. When in the state of shame, the patient tends to freeze psychologically. The precarious management of shame is further complicated by the patient's transference and the therapist's countertransference that arises when a bright physician-patient seems incapable (or willfully resistant) to the self-examination necessary for recovery.

Working with addicted physicians requires understanding of the dynamics of addiction and the distinct but highly interactive elements between addiction and the personality. Inexperienced or overly biased treatment providers tend to label the psychologic effects of addiction as personality issues or, conversely, they view long-standing personality dynamics in the physician-patient as addictive thoughts and actions. A balanced understanding requires a healthy respect for both schools of thought. Addiction uses the specific personality dynamics of the physician-patient to serve its own ends, exaggerating and driving maladaptive forces to ensure its own survival. And conversely, the addictive process also serves complicated internal and interpersonal pathology. It is tempting to establish a cause and effect relationship between nonaddiction psychiatric disorders and the disease of addiction itself. Such a path often colludes with the patient's denial system. A more powerful viewpoint is to envision a patient's addiction and their Axis I and II psychiatric problems as distinct disorders that are independent but most certainly interactive.

Social and legal issues only further confound the type and course of treatment. Because of all the aforementioned issues treatment is, by its nature, very different in physicians. Medical boards, the general public, PHPs, and the physician him- or herself have low tolerance for the potential public harm that can occur when a physician becomes addicted; they are exquisitely intolerant of multiple relapses. This flies in the face of the nature of addiction as a disease characterized by relapse and remission. The societal pressure to "have a perfect recovery" creates a maladaptive alliance with the physician-patient's own perfectionism (62).

Characteristics of the Treatment Setting The treatment of physicians involves a prolonged continuum of care. When a physician leaves his or her initial treatment setting and returns to work, this is described by the unfortunate and inaccurate vernacular of having "completed treatment." In fact, what physicians are asked to do in the second phase of treatment is in many ways more comprehensive care than many patients receive during their primary treatment. This "post-treatment" monitoring commonly involves weekly group therapy sessions, peer support groups, after-care groups, individual counseling, self-help group attendance, drug testing, and worksite monitor reports for 5 years or more.

The confluence of known difficulties engaging physicians in treatment, the public demand for safety, and liability issues involved in allowing a physician to work while in outpatient addiction treatment have promoted physician-specific, long-term residential addiction treatment programs. A paucity of literature exists about the efficacy of less intensive treatment, but fair results have been reported by Dilts (76) and Reading (77). Smith and Smith (78) reported a small cohort of physicians treated in low- and high-intensity care, with substantively better results when longer-term residential care was employed. McLellan et al. (36), reviewing 16 state PHPs over 5 years, noted that 78% of physicians who required treatment went to residential treatment for 30 to 90 days, followed by less intensive outpatient treatment. The remaining 22% of treated physicians went directly to outpatient treatment. Hospitals, malpractice carriers, regulatory boards, health insurance companies, and family and friends have expectations of continuous abstinence. Most medical boards and, increasingly, malpractice insurance companies (who in many states have become a more powerful threat), penalize a physician if he relapses, even a single time. Owing to the research (albeit limited) on the effectiveness of residential treatment and the penalty placed upon relapsing physicians, most physician patients are encouraged to attend longer treatment programs than their nonphysician brethren (79).

Skipper (79) outlined the treatment of the impaired health professional. He reported that all physician-specialized treatment programs use a 12-step philosophy as the core component of treatment. Such programs have proven effectiveness with physicians (80). Studies show that if abstinence is the desired outcome point, consistent involvement with 12-step meetings produces the best results (81). All physician treatment programs reviewed by Skipper (70) utilize family therapy, and most offer a brief psychoeducational family program sometime in the physician's treatment (1). Family participation also leads to a better outcome (82). Family members move through their own denial of the significance of the problem, anger at the physician-patient, and fear of loss of prestige and financial security. The initial goal of family treatment is to redirect the hostility away from the patient (or the treatment program and PHP) toward healthy and constructive family dynamics, focused on relapse prevention.

Physician-specific groups allow self-disclosure and sharing of alcohol and drug-related behaviors that risked or caused patient harm. Such violations of the Hippocratic Oath generate shame. Once articulated, such lapses are best linked to the addictive disease and away from the core self. Physician-specific groups serve a different, more pragmatic, but equally important purpose. Most physicians have work-related triggers (e.g., drug access at work, prescription pads, and locations in the office or hospital where use occurred). Specific trigger management skills are discussed, and medically specific relapse prevention plans are developed in these physician-specific groups. On this practical level, physician-specific groups also address the myriad other issues facing physicians when returning to practice, such as the difficulties of seeing their patients in A.A., Drug Enforcement Agency prescribing restrictions, and continued management of drugs and prescriptions in the office or hospital.

There is an increasing body of evidence for the safe and effective use of pharmacologic adjuncts in the treatment of alcoholism. Most physician treatment programs use one or more medications including disulfiram, naltrexone, acamprosate, and/or topiramate. Of special note is the use of the opioid blocker naltrexone in opioid-addicted physicians who, upon return to practice, have continued easy access to opioids.

It could be argued that monthly injectable naltrexone is especially desirable because the monitoring program is assured that the drug is continuously "on board." Alternatives such as monitoring urine for the presence of naltrexone or observed administration of oral doses of naltrexone may also be used but provide less assurance. Ultimately, long-term monitoring of physicians may be the most essential component of treatment and critical for sustained recovery. Monitoring and support groups are commonly provided by PHPs or occasionally by the treatment center itself.

Physician Health Programs

History The importance of PHPs in supporting and promoting early detection and proper evaluation and treatment of physicians cannot be overstated. The heart of the physician's health movement can be traced back to the founding of International Doctors in Alcoholics Anonymous (IDAA) by Clarence Pearson, in 1949. IDAA has grown from 24 physicians, meeting in Pearson's garage in Cape Vincent, New York, to an international organization attracting thousands of physicians and other doctorate-level individuals in recovery from addiction. On the regulatory side, the Federation of State Medical Boards called for a model probation and rehabilitation process for addicted physicians in 1958. However, no meaningful change occurred until 1973 with the publication of the watershed JAMA article: "The sick physician. Impairment by psychiatric disorders, including alcoholism and drug dependence" (83). The AMA held its first conference on physician impairment in 1975. State medical societies organized committees on physician impairment. The American and Canadian Medical Associations have jointly sponsored conferences on physician impairment every other year since 1975. Concern from medical organizations, governing bodies, and hospital regulatory boards resulted in the state-by-state emergence of PHPs over a period of 25 years. By 2007, almost every state in the United States has some type of PHP, ranging from one employee with a $20,000 budget to a 1.5 million dollar budget and 19 full-time employees (84). In 2007, more than 9,000 physicians were in monitoring by PHPs programs across the United States (84).

Structure PHPs have widely different organizational structures and lines of authority. More than half (54%) of PHPs are nonprofit foundations. Others are part of their respective state medical association (35%) or the licensing board itself (13%) (84). All PHPs have written agreements that guide their interaction with their state licensing boards. Most (59%) of PHPs evaluated in the McLellan et al. study (86) have specific laws that sanction their actions and guide their operation. PHPs have evolved from two distinct sources. Some PHPs have descended from committees of medical board itself and have evolved, with varying degrees of autonomy, from that board. Other PHPs emerged from a state medical society or other concerned physician groups. The independent evolution of state PHPs coalesced into a federation in 1990. Many state medical boards continue to actively monitor some physicians while referring others to the state PHP. Interestingly enough, one comparison study of a state (Oregon) with both programs noted that "voluntary diversion program for appropriately selected physicians may enhance earlier referral and intervention."

Activities

Education and Referral Most PHPs provide education about all types of physician impairment (including substance use disorders) and train local hospitals and physician organizations on techniques to help identify and report suspected impairment. Even more importantly, these educational programs offered by PHPs afford the PHP staff the chance to personally meet and network with medical leadership throughout their state. This public relations/training effort carried out by PHPs is important because it helps individuals understand and trust the supportive goal of the PHP, which in turn promotes early referral. Health care organizations have shown increased interest in these issues thanks to the recent Joint Commission standard (currently MS 4.80), which mandates that "the medical staff implements a process to identify and manage matters of individual health for licensed independent practitioners. This identification process is separate from actions taken for disciplinary purposes" (67).

Addiction continues to be the most commonly identified problem addressed by many PHPs (26), but most PHPs address other psychiatric disorders, behaviorally disruptive physicians, and physicians who suffer from other compulsive, addiction-related disorders such as gambling and sexual misbehaviors. All PHPs offer consultation about a potential impairment, coordinate intake into treatment, and monitor physicians after treatment through statewide systems. Some PHPs offer initial assessment and triage and ongoing therapy groups for the physicians in their state.

PHPs have become more professional, with credibility provided by their expertise, affiliation with the FSPHP, and other medical organizations, such as the American Medical Association (AMA) and the Federation of State Medical Boards. As professionalism has increased, so has their finesse and ability to carry out educational programs, expanding to a broader range of topics (stress and burnout, sexual misconduct, appropriate prescribing, etc.). The core concept of PHPs has become clear: "to detect problems that lead to impairment and to intervene and encourage physicians to obtain assistance prior to damaging their careers or harming patients" (66). Sophistication in dealing with addicted physicians has increased, in partnership with expert evaluators and treatment providers. Follow-up monitoring has become much more sophisticated with additional monitoring tools (hair testing, flexible variations in drug testing, new tests for alcohol, devices for monitoring alcohol, and so on). New software options are making tracking of physicians, obtaining reports through online reporting, and real-time tracking of reports more efficient.

Abstinence Monitoring All PHPs track the abstinence status of their recovering physicians. All programs use random witnessed body fluid analysis (most frequently through urine drug screens but often including hair and blood analysis) through an organized monitoring program. Screens commonly taper in frequency over the course of monitoring, for a period of 5 or more years (36). The physician is mandated to call in or check electronically each day to see whether he or she has to provide a sample for assay. Several providers have arisen to provide the call-in service as well as billing and tracking of the screens. Urine screening in physician populations requires considerable expertise and accuracy. Addicted physicians can use their knowledge to evade detection. Most physician drug panels test for 20 to 25 drugs, including a wide variety of opioids (84). Specialty screens for fentanyl, alfentanil, and sufentanil are necessary in recovering physicians who have access to such compounds. Hair testing can be important in this regard because fentanyl and its congeners have very brief half-lives but are readily detected in hair for weeks or months. Physicians also occasionally abuse more unusual drugs (ketamine, propofol, and dextromethorphan); these physicians need assessment panels specifically designed for them.

More recently, PHPs began more sensitive testing for alcohol use by assaying for ethylglucuronide (EtG), a liver metabolite of alcohol (85,87). False-positive test results for EtG have been reported, solely owing to the sensitivity of the test. The two most common culprits in false-positives are incidental ingestion of ethanol-containing mouthwash and topical application of ethanol-based hand sanitizers (especially if inhaled). Physicians under monitoring should be counseled to avoid these compounds.

Recovery Support In addition to urine monitoring, most state PHPs provide support or therapy groups. Some PHPs provide group-facilitated psychotherapy, while others provide Caduceus groups that are peer-led groups similar to 12-step meetings but often discussing an issue or concern of a given group member. Unlike Alcoholics Anonymous meetings, direct feedback is encouraged. Newcomers often obtain recovery sponsors or guidance from more senior physicians. All long-term sobriety studies of physicians underscore the importance of 12-step meetings (primarily A.A. and N.A.) as a central part of recovery. In a study of 100 physicians with an average of 33.4 months after treatment admission, Galanter et al. (80) noted, "A.A. was apparently perceived by respondents as the most potent element of their recovery."

Relapse Significant consequences to the physician and the public result from relapse. PHPs have developed models of assessing relapse severity. DuPont et al. (84) describe three categories of relapse derived from the earlier work of one of the authors (Skipper) and based upon severity:

- A **Level I relapse** consisted of missing therapy meetings, support groups, dishonesty, or other behavioral infraction.
- A **Level II relapse** involved the reuse of drugs or alcohol but outside the context of medical practice.
- A **Level III relapse** involved drug or alcohol use within the context of practice.

Hankes (89,90) has developed a more extensive relapse management decision tree for the Washington State PHP that classifies relapse and provides decision support for managing seven distinct categories of relapse. It is common for physicians in the first year after treatment to have a brief relapse or slip. If the slip is short-lived, the physician can often be placed in short-term relapse prevention programming, be directed to reintegrate with 12-step meetings, and occasionally begin self-exploration in psychotherapy. Slips (and the resultant treatment) often deepen the physicians' acceptance of their disease and solidify recovery. If managed properly, singular slips are most often helpful in the long run and are not indicators of failed treatment.

Should a physician have a more extensive relapse, he or she should engage in the following:

- An evaluation of the physician's ability to practice until he or she is more stable in recovery
- A longer and tighter monitoring contract
- A reexamination of the patient's psychiatric status, to determine whether an occult mood disorder or other addictive process or past unaddressed trauma is present.
- A reassessment of the patient's family dynamics and support system
- An evaluation of the physician's safety to practice
- A determination of the need to repeat primary residential treatment (or to treat other elements of the addiction or other psychiatric disorder)
- Consideration to add relapse prevention medications

Relapse is part of the disease of addiction. Physicians who have difficulty maintaining abstinence should be removed from the workforce until treatment providers with experience in physician recovery feel that the physician is safe to return. The point in time when a physician is safe to practice is best determined by a joint decision of the physician's treatment provider and the monitoring PHP. All stakeholders must be prudent about when to return physicians to their safety-sensitive occupations.

Treatment Outcome Data Physicians have been the subject of multiple outcome studies focused on the efficacy of extended, multimodal addiction treatment and monitoring. Most addiction treatment outcomes studies are plagued by a high percentage of subjects being lost to follow-up. But, owing to the leverage of medical licensure, physician-based studies have excellent follow-up rates. Physicians appear to have responded very well to their unique treatment and monitoring process. More sophisticated outcome analyses (36,90) have sought to define why physician treatment is so successful and from there identifying which components of the physician treatment process can be generalized to the public at large.

Gallegos et al. (91) reported a 77% sustained abstinence rate in physicians followed for 5 years. In the North Carolina PHP, Ganley et al. (92) noted 65% of physicians had a good outcome (as defined by completing an aftercare contract), and another 26% had a good outcome with complications (e.g., relapsed but eventually completed a monitoring contract) in a 6-year study from 1995 to 2000, resulting in a 91% good outcome. In 2002, Lloyd (93) reported an impressive follow-up of alcoholic physicians in the United Kingdom over 21 years, noting a mean sustained duration of abstinence of 17.6 years abstinence in 68 of 80 physicians reporting. He conservatively scored the 20% lost to follow-up as negative outcomes, and even with this, he noted that 73% of the physicians in his study of 80 physicians were in recovery. Knight et al. (94), reporting on the Massachusetts Medical society's 10-year data between 1993 and 2003, cited 75% program completion (albeit some with multiple contract periods). Successful completion required continuous and complete abstinence for a contract period. Eight percent relapsed, and 17% did not complete a contract for other reasons. They noted that the time to relapse was shorter for women. Medical board involvement in the oversight of the physician was associated with a positive outcome.

Domino et al. (90) noted that 25% of physicians in the Washington state PHP (1991 to 2001) had at least one relapse. Family history, comorbid psychiatric disorder, and a previous relapse increased the probability of relapse. The use of major opioids increased the probability of relapse but only in the presence of a comorbid psychiatric disorder. McLellan et al. (36) evaluated the outcomes among 904 addicted physicians treated in 16 PHPs and found 78% were continuously abstinent throughout the 5- to 7-year period of evaluation; more than 90% of those physicians were still practicing medicine. Among those physicians who did relapse, 74% had only one episode of alcohol or drug use.

Controversies

Privacy and Safety Conflict Physician treatment and abstinence monitoring is troubled by the conflict between the physician-patient's need for privacy and the public's need for safety. Add to this a stigmatized view of addiction; the result is that the addicted physician has become in many ways the "whipping boy" of physician impairment. Many other problems among physicians can and do lead to mistakes and patient harm (e.g., sleep deprivation, overwork, poor communication with hospital staff, intemperate affairs), but they are not as directly addressed and do not receive a fraction of the public or regulatory board outcry or concern. Ironically, confidentiality for treatment of physician mental illness, including substance use disorders, actually increases patient safety by encouraging early referral and safe passage into treatment. Strong privacy laws that protect substance abuse records draw addicted patients (physicians or not) into treatment earlier in the course of their disease.

Conversely, many states have laws that mandate that care givers report physician impairment or restriction of clinical privileges. Physicians who suffer from addiction diseases do become impaired. When a concerned individual reports an addicted physician owing to real or potential impairment, the physician-patient's right to privacy is at times violated through the reporting of the real or potential impairment, and thus privacy is lost. Some states mandate that treatment providers report physicians to the medical board, regardless of whether impairment has been proven, and automatic board action ensues. Although this may superficially appear to protect patients, an excessively broad mandate for reporting actually decreases the probability that a physician will be referred for assessment. If the perceived consequences of referral are sufficiently prejudicial, referral will not occur until a major incident occurs. In some states, regulatory boards allow PHP intercession, holding off disciplinary proceedings as long as the physician effectively addresses his disease in an appropriate and structured manner. If regulatory boards tilt in favor of law enforcement over treatment, colleagues and care providers become more reluctant to report. In this case, the physician's care providers hide behind the confidentiality of their profession and lose the benefit of the organized monitoring and peer support provided by a PHP. The structure of PHPs facilitates a proper balance in the privacy/safety conflict. They hold the awkward middle ground between their medical board and treatment providers. PHPs provide limited confidentiality if the physician does not pose a threat to public safety but report to the medical board should a patient become uncooperative or a risk.

Is Monitored Recovery the Same as Self-Guided Recovery? Physicians frequently enter treatment to retain their medical license. One intent of treatment is to shift the physician from this external driver to an internalized state of recovery as a lifetime's work. During treatment and monitoring, physicians do not easily make this shift and many are held in a drug free state by the threat of drug screens and behavioral monitoring. Their addictive illness is in stasis, but many of these physicians are not self-motivated to recovery. Such physicians have a high probability of returning to alcohol and other drug use when and if monitoring is discontinued. In this "monitoring-induced, disease stasis syndrome," the individual has made an internal commitment to abstinence only as a temporary means to an end. Such physicians are compliant and assume a false persona of acceptance to their treatment providers, monitors, and PHP personnel.

This false recovery is a by-product of external pressure and the intense treatment and monitoring that physicians undergo. Treatment providers should avoid pressuring patients to conform, should encourage patients to verbalize their resistance and dissatisfaction with treatment, and praise honest self-disclosure, especially if the patient is describing how he or she is stuck in the process of change. It should not be a cardinal sin in treatment for a patient to admit to the wish that never quite goes away—that is, to drink or use drugs in a controlled and sociable manner. Psychodynamic psychotherapy may help such individuals integrate how past survival techniques of false compliance to authority figures are at play in their relationship with the current authority figures in their treatment and monitoring programs. In the meantime, monitoring holds the physician behaviorally accountable and, if properly framed as appropriate supportive care for a chronic relapsing illness, is not only justifiable but good medicine.

Can Physicians Return to Practice on Opioid Maintenance? All addiction treatment programs in the United States that specialize in physicians consider complete abstinence from addicting drugs to be the end goal of treatment (84). Despite aggressive treatment, a small percentage of physicians are unable to maintain sobriety. In such cases, should physicians be treated using opioid agonist treatment with methadone or buprenorphine? And should such a physician on a maintenance opioid agonist be allowed to practice?

Poor outcome data from abstinence-based treatment for opioid-dependent patients in the general population arise primarily from studies of heroin treatment. Physicians, on the other hand, have very high sustained success rates using an abstinence-based model when coupled with the additional assistance of well-designed continuing care and licensure leverage. Some have claimed that it would be malpractice to treat physicians with maintenance therapy considering their very high abstinence success rates. Others cite studies that have examined patients on chronic opioid maintenance therapy and show neither cognitive deficits nor significant motor impairments once therapeutic stable doses are achieved. Proponents of opioid agonist treatment therefore argue that in selected cases, when abstinence-based treatment has failed (often repeatedly), opioid agonist maintenance therapy is not only justified but also safe.

A large study of 904 physicians from 16 PHPs (36) found only one addicted physician was reported to be on maintenance opiates. More recently, Skipper (66) surveyed PHPs and reported that 14 of the 36 PHP respondents indicated they were following-up at least one physician on maintenance opioid-agonist medication. When contacted, each state indicated that the number of cases they had were few and usually involved complex pain issues.

Medical-legal issues come into the picture when addicted physicians are maintained on opioid medications. Gray (95) states, "At least one major statewide malpractice carrier has indicated that they will not insure an addicted physician if he is on opioid maintenance therapy, due to the difficulties in defending such a physician in a malpractice case." Opioid agonist treatment does occur in the treatment of physicians, but there is no clear consensus on which cases need opioid agonist treatment. Research assessing physicians who work while receiving opioid agonist treatment does not exist.

This issue becomes more complex when one considers cases of opioid-addicted physicians who suffer from chronic, nonmalignant pain. The opioids may be necessary to maintain the quality of life in such an individual. However, that same individual may have a history of inappropriate opioid use or even diversion of opioids from patients. In this case, the PHP and treatment providers are balancing the physician's need for pain control with the safety of the public and the fear of reprisal by an uninformed public. The decision about a physician's ability to practice in such situations should be approached with caution and a complete knowledge of the research and experience in this area.

Are Opioid-Addicted Anesthesiologists Safe to Return to their Profession? Multiple conflicting studies debate the outcome of opioid-dependent anesthesiologists returning to the operating room. Menk et al. (96) reported a successful reentry rate of only 34% for parenteral opioid–using anesthesiologists versus 70% for nonopiate abusers. They reported 26 deaths in this group, half attributed to relapse. This oft quoted 1990 study promulgated a pessimistic view of anesthesiologists returning to work but has been criticized because it was essentially an opinion survey of anesthesia training directors. Of the 159 anesthesia training programs surveyed, 113 responded, providing 180 case reports, with most programs providing only a single case report of a resident having been addicted. Critics contend that if most programs reported only a single case, it is likely such reports were skewed toward disasters. Collins et al. (97) also surveyed anesthesiology residencies in 2001, noting that 50% of treated anesthesiologists remained in anesthesiology after treatment, with 91% completing training and 9% dying of relapse-related incidences.

Paris and Canavan (98) compared 32 anesthesiologists with 36 physician controls for an average of 7.5 years; they showed no difference in the relapse rates between these two groups. When stratified by residents versus attending physicians, no significance was found. Domino et al. (90) examined the risk of relapse over 11 years and 256 participants in a Washington State PHP, including 32 anesthesiologists. The relapse rate for anesthesiologists was not statistically significantly different than other physicians. Additionally, there was not a single episode of patient harm or death from overdose by any anesthesiologist in this study. A similar report from Pelton (99) involving 255 physicians who had participated in the California Diversion Program over 10 years showed no difference in relapse rates for anesthesiologists.

Domino et al. (90), evaluating physicians in the Washington State PHP, noted that fentanyl users had a slightly lower incidence of relapse than other major opioid users. Anesthesiologists who returned to the practice of anesthesiology did have an increased risk of relapse when compared to those who did not return, although they caution that their numbers are small and the significance uncertain. Major opioid users had a higher risk of relapse as did physicians with an existing comorbid psychiatric disorder or a family history of addiction. They conclude that anesthesiologists who use major opioids and do not have other risk factors (family history, comorbid psychiatric disorder, and history of relapse) are good candidates to return to the practice of anesthesiology.

It is of significance to note that the studies that followed anesthesiologists under close monitoring in PHPs or regulatory boards—Donovan, Washington State (90); Paris and Canavan (98); Pelton, New Jersey, (99); California—describe outcomes of anesthesiologists that are similar to other physicians, whereas studies that based upon a survey of the memories of anesthesiology program directors (where patients had uncertain treatment and monitoring) describe poor, and at times life terminating, outcomes. No study has cross-correlated relapse rate with type or length of treatment or the use of opioid-blocking agents such as maintenance naltrexone. Continued studies that include the use of opioid antagonists are needed. As a result of this conflicting research, some residencies lean toward retraining a resident in an alternative field once addiction to major opioids occurs.

What Happens when a Physician Relapses? Addiction is recognized as a disease characterized by periods of recovery alternating with relapse. Physician-patients are expected not to relapse, placing another burden of perfectionism upon a cohort of already perfectionist and harshly self-judging individuals. For many physicians, the experience of recovery feels more like a jail of perfectionism than a journey of accepting one's imperfections. The consequence of relapse for any addict entails a loss of self-efficacy. For the physician, it involves a loss of livelihood and facing possible board or legal sanctions. Physicians early in their recovery often experience a brief "discovery" relapse (a return to drug use where the individual's relapse experience validates and internalizes a heretofore poorly accepted diagnosis) (89,90). PHPs are familiar with such occurrences; medical boards and the public at large are not. Research into and standardization of interventions in the event of an early recovery relapse should improve outcomes and at the same time increase public trust.

CONCLUSION

Physicians were the first professional group to address addiction in their profession; this leadership continues today. Addiction in physicians follows a similar course as in the public at large, with several notable exceptions. The access to potent drugs is one of the most important of these exceptions. The identification, evaluation, and treatment of the chronic disease of addiction in this population in some ways sets the gold standard for the care of addiction, with many possible applications for the treatment of addiction in the public at large. Despite the exemplary care and self-monitoring by the physician community, physicians are punished for being ill. The treatment of physicians is different, partly driven by public outcry for complete remission in a disease that is chronic and relapsing by nature. PHPs are integral and imperative elements in the comprehensive disease management of physician addiction; they increase the long-term prognosis for physicians who suffer from addictive disease. Controversies in the management of addiction in physicians abound and call for further research in this interesting and complex population.

REFERENCES

1. O'Connor PG, Spickard A. Physician impairment by substance abuse. *Med Clin North Am* 1997;81(4):1037–1052.
2. Centrella M. Physician addiction and impairment—current thinking: a review. *J Addict Dis* 1994;13(1):91–105.
3. Collins GB. Drug and alcohol use and addiction among physicians. In: Miller, NS., ed. *Comprehensive handbook of drug and alcohol addiction.* New York: Marcel Dekker, 1991:947–966.
4. Bissell L, Hankes L. Health professionals. In: Lowinson J, Ruiz P, Millman RB, eds. *Substance abuse: a comprehensive textbook,* 3rd ed. Baltimore: Lippincott Williams & Wilkins, 1997:897–908.
5. Flaherty JA, Richman JA. Substance use and addiction among medical students, residents and physicians. *Psychiatr Clin North Am* 1993;16(1): 189–197.
6. Bissell L, Haberman PW. *Alcoholism in the professions.* New York: Oxford Press, 1984.
7. Angres DH, Talbott, GD, Bettinardi-Angres, K. *Healing the healer: the addicted physician.* Madison, CT: Psychosocial Press, 1998.
8. Nace EP. *Achievement and addiction: a guide to the treatment of professionals.* New York: Brunner/Mazel, 1995.
9. Coombs RH. *Drug impaired professionals.* Cambridge, MA: Harvard University Press, 1997.
10. McAuliffe WE, Rohman M, Breer P, et al. Alcohol use and abuse in random samples of physicians and medical students. *Am J Public Health* 1991;81(2):177–181.
11. Kessler RC, Berglund, P, Demler O, et al. Lifetime prevalence and age-of-onset distributions of DSM-IV disorders in the national comorbidity survey replication. *Arch Gen Psychiatry* 2005;62:593–602.
12. Niven RG, Hurt RD, Morse RM, et al. Alcoholism in physicians. *Mayo Clin Proc* 1984;59:12–16.
13. McAuliffe WE, Rohman M, Santangelo S, et al. Psychoactive drug use among practicing physicians and medical students. *N Engl J Med* 1986;315:805–810.
14. Lutsky I, Hopwood M, Abram SE, et al. Use of psychoactive substances in three medical specialties: anesthesia, medicine, and surgery. *Can J Anesth.* 1994;41(7):561–567.
15. Hughes PH, Storr CL, Brandenburg NA, et al. Physician substance use by medical specialty. *J Addict Dis* 1999;18(2):23–37.
16. Hughes PH, Baldwin DC, Sheehan, DV, et al. Resident physician substance use, by specialty. *Am J Psychiatry* 1992;149(10):1348–1354.
17. Hughes PH, Brandenburg N, Baldwin, DC, et al. Prevalence of substance abuse among U.S. physicians. *JAMA* 1992;267:2333–2339.
18. Hughes PH, Conard SE, Baldwin DC, et al. Resident physician substance use in the United States. *JAMA* 1991;265(16):2069–2073.
19. Clark DC, Daugherty SR, Baldwin DC, et al. Assessment of drug involvement: applications to a sample of physicians in training. *Addiction* 1992;87(12):1649–1662.
20. Valliant GE, Brighton JR, McArthur C. Physicians' use of mood altering drugs: a 20 year follow-up report. *N Engl J Med* 1970;282:365–370.
21. Mangus RS. Hawkons CE, Miller MJ. Tobacco and Alcohol Use Among 1996 Medical School Graduates. *JAMA* 1998;280(13):1192–1193.
22. Valliant GE. Physician, cherish thyself: the hazards of self prescribing. *JAMA* 1992;267:2373–2374.
23. Baldwin DC, Hughes PH. Conard SE, et al. Substance use among senior medical students: a survey of 23 medical schools. *JAMA* 1991;265: 2074–2078.
24. Clark DC, Eckenfels EJ, Daughterty SR, et al. Alcohol-use patterns through medical school: a longitudinal study of one class. *JAMA* 1987;257:2921–2926.
25. Morrison J, Wickersham P. Physicians disciplined by a state medical board. *JAMA* 1998;279(23):1889–1893.
26. Clay SW, Conatser RR. Characteristics of physicians disciplined by the State Medical Board of Ohio. *J Am Osteopath Assoc* 2003;103(2): 81–88.
27. Berry AJ and the Task Force on Chemical Dependence. Model curriculum on drug abuse and addiction for residents in anesthesiology. The American Society of Anesthesiologists, http://www.asahq.org/clinical/curriculum.pdf, 1998.
28. Talbott G, Gallegos K, Wilson P, Porter T. The Medical Association of Georgia's impaired physicians' program: review of the first 1,000 physicians—analysis of specialty. *JAMA* 1987;257:2927–2930.
29. Earley PH, Weaver G. Manuscript in preparation (2008).
30. McGovern MP, Angres DH, Uziel-Miller ND, et al. Female physicians and substance abuse, comparisons with male physicians presenting for assessment. *J Subst Abuse Treat* 1998;15(6):525–533.

31. Smart D. *Physician characteristics and distribution in the U.S.* 2006. Chicago: American Medical Association Press.
32. Bissell L, Jones RW. The alcoholic physician: a survey. *Am J Psychiatry* 1976;133:1142–1146.
33. Wunsch MJ, Knisely JS, Cropsey KL. Women physicians and addiction. *J Addict Dis* 2007;26(2):35–43.
34. Moore RD. Youthful precursors of alcohol abuse in physicians. *Am J Med* 1990;88:332–336.
35. True WR, Xian H, Scherrer JF, et al. Common genetic vulnerability for nicotine and alcohol dependence in men. *Arch Gen Psychiatry* 1999;56: 655–661.
36. McLellan AT, Skipper GS, Campbell M, et al. Five year outcomes in a cohort study of physicians treated for substance use disorders in the United States. *British Medical Journal* 2008;337:1154–1156.
37. Zeldow P, Daughtery S. Personality profiles and specialty choices of students from two medical school classes. *Acad Med* 1991;66(5):283–287.
38. Hyde GL, Wolf J: Alcohol and drug use by surgery residents. *J Am Coll Surg* 1995;181:1–5.
39. Yufit R, Pollock G, Wasserman E. Medical specialty choice and personality. *Arch Gen Psychiatry* 1969;20:89–99.
40. McAuliffe W. Risk factors in drug impairment in random samples of physicians and medical students. *Int J Addict* 1987;22(9):825–841.
41. Gold MS, Melker RJ, Dennis DM, et al. Fentanyl abuse and dependence further evidence for second hand exposure hypothesis. *J Addict Dis* 2006;25(1):15–21.
42. McAuliffe P, Gold MS, Bajpai M. Second-hand exposure to aerosolized intravenous anesthetics propofol and fentanyl may cause sensitization and subsequent opiate addiction among anesthesiologists and surgeons. *Med Hypoth* 2006;66(5):874–882.
43. Skipper GS. Tramadol abuse and dependence among physicians [letter]. *JAMA* 2004;292(15):1818–1819.
44. Wischmeyer E, Johnson BR, Wilson JE, et al. A survey of propofol abuse in academic anesthesia programs. *Anesth Analg* 2007;105:1066–1071.
45. Moore NN, Bostwick JM. Ketamine dependence in anesthesia providers. *Psychosomatics* 1999;40:356–359.
46. McAuliffe W, Rohman M, Wechsler H. Alcohol, substance use, and other risk-factors of impairment in a sample of physicians-in-training. *Adv Alcohol Subst Abuse* 1984;4(2):67–87.
47. Higgins Roche BT. *Substance abuse policies for anesthesia.* Winston-Salem, NC: All Anasthesia, 2007.
48. Udel MM. Chemical abuse/dependence: physicians' occupational hazard. *J Med Assoc Georgia* 1984;73:775–778.
49. Green RC, Carroll GJ, Buxton WD. Drug addiction among physicians. The Virginia experience. *JAMA* 1976;236:1372–1375.
50. American Medical Association Council on Scientific Affairs. Results and implications of the American Medical Association-American Psychiatric Association Physician Mortality Project. *JAMA* 1987;257:2949–2953.
51. Brewin CR, Firth-Cozens J. Dependency and self-criticism as predictors of depression in young physicians. *J Occup Health Psychol* 1997;2(3): 242–246.
52. Angres DA, McGovern MP, Shaw MF. Psychiatric comorbidity and physicians with substance use disorders: a comparison between the 1980s and 1990s. *J Addict Dis* 2003;22(3):79–87.
53. Savage, SR. Addiction and pain: assessment and treatment issues. *Clin J Pain* 2002;18(Suppl 4):S28–S38.
54. Volpicelli J, Balaraman G, Hahn J, et al. The role of uncontrollable trauma in the development of PTSD and addiction. *Alcohol Res Health* 1999;23(4):256–262.
55. Norman SB, Tate SR. Anderson KG, et al. Do trauma and PTSD symptoms influence addiction relapse context? *Drug Alcohol Depend* 2007; 90:89–96.
56. Benzer DG. Healing the Healer: a primer on physician impairment. *Wisc Med J* 1991;90(2):70–79.
57. Talbot GD, Benson EB. Impaired physicians—the dilemma of identification. *Postgrad Med* 1980;68(6):56–64.
58. Valliant GE, Sobowale NC, McArthur C. Some psychological vulnerabilities of physicians. *N Engl J Med* 1972;287:372–372.
59. Johnson RP, Connelly JC. Addicted physicians: a closer look. *JAMA* 1981;245(3):253–257.
60. Nace EP. *Achievement and addiction: a guide to the treatment of professionals.* New York: Brunner/Mazel, 1995:66–69.
61. Jex SM. Relations among stressors, strainers, and substance use in physicians. *Int J Addict* 1992;27(8):979–994.
62. Gabbard GO. The role of compulsiveness in the normal physician. *JAMA* 1985;254(20):2926–2929.
63. Khantzian EJ. The injured self, addiction, and our call to medicine: understanding and managing addicted physicians. *JAMA* 1985;254(2): 249–252.
64. Talbott GD, Wright C. Chemical dependency in health care professionals. *Occup Med State Art Rev* 1987;2(3):581–591.
65. Fleming MF. Physician impairment: options for intervention. *Am Fam Phys* 1994;50(1):41–44.
66. Skipper GE. Personal communication, 2008.
67. Joint Commission on the Accreditation of Healthcare Organizations. *Comprehensive accreditation manual for hospitals.* 2006. *Comprehensive Accreditation Manual for Hospitals (CAMH): The Official Handbook* Chicago: Joint Commission, 2008
68. Physician Health Services of the Massachusetts Medical Society corporation. *JCAHO Requirement—MS.4.80 LIP HEALTH.* http://www.massmed.org/Content/NavigationMenu6/JCAHORequirement/JCAHO_Requirement_M.htm.
69. Igartua KJ. the impact of impaired supervisors on residents. *Acad J Psychiatry* 2000;24(4):199–194.
70. Reuben DB, Noble S. House officer responses to impaired physicians. *JAMA* 1990;263(7):958–960.
71. Federation of State Physician Health Programs, Inc. *The 2005 physician health program guidelines.* Appendix I 22–26.
72. Schneck SA. "Doctoring" doctors and their families. *JAMA* 1998;280(23):2039–2042.
73. Fayne M, Silvan M. Treatment issues in the group psychotherapy of addicted physicians. *Psychiatr Q* 1999;70(2):123–135.
74. Stoudemire A, Rhoads JM. When the doctor needs a doctor: special considerations for the physician-patient. *Ann Intern Med* 1983;98(1): 654–659.
75. Sifneos P, Apfel-Savitz R, Frankl F. The phenomenon of "alexithymia." *Psychother Psychosom* 1977;28:47–57.
76. Dilts S. The Colorado Physician Health Program: observations at 7 years. *Am J Addict* 1994;3(4):337–345.
77. Reading EG. Nine years experience with chemically dependent physicians: the New Jersey Experience. *Maryland Med J* 1992;41(4): 325–329.
78. Smith PC, Smith JD. Treatment outcomes of impaired physicians in Oklahoma. *J Okla State Med Assoc* 1991;84(12):599–603.
79. Skipper GE. Treating the chemically dependent health professional. *J Addict Dis* 1997;16(3):67–73.
80. Galanter M, Talbott GD, Gallegos K, et al. Combined Alcoholics Anonymous and professional care for addicted physicians. *Am J Psychiatry* 1990;147(1):64–68.
81. Florentine R, Hillhouse MP. Drug treatment and 12-step program participation. The effects of integrated recovery activities. *J Subst Abuse Treat* 2000;18:64–74.
82. Enders LE, Mercire JM. Treating chemical dependency: the need for including the family. *Int J Addict* 1993;28:507-519.
83. The sick physician. Impairment by psychiatric disorders, including alcoholism and drug dependence. *JAMA* 1973;223:684–687.
84. DuPont RL, McLellan AT, Carr G. How are addicted physicians treated and managed? The structure and function of physician health programs in the United States, 2008 (in submission).
85. Skipper GE, Weinmann W, Thierauf A, et al. Ethyl glucuronide: a biomarker to identify alcohol use by health professionals recovering from substance use disorders. *Alcohol Alcohol* 2004;39(5):445–449.
86. Nelson HD, Matthews AM Girard DE, et al. Substance-impaired physicians probationary and voluntary treatment programs compared. *West J Med* 1996;165:31–36.

87. Wurst FM, Skipper GE, Weinmann W. Ethyl glucuronide—the direct ethanol metabolite on the threshold from science to routine use. *Addiction* 2003;98(Suppl 2):51–61.
88. Fletcher CE, Ronis DL. Satisfaction of impaired health care professionals with mandatory treatment and monitoring. *J Addict Dis* 2005;24(3): 61–75.
89. Earley PH, Gallegos K, Howell E, et al. Georgia Composite State Board of Medical Examiners: guidelines for problem physicians. 1995.
90. Domino, KB, Hornbein TF, Polissar NL, et al. Risk factors for relapse in health care professionals with substance use disorders. *JAMA* 2005; 293(12):1453–1460.
91. Gallegos KV, Lubin BH, Bowers C, et al. Relapse and recovery: five to ten year follow-up study of chemically dependent physicians—the Georgia experience. *Maryland Med J* 1992;41(4):315–319.
92. Ganley OH, Pendergast WJ, Wilkerson MW, et al. Outcome study of substance impaired physicians and physician assistants under contract with the North Carolina physicians health program for the period 1995–2000. *J Addict Dis* 2005;24(1):1–12.
93. Lloyd G. One hundred alcoholic doctors: a 21-year follow-up. *Alcohol Alcohol* 2002;37(4):370–374.
94. Knight JR, Sanchez LT, Sherritt L, et al. Outcomes of a monitoring program for physicians with mental and behavioral health problems. *J Psychiatr Pract* 2007;13(1):25–32.
95. Gray R. Personal communication, 2007.
96. Menk EJ, Baumgarten RK, Kinsley CP. Success of reentry into anesthesiology training programs by residents with a history of substance abuse. *JAMA* 1990;263(22):3060–3062.
97. Collins GB, McAllister MS, Jensen M, et al. Chemical dependency treatment outcomes of residents in anesthesiology: results of a survey. *Anesth Analg* 2005;101:1457–1462.
98. Paris RT, Canavan DI. Physician substance abuse impairment: anesthesiologists versus other specialties. *J Addict Dis* 1999;18(1):1–7.
99. Pelton C, Ikeda RM. The California Physicians Diversion Program's experience with recovering anesthesiologists. *J Psychoactive Drugs* 1991;23(4):427–431.
100. Shore J. The Oregon experience with impaired physicians on probation—an eight year follow-up. *JAMA* 1987;257:2931–2934.
101. Myers T, Weiss E. Substance use by interns and residents: an analysis of personal, social, and professional differences. *Br J Addict* 1987;82: 1091–1099.

SECTION 6

Management of Intoxication and Withdrawal

CHAPTER 41

Tara M. Wright, MD
Jeffrey S. Cluver, MD
Hugh Myrick, MD

Management of Intoxication and Withdrawal: General Principles

Recognition of intoxication and withdrawal states is critical for the appropriate management of individuals with addiction disorders. In addition to being able to recognize the unique intoxication and withdrawal states of particular substances of abuse, the treatment of patients who are under the influence of, or experiencing withdrawal from, substances of abuse requires an understanding of many variables. These variables include an appreciation of the natural history and variants of such syndromes, a complete assessment of the patient's individual medical, psychiatric, and social issues, and a knowledge of the uses and limitations of a variety of behavioral and pharmacologic interventions. All therapies must be individualized to each patient's needs and adjusted to reflect the patient's response to treatment.

This chapter will serve as an introduction to the identification and management of intoxication and withdrawal states, with the management of specific substances to be reviewed in subsequent chapters in this section.

INTOXICATION STATES

Intoxication is the result of being under the influence of, and responding to, the acute effects of alcohol or another drug of abuse. It typically includes feelings of pleasure, altered emotional responsiveness, altered perception, and impaired judgment and performance. The recognition of intoxication states is of paramount importance in the appropriate treatment of substance abusing patients. Intoxication states can range from euphoria or sedation to life-threatening emergencies when overdose occurs. Typically, each substance of abuse has a set of signs and symptoms that are seen during intoxication. Identification and treatment of intoxication can lead to appropriate management of withdrawal phenomenon and provide an avenue for entry into treatment. The initial challenge to the clinician, however, is diagnosis, because intoxication can mimic many psychiatric and medical conditions.

Identification and Management of Intoxication

The identification of intoxication begins with the collection of patient data through a patient history, physical examination, and laboratory screening. Of immediate concern is life-threatening intoxication or overdose. Thus, the first priority is general supportive care and resuscitative actions. It is important to determine not only the severity of the substance ingestion, but also the patient's level of consciousness, the substances involved, and any complicating medical disorders. Often, more than one substance of abuse is involved, and it is critical to know what substances have been ingested, as well as how much of each substance.

Historical information regarding substance use usually can be obtained from the patient. Questions regarding the quantity and frequency of substance use provide valuable information to the clinician. Discovering chronic patterns of substance use may aid in subsequent referral to addiction treatment. Acute intoxication may impede an individual's ability to provide such information. In these cases, the patient's companions or family may be able to provide important information.

Standardized questionnaires for self-administration by the patient or for use by the physician are designed to elicit answers related to alcohol use (see the discussion of screening and assessment instruments in Section 3 of this book). Toxicology screens provide valuable information regarding the type or types of substances used. When screening for substances of abuse, urine is the most widely used specimen because of the ease with which a sample is obtained, the relatively high concentrations of drugs and metabolites present in urine, and the stability of metabolites when frozen (1). Drug screens can aid in the differential diagnosis when atypical symptoms are present. Such screening can be particularly helpful in cases where little clinical history is available. Having knowledge of the particular sensitivities, specificities, and cross-reactivities of the particular urine drug screen being used is of vital importance to the appropriate interpretation of the urine drug screen. In addition, one must have an understanding of the usual duration of detectability of particular substances. However, the duration of detectability can be significantly impacted by the amount of substance ingested, individual rates of metabolism and excretion, as well as fluid ingestion of the individual.

Screening for alcohol is most frequently accomplished by breathalyzer or blood alcohol levels; however, urine tests are also available which detect metabolites of alcohol. Laboratory assays that measure increases in liver enzymes—such as gamma-glutamyl transpeptidase, aspartate aminotransferase, and alanine aminotransferase—can be helpful in identifying alcohol use. Although alcohol is not the only cause of an increase in gamma-glutamyl transpeptidase, and gamma-glutamyl transpeptidase frequently does not increase in younger drinkers, this assay is a reliable predictor of drinking behavior. A biologic assay to monitor alcohol intake involves percent carbohydrate-deficient transferrin, which is a more sensitive and specific indicator of heavy alcohol consumption (2,3).

WITHDRAWAL STATES

Substance withdrawal has been defined by the American Psychiatric Association as "the development of a substance-specific maladaptive behavioral change, usually with uncomfortable physiological and cognitive consequences, that is the result of a cessation of, or reduction in, heavy and prolonged substance use" (4). The signs and symptoms of withdrawal usually are the opposite of a substance's direct pharmacologic effects. Substances in a given pharmacologic class produce similar withdrawal syndromes; however, the onset, duration, and intensity are variable, depending on the particular agent used, the duration of use, and the degree of neuroadaptation.

Evidence for the cessation of or reduction in use of a substance may be obtained by history or toxicology. Additionally, the clinical picture should not correspond to any of the organic mental syndromes, such as organic hallucinosis (4). Withdrawal may, however, be superimposed on any organic mental syndrome. Therefore, a thorough physical examination is necessary, including appropriate laboratory analysis of basic organ functions.

The term *detoxification* implies a clearing of toxins. However, for individuals with physiologic substance dependence, detoxification is defined as the management of the withdrawal syndrome.

Goals of Detoxification Detoxification includes a set of interventions by which a substance an individual is physically dependent on is eliminated from the body. Detoxification seeks to minimize the physical harm caused by the abuse of substances. The American Society of Addiction Medicine lists three immediate goals for detoxification of alcohol and other substances: 1) "to provide a safe withdrawal from the drug(s) of dependence and enable the patient to become drug-free"; 2) "to provide a withdrawal that is humane and thus protects the patient's dignity"; and 3) "to prepare the patient for ongoing treatment of his or her dependence on alcohol or other drugs" (5). Furthermore, it comprises three essential and sequential steps: evaluation, stabilization, and fostering patient readiness for and entry into treatment (6). It is important to distinguish detoxification from substance abuse treatment. *Substance abuse treatment/rehabilitation* involves a constellation of ongoing therapeutic services ultimately intended to promote recovery for substance abuse patients (6). Detoxification may be the first step in this process.

Many risks are associated with withdrawal, some of which are influenced by the setting in which detoxification occurs. For example, in persons who are severely dependent on alcohol, an abrupt, untreated cessation of drinking may result in marked hyperautonomic signs, seizures (which may be recurrent), withdrawal delirium, or even death. Other sedative-hypnotics also can produce life-threatening withdrawal syndromes. Withdrawal from opioids and stimulants produces severe discomfort, but generally is not life-threatening. It may, however, present a danger to those who are debilitated by advanced HIV disease, medical sequelae of addiction, advanced age, coronary artery disease, and other medical problems. Moreover, risks to the patient and society are not limited to the severity of the patient's physical disturbance, particularly when the detoxification is conducted in an outpatient setting. Outpatients experiencing withdrawal symptoms may self-medicate with alcohol or other drugs that can interact with withdrawal medications in an additive fashion or precipitate overdose.

A caring staff, a supportive environment, sensitivity to cultural issues, confidentiality, and the selection of appropriate detoxification medications (as needed) are important components of a humane withdrawal. However, staff must be clear in their treatment goals and set firm boundaries, as well as be sympathetic and have experience in dealing with difficult behaviors that often accompany detoxification. Supportive others (family members, friends, or employers) should be enlisted whenever possible to assist in the care of the patient during outpatient detoxification.

During detoxification, patients may form therapeutic relationships with treatment staff and other patients, providing an opportunity to explore alternatives to an alcohol- or drug-using lifestyle. Detoxification is therefore an opportunity to offer patients information and to motivate them for longer-term treatment. Unfortunately, managed care organizations and other third-party payers often regard detoxification as separate from other phases of alcohol and other drug treatment as though detoxification occurs in isolation from such treatment. In clinical practice, this separation cannot exist; detoxification is but one component of a comprehensive treatment strategy.

General Principles of Management Some detoxification procedures are specific to particular drugs, whereas others are based on general principles of treatment and are not drug-specific. The general principles are presented here; subsequent chapters address specific treatment protocols for each class of drugs.

There is a risk of serious adverse consequences for some patients who undergo withdrawal. As such, an initial medical assessment is important to determine the need for medication and medical management. Such an assessment should include evaluation of predicted withdrawal severity and medical or psychiatric comorbidity. Although the severity of a given patient's withdrawal cannot always be predicted with accuracy, helpful information includes the amount and duration of alcohol or other drug use, the severity of the patient's prior withdrawal experiences (if any), and the patient's medical and psychiatric history. A history of complicated withdrawal should alert the practitioner to the likely possibility of future complicated withdrawals. The kindling hypothesis has been well supported in alcohol research, such that a history of alcohol withdrawal seizures is a strong indicator of future alcohol withdrawal seizures (7). A widely used instrument in clinical and research settings for the initial assessment and ongoing monitoring of alcohol withdrawal is the Clinical Institute Withdrawal Assessment of Alcohol–revised. The Clinical Institute Withdrawal Assessment of Alcohol–revised is a short test that rates the severity of withdrawal, as observed by the clinician. In general, low scores (≤9) suggest that pharmacotherapy may not be required, whereas high scores (≥10) indicate a greater risk of seizures and delirium tremens.

Every means possible should be used to ameliorate the patient's withdrawal signs and symptoms. Medication should not be the only component of treatment, because psychologic support is extremely important in reducing the patient's distress during detoxification.

The duration of detoxification is not a clearly defined, discrete period. Because detoxification often requires a greater intensity of services than other types of treatment, there is a practical value in defining a period during which a person is "in detoxification." The detoxification period usually is defined as the time during which the patient receives detoxification medications, even though some signs and symptoms may persist for a much longer period. Another way of defining the detoxification period is by measuring the duration of withdrawal signs or symptoms. However, the duration of these symptoms may be difficult to determine in a correctly medicated patient, because symptoms of withdrawal are largely suppressed by the medication.

Another problem in defining the duration of detoxification is the fact that many patients may have prolonged withdrawal signs or symptoms, or "protracted abstinence syndrome." Symptoms of the syndrome include disturbances of sleep, anxiety, irritability, and mood instability. The very existence of the protracted abstinence syndrome has been the subject of considerable controversy; however, there is increasing evidence in the literature supporting its existence. The protracted abstinence syndrome is hypothesized to be a period when individuals are at heightened risk of relapse (8).

Physicians often find it difficult to distinguish symptoms caused by drug withdrawal from those caused by a patient's underlying mental disorder, if one is present. The signs and symptoms of protracted withdrawal thus are not as predictable as those of acute withdrawal, which produces measurable signs that researchers can study in animals under controlled laboratory conditions; protracted withdrawal, on the other hand, often is confined to distress symptoms for which there are no animal models. The plan of care for detoxification should be individualized to account for the considerable variation among patients in terms of signs and symptoms of withdrawal. The best outcomes are obtained by tailoring the detoxification regimen to meet the needs of individual patients. The initial plan of care for detoxification should be adjusted to reflect the patient's response to the treatment provided.

Pharmacologic Management There are two general strategies for pharmacologic management of withdrawal: suppressing withdrawal through use of a cross-tolerant medication, and reducing signs and symptoms of withdrawal through alteration of another neuropharmacologic process. Either or both may be used to manage withdrawal syndromes effectively. To suppress withdrawal with cross-tolerant medication, a longer acting medication typically is used to provide a milder, controlled withdrawal. Examples include use of methadone for opioid detoxification and diazepam for alcohol detoxification. Medications that are not cross-tolerant are used to treat specific signs and symptoms of withdrawal. Examples include use of clonidine for opioid or alcohol withdrawal.

Detoxification alone rarely constitutes adequate treatment. The provision of detoxification services without continuing treatment at an appropriate level of care constitutes less than optimal use of limited resources. The maintenance of abstinence can be a very difficult goal to achieve: it has been estimated that approximately 50% of alcohol-dependent patients relapse within 3 months of detoxification. The appropriate level of care and content of treatment following detoxification must be clinically determined, based on the patient's individual needs. Biopsychosocial factors to be considered in determining the continuing treatment plan include medical and psychiatric conditions, motivation, relapse potential, and available support systems. These factors correspond to the dimensions of illness described in the American Society of Addiction Medicine (ASAM) Patient Placement Criteria for the Treatment of Substance-Related Disorders, 2nd edition–revised (ASAM PPC-2R) (9).

Detoxification Settings The initial assessment should facilitate the selection of the appropriate level of care for detoxification. In determining the most appropriate setting, the practitioner should match the patients' clinical needs with the least restrictive and most cost-effective setting (6). Detoxification may take place in a variety of inpatient and outpatient settings. Multiple instruments have been designed to facilitate selection of an appropriate level of care. The ASAM PPC-2R contains detailed guidelines for matching patients to an appropriate intensity of services for detoxification. Detoxification is conducted in both inpatient and outpatient settings. Both types of settings initiate recovery programs that may include referrals for problems such as medical, legal, psychiatric, and family issues.

Inpatient Detoxification Inpatient detoxification is offered in medical hospitals, psychiatric hospitals, and medically managed residential treatment programs. It allows 24-hour supervision, observation, and support for patients who are intoxicated or experiencing withdrawal. The primary emphasis in this setting should be placed on ensuring that the patient is medically stable (including the initiation and tapering of medications used for the treatment of substance use withdrawal), assessing for adequate biopsychosocial stability (and quickly intervening if this is lacking), and linking the patient to appropriate inpatient and outpatient services once it is medically safe to do so (6). As described by Alling (10), inpatient detoxification may have several advantages to outpatient detoxification. First, the inpatient detoxification restricts the patient's access to substances of abuse. Second, inpatient detoxification allows the clinician to closely monitor the patient for serious withdrawal symptoms and adjust medications as indicated. Such monitoring is especially important if the patient is dependent on high doses of alcohol or other sedative-hypnotic drugs. Finally, detoxification in an inpatient facility can be accomplished more rapidly than in an outpatient setting.

In the case of detoxification from alcohol, about 20% of those undergoing treatment for alcohol withdrawal must be treated as inpatients. Relative indications for inpatient treatment include a history of alcohol withdrawal seizures or delirium, pregnancy, medical or psychiatric illness, or lack of a reliable support system (11,12). Inpatient care of alcohol withdrawal can be 10 to 20 times as expensive as outpatient care. Generally, therefore, it is reserved for those expected to have severe withdrawal symptoms and to require a more intensive level of care (such as patients with a history of severe withdrawal symptoms).

Outpatient Detoxification Outpatient detoxification usually is offered in community mental health centers, methadone maintenance programs, addiction treatment programs, and private clinics. Essential components to a successful outpatient detoxification include a positive and helpful social support network and regular accessibility to the treatment provider (6). Medical and nursing personnel involved must be readily available to evaluate and confirm that detoxification in the less supervised setting is safe. They must be able to interpret the signs and symptoms of alcohol and other drug intoxication and withdrawal, have knowledge of the appropriate treatment and monitoring of these conditions, and have the ability to facilitate the individual's entry into treatment (6). Alling (10) cites several advantages of outpatient detoxification. First, it is much less expensive than inpatient treatment. Second, the patient's life is not disrupted to the degree that it is during inpatient treatment. Finally, the patient does not undergo the abrupt transition from a protected inpatient setting to the everyday home and work settings.

Emergency departments are important components of outpatient detoxification as they often serve as a gateway to detoxification services. Detoxification programs may rely on emergency department staff to assess and initiate treatment for patients with medical conditions or medical complications that occur during detoxification. For social model programs, emergency departments often serve as a safety net for patients who need medical treatment. For the substance-abusing individual who has overdosed or who is experiencing a medical complication of abuse, the emergency department may be the initial point of contact with the health care system and serve as a source of case identification and referral to detoxification. Many patients experiencing alcohol withdrawal seizures present initially to an emergency department where they are taken after a seminal episode.

Considerations in Selecting a Setting The best detoxification setting for a given patient may be defined as the least restrictive, least expensive setting in which the goals of detoxification can be met. The ability to meet this standard assumes that treatment choices always are based primarily on a patient's clinical needs. A comprehensive evaluation of the patient often indicates what therapeutic goals might be achieved realistically during the time allotted for the detoxification process.

Treatment providers should consider detoxification settings and patient matching within the context of a fundamental principle of high-quality patient care. This principle is that the patient's needs should drive the selection of the most appropriate setting. The severity of the patient's withdrawal symptoms and the intensity of care required to ensure appropriate management of these symptoms are of primary importance. Pressures to achieve cost savings are having a significant effect on the selection of treatment settings for detoxification. Many insurance companies, managed care organizations, and other payers have adopted stringent policies concerning reimbursement for alcohol and other drug detoxification services. These policies govern not only the setting in which the services are provided, but also the maximum number and duration of detoxification episodes that are covered benefits. Such policies give insufficient weight to the variety of factors that affect the selection of a setting in which the patient has the greatest likelihood of achieving satisfactory detoxification. Some persons in need of detoxification, for example, may not be appropriate candidates for outpatient detoxification because of environmental impediments such as a spouse who is using alcohol or other drugs. Such a patient may be more appropriately detoxified in a residential setting such as a recovery house or other residential environment that is free of alcohol and other drug use. Panelists convened by the federal Center for Substance Abuse Treatment expressed concern that important clinical decisions often are driven by economic rather than clinical considerations (5,6). They affirmed that the dominant principle in patient placement is that detoxification is cost-effective only if it is appropriate to the needs of the individual patient.

Use of the ASAM Patient Placement Criteria The ASAM PPC-2R is intended for use as a clinical tool for matching patients to appropriate levels of care (see Chapter 27). The criteria reflect a clinical consensus of adult and adolescent treatment specialists and incorporate the results of a comprehensive peer review by professionals in addiction treatment. The ASAM criteria describe levels of treatment that are differentiated by the following characteristics: (i) degree of direct medical management provided, (ii) degree of structure, safety, and security provided, and (iii) degree of treatment intensity provided.

The ASAM criteria offer a variety of options on the premise that each patient should be placed in a level of care that has the appropriate resources (staff, facilities, and services) to assess and treat that patient's substance use disorder. The ASAM patient placement criteria are routinely under review to maximize their utility. As such, a draft supplement to the ASAM Patient Placement Criteria on Pharmacotherapies for Alcohol Use Disorders was distributed for field review and comment at the American Society of Addiction Medicine's Annual Medical Scientific Conference in April 2007. At the time of this writing, this supplement is only for field review and not yet an approved ASAM document.

Relapse Many individuals undergo detoxification more than once, and some do so many times. When recently dependent persons return for repeat detoxification, it generally is with a more realistic expectation of what is needed to remain free from alcohol and other drugs. O'Brien et al. (13) point out that compliance and relapse in addictive disease are comparable to rates of relapse in other illnesses, such as diabetes and hypertension. Therefore they recommend comparable long-term treatment. Although addicted persons are at increased risk of relapse at certain points in their recovery, relapse can occur at any time. The relapsed patient is an appropriate candidate for detoxification and continuing treatment, including relapse prevention education.

SPECIAL POPULATIONS

Although researchers have not yet thoroughly evaluated withdrawal strategies for certain populations, patients in several groups clearly require special consideration.

Pregnant and Nursing Women Special concerns attend detoxification during pregnancy. For example, withdrawal from opioids can result in fetal distress, which can lead to premature labor or miscarriage. On the other hand, opioid agonist treatment, coupled with good prenatal care, is generally associated with good maternal and fetal outcomes. Methadone maintenance has generally been accepted as the standard approach to the opioid-dependent pregnant woman, and buprenorphine may also be useful, particularly as it may be less likely to cause neonatal abstinence syndrome (14,15). It should be noted, however, that both of these medications are classified as pregnancy category C. Although offspring of women on opioid maintenance therapy tend to have a lower birth weight and smaller head circumference than drug-free newborns, no developmental differences at 6 months of age have been documented. Clonidine (frequently used in opioid detoxification) also is a pregnancy category C medication.

Federal panels recommend that all pregnant and nursing women be advised of the potential risks of drugs that are excreted in breast milk (5,16). Nevertheless, they advise that detoxification protocols should not be modified for nursing women unless there is specific evidence that the detoxification medication enters the breast milk in amounts that could be harmful to the nursing infant (5,16). (See Chapter 81.) These decisions often must include weighing the risks and benefits to both the mother and infant. For instance, the American Academy of Pediatrics (17) categorizes benzodiazepines as "drugs for which the effect on nursing infants is unknown, but may be of concern." The addiction provider should coordinate treatment decisions with obstetrician or pediatrician in these cases.

Persons who are HIV-Positive Substance abuse increases the risk of contracting HIV through the use of contaminated needles and risky sexual behavior. In addition, substance abuse treatment can help reduce the transmission of HIV by reducing these behaviors (18). Substance use disorders and HIV/AIDS interact with one another in a complex manner. The presence of an alcohol or drug addiction can certainly impede compliance with an individual's medication regimen for the treatment of HIV (18). A diagnosis of HIV infection does not change the indications for detoxification medications, which can be used in HIV-positive persons in the same way they are used in uninfected patients. A federal panel advises that, if deemed appropriate, the detoxification process need not be altered by the presence of HIV infection (5,19,20). However, the treatment provider does need to be aware of the possible drug interactions between antiretroviral agents used to treat HIV and medications used in detoxification and adjust dosages accordingly (18).

Patients with Other Medical Conditions

Neurologic Disorders Brain-injured patients are at risk for seizures (5). If an alcohol- or other drug-abusing patient who has sustained trauma to the head becomes delirious, the cause of the delirium should be investigated. Slower medication tapers should be used in patients with seizure disorders (5). Doses of anticonvulsant medications should be stabilized before sedative-hypnotic withdrawal begins. The treatment of individuals with past alcohol or sedative-hypnotic withdrawal seizures is controversial. In such a situation, the use of anticonvulsant agents (carbamazepine, valproate) should be considered, either alone or in combination with benzodiazepines.

Cardiovascular Disorders Patients with cardiac disease require continued clinical assessment. Underlying cardiac disease may be worsened by the symptoms of autonomic arousal (elevated blood pressure, increased pulse and sweating) as seen in alcohol, sedative, and opioid withdrawal (6). Because of this, it may be necessary to withdraw the medication at a slower than normal rate. Treatment providers also should be alert to the possibility of interactions between cardiac medications and the agents used to manage detoxification.

Hepatic or Renal Disorders Severe liver or renal disease can slow the metabolism of both the drug of abuse and the detoxification medication. Use of shorter acting detoxification drugs and a slower taper are appropriate for such patients, but require precautions against drug accumulation and oversedation (6).

Chronic Pain Patients who experience pain and receive opioids may not require detoxification from prescribed medications unless they meet the DSM-IV criteria for opioid abuse or dependence (5). However, treatment providers should exercise caution when prescribing medications for chronic pain in patients who have a history of addictive disorders. In a large secondary data analysis of chronic users of opioids for chronic non-cancer pain, a diagnosis of nonopioid substance abuse was the strongest predictor of opioid abuse/dependence (21). Mental health disorders were also moderately strong predictors of opioid abuse/dependence in this group (21). General principles when using opioids in the treatment of chronic pain include comprehensive follow-up, using adjunctive interventions where necessary, regular prescription pickup, appropriate screening for use and abuse, and a limitation on the number of physicians and pharmacists providing treatment (22). Also, when indicated, any patient who has taken opioids or sedative-hypnotics for a prolonged period should be weaned from them gradually.

Patients with Psychiatric Comorbidities It is difficult to accurately assess underlying psychopathology in a patient who is undergoing detoxification (5). Drug toxicity or organic psychiatric symptoms (particularly with amphetamines, cocaine, hallucinogens, or phencyclidine) can mimic psychiatric disorders. For this reason, thorough psychiatric evaluation should be conducted after 2 to 3 weeks of abstinence. At the time patients are evaluated for detoxification, some with underlying psychiatric disorders already may be prescribed antidepressants, neuroleptics, anxiolytics, or lithium. Although staff at some treatment programs may believe that such patients should discontinue all psychoactive medications, a federal panel has advised that this course of action may not be in the best interest of the patient (5). Abrupt cessation of psychotherapeutic medications may cause withdrawal symptoms or reemergence of symptoms of the underlying psychopathology. Thus decisions about discontinuing the medication should be deferred temporarily. If, however, the patient has been abusing the prescribed medication or the psychiatric condition clearly was caused by the patient's alcohol or other drug abuse, the rationale for discontinuing the medication is more compelling. Individuals who use both sedative-hypnotics and alcohol pose a real challenge for detoxification, which generally should be conducted in an inpatient setting and over a prolonged period.

During detoxification, some patients decompensate into psychosis, depression, or severe anxiety. In such cases, careful evaluation of the withdrawal medication regimen is of paramount importance. Anxiety symptoms can cause an overestimation of withdrawal severity on the Clinical Institute Withdrawal Assessment of Alcohol–revised and therefore result in overuse of medication for withdrawal. If the decompensation is the result of inadequate dosing with the withdrawal medication, the appropriate response is to increase that medication. If the dose of the withdrawal medication appears to be adequate, other medications may need to be added. Before selecting that alternative, however, it is important to consider the potential side effects of the additional medication and the possibility of interaction with the withdrawal medication. If withdrawal medications are adequate and appropriate but the patient continues to decompensate, nonaddicting psychotropic medications (such as antipsychotics, anticonvulsants, or antidepressants) may be indicated for the treatment of psychoses, depression, or anxiety emerging during withdrawal. After detoxification is completed, the patient's need for medications should be reassessed. A trial period with no medications may be indicated.

Adolescents Adolescents in detoxification pose somewhat different clinical issues than do adults. Patterns of use, negative consequences, context, and control of use may all be unique in adolescents in comparison to adults. Physical dependence is often not as severe in the adolescent compared with the adult, and the adolescent patient's response to detoxification usually is more rapid than that of the adult (5,23). Inquiring about academic performance, school attendance, and disciplinary problems can be particularly important to help the practitioner ascertain the adolescent's risk of a substance use disorder. Behavioral problems may be more indirect, and the potential for suicide needs to be evaluated carefully. Substance abuse, particularly when comorbid with depression, contributes to an increased rate of suicide in this age group. Adolescents who are undergoing detoxification need a structured environment that is nurturing and supportive. This is especially important because adolescents are notorious for leaving treatment against medical advice. Also, adolescents should be housed separately from adults. Decisions about involving the family in treatment should be made on a case-by-case basis and should reflect an assessment of family functioning. Note that federal regulations allow methadone detoxification of adolescents, but state regulations vary. Methadone detoxification is rare in this age group. Buprenorphine has been investigated for detoxification in adolescents with opioid dependence.

Older Adults Possible factors that may impact the treatment of intoxication and withdrawal in older adults include the increased likelihood of medical comorbidities with multiple prescribed medications and prescribing physicians, greater access to prescription medications (which may be abused) and possible impaired mobility from either social isolation or general medical conditions resulting in difficulty accessing clinic- or office-based treatment. It is essential to conduct a complete assessment and careful monitoring of the patient for comorbid conditions, such as respiratory or cardiac disease or diabetes (24). Because the aging patient may be taking a number of prescription and over-the-counter drugs, the possibility of drug interactions cannot be ignored. For these reasons, detoxification in a medically monitored or medically managed setting often is required (5). The cumulative effects of years of drinking may lead to more severe withdrawal symptoms in elderly persons (25), so the shorter-acting benzodiazepines may be of more clinical utility in this population given their lower risk of oversedation. It may be necessary to reduce the doses of detoxification medications because of older patients' slowed metabolism or coexisting medical disorders.

Persons in Criminal Justice Settings Persons who are incarcerated or in detention in holding cells or elsewhere should be assessed for dependence on alcohol or other drugs because untreated withdrawal from alcohol and sedative hypnotics can be life-threatening. Prevalence of dependence in these settings is higher than in the general population because an estimated 70% of people arrested for violent offenses test positive for substances. According to data from the Arrestee Drug Abuse Monitoring program in 2000, 64% of male arrestees tested positive for at least one of five illicit drugs (cocaine, opioids, marijuana, methamphetamines, and PCP) and 36% reported heavy drinking in the 30 days before arrest (26). It is therefore critical that criminal justice and treatment staff be trained to detect signs and symptoms of substance abuse and to refer clients for appropriate medical treatment in cases of acute intoxication or withdrawal (27).

Although heroin withdrawal is not life threatening to a healthy individual, it can be very difficult for the individual and should be treated appropriately. Patients who have been on opioid agonist treatment before being incarcerated should continue to receive their usual dose of medication. Opioid agonist treatment should be discontinued as gradually as possible if the jurisdiction or setting does not allow patients to receive these medications while incarcerated. Individuals who are on methadone maintenance may experience severe withdrawal symptoms if the medication is stopped abruptly. Indeed, methadone abstinence symptoms may persist for weeks or months and include severe vomiting and diarrhea, which can lead to complications. Pain may be severe and intractable. Detoxification protocols need not be modified for incarcerated persons, except to the extent that state laws restrict the use of methadone or buprenorphine in criminal justice settings. In such cases, linkages with local methadone detoxification programs are advised.

In caring for incarcerated patients, the physician needs to be aware that in some settings, there is an underground market for psychoactive medications. Patients may try to deceive caregivers about their dependence to obtain drugs for sale to others. For this reason, prison medical staff need special training in patient assessment and detoxification (28).

CONCLUSIONS

The recognition and treatment of intoxication and withdrawal states represent important initial steps in the treatment of alcohol or other drug addiction. The primary goal of managing intoxication and withdrawal states is the prevention of morbidity and mortality. Whereas the treatment of intoxication often takes place in a medical setting, the treatment of withdrawal can occur in either an inpatient or an outpatient setting. Many variables must be taken into consideration in providing optimum care to patients who are undergoing treatment of withdrawal states. The ASAM PPC-2R can aid the clinician in matching patients to the appropriate levels of care for ongoing treatment of their addictive disorders.

REFERENCES

1. Council on Scientific Affairs. Scientific issues in drug testing. Council on Scientific Affairs. *JAMA* 1987;257:3110–3114.
2. Litten RZ, Allen JP, Fertig JB. Gamma-glutamyltranspeptidase and carbohydrate-deficient transferrin-alternative measures of excessive alcohol consumption. *Alcohol Clin Exp Res* 1995;19:1541–1546.
3. Hock B, Schwarz M, Domke I, et al. Validity of carbohydrate-deficient transferrin (%CDT), gamma-glutamyltransferase (gamma-GT) and mean corpuscular erythrocyte volume (MCV) as biomarkers for chronic alcohol abuse: a study in patients with alcohol dependence and liver disorders of non-alcoholic and alcoholic origin. *Addiction* 2005;100: 1477–1486.
4. American Psychiatric Association. *Diagnostic and statistical manual of mental disorders*, 4th ed. Washington, DC: American Psychiatric Press, 1994.
5. Center for Substance Abuse Treatment. *Detoxification from alcohol and other drugs* (Treatment Improvement Protocol Series, Number 19). Rockville, MD: Substance Abuse and Mental Health Services Administration, 1995.
6. Center for Substance Abuse Treatment. *Detoxification and substance abuse treatment* (Treatment Improvement Protocol Series, Number 45). Rockville, MD: Substance Abuse and Mental Health Services Administration, 2006.
7. Brown ME, Anton RF, Malcolm R, et al. Alcohol detoxification and withdrawal seizures: clinical support for a kindling hypothesis. *Biol Psychiatry* 1988;23:507–514.
8. Aston-Jones G, Harris GC. Brain substrates for increased drug seeking during protracted withdrawal. *Neuropharmacology* 2004;47(Suppl 1):167–179.
9. Mee-Lee D, Shulman G, Fishman M, et al. *Patient placement criteria for the treatment of substance-related disorders*, 2nd ed.–revised (ASAM PPC-2R). Chevy Chase, MD: American Society of Addiction Medicine, 2001.
10. Alling FA. Detoxification and treatment of acute sequelae. In: Lowinson JH, Ruiz P, Millman RB, eds. *Substance abuse: a comprehensive textbook*. Baltimore, MD: Williams & Wilkins, 1992:402–415.

11. Saitz R, O'Malley SS. Pharmacotherapies of alcohol abuse. Withdrawal and treatment. *Med Clin N Am* 1997;81:881–907.
12. Myrick H, Anton R. Clinical management of alcohol withdrawal. *CNS Spectrums* 2000;5:22–32.
13. O'Brien CP, Childress AR, McLellan AT. *Conditioning factors may help to understand and prevent relapse in patients who are recovering from drug dependence* (NIDA Research Monograph Number 106). Rockville, MD: National Institute on Drug Abuse, 1991.
14. Jarvis MA, Schnoll SH. Methadone treatment during pregnancy. *J Psychoactive Drugs* 1994;26:155–161.
15. American Psychiatric Association. *Substance use disorders practice guideline, quick reference guide*, 2006. Available at: www.psych.org/psych_pract/treatg/pg/prac_guide.cfm. Accessed November 8, 2007.
16. Center for Substance Abuse Treatment. *Pregnant, substance-using women* (Treatment Improvement Protocol Series, Number 2). Rockville, MD: Substance Abuse and Mental Health Services Administration, 1993.
17. American Academy of Pediatrics, Committee on Drugs. Transfer of drugs and other chemicals into human milk. *Pediatrics* 2001;108:776–789.
18. Center for Substance Abuse Treatment. *Substance abuse treatment for persons with HIV/AIDS* (Treatment Improvement Protocol Series, Number 37). Rockville, MD: Substance Abuse and Mental Health Services Administration, 2000.
19. Center for Substance Abuse Treatment. *Treatment for HIV-infected alcohol and other drug abusers* (Treatment Improvement Protocol Series, Number 15). Rockville, MD: Substance Abuse and Mental Health Services Administration, 1993.
20. Center for Substance Abuse Treatment. *Screening for infectious diseases among substance abusers* (Treatment Improvement Protocol Series, Number 6). Rockville, MD: Substance Abuse and Mental Health Services Administration, 1993.
21. Edlund MJ, Steffick D, Hudson T, et al. Risk factors for clinically recognized opioid abuse and dependence among veterans using opioids for chronic non-cancer pain. *Pain* 2007;129:355–362.
22. Ballantyne JC, LaForge KS. Opioid dependence and addiction during opioid treatment of chronic pain. *Pain* 2007;129:235–255.
23. Center for Substance Abuse Treatment. *Treatment of adolescents with substance use disorders* (Treatment Improvement Protocol Series, Number 32). Rockville, MD: Substance Abuse and Mental Health Services Administration, 1999.
24. Wartenberg AA, Nirenberg TD. Alcohol and drug abuse in the older patient. In: Reichel W, ed. *Care of the elderly: clinical aspects of aging*, 4th ed. Baltimore, MD: Williams & Wilkins, 1995:133–141.
25. Anton RF, Becker HC. Pharmacology and pathophysiology of alcohol withdrawal. In: Kranzler HR, ed. *Handbook of experimental pharmacology, volume 114: the pharmacology of alcohol abuse*. New York: Springer-Verlag, 1995:315–367.
26. Taylor BG, Fitzgerald N, Hunt D, et al. *ADAM preliminary 2000 findings on drug use & drug markets: adult male arrestees*. Washington, DC: U.S. Department of Justice, Office of Justice Programs, National Institute of Justice, 2001.
27. Center for Substance Abuse Treatment. *Substance abuse treatment for adults in the criminal justice system* (Treatment Improvement Protocol Series, Number 44) Rockville, MD: Substance Abuse and Mental Health Services Administration, 2005.
28. Center for Substance Abuse Treatment. *Planning for alcohol and other drug abuse treatment for adults in the criminal justice system* (Treatment Improvement Protocol Series, Number 17). Rockville, MD: Substance Abuse and Mental Health Services Administration, 1994.

CHAPTER 42

Michael F. Mayo-Smith, MD, MPH

Management of Alcohol Intoxication and Withdrawal

Management of alcohol intoxication and withdrawal is one of the clinical issues most frequently encountered by specialists in addiction medicine. Effective approaches, with a strong scientific basis, have been developed to reduce the incidence of serious complications.

ALCOHOL INTOXICATION

Clinical Picture As blood alcohol concentration rises, so too does the clinical effect on the individual (Table 42.1) (1). At a blood alcohol concentration between 20 mg% and 99 mg%, loss of muscular coordination begins. Changes in mood, personality, and behavior accompany these blood alcohol levels. As the blood alcohol level rises to the range of 100 mg% to 199 mg%, neurologic impairment occurs, accompanied by prolonged reaction time, ataxia, incoordination, and mental impairment. At a blood alcohol level of 200 mg% to 299 mg%, very obvious intoxication is present, except in those with marked tolerance. Nausea and vomiting, as well as marked ataxia, may occur. As the level rises to 300 mg% to 399 mg%, hypothermia may occur, along with severe dysarthria and amnesia, with Stage I anesthesia. At blood alcohol levels between 400 mg% and 799 mg%, the onset of alcoholic coma occurs. The precise level at which this occurs depends on tolerance; some persons experience coma at levels of 400 mg%, whereas others do not experience it until the level approaches 600 mg%. Serum levels of alcohol between 600 mg% and 800 mg% often are fatal. Progressive obtundation develops, accompanied by decreases in respiration, blood pressure, and body temperature. The patient may develop urinary incontinence or retention, while reflexes are markedly decreased or absent. Death may occur from the loss of airway protective reflexes (with subsequent airway obstruction by the flaccid tongue), from pulmonary aspiration of gastric contents, or from respiratory arrest arising from profound central nervous system depression.

Management The medical management of alcohol intoxication and overdose is supportive. The most important goal of management of alcohol intoxication is to prevent harm to the patient, from severe respiratory depression, and to protect the airway against aspiration. Even with very high blood alcohol levels, survival is probable as long as the respiratory and cardiovascular systems can be supported.

As with all patients with impaired consciousness, intravenous glucose should be given if rapid testing of blood glucose is not immediately available, as well as intravenous thiamine. These are of particular importance in alcohol intoxication as ethanol can impair gluconeogenesis, with an increased risk of hypoglycemia, and chronic alcoholism places the individual at increased risk of thiamine deficiency.

It also is important to assess whether the patient has ingested other drugs in addition to alcohol, because these may further suppress the central nervous system and alter the approach to treatment. Alcohol is rapidly absorbed into the bloodstream, so induction of emesis or gastric lavage usually is not indicated unless a substantial ingestion has occurred within the preceding 30 to 60 minutes, or unless other drug ingestion is suspected. Ipecac-induced emesis may be useful at the scene (e.g., with children at home) if it can be given within a few minutes of exposure. Similarly, gastric lavage is indicated only if the patient presents in the emergency department soon after ingestion. Activated charcoal does not efficiently absorb ethanol, but may be given if other toxins have

TABLE 42.1 Clinical Effects of Alcohol

Blood alcohol level mg%	Clinical manifestations
20–99	Loss of muscular coordination Changes in mood, personality, and behavior
100–199	Neurologic impairment with prolonged reaction time, ataxia, incoordination, and mental impairment
200–299	Very obvious intoxication, except in those with marked tolerance Nausea, vomiting, marked ataxia
300–399	Hypothermia, severe dysarthria, amnesia, Stage I anesthesia
400–799	Onset of alcoholic coma, with precise level depending on degree of tolerance Progressive obtundation, decreases in respiration, blood pressure, and body temperature Urinary incontinence or retention, reflexes markedly decreased or absent
600–800	Often fatal because of loss of airway protective reflexes from airway obstruction by flaccid tongue, from pulmonary aspiration of gastric contents, or from respiratory arrest from profound central nervous system obstruction

been ingested. Enhancement of elimination has a very limited role to play.

More than 90% of alcohol is oxidized in the liver and, at the levels seen clinically, the rate of oxidation follows zero-order kinetics; that is, it is independent of time and concentration of the drug. Elimination thus occurs at a fixed rate, with the level falling at a rate of about 20 mg/dL/hour. In extreme cases of alcohol intoxication, hemodialysis can be used, because it efficiently removes alcohol, but it is needed only rarely because supportive care usually is sufficient. Hemoperfusion and forced diuresis are not effective. At present, there is no known agent that is effective as an alcohol antagonist, reversing the effects of alcohol in the same manner that naloxone reverses opiate intoxication. Benzodiazepine antagonists such as flumazenil do not block or reverse alcohol intoxication.

The acutely intoxicated patient may exhibit some agitation as part of the intoxication syndrome. This is best managed nonpharmacologically. Support and reassurance can go a long way in dealing with agitation in an acutely intoxicated patient. On rare occasions, if pharmacologic intervention is needed to manage a mildly or moderately intoxicated individual's behavior in a medical setting, intramuscular administration of a rapid onset, short-acting benzodiazepine (such as lorazepam), alone or in combination with a neuroleptic agent such as haloperidol, can be useful. Caution must be exercised in regard to a potential synergistic response between the alcohol already in the patient's system and an exogenously administered sedative hypnotic, so this approach should be used only as a last resort and not in individuals with high blood alcohol levels.

HANGOVER

Hangover is a constellation of unpleasant physical and mental symptoms that occur after a bout of heavy alcohol intake. Headache, malaise, diarrhea, nausea, and difficulty concentrating are the most common symptoms, often accompanied by sensitivity to light or sound, sweating, and anxiety. About 75% of individuals who drink to intoxication report experiencing a hangover at least some of the time. The primary alcohol-related morbidity in light-to-moderate drinkers is hangover. Because light-to-moderate drinkers make up most of the workforce, the greatest cost incurred by alcohol in the workplace is the decreased productivity as a result of hangover induced absenteeism or poor job performance. In addition to the personal discomfort, hangover increases risk for injury and poor job performance. Patients with hangover have diminished visual-spatial skills and dexterity with impairment demonstrated in pilots, automobile drivers, and skiers. There are also adverse effects on managerial skills and tasks (2).

The pathophysiology of hangover is not completely understood. In part it is believed to be the effect of the intermediate product of ethanol metabolism, acetaldehyde. In addition congeners, byproducts of individual alcohol preparations found primarily in dark liquors such as brandy, whiskey, wine, and tequila, appear to play a role because they increase the frequency and severity of hangover. Clear liquors, such as rum, vodka, and gin, cause hangover less frequently (2,3). Dehydration, electrolyte imbalance, disruption of sleep and other biologic rhythms, increased physical activity while intoxicated, hypoglycemia, and the many hormonal disruptions caused by alcohol may also play contributing roles (3). Patients with hangover have a diffuse slowing on electroencephalography which persists up to 16 hours after blood alcohol levels become undetectable (2).

Although many interventions have been tried to alleviate hangover symptoms, to date none has clearly demonstrated effectiveness in rigorous investigations (4). Conservative management offers the best course of treatment, and symptoms generally resolve over 8 to 24 hours. Attentiveness to the quantity and quality of alcohol consumed can have a significant effect on preventing hangover. Asking patients about their hangover experiences offers an opportunity for education on a common cause of physical, psychiatric, and occupational consequences.

ALCOHOL WITHDRAWAL

Clinical Presentation *"If the patient be in the prime of life and if from drinking he has trembling hands, it may be well to announce beforehand either delirium or convulsions"* (Hippocrates, circa 400 BC). The relationship of heavy alcohol intake to certain syndromes has been recognized since ancient times. However, it was not until the 18th century that the clinical manifestations of alcohol withdrawal were clearly delineated. As is evident in the writings of Sutton, the vivid descriptions of severe withdrawal written at that time remain relevant today:

> *It is preceded by tremors of the hands, restlessness, irregularity of thought, deficiency of memory, anxiety to be company, dreadful nocturnal dreams when the quantity of liquor through the day has been insufficient: much diminution of appetite, especially an aversion to animal food; violent vomiting in the morning and excessive perspiration from trivial causes. Confusion of thought arises to such height that objects are seen of the most hideous forms, and in positions that it is physically impossible they can be so situated; the patients generally sees flies or other insects; or pieces of money which he anxiously desires to possess. . . .*

For the most part, clinicians believed that these symptoms were a consequence of alcohol itself. It was not until the second half of the 20th century that their relationship to the cessation of chronic alcohol intake—a relationship taken for granted today—was established. In 1953, Victor and Adams reported their careful observations of 286 consecutive alcohol dependent patients admitted to an inner city hospital, revealing the consistent relationship of the cessation of alcohol to the emergence of clinical symptoms (5). Their findings were supported in 1955 by a study by Isbell and colleagues, in which 10 former morphine-addicted individuals were given large quantities of alcohol for 7 to 87 days and then withdrawn abruptly without sedation (6). Over the next two decades, the concept of an alcohol withdrawal syndrome was firmly established by further animal and human studies, and diagnostic criteria based on empirical observation were developed. Today manifestations of alcohol withdrawal are generally categorized in clinical practice as including the common *alcohol withdrawal syndrome* as well as more severe manifestations of hallucinations, seizures, and delirium.

Alcohol Withdrawal Syndrome The current understanding of the alcohol withdrawal syndrome is reflected in the diagnostic criteria of the *Diagnostic and Statistical Manual of Mental Disorders,* 4th edition, listed in Table 42.2 (7). In those with physiologic dependence on alcohol, the clinical manifestations of alcohol withdrawal begin 6 to 24 hours after the last drink, sometimes arising before the blood alcohol level has returned to zero. Early withdrawal signs and symptoms include anxiety, sleep disturbances, vivid dreams, anorexia, nausea, and headache. Physical signs include tachycardia, elevation of blood pressure, hyperactive reflexes, sweating, and hyperthermia. A tremor, best brought out by extension of the hands or tongue, may appear. This tremor has a rate of six to eight cycles per second and appears on electromyography to be an exaggeration of normal physiologic tremor. The severity of these symptoms varies greatly among individuals, but in a majority they are mild and transient, passing within 1 to 2 days (8–10).

Hallucinations In mild alcohol withdrawal, patients may experience perceptual distortions of a visual, auditory, and tactile nature. Lights may seem too bright or sounds too loud and startling. A sensation of "pins and needles" may be experienced. In more severe cases of withdrawal, these misperceptions may develop into frank hallucinations. Visual hallucinations are most common and frequently involve some type of animal life, such as seeing a dog or rodent in the room. Auditory hallucinations may begin as unformed sounds (such as clicks or buzzing) and progress to formed voices. In contrast to the auditory hallucinations of schizophrenia, which may be of religious or political significance, these voices often are of friends or relatives and frequently are accusatory in nature. Tactile hallucinations may involve a sensation of bugs or insects crawling on the skin. In milder cases of withdrawal, the patient's sensorium is otherwise clear and the patient retains insight that the hallucinations are not real. In more severe withdrawal, this insight may be lost.

Alcohol Withdrawal Seizures Grand mal seizures are another manifestation of alcohol withdrawal. Withdrawal seizures occurred in 23% of the patients studied by Victor and Adams, in 33% of the patients in Isbell's study who drank for 48 to 87 days, and in 11% of placebo-treated patients who were enrolled in prospective controlled studies examining the effectiveness of benzodiazepines in symptomatic withdrawal (5,6,11). Withdrawal seizures usually begin within 8 to 24 hours after the patient's last drink and may occur before the blood alcohol level has returned to zero. Most are generalized major motor seizures, occurring singly or in a burst of several seizures over a period of 1 to 6 hours. Although <3% of withdrawal seizures evolve into status epilepticus, alcohol withdrawal has been found to be a contributing cause in up to 15% of status epilepticus patients (12). Seizures peak 24 hours after the last drink, corresponding to the peak of withdrawal-induced electroencephalogram (EEG) abnormalities, which include increased amplitude, a photomyoclonic response, and spontaneous paroxysmal activity. These EEG abnormalities are transient, in keeping with the brevity of the convulsive attacks. Except for this brief period after withdrawal, the incidence of EEG abnormalities in patients with withdrawal seizures is not greater than in the normal population. The risk of withdrawal seizures appears to be in part genetically determined and is increased in patients with a history of prior withdrawal seizures

TABLE 42.2 DSM-IV-TR Diagnostic Criteria for 291.81 Alcohol Withdrawal

A. Cessation of (or reduction in) alcohol use that has been heavy and prolonged.
B. Two (or more) of the following, developing within several hours to a few days after Criterion A:
  (1) autonomic hyperactivity (e.g., sweating or pulse rate >100)
  (2) increased hand tremor
  (3) insomnia
  (4) nausea or vomiting
  (5) transient visual, tactile, or auditory hallucinations or illusions
  (6) psychomotor agitation
  (7) anxiety
  (8) grand mal seizures
C. The symptoms in Criterion B cause clinically significant distress or impairment in social, occupational, or other important areas of functioning.
D. The symptoms are not due to a general medical condition and are not better accounted for by another mental disorder.

The following specifier may be applied to a diagnosis of alcohol withdrawal.

With Perceptual Disturbances. This specifier may be noted in the rare instance when hallucinations with intact reality testing or auditory, visual, or tactile illusions occur in the absence of a delirium. *Intact reality testing* means that the person knows that the hallucinations are induced by the substance and do not represent external reality. When hallucinations occur in the absence of intact reality testing, a diagnosis of substance-induced psychotic disorder, with hallucinations, should be considered.

DSM-IV-TR Diagnostic Criteria for Alcohol Withdrawal Delirium

A. Disturbance of consciousness (i.e., reduced clarity of awareness of the environment) with reduced ability to focus, sustain, or shift attention.
B. A change in cognition (such as memory deficit, disorientation, language disturbance) or the development of a perceptual disturbance that is not better accounted for by a preexisting, established, or evolving dementia.
C. The disturbance develops over a short period (usually hours to days) and tends to fluctuate during the course of the day.
D. There is evidence from the history, physical examination, or laboratory findings that the symptoms in Criteria A and B developed during, or shortly after, an alcohol withdrawal syndrome.

Note: This diagnosis should be made instead of a diagnosis of substance withdrawal only when the cognitive symptoms are in excess of those usually associated with the withdrawal syndrome and when the symptoms are sufficiently severe to warrant independent clinical attention.
From American Psychiatric Association. *Diagnostic and statistical manual of mental disorders*, 4th ed., text rev. Washington, DC: American Psychiatric Association, copyright © 2000.

or in those who are undergoing concurrent withdrawal from benzodiazepines or other sedative-hypnotic drugs.

There also is evidence that the risk of seizures increases as an individual undergoes repeated withdrawals (13). This association has been described as a "kindling effect," which refers to animal studies demonstrating that repeated subcortical electrical stimulation is associated with increases in seizure susceptibility (14). Animal studies have supported this kindling hypothesis in alcohol withdrawal, demonstrating that submitting animals to repeated alcohol withdrawal episodes increases their risk of withdrawal seizures. There is emerging evidence that this effect occurs in humans as well (15–20).

Alcohol Withdrawal Delirium Withdrawal is highly individualized in both severity and duration. For up to 90% of patients, withdrawal does not progress beyond the mild to moderate symptoms described previously, peaking between 24 and 36 hours and gradually subsiding. In other patients, however, manifestations can include delirium. The diagnostic criteria for alcohol withdrawal delirium are shown in Table 42.2. In the classic cases of withdrawal delirium the manifestations of withdrawal steadily worsen and progress into a severe life-threatening delirium accompanied by an autonomic storm: hence the term *delirium tremens* (DTs). DTs generally appear 72 to 96 hours after the last drink. In their classic presentation, DTs are marked by all the signs and symptoms of mild withdrawal but in a much more pronounced form, with the development of marked tachycardia, tremor, diaphoresis, and fever. The patient develops global confusion and disorientation to place and time. The patient may become absorbed in a separate psychic reality, often believing himself or herself to be in a location other than the hospital, and misidentifies staff as personal acquaintances. Hallucinations are frequent, and the patient may have no insight into them. Without this insight, they can be extremely frightening to the patient, who may react in a way that poses a threat to his own or the staff's safety. Marked psychomotor activity may develop, with severe agitation in some cases or continuous low level motor activity in others, so that activities such as efforts to get out of bed can last for hours. Severe disruption of the normal sleep-wake cycle also is common, and may be marked by the absence of clear sleep for several days. The duration of the delirium is variable, but averages 2 to 3 days in most studies (21). In some cases, the delirium is relatively brief, lasting only a few hours before the patient regains orientation. In other cases, the patient remains delirious for several days, with reports of periods as long as 50 days before the confusion clears (22). Before the development of effective treatment, mortality in DTs was substantial. With the development of effective therapy, including intensive care, death from DTs is an unusual event (21).

Because the clinical syndrome of delirium has become more carefully and broadly studied, and standard diagnostic criteria developed, it is becoming apparent that many cases of delirium during alcohol withdrawal occur without the autonomic storm associated with classically described DTs. Although the terms *alcohol withdrawal delirium* and *DTs* are often used interchangeably (7), many cases of delirium in alcohol withdrawal are mild and transient. In one retrospective chart review of 284 patients undergoing withdrawal, 20 patients were identified as meeting DSM IV-R criteria for alcohol withdrawal delirium, only 3 had the syndrome of DTs (23). This is an area needing further investigation, including the role that treatment with sedative hypnotics or concurrent medical illness may play in the development of mild delirium in alcohol withdrawal.

Alcohol Withdrawal Severity Scales Because alcohol withdrawal involves a constellation of nonspecific findings, efforts have been made to develop structured withdrawal severity assessment scales to objectively quantify the severity of withdrawal. Several such scales have been published in the literature (24,25). The most extensively studied and best known is the Clinical Institute Withdrawal Assessment-Alcohol, or CIWA, and a shortened version known as the CIWA-A Revised, or CIWA-Ar (Table 42.3) (26). The CIWA-Ar has well documented reliability, reproducibility, and validity based on comparisons to ratings of withdrawal severity by experienced clinicians. The CIWA-Ar and similar scales require 2 to 5 minutes to complete and have proved useful in a variety of settings, including detoxification units, psychiatric units, medical/surgical wards, and intensive care units. Such scales allow rapid documentation of the patient's signs and symptoms and provide a simple summary score that facilitates accurate and objective communication among staff. In the case of the CIWA-Ar, a score ≤9 indicates mild withdrawal, a score of 10 to 18 moderate withdrawal, and a score >18 severe withdrawal.

A careful analysis of symptoms recorded using withdrawal scales found that patients segregated into distinct clinical groups. Approximately 20% had no significant withdrawal symptoms (8). Another 20% had only vegetative (physical) signs, such as tremor and sweating, but no psychologic symptoms. The largest group, approximately 40%, had both vegetative and mild to moderate psychologic symptoms, primarily anxiety. The last group, about 20% of patients, had both vegetative and severe psychologic symptoms with either disorientation, delirium, or hallucinations. As indicated previously, relatively few patients in alcohol withdrawal experience the adrenergic and clinical manifestations of delirium tremens.

Predictors of Severe Withdrawal Withdrawal scales can also contribute to appropriate triage of patients as it has been shown that high scores early in the course are predictive of the development of seizures and delirium. Those with low scores on withdrawal scales over the first 24 hours have consistently been found to be at little or no risk for severe withdrawal. Other risk factors for severe withdrawal include a history of prior DTs or withdrawal seizures. Marked autonomic hyperactivity, commonly measured as elevated heart rate on admission, elevated blood alcohol level of 100 mg/dL or higher at the time of admission, serum electrolyte abnormalities, and medical comorbidity, particularly infection, are other clinical findings associated with an increased rate of DTs or severe withdrawal. Characteristics that have not been useful in triaging patients include amount of daily intake, duration of heavy drinking, age, and gender. At least one rating system has been developed combining multiple items to predict the severity of withdrawal (9). This and other studies were able to identify patients at low risk for severe withdrawal with high reliability.

Pathophysiology Goldstein and Goldstein proposed in 1961 that dependency develops as a cell or organism makes homeostatic adjustments to compensate for the primary effect of a drug (27). As described in Section 10 of this book, the primary effect of alcohol on the brain is depressant. With chronic exposure, there are compensatory adjustments to this chronic depressant effect, with downregulation of inhibitory systems and upregulation of excitatory systems. With abrupt abstinence from alcohol, these relative deficiencies in inhibitory influences and relative excesses in excitatory influences are suddenly unmasked, leading to the appearance of withdrawal phenomena. The withdrawal symptoms last until the body readjusts to the absence of the alcohol and establishes a new equilibrium.

Two neurotransmitter systems appear to play a central role in the development of alcohol withdrawal syndrome. Alcohol exerts its effects in part by directly or indirectly enhancing the effect of GABA, a major inhibitory neurotransmitter. GABA mediates typical sedative-hypnotic effects such as sedation, muscle relaxation, and a raised seizure threshold. Chronic alcohol intake leads to an adaptive suppression of GABA activity. A sudden relative deficiency in GABA neurotransmitter activity is produced with alcohol abstinence, and is believed to contribute to the anxiety, increased psychomotor activity, and predisposition to seizures seen in withdrawal. Although alcohol enhances the effect of GABA, it inhibits the sensitivity of autonomic adrenergic systems, with a resulting upregulation with chronic alcohol intake. The discontinuation of alcohol leads to rebound over activity of the brain and peripheral noradrenergic systems. Increased sympathetic autonomic activity contributes to such acute manifestations as tachycardia, hypertension, tremor, diaphoresis, and anxiety (28).

A second neurotransmitter, norepinephrine, also seems to be important in alcohol withdrawal presentations. Norepinephrine's metabolites are elevated in plasma, urine, and cerebral spinal fluid during withdrawal; levels of metabolites correlate

TABLE 42.3 Clinical Institute Withdrawal Assessment of Alcohol Scale, Revised (CIWA-Ar)

Patient: ______ Date: ______ Time: ______

(24 hour clock, midnight = 00:00)

Pulse or heart rate, taken for 1 minute: ______ Blood pressure: ______

Nausea and Vomiting: Ask "Do you feel sick to your stomach? Have you vomited?" Observation.

0 No nausea and no vomiting
1 Mild nausea with no vomiting
2
3
4 Intermittent nausea with dry heaves
5
6
7 Constant nausea, frequent dry heaves and vomiting

Tactile Disturbances: Ask "Have you any itching, pins and needles sensations, any burning, any numbness, or do you feel bugs crawling on or under your skin?"
Observation.

0 None
1 Very mild itching, pins and needles, burning or numbness
2 Mild itching, pins and needles, burning or numbness
3 Moderate itching, pins and needles, burning or numbness
4 Moderately severe hallucinations
5 Severe hallucinations
6 Extremely severe hallucinations
7 Continuous hallucinations

Tremor: Arms extended and fingers spread apart.
Observation.

0 No tremor
1 Not visible, but can be felt fingertip to fingertip
2
3
4 Moderate, with patient's arms extended
5
6
7 Severe, even with arms not extended

Auditory Disturbances: Ask "Are you more aware of sounds around you? Are they harsh? Do they frighten you? Are you hearing anything that is disturbing to you? Are you hearing things you know are not there?"
Observation.

0 Not present
1 Very mild harshness or ability to frighten
2 Mild harshness or ability to frighten
3 Moderate harshness or ability to frighten
4 Moderately severe hallucinations
5 Severe hallucinations
6 Extremely severe hallucinations
7 Continuous hallucinations

Paroxysmal Sweats: Observation.

0 No sweat visible
1 Barely perceptible sweating, palms moist
2
3
4 Beads of sweat obvious on forehead
5
6
7 Drenching sweats

TABLE 42.3 Clinical Institute Withdrawal Assessment of Alcohol Scale, Revised (CIWA-Ar) (*Continued*)

Visual Disturbances: Ask "Does the light appear to be too bright? Is its color different? Does it hurt your eyes? Are you seeing anything that is disturbing to you? Are you seeing things you know are not there?"
Observation.
0 Not present
1 Very mild sensitivity
2 Mild sensitivity
3 Moderate sensitivity
4 Moderately severe hallucinations
5 Severe hallucinations
6 Extremely severe hallucinations
7 Continuous hallucinations

Anxiety: Ask "Do you feel nervous?"
Observation.
0 No anxiety, at ease
1 Mild anxious
2
3
4 Moderately anxious, or guarded, so anxiety is inferred
5
6
7 Equivalent to acute panic states as seen in severe delirium or acute schizophrenic reactions

Headache, Fullness in Head: Ask "Does your head feel different? Does it feel like there is a band around your head?" Do not rate for dizziness or lightheadedness. Otherwise, rate severity.
0 Not present
1 Very mild
2 Mild
3 Moderate
4 Moderately severe
5 Severe
6 Very severe
7 Extremely severe

Agitation: Observation.
0 Normal activity
1 Somewhat more than normal activity
2
3
4 Moderately fidgety and restless
5
6
7 Paces back and forth during most of the interview, or constantly thrashes about

Orientation and Clouding of Sensorium: Ask "What day is this? Where are you? Who am I?"
0 Oriented and can do serial additions
1 Cannot do serial additions or is uncertain about date
2 Disoriented for date by no more than 2 calendar days
3 Disoriented for date by more than 2 calendar days
4 Disoriented for place/or person
Total CIWA-Ar score ______
Rater's initials ______
Maximum possible score: 67

The CIWA-Ar is not copyrighted and may be reproduced freely. This assessment for monitoring withdrawal symptoms requires approximately 5 minutes to administer. The maximum score is 67 (see instrument). Patients scoring <10 do not usually need additional medication for withdrawal.
Sullivan JT, Sykora K, Schneiderman J, et al. Assessment of alcohol withdrawal: the revised Clinical Institute Withdrawal Assessment for Alcohol scale (CIWA-Ar). *Br J Addict* 1989;84:1353–1357.

significantly with the sympathetic nervous system signs of withdrawal (29). Research has identified a large number of other neural effects of chronic alcohol intake, including effects on serotonergic systems, neuronal calcium channels, glutamate receptors, cyclic AMP systems, and the hypothalamic-pituitary adrenal neuroendocrine axis and these too may play a role in the pathophysiology of withdrawal (28).

Genetics The role of genetics in alcohol withdrawal is a topic of active investigation. In animal models, the development of selectively bred strains demonstrates that severity of withdrawal and risk of seizures are strongly influenced by genotype. Investigations in humans have focused on genes regulating neurotransmitter systems. Several studies have found an association of the A9 allele, which affects central dopamine functions, with severity of alcohol withdrawal, alcohol withdrawal seizures, and delirium tremens (30–32). To date, no relationship with genes involved in the serotonin, GABAergic or opioidergic systems have been found (33). Although these findings are not of immediate clinical use, genetic studies may shed light on basic pathophysiology and at some point assist in identifying high-risk individuals who may benefit from tailored therapy.

Role of Alcohol Withdrawal in Diagnostic Classification When DSM-IIIR moved to a broad definition of dependence, it removed any requirement for physiologic components, tolerance and withdrawal, for a diagnosis of alcohol dependence. This was done without intensive study of what effect would occur if neither was required for a diagnosis. DSM-IV did add a request to subtype dependence into groups with and without physiologic components. Intervening studies have shown that approximately 60% of individuals meeting DSM-IV criteria for alcohol dependence report withdrawal symptoms, another 35% tolerance without withdrawal symptoms, and only 5% report neither. Of the seven DSM-IV dependence items, withdrawal symptoms has been most strongly associated with an increased number of alcohol-related problems, higher number of drinks per occasion, and future difficulties (34). Alternative approaches to DSM-IV have been proposed which reinstitute withdrawal as a required feature, with evidence that such approaches offer better validity and better discrimination between the dependence and abuse classifications (35). The role of withdrawal in the diagnostic taxonomy of alcohol use disorders continues to be investigated and debated.

MANAGEMENT OF ALCOHOL WITHDRAWAL SYNDROMES

General Principles The primary goals of the treatment of alcohol withdrawal syndromes are to first assure clinical stability of the patient and secondarily encourage ongoing treatment (e.g., rehabilitation) of a patient's alcohol misuse. The first step in managing the patient with alcohol withdrawal is to perform an assessment for the presence of medical and psychiatric problems. Chronic alcohol intake is associated with the development of many acute and chronic medical problems. The clinician needs to determine whether there are acute conditions that require hospital treatment or chronic conditions that may alter the approach to management of withdrawal because they could be exacerbated significantly by the development of withdrawal or its treatment. Pertinent laboratory tests generally include complete blood count, electrolytes, magnesium, calcium, phosphate, liver enzymes, urine drug screen, pregnancy test (when appropriate), and Breathalyzer or blood alcohol level. Others, depending on suspected co-occurring conditions, may include skin test for tuberculosis, chest x-ray, electrocardiogram, and tests for viral hepatitis, other infections, or sexually transmitted diseases. General management also involves maintaining adequate fluid balance, correction of electrolyte deficiencies, and attendance to the patient's nutritional needs. Patients in early withdrawal often are overhydrated so that aggressive hydration usually is not necessary unless there have been significant fluid losses from vomiting or diarrhea. Supportive care and reassurance from health care personnel are important elements of comfortable detoxification and help to facilitate continuing treatment. Supportive nonpharmacologic care is an important and useful element in the management of all patients undergoing withdrawal. Simple interventions such as reassurance, reality orientation, monitoring of signs and symptoms of withdrawal, and general nursing care are effective.

There has been interest in the possible value of complementary and alternative medicine for alcohol withdrawal. Controlled trials of acupuncture have not demonstrated effectiveness, whereas massage therapy did reduce alcohol withdrawal scores (36–38). It is important to note that all these supportive measures do not prevent the development of major complications such as seizures and are not adequate by themselves to manage the patient with severe withdrawal or delirium, in which case pharmacologic intervention is required.

Pharmacologic Management of Uncomplicated Withdrawal Syndrome The medical literature on the pharmacologic management of alcohol withdrawal has been comprehensively reviewed as part of the American Society of Addiction Medicine's evidence-based Clinical Practice Guidelines efforts (11). This review of the evidence indicated that the cornerstone of pharmacologic management of withdrawal is the use of benzodiazepines, a conclusion supported by other more recent systematic reviews (39,40).

Benzodiazepines Benzodiazepines are pharmacologically cross-tolerant with alcohol and have the similar effect of enhancing the effect of GABA-induced sedation. A specific benzodiazepine receptor site has been identified on the GABA receptor complex. It is believed that the provision of benzodiazepines alleviates the acute deficiency of GABA neurotransmitter activity that occurs with sudden cessation of alcohol intake. Well-designed studies consistently have shown that benzodiazepines are more effective than placebo in reducing the signs and symptoms of withdrawal.

Meta-analysis of prospective placebo-controlled trials of patients admitted with symptomatic withdrawal have shown a highly significant reduction in seizures, with a risk reduction of 7.7 seizures per 100 patients treated, as well as in delirium, with a risk reduction of 4.9 cases of delirium per 100 patients treated. Trials comparing different benzodiazepines indicate that all are similarly efficacious in reducing signs and symptoms of withdrawal. However, longer-acting agents such as diazepam and chlordiazepoxide may be more effective in preventing seizures. Longer-acting agents also may contribute to an overall smoother withdrawal course, with a reduction in breakthrough or rebound symptoms. On the other hand, pharmacologic data and clinical experience suggest that longer-acting agents can pose a risk of excess sedation in some patients, including elderly persons and patients with significant liver disease. In such patients, shorter-acting agents such as lorazepam or oxazepam may be preferable.

Another consideration in the choice of benzodiazepine is the rapidity of onset. Certain agents with rapid onset of action (such as diazepam, alprazolam, and lorazepam) demonstrate greater abuse potential than do agents with a slower onset of action (such as chlordiazepoxide and oxazepam). This consideration may be of relevance in an outpatient setting or for patients with a history of benzodiazepine or other substance abuse. However, when rapid control of symptoms is needed, medications with faster onset offer an advantage. A final consideration in the choice of benzodiazepine is cost, as these agents vary considerably in price. Given the evidence of equal efficacy, if a particular agent is available to a practitioner or program at a lower cost, cost is a legitimate factor to consider.

Studies have indicated that nonbenzodiazepine sedative-hypnotics also are effective in reducing the signs and symptoms of withdrawal, but nonbenzodiazepine agents have not been as extensively studied, and the size of studies with them is not adequate to draw conclusions as to their degree of effectiveness in reducing seizures and delirium. Benzodiazepines have a greater margin of safety, with a lower risk of respiratory depression, as well as overall lower abuse potential than do the nonbenzodiazepine agents. Phenobarbital, a long-acting barbiturate, still is used by some programs, as it is long-acting, has well-documented anticonvulsant activity, is inexpensive, and has low abuse liability.

Determining the Dosing Schedule In the majority of studies examining the effectiveness of various medications for withdrawal, the medications were given in fixed amounts at scheduled times (such as chlordiazepoxide 50 mg every 6 hours) and were given for periods of 5 to 7 days. However, it has been shown that many patients can go through withdrawal with only minor symptoms even though they receive little or no medication (10). An alternative to giving medication on a fixed schedule is known as symptom triggered therapy. In this approach, the patient is monitored through use of a structured assessment scale and given medication only when symptoms cross a threshold of severity. Well-designed studies have demonstrated that this approach is as effective as fixed-dose therapy, but leads to the administration of significantly less medication and a significantly shorter duration of treatment (10).

Symptom triggered therapy also facilitates the delivery of large amounts of medication quickly to patients who evidence rapidly escalating withdrawal and thus reduces the risk of undertreatment that may arise with the use of fixed doses. For programs specializing in the management of addiction, use of a symptom-triggered approach with the utilization of a severity scale offers significant advantages. However, there may be situations in which the provision of fixed doses remains appropriate. For example, with patients admitted to general medical or surgical wards, the nursing staff may not have the training or experience to implement the regular use of scales to monitor patients. In certain patients, such as those with severe coronary artery disease, the clinician may wish to prevent the development of even minor symptoms of withdrawal. Finally, because a history of past withdrawal seizures is a risk factor for seizures during a withdrawal episode, and because withdrawal seizures usually occur early in the course of withdrawal, some practitioners administer fixed doses to patients with a history of withdrawal seizures. Whenever fixed doses are given, it is very important that allowances be made to provide additional medication if the fixed dose should prove inadequate to control symptoms.

Treatment should allow for a degree of individualization so that patients can receive large amounts of medication rapidly if needed. In all cases, medications should be administered by a route that has been shown to have reliable absorption. Therefore, the benzodiazepines should be administered orally or, when necessary, intravenously. An exception is lorazepam, which has good intramuscular and sublingual absorption. In the past, intramuscular administration was commonly used. However, for most agents intramuscular absorption is extremely variable, leading to problems when rapid control of symptoms is necessary and also with delayed appearance of oversedation when large amounts are administered. Examples of some treatment regimens consistent with current recommendations are shown in Table 42.4.

Anticonvulsants Carbamazepine has been widely used in Europe for alcohol withdrawal and has been shown to be equal in efficacy to benzodiazepines for patients with mild to moderate withdrawal. Fixed, tapering doses of carbamazepine are without significant toxicity when used in 5- to 7-day protocols for alcohol withdrawal and are associated with less psychiatric distress, a faster return to work, less rebound symptoms, and reduced posttreatment drinking (41). When compared with placebo, there is significantly less use of benzodiazepines for breakthrough symptoms. Carbamazepine does not potentiate the central nervous system and respiratory depression caused by alcohol, does not inhibit learning (an important side effect of larger doses of benzodiazepines), and has no abuse potential. It has well-documented anticonvulsant activity and prevents

TABLE 42.4 Examples of Specific Pharmacologic Treatment Regimens

Monitoring

Monitor the patient every 4 to 8 hours using the CIWA-Ar until the score has been below 8–10 for 24 hours; use additional assessments as needed.

Symptom-Triggered Medication Regimens

Administer one of the following medications every hour when the CIWA-Ar is >8–10:

_ Chlordiazepoxide 50–100 mg
_ Diazepam 10–20 mg
_ Oxazepam 30–60 mg
_ Lorazepam 2–4 mg

(Other benzodiazepines may be used at equivalent substitutions.)

Repeat the CIWA-Ar 1 hour after every dose to assess need for further medication.

Structured Medication Regimens

The physician may feel that the development of even mild to moderate withdrawal should be prevented in certain patients (for example, in a patient experiencing a myocardial infarction) and thus may order medications to be given on a predetermined schedule. One of the following regimens could be used in such a situation:

– Chlordiazepoxide 50 mg every 6 hours for four doses, then 25 mg every 6 hours for eight doses.
– Diazepam 10 mg every 6 hours for four doses, then 5 mg every 6 hours for eight doses.
– Lorazepam 2 mg every 6 hours for four doses, then 1 mg every 6 hours for eight doses.

(Other benzodiazepines may be substituted at equivalent doses.)

– Carbamazepine 300–400 mg twice daily on day 1, tapering to 200 mg as single dose on day 5.

It is very important that patients receiving medication on a predetermined schedule be monitored closely and that additional benzodiazepine be provided should the doses given prove inadequate.

Agitation and Delirium

For the patient who displays increasing agitation or hallucinations that have not responded to oral benzodiazepines alone, one of the following medications may be used:

– Haloperidol 2–5 mg intramuscularly alone or in combination with 2–4 mg of lorazepam.
– Intravenous diazepam given slowly every 5 minutes until the patient is lightly sedated. Begin with 5 mg for two doses. If needed, increase to 10 mg for two doses, then 20 mg every 5 minutes. Given the risk of respiratory depression, the patient on this regimen should be closely monitored, with equipment for respiratory support immediately available.

(Other phenothiazines and benzodiazepines may be substituted at equivalent doses.)

Data from ASAM. Addiction medicine essentials: Clinical Institute Withdrawal Assessment of Alcohol Scale, revised (CIWA-Ar), 2001. Stuppaeck CH, Barnas C, Falk M, et al. Assessment of the alcohol withdrawal syndrome—validity and reliability of the translated and modified Clinical Institute Withdrawal Assessment for Alcohol scale (CIWA-A). *Addiction* 1994;89(10):1287–1292.

alcohol withdrawal seizures in animal studies. Although the evidence base is smaller, use of tapering doses of sodium valproate could be used in similar fashion. Both of these medications may also be used as adjuncts to benzodiazepine-based regimens in patients who have a history of recurrent withdrawal seizures, with prominent mood lability during withdrawal or with concurrent benzodiazepine withdrawal. However, studies of adequate size to assess the efficacy of these agents in preventing withdrawal seizures or delirium are not yet available. They are available only in oral form, making it difficult to titrate doses rapidly for the more symptomatic or rapidly worsening patient. For these reasons, patients treated with carbamazepine or sodium valproate should be monitored using withdrawal scales and receive benzodiazepines should more severe withdrawal symptoms emerge. Both these agents have interactions with other drugs and have hepatic and hematologic toxicities, and thus must be used carefully, if at all, in patients with certain comorbid medical and psychiatric disorders.

The routine use of phenytoin has been advocated as a method to prevent the occurrence of withdrawal seizures, and there is some evidence from early trials that it may be effective for this purpose. However, more recent, methodologically sound trials have failed to show evidence that phenytoin is effective in preventing recurrent withdrawal seizures. Moreover, studies have shown that appropriately used benzodiazepines are extremely effective in preventing withdrawal seizures and that the addition of phenytoin does not lead to improved outcomes so its use has been largely abandoned.

Anticonvulsants such as gabapentin and vigabatrin show promise for use in alcohol withdrawal as they may have fewer side effects and a better safety profile than carbamazepine and sodium valproate. Controlled trials are underway, and until results are available their use should remain investigational.

Other Agents Beta-adrenergic blocking agents, such as atenolol and propranolol, as well as centrally acting alpha-adrenergic agonists, such as clonidine, also are effective in ameliorating symptoms in patients with mild to moderate withdrawal, primarily by reducing the autonomic nervous system manifestations of withdrawal. However, these agents do not have known anticonvulsant activity, and the studies to date have not been large enough to determine their effectiveness in reducing seizures or delirium. Beta blockers pose a particular problem in this regard because delirium is a known, albeit rare, side effect of these drugs. In addition, there is concern that selective reduction in certain manifestations of withdrawal may mask the development of other significant withdrawal symptoms and make it difficult to utilize withdrawal scales to guide therapy. Neuroleptic agents, including the phenothiazines and the butyrophenone haloperidol, demonstrate some effectiveness in reducing the signs and symptoms of withdrawal and for a time were used extensively for that purpose. However, these agents are less effective than benzodiazepines in preventing delirium and actually lead to an increase in the rate of seizures. Neuroleptic agents are widely used to calm agitated patients and are useful for this purpose in the setting of alcohol withdrawal as well. They should not be used alone, but always in conjunction with a benzodiazepine; moreover, neuroleptic agents with less effect on the seizure threshold, such as haloperidol, should be selected. It long has been recognized that magnesium levels often are low during alcohol withdrawal. Closer study has found that magnesium levels usually are normal at admission, but then drop during the course of withdrawal, before spontaneously returning to normal as symptoms subside. Only one randomized trial of magnesium during withdrawal has been performed, and that study found no difference in severity of withdrawal or rate of seizures, even after adjustment for magnesium levels. Providing supplemental oral magnesium to patients with a documented low magnesium level is without significant risk, but routine administration of magnesium, either oral or intramuscular, for withdrawal is no longer recommended.

Case series describing oral or intravenous alcohol for the prevention or treatment of withdrawal symptoms continue to be published in the surgical literature, but no well-designed controlled trials evaluating the safety or relative efficacy of this approach—either compared with placebo or to benzodiazepines—have been performed (11,42,43). Despite the relative lack of evidence of oral and intravenous alcohol for the management of alcohol withdrawal, several hospitals continue to use intravenous or oral alcohol in the management of alcohol withdrawal. (44,45). Intravenous alcohol infusions require close monitoring because of the potential toxicity of alcohol. As a pharmacologic agent, ethyl alcohol has numerous adverse effects, including its well known hepatic, gastrointestinal, and neurologic toxicities, as well as its effects on mental status and judgment. Given the proven efficacy and safety of other agents, the use of oral or intravenous alcohol for alcohol detoxification is generally discouraged.

Thiamine A final agent with an important role in the management of patients withdrawing from alcohol is thiamine. Alcohol-dependent patients are at risk for thiamine deficiency, which may lead to Wernicke disease and the Wernicke-Korsakoff syndrome. Wernicke disease is an illness of acute onset characterized by the triad of mental disturbance, paralysis of eye movements, and ataxia. The ocular abnormality usually is weakness or paralysis of abduction (sixth nerve palsy), which invariably is bilateral, although rarely symmetric. It is accompanied by diplopia, strabismus, and nystagmus. The ataxia primarily affects gait and stance. Mental status changes typically involve a global confusional-apathetic state but, in some patients, a disproportionate disorder of retentive memory is apparent. Wernicke disease is a neurologic emergency that should be treated by the immediate parenteral administration of thiamine, with a dose of 50 mg intravenously and 50 mg intramuscularly. Delay in provision of thiamine increases the risk of permanent memory damage.

The provision of intravenous glucose solutions may exhaust a patient's reserve of B vitamins, acutely precipitating Wernicke disease. Therefore, intravenous glucose always should be accompanied by the administration of thiamine in the alcohol dependent patient. Ocular palsies may respond within hours, whereas the gait and cognitive problems of Wernicke improve more slowly. As the apathy, drowsiness, and confusion recede, the patient may be left with a sometimes permanent defect in retentive memory and learning known as Korsakoff psychosis. To reduce the risk of these sequelae, all patients presenting with alcohol withdrawal should receive 50 to 100 mg of thiamine at the time of presentation, followed by oral supplementation for several weeks. Patients with symptoms of Wernicke disease, those who are to receive glucose-containing intravenous solutions, and those at high risk of malnutrition should receive their initial dose parenterally.

Management of the Patient after a Withdrawal Seizure The patient who presents after experiencing a withdrawal seizure raises a number of management issues. It is important to recognize that not all seizures in alcohol-dependent patients are the result of withdrawal. In epidemiologic studies, the rate of epilepsy and seizures rises in parallel with the amount of an individual's alcohol intake. Alcohol dependent patients are at higher risk for seizures unrelated to withdrawal. A careful history of the temporal relationship of alcohol intake to the seizure should be obtained, and the diagnosis of withdrawal seizure should be made only if there is a clear history of a marked decrease or cessation of drinking in the 24 to 48 hours preceding the seizure. All patients who present with their first seizure warrant a thorough neurologic examination and brain imaging, with lumbar puncture and EEG also appropriate in many cases. Patients who are known to have a history of withdrawal seizures and who present with a seizure that can be attributed clearly to withdrawal may not require a full repeat evaluation. If the seizure was generalized and without focal elements, and if a careful neurologic examination reveals no evidence of focal deficits, there is no suspicion of meningitis and there is no history of recent major head trauma, additional testing has an extremely low yield and may be safely omitted. There is a 6- to 12-hour period during which there is an increased risk of seizures. Withdrawal seizures often are multiple, with a second seizure occurring in one case out of four. For the patient who presents with a withdrawal seizure, rapid treatment is indicated to prevent further episodes. The parenteral administration of a rapid-acting benzodiazepine such as diazepam or lorazepam is effective (46). Several studies have shown that phenytoin is no more effective than placebo in preventing recurrent seizures (47). Initial treatment should be followed by oral doses of long-acting benzodiazepines over the ensuing 24 to 48 hours. Early studies indicated that a withdrawal seizure placed the patient at increased risk for progression to DTs so close monitoring is warranted.

Management of the Patient with Delirium The patient who progresses to delirium raises a number of special management issues. Older studies showed a mortality rate of up to 30% in DTs but, with modern care, mortality has been reduced to <1% (10). The principles of successful treatment involve adequate sedation and meticulous supportive medical care. Such patients require close nursing observation and supportive care, which frequently necessitates admission to an intensive care unit. Careful management of fluids and electrolytes is important, given the patient's inability to manage his own intake and the presence of marked autonomic hyperactivity. Delirium often is encountered in patients admitted for acute medical problems whose alcohol dependence was not recognized and whose withdrawal was not adequately treated. A high index of suspicion for the development of infection—whose presenting signs may be masked by the fever, tachycardia, and confusion of the underlying delirium—is essential, as is careful management of coexisting medical conditions. The use of cross-tolerant sedative-hypnotics has been shown to reduce mortality in DTs and is recommended (21). However, such medications have not been shown to reverse the delirium or reduce its duration. The goal is to sedate the patient to a point of light sleep. This will control the patient's agitation, preventing behavior posing a risk to himself or herself and to staff, and allow staff to provide necessary supportive medical care.

The use of intravenous benzodiazepines with rapid onset, such as diazepam, has been shown to provide more rapid control of the patient's symptoms. An example of a widely used regimen is given in Table 42.4. The main complication of therapy with diazepam is respiratory depression. Whenever this approach is used, providers should have equipment and personnel immediately available to provide respiratory support if needed. One advantage of diazepam is that its peak onset occurs within 5 minutes of intravenous administration. This allows the provider to deliver repeat boluses and titrate sedation quickly without fear of a delayed appearance of oversedation. Once established, delirium can be expected to last for a number of hours, so diazepam offers another advantage in that its longer half-life helps maintain sedation with less chance of breakthrough agitation. Large doses of benzodiazepines may be needed to control the agitation of patients in DTs, with hundreds and even thousands of milligrams of diazepam or its equivalent used over the course of treatment. The practitioner should not hesitate to use whatever amounts are needed to control the agitation, while keeping in mind the possible build up of long acting metabolites especially in patients with impaired hepatic function or the elderly.

There have been reports of the use of continuous intravenous drips of short-acting agents such as lorazepam or midazolam (21). Existing evidence suggests that this approach is no more effective than the use of boluses of longer-acting agents and is extremely expensive (21). In the agitated patient, benzodiazepines can be supplemented with the addition of neuroleptic agents such as haloperidol. As has been discussed, such agents should not be used alone. Also, neuroleptic agents with less effect on seizure threshold, such as haloperidol, should be used. In patients whose withdrawal is not readily controlled with oral benzodiazepines and who are beginning to demonstrate signs of agitation, intramuscular administration of a combination of lorazepam and a neuroleptic such as haloperidol often is effective in calming the patient, thus avoiding the need to use intravenous administration.

COMMON TREATMENT ISSUES

Location of Treatment Services As both research and clinical experience demonstrated that pharmacologic therapy can significantly reduce the incidence of major complications associated with alcohol withdrawal, it became common practice to admit patients to inpatient units to provide 3 to 7 days of medication. However, such intensive—and expensive—therapy is not necessary for many patients, and increasing interest has been shown in managing withdrawal on an outpatient basis. All patients presenting for management of withdrawal should undergo a comprehensive history and medical evaluation. For patients with only mild withdrawal symptoms, no history of seizures or DTs, and no concurrent significant medical or psychiatric problems, management on an outpatient basis is reasonable (48,49). Such patients should have a responsible individual to monitor them, they should be seen on a daily basis until they have stabilized, and ready access, including transportation, to emergency medical services should be available. In addition, many programs are concentrating on sharply reducing the length of stay for patients undergoing withdrawal. Patients may be treated in an observation unit or admitted for a 1-day stay. If significant withdrawal symptoms do not develop, and the withdrawal is easily controlled with little or no medication, patients can be discharged or transferred to an intensive outpatient rehabilitation program. Patients who experience severe withdrawal symptoms, however, need continuous close monitoring and nursing support (50).

Patients Admitted for Medical/Surgical Treatment Studies have shown that about 20% of patients admitted to the hospital have alcohol use disorders, and the rate among those admitted for acute trauma or for problems related to high alcohol intake, such as head and neck cancers, is even higher. Thus hospital admission is a frequent precipitating event for alcohol withdrawal. Screening for alcohol problems should be universal at the time of hospital admission, but is not yet common practice. Patients thus may develop withdrawal that goes unrecognized or becomes far advanced before being recognized and treated. Withdrawal has been shown to contribute to higher postoperative complications, mortality, and length of stay (51). Unfortunately, it is all too common to proceed with elective surgery despite knowledge of active alcohol use disorders. Such patients should be screened for alcohol problems and undergo medically managed withdrawal before proceeding with surgery.

Current management strategies for alcohol withdrawal rely on quantitative assessment of withdrawal severity and were developed in patients presenting specifically for alcohol withdrawal. However, signs and symptoms of withdrawal are very nonspecific and thus they can be difficult to differentiate from manifestations of acute medical conditions. Furthermore, critically ill patients, who may have impaired consciousness or be on ventilators, cannot provide much of the information required to assess severity of withdrawal. Nevertheless use of alcohol withdrawal scales in general medical/surgical patients have been studied and found to be valuable in selected patients (52). Low withdrawal scales can be interpreted with confidence as indicating the absence of significant withdrawal. However, high scores have many causes, and must be interpreted with caution. Given the frequency of alcohol problems in hospitalized patients, instituting standard screening, assessment, and management protocols is appropriate and has been found to be helpful. Patients requiring more than small amounts of medication for withdrawal symptoms need individualized assessment by clinicians experienced in the management of withdrawal.

Alcohol Withdrawal in U.S. Jails Another event that frequently precipitates alcohol withdrawal is arrest and incarceration. In 1997, surveys showed that of the 11 million individuals arrested, approximately 1.2 million were alcohol dependent. Unfortunately, at the same time, only 28% of jail administrators reported that their institutions ever provided medically managed withdrawal for arrestees, despite the ruling of the U.S. Supreme Court that failure to provide proper medical care amounts to a violation of the Eighth Amendment of the U.S. Constitution proscribing cruel and unusual punishment. Overall in 1997, 750,000 arrestees were at risk for untreated alcohol withdrawal (53). Because this situation has not changed significantly in the intervening years, it is not surprising that inadequately treated alcohol withdrawal has been shown to contribute to deaths among newly arrested individuals. American Society of Addiction Medicine has issued a public policy statement on appropriate detoxification services for individuals incarcerated in prisons and jails, which recommends that incarcerated individuals should receive appropriate screening and medical care to manage withdrawal syndromes (54). That this population is at high risk should be kept in mind as health care professionals encounter patients referred from jails with possible withdrawal symptoms.

CONCLUSIONS

It is important to remember that successful management of alcohol withdrawal is only the first—and sometimes the most easily achieved—step toward the primary goal of treating the patient's underlying addiction to alcohol. The underlying goals of the management of alcohol intoxication and withdrawal are to assure the stability and safety of the patient and encourage ongoing treatment of their alcohol misuse. Development of a plan to engage the patient in treatment is a critical component of withdrawal and must not be overlooked.

REFERENCES

1. Naranjo CA, Bremner KE. Behavioural correlates of alcohol intoxication. *Addiction* 1993;88:25–35.
2. Wiese JG, Shlipak MG, Browner WS. The alcohol hangover. *Ann Intern Med* 2000;132:897–902.
3. Swift R, Davidson D. Alcohol hangover: mechanisms and mediators. *Alcohol Health Res World* 1998;22:54–60.
4. Pittler MH, Verster JC, Ernst E. Interventions for preventing and treating alcohol hangover: systematic review of randomized controlled trials. *Br Med J* 2005;331:1515–1518.
5. Victor M, Adams RD. Effect of alcohol on the nervous system. *Res Publication Assoc Res Nervous Mental Dis* 1953;32:526–523.
6. Isbell H, Fraser HF, Wikler A, et al. An experimental study of the etiology of "rum fits" and delirium tremens. *Q J Studies Alc* 1955;16:1–33.
7. American Psychiatric Association. *Diagnostic and statistical manual of mental disorders,* 4th ed. (DSM-IV). Washington, DC: American Psychiatric Press, 1994.
8. Driessen M, Lange W, Junghanns, et al. Proposal of a comprehensive clinical typology of alcohol withdrawal—a cluster analyses approach. *Alcohol Alcohol* 2005;40:301–313.
9. Wetterling T, Weber B, Depfenhart M, et al. Development of a rating scale to predict severity of alcohol withdrawal syndrome. *Alcohol Alcohol* 2006;41:611–615.
10. Saitz R, Mayo-Smith MF, Roberts MS, et al. Individualized treatment for alcohol withdrawal: a randomized double blind controlled trial. *JAMA* 1994;272:519–523.
11. Mayo-Smith MF, Cushman P, Hill AJ, et al. Pharmacological management of alcohol withdrawal: a meta-analysis and evidence-based practice guideline. *JAMA* 1997;278:144–151.
12. Alldredge BK, Lowenstein DH. Status epilepticus related to alcohol abuse. *Epilepticus* 1993;34:1033–1037.
13. Booth BM, Blow FC. The kindling hypothesis: further evidence from a U.S. national study of alcoholic men. *Alcohol Alcoholism* 1993;28: 593–598.
14. Ballenger JC, Post RM. Kindling as a model for alcohol withdrawal syndromes. *Br J Psychiatry* 1978;133:1–14.
15. Womer TM. Relative kindling effect of readmissions in alcoholics. *Alcohol Alcohol* 1996;31:375–80. http://www.ncbi.nlm.nih.gov/pubmed/8879284?ordinalpos=2&itool=EntrezSystem2.PEntrez.Pubmed.Pubmed_ResultsPanel.Pubmed_DefaultReportPanel.Pubmed_RVDocSum
16. Linnoila M, Mefford I, Nutt D, et al. NIH conference. Alcohol withdrawal and noradrenergic function. *Ann Intern Med* 1987;107:875–89. http://www.ncbi.nlm.nih.gov/pubmed/2825572?ordinalpos=1&itool=EntrezSystem2.PEntrez.Pubmed.Pubmed_ResultsPanel.Pubmed_DefaultReportPanel.Pubmed_RVDocSum

17. Ballenger JC, Post RM. Kindling as a model for alcohol withdrawal syndromes. *Br J Psychiatry* 1978;133:1–14. http://www.ncbi.nlm.nih.gov/pubmed/352467?ordinalpos=3&itool=EntrezSystem2.PEntrez.Pubmed.Pubmed_ResultsPanel.Pubmed_DefaultReportPanel.Pubmed_RVDocSum
18. Brown ME, Anton RF, Malcolm R, et al. Alcohol detoxification and withdrawal seizures: clinical support for a kindling hypothesis. *Biol Psychiatry* 1988;23:507–514. http://www.ncbi.nlm.nih.gov/pubmed/3345323?ordinalpos=20&itool=EntrezSystem2.PEntrez.Pubmed.Pubmed_ResultsPanel.Pubmed_DefaultReportPanel.Pubmed_RVDocSum
19. Pinel JP. Alcohol withdrawal seizures: implications of kindling. *Pharmacol Biochem Behav* 1980;13 Suppl 1:225–31. http://www.ncbi.nlm.nih.gov/pubmed/7017761?ordinalpos=5&itool=EntrezSystem2.PEntrez.Pubmed.Pubmed_ResultsPanel.Pubmed_DefaultReportPanel.Pubmed_RVDocSum
20. Becker HC. The alcohol withdrawal "kindling" phenomenon: clinical and experimental findings. *Alcohol Clin Exp Res* 1996;20(8 Suppl):121A–124A. http://www.ncbi.nlm.nih.gov/pubmed/8947249?ordinalpos=2&itool=EntrezSystem2.PEntrez.Pubmed.Pubmed_ResultsPanel.Pubmed_DefaultReportPanel.Pubmed_RVDocSum
21. Mayo-Smith MF, Beecher LH, Fischer TL, et al. Management of alcohol withdrawal delirium: an evidence-based practice guideline. *Arch Intern Med* 2004;164:1405–1412.
22. Wolf KM, Shaughnessy AF, Middleton DB. Prolonged delirium tremens requiring massive doses of medication. *J Am Board Family Pract* 1993;6:502–504.
23. Kraemer KL, Mayo-Smith MF, Calkins DR. Impact of age on the severity, course and complications of alcohol withdrawal. *Arch Intern Med* 1997;157:2234–2241.
24. Gross M, Lewis E, Nagarajan M. An improved quantitative system for assessing the acute alcoholic psychoses and related states (TSA and SSA). In: Gross M, editor, alcohol intoxication and withdrawal: experimental studies. New York. Plenum; 1973;365–376.
25. Sullivan JT, Sykora K, Schneiderman J, et al. Assessment of alcohol withdrawal: the revised clinical institute withdrawal assessment for alcohol scale (CIWA-Ar). *Br J Addict* 1989;84:1353–1357. http://www.ncbi.nlm.nih.gov/pubmed/2597811?ordinalpos=2&itool=EntrezSystem2.PEntrez.Pubmed.Pubmed_ResultsPanel.Pubmed_DefaultReportPanel.Pubmed_RVDocSum
26. Stuppaeck CH, Barnas C, Falk M, et al. Assessment of the alcohol withdrawal syndrome–validity and reliability of the translated and modified Clinical Institute Withdrawal Assessment for Alcohol scale (CIWA-A). *Addiction* 1994;89:1287–1292. http://www.ncbi.nlm.nih.gov/pubmed/7804089?ordinalpos=1&itool=EntrezSystem2.PEntrez.Pubmed.Pubmed_ResultsPanel.Pubmed_DefaultReportPanel.Pubmed_RVDocSum
27. Goldstein DB, Goldstein A. Possible role of enzyme inhibition and repression in drug tolerance and addiction. *Biochem Pharmacol* 1961;8:48.
28. De Witte P, Pinto E, Ansseau, et al. Alcohol and withdrawal: from animal research to clinical issues. *Neurosci Behav Rev* 2003;27:189–197.
29. Hawley RJ, Major LF, Schulman EA et al. Cerebrospinal fluid 3-methoxy-4-hydroxyphenylglycol and norepinephrine levels in alcohol withdrawal: correlations with clinical signs. *Arch Gen Psych* 1985;42:1056–1062.
30. Gorwood P, Limosin F, Batel P, et al. The A9 allele of the DAT gene is associated with delirium tremens and alcohol-withdrawal seizure. *Biol Psychol* 2003;53:85–92.
31. Sander T, Harms H, Podschus J, et al. Allelic association of a dopamine transporter gene polymorphism in the alcohol dependence with withdrawal seizures or delirium. *Biol Psychiatry* 1997;41:299–304.
32. Limosin F, Loze JY, Boni C, et al. The A9 allele of the dopamine transporter gene increases the risk of visual hallucinations during alcohol withdrawal in alcoholic women. *Neurosci Lett* 2004;362:91–94.
33. Schmidt LG, Sander T. Genetics of alcohol withdrawal. *Eur Psychiatry* 2000;15:135–139.
34. Schuckit MA, Danko GP, Smith TL, et al. A 5-year prospective evaluation of DSM-IV alcohol dependence with and without a physiological component. *Alcohol Clin Exp Res* 2003;27:818–825.
35. de Bruijn C, van den Brink W, de Graaf R, et al. The craving withdrawal model for alcoholism: towards DSM-V. Improving the discriminant validity of alcohol use disorder diagnosis. *Alcohol Alcohol* 2005;40:308–313.
36. Trumpler F, Oez S, Stahli P, et al. Acupuncture for alcohol withdrawal: a randomized controlled trial. *Alcohol Alcohol* 2003;38:369–375.
37. Kunz S, Schulz M, Lewitzky M, et al. Ear acupuncture for alcohol withdrawal in comparison with aromatherapy: a randomized controlled trial. *Alcohol Clin Exp Res* 2007;31:436–442.
38. Reader M, Young R, Connor JP. Massage therapy improves the management of alcohol withdrawal syndrome. *J Alt Comp Med* 2005;11:311–313.
39. Holbrook AM, Crowther R, Lotter A, et al. Meta-analysis of benzodiazepine use in the treatment of acute alcohol withdrawal. *CMAJ* 1999;160:649–655.
40. Ntais C, Pakos E, Kyzas P, et al. Benzodiazepines for alcohol withdrawal. *Cochr Database System Rev* 2005; Art No.:CD005063. DOI: 10.1002/14651858.CD005063.pub2.
41. Malcolm R, Myrick H, Brady KT, et al. Update on anticonvulsants for the treatment of alcohol withdrawal. *Am J Addict* 2001;10:16S–23S.
42. Craft PP, Foil MB, Cunningham PR, et al. Intravenous ethanol for alcohol detoxification in trauma patients. *South Med J* 1994;87:47–54. http://www.ncbi.nlm.nih.gov/pubmed/8284718?ordinalpos=3&itool=EntrezSystem2.PEntrez.Pubmed.Pubmed_ResultsPanel.Pubmed_DefaultReportPanel.Pubmed_RVDocSum
43. DiPaula B, Tommasello A, Solounias B, et al. An evaluation of intravenous ethanol in hospitalized patients. *J Subst Abuse Treat* 1998;15:437–442.
44. Smoger SH, Looney SW, Blondell RD, et al. Hospital Use of Ethanol Survey *HUES: preliminary results. *J Addict Dis* 2002;21:65–73.
45. Rosenbaum M, McCarty T. Alcohol prescription by surgeons in the prevention and treatment of delirium tremens: historic and current practice. *Gen Hosp Psychiatry* 2002;24:257–259.
46. D'Onofrio G, Rathlev NK, Ulrich AS, et al. Lorazepam for the prevention of recurrent seizures related to alcohol. *N Engl J Med* 1999;340:915–919.
47. Rathlev NK, D'Onofrio G, Fish SS, et al. The lack of efficacy of phenytoin in prevention of recurrent alcohol related seizures. *Ann Emerg Med* 1994;23:513–518.
48. Hayashida M, Alterman AI, McLellan T, et al. Comparative effectiveness and costs of inpatient and outpatient detoxification of patients with mild-to-moderate alcohol withdrawal syndrome. *N Engl J Med* 1989;320(6):358–365.
49. Soyka M, Horak M. Outpatient alcohol detoxification: implementation efficacy and outcome effectiveness of a model project. *Eur Addict Res* 2004;10:180–187.
50. Mee-Lee D, Shulman GD, Fishman M, et al, eds. *ASAM patient placement criteria for treatment of substance-related disorders*, 2nd ed.-rev. Chevy Chase, MD: American Society of Addiction Medicine, 2001.
51. Spies C, Tennesen H, Andreasson S, et al. Perioperative morbidity and mortality in chronic alcoholic patients. *Alcoholism Clin Exp Res* 2001;5:164S–170S.
52. Jaeger TM, Lohr RH, Pankratz VS. Symptom-triggered therapy for alcohol withdrawal syndrome in medical inpatients. *Mayo Clin Proc* 2001;76:695–710.
53. Fiscella K, Pless N, Meldrum S, et al. Benign neglect or neglected abuse: drug and alcohol withdrawal in U.S. jails. *J Law, Med Ethics* 2004; 32:129–136.
54. Public Policy Statement on Access to Appropriate Detoxification Services for Persons Incarcerated in Prisons and Jails. American Society of Addiction Medicine, Chevy Chase, MD, 2005.

CHAPTER 43

William E. Dickinson, DO, FASAM, FAAFP
Steven J. Eickelberg, MD, FASAM

Management of Sedative-Hypnotic Intoxication and Withdrawal

Sedative-hypnotic medications decrease activity, moderate excitement, exert a calming effect, produce drowsiness, and facilitate sleep. They are among the most widely used prescription drugs in the United States. Misuse of and dependence on these drugs have occurred since their introduction. Sedative-hypnotics stimulate the inhibitory neurotransmitters in the GABA receptors. Although all sedatives and hypnotics have mild stimulant properties at low doses, their primary effect is to inhibit central nervous system function. Drugs in this class that are commonly associated with severe withdrawal states (in addition to alcohol) include methaqualone, glutethimide, phenobarbital, and short-acting benzodiazepines such as alprazolam and triazolam. Sedative drugs associated with less severe clinical withdrawal states include meprobamate and chlordiazepoxide.

SEDATIVE-HYPNOTIC INTOXICATION AND OVERDOSE

Clinical Picture The signs and symptoms of sedative-hypnotic intoxication and overdose are similar for the various drugs in the class (Table 43.1). The patient with mild to moderate toxicity presents with slurred speech, ataxia, and uncoordination similar to that seen with alcohol intoxication. On occasion, particularly in the older adults, a paradoxical agitated confusion and even delirium may be produced. At more severe stages of intoxication, stupor and coma develop. With the older nonbenzodiazepine agents, toxicity may progress, ultimately leading to fatal respiratory arrest or cardiovascular collapse. Overdose with these older agents also may be associated with a variety of agent-specific clinical manifestations, such as bullous skin lesions with barbiturates ("barb blisters"), details of which can be found in textbooks on toxicologic emergencies (1).

An additional problem with several of the older sedative-hypnotics is that, with regular use, tolerance may develop to the drugs' therapeutic effects, but not to their lethal effects. The maintenance dose then may approach the lethal dose and the therapeutic index decreases. Toxicity and overdose thus can occur with only small increases over the individual's regular intake.

On the other hand, benzodiazepines rarely lead to death when ingested by themselves. A lethal dose has not been established for any of the benzodiazepines and there are very few well-documented cases of death from ingestion of benzodiazepines alone. The few deaths that have occurred all involved short-acting, high-potency benzodiazepines such as alprazolam and triazolam (2) or administration of benzodiazepines by an intravenous route. However, inappropriate intramuscular use of chlordiazepoxide can lead to erratic absorption, producing respiratory compromise. The benzodiazepines are free of toxic effects on peripheral (non-central nervous system) organ systems in either long-term use or acute overdose.

Despite their safety, benzodiazepines continue to be a major cause of overdose and continue to pose a significant problem because, although safe by themselves, they act synergistically with other agents when ingested in combination. Mixed overdoses—such as those involving benzodiazepines in combination with alcohol, major tranquilizers, antidepressants, or opiates—can be fatal. This result is true for the nonbenzodiazepine agents as well.

Management Assessment and maintenance of the airway and, when necessary, ventilatory support, form the cornerstone in managing sedative-hypnotic overdose. Many of the benzodiazepine agents slow gut motility and some—such as

TABLE 43.1 Diagnosis of Sedative-Hypnotic Overdose

History
- Sedative-hypnotic use (ask about drug, amount, time of last use)
- Polydrug abuse
- Use multiple sources of information (family, hospital records, etc.)

Physical Examination
- Central nervous system depression
- Respiratory depression

Laboratory Tests
- Rule out hypoglycemia, acidemia, and fluid and electrolyte abnormalities
- Toxicology screens for sedative-hypnotics and other drugs

phenobarbital, meprobamate, glutethimide, and ethchlorvynol—can form concretions in the stomach. Therefore, evacuation of the gastrointestinal tract with a large-bore orogastric tube is the next step, provided an active gag reflex is elicited or the airway is protected by intubation. A slurry of 1.0 g/kg activated charcoal, together with a dose of cathartic, should be given. Repeated doses of activated charcoal, at 0.5 to 1.0 g/kg every 2 to 4 hours (or a similar amount delivered by slow continuous nasogastric infusion) may be helpful, particularly for barbiturate or other nonbenzodiazepine ingestions. Some of these agents have an extensive enterohepatic circulation, and repeated doses of charcoal have been shown to speed their elimination.

Alkalization of the urine also may be helpful in eliminating phenobarbital, but forced diuresis has not been shown to be helpful for any drugs in the class. In extreme cases, hemoperfusion may have a role. Measurement of serum levels can be helpful in documenting the identity and amounts of agents ingested, as well as in tracking levels over time. However, immediate clinical management is based on the patient's condition rather than serum levels.

Flumazenil is a competitive benzodiazepine receptor antagonist with very weak agonist properties at the benzodiazepine receptor (3). It can reverse the sedative effects of benzodiazepines, but not of the other agents or alcohol. Overall, it has found a role in reversing the effects of short-acting benzodiazepines, such as midazolam, after medical procedures. It also may be used when benzodiazepines have been ingested alone as an overdose. In such settings, slow intravenous titration in amounts not exceeding 1 mg is recommended, with monitoring for the recurrence of sedation. The effects of flumazenil are short-lived, and symptoms may return in 30 to 60 minutes. Moreover, its use has been associated with seizures and cardiac arrhythmias. These adverse effects are more likely to occur when it is administered rapidly in large amounts and in patients who have ingested a sedative-hypnotic in combination with a substance capable of causing seizures, such as a tricyclic antidepressant (4). Persons who are physiologically dependent on benzodiazepines are at high risk of seizures when they are given flumazenil. Flumazenil thus has not found a role as part of the standard "coma cocktail" (containing thiamine, glucose, and naloxone) because it produces a rapid benzodiazepine withdrawal. Its use in mixed overdoses or in patients who have used benzodiazepines chronically is limited because of the risk of adverse effects.

SEDATIVE-HYPNOTIC WITHDRAWAL

Overview The use of most sedative, hypnotic, or anxiolytic agents can result in the development of psychologic dependence, physical dependence, or addiction. (In this chapter, "dependence" is used to refer to the host's neurophysiological adaptation to regular or chronic sedative-hypnotic use. The definition of dependence includes adaptation to substance use that leads to an abstinence syndrome with the abrupt and, at times, tapered cessation of use.) Withdrawal is tantamount to, and is defined by, the signs and symptoms contained within the abstinence syndrome. This syndrome can occur with both high- and low-dose use—even use at therapeutic levels monitored by a physician. The development of dependence to sedative-hypnotic compounds is similar across the classes of the benzodiazepines, the barbiturates, and the nonbarbiturate/nonbenzodiazepine agents.

All of the sedative-hypnotic agents covered in this chapter are substances that currently, or in the recent past, have enjoyed widespread use. All possess well-documented, clinically important dependence and withdrawal characteristics. Marked similarities exist between the withdrawal syndromes seen with the benzodiazepines, the barbiturates, and the nonbarbiturate/nonbenzodiazepine agents, all of which resemble acute alcohol withdrawal syndrome in many ways. This resemblance is related to the properties of the binding site in the brain (the GABA receptor). Differences in withdrawal syndrome characteristics among sedative-hypnotic compounds primarily reflect differences in the rate at which dependence is induced, the rapidity with which symptoms occur on discontinuation of the drug, and the severity of those symptoms.

A clinically significant withdrawal syndrome is most apt to occur after discontinuation of daily therapeutic dose (low dose) use of a sedative-hypnotic for at least 4 to 6 months or, at doses that exceed two to three times the upper limit of recommended therapeutic use (high dose), for more than 2 to 3 months. The time course and severity of the sedative-hypnotic withdrawal syndrome reflects the influences of three pharmacologic factors: (i) dose, (ii) duration of use, and (iii) duration of drug action (Fig. 43.1). (For the purposes of this discussion, duration of drug action is directly related to the elimination half-life at steady-state conditions.) Withdrawal severity has been related to dose and duration of treatment. Latency to onset of withdrawal is related to the elimination half-life (5).

Clinical research with benzodiazepines has identified additional drug and host factors that influence the onset and

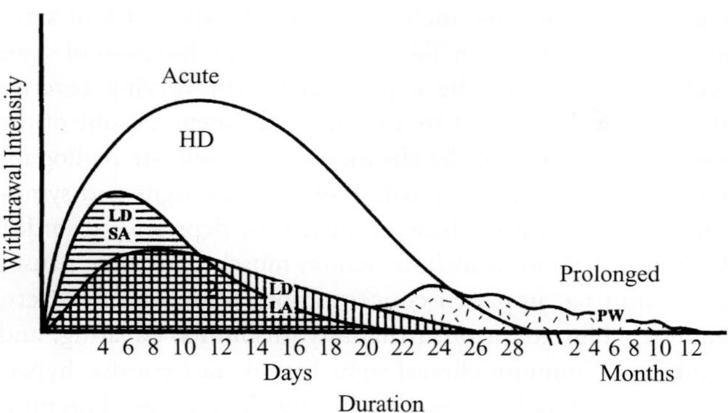

FIGURE 43.1. Time-course of sedative-hypnotic withdrawal. Time course and potential withdrawal intensity as influenced by dose and duration of drug action. HD = high dose; LD = low or therapeutic dose; SA = short-acting; LA = long-acting; PW = prolonged withdrawal.

severity of the withdrawal syndrome; these factors are elaborated on in the following sections.

Signs and Symptoms of Discontinuation The spectrum of signs and symptoms that are experienced most often during the course of withdrawal are summarized in Table 43.2. Considerable variation exists among patients in terms of the signs and symptoms of the abstinence syndrome. Although Figure 43.1 appears to indicate that withdrawal follows a smooth and predictable course, most patients experience significant moment-to-moment quantitative and qualitative variations in their signs and symptoms. Petursson (6) and Salzman (7) reviewed the frequency of various symptoms of benzodiazepine withdrawal. Anxiety, insomnia, restlessness, agitation, irritability, and muscle tension were very frequent. Less frequent were nausea, diaphoresis, lethargy, aches and pains, coryza, hyperacusis, blurred vision, nightmares, depression, hyperreflexia, and ataxia. Psychosis, seizures, confusion, paranoid delusions, hallucinations, and persistent tinnitus were uncommon. The areas under the curves in Figure 43.1 outline the potential time course and withdrawal severity characteristics. The multitude of signs and symptoms outlined in Table 43.2 illustrates that, in the absence of the knowledge that a patient is withdrawing from a sedative-hypnotic, a number of medical or psychiatric differential diagnoses would be entertained to explain the patient's condition.

Benzodiazepines Benzodiazepine use, dependence, and withdrawal are much more thoroughly researched than other classes of sedative-hypnotic compounds. Soon after chlordiazepoxide (Librium, 1960) and diazepam (Valium, 1961) became available commercially, clinical reports were published documenting a high-dose discontinuation withdrawal syndrome with severe characteristics (seizures, depression, delirium, psychosis) (8,9). Reports of a withdrawal syndrome after discontinuation of long-term use of benzodiazepines at therapeutic doses were published within the following decade (10,11). It now is well established that benzodiazepine dependence, withdrawal, and difficulties in discontinuing chronic benzodiazepine use are influenced by multiple pharmacologic and host factors (as discussed later in this chapter).

Barbiturates Reports in the medical literature evidenced an emerging awareness of barbiturate dependence and an abstinence syndrome as early as the 1940s. The first American article (12) directly addressing the barbiturate withdrawal syndrome was followed by a clinical study that chronicled the signs and symptoms of the barbiturate abstinence syndrome (13). Further studies quantified, with high-dose use, the duration of barbiturate ingestion necessary for the appearance of mild, moderate, and severe withdrawal symptoms (14,15). The first evidence that an abstinence syndrome could occur after long-term therapeutic (low-dose) barbiturate use was published nearly two decades later (16,17).

Treatment of barbiturate withdrawal with barbiturate substitution was reported as early as 1953 (15). In 1970 and 1971, Smith and Wesson reported on a protocol that employs phenobarbital substitution, stabilization, and tapering to treat barbiturate dependence. Their technique remains the "gold standard" for the management of all sedative-hypnotic classes or mixed sedative-hypnotic withdrawal.

Nonbarbiturate/Nonbenzodiazepine Agents The medical literature contains case reports documenting the full spectrum of sedative-hypnotic withdrawal signs and symptoms from this

TABLE 43.2 Clinical Manifestations of Sedative-Hypnotic Withdrawal

Vital Signs
- Tachycardia
- Hypertension
- Fever

Central Nervous System
- Agitation
- Anxiety
- Delirium
- Hallucinations
- Insomnia
- Irritability
- Nightmares
- Sensory disturbances
- Tremor

Ears
- Tinnitus

Gastrointestinal
- Anorexia
- Diarrhea
- Nausea

High-Dose (Severe) Withdrawal
- Seizures
- Delirium
- Death

group of compounds. Of greatest concern is the multitude of reports documenting severe withdrawal syndromes, marked by delirium, psychosis, hallucinations, hyperthermia, cardiac arrests, and death (18–25).

Benzodiazepine Discontinuation The signs and symptoms experienced after the discontinuation of benzodiazepine use have been described as falling into four categories: (i) symptom recurrence or relapse, (ii) rebound, (iii) pseudowithdrawal, and (iv) true withdrawal.

Symptom recurrence or relapse is characterized by the recurrence of symptoms (such as insomnia or anxiety) for which the benzodiazepine initially was taken. The symptoms may be similar in character to the condition that existed before drug treatment. Relapse may occur after discontinuation, with or without the prior existence of benzodiazepine dependence. Reemergence of symptoms is quite common, exceeding 60% to 80% for anxiety and insomnia disorders (26,27). Symptom recurrence can present rapidly or slowly over days to months after drug discontinuation.

This pattern can have important implications for routine reassessment of the need for continued benzodiazepine use. The need for the benzodiazepine is reevaluated, with attention given to dose and duration. When the need is diminished or eliminated, so should be the benzodiazepine.

Rebound is marked by the development of symptoms, within hours to days of drug discontinuation, which are qualitatively similar to the disorder for which the benzodiazepine initially was prescribed. However, the symptoms are transiently more intense than they were before drug treatment. Insomnia and anxiety disorders are the best-studied examples (28). Rebound symptoms are of short duration and are self-limited (27), which distinguishes this syndrome from recurrence.

Pseudowithdrawal and overinterpretation of symptoms may occur when expectations of withdrawal lead to the experiencing of abstinence symptoms. This effect has been observed in study patients who discontinued placebo medication or continued benzodiazepine use but believed that the benzodiazepine had been discontinued (29). In addition, expectations of symptoms often are negatively influenced by concerns registered in the media or by friends or physicians.

True withdrawal is marked by the emergence of psychologic and somatic signs and symptoms after the discontinuation of benzodiazepines in an individual who is physically dependent on the drug. The withdrawal syndrome can be suppressed by the reinstitution of the discontinued benzodiazepine or another cross-tolerant sedative-hypnotic. Withdrawal from benzodiazepines results from a reversal of the neuroadaptive changes in the central nervous system that were induced by chronic benzodiazepine use. Withdrawal reflects a relative temporal and temporary diminution of central nervous system GABAergic neuronal inhibition coupled with an increased glutamate response to balance the benzodiazepine-induced GABA release.

There is considerable individual variation over time among patients who discontinue benzodiazepines. The benzodiazepine withdrawal syndrome includes any of the spectrum of signs and symptoms listed in Table 43.2. Any combination of signs and symptoms may be experienced with varying severity throughout the initial 1 to 4 weeks of abstinence. None of the signs or symptoms of the abstinence syndrome are pathognomonic of benzodiazepine withdrawal. Many signs and symptoms are identical to those of anxiety or depressive disorder. Common symptoms include tremor, muscle twitching, nausea and vomiting, impaired concentration, restlessness, anxiety, anorexia, blurred vision, irritability, insomnia, sweating, and weakness. Common clinical signs include tachycardia, hypertension, hyperreflexia, mydriasis, and diaphoresis. The presence of neuropsychiatric symptoms—including perceptual distortions and hypersensitivity to light, sound, and touch—are common. Many believe these "sensory-perceptual symptoms" are most indicative of neurophysiologic withdrawal, but they rarely occur in the absence of some of the aforementioned adrenergic or anxiety symptoms. Lack of clinical signs should not be considered tantamount to the absence of a withdrawal syndrome.

The clinical withdrawal picture can consist primarily of subjective symptoms, accompanied by few or no concurrently observable hyperadrenergic signs or vital sign fluctuations (as seen with acute alcohol withdrawal).

These discontinuation syndromes often occur in combination. For example, considerable overlap exists between the symptoms of recurrence in anxiety and insomnia disorders and the signs and symptoms of rebound and withdrawal. Clinical techniques that treat, minimize, and attenuate benzodiazepine abstinence symptoms also effectively alleviate rebound. As a result, attention to sorting out rebound from withdrawal is unnecessary (if not impossible). However, symptom recurrence or relapse is common. Clinicians must be attuned to the emergence or persistence of clinically important symptoms of relapse during and after the period of acute withdrawal.

Prolonged Withdrawal Some physicians report (30–32), and clinical experience confirms, that a small proportion of patients, after long-term benzodiazepine use, experience a prolonged syndrome of withdrawal. The signs and symptoms may persist for weeks to months after discontinuation. The syndrome is notable for its irregular and unpredictable day-to-day course and qualitative and quantitative differences in symptoms from both the prebenzodiazepine use state and the acute withdrawal period. Patients with prolonged withdrawal often experience slowly abating—albeit characteristic waxing and waning—symptoms of insomnia, perceptual disturbances, tremor, sensory hypersensitivities, and anxiety.

Role of the GABA-Benzodiazepine Receptor Complex Benzodiazepine action in the central nervous system is mediated by the gamma-aminobutyric-acid-benzodiazepine-receptor-complex (GABA-BDZ-R-complex) (33,34), primarily the $GABA_A$ receptor (35). Work by numerous investigators has shown that GABA is the primary central nervous system inhibitory neurotransmitter. Activation of the

GABA receptor induces the opening of a neuronal, membrane-bound chloride ion channel, located within the GABA-BDZ-R-complex. Neuronal inhibition results from neuronal membrane hyperpolarization secondary to the flow of chloride ions down the electrochemical gradient into the neuron. Benzodiazepines bind allosterically to a "benzodiazepine receptor" the $GABA_A$ receptor composed primarily of subunits gamma 2 and alpha 1, 2, 3, and 5 (35) located on the GABA-BDZ-R-complex. $GABA_A$ receptors with alpha 4 and 6 subtypes were found to be diazepam insensitive. The $GABA_A$ receptor with alpha 1, beta 2, and gamma 2 subunits is the most common type (43%) found in the rat brain (35). Benzodiazepines positively modulate and influence the GABA-chloride channel relationship.

A series of studies by Miller and colleagues (36–39) illustrated that, in mice, behavioral tolerance and discontinuation syndromes are temporally associated with molecular/receptor level adaptations. The investigators reported that, as tolerance to the ataxia-inducing effects of lorazepam developed behaviorally, benzodiazepine and GABA receptors were downregulated (through decreased receptor number, decreased GABA-receptor function, and diminished protein synthesis for GABA receptors). After lorazepam was administered for 4 weeks, it was abruptly discontinued. Concurrent with signs of withdrawal, GABA-receptors were upregulated, and GABA-receptor complex function was enhanced (as evidenced by greater affinity for GABA, increased affinity of the benzodiazepine receptor for benzodiazepines, increased benzodiazepine receptor number).

The rate of onset of behavioral tolerance to alprazolam and clonazepam followed by an abstinence syndrome after abrupt discontinuation was similarly computed and then compared with lorazepam in a subsequent report (39). Tolerance and withdrawal developed more rapidly with alprazolam (4 days for tolerance; 2 days for withdrawal) than with lorazepam and clonazepam, which were similar (7 days for tolerance; 4 days for withdrawal) (36,37,39). These studies also demonstrated that tolerance is primarily a pharmacodynamic, neuroadaptive phenomenon (brain and plasma levels remained constant throughout the period of chronic administration).

The amino acid L-glutamate is the major excitatory neurotransmitter in the central nervous system. Glutamate receptors have been classified into two groups; the N-methyl-D-aspartate (NMDA) receptors and non-NMDA receptors AMPA (alpha-amino3-hydoxy-5-methyl 4 isoxazole propionic acid) and kainate. Neuronal plasticity between excitation and inhibition is a balance of GABAergic inhibition and glutamatergic excitation. Benzodiazepine administration increases the inhibition effect of the GABA system while also beginning a compensatory excitation effect of the glutamate system as a counterbalancing response. The continued or increased use of benzodiazepines results in a new balance of these neuronal systems. When the benzodiazepine is lessened or stopped, the increased activity of the glutamate system is seen. Thus rebound anxiety, increased muscle tone, sensory disturbances, tremors, and seizures can be related to the increased glutamate activity. Interestingly, NMDA receptors are known to influence excitotoxity and neuronal damage and are associated with epilepsy and Alzheimer disease (35).

File (40) comments that it is premature to link our current observations of neurochemical changes to behavior etiologically, because multiple potential explanations exist. Events may be independent yet occur simultaneously, reflect neuroadaptive changes resulting from compensatory mechanisms, or be causally linked. Despite numerous unanswered questions, it is apparent that the primary neuroadaptive response occurs at the GABA-BDZ-R-complex. This system then influences changes in other neurotransmitter systems especially the glutamate system depending on the neuroanatomic location of the GABA-BDZ-R-complex. The benzodiazepine discontinuation syndrome subsequently is influenced, if not mediated, by both the GABA and glutamate systems and potentially numerous other neurotransmitter systems.

Pharmacologic Characteristics Affecting Withdrawal Pharmacologic factors are primarily responsible for the relationship between various benzodiazepines and the differing clinical manifestations of benzodiazepine withdrawal syndrome.

Pharmacokinetics Benzodiazepine pharmacokinetics determine the onset of discontinuation symptoms following chronic use. Cessation of use is followed by declining blood levels of drug at receptor sites, brain, blood, and peripheral tissues, with the rate of decline determined primarily by the elimination half-life. The onset, duration, and severity of the withdrawal syndrome correlate with declining serum levels of drug (8,36–38,41,42).

Onset of withdrawal from short-acting benzodiazepines (such as lorazepam, oxazepam, triazolam, alprazolam, and temazepam) occurs within 24 hours of cessation (43), with peak severity of withdrawal occurring within 1 to 5 days after cessation (43,44). With long-acting benzodiazepines (such as diazepam, chlordiazepoxide, and clonazepam), onset of withdrawal occurs within 5 days of cessation (26,43) and withdrawal severity peaks at 1 to 9 days (44).

Duration of acute withdrawal, from the temporal onset to the resolution of symptoms, can be as long as 7 to 21 days for short-acting and 10 to 28 days for long-acting benzodiazepines. While there is a difference in the type or number of withdrawal symptoms after discontinuation of short- or long-acting benzodiazepines (43,44), withdrawal symptoms from short-acting benzodiazepines are experienced as being more intense than those associated with long-acting drugs, and are of more rapid onset after abrupt discontinuation (41,43,44).

Dose and Duration of Use Higher doses and longer use place patients at greater risk for increased withdrawal severity. Daily benzodiazepine use for 10 days or less can lead to transient insomnia when the medications are stopped. A withdrawal syndrome can follow discontinuation of short-term (<2 to 3 months') low-dose therapeutic use, but most symptoms, if present at all, are rated as mild (such as insomnia) and are easily managed. Vorma et al. (45) found that subjects with lower benzodiazepine doses and no previous withdrawal attempts were more successful with discontinuation. On discontinuation of long-term (>1 year) therapeutic (low-dose) use, withdrawal is common and is accompanied by moderate to severe symptoms in 20% to 100% of patients (43,44). Discontinuation of high-dose (more than four or five times the high end of the therapeutic range for longer than 6 to 12 weeks) benzodiazepine use leads to moderate withdrawal in all patients, and severe withdrawal signs and symptoms in most patients (46).

Beyond 1 year of continuous benzodiazepine therapy, the duration of use becomes a less important factor in the severity of withdrawal (47). Use beyond 1 year may, however, predispose patients to prolonged withdrawal sequelae.

Potency Tolerance to the sedative and hypnotic effects develops most rapidly to shorter acting, higher potency benzodiazepines (such as triazolam and alprazolam). Withdrawal from these agents may be more intense and require more aggressive attention and longer periods of medical monitoring than is the case with other benzodiazepines (48,49).

Host Factors Affecting Withdrawal In addition to the aforementioned pharmacologic influences, host factors are implicated in patients' susceptibility to dependence and in the difficulty they encounter in discontinuing benzodiazepines after they become dependent. Clinically important patient factors include the following.

Psychiatric Comorbidity The primary clinical indication for benzodiazepine use involves treatment of the highly prevalent conditions of insomnia, anxiety, thought, and mood disorders. It follows that patients with chronic psychiatric disorders who are maintained on benzodiazepines for more than 3 to 6 months will, in addition to their psychiatric condition (adequately treated or not), also be physically dependent on the benzodiazepine. Numerous benzodiazepine discontinuation studies highlight the high (40% to 100%) prevalence of active concurrent psychiatric disorders seen at intake of study participants (43,44,47,49,50). Most of these studies demonstrate a correlation between the patients' degree of psychopathology and their withdrawal symptom severity and difficulty in discontinuing use.

Rickels and colleagues (43) reported on 119 patients discontinuing long-term, therapeutic-dose use. They noted a 90% prevalence of initial, active psychopathology with diagnoses that included generalized anxiety disorder (44%), panic disorder (27%), depression (14%), and other (7%). Patients with greater psychopathology required more support and assurance. The intensity of the withdrawal syndrome was seen as partially a function of the degree of psychopathology and other premorbid personality variables.

Rickels and colleagues (47) also studied abrupt and tapered discontinuation of long-term, therapeutic-dose benzodiazepine use. They found that 79% to 84% of patients had clinically significant, active symptoms of anxiety and or depression at intake (primary psychiatric diagnoses included generalized anxiety disorder, panic disorder, and major depression). They reported significantly greater withdrawal severity in patients diagnosed with more initial psychopathology, dependent personality disorder, or neuroticism. Patients with panic disorder were more vulnerable to withdrawal than patients with generalized anxiety disorder (51).

Increased withdrawal symptoms also have been associated with high initial anxiety or depression and decreased educational level (52). Clinicians conducting benzodiazepine discontinuation thus must obtain psychiatric histories while remaining vigilantly watchful for, and prepared to manage, the emergence or reemergence of psychiatric disorders. Clinicians also must be aware that patients with psychiatric symptoms or disorders often experience more severe withdrawal symptoms and have greater difficulty discontinuing use. The reduction of fear and anxiety symptoms during withdrawal was the best predictor of a patient's success for achieving and maintaining abstinence (53).

Concurrent Use of Other Substances Concurrent regular use of other dependence-producing substances increases the complexity of the benzodiazepine abstinence syndrome and the clinical situation as a whole. Additional sedative-hypnotic substance use contributes to a withdrawal syndrome of increased severity and less predictable course. For example, opioid substance withdrawal contributes an additional cluster of signs and symptoms. Anxiety, agitation, irritation, hyperarousal, and the adrenergic components of opioid and benzodiazepine withdrawal are additive, often overlap, and lead to an exacerbation of symptoms. Psychomotor stimulant withdrawal symptoms contribute factors from the opposite end of the withdrawal spectrum (for example, apathy, hypersomnia, and lethargy). When stimulant withdrawal is combined with sedative-hypnotic withdrawal, the clinical picture is variable, with hypersomnolence and lethargy mixed with symptoms of severe agitation, depression, irritability, and somatosensory hypersensitivity. Initial hypersomnolence and lethargy can mask symptoms of benzodiazepine withdrawal, particularly involving benzodiazepines with a longer half-life.

Several factors underscore the need for clinicians to be aware of the high cooccurrence of alcoholism, anxiety disorders, or benzodiazepine dependence and their potential influence on the benzodiazepine withdrawal syndrome:

- A high percentage of alcohol-dependent patients use benzodiazepines regularly, ranging from 29% (54) to 33% (55) to 76% (56).
- The rate of comorbid alcohol abuse and anxiety disorders is reported to be 18% to 19% (57).
- Alcohol-dependent patients have a high propensity for dependence on benzodiazepines (56,58).

Moderate alcohol use (exceeding one beer or drink per day) is a more significant predictor of benzodiazepine withdrawal severity than dose or half-life of the drug (47). Patients with high-dose benzodiazepine use who present for inpatient addiction treatment exhibit a high rate (70% to 96%) of concurrent dependence on other substances (49,55). Almost all of these patients reported histories of dependence on other substances. DuPont (59) reported that >20% of patients newly admitted to inpatient addiction treatment reported using benzodiazepines at least weekly, 73% of heroin users reported greater than weekly use, and >15% of heroin users used benzodiazepines daily (60).

It is uncommon for patient with drug addictions to use a benzodiazepine as an initial or primary drug of use (61). Instead, benzodiazepines are used in combination with other psychoactive drugs. In addition, a high rate of benzodiazepine use in methadone maintenance clinics is supported by numerous clinical surveys.

Consequently, clinicians must be aware of, and suspect, benzodiazepine use in patients with any substance use disorders. Conversely, in high-dose benzodiazepine users, other substance use must be assumed until ruled out.

Family History of Alcohol Dependence Mood changes associated with lability or benzodiazepine abuse (and increased propensity to develop dependence) have been reported after controlled clinical administration of diazepam and alprazolam in adult sons of patients with severe alcohol dependence (56,62,63). Similar findings with alprazolam were reported recently in adult daughters of patients with alcohol dependence (64). This predisposition to abuse benzodiazepines is important, because at least one study implicates a linkage of paternal history of alcoholism with increased withdrawal severity in patients discontinuing alprazolam use (48).

Concurrent Medical Conditions Benzodiazepine withdrawal should be avoided during acute medical or surgical conditions because the physiologic stress of withdrawal can adversely and unnecessarily affect the course of the medical condition. On the other hand, continued benzodiazepine use rarely has a negative effect on acute medical conditions. In an acute medical situation, the goal of therapy for a patient dependent on benzodiazepines is to provide adequate stabilization of the benzodiazepine dose so as to prevent withdrawal.

Clinicians need to be secure in their understanding of the indications for discontinuing long-term benzodiazepine use in patients with chronic medical conditions. This understanding is particularly critical when evaluating the discontinuation of sedative-hypnotics in patients with conditions that are significantly influenced by adrenergic and psychologic stress factors (such as cardiac arrhythmia, asthma, systemic lupus erythematosus, and inflammatory bowel disease). The risks of exacerbating the medical condition through acute withdrawal or a protracted withdrawal course may outweigh the longer term benefits of benzodiazepine discontinuation.

In general, patients with chronic medical conditions experience benzodiazepine withdrawal more severely than others. Clinicians and patients must be aware that, during withdrawal, difficulties in managing the medical condition (diabetes, cardiovascular disease, thyroid disease, and arthritis) may emerge. The rate of discontinuation is an important factor. Slower rates can improve the success of detoxification. Achieving lower doses of benzodiazepine use is an acceptable intermediate (and, in some patients, final) goal. It is important to stabilize both the patient's physical and psychologic health at reduced benzodiazepine levels before proceeding with further reductions.

Age The use of anxiolytics peaks between the ages of 50 and 65, whereas the use of hypnotics is most frequent in the oldest age range (5). Hepatic microsomal enzyme oxidase system efficiency decreases with age. Elderly patients may have elimination half-lives that are two to five times slower than the rate in younger adults for benzodiazepines eliminated through the microsomal enzyme oxidase system (all benzodiazepines except for lorazepam, temazepam, and oxazepam). The withdrawal syndrome for elderly persons who are discontinuing oxidatively metabolized benzodiazepines may be quite prolonged or approach the severity of high-dose withdrawal secondary to the pharmacokinetic factors of aging. The withdrawal course can become especially pernicious after discontinuation of long-acting benzodiazepines that are metabolized to sedative-hypnotic compounds with longer elimination half-lives (such as diazepam, chlordiazepoxide, and flurazepam). In general, younger age is associated with favorable withdrawal outcomes (65).

Gender Worldwide, women are prescribed benzodiazepines twice as often as men; hence, twice as many women as men are likely to become dependent (66). Possibly compounding this trend are reports that female gender is a significant predictor of increased withdrawal severity in patients undergoing tapered cessation of long-term, therapeutic benzodiazepine use (47). However, gender has not been implicated as an influential factor in abrupt cessation of long-term, therapeutic-dose use (44).

PATIENT EVALUATION AND MANAGEMENT

Evaluation and Assessment Evaluating patients for benzodiazepine cessation and detoxification requires a combination of clinical, diagnostic, consultation and liaison, counseling, and pharmacologic management skills. To be effective, the clinician must be flexible and able to tolerate ambiguities and variations in the course of withdrawal, while supporting the patient (who generally experiences significant apprehension and anxiety). Clinical evaluation and assessment of the patient typically include the following steps.

Step 1 Determine the reasons the patient or referral source is seeking evaluation of sedative-hypnotic use and/or discontinuation. Determine the indications for the patient's drug use. A discussion with the referring physician should be standard practice. Discussion with any other referring person or close family members often is helpful. Seek evidence to answer the question as to whether the patient's use is improving his or her quality of life or causing significant disability or exacerbating the original condition. Discuss the patient's expectations.

Step 2 Take a sedative-hypnotic use history, including, at a minimum, the dose, duration of use, substances used, and the patient's clinical response to sedative-hypnotic use at present and over time. The history should include attempts at abstinence (including previous detoxifications), symptoms experienced with changing the dose, and reasons for increasing or decreasing the dose. The history should include behavioral responses to sedative-hypnotic use and adverse or toxic side effects. For long-term users, a determination of the current pharmacologic efficacy and clinical efficacy should be sought.

Step 3 Elicit a detailed accounting of other alcohol or psychoactive drug use, including medical and non-medical, prescribed and over-the-counter drugs, current and past, as well as the sequelae of such use. In addition to prior withdrawal experiences, the history also should include prior periods of abstinence and abstinence attempts.

Step 4 Take a psychiatric history, including current and past psychiatric diagnoses, hospitalizations, suicide attempts, treatment, psychotherapy, and therapists (names and locations). Ask if alcohol or other drugs were used during or near the time any psychiatric diagnoses were made. Ask if the evaluator was aware of the patient's alcohol or drug use. A Minnesota Multiphasic Personality Inventory may be helpful for the dependence subscale scores. Early taper dropouts had higher Minnesota Multiphasic Personality Inventory dependence subscale scores than did late taper dropouts and completers of a taper (67). Personality assessments may help identify patients who may be more suitable to attempt withdrawal. High levels of dependency, passivity, neuroticism, and harm avoidance on the Minnesota Multiphasic Personality Inventory contributed to increased withdrawal severity (68).

Step 5 Take a family history of substance use, psychiatric, and medical disorders.

Step 6 Take a medical history of the patient, including illnesses, trauma, surgery, medications, allergies, and history of loss of consciousness, seizures, or seizure disorder.

Step 7 Take a psychosocial history, including current social status and support system.

Step 8 Perform a physical and mental status examination.

Step 9 Conduct a laboratory urine drug screen for substances of abuse. An alcohol Breathalyzer test (if available) often is helpful in providing immediate evidence of alcohol use that was not disclosed in the history. Remember that these are therapeutic tools. Trust the patient, but check the urine. Depending on the patient's profile, a complete blood count, blood chemistry panel, liver enzymes, viral hepatitis panel, HIV test, tuberculosis test, pregnancy test, or electrocardiogram test may be indicated.

Step 10 Complete an individualized assessment, taking into account all aspects of the patient's presentation and history and, in particular, focusing on factors that would significantly influence the presence, severity, and time course of withdrawal.

Step 11 Arrive at a differential diagnosis, including a comprehensive list of diagnoses that have been considered. This greatly aids clinical management decisions as the patient's symptoms diminish, emerge, or change in character during and after drug cessation.

Step 12 Determine the appropriate setting for detoxification.

Step 13 Determine the most efficacious detoxification method. In addition to proven clinical and pharmacologic efficacy, the method selected should be one that the physician and clinical staff in the detoxification setting are comfortable with and experienced in administering.

Step 14 Obtain the patient's informed consent.

Step 15 Initiate detoxification. Ongoing physician involvement is central to appropriate management of detoxification. Subsequent to the patient assessment, development of the treatment plan, and obtaining patient consent, the individualized discontinuation program should be initiated. The physician closely monitors and flexibly manages (adjusting as necessary) the dosing or detoxification strategy to provide the safest, most comfortable and efficacious course of detoxification. To achieve optimal results, the physician and patient will need to establish a close working relationship. A withdrawal contract is a useful tool.

Management Strategies for discontinuation fall into two categories: minimal intervention and systematic discontinuation. Minimal intervention delivers simple advice to discontinue the benzodiazepine. This can be done as part of an office visit, in a letter to the patient, or in a group setting. Several studies have investigated this tool and have found it effective in fostering benzodiazepine discontinuation. Oude Voshaar et al. (69) surveyed 29 articles and reported an improved odds ratio for discontinuation of 2.8 to 1 by using a simple letter or group information session. After receiving a letter with advice to quit gradually, 49% (53/109) of patients using benzodiazepines in 30 general practice clinics maintained abstinence for more than 2 years (819 days ± 100 days) (70). Cormack and colleagues (71) showed a two thirds reduction in the benzodiazepine dose used by using a letter advising the gradual reduction of the benzodiazepine. Minimal interventions are more effective in low dose users.

Systematic Discontinuation For patients who are dependent on sedative-hypnotics, there are two primary options for the detoxification process: tapering or substitution and tapering. Gradual dose reduction (tapering) is the most widely used and most logical method of benzodiazepine discontinuation. The taper method is indicated for use in an outpatient ambulatory setting, patients with therapeutic-dose benzodiazepine dependence, patients who are dependent only on benzodiazepines, and patients who can reliably present for regular clinical follow-up during and after detoxification (42,54,61,67,72–75).

Tapering With the taper method, the patient is slowly and gradually weaned from the benzodiazepine on which he or she is dependent, using a fixed-dose taper schedule. The dose is decreased on a weekly to every-other-week basis. The rate of discontinuation for long-term users (>1 year) should not exceed 5 mg diazepam equivalents per week (12.5 mg chlordiazepoxide or 15 mg phenobarbital equivalents) or 10% of the current (starting) dose per week, whichever is smaller. The first 50% of the taper is usually smoother, quicker, and less symptomatic than the last 50% (44,67). For the final 25% to 35% of the taper, the rate or dose reduction schedule should be slowed to half the previous dose reduction per week and the reduction accomplished at twice the original tapering interval. If symptoms of withdrawal occur, the dose should be increased slightly until the symptoms resolve and the subsequent taper schedule commenced at a slower rate.

Some patients may want to accelerate the reduction. This acceleration is better tolerated and can be encouraged early in the reduction (67). As a general rule, patients tolerate more dose reduction and with shorter intervals early in the tapering process and then require decreased dose reduction over longer intervals as the taper progresses and the dose is reduced. A common error is trying to push the taper process too quickly (75,76).

Brief office visits should be conducted at least weekly to facilitate regular assessment of the patient for withdrawal symptoms, general health, taper compliance, and use of supportive therapy. Standardized advice from the physician doing the taper is an essential component (77). Taper medications should be closely controlled by prescribing an amount sufficient only for the time until the next visit. The prescriber should give a clear message to the patient that lost, misplaced, or stolen medication will not be replaced. A withdrawal contract between the clinician and the patient is advisable. A copy of the written schedule of daily doses, covering multiple weeks to months, may help the patient adhere to the reduction plan.

Patients who are unable to complete a simple taper program should be reevaluated and, if indicated, an alternative detoxification method chosen. Some patients may require a substitution and taper program or a period of hospitalization to receive more intensive monitoring and support to complete drug discontinuation.

Substitution and Taper Substitution and taper methods employ cross-tolerant long-acting benzodiazepines (such as chlordiazepoxide or clonazepam) or phenobarbital to substitute, at equipotent doses, for the sedative-hypnotics on which the patient is dependent (Table 43.3). Chlordiazepoxide, clonazepam, and phenobarbital are the most widely used substitution agents for a number of important reasons.

- At steady state, there is negligible interdose serum level variation with these drugs; with tapering, a more gradual reduction in serum levels, reducing the risk of that withdrawal symptoms will emerge; and
- Each of the drugs has a low abuse potential (phenobarbital is lowest, followed by clonazepam and then chlordiazepoxide).

Phenobarbital offers the added advantage of rarely inducing behavioral disinhibition and possesses broad clinical efficacy in the management of withdrawal from all classes of sedative-hypnotic agents. Clinical experience shows that phenobarbital is most useful and effective in patients with polysubstance dependence, high-dose dependence, and in patients with unknown dose or erratic "polypharmacy" drug use.

If impaired hepatic function or elevated liver tests are present, then oxazepam may be a good substitute (61).

TABLE 43.3 Sedative-Hypnotic Withdrawal Substitution Dose Conversions

Drug	Dose equal to 30 mg of phenobarbital (mg)
Benzodiazepines	
Alprazolam (Xanax)	0.5–1
Chlordiazepoxide (Librium)	25
Clonazepam (Klonopin)	1–2
Clorazepate (Tranxene)	7.5
Diazepam (Valium)	10
Estazolam (ProSom)	1
Flurazepam (Dalmane)	15
Lorazepam (Ativan)	2
Oxazepam (Serax)	10–15
Quazepam (Doral)	15
Temazepam (Restoril)	15
Triazolam (Halcion)	0.25
Barbiturates	
Pentobarbital (Nembutal)	100
Secobarbital (Seconal)	100
Butalbital (Fiorinal)	100
Amobarbital (Amytal)	100
Phenobarbital	30
Nonbarbiturates-nonbenzodiazepines	
Ethchlorvynol (Placidyl)	500
Glutethimide (Doriden)	250
Methyprylon (Noludar)	200
Methaqualone (Quaalude)	300
Meprobamate (Miltown)	1,200
Carisoprodol (Soma)	700
Chloral hydrate (Noctec)	500

Lorazepam could be considered, but its abuse liability is much higher than that of oxazepam (60).

Uncomplicated Substitution and Taper This method is used in outpatient settings for patients who are discontinuing use of short half-life benzodiazepines or for those who are unable to tolerate gradual tapering.

1. Calculate the equivalent dose of chlordiazepoxide, clonazepam, or phenobarbital using the Substitution Dose Conversion Table (Table 43.3). Individual variation in clinical responses to "equivalent" doses can vary, so close clinical monitoring of patient response to substitution is necessary. Adjustments to the initially calculated dose schedule are to be expected.
2. Provide the substituted drug in a divided dose. For chlordiazepoxide, oxazepam, or phenobarbital, give three to four doses per day. For clonazepam, two to three doses per day usually are sufficient.
3. While the substituted agent is achieving steady state levels on a fixed dose schedule, provide the patient with as-needed (PRN) doses of the benzodiazepine he or she has been using. This will help to suppress breakthrough symptoms of withdrawal. Do this for the first week only, then discontinue PRN drug dosing.
4. Stabilize the patient on an adequate substitution dose (same dose on consecutive days without the need for regular PRN doses). This usually is accomplished within 1 week.
5. Gradually reduce the dose. The dose is decreased on a weekly to every-other-week basis, as in the simple taper model. The rate of discontinuation is 5 mg diazepam equivalents per week (or 12.5 mg chlordiazepoxide equivalents or 15 mg phenobarbital equivalents), as shown in Table 43.3; or 10% of the current (starting) dose per week. The first half of the taper usually is smoother, quicker, and less symptomatic than the latter half.
6. For the final 25% to 35% of the taper, the rate, or dose reduction should be slowed. If symptoms of withdrawal occur, hold the taper for 3 to 4 days to stabilize the patient, then resume the process. Some patients may wish to accelerate the reduction. This is better tolerated early in the taper. Care should be taken not to push the taper too quickly.
7. Support the patient with short but frequent visits, as described above. Taper medication should be closely controlled by prescribing only enough medication for the time period until the next visit.

Sedative-Hypnotic Tolerance Testing This method is employed when the degree of dependence is difficult to determine. Such a situation is common in high-dose, erratic-dose, illicit source, polysubstance, or alcohol plus sedative-hypnotic use. Testing is best done in a setting that offers 24-hour medical monitoring. Pentobarbital is used because of its rapid onset of action, short half-life, ease with which signs of toxicity can be monitored, and ease with which it can be replaced by phenobarbital after the patient has been stabilized.

1. A 200-mg pentobarbital dose is given orally every 2 hours for up to 24 to 48 hours.
2. Doses are held for signs of toxicity (intoxication), which develop in the following progression at increasing serum levels: fine lateral sustained nystagmus, coarse nystagmus, slurred speech, ataxia, and somnolence. Doses are held with the development of coarse nystagmus and slurred speech and subsequently resumed with the resolution of the signs of toxicity.
3. After 24 to 48 hours, the total amount of administered pentobarbital is divided by the number of days it was administered. This amount is the 24-hour stabilizing dose.
4. The stabilizing dose is administered in divided doses over the next 24 hours to ensure adequate substitution. The patient's response determines the indications for upward or downward adjustments in the dose.
5. After the patient is stable on a consistent dose for 24 hours, phenobarbital is substituted for pentobarbital with 30 mg of phenobarbital substituting for 100 mg of pentobarbital (Table 43.3).
6. A gradual dose reduction of phenobarbital is conducted, as described under Substitution and Tapering above.

Withdrawal Emergence PRN Phenobarbital Substitution This procedure is best used in a 24-hour medically monitored setting. It provides the smoothest and most effective treatment for sedative-hypnotic withdrawal for patients who are unable to complete outpatient tapering regimens, or who are high-dose users, polysubstance-dependent, and experiencing considerable comorbid psychopathology.

1. Signs and symptoms of withdrawal are treated PRN with 30 to 60 mg of phenobarbital every 1 to 4 hours. The period of PRN dosing is determined by the elimination of most withdrawal signs and symptoms and is influenced by the duration of action of the substances the patient is discontinuing.
2. The patient is monitored hourly to ensure adequate dosing and to prevent oversedation. Ideally, a balance is achieved between the signs and symptoms of withdrawal and those of phenobarbital intoxication.
3. When the patient has received similar 24-hour phenobarbital dose totals for 2 consecutive days, the total dose for those 2 days is divided by 2 to arrive at the stabilizing dose.
4. The stabilizing dose is given in divided-dose increments over the next 24 hours, which may require medication administration every 3 to 4 hours for patients with high tolerance.
5. After the patient is stabilized, a gradual taper is initiated, as described previously.

Patients often can be transferred from an inpatient setting to an intensive (medically monitored) outpatient program after they are stabilized and well established on the tapering portion of the protocol.

Appropriate Clinical Setting Patients who have polysubstance dependence (including sedatives and hypnotics), mixed alcohol with other sedative-hypnotic use, high-dose hypnotic sedative use, erratic behavior, incompatible use histories, involvement with illicit sources, and extensive mental health issues are best served in an inpatient facility that offers 24-hour medical monitoring.

Adjunctive Withdrawal Management Measures

Anticonvulsants Since the 1980s, anticonvulsants have been studied and used to treat hypnotic sedative withdrawal, especially benzodiazepine withdrawal. The use of anticonvulsants grew from the success of treating certain psychiatric disorders and the improved understanding of kindling mechanisms for withdrawal. Some anticonvulsants were also beneficial in treating alcohol withdrawal and cocaine intoxication. There appears to be no addiction potential with anticonvulsants and this is a great advantage (78).

Carbamazepine Carbamazepine's actions have been associated with the neurotransmitters serotonin, GABA, excitatory amino acids, and glutamate (78–81). Adjunctive carbamazepine therapy is not widely used, although clinical protocols and patient selection for this method have been studied. Initial reports on small clinical trials using carbamazepine showed encouraging but mixed effectiveness and utility (51,82–86). Pages and Ries (87) reviewed further use of carbamazepine and found it to be an effective adjunct. Schweizer and colleagues (85) studied 40 patients with a history of difficulty discontinuing long-term therapeutic benzodiazepines. Significantly more patients treated with carbamazepine were benzodiazepine-free at 5 weeks. Patients receiving carbamazepine (but not the clinicians evaluating them) reported a larger reduction in withdrawal severity compared with patients taking placebo.

Ries and colleagues (83) and Pages and Ries (87) reported protocols for the use of carbamazepine: 600 mg/day (usually 200 mg three times per day) is used alone or in combination with a 3-day benzodiazepine taper. Chlordiazepoxide is useful because of its longer half-life and low abuse potential. Phenobarbital can be added PRN to this protocol for breakthrough withdrawal symptoms.

Carbamazepine is continued for a minimum of 2 to 3 weeks after the 3-day benzodiazepine taper is completed and can be tapered to monitor for return of withdrawal symptoms. Elderly patients who are discontinuing benzodiazepines have been treated successfully with carbamazepine at doses of 400 to 500 mg/day.

Adverse consequences of carbamazepine use can include gastrointestinal upset, neutropenia, thrombocytopenia, and hyponatremia, necessitating initial and ongoing laboratory evaluation and monitoring.

Sodium Valproate Reports indicate that sodium valproate is effective in attenuating the benzodiazepine withdrawal syndrome. Valproate possesses GABAergic actions and anticonvulsant effects (88,89). Valproate also may suppress NMDA and reduce L-glutamate responses (81,88,90). Rickels et al. (91) found that although valproate did not reduce acute withdrawal severity, valproate-treated patients were 2.5 times more likely to be benzodiazepine-free at 5 weeks after taper, compared with a placebo group.

Valproate doses of 250 mg three times per day (250 mg two times per day if older than age 60) can be used in combination with a 3-day benzodiazepine taper. Chlordiazepoxide is a useful choice because of its long half-life and low abuse potential. Calculate the equivalent chlordiazepoxide dose for the amount of current benzodiazepine being discontinued. Give one half to two thirds of this dose spaced equally over the first day (24 hours); one third spaced equally over the second day (second 24 hours); and 10% to 20% spaced equally over the third day (third 24 hours). Phenobarbital can be used for breakthrough withdrawal symptoms. Valproate is continued for a minimum of 2 to 3 weeks after the 3-day benzodiazepine taper is completed. Longer treatment may improve the proportion of patients who remain benzodiazepine-free. Valproate can be tapered to monitor for return of withdrawal symptoms.

Valproate has been used to treat anxiety. It has fewer side effects than carbamazepine. It can be used both inpatient and outpatient. For these reasons, further studies may strengthen the role of valproate in the treatment of benzodiazepine withdrawal. Side effects (including elevated liver function tests, thrombocytopenia, bone marrow suppression, and pancreatitis), drug reactions (including rash and erythema multiforme), gastric upset, and behavioral changes require close monitoring.

Gabapentin, topiramate, and lamotrigine have been tried in several small studies. There is little evidence at this time from which to draw any conclusions. More studies are needed (78,92–94).

Flumazenil is useful for complications of acute intoxication with benzodiazepines as discussed earlier in this chapter. Caution must be used as it is capable of causing marked withdrawal symptoms and seizures. Flumazenil is not useful as an adjunct to tapering. Because of its weak agonist properties, it may be useful to reduce cravings after the tapering is complete (95). Flumazenil's antagonist properties may help prevent relapse but no studies support this indication.

Propranolol Tyrer and colleagues (41) clearly demonstrated that propranolol alone does not affect the rate of successful benzodiazepine discontinuation or the incidence of withdrawal symptoms for discontinuation of chronic benzodiazepine use. However, propranolol treatment did diminish the severity of adrenergic signs and symptoms of withdrawal. Propranolol is not cross-tolerant with sedative-hypnotic drugs and should not be used as the sole therapeutic agent in managing sedative-hypnotic withdrawal. Propranolol can be used, in doses of 60 to 120 mg/day, divided three or four times per day, as an adjunct to one of the aforementioned withdrawal methods. However, clinicians need to be mindful that propranolol treatment will diminish some of the very symptoms and signs that are monitored to determine substitution doses.

Clonidine Clonidine has been shown to be ineffective in treating benzodiazepine withdrawal. Doses sufficient to decrease serum levels of norepinephrine metabolites had minimal attenuating effect on the benzodiazepine withdrawal syndrome. One significant result of this study was the demonstration that increased norepinephrine activity plays a small role in the overall benzodiazepine withdrawal syndrome.

Buspirone Buspirone is a nonbenzodiazepine anxiolytic drug that is not cross-tolerant with benzodiazepines or other sedative-hypnotic drugs. Schweizer and colleagues (96) and Ashton et al. (97) demonstrated that buspirone substitution in patients undergoing abrupt or gradual benzodiazepine discontinuation failed to protect against the symptoms of withdrawal.

Trazodone Trazodone is useful in the management of benzodiazepine withdrawal. Trazodone decreased anxiety in benzodiazepine-tapered patients (98). Trazodone improved patients' ability to remain benzodiazepine-free after a 4-week taper of the benzodiazepine. In one study, two thirds of the patients treated with trazodone, compared with 31% of patients treated with placebo, were benzodiazepine-free at 5 weeks after taper (91). Trazodone can be used to improve sleep during benzodiazepine tapering and when benzodiazepine-free. Side effects may include dry mouth, morning hangover, drowsiness, dizziness, and priapism.

Cognitive-Behavioral Therapy Two studies (99,100) demonstrate that, in patients with panic disorder, adding cognitive-behavioral therapy to alprazolam discontinuation improved the rate of successful alprazolam discontinuation. Spiegel and colleagues (99) reported that patients in the combined taper and cognitive-behavioral therapy groups had greater rates of abstinence from alprazolam at 6 months than did those who underwent taper alone. A cognitive group approach improved attrition rates and long term outcomes for benzodiazepine withdrawal (101). Oude Voshaar et al. (102) reported that adding cognitive behavioral group therapy did not improve benzodiazepine discontinuation success.

Patients must maintain abstinence from benzodiazepines in spite of recurrences of the symptoms of the disorder that led to benzodiazepine use. Benzodiazepine tapering must be completed before psychologic treatment concludes. Cognitive behavioral treatment can support the withdrawal taper and help with exacerbations of the initial disorder (103).

Prolonged Benzodiazepine Withdrawal Some physicians report (30–32), and clinical experience confirms, that a small proportion of patients, after long-term benzodiazepine use, experience a prolonged syndrome in which withdrawal signs and symptoms persist for weeks to months after discontinuation. This prolonged withdrawal syndrome is noted for its irregular and unpredictable day-to-day course and qualitative and quantitative differences in symptoms from both the prebenzodiazepine use state and the acute withdrawal period. Patients with prolonged withdrawal often experience slowly abating, albeit characteristic, waxing and waning symptoms of insomnia, perceptual disturbances, tremor, sensory hypersensitivities, and anxiety.

Smith and Wesson (30) propose that protracted symptoms reflect long-term receptor site adaptations. Higgitt and Fonagy (104) propose that a comprehensive etiologic model of the prolonged syndrome must include a psychologic component that can be explained through cognitive and behavioral models. They observe that many patients with persistent withdrawal symptoms resemble patients with somatization disorders. The patients often experience acute withdrawal more severely and may be "sensitized to anxiety." In addition to a potential lack of effective coping mechanisms away from benzodiazepines, such patients often possess a perceptual or cognitive style that leads to apprehensiveness, body sensation amplification and mislabeling, and misinterpretation.

Management Before entertaining the existence of a prolonged withdrawal syndrome, physicians must rule out psychiatric conditions. A distinguishing characteristic of protracted withdrawal from anxiety disorders is the gradual diminution and eventual resolution of symptoms with benzodiazepine withdrawal.

Propranolol in doses of 10 to 20 mg four times per day often is helpful in attenuating anxiety or tremors. Lower doses of sedating antidepressant medications—such as trazodone, amitriptyline, imipramine, or doxepin—are helpful in treating insomnia. Frequent clinical follow-up for education, supportive psychotherapy, and regular reassurance are strongly advised. Frequent reassessment of the working diagnosis is recommended.

COMMON TREATMENT ISSUES

Formal treatment is indicated for nearly all patients with substance use and addictive disorders. Among sedative-hypnotic users, treatment most often is indicated for polysubstance users, high-dose users, or patients in whom addiction is diagnosed. The support, education, and recovery training available in most treatment programs are valuable to many patients who are dependent on sedative-hypnotics. On the other hand, patients with long-term, therapeutic use problems should not be coerced to participate in programs designed to treat addictive disorders, as they often feel out of place and unable to relate to their peers.

Participation in specific components of treatment, tailored to each patient's individual needs, can be helpful and nonthreatening. Patients who choose to participate in treatment often discover an immense source of support and encouragement, in addition to learning and practicing coping skills that facilitate drug discontinuation and abstinence.

Prevention The best prevention for licit (prescribed) benzodiazepine dependence is careful prescribing (74,75). In England, the Committee on the Review of Medicines reported in 1980 that the hypnotic effect of benzodiazepines diminishes after 3 to 14 days and the anxiolytic effect diminishes after 4 months (11). A good understanding of the mental health disorders with anxiety symptoms and their psychologic and pharmacologic therapies is important. Knowledge of a patient's and their family's chemical dependency history is also important. Benzodiazepines are rarely the first-line treatment for any of the anxiety disorders. Cognitive behavioral therapy, group therapy, relaxation therapy, stress management, structured problem solving, selective serotonin reuptake inhibitors, tricyclic antidepressants, and buspirone are all potential options that should be employed as appropriate based on the level of severity. If used, benzodiazepines should be closely monitored for effectiveness and duration. A plan to reassess or taper the benzodiazepine when it is first given is wise. Reevaluate the need for the benzodiazepine when the initial indication has changed or the patient shows improvement (75,105). A benzodiazepine taper should be strongly considered in the long-term management of chronic anxiety with benzodiazepines even if it is only useful to determine whether continued treatment is required or not (67).

REFERENCES

1. Osborn H, Goldfrank LR. Sedative-hypnotic agents. In: LR Goldfrank, NE Flemenbaum, Lewin NA, et al., eds. *Toxicologic emergencies*. Norfolk, CT: Appleton & Lange, 1994:787–804.
2. Litovitz T. Fatal benzodiazepine toxicity. *Am J Emerg Med* 1987;5: 472–473.
3. Howland MA 1994;. Flumazenil. In: LR Goldfrank, NE Flemenbaum, Lewin NA, et al., eds. *Toxicologic emergencies*. Norfolk, CT: Appleton & Lange, 1994:805–810.
4. Spivey WH. Flumazenil and seizures: analysis of 43 cases. *Clin Therap* 1992;14:292–305.
5. Woods J, Katz J, Winger G. Benzodiazepines: use, abuse and consequences. *Pharmacol Rev* 1992;44(2):151.
6. Petursson H. The benzodiazepine withdrawal syndrome. *Addiction* 1994;89:1455–1459.
7. Salzman C. The benzodiazepine controversy: therapeutic effects versus dependence, withdrawal and toxicity. *Psychopharmacology* 1997;4: 279–282.
8. Hollister LE, Motzenbecker FP, Degan RO. Withdrawal reactions for chlordiazepoxide (Librium). *Psychopharmacologia* 1961;2:63–68.
9. Essig CF. Newer sedative drugs that can cause states of intoxication and dependence of barbiturate type. *JAMA* 1966;196(8):126–129.
10. Covi L, Park LC, Lipman RS. Factors affecting withdrawal response to certain minor tranquilizers. In: Cole JO, Wittenborn JR, eds. *Drug abuse: social and pharmacological aspects*. Springfield, IL: Charles C Thomas, 1973:93–108.
11. Lader M. History of benzodiazepine dependence. *J Subst Abuse Treatment* 1991;8:53–59.
12. Isbell H. Addiction to barbiturates and the barbiturate abstinence syndrome. *Ann Intern Med* 1950;33:108–121.
13. Isbell H, Altschul S, Kornetsky CH, et al. Chronic barbiturate intoxication: an experimental study. *Arch Neurol Psychiatry* 1950;64:1–28.
14. Fraser HF, Wikler A, Essig CF, et al. Degree of physical dependence induced by secobarbital or phenobarbital. *JAMA* 1958;166:126–129.
15. Isbell H, White WM. Clinical characteristics of addictions. *Am J Med* 1953;14:558–565.
16. Covi L, Lipman RS, Pattison JH, et al. Length of treatment with anxiolytic sedatives and response to their sudden withdrawal. *Acta Psych Scand* 1973;49:51–64.
17. Epstein RS. Withdrawal symptoms from chronic use of low-dose barbiturates. *Am J Psychiatry* 1980;137(1):107–108.
18. Essig CF. Addiction to nonbarbiturate sedative and tranquilizing drugs. *Clin Pharmacol Therap* 1964;5(3):334–343.
19. Sadwin A, Glen RS. Addiction to glutethimide (Doriden). *Am J Psychiatry* 1958;115:469–470.
20. Lloyd EA, Clark LD. Convulsions and delirium incident to glutethimide (Doriden). *Dis Nerv Sys* 1959;20:1–3.
21. Phillips RM, Judy FR, Judy HE. Meprobamate addiction. *Northwest Med* 1957;56:453–454.
22. Swanson LA, Okada T. Death after withdrawal of meprobamate. *JAMA* 1963;184:780–781.
23. Flemenbaum A, Gumby B. Ethchlorvynol (Placidyl) abuse and withdrawal. *Dis Nerv Sys* 1971;32:188–191.
24. Swartzburg M, Lieb J, Schwartz AH, et al. Methaqualone withdrawal. *Arch Gen Psychiatry* 1973;29:46–47.
25. Vestal R, Rumack B. Glutethimide dependence: phenobarbital treatment. *Ann Intern Med* 1974;80:670–673.
26. Rickels K, Case WG, Downing RW, et al. One-year follow-up of anxious patients treated with diazepam. *J Clin Psychopharmacol* 1986;6: 32–36.
27. Greenblatt DJ, Miller LG, Shader RI. Benzodiazepine discontinuation syndromes. *J Psychiatr Res* 1990;24(Suppl):73–79.
28. Rickels K, Fox IL, Greenblatt DJ. Clorazepate and lorazepam: clinical improvement and rebound anxiety. *Am J Psychiatry* 1988;145:312–317.
29. Winokur A, Rickels K. Withdrawal and pseudowithdrawal reactions from diazepam therapy. *Arch Clin Psychiatry* 1981;42:442–444.
30. Smith DE, Wesson DR. Benzodiazepine dependency syndromes. *J Psychoactive Drugs* 1983;15:85–95.
31. Smith DE, Seymour RB. Benzodiazepines. In: NS Miller, ed. *Comprehensive handbook of drug and alcohol addiction*. New York: Marcel Dekker, 1991:405–426.
32. Landry MJ, Smith DE, McDuff DR, et al. Benzodiazepine dependence and withdrawal: identification and medical management. *J Am Bd Fam Pract* 1992;5:167–176.
33. Haefly W. Possible involvement of GABA in the central actions of benzodiazepines. In: Costa E, Greengard P, eds. *Mechanisms of action of benzodiazepines*. New York: Raven Press, 1975:162–202.
34. Costa E, Guidotti A, Mao C. Evidence for the involvement of GABA in the actions of benzodiazepines: studies on rat cerebellum. In: Costa E, Greengard P, eds. *Mechanisms of action of benzodiazepines*. New York: Raven Press, 1975:141–161.
35. Allison C, Pratt JA. Neuroadaptive processes in GABAergic and glutamatergic systems in benzodiazepine dependence. *Pharmacol Therap* 2003;98:171–195.
36. Miller L, Greenblatt DJ, Barnhill JG, et al. Chronic benzodiazepine administration I: tolerance is associated with benzodiazepine receptor down regulation and decreased GABAA receptor function. *J Pharmacol Exp Ther* 1988;246:170–176.
37. Miller L, Greenblatt DJ, Roy RB, et al. Chronic benzodiazepine administration II: Discontinuation syndrome is associated with up regulation of $GABA_A$ receptor complex binding and function. *J Pharmacol Exp Ther* 1988;146:177–281.
38. Miller L, Greenblatt DJ, Roy RB, et al. Chronic benzodiazepine administration III: Up regulation of GABAA receptor complex binding and function associated with chronic benzodiazepine agonist administration. *J Pharmacol Exp Ther* 1989;248:1096–1101.
39. Miller L. Chronic benzodiazepine administration: from patient to gene. *J Clin Pharmacol* 1991;31:492–495.
40. File SE. The biology of benzodiazepine dependence. In: Hallstrom C, ed. *Benzodiazepine dependence*. New York: Oxford University Press, 1993:95–118.
41. Tyrer P, Rutherford D, Huggett. Benzodiazepine withdrawal symptoms and propanolol. *Lancet* 1981;1:520–522.
42. Schweizer E, Rickels K. Benzodiazepine dependence and withdrawal: a review of the syndrome and its clinical management. *Acta Psychiatr Scand* 1998;393(Suppl):95–101.

43. Rickels K, Case WG, Schweizer E, et al. Low-dose dependence on chronic benzodiazepine users: a preliminary report. *Psychopharmacol Bull* 1986;22:407–415.
44. Schweizer E, Rickels K, Case G, et al. Long-term therapeutic use of benzodiazepines: effects of gradual taper. *Arch Gen Psychiatry* 1990;47:908.
45. Vorma H, Naukkarinen HH, Sarna SJ, et al. Predictors of benzodiazepine discontinuation in subjects manifesting complicated dependence. *Subst Use Misuse* 2005;40:449–510.
46. Hollister LE, Bennett LL, Kimbell I, et al. Diazepam in newly admitted schizophrenics. *Dis Nerv Sys* 1961;24:746–750.
47. Rickels K, Schweizer E, Case WG, et al. Long-term therapeutic use of benzodiazepines. I. Effects of abrupt discontinuation. *Arch Gen Psychiatry* 1990;47:899–907.
48. Dickinson W, Rush PA, Radcliffe AB. Alprazolam use and dependence: a retrospective analysis of 30 cases of withdrawal. *West J Med* 1990; 152(5):604–608.
49. Malcolm R, Brady TK, Johnston AL, et al. Types of benzodiazepines abused by chemically dependent inpatients. *J Psychoact Drugs* 1993; 25(4):315–319.
50. Romach M, Busto U, Somer GR, et al. Clinical aspects of chronic use of alprazolam and lorazepam. *Am J Psychiatry* 1995;152:1161–1167.
51. Klein RL, Colin V, Stolk J, et al. Alprazolam withdrawal in patients with panic disorder and generalized anxiety disorder: vulnerability and effect of carbamazepine. *Am J Psychiatry* 1994;151:1760–1766.
52. Woods J, Winger G. Current benzodiazepine issues. *Psychopharmacology* 1995;118:107–115.
53. Bruce TJ, Spiegel DA, Gregg SF, et al. Predictors of alprazolam discontinuation with and without cognitive behavioral therapy in panic disorder. *Am J Psychiatry* 1995;152:8:1156–1160.
54. Busto U, Sellers E. Anxiolytics and sedative/hypnotics dependence. *Br J Addict* 1991;86:1647–1652.
55. Busto U, Simpkins J, Sellers EM. Objective determination of benzodiazepine use and abuse in alcoholics. *Br J Addict* 1983;78:429–435.
56. Ciraulo DA, Barnhill JG, Greenblatt DJ, et al. Abuse liability and clinical pharmacokinetics of alprazolam in alcoholic men. *J Clin Psychiatry* 1988;49:333–337.
57. Regier DA, Farmer ME, Raes DS, et al. Comorbidity of mental disorders with alcohol and other drug abuse. Results from the epidemiologic catchment area (ECA) study. *JAMA* 1990;264(19):2511–2518.
58. Sellers E, Ciraulo DA, DuPont RL, et al. Alprazolam and benzodiazepine dependence. *J Clin Psychiatry* 1993;54(Suppl 10):64–75.
59. DuPont RL. Abuse of benzodiazepines: the problems and solutions. *Am J Alcohol Drug Abuse* 1988;14S:1–69.
60. Griffiths R, Wolf B. Relative abuse liability of different benzodiazepines in drug abusers. *J Clin Psychopharmacol* 1990;10(4):237.
61. Smith DE, Landry M. Benzodiazepine dependency discontinuation: focus on the chemical dependency detoxification setting and benzodiazepine-polydrug abuse. *J Psychiatric Res* 1990;24(Suppl 2):145–156.
62. Cowley DS, Roy-Byrne PP, Hommer DW et al. (1991). Sensitivity to benzodiazepines in sons of alcoholics. *Biological Psychiatry* 29: 104–112.
63. Cowley DS, Roy-Byrne PP, Gordon C, et al. Response to diazepam in sons of alcoholics. *Alcohol Clin Exp Res* 1992;16:1057–1063.
64. Ciraulo DA, Sarid-Segal O, Knapp C, et al. Liability to alprazolam abuse in daughters of alcoholics. *Am J Psychiatry* 1996;153:956–958.
65. Ashton H. Benzodiazepine withdrawal: outcome in 50 patients. *Br J Addict* 1987;665–671.
66. Gabe J. Women and tranquilizer use: a case study in the social politics of health and health care. In: Hallstrom C, ed. *Benzodiazepine dependence*. New York: Oxford University Press, 1993:350–363.
67. Rickels K, DeMartinis N, Rynn M, et al. Pharmacologic strategies for discontinuing benzodiazepine treatment. *J Clin Psychopharmacol* 1999; 19(6 Suppl 2):12S–16S.
68. Schweizer E, Rickels K, DeMartinis N, et al. The effect of personality on withdrawal severity and taper outcome in benzodiazepine dependent patients. *Psychol Med* 1998;28:713–720.
69. Voshaar RC, Couvee JE, van Balkom AJ, et al. Strategies for discontinuing long-term benzodiazepine use. *Br J Psychiatry* 2006;189:213–220.
70. Oude Voshaar RC, Gorgels W, Mol A, et al. Predictors of relapse after discontinuation of long-term benzodiazepine use by minimal intervention: a 2-year follow-up study. *Fam Pract* 2003;20:370–372.
71. Cormack MA, Sweeney KG, Hughes-Jones H, et al. Evaluation of a easy, cost effective strategy for cutting benzodiazepine use in general practice. *Br J Gen Pract* 1994;44:5–8.
72. Ashton H. Protracted withdrawal syndromes from benzodiazepines. *J Substance Abuse Treatment* 1991;8:19–28.
73. Alexander B, Perry P. Detoxification from benzodiazepines: schedules and strategies. *J Substance Abuse Treatment* 19918:9–17.
74. Higgitt AC, Lader MH, Fonagy P. Clinical management of benzodiazepine dependence. *Br Med J* 1985;291:688–690.
75. Edwards JG, Cantopher T, Olivieri S. Benzodiazepine dependence and the problems of withdrawal. *Postgrad Med J* 1990;66(Suppl 2):S27–S35.
76. Cantopher T, Olivieri S, Cleave N, et al. Chronic benzodiazepine dependence: a comparative study of abrupt withdrawal under propranolol cover versus gradual withdrawal. *Br J Psychiatry* 1990;156: 406–411.
77. Vicens C, Fiol F, Llobera J, et al. Withdrawal from long term benzodiazepine use: randomized trial in family practice. *Br J Gen Prac* 2006;56: 958–963.
78. Zullino DF, Khazaal Y, Hättenschwiler J, et al. Anticonvulsant drugs in the treatment of substance withdrawal. *Drugs Today* 2004;40(7): 603–619.
79. Granger P, Biton B, Faure C, et al. Modulation of the gamma-aminobutyric acid type A receptor by the antiepileptic drugs carbamazepine and phenytoin. *Mol Pharmacol* 1995;47:1189–1196.
80. Elphick M, Yang D, Cowen PJ. Effects of carbamazepine on dopamine- and serotonin-mediated neuroendocrine responses. *Arch Gen Psychiatry* 1990;47:135–140.
81. Lampe H, Bigalke H. Carbamazepine blocks NMDA-activated currents in cultured spinal cord neurons. *NeuroReport* 1990;1:26–28.
82. Klein E, Uhde TW, Post RM. Preliminary evidence for the utility of carbamazepine in alprazolam withdrawal. *Am J Psychiatry* 1986;143: 235–236.
83. Ries RK, Roy-Byrne PP, Ward NG, et al. Carbamazepine treatment for benzodiazepine withdrawal. *Am J Psychiatry* 1989;146(4):536–537.
84. Garcia-Borresuerro D. Treatment of benzodiazepine withdrawal symptoms with carbamazepine. *Psychiatry Cli Neurosci* 1990;241:145–150.
85. Schweizer E, Rickels K, Case G, et al. Carbamazepine treatment in patients discontinuing long-term benzodiazepine therapy. *Arch Gen Psychiatry* 1991;48:448.
86. Galpern W, Miller LG, Greenblatt DJ, et al Chronic benzodiazepine administration IX. Attenuation of alprazolam discontinuation effects by carbamazepine. *Biochem Pharmacol* 1991;42:S99–S104.
87. Pages K, Ries R. Use of anticonvulsants in benzodiazepine withdrawal. *Am J Addictions* 1998;7(3):198.
88. Harris J, Roache J, Thornton J. A role for valproate in the treatment of sedative-hypnotic withdrawal and for relapse prevention. *Alcohol Alcohol* 2000;35(4):319–323.
89. Apelt S, Emrich H. Letter. *Am J Psychiatry* 1990;147(7):950–951.
90. Zeise M, Kasparow S, Zieglgansberger W. Valproate suppresses N-methyl-D-aspartate-evoked, transient depolarizations in the rat neocortex in vitro. *Brain Res* 1991;544:345–348.
91. Rickels K, Schweizer E, Garcia-Espana F, et al. Trazodone and valproate in patients discontinuing long-term benzodiazepine therapy; effects on withdrawal symptoms and taper outcome. *Psychopharmacology* 1999; 141:1–5.
92. Cheseaux M, Monnat M, Zullino DF. Topiramate in benzodiazepine withdrawal. *Hum Psychopharmacol Clin Exp* 2003;18:375–377.
93. White HS, Brown SD, Woodhead JH, et al. Topiramate modulates GABA-evoked currents in murine cortical neurons by a nonbenzodiazepine mechanism. *Epilepsia* 2000;41(Suppl 1):S17–S20.
94. Michopoulos I, Douzenis A, Christodoulou C, et al. Topiramate use in alprazolam addiction. *World J Biol Psychiatry* 2006;7(4):265–267.

95. Gerra G, Zaimovic A, Giusti F, et al. Intravenous flumazenil versus oxazepam tapering in the treatment of benzodiazepine withdrawal: a randomized, placebo-controlled study. *Addict Biol* 2002;7:385–395.
96. Schweizer E, Rickels K. Failure of buspirone to manage benzodiazepine withdrawal. *Am J Psychiatry* 1986;143(12):1590–1592.
97. Ashton CH, Rawlins MD, Tyrer SP. A double-blind placebo-controlled study of Buspirone in diazepam withdrawal in chronic benzodiazepine users. *Br J Psychiatry* 1990;157:232–238.
98. Annsseau M, DeRoeck J. Trazodone in benzodiazepine dependence. *J Clin Psychiatry* 1993;May:189–191.
99. Spiegel DA, Bruce TJ, Gregg SF, et al. Does cognitive behavioral therapy assist slow-taper alprazolam discontinuation in panic disorder? *Am J Psychiatry* 1994;151:876–881.
100. Otto MN, Pollack MH, Sachs GS, et al. Discontinuation of benzodiazepine treatment: efficacy of cognitive behavioral therapy for patients with panic disorder. *Am J Psychiatry* 1993;150:1485–1490.
101. Higgitt AC, Golombok S, Fonagy R. Group treatment of benzodiazepine dependence. *Br J Addict* 1987;82:517–532.
102. Oude Voshaar RC, Gorgels WJMJ, Mol AJ, et al. Tapering off long-term benzodiazepine use with or without group cognitive-behavioral therapy: three-condition, randomized controlled trial. *Br J Psychiatry* 2003;182: 498–504.
103. Spiegel DA. Psychological strategies for discontinuing benzodiazepine treatment. *J Psychopharmacol* 1999;19(6)(Suppl 2):17S–22S.
104. Higgitt A, Fonagy P. Benzodiazepine dependence syndromes and syndromes of withdrawal. In: Hallstrom C, ed. *Benzodiazepine dependence*. New York: Oxford University Press, 1983:58–70.
105. Norman TR, Ellen SR, Burrows GD. Benzodiazepines in anxiety disorders: managing therapeutics and dependence. *Med J Aust* 1997;167(9): 490–495.

SUGGESTED READINGS

American Psychiatric Association (APA). *Diagnostic and statistical manual of mental disorders, 4th ed.* Washington, DC: American Psychiatric Press, 1994.

Barter G, Cormack M. The long-term use of benzodiazepines; patients' views, accounts and experiences. *Fam Pract* 1996;13(6):491.

Denis C, Fatséas M, Lavie E, et al. Pharmacological interventions for benzodiazepine mono-dependence management in outpatient settings. Cochrane Database of Systematic Reviews 2006, Issue 3 Art No. CD005194. DOI: 10.1002/14651858.CD005194.pub2.

Griffiths R. [Commentary on a review by Woods and Winger] Benzodiazepines: long-term use among patients is a concern and abuse among polydrug abusers is not trivial. *Psychopharmacology* 1995;118:116–117.

King M, Gabe J, Williams P, et al. Long term use of benzodiazepines: the views of patients. *Br J Gen Pract* 1990;10:194–196.

Lader R. Guidelines for the prevention and treatment of benzodiazepine dependence: summary of a report from the Mental Health Foundation. *Addiction* 1993;88:1707–1708.

Miller L, Galpern WR, Greenblatt DJ, et al. Chronic benzodiazepine administration IV: a partial agonist produces behavioral effects without tolerance or receptor alternations. *J Pharmacol Exp Ther* 1990;254:33–38.

Mol AJ, Oude Voshaar RC, Gorgels WJ, et al. The absence of benzodiazepine craving in a general practice benzodiazepine discontinuation trial. *Addict Behav* 2005;31:211–222.

Ries RK. Benzodiazepine withdrawal: clinicians' ratings of carbamazepine treatment versus traditional taper methods. *J Psychoact Drugs* 1991;23(1): 73–76.

Roy-Byrne P, Ward N, Donnelly P. Valproate in anxiety and withdrawal syndromes. *J Clin Psychiatry* 1989;50(Suppl):44.

CHAPTER 44

Jeanette M. Tetrault, MD
Patrick G. O'Connor, MD, MPH

Management of Opioid Intoxication and Withdrawal

Opioids include substances that are derived directly from the opium poppy (such as morphine and codeine), the semisynthetic opioids (such as heroin), and the purely synthetic opioids (such as methadone and fentanyl).

These compounds share several pharmacologic effects, including sedation, respiratory depression, and analgesia, and common clinical features of intoxication and withdrawal. This chapter reviews the clinical features of opioid intoxication and withdrawal.

Although all drugs in the class are associated with clinical withdrawal syndromes, those most commonly encountered in clinical practice include heroin, methadone, morphine, oxycodone, codeine, hydrocodone, and meperidine (1).

OPIOID INTOXICATION AND OVERDOSE

Clinical Picture The prevalence of opioid use in the United States continues to increase. According to the results of the National Survey on Drug Use and Health, among individuals 12 years of age or older, self-reported lifetime heroin use has increased from 1.2% in 2000 to 1.5% in 2005. Similarly, the lifetime nonmedical use of prescription opioids among individuals 12 years of age and older has increased from 8.6% in 2000 to 13.4% in 2005 (1). Opioid intoxication and overdose may present in a variety of settings. Although mild-to-moderate intoxication (as evidenced by euphoria or sedation) usually is not life-threatening, severe intoxication or overdose is a medical emergency that causes many preventable deaths and thus requires immediate attention (2). In a retrospective analysis of consecutive cases of presumed opioid overdose in patients initially managed by emergency medical services personnel in an urban setting, 16% either were dead or in full cardiopulmonary arrest at the time of the initial emergency medical services evaluation (3). As the prevalence of opioid use has increased in the United States, the incidence of opioid overdose has increased as well. For example, one population-based study performed in King County, WA, demonstrated a 134% increase in the number of opioid overdose deaths between 1990 and 1999 (4). Using data from the Office of the Chief Medical Examiner in New York City, Bryant et al. showed during this same time period, although the proportion of accidental methadone overdose deaths remained stable, the proportion of accidental deaths due to heroin overdose increased significantly (5). Accidental overdose may occur in a variety of settings. A recent epidemic of more than 1,000 accidental overdoses occurred in several U.S. cities where heroin was mixed with more potent opioids (e.g., fentanyl) or experienced heroin users began to use more potent opioids such as fentanyl. This epidemic, occurring in 2005 in Chicago, Detroit, Philadelphia, and rural areas along the East coast, was unlike prior epidemics of its kind because it had far reaching geographic effects (6).

Increases in opioid overdose deaths have been seen outside the United States as well (7). Despite these increases, opioid overdose can be treated successfully, if patients present in a timely manner and general principles of overdose management (as well as specific therapies for opioid overdose) are employed. In a retrospective analysis in Finland, the survival to hospital discharge rate of cardiopulmonary arrest after heroin overdose (16%) was found to be similar to that of other poisonings (11%) (8).

Nonfatal opioid overdose is an additional cause of significant morbidity and the true prevalence may not be well understood because many nonfatal overdoses are not brought to medical attention (9). The prevalence of nonfatal overdose ranged from 10% to 69% as reported in recent literature (9–11). The factors associated with nonfatal opioid overdose include injection as the route of administration, sporadic heroin use, needing help with injection, prior overdose, and polydrug use.

The pharmacologic actions responsible for opioid intoxication and overdose involve a specific set of opioid receptors, particularly those in the central nervous system (CNS) (12,13). These opioid receptors include the mu, kappa, and delta types, which also interact with endogenous substances, including the endorphins (14). Of primary concern in the management of overdose are interactions with mu receptors in the CNS, which can lead to sedation and respiratory depression. The mechanism of respiratory depression with opioids presumably is direct suppression of respiratory centers in the brain stem and medulla (12).

The level of tolerance to opioids can have a significant effect on an individual's risk of opioid overdose. In addition, tolerance to respiratory depression may be slower than tolerance to euphoric effects, thus explaining why overdose occurs so often, even among "experienced" opioid users (15). Detoxified patients or those who have experienced intentional or unintentional abstinence from opioids for any reason (e.g., incarceration) may be particularly susceptible to death from heroin overdose (16). Nonfatal overdose is also common among recently detoxified patients occurring in 27% of a cohort of 201 opioid dependent patients followed for 2 years after detoxification. Among this group, prior overdose attempts and depressive symptoms were shown to be risk factors for nonfatal overdose (17). Although injecting opioids may be the route of administration associated with the highest risk of overdose, increasingly popular noninjection routes are associated with significant risk as well (18).

Diagnosis As with most clinical challenges, evaluation of opioid intoxication begins with the collection of patient data through a detailed history and physical examination (Table 44.1). An important issue in the patient with moderate to severe respiratory depression is the immediate institution of pharmacologic and supportive therapies to ameliorate morbidity and prevent mortality.

TABLE 44.1 Diagnosis of Opioid Overdose

History
- Opioid use (ask about drug, amount, time of last use)
- Polydrug abuse
- Use multiple sources of information (family, hospital records, etc.)

Diagnosis
- Altered level of consciousness plus one of the following:
  - Respiratory depression (respiratory rate <12/min)
  - Miotic pupils
  - Circumstantial evidence of opioid use (i.e., needle tracks)

Laboratory Tests
- Rule out hypoglycemia, acidemia, and fluid and electrolyte abnormalities
- Toxicology screens for opioids and other drugs

When available, historical information can be obtained concerning opioid use (including the specific drug, amount, and time of last use), either directly from the patient or from friends and family members, this information can supplement available hospital records. In addition to opioid abuse, it is important to ask about use of other drugs or alcohol because of the likelihood of polydrug abuse (19,20). Identification of polydrug use has important implications for patient management; for example, identification of the frequent co-occurrence of heroin and benzodiazepine overdose may indicate the need for additional therapy directed at reversing the benzodiazepine component of the overdose with flumazenil (21). This also is true in cases of suspected opioid overdose in children who are at high risk of co-occurring opioid and benzodiazepine toxicity and who thus may require management of both on presentation for medical care (22). Polydrug overdose often accounts for significant morbidity and mortality. In one retrospective study, more than half of all drug overdose deaths were a result of polydrug overdose with opiates, alcohol, and cocaine (23).

Physical examination of the intoxicated patient may find CNS and respiratory depression, as well as myosis and direct evidence of drug use, such as needle tracks or soft-tissue infection. The heroin overdose syndrome, described as a triad of abnormal mental status, depressed respiration, and miotic pupils, has a sensitivity of 92% and a specificity of 76% for the diagnosis of heroin overdose (2). Additional evidence supports the use of clinical characteristics in the diagnosis of heroin overdose. In a study of 730 patients in Los Angeles receiving naloxone for suspected heroin overdose, the presence of one of the three clinical signs—respirations <12 per minute, presence of pinpoint pupils, and circumstantial evidence of opioid use—had a sensitivity of 92% and a specificity of 76%, whereas the sensitivity of naloxone response was 88% and specificity was 86% (24). The laboratory can also provide important supportive information in the evaluation of opioid intoxication.

In addition, acute mental status changes from HIV-related opportunistic infections may mimic those of opioid intoxication (25). Patients who present with symptoms of such intoxication also may have other important causes of depressed mental status, such as hypoglycemia, acidemia or other fluid and electrolyte disorders or complications from end-stage liver disease. Thus toxicology screening should be performed immediately in emergency settings (26). Urine toxicology is preferred, because urine contains higher concentrations of drugs and their metabolites than serum. Results usually are qualitative, indicating only the presence or absence of specific substances. Even when the results of toxicologic screening are not available until after acute management has been initiated, drug screening may support the diagnosis of drug intoxication and also may reveal the presence of other drugs not suspected on initial evaluation. Benzodiazepine abuse is common among patients with opioid dependence, and some benzodiazepines (such as alprazolam) may not be readily detectable by standard urine techniques. Alternative approaches involving the examination of serum may be useful in documenting benzodiazepine abuse (27).

Kellerman et al. (28) examined the effects of drug screening on suspected overdose in a study of 405 adult patients who presented to an emergency department. Although initial clinical management did not change significantly on the basis of the toxicology results, implications for treatment beyond the acute event were noted. Poor follow-up of drug screening also was demonstrated in a study of alcohol intoxication in patients injured in motor vehicle crashes. In that study, none of 47 patients who had alcohol levels between 200 and 500 mg/dL were referred for a substance abuse follow-up visit (29). Thus toxicology screening is useful not only for acute management, but also for planning care after discharge from the acute setting (30). Referral to drug treatment programs from the emergency department may be an effective mechanism to link opioid-dependent patients, who otherwise may not interface with the medical system, with available treatment programs (31).

Opioid use and overdose also may be complicated by the effects of substances employed to "cut" drugs purchased on the street. Along with inert substances present to add bulk, active substances—including dextromethorphan, lidocaine, and scopolamine—may be present. One report of overdoses that contained significant amounts of scopolamine documented the potential clinical importance of this problem (32).

Although the classic "triad" of respiratory depression, coma, and pinpoint pupils usually alerts clinicians to the possibility of opioid overdose, atypical presentations may cause some initial confusion. In a study of 43 hospitalized patients who received naloxone for a clinically suspected narcotic overdose, only 2 overdose patients had the classic triad, suggesting that a high index of suspicion should be maintained in certain patients who may have atypical presentations (33).

Management In a case of suspected opioid intoxication, general supportive management must be instituted simultaneously with the specific antidote, naloxone (Table 44.2) (2). Adult basic life support and adult advanced cardiac life support need to be available (34). The physician needs to assure that an adequate airway is established and that respiratory and cardiac function are appropriately assessed and managed. Adequate intravenous access is essential so that fluids and pharmacologic agents can be administered as needed. Finally, frequent monitoring of vital signs and cardiorespiratory status is required until it is clearly established that the opioid and any other intoxicating substances have been cleared from the patient's system.

In the course of managing patients with suspected opioid overdose, clinicians need to be aware of the cooccurrence of acute medical problems and the exacerbation of chronic medical problems often seen in this population (25,35). For example, prolonged hypoxia in overdose survivors can result in rhabdomyolysis and myocardial infarction (36). Other issues, such as acute infections, trauma, and chronic liver disease (including chronic hepatitis C) may have major implications for management of the overdose patient (35).

TABLE 44.2 Management of Opioid Overdose

Initial Approach
- Assessment of ventilation
  - For patients with adequate ventilation:
    - Monitor until normal level of arousal
  - For patients with inadequate ventilation:
    - Supportive ventilation with 100% oxygenation
    - Naloxone hydrochloride: 0.4 to 0.8 mg initially, repeated as necessary
    - Consider mechanical ventilation if persistent respiratory depression despite naloxone or if inadequate oxygenation
- Assessment of perfusion
- Intravenous access and fluids
- Assessment for comorbid conditions

For patients with a complete naloxone response
- Observe for 2 to 3 hours after response if no other complications
- Repeat naloxone if clinically significant sedation recurs
- Chest x-ray for patients with pulmonary symptoms
- Referral for substance abuse treatment

For patients with incomplete naloxone response
- Trial of 2 mg dose of naloxone
- Consider polysubstance overdose or alternative diagnosis
- Referral for substance abuse treatment if polysubstance overdose a consideration

Pharmacologic Therapies Generally, when a patient presents to an emergency department with myosis and respiratory depression, pharmacologic therapy for opioid dependence should be instituted immediately (2). However, if the patient is breathing without assistance, specific pharmacotherapy should be withheld and the patient monitored (2). Naloxone hydrochloride, a pure opioid antagonist, can effectively reverse the CNS effects of opioid intoxication and overdose. An initial intravenous dose of 0.4 to 0.8 mg will quickly reverse neurologic and cardiorespiratory depression. The onset of action of intravenously administered naloxone, as manifested by antagonism of opioid overdose, is approximately 2 minutes. Although intravenous naloxone should work more rapidly than subcutaneous naloxone, one study demonstrated that the subcutaneous route may be just as effective for managing patients before they arrive in the emergency department; additionally, the slower absorption time of the subcutaneous route may compensate for the delay in establishing adequate intravenous access (37).

Overdose with opioids that are more potent (such as fentanyl) or longer acting (such as methadone) may require higher doses of naloxone given over longer periods of time, as by ongoing naloxone infusion (38). In patients who do not respond to multiple doses of naloxone, alternative causes of the failure to respond must be considered. Along with the need to monitor patients for continued naloxone requirements, another important consideration to anticipate in administering naloxone is the possibility of initiating a significant withdrawal syndrome.

Follow-Up Care Pharmacologic management of acute opioid overdose is relatively straightforward compared to the challenge of engaging opioid-dependent patients into medical care and addiction treatment once the overdose event has resolved. In one study of 924 injection drug users in Baltimore, MD, 368 (40%) reported ever having an overdose. Twenty-six percent of the patients with an overdose sought drug treatment within 30 days after the event; the most common reason for seeking treatment was noted to be speaking with someone about treatment options at the time of the overdose. Multiple "missed opportunities" were noted: 87% of overdose patients treated by emergency medical services, 74% of overdose patients treated in the emergency room, and 57% of overdose patients hospitalized denied receiving drug treatment information from the medical staff (39). Despite these and similar findings, clinicians who manage overdose patients should establish the need for ongoing addiction treatment as the major goal of patient management while caring for overdose-related complications.

For medical personnel, two common questions concern which patients seen in the emergency department can be discharged and when they can be discharged. Clearly, patients with major acute medical or psychiatric comorbidities, including suicidal ideation, should be hospitalized for further treatment. In the absence of these issues, resolution of the symptoms of intoxication and establishment of follow-up referrals for addiction, medical, and psychiatric care are necessary before a patient can be discharged safely. In a study of 573 emergency department patients, a group of investigators developed a clinical prediction rule to identify patients with opioid overdose who could be safely discharged 1 hour after naloxone administration. The authors reported that patients who can be safely discharged are those who can mobilize as usual, have oxygen saturation on room air of >92%, have a respiratory rate >10 breaths/minute and <20 breaths/minute, have a temperature of >35.0°C and <37.5°C, have a heart rate >50 beats/minute and <100 beats/min, and have a Glasgow Coma Scale score of 15. Such patients are at lower risk of adverse events (40).

Recent evidence suggests that naloxone also may have a role in the prevention and treatment of opioid overdose when used in the community by drug users themselves. This concept is based on the fact that most users of illicit opiates have witnessed overdoses and many have witnessed overdose-related deaths (41). A recent systematic review noted that although the literature regarding take-home naloxone remains descriptive, there is some evidence to suggest its efficacy in reducing heroin overdose mortality (42). Clearly, this concept is complicated by a number of logistic, medicolegal, ethical, and other problems that would need to be addressed. However, the approach may warrant further research, possibly including controlled clinical trials (43,44).

OPIOID WITHDRAWAL

The opioid abstinence syndrome is characterized by two phases (45,46). In the initial phase, opioid-dependent patients experience acute withdrawal. This is followed by the more chronic signs of a protracted abstinence syndrome. Current pharmacotherapeutic strategies are based on this duality.

Acute Withdrawal In the initial opioid withdrawal phase, the patient typically experiences a range of symptoms for various lengths of time. Such symptoms include gastrointestinal distress (such as diarrhea and vomiting), thermoregulation disturbances, insomnia, muscle and joint pain, and marked anxiety and dysphoria. Although these symptoms generally include no life-threatening complications (unlike alcohol withdrawal syndrome), the acute withdrawal syndrome causes marked discomfort, often prompting continuation of opioid use even in the absence of any opioid-associated euphoria.

Chronic Dependence and Protracted Abstinence

In patients with a chronic history of opiate dependence, acute withdrawal, and detoxification are only the beginning of treatment. Himmelsbach (45), reporting on 21 prisoners addicted to morphine, observed that "physical recovery requires not less than six months of total abstinence." Factors he measured included temperature, sleep, respiration, weight, basal metabolic rate, blood pressure, and hematocrit. The times required for return to baseline ranged from 1 week to about 6 months. Martin and Jasinski (46) reported in a subsequent study that this phase persisted for 6 months or more after withdrawal and that it was associated with "altered physiological function." They found decreased blood pressure, decreased heart rate and body temperature, myosis, and a decreased sensitivity of the respiratory center to carbon dioxide, beginning about 6 weeks after withdrawal and persisting for 26 or more weeks. They also found increased sedimentation rates (which persisted for months) and electroencephalogram changes.

Martin and Jasinski also postulated a relationship between the protracted abstinence syndrome and relapse. Based on similar observations, Dole (47) concluded that "human addicts almost always return to use narcotics" after hospital detoxification. In his article, he reviewed the relative importance of metabolic and conditioned factors in relapse and concluded that the underlying drive is metabolic, arguing that "psychological factors are only triggers for relapse."

The concept of protracted abstinence has been controversial (48), but remains a useful model for scientific hypothesis testing and development of new therapeutic approaches (49). Accordingly, Dole recommended methadone maintenance treatment, even though "it does establish physical dependence." Because, as Dole pointed out, methadone continues physical dependence, protracted abstinence may continue to be a problem whenever detoxification from opioids is undertaken. However, it is hoped that the development of pharmacologic agents may prove to ameliorate this problem in the future.

In addition to biologic considerations, psychosocial concomitants of opioid dependence also necessitate longer, more specialized adjunct treatments for these additional problems.

Clinical Picture Withdrawal from opioids results in a specific constellation of symptoms. Although some opioid withdrawal symptoms overlap withdrawal from sedative-hypnotics, opioid withdrawal generally is considered less likely to produce severe morbidity or mortality. Clinical phenomena associated with opioid withdrawal include neurophysiologic rebound in the organ systems on which opioids have their primary actions (50). Thus the generalized CNS suppression that occurs with opioid use is replaced by CNS hyperactivity.

The severity of opioid withdrawal varies with the specific opioid used and the dose and duration of drug use. In addition, route of administration appears to be important as well. Data from one study suggest that injection drug use is associated with significantly higher withdrawal symptom scores than was inhaled opioid use for comparable heroin doses (51). The time to onset of opioid withdrawal symptoms depends on the half-life of the drug being used. For example, withdrawal may begin 4 to 6 hours after the last use of heroin, but up to 36 hours after the last use of methadone (50).

Neuropharmacologic studies of opioid withdrawal have supported the clinical picture of CNS noradrenergic hyperactivity (50,52). Therapies to alter the course of opioid withdrawal (such as clonidine) are designed to decrease this hyperactivity, which occurs primarily at the locus ceruleus (53,54). Evidence for the role of noradrenergic hyperactivity in opioid withdrawal has been provided by studies showing elevated norepinephrine metabolite levels (55).

Diagnosis Opioid withdrawal involves a constellation of clinical manifestations. Several clinical tools are available to measure the severity of opioid withdrawal. One such tool is the Clinical Opiate Withdrawal Scale (Table 44.3) (56). Other validated scales can also be employed for assessment. These include the 10-item Short Opioid Withdrawal Scale, which takes less than a minute to administer (57), the 16-item Subjective Opioid Withdrawal Scale, and the 13-item Objective Opioid Withdrawal Scale (58). Early findings may include abnormalities in vital signs, including tachycardia and hypertension. Bothersome CNS system symptoms include restlessness, irritability, and insomnia. Opioid craving also occurs in proportion to the severity of physiologic withdrawal symptoms. Pupillary dilation can be marked. A variety of cutaneous and mucocutaneous symptoms (including lacrimation, rhinorrhea, and piloerection—also known as "gooseflesh") can occur as well. Patients frequently report yawning and sneezing. Gastrointestinal symptoms, which initially may be mild (anorexia), can progress in moderate to severe withdrawal to include nausea, vomiting, and diarrhea. This combination of uncomfortable symptomatology and intense craving frequently leads to relapse to drug use.

As with the onset of withdrawal, the duration also varies with the half-life of the drug used and the duration of drug use. For example, the meperidine abstinence syndrome may peak within 8 to 12 hours and last only 4 to 5 days (50), whereas heroin withdrawal symptoms generally peak within 36 to 72 hours and may last for 7 to 14 days (47).

A protracted abstinence syndrome has been described, in which a variety of symptoms may last beyond the typical acute withdrawal period (59). Findings in prolonged and protracted abstinence may include mild abnormalities in vital signs and continued craving (60). Despite the extensive literature on protracted withdrawal, a universal definition and diagnostic criteria are lacking, making diagnosis difficult in individual patients (48).

Management As in the management of opioid intoxication and overdose, management of opioid withdrawal involves a combination of general supportive measures and specific pharmacologic therapies. It is very important for the physician to do a thorough evaluation to rule out other medical problems that may be complicating the opioid withdrawal. The choice of pharmacotherapy used to treat withdrawal may be influenced by the presence and severity of a patient's underlying medical comorbidities (30).

In addition to assessment of general health problems, it is important to obtain objective information to help guide the management of patients undergoing opioid withdrawal. Thus a physical examination should be performed to detect specific findings consistent with withdrawal to establish the diagnosis.

General supportive measures for managing withdrawal include providing a safe environment and adequate nutrition, as well as reassuring patients that their symptoms will be taken seriously. The decision as to whether to perform opioid detoxification on an outpatient or inpatient basis depends on the presence of comorbid medical and psychiatric problems, the availability of social supports (such as family members to provide monitoring and transportation), and the presence of polydrug abuse. The preferred method of detoxification also may affect this decision; for example, methadone detoxification has been restricted by federal legislation to inpatient settings or specialized licensed outpatient drug treatment programs (61), although more recent federal initiatives may allow some opioid-based treatments to be used under less restricted circumstances (62,63).

In the course of managing opioid withdrawal, clinicians also need to be able to address medical problems seen in this population (25,35). Issues such as acute bacterial infections, HIV, and hepatitis C (HCV)-related problems may complicate withdrawal presentation and management. For instance, some studies suggest diminished expression of endogenous interferon-α and enhanced HCV viral replication in patients both using and withdrawing from opioids suggesting that opioid use and withdrawal favors HCV persistence in hepatocytes

TABLE 44.3 Clinical Opiate Withdrawal Scale

Resting pulse rate: (record beats/min)
Measured after patient is sitting or lying for 1 min
0 Pulse rate 80 or below
1 Pulse rate 81–100
2 Pulse rate 101–120
4 Pulse rate >120

Sweating: *over past half hour not accounted for by room temperature or patient activity.*
0 No report of chills or flushing
1 Subjective report of chills or flushing
2 Flushed or observable moistness on face
3 Beads of sweat on brow or face
4 Sweat streaming off face

Restlessness: *Observation during assessment*
0 Able to sit still
1 Reports difficulty sitting still, but is able to do so
3 Frequent shifting or extraneous movements of legs/arms
5 Unable to sit still for more than a few seconds

Pupil size:
0 Pupils pinned or normal size for room light
1 Pupils possibly larger than normal for room light
2 Pupils moderately dilated
5 Pupils so dilated that only the rim of the iris is visible

Bone or joint aches: *If patient was having pain previously, only the additional component attributed to opiates withdrawal is scored*
0 Not present
1 Mild diffuse discomfort
2 Patient reports severe diffuse aching of joints/muscles
4 Patient is rubbing joints or muscles and is unable to sit still because of discomfort

Runny nose or tearing: *Not accounted for by cold symptoms or allergies*
0 Not present
1 Nasal stuffiness or unusually moist eyes
2 Nose running or tearing
4 Nose constantly running or tears streaming down cheeks

GI Upset: *over last half hour*
0 No GI symptoms
1 Stomach cramps
2 Nausea or loose stool
3 Vomiting or diarrhea
5 Multiple episodes of diarrhea or vomiting

Tremor: *observation of outstretched hands*
0 No tremor
1 Tremor can be felt, but not observed
2 Slight tremor observable
4 Gross tremor or muscle twitching

Yawning: *Observation during assessment*
0 No yawning
1 Yawning once or twice during assessment
2 Yawning three or more times during assessment
4 Yawning several times/min

Anxiety or Irritability:
0 None
1 Patient reports increasing irritability or anxiousness
2 Patient obviously irritable anxious
4 Patient so irritable or anxious that participation in the assessment is difficult

Gooseflesh skin:
0 Skin is smooth
3 Piloerection of skin can be felt or hairs standing up on arms
5 Prominent piloerection

Total scores

Score:
5–12 = mild
13–24 = moderate
25–36 = moderately severe
>36 = severe withdrawal

Adapted from "Flowsheet for measuring symptoms during buprenorphine induction." Available at: www.naabt.org. Accessed November 1, 2007.

(64), whereas other studies suggest that intravenous drug use (IDU) increases cytokine response in patients coinfected with HIV and HCV(65).

Pharmacologic Therapies Several pharmacologic therapies have been developed to assist patients through a safer, more comfortable opioid withdrawal. These therapies involve the use of opioid agonists (such as methadone); an alpha-2 adrenergic agonist (such as clonidine); an opioid antagonist (such as naltrexone or naloxone) in combination with clonidine, with sedation, or with general anesthesia; or a mixed opioid agonist/antagonist (buprenorphine) (66).

Slow Methadone Detoxification Clinically, it is important to distinguish between withdrawal from short-acting opioids such as heroin (plasma half-life of morphine, the main metabolite: 3 to 4 hours) and long-acting opioids such as methadone (plasma half-life: 13 to 47 hours). For short-acting opioids, the natural course of withdrawal generally is relatively brief, but more intense and associated with a higher degree of discomfort than with equivalent doses of long-acting opioids. However, there is considerable individual variation, so that strong early withdrawal symptoms from methadone are possible, as are delayed severe heroin withdrawal symptoms.

One treatment strategy employing this general principle is to stabilize patients dependent on heroin with methadone, then gradually decrease the methadone dose over months rather than days. Initially, methadone may be given in 5-mg increments as the physical signs of abstinence begin to appear (67), up to a total of 10 to 20 mg over the first 24 hours. Larger methadone doses are required to treat patients who use heroin of greater purity and who have larger opioid habits; for such patients, a routine starting dose might be 30 mg rather than 5 mg. This treatment strategy can only be employed by facilities licensed to prescribe methadone for the treatment of opioid dependence.

The protocol for slow methadone detoxification is similar to the strategy used for withdrawal from methadone maintenance treatment. After a stabilizing dose has been reached, methadone is tapered by 20% a day for inpatients, leading to a 1- to 2-week procedure. Alternatively, the dose is tapered by 5% per day for outpatients, in a gradual cessation phase lasting as long as 6 months (68). Senay et al. (69) studied the effects of rapid (reductions of 10% of initial dose per week) and gradual (3% per week) outpatient cessation under double-blind conditions. They found that the 10% weekly decrements were associated with higher dropout rates, increased illicit opioid use, and elevated levels of subjective distress. The authors recommended a dose-tapering rate of about 3% per week from methadone maintenance.

On such a regimen, successful detoxification can be achieved by as many as 80% of inpatients and 40% of outpatients, when success is measured in terms of completion of detoxification and a withdrawal-free naloxone challenge test. The longer duration of the procedure and the greater discomfort make the outpatient detoxification with methadone especially vulnerable to patient dropout and continuing illicit opioid use. One study showed that even when coupled with enhanced psychosocial counseling, patients enrolled in 6-month methadone detoxification programs demonstrated greater illicit opioid use and greater drug-related HIV-risk behaviors than patients enrolled in methadone maintenance (70).

Clonidine Detoxification Gold et al. (53) reported amelioration of opioid withdrawal symptoms by use of clonidine and postulated that both morphine and clonidine blocked activation of the locus ceruleus, a major noradrenergic nucleus that shows increased activity during opioid withdrawal. Although opioids exert their effect through opiate receptors, clonidine activates alpha-2 adrenergic receptors. Consequently, clonidine does not possess the potential for physical dependence and abuse seen with opioids.

In a subsequent outpatient study (71), clonidine was reported to "reduce or eliminate most of the commonly reported withdrawal symptoms," including lacrimation, rhinorrhea, restlessness, muscle pain, joint pain, and gastrointestinal symptoms. However, symptoms such as lethargy and insomnia persisted. Sedation and dizziness from orthostatic hypotension were reported as the most significant side effects of clonidine. Though clonidine has been shown to be useful to decrease symptoms associated with opioid withdrawal, its use for this purpose is considered off-label.

The protocol involved administering 0.1 mg of clonidine every 4 to 6 hours as needed for withdrawal discomfort on the first day, followed by an increase in clonidine by 0.1 or 0.2 mg/day, to a maximum of 1.2 mg, according to each patient's blood pressure and withdrawal symptoms. The average maximum dose used in the study was 0.8 mg. Toward the end of the detoxification period (days 5 to 7 in heroin detoxification), the clonidine dose was tapered by 0.1 to 0.2 mg daily to avoid rebound hypertension, headaches, and the reemergence of withdrawal symptoms. Success was defined as becoming opiate-free in 10 days and undergoing a naloxone challenge without opioid withdrawal. In this study (71), 80% of methadone-maintained patients (taking 5 to 40 mg per day), but only 36% of heroin-dependent patients were successfully detoxified.

Another study (72) confirmed the 80% completion rate for clonidine-assisted methadone detoxification, but found that withdrawal symptoms of anxiety, restlessness, insomnia, and muscle aches were the most resistant to clonidine treatment. In an outpatient study comparing a slow methadone taper (at 1-mg decrements, beginning with a 20-mg daily methadone dose) with a clonidine detoxification over 10 to 13 days, Kleber et al. (73) demonstrated equal effectiveness, with 40% of subjects successfully completing detoxification. In a 6-month follow-up, about one third of the subjects in each group had maintained abstinence. However, the authors noted that clonidine offered some advantages for outpatient detoxification, in that it poses minimal risk of diversion to illicit use, is not a controlled substance and therefore is more widely available to general physicians, and shortens the detoxification period from 20 days (for the methadone taper) to 10 to 13 days.

Some reports suggest that clonidine does not induce euphoria (53), whereas other reports suggest reinforcing properties associated with this drug in animals (74). The reinforcing properties are relatively weak (75) and are not morphine-like in animals. Although there have been case reports of street abuse (76,77), this has not become a widespread problem.

Lofexidine, an analogue of clonidine that also is an agonist at the alpha-2 noradrenergic receptor, has shown promise as a detoxification agent. It generally is reported to be as effective as clonidine (78–81), but more economic and with fewer side effects. This medication is not available for use in the United States, but is undergoing clinical trials as an opiate detoxification agent.

Combined Clonidine and Naltrexone Treatment Although clonidine alone "ameliorates signs and symptoms, it does not alter the time course of opiate withdrawal" (82). The authors found that addition of the opioid antagonist naltrexone to clonidine shortened the duration of withdrawal without increasing patient discomfort. However, the small naltrexone doses used in this study were clinically impractical, because they were not commercially available. Vining et al. (83) compared two rapid outpatient opioid detoxifications (over 4 and 5 days), using clonidine and naltrexone. In that study, the smallest naltrexone dose was 12.5 mg, or one-quarter of a scored 50-mg naltrexone tablet. In the 4-day protocol, subjects underwent a naloxone challenge test, followed by clonidine therapy administered three times a day. The first naltrexone dose (12.5 mg) was given the afternoon of the first day, after preloading with clonidine at 0.2 to 0.3 mg. Naltrexone was increased to 25 mg on the second day, 50 mg on the third day, and 100 mg on the fourth day. Clonidine was given at 0.1 to 0.3 mg three times per day, as needed, for the first 3 days, and three times at 0.1 mg on the fourth day. The authors reported that 75% of patients successfully completed detoxification and were discharged on maintenance doses of naltrexone. There was no difference in withdrawal symptoms or severity between the 4- and 5-day protocols. Most patients reported that withdrawal was "relatively comfortable." Persistent symptoms included anxiety, restlessness, insomnia, joint pain, and muscle aches. Diazepam 10 mg twice a day on days 1 and 2 was found to be very effective for persistent restlessness and muscle aches. In addition, clonidine lowered blood pressure significantly, but resulted in no clinical problems. In summary, the authors found that combined clonidine and naltrexone therapy had the advantage of "being more rapid and probably more successful in the outpatient setting." The completion rate of 75% (compared with 40% for methadone or clonidine alone) is another significant advantage. Finally, the initiation of naltrexone during withdrawal eased the patients' transition into naltrexone maintenance treatment. A review of clonidine detoxification compared with clonidine and naltrexone detoxification is available in the Cochrane Database (84). Given the intensive approach to this rapid method of detoxification, it has been suggested that only clinicians with significant experience in treatment of opioid withdrawal should offer this intervention.

Buprenorphine Detoxification Buprenorphine is a high-affinity, partial agonist at the mu opioid receptor. Buprenorphine and buprenorphine/naloxone were approved by the U.S. Food and Drug Administration in October 2002 as a pharmacotherapy for opioid dependence (62,85,86). Additionally, the passage of the Drug Addiction and Treatment Act of 2000 allowed physicians with advanced training to provide treatment (i.e., buprenorphine) for opioid dependence in an office-based setting (62). Despite its higher unit-dose cost compared with methadone, buprenorphine has expanded access to opioid agonist treatment, reduced the disparity between the number of opioid-dependent individuals and the number of treatment slots available to them, and facilitated general medical care of addicted individuals (87–89).

For more information regarding buprenorphine development studies, please see Chapter 48.

Clinical research over the past 15 years has established that buprenorphine (hereafter, this term includes both buprenorphine mono and buprenorphine/naloxone combination products) is a safe and effective alternative to methadone (90–99) and levomethadyl acetate hydrochloride (LAAM, which was recently removed from the European market and no longer manufactured in the United States secondary to QT prolongation and fatal arrhythmias) (100) for opioid agonist maintenance treatment. A recent Cochrane systematic review (101) of 18 studies (14 randomized clinical trials) of the use of buprenorphine for opioid withdrawal found that buprenorphine treatment was superior to clonidine and as effective as methadone for ameliorating withdrawal symptoms, treatment retention, and treatment completion. It was also noted in this review that the duration of withdrawal symptoms may be significantly less with buprenorphine compared with methadone (101). These findings were supported by a subsequent multicenter randomized clinical trial of a 13-day detoxification program using buprenorphine/naloxone versus clonidine. In this study of 113 inpatients and 231 outpatients, 77% of inpatients receiving buprenorphine/naloxone versus 22% of inpatients receiving clonidine and 29% of outpatients receiving buprenorphine/naloxone versus 5% of outpatients receiving clonidine achieved the study combined end point of treatment retention and opioid-free urine at study completion (102).

Treatment with buprenorphine also produces significant and substantial improvements in psychosocial functioning over time (103). Buprenorphine also has unique features that permit novel uses, which may alter current strategies for maintenance and detoxification (85,104). In particular, buprenorphine's ceiling on agonist activity reduces the danger of overdose, may limit its abuse liability (105–107), and has low toxicity even at high intravenous doses (108,109), thereby increasing the dose range over which it may be administered safely.

Buprenorphine also can produce sufficient tolerance to block the effects of exogenously administered opioids (107, 110,111), suggesting that it reduces illicit opioid use.

Buprenorphine's slow dissociation from mu opioid receptors results in a long duration of action (ideal for a maintenance medication) and also diminishes withdrawal signs and symptoms on discontinuation (112–117), making it particularly useful for opioid detoxification.

Emerging literature suggest that buprenorphine is effective for the treatment of opioid withdrawal. One study randomly assigned 45 heroin-dependent patients to buprenorphine (2 mg) or methadone (30 mg) for 3 weeks, followed by a taper over a 4-week period, and found that the two approaches produced equivalent results (90). Another study compared a gradual (36-day) with a more rapid (12-day) buprenorphine taper (initially 8 mg) and found that the gradual approach was superior (112). A pilot study comparing single dose buprenorphine of 32 mg to a 3-day buprenorphine detoxification found that these two approaches were similar in terms of treatment completion (118). A study that compared a 3-day course of buprenorphine (3 mg) to a 5-day course of clonidine found these approaches were equivalent (114), although another study found that a longer course of buprenorphine (13 days) was superior to clonidine (102). A larger study (119) compared 162 heroin-dependent patients detoxified in a primary care setting who were randomized to three 8-day treatment protocols: clonidine, combined clonidine and naltrexone, and buprenorphine. Participants in the combined clonidine and naltrexone group and the buprenorphine group were more likely to complete detoxification than the clonidine group, whereas the buprenorphine group experienced less severe withdrawal symptoms than the other two groups.

Buprenorphine's unique properties also make it a promising alternative to methadone for use in special populations and treatment settings. Several pilot studies have shown buprenorphine to be effective for the treatment of opioid dependence among patients with HCV (120), HIV (121), and HIV/HCV coinfection (122). The results of two recently completed retrospective cohort studies found that using a short-term buprenorphine taper as a bridge to long-term residential treatment facilitated treatment completion (123,124). Another study found that the use of buprenorphine in an emergency department setting for the treatment of opioid withdrawal was not associated with any adverse outcomes and did not increase drug-related return visits (125).

In conclusion, buprenorphine is more effective than clonidine in reducing symptoms of withdrawal, retaining patients in treatment, and allowing patients to reach treatment completion. Additionally, it is as effective as methadone in tapering doses for the treatment of opioid withdrawal, although withdrawal symptoms may resolve more quickly with buprenorphine than with methadone. Gradual buprenorphine taper appears to be more effective than rapid taper to treat opioid withdrawal. Finally, buprenorphine is an attractive alternative to methadone for use in special treatment populations and settings. More research is needed to compare the effectiveness of different detoxification regimens with optimize buprenorphine dose-tapering schedules.

Rationale for Methadone-to-Buprenorphine Transfer

It is anticipated that some patients will need to, or seek to, be transferred from methadone to buprenorphine for maintenance or detoxification. This demand will be driven by several factors. First, there is the unique pharmacology of buprenorphine, leading to its more favorable safety profile and longer duration of action (thus, permitting less frequent dosing) relative to methadone (104,126–128).

Second, given its status as a novel treatment option (which may differentially attract or retain novelty-seeking individuals (129), buprenorphine may engender less fear of stigma than methadone. Buprenorphine may also be administered in office-based settings and patients may prefer this setting, rather than methadone treatment settings, for their ongoing opioid agonist maintenance treatment. Third, because of its enhanced safety, buprenorphine may be used effectively in office-based primary care (that is, outside the domain of standard narcotic treatment programs) (119,130). As such, it is appropriate as an early intervention strategy for those with short addiction histories (for example, adolescents) or with less physical dependence.

Buprenorphine can produce withdrawal discomfort among opioid-dependent volunteers under certain conditions (85,131). Low buprenorphine doses may provide too-little agonist effect (that is, insufficient relief from withdrawal syndrome) relative to the maintenance opioid (methadone). Alternatively, buprenorphine may directly precipitate withdrawal discomfort. Among individuals maintained on the long-acting, full mu opioid agonist methadone, the high-affinity partial mu agonist buprenorphine is capable of abruptly reducing the extent of mu opioid receptor stimulation. This would be expected to reduce opioid agonist symptoms or increase withdrawal symptoms.

This principle has been amply demonstrated in humans: Partial mu opioid agonists such as nalorphine and butorphanol (132,133) can, in methadone-maintained individuals, abruptly precipitate opioid withdrawal signs and symptoms that are functionally similar to those produced by the antagonist naloxone. Obviously, it would be ideal to avoid (or at least minimize) this problem because this discomfort may translate into attrition and relapse. It has been suggested that inducting patients dependent on shorter acting opioids (i.e., heroin) should occur 6 to 12 hours after the last heroin use (85). However, transferring patients from a longer acting agonist such as methadone to buprenorphine without producing significant withdrawal discomfort, attrition, or relapse to drug use, has been shown to be more challenging, as discussed next.

Studies Assessing Methadone-to-Buprenorphine Transfer (Inpatient and Outpatient) Several studies have attempted to address the issue of transitioning patients from methadone to buprenorphine for treatment of opioid withdrawal. Several early studies looked at the effect buprenorphine in methadone maintained research volunteers. Four programmatic studies examined the effect of time interval between the last methadone maintenance dose and the initial buprenorphine dose (132,134–136). Most subjects in the four studies were maintained on methadone 30 mg/day. When buprenorphine was administered to the volunteers, buprenorphine significantly increased opioid withdrawal effects at two hours post-methadone (134), but not at 20 to 22 hours (132,134), nor at 40 hours (136). Walsh et al. (136) systematically addressed whether methadone maintenance dose influences the response to buprenorphine when 2 mg, 4 mg, or 8 mg of buprenorphine is administered sublingually 40 hours after last methadone dose. Testing was done in a closed facility and all 13 subjects were exposed to each of the study conditions. One group of volunteers in that study was maintained on 60 mg/day and a second group of volunteers was maintained on 30 mg/day. The first group of volunteers received 60 mg and, in these individuals, buprenorphine precipitated a dose-dependent increase in opioid withdrawal symptoms. In contrast, buprenorphine did not precipitate significant increases in opioid withdrawal in the second group of volunteers, who received 30 mg. This study was limited by lack of either random assignment to different groups (between-subject design) or, alternatively, a within-subject controlled design.

Three studies (134–136) have directly addressed whether buprenorphine dose-dependently precipitates opioid withdrawal in methadone-maintained volunteers. This variable can be interpreted as reflecting the degree of antagonist (or partial agonist) capacity of the challenge drug. In the studies by Strain et al. (134,135), buprenorphine (five active doses from 0.5 to 8 mg intramuscularly) precipitated mild withdrawal at the 2-hour interval. However, withdrawal severity was not dose-related.

Several studies have directly examined a full medication transfer from methadone to buprenorphine. Kosten and Kleber (137) reported the first outpatient trial of the methadone-to-buprenorphine (sublingual liquid) transition. In this open-label study, there were 16 volunteers. However, only half were methadone-maintained (25 mg/day), whereas the other half were using heroin. The eight methadone patients were assigned to receive 2 mg (n = 4), 4 mg (n = 2), or 8 mg (n = 2) per day. Patients were inducted onto buprenorphine within 24 hours after their last methadone dose. Therefore the dosing parameters of this study are comparable to the inpatient challenge studies of Preston et al. (138) and Strain et al. (135). The investigators reported that most patients completed the protocol. However, one patient exhibited persistent withdrawal symptoms and four patients reported headaches during the initial transfer period. Overall, heroin use was relatively low, with 78% of all samples testing drug-free. Across the entire sample (n = 16), withdrawal symptoms were highest on the first two test days. Withdrawal symptom ratings varied by buprenorphine dose, but were not dose-dependent. Limitations of this study include the open-label design, small group, and attendant problems of data interpretation (for example, lack of dose-dependent changes in the dependent measures).

In an open-label study, Banys et al. (139) examined the ability of sublingual liquid buprenorphine to suppress opioid withdrawal 26 to 31 hours after discontinuing methadone. Fifteen participants were allowed to take three low doses of buprenorphine over several hours (0.15 mg at baseline, then 0.15 mg 1 hour later, and 0.3 mg 2 hours later) in an effort to relieve withdrawal signs and symptoms. There were substantial individual differences reported in the ability of buprenorphine to suppress opioid withdrawal. Six subjects reported relief with buprenorphine, four subjects reported partial relief, and five subjects reported no relief at all. In short, these buprenorphine doses provided inadequate agonist effect to offset methadone abstinence symptoms.

Lukas et al. (140) conducted the first double-blind, double-dummy pilot study of three males—maintained on three different methadone doses (25, 58, and 60 mg/day)—who were switched abruptly to buprenorphine 2 mg subcutaneously. Physiologic (including electroencephalogram), behavioral, and subjective ratings were collected during methadone stabilization, the abrupt transfer, buprenorphine stabilization, then detoxification. They found that buprenorphine did not fully substitute for methadone during the transfer: Withdrawal signs and symptoms peaked within the first several days of buprenorphine (depending on the measure) and abated during buprenorphine stabilization. The authors did not report any differences between subjects during substitution of buprenorphine for methadone (that is, no effect of moderate [n = 2] vs. low [n = 1] methadone dose), which could have been due to the very small sample size.

Another published study of the methadone-to-buprenorphine (sublingual liquid) full transfer is a within-subject, double-blind, double-dummy procedure with inpatient volunteers (141). A moderate methadone maintenance dose (60 mg) was tapered over a few days (40 mg, 30 mg, 30 mg, then 0 mg) before initiating buprenorphine (4 mg on day 1, followed by 8 mg). As with Kosten and Kleber (137), the protocol of Levin et al. (141) demonstrated some qualified success, in that 79% (15 of 19) of participants who began the dose-taper completed the transfer. In the Levin study, the 1-day methadone placebo—which produced a 48-hour interval between the last active methadone dose and the first active buprenorphine dose—significantly increased opioid withdrawal symptoms to a "moderate" level. Peak withdrawal symptom scores occurred just before the first buprenorphine dose. Opioid withdrawal symptoms remained elevated, but were not significantly worsened, by the first two buprenorphine daily doses (4 mg, then 8 mg). Withdrawal symptoms gradually were suppressed by subsequent daily doses of buprenorphine (8 mg) and returned to baseline during buprenorphine stabilization (8 mg/day). Thus, the initial buprenorphine doses might have been too low, because they did not rapidly suppress methadone abstinence withdrawal symptoms (139). The authors reported that the participants who dropped out cited an "inability to tolerate the withdrawal symptoms." A second limitation is that there was no control group against which to evaluate the methadone dose-taper. (However, the within-subject design did permit analysis of symptom changes over time.) In addition, individuals were given access to, and used, significant amounts of ancillary medications (mean oxazepam dose of 45 mg/day and mean clonidine dose of 0.3 mg/day) to alleviate withdrawal discomfort during the transfer period. For this reason, this study cannot be compared directly with previous studies, which did not permit use of these medications. It also is difficult to extrapolate this study to outpatient conditions.

In a recent small double-blind, double-dummy pilot study (142), five male heroin-dependent outpatient volunteers were transferred from methadone 60 mg (with one intervening 45-mg dose) to the buprenorphine sublingual tablet. Subjective effects and vital signs were collected before the transfer (methadone 60 mg and 45 mg), and on buprenorphine days 1 and 2 (8 mg/day), and days 7 and 8 (16 mg/day). The 1-day methadone dose-taper did not significantly alter opioid withdrawal or agonist symptoms. On transfer day 1, buprenorphine significantly increased withdrawal symptoms and decreased agonist symptoms and dose preference, as compared to methadone stabilization. On buprenorphine transfer day 2, withdrawal symptoms and blood pressure were elevated, but agonist symptoms and dose preference did not significantly differ from methadone stabilization levels. The amount of self-reported heroin use decreased from before methadone stabilization and did not increase during the transfer. One week later, buprenorphine 16-mg doses increased agonist effects. Therefore, a 1-day methadone dose-taper to 45 mg was well tolerated relative to 60 mg/day stabilization and the transition from methadone 45 mg to buprenorphine 8-mg tablet resulted in a time-related (throughout the same day) increase in opioid withdrawal symptoms, which peaked during the evening (about 6 to 18 hours) after the first buprenorphine 8-mg dose. This suggests that, in practice, peak symptoms might occur outside the clinical setting, thereby increasing the probability of heroin use. Importantly, the protocol used in this pilot study was able to shorten the duration of withdrawal discomfort to about one day, relative to the results of Levin et al. (141).

In another more recent study conducted in Sydney, Australia, Breen et al. (143) investigated the efficacy of three different transfer regimens from methadone to buprenorphine: (1) among patients maintained on 30 to 40 mg of methadone transfer at a fixed dose of 30 mg, (2) among patients maintained on 30 to 40 mg of methadone transfer at a variable dose when uncomfortable, or (3) transfer at entry dose provided entry dose is less than 30 mg. They found no difference in withdrawal severity between the "transfer at a fixed-dose dose" group or the "transfer when uncomfortable" group. Those patients transferred on less than 30 mg reported significantly less withdrawal discomfort. All but one patient stabilized on buprenorphine treatment, 75% of patients were successfully tapered to 0 mg of buprenorphine, and 31% of patients were not using heroin or methadone at 1-month follow-up.

Another recent study among four pregnant inpatients noted that transition from 65 to 85 mg of methadone to 12 to 28 mg of buprenorphine ("mono" formulation), with a 5-day bridge using immediate release morphine, was safe and effective for both mother and fetus (144). The authors suggest that although withdrawal symptoms occurred during the buprenorphine induction, the intensity of the withdrawal symptoms may be lessened by the dose and frequency of buprenorphine administration.

Finally, Rosado et al. showed that patients maintained on 100 mg of methadone showed significant between subject variability to the antagonistic effects of buprenorphine when administered 24 hours after the last dose of methadone (145).

These preliminary results suggest that it is feasible to transfer outpatients on methadone 30 to 60 mg/day to the buprenorphine 8 mg/day sublingual tablet, although refinements are needed to improve the tolerability and clinical efficacy of this protocol. The data presented here imply that lower methadone doses at the time of transfer and higher buprenorphine doses for induction may be useful in suppressing residual withdrawal symptoms and initiating heroin abstinence in some individuals immediately after the transfer, and also may be preferred. For more information please see Chapter 9.

Buprenorphine in Agonist-to-Antagonist Treatment

Buprenorphine has been used in several experimental studies (90,137,146) as a transitional agent between agonists (such as methadone or heroin) and antagonists (such as naloxone or naltrexone). In one study, Kosten and Kleber (137) substituted buprenorphine at 2, 4, and 8 mg for 20 mg to 30 mg of methadone or heroin for 1 month without precipitating substantial withdrawal symptoms. After chronic administration, buprenorphine produces less physical dependence than do pure agonists, as suggested by the minimal withdrawal symptoms that occur when buprenorphine is stopped, and by the use of relatively higher antagonist doses that are needed to precipitate withdrawal in buprenorphine-maintained volunteers (147). After 1 month of buprenorphine stabilization, the drug was abruptly discontinued and a small dose of naltrexone given 24 hours later. The investigators observed that the transition to buprenorphine generally was well-tolerated. The subsequent abrupt discontinuation of buprenorphine was associated with "minimal withdrawal" in the 2-mg and 4-mg buprenorphine groups, and a low dose of naltrexone (1 mg) did not precipitate withdrawal. However, subjects in the 8-mg group reported a more substantial increase in withdrawal symptoms when buprenorphine was stopped.

Because of these properties, Kosten examined whether buprenorphine might facilitate the transition from opioid agonists to antagonists in a three-step process: (i) buprenorphine substitution for agonists such as methadone, (ii) buprenorphine induced reduction in physical dependency, and (iii) discontinuation of buprenorphine with rapid introduction of naltrexone.

In a study testing that hypothesis, Kosten et al. (148) used intravenous naloxone to challenge five opioid-addicted patients who were maintained on 3-mg sublingual buprenorphine. Induction onto naltrexone was attempted in all of those patients who completed 30 days on buprenorphine. The buprenorphine discontinuation and induction onto naltrexone included blinded discontinuation of the buprenorphine, followed by double-blind, placebo-controlled challenges with high-dose naloxone. Five male opioid-addicted patients maintained on buprenorphine 3 mg sublingually for 1 month as outpatients were abruptly discontinued from buprenorphine by blinded, placebo substitution and enlisted in a placebo-controlled, double-blind challenge with intravenous naloxone at 0.5 mg/kg. The naloxone was given over a 20-minute period using a 10 mg/mL solution. Significant withdrawal symptoms were precipitated. However, the severity of withdrawal was about two thirds the severity for methadone patients (Abstinence Rating Scale = 22; SD = 9.3) and less than one third of the full Abstinence Rating Scale score of 45. Moreover, 5 hours after this naloxone challenge, withdrawal symptoms were at baseline levels, and oral naltrexone was given at either 12.5 mg or 25 mg without precipitating further withdrawal symptoms. The authors felt that the withdrawal syndrome was milder for buprenorphine than for pure opioid agonists, "suggesting a partial resetting of the opioid receptors by the antagonist activity of buprenorphine."

In some situations, combination drug treatment may facilitate greater patient acceptance of agonist-antagonist switching. Thus Gerra et al. (149) have shown that the early use of naltrexone during detoxification in combination with benzodiazepines and clonidine facilitated naltrexone acceptance by patients. Umbricht et al. (150), in a study comparing buprenorphine taper alone and buprenorphine with naltrexone, suggested that the combination treatment may reduce the severity of withdrawal symptoms.

The use of buprenorphine stabilization of opioid addicts before switching to naltrexone has the advantage of psychosocial stabilization prior to detoxification. This approach thus may represent a compromise approach between acute detoxification and long-term treatment of chronic dependence.

McCambridge et al. (78) recently published a cohort study with double-blind allocation of treatment assignment of detoxification of opioid dependent inpatients with either a 6-day detoxification with lofexidine + naloxone, lofexidine + placebo naloxone, or a 10-day methadone taper. They found that lofexidine + naloxone was a superior treatment strategy for nonopioid-abstinent patients during follow-up in terms of duration to first opioid use. These data suggest that detoxification with nonopioid medications may be superior to detoxification using opioid medications. Patients with long drug use histories or using high doses of opiates, where transition to nonopioid treatments may be uncomfortable, may require a combined protocol that places methadone- or heroin-dependent patients on buprenorphine for several weeks to stabilize and engage them in the psychosocial aspects of treatment. This could be followed by rapid transition to naltrexone, using clonidine to relieve any withdrawal symptoms caused by stopping the buprenorphine. Such combination approaches are reviewed in an article by Stine and Kosten (151). These generally have been small pilot studies. Larger clinical trials of buprenorphine-to-naltrexone transitions, with and without clonidine, are needed and have potential to lead to shorter, more cost-effective treatment alternatives (to long-term maintenance) for patients who need more treatment than brief detoxification.

Role of Anesthesia Assisted Ultrarapid Opioid Detoxification Please see sidebar regarding ultrarapid opioid detoxification.

Follow-Up Care As with the management of opioid overdose, medical detoxification is an important first step in the treatment of opioid addiction. It must be made clear that detoxification alone, without plans for ongoing drug treatment, is not adequate to manage patients (30). Thus, at the initiation of detoxification, arrangements for ongoing treatment need to be assured.

Role of Detoxification in the Treatment of Opioid Dependence In general, detoxification programs focus solely on one aspect of opioid dependence (i.e., treatment of withdrawal) and often lack appropriate linkages to ongoing treatment services (152). Therefore, this approach to the treatment of opioid dependence may not be successful for some patients, especially those with chronic, relapsing opioid dependence. A systematic review of five studies looking at the addition of psychosocial interventions to opioid substitution detoxification treatment found that addition of psychosocial interventions improved treatment retention, abstinence from drugs, and adherence to clinic visits (153). Opioid maintenance treatment, on the other hand, is effective for the ongoing treatment of opioid-dependent patients (154). Further research into detoxification-based treatments need to take into account relapse prevention services.

CONCLUSIONS

The management of opioid intoxication and withdrawal requires that physicians be familiar with the basic pharmacologic properties of opioids and the clinical manifestations of opioid overdose and withdrawal. Specific pharmacotherapies may be useful in the management of opioid intoxication and withdrawal. Patients experiencing intoxication and withdrawal require careful evaluation and supportive management. Health care provider engagement in opioid intoxication and withdrawal treatment is critical to encourage further prevention and treatment of opioid misuse.

REFERENCES

1. Substance Abuse and Mental Health Services Administration (2006). Results from the 2005 National Survey on Drug Use and Health: National Finding (Office of Applied Studies, NSDUH Series H=30, DHHS Publication No. SMA 06=4194). Rockville, MD.
2. Sporer KA. Acute heroin overdose. *Ann Intern Med* 1999;130:584–590.
3. Sporer KA, Firestone J, Isaacs SM. Out-of-hospital treatment of opioid overdoses in an urban setting [see comment]. *Acad Emerg Med* 1996; 3:660–667.
4. Unintentional opiate overdose deaths—King County, Washington, 1990–1999 MMWR *Morb Mortal Wkly Rep* 2000;49:636–640.
5. Bryant WK, Galea S, Tracy M, et al. Overdose deaths attributed to methadone and heroin in New York City, 1990–1998. *Addiction* 2004; 99:846–854.
6. Substance Abuse and Mental Health Services Administration. *Consultation and debriefing meeting on the response to Fentanyl-related overdoses and deaths—lessons for dealing with future outbreaks.* Washington, DC: Substance Abuse and Mental Health Services Administration, 2007.
7. Hall W, Darke S. Trends in opiate overdose deaths in Australia 1979–1995. *Drug Alcohol Depend* 1998;52:71–77.
8. Boyd JJ, Kuisma MJ, Alaspaa AO, et al. Outcome after heroin overdose and cardiopulmonary resuscitation. *Acta Anaesthesiol Scand* 2006;50:1120–1124.
9. Warner-Smith M, Darke S, Day C. Morbidity associated with non-fatal heroin overdose [see comment]. *Addiction* 2002;97:963–967.
10. Brugal MT, Barrio G, De LF, et al. Factors associated with non-fatal heroin overdose: assessing the effect of frequency and route of heroin administration. *Addiction* 2002;97:319–327.
11. Kerr T, Fairbairn N, Tyndall M, et al. Predictors of non-fatal overdose among a cohort of polysubstance-using injection drug users. *Drug Alcohol Depend* 2007;87:39–45.
12. Martin WR. Pharmacology of opioids. *Pharmacol Rev* 1983;35: 283–323.
13. Jaffe JH, Martin WR. Opioid analgesics and antagonists. In: Gilman AG, AS Nies AS, P Taylor P, ed. *Goodman and Gilman's the pharmacological basis of therapeutics.* New York: Pergamon Press, 1990:485–521.

14. Bozarth MA, Wise RA. Anatomically distinct opiate receptor fields mediate reward and physical dependence. *Science* 1984;224:516–517.
15. White JM, Irvine RJ. Mechanisms of fatal opioid overdose [see comment]. *Addiction* 1999;94:961–972.
16. Tagliaro F, De Battisti Z, Smith FP, et al. Death from heroin overdose: findings from hair analysis, *Lancet* 1998;351:1923–1925.
17. Wines JD, Jr., Saitz R, Horton NJ, et al. Overdose after detoxification: a prospective study. *Drug Alcohol Depend* 2007;89:161–169.
18. Darke S, Ross J. Fatal heroin overdoses resulting from non-injecting routes of administration, NSW, Australia, 1992–1996. *Addiction* 2000; 95:569–573.
19. Gould LC, Kleber HD. Changing patterns of multiple drug use among applicants to a multimodality drug treatment program. *Arch Gen Psychiatry* 1974;31:408–413.
20. Kosten TR, Gawin FH, Rounsaville BJ, et al. Cocaine abuse among opioid addicts: demographic and diagnostic factors in treatment. *Am J Drug Alcohol Abuse* 1986;12:1–16.
21. Dunton AW, Schwam E, Pitman V, et al. Flumazenil: U.S. clinical pharmacology studies. *Eur J Anaesthesiol Suppl* 1988;2:81–95.
22. Perry HE, Shannon MW. Diagnosis and management of opioid- and benzodiazepine-induced comatose overdose in children. *Curr Opin Pediatr* 1996;8:243–247.
23. Coffin PO, Galea S, Ahern J, et al. Opiates, cocaine and alcohol combinations in accidental drug overdose deaths in New York City, 1990–1998. *Addiction* 2003;98:739–747.
24. Hoffman JR, Schriger DL, Luo JS. The empiric use of naloxone in patients with altered mental status: a reappraisal. *Ann Emerg Med* 1991;20:246–252.
25. O'Connor PG, Selwyn PA, Schottenfeld RS. Medical care for injection-drug users with human immunodeficiency virus infection [see comment]. *N Engl J Med* 1994;331:450–459.
26. Council on Scientific Affairs (CSA). Scientific issues in drug testing. *JAMA* 1987;257:3110–3114.
27. Rogers WO, Hall MA, Brissie RM, et al. Detection of alprazolam in three cases of methadone/benzodiazepine overdose. *J Forensic Sci* 1997; 42:155–156.
28. Kellermann AL, Fihn SD, LoGerfo JP, et al. Impact of drug screening in suspected overdose. *Ann Emerg Med* 1987;16:1206–1216.
29. Chang G, Astrachan BM. The emergency department surveillance of alcohol intoxication after motor vehicle accidents. *JAMA* 1988;260: 2533–2536.
30. O'Connor PG, Samet JH, Stein MD. Management of hospitalized intravenous drug users: role of the internist. *Am J Med* 1994;96:551–558.
31. D'Onofrio G, Becker B Woolard RH. The impact of alcohol, tobacco, and other drug use and abuse in the emergency department. *Emerg Med Clin N Am* 2006;24:925–967.
32. Scopolamine poisoning among heroin users—New York City, Newark, Philadelphia, and Baltimore, 1995 and 1996. *Morbid Mortal Wkly Rep* 1996;45:457–460.
33. Whipple JK, Quebbeman EJ, Lewis KS, et al. Difficulties in diagnosing narcotic overdoses in hospitalized patients. *Ann Pharmacother* 1994; 28:446–450.
34. American Heart Association. Guidelines for cardiopulmonary resuscitation and emergency cardiac care. Emergency Cardiac Care Committee and Subcommittees, American Heart Association. Part II. Adult basic life support [see comment]. *JAMA* 1992;268:2184–2198.
35. Cherubin CE, Sapira JD. The medical complications of drug addiction and the medical assessment of the intravenous drug user: 25 years later [see comment]. *Ann Intern Med* 1993;119:1017–1028.
36. Melandri R, Re G, Lanzarini C, et al. Myocardial damage and rhabdomyolysis associated with prolonged hypoxic coma following opiate overdose. *J Toxicol Clin Toxicol* 1996;34:199–203.
37. Wanger K, Brough L, Macmillan I, et al. Intravenous vs. subcutaneous naloxone for out-of-hospital management of presumed opioid overdose [see comment]. *Acad Emerg Med* 1998;5:293–299.
38. LoVecchio F, Pizon A, Riley B, et al. Onset of symptoms after methadone overdose. *Am J Emerg Med* 2007;25:57–59.
39. Pollini RA, McCall L, Mehta SH, et al. Non-fatal overdose and subsequent drug treatment among injection drug users. *Drug Alcohol Depend* 2006;83:104–110.
40. Christenson J, Etherington J, Grafstein E, et al. Early discharge of patients with presumed opioid overdose: development of a clinical prediction rule [see comment]. *Acad Emerg Med* 2000;7: 1110–1118.
41. Strang J, Powis B, Best D et al. Preventing opiate overdose fatalities with take-home naloxone: pre-launch study of possible impact and acceptability [see comment]. *Addiction* 1999;94:199–204.
42. Baca CT, Grant KJ. Take-home naloxone to reduce heroin death. *Addiction* 2005;100:1823–1831.
43. Sporer KA, Kral AH. Prescription naloxone: a novel approach to heroin overdose prevention. *Ann Emerg Med* 2007;49:172–177.
44. Darke S, Hall W. The distribution of naloxone to heroin users. *Addiction* 1997;92:1195–1199.
45. Himmelsbach CK. Clinical studies of drug addiction: physical dependence, withdrawal and recovery. *Arch Intern Med* 1942;69:776–772.
46. Martin WR, Jasinski DR. Physiologic parameters of morphine dependence in man—tolerance, early abstinence, protracted abstinence. *Psychiatry Dig* 1970;31:37 passim.
47. Dole VP. Narcotic addiction, physical dependence and relapse. *N Engl J Med* 1972;286:988–992.
48. Satel SL, Kosten TR, Schuckit MA, et al. Should protracted withdrawal from drugs be included in DSM-IV? [see comment]. *Am J Psychiatry* 1993;150:695–704.
49. Stine S, Kosten T. Reduction of opiate withdrawal-like symptoms by cocaine abuse during methadone and buprenorphine maintenance. *Am J Drug Alcohol Abuse* 1994;20:445–458.
50. Jaffe JH. Drug addiction and drug abuse. In: Gilman AG, Nies AS, Taylor P, eds. *Goodman and Gilman's the pharmacological basis of therapeutics*. New York: Pergamon Press, 1990:522–573.
51. Smolka M, Schmidt LG. The influence of heroin dose and route of administration on the severity of the opiate withdrawal syndrome. *Addiction* 1999;94:1191–1198.
52. Gunne LM. Noradrenaline and adrenaline in the rat brain during acute and chronic morphine administration and during withdrawal. *Nature* 1959;184:1950–1951.
53. Gold M, Redmond DE, Kleber HD. Clonidine blocks acute opiate withdrawal symptoms. *Lancet* 1978;2:599–600.
54. Aghajanian GK. Tolerance of locus coeruleus neurones to morphine and suppression of withdrawal response by clonidine. *Nature* 1978;276: 186–188.
55. Crawley JN, Laverty RN, Roth RH. Clonidine reversal of increased norepinephrine metabolite levels during morphine withdrawal. *Eur J Pharmacol* 1979;57:247–255.
56. Wesson DR, Ling W. The Clinical Opiate Withdrawal Scale (COWS). *J Psychoactive Drugs* 2003;35:253–259.
57. Gossop M. The development of a Short Opiate Withdrawal Scale (SOWS). *Addict Behav* 1990;15:487–490.
58. Handelsman L, Cochrane KJ, Aronson MJ, et al. Two new rating scales for opiate withdrawal. *Am J Drug Alcohol Abuse* 1987;13:293–308.
59. Schuckit MA. Opiates and other analgesics. In: *Drug and alcohol abuse: a clinical guide to diagnosis and treatment*. New York: Plenum Publishing Company, 1988:118–142.
60. Wen HL, Ho WK, Wen PY. Comparison of the effectiveness of different opioid peptides in suppressing heroin withdrawal. *Eur J Pharmacol* 1984;100:155–162.
61. Methadone: rules and regulations. *Fed Reg* 1989;54:8954.
62. Fiellin DA, O'Connor, PG. New federal initiatives to enhance the medical treatment of opioid dependence. *Ann Intern Med* 2002;137: 688–692.
63. O'Connor PG. Treating opioid dependence—new data and new opportunities [see comment]. *N Engl J Med* 2000;343:1332–1334.
64. Wang C-Q, Li Y, Douglas SD, et al. Morphine withdrawal enhances hepatitis C virus replicon expression [see comment]. *Am J Pathol* 2005; 167:1333–1340.

65. Graham CS, Wells A, Edwards EM, et al. Effect of exposure to injection drugs or alcohol on antigen-specific immune responses in HIV and hepatitis C virus coinfection. *J Infect Dis* 2007;195:847–856.
66. O'Connor PG, Fiellin DA. Pharmacologic treatment of heroin-dependent patients. *Ann Intern Med* 2000;133:40–54.
67. Jackson AH, Shader RI. Guidelines for the withdrawal of narcotic and general depressant drugs. *Dis Nervous Syst* 1973;34:162–166.
68. Margolin A, Kosten TR. Opioid detoxification and maintenance with blocking agents. In: Miller, N, ed. *Comprehensive handbook of drug and alcohol addiction.* New York: Marcel Dekker, 1991:1127–1141.
69. Sena, EC, Dorus W, Goldberg F, et al. Withdrawal from methadone maintenance. Rate of withdrawal and expectation. *Arch Gen Psychiatry* 1977;34:361–367.
70. Sees KL, Delucchi KL, Masson C, et al. Methadone maintenance vs. 180-day psychosocially enriched detoxification for treatment of opioid dependence: a randomized controlled trial [see comment]. *JAMA* 2000; 283:1303–1310.
71. Washton AM, Resnick RB. Clonidine for opiate detoxification: outpatient clinical trials. *Am J Psychiatry* 1980;137:1121–1122.
72. Charney DS, Sternberg DE, Kleber HD, et al. The clinical use of clonidine in abrupt withdrawal from methadone. Effects on blood pressure and specific signs and symptoms. *Arch Gen Psychiatry* 1981;38:1273–1277.
73. Kleber HD, Riordan CE. Rounsaville B, et al. Clonidine in outpatient detoxification from methadone maintenance. *Arch Gen Psychiatry* 1985;42:391–394.
74. Asin KE, Wirtshafter D. Clonidine produces a conditioned place preference in rats. *Psychopharmacology* 81985;5:383–385.
75. Davis WM, Smith SG. Catecholaminergic mechanisms of reinforcement: direct assessment by drug-self-administration. *Life Sci* 1977;20:483–492.
76. Beuger M, Tommasello A, Schwartz R, et al. Clonidine use and abuse among methadone program applicants and patients. *J Subst Abuse Treat* 1998;15:589–593.
77. Lauzon P. Two cases of clonidine abuse/dependence in methadone-maintained patients. *J Subst Abuse Treat* 1992;9:125–127.
78. McCambridge J, Gossop M, Beswick T, et al. In-patient detoxification procedures, treatment retention, and post-treatment opiate use: comparison of lofexidine + naloxone, lofexidine + placebo, and methadone. *Drug Alcohol Depend* 2007;88:91–95.
79. Lin SK, Strang J, Su LW, et al. Double-blind randomised controlled trial of lofexidine versus clonidine in the treatment of heroin withdrawal. *Drug Alcohol Depend* 1997;48:127–133.
80. Carnwath T, Hardman J. Randomised double-blind comparison of lofexidine and clonidine in the out-patient treatment of opiate withdrawal. *Drug Alcohol Depend* 1998;50:251–254.
81. Bearn J, Gossop M, Strang J. Accelerated lofexidine treatment regimen compared with conventional lofexidine and methadone treatment for inpatient opiate detoxification. *Drug Alcohol Depend* 1998;50:227–232.
82. Kleber HD, Topazian M, Gaspari J, et al. Clonidine and naltrexone in the outpatient treatment of heroin withdrawal. *Am J Drug Alcohol Abuse* 1987;13:1–17.
83. Vining E, Kosten TR, Kleber HD. Clinical utility of rapid clonidine-naltrexone detoxification for opioid abusers. *Br J Addict* 1988;83:567–575.
84. Gowing L, Ali R, White J. Opioid antagonists and adrenergic agonists for the management of opioid withdrawal. *Cochrane Database System Rev* 2000; CD002021. [Update in *Cochrane Database Syst Rev* 2002;(2):CD002021; PMID: 12076431.]
85. Bickel WK, Amass L. Buprenorphine treatment of opioid dependence: a review, *Exp Clin Psychopharmacol* 1995;3:477–489.
86. Ling W, Rawson RA, Compton MA. Substitution pharmacotherapies for opioid addiction: from methadone to LAAM and buprenorphine. *J Psychoactive Drugs* 1994;26:119–128.
87. Lewis DC. Access to narcotic addiction treatment and medical care: prospects for the expansion of methadone maintenance treatment [see comment]. *J Addict Dis* 1999;18:5–21.
88. NIH Consensus Panel. NIH Consensus Panel recommends expanding access to and improving methadone treatment programs for heroin addiction. *Eur Addict Res* 1999;5:50–51.
89. Rounsaville BJ, Kosten TR. Treatment for opioid dependence: quality and access [see comment]. *JAMA* 2000;283:1337–1339.
90. Bickel WK, Stitzer ML., Bigelow GE, et al. A clinical trial of buprenorphine: comparison with methadone in the detoxification of heroin addicts. *Clin Pharmacol Ther* 1988;43:72–78.
91. Johnson RE, Jaffe JH, Fudala PJ. A controlled trial of buprenorphine treatment for opioid dependence [see comment]. *JAMA* 1992;267: 2750–2755.
92. Strain EC, Stitzer ML, Liebson IA, et al. Comparison of buprenorphine and methadone in the treatment of opioid dependence. *Am J Psychiatry* 1994;151:1025–1030.
93. Ling W, Wesson DR, Charuvastra C, et al. A controlled trial comparing buprenorphine and methadone maintenance in opioid dependence. *Arch Gen Psychiatry* 1996;53:401–407.
94. Ling W, Charuvastra C, Collins JF, et al. Buprenorphine maintenance treatment of opiate dependence: a multicenter, randomized clinical trial. *Addiction* 1998;93:475–486.
95. Uehlinger C, Deglon J, Livoti S, et al. Comparison of buprenorphine and methadone in the treatment of opioid dependence. Swiss multicentre study. *Eur Addict Res* 1998;4(Suppl 1):13–18.
96. Liu Z, Cai Z, Wang XP, et al. Rapid detoxification of heroin dependence by buprenorphine. *Chung Kuo Yao Li Hsueh Pao* 1997;18:112–114.
97. Bouchez J, Beauverie P, Touzeau D. Substitution with buprenorphine in methadone- and morphine sulfate-dependent patients. Preliminary results. *Eur Addict Res* 1998;4(Suppl 1):8–12.
98. Amass L, Kamien JB, Branstetter SA. A controlled comparison of the buprenorphine-naloxone tablet and methadone for opioid maintenance treatment: interim results. In: Harris L, ed. *Problems of drug dependence 1999 (NIDA Research Monograph).* Rockville, MD: National Institute on Drug Abuse, 2001.
99. Galante, M, Dermatis H, Resnick R, et al. Short-term buprenorphine maintenance: treatment outcome. *J Addict Dis* 2003;22:39–49.
100. Chutuape MA, Johnson RE, Strain EC. Controlled clinical trial comparing maintenance treatment efficacy of buprenorphine (buprenorphine), levomethadoneadoneadyl acetate (LAAM) and methadone. In: Harris L, ed. *Problems of drug dependence 1998 (NIDA Research Monograph No. 179).* Rockville, MD: National Institute on Drug Dependence, 1999.
101. Gowing L, Ali R, White J. Buprenorphine for the management of opioid withdrawal. *Cochrane Database Syst Rev* 2006; CD002025 [update of *Cochrane Database Syst Rev* 2004;(4):CD002025; PMID: 15495026].
102. Ling W, Amass L, Shoptaw S, et al. A multi-center randomized trial of buprenorphine-naloxone versus clonidine for opioid detoxification: findings from the National Institute on Drug Abuse Clinical Trials Network [see comment]. *Addiction* 2005;100:1090–1100. [Erratum: *Addiction* 2006;101(9):1374.]
103. Strain EC, Stitzer M., Liebson IA, et al. Buprenorphine versus methadone in the treatment of opioid dependence: self-reports, urinalysis, and addiction severity index. *J Clin Psychopharmacol* 1996;16:58–67.
104. Amass L, Kamien JB, Mikulich SK. Thrice-weekly supervised dosing with the combination buprenorphine-naloxone tablet is preferred to daily supervised dosing by opioid-dependent humans. *Drug Alcohol Depend* 2001;61:173–181.
105. Fiellin DA, Friedland GH, Gourevitch MN. Opioid dependence: rationale for and efficacy of existing and new treatments. *Clin Infect Dis* 2006;43(Suppl 4):S173–S177.
106. Walsh SL, Preston KL, Stitzer ML, et al. Clinical pharmacology of buprenorphine: ceiling effects at high doses. *Clin Pharmacol Ther* 1994;55:569–580.
107. Walsh SL, Preston KL, Bigelow GE, et al. Acute administration of buprenorphine in humans: partial agonist and blockade effects. *J Pharmacol Exp Ther* 1995;274:361–372.
108. Lange WR, Fudala PJ, Dax EM, et al. Safety and side-effects of buprenorphine in the clinical management of heroin addiction. *Drug Alcohol Depend* 1990;26:19–28.
109. Huestis MA, Umbricht A, Preston KL. Safety of buprenorphine: no clinically relevant cardio-respiratory depression at high IV doses. In: Harris L, ed. *Problems of drug dependence (NIDA Research Monograph No. 179).* Rockville, MD: National Institute on Drug Abuse, 1999.

110. Bickel WK, Stitzer ML, Bigelow GE, et al. Buprenorphine: dose-related blockade of opioid challenge effects in opioid dependent humans. *J Pharmacol Exp Ther* 1988;247:47–53.
111. Rosen MI, Wallace EA, McMahon T J, et al. Buprenorphine: duration of blockade of effects of intramuscular hydromorphone. *Drug Alcohol Depend* 199435:141–149.
112. Amass L, Bickel WK, Higgins ST, et al. A preliminary investigation of outcome following gradual or rapid buprenorphine detoxification. *J Addict Dis* 1994;13:33–45.
113. Bickel WK, Amass L, Higgins ST, et al. Effects of adding behavioral treatment to opioid detoxification with buprenorphine. *J Consult Clin Psychol* 1997;65:803–810.
114. Cheskin LJ, Fudala PJ, Johnson RE. A controlled comparison of buprenorphine and clonidine for acute detoxification from opioids. *Drug Alcohol Depend* 1994;36:115–121.
115. Fudala PJ, Jaffe JH, Dax EM, et al. Use of buprenorphine in the treatment of opioid addiction. II. Physiologic and behavioral effects of daily and alternate-day administration and abrupt withdrawal. *Clin Pharmacol Ther* 41990;7:525–534.
116. Jasinski DR, Johnson RE, Kocher TR. Clonidine in morphine withdrawal. Differential effects on signs and symptoms. *Arch Gen Psychiatry* 1985;42:1063–1066.
117. Seow SS, Quigley AJ, Ilett KF, et al. Buprenorphine: a new maintenance opiate? *Med J Aust* 1986;144:407–411.
118. Hopper JA, Wu J, Martus W, et al. A randomized trial of one-day vs. three-day buprenorphine inpatient detoxification protocols for heroin dependence. *J Opioid Manage* 2005;1:31–35.
119. O'Connor PG, Carroll KM, Shi JM, et al. Three methods of opioid detoxification in a primary care setting. A randomized trial. *Ann Intern Med* 1997;127:526–530.
120. Belfiori B, Chiodera A, Ciliegi P, et al. Treatment for hepatitis C virus in injection drug users on opioid replacement therapy: a prospective multicentre study. *Eur J Gastroenterol Hepatol* 2007;19:731–732.
121. Sullivan LE, Barry D, Moore BA, et al. A trial of integrated buprenorphine/naloxone and HIV clinical care. *Clin Infect Dis* 2006;43(Suppl 4):S184–S190.
122. Kresina TF, Eldred L, Bruce RD, et al. Integration of pharmacotherapy for opioid addiction into HIV primary care for HIV/hepatitis C virus-co-infected patients. *AIDS* 2005;19(Suppl 3):S221–S226.
123. Brigham GS, Amass L, Winhusen T, et al. Using buprenorphine short-term taper to facilitate early treatment engagement. *J Subst Abuse Treat* 2007;32:349–356.
124. Collins ED, Horton T, Reinke K, et al. Using buprenorphine to facilitate entry into residential therapeutic community rehabilitation. *J Subst Abuse Treat* 2007;32:167–175.
125. Berg ML, Idrees U, Ding R, et al. Evaluation of the use of buprenorphine for opioid withdrawal in an emergency department. *Drug Alcohol Depend* 2007;86:239–244.
126. Bickel WK, Amass L, Crean JP, et al. Buprenorphine dosing every 1, 2, or 3 days in opioid-dependent patients. *Psychopharmacology* 1999;146: 111–118.
127. Fudala PJ, Bridge TP, Herbert S, and The Buprenorphine+Naloxone Collaborative Study Group. A multisite efficacy evaluation of a buprenorphine+naloxone product for opiate dependence treatment. In: Harris L, ed. *Problems of drug dependence 1998 (NIDA Research Monograph 179)*. Rockville, MD: National Institute on Drug Abuse, 1998.
128. Schottenfeld RS, Pakes J, O'Connor PG, et al. Thrice weekly versus daily buprenorphine maintenance. *Biol Psychiatry* 2000;47: 1072–1079.
129. Helmus TC, Downey KK, Arfken CL, et al. Novelty seeking as a predictor of treatment retention for heroin dependent cocaine users. *Drug Alcohol Depend* 2001;61:287–295.
130. O'Connor PG, Kosten TR. Rapid and ultrarapid opioid detoxification techniques [see comment]. *JAMA* 1998;279:229–234.
131. Johnson RE, Cone EJ, Henningfield JE, et al. Use of buprenorphine in the treatment of opiate addiction. I. Physiologic and behavioral effects during a rapid dose induction. *Clin Pharmacol Ther* 1989;46: 335–343.
132. Preston KL, Bigelow GE, Liebson IA. Buprenorphine and naloxone alone and in combination in opioid-dependent humans. *Psychopharmacology* 1988;94:484–490.
133. Preston KL, Bigelow GE, Liebson IA. Antagonist effects of nalbuphine in opioid-dependent human volunteers. *J Pharmacol Exp Ther* 1989; 248:929–937.
134. Strain EC, Preston KL, Liebson IA, et al. Acute effects of buprenorphine, hydromorphone and naloxone in methadone-maintained volunteers. *J Pharmacol Exp Ther* 1992;261:985–993.
135. Strain EC, Preston KL, Liebson IA, et al. Buprenorphine effects in methadone-maintained volunteers: effects at two hours after methadone. *J Pharmacol Exp Ther* 1995;272:628–638.
136. Walsh SL, June HL, Schuh KJ, et al. Effects of buprenorphine and methadone in methadone-maintained subjects. *Psychopharmacology* 1995;119:268–276.
137. Kosten TR, Kleber HD. Buprenorphine detoxification from opioid dependence: a pilot study. *Life Sci* 1988;42:635–641.
138. Preston KL, Bigelow GE, Liebson IA. Butorphanol-precipitated withdrawal in opioid-dependent human volunteers. *J Pharmacol Exp Ther* 1988;246:441–448.
139. Banys P, Clark HW, Tusel DJ, et al. An open trial of low dose buprenorphine in treating methadone withdrawal. *J Subst Abuse Treat* 1994;11: 9–15.
140. Lukas SE, Jasinski DR, Johnson RE. Electroencephalographic and behavioral correlates of buprenorphine administration. *Clin Pharmacol Ther* 198436:127–132.
141. Levin FR, Fischman MW, Connerney I, et al. A protocol to switch high-dose, methadone-maintained subjects to buprenorphine. *Am J Addict* 1997;6:105–116.
142. Greenwald MK, Schuh KJ, Stine SM. Transferring methadone-maintained outpatients to the buprenorphine sublingual tablet: a preliminary study. *Am J Addict* 2003;12:365–374.
143. Breen CL, Harris SJ, Lintzeris N, et al. Cessation of methadone maintenance treatment using buprenorphine: transfer from methadone to buprenorphine and subsequent buprenorphine reductions. *Drug Alcohol Depend* 2003;71:49–55.
144. Jones HE, Suess P, Jasinski DR, et al. Transferring methadone-stabilized pregnant patients to buprenorphine using an immediate release morphine transition: an open-label exploratory study. *Am J Addict* 2006;15: 61–70.
145. Rosado J, Walsh SL, Bigelow GE, et al. Sublingual buprenorphine/naloxone precipitated withdrawal in subjects maintained on 100 mg of daily methadone. *Drug Alcohol Depend* 2007;90:261–269.
146. Kosten TR, Morgan C, Kleber HD. Phase II clinical trials of buprenorphine: detoxification and induction onto naltrexone *(NIDA Research Monograph)*. Rockville, MD: National Institute on Drug Abuse, 1992;121:101–119.
147. Eissenberg T, Greenwald MK, Johnson RE, et al. Buprenorphine's physical dependence potential: antagonist-precipitated withdrawal in humans. *J Pharmacol Exp Ther* 1996;276:449–459.
148. Kosten TR, Krystal JH, Charney DS, et al. Rapid detoxification from opioid dependence [see comment]. *Am J Psychiatry* 1989;146:1349.
149. Gerra G, Zaimovic A, Rustichelli P, et al. Rapid opiate detoxication in outpatient treatment: relationship with naltrexone compliance. *J Subst Abuse Treat* 2000;18:185–191.
150. Umbricht A, Montoya ID, Hoover DR, et al. Naltrexone shortened opioid detoxification with buprenorphine. *Drug Alcohol Depend* 1999;56:181–190.
151. Stine SM, Kosten TR. Use of drug combinations in treatment of opioid withdrawal. *J Clin Psychopharmacol* 1992;12:203–209.
152. O'Connor PG. Methods of detoxification and their role in treating patients with opioid dependence [see comment]. *JAMA* 2005;294:961–963.
153. Amato L, Minozzi S, Davoli M, et al. Psychosocial and pharmacological treatments versus pharmacological treatments for opioid detoxification. *Cochrane Database Syst Rev* 2004;CD005031.
154. National Consensus Development Panel on Effective Medical Treatment of Opiate Addiction. Effective medical treatment for opiate addiction. *JAMA* 1998;280:1936–1943.

Ultrarapid Opiate Detoxification

Susan M. Stine, MD, PhD, and Thomas R. Kosten, MD

A controversial treatment approach, which has arisen from use of the clonidine-naltrexone combination, is ultrarapid inpatient detoxification from opiates (UROD) using sedatives and anesthetics in combination with opiate antagonists. Streel and Verbanch (1) have reviewed the small number of animal studies relevant to UROD that have been conducted. Ultrarapid opiate detoxification was first described clinically in a study of 12 opiate-dependent patients who were given naloxone while under general anesthesia (2). Loimer and associates (3) also reported a protocol involving barbiturate anesthesia with methohexitone (100 mg intravenous pretreatment, followed by 400 mg intravenously) and naltrexone (10 mg intravenously). This protocol allowed the completion of the detoxification of patients from opiates in 48 hours, but required intensive medical treatment (involving intubation and artificial ventilation), incurred the risks of anesthesia, and did not lead to long-term abstinence; therefore, it has been controversial. Studies after the first reports of this technique (4,5) used various approaches to both the detoxification and the sedation or general anesthesia. These studies generally were small and methodologically limited, did not compare ultrarapid detoxification to other methods, and provided little long-term follow-up, as reviewed by O'Connor and Kosten (4). This led many clinicians to raise serious questions about the widespread use of this procedure.

As reviewed by O'Connor and Fiellin (6), two studies demonstrated that substantial withdrawal symptoms persist well beyond the detoxification period (5,7). In addition, the expense of this procedure (up to $7,500), the additional risk associated with general anesthesia, and safety concerns (8,9) limit its usefulness in clinical practice (4). General anesthesia with intubation, however, was designed to avoid the risk of vomiting and aspiration, which occurs with sedation. In at least one instance, safety concerns led to the termination of a clinical program that provided ultrarapid detoxification (10). Although many investigators suggested early in the study of this method that the procedure should be limited to clinical trials until its safety and efficacy could be established (11), interest in this procedure and consumer demand for it continued to be intense, and a few later studies were relatively encouraging. Albanese et al. (12) evaluated 6-month outcome data for 93 men and 27 women treated with ultrarapid detoxification, followed by naltrexone maintenance and an aftercare program. Outcome was assessed through urine drug screens, report from a significant other, or report from a therapist. All of the study groups were reported to be relapse-free. However, this study is limited by lack of a prospective randomized controlled design.

Long-term outcome is widely considered to be the true test of a treatment method. The outcome after longer term follow-up tends to be similar with all methods of detoxification in most studies examining this issue. For example, in one study in which detoxified patients were followed by telephone interview, only 10% continued naltrexone maintenance therapy for 7 months (13). Another study by these investigators (14) suggested that naltrexone maintenance and counseling after rapid detoxification may be as effective as intensive inpatient detoxification and counseling. In one study, which followed patients for 30 months (15), 16 patients were detoxified with UROD and prospectively evaluated. After a period of at least 30 months, the 16 patients were still alive and were regularly monitored. Only 2 of the 16 never relapsed after UROD and reported total opiate abstinence. Fourteen patients relapsed; 12 of these received methadone treatment and 2 were still using heroin. A study by Hensel and Kox (16) reported follow-up data from 72 opioid-dependent patients (whose drugs of abuse had included morphine, codeine, heroin, and methadone), who were detoxified with propofol general anesthesia using the ultrarapid method and subsequently treated with long-term naltrexone maintenance and a supportive psychotherapy program. At 12 months, 49 patients (68%) were abstinent from opiates, 17 had relapsed, and 6 were lost to follow-up. The investigators reported that patients who had been receiving methadone had more withdrawal symptoms than did those who were ingesting other opioids. This study also had design limitations related to the absence of an open trial and lack of random assignment to a comparison group. A study that compared ultrarapid detoxification with 30-day inpatient detoxification (17) concluded that ultrarapid detoxification was less effective. In this study, 81 of 87 patients who were detoxified in 30 days and 82 of 139 patients who were detoxified by ultrarapid detoxification were interviewed by telephone 12 to 18 months after their participation in the program. Interview results suggested that ultrarapid detoxification was more expensive and less effective than traditional treatment. Although this study was limited by its retrospective design and lack of randomized assignment, it does support longer term biopsychosocial treatment alternatives over rapid detoxification.

Most review articles, such as O'Connor and Fiellin (6) and O'Connor and Kosten (4), have similar conclusions. Cautiously more positive conclusions are found in a later

Ultrarapid Opiate Detoxification *(continued)*

review by Fontaine at al. (18) of the history of UROD procedures; the article discusses its advantages and limits. The authors searched the MEDLINE database between 1966 and 2000 using the terms "ultra-rapid opioid detoxification, rapid opioid detoxification under anesthesia, naloxone, naltrexone, and opioid-related disorders." It must be noted that only three studies in that review included a control group and two used a randomized design. Three studies reported a follow-up beyond 30 days. The authors concluded that the limitation of available literature, the cost and the risks of this technique, and the lack of long-term treatment outcomes obtained from rigorous clinical trials, among other things, all called for further assessments. The authors of this review further concluded that UROD represents a potentially safe and effective treatment for opiate-addicted patients, but more rigorous research methods are needed to render this procedure entirely valid. Another review of the state of UROD as a viable treatment modality has been presented by Singh and Basu (19). These authors conclude that, although useful in some respects (especially in completion rates for detoxification and subsequent induction onto naltrexone maintenance), the justification of this procedure lies in the resolution of the ethical conflicts surrounding the procedure and conduction of methodologically sound long-term studies to demonstrate greater efficacy over routine/standard detoxification procedures beyond the short-term detoxification period. In the most recent review on this topic from the Cochrane Database Review, Gowing et al. (20) analyzed results of controlled trials comparing antagonist-induced withdrawal under heavy sedation or anesthesia with another form of treatment, or a different regime of anesthesia-based antagonist-induced withdrawal. Heavy sedation compared with light sedation did not confer additional benefits in terms of less severe withdrawal or increased rates of commencement on naltrexone maintenance treatment. The reviewers concluded that, because the adverse events are potentially life-threatening, the value of antagonist-induced withdrawal under heavy sedation or anesthesia is not supported and the high cost of anesthesia-based approaches, both in monetary terms and use of scarce intensive care resources, suggest that this form of treatment should not be pursued.

Scientifically well-designed clinical trials have been rare. One well-designed prospective, randomized trial of anesthesia-assisted detoxification using rapid antagonist induction for heroin dependence compared with two alternative detoxification and antagonist induction methods was published by Collins et al. (21). This randomized study enrolled 106 treatment-seeking heroin-dependent patients, ages 21 through 50 years, who were randomly assigned to one of three inpatient withdrawal treatments over 72 hours followed by 12 weeks of outpatient naltrexone maintenance with relapse prevention psychotherapy. Intervention methods were: anesthesia-assisted rapid opioid detoxification with naltrexone induction, buprenorphine-assisted rapid opioid detoxification with naltrexone induction, and clonidine-assisted opioid detoxification with delayed naltrexone induction. Mean withdrawal severities were comparable across the three treatments. Compared with clonidine-assisted detoxification, the anesthesia- and buprenorphine-assisted detoxification interventions had significantly greater rates of naltrexone induction (94% anesthesia, 97% buprenorphine, and 21% clonidine), but the groups did not differ in rates of completion of inpatient detoxification. Treatment retention over 12 weeks was not significantly different among groups. The anesthesia procedure was associated with three potentially life-threatening adverse events. The authors concluded that the study did not support using general anesthesia for heroin detoxification and rapid opioid antagonist induction. Another randomized study of detoxification under anesthesia evaluating its effectiveness compared with traditional detoxification procedures and including long-term follow-up observations was conducted by Favrat et al. (22). Participants included 70 patients with opiate monodependence requesting detoxification: 36 randomized to UROD (treatment as allocated received by 26) and 34 randomized to classical clonidine detoxification (treatment as allocated received by 21). They found that although the detoxification success rate and abstinence after 3 months were slightly better for the UROD procedure compared with clonidine treatment, these differences were not statistically significant and disappeared completely after 6 and 12 months.

CONCLUSIONS

Ultrarapid opiate detoxification remains controversial and the current literature does not support its general use. Recent research has included a few more studies with a stronger scientific design (randomized prospective controlled clinical trials). Overall, most reviews and the few well-designed clinical trials conclude that the approach presents increased risks of adverse events compared to other available methods. Possible justifications for UROD despite increased risks include that it may be the only treatment acceptable to certain otherwise healthy patients who are unwilling to interrupt their work or personal schedules for longer term detoxification. It also may facilitate rapid

(continued)

Ultrarapid Opiate Detoxification *(continued)*

induction to and maintenance on naltrexone. However, the risks remain considerable and much research remains to be done in appropriate subpopulations on long-term outcomes with the application of an appropriate risk versus benefit analysis.

REFERENCES

1. Streel E, Verbanck P. Ultra-rapid opiate detoxification: from clinical applications to basic science. *Addict Biol* 2003;8(2):141–146.
2. Loimer N, Schmid R, Presslich O, et al. Naloxone treatment for opiate withdrawal syndrome [letter]. *Br J Psychiatry* 1988;153: 851–852.
3. Loimer N, Schmid R, Lenz K, et al. Acute blocking of naloxone-precipitated opiate withdrawal symptoms by methohexitone. *Br J Psychiatry* 1990;157:748–752.
4. O'Connor PG, Kosten TR. Rapid and ultra-rapid opioid detoxification techniques. *JAMA* 1998;279(3):129–134.
5. Scherbaum N, Klein S, Kaube H, et al. Alternative strategies of opiate detoxification: evaluation of the so-called ultra-rapid detoxification. *Pharmacopsychiatry* 1998;31(6):205–209.
6. O'Connor PG, Fiellin DA. Pharmacologic treatment of heroin-dependent patients. *Ann Intern Med* 2000;133(1):40–54.
7. Cucchia AT, Monnat M, Spagnoli J, et al. Ultra-rapid opiate detoxification using deep sedation with oral midazolam: short and long-term results. *Drug Alcohol Depend* 1998;52(3):243–250.
8. San L, Puig M, Bulbena A, et al. High risk of ultrashort noninvasive opiate detoxification [letter]. *Am J Psychiatry* 1995;152(6):956.
9. Pfab R, Hirtl C, Zilker T. Opiate detoxification under anesthesia: no apparent benefit, but suppression of thyroid hormones and risk of pulmonary and renal failure. *J Toxicol Clin Toxicol* 1999;37(1):43–50.
10. Zielbauer P. State knew of risky heroin treatment before patient deaths. *New York Times* October 31, 1999:41.
11. Strang J, Bearn J, Gossop M. Opiate detoxification under anaesthesia [editorial] [see comments]. *Br Med J* 1997;315(7118):1249–1250.
12. Albanese AP, Gevirtz C, Oppenheim B, et al. Outcome and six-month follow-up of patients after ultra rapid opiate detoxification (UROD). *J Addict Dis* 2000;19(2):11–28.
13. Rabinowitz J, Cohen H, Tarrasch R, et al. Compliance to naltrexone treatment after ultra-rapid opiate detoxification: an open label naturalistic study. *Drug Alcohol Depend* 1997;47(2):77–86.
14. Rabinowitz J, Cohen H, Atias S. Outcomes of naltrexone maintenance following ultra rapid opiate detoxification versus intensive inpatient detoxification. *Am J Addict* 2002;11(1):52–56.
15. Bochud TC, Favrat B, Monnat M, et al. Ultra-rapid opiate detoxification using deep sedation and prior oral buprenorphine preparation: long-term results. *Drug Alcohol Depend* 2003;69(3):283–288.
16. Hensel M, Wolter S, Kox WJ. EEG controlled rapid opioid withdrawal under general anaesthesia. *Br J Anaesth* 2000;84(2):236–238.
17. Lawental E. Ultra rapid opiate detoxification as compared to 30-day inpatient detoxification program—a retrospective follow-up study. *J Subst Abuse* 2000;11(2):173–181.
18. Fontaine E, Godfroid IO, Guillaume R. Ultra-rapid detoxification of opiate dependent patients: review of the literature, critiques and proposition for an experimental protocol, *Encephale* 2001;27(2): 187–193.
19. Singh J, Basu D. Ultra-rapid opioid detoxification: current status and controversies. *J Postgrad Med* 2004;50(3):227–232.
20. Gowing L, Ali R, White J. Opioid antagonists under heavy sedation or anaesthesia for opioid withdrawal. *Cochrane Database Syst Rev* 2006;(2):CD002022.
21. Collins ED, Kleber HD, Whittington RA, et al. Anesthesia-assisted vs. buprenorphine- or clonidine-assisted heroin detoxification and naltrexone induction: a randomized trial. *JAMA* 2005;294(8):903–913.
22. Favrat B, Zimmermann G, Zullino D, et al. Opioid antagonist detoxification under anesthesia versus traditional clonidine detoxification combined with an additional week of psychosocial support: a randomized clinical trial. *Drug Alcohol Depend* 2006;81(2):109–116.

CHAPTER 45

Jeffery N. Wilkins, MD
Itai Danovitch, MD
David A. Gorelick, MD, PhD

Management of Stimulant, Hallucinogen, Marijuana, Phencyclidine, and Club Drug Intoxication and Withdrawal

This chapter reviews the treatment of acute intoxication and withdrawal states associated with the use of stimulants such as cocaine and methamphetamine (including their smokable forms "crack" and "ice"); hallucinogens such as lysergic acid diethylamide (LSD); marijuana; dissociative anesthetics such as phencyclidine (PCP), ketamine, and dextromethorphan (DXM); "club drugs" such as 3,4-methylenedioxymethamphetamine (MDMA or "Ecstasy") and gamma-hydroxybutyrate (GHB); and common herbal drugs of abuse. It also reviews the treatment of the serotonin syndrome and withdrawal from multiple drugs. Psychiatric and medical complications are considered separately because they often are treated with different modalities and in different settings (for example, in psychiatric versus medical emergency departments). Not all of the substances reviewed here have clinically distinct intoxication or withdrawal syndromes nor are there pharmacologic treatments for all such syndromes.

Successful treatment of acute intoxication, overdose, or withdrawal can facilitate entry into addiction treatment by reducing uncomfortable withdrawal symptoms that negatively reinforce drug-taking. Even when successful, these early stages of treatment often are followed by relapse to substance use, with patients reentering a "revolving door" of repeated detoxification programs. Short-term treatment of acute intoxication or withdrawal does not obviate the need for long-term treatment of addiction.

Pharmacologic treatment of drug intoxication and overdose generally follows one of three approaches: increased clearance of drug from the body, either by increasing catabolism, increasing excretion, or both (1); blockade of the neuronal site to which the drug binds to exert its effect (as through the use of naloxone to block the mu-opioid receptor in the treatment of opiate overdose); and counteracting effects of the drug through alternative neuropharmacologic action.

Pharmacologic treatment of any drug withdrawal syndrome generally follows one of two approaches: suppression by a cross-tolerant medication from the same pharmacologic class—usually a longer-acting one to provide a milder, controlled withdrawal (as in the use of the opioid methadone for opiate detoxification)—and reducing the signs and symptoms of withdrawal by targeting the neurochemical or receptor systems that mediate withdrawal (as in the use of the nonopiate clonidine to treat opiate withdrawal).

The application of these pharmacologic treatment approaches to the drugs reviewed in this chapter is limited. There may be no practical method for altering drug clearance (as with marijuana), or no specific drug receptor sites have been identified. Even when a receptor site has been identified, there may not yet exist a clinically useful antagonist. Finally, current understanding of the neuropharmacologic processes that mediate intoxication or withdrawal may be too limited to suggest appropriate pharmacologic interventions. Thus clinical stabilization, supportive management, and palliation of symptoms often remain the mainstays of treatment.

STIMULANTS

Stimulant Intoxication The acute psychologic and medical effects of cocaine, amphetamines, and other stimulants are attributable principally to increases in catecholamine neurotransmitter activity. Enhanced catecholamine activity occurs through blockade of the presynaptic neurotransmitter reuptake pumps (as by cocaine) and by presynaptic release of catecholamines (as by amphetamines) (2,3) (see also Chapter 10). The resulting stimulation of brain reward circuits (the corticomesolimbic dopamine circuit) is thought to mediate the desired (and addicting) psychologic effects of stimulants. The resulting stimulation of the sympathetic nervous system leads to peripheral vasoconstriction (with organ ischemia), increased heart rate, and lowered seizure threshold, among other adverse effects. Table 45.1 lists acute medical complications of stimulant intoxication.

Blockade of presynaptic catecholamine reuptake sites or postsynaptic receptors should, in principle, be an effective treatment for stimulant intoxication. Several medications have shown promise in attenuating the acute subjective effects of stimulants; for example, bupropion (4), aripiprazole (5), risperidone (6), topiramate (7), and modafinil (8).

Another method of attenuating the effects of stimulant intoxication might be to decrease drug availability in the central nervous system (CNS) by binding it peripherally with antidrug antibodies or by increasing its catabolism (1). The latter approach could be implemented with catalytic antibodies or with the endogenous cocaine-metabolizing enzyme butyrylcholinesterase (BChE, E.C. 3.1.1.8) or other esterases.

Table 45.2 gives an overview of treatment for the acute psychiatric and medical complications of stimulant intoxication.

Psychologic and Behavioral Effects of Stimulant Intoxication The initial desired effects of stimulant intoxication include increased energy, alertness, and sociability; elation; euphoria; and decreased fatigue, need for sleep, and appetite (9). At this stage, users do not seek or need treatment. With high-dose or repeated use, stimulant intoxication usually progresses to unwanted effects such as anxiety, irritability, interpersonal sensitivity, hypervigilance, suspiciousness, grandiosity, impaired judgment, stereotyped behavior, and psychotic symptoms such as paranoia and hallucinations. In some case series, more than half of chronic stimulant users reported psychotic symptoms (10–12). However, these results may reflect selection bias among users who come to medical or research attention. Stimulant users typically remain alert and oriented, but the delusional state may impair judgment, cognition, and attention.

Patients with stimulant-induced psychoses may closely resemble those with acute schizophrenia and may be misdiagnosed as such (12–14). Cocaine-induced psychosis may differ from acute schizophrenic psychosis in having less thought disorder and bizarre delusions and fewer negative symptoms such as alogia and inattention (12). Stimulant-induced hallucinations may be auditory, visual, or somatosensory (10,15,16).

TABLE 45.1 Acute Medical Complications of Stimulant Intoxication

Organ system	Medical effects
Head, Ears, Eyes, Nose, Throat	Pupil dilation; headache; bruxism
Pulmonary*	Hyperventilation, dyspnea; cough; chest pain; wheezing; hemoptysis; acute exacerbation of asthma; barotrauma (pneumothorax, pneumomediastinum) pulmonary edema
Cardiovascular	Tachycardia; palpitations; increased blood pressure; arrhythmia; chest pain; myocardial ischemia or infarction; ruptured aneurysm; cardiogenic shock
Neurologic	Headache; agitation; psychosis; tremor, hyperreflexia; small muscle twitching; tics; stereotyped movements; myoclonus; seizures; cerebral hemorrhage or infarct (stroke); cerebral edema
Gastrointestinal	Nausea, vomiting; mesenteric ischemia; bowel infarction or perforation
Renal	Diuresis; myoglobinuria; acute renal failure
Body temperature	Mild fever; malignant hyperthermia
Other	Rhabdomyolysis

*All pulmonary complications except hyperventilation and pulmonary edema come primarily from the smoked route of administration.

Sources: Ghuran A, Nolan J. Recreational drug misuse: issues for the cardiologist. *Heart* 2000;83:627–633; Neiman J, Haapaniemi HM, Hillblom M. Neurological complications of drug abuse: pathophysiological mechanisms. *Eur J Neurol* 2000;7:595–606; Schuckit MA. *Drug and alcohol abuse. A clinical guide to diagnosis and treatment,* 6th ed. New York: Springer, 2006. Tashkin DP. Airway effects of marijuana, cocaine, and other inhaled illicit agents. *Curr Opin Pulm Med* 2001;7:43–61.

TABLE 45.2 Treatment of Acute Stimulant Intoxication

Clinical problem	Moderate syndrome	Severe syndrome
Anxiety; agitation	Provide reassurance; place in a quiet, nonthreatening environment	Diazepam (10–30 mg PO, 2–10 mg IM, IV); or lorazepam (2–4 mg PO, IM, IV); may repeat every 1–3 h
Paranoia; psychosis	Place in a quiet, nonthreatening environment; benzodiazepines for sedation	High-potency antipsychotic (e.g., haloperidol) or second-generation antipsychotic
Hyperthermia	Monitor body temperature; place in a cool room	If temperature >102°F (oral), use external cooling with cold water, ice packs, hypothermic blanket; if >106°F, use internal cooling; epigastric lavage with iced saline
Seizures	Diazepam (2–20 mg IV, <5 mg/min); or lorazepam (2–8 mg)	For status epilepticus: IV diazepam or phenytoin (15–20 mg/kg IV, <150 mg/min; or phenobarbital (25–50 mg IV)
Hypertension	Monitor blood pressure closely; benzodiazepines for sedation	If diastolic >120 for 15 minutes, give phentolamine (2–10 mg IV over 10 min)
Cardiac arrhythmia	Monitor electrocardiogram, vital signs; benzodiazepines for sedation	As appropriate for specific rhythm, based on advanced cardiac life support criteria
Myocardial infarction	Benzodiazepines for sedation; supplemental oxygen; sublingual nitroglycerin for vasodilation; aspirin for anticlotting; morphine for pain	Give nitrates IV for coronary artery dilation; phentolamine (2–10 mg IV) to control blood pressure; thrombolysis, angioplasty (if clot confirmed and no hemorrhage)
Rhabdomyolysis	IV hydration to maintain urine output >2 mL/kg/hr	Force diuresis with aggressive intravenous hydration
Increased urinary drug excretion	Cranberry juice (8 oz TID) or ammonium chloride (500 mg PO every 3–4 h) until urine pH <6.6 (if renal and hepatic function are normal)	Same as for moderate intoxication
Recent (few hours) oral drug ingestion	Activated charcoal orally or gastric lavage via nasogastric tube (if patient is awake and cooperative)	Gastric lavage via nasogastric tube after endotracheal intubation (if patient is unconscious)

Tactile hallucinations are especially typical of stimulant psychosis, such as the sensation of something crawling under the skin (formication). Specific genetic variations may account for some differences in individual vulnerability to stimulant-induced psychosis (10,17). Panic reactions are common, and may evolve into a panic disorder (18). This may be exacerbated by anxiety elicited by the physiologic symptoms commonly associated with stimulant use, such as palpitations and hyperventilation.

Very severe stimulant intoxication may produce an excited delirium or organic brain syndrome that can be fatal (19,20). Patients should be evaluated promptly for an acute neurologic lesion (e.g., intracranial bleeding) or a preexisting neuropsychiatric condition and treated aggressively (21,22).

Management of Psychologic and Behavioral Effects of Stimulant Intoxication The initial clinical evaluation should include a drug use history and drug toxicology to confirm stimulant intoxication. As the patient's condition permits, further evaluation should rule out other potential medical (hyperthyroidism, hypoglycemia) or neuropsychiatric (panic or bipolar affective disorder) conditions (23). The initial treatment approach is nonpharmacologic (24,25). The patient should be observed in a quiet environment with minimal sensory stimulation to avoid exacerbating symptoms. Treatment staff should interact in a calm and confident manner, using the "ART" approach developed at the Haight Ashbury Free Clinic in San Francisco: *A*cceptance of the patient's immediate needs (such as pain relief or use of the bathroom), *R*eassurance that the condition is due to the drug and likely will dissipate within a few hours, and *T*alkdown, to provide reality orientation and avoid hostility. All procedures should be explained to the patient before initiation. Physical restraints to control agitation or violent behavior should be avoided unless absolutely necessary. The use of restraints can increase risk of hyperthermia and rhabdomyolysis, with resulting severe medical complications (25,26).

If medication is needed, most experts prefer benzodiazepines (such as diazepam [10 to 30 mg PO or 2 to 10 mg IM or IV] or lorazepam [2 to 4 mg PO, IM, or IV]) over antipsychotics to control severe agitation, anxiety, or psychotic symptoms (18,27), although there are very few controlled clinical trials (28). The former protect against the CNS and cardiovascular toxicities of cocaine, whereas the latter may worsen the sympathomimetic and cardiovascular effects, lower the seizure threshold, and increase the risk of hyperthermia. Parenteral benzodiazepine dosing may be repeated every 5 to 10 minutes until light sedation is achieved. If an antipsychotic is needed to control psychosis, a high-potency agent such as droperidol, haloperidol (5 to 10 mg PO, IM, or IV), or risperidone (2 to 4 mg PO) is preferred because of its minimal anticholinergic activity. Anticholinergic activity should be avoided because it may contribute to delirium and hyperthermia (by impairing heat dissipation from sweating). Chlorpromazine (29) and haloperidol (30) have been used safely in treating children with severe amphetamine poisoning. There is little evidence to guide treatment with second-generation antipsychotics, such as ziprasidone, risperidone, quetiapine, and olanzapine. Aripiprazole has been suggested as a promising medication because of its partial dopamine agonism (31).

A psychotic or agitated patient who has not responded to initial treatment should be hospitalized until the episode has resolved. This usually occurs within a few days if no more stimulants are ingested (18). Psychiatric symptoms that persist beyond a few days suggest an etiology other than stimulant use (24,32,33). Transient psychotic symptoms during periods of abstinence ("flashbacks") have also been reported among methamphetamine users (34).

Medical Effects of Stimulant Intoxication Mild stimulant intoxication (the state desired by users) may be accompanied by one or more self-limiting physiologic effects such as restlessness, sinus tachycardia, hyperventilation, mydriasis, bruxism, headache, diaphoresis, or tremor. These do not usually bring the individual to medical attention or require treatment. Higher doses or repeated use are associated with more serious medical events, including nausea and vomiting, acute coronary syndrome (unstable angina or myocardial infarction) (usually resulting in chest pain), cardiac tachyarrhythmia, hypertension, seizures, stroke, hyperthermia, or rhabdomyolysis (35–39). Acute medical complications associated with acute stimulant intoxication are summarized in Table 45.1.

Stimulant use should be high on the list of possible diagnoses for any younger patient presenting with one of these events, especially in the absence of other risk factors (40). Urine or blood samples for toxicologic analysis should be obtained to determine what drugs, if any, the patient has ingested recently. Even if an apparently adequate history has been obtained, the patient or collateral informants may not know the true content of any street drugs that have been used. A history of stimulant use within the preceding 96 hours or a positive toxicology test is highly suggestive. The actual blood cocaine concentration has little prognostic significance (41).

Nontraumatic chest pain is a common presenting complaint among stimulant users who seek acute medical care. The differential diagnosis includes acute coronary syndrome, acute aortic dissection, pneumothorax or pneumomediastinum (especially among drug smokers), endocarditis or pneumonia (especially among injection drug users), pulmonary embolus, myocarditis or cardiomyopathy, or musculoskeletal pain after a seizure (42,43). About 1% to 6% of patients with cocaine-associated chest pain and up to one fourth of those with methamphetamine-associated chest pain will have an acute myocardial infarction (43,44). The risk for infarction is greatest during the first 1 to 3 hours after cocaine use, then declines rapidly (44). Concurrent use of multiple stimulants (e.g., cocaine and methamphetamine) may enhance cardiotoxicity (39), whereas concurrent use of opiates (such as "speedballing") may mask the diagnosis (45).

The electrocardiogram is not always helpful diagnostically because of its low sensitivity and positive predictive value (36% and 18%, respectively, in one study) and the high frequency (more than one third in some studies) of benign early repolarization among patients presenting with cocaine-associated chest pain (46). The best laboratory test for acute myocardial infarction is serial blood levels of cardiac troponin I (44,46). Its high specificity (around 95%) for acute myocardial infarction is not affected by recent cocaine use because it does not cross-react with skeletal muscle troponin. In contrast, myoglobin and creatine kinase levels may be elevated due to cocaine-associated rhabdomyolysis.

Patients who present with nontraumatic stimulant-associated chest pain usually should be observed for 9 to 12 hours while undergoing evaluation (47). Delayed complications are rare, so resolution of symptoms with a negative evaluation warrants discharge. Patients who have persistent chest pain despite standard treatment, hypotension, congestive heart failure, or cardiac arrhythmia require hospitalization for further evaluation and treatment. Even patients with confirmed acute myocardial infarction have a favorable prognosis, possibly because of their relatively young age and good underlying health (35,44).

Rhabdomyolysis may be due to a direct effect of the drug, hyperthermia, excessive muscle activity, or trauma (25). The usual symptoms of myalgia and muscle tenderness and swelling often are absent in rhabdomyolysis associated with stimulants. The diagnosis is suggested by a plasma CK level greater than five times' normal (with other tissue sources ruled out) and a urine dipstick positive for heme but without red blood cells (indicating free myoglobin [or hemoglobin] in the urine).

Management of Medical Effects of Stimulant Intoxication The first priority in the management of severe acute stimulant intoxication is maintenance of basic life support functions (27). Vital signs, hydration status, and neurologic status should be monitored closely. Activated charcoal or gastric lavage with isotonic saline may be helpful if a large amount of stimulant has been taken orally within the preceding hour (18,25). This can be done by oral intake or via nasogastric tube in the awake, cooperative patient. Activated charcoal (50 to 100 g orally) may be just as effective as gastric lavage and minimizes the risk of aspiration. Ipecac-induced vomiting is not recommended.

Severe hypertension (e.g., diastolic blood pressure >120) that lasts >15 minutes should be treated promptly to avoid

CNS hemorrhage (18). Rhabdomyolysis should be treated vigorously with intravenous fluid to maintain a urine output of >2 mL/kg/hour to avoid myoglobinuric renal failure (18,25). Maintenance of urine pH >5.6 with sodium bicarbonate (1 mmol/kg IV) helps to prevent the dissociation and precipitation of myoglobin.

Benzodiazepines in sedative doses are the initial treatment of choice for both acute cardiovascular and CNS toxicity from stimulants (25,35,48). Hypertension or tachycardia that does not respond to sedation alone may be treated with an alpha-adrenergic blocker such as phentolamine (2 to 10 mg IV over 10 minutes). Beta-adrenergic blockers such as propranolol or esmolol are contraindicated because of the risk of unopposed alpha-adrenergic stimulation by the stimulant, resulting in vasoconstriction and worsening hypertension (44,46). The combined alpha- and beta-adrenergic blocker labetalol actually shows little alpha-adrenergic antagonism in clinical practice and also should be avoided (35). If alpha-adrenergic blockade is ineffective, direct vasodilation with sodium nitroprusside infusion (0.25 to 10 μg/kg/min) or nitroglycerin (5 to 100 μg IV) can be used. There is no evidence that rapid lowering of blood pressure compromises peripheral (including cerebral) circulation in an otherwise intact patient. Calcium channel blockers may reduce vasospasm, but their role remains unclear (42). They enhance CNS toxicity in animal studies, have shown inconsistent effects in case series, and may accelerate gastrointestinal drug absorption (e.g., after rupture of cocaine packets ingested by "bodypackers") (35).

Treatment of cocaine-induced cardiac tachyarrhythmias begins with correction of any exacerbating conditions such as myocardial ischemia, hypoxia, electrolyte abnormalities, or acid-base disturbance (44,46,47). Arrhythmias occurring several hours after cocaine use are usually secondary to myocardial ischemia. Standard arrhythmia management is usually appropriate, including use of lidocaine. Arrhythmias occurring immediately after cocaine use are usually from the sodium channel blocking action of cocaine. These may respond to sodium bicarbonate. Lidocaine (which also blocks sodium channels) should be used cautiously in this context because of animal studies suggesting it may exacerbate cocaine-associated arrhythmias and seizures. Class IA antiarrhythmic medications (such as quinidine, procainamide, or disopyramide) should be avoided because of their potential additive effect on QRS and QT interval prolongation. There are no data on the use of amiodarone for cocaine-associated arrhythmias. Treatment of cardiac arrest is the same as for non–cocaine users; the outcome may be more favorable than for drug-free patients (49).

The treatment of stimulant-associated acute coronary syndrome largely resembles that for the nondrug-associated syndrome, with the exception of avoiding use of beta-adrenergic blockers and labetalol (47,50). Initial treatment includes oxygen, benzodiazepine for sedation, morphine for pain, sublingual nitroglycerin for vasodilation, and aspirin for antiplatelet action, while evaluation is continuing. Further treatment can include phentolamine or intravenous nitrates (10 μg/kg/min) to lower blood pressure and reverse coronary artery vasoconstriction. The role of calcium channel blockers is not well defined (44,46). They may be useful in patients who have not responded to benzodiazepines and nitroglycerin.

Both fibrinolytic therapy and percutaneous transluminal coronary angioplasty have a role in the treatment of confirmed myocardial infarction (44). Fibrinolysis should be used cautiously because of the increased risk of intracranial hemorrhage in cocaine users. Both fibrinolysis and angioplasty have been safely and effectively used in nonhemorrhagic patients with focal lesions confirmed by coronary angiography in whom blood pressure was well controlled (51,52).

Elevated body temperature (>102°F orally) should be managed aggressively to avert hyperthermic crisis (as by cold water sponging, cooling blankets, ice packs, ice water gastric lavage, or cold peritoneal lavage) (18,25). Untreated hyperthermia may result in rhabdomyolysis and renal failure.

Intravenous benzodiazepines (diazepam 5 to 10 mg or lorazepam 2 to 10 mg over 2 minutes, repeated as needed) are recommended to control seizures stemming from stimulant intoxication (25). Fosphenytoin (15 to 20 mg/kg at 100 to 150 mg/minute) or phenobarbital (15 to 20 mg/kg over 20 minutes) also can be used. However, the latter may cause hypotension or prolonged sedation.

Excretion of amphetamine can be increased by acidifying the urine to pH <6.6 (as with 500 mg of oral ammonium chloride every 3 to 4 hours), which inhibits renal reabsorption of amphetamine (53). The actual clinical usefulness of this maneuver is uncertain (9). Acidification is contraindicated in the presence of myoglobinuria, if renal or hepatic function is abnormal, or in overdose situations, when plasma acidification may compromise cardiovascular function (32).

Stimulant Withdrawal Abrupt cessation of stimulant use is associated with depression, anxiety, fatigue, difficulty concentrating, anergia, anhedonia, increased drug craving, increased appetite, hypersomnolence, and increased dreaming (because of increased REM sleep) (54–57). The initial period of intense symptoms is commonly termed the "crash," but most symptoms are mild and self-limited, resolving within 1 to 2 weeks without treatment.

One early study of cocaine addicts in outpatient treatment described a triphasic withdrawal syndrome lasting several weeks, but this pattern has not been found in subsequent inpatient or outpatient studies of cocaine withdrawal (54,56–58).

Hospitalization for stimulant withdrawal is rarely indicated on medical grounds and has not been shown to improve the short-term outcome for stimulant addiction (59,60). Pharmacologic treatment has focused more on long-term treatment of addiction than on short-term treatment of acute withdrawal (61,62). Most clinical trials that used medication during the early withdrawal period have continued to use such medication for at least several weeks, with the additional goal of treating the addiction itself (Chapter 51).

Medical Effects of Stimulant Withdrawal The first week of stimulant withdrawal has been associated with myocardial ischemia (63), possibly because of coronary vasospasm. Other medical effects of stimulant withdrawal are relatively minor, including nonspecific musculoskeletal pain, tremors, chills, and involuntary motor movement (64). These rarely require specific medical treatment.

Management of Stimulant Withdrawal The stimulant withdrawal syndrome has been hypothesized to be the result of decreased levels of brain dopamine activity resulting from chronic stimulant exposure. This so-called "dopamine deficiency" hypothesis of withdrawal has not been consistently supported by clinical studies (58,65,66), but has generated use of dopamine agonists to treat cocaine withdrawal. Most commonly used are bromocriptine and amantadine, although neither has been evaluated in an adequate controlled clinical trial.

The dopamine amino acid precursor L-dopa was effective in reducing cocaine withdrawal symptoms in one small inpatient case series (67). The antidepressant reboxetine, a selective norepinephrine reuptake inhibitor not marketed in the United States, substantially reduced withdrawal symptoms in small case series of amphetamine (68) and cocaine (69) users. Inhaled nitrous oxide was effective in reducing acute cocaine withdrawal symptoms in a small single-blind study (70). The antidepressant amineptine, a norepinephrine/dopamine reuptake inhibitor withdrawn from the market because of abuse liability, significantly reduced amphetamine withdrawal symptoms in two small controlled clinical trials. No controlled clinical trial has directly compared the benefits of medication versus a supportive milieu.

Symptoms of stimulant withdrawal are best treated supportively with rest, exercise, and a healthy diet (18,24). Short-acting benzodiazepines such as lorazepam may be helpful in selected patients who develop agitation or sleep disturbance. Severe (suicidal ideation) or persistent (>2 to 3 weeks) depression may require antidepressant treatment (18) and psychiatric admission. The risk of relapse is high during the early withdrawal period, in part because drug craving is easily triggered by encounters with drug-associated stimuli. This issue is better addressed by psychosocial treatment, such as supportive therapy, cognitive-behavioral therapy, relapse prevention, and contingency management, than by medication.

Administration of a cross-tolerant or similarly acting stimulant has not been systematically evaluated as a short-term treatment for stimulant withdrawal (24). A recent double-blind, placebo-controlled pilot inpatient study found that one week of modafinil (200 mg daily) improved retention but did not reduce methamphetamine withdrawal symptoms (71).

HALLUCINOGENS

Hallucinogen Intoxication Hallucinogens fall into two different chemical groups: serotonin- or tryptamine-related (including LSD, psilocybin, or N,N-dimethyltryptamine) and the phenylethylamine or amphetamine-related (including 3,4,5-trimethoxyphenylethylamine [mescaline], 3,5-dimethoxy-4-methylamphetamine [DOM, STP], or 3,4,5-trimethoxyamphetamine). All share enough clinical similarities with LSD to be classified as LSD-like hallucinogens (72,73) (see also Chapter 14). 3,4-methylenedioxymethamphetamine (MDMA, "Ecstasy") has characteristics of both a hallucinogen and a stimulant and is considered below (see also Chapter 14). Phencyclidine (PCP) and its close analogue ketamine are dissociative anesthetics which are abused for their hallucinogenic effects. They are considered in their own section below (see also Chapter 15).

Psychologic and Behavioral Effects of Hallucinogen Intoxication The acute psychologic and behavioral effects of hallucinogen intoxication are summarized in Table 45.3. The subjective experience is influenced greatly by set and setting; that is, the expectations and personality of the user, coupled with the environmental and social conditions of use. Mood can vary from euphoria and feelings of spiritual insight to depression, anxiety, and terror. Perception usually is intensified and distorted, with alterations in the sense of time, space, and body boundaries. Hallucinations (especially visual and auditory) are common. Cognitive function may range from clarity to confusion and disorientation, although reality testing usually remains intact.

A "bad trip" (74) usually takes the form of an anxiety attack or panic reaction, with the user feeling out of control (75,76). An experience of depersonalization may precipitate the fear of losing one's mind permanently. Panic reactions are more common in those who have limited experience with hallucinogens, but previous "positive" experiences provide no protection against an adverse reaction (77). Hallucinogens may trigger a transient psychosis even in psychologically normal users; however, a true psychotic episode is rare. Hallucinogen-induced psychosis may resemble acute paranoid schizophrenia (77). The two usually can be distinguished because patients with schizophrenia tend to have auditory (rather than visual) hallucinations and a history of prior mental illness. Hallucinogen users, unlike patients with schizophrenia, usually retain at least partial insight that their psychosis is drug-related.

Hallucinogen ingestion may result in an acute toxic delirium that is characterized by delusions, hallucinations, agitation, confusion, paranoia, and inadvertent suicide attempts (e.g., attempts to fly or perform other impossible activities).

Medical Effects of Hallucinogen Intoxication Acute medical complications of hallucinogen intoxication are summarized in Table 45.4. Complications that require treatment are rare in the absence of overdose (74,75). Dizziness, paresthesias, headache, nausea, or tremor may occur. Body temperature should be monitored and any elevation treated promptly. Dry skin, increased muscle tone, agitation, and seizures are warning signs of a potential hyperthermic crisis. Patients may not respond to anticonvulsant medication until body temperature is lowered.

TABLE 45.3 Acute Psychologic and Behavioral Effects of Intoxication with LSD, Marijuana, Phencyclidine (PCP), or MDMA

Effects	LSD	Marijuana	Phencyclidine	MDMA
"Abnormal" overall behavior and appearance	XX	X	XXX	X
Disoriented to person, place, time, or situation	XX	None	XX	None
Impaired memory	X	XX	XX	X
Inappropriate affect	XXX	X	XXX	XX
Depressed mood	XX	X	XX	X
Overly elated mood	XXX	XX	XX	XXX
Confused, disorganized thinking	XX	XX	XXX	X
Hallucinations	XXX	X	XXX	X
Delusions	X/XXX	XXX	XX	?
Bizarre behavior	XXX	X	XXX	?
Suicidal or danger to self	XX	XX	XX	?
Homicidal or danger to others	XX	X	XXX	X
Poor judgment	X/XXX	XXX	XXX	XX

Relative weighting: X = mild; XX = moderate; XXX = marked; / = common/rare; ? = insufficient research.
MDMA, 3,4-methylenedioxymethamphetamine.

Sources: Abraham HD, Aldridge AM, Gogia P. The psychopharmacology of hallucinogens. *Neuropsychopharmacology* 1996;14:285–298; Brust JCM. Acute neurologic complications of drug and alcohol abuse. *Neurol Clin N Am* 1998;16(2):503–519; Frecska E, Luna LE. The adverse effects of hallucinogens from intramural perspective. *Neuropsychopharmacol Hung* 2006;8:189–200.

Oral LSD is rapidly absorbed, so that ipecac-induced vomiting or gastric lavage usually are not helpful and may exacerbate the patient's psychologic distress. There is no evidence that LSD binds to charcoal. Gastric lavage may be useful in psilocybin ingestion, or when there is doubt as to the identity of the ingested mushrooms (78).

Management of Hallucinogen Intoxication Initial treatment is nonpharmacologic. The patient should be placed in a quiet environment with minimal sensory stimulation, but should be observed because of the risk of unintended self-injury (as the result of delusions or hallucinations) or of suicide (as the result of depression). The presence of a familiar person usually is comforting. Unless the patient presents in an acutely agitated or threatening state, physical restraints are contraindicated because they may exacerbate anxiety and increase the risk of rhabdomyolysis associated with muscle rigidity or spasms. The use of "gentle restraints" in combination with muscle massage and individualized counseling may be helpful (79).

The "talk-down" or reassurance technique may be helpful. The clinician, in a concerned and nonjudgmental manner, discusses the patient's anxiety reaction, stressing that the drug's effects are temporary and that the patient will recover completely.

For patients who do not respond to reassurance alone, oral benzodiazepines such as lorazepam (1 to 2 mg) or diazepam (10 to 30 mg) are the drugs of choice (80). When oral medication is too slow, or the patient will not take oral medication, intramuscular lorazepam (2 mg, repeated hourly as needed) may be effective. If benzodiazepines are insufficient, a high-potency antipsychotic such as haloperidol (5 to 10 mg orally or 2 mg intramuscularly) may be needed. The role of second generation anti-psychotics in this situation remains unclear, but 5-HT_{2A} receptor antagonism may be a useful property (75). Phenothiazines should be avoided because they have been associated with poor outcomes (81) and may exacerbate unsuspected anticholinergic poisoning.

Patients usually recover sufficiently after several hours and may be released into the care of a responsible relative or friend. If psychosis does not resolve within 1 or 2 days, ingestion of a longer-acting drug such as PCP or DOM should be suspected (18). Symptoms that persist beyond a few days raise the strong likelihood of a pre-existing or concurrent psychiatric or neurologic condition. Psychiatric problems that last more than a month probably are related to preexisting psychopathology.

Treatment for hallucinogen-induced delirium generally follows the guidelines for simple intoxication: Isolate the patient and minimize sensory input until effects of the drug have worn off. Reassurance that the delirium will abate as the drug is metabolized also may be helpful. Pharmacologic treatment is not necessary in most cases and may confuse the clinical picture. If medication is needed, a drug with few anticholinergic properties is preferred for the reasons listed above; for example, diazepam may be given 15 to 30 mg orally, repeating 5 to 20 mg every 3 to 4 hours as needed.

Hallucinogen Withdrawal Withdrawal symptoms, including fatigue, irritability, and anhedonia, are reported by about 10% of hallucinogen users (82), but there is no evidence to suggest a clinically significant hallucinogen withdrawal syndrome (64,77). The rapid development of tolerance (within 3 to 4 days) may explain in part why use of LSD-like drugs generally is intermittent. There is no role for medication in the treatment of hallucinogen withdrawal.

TABLE 45.4 Acute Medical Complications of Intoxication with LSD, MDMA, Marijuana, or Phencyclidine (PCP)

Organ system	LSD	MDMA	Marijuana	PCP (Stage I)	PCP (Stage II)	PCP (Stage III)
Head, Eyes, Ears, Nose, Throat	Pupil dilation	Bruxism; headache; trismus; dry mouth	Pupil constriction; conjunctival injection; headache	Horizontal nystagmus; lid reflex lost; variable pupil size; laryngeal/pharyngeal reflexes hyperactive; ↑ tearing; ↑ saliva	Corneal reflex lost; disconjugate gaze; pupils mid-position and reactive; laryngeal/pharyngeal reflexes diminished; ↑ tearing; ↑ saliva	"Eyes open" coma; pupil dilation; laryngeal/pharyngeal reflexes absent; ↑ tearing; ↑ saliva
Skin	Piloerection; diaphoresis	Diaphoresis; flushing		Diaphoresis; flushing	Diaphoresis; flushing	Diaphoresis; flushing
Pulmonary			Mild tachypnea	Moderate tachypnea	Periodic breathing; apnea, pneumonia, edema	
Cardiovascular	↑ HR; ↑ BP	↑ HR; ↑ BP (rarely, ↓ BP)	↑ HR, ↓ BP orthostatic hypotension	Mildly ↑ HR, BP	Moderately ↑ HR, BP	Greatly ↑ HR, BP; high-output cardiac failure
Neurologic	Hyperreflexia; tremors; seizures	Tremor; trismus; ↑ muscle tone	Tremor; ↓ coordination; ataxia	Conscious; muscle rigidity; repetitive movements; hyperreflexia	Stupor to mild coma; tonic-clonic seizures; deep pain response intact; muscle rigidity; muscle twitching	Deep coma; tonic-clonic seizures; stroke; deep pain response absent; generalized myoclonus, opisthotonus, or decere brate posturing; deep tendon reflexes absent
Gastrointestinal	Nausea; vomiting	Nausea; ↓ appetite	↑ Appetite	Nausea; vomiting	Protracted vomiting	
Renal	Urinary retention	Acute renal failure	Urinary retention	Acute renal failure		
Body temperature	↑ or ↓	↑ (Possible malignant hyperthermia)		Mild ↑	Moderate ↑	Possible malignant hyperthermia
Other		Rhabdomyolysis		Rhabdomyolysis		

MDMA, 3,4-methylenedioxymethamphetamine; HR, heart rate; BP, blood pressure.

Sources: Brust JCM. Acute neurologic complications of drug and alcohol abuse. *Neurol Clin N Am* 1998;16(2):503–519; Frecska E, Luna LE. The adverse effects of hallucinogens from intramural perspective. *Neuropsychopharmacol Hung* 2006;8:189–200; Ghuran A, Nolan J. Recreational drug misuse: issues for the cardiologist. *Heart* 2000;83:627–633; Kalan H. The pharmacology and toxicology of "ecstasy" (MDMA) and related drugs. *Canad Med Assoc J.* 2001;165(7):917–926; Schuckit MA. *Drug and alcohol abuse. A clinical guide to diagnosis and treatment,* 6th ed. New York: Springer, 2006; Selden BS, Clark RF, Curry SC. Marijuana. *Emerg Med Clin North Am* 1990;8(3):527–539.

MARIJUANA

Marijuana Intoxication The major psychologic and physiologic effects of marijuana are mediated by the interaction of delta-9-tetrahydrocannabinol (THC) with specific cannabinoid (CB1) receptors on nerve cells (83,84), the regional distribution of which in the human brain is consistent with the known effects of marijuana (85). Other cannabinoids found in marijuana (e.g., cannabidiol, cannabichromene) do not produce the typical marijuana effects (86). In animal and human studies, acute THC effects are reduced or blocked by CB1 receptor antagonists (87).

Psychologic and Behavioral Effects of Marijuana Intoxication The initial—usually desired—psychologic effects of marijuana intoxication include relaxation, euphoria, slowed time perception, altered (often intensified) sensory perception, increased awareness of the environment, and increased appetite (88). Undesired effects may include impaired concentration, anterograde amnesia (89) and motor incoordination (90). As with hallucinogens, psychologic set and social setting and prior experience with the drug can substantially influence the quality of the experience. Higher doses, repeated use, or a stressful setting are associated with adverse effects such as hypervigilance, anxiety, paranoia, derealization and depersonalization (commonly associated with altered time sense), acute panic (associated with anxiety), illusions or hallucinations (usually auditory or visual), psychosis, or delirium (74,91–93). Acute marijuana-associated psychosis can be difficult to distinguish from schizophrenic psychosis other than by its transient time course (94). Marijuana-associated psychosis may be more likely to exhibit derealization/depersonalization experiences and visual, rather than auditory, hallucinations. Preexisting psychopathology increases the risk of adverse events such as panic attack or psychosis (95). Table 45.3 summarizes the acute adverse psychologic effects of marijuana intoxication.

In addition, marijuana use is probably an independent risk factor for subsequent development of a psychotic disorder (96,97). Oral ingestion of marijuana can produce the same adverse reactions as does smoking, including psychosis (98,99).

Medical Effects of Marijuana Intoxication The acute physiologic effects of oral or smoked marijuana intoxication include conjunctival injection ("red eye"), tachycardia (sometimes with palpitations), orthostatic hypotension (sometimes resulting in syncope), and dry mouth (Table 45.4). Neurologic signs include poor motor coordination, head jerks, and impairment of smooth pursuit eye movements (90). These generally are mild, self-limiting, and do not require medical treatment (88). There are no well-established cases of human fatalities from exclusively marijuana overdose (92), although several cases of possible acute cardiovascular death have been reported (100) and marijuana smoking has been associated with atrial fibrillation and other tachyarrhythmias (101,102). Intravenous use of marijuana, although rare, can be associated with cardiovascular shock and renal failure (103).

Management of Marijuana Intoxication Adverse effects of marijuana intoxication tend to be self-limited and often can be managed without medication. The patient should be kept in a quiet environment and offered supportive reassurance. If immediate pharmacologic intervention is needed to control severe agitation or anxiety, benzodiazepines are preferred to antipsychotics, although there are no controlled studies to confirm this. Psychosis usually responds to low doses of second-generation antipsychotics (93).

Several selective cannabinoid CB1 receptor antagonists are in clinical development (see Chapter 13). One of them, rimonabant (developed for weight loss), has been shown to block the acute psychologic and cardiovascular effects of smoked marijuana (104). Should this or a similar compound prove safe and effective, it could be used to treat acute marijuana intoxication in the same way that naloxone acts on opiate intoxication.

Marijuana Withdrawal Acute marijuana withdrawal, although not a recognized syndrome in the DSM-IV-TR (105), is reported by up to one third of heavy marijuana users in the community and more than half of those seeking treatment for marijuana dependence (106). Symptoms are primarily psychologic, including irritability, anxiety, depression, restlessness, anorexia, insomnia, and vivid or disturbing dreams. Much less common are physical symptoms such as gastrointestinal distress, diaphoresis, chills, nausea, shakiness, and muscle twitches. The syndrome is often relatively mild and has been compared to tobacco withdrawal (107). It can serve as a negative reinforcer for relapse among users trying to maintain abstinence (106,108).

Management of Marijuana Withdrawal Marijuana withdrawal rarely requires treatment for intrinsic medical or psychiatric reasons. Treatment might be warranted to reduce the risk of relapse in persons trying to abstain, but there are no clinical trials addressing this issue (109). In non–treatment-seeking research subjects, agonist substitution with oral synthetic THC (dronabinol) does substantially suppress withdrawal symptoms (110), whereas the antidepressants bupropion and nefazodone and the anticonvulsant divalproex sodium are not effective (109).

DISSOCIATIVE ANESTHETICS

Phencyclidine, Ketamine, and Dextromethorphan Intoxication PCP and its analogue ketamine are dissociative anesthetics; the latter is still legally marketed (27,111, 112). In recent years, ketamine has developed greater popularity as a substance of abuse and "club drug" (112,113). The spectrum of psychiatric complications from ketamine intoxication appears similar to that from PCP, but there are few published data on the treatment of ketamine intoxication.

The related drug dextromethorphan (DXM) is widely available as an ingredient in over-the-counter cough and cold medicines (114). At the recommended antitussive dose of 15 to 30 mg every 6 to 8 hours, adverse reactions are rare. However, about 5% to 10% of Caucasians are unable to demethylate DXM to dextrorphan (an active metabolite) because of deficit in the liver cytochrome P450 CYP 2D6 isozyme. These individuals are less prone to acute adverse effects when using DXM (114).

The main effects of PCP and ketamine are mediated by their action as noncompetitive antagonists of the NMDA-glutamate excitatory amino acid neurotransmitter receptor, although direct effects on other neurotransmitter systems (such as dopamine) may occur at high doses (111,115) (see Chapter 15). In addition to NMDA antagonism, DXM has activity at the sigma receptor, which likely mediates its therapeutic effects as a cough suppressant.

Psychologic and Behavioral Effects of Dissociative Anesthetic Intoxication Dissociative anesthetics produce a range of intoxicated states that can be grouped into three stages (111): Stage I—conscious, with psychologic effects but (at most) mild physiologic effects; Stage II—stuporous or in a light coma, yet responsive to pain; and Stage III—comatose and unresponsive to pain. Table 45.3 summarizes the acute psychologic and behavioral effects of PCP intoxication and overdose. The time course of psychologic effects is highly variable and unpredictable, so that even a recovering patient should be kept under observation until all symptoms have resolved (typically at least 12 hours) (116,117). Patients may "emerge" from one stage of intoxication to the next; that is, a stuporous or comatose patient in Stage II or III may enter Stage I and become agitated and delirious (118,119). Similarly, a conscious patient in Stage I may suddenly become comatose (116). The entire clinical episode may require up to 6 weeks to resolve (18).

The psychiatric manifestations of Stage I intoxication can resemble a variety of psychiatric syndromes, making differential diagnosis difficult in the absence of toxicology results or a history of recent PCP, ketamine, or DXM intake. Common syndromes seen in treatment settings include delirium, psychosis without delirium, catatonia, hypomania with euphoria, and depression with lethargy. Agitated or bizarre behavior, with increased risk of violence, can occur with any psychiatric presentation (32,111). Because of the analgesic effect of PCP, patients may not report the existence of even serious injuries (which may be self-inflicted) (74).

Clinically significant psychological and behavioral effects of DXM begin to occur at approximately five times the therapeutic dose. These effects can be grouped into four dose-dependent plateaus (Table 45.5).

TABLE 45.5 Psychologic and Behavioral Effects of Dextromethorphan Intoxication

Plateau	Dose (mg)	Behavioral effects
First	100–200	Mild stimulation
Second	200–400	Euphoria and hallucinations Distorted visual perceptions
Third	300–600	Loss of motor coordination Disorientation
Fourth	500–1,500	Depersonalization Dissociative sedation
Toxicity	Variable	Hyperexcitability, lethargy, ataxia, diaphoresis, hypertension, and nystagmus

Sources: Schwartz RH. Adolescent abuse of dextromethorphan. *Clin Pediatr,* 2005; 44(7): 565–568. http://www.deadiversion.usdoj.gov/drugs_concern/dextro_m/dextro_m.htm (accessed January 31, 2008).

Medical Effects of Dissociative Anesthetic Intoxication Intoxication at the mild Stage I desired by users is associated with few serious medical complications (Table 45.4) (111). Common medical effects at this stage include nystagmus (especially horizontal), tachycardia, increased blood pressure, ataxia, dysarthria, numbness, increased salivation, and hyperreflexia (74). Higher stages are associated with severe medical effects (Table 45.4), including hypertension, stroke, cardiac failure, seizures, rhabdomyolysis, acute renal failure, coma, and death (27).

The acute effects of ketamine tend to be less severe and of shorter duration than those of PCP, possibly due to its shorter half-life (120). Nystagmus occurs less often than with PCP.

Management of Psychologic and Behavioral Effects of Dissociative Anesthetic Intoxication Treatment of intoxication with dissociative anesthetics is largely supportive and aimed at controlling or reversing specific signs and symptoms (116). No clinically useful antagonist is yet available. The anticonvulsant lamotrigine (300 mg daily), which inhibits glutamate release, was found to reduce the psychologic and cognitive effects of ketamine in a small experimental trial (121). Mild Stage I intoxication is best treated without medication. The patient should be isolated in a quiet room with unobtrusive observation and minimal external stimuli. Frequent or intrusive contact or aggressive medical intervention may worsen the situation and should be avoided. Reassuring, reality-oriented communication ("talking down") rarely works with such patients (74). Urine acidification and diuretics may increase renal clearance of PCP, but are of doubtful clinical utility at this level of intoxication and may exacerbate myoglobinuric renal failure (27,122). Cranberry juice, commonly used as a urine acidifier in the non-medical setting, never has been clearly shown to decrease urine pH (123). Benzodiazepines should be used if medication is needed to control severe anxiety, agitation, or psychotic behavior (27), although they may delay renal clearance of PCP at high doses (118).

If benzodiazepines are insufficient to control psychosis, high-potency first-generation antipsychotics, such as haloperidol or droperidol, or second-generation antipsychotics, such as risperidone or olanzapine, may be used (124,125). They are less likely than other antipsychotics to produce anticholinergic or cardiovascular side effects that may exacerbate PCP's own anticholinergic and cardiovascular effects. No clinical trials have directly compared the efficacy and safety of first- versus second-generation antipsychotics or of benzodiazepines versus antipsychotics.

Management of Medical Effects of Dissociative Anesthetic Intoxication The mild medical effects commonly associated with Stage I intoxication usually do not need specific medical treatment.

Tachycardia and hypertension can be treated with adrenergic-blockers such as labetalol, or calcium channel blockers such as verapamil, although there are no controlled trials to substantiate their efficacy. Severe hypertension can be treated with IV nitroprusside (27).

Stage II and III intoxication are medical emergencies that require treatment in a comprehensive medical setting to maintain life support functions until the drug has been eliminated from the body (111). Tables 45.6 and 45.7 summarize medical treatment for acute PCP intoxication. In this context, increasing the renal clearance of PCP with forced diuresis and urine acidification (pH <5) may be helpful (73), although this may exacerbate myoglobinuric renal failure (27). This can be done by administering ammonium chloride—2.75 mEq/kg in 60 mL of saline every 6 hours through a nasogastric tube and 2 g of IV ascorbic acid in 500 mL of IV fluid every 6 hours (126). IM ascorbic acid also has been used successfully (127). Caution should be exercised to avoid causing metabolic acidosis, especially in the presence of drugs such as barbiturates and salicylates, whose renal clearance is delayed by acidification. Activated charcoal may be helpful, but induced vomiting or gastric lavage are not (12,27,128). Dialysis is not helpful because these agents have a large volume of distribution.

Another pharmacokinetic approach currently undergoing animal testing is administration of anti-PCP monoclonal antibody binding fragments (1). These antibody fragments bind to PCP molecules in the body and prevent them from entering the brain, thereby reducing the acute effects of a PCP dose. Further research is needed to establish the safety and efficacy of this antibody approach in humans.

DXM is marketed as part of multi-ingredient cough or cold preparations. Thus toxicity may result from these other ingredients (e.g., acetaminophen, pseudoephedrine, phenylephrine, guaifenesin, antihistamines) (129). The evaluation and treatment of patients with suspected DXM overdose must attend to the possibility of acetaminophen or other concomitant toxicity.

Dissociative Anesthetic Withdrawal Although a dissociative anesthetic withdrawal syndrome is not recognized in the DSM-IV-TR, about one fourth of heavy PCP users report withdrawal symptoms (82), including depression, anxiety, irritability, hypersomnolence, diaphoresis, and tremor (74,130), although it is not clear to what extent these represent a true withdrawal syndrome. DXM withdrawal has been associated with craving, dysphoria, and insomnia (131). Tricyclic antidepressants such as desipramine may reduce the psychologic symptoms associated with discontinuation of PCP use, but there is no evidence that such treatment improves the outcome of PCP addiction (130,132). The efficacy of selective serotonin reuptake inhibitors, which would be safer in this context, is unknown.

Prolonged Psychiatric Sequelae Hallucinogens and dissociative anesthetics (e.g., PCP) have the potential to trigger psychiatric sequelae that last beyond the period of acute intoxication, including prolonged states of anxiety, depression, or psychosis. The risk of a prolonged psychiatric reaction appears to depend on several factors: the patient's premorbid psychopathology, the number of prior exposures to the drug, and a history of polydrug use (80). Prolonged reactions occasionally are reported in apparently well-adjusted individuals who

TABLE 45.6 Procedures for Managing Acute Phencyclidine (PCP) Intoxication

Procedure	Stage I	Stage II	Stage III
Monitor level of consciousness	Yes	Yes	Yes
Monitor vital signs	Yes	Yes	Yes
Collect blood and urine samples for toxicology	Yes	Yes	Yes
Lower body temperature	Loosen clothing	Sponging, ice packs	Sponging, ice packs
Catheterize urinary bladder	No	Yes	Yes
Gastric lavage	No	Sometimes	Yes
Oral suctioning	Rarely	Gently, as needed	Yes
Tracheal suctioning	No	Sometimes	Yes
Insert nasogastric tube	No	Sometimes	Yes
Neuromuscular blockade and mechanical ventilation	No	Sometimes	Sometimes

Source: Milhorn TH. Diagnosis and management of phencyclidine intoxication. *Am Fam Phys* 1991;43(4):1293–1302.

TABLE 45.7 Medications for Treating Acute Phencyclidine (PCP) Intoxication

Medication	Stage I Conscious	Stage II Stuporous to unconscious; deep pain response intact	Stage III Unconscious; unresponsive to deep pain
Syrup of ipecac	Not indicated	Not indicated	Not indicated
Activated charcoal	Not indicated	If needed	50–150 g initially, then 30–40 g every 6–8 h
Diazepam	For agitation: 10–30 mg orally or 2.5 IV, up to 25 mg total	For muscle rigidity: same dosage, IM or IV, as for agitation in Stage I	For muscle rigidity: same as for Stage II. For status epilepticus: 5–10 mg IV, to 30 mg total
Lorazepam	For agitation: 2–4 mg IM as needed	Not indicated	Not indicated
Haloperidol	For psychosis: 5–10 mg	Not indicated	Not indicated
Ascorbic Acid	Not indicated	For urine pH <5.5: 0.5–1.5 g every 4–6 h as needed	As for Stage II
Hydralazine	Not indicated	For hypertension: 5–10 mg IV	For hypertension: 10–20 mg IV
Propranolol	Not indicated	For hypertension: 1 mg IV every 30 min as needed up to 8 mg total	As for Stage II
Furosemide	Not indicated	For increased urinary output: 20–40 mg IV every 6 h	As for Stage II
Aminophylline	Not indicated	For bronchospasm: 250 mg IV	As for Stage II

Source: Milhorn TH. Diagnosis and management of phencyclidine intoxication. *Am Fam Phys* 1991;43(4):1293–1302.

have no obvious risk factors. Prolonged psychotic reactions to PCP are almost always associated with premorbid psychopathology (133,134).

Treatment of prolonged anxiety or depression usually is psychosocial, but may involve medication if symptoms become sufficiently severe. Treatment of prolonged psychosis essentially follows guidelines for treatment of chronic functional psychosis. Patients may present with wide-ranging symptomatology: apathy, insomnia, hypomania, dissociative states, formal thought disorder, hallucinations, delusions, and paranoia. An observation period of at least several days with no or minimal medication (such as sedatives) is helpful to ensure an accurate diagnosis.

The term "flashback" (hallucinogen persisting perception disorder in DSM-IV-TR) has been given to brief episodes (often lasting a few seconds) in which perceptual aspects of a previous hallucinogenic drug experience are unexpectedly re-experienced after acute intoxication has resolved. Flashbacks are associated principally with LSD, although they can occur after use of other hallucinogens, MDMA, PCP, and, occasionally, marijuana (72,135,136). Flashbacks can precipitate considerable anxiety, particularly if the original drug experience had negative overtones. Re-experience of perceptual effects may be accompanied by somatic and emotional components of the original experience. Flashbacks may occur spontaneously or be triggered by stress, exercise, another drug (such as marijuana), or a situation reminiscent of the original drug experience.

Flashbacks usually are brief and self-limiting. Treatment may involve no more than alleviating anxiety with supportive reassurance. Over time, flashbacks tend to decrease in frequency, duration, and intensity, as long as no further hallucinogens are taken (80).

There have been no clinical trials of pharmacologic treatment for flashbacks (135,136). Benzodiazepines are helpful in treating secondary anxiety. Small case series suggest that clonazepam, clonidine, and haloperidol may be helpful, whereas case reports suggest that phenothiazines, risperidone, and selective serotonin reuptake inhibitors may worsen the condition.

INHALANTS

Inhalant Intoxication Inhalant intoxication produces initial euphoria or "rush," followed by lightheadedness, excitability, and perceptual changes (137,138). Significant mood changes or cognitive impairment are rare. Higher doses or more prolonged exposure may cause dizziness, slurred speech, and motor incoordination, followed by drowsiness and headache. Intoxicated users rarely seek medical attention, in part because exposure tends to be self-limited and the duration of effect from a single exposure is usually only a few minutes.

There is no specific treatment for inhalant intoxication (138). The patient should be assessed, stabilized, and monitored (especially cardiopulmonary status and hydration) in accordance with their clinical condition. Inhalants may sensitize the myocardium, so pressor medications and bronchodilators are relatively contraindicated.

Inhalant Withdrawal Inhalant withdrawal is primarily associated with drug craving and occasional tachycardia and diaphoresis (137). Prominent psychologic or physical symptoms are rare. There is no specific treatment for inhalant withdrawal (138).

CLUB DRUGS

"Club drugs" are a pharmacologically heterogeneous group of drugs associated with a youth subculture that revolves around late-night dance parties known as "raves" or "trances" (113,139). The illicit use of these substances was popularized in this setting because of their perceived ability to enhance the sensory experience and allow for long periods of dancing to repetitive music. Common club drugs include MDMA ("Ecstasy"), an amphetamine analogue with stimulant and hallucinogenic properties, as well as GHB and flunitrazepam (Rohypnol), both of which are CNS depressants. Pharmacologic interactions from the concurrent use of multiple club drugs substantially increase the risk of toxicity (140).

MDMA ("ECSTASY")

"Ecstasy" is the common street name for 3,4-methylenedioxymethamphetamine (MDMA) (see Chapter 14). Related amphetamine analogues such as 3,4-ethylenedioxyethylamphetamine ("Eve"), 3,4-methylenedioxyamphetamine, and N-methyl-1-(3,4-methylenedioxyphenyl)-2-butanamine may also be present in street preparations. The effects of MDMA are those of a stimulant combined with a mild hallucinogen. "Herbal Ecstasy" often refers to preparations containing the stimulant ephedrine. "Liquid Ecstasy" is a street name for GHB (see the following section).

MDMA often is taken concurrently with other drugs, such as LSD (in a combination called "candyflipping"), for enhanced effect. Dextromethorphan (available in over-the-counter cough medicines) is a frequent concomitant drug, and may be substituted for MDMA in street preparations (141). "Stacking" refers to the practice of taking multiple MDMA doses over a short period, often alternating with other drugs to enhance the experience. For example, amphetamine or cocaine may be used initially to augment the experience, followed later by a CNS depressant, such as alcohol, marijuana, or GHB, to temper the "coming down" (113). Menthol, camphor, or ephedrine may be applied to the nasal mucosa or chest wall to enhance the drug experience (139).

MDMA has good oral bioavailability and readily crosses the blood–brain barrier (139,142). The onset of action is within 30 minutes and peak plasma concentrations are achieved in one to three hours (139,143). The elimination half-life is 7 to 8 hours. Because MDMA is a weak acid, this is delayed to 16 to 31 hours with alkaline urine. MDMA is metabolized by several hepatic microsomal enzymes, chiefly CYP2D6.

Individuals who are genetically deficient in CYP2D6 (up to 10% of whites) are theoretically at increased risk of developing MDMA toxicity (144), though some studies suggest this risk is minimal (145).

MDMA appears to have nonlinear kinetics because the higher affinity enzymes become saturated at relatively low drug concentrations (142). This results in disproportionately large increases in drug concentrations in response to small increases in dose (144) and may account for the poor correlation between plasma concentration and toxicity (146). A major MDMA metabolite is methylenedioxyamphetamine (MDA), which also is pharmacologically active and has a longer elimination half-life of 16 to 38 hours (147).

MDMA Intoxication The diagnosis of MDMA intoxication is made by history of drug intake and/or analysis of unused drug. Most signs and symptoms are not specific to MDMA, but resemble those of stimulants or hallucinogens. MDMA is not detected by routine urine or blood drug screens, which may be positive for amphetamines (products of MDMA metabolism) (139).

Gastric lavage with activated charcoal may be helpful within the first hour after ingestion, especially if other drugs also have been taken. Induced emesis is not recommended because of the risk of CNS depression (139). Acidification of urine would quicken MDMA elimination, but usually is contraindicated because it would increase the risk of metabolic acidosis and exacerbate renal toxicity from rhabdomyolysis (139).

Psychologic and Behavioral Effects of MDMA Intoxication Low to moderate oral doses of MDMA (50 to 150 mg) typically produce an intense initial effect (known as "coming on" or "rush"), especially if taken on an empty stomach, that may last 30 to 45 minutes (113). These desired effects include increased wakefulness and energy, euphoria, increased sexual desire and satisfaction, heightened sensory perception, sociability, and increased empathy and sense of closeness to others (139,142,148,149). The initial phase is followed by several hours of less intense experience ("plateau"), during which repetitive dancing is common. Users start to "come down" 3 to 6 hours after ingestion (113).

Undesired effects may occur with repeated use or at higher doses (150). These include hyperactivity, fatigue, insomnia, anxiety, agitation, impaired decision making, flight of ideas, hallucinations, depersonalization, derealization, and bizarre or reckless behavior. Some users develop panic attacks, brief psychotic episodes, or delirium, which usually resolve rapidly as the drug effect wears off (151). Initial treatment should be the same as for hallucinogen intoxication: placement in a quiet, reassuring environment, with observation to reduce the risk of unintended self-injury. Physical restraints are contraindicated because they may exacerbate anxiety and increase the risk of rhabdomyolysis. If severe or persisting symptoms require medication, benzodiazepines are preferred. Antipsychotics should be avoided as much as possible because they may increase the risk of hyperthermia and seizures. A high-potency antipsychotic such as haloperidol should be used if necessary. The role of second-generation antipsychotics remains unclear. A few users may develop persisting depression or recurrent psychotic symptoms or panic attacks, which require psychiatric treatment.

Medical Effects of MDMA Intoxication The acute physical effects of MDMA at low to moderate doses resemble those of a stimulant: increased muscle tension, jaw clenching, tooth grinding (bruxism), restlessness, insomnia, ataxia, headache, nausea, decreased appetite, dry mouth, dilated pupils, and increased heart rate and blood pressure (139,142,148,149). Doses >200 mg are associated with life-threatening toxicities that can be grouped into four major syndromes (152). Most dangerous is hyperthermia, which results from a combination of increased physical activity (as through vigorous dancing), warm environment (as in a crowded, poorly ventilated dance club), and disruption of thermoregulation by the drug, often exacerbated by dehydration (153). The syndrome may resemble that of severe heatstroke. The high body temperature causes rhabdomyolysis (with resulting myoglobinuria and renal failure), liver damage, or disseminated intravascular coagulation (resulting in hemorrhage). Treatment is based on early recognition, close monitoring of serum creatinine kinase levels (to detect rhabdomyolysis), and reversal of the hyperthermia. Core body temperatures >102°F call for urgent measures such as ice-water sponging, gastric or bladder lavage with cool liquids, and intravenous infusion of chilled saline. Muscle paralysis with intubation may be required for refractory, ongoing rhabdomyolysis. Rhabdomyolysis treatment includes vigorous hydration and alkalinization of the urine to minimize myoglobin precipitation in the renal tubules.

Benzodiazepines help control both the hyperthermia and agitation. Antipsychotics should be avoided because they interfere with heat dissipation and lower the seizure threshold. Recent case series suggest that dantrolene (1 mg/kg IV) may be helpful. Because of similarities between MDMA toxicity and the serotonin syndrome (see the following section), serotonin antagonists such as methysergide and cyproheptadine have been used successfully.

Acute hepatic toxicity from MDMA may be related to metabolism into reactive intermediaries that deplete hepatic glutathione, resulting in cell death (142,147). The clinical picture can vary from a mild hepatitis (marked by enlarged, tender liver and elevated serum liver enzymes) that resolves spontaneously over several weeks to fulminant liver failure requiring transplantation. Liver toxicity may be exacerbated by hyperthermia.

Acute cardiovascular toxicity from MDMA is the result of increased catecholamine activity (142,154). This may cause hypertension, with risk of blood vessel rupture and hemorrhage, or tachycardia and cardiac arrhythmia. The preferred treatment is an adrenergic antagonist with both alpha and beta blocking activity, combined with a vasodilator such as nitroglycerin or nitroprusside if needed to control blood pressure. A pure beta-adrenergic blocker should be avoided because of the remaining unopposed alpha-adrenergic stimulation, resulting in vasoconstriction and worsening hypertension. Hypertensive crisis unresponsive to mixed adrenergic blockers and vasodilators should be treated with an alpha-adrenergic antagonist such as phentolamine (35). Cardiac ischemia or arrhythmia should be treated by standard clinical protocols. Agitation should be controlled with a short-acting benzodiazepine such as lorazepam.

In addition to direct MDMA-mediated neurotoxicity (155), acute toxicity can result from hyponatremia ("water intoxication"), which may cause seizures and intracranial fluid shifts that compress the brain stem into the foramen magnum (142). The hyponatremia is caused by loss of sodium in sweat (as during vigorous dancing in a warm environment) and hemodilution from drinking large amounts of water and the antidiuretic effect of MDMA. The conservative initial treatment is fluid restriction. Profound hyponatremia has been treated with hypertonic saline solution (156). Intravenous benzodiazepines should be used to control seizures.

MDMA Withdrawal Symptoms during the first few days after MDMA use may resemble a mild form of stimulant withdrawal or "crash," with depression, anxiety, fatigue, and difficulty concentrating (113,142). These usually resolve without treatment.

Medical Effects of MDMA Withdrawal There is no evidence of a physically prominent or distinctive withdrawal syndrome associated with MDMA that would require specific pharmacologic treatment. Users may complain of muscle pain and stiffness in the jaw, neck, lower back, and limbs for the first 2 to 3 days after use (142), which may be the result of MDMA-induced muscle tension and the vigorous dancing often associated with MDMA use. There is some evidence of increased variability of heart rate and blood pressure for several days after MDMA use.

GAMMA-HYDROXYBUTYRATE (GHB)

GHB (or "liquid Ecstasy") is a naturally occurring metabolite of the neurotransmitter gamma-aminobutyric acid (GABA) (see sidebar, Chapter 8). It is approved for the treatment of narcolepsy (Xyrem, schedule III) (111–112), but is also used recreationally (139,157). GHB became popular in the late 1980s in part because of its reputed aphrodisiac, disinhibitory, and amnestic effects (140), short duration of action, absence of "hangover," and nondetectability by standard drug screens.

The legal precursors gamma-butyrolactone (GBL, an industrial solvent found in floor strippers and some household products) and 1,4-butanediol (1,4-BD), which are readily metabolized to GBH in the body, are also used recreationally (158).

GHB is taken orally as a liquid or in a powder mixed into drinks. A typical dose is one to three teaspoons or capfuls. GHB is rapidly absorbed from the gastrointestinal tract and readily crosses the blood–brain barrier. Effects begin within 15 minutes of ingestion and last 2 to 4 hours. The blood elimination half-life is about 30 minutes, largely because of rapid redistribution into other tissues.

GHB Intoxication The diagnosis of GHB intoxication is based on clinical suspicion, a history of drug intake, or analysis of unused drug. The signs and symptoms are not specific for GHB, but resemble those of any CNS depressant. GHB is not detected by routine drug toxicology assays.

There is no proven antidote for GHB intoxication. Physostigmine, naloxone, and flumazenil have reversed some GHB effects in small case series or animal studies (159), but should be considered experimental. Gastric lavage usually is not helpful because of rapid gastrointestinal absorption, but activated charcoal may be.

Psychologic and Behavioral Effects of GHB Intoxication The desired acute effects of GHB at low oral doses (<20 mg/kg) include relaxation, euphoria, sedation, disinhibition, sociability, and anterograde amnesia (112,160). Higher doses produce somnolence, confusion, and hallucinations (161). Unintended overdose may occur because of GHB's very steep dose-response curve and the great variability in potency of street preparations. First-time users often underestimate the potency of GHB. The effects are prolonged and intensified when taken with other CNS depressants, such as alcohol. Patients recovering from acute GHB intoxication may wake up abruptly with a clear sensorium, or may go through a brief period of agitation and combativeness.

Medical Effects of GHB Intoxication Low to moderate oral doses of GHB may cause headache, dizziness, ataxia, hypotonia, and vomiting (112,139,157). Higher doses (>30 mg/kg) may cause incontinence, myoclonic movements, bradycardia, hypotension, hypothermia, generalized tonic-clonic seizures, and coma (27,162). Most patients recover completely within several hours with supportive care and do not require intubation (163). However, death may result from respiratory depression, so that intubation and mechanical ventilation may be indicated in severe cases. Seizures should be controlled with benzodiazepines, symptomatic bradycardia with atropine, and symptomatic hypotension with intravenous saline (27). Similar adverse effects occur with GBL and 1,4-BD (164).

GHB Withdrawal Cessation of chronic GHB or GBL use leads to a discrete withdrawal syndrome resembling that of sedative-hypnotic withdrawal. Anxiety, restlessness, insomnia, tremor, nystagmus, tachycardia, and hypertension usually appear 2 to 12 hours after the last dose (112,165). Mild symptoms usually resolve gradually over 1 to 2 weeks. More severe withdrawal may cause delirium with hallucinations, psychosis, agitation, and autonomic instability. GHB withdrawal seizures have not been reported.

Most cases of GHB withdrawal can be effectively managed through use of a long-acting benzodiazepine, tapering the dose after the symptoms have been controlled (as for sedative-hypnotic withdrawal) (112,166). Severe cases may require high doses (several hundred milligrams) or parenteral administration. Patients unresponsive to benzodiazepines may benefit from barbiturates, a mood stabilizer such as gabapentin, or low-dose antipsychotics (112).

HERBS OF ABUSE

Herbs are plants used for medicinal, culinary, or spiritual purposes. Many herbs contain psychoactive compounds with stimulant, anxiogenic, anxiolytic, hallucinogenic, euphoric, or dissociative effects (167,168). These properties have long been recognized in many indigenous cultures.

The psychoactive profile of herbs, combined with the fact that production, sale, and purchase of most herbs is largely unregulated, has contributed to a growing market for their recreational use (169). Internet distribution of herbs makes them widely available to minors (170). The perception that herbs are safer than illicit drugs, coupled with the absence of clearly established dosing parameters, may contribute to their misuse. Routine toxicology screens do not detect many of these substances, so that identifying specific intoxication syndromes may be challenging. If a patient is unable to provide pertinent history, accurate diagnosis may rest on collateral information from family, friends, and first responders, in addition to a thorough clinical examination.

Intoxication Herbs of abuse often contain multiple psychoactive compounds, so that intoxication syndromes may not fit neatly into distinctive classifications. For clarity, herbs of abuse may be categorized as predominantly hallucinogenic or stimulating. Table 45.8 describes basic characteristics of some of the commonest herbs of abuse.

Hallucinogenic herbs achieve their psychotomimetic effects principally through activity at serotonergic or cholinergic receptors (see Chapter 14). Stimulating herbs generally augment the activity of norepinephrine, dopamine, or acetylcholine (see Chapter 10). Thus the manifestations and management of intoxication syndromes for this varied group of substances generally follow that for hallucinogen and stimulant intoxication (see relevant sections presented previously).

Management of Psychologic, Behavioral, and Medical Effects Management of intoxication with hallucinogenic herbs is largely supportive because most symptoms, including psychosis, are self-limited. The goal is to maintain safety, preventing patients from physically harming themselves or others. A quiet environment, with calm counseling and guidance, often avoids the need for pharmacologic interventions. Medications with anticholinergic properties are usually avoided to minimize the possibility of exacerbating substance-induced delirium. Physical restraints should be avoided because they increase psychologic distress and may contribute to rhabdomyolysis. Patients who are agitated, in severe panic, or having distressing psychotic symptoms may be relieved by benzodiazepines (e.g., lorazepam 2 mg PO/IM every 1 to 2 hours,

TABLE 45.8 Common Herbal Drugs of Abuse

Herb	Street names	Predominant psychoactive compound	Predominant mechanism of action	Typical duration of action	Dosage at which toxicity becomes more prominent	Urine toxicology screen
Salvia divinorum	Magic mint; Sally-D; Ska	Salvinorin A	Kappa opioid agonist	15 min	>500 μg	Negative
Myristica fragrans	Nutmeg	Myristicin, elemicin, safrole	MAO inhibition, serotonergic	24–72 h	>20 g (5 teaspoons)	Negative
Lophophora williamsii	Peyote; buttons; mescal	Mescaline	Serotonergic; dopaminergic	1–12 h	400–500 mg (6–12 buttons)	Negative
Psilocybe mushrooms	Magic mushrooms, shrooms	Psilocybin, psilocin	Serotonergic	2–6 h	>50 mg (>5 g mushrooms)	Negative
Amanita muscaria	Fly agaric	Ibotenic acid, muscimol	Glutamatergic GABAergic	0.5–3 h	(100 g dried mushrooms)	Negative
Ayahuasca (mixture of various plants)	Huasca, yage, brew, daime	DMT + MAO inhibitor	Serotonergic; anticholinergic	20–60 min	Varies	Negative
Ipomea violacea	Morning glory	LSA	Serotonergic	6–10 h	3–6 gm (25–200 seeds)	Negative
Argyremia nervosa	Hawaiian baby	LSA	Serotonergic	6–10 h	3–6 gm (5–10 seeds)	Negative
Datura stramonium	Jimsonweed, loco-weed, stink weed	Atropine, scopolamine, hyoscyamine	Anticholinergic	1 hr-several days	Varies	Negative
Ephedra species	Ma-huang, herbal ecstasy	Ephedrine, pseudoephedrine	Sympathomimetic	6 h	>8 mg at one time, or >100 mg	MA+
Pausinystalia yohimbe	Yohimbine	Yohimbine	Adrenergic, serotonergic	3–4 h	>35 mg	Negative
Catha edulis	Khat; qat	Cathinone, cathine	Sympathomimetic	1–4 h	>100 mg	Negative
Areca catechu	Betel nut	Arecoline	Cholinergic	2–17 min	Varies	Negative

Sources: Halpern JH. Hallucinogens and dissociative agents naturally growing in the United States. *Pharmacol Ther* 2004;102:131–138; Richardson WH, Slone CM, Michels JE. Herbal drugs of abuse: an emerging problem. *Emerg Med Clin N Am* 2007;254:35–57.

DMT, N,N-dimethyltryptamine; GABA, γ-aminobutyric acid; LSA, lysergic acid hydroxyethylamide; MA, methamphetamine; MAO, monoamine oxidase.

titrated to mild sedation). In cases where predisposing factors or heavy chronic use contribute to prolonged psychotic symptoms, antipsychotic agents may be useful.

Management of intoxication with stimulant herbs is similar to that with hallucinogenic herbs, except that the former are more likely to generate hyperexcitable, agitated, and psychotic states. Patients with unstable vital signs should be closely monitored, including cardiac function, blood pressure, and body temperature. Beta-adrenergic blockers are generally avoided due to concern about unopposed alpha-adrenergic activity.

With one exception, there are no specific antidotes to intoxication with psychoactive herbs. Intoxication with herbs having anticholinergic activity (e.g., jimsonweed) has been successfully treated with physostigmine, a short-acting acetylcholinesterase inhibitor (167). Severe intoxication with betel nut, which has cholinergic activity, can be treated with atropine, a cholinergic antagonist.

Withdrawal Most users of psychoactive herbs do not consume large enough amounts for long enough periods to develop physical dependence or a withdrawal syndrome. Some users of khat and betel nuts do experience a withdrawal syndrome, often including irritability, fatigue, and rhinorrhea (167). Protracted withdrawal symptoms (e.g., psychosis, depression, anxiety), should be treated symptomatically while the patient is evaluated for an underlying psychiatric disorder.

FLUNITRAZEPAM

Flunitrazepam (Rohypnol, also known as "roofies" or the "date rape pill") is a potent, fast-acting benzodiazepine that frequently causes anterograde amnesia (121,158). It is legally manufactured and marketed in Europe and Latin America, but is illegal in the United States because of its association with date rape. Flunitrazepam is difficult to detect with routine toxicology screens because of its low concentration.

Flunitrazepam Intoxication Flunitrazepam intoxication resembles intoxication with other benzodiazepines, and features sedation, disinhibition, anterograde amnesia, confusion, ataxia, bradycardia, hypotension, and respiratory depression (see Chapter 43). Overdose rarely is life-threatening unless the drug is combined with another CNS depressant, such as alcohol. Treatment is supportive; activated charcoal and gastric lavage may be helpful. When respiratory depression or circulatory compromise are severe, the benzodiazepine antagonist flumazenil (Romazicon) may be used, albeit cautiously. Flumazenil precipitates acute withdrawal in patients who are physically dependent on benzodiazepines and lowers the seizure threshold, thus increasing the risk of withdrawal seizures. Flumazenil is effective for about 20 minutes, so that repeated dosing is necessary to avoid re-sedation by flunitrazepam.

Flunitrazepam Withdrawal A typical sedative-hypnotic withdrawal syndrome can develop after cessation of chronic flunitrazepam use. Withdrawal symptoms can develop up to 36 hours after the last dose and include anxiety, restlessness, tremors, headache, insomnia, and paraesthesias. Treatment of withdrawal involves supportive measures and substitution with cross-tolerant medications such as lorazepam or clonazepam, followed by gradual tapering.

SEROTONIN SYNDROME

The serotonin syndrome may account for some of the severe complications associated with intoxication and overdose on amphetamines or MDMA, especially when these are used concurrently with other drugs or medications that increase serotonergic activity (171). The serotonin syndrome is a triad of signs and symptoms, consisting of mental status changes (e.g., anxiety, confusion, agitation, lethargy, delirium, coma), autonomic hyperactivity (e.g., low-grade fever, tachycardia, diaphoresis, nausea, vomiting, diarrhea, dilated pupils, abdominal pain, hypertension, tachypnea), and neuromuscular abnormalities (e.g., myoclonus, nystagmus, hyperreflexia, rigidity, trismus, tremor) (172,173). The clinical presentation is highly variable, making diagnosis difficult, but neuromuscular signs are usually prominent.

The differential diagnosis includes neuroleptic malignant syndrome (with which it is most commonly confused), sepsis, heat stroke, delirium tremens, and sympathomimetic or anticholinergic poisoning. Patients with neuroleptic malignant syndrome differ from those with serotonin syndrome in that they are more likely to present with extrapyramidal signs and autonomic instability and rarely present with the neuromuscular changes common in serotonin syndrome.

The serotonin syndrome is the result of excessive stimulation of 5-HT_{2A}, possibly with some contribution also from 5-HT_{1A}, receptors. This can occur through several different pathways: activation of serotonin receptors by agonists, enhanced release of serotonin (by MDMA or amphetamines), decreased presynaptic serotonin reuptake (by cocaine or selective serotonin reuptake inhibitor antidepressants), decreased serotonin metabolism (by amphetamines or monoamine oxidase inhibitors), and increased serotonin synthesis. The serotonin syndrome is most commonly seen after ingestion of two or more drugs with such actions, but also may occur with a single drug.

The onset of the serotonin syndrome may be within minutes to hours of medication initiation, increase in dose, or overdose. Laboratory abnormalities are nonspecific, but elevated creatine phosphokinase, liver transaminases, white blood cell count, serum bicarbonate, and evidence of disseminated intravascular coagulation may occur in severe cases. In severe cases, or in the absence of appropriate diagnosis and treatment, there may be progression to rhabdomyolysis, hyperthermia, renal failure, disseminated intravascular coagulation, and death.

Effective treatment of the serotonin syndrome requires early identification, immediate discontinuation of all serotonergic medications, close monitoring, and supportive care, usually including intravenous hydration (172,173). Such treatment usually results in a benign, self-limited course; many cases resolve within 24 hours. Muscle rigidity and spasm should be controlled with benzodiazepines to prevent rhabdomyolysis. Severe forms of the syndrome may require more aggressive measures, including neuromuscular blocking agents, mechanical ventilation, and external cooling. Treatment with a 5-HT_{2A} receptor antagonist (e.g., cyproheptadine, olanzapine, chlorpromazine) has been effective in case series, but has not yet been evaluated in controlled clinical trials.

WITHDRAWAL FROM MULTIPLE DRUGS

Multiple Sedative-Hypnotics Withdrawal from dependence on multiple sedative-hypnotic agents, including alcohol, is best managed in the same way as withdrawal from a single such drug: by using tapering dosages of a single, longer-acting sedative-hypnotic (18,174). It usually is safest to focus on managing withdrawal of the longer-acting drug. The time course of withdrawal from multiple sedative-hypnotics is more unpredictable than from single drugs; for example, there may be a bimodal time course of symptomatology if one drug is short-acting and the other is longer-acting. The rate at which the dose is tapered usually should not exceed 10% per day. Successful withdrawal may be facilitated by use of an anticonvulsant such as carbamazepine (175), although such use has not been evaluated in multiple drug withdrawal.

Sedative-Hypnotics with Other Drugs In the pharmacologic management of patients withdrawing from both sedative-hypnotics and CNS stimulants, it is preferable to treat the sedative-hypnotic withdrawal first, because this poses the greatest difficulty and medical risk. For concurrent addiction to sedative-hypnotics and opiates, concurrent pharmacologic treatment is recommended (18,174). The patient may be stabilized on an opiate (preferably oral methadone, although codeine can be used if methadone is not available) at the same time that the sedative-hypnotic dose is tapered by 10% per day. After the sedative-hypnotic withdrawal is completed, opiate withdrawal can begin. Clonidine has been suggested as adjunctive treatment for such mixed sedative-hypnotic and opiate withdrawal, because it can alleviate withdrawal symptoms from both drug classes, but this has not been evaluated systematically.

POPULATION-SPECIFIC CONSIDERATIONS

Neonates Neonatal drug exposure is a substantial public health problem. Many drugs of abuse are readily transferred from the maternal circulation across the placenta to the fetus. Thus, perinatal drug use by the mother raises the possibility of drug intoxication or withdrawal in the newborn (176–178). Obtaining an accurate maternal drug use history for the period preceding delivery is essential. Meconium is the most accurate substrate for neonatal toxicology through the third to fourth day of life, but such testing is not widely available.

Neonatal signs and symptoms of drug intoxication or withdrawal often are nonspecific, including sedation, irritability, restlessness, hypertonia, hyperreflexia, tremors, poor feeding, abnormal sleep patterns, respiratory difficulty, and seizures. Stimulants (such as cocaine), marijuana, LSD, and PCP all have been associated with a neonatal withdrawal syndrome, although one that usually is less intense than the opiate withdrawal syndrome (179).

Perinatal use of stimulants by the mother can be associated with either bradycardia or tachycardia in the newborn (180). The additive cardiovascular effects of the stimulant and the normal catecholamine surge during labor may cause fetal distress and retard delivery (181). These cardiac effects usually resolve as the drug is eliminated from the body. Neonatal stimulant intoxication may be associated with irritability, tremors, hyperactivity, abnormal movements, excessive sucking, and high-pitched and excessive crying for 1 to 2 days, followed by a period of lethargy and hyporeactivity (181–183).

Treatment of drug-exposed newborns is largely supportive, with avoidance of overstimulation. Pharmacologic treatment should be used cautiously because it has its own potential for morbidity. Phenobarbital is the preferred medication for newborns with nonopiate drug withdrawal who do require pharmacologic treatment, as when seizures are a factor. A loading dose of 5 mg/kg/day is given until withdrawal is controlled, with adjustments of 10% to 20% every 2 to 3 days based on the response. Phenobarbital has a long half-life, so plasma concentrations should be checked periodically to avoid drug accumulation and overtreatment.

Older Adults Rates of illicit drug use by the elderly are low, but may be increasing (184). There is little published data on the treatment of drug intoxication or withdrawal in this age group. The elderly may be more susceptible to confusion and disorientation during withdrawal and to medication-induced delirium. The recommended dosing approach is "start low and go slow"; that is, start medication at a lower dose and increase the dose in smaller increments than would be used in younger individuals.

Adolescents Adolescence is the common age of onset for illegal drug use and abuse (185) and the developing adolescent brain may be especially vulnerable to the neurobiologic effects of drugs (186). Adolescents experience symptoms of drug withdrawal similar to those in adults, including physical symptoms (187). There are few published data on the treatment of drug intoxication or withdrawal in adolescents (188,189).

Women Women often differ from men in their response to psychoactive drugs and to drug abuse treatment (190), but there has been little systematic study of gender differences in the treatment of drug intoxication and withdrawal. Limited anecdotal evidence suggests that pharmacologic treatment for women is similar to that for men, taking into account possible gender differences in medication pharmacokinetics. Two topics requiring further research are the influence of the menstrual cycle on intoxication and withdrawal and their treatment and the effects of intoxication and withdrawal and their treatment on pregnancy and the fetus.

ACKNOWLEDGMENTS: *Dr. Gorelick is supported by the Intramural Research Program, National Institutes of Health, National Institute on Drug Abuse.*

REFERENCES

1. Gorelick DA. Pharmacokinetic approaches to treatment of drug addiction. *Exp Rev Clin Pharmacol* 2008;1:277–290.
2. Johanson CE, Fischman MW. The pharmacology of cocaine related to its abuse. *Pharmacol Rev* 198941:3–52.
3. Sulzer D, Sonders MS, Poulsen NW, et al. Mechanisms of neurotransmitter release by amphetamines: a review. *Prog Neurobiol* 2005;75(6):406–433.
4. Newton TF, Roache JD, De La Garza R 2nd, et al. Bupropion reduces methamphetamine-induced subjective effects and cue-induced craving. *Neuropsychopharmacology* 2006;31(7):1537–1544.
5. Lile JA, Stoops WW, Vansickel AR, et al. Aripiprazole attenuates the discriminative-stimulus and subject-rated effects of D-amphetamine in humans. *Neuropsychopharmacology* 2005;30(11):2103–2114
6. Rush CR, Stoops WW, Hays LR, et al. Risperidone attenuates the discriminative-stimulus effects of d-amphetamine in humans. *J Pharmacol Exp Ther* 2003;306(1):195–204.

7. Johnson BA, Roache JD, Ait-Daoud N, et al. Effects of acute topiramate dosing on methamphetamine-induced subjective mood. *Int J Neuropsychopharmacol* 2007;10(1):85–98.
8. McGregor C, Srisurapanont M, Mitchell A, et al. Symptoms and sleep patterns during inpatient treatment of methamphetamine withdrawal: a comparison of mirtazapine and modafinil with treatment as usual. *J Subst Abuse Treat* 2008;35(3):334–342.
9. Romanelli F, Smith KM. Clinical effects and management of methamphetamine abuse. *Pharmacotherapy* 2006;35(3):334–342.
10. Cubells JF, Kranzler HR, McCance-Katz E, et al. A haplotype at the DBH locus, associated with low plasma dopamine beta-hydroxylase activity, also associates with cocaine-induced paranoia. *Mol Psychiatry* 2000;5(1):56–63.
11. Hall W, Hando J, Darke S, et al. Psychological morbidity and route of administration among amphetamine users in Sydney, Australia. *Addiction* 1996;91(1):81–87.
12. Thirthalli J, Benegal V. Psychosis among substance users. *Curr Opin Psychiatry* 2006;19:239–245.
13. Harris D, Batki SL. Stimulant psychosis: symptom profile and acute clinical course. *Am J Addict* 2000;9(1):28–37.
14. Rosse RB, Collins Jr JP, Fay-McCarthy M, et al. Phenomenologic comparison of the idiopathic psychosis of schizophrenia and drug-induced cocaine and phencyclidine psychoses: a retrospective study. *Clin Neuropharmacol* 1994;17(4):359–369.
15. Ujike H, Sato M. Clinical features of sensitization to methamphetamine observed in patients with methamphetamine dependence and psychosis. *Ann N Y Acad Sci* 2004;1025:279–288.
16. Mahoney JJ III, Kalechstein AD, De La Garza R, et al. Presence and persistence of psychotic symptoms in cocaine- versus methamphetamine-dependent participants. *Am J Addict* 2008;17(2):83–98.
17. Matsuzawa D,Hashimoto K, Miyatake R, et al. Identification of functional polymorphisms in the promoter region of the human PICK1 gene and their association with methamphetamine psychosis. *Am J Psychiatry* 2007;164:1105–1114.
18. Schuckit MA. *Drug and alcohol abuse. A clinical guide to diagnosis and treatment,* 6th ed. New York: Springer, 2006.
19. Karch SB, Stephens BG. Drug abusers who die during arrest or in custody. *J Roy Soc Med* 1999;92:110–113.
20. Ruttenber AJ, McAnally HB, Wetli CV. Cocaine-associated rhabdomyolysis and excited delirium: different stages of the same syndrome. *Am J Forensic Med Pathol* 1999;20(2):120–127.
21. Miyashita T, Hayashi T, Ishida Y, et al. A fatal case of pontine hemorrhage related to methamphetamine abuse. *J Forensic Leg Med* 2007; 14(7):444–447.
22. McGee SM, McGee DN, McGee MB. Spontaneous intracerebral hemorrhage related to methamphetamine abuse: autopsy findings and clinical correlation. *Am J Forensic Med Pathol* 2004;25(4):334–337.
23. Brady WJ Jr, Duncan CW. Hypoglycemia masquerading as acute psychosis and acute cocaine intoxication. *Am J Emerg Med* 1999;17(3): 318–319.
24. Ling W, Rawson R, Shoptaw S, Ling W. Management of methamphetamine abuse and dependence. *Curr Psychiatry Rep* 2006;8(5):345–354.
25. Roth BA, Benowitz NL, Olson KR. Emergency management of drug abuse-related disorders. In: Karch SB, ed. *Drug abuse handbook.* Boca Raton, FL: CRC Press, 1998:567–639.
26. Mohr WK, Petti TA, Mohr BD. Adverse effects associated with physical restraint. *Can J Psychiatry* 2003;48(5):330–337.
27. Mokhlesi B, Garimella PS, Joffe A, et al. Street drug abuse leading to critical illness. *Intensive Care Med* 2004;30:1526–1536.
28. Srisurapanont M, Kittirattanapaiboon P, Jarusuraisin N, Treatment for amphetamine psychosis. *Cochrane Database Syst Rev* 2001;CD003026.
29. Callaway CW, Clark RF. Hyperthermia in psychostimulant overdose. *Ann Emerg Med* 1994;24:68–75.
30. Ruha AM, Yarema. Pharmacologic treatment of acute pediatric methamphetamine toxicity. *Pediatr Emerg Care* 2006;22(12):782–785.
31. Stoops WW, Lile JA, Lofwall MR, et al. The safety, tolerability, and subject-rated effects of acute intranasal cocaine administration during aripiprazole maintenance. *Am J Drug Alcohol Abuse* 2007;33:769–776.
32. Hurlbut KM. Drug-induced psychoses. *Emerg Med Clin N Am* 1991; 9(1):31–52.
33. Satel SL, Seibyl JP, Charney DS. Prolonged cocaine psychosis implies underlying major psychopathology. *J Clin Psychiatry* 1991;52(8): 349–350.
34. Yui K, Goto K, Ikemoto S. The role of noradrenergic and dopaminergic hyperactivity in the development of spontaneous recurrence of methamphetamine psychosis and susceptibility to episode recurrence. *Ann N Y Acad Sci* 2004;1025:296–306.
35. Ghuran A, Nolan J. Recreational drug misuse: issues for the cardiologist. *Heart* 2000;83:627–633.
36. Neiman J, Haapaniemi HM, Hillblom M. Neurological complications of drug abuse: pathophysiological mechanisms. *Eur J Neurol* 2000;7: 595–606.
37. Nzerue CM, Hewan-Lowe K, Riley Jr LJ. Cocaine and the kidney: a synthesis of pathophysiologic and clinical perspectives. *Am J Kidney Dis* 2000;35(5):783–795.
38. Richards JR, Johnson EB, Stark RW, et al. Methamphetamine abuse and rhabdomyolysis in the ED: a 5-year study. *Am J Emerg Med* 1999; 17:681–685.
39. Darke S, Kaye S, McKetin R, et al. Major physical and psychological harms of methamphetamine use. *Drug Alcohol Rev* 2008;27:253–262.
40. Pozner CN, Levine M, Zane R. The cardiovascular effects of cocaine. *J Emerg Med* 2005;29:173–178.
41. Blaho K, Logan B, Winbery S, et al. Blood cocaine and metabolite concentrations, clinical findings, and outcome of patients presenting to an ED. *Am J Emerg Med* 2000;18(5):593–598.
42. Hahn I-H, Hoffman RS. Cocaine use and acute myocardial infarction. *Emerg Med Clin N Am* 2001;19(2):493–510.
43. Kaye S, McKetin R, Duflou J, et al. Methamphetamine and cardiovascular pathology: a review of the evidence. *Addiction* 2007;102: 1204–1211.
44. McCord J, Jneid H, Hollander JE, et al. Management of cocaine-associated chest pain and myocardial infarction: a scientific statement from the American Heart Association Acute Cardiac Care Committee of the Council on Clinical Cardiology. *Circulation* 2008;117:1897–1907.
45. Attaran R, Ragavan D, Probst A. Cocaine-related myocardial infarction: concomitant heroin use can cloud the picture. *Eur J Emerg Med* 2005; 12:199–201.
46. Jones JH, Weir WB. Cocaine-induced chest pain. *Clin Lab Med* 2006;26:127–146, viii.
47. Hollander JE, Henry TO. Evaluation and management of the patient who has cocaine-associated chest pain. *Cardiol Clin* 2006;24: 103–114.
48. Baumann BM, Perrone J, Hornig SE, et al. Randomized, doubleblind, placebo-controlled trial of diazepam, nitroglycerin, or both for treatment of patients with potential cocaine-associated acute coronary syndromes. *Acad Emerg Med* 2000;7:878–885.
49. Hsue PY, McManus D, Selby V, et al. Cardiac arrest in patients who smoke crack cocaine. *Am J Cardiol* 2007;99:822–824.
50. Sen A, Fairbairn T, Levy F. Best evidence topic report. Beta-blockers in cocaine induced acute coronary syndrome. *Emerg Med J* 2006;23: 401–402.
51. Shah DM, Dy TC, Szto GY, et al. Percutaneous transluminal coronary angioplasty and stenting for cocaine-induced acute myocardial infarction: a case report and review. *Catheter Cardiovasc Interv* 2000;49: 447–451.
52. Kontos MC, Jesse RL, Tatum JL, et al. Coronary angiographic findings in patients with cocaine-associated chest pain. *J Emerg Med* 2003; 24(1):9–13.
53. Jenkins AJ, Cone EJ. Pharmacokinetics: drug absorption, distribution, and elimination. In: Karch SB, ed. *Drug abuse handbook.* Boca Raton, FL: CRC Press, 1998:151–201.
54. Coffey SF, Dansky BS, Carrigan MH, et al. Acute and protracted cocaine abstinence in an outpatient population: a prospective study of mood, sleep and withdrawal symptoms. *Drug Alcohol Depend* 2000;59: 277–286.

55. Cottler LB, Shillington AM, Compton III WM, et al. Subjective reports of withdrawal among cocaine users: recommendations for DSM-IV. *Drug Alcohol Depend* 1993;33:97–104.
56. Lago JA, Kosten TR. Stimulant withdrawal. *Addiction* 1994;89: 1477–1481.
57. McGregor C, Srisurapanont M, Jittiwutikarn J, et al. The nature, time course and severity of methamphetamine withdrawal. *Addiction* 2005; 100:1320–1329.
58. Satel SL, Price LH, Palumbo JM, et al. Clinical phenomenology and neurobiology of cocaine abstinence: a prospective inpatient study. *Am J Psychiatry* 1991;148:1712–1716.
59. Mulvaney FD, Alterman AI, Boardman CR, et al. Cocaine abstinence symptomatology and treatment attrition. *J Subst Abuse Treatment* 1999;16(2):129–135.
60. Rosenblum A, Foote J, Magura S, et al. Follow-up of inpatient cocaine withdrawal for cocaine-using methadone patients. *J Subst Abuse Treatment* 1996;13(6):467–470.
61. Karila L, Gorelick D, Weinstein A, et al. New treatments for cocaine dependence: a focused review. *Int J Neuropsychopharmacol* 2008;11: 425–438.
62. Vocci FJ, Appel NM. Approaches to the development of medications for the treatment of methamphetamine dependence. *Addiction* 2007; 102(Suppl 1):96–106.
63. Nademanee K, Gorelick DA, Josephson MA, et al. Myocardial ischemia during cocaine withdrawal. *Ann Intern Med* 1989;111:376–380.
64. Khantzian EJ, McKenna GJ. Acute toxic and withdrawal reactions associated with drug use and abuse. *Ann Intern Med* 1979;90:361–372.
65. Gill K, Gillespie HK, Hollister LE. Dopamine depletion hypothesis of cocaine dependence: a test. *Hum Psychopharmacol* 1991;6:25–29.
66. Volkow ND, Fowler JS, Wolf AP. Effects of chronic cocaine abuse on postsynaptic dopamine receptors. *Am J Psychiatry* 1992;147:719–724.
67. Wolfsohn R, Angrist B. A pilot trial of levodopa/carbidopa in early cocaine abstinence. *J Clin Psychopharmacol* 1990;10:440–442.
68. Cox D, Bowers R, McBride A. Reboxetine may be helpful in the treatment of amphetamine withdrawal. *Br J Clin Pharmacol* 2004;58: 100–101.
69. Farina B, di Giannantonio M. Reboxetine in cocaine withdrawal treatment: a three cases report. *Drug Alcohol Rev* 2003;22:373–374.
70. Gillman MA, Lichtigfeld FJ, Harker N. Psychotropic analgesic nitrous oxide for acute cocaine withdrawal in man. *Int J Neurosci* 2006;116: 847–857.
71. Lee N, Pennay A, Hester R. Randomized placebo-controlled trial of modafinil for methamphetamine withdrawal: results of an Australian pilot study. College on Problems of Drug Dependence Annual Meeting, San Juan, Puerto Rico, 2008.
72. Abraham HD, Aldridge AM, Gogia P. The psychopharmacology of hallucinogens. *Neuropsychopharmacology* 1996;14:285–298.
73. Halpern JH. Hallucinogens: an update. *Curr Psychiatry Rep* 2003;5: 347–354.
74. Brust JCM. Acute neurologic complications of drug and alcohol abuse. *Neurol Clin N Am* 1998;16(2):503–519.
75. Frecska E, Luna LE. The adverse effects of hallucinogens from intramural perspective. *Neuropsychopharmacol Hung* 2006;8:189–200.
76. Kulig K. LSD. *Emerg Med Clin N Am* 1990;8(3):551–558.
77. Pechnick RN, Ungerleider JT. Hallucinogens. In: Lowinson JH, Ruiz P, Millman RB, et al., eds. *Substance abuse: a comprehensive textbook,* 3rd ed. Baltimore, MD: Williams & Wilkins, 1997:230–238.
78. Schwartz RH, Smith DE. Hallucinogenic mushrooms. *Clin Pediatr* 1988;27(2):70–73.
79. Miller PL, Gay GR, Ferris KC, et al. Treatment of acute adverse psychedelic reactions: "I've tripped and I can't get down." *J Psychoactive Drugs* 1992;24(3):277–279.
80. Strassman RJ. Adverse reactions of psychedelic drugs: a review of the literature. *J Nerv Ment Dis* 1984;172(10):577–595.
81. Leikin JB, Krantz AJ, Zell-Kanter M, et al. Clinical features and management of intoxication due to hallucinogenic drugs. *Med Toxicol Adv Drug Exp* 1989;4(5):324–350.
82. Cottler LB, Schuckit MA, Helzer JE, et al. The DSM-IV field trial for substance use disorders: major results. *Drug Alcohol Depend* 1995;38: 59–69.
83. Gomez-Ruiz M, Hernandez M, De MR, et al. An overview on the biochemistry of the cannabinoid system. *Mol Neurobiol* 2007;36:3–14.
84. Gonzalez R. Acute and non-acute effects of cannabis on brain functioning and neuropsychological performance. *Neuropsychol Rev* 2007;17: 347–361.
85. MacKie K. Distribution of cannabinoid receptors in the central and peripheral nervous system. *Handb Exp Pharmacol* 2005:299–325.
86. Ilan AB, Gevins A, Coleman M, et al. Neurophysiological and subjective profile of marijuana with varying concentrations of cannabinoids. *Behav Pharmacol* 2005;16:487–496.
87. Huestis MA, Boyd SJ, Heishman SJ, et al. Single and multiple doses of rimonabant antagonize acute effects of smoked cannabis in male cannabis users. *Psychopharmacology (Berl)* 2007;194:505–515.
88. Grotenhermen F. The toxicology of cannabis and cannabis prohibition. *Chem Biodivers* 2007;4:1744–1769.
89. Ranganathan M, D'Souza DC. The acute effects of cannabinoids on memory in humans: a review. *Psychopharmacology (Berl)* 2006;188(4): 425–444.
90. Papafotiou K, Carter JD, Stough C. The relationship between performance on the standardised field sobriety tests, driving performance and the level of Delta9-tetrahydrocannabinol (THC) in blood. *Forensic Sci Int* 2005;155:172–178.
91. Johns A. Psychiatric effects of cannabis. *Br J Psychiatry* 2001;178: 116–122.
92. Kalant H. Adverse effects of cannabis on health: an update of the literature since 1996. *Prog Neuropsychopharmacol Biol Psychiatry* 2004;28: 849–863.
93. Leweke FM, Gerth CW, Klosterkotter J. Cannabis-associated psychosis: current status of research. *CNS Drugs* 2004;18:895–910.
94. Nunez LA, Gurpegui M. Cannabis-induced psychosis: a cross-sectional comparison with acute schizophrenia. *Acta Psychiatr Scand* 2002;105: 173–178.
95. Szuster RR, Pontius EB, Campos PE. Marijuana sensitivity and panic anxiety. *J Clin Psychiatry* 1988;49:427–429.
96. Moore TH, Zammit S, Lingford-Hughes A, et al. Cannabis use and risk of psychotic or affective mental health outcomes: a systematic review. *Lancet* 2007;370(9584):319–328.
97. Semple DM, McIntosh AM, Lawrie SM. Cannabis as a risk factor for psychosis: systematic review. *J Psychopharmacol* 2005;19(2):187–194.
98. Andre C, Jaber-Filho JA, Bento RM, et al. Delirium following ingestion of marijuana present in chocolate cookies. *CNS Spect* 2006;11: 262–264.
99. Favrat B, Menetrey A, Augsburger M, et al. Two cases of "cannabis acute psychosis" following the administration of oral cannabis. *BMC Psychiatry* 2005;5:17.
100. Bachs L, Morland H. Acute cardiovascular fatalities following cannabis use. *Forensic Sci Int* 2001;124:200–203.
101. Aryana A, Williams MA. Marijuana as a trigger of cardiovascular events: speculation or scientific certainty? *Int J Cardiol* 2007;118:141–144.
102. Korantzopoulos P, Liu T, Papaioannides D, et al. Atrial fibrillation and marijuana smoking. *Int J Clin Pract* 2008;62:308–313.
103. Perez JA, Jr. Allergic reaction associated with intravenous marijuana use. *J Emerg Med* 2000;18:260–261.
104. Huestis MA, Boyd SJ, Heishman SJ, et al. Single and multiple doses of rimonabant antagonize acute effects of smoked cannabis in male cannabis users.). *Psychopharmacology (Berl)* 2007;194(4):505–515.
105. American Psychiatric Association (APA). *Diagnostic and statistical manual of mental disorders,* 4th ed–text rev. Washington, DC: American Psychiatric Press, 2000.
106. Budney AJ, Hughes JR. The cannabis withdrawal syndrome. *Curr Opin Psychiatry* 2006;19:233–238.
107. Vandrey RG, Budney AJ, Hughes JR, et al. A within-subject comparison of withdrawal symptoms during abstinence from cannabis, tobacco, and both substances. *Drug Alcohol Depend* 2008:92, 48–54.

108. Copersino ML, Boyd SJ, Tashkin DP, et al. Cannabis withdrawal among non-treatment-seeking adult cannabis users. *Am J Addict* 2006; 15:8–14.
109. Nordstrom BR, Levin FR. Treatment of cannabis use disorders: a review of the literature. *Am J Addict* S2007;16(5):331–342.
110. Budney AJ, Vandrey RG, Hughes JR, et al. Oral delta-9-tetrahydrocannabinol suppresses cannabis withdrawal symptoms. *Drug Alcohol Depend* 2007;86:22–29.
111. Gorelick DA, Balster RL. Phencyclidine (PCP). In: Bloom FE, Kupfer DJ, eds. *Psychopharmacology: the fourth generation of progress.* New York: Raven Press, 1995:1767–1776.
112. Britt GC, McCance-Katz EF. A brief overview of the clinical pharmacology of "club drugs." *Subst Use Misuse* 2005;40:1189–1201.
113. Rome ES. It's a rave new world: rave culture and illicit drug use in the young. *Cleve Clin J Med* 2001;68(6):541–550.
114. Williams JF, Kokotailo PK. Abuse of proprietary (over-the-counter) drugs. *Adolesc Med Clin* 12006;7:733–750.
115. Jentsch JD, Roth RH. The neuropsychopharmacology of phencyclidine: from NMDA receptor hypofunction to the dopamine hypothesis of schizophrenia. *Neuropsychopharmacology* 1999;20:201–225.
116. Baldridge EB, Bessen HA. Phencyclidine. *Emerg Med Clin N Am* 1990; 8(3):541–550.
117. Woolf DS, Vourakis C/ Bennett G. Guidelines for management of acute phencyclidine intoxication. *Crit Care Update* 1980;7(6):16–24.
118. Milhorn TH. Diagnosis and management of phencyclidine intoxication. *Am Fam Phys* 1991;43(4):1293–1302.
119. Rappolt RT, Gay GR, Farris RD. Phencyclidine (PCP) intoxication: diagnosis in stages and algorithms of treatment. *Clin Toxicol* 1980;16: 509–529.
120. Wolff K, Winstock AR. Ketamine: from medicine to misuse. *CNS Drugs* 2006;20:199–218.
121. Anand A, Charney DS, Oren DA, et al. Attenuation of the neuropsychiatric effects of ketamine with lamotrigine. *Arch Gen Psychiatry* 2000; 57:270–276.
122. Gorelick D, Wilkins J, Wong C. *Diagnosis and treatment of chronic phencyclidine abuse.* NIDA Research Monograph 64. Rockville, MD: National Institute on Drug Abuse, 1986:218–228.
123. Soloway MS, Smith RA. Cranberry juice as a urine acidifier. *JAMA* 1988;260:1465.
124. Giannini AJ, Underwood NA, Condon M. Acute ketamine intoxication treated by haloperidol: a preliminary study. *Am J Therap* 2000;7: 389–391.
125. Carls KA, Ruehter VL. An evaluation of phencyclidine (PCP) psychosis: a retrospective analysis at a state facility. *Am J Drug Alcohol Abuse* 2006;32:673–678.
126. Weiss RD, Greenfield SF, Mirin SM. Intoxication and withdrawal syndromes. In: Hyman SE, ed. *Manual of psychiatric emergencies.* Boston, MA: Little, Brown & Co., 1994:279–293.
127. Giannini AJ, Loiselle RH, DiMarzio LR, et al. Augmentation of haloperidol by ascorbic acid in phencyclidine intoxication. *Am J Psychiatry* 1987;144:1207–1209.
128. Chyka PA, Erdman AR, Manoguerra AS, et al. Dextromethorphan poisoning: an evidence-based consensus guideline for out-of-hospital management. *Clin Toxicol (Phila)* 2007;45(6):662–677.
129. Kirages TJ, Sulé HP, Mycyk MB. Severe manifestations of coricidin intoxication. *Am J Emerg Med* 2004;22(7):624–625.
130. Tennant FS, Rawson RA, McCann M. Withdrawal from chronic phencyclidine dependence with desipramine. *Am J Psychiatry* 1981;138: 845–847.
131. Miller SC. Dextromethorphan psychosis, dependence and physical withdrawal. *Am J Emerg Med* 2005;13(2):174–176.
132. Giannini AJ, Loiselle RH, Graham BH. Behavioral response to buspirone in cocaine and phencyclidine withdrawal. *J Subst Abuse Treatment* 1993;10:523–527.
133. Erard R, Luisada PV, Peele R. The PCP psychosis: prolonged intoxication or drug precipitated functional illness? *J Psychedelic Drugs* 1980;12(3-4):235–250.
134. Gwirtsman HE, Winkop W, Gorelick DA, et al. Phencyclidine intoxication: Incidence, clinical patterns, and course of treatment. *Res Commun Psychol Psychiatry Behav* 1984;9:405–410.
135. Halpern JH, Pope HG, Jr. Hallucinogen persisting perception disorder: what do we know after 50 years? *Drug Alcohol Depend* 2003;69: 109–119.
136. Lerner AG, Gelkopf M, Skladman I, et al. Flashback and Hallucinogen Persisting Perception Disorder: clinical aspects and pharmacological treatment approach. *Isr J Psychiatry Relat Sci* 2002;39:92–99.
137. Kono J, Miyata H, Ushijima S, et al. Nicotine, alcohol, methamphetamine, and inhalant dependence: a comparison of clinical features with the use of a new clinical evaluation form. *Alcohol* 2001;24:99–106.
138. Williams JF, Storck M. Inhalant abuse. *Pediatrics* 2007;119:1009–1017.
139. Doyon S. The many faces of ecstasy. *Curr Opin Pediatr* 2001;13: 170–178.
140. Wu LT, Schlenger WE, Galvin DM. Concurrent use of methamphetamine, MDMA, LSD, ketamine, GHB, and flunitrazepam among American youths. *Drug Alcohol Depend* 2006;84(1):102–113.
141. Baggott M, Heifets B, Jones R, et al. Chemical analysis of ecstasy pills. *JAMA* 2000;284(17):2190.
142. Kalant H. The pharmacology and toxicology of "ecstasy" (MDMA) and related drugs. *Can Med Assoc J* 2001;165(7):917–928.
143. Oesterheld JR, Armstrong SC, Cozza KL Ecstasy: pharmacodynamic and pharmacokinetic interactions. *Psychosomatics* 2004;45(1):84–87.
144. de la Torre R, Farre M, Ortuno J, et al. Non-linear pharmacokinetics of MDMA ('Ecstasy') in humans. *Br J Clin Pharmacol* 2000;49: 104–109.
145. Yang J, Jamei M, Heydari A, et al. Implications of mechanism-based inhibition of CYP2D6 for the pharmacokinetics and toxicity of MDMA. *J Psychopharmacol* 2006;20(6):842–849.
146. Henry JA, Jeffreys CJ, Dawling S. Toxicity and deaths from 3,4-methylenedioxymethamphetamine ("Ecstasy"). *Lancet* 1992;340: 384–387.
147. Monks TJ, Jones DC, Bai F, et al. The role of metabolism in 3,4-(+)-methylenedioxyamphetamine and 3,4-(+)-methylenedioxymethamphetamine (ecstasy) toxicity. *Ther Drug Monit* 2004;26(2):132–136.
148. Burgess C, O'Donohoe A, Gill M. Agony and ecstasy: a review of MDMA effects and toxicity. *Eur Psychiatry* 2000;15:287–294.
149. El-Mallakh RS, Abraham HD. MDMA (Ecstasy). *Ann Clin Psychiatry* 2007;19:45–52.
150. Baylen CA, Rosenberg H. A review of the acute subjective effects of MDMA/ecstasy. *Addiction* 2006;101(7):933–947.
151. Vecellio M, Schopper C, Modestin J. Neuropsychiatric consequences (atypical psychosis and complex-partial seizures) of ecstasy use: possible evidence for toxicity-vulnerability predictors and implications for preventative and clinical care. *J Psychopharmacol* 2003;17(3):342–345.
152. Schifano F. A bitter pill. Overview of ecstasy (MDMA, MDA) related fatalities. *Psychopharmacology (Berl)* 2004;173(3–4):242–248.
153. Green AR, O'shea E, Colado MI. A review of the mechanisms involved in the acute MDMA (ecstasy)-induced hyperthermic response. *Eur J Pharmacol* 2004;500(1-3):3–13.
154. Lai TI, Hwang JJ, Fang CC, et al. Methylene 3,4-dioxymethamphetamine-induced acute myocardial infarction. *Ann Emerg Med* 2003;42(6):759–762.
155. Cadet JL, Krasnova IN, Jayanthi S, et al. Neurotoxicity of substituted amphetamines: molecular and cellular mechanisms. *Neurotox Res* 2007; 11(3–4):183–202.
156. Halachanova V, Sansone RA, McDonald S. Delayed rhabdomyolysis after ecstasy use. *Mayo Clin Proc* 2001;76(1):112–113.
157. Shannon M, Quang LS. Gamma-hydroxybutyrate, gammabutyrolactone, and 1,4-butanediol: a case report and review of the literature. *Pediatr Emerg Care* 2000;16(6):435–440.
158. Ricaurte GA, McCann UD. Recognition and management of complications of new recreational drug use. *Lancet* 2005;365:2137–2145.
159. Caldicott D, Kuhn M. Gamma-hydroxybutyrate overdose and physostigmine: teaching new tricks to an old drug. *Ann Emerg Med* 2001;37(1):99–102.

160. Sumnall HR, Woolfall K, Edwards S, et al. Use, function, and subjective experiences of gamma-hydroxybutyrate (GHB). *Drug Alcohol Depend* 2008;92:286–290.
161. Miotto K, Darakjian J, Basch J, et al. Gamma-hydroxybutyric acid: patterns of use, effects and withdrawal. *Am J Addict* 2001;10(3):232–241.
162. Gonzalez A, Nutt DJ. Gamma hydroxy butyrate abuse and dependency. *J Psychopharmacol* 2005;19(2):195–204.
163. Mason PE, Kerns WP 2nd. Gamma hydroxybutyric acid (GHB) intoxication. *Acad Emerg Med* 2002;9(7):730–739.
164. Zvosec D, Smith S, McCutcheon JR, et al. Adverse events, including death, associated with the use of 1,4-butanediol. *N Engl J Med* 2001; 344(2):87–94.
165. Tarabar AF, Nelson LS. The gamma-hydroxybutyrate withdrawal syndrome. *Toxicol Rev* 2004;23(1):45–49.
166. McDonough M, Kennedy N, Glasper A, et al. Clinical features and management of gamma-hydroxybutyrate (GHB) withdrawal: a review. *Drug Alcohol Depend* 2004;75(1):3–9.
167. Richardson WH, Slone CM, Michels JE. Herbal drugs of abuse: an emerging problem. *Emerg Med Clin N Am* 2007;254:35–57.
168. Halpern JH. Hallucinogens and dissociative agents naturally growing in the United States. *Pharmacol Ther* 2004;102:131–138.
169. Dennehy CE, Tsourounis C, Miller AE. Evaluation of herbal dietary supplements marketed on the internet for recreational use. *Ann Pharmacother* 2005;39(10):1634–1639.
170. Yussman SM, Wilson KM, Klein JD. Herbal products and their association with substance use in adolescents. *J Adolesc Health* 2006;38(4):395–400.
171. Silins E, Copeland J, Dillon P. Qualitative review of serotonin syndrome, ecstasy (MDMA) and the use of other serotonergic substances: hierarchy of risk. *Aust N Z J Psychiatry* 2007;41(8):649–655.
172. Boyer EW, Shannon M. The serotonin syndrome. *N Engl J Med* 2005; 352(11):1112–1120.
173. Christensen RC. Identifying serotonin syndrome in the emergency department. *Am J Emerg Med* 2005;23(3):406–408.
174. Gorelick DA, Wilkins JN. Special aspects of human alcohol withdrawal. In: Galanter M, ed. *Recent developments in alcoholism,* vol. 4. New York: Plenum Press, 1986:283–305.
175. Zullino DF, Khazaal Y, Hattenschwiler J, et al. Anticonvulsant drugs in the treatment of substance withdrawal. *Drugs Today (Barc)* 2004;40:603–619.
176. Kuschel C. Managing drug withdrawal in the newborn infant. *Semin Fetal Neonatal Med* 2007;12:127–133.
177. Oei J, Lui K. Management of the newborn infant affected by maternal opiates and other drugs of dependency. *J Paediatr Child Health* 2007;43:9–18.
178. Rayburn WF. Maternal and fetal effects from substance use. *Clin Perinatol* 2007;34:559–71, vi.
179. Greene CM, Goodman MH. Neonatal abstinence syndrome: strategies for care of the drug-exposed infant. *Neonatal Netw* 2003;22(4): 15–25.
180. Smith LM, Lagasse LL, Derauf C, et al. Prenatal methamphetamine use and neonatal neurobehavioral outcome. *Neurotoxicol Teratol* 2008;30(1): 20–28.
181. Wagner CL, Katkaneni LD, Cox TH, et al. The impact of prenatal drug exposure on the neonate. *Obst Gynecol Clin N Am* 1998;25(1):169–194.
182. Kandall SR. Treatment strategies for drug-exposed neonates. *Clin Perinatol* 1999;26(1):231–243.
183. Chomchai C, Na Manorom N, Watanarungsan P, et al. Methamphetamine abuse during pregnancy and its health impact on neonates born at Siriraj Hospital, Bangkok, Thailand. *Southeast Asian J Trop Med Public Health* 2004;35(1):228–231.
184. Simoni-Wastila L, Yang HK. Psychoactive drug abuse in older adults. *Am J Geriatr Pharmacother* 2006;4(4):380–394.
185. Kessler RC, Amminger GP, Gguilar-Gaxiola S, et al. Age of onset of mental disorders: a review of recent literature. *Curr Opin Psychiatry* 2007;20:359–364.
186. Schepis TS, Adinoff B, Rao U. Neurobiological processes in adolescent addictive disorders. *Am J Addict* 2008;17:6–23.
187. Stewart DG, Brown SA. Withdrawal and dependency symptoms among adolescent alcohol and drug abusers. *Addiction* 1995;90:627–635.
188. Bukstein OG, Bernet W, Arnold,V, et al. Practice parameter for the assessment and treatment of children and adolescents with substance use disorders. *J Am Acad Child Adolesc Psychiatry* 2005;44:609–621.
189. Fournier ME, Levy S.. Recent trends in adolescent substance use, primary care screening, and updates in treatment options. *Curr Opin Pediatr* 2006;18:352–358.
190. Becker JB, Hu M. Sex differences in drug abuse. *Front Neuroendocrinol* 2008;29:36–47.

SECTION 7

Pharmacologic Interventions

CHAPTER 46

Henry R. Kranzler, MD
Domenic A. Ciraulo, MD
Jerome H. Jaffe, MD

Medications for Use in Alcohol Rehabilitation

In this chapter, we review the literature on the use of medications to reduce drinking or prevent relapse in heavy drinkers (many of whom meet criteria for alcohol abuse or dependence). Rather than reviewing the literature exhaustively, the focus of the chapter is on developments of current interest to the clinician or that are likely to yield important clinical advances in the future. We also refer the reader to a number of other recent reviews that augment the information provided here (1–5).

The first major approach to the use of medications in the rehabilitation treatment of alcohol dependence involves direct efforts to reduce or stop drinking behavior by producing adverse effects when alcohol is consumed or by modifying the neurotransmitter systems that mediate alcohol reinforcement. Table 46.1 lists the four medications or formulations that use this approach and are approved by the U.S. Food and Drug Administration (FDA) for the treatment of alcohol dependence. The table also shows the year of FDA approval, the presumed mechanism of action, and the approved dosage for each of these. The medications are discussed individually in the sections that follow. The second main approach to the treatment of alcohol dependence involves the treatment of persistent psychiatric symptoms, which aims to stop or reduce drinking by modifying the motivation to use alcohol to "self-medicate" such symptoms. Medications for which this rationale underlies their use in the treatment of alcohol dependence are discussed in the latter part of this chapter.

MEDICATIONS USED TO REDUCE OR STOP DRINKING

Alcohol-Sensitizing Agents Alcohol-sensitizing agents alter the body's response to alcohol, thereby making its ingestion unpleasant or toxic. Disulfiram (Antabuse) is the only alcohol sensitizing medication approved in the United States for the treatment of alcohol dependence and that is widely used clinically. Consequently, we will focus on that agent here.

Disulfiram inhibits the enzyme aldehyde dehydrogenase, which catalyzes the oxidation of acetaldehyde to acetic acid. The ingestion of alcohol while this enzyme is inhibited elevates the blood acetaldehyde concentration, resulting in the disulfiram-ethanol reaction (DER). The intensity of the DER varies both with the dose of disulfiram and the volume of alcohol ingested. Symptoms and signs of the DER include warmness and flushing of the skin, especially that of the upper chest and face; increased heart rate; palpitations; and decreased blood pressure. They may also include nausea, vomiting, shortness of breath, sweating, dizziness, blurred vision, and confusion. Most DERs are self-limited, lasting about 30 minutes. Occasionally, the DER may be severe, with marked tachycardia, hypotension, or bradycardia; rarely, it may result in cardiovascular collapse, congestive failure, and convulsions. Although severe reactions are usually associated with high doses of disulfiram (over 500 mg/day), combined with more than 2 ounces of alcohol, deaths have occurred with lower dosage and after a single drink (6–9). Concern over the potential for such effects may limit clinicians' willingness to prescribe disulfiram.

The efficacy of alcohol sensitizing agents in the prevention of relapse in alcohol-dependent individuals remains to be demonstrated in placebo-controlled, double-blind studies. However, in selected samples of such individuals with whom special efforts, such as supervised administration, are made to ensure compliance, these medications may be useful. As discussed in the following section, disulfiram may also limit the severity of relapse when it occurs. There are no guidelines that

TABLE 46.1 Medications Approved by the U.S. Food and Drug Administration for the Treatment of Alcohol Dependence

Medication	Year approved	Description
Disulfiram (Antabuse)	1949	Aversive medication; after ingestion, alcohol consumption leads to a variety of aversive symptoms. Approved dosage is 250 mg/day.
Naltrexone (ReVia)	1994	Orally bioavailable opioid antagonist that decreases the reinforcing effects of alcohol. Most robust effects clinically are to reduce risk of heavy drinking. Approved dosage is 50 mg/day.
Acamprosate (Campral)	2004	GABA-receptor agonist and NMDA-receptor modulator. Most robust effects clinically are to maintain abstinence. Approved dosage is 1998 mg/day.
Long-acting naltrexone (Vivitrol)	2006	Injectable formulation that produces detectable plasma concentrations for 30 days. May help to improve adherence with oral formulation. Approved dosage is 380 mg/month.

can be offered either to identify patients for whom disulfiram is most likely to have a beneficial effect or to match specific psychosocial interventions with particular patients to enhance compliance.

Pharmacology of Disulfiram (Antabuse) Disulfiram is almost completely absorbed orally. Because it binds irreversibly to aldehyde dehydrogenase, renewed enzyme activity requires the synthesis of new enzyme, so that the potential exists for a DER to occur at least 2 weeks from the last ingestion of disulfiram. Consequently, alcohol should be avoided during this period.

Disulfiram commonly produces a variety of adverse effects, including drowsiness, lethargy, and fatigue (10). Although more serious adverse effects, such as optic neuritis, peripheral neuropathy, and hepatotoxicity occur rarely, patients treated with disulfiram should be monitored regularly for visual changes and symptoms of peripheral neuropathy and the medication discontinued if they appear. Further, the patient's liver enzymes should be monitored at quarterly intervals to identify hepatotoxic effects, which may also warrant discontinuation of the medication. Psychiatric effects of disulfiram are uncommon and probably occur only at higher dosages of the drug, which may result in the inhibition by disulfiram of a variety of enzymes in addition to aldehyde dehydrogenase. For example, disulfiram inhibits dopamine beta-hydroxylase, which increases dopamine concentrations, which in turn can exacerbate psychotic symptoms in patients with schizophrenia and rarely result in psychotic or depressive symptoms among individuals without a psychotic disorder. Such symptoms should also lead to discontinuation of the medication.

Disulfiram is administered orally. There is a correlation between the risk of most adverse effects and dosage, although the risk of hepatic injury does not appear to be related to dose. This concern about dosage-related adverse events has resulted in the daily dosage prescribed in the United States being limited to 250 to 500 mg/day. However, efforts to titrate the dosage of disulfiram in relation to a challenge dose of ethanol have shown that some patients require in excess of 1 g/day of disulfiram to reach blood levels sufficient to produce a DER (11).

Clinical Use of Disulfiram Given its intuitive appeal, disulfiram has long been used in the rehabilitation of alcohol-dependent patients (12), despite a lack of methodologically sound evaluations demonstrating its efficacy in the prevention of relapse.

Its approval for use by the FDA preceded the implementation of rigorous requirements for efficacy that now must be satisfied for a medication to be marketed in the United States. In the controlled studies conducted, the difference in outcome between subjects receiving disulfiram and those given placebo has generally been modest.

The largest and most methodologically sound study of disulfiram was a multicenter trial conducted by the Veterans Administration Cooperative Studies Group. In that 1-year study, more than 600 male alcohol-dependent patients were randomly assigned to receive either 1 mg of disulfiram per day, 250 mg/day, or an inactive placebo (13). Patients assigned to the two disulfiram groups were told they were receiving the medication, but neither patients nor staff knew the dosage. Results showed that greater compliance with the medication regimen (in all three groups) was associated with a greater likelihood of complete abstinence. Among patients who resumed drinking, those in the group receiving 250 mg of disulfiram reported significantly fewer drinking days than patients in either of the other two groups. Based on these findings, it appears that disulfiram may be helpful in reducing the frequency of drinking in men who cannot remain abstinent, though given the large number of statistical analyses, it is possible that this finding arose by chance (13).

Disulfiram may be of clinical value in selected samples of alcohol-dependent patients with whom special efforts are made to ensure compliance. Specific behavioral efforts to enhance compliance with disulfiram (as well as other medications for the treatment of alcohol dependence) include contracting with the patient and a significant other to work together to ensure compliance, and the provision to the patient of incentives, regular reminders and other information, and behavioral training and social support (14). A trial program of stimulus control training, role playing, communication skills training, and recreational and vocational counseling improved outcome in disulfiram-treated patients compared with those receiving placebo (15). Supervision of patients being treated with disulfiram may be an essential element in ensuring compliance and enhancing the beneficial effects of the medication (16). In a 6-month study, Chick et al. (17) randomly assigned patients to receive disulfiram 200 mg/day or vitamin C 100 mg/day (ingested under the supervision of an individual chosen by the patient) as an adjunct to outpatient alcohol treatment. Treatment with disulfiram significantly increased abstinent days and decreased total drinks consumed, effects that were confirmed by parallel changes in levels of the hepatic enzyme γ-glutamyltranspeptidase.

In deciding whether disulfiram should be used in alcohol rehabilitation, patients should be made aware of the hazards of the medication, including the need to avoid over-the-counter preparations with alcohol and drugs that can interact with disulfiram and the potential for a DER to be precipitated by alcohol used in food preparation. The administration of disulfiram to anyone who does not agree to use it, does not seek to be abstinent from alcohol, or who has any psychologic or medical contraindications is not recommended. Given its potential to produce serious adverse effects when combined with alcohol, disulfiram cannot be recommended for use as part of a moderation approach to alcohol treatment.

Medications that Directly Reduce Alcohol Consumption Several neurotransmitter systems appear to influence the reinforcing or discriminative stimulus effects of ethanol: endogenous opioids; catecholamines, especially dopamine; serotonin (5-HT), and excitatory amino acids (e.g., glutamate) (see references 1 and 4 for detailed reviews of the literature on the role of these various neurotransmitter systems in alcohol effects). Although these systems function interactively to influence drinking behavior, many of the medications that have been employed to treat alcohol dependence affect neurotransmitter systems relatively selectively. Consequently, these systems will be discussed individually here.

Opioidergic Agents Naltrexone, and to a lesser extent, nalmefene, both of which are opioid antagonists with no intrinsic agonist properties, have been studied for the treatment of alcohol dependence. In 1984, naltrexone was approved by the FDA for the treatment of opioid dependence; in 1994, it was approved for the treatment of alcohol dependence. Nalmefene is approved in the United States as a parenteral formulation for the acute reversal of opioid effects (e.g., after opioid overdose or analgesia).

Naltrexone The approval by the FDA of naltrexone for alcohol dependence was based on the results of two single-site studies, which showed it to be efficacious in the prevention of relapse to heavy drinking (18,19). In a 12-week trial in a sample of alcohol-dependent veterans, Volpicelli et al. (18) found naltrexone to be well tolerated and to result in significantly less craving for alcohol and fewer drinking days than placebo. Among patients who drank, naltrexone also limited the progression from initial sampling of alcohol to a relapse to heavy drinking, presumably because of their experiencing less euphoric effects of alcohol, suggesting that naltrexone blocked the endogenous opioid system's contribution to alcohol's "priming effect" (20).

The efficacy of combining naltrexone with either supportive or cognitive-behavioral therapy (CBT) in ambulatory alcohol-dependent patients was studied by O'Malley et al. (19). This 12-week trial showed the medication to be well tolerated and to be superior to placebo in increasing the rate of abstinence and reducing the number of drinking days and relapse events, and the severity of alcohol-related problems. There was an interaction effect of medication and therapy. The cumulative rate of abstinence was highest for patients treated with naltrexone and supportive therapy. However, for patients who drank, those who received naltrexone and coping skills therapy were least likely to relapse to heavy drinking.

Analysis of the potential mediating variables in these effects showed that naltrexone reduced craving for alcohol, alcohol's reinforcing properties, the experience of intoxication, and the chances of continued drinking following a slip (21). During a 6-month, posttreatment follow-up period, the effects of naltrexone diminished gradually over time, suggesting that patients may benefit from treatment with naltrexone for longer than 12 weeks (22).

Many, but not all, subsequent studies of naltrexone have provided support for its use in alcohol treatment. The literature on naltrexone treatment of alcohol dependence has been reviewed in detail in a number of meta-analyses (23–26). The two meta-analyses that included the largest number of studies (25,26) show a clear advantage for naltrexone over placebo on a number of drinking outcomes.

Bouza et al. (25) included 19 studies of naltrexone and a total of 3,205 participants with alcohol dependence. The large majority of these studies were of short duration (i.e. ≤12 weeks). Using relapse as an outcome, these studies yielded a highly significant odds ratio (OR) of 0.62 (95% confidence interval [CI] 0.52–0.75), reflecting a 38% lower likelihood of relapse with naltrexone treatment ($p < 0.00001$). The likelihood of total abstinence also favored naltrexone (OR 1.26; 95% CI 0.97–1.64), though it did not reach statistical significance ($p = 0.08$). Outcomes identified as secondary by this meta-analysis, including time to relapse, percentage of drinking days, number of drinks per drinking day, days of abstinence, total alcohol consumption during treatment, and levels of gamma-glutamyl transpeptidase and aspartate aminotransferase, also showed a significant advantage for the naltrexone-treated group.

The meta-analysis by Srisurapanont and Jarusuraisin (26) included a total of 2,861 subjects from 24 randomized, controlled trials. In the short term, naltrexone significantly decreased risk of relapse to heavy drinking (relative risk [RR] 0.64, 95% CI 0.51–0.82), but did not reduce the likelihood of a return to any drinking (RR 0.91, 95% CI 0.81–1.02). Treatment with naltrexone significantly increased adverse effects, roughly doubling the likelihood of reports of nausea and dizziness, and increasing the risk of fatigue by about one third compared with placebo. However, naltrexone treatment did not significantly affect the rate of premature discontinuation of treatment (RR 0.85, 95% CI 0.70–1.01).

Follow-up studies of patients treated with naltrexone or placebo for 12 weeks (22,27) or 4 months (28) have shown that the medication group differences are no longer significant at posttreatment follow-up. These findings suggest that treatment with naltrexone is warranted for longer than 4 months, though the optimal duration of treatment is unknown.

An alternate approach to the use of naltrexone based on its efficacy in reducing the risk of heavy drinking among patients who continue to drink was evaluated in a study that compared the effects of naltrexone 50 mg with those of placebo in an 8-week study of problem drinkers (29). In this study, patients were randomly assigned to receive study medication either on a daily basis or for use targeted to situations identified by the patients as being high-risk for heavy drinking (with the number of tablets available for use by patients in the targeted conditions decreasing over the course of the trial). Irrespective of whether they received naltrexone or placebo, patients who were trained and encouraged to use targeted treatment showed a reduced likelihood of any drinking. There was also a 19% reduction in the likelihood of heavy drinking with naltrexone treatment, suggesting that naltrexone may be useful in reducing heavy drinking, among patients who want to reduce their drinking to safe levels.

Targeted naltrexone was also used by Heinala et al. (30), who compared 50 mg/day of the medication with placebo, paired with either coping skills or supportive therapy. During an initial 12 weeks of treatment, this study showed an advantage for naltrexone in preventing relapse to heavy drinking, but only when combined with coping skills therapy. During a subsequent 20-week period, subjects were told to use the medication only when they craved alcohol (i.e., targeted treatment). The beneficial effect of naltrexone on the risk of relapse was generally sustained during the period of targeted treatment. Based on these findings, it appears that targeted medication administration may be useful both for the initial treatment of problem drinking and for maintenance of the beneficial effects of an initial period of daily naltrexone.

O'Malley et al. (31) conducted a sequence of randomized trials in which subjects with alcohol dependence were first treated with 10 weeks of open-label naltrexone 50 mg, combined with either CBT or primary care management (PCM; a less intensive, supportive approach). Treatment responders from the PCM group and from the CBT group continued in separate 24-week, placebo-controlled studies of maintenance naltrexone. No difference was observed with respect to persistent heavy drinking, with more than 80% of both groups having a positive outcome. However, the percentage of days abstinent declined more over time for the PCM group. In the follow-up studies, there was a greater maintenance response for naltrexone than placebo when combined with PCM, but the advantage for naltrexone did not reach significance when combined with CBT. These findings suggest that the beneficial effects of treatment with naltrexone can be maintained during an extended period through the use of either a more intensive, skills-oriented treatment (i.e., CBT) or a less intensive, supportive treatment combined with continued naltrexone administration.

Poor compliance with oral naltrexone has been shown to reduce the potential benefits of the medication (32). This has generated interest in the development and evaluation of long-acting injectable formulations of the medication. The rationale behind this approach is that monthly, compared with daily, administration would improve medication adherence and that parenteral administration would increase bioavailability by avoiding first-pass metabolism. In addition to the formulations evaluated in published studies, which are reviewed in the following sections, there are long-acting naltrexone formulations that are under development for use in the United States, Europe, and Australia.

In a pilot study, alcohol-dependent patients treated with a subcutaneous depot formulation of naltrexone had detectable plasma concentrations of the medication for more than 30 days after the injection (33). In this study, naltrexone was superior to placebo in reducing the frequency of heavy drinking. Two long-acting naltrexone formulations administered intramuscularly have also been tested for safety and efficacy in alcohol-dependent patients. In the first study, naltrexone depot (at a dosage of 300 mg in the first month and then 150 mg monthly for 2 months) was administered in a 12-week, placebo-controlled trial in 315 patients who also received motivational enhancement therapy (34). Although naltrexone did not reduce the risk of heavy drinking, it significantly delayed the onset of any drinking, increased the total number of abstinent days, and doubled the likelihood of abstinence during the 12-week study period. Two dosage strengths of a second formulation were evaluated over 6 months of treatment in combination with a low-intensity psychosocial intervention in more than 600 alcohol-dependent adults who received 6 monthly injections of either long-acting naltrexone (380 mg or 190 mg), or matching volumes of placebo. Abstinence from alcohol was not required for study participation. The medication and the injections were well tolerated. Compared with placebo, treatment with the 380-mg naltrexone formulation reduced the event rate of heavy drinking by 25%, a statistically significant effect. The 17% reduction in the rate of heavy drinking produced by the 190-mg formulation did not reach statistical significance. On the basis of these findings, the FDA approved long-acting naltrexone for monthly administration at a dosage of 380 mg. Because the analysis also showed that the most robust effects of the medication were seen in patients who were abstinent (by choice) for at least a week before randomization, the package insert states that the medication should be used only in alcohol-dependent patients who are abstinent at treatment initiation.

A secondary analysis of data from this study examined efficacy in the subgroup of 82 patients with 4 days or more of voluntary abstinence before treatment initiation (35). This shorter period of abstinence made it possible to include a larger percentage of the study sample in the analysis than was possible initially with the use of a 7-day interval. In this study, there was a significant advantage for the 380-mg formulation compared with placebo on a number of self-report outcome measures, including greater likelihood of total abstinence (32% vs. 11%), greater median time to a first drinking day (41 days vs. 12 days), greater median time to a first heavy drinking day (>180 days vs. 20 days), lower median number of drinking days per month (0.7 vs. 7.2), and lower median heavy drinking days per month (0.2 days vs 2.9 days). There was also a significantly greater improvement in gamma-glutamyl transpeptidase levels in the 380-mg naltrexone group. Outcomes for the 190-mg group were generally intermediate between the high-dose and placebo groups.

Clinical Considerations in the Use of Naltrexone The clinical use of naltrexone is relatively straightforward, despite the presence of a "black-box" warning in the label concerning hepatotoxicity. The medication should be prescribed at the time that psychosocial treatment is initiated. Because of adverse effects of the medication that could compound the adverse effects of alcohol withdrawal, the initiation of naltrexone therapy is probably best delayed until after the acute withdrawal period. Initial testing for liver enzyme abnormalities is warranted to avoid prescribing the medication in the context of extreme elevations. Ongoing monitoring is required only if symptoms warrant it, because the consistent effect of naltrexone in studies of alcohol dependence have been to decrease liver enzyme concentrations.

Oral naltrexone should be administered initially at a dosage of 25 mg/day to minimize adverse effects. The dosage can then be increased in 25 mg increments every 3 to 7 days to a maximum dosage of 150 mg/day using desire to drink or another symptom that the patient identifies as reflective of risk of relapse to heavy drinking. It should be noted, however, that there is no clear evidence that a higher dosage is more efficacious than the FDA-approved dosage of 50 mg/day. Nausea and other gastrointestinal symptoms are most common early in treatment, as are neuropsychiatric symptoms (e.g., headache, dizziness, lightheadedness, weakness) and are usually transient. Delaying or avoiding a dosage increase can be used to address more persistent adverse events. In a few patients, flulike symptoms occur and the patient may not be willing to consider options other than discontinuation.

Long-acting naltrexone is only available as a 380-mg dose, which should be administered intramuscularly in the buttock every 4 weeks. The medication is approved for use in patients who are abstinent from alcohol and who are also receiving psychosocial treatment. Adverse effects with this formulation are similar to those of the oral medication, though pain and inflammation at the injection site may also occur. Local interventions, such as warm compresses, and nonsteroidal anti-inflammatory medications can be used to treat such injection site reactions.

Nalmefene Nalmefene has also been evaluated as a treatment for alcohol dependence. As with naltrexone, nalmefene is an opioid antagonist without agonist properties. Nalmefene's affinity for the μ- and κ-opioid receptors is similar to that of naltrexone, though its affinity for the δ-opioid receptor is greater than that of naltrexone (36). A pilot study of nalmefene 40 mg/day showed it to be superior to both 10 mg/day of the medication and placebo in the prevention of relapse to heavy drinking in alcohol-dependent patients (37). A subsequent study showed no difference between nalmefene 20 mg/day or 80 mg/day. However, when combined, the nalmefene-treated subjects reported significantly less heavy drinking than the placebo group (38). A 12-week, multisite, dose-ranging study compared placebo with 5, 20, or 40 mg of nalmefene in a sample of recently abstinent outpatient alcohol-dependent patients (39). In this study, all subjects showed a reduction in self-reported heavy drinking days and on biological measures of drinking, with no difference between the active medication and placebo groups on these measures. Recently, targeted nalmefene (where subjects were encouraged to use 10 to 40 mg of the medication when they believed drinking to be imminent) was combined with a minimal psychosocial intervention in a multicenter, placebo-controlled, randomized trial (40). Nalmefene was superior to placebo in reducing heavy drinking days, very heavy drinking days, and drinks per drinking day and in increasing abstinent days. Further, after 28 weeks of treatment, when a subgroup of nalmefene-treated subjects was randomized to a withdrawal extension, patients assigned to receive placebo were more likely to return to heavier drinking.

Summary There now exists abundant evidence of the efficacy of opioid antagonists (particularly naltrexone) for the treatment of alcohol dependence. In unselected samples of patients, these medications exert a modest overall effect. There is growing evidence, however, that naltrexone may be of particular utility in subgroups of patients, so that the ready identification of patients who are more likely to respond to treatment is of great clinical interest. In an effort to identify genetic predictors of naltrexone response, three studies (41–43) have examined the moderating effect of a polymorphism (A118G or Asn40Asp) in the gene encoding the μ-opioid receptor on naltrexone treatment response in alcohol dependent subjects. A similar study was conducted in a sample of non–treatment-seeking heavy drinkers (44). Of these studies, two have shown an effect of the polymorphism in predicting naltrexone response (41,43) and two have not (42,44). Although this approach is promising, further research is needed to resolve these discrepant findings. In addition, the optimal dosage and duration of treatment and the relative benefit accruing to combining the medication with different types and intensities of psychosocial treatment are important clinical questions that have not yet been adequately addressed. New approaches to the use of naltrexone, including targeted administration and long-acting injectable formulations, may enhance the clinical utility of the medication.

Acamprosate Acamprosate (calcium acetylhomotaurinate) is an amino acid derivative that increases gamma-aminobutyric acid (GABA) neurotransmission and also has complex effects on excitatory amino acid (i.e., glutamate) neurotransmission, which is most likely the effect that is important for its therapeutic effects in alcohol dependence. Acamprosate was first shown in a single-site study to be twice as effective as placebo in reducing the rate at which alcohol-dependent patients returned to drinking (45). The medication has been studied extensively in Europe, and three of the European studies provided the basis for the approval of acamprosate by the FDA for clinical use in the United States (46).

Meta-analyses from the European studies provide consistent evidence of the efficacy of acamprosate in the treatment of alcohol dependence (23,25,47,48). The magnitude of the advantage accruing to treatment with acamprosate over placebo in those studies varied as a function of the outcomes examined, but were in the small range of effect sizes. A meta-analysis of continuous abstinence showed a significant advantage for acamprosate over placebo, and although the effects were modest, they increased progressively as treatment duration increased from 3 to 6 and then to 12 months (48).

Chick et al. (47) sought to determine whether treatment with acamprosate reduces the severity of relapse for patients in abstinence-oriented treatment who fail to abstain completely. Among patients who relapsed to drinking, acamprosate treatment was significantly associated with less quantity and frequency of drinking than placebo at follow-up periods as long as 1 year. Acamprosate also reduced the risk of heavy drinking (i.e., five or more drinks/day).

In a study that has implications for the use of acamprosate in combination with disulfiram, a multicenter trial was conducted in which patients were randomly assigned to receive acamprosate or placebo, with stratification for those who voluntarily were using disulfiram. Acamprosate was found to be superior to placebo on measures of total abstinence and on cumulative abstinent days (49). The group treated with acamprosate and disulfiram showed a significantly greater percentage of abstinent days than any of the other three groups. However, because the design was not fully randomized, more rigorous studies of this combination therapy are needed to evaluate the validity of these findings.

In summary, studies in more than 4,000 patients in Europe provide evidence of a beneficial effect of acamprosate in the prevention of relapse to drinking and in the reduction of drinking among patients who relapse. Based on the evidence of its efficacy, the FDA approved the medication for clinical use in the United States (46). However, two multicenter trials conducted in the United States, the first being a multicenter trial of two active dosages of acamprosate (50) and the second being the COMBINE (Combining Medications and Behavioral Interventions for Alcoholism) Study (28), the largest alcohol treatment trial to date (described in the following section), failed to show an advantage of acamprosate over placebo on an intent-to-treat basis. This raises the question of the factors that distinguish alcohol pharmacotherapy trials in Europe from those in the United States. Differences in features of study design (e.g., European studies required a lengthier period of abstinence) and of the samples studied (e.g., European subjects were heavier drinkers) may explain these discrepant findings.

Clinical Considerations in the Use of Acamprosate
Acamprosate is FDA-approved at a dosage of 1998 mg/day (i.e., two 333-mg capsules three times per day) in patients who are abstinent from alcohol and receiving psychosocial treatment. The most common adverse effects of the drug are generally mild and transient and include gastrointestinal (e.g., diarrhea, bloating) and dermatologic (e.g., pruritus) complaints. In contrast to disulfiram and naltrexone, which are metabolized in the liver, acamprosate is excreted unmetabolized, so that renal function is the rate-limiting factor in the drug's elimination. Evaluation of renal function prior to initiation of the drug is warranted, particularly in individuals who have a history or are otherwise at risk of renal disease and in the elderly.

Studies Comparing Acamprosate with Naltrexone and the Two Medications Combined Two placebo-controlled studies have directly compared treatment with acamprosate, naltrexone, and acamprosate and naltrexone combined. In the first study, a 12-week trial in 160 patients, all three active medication groups (naltrexone, acamprosate, and the two medications combined) were significantly more efficacious than placebo (51). In that study, although the rate of relapse of the combined medication group was significantly lower than that in either the placebo or acamprosate groups, it was not statistically better than naltrexone alone.

The COMBINE Study, a 4-month, multicenter study, placebo-controlled study conducted at 11 sites in the United States, compared naltrexone, acamprosate, and their combination in a sample of nearly 1,400 abstinent alcohol-dependent subjects. The design of the study was complex, insofar as two different behavioral interventions (medical management or an intensive behavioral treatment) were combined with naltrexone (100 mg/day), acamprosate 3 g/day), naltrexone and acamprosate, or placebo, so that eight groups received study medication. Further, to evaluate the effects of placebo treatment, a ninth group, which received an intensive behavioral treatment but no medication, was also included. Overall, when on study treatment, subjects significantly increased the percentage of abstinent days. Groups receiving naltrexone and medical management; intensive behavioral treatment, medical management, and placebo; and naltrexone, intensive behavioral treatment, and medical management had a significantly greater percentage of days abstinent than the group receiving placebo and medical management. Naltrexone also reduced the risk of a heavy drinking day in the group receiving medical management but not intensive psychotherapy. In addition to showing a modest advantage for the use of either naltrexone or intensive behavioral treatment, it is noteworthy that the study failed to show an advantage for acamprosate over placebo, either alone or when added to naltrexone on any of the drinking outcomes. The study also showed evidence of a placebo response among individuals receiving the intensive behavioral intervention, in that those that received neither an active nor a placebo medication showed significantly less improvement than those who were treated with placebo. It should be noted that published meta-analyses do not include data from the COMBINE Study, of clear relevance because it is among the largest studies of either naltrexone or acamprosate.

Anticonvulsants Of growing interest is the use of anticonvulsants for the treatment of alcohol dependence. The efficacy of this class of medications for the treatment of alcohol dependence was initially demonstrated in placebo-controlled studies of carbamazepine (52), divalproex (53), and topiramate (54), with a multicenter study (55) confirming the efficacy of topiramate for this indication. Although these medications have different mechanisms of action, it is likely that they exert beneficial effects in alcohol dependence through their actions as glutamate antagonists and GABA agonists, helping to normalize the abnormal activity in these neurotransmitter systems seen following chronic heavy drinking.

In a 12-month pilot study, Mueller et al. (52) found carbamazepine to be superior to placebo in increasing the time to the first heavy drinking day and in reducing drinks/drinking day and the number of consecutive days of heavy drinking. In a 12-week, double-blind pilot study, Brady et al. (53) found that a significantly lower percentage of patients receiving divalproex than placebo relapsed to heavy drinking. There was also a significantly greater decrease in irritability in the divalproex-treated group.

Johnson et al. (54) initially conducted a single-site, 12-week, placebo-controlled study of topiramate, with the dosage gradually increased over 8 weeks to a maximum of 300 mg. Topiramate-treated patients showed significantly greater reductions than placebo-treated patients in drinks/day, drinks/drinking day, drinking days, heavy drinking days, and γ-glutamyltranspeptidase levels. Based on these findings, a subsequent multicenter study was conducted (55), which showed many of the same effects on drinking as the single-site study, though topiramate was not as well tolerated as it was in the initial trial. The authors interpreted these findings to reflect the more rapid dose titration (to a maximum of 300 mg, but over 6 weeks).

The most common adverse effect of topiramate compared to placebo is numbness and tingling (which is secondary to the commonly observed metabolic acidosis produced by the antagonism by topiramate of carbonic anhydrase), with other common side effects including a change in the sense of taste, tiredness/sleepiness, fatigue, dizziness, loss of appetite, nausea, diarrhea, weight decrease, and difficulty concentrating, with memory, and in word finding. Of clinical concern also are suicidal thoughts or actions, which have been reported uncommonly, but at a frequency greater than that seen with placebo treatment. Other adverse effects of topiramate that are less likely to occur but potentially serious are renal calculi and acute secondary glaucoma.

These findings provide clear support for the efficacy of this anticonvulsant for the treatment of alcohol dependence and suggest that the use of topiramate for this purpose should include a slowly increasing dosage. Additional research focusing on the optimal rate of dosage increase and the minimal dosage that is efficacious in alcohol dependence is warranted.

Baclofen This GABA-B receptor agonist has been approved as an antispasmodic for more than 30 years and has recently been studied as a treatment for alcohol dependence. In a small trial, Addolorato et al. (56) randomly assigned recently abstinent alcohol-dependent individuals to receive up to 30 mg/day of the medication or placebo divided into three daily doses. The medication was well tolerated and the baclofen-treated group was more likely to remain abstinent over the 1-month treatment period (also showing a greater number of cumulative abstinence days) than the placebo group. More recently, these investigators (57) evaluated the efficacy of baclofen in a sample of 84 alcohol-dependent patients with liver cirrhosis. Baclofen-treated patients were significantly more likely than placebo-treated patients to maintain abstinence (71% vs. 29%), with a concomitant doubling of abstinence days in the baclofen group. The medication was well tolerated and the baclofen group showed a nonsignificantly lower rate of study dropout than the placebo group (14% vs. 31%).

There is, however, evidence of misuse, overdose, and other complications (e.g., withdrawal reactions, including delirium) associated with baclofen (58,59), which underscores the need for more research on this medication before it can be recommended as a safe and efficacious treatment for alcohol dependence.

Serotonergic Agents A variety of serotonin reuptake inhibitors (SRIs) have been studied for their effects on alcohol consumption in humans, with fluoxetine and citalopram being the SRIs that have been studied the most (60). However, interest in this area of investigation has flagged in recent years because of inconsistent findings. Studies of the effects of SRIs on drinking behavior have been conducted in diverse subject samples. A recent meta-analysis (61) concluded that there was, overall, no benefit to the use of any antidepressant in alcohol-dependent patients without comorbid depression. An alternate interpretation is that these medications have differential effects in subgroups of alcohol-dependent patients, benefiting some and worsening the outcome of others, such that, in unselected groups of patients, they may have a null effect. Efforts to identify the features that differentiate these subgroups have yielded evidence of interactive effects with serotonergic medications.

Alcohol Dependence Subtypes Adapting an approach first used by Kranzler et al. (62), Pettinati et al. (63) found that low risk/severity alcohol-dependent patients (i.e., those with later age of onset) drank on fewer days and were more likely to be completely abstinent in the 12-week treatment trial when treated with sertraline compared with placebo. In a 6-month posttreatment follow-up of these patients (64), the beneficial effects of sertraline treatment persisted in this subgroup. Chick et al. (65) also found an effect with fluvoxamine that was similar to that observed with fluoxetine (62). Specifically, among early-onset drinkers, fluvoxamine was associated with worse outcome than placebo.

Using a subtyping approach, Johnson et al. (66) found that ondansetron (a 5-HT_3 receptor antagonist) selectively reduced drinking among patients with early onset of problem drinking (i.e., before age 25; early-onset alcohol-dependent patients). Specifically, ondansetron was superior to placebo on the proportion of days abstinent and on the intensity of alcohol intake. In contrast, late-onset alcohol-dependent patients showed effects of ondansetron on drinking behavior that were comparable to those of placebo. In a subsequent 8-week, open-label study of ondansetron, early-onset alcohol-dependent patients had a significantly greater decrease in drinks per day, drinks per drinking day, and alcohol-related problems than late-onset alcohol-dependent patients (29). Prospective studies are needed to evaluate whether there is a clearer role for the serotonergic medications in the treatment of heavy drinking or alcohol dependence in individuals differentiated by alcohol dependence subtype.

MEDICATIONS TO TREAT COOCCURRING PSYCHIATRIC SYMPTOMS OR DISORDERS IN ALCOHOL-DEPENDENT PATIENTS

Although most alcohol-dependent patients report a reduction in mood or anxiety symptoms following acute withdrawal, for some, these symptoms may persist for months. Even among patients without substantial symptoms of alcohol withdrawal, persistent, low-level mood or anxiety symptoms may develop, a condition that has been called "subacute withdrawal." In a substantial minority of patients these symptoms may reflect diagnosable psychiatric disorders. Although medications (e.g., SRIs) are often prescribed during the postwithdrawal period in hopes of relieving these symptoms, there is not good evidence that the treatment of persistent or subacute withdrawal symptoms that do not meet diagnostic criteria for a co-occurring psychiatric disorder results in better outcome in alcohol-dependent patients.

Many of the early studies of the efficacy of medications to treat mood disturbances targeted symptoms of depression and anxiety in unselected groups of alcohol-dependent patients after withdrawal. These and other methodologic limitations in these studies make the failure to demonstrate an advantage over control conditions through reductions in either psychiatric symptoms or drinking behavior difficult to interpret (67). Over the past 10 to 15 years, there has been renewed interest in the incidence and prevalence of co-occurring psychiatric disturbances among patients with alcohol abuse/dependence (68). Community studies have shown high rates of co-occurrence of psychiatric disorders in alcohol-dependent individuals in the community (69–73). Further, the majority of such individuals who seek treatment meet lifetime criteria for one or more psychiatric disorders in addition to alcohol dependence, most commonly mood disorders, drug dependence, antisocial personality disorder, and anxiety disorders (74–76).

Antidepressants, benzodiazepines and other anxiolytics, antipsychotics, and lithium have been used to treat anxiety and depression in the postwithdrawal state. Although in general, the indications for use of these medications in alcohol-dependent patients are similar to those for patients with psychiatric illness who do not have alcohol dependence, careful differential diagnosis is warranted to identify patients for whom the symptoms can be ascribed to substance use. Further, the choice of medications should take into account the increased potential for adverse effects when prescribed to individuals who are actively drinking heavily. Adverse effects can result from pharmacodynamic interactions with medical disorders that commonly occur in the course of alcohol dependence, as well as from pharmacokinetic interactions with medications prescribed to treat these disorders (77).

Antidepressant Treatment of Unipolar Depression and Alcohol Dependence A majority of the studies in a meta-analysis that included 14 prospective, parallel-group, double-blind, randomized, placebo-controlled trials of antidepressants for a co-occurring substance use disorder and unipolar depression focused on alcohol dependence (78). Eight studies (six of which were in alcohol-dependent patients) showed a significant or near-significant advantage for the active medication over placebo in reducing symptoms of depression. The pooled effect size on the standardized difference between means on the Hamilton Depression Rating Scale was 0.38 (95% CI 0.18–0.58), a small-to-moderate effect. Studies with a placebo response rate greater than 25% showed no advantage for the active medication, whereas those with a smaller placebo response rate yielded effects in the moderate-to-large range. Allowing a week of abstinence to transpire before making a diagnosis of depression predicted a better antidepressant response. In contrast, a larger proportion of women in the study sample, the use of SRIs (vs. tricyclic or other antidepressants) and a concurrent psychosocial intervention were associated with a poorer medication response. Studies that showed a moderate effect of the medication on depression scores also showed moderate reductions in substance use, whereas smaller effects on depressive symptoms were associated with no beneficial effects on substance use.

Subsequent to the analysis by Nunes and Levin (78), there have been studies of pharmacotherapy for co-occurring alcohol dependence and depression. Hernandez-Avila et al. (79) compared nefazodone with placebo in alcohol-dependent subjects with current major depression. Although there were greater reductions in anxiety and depressive symptoms in the nefazodone group, the effects did not reach statistical significance, potentially because of the small sample size. Nonetheless, nefazodone-treated subjects reduced the frequency of heavy drinking days and total number of drinks more than did placebo-treated subjects. The occurrence of a limited number of reported cases of idiosyncratic hepatic failure during nefazodone treatment limits the drug's clinical utility.

Kranzler et al. (80) conducted a multicenter trial of sertraline in 328 patients with co-occurring major depressive disorder and alcohol dependence. After a 1-week, single-blind, placebo lead-in period, patients were randomly assigned to receive 10 weeks of treatment with sertraline or placebo. Randomization was stratified, based on whether initially elevated depression scores declined with the cessation of heavy drinking. Both depressive symptoms and alcohol consumption decreased substantially over time in both groups, with no reliable medication group differences on depressive symptoms or drinking behavior in either group. The high placebo response rate may have contributed to the null findings.

In summary, there is evidence that most episodes of post-withdrawal depression will remit without specific treatment if abstinence from alcohol is maintained for a period of days or weeks (81,82). However, persistent depression requires treatment. SRIs and newer generation antidepressants have become the first-line treatment of depression because they have a favorable adverse-event profile. These medications do not have the anticholinergic, hypotensive, or sedative effects of the tricyclic antidepressants, nor do they have the adverse cardiovascular effects, which in overdose can be lethal. However, SRIs can exacerbate the tremor, anxiety, and insomnia often experienced by recently detoxified alcohol-dependent patients, and may slightly increase the risk of gastrointestinal bleeding (particularly in combination with nonsteroidal anti-inflammatory drugs or aspirin). Furthermore, the findings of Nunes and Levin (78) suggest that for the treatment of depression among patients with a substance use disorder, SRIs may be less efficacious than tricyclic or other types of antidepressants.

Mood-Stabilizer Treatment of Bipolar Disorder and Alcohol Dependence

Bipolar disorder co-occurs commonly with alcohol dependence. The presence of comorbid alcohol dependence is associated with an increased rate of mixed or dysphoric mania and rapid cycling, as well as greater bipolar symptom severity, suicidality, and aggressivity (83). However, controlled trials of medication to treat these comorbid disorders are difficult to conduct. A placebo-controlled trial of divalproex sodium in this patient group showed that the drug significantly decreased the proportion of heavy drinking days (corroborated by a decrease in the concentration of gamma-glutamyl transpeptidase), whereas manic and depressive symptoms improved equally in both groups.

Treatment of Cooccurring Anxiety Disorders and Alcohol Dependence

Benzodiazepines and Other Anxiolytics

Benzodiazepines (BZs) are widely used and generally considered to be acceptable treatment for acute alcohol withdrawal. In contrast, most nonmedical personnel involved in the treatment of alcoholism oppose the use of medications that can induce dependence to treat the anxiety, depression, and sleep disturbances that can persist for months after withdrawal. The relative merits of the use of BZs in alcohol-dependent and other substance abuse patients during the postwithdrawal period for the management of anxiety or insomnia have also been debated in the medical literature (84,85).

Despite the risks that the use of BZs may create in alcohol-dependent patients beyond the period of acute withdrawal (e.g., physical dependence or overdose), judicious use of the drugs in this setting may be justified. Early relapse, which commonly disrupts alcohol rehabilitation, can result from protracted withdrawal-related symptoms (e.g., anxiety, depression, insomnia). To the extent that these symptoms can be suppressed by low doses of BZs, retention in treatment could be increased (86). Moreover, for some patients, BZ dependence, if it does occur, may be more benign than alcohol dependence.

The controversy surrounding this approach to alcohol treatment stems from the fact that these potential benefits must be weighed against the risk both of overdose and of physical dependence on BZs. Although these drugs alone are comparatively safe, even in overdose, their combination with other brain depressants (including alcohol) can be lethal. Although there is little doubt that alcohol-dependent individuals are more vulnerable to develop dependence on the BZs than the average person, the potential for abuse and dependence may be lower than is generally believed (87–89). However, dependence on both alcohol and BZs may increase depressive symptoms (81) and co-occurring alcohol and BZ dependence may be more difficult to treat than alcoholism alone (90).

The BZs currently available for clinical use vary pharmacokinetically, and in their acute euphoriant effects and the frequency with which they are reported to cause dependence. Diazepam, lorazepam, and alprazolam may have greater abuse potential than chlordiazepoxide or clorazepate (91). Similarly, oxazepam was reported to produce low levels of abuse (87). Jaffe et al. (92) found that, when administered to recently withdrawn alcohol-dependent patients, halazepam produces minimal euphoria even at a supratherapeutic dosage. Partial agonist compounds at the BZ receptor complex may offer an advantage over approved BZs for use in alcohol-dependent individuals, though there is no literature as yet that addresses this question.

Buspirone, a non-BZ anxiolytic, exerts its effects largely via its partial agonist activity at serotonergic autoreceptors. Although comparable in efficacy to diazepam in the relief of anxiety and associated depression in outpatients with moderate-to-severe anxiety (93,94), buspirone is less sedating than diazepam or clorazepate, does not interact with alcohol to impair psychomotor skills, and does not have abuse liability (95–97). This pharmacologic profile makes buspirone more suitable than BZs to treat anxiety symptoms among alcohol-dependent patients. In contrast to BZs, however, buspirone does not have acute anxiolytic effects, is not useful in the treatment of alcohol withdrawal, and is not useful for treating the insomnia that is commonly reported by alcohol-dependent patients during acute and protracted withdrawal.

Results from three of four placebo-controlled, double-blind trials of buspirone to treat anxiety symptoms among alcohol-dependent patients have shown the drug to be superior to placebo in increasing treatment retention and reducing anxiety symptoms and measures of drinking (98–101). Although buspirone appears to be useful in the treatment of anxiety symptoms in alcohol-dependent patients, it has not been possible to identify clinical features that differentiate individuals for whom buspirone may be most efficacious from those who are not responsive to the medication.

SUMMARY AND CONCLUSIONS

Although BZs play a central role in the treatment of alcohol withdrawal, the use of medications that have been approved for alcohol rehabilitation remains very limited, even among addiction physicians. A survey of nearly 1,400 members of the American Society of Addiction Medicine and the American Academy of Addiction Psychiatry (102) showed that they prescribed disulfiram to only 9% of their alcohol-dependent patients and naltrexone was prescribed only slightly more frequently (i.e., to 13% of patients). In contrast, antidepressants were prescribed to 44% of alcohol-dependent patients. Although nearly all of these physicians had heard of disulfiram and naltrexone, their self-reported level of knowledge of these medications was much lower than that for antidepressants and BZs.

Although continuing developments in the United States, Europe, and Australia suggest that medications may eventually become a key element in alcohol treatment, many clinical questions must be considered before medications are likely to be widely employed for this indication. In addition to the issues discussed earlier in regard to specific agents (e.g., What is the optimal duration of naltrexone treatment?), the safety and efficacy of medications to treat alcohol dependence must be examined with adequate statistical power in women, in different ethnic/racial groups and in adolescent and geriatric samples. In addition, studies of cost-effectiveness, cost-benefit, and quality of life must support the routine coverage of pharmacological treatments for alcohol dependence under standard medical insurance plans.

The treatment of psychiatric symptoms that co-occur with alcohol dependence, which can augment efforts at relapse prevention, has been studied in some detail (68). However, the literature remains mixed with respect to the efficacy of specific interventions. Anxiolytics that are low in abuse potential, such as buspirone, and antidepressants with benign side effect profiles, such as the newer generation drugs that may reduce ethanol intake, warrant careful evaluation in the treatment of anxious and depressed alcohol-dependent patients.

However, even if medications that are prescribed to alcohol-dependent patients with persistent co-occurring mood and anxiety symptoms ameliorate those symptoms, they will not necessarily reduce alcohol consumption after a significant degree of alcohol dependence develops. This is likely to hold true even if pathologic mood states were important in the initiation of heavy drinking (68,103). That is, the neuroadaptive changes and the complex learning that characterize the dependence syndrome (104) are not likely to resolve because one major contributing factor is brought under control. The challenge for practitioners treating alcohol dependence is to combine efficacious medications with empirically-based psychologic interventions and self-help group participation for those patients willing and able to incorporate these elements into their treatment.

The medications that have been most widely studied in alcohol rehabilitation are disulfiram, naltrexone, and acamprosate. Results from the COMBINE Study, trials of depot naltrexone formulations, and of topiramate have provided important new information on the use of these medications in alcohol rehabilitation. As the research literature on the use of medications to treat alcohol dependence grows, it will be possible to assess the utility of different medication combinations and a variety of psychotherapies. There are also ongoing efforts to match medications with specific subgroups of alcohol-dependent patients, based on clinical or genetic characteristics, and these are beginning to bear fruit.

The use of medications in patients who are actively participating in self-help groups may be particularly challenging. Although members of abstinence-oriented groups such as Alcoholics Anonymous may be willing to work with physicians when they prescribe disulfiram, the use of which is supportive of their goal of total abstinence, they may be less supportive of other medications that aim to reduce drinking and its associated medical, psychologic, and social harm.

As evidence has accumulated showing that a growing number of medications are efficacious for the treatment of alcohol dependence, the therapeutic options available to physicians in treating these patients have increased. Nonetheless, many of these developments have not been translated to widespread changes in treatment. The major challenge to medications development will be to identify new medications that are efficacious and well tolerated, as well as the patient and treatment factors that can be used to optimize effectiveness. Because all three medications that are FDA-approved for the treatment of alcohol dependence have demonstrated efficacy in some patients, these medications should be considered a first-line treatment in alcohol-dependent patients, to be used in combination with behavioral treatment. Given limited data on how to choose which of the efficacious medications is appropriate for any given patient, the choice can be made based on physician and patient preference.

REFERENCES

1. Kranzler H, Ciraulo D. *Clinical manual of addiction psychopharmacology.* Washington, DC: American Psychiatric Press, Inc., 2005:1–54.
2. Heilig M, Egli M. Pharmacological treatment of alcohol dependence: target symptoms and target mechanisms. *Pharmacol Ther* 2006;111: 855–876.
3. Petrakis IL. A rational approach to the pharmacotherapy of alcohol dependence. *J Clin Psychopharmacol* 2006;26(Suppl 1):S3–S12.
4. Johnson BA. Update on neuropharmacological treatments for alcoholism: scientific basis and clinical findings. *Biochem Pharmacol* 2008;75:34–56.
5. Soyka M, Kranzler H, Berglund M, et al. Guidelines for biological treatment of substance use and related disorders, part 1: alcoholism. *World J Biol Psychiatry* 2008;9:6–23.
6. Lindros KO, Stowell A, Pikkarainen P, et al. The disulfiram (Antabuse)-alcohol reaction in male alcoholics: its efficient management by 4-methylpyrazole. *Alcohol Clin Exp Res* 1981;5:528–530.
7. Peachey JE, Brien JF, Roach CA, et al. A comparative review of the pharmacological and toxicological properties of disulfiram and calcium carbimide. *J Clin Psychopharmacol* 1981;1:21–26.
8. Peachey JE, Maglana S, Robinson GM, et al. Cardiovascular changes during the calcium carbimide-ethanol interaction. *Clin Pharmacol Ther* 1981;29:40–46.
9. Sellers EM, Naranjo CA, Peachey JE. Drug therapy: drugs to decrease alcohol consumption. *N Engl J Med* 1981;305:1255–1262.
10. Chick J. Safety issues concerning the use of disulfiram in treating alcohol dependence. *Drug Saf* 1999;20:427–435.
11. Brewer C. How effective is the standard dose of disulfiram? A review of the alcohol-disulfiram reaction in practice. *Br J Psychiatry* 1984;144: 200–202.
12. Favazza AR, Martin P. Chemotherapy of delirium tremens: a survey of physicians' preferences. *Am J Psychiatry* 1974;131:1031–1033.
13. Fuller RK, Branchey L, Brightwell DR, et al. Disulfiram treatment of alcoholism. A Veterans Administration cooperative study. *JAMA* 1986; 256:1449–1455.
14. Allen JP, Litten RZ. Techniques to enhance compliance with disulfiram. *Alcohol Clin Exp Res* 1992;16:1035–1041.
15. Azrin NH, Sisson RW, Meyers R, et al. Alcoholism treatment by disulfiram and community reinforcement therapy. *J Behav Ther Exp Psychiatry* 1982;13:105–112.
16. Brewer C, Meyers RJ, Johnsen J. Does disulfiram help to prevent relapse in alcohol abuse? *CNS Drugs* 2000;14:329–341.
17. Chick J, Gough K, Falkowski W, et al. Disulfiram treatment of alcoholism. *Br J Psychiatry* 1992;161:84–89.
18. Volpicelli JR, Alterman AI, Hayashida M, et al. Naltrexone in the treatment of alcohol dependence. *Arch Gen Psychiatry* 1992;49:876–880.
19. O'Malley SS, Jaffe AJ, Chang G, et al. Naltrexone and coping skills therapy for alcohol dependence. A controlled study. *Arch Gen Psychiatry* 1992;49:881–887.
20. Volpicelli JR, Watson NT, King AC, et al. Effect of naltrexone on alcohol "high" in alcoholics. *Am J Psychiatry* 1995;152:613–615.
21. O'Malley SS, Jaffe AJ, Rode S, et al. Experience of a "slip" among alcoholics treated with naltrexone or placebo. *Am J Psychiatry* 1996;153: 281–283.
22. O'Malley SS, Jaffe AJ, Chang G, et al. Six-month follow-up of naltrexone and psychotherapy for alcohol dependence. *Arch Gen Psychiatry* 1996;53:217–224.
23. Kranzler HR, Van Kirk J. Efficacy of naltrexone and acamprosate for alcoholism treatment: a meta-analysis. *Alcohol Clin Exp Res* 2001;25: 1335–1341.
24. Streeton C, Whelan G. Naltrexone, a relapse prevention maintenance treatment of alcohol dependence: a meta-analysis of randomized controlled trials. *Alcohol Alcohol* 2001;36:544–552.
25. Bouza C, Angeles M, Munoz A, et al. Efficacy and safety of naltrexone and acamprosate in the treatment of alcohol dependence: a systematic review. *Addiction* 2004;99:811–828.
26. Srisurapanont M, Jarusuraisin N. Naltrexone for the treatment of alcoholism: a meta-analysis of randomized controlled trials. *Int J Neuropsychopharmacol* 2005;8:267–280.
27. Anton RF, Moak DH, Latham PK, et al. Posttreatment results of combining naltrexone with cognitive-behavior therapy for the treatment of alcoholism. *J Clin Psychopharmacol* 2001;21:72–77.
28. Anton RF, O'Malley SS, Ciraulo DA, et al. Combined pharmacotherapies and behavioral interventions for alcohol dependence: the COMBINE study: a randomized controlled trial. *JAMA* 2006;295: 2003–2017.
29. Kranzler HR, Armeli S, Tennen H, et al. Targeted naltrexone for early problem drinkers. *J Clin Psychopharmacol* 2003;23:294–304.
30. Heinala P, Alho H, Kiianmaa K, et al. Targeted use of naltrexone without prior detoxification in the treatment of alcohol dependence: a factorial double-blind, placebo-controlled trial. *J Clin Psychopharmacol* 2001;21:287–292.
31. O'Malley SS, Rounsaville BJ, Farren C, et al. Initial and maintenance naltrexone treatment for alcohol dependence using primary care vs. specialty care: a nested sequence of 3 randomized trials. *Arch Intern Med* 2003;163:1695–1704.
32. Volpicelli JR, Rhines KC, Rhines JS, et al. Naltrexone and alcohol dependence. Role of subject compliance. *Arch Gen Psychiatry* 1997;54: 737–742.
33. Kranzler HR, Modesto-Lowe V, Nuwayser ES. Sustained-release naltrexone for alcoholism treatment: a preliminary study. *Alcohol Clin Exp Res* 1998;22:1074–1079.
34. Kranzler HR, Wesson DR, Billot L. Naltrexone depot for treatment of alcohol dependence: a multicenter, randomized, placebo-controlled clinical trial. *Alcohol Clin Exp Res* 2004;28:1051–1059.
35. O'Malley SS, Garbutt JC, Gastfriend DR, et al. Efficacy of extended-release naltrexone in alcohol-dependent patients who are abstinent before treatment. *J Clin Psychopharmacol* 2007;27:507–512.
36. Emmerson PJ, Liu MR, Woods JH, et al. Binding affinity and selectivity of opioids at mu, delta and kappa receptors in monkey brain membranes. *J Pharmacol Exp Ther* 1994;271:1630–1637.
37. Mason BJ, Ritvo EC, Morgan RO, et al. A double-blind, placebo-controlled pilot study to evaluate the efficacy and safety of oral nalmefene HCl for alcohol dependence. *Alcohol Clin Exp Res* 1994;18:1162–1167.
38. Mason BJ, Salvato FR, Williams LD, et al. A double-blind, placebo-controlled study of oral nalmefene for alcohol dependence. *Arch Gen Psychiatry* 1999;56:719–724.
39. Anton RF, Pettinati H, Zweben A, et al. A multi-site dose ranging study of nalmefene in the treatment of alcohol dependence. *J Clin Psychopharmacol* 2004;24:421–428.
40. Karhuvaara S, Simojoki K, Virta A, et al. Targeted nalmefene with simple medical management in the treatment of heavy drinkers: a randomized double-blind placebo-controlled multicenter study. *Alcohol Clin Exp Res* 2007;31:1179–1187.
41. Oslin DW, Berrettini W, Kranzler HR, et al. A functional polymorphism of the mu-opioid receptor gene is associated with naltrexone response in alcohol-dependent patients. *Neuropsychopharmacology* 2003;28: 1546–1552.
42. Gelernter J, Gueorguieva R, Kranzler HR, et al. Opioid receptor gene (OPRM1, OPRK1, and OPRD1) variants and response to naltrexone treatment for alcohol dependence: results from the VA Cooperative Study. *Alcohol Clin Exp Res* 2007;31:555–563.

43. Anton RF, Oroszi G, O'Malley S, et al. An evaluation of mu-opioid receptor (OPRM1) as a predictor of naltrexone response in the treatment of alcohol dependence: results from the Combined Pharmacotherapies and Behavioral Interventions for Alcohol Dependence (COMBINE) study. *Arch Gen Psychiatry* 2008;65:135–144.
44. Mitchell JM, Fields HL, White RL, et al. The Asp40 mu-opioid receptor allele does not predict naltrexone treatment efficacy in heavy drinkers. *J Clin Psychopharmacol* 2007;27:112–115.
45. Lhuintre JP, Daoust M, Moore ND, et al. Ability of calcium bis acetyl homotaurine, a GABA agonist, to prevent relapse in weaned alcoholics. *Lancet* 1985;1:1014–1016.
46. Kranzler HR, Gage A. Acamprosate efficacy in alcohol-dependent patients: reanalysis of results from 3 pivotal trials. *Am J Addict* 2008;17: 70–76.
47. Chick J, Lehert P, Landron F. Does acamprosate improve reduction of drinking as well as aiding abstinence? *J Psychopharmacol* 2003;17: 397–402.
48. Mann K, Lehert P, Morgan MY. The efficacy of acamprosate in the maintenance of abstinence in alcohol-dependent individuals: results of a meta-analysis. *Alcohol Clin Exp Res* 2004;28:51–63.
49. Besson J, Aeby F, Kasas A, et al. Combined efficacy of acamprosate and disulfiram in the treatment of alcoholism: a controlled study. *Alcohol Clin Exp Res* 1998;22:573–579.
50. Mason BJ, Goodman AM, Chabac S, et al. Effect of oral acamprosate on abstinence in patients with alcohol dependence in a double-blind, placebo-controlled trial: the role of patient motivation. *J Psychiatr Res* 2006;40:383–393.
51. Kiefer F, Jahn H, Tarnaske T, et al. Comparing and combining naltrexone and acamprosate in relapse prevention of alcoholism: a double-blind, placebo-controlled study. *Arch Gen Psychiatry* 2003;60:92–99.
52. Mueller TI, Stout RL, Rudden S, et al. A double-blind, placebo-controlled pilot study of carbamazepine for the treatment of alcohol dependence. *Alcohol Clin Exp Res* 1997;21:86–92.
53. Brady KT, Myrick H, Henderson S, et al. The use of divalproex in alcohol relapse prevention: a pilot study. *Drug Alcohol Depend* 2002;67: 323–330.
54. Johnson BA, Ait-Daoud N, Bowden CL, et al. Oral topiramate for treatment of alcohol dependence: a randomised controlled trial. *Lancet* 2003;361:1677–1685.
55. Johnson BA, Rosenthal N, Capece JA, et al. Topiramate for treating alcohol dependence: a randomized controlled trial. *JAMA* 2007;298: 1641–1651.
56. Addolorato G, Caputo F, Capristo E, et al. Baclofen efficacy in reducing alcohol craving and intake: a preliminary double-blind randomized controlled study. *Alcohol Alcohol* 2002;37:504–508.
57. Addolorato G, Leggio L, Ferrulli A, et al. Effectiveness and safety of baclofen for maintenance of alcohol abstinence in alcohol-dependent patients with liver cirrhosis: randomised, double-blind controlled study. *Lancet* 2007;370:1915–1922.
58. Perry HE, Wright RO, Shannon MW, et al. Baclofen overdose: drug experimentation in a group of adolescents. *Pediatrics* 1998;101: 1045–1048.
59. Leo RJ, Baer D. Delirium associated with baclofen withdrawal: a review of common presentations and management strategies. *Psychosomatics* 2005;46:503–507.
60. Pettinati HM, Kranzler HR, Madaras J. The status of serotonin-selective pharmacotherapy in the treatment of alcohol dependence. *Recent Dev Alcohol* 2003;16:247–262.
61. Torrens M, Fonseca F, Mateu G, et al. Efficacy of antidepressants in substance use disorders with and without comorbid depression. A systematic review and meta-analysis. *Drug Alcohol Depend* 2005;78:1–22.
62. Kranzler HR, Burleson JA, Brown J, et al. Fluoxetine treatment seems to reduce the beneficial effects of cognitive-behavioral therapy in type B alcoholics. *Alcohol Clin Exp Res* 1996;20:1534–1541.
63. Pettinati HM, Volpicelli JR, Kranzler HR, et al. Sertraline treatment for alcohol dependence: interactive effects of medication and alcoholic subtype. *Alcohol Clin Exp Res* 2000;24:1041–1049.
64. Dundon W, Lynch KG, Pettinati HM, et al. Treatment outcomes in type A and B alcohol dependence 6 months after serotonergic pharmacotherapy. *Alcohol Clin Exp Res* 2004;28:1065–1073.
65. Chick J, Aschauer H, Hornik K. Efficacy of fluvoxamine in preventing relapse in alcohol dependence: a one-year, double-blind, placebo-controlled multicentre study with analysis by typology. *Drug Alcohol Depend* 2004;74:61–70.
66. Johnson BA, Roache JD, Javors MA, et al. Ondansetron for reduction of drinking among biologically predisposed alcoholic patients: a randomized controlled trial. *JAMA* 2000;284:963–971.
67. Ciraulo DA, Jaffe JH. Tricyclic antidepressants in the treatment of depression associated with alcoholism. *J Clin Psychopharmacol* 1981;1: 146–150.
68. Kranzler H, Tinsley J. *Dual diagnosis: substance abuse and comorbid medical and psychiatric disorders.* New York: Marcel Dekker; 2004.
69. Regier DA, Farmer ME, Rae DS, et al. Comorbidity of mental disorders with alcohol and other drug abuse. Results from the Epidemiologic Catchment Area (ECA) Study. *JAMA* 1990;264:2511–2518.
70. Kessler RC, McGonagle KA, Zhao S, et al. Lifetime and 12-month prevalence of DSM-III-R psychiatric disorders in the United States. Results from the National Comorbidity Survey. *Arch Gen Psychiatry* 1994;51:8–19.
71. Kessler RC, Crum RM, Warner LA, et al. Lifetime co-occurrence of DSM-III-R alcohol abuse and dependence with other psychiatric disorders in the National Comorbidity Survey. *Arch Gen Psychiatry* 1997;54: 313–321.
72. Grant BF, Harford TC. Comorbidity between DSM-IV alcohol use disorders and major depression: results of a national survey. *Drug Alcohol Depend* 1995;39:197–206.
73. Grant BF, Dawson DA, Stinson FS, et al. The 12-month prevalence and trends in DSM-IV alcohol abuse and dependence: United States, 1991–1992 and 2001–2002. *Drug Alcohol Depend* 2004;74:223–234.
74. Powell BJ, Penick EC, Othmer E, et al. Prevalence of additional psychiatric syndromes among male alcoholics. *J Clin Psychiatry* 1982;43: 404–407.
75. Hesselbrock MN, Meyer RE, Keener JJ. Psychopathology in hospitalized alcoholics. *Arch Gen Psychiatry* 1985;42:1050–1055.
76. Ross HE, Glaser FB, Germanson T. The prevalence of psychiatric disorders in patients with alcohol and other drug problems. *Arch Gen Psychiatry* 1988;45:1023–1031.
77. Sullivan L, O'Connor P. Medical disorders in substance abuse patients. In: Kranzler H, Tinsley J, eds. *Dual diagnosis and psychiatric treatment: substance abuse and comorbid disorders,* 2nd ed. New York: Marcel Dekker, 2004:515–553.
78. Nunes EV, Levin FR. Treatment of depression in patients with alcohol or other drug dependence: a meta-analysis. *JAMA* 2004;291:1887–1896.
79. Hernandez-Avila CA, Modesto-Lowe V, Feinn R, et al. Nefazodone treatment of comorbid alcohol dependence and major depression. *Alcohol Clin Exp Res* 2004;28:433–440.
80. Kranzler HR, Mueller T, Cornelius J, et al. Sertraline treatment of co-occurring alcohol dependence and major depression. *J Clin Psychopharmacol* 2006;26:13–20.
81. Schuckit M. Alcoholic patients with secondary depression. *Am J Psychiatry* 1983;140:711–714.
82. Brown SA, Schuckit MA. Changes in depression among abstinent alcoholics. *J Stud Alcohol* 1988;49:412–417.
83. Frye MA, Salloum IM. Bipolar disorder and comorbid alcoholism: prevalence rate and treatment considerations. *Bipolar Disord* 2006;8:677–685.
84. Ciraulo DA, Nace EP. Benzodiazepine treatment of anxiety or insomnia in substance abuse patients. *Am J Addict* 2000;9:276–279; discussion 280–274.
85. Posternak MA, Mueller TI. Assessing the risks and benefits of benzodiazepines for anxiety disorders in patients with a history of substance abuse or dependence. *Am J Addict* 2001;10:48–68.
86. Kissin B. Medical management of the alcoholic patient. Kissin B, Begleiter H (eds). *The biology of alcoholism—vol. 5. Treatment and rehabilitation of the chronic alcoholic, vol. 5.* New York: Plenum Press, 1977:55–103.

87. Bliding A. The abuse potential of benzodiazepines with special reference to oxazepam. *Acta Psychiatr Scand Suppl* 1978:111–116.
88. Marks J. *The benzodiazepines: use, misuse, abuse.* Lancaster, UK: MTP Press Ltd., 1978.
89. Ciraulo DA, Barnhill JG, Jaffe JH, et al. Intravenous pharmacokinetics of 2-hydroxyimipramine in alcoholics and normal controls. *J Stud Alcohol* 1990;51:366–372.
90. Sokolow L, Welte J, Hynes G, et al. Multiple substance use by alcoholics. *Br J Addict* 1981;76:147–158.
91. Wolf B, Iguchi MY, Griffiths RR. Sedative/tranquilizer use and abuse in alcoholics currently in outpatient treatment: incidence, pattern and preference. In: Harris L, ed. *Problems of drug dependence 1989* (NIDA Research Monograph 95). Washington, DC: U.S. Government Printing Office, 1990:376–377.
92. Jaffe JH, Ciraulo DA, Nies A, et al. Abuse potential of halazepam and of diazepam in patients recently treated for acute alcohol withdrawal. *Clin Pharmacol Ther* 1983;34:623–630.
93. Goldberg HL, Finnerty RJ. Comparative efficacy of tofisopam and placebo. *Am J Psychiatry* 1979;136:196–199.
94. Jacobson AF, Dominguez RA, Goldstein BJ, et al. Comparison of buspirone and diazepam in generalized anxiety disorder. *Pharmacotherapy* 1985;5:290–296.
95. Seppala T, Aranko K, Mattila MJ, et al. Effects of alcohol on buspirone and lorazepam actions. *Clin Pharmacol Ther* 1982;32:201–207.
96. Mattila MJ, Aranko K, Seppala T. Acute effects of buspirone and alcohol on psychomotor skills. *J Clin Psychiatry* 1982;43:56–61.
97. Griffith JD, Jasinski DR, Casten GP, et al. Investigation of the abuse liability of buspirone in alcohol-dependent patients. *Am J Med* 1986;80: 30–35.
98. Tollefson GD, Montague-Clouse J, Tollefson SL. Treatment of comorbid generalized anxiety in a recently detoxified alcoholic population with a selective serotonergic drug (buspirone). *J Clin Psychopharmacol* 1992; 12:19–26.
99. Malcolm R, Anton RF, Randall CL, et al. A placebo-controlled trial of buspirone in anxious inpatient alcoholics. *Alcohol Clin Exp Res* 1992; 16:1007–1013.
100. Kranzler HR, Burleson JA, Del Boca FK, et al. Buspirone treatment of anxious alcoholics. A placebo-controlled trial. *Arch Gen Psychiatry* 1994; 51:720–731.
101. Bruno F. Buspirone in the treatment of alcoholic patients. *Psychopathology* 1989;22(Suppl 1):49–59.
102. Mark TL, Kranzler HR, Song X, et al. Physicians' opinions about medications to treat alcoholism. *Addiction* 2003;98:617–626.
103. Meyer RE. How to understand the relationship between psychopathology and addictive disorders: another expample of the chicken and the egg. In: Meyer RE, ed. *Psychopathology and addictive disorders.* New York: Guilford Press, 1986 pp. 3–16.
104. Edwards G, Gross MM. Alcohol dependence: provisional description of a clinical syndrome. *Br Med J* 1976;1:1058–1061.

CHAPTER 47

Jeffrey S. Cluver, MD
Tara M. Wright, MD
Hugh Myrick, MD

Pharmacologic Interventions for Sedative-Hypnotic Addiction

INTRODUCTION

Sedative-hypnotic agents have been utilized for centuries because of their ability to induce sleep. Most of the drugs in this class of medications have a mechanism of action in the central nervous system (CNS) that leads to their anxiolytic and sleep-inducing properties. Prior to 1900, agents such as chloral hydrate, bromide, paraldehyde, and sulford were used. The first barbiturate (*barbital*, a derivative of barbituric acid) was introduced in 1903 and soon became popular because of its ability to induce sleep and decrease anxiety. Phenobarbital was introduced in 1912, and in addition to the effects seen with barbital, this medication was also shown to have anticonvulsant properties. Despite safety and abuse issues, such as its narrow therapeutic index, tolerance, and drug interactions, phenobarbital proved to be a popular medication, and thousands of derivative compounds were developed. Today there are <20 barbiturates that are available, and their clinical use has been largely supplanted by benzodiazepines.

The first benzodiazepine was synthesized in 1957. Chlordiazepoxide (Librium), and the other benzodiazepines that followed, were found to be useful in the treatment of anxiety and sleep. Although the properties of benzodiazepines and barbiturates are similar, the relative safety and tolerability of the benzodiazepines has led to their more widespread and lasting use. Medications in the benzodiazepine class all share a similar structure and bind to the same receptor site on the γ-aminobutyric acid (GABA) receptor.

Barbiturates are now often categorized with other sedative-hypnotics, keeping in mind that barbiturates also act on the GABA receptor by binding to a different subunit than the benzodiazepines. Other relatively new additions to this category of medications are the imidazopyridine derivatives (zolpidem, and others), zaleplon, and eszopiclone. These medications are chemically distinct from benzodiazepines, but they also bind to the GABA receptor, at the omega subunit.

In Table 47.1, currently available sedative-hypnotic agents are listed. It has been reported that individuals with a history of substance abuse have reactions similar to those of these newer compounds and traditional benzodiazepines (1,2), and self-administration in laboratory animals has also been seen (3). Benzodiazepines and other sedative-hypnotics are often used in conjunction with other substances of abuse to enhance the effects of the other substances or to help an individual cope with unpleasant side effects of other drug use or withdrawal. Additionally, alone or when used with other CNS depressants, benzodiazepines and sedative-hypnotics can lead to respiratory depression, coma, and death. In this chapter, we will focus on the management of individuals with dependence on these medications, especially in the context of withdrawal.

PHARMACOLOGY

As mentioned previously, the effects of benzodiazepines and other sedative-hypnotics are mediated by their binding to the GABA receptor. GABA receptors are distributed widely

TABLE 47.1 Classes of Sedative-Hypnotic Drugs: Drug Classes, Nonproprietary Names, and Trade Names

Benzodiazepines	Barbiturates	Miscellaneous
Alprazolam (Xanax)	Amobarbital (Amytal)	Chloral hydrate (Noctec, others)
Chlordiazepoxide (Librium, others)	Aprobarbital (Alurate)	Eszopiclone (Lunesta)
Clonazepam (Klonopin, others)	Butabarbital (Butisol Sodium, others)	Ethchlorvynol (Placidyl)
Clorazepate (Tranxene, others)	Butalbital	Ethinamate (Valmid)
Diazepam (Valium, others)	Mephobarbital (Mebaral)	Glutethimide (Doriden, others)
Flurazepam HCl (Dalmane, others)	Pentobarbital (Nembutal)	Meprobamate (Miltown, others)
Lorazepam (Ativan, others)	Phenobarbital (Luminal Sodium, others)	Methyprylon (Noludar)
Oxazepam (Serax, others)	Secobarbital (Seconal Sodium)	Paraldehyde (Paral)
Temazepam (Restoril, others)	Talbutal (Lotusate)	Zaleplon (Sonata)
Triazolam (Halcion)	—	Zolpidem (Ambien)

throughout the brain and are so-named because they bind gamma aminobutyric acid, the major inhibitory neurotransmitter in the CNS. There are specific receptor subunits that are allosterically bound to the GABA receptor, and these medications act as agonists by increasing the ability of the inhibitory neurotransmitter gamma aminobutyric acid to bind to and activate the GABA-A receptor. When an agonist such as a benzodiazepine or barbiturate binds to the GABA receptor, the receptor opens its chloride channel, which then decreases neuronal excitability. Clinically this leads to the effects of decreased anxiety, increased sedation, muscle relaxation, and increased seizure threshold. The toxic effects of these compounds are caused by excessive opening of chloride channels and can lead to respiratory depression, coma, and death. One essential difference between benzodiazepines and barbiturates is that high doses of barbiturates lead to excessive activity of GABA at the GABA-A receptor (which directly leads to respiratory depression), whereas high doses of benzodiazepines do not. Among the sedative-hypnotic agents, there are important differences in the onset of activity, half-life of the medication, presence of active metabolites, and specificity of the clinical effects.

Although benzodiazepines and other sedative-hypnotics are agonists at the GABA receptor, there are also inverse agonists (such as betacarboline) that bind to the GABA receptor but cause the chloride channels to close. Such inverse agonists can cause increased anxiety and lower the seizure threshold. A compound with a high affinity for the GABA receptor that does not exert an agonist or inverse agonist effects is flumazenil. This medication was developed and marketed to reverse the effects of benzodiazepines, including sedation and respiratory depression.

DEFINITIONS OF ABUSE AND DEPENDENCE

It is worth taking a moment to clarify several definitions, especially when discussing this class of medications. *Physical dependence* can be defined as an altered homeostasis at several levels of drug effect and activity. Discontinuation of the drug in this state leads to symptoms resulting from a disruption of this homeostasis. *Tolerance* can be defined as a decreased pharmacologic effect after repeated or prolonged exposure to the drug so that higher doses are needed to achieve the same initial clinical effects. Both physical dependence and tolerance are inevitable with prolonged and regular use of medications in the class of benzodiazepines and other sedative-hypnotics. Drug *misuse* generally refers to inappropriate use of a medication such as the use of a higher dose than prescribed. DSM-IV substance dependence is a syndrome that is associated with an apparent loss of control over the use of a drug, a preoccupation with obtaining the drug, and continued use despite negative consequences. This condition is largely seen in drugs with reinforcing properties, such as the ability to produce euphoria or other positive subjective experiences. Clarification of these definitions is important, as physical dependence should not be equated with, or imply, the syndrome of DSM-IV dependence, although the two often coexist. Similarly, the misuse of a medication does not directly imply dependence, as may be the case in patients with severe anxiety disorders who do not achieve relief with their initially prescribed doses.

ISSUES OF ABUSE AND DEPENDENCE

Benzodiazepines have largely replaced barbiturates and other sedative hypnotics in clinical settings, owing to their preferred pharmacologic profile. Overall there has been a trend toward decreased use of benzodiazepines and other sedative-hypnotics, but their use is still widespread. In1999, about 100 million prescriptions were written for benzodiazepines in the United States (4) and just more than 12% of individuals over the age of 12 report lifetime abuse of benzodiazepines and sedative-hypnotic medications (5). These medications are often initially prescribed for the treatment of anxiety disorders and insomnia, but their misuse (use at high doses or more frequent intervals) often leads to euphoria and disinhibition, making them desirable as drugs of abuse.

Laboratory studies involving rats and nonhuman primates demonstrate that many sedative-hypnotics are self-administered, although the benzodiazepines appear to be less reinforcing than barbiturates (6). Although there have been human studies that have demonstrated the reinforcing effects of the benzodiazepines, there are notable differences among the compounds that correlate with the agents' onset of action. Lorazepam, alprazolam, and diazepam all appear to have a greater potential for abuse, based on their inherent properties (i.e., their lipophilic properties and therefore more rapid onset of action). It is also important to note that other human studies have demonstrated that benzodiazepines do not have reinforcing effects in most individuals (7), thus suggesting that some individuals may have a vulnerability that leads to abuse.

Misuse and abuse of benzodiazepines and sedative-hypnotics is commonly seen in individuals with other substance use disorders (8). In this context, sedative-hypnotics are often used to enhance the effects of other drugs and alleviate unpleasant side effects from use of or withdrawal from other substances. Benzodiazepines and other sedative hypnotics may also be misused or abused when individuals who abuse many substances cannot obtain their substance of choice. Dependence does not often develop in this population, as the use of these substances is more likely to be intermittent and combined with other substances. The majority of patients who develop benzodiazepine and sedative-hypnotic dependence were initially being treated for problems with sleep and anxiety disorders. Individuals seeking treatment for anxiety disorders, sleep disorders, and depression are at higher risk for developing sedative-hypnotic dependence if they have a history of substance use disorders. A family history of substance use disorders also places an individual at higher risk for developing dependence. The issue of alcohol abuse and dependence warrants special caution because of the potential for dangerous interactions. The assumption that all individuals with alcohol abuse or dependence have a propensity for abusing benzodiazepines or becoming dependent has been challenged (9), but the use of these medications should be closely monitored in this population.

INTERVENTIONS

In general, there are two clear indications for pharmacologic intervention in individuals who are taking benzodiazepines and other sedative hypnotics and meet criteria for abuse or dependence. In a state of intoxication, a patient may require monitoring and even intervention to ensure a safe recovery. In patients experiencing acute withdrawal, pharmacologic management is often recommended because of the risk of serious consequences, including seizures and delirium tremens. The decision as to whether a benzodiazepine or other sedative hypnotic should be continued is also important to consider in any patient who is prescribed these medications. In general, if there is a clear diagnosis, benefit from the treatment, minimal side effects, and no evidence of abuse or misuse, then the medication should be continued. Sedative-hypnotics are commonly recommended for the shortest period of time possible, and these medications are often seen as short-term therapies that should be discontinued as soon as the clinical situation permits. Guidelines for benzodiazepine prescribing have been published by the American Psychiatric Association (10).

MANAGEMENT OF INTOXICATION

The signs and symptoms of benzodiazepine and sedative-hypnotic intoxication are very similar to those of alcohol intoxication. Severe intoxication can lead to respiratory depression, coma, and death, especially with the barbiturates and other older, nonbenzodiazepine agents. Benzodiazepine intoxication, even in the situation of an overdose, rarely leads to death, unless the benzodiazepines are combined with other CNS depressants. The management of acute intoxication is mostly supportive, with special attention to airway management, as respiratory depression is the most likely cause of death in overdose. In overdose, it is also critical to know what other psychoactive agents (especially CNS depressants) may have been acutely or chronically ingested. Flumazenil can be used in the case of benzodiazepine intoxication, but its use is limited by the risk of precipitating withdrawal symptoms, including seizures if this is not used with caution.

WITHDRAWAL

Withdrawal symptoms are most often seen in patients who abruptly discontinue taking benzodiazepines and other sedative-hypnotics. Withdrawal may be precipitated unintentionally when an individual stops taking a prescribed medication or is unable to obtain the sedative-hypnotic from illicit sources. Withdrawal may also be initiated by a provider owing to concerns of misuse, abuse, psychologic dependence, or other substance use disorders. In some cases, the decision is made to stop benzodiazepines because of side effects, such as memory impairment or behavioral problems. Individuals are likely to develop withdrawal symptoms when they have been taking high doses of sedative-hypnotics or if they have been taking low or moderate doses for a prolonged period of time (6).

Although withdrawal symptoms are similar to those seen in alcohol withdrawal (Table 47.2), the signs and symptoms of withdrawal manifest differently in each patient, because of characteristics like age and overall state of health and the properties of the unique pharmacologic properties of each medication. The half-life of the medication is of particular importance, especially when discussing the onset of withdrawal symptoms. The withdrawal from agents with short half-lives usually begins within 12 to 24 hours and reaches peak intensity within 1 to 3 days. With longer-acting agents, withdrawal

TABLE 47.2 Sedative-Hypnotic Withdrawal Symptoms

Mild	Moderate	Severe
• Anxiety • Insomnia • Dizziness • Headache • Anorexia • Perceptual hyperacusis • Irritability • Agitation	• Panic • Decreased concentration • Tremor • Sweating • Palpitations • Perceptual distortions • Muscle aches • GI upset • Insomnia • Elevated vital signs • Depression	• Hypothermia • Vital sign instability • Muscle fasciculations • Seizures • Delirium • Psychosis

symptoms may begin later and not peak until 4 to 7 days after discontinuation. Symptoms may then continue for several more days or even weeks, depending on the half-life of drug.

Another common occurrence during withdrawal is the reemergence of symptoms of anxiety and insomnia, which has been found to occur in 60% to 80% of benzodiazepine-dependent patients who were initially treated for these disorders (11). Initially, these rebound symptoms are perceived to be more severe and intense than the original symptoms but within several weeks return to pretreatment levels. Although there is some debate as to the validity of the "protracted abstinence syndrome," these symptoms are thought to persist for weeks to months, and even years. Smith and Wesson (12) suggest that receptor-mediated changes lead to worsening withdrawal symptoms when patients are tapered from the remaining low-dose medication. Prolonged or protracted withdrawal symptoms may include anxiety, sensitivity to light, sound, touch (13), and tinnitus (14). In contrast to symptom reemergence, protracted withdrawal symptoms often wax and wane and slowly resolve with continued abstinence.

It has been estimated that up to 50% (15) of regular benzodiazepine users will experience clinically significant signs of withdrawal with sudden discontinuation. The duration of treatment necessary to cause withdrawal symptoms is unclear. Some sources suggest that it may take as little as 4 to 6 weeks (16), whereas rebound insomnia has been seen after just 2 weeks of daily drug use (17).

MANAGEMENT OF WITHDRAWAL

The decision to discontinue or taper sedative-hypnotic drugs should be discussed at length with patients, with education provided about the reasons for discontinuation, the signs and symptoms that they are likely to experience, and the risks and benefits of the available withdrawal strategies. There are several strategies that may be employed in the management of sedative-hypnotic withdrawal. The most common approach is to slowly taper a medication over a prolonged period to minimize the withdrawal symptoms. This can be safely completed in an outpatient setting. Another treatment that has been used with success involves the use of phenobarbital in the setting of an acute medically supervised withdrawal. More acute and rapid medically supervised withdrawals have also been done with benzodiazepines, similar to the approach taken in alcohol withdrawal treatment. These later two options require close observation and monitoring and thus should be undertaken only in an inpatient setting. Lastly, the emerging use of anticonvulsants for the treatment of alcohol withdrawal suggests that there may be a role for the use of similar agents in the treatment of sedative-hypnotic withdrawal (18–20).

The most straightforward approach is to initiate a taper that uses decreasing doses of the therapeutic agent over the course of 6 to 12 weeks (21). This is most often used in settings of long-term use and physical dependence, where there is not an urgent need to discontinue the current medication. Although this method could be used in settings where there are issues of misuse, abuse, or the DSM-IV syndrome of dependence, this approach is not recommended because it would provide the patient with continued doses of the drug for a period of weeks to months. For this strategy to be effective, the patient must be able to follow complex dosing regimens, adhere to regular follow-up appointments, and be free of other active substance use disorders. It is recommended that as lower doses are achieved, the dose reduction at each stage should be more modest, especially if short-half-life drugs are being prescribed. More frequent dosing intervals can also be used in the later stages to help prevent the emergence of any withdrawal symptoms.

There is an increased likelihood of withdrawal symptoms with medications with a short half-life, even during prolonged tapers. Thus, another withdrawal strategy is to convert the therapeutic agent to an equivalent dose of a longer-acting agent and then gradually reduce the dose of the latter, using the principles described earlier. Agents such as clonazepam (22) and chlordiazepoxide are especially good choices given their slower onset of action and therefore relatively limited abuse potential.

Short-acting benzodiazepines, such as the triazolobenzodiazepines alprazolam and triazolam, warrant special consideration. These agents may have a higher binding affinity at a subpopulation of benzodiazepine GABA receptors that are not targeted by other benzodiazepines (23). Because of this, other benzodiazepines may not have fully effective cross-tolerance and therefore may be less effective when they are used for tapering and withdrawal. There are case reports that suggest that clonazepam can be used effectively for the treatment of triazolobenzodiazepine withdrawal (22), whereas others have reported distinct withdrawal symptoms with alprazolam (24).

Another option for withdrawal treatment is the use of phenobarbital. Smith and Wesson (25,26) elucidated a protocol for utilizing phenobarbital for medically supervised withdrawal by converting patients from other sedative-hypnotics to equivalent phenobarbital doses. The starting daily dose of phenobarbital should be based on the patient's drug use during the previous month. In cases when this is not known, a pentobarbital challenge test (27) can be used to determine the starting dose. (The maximum starting dose is 500 mg daily.) The daily dose should be administered in divided doses, three times a day, and then tapered by 30 mg a day. Signs of phenobarbital intoxication are similar to those seen with other sedative hypnotics and include slurred speech, ataxia, and nystagmus. If signs and symptoms of intoxication are present, then the total daily dose should be decreased by 50% or more and the patient reassessed at frequent intervals until the intoxication resolves.

Another strategy for the treatment of withdrawal is the use of carbamazepine. This anticonvulsant has been shown to be as effective as oxazepam in the treatment of alcohol withdrawal (28), and two open-label studies also demonstrated the effectiveness of this agent in the management of complicated benzodiazepine withdrawal (29,30). One multisite, placebo-controlled study suggested that carbamazepine could also be effective for the treatment of alprazolam withdrawal, but the findings were limited by a high dropout rate. On the basis of initial studies, the suggested dosing of carbamazepine is in the range of 200 mg three times a day for 7 to 10 days. Clinical experience suggests that this strategy is effective, but because of the potential for serious adverse events during sedative-hypnotic withdrawal, patients should be monitored closely, and benzodiazepines should be used as needed, especially for elevated vital signs or other uncontrolled symptoms. Carbamazepine has the distinct advantage of having low abuse potential and limited cognitive side effects, especially during short-term use. These properties make carbamazepine an attractive option in patients who are beginning a treatment program while also undergoing medically supervised withdrawal.

Studies have also shown gabapentin and divalproex to be effective in the treatment of alcohol withdrawal in patients who experience mild to moderate symptoms (18). Though these medications have not been directly studied in the context of sedative-hypnotic withdrawal, there is reason to suggest that these agents could be used in this context. The activity of alcohol and other sedative-hypnotics, especially benzodiazepines, are similar as they act at a common receptor. Both gabapentin and divalproex compare favorably to carbamazepine in terms of research supporting their use in the treatment of alcohol withdrawal. This suggests that these agents would also be efficacious in the treatment of the symptoms of sedative-hypnotic withdrawal.

TREATMENT SETTING

While discussing with the patient the pharmacologic strategy for the treatment of withdrawal, a decision must also be made regarding the setting in which the withdrawal will be treated. Though inpatient treatment is often optimal because of the close observation and controlled environment, this is often not feasible in today's health care system. Therefore, inpatient treatment of withdrawal should be limited to cases in which the patient is medically compromised or a high risk of the patient's developing severe symptoms, such as seizures, exists. This may be the case in patients who have been taking high doses of sedative-hypnotics for a long period and who require a rapid medically supervised withdrawal. Medically supervised withdrawal on an inpatient basis may also be appropriate if the patient has been taking multiple sedative-hypnotics or is alcohol-dependent. Patients who have a history of experiencing severe withdrawal when they have previously stopped using sedative-hypnotics are also at high risk for having their withdrawal complicated by serious side effects.

Medically supervised outpatient withdrawal is reasonable if the patient does not appear to be at risk for severe withdrawal, especially if the method of slowly reducing the sedative-hypnotic dose can be utilized. If outpatient management is undertaken, the patient should be given clear instructions and close follow-up appointments. If a gradual dose reduction approach is employed, it is recommended that the patient be seen each time there is a dose reduction; if this is not possible, there should be a mechanism by which the patient can access the provider to address any questions or concerns. It is preferable for the patient to have some level of supervision by friends or family, but this is not always possible.

POSTWITHDRAWAL TREATMENT

Medically supervised withdrawal should not be seen as definitive treatment in the case of sedative-hypnotic dependence. This is the first step in the management of patients who often have other substance use disorders, anxiety and sleep disorders and other co-occurring medical and psychiatric disorders. In the case of other substance use disorders, a treatment plan should include co-occurring medically supervised withdrawal from other substances and substance abuse treatment in an appropriate setting. When treating patients with underlying anxiety and sleep disorders, other pharmacologic and psychotherapeutic treatments, particularly cognitive behavioral therapy, should be initiated to counter any reemerging symptoms that may be experienced after withdrawal. Co-occurring psychiatric disorders should also be addressed during or soon after withdrawal. Failure to stabilize anxiety, sleep, or other co-occurring conditions will likely lead to higher rates of relapse owing to patient discomfort, limited compliance, and inability to effectively engage in the early stages of rehabilitative treatment.

CONCLUSIONS

Sedative-hypnotic medications have been used for many years for a variety of disorders and symptoms. Today, benzodiazepines are by far the most commonly used sedative-hypnotics, and their use is widespread. The appropriate use of benzodiazepines requires a clear understanding of the medications, an accurate diagnosis and treatment plan, and close monitoring. Most users of sedative-hypnotic medications take their medications as prescribed and do not misuse, abuse, or develop dependence. Physical dependence may be unavoidable in cases of prolonged use; therefore, benzodiazepines should be prescribed for the shortest period of time that is clinically reasonable. In most cases, tapering of the drug over several weeks is an effective way to avoid withdrawal symptoms. Potential withdrawal signs and symptoms should be initially discussed with patients before treatment is initiated. In other cases, a more rapid withdrawal is needed, often because of misuse, abuse, a syndrome of DSM-IV dependence, or other substance use disorders. Prescribers must be aware of the risks inherent in prescribing benzodiazepines and other sedative-hypnotics, but they should be careful not to withhold treatment when appropriate. If providers and patients are well informed and openly discuss the risks and benefits of these medications and they are prescribed at reasonable doses, sedative-hypnotics can be used safely and effectively for the treatment of a number of otherwise disabling conditions.

REFERENCES

1. Rush CR, Frey JM, Griffiths RR. Zalpedom and triazolam in humans: Acute behavioral effects and abuse potential. *Psychopharmacology* 1999; 145:39–51.
2. Rush CR, Griffiths RR. Zolpidem, triazolam, and temazepam: Behavioral and subject-related effects in normal volunteers. *J Clin Psychopharmacol* 1996;16:146–157.
3. Griffiths RR. Zolpidem behavioral pharmacology in baboons: Self-injection, discrimination, tolerance, and withdrawal. *J Pharmacol Exp Ther* 1992;260:1199–1208.
4. U.S. Drug Enforcement Administration. *Benzodiazepines*. Accessed February 29, 2008, from www.dea.gov/concern/benzodiazepines.html.
5. Substance Abuse and Mental Health Services Administration. *2006 National Survey on Drug Use and Health*.
6. Griffiths RR, Sannerud CA. Abuse and dependence on benzodiazepines and other anxiolytic/sedative drugs. In: Meltzer HY, Coyle JT (eds.). *Psychopharmacology: The third generation of progress,* 2nd ed. New York: Raven Press, 1987:1535–1541.
7. Chutuape MA, de Wit H. Relationship between subjective effects and drug preferences: Ethanol and diazepam. *Drug Alcohol Depend* 1994;34: 243–251.
8. Malcolm R, Brady KT, Johnson AL, et al. Types of benzodiazepines abused by chemically dependent inpatients. *J Psychoactive Drugs* 1993;25: 315–319.
9. Ciraulo DA, Sands BF, Shader RI. Critical review of liability for benzodiazepine abuse among alcoholics. *A J Psychiatry* 1988;145:1501–1506.
10. American Psychiatric Association. Benzodiazepine dependence, toxicity, and abuse. Washington, DC: American Psychiatric Association Press, 1990.
11. Greenblatt DJ, Miller LG, Shader RI. Benzodiazepine discontinuation syndromes. *J Psychiatric Res* 1990;24 (Suppl 2):73–79.
12. Smith DE, Wesson DR. Benzodiazepines and other sedative-hypnotics. In: Galanter M, Kleber H (eds.). *American Psychiatric Press textbook of substance abuse treatment,* 1st ed. Washington, DC: American Psychiatric Press, 1995.
13. Lader M. Drug development optimization—benzodiazepines. *Agents Actions Supplements* 1990;29:59–69.
14. Busto U, Fornazzari L, Naranjo CA. Protracted tinnitus after discontinuation of long-term therapeutic use of benzodiazepines. *J Clin Psychopharmacol* 1988;8:359–362.
15. Tyrer P. Benzodiazepine dependence: A shadowy diagnosis. *Biochem Soc Symp* 1993;59:107–119.
16. Fontaine R, Chouinard G, Annable L. Rebound anxiety in anxious patients after abrubt withdrawal of benzodiazepine treatment. *A J Psychiatry* 1984;141:848–852.
17. Bixler EO, Kales JD, Kales A, et al. Rebound insomnia and elimination half-life: Assessment of individual subject response. *J Clin Pharmacol* 1985;25:115–124.
18. Myrick H, Malcolm R, Anton RF. The use of anticonvulsants in the treatment of addictive disorders. *Prim Psychiatry* 2003;10:59-63.
19. Denis C, Fatséas M, Lavie E, Auriacombe M. Pharmacological interventions for benzodiazepine mono-dependence management in outpatient settings. *Cochrane Review*, 2006.
20. Malcolm R, Myrick H, Brady KT, Ballenger JC. Update on anticonvulsants for the treatment of alcohol withdrawal. *Am J Addict* 2001;(Suppl 10):16–23.
21. Voshaar RC, Couvee JE, van Balkom AJ, Mulder PG, Zitman FG. Strategies for discontinuing long-term benzodiazepine use: Meta-analysis. *Br J Psychiatry* 2006;189:213–220.
22. Herman JB, Rosenblum JF, Brotman AW. The alprazolam to clonazepam switch for the treatment of panic disorder. *J Clin Psychopharmacol* 1987;7:175–178.
23. Brown JL, Hughes KJ. A review of alprazolam withdrawal. *Drug Intell Clin Pharm* 1986;20:837–884.
24. Rashi K, Patrissi G, Cook B. Alprazolam found to have serious side effects. *Psychiatr News* 1988;23:14.
25. Smith D, Wesson D. A new method for treatment of barbiturate dependence. *JAMA* 1970;213:294–295.
26. Smith D, Wesson D. A phenobarbital technique for withdrawal of barbiturate abuse. *Arch Gen Psychiatry* 1971;24:56–60.
27. Jackson AH, Shader RI. Guidelines for the withdrawal of narcotic and general depressant drugs. *Dis Nerv Syst* 1973;34:162.
28. Malcolm R, Ballenger JC, Sturgis E, et al. A double blind controlled trial of carbamazepine in alcohol withdrawal. *Am J Psychiatry* 1989;146: 617–621.
29. Klein E, Uhde TW, Post RM. Preliminary evidence for the utility of carbamazepine in alprazolam withdrawal. *Am J Psychiatry* 1986;143: 235–236.
30. Ries RK, Roy-Byrne PP, Ward NG, et al. Carbamazepine treatment for benzodiazepine withdrawal. *Am J Psychiatry* 1989;146:536–537.

CHAPTER 48

Susan M. Stine, MD, PhD
Thomas R. Kosten, MD

Pharmacologic Interventions for Opioid Dependence

This chapter first provides a brief overview of the main pharmacologic agents for treating opioid dependence. Second, it provides a brief overview of pharmacologic approaches to medically assisted withdrawal and, finally, this chapter focuses on long-term pharmacologic (maintenance) treatments.

OVERVIEW OF PHARMACOLOGIC INTERVENTIONS

The principal opioid medications used to treat opioid dependence covered in this chapter are the mu-receptor antagonists naloxone and naltrexone, the full agonists methadone and levo-alpha-acetylmethadol (LAAM), the partial agonist buprenorphine, and the nonopioid α-adrenergic agonists clonidine and lofexidine.

Opioid Antagonists

Naloxone Naloxone is a short-acting, parenterally administered full opioid antagonist medication used to counter the life-threatening depression of the central nervous and respiratory systems caused by opioid overdose. It is a competitive antagonist with an extremely high affinity for μ-opioid receptors, and its rapid displacement of any opioid agonists and blockade of the μ-opioid receptors often produces rapid onset of withdrawal symptoms. Naloxone also has antagonist action, though with a lower affinity, at κ- and δ-opioid receptors. Naltrexone is structurally similar but has a slightly increased affinity for κ-opioid receptors over naloxone and can be administered orally with a longer duration of action than naloxone.

Naltrexone Naltrexone is a synthetic congener of oxymorphone with no opioid agonist properties. Naltrexone hydrochloride differs in structure from oxymorphone in that the methyl group on the nitrogen atom is replaced by a cyclopropylmethyl group. Naltrexone hydrochloride is a competitive opioid antagonist and reversibly blocks the subjective effects of opioids. Although naltrexone has few, if any, intrinsic actions besides its opioid blocking properties (1), it produces some pupillary constriction, by an unknown mechanism (2). The administration of naltrexone is not associated with the development of tolerance or dependence. In subjects physically dependent on opioids, naltrexone will precipitate withdrawal symptoms. Clinical studies indicate that 50 mg of naltrexone hydrochloride will block the pharmacologic effects of 25 mg of intravenously administered heroin for periods as long as 24 hours. Other data suggest that doubling its dose provides blockade for 48 hours, and tripling its dose provides blockade for about 72 hours.

Opioid Full and Partial Agonists

Methadone Methadone is an orally active, long-acting synthetic opioid that was recognized in the 1960s as having the potential to treat opioid dependence. A clinical pharmacology study demonstrated that increasing doses of methadone affected abstinence signs and symptoms and reduced drug craving. Doses of methadone ranging from 80 to 120 mg/day produced a tolerance to the effects of intravenously administered heroin, hydromorphone, and methadone. The term *agonist blockade* was coined to describe this phenomenon.

LAAM LAAM is the α-acetyl congener of methadone. Its principal difference from methadone is its longer half-life and its conversion to the active metabolites norLAAM and dinor-LAAM. It is approved by U.S. Food and Drug Administration (FDA) for opioid maintenance treatment in opioid treatment programs but is no longer marketed owing to low demand in the wake of reports of an association with cardiac arrhythmias (torsades de pointes).

Buprenorphine Buprenorphine is a high-affinity mu opioid partial agonist and κ-opioid antagonist that the FDA approved as a pharmacotherapy for opioid dependence in October 2002 (3,4). The introduction of buprenorphine as an agent for the treatment of opioid dependence is of intense scientific interest and great public health significance. Despite its higher unit-dose cost compared to methadone, buprenorphine has expanded access to opioid dependence treatment owing to its availability in office-based practice. This could reduce the disparity between the number of opioid-dependent individuals and the number of treatment slots available to them and facilitate general medical care of dependent individuals (5–7).

Nonopioid Agonists: α-Adrenergic Agents

Clonidine Clonidine is a centrally acting α-adrenergic receptor agonist with more affinity for α_2 than α_1 receptors. It decreases adrenergic neurotransmission from the locus coeruleus through feedback inhibition. The medication is FDA-approved for treatment of hypertension but is used off label for the medical management of opioid withdrawal. Many of the autonomic symptoms of opioid withdrawal result from the loss of opioid suppression of the locus ceruleus system during the abstinence syndrome. The use of clonidine in the management of opioid withdrawal has been hampered by side effects of sedation and hypotension.

Lofexidine Lofexidine is also a centrally acting α_2-adrenergic agonist, which has not yet been approved by the FDA but is used in Europe. It is associated with less of the hypotension that limits the use of clonidine for withdrawal treatment and therefore is currently being studied in clinical trials for the medical management of withdrawal.

ABSTINENCE SYNDROMES AND MEDICALLY SUPERVISED WITHDRAWAL

The opioid abstinence syndrome is characterized by two phases (8): a relatively brief initial phase in which opioid-dependent patients experience acute withdrawal followed by a protracted abstinence (PA) syndrome. Current pharmacotherapeutic strategies are designed to address these two distinct phases, acute withdrawal and protracted withdrawal. The acute withdrawal syndrome lasts from 5 to 14 days and consists of a wide range of symptoms. Symptoms include gastrointestinal distress (such as diarrhea and vomiting), disturbances in thermal regulation, insomnia, muscle pain, joint pain, marked anxiety, and dysphoria. Although these symptoms generally include no life-threatening complications, the acute withdrawal syndrome causes marked discomfort, often prompting continuation of opioid use, even in the absence of any opioid-associated euphoria. Longer-term, PA symptoms are discussed in this chapter under long-term treatments.

Medically supervised withdrawal is discussed briefly next and in greater detail in Chapter 45.

Opioid Agonists and Partial Agonists Opioid-based medically supervised withdrawal is based on the principle of cross-tolerance, in which one opioid is replaced with another that is slowly tapered. Methadone is used because it has a long half-life and can be administered once daily. Withdrawal from heroin is usually managed with initial dosages of methadone in the range of 15 to 30 mg/day (9). Although this dosage is generally adequate to control symptoms in many heroin users over a 24-hour period, additional methadone can be given as required on the basis of clinical findings. However, a simple conversion of short-acting prescription medications into an equivalent dosage of methadone can lead to overdose as the methadone accumulates over the first several days of dosing. Thus, any methadone dose over about 40 mg daily should involve careful and slow dosage increases over at least several days. Various guidelines that are available for conversion from short-acting opioids to methadone typically suggest giving half of the calculated equivalent methadone dose to any patient with a calculated dose of more than 50 mg daily of methadone. In acute medical settings, this starting dosage should be maintained through the second or third day after the peak dose is attained and then the methadone can be slowly tapered by approximately 10% to 15% per day. Longer-term opioid medically supervised withdrawal using methadone is often available through drug treatment programs. Although a licensed physician can perform supervised methadone withdrawal in an inpatient medical setting, outpatient withdrawal using methadone must be performed in a federally licensed opioid treatment program.

Buprenorphine has been studied as a treatment for opioid withdrawal. Buprenorphine's slow dissociation from mu opioid receptors results in a long duration of action (ideal for a maintenance medication) and also has milder withdrawal signs and symptoms on discontinuation than full agonists (10–15), making it particularly useful for medically supervised withdrawal from opioids. Such qualities may make buprenorphine an advance in medically supervised withdrawal treatment by permitting accelerated withdrawal without significant distress. An early study randomly assigned 45 heroin-dependent patients to buprenorphine (2 mg) or methadone (30 mg) for 3 weeks, followed by tapering over a 4-week period, and found both approaches to be equivalent (16). Another study that compared a gradual (36-day) to a more rapid (12-day) buprenorphine taper (initially 8 mg) found the gradual approach to be superior (10). A study that compared a 3-day course of buprenorphine (3 mg) to a 5-day course of clonidine reported that these approaches were equivalent (11), although another study found that a longer course of buprenorphine (10 days) was superior to clonidine (17). A larger study (18) of

162 heroin-dependent patients withdrawn in a primary care setting randomly assigned the patients to three 8-day treatment protocols: clonidine, combined clonidine and naltrexone, and buprenorphine. Participants in the combined clonidine and naltrexone group and the buprenorphine group were more likely to complete medically supervised withdrawal than the clonidine group, whereas the buprenorphine group experienced less severe withdrawal symptoms than the other two groups. Another study provided further evidence that step-down medically supervised withdrawal using buprenorphine minimizes withdrawal symptoms, thus reducing the need for concurrent medication (19). The clinical effectiveness of buprenorphine/naloxone and clonidine for medically supervised opioid withdrawal in inpatient and outpatient community treatment programs was investigated in the first studies of the National Institute of Drug Abuse Clinical Trials Network (20). Opioid-dependent individuals seeking short-term treatment were randomly assigned, in a 2:1 ratio favoring buprenorphine/naloxone, to a 13-day medically supervised withdrawal using buprenorphine/naloxone or clonidine. A total of 113 inpatients (77 buprenorphine/naloxone, 36 clonidine) and 231 outpatients (157 buprenorphine/naloxone, 74 clonidine) participated. Primary outcome measures included the proportion of subjects in each condition who both were retained in the study for the entire duration and provided an opioid-free urine sample on the last day. Secondary outcome measures included use of ancillary drugs, number of side effects, and withdrawal and craving ratings. A total of 59 of the 77 (77%) inpatients assigned to buprenorphine/naloxone achieved treatment success compared to 8 of the 36 (22%) assigned to clonidine. Forty-six of the 157 (29%) outpatients assigned to buprenorphine/naloxone achieved treatment success, compared to 4 of the 74 (5%) assigned to clonidine. Thus, several studies have supported the benefits of buprenorphine and buprenorphine/naloxone for medically supervised opioid withdrawal.

The optimum dose of buprenorphine for acute inpatient heroin withdrawal has not been determined. A randomized, double-blind, double-dummy pilot study conducted by Oreskovich et al. (21) compared two buprenorphine sublingual-tablet dosing schedules to oral clonidine. Heroin users ($N = 30$) who met DSM-IV criteria for opioid dependence and achieved a Clinical Opiate Withdrawal Scale (COWS) score of 13 (moderate withdrawal), were randomly assigned to receive higher-dose buprenorphine (HD, 8-8-8-4-2 mg/day on days 1 to 5); lower-dose buprenorphine (LD, 2-4-8-4-2 mg/day on days 1 to 5); or clonidine (C, 0.2-0.3-0.3-0.2-0.1 mg QID on days 1 to 5). COWS scores were obtained four times daily. Twenty-four hours after random placement, the percentages of subjects who achieved suppression of withdrawal, as defined by four consecutive COWS scores <12, were: C = 11%, LD = 40%, and HD = 60%. COWS scores over the course of 5 days were lower in both LD and HD compared to C. Similar analyses examining scores over time on the Adjective Rating Scale for Withdrawal (ARSW) and on a Visual Analog Scale of Opiate Craving (VAS) indicated an overall treatment effect on the VAS accounted for by a significant difference between HD and C but no overall treatment effect on the ARSW. Both HD and LD regimens were found safe and efficacious treatments for supervised opioid withdrawal, but HD demonstrated superiority to C, including a lesser severity of withdrawal symptoms at both doses of buprenorphine and decreased craving at the higher dose.

Nonopioid Medication Treatments

The α-adrenergic agents are widely used in medically supervised withdrawal, especially in clinical settings that do not have availability of controlled substances. Nonopioid methods of medically supervised opioid withdrawal have focused primarily on clonidine, an α_2-adrenergic agonist. This approach is based on the discovery that one important mechanism underlying opioid withdrawal is noradrenergic hyperactivity (22). Therefore, α_2-adrenergic agonists act centrally at the locus coeruleus via presynaptic receptors to moderate the symptoms of noradrenergic hyperactivity during medically supervised opioid withdrawal. Discovery of the capacity of the α_2-adrenergic agonist, clonidine, to ameliorate some signs and symptoms of withdrawal led to widespread use of this drug as a nonopioid alternative for managing withdrawal (23) as well as interest in developing other α_2-adrenergic agonists for this indication.

Clonidine

Early clinical studies demonstrated that clonidine diminished withdrawal symptoms in patients who were withdrawn from methadone (24,25). Clonidine seems to be most effective in suppressing autonomic signs and symptoms of opioid withdrawal but is less effective for subjective withdrawal symptoms (26). Initial daily doses of up to 1.2 mg per 24 hours in divided doses are commonly suggested. For example, a regimen of 0.1 to 0.2 mg every 4 hours has been used in two clinical trials for heroin withdrawal, with careful monitoring of blood pressure. Because it may be less effective in managing subjective withdrawal symptoms, adjuvant therapy (nonsteroidal anti-inflammatory drugs for myalgia, benzodiazepines for insomnia, and antiemetics) may be needed (27,28). In addition, in a randomized trial that included 55 patients who received clonidine in a primary care setting, 65% of patients underwent successful medically supervised withdrawal (28). In another study that examined predictors of successfully completed supervised withdrawal using clonidine, patients who completed withdrawal were more likely to be heroin smokers (rather than intravenous users) and to have abstained from opioids for a longer time before presenting for treatment (29).

Lofexidine and Other α_2-Adrenergic Agonists

The use of clonidine in the management of opioid withdrawal has been hampered by side effects of sedation and hypotension. This in turn has led to the investigation of the effectiveness of other α_2-adrenergic agonists—lofexidine, guanfacine and guanabenz acetate—in the management of opioid withdrawal, the aim being to find a drug that has clonidine's capacity to ameliorate the signs and symptoms of opioid withdrawal but with fewer side effects.

Lofexidine, a centrally acting α_2-adrenergic agonist, has, after clonidine, been the most used and investigated α_2-adrenergic treatment for opioid withdrawal, although it has not yet been approved by the FDA. In a randomized trial that compared lofexidine to methadone in 86 opioid addicts, lofexidine-treated patients had more severe withdrawal symptoms from days 3 to 7 and again on day 10 but had similar symptoms thereafter. Rates of treatment completion did not significantly differ (30). In two randomized, double-blind trials that compared lofexidine with clonidine in patients dependent on methadone (31) and heroin (32), both agents effectively reduced withdrawal symptoms. Patients treated with lofexidine experienced fewer side effects, especially hypotension. Finally, one study suggested that a 5-day lofexidine regimen decreased symptoms of opioid withdrawal more rapidly than a 10-day regimen (33). A large multicenter randomized clinical efficacy trial comparing lofexidine to placebo for opioid detoxification has recently been completed and found substantial efficacy for lofexidine in symptom reduction and patient retention (34). A Cochrane review (35) reviewed 22 major studies of nonopioid management involving 1,709 participants. Eighteen of these were randomized controlled trials either comparing treatment with an α_2-adrenergic agonist with reducing doses of methadone (12 studies) or comparing one α_2-adrenergic agonist compared with another or with placebo. Compared with reducing doses of methadone, withdrawal intensity appears similar to or marginally greater with α_2-adrenergic agonists, though signs and symptoms of withdrawal occur and resolve earlier in treatment. Participants stay in treatment longer with methadone. No significant difference was detected in rates of completion of withdrawal with adrenergic agonists compared to methadone, or clonidine compared to lofexidine. Clonidine is associated with more adverse effects (low blood pressure, dizziness, dry mouth, lack of energy) than reducing doses of methadone. Lofexidine does not reduce blood pressure to the same extent as clonidine, but is otherwise similar to clonidine. Overall, the authors concluded that the management of withdrawal from heroin or methadone using the α_2-adrenergic agonists clonidine or lofexidine showed no significant difference in efficacy from reducing doses of methadone over a period of around 10 days.

Medication Combinations, Rapid and Ultrarapid Opioid Detoxification Because most opioid and nonopioid approaches to medically supervised withdrawal require a prolonged time frame of a week or more, "rapid" and "ultrarapid" opioid withdrawal protocols have been developed (36,37). These "rapid" protocols use an opioid antagonist (e.g., naloxone or naltrexone) to cause an accelerated withdrawal response, with the goal of completing withdrawal in shorter periods from 8 days to as little as 2 or 3 days. In addition to an opioid antagonist, rapid approaches use pharmacotherapies (e.g., clonidine and sedation) to minimize the acute withdrawal symptoms experienced when opioid antagonists are administered. Because withdrawal is completed more quickly, the combination rapid approach has been proposed to have the advantage of minimizing the risk for relapse and allowing patients to enter continued treatment with naltrexone maintenance more rapidly. These methods have not been in widespread use, however. Ultrarapid methods are similar in pharmacologic approach to the rapid method but use general anesthesia and complete the procedure in several hours. This method is not recommend because of the risks of general anesthesia and because the long-term efficacy is not superior to use of buprenorphine or clonidine (38). Ultrarapid approaches to medically assisted withdrawal are discussed in more detail elsewhere in this text (see sidebar on page 604 of this text).

LONG-TERM TREATMENTS FOR OPIATE DEPENDENCE

Dependence and Protracted Abstinence In patients with a history of opioid dependence, acute withdrawal and medically supervised withdrawal are only the beginning of treatment. Himmelsbach (39), reporting on 21 prisoners dependent on morphine, observed that "physical recovery requires not less than six months of total abstinence." Factors he measured included temperature, sleep, respiration, weight, basal metabolic rate, blood pressure, and hematocrit. The times required for return to baseline ranged from 1 week to about 6 months. Martin and Jasinski (8) reported in a subsequent study that the period of PA persisted for 6 months or more after withdrawal and that it was associated with "altered physiological function." They found decreased blood pressure, decreased heart rate and body temperature, miosis, and a decreased sensitivity of the respiratory center to carbon dioxide, beginning about 6 weeks after withdrawal and persisting for 26 to 30 or more weeks. They also found increased sedimentation rates (which persisted for months) and electroencephalograph EEG changes. Martin and Jasinski (8) postulated a relationship between the PA syndrome and relapse. Based on similar observations, Dole (40) concluded that "human addicts almost always return to use of narcotics" after medically supervised withdrawal in the hospital. In his paper, Dole reviewed the relative importance of metabolic and conditioned factors in relapse and concluded that the underlying drive is metabolic, arguing that "psychological factors are only triggers for relapse." More recently, Prosser et al. (41) tested the hypothesis that former heroin users who have withdrawn from methadone maintenance therapy (MMT) and are drug-free have less pronounced cognitive impairment than patients continuing long-term MMT. Both methadone-maintained and -abstinent subject groups performed worse than controls on tasks that measured verbal function, visual-spatial analysis and memory, and resistance to distractibility. Both patients receiving MMT and former heroin users in prolonged abstinence exhibited a similar degree of cognitive impairment. In another study, Shi et al., (42) compared PA symptoms between drug-free and methadone-maintained former heroin users after similar lengths of heroin abstinence. Seventy former heroin users were included in one of four groups: in days 15 to 45 of short-term MMT; in months 5 to 6 of MMT (long-term MMT); opioid-free for 15 to 45 days after methadone-assisted heroin detoxification (short-term post-methadone); and opioid-free for 5 to 6 months after methadone-assisted heroin withdrawal (long-term post-methadone). Analysis of protracted abstinence symptoms during the study allowed the investigators to conclude that long-term methadone maintenance reduces PA symptoms of heroin abstinence and cue-induced craving.

The concept of PA has been controversial (43) but remains a useful model for scientific hypothesis testing and development of new therapeutic approaches (44). Accordingly, Dole (40) recommended methadone maintenance treatment, even though "it does establish physical dependence." Because, as Dole pointed out, methadone continues physical dependence, PA may remain a problem at a later time when medically supervised withdrawal from methadone is undertaken. In addition to biologic considerations, psychosocial concomitants of opioid dependence also necessitate longer, more specialized adjunct treatments for these and additional problems. Fortunately, the recent development of new pharmacologic agents may help to address these problems.

Naltrexone Maintenance Treatment Naltrexone is a long-acting, orally effective, predominantly μ-opioid antagonist that provides complete blockade of μ-opioid receptors when taken at least three times a week for a total weekly dose of about 350 mg (45). Because the reinforcing properties of opioids are completely blocked, naltrexone is theoretically an ideal maintenance agent in the rehabilitation of opioid-dependent patients who can successfully complete withdrawal and maintain abstinence from opioids. However, this optimistic theoretical perspective is contradicted by clinical reality, as reflected in treatment retention rates of only 20% to 30% over 6 months. Multiple factors appear to account for such poor retention (46). Opioid antagonists, unlike methadone, do not provide any opioid effect. Therefore, if antagonists are stopped, there is no immediate reminder in the form of withdrawal. In addition, craving for opioids may continue during naltrexone treatment. A meta-analysis of multiple studies did not provide strong support for naltrexone treatment of opioid dependence (47). Nevertheless, for some patients (such as health care professionals, business executives, or probation referrals) for whom there is an external incentive to comply with naltrexone therapy and to remain opioid abstinent, naltrexone has been very effective (48).

A pharmacologic approach to patient noncompliance may be the availability of an injectable, long-acting preparation of naltrexone, which would eliminate the need for daily intake. Comer et al. (49,50) found that a depot naltrexone formulation significantly reduced opiate use and reinforcement. New, long-lasting injectable naltrexone formulations such as Vivitrol (approved for treatment of alcohol dependence) have not been tested in opioid-dependent patients but may in the future provide new options for naltrexone treatment. Other supportive measures to increase compliance include family therapy and several behavior modification approaches (45). Clinically, naltrexone is initiated after acute withdrawal from opioids. There should be at least a 5- to 7-day opioid-free period for the short-acting opioids and a 7- to 10-day period for the long-acting agents. This, of course, does not apply to withdrawal treatments using the naltrexone-clonidine combination (see Section 6, "Management of Intoxication and Withdrawal"). The initial dose of naltrexone used generally is 25 mg on the first day, followed by 50 mg daily or an equivalent of 350 mg weekly, divided into three doses (100, 100, and 150 mg). The principal reason for the reduced dose on day 1 is the potential for gastrointestinal side effects, such as nausea and vomiting. This occurs in about 10% of patients taking naltrexone. In most cases, gastrointestinal upset is relatively mild and transient but, in some cases, it may be so severe as to cause discontinuation of the naltrexone. The most serious (but far less frequent) potential side effect of naltrexone is liver toxicity; however, 50 mg daily has been given safely to opioid dependent individuals (51). Liver toxicity, in the rare instances it occurs, appears to be limited in extent in that it resolves when naltrexone is discontinued and does not progress to liver failure. The enzyme dihydrodiol dehydrogenase appears to catalyze the metabolism of naltrexone to the active metabolite, 6-β naltrexol. When administered orally, naltrexone has an average plasma half-life of 4 hours, whereas 6-β naltrexol has an average half-life of 13 hours after oral administration of the parent drug. In summary, though naltrexone has not lived up to expectations, for selected, motivated patients who are opioid-dependent, it may represent a very effective form of maintenance pharmacotherapy.

Methadone Maintenance Treatment The initial pharmacologic rationale for long-term methadone maintenance was its ability to relieve the PA syndrome and to block heroin euphoria (40,52). However, an equally important benefit of longer-term maintenance has proved to be the opportunity it affords for psychosocial stabilization in the context of symptom relief. Good treatment retention, improved psychosocial adjustment, and reduced criminal activity are among the benefits reported (40,53). No serious side effects are associated with continued methadone use (46) with the exception of hypogonadism in men and risk of QT prolongation and exceedingly rare but potential subsequent progression to torsades de pointes (54). Minor side effects, such as constipation, excess sweating, drowsiness, and decreased sexual interest and performance have been noted. In addition, neuroendocrine studies have shown normalization of stress hormone responses and reproductive functioning (both of which are significantly disrupted in heroin users) after several months of stabilization on methadone (55). (For a detailed discussion of methadone maintenance, see Chapter 50).

A series of large-scale studies have demonstrated that patients maintained on doses of 60 mg or more of methadone a day had better treatment outcomes than those maintained on lower doses and that doses below 60 mg appear to be inadequate for most patients (56–62). These studies also confirm that medical decisions should not be based on public biases but on scientific knowledge and clinical evaluation. In particular, the study by Ball and Ross (59) showed that opioid use was directly related to methadone dose levels and that the effectiveness of methadone was even greater for patients on a 70-mg dose and was still more pronounced for patients on 80 mg a day or more. A recent factor mandating higher doses is the current purity of street heroin: Opioid cross-tolerance implies that the amount of heroin needed to produce euphoria would be prohibitively expensive for someone maintained on a sufficiently high dose of methadone. However, today's high-purity street heroin has required even higher methadone doses to achieve cross-tolerance (63). High doses and pure street drugs also may increase the risk of toxicity if patients try to override the cross-tolerance with illicit heroin, as tolerance to respiratory depression may not be as complete as that to euphoria. The functional biologic distinction between these pharmacologic effects in animal and binding studies can perhaps be explained by receptor theory (64). Classic pharmacologic studies have long implied the existence of multiple subtypes of mu opioid receptors. More recently, a number of variants of the cloned mu opioid receptor have been described (64). These variants all show the same selectivity for mu opioids, confirming their classification as mu opioid receptors. Yet, they differ in their functional activation by opioids as well as in their localization within cells and regions in the brain. These multiple mu opioid receptors may help explain the range of responses seen clinically among patients for the various opioid drugs.

Many diverse factors may, in theory, significantly modify the pharmacologic effectiveness of methadone. Three types of factors that have been shown to significantly modify the metabolic breakdown of methadone in the body, and thus potentially its pharmacologic effectiveness, are (1) chronic diseases, including chronic liver disease, chronic renal disease, and possibly other diseases; (2) medication interactions, including interactions of methadone with rifampin and phenytoin, carbamazepine in humans, possibly with ethanol and disulfiram and, also, by inference from animal studies, interactions of methadone with phenobarbital, diazepam, desipramine, and other drugs, as well as with estrogen steroids, cimetidine, and antiviral agents used in treatment of HIV (65); and (3) altered physiologic states, especially pregnancy. The liver in particular may play a central role in several aspects of methadone disposition, involving not only methadone metabolism and clearance but also storage and subsequent release of unchanged methadone. In a study by Kreek et al. (66), unchanged methadone persisted in the liver for up to 6 weeks, and methadone disposition was significantly altered only in a patient subgroup with moderately severe but compensated cirrhosis. These factors have been reviewed in detail by Kreek (67) and Stine (68). Of the multiple medical problems that result from direct and/or indirect effects of opioid use, chronic liver disease is the most common. For example, 50% to 60% of all heroin-dependent persons entering methadone maintenance have biochemical evidence of chronic liver disease, either secondary to infection (hepatitis B and C) or alcohol-induced liver disease. Chronic liver disease in all its forms has major implications for medication use. For example, opioid medications for treatment of dependence (such as methadone, LAAM, and buprenorphine); medications (such as isoniazid and rifampin) that are prescribed for other prevalent diseases in drug users, such as tuberculosis; as well as some antibiotics (such as trimethoprim-sulfamethoxazole) and some antiretroviral agents (such as didanosine) may have hepatotoxic effects (67,69–71). Other diseases co-occurring with chronic opioid dependence that can affect maintenance pharmacotherapy are bacterial infections and tuberculosis, particularly drug-resistant and "extrapulmonary" manifestations of tuberculosis in HIV-infected individuals (72–75). Interactions of HIV antiretroviral medications with opioid maintenance treatment may also be problematic. These are discussed further below (page 661). (See also Chapter 77 page 1057 in this volume for HIV issues).

The duration of methadone maintenance treatment warrants mention. In general, for successful rehabilitation, length of treatment with methadone is best seen in terms of years rather than months. For many patients, 5 to 10 years—or even a lifetime—of methadone maintenance may be required. At about a year of treatment the pharmacologic component of PA may still present a problem, but ongoing therapeutic support in a context of psychosocial stability may render this problem more manageable. The importance of psychosocial treatment as an adjunct to methadone pharmacotherapy has been emphasized in the field since the Ball and Ross study (59).

From an organizational and public health perspective, early treatment termination, illicit use of nonopioid substances (such as cocaine or alcohol), and diversion of the take-home dose of methadone to the illicit market remain significant issues for most methadone maintenance programs. Although concurrent substance use also is a problem (initially, 20% to 50% of methadone patients use cocaine, and 25% to 40% abuse alcohol), several effective treatment interventions have been developed, including behavioral approaches and pharmacologic interventions. Diversion of take-home doses is of concern to every methadone maintenance program, though its impact on illicit opioid use remains small (methadone accounts for about 4% of opioids used on the street). Hospital emergency department visits involving methadone rose 176% from 1995 to 2002. The rise from 2000 to 2002 was 50%, according to the Drug Abuse Warning Network of the Substance Abuse and Mental Health Services Administration (SAMHSA). The SAMHSA convened a panel in May 2003 to determine whether its methadone regulations were allowing diversion of methadone from clinics or whether the rise of methadone mentions in hospital emergency rooms and reports of deaths were due to methadone's coming from other sources. The panel—state and federal experts, researchers, epidemiologists, pathologists, toxicologists, medical examiners, coroners, pain management specialists, addiction medicine specialists, and others—concluded that the methadone from reported deaths came from sources other than opioid treatment programs (SAMSHA News, Mar-Apr, 2004 Vol. 12).

Levo-Alpha-Acetylmethadol Maintenance Treatment Initial studies of LAAM were performed in the 1970s with a dosing regimen of three times a week. Its duration of action is up to three days, which made a three-times-a-week dosing schedule possible. The principal disadvantage of such a long duration of action is the time necessary to reach a steady state and to stabilize the patient at an appropriate comfort level (77,78). The long action of LAAM solved some clinical problems that seemed to undermine the efficacy of methadone in some patients. For example, patients who apparently metabolize methadone quickly, requiring split dosing; patients unable for miscellaneous reasons (e.g., child care needs, employment) to attend daily dispensing clinic; and patients who presented medication diversion risks were able to be successfully treated with LAAM (79). A dose effect of LAAM on illicit opiate use was reported, with the 100/100/140 mg thrice-weekly regimen giving the greatest reduction in opiate use. The FDA issued a "black box" warning for LAAM because of postmarketing surveillance reports of QTc prolongation in electrocardiograms (ECGs), with several reports of torsades de pointes, a polymorphic life-threatening ventricular arrhythmia. As a result, LAAM was removed from the market in Europe and has been withdrawn by the manufacturer in the United States. Although production has been discontinued by the manufacturer, the medication remains FDA-approved, and many physicians feel that it addresses a needed niche (80). The development of buprenorphine, however, has provided an additional option for patients requiring a longer-lasting pharmacotherapy agent.

Buprenorphine Maintenance Treatment Buprenorphine is a mu opioid partial agonist that was originally marketed as a parenterally administered analgesic product. Investigators conducting an abuse liability study in human volunteers reported that subcutaneously administered buprenorphine had fewer subjective effects than morphine, a lesser withdrawal syndrome, and an ability to block the subjective responses of up to 120 mg doses of morphine. Subsequent work established that the sublingual route was preferable to oral dosing because of high first-pass effects. The first outpatient treatment study compared 8 mg of sublingual buprenorphine liquid to 20 and 60 mg doses of orally administered methadone in a randomized, double-blind, double-dummy study. Retention and decreased illicit opioid use in the buprenorphine group were superior to the response seen in the group that was receiving 20 mg/day of methadone. A study conducted with a liquid formulation was performed in a multisite trial in which opioid dependent individuals were randomly assigned to 1, 4, 8, and 16 mg/day of buprenorphine. The comparison was the effects of 1 mg/day versus 8 mg/day on illicit opioid use, retention, and opioid craving. The 8 mg/day dose group had significant reductions in illicit opioid use, reduced craving, and had better retention. Subsequent to the study by Ling et al. (4), it was decided to develop a sublingual tablet and to add naloxone, an opioid antagonist, to one of the formulations. The rationale for adding naloxone was to produce a less abusable, less divertible tablet. The dose ratio of buprenorphine to naloxone was chosen from data gathered in clinical pharmacology studies in opioid-dependent subjects maintained with morphine, methadone, or buprenorphine. In the first study, the subjects maintained on a dosage of 60 mg/day of morphine sulfate were randomly administered one of six medication treatments intravenously in a counterbalanced order: morphine, buprenorphine, buprenorphine/naloxone at 8:1, buprenorphine/naloxone at 4:1, buprenorphine/naloxone at 2:1, and placebo. Subjective measures of positive and negative effects were assessed for the first hour after dosing. The 4:1 ratio was chosen because it produced significant attenuation of buprenorphine's effects without producing significant withdrawal signs. The 2:1 ratio was aversive because it produced withdrawal on four measures and was the only dose combination for which the subjects would not pay money. A randomized, double-blind comparison of the effects of tablet formulations of 16 mg/day of buprenorphine at 16/4, buprenorphine/ naloxone or placebo, was carried out in a multicenter trial. The placebo-controlled portion of the trial lasted 1 month. Subjects in either buprenorphine dose group had reduced opioid use and reduced craving versus the placebo group. Thereafter, all subjects were given open-label buprenorphine/naloxone for 11 months. Other subjects participating at new sites were given 1 year of open-label buprenorphine/naloxone. Most phase 1 and phase 2 medication development studies with buprenorphine have been conducted using parenteral and sublingual (s.l.) liquid formulations, and the s.l. liquid has been extensively studied in phase 3 clinical trials. The buprenorphine s.l. tablet is available in two forms. One formulation (Subutex) contains only buprenorphine (the "mono" tablet). The second formulation (Suboxone) contains buprenorphine and the opioid antagonist naloxone in a 4:1 ratio, which is designed to discourage illicit diversion and intravenous use. The "mono" form would be employed in the clinical setting under direct observation, whereas the "combo" form would be suitable for take-home use. Pharmacokinetic studies have found that the buprenorphine s.l. liquid formulation differs in bioavailability from the s.l. tablet (81,83). The tablet has been shown to produce blood levels that are about 50% to 60% those achieved with the liquid. Based on the findings of Compton et al, (84) that repeated administration of the tablet achieves about 70% bioequivalence to the solution, clinicians should prescribe a little less than 16 mg in tablet form to achieve bioequivalence to the 8 mg solution. Thus, tablet doses used in clinical practice probably will exceed those shown to be effective in past controlled studies with the sublingual solution. Clinical research over the past 15 years has established that buprenorphine (and buprenorphine with naloxone) is a safe and effective alternative to methadone (85–93), and LAAM (94) for opioid agonist maintenance treatment. Treatment with buprenorphine produces significant and substantial improvements over time in psychosocial functioning (95).

Buprenorphine also has unique features that permit novel uses, which may alter current strategies for maintenance and medically supervised withdrawal (96). In particular, buprenorphine's ceiling on agonist activity reduces the danger of overdose and may limit its abuse liability (97,98), and buprenorphine has low toxicity even at high intravenous doses (99,100), thereby increasing the dose range over which it may be administered safely. Buprenorphine appears less likely than methadone to prolong the QT interval on the ECG (101,102). Buprenorphine also can produce sufficient tolerance to block the effects of exogenously administered opioids (98,103,104), suggesting that it may help to reduce illicit opioid use. A transdermal and a depot formulation of buprenorphine have been developed that may provide extended relief from opioid withdrawal, reduce required clinic visits and improve adherence, while having less potential for diversion and abuse (105).

Office-Based Treatment Office-based treatment of opioid dependence with a sublingual-tablet formulation of buprenorphine and naloxone has been implemented. The final labeling study was a 4-week, multicenter, randomized, placebo-controlled trial that assigned 326 opiate-dependent persons to one of three daily office-based treatment options: sublingual buprenorphine (16 mg) and naloxone (4 mg) tablets; buprenorphine alone (16 mg); or placebo (106). The primary outcome measures were the percentage of urine samples negative for opioids and the subjects' self-reported craving for opioids. Safety data were obtained on 461 opiate-dependent persons who participated in an open-label study of buprenorphine and naloxone (at daily doses of up to 24 mg and 6 mg, respectively) and another 11 persons who received this combination only during the trial. The proportion of urine samples that were negative for opioids was greater in the combined-treatment and buprenorphine groups (17.8% and 20.7%, respectively) than in the placebo group (5.8%; $p < 0.001$ for both comparisons); the active-treatment groups also reported less opioid craving ($p < 0.001$ for both comparisons with placebo). Rates of adverse events were similar in the active-treatment and placebo groups. During the open-label phase, the percentage of urine samples negative for opioids ranged from 35.2% to 67.4%. Results from the open-label follow-up study indicated that the combined treatment was safe and well tolerated. The investigators concluded that buprenorphine and naloxone in combination and buprenorphine alone are safe and reduce the use and craving for opioids in an office-based setting.

Buprenorphine Induction and Stabilization

Buprenorphine can produce withdrawal discomfort among opioid-dependent volunteers under certain conditions, which may be due to more than one mechanism (3,107). Low buprenorphine doses may provide too-little agonist effect (that is, insufficient substitution) relative to the maintenance opioid (such as heroin). In this case, raising the buprenorphine dose may or may not surmount this problem. Put another way, the partial agonist profile of buprenorphine may limit its ability to suppress opioid abstinence signs and symptoms. Alternatively, buprenorphine may directly precipitate withdrawal discomfort, in which case higher doses could be expected to aggravate the problem. Individuals maintained on the long-acting, full mu opioid agonist methadone can experience withdrawal symptoms, when given the high-affinity partial mu-agonist buprenorphine, which abruptly reduces the extent of μ-opioid receptor stimulation. This principle has been amply demonstrated in humans: Partial mu opioid agonists such as nalorphine and butorphanol (108,109) can, in methadone-maintained individuals, abruptly precipitate opioid withdrawal signs and symptoms that are functionally similar to those produced by the antagonist naloxone. Obviously, it would be ideal to avoid (or at least minimize) this problem because this discomfort may translate into attrition and relapse. It is important to note that, among individuals maintained on shorter-acting μ-opioid agonists such as morphine (relative to the longer-acting agonist methadone), buprenorphine administered alone did not precipitate a significant opioid withdrawal syndrome provided those individuals have abstained from opioid use long enough to enter a state of early opioid withdrawal (110–113). Bickel and Amass (3) proposed tentative guidelines for inducting heroin-dependent patients onto buprenorphine, which involve considering the amount of heroin used and maintaining a sufficient interval (at least 12 hours) between the last heroin use and the first buprenorphine dose. They recommended that the induction dose of buprenorphine be administered when patients are beginning to experience opioid withdrawal, so that buprenorphine can suppress those symptoms. Clinical experience with administering initial doses of buprenorphine to heroin-dependent patients suggests that an interval of 6 hours probably is sufficient to minimize the risk of precipitated withdrawal.

The general guidelines for beginning opioid treatment medication are published in the CSAT Treatment Improvement Publications (TIPs) 43 (for opioid treatment in opioid treatment programs [OTPs]) and 40 (for buprenorphine) (114). After physical assessment to rule out any acute, life-threatening condition, including the presence of sedatives such as benzodiazepines or alcohol (that might have abstinence or intoxication symptoms masked or worsened by buprenorphine treatment), treatment with buprenorphine should begin when there are no signs of opioid intoxication or sedation and some beginning signs of opioid withdrawal. Awaiting signs of withdrawal before administering the first dose is especially important for buprenorphine induction because, as described, buprenorphine can precipitate withdrawal in some circumstances (115). Precipitated withdrawal usually is more sudden and can be more severe and uncomfortable than naturally occurring withdrawal. The typical first dose of buprenorphine is 4 mg, and a sublingual tablet should be observed to have dissolved completely under the tongue. After the first dose, patients should wait in an observation area and be checked 30 to 60 minutes later for acute adverse effects. If same-day dosing adjustments must be made, patients should wait 2 to 4 more hours after the additional dosing, for further evaluation when peak effects are achieved.

If withdrawal symptoms persist after 2 to 4 hours, the initial dose can be supplemented with up to 4 mg for a maximum first day dose of 8 mg of buprenorphine (116). The first day's dose should be followed by dosage increases over subsequent days until withdrawal symptoms are suppressed within about 2 hours after taking the medication and lasting until the next day's dosing when using once-daily dosing. For most patients undergoing induction with the combination tablet, the initial target dose after induction should be 12 to 16 mg of buprenorphine in a 4-to-1 ratio to naloxone (i.e., 12/3 to 16/4 mg [buprenorphine/naloxone]). Bringing patients to this target dosage may be achieved over the first 3 days of treatment by doubling the dose each successive day after initial administration. An initial dose of 4/1 mg (buprenorphine/naloxone) is recommended, followed in 2 to 4 hours with an additional 4/1 mg if indicated. The dosage should be increased on subsequent days to the target dosage (ranging from 12/3 to 16/4 mg/day). During dose induction, patients may need to visit their OTP or physician's office daily for dose adjustments and clinical monitoring. Further information and guidelines for buprenorphine induction and use can be found in TIP 40, *Clinical Guidelines for the Use of Buprenorphine in the Treatment of Opioid Addiction* (114). These CSAT clinical guidelines address the pharmacology and physiology of opioids, opioid addiction, and treatment with buprenorphine; describe patient assessment and the choice of opioid addiction treatment options; provide detailed treatment protocols for opioid withdrawal and maintenance therapy with buprenorphine; and include information on the treatment of special populations, e.g., pregnant women, adolescents, and polysubstance users. The pharmacologil complexity of transferring methadone-maintained patients to buprenorphine maintenance is discussed further later.

Special considerations are needed for patients inducted onto buprenorphine after treatment with or nonmedical use of long half-life full agonist opioid medications such as methadone. Three national evaluations of the buprenorphine-naloxone combination tablet (Suboxone) found that direct induction with buprenorphine alone was effective for most people who were opioid-addicted. However, buprenorphine tablets without naloxone (often called "monotherapy") may be used during the first 2 days of induction for patients attempting to transfer from a longer-acting opioid such as sustained-release morphine or methadone (117,118) to avoid any possibility that these patients would experience withdrawal effects from any naloxone absorbed from the combination tablets—an unlikely phenomenon due to the low sublingual absorption of naloxone.

SPECIAL ISSUES IN MAINTENANCE TREATMENT

Opioid Maintenance Treatment during Pregnancy

Opioid misuse during pregnancy is a serious and growing concern in the United States and around the world and is often associated with a multitude of environmental and medical factors contributing to adverse consequences for both the mother and her infant, including high rates of infection, premature delivery, and low birth weight, which is an important risk factor for later developmental delay (119–127). The pharmacologic management of opioid dependence in pregnant women is a complex clinical problem. The increasing prevalence of nonmedically used analgesics in the general population and women of child bearing age has made the focus on this problem especially urgent. The pattern of increased nonmedical use of analgesics seen in the general population has also been found for pregnant women, with self-reported nonmedical use increasing from 51,900 in 1993 to an average of 109,000 in 2002 to 2004 (128).The current literature suggests that children of opioid-dependent women might be at risk for poor outcomes not only because of opioid drug exposure, but also because of concomitant alcohol and tobacco exposure and numerous factors related to the care giving environment (129,130). Treatment options studied include methadone maintenance (131,132), antagonist maintenance (133) (i.e., naltrexone), and medication-assisted withdrawal (134). Methadone maintenance has been the recommended standard of care over no treatment or medication-assisted withdrawal. This recommendation is based on longer durations of maternal drug abstinence, better obstetrical care compliance, avoidance of associated risk behaviors, reductions in fetal illicit drug exposure, and enhanced neonatal outcomes (i.e., heavier birth weight) (131). Methadone is the oldest, most widely used medication prescribed during pregnancy (132), and in comparison to infants from heroin-abusing mothers, infants from methadone-treated mothers have increased fetal growth, reduced fetal mortality, decreased risk of HIV infection, decreased risk of pre-eclampsia and fetal exposure to rapid and unpredictable cycles of heroin-induced highs and withdrawal, and an increased likelihood of the infant being discharged to his or her parents (125,135). Moreover, for pregnant women under conditions where nonmedication-assisted and methadone treatment were both available, methadone is associated with longer treatment retention (136–139) and less relapse (135). Studies examining the consequences of prenatal methadone exposure on later development have produced inconsistent results (140–147) that could be due to a number of confounding factors and are complicated by significant study attrition (140). One long-term follow-up study of 27 children who had been exposed to methadone in utero found no cognitive impairment in the preschool years (119). Overall, prenatal exposure to methadone provided as a part of comprehensive treatment does not appear to be associated with developmental or cognitive impairments (140).

Nevertheless, methadone use at the usually effective clinical doses during pregnancy is considered controversial by many practitioners because of the associated neonatal abstinence syndrome (NAS). Although newborns of methadone-maintained women may experience opioid withdrawal symptoms, these are readily treated without damaging consequences (140). Generally, 50% to 81% of neonates prenatally exposed to methadone show some signs of NAS (120,148). In a retrospective review of pregnancies that were maintained on methadone therapy in one hospital (120), 100 mother/neonate pairs on methadone therapy were identified. Women who received an average methadone dose of >80 mg were similar to women maintained on dosages of ≤80 mg in having infants with similar neonatal abstinence scores, needs for neonatal treatment for withdrawal, and similar duration of withdrawal, when it occurred in the neonate. The authors concluded that maternal methadone dosage does not correlate with neonatal withdrawal; therefore, maternal benefits of effective methadone dosing are not offset by neonatal harm. However, another study addressing maternal maintenance dose found that NAS was related to the mother's dose of methadone. It reported that opioid-dependent pregnant patients receiving mean methadone doses of 132 mg methadone had less illicit drug use at delivery, but their neonates had no more severe NAS than expectant mothers receiving mean doses of 62 mg of methadone (149). Hence, pregnant women should receive appropriate methadone doses to treat their addiction, but concerns regarding greater NAS severity associated with larger methadone should not be the primary factor in determining dose (150).

Similar to research with methadone, large, definitive randomized controlled trials of buprenorphine in pregnant women have not been conducted. There have been 31 published reports of buprenorphine exposure during pregnancy that were reviewed and summarized by Jones et al. (150). Of note, two small-scale, randomized, double-blind controlled trials were completed using similar methodology to obtain safety and efficacy data comparing methadone and buprenorphine in pregnant women (151–153). In addition, the literature includes 10 prospective studies and 18 reports summarizing case-report data. Overall, the studies report approximately 522 neonates prenatally exposed to buprenorphine, with a wide range of therapeutic doses, from 0.4 to 24 mg sublingual tablets per day. Generally, the pregnancies were uneventful, without physical teratogenic effects, and with low rates of prematurity, suggesting that buprenorphine is relatively safe and effective in this population. Clearly, conclusions from data on the prenatal exposure to buprenorphine are limited by methodologic challenges (e.g., varied dose ranges, lengths of exposure, care settings). Many published reports omitted information regarding concomitant drug use, including licit drugs of abuse (nicotine, alcohol), prescribed medications (e.g., benzodiazepines, antidepressants), and illicit drugs that could impact the expression of NAS. The most glaring omission is the insufficient detail regarding medication used to treat ensuing NAS, as well as the criteria for initiation, maintenance, and weaning of NAS medication. Moreover, the scoring systems used to assess NAS treatment efficacy vary widely across all reports (e.g., Finnegan [154] or modifications of this scale and Lipsitz [155]), and thus limit the ability to compare studies. Despite significant variability in the instruments and scoring methods used, the literature suggests that buprenorphine exposure is also associated with NAS, half the cases of which require pharmacotherapy. The pregnancy, birth and NAS outcomes are also confounded by other drug use in 86% of the reports. Although considerable individual variability exists, the NAS timing observed to date has an apparent onset within the first 12 to 48 hours, peaks within approximately 66 to 96 hours, and lasts approximately 120 to 168 hours. The exception to this has been the few infants who were reported to exhibit withdrawal signs for 6 to 10 weeks after delivery. Such a protracted withdrawal syndrome may be due to both the NAS medication and the regimen used to treat withdrawal rather than a direct effect of buprenorphine. To date, only one report has found a correlation between buprenorphine dose and the severity of the NAS (156). Other recent reports (151,153) and one that included a large sample size (157) have reported no correlation.

Although there are hundreds of published papers on methadone treatment of substance-abusing pregnant women, and more than 31 published reports documenting perinatal buprenorphine exposure, much of the literature has methodologic limitations. These include the fact that studies are frequently open-label, retrospective, of small sample sizes, and lack appropriate controls (e.g., prospective data collection, randomization, blind dosing and data collection, systematic collection of data). Only two previous small sample–sized RCTs comparing methadone and buprenorphine (151,153) have been completed. The need for a large multisite clinical trial enrolling a diverse sample of pregnant opioid-dependent women in order to conclusively determine each medication's safety and efficacy is currently being addressed by the Maternal Opioid Treatment: Human Experimental Research study in progress (150). This is a double-blind, double-dummy; randomized, stratified, parallel group design. Its current methods and procedures were based on extensive pilot research examining the safety and feasibility of studying these medications in pregnant women and their neonates (152,153). Participants are 18 to 41 years of age, pregnant with estimated gestational age between 6 and 30 weeks, currently opioid-dependent according to the E module of the Structured Clinical Interview for DSM-IV SCID I (158), or have a history of opioid dependence and being at risk for relapse (159) and have opioid-positive urine sample results. Buprenorphine without naloxone was selected for this trial to minimize risks of side effects, to obtain scientific information on effects of buprenorphine alone before adding other medications, and to avoid possible maternal and fetal hormonal effects suggested by animal data after naloxone exposure (160,161). A flexible dose range of 2 to 32 mg of buprenorphine estimated to be equivalent to the methadone flexible dosing range of 20 to 140 mg methadone is used based on reported clinical trial data (162–164). Based on the results of the pilot study (153), five primary outcome measures were selected for examination, given their importance to the health and well-being of the child and the cost of this illness to society: (i) NAS; (ii) number of neonates requiring treatment; (iii) amount of medication needed to treat NAS; (iv) head circumference; and (v) length of hospital stay. The pilot study results as well as preliminary results from the literature led to the hypothesis that buprenorphine will produce a superior outcome for all five variables. Maternal outcomes, objective and self-reported drug use changes in psychosocial functioning, the adequacy of the medication, side effects, and adverse events during the study are hypothesized to be equivalent.

Interactions of Opioid Maintenance and Human Immunodeficiency Virus and Acquired Immunodeficiency Syndrome Pharmacotherapy In response to concerns about HIV and drug injection as a mode of transmission, methadone maintenance has been accorded renewed attention. Given that there are more than a million chronic intravenous heroin users in the United States, the magnitude of this problem becomes clear. Prevalence studies in New York City from 1984 to 1985 found that <10% of methadone-maintained patients who entered treatment before 1978 were HIV-positive, compared to more than half of heroin-dependent patients who were not in treatment (165). Similarly, a prospective study in Philadelphia found an HIV seroconversion rate four times higher in active intravenous heroin users than in methadone-maintained patients (166). Other studies documented a dramatically reduced HIV seroprevalence rate for patients who were successfully maintained on methadone, as compared to active injecting drug users (167–169). Methadone maintenance thus appears to be extremely effective in reducing injection-related risk factors for HIV.

The introduction of new antiretroviral agents and highly active antiretroviral therapy (HAART) created a new therapeutic era for HIV-infected patients but also has introduced new complexities related to potential drug toxicities and interactions. Preclinical studies of antiretroviral medications and opioids indicate that drug interactions are likely to occur as methadone and buprenorphine are both primarily metabolized by hepatic cytochrome CYP 450 3A4 (170,171). A number of antiretroviral medications have been shown in preclinical studies to inhibit or induce the activity of this same enzyme.

Methadone has been associated with several clinically important adverse drug interactions with HIV medications. A study of possible interactions between methadone and zidovudine (Azidothymidine, or AZT) has shown that serum levels of methadone are not affected by this drug, but that some patients who receive methadone maintenance treatment may show a potentially toxic increase in serum levels of AZT (65). However, the authors caution against making changes in the dose of AZT; instead, they suggest careful clinical monitoring for signs of dose-related AZT toxicity. Another possible complication when an antiretroviral medication that can induce methadone metabolism is discontinued is cardiac arrhythmia due to increased methadone exposure after reversal of methadone metabolism induction leads to increased methadone exposure (172). It has been recommended that after the medication that is inducing CYP 450 3A enzymes is stopped, the methadone dose should be tapered over 1 to 2 weeks to re-establish the previous therapeutic dose of methadone (i.e., that dose on which the patient was stable before starting the HAART regimen) (173). A recent review citing numerous case reports, chart reviews, and pharmacokinetic studies (174) observed that many HAART drugs compete with methadone for metabolizing enzymes thus requiring dose changes for methadone during concomitant treatment for HIV.

Buprenorphine has been studied in combination with antiretroviral medications more recently. To date, reductions in buprenorphine concentrations resulting from drug interactions have not been associated with opioid withdrawal. A study examining drug interactions between buprenorphine and the nonnucleoside reverse-transcriptase inhibitors efavirenz (EFV) and delavirdine (DLV) (175) found that buprenorphine did not alter antiretroviral pharmacokinetics. Adjustments of doses of either buprenorphine or EFV or DLV are not likely to be necessary when these drugs are administered for the treatment of opioid dependence and HIV disease. They also examined drug interactions between buprenorphine and the protease inhibitors (PIs) nelfinavir (NFV), ritonavir (RTV), and lopinavir/ritonavir (LPV/R). The authors concluded that buprenorphine had no significant effects on the PI AUC. Adjustments of doses of buprenorphine or NFV, LPV/R, or RTV are not likely to be necessary when these drugs are administered for the treatment of opioid dependence and HIV disease (176). Further, Bruce et al. (177) have reviewed the current state of knowledge regarding specific interactions between buprenorphine and antiretrovirals and found that drug interactions between buprenorphine/naloxone and antiretrovirals to date show a drug interaction profile with antiretroviral therapies that is much more promising than that of methadone.

Though pharmacologically buprenorphine may present fewer medication interaction problems, the outpatient office setting may not be the most therapeutic with respect to medication adherence. Opioid treatment programs are ideal sites to support adherence to treatment of HIV and other infectious diseases. Resistance to antiretroviral drugs is one of the greatest limitations to effective long-term therapy for HIV infection—a problem alleviated by the development of carefully selected, sequential combination HAART regimens (178). This strategy depends on careful adherence of 90% or greater, in order to maintain efficacy. Drug abuse treatment programs, irrespective of modality, are associated with improved adherence to antiretroviral therapies among drug users (179). MMT, in particular, has been shown to be associated with HAART adherence and improved HIV treatment outcomes among HIV/HCV co-infected injection drug users (180). It should also be mentioned in this context that a similar situation exists for tuberculosis wherein incomplete chemoprophylaxis and treatment are major causes of the resurgence of this disease, often drug-resistant, among drug users. Adherence to and completion of directly observed antituberculosis therapy can be attained by drug users in treatment, even despite ongoing drug misuse (181).

In conclusion, opioid maintenance treatment has multiple beneficial effects on clinical status in patients with HIV infection, primarily as a result of improving adherence to treatment and decreasing risky behavior. Both methadone and buprenorphine treatments are compatible with HIV HAART treatment. The complexity of multiple-agent antiretroviral treatment complicates the use of methadone owing to pharmacokinetic interactions, but these can be managed by appropriate dose adjustments. The choice of opioid pharmacotherapy agent should be based on individual clinical needs. Though buprenorphine has fewer clinically significant drug interactions with antiretroviral medications than methadone, some patients may respond better to a full agonist in an opioid treatment program. However, if there are no contraindications, patients needing HAART may benefit from a trial of buprenorphine treatment. A trial of buprenorphine may be best managed in an opioid treatment program or by physicians who provide HAART treatment and are also qualified to prescribe buprenorphine (182).

Methadone-to-Buprenorphine Transfer Some patients will be transferred from methadone to buprenorphine for maintenance or medically supervised withdrawal. This clinical decision may be driven by several possible factors. First, there is the unique pharmacology of buprenorphine, leading to its more favorable safety profile and longer duration of action (thus permitting less-frequent dosing) relative to methadone (12,183–185). Second, given its status as a novel treatment option (which may differentially attract or retain novelty-seeking individuals (186), buprenorphine may engender less fear of stigma than methadone. Third, owing to its availability in office-based primary care—outside the domain of standard opioid treatment programs (18,36,187)—buprenorphine is more accessible over a wide geographic area. It also may be more appropriate as an early intervention strategy for those with short dependence histories (e.g., adolescents), or with less physical dependence. However, if a patient is stable on methadone, the advisability of transfer to buprenorphine requires careful scrutiny of the factors motivating the request. Furthermore, transferring patients from a longer-acting agonist such as methadone to buprenorphine without producing significant withdrawal discomfort, attrition, or relapse to drug use, has been shown to be more challenging than transfer from a shorter-acting opiate.

Studies of transfer from methadone to buprenorphine are limited to small studies, including human laboratory studies, but these results offer some evidence on which to base clinical treatment in both inpatient and outpatient settings. These studies support an important role for agonist maintenance dose and interval between full and partial agonist administration in determining precipitated withdrawal symptoms. Several clinical studies have investigated switching methadone-maintained research volunteers to buprenorphine. Four programmatic studies examined the effect of time interval between the last methadone maintenance dose and the initial buprenorphine dose (108,188–190). Most subjects in the four studies were maintained on methadone at 30 mg/day. When buprenorphine was administered to the volunteers, buprenorphine significantly increased opioid withdrawal effects at 2 hours after methadone (188) but not at 20 to 22 hours (108,188), nor at 40 hours (190). Results from another study in which buprenorphine was administered intravenously at about a 20-hour interval (81) also are consistent with these data. Walsh and June (190) systematically addressed whether methadone maintenance dose influences the response to buprenorphine. In that study, one group of volunteers was maintained on 30 mg/day, and a second group of volunteers was maintained on 60 mg/day. The 60-mg group experienced increased opioid withdrawal symptoms from buprenorphine whereas the 30-mg group had minimal symptoms. Two additional studies by this research team (191,192) also addressed whether buprenorphine dose-dependently precipitates opioid withdrawal in methadone-maintained volunteers. In these studies buprenorphine (five intramuscular active doses from 0.5 to 8 mg) precipitated mild withdrawal at the 2-hour interval, but withdrawal severity was not dose-related. Five studies have directly examined a full medication transfer. Kosten and Kleber (191) reported the first outpatient trial of the methadone-to-buprenorphine (using s.l. liquid) transition. In this open-label study, eight heroin-using and eight methadone-maintained (25 mg/day) volunteers were assigned to receive 2 mg (n = 4), 4 mg (n = 2), or 8 mg (n = 2) per day within 24 hours after their last methadone dose in those on methadone. Across the entire sample (N = 16), withdrawal symptoms were not buprenorphine-dose-dependent and were highest on the first two test days, but most patients completed the protocol, and later heroin use was relatively low, with 78% of all samples testing drug-free. In an open-label study, Banys (192) examined the ability of s.l. liquid buprenorphine to suppress opioid withdrawal 26 to 31 hours after discontinuing methadone. Fifteen participants took three low doses of buprenorphine over several hours (0.15 mg, 0.15 mg 1 hour later, then 0.3 mg 2 hours later) to relieve withdrawal signs and symptoms. In six subjects, a low dose of 0.15 to 0.30 mg resulted in the disappearance of subjective and objective withdrawal symptoms within 10 minutes to 2.5 hours. Four others had brief, partial relief of symptoms. Five subjects failed to experience any relief of withdrawal symptoms after a total of 0.6 mg buprenorphine administered over 3 hours. Lukas (193) conducted the first double-blind, double-dummy pilot study of three males—maintained on three different methadone doses (25, 58 and 60 mg/day)—who were switched abruptly to buprenorphine 2 mg/day, subcutaneously with physiologic (including EEG), behavioral, and subjective ratings collected. They found that buprenorphine did not fully substitute for methadone during the transfer. In a within-subject, double-blind, double-dummy procedure with inpatient volunteers, Levin et al. (194) tapered a moderate methadone maintenance dose (60 mg) over a few days (40 mg, 30 mg, 30 mg, then 0 mg) before initiating buprenorphine (4 mg on day 1 followed by 8 mg). Like Kosten and Kleber (191), the protocol of Levin et al. (194) demonstrated some qualified success, in that 79% (15 of 19) of participants who began the dose-taper completed the transfer even though opioid withdrawal symptoms remained elevated, after the first two buprenorphine daily doses

(4 mg, then 8 mg). Withdrawal symptoms gradually were suppressed by subsequent daily doses of buprenorphine (8 mg) and returned to baseline during buprenorphine stabilization (8 mg/day). In another small double-blind, double-dummy pilot study (195), five male heroin-dependent outpatient volunteers were transferred from methadone 60 mg (via one intervening 45 mg dose) to the buprenorphine s.l. tablet. Subjective effects and vital signs were collected before the transfer (methadone 60 mg and 45 mg), on buprenorphine days 1 and 2 (8 mg/day), and on days 7 and 8 (16 mg/day). The 1-day methadone dose-taper did not significantly alter opioid withdrawal, but the protocol used in this pilot study was able to shorten the duration of withdrawal discomfort to about 1 day, relative to the results of Levin et al. (194). These preliminary results suggest that it is feasible to transfer outpatients on methadone 60 mg/day to the buprenorphine 8 mg/day s.l. tablet. The authors suggest that if the first daily transfer dose of buprenorphine does precipitate withdrawal, it may be useful to consider increased subsequent buprenorphine doses to suppress this withdrawal.

More recently, a study by Breen et al. (196) investigated the response of 23 opioid-dependent patients receiving high and intermediate doses of methadone between 30 and 70 mg/day when transferred to buprenorphine at doses between 12 to 16 mg/day. After the last morning dose of methadone, buprenorphine was substituted in doses increasing from 4 mg to a maximum of 16 mg, with adjunctive lofexidine (maximum of 2.4 mg/day). All except two patients successfully completed transfer to buprenorphine. Average stabilization dose of buprenorphine for the sample who completed transfer was 14.0 mg/day (SD, 2.3), and average daily lofexidine dose during transfer was 0.57 mg (SD, 0.39). The high-dose group (50 to 70 mg/day; n = 11) used significantly more lofexidine to complete transfer compared to the intermediate dose (30 to 49 mg/day; n = 10) group. Higher opioid withdrawal symptoms measured by the Short Opiate Withdrawal Scale (SOWS) were found in the high-dose group during the first and last day of buprenorphine stabilization, but average SOWS scores for the whole of the period of transfer were not significantly different between groups. This study suggested that transfer to buprenorphine is relatively uncomplicated from daily methadone doses of 30 to 70 mg in an inpatient setting and may be facilitated by use of lofexidine. Glasper et al. (197) conducted a study that showed that transfer from methadone to buprenorphine can safely occur from doses of around 30 mg of methadone. Patients on methadone doses between 30 and 40 mg were randomly assigned to transfer to buprenorphine using a fixed dose (transfer at 30 mg methadone) or a variable-dose induction (transfer when the methadone dose was sufficiently low to be "uncomfortable"). A third group of patients with methadone doses <30 mg were transferred to buprenorphine at their entry methadone dose. Fifty-one patients were inducted into buprenorphine using the same dosing protocol with the first dose of 4 mg buprenorphine. After stabilization on buprenorphine, patients gradually reduced the buprenorphine dose to 0 mg. Withdrawal severity and drug use were monitored. Severity of withdrawal during transfer to buprenorphine did not significantly differ between the transfer at 30 mg and transfer using the uncomfortable methadone-dosing protocol. Those on doses of <30 mg reported significantly less withdrawal discomfort than either of these other two groups during transfer to buprenorphine. All but one patient stabilized on buprenorphine. Thirty-eight of the 51 patients inducted into buprenorphine reached 0 mg. Rosado et al. (198) conducted a study to test the acute effects of sublingual buprenorphine/naloxone tablets in volunteers with a higher level of physical dependence. The goal was to identify a dose that would precipitate withdrawal. In phase 1, sublingual buprenorphine/naloxone at four different doses (4/1, 8/2, 16/4, 32 mg/8 mg), or intramuscular naloxone (0.2 mg) or placebo were administered to volunteers on 100 mg of oral methadone. Then in phase 2, they split this buprenorphine/naloxone dose to determine whether withdrawal could be attenuated using this split dose. The conditions again were methadone, placebo, naloxone, 100% of the buprenorphine/naloxone dose that precipitated withdrawal in phase 1, and 50% of this dose administered twice during a session. Six subjects did not complete the study. Of the 10 who completed, 3 tolerated up to 32 mg/8 mg of buprenorphine/naloxone without evidence of precipitated withdrawal. For the seven completing both phases, split doses generally produced less precipitated withdrawal as compared to full doses. The authors concluded that low, repeated doses of buprenorphine/naloxone (e.g., 2 mg/0.5 mg) may be an effective strategy for safely dosing this medication in persons with higher levels of physical dependence.

In conclusion a multitude of small clinical studies now show that methadone to buprenorphine transfer is feasible over a range of starting methadone doses. Owing to variable designs and individual differences among volunteers, a single recommended protocol is not currently available. Recommendations from CSAT (TIP 40) for patients taking methadone are to taper methadone to 30 mg or less per day for 1 week or more before initiating buprenorphine. Induction should not begin until at least 24 hours after the last dose of methadone and should start at 2 mg of the monotherapy formulation. If signs or symptoms of withdrawal are seen after the first dose, a second dose of 2 mg should be administered and repeated, if necessary, to a maximum of 8 mg buprenorphine on day 1. More recently, still in the absence of large clinical trials, a Physician Clinical Support System (PCSS) guidance (PCSS 2006) recommends tapering to 20 or 30 mg of methadone, obtaining a COWS of 15 to quantify withdrawal, and starting buprenorphine at 2 mg, continuing to dose until the patient is comfortable at up to 32 mg on day 1. If withdrawal is precipitated, management with ancillary medications is advised. Discomfort may persist for up to 96 hours but usually after 3 to 5 days the patient will be stable and comfortable. Nevertheless, patients on moderate to high doses of methadone (>60 to 100 mg) may not be able to taper without discomfort and a risk of relapse. For these patients, recent data suggest that induction onto buprenorphine/naloxone might still be possible directly from methadone starting with 2/0.5 mg buprenorphine/naloxone tablets.

In addition to clarifying the best strategy for minimizing symptoms during the transfer, larger clinical trials are needed to answer questions concerning short- and long-term clinical outcomes after methadone to buprenorphine transfer. A related relevant clinical need is identification of clinical profiles of patients responding differentially to methadone versus buprenorphine (pharmacotherapy treatment matching).

Buprenorphine in Agonist-to-Antagonist Treatment Buprenorphine has been used in several experimental studies (103,191,199) as a transitional agent between agonists (such as methadone or heroin) and antagonists (such as naloxone or naltrexone). In one study, Kosten and Kleber (191) substituted buprenorphine at 2, 4, and 8 mg for 20 to 30 mg of methadone or heroin for 1 month without precipitating substantial withdrawal symptoms, though buprenorphine may act as an opioid antagonist at doses as low as 8 mg. After chronic administration, buprenorphine produces less physical dependence than do pure agonists, as suggested by the less severe withdrawal symptoms that occur when stopping buprenorphine compared to short-acting opiates or methadone and by the need for relatively higher antagonist doses to precipitate withdrawal in buprenorphine than methadone-maintained volunteers (200). After 1 month of buprenorphine stabilization, the drug was abruptly discontinued, and a small dose of naltrexone was given 24 hours later. The investigators observed that the transition to buprenorphine generally was well tolerated. The subsequent abrupt discontinuation of buprenorphine was associated with "minimal withdrawal" in the 2- and 4-mg buprenorphine groups, and a low dose of naltrexone (1 mg) did not precipitate withdrawal. However, subjects in the 8-mg group reported a more substantial increase in withdrawal symptoms when buprenorphine was stopped. Because of these properties, Kosten and Kleber examined whether buprenorphine might facilitate the transition from opioid agonists to antagonists in a three-step process: (i) buprenorphine substitution for agonists such as methadone, (ii) buprenorphine-induced reduction in physical dependence, and (iii) discontinuation of buprenorphine with rapid introduction of naltrexone. In a study testing that hypothesis, Kosten (199) used intravenous naloxone to challenge five opioid-dependent patients who were maintained on 3 mg s.l. buprenorphine. Induction into naltrexone was attempted in all of those patients who completed 30 days on buprenorphine. Five male opioid-dependent patients maintained on buprenorphine 3 mg sublingually for 1 month as outpatients were abruptly discontinued from buprenorphine by blinded, placebo substitution and enlisted in a placebo-controlled, double-blind challenge with intravenous naloxone at 0.5 mg/kg. The naloxone was given over a 20-minute period using a 10-mg/ml solution. Significant withdrawal symptoms were precipitated. Moreover, 5 hours after this naloxone challenge, withdrawal symptoms were at baseline levels, and oral naltrexone was given at either 12.5 mg or 25 mg without precipitating further withdrawal symptoms. The authors believed that the withdrawal syndrome was milder for buprenorphine than for pure opioid agonists, "suggesting a partial resetting of the opioid receptors by the antagonist activity of buprenorphine." In some situations, combination drug treatment may facilitate greater patient acceptance of agonist-antagonist switching. Thus, Fudala et al. (106) have shown that the early use of naltrexone during medically supervised withdrawal in combination with benzodiazepines and clonidine facilitated naltrexone acceptance by patients. Johnson (107), in a study comparing buprenorphine taper alone and buprenorphine with naltrexone, suggested that the combination treatment may reduce the severity of withdrawal symptoms. The use of buprenorphine to stabilize opioid dependent patients before switching them to naltrexone has the advantage of psychosocial stabilization prior to medically supervised withdrawal. This approach may represent a compromise between acute medically supervised withdrawal and long-term treatment of chronic dependence. The foregoing techniques (clonidine/naltrexone and buprenorphine/naltrexone) may be combined in a clinical protocol that places methadone patients or heroin-dependent patients on buprenorphine for several weeks to stabilize and engage them in the psychosocial aspects of treatment. This could be followed by rapid transition to naltrexone, using clonidine to relieve any withdrawal symptoms caused by stopping the buprenorphine. Such combination approaches are reviewed in Stine (68). These generally have been small pilot studies.

SUMMARY

Opioid dependence is unique among substance use disorders in having multiple available pharmacotherapy options for treatment. In addition to full and partial agonist treatments available for medically assisted withdrawal, this treatment remains an area of active research as development of nonopioid medications, especially α_2-adrenergic agonists and combination treatments continues. Evidence to date does not support differences in efficacy among these various methods of medically assisted withdrawal but supports the common occurrence of relapse after withdrawal using any method. Therefore, as a chronic relapsing disorder, opioid dependence is primarily treated with long-term pharmacotherapies. Antagonist maintenance is not widely accepted but may have increased utility with the availability of new depot formulations, another current research question. Full agonist treatments are the most extensively used and researched for efficacy. Although methadone is available only in specialized and licensed opioid treatment program settings, buprenorphine is available in medical offices across the United States. Multiple head-to-head studies have shown equivalent efficacy of buprenorphine to moderate doses of methadone. Identification of patients who benefit differentially from methadone versus buprenorphine treatments is a topic for active clinical research. Other clinical issues that continue to be studied include nonopioid medication interactions with various full and partial opioid agonists, uses of combination medications for transitions from full agonists to partial agonists such as buprenorphine or to antagonists such as naltrexone, and using full versus partial opioid agonists in special populations (i.e., pregnant women).

ACKNOWLEDGMENTS: *This work was supported by National Institute on Drug Abuse Grants RO1-DA015832 (SMS), R01-DA05626 (TRK), K05-DA0454 (TRK), and P50-DA09250 and 18197, and the Veterans Affairs Mental Illness Research, Education and Clinical Center. Special thanks are also due to Robert A Hollenbeck, PhD, for editorial assistance.*

REFERENCES

1. Rea F, Bell JR, Young MR, Mattick RP. A randomised, controlled trial of low dose naltrexone for the treatment of opioid dependence. *Drug Alcohol Depend* 2004;75(1):79–88.
2. Walsh SL, Chausmer AE, Strain EC, Bigelow GE. Evaluation of the mu and kappa opioid actions of butorphanol in humans through differential naltrexone blockade. *Psychopharmacology (Berl)* 2008;196(1):143–55.
3. Bickel WK, Amass L. Buprenorphine treatment of opioid dependence: a review. *Exp Clin Psychopharmacol* 1995;3:477–489.
4. Ling W, Rawson RA, Compton MA. Substitution pharmacotherapies for opioid addiction: from methadone to LAAM and buprenorphine. *J Psychoactive Drugs* 1994;26(2):119–128.
5. Lewis DC. Access to narcotic addiction treatment and medical care: prospects for the expansion of methadone maintenance treatment. *J Addict Dis* 1999;18:5–21.
6. National Institutes of Health Consensus Panel. NIH Consensus Panel recommends expanding access to and improving methadone treatment programs for heroin addiction. *Eur Addict Res* 1999;5:50–51.
7. Rounsaville B, Kosten TR. Treatment for opioid dependence: quality and access. *JAMA* 2000;283:1337–1339.
8. Martin WR, Jasinski DR. Physiological parameters of morphine dependence in man: tolerance, early abstinence, protracted abstinence. *J Psychiatr Res* 1969;7:9–17.
9. Fultz JM, Senay EC. Guidelines for the management of hospitalized narcotics addicts. *Ann Intern Med* 1975;82(6):815–818.
10. Amass L, Bickel WK, Higgins ST, et al. A preliminary investigation of outcome following gradual or rapid buprenorphine detoxification. *J Addict Dis* 1994;13(3):33–45.
11. Cheskin LJ, Fudala PJ, Johnson RE. A controlled comparison of buprenorphine and clonidine for acute detoxification from opioids. *Drug Alcohol Depend* 1994;36(2):115–121.
12. Fudala PJ, Jaffe JH. Use of buprenorphine in the treatment of opioid addiction: II. Physiologic and behavioral effects of daily and alternate-day administration and abrupt withdrawal. *Clin Pharmacol Ther* 1990; 47:525–534.
13. Jasinski DR, Pevnick JS, Griffith JD. Human pharmacology and abuse potential of the analgesic buprenorphine. *Arch Gen Psychaitry* 1978;35: 501–516.
14. Seow SS, Quigley AJ, Ilett KF, et al. Buprenorphine: a new maintenance opiate. *Med J Austria* 1986;144(8):407–411.
15. Greenwald M, Johanson CE, Bueller J, et al. Buprenorphine duration of action: mu-opioid receptor availability and pharmacokinetic and behavioral indices. *Biol Psychiatry* 2007;61(1):101–110.
16. Bickel WK, Stitzer MI. A clinical trial of buprenorphine: comparison with methadone in the detoxification of heroin addicts. *Clin Pharmacol Ther* 1988;43:72–78.
17. Nigam AK, Ray R, Tripathi BM. Buprenorphine in opiate withdrawal: a comparison with clonidine. *J Subst Abuse Treat* 1993;10(4): 391–394.
18. O'Connor P, Carroll K, Shi JM, et al. Three methods of opioid detoxification in a primary care setting. A randomized trial. *Ann Intern Med* 1997;127(7):526–530.
19. Vignau J. Preliminary assessment of a 10-day rapid detoxification programme using high dosage buprenorphine. *Eur Addict Res* 1998; 4(Suppl 1):29–31.
20. Ling W, Amass L, Shoptaw S, et al., Buprenorphine Study Protocol Group. A multi-center randomized trial of buprenorphine-naloxone versus clonidine for opioid detoxification: findings from the National Institute on Drug Abuse Clinical Trials Network. *Addiction* 2005;100(8): 1090–1100.
21. Oreskovich MR, Saxon AJ, Ellis ML, et al. A double-blind, double-dummy, randomized, prospective pilot study of the partial mu opiate agonist, buprenorphine, for acute detoxification from heroin. *Drug Alcohol Depend* 2005;77(1):71–79.
22. Gold MS, Redmond DE, Kleber HD. Noradrenergic hyperactivity in opiate withdrawal supported by clonidine reversal of opiate withdrawal. *Am J Psychiatry* 1979;136(1):100–102.
23. Gossop M. Clonidine and the treatment of the opiate withdrawal syndrome. *Drug Alcohol Depend.* 1988;21(3):253–259.
24. Charney DS, Sternberg DE, Kleber HD, et al. The clinical use of clonidine in abrupt withdrawal from methadone. Effects on blood pressure and specific signs and symptoms. *Arch Gen Psychiatry* 1981;38(11): 1273–1277.
25. Kleber HD, Riordan CE, Rounsaville B, et al. Clonidine in outpatient detoxification from methadone maintenance. *Arch Gen Psychiatry* 1985;42(4):391–394.
26. Rosen MI, McMahon TJ, Hameedi FA, et al. Effect of clonidine pretreatment on naloxone-precipitated opiate withdrawal. *J Pharmacol Exp Ther* 1996;276(3):1128–1135.
27. O'Connor PG, Waugh ME, Carroll KM, et al. Primary care-based ambulatory opioid detoxification: the results of a clinical trial. *J Gen Intern Med* 1995;10(5):255–260.
28. O'Connor PG, Carroll KM, Shi JM, et al. Three methods of opioid detoxification in a primary care setting. A randomized trial. *Ann Intern Med* 1997;127(7):526–530.
29. McCann MJ, Miotto K, Rawson RA, et al. Outpatient non-opioid detoxification for opioid withdrawal. Who is likely to benefit. *Am J Addict* 1997;6(3):218–223.
30. Bearn J, Gossop M, Strang J. Randomised double-blind comparison of lofexidine and methadone in the in-patient treatment of opiate withdrawal. *Drug Alcohol Depend* 1996;43(1-2):87–91.
31. Kahn A, Mumford JP, Rogers GA, Beckford H. Double-blind study of lofexidine and clonidine in the detoxification of opiate addicts in hospital. *Drug Alcohol Depend.* 1997;44(1):57–61.
32. Lin SK, Strang J, Su LW, Tsai CJ, Hu WH. Double-blind randomised controlled trial of lofexidine versus clonidine in the treatment of heroin withdrawal. *Drug Alcohol Depend* 1997;48(2):127–133.
33. Bearn J, Gossop M, Strang J. Accelerated lofexidine treatment regimen compared with conventional lofexidine and methadone treatment for in-patient opiate detoxification. *Drug Alcohol Depend* 1998;50(3): 227–232.
34. Yu E, Miotto K, Akerele E, et al. A Phase 3 placebo-controlled, double-blind, multi-site trial of the alpha-2-adrenergic agonist, lofexidine, for opioid withdrawal. *Drug Alcohol Depend* 2008;97(1-2):158–168.
35. Gowing L, Farrell M, Ali R, White J. Alpha2 adrenergic agonists for the management of opioid withdrawal. *Cochrane Database Syst Rev* 2004; 4:CD002024.
36. O'Connor P, Kosten TR. Rapid and ultrarapid opioid detoxification techniques [see comments]. *JAMA* 1998;279(3):229–234.
37. Collins ED, Kleber HD, Whittington RA, Heitler NE. Anesthesia-assisted vs. buprenorphine- or clonidine-assisted heroin detoxification and naltrexone induction: a randomized trial. *JAMA* 2005;294(8): 903–913.
38. Gowing L, Ali R. The place of detoxification in treatment of opioid dependence. *Curr Opin Psychiatry* 2006;19(3):266–270.
39. Himmelsbach CK. Clinical studies of drug addiction: physical dependence, withdrawal and recovery. *Arch Intern Med* 1942;69:766–772.
40. Dole VP. Narcotic addiction, physical dependence and relapse. *N Engl J Med* 1972;286:988–992.

41. Prosser J, Cohen LJ, Steinfeld M, et al. Neuropsychological functioning in opiate-dependent subjects receiving and following methadone maintenance treatment. *Drug Alcohol Depend* 2006;84(3):240–247.
42. Shi J, Zhao LY, Epstein DH, et al. Long-term methadone maintenance reduces protracted symptoms of heroin abstinence and cue-induced craving in Chinese heroin abusers. *Pharmacol Biochem Behav* 2007; 87(1):141–145.
43. Satel S, Kosten T. Should protracted withdrawal from drugs be included in DSM-IV? [see comments]. *American Journal of Psychiatry.* 1993; 150(5):695–704.
44. Stine S, Kosten T. Reduction of opiate withdrawal-like symptoms by cocaine abuse during methadone and buprenorphine maintenance. *Am J Drug Alcohol Abuse.*1994;20(4):445–458.
45. Kosten TR, Kleber HD. Strategies to improve compliance with narcotic antagonists. *Am J Drug Alcohol Abuse* 1984;10:249–266.
46. Kleber HD. Treatment of narcotic addicts. *Psychiatr Med* 1987;3: 389–418.
47. Minozzi S, Amato L, Vecchi S, et al. Oral naltrexone maintenance treatment for opioid dependence. *Cochrane Database Syst Rev* 2006;25; (1):CD001333.
48. Washton AM, Gold MS, Pottash AC. Naltrexone in addicted physicians and business executives. *NIDA Res Monogr* 1984;55:185–190.
49. Comer SD, Collins ED. Depot naltrexone: long-lasting antagonism of the effects of heroin in humans. *Psychopharmacology (Berl)* 2002;159(4): 351–360.
50. Comer SD, Sullivan MA, Yu E, et al. Injectable, sustained-release naltrexone for the treatment of opioid dependence: a randomized, placebo-controlled trial. *Arch Gen Psychiatry* 2006;63(2):210–218.
51. Brahen LS, Capone TJ, Capone DM. Naltrexone: lack of effect on hepatic enzymes. *J Clin Pharmacol* 1988;28:64–70.
52. Kosten TR. Current pharmacotherapies for opioid dependence. *Psychopharmacol Bull* 1990;26:69–74.
53. Cooper JR, Altman F, Brown B, et al. *Research on the treatment of narcotic addiction: state of the art.* Rockville, MD: National Institute on Drug Abuse, 1983.
54. Bliesener N, Albrecht S, Schwager A, et al. Plasma testosterone and sexual function in men receiving buprenorphine maintenance for opioid dependence. *J Clin Endocrinol Metab* 2005;90(1):203–206.
55. Kreek MJ. Medical management of methadone-maintained patients. In: Lowinson JH, and Ruiz P, eds. *Substance abuse: clinical problems and perspectives.* Baltimore: Williams & Wilkins, 1981:660–673.
56. Hartel D, Selwyn PA, Schoenbaum EE, et al. Methadone maintenance treatment and reduced risk of AIDS and AIDS-specific mortality in intravenous drug users [Abstract 8526]. 4th International Conference on AIDS, Stockholm, Sweden, June, 1988.
57. Hartel D, Schoenbaum EE, Selwyn PA, et al. Temporal patterns of cocaine use and AIDS in intravenous drug users in methadone maintenance [Abstract]. 5th International Conference on AIDS, Stockholm, Sweden, June, 1989.
58. Hartel D. Cocaine use, inadequate methadone dose increase risk of AIDS for IV drug users in treatment. *NIDA Notes* 1989–1990;5(1).
59. Ball JC, Ross A. *The effectiveness of methadone maintenance treatment.* New York: Springer-Verlag, 1991.
60. Caplehorn JRM, Bell J. Methadone dosage and retention of patients in maintenance treatment. *Med J Aust* 1991;154:195–199.
61. Strain EC, Bigelow GE, Liebson IA Stitzer ML. Moderate- vs. high-dose methadone in the treatment of *opioid* dependence: a randomized trial. *JAMA* 1999;281(11):1000–1005.
62. Johnson RE, Chutuape MA, Strain EC, et al. A comparison of levomethadyl acetate, buprenorphine, and methadone for opioid dependence. *N Engl J Med* 2000;343(18):1290–1297.
63. Donny EC, Brasser SM, Bigelow GE, et al. Methadone doses of 100 mg or greater are more effective than lower doses at suppressing heroin self-administration in opioid-dependent volunteers. *Addiction* 2005;100 (10):1496–1509.
64. Pasternak GW. Molecular biology of opioid analgesia. *J Pain Symptom Manage* 2005;29(5 Suppl):S2–S9.
65. Friedland A, Schwartz E, Brechbuhl AB, et al. Pharmacokinetic interactions of zidovudine and methadone in intravenous drug using patients with HIV infection. *J Acquir Immune Defic Syndr* 1992;5:619–626.
66. Kreek MJ, Oratz M, Rothschild MA. Hepatic extraction of long and short-acting narcotics in the isolated perfused rabbit liver. *Gastroenterology* 1978;75:88–94.
67. Kreek MJ. Factors modifying the pharmacological effectiveness of methadone. NIDA Monograph Series. Rockville, MD: National Institute on Drug Abuse, 1986.
68. Stine SM. New developments in methadone treatment and matching treatments to patient. In: Stine SM, Kosten TR, eds. *New treatments for opiate dependence.* New York: Guilford Press, 1997:121–172.
69. O'Connor PG, Selwyn PA, Schottenfeld RS Medical care for injection drug users with human immunodeficiency virus infection. *N Engl J Med* Aug 1994;331:450–459.
70. Sawyer RC, Brown LS, Narong PG, et al. Evaluation of a possible pharmacological interaction between rifampin and methadone in HIV seropositive injecting drug users [Abstract]. In: *Abstracts of the Ninth International Conference on AIDS/Fourth STD World Congress, Berlin, Germany, June 6–11.* London: Wellcome Foundation, 1993:501.
71. Schwartz EL, Brechbuhl AB, Kahl P, et al. Altered pharmacokinetics of zidovudine in former IV drug-using patients receiving methadone. In: *Abstracts of the Sixth International Conference on AIDS, San Francisco, June 20–24, vol 3* [Abstract]. San Francisco: University of California, 1990:194.
72. Braun MM, Byers RH, Heyward WL, et al. Acquired immunodeficiency syndrome and extrapulmonary tuberculosis in the United States. *Arch Intern Med* 1990;150:1913–1916.
73. Barnes PF, Bloch AB, Davidson PT, et al. Tuberculosis in patients with human immunodeficiency virus infection. *N Engl J Med* 1991: 1644–1650.
74. Small PM, Shafer RW, Hopewell PC, et al. Exogenous re-infection with multi-drug-resistant Mycobacterium tuberculosis in patients with advanced HIV infection. *N Engl J Med* 1993;328:1137–1144.
75. Centers for Disease Control and Prevention. Nosocomial transmissions of multidrug-resistant tuberculosis among HIV-infected persons—Florida and New York, 1988–1991. *MMWR* 1991;40:585–602.
76. D'Aunno T, Pollack HA. Changes in methadone treatment practices: results from a national panel study. *JAMA.* 2002;288(7):850–856, 1988–2000.
77. Schwetz BA. From the U.S. Food and Drug Administration. *JAMA* 2001; 285(21):2705.
78. Deamer RL, Wilson DR, Clark DS, et al. Torsades de pointes associated with high dose levomethadyl acetate (ORLAAM). *J Addict Dis* 2001;20(4):7–14.
79. Cone EJ, Preston KL. Toxicologic aspects of heroin substitution treatment. *Ther Drug Monit* 2002;24(2):193–198.
80. Newcombe DA, Bochner F, White JM, Somogyi AA. Evaluation of levo-alpha-acetylmethadol (LAAM) as an alternative treatment for methadone maintenance patients who regularly experience withdrawal: a pharmacokinetic and pharmacodynamic analysis. *Drug Alcohol Depend* 2004;76(1):63–72.
81. Mendelson J, Upton RA, Everhart ET, et al. Bioavailability of sublingual buprenorphine. *J Clin Pharmacol* 1997;37(1):31–37.
82. Nath RP, Upton RA. Buprenorphine pharmacokinetics: relative bioavailability of sublingual tablet and liquid formulations. *J Clin Pharmacol* 1999;39(6):619–623.
83. Schuh KJ, Johanson CE. Pharmacokinetic comparison of the buprenorphine sublingual liquid and tablet. *Drug Alcohol Depend* 1999;56:55–60.
84. Compton P, Ling W, Moody D, Chiang N. Pharmacokinetics, bioavailability and opioid effects of liquid versus tablet buprenorphine. *Drug Alcohol Depend* 2006;82(1):25–31.
85. Bickel WK, Stitzer MI. A clinical trial of buprenorphine: comparison with methadone in the detoxification of heroin addicts. *Clin Pharmacol Ther* 1988;43:72–78.
86. Johnson RE, Jaffe JH, Fudala PJ. A controlled trial of buprenorphine treatment for opioid dependence. *JAMA* 1992;267:2750–2755.

87. Strain EC, Stitzer ML. Comparison of buprenorphine and methadone in the treatment of opioid dependence. *American Journal of Psychiatry.* 1994;151(7):1025–1030.
88. Ling W, Wesson DR, Charuvastra C, et al. A controlled trial comparing buprenorphine and methadone maintenance in opioid dependence. *Arch Gen Psychaitry* 1996;53:401–407.
89. Ling W, Charuvastra C, Collins JF, et al. Buprenorphine maintenance treatment of opiate dependence: a multicenter, randomized clinical trial. *Addiction* 1998;93(4):475–486.
90. Uehlinger C, Deglon J, Livoti S, et al. Comparison of buprenorphine and methadone in treatment of opioid dependence. Swiss multicenter study. *Eur Addict Res* 1998;4(Suppl 1):13–18.
91. Liu Z, Cai Z. Rapid detoxification of heroin dependence by buprenorphine. *Chung Kuo Yao Li Hsueh Pao* 1997;18(2):112–114.
92. Bouchez J, Beauverie P, Touzeau D. Substitution with buprenorphine in methadone- and morphine sulfate–dependent patients. Preliminary results. *Eur Addict Res* 1998;4(Suppl)1:8–12.
93. Amass L, Kamien JB. A controlled comparison of the buprenorphine-naloxone tablet and methadone for opioid maintenance treatment: Interim results. In: Harris LS, ed. *Problems of drug dependence 1999.* NIDA Research Monograph Series. Bethesda: National Institute on Drug Abuse, 2001.
94. Chutuape MA, Johnson RE, Strain EC, et al. Controlled clinical trial comparing maintenance treatment efficacy of buprenorphine (buprenorphine), levomethadoneadoneadyl acetate (LAAM) and methadone (m). In: Harris LS, ed. *Problems of drug dependence1998* (NIDA Research Monograph 179). Rockville, MD: National Institute on Drug Abuse, 1999:74.
95. Strain EC Stitzer ML. Buprenorphine versus methadone in the treatment of opioid dependence: self-reports, urinalysis, and Addiction Severity Index. *J Clin Psychopharmacol* 1996;16:58–67.
96. Bickel WK, Amass L. Buprenorphine treatment of opioid dependence: a review. *Exp Clin Psychopharmacol* 1995;3:477–489.
97. Walsh SL, Preston KL. Clinical pharmacology of buprenorphine: ceiling effects at high doses. *Clin Pharmacol Ther* 1994;55:569–580.
98. Walsh SL, Preston KL. Acute administration of buprenorphine in humans: partial agonist and blockade effects. *J Pharmacol Exp Ther* 1995;274:361–372.
99. Lange WR. Safety and side effects of buprenorphine in the clinical management of heroin addiction. *Drug Alcohol Depend* 1990;26:19–28.
100. Huestis MA, Umbricht A, Preston KL, et al. Safety of buprenorphine: no clinically relevant cardio-respiratory depression at high IV doses. In: Harris LS, ed. *Problems of drug dependence 1998* (NIDA Research Monograph 179). Rockville, MD: National Institute on Drug Abuse, 1999:62.
101. Fanoe S. Syncope and QT prolongation among patients treated with methadone for heroin dependence in the city of Copenhagen. *Heart* 2007;93(9):1051–1055. Epub March 7, 2007.
102. Wedam EF, Bigelow GA, Johnson RE, et al. QT-interval effects of methadone, levomethadyl, and buprenorphine in a randomized trial. *Arch Intern Med* 167(22):2469–2475.
103. Bickel WK. Buprenorphine: dose-related blockade of opioid challenge effects in opioid dependent humans. *J Pharmacol Exp Ther* 1988b;247: 47–53.
104. Rosen MI, Wallace EA, McMahon TJ, et al. Buprenorphine: duration of blockade of effects of intramuscular hydromorphone. *Drug Alcohol Depend* 1994;35:569–580.
105. Lanier RK, Umbricht A, Harrison JA, et al. Evaluation of a transdermal buprenorphine formulation in opioid detoxification. *Addiction* 2007; 102(10):1648–1656.
106. Fudala PJ, Bridge TP, Herbert S, et al. A multisite efficacy evaluation of a buprenorphine/naloxone product for opiate dependence treatment. NIDA Research Monograph 179. Rockville, MD: National Institute on Drug Abuse, 1998:105.
107. Johnson RE. A controlled trial of buprenorphine in the treatment of heroin addiction: I. Physiological and behavioral effects during a rapid dose induction. *Clin Pharmacol Ther* 1989;46:335–343.
108. Preston KL, Bigelow GE, Liebson IA. Buprenorphine and naloxone alone and in combination in opioid-dependent humans. *Psychopharmacology* 1988b;94:484–490.
109. Preston KL, Bigelow GE, Liebson IA. Antagonist effects of nalorphine in opioid-dependent human volunteers. *J Pharmacol Exp Ther* 1989; 248:929–937.
110. Fudala PJ, Bridge TP, Herbert S, et al., Buprenorphine/Naloxone Collaborative Study Group. Office-based treatment of opiate addiction with a sublingual-tablet formulation of buprenorphine and naloxone. *N Engl J Med* 2003;349(10):949–958.
111. Mendelson J. Buprenorphine and naloxone interactions in opiate-dependent volunteers. *Clin Pharmacol Ther.* 1996;60:105–114.
112. Mendelson J. Buprenorphine and naloxone combinations: the effects of three dose ratios in morphine stabilized, opiate-dependent volunteers. *Psychopharmacology (Berl)* 1999;141:37–46.
113. Walsh SL. Effects of buprenorphine and methadone in methadone-maintained subjects. *Psychopharmacology (Berl)* 1995;119:268–276.
114. Center for Substance Abuse Treatment. Clinical guidelines for the use of buprenorphine in the treatment of opioid addiction. Treatment Improvement Protocol Series 40. DHHS Publication No. (SMA) 04-3939. Rockville, MD: Substance Abuse and Mental Health Services Administration, 2004a.
115. Johnson RE, Strain EC. Other medications for opioid dependence. In: Strain EC, Stitzer ML, eds. *Methadone treatment for opioid dependence.* Baltimore: Johns Hopkins University Press, 1999:281–321.
116. Johnson RE, Strain EC, Amass L. Buprenorphine: how to use it right. *Drug Alcohol Depend* 2003;70(Suppl):S59–S77.
117. Amass L, Kamien JB, Mikulich SK. Efficacy of daily and alternate-day dosing regimens with the combination buprenorphine-naloxone tablet. *Drug Alcohol Depend* 2000;58:143–152.
118. Amass L, Kamien JB, Mikulich SK. Thrice-weekly supervised dosing with the combination buprenorphine-naloxone tablet is preferred to daily supervised dosing by opioid-dependent humans. *Drug Alcohol Depend* 2001;61:173–181.
119. Kaltenbach K, Finnegan L. Children exposed to methadone *in utero*: cognitive ability in preschool years. NIDA Research Monograph 81. Rockville, MD: National Institute on Drug Abuse, 1988.
120. Berghella V, Lim PJ, Hill MK, et al. Maternal methadone dose and neonatal withdrawal. *Am J Obstet Gynecol* 2003;189(2):312–317.
121. Alroomi LG. Maternal narcotic abuse and the newborn. *Arch Dis Child* 1998;63:81–83.
122. Connaughton JF, Reeser D, Finnegan LF. Pregnancy complicated by drug addiction. In: Bolognese R, Schwartz RH, eds. *Perinatal medicine: management of the high risk fetus and neonate.* Baltimore: Williams & Wilkins, 1977:259–272.
123. Glass L. Narcotic withdrawal in the newborn. *Am Fam Physician* 1972;6:75–78.
124. Hulse GK. The relationship between maternal use of heroin and methadone and infant birth weight. *Addiction* 1997;92:1571–1579.
125. Kandall SR, Albin S, Gartner LM, et al. The narcotic-dependent mother: fetal and neonatal consequences. *Early Hum Dev* 1977;1:159–169.
126. Messinger DS. The maternal lifestyle study: cognitive, motor, and behavioral outcomes of cocaine-exposed and opiate-exposed infants through three years of age. *Pediatrics* 2004;113:1677–1685.
127. Naeye RL. Fetal complications of maternal heroin addiction: abnormal growth, infections, and episodes of stress. *J Pediatr* 1973;83:1055–1061.
128. Substance Abuse and Mental Health Services Administration. *National Survey on Drug Use and Health from 2004 and 2005* [data files SAMHSA Web site]. September 8, 2005 and September 7, 2006.
129. Lifschitz MH, Wilson GS, Smith EO, et al. Factors affecting head growth and intellectual function in children of drug addicts. *Pediatrics* 1985;75:269–274.
130. Lester BM, Andreozzi L, Appiah L. Substance use during pregnancy: time for policy to catch up with research. *Harm Reduction J* 2004; 1:5–49.
131. Kaltenbach K. Opioid dependence during pregnancy: effects and management. *Obstet Gynecol Clin North Am* 1998;25:139–151.

132. Jones HE, Tuten M. Specialty treatment for women. In: Strain EC, and Stitzer M, eds. *Methadone treatment for opioid dependence.* Baltimore: Johns Hopkins University Press, 2006:455–484.
133. Hulse G, O'Neil G. Using naltrexone implants in the management of the pregnant heroin user. *Aust N Z J Obstet Gynaecol* 2002;42:569–573.
134. Dashe JS, Jackson GL, Olscher DA, et al. Opioid detoxification in pregnancy. *Obstet Gynecol* 1998;92:854–858.
135. Finnegan LP. Treatment issues for opioid-dependent women during the perinatal period. *J Psychoactive Drugs* 1991;23:191–201.
136. Jones HE, Haug N, Silverman K, et al. The effectiveness of incentives in enhancing treatment attendance and drug abstinence in methadone-maintained pregnant women. *Drug Alcohol Depend* 2001;61:297–306.
137. Laken MP. Effects of case management on retention in prenatal substance abuse treatment. *Am J Drug Alcohol Abuse* 1996;22:439–448.
138. Svikis DS. Attendance incentives for outpatient treatment: effects in methadone- and nonmethadone-maintained pregnant drug dependent women. *Drug Alcohol Depend* 1997;48:33–41.
139. Finnegan LP, Kaltenbach K. Neonatal abstinence syndrome. In: Hoekelman RA, Friedman SB, Nelson NM, et al., eds. *Primary pediatric care,* 2nd ed. St. Louis: Mosby, 1992:1367–1378.
140. Kaltenbach K. Exposure to opiates: behavioral outcomes in preschool and school age children. In: Wetherington CL, Smeriglio VL, Finnegan LP, eds. *Behavioral studies of drug-exposed offspring: methodological issues in human and animal research.* Rockville, MD: NIDA Monograph 164 DHHS pub no. 96-4105,1996:230–241.
141. Hans SL. Developmental consequences of prenatal exposure to methadone. *Ann N Y Acad Sci.* 1989;562:195–207.
142. Rosen TS. Children of methadone-maintained mothers: follow-up to 18 months of age. *J Pediatr* 1982;101:192–196.
143. Strauss ME, Starr RH, Ostrea EM, et al. Behavioral concomitants of prenatal addiction to narcotics. *J Pediatr* 1976;89:842–846.
144. Chasnoff IJ, Schnoll SH, Burns WJ, et al. Maternal non-narcotic substance abuse during pregnancy: effects on infant development. *Neurobehav Toxicol Teratol* 1984;6:277–280.
145. Kaltenbach K, Finnegan LP. Developmental outcome of infants exposed to methadone in utero: a longitudinal study. *Pediatr Res* 1986;20:57.
146. Rosen TS, Johnson HL. Long term effects of prenatal methadone maintenance. In: Pinkert TM, ed. *Current research on the consequences of maternal drug abuse.* NIDA Monograph 59. DHHS Pub no. ADM 85-1400. Washington, DC: Government Printing Office, 1985.
147. Wilson GS, Desmond MM, Wait RB. Follow-up of methadone-treated and untreated narcotic-dependent women and their infants: health, developmental, and social implications. *J Pediatr* 1981;98:716–722.
148. Johnson RE, Jones HE, Fischer G. Use of buprenorphine in pregnancy: patient management and effects on the neonate. *Drug Alcohol Depend* 2003;70:S87–S101.
149. McCarthy JJ. High-dose methadone maintenance in pregnancy: maternal and neonatal outcomes. *Am J Obstet Gynecol* 2005;193: 606–610.
150. Jones HE, Martin PR, Heil SH, et al. Treatment of opioid-dependent pregnant women: clinical and research issues. *J Subst Abuse Treat;* 2008 Oct; 35(3):245–259.
151. Fischer G. Methadone versus buprenorphine in pregnant addicts: a double-blind, double-dummy comparison study. *Addiction* 2006;101: 275–281.
152. Jones HE, Johnson RE, Jasinski DR, et al. Randomized controlled study transitioning opioid-dependent pregnant women from short-acting morphine to buprenorphine or methadone. *Drug Alcohol Depend* 2005a;78:33–38.
153. Jones HE, Johnson RE, Jasinski DR, et al. Buprenorphine versus methadone in the treatment of pregnant opioid-dependent patients: effects on the neonatal abstinence syndrome. *Drug Alcohol Depend* 2005b;79:1–10.
154. Finnegan LP, Kron RE, Connaughton JF, et al. Assessment and treatment of abstinence in the infant of the drug-dependent mother. *Int J Clin Pharmacol Biopharm* 1975;12:19–32.
155. Lipsitz PJ. A proposed narcotic withdrawal score for use with newborn infants: a pragmatic evaluation of its efficacy. *Clin Pediatr (Phila)* 1975;14:592–594.
156. Marquet P, Lavignasse P, Gaulier JM, et al. Case study of neonates born to mothers undergoing buprenorphine maintenance treatment. In: Kintz P, Marquet P, eds. *Buprenorphine therapy of opiate addiction.* Totowa, NJ: Humana Press, 2002:123–135.
157. Lejeune C, Simmat-Durand L Gourarier L, et al. Prospective multicenter observational study of 260 infants born to 259 opiate-dependent mothers on methadone or high-dose buprenophine substitution. *Drug Alcohol Depend* 2006;82:250–257.
158. First MB. *Structured clinical interview for DSM-IV Axis I disorders.* New York: Biometrics Research, New York State Psychiatric Institute, 1996.
159. Department of Health and Human Services. *Federal guidelines for opioid agonists, 2001.* Washington, DC: Author, 2001.
160. Brunton PJ. Endogenous opioids and attenuated hypothalamic-pituitary-adrenal axis responses to immune challenge in pregnant rats. *J Neurosci* 2005;25:5117–5126.
161. Douglas AJ. Reduced activity of the noradrenergic system in the paraventricular nucleus at the end of pregnancy: implications for stress hyporesponsiveness. *J Neuroendocrinol* 2005;17:40–48.
162. Johnson RE, Jaffe JH, Fudala PJ. A controlled trial of buprenorphine treatment for opioid dependence. *JAMA* 1992;267:2750–2755.
163. Ling W. A controlled trial comparing buprenorphine and methadone maintenance in opioid dependence. *Arch Gen Psychiatry* 1996;53: 401–407.
164. Strain EC, Stitzer ML, Liebson IA, et al. Comparison of buprenorphine and methadone in the treatment of opioid dependence. *Am J Psychiatry* 1994;151:1025–1030.
165. Des DC, Friedman SR, Woods J, et al. HIV infection among intravenous drug users: Epidemiology and emerging public health perspectives. In: Lowinson JH, Ruiz P, Millman RB, eds. *Substance abuse: a comprehensive textbook..* Baltimore: Williams & Wilkins, 1992:734–743.
166. Metzger DS, Woody GE, McLellan AT, et al. Human immunodeficiency virus seroconversion among intravenous drug users in- and out-of-treatment: an 18 month prospective follow-up. *J Acquir Immune Defic Syndr* 1993;6:1049–1056.
167. Barthwell A, Senay E, Marks R, et al. Patients successfully maintained with methadone escaped human immunodeficiency virus infection. *Arch Gen Psychaitry* 1989;46:957–958.
168. Novick DM, Joseph H, Croxson TS, et al. Absence of antibody to human immunodeficiency virus in long-term, socially rehabilitated methadone maintenance patients. *Arch Intern Med* 1990;150:97–99.
169. Tidone L, Sileo F, Goglio A, et al. AIDS in Italy. *Am J Drug Alcohol Abuse* 1987;13(4):485–486.
170. Iribarne C, Picart D, Dréano Y, et al.. Involvement of cytochrome P450 3A4 in N-dealkylation of buprenorphine in human liver microsomes. *Life Sci* 1997;60(22):1953–1964.
171. Moody DE, Alburges ME, Parker RJ, et al. The involvement of cytochrome P450 3A4 in the N-demethylation of L-alpha-acetylmethadol (LAAM), norLAAM, and methadone. *Drug Metab Dispos* 1997;25(12):1347–1353.
172. Krantz MJ, Kutinsky IB, Robertson AD, Mehler PS. Dose-related effects of methadone on QT prolongation in a series of patients with torsades de pointes. *Pharmacotherapy* 2003;23(6):802–805.
173. Rainey PM, Friedland G, McCance-Katz EF, et al. Interaction of methadone with didanosine and stavudine. *J Acquir Immune Defic Syndr* 2000;24(3):241–248.
174. http://www.tthhivclinic.com./interact_tables.html, Drug Interaction Tables: Antiretroviral-Methadone Interactions. Prepared by: Tony Antoniou St. Michael's Hospital & Alice Tseng, Toronto General Hospital, Toronto, July 30, 2007.
175. McCance-Katz EF, Moody DE, Morse GD, et al. Interactions between buprenorphine and antiretrovirals: I. The nonnucleoside reverse-transcriptase inhibitors efavirenz and delavirdine. *Clin Infect Dis* 2006;43 (Suppl 4):S224–S234.

176. McCance-Katz EF, Moody DE, Smith PF, et al. Interactions between buprenorphine and antiretrovirals: II. The protease inhibitors nelfinavir, lopinavir/ritonavir, and ritonavir. *Clin Infect Dis* 2006;43(Suppl 4): S235–S246.
177. Bruce RD, McCance-Katz E, Kharasch ED, et al. Pharmacokinetic interactions between buprenorphine and antiretroviral medications. *Clin Infect Dis* 2006;43(Suppl 4):S216–S223.
178. de Béthune MP, Hertogs K. Screening and selecting for optimized antiretroviral drugs: rising to the challenge of drug resistance. *Curr Med Res Opin* 2006;22(12):2603–2612.
179. Kapadia F, Vlahov D, Wu Y, et al. Impact of drug abuse treatment modalities on adherence to ART/HAART among a cohort of HIV seropositive women. *Am J Drug Alcohol Abuse* 2008;34(2):161–170.
180. Palepu A, Tyndall MW, Joy R, et al.. Antiretroviral adherence and HIV treatment outcomes among HIV/HCV co-infected injection drug users: the role of methadone maintenance therapy. *Drug Alcohol Depend* 2006;84(2):188–194. Epub Mar 20, 2006.
181. Gourevitch MN, Wasserman W, Panero MS, Selwyn PA. Successful adherence to observed prophylaxis and treatment of tuberculosis among drug users in a methadone program. *J Addict Dis* 1996;15(1):93–104.
182. Physician Clinical Support System. *PCSS guidance: transfer from methadone to buprenorphine*. PCSSproject@asam.org | www.PCSSmentor.org, 2008.
183. Bickel W, Amass L, Crean JP, et al. Buprenorphine dosing every 1, 2, or 3 days in opioid-dependent patients. *Psychopharmacology* 1999;146 (2):111–118.
184. Petry NM, Bickel WK, Badger GJ. A comparison of four buprenorphine dosing regimens in the treatment of opioid dependence. *Clin Pharmacol Ther* 1999;66:306–314.
185. Schottenfeld RS, Pakes J, O'Connor P, et al. Thrice weekly versus daily buprenorphine maintenance. *Biol Psychiatry* 2000;47:1072–1079.
186. Helmus TC, Downey KK, Arfken CL, et al. Novelty seeking as a predictor of treatment retention for heroin dependent cocaine users. *Drug Alcohol Depend* 2001;61(3):287–295.
187. Amass L, Ling W, Freese TE, et al. Bringing buprenorphine-naloxone detoxification to community treatment providers: the NIDA Clinical Trials Network field experience. *Am J Addict* 2004;13 Suppl 1:S42–S66.
188. Strain EC. Acute effects of buprenorphine, hydromorphone and naloxone in methadone-maintained volunteers. *J Pharmacol Exp Ther* 1992; 261:985–993.
189. Strain EC, Preston KL, Liebson IA, et al. Buprenorphine effects in methadone-maintained volunteers: effects at two hours after methadone. *J Pharmacol Exp Ther* 1995;272:628–638.
190. Walsh SL, June HL. Effects of buprenorphine and methadone in methadone-maintained subjects. *Psychopharmacology (Berl)* 1995;119: 268–276.
191. Kosten TR, Kleber HD. Buprenorphine detoxification from opioid dependence: a pilot study. *Life Sci* 1988;42:611–635.
192. Banys P. An open trial of low dose buprenorphine in treating methadone withdrawal. *J Subst Abuse Treat* 1994;11:9–15.
193. Lukas SE. Electroencephalographic and behavioral correlates of buprenorphine administration. *Clin Pharmacol Ther* 1984;36: 127–132.
194. Levin FR, Fischman MW, Connerney I, et al. A protocol to switch high-dose, methadone-maintained subjects to buprenorphine. *Am J Addict* 1997;6:105–116.
195. Greenwald MK. Transferring heroin-dependent outpatients stabilized on moderate-dose methadone to the buprenorphine sublingual tablet: a preliminary study. *Am J Addict* 2003;12(4):365–374.
196. Breen CL, Harris SJ, Lintzeris N, et al. Cessation of methadone maintenance treatment using buprenorphine: transfer from methadone to buprenorphine and subsequent buprenorphine reductions. *Drug Alcohol Depend* 2003;71(1):49–55.
197. Glasper A, Reed LJ, de Wet CJ, Gossop M, Bearn J. Induction of patients with moderately severe methadone dependence onto buprenorphine. *Addict Biol* 2005;10(2):149–155.
198. Rosado J, Walsh SL, Bigelow GE, Strain EC. Sublingual buprenorphine/naloxone precipitated withdrawal in subjects maintained on 100 mg of daily methadone. *Drug Alcohol Depend* 2007;90(2-3):261–269.
199. Kosten TR. Rapid detoxification from opioid dependence. *American Journal of Psychiatry*. 1989;146:1349.
200. Eissenberg T. Buprenorphine's physical dependence potential: antagonist-precipitated withdrawal in humans. *J Pharmacol Exp Ther* 1996; 276(2):449–459.

CHAPTER 49

Judith Martin, MD
Joan E. Zweben, PhD
J. Thomas Payte, MD

Opioid Maintenance Treatment

Of an estimated 1 million opioid-dependent persons in the United States, approximately 260,000 are involved in opioid maintenance treatment (OMT), making it the largest single treatment intervention for this population (1). Forty years of extensive research, clinical experience and attention to public health concerns—combined with an extensive educational effort—have made OMT more available to those who need it. In the United States, there are 1,069 specially licensed opioid treatment programs (OTPs) that offer counseling, testing, and maintenance pharmacotherapy using methadone, with daily dispensing and strictly regulated take-home medication for selected patients (2). Since 2002, office-based maintenance using sublingual buprenorphine has been available in the United States. A few OTPs also dispense buprenorphine as a second treatment option. This chapter focuses on maintenance pharmacotherapy in the context of the licensed OTP and is mostly about methadone maintenance. During the 1990s, several major scientific bodies examined the evidence regarding treatment benefits and access barriers; they concluded that OMT is effective and that barriers to obtaining it need to be reduced (3,4).

Since 1995, there has been an enormous upsurge in nonmedical use of prescription opioids and sedatives. The National Survey on Drug Use and Health (NSDUH) reports 1.6 million persons were regularly abusing or addicted to prescription opioids in 2006, with an additional 323,000 persons with heroin abuse or dependence (5). In some areas, nonmedical use of oxycodone and hydrocodone have overtaken heroin as drugs of abuse leading to OTP admissions (6). The parallel upsurge in nonmedical abuse of sedative medications is particularly dangerous for opioid-maintained patients, as the combination of benzodiazepines and opioids can be deadly.

Physicians often are unaware of the discrepancy between the benefits of maintenance treatment documented by scientific research and the public's perceptions of such treatment; for this reason, it is necessary to begin with a description of the context in which OMT takes place.

HISTORY AND CONTEXT OF OMT

The modern use of opioids as a maintenance pharmacotherapy began with the use of methadone by Dole and Nyswander in the 1960s (7). Negative attitudes toward OMT have been common since that time among physicians, other treatment staff, patients, and the general public. These attitudes often stem from the perception that methadone treatment is "just substituting one addicting drug for another." Rather than a simple substitution or replacement for illicit opioids, OMT involves a stabilization or correction of a possible lesion or defect in the endogenous opioid system (8,9). The neurobiologic mechanism remains poorly understood. This intervention, by reducing opioid craving and preventing opioid withdrawal, reduces the likelihood of injection drug use, frees the patient from preoccupation with obtaining illicit opioids, and enhances overall function, thus enabling the patient to make use of available psychosocial interventions.

Methadone maintenance has been shown to decrease mortality, reduce illicit drug use, reduce seroconversion to HIV, reduce criminal activity and increase engagement in socially productive activities (10–13). Nevertheless, a set of regulatory requirements unmatched by anything in medicine continues to contribute to the stigmatization of methadone as a treatment modality and creates many barriers to providing treatment to those who need it. Despite the 2001 reduction in regulatory barriers at the federal level (14), methadone continues to remain separate from the medical mainstream of care and poorly understood by clinicians not involved in its daily application.

Negative attitudes affect OMT in a variety of ways (15). Physicians in other medical settings sometimes refuse to treat a patient who discloses that he or she is receiving maintenance pharmacotherapy. Occasionally, patients are told that they must withdraw from maintenance pharmacotherapy to receive treatment for other medical conditions. A physician may withhold medication needed for symptomatic relief, thus causing unnecessary discomfort and pain. Contrary to common beliefs, many opioid dependent patients enter OMT with great ambivalence and want to discontinue maintenance therapy as soon as possible. Indeed, the initial hope of many practitioners, policy makers, and regulators was that methadone could be used to transition patients to a drug-free lifestyle and then be withdrawn. This has not proved to be the case. Early studies suggest that only 10% to 20% of patients who discontinue methadone are able to remain abstinent (16), a range consistent with clinical impressions and the findings of subsequent studies (12,17–19). This range is similar to that seen with many chronic medical conditions for which control requires the ongoing use of medication.

UNIQUE ASPECTS OF OPIOID DEPENDENCE

Though this chapter focuses on medical aspects of OMT, it is commonly accepted that addictive disorders are complex phenomena that involve the interaction of biological, psychosocial, and cultural variables, all of which need to be addressed if treatment is to be effective. As a medical modality based on proper use of opioid agonist medication, it should be clear that the medication itself is central to OMT as a treatment modality. Much of the destructive behavior of treatment professionals results from inappropriate expectations, particularly the belief that addicted persons could avoid drug use if they were sufficiently motivated. Vincent Dole, a pioneer in developing methadone treatment, always held the view that there is something unique about opioid addiction that makes it difficult for patients to remain free of illicit heroin use for extended periods of time. Prior to the discovery of the opioid receptor system, Dole and Nyswander (20) postulated the existence of a "metabolic disease," a view supported and refined by subsequent biomedical research. Dole won the Albert Lasker Clinical Medicine Research Award in 1988 for his work in this area. He summarized his views in a paper in the *Journal of the American Medical Association* (9), in which he wrote:

> *It is postulated that the high rate of relapse of addicts after detoxification from heroin use is due to persistent derangement of the endogenous ligand narcotic receptor system and that methadone in an adequate daily dose compensates for this defect. Some patients with long histories of heroin use and subsequent rehabilitation on a maintenance program do well when the treatment is terminated. The majority, unfortunately, experience a return of symptoms after maintenance is stopped. The treatment, therefore, is corrective but not curative for severely addicted persons. A major challenge for future research is to identify the specific defect in receptor function and to repair it. Meanwhile, methadone maintenance provides a safe and effective way to normalize the function of otherwise intractable opiate addicts.*

In Dole's view, the persistent receptor disorder is the result of chronic opiate use, leading to down-regulation of the modulating system and possibly also to suppression of the endogenous ligands. Goldstein (8) supported the concept of a metabolic disease as well as a genetic predisposition to that disease. Goldstein suggested that genetic influence carries an exceptional vulnerability to the disease in the presence of certain environmental influences. Kreek (21) suggested that multiple genes may account for different degrees of vulnerability to developing addiction. Other research also supports the view that heroin addiction has a genetic component (22–26). Further research is needed to define the metabolic disease process and the respective roles of genetic predisposition and environmental exposure.

Positron emission tomography scans that look at cerebral metabolism in opiate-dependent patients suggest that methadone maintenance at least partly normalizes cerebral glucose metabolism, as compared with patients withdrawn from methadone and in sustained remission (27). Magnetic resonance spectroscopy comparing methadone maintained patients with different elapsed treatment times showed a nearly normal phosphorus metabolism profile in those patients who had been in treatment long term, suggesting healing at the neurochemical level over time (28). A key question for future research remains whether it is possible to restore normal functioning without maintenance therapy and, if so, how to accomplish this function.

CLINICAL ISSUES IN MAINTENANCE PHARMACOTHERAPY

Goals of Pharmacotherapy of Opioid Dependence

Kreek (21) outlined the goals of treatment and the properties of desirable opioid agonist medications as follows:

1. Prevention or reduction of withdrawal symptoms
2. Prevention or reduction of opioid craving

3. Prevention of relapse to use of addictive opioids
4. Restoration to or toward normalcy of any physiologic function disrupted by chronic opioid use

Profile of Potential Psychotherapeutic Agents

Characteristics of potential psychotherapeutic agents can be defined as follows:

1. Such medications are effective after oral administration.
2. They have a long biologic half-life (>24 hours).
3. They have minimal side effects during chronic administration.
4. They are safe (that is, they lack true toxic or serious adverse effects).
5. They are efficacious for a substantial proportion of persons with the disorder. Methadone and buprenorphine generally evince these characteristics.

MAINTENANCE TREATMENT USING METHADONE

Heroin Versus Methadone The opioid-dependent person who is actively misusing heroin or other short-acting opioids typically experiences rapid and wide swings from a brief pleasure usually characterized by sedation, fading into a period of normalcy and alertness, which can be described as the "comfort zone." This period is followed by the beginnings of subjective withdrawal, sometimes called *craving*, which soon develops into the full objective withdrawal syndrome typical of opioid addiction. (Symptoms of opioid withdrawal are described in Chapter 45, "Management of Stimulant, Hallucinogen, Marijuana, Phencyclidine, and Club Drug Intoxication and Withdrawal.") This cycle is particularly evident in the patient who engages in injection or inhalation of potent short-acting opioids such as heroin. A full cycle from "sick" to "high" to "normal" to "sick" can occur repeatedly throughout the day (Fig. 49.1). The sensation of the "rush" is associated with a very rapid increase in blood levels, to a point somewhat above the therapeutic window. The pleasure is experienced during the time that drug levels remain above the therapeutic window (Fig. 49.2). Methadone, regularly administered at steady state, is present at levels sufficient to maintain alertness without craving or drug preoccupation (comfort zone or therapeutic window) throughout the dosing interval—usually 24 hours.

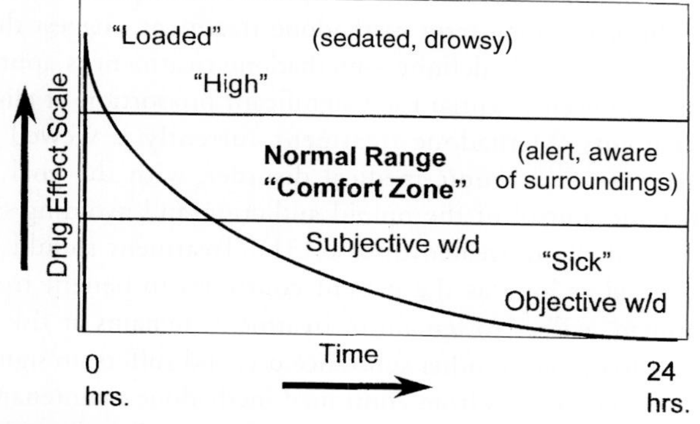

FIGURE 49.1. Heroin-simulated 24-hour dose-response.

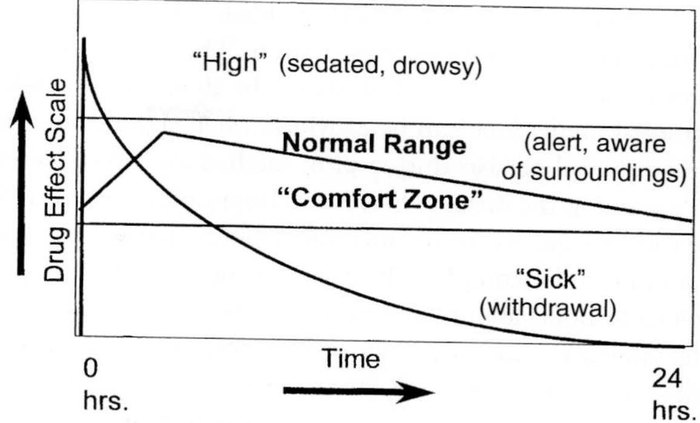

FIGURE 49.2. Methadone 24-hour . . . at steady-state.

With the next maintenance dose, there is a gradual rise in blood level, reaching a peak at 3 to 4 hours. Typically, the peak level is less than two times the trough level. There is a gradual decline over the rest of the 24-hour period, back to the trough level. When the patient is on the correct dose at steady state, at no time does the rate or extent of change in blood levels cause a sensation of being high or result in withdrawal symptoms.

Induction Although most patients eventually will need 80 to 120 mg/day of methadone to achieve stability (13), and although adequately high doses are needed to provide stability and retention in treatment (29), the starting dose must be much lower, and the eventual steady state is reached slowly, sometimes over weeks. The first several doses require careful evaluation and adjustment. This phase is usually called *induction* and is the most critical phase of treatment. As treatment is made more available, an understanding of the pitfalls of this time of early treatment has become evident. Even though methadone maintenance has been shown to reduce mortality, including overdose mortality (30,31), several studies have reported deaths during the first 10 to 14 days of treatment, particularly when induction doses are high and when the patient is also ingesting sedatives (32–36). About 42% of drug-related deaths during treatment occurred during the first week of OMT (37). In an Australian survey, patients were reported to be 6.7 times more likely to die during induction as compared to untreated heroin users (38). The mean induction dose was more than 50 mg among those who had died. Such deaths also occur in the United States, though the maximum first dose is set at 30 mg by regulation. Variability in methadone metabolism, discussed later in the section on drug interactions, may be implicated.

Initial Dose In most cases, patients being evaluated for admission to OMT have developed significant tolerance to opioids and demonstrate objective signs of withdrawal as a sign of current opioid physical dependence. The response to the initial dose of agonist medication provides valuable information about tolerance levels and the target "therapeutic window." Significant relief during peak (2 to 4 hours) is evidence that the dose is in the range of the established level of tolerance and may not require further escalation. The absence of relief suggests that the dose is well short of the therapeutic window. Additional methadone can be provided when significant objective withdrawal persists during peak methadone levels. Patients who present at the dosing window 24 hours after their very first dose can be expected to be uncomfortable as tissue stores accumulation is still incomplete. If they were comfortable during the first 4 to 12 hours after their dose, they probably need more time at the same dose, and not a higher daily dose. The initial dose of methadone is no more than 30 mg in most cases and may be lower in patients in whom low tolerance might be expected (e.g., recent relapse after a significant period of abstinence, or addiction to lower-potency opioids such as hydrocodone or codeine, or in opium smokers). Under federal regulations (14), the first dose is limited to no more than 30 mg, and a total dose of no more than 40 mg on the first treatment day unless the program physician documents in the patient's record that 40 mg did not suppress opioid abstinence symptoms.

Stabilization and Steady State After the initial dose, the induction phase allows for subsequent careful adjustments of the dose to achieve elimination of drug craving and prevention of withdrawal while avoiding the risk of intoxication or overdose associated with accumulation of methadone (39,40), The induction phase can be considered to last until the patient has been on a stable dose for 4 to 5 days (half-lives). The safe and effective introduction of methadone requires an understanding of steady-state pharmacologic principles. In general, steady-state levels are reached after a drug is administered for four to five half-lives (methadone has an average half-life of 24 to 36 hours). The clinical significance is that, with daily dosing, a significant portion of the previous dose remains in tissue stores, resulting in increased peak-and-trough methadone levels after the second and subsequent doses. Thus, the levels of methadone increase daily, even without an increase in dose. The rate of increase levels off as steady state is achieved at four to five half-lives, that is, three to seven days (Fig. 49.3). Further dose changes every 3 to 7 days may be needed to achieve the maintenance dose. Dose adjustments can be done in 5- to 10-mg increments for highly tolerant patients. Liquid medication allows dose adjustments by smaller increments for less tolerant patients.

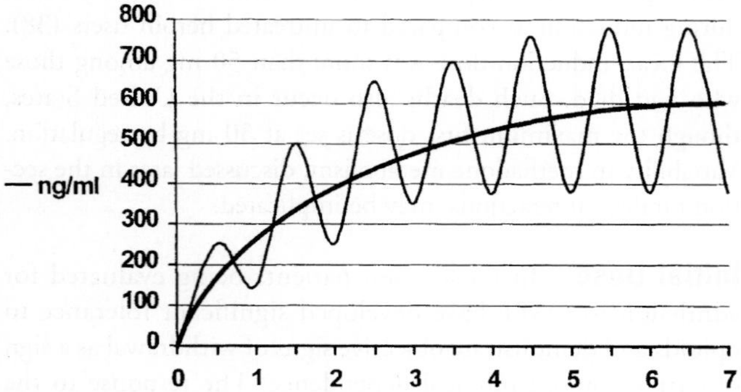

FIGURE 49.3. Steady-state simulation—maintenance pharmacology attained after 4 to 5 half-times, 1 dose/half-life.

Maintenance Once a stable dose is established, based on the presence of desired clinical effects, elimination of craving, and prevention of withdrawal, the maintenance phase begins. Maintenance continues until such a time that there is a reason to alter the treatment. Most methadone maintained patients do well on a dose range of 80 to 120 mg/day (13), though some patients require less and some require more. Patients are often able to remain at their maintenance dose for years with no need to adjust it. Tolerance appears to remain stable with no need to escalate the dose, as would be the case for short-acting opioid analgesics. Endocytosis of mu-opioid receptors and *N*-methyl D-aspartate receptor antagonism are unique characteristics of methadone itself which may contribute to this stabilizing feature (41–44).

Duration and Dose Dose level and duration of treatment are individualized clinical decisions. For most patients in methadone maintenance, a chronic care approach is most appropriate. In the early 1970s, efforts to limit the duration of treatment and to cap the dose occurred initially at the federal level and later were initiated by some individual state methadone authorities (45). There is no scientific or clinical basis for an arbitrary dose ceiling on methadone, although QT prolongation has been seen in the electrocardiograms of patients receiving high doses of methadone (39). Methadone doses of 80 to 100 mg have greater benefits than doses below 50 in heroin-dependent patients (46–49). Based on an extensive review of the research literature on the prognosis of patients who have been withdrawn from methadone, as well as the safety of continued maintenance treatment, the American Society of Addiction Medicine supports the principle that methadone maintenance treatment is most effective as a long-term modality (50). Once dose has been determined to be adequate, daily dose remains constant, and appropriate behavioral and psychosocial interventions can be effective.

The known risks of discontinuing methadone treatment, with predictable relapse to injected heroin use, become increasingly critical when viewed in the context of the HIV epidemic. These risks, when compared to the proven safety and efficacy of long-term methadone treatment, suggest that long-term—even indefinite—methadone treatment is appropriate and even essential for a significant proportion of eligible patients. Methadone treatment currently is viewed as treatment of a chronic medical disorder, with the goal of achieving control of the opioid addiction and avoiding the ravages of the untreated disease (51). Treatment should be continued as long as the patient continues to benefit from treatment, wishes to remain in treatment, remains at risk of relapse to opioid or other substance use, and suffers no significant adverse effects from continued methadone maintenance treatment and as long as continued treatment is indicated in the professional judgment of the physician (52). Patients receiving methadone do seek to discontinue maintenance for nonmedical but very real and practical reasons (for example, transportation or scheduling difficulties) and to escape continued disruption of their lives associated with the burdensome restrictions, regulations, and structure of the treatment delivery system. For patients who attempt withdrawal, it is important for practitioners to provide encouragement along with the best medical and supportive treatment available, without fostering unrealistic expectations or unnecessary guilt, and to provide a means for rapid readmission to methadone treatment in the event of relapse or impending relapse to the use of illicit opiates (50).

Techniques to Ensure Adequacy of Dose In most cases, clinical observation and patient reporting are adequate to make appropriate dose determinations.

Blood Levels in Dose Determination Mean, random, or trough levels of methadone do not define an adequate dose. The clinical utility of blood levels is based on peak and trough values to define a rate of change, or a peak-to trough ratio. In the methadone clinic setting, patients occasionally experience problems in maintaining stability on a given dose of methadone. Statements such as "My dose isn't holding me," "I wake up sick every morning," "My dose only lasts a few hours," "I have drug hunger every night," or "I get sleepy at work but start getting sick by bedtime" are not uncommon in patients receiving methadone. These clinical problems may not respond to simple dose adjustments and may suggest wide fluctuations over the dosing interval (rapid metabolism). As early as 1978, it was suggested that serial methadone levels could result in dramatic clinical improvement, with a "flattening of the curve" associated with a divided dose regimen in those methadone maintenance patients who were experiencing problems on a single daily dose (53). Researchers in the early 1980s compared 24-hour methadone serum levels in two groups of patients, all of whom received 80 mg/day. One of the groups was composed of patients who were doing very well in treatment, while the patients in the other group were doing poorly in terms of drug use and compliance. The results showed the stable group to have a mean serum level of 410 ng/mL at 24 hours, whereas the poor performers had a mean of 101 ng/mL (54). It has become clear that the same dose may vary in efficacy among individuals and that patients may be doing poorly as a result of inadequate dosing. Several researchers support blood levels >150 to 200 ng/mL at all times for optimum results (9,55,56). There is growing consensus that levels above 400 ng/mL can represent an optimum level in providing adequate cross-tolerance to make ordinary doses of intravenous heroin ineffective (nonreinforcing) during methadone treatment (57). Methadone peak, trough, and mean levels, and the rate of elimination (half-life) can be influenced by several factors. Individual differences in the metabolism of methadone, poor absorption, changes in urinary pH, effects of concomitant medications, diet, and even vitamins are among the possible factors that can influence the 24-hour dose-response curve of methadone. Pregnancy, particularly during the third trimester, is associated with significant decrease in trough methadone levels, suggesting increased rates of metabolism of methadone (58). Blood level assays can be very useful in evaluating suspected drug interactions. Blood levels can help identify patients who may benefit from a divided-dose regimen or demonstrate the effectiveness of a divided-dose regimen.

Procedure for Obtaining Blood Levels Ideally, peak blood levels should be drawn at 3 (2 to 4) hours after a dose and trough levels at 24 hours. Patients already on a divided dose, such as every 12 hours, should have 2- to 3-hour and 12-hour specimens. A trough level alone is of little clinical value unless it is extremely low or very high. Blood levels are interpreted in the context of a clinical presentation for which the laboratory values can supplement clinical judgment. The peak level at 2 to 4 hours should be no more than twice the trough level. A peak/trough ratio of 2 or less is ideal (peak/trough = ratio). Ratios >2 suggest rapid metabolism. The rate of change is of greater clinical significance than the actual levels. For example, a patient with a 24-hour level of 350 ng/mL after a peak of 1,225 ng/mL (1,225/350 = 3.5, indicating rapid metabolism) may be experiencing early opioid withdrawal, whereas a patient with a trough of 150 ng/mL and a peak of 250 ng/mL (250/150 = 1.7, indicating a normal metabolism) may be quite comfortable. No particular blood level should be considered "therapeutic" outside of the clinical context.

Methadone-Drug Interactions Clinical experience suggests that concomitant medications can either induce or inhibit CYP450 activity on methadone metabolism (59). Drugs that stimulate or induce CYP450 activity can precipitate opioid withdrawal by accelerating metabolism, thus shortening duration and diminishing intensity of the effect of methadone. For example, addition of rifampicin, phenytoin, carbamazepine, phenobarbital, nevirapine, or efavirenz may result in onset of withdrawal symptoms and require dose adjustments of the methadone. Considerable flexibility in dosing may be required to stabilize some patients whose metabolism has been altered by drug interactions or naturally occurring altered rates of metabolism. Other drugs such as cimetidine, ciprofloxacin, fluconazole, erythromycin, and fluvoxamine may inhibit this enzyme activity, slowing the metabolism and extending the duration of the drug effect. Metabolism of methadone is largely a function of enzyme activity in the liver, and intestinal enzymatic activity has also been observed to be clinically relevant. Multiple enzymes may affect methadone metabolism in vivo (60). Liver 3A4 activity *in vitro* is shown to influence methadone metabolism (61). Methadone exists as a racemic mixture of R and S isomers. Genetic variability in CYP 2D6 activity may affect clinical status by affecting metabolism of the R-methadone isomer (62,63) and may also affect toxicity (64). Enzymatic activity of intestinal CYP2B6 is stereoselective and may be important in clinical effects and drug interactions (65). A 17-fold variability between patients in their methadone metabolism is shown, mostly due to activity of various enzymes (66).

Methadone and QT Interval Several case series have been published showing that methadone treatment is associated with prolongation of the QT interval on the electrocardiogram and possible consequent cardiac arrhythmia (Torsade des Pointes or TdP) (67,68).

In vitro study of hERG K+ channels confirms that methadone at therapeutic doses can affect cardiac conduction (69). Genomics of CYP2B6 were shown to be associated with QT interval, and *in vitro* studies suggest that most of this prolongation is due to the non-therapeutic S-methadone enantiomer (70). Interviews of patients receiving methadone treatment found an association between longer QT and retrospective self-report of syncopal episodes (71).

In 2006 the FDA published a 'black box' warning that included QT interval prolongation and risk of arrhythmia. Although this warning was aimed at patients on high doses for pain treatment, clinicians in OTPs are becoming more aware of this risk.

Two studies look at QT interval in the methadone clinic setting. Martell et.al. performed electrocardiograms on 160 patients admitted to methadone treatment at baseline, and again after six months and 12 months of treatment. The study found that admission to methadone treatment prolonged the QTc an average of 10 msec at 12 months and that the prolongation correlated with serum levels of methadone (72). Peles et al. measured QT in 138 patients already on stable doses of methadone and found that three of them had QTc >500 msec and during the study two of those patients died, although the deaths were not judged to be cardiac. An additional 19 patients, all with doses >120 mg, had QTc >450 msec (73). Both of these studies give an overall prevalence of prolonged QT interval (≥500 msec) of around 2% in the OTP. Another recent study found that 23% of methadone patients had a QTc >470 msec (women) or 490 msec (men) but did not find frequent QTc prolongation among patients treated with buprenorphine (74). Physicians remain under-aware of cardiac safety concerns about methadone (75), but many are adapting to this information in various ways. There are no clear data to guide any intervention. Some clinics are offering cardiograms and are screening patients for cardiac risk. Risk-benefit discussion with patients includes a review of other medications that might contribute additional cardiac risk. In general, it is considered that almost certain relapse to uncontrolled opioid use is more risky than the rare occurrence of an arrhythmia. However, coordination of care with outside physicians to monitor use of other medications or transfer to buprenorphine treatment might in some cases be indicated (74). Hospitalized patients receiving methadone may have particularly high risk of TdP (76). The Center for Substance Abuse Treatment (CSAT) is convening a consensus panel on this topic, and the final iteration of the consensus panel's recommendations is pending as of this writing.

Methadone-Related Deaths of Persons Not in Treatment The increase in methadone abuse parallels the increase in prescription analgesic abuse noted since 1995, with associated mortality from nonmedical ingestion of methadone, in particular a dramatic increase in mortality by ingestion of diverted methadone intended for pain treatment. Deaths from methadone overdoses exceeded deaths from heroin in some states by 2002 (77). In 2003 the CSAT published an analysis of an increase in deaths related to methadone in the United States, and in 2007 a second review (78). Most of these deaths involved diverted methadone intended for pain treatment and were not patients in maintenance treatment, nor did it appear that the methadone was diverted from that dispensed at the OTPs. Most of these deaths also involve multiple medications, usually including sedative medication. These observations are similar to observations of increased diversion-related deaths after ingesting methadone in other countries where OMT was initiated (79–81).

Levo Alpha Acetyl Methadol Levo alpha acetyl methadol (LAAM) was developed in 1948. By 1952, it had been observed to suppress opioid withdrawal for more than 72 hours (82). LAAM was evaluated in opioid addiction in the late 1960s and 1970s, ignored in the 1980s, and resurrected in 1990 by the Medications Development Division of the National Institute on Drug Abuse (83). LAAM was approved for use in the treatment of opioid addiction by the U.S. Food and Drug Administration (FDA) in 1993 (84). After several cases of the arrhythmia Torsade des Pointes were reported, the FDA placed a black-box QT warning label on LAAM, and subsequently the pharmaceutical company withdrew LAAM from the market. As of this writing it remains unavailable in the United States, though still approved as an opioid agonist medication for OMT.

MAINTENANCE TREATMENT USING BUPRENORPHINE

Buprenorphine is a partial mu-opioid agonist. In October 2002, the FDA approved two sublingual tablet formulations of buprenorphine for treatment of opioid dependence. One formulation, a combination of buprenorphine and naloxone in a 4:1 ratio, is designed to discourage injected diversion and misuse. Naloxone is an opioid antagonist that is not significantly bioavailable when taken sublingually or when swallowed. When injected into actively using opioid-dependent subjects who are blinded, the combination was not judged to be desirable or to be different from antagonist in the first hour after injection (85,86). This buprenorphine/naloxone tablet is the preferred formulation for outpatient use as an effort to minimize diversion. The other sublingual formulation contains only buprenorphine and is used in controlled settings, such as inpatient medically supervised withdrawal, or in pregnancy. Sublingual buprenorphine/naloxone maintenance treatment is usually offered in office-based settings, and such treatment is discussed in Chapter 50, "Special Issues in Office-Based Opioid Treatment." Sublingual buprenorphine is listed as an opioid treatment medication under federal regulations that govern OTP licensure.

Pharmacology of Sublingual Buprenorphine

Buprenorphine has slow onset and long duration of action, conferring similar maintenance benefits as discussed earlier for methadone. Its peak effect is 2 to 4 hours after sublingual administration, and its duration is 72 hours. As a partial mu agonist, buprenorphine has a maximal dose-effect ceiling that is well below significant respiratory depression. This safety profile led to its DEA schedule III, allowing office-based use under the restrictions of the Drug Addiction Treatment Act of 2000 (87). (See Chapter 50, "Special Issues in Office-Based Opioid Treatment.")

Induction and Precipitated Withdrawal Buprenorphine is a partial agonist with strong receptor attachment. Relative to a displaced full agonist, its activity can be felt as the rapid onset of (relative) opioid withdrawal by the patient unless the first dose is clinically well timed. The first dose should be given when the patient is already in obvious opioid withdrawal. When opioid withdrawal is already present, the onset of activity will be felt as agonist, with relief of withdrawal. Contrary to methadone, induction doses are not set by regulation, though clinical guidelines and physician training courses recommend 2 to 4 mg of sublingual buprenorphine/naloxone as a first dose, with first-day maximum of 8 mg (88). One Italian study found that higher induction doses were associated with better engagement in ongoing care (89).

Buprenorphine Dose Adjustment The dose can be rapidly titrated over the first 3 days to control withdrawal. Average daily doses are 16 to 20 mg. One labeled imaging study showed opioid receptors to be fully occupied at doses of 16 mg (90). Because of the partial agonist ceiling effect, no additional maintenance benefit is expected in doses above 32 mg/day. Sublingual buprenorphine/naloxone is usually prescribed as a single daily dose. In cases requiring supervised dosing, it can be given every other day, or three times a week, while keeping the total weekly dose unchanged (91,92).

Buprenorphine Medication Interactions Compared to methadone, buprenorphine may confer advantages when certain HIV medications are used (93) and in cases of QT prolongation with methadone (74,94). Even though it is metabolized by the liver in a manner similar to that of methadone, by CY450 3A4, the presence of an active metabolite—nor-buprenorphine—and the strong receptor attachment make this medication less dependent than methadone on blood level and tissue stores.

Federal Regulations and Sublingual Buprenorphine When dispensed in the OTP, sublingual buprenorphine/naloxone is subject to the same regulations as methadone. When prescribed in the office-based setting, there are certain restrictions set forth in the Drug Addiction Act of 2000 (87). This law provides for a waiver to the 1914 Harrison Act that forbids prescription of a narcotic to an addicted person. The qualifying physician notifies the Secretary of Health and Human Services of his or her intent to prescribe, after which the DEA assigns to the physician a second DEA number that is specifically for use under DATA 2000. There are restrictions on census and type of medication and rules on storage and record keeping. The DATA 2000 restrictions do not apply when buprenorphine or buprenorphine/naloxone are dispensed at clinics under their OTP license. In those cases, the same federal regulatory restrictions apply to both buprenorphine and methadone.

The inception of office-based treatment of opioid dependence prompted a nationwide government-sponsored mentoring network, the Physician Clinical Support System, that provides community clinicians with access to addiction specialist advice.

Diversion and Abuse of Buprenorphine An investigation of the effects of DATA 2000 was carried out in 2005. No serious adverse events were found by the introduction of sublingual buprenorphine/naloxone in the office-based setting. That study showed that most of the patients treated with buprenorphine listed prescription pain relievers as their primary opioid of abuse (95). In view of the serious increase in nonmedical usage of prescription opioids, it is hoped that buprenorphine/naloxone may provide a timely treatment for those who become addicted and who might not otherwise seek out a methadone clinic.

Wherever buprenorphine treatment has been introduced, there has been diversion and abuse of the medication, including injected use (96,97). One study in the United States showed that diverted buprenorphine/naloxone is being used mostly for relief of withdrawal and rarely as a primary drug of abuse (98).

Choice between Methadone and Buprenorphine

Though both medications were shown comparable in various outcomes (99,100), systematic reviews suggest that methadone is superior in retaining patients (101). In the United States, site of care and level of care, local availability or cost may determine which medication is applicable for a given patient. An interesting blinded study showed that a "stepped" approach of starting patients on buprenorphine and transferring those who did not stabilize onto methadone had identical outcomes to directly admitting patients to methadone treatment. In this study, 46% of patients did well on buprenorphine (102). Comparison studies in specific clinical areas such as pregnancy (103,104), cardiac risk (71), and medication interactions may eventually lead to more patient-tailored medication choices. A randomized study of liver function and a randomized, blinded study of treatment during pregnancy compare the two medications and are currently under way in the United States.

Observed Doses and Take-Home Medication in OMT As the patient who is on maintenance surfaces from his or her addiction and begins to work on major life changes, the need for daily visits to the dispensing window and for regular counseling can change as well. Patients who do well and who improve according to specified criteria set out in federal regulations can earn take-home medications for unsupervised dosing. The criteria include adherence to treatment, stability of home environment, involvement in productive activity, abstinence from drugs of abuse, and resolution of any legal problems. As of May 2001, the guidelines governing methadone treatment started to allow patients to take home up to six doses a week after 9 months, 2 weeks of medication after the first year, and 30-day doses after the second year of treatment (14). Some states have additional, more stringent regulations. The same observed dosing requirements apply to sublingual buprenorphine dispensed under OTP license but not if prescribed by a physician and dispensed at a retail pharmacy. In buprenorphine dispensed from an OTP, the nurse or pharmacist observes the proper placement of the tablet(s) under the tongue. Some OTPs have the patient wait until tablets have completely dissolved. As mentioned earlier, alternate-day or thrice-weekly dosing is an option for the buprenorphine-maintained patient who is not stable enough to have take-out doses (91,92).

Monthly observed dosing at the OTP, with carry-out of the remaining doses for the month, is as close as most methadone maintenance patients come to receiving their medication in a fashion similar to that in other well-controlled medical conditions. Methadone medical maintenance (MMM) and Office-Based Opioid Treatment (OBOT) with methadone remain a rarity in the United States.

Methadone Medical Maintenance Methadone medical maintenance (MMM), designed for "stable, recovered" patients on methadone, is an effort to release the patient from burdensome attendance in an OTP by allowing a physician who is affiliated with the clinic, but in office practice, to prescribe or administer the maintenance medication. In April 2000, the CSAT circulated draft guidelines describing medical maintenance. These guidelines were developed after more than 10 years of pilot projects showed that this approach to care works and that it improves the quality of life for patients (105). As of 2008, these guidelines remain in draft format, and MMM is still rarely used. Physicians interested in offering integrated treatment in an office setting are doing so under the Drug Addiction Treatment Act of 2000, the legislation enabling use of sublingual preparations of buprenorphine, discussed in Chapter 50, "Special Issues in Office-Based Opioid Treatment."

Medical maintenance generally refers to attendance that is reduced to one or two visits per month, with a minimum number of supportive services and is offered to selected stable patients. Two models have emerged. The first was designed by Des Jarlais and colleagues (106) as a feasibility study and subsequently was reported by Novick. According to the model, medical maintenance is defined as the treatment of rehabilitated methadone maintenance patients in a general medical setting rather than a licensed clinic. Selection criteria called for a minimum of 5 years in treatment, with essentially perfect compliance for a period of 3 years. Results are excellent in terms of enhanced retention and reduced rates of addictive disorder or lost medication (107–109). The other model, developed by Senay, differs in several ways. Admission to the study was based on performance rather than time in treatment, with only 6 months of excellent performance required. The reduced attendance and services were provided in a methadone program, with continued periodic counseling and urine drug screens. The Senay model also demonstrated an excellent treatment outcome (110,111). An obvious advantage to both models is a reduced level or intensity of care and cost of treatment, thus freeing resources for patients just entering treatment, while stable rehabilitated patients benefit from ongoing methadone treatment with a minimum of cost and disruption of their lives. As mentioned earlier, many patients risk their abstinence and, in an AIDS epidemic, their lives, in an effort to withdraw from methadone for nonmedical reasons. For those who are attempting to free themselves from OTP constraints rather than from the effects of daily medication, medical maintenance could be an acceptable solution. Current regulations require a federal waiver for medical maintenance. A 2001 study randomly assigning patients to either office- or OTP-based methadone showed no difference in clinical outcomes and improved patient and physician satisfaction (112). Office-based maintenance with sublingual buprenorphine is becoming more available as physicians become trained and experienced.

PAIN MANAGEMENT

A full discussion of the treatment of addiction patients who have pain is presented in Chapter 94, "Treating Co-morbid Pain and Addiction." Patients on OMT require special consideration because of their baseline maintenance opioid. They will be tolerant to additional opioids, and if non-opioid approaches are not effective, they may need unusually high and frequent doses of opioids to manage their pain.

Acute Pain In cases of acute pain associated with surgery, trauma, or dental work, the physicians or dentists involved often—incorrectly—assume that the maintenance dose of methadone also will relieve any ensuing pain from the injury or procedure. The current emphasis on proper pain control in medical settings has improved patient care, and patients are more likely to be treated according to their symptoms and function rather than their maintenance dose. Several points should be kept in mind. First, single daily doses of methadone may be effective in controlling addiction, but multiple daily doses may be required for analgesia. Second, long-term use of methadone and possibly buprenorphine as well, is associated with hyperalgesia (113–115). Tolerance and hyperalgesia combined means that patients in OMT who require opioids for pain management may need very high doses of opioids. Morphine, hydromorphone, fentanyl, oxycodone, hydrocodone, codeine, and other agonist drugs may be appropriate for methadone maintained patients as part of pain management when additional opioids are required. Mixed agonist-antagonists (pentazocine, butorphanol, nalbuphine) and partial agonists (buprenorphine) must not be used in methadone-maintained patients, as they will precipitate an opioid withdrawal syndrome. Meperidine and propoxyphene should be avoided because of the risk of seizures at the higher doses required to produce analgesia in methadone maintained patients.

In summary, for methadone-maintained patients who require opioids for acute pain management: (1) Continue maintenance treatment without interruption and use non-opioid pain treatments whenever possible; (2) provide adequate individualized doses of opioid agonists, which must be titrated to the desired analgesic or functional effect; and (3) doses should be given more frequently and on a fixed schedule rather than "as needed for pain." Although not thoroughly documented, it is probably best to choose agonists different from those previously abused.

Chronic Pain More than 30% of OMT patients report chronic, severe pain (116). Compared to those who primarily misuse heroin, patients admitted to the OTP for prescription opioid abuse may have higher prevalence of pain (6,117). The historical separation of pain treatment from addiction treatment in American medicine gets in the way of properly managing patients with chronic pain and who are on maintenance opioids. The OTP physician can sometimes bridge this gap by coordinating care with the patient's primary care or pain specialist. For example, in a patient with chronic nonmalignant pain who is able to comply with the regulatory criteria for take-home medication, the OTP physician can order a divided dose of methadone, and the outside physician can prescribe short-acting rescue medication. This might improve baseline pain control without the patient's needing multiple sources of long-acting medication.

PREGNANCY AND OPIOID AGONIST TREATMENT

Agonist treatment during pregnancy remains a controversial and emotionally charged topic. This is largely attributable to the neonatal opioid withdrawal syndrome (neonatal abstinence syndrome), which is the most visible and dramatic sequela of physical dependence in the neonate. Efforts to treat, prevent, and minimize neonatal opioid withdrawal have predominated since the results of the first 13 pregnancies were reported in 1969 (118). Neonatal withdrawal is monitored in the hospital for several days after birth. The Finnegan scale of infant withdrawal is used to determine whether treatment becomes necessary (119). In a case series of 80 women in California who were treated with methadone maintenance, only 45% of the infants needed treatment, with no difference between low and high doses of methadone dose (120). An interesting feature noted in this case series was better outcomes in women who became pregnant during their methadone maintenance treatment (121). Except for HIV-positive mothers, breastfeeding by patients on OMT is encouraged (122). Preliminary studies comparing methadone to sublingual buprenorphine during pregnancy suggest that buprenorphine may eventually offer a second choice (103,104). Neonatal withdrawal still must be monitored for several days after birth. Methadone and buprenorphine are category C medications, though there is more experience with the use of methadone in pregnancy. Clinicians face a clinical decision regarding starting or continuing buprenorphine maintenance in pregnant patients when methadone treatment is not an option.

Opioid maintenance remains the treatment of choice for pregnant, opioid-dependent patients. Maternal medically supervised withdrawal during pregnancy is technically possible (123). There is concern that it would result in potentially dangerous intrauterine fetal distress. For this reason, medically supervised withdrawal of pregnant patients is usually done in the hospital with fetal monitoring. The main practical consideration of medically supervised withdrawal during pregnancy is relapse. Treatment during pregnancy is addressed in detail in Chapter 81, "Alcohol and Other Drug Use During Pregnancy: Management of the Mother and Child."

NEEDLE-RELATED COMORBIDITY

Of heroin-addicted patients admitted to OMT in 2005, 63% were injection drug users (IDUs) (124). Infections related to needle use are a main source of comorbidity and death in the OMT population. Infectious comorbidity is discussed in detail in Chapter 77, "HIV, TB, and Other Infectious Diseases Related to Alcohol and Other Drug Use."

Acute skin infections at the site of injection may form an abscess that responds to incision and drainage or may worsen and produce cellulitis requiring systemic or parenteral antimicrobials. One particularly lethal and disfiguring infection is necrotizing fasciitis (125). Clusters of botulism cases have been found in areas where the less processed "black tar" heroin is used, and the epidemiology suggests that the toxin is already present in the injected drug itself (126,127). Endocarditis should be ruled out in IDU patients who present with a fever and heart murmur.

Human Immunodeficiency Virus Between 15% and 20% of long-term injection drug users are positive for the human immunodeficiency virus (HIV) (128,129), so maintenance patients are routinely screened and if necessary treated with antiretrovirals. Participation in opioid maintenance treatment is useful in prevention of HIV (11,130). Methadone maintenance treatment is associated with fewer high-risk behaviors, such as unsafe injection practices or having multiple sexual partners (131). Patients at risk for injection drug use who were maintained on buprenorphine had higher adherence to their antiretroviral regimen than those not in treatment (132).

Dose adjustments may become necessary in patients on methadone or buprenorphine maintenance who begin highly active antiretroviral treatment (HAART) for HIV (93,133). HIV-related conditions usually require coordination with specialty clinics. OMT clinicians can support medication adherence to complicated HAART treatment (134).

Hepatitis C Virus Novick (135) reported Hepatitis C virus (HCV) positivity rates of 66% to 88% of all injection drug users, with 77% in persons using for 1 year or less and 94% in persons who had injected drugs for at least 10 years. HCV becomes chronic in 85% of infected persons but progresses slowly. Cirrhosis is seen in 20% to 30% and also develops slowly—in most cases, over 10 to 20 years. Approximately 50% to 75% of acute HCV infections in adults are asymptomatic. If symptoms are present, they are often nonspecific. Tong and El-Farra (136) described the course of HCV infection in 125 patients with a history of injection drug use. The mean age at which drug use was initiated was 23.1 years, with presentation to a tertiary care center in California occurring approximately 20 years later (139). The most common presenting symptoms were fatigue, abdominal pain, anorexia, and weight loss. The initial workup indicated 26% had chronic hepatitis, 37% had chronic active hepatitis, 36% had cirrhosis, and 0.8% had hepatocellular carcinoma. Alcohol use increases the severity of the disease (135).

Testing and staging of hepatitis C are becoming available for IDU patients, and those admitted to opioid maintenance treatment are often able to report their status.

OTP programs are developing educational interventions to encourage health practices (such as complete elimination of alcohol) that are likely to prolong the period of good health (137,138) Patients with hepatitis C should be vaccinated against hepatitis A and hepatitis B if they are not immune, or if serologic status cannot be determined. Advocacy will be needed to ensure that patients have access to emerging treatments and better access to liver transplantation when necessary (139).

When patients need treatment for hepatitis C, the standard care includes a weekly pegylated interferon injection and oral ingestion of ribavirin several times a day. Most IDUs require a year of treatment, depending on genotype. Patients on OMT can expect excellent results in treatment, with sustained remission in 54% (140). Clinicians in the OTP may find themselves either supporting or providing this care onsite.

PATIENTS WITH CO-OCCURRING PSYCHIATRIC DISORDERS

The high rate of co-occurring psychiatric and addictive disorders (141–143) obligates treatment providers to equip themselves to address both problems. It can be difficult to differentiate substance-induced disorders from independent conditions at intake, but it is noteworthy that symptoms can diminish rapidly upon initiation of methadone maintenance, especially within the first month (144,145). Nonetheless, many patients will remain with psychiatric conditions that need to be addressed. A recent study confirmed that patients with co-occurring psychiatric disorders remained in treatment longer, but those with severe subjective distress had more negative outcomes (146).

Woody and colleagues (147) examined the efficacy of two kinds of professional psychotherapy and drug abuse counseling typically provided in methadone programs as a function of global psychiatric status ratings of the patients. They found that low-severity patients benefited from both drug abuse counseling (focused on current life problems) and psychotherapy (employing supportive-expressive and cognitive behavioral approaches). Patients with high levels of psychiatric symptoms were lower in all areas of pretreatment functioning and did not improve as much as did patients with less severe problems. However, the addition of psychotherapy did maximize their improvement in many areas. Professionally trained therapists, integrated into the ongoing program, improved outcome for these difficult patients.

Depression and dysthymia are common co-occurring disorders in the treatment-seeking population (148). Psychosocial stress and the discomforts of withdrawal may contribute to temporarily low mood as well. Life crises and depressive symptoms posed a substantial risk of relapse, which lessened for those who remained in treatment (149). Studies of antidepressants with this population have produced mixed results, indicating a need to determine how to select opiate-dependent patients most likely to benefit (145). These authors recommended research on integrated models of care in which treatment algorithms are developed to determine the efficacy and cost-effectiveness of both medication and psychosocial interventions.

Anxiety disorders also are common, with symptoms abating with a combination of an adequate methadone dose and the provision of counseling or psychotherapy over a period of time (150). Posttraumatic stress disorder (PTSD) is common in methadone patients, and though it may be associated with greater drug abuse severity (151), PTSD does not necessarily worsen the outcome of substance abuse treatment. Trafton and colleagues (152) found differences in PTSD patients compared to those without, including a longer history of drug use at intake, but these did not negatively influence outcomes. Patients with PTSD received higher doses of medication, attended more psychosocial treatment sessions, and had better treatment retention. However, their PTSD symptoms did not improve with substance abuse treatment alone. Seeking Safety represents a manualized intervention for early recovery stabilization of patient with PTSD and substance abuse (153). It has been widely disseminated and shows good levels of acceptance by patients and counselors.

Sleep disorders are often overlooked and appear to be common in those with psychiatric disorders, chronic pain, benzodiazepine abuse, and whose methadone dose is high

(154). Schizophrenia is relatively uncommon in opioid treatment patients (155,156), though most programs have some patients with the disorder. Based on historical references and clinical observations, some clinicians have proposed that opioids have antipsychotic properties (157,158). Clinicians have described a subgroup of patients, such as the one who referred to methadone as his "sanity syrup," who appear calmed and stabilized by the medication; when their doses drop, they become disorganized. It also is likely that the high degree of structure characteristic of many treatment programs has a beneficial effect on these patients by providing a sense of safety and security.

It is common to find reports of personality disorders, particularly antisocial personality disorder, in the heroin-using population. Effective treatments are being developed, even for this difficult group. Ball studied methadone patients with at least one personality disorder who were receiving two different forms of psychotherapy and who showed significant reductions in various severity indicators, including psychiatric symptoms and psychosocial impairment (159).

It is important to view a personality disorder diagnosis with caution. Criteria in editions of the Diagnostic and Statistical Manual of Mental Disorders before the DSM-IV(160) failed to distinguish behaviors characteristic of alcohol and drug users from personality traits that were more enduring. The self-preoccupation of the opioid agonist treatment patient in the stabilization phase (comparable to other patients who are newly abstinent or in early recovery) was too readily interpreted as narcissistic preoccupation characteristic of personality disorder. In addition, symptoms of posttraumatic stress disorder can be mistaken for personality disorder. As clinicians come to understand the high prevalence of emotional trauma in addicted persons, they will note that apparent lack of feelings and/or interpersonal connection may represent numbing symptoms (for example, feelings of detachment or estrangement, restricted range of emotions) seen in PTSD. It is important to be attentive to these potential confusions because personality disorder—and especially antisocial personality disorder—carries a poor prognosis and often evokes negative staff attitudes. It is advisable to be wary of psychiatric disorders diagnosed at or shortly after admission, because many patients look more pathologic than they will after their medication has been stabilized and they have begun to make use of psychosocial services.

PSYCHOSOCIAL INTERVENTIONS

Psychosocial interventions are considered integral to good treatment in a methadone program, and requirements for this are written into regulations. Many individual studies support this view, but a rigorous analysis finds flaws in the research that make it difficult to draw definitive conclusions. In a Cochrane review published in 2004, Amato and colleagues (161) offer evidence from the 12 of 77 studies that met their inclusion criteria that adding any psychosocial support to standard methadone treatment significantly reduces heroin use during treatment (164). The trials were heterogeneous, both in the interventions studied and the way outcomes were assessed, making it difficult to do a meta-analysis on outcomes for key issues. The short duration of the studies also made it impossible to assess outcomes such as mortality. Large, multisite studies with standardized interventions would be needed to determine the added value of psychosocial interventions. Inasmuch as medication makes other changes possible but does not in itself produce them, it is important to preserve the capacity of programs to provide a broad spectrum of care.

Physicians who work in clinics focused on opioid maintenance pharmacotherapy typically find that counseling and case management vary widely in quality and comprehensiveness. In many states, the introduction of methadone was permitted only if accompanied by a serious rehabilitative effort, but recent changes in funding have undermined efforts to maintain comprehensive services. Clinic-based buprenorphine treatment offers the same intensity of psychosocial interventions as methadone maintenance; however, most buprenorphine maintenance is carried out in nonclinic settings with variable availability of counseling. Integration of psychosocial care with buprenorphine maintenance medication is beneficial in reducing drug abuse and improving retention (89,163), though the optimal intensity of such care is harder to determine (163).

In many OTPs, psychosocial interventions are provided by counselors, who range widely in educational level and professional training. The counselor's task is to identify and address specific problems in the areas of drug use, physical health, interpersonal relationships (including family interaction), psychologic problems, and educational or vocational goals (164). Short- and long-term treatment plans provide structure for the counseling sessions and a tool by which to monitor the patient's progress and quality of care. The counselor often serves as a case manager as well, initiating screening for medication and other program services; attending to issues concerning program rules, privileges, and policies; and providing links to other agencies. Clinics that have access to professionally trained staff may offer psychotherapy to selected patients. Typically, this access is found in programs involved in research or professional training.

An increasing number of intervention strategies are being disseminated in forms that make onsite counselor training easier. (Materials are available from both the SAMHSA/CSAT and NIDA Web sites.) Many of these have been supported in random-assignment controlled trials, though not necessarily with methadone patients. Given the growing emphasis on evidence-based interventions, it is important to understand that many have not been extensively tested under real-world conditions, and there is insufficient information about the costs of implementation compared to the benefits achieved. Nonetheless, specific interventions have great potential to improve engagement, retention and outcomes and to reduce clinician frustration. Treatment programs rarely rely on one particular intervention alone, and it is the program's ability to integrate various elements that is likely to bring success.

Motivational enhancement strategies and a variety of forms of cognitive-behavioral therapy (CBT) are available in manualized form, some with accompanying DVD materials. The Treatment Improvement Protocol (TIP 35) is available to download or in a printed version at no charge from the Center for Substance Abuse Treatment *(/www.ncbi.nlm.nih.gov/books)*. Buprenorphine-specific training for counselors is also available online *(http:// www.danyalearningcenter.org)*.

This set of strategies can strengthen the physician's and counselor's ability to address a range of issues. Many maintenance patients start treatment but are not fully committed to giving up alcohol, heroin, and other drugs. Important public health benefits have been documented even when they do not commit themselves fully. However, supportive long-term work in the context of a good therapeutic alliance can shift the goals for many patients in time. Studies have documented continuing improvement over a period of years (165).

Motivational enhancement strategies (166,167) offer an alternative to harsh confrontation and encourage counselors to meet patients wherever they are prepared to begin and to move forward from there. CBT takes a variety of forms. These include what are called early recovery and relapse prevention skills *(www.matrixinstitute.org)*. Though the Matrix manuals focus on stimulant use, the strategies are applicable to opiate users with modest changes. Contingency management (168), community reinforcement, and node-link mapping are described in TIP #42, also available at no charge from SAMHSA/CSAT (169).

The provision of comprehensive services is supported by recent research (170–173). McLellan and colleagues (16,162,174,175) have demonstrated that the addition of enhanced onsite professional services led to better results than basic counseling alone. Quality, quantity, and the match between the patient's specific problem areas (e.g., vocational, family, or psychiatric) and the services offered all led to demonstrably better outcomes in a variety of populations (175,176). A quality assurance process that monitors and encourages a close fit between the patient's needs and the services delivered is likely to produce the best outcome, in contrast to a single approach in which most patients receive a similar mix of services.

Phased programs allow treatment to be individualized within a highly structured, systematic process that allows the patient to move forward, achieving tangible markers of progress. Hoffman and Moolchan (177) described one such model, divided into three phases: intensive stabilization, commitment, and rehabilitation. More recently, TIP #42 described goals, strategies and indications for transition to a new phase in a phased approach to both heroin detoxification and methadone maintenance. Staff/patient ratios can be adjusted according to the levels of support and assistance required by the patient at each stage, and specific activities can be tailored to the individual's needs. Services can be provided onsite or through a network of referral sources in the community. In the later stages, the patient can be tracked into a tapering phase or a medical maintenance phase, with a reinforcement phase used as follow-up.

Other approaches address problems at the systems level. The NIATx *(https://www.niatx.net)* offers a model for process improvement that allows agency managers and staff identify areas where there are problems and solve them step by step.

GROWTH, CONTROVERSY, AND FUTURE CHALLENGES

Any physician who becomes involved in the treatment of an OMT patient has an important task beyond that of medical practitioner: education and advocacy. A few minutes spent educating family members, clinical providers, employers, and others can have a major effect on reducing stigma and improving the way in which the patient is treated in a variety of systems of care. The patient who feels that his or her physician is knowledgeable and concerned will make a far greater effort to comply with that physician's treatment recommendations. An issue that merits attention, though there is little literature on the subject, involves middle-class individuals who use illicit opiates but who would not consider seeking treatment in the system that currently delivers OMT. The CSAT-sponsored evaluation of the buprenorphine DATA 2000 waiver program suggests that as of 2005, office-based treatment with sublingual buprenorphine addresses a younger, better-educated group of patients more likely to misuse prescription opioids (178). Clinical trials of buprenorphine have shown it to be effective and safe in office-based practice as a maintenance medication (98,99). Also, work is under way on office-based use of methadone (office-based opioid treatment, or OBOT) to expand treatment capacity. CSAT is evaluating several such projects around the country. OBOT with methadone currently is available and successful in several nations outside the United States, including Canada. (See Chapter 50, "Special Issues in Office-Based Opioid Treatment" for full discussion of OBOT.)

OVERSIGHT AND REGULATORY CHALLENGES

Since the early 1970s, methadone maintenance and withdrawal treatment have been influenced by regulations promulgated by the FDA, in consultation with the National Institute on Drug Abuse (NIDA) and the U.S. Drug Enforcement Administration. In addition, some states have adopted their own regulations, most of which are based on federal regulations but may be more restrictive in their provisions. There is little question that these regulations, in their current form, have failed to ensure the quality of patient care and have had some unintended consequences (3,178,180). A 1995 report by the Institute of Medicine estimated that only 18% to 36% of heroin users were enrolled in methadone treatment in that year (3). A consensus statement issued in 1998 by the National Institutes of Health supported the chronic disease model of opiate addiction and pointed to methadone maintenance as the best available treatment (4). Since then, efforts to improve access to treatment have taken several forms.

The most significant is a transition of primary federal oversight responsibilities from the FDA to the CSAT. Major revisions of regulations, guidelines, and standards are part of this transition, which implements revised federal regulations published in May 2001 (14). Existing programs became accredited as of 2003, and new ones are required to do so within 9 months. Accrediting bodies include state agencies and private accreditation organizations.

The CSAT has published Guidelines for the Accreditation of Opioid Treatment Programs. Changes involving more flexibility in take-home unsupervised dosing and the elimination of artificial barriers to admission to methadone maintenance programs have the potential to make medical decisions part of everyday life in treatment programs. In addition, some previously regulated areas are to be incorporated into clinic-specific policies and procedures. For example, each clinic must have policies to reduce diversion of medication. In the past, regulations that attempted to thwart diversion might have dictated use of liquid medications, locked boxes, and inspection of returned bottles, leaving none of the decisions to clinic policy. Another area is the requirement for continued performance evaluation. Each clinic is to designate the outcome measures to be followed, reflecting the clinic's own philosophy of care and based on current research about opiate addiction. This task has the potential to put decisions about delivery of care into the hands of clinic administrators rather than regulatory bodies. Although these changes have been made at the federal level, many states still have not changed their regulations to come into conformance with them, so it remains to be seen when and how much clinical ground actually is won.

An urgent need to increase access to treatment while improving and ensuring the quality of that treatment drives the need for restructuring. However, the rapid rise of methadone-associated deaths has created a new context for efforts to reduce barriers. Although the majority of these deaths are related to pain management rather than clinic practices, deaths due to poor management of the induction period have been documented (181). Extensive efforts to train physicians more systematically are underway.

In this context, two other changes deserve mention. DATA 2000—the law enabling office-based buprenorphine maintenance—contains specific requirements for training, and courses in the use of buprenorphine have been offered to physicians around the country.

REFERENCES

1. SAMHSA. *National Survey of Substance Abuse Treatment Services (N-SSATS), for 2006.* Retrieved November 12, 2007, from http://wwwdasis.samhsa.gov.
2. SAMHSA. http://www.drugabusestatistics.samhsa.gov/2k6/OTP/OTP.pdf. Facilities operating opioid treatment programs: 2005: The DASIS Report. In: *The DASIS report: Drug and Alcohol Services Information System.* Rockville, MD: Office of Applied Studies, 2006.
3. Rettig R, Yarmolinsky A, eds. *Institute of Medicine—Federal Regulation of Methadone Treatment.* Washington, DC: National Academy Press, 1995.
4. National Institutes of Health-Centers for Disease Control. *Effective medical treatment of heroin addiction. NIH Consensus Statement.* Bethesda, MD: National Institutes of Health, 1997.
5. Substance Abuse and Mental Health Services Administration. http://www.oas.samhsa.gov/nsduh/2k6nsduh/2k6Results.pdf. *Results from the 2006 National Survey on Drug Use and Health: National findings.* Washington, DC: Office of Applied Studies, 2007.
6. Rosenblum, A., et al. Prescription opioid abuse among enrollees into methadone maintenance treatment. *Drug Alcohol Depend* 2007;90(1): 64–71.
7. Dole VP, Nyswander M. A medical treatment for diacetylmorphine (heroin) addiction—a clinical trial with methadone hydrochloride. *JAMA* 1965;193(8):646–650.
8. Goldstein A. Heroin addiction: Neurobiology, pharmacology, and policy. *J Psychoactive Drugs* 1991;23(2):123–33.
9. Dole VP. Implications of methadone maintenance for theories of narcotic addiction (see comments). *JAMA* 1988;260(20):3025–3029.
10. Gronbladh LL, Ohlund S, Gunne LM. Mortality in heroin addiction: Impact of methadone treatment. *Acta Psychiatr Scand* 1990;82(3): 223–227.
11. Ball JC, et al. Reducing the risk of AIDS through methadone maintenance treatment. *J Health Soc Behav* 1988;29(3):214–226.
12. Ball JC, Ross A. The effectiveness of methadone maintenance treatment. New York: Springer-Verlag, 1991:283.
13. Joseph H, Stancliff S, Langrod J. Methadone Maintenance Treatment (MMT): A review of historical and clinical issues. *Mount Sinai J Med* 2000;67(5-6):347–364.
14. *Code of Federal Regulations, 42 part 8,* 2001. Retrieved November 28, 2008. http://ecfr.gpoaccess.gov/cgi/t/text/text-idx?c=ecfr&tpl=/ecfrbrowse/Title42/42cfr8_main-02.tpl.
15. Zweben JE, Payte JT. Methadone maintenance in the treatment of opioid dependence. A current perspective. *West J Med* 1990;152(5): 588–599.
16. McLellan AT. Patient characteristics associated with outcome. In: Cooper JR, et al. (eds.). research on the treatment of narcotic addiction: state of the art. Rockville, MD: National Institute on Drug Abuse Treatment, Monograph Series, 1983:500–529.
17. Magura S, Rosenblum A. Leaving methadone treatment: lessons learned, lessons forgotten, lessons ignored. *Mount Sinai J Med* 2001; 68(1):62–74.
18. O'Connor PG. Methods of detoxification and their role in treating patients with opioid dependence. *JAMA* 2005;294(8):961–963.
19. Mattick RP, et al. Methadone maintenance therapy versus no opioid replacement therapy for opioid dependence. *Cochrane Database Syst Rev* 2003;CD002209.
20. Dole VP, Nyswander ME. Heroin addiction—a metabolic disease. *Arch Intern Med* 1967;120(1):19–24.
21. Kreek MJ. Rationale for maintenance pharmacotherapy of opiate dependence. In: O'Brien CP, Jaffee JH eds. *Addictive states.* New York: Raven Press, 1992:205–230.
22. Merikangas KR, et al. Familial transmission of substance use disorders. *Arch Gen Psychiatry* 1998;55:973–979.
23. Pickens RW. Genetic and other risk factors in opiate addiction. In: *Effective medical treatment of heroin addiction.* Bethesda, MD: National Institutes of Health,William H. Natcher Conference Center, 1997.
24. Tsuang MT, et al. Co-occurrence of abuse of different drugs in men. *Arch Gen Psychiatry* 1998;55:967–972.
25. Kreek MJ. Methadone-related opioid agonist pharmacotherapy for heroin addiction. History, recent molecular and neurochemical research and future in mainstream medicine. Ann NY Acad Sci 2000;909: 186–216.
26. Gelernter J, et al. Genomewide linkage scan for opioid dependence and related traits. *Am J Hum Genet* 2006;78(5):759–769.
27. Galynker II, et al. Cerebral metabolism in opiate-dependent subjects: effects of methadone maintenance. *Mount Sinai J Med* 2000;67 (5-6):381–387.

28. Kaufman M, et al. Cerebral phosphorus metabolite abnormalities in opiate-dependent polydrug abusers in methadone maintenance. *Psychiatry Res* 1999;90(3):143–152.
29. Caplehorn JR, et al. Retention in methadone maintenance and heroin addicts' risk of death. *Addiction* 1994;89(2):203–209.
30. Langendam M, et al. The impact of harm-reduction-based methadone treatment on mortality among heroin users. *Am J Public Health* 2001;91(5):774–780.
31. Fugelstad A, et al. Mortality among HIV-infected intravenous drug addicts in Stockholm in relation to methadone treatment. *Addiction* 1995;90(5):711–716.
32. Wagner-Servais D, Erkens M. Methadone-related deaths associated with faulty induction procedures. *J Maint Addict* 2003;2(3):57–67.
33. Drummer OH, et al. Methadone toxicity causing death in ten subjects starting on a methadone maintenance program. *Am J Forensic Med Pathol* 1992;13(4):346–350.
34. Caplehorn JR, Drummer OH. Fatal methadone toxicity:Signs and circumstances, and the role of benzodiazepines. *Aust N Z J Public Health* 2002;26(4):358–362; discussion 362–363.
35. Wu CH, Henry JA. Deaths of heroin addicts starting on methadone maintenance. *Lancet* 1990;335(8686):424.
36. Vormfelde SV, Poser W. Death attributed to methadone. *Pharmacopsychiatry* 2001;34(6):217–222.
37. Zador D, Sunjic S. Deaths in methadone maintenance treatment in New South Wales, Australia 1990–1995. *Addiction* 2000;95(1):77–84.
38. Caplehorn JR, Drummer OH. Mortality associated with New South Wales methadone programs in 1994: Lives lost and saved. *Med J Aust* 1999;170(3):104–109.
39. Kaufman J, Payte JT, McLellan AT. Treatment standards and optimal treatment. In: Rettig RA, Yarmolinski A (eds.). *Federal regulation of methadone treatment*. Washington, DC: National Academy Press, 1995:185–216.
40. Payte JT, Khuri ET. Principles of methadone dose determination. In: Parrino M ed. *CSAT State Methadone Treatment Guidelines*. Rockville, MD: U.S. Department of Health and Human Services, 1993:47–58.
41. Inturrisi C. Pharmacology of methadone and its isomers. *Minerva Anest* 2005;71(7–8):435–437.
42. Koch T, et al. Receptor endocytosis counteracts the development of opioid tolerance. *Mol Pharmacol* 2005;67(1):280–287.
43. Finn A, Whistler J. Endocytosis of the mu opioid receptor reduces tolerance and a cellular hallmark of opiate withdrawal. *Neuron* 2001;32(5):829–839.
44. He L, Whistler J. The biochemical analysis of methadone modulation on morphine-induced tolerance and dependence in the rat brain. *Pharmacology* 2007;79(4):193–202.
45. Courtwright D, Joseph H, DesJarlais D. Methadone maintenance: Interview with Vincent Dole. In: *Addicts who survived: An oral history of narcotic use in America, 1923–1965*. Knoxville: University of Tennessee Press, 1989:331–343.
46. Amato L, et al. An overview of systematic reviews of the effectiveness of opiate maintenance therapies: Available evidence to inform clinical practice and research. *J Subst Abuse Treat* 2005;28(4):321–329.
47. Strain E, et al. Moderate- vs. high-dose methadone in the treatment of opioid dependence: a randomized trial. *JAMA* 1999;281(11):1000–1005.
48. Caplehorn JR, et al. Methadone dose and heroin use during maintenance treatment. *Addiction* 1993;88(1):119–124.
49. Strain EC, et al. Dose-response effects of methadone in the treatment of opioid dependence. *Ann Intern Med* 1993; 119(1):23–27.
50. American Society of Addiction Medicine. *American Society of Addiction Medicine Policy Statement on Methadone Treatment*. Washington, DC: American Society of Addiction Medicine, 1991.
51. Hser Y-I, et al. A 33-year follow-up of narcotics addicts. *Arch Gen Psychiatry* 2001;58:503–508.
52. Payte JT, Khuri ET. Treatment duration and patient retention. In: Parrino MW ed. *State methadone treatment guidelines*. Rockville, MD: U.S. Department of Health and Human Services, 1993:119–124.
53. Walton RG, Thornton TL, Wahl GF. Serum methadone as an aid in managing methadone maintenance patients. *Int J Addict* 1978;13(5):689–694.
54. Tennant FS Jr, et al. Methadone plasma levels and persistent drug abuse in high dose maintenance patients. *NIDA Res Monogr* 1984;49(8):262–268.
55. Holmstrand J, Anggard E, Gunne LM. Methadone maintenance: Plasma levels and therapeutic outcome. *Clin Pharmacol Ther* 1978;23(2):175–180.
56. Loimer N, Schmid R. The use of plasma levels to optimize methadone maintenance treatment. *Drug Alcohol Depend* 1992;30(3):241–246.
57. Loimer N, et al. Psychophysiological reactions in methadone maintenance patients do not correlate with methadone plasma levels. *Psychopharmacology (Berlin)* 1991;103(4):538–540.
58. Pond SM, et al. Altered methadone pharmacokinetics in methadone-maintained pregnant women. *J Pharmacol Exp Ther* 1985;233(1):1–6.
59. Grudzinskas CV, et al. Problems of drug dependence, 1995: Proceedings of the 57th annual scientific meeting of the college on problems of drug dependence, inc, Symposium IX. The documented role of pharmacogentics in the identification and administration of new medications for treating drug abuse. *NIDA Res Monogr* 1996;162:60–63.
60. Kharasch E, et al. Role of hepatic and intestinal cytochrome P450 3A and 2B6 in the metabolism, disposition, and miotic effects of methadone. *Clin Pharmacol Ther* 2004;76(3):250–269.
61. Moody D, et al. The involvement of cytochrome P450 3A4 in the N-demethylation of L-alpha-acetylmethadol (LAAM), norLAAM, and methadone. *Drug Metab Disp* 1997;25(12):1347–1353.
62. Perez de los Cobos J, et al. Association of CYP2D6 ultrarapid metabolizer genotype with deficient patient satisfaction regarding methadone maintenance treatment. *Drug Alcohol Depend* 2007;89(2–3):190–194.
63. Eap C, et al. Cytochrome P450 2D6 genotype and methadone steady-state concentrations. *J Clin Psychopharmacol* 2001;21(2):229–234.
64. Wong S, et al. Pharmacogenomics as an aspect of molecular autopsy for forensic pathology/toxicology: Does genotyping CYP 2D6 serve as an adjunct for certifying methadone toxicity? *J Forensic Sci* 2003;48(6):1406–1415.
65. Totah R, et al. Enantiomeric metabolic interactions and stereoselective human methadone metabolism. *J Pharmacol Exp Ther* 2007;321(1):389–399.
66. Eap C, Buclin T, Baumann P. Interindividual variability of the clinical pharmacokinetics of methadone: implications for the treatment of opioid dependence. *Clin Pharm* 2002;41(14):1153–1193.
67. Walker P, Klein D, Kasza L. High dose methadone and ventricular arrhythmias: a report of three cases. *Pain* 2003;103:321–324.
68. Krantz M, et al. Torsade de pointes associated with very-high-dose methadone. *Ann Intern Med* 2002;137(6):501–504.
69. Katchman A, et al. Influence of opioid agonists on cardiac human ether-a-go-go-related gene K(+) currents. *J Pharmacol Exp Ther* 2002;303(2):688–694.
70. Eap C, et al. Stereoselective block of hERG channel by (S)-methadone and QT interval prolongation in CYP2B6 slow metabolizers. *Clin Pharmacol Ther* 2007;81(5):719–728.
71. Fanoe S, et al. Syncope and QT prolongation among patients treated with methadone for heroin dependence in the city of Copenhagen. *Heart* 2007;93(9):1051–1055.
72. Martell B, et al. Impact of methadone treatment on cardiac repolarization and conduction in opioid users. *Am J Cardiol* 2005;95:915–918.
73. Peles E, et al. Corrected-QT intervals as related to methadone dose and serum level in methadone maintenance treatment (MMT) patients: a cross-sectional study. *Addiction* 2007;102(2):289–300.
74. Wedam E, et al. QT-Interval effects of methadone, levomethadyl, and buprenorphine in a randomized trial. *Arch Intern Med* 2007;167(22):2469–2475.
75. Krantz M, et al. Physician awareness of the cardiac effects of methadone:results of a national survey. *J Addict Dis* 2007;26(4):79–85.

76. Ehret G, et al. Drug-induced long QT syndrome in injection drug users receiving methadone:high frequency in hospitalized patients and risk factors. *Arch Intern Med* 2006;166(12):1280–1287.
77. Goldberger B, Frost-Pineda K, Gold M. Methadone related deaths exceed heroin in the state of Florida. *J Addict Dis* 2003;22(2): 140(34A).
78. Center for Substance Abuse Treatment. *Methadone-Associated Mortality: Report of a National Assessment, May 8-9, 2003.* SAMHSA Publication No. 04-3904. Rockville, MD: Center for Substance Abuse Treatment, Substance Abuse and Mental Health Services Administration, 2004.
79. Heinemann A, et al. Methadone-related fatalities in Hamburg 1990–1999: implications for quality standards in maintenance treatment? *Forensic Sci Int* 2000;113(1-3):449–455.
80. Ward M, Barry J. Opiate-related deaths in Dublin. *Ir J Med Sci* 2001;170(1):35–37.
81. Williamson PA, et al. Methadone-related overdose deaths in South Australia, 1984–1994. How safe is methadone prescribing? *Med J Aust* 1997;166(6):302–305.
82. Fraser HF, Isbell H. Actions and addiction liabilities of alpha-acetylmethadol in man. *J Pharmacol Exp Ther* 1952;105:458–465.
83. Fudala PJ, et al. Levomethadyl acetate (LAAM) for the treatment of opioid dependence: a multisite, open-label study of LAAM safety and an evaluation of the product labeling and treatment regulations. *J Maint Addict* 1997;1(2):9–39.
84. Marion IJ, ed. *LAAM in the treatment of opiate addiction.* Treatment Improvement Protocol (TIP) Series #22. Rockville, MD: Center for Substance Abuse Treatment, U.S. Department of Health and Human Services, 1995.
85. Mendelson J, et al. Buprenorphine and naloxone interactions in opiate-dependent volunteers. *Clin Pharmacol Ther* 1996;60(1):105–114.
86. Mendelson J, et al. Buprenorphine and naloxone combinations: the effects of three dose ratios in morphine-stabilized, opiate-dependent volunteers. *Psychopharmacology (Berlin)* 1999;141(1):37–46.
87. DATA 2000 http://buprenorphine.samhsa.gov/fulllaw.html. Public law 106–310, title XXXV, Section 3502 of the Children's Health Act of 2000.
88. Fiellin DA, et al. Consensus statement on office-based treatment of opioid dependence using buprenorphine. *J Subst Abuse Treat* 2004;27: 153–159.
89. Leonardi C, et al. Multi-centre observational study of buprenorphine use in 32 Italian drug addiction centres. *Drug Alcohol Depend* 2008; 94(1-3):125–132.
90. Zubieta J, et al. Buprenorphine-induced changes in Mu-opioid receptor availability in male heroin-dependent volunteers: a preliminary study. *Neuropsychopharmacology* 2000;23(3):326–334.
91. Amass L, Kamien J, Mikulich S. Efficacy of daily and alternate-day dosing regimens with the combination buprenorphine-naloxone tablet. *Drug Alcohol Dep*end 2000;58:143–152.
92. Amass L, Kamien J, Mikulich S. Thrice-weekly supervised dosing with the combination buprenorphine-naloxone tablet is preferred to daily supervised dosing by opioid-dependent humans. *Drug Alcohol Depend* 2001;61:173–181.
93. Bruce R, et al. Pharmacokinetic interactions between buprenorphine and antiretroviral medications. *Clin Infect Dis* 2006;43(Suppl 4): S216–S223.
94. Krantz M, Garcia J, Mehler P. Effects of buprenorphine on cardiac repolarization in a patient with methadone-related torsade de pointes. *Pharmacotherapy* 2005;25(4):611–614.
95. Kissin W, et al. Experiences of a national sample of qualified addiction specialists who have and have not prescribed buprenorphine for opioid dependence. *J Addict Dis* 2006;25(4):91–103.
96. Aitken C, Higgs P, Hellard M. Buprenorphine injection in Melbourne, Australia—an update. *Drug Alcohol Rev* 2008;27(2):197–199.
97. Hakansson A, et al. Buprenorphine misuse among heroin and amphetamine users in Malmo, Sweden: purpose of misuse and route of administration. *Eur Addict Res* 2007;13(4):207–215.
98. Cicero T, Surratt H, Inciardi J. Use and misuse of buprenorphine in the management of opioid addiction. *J Opioid Manag* 2007;3(6): 302–308.
99. Johnson RE, Chutuape MA, et al. A comparison of levomethadyl acetate, buprenorphine and methadone for opioid dependence. *N Engl J Med* 2000;343: 1290–1295.
100. Ling W, et al. A controlled trial comparing buprenorphine and methadone maintenance in opioid dependence. *Arch Gen Psychiatry* 1996;53(5):401–407.
101. Mattick R, et al. Buprenorphine maintenance versus placebo or methadone maintenance for opioid dependence. *Cochrane Database Syst Rev* 2004:CD002207.
102. Kakko J, et al. A stepped care strategy using buprenorphine and methadone versus conventional methadone maintenance in heroin dependence: a randomized controlled trial. *Am J Psychiatry* 2007; 164(5):797–803.
103. Jones H, et al. Buprenorphine versus methadone in the treatment of pregnant opioid-dependent patients: effects on the neonatal abstinence syndrome. *Drug Alcohol Depend* 2005;79(1):1–10.
104. Lejeune C, et al. Prospective multicenter observational study of 260 infants born to 259 opiate-dependent mothers on methadone or high-dose buprenophine substitution. *Drug Alcohol Depend* 2006;82(3): 250–257.
105. Salsitz EA, et al. Methadone medical maintenance (MMM): treating chronic opioid dependence in private medical practice—a summary report (1983–1998). *Mount Sinai J Med* 2000;67(5–6):388–397.
106. Des Jarlais DC, et al. Medical maintenance feasibility study. *NIDA Res Monogr* 1985;58(10):101–110.
107. Novick DM, et al. Methadone maintenance patients in general medical practice. A preliminary report. *JAMA* 1988;259(22):3299–3302.
108. Novick DM, et al. Outcomes of treatment of socially rehabilitated methadone maintenance patients in physicians' offices (medical maintenance): follow-up at three and a half to nine and a fourth years. *J Gen Intern Med* 1994;9(3):127–130.
109. Novick DM, Joseph H. The treatment of chronic opiate dependence in general medical practice. *J Subst Abuse Treat* 1991;8:233–239.
110. Senay EC, et al. Medical maintenance: a pilot study. *J Addict Dis* 1993;12(4):59–76.
111. Senay EC, et al. Medical maintenance: an interim report. *J Addict Dis* 1994;13(3):65–69.
112. Fiellin DA, et al. Methadone maintenance in primary care: a randomized controlled trial. *JAMA* 2001;286(14):1724–1731.
113. Compton P, Charuvastra VC, Ling W. Pain intolerance in opioid-maintained former opiate addicts: effect of long-acting maintenance agent. *Drug Alcohol Depend* 2001;63:139–146.
114. Compton P, McCaffrey M. Controlling pain: treating acute pain in addicted patients. *Nursing* 2001;2001(1):17.
115. Koppert W, et al. Different profiles of buprenorphine-induced analgesia and antihyperalgesia in a human pain model. *Pain* 2005;118(1–2): 15–22.
116. Rosenblum A. Prevalence and characteristics of chronic pain among chemically dependent patients in methadone maintenance and residential treatment facilities. *JAMA* 2003;289(18):2370–2378.
117. Brands B, et al. Prescription opioid abuse in patients presenting for methadone maintenance treatment. *Drug Alcohol Depend* 2004; 73:199–207.
118. Wallach RC, Jerez E, Blinick G. Pregnancy and menstrual function in narcotics addicts treated with methadone. The Methadone Maintenance Treatment Program. *Am J Obstet Gynaecol* 1969;105(8): 1226–1229.
119. Finnegan LP, et al. Neonatal abstinence syndrome: assement and management. *Addict Dis:* 1975;2(1): 141–158.
120. McCarthy J, et al. High-dose methadone maintenance in pregnancy: maternal and neonatal outcomes. *Am J Obstet Gynaecol* 2005;193(3): 606–610.
121. McCarthy J, et al. Outcomes of neonates conceived on methadone maintenance therapy. *J Subst Abuse Treat* 2007, in press.
122. Jansson L, Velez M, Harrow C. Methadone maintenance and lactation: a review of the literature and current management guidelines. *J Hum Lact* 2004;20(1):62–71.

123. Luty J, Nikolaou V, Bearn J. Is opiate detoxification unsafe in pregnancy? *J Subst Abuse Treat* 2003;24(4):363–367.
124. Substance Abuse and Mental Health Services Administration, Office of Applied Studies. *Treatment Episode Data Set (TEDS) Highlights—2005: National Admissions to Substance Abuse Treatment Services*, 2006. http://www.oas.samhsa.gov/TEDS2K6highlights/toc.cfm.
125. Smolyakov R, et al. Streptococcal septic arthritis and necrotizing fasciitis in an intravenous drug user couple sharing needles. *Israel Medical Association Journal* 2002;4: 302–303.
126. Werner SB, et al. Wound botulism in California, 1951–1998: recent epidemic in heroin injectors. *Clin Infect Dis* 2000;31:1018–1024.
127. Anderson MW, Sharma K, Feeney CM. Wound botulism associated with black tar heroin. *Acad Emerg Med* 1997;4:805–809.
128. Hagan H, Jarlais DCD. HIV and HCV infection among injecting drug users. *Mount Sinai J Med* 2000;67(5-6):423–428.
129. Appel PW, Joseph H, Richman B. Causes and rates of death among methadone maintenance patients before and after the onset of the HIV/AIDS epidemic. *Mount Sinai J Med* 2000;67(5-6):444–451.
130. Sullivan L, et al. Decreasing international HIV transmission: the role of expanding access to opioid agonist therapies for injection drug users. *Addiction* 2005;100(2):150–158.
131. Gowing L, et al. Brief report: methadone treatment of injecting opioid users for prevention of HIV infection. *J Gen Intern Med* 2006;21(2): 193–195.
132. Moatti J, et al. Adherence to HAART in French HIV-infected injecting drug users: the contribution of buprenorphine drug maintenance treatment. The Manif 2000 study group. *AIDS* 2000;14(2):151–155.
133. Gourevitch MN, Friedland GH. Interactions between methadone and medications used to treat HIV infection: A review. *Mount Sinai J Med* 2000;67(5-6):429–436.
134. Haug N, et al. HAART adherence strategies for methadone clients who are HIV-positive: a treatment manual for implementing contingency management and medication coaching. *Behav Mod* 2006;30(6): 752–781.
135. Novick DM. The impact of hepatitis C virus infection on methadone maintenance treatment. *Mount Sinai J Med* 2000;67(5-6):437–443.
136. Tong MJ, El-Farra NS. Clinical sequelae of hepatitis C acquired from injection drug use. *West J Med* 1996;164:399–404.
137. Strauss S, et al. Drug treatment program patients' hepatitis C virus (HCV) education needs and their use of available HCV education services. *Health Serv Res* 2007;7:39.
138. Galindo L, et al. Education by peers is the key to success. *Int J Drug Policy* 2007;18(5):411–416.
139. Koch M, Banys P. Liver transplantation and opioid dependence. *JAMA* 2001;285:1056–1058.
140. Sylvestre D. Treating hepatitic c in methadone maintenance patients: an interim analysis. *Drug Alcohol Depend* 2002;67(2):117–123.
141. Regier DA, et al. Comorbidity of mental disorders with alcohol and other drug abuse. *JAMA* 1990;264(19):2511–2518.
142. Kessler RC, et al. Lifetime and 12 month prevalence of DSM-III-R psychiatric disorders in the United States. *Arch Gen Psychiatry* 1994; 51:8–19.
143. Brooner R, et al. Psychiatric and substance use comorbidity among treatment-seeking opioid abusers. *Arch Gen Psychiatry* 1997;54(1):71–80.
144. Gossop M, Marsden J, Stewart D. Remission of psychiatric symptoms among drug misusers after drug dependence treatment. *J Nerv Ment Dis* 2006;194(11):826–832.
145. Nunes EV, Sullivan MA, Levin FR. Treatment of depression in patients with opiate dependence. *Biol Psychiatry* 2004;56(10):793–802.
146. Gelkopf M, et al. Does psychiatric comorbidity affect drug abuse treatment outcome? A prospective assessment of drug abuse, treatment tenure and infectious diseases in an Israeli methadone maintenance clinic. *Isr J Psychiatry Relate Sci* 2006;43(2):126–136.
147. Woody GE, et al. Psychotherapy for substance abuse. *Psychiatric Clin North Am* 1986;9(3):547–562.
148. Rounsaville BJ, Kleber HD. Untreated opiate addicts: how do they differ from those seeking treatment? *Arch Gen Psychiatry* 1985;42: 1072–1077.
149. Kosten TR, Rounsaville BJ, Kleber HD. A 2.5 year follow-up of depression, life crises, and treatment effects on abstinence among opioid addicts. *Arch Gen Psychiatry* 1986;43:733–738.
150. Musselman DL, Kell MJ. Prevalence and improvement in psychopathology in opioid dependent patients participating in methadone maintenance. *J Addict Dis* 1995;14(3):67–82.
151. Clark HW, et al. Violent traumatic events and drug abuse severity. *J Subst Abuse Treat* 2001;20:121–127.
152. Trafton JA, Minkel J, Humphreys K. Opioid substitution treatment reduces substance use equivalently in patients with and without posttraumatic stress disorder. *J Stud Alcohol* 2006;67(2):228–235.
153. Zlotnick C, et al. A cognitive-behavioral treatment for incarcerated women with substance abuse disorder and posttraumatic stress disorder: findings from a pilot study. *J Subst Abuse Treat* 2003;25(2):99–105.
154. Peles E, Schreiber S, Adelson M. Variables associated with perceived sleep disorders in methadone maintenance treatment (MMT) patients. *Drug Alcohol Depend* 2006;82(2):103–110.
155. O'Brien CP, Woody GE, McLellan AT. Psychotherapeutic approaches in the treatment of drug abuse. *NIDA Res Monogr* 1984;51(38):129–138.
156. Rounsaville BJ, et al. The heterogeneity of psychiatric diagnosis in treated opiate addicts. *Arch Gen Psychiatry* 1982;39:161–169.
157. Comfort A. Morphine as an antipsychotic. *Lancet* 1977;2(8035):448–449.
158. Verebey K., ed. Opioids in mental illness: theories, clinical observations, and treatment possibilities. *Ann N Y Acad Sci* 1982;398:1–510.
159. Ball SA. Comparing individual therapies for personality disordered opioid dependent patients. *J Personal Dis* 2007;21(3):305–321.
160. American Psychiatric Association. *Diagnostic and statistical manual of mental disorders*, 4th ed. Washington DC: American Psychiatric Association, 1994.
161. Amato L, et al. Psychosocial combined with agonist maintenance treatments versus agonist maintenance treatments alone for treatment of opioid dependence. *Cochrane Database Syst Rev* 2004(4):CD004147.
162. McLellan AT, et al. The effects of psychosocial services in substance abuse treatment. *JAMA* 1993;269(15):1953–1959.
163. Fiellin D, et al. Counseling plus buprenorphine-naloxone maintenance therapy for opioid dependence. *N Engl J Med* 2006;355(4):365–374.
164. Zweben JE. Counseling issues in methadone maintenance treatment. *J Psychoactive Drugs* 1991;23(2):177–190.
165. Ball J, Ross A. *The effectiveness of methadone maintenance treatment*. New York: Springer-Verlag, 1991.
166. Miller WR, et al. *Motivational Enhancement Therapy Manual*. Project Match Monograph Series #2. Rockville, MD: U.S. Department of Health and Human Services, 1994.
167. Miller WR, Rollnick S. *Motivational interviewing: preparing people to change addictive behavior*. New York: Guilford Press, 1991.
168. Epstein DH, Preston KL. *Opioids*. In: Higgins ST, Silverman K, Heil SH (eds.). *Contingency management in substance abuse treatment*. New York: The Guilford Press, 2008.
169. Batki SL, et al. *Medication-assisted treatment for opioid addiction in opioid treatment programs*. Treatment Improvement Protocol, vol. 43. Rockville, MD: U.S. Department of Health and Human Services, 2005.
170. Weisner C, et al. Integrating primary medical care with addiction treatment: a randomized controlled trial. *JAMA* 2001;286(14):1715–1723.
171. Friedmann P, et al. Effect of primary medical care on addiction and medical severity in substance abuse treatment programs. *J Gen Intern Med* 2003;18(1):1–8.
172. Saitz R, et al. Primary medical care and reductions in addiction severity: a prospective cohort study. *Addiction* 2005;100(1):70–78.
173. Saxon A, et al. Randomized trial of onsite versus referral primary medical care for veterans in addictions treatment. *Med Care* 2006;44(4): 334–342.
174. McLellan AT, et al. Similarity of outcome predictors across opiate, cocaine, and alcohol treatments:role of treatment services. *J Consult Clin Psychol* 1994;62(6):1141–1158.
175. McLellan AT, et al. Problem-service 'matching' in addiction treatment. A prospective study in 4 programs (see comments). *Arch Gen Psychiatry* 1997;54(8):730–735.

176. McLellan AT, et al. Supplemental social services improve outcomes in public addiction treatment. *Addiction* 1998;93(10):1489–1499.
177. Hoffman JA, Moolchan ET. The phases-of-treatment model for methadone maintenance: implementation and evaluation. *J Psychoactive Drugs* 1994;26(2):181–197.
178. Kissin W, et al. Experiences of a national sample of qualified addiction specialists who have and have not prescribed buprenorphine for opioid dependence. *J Addict Dis* 2006;25(4):91–103.
179. Dole VP. Hazards of process regulations. The example of methadone maintenance. *JAMA* 1992;267(16):2234–2235.
180. Dole VP. On federal regulation of methadone treatment [see comments]. *JAMA* 1995;274(16):1307.
181. Center for Substance Abuse Treatment, Methadone-Associated Mortality: report of national assessment, May 8-9, 2003. Center for Substance Abuse Treatment, Substance Abuse and Mental Health Services Administration: Rockville, MD. SAMHSA 04-3904.

CHAPTER 50

Andrew J. Saxon, MD

Special Issues in Office-Based Opioid Treatment

Current interest in office-based approaches to the treatment of opioid addiction springs from a recognition that the numbers and needs of opioid-dependent individuals continue to overwhelm the capacity of the existing treatment system. Many such individuals cannot gain access to opioid agonist therapy, which is the most effective intervention yet devised for this disorder (1). Meanwhile, indicators of opioid-related health care costs and criminal justice contacts continue to surge (2,3), as do the number of opioid-related deaths (4). Many opioid-dependent individuals also have unique and serious medical and psychiatric problems that the existing treatment system cannot always address and that contribute to morbidity and mortality (1). Office-based opioid therapy (OBOT) offers one potential avenue and has made substantial inroads in the drive to ameliorate this unsatisfactory situation.

This chapter reviews some of the historic and regulatory events that shaped our current treatment system and account for some of the ongoing gaps in services for opioid-dependent individuals. Office-based treatment effectively fills some of these gaps, in part because office-based treatment encompasses two distinct treatment paradigms. First, OBOT offers a less structured, more flexible, and more personalized form of intervention for opioid-dependent patients who have succeeded in the traditional treatment system of opioid agonist clinics licensed by the Center for Substance Abuse Treatment of the Substance Abuse and Mental Health Services Administration but who need to continue in pharmacotherapy. Second, OBOT provides an alternative route of entry into treatment for opioid-dependent individuals who, for a variety of reasons, have not had access to adequate treatment or to reengagement in treatment for individuals who have not achieved their goals in the traditional treatment system.

A summary of the evidence for the benefits of transferring selected, stable methadone-treated patients into office-based settings precedes a synopsis of efforts to apply and evaluate the office-based approach for less stable patients newly entering treatment. Results of these investigations of office-based treatment then guide a discussion of clinical issues pertinent to conducting office-based treatment with opioid-dependent patients.

EPIDEMIOLOGIC AND REGULATORY ISSUES

During the first few years of the 21st century, the purity of heroin sold in the United States continued to increase, while the price decreased (5). Heroin-related emergency department visits have increased from 33,900 in 1990 to 164,572 in 2005 (6). Heroin-related overdose deaths reported to the Drug Abuse Warning Network increased from 2,300 in 1991 to 4,330 in 1998 (7,8). Heroin overdose deaths are no longer reported on a nationwide basis but rather by metropolitan and state areas. As of 2003, these death were still occurring in large numbers (4). Overdose accounts for only half the overall observed mortality in heroin users, who exhibit mortality rates 6 to 20 times those of age-matched populations (9,10).

A subset of the heroin-using population engages in repeated criminal activity (11). The Arrestee Drug Abuse Monitoring Program (12) provides urine toxicology results for the year 2003 for 22,666 male arrestees in 39 sites around the country and 3,664 female arrestees in 25 sites. These data show that, in 2003, adult male arrestees tested positive for recent opiate use at a median site rate of 5.8%. Female arrestees tested positive for recent opiate use at a rate of 6.6%.

The past decade has also seen a surge in the illicit use of and problems with prescription opioid medications. In 2005, the number (196,225) of emergency room visits related to nonmedical use of prescription opioids exceeded the number for heroin (6). Large numbers of overdoses on prescription opioids have also been noted (4). In 2006, as many people abused OxyContin in the past month (0.3 million) as used heroin, and 5.2 million abused some type of pain reliever (primarily hydrocodone and oxycodone) in the past month (13).

Despite these trends, most opioid-dependent individuals cannot access adequate treatment services. In 2005, approximately 254,000 individuals entered treatment for heroin dependence, but only 30% received medication-assisted treatment. Similarly, 67,000 entered treatment for dependence on other opioids, but only 20% received medication-assisted treatment. These data reflect a circumstance that has been prevalent throughout the past 100 years.

The mobilization of office-based treatment as a response to this problem does not represent a true innovation but rather a return to a once commonly used strategy. Thousands of untreated opioid-dependent individuals also worried society in the early part of the 20th century. Before the Harrison Narcotic Act was enacted in 1914 (see Chapter 22, "Addiction Medicine in America: Its Birth and Early History (1750–1935) with a Modern Postscript"), no legal restrictions limited the right of physicians to prescribe opioid medications for the care of patients considered addicted. Although controversy raged then, as it does now, about how best to handle opioid-dependent individuals, many experts of that generation already had recognized the high likelihood that opioid-dependent patients would resume opioid use after enforced withdrawal. Physicians in many areas of the country thus viewed opioid addiction as a medical disorder; they advocated and practiced the ongoing prescribing of opioids from their offices as a reasonable and apparently useful way to manage the problem.

Most of these physicians conducted this part of their work in a responsible way. A minority may have allowed their practices to become conduits for controlled substances out of a profit motive without always providing adequate medical care. On the basis of a small number of reports of this type of inappropriate prescribing, concern about the safety and wisdom of prescribing opioids to opioid-dependent individuals increased in the medical profession itself as well as among regulators and the general public. In 1919, the U.S. Supreme Court ruled that the Harrison Act disallowed such prescribing to opioid-dependent individuals for "maintenance" purposes (14). This decision effectively ended the first era of office-based treatment for opioid addiction.

Such a wholesale shift in policy left patients without access to the opioids on which they depended. Many municipalities responded by creating publicly funded and administered opioid maintenance clinics (14). For example, when New York City experienced one of its waves of heroin addiction after World War I, a clinic under the auspices of the city health department treated 8000 heroin-dependent patients with prescribed heroin (15). These pioneer efforts at agonist pharmacotherapy ended within a few years when the Narcotic Division of the Federal Prohibition Unit shut down these maintenance clinics as violators of the Harrison Act (14). Thus, from the 1920s onward, physicians were actively discouraged from treating heroin-dependent individuals and, indeed, medical school curricula provided no training to physicians in this regard. In essence, opioid addiction was reconceptualized as a criminal justice rather than a medical problem. Convicted violators of federal narcotics laws caused an overload in the federal penal system, so Congress established federal narcotics hospitals at Lexington, KY, and Forth Worth, TX, in the 1930s. Despite high recidivism rates, these isolated facilities remained the only treatment option for opioid-dependent individuals until the advent of methadone maintenance 30 years later (14).

In some respects, the severance of opioid addiction treatment from the general practice of medicine actually was exaggerated in the 1970s when opioid agonist therapy, in the form of methadone maintenance, once again was permitted and, to some extent, promulgated. Federal methadone regulations (21 CFR Part 291) promulgated in 1972 and the Narcotic Addict Treatment Act of 1974 mandated a closed distribution system for methadone, with special licensing by both federal and state authorities. These regulations effectively made it illegal for physicians not associated with a licensed program to treat opioid-dependent patients with agonist pharmacotherapy in an office setting. Until very recently, a private physician would have to obtain an additional registration from the U.S. Drug Enforcement Administration, annual certification by the U.S. Department of Health and Human Services, and approval by state drug authorities to provide opioid agonist therapy (16). Only a small number of physicians around the country have been willing to negotiate this bureaucratic maze. As a result, the only option for patients who desired opioid agonist pharmacotherapy was to enroll in a specialized, licensed methadone treatment program. Once again, most practicing physicians were deprived of exposure to and experience in treating opioid-dependent patients.

The divergence between mainstream medicine and opioid addiction treatment has had some unfortunate consequences. Opioid addiction causes considerable medical morbidity (see Chapter 94, "Non-Opioid Treatments in the Management of Pain") as a consequence of drug effects and intravenous route of administration (17). Medical problems common in users of illicit opiates include infectious diseases such as pneumonia, tuberculosis, endocarditis, as well as sexually transmitted diseases (18); soft-tissue infections (19); bone and joint infections (20); central nervous system infections (21); and viral hepatitis (22), particularly hepatitis C (23). In addition, HIV infection and AIDS pose a massive problem among intravenous drug users (22,24). Non-infectious problems also typically occur in the lungs (25), the central and peripheral nervous systems (21), the vascular system (19), and the musculoskeletal system (19). Licensed opioid agonist treatment programs often lack the resources to provide comprehensive medical care (16), with the result that comorbid medical disorders may be unattended, delaying care and driving up its ultimate cost. Total health care costs related to heroin addiction have reached $1.2 billion annually (2).

Similarly, a high prevalence of Axis I psychiatric comorbidity, particularly mood and anxiety disorders, is seen among patients who are addicted to opioids (26,27), and licensed programs typically cannot provide the treatment these conditions require (16).

As the divide between general medical practice and opioid agonist treatment is bridged, patients have improved access to simultaneous care for these serious comorbid medical and psychiatric conditions.

Many potential patients who need and desire opioid agonist treatment and are willing to enroll in licensed programs cannot overcome the barriers to entry. Geography creates an impossible hurdle for some. Six states (Idaho, Mississippi, Montana, North Dakota, South Dakota, and Wyoming) do not offer licensed opioid agonist treatment. New Hampshire instituted its first program in 2000. West Virginia instituted its first program in 2001. Vermont instituted its first program in 2002. In states that do offer such programs, the licensed clinics, by virtue of economic necessity and neighborhood acceptance, tend to be sited primarily in urban locations (16,28). Even within larger metropolitan areas, specific neighborhoods or communities can bar licensed clinics (16,29). A few patients who reside in states or communities without opioid agonist clinics or in rural areas invest considerable effort in traveling to other states or cities to obtain treatment; most who cannot afford the time or cost simply must forgo it (28).

Inadequate treatment capacity creates another barrier for potential patients who do live in reasonable proximity to a licensed clinic (30). Many clinics have waiting lists that discourage potential patients from even attempting entry (31). Many more potential patients lack the financial resources to pay for their treatment (31). Although OBOT does not necessarily cost less than treatment in a licensed clinic, insurance companies and managed care organizations frequently reimburse at least some of the expense of physician office visits, particularly if comorbid conditions are addressed (30).

Finally, the very nature of licensed opioid agonist treatment clinics, with the potential to be recognized and stigmatized by passersby, waiting lines for medication administration, rigid attendance policies, and lack of privacy, deters some potential patients (32).

Many of the latter concerns pertain most directly to long-term, stable patients who have achieved a measure of rehabilitation in opioid agonist treatment. Such patients have ceased illicit drug use and, in most cases, have employment and family responsibilities (30,33). To make their schedules accommodate frequent clinic visits with waits for medication, to hold up their travel plans to obtain regulatory approval, and to bring them to a locale where unstable patients with residual drug use congregate may undermine rather than support their rehabilitation (30,33). In addition, many of these rehabilitated patients already have derived maximum benefit from counseling and other services available at licensed clinics. Moving stable patients out of the restrictive clinic setting while continuing their agonist pharmacotherapy would permit reallocation of clinic resources to patients who most need them.

Three important developments have now altered the landscape. Since March 2000, the licensed opioid agonist treatment programs can apply for exceptions so that stable, long-term patients can enter methadone medical maintenance and have visits to obtain medication less frequently than once per week. The Children's Health Act of 2000, signed into law in October 2000, included a provision waiving the requirements of the Narcotic Addict Treatment Act to permit qualified physicians to dispense or prescribe Schedule III, IV, or V narcotic drugs or combinations of such drugs that are approved by the FDA for the treatment of opioid addiction. This change, termed the *Drug Addiction Treatment Act*, allows qualified physicians to prescribe certain opioid agonist medications in an office-based setting. In October 2002, the FDA approved buprenorphine and buprenorphine + naloxone for the treatment of opioid dependence. These medications were placed in Schedule III and so are available for use in OBOT.

Clearly, our current treatment system cannot accommodate all the opioid-dependent individuals who want or need treatment. A century ago, office-based treatment met with some success in the United States. The current resurrection of office-based treatment has helped to remove geographic, social, and regulatory barriers for both new and rehabilitated patients and thus make opioid agonist treatment more widely available. Because of the divide between opioid agonist treatment and general medical practice, some physician education and training in management of opioid-dependent patients with pharmacotherapy has been necessary, has been delivered, and will continue to occur. Considerable data, described in detail in the subsequent text, offer instruction to physicians.

RESEARCH ISSUES

Research Related to Stable, Long-Term Patients in Office-Based Practice Several investigations have demonstrated the general safety and utility of transferring patients who have achieved specified degrees of stability through initial treatment in a licensed methadone clinic into an office-based setting (Table 50.1). The concept of transferring stable methadone patients to office-based practice originated with Novick and colleagues of New York City, who have used this procedure since 1983 and have documented their findings in several reports over the years (34–36).

A summary of their work describes outcomes for 158 total patients (33). Stringent standards were set for patients to participate in the program. Until 1996, patients were required to have completed 5 years of methadone treatment; this requirement subsequently was reduced to 4 years, though all patients actually accepted had at least 6 years of methadone treatment. At the time of entry, all participants had to have at least 3 years without illicit drug use, excessive alcohol use, or criminal activity. All had to verify employment or other productive activity. Additional criteria addressed the need for financial, emotional, and social stability. Patients who met the criteria were transferred from their methadone programs to the care of internists

TABLE 50.1 Studies of Stable Methadone-Treated Patients Transferred to Office-Based Opioid Therapy

Author	Year	Method	Requirements for entry	N	Methadone dose (take-home)	Protocol retention	Use of illicit opiates	Use of other illicit substances
Salsitz et al.	2000	Naturalistic program evaluation	Employment; 4–5 years on methadone; 3 years no illicit use	158	Mean = 60 mg (30-day supply)	83.5%; median retention = 13.8 years	None	15/158 excessive cocaine use
Schwartz et al.	1999	Naturalistic program evaluation	Employment; 5 years on methadone; 5 years no illicit use	21	Mean = 71.4 mg (28-day supply)	71.4% over 12 years	None	2/21-1 cocaine positive UA;1/21-1 positive barb UA
Merrill	2005	Naturalistic program evaluation	1 year on methadone; 1 year no illicit use; responsible with take-home medications	30	Mean = 63 mg (30-day supply)	93.3% 12 months	445 of 449 (99%) of collected specimens negative. Type of positive not specified.	445 of 449 (99%) of collected specimens negative. Type of positive not specified
Senay et al.	1993	Randomized clinical trial: medical mainten-ance vs. control	Employment; 1 year on methadone; 6 months no illicit use	130	N/A (14-day supply)	73% reached 1 year for both conditions	2 experi-mental 1 control	14 experi-mental; 8 control
Fiellin et al.	2001	Randomized clinical trial: office-based vs. clinic treatment	Stable income, > 1 year on methadone; 1 year free of illicit opioid use; no dependence on other substances	22 office; 24 standard	Mean = 69 mg office (7-day supply); mean =70 mg standard (2–7 day supply)	82% office; 79% standard over 6 months	55% office; 42% standard	Cocaine use: 27% office; 25% standard
King et al.	2006	Randomized clinical trial: office-based vs. monthly clinic pick-up vs. clinic	Employment; 1 year on methadone; 1 year free of illicit substance use;2 years of no problems	32 office; 33 monthly pick-up; 27 routine clinic care	Mean = 65 mg (28-day supply vs. 3–7 day supply)	92% office; 79% monthly clinic; 82% routine clinic over 12 months	0.4% office; 2.3% monthly clinic; 1.3% routine clinic. Type of substance not specified.	0.4% office; 2.3% monthly clinic; 1.3% routine clinic. Type of substance not specified.

or family physicians in a hospital-based practice. The physicians, most of whom had little familiarity with treating opioid addiction, received specific training from physicians with experience in methadone agonist treatment. The average methadone dose at entry was 60 mg/day. Patients attended two office visits in the first month and then advanced to a monthly reporting and dosing schedule. At each office visit, they provided a specimen for urine toxicology screening and took a dose of methadone under observation to confirm tolerance. They received annual physical examinations from their office-based provider along with routine medical care as needed.

To remain in compliance with the office-based program, patients had to avoid methadone misuse or loss, avoid illicit drug use, attend all appointments, pay fees, and maintain acceptable office comportment. Only 26 patients (16.5%) ever failed to meet these standards, 15 for uncontrollable use of cocaine and 11 for other violations. Eighteen of the "failed patients" returned to their clinics of origin. Patients had a projected median retention time of 13.8 years in office-based treatment. During the years of this investigation, 12 subjects voluntarily and successfully tapered off methadone. Of 99 active patients, 27 required dose increases, while 10 achieved dose reductions.

A retrospective analysis detected several differences between successful and unsuccessful office-based patients. Successful patients were more likely to be married or in stable relationships, were more likely to have had multiple prior treatment episodes in traditional methadone programs, and had more total years of treatment in traditional methadone programs before entering office-based treatment.

A similar, though smaller, uncontrolled trial was conducted in Baltimore by Schwartz and colleagues (30). The sample consisted of 21 patients enrolled during a 4-month period in 1985 and 1986. This program required that patients have at least 5 years' documented abstinence from illicit drug use in a traditional methadone program and a record of no alcohol misuse. Patients also were required to have self-supporting employment and emotional and social stability. Those who used psychotropic medications for psychiatric disorders were excluded. All patients transferred to the private office practice were under the care of a single physician. For the first 6 months, patients visited the office every 2 weeks, at which time they gave a urine specimen, had a brief interview with the physician, and received a 14-day supply of methadone. They subsequently advanced to visits every 28 days and a 28-day supply of medication. Only minor medical problems were addressed by the primary practitioner, with most health care services delivered by outside referral. Average methadone dose over the course of the project was 71.4 mg/day. To remain in compliance with the office-based program, patients had to avoid methadone misuse or loss, have accurate return of outstanding medication doses during a "call-back" procedure, avoid illicit drug or alcohol use, attend all appointments, and avoid legal problems leading to arrest.

During 12 years of follow-up, six patients (28.6%) failed to comply and were transferred back to their original methadone program: two for legal problems, three for positive urine tests, and one for a combination of problems. Of all urine specimens collected, only 0.5% showed any positive results. Not a single patient failed any of the 65 random medication call-backs conducted.

A third uncontrolled trial of the transfer of stable clinic-treated patients to an office-based setting was conducted in Seattle (37). The two programs described earlier gained permission to provide methadone treatment outside the established guidelines by obtaining an Investigational New Drug approval by the FDA to conduct research. The Seattle program was the first to obtain extensive FDA waivers to establish a clinical program allowing stabilized patients to receive methadone in a medical setting, with extended take-home privileges. Thirty-one patients who attended the licensed methadone clinic no more often than three times a week and who had 12 months of clinical stability (demonstrating responsibility with take-home medication, no urine drug tests positive for illicit drugs, consistent clinic attendance, and psychiatric stability) were transferred to an internal medicine clinic in a public hospital for primary medical care and methadone treatment. General internal medicine specialists cared for the patients after attending several training sessions on opioid addiction and agonist therapy. Ongoing counseling beyond physician visits was not required but was available through the licensed clinic. Trained pharmacists dispensed the medication through a satellite hospital pharmacy in the medical clinic.

Patients who demonstrated stability in office-based care could be advanced to monthly medication pick-ups. Subjects supplied monthly urine toxicology specimens and had to comply with periodic medication call-backs. Patients who required intensive monitoring or treatment could be returned immediately to the licensed methadone clinic. Twelve-month results showed that 28 of 30 patients were still in office-based treatment, with two patients choosing to leave the program voluntarily. Only two patients provided any drug-containing urine toxicology specimens, and 99% of collected specimens were negative.

An additional recent retrospective study of 127 methadone patients transferred to an office-based setting had similar positive results (38).

Although the investigations described certainly suggest that most highly stable methadone patients can safely transfer to office-based care, the lack of control groups in these open trials precludes conclusions about whether fewer subjects would deteriorate if they remained in traditional methadone clinics. A few controlled investigations of stable methadone patients in office-based practice have been completed. The largest of these controlled trials, although a very worthwhile study that addressed many of the concerns pertinent to office-based practice, did not represent, in the strictest sense, a trial of office-based practice because of the methodology employed. In the study, Senay and colleagues (39) worked with a group of 130 patients who had received at least 1 year of methadone treatment, who had 6 months of negative urine toxicologies, steady employment or productive activity, no arrests, general program compliance, and no current legal involvement. Patients were assigned randomly to either an experimental (two of three subjects) or a control condition (one of three subjects). The experimental condition consisted of a monthly visit with a physician; observed ingestion of methadone every 14 days, with 13 take-home doses for use between visits; three random urine toxicology screens per year; and random medication call-backs. Patients were required to attend at least one counseling session and leave one nonrandom urine specimen per month in their clinic of origin. Thus, the experimental subjects did continue ongoing contact with their traditional methadone programs, a situation not typical of most office-based paradigms. The control subjects remained in their clinics of origin for 6 months and then entered the experimental program. The report of this study did not provide methadone dose levels. Subjects continued in either the experimental or control conditions if they provided negative urine specimens, paid their fees, and refrained from criminal activity or lateness. During the first 6 months, 89% of experimental and 85% of control subjects remained in the program. At 1 year, 73% of both groups remained. Of the patients removed from the program, 70% were for positive urine specimens, and 30% were for other causes. Removal rates did not differ by condition. The report of this study does not mention the results of the medication call-backs. The advantages of this study derive from its randomized, controlled methodology and from its enrollment of subjects who had far less time in traditional methadone programs and less stable time than did the subjects in the studies described earlier by Salsitz and colleagues (33) or Schwartz and colleagues (30). Obviously, subjects of the type in the Senay (39) study comprise a much larger proportion of typical methadone clinic populations than do the exceedingly stable patients in the other studies. The disadvantage of the Senay study resides in the fact that all subjects continued some attendance and counseling at their clinics of origin. Hence, the study really only demonstrates that most moderately stable methadone patients can manage adequately with observed ingestion of medication only once every 14 days and monthly contact with a physician, but it conveys little about office-based practice independent of a traditional methadone program.

Two small controlled studies have, however, assessed office-based practice for stable methadone patients without confounds from ongoing clinic involvement. In one study (40), 46 patients already receiving methadone agonist therapy at a licensed treatment program were randomly assigned to be transferred to office-based treatment with an internal medicine physician (n = 22) or to remain in standard clinic treatment (n = 24). Eligibility requirements for participants included more than a year of methadone treatment; 1 year's abstinence from use of illicit opiates, as reflected by negative monthly random urine specimens; no current evidence of dependence on other substances; no significant medical or psychiatric conditions that could be compromised by the transfer; a source of legal income; and stable housing. Of note is the fact that only slightly more than 10% of the clinic's total population met these criteria, which clearly are less stringent than those employed in the studies by Salsitz and colleagues (33) and Schwartz and colleagues (30). The average methadone dose for the subjects assigned to the office-based treatment condition was 69 mg. The average dose for those assigned to remain in standard clinic treatment was 70 mg. The six physicians who provided the office-based treatment and their staff members received training in management of patients on opioid agonist therapy.

Subjects assigned to office-based treatment received a weekly supply of methadone from the physician's office. They had an initial 1-hour office visit in which a history and physical were performed. They subsequently met with their physician monthly. Subjects assigned to remain in standard clinic treatment came to the clinic one to three times a week to pick up their methadone. All subjects provided monthly urine specimens and quarterly hair specimens for toxicologic analysis. If a patient's urine was positive for opiates or cocaine or negative for methadone, a repeat urine specimen was obtained within 1 week. If this repeat specimen also tested positive for opiates or cocaine or negative for methadone, patients were considered out of compliance with the protocol, removed from the study, and transferred back to routine care. During a 6-month follow-up interval, 18% of the office-based subjects and 21% of the standard clinic subjects violated the study criteria and were transferred back to routine care. By either urinalysis, hair toxicology, or self-report, 55% of office-based and 42% of standard clinic subjects had evidence of illicit opiate use, and 27% and 25%, respectively, had evidence of cocaine use.

Hair toxicology testing at baseline in this study allowed for some valuable observations. Though all subjects had submitted 12 consecutive negative monthly urine specimens before entering the study, hair testing found evidence of illicit drug use in the preceding 90 days by 44% of the subjects. Though the failure of monthly urine testing to detect all substance use does not come as a surprise (41), positive hair testing at baseline did act as a predictor of substance use during follow-up. Among those with positive hair toxicology at baseline, 90% had evidence of illicit use during follow-up. In contrast, only 20% of those with negative baseline hair toxicology had such evidence at follow-up.

In another controlled study (42,43), 98 subjects who were receiving methadone treatment were randomly assigned to one of three conditions: (i) medication pick-up every 28 days in a physician's office away from the licensed treatment program, (ii) medication pick-up every 28 days, with a monthly physician visit at the licensed treatment clinic, or (iii) continued routine clinic care, with medication pick-up once or twice a week at the clinic. Of those randomly assigned, six declined further participation after receiving their treatment assignment and were terminated from the study. Eligibility requirements for participants included continuous methadone treatment and absence of any positive monthly urine specimens over the preceding 12 months, full-time employment, and no failed medication recalls or problems handling medication over the preceding 24 months. About 25% of patients from two different clinics met these criteria. The average methadone dose was 65 mg/day. The four physicians who provided the office-based treatment had previous experience treating patients with methadone agonist therapy. All subjects received a single 20-minute counseling session per month. The 28-day pick-up subjects received counseling from their physicians. The routine care subjects received counseling from clinic counselors. All subjects submitted to a monthly random medication recall procedure. All subjects gave two urine specimens per month. The 28-day pick-up subjects provided a routine, nonrandom specimen at the time of their scheduled physician visits and also produced a random urine specimen at the time of the medication recall. The routine care patients gave a routine random urine specimen once a month, just as did the other clinic patients, and provided a second random specimen at the time of their medication recall. An innovative stepped-care counseling intensification procedure was used so that subjects who exhibited problems such as a positive urine specimen or failed medication recall could be transferred back to the clinic for five weekly medication visits until they again attained stability. They would then resume treatment in their assigned research condition. Treatment retention at 12 months was 82% for routine clinic care, 79% for clinic-based medical maintenance, and 92% for office-based medical maintenance. Only 12 patients submitted positive urine specimens over 12 months (9 had one positive, 2 had two positives; and 1 had repeated positive specimens for cocaine and benzodiazepines), while nearly 30% of patients failed at least one medication recall. These problems resulted in 33 subjects' (36%) entering intensified counseling. The three groups did not differ significantly in the likelihood that patients would experience any negative outcome.

Consideration of the overall data obtained from patients who have achieved some measure of stability on methadone therapy delivered in a clinic setting show fairly convincingly that most can transfer successfully to office-based care. In addition, in virtually all cases, patients who fail in office-based treatment because of substance relapse or rule violations can be returned to routine clinic care to receive intensified counseling and monitoring without undue harm. The controlled studies also suggest that relapse or other problems in previously stable patients in office-based practice occur at rates no greater than those of similarly stable patients who remain in routine clinic care.

Research Related to Patients Entering Directly into Office-Based Practice Though policies and attitudes in the United States have, until 2000, steered practitioners away from the idea of bringing unstable opioid dependent individuals directly into office-based treatment, other countries have, out of necessity and an innovative spirit, embraced this concept more quickly (Table 50.2).

For example, in Scotland, most patients who receive methadone have it prescribed in general practitioners' offices and ingest it in community pharmacies (44–48). These general practitioners receive training specific to this endeavor (45). A 1-year follow-up of 204 opioid-dependent patients who entered such a paradigm in 1996 has been reported by Hutchinson and colleagues (45). A total of 58 general practitioners provided treatment to these patients. The study report does not specify the frequency or content of office visits, so practitioners presumably arranged their interventions on an individualized basis. The report also does not explicitly mention the frequency with which methadone doses were taken under observation, but it implies that this occurred on a daily or near-daily basis. Methadone dose levels are reported only for the 50 subjects who remained in continuous treatment for 12 months and who completed follow-up interviews. These subjects began at an average dose of 43 mg and increased to an average dose of 65 mg at 12 months. Follow-up interviews at 12 months were completed with 119 subjects (58.3%). Predictors of failure at follow-up included prostitution, unstable living arrangements, higher proportion of drug-using associates, higher daily drug expenditures, a higher level of benzodiazepine use, and a higher proportion of income from illegal sources. Among the 119 subjects followed up, 50 (42.4%) remained continuously on methadone for 12 months, 34 (28.8%) interrupted and then resumed methadone treatment, and 35 stopped methadone treatment. In the group who stopped treatment, 39% did so because of imprisonment, 33% did so because they were taking other drugs or misbehaving in the pharmacy, and 27% left voluntarily because they disliked the program. In one analysis, the researchers imputed missing data for follow-up failures by carrying forward their baseline values. In this analysis, daily opiate injecting for the entire cohort declined from 80% at baseline to 43% at 12 months, the mean daily amount spent on drugs declined from £63 to £38, and the mean number of acquisitive crimes in the preceding month declined from 18 to 11. Another analysis that examined subjects followed up at 12 months compared 50 subjects who remained continuously on methadone with 57 subjects who interrupted methadone treatment during the first 6 months. Only 2% of those who remained continuously on methadone reported daily opiate injecting at 12 months as compared with 21% of those with interrupted treatment. Continuous treatment subjects were spending a daily mean of £4 on drugs at 12 months, compared with £16 for those with interrupted treatment. Continuous treatment subjects committed a mean of three acquisitive crimes in the preceding month, compared with five for those with interrupted treatment.

England also has had a policy since the 1980s of encouraging opioid-dependent individuals to get methadone treatment through office-based treatment by general practitioners (49). A nonrandomized comparison study evaluated subjects who began methadone in 1995, either in a specialist drug clinic (n = 297) or with a general practitioner (n = 155). Training required for general practitioners was not specifically mentioned. At baseline, the two groups were similar in illicit drug use except that the specialist clinic group had greater use of amphetamines. The mean initial methadone dose was

TABLE 50.2 Studies of Patients Admitted Directly to Office-Based Opioid Treatment

Author	Year	Method	Requirements for entry	N	Medication dose (take-home)	Protocol retention	Use of illicit opioids	Use of other illicit substances
Hutchinson et al.	2000	Naturalistic program evaluation	Opioid dependence	204	Methadone; mean initial dose= 43 mg	42.4% of 119 followed up at 12 months	2% daily heroin for subjects in continuous treatment	0% daily benzodiazepine for subjects in continuous treatment
Gossop et al.	1999	Non-randomized comparison: GP office vs. clinic	Opioid dependence	155-GP; 297 clinic	Methadone; mean initial dose = 51 mg (GP) or 48 mg (clinic)	6 months: 66% GP; 60% clinic	< 10 days heroin use per month, both groups	Reduced significantly and equally for both groups
Vignau & Brunelle	1998	Non-randomized comparison: GP office vs. clinic	Opioid dependence	32-GP; 37 clinic	Buprenorphine; mean = 5.9 mg/d (GP) or 6.6 mg/d (clinic)	6 months:70% GP; 60% clinic	N/A	N/A
O'Connor et al.	1998	Randomized clinical trial: Primary care clinic vs. drug clinic treatment	Opioid dependence	23 in each condition	Buprenorphine: 22 mg Mon/Wed; 40 mg Fri	12 weeks: 78% primary care; 52% drug clinic	63% positive UAs primary care; 85% drug clinic	33% cocaine positive UAs both conditions
Fudala et al.	2003	Randomized clinical trial: Buprenorphine vs. buprenorphine + naloxone vs. placebo	Opioid dependence	326 randomized subjects	Buprenorphine 16 mg/d vs. Buprenorphine + naloxone 16/4 mg/d vs. placebo (on weekends or holidays)	4 weeks: Buprenorphine 86%; Buprenorphine + naloxone 82%; Placebo 75%	% Negative Urine Specimens: Bupreorphine 20.7%; Buprenorphine + naloxone 17.8%; Placebo 5.8%	Cocaine 40%–45%; Benzodiazpines, 10%; no significant differences across groups.
Walsh	2007	Naturalistic study	Opioid dependence	582	Buprenorphine + naloxone 2/0.5 mg/d to 24/6 mg/d (weekly to every 4 weeks)	62% at 16 weeks; 32% at 52 weeks	29.6% UAs positive at 3 months, 23.6% at 6 months, 19.0% at 12 months	Not reported
Fiellin et al.	2006	Randomized Clinical Trial: Standard medical management with once vs. thrice weekly buprenorphine + naloxone dispensing vs. enhanced medical management with thrice weekly dispensing	Opioid Dependence	166 randomized subjects	Buprenorphine + naloxone 16/4 to 24/6 mg/d (once or thrice weekly dispensing)	39%–48% retention at 24 weeks with no significant difference across groups	40%–44% negative urine specimens with no difference across groups	71.1%–75.5% negative specimens for cocaine with no difference across groups.

Alford et al.	2007	Retrospective chart review	Opioid Dependence	41 housed, 44 homeless	Buprenorphine, dose not given (1- to 4-week supply of take-homes)	Mean = 9 months both groups	4% positive urines both groups at 12 months.	8% positive urines both groups at 12 months
Magura et al.	2007	Retrospective chart review	Receiving buprenorphine in 1 of 6 offices in New York City	86	Buprenorphine median dose = 15 mg	Median = 8 months	8% estimated to be using at data collection end point.	16% estimated using at data collection end point.
Mintzer et al.	2007	Chart abstraction	Receiving buprenorphine + naloxone in 1 of 3 primary care practices in Boston	99	Buprenorphine + naloxone mean dose = 15.4 mg/d	Abstinent patients mean = 169 days; nonabstinent mean = 62 days	54% judged abstinent at 6 months	54% judged abstinent at 6 months

51 mg (standard deviation [SD] = 18.7) for the general practitioner group and 48 mg (SD = 19.1) for the specialist clinic group. General practitioners prescribed less than daily dispensing for 43% of their patients, while specialist clinics allowed less than daily dispensing for only 25% of their patients. Only 14% of general practitioners required that methadone administration (at retail pharmacies) be supervised. Frequency of office visits with general practitioners was not specified. Follow-up at 6 months was achieved with 76% of the original sample.

At 6 months, 66% of general practitioner patients and 60% of specialized clinic patients remained in treatment. In both groups, heroin use was reduced, on average, from more than 19 days per month at baseline to fewer than 10 days per month at follow-up; there was no significant difference between groups. All other substance use was reduced significantly and similarly for both groups. Drug injecting decreased among the general practitioner group from 53% to 41% and among the specialist clinic group from 66% to 53%. Non-drug-related crime fell among both groups but significantly more so among the general practitioner group.

France did not offer agonist pharmacotherapy to opioid-dependent individuals until the introduction of methadone at specialist addiction centers in 1995 (50). Shortly thereafter, buprenorphine became available in France for the treatment of opioid addiction, and general practitioners, regardless of their training, gained permission to prescribe it for this indication (50,51). Today, general practitioners in France can prescribe up to 28 days' supply of take-home medications and a maximum daily buprenorphine dose of 16 mg. About 65,000 patients per year have received buprenorphine in this office-based paradigm (52). A nonrandomized comparison study examined outcomes for opioid-dependent patients in France who were treated with buprenorphine by general practitioners (n = 32), compared with patients treated with buprenorphine at specialized addiction centers (n = 37) (50). The general practitioners had a fixed frequency of consultations, although the report does not specify the frequency. General practitioners performed urine testing weekly, required cannabis abstinence, and could arrange psychosocial services but did not necessarily have such services available. The addiction centers had a variable frequency of consultations, had no systematic frequency of urine testing, did not require cannabis abstinence, but had psychosocial services directly available. Apparently, subjects self-selected their own treatment venues.

The two groups differed at baseline on important variables. The patients treated in the addiction centers were older, less likely to be employed, had more polydrug use, experienced many more episodes of overdose, and were more likely to be injecting heroin. Doses of buprenorphine (5.9 mg/day for the general practitioner group versus 6.6 mg/day in the addiction center group) were relatively low in both groups. Treatment retention at 180 days was approximately 70% in the general practitioner group and about 60% in the addiction center group. Addiction Severity Index scores improved similarly for both groups from baseline to 90 days.

The first U.S. study to evaluate a quasi-office-based approach to opioid-dependent individuals just entering treatment also used buprenorphine as an agonist pharmacotherapeutic agent (53). Potential subjects with other drug or alcohol addiction, recent cocaine use, or complex medical or psychiatric comorbidities were excluded. Subjects were assigned randomly to receive 12 weeks of buprenorphine pharmacotherapy, either in a primary care setting or in a drug treatment setting that typically provided methadone treatment. The primary care setting was housed in a clinic designed to handle the primary care needs of substance users and psychiatric patients. Physicians in the primary care setting relied on a manual-guided clinical management protocol. Subjects assigned to the primary care setting (n = 23) received an initial 1-hour visit with a primary care provider, who recorded a substance use and medical history, created a treatment plan, made a referral to group psychotherapy, and prescribed buprenorphine. The subjects then saw their primary care provider in weekly 20-minute sessions. Group therapy conducted by a primary care nurse practitioner occurred weekly for 50 minutes, with a self-help focus on promoting abstinence.

Subjects assigned to the drug treatment setting (n = 23) received a standard set of services, including individualized substance abuse counseling and weekly relapse prevention group therapy. In both settings, subjects attended 5 days during week 1, with a buprenorphine dose escalation beginning at 2 mg and doubling daily until the dose reached 32 mg on day 5. From weeks 2 through 12, subjects attended clinic three times a week and received observed buprenorphine doses of 22 mg on Mondays and Wednesdays and 40 mg on Fridays. Thus, this study avoided prescribing take-home medications. Subjects in both settings also gave urine specimens three times a week. Patients were terminated from the study for missing three consecutive medication doses or for failure to attend group therapy. Successful completion of 12 weeks of treatment was observed for 78% of the subjects in primary care, compared with 52% of the subjects in drug treatment. Urine specimens were positive for opiates in 63% of urine specimens provided by primary care subjects, compared with 85% of drug treatment subjects. Primary care subjects showed a decreasing trend of opiate-positive specimens over time, whereas drug treatment subjects did not. Roughly a third of urine specimens in both groups tested positive for cocaine (53).

This study lends some support to the notion that treatment-seeking opioid-dependent patients can derive as much benefit from treatment in an office-based setting as from a drug treatment setting. Nevertheless, the researchers themselves properly note several aspects of the study design that limit its applicability to a true office-based setting. The primary care setting in this study required many more visits and more observed medication administration than would be practical in a typical office-based practice. The clinic used for the primary care setting had much more familiarity and expertise with substance-using patients than would most office-based settings. The study excluded patients with the medical and psychiatric complications commonly seen in opioid-dependent treatment seekers.

Another, much larger U.S. study also examined a quasi-office-based approach for opioid-dependent patients just entering treatment (54). This study differed from the others in that it did not compare an office-based with a clinic approach, but rather compared different medication strategies within a quasi-office-based setting. In this randomized, double-blind, placebo-controlled, multicenter trial, 326 subjects were randomly assigned to receive either (i) buprenorphine 16 mg/day, (ii) buprenorphine 16 mg + naloxone 4 mg/day, or (iii) placebo. Medication was administered in office-based settings affiliated with Veterans Affairs Medical Centers. Subjects received their doses 5 days a week, with take-home medications given for weekends and holidays. The trial was terminated early because of the demonstrated efficacy of buprenorphine + naloxone compared with placebo. Subjects treated with either buprenorphine alone or buprenorphine + naloxone had a greater proportion of urine specimens that were negative for opiates than did the subjects given placebo. The rate of adverse events was manageable and comparable between the two active treatments.

The largest study yet conducted of office-based treatment, A Multicenter Safety Trial of Buprenorphine + Naloxone for the Treatment of Opiate Dependence, consisted of an uncontrolled, naturalistic investigation that examined outcomes for 582 opioid-dependent individuals newly entering office-based treatment. Patients were not excluded for psychiatric or medical problems (other than pregnancy, because buprenorphine + naloxone is not approved for use in pregnant patients), as long as the treating physician could manage the problems on her or his own or by appropriate referral. Patients were treated by 38 physicians in seven states with buprenorphine + naloxone, in doses ranging from 2 mg/0.5 mg to 24 mg/6 mg/day. Medications were dispensed by institutional and community pharmacies. Physicians and pharmacists involved in the study received at least 8 hours of training in the pharmacology of buprenorphine + naloxone and issues pertinent to office-based treatment of opioid addiction. Treatment lasted up to a year. Patients were seen by the physicians at least twice in the first week of treatment, at least weekly during weeks 2 through 12 of treatment, at least biweekly from weeks 13 to 26, and monthly thereafter until week 52. For stable patients, medication dispensing followed a pattern similar to the office visits, so that in the final 6 months of treatment, patients could have monthly medication pick-ups. Urine toxicology screens were obtained onsite at each office visit. Relapse prevention counseling was available and encouraged but not required. Patients who became stable early in treatment had the option to taper the dose of buprenorphine + naloxone between weeks 7 and 9 and to complete treatment at that time.

The majority of patients (97.6%) were successfully inducted with the buprenorphine–naloxone combination. Most patients received 4 mg (22%), 8 mg (33%), or 16 mg (18%) on their first day. The most common maintenance doses prescribed to patients were 8 mg (11%), 16 mg (26%), and 24 mg (29%). The 16-week completion/retention rate was 362 (62%), with 189 patients (32.5%) completing either a supervised withdrawal or 52 full weeks of treatment. Patients demonstrated a significant decrease in percent of opioid positive urines over time. There was significant improvement in composite scores for drug, legal, and family/social domains of the Addiction Severity Index. A significant reduction in HIV risk behavior was also seen (55). Four recent smaller uncontrolled studies of patients treated for opioid dependence with buprenorphine + naloxone showed outcomes quite similar to those found in the multicenter safety study (56–59).

Finally, as mandated by the Drug Addiction Treatment Act, the Substance Abuse and Mental Health Services Administration conducted a 3-year evaluation of the impact of buprenorphine availability between 2002 and 2005 (60). Among the data sources used for this evaluation were surveys of 959 addiction medicine specialists (80% response rate), surveys of 1,837 physicians who had obtained a waiver to prescribe buprenorphine (86% response rate) and telephone interviews with 433 buprenorphine-treated patients recruited through prescribing physicians' offices or clinics. The results showed that about half the patients receiving buprenorphine had never previously received opioid agonist treatment. More than half the patients surveyed were not users of heroin and were dependent on prescription opioids. Both the patients and the physicians overwhelmingly believed that buprenorphine was effective. At 6 months after treatment initiation, more than 70% of patients remained in treatment or had completed treatment, and 81% were abstinent from nonprescribed opioids. Increases in employment and decreases in criminal activity occurred among the patient group. Opioid agonist treatment became available in geographic locations previously not served.

All of these early evaluations of direct entry to office-based treatment for opioid addiction support its viability as a treatment option and show its acceptance by patients, physicians, and pharmacists. Treatment retention in these office-based investigations did not fall markedly below—nor did illicit opiate use rise strikingly above—rates reported in recent clinic-based investigations of opioid agonist treatment, even though the European studies discussed here used doses of agonist medications that currently would be considered less than optimal.

CLINICAL ISSUES

Though the totality of clinical experience with office-based treatment remains somewhat limited, it has increased considerably in the past few years, and the body of evidence reviewed previously does encourage some synthesis of relevant ideas and recommendations related to clinical practice in an office setting. Again, it makes sense to divide this discussion into two segments: one most pertinent to care of long-term, stable patients who are transferred from a licensed program to office-based care and one focused on management of patients who are admitted directly to an office-based setting.

Patient assessment and appropriate selection of patients for transfer from clinic-based to office-based care obviously are key elements of this paradigm. A comparison of the various studies discussed earlier gives rise to the expected impression that more stringent selection criteria with more required time and stability in clinic-based treatment lead to better success after transfer to office-based treatment. When several years of treatment and stability are required (30,33), patients exhibit no illicit opioid use and minimal other substance use and most remain in the protocol for many years. Within the group of subjects in the study by Salsitz and colleagues (33), more episodes of methadone treatment and longer time in treatment were associated with a greater likelihood of a good outcome after transfer to office-based care. When less stringent selection criteria are used (39,40), illicit drug use is more likely to manifest in the office-based setting. The hair toxicology performed in the Connecticut study (40) also provides insights into this issue. Hair testing detected illicit substance use for some subjects who were believed by their program to be substance-free on the basis of monthly urine screens. Positive hair testing at baseline in that study clearly predicted substance use during the experimental paradigm for subjects in either office-based or standard clinic care. Because hair testing remains unavailable in most clinical settings, an alternative might be to obtain weekly or more frequent urine screens for some period before the anticipated transfer of any apparently stable patient from a licensed clinic to office-based care.

How thoroughly to assess and how stringently to screen patients for potential transfer to office-based care also depends on how much illicit substance use would be tolerated in the office-based setting. The programs thus far reported in the literature and reviewed here tolerated very little use before initiating protective transfer of the patient back to standard clinic care. In view of the fact that patients in office-based methadone treatment may have substantial quantities of take-home methadone doses in their possession, this conservative approach toward illicit drug use makes sense. Safety concerns would dictate that patients who are using illicit drugs should not have any (or have only a negligible supply of) take-home methadone to minimize the potential for overdose. Also, patients who use illicit drugs may pose a greater risk of diverting methadone to raise cash to buy drugs. Nevertheless, the controlled studies indicate that substance use did not differ on the basis of treatment in office-based versus standard clinic care (40).

What remains unknown is whether patients transferred to office-based care who experience more than a few brief episodes of substance use will continue to deteriorate in office-based care and need protective transfer back to standard clinic care or whether such relapses could be contained as effectively within the office-based setting, presuming a practical mechanism exists to limit the number of take-home doses of methadone provided until stability is regained. The report by Salsitz and colleagues (33) described the need for termination of 15 patients with serious abuse of cocaine who could not be treated within private practice, but it does not specify what measures might be taken within an office-based setting to address this type of problem. The stepped care intensification procedure used in the study by King and colleagues (42) offered one model for handling instability in the office-based setting that does not preclude rapid return to office-based care. Future studies could help to answer this question through controlled trials that randomly assign office-based patients undergoing a substance use relapse either to stay in office-based care or to receive protective transfer back to standard clinic care.

Further, office-based practitioners no doubt vary in their ability to tolerate and manage relapse. Some may feel very uncomfortable and immediately wish to transfer the patient back to standard clinical care, while others may prefer to intensify services in other ways, as through an increased number of office visits, a referral to counseling or self-help groups, or an increase in the methadone dose.

Concerns about relapse lead directly to a consideration of techniques for monitoring stable patients in office-based practice. All the studies described used urine testing, which would be common practice in licensed agonist treatment clinics. With the exception of the study by Senay and colleagues (39), these studies typically tested urine specimens at least monthly, often in a nonrandom fashion. In the study by Fiellin and colleagues (40), subjects who provided a specimen that was positive for drugs were required to give another specimen within the following week. The study by King and colleagues (42) used a monthly, random medication call-back schedule that also required subjects to give a random urine specimen. Rates of illicit drug use were lower in this study than in the study by Fiellin and colleagues (40), even though the subject populations appear to be relatively similar. Despite the dangers of comparing results across different studies, these observations lead to speculation that the random nature of the call-back procedures in the King (42) study may have deterred some illicit drug use. Although the regular and frequent call-back procedure used in that study might prove somewhat cumbersome in a purely clinical setting, the data argue for physicians who provide opioid agonist treatment in an office-based setting to institute some type of call-back procedure. The office-based subjects in the King (42) study were highly satisfied with their treatment, even though the call-back procedures meant that they had to visit their physician's office twice rather than once a month. A call-back procedure obviously also helps to minimize the risk of inappropriate or excessive medication use or diversion.

A monitoring plan that would be practical in an office-based setting would involve monthly nonrandom urine specimens at the time of scheduled office visits; a few unscheduled call-backs per year, with medication checks and provision of random urine specimens; and a very quick call-back after any positive urine specimen to obtain a repeat specimen within a few days. The latter part of the plan dictates that the physician must use a toxicology laboratory with a rapid turnaround time and must remain vigilant and act on positive test results as soon as they are received from the lab. Alternatively, with the technology to conduct onsite urine testing now readily available, an office setting with that capacity could detect illicit drug use at the time of the office visit. A more frequent medication pick-up schedule could be instituted immediately, along with plans to return for repeat urine monitoring.

The clinical management of methadone pharmacotherapy clearly encompasses another major component of office-based treatment for transferred patients. A substantial number of subjects in the investigation by Salsitz and colleagues (33) required methadone dose changes. Physicians who treat patients with methadone in office-based practice need to remain alert to the need for alterations in medication dose. Methadone stereoisomer plasma concentrations can change over time in response to a variety of somewhat unpredictable environmental factors, and such changes could lead to variations in clinical medication effects (61,62). Thus, physicians should frequently inquire about symptoms such as rhinorrhea, lacrimation, chills, nausea, diarrhea, muscle aches, and insomnia and assess whether these symptoms could be related to opioid withdrawal. They should query patients about thoughts of drug use or cravings. If such symptoms are occurring, an increase in the methadone dose should be given serious consideration. Similarly, physicians should ask about possible methadone side effects (such as constipation, excess sedation, or lowered libido) that may suggest the need for a reduction in methadone dose. In the absence of serious side effects or serious risk of relapse to drug use, the patient's wishes about dose changes often serve as the best guide to clinical decision making (63).

Psychosocial interventions form another potentially valuable element of office-based treatment for transferred patients. It would be expected, in general, that such interventions would be brief and might be minimal or unnecessary for the highly stable, long-term patients seen in the studies by Salsitz and colleagues (33) and Schwartz and colleagues (30). In the context of an office visit, it would be desirable for the physician to ask about the patient's drug and alcohol use and cravings; how the patient is doing at work and/or with family or child care responsibilities, financial and housing circumstances; about psychiatric and medical status; and about use of leisure time. In most cases, long-term patients will indicate in a few words that they have maintained stability in these areas of their lives. In the event that a patient acknowledges some problem or added stress, a few moments to delineate the scope of the difficulty, express concern and empathy, and provide support, advice, and encouragement may suffice to assist the patient in coping with mild or moderate distress. If the problem seems more severe, the office-based physician must either arrange more frequent sessions with the patient or have ready access to referral to counseling resources. Some of the office-based paradigms described earlier (37,42) had ongoing arrangements for temporary intensification of counseling services at the original licensed treatment program.

The clinical management of unstable, opioid-dependent patients newly entering office-based treatment poses some challenges that overlap those of already stabilized clinic patients, but also some that are distinct. Patients who enter directly into office-based care exhibit marked reductions in substance use, risk behavior, and criminality; also, they have much higher rates of drop-out and drug use than do stable patients. Even in the study by O'Connor and colleagues (53), which excluded subjects with recent cocaine use or serious psychiatric or medical problems, rates of dropout and substance use were substantial. With the exception of that study, most investigations of direct entry into office-based treatment have applied no exclusions to admission, so little direct scientific information exists to guide patient selection. To a great extent, then, patient selection for direct entry into office-based treatment must rely on the specific areas of expertise and clinical skills of the treating physician. Through thorough assessment, including a complete history and physical examination, the physician should ascertain whether he or she can comfortably manage—either by direct care and/or by adequate referral networks—the combination of substance use problems, general medical problems, psychiatric problems, and life crises likely to arise in the treatment of each patient. Physicians should exercise caution and refer patients who are not good candidates for their practice settings to licensed treatment programs. Although the early evidence suggests that some patients who enter directly into office-based opioid agonist therapy have a smooth treatment course, many certainly remain unstable for some time. Physicians who accept patients directly into office-based treatment will have to be able to tolerate and deal with some serious and unexpected clinical events.

As with stable, transferred patients, appropriate monitoring strategies will help the physician to stabilize patients newly entering office-based treatment. Again, no solid scientific data are available to guide precise techniques or monitoring schedules. Urine toxicology testing and periodic medication call-backs, coupled with regular clinical evaluation, likely will continue to serve as the mainstays of monitoring.

Medication-dispensing schedules allow another method of managing instability. For transferred, stable patients, weekly or more frequent dispensing schedules make no sense because such patients could obtain equivalent schedules at licensed clinics. For newly entering patients, conversely, tight control of medication dispensing, when practical, likely enhances the patient's progress toward stability. Buprenorphine and buprenorphine + naloxone are the only agonist medications approved for the treatment of patients directly entering office-based care in the United States. Although daily observation of medication ingestion would not be practical in most office-based settings, buprenorphine can be administered effectively three times a week (53), a schedule that probably is feasible in some office-based settings and/or their affiliated community pharmacies.

Monitoring and dispensing schedules will vary much more for newly entering patients, with more intensity of services expected initially, later decreasing as indicators of stability appear. Such indicators would include generally compliant behavior; regular, timely attendance at scheduled office visits; successful compliance with medication call-backs; negative urine toxicology tests; productive use of time; supportive interpersonal relationships; and the absence of criminal justice involvement. As such signs of stability appear, medication dispensing can be liberalized from three times a week to once a week, biweekly, or monthly, with an appropriate number of take-home doses. The frequency of scheduled office visits, urine testing, and medication call-backs can be adjusted in a similar fashion. If signs of instability reappear, any or all of these monitoring techniques can be readjusted for greater frequency.

As in the treatment of stable, transferred patients, careful pharmacotherapy of newly entering patients can contribute to their stability. The physician needs considerable skill to prescribe buprenorphine, particularly in view of its potential to precipitate opioid withdrawal during induction of patients with high levels of physical dependence (64–66). This characteristic of buprenorphine generally dictates initiation of pharmacotherapy at low doses, followed by dose escalation as soon as the patient demonstrates medication tolerance. Throughout the course of treatment, as in the care of transferred patients, the physician will need to be alert to the signs and symptoms described earlier and be ready to adjust the dose.

The potential for medication diversion plays into decisions about medication dose and frequency of dispensing. Certainly, diversion poses a danger to the community by increasing the supply of illicit opioids. In addition, diversion by a patient undermines and endangers the patient's efforts toward achieving a stable recovery from opioid dependence. The presence of illicit methadone and buprenorphine in the community lets us know that some diversion is indeed occurring. Scant firm data exist on the frequency or the patient characteristics and behaviors associated with diversion. Failing a medication call-back or request for early refills because of purported lost or stolen medication offer some obvious warning signs. Other more subtle but certainly not pathognomonic signs might be a sudden unexplained increase in disposable income or a sudden request for a dose increase in a previously stable patient without an apparent explanation for instability. Physicians can deal with the risk of diversion first by exercising preventive measures. They should convey to patients at the outset of treatment, preferably in a written agreement, that being prescribed opioid medications entails a lot of responsibility and that diversion will not be tolerated. Loss of take-home medication or even discontinuation of treatment could be a consequence for diversion. Faced with these strictures, those patients who might actually consider diversion will desist for fear of losing their treatment. Medication call-backs, as noted earlier, also serve as a strong bulwark against diversion. If patients know that they will have to account for all outstanding medication, diversion will be deterred. If diversion is suspected, a call-back should be implemented. If the patient fails the call-back, appropriate interventions depend on the specific circumstances of the patient and the practice. At the very least, the amount of medication dispensed at any one time should be drastically reduced. Some physicians might want to consider discontinuation of office-based treatment and referral to a licensed opioid treatment program if available. Repeated episodes of diversion clearly indicate that office-based treatment is not an appropriate setting and argue for transfer to a more structured, licensed program.

Psychosocial treatments may be even more important to patients who are newly entering office-based treatment than to stable patients who already have received regular counseling at a licensed program. Scant scientific data are available to provide reliable instruction as to the optimal modality or frequency of psychosocial treatments for these patients. The uncontrolled studies conducted in Britain did not evaluate the variety of psychosocial treatments prescribed by physicians. The study by O'Connor and colleagues (53) used weekly physician visits and weekly group therapy—an intensity of psychosocial services that might not be available or reimbursable in most clinical settings. Studies of various intensities of psychosocial services in licensed methadone programs (67–69) do offer some illumination on this point: Patients who receive minimal psychosocial services do not fare as well as do those who receive moderate or high levels of services; however, the lower cost-effectiveness of more intensive services may nullify any slight advantage they hold over moderate services (67,70). One recent controlled study of the efficacy of weekly extended medical management counseling (45-minute sessions) compared to weekly standard medical management counseling (20-minute sessions) found no advantage of the extended counseling (71). In the absence of any more definitive information, these findings would argue for the value of at least monthly counseling for a patient newly entering office-based treatment. If the physician does not wish to provide this service, ancillary office staff or an outside counselor to whom patients are referred could do so. The intensity of psychosocial services then could be titrated to the response of each individual patient.

Many of the studies summarized here used some form of brief physician training before the physician engaged in office-based care of opioid-dependent patients. As with many aspects of OBOT, little empirical evidence exists to specify the optimal training method. Practicing physicians have limited amounts of time in their schedules for training, so a brief course makes sense. At present, physicians are eligible to practice office-based treatment of opioid addiction on completion of 8 hours of formal training. Expert consensus suggests that appropriate training should consist of most of the following topics: (a) overview of opioid dependence and rationale for agonist treatment; (b) legislation permitting office-based treatment; (c) general opioid pharmacology; (d) pharmacology of buprenorphine and buprenorphine + naloxone; (v) efficacy and safety of buprenorphine; (e) clinical use of buprenorphine including induction, stabilization, and withdrawal; (f) patient assessment and selection; (g) office management, including treatment agreements, urine testing, record keeping, and confidentiality; (h) co-occurring psychiatric and medical disorders; (i) psychosocial treatments; and (j) special populations including adolescents, pregnancy, and patents with pain.

CONCLUSIONS

Patients who are addicted to opioids have posed a perennial challenge to the health care system. In recent decades, the system has tried to meet the challenge by providing opioid agonist pharmacotherapy at licensed treatment programs. This approach has greatly improved the outcomes and lives of many patients but has failed to accommodate many others because of inadequate capacity and because, for some individuals, attendance at such a program creates undue hardships. Good scientific data now show that transfer of patients who have 1 or 2 years of demonstrated stability in a licensed methadone program to office-based care leads to outcomes comparable to those obtained if the patients had continued at a licensed clinic. If such patients become unstable in office-based care, they can be transferred safely back to clinic care.

Many such patients prefer office-based care and have more time for productive activities when receiving treatment in an office setting. Moreover, transferring such patients to office-based care opens treatment slots in methadone clinics to previously untreated patients. Now that several thousand patients have been treated in office settings, the appropriate management techniques (including patient selection, monitoring, and pharmacotherapy) have been reasonably well established.

Early evidence from studies of office-based care of opioid-dependent patients newly entering treatment likewise suggests that such care is reasonable for many such patients and that their short-term outcomes appear nearly equivalent to those achieved with similar patients in traditional licensed programs. Although this approach holds a great deal of promise, implementation of optimal management techniques awaits completion of additional rigorous research.

As more knowledge accrues about office-based treatment of opioid addiction and as it becomes a more widespread practice, a number of positive "ripple effects" likely will ensue. The "treatment gap" should narrow as more patients who live in a variety of locations and have varying needs gain access to opioid agonist treatment. The medical and addiction treatment systems will reintegrate. Not only will medical and psychiatric comorbidities be attended to more fully but physicians may become more willing to address substance use problems other than opioid addiction. Society in general will benefit from reductions in crime and its associated costs, from an increased engagement in the workforce by previously unemployable individuals and, possibly, from an overall decline in health care expenditures.

REFERENCES

1. National Consensus Development Panel on Effective Medical Treatment of Opiate Addiction (Consensus Development Panel). Effective medical treatment of opiate addiction. *JAMA* 1998; 280(22):136–143.
2. Mark TL, Woody GE, Juday T, et al. The economic costs of heroin addiction in the United States. *Drug Alcohol Depend* 2001;61(2):195–206.
3. Masson CL, Sorensen JL, Batki SL, et al. Medical service use and financial charges among opioid users at a public hospital. *Drug Alcohol Depend* 2002;66(1):45–50.
4. Office of Applied Studies, Substance Abuse and Mental Health Services Administration. *Drug Abuse Warning Network, 2003: Area Profiles of Drug-Related Mortality*. Rockville, MD: Substance Abuse and Mental Health Services Administration, 2005.
5. Guevara RE. *Statement of Rogelio E. Guevara, chief of operations, Drug Enforcement Administration, before House Committee on Government Reform*. Washington, DC: House Committee on Government Reform, 2002.
6. Office of Applied Studies, Substance Abuse and Mental Health Services Administration. *Drug Abuse Warning Network, 2005: National estimates of drug-related emergency department visits*. Rockville, MD: Substance Abuse and Mental Health Services Administration, 2007a.
7. Substance Abuse and Mental Health Services Administration (SAMHSA). Press release, July 22, 1999. Retrieved from http://www.samhsa.gov/press/99/990722nr.htm.
8. Substance Abuse and Mental Health Services Administration (SAMHSA). *Mortality Data from the Drug Abuse Warning Network*, 1998. Retrieved from http://www.samhsa.gov/oas/dawn.htm#mecomp. Accessed July 11, 2008.
9. Barnett PG. The cost-effectiveness of methadone maintenance as a health care intervention. *Addiction* 1999;94(4):479–488.
10. Darke S, Zador D. Fatal heroin "overdose": A review. *Addiction* 1996;91(12):1765–1772.
11. Hanlon TE, Nurco DN, Kinlock TW, et al. Trends in criminal activity and drug use over an addiction career. *Am J Drug Alcohol Abuse* 1990;16(3-4):223–238.
12. Zang Z. *Drug and alcohol use and related matters among arrestees 2003*. National Institute of Justice. Retrieved September 29, 2007, from http://www.ncjrs.gov/nij/adam/ADAM2003.pdf.
13. Office of Applied Studies, Substance Abuse and Mental Health Services Administration. *Results from the 2006 National Survey on Drug Use and Health: National Findings*. Rockville, MD: Substance Abuse and Mental Health Services Administration, 2007b.
14. Musto DF. *The American disease*. New York: Oxford University Press, 1987.
15. Wren CS. Holding an uneasy line in the long war on heroin: methadone emerged in city now debating it. *New York Times* October 3, 1998.
16. Cooper JR. Including narcotic addiction treatment in an office-based practice. *JAMA* 1995;273(20):1619–1620.
17. Cushman P. The major medical sequelae of opioid addiction. *Drug Alcohol Depend* 1980;5:239–254.
18. Haverkos HW, Lange WR. Serious infections other than human immunodeficiency virus among intravenous drug abusers. *J Infect Dis* 1990; 161:894–902.
19. Makower RM, Pennycock AG, Moulton C. Intravenous drug abusers attending an inner city accident and emergency department. *Arch Emerg Med* 1992;9:32–39.
20. Chandrasekar PH, Narula AP. Bone and joint infections in intravenous drug abusers. *Rev Infect Dis* 1986;6:904–911.
21. Rubin AM. Neurologic complications of intravenous drug abuse. *Hosp Pract* 1987;22:279–288.
22. Chamot E, de Saussure PH, Hirschel B, et al. Incidence of hepatitis C, hepatitis B and HIV infections among drug users in a methadone maintenance programme [letter]. *AIDS* 1992;6:430–431.
23. Dieperink E, Willenbring M, Ho SB. Neuropsychiatric symptoms associated with hepatitis C and interferon alpha: A review. *Am J Psychiatry* 2000;157:867–876.
24. Selwyn PA, Alcabes P, Hartel D. Clinical manifestations and predictors of disease progression in drug users with human immunodeficiency virus infection. *N Engl J Mede* 1992;327:1697–1703.
25. O'Donnell AE, Pappas LS. Pulmonary complications of intravenous drug abuse, experience at an inner city hospital. *Chest* 1988;94:251–253.
26. Brooner RK, King VL, Kidorf M, et al. Psychiatric and substance use comorbidity among treatment-seeking opioid abusers. *Arch Gen Psychiatry* 1997;54(1):71–80.
27. Mason BJ, Kocsis JH, Melia D, et al. Psychiatric comorbidity in methadone maintained patients. *J Addict Dis* 1998;17(3):75–89.

28. Wren CS. Ex-addicts find methadone more elusive than heroin. *New York Times* February 2, 1997.
29. Roane KR. Legislation for those with a methadone clinic next door. *New York Times* April 6, 1997.
30. Schwartz RP, Brooner RK, Montoya ID, et al. A 12-year follow-up of a methadone medical maintenance program. *Am J Addict* 1999;8(4): 293–299.
31. Modie N. More heroin addicts may be offered treatment. *Seattle Post-Intelligencer* December 8, 1999.
32. Hunt DE, Lipton DS, Goldsmith DS, et al. "It takes your heart": the image of methadone maintenance in the addict world and its effect on recruitment into treatment. *Int J Addict* 1985;20(11–12):1751–1771.
33. Salsitz EA, Joseph H, Fran B, et al. Methadone medical maintenance (MMM): treating chronic opioid dependence in private medical practice—a summary report (1983–1998). *Mount Sinai J Med* 2000; 67(5–6):388–397.
34. Novick DM, Pascarelli EF, Joseph H, et al. Methadone maintenance patients in general medical practice. A preliminary report. *JAMA* 1988;259(22):3299–3302.
35. Novick DM, Joseph H. Medical maintenance: the treatment of chronic opiate dependence in general medical practice. *J Subst Abuse Treat* 1991; 8(4):233–239.
36. Novick DM, Joseph H, Salsitz EA, et al. Outcomes of treatment of socially rehabilitated methadone maintenance patients in physicians' offices (medical maintenance): follow-up at three and a half to nine and a fourth years. *J Gen Intern Med* 1994;9(3):127–130.
37. Merrill, JO, Jackson, TR, Schulman, BA, et al. Methadone medical maintenance in primary care. An implementation evaluation. *J Gen Intern Med* 2005;20(4):344–349.
38. Harris KA Jr., Arnsten JH, Joseph H, et al. A 5-year evaluation of a methadone medical maintenance program. *J Subst Abuse Treat* 2006; 31(4):433–438.
39. Senay EC, Barthwell AG, Marks R. et al. Medical maintenance: a pilot study. *J Addict Dis* 1993;12(4):59–76.
40. Fiellin DA, O'Connor PG, Chawarski M, et al. Methadone maintenance in primary care: a randomized controlled trial. *JAMA* 2001;286: 1724–1731.
41. Saxon AJ, Calsyn DA, Haver VM, et al. A nationwide survey of urinalysis practices of methadone maintenance clinics. Utilization of laboratory services. *Arch Pathol Lab Mede* 1990;114(1):94–100.
42. King VL, Stoller KB, Hayes M, et al. A multicenter randomized evaluation of methadone medical maintenance. *Drug Alcohol Depend* 2002; 65(2):137–148.
43. King VL, Kidorf MS, Stoller KB, et al. A 12-month controlled trial of methadone medical maintenance integrated into an adaptive treatment model. *J Subst Abuse Treatment* 2006;31(4):385–393.
44. Gruer L, Wilson P, Scott R, et al. General practitioner centered scheme for treatment of opiate dependent drug injectors in Glasgow. *Br Med J* 1997;314(7096):1730–1735.
45. Hutchinson SJ, Taylor A, Gruer L, et al. One-year follow-up of opiate injectors treated with oral methadone in a GP-centred programme. *Addiction* 2000;95(7):1055–1068.
46. Peters AD, Reid MM. Methadone treatment in the Scottish context: outcomes of a community-based service for drug users in Lothian. *Drug Alcohol Depend* 1998;50(1):47–55.
47. Weinrich M, Stuart M. Provision of methadone treatment in primary care medical practices: Review of the Scottish experience and implications for U.S. policy. *JAMA* 2000;283(10):1343–1348.
48. Wilson P, Watson R, Ralston GE. Methadone maintenance in general practice: patients, workload, and outcomes. *Br Med J* 1994;309(6955): 641–644.
49. Gossop M, Marsden J, Stewart D, et al. Methadone treatment practices and outcome for opiate addicts treated in drug clinics and in general practice: results from the National Treatment Outcome Research Study. *Br J Gen Pract* 1999;49(438):31–34.
50. Vignau J, Brunelle E. Differences between general practitioner- and addiction-centre-prescribed buprenorphine substitution therapy in France. *Eur Addict Res* 1998;4(Suppl 1):24–28.
51. Moatti JP, Souville M, Escaffre N, et al. French general practitioners' attitudes toward maintenance drug abuse treatment with buprenorphine. *Addiction* 1998;93(10):1567–1575.
52. Auriacombe M, Fatseas M, Dubernet J, et al. French field experience with buprenorphine. *Am J Addict* 2004;13(Suppl 1):S17–S28.
53. O'Connor PG, Oliveto AH, Shi JM, et al. A randomized trial of buprenorphine maintenance for heroin dependence in a primary care clinic for substance users versus a methadone clinic. *Am J Med* 1998; 105(2):100–105.
54. Fudala PJ, Bridge TP, Herbert S, et al. Office-based treatment of opiate addiction with a sublingual-tablet formulation of buprenorphine and naloxone. *N Engl J Med* 2003;349(10):949–958.
55. Walsh R. Personal communication, 2007.
56. Alford DP, LaBelle CT, Richardson JM, et al. Treating homeless opioid dependent patients with buprenorphine in an office-based setting. *J Gen Intern Med* 2007;22(2):171–176.
57. Magura S, Lee SJ, Salsitz EA, et al. Outcomes of buprenorphine maintenance in office-based practice. *J Addict Dis* 2007;26(2):13–23.
58. Mintzer IL, Eisenberg M, Terra M, et al. Treating opioid addiction with buprenorphine-naloxone in community-based primary care settings. *Ann Fam Med* 2007;5(2):146–150.
59. Stein MD, Cioe P, Friedmann PD. Buprenorphine retention in primary care. *J Gen Intern Med* 2005;20(11):1038–1041
60. Center for Substance Abuse Treatment. *The SAMHSA Evaluation of the Impact of the DATA Waiver Program*. Rockville, MD: Westat, 2006.
61. Eap CB, Bertschy G, Baumann P, et al. High interindividual variability of methadone enantiomer blood levels to dose ratios [letter]. *Arch Gen Psychiatry* 1998;55(1):89–90.
62. Rostami-Hodjegan A, Wolff K, Hay AW, et al. Population pharmacokinetics of methadone in opiate users: characterization of time-dependent changes. *Br J Clin Pharmacol* 1999;48(1):43–52.
63. Maddux JF, Desmond DP, Vogtsberger KN. Patient-regulated methadone dose and optional counseling in methadone maintenance. *Am J Addict* 1995;4(1):18–32.
64. Jacobs EA, Bickel WK. Precipitated withdrawal in an opioid-dependent outpatient receiving alternate-day buprenorphine dosing [letter]. *Addiction* 1999;94(1):140–141.
65. Strain EC, Preston KL, Liebson IA, et al. Buprenorphine effects in methadone-maintained volunteers: effects at two hours after methadone. *J Pharmacol Exp Ther* 1995;272(2):628–638.
66. Walsh SL, Preston KL, Bigelow GE, et al. Acute administration of buprenorphine in humans: partial agonist and blockade effects. *J Pharmacol Exp Ther* 1995;274(1):361–372.
67. Avants SK, Margolin A, Sindelar JL, et al. Day treatment versus enhanced standard methadone services for opioid-dependent patients: a comparison of clinical efficacy and cost. *Am J Psychiatry* 1999;156(1): 27–33.
68. Calsyn DA, Wells EA, Saxon AJ, et al. Contingency management of urinalysis results and intensity of counseling services have an interactive impact on methadone maintenance treatment outcome. *J Addict Dis* 1994;13(3):47–63.
69. McLellan AT, Arndt IO, Metzger DS, et al. The effects of psychosocial services in substance abuse treatment. *JAMA* 1993;269(15): 1953–1959.
70. Kraft MK, Rothbard AB, Hadley TR, et al. Are supplementary services provided during methadone maintenance really cost-effective? *Am J Psychiatry* 1997;154(9):1214–1219.
71. Fiellin, DA, Pantalon, MV, Chawarski, MC, et al. Counseling plus buprenorphine-naloxone maintenance therapy for opioid dependence. *N Engld J Med* 2006;355(4):365–374.

SUGGESTED READINGS

Salsitz EA, Joseph H, Fran B, et al. Methadone medical maintenance (MMM): treating chronic opioid dependence in private medical practice—a summary report (1983–1998). *Mount Sinai J Med* 2000;67(5–6): 388–397.

King VL, Kidorf MS, Stoller KB, et al. A 12-month controlled trial of methadone medical maintenance integrated into an adaptive treatment model. *J Subst Abuse Treatment* 2006;31(4):385–393.

Fudala PJ, Bridge TP, Herbert S, et al. Office-based treatment of opiate addiction with a sublingual-tablet formulation of buprenorphine and naloxone. *N Engl J Med* 2003;349(10):949–958.

Mintzer IL, Eisenberg M, Terra M, et al. Treating opioid addiction with buprenorphine-naloxone in community-based primary care settings. *Ann Fam Med* 2007;5(2):146–150.

Fiellin DA, Moore BA, Sullivan LE, et al. Long-term treatment with buprenorphine/naloxone in primary care: results at 2-5 years. *Am J Addict* 2008;17:116–20.

CHAPTER 51

David A. Gorelick, MD, PhD

Pharmacologic Interventions for Cocaine, Methamphetamine, and Other Stimulant Addiction

Stimulants such as cocaine and amphetamines are the second most widely used illegal drugs in the United States, surpassed only by cannabis. In 2006, more than 2 million Americans were estimated to have abuse or dependence on stimulants (1.7 million on cocaine) (1). More than 400,000 patients who reported a stimulant as their primary drug of abuse were admitted to publicly funded substance abuse treatment programs in 2005 (2). Despite this clinical need, there is no well-established, broadly effective pharmacotherapy for stimulant dependence. Both clinical and scientific interest in pharmacologic treatment continues to be stimulated by the often disappointingly low success rates and short duration of efficacy of current psychosocial treatment approaches (3,4).

This chapter reviews the current state of pharmacologic treatment of stimulant dependence, including choice of medication and medications for use in special treatment situations, such as patients with mixed addictions or psychiatric comorbidities. Emphasis is given to the use of medications in clinical practice, rather than to laboratory studies or preclinical pharmacology. (For more information about the pharmacology of stimulant dependence, see Section 2, Chapter 10.)

Much of the clinical and clinical research literature deals with cocaine; the remainder deals with the amphetamines. These two classes of stimulants are considered separately. The extent to which findings related to cocaine dependence can be extrapolated to other stimulant addictions remains unclear.

COCAINE DEPENDENCE

Goals of Treatment The goals of pharmacologic treatment of cocaine dependence are the same as for any other treatment modality; that is, to help patients abstain from cocaine use and regain control of their lives. The behavioral mechanisms by which medication achieves these goals are poorly understood and can vary across patients and medications. In theory, medication could shift the balance of reinforcement away from cocaine taking in favor of other behaviors through several mechanisms: (1) by reducing or eliminating the positive reinforcement from taking a cocaine dose (for example, by reducing the euphoria or "high"), (2) by reducing or eliminating a subjective state (such as "craving") that predisposes to taking cocaine, (3) by reducing or eliminating negative reinforcement from taking a cocaine dose (as by reducing withdrawal-associated dysphoria), (4) by making cocaine-taking aversive, or (5) by increasing the positive reinforcement obtained from non-cocaine-taking behaviors. Currently available medications are considered to act by one or more of the first three mechanisms, and these mechanisms are the focus of research in medications development. No research addresses the fourth mechanism (which would be analogous to use of disulfiram in treating alcohol dependence). The fifth mechanism is crucial to successful treatment because it ensures that other behaviors are reinforced to replace cocaine taking as the latter is extinguished, but such medications do not exist. In current practice, this mechanism is engaged by psychosocial interventions that address issues such as vocational rehabilitation, the patient's social network, and use of leisure time.

Because of the importance of this mechanism, as well as other factors such as medication adherence, medication almost never is used without some psychosocial treatment component. Few controlled clinical trials explicitly compare the efficacy of medication use with varying (or no) psychosocial treatments (5,6), so the relative contributions of pharmacologic and psychosocial treatments are largely unknown. The type, intensity, and duration of psychosocial treatment that should accompany pharmacologic treatment are questions with little data to guide clinical decision making. At a minimum, one would expect that addressing psychosocial factors that influence medication adherence would improve treatment outcome.

Pharmacologic Mechanisms At least four pharmacologic approaches are potentially useful in the treatment of cocaine dependence (7). These approaches are (1) substitution treatment with a cross-tolerant stimulant (analogous to methadone maintenance treatment of opioid dependence), (2) treatment with an antagonist medication that blocks the binding of cocaine at its site of action (true pharmacologic antagonism, analogous to naltrexone treatment of opioid dependence), (3) treatment with a medication that functionally antagonizes the effects of cocaine (as by reducing the reinforcing effects of or craving for cocaine), and (4) alteration of cocaine pharmacokinetics so that less drug reaches or remains at its site(s) of action in the brain.

No medication currently is approved by the U.S. Food and Drug Administration (FDA) or any other national health authority for the treatment of cocaine dependence, chiefly because no medication has met the scientifically rigorous standard of consistent, statistically significant efficacy in replicated, controlled clinical trials. Most current clinical and research attention has focused on the second and third approaches mentioned above: reducing or blocking cocaine's actions, either directly at its neuronal binding site (true pharmacologic antagonism) or indirectly by otherwise reducing its reinforcing effects. The first approach has been evaluated in a small number of clinical trials, with mixed results. The fourth approach has shown promise in animal studies and early phase II clinical trials (8).

Cocaine has two major neuropharmacologic actions: blockade of presynaptic neurotransmitter reuptake pumps, resulting in psychomotor stimulant effects, and blockade of sodium ion channels in nerve membranes, resulting in local anesthetic effects.

Cocaine's positively reinforcing effects derive from its blockade of the dopamine reuptake pump, causing presynaptically released dopamine to remain in the synapse and enhancing dopaminergic neurotransmission (9). Cocaine's local anesthetic effects are believed to contribute to cocaine-induced kindling, the phenomenon by which previous exposure to cocaine sensitizes the individual so that later exposure to low doses produces an enhanced response.

CHOICE OF MEDICATION

Antidepressants

Heterocyclic Antidepressants Tricyclic and other heterocyclic antidepressants are the most widely used and best-studied class of medications for the treatment of cocaine dependence. Their use is based both on the clinical observation of frequent depressive symptoms among cocaine-dependent individuals seeking treatment (see further for treatment of patients with comorbid depression) and on their pharmacologic mechanism of increasing biogenic amine neurotransmitter activity in synapses. Such increase is achieved primarily by inhibiting presynaptic neurotransmitter reuptake pumps.

Desipramine inhibits norepinephrine reuptake, with some action on serotonin reuptake. It was the first medication found effective in an outpatient, double-blind, controlled clinical trial—a finding that received wide publicity even before the complete study was published in a peer-reviewed journal. As a result, desipramine is the best-studied of the tricyclic antidepressants, with more than a half dozen controlled clinical trials in the published literature (10–12). Typical doses are 150 to 300 mg/day (about 2.5 mg/kg), similar to those used in the treatment of depression. Meta-analysis suggests a non-significant trend toward efficacy but with substantial heterogeneity across studies (10).

Differences in patient characteristics, concomitant treatment, and desipramine plasma concentrations may account for some of the variability in efficacy of desipramine. For example, patients with depression (13) and without antisocial personality disorder (14) may respond best to desipramine. Patients dually dependent on cocaine and opiates may do better on desipramine if their opioid dependence is treated with buprenorphine rather than methadone (12) or if they receive contingency management treatment along with medication (12). There is limited evidence that patients with steady-state desipramine plasma concentrations above 200 ng/mL have poorer outcomes (15), with better outcomes at concentrations around 125 ng/mL (11).

Experience with other heterocyclic antidepressants has shown limited evidence for efficacy. Reboxetine and maprotiline, which block norepinephrine reuptake, were effective in small open-label trials (16,17). Imipramine, the precursor of desipramine, which blocks serotonin reuptake much more than norepinephrine reuptake, showed no efficacy in two controlled clinical trials, except in subjects who used intranasal cocaine (18,19). Nefazodone and venlafaxine, which block both serotonin and norepinephrine reuptake, were not effective in controlled clinical trials (20–22). Mirtazapine, which increases brain serotonin and norepinephrine activity by blocking autoregulatory α_2-adrenergic and 5-HT_2 receptors, showed some benefit in a small open-label trial (23).

No unexpected or medically serious side effects have been reported in published clinical trials of heterocyclic antidepressants. However, patients who relapse to cocaine use while still on antidepressant medications could, in theory, be at increased risk of cardiovascular side effects. Both cocaine and the tricyclics have quinidine-like membrane effects that, when superimposed, could lead to cardiac arrhythmias. The concurrent administration of cocaine and desipramine (blood levels above 100 ng/mL) to research volunteers has produced additive increases in heart rate and blood pressure (24).

Selective Serotonin Reuptake Inhibitors Antidepressants that selectively block the presynaptic serotonin reuptake pump have attracted interest because of the role of serotonin and its receptors in modulating dopaminergic brain reward circuits and the behavioral effects of cocaine (25,26) (see Section 2, Chapter 10). Several controlled clinical trials have not found any advantage for fluoxetine (20, 40, or 60 mg/day) (10), paroxetine (20 mg/day) (22), or sertraline (100 mg/day) (27) over placebo, although treatment retention was improved in two of the studies. A recent clinical trial found citalopram (20 mg/day) significantly better than placebo (28). That study, unlike previous studies, used contingency management in addition to cognitive-behavioral therapy, suggesting the importance influence of psychosocial treatment on medication efficacy.

Monoamine Oxidase Inhibitors The rationale for use of monoamine oxidase (MAO) inhibitors lies in their effect of increasing brain levels of biogenic amine neurotransmitters by inhibiting a major catabolic enzyme. Limited open-label experience with phenelzine, at antidepressant doses of 30 to 90 mg/day, suggests that this medication can reduce cocaine and other stimulant use (29–31). However, its clinical usefulness may be limited by the need for dietary and concomitant medication restrictions to avoid precipitating a hypertensive crisis, as well as by the theoretical possibility of potentiating cocaine-induced effects should the patient relapse to cocaine use while still taking the medication. Some researchers have argued that fear of such an aversive, potentially life-threatening reaction is what motivates abstinence while taking an MAO inhibitor (29), making the mechanism of action analogous to that of disulfiram for alcohol dependence.

Current research is focusing on selective MAO inhibitors that act only on MAO type B, the predominant type in the brain, while sparing MAO type A, the predominant type in the gastrointestinal tract. It is inhibition of MAO in the gastrointestinal tract that produces a hypertensive crisis ("cheese reaction") after ingestion of tyramine-containing foods or certain catecholaminergic medications. Selegiline, marketed for the treatment of parkinsonism and, in the transdermal form, for treatment of depression, is fairly selective for MAO type B at recommended doses (10 mg/day for parkinsonism, 12 mg/day for depression) and is being studied as a treatment for cocaine dependence. A recent multisite controlled clinical trial using selegiline administered via a skin patch (selegiline transdermal system) found no evidence for efficacy (32).

Other Antidepressants Bupropion has attracted interest because it is a weak inhibitor of monoamine reuptake and has some stimulant-like behavioral effects in animals. Two controlled clinical trials in methadone-maintained, cocaine-dependent patients found no significant effect on cocaine use, except in subjects also receiving contingency management treatment (33,34).

Ritanserin, a 5-HT_2 receptor antagonist developed as an antidepressant, attracted interest because it reduced cocaine self-administration in some (but not all) animal studies. However, two controlled clinical trials found ritanserin no better than placebo in reducing cocaine use (35,36).

Dopamine Agonists (anti-Parkinson Agents) A variety of direct and indirect dopamine agonist medications have been evaluated, based on the dopamine depletion hypothesis of cocaine dependence (37), although the data supporting the hypothesis in human subjects are equivocal (38). Dopamine agonists, by stimulating synaptic dopamine activity, would ameliorate the effects of decreased dopamine activity caused by cessation of cocaine use; these include anhedonia, anergia, depression, and cocaine craving. In rats, dopamine receptor agonists such as bromocriptine and lisuride reduce cocaine self-administration and reverse the reduced metabolic rate and elevated intracranial self-stimulation threshold produced in dopaminergic mesocorticolimbic brain regions after cessation of chronic cocaine administration (39). Bromocriptine, pergolide, and amantadine, all marketed for the treatment of parkinsonism (another dopamine deficiency condition), are the most commonly studied dopamine agonist medications (40).

Findings with direct dopamine receptor agonists (primarily at the D_2 subtype) are inconsistent. Of two small (7 and 29 patients, respectively), short-term (10 and 15 days, respectively) uncontrolled trials with bromocriptine, one found a decrease in cocaine use (41), whereas the second found no significant change (42). A larger (69 patients) controlled clinical trial found that bromocriptine (started during inpatient treatment) did not significantly reduce relapse to cocaine use during subsequent outpatient treatment (43). Three controlled clinical trials of pergolide (a mixed D_1/D_2 agonist) found it no better or worse than placebo (44–46). A controlled clinical trial of pramipexole found it no better than placebo (22). In contrast, a controlled clinical trial of cabergoline (47) and an open-label trial of ropinirole (48) found them effective.

Amantadine is an indirect dopamine agonist that acts by releasing dopamine presynaptically. It also is a weak antagonist at the N-methyl-D-aspartate glutamate receptor. Only one of more than half-a-dozen controlled clinical trials found amantadine (200–400 mg/day) better than placebo (40,49,50). An initial finding of benefit among outpatients with more severe cocaine withdrawal symptoms was not replicated in a larger trial (50).

The amino acid L-DOPA, a precursor for the synthesis of catecholamines that is used in the treatment of parkinsonism, has been used to increase brain dopamine levels in the treatment of cocaine dependence, both alone and in combination with carbidopa, a peripheral amino acid decarboxylase inhibitor that prevents systemic side effects by blocking the conversion of L-DOPA to dopamine outside the brain. Three controlled clinical trials found no advantage of L-DOPA/carbidopa over placebo (47,51). A fourth controlled clinical trial found a medication advantage over placebo only in subjects also receiving contingency management treatment (5).

L-tyrosine, the amino acid precursor of L-DOPA, reduced cocaine craving in a small (12 patients) double-blind study of inpatients (52), but was not effective in reducing cocaine use in two outpatient clinical trials at 2 g every eight hours (open-label) or 800 or 1,600 mg twice a day (double-blind) (53,54).

Disulfiram Disulfiram can be considered a functional dopamine agonist because it blocks the conversion of dopamine to norepinephrine by the enzyme dopamine-β-hydroxylase, thereby increasing dopamine concentrations (55). Interest in disulfiram as a treatment for cocaine dependence initially was generated by suggestions of its efficacy in patients with concurrent cocaine and alcohol dependence, a common comorbidity (56). Three controlled clinical trials in cocaine-dependent patients without alcohol dependence (but with, in two studies, concurrent opioid dependence treated with methadone or buprenorphine) found disulfiram (250 mg/day) significantly better than placebo in promoting cocaine abstinence (57–59). A retrospective pooled analysis of two of these studies found that men treated with disulfiram had better outcomes than women (60). However, a recent unpublished controlled clinical trial found that women did better than men at the usual disulfiram dose of 250 mg daily (61). Both genders did more poorly at lower disulfiram doses (62.5 or 125 mg daily).

Though disulfiram has been well tolerated in clinical trials, where subjects are screened for medical and psychiatric comorbidity, questions have been raised about its safety in routine clinical practice (62). An early human laboratory study found that pretreatment with disulfiram (250 mg daily for 3 days) significantly prolonged cocaine's plasma half-life, increased plasma cocaine concentrations, and potentiated the tachycardic and hypertensive effects of intranasal cocaine (1 or 2 mg/kg) (63). A more recent human laboratory study also found that disulfiram (250 mg daily for 4–6 days) decreased cocaine clearance but found no potentiation of the cardiovascular effects of intravenous cocaine (0.25 or 0.5 mg/kg) (64). Disulfiram did significantly reduce the positive subjective response to cocaine. These findings suggest that disulfiram may be a promising new treatment for cocaine dependence, although raising a caution about potential adverse drug interactions should patients use cocaine while on the medication.

Stimulants By analogy with methadone maintenance treatment of opioid dependence or nicotine replacement treatment of tobacco dependence, maintenance treatment of cocaine-dependent patients with stimulant medication might be clinically beneficial in reducing cocaine craving and use (67). As with methadone, advantages might include use of the less medically risky oral route of administration (vs. injected or smoked cocaine), use of pure medication of known potency (thus avoiding contaminant effects or inadvertent overdose), and use of a medication with slower onset and longer duration of action (thus avoiding "rush"/ "crash" cycling) (65).

Several orally active psychomotor stimulants marketed for the treatment of attention deficit/hyperactivity disorder (ADHD) and narcolepsy or as appetite suppressants (anorexiants) have been used to test the substitution approach (40,66,67). Two small controlled clinical trials with sustained release d-amphetamine found significant reductions in cocaine use at 30 to 60 mg daily, with no difference from placebo at lower doses (15–30 mg). A trial using immediate release d-amphetamine (20–60 mg daily) found no effect. Two controlled clinical trials using methylphenidate (90 mg daily) found no significant effect on cocaine use. One of these trials included patients with comorbid ADHD; ADHD symptoms were improved by the medication. None of these studies reported significant adverse effects, suggesting that stimulant substitution treatment might be safe in cocaine-using patients.

Several marketed stimulants with less abuse potential (classified as Schedule IV controlled substances) have yielded disappointing results. Diethylpropion (up to 75 mg/day for 2 weeks) did not reduce cocaine craving (both spontaneous and cocaine-cue elicited) among inpatients in a double-blind trial (68). Mazindol was ineffective in three double-blind outpatient studies (at 1, 2, or 2–4 mg/day) (69–71).

Modafinil, used for the treatment of excessive sleepiness in narcolepsy, obstructive sleep apnea, and shift work sleep disorder, can be considered a weak stimulant (Schedule IV). Its mechanisms of action are unclear but include some blockade of presynaptic dopamine transporters as well as increases in brain glutamate release and decreases in GABA release (72). A small phase II clinical trial found that 400 mg daily significantly reduced cocaine use (73). A recent multi-site clinical trial found no significant reduction in cocaine use in the study sample as a whole (74). However, in the subgroup of subjects without alcohol dependence, both 200 mg and 400 mg daily of modafinil significantly increased the percentage of abstinent days. Modafinil was safe and well tolerated. It does not appear to evoke cocaine craving or itself produce euphoria (72,75). In phase I human laboratory studies, modafinil does not potentiate the effects of cocaine (76), nor does it alter cocaine pharmacokinetics, except for a decrease in the area under the cocaine plasma concentration-time curve over the first 3 hours after intravenous cocaine administration (77). These findings suggest that modafinil could be safely used in cocaine-using patients.

In principle, cocaine itself, in a slow-onset formulation or route of administration, might be used for agonist maintenance treatment (78,79), in the same way that slow-onset transdermal or transbuccal nicotine is used to treat dependence to rapid-onset smoked nicotine (cigarettes). Oral cocaine salt capsules (100 mg four times a day) significantly attenuated the response to an intravenous cocaine challenge (25 mg) (79) and reduced coca paste smoking in an open-label series of 18 patients in Lima, Peru (where oral cocaine products are legal) (80). A larger series of 200 patients treated with coca tea, also in Lima, reported that almost 80% reduced their cocaine smoking (80). A case series of 50 coca paste smokers in La Paz, Bolivia, reported that chewing 100 to 200 g of coca leaf per week for a mean of 2 years substantially improved the mental health of one-third of the patients and improved the socioeconomic functioning of almost half (data on cocaine smoking was not reported) (81).

Antipsychotics The older (so-called first-generation) antipsychotics, which are potent dopamine receptor antagonists (chiefly D2 [postsynaptic] subtype), do not appear to significantly alter cocaine craving or use, as evidenced by clinical experience with patients with schizophrenia who abuse cocaine while receiving chronic antipsychotic treatment (82–84). Greater efficacy was hoped for from the newer "second-generation" antipsychotics, in part because of their broader spectrum of receptor binding (that is, to dopamine D1 and serotonin). However, this promise has not been confirmed in clinical trials of cocaine users without comorbid psychiatric disorders (85). A small open-label trial of olanzapine in 21 patients dually dependent on cocaine and opioids (being treated with methadone) reported a decrease in cocaine use in 53.2% of patients (86). However, two more recent controlled clinical trials reported no significant advantage for olanzapine over placebo (87,88). Two controlled clinical trials using oral risperidone (89,90) and one using long-acting injectable risperidone (91) also found no advantage over placebo.

Caution should be exercised when prescribing any antipsychotic to cocaine users because of their potential vulnerability to the neuroleptic malignant syndrome, based on their presumed cocaine-induced dopamine depletion (92). Cocaine or amphetamine users may also be at elevated risk of antipsychotic-induced movement disorders (93–96).

Anticonvulsants Anticonvulsants have been tried in the treatment of cocaine dependence because they block the development of cocaine-induced kindling in animals. Kindling (increased neuronal sensitivity to a drug because of prior intermittent exposure) has been hypothesized as a neurophysiologic mediator of cocaine craving in humans (97). At the neurotransmitter level, anticonvulsants might be effective because they increase inhibitory GABA activity and/or decrease excitatory glutamate activity in the brain, both actions that would decrease the response to cocaine in the dopaminergic corticomesolimbic brain reward circuit (7,98,99).

Carbamazepine has been the most-studied anticonvulsant, but the promise of early open-label studies has not been confirmed in controlled trials. Four of five double-blind outpatient trials found no significant effect on cocaine use (100). Gabapentin was found ineffective in three controlled clinical trials (101–103), as were lamotrigine (101) and valproic acid (88) in single trials.

Several other anticonvulsants have shown more promising results. Tiagabine, which increases GABA activity by blocking its presynaptic reuptake, significantly reduced cocaine use in two controlled clinical trials at doses of 12 or 24 mg daily (103,104) but had no effect in a third trial at 20 mg daily (105). All three trials used concomitant cognitive-behavioral therapy. Topiramate, which decreases glutamate activity by blocking AMPA-type glutamate receptors and increases GABA activity (by an unknown mechanism), significantly reduced cocaine use in a controlled clinical trial at up to 200 mg daily, in conjunction with cognitive-behavioral therapy (106). Vigabatrin (γ-vinyl-GABA), which increases GABA activity by inhibiting the breakdown of GABA by GABA-transaminase, reduced cocaine use in three open-label studies (107–109). Vigabatrin is not marketed in the United States because of ophthalmological side effects, but none were observed during these short-term studies. Phenytoin (300 mg daily) significantly reduced cocaine use in one controlled clinical trial, especially at serum concentrations above 6.0 μg/mL (110).

Baclofen, an antispasmotic rather than anticonvulsant, increases GABA activity by acting as an agonist at $GABA_B$ receptors. One controlled clinical trial found that baclofen (60 mg daily) did not significantly reduce cocaine use, except in the subgroup of subjects with heavier cocaine use (111).

Nutritional Supplements and Herbal Products

Nutritional Supplements The use of amino acid mixtures, either alone or with other nutritional supplements (vitamins and minerals), has been widely publicized in the drug abuse treatment field, encouraged by their freedom from the regulations imposed on prescription medications and their perceived safety and absence of side effects. Proprietary mixtures, including tyrosine (the amino acid precursor of L-DOPA) and L-tryptophan (the amino acid precursor of serotonin), have been marketed with claims of efficacy (112), but a double-blind, 28-day cross-over study found no significant effect of tyrosine and tryptophan (1 gram of each daily) on cocaine craving or withdrawal symptoms (113). A more recent controlled clinical trial found L-tryptophan, even when coupled with contingency management treatment, no better than placebo in reducing cocaine use (114). L-carnitine (500 mg/day) plus coenzyme Q10 (200 mg/day) was no better than placebo in an 8-week controlled clinical trial (88). A small controlled clinical trial found magnesium L-aspartate (732 mg daily), an easily absorbed form of magnesium, no better than placebo (115).

Herbal Products Various herbal and plant-derived products have been touted as treatments for drug abuse, but few have undergone controlled clinical evaluation. One that has received substantial publicity, but not yet clinical evaluation, is ibogaine, an indole alkaloid found in the root bark of the West African shrub *Tabernanthe iboga*. This compound has been claimed to suppress cocaine (and opioid and alcohol) withdrawal and craving for several months after a single oral dose (116). Ginkgo biloba (120 mg/day for 8 weeks) was no better than placebo in a controlled clinical trial (117).

Calcium Channel Blockers Calcium channel blockers have been suggested as treatment for cocaine dependence because of their effects on neurotransmitter release and inhibition of cocaine's psychological effects in some, but not all, studies of human research volunteers (118). However, amlodipine showed no efficacy in a controlled clinical trial (118).

Other Medications A wide variety of other medications have been evaluated for the treatment of cocaine dependence, often on the basis of promising case reports or animal studies suggesting that they influenced the reinforcing effects of cocaine.

Ondansetron, a $5\text{-}HT_3$ receptor antagonist used to reduce nausea and vomiting, significantly reduced cocaine use in a small-scale controlled clinical trial (119). The effect was significant only at the highest dose (4 mg twice daily).

Naltrexone, a mu-opioid receptor antagonist marketed for the treatment of alcohol dependence and opioid dependence, showed some efficacy at 50 mg/day in cocaine-dependent outpatients without alcohol or opioid dependence but only when combined with relapse prevention therapy (120).

Numerous medications have been found no better than placebo in (usually small-scale) controlled clinical trials. These include mecamylamine, a nicotinic cholinergic receptor antagonist (121); donepezil, an acetylcholinesterase inhibitor (27); propranolol, a beta-adrenergic receptor antagonist (50); reserpine, a depleter of presynaptic monoamine neurotransmitters (122); hydergine, an agonist at dopamine and serotonin receptors and antagonist at alpha-adrenergic receptors that stimulates blood flow (47); pentoxifylline, a phosphodiesterase inhibitor (22); riluzole, an inhibitor of glutamate release (22); celecoxib, a nonsteroidal anti-inflammatory drug (123); lithium (124); and dehydroepiandrosterone (DHEA), an endogenous steroid precursor of androstenedione, itself a precursor of androgenic and estrogenic hormones (125). DHEA is also a sigma-1 receptor agonist.

Medication Combinations Concurrent use of two different medications is being studied in the hope that such combinations will enhance efficacy while minimizing side effects, either by acting on a single neurotransmitter system by two different mechanisms or by acting on two different neurotransmitter systems. Concurrent open-label use of the dopaminergic agents bupropion and bromocriptine in cocaine-dependent outpatients has been found safe, albeit with little suggestion of efficacy (126). Concurrent use of pergolide (a dopamine D_1/D_2 receptor agonist) and haloperidol (a dopamine D_2 receptor antagonist), designed to produce relatively pure D_1 agonist action, also found little evidence of efficacy (127), as did combined use of amantadine and propranolol (50).

The combined use of the dopamine releaser phentermine and the serotonin releaser fenfluramine, each marketed as an appetite suppressant, received substantial publicity during the 1990s as the so-called "phen-fen" treatment for obesity and addictive disorders. This medication combination had mixed results in the outpatient treatment of cocaine dependence (128). The combination no longer is available since the withdrawal of fenfluramine because of its association with primary pulmonary hypertension and valvular heart disease (129). Combinations that replace fenfluramine with a selective serotonin reuptake inhibitor (SSRI) such as fluoxetine have not been systematically evaluated.

A proprietary combination of intravenous flumazenil (a benzodiazepine receptor antagonist) and oral gabapentin and hydroxyzine (a histamine antagonist) substantially reduced methamphetamine use in an open-label trial (130). Controlled clinical trials are currently underway.

Other Physical Treatments Acupuncture is an ancient Chinese treatment that involves mechanical (with needles), thermal (moxibustion), or electrical (electroacupuncture) stimulation of specific points on the body surface (131). The mechanism of action is unknown; speculation has included stimulation of endogenous opioid systems. Acupuncture of the outer ear (auricular) has enjoyed growing popularity as a treatment for drug withdrawal, especially using five standard locations recommended by the National Acupuncture Detoxification Association (NADA): kidney, liver, lung, shen men, and sympathetic. Meta-analyses of nine published studies (six using the NADA locations) did not find a significant benefit of active acupuncture over sham treatment (132,133).

Transcranial magnetic stimulation (TMS) involves activation of brain cells by magnetic fields generated by electromagnetic coils placed on the scalp. Repetitive TMS (rTMS) is being evaluated as a treatment for depression and other neuropsychiatric disorders (134). Single and multiple sessions of rTMS of the prefrontal cortex (either right or left) have been reported to reduce cocaine craving (135,136).

AMPHETAMINE DEPENDENCE

Many of the medications evaluated for the treatment of cocaine dependence have also been studied for the treatment of amphetamine dependence, often for the same pharmacologic rationale (137,138). As with cocaine dependence, most controlled clinical trials do not show efficacy.

The most promising approaches to date appear to be agonist substitution with stimulants and enhancement of GABA activity. Two of three controlled clinical trials with d-amphetamine (one using a sustained release formulation) found a significant reduction in amphetamine use compared with placebo (67). There were no significant adverse events in any study. Slow-release methylphenidate (54 mg daily) reduced amphetamine use significantly more than did placebo in one controlled clinical trial (139). Modafinil (200 mg twice daily) reduced amphetamine use in a case report (140), and is currently undergoing a controlled clinical trial.

Vigabatrin (γ-vinyl-GABA), an anticonvulsant that increases GABA activity by inhibiting the breakdown of GABA by GABA-transaminase, substantially reduced methamphetamine use in two open-label trials (108,109). Vigabatrin is not marketed in the United States because of ophthalmologic side-effects, but none were observed during these short-term studies. Baclofen, an antispasmotic that increases GABA activity by acting as an agonist at $GABA_B$ receptors, had no overall effect on methamphetamine use in a controlled clinical trial but did significantly reduce use in a subgroup of highly medication-adherent subjects (141). Gabapentin, an anticonvulsant with an unknown mechanism of action, was no different from placebo, even in the adherent subgroup.

Other medications showing promise in early trials include naltrexone (142), bupropion, and risperidone. The antidepressant bupropion showed no overall efficacy in two controlled clinical trials but did significantly reduce methamphetamine use in the subgroup of subjects with lower levels of methamphetamine use (143,144). The antipsychotic risperidone, either oral or long-acting injectable, reduced methamphetamine use in two open-label trials (145,146). Another second-generation antipsychotic, aripiprazole (15 mg daily), showed no efficacy in a small controlled clinical trial (139).

Medications not showing efficacy in the treatment of amphetamine dependence in clinical trials include tricyclic antidepressants (e.g., imipramine, desipramine), selective serotonin reuptake inhibitors (e.g., fluoxetine, sertraline, paroxetine), ondansetron (a 5-HT_3 receptor antagonist) (147), and the calcium channel blocker amlodipine (137,138,148).

SPECIAL TREATMENT SITUATIONS

Mixed Dependence

Opioid Dependence Concurrent opioid use, including dependence, is a common clinical problem among cocaine-dependent individuals. Some individuals use cocaine and opioids simultaneously (as in the so-called speedball) to enhance the drugs' subjective effects. Up to 20% or more of opioid-dependent patients in methadone maintenance treatment also use cocaine for a variety of reasons, including continuation of prior polydrug abuse, replacement for the "high" no longer obtained from opioids, self-medication for the sedative effects of high methadone doses, or attenuation of opioid withdrawal symptoms (149,150). Three different pharmacologic approaches have been used for the treatment of such dual cocaine and opioid dependence: (1) adjustment of methadone dose, (2) maintenance with another opioid medication, and (3) addition of medication targeting the cocaine dependence.

Higher methadone doses (usually 60 mg or more daily) generally are associated with less opioid use by patients in methadone maintenance. This relationship also holds in general for cocaine use among patients in methadone maintenance (151,152), although exceptions have been reported (153). Increasing the methadone dose as a contingency in response to cocaine use can be effective in reducing such use (and more so than decreasing the methadone dose in response to a cocaine-positive urine sample) (151,154).

Buprenorphine is a partial opioid agonist (mu-receptor agonist/kappa-receptor antagonist) used for the agonist substitution treatment of opioid dependence (155). Advantages over methadone (a pure mu-receptor agonist) include a milder withdrawal syndrome and higher therapeutic index (that is, safety in overdose). Some (but not all) studies in patients concurrently dependent on both opioids and cocaine suggest that cocaine use (as well as opioid use) is reduced at higher buprenorphine doses (16–32 mg daily) (156–158). Making buprenorphine dosing partially dependent on cocaine-free urine samples can also reduce cocaine use in opioid-dependent patients (159).

Non-opioid medications for the treatment of cocaine dependence frequently are evaluated in methadone- or buprenorphine-maintained, opioid-dependent outpatients because the opioid agonist maintenance component substantially enhances treatment retention and adherence, making medication trials easier to conduct and complete. A variety of the medications discussed earlier, including desipramine, fluoxetine, amantadine, bromocriptine, disulfiram, and bupropion, have been studied in opioid-maintained, cocaine-dependent patients. There is no evidence that such maintenance treatment significantly influences medication efficacy, but no studies have explicitly and directly addressed this issue.

Alcohol Dependence Alcohol dependence is a common problem among cocaine-dependent individuals, both in the community and in treatment settings, with rates of comorbidity as high as 90% (160). Alcohol use by cocaine-dependent patients is associated with poorer treatment outcome (160,161), which can be related to a variety of factors, including production of the toxic psychoactive metabolite cocaethylene (162), stimulation of cocaine craving by alcohol (160), or alteration of medication metabolism by the hepatic effects of alcohol.

Two medications used in the treatment of alcohol dependence have been studied in the treatment of outpatients concurrently dependent on cocaine and alcohol. Disulfiram substantially decreased both cocaine and alcohol use in two clinical trials (163,164) and a small case series (165) but not in a third clinical trial (166). Naltrexone, a mu-opioid receptor antagonist marketed for the treatment of alcohol dependence and opioid dependence, also substantially decreased both cocaine and alcohol use at 150 mg daily (56,167) but not at 50 mg daily (168–170) or 100 mg daily (166,171), the doses more typically used in treatment of alcohol or opioid dependence. Combined treatment with both disulfiram (250 mg daily) and naltrexone (100 mg daily) significantly improved abstinence from cocaine and alcohol (166).

Psychiatric Comorbidities Treatment-seeking, cocaine-dependent individuals have high rates of psychiatric comorbidity (that is, psychiatric diagnoses other than another substance use disorder), with rates as high as 65% for lifetime disorders and 50% for current disorders (172,173). The most common comorbid disorders tend to be major depression, bipolar spectrum, phobias, and posttraumatic stress disorder (174). Personality disorders are common among treatment-seeking, cocaine-dependent individuals, with rates in this population as high as 69% (175). The most common of these is antisocial personality disorder (176).

Depression Antidepressants appear to vary in their efficacy for reducing cocaine use among patients with comorbid major depression, although there have been few direct comparisons or controlled clinical trials (177,178). Desipramine, imipramine, and bupropion have usually, but not always (179,180), been found effective, whereas SSRIs (e.g., fluoxetine) are usually not effective. Venlafaxine (150 mg daily) and nefazodone (200 mg twice daily) have shown some efficacy in small clinical trials (181,182).

Bipolar Disorder Both anticonvulsant "mood stabilizers" and antipsychotics have been used to treat comorbid bipolar disorder and cocaine dependence. Case series and open-label trials suggest that anticonvulsants such as valproate, divalproex, lamotrigine, and carbamazepine have some efficacy in reducing cocaine use in dually diagnosed patients (183–187) and are more effective than lithium (124). Combining lithium with an anticonvulsant may be helpful in treatment-resistant patients (184).

The second-generation antipsychotics have generated mixed results in cocaine-dependent patients with comorbid bipolar disorder. Quetiapine reduced cocaine use in one of two clinical trials (188,189); risperidone reduced cocaine use in one trial (189). Switching treated patients to aripiprazole did not reduce their cocaine use (190).

One controlled clinical trial found that adding citicoline, a precursor in the biosynthesis of cell membranes, to existing medication was better than adding placebo in reducing cocaine use by dually diagnosed patients (191).

Attention Deficit/Hyperactivity Disorder Up to one-fourth of cocaine-dependent adults have either adult ADHD or a history of childhood ADHD (192,193). Stimulant and dopaminergic medications are the mainstay of treatment for ADHD, suggesting that some of these patients may be self-medicating their ADHD with cocaine. Case series and clinical trials generally find that such medications successfully treat ADHD symptoms and reduce cocaine use in adults: dextroamphetamine (up to 60 mg/day), methamphetamine (15 mg/day), and bupropion (up to 100 mg three times a day) (194–196). However, one of two recent controlled clinical trials with sustained-release methylphenidate found no significant reduction in cocaine use (197,198), as did a controlled clinical trial with immediate release methylphenidate (199). A recent controlled clinical trial with sustained-release bupropion also found no significant decrease in cocaine use (197).

Schizophrenia Although schizophrenia is not a common comorbid psychiatric disorder among cocaine-dependent individuals, cocaine use and abuse are common among treatment-seeking patients with schizophrenia (200). Clinical experience indicates that first-generation antipsychotics, at doses that are effective in the treatment of schizophrenia, do not significantly alter cocaine craving or use (201,202). One exception may be flupenthixol, a mixed dopamine D_1/D_2 receptor and 5-HT_{2A} receptor antagonist that is not marketed in the U.S. (203). Depot flupenthixol (40 mg of decanoate intramuscularly every 2 weeks) reduced cocaine use and improved psychopathology in a small case series of cocaine-using patients with schizophrenia (204).

Several case series and open-label trials suggest that the second generation antipsychotics, including clozapine, olanzapine, quetiapine, risperidone, and aripiprazole, may be more effective in reducing cocaine and other drug use among patients with schizophrenia (201,202). However, two head-to-head controlled clinical trials found no difference between olanzapine and haloperidol in reducing cocaine use, with each medication reducing cocaine craving in one of the trials (205,206). A controlled clinical trial comparing olanzapine and risperidone found a trend favoring greater reduction in cocaine use by olanzapine (207).

Use of cocaine or amphetamines can exacerbate or provoke anti-psychotic-induced movement disorders (93,94) and increase vulnerability to the neuroleptic malignant syndrome (92).

Medical Comorbidities Few data have been systematically or prospectively collected to guide the pharmacotherapy of cocaine dependence in medically ill patients, making this an important issue for future clinical research. Prudent clinical practice would require a careful medical evaluation of any patient before starting medication, with special attention to medical conditions common in cocaine-dependent individuals. Such conditions would include viral hepatitis and alcoholic liver disease, which might alter the metabolism of prescribed medications, and HIV infection. The presence of the latter necessitates caution in prescribing medications with a known potential for inhibiting immune function. Clinical experience suggests that buprenorphine (208,209) and bupropion can be used safely in HIV-positive patients (210), although anti-retroviral medications may decrease bupropion plasma concentrations (211).

Gender-Specific Issues Women tend to be excluded from or underrepresented in many clinical trials of cocaine dependence pharmacotherapy (212), in part because of concern, embodied in former FDA regulations, over risk to the fetus and neonate should a female subject become pregnant. Thus, there is a substantial lack of information about gender-specific issues of pharmacotherapy in general and the pharmacotherapy of cocaine dependence in particular (213,214). This situation should improve in the future because current FDA and National Institutes of Health regulations require appropriate representation of women in clinical trials. Meanwhile, clinicians must deal on an *ad hoc* basis with the treatment implications of possible gender differences in medication pharmacokinetics (such as those resulting from differences in body mass and composition) and in pharmacodynamics (such as those related to the menstrual cycle or exogenous hormones such as oral contraceptives).

In the absence of directly relevant and systematically collected data, caution should be used when prescribing medications to pregnant women with stimulant dependence and to those with pregnancy potential, keeping in mind both the risks of medication and the risks of continued stimulant use. Some medications proposed for the treatment of cocaine dependence (such as tricyclic antidepressants, bupropion, and buprenorphine) appear to have little potential for morphologic teratogenicity or disruption of pregnancy, although there are little or no data on behavioral teratogenicity. Some medications do pose at least slight risk, such as amantadine (associated with pregnancy complications), lithium (associated with cardiac malformations and neonatal toxicity), anticonvulsants (associated with increased risk of congenital malformations), and antipsychotics (which can be associated with nonspecific congenital anomalies and neonatal withdrawal).

Some medications (e.g., disulfiram, naltrexone) may generate different treatment responses in men versus women (56,60). The reasons for such gender differences are poorly understood but may include differences in medication pharmacokinetics, hormonal interactions, or subjects' psychological or socioeconomic status.

Age Although adolescents make up a substantial minority of heavy cocaine users, they have been largely excluded from clinical trials of cocaine pharmacotherapies because of legal and informed consent considerations. On the basis of the scarcity of published case reports, it appears that medication is not often used in the treatment of adolescent cocaine dependence.

FUTURE PROSPECTS

Future progress in pharmacologic treatment for cocaine dependence is likely to come from development of new medications with novel or more selective mechanisms of action. New medications should evolve from an improved understanding of the neuropharmacology of cocaine dependence and animal studies of the interactions of cocaine with novel compounds (7,98,99).

Preclinical studies with compounds that bind to the same presynaptic dopamine transporter site as does cocaine (thereby keeping cocaine from acting), but which do not themselves produce robust reinforcing effects (because of slow onset of effect and tight, long-lasting binding), suggest that such compounds may be useful as functional cocaine "antagonists" (215). One such compound, vanoxerine (GBR-12909), has already been in phase I human trials, although safety concerns may limit its development. Manipulation of brain dopamine activity with selective dopamine receptor ligands, especially for the D_3 type, has attenuated the rewarding effects of cocaine in several animal studies (216) and awaits the development of compounds suitable for clinical trials. Medications that presynaptically release both dopamine and serotonin have also shown promise in animal studies (217).

Animal studies suggest that chronic cocaine use results in lower basal levels of glutamate in the nucleus accumbens, resulting in an exaggerated glutamate response to cocaine, which may mediate strong cocaine-seeking behavior (218). N-acetylcysteine, used as a mucolytic in the treatment of cystic fibrosis and to treat acetaminophen toxicity, increases basal glutamate levels. It reduced spontaneous and cue-elicited cocaine craving in a controlled clinical trial (219) and substantially reduced cocaine use in an open-label outpatient trial (220). Controlled clinical trials are currently underway.

Cocaine administration, like stress, activates the hypothalamic-pituitary-adrenal (HPA) axis, and stress may play a role in relapse to cocaine use after abstinence (99). These observations have stimulated interest in corticotrophin-releasing factor receptor antagonists, some of which reduce cocaine self-administration in animals (221).

The endogenous cannabinoid (endocannabinoid) brain neurotransmitter system appears to modulate the dopaminergic reward system (99). Blockade of cannabinoid CB_1 receptors inhibits relapse to cocaine self-administration after abstinence in animals. Several CB_1 receptor antagonists (or inverse agonists) are available for clinical research.

The failure of existing medications to show consistent efficacy in the treatment of cocaine dependence has prompted growing interest in pharmacokinetic approaches: that is, preventing ingested cocaine from entering the brain and/or enhancing its elimination from the body (8). The former approach could be implemented by active or passive immunization to produce binding antibodies that keep cocaine from crossing the blood-brain barrier. The latter approach could be implemented by administration of an enzyme (e.g., butyrylcholinesterase) that catalyzes cocaine hydrolysis or by immunization with a catalytic antibody. These pharmacokinetic approaches already have shown promise in attenuating cocaine's behavioral effects in animals. An anti-cocaine vaccine (that is, active immunization against cocaine) has shown promise in significantly reducing cocaine use in a phase II controlled clinical trial. Further work is needed to increase the consistency of the antibody response and lengthen the duration that antibody concentrations remain high enough to block cocaine use.

CONCLUSIONS

The absence of any medication that meets FDA standards for efficacy and safety leaves physicians with little clear-cut guidance for pharmacologic treatment of stimulant dependence. Among existing medications marketed for other indications, none has yet been proved broadly effective in replicated controlled clinical trials. Disulfiram appears the most promising, especially for patients with comorbid alcohol abuse. Tricyclic antidepressants such as desipramine and imipramine (but not SSRIs such as fluoxetine) may be of use in patients with milder dependence or with comorbid depression. Anticonvulsants such as topiramate, tiagabine, and phenytoin (but not carbamazepine or gabapentin) have shown promise in controlled clinical trials and warrant further evaluation. The stimulant maintenance approach also warrants further evaluation using medications with low abuse potential (for example, modafinil or sustained-release methylphenidate or amphetamine), or perhaps even a slow-onset (for example, oral or transdermal) form of cocaine itself.

More sophisticated patient-treatment matching could enhance the efficacy of current medications by taking into account both patient characteristics that can influence treatment response (for example, severity of dependence, psychiatric comorbidity, or concomitant medications) and characteristics of the psychosocial treatment accompanying the medication (222). For example, a few studies suggest that some medications (e.g., bupropion, L-DOPA, SSRIs) that are not effective when used with drug abuse counseling or cognitive-behavioral therapy may be effective when combined with contingency management treatment (5,28,34).

Improved understanding of the neurobiology of dependence should lead to new and more effective medications in the future, possibly acting by manipulation of the glutamate or endocannabinoid systems or HPA axis or by a pharmacokinetic mechanism. Regardless of which medications show promise in the future, their adoption into clinical practice should be guided by acceptable scientific proof of efficacy and safety, based on data from replicated, well-designed, controlled clinical trials. Clinicians should also keep in mind the distinctions between efficacy (treatment works in a research setting in a selected research population getting close attention) and effectiveness (treatment works in a heterogeneous population in a realistic clinical environment) and between a statistically significant and clinically meaningful treatment effect (223).

ACKNOWLEDGMENT: *Dr. Gorelick is supported by the Intramural Research Program, National Institutes of Health, National Institute on Drug Abuse.*

REFERENCES

1. Substance Abuse and Mental Health Services Administration, Office of Applied Studies (2007). *Results from the 2006 National Survey on Drug Use and Health: National Findings* (Office of Applied Studies, NSDUH Series H-32, DHHS Publication No. SMA 07-4293). Rockville, MD.
2. Substance Abuse and Mental Health Services Administration, Office of Applied Studies (2008). *Treatment Episode Data Set (TEDS): 2005. Discharges from Substance Abuse Treatment Services,* DASIS Series: S-41, DHHS Publication No. (SMA) 08-4314, Rockville, MD.
3. Knapp WP, Soares BG, Farrel M, Lima MS. Psychosocial interventions for cocaine and psychostimulant amphetamines related disorders. *Cochrane Database Syst Rev* 2007:CD003023.
4. Lee NK, Rawson RA. A systematic review of cognitive and behavioural therapies for methamphetamine dependence. *Drug Alcohol Rev* 2008; 27:309–317.
5. Schmitz JM, Mooney ME, Moeller FG, et al. Levodopa pharmacotherapy for cocaine dependence: choosing the optimal behavioral therapy platform. *Drug Alcohol Depend* 2008;94:142–150.
6. Carroll KM, Kosten TR, Rounsaville BJ. Choosing a behavioral therapy platform for pharmacotherapy of substance users. *Drug Alcohol Depend* 2004;75:123–134.
7. Gorelick DA, Gardner EL, Xi ZX. Agents in development for the management of cocaine abuse. *Drugs* 2004;64:1547–1573.
8. Gorelick, DA. Pharmacokinetic approaches to treatment of drug addiction. *Expert Rev Clin Pharmacol* 2008;1(2):277–290.
9. Howell LL, Kimmel HL. Monoamine transporters and psychostimulant addiction. *Biochem Pharmacol* 2008;75:196–217.
10. Lima MS, Reisser AA, Soares BG, Farrell M. Antidepressants for cocaine dependence. *Cochrane Database Syst Rev* 2003:CD002950.
11. Kosten T, Oliveto A, Feingold A, et al. Desipramine and contingency management for cocaine and opioid dependence in buprenorphine maintained patients. *Drug Alcohol Depend* 2003;70:315–325.
12. Kosten T, Sofuoglu M, Poling J, Gonsai K, Oliveto A. Desipramine treatment for cocaine dependence in buprenorphine- or methadone-treated patients: baseline urine results as predictor of response. *Am J Addict* 2005;14:8–17.
13. Ziedonis DM & Kosten TR. Pharmacotherapy improves treatment outcome in depressed cocaine addicts. *J Psychoactive Drugs* 1991;23(4): 417–425.
14. Arndt IO, McLellan AT, Dorozynsky L, et al. Desipramine treatment for cocaine dependence. *J Nerv Ment Dis* 1994;182:(3)151–156.
15. Khalsa ME, Gawin FH, Rawson R, et al. A desipramine ceiling in cocaine abusers. *Problems of Drug Dependence, 1992 (NIDA Research Monograph 132).* Rockville, MD: National Institute on Drug Abuse, 1993:18.
16. Brotman AW, Witkie SM, Gelenberg AJ, et al. An open trial of maprotiline for the treatment of cocaine abuse. *J Clin Psychopharmacol* 1988;8:125–127.
17. Szerman N, Peris L, Mesias B, et al. Reboxetine for the treatment of patients with Cocaine Dependence Disorder. *Hum Psychopharmacol* 2005;20:189–192.
18. Nunes EV, McGrath PJ, Quitkin FM, et al. Imipramine treatment of cocaine abuse possible boundaries of efficacy. *Drug Alcohol Depend* 1995;39:185–195.
19. Galloway GP, Newmeyer J, Knapp T, Stalcup SA, Smith D. Imipramine for the treatment of cocaine and methamphetamine dependence. *J Addict Dis* 1994;13:201–216.
20. Specker S, Crosby R, Borden J, et al. Nefazodone in the treatment of females with cocaine abuse. *Drug Alcohol Depend* 2000;60(Suppl 1):S179.
21. Passos SR, Camacho LA, Lopes CS, dos Santos MA. Nefazodone in outpatient treatment of inhaled cocaine dependence: a randomized double-blind placebo-controlled trial. *Addiction* 2005;100:489–494.
22. Ciraulo DA, Sarid-Segal O, Knapp CM, et al. Efficacy screening trials of paroxetine, pentoxifylline, riluzole, pramipexole and venlafaxine in cocaine dependence. *Addiction* 2005;100(Suppl 1):12–22.
23. Zueco Perez PL. Mirtazapine in the treatment of cocaine-dependence in patients with methadone. *Actas Esp Psiquiatr* 2002;30:337–342.
24. Fischman MW, Foltin RW, Nestadt G, et al. Effects of desipramine maintenance on cocaine self-administration by humans. *J Pharmacol Exp Ther* 1990;253(2):760–770.
25. Filip M, Frankowska M, Zaniewska M, Golda A, Przegalinski E. The serotonergic system and its role in cocaine addiction. *Pharmacol Rep* 2005;57:685–700.
26. Muller CP, Huston JP. Determining the region-specific contributions of 5-HT receptors to the psychostimulant effects of cocaine. *Trends Pharmacol Sci* 2006;27:105–112.
27. Winhusen TM, Somoza EC, Harrer JM, et al. A placebo-controlled screening trial of tiagabine, sertraline and donepezil as cocaine dependence treatments. *Addiction* 2005;100(Suppl 1):68–77.
28. Moeller FG, Schmitz JM, Steinberg JL, et al. Citalopram combined with behavioral therapy reduces cocaine use: a double-blind, placebo-controlled trial. *Am J Drug Alcohol Abuse* 2007;33:367–378.
29. Brewer C. Treatment of cocaine abuse with monoamine oxidase inhibitors. *Br J Psychiatry* 1993;163:815–816.
30. Maletzky BM. Phenelzine as a stimulant drug antagonist. *Int J Addict* 1977;12(5):661–665.
31. Golwyn DH. Cocaine abuse treated with phenelzine. *Int J Addict* 1988;23:897–905.
32. Elkashef A, Fudala PJ, Gorgon L, et al. Double-blind, placebo-controlled trial of selegiline transdermal system (STS) for the treatment of cocaine dependence. *Drug Alcohol Depend* 2006;85:191–197.
33. Margolin A, Kosten TR, Avants SK, et al. A multicenter trial of bupropion for cocaine dependence in methadone maintained patients. *Drug Alcohol Depend* 1995;40:125–131.
34. Poling J, Oliveto A, Petry N, et al. Six-month trial of bupropion with contingency management for cocaine dependence in a methadone-maintained population. *Arch Gen Psychiatry* 2006;63:219–228.
35. Cornish JW, Maany I, Fudala PJ, et al. A randomized, double-blind, placebo-controlled study of ritanserin pharmacotherapy for cocaine dependence. *Drug Alcohol Depend* 2001;61:183–189.

36. Johnson BA, Chen YR, Swann AC, et al. Ritanserin in the treatment of cocaine dependence. *Biol Psychiatry* 1997;42:932–940.
37. Dackis CA, Gold MS. Pharmacological approaches to cocaine addiction. *J Subst Abuse Treat* 1985;2:139–145.
38. Gorelick DA. Pharmacological treatment of cocaine addiction. *Einstein Q J Biol Med* 1999;16:61–69.
39. Pulvirenti L, Koob GF. Lisuride reduces intravenous cocaine self-administration in rats. *Pharmacol Biochem Behav* 1994;47(4):819–822.
40. Soares BG, Lima MS, Reisser AA, Farrell M. Dopamine agonists for cocaine dependence. *Cochrane Database Syst Rev* 2003:CD003352.
41. Tennant FS, Sagherian AA. Double-blind comparison of amantadine and bromocriptine for ambulatory withdrawal from cocaine dependence. *Arch Intern Med* 1987;147:109–112.
42. Moscovitz H, Brookoff D, Nelson L. A randomized trial of bromocriptine for cocaine users presenting to the emergency department. *J Gen Intern Med* 1993;8:1–4.
43. Gorelick DA, Wilkins JN. Bromocriptine treatment for cocaine addiction: association with plasma prolactin levels. *Drug Alcohol Depend* 2006;81:189–195.
44. Levin FR, McDowell D, Evans SM, et al. Pergolide mesylate for cocaine abuse: a controlled preliminary trial. *Am J Addict* 1999;8:120–127.
45. Malcolm R, Herron J, Sutherland SE, et al. Adverse outcomes in a controlled trial of pergolide for cocaine dependence. *J Addict Dis* 2001;20:81–92.
46. Focchi GR, Leite MC, Andrade AG, Scivoletto S. Use of dopamine agonist pergolide in outpatient treatment of cocaine dependence. *Subst Use Misuse* 2005;40:1169–1177.
47. Shoptaw S, Watson DW, Reiber C, et al. Randomized controlled pilot trial of cabergoline, hydergine and levodopa/carbidopa: Los Angeles Cocaine Rapid Efficacy Screening Trial (CREST). *Addiction* 2005;100(Suppl 1):78–90.
48. Meini M, Capovani B, Sbrana A, et al. A pilot open-label trial of ropinirole for cocaine dependence. *Am J Addict* 2008;17:165–166.
49. Shoptaw S, Kintaudi PC, Charuvastra C, Ling W. A screening trial of amantadine as a medication for cocaine dependence. *Drug Alcohol Depend* 2002;66:217–224.
50. Kampman KM, Dackis C, Lynch KG, et al. A double-blind, placebo-controlled trial of amantadine, propranolol, and their combination for the treatment of cocaine dependence in patients with severe cocaine withdrawal symptoms. *Drug Alcohol Depend* 2006;85:129–137.
51. Mooney ME, Schmitz JM, Moeller FG, Grabowski J. Safety, tolerability and efficacy of levodopa-carbidopa treatment for cocaine dependence: two double-blind, randomized, clinical trials. *Drug Alcohol Depend* 2007;88:214–223.
52. Cold JA. NeuRecover-DA in the treatment of cocaine withdrawal and craving, a pilot study. *Clin Drug Invest* 1996;12:1–7.
53. Galloway GP, Frederick SL, Thomas S, et al. A historically controlled trial of tyrosine for cocaine dependence. *J Psychoactive Drugs* 1996;28:305–309.
54. Thomas HM, Campbell J, Laster L, et al. Efficacy of two doses of tyrosine in retaining crack cocaine abusers in outpatient treatment. *Prob Drug Depend 1995 (NIDA Research Monograph 162)*. Rockville, MD: National Institute on Drug Abuse, 1996:148.
55. Suh JJ, Pettinati HM, Kampman KM, O'Brien CP. The status of disulfiram: a half of a century later. *J Clin Psychopharmacol* 2006;26: 290–302.
56. Pettinati HM, Kampman KM, Lynch KG, et al. Gender differences with high-dose naltrexone in patients with co-occurring cocaine and alcohol dependence. *J Subst Abuse Treat* 2008;34:378–390.
57. George TP, Chawarski MC, Pakes J, et al. Disulfiram versus placebo for cocaine dependence in buprenorphine-maintained subjects: a preliminary trial. *Biol Psychiatry* 2000;47:1080–1086.
58. Petrakis IL, Carroll KM, Nich C, et al. Disulfiram treatment for cocaine dependence in methadone-maintained opioid addicts. *Addiction* 2000; 95:219–228.
59. Carroll KM, Fenton LR, Ball SA, et al. Efficacy of disulfiram and cognitive behavior therapy in cocaine-dependent outpatients: a randomized placebo-controlled trial. *Arch Gen Psychiatry* 2004;61:264–272.
60. Nich C, Cance-Katz EF, Petrakis IL, et al. Sex differences in cocaine-dependent individuals' response to disulfiram treatment. *Addict Behav* 2004;29:1123–1128.
61. Mancino MJ, Feldman Z, Oliveto A. Gender differences in response to disulfiram treatment for cocaine dependence in methadone-stabilized opioid- and cocaine-dependent individuals. Presented at College on Problems of Drug Dependence annual meeting, San Juan, PR, June 2008.
62. Malcolm R, Olive MF, Lechner W. The safety of disulfiram for the treatment of alcohol and cocaine dependence in randomized clinical trials: guidance for clinical practice. *Expert Opin Drug Saf* 2008;7: 459–472.
63. McCance-Katz EF, Kosten TR, Jatlow P. Chronic disulfram treatment effects on intranasal cocaine administration: initial results. *Biol Psychiatry* 1998;43:540–543.
64. Baker J, Jatlow P, Pade P, Ramakrishnan V, McCance-Katz EF. Acute cocaine responses following cocaethylene infusion. *Am J Drug Alcohol Abuse* 2007;33:619–625.
65. Lile JA. Pharmacological determinants of the reinforcing effects of psychostimulants: relation to agonist substitution treatment. *Exp Clin Psychopharmacol* 2006;14:20–33.
66. Castells X, Casas M, Vidal X, et al. Efficacy of central nervous system stimulant treatment for cocaine dependence: a systematic review and meta-analysis of randomized controlled clinical trials. *Addiction* 2007;102:1871–1887.
67. Shearer J. The principles of agonist pharmacotherapy for psychostimulant dependence. *Drug Alcohol Rev* 2008;27:301–308.
68. Alim TN, Rosse RB, Vocci FJ Jr, et al. Diethylpropion pharmacotherapeutic adjuvant therapy for inpatient treatment of cocaine dependence: a test of the cocaine-agonist hypothesis. *Clin Neuropharmacol* 1995;18: 183–195.
69. Kosten TR, Steinberg M, Diakogiannis IA. Crossover trial of mazindol for cocaine dependence. *Am J Addict* 1993;2:161.
70. Margolin A, Avants SK, Kosten TR. Mazindol for relapse prevention to cocaine abuse in methadone-maintained patients. *Am J Drug Alcohol Abuse* 1995;21:469–481.
71. Stine SM, Krystal JH, Kosten TR, et al. Mazindol treatment for cocaine dependence. *Drug Alcohol Depend* 1995;39:245–252.
72. Ballon JS, Feifel D. A systematic review of modafinil: potential clinical uses and mechanisms of action. *J Clin Psychiatry* 2006;67:554–566.
73. Dackis CA, Kampman KM, Lynch KG, Pettinati HM, O'Brien CP. A double-blind, placebo-controlled trial of modafinil for cocaine dependence. *Neuropsychopharmacology* 2005;30:205–211.
74. Elkashef A. Modafinil for cocaine dependence, results from NIDA/DPMC multisite trial. Presented at College on Problems of Drug Dependence annual meeting, Quebec City, Canada, June 2007.
75. O'Brien CP, Dackis CA, Kampman K. Does modafinil produce euphoria? *Am J Psychiatry* 2006;163:1109.
76. Malcolm R, Swayngim K, Donovan J, et al. Modafinil and cocaine interactions. *Am J Drug Alcohol Abuse* 2006;32:577–587.
77. Donovan JL, DeVane CL, Malcolm RJ, et al. Modafinil influences the pharmacokinetics of intravenous cocaine in healthy cocaine-dependent volunteers. *Clin Pharmacokinet* 2005;44:753–765.
78. Gorelick DA. The rate hypothesis and agonist substitution approaches to cocaine abuse treatment. *Adv Pharmacol* 1998;42:995–997.
79. Walsh SL, Haberny KA, Bigelow GE. Modulation of intravenous cocaine effects by chronic oral cocaine in humans. *Psychopharmacology* 2000;150:361–373.
80. Llosa T, Llosa L. Oral cocaine as agonist therapy in cocaine dependence. Presented at College on Problems of Drug Dependence annual meeting, Orlando, FL, June 2005.
81. Hurtado-Gumucio J. Coca leaf chewing as therapy for cocaine maintenance. *Ann Med Interne (Paris)* 2000;151(Suppl B):B44–B48.
82. Brady K, Anton R, Ballenger JC, et al. Cocaine abuse among schizophrenic patients. *Am J Psychiatry* 1990;147:1164–1167.
83. Farren CK, Hameedi FA, Rosen MA, et al. Significant interaction between clozapine and cocaine self-administration by humans. *Drug Alcohol Depend* 2000;59:153–163.

84. Ohuoha DC, Maxwell JA, Thomson LE 3rd, et al. Effect of dopamine receptor antagonists on cocaine subjective effects: a naturalistic case study. *J Subst Abuse Treat* 1997;14:249–258.
85. Amato L, Minozzi S, Pani PP, Davoli M. Antipsychotic medications for cocaine dependence. *Cochrane Database Syst Rev* 2007:CD006306.
86. Bano MD, Mico JA, Agujetas M, Lopez ML, Guillen JL. Olanzapine efficacy in the treatment of cocaine abuse in methadone maintenance patients. Interaction with plasma levels. *Actas Esp Psiquiatr* 2001;29: 215–220.
87. Kampman KM, Pettinati H, Lynch KG, Sparkman T, O'Brien CP. A pilot trial of olanzapine for the treatment of cocaine dependence. *Drug Alcohol Depend* 2003;70:265–273.
88. Reid MS, Casadonte P, Baker S, et al. A placebo-controlled screening trial of olanzapine, valproate, and coenzyme Q10/L-carnitine for the treatment of cocaine dependence. *Addiction* 2005;100(Suppl 1):43–57.
89. Grabowski J, Rhoades H, Silverman P, et al. . Risperidone for the treatment of cocaine dependence: randomized, double-blind trial. *J Clin Psychopharmacol* 2000;20:305–310.
90. Grabowski J, Rhoades H, Stotts A, et al. Agonist-like or antagonist-like treatment for cocaine dependence with methadone for heroin dependence: two double-blind randomized clinical trials. *Neuropsychopharmacology* 2004;29:969–981.
91. Loebl T, Angarita GA, Pachas GN, et al. A randomized, double-blind, placebo-controlled trial of long-acting risperidone in cocaine-dependent men. *J Clin Psychiatry* 2008;69:480–486.
92. Akpaffiong MJ, Ruiz P. Neuroleptic malignant syndrome: a complication of neuroleptics and cocaine abuse. *Psychiatr Q* 1991;62:299–309.
93. Decker KP, Ries RK. Differential diagnosis and psychopharmacology of dual disorders. *Psychiatr Clin North Am* 1993;16(4):703–718.
94. van Harten PN, van Trier JCAM, Horwitz EH, et al. Cocaine as a risk factor for neuroleptic-induced acute dystonia. *J Clin Psychiatry* 1998;59:128–130.
95. Henderson JB, Labbate L, Worley M. A case of acute dystonia after single dose of aripiprazole in a man with cocaine dependence. *Am J Addict* 2007;16:244.
96. Duggal HS. Cocaine use as a risk factor for ziprasidone-induced acute dystonia. *Gen Hosp Psychiatry* 2007;29:278–279.
97. Halikas JA, Kuhn KL. A possible neurophysiological basis of cocaine craving. *Ann Clin Psychiatry* 1990;2:79–83.
98. Kalivas PW. Neurobiology of cocaine addiction: implications for new pharmacotherapy. *Am J Addict* 2007;16:71–78.
99. Karila L, Gorelick D, Weinstein A, et al. New treatments for cocaine dependence: a focused review. *Int J Neuropsychopharmacol* 2008;11: 425–438.
100. Minozzi S, Amato L, Davoli M, et al. Anticonvulsants for cocaine dependence. *Cochrane Database Syst Rev* 2008:CD006754.
101. Berger SP, Winhusen TM, Somoza EC, et al. A medication screening trial evaluation of reserpine, gabapentin and lamotrigine pharmacotherapy of cocaine dependence. *Addiction* 2005;100(Suppl 1):58–67.
102. Bisaga A, Aharonovich E, Garawi F, et al. A randomized placebo-controlled trial of gabapentin for cocaine dependence. *Drug Alcohol Depend* 2006;81:267–274.
103. Gonzalez G, Desai R, Sofuoglu M, et al. Clinical efficacy of gabapentin versus tiagabine for reducing cocaine use among cocaine dependent methadone-treated patients. *Drug Alcohol Depend* 2007;87:1–9.
104. Gonzalez G, Sevarino K, Sofuoglu M, et al. Tiagabine increases cocaine-free urines in cocaine-dependent methadone-treated patients: results of a randomized pilot study. *Addiction* 2003;98:1625–1632.
105. Winhusen T, Somoza E, Ciraulo DA, et al. A double-blind, placebo-controlled trial of tiagabine for the treatment of cocaine dependence. *Drug Alcohol Depend* 2007;91:141–148.
106. Kampman KM, Pettinati H, Lynch KG, et al. A pilot trial of topiramate for the treatment of cocaine dependence. *Drug Alcohol Depend* 2004;75: 233–240.
107. Brodie JD, Figueroa E, Dewey SL. Treating cocaine addiction: from preclinical to clinical trial experience with gamma-vinyl GABA. *Synapse* 2003;50:261–265.
108. Brodie JD, Figueroa E, Laska EM, Dewey SL. Safety and efficacy of gamma-vinyl GABA (GVG) for the treatment of methamphetamine and/or cocaine addiction. *Synapse* 2005;55:122–125.
109. Fechtner RD, Khouri AS, Figueroa E, et al. Short-term treatment of cocaine and/or methamphetamine abuse with vigabatrin: ocular safety pilot results. *Arch Ophthalmol* 2006;124:1257–1262.
110. Crosby RD, Pearson VL, Eller C, et al. Phenytoin in the treatment of cocaine abuse: a double-blind study. *Clin Pharmacol Ther* 1996;59: 458–468.
111. Shoptaw S, Yang X, Rotheram-Fuller EJ, et al. Randomized placebo-controlled trial of baclofen for cocaine dependence: preliminary effects for individuals with chronic patterns of cocaine use. *J Clin Psychiatry* 2003;64:1440–1448.
112. Blum K, Allison D, Trachtenberg MC, et al. Reduction of both drug hunger and withdrawal against advice rate of cocaine abusers in a 30-day inpatient treatment program by the neuronutrient tropamine. *Curr Ther Res* 1988;43:1204–1214.
113. Chadwick MJ, Gregory DL. A double-blind amino acids, L-tryptophan and L-tyrosine, and placebo study with cocaine-dependent subjects in an inpatient chemical dependency treatment center. *Am J Drug Alcohol Abuse* 1990;16:275–286.
114. Jones HE, Johnson RE, Bigelow GE, et al. Safety and efficacy of L-tryptophan and behavioral incentives for treatment of cocaine dependence: a randomized clinical trial. *Am J Addict* 2004;13: 421–437.
115. Margolin A, Kantak K, Copenhaver M, Avants SK. A preliminary, controlled investigation of magnesium L-aspartate hydrochloride for illicit cocaine and opiate use in methadone-maintained patients. *J Addict Dis* 2003;22:49–61.
116. Szumlinski KK, Maisonneuve IM, Glick SD. Iboga interactions with psychomotor stimulants: panacea in the paradox? *Toxicon* 2001;39: 75–86.
117. Kampman K, Majewska MD, Tourian K, et al. A pilot trial of piracetam and ginkgo biloba for the treatment of cocaine dependence. *Addict Behav* 2003;28:437–448.
118. Malcolm R, LaRowe S, Cochran K, et al. A controlled trial of amlodipine for cocaine dependence:a negative report. *J Subst Abuse Treat* 2005; 28:197–204.
119. Johnson BA, Roache JD, Daoud N, et al. A preliminary randomized, double-blind, placebo-controlled study of the safety and efficacy of ondansetron in the treatment of cocaine dependence. *Drug Alcohol Depend* 2006;84:256–263.
120. Schmitz JM, Stotts AL, Rhoades HM, et al. Naltrexone and relapse prevention treatment for cocaine-dependent patients. *Addict Behav* 2001;26:167–180.
121. Reid MS, Angrist B, Baker SA, et al. A placebo controlled, double-blind study of mecamylamine treatment for cocaine dependence in patients enrolled in an opiate replacement program. *Subst Abuse* 2005; 26:5–14.
122. Winhusen T, Somoza E, Sarid-Segal O, et al. A double-blind, placebo-controlled trial of reserpine for the treatment of cocaine dependence. *Drug Alcohol Depend* 2007;91:205–212.
123. Reid MS, Angrist B, Baker S, et al. A placebo-controlled screening trial of celecoxib for the treatment of cocaine dependence. *Addiction* 2005;100(Suppl 1):32–42.
124. Nunes EV, McGrath PJ, Wager S, et al. Lithium treatment for cocaine abusers with bipolar spectrum disorders. *Am J Psychiatry* 1990;147(5): 655–657.
125. Shoptaw S, Majewska MD, Wilkins J, et al. Participants receiving dehydroepiandrosterone during treatment for cocaine dependence show high rates of cocaine use in a placebo-controlled pilot study. *Exp Clin Psychopharmacol* 2004;12:126–135.
126. Montoya ID, Preston K, Rothman R, et al. Open-label pilot study of bupropion plus bromocriptine for treatment of cocaine dependence. *Am J Drug Alcohol Abuse* 2002;28:1–8.
127. Malcolm R, Moore JA, Brady KT, et al. Pergolide/haloperidol for the treatment of cocaine dependence. *Problems of Drug Dependence, 1999*

(NIDA Research Monograph 180). Rockville, MD: National Institute on Drug Abuse, 1999:165.

128. Kampman KM, Rukstalis M, Pettinati H, et al. The combination of phentermine and fenfluramine reduced cocaine withdrawal symptoms in an open trial. *J Subst Abuse Treat* 2000;19:77–79.
129. Connolly HM, McGoon MD. Obesity drugs and the heart. *Curr Prob Cardiol* 1999;24:745–792.
130. Urschel HC, III, Hanselka LL, Gromov I, White L, Baron M. Open-label study of a proprietary treatment program targeting type A gamma-aminobutyric acid receptor dysregulation in methamphetamine dependence. *Mayo Clin Proc* 2007;82:1170–1178.
131. Margolin A. Acupuncture for substance abuse. *Curr Psychiatry Rep* 2003;5:333–339.
132. Gates S, Smith LA, Foxcroft DR. Auricular acupuncture for cocaine dependence. *Cochrane Database of Syst Rev* 2006:CD005192.
133. Mills EJ, Wu P, Gagnier J, Ebbert JO. Efficacy of acupuncture for cocaine dependence: a systematic review & meta-analysis. *Harm Reduction J* 2005;2:4.
134. Ridding MC, Rothwell JC. Is there a future for therapeutic use of transcranial magnetic stimulation? *Nat Rev Neurosci* 2007;8:559–567.
135. Camprodon JA, Martinez-Raga J, onso-Alonso M, Shih MC, Pascual-Leone A. One session of high frequency repetitive transcranial magnetic stimulation (rTMS) to the right prefrontal cortex transiently reduces cocaine craving. *Drug Alcohol Depend* 2007;86:91–94.
136. Politi E, Fauci E, Santoro A, Smeraldi E. Daily sessions of transcranial magnetic stimulation to the left prefrontal cortex gradually reduce cocaine craving. *Am J Addict* 2008;17:345–346.
137. Ling W, Rawson R, Shoptaw S, Ling W. Management of methamphetamine abuse and dependence. *Curr Psychiatry Rep* 2006;8:345–354.
138. Hill KP, Sofuoglu M. Biological treatments for amphetamine dependence: recent progress. *CNS Drugs* 2007;21:851–869.
139. Tiihonen J, Kuoppasalmi K, Fohr J, et al. A comparison of aripiprazole, methylphenidate, and placebo for amphetamine dependence. *Am J Psychiatry* 2007;164:160–162.
140. Camacho A, Stein MB. Modafinil for social phobia and amphetamine dependence. *Am J Psychiatry* 2002;159:1947–1948.
141. Heinzerling KG, Shoptaw S, Peck JA, et al. Randomized, placebo-controlled trial of baclofen and gabapentin for the treatment of methamphetamine dependence. *Drug Alcohol Depend* 2006;85: 177–184.
142. Jayaram-Lindstrom N, Hammarberg A, Beck O, Franck J. Naltrexone for the treatment of amphetamine dependence: A randomized placebo-controlled trial. *Am J Psychiatry* 2008;165:11:1442–1448.
143. Elkashef AM, Rawson RA, Anderson AL, et al. Bupropion for the treatment of methamphetamine dependence. *Neuropsychopharmacology* 2008;33:1162–1170.
144. Shoptaw S, Heinzerling KG, Rotheram-Fuller E, et al. Randomized, placebo-controlled trial of bupropion for the treatment of methamphetamine dependence. Presented at College on Problems of Drug Dependence annual meeting, San Juan, PR, June 2008.
145. Meredith CW, Jaffe C, Yanasak E, Cherrier M, Saxon AJ. An open-label pilot study of risperidone in the treatment of methamphetamine dependence. *J Psychoactive Drugs* 2007;39:167–172.
146. Saxon AJ, Meredith CW, Jaffe C, et al. Changes in addiction severity in an open trial of long-acting injectable risperidone for methamphetamine dependence. Presented at College on Problems of Drug Dependence annual meeting, San Juan, PR, June 2008.
147. Johnson BA, it-Daoud N, Elkashef AM, et al. A preliminary randomized, double-blind, placebo-controlled study of the safety and efficacy of ondansetron in the treatment of methamphetamine dependence. *Int J Neuropsychopharmacol* 2008;11:1–14.
148. Srisurapanont M, Jarusuraisin N, Kittirattanapaiboon P. Treatment for amphetamine dependence and abuse. *Cochrane Database Syst Rev* 2001:CD003022.
149. Grella CE, Anglin MD, Wugalter SE. Patterns and predictors of cocaine and crack use by clients in standard and enhanced methadone maintenance treatment. *Am J Drug Alcohol Abuse* 1997;23:15–42.
150. Dobler-Mikola A, Hattenschwiler J, Meili D, et al. Patterns of heroin, cocaine, and alcohol abuse during long-term methadone maintenance treatment. *J Subst Abuse Treat* 2005;29:259–265.
151. Tennant F, Shannon J. Cocaine abuse in methadone maintenance patients is associated with low serum methadone concentrations. *J Addict Dis* 1995;14:67–74.
152. Peles E, Kreek MJ, Kellogg S, Adelson M. High methadone dose significantly reduces cocaine use in methadone maintenance treatment (MMT) patients. *J Addict Dis* 2006;25:43–50.
153. Grabowski J, Rhoades H, Elk R, et al. Methadone dosage, cocaine, and opiate abuse. *Am J Psychiatry* 1993;150(4):675.
154. Stine SM, Freeman M, Burns B. Effect of methadone dose on cocaine abuse in a methadone program. *Am J Addict* 1992;1(4):294–303.
155. Mattick RP, Kimber J, Breen C, Davoli M. Buprenorphine maintenance versus placebo or methadone maintenance for opioid dependence. *Cochrane Database Syst Rev* 2008:CD002207.
156. Schottenfeld R, Pakes J, Ziedonis D, et al. Buprenorphine: dose-related effects on cocaine and opioid use in cocaine-abusing opioid-dependent humans. *Biol Psychiatry* 1993;34:66–74.
157. Montoya ID, Gorelick DA, Preston KL, et al. Randomized trial of buprenorphine for treatment of concurrent opiate and cocaine dependence. *Clin Pharmacol Ther* 2004;75:34–48.
158. Schottenfeld RS, Chawarski MC, Pakes JR, et al. Methadone versus buprenorphine with contingency management or performance feedback for cocaine and opioid dependence. *Am J Psychiatry* 2005;162:340–349.
159. Gross A, Marsch LA, Badger GJ, Bickel WK. A comparison between low-magnitude voucher and buprenorphine medication contingencies in promoting abstinence from opioids and cocaine. *Exp Clin Psychopharmacol* 2006;14:148–156.
160. Gorelick DA. Alcohol and cocaine: clinical and pharmacological interactions. *Recent Dev Alcohol* 1992;11:37–56.
161. Carroll KM, Nich C, Ball SA, et al. Treatment of cocaine and alcohol dependence with psychotherapy and disulfiram. *Addiction* 1998;93: 713–728.
162. Pennings EJ, Leccese AP, Wolff FA. Effects of concurrent use of alcohol and cocaine. *Addiction* 2002;97:773–783.
163. Carroll KM, Nich C, Ball SA, et al. One-year follow-up of disulfiram and psychotherapy for cocaine-alcohol users: sustained effects of treatment. *Addiction* 2000;95:1335–1349.
164. Higgins ST, Budney AJ, Bickel WK, et al. Disulfiram therapy in patients abusing cocaine and alcohol. *Am J Psychiatry* 1993;150(4):675–676.
165. Grassi MC, Cioce AM, Giudici FD, Antonilli L, Nencini. Short-term efficacy of disulfiram or naltrexone in reducing positive urinalysis for both cocaine and cocaethylene in cocaine abusers: a pilot study. *Pharmacol Res* 2007;55:117–121.
166. Pettinati HM, Kampman KM, Lynch KG, et al. A double blind, placebo-controlled trial that combines disulfiram and naltrexone for treating co-occurring cocaine and alcohol dependence. *Addict Behav* 2008;33:651–667.
167. Oslin DW, Pettinati HM, Volpicelli JR, et al. The effects of naltrexone on alcohol and cocaine use in dually addicted patients. *J Subst Abuse Treat* 1999;16:163–167.
168. Carroll KM, Ziedonis D, O'Malley S, et al. Pharmacologic interventions for alcohol- and cocaine-abusing individuals. *Am J Addict* 1993;2(1): 77–79.
169. Hersh D, Van Kirk JR, Kranzler HR. Naltrexone treatment of comorbid alcohol and cocaine use disorders. *Psychopharmacology* 1998;139: 44–52.
170. Schmitz JM, Stotts AL, Sayre SL, DeLaune KA, Grabowski J. Treatment of cocaine-alcohol dependence with naltrexone and relapse prevention therapy. *Am J Addict* 2004;13:333–341.
171. Schmitz JM, Grabowski J, Green C, Herin D, Lindsay J. High-dose naltrexone therapy for cocaine-alcohol dependence. Presented at College on Problems of Drug Dependence annual meeting, San Juan, PR, June 2008.
172. Rounsaville BJ, Anton SF, Carroll K, et al. Psychiatric diagnoses of treatment-seeking cocaine abusers. *Arch Gen Psychiatry* 1991;48:43–51.

173. Thevos AK, Brady KT, Grice D, et al. A comparison of psychopathy in cocaine and alcohol dependence. *Am J Addict* 1993;2:279–286.
174. Conway KP, Compton W, Stinson FS, Grant BF. Lifetime comorbidity of DSM-IV mood and anxiety disorders and specific drug use disorders: results from the National Epidemiologic Survey on Alcohol and Related Conditions. *J Clin Psychiatry* 2006;67:247–257.
175. Weiss RD, Mirin SM, Griffin ML, et al. Personality disorders in cocaine dependence. *Comprehensive Psychiatry* 1993;34:145–149.
176. Compton WM, Conway KP, Stinson FS, Colliver JD, Grant BF. Prevalence, correlates, and comorbidity of DSM-IV antisocial personality syndromes and alcohol and specific drug use disorders in the United States: results from the National Epidemiologic Survey on Alcohol and Related Conditions. *J Clin Psychiatry* 2005;66:677–685.
177. Rounsaville BJ. Treatment of cocaine dependence and depression. *Biol Psychiatry* 2004;56:803–809.
178. Nunes EV, Levin FR. Treatment of depression in patients with alcohol or other drug dependence: a meta-analysis. *JAMA* 2004;291: 1887–1896.
179. Gonzalez G, Feingold A, Oliveto A, Gonsai K, Kosten TR. Comorbid major depressive disorder as a prognostic factor in cocaine-abusing buprenorphine-maintained patients treated with desipramine and contingency management. *Am J Drug Alcohol Abuse* 2003;29: 497–514.
180. McDowell D, Nunes EV, Seracini AM, et al. Desipramine treatment of cocaine-dependent patients with depression:a placebo-controlled trial. *Drug Alcohol Depend* 2005;80:209–221.
181. McDowell DM, Levin FR, Seracini AM, et al. Venlafaxine treatment of cocaine abusers with depressive disorders. *Am J Drug Alcohol Abuse* 2000;26:25–31.
182. Ciraulo DA, Knapp C, Rotrosen J, et al. Nefazodone treatment of cocaine dependence with comorbid depressive symptoms. *Addiction* 2005;100(Suppl 1):23-31.
183. Brown ES, Suppes T, Adinoff B, et al. Drug abuse and bipolar disorder: comorbidity or misdiagnosis? *J Affect Dis* 2001;65:105–115.
184. Goldberg JF, Garno JL, Leon AC, et al. A history of substance abuse complicates remission from acute mania in bipolar disorder. *J Clin Psychiatry* 1999;60:733–740.
185. Sattar SP, Petty F. Valproate in the treatment of bipolar disorder and comorbid substance abuse: a 24-week open label trial. *Am J Addict* 2008; 17:329.
186. Salloum IM, Douaihy A, Cornelius JR, et al. Divalproex utility in bipolar disorder with co-occurring cocaine dependence: a pilot study. *Addict Behav* 2007;32:410–415.
187. Brown ES, Perantie DC, Dhanani N, et al. Lamotrigine for bipolar disorder and comorbid cocaine dependence: a replication and extension study. *J Affect Disord* 2006;93:219–222.
188. Brown ES, Nejtek VA, Perantie DC, Bobadilla L. Quetiapine in bipolar disorder and cocaine dependence. *Bipolar Disord* 2002;4:406–411.
189. Nejtek VA, Avila M, Chen LA, et al. Do atypical antipsychotics effectively treat co-occurring bipolar disorder and stimulant dependence? A randomized, double-blind trial. *J Clin Psychiatry* 2008;e1–e10.
190. Brown ES, Jeffress J, Liggin JD, Garza M, Beard L. Switching outpatients with bipolar or schizoaffective disorders and substance abuse from their current antipsychotic to aripiprazole. *J Clin Psychiatry* 2005;66: 756–760.
191. Brown ES. A randomized, placebo-controlled trial of citicholine add-on therapy in outpatients with bipolar disorder and cocaine dependence. *Biol Psychiatry* 2007;61:565.
192. Schubiner H. Substance abuse in patients with attention-deficit hyperactivity disorder: therapeutic implications. *CNS Drugs* 2005;19: 643–655.
193. Kollins SH. A qualitative review of issues arising in the use of psychostimulant medications in patients with ADHD and co-morbid substance use disorders. *Curr Med Res Opin* 2008;24:1345–1357.
194. Castaneda R, Levy R, Hardy M, et al. Long-acting stimulants for the treatment of attention-deficit disorder in cocaine-dependent adults. *Psychiatr Serv* 2000;51:169–171.
195. Downey KK, Schubiner H, Schuster CR. Double-blind placebo controlled stimulant trial for cocaine-dependent ADHD adults. *Prob Drug Depend, 1999 (NIDA Research Monograph 180).* Rockville, MD: National Institute on Drug Abuse, 1999:116.
196. Levin FR, Evans SM, McDowell DM, et al. Methylphenidate treatment for cocaine abusers with adult attention-deficit/hyperactivity disorder: a pilot study. *J Clin Psychiatry* 1998;59:300–305.
197. Levin FR, Evans SM, Brooks DJ, et al. Treatment of methadone-maintained patients with adult ADHD: double-blind comparison of methylphenidate, bupropion and placebo. *Drug Alcohol Depend* 2006; 81:137–148.
198. Levin FR, Evans SM, Brooks DJ, Garawi F. Treatment of cocaine dependent treatment seekers with adult ADHD: double-blind comparison of methylphenidate and placebo. *Drug Alcohol Depend* 2007;87: 20–29.
199. Schubiner H, Saules KK, Arfken CL, et al. Double-blind placebo-controlled trial of methylphenidate in the treatment of adult ADHD patients with comorbid cocaine dependence. *Exp Clin Psychopharmacol* 2002;10:286–294.
200. Buckley PF. Prevalence and consequences of the dual diagnosis of substance abuse and severe mental illness. *J Clin Psychiatry* 2006;67(Suppl 7): 5–9.
201. Green AI. Treatment of schizophrenia and comorbid substance abuse: pharmacologic approaches. *J Clin Psychiatry* 2006;67(Suppl 7):31–35.
202. San L, Arranz B, Martinez-Raga J. Antipsychotic drug treatment of schizophrenic patients with substance abuse disorders. *Eur Addict Res* 2007;13:230–243.
203. Soyka M & De Vry J. Flupenthixol as a potential pharmacotreatment of alcohol and cocaine abuse/dependence. *Eur Neuropsychopharmacol* 2000; 10:325–332.
204. Levin FR, Evans SM, Coomaraswammy S, et al. Flupenthixol treatment for cocaine abusers with schizophrenia: a pilot study. *Am J Drug Alcohol Abuse* 1998;24:343–360.
205. Sayers SL, Campbell EC, Kondrich J, et al. Cocaine abuse in schizophrenic patients treated with olanzapine versus haloperidol. *J Nerv Ment Dis* 2005;193:379–386.
206. Smelson DA, Ziedonis D, Williams J, et al. The efficacy of olanzapine for decreasing cue-elicited craving in individuals with schizophrenia and cocaine dependence: a preliminary report. *J Clin Psychopharmacol* 2006; 26:9–12.
207. Akerele E, Levin FR. Comparison of olanzapine to risperidone in substance-abusing individuals with schizophrenia. *Am J Addict* 2007;16: 260–268.
208. Sullivan LE, Bruce RD, Haltiwanger D, et al. Initial strategies for integrating buprenorphine into HIV care settings in the United States. *Clin Infect Dis* 2006;43(Suppl 4):S191–S196.
209. Carrieri MP, Vlahov D, Dellamonica P, et al. Use of buprenorphine in HIV-infected injection drug users: negligible impact on virologic response to HAART. The Manif-2000 Study Group. *Drug Alcohol Depend* 2000;60:51–54.
210. Avants SK, Margolin A, DePhilippis D, et al. A comprehensive pharmacologic-psychosocial treatment program for HIV-seropositive cocaine- and opioid-dependent patients. *J Subst Abuse Treat* 1998; 15:261–265.
211. Hogeland GW, Swindells S, McNabb JC, et al. Lopinavir/ritonavir reduces bupropion plasma concentrations in healthy subjects. *Clin Pharmacol Ther* 2007;81:69–75.
212. Gorelick DA, Montoya ID, Johnson EO. Sociodemographic representation in published studies of cocaine abuse pharmacotherapy. *Drug Alcohol Depend* 1998;49:89–93.
213. Helmbrecht GD, Thiagarajah S. Management of addiction disorders in pregnancy. *J Addict Med* 2008;2(1):1–16.
214. Rayburn WF, Bogenschutz MP. Pharmacotherapy for pregnant women with addictions. *Am J Obstet Gynecol* 2004;191:1885–1897.
215. Rothman RB, Baumann MH, Prisinzano TE, Newman AH. Dopamine transport inhibitors based on GBR12909 and benztropine as potential

medications to treat cocaine addiction. *Biochem Pharmacol* 2008;75: 2–16.

216. Xi ZX, Gardner EL. Pharmacological actions of NGB 2904, a selective dopamine D3 receptor antagonist, in animal models of drug addiction. *CNS Drug Rev* 2007;13:240–259.
217. Rothman RB, Blough BE, Baumann MH. Dual dopamine/serotonin releasers as potential medications for stimulant and alcohol addictions. *AAPS J* 2007;9:E1–E10.
218. LaRowe SD, Mardikian P, Malcolm R, et al. Safety and tolerability of N-acetylcysteine in cocaine-dependent individuals. *Am J Addict* 2006; 15:105–110.
219. LaRowe SD, Myrick H, Hedden S, et al. Is cocaine desire reduced by N-acetylcysteine? *Am J Psychiatry* 2007;164:1115–1117.
220. Mardikian PN, LaRowe SD, Hedden S, et al. An open-label trial of N-acetylcysteine for the treatment of cocaine dependence: a pilot study. *Prog Neuropsychopharmacol Biol Psychiatry* 2007;31: 389–394.
221. Specio SE, Wee S, O'Dell LE, et al. CRF(1) receptor antagonists attenuate escalated cocaine self-administration in rats. *Psychopharmacology (Berl)* 2008;196:473–482.
222. Carroll KM, Rounsaville BJ, Gordon LT, et al. Psychotherapy and pharmacotherapy for ambulatory cocaine abusers. *Arch Gen Psychiatry* 1994;51:177–187.
223. Miller WR, Manuel JK. How large must a treatment effect be before it matters to practitioners? An estimation method and demonstration. *Drug Alcohol Rev* 2008:1–5.

CHAPTER 52

Richard D. Hurt, MD, FASAM
Jon O. Ebbert, MD
J. Taylor Hays, MD

Pharmacologic Interventions for Tobacco Dependence

Tobacco has been used since the earliest recorded history of the Western hemisphere, but cigarettes were not mass produced and marketed until the early part of the 20th century. The resulting annual consumption increased from less than 4 billion cigarettes in 1905 to more than 100 billion 20 years later (1) peaking in the mid-1960s when Americans consumed more than 600 billion cigarettes annually. The epidemic of tobacco-caused diseases emerged in the mid-20th century and has spread throughout the world. In 2000, about 5 million people died of tobacco-related diseases and an estimated 10 million annual tobacco-related deaths are expected to occur by 2030 (2,3). The tobacco industry responded to these staggering figures by denying the relationship of cigarettes to disease and mounting a public relations campaign to deceive the public (4). The common thread woven through the history of the major tobacco companies is their pursuit of a highly sophisticated and efficient nicotine delivery device which they perfected in the modern cigarette. Smoking one cigarette results in a high level of occupancy of the $\alpha_4\beta_2$ nicotinic acetylcholine receptors in the central nervous system, and three cigarettes completely saturate these receptors for as long as 3 hours (5). Craving reduction requires virtually complete receptor saturation. Clinicians need to understand this important background information that places into context two important facts regarding treatment for tobacco use and dependence: the efficient and rapid delivery of nicotine by cigarettes is a key factor in the development of tobacco dependence, and nicotine replacement products commonly used to treat tobacco dependence are relatively inefficient in delivering nicotine and deliver much lower concentrations compared with cigarettes. Nicotine replacement products as well as other non-nicotine medications are indicated to treat tobacco dependence.

The U.S. Food and Drug Administration (FDA) has now approved seven products for the treatment of tobacco dependence in the United States, all of which are considered first-line medications in the U.S. Public Health Service (USPHS) Guideline "Treating Tobacco Use and Dependence – 2008" (6). The authors of the 2008 guideline note substantial progress has been made since the first guideline was published in 1996. The guideline points to the increased coverage of tobacco dependence treatments by health plans, Medicare and Medicaid. The Joint Commission now requires interventions for smokers with the diagnosis of acute myocardial infarction, congestive heart failure, or pneumonia *(www.coreoptions.com/new_site/jcahocore.html)*. In addition, the guideline highlights that progress has been made in disseminating treatment options. Telephone quitlines have been particularly effective in providing wide access to counseling and many quitlines provide nicotine replacement at no cost to the smoker (7). Finally, the guideline states that unless there are contraindications, medications should be considered for all smokers who want to quit and that counseling adds significantly to the effectiveness of medications. Because pharmacotherapy has been established as a cornerstone of treatment of the tobacco-dependent patient, research and development of new medications is likely to continue.

PATHOPHYSIOLOGY OF TOBACCO DEPENDENCE

Nicotine has complex and wide-ranging effects on the central nervous system. Nicotine binds to and causes conformational changes in nicotinic acetylcholine receptors. Nicotinic acetylcholine receptors are located in all areas of the human brain and, when stimulated, cause the release of dopamine, norepinephrine, glutamate, vasopressin, serotonin, gamma-aminobutyric acid (GABA), beta-endorphins, and other neurotransmitters. High concentrations of nicotinic acetylcholine receptors exist in the mesolimbic dopamine system and locus ceruleus (8). The former is important in pleasure and reward and the latter is important for cognitive function. Although not completely understood, upregulation of the high affinity $\alpha_4\beta_2$ nicotinic acetylcholine receptor is critical for the development of tolerance to and dependence on nicotine (9). Repeated exposure to high concentrations of nicotine causes upregulation of the $\alpha_4\beta_2$ nicotinic acetylcholine receptors, leading to an absolute increase in their numbers (9,10). Neuroadaptation of the mesolimbic system in smokers and its target neurons in the nucleus accumbens may be longer lasting than previously thought, which could explain the observation that cravings to smoke last for months after a smoker stops smoking (11).

In the mesolimbic system, the so-called "reward center," nicotine causes the release of dopamine believed to be associated with nicotine's positive reinforcing effects and a critical mediator of addiction (8,15). The mesolimbic system area is also involved with the positive reinforcing effects of amphetamines, cocaine, and opiates (12–14). Nicotine-induced dose-dependent increases in feelings of pleasure have been observed to occur simultaneously with increases in the functional magnetic resonance imaging of neuronal activity in the nucleus accumbens, amygdala, cingulate, and frontal lobes (16). Because dopaminergic transmission within the nucleus accumbens is modulated by GABA, it has been postulated that GABA-transaminase inhibitors such as gamma vinyl GABA might inhibit nicotine-induced increases in dopamine by increasing levels of GABA in the nucleus accumbens (17). In laboratory animals, self-administered intravenous nicotine increases the sensitivity of brain reward systems and imprints an indelible memory of its effects in reward systems, an action that appears unique to nicotine among drugs of abuse (18). This may partially explain the rapid relapse to former levels of smoking that frequently follows a smoker having a few cigarettes after a prolonged period of smoking abstinence.

Tobacco dependence in smokers has been hypothesized to have a genetic component as well (19). Accumulating data support the role of genetic factors in smoking initiation, progression to tobacco dependence, and continued smoking (20). Twin studies have confirmed an inherited component for tobacco use and dependence, and familial transmission of smoking behavior has been observed across three generations of families (21). Multiple genetic polymorphisms have been hypothesized to exist relating to dopamine release, dopamine transmission, dopamine receptors, and nicotine metabolism that are important inherited factors influencing the initiation and perpetuation of tobacco use (22,23). Evidence suggests that two single-nucleotide polymorphisms in CHRNA4 (gene coding for the α4 subunit of nicotinic acetylcholine receptors) are biologically functional and associated with tobacco dependence phenotypes (24). However, substance dependence is complex and involves multiple genetic and environmental risk factors (25). Indeed the evidence for a contribution of specific genes to smoking behavior remains modest (26). Further work is needed to study the spectrum of heritable traits that influence genetic susceptibility to tobacco dependence.

Genetic factors may also have implications for treatment. Studies of the dopamine D4 receptor gene demonstrate that genetic variants related to relatively decreased dopaminergic tone in the mesocorticolimbic system are associated with relapse to smoking after a quit attempt (27). As this research advances, it will be important to address the practical, economic, ethical, and social barriers to the translation of genetics research on tobacco dependence treatment into clinical practice (28).

MEASURING NICOTINE EXPOSURE

One approach to the therapeutic use of nicotine replacement therapy (NRT) for the treatment of tobacco dependence is to determine the patient's level of nicotine exposure. After this exposure is determined, a nicotine replacement dose approximating the dose the individual receives from smoking can be prescribed. However, several factors make this task difficult. Smokers exposed to the same amount of nicotine through inhaled tobacco smoke have marked interindividual differences in venous nicotine concentrations (29,30). Cigarette smoking produces initial arterial nicotine concentrations that are several-fold higher than concomitant venous nicotine levels (31). In addition, nicotine has a short half-life (i.e., 120 minutes) and, with smoking, tends to have peaks and troughs in both the venous and the arterial circulation. For these reasons, a non-nicotine biologic measure is needed to estimate nicotine exposure.

Cotinine, the major metabolite of nicotine, has a half-life of 18 to 20 hours and can be used to quantify an individual's exposure to nicotine. Venous nicotine concentrations (albeit less than arterial levels) reflect acute nicotine exposure, whereas cotinine reflects nicotine exposure over 2 to 3 days. Minor tobacco alkaloids such as nornicotine, anatabine, and anabasine can be measured in the urine of tobacco users (32–34). Anabasine is a tobacco alkaloid that is not a metabolic product of nicotine. Anabasine is present in the urine of tobacco users but not in the urine of patients using NRT. Anabasine thus can be especially useful in distinguishing abstinent tobacco users who are using NRT from those who are continuing to use tobacco. This has become especially important for adjudicating tobacco abstinence in lung or heart transplant candidates as many transplant surgeons insist on such patients being abstinent from tobacco before being placed on a transplant list.

NRT

According to the USPHS Clinical Practice Guideline, every patient who is willing to make an attempt to stop smoking should be offered counseling and medications (6). The guideline states that approved medications should be used in all patients except groups in whom efficacy is not established (i.e., adolescent smokers) or in the presence of contraindications. Clinical trials have shown that adding pharmacotherapy to a behavioral intervention generally doubles smoking abstinence rates and that the combination of medication and counseling is more effective than either alone. Thus counseling and medication should be routinely provided to patients who are prepared to make a quit attempt. Because of its demonstrated efficacy in multiple clinical trials, NRT remains a mainstay of pharmacotherapy for the treatment of tobacco dependence.

To date, the FDA has approved five nicotine replacement products: nicotine gum, nicotine patches, nicotine nasal spray, a nicotine vapor inhaler, and nicotine lozenges. The nicotine gum, patches and lozenges are available over-the-counter; the nasal spray and inhaler are available by prescription only. Physicians who prescribe NRT for tobacco dependence should individualize the dose and duration of treatment and schedule follow-up office visits or telephone calls to monitor patient response. The dose and duration of therapy should be based on the patient's subjective need for relief of withdrawal symptoms and support of smoking abstinence.

The 2008 USPHS Guideline shows increasing efficacy with total contact time of up to 90 minutes and four to eight sessions (odds ratio [OR] 1.9) compared with a single session, whereas >8 sessions with an OR = 2.3 produces an average smoking abstinence rate of almost 25%.

Nicotine Gum Nicotine gum is available as an over-the-counter product, in both the 2- and 4-mg doses and has been shown to be effective as monotherapy or in combination with other NRT. Venous nicotine concentrations achieved through the proper use of nicotine gum are relatively low compared with those produced by smoking cigarettes (35). The 4-mg dose is indicated for use in smokers who are more dependent (36,37) and is recommended for those who smoke 25 or more cigarettes per day. Patients should be instructed to bite into a piece of nicotine gum a few times until a mild tingling or peppery taste indicates nicotine release. The patient then should "park" the gum between the cheek and gum for several minutes before chewing it again. This cycle allows for buccal absorption and should be repeated over a period of 30 minutes per piece of gum. Because the absorption of nicotine is lowered by a more acidic pH, patients should be instructed not to drink beverages or eat for several minutes before and while using the gum. When nicotine gum is used as a single agent, most patients should use a minimum of 10 to 15 pieces per day to achieve initial smoking abstinence. The most common adverse effects of nicotine gum are nausea and indigestion, which can be minimized with the proper "chew-and-park" technique. Other adverse effects reported include gingival soreness and mouth ulcerations.

Nicotine Lozenge The nicotine lozenge is available in the United States as an over-the-counter product. The nicotine lozenge is available in 2- and 4-mg doses, with the latter for use in "high" dependence smokers (i.e., time to first cigarette of the day <30 minutes after arising) (37). Although the method of delivery (transbuccal) is similar to that of nicotine gum, the lozenge is simpler to use and likely will demonstrate improved patient compliance. As with the other short-acting NRT products, it can be used alone or in combination with other NRT.

Nicotine Patch Nicotine patch therapy was introduced in 1991 and delivers a steady dose of nicotine for 24 hours after a single application. The once-daily dosing requires little effort on the part of the patient, which enhances compliance. Nicotine patches are available without a prescription in doses of 7, 14, and 21 mg, which deliver nicotine over 24 hours. In almost every randomized clinical trial performed to date, the nicotine patch has been shown to be effective compared with placebo usually with a doubling of the stop rate.

Standard-dose nicotine patch therapy is 21 mg/24 hours. Most regimens continue this dose for several weeks before tapering over a period of weeks. However, the standard dose patch approach is not effective in all smokers. In fact, it has been shown that a standard dose (21 mg/24 hours) of nicotine patch therapy achieves a median serum cotinine level of only 54% of the cotinine concentrations achieved through smoking (29,39). There is a dose-response for nicotine patch therapy particularly among lighter smokers with lower baseline cotinine concentrations, suggesting that their nicotine replacement needs are more adequately met than those of heavier smokers (40).

Because of the observation that many patients are underdosed with standard nicotine patch doses, studies have been conducted assessing the efficacy of higher doses. Use of high doses of nicotine patch therapy (i.e., doses >21 mg/day) are appropriate for smokers who previously failed single-dose patch therapy or for those whose nicotine withdrawal symptoms are not relieved sufficiently with standard therapy (41). This approach can be especially important for heavy smokers because they will be significantly underdosed with single-dose patch therapy (29). High-dose nicotine patch therapy has been shown to be safe and well tolerated in patients who smoke more than 20 cigarettes per day (29,42). It should be noted, however, that the 2008 USPHS Guideline Panel concluded that high-dose nicotine patch therapy did not appear to produce benefit above and beyond that of standard-dose nicotine patch therapy. However, the panel observed that if the patient is severely addicted the clinician may consider higher than the FDA-recommended dose and that higher doses have been shown to be effective in highly dependent smokers.

By employing the concept of therapeutic drug monitoring, clinicians can use serum cotinine concentrations to tailor the nicotine replacement dose so that it approaches 100% replacement. A baseline cotinine concentration is obtained while the smoker is smoking his or her usual number of cigarettes. An initial nicotine patch dose based on the baseline cotinine concentration (or cigarettes per day) is prescribed. After the patient reaches steady state (>3 days of nicotine patch therapy and not smoking), the serum cotinine concentration is

TABLE 52.1 Nicotine Patch Dose Based on Baseline (while Smoking) Blood Cotinine Concentration

Cotinine in ng/mL	Nicotine patch dose
<200	14–21 mg/day
200–300	21–42 mg/day
>300	≥42 mg/day

TABLE 52.2 Recommended Initial Dosing of Nicotine Patch Therapy Based on Number of Cigarettes Smoked Daily

Cigarettes per Day	Patch dose (mg/d)*
<10	7–14
10–20	14–21
21–40	21–42
>40	42+

*Nicotine patches are available in the following doses: 7, 14, and 21 mg.

rechecked and the replacement dose can be adjusted to achieve a steady-state cotinine level that approaches the baseline level. Percentage replacement for a given dose of nicotine patch therapy can be expressed as follows:

Percentage replacement = (steady-state serum cotinine ÷ baseline serum cotinine) × 100%. Table 52.1 shows the recommended initial dosing of nicotine patch therapy based on serum cotinine concentrations. Higher percentage replacement has been shown to reduce nicotine withdrawal symptoms (29), but the efficacy for long-term smoking abstinence of such an approach has not been completely established (29,43–45). Nevertheless, this concept can be used to titrate more precisely the dose to achieve higher concentrations of nicotine replacement in the more highly addicted patient.

For special populations in whom a need to use the lowest possible effective dose exists (e.g., pregnant women), therapeutic drug monitoring with cotinine can be used to maintain nicotine replacement levels close to baseline. Individualizing the nicotine patch dose is warranted because of interindividual variability of baseline nicotine and cotinine concentrations among smokers who smoke a similar number of cigarettes per day. Interindividual variability also exists in steady-state serum cotinine concentrations achieved while receiving nicotine patch therapy during smoking abstinence (29,46). Serum cotinine is the test of choice for calculating the percentage replacement, even though urine nicotine or cotinine can be used (47,48). Blood can be drawn at any time of the day for this assessment (47). If serum cotinine testing is not available, the replacement dose can be estimated based on the number of cigarettes smoked per day.

Table 52.2 shows the recommended initial dosing of nicotine patch therapy based on the number of cigarettes smoked per day, which has been shown to correlate with the cotinine concentrations shown in Table 52.1.

After initiation of nicotine patch therapy on the stop date, the patient should have a follow-up visit or a telephone counseling session within the first 2 weeks and periodically thereafter. Abstinence from smoking during the first 2 weeks of patch therapy has been shown to be highly predictive of long-term abstinence (40,49). Thus the first 2 weeks of nicotine patch therapy are critical. Alterations in therapy at follow-up depend on relief of withdrawal symptoms and how well the patient is maintaining smoking abstinence. If the patient continues to smoke at all during the first 2 weeks, the treatment must be changed either by changing the nicotine patch dose, adding additional pharmacotherapy, or intensifying behavioral counseling. Nicotine patch doses should be increased for patients experiencing pronounced withdrawal symptoms such as irritability, anxiety, loss of concentration, or craving, or for patients who do not achieve 100% replacement based on the second serum cotinine concentration. Although various nicotine patches have quite comparable pharmacokinetic profiles, differences between brands exist leading to higher percentage replacement (50). Thus measuring cotinine is a more accurate method of assessing the adequacy of nicotine replacement and avoiding "over replacement." Most patients use the nicotine patch for 4 to 8 weeks, but it is safe to use it longer if needed to maintain abstinence. Optimal length of treatment has not been determined.

Side effects of nicotine patch therapy are relatively mild and include localized skin reactions at the patch site. Such reactions generally begin to occur about 4 weeks after initiation of patch therapy. Lesions vary from erythema to erythema plus vesicles. Topical corticosteroid therapy sometimes is helpful in controlling these local symptoms. Rotation of the patches to different sites of the skin helps to reduce the frequency of this side effect. In rare instances, a generalized skin eruption can occur requiring that nicotine patch therapy be discontinued. Although sleep disturbance is another side effect that has been attributed to nicotine patch therapy, it often is difficult to ascertain whether this is attributable to nicotine withdrawal or to the administration of nicotine during the evening hours. In a sleep study of smokers who were trying to stop, the best quality of sleep was observed in those who stopped smoking while receiving a 22 mg/24 hours nicotine patch dose compared with placebo (51). If there is a concern that nicotine patch therapy is causing sleep disturbance, the patch can be removed at night to see if the sleep disturbance resolves. Shortly after nicotine patches reached the market, some concern was expressed in the lay press that smokers might be at increased risk of myocardial infarction if they continued to smoke while using the patch. This exposure in the press led to hearings at the FDA, which concluded that there is no cause for concern. Subsequent studies have shown no adverse effects in smokers with a history of coronary artery disease receiving the 14- or 21-mg patch doses (52,53), nor were there adverse effects on lipids or markers of homeostasis in nonsmokers who received nicotine patch therapy (54). Nicotine patch doses up to 63 mg/day were not associated with short-term adverse cardiovascular effects in smokers (55). Standard nicotine patch doses have been shown to reduce exercise-induced myocardial ischemia (assessed by exercise thallium studies) in smokers who were trying to stop smoking (56). Experimentally, nicotine patch doses of up to 44 mg/day for four weeks have not adversely affected the early patency of coronary artery bypass grafts in dogs (57). Despite the fact that NRT product labeling continues to carry a caution for their use in smokers with coronary heart disease, the 2008 Guideline Panel asserts that separate analyses have now documented the lack of association between nicotine patch therapy and acute cardiovascular events (58–61).

Nicotine Nasal Spray Nicotine nasal spray delivers nicotine directly to the nasal mucosa and has been observed to be effective for achieving smoking abstinence (62). This device delivers nicotine more rapidly than other therapeutic nicotine replacement delivery systems and reduces withdrawal symptoms more quickly than nicotine gum (63,64). The reduction in withdrawal symptoms may be partially attributable to the rapidity with which nicotine is absorbed from the nasal mucosa and the resulting arterial venous differences in the plasma concentration of nicotine (65). Each spray contains 0.5 mg of nicotine, and one dose is one spray in each nostril (a total of 1 mg). Recommended dosing is one to two doses per hour, not to exceed five doses per hour or 40 doses per day. When using the nicotine nasal spray as a single agent, most patients initially use 12 to 16 doses per day. The recommended length of treatment is up to 12 weeks of *ad lib* use, followed by a tapering schedule. The nicotine nasal spray can be used in combination with other nicotine replacement products or with bupropion sustained release (SR). Patients should be instructed to spray against the lower nasal mucosa and not to sniff the spray into the upper nasal passages or to attempt to inhale it. The most common adverse side effects are rhinorrhea, nasal and throat irritation, watery eyes, and sneezing. These irritant side effects decrease significantly within the first week of use independent of dose (66). Because the nicotine nasal spray is a more rapid delivery device than other nicotine replacement products, there was early concern that the spray could have long-term abuse liability (67), a concern that was later dispelled (68). Nicotine nasal spray should be used with caution in patients with reactive airway disease.

Nicotine Inhaler The nicotine vapor inhaler has also been shown to be effective for increasing smoking abstinence (69). This device is a plastic holder into which a cartridge containing a cotton plug impregnated with 10 mg of nicotine is inserted. The device delivers a nicotine vapor that is absorbed across the oral mucosa. Although the device is called an inhaler, this is a misnomer because little of the nicotine vapor reaches the pulmonary alveoli even with deep inhalations (70). So the inhaler does not provide high arterial levels of nicotine in the manner of cigarettes (71,72). When the nicotine inhaler is used as a single therapy, efficacy is increased when more than six cartridges per day are used. Nicotine replacement levels based on serum cotinine concentrations vary from 43% to more than 60%, depending on the number of nicotine cartridges used per day with six cartridges associated with higher levels of replacement and improved abstinence rates (69,73). The recommended initial dose of the nicotine inhaler when used alone is 6 to 16 cartridges per day. The recommended length of treatment is approximately 12 weeks followed by a tapering schedule, although the inhaler could be used longer. This device requires frequent puffing to deliver substantial amounts of nicotine and to some smokers the puffing mimics some of the behavior of smoking. Because it is a unique delivery device, the nicotine inhaler lends itself to being used in combination with other nicotine replacement products or bupropion SR. Adverse effects generally are mild and most often involve mouth or throat irritation, with occasional coughing.

Summary All of the approved nicotine replacement products discussed have been proven to be effective in randomized, placebo-controlled trials, with a doubling of the stop rate in the active treatment group. They have also proven to be remarkably safe. As the number and availability of such products have increased so, too, has the number of attempts to stop smoking by U.S. smokers (74). Although all of the nicotine replacement products seem to be equally effective, differences in compliance exist with the recommended dose. However, no notable differences between the products exist when used at standard doses, nor are there different effects on withdrawal symptom discomfort, perceived helpfulness, and general efficacy (75). Nicotine products are contraindicated in patients with hypersensitivity to nicotine.

NON-NICOTINE PRODUCTS

Bupropion SR The relationship between smoking and depression has been well-documented. Smokers are more likely than nonsmokers to have a history of major depression (76–78). During the course of an attempt to stop smoking, many smokers develop a depressed affect and some become overtly depressed (79–82). The development of a depressed affect during an attempt to stop smoking is associated with relapse to smoking (83,84). This association has raised the question of the role antidepressants might play in treating tobacco dependence and has led to the study of the efficacy of antidepressants in treating smokers. Among the antidepressants evaluated, bupropion is the first non-nicotine pharmacologic treatment approved for the treatment of tobacco dependence. Bupropion is a monocyclic antidepressant that inhibits the reuptake of both norepinephrine and dopamine (85). Dopamine release in the mesolimbic system and the nucleus accumbens is thought to be the basis for the reinforcing properties of nicotine and other drugs of addiction (86–88).

Bupropion does not appear to work through its antidepressant activity. Rather, the efficacy of bupropion in smoking cessation is hypothesized to stem from its dopaminergic activity on the pleasure and reward pathways in the mesolimbic system and nucleus accumbens. Bupropion also has been shown to have an antagonist effect on nicotinic acetylcholine receptors (89,90). Thus its mechanism of action likely is multifactorial.

Bupropion SR has been shown to be effective and exhibits a significant dose-response effect (91). The smoking abstinence rates for the 150- and 300-mg treatment groups were significantly higher than placebo at end-of-treatment and 1 year. In addition, an attenuation of weight gain was observed during the treatment phase for subjects continuously abstinent while receiving the 300 mg/day dose. However, the attenuation of weight gain did not persist at 1-year follow-up. Bupropion SR has also been shown to be effective in subpopulations of smokers including those with coronary disease, chronic obstructive pulmonary disease or who have previously failed to achieve long-term smoking abstinence after an initial course of bupropion SR (92–94). Treatment with bupropion SR alone or in combination with the nicotine patch resulted in a significantly higher long-term rate of abstinence from smoking than did use of either the nicotine patch alone or placebo (95). Smoking abstinence rates were higher with combination therapy than with bupropion SR alone, but the differences were not statistically significant. However, the 2008 USPHS Guidelines concluded that additional studies now show evidence of efficacy for the combined used of bupropion SR and nicotine patch therapy (6).

Treatment with bupropion SR should be initiated about 1 week before the patient's stop date at an initial dose of 150 mg/day for 3 days then 150 mg twice daily. The usual length of treatment is 6 to 12 weeks, but bupropion SR can be used safely for much longer. As with other antidepressants, a small risk (0.1%) of seizures is associated with this medication. Therefore bupropion SR is contraindicated in patients who have a history of seizures, serious head trauma with skull fracture or a prolonged loss of consciousness, an eating disorder (i.e., anorexia nervosa or bulimia), or concomitant use of medications that lower the seizure threshold.

The most common adverse side effects are insomnia and dry mouth. Cardiovascular and sexual adverse effects are uncommon. Treatment-emergent hypertension can occur rarely during treatment with bupropion SR, especially when it is used in combination with nicotine patch therapy.

In an assessment of predictors of successful tobacco dependence treatment outcomes, bupropion SR was observed to be effective independent of all other characteristics. However, lower smoking rate, prior abstinence from smoking for brief periods (<24 hours) or long periods (>4 weeks), and male gender all were predictors of better outcome independent of the bupropion SR dose. Further, bupropion SR appears to be equally effective in smokers with or without a history of depression or in recovering alcohol-dependent and non–alcohol-dependent individuals (97). Bupropion SR has been evaluated as an agent for relapse prevention in an open-label study with more than 700 smokers who received bupropion SR (300 mg/day) treatment for 7 weeks. Subjects who were abstinent from smoking at the end of the open-label period were assigned randomly to active or placebo bupropion SR for the remainder of the year and followed for a subsequent year (98). Smoking abstinence rates were significantly higher in the bupropion SR group compared with placebo at the end-of-medication (week 52) and at week 78, but not at 104 weeks. The median time to relapse was significantly longer for subjects who received bupropion SR compared with placebo, and significantly less weight gain in the bupropion SR group was observed compared with placebo at weeks 52 and 104. As with the dose-response study, the best overall predictor of successful relapse prevention was assignment to bupropion SR (99). This medication effect was independent of any predictor except older age and no or minimal weight gain during the open-label phase. Predictors of successful relapse prevention included lower baseline smoking rates, a Fagerström Test for Nicotine Dependence (FTND) score lower than 6 (Table 52.3), and initiation of smoking at an older age.

As with the dose-response study, the extended use of bupropion SR for relapse prevention is effective for smokers

TABLE 52.3 Items and Scoring for the Fagerström Test for Nicotine-Dependence Questions (Answers and Points)

1. **How soon after you wake up do you smoke your first cigarette?**
   Within 5 min 3
   6–30 min 2
   31–60 min 1
   After 60 min 0
2. **Do you find it difficult to refrain from smoking in places where it is forbidden (in church, at the library, in cinema, etc.)?**
   Yes 1, No 0
3. **Which cigarette would you hate most to give up?**
   The first one in the morning 1
   All others 0
4. **How many cigarettes per day do you smoke?**
   10 or less 0
   11–20 1
   21–30 2
   31 or more 3
5. **Do you smoke more frequently during the first hours after waking**
   Yes 1
   Than during the rest of the day? No 0
6. **Do you smoke if you are so ill that you are in bed most of the day? Yes 1, No 0**

From Fagerström KO. Measuring degree of physical dependence to tobacco smoking with reference to individualization of treatment. *Addict Behav* 1978;3:235–241.

with or without a history of depression (100). However, in a community-based study, bupropion SR was not shown to be effective in preventing relapse to smoking in smokers who stopped smoking with tailored nicotine patch therapy (101).

Because of the high prevalence of a history of depression in smokers, clinicians often encounter smokers who want to stop smoking but already are being treated with an antidepressant. The question arises whether to discontinue the current antidepressant before starting bupropion SR or to simply add bupropion SR to the regimen. No drug-drug interactions exist to preclude the use of bupropion SR with either selective serotonin reuptake inhibitors (SSRIs) or tricyclic antidepressants. Thus, adding bupropion SR to an SSRI is preferable to discontinuing that medication and using bupropion SR only. Although one study showed no serious adverse effects (102); patients receiving two antidepressants should be monitored for side effects. The use of monoamine oxidase inhibitors (MAOIs) is a contraindication for use of bupropion SR.

Summary Bupropion SR has utility in the general smoking population as well as in subpopulations with tobacco-caused diseases, attenuates weight gain associated with stopping smoking, and may be used to prevent smoking relapse.

Varenicline The newest first-line drug for treating tobacco dependence is varenicline. Varenicline is a partial nicotine agonist/antagonist that selectively binds to the $\alpha_4\beta_2$ nicotinic acetylcholine receptor. Varenicline both blocks nicotine from binding to the receptor (antagonist effect) (103) and stimulates (agonist effect) receptor-mediated activity leading to the release of dopamine which reduces craving and nicotine withdrawal symptoms. Varenicline is rapidly absorbed after one administration and reaches peak serum concentration in 4 hours and steady-state serum concentrations after 4 days. Varenicline is not metabolized, is excreted virtually unchanged in the urine and has a half-life of approximately 17 hours.

Two pivotal trials comparing varenicline 1 mg twice daily to placebo or bupropion SR have been conducted (104,105). In these studies, varenicline was more effective for achieving smoking abstinence compared to placebo or bupropion SR with end-of-treatment continuous smoking abstinence rates of 44% versus 30% for bupropion SR and 18% for placebo. The end-of-treatment 7-day point prevalence smoking abstinence rates were approximately 50% for varenicline versus 35% for bupropion SR and 20% for placebo. The third pivotal trial showed that an additional 12 weeks of varenicline was effective in maintaining smoking abstinence in smokers who had stopped smoking after 12 weeks of open-label varenicline treatment with 70% treated with varenicline being continuously abstinent from smoking from week 13 to 24 compared with 50% assigned to placebo ($p < 0.001$) (106). Finally, the long-term safety of varenicline has been evaluated in a placebo-controlled trial in 251 smokers receiving varenicline or placebo for 52 weeks (107). This study also demonstrated that at 52 weeks, 37% of smokers treated with varenicline were abstinent from smoking compared with 8% in the placebo group. One serious adverse event was reported in one subject in this study (i.e., subcapsular cataracts).

Varenicline has not been studied systematically in combination with other medications to treat tobacco dependence. If used in combination with NRT there is an increased risk that nausea will occur. Varenicline is not recommended for use in combination with NRT; however, some patients may need short-acting NRT for nicotine withdrawal symptom control, especially in the first few days/weeks of varenicline therapy. Bupropion SR and varenicline have different mechanisms of action and no drug interactions between these drugs are likely. This suggests that the combination of these drugs may prove beneficial and would have an acceptable side effect profile. Clinical trials assessing this combination are ongoing. However, no clinical trial data to support this treatment approach are available.

The most frequent adverse effect of varenicline is nausea reported by approximately 30% of the participants in the three studies mentioned earlier. However, the nausea was most often mild to moderate, and participant dropouts related to nausea were infrequent (<3%). In a comparison study of varenicline versus NRT in smokers with or without mental illness, varenicline showed better smoking abstinence outcomes compared with NRT and was equally effective and safe in smokers with or without a mental illness (108). In February 2008, the FDA issued a public health advisory because of reports of suicidal thoughts and aggressive and erratic behavior in a patient who have taken varenicline. In addition, some case reports have suggested that varenicline could exacerbate psychiatric symptoms in individuals with severe mental illness, so these types of patients should be monitored carefully when on varenicline. The only contraindication to its use is an allergy to varenicline.

Nortriptyline Nortriptyline is a tricyclic antidepressant recommended as a second-line drug for treating tobacco dependence (6). Randomized clinical trials have demonstrated that nortriptyline significantly increases smoking abstinence rates compared with placebo (109,110). In these studies, the maximal dose range was 75 to 100 mg/day, and the length of treatment was 8 to 12 weeks. Systematic reviews demonstrate the efficacy of nortriptyline in contrast to SSRIs, which have not been shown to help smokers stop (111,112). Nortriptyline seems to be as efficacious as bupropion in treating smokers with chronic obstructive pulmonary disease (113).

The most common adverse effects with nortriptyline are sedation and dry mouth. Nortriptyline is thought to be as effective as bupropion SR in helping smokers to stop smoking and that the mechanism of action of each is independent of their antidepressant effects (111). Nortriptyline produces higher smoking abstinence rates than placebo independent of a history of depression. However, increases in negative affect after quitting smoking have been observed to be attenuated by nortriptyline (109). In addition, it appears that nortriptyline is effective at plasma concentrations lower than those found for the treatment of depression (111) and prolonged treatment with more intensive psychologic treatment can produce higher smoking abstinence rates (114). Nortriptyline is contraindicated in combination with an MAOI (monamine oxidase inhibitor) or within 14 days of discontinuing one, nortriptyline allergy, or in the acute recovery phase after a myocardial infarction.

Clonidine Clonidine is a centrally acting alpha-agonist that can be used as a second-line drug (6) and is available in both oral or transdermal forms. The transdermal form is easier to use with a recommended dose of 0.2 mg/day for 3 to 10 weeks. The clonidine patch should be initiated a week before the patient's stop date and changed weekly thereafter. Common side effects include dry mouth and drowsiness. The only contraindication to its use is a clonidine allergy.

COMBINATION PHARMACOTHERAPIES

The 2008 USPHS Guideline states that certain combinations of first-line medications have been shown to be effective. Long-term (>14 weeks) nicotine patch therapy combined with nicotine gum or nicotine nasal spray, nicotine patch therapy plus nicotine inhaler, and nicotine patch therapy plus bupropion SR are cited as examples. Combining bupropion with the nicotine inhaler provides a better treatment effect than either alone (115). However, the expert panel points out that the use of combinations of medications may be based on considerations other than smoking abstinence. Withdrawal symptom control is an important consideration, as is patient experience or preference. Whether the superiority of combination therapy is due to the use of two types of delivery systems or to the fact that two delivery systems tend to produce higher blood nicotine levels remains unclear. Combination pharmacotherapy or higher than usual doses of nicotine replacement therapy effectively relieve withdrawal symptoms, especially in more dependent smokers.

UNPROVEN PHARMACOTHERAPIES

Anxiolytics have not been shown to be effective in helping patients stop smoking (116). Specifically, buspirone has not been shown to have efficacy in a placebo-controlled trial (117). Antidepressants other than bupropion and nortriptyline have been tested and generally have been found to be ineffective in producing long-term abstinence from smoking. Doxepin was reported to be effective in one small clinical trial, which has not been replicated (118). The SSRIs fluoxetine, sertraline, and paroxetine have been tested and show no long-term benefit, nor did the MAOI (monoamine oxidase inhibitor) moclobemide or the atypical antidepressant venlafaxine (111). Fluoxetine was not observed to enhance nicotine inhaler therapy (119). Paroxetine has been tested in combination with nicotine patch therapy and showed no added value in improving abstinence rates (120). The antihypertensive mecamylamine was shown to have efficacy in a small trial of smokers (121). Despite the theoretical role that dopamine plays as a critical mediator of the reinforcing effects of nicotine, administration of carbidopa/levodopa in doses used to treat Parkinson disease showed no efficacy compared with placebo (122). Finally, naltrexone did not demonstrate efficacy compared with placebo in clinical trial using naltrexone and the nicotine patch (123); however, other studies suggest that it may have some short-term effects (124,125). The 2008 USPHS Guideline analysis concluded that naltrexone treatment does not increase the likelihood of producing smoking abstinence compared with placebo.

CLINICAL DECISIONS ABOUT PHARMACOTHERAPY

In clinical medicine, we base our clinical decision making for medication selection and dosing on the published literature, but also on our clinical experience. As has long been recognized by clinicians, limitations exist to standard or fixed-dose regimens with most drugs used in clinical practice today. As a result, clinicians use their clinical skills and knowledge of pharmacotherapy to individualize drug dosing for patients. These same skills and knowledge should be applied to medications used to treat tobacco dependence.

Although each of the FDA-approved products has been shown to be effective compared with placebo in randomized clinical trials, we rarely use nicotine gum, nicotine inhaler, nicotine lozenge, or nicotine nasal spray alone. From a practical standpoint, we view nicotine patch therapy, bupropion SR, or varenicline as the foundation on which to begin building a patient's pharmacotherapeutic regimen and will often use one of these treatments as stand-alone therapy in treating patients with tobacco dependence or those who achieve initial smoking abstinence with one of these products. Depending on the patient, we may use nicotine patch therapy in combination with bupropion SR. We then use the shorter acting NRT products as needed by the patient to control intermittent withdrawal symptoms or cravings. Similarly, we offer short-acting NRT with varenicline for the purpose of withdrawal symptom relief. Much of this clinical decision making is based on the patient's experience and the patient's preference. For patients with more severe tobacco dependence, such as those treated in our residential treatment program, we usually use combination therapy and often use three or more products simultaneously.

The 2008 USPHS Guideline observes that there is stronger evidence that counseling is an effective tobacco dependence treatment strategy and that counseling adds significantly to the efficacy of the approved medications. Practical counseling (problem solving/skills training) and social support delivered as part of treatment are especially effective. Individual, group and proactive telephone counseling are effective, and efficacy increases with treatment intensity and duration (dose response). Finally, the guideline states that the combination of counseling and medication is more effective than either alone thus both should be routinely offered to smokers.

Self-Help Materials and Longer Term Pharmacotherapy for Relapse Prevention Although self-help materials have not been shown to be effective in initiating abstinence from smoking, specific self-help materials, such as the National Cancer Institute's *Forever Free*, have been effective in helping smokers maintain smoking abstinence (126). Longer use of pharmacotherapy is useful in some patients to maintain smoking abstinence long enough to stabilize the initial treatment effect. The optimal length of pharmacotherapy has not been established for any of the available medications. Two studies in which bupropion SR was administered for approximately 12 months to smokers abstinent from smoking at the end of a short course of pharmacotherapy showed mixed results (98,101). Prolonged nicotine patch therapy (5 months) combined with nicotine nasal spray for 1 year also seems to prevent smoking relapse (127). Although the study was designed to assess safety, varenicline given for 52 weeks showed an impressive smoking abstinence rate of 37% compared with placebo (8%) (107).

CONCLUSIONS

Progress has been made in recent years in treating tobacco dependence. Seven FDA-approved medications exist, three of which are readily available as over-the-counter products. An evidence-based guideline published by the USPHS in 2008 extends our understanding of effective treatments and encourages clinicians to be more persistent in recognizing tobacco users and more aggressive with treatment. The guideline outlines the potential use of the approved medications as first-line drugs and two additional medications as second-line drugs. The guideline encourages the use of combinations of these medications when appropriate. New and more effective pharmacotherapies are needed to further decrease the death and disability caused by cigarette smoking. More intensive behavioral treatments such as residential treatment for more severely dependent smokers may be indicated (128).

REFERENCES

1. McNally WD. The tar in cigarette smoke and its possible effects. *Am J Cancer* 1932;162:1502–1514.
2. Ezzati M, Lopez AD. Estimates of global mortality attributable to smoking in 2000. *Lancet* 2003;362:847–852.
3. Peto R, Lopey AD, Boreham J, et al. Mortality from Smoking in Developed Countries 1950–2000. Indirect estimate from National Vital Statistics. Oxford, UK, Oxford University Press, 1994.
4. Hurt RD, Robertson CR. Prying open the door to the tobacco industry's secrets about nicotine: The Minnesota Tobacco Trial. *JAMA* 1998;280: 1173–1181.
5. Brody AL, Mandelkern MA, London ED. Cigarette smoking saturates brain alpha 4 beta 2 nicotinic acetylcholine receptors. *Arch Gen Psychiatry* 2006;63(8):907–915.
6. Fiore MC, Jaen CR, Baker TB, et al. U.S. Public Health Service Guideline. *Treating tobacco use and dependence,* 2008.
7. Swartz SH, Cowan TM, Klayman JE, et al. Use and effectiveness of tobacco telephone counseling and nicotine therapy in Maine. *Am J Prev Med* 2005;29(4):288–294.
8. Watkins SS, Koob GF, Markou A. Neural mechanisms underlying nicotine addiction: acute positive reinforcement and withdrawal. *Nicotine Tob Res* 2000;2(1):19–37.
9. Balfour DJK. The neurochemical mechanisms underlying nicotine tolerance and dependence. In: Pratt JA, ed. *The biological basis of drug tolerance and dependence.* London, UK: Academic Press, 1991:121–151.
10. Perry DC, Dávila-Garcia MI, et al. Increased nicotinic receptors in brains from smokers: membrane binding and autoradiography studies. *J Pharmacol Exp Ther* 1999;289(3):1545–1952.
11. Hope BT, Nagarkar D, Leonard S, et al. Long-term upregulation of protein kinase A and adenylate cyclase levels in human smokers. *J Neurosci* 2007;27(8):1964–1972.
12. Clarke PB. Nicotine dependence—mechanisms and therapeutic strategies. *Biochem Soc Symp*1993;59:83–95.
13. DiChaiara G, Imperato A. Drugs abused by humans preferentially increase synaptic dopamine concentrations in the mesolimbic system of freely moving rates. *Proc Natl Acad Sci U S A* 1988;85(14):5274–5278.
14. Ponieri FE, Tanda G, Orzi F, et al. Effects of nicotine on the nucleus accumbens and similarity to those of addictive drugs. *Nature* 1996; 382:255–257.
15. Dichaiara G. Role of dopamine in the behavioral actions of nicotine related to addiction. *Eur J Pharmacol* 2000;393(1–3):295–314.
16. Stein EA, Pankoewicz J, Harsch HH, et al. Nicotine-induced limbic cortical activation in the human brain: a functional MRI study. *Am J Psychiatry* 1998;155(8):1009–1015.
17. Dewey SL, Brodie JD, Gerasimov M, et al. A pharmacologic strategy for the treatment of nicotine addiction. *Synapse* 1999;31(1):76–86.
18. Kenny PJ, Markou A. Conditioned nicotine withdrawal profoundly decreases the activity of brain reward system. *J Neurosci* 2005;25(26): 6208–6212.
19. Carmelli D, Swan GE, Robinette D. Genetic influence on smoking. A study of male twins. *N Engl J Med* 1992;327:829–833.
20. Schnoll RA, Johnson TA, Lerman C. Genetics and smoking behavior. *Curr Psychiatry Rep* 2007;9(5):349–357.
21. Cheng LS, Swan GE, Carmelli D. A genetic analysis of smoking behavior in family members of older adult males. *Addiction* 2000;95(3): 427–435.
22. Lerman C, Caporaso NE, Audrain J, et al. Evidence suggesting the role of specific genetic factors in cigarette smoking. *Health Psychol* 1999; 18(1):14–20.
23. Sabol SZ, Nelson ML, Fisher C, et al. A genetic association for cigarette smoking behavior. *Health Psychol* 1999;18(1):7–13.
24. Hutchison KE, Allen DL, Filbey FM. CHRNA4 and tobacco dependence: from gene regulation to treatment outcome. *Arch Gen Psychiatry* 2007;64(9):1078–1086.
25. Kendler KS, Neale MC, Sullivan P, et al. A population-based twin study in women of smoking initiation and nicotine dependence. *Psychol Med* 1999;29(2):299–308.
26. Munafo M, Clark T, Johnstone E, et al. The genetic basis for smoking behavior: a systematic review and meta-analysis. *Nicotine Tob Res* 2004;6(4):583–597.
27. David SP, Munafo MR, Murphy MF, et al. Genetic variation in the dopamine D4 receptor (DRD4) gene and smoking cessation: follow-up of a randomized clinical trial of transdermal nicotine patch. *Pharmcogenomics J* 2008;8(2):122–128.
28. Schnoll RA, Johnson TA, Lerman C. Genetics and smoking behavior. *Curr Psychiatry Rep* 2007;9(5):349–357.
29. Dale LC, Hurt RD, Offord KE, et al. High-dose nicotine patch therapy. Percentage of replacement and smoking cessation. *JAMA* 1995;274(17): 1353–1358.
30. Gourlay SG, Benowitz NL. Arteriovenous differences in plasma concentration of nicotine and catecholamines and related cardiovascular effects after smoking, nicotine nasal spray and intravenous nicotine. *Clin Pharmacol Therap* 1997;62(4):453–463.
31. Henningfield JE, Stapleton JM, Benowitz NL, et al. Higher levels of nicotine in arterial than in venous blood after cigarette smoking. *Drug Alcohol Depend* 1993;33(1):23–29.

32. Jacob PI, Yu L, Shulgin AT, et al. Minor tobacco alkaloids as biomarkers for tobacco use: comparison of users of cigarettes, smokeless tobacco, cigars, and pipes. *Am J Public Health* 1999;89(5):731–736.
33. Moyer TP, Charlson JR, Enger RJ, et al. Simultaneous analysis of nicotine, nicotine metabolites, and tobacco alkaloids in serum or urine by tandem mass spectrometry, with clinically relevant metabolic profiles. *Clin Chem* 2002;48(9):1460–1471.
34. Jacob P, Hatsukami D, Severson H, et al. Biomarkers and prevention. *Cancer Epidemiol* 2002;11:1688–1673, 2002.
35. Russell MAH, Raw M, Jarvis MJ. Clinical use of nicotine chewing gum. *Br Med J* 1980;280:1599–1602.
36. Glover ED, Sachs DPL, Stitzer ML, et al. Smoking cessation in highly dependence smokers with 4 mg nicotine polacrilex. *Am J Health Behav* 1996;20(5):319–332.
37. Sachs DPL. Effectiveness of the 4 mg dose of nicotine polacrilex for the initial treatment of high-dependent smokers. *Arch Intern Med* 1995; 155:1973–1980.
38. Shiffman S, Dresler, CM, Hajek P, et al. Efficacy of a nicotine lozenge for smoking cessation. *Arch Intern Med* 2002;162:1267–1276.
39. Hurt RD, Dale LC, Offord KP, et al. Serum nicotine and cotinine levels during nicotine patch therapy. *Clin Pharmacol Therap* 1993;54(1):98–106.
40. Hurt RD, Dale LC, Fredrickson PA, et al. Nicotine patch therapy for smoking cessation combined with physician advice and nurse follow-up—one-year outcome and percentage nicotine replacement. *JAMA* 1994;271(8):595–600.
41. Hughes JR. Treatment of nicotine dependence. Is more better? (editorial). *JAMA* 1995;274(17):1390–1391.
42. Fredrickson PA, Hurt RD, Lee GM. High dose transdermal nicotine therapy for heavy smokers: safety, tolerability and measurement of nicotine and cotinine levels. *Psychopharmacology* 1995;122:215–222.
43. Hughes JR, Lesmes GR, Hatsukami DK, et al. Are higher doses of nicotine replacement more effective for smoking cessation? *Nicotine Tob Res* 1999;1(2):169–174.
44. Jorenby DE, Smith SS, Fiore MC, et al. Varying nicotine patch dose and type of smoking cessation counseling. *JAMA* 1995;274(17):1347–1352.
45. Tonnesen P, Paeletti P, Gustavsson G, et al. Higher dosage nicotine patches increase one-year smoking cessation rates: results from the European CEASE trial. Collaborative European Anti-Smoking Evaluation. European Respiratory Society. *Eur Respir J* 1999;13(2):238–246.
46. Hurt RD, Dale LC, Offord KP, et al. Serum nicotine and cotinine levels during nicotine-patch therapy. *Clin Pharmacol Ther* 1993; Jul;54(1):98–106.
47. Lawson GM, Hurt RD, Dale LC, et al. Application of serum nicotine and plasma cotinine concentrations to assessment of nicotine replacement in light, moderate, and heavy smokers undergoing transdermal therapy. *J Clin Pharmacol* 1998;38(6):502–509.
48. Lawson GM, Hurt RD, Dale LC, et al. Application of urine nicotine and cotinine excretion rates to assessment of nicotine replacement in light, moderate, and heavy smokers undergoing transdermal therapy. *J Clin Pharmacol* 1998;38(6):510–516.
49. Kenford SL, Fiore MC, Joreny DE, et al. Predicting smoking cessation. Who will quit with and with the nicotine patch. *JAMA* 1994;271(8): 589–594.
50. Gariti P, Alterman AI, Barber W, et al. Cotinine replacement levels for a 21 mg/day transdermal nicotine patch in an outpatient treatment setting. *Drug Alcohol Depend* 1999;54(2):111–116.
51. Wetter DW, Fiore MC, Baker TB, et al. Tobacco withdrawal and nicotine replacement influence objective measures of sleep. *J Conslt Clin Psychol* 1995;63(4):658–667.
52. Joseph AM, Norma SM, Ferry LH, et al. The safety of transdermal nicotine as an aid to smoking cessation in patients with cardiac disease. *N Engl J Med* 1996;335(24):1792–1798.
53. Working Group for the Study of Transdermal Nicotine in Patients with Coronary Artery Disease. Nicotine replacement therapy for patients with coronary artery disease. *Arch Intern Med* 1994;154:989–995.
54. Thomas GAO, Davies SV, Rhodes J, et al. Is transdermal nicotine associated with cardiovascular risk? *J Roy Coll Phys London* 1995;29(5): 392–396.
55. Zevin S, Jacob P, Benowitz NL Dose-related cardiovascular and endocrine effects of transdermal nicotine. *Clin Pharmacol Therap* 1998; 54:87–95.
56. Mahmarian JJ, Moye LA, Nasser GA, et al. Nicotine patch therapy in smoking cessation reduces the extent of exercise-induced myocardial ischemia. *Am Coll Cardiol* 1997;30(1):125–130.
57. Clouse WD, Yamaguchi H, Phillips MR, et al. Effects of transdermal nicotine treatment on structure and function of coronary artery bypass grafts. *J Appl Physiol* 2000;89:1213–1223.
58. Frishman WH, Ky T, Ismail A. Tobacco smoking, nicotine, and nicotine and non-nicotine replacement therapies. *Heart Dis* 2001;3:365–377.
59. Haustein KO, Krause J, Haustein H, et al. Effects of cigarette smoking or nicotine replacement on cardiovascular risk factors and parameters of haemoreheology. *J Intern Med* 2002;252:130–139.
60. McRobbie H, Hajek P. Nicotine replacement therapy in patients with cardiovascular disease: guidelines for health professionals. *Addiction* 2001;96:1547–1551.
61. Mohiuddin SM, Mooss AN, Hunter CB, et al. Intensive smoking cessation intervention reduces mortality in high-risk smokers with cardiovascular disease. *Chest* 2007;131:445–452.
62. Schneider NG, Olmstead R, Mody FV, et al. Efficacy of a nicotine nasal spray in smoking cessation: a placebo-controlled, double-blind trial. *Addiction* 1995;90(12):1671–1682.
63. Hurt RD, Offord KP, Croghan GA. Temporal-effects of nicotine nasal spray and gum on nicotine withdrawal symptoms. *Psychopharmacology* 1998;140:98–104.
64. Schneider NG, Lunell E, Olmstead RE, et al. Clinical pharmacokinetics of nasal nicotine delivery: a review and comparison to other nicotine systems. *Clin Pharmacokin* 1996;31(1):65–80.
65. Gourlay SG, Benowitz NL. Arteriovenous differences in plasma concentration of nicotine and catecholamines and related cardiovascular effects after smoking, nicotine nasal spray, and intravenous nicotine. *Clin Pharmacol Therap* 1997;62(4):453–463.
66. Hurt RD, Dale LC, Croghan GA, et al. Nicotine nasal spray for smoking cessation: pattern of use, side effects, relief of withdrawal symptoms, and cotinine levels. *Mayo Clin Proc* 1998;73:118–125.
67. Sutherland G, Stapleton JA, Russell MA, et al. Randomized controlled trial of nasal nicotine spray in smoking cessation. *Lancet* 1992;340: 324–329.
68. Schuh KJ, Schuh LM, Henningfield JE, et al. Nicotine nasal spray and vapor inhaler: abuse liability assessment. *Psychopharmacology* 1997; 130(4):352–361.
69. Leischow SJ, Nilsson F, Franzon M, et al. Efficacy of the nicotine inhaler as an adjunct to smoking cessation. *Am J Health Behav* 1996;20(5): 364–371.
70. Bergstrom M, Nordberg A, Lunell E, et al. Regional deposition of inhaled 11C-nicotine vapor in the human airway as visualized by positron emission tomography. *Clin Pharmacol Therap* 1995;57(3):309–317.
71. Lunell E, Bergstrom M, Antoni G, et al. Nicotine deposition and body distribution from a nicotine inhaler and a cigarette studied with positron emission tomography [letter to editor]. *Clin Pharmacol Therap* 1996; 59(5):593–594.
72. Lunell E, Molander L, Ekberg K, et al. Site of nicotine absorption from a vapour inhaler—comparison with cigarette smoking. *Eur J Clin Pharmacol* 2000;55(10):737–741.
73. Hjalmarson A, Nilsson F, Sjostrom L, et al. The nicotine inhaler in smoking cessation. *Arch Internl Med* 1997;157:1721–1728.
74. Burton SL, Gitchell JG, Shiffman S. Use of FDA-approved pharmacologic treatments for tobacco dependence—United States, 1984–1998. *MMWR Morbid Mortal Wkly Rep* 2000;49(29):665–668.
75. Hajek P, West R, Foulds J, et al. Randomized comparative trial of nicotine polacrilex, a transdermal patch, nasal spray, and an inhaler. *Arch Intern Med* 1999;159:2033–2038.
76. Anda RF, Williamson DF, Escobedo LG, et al. Depression and the dynamics of smoking: a national perspective. *JAMA* 1990;264:1541–1545.
77. Glassman AH, Helzer JE, Covey LS, et al. Smoking, smoking cessation, and major depression. *JAMA* 1990;264:1546–1549.

78. Hall SM, Munoz R, Reus V. Smoking cessation, depression and dysphoria. *NIDA Res Monogr* 1991;105:312–313.
79. Borrelli B, Niaura R, Keuthen NJ, et al. Development of major depressive disorder during smoking cessation treatment. *J Clin Psychiatry* 1996;57:534–538.
80. Covey LS, Glassman AH, Stetner F. Depression and depressive symptoms in smoking cessation. *Comp Psychiatry* 1990;31:350–354.
81. Glass RM. Blue mood, blackened lungs: depression and smoking [editorial]. *JAMA* 1990;264:1583–1584.
82. Tsoh JY, Humfleet GL, Munoz RF, et al. Development of major depression after treatment for smoking cessation. *Am J Psychiatry* 2000;157:368–374.
83. Hall SM, Munoz RD, Reus VI. Cognitive-behavioral intervention increases abstinence rates for depressive-history smokers. *J Consult Clin Psychol* 1994;62(1):141–146.
84. Shiffman S. Relapse following smoking cessation: a situational analysis. *J Consult Clin Psychol* 1982;50:71–86.
85. Ascher JA, Cole JO, Colin JN, et al. Bupropion: a review of its mechanism of antidepressant activity. *J Clin Psychiatry* 1995;56(9):395–401.
86. Clarke PB. Nicotine dependence—mechanisms and therapeutic strategies. *Biochem Soc Symp* 1993;59:83–95.
87. DiChiara G, Imperato A. Drugs abused by humans preferentially increase synaptic dopamine concentrations in the mesolimbic system of freely moving rats. *Proc Natl Acad Sci U S A* 1988;85(14):5274–5278.
88. Pontieri FE, Tanda G, Orzi F, et al. Effects of nicotine on the nucleus accumbens and similarity to those of addictive drugs. *Nature* 1996;382:255–257.
89. Fryer JD, Lukas RJ. Noncompetitive functional inhibition at diverse human nicotinic acetylcholine receptor subtypes by bupropion phencyclidine and ibogaine. *J Pharmacol Exp Therap* 1999;288(1):88–92.
90. Slemmer JE, Martin BR, Damaj MI. Bupropion is a nicotinic antagonist. *J Pharmacol Exp Ther* 2000;295(1):321–327.
91. Hurt RD, Sachs DPL, Glover E, et al. A comparison of sustained-release bupropion and placebo for smoking cessation. *N Engl J Med* 1997;337:1195–1202.
92. Gonzales DH, Nides MA, Ferr LH, et al. Bupropion SR as an aid to smoking cessation in smokers treated previously with bupropion: a randomized placebo-controlled study. *Clin Pharm Ther* 2001;69(6):438–444.
93. Tashkin D, Kanner R, Bailey W, et al. Smoking cessation in patients with chronic obstructive pulmonary disease: a double-blind, placebo-controlled, randomized trial. *Lancet* 2001;357(9268):1571–1575.
94. Tonstad S, Frasang C, Klaene G, et al. Bupropion SR for smoking cessation in smokers with cardiovascular disease: a multicentre, randomized study. *Eur Heart J* 2003;24(10):945–955.
95. Jorenby DR, Leischow SJ, Nides M, et al. A controlled trial for sustained-release bupropion, a nicotine patch, or both for smoking cessation. *N Engl J Med* 1999;340(9):685–691.
96. Dale LC, Glover ED, Sachs DPL, et al. Bupropion for smoking cessation: predictors of successful outcome. *Chest* 2001;119:1357–1364.
97. Hayford KE, Patten CA, Rummans RA, et al. Efficacy of bupropion for smoking cessation in smokers with a former history of major depression or alcoholism. *Br J Psychiatry* 1999;174:173–178.
98. Hays JT, Hurt RD, Rigotti N, et al. A randomized controlled trial of sustained-release bupropion for pharmacologic relapse prevention following smoking cessation. *Ann Intern Med* 2001;135(6):423–433.
99. Hurt RD, Wolter TD, Rigotti N, et al. Bupropion for pharmacologic relapse prevention to smoking: predictors of outcome. *Addict Behav* 2001;26:1–15.
100. Cox LS, Patten CA, Niaura RS, et al. Efficacy of bupropion for relapse prevention in smokers with and without a past history of major depression. *J Gen Intern Med* 2004;19(8):828–834.
101. Hurt RD, Krook JE, Croghan IT, et al. Nicotine patch therapy based on smoking rate followed by bupropion for prevention of relapse to smoking. *J Clin Oncol* 2003;21(5):914–920.
102. Chengappa KNR, Kambhampati RK, Perkins KA, et al. Bupropion SR as a smoking cessation treatment in remitted depressed patients maintained on selective serotonin reuptake inhibitor antidepressants. *J Clin Psychiatry* 2001;62(7):503–508.
103. Rollema H, Chambers LK, Coe JW, et al. Pharmacological profile of the $\alpha_4\beta_2$ nicotinic acetylcholine receptor partial agonist varenicline, an effective smoking cessation aid. *Neuropharm* 2007;52(3):985–994.
104. Jorenby, DE, Hays JT, Rigotti, NA, et al. Efficacy of varenicline, an $\alpha_4\beta_2$ nicotinic acetylcholine receptor partial agonist, vs. placebo or sustained-release bupropion for smoking cessation. *JAMA* 2006;296(1):56–63.
105. Gonzales D, Rennard SI, Nides M, et al. Varenicline, an $\alpha_4\beta_2$ nicotinic acetylcholine receptor partial agonist, vs. sustained-release bupropion and placebo for smoking cessation. *JAMA* 2006;296(1):47–55.
106. Tonstad S, Tonnesen P, Hajek P, et al. Effect of maintenance therapy with varenicline on smoking cessation; a randomized controlled trial. *JAMA* 2006;296(1):64–71.
107. Williams KE, Reeves KR, Billing CB, et al. A double-blind study evaluating the long-term safety of varenicline for smoking cessation. *Curr Med Res Opin* 2007;23(4):793–801.
108. Stapleton JA, Watson L, Spirling LI, et al. Varenicline in the routine treatment of tobacco dependence: a pre-post comparison with nicotine replacement therapy and an evaluation in those with mental illness. *Addiction* 2007;103(1):146–154.
109. Hall SM, Reus V, Munoz R, et al. Nortriptyline and cognitive-behavioral therapy in the treatment of cigarette smoking. *Arch Gen Psychiatry* 1998;55:683–690.
110. Prochazka AV, Weaver MJ, Keller RT, et al. A randomized trial of nortriptyline for smoking cessation. *Arch Intern Med* 1998;158:2035–2039.
111. Hughes JR, Stead LF, Lancaster T. Antidepressants for smoking cessation. *Cochrane Database Syst Rev* 2007;Jan 24(1):CD000031. Review.
112. Mooney ME, Reus VI, Gorecki J, et al. Therapeutic drug monitoring of nortriptyline in smoking cessation: a multistudy analysis. *Clin Pharmacol Ther* 2008;83(3):436–442.
113. Wagena EJ, Knipschild PG, Huibers MJH, et al. Efficacy of bupropion and nortriptyline for smoking cessation among people at risk for or with chronic obstructive pulmonary disease. *Arch Intern Med* 2005;165(19):2286–2292.
114. Hall SM, Humfleet GL, Reus VI, et al. Extended nortriptyline and psychological treatment for cigarette smoking. *Am J Psychiatry* 2004;161(11):2100–2107.
115. Croghan IT, Hurt RD, Dakhil SR, et al. Randomized comparison of a nicotine inhaler and bupropion for smoking cessation and relapse prevention. *Mayo Clin Proc* 2007;82(2):186–195.
116. Hughes JR, Stead LF, Lancaster T. Anxiolytics and antidepressants for smoking cessation (Cochrane Review). *Cochrane Database Syst Rev* 2000(2):CD000031. Review. Update in: *Cochrane Database Syst Rev* 2000(4):CD000031, 1999.
117. Schneider NG, Olmstead RE, Steinberg C, et al. Efficacy of buspirone in smoking cessation: a placebo-controlled trial. *Clin Pharmacol Therap* 1996;60:568–575.
118. Edwards NB, Murphy JK, Downs AD, et al. Doxepin as an adjunct to smoking cessation: a double-blind pilot study. *Am J Psychiatry* 1989;146(3):373–376.
119. Blondal T, Gudmundsson LJ, Tomasson K, et al. The effects of fluoxetine combined with nicotine inhalers in smoking cessation—a randomized trial. *Addiction* 1999;94(7):1007–1015.
120. Killen JD, Fortmann SP, Schatzberg AF, et al. Nicotine patch and paroxetine for smoking cessation. *J Consult Clin Psychol* 2000;68(5):883–889.
121. Rose JE, Behm FM, Westman ED, et al. Mecamylamine combined with nicotine skin patch facilitates smoking cessation beyond nicotine patch treatment alone. *Clin Pharmacol Therap* 1994;56(1):86–99.
122. Hurt RD, Ahlskog E, Croghan GA, et al. Carbidopa/levodopa for smoking cessation: a pilot study with negative results. *Nicotine Tobacco Res* 2000;2:71–78.
123. Wong GY, Wolter TD, Croghan GA, et al. A randomized trial of naltrexone for smoking cessation. *Addiction* 1999;94(8):1227–1237.
124. Brauer LH, Behm FM, Westman Ed, et al. Naltrexone blockade of nicotine effects in cigarette smokers. *Psychopharmacology* 1999;143(4):339–346.

125. Covey LS, Glassman AH, Stetner F. Naltrexone effects on short-term and long-term smoking cessation. *J Addict Dis* 1999;18(1):31–40.
126. Brandon TH, Meade CD, Herzog TA, et al. Efficacy and cost-effectiveness of a minimal intervention to prevent smoking relapse: dismantling the effects of amount of content versus contact. *J Consult Clin Psychol* 2004;72(5):797–808.
127. Blondal T, Gudmundsson LJ, Olafsdottir I, et al. Nicotine nasal spray with nicotine patch for smoking cessation: randomized trial with six year follow up. *BMJ* 1999;318(7179):285–288.
128. Hays JT, Wolter TD, Eberman KM, et al. Residential (inpatient) treatment compared with outpatient treatment for nicotine dependence. *Mayo Clin Proc* 2001;76(2):124–133.

CHAPTER 53

Jeffery N. Wilkins, MD
Mark Hrymoc, MD
David A. Gorelick, MD, PhD

Pharmacologic Interventions for Other Drug and Multiple Drug Addictions

Pharmacologic treatment of individuals with addiction can follow at least five different strategies (1). Patients can be given medications with pharmacologic actions similar to those of the target drug (e.g., cross-tolerant agonists), with the goal of substitution (as when methadone is employed for opioid dependence or nicotine for tobacco dependence). A second approach is to use antagonists or receptor blockers, with the goal of preventing or blunting the action of the target drug (as when the opiate receptor antagonist naltrexone is used in the treatment of opioid dependence). A third approach uses medications that alter neural mechanisms mediating reinforcement or drug craving (other than by acting at the same drug receptor). A fourth approach is pharmacokinetic (i.e., to reduce drug concentration at its site of action by increasing drug metabolism or decreasing its crossing of the blood–brain barrier) (2). A fifth approach is to use medication to produce a conditioned aversion to the drug, with the goal of reducing or reversing the reinforcing qualities of the target drug (such as disulfiram in the treatment of alcoholism).

This chapter focuses on pharmacologic therapies for the following single substances: marijuana, anabolic steroids, phencyclidine (PCP), hallucinogens (such as lysergic acid diethylamide [LSD], 3,4-methylenedioxymethamphetamine [MDMA, "Ecstasy"], N,N-dimethyltryptamine [DMT], and mescaline), and inhalants (volatile substances, including solvents), as well as the following mixed addictions: nicotine with other drugs, opiates with other drugs (alcohol, cocaine), and cocaine with PCP. Few of the potential treatment strategies listed here have been tried with these drugs. In almost all cases, the pharmacologic treatments described must be considered experimental or unproven, in that they lack any rigorous clinical data (as from controlled clinical trials) to support their use. Therefore, in most cases, the mainstay of treatment is psychosocial modalities (see Section 8).

This chapter includes a discussion of the potential use of hallucinogenic drugs as pharmacologic agents in the treatment of addiction and other psychiatric disorders. This use of hallucinogens received considerable attention in the 1950s and 1960s, then waned for a variety of social, legal, and ethical reasons. It has recently gained renewed attention.

MARIJUANA

There is no recognized or proven role for pharmacotherapy in the short- or long-term treatment of marijuana abuse or dependence. No medication has any substantial body of clinical experience to support its use (3,4). Controlled clinical trials have failed to show efficacy for divalproex, bupropion, or nefazodone. A small open-label trial found that buspirone (up to 60 mg/day for 12 weeks) reduced marijuana use (5), whereas an open-label trial of atomoxetine showed no efficacy (6).

Current research in cannabinoid pharmacology is opening new opportunities for pharmacologic treatment (7) (see also Section 2, Chapter 13). In particular, the development of specific agonists or antagonists for the cannabinoid CB1 receptor (which mediates the psychoactive effects of marijuana) could lead to a pharmacologic treatment for marijuana abuse, using the strategy either of cross-tolerant agonist substitution or of receptor blockade. Agonist substitution with oral synthetic Δ9-tetrahydrocannabinol (dronabinol; Marinol) suppresses cannabis withdrawal in human laboratory studies and outpatient settings. A recent case report found that dronabinol reduced cannabis use in two outpatients (8). Clinical trials evaluating agonist substitution with dronabinol are currently under way. The CB1 receptor antagonist rimonabant (developed for the treatment of obesity and the metabolic syndrome, but no larger marketed) blocks the physiologic and psychologic effects of marijuana in animals and humans (9). CB1 receptor antagonists might be used to treat marijuana abuse in the way that naltrexone, a mu-opioid receptor antagonist, is used to treat opioid abuse.

ANABOLIC STEROIDS

There is no established medication for the treatment of anabolic steroid abuse (10,11,11a). Two pharmacologic treatment approaches have been suggested: hormonal treatments to restore hypothalamic-pituitary-gonadal dysfunction caused by use of steroids, and medications to relieve specific psychiatric symptoms associated with steroid withdrawal. Neither approach has been systematically evaluated for efficacy or safety.

The first approach could be implemented with tapering doses of a long-acting steroid such as testosterone enanthate (for example, 200 to 400 mg intramuscularly initially, tapering by 50 to 100 mg every 1 to 2 weeks). This approach could be considered analogous to treating heroin withdrawal with a long-acting opiate such as methadone. Other possible treatments include human chorionic gonadotropin or synthetic forms of luteinizing hormone-releasing hormone to stimulate testosterone production, or anti-estrogenic agents such as clomiphene (e.g., 50 mg twice per day for 10 to 14 days) to reduce the elevated estradiol levels associated with anabolic steroid use.

The second approach uses standard psychotropic medications to target the depression, irritability, and aggression often associated with anabolic steroid use, although these symptoms often resolve without medication. The selective serotonin reuptake inhibitor (SSRI) antidepressants are most often used. The use of tricyclic antidepressants has been discouraged by some on theoretical grounds because their cardiovascular and anticholinergic effects might exacerbate the cardiotoxicity and urinary retention (because of prostatic hypertrophy) associated with anabolic steroid use. Low-dose neuroleptics (such as phenothiazine-equivalent doses of about 200 mg daily) have been reported effective for managing steroid-induced psychosis, hostility, and agitation.

PHENCYCLIDINE

PCP is a synthetic dissociative anesthetic that gained popularity as an abused drug in the 1960s and no longer is legally available in the United States (see Section 2, Chapter 15). A synthetic analogue, ketamine, still is used clinically and marketed legally in the United States, although it also is subject to abuse (12). There is little systematic experience with pharmacologic treatment of PCP addiction. Almost all published studies involve psychosocial treatment approaches, which usually have poor long-term success rates (13–15). Both the tricyclic antidepressant desipramine and the anxiolytic buspirone have significantly improved psychologic symptoms such as depression in small outpatient-controlled clinical trials, but neither medication significantly reduced PCP use when compared with a double-blind placebo (16,17). A monoclonal anti-PCP antibody is in preclinical development (2). There is no published experience with pharmacologic treatment of ketamine abuse (12).

PCP in Combination with Cocaine or Marijuana

PCP often is smoked with cocaine ("space basing") or marijuana ("primos"). There is very little literature on the treatment of these dual addictions, and no clinical trial has shown any medication to be effective. The antidepressant desipramine has been used because of its possible effectiveness in the treatment of separate PCP or cocaine addiction. In a double-blind study of 20 chronic PCP/cocaine users, desipramine (200 mg/day) significantly reduced symptoms associated with withdrawal, but had less effect on actual drug use (18).

INHALANTS

Inhalants are a heterogeneous group of volatile abused substances that include adhesives, aerosols, solvents, anesthetics (including nitrous oxide), gasoline, cleaning agents, and nitrites (19–21) (see Section 2, Chapter 16). Because these agents usually are marketed legally for commercial purposes, they generally are inexpensive and readily available. Many inhalant abusers entering treatment have co-occurring psychiatric and addictive disorders, typically involving alcohol and marijuana, that can complicate treatment. The mainstay of treatment is psychosocial, including techniques such as cognitive-behavioral therapy, multisystem and family therapy, 12-step facilitation, and motivational enhancement. There is little published experience with pharmacologic treatment, probably related to the overrepresentation of minors in the population of users. Single case reports suggest some benefit from buspirone (22), lamotrigine (23), or risperidone (24). Pharmacologic treatment of associated or comorbid psychiatric conditions may be effective (e.g., antipsychotics for psychosis) (25).

NICOTINE WITH OTHER DRUGS

There is substantial comorbidity between nicotine dependence and other substance use disorders. Among U.S. adults with current nicotine dependence, 8.2% have a current (non-alcohol) drug use disorder (26), an odds ratio of 3.2 for having a drug use disorder compared with those without nicotine dependence, after adjusting for sociodemographic characteristics and other psychiatric disorders (27). Conversely, 52.4% of those with a current drug use disorder are nicotine dependent. Comorbidity rates may exceed 70% among patients in treatment (28). Tobacco-related diseases are a substantial cause of morbidity and mortality among drug users, and many drug abuse treatment patients are interested in smoking cessation (29). Most studies find that smoking cessation treatment does not adversely influence the outcome of drug abuse treatment (29,30) and that patients with substance use disorders are interested in (31) and can respond well to smoking cessation treatment (32). Therefore it makes good clinical sense to screen for and treat nicotine dependence in this population. Limited evidence suggests that polydrug abusers (e.g., alcohol + stimulants + cannabis) may respond better to the combination of nicotine replacement + bupropion than to either treatment alone (34).

Nicotine and Alcohol Almost 3% of the U.S. adult population has current nicotine dependence and an alcohol use disorder (35), a comorbidity rate that may be influenced by neurobiologic and neurocognitive effects of concurrent tobacco and alcohol use (36). Among adults with nicotine dependence, 22.8% have an alcohol use disorder (26). The odds ratio is 4.4 for an alcohol use disorder among those with nicotine dependence compared with those without nicotine dependence. Conversely, among adults with an alcohol use disorder, 34.5% have nicotine dependence (26), an odds ratio of 2.7 for having nicotine dependence compared with those without an alcohol use disorder, after controlling for sociodemographic characteristics and other psychiatric disorders (37).

Tobacco-related diseases are a greater cause of morbidity and mortality in patients with alcohol use disorders than are alcohol-related medical conditions (31,38), highlighting the importance of smoking cessation treatment for this population. Cigarette smokers with a current alcohol use disorder (but not those in remission) tend to have more severe nicotine dependence, and so may need more intensive treatment, including higher doses of medication (39). Most, but not all, studies suggest that nicotine and alcohol dependence can be successfully treated at the same time without adversely affecting outcome (31,40).

There is limited evidence from controlled clinical trials that nicotine replacement therapy (e.g., nicotine patch) may be more effective than naltrexone in reducing cigarette smoking by alcohol-dependent patients (41). Higher than usual doses of both medications may be needed to achieve efficacy. Topiramate (up to 300 mg/day) reduced alcohol use and cigarette smoking in one clinical trial (42). There are preclinical data that varenicline, a nicotine partial agonist, can decrease alcohol seeking and consumption in animals (43).

Nicotine and Opioids More than three fourths of individuals with opioid dependence (including patients in methadone maintenance treatment) smoke cigarettes (28,30,44). Opiate drugs themselves, including methadone, may acutely increase cigarette smoking (28,44). Limited evidence suggests that nicotine replacement therapy, with or without bupropion, can be effective for smoking cessation in patients on methadone maintenance (45–47). Treatment outcomes are improved with concurrent psychosocial treatment (e.g., cognitive therapy or contingency management).

OPIOIDS WITH OTHER DRUGS

Opioids and Alcohol Heavy drinking, alcohol abuse, or alcohol dependence occur in one third or more of opioid-dependent individuals, including those in methadone maintenance treatment, and is associated with poor treatment outcome (48–51). There does not appear to be a strong association between methadone dose and alcohol use (49,52). Naltrexone, a mu-opioid receptor antagonist marketed for the treatment of both opioid and alcohol dependence (53), and which is available in a long-acting depot formulation to improve treatment adherence, seems a plausible treatment option (41), but was associated with worsening depression in one case report (54). Buprenorphine, a partial mu-opioid receptor agonist marketed for the treatment of opioid dependence, reduces alcohol intake in animal studies (55), but has not yet been evaluated for this in clinical trials. Disulfiram, at typical doses used to treat alcohol dependence, can be effective in reducing alcohol intake among patients in methadone maintenance (56). The careful medication monitoring and incentives for compliance that are possible in a methadone maintenance program could make disulfiram treatment more effective than it is in other treatment settings. Other medications being studied for the treatment of dually dependent patients include acamprosate (marketed for the treatment of alcohol dependence) and memantine (an NMDA receptor antagonist marketed for the treatment of dementia) (41).

Opioids and Cocaine Cocaine use is common among opioid addicts and is associated with greater opioid use, even among those in methadone maintenance treatment (57–59). A popular pattern involves simultaneous use of the two drugs ("speed balling") (59), which is said to provide a qualitatively better subjective experience ("high") than either drug alone (60). For patients already in methadone maintenance, increasing the methadone dose (usually to >60 mg/day) can reduce both opioid and cocaine use (41,61). The mu-opioid receptor antagonist naltrexone, marketed for the treatment of both opioid and alcohol dependence, has shown modest success in reducing cocaine use in patients without opioid dependence (62,63), but has not been evaluated in patients addicted to both opioids and cocaine.

Buprenorphine is a partial mu-opioid receptor agonist marketed as a parenteral analgesic and for the treatment of opioid dependence (as a sublingual tablet). High-dose buprenorphine (8 to 16 mg/day as sublingual liquid, equivalent to 16 to 32 mg/day as sublingual tablet) reduces both cocaine and opioid use in dually dependent patients (64), whereas lower doses do not (65,66).

HALLUCINOGENS

Hallucinogens are a varied group of plant-derived alkaloids and synthetic compounds that have in common the ability to produce sensory, perceptual, and cognitive changes without impairing attention or level of consciousness (i.e., with a clear sensorium) (67) (see Section 2, Chapter 14). They include compounds that influence serotonergic neurotransmission, such as LSD, psilocybin, and DMT, and those that influence catecholaminergic neurotransmission (such as mescaline and amphetamine analogues like MDMA).

At present, no pharmacologic treatment is available for the treatment of hallucinogen abuse (67–69). Several retrospective case reports suggest that long-term treatment with monoamine oxidase inhibitors (such as phenelzine) or SSRI antidepressants (fluoxetine, sertraline) can reduce the acute psychologic effects of LSD, whereas treatment with tricyclic antidepressants (imipramine, desipramine) or lithium may enhance LSD effects (70).

Single doses of the SSRI antidepressant citalopram or the 5-$HT_{2A/C}$ receptor antagonist ketanserin attenuated many of the acute psychologic effects of MDMA in human experimental studies (71,72), whereas a dose of the dopamine D_2 receptor antagonist haloperidol attenuated only the mania-like mood effect (73). These findings suggest that medications affecting serotonergic neurotransmission are a promising area for development of pharmacologic treatments for hallucinogen abuse.

The mainstay of treatment remains psychosocial intervention, which can require residential treatment in patients with severe personality disorganization. Prolonged psychotic reactions appear to occur chiefly in individuals who have preexisting psychiatric disorders; these can be difficult to distinguish from hallucinogen-induced precipitation or exacerbation of a preexisting psychotic disorder such as schizophrenia (74). Regardless of etiology, such psychotic reactions can require treatment with antipsychotic medication (68,74). Low doses of a high-potency neuroleptic have been recommended (such as 2 to 5 mg haloperidol) (75).

LSD use has been associated with perceptual abnormalities, such as illusions, distortions, and hallucinations, persisting or recurring intermittently for long periods (up to years) after the last LSD use (hallucinogen persisting perception disorder in DSM-IV) (67,75a,76). When these abnormalities occur after a period of normal perceptual functioning, they are termed *flashbacks*. Case reports suggest that sertraline, naltrexone, clonidine, or benzodiazepines can be helpful in the treatment of both persisting perceptual abnormalities and flashbacks, while antipsychotics (e.g., haloperidol, risperidone) and SSRIs have been reported to worsen the condition (76). These perceptual disorders can be associated with secondary depression or anxiety disorders such as panic and agoraphobia. In such cases, treatment with benzodiazepines or SSRI antidepressants has been reported to be helpful (68).

HALLUCINOGENS AS PHARMACOLOGIC TREATMENT FOR ADDICTION AND OTHER PSYCHIATRIC DISORDERS

Hallucinogens have also been called "empathogens" or "entheogens" because of their apparent ability to increase sociability, foster introspection and spiritual experiences, and reduce fear and anxiety. These characteristics sparked a flurry of research interest during the 1960s and early 1970s in hallucinogens as potential aids to psychotherapy for addiction and other psychiatric disorders (77,78). Increasing recreational use of hallucinogens outside the medical setting led to increased reports of adverse reactions, misuse, and abuse. Research with hallucinogens was criticized for lack of scientific rigor, inadequate controls, and poor follow-up. These concerns led many countries to place hallucinogens under strict regulatory controls (e.g., reclassification in Schedule I of the U.S. Controlled Substances Act). These actions stopped virtually all clinical research with hallucinogens for more than two decades (79). Since the early 1990s, there has been a revival of research interest in these compounds as potential aids in psychotherapy for a variety of psychiatric disorders, especially anxiety (80–82).

MDMA MDMA (3,4-methylenedioxmethamphetamine, "Ecstasy") is an amphetamine analogue with stimulant and hallucinogenic properties (see Section 2, Chapter 14). It was reclassified into Schedule 1 in 1985. Several controlled clinical trials of MDMA-assisted psychotherapy for posttraumatic stress disorder or anxiety associated with advanced-stage cancer are under way in the United States, Israel, and Switzerland (*www.clinicaltrials.gov*); studies in Norway and Spain are planned. Typical MDMA dosing is 125 mg, followed by 62.5 mg 2 to 3 hours later.

LSD LSD was synthesized by Albert Hoffman in 1938. Within 4 years of its discovery, it was marketed as an adjunct to psychotherapy (83). Over the following decades, it was used clinically as a pharmacologic treatment for a variety of psychiatric disorders, including depression, anxiety, alcoholism, and drug abuse (67,84,85). Other hallucinogens such as mescaline, psilocybin, and DMT also were used, but to a much lesser extent. Because hallucinogens were considered to induce a temporary "model" psychosis, it was hoped that study of their effects might unlock some of the neurochemical mysteries of psychiatric disorders (86). The literature accompanying LSD recommended that psychiatrists take it themselves to better understand the subjective experiences of their schizophrenic patients.

LSD was given orally as a psychiatric treatment in two ways: one or two high doses (usually 200 to 800 μg), with or without formal psychotherapy, to generate a cathartic or transforming emotional experience (this so-called psychedelic approach was popular in North America), or multiple low doses (usually 25 to 200 μg) as an adjunct to psychotherapy to break down therapeutic resistance and enhance access to unconscious material (the so-called psycholytic approach, popular in Europe) (85). This use in medical and research settings appeared safe, with low rates of psychosis and suicidality and little or no potential for addiction or overdose (85,87).

LSD is one of the more frequently studied pharmacologic treatments for alcohol dependence, albeit with no published studies since the early 1970s (67,87). Indeed, even the famed Bill Wilson, one of the originators of Alcoholics Anonymous, took LSD in this capacity (88). Most studies had serious methodologic flaws, such as no control or comparison groups, poorly characterized patient samples, and vaguely defined or unspecified outcome measures. At least nine randomized, controlled trials have been published, all of which used the psychedelic approach. Only three trials (two double-blind) found significantly more improvement in the LSD group than in the comparison group at follow-up intervals of 2 to 12 months. In two of the three studies, the advantage of LSD treatment no longer was present after 6 or 12 months. No controlled trials have evaluated the psycholytic approach, so its efficacy remains undetermined.

One open-label study found that LSD-assisted psychotherapy was better than conventional weekly group psychotherapy in promoting abstinence among opioid-dependent patients (84). More recently, there have been case reports of the beneficial effects of LSD for cluster headaches (89).

Psilocybin Psilocybin is one of the psychoactive compounds in the hallucinogenic mushrooms of the *Psilocybe* genus. Psilocybin showed efficacy in a recent open-label study of obsessive-compulsive disorder (89a) and in several cases of cluster headaches (89). Two clinical trials of psilocybin for relief of anxiety in advanced-stage cancer patients are under way (*www.clinicaltrials.gov*).

Ketamine Ketamine is marketed as a dissociative anesthetic and is also used as an analgesic (12). A controlled clinical trial of high-dose ("psychedelic-dose") ketamine-assisted psychotherapy found a higher rate of abstinence and less craving for heroin over a 2-year follow-up period compared with low-dose ketamine (90). A second randomized trial found better outcomes after three ketamine-assisted psychotherapy sessions than after one (91). A clinical trial in patients with alcohol dependence also had positive results (92). Intravenous ketamine has been shown to produce rapid (within 2 hours) and robust antidepressant effects in patients with treatment-resistant depression (93).

Ibogaine Ibogaine is a psychoactive alkaloid derived from the West African plant *Tabernanthe iboga*. In animals, it blocks the drug-induced release of dopamine in the nucleus accumbens caused by cocaine, opioids, and nicotine (94). Open-label case series suggest that single high doses (1 g or more) alleviate withdrawal symptoms, reduce drug craving, and produce long-term (>3 months) abstinence in patients with cocaine, heroin, and polydrug dependence (95). No clinical trials have been conducted because of concern over ibogaine's neurotoxicity. At least eight deaths have been associated with ibogaine administration (96). This has generated interest in the ibogaine metabolite noribogaine and the structural analogue 18-methoxycoronaridine (18-MC), which appear to be less toxic in animals.

CONCLUSIONS

This chapter reviewed approaches to pharmacologic treatment of addiction to several individual drugs of abuse, including marijuana, anabolic steroids, PCP, inhalants, and hallucinogens, as well as to some common mixed addictions, including nicotine or opiates with alcohol and other drugs, and cocaine with PCP. In most cases, there is little or no published literature to guide the choice of pharmacologic treatment and no clinical trials to support the efficacy of any treatment.

Thus the mainstay of treatment for marijuana, anabolic steroid, PCP, hallucinogen, or inhalant abuse is psychosocial interventions. The use of pharmacologic treatments remains a question for which the physician must rely almost exclusively on his or her own experience and judgment, with very little help from the medical or scientific literature. Future research may alter this situation and spur the development of effective new pharmacologic treatments. Two intriguing areas now gaining attention are compounds that interact with cannabinoid CB1 receptors in the brain (such as specific "marijuana antagonists") and the use of psychedelic drugs in the treatment of addiction and other psychiatric disorders.

ACKNOWLEDGMENTS: *Dr. Gorelick is supported by the Intramural Research Program, National Institutes of Health, National Institute on Drug Abuse.*

REFERENCES

1. Gorelick DA, Gardner EL, Xi ZX. Agents in development for the management of cocaine abuse. *Drugs* 2004;64:1547–1573.
2. Gorelick DA. Pharmacokinetic approaches to treatment of drug addiction. *Exp Rev Clin Pharmacol* 2008;1(2):277–290.
3. Nordstrom BR, Levin FR. Treatment of cannabis use disorders: a review of the literature. *Am J Addict* 2007;16:331–342.
4. Benyamina A, Lecacheux M, Blecha L, et al. Pharmacotherapy and psychotherapy in cannabis withdrawal and dependence. *Expert Rev Neurother* 2008;8:479–491.
5. McRae AL, Brady KT, Carter RE. Buspirone for treatment of marijuana dependence: a pilot study. *Am J Addict* 2006;15:404.
6. Tirado CF, Goldman M, Lynch K, et al. Atomoxetine for treatment of marijuana dependence: a report on the efficacy and high incidence of gastrointestinal adverse events in a pilot study. *Drug Alcohol Depend* 2008;94:254–257.
7. Pacher P, Batkai S, Kunos G. The endocannabinoid system as an emerging target of pharmacotherapy. *Pharmacol Rev* 2006;58 389–462.
8. Levin FR, Kleber HD. Use of dronabinol for cannabis dependence: two case reports and review. *Am J Addict* 2008;17:161–164.
9. Huestis MA, Boyd SJ, Heishman SJ, et al. Single and multiple doses of rimonabant antagonize acute effects of smoked cannabis in male cannabis users. *Psychopharmacology (Berl)* 2007;194:505–515.
10. Brower KJ. Anabolic steroid abuse and dependence. *Curr Psychiatry Rep* 2002;4:377–387.
11. Trenton AJ, Currier GW. Behavioural manifestations of anabolic steroid use. *CNS Drugs* 2005;19:571–595.
11a. Talih F, Fattal O, Malone D, Jr. Anabolic steroid abuse: psychiatric and physical costs. *Cleve Clin J Med* 2007;74: 341–352.
12. Wolff K, Winstock AR. Ketamine: from medicine to misuse. *CNS Drugs* 2006;20:199–218.
13. Daghestani AN, Schnoll SH. Phencyclidine abuse and dependence. In: American Psychiatric Association Task Force on Treatment of Psychiatric Disorders *Treatments of psychiatric disorders, vol. 2.* Washington, DC: American Psychiatric Press, 1989:1209–1218.
14. Gorelick DA, Wilkins JN. Inpatient treatment of PCP abusers and users. *Am J Drug Alcohol Abuse* 1989;15:1–12.

15. Gorelick DA, Wilkins JN, Wong C. Outpatient treatment of PCP abusers. *Am J Drug Alcohol Abuse* 1989;15:367–374.
16. Giannini AJ, Loiselle RH, Graham BH. Behavioral response to buspirone in cocaine and phencyclidine withdrawal. *J Subst Abuse Treatment* 1993;10:523–527.
17. Giannini AJ, Malone DA, Giannini MC, et al. Treatment of depression in chronic cocaine and phencyclidine abuse with desipramine. *J Clin Pharmacol* 1986;26(3):211–214.
18. Giannini AJ, Loiselle RH, Giannini MC. Space-based abstinence: alleviation of withdrawal symptoms in combinative cocaine-phencyclidine abuse. *Clin Toxicol* 1987;25(6):493–500.
19. Brouette T, Anton R. Clinical review of inhalants. *Am J Addict* 2001;10: 79–94.
20. Williams JF, Kokotailo PK. Abuse of proprietary (over-the-counter) drugs. *Adolesc Med Clin* 2006;17:733–750.
21. Williams JF, Storck M, and the Committee on Substance Abuse and Inhalant Abuse. Inhalant abuse. *Pediatrics* 2007;119(5):1009–1017.
22. Niederhofer H. Treating inhalant abuse with buspirone. *Am J Addict* 2007;16:69.
23. Shen YC. Treatment of inhalant dependence with lamotrigine. *Prog Neuropsychopharmacol Biol Psychiatry* 2007;31:769–771.
24. Misra LK, Kofoed L, Fuller W. Treatment of inhalant abuse with risperidone. *J Clin Psychiatry* 1999;60:620.
25. Hernandez-Avila CA, Ortega-Soto HA, Jasso A, et al. Treatment of inhalant-induced psychotic disorder with carbamazepine versus haloperidol. *Psychiatr Serv* 1998;49:812–815.
26. Grant BF, Hasin DS, Chou SP, et al. Nicotine dependence and psychiatric disorders in the United States: results from the National Epidemiologic Survey on Alcohol and Related Conditions. *Arch Gen Psychiatry* 2004;61:1107–1115.
27. Compton WM, Thomas YF, Stinson FS, et al. Prevalence, correlates, disability, and comorbidity of DSM-IV drug abuse and dependence in the United States: results from the National Epidemiologic Survey on Alcohol and Related Conditions. *Arch Gen Psychiatry* 2007;64:566–576.
28. Kalman D, Morissette SB, George TP. Co-morbidity of smoking in patients with psychiatric and substance use disorders. *Am J Addict* 2005; 14:106–123.
29. Richter KP, Arnsten JH. A rationale and model for addressing tobacco dependence in substance abuse treatment. *Subst Abuse Treat Prev Policy* 2006;1:23.
30. Sullivan MA, Covey LS. Current perspectives on smoking cessation among substance abusers. *Curr Psychiatry Rep* 2002;4:388–396.
31. Gulliver SB, Kamholz BW, Helstrom AW. Smoking cessation and alcohol abstinence: what do the data tell us? *Alcohol Res Health* 2006;29:208–212.
32. Gershon Grand RB, Hwang S, et al. Short-term naturalistic treatment outcomes in cigarette smokers with substance abuse and/or mental illness. *J Clin Psychiatry* 2007;68:892–898.
33. Hall SM. Nicotine interventions with comorbid populations. *Am J Prev Med* 2007;33:S406–S413.
34. Saxon AJ, Baer JS, Davis TM, et al. Smoking cessation treatment among dually diagnosed individuals: preliminary evaluation of different pharmacotherapies. *Nicotine Tob Res* 2003;5:589–596.
35. Falk DE, Yi HY, Hiller-Sturmhofel S. An epidemiologic analysis of co-occurring alcohol and tobacco use and disorders: findings from the National Epidemiologic Survey on Alcohol and Related Conditions. *Alcohol Res Health* 2006;29:162–171.
36. Durazzo TC, Gazdzinski S, Meyerhoff DJ. The neurobiological and neurocognitive consequences of chronic cigarette smoking in alcohol use disorders. *Alcohol Alcohol* 2007;42:174–185.
37. Hasin DS, Stinson FS, Ogburn E, et al. Prevalence, correlates, disability, and comorbidity of DSM-IV alcohol abuse and dependence in the United States: results from the National Epidemiologic Survey on Alcohol and Related Conditions. *Arch Gen Psychiatry* 007;64: 830–842.
38. Littleton J, Barron S, Prendergast M, et al. Smoking kills (alcoholics)! Shouldn't we do something about it? *Alcohol Alcohol* 2007;42:167–173.
39. Hughes JR, Kalman D. Do smokers with alcohol problems have more difficulty quitting? *Drug Alcohol Depend* 2006;82:91–102.
40. Kodl M, Fu SS, Joseph AM. Tobacco cessation treatment for alcohol-dependent smokers: when is the best time? *Alcohol Res Health* 2006;29: 203–207.
41. Kenna GA, Nielsen DM, Mello P, et al. Pharmacotherapy of dual substance abuse and dependence. *CNS Drugs* 2007;21:213–237.
42. Johnson BA, it-Daoud N, Akhtar FZ, et al. Use of oral topiramate to promote smoking abstinence among alcohol-dependent smokers: a randomized controlled trial. *Arch Intern Med* 2005;165:1600–1605.
43. Steensland P, Simms JA, Holgate J, et al. Varenicline, an alpha4beta2 nicotinic acetylcholine receptor partial agonist, selectively decreases ethanol consumption and seeking. *Proc Natl Acad Sci U S A* 2007;104 (30):12518–12523.
44. Richter KP, Hamilton AK, Hall S, et al. Patterns of smoking and methadone dose in drug treatment patients. *Exp Clin Psychopharmacol* 2007;15:144–153.
45. Reid MS, Fallon B, Sonne S, et al. Smoking cessation treatment in community-based substance abuse rehabilitation programs. *J Subst Abuse Treat.* 2008;35:68–77.
46. Richter KP, McCool RM, Catley D, et al. Dual pharmacotherapy and motivational interviewing for tobacco dependence among drug treatment patients. *J Addict Dis* 2005;24:79–90.
47. Shoptaw S, Rotheram-Fuller E, Yang X, et al. Smoking cessation in methadone maintenance. *Addiction* 2002;97:1317–1328.
48. Backmund M, Schutz CG, Meyer K, et al. Alcohol consumption in heroin users, methadone-substituted and codeine-substituted patients—frequency and correlates of use. *Eur Addict Res* 2003;9(1):45–50.
49. Srivastava A, Kahan M, Ross S. The effect of methadone maintenance treatment on alcohol consumption: a systematic review. *J Subst Abuse Treat* 2008;34:215–223.
50. Stenbacka M, Beck O, Leifman A, et al. Problem drinking in relation to treatment outcome among opiate addicts in methadone maintenance treatment. *Drug Alcohol Rev* 2007;26:55–63.
51. Teplin D, Raz B, Daiter J, et al. Screening for alcohol use patterns among methadone maintenance patients. *Am J Drug Alcohol Abuse* 2007;33:179–183.
52. Dobler-Mikola A, Hattenschwiler J, Meili D, et al. Patterns of heroin, cocaine, and alcohol abuse during long-term methadone maintenance treatment. *J Subst Abuse Treat* 2005;29:259–265.
53. Roozen HG, de Waart R, van der Windt DA, et al. A systematic review of the effectiveness of naltrexone in the maintenance treatment of opioid and alcohol dependence. *Eur Neuropsychopharmacol* 2006;16:311–323.
54. Schurks M, Overlack M, Bonnet U. Naltrexone treatment of combined alcohol and opioid dependence: deterioration of co-morbid major depression. *Pharmacopsychiatry* 2005;38:100–102.
55. Ciccocioppo R, Economidou D, Rimondini R, et al. Buprenorphine reduces alcohol drinking through activation of the nociceptin/orphanin FQ-NOP receptor system. *Biol Psychiatry* 2007;61:4–12.
56. Liebson I, Bigelow G, Flamer R. Alcoholism among methadone patients: a specific treatment method. *Am J Psychiatry* 1973;130:483–485.
57. DeMaria PA Jr, Sterling R, Weinstein SP. The effect of stimulant and sedative use on treatment outcome of patients admitted to methadone maintenance treatment. *Am J Addict* 2000;9:145–153.
58. Grella CE, Anglin MD, Wugalter SE. Patterns and predictors of cocaine and crack use by clients in standard and enhanced methadone maintenance treatment. *Am J Drug Alcohol Abuse* 1997;23:15–42.
59. Leri F, Bruneau J, Stewart J. Understanding polydrug use: review of heroin and cocaine co-use. *Addiction* 2003;98:7–22.
60. Walsh SL, Sullivan JT, Preston KL, et al. Effects of naltrexone on response to intravenous cocaine, hydromorphone and their combination in humans. *J Pharmacol Exper Ther* 1996;279:524–538.
61. Peles E, Kreek MJ, Kellogg S, et al. High methadone dose significantly reduces cocaine use in methadone maintenance treatment (MMT) patients. *J Addict Dis* 2006;25:43–50.

62. Schmitz JM, Stotts AL, Rhoades HM, et al. Naltrexone and relapse prevention treatment for cocaine-dependent patients. *Addictive Behavior* 2001;26(2):167–180.
63. Grassi MC, Cioce AM, Giudici FD, et al. Short-term efficacy of disulfiram or naltrexone in reducing positive urinalysis for both cocaine and cocaethylene in cocaine abusers: a pilot study. *Pharmacol Res* 2007; 55:117–121.
64. Montoya ID, Gorelick DA, Preston KL, et al. Randomized trial of buprenorphine for treatment of concurrent opiate and cocaine dependence. *Clin Pharmacol Thera.* 2004;75(1):34–48.
65. Compton PA, Ling W, Charuvastra VC, et al. Buprenorphine as a pharmacotherapy for cocaine abuse: a review of the evidence. *J Addict Dis* 1995;14(3):97–114.
66. Schottenfeld RS, Pakes JR, Oliveto A, et al. Buprenorphine vs. methadone maintenance treatment for concurrent opioid dependence and cocaine abuse. *Arch Gen Psychiatry* 1997;54(8):713–20.
67. Abraham HD, Aldridge AM, Gogia P. The psychopharmacology of hallucinogens. *Neuropsychopharmacology* 1996;14:285–298.
68. Smith DE, Seymour RB. LSD: history and toxicity. *Psychiatr Ann* 1994;24(3):145–147.
69. El-Mallakh RS, Abraham HD. MDMA (Ecstasy). *Ann Clin Psychiatry* 2007;19:45–52.
70. Bonson KR. Murphy DL. Alterations in responses to LSD in humans associated with chronic administration of tricyclic antidepressants, monoamine oxidase inhibitors or lithium. *Behav Brain Res* 1996;73: 229–233.
71. Liechti ME, Baumann C, Gamma A, et al. Acute psychological effects of 3,4-methylenedioxymethamphetamine (MDMA, "ecstasy") are attenuated by the serotonin uptake inhibitor citalopram. *Neuropsychopharmacology* 2000;22(5):513–521.
72. Liechti M, Saur MR, Gamma A, et al. Psychological and physiological effects of MDMA ("Ecstasy") after pretreatment with the 5-HT_2 antagonist ketanserin in healthy humans. *Neuropsychopharmacology* 2000; 23(4):396–404.
73. Liechti M, Vollenweider FX. Acute psychological and physiological effects of MDMA ("Ecstasy") after haloperidol pretreatment in healthy humans. *Eur Neuropsychopharmacol* 2000;10(4):289–295.
74. Boutros NN, Bowers MB Jr. Chronic substance-induced psychotic disorders: state of the literature. *J Neuropsychiat Clinl Neurosci* 1996;8:262–269.
75. Giannini AJ. Inward the mind's I: description, diagnosis, and treatment of acute and delayed LSD hallucinations. *Psychiatr Ann* 1994;24(3): 134–136.
75a. American Psychiatric Association. *Diagnostic and statistical manual of mental disorders, 4th ed. (DSM-IV).* Washington, DC: American Psychiatric Association, 1994.
76. Halpern JH, Pope HG, Jr. Hallucinogen persisting perception disorder: what do we know after 50 years? *Drug Alcohol Depend* 2003;69: 109–119.
77. Dyck E. Flashback: psychiatric experimentation with LSD in historical perspective. *Can J Psychiatry* 2005;50:381–388.
78. Halpern JH. The use of hallucinogens in the treatment of addiction. *Addict Res* 1996;4:177–189.
79. Gouzoulis-Mayfrank E, Hermle L, Thelen BM et al. History, rationale and potential of human experimental hallucinogenic drug research in psychiatry. *Pharmacopsychiatry* 1998;31(Suppl 2):63–68.
80. Moreno FA, Delgado PL. Hallucinogen-induced relief of obsessions and compulsions. *Am J Psychiatry* 1997;154(7):1037–1038.
81. Riedlinger TJ, Riedlinger JE. Psychedelic and entactogenic drugs in the treatment of depression. *J Psychoactive Drugs* 1994;26(1):41–55.
82. Halpern JH. Hallucinogens: an update. *Curr Psychiatry Rep* 2003;5: 347–354.
83. Ulrich RF, Patten BM. The rise, decline, and fall of LSD. *Perspect Biol Med* 1991;34(4):561–578.
84. Savage C, McCabe L. Residential psychedelic (LSD) therapy for the narcotic addict: a pilot study. *Arch Gen Psychiatry* 1973;28(6):808–814.
85. Strassman RJ. Hallucinogenic drugs in psychiatric research and treatment. *J Nerv Ment Dis* 1995;183:127–138.
86. Vollenweider FX. Advances and pathophysiological models of hallucinogenic drug actions in humans: a preamble to schizophrenia research. *Pharmacopsychiatry* 1998;31(Suppl):92–103.
87. Mangini M. Treatment of alcoholism using psychedelic drugs: a review of the program of research. *J Psychoactive Drugs* 1998;30(4):381–418.
88. Alcoholics Anonymous World Services. *"Pass it on": the story of Bill Wilson and how the A.A. message reached the world.* New York: Alcoholics Anonymous World Services, Inc., 1984.
89. Sewell RA, Halpern JH, Pope, Jr., HG. Response of cluster headache to psilocybin and LSD. *Neurology* 2006;66:1920–1922.
89a. Moreno FA, Wiegand CB, Taitano EK. Safety, tolerability, and efficacy of psilocybin in 9 patients with obsessive-compulsive disorder. *J Clin Psychiatry* 2006;67(11):1735–1740.
90. Krupitsky E, Burakov A, Romanova T, et al. Ketamine psychotherapy for heroin addiction: immediate effects and two-year follow-up. *J Subst Abuse Treat* 2002;23:273–283.
91. Krupitsky EM, Burakov AM, Dunaevsky IV, et al. Single versus repeated sessions of ketamine-assisted psychotherapy for people with heroin dependence. *J Psychoactive Drugs* 2007;39:13–19.
92. Krupitsky EM, Grinenko AY. Ketamine psychedelic therapy (KPT): a review of the results of ten years of research. *J Psychoactive Drugs* 1997; 29(2):165–183.
93. Maeng S, Zarate CA, Jr. The role of glutamate in mood disorders: results from the ketamine in major depression study and the presumed cellular mechanism underlying its antidepressant effects. *Curr Psychiatry Rep* 2007;9:467–474.
94. Werneke U, Turner T, Priebe S. Complementary medicines in psychiatry: review of effectiveness and safety. *Br J Psychiatry* 2006;188:109–121.
95. Vastag B. Addiction research. Ibogaine therapy: a 'vast, uncontrolled experiment'. *Science* 2005;308:345–346.
96. Maas U, Strubelt S. Fatalities after taking ibogaine in addiction treatment could be related to sudden cardiac death caused by autonomic dysfunction. *Med Hypotheses* 2006;67:960–964.

SECTION 8

Behavioral Interventions

CHAPTER 54

James O. Prochaska, PhD

Enhancing Motivation to Change

What motivates people to take action? The answer to this key question depends on what type of action is to be taken. What moves people to start therapy? What motivates them to continue therapy? What moves people to progress in therapy, or to continue to progress after therapy? Answers to these questions can provide better alternatives to one of the field's most pressing concerns: What types of therapeutic interventions would have the greatest effect on the entire population at risk for or experiencing addictive disorders?

What motivates people to change? The answer to this question depends in part on where they start. What motivates people to begin thinking about change can be different from what motivates them to begin preparing to take action. Once prepared, different forces can move people to take action. Once action is taken, what motivates people to maintain that action? Conversely, what causes people to regress or relapse to their addictive behaviors?

Fortunately, the answers to this complex set of questions may be simpler, or at least more systematic, than the questions themselves. To appreciate the answers, it is helpful to begin with the author's model of change (1–3).

THE STAGES OF CHANGE

Change is a process that unfolds over time through a series of stages: precontemplation, contemplation, preparation, action, maintenance, and termination.

Precontemplation is a stage in which the individual does not intend to take action in the foreseeable future (usually measured as the next 6 months). The individual may be at this stage because he or she is uninformed or underinformed about the consequences of a given behavior. Or he or she may have tried to change a number of times and become demoralized about his or her ability to do so. Individuals in both categories tend to avoid reading, talking, or thinking about their high-risk behaviors. In other theories, such individuals are characterized as "resistant" or "unmotivated" or "not ready" for therapy or health promotion programs. In fact, traditional treatment programs were not ready for such individuals and were not motivated to match their needs.

Individuals who are in the precontemplation stage typically underestimate the benefits of change and overestimate its costs, but are unaware that they are making such mistakes. If they are not conscious of making such mistakes, it is difficult for them to change. As a result, many remain "stuck" in the precontemplation stage for years, with considerable resulting harm to their bodies, themselves, and others. There appears to be no inherent motivation for people to progress from one stage to the next. The stages are not like stages of human development, in which children have inherent motivation to progress from crawling to walking, even though crawling works very well and even though learning to walk can be painful and embarrassing. Instead, two major forces can move people to progress.

The first is *developmental events*. In the author's research, the mean age of smokers who reach long-term maintenance is 39 years. Those who have passed 39 recognize it as an age to reevaluate how one has been living and whether one wants to die from that lifestyle or whether one wants to enhance the quality and quantity of the second half of life. The other naturally occurring force is *environmental events*. A favorite example is a couple who were both heavy smokers. Their dog of many years died of lung cancer. This death eventually moved the wife to quit smoking. The husband bought a new dog. So, even the same events can be processed differently by different people.

A common belief is that people with addictive disorders must "hit bottom" before they are motivated to change. So family, friends, and physicians wait helplessly for a crisis to occur. But how often do people turn 39 or have a dog die? When individuals show the first signs of a serious physical illness, such as cancer or cardiovascular disease, those around them usually become mobilized to help them seek early intervention. Evidence shows that early interventions often are lifesaving, and so it would not be acceptable to wait for such a patient to "hit bottom." In opposition to such a passive stance, a third force that has been created to help patients with addictions progress beyond the precontemplation stage is called *planned interventions*.

Contemplation is a stage in which an individual intends to take action within the ensuing 6 months. Such a person is more aware of the benefits of changing, but also is acutely aware of the costs. When an addicted person begins to seriously contemplate giving up a favorite substance, his or her awareness of the costs of changing can increase. There is no free change. This balance between the costs and benefits of change can produce profound ambivalence, which may reflect a type of love-hate relationship with an addictive substance, and thus can keep an individual stuck at the contemplation stage for long periods of time. This phenomenon often is characterized as "chronic contemplation" or "behavioral procrastination." Such individuals are not ready for traditional action-oriented programs.

Preparation is a stage in which an individual intends to take action in the immediate future (usually measured as the ensuing month). Such a person typically has taken some significant action within the preceding year. He or she generally has a plan of action, such as participating in a recovery group, consulting a counselor, talking to a physician, buying a self-help book, or relying on a self-change approach. It is these individuals who should be recruited for action oriented treatment programs.

Action is a stage in which the individual has made specific, overt modifications in his or her lifestyle within the preceding 6 months. Because action is observable, behavior change often has been equated with action. But in the Transtheoretical Model (TTM), action is only one of six stages. In this model, not all modifications of behavior count as action. An individual must attain a criterion that scientists and professionals agree is sufficient to reduce the risk of disease. In smoking, for example, only total abstinence counts. With alcoholism and alcohol abuse, many believe that only total abstinence can be effective, whereas others accept controlled drinking as an effective action.

Maintenance is a stage in which the individual is working to prevent relapse, but does not need to apply change processes as frequently as one would in the action stage. Such a person is less tempted to relapse and is increasingly confident that he or she can sustain the changes made. Temptation and self-efficacy data suggest that maintenance lasts from 6 months to about 5 years.

One of the common reasons for early relapse is that the individual is not well prepared for the prolonged effort needed to progress to maintenance. Many persons think the worst will be over in a few weeks or a few months. If, as a result, they ease up on their efforts too early, they are at great risk of relapse.

To prepare such individuals for what is to come, they should be encouraged to think of overcoming an addiction as running a marathon rather than a sprint. They may have wanted to enter the 100th running of the Boston Marathon, but they know they would not succeed without preparation and so would not enter the race. With some preparation, they might compete for several miles but still would fail to finish the race. Only those who are well prepared could maintain their efforts mile after mile. Using the Boston Marathon metaphor, people know they have to be well prepared if they are to survive Heartbreak Hill, which runners encounter at about mile 20. What is the behavioral equivalent of Heartbreak Hill? The best evidence available suggests that most relapses occur at times of emotional distress. It is in the presence of depression, anxiety, anger, boredom, loneliness, stress, and distress that humans are at their emotional and psychological weak point.

How does the average person cope with troubling times? He or she drinks more, eats more, smokes more, and takes more drugs to cope with distress (4). It is not surprising, therefore, that persons struggling to overcome addictive disorders will be at greatest risk of relapse when they face distress without their substance of choice. Although emotional distress cannot be prevented, relapse can be prevented if patients have been prepared to cope with distress without falling back on addictive substances.

If so many Americans rely on oral consumptive behavior as a way to manage their emotions, what is the healthiest oral behavior they could use? Talking with others about one's distress is a means of seeking support that can help prevent relapse. Another healthy alternative is exercise. Physical activity helps manage moods, stress, and distress. Also, 60 minutes per week of exercise can provide a recovering person with more than 50 health and mental health benefits (5). Exercise thus should be prescribed to all sedentary patients with addictions. A third healthy alternative is some form of deep relaxation, such as meditation, yoga, prayer, massage, or deep muscle relaxation. Letting the stress and distress drift away from one's muscles and one's mind helps the patient move forward at the most tempting of times.

Termination is a stage at which individuals have zero temptation and 100% self-efficacy. No matter whether they are depressed, anxious, bored, lonely, angry, or stressed, such persons are certain they will not return to their old unhealthy habits as a method of coping. It is as if they never acquired the habit in the first place. In a study of former smokers and alcoholics, fewer than 20% of each group had reached the stage of no temptation and total self-efficacy (6). Although the ideal is to be cured or totally recovered, it is important to recognize that, for many patients, a more realistic expectation is a lifetime of maintenance.

USING THE STAGES OF CHANGE MODEL TO MOTIVATE PATIENTS

The stages of change model can be applied to identify ways to motivate more patients at each phase of planned interventions for the addictions. The five phases are 1) recruitment, 2) retention, 3) progress, 4) process, and 5) outcomes.

Recruitment Too few studies have paid attention to the fact that professional treatment programs recruit or reach too few persons with addictions. Across all diagnoses in the *Diagnostic and statistical manual of mental disorders, 4th edition* (7), fewer than 25% of persons with addictive disorders enter professional treatment in their lifetimes (8,9). With smoking, the deadliest of addictions, fewer than 10% ever participate in a professional treatment program (10).

Given that addictive disorders are among the costliest of contemporary conditions, it is crucial to motivate many more persons to participate in appropriate treatment. These conditions are costly to the addicted individuals, their families and friends, their employers, their communities, and their health care systems. Health professionals no longer can treat addictive disorders just on a case basis; instead, they must develop programs that can reach addicted persons on a population basis.

Governments and health care systems are seeking to treat addictive disorders on a population basis. But when they turn to the largest and best clinical trials of addiction therapies, they find less than completely positive outcomes (11–14). Whether the trials were conducted in work sites, schools, or entire communities, the results are remarkably similar: No significant effects compared with the control conditions.

If we examine more closely one of these trials, the Minnesota Heart Health Study, we can find hints of what went wrong (15). With smoking as one of the targeted behaviors, nearly 90% of the smokers in treated communities reported seeing media stories about smoking, but the same was true with smokers in the control communities. Only about 12% of smokers in the treatment and control conditions said their physicians talked to them about smoking in the preceding year. If one looks at what percentage participated in the most powerful behavior change programs (clinics, classes, and counselors), it is apparent that only 4% of smokers participated in the past 5 years of planned interventions. Even when state-of-the-science smoking cessation clinics are offered at no charge, only 1% of smokers are recruited (16). There simply will be little effect on the health of the nation if our best treatment programs reach so few persons with the deadliest of addictions.

How can more people with addictive disorders be motivated to seek the appropriate help? By changing both paradigms and practices. There are two paradigms that need to be changed. The first is an action-oriented paradigm that construes behavior change as an event that can occur quickly, immediately, discretely, and dramatically. Treatment programs that are designed to have patients immediately quit abusing substances are implicitly or explicitly designed for the portion of the population in the preparation stage.

The problem is that, with most unhealthy behaviors, fewer than 20% of the affected population is prepared to take action. Among smokers in the United States, for example, about 40% are in the precontemplation stage, 40% in the contemplation stage, and 20% in the preparation stage (17). Among college students who abuse alcohol, about 85% are in the precontemplation stage, 10% in the contemplation stage, and 5% in the preparation stage.

When only action-oriented interventions are offered, fewer than 20% of the at-risk population is being recruited. To meet the needs of the entire addicted population, interventions must meet the needs of the 40% in the precontemplation and the 40% in the contemplation stages.

In the most recent clinical guidelines for the treatment of tobacco, however, there were only evidence-based programs for motivated smokers in the preparation stage (18). In spite of there being more than 6,000 studies on tobacco, research had excluded the vast majority from treatment studies.

By offering stage-matched interventions and applying proactive or outreach recruitment methods in three large-scale clinical trials, the author and others have been able to motivate 80% to 90% of smokers to enter a treatment program (19,20). Comparable participation rates were generated with college students who abuse alcohol, even though 75% were in the precontemplation stage (21). These results represent a quantum increase in our ability to move many more people to take the action of starting therapy.

A treatment program for problem gamblers in Windsor, Ontario, used creative communications to let their prospective population know wherever they are, the program can work with them. This program had generous support of 2% of earnings from local casinos, but they were not reaching many people. So, on the back of city buses, they placed ads with a traffic light logo: red light not ready, yellow light getting ready and green light ready. Not only did they dramatically increase their recruitment, some clients would take pride in saying, "Hey, there goes my bus!"

The second paradigm change that is required is movement from a passive-reactive approach to a proactive approach. Most professionals have been trained to be passive-reactive: to passively wait for patients to seek their services and then to react. The problem with this approach is that most persons with addictive disorders never seek such services.

The passive-reactive paradigm is designed to serve populations with acute conditions. The pain, distress, or discomfort of such conditions can motivate patients to seek the services of health professionals. But the major killers today are chronic lifestyle disorders such as the addictions. To treat the addictions seriously, professionals must learn how to reach out to entire populations and offer them stage-matched therapies.

There are a growing number of national disease management and disease prevention companies who train health professionals in these new paradigms. Thousands of nurses, counselors, and health coaches have been trained to proactively reach out by telephone to interact at each stage of change with entire patient and employee populations with high-risk behaviors including smoking, alcohol abuse, and obesity.

What happens if professionals change only one paradigm and proactively recruit entire populations to action-oriented interventions? This experiment has been tried in one of the largest U.S. managed care organizations (16). Physicians spent

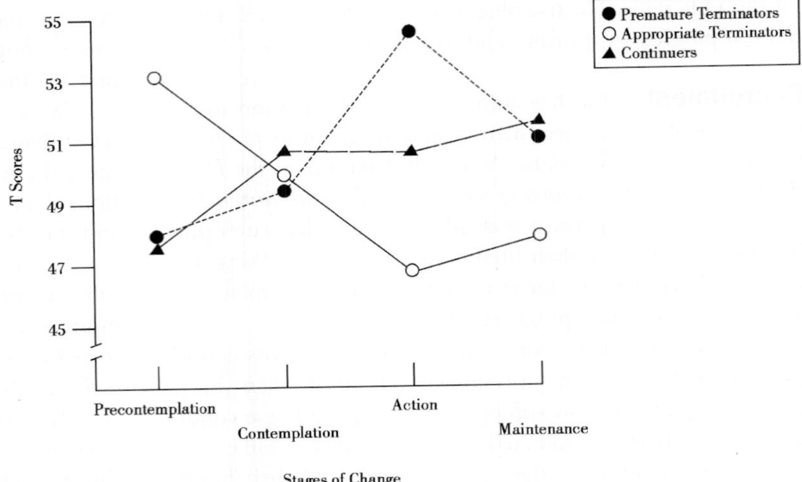

FIGURE 54.1. Pretherapy stage profiles for premature terminators, appropriate terminators, and continuers. (Data from Brogan ME, Prochaska JO, Prochaska JM. Predicting termination and continuation status in psychotherapy using the Transtheoretical Model. *Psychotherapy* 1999;36:105–113.)

time with every smoker in an effort to persuade him or her to enroll in a state-of-the-art action-oriented clinic. If that did not work, nurses spent up to 10 minutes encouraging the smoker to enroll, followed by 12 minutes with a health educator and a counselor call to the home. The base rate was 1% participation.

This most intensive recruitment protocol motivated 35% of smokers in precontemplation to enroll. However, only 3% actually entered the program, 2% completed it, and none showed improved outcomes. From a combined contemplation and preparation group, 65% enrolled, 15% entered the program, 11% completed it, and some had an improved outcome.

In the face of this evidence, there may be several answers to the question: What can move a majority of people to enter a professional treatment program for an addictive disorder? One is the availability of professionals who are motivated and prepared to proactively reach out to entire populations and offer them interventions that match whatever stage of change they are in.

Retention What motivates patients to continue in therapy? Or conversely, what moves clients to terminate counseling quickly and prematurely, as judged by their counselors? A meta-analysis of 125 studies found that nearly 50% of clients drop out of treatment (22). Across studies, there were few consistent predictors of premature termination. Although addictive disorder, minority status, and lower education predicted a higher percentage of dropouts, these variables did not account for much of the variance.

At least five studies are available on dropouts from a stage model perspective on addictive disorder, smoking, obesity, and a broad spectrum of psychiatric disorders. These studies found that stage-related variables were more reliable predictors than demographics, type of problem, severity of problem, and other problem-related variables. Figure 54.1 presents the stage profiles of three groups of patients with a broad spectrum of psychiatric disorders (2,23). In that study, the investigators were able to predict 93% of the three groups: premature terminators, early but appropriate terminators, and those who continued in therapy (23).

Figure 54.1 shows that the before-therapy profile of the entire group who dropped out quickly and prematurely (40%) was a profile of persons in the precontemplation stage. The 20% who finished quickly but appropriately had a profile of patients who were in the action stage at the time they entered therapy. Those who continued in long-term treatment were a mixed group, with most in the contemplation stage.

The lesson is clear: Persons in the precontemplation stage cannot be treated as if they are starting in the same place as those in the action stage. If they are pressured to take action when they are not prepared, they simply will leave therapy.

For patients in the action stage who enter therapy, what would be an appropriate approach? One alternative would be to provide relapse prevention strategies like those described by Dr. Alan Marlatt. But would relapse prevention strategies make any sense with the 40% of patients who enter in the precontemplation stage? What might be a good match for them? Experience suggests a dropout prevention approach, because such patients are likely to leave early if they are not helped to continue.

With patients who begin therapy in the precontemplation stage, it is useful for the therapist to share key concerns: "I'm concerned that therapy may not have a chance to make a significant difference in your life, because you may be tempted to leave early." The therapist then can explore whether the patient has been pressured to enter therapy. How do such patients react when someone tries to pressure or coerce them into quitting an addiction when they are not ready? Can they tell the therapist if they feel pressured or coerced? It is only feasible to encourage them to take steps when they are most ready to succeed.

The author and others have conducted four studies with stage-matched interventions in which retention rates of persons entering interventions in the precontemplation stage can be examined. What is clear is that, when treatment is matched to stage, persons in the precontemplation stage will remain in

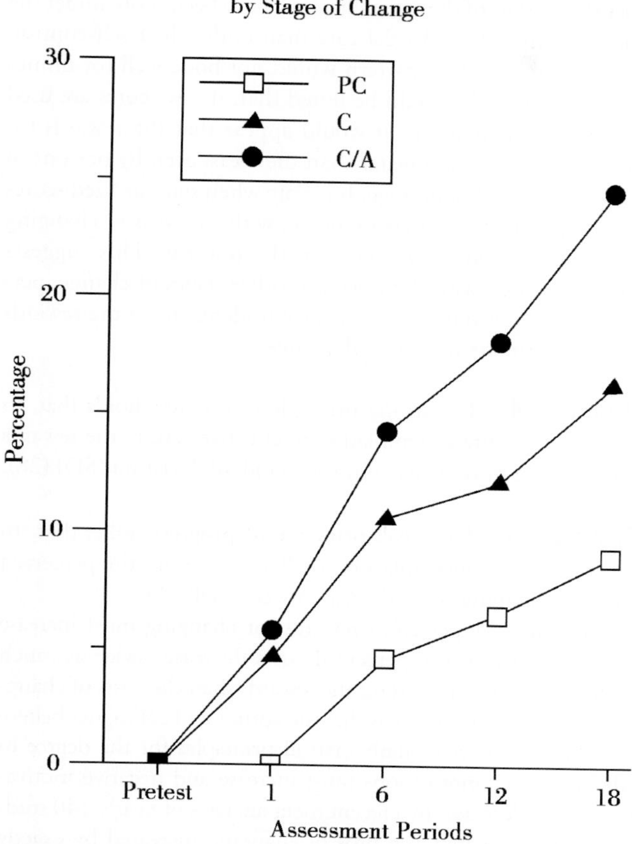

FIGURE 54.2. Percentage of smokers who maintained abstinence over 18 months. Note: Groups were in the following stages at the time of entry into treatment: Precontemplation (PC), Contemplation (C), and Preparation (C/A) ($n = 570$).

treatment at the same rates as those who start in the preparation stage (19,20). This result was consistent in clinical trials in which patients were recruited proactively (the therapist reached out with an offer of help), as well as in trials in which patients were recruited reactively (they asked for help). What motivates people to continue in therapy? Receiving treatments that match their stage of readiness to change.

Another strategy is to begin therapy with a single session of Motivational Interviewing. Connors et al. (24) found that a single session reduced dropouts from their intensive alcohol treatment program from 75% to 50%. A session of role induction designed to prepare people for what to expect from therapy made no difference, even though clinically it has been most widely used to try to prevent premature dropout.

Progress What moves people to progress in therapy and to continue to progress after therapy? Figure 54.2 presents an example of what is called the *stage effect.* The stage effect predicts that the amount of successful action taken during and after treatment is directly related to the stage at which the person entered treatment (2). In the study cited, interventions with smokers ended at 6 months. The group of smokers who started in the precontemplation stage showed the least amount of effective action, as measured by abstinence at each assessment point. Those who started in the contemplation stage made significantly more progress, whereas those who entered treatment already prepared to take action were most successful at every assessment.

The stage effect has been found across a variety of problems and populations, including rehabilitative success for brain injury and recovery from anxiety and panic disorders after random assignment to placebo or effective medication (25,26). In the latter clinical trial, the psychiatrist leading the trial concluded that patients need to be assessed for their stage of readiness to benefit from medication and to be helped through the stages so that they are well prepared before being placed on the medication.

One strategy for applying the stage effect clinically involves setting realistic goals for brief encounters with patients at each stage of change. A realistic goal is to help patients progress one stage in brief therapy. If a patient moves relatively quickly, he or she may be able to progress two stages. The results to date indicate that, if a patient progresses one stage in one month, the likelihood of his or her taking effective action by 6 months is doubled. If the patient progresses two stages, the likelihood that he or she will take effective action increases three to four times (19). Setting realistic goals thus can enable many more people to enter therapy, continue in therapy, progress in therapy, and continue to progress after therapy.

One result for health professionals trained in this approach to the addictions can be a dramatic increase in the morale of the health professionals involved (personal communication). They can see progress with most of their patients, where they once saw failure when immediate action was the only criterion for success. They are much more confident that they have treatments that can match the stages of all of their patients rather than the small number who are prepared to take immediate action.

A lesson here is that the models of therapy selected should be good for the mental health of the therapist as well as the patient. After all, the professional is engaged in therapy for a lifetime, while most patients are involved for only a brief time.

As managed care organizations move to briefer and briefer therapies for addictions and other disorders, there is a danger that most health professionals will feel pressured to produce immediate action. If this pressure is transferred to patients who are not prepared for such action, most patients will not be reached or not retained in treatment. A majority of patients can be helped to progress in treatment through relatively brief encounters, but only if realistic goals are set for both patient and therapist. Otherwise, there is a risk of demoralizing and demotivating both patient and therapist. Given the vast public health needs described above, another misuse of the model is for managed care organizations or health professionals to limit treatment only to patients who are prepared to take immediate action.

Process To help motivate patients to progress from one stage to the next, it is necessary to know the principles and processes of change that can produce such progress.

Principle 1 The rewards for changing must increase if patients are to progress beyond precontemplation. In a review of 12 studies, all showed that the perceived benefits were higher in the contemplation than in the precontemplation stage (27). This pattern held true across 12 problem behaviors: use of cocaine, smoking, delinquency, obesity, inconsistent condom use, unsafe sex, sedentary lifestyles, high-fat diets, sun exposure, radon testing, mammography screening, and physicians practicing behavioral medicine.

A technique that can be used in population-based programs involves asking a patient in the precontemplation stage to describe all the benefits of a change such as quitting smoking or starting to exercise. Most persons can list four or five. The therapist can let the patient know that there are 8 to 10 times that number, and challenge the patient to double or triple the list for the next meeting. If the patient's list of benefits of exercise begins to indicate many more motives, such as a healthier heart, healthier lungs, more energy, healthier immune system, better moods, less stress, better sex life, and enhanced self-esteem, he or she will be more motivated to begin to seriously contemplate such a change.

Principle 2 The "cons" of changing must decrease if patients are to progress from contemplation to action. In 12 of 12 studies, the author and colleagues found that the perceived costs of changing were lower in the action than in the contemplation stage (27).

Principle 3 The relative weight assigned to benefits and costs must cross over before a patient will be prepared to take action. In 12 of 12 studies, the costs of changing were assessed as higher than the rewards in the precontemplation stage, but in 11 of 12, the rewards were assessed as higher than the costs in the action stage. The sole exception involved quitting cocaine. In that study, a large percentage of treatment was delivered to inpatients. We interpret this exception to mean that the actions of these patients may have been more under the social control of residential care than under their self-control. At a minimum, their pattern would not bode well for immediate discharge. It should be noted that, if raw scores are used to assess these patterns, it would appear that the rewards for changing are seen as greater than the costs, even by persons in the precontemplation stage. It is only when standardized scores are used that clear patterns emerge, with the costs of changing always perceived as greater than the rewards. This suggests that, compared with their peers at other stages of change, persons in the precontemplation stage underestimate the rewards and overestimate the costs of change.

Principle 4 The strong principle of progress holds that, to progress from precontemplation to effective action, the rewards for changing must increase by one standard deviation (SD) (28).

Principle 5 The weak principle of progress holds that, to progress from contemplation to effective action, the perceived costs of changing must decrease by one-half SD.

Because the perceived rewards for changing must increase twice as much as the perceived costs decrease, twice as much emphasis must be placed on the rewards than the costs of changing. What is striking here is that the author and colleagues believe they have discovered mathematical principles for the degree to which positive motivations must increase and negative motivations must decrease. In a recent meta-analyses of nearly 140 studies on 48 behaviors, the pros of changing increased by exactly 1.00 SD, whereas the cons decreased by 0.54 SD (29). Such principles can produce much more sensitive assessments to guide interventions, giving therapists and patients feedback for when therapeutic efforts are producing progress, and when they are failing. Together, they can modify methods if movement is needed for the patient to become adequately prepared for action.

Principle 6 It is important to match particular processes of change with specific stages of change. Table 54.1 presents the empirical integration found between processes and stages of

TABLE 54.1 Stages of Change in Which Change Processes are Emphasized

	Stages of Change				
	Precontemplation	**Contemplation**	**Preparation**	**Action**	**Maintenance**
Processes	Consciousness raising Dramatic relief Environmental reevaluation				
		Self-reevaluation			
			Self-liberation		
				Contingency management Helping relationships Counterconditioning Stimulus control	

change. Guided by this integration, the following processes would be applied to patients in the precontemplation stage.

1. *Consciousness raising* involves increased awareness of the causes, consequences, and responses to a particular problem. Interventions that can increase awareness include observations, confrontations, interpretations, feedback, and education. Some techniques, such as confrontation, pose considerable risk in terms of retention and are not recommended as highly as motivational enhancement methods such as personal feedback about the current and long-term consequences of continuing the addictive behavior. Increasing the costs of not changing is the corollary of raising the rewards for changing. So consciousness-raising should be designed to increase the perceived rewards for changing.

2. *Dramatic relief* involves emotional arousal about one's current behavior and the relief that can come from changing. Fear, inspiration, guilt, and hope are some of the emotions that can move persons to contemplate changing. Psychodrama, role-playing, grieving, and personal testimonies are examples of techniques that can move people emotionally. It should be noted that earlier literature on behavior change concluded that interventions such as education and fear arousal did not motivate behavior change. Unfortunately, many interventions were evaluated in terms of their ability to move people to immediate action. However, processes such as consciousness raising and dramatic relief are intended to move people to the contemplation rather than the action stage. Therefore their effectiveness should be assessed according to whether they lead to the expected progress.

3. *Environmental reevaluation* combines both affective and cognitive assessments of how an addiction affects one's social environment and how changing would affect that environment. Empathy training, values clarification, and family or network interventions can facilitate such reevaluation. For example, a brief media intervention aimed at a smoker in precontemplation might involve an image of a man clearly in grief saying, "I always feared that my smoking would lead to an early death. I always worried that my smoking would cause lung cancer. But I never imagined it would happen to my wife." Beneath his grieving face appears this statistic: "50,000 deaths per year are caused by passive smoking". In 30 seconds, this message achieves consciousness raising, dramatic relief, and environmental reevaluation.

4. *Self-reevaluation* combines both cognitive and affective assessments of an image of one's self free from addiction. Imagery, healthier role models, and values clarification are techniques that can move individuals in this type of intervention. Clinically, patients first look back and reevaluate how they have lived as addicted individuals. As they progress into the preparation stage, they begin to develop a focus on the future as they imagine how life could be if they were free of addiction.

5. *Self-liberation* involves both the belief that one can change and the commitment and recommitment to act on that belief. Techniques that can enhance such willpower include public rather than private commitments. Motivational research also suggests that individuals who have only one choice are not as motivated as if they have two choices (30). Three choices are even better, but four choices do not seem to enhance motivation. Wherever possible, then, patients should be given three of the best choices for applying each process. With smoking cessation, for example, there are at least three good choices: quitting "cold turkey," using nicotine replacement therapy, and using nicotine fading. Asking clients to choose which alternative they believe would be most effective for them and which they would be most committed to can enhance their motivation and their self-liberation.

6. *Counterconditioning* requires the learning of healthier behaviors that can substitute for addictive behaviors. Counterconditioning techniques tend to be quite specific to a particular behavior. They include desensitization, assertion, and cognitive counters to irrational self-statements that can elicit distress.

7. *Contingency management* involves the systematic use of reinforcements and punishments for taking steps in a particular direction. Because successful self-changers rely much more on reinforcement than punishment, it is useful to emphasize reinforcements for progressing rather than punishments for regressing. Contingency contracts, overt and covert reinforcements, and group recognition are methods of increasing reinforcement and incentives that increase the probability that healthier responses will be repeated. To prepare patients for the longer term, they should be taught to rely more on self-reinforcements than social reinforcements. Clinical experience shows that many patients expect much more reinforcement and recognition from others than they actually receive. Relatives and friends may take action for granted. Average acquaintances typically generate only a few positive consequences early in the action stage. Self-reinforcements obviously are much more under self-control and can be given more quickly and consistently when temptations to lapse or relapse are resisted.

8. *Stimulus control* involves modifying the environment to increase cues that prompt healthy responses and decrease cues that lead to relapse. Avoidance, environmental reengineering (such as removing addictive substances and paraphernalia), and attending self-help groups can provide stimuli that elicit healthy responses and reduce the risk of relapse.

9. *Helping relationships* combine caring, openness, trust, and acceptance, as well as support for changing. Rapport building, a therapeutic alliance, counselor calls, buddy systems, sponsors, and self-help groups can be excellent resources for social support. If patients become dependent on such support to maintain change, the support will need to be carefully faded, lest termination of therapy becomes a condition for relapse.

Competing theories of therapy have implicitly or explicitly advocated alternative processes of enhancing motivation for change. Is it ideas or emotions that move people? Is it values, decisions, or dedication? Do contingencies incentivize humans, or is behavior determined by environmental conditions or habits? Or is it the therapeutic relationship that is the common healer across all therapeutic modalities?

The answer to each of these questions is "yes." Therapeutic processes originating from competing theories can be compatible when they are combined in a stage-matched paradigm. With patients in earlier stages of change, motivation can be enhanced through more experiential processes that produce healthier cognitions, emotions, evaluations, decisions, and commitments. In later stages, it is possible to build on such solid preparation and motivation by emphasizing more behavioral processes that can help condition healthier habits, reinforce these habits, and provide physical and social environments that support healthier lifestyles freer from addictions.

Outcomes What is the result when all of these principles and processes of change are combined to help patients and entire populations move toward action on their addictions? A series of clinical trials applying stage-matched interventions offers lessons about the future of behavioral health care generally and treatment of the addictions specifically.

In a large-scale clinical trial, the author and colleagues compared four treatments: 1) a home-based action-oriented cessation program (standardized), 2) stage-matched manuals (individualized), 3) a computerized expert system plus manuals (interactive), and 4) counselors plus an expert system and manuals (personalized). Patients (739 smokers) were randomly assigned by stage to one of the four treatments (31).

In the expert system condition, participants completed 40 questions by mail or telephone. Their responses were entered into a central computer, from which feedback reports were generated. These reports informed participants about their stage of change, the benefits and costs of changing, and change processes appropriate to their stages of change. At baseline, participants were given positive feedback on what they were doing correctly and guidance on which principles and processes they needed to apply to progress. In two progress reports delivered over the following 6 months, participants also received positive feedback on any improvement in any of the variables relevant to progress. Thus demoralized and defensive smokers could begin to progress without having to quit and without having to work too hard. Smokers in the contemplation stage could begin to take small steps, such as delaying their first cigarette in the morning for an additional 30 minutes. They could choose small steps that would increase their self-efficacy and help them become better prepared for quitting.

In the personalized condition, smokers received four proactive counselor calls over the 6-month intervention period. Three of the calls were based on the expert system's reports. Counselors reported much more difficulty in interacting with participants without any progress data. Without scientific assessments, it was more difficult for both patients and counselors to know whether any significant progress had occurred since their last interaction.

Figure 54.3 presents point-prevalence abstinence rates for each of the four treatment groups over 18 months, with treatment ending at 6 months. Results with the two self-help manual conditions were parallel for 12 months, but the stage-matched manuals achieved better results at 18 months. This is an example of a *delayed action effect*, which often is observed with stage-matched programs and which others have

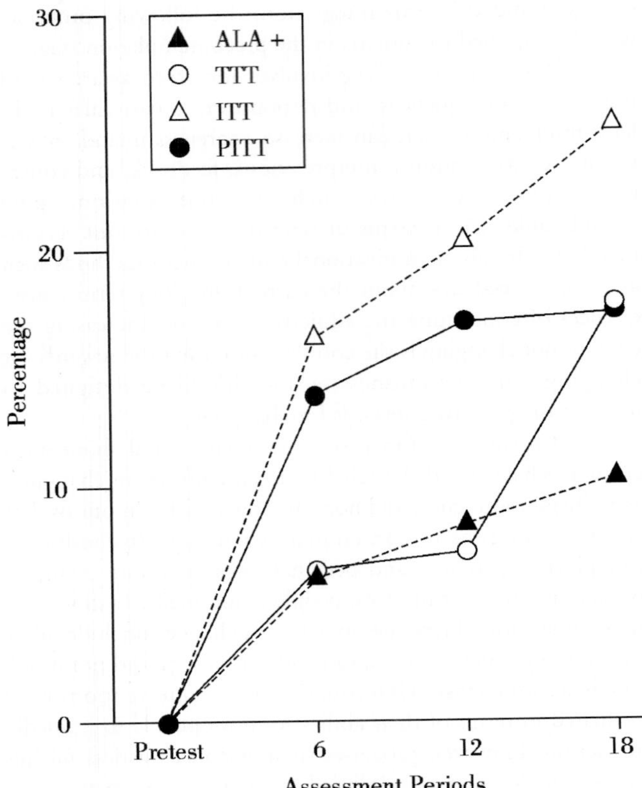

FIGURE 54.3. Point-prevalence abstinence (%) for four treatment groups at pretest and at 6, 12, and 18 months. ALA+, standardized manuals; TTT, individualized stage-matched manuals; ITT, interactive computer reports; PITT, personalized counselor calls.

observed with self-help programs. It takes time for participants in early stages to progress all the way to action. Therefore some treatment effects as measured by action will be observed only after considerable time has elapsed. But it is encouraging to find treatments producing therapeutic effects months and even years after active treatment has ended. The expert system alone and expert system-plus-counselor conditions produced comparable results for 12 months.

Then, the effects of the counselor condition flattened out, whereas the expert system condition effects continued to increase. Potential reasons for the delayed differences between these conditions include the possibility that participants in the personalized condition may have become somewhat dependent on the social support and social control of the counselor calling. The last call occurred after the 6-month assessment, and benefits would be observed at 12 months. Termination of the counselor calls could result in no further progress because of the loss of social support and control. The classic pattern in smoking cessation clinics is rapid relapse that begins as soon as treatment is terminated. Some of this rapid relapse could well be due to the sudden loss of social support or social control provided by the counselors and other participants when active treatment ends.

The next test was to demonstrate the efficacy of the expert system when applied to an entire population recruited proactively. With more than 80% of 5,170 smokers participating and less than 20% in the preparation stage, this study demonstrated significant benefits of the expert system at each 6-month follow-up (20). Moreover, the advantages over proactive assessment alone increased at each followup for the full 2 years assessed. The implications here are that expert system interventions in a population can continue to demonstrate benefits long after the intervention has ended.

The efficacy of the expert system intervention was demonstrated again in a health maintenance organization (HMO) population of 4,000 smokers, with 85% participation (19). In the first population-based study, the expert system was 34% more effective than assessment alone; in the second, it was 31% more effective. These differences were clinically significant as well. Although working on a population basis, the investigators were able to show a level of success normally found only in intensive clinic-based programs with low participation rates of more carefully selected samples of smokers. The implication is that, after expert systems are developed and show effectiveness with one population, they can be transferred to, and show replicable results in, other populations.

A recent meta-analysis of 54 studies on computer-based interventions across a broad range of behaviors has found that tailoring treatment on each of the TTM variables (stage, pros and cons, processes or self-efficacy) produces greater effects than treatments that do not tailor on these variables. Tailoring on some treatment variables, such as perceived susceptibility to negative consequences, produced worse effects. Some other theoretical variables, such as social norms and behavior intentions, made no difference (32).

Enhancing Interactive Interventions In recent benchmarking research, the author and colleagues have been attempting to create enhancements to the expert system to produce even better outcomes. In the first enhancement, which involved a study of an HMO population, a personal digital assistant designed to bring the behavior under stimulus control was added (19). However, this action-oriented intervention did not enhance the study outcomes on a population basis. In fact, the original expert system alone was twice as effective as the system plus the personal digital assistant enhancement. This result suggests that more is not necessarily better and providing interventions that are mismatched to stage can make outcomes markedly worse.

Counselor Enhancements In the HMO population, counselors plus expert system computer-based interventions were outperforming expert systems alone at 12 months. But at 18 months, results for the counselor enhancement had declined, whereas those for the expert systems alone had increased. Both interventions were producing identical outcomes of 23.2% abstinence, which are excellent for an entire population. Why did the effect of the counselor condition drop after the intervention? A leading hypothesis is that patients can become dependent on counselors for social support and social monitoring. Withdrawing those social influences may place such patients at increased risk of relapse. The expert system, in contrast, tends to maximize self-reliance. In a current clinical trial, the author and colleagues are "fading out" the counselor intervention over time in an effort to minimize dependence on the counselor. If fading is effective, it will have implications for how counseling should be terminated: gradually over time rather than suddenly.

It seems clear that the most powerful change programs will combine the personalized benefits of counselors and consultants with the individualized, interactive, and databased benefits of expert system computer-based interventions. However, studies have not demonstrated that the more costly counselors, who have been the most powerful change agents, actually add value over expert system interventions alone. These findings have clear implications for the cost-effectiveness of expert systems for entire populations in need of health promotion programs.

Interactive versus Noninteractive Interventions
Another important goal of the HMO study was to assess whether an interactive intervention (specifically, a computer-based expert system) is more effective than noninteractive communications (such as self-help manuals) when the results are adjusted to control for the number of intervention contacts (33). At 6, 12, and 18 months for groups of smokers receiving a series of one, two, three, or six interactive versus noninteractive contacts, the interactive interventions (expert system) outperformed the noninteractive manuals. The difference at 18 months was at least 5%—a difference between treatment conditions assumed to be clinically significant. These results clearly support the hypothesis that interactive interventions will outperform the same number of noninteractive interventions.

These results support the assumption that the most powerful health promotion programs for entire populations will be interactive. Reports in the clinical literature support the hypothesis that interactive interventions such as behavioral counseling produce better long-term abstinence rates (20% to 30%) than do noninteractive interventions such as self-help manuals (10% to 20%). In assessing these results, it should be kept in mind that traditional action-oriented programs were implicitly or explicitly recruiting for populations of individuals in the preparation stage, whereas the studies cited here involved proactively recruited smokers, of whom fewer than 20% were in the preparation stage. Even so, long-term abstinence rates were in the 20% to 30% range for the interactive interventions and in the 10% to 20% range for noninteractive interventions. The implications are clear. Providing interactive interventions through the use of computer-based expert systems is likely to produce better outcomes than relying on noninteractive communications such as newsletters, media, or self-help manuals.

Multiple Behaviors A series of studies applied our best practice of TTM-tailored expert systems plus a stage-based self-help manual for multiple behaviors. Consistent across all studies was that the TTM treatments produced significant impacts on multiple behaviors (34–36). The studies also produced abstinence rates for smoking cessation that were in the same narrow 24% range found when the single behavior of smoking was treated. This is the first body of research that has demonstrated that multiple-behavior treatments can be as effective as treating single behaviors, but the impacts are greater because more behaviors are treated effectively. The other treated behaviors, such as diet and prevention of skin cancer, were even more effective, with the percentages in the action-maintenance stage at long-term follow-up ranging from 35% to 40%.

With male perpetrators of partner violence, TTM-tailored treatments were added to the best practice of mandatory 6-month weekly group therapy. At the 6-month follow-up with the first 200 participants, the addition of the TTM tailoring produced significant reduction in a variety of physical and emotional abuse behaviors compared with the weekly group counseling alone. With the addition of TTM tailoring, only 3% of the female partners of the perpetrators had been beaten in the past 6 months compared to 23% of the women whose partners received only the group therapy (37). With the TTM treatment, about twice as many perpetrators (most of whom also had addiction problems) had progressed to the action or maintenance stage at the 6-month assessment. Particularly encouraging was that more than twice as many of the perpetrators in the TTM treatment had voluntarily sought additional therapy.

CONCLUSIONS

It seems clear that the future of health promotion programs lies in stage-matched, proactive, interactive interventions. Much greater effects can be generated through the use of proactive programs because participation rates are increased, even if efficacy rates are lower. But proactive programs also can produce outcomes comparable to those of traditional reactive programs. Although it is counterintuitive to suggest that outcomes for groups that are proactively recruited can match those of individuals who reach out for help, that is what informal comparisons strongly suggest. For example, in a comparison of results at 18-month follow-up for all subjects who received three expert system interventions in a study of reactive intervention and a study of proactive intervention, the abstinence curves were remarkably similar (20,32). The results with the counseling plus expert system conditions were even more impressive. Proactively recruited smokers, working with both counselors and the expert system, achieved higher rates of abstinence at each follow-up than did the smokers who had called for help. These results are partially attributable to the fact that the proactive counseling protocol has been revised and, it is to be hoped, improved on the basis of previous data and experience. But the point is that if it is possible to reach out and offer people improved behavior-change programs that are appropriate for their stage of readiness to change, it ought to be possible to produce efficacy or abstinence rates at least equal to those seen with individuals who reach out for help. Unfortunately, there is no experimental design that would make it possible to assign study subjects randomly to proactive versus reactive recruitment programs. Thus one is left with informal but provocative comparisons.

Results with multiple behavior interventions using some type of TTM tailoring and proactive recruitment have found as good effects as when smoking alone is treated. The results with the other treated behaviors were even better.

If these results continue to be replicated, therapeutic programs will be able to produce unprecedented effects on entire populations. To do so will require scientific and professional shifts: 1) from an action paradigm to a stage paradigm, 2) from reactive to proactive recruitment, 3) from expecting participants to match the needs of programs to having programs match the needs of patients, 4) from single to multiple behavior interventions, and 5) from clinic-based to population-based programs that apply individualized and interactive intervention strategies.

REFERENCES

1. Prochaska JO, DiClemente CC. Stages and processes of self-change of smoking: Toward an integrative model of change. *J Consult Clin Psychol* 1983;51:390–395.
2. Prochaska JO, DiClemente CC, Norcross JC. In search of how people change: applications to the addictive behaviors. *Am Psychol* 1992;47: 1102–1114.
3. Prochaska JO, Norcross JC, DiClemente CC. *Changing for good.* New York: William Morrow, 1994.
4. Mellinger GD, Balter MB, Uhlenhuth EH, et al. Psychic distress, life crisis, and use of psychotherapeutic medications: National Household Survey Data. *Arch Gen Psychiatry* 1978;35:1045–1052.
5. Reed G. *Measuring stage of change for exercise.* Unpublished doctoral dissertation, University of Rhode Island, 1995.
6. Snow MG, Prochaska JO, Rossi JS. Stages of change for smoking cessation among former problem drinkers: a cross-sectional analysis. *J Substance Abuse* 1992;4:107–116.
7. American Psychiatric Association (APA). *Diagnostic and statistical manual of mental disorders, 4th edition (DSM-IV).* Washington, DC: American Psychiatric Press, 1994.
8. Veroff J, Douvan E, Kulka RA. *The inner America.* New York: Basic Books, 1981.
9. Veroff J, Douvan E, Kulka RA. *Mental health in America.* New York: Basic Books, 1981.
10. U.S. Department of Health and Human Services (DHHS). *The health benefits of smoking cessation: a report of the Surgeon General.* Washington, DC: U.S. Government Printing Office; 1990.
11. Luepker RV, Murray DM, Jacobs DR, et al. Community education for cardiovascular disease prevention: risk factor changes in the Minnesota Heart Health Program. *Am J Public Health* 1994;84:1383–1393.
12. COMMIT Research Group. COMMunity Intervention Trial for smoking cessation (COMMIT): I. Cohort results from a four-year community intervention. *Am J Public Health* 1995;85:183–192.
13. Glasgow RE, Terborg JR, Hollis JF, et al. Take Heart: results from the initial phase of a work-site wellness program. *Am J Public Health* 1995;85:209–216.
14. Ennett ST, Tabler NS, Ringwolt CL, et al. How effective is drug abuse resistance education? A meta-analysis of Project DARE outcome evaluations. *Am J Public Health* 1994;84:1394–1401.
15. Lando HA, Pechacek TF, Pirie PL, et al. Changes in adult cigarette smoking in the Minnesota Heart Health Program. *Am J Public Health* 1995; 85:201–208.
16. Lichtenstein E, Hollis J. Patient referral to smoking cessation programs: who follows through? *J Fam Pract* 1992;34:739–744.

17. Velicer WF, Fava JL, Prochaska JO, et al. Distribution of smokers by stage in three representative samples. *Prevent Med* 1995;24:401–411.
18. Fiore MC, Bailey WC, Cohen SJ, et al. *Treating tobacco use and dependence: clinical practice guideline.* Rockville, MD: U.S. Department of Health and Human Services, Public Health Service, 2000.
19. Prochaska JO, Velicer WF, Fava JL, et al. Counselor and stimulus control enhancements of a stage-matched expert system for smokers in a managed care setting. *Preventive Medicine* 2000;32:39–46.
20. Prochaska JO, Velicer WF, Fava JL et al. Evaluating a population-based recruitment approach and a stage-based expert system intervention for smoking cessation. *Addict Behav* 2002;26:583–602.
21. Laforge RG, Gomes SO, Cottrill SD, et al. Baseline results of proactive telephone recruitment of college drinkers in the College-Based Alcohol Risk Reduction (C-BARR) trial. [Abstract]. *Alcohol Clin Exp Res* 25(5):147A, 2001.
22. Wierzbicki M, Pekarik G. A meta-analysis of psychotherapy dropout. *Prof Psychol Res Pract* 1993;29:190–195.
23. Brogan ME, Prochaska JO, Prochaska JM. Predicting termination and continuation status in psychotherapy using the Transtheoretical Model. *Psychotherapy* 1999;36:105–113.
24. Connors G, Walitzer K, Dermen K. Preparing clients for alcoholism treatment: effects on treatment participation and outcomes. *J Consult Clin Psychol* 2002;70:1161–1169.
25. Beitman BD, Beck NC, Deuser W, et al. Patient stages of change predicts outcome in a panic disorder medication trial. *Anxiety* 1994;1:64–69.
26. Lam CS, McMahon BT, Priddy DA et al. Deficit awareness and treatment performance among traumatic head injury adults. *Brain Inj* 1988; 2:235–242.
27. Prochaska JO, Velicer WF, Rossi JS, et al. Stages of change and decisional balance for twelve problem behaviors. *Health Psychol* 1994;13: 39–46.
28. Prochaska JO. Strong and weak principles for progressing from Precontemplation to Action based on twelve problem behaviors. *Health Psychol* 1994;13:47–51.
29. Hall KL, Rossi JS. Meta-analytic examination of the strong and weak principles across 48 health behaviors. *Prevent Med* 2008;46(3):266– 274.
30. Miller WR. Motivation for treatment: a review with special emphasis on alcoholism. *Psychol Bull* 1985;98:84–107.
31. Prochaska JO, DiClemente CC, Velicer WF, et al. Standardized, individualized, interactive and personalized self-help programs for smoking cessation. *Health Psychol* 1993;12:399–405.
32. Noar SM, Benac C, Harris M. Does tailoring matter? Meta-analytic review of tailored print health behavior change interventions. *Psychol Bull* 2007;133(4):673–693.
33. Velicer WF, Prochaska JO, Fava JL, et al. Interactive versus noninteractive and dose response relationships for stage matched smoking cessation programs in a managed care setting. *Health Psychol* 1999;18:1–8.
34. Jones H, Edwards L, Vallis MT, et al. Changes in diabetes self-care behaviors make a difference to glycemic control: the diabetes stages of change (DiSC) study. *Diabetes Care* 2003;26:732–737.
35. Prochaska JO, Velicer WF, Redding CA, et al. Multiple risk expert systems interventions: impact of simultaneous stage-matched expert system interventions for smoking, high-fat diet and sun exposure in a population of parents. *Health Psychol* 2004;23:503–516.
36. Prochaska JO, Velicer WF, Redding CA, et al. Stage-based expert systems to guide a population of primary care patients to quit smoking, eat healthier, prevent skin cancer and receive regular mammograms. *Prevent Med* 2005;41:406–416.
37. Levesque DA, Driskell MM, Prochaska JM, Prochaska JO. Acceptability of a stage-matched expert system intervention for domestic violence offenders. *Violence and victims. Violence Vict* 2008;23(4):432–435.

CHAPTER 55

Dennis C. Daley, PhD
Antoine Douaihy, MD
Roger D. Weiss, MD
Delinda E. Mercer, PhD

Group Therapies

Group therapies are used widely in the treatment of substance use disorders (SUDs) in short-term residential rehabilitation, long-term therapeutic community, partial hospital, intensive outpatient, drug-free outpatient, and aftercare programs. In fact, the most common treatment modality for SUDs is "group therapy," a term that holds several meanings (1). Recently, the term *group therapy* has been incorporating more didactic cognitive-behavioral skills and psychoeducational approaches (1). For structured treatment programs such as residential, therapeutic community, partial hospital, or intensive outpatient programs, group therapies often are the principal modality of clinical intervention. In these contexts, groups are used to address early recovery issues such as initiating abstinence and engaging the patient in a recovery process (2–7), anger management (8), and co-occurring psychiatric disorders (9–12). Group therapies also are widely used in the treatment of specific clinical populations, particularly women (13); alcoholics (14,15); persons in the criminal justice system (16,17); those dependent on marijuana (18), cocaine (3,19,20), methamphetamine (21), or opiates (22); and families of substance abusers (23).

This chapter provides an overview of group therapies. It reviews the goals and types of group therapies as they are used to treat SUDs. It also provides a discussion on treatment outcome studies examining the effectiveness of group therapies for SUDs and their limitations. It also reviews the group therapies in the context of co-occurring disorders. Training and supervision issues are discussed.

GOALS OF GROUP THERAPIES

The ultimate goal of addiction treatment is to enable an individual to achieve and maintain lasting abstinence, but the immediate goals are to reduce drug or alcohol abuse, improve the individual's ability to function, and minimize the medical and psychosocial complications of addiction. Individuals in treatment for addiction will also need to change their behaviors to adopt a healthier lifestyle. Group therapies help patients achieve these goals by creating a milieu in which members of a group can bond with each other, thus reducing the stigma associated with addiction and the humiliation of having lost control of one's own behavior (4). The specific ways in which groups can help achieve this include providing education on addiction, recovery, and relapse; resolving ambivalence by overcoming denial and enhancing motivation to change; evoking hope and optimism for change; providing an opportunity to give and receive feedback from peers; teaching recovery skills to manage the addictive disorder over the long term; understanding and resolving problems contributing to or resulting from the addiction disorder, rather than avoiding such problems; providing a context in which the patient can identify with others and give and receive support; creating an experience of positive membership in a recovery-oriented group in which feelings, thoughts, and conflicts can be freely expressed; preparing the patient for involvement in long-term recovery; and facilitating the patient's interest in participating in self-help programs in addition to treatment groups (3,24–27). Treatment groups provide a context in which addicted persons can gain support, encouragement, feedback, and confrontation from peers who understand from personal experience how addicted individuals think, feel, and act, including the manipulations, schemes, and diversions they sometimes use to rationalize their substance use and other maladaptive behaviors (4,7).

ORGANIZATION OF GROUP THERAPIES

Group therapies vary in their theoretical underpinnings, structure, format, rules, number and duration of sessions, clinical focus, size, types of patients accepted, requirements for abstinence, approach to the group model, relative focus on content or process, and role of the group leader. For example, psychoeducational groups are more structured and content-focused, depend on the leader to facilitate discussion of educational material, and can accommodate larger numbers of patients than therapy groups. Therapy groups usually are limited to 6 to 12 persons, with the content of discussions determined by the participants. Leaders are less verbally active in these groups and serve more as facilitators of members' exploration of problems and sharing of support and feedback. Although some groups incorporate principles and information from self-help groups such as Alcoholics Anonymous (AA), Narcotics Anonymous (NA), Cocaine Anonymous (CA), or Crystal Meth Anonymous (CMA) therapy groups differ from self-help groups in their focus on in-depth exploration of psychologic, interpersonal, and intrapsychic issues. Structured inpatient, residential, partial hospital, and intensive outpatient treatment programs can last from several days to a year, thus exposing patients to considerable heterogeneity in the number of group sessions they receive. For example, a large multisite study of outpatient treatment for cocaine addiction (28) offered 39 individual sessions to patients in three of the four treatment conditions, in addition to 24 group counseling sessions, over a period of 6 months of active treatment and three additional monthly individual booster sessions.

Types of Group Therapies Although many different types and structures of group treatments are available for the treatment of substance use disorders, many of the problems or issues addressed are similar (Table 55.1). Group therapists or

TABLE 55.1 Issues Commonly Addressed in Recovery Groups

Physical/Lifestyle Issues	Understanding Addiction and Recovery
Tolerance, physical withdrawal, and the need for detoxification	Understanding addiction (etiology, symptoms, effects)
Craving management	Effects of specific substances (e.g., alcohol, cocaine, marijuana)
Medications for addiction and for co-occurring disorders	Acceptance of addiction
Medical problems including pain issues	Stages of change
HIV/AIDS, hepatitis C virus, and hepatitis B virus	Motivation to change and motivational struggles such as ambivalence
Sexuality issues	Tips for quitting alcohol or drug use
Importance of exercise, rest, relaxation, and nutrition in recovery	Pros and cons of change
Types and purposes of treatment	Pros and cons of abstinence
Defining personal goals/values	Denial and other defenses
Structuring time	Phases of recovery and domains of recovery (physical, psychologic, family, social, spiritual)
Engaging in non–substance-using activities	Risky behaviors (such as sharing needles and equipment)
Achieving balance in life	Other nonsubstance addictions
Regular use of recovery tools in daily life	Family/Interpersonal/Social Domains
Psychological/Behavioral/Spiritual Issues	Effects of addiction on family and interpersonal relationships
Understanding and identifying feelings and their connections to relapse	Role of the family, concerned significant others in treatment/recovery
Managing anxiety	Resolving marital or family conflicts
Managing depression	Making amends to family or others
Managing feelings of emptiness	Managing high-risk people, places, and events
Managing boredom	Engaging in healthy leisure interests
Reducing shame and guilt	Addressing social life and relationship conflicts
Grief and loss issues	Resisting social pressures to drink alcohol or use other drugs
Self-esteem	Presenting a history of addiction disorders to the employer
Self-defeating and therapy-sabotaging behaviors	Facing versus avoiding interpersonal conflicts
Psychiatric comorbidities	Learning to ask for help and support
Relapse and personal growth	Love and intimacy
High risk factors or dangerous situations for relapse	Self-help programs in recovery
Relapse warning signs	The Twelve Steps
Relapse setups	Recovery clubs
Lapse/relapse interruption	
Spirituality	
Meditation and prayer	

counselors employ a variety of techniques, such as providing education, eliciting support and feedback from members, confronting problematic behaviors, clarifying problems and feelings, helping the group remain focused, facilitating participant self-disclosure, teaching coping skills, and integrating experiential strategies relevant to the problems or issues being discussed (for example, using role-play to address interpersonal issues or conflicts, or monodramas to address internal conflicts). Group therapies for substance use disorders generally fall into one of the following categories.

Milieu Groups Milieu groups are offered in residential programs and usually involve a group meeting to start or end the day. A community group may review the upcoming day's schedule, discuss issues pertinent to the community of patients, ask each patient to state a goal for the day, or have patients listen to and reflect on the reading of the day (e.g., an inspirational reading from a recovery book such as *24 Hours a Day*). A wrap-up group may review the day's activities and provide participants a chance to reflect on experiences and insights from the day's treatment activities.

Psychoeducational Groups Psychoeducational groups provide information about specific topics related to addiction and recovery, and help patients begin to learn how to cope with the challenges of recovery (e.g., how to resist social pressure to use substances or how to reduce boredom). These groups use a combination of lectures, discussions, educational videos, behavioral rehearsals, and completion of written assignments such as a recovery workbook or personal journal.

Skill Groups Skill groups are aimed at helping patients develop or improve their intrapersonal and interpersonal skills. For example, these groups teach problem-solving methods and stress management, cognitive, and relapse prevention strategies.

Therapy or Counseling Groups These groups are less structured and often give the participants an opportunity to create their own agenda. Any of the issues presented in Table 56.1 can be discussed. These groups focus more on insight and raising self-awareness than on education or skill development. Some clinics provide gender-specific therapy or counseling groups so that women and men can work separately on their concerns and problems.

More extensive discussions of various group approaches for addiction, such as interactional group therapy (24,25), modified dynamic group therapy (3,29), cognitive-behavioral (3), psychoeducational, and problem-solving (30), skills training (14), and recovery stage-specific groups (4,7) can be found in texts elsewhere (12).

Format of Group Therapy Sessions Five common models of group therapy were identified by Stinchfield et al. (31): the group educational model, in which the group leader serves as an educator on substance abuse and its risks; recovery skills training also educationally based teaching relapse prevention skills; the group process model; the check-in group, consisting of brief individual interventions conducted within a group framework; and groups addressing other issues such as anger management or parenting skills. Some groups incorporate elements of all models. Group sessions usually last from 60 to 90 minutes. Groups can be limited to a specific number of sessions or be open-ended, so that the patient can attend for as long as needed. Programs vary in the frequency of sessions as well. For example, the Matrix model of addiction treatment, developed by Rawson et al. (32), offered 20 individual sessions during the first 6 months of an intensive outpatient program that included many group sessions. In a variation of this model, three individual sessions are provided to patients during the course of a 16-week treatment episode (21). The Washton structured outpatient model involves group therapy two to four times each week in combination with weekly individual counseling sessions (20). Interestingly, the last model explicitly acknowledges that, "although group therapy is the core treatment modality for most patients, some are not able to tolerate group as a result of psychiatric and/or interpersonal impairment. Treatment for these patients can consist of individual therapy two to three times a week."

Recovery Group Sessions In the cocaine collaborative study in which the authors participated, patients attended 90-minute Recovery Group sessions each week for 12-weeks (28,30,33). Each session focused on a specific topic relevant to early or middle recovery. At every session, patients were encouraged to abstain from all substances, seek and use a sponsor, participate in self-help groups, and use the "tools" of recovery (e.g., talking about versus acting on strong cravings, reaching out for support, and the like). Patients were encouraged to socialize with each other before the start of the session while the group leader administered a Breathalyzer test. Each group session began with a check-in period (10 to 20 minutes), during which time patients briefly reported any substance use, strong cravings, or "close calls." This was followed by a review of the topic for the session, lasting 40 to 60 minutes. Although the group leader had a specific curriculum for each meeting, the session was conducted in a way that encouraged patients to relate to the material in a personal way. Each session provided materials from a workbook that contained information about the topic and several questions for the patients to complete to relate the material to their own lives. During these discussions, patients were encouraged to ask questions, share personal experiences related to the psychoeducational material, give each other feedback, and identify strategies to manage their problems in recovery.

Each session ended with a brief review of patients' plans for the coming week (10 to 15 minutes). Patients could discuss self-help meetings and other steps they could take toward recovery. Just before the session closed, patients recited the Serenity Prayer of AA. Topics of Phase 1 therapy sessions included the following.

Session 1—Understanding Addiction Addiction was defined as a biopsychosocial disorder in which multiple factors contributed to its development and maintenance.

Symptoms of addiction were reviewed in terms of the *Diagnostic and statistical manual of mental disorders, 4th edition* (34), with a focus on compulsive use, impaired control, continued use despite negative consequences, tolerance changes, withdrawal syndrome, and psychosocial impairment.

Sessions 2 and 3—The Process of Recovery Effects of addiction on all areas of functioning and the concept of denial were reviewed. Recovery was defined as a long-term process of abstinence and change involving multiple domains: physical, psychologic, family, social, and spiritual. Each patient identified and discussed one area of change and a plan to achieve such change. Feedback was elicited from peers about the plan.

Sessions 4 and 5—Social and Interpersonal Issues in Recovery The group discussed cravings, internal and external triggers, and enabling behaviors on the part of other people in the patient's life. Major emphasis was given to identifying and learning to manage direct and indirect social pressures to engage in substance use (people, places, events, and things). The effects of addiction on family and relationships and activities are described, and patients discussed strategies to address interpersonal problems in early recovery. Finally, components of healthy relationships were discussed.

Sessions 6 and 7—Self-Help Groups and Support Systems The importance of participating in Twelve-Step programs of AA, NA, and CA was emphasized in all group sessions; these two sessions provided specific information on types of meetings, sponsorship, the Twelve Steps, and other tools of recovery. Barriers and negative perceptions or experiences with self-help programs were discussed, as were the benefits of self-help programs. Discussions also addressed sources of support outside AA, NA, CMA, and CA (e.g., family, friends, recovery clubs, and organizations); barriers to asking for help; and ways to actually ask others for help.

Sessions 8 and 9—Managing Feelings in Recovery These sessions focused on understanding the connection between feelings and substance use and becoming aware of "high-risk" emotional states associated with relapse. Strategies to manage feelings were reviewed, and patients were asked to develop a plan to address one emotional state they felt was a problem for them (such as anger, anxiety, boredom, depression, or loneliness).

An entire session focused on understanding and dealing with guilt and shame, as these feelings are so common among patients in early recovery.

Sessions 10, 11, and 12—Relapse Prevention and Maintenance Relapse was defined as both a process and an event, with both obvious and covert warning signs. These sessions focused on helping patients identify and manage warnings of relapse, as well as individual high-risk situations. Common risk factors identified in research studies were reviewed to help patients learn to anticipate and prepare to address them. Strategies for maintaining recovery over time and using the tools of recovery on a daily basis also were discussed.

Phase 2: Problem-Solving Groups Phase 2 groups met for 90 minutes weekly for 12 sessions after completing Phase 1. The goals were to help patients identify, rank, and discuss their problems in recovery and identify strategies to manage these problems to reduce relapse risk. Sessions provided an opportunity for patients to give and receive support and feedback from peers. After the check-in period—in which patients reported on any episodes of use, strong cravings, or close calls—they were asked to identify a problem or recovery issue for discussion in the group. Often, more than one member would identify a similar problem or issue for discussion. The issues and problems reviewed in the psychoeducational groups were revisited frequently. Issues discussed often involved struggles with motivation to change or remain abstinent; persistent obsessions; compulsions and close calls to use cocaine or other substances; actual lapses or relapses; boredom with sobriety; upsetting emotional states (e.g., anxiety, anger, depression); concerns or experiences with self-help programs; the Twelve Steps or a sponsor; interpersonal problems and pressures to use substances; financial, job, and lifestyle problems; other addictions; and spirituality. At the end of each session, patients were asked to state their plans for the coming week in terms of attendance at self-help meetings or other steps they could take to aid their recovery or resolve a problem.

Group Process Issues In both Phases 1 and 2, group counselors had to attend to the group process to keep the group focused and productive. This attention required counselors to engage quiet members in discussions and facilitate their self-disclosure and to limit or redirect members who talked too much and tried to dominate group discussions, listened poorly to fellow group members, or tried to use the group to obtain individual therapy from the leader. Counselors kept the group from going off on unrelated tangents or talking in generalities, balanced the discussions between problems and coping strategies, facilitated group members' sharing of support and feedback, and addressed impasses or problems in the group. In Phase 1 groups, the counselor had to ensure that the curriculum for each session was covered, because this was viewed as an important part of treatment.

Obstacles to Group Therapy Other researchers who have written about group treatments identify problems with group participants that create obstacles to treatment. Washton (4) reports the following problems among members of therapy groups: lateness and absenteeism, intoxication, hostility and chronic complaining, silence and lack of participation, terse and superficial presentations, factual reporting and focusing on externals, proselytizing and hiding behind AA, and playing cotherapist. In his classic text on group psychotherapy, Yalom (24) identified a number of "recurring behavioral constellations" that occur in the treatment group. He identified these constellations as monopolist, schizoid, silent, boring, help-rejecting complainer, self-righteous moralist, psychotic, narcissistic, and borderline. Because the problems affect the group as a whole, the leader must have strategies to address any that arise in the course of a group session. For example, if a member consistently rejects the advice or feedback of other group members, the group leader can point out this pattern and engage the group in a discussion of why this pattern is occurring. The members who offer help and support only to have their attempts rejected can be asked to talk about what this feels like so that the member who rejects their help is aware of the impact this behavior has on others.

Family Psychoeducational Workshops Family psychoeducational workshops (FPWs) and other family programs often are used to educate the family, provide support, help reduce the family's burden, increase helpful behaviors, and decrease unhelpful behaviors (3,21,35–37). FPWs are semistructured sessions in which specific information is provided to patients and families in the context of a group of families. Support is provided, and families are encouraged to share their questions, concerns, and feelings.

Strong affect always is present in these workshops, and some sharing of emotion is necessary. However, encouraging families to share their emotions too much can be counterproductive, so education and support are the main areas of focus. Thus the group leader must be careful not to allow the group to become a venue for sharing deep-seated emotions. Interactive discussion is encouraged because it increases participants' understanding of addiction and recovery. The specific material covered in FPWs depends on the amount of time available. Possibilities include the following.

- *An overview of substance abuse and dependence:* Prevalence, symptoms, causes, and basic concepts (such as various degrees of substance use problems, denial, obsession, compulsion, tolerance, and psychiatric comorbidity).
- *Effects of SUDs:* The effects on the individual, the family system, and specific family members, including children.
- *An overview of recovery:* Recovery issues for the affected person (physical, psychologic or emotional, social, family, spiritual, other) and how to measure outcomes.
- *An overview of treatment resources:* Treatment resources and approaches for the affected individual.
- *How the family can help:* Enabling behaviors for the family to avoid and behaviors that are helpful in supporting the addicted family member's recovery.
- *Family recovery issues:* How the family member can recover from the adverse effects of addiction and involvement in a close relationship with an addicted member.
- *Self-help programs:* Programs available for addicted individuals and their family members, how such programs can help the family, and how to access them.
- *Relapse:* Warning signs of relapse, the importance of relapse prevention planning, how the family can be involved, and how to deal with an actual lapse or relapse of an addicted family member.

In the Cocaine Collaborative Study (33), the authors offered a single FPW during the first month of treatment. The purpose of the session was to educate families about the study, to seek their help in supporting the patients' compliance with treatment, and to provide education about addiction, recovery, their effect on the family, and community resources available to the family.

The role of interpersonal processes and social support is a critical component of relapse prevention (38). This underscores the value of involving family members in supporting the patient's recovery efforts through their participation in FPW sessions.

EMPIRICAL VALIDATION OF GROUP THERAPIES

Recent years have witnessed a number of studies that have compared different models of psychotherapy or counseling for addiction disorders (39,40). Most studies funded by the National Institute on Drug Abuse and the National Institute on Alcohol Abuse and Alcoholism involve individual or pharmacotherapeutic interventions. Despite the widespread use of group therapies in addiction treatment, controlled trials of group interventions have been somewhat limited, and many studies report results from "programs" that involve multiple components (i.e., individual plus group, multiple types of group treatments, or group plus other services). A recent paper reviewed 24 prospective treatment outcome studies comparing group therapy with one or more treatment conditions. The results of the studies were mixed, varying on the nature of the research design, the population studied, and the format of treatment (content, intensity, and length). The findings showed three important patterns: additional specialized group therapy can enhance the effectiveness of "treatment as usual," no differences were found between group and individual modalities, and no single type of group therapy demonstrated any consistent superiority in efficacy (41). The content of the group (whether skilled-based or interpersonal) did not make a difference (41). The authors concluded that the most notable finding of that study was the paucity of research on this topic. However, researchers and clinicians agree on the importance of group therapies, and groups remain one of the principal modalities of treatment in most residential, therapeutic community, partial hospital, intensive outpatient, and aftercare programs. Some manual-based group treatments do exist for specific subpopulations of women with SUDs (42,43). No randomized controlled trial has compared single-gender, women-focused substance abuse group therapy with standard mixed-gender group treatment for women with SUDs (44) until recently. A stage I randomized controlled trial of a new, manual-based, women-focused, single-gender group therapy compared with a manual-based mixed-gender group treatment demonstrated effectiveness. Although in-treatment improvement in substance abuse outcomes was not different between the two treatments, the Women's Recovery Group demonstrated continued improvement in substance abuse outcomes 6-month post-treatment compared with the mixed-gender group drug counseling (GDC). A women-focused, single-gender group treatment may have a positive impact on longer term clinical outcomes among women with SUDs (45).

A recent pilot study sought to evaluate a women's manual-based substance use disorder recovery model. Participants were opioid-dependent women in a methadone maintenance treatment program who received 12 sessions of the gender-based model in group format over 2 months. The findings indicated significant improvements in drug use (verified by urinalysis), impulsive-addictive behavior, global improvement, and knowledge of the treatment concepts. Patients' high attendance rate (87% of available sessions) and strong treatment satisfaction additionally support the potential use of this treatment model (46). The interest in researching various models of psychotherapy has led to the development of treatment manuals that describe the various psychotherapeutic approaches. Psychotherapy outcomes studies have found that such manuals have an important, positive effect on the quality of both research and clinical practice. In fact, the use of treatment manuals has become a standard practice in research studies because they help ensure that therapists or counselors are providing treatment in a defined, measurable way. This practice also appears to reduce the variance among therapists providing what is nominally the same treatment.

Adherence to Group Sessions and Treatment Dropout Most randomized clinical trials on addiction treatment showed significant reductions in drug use, improved health, and reduced social pathology (47). Patients who comply with sessions and attend a sufficient number of sessions show better outcomes than those who drop out prematurely. However, two of the major problems in the treatment of addictive disorders and cooccurring psychiatric disorders are poor adherence with session attendance or medications and early termination (48). Integrated supportive group therapy in a randomized trial has shown a differential effect on treatment retention in subjects with severe mental disorders and substance use disorders (49).

Reasons for Dropping Out of Group Treatment In the National Institute on Drug Abuse Collaborative Cocaine Treatment Study (33), patients were assessed to learn the reasons for early termination of treatment. The reasons most commonly cited were time problems (42.7%), the relapse to use or the desire to use (30.7%), not finding group sessions helpful (29.3%), wanting a different treatment, such as individual therapy (30.7%), improvement in the problem (18.7%), other unspecified reasons (18.7%), unwillingness to participate in treatment (16%), and need for hospitalization (13.3%).

Limitations of Research Although evidence suggests that group treatments are effective for SUDs, limitations to the research conducted on group treatments arise from two sources: variations in content and differences in process. A level of interaction and complexity must be taken into consideration, over and above the content of the intervention and the counselor's skill in conducting it. Very often, group programs are studied rather than a single group intervention. For example, studies of intensive outpatient programs often evaluate a comprehensive program that involves several different types of groups that together make up the intensive outpatient program. Therefore it is unclear how much each type of group actually contributes to the treatment outcome. In addition, studies sometimes involve a combination of group and individual treatments, making it difficult to determine how much each intervention contributes to the outcome.

The discrepancy between the widespread clinical application of group therapy and the limited research on this topic stems from the inherent difficulties in conducting meaningful research on group therapy (41).

GROUP THERAPIES FOR CO-OCCURRING DISORDERS

Community surveys and clinical studies document high rates of co-occurring psychiatric and substance use disorders (50–52). Group therapy appears to be helpful to patients with such co-occurring disorders. Considerable clinical research supports the use of various group treatments for so-called "dual diagnosis" patients, including those with chronic and persistent mental disorders (10,53,54). Several investigators have developed and are testing in clinical trials the effects of manual-driven group treatments. Najavits et al. (55,56) developed a cognitive-behavioral therapy (CBT) model for women with posttraumatic stress disorder (PTSD). Their CBT protocol involves 24 weekly group sessions, which are divided into "units" dealing with problems that are frequently encountered. An introductory unit of two sessions provides education on PTSD and SUDs and introduces the women to community resources and self-help programs. A behavioral unit of seven sessions teaches skills to manage the SUD and PTSD, addressing issues such as setting a daily schedule, structuring time, nurturing the self, learning to ask for help and support from others, identifying and managing triggers for both disorders, managing ambivalence about change, and learning to deal with life stressors. A unit of six sessions teaches cognitive strategies, such as changing maladaptive thoughts or cognitive distortions associated with SUD or PTSD. A unit of six sessions focuses on improving communication skills and interpersonal relationships. (This unit also addresses issues such as self-protection in relationships, rebuilding trust, and healthy relationship thinking.) The final unit of three sessions reviews the experience of group and termination issues with a focus on ongoing supports, knowing how to judge progress or deterioration, and the importance of a continuing care plan. At the time the group treatment contract is signed an interview is conducted with each patient before he or she enters the group, and ways to benefit from this treatment are reviewed. An individual

HIV counseling session is provided to each patient within the first 3 weeks of treatment, at which time an HIV risk assessment is completed and education and counseling on HIV issues are provided. Homework assignments and action techniques such as role-play are used throughout this protocol.

A study of 17 women enrolled in this treatment program found major improvements in substance use, trauma-related symptoms, suicide cognitions about substance use, and didactic knowledge of topics covered in treatment sessions (56). Although this finding suggests that group treatment can be helpful to substance-abusing women with PTSD, the results are tentative because of the lack of a control group. Hien et al.'s subsequent study showed this to be no better than relapse prevention treatment (42).

A recent randomized clinical trial evaluated the efficacy of a 12-session cognitive behavioral group therapy for alcohol-dependent males with cooccurring interpersonal violence. The findings were impressive. There was a significant difference between participants in the integrated approach (substance abuse-domestic violence) versus the Twelve-Step Facilitation group on alcohol use outcomes. The group assigned to substance abuse-domestic violence reported using alcohol significantly fewer days as compared with the Twelve-Step Facilitation group. Regarding physical violence, there was a trend for participants in the substance abuse-domestic violence condition to achieve a greater reduction in the frequency of violent behaviors across time compared with individuals in the Twelve-Step Facilitation group (57).

Weiss et al. (58) sequentially (although not randomly) assigned 45 patients having both bipolar disorders and SUD to one of two conditions: integrated cognitive-behavioral model of group treatment or monthly assessments. All patients also received treatment as usual, including pharmacotherapy. The study found that patients participating in the integrated group therapy addressing both disorders simultaneously had significantly better substance abuse outcomes. Following these findings, Weiss et al. (59) undertook a randomized controlled trial with 3 months of posttreatment follow-up, to compare the efficacy of integrated group therapy (IGT) versus an active treatment, GDC, which is an adaptation of the model used in the National Institute on Drug Abuse Collaborative Cocaine Treatment Study (28,60).

Both IGT and GDC are manual-driven treatments that involve 20 weekly group sessions lasting 1 hour each. IGT focuses on issues pertinent both to substance use and bipolar illness, whereas GDC focuses solely on SUD. GDC patients address psychiatric issues in separate sessions with a mental health professional. The IGT was more successful at reducing substance use than GDC. In addition, integrated group therapy had better substance use outcomes than GDC despite more subclinical mood symptoms. IGT seems to be well accepted by patients and has promising results for patients with cooccurring bipolar disorder and SUD. In an uncontrolled quality improvement study of 117 patients who participated in an integrated dual-diagnosis intensive outpatient program (9), there was a steady weekly decrease in mean scores for the Beck Anxiety Inventory, Beck Depression Inventory, and Addiction Severity Index from baseline to week 4. The mean rating of both Beck Anxiety Inventory and Beck Depression Inventory scores declined from "moderate" to "mild" by week 4, and the mean Addiction Severity Index scored was 58% lower at week 4 than at baseline (9). More studies have been evaluating group interventions for patients with co-occurring psychotic disorders and SUDs. A review of 36 studies assessing group interventions for that population concluded that the most encouraging interventions include the following features: assertive outreach, integration within the treatment setting, motivational interviewing (MI) for substance abuse, and follow-up longer than one year to attain clinically significant reductions in substance use over time (61). Short-term results from a randomized controlled trial among people with psychotic disorders, which used group motivational interviewing and CBT within a harm minimization paradigm over six 90-minute sessions, showed that compared to a control group that received a single hour-long session of education regarding drug use, the motivational interviewing/CBT group intervention condition did significantly better in terms of reductions in global psychopathology, drug use, severity of dependence, in to addition a lower rate of hospitalization at 3 months after intervention (62). Bradley et al. (63) evaluated an open-ended outpatient group intervention (in the context of a service evaluation project with clinicians administered ratings), incorporating the features reported in the previous study (61), consisting of motivational interviewing and CBT, among patients with psychosis and substance use disorders. This group intervention was conducted in a rural setting and with groups led by clinicians from mental health and drug and alcohol services, including coleaders who were not originators of the intervention model. Compared with baseline, the group intervention was associated with significant improvements in substance use, symptomatology, treatment noncompliance, and overall functioning.

Group motivational interviewing in a nonrandomized, but sequentially assigned study showed promising results when added to standard treatment for dually diagnosed psychiatric inpatients, leading to improved treatment outcomes. Of those patients who attended aftercare and who used alcohol or drugs, those who participated in group motivational interviewing were more adherent to treatment sessions, used less alcohol, and engaged in less binge drinking at follow-up compared with those in the control group (64).

The Need for Physician Support Physicians and other addiction professionals who do not provide group therapies can play a significant role in supporting and facilitating patients' participation in groups. First, they can educate, encourage, and persuade patients to participate in groups as part of their overall treatment program. It is helpful for all clinical staff members to give patients a consistent message about the value of groups. The physician can use his or her status as a healer to help the patient make a decision to participate and not underestimate his or her influence, given the power of even brief interventions on drug use behaviors (65). Second, the physician can monitor and discuss the patient's group participation. This task allows the physician to identify and resolve any barriers related to the patient's continued participation, to understand the reasons for poor adherence or early dropout, and to help the patient reengage in group. Third, the physician can collaborate with group therapists about patients' clinical status or problems with adherence. A physician may also see a patient for management of withdrawal, for management of a cooccurring psychiatric disorder, or for medication management. If, during such a visit, the physician learns that the patient is not adhering to the plan to attend or participate actively in group therapy, the physician can facilitate a discussion with the group leader or even hold a joint meeting with the patient and group therapist to try to resolve the problem. Again, the message the patient receives from this collaboration is that the group is an important part of the overall treatment plan and is valued by the physician.

COUNSELOR TRAINING AND SUPERVISION

Counselor Training To provide effective group treatment, it is necessary for counselors or therapists to be familiar with and skillful in addiction treatment and group therapy. It goes without saying that training in these areas is necessary when one is beginning in the field and that ongoing training and supervision help to keep counselors abreast of current developments in the field and enthusiastic about their work.

The knowledge base that one should have to provide competent addiction treatment involves knowledge of the effects of the various drugs of abuse and which drugs are commonly used in combination and their interactions, as well as the medical, psychologic, social, family, and spiritual consequences of addiction. It also is necessary to understand the processes of recovery and relapse and the strategies or tools that can help the recovering person to manage the recovery process. The clinician should be familiar with the Twelve Step self-help approach of AA or NA for addiction recovery and with alternative self-help resources for patients who are not comfortable with Twelve-Step programs. In terms of group counseling or therapy, counselors should have an understanding of counseling theory and experience in counseling individual patients. Such understanding and experience are necessary because situations can arise in any group that requires the group counselor to intervene in a therapeutic way with an individual while continuing to conduct the group. Conducting groups thus involves an additional level of complexity compared with working with individuals, in that the group leader must be able to understand and respond to individual as well as group dynamics or group process issues simultaneously. This ability involves understanding the ongoing process that is a key part of the group experience. "Group process" refers to the attitudes and interaction of the group members and leaders (30). It also is important for the counselor to be familiar with the stages of groups: the beginning, the middle or working stage, and the ending or closing stage. The group leader should be familiar with the kinds of interventions he or she will use most often and how to deal with problem situations that occur most commonly in groups. Basic intervention skills include active listening, clarification and questioning, information giving, summarization, encouraging and supporting, modeling, eliciting feedback, and addressing problems that commonly arise (e.g., a member who dominates the group, resistant members who are reluctant to participate, a member who tries to assume the role of the leader, mutually hostile members, insensitive or destructive feedback, and members who try to challenge the leader).

Counselor Supervision Supervision is a very important, meaningful part of the practice of group treatment, yet it often is overlooked or provided in a less than optimal manner. Generally speaking, it is always a good idea to provide the group counselor with access to someone who has more experience and expertise in the field, to whom the counselor can bring any problems as they emerge. It also is important to communicate that supervision is not primarily about evaluation of the counselor's work, but rather an opportunity for the counselor to air problems, hone his or her skills, and continue to learn.

Counselors in the cocaine collaborative study protocol received ongoing supervision that involved weekly meetings or telephone conversations with their supervisor. The goals of supervision were to ensure that the group sessions conformed to the research protocol and that the best possible clinical treatment was being delivered. Because this study was for comparative research, adherence to the counseling approach was of utmost importance. For this reason, an adherence scale was developed in conjunction with the group drug counseling manual and was used by the supervisors to rate videotaped group sessions. An adherence scale provides specific operational definitions of desired interventions. These definitions make it clear to counselors what interventions should be incorporated into their work and make it easy for supervisors to point out strengths and deficiencies when giving feedback.

Adherence scales associated with a treatment manual can be a useful tool for both research and clinical purposes, in that they allow researchers to assess whether therapists are following the specified treatment manual. They are helpful in showing that treatments can be differentiated from one another and in assessing the extent to which counselors incorporate techniques from other treatments. Moreover, they are useful clinically in training and supervision of a particular model of treatment.

Counselor Satisfaction It is important that counselors feel satisfied with the group approach they are providing and with the clinical environment in which they work. When counselors are dissatisfied, burnout, indifferent treatment, and departures from appropriate counseling behavior often result. Dissatisfied counselors also tend to feel less positive about their work and to express less confidence in their patients' ability to achieve recovery; such feelings can undermine the patients' own perception of their ability to recover.

LIMITATIONS OF GROUP THERAPIES

Although group therapies offer many benefits, they also have some limitations with which the clinician should be familiar. One of the most common is an overemphasis on group treatment at the expense of individual treatment. As part of an ongoing quality improvement effort, one of the authors (D.D.) has met with small focus groups of patients (totaling more than 1,000 over a period of several years) in a broad range of addiction and dual diagnosis inpatient, partial hospital, and outpatient treatment programs to inquire about what they liked and disliked about treatment. Although most patients participating in group treatment were able to articulate benefits of the group, a consistent criticism heard over many years has been a concern that they did not receive any or enough individual therapy. Patients often reported that there were certain types of problems or issues that they would not discuss in group sessions and that they preferred the privacy and confidentiality afforded by an individual counseling or therapy session.

Examples that patients reported of the personal problems difficult to disclose in group sessions included experiences as a victim or perpetrator of violence, sexual abuse, child abuse, some types of deviant behaviors, the presence of certain psychiatric symptoms, and conflicts related to sexual identity or behaviors. Confidentiality issues were cited as another reason for reluctance to disclose personal information in some group sessions. This was particularly true of patients who participated in a group session in which another member was from the same neighborhood or shared mutual friends. Patients who had difficulty with assertiveness or disclosing personal problems reported that it was easy for them to blend into the background in a group. Although this felt "safe," the patients recognized that this feeling led to less than optimal gain from group therapy. Some patients described attending group sessions in which the leader did not control participants who talked too much or who listened poorly to others, or leaders who did not engage quiet members in group discussions. Social anxiety or phobias are common among patients with SUDs (66). Daley and Salloum (67) administered the Davidson Brief Social Phobia questionnaire to 128 outpatients and found that more than one third reported high levels of social anxiety and avoidance behavior. Specifically, patients reported high levels of anxiety about speaking at AA or NA meetings or in a group therapy session. As a result of social anxiety, patients may choose to limit participation in therapy or self-help group discussions, miss group sessions, or drop out prematurely. They often do so without discussing their reasons with a therapist, counselor, or sponsor.

CONCLUSIONS

The research literature and clinical experience suggest a number of points that are important to an understanding of group therapies for SUDs. First, group therapies play a critical role in addiction treatment and should be supported by all clinicians, regardless of whether they actually provide group sessions themselves. Second, different group therapies can be used, depending on a given patient's progress in relation to the stages of change and the treatment context. Third, a combination of group and individual treatment probably is optimal. (This issue is important because group therapy is the primary and often sole modality offered by many addiction treatment programs.) Integrated group interventions appear to be a promising approach for patients with cooccurring psychiatric disorders. Fourth, careful staff training and ongoing supervision appear to enhance the effectiveness of group therapies. Traditional addiction counseling may be very effective, but only when it is supported by good clinical supervision and opportunities for ongoing training. Fifth, patients who participate in group therapies often benefit from pharmacotherapies as well. Considerable research indicates that a combination of behavioral treatments and medications improve treatment outcomes (39,68). Sixth, self-help programs and group therapies are different in their purpose and structure. Group therapies can encourage self-help attendance, provide education, and explore experiences and resistances. Therapy groups are different from self-help programs in that they are designed to explore psychologic, personal, and interpersonal issues in a safe environment in which self-disclosure, self-awareness, and self-change are encouraged and valued. Seventh, treatment personnel must be sensitive to the fact that SUDs are debilitating, chronic, and relapsing in nature and cause many problems for the individual, the family and society. As with other chronic disorders, they require ongoing management. Professional group therapy is one approach to initiating and continuing this process to the maintenance phase of recovery.

REFERENCES

1. National Institute on Drug Abuse, National Institute on Alcohol Abuse and Alcoholism. Request for applications for group therapy for individuals in drug abuse or alcoholism treatment [No. RFA-DA-04-008]. Washington, DC: Department of Health and Human Services, 2003.
2. The Matrix Center. *The neurobehavioral treatment model volume II: group sessions.* Beverly Hills, CA: Matrix Center, 1989.
3. McAuliffe WE, Albert J. *Clean start: an outpatient program for initiating cocaine recovery.* New York: Guilford Press, 1992.
4. Washton AM. Outpatient group therapy at different stages of substance abuse treatment: preparation, initial abstinence, and relapse prevention. In: Brook DW, Spitz HI, eds. *Group psychotherapy of substance abuse.* New York: Haworth Medical Press, 2002:99–1194.
5. Daley DC, Marlatt GA. *Managing your drug or alcohol problem: therapist guide.* San Antonio, TX: The Psychological Corporation, 1997.
6. Schmitz JM, Oswald LM, Jacks SD, et al. Relapse prevention treatment for cocaine dependence: group vs. individual format. *Addict Behav* 1997;22(3):405–418.
7. Washton AM. Group therapy for substance abuse: a clinician's guide to doing what works. In: Coombs R, ed. *Addiction recovery tools.* Thousand Oaks, CA: Sage Publications, 2001:239–256.
8. Reilly PM, Shropshire MS. Anger management group treatment for cocaine dependence: preliminary outcomes. *Am J Drug Alcohol Abuse* 2000;26(2):161–177.
9. Daley DC, Thase ME. *Dual disorders recovery counseling: integrated treatment for substance use and mental health disorders.* Independence, MO: Herald House/Independence Press, 2000.

10. Daley DC, Moss HB. *Dual disorders: counseling clients with chemical dependency and mental illness*, 3rd ed. Center City, MN: Hazelden, 2002.
11. Najavits LM, Weiss RD, Liese BS. Group cognitive-behavioral therapy for women with PTSD and substance use disorder. *J Subst Abuse Treatment* 1995;13(1):13–22.
12. Rosenthal RN. Group treatments for schizophrenic substance abusers. In: Brook DW, Spitz HI, eds. *The group psychotherapy of substance abuse*. New York: The Haworth Press, Inc., 2002.
13. Covington SS. *A woman's journal*. San Francisco, CA: Jossey- Bass Publishers, 1999.
14. Monti PM, Abrams DB, Kadden RM, et al. *Treating alcohol dependence*. New York: Guilford Press, 1989.
15. Yalom ID, Bloch S, Bond G, et al. Alcoholics in interactional group therapy: an outcome study. *Arch Gen Psychiatry* 1978;35:419–425.
16. Peters RH, Hills HA. Community treatment and supervision strategies for offenders with co-occurring disorders: what works? In: Latessa E, ed. *Strategic solutions: the international community corrections association examines substance abuse*. Lanham, MD: American Correctional Association, 1999:81–137.
17. Gorski TT, Kelly JM. *Counselor's manual for relapse prevention with chemically dependent criminal offenders*. Rockville, MD: Substance Abuse and Mental Health Services Administration, 1996.
18. Roffman RA, Stephens RS, Simpson EE. Relapse prevention with adult chronic marijuana smokers. In: DC Daley, ed. *Relapse: conceptual, research and clinical perspectives*. Binghamton, NY: Haworth Press, 1988:241–257.
19. Gottheil E, Weinstein SP, Sterling RC, et al. A randomized controlled study of the effectiveness of intensive outpatient treatment for cocaine dependence. *Psychiatr Serv* 1998;49(6):782–787.
20. Malik R, Washton AM, Stone-Washton N. Structured outpatient treatment. In: Washton AM, ed. *Psychotherapy and substance abuse: a practitioner's handbook*. New York: Guilford Press, 1995:285–294.
21. Obert JL, McCann MJ, Marinelli-Casey P, et al. The matrix model of outpatient stimulant abuse treatment: history and description. *J Psychoactive Drugs* 2000;32(2):157–164.
22. National Institute on Drug Abuse (NIDA). *Addict aftercare: recovery training and self-help, 2nd ed*. Rockville, MD: NIDA, 1994.
23. Vannicelli M. Group psychotherapy with substance abusers and family members. In: Washton AM, ed. *Psychotherapy and substance abuse: a practitioner's handbook*. New York: Guilford Press, 1995:337–356.
24. Yalom ID. *The theory and practice of group psychotherapy*. New York: Basic Books, 1985.
25. Flores PJ. *Group psychotherapy with addicted populations*. New York: Haworth Press, 1988.
26. Daley DC, Mercer D, Carpenter G. *Group drug counseling manual*. Holmes Beach, FL: Learning Publications, Inc., 1998.
27. Washton AM. Structured outpatient group treatment. In: Lowinson JH, Ruiz P, Millman RB, et al., eds. *Substance abuse: a comprehensive textbook, 3rd ed*. Baltimore, MD: Williams & Wilkins, 1997:440–447.
28. Crits-Christoph P, Siqueland L, Blaine J, et al. The National Institute on Drug Abuse Collaborative Cocaine Treatment Study: rationale and methods. *Arch Gen Psychiatry* 1997;54:721–726.
29. Khantzian EJ, Halliday KS, McAuliffe WE. *Addiction and the vulnerable self: modified dynamic group therapy for substance abusers*. New York: Guilford Press, 1990.
30. Daley DC, Mercer D,& Carpenter G. *Group drug counseling manual*. Holmes Beach, FL: Learning Publications, Inc., 1998.
31. Stinchfield R, Owen PL, Winters KC. Group therapy for substance abuse: a review of the empirical research. In: Fuhriman A, Burlingame G, eds. *Handbook of group psychotherapy: an empirical and clinical synthesis*. New York: Wiley, 1994:458–488.
32. Rawson RA, Shoptaw SJ, Obert JL, et al. An intensive outpatient approach for cocaine abuse treatment. *J Subst Abuse Treatment* 1995; 12(2):117–127.
33. Daley DC, Mercer D, Carpenter G. *Group drug counseling participant recovery workbook*. Holmes Beach, FL: Learning Publications, Inc., 1998.
34. American Psychiatric Association. *Diagnostic and statistical manual of mental disorders, 4th ed. (DSM-IV)*. Washington, DC: American Psychiatric Press, 1994.
35. Anderson CM, Reiss DJ, Hogarty GE. *Schizophrenia and the family*. New York: Guilford Press, 1986.
36. Daley DC, Bowler K, Cahalane H. Approaches to patient and family education with affective disorders. *Pat Ed Counsel* 1992;19:163–174.
37. Washton AM, ed. *Psychotherapy and substance abuse: a practitioner's handbook*. New York: Guilford Press, 1995.
38. Stanton M. Relapse prevention needs more emphasis on interpersonal factors. *Am Psychol* 2005;60(4):340–341.
39. National Institute on Alcohol Abuse and Alcoholism (NIAAA). Highlights from the 10th Special Report to Congress. *Alcohol Res Health* 2000;24(1).
40. National Institute on Drug Abuse (NIDA). *Principles of drug addiction treatment: a research-based guide*. Rockville, MD: NIDA, 1999.
41. Weiss RD, Jaffee WB, de Menil VP, et al. Group therapy for substance use disorders: what do we know? *Harv Rev Psychiatry* 2004;12:339–350.
42. Hien DA, Cohen LR, Miele GM, et al. Promising treatments for women with comorbid PTSD and substance use disorders. *Am J Psychiatry* 2004;161:1425–1432.
43. Killeen T, Brady K. Parental stress and child behavioral outcomes following substance abuse residential treatment: follow-up at 6 and 12 months. *J Subst Abuse Treatment* 2000;19(1):23–29.
44. Greenfield SF, Brooks AJ, Gordon SM, et al. Substance abuse treatment, entry, retention, and outcome in women: a review of the literature. *Drug Alcohol Depend* 2007;86:1–21.
45. Greenfield SF, Trucco EM, McHugh RK, et al. The Women's Recovery Group Study: a stage I trial of women-focused group therapy for substance use disorders versus mixed-gender group drug counseling. *Drug Alcohol Depend* 2007;90:39–47.
46. Najavits LM, Rosier M, Nolan AL, et al. A new gender-based model for women's recovery from substance use disorder: results of a pilot outcome study. *Am J Drug Alcohol Abuse* 2007;33(1):5–11.
47. McLellan AT, Lewis DC, O'Brien CP, et al. Drug dependence, a chronic medical illness: implications for treatment, insurance, and outcomes evaluation. *JAMA* 2000;284(13):1689–1695.
48. Daley DC, Zuckoff A. *Improving treatment compliance: counseling and system strategies for substance use and dual disorders*. Center City, MN: Hazelden, 1999.
49. Hellerstein DJ, Rosenthal RN, Miner CR. A prospective study of integrated outpatient treatment for substance-abusing schizophrenic patients. *Am J Addict* 1995;4:33–42.
50. Robins LN, Regier DA. *Psychiatric disorders in America*. New York: Free Press, 1991.
51. Kessler RC, McGonagle KA, Zhao S, et al. Lifetime and 12-month prevalence of DSM-IIIR psychiatric disorders in the United States. Results from the National Comorbidity Survey. *Arch Gen Psychiatry* 1994;41:8–19.
52. O'Connell D, Beyer E, eds. *Managing the dually diagnosed patient, 2nd ed*. New York: Haworth Press, 2002.
53. Minkoff K, Drake RE. *Dual diagnosis of major mental illness and substance disorder*. San Francisco, CA: Jossey-Bass, 1991.
54. Montrose K, Daley D. *Celebrating small victories: a primer of approaches and attitudes for helping clients with dual disorders*. Center City, MN: Hazelden, 1995.
55. Najavits LM, Weiss RD, Shaw SR, et al. A clinical profile of women with posttraumatic stress disorder and substance dependence. *Psychol Addict Behav* 1998;13(2):98–104.
56. Najavits LM, Weiss RD. "Seeking safety" outcome of a new cognitive-behavioral psychotherapy for women with posttraumatic stress disorder and substance dependence. *J Traum Stress* 1998;11:437–456.
57. Eaton CJ, Mandel DL, Hinkele KA, et al. A cognitive behavioral therapy for alcohol-dependent domestic violence offenders: an integrated substance abuse-domestic violence treatment approach (SADV). *Am J Addict* 2007;16(1):24–31.

58. Weiss RD, Griffin ML, Greenfield SF, et al. Group therapy for patients with bipolar disorder and substance dependence: results from a pilot study. *J Clin Psychiatry* 2000;61:361–367.
59. Weiss RD, Griffin ML, Kolodziej ME, et al. A randomized trial of integrated group therapy versus group drug counseling for patients with bipolar disorders and substance dependence. *Am J Psychiatry* 2007; 164:100–107.
60. Daley DC, Mercer D, Carpenter G. *Group drug counseling for cocaine dependence. Therapy manuals for addiction, manual 4.* Bethesda, MD: National Institute on Drug Abuse, 2002.
61. Drake R, Mercer-McFadden C, Mueser KT. Review of integrated mental health and substance abuse treatment for patients with dual diagnosis. *Schiz Bull* 1998;24:589–608.
62. James W, Preston NJ, Koh G, et al. A group intervention which assists patients with dual diagnosis reduces their drug use: a randomized controlled trial. *Psychol Med* 2004;34:983–990.
63. Bradley AC, Baker A, Lewin TJ. Group intervention for co-existing psychosis and substance use disorders in rural Australia: outcomes over 3 years. *Aust N Z J Psychiatry* 2007;41(6):501–508.
64. Santa Ana EJ, Wulfert E, Nietert PJ. Efficacy of group motivational interviewing for psychiatric inpatients with chemical dependence. *J Consult Clin Psychol* 2007;75(5):816–822.
65. Fleming MF, Mundt MP, French MT, et al. Brief physician advice for problem drinkers: long-term efficacy and benefit cost-analysis. *Alcohol Clin Exp Res* 2002;26(1):36–43.
66. Myrick H, Brady KT. Social phobia in cocaine-dependent individuals. *Am J Addict* 1997;6(2):99–104.
67. Daley DC, Salloum IM. *Social anxiety among dual diagnosis outpatients.* Unpublished data, 1996.
68. National Institute on Drug Abuse (NIDA). Study sheds new light on the state of drug abuse treatment nationwide. *NIDA Notes* 1997;12 (5):1–8.

CHAPTER 56

Bruce J. Rounsaville, MD
Kathleen M. Carroll, PhD
Sudie E. Back, PhD

Individual Psychotherapy

This chapter focuses on those aspects of individual therapy that are unique to the one-to-one format of treatment delivery. The chapter presents guidelines on individual therapy that are applicable to those dependent on alcohol as well as other drugs. The chapter emphasizes a review of research findings relative to illicit drugs because the extensive literature on psychosocial treatments for patients with alcoholism has been reviewed elsewhere (1–4).

The history of individual psychotherapy for addiction disorders has been one of importation of methods first developed to treat other conditions. Thus, when psychoanalytic and psychodynamic therapies were the predominant modality for treating most mental disorders, published descriptions of the dynamics of substance abuse or of therapeutic strategies arose from using this established general modality to treat the special population of individuals with addictive disorders (5). Similarly, with the development of behavioral techniques, client-centered therapies, and cognitive behavioral treatments, earlier descriptions based on other types of patients were followed by discussions of the special modifications needed to treat addiction disorders.

Psychosocial treatment approaches that have originated with treating addiction disorders, such as Alcoholics Anonymous (AA) and therapeutic communities, have emphasized large- and small-group treatment settings. Although always present as a treatment option, individual psychotherapy has not been the predominant treatment modality for drug abusers since the 1960s, when inpatient Twelve Step–informed milieu therapy, group treatments, methadone maintenance, and therapeutic community approaches came to be the fixtures of addictive disorder treatment programs.

In fact, these newer modalities derived their popularity from the failures of dynamically informed ambulatory individual psychotherapy when it was used as the sole treatment for addictive disorders. There are several reasons why this approach was poorly suited to the needs of addicted patients when it was offered as the sole ambulatory treatment.

First, the lack of emphasis on symptom control and the lack of structure in the therapist's typical stance allowed the patients' continued drug or alcohol use to undermine the treatment. Therapists did not develop methods for addressing patient's needs for coping skills because this removal of symptoms was seen as palliative and likely to result in symptom substitution. As a result, substance use often continued unabated while the treatment focused on underlying dynamics. The major strategy that is now common to all currently practiced psychotherapies for addictive disorders is to place primary emphasis on controlling or reducing drug use, while pursuing other goals only after such use has been at least partly controlled. This means that either the individual therapist uses techniques designed to help the patient stop alcohol or drug use as a central part of the treatment, or the therapy is practiced in the context of a comprehensive treatment program in which other aspects of the treatment curtail the patient's use of alcohol or other drugs (e.g., pharmacotherapy or residential treatment).

A second major misfit between individual dynamic therapy and addiction disorders is its anxiety-arousing nature coupled with the lack of structure provided by the neutral therapist. Because patients with addiction frequently react to increased anxiety or other dysphoric affects by resuming substance use, it is important to introduce anxiety-arousing aspects of treatment only after a strong therapeutic alliance has been developed or within the context of other supportive structures (e.g., an inpatient unit, a strong social support network, or methadone maintenance) that guard against relapse to substance use when the patient experiences heightened anxiety and dysphoria in the context of therapeutic exploration.

Individual psychotherapy has become a resurgent approach since the 1980s, as the limitations of other modalities have become apparent (for example, methadone maintenance without ancillary services) (6,7), and necessary modifications in technique have been made to address the factors underlying earlier failures. A major development in recent years is the growing list of individual psychotherapies for addictive disorders that have demonstrated efficacy in rigorously conducted randomized clinical trials (8–10).

Two key research developments have encouraged renewed interest in individual psychotherapies. The first development was the publication of results of Project MATCH, a landmark multisite clinical trial in which 3 months of treatment with one of three individual psychotherapies—motivational enhancement treatment (11), Twelve-Step facilitation (TSF) (12), and cognitive-behavioral therapy (CBT) (13)—was followed by marked and sustained reductions in alcohol consumption (14,15). To illustrate, in all three conditions, patients, on average, entered treatment drinking more than 80% of days, rapidly reduced their consumption to less than 15% of days, and kept those levels down at follow-up visits over 3 years.

The second development was the growing evidence for the efficacy of brief psychotherapies (1,4,16,17). This approach includes brief advice to nondependent, heavy substance users in medical settings (18,19). There also was mounting evidence for the efficacy of four or fewer sessions of motivational enhancement treatment, one of the three treatments included in Project MATCH.

To encourage more widespread use of efficacious treatments, the National Institute on Drug Abuse (NIDA), the National Institute on Alcohol Abuse and Alcoholism, and the Center for Substance Abuse Treatment disseminated training manuals for many of these treatments, either through the Internet from their Web sites (*www.nida.nih.gov or www.niaaa.nih.gov*) or in a printed format that can be ordered through the National Clearinghouse on Alcohol and Drug Abuse Information (P.O. Box 2345, Rockville, MD 20847).

WHEN IS PSYCHOTHERAPY INDICATED?

Some form of behavioral therapy should be considered as a treatment option for all patients who seek help for a substance use disorder. Treatment seekers represent only about 20% of community members who meet the criteria for current substance use disorders (20), and they are likely to represent the more severe end of the spectrum, as most of those who seek treatment do so only after numerous unsuccessful attempts to stop or reduce drug use on their own (21). The alternatives to psychotherapy are either pharmacologic or structural (as through sequestration from access to drugs and alcohol in a residential setting), and both treatments have limited effectiveness if not combined with psychotherapy or counseling. Removal from the substance-using setting is a useful and, sometimes, necessary part of treatment, but it seldom is sufficient in itself, as demonstrated by the high relapse rates typically seen from residential detoxification programs or incarceration during the year after the patient's return to his or her community (22,23).

Psychotherapy and Pharmacotherapy The most powerful and commonly used pharmacologic approaches to drug abuse are maintenance on an agonist that has an action similar to that of the abused drug (e.g., methadone for opioid addicts or nicotine gum for cigarette smokers), use of an antagonist that blocks the effect of the abused drug (e.g., naltrexone for opioid addicts), the use of an aversive agent that provides a powerful negative reinforcement if the drug is used (e.g., disulfiram for alcohol addicted patients), or the use of agents that reduce the desire to use the substance (e.g., naltrexone and acamprosate for alcohol addicted patients). Although all of these agents are widely used, they seldom are employed without adjunctive psychotherapy, because, for example, naltrexone maintenance alone for opioid dependence is plagued by high rates of premature dropout (24,25), and disulfiram use without adjunctive psychotherapy has not been shown to be superior to placebo (26–28).

In particular, the large body of literature on the effectiveness of methadone maintenance points to the success of methadone maintenance in retaining opioid addicts in treatment and reducing their illicit opioid use and illegal activity (6). However, there is a great deal of variability in success rates across different methadone maintenance programs, which is at least partially the result of wide variations in the provision and quality of psychosocial services (6).

The shortcomings of even powerful pharmacotherapies delivered without psychotherapy were convincingly demonstrated by McLellan et al. at the Philadelphia Veterans Affairs medical center (29). In a 24-week trial, 92 opioid-addicted patients were randomly assigned to receive either methadone maintenance alone, without psychosocial services; methadone maintenance with standard psychosocial services, which included regular individual meetings with a counselor; and enhanced methadone maintenance, which included regular counseling plus access to onsite psychiatric, medical, employment, and family therapy. In terms of drug use and psychosocial outcomes, the best outcomes were seen in the enhanced methadone maintenance condition, with intermediate outcomes for the standard methadone services condition, and poorest outcomes for the methadone alone condition. Although a few patients did reasonably well in the methadone alone condition, 69% had to be transferred out of that condition within 3 months of initiation of the study inception because their substance use did not improve or even worsened or because they experienced significant medical or psychiatric problems that required a more intensive level of care.

The results of this study suggest that, although methadone maintenance alone can be sufficient for a small subgroup of patients, the majority will not benefit from a purely pharmacologic approach, and the best outcomes are associated with higher levels of psychosocial treatments. Even when the principal treatment is seen as pharmacologic, psychotherapeutic interventions are needed to complement the pharmacotherapy by enhancing the motivation to stop substance use by taking the prescribed medications, providing guidance for the use of prescribed medications and management of side effects, maintaining motivation to continue taking the prescribed medications after the patient achieves an initial period of abstinence, providing relationship elements to prevent premature termination, and helping the patient to develop the skills to adjust to a life without drug and alcohol use.

The elements that psychotherapy can offer to complement pharmacologic approaches are likely to be needed even if "perfect" pharmacotherapies become available. This is because the effectiveness of even the most powerful pharmacotherapies is limited by patients' willingness to comply with them, and the strategies found to enhance compliance with pharmacotherapies (monitoring, support, encouragement, education) are inherently psychosocial. Moreover, the provision of a clearly articulated and consistently delivered psychosocial treatment in the context of a primarily pharmacologic treatment is an important strategy for reducing noncompliance and attrition, thereby enhancing outcomes in clinical research and clinical treatment (30).

Moreover, the importance of psychotherapy and psychosocial treatments is reinforced by recognition that the repertoire of pharmacotherapies available for treatment of drug addicts is limited to a handful, with the most effective agents limited in their utility to treatment of opioid dependence (31–34) and alcohol dependence (27,35–38). Effective pharmacotherapies for dependence on cocaine, marijuana, hallucinogens, sedative-hypnotics, and stimulants have not yet been developed, and behavioral therapies remain the principal approaches for the treatment of these classes of drugs (33,39).

Although the foregoing has emphasized the need for psychotherapy to enhance the effectiveness of pharmacotherapy, this section would not be complete without considering the role of pharmacotherapy to enhance the efficacy of psychotherapy. These two treatments have different mechanisms of action and targeted effects that can counteract the weaknesses of either treatment alone. Psychotherapies effect change by psychologic means in psychosocial aspects of drug abuse, such as motivation, coping skills, dysfunctional thoughts, or social relationships. Their weaknesses include limited effects on the physiologic aspects of drug use or withdrawal. Also, the effects of behavioral treatments tend to be delayed, requiring practice, repeated sessions, and a "working through" process. In contrast, the relative strengths of pharmacologic treatments are their rapid actions in reducing immediate or protracted withdrawal symptoms, drug craving, or the rewarding effects of continued drug use. In effect, pharmacotherapies for drug dependence reduce the patients' immediate access to and preoccupation with drugs, freeing the patient to address other concerns such as long-term goals or interpersonal relationships. Dropout from psychotherapy is reduced because drug urges and relapse are mitigated by the effects of the medication. Greater duration of abstinence can further enhance the effects of psychotherapy because substance-related effects on attention and mental acuity are prevented, maximizing new learning that therapy can induce. Because of the complementary actions of psychotherapies and pharmacotherapies, combined treatment has a number of potential advantages. As reviewed later, research evidence on combined treatment is sparse but generally supportive of this approach. Although factors such as cost and patient acceptance can limit use of combined approaches, it is important to note that no studies have shown that combined treatments are less than effective with either psychotherapy or pharmacotherapy alone.

Individual versus Group Therapy If psychotherapy is necessary for at least a substantial number of treatment-seeking drug addicts, when is individual therapy a better choice than other modalities such as family therapy or group therapy? Because group therapy has become the modal format for psychotherapy of drug addicts, evaluation of the role of individual therapy should take the strengths and weaknesses of group therapy as its starting point.

A central advantage of group over individual psychotherapy is economy, which is a major consideration in an era of generally skyrocketing health care costs and increasingly curtailed third-party payments for the treatment of addictive disorders. Groups typically have a minimum of six members and a maximum of two therapists, yielding at least a threefold increase in the number of patients treated per therapist hour. Although the efficacy of group versus individual therapy has only rarely been systematically studied with drug addicts, no evidence is available from other populations that individual psychotherapy yields superior benefits (40).

In addition to the general concept that group therapy can be just as effective as but less expensive than individual therapy (41), there are aspects of group therapy that can be argued to make this modality more effective than individual treatment of drug addicts. For example, given the social stigma attached to having lost control of substance use, the presence of other group members who acknowledge having similar problems can provide comfort. Related to this aspect, other group members who are farther along in their recovery from addiction can act as models to illustrate that attempting to stop drug and alcohol use is not a futile effort. These more experienced group members can offer a wide variety of coping strategies that go beyond the repertoire known even by the most skilled individual therapist. Moreover, group members frequently can act as "buddies" who offer continued support outside of the group sessions in a way that most professional therapists do not.

Finally, the "public" nature of group therapy, with its attendant aspects of confession and forgiveness, coupled with the pressure to publicly confess future slips and transgressions, provides a powerful incentive to avoid relapse. The ability to publicly declare the number of days sober, coupled with the fear of having to publicly admit to "falling off the wagon," are strong forces that push an addict toward recovery. This public affirmation or shaming can be all the more crucial in combating a disorder that is characterized by a failure of internalized mechanisms of control. Drug addicts have been characterized as having poorly functioning internal self-control mechanisms (42,43), and the group process—with many eyes watching—provides a robust source of external control. Moreover, because the group is composed of recovering addicts, members may be better able to detect each other's attempts to conceal relapse or early warning signals for relapse than would an individual therapist who may not have personal experience with an addictive disorder.

Given these strengths of group therapy, what are the advantages of individual therapy that can justify its greater expense? First, a key advantage of individual therapy is that it provides privacy. Although self-help groups such as AA attempt to protect the confidentiality of group members by asking for first names only, and routine group therapy procedures involve instructions to members to keep identities of individuals and the contents of sessions confidential, participation in group therapy always risks a breach in confidentiality, especially in small communities. Although publicly admitting to one's need for help can be a key element of the recovery process, it is a step that is very difficult to take, particularly when the problems associated with substance use have not yet become severe. Public knowledge of drug and alcohol use still can ruin careers and reputations.

Second, the individualized pace of individual therapy allows the therapist more flexibility to address the patient's problems as they arise, whereas group therapy can be out of sync with some members while suiting the needs of the majority. This situation is particularly an issue for open groups that add new members throughout the life of the group, necessitating repetition of many therapeutic elements so as to acquaint new members with the group's history and to address the needs of individuals who have just begun treatment.

Third, from the patient's point of view, individual therapy allows a much higher percentage of therapy time to concentrate on issues that are uniquely relevant to that individual. Members of therapy groups usually have the experience of spending many hours discussing issues that are not problems for them, and the individual tailoring of therapy sessions to fit particular needs ultimately can be more efficient.

Fourth, logistical issues make individual therapy more practical in many settings. Given the decentralization of much mental health service delivery, individual therapy is most feasible for many mental health professionals or medical practitioners who do not have a caseload of addicts large enough to conduct group treatment. If group therapy is to be started with a new group, it can be many weeks before enough members are screened to be entered into a new group, resulting in patients' discouragement and high dropout rates while awaiting the onset of treatment. If group therapy involves rolling admission to an ongoing group, this situation can present formidable obstacles to joining. Also, unless group therapy is offered in the context of a large clinic or practice with many ongoing groups, scheduling can be very difficult for those patients whose employer is not apprised of the need for treatment.

Fifth, the process and structure of individual therapy can confer unique advantages in dealing with some kinds of problems presented by patients. For example, individual therapy can be more conducive to the development of a deepening relationship between the patient and therapist over time, which can allow exploration of relationship elements not possible in group therapy. Alternatively, patients with particular personality disorders, such as borderline or schizoid patients, may be unable to get involved with other group members, as can patients who are so shy that they cannot bring themselves to attend group sessions.

SPECIALIZED KNOWLEDGE NECESSARY FOR THERAPY WITH ADDICTED PATIENTS

This section bases its recommendations on the supposition that most individual psychotherapists who attempt to work with addicts obtained their first psychotherapy experience and training with other groups of patients, such as those typically seen at inpatient or outpatient general psychiatric clinics. This supposition is based on the status of addiction treatment as a subspecialty placement within training programs for the major professions that practice psychotherapy, including psychologists, psychiatrists, and social workers. Thus, to treat addicts, the task for the typical psychotherapist is to acquire necessary new knowledge and modify already learned skills.

Pharmacology, Use Patterns, Consequences, and Course of Addiction The principal areas of knowledge to be mastered by the beginning therapist are pharmacology, use patterns, consequences, and course of addiction for the major types of abused substances. For therapy to be effective, it is useful not only to obtain the textbook knowledge about frequently abused drugs but also to become familiar with street knowledge about drugs (e.g., slang names, favored routes of administration, prices, and availability) and the clinical presentation of individuals when they are intoxicated or experiencing withdrawal from the various abused drugs. This knowledge has many important uses in the course of individual therapy.

First, it fosters a therapeutic alliance by allowing the therapist to convey an understanding of the addict's problems and the world in which the addict lives. This issue is especially important when the therapist is from a different racial or social background from the patient. In engaging the patient in treatment, it is important to emphasize that the patient's primary presenting complaint is likely to be substance abuse, even if many other issues also are amenable to psychotherapeutic interventions. Hence, if the therapist is not comfortable and familiar with the nuances of problematic drug and alcohol use, it can be difficult to forge an initial working alliance. Moreover, by knowing the natural history of addiction and the course of drug and alcohol effects, the clinician can be guided in helping the patient anticipate problems that will arise in the course of initiating abstinence. For example, knowing the typical type and duration of withdrawal symptoms can help the addict recognize their transient nature and develop a plan for successfully completing an ambulatory detoxification.

Second, knowledge of drug actions and withdrawal states is crucial for diagnosing comorbid psychopathology and for helping the addict to understand and manage dysphoric affects. It has been observed in clinical situations and demonstrated in laboratory conditions (44–46) that most abused drugs, such as opioids or cocaine, are capable of producing constellations of symptoms that mimic psychiatric syndromes, such as depression, mania, anxiety disorders, or paranoia. Many of these symptomatic states are completely substance-induced and resolve spontaneously when such use is stopped. It often is the therapist's job to determine whether or not presenting symptoms are part of an enduring, underlying psychiatric condition or a transient, drug-induced state. If the former, then simultaneous treatment of the psychiatric disorder is appropriate; if the latter, reassurance and encouragement to maintain abstinence usually are the better course.

This need to distinguish transient substance-induced affects from enduring attitudes and traits also is an important psychotherapy task. Affective states have been shown to be linked closely with cognitive distortions, as Beck et al. (47) have demonstrated in their delineation of the cognitive distortions associated with depression. While experiencing depressive symptoms, a patient is likely to have a profoundly different view of himself or herself, the future, the satisfactions available in life, and his or her important interpersonal relationships. These views are likely to change radically with remission of depressive symptoms, even if the remission of symptoms is induced by pharmacotherapy and not by psychotherapy or actual improvement in life circumstances (48,49). Because of this tendency for substance-related affective states to greatly color the patient's view of self and world, it is important for the therapist to be able to recognize these states so that the associated distorted thoughts can be recognized as such rather than being taken at face value. Moreover, it is important that the patient also be taught to distinguish between sober and substance-affected conditions and to recognize when, in the colloquial phrase, it is "the alcohol talking" and not the person's more enduring sentiments.

Third, learning about drug and alcohol effects is important in detecting when patients have relapsed or come to sessions intoxicated. It is very rarely useful to conduct psychotherapy sessions when the patient is intoxicated and, when this happens, the session should be rescheduled for a time when the patient can participate while sober. For patients with alcoholism, noticing the smell of alcohol or using a Breathalyzer is a useful technique for detecting intoxication. A number of inexpensive and rapid urine tests are commercially available that can be used in the office to detect recent drug use. Samples also can be sent to commercial laboratories for verification. The clinician then must rely on his or her own clinical skills to determine whether or not the patient is drug free and able to participate fully in the psychotherapy.

Other Treatment and Self-Help Group Philosophies and Techniques A second area of knowledge to be mastered by the psychotherapist is an overview of treatment philosophies and techniques for the range of treatments and self-help groups that are available to substance-using patients. As noted previously, the early experience of attempting individual psychotherapy as the sole treatment of the more severe types of drug addiction was marked by failure and early dropout. Hence, for many addicts, individual psychotherapy is best conceived as a component of a multifaceted program of treatment to help the patient overcome a chronic, relapsing condition. In fact, one function of individual psychotherapy can be to help the patient choose which additional therapies to employ in his or her attempt to stop using alcohol or other drugs. Thus, even when the therapist is a solo practitioner, he or she should know when detoxification is necessary, when inpatient treatment is appropriate, and what pharmacotherapies are available.

Another major function of knowing about the major alternative treatment modalities for addicts is to be alert to the possibility that different treatments can provide contradictory recommendations that may confuse the patient or foster the patient's attempts to sabotage treatment. Unlike a practitioner whose treatment is likely to be sufficient in itself, the individual psychotherapist does not have the option of simply instructing the patient to curtail other treatments or participation in self-help groups while individual treatment is taking place. Rather, it is vital that the therapist attempt to adjust his or her own work to bring the psychotherapy into accord with other treatments.

A commonly occurring set of conflicts arises between the treatment goals and methods employed by professional therapists and those of Twelve Step self-help movements such as AA, Cocaine Anonymous (CA), and Narcotics Anonymous. For example, the recovery goal for many who use a Twelve Step approach is a life of complete abstinence from psychotropic medications. This approach may conflict with professional advice when the therapist recommends use of psychopharmacologic treatments for co-occurring psychiatric disorders such as depression, mania, or anxiety. Although the Twelve Step literature supports use of appropriately prescribed medications of all kinds, many individual members draw the line at prescribed psychotropic medications. In the face of disapproval from fellow members, patients may prematurely discontinue psychotropic medications and experience relapse of psychologic symptoms, with consequent return to substance use.

To avoid this situation, it is important for the therapist who recommends or prescribes psychotropic medications to warn the patient about the apparent contradiction between the Twelve Step admonition to lead a drug-free life and the clinician's use of prescribed psychotropic medications. One way to approach this issue is to describe the psychiatric condition for which the medications are prescribed as a disease separate from the addictive disorder and to impress on the patient that medications are as necessary for the treatment of this separate condition as insulin would be for diabetes. That the medications are intended to affect brain functioning and attendant mental symptoms, whereas insulin affects other parts of the body, is less important than the concept that two diseases are present and not one.

A second common area of conflict between some forms of psychotherapy and the Twelve Step philosophy is the role played by family members. The Al-Anon approach tends to suggest that family members get out of the business of attempting to control the addict's use of drugs and alcohol. Separate meetings are held for family members and addicts. In contrast, many therapists encourage involvement of family members in dealing with family dynamics that can foster substance use or in acting as adjunctive therapists (50). As with the use of psychotropic medications, the major way to prevent a patient's confusion is to anticipate the areas of contradictory advice and to provide a convincing rationale for the therapist's recommendations. In doing so, it is advisable to acknowledge that different strategies appear to work for different individuals and that alternative approaches may be employed sequentially if the initial plan fails.

COMMON ISSUES AND STRATEGIES

This section reviews issues that must be addressed, if not emphasized, for individual psychotherapy to be effective. As noted in reviewing the difficulties encountered by early psychodynamic practitioners, the central modification that is required of psychotherapists is to be aware that the patient being treated is an addict. Hence, even when attempting to explore other issues in depth, the therapist should devote at least a small part of every session to monitoring the patient's most recent successes and failures in controlling or curtailing substance use and be willing to interrupt other work to address slips and relapses as they occur.

Implicit in the need to remain focused on the patient's substance use is the recognition that psychotherapy with these patients entails a more active therapist stance than does treatment of patients with other psychiatric disorders, such as depression or anxiety. This need is related to the fact that the principal symptom of substance abuse—compulsive use—is at least initially gratifying, whereas it is the long-term consequences of substance use that induce pain and the desire to stop. In contrast, the principal symptoms of depression or anxiety disorders are inherently painful and alien. Because of this key difference, psychotherapy with addicts typically requires both empathy and structured limit-setting, whereas the need for limit-setting is less marked in psychotherapy with depressed or anxious patients.

Beyond these key elements, this section also elaborates on the following set of psychotherapy tasks: enhancing motivation to stop drug use, teaching coping skills, changing reinforcement contingencies, fostering management of painful affects, improving interpersonal functioning, and enhancing social supports. Although different schools of thought about therapeutic action and behavior change can vary in the degree to which emphasis is placed on the various tasks, some attention to each area is likely to be part of any successful treatment.

Enhancing Motivation Addicts often enter treatment not with the goal to stop, but rather to return to the days when drug and alcohol use was enjoyable (51). The natural history of substance abuse (21,23,52,53) typically is characterized by an initial period of episodic use lasting months to years in which substance-related consequences are minimal and use is perceived as beneficial. Even at the time of treatment-seeking, which usually occurs only after substance-related problems have become severe, patients usually can identify many ways in which they want or feel the need for drugs or alcohol and have difficulty developing a clear picture of what life without these substances might be like. To be able to achieve and maintain abstinence or controlled use, such patients need a clear conception of their treatment goals. Several investigators (54,55) have postulated stages in the development of addicts' thinking about stopping use, beginning with precontemplation, moving through contemplation, and culminating with determination as the ideal cognitive set with which to derive the greatest benefit from treatment.

Regardless of the treatment type, an early task for psychotherapists is to gauge the patient's level of motivation to stop his or her substance use by exploring the patient's treatment goals. In this task, it is important to challenge overly quick or glib assertions that the patient's goal is to stop using substance altogether. One way to approach the patient's likely ambivalence is to attempt an exploration of the patient's perceived benefits from use of alcohol or drugs, or his or her perceived need for them. To obtain a clear report of the patient's positive attitudes toward substance use, it may be necessary to elicit details of the patient's early involvement with drugs and alcohol. After the therapist has obtained a clear picture of the patient's perceived needs and desires, it is important to counter these perceptions by exploring the advantages of a drug-free life.

As noted earlier, although virtually all types of psychotherapy for addiction addresses the issue of motivation and goal-setting to some extent, motivational therapy or interviewing (56) makes this the sole initial focus of treatment. Motivational approaches, which usually are quite brief (e.g., two to four sessions) are based on principles of motivational psychology and are designed to produce rapid, internally motivated change by seeking to maximize patients' motivational resources and commitment to abstinence. Active ingredients of these approaches are hypothesized to include objective feedback of personal risk or impairment, emphasis on personal responsibility for change, clear advice to change, a menu of alternative change options, therapist empathy, and facilitation of patient self-efficacy (11,57). Motivational approaches have substantial empirical evidence supporting their effectiveness with alcohol-addicted patients (1,4,17), but have comparatively recently been evaluated for drug-abusing populations (58–61).

One major controversy in this area is whether controlled use can be an acceptable alternative treatment goal to abstinence from all psychoactive drugs. Many, if not most, patients enter treatment with a goal of controlled use, especially of alcohol (62), and failure to address the patient's presenting goal may result in failure to engage the patient. At the heart of the issue is whether or not drug abuse is seen as a categorical disease, for which the only treatment is abstinence, or as a set of habitual dysfunctional behaviors that are aligned along a continuum of severity (63,64). For illicit drugs of abuse (such as cocaine or heroin), it is unwise for a clinician to take a position that advocates any continued use, because such a stance allies the therapist with illegal and antisocial behavior. Even advocates of controlled use as an acceptable treatment goal usually acknowledge that patients with more severe dependence should seek an abstinence goal. In practice, the therapist cannot force the patient to seek any goal that the patient does not choose. The process of arriving at an appropriate treatment goal frequently involves allowing the patient to make several failed attempts to achieve a goal of controlled use. This initial process may be necessary to convince the patient that a goal of abstinence is more appropriate.

Teaching Coping Skills The most enduring challenge in treating patients with addiction is to help the patient avoid relapse after achieving an initial period of abstinence (65). A general tactic for avoiding relapse is to identify specific circumstances that increase an individual's likelihood of resuming substance use and to help the patient anticipate and practice strategies (e.g., refusal skills, recognizing and avoiding cues for craving) for coping with these high-risk situations. Approaches that emphasize the development of coping skills include CBT (13,65–67), in which a systematic effort is made to identify high-risk situations and master alternative behaviors, as well as coping skills intended to help the patient avoid drug use when these situations arise. A postulate of this approach is that proficiency in coping skills that are generalizable to a variety of problem areas will help foster durable change. Evidence is emerging that points to the durability and in some cases the delayed emergence of effects of coping skills treatments (68–72). For other approaches, enumeration of risky situations and development of coping skills is less structured (73,74) and embedded in a more general exploration of patients' wishes and fears.

Changing Reinforcement Contingencies Edwards et al. (64,75) have noted that a key element of deepening dependence on alcohol or other drugs is the rise of substance-related behavior to the top of an individual's list of priorities. As dependence deepens, it can take precedence over concerns about work, family, friends, possessions, and health. As compulsive use becomes a part of every day, previously valued relationships or activities may be given up, so that the rewards available in daily life are narrowed progressively to those derived from use of the substance. When such use is ended, its absence may leave the patient with a need to fill the time that had been spent using drugs or alcohol and to find rewards to substitute for those derived from their use.

The ease with which the patient can rearrange priorities is related to the level of achievement before he or she became involved with alcohol or drugs and the degree to which substance use destroyed or replaced valued relationships, jobs, or hobbies. Because the typical course of illicit drug use entails initiation of compulsive use between the ages of 12 and 25 years (76,77), many patients come to treatment without having achieved satisfactory adult relationships or vocational skills. In such cases, achieving a drug- and alcohol-free life may require a lengthy process of vocational rehabilitation and development of meaningful relationships. Individual psychotherapy can contribute importantly to this process by helping maintain the patient's motivation throughout the recovery process and by helping the patient to explore factors that have interfered with achievement of rewarding ties to others. An example of an approach that actively changes reinforcement contingencies is the one developed by Higgins et al. (78,79), which incorporates positive incentives for abstinence into a community reinforcement approach (80).

Fostering Management of Painful Affects Marlatt and Gordon (81) demonstrated that dysphoric affects are the most commonly cited precipitant for relapse, and many psychodynamic clinicians (42,43) have suggested that failure of affect regulation is a central dynamic underlying the development of compulsive alcohol or drug use. Moreover, surveys of psychiatric disorders in treatment-seeking and community populations concur in demonstrating high rates of depressive disorders among drug users (82–85).

A key element in developing ways to handle powerful dysphoric affects is learning to recognize and identify the probable cause of such feelings. The difficulty in differentiating among negative emotional states has been identified as a common characteristic among addicted patients (42,43). To foster the development of mastery over dysphoric affects, most psychotherapies include techniques for eliciting strong affects within a protected therapeutic setting and then enhancing the patient's ability to identify, tolerate, and respond appropriately to them. Given the demonstrated efficacy of pharmacologic treatments for affective and anxiety disorders (86) and the high rates of these disorders seen in treatment-seeking populations, the individual psychotherapist should be alert to the possibility that a patient may benefit from combined treatment with psychotherapy and medications.

Moreover, as evidence points to the difficulty many patients face in articulating strong affect (87), which can have an effect of treatment response (88), clinicians should be alert to the need to assess and address difficulties in expression of affect and cognition when working with addicted patients in psychotherapy.

Improving Interpersonal Functioning and Enhancing Social Supports A consistent finding in the literature on relapse is the protective influence of an adequate network of social supports (89,90). Gratifying friendships and intimate relationships provide a powerful source of rewards to replace those obtained from drug and alcohol use, and the threat of losing those relationships can furnish a strong incentive to maintain abstinence. Typical issues presented by addicted patients are the loss of or damage to valued relationships that occurred when alcohol or drug use became the individual's principal priority, failure to have achieved satisfactory relationships even before having initiated substance use, and inability to identify friends or intimates who are not, themselves, engaged in substance abuse. For some types of psychotherapy (such as interpersonal therapy and supportive-expressive treatment), working on relationship issues is the central focus of the work, whereas, for others, this aspect is implied in other therapeutic activities such as identifying risky and protective interpersonal situations (65).

A major potential limitation of individual psychotherapy as the sole treatment for alcohol or drug dependence is its failure to provide adequate social supports to patients who lack a supportive social network of friends who are not engaged in substance abuse. Individual psychotherapy can fill only one to several hours per week of a patient's time.

Again, although most approaches address these issues to some degree in the course of treatment, approaches that emphasize the development of a strong relationship with persons who are not substance users are traditional counseling, TSF (12), and other approaches that underline the importance of involvement in self-help groups. Self-help groups offer a fully developed social network of welcoming individuals who are understanding and committed to leading a substance-free life. Moreover, in most urban and suburban settings, self-help meetings are held daily or several times a week, and a sponsor system is available to provide the recovering person with individual guidance and support on a 24-hour basis, if needed. For psychotherapists who working with addicted patients, encouraging patients to become involved in self-help groups can provide a powerful source of social support that protects the patient from relapse while the work of therapy progresses.

EFFICACY RESEARCH

As noted previously, early efforts to engage and treat drug users with dynamically oriented individual psychotherapy as the sole treatment were marked by failure. These failures led researchers to focus increasingly on the evaluation of psychotherapy as a treatment for addiction in terms of the context in which individual psychotherapy is delivered most effectively as well as the types of patients most likely to benefit from individual psychotherapy. Hence the following section reviews empiric evidence for the effectiveness of individual psychotherapy by substance of abuse and treatment setting. The section reviews findings from the growing number of studies that have used rigorous methodologies associated with the technology model of psychotherapy research (91,92). Akin to specification of the formulation and dosage of medications in pharmacotherapy trials, this approach has generated methods for specifying the techniques to be evaluated, for training therapists to use these techniques consistently, and for monitoring the dose and delivery of these techniques over the course of clinical trials. These methodologic features include random assignment to treatment conditions, specification of treatments in manuals, selection of well-trained therapists committed to the type of approach they conduct in the trial, extensive training of therapists, ongoing monitoring of therapy implementation, multidimensional ratings of outcome by independent evaluators blind to the study treatment received by the patient, and adequate sample sizes.

In this review, the authors have focused on studies of opiate- and cocaine-addicted patients because the more extensive literature on psychosocial treatments of alcohol has received detailed review elsewhere (2,4).

Individual Psychotherapy for Opioid Dependence

Opioid Agonist Therapy Only a few studies have evaluated the efficacy of formal psychotherapy to enhance outcomes with agonist treatments. The landmark study in this area was done by Woody et al. (93) and was also replicated in community settings (94). Although the original study is now nearly 20 years old, it is reviewed here because it remains an impressive demonstration of the benefits and role of psychotherapy in the context of methadone maintenance. In the study, a total of 110 opiate-addicted patients entering a methadone maintenance program were randomly assigned to one of three treatments: drug counseling alone, drug counseling plus supportive-expressive psychotherapy (SE), which is a short-term dynamic approach, or drug counseling plus cognitive psychotherapy, a structured cognitive approach. After a 6-month course of treatment, although the SE and cognitive psychotherapy groups did not differ significantly from each other on most measures of outcome, subjects who received either form of professional psychotherapy evidenced greater improvement in more outcome domains than the subjects who received drug counseling alone (93). Moreover, gains made by the subjects who received professional psychotherapy were sustained over a 12-month follow-up period, whereas subjects who received drug counseling alone evidenced some attrition of gains (95). The study also demonstrated differential responses to psychotherapy as a function of patient characteristics, which can point to the best use of psychotherapy (relative to drug counseling) when resources are scarce: although methadone-maintained opiate-addicted patients with lower levels of psychopathology tended to improve regardless of whether they received professional psychotherapy or drug counseling, those with higher levels of psychopathology tended to improve only if they received psychotherapy.

Contingency Management Several studies have evaluated the use of contingency management to reduce the use of illicit drugs in patients with addiction who are maintained on methadone. In these studies, a reinforcer (reward) is provided to patients who demonstrate specified target behaviors such as providing drug-free urine specimens, accomplishing specific treatment goals, or attending treatment sessions. For example, offering methadone take-home privileges contingent on reduced drug use is an approach that capitalizes on an inexpensive reinforcer that is potentially available in all methadone maintenance programs. Stitzer et al. (96–98) have done extensive work in evaluating methadone take-home privileges as a reward for decreased illicit drug use. In a series of well-controlled trials, these researchers demonstrated the relative benefits of positive (e.g., rewarding desired behaviors such as abstinence) compared with negative (e.g., punishing undesired behaviors such as continued drug use through discharges or dose reductions) contingencies (96), the attractiveness of take-home privileges over other incentives available within methadone maintenance clinics (97), and the relative effectiveness of rewarding drug-free urine specimens compared with other target behaviors (99).

Silverman et al. (100,101), drawing on the compelling work of Higgins et al. (described later), evaluated a voucher-based contingency management system to address concurrent illicit drug use (typically cocaine) among methadone-maintained opioid-addicted patients. In this approach, urine specimens are required three times a week to systematically detect all episodes of drug use. Abstinence, verified through drug-free urine screens, is reinforced through a voucher system in which patients receive points redeemable for items consistent with a drug-free lifestyle that are intended to help the patient develop alternate reinforcers to drug use (e.g., movie tickets and sporting goods). In a very elegant series of studies, Silverman et al. (100,101) have demonstrated the efficacy of this approach in reducing illicit opioid and cocaine use and producing a number of treatment benefits in this very difficult population.

Behavioral Therapies Opioid antagonist treatment (naltrexone) offers many advantages over methadone maintenance, including the fact that it is nonaddicting and can be prescribed without concerns about diversion, has a benign side effect profile, and can be less costly in terms of demands on professional time and of patient time than the daily or near-daily clinic visits required for methadone maintenance (102). Most important are the behavioral aspects of treatment, as unreinforced opiate use allows extinction of relationships between cues and drug use. Although naltrexone treatment is likely to be attractive only to a minority of opioid-addicted patients (31), naltrexone's unique properties make it an important alternative to methadone maintenance and other agonist approaches.

However, naltrexone has not, despite its many advantages, fulfilled its promise. Naltrexone treatment programs remain comparatively rare and underutilized as compared with methadone maintenance programs (102). This situation is largely due to problems with retention, particularly during the induction phase, when an average of 40% of patients drop out during the first month of treatment and 60% drop out by 3 months (31). In the 1970s, several preliminary evaluations of behavioral interventions used to address naltrexone's weaknesses, including providing incentives for compliance with naltrexone (103,104) and the addition of family therapy to naltrexone treatment (105), suggested the promise of these strategies. However, the interventions were not widely adopted, compliance remained a major problem, and naltrexone treatment and research dropped off considerably until the past few years, when the need for alternatives to methadone maintenance stimulated a modest revival of interest in naltrexone.

Some of the most recent promising data about strategies to enhance retention and outcome in naltrexone treatment has come from investigations of contingency management approaches. Preston et al. (106) found improved retention and naltrexone compliance with an approach that provided vouchers for naltrexone compliance, as compared with standard naltrexone treatment that did not provide vouchers. Carroll et al. (107,108) found that reinforcement of naltrexone compliance and drug-free urine specimens, alone or in combination with family involvement in treatment, improved retention and reduced drug use among recently detoxified opioid-dependent individuals.

Individual Psychotherapy for Cocaine Dependence Compared with the results of trials evaluating pharmacologic treatment of cocaine dependence, evaluations of behavioral therapies—particularly contingency management, CBT, and manualized disease-model approaches—have been much more promising (8,109). Because of the lack of an effective pharmacologic platform for cocaine dependence (analogous to methadone maintenance for the treatment of opioid dependence), behavioral therapies for cocaine-dependent individuals have had to focus on key outcomes such as retention and the inception and maintenance of abstinence, rather than placing initial emphasis on secondary psychosocial problems (e.g., family, psychologic, legal problems). Major findings from randomized controlled trials evaluating each of these treatments for adult cocaine-dependent groups are summarized here.

Contingency Management Perhaps the most exciting findings pertaining to the effectiveness of behavioral treatments for cocaine dependence have been the reports by Higgins et al. (79,110–112) on the use of behavioral incentives for abstinence, as described earlier. The strategy of Higgins has four organizing features that are grounded in principles of behavioral pharmacology: 1) drug use and abstinence must be swiftly and accurately detected, 2) abstinence is positively reinforced, 3) drug use results in loss of reinforcement, and 4) emphasis is placed on the development of reinforcers to compete with drug use (78). In this approach, urine specimens are required three times weekly to systematically detect all episodes of drug use. Abstinence, verified through drug-free urine screens, is reinforced through a voucher system in which patients receive points redeemable for items consistent with a drug-free lifestyle (such as movie tickets and sporting goods).

In a series of well-controlled clinical trials, Higgins has demonstrated high acceptance, retention, and rates of abstinence for patients receiving this approach, as compared with standard counseling oriented toward Twelve Step programs (79,110). Rates of abstinence do not decline substantially when less valuable incentives are substituted for the voucher system (110). The value of the voucher system itself, as opposed to other program elements, in producing good outcomes was demonstrated by comparing the behavioral system with and without the vouchers (113). Although the strong effects of this treatment declined somewhat after the contingencies were terminated, the voucher system has been shown to have durable effects (111). Moreover, the efficacy of a variety of contingency management procedures (including vouchers, direct payments, and free housing) have been replicated in other settings and samples, including cocaine-dependent individuals within methadone maintenance (100,101), homeless persons with addiction (114), freebase cocaine users (115), and pregnant drug users (116).

These findings are of great importance because contingency management procedures are potentially applicable to a wide range of target behaviors and problems, including treatment retention and compliance with pharmacotherapy (such as retroviral therapies for individuals with HIV). For example, Iguchi et al. (99) showed that contingency management can be used effectively to reinforce desired treatment goals (e.g., looking for a job) in addition to abstinence.

Nevertheless, despite the very compelling evidence of the effectiveness of these procedures in promoting retention in treatment and reducing cocaine use, the procedures rarely are used in clinical treatment programs. One major impediment to broader use is the expense associated with the voucher program; average earnings for patients are about $600 (79,113,117). Recently developed low-cost contingency management (CM) procedures may be a way to bring these effective approaches into general clinical use. In a recently completed study, Petry et al. (118,119) demonstrated that a variable ratio schedule of reinforcement that provides access to large reinforcers (but at low probabilities) is effective in retaining subjects in treatment and reducing substance use. Rather than earning vouchers, subjects earn the chance to draw from a bowl and win prizes of varying magnitudes. The prizes range from small $1 prizes (bus tokens, McDonald's coupons) to large $20 prizes (portable radios, watches, and phone cards), to jumbo $100 prizes (e.g., small televisions). This system is far less expensive than the standard voucher system, because only a proportion of behaviors are reinforced with a prize. In a study of 42 alcohol-dependent veterans who were randomly assigned to standard treatment or standard treatment plus CM, 84% of the CM subjects were retained in treatment throughout an 8-week period, compared with 22% of standard treatment subjects. By the end of the treatment period, 69% of those receiving CM had not experienced a relapse to alcohol use, but only 39% of those receiving standard treatment were abstinent (119), with similar findings among cocaine abusers (118).

CBTs Another behavioral approach that was shown to be effective in treating cocaine abusers is CBT. This approach is based on social learning theories on the acquisition and maintenance of substance use disorders (120). Its goal is to foster abstinence by helping the patient master an individualized set of coping strategies as an effective alternative to substance use. Typical skills include fostering the patient's resolve to stop using cocaine and other substances by exploring positive and negative consequences of continued use, functional analysis of substance use (i.e., understanding substance use in relationship to its antecedents and consequences), development of strategies for coping with cocaine craving, identification of seemingly irrelevant decisions that could culminate in high-risk situations, preparation for emergencies and coping with a relapse to substance use, and identifying and confronting thoughts about substance use.

A number of randomized clinical trials among several diverse cocaine-dependent populations have demonstrated that compared with other commonly used psychotherapies for cocaine dependence, CBT appears to be particularly more effective with more severe cocaine users or those with comorbid disorders (121–126); CBT is significantly more effective than less intensive approaches that have been evaluated as control conditions (127,128); and CBT is as or more effective than manualized disease-model approaches (124,127). Moreover, CBT appears to be a particularly durable approach, with patients continuing to reduce their cocaine use even after they leave treatment (68–70,72).

Manualized Disease-Model Approaches Until very recently, treatment approaches based on disease models were widely practiced in the United States, but virtually no well-controlled randomized clinical trials had evaluated their efficacy alone or in comparison with other treatments. Thus another important finding emerging from randomized clinical trials that has great significance for the treatment community is the effectiveness of manualized disease-model approaches. One such approach is TSF (12), a manual-guided, individual approach that is intended to be similar to widely used approaches that emphasize principles associated with disease models of addiction and has been adapted for use with cocaine-dependent individuals (129). Although this treatment has no official relationship with AA or CA, its content is intended to be consistent with the Twelve Steps of AA, with primary emphasis given to Steps 1 through 5 and the concepts of acceptance (e.g., to help the patient accept that he or she has the illness, or disease, of addiction) and surrender (e.g., to help the patient acknowledge that there is hope for sobriety through accepting the need for help from others and a "Higher Power"). In addition to abstinence from all psychoactive substances, a major goal of the treatment is to foster active participation in self-help groups. Patients are actively encouraged to attend AA or CA meetings, become involved in traditional fellowship activities, and maintain journals of their self-help group attendance and participation.

In a comparison of TSF, CBT, and clinical management (a supportive approach in which patients received comparable empathy, support, and other "common elements" of psychotherapy but none of the unique "active ingredients" of TSF or CBT) for alcohol- and cocaine-dependent individuals, TSF was found to be significantly more effective than clinical management and was comparable to CBT in reducing cocaine use (127). In addition, a 1-year follow-up suggested that gains from treatment were maintained for subjects who received TSF or CBT, who reported continuing to reduce their cocaine use throughout the follow-up period, compared with subjects who received clinical management. Moreover, there was a strong relationship between the attainment of significant periods of abstinence during treatment and abstinence during follow-up, which emphasizes that the inception of abstinence, even for comparatively brief periods, is an important goal of treatment (68,111).

More recently, the NIDA Collaborative Cocaine Treatment Study, a multisite randomized trial of psychotherapeutic treatments for cocaine dependence (130,131), suggested the effectiveness of a similar approach: individual drug counseling (132). In that study, 487 cocaine-dependent participants in four sites were randomly assigned to one of four manual-guided treatment conditions: cognitive therapy (133) plus group drug counseling; SE therapy, a short-term psychodynamically oriented approach (73) plus group drug counseling; individual drug counseling plus group drug counseling; or group drug counseling alone. The treatments offered were intensive (36 individual and 24 group sessions over 24 weeks, for a total of 60 sessions) and were met with comparatively poor retention, with patients on average completing less than half the sessions offered, with higher rates of retention for subjects assigned to cognitive therapy or SE therapy (130). On the whole, outcomes were good, with all groups significantly reducing their cocaine use from baseline; however, the best cocaine outcomes were seen for subjects who received individual drug counseling (a related point is that this study suggests that psychodynamic and cognitive approaches, which rarely have been studied with this population, may not be optimal initial approaches for general populations of cocaine users) (134).

Considered together with the findings of Project MATCH (14,135), TSF was found to be comparable to CBT and MET in reducing alcohol use among 1,726 alcohol-dependent individuals. The findings from these studies offer compelling support for the efficacy of manual-guided disease-model approaches. This finding has important clinical implications because these approaches are similar to the dominant model applied in most community treatment programs (136) and thus can be more easily mastered by "real-world" clinicians than approaches such as CM or CBT—treatments whose theoretical underpinnings may not be perceived highly compatible with disease-model approaches (although such incompatibility has yet to be demonstrated) (137).

Moreover, it is critical to recognize that the evidence supporting disease-model approaches has emerged from well-conducted clinical trials in which therapists were selected on the basis of their expertise in this approach and were trained and closely supervised so as to foster high levels of adherence and competence in delivering the treatments, and it remains to be seen whether these approaches will be as effective when applied under less-than-ideal conditions. Likewise, these professional, individual approaches should be distinguished from merely referring patients to self-help meetings. It is of note that a large randomized trial that directly compared referral to self-help with professional treatments found poorer outcomes with high rates of treatment utilization for the patients referred to self-help compared with inpatient treatment (138).

Individual Psychotherapy for Marijuana Dependence Although marijuana is the most commonly used illicit substance, treatment of marijuana abuse and dependence is a comparatively understudied area to date, in part because comparatively few individuals present for treatment with a primary complaint of marijuana abuse or dependence. No effective pharmacotherapies for marijuana dependence exist, and only a few controlled trials of behavioral approaches have been completed. Stephens et al. (139,140) compared a delayed-treatment control group with a two-session motivational approach and to an intensive (14-session) relapse prevention approach and found better marijuana outcomes for the two active treatments compared with the delayed-treatment control group, but found no significant differences between the brief and the more intensive treatment. More recently, a replication and extension of that study, involving a multisite trial of 450 marijuana-dependent patients, compared three approaches: 1) a delayed treatment control, 2) a two-session motivational approach, and 3) a nine-session combined motivational/coping skills approach. Results suggested that both active treatments were associated with significantly greater reductions in marijuana use than the delayed treatment control through a 9-month follow-up period (141). Moreover, the nine-session intervention was significantly more effective than the two-session intervention, and this effect also was sustained through the 9-month follow-up period. Budney et al. have extended the application of contingency management to marijuana users, and recently reported that adding voucher-based incentives to coping skills and motivational enhancement improves outcomes during treatment for marijuana dependence (142).

CONCLUSIONS

The empirical evidence reviewed here and the literature on behavioral treatments of alcoholism reviewed elsewhere (2,4) suggest the following.

- To date, most studies suggest that individual psychotherapy is superior to control conditions as a treatment for patients with substance use disorders. This finding is consistent with the bulk of findings from psychotherapy efficacy research in areas other than substance use, which suggests that the effects of many psychotherapies are clinically and statistically significant and are superior to no treatment and placebo conditions.

- No particular type of individual psychotherapy was found to be consistently superior as a treatment for substance use disorders.
- The effects of even comparatively brief psychotherapies appear to be durable among patients with substance use disorders.

Ongoing Development of Innovative Behavioral Therapies Our review of rigorously conducted efficacy research on psychotherapies for substance use disorders provides support for the use of a number of innovative approaches: SE treatment for methadone-maintained opioid-addicted patients, CBT for cocaine and marijuana dependence, and contingency management for a wide range of substance use disorders.

This growing list of empirically validated treatments is attributable, in part, to the behavioral therapies initiative begun in the early 1990s by NIDA (143). That initiative was begun to encourage development and testing of new and improved psychotherapies for persons with addiction disorders. Although strong evidence suggests that addiction treatment works, the field needs better methods, because too few addicts enter treatment, complete treatment, and achieve lasting improvement. Novel treatment ideas can come from any source, but widespread adoption of new methods should be reserved for those treatments with proven efficacy.

The behavioral therapies initiative was instituted to promote the process of moving new treatments from the stage in which they represent "good ideas" to one in which they are shown to be effective, are fully specified in training manuals, and are ready for use in community programs. This process is guided by a new stage model of behavioral therapies research (144), demarcating three divisions in a rigorous scientific process that leads from initial innovation through efficacy research to effectiveness research. Stage I consists of pilot/feasibility testing, manual writing, training program development, and adherence/competence measure development for new and untested treatments. Stage II initially consists of randomized clinical trials (RCTs) to evaluate efficacy of manualized and pilot-tested treatments that have shown promise or efficacy in earlier studies. Stage II research also can address mechanisms of action or effective components of treatment for approaches with evidence of efficacy derived from RCTs. Stage III consists of studies to evaluate transportability of treatments whose efficacy has been demonstrated in at least two RCTs (145,146). Key Stage III research issues revolve around generalizability (i.e., will this treatment maintain effectiveness with different practitioners, patients, and settings?), implementation issues (i.e., what kinds of training by what kinds of trainers are necessary to train what kinds of clinicians to learn a new technique?), cost-effectiveness issues (i.e., compared with the costs of learning and implementing this treatment, what are the savings, particularly in comparison to existing methods?), and consumer/marketing issues (i.e., how acceptable is a new treatment to clinicians, patients, and payers outside of research settings?).

The stage model was developed in an attempt to bridge the gap (147) between research and practice in the treatment of addiction. Although psychotherapies are widely practiced, the types of treatments most widely used have not been shown to be effective in RCTs. Conversely, comparatively few practitioners use the empirically validated treatments listed previously. This gap is attributable, in part, to bottlenecks at Stage I and Stage III.

At the front end, creative clinicians have proffered many new treatments, but few of the originators have had an opportunity to prove their efficacy of their treatments in clinical trials. As a result, many promising, potentially effective treatments have been ignored. By following guidelines for Stage I research (144), clinicians can move their treatments to a stage at which efficacy testing can take place.

Another bottleneck occurs after a treatment is shown to be efficacious in rigorous clinical trials, but before community programs are ready to adopt the new treatments. The role of Stage III research is to answer important questions about a new treatment's effectiveness and cost-effectiveness in real-world settings. In addition to articulating the stage model, NIDA has taken a major role in Stage III research by developing the National Drug Abuse Treatment Clinical Trials Network. The Clinical Trials Network is a network of academically based regional research and training centers that are linked in partnership with clinical treatment programs to provide the infrastructure for large-scale trials to evaluate the effectiveness of promising pharmacologic or behavioral treatments in representative community settings. NIDA's Clinical Trials Network plays a unique role for behavioral treatments. Unlike medication treatments that are distributed for profit by commercial pharmaceutical manufacturers, behavioral treatments have no organizational resources or advocates to promote their dissemination into community practice.

From the preceding summary, it is clear that the empirical literature offers only the most general sort of guidance about the choice of which individual psychotherapy is likely to be useful for a particular patient and when in the course of treatment it should be offered. Hence the following recommendations are made on the basis of clinical experience rather than research evidence. With this caveat, it is suggested that individual psychotherapy may have the following uses: as an initial treatment or an introduction into treatment, to treat patients with low levels of substance dependence, to treat patients who failed in other modalities, to complement other ongoing treatment modalities for selected patients, and to help the patient solidify gains after achievement of stable abstinence (148).

Psychotherapy as Initial Treatment As noted previously, a key advantage of individual therapy is the privacy and confidentiality it affords. This aspect can make individual therapy or counseling an ideal setting in which to clarify the treatment needs of patients who are in early stages (i.e., contemplation, precontemplation) of thinking about changing their patterns of substance use (55). Notably, the growing evidence for the efficacy of brief (two to four sessions) motivational interviewing approaches suggests that this can be sufficient for certain patients (149). For individuals with severe dependence who deny the seriousness of their involvement, a course of individual therapy in which the patient is guided to a clear recognition of the problem can be an essential first step toward more intensive approaches such as residential treatment or methadone maintenance. An important part of this process may involve allowing the patient to fail one or more times at strategies that have a low probability of success, such as attempting to cut down on substance use without stopping or attempting outpatient detoxification.

A general principle underlying this process is the successive use of treatments that involve greater expense or patient involvement only after less intensive approaches have been shown to fail. Hence brief individual treatment may be sufficient alone or may serve a cost-effective triage function.

Psychotherapy for Patients with Mild to Moderately Severe Substance Dependence Although less studied with non alcohol-using drug abusers, the drug-dependence syndrome concept (75) has received considerable attention in the study of alcoholism. This concept, first described by Edwards and Gross (64), suggests that drug dependence is best understood as a constellation of cognitions, behaviors, and physical symptoms that underlie a pattern of progressively diminished control over drug use. This dependence syndrome is conceived to be aligned along a continuum of severity, with higher levels of severity associated with poorer prognosis and the need for more intensive treatment, and lower levels of severity requiring less intensive interventions. The dependence syndrome construct has generated a large empiric literature, suggesting its validity with alcohol-addicted patients (63). Moreover, several scales have been developed for gauging the severity of alcohol dependence (150). Generally, measures of quantity and frequency of alcohol use show a high correlation with dependence severity, and similar quantity/frequency indices for other drugs of abuse can be an adequate gauge of dependence severity. Evidence from studies of individuals who are mildly to moderately dependent on alcohol has indicated that a brief course of psychotherapy is sufficient for many to achieve substantial reductions in or abstinence from drinking (1,4,16,17). Although these findings have yet to be replicated with other types of substance use disorders, they are likely to be generalizable.

Psychotherapy for Patients Who Failed in Other Therapies Although numerous predictors of outcomes for addiction treatment have been identified (151), only a few are robust and still fewer have been evaluated in terms of the issue of matching patients to treatments (152). As a result, the choice of treatment often involves a degree of trial and error. Each type of treatment has its strengths and weaknesses, which can result in a better or worse "fit" for a particular patient. For example, individual therapy is more expensive but more private than group therapy, more enduring and less disruptive to normal routine than residential treatment, and less troubled by side effects and medical contraindications than pharmacotherapies. Each of these advantages may be crucial to a patient who has responded poorly to other therapeutic approaches.

Psychotherapy as Ancillary Treatment In considering psychotherapy as part of an ongoing comprehensive program of treatment, it is useful to distinguish between treatment of patients with alcoholism and opioid-addicted patients, for which powerful pharmacologic approaches are available, and treatment of other drugs of abuse, for which strong alternatives to behavioral approaches are not yet available (33,39). For patients with alcoholism, naltrexone, acamprosate, and disulfiram have strong potential for improving treatment outcome and reducing relapse rates. However, the effectiveness of disulfiram in the absence of a strong psychosocial treatment was no greater than placebo (27), and most studies demonstrating the efficacy of naltrexone and acamprosate have been done in the context of a comparatively intense psychosocial intervention (36–38,71,153,154). For opioid-dependent patients, the modal treatment approach remains methadone maintenance, which is used with the majority of those in treatment, whereas an alternative pharmacotherapy, naltrexone, can be highly potent for the minority who choose this approach. Because of their powerful and specific pharmacologic effects, either to satisfy the need for opioids or to prevent illicit opioids from yielding their desired effect, these agents—provided that they are delivered with at least minimal counseling—can be sufficient for many opioid addicts (29). The choice of those who might benefit from additional individual psychotherapy may be guided by the unique but robust empiric findings of Woody et al. (155,156) and McLellan (157,158), which suggest that psychotherapy is most likely to be of benefit to those opioid addicts with higher levels of psychiatric symptoms. Because the benefits of psychotherapy can be maximized when instituted relatively soon after the patient enters treatment, assessment instruments such as the ASI (159) can be used to quickly identify those with psychopathology or depression, alerting staff to the need to refer the client for psychotherapy.

For nonopioid drugs of abuse, an active search for effective pharmacotherapies is under way. In the interim, the mainstay of treatment for such patients remains some form of psychosocial treatment offered in a group, family, residential, or individual setting. For cocaine use, forms of treatment that currently have the strongest levels of empirical support for general groups of cocaine users include contingency management and cognitive behavioral therapy. However, there is as yet no strong empirical evidence as to the optimal duration of treatment, nor are there clear guidelines for matching patients to treatment.

For other types of drug abuse, in the absence of empirically validated guidelines, the choice of individual psychotherapy can be based on such factors as expense, logistical considerations, patient preference, or the clinical fit between the patient's presenting picture and the treatment modality (e.g., family therapy is ruled out for those without families).

Psychotherapy after Achievement of Sustained Abstinence As noted earlier, an individual who experiences frequent relapses or who is only tenuously holding onto abstinence can be a poor candidate for certain types of psychotherapy, particularly those that involve bringing into focus painful and anxiety-provoking clinical material as an inevitable part of helping the patient to master his or her dysphoric affects or avoid recurrent failures in establishing enduring intimate relationships. In fact, some arousal of anxiety or frustration may occur with most types of psychotherapy, even those that are conceived as being primarily supportive. Because of this situation, individual psychotherapy may be effective for many individuals only after they have achieved abstinence through some other treatment approach, such as residential treatment, methadone maintenance, or group therapy. Given the vulnerability of these patients to relapse (which can extend over a lifetime), and the frequency with which dysphoric affects or interpersonal conflict are noted as precipitants of relapse (81), individual psychotherapy may be particularly indicated for those whose psychopathology or disturbed interpersonal functioning is found to endure after the achievement of abstinence. Given findings pointing to the delayed emergence of effects of individual psychotherapy for both cocaine and opioid users, psychotherapy aimed at these enduring issues can be helpful not only for such problems independent of their relationship to drug use, but also as a form of insurance against the likelihood that these continuing problems eventually will lead to relapse.

REFERENCES

1. Babor TF. Avoiding the horrid and beastly sin of drunkenness: does dissuasion make a difference? *J Consult Clin Psychol* 1994;62:1127–1140.
2. Institute of Medicine. *Broadening the Base of treatment for alcohol problems.* Washington, DC: National Academy Press, 1990.
3. Miller WR, Heather N. *Treating addictive behaviors,* 2nd ed. New York: Plenum, 1998.
4. Miller WR, Wilbourne PL. Mesa Grande: a methodological analysis of clinical trials of treatments for alcohol use disorders. *Addiction* 2002;97: 265–277.
5. Blatt SJ, McDonald C, Sugarman A, et al. Psychodynamic theories of opiate addiction: new directions for research. *Clin Psychol Rev* 1984;v 4:159–189.
6. Ball JC, Ross A. *The effectiveness of methadone maintenance treatment.* New York: Springer-Verlag, 1991.
7. Dole VP, Nyswander ME, Warner A. Methadone maintenance treatment: a ten-year perspective. *JAMA* 1976;235:2117–2119.
8. DeRubeis RJ, Crits-Christoph P. Empirically supported individual and group psychological treatments for adult mental disorders. *J Consult Clin Psychol* 1998;66:37–52.
9. Leshner AI. Science-based views of drug addiction and its treatment. *JAMA* 1999;282:1314–1316.
10. McLellan AT, McKay JR. The treatment of addiction: what can research offer practice? In Lamb S, Greenlick MR, McCarty D, eds. *Bridging the gap between practice and research: forging partnerships with community based drug and alcohol treatment.* Washington, DC: National Academy Press, 1998:147–185.
11. Miller WR, Zweben A, DiClemente CC, et al. *Motivational enhancement therapy manual: a clinical research guide for therapists treating individuals with alcohol abuse and dependence.* Rockville, MD: NIAAA, 1992.
12. Nowinski J, Baker S, Carroll KM. *Twelve-step facilitation therapy manual: a clinical research guide for therapists treating individuals with alcohol abuse and dependence.* Rockville, MD: NIAAA, 1992.
13. Kadden R, Carroll KM, Donovan D, et al. *Cognitive-behavioral coping skills therapy manual: a clinical research guide for therapists treating individuals with alcohol abuse and dependence.* Rockville, MD: NIAAA, 1992.
14. Project MATCH Research Group. Matching Alcohol Treatments to Client Heterogeneity: Project MATCH posttreatment drinking outcomes. *J Stud Alcohol* 1997;58:7–29.
15. Project MATCH Research Group. Matching alcoholism treatments to client heterogeneity: Project MATCH three-year drinking outcomes. *Alcohol Clin Exp Res* 1998;22:1300–1311.
16. Bien TH, Miller WR, Tonigan JS. Brief interventions for alcohol problems: a review. *Addiction* 1993;88:315–335.
17. Wilk AI, Jensen NM, Havighurst TC. Meta-analysis of randomized controlled trials addressing brief interventions in heavy alcohol drinkers. *J Gen Intern Med* 1997;12:274–283.
18. Babor TF, Grant M, Acuda W, et al. A randomized clinical trial of brief interventions in primary care: Summary of a WHO project. *Addiction* 1994;89:657–660.
19. WHO Brief Intervention Study Group. A randomized cross-national clinical trial of brief interventions with heavy drinkers. *Am J Public Health* 1996;86: 948–955.
20. Norquist G, Regier DA. The epidemiology of psychiatric disorders and the de facto mental health care system. *Annu Rev Med* 1996;47:473–479.
21. Robins LN. Addicts' careers. In: Dupont RI, Goldstein A, O'Donnell J, et al., eds. *Handbook on drug abuse.* Rockville, Maryland: NIDA, 1979.
22. Simpson DD, Joe GW, Bracy SA. Six-year follow-up of opioid addicts after admission to treatment. *Arch Gen Psychiatry* 1982;39:1318–1326.
23. Valliant GE Twelve-year follow-up of New York addicts. *Am J Psychiatry* 1966;122:727–737.
24. Kleber HD, Kosten TR. Naltrexone induction: psychologic and pharmacologic strategies. *J Clin Psychiatry* 1984;45:29.
25. Kosten TR, Rounsaville BJ, Kleber HD. A 2.5 year follow-up of depression, life events, and treatment effects on abstinence among opioid addicts. *Arch Gen Psychiatry* 1986;43:733–738.
26. Chick J, Gough K, Falkowski W, et al. Disulfiram treatment of alcoholism. *Br J Psychiatry* 1992;161:84–89.
27. Fuller RK, Branchey L, Brightwell DR, et al. Disulfiram treatment of alcoholism: a Veterans Administration cooperative study. *JAMA* 1986;256: 1449–1455.
28. Ling W, Weiss DG, Charuvastra VC, et al. Use of disulfiram for alcoholics in methadone maintenance programs: a Veterans Administration Cooperative Study. *Arch Gen Psychiatry* 1983;40:851–854.
29. McLellan AT, Arndt IO, Metzger D, et al. The effects of psychosocial services in substance abuse treatment. *JAMA* 1993;269:1953–1959.
30. Carroll KM. Manual guided psychosocial treatment: a new virtual requirement for pharmacotherapy trials? *Arch Gen Psychiatry* 1997;54: 923–928.
31. Greenstein RA, Fudala PJ, O'Brien CP. Alternative pharmacotherapies for opiate addiction. In: Lowinson JH, Ruiz P, Millman RB, et al., eds. *Comprehensive textbook of substance abuse,* 3rd ed. New York: Williams & Wilkins, 1997:415–425.
32. Lowinson II, Marion IJ, Joseph H, et al. Methadone maintenance. In Lowinson JH, Ruiz P, Millman RB, eds. *Substance Abuse: A Comprehensive Textbook,* 2E. Baltimore, Williams & Wilkins, 1992:550–561.
33. O'Brien CP. A range of research-based pharmacotherapies for addiction. *Science* 1997;278:66–70.
34. Senay E. Methadone maintenance. In Karasu TB, ed. *Treatments of psychiatric disorders.* Washington, DC: American Psychiatric Association Press, 1989:1341–1358.
35. O'Malley SS, Jaffe AJ, Chang G, et al. Naltrexone and coping skills therapy for alcohol dependence: a controlled study. *Arch Gen Psychiatry* 1992;49:881–887.
36. Sass H, Soyka M, Mann K, et al. Relapse prevention by acamprosate. *Arch Gen Psychiatry* 1996;53:673–680.

37. Volpicelli JR, Alterman AI, Hayashida M, et al. Naltrexone in the treatment of alcohol dependence. *Arch Gen Psychiatry* 1992;49: 876–880.
38. Whitworth AB, Fischer F, Lesch OM. Comparison of acamprosate and placebo in long-term treatment of alcohol dependence. *Lancet* 1996;347:1438–1442.
39. Kosten TR, McCance-Katz EF. New pharmacotherapies. In: Oldham JM, Riba MB, eds. *American psychiatric press review of psychiatry* (vol. 14). Washington: American Psychiatric Press, Inc., 1995:105–126.
40. Smith M, Glass C, Miller T. *The benefits of psychotherapy*. Baltimore: Johns Hopkins Press, 1980.
41. Marques AC, Formigoni ML. Comparison of individual and group cognitive behavioral therapy for alcohol and/or drug dependent patients. *Addiction* 2001;96:835–846.
42. Khantzian EJ. The self-medication hypothesis of addictive disorders: focus on heroin and cocaine. *Am J Psychiatry* 11985;42:1259–1264.
43. Wurmser L. *The hidden dimension: psychopathology of compulsive drug use*. New York: Jason Aronson, 1979.
44. Gawin FH, Ellinwood EH. Stimulants: actions, abuse, and treatment. *N Engl J Med* 1988;318:1173–1183.
45. Mendelson JH, Mello NK. Experimental analysis of drinking behavior in chronic alcoholics. *Ann N Y Acad Sci* 1966;133:828–845.
46. Mirin SR, Meyer RE, McNamme B. Psychopathology and mood duration in heroin use: acute and chronic effects. *Arch Gen Psychiatry* 1980; 33:1503–1508.
47. Beck AT, Rush AJ, Shaw BF, et al. *Cognitive therapy of depression*. New York: Guilford, 1979.
48. Raimo EB, Schuckit MA. Alcohol dependence and mood disorders. *Addict Behav* 1998;23:933–946.
49. Schuckit MA, Smith TL, Danko GP., et al. Five year clinical course associated with DSM-IV alcohol abuse or dependence in a large group of men and women. *Am J Psychiatry* 2001;158:1084–1090.
50. Stanton MD, Shadish WR. Outcome, attrition, and family-couples treatment for drug abuse: a meta-analysis and review of the controlled, comparative studies. *Psychol Bull* 1997;122:170–191.
51. Cummings N. Turning bread into stones: our modern anti-miracle. *Am Psychol* 1979;34:1119–1129.
52. Hser Y, Hoffman V, Grella CE, et al. A 33-year follow-up of narcotics addicts. *Arch Gen Psychiatry* 2001;58:503–508.
53. Valliant GE. A long-term follow-up of male alcohol abuse. *Arch Gen Psychiatry* 1996;53:243–249.
54. Prochaska JO, DiClemente CC. Transtheoretical therapy: toward a more integrative model of change. *Psychother Theory Res Pract* 1982;19: 276–288.
55. Prochaska JO, DiClemente CC, Norcross JC. In search of how people change: applications to addictive behaviors. *Am Psychol* 1992;47: 1102–1114.
56. Miller WR, Rollnick S. *Motivational interviewing: preparing people for change,* 2nd ed. New York: Guilford Press, 2002.
57. Miller WR. Rediscovering fire: small interventions, large effects. *Psychol Addict Behav* 2000;14:6–18.
58. Carroll KM, Libby B, Sheehan J, et al. Motivational interviewing to enhance treatment initiation in substance abusers: an effectiveness study. *Am J Addict* 2001;10:335–339.
59. Saunders B, Wilkinson C, Philips M. The impact of a brief motivational intervention with opiate users attending a methadone programme. *Addiction* 1995;90:415–424.
60. Stotts AL, Schmitz JM, Rhoades HM, et al. Motivational interviewing with cocaine-dependent patients: a pilot study. *J Consult Clin Psychol* 2001;69:858–862.
61. Swanson AJ, Pantalon MV, Cohen KR. Motivational interviewing and treatment adherence among psychiatric and dually diagnosed patients. *J Nerv Ment Dis* 1999;187:630–635.
62. Sanchez-Craig M, Wilkinson DA. Treating problem drinkers who are not severely dependent on alcohol. *Drugs Society* 1986;1:39–67.
63. Edwards G. The alcohol dependence syndrome: a concept as stimulus to enquiry. *Br J Addict* 1986;81:171–183.
64. Edwards G, Gross MM. Alcohol dependence: provisional description of a clinical syndrome. *Br Med J* 1976;1:1058–1061.
65. Marlatt GA, Gordon JR. *Relapse prevention: maintenance strategies in the treatment of addictive behaviors*. New York: Guilford, 1985.
66. Carroll KM. *A cognitive-behavioral approach: treating cocaine addiction*. Rockville, MD: NIDA, 1998.
67. Monti PM, Rohsenow DJ, Abrams DB, et al. *Treating alcohol dependence: a coping skills training guide in the treatment of alcoholism*. New York: Guilford Press, 1989.
68. Carroll KM, Nich C, Ball SA, et al. One year follow-up of disulfiram and psychotherapy for cocaine-alcohol abusers: sustained effects of treatment. *Addiction* 2000;95:1335–1349.
69. Carroll KM, Rounsaville BJ, Nich C, et al. One year follow-up of psychotherapy and pharmacotherapy for cocaine dependence: delayed emergence of psychotherapy effects. *Arch Gen Psychiatry* 1994;51:989–997.
70. McKay JR, Alterman AI, Cacciola JS, et al. Continuing care for cocaine dependence: comprehensive 2-year outcomes. *J Consult Clin Psychol* 1999;63:70–78.
71. O'Malley SS, Jaffe AJ, Chang G, et al. Six month follow-up of naltrexone and psychotherapy for alcohol dependence. *Arch Gen Psychiatry* 1996;53:217–224.
72. Rawson RA, Huber A, McCann MJ., et al. A comparison of contingency management and cognitive-behavioral approaches during methadone maintenance for cocaine dependence. *Arch Gen Psychiatry* 2002;59: 817–824.
73. Luborsky L. *Principles of psychoanalytic psychotherapy: a manual for supportive-expressive treatment*. New York: Basic Books, 1984.
74. Rounsaville BJ, Gawin FH, Kleber HD. Interpersonal psychotherapy adapted for ambulatory cocaine abusers. *Am J Drug Alcohol Abuse* 1985;11:171–191.
75. Edwards G, Arif A, Hodgson R. Nomenclature and classification of drug and alcohol related problems. *Bull WHO* 1981;59:225–242.
76. Kandel D, Faust R. Sequence and stages in patterns of adolescent drug use. *Arch Gen Psychiatry* 1975;32:923–932.
77. Kandel DB, Yamaguchi K, Chen K. Stages of progression in drug involvement from adolescence to adulthood. *J Stud Alcohol* 1992;53: 447–457.
78. Budney AJ, Higgins ST. *A Community reinforcement plus vouchers approach: treating cocaine addiction*. Rockville, MD: NIDA, 1998.
79. Higgins ST, Delany DD, Budney AJ, et al. A behavioral approach to achieving initial cocaine abstinence. *Am J Psychiatry* 11991;48: 1218–1224.
80. Azrin NH. Improvements in the community-reinforcement approach to alcoholism. *Behav Res Ther* 1976;14:339–348.
81. Marlatt GA, Gordon GR. Determinants of relapse: implications for the maintenance of behavior change. In: Davidson PO, Davidson SM, eds. *Behavioral medicine: changing health lifestyles*. New York: Brunner/Mazel, 1980:410–452.
82. Khantzian EJ, Treece C. DSM-III psychiatric diagnosis of narcotic addicts. *Arch Gen Psychiatry* 41985;2:1067–1071.
83. Regier DA, Farmer ME, Rae DS, et al. Comorbidity of mental disorders with alcohol and other drug abuse. Results from the Epidemiologic Catchment Area (ECA) study. *JAMA* 1990;264:2511–2518.
84. Rounsaville BJ, Anton SF, Carroll KM, et al. Psychiatric diagnosis of treatment seeking cocaine abusers. *Arch Gen Psychiatry* 1991;48:43–51.
85. Rounsaville BJ, Weissman MM, Kleber HD, et al. Heterogeneity of psychiatric diagnosis in treated opiate addicts. *Arch Gen Psychiatry* 1982;39: 161–166.
86. Beckman EE, Leber WR. *Handbook of depression: treatment, assessment and research*. Homewood, IL: Dorsey Press, 1985.
87. Keller DS, Carroll KM, Nich C, et al. Differential treatment response in alexithymic cocaine abusers: findings from a randomized clinical trial of psychotherapy and pharmacotherapy. *Am J Addict* 1995;4:234–244.
88. Taylor GJ, Parker JD, Babgby RM. A preliminary investigation of alexithymia in men with psychoactive substance dependence. *Am J Psychiatry* 1990;147:1228–1230.
89. Galanter M. *Network Therapy for alcohol and drug abuse: a new approach in practice*. New York: Basic Books, 1993.

90. Longabaugh R, Beattie M, Noel R, et al. The effect of social support on treatment outcome. *J Stud Alcohol* 1993;54:465–478.
91. Carroll KM, Rounsaville BJ. Can a technology model be applied to psychotherapy research in cocaine abuse treatment? In: Onken LS, Blaine JD, eds. *Psychotherapy and counseling in the treatment of drug abuse.* Rockville, MD: NIDA, 1991:91–104.
92. Waskow IE. Specification of the technique variable in the NIMH Treatment of Depression Collaborative Research Program. In: Williams JBW, Spitzer RL, eds. *Psychotherapy research: where are we and where should we go?* New York: Guilford, 1984.
93. Woody GE, Luborsky L, McLellan AT, et al. Psychotherapy for opiate addicts: does it help? *Arch Gen Psychiatry* 1983;40:639–645.
94. Woody GE, McLellan AT, Luborsky L, et al. Psychotherapy in community methadone programs: a validation study. *Am J Psychiatry* 1995;152: 1302–1308.
95. Woody GE, McLellan AT, Luborsky L, et al. Twelve-month follow-up of psychotherapy for opiate dependence. *Am J Psychiatry* 1987;144:590–596.
96. Stitzer ML, Bickel WK, Bigelow GE, et al. Effect of methadone dose contingencies on urinalysis test results of polydrug abusing methadone maintenance patients. *Drug Alcohol Depend* 1986;18:341–348.
97. Stitzer ML, Bigelow GE. Contingency management in a methadone maintenance program: Availability of reinforcers. *Int J Addict* 1978;13: 737–746.
98. Stitzer ML, Iguchi MY, Felch LJ. Contingent take-home incentives: effects on drug use of methadone maintenance patients. *J Consult Clin Psychol* 1992;60:927–934.
99. Iguchi MY, Lamb RJ, Belding MA, et al. Contingent reinforcement of group participation versus abstinence in a methadone maintenance program. *Exp Clin Psychopharmacol* 1996;4:1–7.
100. Silverman K, Higgins ST, Brooner RK, et al. Sustained cocaine abstinence in methadone maintenance patients through voucher-based reinforcement therapy. *Arch Gen Psychiatry* 1996;53:409–415.
101. Silverman K, Wong CJ, Umbricht-Schneiter A, et al. Broad beneficial effects of cocaine abstinence reinforcement among methadone patients. *J Consult Clin Psychol* 1998;66:811–824.
102. Rounsaville BJ. Can psychotherapy rescue naltrexone treatment of opioid addiction? In Onken LS, Blaine JD, eds. *Potentiating the efficacy of medications: integrating psychosocial therapies with pharmacotherapies in the treatment of drug dependence.* Rockville, MD: NIDA, 1995:37–52.
103. Grabowski J, O'Brien CP, Greenstein RA, et al. Effects of contingent payments on compliance with a naltrexone regimen. *Am J Drug Alcohol Abuse* 1979;6:355–365.
104. Meyer RE, Mirin SM, Altman JL, et al. A behavioral paradigm for the evaluation of narcotic antagonists. *Arch Gen Psychiatry* 1976;33:371–377.
105. Anton RF, Hogan I, Jalali B, et al. Multiple family therapy and naltrexone in the treatment of opioid dependence. *Drug Alcohol Depend* 1981; 8:157–168.
106. Preston KL, Silverman K, Umbricht A, et al. Improvement in naltrexone treatment compliance with contingency management. *Drug Alcohol Depend* 1999;54:127–135.
107. Carroll KM, Ball SA, Nich C, et al. Targeting behavioral therapies to enhance naltrexone treatment of opioid dependence: efficacy of contingency management and significant other involvement. *Arch Gen Psychiatry* 2001;58:755–761.
108. Carroll KM, Sinha R, Nich C, et al. Contingency management to enhance naltrexone treatment of opioid dependence: a randomized clinical trial of reinforcement magnitude. *Exp Clin Psychopharmacol* 2002;10:54–63.
109. Van Horn DH, Frank AF. Psychotherapy for cocaine addiction. *Psychol Addict Behav* 1998;12:47–61.
110. Higgins ST, Budney AJ, Bickel WK, et al. Achieving cocaine abstinence with a behavioral approach. *Am J Psychiatry* 1993;150:763–769.
111. Higgins ST, Wong CJ, Badger GJ., et al. Contingent reinforcement increases cocaine abstinence during outpatient treatment and one year follow-up. *J Consult Clin Psychol* 2000;68:64–72.
112. Petry NM. A comprehensive guide to the application of contingency management procedures in clinical settings. *Drug Alcohol Depend* 2000; 58:9–25.
113. Higgins ST, Budney AJ, Bickel WK, et al. Incentives improve outcome in outpatient behavioral treatment of cocaine dependence. *Arch Gen Psychiatry* 1994;51:568–576.
114. Milby JB, Schumacher JE, Raczynski JM, et al. Sufficient conditions for effective treatment of substance abusing homeless persons. *Drug Alcohol Depend* 1996;43:39–47.
115. Kirby KC, Marlowe DB, Festinger DS, et al. Schedule of voucher delivery influences initiation of cocaine abstinence. *J Consult Clin Psychol* 1998;66:761–767.
116. Svikis DS, Haug NA, Stitzer ML. Attendance incentives for outpatient treatment: effects in methadone- and nonmethadone maintained pregnant drug dependent women. *Drug Alcohol Depend* 1997;25:33–41.
117. Higgins ST, Silverman K. *Motivating behavior change among illicit-drug abusers.* Washington, DC: American Psychological Association, 1999.
118. Petry NM, Martin B. Low-cost contingency management for treating cocaine- and opioid abusing methadone patients. *J Consult Clin Psychol* 2002;70:398–405.
119. Petry NM, Martin B, Cooney JL, et al. Give them prizes and they will come: contingency management treatment of alcohol dependence. *J Consult Clin Psychol* 2000;68:250–257.
120. Carroll KM. Behavioral and cognitive behavioral treatments. In: McCrady BS, Epstein EE, eds. *Addictions: a comprehensive guidebook.* New York: Oxford University Press, 1999:250–267.
121. Carroll KM, Nich C, Rounsaville BJ. Differential symptom reduction in depressed cocaine abusers treated with psychotherapy and pharmacotherapy. *J Nerv Ment Dis* 1995;183:251–259.
122. Carroll KM, Rounsaville BJ, Gawin FH. A comparative trial of psychotherapies for ambulatory cocaine abusers: relapse prevention and interpersonal psychotherapy. *Am J Drug Alcohol Abuse* 1991;17:229–247.
123. Carroll KM, Rounsaville BJ, Gordon LT, et al. Psychotherapy and pharmacotherapy for ambulatory cocaine abusers. *Arch Gen Psychiatry* 1994;51:177–197.
124. Maude-Griffin PM, Hohenstein JM, Humfleet GL, et al. Superior efficacy of cognitive-behavioral therapy for crack cocaine abusers: main and matching effects. *J Consult Clin Psychol* 1998;66:832–837.
125. McKay JR, Alterman AI, Cacciola JS, et al. Group counseling versus individualized relapse prevention aftercare following intensive outpatient treatment for cocaine dependence. *J Consult Clin Psychol* 1997;65:778–788.
126. Rosenblum A, Magura S, Palij M, et al. Enhanced treatment outcomes for cocaine-using methadone patients. *Drug Alcohol Depend* 1999;54:207–218.
127. Carroll KM, Nich C, Ball SA, et al. Treatment of cocaine and alcohol dependence with psychotherapy and disulfiram. *Addiction* 1998;93: 713–728.
128. Monti PM, Rohsenow DJ, Michalec E, et al. Brief coping skills treatment for cocaine abuse: substance abuse outcomes at three months. *Addiction* 1997;92:1717–1728.
129. Nowinski J, Baker SM. *The Twelve Step Facilitation Handbook.* San Francisco: Jossey Bass, 1998.
130. Crits-Christoph P, Siqueland L, Blaine J D, et al. Psychosocial treatments for cocaine dependence: results of the National Institute on Drug Abuse Collaborative Cocaine Study. *Arch Gen Psychiatry* 1999;56:495–502.
131. Crits-Christoph P, Siqueland L, McCalmont E, et al. Impact of psychosocial treatments on associated problems of cocaine-dependent patients. *J Consult Clin Psychol* 2001;69:825–830.
132. Mercer DE, Woody GE. *An individual drug counseling approach to treat cocaine addiction: the collaborative cocaine treatment study model.* Rockville, MD: NIDA, 1999.
133. Beck AT, Wright FD, Newman CF, et al. *Cognitive therapy of substance abuse.* New York: Guilford Press, 1993.
134. Carroll KM. Old psychotherapies for cocaine dependence....revisited. *Arch Gen Psychiatry* 1999;56:505–506.
135. Project MATCH Research Group. Matching alcoholism treatments to client heterogeneity: treatment main effects and matching effects on drinking during treatment. *J Stud Alcohol* 1998;59:631–639.
136. Horgan CM, Levine HJ. The substance abuse treatment system: what does it look like and whom does it serve? In: Lamb S, Greenlick MR, McCarty D, eds. *Bridging the gap between practice and research: forging*

partnerships with community-based drug and alcohol treatment. Washington, DC: National Academy Press, 1999:186–197.

137. Morgenstern J, Morgan TJ, McCrady BS, et al. Manual-guided cognitive behavioral therapy training: a promising method for disseminating empirically supported substance abuse treatments to the practice community. *Psychol Addict Behav* 2001;15:83–88.
138. Walsh DC, Hingson RW, Merrigan DM, et al. A randomized trial of treatment options for alcohol-abusing worker. *N Engl J Med* 1991; 325:775–782.
139. Stephens R, Roffman RA, Curtin L. Comparison of extended versus brief treatments for marijuana use. *J Consult Clin Psychol* 2000;68: 898–908.
140. Stephens R, Roffman RA, Simpson EE. Treating adult marijuana dependence: a test of the relapse prevention model. *J Consult Clin Psychol* 994;62:92–99.
141. MTP Research Group. Brief treatments for camabis dependence: findings from a randomized multisite trial. *Clin. Psychology* 2004;72:455–466.
142. Budney AJ, Higgins ST, Radonovich KJ, et al. Adding voucher-based incentives to coping skills and motivational enhancement improves outcomes during treatment for marijuana dependence. *J Consult Clin Psychol* 2000;68:1051–1061.
143. Onken LS, Blaine JD, Battjes R. Behavioral therapy research: a conceptualization of a process. In: Hennegler SW, Amentos R, eds. *Innovative approaches for difficult to treat populations.* Washington, DC: American Psychiatric Press, 1997:477–485.
144. Rounsaville BJ, Carroll KM, Onken LS. A stage model of behavioral therapies research: getting started and moving on from Stage I. *Clin Psychol Sci Pract* 2001;8:133–142.
145. Carroll KM, Nuro KF. One size can't fit all: a stage model for psychotherapy manual development. *Clin Psychol Sci Pract* 2002;9: 396–406.
146. Carroll KM, Rounsaville BJ. Bridging the gap: a hybrid model to link efficacy and effectiveness research in substance abuse treatment. *Psychiatr Serv* 2003;54(3):333–339.
147. Institute of Medicine. *Bridging the gap between practice and research: forging partnerships with community-based drug and alcohol treatment.* Washington, DC: National Academy Press, 1998.
148. Rounsaville BJ, Kleber HD. Psychotherapy/counseling for opiate addicts: strategies for use in different treatment settings. *Int J Addiction* 1985;20:869–896.
149. Miller WR, Brown JM. Simpson TL, et al. What works? A methodological analysis of the alcohol treatment literature. In: Hester RK, Miller WR, eds. *Handbook of alcoholism treatment approaches: effective alternatives.* Boston, MA: Allyn & Bacon, 1995:12–44.
150. Sobell LC, Toneatto T, Sobell MC. Behavioral assessment and treatment planning for alcohol, tobacco, and other drug problems: current status with an emphasis on clinical applications. *Behav Ther* 1994;25: 533–580.
151. McLellan AT, Alterman AI, Metzger DS, et al. Similarity of outcome predictors across opiate, cocaine, and alcohol treatments: role of treatment services. *J Consult Clin Psychol* 1994;62:1141–1158.
152. McLellan AT, Luborsky L, Woody GE, et al. Predicting response to alcohol and drug treatments: role of psychiatric severity. *Arch Gen Psychiatry* 1983;40:620–625.
153. Anton RF, Moak DH, Waid LR, et al. Naltrexone and cognitive-behavioral therapy for the treatment of outpatient alcoholics: results of a placebo-controlled trial. *Am J Psychiatry* 1999;156:1758–1764.
154. Krystal JH, Cramer JA, Krol WF, et al., and for the Naltrexone Cooperative Study 425 Group. Naltrexone in the treatment of alcohol dependence. *N Engl J Med* 2001;345:1734–1739.
155. Woody GE, McLellan AT, Luborsky L, et al. Severity of psychiatric symptoms as a prediction of benefits from psychotherapy: the Veterans Administration-Penn study. *Am J Psychiatry* 1984;141:1172–1177.
156. Woody GE, McLellan At, Luborsky L, et al. Sociopathy and psychotherapy outcome. *Arch Gen Psychiatry* 1985;42:1081–1086.
157. McLellan AT, Grissom GR, Zanis D, et al. Problem-service "matching" in addiction treatment: a prospective study in four programs. *Arch Gen Psychiatry* 1997;54:730–735.
158. McLellan AT, O'Brien CP, Kron R, et al. Matching substance abuse patients to appropriate treatments: a conceptual and methodological approach. *Drug Alcohol Depend* 1980;5:189–195.
159. McLellan AT, Luborsky L, Woody GE, et al. An improved diagnostic evaluation instrument for substance abuse patients: the Addiction Severity Index. *J Nerv Ment Dis* 1980;168:26–33.

CHAPTER 57

Stephen T. Higgins, PhD
Jennifer W. Tidey, PhD
Randall E. Rogers, PhD

Contingency Management and the Community Reinforcement Approach

Contingency-management (CM) interventions and community reinforcement approach (CRA) therapy for treating substance use disorders (SUDs) are based in the conceptual framework of learning and conditioning theory. Especially fundamental to these treatment approaches is operant conditioning, which is the study of how systematically applied environmental consequences increase (i.e., reinforce) or decrease (i.e., punish) the frequency and patterning of voluntary behavior (1).

In this chapter, we describe how SUDs are conceptualized within an operant framework, describe the treatments, and review controlled studies on the efficacy of CM and CRA in the treatment of SUDs. These interventions have been researched most extensively with regard to treating alcohol, cocaine, and opioid dependence, each of which is addressed in this chapter. More recently, CM and CRA have been extended to other forms of SUDs and to special populations (2). Those advances are reviewed as well. The review is restricted to controlled studies published in peer-reviewed journals. The only exceptions are where an uncontrolled study is mentioned as the first in a series of studies that included a controlled trial.

HISTORICAL PERSPECTIVE

Studying and conceptualizing SUDs within an operant conditioning framework began in earnest in the 1960s and early 1970s (3). Convergent evidence from studies conducted with laboratory animals residing in highly controlled experimental chambers, humans with SUDs residing in medically supervised hospital settings, and humans seeking treatment for SUDs demonstrated the operant nature of drug use. In the studies with laboratory animals, for example, subjects fitted with intravenous catheters readily learned arbitrary behavioral responses such as pressing a lever or pulling a chain when the only consequence for doing so was the delivery of an injection of a commonly abused drug (e.g., morphine or cocaine). Effects are pharmacologically specific in that injections of drugs that humans rarely abuse (e.g., chlorpromazine) or saline failed to generate or maintain responding. In some instances, the reinforcing effects of the commonly abused drugs were so robust that they promoted in these laboratory animals the dangerous extremes in consumption characteristic of humans with SUDs. Monkeys given unconstrained opportunities to self-administer intravenous cocaine, for example, would consume the drug to the exclusion of basic sustenance, and barring experimenter intervention, to the point of death (4). Substitute saline for the cocaine and the animals would readily discontinue giving themselves injections (i.e., responding extinguished). A robust body of evidence demonstrated that the drugs that humans commonly abuse function as unconditioned positive reinforcers much as do food, water, and sex.

The residential studies of humans with SUDs often examined the sensitivity of drug use to systematically administered environmental consequences. An elegant series of studies, for example, demonstrated the operant nature of alcohol use among severe alcoholics (5). In this programmatic series of studies, alcoholics resided on an inpatient unit where they were permitted to purchase and consume alcoholic drinks. Abstinence from voluntary drinking increased when (1) access to an alternative reinforcer (enriched environment) was made available contingent on doing so, (2) monetary reinforcement was provided contingent on abstinence from drinking, (3) the amount of work required to obtain drinks was increased, or (4) brief periods of social isolation were imposed contingent upon drinking. The studies provided strong evidence that even among individuals with diagnosed severe SUDs, drug use was sensitive to environmental consequences.

Initial studies with treatment seekers typically involved small-sample demonstrations that systematically applied consequences could improve treatment outcome. In a controlled case study, for example, breath samples were collected twice weekly on a quasi-random schedule from a male with severe alcoholism (6). Baseline observations demonstrated a high-rate of drinking. During the intervention period, the patient received a $3.00 coupon book contingent on randomly scheduled alcohol-negative breath samples. Coupons could be exchanged for goods at a hospital commissary. After a discernible increase in the rate of negative breath tests during the period of contingent coupon delivery, the contingency was removed, and booklets were delivered independent of breath results. Under that condition, the frequency of negative specimens decreased towards baseline levels. Reimposing the contingency again increased the frequency of alcohol-negative breath results. Around this same time, several studies were reported suggesting that allowing participants to earn back monetary deposits contingent on objective verification of smoking abstinence improved outcomes among those trying to quit cigarette smoking (7,8). These studies illustrated the clinical implications of the emerging body of evidence supporting the operant nature of SUDs.

Such studies provided the empirical foundation for a conceptual model wherein drug use is considered a normal, learned behavior that falls along a continuum ranging from little use and few problems to excessive use and many untoward effects (9). The same principles of learning and conditioning are assumed to operate across this continuum. Within this framework, all physically intact humans are considered to possess the necessary neurobiologic systems to experience drug-produced reinforcement and hence to develop drug use and SUDs. Genetic or acquired characteristics (e.g., family history of alcoholism, other psychiatric disorders) are recognized as factors that affect the probability of developing SUDs but are not deemed to be necessary for the problem to emerge.

TREATMENT MODEL

Within an operant conceptual framework, reinforcement derived from drug use and the associated lifestyle is deemed to have monopolized the behavioral repertoire of the user. Treatments developed within this framework are designed to reorganize the user's environment to systematically increase the rate of reinforcement obtained while abstinent from drug use and reduce or eliminate the rate of reinforcement obtained through drug use and associated activities. Primary emphasis is placed on decreasing drug use by systematically increasing the availability and frequency of alternative reinforcing activities either through relatively contrived sources of reinforcement as in CM interventions or more naturalistic sources as in CRA therapy (10). Additionally, arranging the environment so that aversive events or the loss of reinforcing events (i.e., punishment procedures) occur as a consequence of drug use also can decrease drug use. As with reinforcement, such aversive procedures can involve relatively contrived (e.g., forfeiture of a large-value incentive) or more naturalistic (e.g., suspension from work) consequences. This distinction between CM and CRA with regard to the former's relying primarily on contrived contingencies and the latter's relying primarily on naturalistic contingencies will become clearer when the treatments are described in greater detail later. By *contrived*, we mean a set of contingencies that are put in place explicitly and exclusively for therapeutic purposes (e.g., earning vouchers exchangeable for retail items contingent on cocaine-negative urine toxicology results). By *naturalistic*, we mean a set of contingencies that are already operating in the natural environment for nontherapeutic purposes but can be used to support the therapeutic process (e.g., teaching a spouse to deliver praise when a patient avoids bars and to withhold praise or express disapproval for going to bars).

Some treatments, such as the CRA + vouchers treatment for cocaine dependence (11,12), are designed to deliver contrived consequences during the initial treatment period, with a transition to more naturalistic sources later in treatment. The rationale for that sequence is that the lifestyle of the user is often so disrupted upon treatment entry that it is largely devoid of effective alternative sources of reinforcement that can compete with the reinforcement derived from drug use. Contrived sources of alternative reinforcement delivered through CM are designed to promote initial abstinence, thereby allowing time for therapists and patient to work towards reestablishing more naturalistic alternatives (e.g., job, stable family life, participation in self-help and other social groups that reinforce abstinence). Of course, it is these naturalistic alternatives that eventually will need to sustain long-term abstinence once the contrived reinforcers are discontinued.

Also important to recognize is that for any number of reasons, some patients may have behavioral repertoires that are too limited to recruit sufficient sources of naturalistic reinforcement to effectively compete with drug use and, as such, these patients will need some form of maintenance treatment involving contrived reinforcement contingencies in order to sustain long-term abstinence. Certainly that is widely recognized with opioid-dependent individuals who often need a maintenance pharmacotherapy in order to sustain long-term abstinence from illicit drug use. Others may need lifelong participation in self-help programs in order to succeed. Such programs might be deemed as falling somewhere around the midpoint on the continuum of contrived versus naturalistic sources of alternative reinforcement (10). The following discussion illustrates how this general strategy is implemented in CM and CRA interventions.

TREATMENT PLANNING

A thorough patient evaluation is an essential first step in effective clinical management of SUDs and that certainly holds true when using CM and CRA interventions. In this section, we outline the assessment practices used in the CRA + vouchers treatment for cocaine dependence to illustrate the type of assessments conducted when using CM and CRA interventions (12). The assessment framework is relatively generic and can be readily applied to other types of SUDs by substituting information specific to cocaine use with pertinent information on whatever other type of SUD is the presenting problem.

Every effort is made to schedule an intake assessment interview as soon as possible after initial patient contact with the clinic. Scheduling the interview within 24 hours of clinic contact significantly reduces attrition between the initial clinic contact and assessment interview, which is a substantial problem among those with SUDs (13). Some patients cannot come in to the clinic within 24 hours, so secondary plans are made to get them in within 72 hours or as soon as is practicable.

Detailed information is collected on drug use, treatment readiness, psychiatric functioning, employment/vocational status, recreational interests, current social supports, family and social problems, and legal issues. The following is a list of instruments that we use to obtain such information, listed in the order in which they are typically administered. Modifications can be readily made to the list depending on the population being treated. We use several patient-rated questionnaires that can be completed upon clinic arrival for an intake assessment. We have clients complete a brief demographics questionnaire. Obtaining a current address and phone number is important, as is a number of someone who will always know the client's whereabouts. This information is important for purposes of during-treatment outreach efforts should the client stop coming to scheduled therapy sessions or need to be contacted for other clinical purposes and for contacting clients for routine posttreatment follow-up evaluations. The Stages of Change Readiness and Treatment Eagerness Scale (SOCRATES) (14) provides information on clients' perception of the severity of their drug use problems and their readiness to engage in behavior to reduce their use. We use three versions of the SOCRATES that refer to specific substances (i.e., cocaine, alcohol, and other drug use), as the patient's motivation to reduce substance use is often drug-specific.

We use an adaptation of the Cocaine Dependency Self-Test (15) to collect information on the type of adverse effects from cocaine use that patients have experienced. Such information can be useful in helping patients problem solve regarding the pros and cons of cocaine use as part of efforts to promote and sustain motivation for change during the course of treatment. A sizeable proportion of patients with illicit-drug use disorders are also problem drinkers, making assessment of that problem essential. As part of our alcohol assessment, we use the Michigan Alcoholism Screening Test (MAST), a widely used brief alcoholism-screening instrument (16), along with a drug-history questionnaire described later. Depressed mood is another common problem among those presenting for treatment for drug use disorders. We use the Beck Depression Inventory (BDI) to screen for depressive symptoms (17). The SCL-90-R (18) is also used to screen for psychiatric symptoms more broadly and is helpful in determining whether a more in-depth psychiatric evaluation is warranted.

A semi-structured drug-history interview developed in our clinic is used to facilitate the collection of information on current and past substance use. Such detailed information is essential for proper treatment planning. The goal in completing a drug use history is to obtain detailed information regarding the duration, severity, and pattern of the patient's drug use. The accuracy of the patient's report of drug use (amount and frequency) is facilitated by the use of an effective technique for reviewing recent use (i.e., the timeline follow-back) (19). Diagnoses of abuse and dependence are made later by master's- or doctorate-level psychologists. We use the Addiction Severity Index (ASI) (20) to assess multiple problems commonly associated with drug use. The ASI provides a quantitative, time-based assessment of problem severity in the following areas: alcohol use, drug use, and employment, medical, legal, family, social, and psychological functioning. The information obtained in this interview is quite useful for developing treatment plans that include lifestyle change goals.

A practical needs assessment questionnaire (developed in our clinic) is used to determine whether the patient has any pressing needs or crises that may interfere with initial treatment engagement (e.g., housing, legal, transportation, or childcare). The intake worker asks specific questions regarding current housing, child care, legal circumstances, medical issues, and other matters that might been of current and serious concern to the client. Detailed information is collected on any identified crisis. The rationale here is to identify matters that may need immediate clinical attention.

If it appears that a medication is indicated, initial steps are taken after the initial intake assessment toward implementing the relevant medical protocols. With the cocaine-dependent population, we routinely use a regimen of clinic-monitored disulfiram therapy to address problem drinking, which also reduces cocaine use (21). More recently we are often using a regimen of clinic-monitored naltrexone therapy as the prevalence of prescription-opioid use has increased.

PRETREATMENT ISSUES

Motivation Within an operant framework, motivation is not thought of as a characteristic of the patient per se but rather as a product of current and past reinforcement contingencies. Thus, the main focus of the interventions is to directly ensure the availability of sufficient reinforcement to promote and sustain therapeutic change. Following, we discuss how that is accomplished.

Rationale for Choice of Treatment The historical and conceptual background information described previously provides the overarching rationale for the use of CM and CRA interventions. CM and CRA have the potential to be useful with virtually any type of SUDs. There is no minimal or maximal intensity or duration of CM or CRA, and thus there is a great deal of flexibility in terms of adapting them to particular forms of SUDs and special populations.

Selection and Preparation of Patients As noted, we know of no particular type of SUD patient for whom CM or CRA is contraindicated. Both have been used effectively across a wide spectrum of patient populations and types of SUDs. Both interventions require a detailed and careful patient orientation. With CM, it is quite common to have patients sign a written contract stipulating all aspects of the CM arrangement so as to avoid any confusion about the contingencies. Brief tests are also commonly administered to ensure that patients understand the contingencies. The vocabulary and other information contained in the contract and tests should be prepared with the potential intellectual limitations of the patient population in mind and plans to surmount potential individual difficulties. For example, reading problems are common among patients with SUDs, and certain patients may need to have written materials read aloud to them.

Therapist Characteristics Therapists typically do not manage CM programs owing to the detailed record keeping involved and the need to biochemically verify abstinence, though there are exceptions. Thus, this section largely pertains to characteristics of CRA therapists. CRA is a manually based intervention, which minimizes the influence of therapist characteristics on outcome. In the series of studies examining CRA + vouchers treatment of cocaine dependence, for example, there have not been any significant therapist effects on outcome noted.

To implement CRA effectively, therapists need to be directive but also flexible, which we believe facilitates treatment retention and progress toward achieving treatment goals. Particularly in the early stages of treatment, therapists try to work around patient schedules and generally make participation in treatment convenient to the patient. Therapists try to be flexible with regard to tardiness to sessions, early departure from sessions, and the time of day that sessions are scheduled and will meet with patients outside the office if necessary. With especially difficult patients, improvements in these areas can be worked on as part of the treatment plan. CRA therapists must exhibit appropriate empathy and good listening skills. They need to convey a sincere understanding of the patient's situation and its inherent difficulties. Throughout treatment, therapists avoid making value judgments and, instead, exhibit genuine empathy and consideration for the difficult challenges that patients face.

CRA requires that therapists and patients develop an active, make-it-happen attitude throughout treatment. Therapists must have good organizational skills, which are important to developing, implementing, monitoring, and adapting treatment plans. Problem-solving skills also are important. Within ethical boundaries, therapists must be committed to doing what it takes to facilitate lifestyle changes on the part of patients. For example, therapists often accompany patients to appointments or job interviews. They initiate recreational activities with patients and schedule sessions at different times of day to accomplish specific goals. They have patients make phone calls from their office. They search newspapers for job possibilities or ideas for healthy recreational activities in which patients might be able to participate. Without question, the amount of direct support that CRA therapists provide to patients can represent a rather significant departure from more traditional forms of substance abuse counseling. However, in CRA, these therapeutic efforts are deemed to be very important for at least three reasons. First, while patients may have the aptitude, they may simply lack certain skills to accomplish important tasks (e.g., effective job searching). Second, early in treatment patients may lack the requisite reinforcement history (i.e., motivation) with certain healthy activities (e.g., attending the local YMCA) to carry through on assigned tasks in the absence of the therapist being present to prompt the response and provide social reinforcement for completing the task. Third, patients may lack the necessary material resources (e.g., transportation or materials for résumé preparation) to complete a task in a timely manner. CRA therapists are committed to overcoming such deficiencies in skills, motivation, or resources in order to facilitate patient movement in the direction of a healthier, non–drug-abusing lifestyle.

TREATMENT AND TECHNIQUE

In this section, we describe basic elements of CM and CRA interventions using the CRA + vouchers treatment for cocaine dependence for illustration purposes.

Contingency Management The efficacy of CM interventions is very much dependent on how they are structured and implemented. Following we provide a brief description of a voucher-based CM intervention. Next we outline 10 features of CM interventions that are important to their efficacy (22).

In the voucher-based CM program, patients sign a written contract stipulating all aspects of the CM interventions. Vouchers exchangeable for retail items are earned contingent on cocaine-negative results in thrice-weekly urine toxicology testing. The program is 12 weeks in duration (on Monday, Wednesday, and Friday). The first cocaine-negative specimen earns a voucher worth $2.50 in purchasing power. The value of each subsequent consecutive cocaine-negative specimen increases by $1.25. The equivalent of a $10 bonus is provided for each three consecutive cocaine-negative specimens. The intent of the escalating magnitude of reinforcement and bonuses is to reinforce continuous cocaine abstinence. A cocaine-positive specimen or failure to submit a scheduled specimen resets the value of vouchers back to the initial $2.50 value. This reset feature is designed to punish relapse to cocaine use after a period of sustained abstinence, with the intensity of the punishment tied directly to the length of sustained abstinence that would be broken. In order to provide patients with a reason to continue abstaining from drug use after a reset, submission of five consecutive cocaine-negative specimens after a cocaine-positive specimen returns the value of points to where they were prior to the reset. Points cannot be lost once earned. If someone is continuously abstinent throughout the 12-week intervention, total earnings would be approximately $997.50. However, because most patients are unable to sustain abstinence throughout the intervention, the average earning is usually about half that maximal amount.

The voucher CM intervention contains most features important to effective CM. First, as was noted, the details of the intervention are carefully explained to patients in the form of a written contract prior to beginning treatment. Second, the response being targeted by the CM intervention—cocaine abstinence—is defined in objective terms (i.e., cocaine-negative urine toxicology results). Third, the methods for verifying that the target response occurred are well specified and objective (urine toxicology testing). Fourth, the schedule for monitoring progress is well specified (each Monday, Wednesday, and Friday). Fifth, the schedule is designed to include frequent opportunities for patients to experience the programmed consequences (thrice weekly). Sixth, the duration of the intervention is stipulated in advance (12 weeks). Seventh, the intervention is focused on a single target (cocaine abstinence). CM interventions that focus on a single target on average produce larger treatment effects than those that target multiple targets (e.g., abstinence from multiple substances) (23). Eighth, the consequences that will follow success and failure to emit the target response are clear (consequences including voucher reinforcement schedule carefully detailed). Ninth, there is minimal delay in delivering designated consequences (urine specimens are analyzed on-site, and vouchers earned are delivered immediately after testing). Delivering the consequence on the same day that occurrence of the target response is verified produces larger treatment effects than delivering the consequence at a later time (23). Tenth, the magnitude of reinforcement that can be earned is relatively substantial (maximal total earnings = $997.50). Larger value incentives on average produce larger treatment effects (23).

Community Reinforcement Approach The CRA component of the CRA + vouchers treatment has seven elements. First, patients are instructed in how to recognize antecedents and consequences of their cocaine use; that is, how to functionally analyze their cocaine use. They are also instructed in how to use that information to reduce the probability of using cocaine. A twofold message is conveyed to the patient: (1) His or her cocaine use is orderly behavior that is more likely to occur under certain circumstances than others, and (2) by learning to identify the circumstances that affect one's cocaine use, plans can be developed and implemented to reduce the likelihood of future cocaine use. In conjunction with functional analysis, patients are taught self-management plans for using the information revealed in the functional analyses to decrease the chances of future cocaine use. Patients are counseled to restructure their daily activities in order to minimize contact with known antecedents of cocaine use, to find alternatives to the positive consequences of cocaine use, and to make explicit the negative consequences of cocaine use.

Second, developing a new social network that will support a healthier lifestyle and getting involved with recreational activities that are enjoyable and do not involve cocaine or other drug use is addressed with all patients. Systematically developing and maintaining contacts with "safe" social networks and participation in "safe" recreational activities remains a high priority throughout treatment for the vast majority of patients. Specific treatment goals are set, and weekly progress on specific goals is monitored. Clearly, plans for developing healthy social networks and recreational activities must be individualized depending on the circumstances, skills and interests of the patient. For those patients who are willing to participate, self-help groups (Alcoholics or Narcotics Anonymous) can be an effective way to develop a new network of associates who will support a sober lifestyle.

Third, various other forms of individualized skills training are provided, usually to address some specific skill deficit that may influence directly or indirectly a patient's risk for cocaine use (e.g., time management, problem solving, assertiveness training, social skills training, and mood management). For example, essential to success with the self-management skills and social/recreational goals discussed is some level of time-management skills. As another example, we implement protocols on controlling depression with those patients whose depression continues after discontinuing cocaine use (24,25).

Fourth, unemployed patients are offered Job Club, which is an efficacious method for assisting chronically unemployed individuals obtain employment (Job Club manual, Azrin and Besalel) (26). The majority of patients who seek treatment for cocaine dependence are unemployed, so this is a service that we offer many of our patients. For others, we assist in pursuing educational goals or new career paths.

Fifth, patients with romantic partners who are not drug abusers are offered behavioral couples therapy, which is an intervention designed to teach couples positive communication skills and how to negotiate reciprocal contracts for desired changes in each other's behavior (27). We attempt to deliver relationship counseling across eight sessions, with the first four sessions delivered across consecutive weeks and the next four delivered on alternating weeks.

Sixth, human immunodeficiency virus/acquired immunodeficiency syndrome (HIV/AIDS) education is provided to all clients in the early stages of treatment, along with counseling directed at addressing any specific needs or risk behavior of the individual patient (28). We address with all clients the potential for acquiring HIV/AIDS from sharing injection equipment and through sexual activity. This involves at least two sessions. First, patients complete an HIV/AIDS knowledge test. They next watch and discuss with their therapist a video on HIV/AIDS. Patients are also provided HIV/AIDS prevention pamphlets and free condoms if desired. The HIV/AIDS knowledge test is repeated and any remaining errors discussed and resolved. Last, patients are given information about testing for HIV and hepatitis B and C and are encouraged to get tested. Those interested in being tested are assisted in scheduling an appointment to do so.

Seventh, all who meet diagnostic criteria for alcohol dependence or report that alcohol use is involved in their use of cocaine are offered disulfiram therapy, which is an integral part of the CRA treatment for alcoholism (29) and decreases alcohol and cocaine use in clients dependent on both substances (21). Patients generally ingest a 250-mg daily dose under clinic staff observation on urinalysis test days and, when possible, under the observation of a significant other (SO) on the other days. Disulfiram therapy is only effective when implemented with procedures to monitor compliance with the recommended dosing regimen. We find that having staff monitor compliance on days that patients attend clinic works very well. Having an SO monitor compliance on the other days can work well if an appropriate person is available to do so at the frequency needed. When that is not possible, we sometimes adopt a practice of having the client ingest a larger dose (500 mg) on days when the patient reports to the clinic and skip dosing on the intervening days.

Use of substances other than tobacco and caffeine is discouraged as well via CRA therapy. Anyone who meets criteria for physical dependence on opiates is referred to an adjoining service located within our clinic for methadone or other opioid replacement therapy (30). We recommend marijuana abstinence because of the problems associated with its abuse, but have found no evidence that marijuana use or dependence adversely affects treatment for cocaine dependence (31). As important, we never dismiss or refuse to treat a patient owing to other drug use. We recommend cessation of tobacco use but usually not during the course of treatment for cocaine dependence. That practice may change as new research begins to demonstrate that smoking cessation can be successfully integrated into simultaneous treatment for other substance abuse or dependence disorders.

Upon completion of the 24 weeks of treatment, patients are encouraged to participate in 6 months of aftercare in our clinic, which involves at least once-monthly brief therapy sessions and urine toxicology screening. More frequent clinic contact is recommended if the therapist or patients deem it necessary.

EMPIRICAL SUPPORT

Contingency Management Interventions

Initial Contingency Management Studies Among the most impressive of the early CM studies on SUDs was a randomized controlled trial conducted with 20 chronic public drunkenness offenders (32). Subjects randomly assigned to the CM group earned housing, employment, medical care, and meals based on sobriety (measured by direct staff observation or blood alchohol level of less than 0.01%), and those in the control group received the same goods and services independent of sobriety status. The intervention produced a fivefold decrease in arrests for subjects in the CM group and no or minimal change for the control group.

Another early approach to treating alcohol use disorders with CM involved reinforcing disulfiram treatment compliance. At least three experimental reports support the efficacy of CM for increasing disulfiram compliance in methadone-maintained patients with alcohol use disorders (33–35). For example, in one well-controlled study (35), alcoholic methadone patients whose daily methadone doses were contingent upon compliance with disulfiram spent 2% of study days drinking, as compared to 21% for the noncontingent control group. Similar results were reported using a controlled case-study design (33).

Despite these impressive results, the use of CM to treat primary alcohol use disorders has largely failed to gain a foothold among the alcohol research or clinical communities. One obstacle is that objectively monitoring alcohol intake using blood alcohol levels (BALs) provides evidence about use only during the few hours preceding the test. Considering that alcohol often is abused in an episodic or binge manner, the absence of a biologic marker with a longer detection duration makes it difficult to reinforce or punish alcohol use. Nevertheless, reports such as those by Miller (32) and Brigham et al. (36) illustrate that this difficulty could be surmounted by relying on a combination of observations by individuals in the subject's natural environment and randomly scheduled BALs. Alternatively, the studies already described illustrate how reinforcing compliance with disulfiram or with other treatment goals can reduce drinking when the contingencies are managed systematically. Overall, CM appears to have more to offer alcohol treatment than currently is being realized. Worth noting is that while the work begun using CM to reinforce disulfiram compliance has not been continued in any programmatic manner, the concept was successfully extended to reinforcing naltrexone compliance among patients with opioid use disorders (31,38) as well as reinforcing adherence to antiretroviral therapies among HIV-positive patients with SUDs (37,39).

Developing Contingency Management as a Treatment for Illicit-Drug Use Disorders Though research on CM among those with primary alcohol use disorders was having difficulty gaining a foothold during the 1970s and 1980s, a concerted body of work emerged on the use of CM to treat illicit-drug use. That work was almost exclusively conducted with patients enrolled in methadone treatment for opioid use disorders.

Though methadone and related substitution therapies are effective at eliminating the use of illicit opioids, a subset of patients continue abusing other nonopioid drugs. A commonly used reinforcer in this area of CM research is the medication take-home privilege, where an extra daily dose of opioid medication is dispensed to the patient for ingestion at home on the following day, thereby granting the patient a break from the grind of having to travel daily to the clinic to ingest the medication under staff supervision (40–44). For example, in what is probably the most rigorous evaluation of the use of contingent medication take-home privileges, Stitzer et al. (44) examined the use of take-home incentives among 54 newly admitted methadone maintenance patients. Half the group received take-home privileges contingent on abstinence from illicit drug use, while the other half received the take-home doses noncontingently. Overall, 32% of the contingent patients

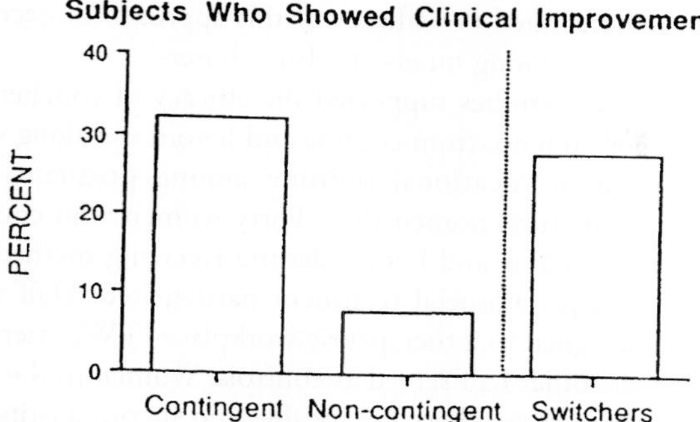

FIGURE 57.1. Improvement in urine test results. Percentages of subjects whose urine test results improved 10% or more from baseline to intervention periods and submitted at least 12 consecutive drug-free tests during the intervention period are shown for the original contingent and noncontingent take-home groups and also for the group of noncontingent subjects who received delayed exposure to the contingent protocol later in treatment. (Reprinted with permission from Stitzer ML, Iguchi MY, Felch LJ. Contingent take-home incentive: effects on drug use of methadone maintenance patients. *J Consult Clin Psychol* 1992;60:927–934.)

achieved sustained periods of abstinence during the intervention (mean, 9.4 weeks; range, 5 to 15 weeks), compared with approximately 10% in the control group (Fig. 57.1). The beneficial effect of contingent take-home delivery was replicated within the group of noncontingent patients who switched over to the contingent intervention after their six-month evaluation in the main study (partial crossover design).

Other consequences in addition to medication take-home privileges were investigated as well. For example, suppression of opiate use during outpatient methadone detoxification was achieved in a study in which the contingent incentive for opiate abstinence was an increase in the methadone dose of up to 20 mg (45). Noncontingent dose increases failed to produce the same degree of abstinence. Another study also using contingent dose changes demonstrated that decreases in poly-drug use could be achieved among methadone maintenance patients when the usual dose was increased above original maintenance levels contingent on drug-free urine toxicology results and also when the usual dose was decreased below original maintenance levels as a consequence of drug-positive urine toxicology results (46).

Voucher-Based Contingency Management as a Treatment for Illicit-Drug Use Disorders The introduction of voucher-based interventions in the 1990s was associated with a substantial increase in research on the use of CM to treat SUDs (47). A major reason why this intervention garnered significant interest was its efficacy with cocaine use disorders. At a time when most clinical trials investigating treatments for cocaine use disorders were consistently producing negative outcomes, a series of controlled trials examining voucher-based CM produced reliably positive outcomes (11,48–52).

The seminal voucher-based procedure was described earlier. The initial two trials involving this intervention combined voucher-based CM with CRA using research designs that did not permit a dissociation of the separate effects of the two interventions (11,48). The first randomized trial designed to isolate the contribution of voucher-based CM to outcome was conducted with 40 cocaine-dependent outpatients who were assigned to receive CRA with or without vouchers (49). Of those, 75% in the group with vouchers completed 24 weeks of treatment, compared to 40% in the group without vouchers. Average duration of continuous cocaine abstinence in the two groups was 11.7 ± 2.0 weeks in the vouchers group versus 6.0 ± 1.5 in the no-vouchers group (Fig. 57.2). At the end of the 24-week treatment period and during follow-up, significant decreases from pretreatment scores were observed in both treatment groups on the ASI family/social and alcohol scales,

MEAN WEEKS OF CONTINUOUS COCAINE ABSTINENCE

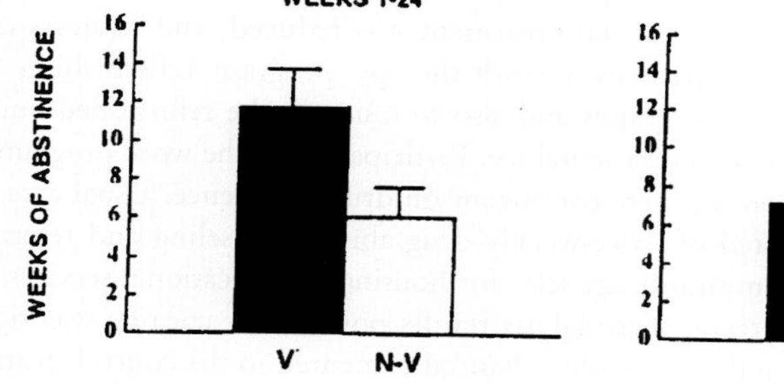

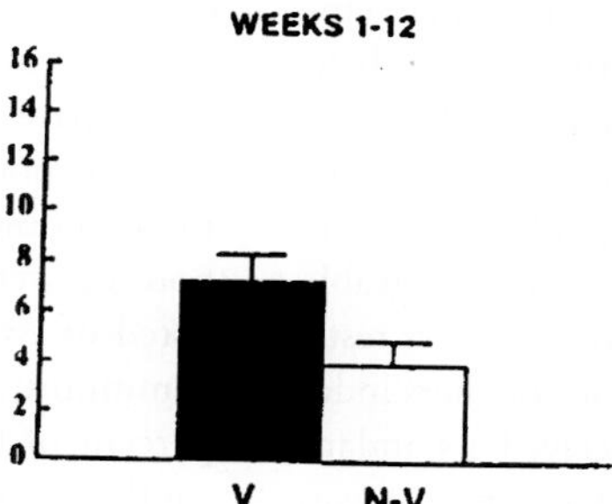

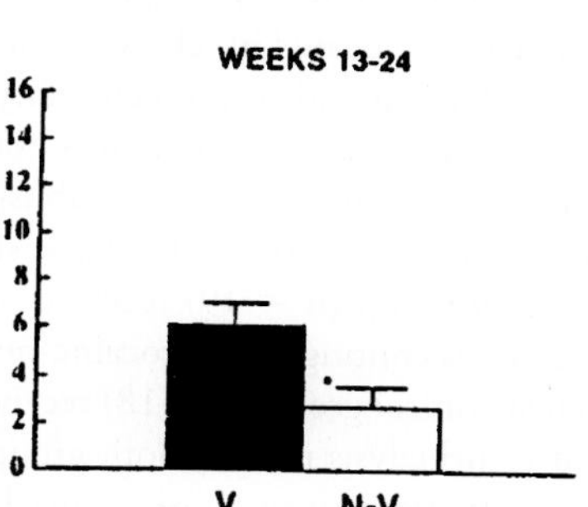

FIGURE 57.2. Mean durations of continuous cocaine abstinence. Mean durations of continuous cocaine abstinence documented via urinalysis testing in each treatment group during weeks 1–24, 1–12, and 13–24 of treatment. Solid and shaded bars indicate the voucher and no-voucher groups, respectively. Error bars represent + standard error of the mean. (Reprinted with permission from Higgins ST, Budney AJ, Bickel WK, et al. Incentives improve treatment retention and cocaine abstinence in ambulatory cocaine-dependent patients. *Arch Gen Psychiatry* 1994;51:568–576.)

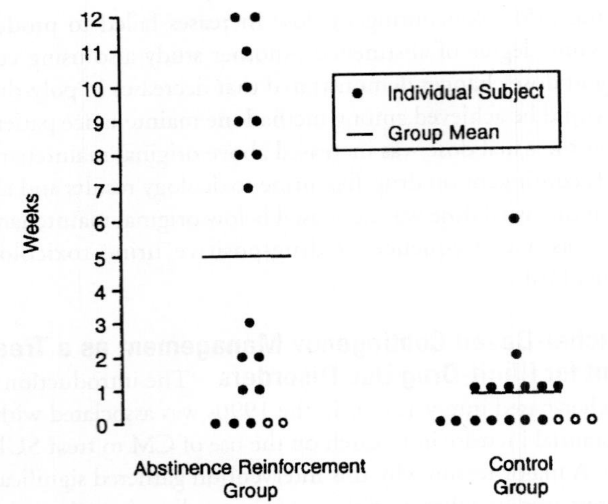

FIGURE 57.3. Point-prevalence abstinence during posttreatment follow-up. Percentage of patients in the two treatment conditions who were cocaine-abstinent at specific posttreatment assessments (i.e., point-prevalence abstinence). Patients were considered abstinent at an assessment period if they reported no cocaine use for the 30 days preceding the assessment and had cocaine-negative urinalysis test results. (Reprinted with permission from Higgins ST, Wong CJ, Badger GJ, et al. Contingent reinforcement increases cocaine abstinence during outpatient treatment and 1 year of follow-up. *J Consult Clin Psychol* 2000;68:64–72.)

with no differences between the groups (50). Both groups also decreased on the ASI drug scale, but the magnitude of change was significantly greater in the voucher than the non-voucher groups, and only the voucher group showed a significant improvement on the ASI psychiatric scale. In more recent randomized trials further examining the efficacy of contingent vouchers when combined with CRA (51,52), positive effects on cocaine abstinence remained discernible through posttreatment follow-up periods extending out to 21 months following discontinuation of the voucher program (Fig. 57.3).

The series of studies by Higgins et al. (52,53) were all conducted in a clinic located in relatively rural Vermont. The seminal study demonstrating the generality of this approach to abusers residing in a large urban area examined the efficacy of the voucher program with cocaine-abusing methadone maintenance patients. During a 12-week study, subjects in the experimental group (n = 19) received vouchers exchangeable for retail items contingent on cocaine-negative urinalysis tests. A matched control group (n = 18) received the vouchers independent of urinalysis results. Both groups received a standard form of outpatient drug abuse counseling. Cocaine use was substantially reduced in the experimental group but remained relatively unchanged in the control group (Fig. 57.4). Use of opiates decreased during the voucher period in the contingent compared to the noncontingent conditions even though the contingency was exclusively on cocaine use. Subsequent randomized trials from this same group (54,55) and others (56) further demonstrated the efficacy of this approach in decreasing cocaine use among inner-city drug abusers.

Subsequent studies supported the efficacy of vouchers in promoting abstinence from cocaine and heroin use along with participation in vocational training among pregnant and recently postpartum women (57). Forty women who continued abusing cocaine and heroin despite receiving methadone and intensive psychosocial treatment participated. Half were randomly assigned to a therapeutic workplace (TW) intervention, and the other half served as controls. Women in the TW condition earned vouchers for cocaine and heroin abstinence and for participating in vocational training. Across a 3-year period, women assigned to the therapeutic workplace sustained cocaine abstinence greater than controls (54% vs. 28% negative) and opiate abstinence greater than controls (60% vs. 37% negative).

An emerging area of investigation that is potentially important to the development of voucher-based CM is focused on combining them with antidepressant therapy with opioid- and cocaine-dependent patients. In a study of desipramine and voucher-based CM, for example, opioid- and cocaine-dependent patients were randomly assigned to one of four conditions: combined desipramine and voucher-based CM; placebo and voucher-based CM; desipramine and noncontingent voucher-based CM; or placebo and vouchers delivered noncontingently (i.e., independent of recent drug use) (58). Vouchers were delivered contingent on abstinence from both opioids and cocaine in the Voucher Based Reinforcement Therapy (VBRT) conditions. Abstinence from cocaine alone and from opioids and cocaine increased more in the desipramine and voucher-based CM condition compared to the other three conditions. A subsequent parallel study examining bupropion reported similar findings (59). This is an interesting area that warrants further investigation.

Among other innovative approaches involving CM in the treatment of cocaine use disorders was one combining day-treatment with access to work therapy and housing contingent on drug abstinence (60). A total of 176 homeless individuals who abused cocaine and other substances were randomly assigned to receive enhanced or usual care. Enhanced care involved 2 months of intensive 5-day-a-week clinic attendance. During the last 4 months of the 6-month treatment, intensity of day-treatment was reduced, and subjects could participate in a work-therapy program refurbishing condemned houses and also to reside in the refurbished housing for a modest rental fee. Participation in the work program and housing were contingent on drug abstinence. Usual care consisted of twice-weekly drug abuse counseling and referral to community agencies for housing and vocational services. The percent of urinalysis results positive for cocaine was significantly less in the enhanced compared to the control treatment across assessments conducted at 2, 6, and 12 months after treatment entry, though by the last assessment cocaine use in the enhanced condition had returned close to levels observed in the usual-care condition. Enhanced care also produced significantly greater reductions than usual care in alcohol use and fewer days of homelessness at the 6- and 12-month assessments.

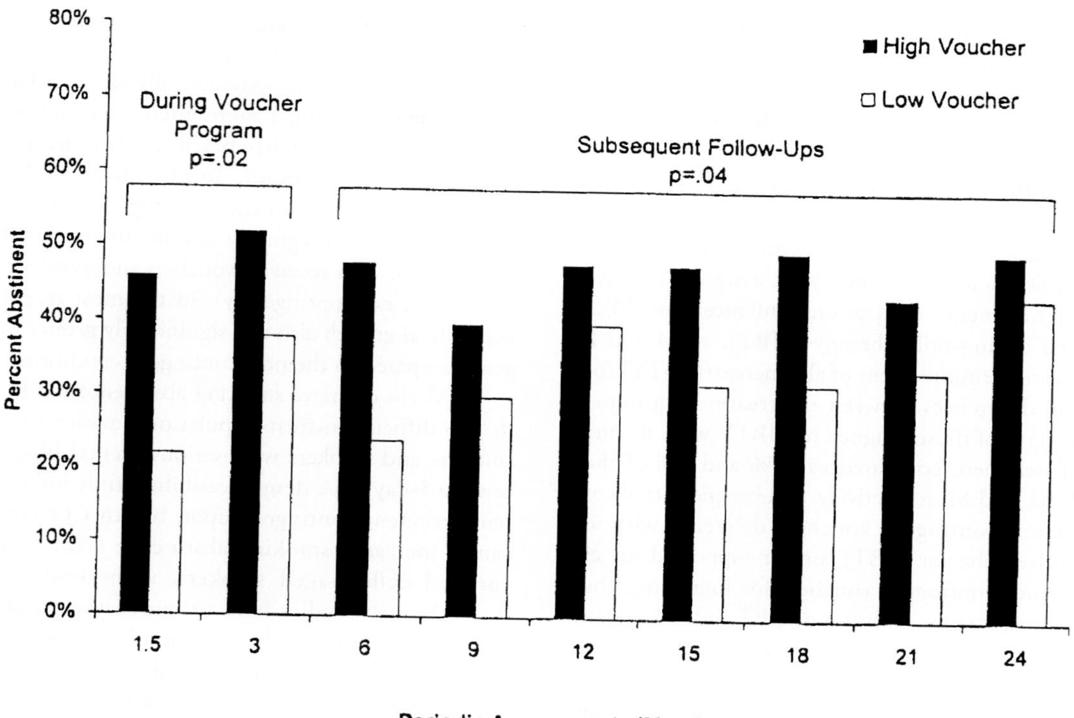

FIGURE 57.4. Longest duration of sustained cocaine abstinence. Longest duration of sustained cocaine abstinence achieved during the 12-week voucher condition. Each data point indicates data from an individual subject and the lines represent group means. Subjects in the reinforcement and control conditions are displayed in the left and right columns, respectively. *Open circles* represent early study drop outs. (Reprinted with permission from Silverman K, Higgins ST, Brooner RK, et al. Sustained cocaine abstinence in methadone maintenance patients through voucher-based reinforcement therapy. *Arch Gen Psychiatry* 1996;53:409–415.)

A follow-up study by this same group of investigators systematically replicated those findings (61). More recent studies have demonstrated the benefits of abstinence-contingent housing on outcomes (62) and the importance of the CM elements to improved outcomes in this multi-component intervention (63).

With the goal of improving chances that voucher-based CM approach could be disseminated to community clinics, Petry et al. (64) developed a variation known as prize-based CM. Rather than reinforce each occurrence of the target response, in this procedure patients earned the opportunity to draw from an urn that contained vouchers of varying value, including many that are of zero value but offer verbal praise, some that are of relatively low monetary value (e.g., $1), still fewer of moderate value ($20), and a very few worth high monetary value (i.e., $100). Rather than exchanging these vouchers for the opportunity to make retail purchases in the community, patients choose among items already available at the clinic that are referred to as prizes. Interestingly, the seminal report on this prize-based procedure represented a return to the use of CM in the treatment of alcohol abuse/dependence (64). Forty-two alcohol-dependent clients entering an intensive outpatient substance abuse clinic were randomly assigned to standard treatment plus CM or standard treatment only. In both groups, patients provided breath samples to a research assistant daily during the 4-week intensive day-program treatment and weekly during 4-week after-care. In the CM group, negative BALs and completion of preselected activities earned patients opportunities to win prizes of varying value. Results from the 8-week trial indicated that retention and abstinence were significantly higher in the CM condition (84% retention, 69% abstinence) than the control condition (22% retention, 39% abstinence).

As important, this prize-based arrangement has been demonstrated to be efficacious for increasing cocaine and other drug abstinence in drug-free and methadone community clinics (65,66). Those studies are very important to efforts at eventually disseminating CM interventions into community clinics. Worth clarifying, though is that there is no evidence that the prize-based arrangement results in better outcomes than a voucher-based program involving lower-than-usual voucher values. Indeed, in two direct comparisons of the prize- and voucher-based procedures with incentive costs at comparable levels, there were no significant difference between the two programs (67,68). There is no evidence that lowering costs with this prize-based arrangement gets around the inverse relationship already mentioned between treatment effect size and reinforcement magnitude in voucher-based CM interventions.

Indeed, as would be expected, effect sizes obtained with the prize-based intervention appear to be smaller than those achieved with more expensive CM interventions in comparable populations (23).

New Directions In an important extension of voucher-based CM, the intervention was extended to treatment of marijuana use disorders. In a seminal randomized controlled trial on this topic, 60 men and women were assigned to one of three, 14-week treatments: motivational enhancement (M), M plus behavioral coping-skills therapy (MBT), or M and BT plus voucher-based reinforcement of abstinence (MBTV) (69). There were no differences between the treatment groups in retention, but 35% of those assigned to MBTV were abstinent at the end of treatment compared to 10% and 5% of those assigned to MBT and M, respectively. A subsequent trial comparing abstinence contingent vouchers delivered with and without cognitive behavior (CBT) further supported the efficacy of abstinence-contingent vouchers for increasing abstinence and showed that the addition of CBT did not enhance outcomes during treatment but may do so after the vouchers are discontinued (70).

A feasibility study demonstrated the sensitivity of marijuana use by 18 non-treatment-seeking outpatients with schizophrenia to monetary incentives for abstinence (71). During two baseline conditions, participants received money independent of their urinalysis results. During three incentive conditions, participants received money incentives varying from $25 to $100 contingent on urine toxicology results indicating marijuana abstinence. Abstinence increased in the contingent compared to the baseline conditions, thereby demonstrating the sensitivity of marijuana use to the reinforcement contingencies. With several individuals, marijuana use was not sensitive to the contingencies, even when the monetary amount was increased to the $100/test value. An important practical question not answered in this initial feasibility study was how much the incentives could have been lowered in value without losing efficacy among those who were sensitive to the incentives. That question merits investigation. A follow-up study in this same population demonstrated similar positive outcomes when abstinence-contingent vouchers rather than cash payments were used among marijuana abusers with serious mental illness (72).

Voucher-based reinforcement of abstinence has been successfully extended to the treatment of pregnant cigarette smokers. In a seminal study (73), 220 pregnant smokers were randomly assigned to a treatment group involving contingent vouchers for abstinence or a control group. Women in both groups received smoking-cessation self-help kits. Those in the treatment group were requested to include an SO in treatment. All participants were telephoned monthly and asked to self-report smoking status. Those in the treatment condition who reported abstinence were invited to the clinic to provide a saliva specimen. If the specimen confirmed abstinence, the participant earned a $50 voucher, and the SO received a voucher as well. A greater percentage of smokers in the treatment than control conditions (32% vs. 9%) were abstinent at 8 months' gestation, and that difference was maintained at the 2-month postpartum assessment (21% vs. 6%).

Those results were systematically replicated and extended in two trials involving a more intense schedule of abstinence monitoring and voucher-based contingent reinforcement (74,75). In both studies, approximately 40% of women assigned to receive abstinence-contingent vouchers were abstinent at an end-of-pregnancy assessment compared to approximately 10% who received vouchers independent of smoking status (i.e., noncontingently). In the most recent study, estimated fetal growth also was significantly greater in the contingent compared to the non-contingent conditions (74).

CM for cigarette smoking abstinence has been extended to two difficult-to-treat populations, adolescent/college-aged smokers and smokers with serious mental illness. In adolescents, a 5-day ABA-design feasibility study indicated that cash reinforcement contingent upon breath CO samples significantly increased smoking abstinence (76). A similar study enrolled college-aged smokers, with similar results (77). Recently, two studies have extended the duration of these interventions. In a study that combined CM with psychosocial treatment for adolescent smokers in a school setting, 28 participants who received a 4-week CM plus CBT intervention had more biochemically-verified abstinence in weeks 1 and 4 compared to those in CBT only (78). Another study examined CM for smoking in 23 adolescent smokers and found that contingently reinforcing smoking reductions for several days prior to an abstinence-based CM trial enhanced CM effects (79).

Schizophrenia is associated with high rates of smoking and low smoking-cessation success. A feasibility study of CM for smoking reductions in this population used an ABA-design in outpatients with schizophrenia who were not seeking treatment for smoking and demonstrated that cash reinforcement of CO reductions significantly reduced smoking (80). These results were systematically replicated, though the addition of nicotine replacement therapy did not enhance the efficacy of the monetary incentives (81). Results from several rigorous laboratory-based studies also support the sensitivity of smoking among schizophrenics to reinforcement contingencies and other environmental manipulations (82,83). Overall, innovations in the use of CM for cigarette smoking include targeting difficult-to-treat populations and incorporating pharmacotherapy or psychotherapy to enhance or prolong the effects of CM.

In another promising extension of CM, 113 patients with methamphetamine use disorders were randomly assigned to 12 weeks of either treatment as usual or treatment as usual plus the fishbowl CM intervention as part of the CTN studies previously described (84). Urine samples were tested for commonly used illicit drugs, and breath samples were tested for alcohol. The reinforcers for drug-negative samples were plastic chips, some of which could be exchanged for prizes. Patients receiving CM in addition to usual treatment submitted significantly more negative samples, and they were abstinent for a longer period of time (5 vs. 3 weeks).

Conclusions There is no longer any question that CM interventions are efficacious. No fewer than three separate meta-analyses specifically examining CM interventions offer overwhelming evidence supporting their efficacy, with effect sizes generally in the moderate range according to Cohen's standard (23,85,86). In a fourth meta-analysis examining the efficacy of psychosocial treatments for SUDs, CM was examined along with relapse prevention therapy, general CBT, and combined CBT and CM (87). The largest effects across the different therapies were obtained with CM.

CM treatments clearly represent an important part of evidence-based treatments for SUDs and, as was amply demonstrated earlier, have developed in many exciting directions during the past three decades. The varied CM applications outlined in this chapter demonstrate the striking effectiveness and versatility of CM interventions, and the feasibility of disseminating them into community treatment clinics and other settings. Though the promise of CM interventions for treating SUDs across a broad range of substances, populations, and settings is clear, more research is needed on how to (1) increase the proportion of patients who have positive outcomes, (2) sustain treatment effects over time, and (3) to continue to develop and refine practical applications that will be used widely in society.

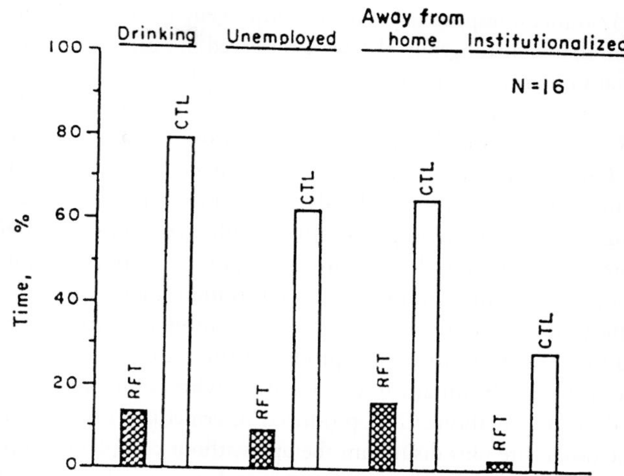

FIGURE 57.5. Comparison of CRA and control groups on key dependent measures. Comparison of the CRA and control groups on key dependent measures during the 6-months of follow-up after hospital discharge: mean percentage of time spent drinking, unemployed, away from home, and institutionalized. (Reprinted with permission from Hunt GM, Azrin NH. A community-reinforcement approach to alcoholism. *Behav Res Ther* 1973;11:91–104.)

Community Reinforcement Approach CRA was developed and most extensively researched in the treatment of alcohol-dependent adults. Subsequently, CRA was extended to the treatment of cocaine- and opioid-dependent adults, adolescents with SUDs, and families of treatment-resistant patients with SUDs. Each of those applications is addressed now.

Initial Study The seminal CRA study was conducted with 16 severe alcoholics admitted to a rural state hospital for treatment of alcoholism (88). These men were divided into eight matched pairs. Pair members were randomly assigned to receive CRA plus standard hospital care or standard care alone. Standard hospital care consisted of 25 one-hour didactic sessions involving lectures on Alcoholics Anonymous, alcoholism, and related medical problems.

CRA was designed to rearrange and improve the quality of the reinforcers obtained by patients through their vocational, family, social, and recreational activities. The goal was for these reinforcers to be available and of high quality when the patient was sober and unavailable when drinking resumed. Plans for rearranging these reinforcers were individualized to conform to each patient's unique situation.

During the 6-month follow-up period after hospital discharge, time spent drinking was 14% for participants in CRA versus 79% for those in standard treatment (Fig. 57.5). Those treated with CRA had superior outcomes on a number of other outcome measures as well.

Further Developing the Community Reinforcement Approach After publication of the seminal study, CRA was subsequently expanded to include disulfiram therapy, with monitoring by an SO to ensure medication compliance. Additionally, counseling directed at crises resolution was added, as was a "buddy" system in which individuals in the alcoholic's neighborhood volunteered to be available to give assistance with practical issues such as repairing cars and the like and a switch from individual to group counseling to reduce cost. This revised intervention was investigated in a study where 20 matched pairs of hospitalized alcoholic men were randomly assigned to receive this "improved" CRA or standard hospital care (89). Standard care included advice to take disulfiram but no steps to ensure medication compliance. During the 6 months after hospital discharge, outcomes achieved with CRA were superior to standard care in terms of percent time spent drinking (2% vs. 55%), time unemployed (20% vs. 56%), time away from family (7% vs. 67%), and time institutionalized (0% vs. 45%). The CRA group spent 90% or more of the time abstinent during a 2-year follow-up period; comparable data were not reported for the standard treatment group.

Another study completed as part of the original CRA series examined the effects of adding the social club previously described to a standard regimen of outpatient counseling (90). The club was designed to have the social atmosphere of a tavern but without alcohol. Individuals had to be abstinent to attend. Forty male and female alcoholics were randomly assigned to a group that was encouraged to attend the social club or to a control group that was not. At 3-month follow-up, drinking in the social-club group decreased from a baseline average of 4.67 ounces of alcohol consumed daily to 0.85 ounces, whereas in the control group, values were 3.56 and

3.32 ounces, respectively. Greater improvements in the social-club than control group also were observed in ratings of behavioral impairment and time spent in heavy-drinking situations.

Azrin et al. (91) also completed a study dissociating the effects of monitored disulfiram therapy from the other aspects of CRA. In a parallel-groups design, 43 male and female alcoholic outpatients were randomly assigned to receive usual care plus disulfiram therapy without compliance support, usual care plus disulfiram therapy involving SOs to support compliance, or CRA in combination with disulfiram therapy and significant-other support. CRA in combination with disulfiram and compliance procedures produced the greatest reductions in drinking, disulfiram in combination with compliance procedures but without CRA produced intermediate results, and the usual care plus disulfiram therapy without compliance support produced the poorest outcome. Interestingly, married patients did equally well with the full CRA treatment or disulfiram plus compliance procedures alone. Only unmarried subjects appeared to need CRA treatment plus monitored disulfiram to achieve abstinence. This was the first full report on the efficacy of CRA with less-impaired outpatients. With these less impaired individuals, treatment group differences were noted on measures of drinking only, whereas in the prior studies with more severe hospitalized alcoholics, differences also were discerned on measures of time institutionalized and employed.

Extending the Community Reinforcement Approach to Treatment of Patients with Cocaine and Opioid-Use Disorders Studies on the use of CRA to treat cocaine use disorders represented, to our knowledge, the first reports on the use of CRA from investigators who were not part of the original investigative team of Azrin et al. As was mentioned, these studies examined a treatment involving CRA in combination with voucher-based CM (CRA + vouchers). The initial two trials involved comparisons of this combined treatment to standard outpatient drug-abuse counseling (11,48). The first trial was 12 weeks in duration, and 28 cocaine-dependent outpatients were assigned as consecutive admissions to their respective treatment conditions. The second trial was 24 weeks in duration, and 38 cocaine-dependent patients were randomly assigned to the same two treatment conditions. Outcomes in both trials were significantly better among those treated with the CRA + voucher treatment than standard drug abuse counseling. In the randomized trial, for example, 58% of patients assigned to CRA + vouchers completed the recommended 24 weeks of treatment compared to 11% of those assigned to drug abuse counseling. Regarding cocaine use, 68% of those assigned to CRA + vouchers were objectively verified to have achieved 8 or more weeks of continuous cocaine abstinence as compared to only 11% of those treated with drug abuse counseling. A randomized controlled trial conducted in Spain using CRA plus a variation of the voucher intervention reported positive improvements in retention and cocaine abstinence as compared to standard care, thereby demonstrating the generality of the CRA + vouchers intervention to communities outside of the United States (92).

As was discussed, subsequent trials on this treatment generally focused on experimentally isolating the contributions of the voucher intervention to outcomes during treatment (49) and posttreatment follow-up (51,52). The exception was a randomized clinical trial designed to isolate the contributions of CRA to the combined effects of the CRA + vouchers intervention (93). In the latter study, 100 cocaine-dependent outpatients were randomly assigned to receive the CRA + vouchers treatment or the vouchers component only. Vouchers were in place for 12 weeks, CRA for 24 weeks, and patients were assessed at least every 3 months for 2 years after treatment entry. Patients treated with CRA + vouchers were retained better in treatment, used cocaine at a lower frequency during treatment but not follow-up, and reported a lower frequency of drinking to intoxication during treatment and follow-up as compared with patients treated with vouchers only. Patients treated with CRA + vouchers also reported a higher frequency of days of paid employment during treatment and 6 months of posttreatment follow-up, decreased depressive symptoms during treatment only, and fewer hospitalizations and legal problems during follow-up. The results provided a strong case that CRA contributed in numerous ways to the positive outcomes observed during treatment and post-treatment follow-up with the CRA + vouchers treatment, while also providing a systematic replication of the seminal findings of Azrin et al.

We know of two trials that have been reported wherein CRA was investigated in the treatment of opioid-dependent patients receiving opioid pharmacotherapy (30,94). The first of those two trials examined whether the CRA + vouchers treatment could improve what are usually poor outcomes with opioid detoxifications (30). Thirty-nine outpatients undergoing a 24-week buprenorphine detoxification were randomly assigned to CRA + vouchers or standard drug abuse counseling. Those assigned to CRA + vouchers were more likely to complete the detoxification protocol (53% vs. 20%) and achieved greater periods of biochemically-confirmed abstinence from illicit-opioid use.

In the second trial (94), 181methadone maintenance patients were randomly assigned to CRA or drug abuse counseling. More patients treated with CRA than drug abuse counseling achieved 3 or more weeks of biochemically-verified abstinence from illicit-opiate use (89% vs. 78%). No other significant differences were reported. Considered together, these two trials are encouraging that CRA delivered alone or in combination with voucher-based CM can improve outcomes above that achieved with standard drug abuse counseling among opioid-dependent patients receiving opioid-substitution detoxification and maintenance therapies.

Extending the Community Reinforcement Approach to Special Populations CRA has been successfully extended to at least two special subpopulations, adolescents and the homeless. The first study with adolescents involved 82 individuals randomly assigned to CRA or supportive counseling (95). The intervention had three major components: stimulus control, urge control, and social control/contracting. The

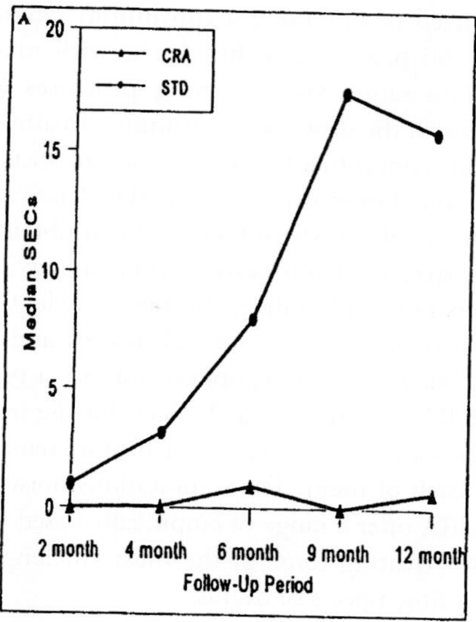

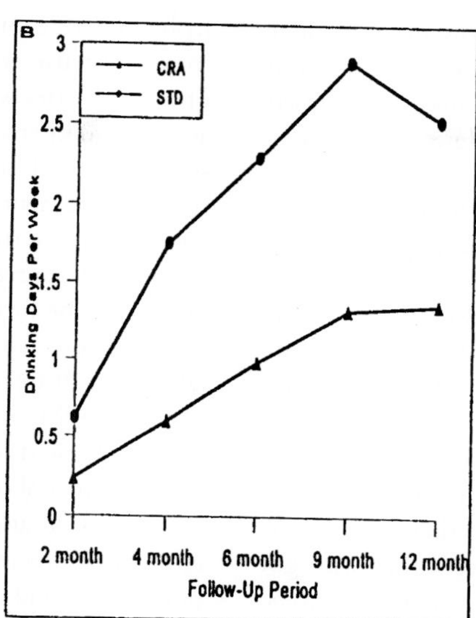

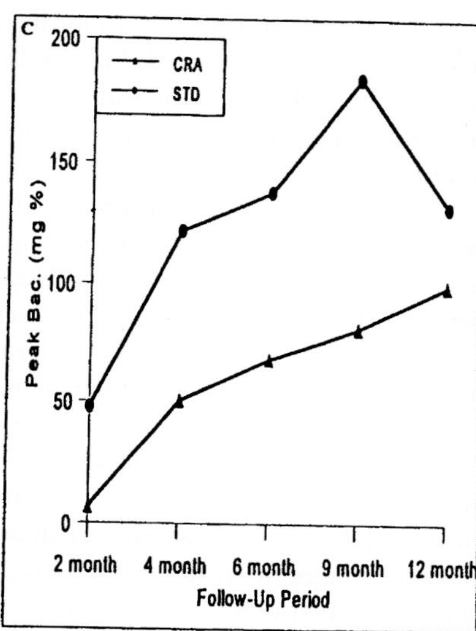

FIGURE 57.6. Comparison of CRA and standard treatment groups on key dependent measures. Comparison of the CRA and standard treatment groups on standard ethanol content **(A)**, drinking days per week **(B)**, and peak blood alcohol concentration **(C)**. (Reprinted with permission from Smith JE, Meyers RJ, Delaney HD. The community reinforcement approach with homeless alcohol-dependent individuals. *J Consult Clin Psychol* 1998;66:541–548.)

stimulus control component involved assisting youth in identifying safe and risky situations for substance use and therapist-assisted problem solving regarding how to increase the amount of time spent in the former and decrease time spent in the latter. Urge control involved teaching youth to recognize the early internal events that were precursors to drug use and how to interrupt them with alternative activities that are incompatible with drug use. Social control/contracting focused on involving parents in providing youth with opportunities to engage in safe activities contingent on youth compliance with activities that are incompatible with substance abuse. Abstinence from drug use in the CRA condition ranged between 37% and 65% across the 12-month study period as compared to 20% in the supportive counseling condition. Measures of attendance at school and employment, family relationships, depression, and time institutionalized were also better in the CRA as compared to the supportive counseling condition. Later follow-up results collected 9 months after completion of the initial study period indicated better outcomes in the CRA compared to the supportive counseling conditions (95).

Adolescent CRA therapy was compared to motivational enhancement therapy plus CBT (MET/CBT) and multidimensional family therapy (MDFT) in a multi-site trial conducted with 300 adolescent cannabis users (96). Therapy was approximately 3 months in duration, and patients were followed up for 1 year. Across that time period, overall percent of patients in recovery was somewhat higher among patients treated with CRA than MET/CBT and MDFT (34%, 23%, and 19%, respectively). That difference was not statistically significant overall, though it was at several of the individual sites.

The use of CRA with homeless individuals was examined in two studies involving adult alcoholics (97) and street-living youth (98). In the study with adults, 106 alcohol-dependent homeless persons were randomly assigned to CRA or standard treatment at a large day shelter. Those treated with CRA showed greater improvement on measures of drinking across five assessments conducted over a one-year period (Fig. 57.6). Both conditions showed marked improvement in employment and housing stability. In the study with youth, 180 individuals between 14 and 19 years who attended an urban community drop-in center were randomly assigned to receive adolescent CRA or usual care. Substance use decreased during a 6-month study period among a larger proportion of those treated with CRA than usual care (37% vs. 17%) as did depression scores (40% vs. 23%) and measures of social stability increased more among those treated with CRA than usual care (58% vs. 13%).

Extending the Community Reinforcement Approach to Assist Relatives of Treatment-Resistant Persons with Substance Use Disorders As part of the original series of studies on CRA, Sisson and Azrin (99) adapted CRA for use with the SOs of treatment-resistant alcoholics. Twelve SOs were randomly assigned to receive either the CRA intervention (n = 7) or a standard program (n = 5) involving group instruction about alcohol and the disease model of alcoholism. The CRA intervention included education about alcohol problems, information and discussion of the positive consequences of not drinking, assistance in involving the alcoholic in healthy activities, increasing the involvement of the SO in social and recreational activities, and training in how to respond to drinking episodes (including dangerous situations) and how to recommend treatment entry to the alcoholic family member. In the control group, none of the alcoholics entered treatment during the 3-month follow-up, and their drinking remained unchanged. In the CRA group, six of seven alcoholics entered treatment, and average drinking decreased from 25 days per month at pretreatment to fewer than 5 days per month after treatment.

A series of subsequent controlled trials have consistently supported the efficacy of CRA in assisting concerned significant others (COSs) to get unmotivated individuals with alcohol use disorders (100) and individuals with illicit-drug use disorders (101,102) to enter treatment. The treatment has come to be referred to as community reinforcement and family training (CRAFT). In the most recent of the trials, for example, 90 COSs of treatment-refusing illicit-drug users were randomly assigned to CRAFT, CRAFT with additional after-care sessions, or Al-Anon and Nar-Anon facilitation therapy (Al-Nar-FT). Percentages of treatment-refusing loved ones who got engaged in treatment after the intervention were 58.6%, 76.7%, and 29.0%, respectively, in CRAFT alone, CRAFT plus afterare, and Al-Nar-FT, respectively.

Conclusions Considered together, the evidence reviewed earlier supporting the efficacy of CRA is quite robust. There has been at least one meta-analysis supporting the efficacy of CRA as a treatment for SUDs (103). The evidence is strong in support of CRA's efficacy in treating alcohol dependence, even when the clinical situation is complicated by homelessness. The evidence is also quite strong regarding the efficacy of CRA combined with voucher-based CM for outpatient treatment of cocaine dependence. Experimental evidence demonstrates that CRA and voucher-based CM each contribute significantly to the positive outcomes achieved with that intervention. The evidence in support of CRA plus vouchers or CRA alone in the treatment of opioid-use disorders is positive but still relatively limited. Studies further evaluating the efficacy of CRA with and without contingent vouchers in this population will be helpful in more fully elucidating how this treatment approach can be utilized to better optimize outcomes during opioid-replacement therapy. The evidence supporting the efficacy of adolescent CRA even when complicated by homelessness is positive and encouraging. Indeed, CRA seems to have much unrealized potential for treatment of special populations with SUDs such as those with serious mental illness or perhaps complications related to other illness (e.g., HIV or other infectious disease). For those who might be interested, therapist manuals are available on the use of CRA to treat alcohol abuse/dependence (104) cocaine dependence (12), and adolescent marijuana abuse (105). Overall, CRA is clearly capable of making substantive contributions to the development of evidence-based treatments for a wide range of different types of SUDs, populations, problems, and settings.

CONCLUSIONS

This chapter has reviewed how within an operant framework drug use is considered a normal, learned behavior that can be fruitfully conceptualized to fall along a continuum ranging from light use with no problems to heavy use with many untoward effects. The same basic learning processes are assumed to operate across the drug-use continuum. Treatment strategies based on this conceptual framework look to weaken the reinforcement obtained from drug use and related activities and to enhance the material and social reinforcement obtained from other sources, especially from participation in activities deemed to be incompatible with a drug-abusing lifestyle. CM and CRA procedures are based on this general strategy and are efficacious in treating alcohol, cocaine, opioid, and other types of SUDs. CM and CRA offer no "magic bullets" for the treatment of these disorders and, as discussed, much more remains to be learned about each of them. Those limitations notwithstanding, CM and CRA offer a range of empirically based and effective strategies for treating some of the most challenging populations and daunting aspects of SUDs.

ACKNOWLEDGMENTS: *Preparation of this chapter was supported by Research Grants DA09378, DA08076, and DA14028 and Training Grant DA07242 from the National Institute on Drug Abuse.*

REFERENCES

1. Mazur JE. *Learning and behavior*, 5th ed. Upper Saddle River, NJ: Prentice-Hall, 2002.
2. Higgins ST, Silverman K, Heil SH, eds. *Contingency management in substance abuse treatment.* New York: The Guilford Press, 2008.
3. Schuster CR, Thompson T. Self-administration of and behavioral dependence on drugs. *Ann Rev Pharmacol* 1969;9:483–502.
4. Aigner TG, Balster RL. Choice behavior in rhesus monkeys: cocaine versus food. *Science* 1978;201:434–435.
5. Bigelow GE, Griffiths R, Liebson I. Experimental models for the modification of human drug self-administration: methodological developments in the study of ethanol self-administration by alcoholics. *Fed Proc* 1975;34:1785–1792.
6. Miller PM, Hersen M, Eisler RM. Relative effectiveness of instructions, agreements, and reinforcement in behavioral contracts with alcoholics. *J Abnorm Psychol* 1974;83:548–553.
7. Elliot R & Tighe T. Breaking the cigarette habit: effects of a technique involving threatened loss of memory. *Psychol Rec* 1968;18:503–513.
8. Winett RA. Parameters of deposit contracts in the modification of smoking. *Psychol Rec* 1973;23:49–60.
9. Higgins ST, Heil SH, Lussier JP. Clinical implications of reinforcement as a determinant of substance use disorders. *Ann Rev Psychol* 2004; 55:431–461.
10. Higgins ST. Some potential contributions of reinforcement and consumer-demand theory to reducing cocaine use. *Addict Behav* 1996;21:803–816.
11. Higgins ST, Delaney DD, Budney AJ, et al. A behavioral approach to achieving initial cocaine abstinence. *Am J Psychiatry* 1991;148:1218–1224.
12. Budney AJ, Higgins ST. *The community reinforcement plus vouchers approach: Manual 2. National Institute on Drug Abuse therapy manuals for drug addiction.* NIH publication #98-4308. Rockville, MD: National Institute on Drug Abuse, 1998.
13. Festinger DS, Lamb RJ, Kirby KC, Marlow DB. The accelerated intake: a method for increasing initial attendance to outpatient cocaine treatment. *J Appl Behav Anal* 1996;29:387–389.
14. Miller WR, Tonigan JS. Assessing drinkers' motivation to change: the Stages of Change Readiness and Treatment Eagerness Scale (SOCRATES). *Psychol Addict Behav* 1996;10:81–89.

15. Washton AM, Stone NS, Hendrickson EC. *Cocaine abuse*. In: Donovan DM, Marlatt GA, eds. *Assessment of addictive behavior*. New York: Guilford Press, 1988:364–389.
16. Selzer ML. The Michigan Alcoholism Screening Test: the quest for a new diagnostic instrument. *Am J Psychiatry* 1971;127:1653–1658.
17. Beck AT, Ward CH, Mendelson M, et al. An inventory for measuring depression. *Arch Gen Psychiatry* 1961;4:561–571.
18. Derogatis LR. Misuse of the symptom checklist 90. *Arch Gen Psychiatry* 1983;40:1152–1153.
19. Sobell LC, Sobell MB. Timeline follow-back: a technique for assessing self-reported alcohol consumption. In: Litten RZ, Allen JP, eds. *Measuring alcohol consumption: psychosocial and biochemical methods*. Totowa, NJ: Humana Press, 1992:41–72.
20. McLellan AT, Luborsky L, Cacciola J, et al. New data from the Addiction Severity Index: reliability and validity in three centers. *J Nerv Ment Dis* 1985;173:412–423.
21. Carroll KM, Nich C, Ball SA, et al. Treatment of cocaine and alcohol dependence with psychotherapy and disulfiram. *Addiction* 1998;93: 713–728.
22. Higgins ST, Silverman K. Contingency management. In: Galanter M, Kleber HD, eds. *Textbook of substance abuse treatment*, 4th ed. Washington, DC: The American Psychiatric Press (in press).
23. Lussier JP, Heil SH, Mongeon JA, et al. A meta-analysis of voucher-based reinforcement therapy for substance use disorders. *Addiction* 2006;101:192–203.
24. Lewinsohn PM, Munoz RF, Youngren MA, Zeiss AM. *Control your depression*. New York: Simon & Schuster, 1986.
25. Munoz RF, Miranda J. *Individual therapy manual for cognitive behavioral treatment for depression*. Santa Monica, CA: RAND Corporation, 2000.
26. Azrin NH, Besalel VA. *Job Club counselor's manual*. Baltimore: University Park Press, 1980.
27. O'Farrel TJ, Fals-Stewart W. Alcohol abuse. In: Sprenkle DH, ed. *Effectiveness research in marriage and family therapy*. Alexandria, VA: American Association for Marriage and Family Therapy, 2002:123–161.
28. Heil SH, Sigmon S, Mongeon JA, Higgins ST. Characterizing and improving HIV/AIDS knowledge among cocaine-dependent outpatients. *Exp Clin Psychopharmacol* 2005;13:238–243.
29. Smith JE, Meyers RJ. The community reinforcement approach. In: Hester R, Miller W, eds, *Handbook of alcoholism treatment approaches: effective alternatives*, 2nd ed. New York: Allyn & Bacon, 1995.
30. Bickel WK, Amass L, Higgins ST, et al. Effects of adding behavioral treatment to opioid detoxification with buprenorphine. *J Consult Clin Psychol* 1997;65:803–810.
31. Budney AJ, Higgins ST, Wong CJ. Marijuana use and treatment outcome in cocaine-dependent patients. *Exp Clin Psychopharmacol* 1996;4:396–403.
32. Miller PM. A behavioral intervention program for chronic public drunkenness offenders. *Arch Gen Psychiatry* 1975;32:915–918.
33. Bickel WK, Rizzuto P, Zielony RD, et al. Combined behavioral and pharmacological treatment of alcoholic methadone patients. *J Subst Abuse* 1989;1:161–171.
34. Liebson IA, Bigelow GE, Flamer R. Alcoholism among methadone patients: a specific treatment model. *Am J Psychiatry* 1973;130:483–485.
35. Liebson IA, Tommasello A, Bigelow GE. A behavioral treatment of alcoholic methadone patients. *Ann Intern Med* 1978;89:342-344.
36. Brigham SL, Rekers GA, Rosen AC, et al. Contingency management in the treatment of adolescent alcohol drinking problems. *J Psychol* 1981; 109:73–85.
37. Carrol KM, Ball SA, Nich C, et al. Targeting behavioral therapies to enhance naltrexone treatment of opioid dependence: efficacy of contingency management and significant other involvement. *Arch Gen Psychiatry* 2001;58:755–761.
38. Preston KL, Silverman K, Umbricht A, et al. Improvement in naltrexone treatment compliance with contingency management. *Drug Alcohol Depend* 1999;54:127–135.
39. Rounsaville BJ, Rosen M, Carroll KM. Medication compliance. In: Higgins ST, Silverman K, Heil SH, eds. *Contingency management in substance abuse treatment*. New York: The Guilford Press, 2008:140–158.
40. Iguchi MY, Stitzer ML, Bigelow GE, Liebson IA. Contingency management in methadone maintenance: effects of reinforcing and aversive consequences on illicit polydrug use. *Drug Alcohol Depend* 1988;22:1–7.
41. Magura S, Casriel C, Goldsmith DS, et al. Contingency contracting with polydrug-abusing methadone patients. *Addict Behav* 1988;13:113–118.
42. Milby JB, Garrett C, English C, et al. Take-home methadone: contingency effects on drug-seeking and productivity of narcotic addicts. *Addict Behav* 1978;3:215–220.
43. Stitzer ML, Bigelow GE. Contingency management in a methadone maintenance program: availability of reinforcers. *Int J Addict* 1978;13:737–746.
44. Stitzer ML, Iguchi MY, Felch LJ. Contingent take-home incentive: effects on drug use of methadone maintenance patients. *J Consult Clin Psychol* 1992;60:927–934.
45. Higgins ST, Stitzer ML, Bigelow GE, Liebson IA. Contingent methadone delivery: effects on illicit-opiate use. *Drug Alcohol Depend* 1986;17:311–322.
46. Stitzer ML, Bickel WK, Bigelow GE, Liebson IA. Effect of methadone dose contingencies on urinalysis test results of polydrug-abusing methadone-maintenance patients. *Drug Alcohol Depend* 1986;18:341–348.
47. Higgins ST, Alessi SM, Dantona RL. Voucher-based incentives: a substance abuse treatment innovation. *Addict Behav* 2002;27:887–910.
48. Higgins ST, Budney AJ, Bickel WK, et al. Achieving cocaine abstinence with a behavioral approach. *Am J Psychiatry* 1993;150:763–769.
49. Higgins ST, Budney AJ, Bickel WK, et al. Incentives improve treatment retention and cocaine abstinence in ambulatory cocaine-dependent patients. *Arch Gen Psychiatry* 1994;51:568–576.
50. Higgins ST, Budney AJ, Bickel WK, et al. Outpatient behavioral treatment for cocaine dependence: one-year outcome. *Exp Clin Psychopharmacol* 1995;3:205–212.
51. Higgins ST, Wong CJ, Badger GJ, et al. Contingent reinforcement increases cocaine abstinence during outpatient treatment and 1-year of follow-up. *J Consult Clin Psychol* 2000;68:64–72.
52. Higgins ST, Heil SH, Dontona RL, et al. Effects of varying the monetary value of voucher-based incentives on abstinence achieved during and following treatment among cocaine-dependent outpatients. *Addiction* 2007;102:271–281.
53. Silverman K, Higgins ST, Brooner RK, et al. Sustained cocaine abstinence in methadone maintenance patients through voucher-based reinforcement therapy. *Arch Gen Psychiatry* 1996;53:409–415.
54. Silverman K, Preston KL, Stitzer ML, Schuster CR. Treatment of cocaine abuse in methadone maintenance patients. In: Higgins ST, Katz JL eds. *Cocaine abuse research: pharmacology, behavior, and clinical application*. San Diego: Academic Press, 1998:363–388.
55. Silverman K, Chutuape MA, Bigelow GE, Stitzer ML. Voucher-based reinforcement of cocaine abstinence in treatment-resistant methadone patients: effects of reinforcer magnitude. *Psychopharmacology* 1999;146:128–138.
56. Kirby KC, Marlowe DB, Festinger DS, et al. Schedule of voucher delivery influences initiation of cocaine abstinence. *J Consult Clin Psychol* 1998;66:761–767.
57. Silverman K, Svikis D, Wong CJ, et al. A reinforcement-based therapeutic workplace for the treatment of drug abuse: three-year abstinence outcomes. *Exp Clin Psychopharmacol* 2002;10:228–240.
58. Kosten T, Olivet A, Feingold A, et al. Desipramine and contingency management for cocaine and opiate dependence in buprenorphine maintained patients. *Drug Alcohol Depend* 2003;70:315–325.
59. Poling J, Oliveto A, Petry N, et al. Six-month trial of bupropion with contingency management for cocaine dependence in a methadone-maintained population. *Arch Gen Psychiatry* 2006;63:219–228.
60. Milby JB, Schumacher JE, Raczynski JM, et al. Sufficient conditions for effective treatment of substance abusing homeless persons. *Drug Alcohol Depend* 1996;43:39–47.
61. Milby JB, Schumacher JE, McNamara C, et al. Initiating abstinence in cocaine abusing dually diagnosed homeless persons. *Drug Alcohol Depend* 2000;60:55–67.
62. Milby JB, Schumacher, JE, Wallace D, et al. To house or not to house: the effects of providing housing to homeless substance abusers in treatment. *Am J Public Health* 2005;95:1259–1265.

63. Milby JE, Schumacher JE, Vuchinich RE, et al. Toward cost-effective initial care for substance-abusing homeless. *J Subst Abuse Treat* 2008;34: 180–191.
64. Petry NM, Martin B, Cooney JL, Kranzler HR. Give them prizes, and they will come: contingency management for treatment of alcohol dependence. *J Consult Clin Psychol* 2000;68:250–257.
65. Petry NM, Peirce JM, Stitzer ML, et al. Prize-based incentives improve outcomes of stimulant abusers in outpatients psychosocial treatment programs: a national drug abuse treatment Clinical Trials Network study. *Arch Gen Psychiatry* 2005;62:1148–1156.
66. Pierce JM, Petry NM, Stiter ML, et al. Effects of lower-cost incentives on stimulant abstinence in methadone maintenance treatment: a national drug abuse treatment Clinical Trials Network study. *Arch Gen Psychiatry* 2006;63:201–208.
67. Petry NM, Alessi SM, Marx J, et al. Vouchers versus prizes: contingency management treatment of substance abusers in community settings. *J Consult Clin Psychol* 2005;73:1005–1014.
68. Petry NM, Alessi SM, Hanson T, Sierra S. Randomized trial of contingent prizes versus vouchers in cocaine-using methadone patients. *J Consult Clin Psychol* 2007;75:983–991.
69. Budney AJ, Higgins ST, Radonovich KJ, Novy PL. Adding voucher-based incentives to coping skills and motivational enhancement improves outcomes during treatment for marijuana dependence. *J Consult Clin Psychol* 2000;68:1051–1061.
70. Budney AJ, Moore BA Higgins S, Rocha HL. Clinical trial of abstinence-based vouchers and cognitive-behavioral therapy for cannabis dependence. *J Consult Clin Psychol* 2006;74:307–316.
71. Sigmon SC, Steingard S, Badger GJ, et al. Contingent reinforcement of marijuana abstinence among individuals with serious mental illness: a feasibility study. *Exp Clin Psychopharmacol* 2000;8:509–517.
72. Sigmon SC, Higgins ST. Voucher-based contingent reinforcement of marijuana abstinence among individuals with serious mental illness. *Subst Abuse Treat* 2006;30:291–295.
73. Donatelle RJ, Prows SL, Champeau D, Hudson D. Randomised controlled trial using social support and financial incentives for high risk regnant smokers: significant other supporter (SOS) program. *Tobac Control* 2000;9(Suppl 3):III67–III69.
74. Heil SH, Higgins ST, Bernstein IM, et al. *Effects of voucher-based incentives on abstinence from cigarette smoking and fetal growth among pregnant women* (in press).
75. Higgins ST, Heil SH, Solomon LJ, et al. A pilot study on voucher-based incentives to promote abstinence from cigarette smoking during pregnancy and postpartum. *Nicotine Tobac Res* 2004;6:1015–1020.
76. Corby EA, Roll JM, Ledgerwood DM, Schuster CR. Contingency management interventions for treating adolescents: a feasibility study. *Exp Clin Psychopharmacol* 2000;8:371–376.
77. Correia CJ, Benson TA. The use of contingency management to reduce cigarette smoking among college students. *Exp Clin Psychopharmacol* 2006;14:171–179.
78. Krishnan-Sarin S, Duhig AM, McKee SA, et al. Contingency management for smoking cessation in adolescent smokers. *Exp Clin Psychopharmacol* 2006;14:306–310.
79. Tevyaw T, Gwaltney C, Tidey JW, et al. Contingency management for adolescent smokers: An exploratory study. *J Child Adolesc Subst Abuse* 2007;16:23–44.
80. Roll JM, Higgins ST, Steingard S,McGinley M. Investigating the use of monetary reinforcement to reduce the cigarette smoking of schizophrenics: a feasibility study. *Exp Clin Psychopharmacol* 1998;6:157–161.
81. Tidey JW, O'Neill SC, Higgins ST. Contingent monetary reinforcement of smoking reductions, with and without transdermal nicotine, in outpatients with schizophrenia. *Exp Clin Psychopharmacol* 2002;10:241–247.
82. Tidey JW, Higgins ST, Bickel WK, Steingard S. Effects of response requirement and the availability of an alternative reinforcer on cigarette smoking by schizophrenics. *Psychopharmacology* 1999;145:52–60.
83. Tidey JW, O'Neill SC, Higgins ST. *Effects of contingent monetary reinforcement and transdermal nicotine on cigarette smoking in schizophrenics* (in press).
84. Roll JM, Petry NM, Stitzer ML, et al. Contingency management for the treatment of methamphetamine use disorders. *Am J Psychiatry* 2006; 163:1993–1999.
85. Griffith JD, Rowan-Szal GA, Roark RR, Simpson DD. Contingency management in outpatient methadone treatment: a meta-analysis. *Drug Alcohol Depend* 2000;58:55–66.
86. Pendergrast M, Podus D, Finney J, et al. Contingency management for treatment of substance use disorders: a meta-analysis. *Addiction* 2006; 101:1546–1560.
87. Dutra L, Stathopoulou G, Basden SL, et al. A meta-analytic review of interventions for substance use disorders. *Am J Psychiatry* 2008;165:179–187.
88. Hunt GM, Azrin NH. A community-reinforcement approach to alcoholism. *Behav Res Ther* 1973;11:91–104.
89. Azrin NH. Improvements in the community-reinforcement approach to alcoholism. *Behav Res Ther* 1976;14:339–348.
90. Mallams JH, Godley MD, Hall GM, Meyers RJ. A social-systems approach to resocializing alcoholics in the community. *J Stud Alcohol* 1982;43:1115–1123.
91. Azrin NH, Sisson RW, Meyers R, Godley M. Alcoholism treatment by disulfiram and community reinforcement therapy. *J Behav Ther Exp Psychiatry* 1982;13:105–112.
92. Secades-Villa R, Garcia-Rodriguez O, Rodriguez AH, et al. Community reinforcement approach plus vouchers for cocaine dependence treatment. *Addicciones* 2007;19:51–57.
93. Higgins ST, Sigmon SC, Wong CJ, et al. Community reinforcement therapy for cocaine-dependent outpatients. *Arch Gen Psychiatry* 2003;60:1043–1052.
94. Abbott PJ, Moore BA, Weller SB, Delaney HD. AIDS risk behavior in opioid dependent patients treated with community reinforcement approach and relationships with psychiatric disorders. *J Addict Dis* 1998;17:33–48.
95. Azrin NH, Acierno R, Kogan ES, et al. Follow-up results of supportive versus behavioral therapy for illicit drug use. *Behav Res Ther* 1996; 34:41–46.
96. Dennis M, Godley SH, Diamond G, et al. The cannabis youth treatment (CYT) study: main findings from two randomized trials. *J Subst Abuse Treat* 2004;27:197–213.
97. Smith JE, Meyers RJ, Delaney HD. The community reinforcement approach with homeless alcohol-dependent individuals. *J Consult Clin Psychol* 1998;66:541–548.
98. Slesnick N, Prestopnik JL, Meyers, RJ, Glassman, M. Treatment outcome for street-living, homeless youth. *Addict Behav* 2007;32:1237–1251.
99. Sisson RW, Azrin AH. Family-member involvement to initiate and promote treatment of problem drinkers. *J Behav Res Ther* 1986;7:15-21.
100. Miller WR, Meyers RJ, Tonigan JS. Engaging the unmotivated in treatment for alcohol problems: a comparison of three strategies for intervention through family members. *J Consult Clin Psychol* 1999;7:688–697.
101. Kirby KC, Marlowe DB, Festinger DS, et al. Community reinforcement training for family and significant others of drug abusers: a unilateral intervention to increase treatment entry of drug users. *Drug Alcohol Depend* 1999;56:85–96.
102. Meyers RJ, Miller WR, Smith JE, Tonigan JS. A randomized trial of two methods for engaging treatment-refusing drug users through concerned significant others. *J Consult Clin Psychol* 2002;70:1182–1185.
103. Roozen GH, Boulogne JJ, van Tulder MW, et al. A systematic review of the effectiveness of the community reinforcement approach in alcohol, cocaine and opioid addiction. *Drug Alcohol Depend* 2004;74:1–13.
104. Meyers RJ, Smith JE. *Clinical guide to alcohol treatment: the community reinforcement approach.* New York: Guilford Press, 1995.
105. Godley SH, Meyers RJ, Smith JE, et al. The adolescent community reinforcement approach (ACRA) for adolescent cannabis users. Rockville, MD: Center for Substance Abuse Treatment, 2001.

CHAPTER 58

Christopher W. Kahler, PhD
Adam M. Leventhal, PhD
Richard A. Brown, PhD

Behavioral Interventions in Smoking Cessation

Smoking is the leading cause of preventable death in the United States (1), resulting in more than 430,000 deaths each year (2) and almost one third of all deaths from cancer (3). Costs of medical care, lost productivity, and forfeited earnings from smoking-related disability are estimated at more than $100 billion per year (4,5). Following significant public health efforts, cigarette smoking among adults in the United States declined from a peak of 42.4% in 1965 to 20.9% in 2005 (6). However, decreases in smoking rates have been relatively slow since 1990 (7,8). About 2.2% of the U.S. population smoke cigars, and rates of smokeless tobacco use are at 2.3% (6).

Smokers are generally well aware of the possible benefits of quitting (9), with more than 70% wanting to quit (10) and 42.5% making a quit attempt in the past year (6). However, only about 4% of those attempting to quit on their own remain abstinent as long as 1 year (11). Rates of success are much higher for those involved in intensive smoking cessation treatments range from about 15% to 30% (12). However, even in those receiving intensive treatment, relapse is the rule rather than the exception, and multiple quit attempts are often needed before individuals are successful in quitting (11,13). Clinicians play a crucial role in assessing tobacco use, encouraging all patients to quit smoking, and providing ongoing assistance for patients attempting to quit and for those relapsing back to smoking.

RELEVANCE FOR ADDICTIONS TREATMENT

Knowledge of assessment, intervention, and treatment of cigarette smoking is especially important for clinicians working with patients who drink alcohol excessively and who are dependent on alcohol or other drugs. There is a robust association between smoking and heavy alcohol use, which extends to alcohol use and other substance use disorders as well (14–18). Approximately 23% of those with nicotine dependence meet criteria for a current alcohol use disorder and 8% meet criteria for a current drug use disorder (19). Conversely, in the general U.S. adult population, 51.4% of men with alcohol dependence and 46.2% of women with alcohol dependence use tobacco daily (18). Rates of smoking are especially high among those in substance abuse treatment with rates of 75% or higher reported in some studies (20–22). Among lifetime smokers in the general population, cessation rates are lower for individuals with a history of alcohol use disorder compared with those without an alcohol use disorder history (15). The relationship between alcohol use disorder history and success in formal smoking cessation treatment is less clear, with some studies (23–26), but not others (27–30) finding that past alcohol use disorder is associated with poor smoking cessation outcome (31). In the general population, current problematic alcohol use has a more clear negative impact on smoking cessation than a history of alcohol problems (14,15,17,32).

There are compelling reasons to address tobacco use in individuals seeking treatment for other addictions. Most notable is that patients who have been treated for alcoholism or other non-nicotine drug dependence are more likely to die from tobacco-related (50.9%) than from alcohol-related causes (34.1%) (22). However, there has traditionally been limited support from addictions treatment staff for smoking cessation programs. Early studies found that fewer than 50% of program personnel encouraged patients to quit smoking, and 40% believed that smoking cessation should *not* be provided within the context of chemical dependency treatment (33,34). These attitudes reflect beliefs that smoking is less harmful than the patients' alcohol or drug use, doubt that alcohol and drug dependent patients can mount a serious effort to quit smoking, or concerns that smoking cessation during chemical dependency treatment will jeopardize abstinence from alcohol or drugs (35). Recent empirical findings have indicated that these concerns are not compelling and should not dissuade staff from encouraging efforts to quit smoking.

Another barrier to integrating tobacco dependence treatment into addictions treatment programs is that a high proportion of staff members in these programs smoke and therefore may be reluctant to counsel patients on quitting smoking (36). Providing resources to staff members to help them quit smoking is one way to address this barrier and to improve the overall health of staff members. There are good models available for integrating smoking cessation treatment into addictions treatment programs that appear promising (37). These include staff training in assessment and treatment of smoking, incorporating tobacco issue into program materials, and implementation of tobacco policies such as smoke-free grounds (36).

Over the past 20 years, several studies have investigated smoking cessation interventions in the context of substance abuse treatment, where about 50% to 80% of all patients indicate an interest or desire to quit smoking (38–42). Smoking abstinence rates achieved in these settings have been low (40,43–47). However, more recent studies that have included nicotine replacement therapy have produced higher smoking abstinence rates (42). The use of pharmacotherapy may be especially important given that alcohol- and drug-dependent individuals tend to smoke more per day and to be more nicotine dependent than those without alcohol and drug problems (35).

Studies have found that inclusion of smoking cessation treatment in other addictions programs does not reduce long-term treatment completion (35). Furthermore, most studies have found that smoking cessation interventions initiated during alcohol treatment (which often mirror those used in other settings) do not harm treatment outcome and may even be associated with better drinking and other substance use outcomes (42,48), although there have been some exceptions (49). In addition, a recent study found that patients who quit smoking on their own after addictions treatment have significantly better drinking outcomes in the 6 months after quitting compared with those who continue smoking (50).

Whether to initiate smoking cessation treatment early in the course of substance abuse treatment or to wait until sobriety has been attained for a few months remains a question. Greater lengths of sobriety from alcohol are positively associated with improved smoking cessation outcomes (51,52), suggesting that individuals with more prolonged recovery are more capable of quitting smoking successfully. Furthermore, the majority of addiction patients' treatment state a preference for treating their alcohol problems before initiating treatment for smoking (39). On the other hand, initiating smoking cessation interventions during addictions treatment increase rates of participation in smoking cessation treatment (49), although smoking abstinence rates between immediate versus delayed smoking interventions do not appear to differ significantly. One potential means of avoiding the risk of tobacco dependence treatment interfering with recovery is to delay intensive treatment until a few weeks of treatment of other addictions have been completed (53). However, more research in this area is needed.

Based on studies on tobacco treatment in substance abuse settings, we recommend that all smokers in addictions treatment be provided at least a brief smoking cessation intervention, including offering pharmacologic aid to cessation, with encouragement to quit smoking as soon as possible. Such direct advice to quit smoking appears at least as effective, if not more effective, than more extensive motivational interventions (54). Especially after smokers in addictions treatment have attained sobriety from alcohol and drugs, it is essential that clinicians clearly advise these patients to quit smoking as soon as possible and provide assistance. Interventions with this population can generally mirror those used with all smokers, which are reviewed in the following sections. However, individuals in recovery also may be likely to rely on principles of 12-step mutual help programs, such as Alcoholics Anonymous, when trying to quit smoking (55).

CHAPTER OVERVIEW

In this chapter, we describe a variety of behavioral interventions that can improve smokers' odds of successfully quitting. We begin by briefly reviewing the history of treatment of tobacco dependence before outlining some general theories of behavior change. We then discuss treatment planning and techniques for working with individuals who intend to quit smoking in the near future and those who do not. We conclude by reviewing considerations for working with specific populations of smokers. In discussing behavioral interventions, we focus primarily on cigarette smoking among adults where research and clinical applications have been most well developed. However, smoking among adolescents and the use of other tobacco products are also serious public health concerns. There are few theoretical reasons to expect that behavioral principles do not apply to equally well to adolescents, although the context of treatment dissemination may require modification (56). Although research in treating adolescents is in its infancy, initial evidence suggests that treatment involving cognitive-behavioral skill enhancement and motivational enhancement are effective for teens, but success rates are especially low (57). Recommendations for treating cigarette smoking in adults generally can be applied to other tobacco products as well (12).

HISTORY OF TREATMENTS FOR NICOTINE DEPENDENCE

Historical records indicate that as early as the mid-1800s, accounts of tobacco dependence were reported. Nineteenth century anti-tobacco organizations branded "tobaccoism" (i.e., habitual tobacco use) a disease that can cause a range of ailments from insanity to cancer (58,59). During this period, cigarettes were considered narcotics because they appeared to have addictive qualities. Despite these early reports of the negative effects of tobacco use, pervasive efforts to develop and disseminate treatments designed to help smokers quit did not come into favor until after the 1960s. At that time, the medical community reached a consensus that smoking is a principle etiologic factor in the development of several harmful conditions, including cancer (60).

Earlier reports estimate that most smokers (>90%) who quit smoking did not use any formal treatment program (61). More recent estimates indicate that approximately 20% to 58% of smokers are using some form of assistance when trying to quit (62–64), which coincides with the advancement and dissemination of treatment methods. Initial treatment efforts mainly involved physicians using unsystematic methods to advise their patients to quit smoking. However, with the medical and scientific community's change in viewing smoking as a "habit" to an "addiction" (65), more substantial, standardized interventions have been developed. For example, early research led to the development of nicotine gum as the first U.S. Food and Drug Administration–approved pharmacologic treatment for nicotine dependence in 1984. This was followed by U.S. Food and Drug Administration approval of transdermal nicotine patches and nicotine nasal spray, and more recently bupropion and varenicline.

With regard to behavioral interventions, systematic study of the factors that increase treatment efficacy (e.g., treatment approach and content, components of intervention, length of sessions, number of sessions, type of practitioner) became prevalent in the 1970s and 1980s (66). Early interventions varied markedly in their approach from systematic brief advice (67) to aversive-smoking strategies (e.g., rapid smoking) (68). More recently, behavioral interventions have focused on skill building techniques to increase smokers' coping resources (69) and enhance smokers' commitment to initiating and maintaining abstinence (70). In addition to content changes, the modality of treatment has also transformed with advancement in technology. Although traditionally behavioral treatments are delivered face-to-face between the provider and patient, interventions delivered through the phone (e.g., telephone counseling) or the Internet have increased in prevalence and have been shown to be effective in enhancing cessation success (71). These modalities may be more cost-effective (72), and may have the potential for reaching a wider range of smokers who may not have otherwise had access to treatment (e.g., rural and poor populations). Future scientific, medical, and technologic developments will likely continue to change the landscape of behavioral interventions for tobacco dependence, potentially increasing their effectiveness as well as their impact on public health.

TREATMENT MODEL

Theory of Change The treatment model we rely on in this chapter is based on a theory of change that proposes that for individuals to change their behavior they must: be motivated or ready to change and have the skills to execute the change in behavior effectively (73,74).

Motivation Motivation (or readiness) to change a behavior is defined as the desire and intention to discontinue an old behavior and initiate a new behavior. Readiness to change is thought to lie along a continuum ranging from very low motivation (i.e., no desire to change) to moderate motivation (i.e., some interest in changing but no current intentions) to very high motivation (i.e., firm intention to change). This conceptualization of motivation is also consistent with the stages of change model, which suggests that smokers move between one of five stages of change: precontemplation, contemplation, preparation, action, and maintenance (75).

Psychological theories argue that people are motivated to cease behaviors that yield low reward and high risk, whereas they are motivated to initiate behaviors that yield high reward and low risk (73,76). Accordingly, motivation to change is thought to be determined by cognitive processes involved in weighing the personal pros versus cons of persisting with the old behavior and weighing the personal pros versus cons of initiating the new behavior. Motivation will be greater if the cons of the old behavior and the pros of the new behavior are *high* and the pros of the old behavior and the cons of the new behavior are *low*.

Motivation is dynamic as it can vary within an individual across time and circumstances (presumably because of changes in the accessibility, salience, and strength of beliefs regarding the relevance of benefits and costs of smoking versus quitting). Based on this framework, behavioral change occurs when there is a transformation in an individual's beliefs toward greater cons for the old behavior and pros for the new behavior or lesser pros for the old behavior and cons for the new behavior. When this shift is sufficiently large, an intention to change will occur. In addition, a particular benefit that is especially relevant to a given individual may have a larger impact on overall motivation than the other pros and cons (e.g., a truck driver may argue that smoking helps pass the time quicker while on the road, which could outweigh all of the other cons of smoking and pros of quitting). Furthermore, the personal relevance of certain pros or cons for a particular individual may change in response to new circumstances (e.g., learning that you have developed lung cancer, your spouse demands that you quit). Therefore external influences that help smokers shift their beliefs regarding the pros and cons of smoking versus quitting may enhance motivation and ultimately result in their initiating a cessation attempt.

Skills According to behavioral theories of behavior change, after an intention to change a behavior has been formed, specific skills are required for the individual to effectively initiate and maintain the new behavior. Therefore the acquisition of new skills is likely to be necessary to promote persistence of the new behavior. In smoking cessation, various factors make it difficult to initiate and maintain the new behavior of abstinence, such as nicotine withdrawal, cigarette cravings, stress, stimuli in the environment that could tempt people to smoke (e.g., ashtrays, lighters), negative moods, and boredom. Especially among individuals making their first quit attempt, these barriers are novel, and they may not know strategies that could maintain abstinence in the face of these barriers. Accordingly, learning "nonsmoking skills" can be helpful to prevent these barriers from impeding cessation. For example, learning strategies of how to anticipate and manage situations that are high risk (e.g., running into my friend who I used to smoke with) may provide individuals with skills necessary to maintain their new behavior (i.e., abstinence) without going back to their old behavior (i.e., smoking).

Behavioral Treatment Cognitive social learning theory provides a useful framework for conceptualizing behavioral treatment of tobacco dependence (77); this theory has also been extended to treatment of other substances such as alcohol where similar processes may operate (78). In this model, smoking or other tobacco use is viewed as a learned behavior acquired through classical and operant conditioning, modeling, and other cognitive processes (79). Through pairing over time, various external and interoceptive stimuli (e.g., drinking coffee, feeling stressed, celebrating at a party) (80) come to be associated with smoking behavior. These stimuli or *antecedents* can then trigger an urge to smoke. After the individual smokes a cigarette (the *behavior*), he or she experiences the rewarding *consequences* (e.g., relaxation), increasing the likelihood of future smoking. Smokers also develop certain expectations about the effects of smoking, which in turn influence on smoking behavior. Positive outcome expectancies (e.g., "smoking will relax me") increase the likelihood of continued smoking, whereas negative outcome expectancies increase the likelihood of quitting (e.g., "smoking increases my risk of heart disease").

The general rationale of behavioral treatment is that through skills training, the automatic chain of events (Antecedent → Behavior → Consequences) leading to smoking can be disrupted, and smoking behavior can be replaced with alternative behaviors. The learning of nonsmoking skills occurs through a series of success experiences. As smokers become more proficient in these skills, their self-efficacy for quitting increases, thereby increasing the likelihood of successful smoking cessation. This general theory provides the core of most intensive behavioral smoking cessation programs.

TREATMENT PLANNING

Clinicians typically initiate counseling with smokers through one of two distinct pathways: clinicians may identify smokers through routine clinical practice in a variety of settings and advise these smokers to quit or smokers may approach clinicians with an interest in quitting smoking and seek specific assistance in doing so. In each of these contexts, the methods of behavioral counseling for those who want to quit would be similar. For those who are not ready to quit, methods for moving smokers towards initiating a quit attempt and for continuing to assess readiness to quit are indicated. Each of these methods is detailed in the section Treatment and Technique. A simple set of procedures for working with patients who smoke is to follow what has been termed the five As of intervention: *Ask* patients whether they use tobacco; *advise* all patients to quit; *assess* willingness to make a quit attempt; *assist* patients in making a quit attempt; and *arrange* follow-up contacts to help prevent relapse (12). These steps are described in more detail in the following sections. In Figure 58.1, we also provide a general schematic for treatment planning with patients who smoke. The figure provides different steps for those who are willing and those who are not willing to quit smoking in the near future. It also highlights the need for continued assessment of smoking status at each stage of intervention.

The first step in effectively treating tobacco use and dependence for any clinician is to assess tobacco use in all patients (12). This assessment would include whether patients had ever smoked, when they last smoked a cigarette, and the typical number of cigarettes they currently smoke per day. Several studies have suggested that tobacco use is not assessed with sufficient regularity by clinicians in position to counsel patients on quitting smoking. For example, less than two thirds of current smokers report that they have been asked about whether they smoke or have been encouraged to quit (12). The enactment of procedures and systems that routinely identify and document smoking status in health care settings is critical, resulting in about three times higher rates of smoking cessation interventions being delivered by clinicians and almost two times higher quit rates among patients who smoke (12). Possible methods of documentation and identification of tobacco users include expanded vital sign sheets that incorporate tobacco use status along with blood pressure, pulse, and temperature, and reminder systems such as chart stickers or prompts on computer records.

The second step in treating tobacco use is to provide clear advice to quit smoking. Smokers report that physician advice to quit smoking is often an important factor in their deciding to make a quit attempt (81,82), and clinical trials have found that brief advice (less than 3 minutes) by a clinician to quit smoking increases the odds of abstinence by about 30% compared with the absence of such advice (12). Therefore smokers should be provided at least a brief intervention at each office visit. Advice is most effective if it is clear ("It is very important for you to quit smoking"), strong ("Quitting smoking is one of the most important things you can do to improve and protect your health"), and personalized ("Smoking increases the risk of heart attacks, which is especially important for you given your family history of heart disease and your high blood pressure").

The third step in treating tobacco use is to assess readiness to quit smoking among those who are actively smoking. (Of course, it is also important to reinforce those past smokers who have quit and to continue to assess smoking status in those patients at later follow-ups.) Patients present with differing levels of motivation for quitting smoking, and intervention

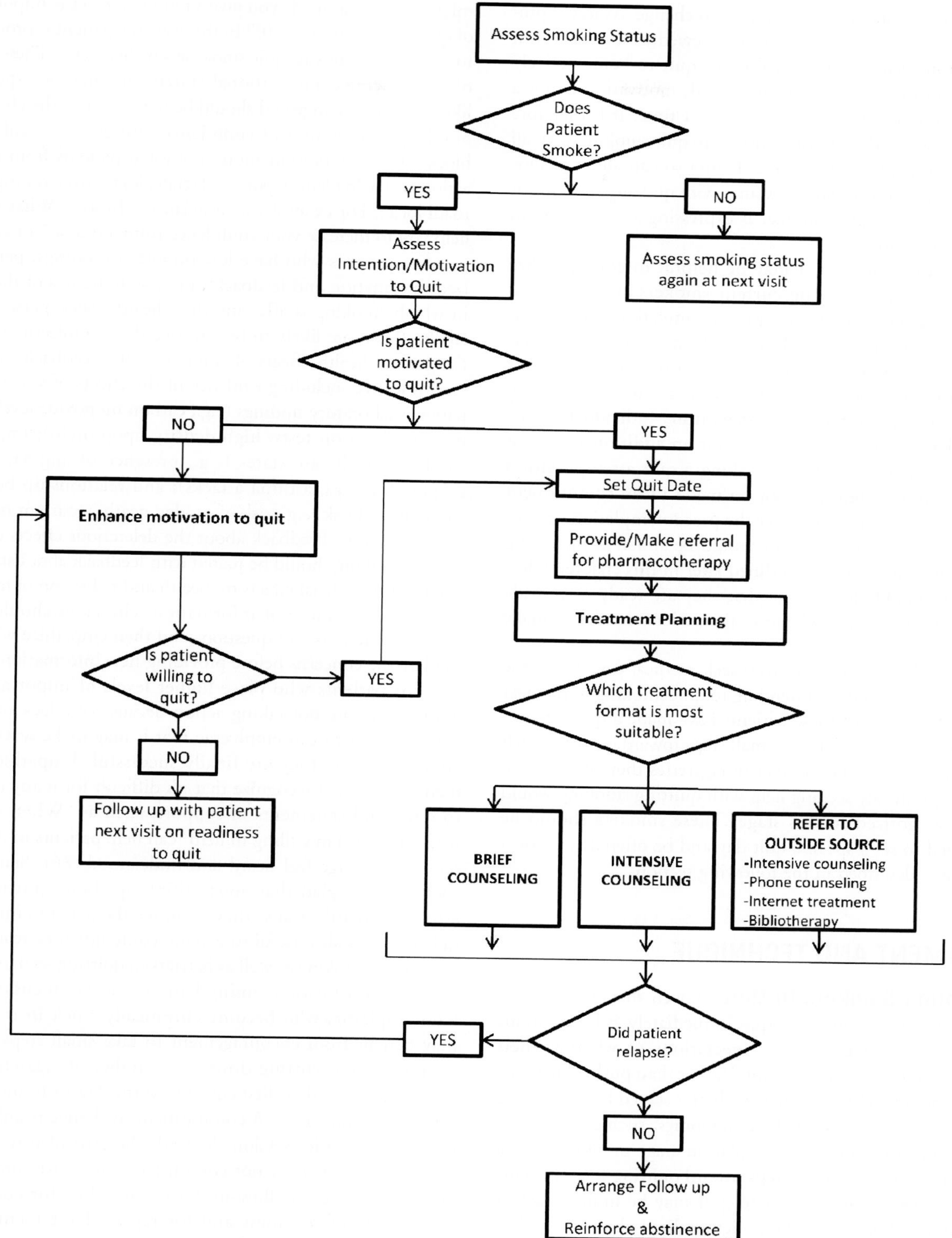

FIGURE 58.1. Schematic for treating cigarette smoking.

should be based on patients' readiness to change. As noted previously, readiness to change can be viewed as a continuum ranging from being entirely willing to quit to being actively involved in quitting (83). In this regard, motivation is not a static trait but a state that fluctuates over time. It is therefore crucial to assess and monitor readiness to quit smoking with all patients who continue to smoke. Doing so can allow a clinician to provide appropriate assistance with quitting smoking at a time in which a given smoker is expressing a willingness to make a quit attempt.

For many clinicians it may be helpful to conceptualize readiness to change among current smokers as falling into three discrete stages of change: precontemplation, contemplation, and preparation (84). Individuals at the precontemplation stage, representing as many as 40% of current smokers seen in a typical medical practice (85), are not considering stopping smoking in the foreseeable future. Individuals in the contemplation stage, who account for an additional 40% of smokers (85), are considering making a quit attempt within the next 6 months but have not yet made a firm commitment to change. For smokers in either the precontemplation or contemplation stages, intervention should be aimed at increasing motivation using methods outlined later in this chapter. Clinicians also should clearly state that they are ready to provide assistance with quitting whenever the patient decides to make a quit attempt.

About 20% of smokers who seek medical care are in the preparation stage and are intending to quit smoking in the next month (85). Many of these patients have made a quit attempt in the past year or have taken small steps toward quitting, such as cutting down on the number of cigarettes they smoke (86). Smokers specifically seeking help with quitting smoking would also be categorized in this stage. These smokers should be encouraged to set a specific quit day and be offered additional assistance as described in the following sections.

TREATMENT AND TECHNIQUE

Motivating Smokers to Quit Given that the majority of smokers are not willing to quit immediately, it is important that clinicians have modest expectations of whether their patients will make a quit attempt. Rather than push all patients to quit smoking, clinicians may be better served by developing strategies to attain intermediate outcomes, such as moving a precontemplator to the contemplation stage or motivating a contemplator to take small steps toward quitting (86). Patients who are unwilling to attempt to quit may be uninformed or underinformed about smoking, demoralized about their ability to change, or defensive and resistant to change (86).

A useful and effective method for exploring readiness to change is to have patients rate on a numeric scale (e.g., from 0 to 10) the importance they place on quitting smoking and the confidence they have in successfully quitting (87). After a patient has provided these ratings, a clinician can inquire further about factors influencing each rating. For example, a clinician might ask "What made you give a rating of 4 to the importance of quitting rather than a 0?" In this way, the patient is prompted to generate reasons to quit smoking on their own. These types of self-generated motivational statements may be especially likely to foster change and should be reinforced by the clinician. Similarly, exploration of confidence ratings can reveal roadblocks that may prevent more motivated patients from taking action and help identify potential strategies for overcoming these roadblocks. For example, a clinician might ask "What would help you to increase your confidence from a 6 to a 7 or an 8?"

For patients who have low importance ratings, personalized information and feedback can raise awareness of the ways in which smoking is affecting their health. Such personalized feedback is more likely to be effective than minilectures about the general health effects of smoking (70). Feedback can take several forms, including evidence of the effects of smoking on patient's laboratory findings (e.g., carbon monoxide levels, pulmonary function tests, high-density lipoprotein); impact of smoking on disease states (e.g., presence of angina, angiographic findings, asthma attacks); and relationship between smoking and risk (e.g., risk of sudden death, recurrent myocardial infarction). Feedback about the deleterious effects of continued smoking should be paired with feedback about smoking cessation's beneficial effects on health and reduction of morbidity. After each piece of information, clinicians should elicit patients' reactions and questions and then empathize with and validate the concerns before providing new information.

For patients who place higher levels of importance on quitting but are not taking action because of a lack of confidence, clinicians can emphasize that it may make several quit attempts before they are finally successful. Empathic statements, such as "I recognize that it's difficult for many patients to quit" and statements of support, such as "When you are ready to quit, I'm willing to help" can help patients in the contemplation stage feel heard and understood (86). Statements such as, "I'm glad that you're thinking about quitting" are especially useful because they reinforce the patient's interest in quitting. It is also useful to explore contemplators' reasons for continued smoking as well as barriers to quitting so that potential solutions for overcoming barriers can be discussed (86). Contemplators who become chronically stuck in this stage may benefit from encouragement to take small steps toward action, such as cutting down the number of cigarettes they smoke, delaying their first cigarette of the day, or trying to quit for just 24 hours (86). A commitment to change is unlikely to occur in one brief session. Instead, the goal of intervention with a patient who is not committed is to move him or her closer to change. Follow-up visits can allow for continued monitoring of readiness and for repeated interventions to enhance motivation and facilitate quitting.

Rationale for the Choice of Behavioral Treatments

All patients who are willing to attempt to quit smoking should be provided assistance, both from physicians and from other health care providers. After it has been established that a smoker intends to quit, a clinician needs to decide, in consultation with the patient, the nature of the assistance that will be provided. Interventions delivered by multiple types of providers increase the likelihood of smoking cessation, suggesting that smoking cessation interventions should be delivered by as many clinicians and types of clinicians as feasible (12). There is also a strong dose-response relationship between the intensity of person-to-person contact and smoking cessation outcome (12). It has been shown that relatively intensive interventions involving four or more sessions lasting 10 or more minutes of duration produce higher rates of smoking abstinence than brief interventions. In fact, increasing the intensity of counseling from less than 3 minutes to 3 to 10 minutes increases quit rates by more than 20%. However, there are a number of obstacles to using these more intensive interventions. First, in many settings, clinician time to deliver extended interventions is simply not available. Clinicians also may not possess the relevant training and experience to conduct such interventions. Patients, too, may be reluctant to commit to coming to counseling on a regular basis. For these reasons, brief clinical interventions with appropriate referral to pharmacotherapy and other resources are often most readily implemented in many clinical settings.

Brief Clinical Interventions The primary component of a brief clinical tobacco intervention is helping the patient create a plan of action for quitting. An important step in this is to review past quit attempts to identify strategies that were successful and to highlight potential obstacles to success. Central to the quit plan is setting a target quit date, ideally within 2 weeks. Setting this quit date allows smokers to plan for quitting and to obtain the necessary support for quitting. Patients should be advised to smoke their last cigarette on the night before their quit date so that they wake up a nonsmoker. It is important to stress that quitting smoking means avoiding smoking completely, because even one puff of a cigarette can prompt further smoking.

As part of a plan to quit smoking, patients should be encouraged to tell their family and friends about their quit date and to elicit support from these people. For those who have smokers in their household, this might necessitate asking these smokers to refrain from smoking in the house or in front of them. Patients also should make sure that they have eliminated all tobacco products and associated cues, such as ashtrays and cigarette lighters. For those who drink alcohol, recommend that they try to avoid drinking alcohol as much as possible while quitting because alcohol use is involved in about one fourth of all lapses to smoking (88–90). Finally, patients should be encouraged to think about their potential triggers for smoking and consider the situations in which they might be likely to relapse. After situations have been identified, the clinician can discuss with the patient potential strategies for handling those high-risk situations.

Additional assistance can be provided in the form of self-help materials or "bibliotherapy." Self-help manuals are important tools that enhance the capacity of the health care provider to provide information and advice. Materials are available through agencies such as the National Cancer Institute, Public Health Service, American Cancer Society, American Heart Association, American Lung Association, and the Office on Smoking and Health. A second appealing and feasible option is to refer patients to state-funded quitlines. Quitlines are now available in all 50 states. They offer from three to six sessions of proactive counseling (i.e., the quitline counselor calls the patient to deliver counseling according to the quitline's protocol), and many offer free nicotine replacement therapy for participants. Proactive telephone counseling has been found to be both efficacious and effective (71,91).

Finally, except where special circumstances exist, all smokers willing to quit should be offered pharmacotherapy along with an explanation that such medication can reduce withdrawal symptoms and increase success rates (12). First-line pharmacotherapies include nicotine replacement therapies (gum, inhaler, nasal spray, lozenge, or patch), varenicline (Chantix), and bupropion SR (Zyban) (See Chapter 52).

Follow-Up For smokers who are attempting to quit, providers should schedule a specific time to connect immediately after quit day to reinforce successes and trouble-shoot difficulties in cessation efforts, including use and potential side effects of medication. Follow-up contacts also provide an opportunity to work with patients who have lapsed to smoking. Clinicians can empathize with patients about the difficulty in staying quit, help patients view a lapse as a learning experience that is part of the normal process of quitting, and encourage patients to continue their efforts to quit.

Intensive Clinical Interventions Intensive clinical interventions involve many of the same components used in brief interventions. However, they add additional components and go into greater depth in specific areas, such as managing alcohol use and coping with high-risk situations. These intensive interventions would be likely to be administered primarily by individuals who specialize in treating tobacco dependence. As noted previously, more intensive counseling tends to produce higher abstinence rates, although evidence for increasing improvements in abstinence rates beyond 90 minutes of counseling is lacking (12). Counseling involving eight or more sessions has shown superiority over counseling of only two to three sessions (12). Many of these intensive interventions may be delivered in group settings to increase economy of delivery and also to enhance the social support provided by other smokers attempting to quit. Although a description of an intensive group behavioral intervention is provided in later sections, more detailed accounts of this intensive intervention are also available (92).

Preparing for Quitting We recommend a "preparation" period before quitting smoking, the length of which can vary according to program needs. There are three key objectives for this period. First, patients' motivation to quit and commitment to the program should be clarified and reinforced. Second, a target quit day should be clearly established to allow patients the time to "mentally prepare" and develop coping strategies for quitting smoking. Third, patients should self-monitor their daily smoking behavior to begin to learn about their smoking triggers (i.e., antecedents).

Enhancing Motivation in Smokers who are Quitting

Even after smokers express an intent to quit smoking in the near future, it remains important for clinicians to work to enhance commitment to quitting. Commitment to quitting is a robust predictor of smoking cessation treatment outcome (93). Smokers may be ambivalent about the prospect of quitting for a variety of reasons. Although acknowledging rational reasons for quitting, they may dread the potential discomfort of quitting, feel that they are attached to smoking and that they are giving up a friend, lack confidence in their ability to quit, feel hopelessly addicted, and continue to question whether the health risks could ever really impact them. This may be especially true of smokers who may have tried in the past to quit and failed. Acknowledging this ambivalence without directly challenging smokers can help diffuse some of its power to undermine commitment. For example, clinicians can use double-sided reflective statements to highlight both sides of ambivalence (70) (e.g., "On the one hand you find that smoking helps you relax and serves as a reward for a hard day's work, but on the other hand you know that it is costing you a lot of money, has made it harder for you to be physically active, and is greatly raising your risk of having a heart attack").

For many smokers, the expected short-term benefits of smoking (e.g., "smoking calms my nerves") override the more distal, negative consequences (e.g., potentially life-threatening illnesses). The challenge is to move smokers from general acceptance of potential negative consequences ("Smoking is dangerous to health") to personalized acceptance ("Smoking is dangerous to my *own* health") (94). Encouraging smokers to consider their smoker's cough and other current physical symptoms is one way to make negative consequences more personally salient. When appropriate, exploring the consequences of illness or premature death of a loved one or what they will miss if they themselves die prematurely also can be a powerful motivator. A concurrent focus on the health benefits of quitting may be especially effective in motivating and sustaining efforts to quit smoking (95). A useful approach to enhance motivation involves having patients write down their specific, self-relevant reasons for wanting to stop smoking and for wanting to continue smoking. Listing reasons to continue smoking may seem contradictory, but can help patients identify likely barriers to quitting. Motivation for quitting smoking needs to be monitored throughout treatment for potential setbacks.

Self-Monitoring of Smoking Behavior Keeping a written record of cigarettes smoked can help increase knowledge about the factors cueing and maintaining smoking behavior. Self-monitoring also interrupts the automatic smoking habit, encouraging patients to think about every cigarette they smoke and why they smoke it. Often this procedure reduces the number of cigarettes smoked per day (96). Preprinted cards or "wrap sheets" can be given to patients to record the time of day and the situation in which each cigarette is smoked (e.g., "talking on the phone"). Assessment of mood at the time of each cigarette also can be useful. The situational notations allow patients to identify antecedents that trigger their smoking.

Patients typically find self-monitoring of their smoking behavior inconvenient. It is important that clinicians present the rationale for self-monitoring clearly and follow through at all sessions by reviewing wrap sheets with patients to highlight the relevance of the information in their quitting efforts. For example, it is useful to ask each patient what they learned about his or her smoking behavior and its patterns over the course of a typical week; specifically, what moods were common triggers of smoking, during which times of the day did the patient smoke most often, and which people or events typically triggered the smoking.

CESSATION STAGE INTERVENTIONS

Self-Management Self-management (sometimes termed *self-control* or *stimulus control*) procedures are a critical component of behavioral smoking interventions. They refer to strategies intended to rearrange environmental cues that "trigger" smoking or to alter the consequences of smoking. Using their wrap sheets, patients develop a list of trigger situations. They then begin to intervene in these situations to break up the smoking behavior chain (situation - urge - smoke) by using one of three general strategies: avoid the trigger situation, alter or change the trigger situation, or use an alternative or substitute in place of the cigarette. Examples of avoiding trigger situations include foregoing a coffee break at work with other smokers, leaving the table after dinner, and avoiding social situations involving alcohol. Altering a trigger situation might involve drinking tea or juice in the morning instead of coffee, watching television in the bedroom (a nonsmoking room) rather than the living room, and putting cigarettes in the trunk of the car before driving. Alternatives or substitutes can be used in conjunction with avoiding or altering trigger situations or in situations that cannot be avoided or altered. Possible alternatives include sugarless candy or gum, cut-up vegetables such as carrot or celery sticks, toothpicks, relaxation techniques in stressful situations, or activities such as needlework that keep hands busy. Patients should choose strategies they think will work for them and then try out different approaches, rejecting those that are not useful until they have successfully managed all or most trigger situations without smoking.

Social Support Positive social support both within (e.g., from the clinician) and outside of treatment has been shown to increase cessation rates (12,97). Social support can be a source of motivation for quitting and of positive reinforcement for maintaining abstinence. Social support also may provide a buffer against stressful life events that might precipitate a relapse. Clinicians should encourage patients' efforts at cessation, communicate care and concern for their well-being, and encourage open discussion about their experiences during quitting. Encouraging patients' to access social support outside of treatment also may be helpful; this might include making specific requests to friends and family members about steps they can take to support patients' abstinence efforts.

Maintenance Because the majority of smokers who initially quit resume smoking within several months of treatment termination (98), maintenance is a critical issue for smoking cessation programs. The most commonly used behavioral maintenance strategies are based on the relapse prevention model (74), the main components of which are described later in this chapter. Research on the effectiveness of relapse prevention components has been mixed with relapse prevention treatments generally outperforming no-treatment controls but rarely outperforming credible alternative treatments (99,100). A notable exception is a study by Stevens and Hollis (101), in which relapse prevention booster sessions produced higher abstinence rates than both social support and no treatment controls. Also, Hall and colleagues (102) found that extended treatment involving an additional 44 weeks of medication, 9 monthly counseling sessions, and between-session check-up telephone calls resulted in better smoking cessation outcomes than an 8-week protocol. This preliminary evidence suggests that extending behavioral treatment and pharmacotherapy may improve cessation outcomes.

Identifying and Coping with High-Risk Situations for Relapse Relapse prevention theory (74) proposes that the ability to cope with "high-risk" situations for relapse determines an individual's probability of maintaining abstinence. High-risk situations often involve at least one of the following elements: negative moods, positive moods, social situations involving alcohol, and being in the presence of smokers. To help patients identify high-risk situations, a clinician can ask, "If you were to slip and smoke a cigarette after quit day, in what situation would it be?" For each high-risk situation, patients can develop a set of strategies for managing the situation without smoking. They should be reminded that these high-risk situations are functionally similar to the trigger situations they have previously addressed and that they can apply similar self-management strategies (i.e., avoid, alter, or use a substitute), as well as other problem-solving skills.

Managing Slips When patients experience a slip to smoking, they often progress to further smoking and relapse. Preventing slips is the best way to achieve smoking abstinence and this point should be stress to all patients. However, in the event that a slip happens, a few steps can be taken to manage the slip and regain abstinence. First, a slip is an important time for clinicians to assess motivation or commitment to quitting. Has motivation changed or is the patient ambivalent about quitting? Does the patient support the goal of quitting completely or does he or she believe that occasional cigarettes are unlikely to be harmful? If motivation is flagging, then use of the motivational interventions described above is appropriate. On the other hand, if motivation remains high, then it is important for the clinician and the patient to review the circumstances of the lapse to figure out what conditions allowed that lapse to occur. The lessons learned from the lapse are reviewed, and plans for avoiding similar lapses in the future can then be made. These plans often involve application of the coping strategies described previously.

Lifestyle Change Marlatt and Gordon (74) discuss the concept of replacing a negative addiction (such as smoking) with a "positive addiction" by increasing participation in activities that are incompatible with smoking and are a source of pleasure. Patients are encouraged to set aside time as often as possible (ideally, on a daily basis) for this purpose. It is in this context that we strongly encourage patients to engage in some type of regular physical exercise. Vigorous exercise has recently been shown to enhance smoking cessation in women (103). Exercise may be a good alternative to dieting for individuals who are concerned about post-cessation weight gain.

SPECIAL POPULATIONS

The interventions described above have been studied most intensively in primary care and other health care settings and in clinical trials of smokers recruited from the community. However, over the past decade, there has been an increasing body of research on methods for enhancing rates of smoking cessation in populations in which smoking rates are especially high and in which cessation rates are particularly low. The literature on treatment of tobacco dependence in traditional addictions treatment programs has been reviewed above. Here we review studies on additional patient groups that have high rates of smoking: heavy, non-alcohol–dependent drinkers, psychiatric patients, and patients with a history of major depressive disorder.

Heavy Drinkers Heavy alcohol use is one risk factor that commonly cooccurs with smoking (14,15,104) and impedes smoking cessation efforts (30). Alcohol consumption is the third leading cause of death in the United States (105), and excessive drinking results in numerous well-documented health, mental health, and social problems (106). The combined effects of excessive drinking and smoking are enormous. For example, smoking and heavy drinking combine to produce especially negative consequences on brain morphology and function (107–112), and smoking negates the cardioprotective effects of regular drinking (113,114). Furthermore, a multiplicative effect operates when smoking is combined with heavy drinking, conferring markedly greater risk for oral, pharyngeal, laryngeal, and esophageal cancers relative to just smoking, just drinking, or neither smoking nor drinking (3,115–117). Cessation of smoking (115,116), as well as cessation of drinking (118), can significantly reduce cancer risk.

A recent clinical trial found that incorporating a brief alcohol intervention into smoking cessation treatment for heavy drinkers, who were not alcohol dependent, led to significantly lower levels of drinking and increased the odds of smoking abstinence (119). However, both effects were relatively small. More research in this area is needed, but it appears that conducting brief alcohol interventions in conjunction with smoking cessation treatment with excessive drinkers is feasible and may benefit both behaviors. The National Institute on Alcohol Abuse and Alcoholism Clinician's Guide provides a set of strategies for conducting brief interventions for heavy drinkers (120). Heavy drinkers are defined as those who have had heavy drinking days in the past year (4+ or 5+ drinks for women and men, respectively) or who drink 8+/15+ drinks per week for women and men, respectively. Steps for brief alcohol intervention include assessing alcohol use and problems, providing clear advice to reduce drinking to those who are drinking at medically unsafe levels, assessing readiness to change drinking, and helping patients set drinking goals and make plans for achieving those goals. Stressing that avoiding heavy drinking may increase the odds of quitting smoking successfully is one way of using motivation to quit smoking to encourage changes in heavy drinking as well.

Psychiatric Patients More than 50% of psychiatric patients smoke, compared with 25% of individuals without psychiatric problems (121). Psychotic disorders, mood disorders, anxiety disorders, and attention deficit hyperactivity disorder are among the most common psychiatric problems among smokers (122). Despite the high prevalence of smoking in this population, evidence from routine psychiatric practice indicates there are low rates of identification and treatment of tobacco dependence among patients treated by psychiatrists (123,124). This disparity may be a result of the paucity of research on what types of approaches are mores effective for treating nicotine dependence in psychiatric patients.

Initial evidence suggests that principles such as motivational enhancement and skill building may be effective in treating nicotine dependence in psychiatric patients (125). Thus we speculate that the general treatment strategies outlined earlier in the chapter may be the most appropriate methods of reducing smoking rates among psychiatric patients. However, certain clinical characteristics of psychiatric patients and contextual factors present only in psychiatric settings should be taken into account when applying behavioral treatments for smoking.

In comparison to psychiatric patients without a nicotine problem, psychiatric patients with tobacco dependence are more likely to have sociodemographic risk factors that could in lead to poorer smoking outcomes including being divorced or separated, disabled, and uninsured, and have fewer years of education (124). Among psychiatric patients, patients who are smokers have more comorbid psychiatric disorders, lower global functioning, and poorer compliance relative to psychiatric comparisons (124). Thus smokers in the psychiatric setting may be encountering the most severe and complex psychosocial problems of any population, which should be considered by clinicians. Despite this, severity and chronicity does not predict whether or not depressed psychiatric patients are willing to accept a combined behavioral-pharmacologic nicotine dependent treatment program (126), nor does severity predict current motivation to quit smoking (127). Thus psychiatric patients who smoke (even those with greater levels of psychosocial problems) would benefit from being offered nicotine dependence treatment.

Another clinical characteristic that may differ in smokers with versus without psychiatric problems is nicotine withdrawal severity. Evidence suggests that smokers with anxiety, depression, and eating disorder symptoms are more likely to experience greater nicotine withdrawal symptoms when discontinuing tobacco use (128,129). Although it is not yet clear whether greater withdrawal may contribute to increase relapse risk in smoking cessation treatment, these findings suggest that psychiatric patients may potentially benefit from increased assessment and treatment to buffer the effects of nicotine withdrawal. Psychiatric patients also are more likely to experience cognitive problems because disorders such as major depression and psychosis often present with disturbance in memory, concentration, and thinking (130). Nonetheless, studies have demonstrated that skill-building and motivational enhancement techniques can be applied to psychiatric patients (125), including those with active psychotic disorders (131,132), though modifications should be made to meet the needs of this population. Modifications may include: ensuring that cognitive processing demands do not exceed patients' capacity; using devices for remembering, such as notices, schedules, and diaries, and for organizing and monitoring the correct order of task behaviors; prompting or using supportive reminder cues, which may be more appropriate than teaching skills or imparting information; and considering the social and financial limitations of individuals with severe mental illness when designing potential rewards and alternate behaviors and strategies to smoking (132–134).

A major contextual issue specific to the inpatient psychiatric setting that should be considered when planning nicotine dependence treatment is the role of smoke breaks in the psychiatric treatment program. An English psychiatric hospital survey found that 60% of staff believed that they should smoke with patients, 54% of staff (and 79% of staff who smoke) also believed that smoking had a therapeutic role, and 93% believed that patients would deteriorate without access to cigarettes (135,136). Although evidence from hospitals that have implemented smoking bans does not support notions that patients' psychiatric status will deteriorate after discontinuing tobacco use (137), it is important to consult with inpatient staff when implementing a tobacco dependence treatment. Relatedly, if cigarettes are used as reinforcers in a psychiatric treatment program, it is important to work with staff to develop alternative reinforcers that can be used promote healthy behaviors.

Behavioral Approaches and Comorbid Mood Problems Increasingly, attention has been paid to the important roles negative affect and depression play in impeding efforts at smoking cessation. Cigarette smoking is disproportionately higher among people with depression than among people in the general U.S. population. In contrast to the national smoking rate of 20.9% in the general population (6), more 30% of patients with current depression are daily smokers (19). Nearly 60% of those with a lifetime history of depression are current or past smokers (17). Conversely, smokers typically exhibit higher rates of major depressive disorder (MDD) (138–140) and depressive symptoms (141–143) than nonsmokers, although exceptions have been noted (144). Lifetime prevalence rates of MDD are particularly high among smokers entering clinic-based smoking treatment, with rates as high as 64% (145).

Several studies have shown that affective distress at the beginning of treatment (146,147) and after quitting (148–150) predicts poor outcome. An association between a history of MDD and poor smoking outcome was not found in an initial meta-analysis of smoking cessation trials published between 1988 and 2000 (145). However, an update of this meta-analysis, including treatment studies published through April 2006, was restricted to only the participants randomized to the placebo or alternative lowest intensity treatment arm of each study to remove the potential influence of any experimental interventions hypothesized to specifically benefit depressive smokers (151). Although there was no difference between groups in short-abstinence, smokers with a history of depression had a 34% lower odds of long-term abstinence (152). Furthermore, a subgroup of depression vulnerable smokers appears to be at heightened risk for failure in smoking treatment. The majority of individuals with depression will experience multiple depressive episodes. Adult smokers with a history of recurrent depression, as compared with those with only a single episode history, show significantly lower abstinence rates after treatment, despite comparable rates of adherence to the interventions (27,153,154). Recurrent depression also has been associated with an inability to quit or reduce smoking among women (144).

Given the negative association between mood problems and abstinence, cessation treatments that provide behavioral strategies for managing depressive symptoms and negative mood have generated substantial interest. Two studies have found significant effects of depression coping skills for smokers with an MDD history; however, in both of these studies, the experimental treatment had greater therapist contact time than the control (155,156). In a study equating for therapist contact, the effect was not replicated (157). Brown and colleagues (27) found that cessation treatment incorporating cognitive-behavioral therapy for depression was particularly efficacious for smokers with recurrent MDD, even when equating for therapist contact time. Subsequent analyses of pooled data from the three studies of Hall and colleagues (155–157) revealed that smokers with recurrent MDD who received cognitive-behavioral depression skills training were 2.4 times more likely to be abstinent at 12-month follow-up compared with recurrent MDD smokers in the control conditions (154). Thus evidence suggests that adding cognitive-behavioral therapy for depression to standard smoking cessation treatment is efficacious for smokers with a history of recurrent MDD, although the mechanism by which this effect is achieved does not appear to be through the reduction of depressive symptoms.

Cognitive-behavioral Treatment for Depression The Coping with Depression course (158–160) can serve as a basis for treatment of comorbid mood problems in smoking cessation (27). The major elements of the treatment include: daily monitoring of mood and factors influencing mood; contracting for achievable, systematic increases in pleasant activities to maintain or improve mood and to prevent the onset of depressive symptoms after cessation; cognitive self-management techniques for reducing negative thoughts and for increasing positive thoughts (160); the antecedents-behavior-consequences technique for identifying and challenging distorted, depressive thoughts (161); and assertiveness training using modeling, role-playing, and homework exercises, including situations involving social pressure to smoke. These treatment elements are readily incorporated into behavioral cessation programs and may be helpful for smokers with a history of recurrent MDD (27). A detailed description of the application of these depression coping skills to smoking cessation is also available (162).

SUMMARY AND CONCLUSIONS

Treating tobacco use and dependence is a high priority for improving public health. Although efficacious behavioral and pharmacologic interventions have been identified, many clinicians do not apply these interventions routinely with smokers and other tobacco users. Increased awareness of the need to assess and intervene with tobacco users, as well as increased knowledge about available treatment options is needed. Behavioral interventions increase smoking cessation rates and should be regularly applied in a range of settings including primary care settings, addictions treatment settings, and psychiatric settings. Combining behavioral interventions with pharmacotherapy produces the highest rates of success in smoking cessation. Nonetheless, rates of sustained smoking cessation are relatively low even when the most intensive interventions are applied. Therefore multiple attempts at quitting are often needed, and clinicians should continue to follow-up with patients who have made a quit attempt to reinforce abstinence and encourage new quit attempts among those who have relapsed (see Fig. 58.1). Although there is some empirical support for specific behavioral interventions to target specific risk factors for poor smoking cessation outcomes, such as current heavy drinking and a history of recurrent MDD, more research in this area is needed to determine whether such targeted interventions can substantially improve overall quit rates.

REFERENCES

1. McGinnis J, Foege W. Actual causes of death in the United States. *JAMA* 1993;270:2207–2212.
2. Centers for Disease Control and Prevention. Smoking-attributable mortality and years of potential life lost—United States, 1984. *MMWR Morb Mortal Wkly Rep* 1997;46:444–451.
3. American Cancer Society. *Cancer facts and figures.* 1999, Atlanta, GA: ACS.
4. Centers for Disease Control and Prevention. Medical-care expenditures attributable to cigarette smoking—United States, 1993. *MMWR Morb Mortal Wkly Rep* 1994;43:469–472.
5. Miller LS, Zhang X, Rice DP, et al. State estimates of total medical care expenditures attributable to cigarette smoking. *Public Health Rep* 1993; 113:447–458.
6. Centers for Disease Control and Prevention. Tobacco use among adults—United States, 2005. *MMWR Morb Mortal Wkly Rep* 2006;55: 1145–1148.
7. Centers for Disease Control and Prevention. Tobacco use—United States, 1990–1999. *MMWR Morb Mortal Wkly Rep* 1999;48:986–993.
8. Centers for Disease Control and Prevention. Cigarette smoking among adults—United States, 2002. *MMWR Morb Mortal Wkly Rep* 2004;53: 427–431.
9. Centers for Disease Control and Prevention. Smokers' beliefs about the health benefits of smoking cessation—20 U.S. communities, 1989. *MMWR Morb Mortal Wkly Rep* 1990;39:653–656.
10. Centers for Disease Control and Prevention. Cigarette smoking among adults—United States, 1993. *MMWR Morb Mortal Wkly Rep* 1994;43: 925–929.
11. Cohen S, Lichtenstein E, Prochaska JO, et al. Debunking myths about self-quitting. *Am Psychol* 1989;44(11):1355–1365.
12. Fiore MC, Bailey WC, Cohen SJ, et al. Treating tobacco use and dependence: clinical practice guideline. Rockville, MD: U.S. Department of Health and Human Services. Public Health Service, 2000.
13. Fiore MC, Bailey WC, Cohen SJ, et al. Smoking cessation: clinical practice guideline—number 18. U.S. Department of Health and Human Services, Public Health Service, Agency for Health Care Policy and Research, Centers for Disease Control and Prevention, 1996.
14. Kahler CW, Strong DR, Papandonatos GD, et al. Cigarette smoking and the lifetime alcohol involvement continuum. *Drug Alcohol Depend* 2008;93:111–120.
15. Dawson DA. Drinking as a risk factor for sustained smoking. *Drug Alcohol Depend* 2000;59(3):235–249.
16. Grant BF. Age at smoking onset and its association with alcohol consumption and DSM-IV alcohol abuse and dependence: results from the national longitudinal alcohol epidemiologic survey. *J Subst Abuse* 1998; 10:59–73.
17. Lasser K, Boyd JW, Woolhandler S, et al. Smoking and mental illness: a population-based prevalence study. *JAMA* 2000;284(20): 2606–2610.
18. Falk DE, Yi HY, Hiller-Sturmhofel S. An epidemiologic analysis of co-occurring alcohol and tobacco use and disorders: findings from the National Epidemiologic Survey on Alcohol and Related Conditions. *Alcohol Res Health* 2006;29(3):162–171.
19. Grant BF, Hasin DS, Chou SP, et al. Nicotine dependence and psychiatric disorders in the United States: results from the national epidemiologic survey on alcohol and related conditions. *Arch Gen Psychiatry* 2004;61(11):1107–1115.
20. Hughes JR. Clinical implications of the association between smoking and alcoholism. In: Fertig J, Fuller R, eds. *Alcohol and tobacco: from basic science to policy, NIAAA research monograph 30.* 1995, Washington, DC: U.S. Government Printing Office, 1995;171–185.
21. Bobo JK. Nicotine dependence and alcoholism epidemiology and treatment. *J Psychoactive Drugs* 1989;21:323–329.
22. Hurt R, Offord K, Croghan I, et al. Mortality following inpatient addictions treatment. Role of tobacco use in a community-based cohort. *JAMA* 1996;276:784.
23. Blondal T, Gudmundsson LJ, Tomasson K, et al. The effects of fluoxetine combined with nicotine inhalers in smoking cessation—a randomized trial. *Addiction* 1999;94(7):1007–1015.
24. Hays JT, Schroeder DR, Offord KP, et al. Response to nicotine dependence treatment in smokers with current and past alcohol problems. *Ann Behav Med* 1999;21(3):244–250.
25. Hughes JR. Treatment of smoking cessation in smokers with past alcohol/drug problems. *J Subst Abuse Treatment* 1993;10:181–187.
26. Hurt RD, Dale LC, Fredrickson PA, et al. Nicotine patch therapy for smoking cessation combined with physician advice and nurse follow-up: one year outcome and percentage of nicotine replacement. *JAMA* 1994;271(8):595–600.
27. Brown RA, Kahler CW, Niaura R, et al. Cognitive-behavioral treatment for depression in smoking cessation. *J Consult Clin Psychol* 2001;69: 471–480.
28. Covey LS, Glassman AH, Stetner F, et al. Effect of history of alcoholism or major depression on smoking cessation. *Am J Psychiatry* 1993;150: 1546–1547.
29. Humfleet G, Munoz R, Sees K, et al. History of alcohol or drug problems, current use of alcohol or marijuana, and success in quitting smoking. *Addict Behav* 1999;24(1):149–514.
30. Murray RP, Istvan JA, Voelker HT, et al. Level of involvement with alcohol and success at smoking cessation in the lung health study. *J Stud Alcohol* 1995;56(1):74–82.
31. Hughes JR, Kalman D. Do smokers with alcohol problems have more difficulty quitting? *Drug Alcohol Depend* 2006;82(2):91–102.
32. Breslau N, Peterson E, Schultz L, et al. Are smokers with alcohol disorders less likely to quit? *Am J Public Health* 1996;86(7):985–990.
33. Bobo JK, Gilchrist LD. Urging the alcoholic client to quit smoking cigarettes. *Addict Behav* 1983;8(3):297–305.
34. Kozlowski LT, Skinner W, Kent C, et al. Prospects for smoking treatment in individuals seeking treatment for alcohol and other drug problems. *Addict Behav* 1989;14:273–278.
35. Gulliver SB, Kamholz BW, AW Helstrom. Smoking cessation and alcohol abstinence: what do the data tell us? *Alcohol Res Health* 2006;29(3): 208–212.
36. Ziedonis DM, Guydish J, Williams J, et al. Barriers and solutions to addressing tobacco dependence in addiction treatment programs. *Alcohol Res Health* 2006;29(3):228–235.
37. Foulds J, Williams J, Order-Connors B, et al. Integrating tobacco dependence treatment and tobacco-free standards into addiction treatment: New Jersey's experience. *Alcohol Res Health* 2006;29(3):236–240.
38. Bobo JK, Gilchrist LD, Schilling RF II, et al. Cigarette smoking cessation attempts by recovering alcoholics. *Addict Behav* 1987;12:209–215.
39. Ellingstad TP, Sobell LC, Sobell MB, et al. Alcohol abusers who want to quit smoking: implications for clinical treatment. *Drug Alcohol Depend* 1999;54(3):259–265.
40. Hurt, RD, KM Eberman, IT Croghan, et al. Nicotine dependence treatment during inpatient treatment for other addictions: a prospective intervention trial. *Alcohol Clin Exp Res* 1994;18(4):867–872.
41. Kozlowski LT, Ferrence RG, Corbit T. Tobacco use: a perspective for alcohol and drug researchers. *Br J Addict* 1990;85:245.
42. Prochaska JJ, Delucchi K, Hall SM. A meta-analysis of smoking cessation interventions with individuals in substance abuse treatment or recovery. *J Consult Clin Psychol* 2004;72(6):1144–1156.
43. Bobo JK, Mcilvain HE, Lando HA, et al. Effect of smoking cessation counseling on recovery from alcoholism: findings from a randomized community intervention trial. *Addiction* 1998;96:877–887.
44. Bobo JK, Slade J, Hoffman AL. Nicotine addiction counseling for chemically dependent patients. *Psychiatric Serv* 1995;46:945–947.
45. Burling TA, Marshall GD, Seidner AL. Smoking cessation for substance abuse inpatients. *J Subst Abuse* 1991;3:269–276.
46. Monti PM, Rohsenow DJ, Colby SM, et al. Smoking among alcoholics during and after treatment: implications for models, strategies, and policy. In: Fertig JB, Allen JP, eds. *Alcohol and tobacco: from basic science to clinical practice.* Bethesda, MD: National Institutes of Health, 1995: 187–206.

47. Burling TA, Burling AS, Latini D. A controlled smoking cessation trial for substance-dependent inpatients. *J Consult Clin Psychol* 2001;69(2): 295–304.
48. Romberger DJ, Grant K. Alcohol consumption and smoking status: the role of smoking cessation. *Biomed Pharmacother* 2004;58(2):77–83.
49. Joseph AM, Willenbring ML, Nugent SM, et al. A randomized trial of concurrent versus delayed smoking intervention for patients in alcohol dependence treatment. *J Stud Alcohol* 2004;65(6):681–691.
50. Friend KB, Pagano ME. Smoking cessation and alcohol consumption in individuals in treatment for alcohol use disorders. *J Addict Dis* 2005; 24(2):61–75.
51. Kalman D, Kahler CW, Tirch D, et al. Twelve-week outcomes from an investigation of high-dose nicotine patch therapy for heavy smokers with a past history of alcohol dependence. *Psychol Addict Behav* 2004;18(1): 78–82.
52. Kalman D, Kahler CW, Garvey AJ, et al. High-dose nicotine patch therapy for smokers with a history of alcohol dependence: 36-week outcomes. *J Subst Abuse Treat* 2006;30(3):213–217.
53. Kodl M, Fu SS, Joseph AM. Tobacco cessation treatment for alcohol-dependent smokers: when is the best time? *Alcohol Res Health* 2006;29 (3):203–207.
54. Rohsenow DJ, Monti PM, Colby SM, et al. Brief interventions for smoking cessation in alcoholic smokers. *Alcohol Clin Exp Res* 2002;26 (12):1950–1951.
55. Bobo JK Davis CM. Cigarette smoking cessation and alcohol treatment. *Addiction* 1993;88(3):405–412.
56. McVea KL. Evidence for clinical smoking cessation for adolescents. *Health Psychol* 2006;25(5):558–562.
57. Sussman S, Sun P, Dent CW. A meta-analysis of teen cigarette smoking cessation. *Health Psychol* 2006;25(5):549–557.
58. Burnham JD. American physicians and tobacco use: two surgeon generals, 1929 and 1964. *Bull Hist Med* 1989;63:1–31.
59. Tate C. *Cigarette wars: the triumph of "the little white slaver."* New York: Oxford University Press, 1999.
60. U.S. Department of Health, Education, and Welfare. *Smoking and health: report of the advisory committee of the Surgeon General of the Public Health Service.* Washington, DC: USDHEW, 1964.
61. USDHHS. *Reducing the health consequences of smoking: 25 years of progress. A report of the Surgeon General.* Rockville, MD: U.S. Department of Health and Human Services, Public Health Service, Centers for Disease Control, Center for Chronic Disease Prevention and Health Promotion, Office on Smoking and Health, 1989.
62. Solberg LI, Boyle RG, Davidson G, et al. Aids to quitting tobacco use: how important are they outside controlled trials? *Prev Med* 2001;33(1):53–58.
63. Willemsen MC, Wiebing M, van Emst A, et al. Helping smokers to decide on the use of efficacious smoking cessation methods: a randomized controlled trial of a decision aid. *Addiction* 2006;101(3):441–449.
64. Zhu S, Melcer T, Sun J, et al. Smoking cessation with and without assistance: a population-based analysis. *Am J Prev Med* 2000;18(4):305–311.
65. USDHHS. *Reducing tobacco use: a report of the Surgeon General.* Atlanta, GA: U.S. Department of Health and Human Services, CDC, National Center for Chronic Disease Prevention and Health Promotion, Office on Smoking and Health, 2000.
66. Kottke TE, Battista RN, GH DeFriese, et al. Attributes of successful smoking cessation in medical practice: a meta-analysis of 39 controlled trials. *JAMA* 1988;259(19):2882–2889.
67. Cummings SR, Coates TJ, RJ Richard, et al. Training doctors in counseling about smoking cessation. *Ann Intern Med* 1989;110:640–647.
68. Lichtenstein E, Harris DE, Birchler GR, et al. Comparison of rapid smoking, warm, smoky air, and attention placebo in the modification of smoking behavior. *J Consult Clin Psychol* 1973;40(1):92–98.
69. Shiffman S, Kassel JD, Gwaltney C. Relapse prevention strategies for smoking. In: *Relapse prevention: maintenance strategies in the treatment of addictive behaviors,* 2nd ed. Marlatt GA, Dennis M, eds. Guilford Press: New York, 2005:92–129.
70. Miller WR, Rollnick S. *Motivational interviewing: preparing people for change.* 2nd ed. New York: Guilford Press, 2002.
71. Stead LF, Perera R, Lancaster T. Telephone counselling for smoking cessation. *Cochrane Database Syst Rev* 2006;3:CD002850.
72. Parker DR, Windsor RA, Roberts MB, et al. Feasibility, cost, and cost-effectiveness of a telephone-based motivational intervention for underserved pregnant smokers. *Nicotine Tob Res* 2007;9(10):1043–1051.
73. Azjen I. From intentions to actions: a theory of planned behavior. In: Kuhl J, Beckman J, ed. *Action-control: from cognition to behavior.* Springer: Heidelberg, 1985.
74. Marlatt GA, Gordon JR. *Relapse prevention: maintenance strategies in the treatment of addictive behaviors.* New York: Guilford Press, 1985.
75. DiClemente CC, Schlundt D, Gemmell L. Readiness and stages of change in addiction treatment. *Am J Addict* 2004;13(2):103–119.
76. Azjen I, Fishbein M. *Understanding attitudes and predicting social behavior.* Englewood Cliffs, NJ: Prentice-Hall, 1980.
77. Bandura A. Self-efficacy: toward a unifying theory of behavioral change. *Psychol Rev* 1977;84(2):191–215.
78. Abrams DB, Niaura RS. Social learning theory. In: Blane HT, Leonard KE, eds. *Psychological theories of drinking and alcoholism.* New York: The Guilford Press, 1987:131–178.
79. Bandura A. *Social foundations of thought and action: a cognitive theory.* Englewood Cliffs, NJ: Prentice Hall, 1986.
80. Niaura RS, Rohsenow DJ, JA Binkoff, et al. Relevance of cue reactivity to understanding alcohol and smoking relapse. *J Abnormal Psychol* 1988;7(2):133–152.
81. Ockene JK, Hosmer DW, Williams JW, et al. Factors related to patient smoking status. *Am J Public Health* 1987;77:356–357.
82. Pederson LL. Compliance with physician advice to quit smoking: a review of the literature. *Prevent Med* 1982;11:71–84.
83. Biener L, Abrams DB. The contemplation ladder: validation of a measure of readiness to consider smoking cessation. *Health Psychol* 1991; 10(5):360–365.
84. Prochaska JO, DiClemente CC. Stages and processes of self-change of smoking: toward an integrative model of change. *J Consult Clin Psychol* 1983;51(3):390–395.
85. Velicer WF, Fava JL, Prochaska JO, et al. Distribution of smokers by stage in three representative samples. *Prev Med* 1995;24(4):401–411.
86. Prochaska JO, Goldstein MG. Process of smoking cessation. Implications for clinicians. *Clin Chest Med* 1991;12(4):727–735.
87. Rollnick S, Mason P, Butler C. *Health behavior change. a guide for practitioners,* ed. London: Churchill Livingstone, 1999.
88. Baer JS, Lichtenstein E. Classification and prediction of smoking relapse episodes: an exploration of individual differences. *J Consult Clin Psychol* 1988;56(1):104–110.
89. Borland R. Slip-ups and relapse in attempts to quit smoking. *Addict Behav* 1990;15:235–245.
90. Shiffman S. Relapse following smoking cessation: a situational analysis. *J Consult Clin Psychol* 1982;50(1):71–86.
91. Pan W. Proactive telephone counseling as an adjunct to minimal intervention for smoking cessation: a meta-analysis. *Health Educ Res* 2006;21 (3):416–427.
92. Brown RA. Intensive behavioral treatments. In Abrams DB, et al, eds. *The tobacco dependence treatment handbook: a guide to best practices.* New York: Guilford, 2003.
93. Kahler CW, Lachance HR, Strong DR, et al. The commitment to quitting smoking scale: initial validation in a smoking cessation trial for heavy social drinkers. *Addict Behav* 2007;32(10):2420–2424.
94. Fishbein M. Consumer beliefs and behavior with respect to cigarette smoking: a critical analysis of the public literature. University of Illinois at Champaign-Urbana, 1977.
95. Brown RA, Emmons KM. Behavioral treatment of cigarette dependence. In: Cocores JA, ed. *The clinical management of nicotine dependence.* New York: Springer-Verlag, 1991:97–118.
96. Abrams DB, Wilson GT. Self-monitoring and reactivity in the modification of cigarette smoking. *J Consult Clin Psychol* 1979;47(2):243–251.
97. Mermelstein R, Cohen S, Lichtenstein E, et al. Social support and smoking cessation and maintenance. *J Consult Clin Psychol* 1986;54(4): 447–453.

98. Hunt WA, Bespalec DA. An evaluation of current methods of modifying smoking behavior. *J Clin Psychol* 1974;30:431–438.
99. Carroll KM. Relapse prevention as a psychosocial treatment: a review of controlled clinical trials. *Exp Clin Psychopharmacol* 1996;4(1):46–54.
100. Ockene JK, Emmons KM, Mermelstein RJ, et al. Relapse and maintenance issues for smoking cessation. *Health Psychol* 2000;19(1):17–31.
101. Stevens VJ, Hollis JF. Preventing smoking relapse, using an individually tailored skills-training technique. *J Consult Clin Psychol* 1989;57(3):420–424.
102. Hall SM, Humfleet GL, Reus VI, et al. Extended nortriptyline and psychological treatment for cigarette smoking. *Am J Psychiatry* 2004;161 (11):2100–2107.
103. Marcus BH, Albrecht AE, King TK, et al. The efficacy of exercise as an aid for smoking cessation in women: a randomized controlled trial. *Arch Intern Med* 1999;159:1229–1234.
104. Ockene JK, A Adams A. Screening and intervention for smoking and alcohol use in primary care settings: similarities, differences, gaps, and challenges. In: Fertig JB, Allen JP, eds. *Alcohol and tobacco: from basic science to clinical practice.* National Institutes of Health: Bethesda, MD, 1995:281–294.
105. Mokdad AH, Marks JS, Stroup DF, et al. Actual causes of death in the United States, 2000. *JAMA* 2004;291(10):1238–1245.
106. NIAAA. *Ninth special report to the U.S. Congress on alcohol and health.* Bethesda, MD: U.S. Department of Health and Human Services, 1997.
107. Durazzo TC, Gazdzinski S, Banys P, et al. Cigarette smoking exacerbates chronic alcohol-induced brain damage: a preliminary metabolite imaging study. *Alcohol Clin Exp Res* 2004;28(12):1849–1860.
108. Gazdzinski S, Durazzo TC, Studholme C, et al. Quantitative brain MRI in alcohol dependence: preliminary evidence for effects of concurrent chronic cigarette smoking on regional brain volumes. *Alcohol Clin Exp Res* 2005;29(8):1484–1495.
109. Meyerhoff DJ, Tizabi Y, Staley JK, et al. Smoking comorbidity in alcoholism: neurobiological and neurocognitive consequences. *Alcohol Clin Exp Res* 2006;30(2):253–264.
110. Gazdzinski S, Durazzo T, Jahng GH, et al. Effects of chronic alcohol dependence and chronic cigarette smoking on cerebral perfusion: a preliminary magnetic resonance study. *Alcohol Clin Exp Res* 2006; 30(6):947–958.
111. Durazzo TC, Rothlind JC, Gazdzinski S, et al. A comparison of neurocognitive function in nonsmoking and chronically smoking short-term abstinent alcoholics. *Alcohol* 2006;39(1):1–11.
112. Durazzo TC, Cardenas VA, Studholme C, et al. Non-treatment-seeking heavy drinkers: Effects of chronic cigarette smoking on brain structure. *Drug Alcohol Depend* 2007;87(1):76–82.
113. Ebbert JO, Janney CA, Sellers TA, et al. The association of alcohol consumption with coronary heart disease mortality and cancer incidence varies by smoking history. *J Gen Intern Med* 2005;20(1):14–20.
114. Schroder H, Marrugat J, Elosua R, et al. Tobacco and alcohol consumption: impact on other cardiovascular and cancer risk factors in a southern European Mediterranean population. *Br J Nutr* 2002;88(3):273–281.
115. Tuyns AJ, Esteve J, Raymond L, et al. Cancer of the larynx/hypopharynx, tobacco and alcohol: IARC international case-control study in Turin and Varese (Italy), Zaragoza and Navarra (Spain), Geneva (Switzerland) and Calvados (France). *Int J Cancer* 1988;41(4): 483–491.
116. Blot WJ, McLaughlin JK, Winn DM. Smoking and drinking in relation to oral and pharyngeal cancer. *Cancer Res* 1988;48:3282–3287.
117. Zambon P, Talamini R, La Vecchia C, et al. Smoking, type of alcoholic beverage and squamous-cell oesophageal cancer in northern Italy. *Int J Cancer* 2000;86(1):144–149.
118. Bosetti C, Franceschi S, Levi F, et al. Smoking and drinking cessation and the risk of oesophageal cancer. *Br J Cancer* 2000;83(5):689–691.
119. Kahler CW, Metrik J, LaChance HR, et al. Addressing heavy drinking in smoking cessation treatment: a randomized clinical trial. *J Consult Clin Psychol* 2008;76:852–862.
120. National Institute on Alcohol Abuse and Alcoholism. Helping patients who drink too much: a clinician's guide. Washington, DC: U.S. Department of Health and Human Services, 2005.
121. Hughes JR, Frances RJ. How to help psychiatric patients stop smoking. *Psychiatr Serv* 1995;46(5):435–436.
122. Williams JM, Ziedonis D. Addressing tobacco among individuals with a mental illness or an addiction. *Addict Behav* 2004;29(6):1067–1083.
123. Himelhoch S, Daumit G. To whom do psychiatrists offer smoking-cessation counseling? *Am J Psychiatry* 2003;160(12):2228–2230.
124. Montoya ID, Herbeck DM, Svikis DS, et al. Identification and treatment of patients with nicotine problems in routine clinical psychiatry practice. *Am J Addict* 2005;14(5):441–454.
125. Hall SM, Tsoh JY, JJ Prochaska, et al. Treatment for cigarette smoking among depressed mental health outpatients: a randomized clinical trial. *Am J Public Health* 2006;96(10):1808–1814.
126. Haug NA, Hall SM, JJ Prochaska, et al. Acceptance of nicotine dependence treatment among currently depressed smokers. *Nicotine Tob Res* 2005;7(2):217–224.
127. Prochaska, JJ, Rossi JS, Redding CA, et al. Depressed smokers and stage of change: implications for treatment interventions. *Drug Alcohol Depend* 2004;76(2):143–151.
128. Pomerleau OF, Pomerleau CS, Mehringer AM, et al. Nicotine dependence, depression, and gender: characterizing phenotypes based on withdrawal discomfort, response to smoking, and ability to abstain. *Nicotine Tob Res* 2005;7(1):91–102.
129. Pomerleau CS, Pomerleau OF, Snedecor SM, et al. Heterogeneity in phenotypes based on smoking status in the Great Lakes Smoker Sibling Registry. *Addict Behav* 2004;29(9):1851–1855.
130. American Psychiatric Association. Diagnostic and statistical manual of mental disorders (4th ed.). Washington, DC: Author, 1994.
131. Evins AE, Cather C, Culhane MA, et al. A 12-week double-blind, placebo-controlled study of bupropion SR added to high-dose dual nicotine replacement therapy for smoking cessation or reduction in schizophrenia. *J Clin Psychopharmacol* 2007;27(4):380–386.
132. Ziedonis DM, George TP. Schizophrenia and nicotine use: report of a pilot smoking cessation program and review of neurobiological and clinical issues. *Schizophr Bull* 1997;23(2):247–254.
133. Addington J. Group treatment for smoking cessation among persons with schizophrenia. *Psychiatr Serv* 1998;49(7):925–928.
134. Washington A, Moll S, Pawlick J. *Smokebusters: an approach to help people with mental illness move closer to a smoke-free lifestyle.* Hamilton: Ontario, 1997.
135. Dickens G, Stubbs J, Popham R, et al. Smoking in a forensic psychiatric service: a survey of inpatients' views. *J Psychiatr Ment Health Nurs* 2005; 12(6):672–678; quiz 678.
136. Dickens GL, Stubbs JH, Haw CM. Smoking and mental health nurses: a survey of clinical staff in a psychiatric hospital. *J Psychiatr Ment Health Nurs* 2004;11(4):445–451.
137. Jochelson K. Smoke-free legislation and mental health units: the challenges ahead. *Br J Psychiatry* 2006;189:479–480.
138. Black DW, Zimmerman M, Coryell WH. Cigarette smoking and psychiatric disorder in a community sample. *Ann Clin Psychiatry* 1999;11 (3):129–136.
139. Glassman AH, Helzer JE, Covey LS, et al. Smoking, smoking cessation, and major depression. *JAMA* 1990;264(12):1546–1549.
140. Breslau N, Johnson EO. Predicting smoking cessation and major depression in nicotine-dependent smokers. *Am J Public Health* 2000;90(7):1122–1127.
141. Anda RF, Williamson DF, Escobedo LG, et al. Depression and the dynamics of smoking: a national perspective. *JAMA* 1990;264(12):1541–1545.
142. Frederick T, Frerichs RR, Clark VA. Personal health habits and symptoms of depression at the community level. *Prev Med* 1988;17(2):173–182.
143. Brown C, Madden PA, Palenchar DR, et al. The association between depressive symptoms and cigarette smoking in an urban primary care sample. *Int J Psychiatry Med* 2000;30(1):15–26.
144. Covey LS, Hughes DC, Glassman AH, et al. Ever-smoking, quitting, and psychiatric disorders: Evidence from the Durham, North Carolina, epidemiologic catchment area. *Tobacco Control* 1994;3:222–227.
145. Hitsman B, Borrelli B, McChargue DE, et al. History of depression and smoking cessation outcome: a meta-analysis. *J Consult Clin Psychol* 2003;71(4):657–663.

146. Kinnunen T, Doherty K, Militello FS, et al. Depression and smoking cessation: Characteristics of depressed smokers and effects of nicotine dependence. *J Consult Clin Psychol* 1996;64(4):791–798.
147. Berlin I, Covey LS. Pre-cessation depressive mood predicts failure to quit smoking: the role of coping and personality traits. *Addiction* 2006;101(12):1814–1821.
148. Covey LS, Glassman AH, Stetner F. Depression and depressive symptoms in smoking cessation. *Compr Psychiatry* 1990;31(July/August):350–354.
149. Ginsberg D, Hall SM, Reus VI, et al. Mood and depression diagnosis in smoking cessation. *Exp Clin Psychopharmacol* 1995;3(4):389–395.
150. West RJ, Hajek P, Belcher M. Severity of withdrawal symptoms as a predictor of outcome of an attempt to quit smoking. *Psychol Med* 1989;19:981–985.
151. Covey L. Comments on "History of depression and smoking cessation outcome: a meta-analysis." *Nicotine Tob Res* 2004;6(4):743–745; author reply 747–749; discussion 751–752.
152. Ziedonis D, Hitsman B, Beckham JC, et al. Tobacco use and cessation in psychiatric disorders: National Institute of Mental Health (NIMH) report. *Nicotine Tob Res.* In press.
153. Covey LS, Glassman AH, Stetner F. Major depression following smoking cessation. *Am J Psychiatry* 1997;154(2):263–265.
154. Haas AL, Munoz RF, Humfleet GL, et al. Influences of mood, depression history, and treatment modality on outcomes in smoking cessation. *J Consult Clin Psychol* 2004;72(4):563–570.
155. Hall SM, Muñoz RF, Reus VI. Cognitive-behavioral intervention increases abstinence rates for depressive-history smokers. *J Consult Clin Psychol* 1994;62(1):141–146.
156. Hall SM, Reus VI, Muñoz RF, et al. Nortriptyline and cognitive-behavioral therapy in the treatment of cigarette smoking. *Arch Gen Psychiatry* 1998;55:683–690.
157. Hall, SM, RF Muñoz, V.I. Reus, et al. Mood management and nicotine gum in smoking treatment: a therapeutic contact and placebo-controlled study. *Journal of Consulting and Clinical Psychology* 1996;64(5): 1003–1009.
158. Brown RA, Lewinsohn PM. *Coping with depression: course workbook.* Eugene, OR: Castalia Press, 1984.
159. Brown RA, Lewinsohn PM. A psychoeducational approach to the treatment of depression: comparison of group, individual, and minimal contact procedures. *J Consult Clin Psychol* 1984;52(5):774–783.
160. Lewinsohn PM, Antonuccio DO, Breckenridge JS, et al. *The coping with depression course: a psychoeducational intervention for unipolar depression.* Eugene, OR: Castalia Press, 1984.
161. Ellis A, Harper RA. *A guide to rational living.* Hollywood, CA: Wilshire, 1961.
162. Brown RA. Comorbidity treatment: Skills training for coping with depression and negative moods. In: Abrams DB, et al, eds. *The tobacco dependence treatment handbook: a guide to best practices.* New York: Guilford, 2003.

CHAPTER 59

Marc Galanter, MD, FASAM

Network Therapy

INTRODUCTION

In recent years there has been considerable progress toward developing psychosocial modalities specific to the treatment of addiction. Indeed, the situation is quite different than it was when Alcoholics Anonymous (AA) emerged in a climate of inadequate physician attention to the rehabilitation of alcoholics. Professionals in the addiction field now have access to a variety of therapeutic techniques. These include variants of cognitive therapy, motivational enhancement, and family and group therapy modalities, all tailored to the needs of the patient with alcohol or drug disorder.

The clinician in office practice, however, often is uncertain as to how to integrate these approaches to meet the needs of a given patient. On the face of it, there is no obvious relationship, for example, between the use of cognitively oriented approaches, such as relapse prevention, and the engagement of family support to secure improved motivation. To address this issue, this chapter examines network therapy (1–3), a multimodal approach that has been disseminated to practitioners and standardized and studied in the clinical research setting.

HISTORICAL PERSPECTIVE

Support for addiction treatment itself has expanded over time, and recognition of the severity of the problem initially led to an increase in resources for inpatient care. Initially, the availability of beds in designated units increased by 62% from 1977 to 1984, with all of the net gain in the private sector (4). The "Minnesota model" for inpatient management (5,6), based on a protracted inpatient stay, became a standard of treatment for many middle-class addicts. The imposition of managed care, however, led to a transition to ambulatory care. The decline in inpatient treatment was also fueled by a lack of support in randomized controlled trials for its relative advantage over ambulatory care.

In early studies, no difference in outcome was found when outpatients were offered individual therapy as a treatment added to medical monitoring alone, nor was insight-oriented therapy found to enhance the effectiveness of outpatient milieu treatment for alcoholism. Early on, Vaillant (7), commented on alcoholism treatment that "The greatest danger of this is wasteful, painful psychotherapy that bears analogy to someone trying to shoot a fish in a pool. No matter how carefully he aims, the refracted image always renders the shot wide of its mark." As conventionally practiced, individual therapy did not appear to be an effective tool for addiction rehabilitation.

New perspectives on ambulatory care soon arose. Evidence mounted for both research-based and clinically based support for the importance of securing abstinence for substance-dependent persons as an initial step in addiction treatment, rather than awaiting results of an exploratory therapy (8–10). This position has been strengthened by the widespread acceptance of AA, which is strongly oriented toward abstinence, and by a recent consensus-based definition of recovery (11). To implement a regimen of abstinence, clinical researchers have developed a number of structured techniques, focusing on cognitive-behavioral change (12,13) and interpersonal support from family and peers (14,15). These approaches can be adapted to an office practice oriented toward individual therapy so as to promote abstinence and effective rehabilitation.

The integrated approach discussed here is called *network therapy* because it draws on the support of a group of family and peers who are introduced into individual therapy sessions. The term derived from the work of Speck and Attneave (16), who used a large support group drawn from the patient's family and social network as a tool for psychiatric management. These networks were used for both psychological and practical aid in addressing acute psychiatric illness so as to avert a hospitalization until the acute symptoms remitted. Once mobilized, the network became available to aid in ambulatory rehabilitation as well.

THE TREATMENT MODEL

To define what this approach must accomplish, it is first necessary to examine some unique characteristics of the substance dependence syndrome.

Psychological Mechanisms For many clinicians, the problems of relapse and loss of control, embodied in the criteria for substance dependence in the DSM-IVR, epitomize the pitfalls inherent in addiction treatment. Because addicted patients typically experience pressure to relapse and ingest alcohol or drugs, they are seen as poor candidates for stable treatment. The concept of "loss of control" has been used to describe addicts' inability to reliably limit consumption once an initial dose is taken. This clinical phenomenon is generally described anecdotally but can be explained mechanistically as well by recourse to the model of conditioned withdrawal. Wikler (17), an early investigator of addiction pharmacology, developed this model to explain the spontaneous appearance of drug craving and relapse. He pointed out that drugs of dependence typically produce compensatory responses in the central nervous system at the same time that their direct pharmacologic effects are felt, and these compensatory effects partly counter the drug's direct action. Thus, when an opiate antagonist is administered to addicts maintained with morphine, latent withdrawal phenomena are unmasked. Similar compensatory effects were observed in alcoholics maintained with alcohol, who evidence evoked response patterns characteristic of withdrawal while still clinically intoxicated (18). A potential addict who has begun to drink or use another drug heavily may be repeatedly exposed to an external stimulus (such as a certain mood state) while drinking. Subsequent exposure to these cues may thereby produce conditioned withdrawal symptoms, subjectively experienced as craving.

Modulations of mood are often the conditioned stimuli for drug seeking, and the substance-abusing individual can become vulnerable to relapse through reflexive response to a specific affective state. Khantzian (19) described such phenomena clinically as *self-medication.* Such mood-related cues, however, are not necessarily mentioned spontaneously by the patient in conventional therapy, because the triggering feeling may not be associated with a memorable event, and the drug use may avert memorable distress.

More dramatic is the phenomenon of *affect regression* (20) observed among addicted patients who were studied in a psychoanalytic context. When addicted subjects sustain narcissistic injury, they are prone to a precipitous collapse of ego defenses followed by intense and unmanageable affective flooding. In the face of such vulnerability, these subjects handle stress poorly and may turn to drugs for relief. This vulnerability can be considered in light of the model of conditioned withdrawal, whereby drug seeking can become an immediate reflexive response to stress, undermining the stability and effectiveness of a patient's coping mechanisms. Drug seeking can occur quite suddenly in patients who have long associated drug use with their attempts to cope with stress.

This model helps to explain why relapse is such a frequent and unanticipated aspect of addiction treatment. Exposure to conditioned cues, ones that were repeatedly associated with drug use, can precipitate reflexive drug craving during the course of therapy, and such cue exposure can also initiate a sequence of conditioned behaviors that lead addicted individuals to relapse unwittingly into drug use.

Social Support A client's social environment and personal relationships are often instrumental in the development of addiction and may be just as important in processes of recovery. In fact, social environmental factors are the most robust predictors of long-term positive outcome (21). Social networks for individuals in treatment can be differentiated into two basic components: the peer-led self-help network, which is inherent in the philosophy of the therapeutic community model, and the natural social network consisting of family and close friends. It has been demonstrated that family involvement in substance abuse treatment is effective in improving outcome, and there are numerous approaches that make use of social network involvement in treatment, including behavioral couples therapy (22), marital therapy (23), and the community reinforcement approach (24,25). Other approaches involve utilizing the social network to encourage the addict to seek treatment using intervention. These include Community Reinforcement and Family Training (CRAFT) (25) and the Johnson Intervention (26). The philosophy of supportive collaterals and the philosophy of social networks have several underlying similarities, in particular those of affiliation. Both approaches seek to discourage the affiliation of the client with negative social supports or those sources that encourage drug use and encourage the clients' affiliation with positive drug-free networks.

Cognitive Behavioral Orientation in Treatment

Network therapy makes use of a variety of empirically tested cognitive-behavioral relapse prevention techniques (12) that are delivered with participation by members of the patient's natural support system (i.e., family and friends). Along with the patient, these supportive others are taught to apply a behavioral model of the nature of addiction to understanding the patient's addiction; to participate in the development of relapse prevention strategies; to assist the therapist in securing patient adherence with medication regimens; and to assist the therapist in securing patient adherence with other parts of the treatment plan, such as in the execution of relapse prevention strategies. In these respects, network therapy shares some of the components of both the community reinforcement approach and behavioral marital therapy (e.g., behavioral skills training, medication monitoring by a significant other).

TREATMENT AND TECHNIQUE

Selection of Patients Network therapy is appropriate for individuals who cannot reliably control their intake of alcohol or drugs once they have taken their first dose; those who have tried to stop and relapsed; and those who have not been willing or able to stop. Individuals whose problems are too severe for the network approach in ambulatory care include those who cannot stop their drug use even for a day or who cannot comply with outpatient detoxification. Conversely, individuals who can be treated with conventional therapy and without a network include those who have demonstrated the ability to moderate their consumption without problems.

The Network's Membership Networks generally consist of three or four members. Once the patient has come for an appointment, establishment of a network is undertaken with active collaboration between the patient and the therapist. The two, aided by those parties who join the network initially, must search for the right balance of members. The therapist, however, must carefully promote the choice of appropriate network members. The network will be crucial in determining the balance of the therapy. This process is not without problems, and the therapist must think strategically of the interactions that may occur among network members. The following case illustrates the nature of the therapist's task:

> *A 25-year-old graduate student had been abusing drugs since high school, in part drawing on funds from his affluent family, who lived in a remote city. At two points in the process of establishing his support network, the reactions of his live-in girlfriend were particularly important. They both agreed to bring in his 19-year-old sister, a freshman at a nearby college. He then mentioned a "friend" of his, a woman whom he had apparently found attractive, even though there was no history of an overt romantic involvement. The expression on his girlfriend's face suggested that she was uncomfortable with this option. The therapist temporarily put aside the idea of the friend and moved on to evaluating the patient's uncle. Initially, the patient was reluctant to include him in the network because he perceived the uncle as a potentially disapproving representative of the parental generation. The therapist and the girlfriend nonetheless encouraged him to accept the uncle as a network member to round out the range of relationships within the group. The uncle was caring and supportive, particularly after he was helped to understand the nature of the addictive process.*

The Network's Task The therapist's relationship to the network is one of a task-oriented team leader rather than of a family therapist oriented toward restructuring relationships. The network is established to implement a straightforward task, that of aiding the therapist to sustain the patient's abstinence. The network must be directed with the same clarity of purpose that a task force is directed in any effective organization. Competing and alternative goals must be implicitly suppressed or at least prevented from interfering with the primary task, but the atmosphere must be kept supportive.

Unlike family members involved in traditional family therapy, network members are not led to expect symptom relief or self-realization for themselves. This approach prevents development of competing goals for the network's meetings. It also protects members from having their own motives scrutinized and thereby supports their continuing involvement without the threat of an assault on their psychologic defenses. Because network members have kindly volunteered to participate, their motives must not be impugned. Their constructive behavior should be commended. Network members should be acknowledged for the contribution they are making to the therapy. They often have a counterproductive tendency to minimize the value of their contribution. The network must therefore be structured as an effective working group with good morale. This approach is illustrated below:

> *A 45-year-old single woman served as an executive in a large family-held business, except when her alcohol problem led her into protracted binges. Her father, brother, and sister were prepared to banish her from the business but decided first to seek consultation. The father was a domineering figure who intruded in all aspects of the business, evoking angry outbursts from his children. The children typically reacted with petulance, provoking him in return. The situation came to a head two months into treatment, when the patient's siblings angrily petitioned the therapist to exclude the father from the network. This presented a problem because the father's control over the business made his involvement important in securing the patient's compliance. Relapse by the patient was still a real possibility. The father implied that he might compromise his son's role in the family business. The father's potentially coercive role, however, was an issue that the group could not deal with easily. The therapist supported the father's membership in the group, pointing out the constructive role he had played in getting the therapy started. It was clear to the therapist that the father could not deal with a situation in which he was not accorded sufficient respect and that there was no place in this network for addressing the father's character pathology directly. The children became less provocative as the group responded to the therapist's pleas for civil behavior.*

Couples A cohabiting couple will provide the first example of how natural affiliative ties can be used to develop a secure basis for rehabilitation. Couples therapy for addiction

Month ____________

Date/day	Time Taken	Therapist Checkoff	Date/day	Time Taken	Therapist Checkoff
1.			17.		
2.			18.		
3.			19.		
4.			20.		
5.			21.		
6.			22.		
7.			23.		
8.			24.		
9.			25.		
10.			26.		
11.			27.		
12.			28.		
13.			29.		
14.			30.		
15.			31.		
16.					

FIGURE 59.1. Format for network member's observation of pill ingestion by the patient.

has been described in both ambulatory and inpatient settings, and good marital adjustment has been found to be associated with a diminished likelihood of dropping out and a positive overall outcome (27). It is recognized, however, that a spouse must be involved in an appropriate way. Constructive engagement should be distinguished from a codependent relationship or overly involved interaction, which is thought to be a problem in recovery. Indeed, couples managed with a behavioral orientation showed greater improvement in alcoholism than those treated with interactional therapy, where attempts were made to engage them in relational change (28). Thus, we will consider here a simple, behaviorally oriented device for making use of the marital relationship: working with a couple to enhance the effectiveness of disulfiram therapy.

The use of disulfiram has yielded relatively little benefit overall in controlled trials when patients are responsible for taking their doses on their own (29). This is largely because this agent is effective only when it is ingested as instructed, typically on a daily basis. Alcoholics who forget to take required doses likely will resume drinking in time. Indeed, such forgetting often reflects the initiation of a sequence of conditioned drug-seeking behaviors.

The involvement of a spouse, however, in observing the patient's consumption of disulfiram has been shown to yield a considerable improvement in outcome (24,30). Patients alerted to taking disulfiram each morning by this external reminder are less likely to experience conditioned drug seeking when exposed to addictive cues and are more likely to comply on subsequent days with the dosing regimen.

The technique also helps in clearly defining the roles in therapy of both the alcoholic-addicted person and spouse, typically the wife, by avoiding the spouse's need to monitor drinking behaviors she cannot control. The spouse does not actively remind the alcoholic-addicted to take each disulfiram dose. She merely notifies the therapist if she does not observe the pill being ingested on a given day (Fig. 59.1). Decisions about managing compliance are then shifted to the therapist, and the couple does not become entangled in a dispute over the patient's attitude and the possibility of secret drinking. By means of this technique, a majority of alcohol-addicted patients in one clinical trial (31) experienced marked improvement and sustained abstinence over the period of treatment.

A variety of other behavioral devices shown to improve outcome can be incorporated into this couples format. For example, it has been found (32) that scheduling the first appointment for as soon as possible after the initial telephone contact improves outcome by diminishing the possibility of an early loss of motivation. Spouses also can be engaged in history taking at the outset of treatment to minimize the introduction of denial into the patient's representation of the illness (33). The initiation of treatment with such a technique is illustrated in the following case report.

A 39-year-old alcoholic man was referred for treatment. Both the patient and his wife were initially engaged by the psychiatrist in a telephone exchange so that all three could plan for the patient to remain abstinent on the day of the first session. They agreed that the wife would meet the patient at his office at the end of the work day on the way to the appointment. This would ensure that cues presented by his friends going out for a drink after work would not lead him to drink. In the session, an initial history was taken from the spouse as well as the patient, allowing her to expand on the negative consequences of the patient's drinking, thereby avoiding his minimizing of the problem. A review of the patient's medical status revealed no evidence of relevant organ damage, and the option of initiating his treatment with disulfiram was discussed. The patient, with the encouragement of his wife, agreed to take his first dose that day, continue under her observation, and then be evaluated by his internist within a few days. Subsequent sessions with the couple were dedicated to dealing with implementation of this plan, and concurrent individual therapy was initiated as well.

Patients who take disulfiram in this manner have acquired a cognitive label to help them avoid a sudden and unanticipated relapse. The potential efficacy of this approach is illustrated by the reaction of a patient who experiences a precipitous collapse of psychologic defenses and potentially relapses. If he or she has been taking disulfiram as described here, knowledge of a potential disulfiram reaction can alert him or her to avoid going out to get a drink. Patients who are maintained with disulfiram, as described, for an initial year of recovery thus have the opportunity to deal in therapy with the issues that precipitate craving, without exposing themselves unduly to the threat of relapse.

It is important to clarify certain aspects of engaging a collateral in the treatment, particularly a spouse. Long-standing conflicts between members of an alcohol-misusing couple should not be allowed to interfere with the disulfiram monitoring. For example, the spouse should not be placed in a role in which he or she must demand compliance. This is why patients are vested with the responsibility of ingesting the disulfiram so that they are clearly seen by their spouse; their role is only to notify the therapist in a telephone message if one does not see the other taking the pill on a given morning. Discussions of compliance per se, therefore, are initiated by the therapist and not by the spouse. In this way, the role of the spouse as enforcer is eliminated.

Typical Networks The therapist's intervening with family and friends to start treatment was introduced by Johnson (34) as one of the early ambulatory techniques in the addiction field. More broadly, the availability of greater social support to patients has been shown to be an important predictor of positive outcome in addiction. In light of this, it is important to consider what would serve as a useful paradigm for using family and social supports in office treatment. This can be used as well to enhance the stability of the technique for disulfiram observation already described. There are two options for stabilizing abstinence: the ecologic and the problem-solving family treatment. The ecologic approach emphasizes the engagement of resources from the patient's family and social environment. It presumes that the pathology is embedded in the broader social context and acknowledges that this context must be used to effect recovery. There are many approaches to treatment that employ this in one form or another, from community reinforcement to social service-based models. Problem-solving family therapy, originally developed by Haley (35) and others, relies on an initial assessment of the principal presenting symptom, and subsequent treatment is directed at the problem itself, rather than primarily at restructuring the family relations. By means of these approaches, the therapist can develop an option that parallels the community reinforcement behavioral approach used in multimodality clinics, as in the following case.

Friends of a 46-year-old alcohol-dependent man sought out consultation to secure his abstinence. At the psychiatrist's suggestion, they brought him along with them to a conjoint session, where he avowed that he could stop drinking on his own. An agreement was made among the network members, the patient and the psychiatrist that they would maintain contact so that they could act together in case the patient's suggested approach did not succeed. Two months later, after the patient had required brief hospitalization for detoxification following a relapse into drinking, members of the network prevailed on him to come for treatment. The patient and network members then agreed that he would participate in individual therapy and would meet with the network and psychiatrist at regular intervals. The patient suffered a relapse six months later; one of the network members consulted the psychiatrist and stayed with the patient in his home for a day to ensure that he would not drink. He and other network members then brought the patient to the psychiatrist's office to reestablish a plan for abstinence.

This case illustrates how members of the network can help to counter the patient's inclination to deny a drinking problem in the initial stages of engagement and during relapse as well. It shows the value of the network in providing the psychiatrist with the means of communicating with a relapsing patient and of assisting in reestablishment of abstinence. As illustrated in the following case vignette, an effective intervention need involve no more than the network members' providing advice in the therapy session. The weight of the patient's relationship with his own chosen network members and his ability to respond to their efforts to help him are potent tools in securing compliance. In the following case, the network members were instrumental in ensuring that the patient would remove himself from conditioned environmental cues for substance use during the period of early abstinence.

A 23-year-old man who had insufflated heroin for a year had recently begun using it intravenously. In a psychiatric consultation that he solicited, he agreed to bring in his uncle, his cousin and a friend for support and to take naltrexone each day under the observation of the uncle. In the ensuing session with this network, he expressed reluctance to move to his parents' house temporarily to provide a setting that would help him avoid friends who would expose him to regular drinking and marijuana use. After discussing the importance of this added security with his network members and the psychiatrist, he concurred with the consensus that he did need the move temporarily. On the basis of their input, he conceded that it was more important at the moment to avoid the drug cues of his peer group than to insist on independence from his parents.

In the network format, a cognitive framework can be provided for each session by starting out with the patient's recounting events related to cue exposure or substance use since the last meeting. Network members then are expected to comment on this report to ensure that all are engaged in a mutual task with correct, shared information. Their reactions to the patient's report are addressed as well, as illustrated below.

An alcoholic man began one of his early network sessions by reporting a minor lapse in abstinence. This was disrupted by an outburst of anger from his older sister. She said that she had "had it up to here" with his frequent unfulfilled promises of sobriety. The psychiatrist addressed this source of conflict by explaining in a didactic manner how behavioral cues affect vulnerability to relapse. This didactic approach was adopted in order to defuse the assumption that relapse is easily controlled and to relieve consequent resentment. He then led members in planning concretely with the patient how he might avoid further drinking cues in the period preceding their next conjoint session.

This case illustrates the importance of maintaining an appropriate therapeutic milieu in the network sessions. In volunteering to participate, members agree to help the patient but not to subject their own motives to scrutiny. In this, the network format therefore differs materially from the systemic family therapy approach, as it avoids subjecting network members to the demands of addressing their own motives. The didactic or intellectualized approach can be helpful in neutralizing excessive anger that may be felt toward the patient, without scrutinizing the reasons for a member's anger.

In addition, the patient himself is expected to help maintain amicable relations with network members to protect the supportive milieu. This is made explicit in both network and individual sessions. For example, if a network member is absent for a few sessions, the patient is expected to discuss the matter with that member and to resolve any outstanding issues in order to promote the member's return. Any difficulty the patient may experience in carrying out this role is viewed as an issue to be addressed in individual sessions. The network, therefore, is conceived of as an active collaboration in which conflicts are minimized to ensure optimal function. When led effectively, members are inclined to be effective team members.

They develop a positive transference toward the therapist and are willing to support the therapist's views.

Complementing Individual Therapy Psychotherapeutic approaches have been found to yield improved outcomes when combined with certain addiction treatments, such as AA, opioid maintenance, and cocaine management techniques (36). In the context of network therapy, individual expressive sessions can complement the abstinence orientation of network meetings if the therapist closely attends to conditioned cues for substance use. Once abstinence is stabilized, network sessions can augment the psychotherapy with support for the patient's general social recovery.

Even after the patient's abstinence is apparently stable, it is important to examine in therapy the patient's thoughts about drinking, dreams related to substance use, and responses to environmental drinking cues. On the one hand, they alert the patient to the need to be aware of the long-term risk of relapse. On the other hand, they provide revealing clues to ongoing conflicts, which may be apparent only in their expression in the symbolism of addiction.

Though network sessions may be terminated before long-term individual therapy comes to an end, it is essential to make clear that the network members should be available if the patient experiences difficulties in the future, as illustrated in the next case vignette.

> *An alcoholic woman had been seen in network and individual sessions for 16 months and had been abstinent for a year. Because of her stability, a final network session was scheduled with her husband and two friends. Discussion there initially focused on her successful recovery, as evidenced by her beginning employment in the previous month. Those present then agreed that any of the network members could contact the therapist if the patient relapsed in the future. The patient indicated that she would discuss any lapse in abstinence with both the network members and the therapist.*

In Contrast to an Intervention The Johnson Institute intervention approach, first developed by Vernon E. Johnson in the 1960s (34), is what people generally mean when they use the term *intervention*. Unlike network therapy, this approach convenes a number of people from the substance abuser's family and close friends who might otherwise constitute members of a network. In a series of preparatory meetings, letters and statements are prepared for the substance abuser describing the compromise to them and to himself because of his addiction. A confrontation is then planned in which the threat is explicitly made of withdrawal of support and personal contact if the patient does not agree to enter treatment—typically in a residential setting.

In some cases of network therapy, distressed family or friends may call and meet for consultation about a reluctant addicted person over whom they are concerned. The network therapist may then meet with those potential network members before an encounter with the addicted person. If the "patient" is reluctant to enter treatment, the collaterals can be instructed to approach him as a group and press him to meet with them and with the therapist, but an aggressive confrontation is not used. The encounter is not meant to be highly confrontational like that employed in a Johnson intervention approach. This network initiation can be applied to engaging patients in both outpatient and inpatient treatment. A similar approach has been formalized in the ARISE format developed by Garret et al. (36). A strategy, however, may have to be worked out with potential network members as to how a patient who is initially reluctant will be pressed to come to treatment, as follows:

> *A 40-year-old man who had managed his family-owned company had devolved into heavy cocaine use. He was now spending much of his time in his apartment ordering the cocaine which he was using on a daily basis by phone. When members of his family came to seek consultation, it emerged that he was sustaining himself with credit card charges from a family-managed account. The therapist said that they should each press him to come in, but inform him as well that his economic resources could be cut back if he did not to come with them to a therapy session. Although the therapist promoted a supportive exchange between the patient and family when they all arrived at a joint session, the patient was under pressure to comply with treatment to assure continuing access to family funds. An exchange ensued in which the patient acknowledged his problem and agreed to come to another network meeting, while seeing the therapist individually. After an individual session followed by another network and individual session, an agreement was reached. He would participate in ongoing therapy, both individually and with the network. Because of implied pressure from network members, the therapist had been able to serve as a mediator in the network sessions, and avoid an unduly defensive response to him on the part of this potential patient.*

Use of Alcoholics Anonymous Use of AA is desirable. For the alcoholic individual, certainly, participation in AA is strongly encouraged. Groups such as Narcotics Anonymous, Pills Anonymous, and Cocaine Anonymous are modeled after AA and play a similarly useful role among drug-abusing individuals. One approach is to tell the patient that he or she is expected to attend at least two AA meetings each week for at least 1 month to familiarize him or her with the program. If after 1 month the patient is quite reluctant to continue and other aspects of the treatment are going well, his or her nonparticipation may have to be accepted.

Some patients are easily convinced to attend AA meetings. Others may be less compliant. The therapist should mobilize the support network as appropriate to continue pressing the patient to give participation in AA a reasonable try.

Principles of Network Treatment The following is a set of guidelines for applying network therapy. It can be adapted to the needs of a given patient and to the relative availability of potential network members.

Begin a Network as Soon as Possible

1. It is important to see the patient promptly, as the window of opportunity for openness to treatment generally is brief. A week's delay can result in loss of motivation or relapse to drinking.
2. If the patient is married, engage the spouse early on, preferably at the time of the first telephone call. Point out that addiction is a family problem. The spouse generally can be enlisted in ensuring that the patient arrives at the office with a day's sobriety.
3. In the initial interview, frame the exchange so that a good case is built for the grave consequences of the patient's addiction, and do this before the patient can introduce his or her system of denial. This approach avoids putting the spouse or other network members in the awkward position of having to contradict a close relative.
4. Make clear that the patient needs to be abstinent, beginning immediately. (A tapered detoxification may be necessary with some drugs, such as the sedative-hypnotics.)
5. An alcoholic patient can be started on disulfiram treatment as soon as possible, in the office at the time of the first visit, if possible. Instruct the patient to continue taking disulfiram under the observation of a network member. Get baseline chemistries concomitantly.
6. Start to build a network for the patient at the first visit, involving the patient's family members and close friends.
7. From the very first meeting, consider how to ensure the patient's sobriety until the next meeting and plan that with the network. Initially, their immediate companionship, a plan for daily AA attendance, and planned activities all may be necessary.

Keep the Network's Agenda Focused

1. *Maintain abstinence:* The patient and the network members should report at the outset of each session any exposure of the patient to alcohol or drugs. The patient and network members should be instructed as to the nature of relapse and should work with the clinician to develop a plan to sustain abstinence. Cues to conditioned drug-seeking should be examined.
2. *Support the network's integrity*: Everyone has a role in this: The patient is expected to ensure that network members keep their meeting appointments and stay involved with the treatment. The therapist sets meeting times and summons the network for any emergency, such as relapse. (The therapist does whatever is necessary to secure stability of the membership if the patient is having trouble doing so.) Members of the network are responsible for attending network sessions and engaging in other supportive activities with the patient.
3. *Secure future behavior*: The therapist should combine any and all modalities necessary to ensure the patient's stability. This may involve establishing a stable, drug-free residence; avoiding substance abusing friends; attending Twelve Step meetings; using medications such as disulfiram or blocking agents; observing urinalysis; and obtaining ancillary psychiatric care. Written agreements may be useful. This may involve a mutually acceptable contingency contract, with penalties for violation of understandings.

End Network Therapy Appropriately

1. Network sessions can be terminated after the patient has been stably abstinent for at least 6 months to 1 year. Before network therapy is stopped, the therapist should discuss with the patient and network the patient's readiness to handle sobriety.
2. An understanding is established with the network members that they will contact the therapist at any point in the future if the patient becomes vulnerable to relapse. The network members can also be summoned by the therapist. These points should be made clear to the patient before termination, in the presence of the network, but they also apply throughout treatment.

RELEVANT RESEARCH

A number of studies have demonstrated the effectiveness of network therapy in treatment and training. Each addressed the technique's validation from a different perspective: a trial in office management; studies of its effectiveness in the training of psychiatry residents and of counselors who work with cocaine-addicted persons; and an evaluation of acceptance of the network approach in an Internet technology transfer course.

An Office-Based Clinical Trial In an initial study, a chart review was conducted involving a series of 60 substance-dependent patients, with follow-up appointments scheduled through the period of treatment and up to 1 year thereafter (31). For 27 patients, the primary drug of dependence was alcohol; for 23, it was cocaine; for 3, it was marijuana; and for 1, it was nicotine. Opiates were the primary drugs of dependence for 6 patients. For all but 8 of the patients, networks were fully established. Of the 60 patients, 46 experienced abstinence for at least 6 months or a marked decrease in drug use to nonproblematic levels. The study demonstrated the viability of establishing networks and applying them in the practitioner's treatment setting.

Treatment by Psychiatry Residents A network therapy training sequence was implemented in a psychiatry residency program and then evaluated the clinical outcomes of a group of cocaine-dependent patients treated by the residents. A training manual was prepared on the network technique, defining the specifics of the treatment in a manner allowing for uniformity in practice. Network therapy tape segments drawn from a library of 130 videotaped sessions were used to illustrate typical therapy situations. A network therapy rating scale was developed to assess the technique's application, with items emphasizing key aspects of treatment (38). The scale was evaluated for reliability in distinguishing two contrasting addiction therapies (Network Therapy and systemic family), and the internal consistency of responses for each of the techniques was high for both the faculty and the resident samples, and both groups consistently distinguished the two modalities. The scale was then used by clinical supervisors as an aid in training and to monitor therapist adherence to the study treatment manual.

The residents worked with a sample of 47 cocaine-addicted patients. Once treatment was initiated, 77% of subjects established a network, with an average of 1.47 collaterals at any given network therapy session. Of the patients who completed a 24-week regimen, 15 of 17 tested negative for cocaine in their last three urine toxicology screenings. Conversely, 4 of 18 subjects of those who attended the first week but did not complete the sequence met this outcome criterion (39). The residents, inexperienced in drug treatment, achieved results similar to those reported for experienced professionals at the time (40–42). These comparisons supported the feasibility of successful training of psychiatry residents new to administration of addiction treatment and the efficacy of the treatment in their hands (43).

Treatment by Addiction Counselors Another study was conducted in a community-based addiction treatment clinic, and the network therapy training sequence was essentially the same as the one applied to the psychiatry residents (44). A cohort of 10 cocaine-dependent patients received treatment in the community program with a format that included network therapy along with the clinic's usual package of modalities. An additional 20 cocaine-dependent patients received treatment as usual and served as control subjects. Network therapy was found to enhance the outcome of the experimental patients. Of the 107 urinalyses conducted in the network therapy group, 88% yielded negative results, but only 66% of the 82 urine samples from the control subjects were negative for cocaine, a significantly lower proportion ($p < 0.05$). The results of this study supported the feasibility of transferring the network technique into community-based settings, with the potential for enhancing outcomes.

Engagement in Buprenorphine Treatment During the initial stages of buprenorphine treatment, patients with opioid addiction, particularly those dependent on heroin, often continue to use heroin intermittently and may also misuse other substances. To minimize this, it is advantageous to initiate buprenorphine treatment with the support of network therapy.

In a recent study, all patients received a standard course of buprenorphine/naloxone tablets (16 mg/40 mg) daily for opioid dependence and underwent random urine toxicologies. They were randomly assigned to one of two treatment groups, network therapy or medication management. Patients in each group were provided the same amount of time overall in therapy sessions. The study consisted of an 18-week trial during which patients were inducted onto buprenorphine and then tapered to zero dose. By the end of the study, the abstinence rate of patients who participated in network therapy was twice that of the patients in the comparison group who received standard medication management (50% vs. 23%), indicating the effectiveness of the network support (45).

For patients who enter treatment with secondary substance abuse, such as cocaine dependence, it is important that a pattern of addictive behavior to the secondary drug also be addressed, as continuation of any misuse of a substance is more likely to be associated with an unsuccessful long-term outcome. Because of this, the network approach can be particularly useful in addressing this latter issue, given the support provided for abstinence from all drugs.

Multi-Site Comparison to Motivational Enhancement The feasibility of treatment in the network modality was demonstrated with the use of a brief training course, video observation, and subsequent supervision (46). Alcohol-dependent patients (N = 742) were then divided among 52 nonphysician therapists and randomly assigned to either of the two treatments. The network approach consisted of eight 50-minute sessions over 12 weeks, whereas the motivational enhancement approach comprised three 50-minute sessions over the same period. An evaluation at 12 months showed equivalent outcome in terms of days abstinent and number of drinks per drinking day (47). Though the network approach involved greater staff time, a calculation of the relative cost saving, as measured by additional factors such as health care costs, social services, and the expense of the criminal justice system when indicated, showed no difference in overall cost of the two approaches (48). When applied as described in this chapter, the open-ended nature of the network commitment may well provide an incremental benefit in maintaining long-term positive availability of support that may not be available with the use of a brief motivational intervention.

Use of the Internet An advertisement was placed in *Psychiatric News,* the newspaper of the American Psychiatric Association, offering an Internet course combining network therapy with the use of naltrexone for the treatment of alcoholism. The material presented on the Internet was divided into three didactic "sessions," followed by a set of questions, with a hypertext link to download relevant references and a certificate of completion. The course took about 2 hours to complete. An assessment was based on 679 sequential counts, representing 240 unique respondents who went beyond the introductory Web page (49). Of these respondents, 154 were psychiatrists, who responded positively to the course. A majority of them responded "a good deal" or "very much" (a score of 3 or 4 on a 4-point scale) to the following statements about the course: "It helped me understand the management of alcoholism treatment" (56%), "It helped me learn to use family or friends in network treatment for alcoholism" (75%), and "It improved my ability to use naltrexone in treating alcoholism" (64%).

CONCLUSIONS

Network therapy is a multimodal approach to rehabilitation in which specific family members and friends are enlisted to provide ongoing support and promote attitude change. Its goal is the prompt achievement of abstinence with relapse prevention and the development of a drug-free adaptation. Network members are part of the therapist's "team" working toward achieving this goal and not subject of treatment themselves. This approach has been shown to be useful in controlled comparisons to other psychosocial modalities. It has also been demonstrated to be successfully adapted for both psychiatric residency training and community-based physicians and nonphysician therapists.

REFERENCES

1. Galanter M. *Network therapy for drug abuse: A new approach in practice.* New York: Basic Books, 1993a.
2. Galanter M. Network therapy for addiction: a model for office practice. *Am J Psychiatry* 1993b;150:28–36.
3. Galanter M. *Network therapy for drug and alcohol abuse* [Expanded edition]. New York: Guilford, 1999.
4. National Institute on Alcohol Abuse and Alcoholism. *Alcoholism and health.* Washington DC: U.S. Government Printing Office, 1987.
5. Cook CCH. The Minnesota Model in the management of drug and alcohol dependency: miracle, method or myth? Part I: The philosophy and the programme. *Br J Addict* 1988;83:625–634.
6. Cook CCH. The Minnesota Model in the management of drug and alcohol dependency: miracle, method or myth? Part II: Evidence and conclusions. *Br J Addict* 1988;83:735–748.
7. Vaillant GE. Dangers of psychotherapy in the treatment of alcoholism. In: Bean MH, Zinberg NE eds. *Dynamic approaches to the understanding and treatment of alcoholism.* New York: Free Press, 1981.
8. Nathan PE, McCrady BS. Bases for the use of abstinence as a goal in the treatment of alcohol abusers. *Drugs Soc* 1986/87;1:109–131.
9. Gitlow SE, Peyser HS. *A practical treatment guide.* New York: Grune & Stratton, 1980.
10. Gallant DM. *A guide to diagnosis, intervention and treatment.* New York: WW Norton, 1987.
11. The Betty Ford Institute Consensus Panel and Belleau C, Dupont RL, Erickson CK, et al. What is recovery? A working definition from the Betty Ford Institute. *J Subst Abuse Treat* 2007;33:221–228.
12. Marlatt GA, Gordon JR eds. *Relapse prevention: Maintenance strategies in the treatment of addictive disorders.* New York: Guilford Press, 1985.
13. Annis HM. A relapse prevention model for treatment of alcoholics. In: Miller WE, Heather N eds. *Treating addictive behaviors: Processes of change.* New York: Plenum Publishing Co., 1986.
14. Stanton MD & Thomas TC eds. *The family therapy of drug abuse and addiction.* New York: Guilford Press, 1982.
15. Kaufman E, Kaufman PN eds. *Family therapy of drug and alcohol abuse.* New York: Gardner Press, 1979.
16. Speck R, Attneave C. *Family networks.* New York: Vintage Books, 1974.
17. Wikler A. Dynamics of drug dependence. *Arch Gen Psychiatry* 1973;28: 611–616.
18. Begleiter H, Porjesz B. Persistence of a subacute withdrawal syndrome following chronic ethanol intake. *Drug Alcohol Depend* 1979;4:353–357.
19. Khantzian EJ. The self-medication hypothesis of addictive disorders: focus on heroin and cocaine dependence. *Am J Psychiatry* 1985;142:1259–1264.
20. Wurmser L. Mrs. Pecksniff's horse? Psychodynamics of compulsive drug use. In: Blaine JD, Julius DS eds. *Psychodynamics of drug dependence* [Research Monograph 12]. Rockville, MD: National Institute on Drug Abuse, 1977.
21. Longabaugh R. Involvement of support networks in treatment. *Recent Dev Alcohol* 2003;16:133–147.
22. Fals-Stewart W, O'Farrell TJ, Feehan M, et al. Behavioral couples therapy versus individual-based treatment for male substance-abusing patients. *J Subst Abuse Treatment* 2000;18:249–254.
23. O'Farrell TJ. Marital therapy in the treatment of alcoholism. In: Jacobson NS, Gurman AS eds. *Clinical handbook of marital therapy.* New York: Guilford Press, 1986:513–535.
24. Azrin NH, Sisson RW, Meyers R, Godley M. Alcoholism treatment by disulfiram and community reinforcement therapy. *J Behav Ther Exp Psychiatry* 1982;13:105–112.
25. Meyers RJ, Smith JE, Lash DN. The community reinforcement approach. *Recent Dev Alcohol* 2003;16:183–195.
26. White RK, Wright DG. *Addiction intervention. Strategies to motivate treatment-seeking behavior.* New York: Haworth Press, 1998.
27. McCrady BS, Stout R, Noel N, et al. Effectiveness of three types of spouse-involved behavioral alcoholism treatment. *Br J Addict* 1991;86: 1415–1424.
28. Fuller RK, Branchey L, et al. Disulfiram treatment of alcoholism: a Veterans Administration cooperative study. *JAMA* 1986;256:1449–1455.
29. O'Farrell TJ, Cutter HSG, Floyd FJ. Evaluating behavioral marital therapy for male alcoholics: effects on marital adjustment and communication before and after treatment. *Behav Ther* 1985;16:147–167.
30. Galanter M. Management of the alcoholic in psychiatric practice. *Psychiatr Ann* 1989;19:266–270.
31. Galanter M. Network therapy for substance abuse: a clinical trial. *Psychotherapy* 1993c;30:251–258.
32. Stark MJ, Campbell BK, Brinkerhoff CV. Hello, may we help you? A study of attrition prevention at the time of the first phone contact with substance-abusing clients. *American J Drug Alcohol Abuse* 1990;15:209–222.
33. Liepman MR, Nierenberg TD, Begin AM. Evaluation of a program designed to help family and significant others to motivate resistant alcoholics to recover. *Am J Drug Alcohol Abuse* 1989;15:209–222.
34. Johnson VE. *How to help someone who doesn't want help.* Minneapolis: Johnson Institute Books, 1986.
35. Haley J. *Problem-solving therapy.* San Francisco: Jossey-Bass, 1977.
36. Carroll K. Manual-guided psychosocial treatment. *Arch Gen Psychiatry* 1997;54:923–928.
37. Garret J, Landau J, Shea R, et al. The ARISE intervention using family and network links to engage addicted persons in treatment. *J Subst Abuse Treat* 1998;15:333–343.
38. Keller DS, Galanter M, Weinberg S. Validation of a scale for network therapy: a technique for systematic use of peer and family support in addiction treatment. *Am J Drug Alcohol Abuse* 1997;23:115–127.
39. Galanter M, Dermatis H, Keller D, et al. Network therapy for cocaine abuse: use of family and peer supports. *Am J Addict* 2002;11:161–166.
40. Carroll KM, Rounsaville BJ, Gordon LT, et al. Psychotherapy and pharmacotherapy for ambulatory cocaine abusers. *Arch Gen Psychiatry* 1994;51:177–187.
41. Higgins ST, Budney AJ, Bickel WK, et al. Achieving cocaine abstinence with a behavioral approach. *Am J Psychiatry* 1993;150:763–769.
42. Shoptaw S, Rawson RA, McCann MJ, et al. The Matrix model of outpatient stimulant abuse treatment: evidence of efficacy. *J Addict Dis* 1994; 13:129–141.
43. Galanter M, Keller DS, Dermatis H. Network therapy for addiction: assessment of the clinical outcome of training. *Am J Drug Alcohol Abuse* 1997a;23:355–367.

44. Keller DS, Galanter M. Technology transfer of network therapy to community-based addictions counselors. *J Subst Abuse Treat* 1999;16: 183–189.
45. Galanter M, Dermatis H, Glickman L, et al. Network therapy: decreased secondary opioid use during buprenorphine maintenance. *J Subst Abuse Treat* 2004;26:313–318.
46. Copello A, Williamson E, Orford J, Day E. Implementing and evaluating social behaviour and network therapy in drug treatment practice in the UK: a feasibility study. *Addict Behav* 2006;31:802–810.
47. UKATT Research Team. Effectiveness of treatment for alcohol problems: findings of the randomised UK alcohol treatment trial (UKATT). *Br Med J* 2005a;331:541–544.
48. UKATT Research Team. Cost effectiveness of treatment for alcohol problems: findings of the randomised UK alcohol treatment trial (UKATT). *Br Med J* 2005b;331:544.
49. Galanter M, Keller DS, Dermatis H. Using the Internet for clinical training: a course on network therapy for substance abuse. *Psychiatr Serv* 1997b;48:999–1000, 1008.

CHAPTER 60

Donald J. Kurth, MD, MBA, MPA, FASAM

Therapeutic Communities

In the TC philosophy, drug or alcohol use is considered a symptom of a complex disorder involving the whole person. Self-destructive and defeating patterns of behavior and thought processes are thought to disrupt both the individual's lifestyle and society's functioning. Though genetic, environmental, and pharmacologic contributions to addiction are recognized, the individual is held fully responsible for his or her own disorder, behavior, and recovery. Addiction is regarded as the symptom, rather than the disorder. The problem is the behavior of the person, not the drug.

The modern addiction therapeutic community (TC) is a powerful therapeutic tool that, over the past several decades, has helped hundreds of thousands of addicts and alcoholics achieve abstinence-based recovery (1). Abstinence rates of more than 90% for many years after treatment are documented in well-established TCs.

Historically, the TC has been used to treat a variety of problems in living, but the modern addiction TC or "concept TC" is a hybrid of self-help and public support geared toward the treatment of addictive and co-occurring psychiatric disorders.

The philosophic foundation of the modern TC is personal responsibility for one's behavior and the belief that change is fully possible if the individual exerts the personal effort to follow the teachings of the program.

Evolving out of Alcoholics Anonymous (AA) in the 1960s, the modern addiction TC still retains many of the underpinnings of the Twelve Step approach to treatment. Drug addiction is viewed as a "whole person" disorder and, therefore, is treated with a holistic approach. Emotions and feelings are considered important and can be explored in depth, but change is based on action. That action is the responsibility of the individual. As in Twelve Step recovery, the individual is not expected to walk this road alone. The community is available to help the addict at every step of the way.

HISTORY AND EVOLUTION

The modern TC is a new application of an ancient concept. The Dead Sea Scrolls found at Qumron document the first TC. The communal practices of an ascetic religious sect, perhaps the Essenes, include the "Rules of Community." The Essene code denounces "the ways of the spirit of falsehood" and speaks of the problems of greed, lying, cruelty, brazen insolence, lust, and "walking the ways of darkness and guile." Righteous and healthy living required strict adherence to the rules and teachings of the community.

Violation of the Rules of Community incurred sanctions resembling, though much harsher than, the sanctions used in the modern addiction TC. For violations such as lying, bearing a grudge, foolish speech or laughter, sleeping during a community meeting, or leaving a community meeting, sanctions could include periods of banishment from the community or limited rations or privileges.

At about the time Jesus walked the earth, a group of healers (therapeutrides) of the "incurable" diseases of the soul lived in Alexandria, Egypt. Philo Judaeus (BC 25 to 45 AD) described the group as professing "an art of medicine for [excessive] pleasures and appetites . . . the immeasurable multitude of passions and vices" (2). As in the modern TC philosophy, diseases of the soul were seen as manifesting themselves through the whole person. Healing was regarded as occurring through some form of community involvement.

The Washingtonians (founded by a group of drinkers) later appeared in the United States as a 19th century precursor to AA. Though the Washingtonians did not survive as a group, several of their methods are still apparent in the modern addiction TC. These include the commitment to abstinence, proselytizing its message to others, and the practice of self-appraisal during group meetings.

The conceptual and organizational lineage of the modern addiction TC began about 1921 with the Oxford Group—also known as The Buchmanites, the First Century Christians Fellowship, and Moral Rearmament (3). A branch of the Oxford Group in Akron, OH evolved into AA in 1935 under the guidance of Bill Wilson and Doctor Bob Smith. A Santa Monica, CA AA group evolved into Synanon in 1958 under the guidance of AA members. From Synanon sprang Daytop Village in New York City, under the guidance of Monsignor William O'Brien. From Daytop, more than 100 other therapeutic communities have developed around the world.

The Oxford Group (or Oxford Movement) began in the second decade of the 20th century as the First Century Christian Fellowship. Founded by Lutheran evangelist minister Frank Buchman, the early Oxford Group preached a return to the purity and innocence of the early church. This spiritual rebirth was to be applied to all forms of human suffering. Though alcoholism and mental illness were not the primary focus of the Oxford Group, they were certainly seen as signs of spiritual deficit and thus were encompassed by the Oxford Group's principles.

The Reverend Buchman headquartered the Oxford Movement in New York City, where Dr. Samuel Shoemaker, pastor of Calvary Episcopal Church, became involved as well. During this period, the philosophies of the Quakers and Anabaptists (precursors to the Mennonites and Amish) began to influence the movement. These early influences carry through to the foundation of the modern addiction TC. Concepts and practices such as the work ethic, mutual concern, and sharing guidance are basic to the TC philosophy. Evangelical values such as honesty, purity, unselfishness, love, making amends for harm done, and working well with others all can be traced to this era (4,5).

The thread continues even today. Though not directly related to the Oxford Group, "Oxford House" is the name of a self-run, self-supported sober-living housing initiative that was begun in Silver Spring, MD in 1975 and now includes more than 450 sober-living houses situated throughout the United States.

The Twelve Steps of AA evolved directly from the Six Steps of the Oxford Group. Together with the Twelve Traditions and the Twelve Concepts, the Twelve Steps embody the principles that guide the individual in recovery. The concepts of confessing to others and making amends and the belief that individual change requires conversion to belief in the group are principles derived directly from the Oxford Group. Other AA principles include admitting one's loss of control over alcohol and surrendering to one's "Higher Power," performing self-examination, seeking help from one's Higher Power in changing one's self, making amends to others, praying in the personal struggle, and helping others to engage in a similar process. Some striking differences are found, however. AA deviated from the Oxford requirement of a religious God by allowing each AA member to develop his or her own concept of a Higher Power. Though AA does not require a Christian god, its principles do stress that one's power to change is derived from a power greater than one's self. Nonsectarian AA, in fact, allows the Higher Power to be the AA group. This concept of the group as Higher Power is further developed in Synanon and later TCs, as it evolved into reliance on self and group process as the medium of individual behavioral change.

Fifteen years before Synanon appeared on the scene in the United States, however, psychiatric hospital TCs began to develop in Great Britain. Pioneered by Maxwell Jones, the first of these appeared as a social rehabilitation unit at Belmont Hospital in England in the mid-1940s. The Jones TC embraced the therapeutic nature of the total environment as a treatment tool (Table 60.1). Though the Jones TC is used today as a viable treatment method in Great Britain, its application to the treatment of addictive disorders occurred only

TABLE 60.1 Characteristics of the Psychiatric (Jones) TC

1. The total organization is seen as affecting therapeutic outcomes.
2. The social organization is useful in creating a milieu that maximizes therapeutic effects and is not simply the background for treatment.
3. A core element is democratization: The social environment provides opportunities for patients to take an active part in the affairs of the institution.
4. All relationships are therapeutic.
5. The qualitative atmosphere of the social environment is therapeutic in that it is balanced between acceptance, control, and tolerance for disruptive activities.
6. Great value is placed on communication.
7. The orientation of the group is toward productive work and a quick return to society.
8. Educational techniques and group pressure are used for constructive purposes.
9. There is a diffusion of authority from staff to patients.

Adapted from DeLeon (6).

in the context of dual-diagnoses patients. Some addictive disorder treatment adaptation of the Jones TC model has occurred in the United States in the Veterans Administration hospitals. There is little data about the efficacy of treatment in this application.

The evolution of Synanon from an AA group resulted in the concepts, program model, and basic practices that have become the essential elements of all modern addiction TCs. Synanon's charismatic founder, Chuck Dederich, integrated his AA experiences with other philosophic, pragmatic, and psychologic influences to create the Synanon program. The unique encounter group process ("the game") evolved from weekly AA meetings. Distinct psychologic changes were evident as a result of this process. The participants recognized this change as a new form of therapy and, within a year, the weekly meetings expanded into a residential community. In August 1959, the organization was officially founded to treat any addict, regardless of the chemical of choice. The name *Synanon* apparently was coined during the confused mumbling of a heroin addict who was having trouble pronouncing the word "seminar," fusing it with the word "symposium." Despite its role in the evolution of the modern TC, Synanon never considered itself a TC but rather an alternative community for teaching and living.

Synanon evolved from AA and, as a result, the precepts of AA are fundamental to Synanon and to all modern addiction TCs. Still, the evolution did occur, and the differences are what created the TC as a distinct approach. Self-help recovery, a belief that the ability to change and heal lies within the individual and a belief that healing occurs as a result of a therapeutic relationship with others who have a similar affliction, all are philosophies common to both programs. The AA traditions and program activities led directly to the TC's individual self-reliance, organizational self-reliance, and its schedule of regular groups and meetings.

The numbering system of AA's Twelve Steps did not carry through to Synanon, but the same stages of recovery are very much a part of the Synanon program and the other modern addiction TCs as well. Steps 1 to 3 are embodied in the TC's early phase recovery, which emphasizes breaking through denial and engaging in the change process. Steps 4 to 9 are seen in the mid-phase recovery period of intense self-examination and socialization. This period involves taking a personal inventory, sharing confession with another person, and making amends. Steps 10 to 12 are reflected in the maturational process and increased autonomy that develop in the reentry phase of the TC. This phase requires continued personal honesty, humbly asking for help to sustain recovery, and actively helping others.

Critical differences, however, define the addiction TC as a new treatment modality. These include the residential setting, organizational structure, and profile of participants, goals, philosophy, and ideologic orientation.

Initially, residents could graduate from Synanon. Soon, however, Synanon (like AA) abandoned the concepts of graduation or completion of the program. In AA, when participants are fully integrated in society, they continue to participate in the program of recovery and continue to attend group meetings. This participation is analogous, perhaps, to continuing to attend church. In the case of 24-hour-a-day residential Synanon, completion of the program signified quite a different situation. All activities of a person's life were to occur within the highly structured hierarchical organization, with no sort of reentry or reintegration back into society as a whole. Synanon embraced AA's Seventh Tradition of fiscal independence with entrepreneurial spirit, developing profit-making businesses as well as pursuing both public and private funding. Though any member could rise within the hierarchy, the management was never democratic but rather oligarchic.

THE DAYTOP MODEL

Monsignor William O'Brien, a young priest, and Dr. Daniel Casriel, a Manhattan psychiatrist, first attempted to apply the concept of a TC specifically to the treatment of drug addiction. With the help of Joseph Shelly, chief probation officer of Brooklyn, NY, and Alexander Basson, a doctoral student who wrote the first grant, funds were obtained from the National Institute on Mental Health to develop an addiction TC.

The new program needed a director, and none of the initial applicants had been willing to take the job. So, Basson called the New York office of AA. A gentleman with no experience in treating drug addiction named Dean Colcord was sent to apply and was hired as the first director of Daytop Lodge (later to become Daytop Village).

Daytop Lodge opened with 25 beds on September 1, 1963, in Staten Island, NY. Dean Colcord had spent 3 weeks visiting the Westport Synanon to learn how it operated. Daytop applied the Synanon program with a strong dose of AA to the public sector treatment of addiction.

The founding of Daytop marked a milestone in the development of the modern TC (Table 60.2).

TABLE 60.2 The Daytop Philosophy

I am here because there is no refuge, finally, from myself. Until I confront myself in the eyes and hearts of others, I am running.
Until I suffer them to share my secrets, I have no safety from them. Afraid to be known, I can know neither myself nor any other,
I will be alone. Where else but in our common ground, can I find such a mirror? Here, together, I can at last appear clearly to myself not as a giant of my dreams nor the dwarf of my fears, but as a person, part of a whole, with my share in its purpose. In this ground, I can take root and grow not alone any more as in death but alive to myself and to others.

Author: Richard Beauvais.

The modern TC rests on a foundation of secular ideology with certain existential assumptions, including the following:

- Self-determination: A core value is self-determination. Each individual is seen as the captain of his or her own ship and the one who determines the path of his or her life.
- Individual responsibility: The TC philosophy holds each individual fully responsible for his or her own behavior. No matter the genetic predisposition or environmental or family influences, each person is seen as fully and completely responsible for his or her own behavior.
- Self-change: The concept of self-change is regarded as possible through personal commitment and adherence to recovery teachings.

FEATURES OF THE MODERN THERAPEUTIC COMMUNITY

The addiction TC is a powerful tool for changing behavior, and its efficacy is well documented in the literature. It is less clear how and why this therapeutic modality is so effective in changing difficult behaviors for which so many other methods are not successful.

Components of a Therapeutic Community Program

Several features characterize TC programs that follow the Daytop Village model and other first-generation therapeutic communities (6) (Table 60.3).

Community Separateness TC-oriented programs have their own identities and are housed in a space or locale that is separated from other agency or institutional programs or units or generally from the drug-related environment. In residential settings, clients remain away from outside influences 24 hours a day for several months before earning the privilege of a brief visit to the outside community. In nonresidential "day treatment" settings, the individual spends 4 to 8 hours a day in the TC environment and is monitored by peers and family while outside the TC. Even in the least restrictive outpatient settings, TC-oriented programs and components are in place. This is designed to help members gradually detach from old networks and relate to the drug-free peers in the program.

A Community Environment The TC environment prominently features communal spaces and collective activities. Walls carry signs declaring the philosophy of the program, the messages of right living and recovery. Cork boards and blackboards are used to identify all participants by name, seniority level, and job function in the program. Daily schedules are posted as well. These visuals display an organizational picture of the program that the individual can relate to and comprehend, thus promoting program affiliation.

Community Activities The TC philosophy holds that, to be effective, treatment and educational services must be provided within a context of the peer community. Thus, with the exception of individual counseling, all activities are programmed in collective formats. These activities include at least one daily meal prepared, served, and shared by all members; a daily schedule of groups, meetings, and seminars; jobs performed in teams; organized recreational/leisure time; and ceremonies and rituals (to mark birthdays, phase/progress graduations, and the like).

TABLE 60.3 Fundamental Changes in TCs after the Founding of Daytop Village

1. Marks the shift from being an alternative community for deviant addicts who presumably could not function in mainstream society to a human services agency preparing individuals for reintegration into a larger society
2. Marks the shift from indefinite tenure in the same residential community to a planned duration of residential stay guided by a treatment plan and protocol
3. Marks the shift from complete or partial private and entrepreneurial sources of support to virtually sole reliance on public funding for operational budgets, necessitating compliance with requirements for accountability and oversight by external boards of directors
4. Marks a de-emphasis of charismatic leaders and increased importance of peer leadership, staff members as role models, and multiple decision makers
5. Marks the inclusion of increasing proportions of nonrecovering staff in primary clinical and administrative roles from varied professional disciplines
6. Develops after-care programs for those who complete the residential phase of treatment
7. Reintegrates AA Twelve Step principles and traditions into the treatment protocol of many residential TCs
8. Includes gradual rapprochement between psychiatric and addiction TC models and methods
9. Adapts the TC for special populations and in special settings such as mental health facilities and correctional institutions
10. Marks the development of a research and evaluation knowledge base by independent and program-based investigative teams
11. Codifies competency requirements for staff training, staff credentialing, and program accreditation
12. Develops regional, national, and international TC organizations
13. Promulgates and disseminates the TC for addictions worldwide through training, program development, technical assistance, and research

Alcoholics Anonymous World Service (Author), Alcoholics Anonymous comes of age: A brief history of AA. New York: Alcoholics Anonymous World Service. 1957.

Staff Rules and Functions Staff members are a mix of self-help professionals who are themselves in recovery and other helping professionals (medical, legal, mental health, and educational), who are integrated through cross-training grounded in the TC perspective and community approach. Professional skills define the function of staff members (e.g., nurse, physician, lawyer, teacher, administrator, case worker, clinical counselor). Regardless of professional discipline or function, however, the generic *role* of all staff members is that of community members who, rather than providers and treaters, are viewed as rational authorities, facilitators, and guides in the self-help community method.

Peers as Role Models Members who demonstrate the expected behaviors and reflect the values and teachings of the community are viewed as role models. Indeed, the strength of the community as a context for social learning relates to the number and quality of its role models. All members of the community are expected to be role models: roommates; older and younger residents; and junior, senior, and directorial staff. TCs require these multiple role models to maintain the integrity of the community and to ensure the spread of social learning effects.

A Structured Day The structure of the program relates to the TC perspective, particularly the view of the client and recovery. Ordered activities conducted in a regular routine counter the characteristically disordered lives in which clients have lived and distract from negative thinking and boredom—factors that are thought to predispose individuals to drug use. Structured activities also are regarded as facilitating the acquisition of self-structure on the part of the individual, as expressed in time management; planning, setting, and meeting goals; and general accountability. Thus, regardless of its length, the day has a formal schedule of therapeutic and educational activities with prescribed formats, fixed times, and routine procedures.

Work as Therapy and Education Consistent with the TC's self-help approach, all clients are responsible for the daily management of the facility (e.g., cleaning, meal preparation and service, maintenance, purchasing, security, scheduling, preparation for group meetings, seminars, activities). In the TC, the various work roles mediate essential educational and therapeutic effects. Job functions strengthen affiliation with the program through participation, provide opportunities for skill development, and foster self-examination and personal growth through performance challenge and program responsibility. The scope and depth of clients' work depends on the program (for example, institutional versus free-standing facility) and client resources (levels of psychologic function, social and life skills).

Phase Format The treatment protocol, or plan of therapeutic and educational activities, is organized into phases that reflect a developmental view of the change process. Emphasis is placed on incremental learning at each phase, so as to move the individual to the next stage of recovery.

Therapeutic Community Concepts Formal and informal curricula are focused on teaching the TC perspective, particularly its self-help recovery concepts and view of right living. The concepts, messages, and lessons are repeated in the various groups, meetings, seminars, and peer conversations, as well as in readings, signs, and personal writings.

Peer Encounter Groups The principal community or therapeutic group is the encounter, though other forms of therapeutic, educational, and support groups are employed as needed. The minimal objective of the peer encounter is similar to TC-oriented programs—to heighten the individual's awareness of specific attitudes or behavior patterns that need to be modified. However, the encounter process can differ in degree of staff direction and intensity, depending on the client subgroups (e.g., adolescents, prison inmates, and the dually diagnosed).

Awareness Training All therapeutic and educational interventions involve raising the individual's awareness of the effects of his or her conduct and attitudes on himself or herself and the social environment and, conversely, the effect of the behaviors and attitudes of others on the individual and his or her environment.

Emotional Growth Training Achieving the goals of personal growth and socialization involves teaching individuals how to identify feelings, express them appropriately, and manage them constructively through the interpersonal and social demands of communal life.

Planned Duration of Treatment The optimal length of a full program involvement must be consistent with the TC goals of recovery and its developmental view of the change process. How long the individual must be involved in the program depends on his or her phase of recovery, though a minimum period of intensive involvement is required to assure internalization of the TC teachings. The duration of treatment of the traditional therapeutic community generally is 12 to 18 months.

Continuity of Care Completion of primary treatment is a stage in the recovery process. It is followed by after-care services, which are an essential component of the TC model. Whether implemented within the main program or separately (as in residential or nonresidential halfway houses or ambulatory settings), the perspective and approach guiding aftercare programming must be *continuous* with that primary treatment in the TC. Thus, the views of right living and self-help recovery and the use of a peer network are essential to enhance the appropriate use of vocational, educational, mental health, social, and other typical aftercare or reentry services.

TABLE 60.4 Indicators of the Presenting Disorder Among Typical TC Clients

A life in crisis
- Clients have a history of out-of-control behavior with respect to drug use, criminality, and often sexuality.
- Clients evidence suicidal potential through overdose.
- Clients are at risk of injury or death through other drug-related means.
- Clients exhibit a high degree of anxiety and fear concerning violence, jail, illness, or death.
- Clients have a history of profound personal losses (financial, relationships, employment).

Inability to maintain abstinence
- Clients are unable to maintain any significant period of drug abstinence or sobriety on their own; characterized by multiple substance use though often having a primary drug of choice.
- Clients have some previous treatment experiences, self-initiated attempts at abstinence, or cycles of short-term medical detoxification.

Social and interpersonal dysfunction
- Clients have a diminished capacity to function responsibly in any social or interpersonal setting.
- Clients are involved in the drug lifestyle (friends, places, activities), have a poor record of maintaining employment or school responsibilities, and have minimal or dysfunctional social relations with parents, spouses, and friends outside the drug lifestyle.
- Clients need a TC that focuses on the broad socialization or habilitation of the individual building these basic skills and fostering the individual's progress through developmental stages that previously were missed.

Antisocial lifestyle
- Clients have criminal histories involving illegal activities, incarceration, and court proceedings: Some were involved with the criminal justice system as juveniles; a considerable number are legally referred to treatment.
- Clients have other characteristics that are highly correlated with drug use, including exploitation, abuse, and violence; attitudes of disaffiliation with mainstream society; and the rejection of absence of prosocial values.

Adapted from Barr (14).

REFERRAL CRITERIA

For the physician in office-based practice, either as an addiction medicine specialist or simply as a perceptive, caring physician willing to address patients' addictive disorders, a question often arises as to which type of treatment is most appropriate for a particular patient. This question may not be easy to answer but may well be the critical step that makes the difference between life and death for that particular human being.

Any one of four specific characteristics would qualify an addict and/or alcoholic for treatment in a TC (Table 60.4). But just what does such a person look like? Though a complete answer to this question could fill a volume or more, a few examples may serve to illustrate the broad outlines of the characteristics that might define a patient as a good candidate for treatment in a therapeutic community.

Case 1 The first example involves a patient who is abusing drugs or alcohol and who has begun to experience negative consequences of those behaviors but still is able to stop such use when the negative consequences are pointed out. For example, a young woman drinks only two or three times a year but has three wine coolers at the office Christmas party and perhaps even a joint offered by a coworker. If stopped for driving under the influence, such an individual may seek help for the problem, either on her own initiative or through a referral from the courts. Such an individual may not in fact be addicted to alcohol or drugs and probably can stop drinking and using on her own if she understands that negative consequences are directly and causally related to her substance use. She certainly does not need to participate in a long-term residential treatment program such as a TC.

Case 2 Another case involves a 44-year-old engineer who began drinking in college and has continued to drink heavily throughout his adult life. His family life may be stressed, but he still is married. His children are adolescents and not home very much. He may have had a DUI arrest 10 years earlier and, as a result, attended AA meetings briefly. But he found that he could not tolerate all the talk about God and Higher Power, so he drifted away from the meetings and continued to drink.

He was regarded as someone with high potential at the time he finished engineering school 20 years earlier, but he has not lived up to those expectations. He is resentful of his employer for not promoting him as he feels he deserves. His employer, on the other hand, is on the verge of firing him because he seems to have trouble making it to work on Mondays, especially after long weekends. He drinks six to eight vodka martinis every day when he gets home from work. However, he generally does not drink in the morning, except on the weekend. He does not consider himself an alcoholic.

Outpatient treatment probably will not be effective for this patient. He already has been to AA and found that it did not apply to his situation. If he is even slightly ready to change, he probably can do very well in hospital-based detoxification followed by inpatient rehabilitation for 30 days or so. This detoxification should be followed by outpatient treatment in either a partial hospitalization or intensive outpatient treatment program, with perhaps the additional support of a sober-living home. Finally, gradual transition back to his own home and work responsibilities over several weeks would give this fellow a good chance to build a strong foundation for a program of recovery that can well last him for the rest of his life.

Again, though his life is beginning to fall apart at the seams, this individual still has a lot going for him. He has a house, family, job, finances, and probably some social life left intact. The rest can be repaired or resurrected simply by adding some consistent sobriety to the equation.

Case 3 A third patient is a 34-year-old dentist who began drinking in high school and smoked a little marijuana as well. He did well in college without working very hard but found that it was easier to study if he used cocaine occasionally for those all-nighters at final exam time. After finishing dental school, he took over his father's dental practice and did well for a few years. After a skiing injury to his back, he began taking prescription Vicodin and later OxyContin for the pain. He has had three surgeries on his back but still has pain.

The state physician diversion program interceded after he was investigated for writing excessive prescriptions for narcotics in the name of his office manager, and he currently is in the state's physician diversion program. He has completed three inpatient treatment programs. The first program was a 1-week detoxification program with outpatient follow-up. That program proved to be barely a bump in the road of the progression of his disease. The second program consisted of inpatient detoxification followed by 4 weeks of inpatient rehabilitation in the standard Twelve Step format. Finally, after urinalysis showed continued opioid use, his license was suspended, and he was referred to a 90-day modified TC program that specializes in treating professionals.

He completed the program and did well for 6 months after treatment. Then he began to use heroin intravenously and again was found out through random urine testing. At this point, his wife and children have left him and he is in the throes of a divorce. He no longer has health insurance, and his car has been repossessed. He is living in an apartment that his father has been paying for from his retirement income. The diversion program is about to revoke his license and discharge him from the program for failure to derive benefit from treatment. This person is an excellent candidate for a residential modern addiction TC. He is at high risk of death. He probably has hepatitis B and C and can contract acquired immunodeficiency syndrome if he continues in his current lifestyle. There is little or nothing left in his life to repair or resurrect. He is in need of a new lifestyle and renovation of his behavior patterns, which is exactly what a TC has to offer. He may be reaching a state of desperation necessary for him to make the commitment needed to succeed in the TC environment.

These examples illustrate the fact that treatment in a TC is not appropriate for every person with a drug or alcohol problem. The commitment of time, money, and surrender to the program is significant. What makes the dentist in Case 3 a good candidate for a TC is clear from that illustration. His life is in crisis, he is unable to maintain abstinence, his social and interpersonal dysfunction has permeated every aspect of his life, and he has begun to display the antisocial lifestyle typical of end-stage addicts.

If such a patient has the good fortune to cross paths with a physician who is perceptive and knowledgeable enough to refer him to an appropriate addiction TC, he may have a chance to survive. In fact, in some ways, he actually may have a better chance than someone such as the engineer in Case 2.

Many patients seem to do better with a little external motivation. In the case of the dentist, the state diversion program may impose some requirements that will help him to remain focused on his recovery while going through the tough times of personal redevelopment in the TC process.

Requirements imposed through probation or parole orders can be helpful as well. Such requirements may sound harsh but are appropriate when balanced with the fact that the patients have a fatal illness and have failed at every other form of therapy. Admission to a TC may be the only defense between the addict and death in the street.

Outcome Studies Hubbard et al. (7) (Fig. 60.1) found that even those who did not achieve complete abstinence showed significant improvement in term of frequency of drug use, illegal activity, full time work, and psychiatric factors. The work of Simpson et al. (8) (Fig. 60.2) showed that longer lengths of stay in residential treatment resulted in dramatically better outcomes over a variety of parameters.

Application to Specific Population Groups Those dealing with specific subpopulations have not overlooked the powerful rate of successful outcome of the therapeutic community. In particular, prison, adolescent, and dually diagnosed persons all have good recovery rates in TC programs. Broader applications are now being evaluated.

CRITICISMS OF THE THERAPEUTIC COMMUNITY MODEL

Critics of TCs generally fall into one of two groups: those who believe that TCs cost too much and those who believe that the treatment is too harsh.

Treatment in a 12- to 18-month residential TC program certainly costs more than attending AA or Narcotics Anonymous meetings. That is why this modality is reserved for those who have failed at lesser forms of treatment, usually on more that one occasion. However, TC treatment costs just a fraction of incarceration—usually about one-third the price per resident

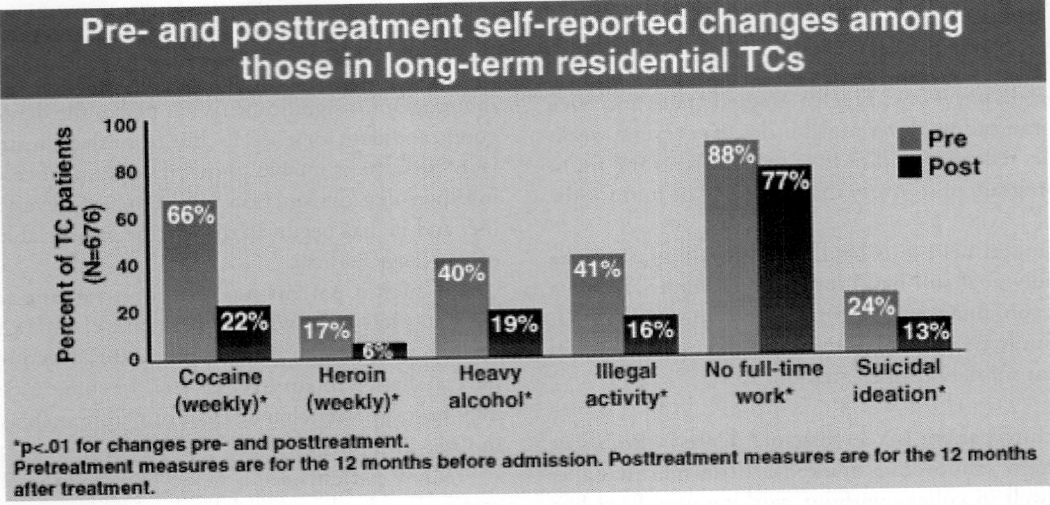

FIGURE 60.1. Pre- and posttreatment self-reported changes among those in long term-residential TCs. (Reprinted with permission from Hubbard RL, Craddock SG, Flynn PM, et al. Overview of one-year follow-up outcomes in the drug abuse treatment outcome study (DATOS). *Psychol Addict Behav* 1997;11:261–278.)

per year. Even that cost is easily recouped by the lower rates of relapse or recidivism in TC programs.

The "rough edges" of TC life have been smoothed over the years in response to public opinion and payer oversight. Still, treatment in the modern addiction TC is the most difficult thing most residents will ever do. Generally, TC treatment is reserved for those who have had multiple treatment failures and who are at high risk of dying of the disease. The goal of the modern addiction TC is to rebuild human lives from the ground up. Some struggle and effort are required to achieve that change.

CONCLUSIONS

The modern addiction TC is a powerful therapeutic tool with broad application to changing human behavior. With roots in ancient times, the TC evolved out of AA into a highly structured, often publicly funded, highly successful therapeutic modality. The Daytop model has developed into a traditional TC agency and has been the progenitor of TC programs around the world. Despite its shortcomings, the TC has returned hundreds of thousands of "hopeless" addicts and alcoholics to useful, productive lives (9–38).

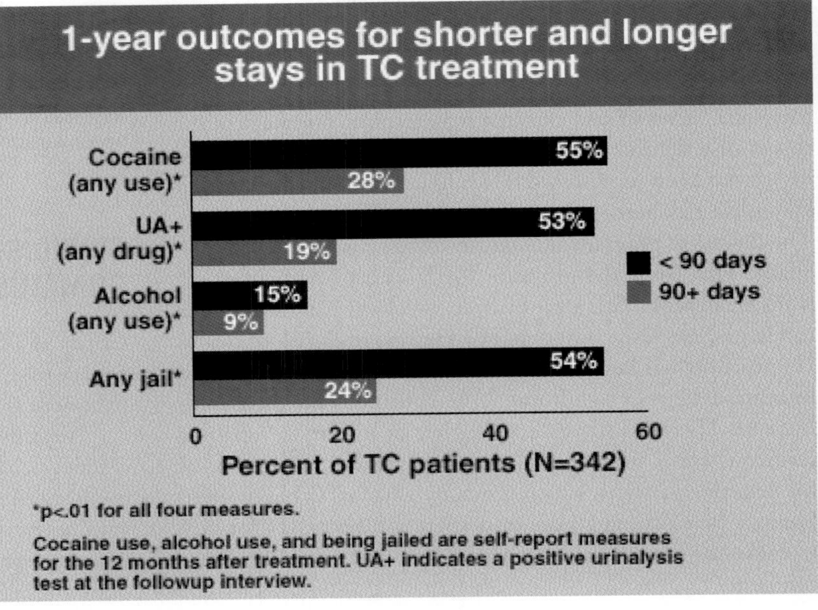

FIGURE 60.2. 1-year outcomes for shorter and longer stays in TC treatment. (Reprinted with permission from Simpson DD, Joe GW, Brown BS. Treatment retention and follow-up outcomes in the Drug Abuse Treatment Outcome Study (DATOS). *Psychol Addict Behav* 1997;11:294–307.)

REFERENCES

1. National Institute on Drug Abuse. What is a therapeutic community? *NIDA Research Report Series—Therapeutic Community*. NIH Publication No. 02-4877. Retrieved from the Internet on July 5, 2008, from http://www.drugabuse.gov/ResearchReports/Therapeutic/Therapeutic2.html.2002.
2. Slater MR. *An historical perspective of therapeutic communities* [thesis proposal to the MSS program, University of Colorado at Denver], 1984.
3. Glaser FB. Some historical and theoretical background of a selfhelp addiction treatment program. *Am J Drug Alcohol Abuse* 1974;1:37–52.
4. Ray R. The Oxford Group Connection (1999). Retrieved from the Internet on January 6, 2009 from http://www.winternet.com/~terrym/oxford.html.
5. Wilson B. *Alcoholics Anonymous comes of age: a brief history of AA*. New York: Alcoholics Anonymous World Services, 1957.
6. DeLeon G. *The therapeutic community: theory, model, and method*. New York: Springer Publishing Co., 2000.
7. Hubbard RL, Craddock SG, Flynn PM, et al. Overview of 1-year follow-up outcomes in the drug abuse treatment outcome study (DATOS), *Psychology of Addictive Behaviors: Special Issue: Drug Abuse Treatment Outcome Study (DATOS)* 1997;11(4):261–278.
8. Simpson DD, Joe GW, Rowan-Szal GA, et al. Treatment retention and follow-up outcomes in the Drug Abuse Treatment Outcome Study (DATOS). *Psychology of Addictive Behaviors,* 1997;11:294–307.
9. Agnew R. The interactive effect of peer variables on delinquency. *Criminology* 1991;29:47–72.
10. Anglin MD, Hser Y. Legal coercion and drug abuse treatment: research findings and social policy implications. In: Inciardi JA, Biden JR, eds. *Handbook of drug control in the United States*. New York: Greenwood Publishing Group, 1990:151–176.
11. Anglin MD, Hser Y. Treatment of drug abuse. In: Tonry M, Wilson JQ, eds. *Crime and justice: an annual review of research*, vol. 13. Chicago: University of Chicago Press, 1990:393–460.
12. Anglin MD, Nugent JF, Ng LKY. Synanon and Alcoholics Anonymous: is there really a difference? *Addict Ther* 1976;1(4):6–9.
13. Bandura A. *Social learning theory*. Englewood Cliffs, NJ: Prentice-Hall, 1977.
14. Barr H. Outcome of drug abuse treatment on two modalities. In: DeLeon G, Ziegenfuss JI, eds. *Therapeutic communities for addictions*. Springfield, IL: Charles C Thomas, 1986:97–108.
15. Barton E. The adaptation of the therapeutic community to HIV/AIDS. In: *Proceedings of the Therapeutic Communities of America, 1992 planning conference: paradigms—past, present and future*. Chantilly, VA, December 6–9, 1994.
16. Bell DC. Connection in therapeutic communities. *Int J Addict* 1994; 29:525–543.
17. Brown BS. Towards the year 2000. Drug use—chronic and relapsing or a treatable condition? *Subst Use Misuse* 1998;33(12):2515–2520.
18. Carroll JFX, McGinley I. Managing MICA clients in a modified Therapeutic Community with enhanced staffing. *J Subst Abuse Treat* 1998; 15(6):565–577.
19. Condelli WS Hubbard RL. Client outcomes from therapeutic communities. In: Tims FM, DeLeon G, Jainchill N, eds. *Therapeutic community: advances in research and application*. NIDA Research Monograph 144. Rockville, MD: National Institute on Drug Abuse, 1994:80–98.
20. DeLeon G. Legal pressure in therapeutic communities. In: Leukefeld CG, Tims FM, eds. *Compulsory treatment of drug abuse: research and clinical practice*. NIDA Research Monograph 86. Rockville, MD: National Institute on Drug Abuse, 1988.
21. Jainchill N. Co-morbidity and therapeutic community treatment. In: Tims FM, DeLeon G, Jainchill N, eds. *Therapeutic community: advances in research and application*. NIDA Research Monograph 144. Rockville, MD: National Institute on Drug Abuse, 1994:209–231.
22. Jainchill N, Battacharya G, Yagelka J. (1995). Therapeutic communities for adolescents. In: Rahdert E, Czechowicz D, eds. *Adolescent drug use: clinical assessment and therapeutic interventions*. NIDA Research Monograph 156. Rockville, MD: National Institute on Drug Abuse, 190–217.
23. Kennard D. *An Introduction to therapeutic communities*. London: Rutledge and Kegan Paul, 1983.
24. Kerr DH. The therapeutic community: a codified concept for training and upgrading staff members working in a residential setting. In: DeLeon G, Ziegenfuss JI, eds. *Therapeutic communities for addictions*. Springfield, IL: Charles C Thomas, 1986:55–63.
25. Kooyman M. *The therapeutic community for addicts: intimacy, parent involvement and treatment outcome*. Amsterdam: Swets and Zeitlinger, 1993.
26. Liberty HI, Johnson BD, Jainchill N, et al. Dynamic recovery: comparative study of therapeutic communities in homeless shelters for men. *J Subst Abuse Treat* 1998;15(5):401–423.
27. Lipton DS. Therapeutic community treatment programming in corrections. In: Hollin CR, ed. *Handbook of offender assessment and treatment*. London: John Wiley & Sons, 1999.
28. Messina NR, Wish ED, Nemes S. Therapeutic community treatment for substance abusers with anti-social personality disorder. *J Subst Abuse Treat* 1999;17(1-2):121–128.
29. Nielsen A, Scarpitti F. Changing the behavior of substance abusers: Factors influencing the effectiveness of therapeutic communities. *J Drug Issues* 1997;27(2):279–298.
30. Nuttbrock LA, Rahav M, Rivera I, et al. Outcomes of homeless mentally ill chemical abusers in community residences and a therapeutic community. *Psychiatr Serv* 1998;49:68–76.
31. Preston CA, Viney LL. Self- and ideal self-perception of drug addicts in therapeutic communities. *Int J Addict* 1984;19(7):805–818.
32. Sacks S, DeLeon G, Bernhardt AI, et al. A modified therapeutic community for homeless mentally ill chemical abusers. In: DeLeon G, ed. *Community as method: therapeutic communities for special populations and special settings*. Westport, CT: Greenwood Publishing Group, 1997:19–37.
33. Silberstein CH, Metzger EI, Galanter M. The Greenhouse: a modified therapeutic community for mentally ill homeless addicts at New York University. In: DeLeon G, ed. *Community as method: therapeutic communities for special populations and special settings*. Westport, CT: Greenwood Publishing Group, 1997:53–65.
34. Stevens SJ, Arbiter N, McGrath R. Women and children: therapeutic community substance abuse treatment. In: DeLeon G, ed. *Community as method: therapeutic communities for special populations and special settings*. Westport, CT: Greenwood Publishing Group, 1997:129–142.
35. Talbot ES. *Therapeutic community experiential training: facilitator's guide*. Kansas City, MO: University of Missouri-Kansas City, Mid-America Technology Transfer Center, 1998.
36. Winick C, Evans JT. A therapeutic community program for mothers and their children. In: DeLeon G, ed. *Community as method: therapeutic communities for special populations and special settings*. Westport, CT: Greenwood Publishing Group, 1997:143–160.
37. Yablonsky L. *The therapeutic community*. New York: Gardner Press, 1989.
38. Zweben JE, Smith DE . Changing attitudes and policies toward alcohol use in the therapeutic community. *J Psychoactive Drugs* 1986;18(3):253–260.
39. DeLeon G. Therapeutic communities for addictions: a theoretical framework. *Int J Addict* 1995;30(12):1603–1645.

Overview of Therapeutic Community Outcome Research

Stanley Sacks, PhD

The effectiveness of community-based therapeutic communities (TCs) in achieving positive outcomes for drug use, criminality, and employment has been documented in a number of single-site (1–7) and multi-site studies employing pre-post designs (8–10). Studies of TC programs have also clarified the contribution of retention to the ultimate effectiveness of TC treatment, finding lower rates of drug use and criminal behavior and higher rates of employment for clients who stayed in programs for longer periods of time (4,11,12).

Three national, multi-site, longitudinal evaluations have made particular contributions to an understanding of the effectiveness of community-based TCs: the Drug Abuse Reporting Program (DARP); the Treatment Outcome Prospective Study (TOPS), and the Drug Abuse Treatment Outcome Study (DATOS). Two of these, the DARP and the TOPS, documented large decreases in opiate use and criminal involvement after treatment (10,12–16). Findings from the DATOS, the most recent and comprehensive of these evaluations, showed major reductions in all types of drug use for TCs and other residential programs, independent of length of exposure to treatment; specifically, reductions of 66% in cocaine and heroin use, of 50% in weekly or more frequent alcohol or marijuana use, of 60% in predatory illegal behavior, and of 50% in suicidal thoughts and/or attempts were documented at 1-year after treatment (9). Even larger reductions were evident for those who stayed in treatment 3 months or longer, and those who successfully completed treatment in a TC had significantly lower levels of cocaine, heroin, and alcohol use; criminal behavior, unemployment; and indicators of depression relative to their functioning prior to entering treatment, improvements that were maintained 5 years later (17–19). A recent National Institute on Drug Abuse publication in the *Research Report Series* reviewed three decades of research into TC treatment, including baseline data from more than 65,000 individuals, and found that participation in a TC was associated with several positive outcomes (20).

The effectiveness of TCs, especially in obtaining reductions in criminality, provided the empirical basis for extending TC models to correctional settings. Randomized studies have shown that therapeutic community services adapted to correctional settings have achieved significantly greater reductions in recidivism to drugs and to crime (21). The most significant reductions (i.e., of greater magnitude and sustained for longer periods of time) in recidivism have been obtained when institutional care was integrated with aftercare, exemplified by TC work-release (22–24) and the post-prison TC (25–28). Recent studies have shown that treatment effects producing lower rates of return to custody may persist for up to 5 years (29). A meta-analytic review of the effectiveness of corrections-based treatment for drug abuse examined intervention programs reported from 1968 to 1996 and concluded that TC programs are effective in reducing recidivism (30,31).

The demonstrated improvement in psychologic well-being during (32–35) and after (36) standard TC treatment provided the rationale for modifying the TC to respond to the concerns of individuals with co-occurring substance use and mental disorders (37). A study of a long-term (1-year) modified TC (MTC) led to findings of significantly more positive outcomes for MTC clients on measures of drug use and employment than were obtained for their counterparts receiving the standard care typically provided to homeless clients (38). In a randomized study conducted in a drug treatment setting, clients showing evidence of co-occurring disorders who received MTC programming achieved more positive mental health outcomes during treatment (significantly greater reductions in symptoms of depression) than those who received standard TC services (39), pointing both to the adaptability of the TC to the needs of particular clients and the importance of making those adjustments in programming. An analysis of economic benefits associated with MTC treatment obtained findings of $5 of benefit for every dollar spent on MTC treatment (40). More recently, the MTC has been introduced in prisons to address the complex needs of offenders with co-occurring mental health and substance use disorders (41) and has also shown significant reductions in reincarceration rates (42) and substance use (43) for those randomly assigned to the MTC compared to those receiving standard mental health treatment services.

In summary, a significant body of research, conducted over more than three decades has demonstrated the effectiveness of community-based TCs and, more recently, of TCs in correctional settings and of MTCs for people with co-occurring disorders. The model is most strongly indicated for very difficult-to-treat individuals who require long-term residential care.

REFERENCES

1. Aron WS, Daily DW. Graduates and splittees from therapeutic community drug treatment programs: a comparison. *Int J Addict* 1976;11(5):1–18.
2. Barr H., Antes D. *Factors related to recovery and relapse in follow-up.* Final Report of Project Activities, Grant. No. 1-H81-DA-01864. Rockville, MD: National Institute on Drug Abuse, 1981.
3. Brooke RC, Whitehead IC. *Drug free therapeutic community.* New York: Human Science Press, 1980.

Overview of Therapeutic Community Outcome Research *(continued)*

4. De Leon G. *The therapeutic community: study of effectiveness.* National Institute on Drug Abuse Research Monograph, DHHS Pub. No. ADM 84-1286. Washington, DC: U.S. Government Printing Office, 1984:20402.
5. De Leon G. Alcohol use among drug abusers: treatment outcomes in a therapeutic community. *Alcohol Clin Exp Res* 1987;11(5):430–436.
6. De Leon G. Psychopathology and substance abuse: what we are learning from research in therapeutic communities. *J Psychoactive Drugs* 1989;21(2):177–187.
7. De Leon G, Rosenthal MS. Treatment in residential communities. In: Karasu TB, ed. *Treatment of psychiatric disorders*, vol. II Washington, DC: American Psychiatric Press, 1989:1379–1396.
8. Hubbard RL, Rachal JV, Craddock SG, Cavanaugh ER. Treatment outcome prospective study (TOPS): client characteristics and behaviors before, during and after treatment. In: Tims FM, Ludford JP, eds. *Drug abuse treatment evaluation: strategies, progress and prospects.* National Institute on Drug Abuse Research Monograph 51, DHHS Pub. No. ADM 84-1329. Washington, DC: U.S. Government Printing Office, 1984:20402.
9. Hubbard RL, Craddock SG, Flynn PM, et al. Overview of 1-year follow-up outcomes in the drug abuse treatment outcome study (DATOS). *Psychol Addict Behav* 1997;11(4):261–278.
10. Simpson DD, Sells SB. Effectiveness of treatment of drug abuse: an overview of the DARP research program. *Adv Alcohol Subst Abuse* 1982;2(1):7–29.
11. Bale RN, Van Stone WW, Kuldau JM, et al. Therapeutic communities vs methadone maintenance. A prospective controlled study of narcotic addiction treatment: design and one-year follow-up. *Arch Gen Psychiatry* 1980;37(2):179–193.
12. Hubbard RL, Marsden ME, Rachal JV, et al. *Drug abuse treatment: a natural study of effectiveness.* Chapel Hill: University of North Carolina Press, 1989.
13. Hubbard RL, Marsden ME, Cavanaugh E, et al. Role of drug abuse treatment in limiting the spread of AIDS. *Rev Infect Dis* 1988;10:377–384.
14. Sells SB, Simpson DD. The case for drug abuse treatment effectiveness, based on the DARP research program. *Br J Addict* 1980;75:117–131.
15. Simpson DD. Treatment for drug abuse: follow-up outcomes and length of time spent. *Arch Gen Psychiatry* 1981;38:875–880.
16. Simpson DD, Sells SB. *Opioid addiction and treatment: a 12-year follow-up.* Malabar, FL: Krieger, 1990.
17. Grella, CE, Joshi V, Hser YI. Follow-up of cocaine-dependent men and women with antisocial personality disorder in DATOS. *J Subst Abuse Treat* 2003;25(3):155–164.
18. Hubbard RL, Craddock SG, Anderson J. Overview of 5-year follow-up outcomes in the Drug Abuse Treatment Outcome Studies (DATOS). *J Subst Abuse Treat* 2003;25(3):125–134.
19. Simpson DD. Introduction to 5-year follow-up treatment outcome studies [editorial]. *J Subst Abuse Treat* 2003;25(3):123–124.
20. National Institute on Drug Abuse. *Therapeutic community.* NIDA Research Report Series, National Institute on Drug Abuse, National Institutes of Health. Retrieved July 18, 2008, from http://www.nida.nih.gov/PDF/RRTherapeutic.pdf.2002.
21. Wexler HK, Falkin GP, Lipton DS. Outcome evaluation of a prison therapeutic community for substance abuse treatment. *Crim Justice Behav* 1990;17(1):71–92.
22. Butzin CA, Martin SS, Inciardi JA. Evaluating components effects of a prison-based treatment continuum. *J Subst Abuse Treat* 2002;22:63–69.
23. Inciardi JA, Surratt HL, Martin SS, Hooper RM. The importance of aftercare in a corrections-based treatment continuum. In: Leukefeld CG, Tims FM, Farabee D, eds. *Treatment of drug offenders: policies and issue.* New York: Springer Publishing, 2002:204–216.
24. Martin SS, Butzin CA, Saum CA, Inciardi JA. Three-year outcomes of TC treatment for drug-involved offenders in Delaware: from prison to work release to aftercare. *Prison J* 1999;79(3):294–320.
25. Griffith JD, Hiller ML, Knight K, Simpson DD. A cost-effectiveness analysis of in-prison TC treatment and risk classification. *Prison J* 1999;79(3):352–368.
26. Hiller ML, Knight K Simpson DD. Prison-based substance abuse treatment, residential aftercare and recidivism. *Addiction* 1999;94(6):833–842.
27. Knight K, Simpson DD, Chatham LR, Camacho LM. An assessment of prison-based drug treatment: Texas' in-prison TC program. *J Offend Rehab* 1997;24(3/4):75–100.
28. Wexler HK, Lowe L, Melnick G, Peters J. Three-year reincarceration outcomes for Amity in-prison and aftercare therapeutic community and aftercare in California. *Prison J* 1999;79(3):321–336.
29. Prendergast ML, Hall EA, Wexler HK, et al. Amity prison-based therapeutic community: five-year outcomes. *Prison J* 2004;84(1):36–60.
30. Lipton DS, Pearson FS, Cleland CM, Yee D. The effects of therapeutic communities and milieu therapy on recidivism. In: McGuire J, ed. *Offender rehabilitation and treatment.* Chichester, UK: Wiley, 2002.
31. Pearson FS, Lipton DS. A meta-analytic review of the effectiveness of corrections-based treatments for drug abuse. *Prison J* 1999;79(4): 384–410.
32. De Leon G, Jainchill N. Male and female drug abusers: social and psychological status 2 years after treatment in a therapeutic community. *Am J Drug Alcohol Abuse* 1981;8(4):465–496.
33. De Leon G, Wexler HK, Jainchill N. The therapeutic community: success and improvement rates five years after treatment. *Int J Addict* 1982;17(4):703–747.
34. Jainchill N, De Leon G. Therapeutic community research: recent studies of psychopathology and retention. In: Buhringer G, Platt JJ, eds. *Drug addiction treatment research: German and American perspectives.* Melbourne, FL: Krieger Publications, 1992:367–388.
35. Sacks S, De Leon G. Modified therapeutic communities for dual disorders: evaluation overview. *Proceedings of Therapeutic Communities of America 1992 Planning Conference, Paradigms: Past, Present, and Future*, December 6–9, 1992, Chantilly, VA.
36. Biase DV, Sullivan AP, Wheeler B. Daytop miniversity–phase 2–college training in a therapeutic community: development of self-concept among drug free addict/abusers. In: De Leon G, Ziegenfuss JT, eds. *Therapeutic community for addictions: readings in theory, research, and practice.* Springfield, IL: Charles C Thomas Publishing, 1986:121–130.
37. Sacks S, Sacks JY, De Leon G. Treatment for MICAs: design and implementation of the modified TC. *J Psychoactive Drugs* [special edition], 1999;31(1):19–30.
38. De Leon G, Sacks S, Staines G, et al. Modified therapeutic community for homeless MICAs: treatment outcomes. *Am J Drug Alcohol Abuse* 2000;26(3):461–480.
39. Rahav M, Rivera JJ, Nuttbrock L, et al. Characteristics and treatment of homeless, mentally ill chemical-abusing men. *J Psychoactive Drugs* 1995;21(1):93–103.
40. French MT, McCollister KE, Sacks S, et al. Benefit-cost analysis of a modified TC for mentally ill chemical abusers. *Eval Program Plan* 2002;25(2):137–148.
41. Sacks S., Sacks JY, Stommel J. Modified TC for MICA inmates in correctional settings: a program description. *Correct Today* (October) 2003;65(6):90–99.
42. Sacks S, Sacks J, McKendrick K, et al. Modified TC for MICA Offenders: crime outcomes. *Behav Sci Law* 2004;22:477–501.
43. Sullivan CJ, McKendrick K, Sacks S, Banks S. Modified therapeutic community treatment for offenders with MICA disorders: substance use outcomes. *Am J Drug Alcohol Abuse* 2007;33(6):823–832.

CHAPTER 61

P. Joseph Frawley, MD
Matthew O. Howard, PhD

Aversion Therapies

AVERSION THERAPY AS PART OF A MULTIMODALITY TREATMENT PROGRAM

Aversion therapy, or counter-conditioning, is a powerful tool in the treatment of alcohol and other drug addiction. Its goal is to reduce or eliminate the "hedonic memory" or craving for a drug and to simultaneously develop a distaste and avoidance response to the substance. Unlike punishments (jail, firings, fines, divorce, hangovers, cirrhosis, and the like), which often are delayed in time from the use episode, aversion therapy relies on the immediate association of the sight, smell, taste, and act of using the substance with an unpleasant or "aversive" experience.

This treatment is not designed to appeal to the logical part of the individual's brain, which often is all too aware of the negative consequences of alcohol and other drug use, but to the part of the brain where emotional attachments are made or broken through experienced associations of pleasure or discomfort. Aversion therapy provides a means of achieving control over injurious behavior for a period of time, during which alternative and more rewarding modes of response can be established and strengthened (1). It is first reported to be used in America by Benjamin Rush, a physician, in 1789 (2).

People need care—behavior needs modification. It is important not to confuse aversion with punishment. In punishment, it is the individual who receives the negative consequence, whereas in aversion therapy the negative consequence is *only* paired with the act of using a drug. This has a very important benefit to self-esteem. While the patient is engaging in positive recovery activities, he or she is receiving immediate positive support for a new way of behaving and thinking. It is only when the patient is engaging in an old behavior—alcohol or drug use—that he or she experiences immediate and consistent discomfort. Hence, self-esteem is rebuilt by separating the drug from the self (3).

In nonaddicted populations, hangovers have been cited as a significant reason to cut down or stop drinking (4). However, the hangover is delayed in time from the actual use of alcohol; thus, for the alcoholic, who drinks for the immediate euphorogenic effects of alcohol, a hangover often is ineffective in producing aversion because it is delayed in time from use of the substance whose immediate effect was experienced as pleasant or euphoric. Moreover, the discomfort of a hangover, though logically understood to be the result of drinking, is blamed on "drinking too much" (weakness) rather than drinking at all (disease). Even worse, alcohol may be used to cure the withdrawal ("hair of the dog"), which ensures that emotionally the patient perceives the alcohol as a solution, not a problem.

Contrary to popular belief, disulfiram (Antabuse) is not an aversion treatment. In aversion therapy for alcohol addiction, alcohol is not absorbed into the system (3). With disulfiram, alcohol must be absorbed and metabolism begun for it to produce its toxic effect (5). Aversion relies on safe but uncomfortable experiences that can be repeated, whereas disulfiram reactions can be life-threatening, even in healthy persons. For this reason, patients today are not given alcohol at the same time that they are prescribed disulfiram. As a result, they have not actually experienced a disulfiram reaction. Thus, disulfiram does not change the way the addict feels about alcohol. He or she may fear the consequence of drinking, just as he or she fears being arrested for drinking and driving; nevertheless, he or she still retains the euphoric recall of past episodes of drinking alcohol and hence the craving for the alcohol itself. Aversion works to eliminate or reduce euphoric recall by recording new negative experiences with the drug (6).

In fact, spontaneous aversions are common, because the capacity to develop aversions is a biological defense mechanism. DeSilva and Rachman (7) published a study of 125 students and hospital employees, 105 (84%) of whom had a history of natural aversions. There were an average of 3.5 aversions per person (females more than males), and 70.1% had been present since childhood.

PRINCIPLES OF CONDITIONING

Ivan Pavlov noted that the repetitive pairing of a bell with food soon led to a "conditioned response" in dogs, who salivated at the sound of the bell alone, even with no food present. This type of pairing or training is called *classical conditioning.*

B. F. Skinner expounded on the observation that the nervous system is so constructed that organisms will reduce or avoid behavior that is consistently paired with negative consequences and will increase behavior that is rewarded. This type of learning is called *operant conditioning.* Both types of learning can be shown to occur in addiction (8). Aversion therapy uses these principles in reversing the drug-rewarded learning and conditioned reflex to seek drugs.

The development of an aversion can be very specific. Inadequate treatment can occur when aversion is developed only to one type of alcoholic beverage (9,10). In professional alcohol addiction treatment, for example, 50% of trials may be with the addict's favorite brand or type of liquor, but the other trials include a range of alcoholic beverages (3,11).

Repetition is an essential part of training and conditioning (12). Adequate trials are needed to develop an aversion (11) and to maintain and reinforce it to prevent extinction (13,14).

Addicts already have been conditioned by the drug prior to entry into treatment. Studies have shown that alcoholics increase the number of swallows and amount of salivation in response to the sight of alcohol, as compared to nonalcoholics (15). Studies of smokers seeking to quit show that those who are least likely to quit have a much larger conditioned drop in pulse (presumably to compensate for the increase in pulse rate caused by smoking) when presented with a cigarette (16). Cocaine-dependent addicts experience progressively steeper drops in skin temperature and increased galvanic skin response (a sign of arousal) when viewing progressively more intense and explicit pictures of cocaine use. These responses can be shown to decay in strength as time away from the drug increases.

The presence of these phenomena suggests that one of the consequences of addiction is that the body becomes conditioned to drink or use drugs in the presence of certain stimuli. This may contribute to the sensation of physical craving experienced by addicts. The availability of drugs such as heroin or cocaine in the environment also influences craving (17–19).

USES OF AVERSION THERAPY

Aversion Therapy in Smoking Cessation It is estimated that more than 80% of smokers wish to quit but feel compelled to continue smoking because of the difficulty of stopping; indeed, the annual spontaneous recovery rate for smokers is less than 5% (20). Sachs (20,21) reviewed modern smoking cessation treatments and concluded that programs that use rapid smoking aversion or satiation had superior outcomes. Rapid smoking or satiation involves smoking cigarettes with inhalations every 6 seconds. Sessions last an average of 15 minutes, and the subject smokes an average of 5 cigarettes (Hall et al., 22). The treatment sessions are usually daily for 5 days with a tapering frequency of booster treatments after that. When compared to the physical effects of normally paced smoking, clients undergoing rapid smoking experience increased burning in the lungs, palpitations, facial flush, headache, and feeling faint or weak (23). Hall et al. (24) and Lando (25) reported in separate studies that the best results were reported by programs in which aversion was combined with several other modalities, including relapse prevention, relaxation training, written exercises, contract management, booster sessions of aversion, and group support. Hall et al. (26) found that skills training (cue-produced relaxation training, commitment-enhanced training, and relapse prevention training) had more of an effect than type of aversive smoking on outcome. Conversely, in a study of 18 patients with cardiopulmonary disease, Hall et al. (22) reported that those in a waiting list control group had no abstinence as compared with those treated with satiation aversion, 50% of whom achieved 2-year abstinence. Their study of 18 patients with cardiopulmonary disease who underwent satiation treatment also found no myocardial ischemia or significant arrhythmia in this group. Five patients with ischemic changes on the treadmill did not experience the changes during the satiation treatment.

Much of the research on aversion therapy for smoking cessation has focused on improved outcomes with aversive smoking (puffing or inhaling smoke from the cigarette in a rapid manner to induce nicotine toxicity, often including nausea) (27). Though nicotine is taken into the system during this treatment, the aversion developed to smoking is adequate to prevent relapse despite the transient presence of nicotine in the bloodstream during treatment. A Cochrane Review of 25 trials of aversions therapy for smoking reported that "the existing studies provide insufficient evidence to determine the efficacy of rapid smoking, or whether there is a dose response to aversive stimulation. Milder versions of aversive smoking seem to lack specific efficacy. Rapid smoking is an unproven method

TABLE 61.1 Percent Abstinence from Alcohol during Specified Follow-Up Periods

Follow-up period	Aversion (%)	Match (%)	*p* Value x^2, 1df
0–6 mos	85	72	0.01
0–12 mos	79	67	0.05

Reprinted with permission from Smith JW, Frawley PJ, Polissar L Six- and twelve-month abstinence rates in inpatient alcoholics treated with either faradic aversion or chemical aversion compared with matched inpatients from a treatment registry. *J Addict Dis* 1997;16(1):5–24.

with sufficient indications of promise to warrant evaluation using modern rigorous methodology" (28). Faradic aversion (mild electrical stimulus applied to the forearm) has been used commercially for smoking cessation since 1972 (29). With faradic aversion, the smoke is not inhaled but merely puffed. Inhaling during faradic aversion may lead to early relapse because of maintenance of the nicotine dependence (30).

One advantage of this form of treatment is that less medically sophisticated staff can supervise the administration of the treatment. In both forms of treatment, patients personally administer the aversive agent (rapid smoking or electrical stimulus) to themselves, while the therapist serves as a coach. In the case of faradic aversion, each time a patient brings a cigarette toward his or her lips, a mild electrical stimulus is administered automatically by a 9-volt battery. The stimulus is activated by a string attached to the smoker's wrist. The therapist also instructs the patient in relapse prevention methods and behavior and dietary changes that help maintain abstinence and achieve comfort during the initial period after smoking cessation. Smith (29) contacted 59% of 556 patients treated with this method in a commercial program and found that 52% had achieved continuous abstinence at 1 year.

Aversion Therapy for Alcohol Addiction The spontaneous recovery rate for alcoholism is influenced by a variety of factors, including severity of problems, age, and the presence of a co-occurring psychiatric disorder (31). Nevertheless, the annual spontaneous recovery rate estimated by Vaillant in his study of the natural history of alcoholism was 2% to 3% (32). In 1949, Voegtlin and Broz (33) published a 10.5-year follow-up of 3,125 patients treated with aversion therapy. One-year abstinence rates of 70% were reported using chemical aversion therapy with minimal counseling.

There are three well-conducted controlled trials of aversion therapy for alcohol dependence. Boland et al. (34) evaluated the 6-month abstinence rates for 50 lower socioeconomic alcoholics, using lithium as a chemical aversive agent. Twenty-five patients given emetic aversion with lithium had 36% total abstinence, as compared to 12% for the 25 patients given control treatment ($p < 0.05$). Cannon et al. (35) divided 20 Veterans Administration patients into three groups and found that there was little difference in outcome between seven patients given chemical aversion and those given control treatment (both groups, however, had extremely high abstinence rates: 170 to 180 days for the chemical aversion group versus 158 to 180 days for the control group). Both did better than seven patients receiving faradic aversion. However, the groups were small, there may have been some ceiling effect, and the subjects had to drink some alcohol during the actual testing sessions, which could counteract any aversion being developed.

In the private sector, Smith et al. (14) compared 249 inpatients receiving aversion therapy as part of a multimodality treatment program with 249 inpatients from a large treatment registry more than 9,000 patients) receiving multimodality treatment but without aversion therapy. All were matched on 17 baseline characteristics. Of the patients receiving aversion therapy, 84.7% had total abstinence from alcohol at 6 months, compared with 72.2% in the control group ($p < 0.01$); at 1 year, 79% of those treated with aversion had maintained abstinence, versus 67% of those without such treatment ($p < 0.05$; Table 61.1). The group showing the greatest benefit from aversion therapy was the daily drinkers (84% vs. 67%; $p < 0.001$).

Though the majority of patients in the study were treated with chemical aversion therapy, a subsample of 28 patients received faradic aversion instead. The decision to prescribe faradic aversion instead of chemical aversion within clinical practice usually is based on the patient's medical condition. If the patient has a medical contraindication to chemical aversion therapy, then faradic is prescribed. Jackson and Smith (36) reported that patients selected in this way had nearly identical abstinence rates. In a more recent study, the same results were found (37). Blake (38) found that alcoholics treated with relaxation training, motivational arousal and faradic aversive conditioning had a 6-month follow-up of 100% and an abstinence rate of 54% and a 12-month follow-up rate of 100% and an abstinence rate of 52%.

Neueberger et al. (39) found 1-year abstinence rates of 50% to 56% in patients treated with chemical aversion therapy. As a replication study, Wiens and Menustik (40) found total abstinence rates of 63% in patients treated with chemical aversion therapy. A meta-analysis by Thurber (41) of six studies on chemical aversion therapy found support for chemical aversion that uses nausea as the unconditioned stimulus (emetine and lithium). These had a significant effect size but not paralysis-inducing drugs (succinyl choline chloride or suxamethonium). He found that aversion accounted for 9% of the variance in outcomes. Caddy and Block (42) review the use of vertigo to produce a nausea aversion, but no outcome study using this method in clinical practice is available.

Garcia and Koelling (43) compared stimulus conditioning in rats, comparing lithium and radiation that produced unconditioned nausea in rats to electric shock to the paw. Rats conditioned with lithium and radiation developed conditioned nausea to a gustatory stimulus but not to an auditory stimulus, whereas rats conditioned with shock to the paw developed conditioned avoidance to an auditory/visual stimulus but not to a gustatory stimulus. These preclinical findings suggest that humans and other organisms may be biologically predisposed to form long-lasting conditioned aversions to consumables such as alcohol and foodstuffs whose consumption is followed by nausea and vomiting.

Nausea Aversion. As reported by Smith (3)

The usual treatment session involves having the patient take nothing except clear liquids by mouth for six hours prior to treatment. This reduces the likelihood of aspiration of solid stomach contents during treatment. The patient, after receiving a full explanation of the treatment procedure, is taken to the treatment room, which is small in size and has shelves containing all types of alcoholic beverages along the walls. It also has cutouts of various liquor ads on the walls. The intent is to have the majority of the patient's visual stimuli associated with alcohol beverages and visual cues for drinking. The patient is then seated in a comfortable chair with an attached large emesis basin. The patient then receives an injection of pilocarpine and ephedrine to induce an autonomic arousal and an oral dose of emetine. The emetic effect begins in approximately five to eight minutes. Prior to that time, the patient is given two 10 oz. glasses of warm water with a small amount of added salt. The water provides a volume of easily vomited material, while the salt content tends to counteract the excessive loss of electrolytes during the procedure. Shortly before the expected onset of nausea, the nurse administering the treatment pours a drink of the patient's preferred alcoholic beverage and mixes it with an equal amount of warm water. The patient then is instructed to smell the beverage, and to take a small mouthful, swish it around in the mouth to get the full flavor of it, and then to spit it out into the basin. This "sniff, swish, and spit" phase is designed to insure that the patient has well-defined visual, olfactory, and gustatory sensations associated with the preferred beverage prior to the onset of the aversive stimulus of nausea. The nausea and vomiting ensue shortly thereafter and the procedure is altered to that of "sniff, swish, and swallow." The alcoholic beverage swallowed is shortly returned as emesis so that no significant amount of alcohol is retained to be absorbed, an event that would negate the treatment. After an intensive conditioning session in the treatment room, lasting 20 to 30 minutes, the patient is returned to the hospital room, where 30 minutes later, another drink of alcoholic beverage is given containing an oral dose of emetine and tartar emetic, which induces a slower-acting residual nausea lasting up to three hours. The average patient receives five treatment sessions, which are given every other day over a 10-day period of time.

Howard (44) has provided a detailed review of the production of nausea and vomiting as treatment progresses. He showed that both nurses and patients reported on a 0 to 3 scale progression from 2.22 and 2.30, respectively, after the first treatment to 2.99 and 3.00, respectively, at the end of the fifth treatment. By the third treatment, more than 95% of patients and nurses reported the production of nausea and vomiting.

Faradic Aversion Therapy for Alcohol. As reported by Smith (3)

During each session, a pair of electrodes is attached to the forearm of the dominant hand and placed approximately two inches (0.05 dm) apart. The electrodes are attached to an electrostimulus machine capable of delivering 1 to 20 mA (DC, constant current). The faradic therapist runs an ascending series of test stimuli to determine the level of stimulus perceived as aversive by the patient on that particular day (there is a relatively wide variance between patients and within the same individual from day to day).

The treatment paradigm consists of pairing an aversive level of electrostimulation with the sight, smell, and taste of alcoholic beverages. At the direction of the therapist (forced choice trial) the patient reaches for a bottle of alcoholic beverage, pours some of it in a glass and tastes it without swallowing. Electrostimulus onset occurs randomly throughout the entire behavior continuum, from reaching for the bottle through tasting the alcoholic beverage. The number of electrostimuli with each trial varies from 1 to 8. An additional 10 free choice trials are designed so that the patient is negatively reinforced, with removal of the aversive stimulus if he or she selects a nonalcoholic choice such as fruit juice. The patient is instructed not to swallow any alcohol at any time throughout the faradic session, and this behavior is closely monitored by the therapist.

Sessions last 20 to 45 minutes, depending on the individual patient. After the aversion conditioning session in the treatment room, the patient returns to his or her room, listens to a relaxation tape, makes a list of positive changes with sobriety, and contrasts them with the negative consequences of continued use.

Covert Sensitization Elkins (45,46) has published on the use of covert sensitization to demonstrate that conditioned nausea responses can be trained in alcoholic patients through the use of imagination and verbal suggestion without the use of an emetic drug. In covert sensitization, patients are helped to imagine personally relevant drinking scenes that emphasize the motivational, sensory, and behavioral precursors and concomitants of alcohol ingestion. The drinking scenes then are paired repeatedly with verbally induced nausea. Most cooperative participants can learn to experience genuine and intense nausea reactions by focusing on the therapist's noxious verbal suggestions; these suggestions prompt recipients to remember and recreate prior feelings and thoughts that have been prominent in their former nausea experiences. Such verbally induced nausea is designated as demand nausea. Repeated presentations of the drinking scenes (i.e., conditioned stimulus or CS) followed by episodes of verbally-induced demand nausea (i.e., unconditioned stimulus or US) can, over extended conditioning trials, produce conditioned aversions to alcohol in a majority of participants. Elkins (45) described behavioral and psychophysical indices that can be used to define individual subject's transition from demand nausea to conditioned nausea, the goal of treatment. Conditioned nausea is nausea as an automatic consequence of the patient's focusing on a drinking scene without any attempted therapist or self-induction of nausea.

Fifty-two patients were entered. Thirty-three were able to develop verbally induced nausea after imagined drinking scenes. It took an average of four CS-US pairings over an average of 1.8 sessions to develop this demand nausea. Of these patients, 23 were able to develop conditioned nausea to either the desire for alcohol or other alcohol-related physical stimuli. It took an average of 13.43 scenes over 4.83 sessions for them to develop conditioned aversion. Of note, the 10 patients who did not develop conditioned nausea had the same number of training sessions compared to those who did (11.79 vs. 11.64) but had more scenes (48.48 vs. 37.82).

Those who developed conditioned nausea had an average of 13.74 months of total abstinence as compared to 4.52 months for those who failed to progress beyond the demand nausea stage or treatment ($p < 0.05$). Elkins suggests that some patients are resistant to developing conditioned nausea to alcohol, despite the ability to develop demand nausea to verbal prompting.

Aversion Therapy for Marijuana Dependence

The spontaneous recovery rate from marijuana dependence is not known and, like that for alcohol and nicotine, probably depends on multiple factors. Chemical aversion using emetine has been used for marijuana dependence. In clinical practice, aversion therapy for marijuana uses faradic aversion. The protocol for faradic aversion is similar to that of the treatment for alcohol, except that it uses a variety of bongs, drug paraphernalia, and visual imagery. An artificial marijuana substitute and marijuana aroma are used in treatment. A 1-year abstinence rate of 84% was reported after 5 days of treatment, combined with three weekly group sessions on self-management techniques (47).

Aversion Therapy for Cocaine-Amphetamine Dependence The spontaneous recovery rate from cocaine or amphetamine dependence is not known. Rawson et al. (48) followed 30 patients who had requested information about stopping cocaine but had not used treatment for an 8-month period; 47% were reported at the follow-up point to be using cocaine at least monthly. No total abstinence figures are available. Frawley and Smith (49) reported the use of chemical aversion for the treatment of cocaine dependence. In this treatment, an artificial cocaine substitute called Articaine was developed from tetracaine, mannitol, and quinine. Patients snorted this substance and paired it with nausea induced by emetine. Of those so treated, 56% were continuously abstinent and 78% currently abstinent (that is, for the prior 30 days) at 6 months after treatment; at 18 months, 38% were continuously abstinent and 75% currently abstinent. For those treated for both alcohol and cocaine, 70% were continuously and currently abstinent from cocaine at 6 months, and 50% were continuously abstinent and 80% currently abstinent at 18 months after treatment.

Frawley and Smith (50) reported a 53% 1-year continuous abstinence rate in 156 cocaine- and/or amphetamine-dependent patients treated with aversion. This was based on a 73% follow-up rate. Outcomes for chemical and faradic aversion were not significantly different. The report also compared patients with both alcohol and cocaine dependencies who were treated with aversion to alcohol only with a later group when aversion was available for cocaine also. The addition of the aversion for cocaine produced statistically significantly improved abstinence rates in this population. The increase in cocaine abstinence in the later group compared to the first (55% vs. 88%) is greater than the decrease on follow-up from the first to the second group (84% vs. 64%). Because of the lower follow-up rate in the second study, this research needs replication.

Elkins et al. (51) reported a well-designed experimental evaluation of three aversion therapy treatments for cocaine dependence. Volunteer participants from the Augusta VA Medical Center (VAMC) Substance Abuse Treatment Program (SATP) were assigned to one of three aversion therapy treatments or to one of two control groups. All accepted participants satisfied the stringent medical criteria that must be met for participation in emetic therapy, the most physically demanding treatment. The additional two experimental treatments were faradic therapy and covert sensitization therapy. Participants were randomly assigned to one of the three aversion therapy groups or to one of the two control conditions—milieu treatment or relaxation therapy. Milieu therapy was the baseline control treatment that was received by all SATP participants. Emetic and faradic therapy participants used realistic placebo cocaine products during their assigned aversion interventions. The covert sensitization subjects imagined cocaine usage in conjunction with verbal nausea induction. The placebo cocaine products included simulated "rocks" of crack cocaine, simulated snortable cocaine, and Psychem, an essence that contains oils that mimic the odor of street cocaine. Each "rock" of smokeable placebo cocaine was prepared from benzocaine, baking soda, and water. Snortable placebo cocaine consisted of 97% mannitol, 1% quinine, and 2% tetracaine in powder form. The quinine was added to simulate the bitter aspect of cocaine, and the tetracaine was added to mimic the "nose deadening" anesthetic properties of snorted cocaine (49). All efforts were made to provide paraphernalia for snorting and smoking the placebo cocaine that resembled each patient's customary paraphernalia. All aversion therapy sessions were completed without any serious side effects. Posttreatment abstinence performance was rigorously tracked during a 6-month follow-up period through telephone queries of the participants and their designated collateral contacts and via in-person contacts that included urine drug screens. Patients lost during follow-up were classified as relapsed.

A major positive outcome of this study is found in the emetic therapy participants' significantly elevated posttreatment abstinence performance. The 57.9% 6-month follow-up abstinence finding for the emetic therapy recipients significantly exceeded the 26.5% 6-month abstinence finding for the milieu control participants. These emetic therapy data are quite encouraging and are consistent with the reported 56% 6-month abstinence rate from the previously discussed clinical trial of emetic therapy for cocaine dependence (49). Covert sensitization produced a significant therapeutic benefit, but its effect did not extend beyond 3 months after treatment. The second major positive outcome is found in the emetic therapy participants' uniquely reported total loss of cravings for cocaine by the end of treatment (discussed in more detail in a later section).

Aversion Therapy for Heroin Addiction Copemann (52) employed a unique approach to aversion therapy by pairing aversive stimuli to cognitive images of heroin use. Patients were asked to verbalize only after they had conjured up a strong mental image. A second part of the treatment asked addicts to conjure images of socially appropriate behavior, involving employment, education, or nondrug entertainment. Latency to verbalization was measured. Copemann found that, at baseline, addicts could rapidly conjure up positive thoughts about heroin use but had significant delays in conjuring up thoughts about rewarding nondrug activities. Subjects were in a halfway house for heroin addicts and received group therapy in conjunction with relaxation therapy in addition to the aversion treatment. A faradic stimulator was used. Once addicts had conjured up drug images, faradic aversion was applied. At other times, addicts were given 15 seconds to conjure images of nondrug socially appropriate behavior to prevent aversion from being applied. With this training over an average of 15 sessions (range, 5 to 25), latency for drug-related images increased, while that for socially appropriate images decreased. Thirty of 50 patients completed the treatment and, at 24 months, 80% (24 of 30) were reported to be drug-free.

Use of Reinforcement (Booster) Aversion Treatments Smith and Frawley (53) followed-up at 1 year on 437 patients of 600 patients treated with chemical and faradic aversion for alcohol, marijuana, or cocaine. One-year complete abstinence rates for alcohol for those who did not return for any reinforcements (n = 51) was 29.4%; for one booster aversion treatment (n = 93), the abstinence rate was 50.5%; the two booster aversions (n = 273) abstinence rate was 68.5%; and for more than two aversions (n = 10), the abstinence rate was 80%. Wiens and Menustik (40) reported that the use of reinforcement aversion treatments (or recaps) was associated with improvement in abstinence at 1 year after treatment: no recaps, 24%; 1 recap, 21%; 2 recaps, 40%; 3 recaps, 27%; 4 recaps, 64%; 5 recaps, 72%; and 6 recaps, 99%. Of note: 144 of 385 (38%) patients received the 6 recaps.

Use of Support Programs and 12-Step Meetings after Receiving Aversion Therapy Beaubrum (54), in a follow-up study of patients, some of whom were offered group emetine aversion and AA follow-up, found that those who went to AA after receiving aversion had a 71% 2-year abstinence as compared to 27% who did AA alone, 18% who did aversions alone, and 23% who did neither. However, these were not random assignments. Smith and Frawley (53) found that those who used some form of support groups after aversion treatment did better than those who did not use such support. The use of any support (n = 232) versus no support (n = 195) is associated with a total abstinence rate of 68.1% versus 48.7% ($p < 0.001$), respectively. Smith and Frawley (53) found an additive effect of the use of reinforcement treatments and support and/or 12-step meetings after completion of a hospital aversion program. Those who did not complete at least two booster aversions and did not go to any support after treatment (n = 79) had a 1-year complete abstinence rate from all drugs of 34.2%. For those who went to support groups but did not receive at least two booster aversions (n = 65), the rate was 52.3%. For those who had at least two booster aversions but did not go to support (n = 116), the abstinence rate was 58.6%. For those who had at least two booster treatments and attended support groups (n = 167), the abstinence rate was 74.3% (Table 61.2). Though total abstinence was associated with use of support groups after treatment, for those with urges to drink, increased support use was negatively associated with abstinence. For those using AA more than once a week with urges (n = 25), the abstinence rate was 20%. For those going once a week (n = 17), the abstinence rate was 35%. For those who were going less than once a week (n = 29), the abstinence rate was 66%. ($p < 0.01$) A similar pattern was found for patients going to Schick Shadel Hospital–sponsored support groups. For those going more than once a week (n = 9), the abstinence rate was 38%. For those going once a week (n = 30), the abstinence rate was 50%. For those going less than once a week (n = 24), the abstinence rate was 63% (p = n.s.; Table 61.3).

EFFECT OF AVERSION ON URGES TO DRINK ALCOHOL

Baker and Cannon (55) studied individual patients and showed evidence for conditioned autonomic responses such as heart rate and skin conductance that increased during the

TABLE 61.2 One-Year Total Abstinence Rates: Use of Reinforcements and Follow-up Support

Condition	1	2	3	4
Number of pts	79	65	116	167
Support group use	No	Yes	No	Yes
Reinforcements	<2	<2	>2	>2
Total abstinence (%)	34.2	52.3	58.6	74.3

Reprinted with permission from Smith JW, Frawley PJ. Treatment outcome of 600 chemically dependent patients treated in a multimodal inpatient program including aversion therapy and pentothal interviews. *J Subst Abuse Treat* 1993;10:359–369.

course of aversion treatment and were related sequentially to the presentation of alcoholic beverages. They also demonstrated reduction of autonomic responses in taste tests to alcoholic beverages but not nonalcoholic beverages. They did note that attentional factors played some role in the autonomic responses. A detailed review of chemical aversion therapy, its rationale, and comparison with other treatments for alcoholism has been presented by Howard et al. (56). They emphasize that it has been shown that patients are able to develop an aversion to alcohol as demonstrated by autonomic markers and patient report and that there is an association between the strength of the aversion and abstinence from alcohol. Elkins (2) notes that a variety of researchers have reported that some patients do not seem to develop aversions. He indicates that animals can be bred to have different susceptibility to the development of taste aversions. In rats, taste aversion–prone animals have lower plasma tryptophan levels than those who are taste aversion–resistant. This line of research may ultimately help identify patients who are more or less able to develop aversions to alcohol.

Howard (44) provided a detailed evaluation of the process of aversion development during treatment. He recruited 94 of 181 patients who were receiving aversion therapy for the first time. Eighty-two of these patients agreed to participate in the study. He found that there were significant differences between pre- and posttreatment responses to patients' desire to drink alcohol ($p < 0.01$), confidence that you will not drink in the next 2 months ($p < 0.01$), confidence that you will be drinking less alcohol at 6 months ($p < 0.01$), difficulty with the ability to cut down drinking ($p < 0.01$), and strength of desire to quit drinking permanently ($p < 0.01$). An alcohol expectancy questionnaire revealed significantly reduced positive expectancies from drinking ($p < 0.001$). Confidence in not drinking in high-risk situations was also significantly improved ($p < 0.001$). Videotaped alcohol olfaction tests that included heart rate response compared the patient's response to the smell of their favorite alcoholic beverage, a nonpreferred beverage, and a nonalcoholic beverage. After treatment, heart rates significantly increased to the alcoholic beverages and were reduced to nonalcoholic beverages ($p < 0.05$). The evaluation of the videotaped aversion response was blinded to condition. The difference between pre- and posttreatment responses was highly significant ($p < 0.001$). An adjective-rating scoring system also showed significant changes between pre- and posttreatment ($p < 0.001$). To document the production of nausea, both patients and nurses provided ratings. By the third treatment session, more than 90% of patients and nurses reported vomiting.

Howard (44) did regression evaluations of up to 17 variables to attempt to identify pretreatment factors that might predict differences in developing an aversion response. He used posttreatment heart rate responses as one measure of conditioned aversion. As the number of lifetime arrests (15% of variance), instances of drug use, negative life events, and family income increased (1% of variance), posttreatment heart rate

TABLE 61.3 Patients with Urges: Association between Support Group Attendance and 1-Yr Abstinence

	Frequency of support group attendance			
	>1/wk	1/wk	<1/wk	*p* Value
AA No. of patients	25	17	29	—
Total abstinence (%)	20	35	66	<0.01
Schick No. patients	8	30	24	
Total Abstinence (%)	38	50	63	n.s.

Reprinted with permission from Smith JW, Frawley PJ. Treatment outcome of 600 chemically dependent patients treated in a multimodal inpatient program including aversion therapy and pentothal interviews. *J Subst Abuse Treat* 1993;10: 359–369.

response to the preferred alcoholic beverage decreased when compared to that of a nonalcoholic beverage ($p < 0.001$). Pre- to posttreatment change in heart rate response to the preferred alcoholic beverage was less in patients who rated themselves as more alcohol-dependent, had driven after having more than three drinks, had more positive life events in the 6 months prior to treatment, and had lower family income. Of interest, those who had had more lifetime nausea and vomiting with drinking had less of a change in heart rate over the treatment session. These associations are of interest, in particular since chemical aversion induces nausea; however, they will need to be replicated.

Howard (44) used two blinded raters in evaluating videotaped aversion responses. One rater found a correlation between greater pretreatment perceived difficulty with cutting down drinking and a stronger videotaped conditioned aversion response ($p < 0.06$). A second rater found a correlation between both, a patient's pretreatment feeling of nausea due to drinking and difficulty with cutting down and a greater conditioned aversion after treatment ($p < 0.01$).

A greater change from pre- to post-aversion response was correlated with pretreatment nausea with thinking about drinking, less confidence in being able to drink less in the next 2 months, high pretreatment alcohol-related positive expectancies, and the lowest level of physical dependence. Posttreatment adjective ratings were also correlated with pretreatment variables. The greater the client's pretreatment level of confidence that he or she would be drinking less alcohol in 6 months, the more negatively the patient rated alcohol after treatment. Patients who more frequently drove after drinking, who had higher levels of pretreatment self-reported efficacy in high-risk situations, who had fathers who were heavier drinkers, and who did not accept the need for total abstinence had more positive adjectives for alcohol after treatment ($p < 0.0001$). The change in adjective rating of the preferred alcoholic beverage was correlated with being a man, having higher pretreatment positive alcohol-related expectancies, and clients with spouses who were lighter drinkers ($p < 0.0001$). If replicated, these findings along with those earlier may help to stratify patients in terms of difficulty with developing aversion and/or evaluating their aversion in a different way.

Relapse to alcohol and drug use is the result of a variety of factors. Patients who report that aversion therapy greatly reduced their urges have the best outcome (49). Smith and Frawley (53) found that at follow-up, patients who reported the loss of all urges to drink after aversion treatment (n = 165) had a total abstinence rate at 1 year from alcohol of 89.7%. Those who reported only the loss of uncontrollable urges (n = 183) had an abstinence rate of 56.8%. Those who reported that they still had urges had an abstinence rate of 6.3%.

Smith and Frawley found no association between the use of support groups during the period of being at risk for relapse and the status of urges to drink. There was an insignificant trend toward more urges with greater support group use. However, there was an association between use of reinforcements and urge to drink. Seventy-six and one-half percent of those who used no reinforcements (n = 51) reported urges to drink, while 54.8% of those who had one reinforcement (n = 93) and 49.8% of those who had at least two reinforcements (n = 283) reported urges ($p < 0.01$).

EFFECT OF AVERSION ON COCAINE CRAVING

Ninety-seven participants within the relaxation training, covert sensitization, faradic treatment, and emetic therapy conditions of the Elkins et al. (51) study provided pre- and postsession subjective ratings of cocaine cravings. The ratings were on a scale of 0 to 10, with 0 representing a complete absence of craving and 10 representing the most extreme craving the participant had ever experienced. Each participant's four craving scores from treatment sessions 1 and 2 were dichotomously classified as either reflecting positive cravings (e.g., at least one score in excess of 0) or no craving (all scores were 0). The same tabulation was applied to the craving scores from sessions 7 and 8. The emetic therapy and faradic therapy participants all reported positive cue-induced cravings for cocaine upon their initial exposure to the placebo cocaine materials. The high rates of craving of the faradic and emetic participants during sessions 1 and 2 exceeded those of the relaxation and covert sensitization subjects; these differences probably occurred because the faradic and emetic participants were exposed to the placebo cocaine products whereas relaxation and covert sensitization participants were not so exposed. The emetic therapy group was the only treatment condition in which every participant's reported cravings were reduced to 0 during the final two treatment sessions. All emetic and faradic therapy participants had reported positive cravings for cocaine during the first two treatment sessions. A comparable pattern of maximum craving loss by emetic therapy participants also was reported in an analysis of a subset of the present data (57). That preliminary data analysis was included in a University of Georgia doctoral dissertation by Patrick S. Bordnick, who had participated in the research study while completing a predoctoral internship in Elkins's VAMC laboratory.

DETERMINANTS OF RELAPSE AFTER AVERSION TREATMENT

In addition to craving, however, relapse may be related to reflex-conditioned responses to drink or use in response to either external cues such as being around others who drink or use drugs or going to parties, or may be in response to internal cues such as negative or positive emotional states (50,58). The development of new, more appropriate responses to these emotional states and a change in the recovering person's associations remain important goals of treatment. Aversion therapy does not interfere with their development but instead enhances the readiness of the patient to avoid the alcohol or drug and thus prepares him or her for new approaches and patterns that do not involve chemicals. Frawley and Smith (50) found that the use of support groups was associated with improved abstinence in patients treated with aversion for cocaine and methamphetamine dependence. Smith and Frawley (53) report that 49.5% of patients who relapsed after aversion treatment did so for one of two reasons: (1) "intrapersonal determinants of relapse" associated with stress from work (9.4%), or marriage/family relationships (17.6%) or (2) "interpersonal determinants of relapse" associated with being around others who were drinking (10.6%) or at a celebration or special event (11.8%). Relapse to the use of cocaine or marijuana showed this trend more strongly. Nearly three of four (72.9%) who relapsed did so in an association with these two factors. Interpersonal factors were the most powerful in inducing relapse. Being around others who were using or pressuring the patient to use was reported as the principal cause for relapse by 34.9% of cases and participation in a celebration or special event in 19% of cases. Intrapersonal factors were not as important in cocaine/marijuana relapse as in alcohol relapse. Marital/family relationship stress accounted for only 11.1% of relapses, and work-related stress accounted for 7.9% of relapses.

SAFETY OF AVERSION THERAPY

Faradic aversion has virtually no unwanted side effects and has been found to be safe for patients with pacemakers and pregnant women (because the current only travels between two electrodes on the arm). To be eligible for chemical aversion therapy, patients must be free of medical contraindications such as esophageal varices, serious coronary artery disease, or active gastrointestinal (GI) pathology. Emetine is given only orally, effectively eliminating the risk of cardiotoxic effects of intramuscular emetine, since very little of the orally administered emetine is absorbed (59,60). Emetine exerts its principal action by irritating the GI mucosa, hence stimulating the afferent vagus nerve to stimulate the vomiting center in the medulla. Oral emetine is effective in stimulating nausea in more than 95% of cases, whereas intramuscular emetine produces nausea only 30% to 40% of the time, probably through excretion in the bile (60,61). Pilocarpine and ephedrine are not used in patients with asthma or serious hypertension, and tartar emetic is held for patients with excessive diarrhea or prolonged nausea. Smith et al. (14,62) found that there was no increased incidence of medical utilization or hospitalization in the 6 months after treatment in a group treated with aversion therapy, as compared to matched controls treated without aversion.

There are some contraindications to covert sensitization, similar to those for chemical aversion; however, with this therapy, emesis can be prevented in most cases. The drawback to covert aversion therapy is that the induction of nausea or other aversive state is not as predictable as with medication and requires more patient preparation (46).

Satiation therapy with nicotine has been studied by Hall et al. (22) in 18 patients (nine men and nine women; average age, 45.8 years) with pulmonary and cardiac disease. Nine had definite or probable cardiac ischemia, but none showed ischemic changes during rapid smoking. Premature ventricular contractions were not increased above baseline by rapid smoking. Wiens et al. (63) have reviewed the outcome of treatment with chemical aversion therapy in patients who were 65 years and older. Seventy-eight of 87 patients (89%) who were admitted were able to complete an initial course of chemical aversion therapy. The report does not indicate that patients had any adverse effects from treatment, though six patients did not complete treatment owing to medical concerns such as pneumonia, chest pain, shortness of breath, other pulmonary problems, and anemia. Two patients had organic brain syndrome or Korsakoff's syndrome, and one patient chose to detox only. Sixty-five percent of the patients who completed the initial treatment were able to stay sober for at least 12 months.

AVERSION THERAPY AS PART OF ESTABLISHED CARE FOR ADDICTIVE DISEASE

Selecting the appropriate treatment for a particular patient involves the patient's having full informed consent. The practitioner needs to counsel the patient about the risks of continuing the addiction and the risks, benefits, and expected outcomes of various methods of treatment. Studies of patients who voluntarily received aversion therapy do not show higher rates of leaving against medical advice than is found in patients in Minnesota Model programs (64–66). Wiens and Menustik (40) reported that of 835 patients admitted in 1978 and 1979 to the Raleigh Hills Program in Oregon, only 52 (6%) did not complete treatment. Hence, for patients seeking aversion therapy in clinical populations, they complete treatment at the same rate as patients seeking alternative established treatments.

Chemical aversion therapy has been reviewed and approved as a treatment for alcoholism by the National Center for Health Services Research and Health Care Technology Assessment (67), the body charged with determining which services should be reimbursable under Medicare. A 1987 Office of the Civilian Health and Medical Programs for the Uniformed Services (OCHAMPUS) demonstration project recommended coverage for chemical aversion therapy for alcoholism (68). A California Medical Association Scientific Advisory Panel approved aversion therapy as appropriate treatment as part of a multimodality program (69). The American Society of Addiction Medicine includes aversion therapy as an appropriate part of treatment for alcoholism and other drug dependencies (70). In a 1987 review, the American Medical Association's Council on Scientific Affairs (71) found that the available research for the efficacy of faradic aversion for alcohol was weak but that there was moderate support for the efficacy of chemical aversion. The Council found some support for both faradic and rapid smoking aversion techniques. However, the report emphasized that there have been few controlled trials. The Office of Technology Assessment of the U.S. Congress found that aversion therapy was effective for some patients under certain conditions (72). As a result of these reviews, aversion therapy has been recognized by both governmental and private agencies as appropriate treatment for patients with addictive disease.

CRITICISMS OF AVERSION THERAPY

Much of the criticism of aversion therapy is similar to criticisms of other forms of addiction treatment and stems from a lack of multiple well-designed controlled trials and the need to identify which treatment is appropriate for a given patient (72,73). Elkins (56) and Wilson (74) have taken up a debate in the literature about aversion therapy. Wilson summarized a variety of criticisms, including (1) greater medical expense than some other forms of treatment, (2) intrusiveness of aversion, and (3) the theoretical framework of aversive conditioning. Howard and Jenson (75) responded to these with a detailed review of the literature and concluded that chemical aversion therapy effectively produces a conditioned aversion and this contributes to the positive treatment outcome. Elkins (2) has also responded to these criticisms and initiated a debate in the literature with Wilson. With regard to intrusiveness, Elkins (2) quotes from Bandura that "The brief discomfort occasioned by a program of aversion therapy is minor compared to the repeated incarceration, social ostracism, serious disruption of family life, and self-condemnation resulting from uncontrollable injurious behavior." He also thoroughly reviews the physiologic and psychologic bases of aversion therapy both from animal and human work. Wilson (76) subsequently responds by agreeing with Elkins on some of his points, but he then outlines the following areas of disagreement: (1) The methodologic problems associated with outcome studies of aversion therapy leave its results in question; (2) he questions whether aversion itself is the cause of improved outcomes as opposed to other unmeasured patient or treatment characteristics; and (3) he advocates that the least intrusive and most cost-effective methods should be used first. Elkins (77) responds that because there are many factors that lead to relapse, emetic therapy should continue to be available as part of multimodal treatment program for alcohol addiction treatment especially given the fact of high rates of relapse with the forms of treatment currently available. Elkins also challenges the concept of aversion's being less cost-effective in that the costs of aversion therapy, which is provided in an inpatient setting, is within the mid-range of costs of other commercially available programs. Moreover, he reports that though there are no commercially available outpatient aversion programs in the United States, there are reports of outpatient aversion therapy in research studies and from other countries.

Though aversion therapy is more expensive than some other forms of treatment, the OCHAMPUS demonstration project did compare costs of OCHAMPUS beneficiaries admitted to the hospital with other forms of treatment and found the average cost to be slightly less for aversion therapy (which may be partially attributable to the shorter length of stay for aversion). The principle that, when treatment outcomes are the same, the least intrusive treatment should be tried first has been raised by Wilson (74) and echoed by Carter (67). As further work is done on patient-treatment matching, patients for whom aversion clearly is more effective should be offered this treatment before less effective but less intrusive treatment. Smith et al. (14) found significantly better outcomes with aversion therapy in males and daily drinkers, and Boland et al. (30) found significantly better outcomes with aversion therapy in indigent male alcoholics. This work should be replicated. The theoretical framework of aversion conditioning as a treatment does not exclude the need to develop alternative modes of behavior as part of a multimodality treatment program. DeSilva and Rachman (7) demonstrated that aversions are common and can persist for a long time. Cannon et al. (6) demonstrated a relationship between the strength of an aversion and the duration of abstinence after treatment.

NEED FOR FURTHER RESEARCH

We were pleased to note that the work by Elkins et al. (51) at the VAMC in Augusta, Georgia, was funded by the National Institute on Drug Abuse (NIDA). Though private hospitals can fund some research, they are not set up to do randomized trials. Drug companies will fund medication trials to help reduce craving and relapse but with the hope to get a patentable compound. Medical treatments are not generally patentable procedures; hence, the private funding for this research is limited. The National Institutes on Alcohol Abuse and Alcoholism conducted a trial to look at three different counseling interventions, which were found to be equivalent in outcome (78). We would like to see more research focused on aversion and its ability to reduce craving and hence relapse.

The emetic therapy recipients of the Elkins et al. (51) cocaine treatment experimental evaluation did more than simply lose their cravings for cocaine; they also developed strong active revulsions for the placebo cocaine materials as well as for cocaine related cues as detailed in that report. However, the revulsions were not measurable by the 0-to-10 cravings scale that was used in the study. Future studies should incorporate bidirectional scales that measure maximum craving at one extreme and maximum revulsion at the other extreme with a neutral zero-craving mid-scale region.

Future research should better characterize the physiologic changes that coincide with the transition from cue-induced cravings to cue-induced revulsion within a course of emetic aversion treatments. A traditional approach could build on the studies of psychophysiologic measurements such as those used during covert sensitization alcoholism treatment (45) and during emetic therapy alcoholism treatments (6,55). However, the dynamically expanding field of brain imaging research is likely to provide the greatest near-term advancements in our basic understanding and possible clinical applications of cue-induced brain-changes that occur during the emetic therapy–induced transition from cocaine cravings to revulsions. Recent studies have reported activations of specific brain regions during cue-induced cravings for cocaine. Elkins et al. (51) have hypothesized that reliable change in brain activation patterns will be revealed by comparisons of the initial episodes of cue-induced cravings that typify the beginning of treatment with those that accompany the late-treatment cue-induced revulsions of successfully conditioned participants. The landmark positron emission tomography (PET) scan findings of Volkow et al. (79), obtained from cocaine-addicted human volunteers, have shown that dopamine in the dorsal striatum is involved in cocaine craving and addiction. The dorsal striatum is a region that has been implicated in habit learning and in action initiation; the dorsal striatum, therefore, is a high-interest area for studies of possible transitions from cravings to revulsions. Based on the PET scan findings of Kilts et al. (80), cue-induced craving to revulsion changes also are likely to be found in brain regions that include the amygdala, the right nucleus accumbens, the dorsal anterior cingulate cortex, the ventral anterior cingulate cortex, and the frontal cortex. An obvious clinical application of such information would be to assess the strength of the attained aversion at the end of treatment. Additionally, the findings could support propitious individually tailored timings of booster treatments.

Functional magnetic resonance imaging (fMRI) also may be well suited to studies of emetic therapy–induced changes of cue-induced cravings to revulsions. The fMRI technology, unlike PET scan technology, does not involve the injection of radioactive compounds; it therefore can be safely used during repeated measures of the same participants across different time periods.

Elkins (2) notes that a variety of researchers have reported that some patients do not seem to develop aversions. Those reports plus his previously described individual differences in conditionability of alcoholic recipients of covert sensitization treatment prompted Elkins and his collaborators to develop and to study lines of selectively-bred taste aversion prone (TAP) and taste aversion resistant (TAR) rats (81–84). Selective breeding has produced a line of TAP rats that have robust taste aversion (TA) conditioning propensities and a line of TAR rats that are extremely resistant to TA learning. The TAP and TAR lines have not been found to differ when tested within any other traditional non-TA learning paradigm. The differences between the two lines, therefore, may be largely confined to line-specific separations of the pool of genes that subserve efficient TA conditionability.

Studies of the TAP-TAR models give promise of leading to identifications of biologic indices to separate conditionable and nonconditionable potential emetic therapy recipients. Additionally, studies of the two lines may support the development of pharmacologic or nutritional interventions to increase the nausea-based conditionability or TAR substance abusers. Two preliminary studies in this area of research include reports of marked cocaine-induced differences in gene expression patterns in the amygdalae of TAP and TAR rats. The subjects received a cocaine injection, and brain tissue was harvested 6 hours later for analysis via an oligonucleotide probe arrays (Affymetrix Corporation Santa Clara, CA). The findings included between-lines differences in cocaine-induced gene expressions of glutamate receptor subunits and transporters (85), in $Ca2+/$ calmodulin-dependent protein kinase subunits (86), and in 5-HT3 receptors and Na+/K+-APTase pump subunits (87). Summaries and references for all published studies reporting the development and characterizations of the TAP and TAR rat lines will be found posted on the Taste Aversion Learning Web site of Dr. Anthony Riley of American University (88–90).

A new treatment for oxycontin dependence has been developed in the Schick Shadel Hospital by Merchant (90). This treatment capitalizes on the use of naltrexone to negate the psychotropic effects of oxycontin. Oxycontin-dependent recipients first are detoxified; they then are started on a daily naltrexone regimen that begins in the morning of the first treatment day. The recipients then use oxycontin in their customary manner during emetic therapy sessions. The treatment has been well received and is being requested by an increasing number of patients. If the clinical follow-up results are consistent with likely therapeutic efficacy, then this innovative treatment clearly will merit a NIDA-type experimental evaluation similar to that previously described for the emetic therapy treatment of cocaine dependence.

CONCLUSIONS

Aversion therapy is an important tool to help patients achieve abstinence from alcohol and other drugs. The knowledgeable clinician should be aware of the risks, benefits, and expected outcomes for this approach to treatment.

ACKNOWLEDGMENT AND DEDICATION: *The authors acknowledge the assistance of James W. Smith, MD, FASAM, who has reviewed the manuscript, and thank him for his insights.*

Dr. Smith utilized aversion therapy in the treatment of addiction over his 42-year career in the field, improved the safety and efficacy of the treatment, and conducted much of the research on aversion therapy. In gratitude for his dedication to the field, the authors dedicate this chapter to his memory. They also thank Dr. Ralph Elkins for his assistance in preparation of the chapter.

REFERENCES

1. Bandura A. *Principles of behavior modification*. New York: Holt, Rinehart and Winston, 1969:509.
2. Elkins RL. An appraisal of chemical aversion (emetic therapy) approaches to alcoholism treatment, *Behav Res Ther* 1991;29(3):387–413.
3. Smith JW. Treatment of alcoholism in aversion conditioning hospitals. In: Pattison EM, Kaufman E, eds. *Encyclopedic handbook of alcoholism*. New York: Gardner Press, 1982:874–884.
4. Smith C, Bookner S, Dreher F. Effects of alcohol intoxication and hangovers on subsequent drinking. *NIDA Research Monograph 90*. Rockville, MD: National Institute on Drug Abuse, 1988:366.
5. Ritchie JM. The aliphatic alcohols. In: Gilman AG, Goodman LS, Gilman A, eds. *The pharmacological basis of therapeutics,* 6th ed. New York: Macmillan, 1980.

6. Cannon DS, Baker TB, Gino A, et al. Alcohol-aversion therapy: relation between strength of aversion and abstinence. *J Consult Clin Psychol* 1986; 54(6):825–830.
7. deSilva P, Rachman S. Human food aversions: nature and acquisition. *J Consult Clin Psychol* 1987;25(6):457–468.
8. Hoeschen LE. The pharmacokinetics and pharmacodynamics of alcohol and drugs of addiction. In: Miller NS, ed. *Comprehensive handbook of drug and alcohol addiction.* New York: Marcel Dekker, 1991:745–746.
9. Lemere F, Voegtlin WL. Conditioned reflex therapy of alcoholic addiction: Specificity of conditioning against chronic alcoholism. *Calif West Med* 1940;53(6):1–4.
10. Quinn JT, Henbest R. Partial failure of generalization in alcoholics following aversion therapy. *Q J Stud Alcohol* 1967;28:70–75.
11. Lemere F, Voegtlin WL, Broz WR, et al. Conditioned reflex treatment of chronic alcoholism: VII. *Dis Nerv System* 1942;3(8):59–62.
12. Schwartz B. *Psychology of learning and behavior: Pavlovian conditioning.* New York: W.W. Norton & Co., 1978:55.
13. Voegtlin WL, Lemere F, Broz WR, et al. Conditioned reflex therapy of chronic alcoholism: IV. A preliminary report on the value of reinforcement. *Q J Stud Alcohol* 1941;2(3):505–511.
14. Smith JW, Frawley PJ, Polissar L. Six- and twelve-month abstinence rates in inpatient alcoholics treated with aversion therapy compared with matched inpatients from a treatment registry. *Alcohol Clin Exp Res* 1991;15(5):862–870.
15. Pomerleau OF, Fertig J, Baker L. et al. Reactivity to alcohol cue in alcoholics and non-alcoholics: implications for a stimulus control analysis of drinking. *Addict Behav* 1983;8:1–10.
16. Niaura R, Abrams D, Demuth B, et al. Responses to smoking-related stimuli and early relapse to smoking. *Addict Behav* 1989;14:419–428.
17. Sherman JE, Zinser MC, Sideroff SI, et al. Subjective dimensions of heroin urges: influence of heroin-related and affectively related stimuli. *Addict Behav* 1989;14:611–623.
18. Weddington WW, Brown BS, Haertzen CA, et al. Changes in mood, craving, and sleep during short-term abstinence reported by male cocaine addicts. *Arch Gen Psychiatry* 1990;47:861–868.
19. Gawin FH, Kleber HD. Abstinence symptomatology and psychiatric diagnosis in cocaine abusers. *Arch Gen Psychiatry* 1986;43:107–113.
20. Sachs DPL. Advances in smoking cessation treatment. *Curr Pulmonol* 1991;12:139–198.
21. Sachs DPL. Cigarette smoking: health effects and cessation strategies. *Clin Geriatr Med* 1986;2(2):337–363.
22. Hall RG, Sachs DPL, Hall SM, Benowitz NL. Two-year efficacy and safety of rapid smoking therapy in patients with cardiac and pulmonary disease. *J Consult Clin Psychol* 1984;52(4):574–581.
23. Glasgow RE, Lichtenstein E, Beaver C, O'Neill K. Subjects reactions to rapid and normal paced aversive smoking. *Addict Behav* 1981;6:53–59.
24. Hall S, Tunstall C, Rugg D, et. al. Nicotine gum and behavioral treatment in smoking cessation. *J Consult Clin Psychol* 1985;53(2):256–258.
25. Lando HA. Successful treatment of smokers with a broad-spectrum behavioral approach. *J Consult Clin Psychol* 1977;45(3):361–366.
26. Hall SM, Rugg D, Tunstall C, Jones RT. Preventing relapse to cigarette smoking by behavioral skill training. *J Consult Clin Psychol* 1984;52(3):372–382.
27. Erickson LM, Tiffany ST, Martin EM, et al. Aversive smoking therapies: a conditioning analysis of therapeutic effectiveness. *Behav Res Ther* 1983;21(60):595–611.
28. Hajek P, Stead LF. Aversive smoking for smoking cessation. *Cochrane Database System Rev* 1997;4: No. CD000546. DOI: 10.1002/14651858.CD000546.pub2.
29. Smith JW. Long-term outcome of clients treated in a commercial stop smoking program. *J Subst Abuse* 1988;5:33–36.
30. Berecz JM. Reduction of cigarette smoking through self-administered aversion conditioning: a new treatment model with implications for public health. *Social Sci Med* 1972;6:57–66.
31. Vaillant GE. *The natural history of alcoholism revisited.* Cambridge, MA: Harvard University Press, 1995:231–277.
32. Vaillant GE. *The natural history of alcoholism: causes, patterns and paths to recovery.* Cambridge, MA: Harvard University Press, 1983:128.
33. Voegtlin WL, Broz WR. The conditioned reflex treatment of chronic alcoholism. X. An analysis of 3,125 admissions over a period of ten and a half years. *Ann Intern Med* 1949;30:580–597.
34. Boland FJ, Mellor CS, Revusky S. Chemical aversion treatment of alcoholism: lithium as the aversive agent. *Behav Res Ther* 1978;16: 401–409.
35. Cannon DS, Baker TB, Wehl CK. Emetic and electric shock alcohol aversion therapy: six- and twelve-month follow-up. *J Consult Clin Psychol* 1981;49(3):360–368.
36. Jackson TR, Smith JW. A comparison of two aversion treatment methods for alcoholism. *J Stud Alcohol* 1978;39(1):187–191.
37. Smith JW, Frawley PJ, Polissar L. Six- and twelve-month abstinence rates in inpatient alcoholics treated with either faradic aversion or chemical aversion compared with matched inpatients from a treatment registry. *J Addict Dis* 1997;16(1):5–24.
38. Blake BG. The application of behaviour therapy to the treatment of alcoholism. *Behav Res Ther* 1965;3:77–85.
39. Neueberger OW, Hasha H, Matarazzo JD, et al. Behavioral-chemical treatment of alcoholism: an outcome replication, *J Stud Alcohol* 1981;42 (9):806–810.
40. Wiens AN, Menustik CA. Treatment outcome and patient characteristics in an aversion therapy program for alcoholism. *Am Psychol* 1983;38(10): 1089–1096.
41. Thurber S. Effect size estimates in chemical aversion treatments of alcoholism. *J Clin Psychol* 1985;41(2):285–287.
42. Caddy GR, Block T. Behavioral treatment methods for alcoholism. *Recent Dev Alcohol* 1983;1:139–165.
43. Garcia J, Koelling RA. Relation of cue consequence in avoidance learning, *Psychosom Sci* 1966; 4:123–131.
44. Howard MO. Pharmacological aversion treatment of alcohol dependence: 1. Production and prediction of conditioned alcohol aversion. *Am J Drug Alcohol Abuse* 2001;27(3):561–585.
45. Elkins RL. Covert sensitization treatment of alcoholism: contributions of successful conditioning to subsequent abstinence maintenance. *Addict Behav* 1980;5:67–89.
46. Elkins RL. Aversion therapy for alcoholism: Chemical, electrical, or verbal imagery? *Int J Addict* 1975;10(2):157-209.
47. Smith JW, Schmeling G, Knowles PL. A marijuana smoking cessation clinical trial utilizing THC-free marijuana, aversion therapy, and self-management counseling. *J Subst Abuse Treat* 1988;5(2):89–98.
48. Rawson RA, Obert JL, McCann MJ, et al. In: Harris LS, ed. *Cocaine treatment outcome: cocaine use following inpatient, outpatient and no treatment* (NIDA Research Monograph 67). Rockville, MD: National Institute on Drug Abuse, 1986:271–277.
49. Frawley PJ, Smith JW. Chemical aversion therapy in the treatment of cocaine dependence as part of a multimodal treatment program: treatment outcome. *J Subst Abuse Treat* 1990;7:21–29.
50. Frawley PJ, Smith JW. One-year follow-up after multimodal inpatient treatment for cocaine and methamphetamine dependence. *J Subst Abuse Treat* 1992;9(4):271–286.
51. Elkins RL, Stoddard JL, Walters PA, Orr TE. Aversion therapy treatment of cocaine dependent persons: an experimental evaluation. *Addict Behav* 2008 (submitted).
52. Copemann CD. Drug addiction: II. An aversive counterconditioning technique for treatment. *Psychol Rep* 1976;38:1271–1281.
53. Smith JW, Frawley PJ. Treatment Outcome of 600 chemically dependent Patients treated in a multimodal inpatient program including aversion therapy and pentothal interviews. *J Subst Abuse Treat* 1993;10:359–369.
54. Beaubrum MH. Treatment of alcoholism in Trinidad and Tobago. *Br J Psychiatry* 1967;113:643–658.
55. Baker TB, Cannon DS. Taste aversion therapy with alcoholics: techniques and evidence of a conditioned response. *Behav Res Ther* 1979;17:229–242.
56. Howard MO, Elkins RL, Rimmele C, Smith JW. Chemical aversion treatment for alcohol dependence. *Drug Alcohol Depend* 1991;29:107– 143.
57. Bordnick PS, Elkins RL, Orr TE, et al. Evaluating the relative effectiveness of three aversion therapies designed to reduce craving among cocaine abusers. *Behav Interv* 2004;19:1–24.

58. Marlatt GA, Gordon JR. Determinants of relapse: implications for the maintenance of behavior change. In: Davidson PO, Davidson SM, eds. *Behavioral medicine: changing health lifestyles.* New York: Bruner/Mazel, 1980.
59. Kattwinkel EE. Death due to cardiac disease following the use of emetine hydrochloride in conditioned-reflex treatment of chronic alcoholism. *JAMA* 1949;240(25):995–997.
60. Loomis TA. *Emetine risk analysis for the Shadel Hospital's aversion therapy program.* Arlington, VA: Drill, Freiss, Hays, Loomis & Shaffer, 1986.
61. Klatskin G, Friedman H. Emetine toxicity in man: studies on the nature of early toxic manifestations, their relation to the dose level, and their significance in determining safe dosage. *Ann Intern Med* 1948;28:892–915.
62. Smith et al. Unpublished data from CATORIII Chemical Abuse/Addiction Treatment Outcome Registry-modification III St. Paul, MN:
63. Wiens AN, Menustik CE, Miller SI, Schmitz RE. Medical-behavioral treatment of the older alcoholic. *Am J Drug Alcohol Abuse* 1982;9(4); 461–475.
64. Smith JW, Frawley PJ. Long-term abstinence from alcohol in patients receiving aversion therapy as part of a multimodal inpatient program. *J Subst AbuseTreat* 1990;7:77–82.
65. Gilmore K. *Hazelden primary residential treatment program: 1983 profile and patient outcome.* Center City, MN: Hazelden Foundation, 1985.
66. Patton M. *The outcomes of treatment: a study of patients admitted to Hazelden in 1976.* Center City, MN: Hazelden Foundation, 1979.
67. Carter E. Chemical aversion therapy for the treatment of alcoholism. *Health technology assessment reports, 4.* Washington, DC: National Center for Health Care Services Research and Health Care Technology Assessment, 1987.
68. Mendes E. Letter to Honorable Jamie L. Whitten, Chairman, Committee on Appropriations, House of Representatives. Washington, DC, 1992.
69. California Medical Association. Scientific Advisory Panels on General and Family Practice and Internal Medicine and the Committee on Alcoholism and Other Drug Dependence. *Medical practice question: is aversion therapy for the treatment of alcoholism considered accepted medical practice or is it investigational?* San Francisco: California Medical Association, 1984.
70. American Society of Addiction Medicine. *Statement on treatment for alcoholism and other drug dependencies.* Chevy Chase, MD: The Society, 1986.
71. American Medical Association. Aversion therapy report of the Council on Scientific Affairs. *JAMA* 1987;258(18):2562–2566.
72. Saxe L, Dovaterty D, Esty K, et al. Research on the effectiveness of alcoholism treatment. *Health technology case study 22: the effectiveness and costs of alcoholism treatment.* Washington, DC: Office of Technology Assessment, U.S. Congress, 1983:43–53.
73. Institute of Medicine. *Broadening the base of treatment for alcohol problems.* Washington, DC: National Academy Press, 1990.
74. Wilson GT. Chemical aversion conditioning as a treatment for alcoholism: a re-analysis. *Behav Res Ther* 1987;25(6):503–516.
75. Howard MO, Jenson JM. Chemical aversion treatment of alcohol dependence: 1. Validity of current criticisms. *Int J Addict* 1990;25(10):1227–1262.
76. Wilson GT. Chemical aversion conditioning in the treatment of alcoholism: further comments. *Behav Res Ther* 1991;5:415–419.
77. Elkins RL. Chemical aversion emetic therapy treatment of alcoholism: further comments. *Behav Res Ther* 1991;5:421–428.
78. Project MATCH Research Group. Matching alcoholism treatments to client heterogeneity: treatment main effects and matching effects on drinking during treatment. *J Stud Alcohol* 1998;59(6):631–639.
79. Volkow ND, Wang GJ, Telang F, et al. Cocaine cues and dopamine in dorsal striatum: mechanism of craving in cocaine addiction. *J Neurosci* 2006;26(24):6583–6588.
80. Kilts CD, Gross RE, Ely TD, Drexler KPG. The neural correlates of cue-induced craving in cocaine-dependent women. *Am J Psychiatry* 2004; 161:223–241.
81. Elkins RL, Walters PA, Orr TE. Continued development and unconditioned stimulus characterization of selectively bred lines of taste aversion prone and resistant rats. *Alcohol Clin Exp Res* 1992;16:928–934.
82. Elkins RL. Separation of taste-aversion-prone and taste-aversion-resistant rats through selective breeding: Implications for individual differences in conditionability and aversion-therapy alcoholism treatment. *Behav Neurosci* 1986;100(1):121–124.
83. Orr TE, Whitford-Stoddard JL, Elkins RL. Taste-aversion-prone TAP rats and taste-aversion-resistant TAR rats differ in ethanol self-administration, but not in ethanol clearance or general consumption. *Alcohol* 2004; 33:1–7.
84. Orr TE, Walters PA, Elkins RL. Differences in free-choice ethanol acceptance between taste-aversion-prone and taste-aversion-resistant rats. *Alcohol Clin Exp Res* 1997;21:1491–1496.
85. Elkins RL, Orr TE, Rausch JL, et al. Cocaine-induced expression differences in glutamate receptor subunits and transporters in amygdalae of taste-aversion-prone and taste-aversion-resistant rats. *Ann N Y Acad Sci* 2003;1003:381–385.
86. Elkins RL, Orr TE, Rausch JL, et al. Cocaine-induced expression differences in PSD-95/SAP-90-associated protein 4 and in Ca2+/Calmodulin-dependent protein kinase subunits in amygdalae of taste-aversion-prone and taste-aversion-resistant rats. *Ann N Y Acad Sci* 2003;1003: 386–390.
87. Elkins RL, Orr TE, Edwards GL, et al. Cocaine-induced expression differences in of 5-HT3 receptors and Na+/K+APTase pump subunits in amygdalae of taste-aversion-prone and taste-aversion-resistant rats. *Ann N Y Acad Sci* 2003;985:519–521.
88. Riley AL, Tuck DL. Conditioned food aversions: a bibliography. *Ann N Y Acad Sci* 1985;443:381–437.
89. Riley AL, Freeman KB. Conditioned taste aversion: an annotated bibliography. http://www.ctalearning.com.
90. Merchant R. Personal communication. Oxycontin emetine aversion treatment. Unpublished treatment protocol, 2008.

CHAPTER 62

Michael R. Liepman, MD, FASAM, DFAPA
Theodore V. Parran, Jr., MD, FACP
Kathleen J. Farkas, PhD, LISW-S, ACSW
Maritza Lagos-Saez, MD

Family Involvement in Addiction, Treatment and Recovery

Many physicians do not assess nor attend to family issues of their patients. This is a grave error in caring for patients with chronic illness in general and addiction disorders in particular. In fact, it is vital to address family issues with the patient who has an alcohol or drug use disorder, or a process addiction (e.g., gambling, sex-addiction, Internet addiction) for the following reasons.

- Addiction disorders are very prevalent, produce a significant amount of morbidity (and, not uncommonly, mortality) in family members, and often are overlooked by physicians and other treatment providers.
- Patient denial or deception might make it difficult for the clinician to initially discover an addiction disorder and later to stay current on the relapse/recovery status of the patient.
- Addiction can be seen as a prototype for chronic illnesses that affect families.
- Addiction disorders overwhelmingly are familial in origin, genetically and environmentally, and heavily cluster in certain families.
- Family members can have a significant impact on the processes of enabling the addiction to progress but also on recognition and recovery.
- Family education and therapy as part of addiction treatment have been shown to have substantial therapeutic value for the addicted patient as well as the other family members.
- A number of simple, straightforward interventions are available to help family members of addicted patients.

For all of these reasons, learning about and addressing family aspects of addiction is valuable to physicians and other caregivers.

DEFINITIONS OF TERMS

The term *family of origin* describes the individual's parents and siblings, and the term *family of procreation* is used to indicate the nuclear family, including the individual's spouse and children. *Extended family* refers to all the known living relatives. *Family with addiction* or *addicted family* describes a family in which at least one (and, not infrequently, more than one) member suffers from an addiction disorder, whereas a *recovering family* refers to a family that has undergone treatment for all of its addiction disorders and codependence and is functioning well and pursuing ongoing recovery support. We do not define *recovered family* because addiction is a chronic condition that can recur in a family without warning at any time; whereas there is effective treatment for such families, there is no known cure. *Codependence* refers to the tendency of family members in an addicted family to become harmfully overinvolved with the addiction process in such a manner that enables the actively addicted person to resist pressures to seek treatment and recover and reduces the level of well-being and functionality of this codependent family member. Codependent family members may even quarrel among themselves over the best way to "help" the addicted person, whereas, in the chaos, the addicted person continues the addiction enjoying support from each of the enablers. An addicted person who is temporarily in remission may stop the addiction behavior for awhile yet might not seriously invest in recovery. This may transiently reduce the strain on the family, but it may not produce any lasting benefits. Family members typically express relief that the addiction behavior has ceased but are devastated when it resumes during the next relapse. Family members may not invest in recovery support for their codependence either, and they might relapse as well. Sometimes the addiction behavior resurfaces in another member of the family such as an adolescent child or a partner.

THE IMPORTANCE OF FAMILY IN ADDICTION

Given that the lifetime prevalence of addiction disorders is quite common, and the tendency of addiction disorders to manifest initially in late adolescence and early adulthood, addiction has a proportionately larger effect on family systems during the prime of family life. At least 25% of the population is part of a family that is affected by an addiction disorder in a first-degree relative. The data also suggest that up to 90% of actively addicted individuals live at home with a family or significant other. If physicians tend to overlook addiction in their patients, they are even more likely to miss the diagnosis of addiction in family members (1). As a result, the attendant dysfunction, morbidity, and risk of mortality can go unrecognized, and the underlying cause of many somatic (e.g., headaches, gastrointestinal complaints, insomnia) and emotional (e.g., depression, anxiety, sexual desire and function) complaints may not be identified and addressed (2,3).

Family attitudes can directly or indirectly encourage or permit the early experimentation with and repetitive use of mood altering substances by children, a risk factor for continuing addiction in later life. For example, one of the most influential predictors of childhood experimentation with tobacco is a parent who smokes. Families that react in an accepting manner to outward display of intoxication in a member during a family ritual such as a party or celebration transmit to their offspring the idea that getting intoxicated is acceptable behavior; families that reject such displays send the opposite message; these messages affect subsequent life decisions including use of intoxicants and partner selection (4,5). Families also can play an important role in discouraging substance abuse by family members and swiftly encouraging an individual to seek treatment and begin recovery. Close parental relationships have been associated with reduced rates of risky alcohol and drug use in young adults (6). Conversely, sheltering the family member from the adverse consequences of his or her substance use and thus enabling continuing addiction is a natural outgrowth of the normal phenomenon of caring and support that takes place to a greater or lesser extent in all families, but it can become distorted by an addiction disorder into impressively pathologic forms (7).

Families often play a role in the progression and perpetuation of addiction behaviors, and family problems are widely recognized as an important risk factor for relapse. Some examples: a teen may offer a drug to a younger sibling or a couple may orient their sexual intimacy around smoking marijuana together. Finally, continued use of mood-altering drugs by family members, or continued interpersonal strife within the family system, can precipitate relapse, especially during the early phases of abstinence or recovery.

FAMILY CONSEQUENCES OF ADDICTION

Transmission of Addictions across Generations and Within Families Addictions are among the most familial of disorders, with strong genetic determinants and significant environmental contributions. Living in a family affected by addiction can lead to induction of alcohol or other drug abuse in additional family members. It has been observed that heterosexual women who are married to or who live with addicted men are more likely to become addicted themselves (8–11); conversely, many heavily drinking women who separate from or divorce addicted partners subsequently reduce their own drinking or drug use or seek treatment. Among urban African American women, early family discipline and family cohesion have been found to be related to abstention and lower rates of drug and alcohol and drug use in adulthood (12).

Pregnant women who abuse substances are at particular risk of poor pregnancy outcome. Alcohol has been implicated in serious teratologic effects known as fetal alcohol effects and fetal alcohol syndrome, which can produce a child with serious health and mental handicaps. However, there are still many misconceptions, held both by professional and lay people, about alcohol use among pregnant women and a need to involve families in detection and treatment efforts among pregnant and postpartum women (13).

Children who grow up in a home where alcohol or other drugs are abused, whether in the open or "under wraps," generally are at increased risk of developing addiction problems themselves. This may be related to genetic predisposition (14–19). Especially the Type II alcoholic with teen onset, severe prognosis, tendency to become involved in many other drugs, likelihood of attention and learning problems, and deviancy related to thrill-seeking and risk-taking have heritability estimates of 80% (20,21). Substance abuse prevention research suggests that smoking and drinking alcohol are two early steps in an adolescent's progression into illicit drug use (22). Exposure to drinking, smoking, and drug use in the home provides behavioral role models, tacit approval, and ease of access to the drugs, all of which encourage early experimentation.

The good news is that children whose parents recover have been shown to thrive. Moos and Billings (23) found that latency-age sons of recovering alcoholic veterans did better at home and school than sons of actively drinking alcoholics and sons of nonalcoholics. Although this may not always be the case, it is reassuring that treatment and recovery for the addicted person may help the whole family.

Social, Psychologic, Physical, and Spiritual Harm

Families can be harmed by the consequences of addiction in ways that include realignment of priorities and deteriorating values, emergence of illness and disability, violence and exposure to other dangers, experience of early losses, and enabling others to become affected by alcohol or other drugs. Family rituals are one way that youngsters learn the values of their ancestors. However, in some families, use of alcohol and drugs may not always adhere to community legal, cultural, or health-related norms. Watching parents and relatives while they recreate, celebrate, or dine together permits children to observe and copy attitudes and behaviors, including those related to drug and alcohol intake, intoxication, coping with consequences, and reacting to those behaviors (4,5).

Alcohol and drug addiction are classified as behavioral disorders. Judgment and moral values are key determinants that govern behavior, but addiction repetitively and unpredictably impairs judgment and disrupts moral values, resulting in erratic and atypical behaviors. As the addicted person becomes progressively more enmeshed in obtaining and using alcohol or other drugs, his or her values are compromised. Dishonesty may surface first as "white lies" to cover up indiscretions, then as stealing, drug dealing, or involvement in other illicit behavior to obtain drugs—sometimes progressing even to more serious criminal activities. Sharing alcohol and other drugs in social situations may lead to early sexual activity, poor choices in sexual partners and when to have sex, failure to use precautions, sexual exploitation or traumatization, trading sex for drugs, promiscuity, and prostitution. Sporadic failures to honor religious, civic, and family responsibilities because of intoxication, withdrawal, or trying to obtain drugs may accumulate to such an extent that the individual appears to shirk responsibility altogether.

Individuals in the recovery community often refer to their addiction as having been a major love relationship with a jealous "significant other," which just happens to be a mood-altering drug. As their relationship with the drug gradually hypertrophies, it crowds out and severely stresses all other major relationships in their lives—particularly their family relationships. Because psychoactive drugs often remain in the body for long periods, an episode of alcohol or other drug use may spill over into times that should have been, or were intended to be, devoted to other activities. In fact, one of the diagnostic criteria for substance abuse is "recurrent substance use resulting in a failure to fulfill major role obligations at work, school or home" (24). As the addiction progresses through development of toxicity, tolerance, dependence, withdrawal, and obsession over acquisition and ingestion, the amount of time spent impaired increases, and the amount of time spent drug-free diminishes. Over time, this individual may become convinced that he or she cannot live or function without it, and family members may likewise incorporate addiction (enabling) related behavior into their lives and become convinced that it is hopeless and can never be resolved (7).

An individual who abuses alcohol or other drugs has a substantially increased risk of illness or disability. Dangers such as traumatic injury and morbidity associated with the psychologic or physiologic effects of alcohol and other drugs increase the risk of hospitalization, permanent disability, and death (25–27). Risk of accidents increases, and family members can be harmed in these accidents. The burden on the family increases during times when the alcohol or drug abusing member is ill or disabled. Interpersonal verbal, physical, and sexual violence often erupts within addicted families, to the extent that addiction is clearly associated with an increased risk of domestic violence. When alcohol or sedative-hypnotics are involved, the anxiolytic effect may numb the awareness of fear of harming loved ones. The amnestic effect of these drugs also may lead to memory blackouts that support denial by preventing recall of prior hurtful acts that were committed under the influence.

Stimulants cause irritability, intensify aggression and expressions of anger, and enhance paranoia sometimes leading to frank psychosis. If both the victim and the perpetrator of violence are intoxicated, they may lack the ability to deescalate the conflict before it becomes dangerous.

Sexual violence has been associated with substance abuse and addiction, and particularly with the use of alcohol and stimulants. The ability of an intoxicated person to remain sensitive to the subtle cues of a willing sexual partner and to heed warnings may be diminished, leading to partner or date rape or to sexual insensitivity (28).

Active addiction carries with it a sevenfold increase in risk of mortality, so death of an addicted family member is all too common. Although some may consider this a welcome opportunity for the family to rid itself of continuing exposure to danger and unhappiness, it tragically deprives children of parents or siblings and parents and grandparents of children and grandchildren and causes grief over loss of a valued family member. Family roles need to shift to adjust to such a loss. Some members may blame themselves or others in the family for the untimely death of the addicted parent, sibling, child, or spouse. Loss of a role model may affect children, and loss of a spouse and sexual partner may lead to more instability, sometimes accompanied by introduction of a new (all too often addicted) spouse/partner, whose presence as stepparent or transient surrogate may be resented and resisted by the children. Loss of a parent or sibling may occur in other ways, as through institutionalization (in prison, mental hospital, foster or group home, or nursing home) as the result of trauma or emotional problems, or through running away from home (29), adolescent pregnancy, and premature marriage, divorce, or separation. Family addiction may lead to other family structural changes as various members remove themselves from an increasingly dysfunctional family (30).

FAMILY ADJUSTMENT TO ADDICTION

Addiction disorders provide a model for understanding the effects and minimizing the impact of any chronic disease on families and individual family members. Such disorders often occur during periods of peak family involvement in the life cycle, are of gradual and insidious onset, involve aberrant behaviors as their earliest symptoms, and feature periods of relapse and remission. As such, addiction disorders alter family "rules, roles, and customs/rituals," and often cause family members to overlook the very existence of the disorder.

The early onset, gradual progression, and intermittent chronic nature of addiction disorders, coupled with the addict's resistance to the constructive influences exerted by family members, often lead other family members to resigned acceptance of the disordered member's addiction as an unchangeable trait of family life (7). This is particularly true in families where the addiction has persisted for a long time (decades or generations). Such families adjust to the chronic condition of addiction so completely that adjusting to recovery may become stressful; they do so by evolving various bizarre or at least self-defeating defensive routines. Knowledge of the stereotypical defense mechanisms that families develop in response to addiction can be helpful to physicians and addiction treatment professionals. Typical defense mechanisms adopted by families include *classic denial* that there is a problem, *minimization* of the magnitude of the problem, *projection* of the problem (i.e., blaming the problem onto others), and *rationalization* or making excuses for the problem (31). Through use of these mechanisms, family members attempt to protect themselves or to reinforce the normalcy and worth of their family system. Addicted families tend to employ *isolation* as a defense to shame, minimizing the amount of potential embarrassment to which they are exposed, while at the same time limiting the exposure of their own members to other healthier family systems (2,32). In fact, families affected by addiction often are not even aware that an addiction disorder is present. If families do not identify addiction as a problem for an individual family member, then they are not able to recognize that addiction also is adversely affecting the family as a system.

All family systems develop typical patterns of interrelating with one another; these patterns have been termed *family rules* and *family roles* (33). The rules have been summarized as "don't talk:" discussing dysfunctional and painful drinking events by the family often is energetically avoided; "don't feel": suppressing feelings is common in addiction affected families, much as it is in addicted individuals; and "don't trust": the disease of addiction almost inevitably results in repeated episodes of irresponsible and erratic behavior. This sort of behavior causes frequent disappointments to others and diminishes their ability to trust in others. The emphasis on the following rules may well provide some protective effect for individual family members, but it does not encourage the development of healthy, intimate, nurturing relationships.

Stereotypical family roles, first described by Wegscheider-Cruse (34), now are widely accepted in popular culture. She postulated that children in families with alcoholism internalize limited and rigid family roles that can stay with them throughout their lives. Her descriptions of those roles (enabler, hero, scapegoat, lost child, mascot) are taught in virtually every treatment program in the United States today. It is important for physicians to be familiar with the roles in order to understand patients' actions within their family systems (2). Individuals may move from one role to another over time, but it is striking how often individuals adapt their behaviors to fit the assigned roles. For example, spouses and other family members may become enablers by acting as though the family's most important priority is helping the active alcoholic or addict to flourish over the short term, even at a substantial long-term cost (35–37). Enablers typically become overinvolved with the addicted family member and align themselves with the addiction, sometimes assisting in defensive activities against others who would apply constructive influences against the addiction (38). Such alignments contribute to the prolongation or chronicity of the addiction disorder.

Cultural factors influence these interactions. In an elegant, yet now dated, ethnographic study that compared Italian American and Irish American Roman Catholic cultures, Ames et al. (39) examined the connection between alcohol abuse by the male alcoholic and domestic violence. The Irish American couples reported that the male did his drinking in a pub and any violent behavior seemed limited to those surroundings. Husbands and wives agreed that episodes of domestic violence would not be tolerated in their marital relationship, despite the rules of the Roman Catholic church concerning divorce. In contrast, the Italian American couples described the male's drinking as limited to the home, where his violence also erupted; both husbands and wives agreed that their marriages would continue despite the violence, "until death do we part." In the United States, where there are myriad cultures of origin and where marriages often bring together couples from different cultures, families may represent an interactive mixture of cultural rules and beliefs as well as acculturation experiences. In families of mixed cultural backgrounds, it is possible for the "rules" about use of alcohol and drugs, or behaviors associated with such use, to have critical protective elements deleted. This extends the notion advanced by Wolin et al. (4,5) that family rituals are influenced by, and promote transmission of, family cultural beliefs to future generations. However, it is also important to note that assimilation and acculturation play a role in the development of family cultural beliefs.

Families have been observed to develop stereotyped repetitive oscillations between behavioral sequences that occur in association with ingestion of alcohol or other drugs and those associated with abstinence (called *family behavioral loops*) (40–42). The results, like the story of Dr. Jekyll and Mr. Hyde, feature transformations under certain circumstances involving drinking or drug use. What is remarkable about such transformations is that, although the addicted person changes the character of his or her behavior, so do the other members of the family (43). The behavioral changes of family members are triggered by conditioned cues that indicate that the addicted person is currently sober or has relapsed.

THE PHYSICIAN'S ROLE WITH ADDICTED FAMILIES

Physicians have a unique opportunity to help families deal effectively with an addiction disorder in a family member. The clinical skills that any concerned physician should employ in dealing with family issues around addiction disorders include:

- screening for (past and present) addiction disorders in the family and educating the family so that they can identify addiction in their family members.

- flagging and addressing family consequences of the addiction.
- identifying the benefits of the addiction to the family.
- helping family members identify and address their enabling behaviors and codependency issues and to make a "family diagnosis of addiction" (that is, morbidity, pain, and suffering in their own lives as a consequence of the addiction).
- working with the family to confront and motivate the addicted persons in the family to seek treatment when needed.
- referring addicted persons for family-oriented treatment.
- referring the family members for the help they need and encouraging their participation in treatment.
- supporting family members during relapse and recovery.

Screening Most families affected by addiction are missed by the health care team. This is due in part to family denial, and in part to families not having recognized the problem themselves. Sometimes, it is not recognized because the right questions never were asked. Given their high prevalence rate and significant effect on all family members, addiction disorders should become part of the routine family history. Simply asking all patients if they have a family history of alcohol or drug problems would improve detection considerably. However, the optimal approach to the family history of addiction is through the use of the family CAGE or f-CAGE (1). The f-CAGE is a clinical tool that permits screening for the symptoms of addiction without requiring that the individuals actually have made the diagnosis themselves. The f-CAGE markedly improves sensitivity and specificity of screening for family addictions.

An added value of adding the f-CAGE to the family interview is that it provides evidence of dysfunction and disability, or pain and suffering on the part of a loved one around his or her use of alcohol or drugs. This can be especially powerful data when it is time to present the diagnosis of a family member's addiction to the person being interviewed. It also is useful in the second task in dealing with addiction in families: helping the family make a diagnosis of addiction in the affected individual.

Another tool that can help in this effort is the use of a questionnaire such as the "Family Drinking Survey" (FDS) (31). The FDS incorporates 32 questions related to the family effects of alcohol or other drugs. The questions are divided into three clinical areas of inquiry: diagnosis of addiction, diagnosis of family addiction (codependency resulting from the significant other's addiction), and enabling traits on the part of the family. The questions that help make the diagnosis of addiction in a family member, when combined with the results of the f-CAGE, can be extremely useful in convincing the family that they do in fact have an addicted member.

The Risk Inventory for Substance Abuse Affected Families is a tool to help physicians and other health professionals who work with children and family services (44). The tool takes about 15 minutes to administer by a trained interviewer. It assesses the dimensions and consequences of substance abuse that make it difficult for parents to care safely and adequately for children. The scales include the areas of commitment to recovery, patterns of substance abuse, ability to meet children's needs, parental well-being, and neighborhood safety.

Flagging and Addressing Family Consequences of Addictions Questions that identify pain and suffering in the family as a result of addiction should be asked to identify consequences of the family illness resulting from the addicted person's disorder and behavior. The FDS identifies issues of family morbidity including self-pity, ruined occasions, arguments, anger or depression, worry, fear for safety, insomnia, and other somatic symptoms. Positive responses to the questions permit the physician to make and present the diagnosis of a family illness. Counseling the family members about family addiction is more effective when it incorporates their own responses on the FDS, because it can identify ways in which the family's quality of life has been diminished by a family member's addiction.

Frequent visits to emergency rooms for injuries and psychosomatic complaints are typical with children of alcoholics and addicts (45). Emotional factors may play a role in help seeking that does not overtly identify the underlying problem of addiction in the family. As physicians watch patients and their families move through transition points in the family life cycle, it is important to use anticipatory guidance in dealing with the stresses of such times to prevent relapses of recovering persons and initiation of new addictions in family members.

Identifying the Benefits of the Addiction to the Family Although there are many negative aspects of addiction, it is the positive aspects that underlie resistance to recovery. Both the individual with the addiction disorder and the family may perceive (often unconsciously) that the addiction somehow makes their lives better. It is this ambivalence towards the addiction that makes it difficult to initiate treatment and recovery and that causes relapses, and ultimately makes families give up on treatment and recovery (7,28,40,46). Understanding how families change with substance use versus abstinence sheds light on family resistance to treatment and recovery.

Helping Family Members Identify and Address Enabling Behaviors and Codependency Issues and Make a "Family Diagnosis" of Addiction The family's adaptation to the addiction behavior serves to enable continuation of the dysfunctional pattern without change. This takes a toll on the addicted individual by permitting the disorder to progress without resistance from the family. It continues to hurt the family, and the demoralized family feels as though it has been tricked into conspiring with the disorder to allow it to resist recovery.

Working with the Family to Confront and Motivate the Addicted Persons in the Family to Seek Treatment when Needed In hospital consultations and in the office, when it becomes apparent that an addiction disorder is active, one may begin by discussing this with the identified patient. Likelihood of change can be enhanced by using motivational interviewing techniques (47). Motivational interviewing offers the opportunity to assess barriers and facilitate change via an array of possible stage-specific goals and outcomes. If resistance is met, widening the net to include family members in the discussion is indicated. Concerns about violations of confidentiality often can be overcome by persuasion that the family already worries that something bad is happening, even if the details are not known. Furthermore, by mentioning that their involvement would improve treatment outcome for self and for the other members of the family, the addicted patient is more likely to grant permission for a family meeting. In inpatient settings at the bedside, rounding during a family visitation often can lead to an opportunity to frankly and openly discuss the reason for the hospitalization (if that is the addiction disorder), which then naturally can lead to dialogue about treatment engagement for the underlying condition. In the office, listening for or asking about family reactions to the addiction behavior and its consequences may lead to the opportunity to invite the partner or other family members in for a conjoint consultation visit to discuss the family's concerns. In cases where the addicted person is extremely defensive, family members may independently approach the physician with a desire to get help for this person. The physician can listen and seek out additional information about what is going on at home that may not have been shared during office visits or hospitalizations. The physician can then refer the family to a family therapist with skills in addiction or to an interventionist who may help the family to engage their addicted member and the whole family in treatment and recovery (36,37,48–52).

It should be noted that the traditional approach often mentioned by members of Alcoholics Anonymous, Narcotics Anonymous, and Al-Anon of waiting until the addicted person hits *rock bottom* before accepting treatment and beginning recovery is suboptimal for several reasons: 1) hitting rock bottom can be very damaging to self and others or, in the worst case, fatal; family is the first to notice the addiction because of all the trouble is causes for the family; 2) it may take a very long time for the individual with addiction disorder to lose enough to accept treatment, successfully complete treatment, and remain sober; 3) significant others may have given up on this person by the time stable and lasting recovery is established; 4) losses that accumulate to eventually motivate engagement in recovery also diminish the resources that person has apply to recovery; 5) family members who give up on the addicted person often do not address their own issues before or after the addicted person does recover; and 6) resentments or termination of relationships may interfere with willingness to volunteer for family treatment when the addicted person engages in recovery.

Often it is a crisis or *last straw* that motivates someone to seek help for their loved one. A Relational Intervention Sequence for Engagement (ARISE) has been developed by Judith Landau et al. (48). This approach is used when someone requests help engaging a person who suffers from an addiction disorder but who is resistant to admitting it is a problem or to getting help. Evolved from the Johnson Institute Intervention (49–52) with the addition of a family systems focus, this approach involves a series of visits with the family (and significant others) including the addicted person if he or she is willing to accept the invitation to attend. Level 1 begins with the first caller over the telephone or at a face-to-face visit at the office or hospital. The approach instills confidence in the *first caller* that something can be done. On the phone, the family members and, if possible, the addicted person can generate a list of who should be invited to participate in the first group meeting, develop a strategy to engage these supporters in this task, facilitate an optimal invitation to the addicted person to attend, craft a *recovery message*, and elicit a commitment from the invitees to attend the first meeting whether or not the addicted person attends; 55% of the time this level of effort is sufficient to engage the addicted person in treatment (53).

If treatment does not begin, level 2 offers a series of group meetings of the support network with or without the addicted person in attendance. Each member of the group is a "significant other" of the patient, and is coached to describe an iconic experience in which the patient's drinking, drug use, or process addiction adversely affected that person. Team members are coached to present the feedback in a nonaccusing manner, focusing mostly on how it made him or her feel. They are not to engage in arguing, blaming, name calling, or other disrespectful behavior. If the addicted person is present, he or she is asked (and reminded if necessary) to listen to all the feedback before responding. Examples of phrases that can be uttered by the team members include: "It's not you, it's the drinking," "It hurts me too much to see you continue in this painful disease," "You did not develop this on purpose, but you've got it," "We care about you, but hate your drinking," "I will not argue; this is what you did, this is when you did it, and this is how it made me feel." There are several common threads in these phrases: exhibiting positive regard toward the individual but negative attitudes toward the addiction behavior; providing data about specific events rather than generalities; validating the disease through statements about the obvious pain of this progressive illness—which destroys families, jobs, finances, legal standing, spirituality, and physical health—thus giving the patient permission to become less defensive; and relieving guilt and reducing defensiveness by acknowledging that patients with addiction disorders did not intend to "catch it," but insisting that they need treatment nonetheless. With the weight of all of this evidence, presented by mutually supportive friends and family members, the "wall of denial" for many patients breaks down sufficiently to encourage the patient to enter a treatment program. By this level, 81% have entered treatment (53).

Even if it is not successful in engaging the index patient in treatment, a family intervention usually alters the family system surrounding the index patient in a positive way by helping family members free themselves from the secrets, isolation, guilt, and fear engendered by the index patient's addiction.

Level 3 involves meetings at which contingencies are crafted by the support group team that will be executed if the addicted person continues to resist treatment and recovery; 2%

of additional cases entered treatment during this level making A Relational Intervention Sequence for Engagement procedure effective for 83% (53). This approach engages the supporters of the addicted person in resisting further enlistment as enablers and builds a confident, cohesive team to put a firm, healing structure into the life of the addicted person. This team must withstand pleading, lying, threats, empty promises, rationalizations, minimization, tricks, and subterfuge to stand firm with its contingencies. Through thick and thin, the team must sustain its commitment to hold the addicted person responsible for his or her behavior, for completing needed treatment and for sustaining recovery.

Referring Addicted Persons for Family-Oriented Treatment Many addiction treatment programs offer some sort of family-oriented care. Sometimes it consists of a psychoeducational multifamily group in which information is presented about the disease concept of addiction disorders and recovery. Often featured is information about genetics and familial transmission of addiction disorders, the impact of growing up in a dysfunctional family with addiction, how Twelve Step support groups enhance recovery of the addicted person (e.g., Alcoholics Anonymous, Narcotics Anonymous) and the significant others (e.g., Al-Anon, Adult Children of Alcoholics Al-Anon, Families Anonymous). Films showing enactments of family approaches to engagement and treatment may be viewed. Family or couples therapy may be offered as indicated to individual families focusing on either recovery only or on broader issues that trouble the family. Single parents whose children are symptomatic or who have been removed may be provided parenting education, parent-child therapy, or reunification therapy. Families with domestic violence may undergo communication and problem solving training or anger management. Although most alcohol and drug treatment programs offer family-oriented aspects in their services, there can be wide variation in attendance policies and family involvement.

Some programs offer variants of empirically tested cognitive-behavioral treatments designed specifically to promote abstinence while improving family function (communication training) (53–55) (see detailed discussion in the following section).

When the addicted person refuses any involvement in formal treatment, there is unilateral family therapy (56) and community reinforcement and family training (57–59), which trains concerned significant others (CSOs) to positively reinforce abstinence, reduced substance use, and recovery behaviors while negatively reinforcing continuing substance abuse.

The community reinforcement and family training procedure when tested in a randomized controlled trial with 130 CSOs of alcoholics found that 64% of their index patients engaged in alcoholism treatment, whereas the Johnson Institute Intervention engaged only 30% and Al-Anon facilitation only 13% (58). These results reflect the dominant themes of Al-Anon: disengage from the alcoholic behavior (stop enabling); abandon hope of influencing the drinking behavior; take care of yourself. The Johnson Intervention CSOs only had 53% (compared with community reinforcement and family training 89%, Al-Anon 95%) completion of their sessions mostly the result of being intimidated by the family coercive confrontation. Two controlled trials with illicit drug abusers engaged 64% and 67% of index patients compared with 17% and 29% in the Twelve Step facilitation condition (59,60). The CSOs seemed to derive substantial benefit (in pre- and post-comparisons on levels of depression and anger as well as relationship characteristics such as happiness, cohesion, and conflict) from whatever treatment condition they were assigned regardless of index patient outcomes (58).

Referring the Family Members for the Help They Need The full range of treatment that individuals or families may require to address the family consequences of addiction is beyond the scope of this chapter. It is important for the physician to be aware of the broad range of treatment resources and to be able to help patients engage in the process.

Bibliotherapy, or recommending that individuals begin to read materials related to families and addiction, often is a good place to start. Materials from Al-Anon are quite useful, as are a number of self-help books and addiction memoirs that discuss family involvement (59,60). For individuals or families who are willing, referral to individual or family counseling or psychoeducational sessions can be extraordinarily helpful.

In making such a referral, the physician needs to communicate with the therapist regarding the family illness and consequences that led to the referral. Otherwise individuals and even whole families can participate in counseling for long periods without ever disclosing the presence of the underlying addiction disorder. It is as important to assess the therapist's knowledge, experience, and skill in working with families who suffer from addiction disorders because it is important to assess the family's motivation for change and ability engage in active treatment. It is important also to communicate to both the therapist and the family your commitment to working as a team member with them to assure that all medical issues will be addressed properly and promptly during the treatment process.

Finally, self-help groups for family members—including Al-Anon, Alateen, Ala-Tot, Tough Love, and Families Anonymous—are available in every part of the country (contact information generally is found in the telephone book or on the Web, or advice from local addiction treatment professionals). Most such groups are organized on the principles and steps of Alcoholics Anonymous, but focus on the recovery tasks of the individual family member who is experiencing pain from another's addiction disorder.

Addressing Enabling Behaviors Another task for physicians to master is that of helping families identify and ultimately alter behaviors that enable the disease of addiction to continue unabated and progress (2). Several questions on the FDS assess family enabling, covering areas such as making excuses for the individual, avoiding situations that may prove embarrassing, trying to limit the family member's drinking or drug use, joining in the drinking or drug use, and altering schedules or habits to accommodate the family member's addiction behavior. Presenting information to help them understand how their actions may actually be sheltering the addicted person from appropriate consequences can be very helpful for families. However, it is important to remember that the identification of enabling behaviors is a late step in family treatment, and is useful only after families have progressed through the core steps discussed earlier.

FAMILY THERAPY FOR ADDICTIONS

Meta-analyses and reviews of studies on family oriented treatment approaches have shown superior rates of engagement, treatment outcome, and participation in aftercare when compared with individual oriented care (63–66). The evidence from the Stanton and Shadish (66) meta-analysis of 1,571 cases involving an estimated 3,500 patients and family members favored family therapy over individual counseling or therapy, peer group therapy, and family psychoeducation. It was effective for adolescents and adults. It can also enhance methadone maintenance and other medication assisted treatments. It promotes higher treatment retention, which improves outcome.

Approaches for Adults with Addiction Problems

Behavioral couples therapy (BCT) is the most extensively researched family approach in the treatment of substance abuse and has been shown effective (64–67). In an extensive review of the literature, Epstein and McCrady (67,68) found empirical support for the effectiveness of behavioral couple therapy; however, Fals-Stewart and Birchler (69) have shown that fewer than 30% of the addiction treatment programs surveyed use BCT. Couples therapy has been shown to be effective in a variety of formats. Based on their extensive review of the literature, Thomas and Corcoran (70) report that overall, all treatment conditions showed reduced substance use for up to 2 years after treatment had ended, although drinking tended to increase as time elapsed. There is limited research on drug-using couples, minority groups, and low-income couples. Although there are numerous other approaches to family therapy in addiction, much can be said for having empirical evidence of efficacy.

BCT works with couples who cohabitate where one of the partners suffers from an addiction disorder. It uses a recovery contract to clearly set out the goals of the treatment and conditions that would indicate relapse. Partners learn to go over the recovery contract daily with a trust discussion about intent to remain sober and verbal reinforcement for doing so. Arguing about past or future relapses is avoided and can be saved for therapy sessions. Providing clean urine drug screens and taking medications to assist in maintaining sobriety (e.g., methadone, buprenorphine, modafinil, disulfiram, naltrexone, acamprosate) in the presence of the partner are used, and progress is recorded on a calendar. Urges and triggers to urges are discussed openly. Relapses are identified by either partner and must be interrupted as soon as possible as specified in the recovery contract.

Once continuing abstinence is maintained, the focus for the therapy shifts to improving the dyadic relationship. Resentments over past mistakes, disloyalties, dishonesties, and the like must be resolved without triggering a relapse. These include increasing "positive feeling, goodwill and commitment to the relationship . . . and teaching communication skills to resolve conflicts . . ." (53, p. 206). The positive feelings are enhanced by three procedures: 1) catch your partner doing something nice (noticing the positive behaviors and reinforcing progress); 2) planning shared rewarding experiences (often leisure time activities that had been neglected or supplanted by the addiction behaviors and fighting); and 3) Caring Day assignment (to perform special acts for each other to demonstrate their love; taking the initiative rather than waiting for the partner to initiate). Communication is enhanced by teaching: good listening skills; directly expressing feelings; daily times to communicate with one another, without aggression or passivity, on feelings, events and problems; and negotiation skills for satisfying desires and needs.

Efficacy of BCT has been established for alcoholism and for drug abuse by two meta-analyses (64,66). It had a moderate effect size indicating a robust advantage over individual oriented treatments in the following areas: frequency and duration of abstinence, happiness in relationships, fewer separations, reduced domestic violence, benefit to the children, improved adherence to recovery medications, and 5:1 benefit:cost ratio. However, Longabaugh et al. (71) found that patients diagnosed with antisocial personality disorder had better outcomes with individual approaches. The work of Holtzworth-Munroe et al. (72) illustrates the need for individual treatment in intimate partner violence. Fichter et al. (73) found that alcoholism relapse was predicted by excessive critical comments by significant others, low warmth, and lesser involvement. These skills can be altered by family relationship enhancement training.

Approaches for Families with Troubled Adolescents

Families with adolescents who require substance abuse treatment present special problems, given the complex issues of adolescent development, substance abuse, and family dynamics. Toumbourou et al. (74) conducted an evaluation of the Behavioral Exchange Systems Training program, which is an 8-week parent group that supports and assists parents in coping with their adolescent's substance use. Parents participating in the Behavioral Exchange Systems Training program showed reductions in mental health symptoms and increases in satisfaction and assertive parenting behaviors. McGillicuddy et al. (75) developed a coping skills training program for parents of substance-abusing adolescents. Skills training was associated with improved parental coping, family communication, and parental reports of their own functioning. Prosocial family therapy is based on theories of risk and protective factors and integrates specific parent training with nonspecific family therapy (76). Prosocial family therapy is designed as a preventive intervention for juvenile offenders and their families.

Brief strategic family therapy has been developed to address not only drug use behavior but also the host of other behavioral problems that cluster with drug abuse such as: oppositional defiance, underachievement and lack of interest and connection with school, aggression and delinquency, sexual risk behaviors, and disinterest in pro-social behaviors (75). The call from the concerned parent immediately leads to scheduling the initial family visit. In a randomized controlled trial with Miami area Hispanic youth, brief strategic family therapy engaged 93% of families compared with 42% using the usual approach (76). Further, 77% of the brief strategic family therapy assigned families remained engaged in treatment for at least eight sessions compared to only 25% of the control families. It is well known that adolescents exposed to group therapy approaches actually get worse as they feed on one another's pathologic attitudes and behaviors, whereas family therapy helps immensely in improving outcome: cannabis use was reduced by 75%, hanging out with antisocial peers dropped by 58%, and acting out improved by 42%, all substantially better than the control group therapy condition (77–79).

Another type of family therapy for adolescents is multidimensional family therapy (MDFT) (80). It addresses expectancies about using intoxicants, parental addiction, and prevention of family relapse. This model uses both individual and family sessions to address the myriad of issues within the addiction affected family. In a three-condition randomized controlled trial, MDFT outperformed adolescent group therapy and family psychoeducation in reducing alcohol and cannabis use (54% vs. 18% and 24%) (81). MDFT was able to sustain a 40% reduction in drinking for a year after treatment, whereas cognitive behavioral therapy could not do so. Another study comparing MDFT with adolescent group therapy showed that MDFT was superior in reducing externalizing symptoms and peer delinquency, and in improving family cohesion and school behavior (82). These teens showed a 71% decrease in drinking alcohol compared to an 18% increase in those attending group therapy!

Multisystemic therapy (MST) for juvenile offenders also has been shown effective in reducing substance use. This approach analyzes the symptomatic behavior in its environmental context, maintains an optimistic positive attitude, and empowers parents and caregivers to influence youth to take progressively more responsibility for their behavior. Treatment may occur at home, in schools, and elsewhere in the youth's environment. One goal is to prevent out-of-home placement. Its efficacy is supported by nine clinical trials, two with substance abusing juvenile offenders (83–85). Treatment retention of families was an incredible 100% for 2 months and 98% for the full 4 months of the program. Cost of treatment was offset by cost of out-of-home placement and hospitalizations. Clinical benefits were evident at 4- and 14-year follow-ups. In the drug court study, enhancement with multisystemic therapy reduced positive urines from 70% to 28%.

The Youth Support Project, which also targets juvenile offenders. Many physicians who treat high-risk families struggle with ways to engage them in treatment interventions. The Youth Support Project was developed especially for high-risk families—those who are difficult to enroll and to retain in addiction treatment (86).

Given the demographic changes in U.S. society and the expected increase in the number of older adults experiencing problems with alcohol and other drugs (87), family therapy approaches for adult children and their older, substance using parents will become increasingly important. Physicians can play a significant role in screening, assessment, and treatment planning for older families because of the increased number of physician services older people use, the greater extent to which they take prescription medications, and gerontologic health models that stress family involvement. Age-appropriate tools, such as the Michigan Alcoholism Screening Test-Geriatric Version improves accuracy in detection among older adults (88). Recent reviews of family approaches in the treatment of alcohol-related problems among older adults show this is an understudied area (89), especially in terms of access to family therapy (90) and outcome research.

SUMMARY

When one encounters a patient suffering from addiction or a family member who has a loved one with addiction, the physician can provide screening, assessment, diagnosis, advice, motivational enhancement, referral, recovery monitoring, and relapse prevention and intervention services. The family may be the key to recognizing the addiction, and family-oriented approaches enhance engagement in treatment, completion of treatment, and sustained participation in aftercare. There is a lot at stake as the family suffers when the addiction is active, but the family also may interfere with treatment and recovery if not helped to work as a unified recovery team. The family also can get help for its own codependency and consequential issues as well contributing to better overall family function and satisfaction. A number of very effective family therapy approaches are described that greatly enhance the success rates with the addicted person as well as improving overall family function. Family-oriented care for addiction disorders should be available in all communities and at all treatment programs to optimize efficacy and reduce overall costs for care and harm to the community.

REFERENCES

1. Frank SH, Graham AV, Zyzanski SJ, et al. Use of the Family CAGE in screening for alcohol problems in primary care. *Arch Fam Med* 1992; 1:209–216.
2. Graham AV. Family issues in substance abuse. *Faculty development program in substance abuse*. Rockville, MD: Center for Substance Abuse Prevention, 1996.
3. McGann KP. Self-reported illnesses in family members of alcoholics. *Fam Med* 1990;22:103–106.
4. Wolin SJ, Bennett LA, Noonan DL. Family rituals and the recurrence of alcoholism over generations. *Am J Psychiatry* 1979;136(4B):589–593.
5. Wolin SJ, Bennett LA, Noonan DL, et al. Disrupted family rituals: a factor in the intergenerational transmission of alcoholism. *J Stud Alcohol* 1980;41:199–214.
6. Padilla-Walker L, Nelson L, Madsen S, et al. The role of perceived parental knowledge on emerging adults' risk behaviors. *J Youth Adolesc* 2008;37:847–859.

7. Steinglass P. Family systems and motivational interviewing: a systemic-motivational model for treatment of alcoholism and other drug problems. *Alcohol Treatment Q* 2008;26:9–29.
8. Klassen AD, Wilsnack SC, Harris TR, et al. *Partnership dissolution and remission of problem drinking in women: findings from a U.S. longitudinal survey.* Presented at the Symposium on Alcohol, Family and Significant Others, Social Research Institute of Alcohol Studies and Nordic Council for Alcohol and Drug Research; Helsinki, Finland; March 1991.
9. Lex BW. Male heroin addicts and their female mates: impact on disorder and recovery. *J Subst Abuse* 1990;2:147–175.
10. Wilsnack SC, Wilsnack RW. Epidemiology of women's drinking. *J Subst Abuse* 1990;3:133–157.
11. Wilsnack SC, Wilsnack RW. Epidemiological research on women's drinking: recent progress and directions for the 1990s. In Gomberg ESL, Nirenberg TD, eds. *Women and substance abuse.* Norwood, NJ: Ablex, 1993:62–99.
12. Doherty E, Green K, Reisinger H. Long-term patterns of drug use among an urban African American cohort: The role of gender and family. *J Urban Health* 2008;85:250–267.
13. Arendt R, Farkas K. Maternal alcohol abuse and fetal alcohol spectrum disorder: a life-span perspective. *Alcohol Treatment Q* 2007;25:3–20.
14. Cadoret RJ, Troughton E, O'Gorman TW, et al. An adoption study of genetic and environmental factors in drug abuse. *Arch Gen Psychiatry* 1986;43:1131–1136.
15. Cloninger CR, Sigvardsson S, Bohman M. Childhood personality predicts alcohol abuse in young adults. *Alcohol Clin Exp Res* 1988;12:494–505.
16. Goodwin DW. Alcoholism and heredity: a review and hypothesis. *Arch Gen Psychiatry* 1979;36:57–61.
17. Heath AC, Cates R, Martin NG, et al. Genetic contribution to risk of smoking initiation: comparisons across birth cohorts and across cultures. *J Subst Abuse* 1993;5:221–246.
18. Reich T, Cloninger CR, Van Eerdewegh P, et al. Secular trends in the familial transmission of alcoholism. *Alcohol Clin Exp Res* 1988;12:458–464.
19. Swan GE, Carmelli D, Rosenman RH, et al. Smoking and alcohol consumption in adult male twins: genetic heritability and shared environmental influences. *J Subst Abuse* 1990;2:39–50.
20. Cloninger CR. Neurogenetic adaptive mechanisms in alcoholism. *Science* 1986;236:410–416.
21. Liepman MR, Calles JL, Kizilbash L, et al. Genetic and nongenetic factors influencing substance use by adolescents. *Adolesc Medic* 2002;13, 375–401.
22. Kandel D, Faust R. Sequence and stages in patterns of adolescent drug use. *Arch Gen Psychiatry* 1975;32:923–932.
23. Moos RH, Billings AG. Children of alcoholics during the recovery process: alcoholic and matched control families. *Addict Behav* 1982;7:155–163.
24. American Psychiatric Association. *Desk reference to the diagnostic criteria from* DSM-IV- TR. Washington, DC: Author, 2000:115.
25. Burant D, Liepman MR, Miller MM. Mental health disorders and their impact on treatment of addictions. In: Fleming MD, Barry KL, eds. *Addictive disorders.* St. Louis: Mosby/Year Book, 1992:315–337.
26. Wartenberg AA, Liepman MR. Medical consequences of addictive behaviors. In: Nirenberg TD, Maisto SA, eds. *Developments in the assessment and treatment of addictive behaviors.* Norwood, NJ: Ablex, 1987:49–85.
27. Wartenberg AA, Liepman MR. Medical complications of substance abuse. In: Lerner WD, Barr MA, eds. *Handbook of hospital-based substance abuse treatment.* New York: Pergamon, 1990:45–65.
28. Nirenberg TD, Liepman MR, Begin AM, et al. The sexual relationship of male alcoholics and their female partners during periods of drinking and abstinence. *J Stud Alcohol* 1990;51:565–568.
29. Casey K. *Children of Eve: the shocking story of America's homeless kids.* Hollywood: Covenant House, 1991.
30. Liepman MR, White WT, Nirenberg TD. Children in alcoholic families. In: Lewis DC, Williams CN, eds. *Providing care for children of alcoholics: clinical and research perspectives.* Pompano Beach, FL: Health Communications, 1986:39–64.
31. Barker LR, Whitfield C, Davis J. Alcoholism. In: Barker LR, Burton JR, Zieve PD, eds. *Principles of ambulatory medicine.* Baltimore: Williams & Wilkins, 1995.
32. Graham AV, Berolzheimer N. Alcohol abuse: a family disease. *Primary Care Clin Office Pract* 1993;20:121–130.
33. Baird MA. Care of family members and other affected persons. In: Fleming MF, Barry KL, eds. *Addictive disorders.* St. Louis: Mosby Year Book, 1992:195–210.
34. Wegscheider-Cruse S. *Another chance: hope and health for the alcoholic family.* Palo Alto, CA: Science and Behavior Books, 1989.
35. Kaufman E. *Substance abuse and family therapy.* New York: Harcourt Brace Jovanovich, 1985:221.
36. Liepman MR. Using family influence to motivate alcoholics to enter treatment: the Johnson Institute Intervention Approach. In: O'Farrell TJ, ed. *Marital and family therapy in alcoholism treatment.* New York: Guilford Press, 1993:54–77.
37. Liepman MR, Wolper B, Vazquez J. An ecological approach for motivating women to accept treatment for chemical dependency. In: Reed BG, Mondanaro J, Beschner GM, eds. *Treatment services for drug dependent women, vol. II.* Rockville, MD: National Institute on Drug Abuse, 1982:1–61.
38. Prochaska JO, DiClemente CC. Towards a comprehensive model of change. In: Miller WR, Heather N, eds. *Treating addictive behaviors: processes of change.* New York: Plenum, 1986:3–27.
39. Bennett LA, Ames GM. *The American experience with alcohol: contrasting cultural perspectives.* New York: Plenum, 1985.
40. Liepman MR, Flachier R, Tareen RS. Family Behavior Loop Mapping: a technique to analyze the grip addictive disorders have on families and to help them to recover. *Alcohol Treatment Q* 2008;26:59–80.
41. Liepman MR, Silvia LY, Nirenberg TD. The use of Family Behavior Loop Mapping for substance abuse. *Fam Relations* 1989;38:282–287.
42. Silvia LY, Liepman MR. Family Behavior Loop Mapping enhances treatment of alcoholism. *Fam Comm Health* 1991;13:72–83.
43. Steinglass P, Davis DI, Berenson D. Observations of conjointly hospitalized "alcoholic couples" during sobriety and intoxication: implications for theory and therapy. *Fam Proc* 1977;16:1–16.
44. Olsen L, Allen D, Azzi-Lessing L. Assessing risk in families affected by substance abuse. *Child Abuse Neglect* 1996;20:833–842.
45. Burd L, Wilson H. Fetal, infant, and child mortality in the context of alcohol use. *Am J Med Genet Part C,* 2004;127:51–58.
46. Liepman MR, Nirenberg TD, Doolittle RH, et al. Family functioning of male alcoholics and their female partners during periods of drinking and abstinence. *Fam Proc* 1989;28:239–249.
47. Miller WR, Rollnick S. *Motivational interviewing,* 2nd ed. New York: Guilford Press, 2002.
48. Landau J, Garrett J. Invitational intervention: the ARISE Model for engaging reluctant alcohol and other drug abusers in treatment. *Alcohol Treatment Q* 2008;26:147–168.
49. Johnson VE. *Intervention: how to help those who don't want help.* Minneapolis: Johnson Institute, 1986.
50. Liepman MR, Nirenberg TD, Begin AM. Evaluation of a program designed to help families and significant others to motivate resistant alcoholics into recovery. *Am J Drug Alcohol Abuse* 1989;15:209–221.
51. Loneck B, Garrett J, Banks S. A comparison of the Johnson Intervention with four other methods of referral to outpatient treatment. *Am J Drug Alcohol Abuse* 1996;22:233–246.
52. Loneck B, Garrett J, Banks S. The Johnson Intervention and relapse during outpatient treatment. *Am J Drug Alcohol Abuse* 1996;22:363–375.
53. Landau J, Stanton MD, Brinkman-Sull D, et al. Outcomes with ARISE approach to engaging reluctant drug- and alcohol-dependent individuals in treatment. *Am J Drug Alcohol Abuse* 2004;30:711–748.
54. Monti PM, Abrams DB, Binkoff JA, et al. Communication skills training, communication skills training with family, and cognitive behavioral mood management training for alcoholics. *J Stud Alcohol* 1990;51:263–270.
55. O'Farrell TJ, Fals-Stewart W. Behavioral couples therapy for alcoholism and other drug abuse. *Alcohol Treatment Q* 2008;26:195–219.
56. Thomas EJ, Santa CA. Unilateral family therapy for alcohol abuse: a working conception. *Am J Family Ther* 1982;10:49–58.
57. Smith JE, Meyers RJ, Austin JL. Working with family members to engage treatment-refusing drinkers: the CRAFT program. *Alcohol Treatment Q* 2008;26:169–193.

58. Miller WR, Meyers RJ, Tonigan JS. Engaging the unmotivated in treatment for alcohol problems: a comparison of three strategies for intervention through family members. *J Consult Clin Psychol* 1999;67:688–697.
59. Kirby KC, Marlowe DB, Festinger DS, et al. Community reinforcement training for family and significant others of drug abusers: a unilateral intervention to increase treatment entry of drug users. *Drug Alcohol Depend* 1999;56:85–96.
60. Meyers RJ, Miller WR, Smith JE, et al. A randomized trial of two methods for engaging treatment-refusing drug users through concerned significant others. *J Consult Clin Psychol* 2002;70:1182–1185.
61. Montgomery, L. *The things between us: a memoir.* New York: The Free Press, 2006.
62. Moyers WC, Ketchum K. *Broken: my story of addiction and redemption.* New York: Viking Press, 2006.
63. Edwards ME, Steinglass P. Family therapy treatment outcomes for alcoholism. *J Marital Family Ther* 1995;21:475–509.
64. O'Farrell TJ, Fals-Stewart W. Family-involved alcoholism treatment: an update. In: Galanter M, ed. *Recent developments in alcoholism, vol. 15: services research in the era of managed care.* New York: Brunner-Routledge, 2001:329–356.
65. Ripley J, Cunion A, Noble N. Alcohol abuse in marriage and family contexts: relational pathways to recovery. *Alcohol Treatment Q* 2006;24:171–184.
66. Stanton MD, Shadish WR. Outcome, attrition, and family-couple treatment for drug abuse: a meta-analysis and review of the controlled, comparative studies. *Psychol Bull* 1997;122:170–191.
67. Epstein E. McCrady B. Couple therapy in the treatment of alcohol problems. In: Gurman AS, Jacobson NS, eds. *Clinical handbook of couple therapy,* 3rd ed. New York: Guilford Press; 2002:597–628.
68. Epstein E, McCrady B. Behavioral couples treatment of alcohol and drug use disorders: current status and innovations. *Clin Psychol Rev* 1998; 18:689–711.
69. Fals-Stewart W, Birchler GR. A national survey of the use of couples therapy in substance abuse treatment. *J Subst Abuse Treatment* 2001;20:277–283.
70. Thomas C, Corcoran J. Empirically based marital and family interventions for alcohol abuse: a review. *Res Social Work Practice* 2001;11:549–575.
71. Longabaugh R, Rubin A, Malloy P, et al. Drinking outcomes of alcohol abusers diagnosed as antisocial personality disorder. *Alcohol Clin Exp Res* 1994;18:778–785.
72. Holtzworth-Munroe A, Meehan J, Rehman U, et al. Intimate partner violence: an introduction for couple therapists. In: Gurman AS, Jacobson NS, eds. *Clinical handbook of couples therapy,* 3rd ed. New York: Guilford Press; 2002:441–465.
73. Fichter MM, Glynn SM, Weyerer S, et al. Family climate and expressed emotion in the course of alcoholism. *Fam Proc* 1997;36:203–221.
74. Toumbourou J, Blyth A, Bamberg J, et al. Early impact of the BEST intervention for parents stressed by adolescent substance abuse. *J Comm Appl Soc Psychol* 2001;11:291–304.
75. McGillicuddy N, Rychtarik R, Duquette J, et al. Development of a skill training program for parents of substance-abusing adolescents. *J Subst Abuse Treatment* 2001;20:59–68.
76. Blechman E, Vryan K. Prosocial family therapy: a manualized preventive intervention for juvenile offenders. *Aggress Violent Behav* 2000;5:343–378.
77. Briones E, Robbins MS, Szapocznik J. Brief strategic family therapy: engagement and treatment. *Alcohol Treatment Q* 2008;26:81–103.
78. Szapocznik J, Perez-Vidal A, Brickman A, et al. Engaging adolescent drug abusers and their families into treatment: a strategic structural systems approach. *J Consult Clin Psychol* 1988;56:552–557.
79. Santisteban D, Coatsworth JD, Perez-Vidal A, et al. Efficacy of brief strategic family therapy in modifying Hispanic adolescent behavior problems and substance use. *J Fam Psychol* 2003;17:121–133.
80. Rowe CL, Liddle HA. Multidimensional family therapy for adolescent alcohol abusers. *Alcohol Treatment Q* 2008;26:105–123.
81. Liddle HA, Dakoff GA, Parker K, et al. Multidimensional family therapy for adolescent substance abuse: results of a randomized clinical trial. *Am J Drug Alcohol Abuse* 2001;27:651–687.
82. Liddle HA, Rowe CL, Henderson C, et al. Early intervention for adolescent substance abuse: pretreatment and posttreatment outcomes of a randomized controlled trial comparing multidimensional family therapy and peer group treatment. *J Psychoactive Drugs* 2004;36:2–37.
83. Henggeler SW, Clingempeel WG, Brondino MJ, et al. Four-year follow-up of multisystemic therapy with substance-abusing and substance-dependent juvenile offenders. *J Am Acad Child Adolesc Psychiatry* 2002;41: 868–874.
84. Henggeler SW, Halliday-Boykins CA, Cunningham PB, et al. Juvenile drug court: enhancing outcomes by integrating evidence-based treatments. *J Consult Clin Psychol* 2006;74:42–54.
85. Sheidow AJ, Henggeler SW. Multisystemic therapy for alcohol and other drug abuse in delinquent adolescents. *Alcohol Treatment Q* 2008;26: 125–145.
86. Dembo R, Cervenka K, Hunter B, et al. Engaging high risk families in community based intervention services. *Aggress Violent Behav* 1999;4: 41–58.
87. Substance Abuse and Mental Health Services Administration (SAMHSA). *Substance abuse among older adults: Treatment Improvement Protocol* (TIP). Series Number 26. Rockville, MD: U.S. Department of Health and Human Services, 2004.
88. Blow F, Brower K, Schulenberg J, et al. The Michigan Alcoholism Screening Test-Geriatric Version (MAST-G): a new elderly-specific screening instrument. *Alcohol Clin Exp Res* 1992;16:372.
89. Stelle C, Scott J. Alcohol abuse by older family members: a family systems analysis of assessment and intervention. *Alcohol Treatment Q* 2007;25: 43–63.
90. Lemke S, Moos R. Prognosis of older patients in mixed-age alcoholism treatment programs. *J Subst Abuse Treatment* 2002;22:33–43.

CHAPTER 63

Kathleen M. Carroll, PhD

Twelve Step Facilitation Approaches

Of the behavioral therapies described in this volume, Twelve Step Facilitation (TSF) is perhaps unique in that it is an approach that had its roots in traditional clinical practice and was then codified and moved into clinical research, as opposed to a scientifically developed treatment then transferred to clinical practice. TSF therapy (1) is a manual-guided treatment that was developed for use in Project MATCH, a major multisite trial of behavioral treatments for alcohol abuse and dependence. TSF was developed specifically to approximate the style of counseling commonly used in treatment programs throughout the United States. Thus its content was intended to be consistent with active involvement in Twelve Step recovery programs such as Alcoholics Anonymous (AA) and with a treatment goal of abstinence from all psychoactive substances. Since its introduction in 1992, utilization and empirically support for this approach has grown steadily. This chapter will describe its historical roots, summarize its use in clinical practice, and briefly review the empirically data regarding its use with substance abusing populations.

HISTORICAL PERSPECTIVE

For many years, treatment based on or related to the Twelve Steps of Alcoholics Anonymous were widely practiced in the clinical community, particularly residential and 90-day programs. In many ways, self-help and Twelve Step–oriented groups formed the foundation of substance abuse treatment in the United States and played a major formative roles in the philosophies of some of the most influential treatment centers and programs, including the Hazelden Foundation, the Betty Ford Center, and many more programs using the Minnesota Model and similar approaches Although there were differences across programs, programs general had two related foci: emphasis on abstinence from all psychoactive substances and encouraging self-help attendance. Although AA has been challenging to study systematically (2) and the quality of research on the effectiveness of self-help has been variable (3), the bulk of the evidence suggests that attendance at self-help groups is associated with better outcomes (see previous work [4,5]).

Recognizing that self-help programs represent an important, broadly available, and inexpensive resource, the defining feature of TSF is to encourage meaningful, long-term involvement with AA and other self-help groups. Because of the importance of including an approach that was representative of the dominant model of clinical practice in Project MATCH (6), and the need for a clear, structured description of these approaches that could be used in a large research protocol, the Project MATCH Steering Committee asked Joe Nowinski, PhD, and Stu Baker, two clinical experts to collaborate with our group at Yale (7) to develop the TSF manual, which was done in close collaboration with experts from the Hazelden Foundation (6,8). After its initial evaluation in Project MATCH, TSF and closely related approaches have been evaluated in several subsequent trials and has extended to populations other than those with alcohol use disorders.

TREATMENT MODEL

TSF is a highly structured, individual, manual-guided approach delivered over the course of 12 to 24 weeks. As described in the manual (1), it consists of a set of core topics (assessment and overview, acceptance, surrender, and getting active), which are to be covered with all patients, as well as a set of elective topics, which can be selected to tailor the treatment to different individuals (people places and things; review of a genogram; enabling, HALT), as well as guidelines for conjoint sessions with family members.

TSF sessions follow a common format in that each session begins with a careful review of the previous week and self-help attendance, as well as review of the patient's recovery journal as well as reactions to an AA-related readings that may have been assigned. Next, the TSF therapist introduces the "recovery topic" for the week from the set of core and elective sessions, to which the bulk of the session is devoted. Finally, sessions end with assignment of the patient's recovery tasks for the weeks (specific self-help meetings and activities to attend, readings and other tasks).

TSF assumes that alcoholism and addiction are progressive diseases of mind, body, and spirit, for which the only effective remedy is abstinence from mood-altering substances, *one day at a time*. TSF adheres to the concepts set forth in the Twelve Steps and Twelve Traditions (9). Core, essential features of TSF include:

- taking a thorough alcohol and substance use history, identifying positive and negative consequences of substance use, and giving feedback as ground work to Step 1.
- providing education about Steps 1, 2, and 3 of AA, as well as explanation of the disease concept of alcoholism and addiction.
- exploring discrepancies between the patient's stated goals and actions in terms of denial.
- identifying "people, places, and things" that could trigger substance use and identification of "people, places, and things" that support recovery.
- encouraging patients to actively work the "Twelve Steps" as the primary goal of treatment.
- supporting the point of view that the best chance of abstinence and health is to accept loss of control and the need to reach out to the fellowship of AA (or NA or CA).

THEORY OF CHANGE

As with AA, which grew out of the experiences of a group of men as they struggled with severe alcohol dependence, TSF has historic, rather than theoretic foundations. In TSF, change is thought to occur through building a meaningful relationship with the fellowship of AA and in following the Twelve Steps of AA. Several authors have pointed out similarities between the processes of change in AA and those of other effective behavioral therapies (10,11). McCrady (11) noted that the key change principles of AA include changing reference groups through group affiliation, articulating a clear treatment goal through commitment to abstinence, and emphasis on spirituality and intra- and interpersonal change parallel those of some aspects of cognitive and behavioral therapies. The theory of change in TSF is, essentially, the process of the Twelve Steps, as the individual moves from acceptance of alcoholism or addiction and the need for complete abstinence, through the need for affiliation with others and a Higher Power, to recognizing and making amends to others. Hence TSF makes no commitment to a particular causal model of addiction; emphasis is placed on the core concepts of loss of control and denial, and emphasizes two themes.

- Spirituality: Belief in a "power greater than ourselves," which is defined individually, by each person and represents faith and hope for recovery.
- Pragmatism: Belief in doing "what works" for the individual, meaning doing whatever it takes in order to avoid taking the first drink.

TREATMENT PLANNING AND EVALUATION

A thorough evaluation of the individuals alcohol and drug use history is an essential feature of TSF, and in fact dominates much of the first session and may extend into several sessions. The goal is to begin the breakdown of the patient's denial system. The comprehensive alcohol and drug history are taken in a particular format to do this, highlighting progressive loss of control over alcohol and drugs, covering age; substance used (amount and frequency); positive and negative consequences of use; major life events.

Therapists introduce this section by advising the patient that completing this history will help them begin to make sense of what has happened in their life in relation to their use of alcohol or drugs and is used as a means for preparing for Step 1 (admitting powerlessness and acknowledging unmanageability). The TSF therapist begins with the age of earliest use, outside the home, and then progresses by looking at different time periods. Typically, the TSF therapist would ask about a period 3 years after the initial use and then ask about subsequent periods of time in 5-year intervals. For example, if a patient were a 28 year old, who started using marijuana at age 12, the TSF therapist would start at 12, then go to age 15, then to age 20 (or late teens), then to age 25 (or early 20s). Finally, the TSF therapist would ask about the past year to get a sense of current use patterns and issues. At each age, the TSF therapist would work across the table, asking about each of the categories. As this is done, patterns usually emerge. The TSF therapist pays particular attention to any increase in the amount and frequency of use and periods of time that the patient abstained from use or attempted to control their use. This information is used to highlight loss of control over alcohol or drugs, which is the hallmark of addiction in TSF.

The TSF therapist also explores positive and negative consequences of substance use. Typically, the relationship with alcohol and drugs starts out very positively with tremendous enjoyment by the patient. However, as use increases in amount and frequency, there is invariably an increase in negative consequences (e.g., spending too much money, problems at work, problems at home, legal problems). These negative consequences are evidence of the "unmanageability" referred to in the first step. Examining major life events at different ages helps to place the patient's relationship with alcohol and drugs in perspective. TSF recognizes that substance use takes place in a social and environmental context and is not an isolated behavior.

After the alcohol and drug use history is completed, the TSF therapist asks the patient to react to what they have observed. For some, this is the first time they have looked at the big picture of how addiction has affected their life. The therapist then underlines evidence of unmanageability by pointing out negative consequences from their addiction in the following areas:

Physical. Health problems, accidents, or injuries the patient may have experienced.

Legal. Arrests, difficulties with child protection agencies, civil problems, law suits, etc.

Social. Loss of friends, family relationship problems, lack of supportive relationships, lack of social skills.

Sexual. Changes in sexual functioning, positive and negative, trading sex for drugs.

Psychologic. Depression, anxiety, shame, and guilt about using despite the intention to remain abstinent.

Financial. Loss of job, effects on job performance, income used to buy drugs or alcohol, indebtedness.

Finally, the TSF therapist asks about loss of control over alcohol or drug use. This includes behaviors such as repeated failed attempts to stop or control use, using alone, preoccupation with drugs or alcohol, and substance substation. Using the evidence offered by the patient, usually the only logical conclusion is that the patient is an alcoholic or drug addict.

The TSF therapist then describes addiction as follows: Alcoholism or addiction is a disease that is chronic (the patient will remain an addict for the remainder of his or her life), progressive, and if left untreated, can be fatal. Because of the nature of the disease, once a person becomes an addict, he or she can never return to safe use of mood-altering substances. The progressive nature of the disease is noted in the patient's history of increasing losses and problems and increasing amounts and frequency of use over time. The good news is that alcoholism and drug dependence are treatable. The therapist emphasizes that what has worked best for most is to abstain from all mood-altering substances, one day at a time. To learn how to do this and to gain support to do this task, the TSF therapist then recommends that the patient make use of Twelve Step recovery programs such as AA. This leads naturally and easily into contracting with the patient about participating in TSF Therapy and beginning to attend self-help meetings.

INDICATIONS FOR TREATMENT

In general, TSF therapy is intended for alcohol and drug users at the higher end of severity—that is, those who meet criteria for alcohol or drug dependence. As described previously, the assumption is that the patient is coming to treatment after incurring significant consequences of substance use and being unable to control or stop use on their own, and thus would meet formal *Diagnostic and statistical manual of mental disorders* criteria for dependence. Thus TSF is not intended for those who are at the earlier stage of addiction or are "at risk" users. It is of note, however, that, contrary to expectations (and a Project MATCH *a priori* hypothesis), level of alcohol involvement did not predict differential response to TSF in Project MATCH (13).

Similarly, although it was predicted that several patient characteristics (gender, psychiatric severity, conceptual level, motivation) would be associated with poorer response to TSF compared with cognitive-behavioral therapy and motivational interviewing, the primary matching hypotheses in Project MATCH did not receive strong empirical support. Thus the data from Project MATCH suggested that TSF was generally appropriate for a wide range of alcohol-dependent individuals; that is, there were few strong contraindications for TSF found in that dataset.

PRETREATMENT ISSUES

Motivation In TSF, motivation, especially lack thereof, is generally interpreted in terms of denial. The goal of treatment is to engage the patient's interest in voluntarily committing to this Twelve Step facilitation program. Hence approaches that use excessive pressure, threat, or coercion toward this are likely to elicit a false commitment from the patient at best. In TSF, the therapist is advised to take a direct, nonjudgmental, and educative approach to confrontation of denial. The history of substance use, along with symptomatology (e.g., tolerance) and an understanding of the process of addiction is relied on consistently as the basis for directly confronting patients with their current situation. The therapist attempts to highlight denial in a direct yet supportive and empathetic way.

Therapist Characteristics In Project MATCH and the other research studies that have evaluated this approach, TSF has been implemented primarily by masters' level therapists with substantial experience in and commitment to Twelve Step programs as a therapeutic intervention, who also had extensive experience treating a broad range of substance abusers. Because the therapist training period for these clinical trials was brief, it was important to select therapists who already had a high level of expertise and experience in this approach, and thus could achieve optimal levels of adherence and competence rapidly. However, a much broader range of therapists can, with appropriate training and supervision, implement this treatment effectively.

In TSF, the therapist uses his/her therapeutic skills to help the patient overcome barriers to becoming actively involved in Twelve Step recovery programs. Skills such as active listening, accurate empathy, problem solving, feedback, and confrontation all have a place in this therapy. A critically important role is to be an educator about Twelve Step programs, and knowledgeable about local meetings, types of meetings, and guidance and advice about how best to access the resources of Twelve Step programs. This may be based on the wisdom found in recovering literature, or slogans, or the stories of other recovering addicts. Last, the therapist provides empathy and a sense of hope for the patient through communicating an understanding of the struggles of early recovery.

TSF requires an active, supportive, and involved presence by the therapist in sessions. Good TSF appears almost conversational in tone. A good session involves give and take between the therapist and the patient. The session, however, is quite focused. The therapist takes an active part in keeping the focus of the session on recovery. Some therapists begin their sessions by asking the patient, "How has your recovery week been?" When faced with the day-to-day struggles of the patient, the therapist refers the patient back to the use of Twelve Step program tools. For example, the therapist frequently suggests also talking a problem over with a sponsor or peer as well as talk about the issue at a meeting.

Last, an effective TSF therapist uses confrontation constructively. The TSF therapist is careful to confront the patient's behavior as it relates to his or her addiction (i.e., denial, avoidance) rather than the person. This means separating the person from the disease and communicating that the patient is a good person who has a disease (addiction) that leads him or her to act in ways that are hurtful toward himself or herself and others.

RELEVANT RESEARCH

For many years, treatments based on the Twelve Steps of AA and Cocaine Anonymous were widely used and had a great deal of popular support in the treatment community, but until recently have had very little empirical support from controlled clinical trials (12,14,15). Recently, however, several rigorous randomized clinical trials have been done that have found strong support for the efficacy of well-defined, manualized, Twelve Step–oriented treatments.

For example, in Project MATCH (16,17), the largest randomized trial of treatments for alcoholism conducted to date, TSF was not significantly different in effectiveness from cognitive-behavioral therapy (CBT) and motivational enhancement therapy (MET), two forms of treatment with strong records of empirical support. Moreover, where there were differences in outcome on some variables (e.g., rates of complete abstinence and negative consequences of drinking), these tended to favor the Twelve Step Facilitation approach over CBT and MET (16–19). TSF has also been associated with higher rates of self-help involvement (20–23), which in turn has been associated with better drinking and drug use outcomes (5,21,24,25).

TSF has also been found to be effective with drug abusers. In a clinical trial of disulfiram and psychotherapy with cocaine and alcohol-dependent subjects, TSF was found to be comparable in effectiveness to CBT in reducing cocaine and alcohol use; moreover, both TSF and CBT were found to be significantly more effective than a psychotherapy control condition, clinical management (26). The effects of TSF in this study were also durable and associated with good outcome up to 1 year after patients completed the 12-week treatment program (27). These findings were similar to those of Wells et al. (28), who demonstrated that TSF was comparable in effectiveness to CBT in a randomized controlled trial with cocaine abusers in a group setting. Finally, Ouimette et al. (29), in a nonrandomized trial, evaluated the effectiveness of Twelve Step and CBT approaches in 15 Veterans Affairs programs in a sample of 3,017 subjects. Participants in both types of treatment programs had good outcomes at 1 year; moreover, patients in the Twelve Step–oriented programs had somewhat higher rates of abstinence.

Despite emerging support for the efficacy of TSF, it has proven challenging to disseminate TSF and other empirically validated treatments to the clinical community. Many clinicians have limited access to comprehensive training in TSF or other empirically validated therapies (30). Although workshops in some empirically supported therapies are more available recently, training sessions are usually quite brief (e.g., workshops of several hours duration) and hence unlikely to produce lasting change in clinician's ability to implement new therapies (31). Moreover, it should not be assumed that counselors, even those espousing a Twelve Step model, can implement TSF without training. Although based on standard counseling models, TSF differs from it in several ways. These include its high emphasis on therapist support, discouragement of aggressive "confrontation of denial" and therapist self-disclosure, and highly focused and structured format.

In this context, Sholomskas and Carroll recently completed a randomized training trial in which predominantly bachelors and masters' level counselors were randomly assigned to one of two training conditions: either the TSF manual (1) or a computer-assisted training method (32). Pre- to posttraining data indicated that the clinicians' ability to implement TSF, as assessed by independent ratings of adherence and skill for five key TSF interventions, was significantly higher after training for those assigned to the computer-assisted training method than for those who were assigned to the manual-only training condition. Those who were assigned to the CD-ROM condition also evidenced greater gains in a knowledge test assessing familiarity with concepts presented in the TSF manual. Moreover, no significant effects of the clinicians' self-reported recovery status were seen on adherence, competence, or knowledge scores (32).

SUMMARY AND CONCLUSIONS

TSF is a professionally delivered, individual, manual guided therapy that is grounded in the principles and Twelve Steps of AA. It is important to note, however, that TSF has no official relationship with, or sanction from, any Twelve Step program. AA does not sponsor or conduct research on alcohol or drug treatment and does not endorse any treatment program. While intended to be consistent with Twelve Step principles, it is important to note that TSF was designed for delivery in research protocols and in clinical settings and thus is a fairly recent addition to the repertoire of behavioral therapies for alcohol and drug use disorders. With that as its basis, TSF received comparatively strong empirical support in Project MATCH, one of the largest alcohol treatment trials ever conducted in the United States, and support is emerging for its use with other patient groups as well.

ACKNOWLEDGMENT: *Sections of this chapter were adapted from Nowinski J, Baker S, Carroll KM. Twelve-step facilitation therapy manual: a clinical research guide for therapists treating individuals with alcohol abuse and dependence. Rockville, MD: NIAAA, 1992.*

REFERENCES

1. Nowinski J, Baker S, Carroll KM. *Twelve-step facilitation therapy manual: a clinical research guide for therapists treating individuals with alcohol abuse and dependence.* Rockville, MD: NIAAA, 1992.
2. Humphreys K. The trials of Alcoholics Anonymous. *Addiction* 2006;101: 617–618.
3. Ferri M, Amato L, Davoli, M. Alcoholics Anonymous and other 12-step programmes for alcohol dependence (review). *Cochrane Libr* 2008;3:1–25.
4. Humphreys K. *Circles of recovery: self-help organizations for addictions.* Cambridge, UK: Cambridge University Press, 2004.
5. Humphreys K, Wing S, McCarty D, et al. Self-help organizations for alcohol and drug problems: toward evidence-based practice and policy. *J Subst Abuse Treat* 2004;26:151–158.
6. Donovan D, Kadden R, DiClemente CC, et al. Issues in the selection and development of therapies in alcoholism treatment matching. *J Studies Alcohol* 1994;(Suppl. 12):138–148.
7. Connors GJ, Tonigan JS, Miller WR. A longitudinal model of intake symptomatology, AA participation and outcome: retrospective study of the project MATCH outpatient and aftercare samples. *J Stud Alcohol* 2001;62(6):817–825.
8. Carroll KM, Kadden R, Donovan D, et al. Implementing treatment and protecting the validity of the independent variable in treatment matching studies. *J Studies Alcohol* 1994;(Suppl 12):149–155.
9. Alcoholics Anonymous-Big Book 4E. *Alcoholic Anonymous World Services* 2002. ISBN-13: 978-1893007178.
10. Longabaugh R, Donovan DM, Karno MP, et al. Active ingredients: how and why evidence-based alcohol behavioral treatment interventions work. *Alcohol Clin Exp Res* 2005;29:235–247.
11. McCrady BS. Alcoholics Anonymous and behavior therapy: can habits be treated as diseases? Can diseases be treated as habits? *J Consult Clin Psychol* 1994;62(6):1159–1166.
12. Morgenstern J, Labouvie E, McCrady BS, et al. Affiliation with Alcoholics Anonymous after treatment: a study of its therapeutic effects and mechanisms of action. *J Consult Clin Psychol* 1997;65:768–777.
13. Babor TF, Del Boca FK, eds. *Treatment matching in alcoholism.* Cambridge: Cambridge University Press, 2003.
14. Miller WR, Brown JM, Simpson TL., et al. What works? A methodological analysis of the alcohol treatment literature. In: Hester RK, Miller WR, eds. *Handbook of alcoholism treatment approaches: effective alternatives.* Boston, MA: Allyn & Bacon, 1995:12–44.
15. Tonigan JS, Toscova R, Miller WR. Meta-analysis of the literature on Alcoholics Anonymous: sample and study characteristics that moderate findings. *J Studies Alcohol* 1996;57:65–72.
16. Project MATCH Research Group. Matching Alcohol Treatments to Client Heterogeneity: Project MATCH posttreatment drinking outcomes. *J Studies Alcohol* 1997;58:7–29.
17. Project MATCH Research Group. Project MATCH secondary a priori hypotheses. *Addiction* 1997;92:1671–1698.
18. Project MATCH Research Group. Matching alcoholism treatments to client heterogeneity: project MATCH three-year drinking outcomes. *Alcohol Clin Exp Res* 1998;22:1300–1311.
19. Project MATCH Research Group. Matching alcoholism treatments to client heterogeneity: treatment main effects and matching effects on drinking during treatment. *J Stud Alcohol* 1998;59:631–639.
20. Bogenschutz MP, Tonigan JS, Miller WR. Examining the effects of alcoholism typology and AA attendance on self-efficacy as a mechanism of change. *J Stud Alcohol* 2006;67(4):562–567.
21. Carroll KM, Nuro KF. One size can't fit all: a stage model for psychotherapy manual development. *Clin Psychol Sci Practice* 2002;9:396–406.
22. Weiss RD, Griffin ML, Gallop RJ, et al. The effect of 12-step self-help group attendance and participation on drug use outcomes among cocaine-dependent patients. *Drug Alcohol Depend* 2005;77:177–184.
23. Weiss RD, Griffin ML, Najavits LM, et al. Self-help activities in cocaine dependent patients entering treatment: results from the NIDA collaborative cocaine treatment study. *Drug Alcohol Depend* 1996;43: 79–86.
24. Brown TG, Seraganian P, Tremblay J, et al. Process and outcome changes with relapse prevention versus 12-Step aftercare programs for substance abusers. *Addiction* 2002;97:677–689.
25. Owen PL, Slaymaker V, Tonigan JS, et al. Participation in alcoholics anonymous: intended and unintended change mechanisms. *Alcohol Clin Exp Res* 2003;27(3):524–532.
26. Carroll KM, Nich C, Ball SA, et al. Treatment of cocaine and alcohol dependence with psychotherapy and disulfiram. *Addiction* 1998;93: 713–728.
28. Wells EA, Peterson PL, Gainey RR, et al. Outpatient treatment for cocaine abuse: a controlled comparison of relapse prevention and Twelve-Step approaches. *Am J Drug Alcohol Abuse* 1994;20:1–17.
29. Ouimette PC, Finney JW, Moos RH. Twelve-Step and cognitive behavioral treatment for substance abuse: a comparison of treatment effectiveness. *J Consult Clin Psychol* 1997;65:230–240.
30. Institute of Medicine. *Bridging the gap between practice and research: forging partnerships with community-based drug and alcohol treatment.* Washington, DC: National Academy Press, 1998.
31. Walters ST, Matson SA, Baer JS., et al. Effectiveness of workshop training for psychosocial addiction treatments: a systematic review. *J Subst Abuse Treatment* 2005;29:283–293.
32. Sholomskas DE, Carroll KM. One small step for manuals: computer-assisted training in twelve-step facilitation. *J Studies Alcohol* 2006;67 (6):939–945.

CHAPTER 64

Zebulon Taintor, MD
Richard N. Rosenthal, MD

Microprocessor Abuse and Internet Addiction

INTRODUCTION

Microprocessors are all around us, serving as prosthetic brains, guides, knowledge sources, calculators, and the like, a technological leap of the late twentieth century that will have profound effects on human functioning in the twenty-first. Microprocessors help us manage many aspects of our lives, and we use them a lot. They can provide much stimulation, but they don't manage our time, our motivations, and our involvements. Some of us use them too much, lose track of time while getting too involved, and become dependent on the stimulation they provide. Some of us have significant negative life consequences as a result of that dependence, not that different from addiction to substances, which in itself is a topic of debate. This chapter is about the use of microprocessors and the problems that can ensue.

The Internet has five major uses that affect clinicians and their patients: (1) source of information on disease, diagnosis, treatments and therapists; (2) support and self-help groups (moderated or not); (3) provision of advice, diagnosis, and counseling whereby the person being helped has not met the helper except over the Internet; (4) obtaining addictive substances, both prescription and nonprescription' and (5) enhanced opportunities for people to do things that would tend to bring them to the attention of a clinician even if they didn't happen to use the Internet (sex, gambling, etc.). Some of these last activities are regarded as addicting in their own right.

"Internet addiction" covers only part of the problems encountered by clinicians in patients who spend too much time using devices built around microprocessors. Consider the accident resulting from instant messaging while driving, the gunshots exchanged over X-Box use, too many hours on the Internet using a souped-up mobile phone, or a person who finds *Second Life* more real than his or her real life. The common denominator is the use of microprocessors in an increasingly wide variety of devices. Thus, the title of this chapter is expanded past "Internet Addiction" and a considerable broadening of situations to be considered. What is clear is that the human problems that are now becoming apparent in the context of microprocessor use are related to the interaction of the novel technology and the people using it, as compared to intrinsic mental disorders that have been around for millennia, such as depression and schizophrenia, or other disorders of compulsive/impulsive behavior such as eating disorders or pathologic gambling.

HISTORICAL PERSPECTIVE

The history that matters is the most recent, as the pace of change has been so fast. The Internet was established in 1969 at the University of Southern California as a way of linking computers for national defense uses. Even early on, computers offered opportunities to impair functioning, even in the absence of the Internet. Weinberg (1) described programmers so immersed in programming they failed to properly document their work. Later, Weitzenbaum (2) described the development of compulsive programmers who had lost the broad view of problem solving, and came to see problems simply as means to interact with the computer. The concept of the impaired computer user was described in 1992 by Kuiper (3), who called them "space cadets," characterized as spending too much time in front of industrial or commercial computers, and having too few other ambitions or interests. Once the Internet became functional in the business community, it didn't take long for it to become an instrument of non-work-related use in the workplace, problematic if not necessarily pathologic. A recent survey of 224 U.S. companies by Greenfield and Davis (4) demonstrated that 60% of companies had disciplined employees about inappropriate Internet use, and 30% had terminated employees owing to Internet behavior. Forty-seven percent of a randomly selected group of workers from the 224 companies surfed non-work-related Web sites more than 3 hours per week and 19% 4 or more hours per week.

Specialized offers to certain customers via e-mail began in 1973, and the first online service among users started in 1979. Use of e-mail for therapy was documented in the 1980s, and simulated patients were developed (e.g., "Eliza" and "Parry") to demonstrate typical psychopathology to those who signed on to interact with them. But widespread use of e-mail skyrocketed in the 1990s as e-mail programs became interoperable and anyone was able to get and send from any of a variety of software programs. The first wave of articles about Internet addiction appeared in the mid 1990s, and the Center for Internet Addiction Recovery was one of dozens of sites set up to help the addicted. A book by its founder, Kimberly Young, PsyD, provides a picture of internet addiction in the late 1990s (5). Text and instant messaging took off as the twenty-first century began with personal digital assistants (PDAs), Blackberrys, and increasingly smart telephones. Currently, it is estimated that 82% of American population has access to the Internet. In large cities, just less than 50% have broadband access (6). More than that have cellular telephones, although the number with Internet and e-mail capability is unknown. Newer models typically include a wide variety of communication modes. Current estimates have 82% of the American population having some sort of computer access. Most use e-mail, which can be used without the Internet or a computer. That handheld devices can be taken anywhere and are used in many places is evidenced by America On Line's Fourth Annual Survey of 4000 e-mail users. It found an increase from 15% (in 2007) to 46% of those describing themselves as "e-mail addicts." E-mail is checked while in bed (67%), the bathroom (59%), while driving (50%, up from 37% last year), and church (15%) (7).

Identity and the Internet are emerging as a separate field of study with the mushrooming growth of programs like Second Life *(www.secondlife.com),* which has more than 12 million regular users. Second Life describes itself as "a 3-D virtual world entirely created by its Residents [who socialize, create, and chat using voice and text chat]. Since opening to the public in 2003, it has grown explosively and today is inhabited by millions of Residents from around the globe. Its world is filled with creations of the Residents, often elaborately and colorfully costumed, often with special powers. Second Life creations can include cities, countries, whatever. Real world commercial interests, such as Sony, BMG Music Entertainment, Sun Microsystems, Nissan, Adidas/Reebok, Toyota, and Starwood Hotels. NYU has placed a virtual film making school in Second Life; The Second Life marketplace uses Linden Dollars, which can be earned in Second Life or bought with, or exchanged for, world currency. Several other sites (Metaverse, Open Life) offer similar fare. All are developing additional features to make their offerings more attractive and enveloping. Participation in alternate realities offers rich material for considering identity choices and psychodynamics. Some people have reported having more success in Second Life than in their real lives (8), while other patients have entered therapy because of Second Life relationships gone awry. One creates an identity for one's self, which often is quite opposite from one's regular self. Second Life uses Linden dollars, which are convertible to regular U.S. dollars. Recently, a bank in Second Life failed via a Ponzi scheme, and the crowd milling around in front seemed to consist of hookers, Mafia types, and many bizarrely dressed unidentifiable characters. They had lost real money; now there are banking regulations.

As any assessment of addiction involves considering risk-taking behavior, it is important for clinicians to understand the current risks that the use of microprocessors offers. One can easily become a victim when participating in e-mail and chat groups wherein others are using false identities, often for a specific purpose such as sexual predation. Technology change has outstripped the legal system's ability to provide basic protections. Even where economic damages can be claimed, such as false information engendering stock price swings, prosecution has been scant. Meanwhile, there are almost daily reports of data security breaches involving thousands of people (see *http://datalossdb.org/*).

DIAGNOSTIC DILEMMAS

There has been an animated discussion of terms such as "Internet addiction," "pathological computer use," "e-mail addiction" (see above), and the like in the popular press, where the concept of addiction is used to describe a much less serious phenomenon than what clinicians usually mean by "addiction." With increasing use of microprocessors, the terms have progressed from being jokes to being taken seriously. In considering whether the microprocessors are a *bona fide* substrate for addictive processes, it is important to present some caveats:

- Using the computer, cell phone, or videogame is not intrinsically illegal, although the media can be used for that purpose.
- Using the computer, cell phone, or videogame is generally normal, prosocial, encouraged behavior.
- There is a learning curve to information acquisition, time management, and social behavior when people experience these new and powerful tools (think about pedestrians walking in city streets holding their cell phones that block their view of oncoming traffic, or listening to iPods, which attenuate their ability to hear important auditory cues from without).

- People can be very engaged in microprocessor use without its being pathological.
- Calling maladaptive microprocessor-related behavior pathological rather than, say, a bad habit may medicalize what is in actuality a social problem.

Unanswered questions thus arise in the context of considering whether Internet addiction is a discrete disorder and whether it is an addiction or some other type of disorder:

- Are most surveys that present high rates of pathological Internet use suffering from selection bias?
- Is the term *Internet addiction* overstated and overgeneralized (i.e., are there too many false positives determined by current screening instruments)?
- Is it the technology or that which it enables that people may become addicted to?
- Does the use of the Internet as a conduit for other disorders such as pathological gambling or compulsive sexual behavior become in itself a substrate for addictive process?

Martin and Petry recently debated whether non-substance-related addiction (i.e. behavioral addictions) were really addictions. In this debate, Martin pointed out that addiction as a process requires transformation of basic survival-oriented drives into misdirected or overly frequent actions that leave less time for more adaptive functioning. In considering whether Internet addiction is a real disorder, an approach different from the DSM-IV polythetic approach may be useful in creating a narrow construct within which to categorize Internet addiction. In a monothetic approach, all criteria must be endorsed in order to give a diagnosis, and it should have high sensitivity for diagnosing true positives. If a monothetic approach can be constructed that has good construct and predictive validity, then expanding out from that may allow a criterion set that has reasonable clinical utility in reducing false negatives. Griffiths, in considering the necessary components of addiction that would subtend diagnostically both chemical and behavioral addictions, identified six necessary domains based on the work of Brown (11,12) in modeling problem gambling behavior: salience, mood modification, tolerance, withdrawal symptoms, conflict, and relapse. This method is interesting, and clinicians who treat patients with chemical addictions will recognize the symptom set in their patients, and thus the economy in the approach:

- Salience: The drug or behavior has gained primacy in a person's life, which can be a cognitive change, dominating the person's mental life, or behaviorally, dominating a person's activity in a compulsive fashion.
- Mood modification: The substance or behavior subjectively gives one a rewarding high or alleviates a negative mood state.
- Tolerance: The person must increase the amount or intensity of the substance or behavior in order to achieve the desired effect.
- Withdrawal symptoms: After stopping or reducing the substance or behavior, the person demonstrates either physical symptoms after, or dysphoria characterized by irritability, mood lability, depressive symptoms, and so on.
- Conflict: The person has conflicts regarding the use of the substance or the behavior that manifests as either interpersonal (e.g., marital strife) or intrapsychic (e.g., guilt).
- Relapse: After a period of abstinence, the use or behavior is reinstated with the same intensity.
- Proponents of a polythetic approach to Internet addiction modeled after DSM-IV Substance Dependence might point out that one of the hallmarks of the modern concept of addiction is the idea of loss of control despite negative consequences, which is embodied in several of the DSM-IV criteria and not included as one of the six necessary domains of the monothetic approach. However, compulsive behavior in the Salience category accounts for the symptom of loss of control.

It may be argued that problem Internet use better fits criteria for DSM-IV disorder groups other than the substance-related disorders (i.e. Internet addiction), which is what is behind the differing nomenclature, such as pathological Internet use, which is modeled after pathological gambling, currently a DSM-IV impulse control disorder (ICD) diagnosis. For example, problem Internet use has been proposed as an OCD spectrum disorder. However, in compulsive disorders such as OCD, the intrusive thoughts or compulsive behaviors are typically ego-dystonic, whereas in pathological Internet use, the preoccupation is ego-syntonic and pleasurable. OCD patients are anxious and full of doubt and tend to avoid risk, which is frequently in contrast to the experience of patients with problem Internet use, who underestimate risk. Shapira et al. (13), using the SCID, Internet use history, and a Yale-Brown Obessive Compulsive Scale modified for Internet use, examined 20 recruited volunteers or referred patients with problematic Internet use characterized as uncontrollable, markedly distressing, time-consuming, or resulting in social, occupational, or financial difficulties and not solely present during hypomanic or manic symptoms. In general, the subjects had, in contrast to patients with compulsive disorders, low levels of distress and resistance to excessive Internet use. Their problem Internet use symptoms were highly impulsive, with all subjects meeting DSM-IV criteria for an ICD not otherwise specified (NOS), whereas only 15% subjects met DSM-IV criteria for OCD based on their problem Internet use. However, this uncontrolled study had a small sample size and a clear selection bias, so generalizing from the results may be problematic. Nonetheless, like pathological gambling, pathological Internet use could be conceived as an ICD, and several authors have proposed this (5,14–16). Hallmarks of ICD are repeated failure to resist impulses that are harmful to self or others and tension or arousal before and pleasure or relief during the act, followed by guilt or self-reproach. However, this may not necessarily be the case in patients with problematic Internet use and will need to be explored with larger epidemiologic studies and more refined research of potential diagnostic criteria. The DSM-V workgroup has been contemplating problematic Internet use as a compulsive-impulsive disorder in the group of impulse control disorders (16). As such, it may be that the placement of what may be considered Internet addiction among the DSM-IV impulse disorders is an artifact of the failure to expand the category of substance-related disorders to broader diagnostic category that includes non-substance-related "behavioral addictions." The monothetic approach to addiction described above supplies one potential model for building that category (10).

Another approach to developing stable and valid criteria for Internet addiction has been to build a bottom-up construct of most frequent symptoms from factor analysis of a group. Pratarelli and Browne (17) conducted a 94-item anonymous survey in college students (N = 524) and demonstrated the non-independent factors: Internet Addiction (preoccupation, external complaints, less sleep, food, exercise, and punctuality) [salience]; Sexual (downloading graphic sexual material); and an Internet Use factor (excessive use for professional, educational, gaming, shopping activities, etc.) When the data were best-fit to a structural equation model, the Addiction factor was primary and causal to Sex and Use factors rather than vice-versa. Charlton (18) performed a factor analysis on 47 variables derived from the six-factor monothetic model of addiction described above (10–12), with added items that evaluated engagement (computer apathy/engagement and computer anxiety/comfort) from data collected from a survey of 404 college and graduate students. The Addiction factor loaded upon all items of the monothetic model behavioral addiction criteria supporting the construct validity of this model of computer addiction. However, the Engagement factor also loaded upon tolerance, euphoria, and cognitive salience, demonstrating that these factors are not unique to addiction. This suggests that high computer engagement is part of the structure of "computer (includes Internet) addiction" but is not necessarily pathologic in and of itself. One can be highly engaged in Internet use without negative consequences. Beard and Wolf (16) describe a woman who is preoccupied by thoughts, desires increased time spent in activity, is unsuccessful or unable to control or cut back interactions, is restless, anxious, or moody when not interacting, and interacts for longer periods than intended. Without a defined substrate, the symptoms seem ominous in the example above, but the high engagement of this woman for her baby is not pathologic, and the authors suggest that additional requirement of impairment in a person's daily functioning (i.e., jeopardized loss of relationship or work/educational opportunity, lied to significant others to conceal extent of Internet involvement, or used so as to escape problems or relieve dysphoria), over and above symptoms of high engagement, is necessary for a diagnosis of Internet Addiction. This find is paralleled in the work of Ko et al. (17), who in establishing a criterion set for adolescent Internet addiction that had high diagnostic accuracy and specificity, as well as good sensitivity, determined three main criteria: characteristic symptoms of Internet addiction not dissimilar from DSM-IV substance dependence symptoms, an exclusion criterion, and functional impairment due to Internet use.

ASSESSMENT

Talking to patients, one can discuss the intensity and impact of their use of microprocessor-containing devices and assign general risk categories based upon the information provided. A simple screening cutoff can begin to establish whether use is "normal" or problematic. From there, it becomes more difficult to establish what one is dealing with, owing to the lack of scientific consensus as to whether certain types of maladaptive microprocessor use rise to the level of disorders, what type of disorders they may be, and what the criteria are for those disorders. As discussed above, functional impairment is a good marker for a clinically relevant misuse of microprocessors (21).

Use: A reasonable time spent accomplishing specific goals using microprocessors, such as a Google search on "pathological computer use" (1,410 sites) or getting back your dog that strayed because the staff at the pound found the chip under his skin with your name and telephone number. Remember that high engagement does not necessarily mean pathology.

Problem use: One can conceptualize this as use with trouble in that the use is causing clinically significant impairment. The issue here is the repeated taking on of undue risk, getting oneself into legal problems, the interference with fulfilling major role obligations, or continuing the microprocessor use in spite of recurring social or interpersonal problems. These parallel the abuse category for the DSM-IV substance-related disorders. Instant messaging (IM) while driving is risk taking and increasingly illegal, yet emerging as more accident-related in some jurisdictions than a handheld cell phone. A mother showed author ZT her initial failure to limit her daughter's IMs to 500/day—one printout showed more than 3,000—"She's here but she's not here."

Dependence: The patient experiences that he or she can't get along without it. Here the problem is the level of functioning. Can we get by without the facts so easily pulled off the Internet? Can you calculate as well or as fast as your spreadsheet? Can you avoid e-mail for a day a week, as is increasingly recommended in the popular press? As with most dependencies, there may be a false sense of being in control and "able to stop any time" when one cannot.

Though some describe addiction as a severe form of dependence, many reserve this term for physiologic dependence, as evidenced by withdrawal symptoms. Symptoms such as nervousness, aggression, agitation, insomnia, anorexia, tremulousness, and depression have been noted after microprocessor deprivation. While one can argue that use of an exogenous substance is necessary to produce the physiological changes of true addiction, it is increasingly evident that the body and brain change in response to the environment. Whereas the brain is composed of chemicals, its final pathway of action is electrical, and input from computers increasingly taps into cerebral rhythms. Virtual reality, use of smell, more sophisticated visual and auditory inputs, and probably other paths into the brain will increase influence on the brain. However, at least one study (22) found surprisingly that the interactive functions of the Internet are not as addictive as other functions such as salience, lack of control or anticipation. Substance addiction can result from buying addictive substances through the Internet, where enforcement has been unsuccessful against thousands of sites offering prescription drugs and a handful of sites openly offering cocaine, heroin, and other illegal substances.

INTERNET CHARACTERISTICS

The Internet offers many advantages over other agents with high liability for abuse and dependence (23), including the following:

- Always available: 24/7, lending itself to impulsive access and marathon sessions
- Convenient: No need to leave home or work (those caught downloading pornography or playing games at work are the tip of the iceberg)
- Inexpensive: Now just the cost of the hookup. Internet addiction was a problem when users were paying $800/month access fees (5). There are no dealers to pay.
- Rewarding: Content-rich, with Web sites consistently present and calculated to please; increasing, mostly benign interactivity; a continuous flow of new sites that offer novelty, more videos everyone is talking about, all developed and distributed at an ever-increasing pace.
- Controllable: The user can go wherever desired and leave at will. Of course, addicts usually feel they can stop at any time. Users can better control others' access to them but still interact.
- Escapist: Sites of interest to the potentially addicted offer a welcoming reality in which all sex partners are attractive and interested and bets are likely to be won. Some women are attracted to the Internet because they can act like men (24), whereas introverts can act like extroverts (25).
- Validating: One can find that which caters to one's interests and tastes, thus verifying that these are legitimate because others feel the same way. The Internet is always at least nonjudgmental, unless one chooses a role-playing mode wherein negative feedback is part of the social context but positive judgments can be found readily.

The Internet may differentially support addictive process as Internet communication is anonymous, isolated from normative feedback, and provides easy access to reinforcing stimuli. Powerful search engines aggregate special interest groups and provide virtual and real communities where fringe behaviors and beliefs are consensually validated (26).

TREATMENT MODEL

Theory of Change Motivation is key. If rewards are the issue, others must be found. If obsessive-compulsive concerns are more important, efforts and medication are directed at developing different habits and thought patterns. Recovery is about learning to avoid triggers for impulsive Internet use, making use of social support for healthy reinforcers found in everyday life, and relearning how to use microprocessors in non-pathologic ways.

TREATMENT PLANNING

Evaluation-Diagnosis Parents are often limited by technological naïveté from understanding what their children may be experiencing and doing, adding a dimension of complication to the evaluation they may present.

Is there a need for a new diagnostic category? Possibly, as incidence estimates for Internet addiction range from 1% to 3% of the American population (27). It is not in the *Diagnostic and Statistical Manual* (DSM) of the American Psychiatric Association, currently being revised. However, the addiction field is used to epidemics of powerfully rewarding substances that die down and become endemic. There seemed to be no end to the crack cocaine epidemic of the 1970s and 1980s—much was made of rats pressing levers to inject cocaine into their brains until they died (23)—but it did end. We have had more than a decade of concern about pathological computer use and use and abuse are increasing.

The diagnostic divides are among addiction, impulse control (non-substance-based reward) and compulsive disorders. The addiction field is familiar with reward mechanisms, dopamine medication, conditioned cues, and the like. Rewards usually are related to content or specific activities, such as pornography, gambling, and so on. Diagnoses related to these specific areas are well established and should be used, although for example, pathologic gambling is classified by DSM-IV as an ICD rather than as an addiction under the substance-related disorders category. There remains a population that compulsively uses devices without seeming to get much gratification. They don't feel good, but not doing it leads to feeling bad. Addiction clinicians will recognize this state of compulsive use that is frequently seen in crack addicts using in spite of the lack of "liking" or heroin addicts shooting up in order to "get straight." Compulsive device users rearrange files, check e-mail too often, get on mailing lists that shower them with trivia, and so on. Frequently they meet criteria for a compulsive disorder.

Rating scales serve as diagnostic aids and, in offering objective data for feedback in motivational approaches, can help patients to realize the extent of their problems. Several are available, but that from the Center for Recovery from Internet Addiction, the Internet Addiction Test (IAT) *(http://netaddiction.com/resources/internet_addiction_test.htm)* is best established, having been filled out by thousands of visitors to its Web site (5). Its 20 questions are answered on a five-point scale (with a sixth alternative: does not apply). A score of 100 is possible, with ranges of 20 to 49 indicating average on-line use, 50 to 79 indicating occasional or frequent problems using the Internet and the "need to assess their full impact on your life." The questions get at staying on longer than intended, neglecting household chores, preferring the excitement of the Internet to intimacy with one's partner, forming new relationships on the Web, others complaining about the amount of time one spends on-line, decreased productivity (grades, school work, job), checking e-mail before something else one needs to do, defensiveness or secretiveness when asked about on-line activities, blocking out disturbing thoughts about one's life with soothing thoughts about the Internet, anticipating going online, thinking life would be empty and joyless without the Internet, irritability if bothered while online, losing sleep because of late night use, preoccupation or fantasies while offline, rationalizing extra time online, attempts to reduce online time, hiding how long online, choosing online versus socializing, and depression and moodiness when offline remedied when online. Many of these items correspond to similar items in the DSM-IV diagnostic categories of substance abuse and substance dependence (APA, 2004). The scale can be used by significant others, who usually insist on treatment for reasons common to other addictions: a sense of losing the loved one whose life has been taken over by the addiction, significant impairment in activities and relationships, all usually minimized by the patient. Widyanto and McMurran (22) recruited 86 participants through the Internet who completed a Web version of the IAT with some added items, Factor analysis of the IAT revealed six factors, which showed good internal consistency and concurrent validity: salience, excessive use, neglecting work, anticipation, lack of control, and neglecting social life.

INDICATIONS FOR TREATMENT

Patients and families understand and feel impairment, so responses to the scale above and issues of morbidity and mortality can help all concerned understand indications for treatment.

Mortality Murder and suicide have been reported after microprocessor deprivation, usually an adolescent killing the depriving parent or demonstrating through suicide that life without the microprocessor is not possible. Many of these cases have occurred in South Korea where Internet and microprocessor use is among the highest in the world. One study found that among 452 South Korean adolescents, Internet addiction identified by the IAT was significantly associated with depressive symptoms (29). Morbidity occurs at several levels. The amount of time spent with microprocessors results in necessary tasks going undone. Real-life social relationships get less time, and what may be thought to be more satisfying relationships are developed on the Internet. Impairment can be difficult to tease out but, as described above, becomes a crucial component of a diagnosis over and above high engagement. The patient is not necessarily a recluse but can document that those hours spent in his room involve communicating with "friends" around the world to play "World of War Craft." Objective observers may rate these relationships less favorably, often reminiscent of an alcoholic's drinking buddies. Managing multiple identities can be taxing, and identity fragmentation occurs if one's Internet persona is markedly different from one's real-life persona. Clinicians have to assess cyber relationships in detail. Some patients present as having lost touch with what is the "true" reality. Impairment may also result from physical activity of prolonged sitting in front of screens, with increased obesity and less exercise. Decreasing use of national parks, 4 million fewer golfers, and a decline in outdoor activities may be related to increasing use of microprocessors. However, inactivity is preferable to accidents that occur while multitasking. The American College of Emergency Physicians (2008, *http://www.emergencycareforyou.org/YourHealth/InjuryPrevention/Default.aspx?id = 1240*) responded to increasing reports of injuries related to being hit or falling while texting by issuing an alert against "text walking." It may seem to be common sense that people should watch where they are walking, but the number of vehicle hits, falls, and running into trees, lamp posts, and other people has become noticeable in emergency rooms across the country.

PRETREATMENT ISSUES

Motivation-Rationale for Choice of Treatment

As with most addictions, motivation prior to engagement in treatment may be scant or absent. Problems are minimalized, rationalized, or denied. A non-confrontational discussion of impairment often helps the patient to gain perspective. This can be done using the principles of motivational interviewing (MI), where the facts about the impact of microprocessor overuse are carefully elicited and then fed back to the patient in a nonjudgmental manner (26). This helps the patient to use his or her native analytic capacity and values in determining that the overuse is actually problematic or impairing and helps to tip the decisional balance toward seeking help to reduce the problem.

An important way station between Internet addiction and returning to the real world is more therapeutic use of the Internet and microprocessors. This is somewhat of a departure from the abstinence-oriented approach of classic addiction treatment. A mother was successful in restricting her daughter's instant messaging from 3,000 per day to 500, then 200. Online support groups are thought to help, but a review of 38 controlled studies of illness (not just Internet addiction) support groups found no robust evidence of effects, in part because most were measuring complex interventions (31).

Selection and Preparation of Patients/Suitability

Unlike the subpopulations that comprise the sufferers of many chemical addictions, microprocessor abusers are technically competent, often innovative, and well-educated (32), which makes them more suitable as a group for clinical interventions. However, the subpopulation has been demonstrated to have high rates of current and lifetime co-occurring mental disorders which tend to have a negative impact upon recovery (13). Retreat into cyberspace may mask co-occurring social phobia and/or other anxiety disorders.

Therapist Characteristics Familiarity with the Internet and uses of microprocessors and technology are important both for understanding patients, expressing empathy, and earning respect and credibility with patients, all of which are associated with better treatment outcomes (33).

Treatment and Technique

Choice and Timing of Interventions When parents or significant others are in control, taking away or restricting access to the microprocessor may increase motivation or result in destructive anger, so clinicians must expect to hear about and perhaps participate in whatever decision is made. However, similar to binge eating and other disorders of compulsive food intake, complete abstinence is usually not a feasible long-term treatment goal, as use of microprocessors is unavoidable in today's world, and non-use is associated with significant vocational and social disadvantage.

General and Stage-Specific Interventions The general plan is reintroduction into the real world, which must be done in stages to ease transitions. It is a desensitization process, with small steps to be taken that will bring about a sense of success and increased self-esteem. Where identity issues predominate, the successful elements of the Internet identity should be characterized, and there should be an open discussion of integrating these into the real-world persona. Therapy should be seen as a rewarding process that helps the patient get in real life what has been available only on the Internet. This is consistent with community reinforcement principles in replacing the rewards of the abused substance with more natural and socially appropriate reinforcers (34). With compulsive patients, the therapist can take responsibility for the compulsive behavior and relieve the patient's anxiety. Medication treatment for co-occurring obsessive-compulsive disorders and/or anxiety can be helpful. Clearly, treating co-occurring mood, anxiety, psychotic, and substance use disorders is likely to be helpful in supporting recovery from involvement of significant others and is key to supporting recovery and reintegration into the real world. Social skills training may also be helpful.

RELEVANT RESEARCH

There is little relevant research because research funding agencies have not yet recognized the problem as deserving much attention (i.e., significant clinical impact, public outcry, or political will). The development and use of the Internet is seen as an enormous technologic advance. More and more material is being made available on the Internet, and its legitimate use is increasing exponentially. There is strong commercial support for Internet use, as the Internet generates huge advertising revenues and is used to sell many products. Complaints about Internet addiction can be seen as spoiling the party. The American Medical Association called in 2007 on the National institutes of Health and the Centers for Disease Control to start research programs in Internet addiction, but no grant programs have been announced as yet. As such, much of the available epidemiologic and treatment outcome research devoted to Internet addiction has been based upon case studies and survey data, of which Internet-based surveys can be driven by the motivation of the responders, and thus subject to selection bias.

Efficacy Studies have reported therapeutic success with escitalopram, a selective serotonin reuptake inhibitor antidepressant (30), but the active treatment phase was open-label. Similarly, a trial of cognitive behavior therapy specifically focused upon Internet addiction demonstrated efficacy in reducing pathologic Internet usage and improving online time management among 114 patients who were screened with the IAT, but this was an uncontrolled study (32). Interestingly, in the prospective case series of recruited and treatment-seeking pathologic Internet users described above (13), there were high rates of current comorbid bipolar depression that responded to anticonvulsant treatment (with or without adjunctive antipsychotic or antidepressant agents) with both normalization of mood and moderate to marked remittance of pathologic Internet use.

Effectiveness-External Validity The usual addiction treatments (AA-type groups and other treatments described in this book) have been reported to be effective in case studies or vignettes, but there are no controlled studies of psychosocial treatments other than CBT. Likely validity for these approaches is derived from recognition of the applicability of the impulse-control/obsessive-compulsive model of addictions to microprocessor abuse but will require controlled trials of standardized interventions in target populations using established and validated diagnostic criteria and outcomes measures.

SUMMARY AND CONCLUSIONS

Use of microprocessors is increasing rapidly as these are placed in a wide variety of communication and amusement devices. These devices are always available, cost little to use, and provide many rewards. About 1% of the U.S. population uses them to the point of abuse, dependency, and addiction. These problems are likely to increase as microprocessor use and power continues to increase. While sharing many commonalities with other addictions, microprocessor abuse differs in that no exogenous substance is involved, patients are technologically savvy and computer-literate, and are able to manipulate their identities in cyberspace.

Even without resorting to a pathology model, current societal adaptation to the use of microprocessors can, at its most extreme, be likened to the London Gin Epidemic, where citizens previously comfortable with a culture that drank beer and ale, frequently to intoxication, had to adapt poorly to a new more potent alcoholic liquid, with disastrous results in a population that was already ripe for social unrest (36). Eventually, the culture moderated its use more globally, leaving the bulk of maladaptive and damaging alcohol-related trajectories to those with alcohol use disorders. It may be that our culture is on a similar path, and in the wake of our corporate learning curve will be those for whom microprocessor is a substance fulfilling its role as a substrate for a pathologic use disorder.(2,13, 27,37–40)

REFERENCES

1. Weinberg, GM. *The psychology of computer programming.* New York: Van Nostrand Reinhold, 1971.
2. Weizenbaum J. *Computer power and human reason.* London: Penguin, 1984.
3. Kuiper D. *Those idiots in the computer room.* Portland: Macadam House, 1992.
4. Greenfield DN, Davis RA. Lost in cyberspace: the Web @ work. Cyberpsychol Behav 2002;5(4):347–353.
5. Young K. *Caught in the net: how to recognize the signs of internet addiction—and a winning strategy for recovery.* New York: John Wiley & Sons, 1998.
6. Sablin B. Broadband report: "Digital Divide" exists in city. *New York Sun,* July 31, 2008, p. 2.
7. Gifford E. AOL Mail Fourth Annual Email Addiction Survey. http://corp.aol.com/press-releases/2008/07/it-s-3-am-are-you-checking-your-email-again, July 30, 2008.
8. Au WJ. *The making of second life: notes from the new world.* New York: HarperCollins, 2008.
9. Martin PR, Petry NM. Are non-substance-related addictions really addictions? *Am J Addict* 2005;14(1):1–7.
10. Griffiths M. Nicotine, tobacco, and addiction. *Nature* 1996;384:18.
11. Brown RIF. Gaming, gambling and other addictive play. In: Kerr JH, Apter MJ, eds. *Adult play: a reversal theory approach* (pp. 101–118). Amsterdam: Swets & Zeitlinger, 1991.
12. Brown RIF. Some contributions of the study of gambling to the study of other addictions. In: Eadington WR, Cornelius JA, eds. *Gambling behavior and problem gambling* (pp. 241–272). Reno: University of Nevada, 1993.
13. Shapira NA, Goldsmith TD, Keck PE Jr, et al. Psychiatric features of individuals with problematic internet use. *J Affect Disord* 2001;66 (2–3):283.
14. Young KS, Rogers RC. The relationship between depression and internet addiction. *Cyber Psychol Behav* 1998;1:25–28.
15. Treuer T. Fabian Z. Furedi J. Internet addiction associated with features of impulse control disorder: is it a real psychiatric disorder?. *J Affect Disord* 2001;66(2–3):283.
16. Dell'Osso B, Altamura AC, Allen A, et al. Epidemiologic and clinical updates on impulse control disorders: a critical review. *Eur Arch Psychiatry Clin Neurosci* 2006;256(8):464–475. Epub 2006 Sept. 7. Review.
17. Pratarelli ME, Browne BL. Confirmatory factor analysis of internet use and addiction. *Cyberpsychol Behav* 2002;5(1):53–64.
18. Charlton JP. A factor-analytic investigation of computer addiction and engagement. *Br J Psychol* 2002;93:329–344.
19. Beard KW, Wolf EM. Modification in the proposed diagnostic criteria for Internet addiction. *Cyberpsychol Behav* 20014(3):377–383.
20. Ko CH, Yen JY, Chen CC, et al. Proposed diagnostic criteria of Internet addiction for adolescents. *J Nerv Ment Dis* 2005;193(11):728–733.
21. Beard KW. Internet addiction: a review of current assessment techniques and potential assessment questions. *Cyberpsychol Behav* 2005;8:7–14.
22. Widyanto L, McMurran M. The psychometric properties of the internet addiction test. *Cyberpsychol Behav* 2004;7(4):443–450.
23. Taintor Z. Internet/computer addiction. In: Lowinson J, Ruiz P, Millman R, Langrod J, eds. *Substance abuse,* 4th ed. New York, Lippincott Williams & Wilkins, 2005:540–548.
24. Grigoradis V. The casual sex revolution: how the Internet took the sting out of sleeping with strangers. *New York Magazine* 2003;13:17–20.
25. Amichai-Hamburger Y, Wainapel G, Fox S. "On the Internet no one knows I'm an introvert": extroversion, neuroticism, and Internet interaction. *Cyberpsychol Behav* 2002;5(2):125–128.
26. Griffiths M. Does Internet and computer "addiction" exist? *Cyberpsychol Behav* 3:211–18, 2000.
27. Aboujaoude E, Koran LM, Gamel N, et al. Potential markers for problematic internet use: a telephone survey of 2,513 adults. *CNS Spectr* 2006;11(10):750–755.
28. Bozarth MA, Wise RA. Toxicity associated with long-term intravenous heroin and cocaine self-administration in the rat. *JAMA* 1985;254(1):81–83.
29. Ha JH, Kim SY, Bae SC, et al. Depression and Internet addiction in adolescents. *Psychopathology* 2007;40(6):424–430. Epub 2007, Aug 20.
30. Miller WR, Rollnick S. *Motivational interviewing: preparing people for change,* 2nd ed. New York: Guilford Press, 2002.
31. Eysenbach GP, et al. Health related virtual communities and electronic support groups: systematic effects of the effects of online peer to peer interactions. *Br Med J* 2004;328:1166–1172.
32. Young K. Cognitive behavior therapy with Internet addicts: treatment outcomes and implications. *Cyberpsychol Behav* 2007;10(5):671–679.
33. Pettinati HM, Monterosso J, Lipkin C, et al. Patient attitudes toward treatment predict attendance in clinical pharmacotherapy trials of alcohol and drug treatment. *Am J Addict* 2003;12(4):324–335.
34. Higgins ST. Some potential contributions of reinforcement and consumer-demand theory to reducing cocaine use. *Addict Behav* 1996;21: 803–816.
35. Dell'Osso B, Hadley S, Allen A, et al. Efficacy of escalitopram in impulsive-compulsive internet usage disorder: an open-label trial followed by a double-blind discontinuation phase. *J Clin Psychiatry* 2008;69(3): 452–456.
36. Coffey TG. Beer Street: Gin Lane. Some views of 18th-century drinking. *Q J Stud Alcohol* 1966;27:669–692.
37. Bostwick JM, Bucci JA. Internet sex addiction treated with naltrexone. *Mayo Clin Proc* 2008;83(2):226–230.
38. Shapira NA, Lessig MC, Goldsmith TD, et al. Problematic internet use: proposed classification and diagnostic criteria. *Depress Anxiety* 2003; 17(4):207–216.
39. Liu CY, Kuo FY. A study of Internet addiction through the lens of the interpersonal theory. *Cyberpsychol Behav* 2007;10(6):799–804.
40. Miller MC. Questions & answers. Is "Internet addiction" a distinct mental disorder? *Harv Ment Health Lett* 2007;24(4):8.

CHAPTER 65

Antoine Douaihy, MD
Dennis C. Daley, PhD
G. Alan Marlatt, PhD
Crystal R. Spotts, MEd

Relapse Prevention: Clinical Models and Intervention Strategies

Longitudinal studies have demonstrated that the treatment of substance use disorders (SUDs) is associated with major reductions in substance use, related problems, and societal costs (1,2). Epidemiologic studies of people with lifetime substance dependence suggest that 58% eventually enter sustained recovery (i.e., no symptoms for the past year) (3). Of the people who eventually achieved a state of sustained recovery, the majority managed to do so after participating in treatment (4). Although most people with a SUD eventually abstain or manage to control their use without professional help (5), many will suffer from a long-lasting chronic condition, whereby they cycle through episodes of lapse, relapse, treatment reentry, and recovery (6). High rates of relapse have led many researchers to conceptualize addiction as a "chronic relapsing illness" (7), and understand relapse prevention (RP) as an iterative process of change rather than as a full inoculation against relapse (8). Numerous approaches and models have been suggested to explain the relapse process.

RP was originally described as an aftercare program for individuals receiving treatment for an alcohol use disorder (9), then later on used to encompass any cognitive-behavioral skills that address variables and risk factors predicting relapse, high-risk situations, and effective coping strategies to assist individuals in maintaining desired behavioral changes. RP strategies have been incorporated into individual and group treatment manuals (10–12). In addition, RP has been incorporated as a component of rehabilitation, partial hospital, and outpatient programs. Focusing on the complexity of the relapse process would help us better understand the challenges of posttreatment change process and identify RP interventions targeting the various pathways in the addiction-recovery cycle.

This chapter summarizes the major tenets of RP including the concepts of lapse, relapse, and recovery. It also provides a summary of the empirical support of RP (efficacy and effectiveness of RP), determinants of relapse, models of RP, and a review of the conceptualization of relapse as a dynamic process. We also present highlights of RP assessment and intervention strategies representing the most common principles espoused in the RP models. An overview of RP for co-occurring disorders is discussed.

LAPSE, RELAPSE, AND RECOVERY

The lack of consensus regarding the conceptualization of relapse has made it difficult to assess treatment outcomes and different estimates of relapse rates. Relapse has been described as a discrete phenomenon and as a process of behavior change (13). It has been initially used to describe in a simplistic way that the person either resumed drinking or using drugs or not resumed drinking or using drugs, or is once again involved in addictive behaviors after a period of abstinence. However, it is not as straightforward as it appears. Relapse denotes meaning that goes beyond the dichotomous outcome. Marlatt has identified a *lapse* as the initial episode of use of a substance after a period of abstinence, a *relapse* as a continued use after the initial slip, "a breakdown or set-back in the person's attempt to change or modify any target behavior," and a *prolapse* as a behavior that is consistent with getting back on track in the direction of positive behavior change (9,14,15). Multiple meanings have emerged to describe the concept of relapse and some of them include the following: daily use for a specific number of sequential days such as hazardous drinking; a consequence of substance use resulting in the need for subsequent treatment (e.g. "recidivism") (16); an "unfolding process in which the resumption of substance use is the last event in a long series of maladaptive responses to internal or external stressors or stimuli" (17); a continuous process defined by a series of transgressive behaviors (18); and a complex multidimensional composite indices of outcome that takes into account the different aspects of return to the addictive behavior, goes beyond the binary classification of abstinence-relapse, and fits better into the concept of "harm reduction" approach in some programs that have nonabstinence goals (19,20).

The definition of relapse has a significant impact on the conceptual and clinical approach to assessment. The ways in which clinicians quantify and qualify relapse determine how they will respond to patient's relapsing behaviors. If a patient is involved in a treatment program that identifies *any drinking* behavior such as one drink after a period of abstinence as a relapse, it is more probable for him or her to engage in heavier drinking behavior, which is explained by the phenomenon of the "abstinence violation effect" (self-blame and loss of perceived control that individuals often experience after the violation of self-imposed rules) (13,14). However, if the same patient's drinking behavior (one drink) receiving treatment in a program that does not convey that this behavior is a relapse, it is more probable for him or her to have an increased awareness of his or her reactions to drinking and may be less vulnerable to the abstinence violation effect. Lapse and relapse may also be defined according to the individual's goals for change. If abstinence is a goal, then a drink may be considered as a lapse; but if the individual maintains harm reduction goals, then a lapse may be defined as harmful consequence of drinking behavior.

A recent study showed that a lapse does not necessarily herald a full-blown relapse in users of tobacco (21). Milby et al. (22) compared behavioral day treatment with the same-day treatment plus abstinent-contingent housing and work in cocaine users and found that these subjects who lapsed were actually less likely to relapse, indicating that the lapse event could be perceived as a crossroads. The different rates of relapse vary between studies and across substances but "relapse is the rule" not the exception as stated by De Leon in a review of addiction treatment outcome research (23). It has become clearer to think of relapse as both a dichotomous outcome and a dynamic process involving a series of prior related events, immediate precipitants, and related consequences as predictors of relapse interfering with behavior change (24–26). The relapse process has been studied in many types of addictions (15,27–29) and it may be highly similar across the different drugs of abuse (30,31). Therefore a dynamic assessment model is necessary to gain a clearer picture of the relapse process and would potentially capture all the elements of relapse and their dynamic interactions across time and in the moment of crisis (16,29,31).

Recovery is defined as a long-term and ongoing process rather than an end point (32). The road to recovery remains anything but linear and smooth, and the outcome anything but predictable (33). Specific areas of change during the process of recovery include physical, psychologic, spiritual, behavioral, interpersonal, sociocultural, familial, and financial (25,34). Recovery tasks and areas of clinical focus are contingent on the stage or phase of recovery the individual is in (35,36). Recovery and relapse are mediated by the severity and damage caused by the SUD, the presence of comorbid psychiatric or medical illness, and the individual's coping skills, motivation, and support system. Although some individuals achieve full recovery, others only achieve partial recovery (37). The latter group is at risk for multiple relapses over time, yet still can benefit from the cumulative effects of multiple treatments. A recent study showed that stable recovery 10 years later among heroin addicts was predicted by self-efficacy and psychologic distress, emphasizing the importance of addressing those factors to enhance the odds of maintaining long-term stable recovery (38).

Recovering from SUD involves gaining information, increasing self-awareness, developing skills for sober living, and following a program of change (25). The program of change may also incorporate psychotherapy, pharmacotherapy, case management, participation in self-help groups including Twelve Step programs, and self-management approaches. As recovery progresses, patients rely more on themselves after initially using their support system, with the goal of improving their overall quality of life. Flynn et al. (39) studied a group of opiate users 5 years after treatment and compared those who were in recovery and those who were not. The subjects in recovery were more likely to benefit from family and friends as a support group and were more likely to agree that their social network did not include people with SUDs. The subjects in recovery were four times more likely to perceive themselves as improving their overall personal growth and ability to lead a fulfilling life.

TREATMENT OUTCOMES AND RELAPSE RATES

Despite advances in treatment, relapse rates are still high (40–43). Substantial research provides good evidence that treatment can be successful, but treatment is not always followed by positive treatment outcomes (44). Multiple variables including amount of drug use at treatment entry, treatment retention and completion, and frequency of participation in Twelve Step program before and throughout treatment have been found to predict treatment outcome (45). Research continues to attempt to differentiate predictors of treatment performance and outcome; for example, in the context of methamphetamine dependence (46). A recent review exploring gender differences in alcohol and substance use relapse showed that, for women, marriage and marital stress were risk factors for alcohol relapse, and, among men, marriage lowered relapse risk (47). In contrast to the lack of gender differences in alcohol relapse rates, this review showed that women appear to be less likely to experience relapse to substance use relative to men.

Even though retention and treatment dosage may predict better outcomes for a given episode of care (48), multiple episodes of care can also be a marker for individuals who have not been responsive to prior treatment and hence have a worse prognosis (45,49). Multiple episodes of care seem to be the norm (50). Treatment episodes may have a cumulative effect on the recovery process (51). Scott et al. (1) recently demonstrated the need to adopt a chronic versus acute care model for substance use that helps better identify targets of interventions designed to shorten the cycle of relapse.

Early studies and reviews of the outcome literature reported rates of relapse of more than 70% among alcohol and drug abusing patients participating in treatment (52,53). Miller and Hester (52) reviewed more than 500 alcoholism outcome studies and reported that three fourths of subjects relapse within 1 year. More recently, McLellan et al. (3) reviewed more than a hundred clinical trials of drug addiction treatments and reported that most studies showed significant reductions in substance use, improved personal heath, and reduced social pathology. In addition, they noted that in 1-year postdischarge follow-up studies, 40% to 60% of individuals discharged from treatment were continuously abstinent and 15% to 30% had not used substances addictively. Those positive outcomes are similar to those seen with other chronic medical illnesses such as diabetes type 2, hypertension, and asthma. Also as with other chronic disorders, persons with SUDs have difficulty adhering to treatment, sometimes drop out early, and may relapse on substance use. Numerous publications by National Institute on Drug Abuse and the Center for Substance Abuse Treatment and the 2000 report to Congress by National Institute on Alcohol Abuse and Alcoholism describe positive outcomes for substance abusers who have received treatment including reduced rates of substance use, reduced medical costs, reduced rates of criminal behaviors, improved psychological functioning, improved employment rates, improved family productivity, and reduced suicidal thoughts and behaviors (32,55–58). Patients who remain in treatment the longest generally have the best outcomes (54,59).

EFFECTIVENESS AND EFFICACY OF RP

Several studies have evaluated the effectiveness and efficacy of RP approaches for SUDs. Chaney et al. (60) provided the first randomized trial of RP techniques in an inpatient population of problem drinkers. The authors concluded that "problem drinkers' responses to situations that present a high risk of relapse could be improved through training." Carroll (61) reviewed randomized controlled trials on the effectiveness of RP among smokers (12 studies), alcohol abusers (6 studies), cocaine abusers (3 studies), opiate addicts (1 study), and other drug abusers (2 studies), using the RP strategies that explicitly cited the work of Marlatt (9). The review examined the relative effectiveness of RP compared with no-treatment controls, attention controls, and an active treatment (interpersonal therapy, supportive therapy). Carroll concluded that there was evidence for the effectiveness of RP compared with no-treatment controls, particularly in the area of smoking cessation. Carroll found less consistent evidence of effectiveness when RP was compared with discussion control groups or to another active treatment. Results from the analysis also indicate that RP may be particularly promising in reducing the severity of relapses when they occur, in enhancing durability of treatment effects, and for patients who demonstrate higher levels of impairment across multiple dimensions (psychopathology and dependence severity). Although RP does not provide full inoculation against relapse, it significantly reduces the negative consequences and damage resulting from a return to substance use. Several studies showed sustained main effects for RP, suggesting that RP may provide continued improvement over a longer period (indicating a "delayed emergence effect" or "sleeper effect"), whereas other treatments' effects may only be short-lived (62–64). These findings of delayed effects of RP suggest a lapse-relapse learning curve, in which there is a higher likelihood of lapse immediately after treatment, but learning new coping skills leads to a decreased probability of relapse over time. Polivy and Herman (65) emphasized the problem of learning new behaviors, and demonstrated that 90% of individuals who attempt to change their behavior struggle with lapses and do not achieve change on their first attempt.

Two large studies comparing the effectiveness of cognitive behavioral substance abuse treatments to other active treatments that emphasize participation in the Twelve Step fellowship have demonstrated no difference between conditions at follow-up. The first study is Project MATCH, a multisite study sponsored by the National Institute on Alcohol Abuse and Alcoholism that compared three different treatments for 1,726 patients diagnosed as alcohol abusers or alcohol dependent (66). Patients were randomly assigned to Cognitive Behavioral Coping Skills Therapy (CBT), Motivational Enhancement Therapy (MET), and Twelve Step Facilitation Therapy (TSF), all of which were delivered over a 12-week period. Patients in all three conditions demonstrated significant improvements from pretreatment through the 1-year posttreatment follow-up. Surprisingly, no statistically significant differences were found in outcome by type of treatment and no matching hypotheses were confirmed. The only significant difference between groups was found in one of nine settings: patients with low psychiatric severity reported more abstinent days after the Twelve Step Facilitation Therapy. Several limitations of this study include the use of a fairly homogenous, high-functioning pool of study participants, participant sample comprised more than 75% males, and not including a control condition to account for usual threats to internal validity. The second large study involved 3,018 substance-abusing patients receiving services at 15 Veteran Affairs Medical Centers across the country (67). Conducted in a naturalistic setting, participants were not randomly assigned to group conditions. Similar to the Project MATCH results, patients in all three conditions (TSF, CBT, or a combination of both) performed equally well at 1-year follow-up. The study used an all-male sample. The study extends MATCH results by illustrating that comparative treatment effectiveness between Twelve Step and CBT holds across illicit substances in addition to alcohol.

There have been two recent meta-analyses of RP. Irvin et al. (68) evaluated the efficacy of Marlatt-based RP across SUDs in a meta-analytic review based on 26 studies representing a sample of 9,504 participants. The authors found a significant overall effect size for reduction in substance use and a much larger effect for improving psychosocial adjustment. Treatment effects were strongest for alcohol and polysubstance use, and weaker for smoking, but all three were significant. The results indicate that certain characteristics of alcohol use are particularly amenable to RP model. The analysis showed that individual, group, and marital modalities were equally effective.

Randomized trials of RP for smoking showed that additional supportive elements such as stress management, emotion regulation techniques, and abstinence "resource renewal" might be needed in addition to RP in a smoking intervention (27,69). Research should focus more on improving and modifying RP techniques in the context of other substances such as cocaine, and opioids. The most recent meta-analysis focused solely on smoking (70) and included 42 studies of controlled trials with at least 6 months of follow-up, most of which used skills training approaches. Although odd ratios were generally positive, they were small and no significant effects were found for behavioral interventions. These findings are in contrast with the strong meta-analytic evidence for the efficacy of interventions consistent with RP for smoking cessation reported in the U.S. Public Health Service's Clinical Practice Guideline (71). These disparate findings may be the result of the analysis using more conservative strategy in evaluating outcomes and most interventions were low intensity and the included studies were not limited to Marlatt-based interventions.

Self-help RP interventions have been most commonly used in the area of smoking cessation. Brandon et al. (72,73) conducted two randomized, controlled trials of self-help relapse prevention intervention for ex-smokers who had quit on their own before study enrollment. The first study found that eight RP booklets (based on the principles of Marlatt) mailed to self-quit ex-smokers over the course of 1 year reduced relapse by two thirds among recent quitters. The follow-up study indicated that efficacy was due to the content of the booklets rather than to the frequency of contact made with participants via the repeated mailings and the intervention was cost-effective relative to other public health interventions.

Recent randomized controlled trials support the reported efficacy of combined CBT-like therapies and naltrexone for alcohol-dependent individuals (74). The Effect of Combined Pharmacotherapies and Behavioral Interventions study suggested that medical management of an alcohol-dependent patient with a physician providing treatment with naltrexone and basic advice and information is as effective as CBT. The trial enrolled 1,383 alcohol-dependent subjects and randomly assigned them to one of eight groups that include naltrexone, acamprosate, or both of the drugs, with or without what was identified as a cognitive-behavioral intervention (CBI). One group received the CBI alone, without placebo. The patients who received a medication received medical management that was fairly rigorous (nine appointments over 16 weeks), during which a physician or a nurse discussed the patient's diagnosis and progress and suggested attendance to Alcoholics Anonymous (AA). Those who got the CBI received up to 20 sessions, which was comparable with a streamlined version of outpatient alcoholism treatment. Subjects receiving medical management with naltrexone, or CBI, or both, fared better on drinking outcomes, whereas acamprosate showed no evidence of efficacy, with or without CBI. Describing it more from a clinical perspective, the percentage of subjects with a good clinical outcome were 58% for those who received only medical management and placebo, 74% for those who received medical management with naltrexone only, 74% for those who received medical management with naltrexone and CBI, and 71% for those who received medical management with placebo and CBI. The subjects were also followed for a year after the 16-week treatment, and although the patterns of efficacy remained much the same, there was appreciable falloff for all groups (75–77).

Maude-Griffin et al. (78) randomized 128 cocaine users to either CBT or TSF to test several *a priori* matching hypotheses. Treatment was delivered in both group and individual sessions. Results suggested that CBT was more effective than TSF overall. CBT was differentially effective for individuals with depression, whereas TSF was more effective for participants with low levels of abstract reasoning skills. In a recently completed trial (79), 121 cocaine-dependent individuals were randomized to one of four conditions in a 2 × 2 factorial design: disulfiram (250 mg daily) + CBT, disulfiram + interpersonal therapy (IPT), which did not include any RP components, placebo + CBT, and placebo + IPT. This study showed that patients assigned to CBT reduced their cocaine use significantly more than those assigned to IPT and patients assigned to disulfiram reduced their cocaine use significantly more than those assigned to placebo. Effects of CBT + placebo were comparable to those of the CBT-disulfiram combination. Although retention was a significant predictor of better drug use outcomes, the CBT × time effect remained statistically significant after controlling for retention.

The literature evaluating the efficacy and effectiveness of RP with stimulant users has been nearly all conducted with cocaine users. Some data support the view that the response to RP treatment is quite comparable between cocaine-dependent individuals and those dependent on methamphetamine (80). Rawson et al. (81) conducted a multisite study with methamphetamine-dependent individuals in an attempt to assess the effectiveness of the Matrix treatment protocol (9,64,81) versus "treatment as usual" in eight community treatment organizations. A total of 978 methamphetamine-dependent individuals were randomly assigned to outpatient treatment with either the Matrix 16-week protocol, or to the treatment approach that was routinely used by the eight treatment organizations. The study provided support for the superior treatment response of methamphetamine users treated with the Matrix approach. These gains were not significantly different at posttreatment follow-up (i.e., not sustained). Clearly, the Matrix treatment approach has positive empirical evidence for treating methamphetamine-dependent individuals when compared to a group of community treatment protocols.

Rawson et al. (64) recently compared group CBT, voucher contingency management (CM), and a CBT/CM in combination with standard methadone maintenance treatment for cocaine-using methadone maintenance patients. During the acute phase of treatment, the CM group had significantly better cocaine use outcomes. However, during the follow-up period, a CBT sleeper effect emerged again, where the CBT group had better outcomes at the 26-week and 52-week follow-up than the CM group. Another study in the context of intensive methadone maintenance showed best 1-year outcomes for the CBT and CM combination (83). No difference has been found in group versus individually delivered CBT/RP (84,85).

The empirical evidence on testing RP strategies (12 studies) for cannabis dependence has also sometimes added other treatment components such as aversion training, MET, contingency reinforcement, and case management. A multisite study involving 450 marijuana-dependent individuals demonstrated that a nine-session individual approach that integrated CBT and Motivational Interviewing (MI) was more effective than a two-session MI approach, which in turn was more effective than a delayed-treatment control (86). The relatively modest long-term outcomes reported in the trials conducted thus far suggest that intervention protocols need to be developed to effectively meet the needs of this population. There are no efficacy studies evaluating RP specifically for abuse of club drugs, hallucinogens, inhalants, and steroids (87).

Several studies included spouses in the RP intervention (88,89). A recent study evaluated conjoint treatments in 90 men with alcohol problems and their female partners. The subjects were randomly assigned to one of the three outpatient conjoint treatments: alcohol behavioral couples therapy (ABCT); ABCT with RP techniques (RP/ABCT) (9); or ABCT with interventions encouraging AA involvement (AA/ABCT). Couples were followed 18 months after treatment. Across the three treatment approaches, drinkers who provided follow-up data maintained abstinence on almost 80% of days during follow-up, with no difference in drinking or marital happiness outcomes between groups. In the RP/ABCT treatment, attendance at posttreatment booster sessions was related to posttreatment abstinence. AA attendance was positively related to abstinence during follow-up treatment in both concurrent and time-lagged analyses (90). Despite strong evidence for efficacy of psychosocial treatments for alcohol use disorders, aggregate rates of continuous abstinence are well below 50% and relapses are more common than abstinence, indicating the need for more efforts to develop efficacious treatments (91).

Despite several limitations to studies on RP, the literature generally favors the efficacy and effectiveness of RP and shows that RP strategies especially as a component of a multimodal treatment approach enhance the recovery of individuals with SUDs.

RELAPSE REPLICATION AND EXTENSION PROJECT

In a series of studies led by the National Institute on Alcohol Abuse and Alcoholism called the Relapse Replication Extension Project (RREP), aspects of RP including Marlatt's taxonomy for relapse determinants were explored. The RREP focused on the identification of high-risk situations and several studies in it showed that the taxonomy had minimal ability to predict drinking outcomes (92,93). The data in the RREP raise significant methodologic problems concerning the predictive validity of Marlatt's (94) relapse taxonomy and coding system (93,95). On the basis of the findings, a major reconceptualization of the relapse taxonomy was recommended (96). Longabaugh et al. (95) suggested a revision of the taxonomy categories to include greater distinction between inter- and intrapersonal determinants of relapse. An expanded model of Marlatt's relapse precipitant taxonomy has been recommended (97). Many of the RREP findings are in fact quite supportive of the original RP model (15). In response to the criticisms provided in the RREP, a new reconceptualization of cognitive behavioral model of relapse that focuses on the dynamic interactions between multiple risk factors and situational determinants was proposed and will be discussed later (31).

DETERMINANTS OF RELAPSE

Marlatt et al. (15) developed a taxonomy of high-risk situations that included three hierarchically arranged levels of categories used in the classification of relapse episodes. The first level distinguishes between the intrapersonal and interpersonal precipitants of relapse. The second level consists of eight subdivisions including five within the intrapersonal category and three within the interpersonal category. The third level of the taxonomy provides a more detailed inspection of five of the eight level two subdivisions. This classification scheme has been found useful in other countries (98,99) and is supported by prospective studies (100,101). It also has been used as the basis of research protocols (102), treatment protocols (103), and patient recovery guides (104,105). In this section, we review the most commonly identified relapse determinants based on Marlatt's relapse taxonomy.

Intrapersonal Determinants Self-efficacy refers to individuals' beliefs in their capabilities to organize and carry out specific courses of action to attain some goal or situation-specific task (106). These beliefs have great influence on self-regulation and the quality of human functioning, because they shape the goals individuals set for themselves, the persistence in reaching those goals, and the effectiveness of problem-solving activities (107). Individuals' sense of efficacy is the result of their cognitive processing from many sources of efficacy information (107). This construct is intimately related to the individual's coping abilities and reflects the degree of confidence that the individual has about being confronted with a high-risk situation and successfully avoiding a lapse. The patient's personal belief in his or her ability to control his or her substance use is a reliable predictor of lapses immediately after treatment (21,108) and over long-term outcomes (109). In general, self-efficacy is a predictor of outcomes across all types of addictions, including gambling, smoking, and drug use (110). Low levels of self-efficacy are predictive of relapse (111). Shiffman et al. (112) found that baseline self-efficacy was as predictive of the first smoking lapse as they were daily self-efficacy measurements, explaining the stability of self-efficacy during abstinence. More evidence from a daily monitoring study showed decreases in self-efficacy preceded a first lapse on the following day and daily variation in self-efficacy predicted transitions from lapse to heavier use (21). Given the relationship between self-efficacy and relapse, self-efficacy should be thoroughly assessed during treatment and appropriately targeted for interventions.

Outcome Expectancies A factor enhancing the likelihood of relapse is the set of cognitive expectancies that individuals develop about the expected outcomes associated with addictive behaviors. Such expectancies are known as outcome expectancies (113). Underlying motives for engaging in addictive behaviors include both a desire to change one's mood and to increase sociability (114). Individuals who developed an addiction typically have developed a set of expectancies that anticipate positive outcomes from engaging in the behavior, serving as a source of motivation to engage in it. Such outcome expectancies are shaped by an individual's past direct and indirect experience with the behaviors related to the addiction, including vicarious learning through the modeling they see early on displayed by parents and later by peers (115). Jones et al. (116) reported that although expectancies are strongly related to outcome, there is little evidence that targeting expectancies in treatment leads to changes in posttreatment consumption. There is a possibility that expectancies influence outcome via their relationship with other relapse predictors. In fact, outcome expectancies may be influencing substance use behavior via the relationship between negative emotional states and beliefs about substances relieving negative affect, particularly among treatment seeking individuals (117,118). Individuals endorsing positive outcome expectancies at the beginning of treatment may benefit from an intervention challenging their expectancies (119).

Craving Although craving has been implicated in general in the relapse process, its role in alcohol relapse remains controversial, because studies examining the relationship of craving to relapse yielded equivocal results (120). Multiple and often conflicting theories, definitions, and measurements have plagued the study of craving. Craving has been described as a cognitive experience focused on the desire to use a substance and is often highly related to expectancies for the desired effect of the substance, whereas an urge has been defined as the behavioral intention or impulse to use a substance. One common finding is that craving is a poor predictor of relapse (121). Drummond et al. (122) proposed that the subjective experience of craving may not directly predict substance use, but relapse may be predicted from the correlates and underlying mechanisms of craving. A recent study assessing the usefulness of craving as a predictor of relapse in 218 adult, alcohol-dependent patients admitted to two separate residential addiction treatment programs showed that days craving reported in the week before discharge predicted alcohol use at 3-month follow-up. Admission spirituality, alcohol-refusal self-efficacy, and depression levels differentiated cravers from noncravers. Patients who crave alcohol in residential treatment may be at higher relapse risk and identified by intake assessments of self-efficacy, depression, and spirituality (123). Another study demonstrated that stress-induced cocaine craving is predictive of cocaine relapse outcomes (124). Mindfulness and meditation may provide a useful antidote to the experience of craving (125,126). The heightened state of present-focused awareness that is encouraged by meditation may directly counteract the conditioned automatic response to use alcohol in response to cravings and urges. In addition, the use of anticraving medications, which is described later, can pharmacologically reduce the experience of craving.

Motivation An important element in determining the likelihood of relapse is the individual's commitment to or motivation for self-improvement (127). The motivation may relate to the relapse process in two distinct ways: the motivation for positive behavior change and the motivation to engage in the problematic behavior. Motivation is judged with regard to a particular action or outcome. The transtheoretical stages of change: precontemplation, contemplation, preparation, action, and maintenance, are measured in relation to a specific behavior or goal (128). Precontemplation represents the lowest level of readiness to change. A person's level of motivation (e.g., desire, self-efficacy, readiness, problem recognition) is action-specific. A person might be quite motivated for change but not for treatment. Polysubstance users commonly show levels of motivation that are different depending on the drug. The most common motivational obstacle to early help seeking is ambivalence. The ambivalence toward change is highly related to self-efficacy and outcome expectancies. Baer et al. (8) indicated that an analysis of relapse needs to examine the interaction between commitment and coping skills. Even well developed coping abilities will not prevent relapse if the individual's commitment to stay clean is low; conversely, strong commitment may be insufficient in the absence of adequate coping skills. Interventions that focus on addressing ambivalence (decisional balance) may increase intrinsic motivation by allowing patients to explore their own values and how they differ from their actual behavioral choices. MI is a person-centered–goal-oriented approach for facilitating change through exploring and resolving ambivalence (129). MI has demonstrated efficacy for reducing alcohol consumption and frequency of drinking in this population. Rohsenow et al. (130) evaluated the effectiveness of MET and group coping skills in cocaine abusers and showed that the motivational intervention had better substance use outcomes with individuals having a low level of initial motivation to change when compared with those with higher levels of initial motivation. Thus it is important to assess commitment and motivation to change and understand that motivation for change is comprised of multiple dimensions that are at best modestly intercorrelated. Interventions designed to enhance commitment to change should be a component of any RP approach.

Coping Based on the cognitive-behavioral model of relapse, the most critical predictor of relapse is the individual's ability to utilize adequate coping strategies in dealing with high-risk situations. The assessment of coping in general (131) and more specifically in relation to relapse is very challenging (132,133). A number of different dimensions of coping need to be considered in the assessment process (16). Coping has been shown to be a critical predictor of substance use treatment outcomes and is often the strongest predictor of behavioral lapses in the moment (134–136). Moos and Holahan (131) highlighted the distinction between approach and avoidance coping. Approach coping may involve attempts to accept, confront, and reframe, as a means of coping, whereas avoidance coping may include distraction from cues or engaging in other activities. Chung et al. (137) predicted 12-month treatment outcomes in alcoholic patients by focusing on the distinction between the behavioral and cognitive components of approach and avoidance coping. Results suggested that avoidance coping, particularly cognitive avoidance coping, was predictive of fewer alcohol (alcohol problem severity and alcohol dependence symptoms), interpersonal, and psychologic problems at the 12-month follow-up. Behavioral approach coping also predicted decreased alcohol problem severity at 12-month follow-up. Coping appears to be a dynamic process (31). The dynamic interaction between coping, self-efficacy, and motivation explains alcohol treatment outcomes (138,139). Coping may be also experienced as inaction. Inaction has been understood as the acceptance of substance cues (140), which can be described as "letting go" and not acting on an urge. This view is consistent with the Buddhist notion of skillful means (140). The focus is not about "doing what is right," but rather the goal is "just do." An example of that coping strategy is the use of "urge surfing" (141). In this strategy, the patient is first taught to label internal sensations and cognitive preoccupation as an urge and to foster an attitude of detachment from the urge. The focus is on identifying and accepting the urge, not attempting to fight it. In a recent study on the effectiveness of a mindfulness meditation technique of the Vipassana tradition in reducing substance use in an incarcerated population, participants reported that accepting the "here and now," "staying in the moment," and being mindful of the urges were helpful coping strategies (142).

Emotional States Earlier studies and several other studies have reported a strong link between negative affect and relapse to substance use (143,144). Baker et al. (145) identified negative affect as the primary motive for drug use. Excessive substance use is motivated by affective regulation both positive and negative. Furthermore, substance use is often reinforcing for patients, leading the individual to engage in future substance use. Oftentimes, substance use provides negative reinforcement via the amelioration of an unpleasant affective state, such as physical withdrawal symptoms (145). Thus clinicians should incorporate strategies to decrease and manage negative emotional states as a part of the RP approach.

Interpersonal Determinants Stanton (146) reviewed the research on the role of social support in lapses and provided an overview of interpersonal dynamics as a high-risk situation for relapse. However, the relationship between interpersonal factors and relapse is not well understood (90,147). Functional social support or the level of emotional support is highly predictive of long-term abstinence across several addictions (148–150). The social support network size, the perceived quality of social support, and the level of support from nonsubstance users have also been shown to predict relapse (149,150). Negative social support in the form of interpersonal conflict and social pressure to use substances has been related to an increased risk of relapse (151). Behavioral marital therapy, which incorporates partner support in treatment goals, has been described as one of the top three empirically supported treatment methods for alcohol problems (152,153).

MODELS OF RP

As discussed previously, most of the RP interventions have a multicomponent character. Treatment studies such as MET, CM, individual and group counseling approaches, and case management typically have included RP modules (10,11). Psychopharmacologic interventions combined with RP are evaluated as a part of an overall treatment strategy to reduce relapse risk and improve abstinence rates (74). Various models of RP are described in the literature, and many of these have been adapted for use in clinical trials (for summaries of various RP models, see references 15 and 104). RP models include the following:

- Marlatt and Gordon's cognitive-behavioral approach (11,154).
- Annis's cognitive-behavioral approach (155), which incorporates concepts of Marlatt's model with Bandura's self-efficacy theory.
- Daley's psychoeducational approach (24), which adapted Marlatt's classification of relapse precipitants to a treatment protocol that can be used in individual or group sessions.
- Gorski's neurologic impairment model, which incorporates elements from the disease model of addiction and relapse, as well as Marlatt's model (154).
- Zackon, McAuliffe, and Chien's recovery training and self-help model (156).
- The Matrix neurobehavioral model of treatment of Rawson et al., which includes RP as a central component of treatment (82,158,159).
- Washton's intensive outpatient model (35,36), which includes significant attention to RP during the third phase of treatment.

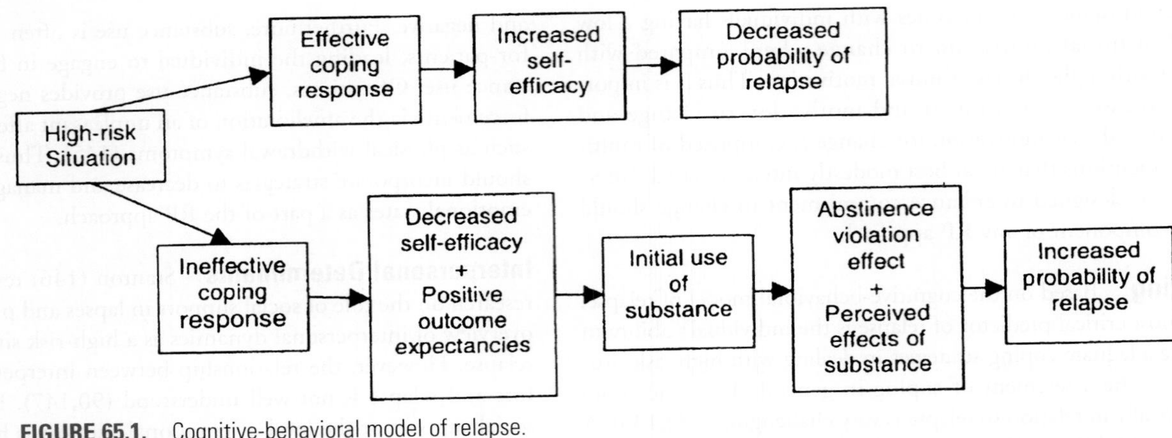

FIGURE 65.1. Cognitive-behavioral model of relapse.

- The coping/social skills training model of Monti et al. (160).
- The Cue Extinction (CE) model developed by Childress et al. (17).

The Cognitive-Behavioral Model of Relapse

Drawing from the taxonomy of high-risk situations, Marlatt proposed the first cognitive-behavioral model of the relapse process (9). Shown in Figure 65.1, the model centers on the individual's response to high-risk situation. The components include the interaction between the person (affect, coping, self-efficacy, outcome expectancies) and environmental risk factors such as social influences, cue exposure, and access to substance. If the individual lacks an adequate coping response or confidence to deal with the situation (low self-efficacy), the tendency is "to give in to temptation." The "decision" to use or not is then mediated by the individual's outcome expectancies for the initial effects of using the substance. The combination of being unable to cope effectively in a high-risk situation and positive outcome expectancies greatly increases the probability that an initial lapse will occur. Whether the first lapse is followed by a full-blown relapse depends in part on the person's attributions as to the cause of relapse and the reactions associated with its occurrence. Individuals who decide to use the substance may be vulnerable to the abstinence violation effect. Persons who experience intense abstinence violation effect such as conflict and self-blame after a lapse go through a motivation crisis (demoralization) that undermine their commitment to abstinence goals. The lapse is more likely to lead to a relapse if the person views it as an irreparable failure. The individual's restorative coping abilities to deal with the negative consequences and emotions, the reaction of friends and family, and the individual's commitment to return to abstinence or moderation/harm reduction should be considered.

The Cognitive-Behavioral Model of Relapse, Revised

Based on previous descriptions of relapse as complex process, Witkiewitz and Marlatt (31) proposed a dynamic model of the relapse process. This model incorporates the temporal dynamic relationships between cognitive (self-efficacy, outcome expectancies, motivation, craving, abstinence violation effect), behavioral (coping strategies), affective (emotional states), and physical (withdrawal) processes, leading up to, and during, a high-risk situation. In every situation, an individual is faced with the challenge of balancing multiple cues and possible consequences. According to the model, the interrelationship between these processes is contextual, but the driving force behind the processes may be traced back to an individual's vulnerability to relapse. As shown in Figure 65.2, this model allows for several configurations of distal and proximal relapse risks. Distal risks (solid lines) are defined as stable predispositions that increase an individual's vulnerability to lapse (years of dependence, family history, social support, and comorbid psychopathology), whereas proximal risks (dotted lines) are immediate precipitants that actualize the statistical probability of a lapse. Connected boxes are hypothesized to be related through reciprocal causation (e.g., coping skills influence drinking behavior, and in turn, drinking influences coping) (161). These feedback loops (indicated by double-headed arrows) allow for the bidirectional interaction between cognitions and lapse, as well as affect and lapse. Coping is shown as directly interrelated with lapse. The difference between a feedback loop and interrelatedness in the model is primarily a consideration of the distinction between the tonic and the phasic processes. The large stripped circle in Figure 65.2 indicates the role of contextual factors, with situational cues (e.g., walking by the liquor store) moderating the relationship between risk factors and substance use behavior (138). The source of support for the model comes from clinical anecdotes and recent empirical studies on the complexity of substance use behavior (31,162–167). Recognizing the complexity of the relapse process may help clinicians see the importance of a comprehensive assessment of domains related to relapse (16). The consideration of how the factors in the domains may interact within a high-risk situation and how changes in proximal risk factors can alter behavior leading up to high-risk situations will enable patients to continually assess their own relapse vulnerability.

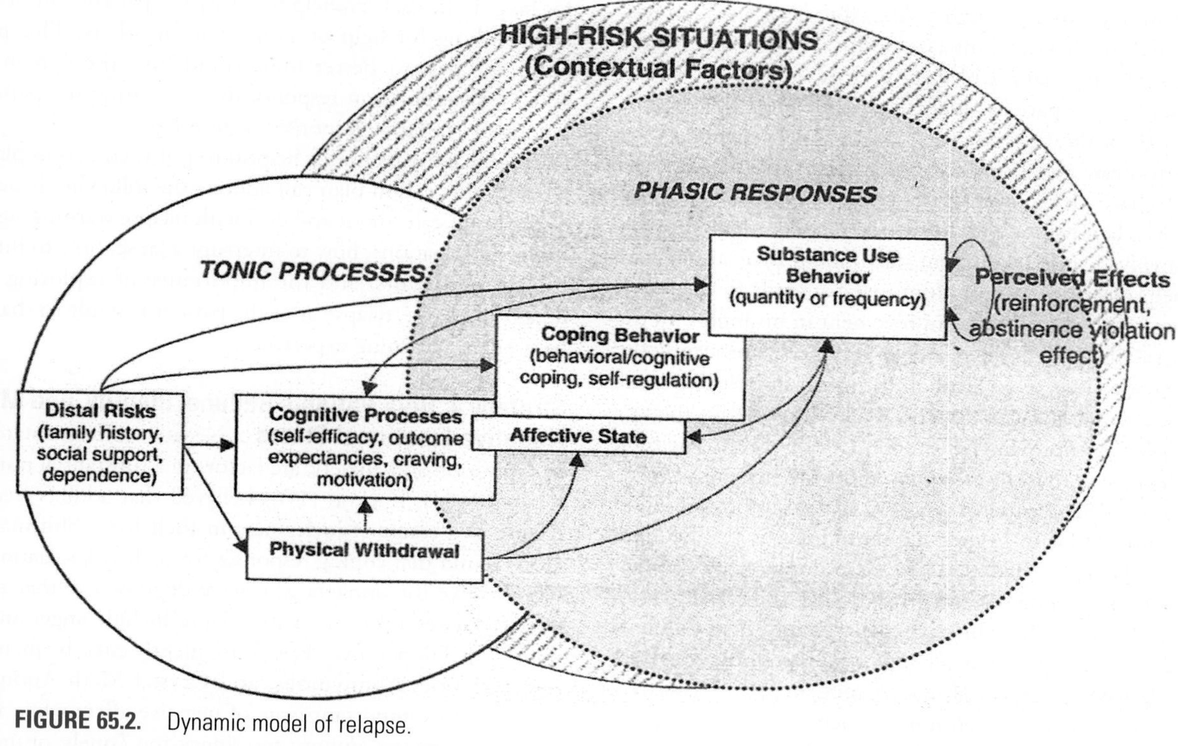

FIGURE 65.2. Dynamic model of relapse.

Clinical RP Interventions to Reduce Lapse and Relapse Risk This section describes practical RP clinical interventions that reflect the models of RP discussed earlier and approaches of numerous clinicians and researchers who have developed specific models of RP or written patient-oriented RP recovery materials. The literature emphasizes individualizing RP strategies, taking into account the patient's level of motivation, severity of substance use, ego functioning, and sociocultural environment. These RP interventions can be provided in individual or group sessions (many RP programs were designed for small groups of participants) (17,36,168,169).

The use of experiential learning or action techniques such as role playing or behavioral rehearsal, metaphors, monodramas, psychodrama, bibliotherapy, use of workbooks, a daily inventory, interactive videos, and homework assignments makes learning an active experience for the patient. Such techniques enhance self-awareness, decrease defensiveness, and encourage behavioral change (7,17,37,104,105,156).

Strategy 1: Help Patients Understand Relapse as a Process and Event, and Learn to Identify Warning Signs The understanding of addiction as a chronic cyclical condition often involving many transitions between lapse, relapse, and recovery helps the patient look at relapse as a process occurring in certain context and understand that early warning signs often precede an actual lapse. Attitudinal, emotional, cognitive, and behavioral changes seem to occur days, weeks, and even longer before resuming the use of substances (24). Warning signs can be conceptualized as links in a relapse chain (25,34). Reviewing with the patient the relapse history, relapse calendar (use of daily inventory that helps identify risk factors, relapse warning signs, or significant life events that could lead to a relapse) is essential. Patients in treatment for the first time can benefit from reviewing common relapse warning signs identified by others in recovery. The clinician can ask the patient to review the relapse experience in detail to learn the connections between thoughts, feelings, events, or situations and relapse to substance use. A survey ($n = 511$) of an RP model developed by one of the authors, as well as a workbook used in conjunction with that program, found that "Understanding the Relapse Process" was the topic rated most useful by patients participating in a residential addiction treatment program (170).

Strategy 2: Help Patients Identify their High-Risk Situations and Develop Effective Cognitive and Behavioral Coping The need to recognize and manage high-risk factors is an essential component of RP. High-risk factors involve intrapersonal and interpersonal situations in which the patient feels vulnerable to substance use (9,171). Relapse is more likely to occur as the result of lack of coping skills than the high-risk situation itself, so the clinician should assess the patient's coping style to identify targets for an intervention (100,172). A person heading for a relapse usually makes a number of mini-decisions over time, each of which brings the person closer to creating a high-risk situation or giving in. These choices are called "apparently irrelevant decisions" and they need to be identified and addressed with patients to decrease lapse risk.

The meaning of specific high-risk factors also varies among patients. RP strategies and interventions therefore need to take into account the nuances of each patient's high-risk factors. For example, two patients identified depression as a serious relapse risk. In the first case, depression was described as the rather common and normal feeling experienced when the patient realized that his drug addiction caused serious problems in his relationships with his wife and children. Getting his family involved in his treatment, facilitating their attendance at self-help meetings, helping him make amends to them and spend time with them led to improvement in his mood. In the second case, the patient's depression worsened significantly the longer she was sober from alcohol. Although she felt that some of the behavioral and cognitive strategies explored in therapy were helpful in improving her mood, it was not until she took an antidepressant that she experienced the full benefits of treatment. Both of these patients reported that an improved mood was a significant factor in their ability to prevent a subsequent relapse to addiction. Marlatt (173), for example, suggested that in addition to teaching patients "specific" RP skills to deal with high-risk factors, the clinician also should use "global" approaches such as problem-solving or skills-training strategies (such as behavioral rehearsal, covert modeling, and assertiveness training), cognitive reframing (such as coping imagery, reframing reactions to lapse/relapse), and lifestyle interventions (such as meditation, exercise, and relaxation).

Strategy 3: Help Patients Enhance Their Communication Skills, Interpersonal Relationships, and Develop a Recovery Social Network McCrady (174) has modified Marlatt's cognitive-behavioral model of RP and applied it to couples in recovery. Daley (170) emphasized the need to involve family or significant others in developing RP plans or intervening in the process of a lapse or relapse. Positive family and social supports generally enhance recovery for the substance-dependent member. Families are more likely to support the recovery of the addicted member if they are engaged in treatment and have an opportunity to ask questions, share their concerns and experiences, learn practical coping strategies, and learn behaviors to avoid (175). This opportunity is more likely to occur if the member with the SUD understands the effect of an addictive disorder on the family and makes amends for some of its adverse effects. Patients can be encouraged to become involved in self-help support groups. Sponsors, other recovering members of self-help groups, personal friends, and employers can become part of an individual's RP network. Following are some suggested steps for helping patients develop a RP network. First, the patient needs to identify whom to include in or exclude from this network. Others who abuse substances, harbor strong negative feelings toward the recovering person, or who generally are not supportive of recovery usually should be excluded. The patient then can determine how and when to ask for support or help. Behavioral rehearsal can help the patient practice ways to make specific requests for support. Rehearsal also helps to increase confidence and clarify thoughts and feelings about reaching out for help. Rehearsal can help to clarify the patient's ambivalence about asking for help or support from others. This process helps the patient better understand how the person being asked for support can respond, thus preparing the patient for potentially negative responses from others.

Some patients find it helpful to put their action plan into writing. The action plan can address the following issues: how to communicate about and deal with relapse warning signs and high-risk situations, how to interrupt a lapse, how to intervene if a relapse occurs, and the importance of exploring all the details of a lapse/relapse after the patient is stable so that it can be used as a learning experience.

Strategy 4: Help Patients Reduce, Identify, and Manage Negative Emotional States Negative affective states, such as depression and anxiety, are factors in a substantial number of relapses (101). Zackon (176) believed that addicts frequently relapse as a result of joylessness in their lives. Shiffman et al. (133) found that coping responses for high-risk situations were less effective for smokers who were depressed. Other negative affective states associated with relapse include anger and boredom (34). The acronym HALT, frequently cited by members of AA, Narcotics Anonymous, and Crystal Meth Anonymous, speaks to this important issue of negative affect when it warns not to become too *H*ungry, too *A*ngry, too *L*onely, or too *T*ired. Interventions that help patients develop appropriate coping skills for managing negative emotional states depend on the issues and needs of the individual.

Strategy 5: Help Patients Identify and Manage Cravings and Cues that Precede Cravings A strong desire or craving for a substance can be triggered by exposure to environmental or internal cues associated with prior use. Cues such as the sight or smell of the substance can trigger cravings that are evidenced in increased thoughts of using and physiologic changes (for example, anxiety). The concept of craving is not clearly defined across autonomic, behavioral, or subjective domains. Further, trials looking at craving and relapse may be measuring different aspects of the phenomenon (122). What is clear is that craving has clinical meaning. CE treatment (17) is one method used to help patients identify drug use triggers and master or learn to control the conditioned response to those triggers. This treatment differs from the traditional focus on "avoiding people, places, and things" and instead involves exposing the patient to specific cues associated with substance use. CE aims to enhance behavioral and cognitive coping skills as well as the patient's confidence in his or her ability to resist the desire to use. Systematic relaxation, behavioral alternatives, visual imagery, and cognitive interventions are used in CE. Several studies have validated CE (177,178). The clinician can provide information about cues and how they trigger cravings for alcohol or other drugs. Monitoring and recording cravings, associated thoughts, and outcomes in a daily log or journal can help patients become more vigilant and prepare them to cope when they occur. Cognitive interventions include changing thoughts about the craving or desire to use, challenging euphoric recall, talking oneself through the craving, thinking beyond the high by identifying negative consequences of using (immediate and delayed) and positive benefits of not using, using Twelve Step recovery slogans, and delaying the decision to use. Behavioral interventions include avoiding, leaving, or changing situations that trigger or worsen a craving; redirecting activities or becoming involved in pleasant activities; obtaining help or support from others by admitting and talking about cravings and hearing how others have survived them; attending self-help support group meetings; or taking medications that reduce craving and increase confidence in the ability to cope.

A new cognitive-behavioral treatment program for the treatment of addiction, Mindfulness-Based Relapse Prevention is in the process of being developed. The overall goal of Mindfulness-Based Relapse Prevention is to develop awareness and nonjudgmental acceptance of thoughts, sensations, and emotional states, through the practice of mindfulness meditation, and to practice these skills as a coping strategy in the face of high-risk trigger situations for relapse (126). One example of how mindfulness meditation can be helpful in preventing relapse is known as "urge surfing" (140). The patient is instructed to "detach" from his or her craving by externalizing and labeling it. Similar to a surfer who must learn to ride the waves so as not to get wiped out, the addicted patient imagines" riding the crest" of an urge or craving, maintaining balance until the crest has finally broken and the wave of feeling subsides. The process of incorporating a mindfulness practice and learning to accept and tolerate urges fits well within RP therapy.

Strategy 6: Help Patients Identify and Challenge Cognitive Distortions Marlatt (172) observed, "the patient's cognitive errors and distortions may increase the probability that an initial slip will develop into a total relapse." Twelve Step programs refer to these patterns as "stinking thinking" and suggest that recovering persons need to alter their thinking if they are to remain alcohol and drug-free. Teaching patients to identify their negative thinking patterns or cognitive errors (for example, black-and-white thinking, overgeneralizing, catastrophizing, jumping to conclusions, and so forth) and to evaluate how these affect recovery and relapse is one strategy. Patients then can be taught to use counter-thoughts to challenge their thinking errors or specific negative thoughts. One way to achieve this is to have the patient discuss or write down specific relapse-related thoughts (for example, "relapse can't happen to me," "I'll never use alcohol or drugs again," "I can control my use of alcohol or other drugs," "a few drinks, tokes, pills, lines won't hurt," "recovery isn't happening fast enough," "I need alcohol or other drugs to have fun," and "my problem is cured"); what is wrong with such thinking in terms of potential effect on relapse; and new self-statements or thoughts that counteract negative thinking (34). Many of the Twelve Step slogans were devised to help alcoholics and drug addicts alter their thinking and survive desires to use substances. Slogans such as "this too will pass," "let go and let God," and "one day at a time" have helped many patients manage thoughts of using.

Strategy 7: Help Patients Work Toward a More Balanced Lifestyle In addition to identifying and managing intrapersonal and interpersonal high-risk relapse factors, patients can benefit from global changes to restore or achieve balance in their lives (172). Development of a healthy lifestyle is seen as important in reducing stress that makes the patient more vulnerable to relapse. Lifestyle can be assessed by evaluating patterns of daily activities, sources of stress, stressful life events, daily hassles and up-lifts, the balance between "wants" (activities engaged in for pleasure or self-fulfillment) and "shoulds" (external demands), health, exercise and relaxation patterns, interpersonal activities, and religious beliefs (172). Working with patients to develop positive habits or substitute indulgences (such as jogging, meditation, relaxation, exercise, hobbies, or creative tasks) for an addictive disorder can help balance their lifestyles (179). Patients with a need for greater adventure or action may become involved in more challenging activities (34).

Strategy 8: Consider the Use of Medications in Combination with Psychosocial Treatments In the treatment of addictions, there are two goals for the use of medications: to help patients attain an initial period of abstinence after treating withdrawal syndromes and to assist patients with RP. There is now a range of medications used for their anticraving effect available for each of the major classes of addictive substances. None of the medications approved for treating alcohol dependence has proven effective without some form of concurrent behavioral therapy. The best use of medications may be in combination with one another and with psychosocial interventions. For example, treatment with both acamprosate and naltrexone has been shown to be efficacious in reducing relapse risk and safe (180,181). Furthermore, studies show that individuals who relapse and fail to be totally abstinent while on these drugs still drink a lot less, which presumably means fewer negative consequences. It was hypothesized that naltrexone would specifically attenuate reward craving and acamprosate would diminish relief craving. Naltrexone seems more indicated in programs geared to controlled consumption (harm reduction) because it showed to reduce the relapse rate but was not associated with a significant change in the abstinence rate, whereas acamprosate seems especially useful in a therapeutic approach targeted at achieving abstinence because it showed to be associated with a significant improvement in abstinence rate (182). The old concept of total abstinence as the only goal to treat alcohol dependence stemmed from two sources: AA and the use of medications such as disulfiram, which makes a person feel sick when she or he drinks (aversive response to alcohol). A survey of AA members' attitudes about taking a medication to help prevent relapse yielded an interesting finding. Only 17% of the 277 AA members surveyed believed they should *not* take a medication; more than 50% of the sample thought medication that helped reduce drinking was a good idea (183). Although many patients may benefit from the use of available medications for the treatment of alcohol dependence, their treatment effects are moderate at best, and some alcoholics fail to respond. This to some degree reflects the heterogeneous nature of the patients and possibly of the illness itself. Clearly, in the treatment of patients with alcohol dependence, one size does not fit all. At present no medication is U.S. Food and Drug Administration–approved for the treatment of stimulant dependence. Three types of U.S. Food and Drug Administration–approved medications are available to treat nicotine dependence: sustained-release bupropion, nicotine replacement therapies, and varenicline. Research showed that the combined effects of the pharmacologic and behavioral treatment are additive for smoking cessation (184). Medications can be of major benefit in preventing relapse to opioid dependence. These medications can provide antagonism to the reinforcing effects of opioid drugs and can provide stable replacement for illegal drugs. These medications include opioid agonist agents such as methadone, a mixed agonist/antagonist buprenorphine, and opioid antagonist such as naltrexone. Despite some clinical trials with good outcomes, medications are still underused by physicians.

Strategy 9: Facilitate the Transition Between Levels of Care for Patients Completing Residential or Hospital-Based Inpatient Treatment (IPT) Programs, or Structured Partial Hospital or Intensive Outpatient Programs Patients can make significant gains in residential or day treatment programs only to have the gains negated because of failure to adhere to ongoing outpatient or aftercare treatment. Interventions used to enhance treatment entry and adherence that also lower the risk of relapse include providing a single session of motivational therapy before discharge from IPT, using telephone or mail reminders of initial treatment appointments, and providing reinforcers for appropriate participation in treatment activities or for providing drug-free urine tests (185). In a quality improvement survey, the authors found that a single motivational therapy session provided to hospitalized psychiatric patients with comorbid SUDs led to a nearly twofold increase in the show rate for the initial outpatient appointment (186). Patients who complied with their initial appointment had a reduced risk of treatment dropout and subsequent psychiatric or substance use relapse.

Strategy 10: Incorporate Strategies to Improve Adherence to Treatment and Medications Numerous studies and reports show that patients who are retained in treatment show better outcomes, including lower relapse rates, than those who drop out early (54,59). Many clinical and systems strategies have been shown to improve adherence to treatment among patients with SUDs and dual disorders (186).

RP FOR CO-OCCURRING DISORDERS

As mentioned previously, relapse process is complex. This is especially true in the context of comorbid psychiatric disorders. Individuals with severe mental illness and SUDs have increased vulnerability for relapse because of many challenges including cognitive and social skills deficits and psychosocial issues. There is a significantly high rate of co-occurring mood and anxiety disorders with SUDs (187). For example, co-occurring PTSD and SUD is common and associated with poorer treatment outcomes than found with SUD only (188,189). Recent evidence suggests that patients with unremitted PTSD are at greater risk than those with remitted PTSD for continued SUD problems and that improvement in PTSD symptoms strongly associated with improvement in alcohol-related symptoms than is the inverse relationship (190). Many cognitive behavioral interventions and other interventions such as mindfulness-based approach targeting this population have been associated with reductions in substance use (191,192). In addition, pharmacologic interventions have been demonstrated to improve outcomes for patients with comorbid depression, bipolar, and SUDs (187,193,194).

CONCLUSIONS

Relapse is a major challenge in the treatment of addictions. The dynamic model of relapse acknowledges the complexity and unpredictable nature of substance use behavior after the commitment to abstinence or a harm reduction goal. An adequate assessment model must be sufficiently comprehensive to include theoretically relevant variables from each of the domains of relapse and different levels of potential predictors. Clinical RP strategies can be used throughout the continuum of care and be integrated with other treatment modalities such as MI and CM, pharmacotherapy, spirituality, mindfulness meditation, and family-based interventions. Future research focusing on a better assessment of the dynamic interplay of relapse factors will add to the understanding of relapse and how to prevent it.

REFERENCES

1. Scott CK, Foss MA, Dennis ML. Pathways in the relapse–treatment–recovery cycle over 3 years. *J Subst Abuse Treatment* 2005; 28:S63–S72.
2. Salomé HJ, French MT, Miller M, et al. Estimating the client costs of addiction treatment: first findings from the Client DATCAP. *Drug Alcohol Depend* 2003;71:195–206.
3. McClellan AT, Lewis DC, O'Brien CP, et al. Drug dependence, a chronic medical illness: implications for treatment, insurance, and outcomes evaluation. *JAMA* 2000;284:1689–1695.
4. Cunningham JA, Lin E, Ross HE, et al. Factors associated with untreated remissions from alcohol abuse or dependence. *Addictive Behav* 2000;25:317–321.
5. Burman S. The challenge of sobriety: natural recovery without treatment and self-help groups. *J Subst Abuse* 1997;9:41–61.
6. Anglin MD, Hser YI, Grella CE, et al. Drug treatment careers: conceptual overview and clinical, research, and policy implications. In: Tims F, Leukefeld C, Platt J, eds. *Relapse and recovery in addictions.* New Haven, CT: Yale University Press, 2001:18–39.
7. Dimeff LA, Marlatt GA. Relapse prevention. In: Hester R, Miller W, eds. *Handbook of alcoholism treatment approaches,* 2nd ed. Boston: Allyn & Bacon, 1995:176–194.
8. Baer JS, Kivlahan, DR, Donovan DM. Integrating skills training and motivational therapies: implications fro the treatment of substance dependence. *J Subst Abuse Treatment* 1999;17(1–2):15–23.

9. Marlatt GA, Gordon JR, eds. *Relapse prevention: maintenance strategies in the treatment of addiction behaviors.* New York: Guildford Press, 1985.
10. National Institute on Alcohol Abuse and Alcoholism (NIAAA). Highlights from the 10th special report to Congress. *Alcohol Res Health* 2000;24.
11. National Institute on Drug Abuse (NIDA). *Group drug counseling for cocaine dependence: the cocaine collaborative model.* Rockville: NIDA, National Institutes of Health, 2001.
12. Rawson RA, Obert JL, McCann MJ, et al. *The Matrix Modal of Intensive Outpatient Alcohol and Drug Treatment.* Center City, MN: Hazelden, 2005.
13. Miller WR. What is a relapse? Fifty ways to leave the wagon. *Addiction* 1996;91:S15–S27.
14. Marlatt GA. Relapse prevention: theoretical rationale and overview model. In Marlatt GA, Gordon G, eds. *Relapse prevention: a self-control strategy for the maintenance of behavioral change.* New York: Guildford, 1985:3–70.
15. Marlatt GA. Taxonomy of high-risk situations for alcohol relapse: evolution and development of a cognitive-behavioral model. *Addiction* 1986;91:S37–S49.
16. Donovan DM. Assessment issues and domains in the prediction of relapse. *Addiction* 1996;91:S29–S36.
17. National Institute on Drug Abuse (NIDA). *Cue extinction techniques: IDA technology transfer package.* Rockville, MD: NIDA, National Institutes of Health, 1993.
18. Larimar ME, Palmer RS, Marlatt GA. Relapse prevention: an overview of Marlatt's cognitive behavioral model. *Alcohol Res Health* 1999;23(2):151–161.
19. Marlatt GA, Witkiewitz K. Harm reduction approaches to alcohol use: health promotion, prevention, treatment. *Addictive Behav* 2002;27: 867–886.
20. Zweben A, Cisler RA. Clinical and methodological utility of a composite outcome measure for alcohol treatment research. *Alcohol Clin Exp Res* 2003;27:1680–1685.
21. Gwaltney CJ, Shiffman S, Balabanis, et al. Dynamic self-efficacy and outcome expectancies: prediction of smoking lapse and relapse. *J Abnorm Psychol* 2005;114(4):661–675.
22. Milby JB, Schumacher JE, Vuchinich RE, et al. Transitions during effective treatment for cocaine-abusing homeless persons: establishing abstinence, lapse, and relapse, and reestablishing abstinence. *Psychol Addictive Behav* 2004;18:250–256.
23. De Leon G. Cocaine abusers in therapeutic community treatment. In: Tims FM, Leukefeld CG, eds. *Cocaine treatment: research and clinical perspectives.* NIDA Research Monograph 135, NIH Publication No. 93-3639. Advances in cocaine treatment. NIDA Technical Review Meeting, Bethesda, MD, 1993:163–189.
24. Daley DC, Marlatt GA. Relapse prevention. In: Lowinson JH, Ruiz P, Millman RB, et al., eds. *Substance abuse: a comprehensive textbook,* 4th ed. Philadelphia: Lippincott, Williams & Wilkins, 2005:772–785.
25. Daley DC, Marlatt GA. Overcoming your alcohol and drug problem: effective recovery strategies. *Therapist guide,* 2nd ed. New York: Oxford University Press, 2006.
26. Wang SJ, Winchell CJ, McCormick CG, et al. Short of complete abstinence: an analysis exploration of multiple drinking episodes in alcoholism treatment trials. *Alcohol Clin Exp Res* 2002;26:1803–1809.
27. Piasecki TM, Fiore MC, McCarthy DE, et al. Have we lost our way? The need for dynamic formulations of smoking relapse proneness. *Addiction* 2002;97(9):1093–1108.
28. Moore BA, Budney AJ. Relapse in outpatient treatment for marijuana dependence. *J Subst Abuse Treatment* 2003;25(2):85–89.
29. Hufford MH, Witkiewitz K, Shields AL, et al. Applying nonlinear dynamics to the prediction of alcohol use disorder treatment outcomes. *J Abnorm Psychol* 2003;112:219–227.
30. Marlatt GA, Witkiewitz K. Relapse prevention for drug and alcohol problems. In: Marlatt GA, Donovan D, eds. *Relapse prevention,* 2nd ed. New York: Guilford, 2005:1–44.
31. Witkiewitz K, Marlatt GA. Relapse prevention for alcohol and drug problems: that was Zen, this is Tao. *Am Psychol* 2004;59:224–235.
32. National Institute on Alcohol Abuse and Alcoholism (NIAAA). *Strategies for facilitating protocol compliance in alcoholism treatment research.* Rockville, MD: NIAAA, 1998.
33. Dimeff AA, Marlatt GA. Preventing relapse and maintaining change in addictive behaviors. *Clin Psychol Sci Pract* 1998;5:513–525.
34. Daley DC, Marlatt GA. Overcoming your alcohol and drug problem: effective recovery strategies. *Client workbook,* 2nd ed. NY: Oxford University Press, 2006.
35. Washton AM. Group therapy: a clinician's guide to doing what works. In: Coombs R, ed. *Addiction recovery tools: a practical handbook.* Newbury Park: Sage Publications, 2001.
36. Washton AM. Outpatient groups at different stages of substance abuse treatment: preparation, initial abstinence, and relapse prevention. In: Brook DW, Spitz HI, eds. *The group therapy of substance abuse.* New York: Haworth Medical Publishing, 2002.
37. Gorski TT, Kelly JM. *Counselor's manual for relapse prevention with chemically dependent criminal offenders.* Rockville, MD: Substance Abuse and Mental Health Services Administration, 1996.
38. Hser YI. Predicting long-term stable recovery from heroin addiction: findings from a 33 year follow-up study. *J Addictive Disord* 2007;26(1): 51–60.
39. Flynn PM, Joe GW, Broome KM, et al. Recovery from opioid addiction in DATOS. *J Subst Abuse Treatment* 2003;25:177–186.
40. Hughes JR, Keely J, Naud S. Shape of the relapse curve and long-term abstinence among untreated smokers. *Addiction* 2004;99:29–38.
41. Medioni J, Berlin I, Mallet A. Increased risk of relapse after stopping nicotine replacement therapies: a mathematical modeling approach. *Addiction* 2005;100:247–254.
42. Shah NG, Galai N, Celentano DD, et al. Longitudinal predictors of injection cessation and subsequent relapse among a cohort of injection drug users in Baltimore, MD, 1988–2000. *Drug Alcohol Depend* 2006;83:147–156.
43. Darke S, Ross J, Teeson M, et al. Factors associated with 12 months continuous heroin abstinence: findings from the Australian Treatment Outcome Study (ATOS). *J Subst Abuse Treatment* 2005;28:255–263.
44. Rawson RA and the Methamphetamine Treatment Project Corporate authors. A multi-site comparison of psychosocial approaches for the treatment of methamphetamine dependence. *Addiction* 2004;99: 708–717.
45. Hser YI, Joshi V, Anglin MD, et al. Predictive post-treatment cocaine abstinence: what works for first-time admissions and treatment repeaters. *Am J Public Health* 1999;89:666–671.
46. Hillhouse MP, Marinelli P, Gonzales R, et al., the Methamphetamine Treatment Project Corporate Authors. Predicting in-treatment performance and post-treatment outcomes in methamphetamine users. *Addiction* 2007;102 (s1):84–95.
47. Walitzer KS, Dearing R. Gender differences in alcohol and substance use relapse. *Clin Psychol Rev* 2006;26:128–148.
48. Simpson DD, Joe GW, Broome KM. A national 5-year follow-up of treatment outcomes for cocaine dependence. *Arch Gen Psychiatry* 2002;59:538–544.
49. Hser YI, Hoffman V, Grella CE, et al. A 33-year follow-up of narcotics addicts. *Arch Gen Psychiatry* 2001;58:503–508.
50. Dennis ML, Scott CK, Funk R, Foss MA. The duration and correlates of addiction treatment careers. *J Subst Abuse Treatment* 2005;28: S51–S62.
51. Hser YI, Anglin MD, Grella C, et al. Drug treatment careers: a conceptual framework and existing research findings. *J Subst Abuse Treatment* 1997;14:543–558.
52. Miller W, Hester R. *Treating the problem drinker: modern approaches. The addictive behaviors treatment of alcoholism, drug abuse, smoking and obesity.* New York: Pergamon Press, 1980.
53. Catalano R, Howard M, Hawkins J, et al. Relapse in the addictions: rates, determinants, and promising prevention strategies. *1988 Surgeon General's report on health consequences of smoking.* Washington, DC:

Office of Smoking and Health, Department of Health and Human Services, 1988.
54. National Institute on Drug Abuse (NIDA). Beyond the therapeutic alliance: keeping the drug dependent individual in treatment. In: Simon Onken L, Blaine JD, Boren JJ, eds. *NIDA Research Monograph 165.* Rockville, MD: NIDA, National Institutes of Health, 1997.
55. Center for Substance Abuse Treatment (CSAT). Treatment succeeds in fighting crime. In: *Substance abuse brief.* Rockville, MD: CSAT, SAMHSA, 1999.
56. Center for Substance Abuse Treatment (CSAT). Substance abuse treatment reduces family dysfunction, improves productivity. In: *Substance abuse brief.* Rockville, MD: CSAT, SAMHSA, 2000.
57. Center for Substance Abuse Treatment (CSAT). Treatment cuts medical costs. In: *Substance abuse brief.* Rockville, MD: CSAT, SAMHSA, 2000.
58. Daley DC, Marlatt GA, Spotts CE. Relapse prevention: clinical models and intervention strategies. In: Graham AW, et al., eds. *Principles of addiction medicine,* 3rd ed. Chevy Chase, MD: American Society of Addiction Medicine, 2003:467–485.
59. National Institute on Drug Abuse (NIDA). Study sheds new light on the state of drug abuse treatment nationwide. *NIDA Notes* 1997;12(5):1–8.
60. Chaney ER, O' Leary MR, Marlatt GA. Skill training with alcoholics. *J Consult Clin Psychol* 1978;46:1092–1104.
61. Carroll KM. Relapse prevention as a psychosocial treatment: a review of controlled clinical trials. *Exp Clin Psychopharmcol* 1996;4:46–54.
62. Goldstein MG, Niaura R, Follick MJ, et al. Effects of behavioral skills training and schedule of nicotine gum administration on smoking cessation. *Am J Psychiatry* 1989;146:56–60.
63. Carroll KM, Rounsaville BJ, Nich C, et al. One-year follow-up of psychotherapy and pharmacotherapy for cocaine dependence. Delayed emergence of psychotherapy effects. *Arch Gen Psychiatry* 1994;51: 989–997.
64. Rawson R, McCann M, Flammino F, et al. A comparison of contingency management and cognitive-behavioral approaches for cocaine and methamphetamine-dependent individuals. *Arch Gen Psychiatry* 2002;59: 817–824.
65. Polivy J, Herman CP. If at first you don't succeed: false hopes of self-change. *Am Psychol* 2002;109:74–86.
66. Project MATCH Research Group. Matching alcoholism treatment to client heterogeneity: post treatment drinking outcomes. *J Studies Alcohol* 1997;58:7–29.
67. Ouimette PC, Finney JW, Moos RH. 12-Step and cognitive behavioral treatment for substance abuse: a comparison of treatment effectiveness. *J Consult Clin Psychol* 1997;65:230–240.
68. Irvin JE, Bowers CA, Dunn ME, et al. Efficacy of relapse prevention: a meta-analytic review. *J Consult Clin Psychol* 1999;67:563–570.
69. Hajek P, Stead LF, West R, et al. Relapse prevention interventions for smoking cessation. *Cochrane Database Syst Rev* 2005(1):CD003999.
70. Lancaster T, Hajek P, Stead L, et al. Prevention of relapse after quitting smoking: a Systematic Review of Trials. *Arch Intern Med* 2006;166: 828–835.
71. Fiore MC, Bailey WC, Cohen SJ, et al. *Treating tobacco use and dependence: clinical practice guideline.* Rockville, MD: U.S. Department of Health and Human Services, Public Health Service, 2000.
72. Brandon TH, Collin BN, Juliano LM, et al. Preventing relapse among former smokers: a comparison of minimal interventions through telephone and mail. *J Consult Clin Psychol* 2000;68(1):103–113.
73. Brandon TH, Meade CD, Herzog S, et al. Efficacy and cost-effectiveness of a minimal intervention to prevent smoking relapse: dismantling the effects of amount of content versus contact. *J Consult Clin Psychol* 2004;72(5):797–808.
74. Anton RF, Moak DH, Latham P, et al. Naltrexone combined with either cognitive behavioral or motivational enhancement therapy for alcohol dependence. *J Clin Psychopharmacol* 2005;25:349–357.
75. Anton RF, O'Malley SS, Ciraulo DA, et al. Combined pharmacotherapies and behavioral interventions for alcohol dependence. *JAMA* 2006;295:2003–2017.
76. The COMBINE Study Group. Testing combined pharmacotherapies and behavioral interventions for alcohol dependence (the COMIBINE study): rationale and methods. *Alcohol Clin Exp Res* 2003;27:1107–1122.
77. The COMBINE Study Group. Testing combined pharmacotherapies and behavioral interventions for alcohol dependence (the COMIBINE study): a pilot feasibility study. *Alcohol Clin Exp Res* 2003;27: 1123–1131.
78. Maude-Griffin PM, Hohenstein JM, et al. Superior efficacy of cognitive-behavioral therapy for crack cocaine abusers: main and matching effects. *J Consult Clin Psychol* 1998;66:832–837.
79. Carroll KM, Fenton LR, Ball S, et al. Efficacy of disulfiram and cognitive-behavioral therapy for cocaine-dependent outpatients. *Arch Gen Psychiatry* 2004;64:264–272.
80. Rawson RA, Huber A, Brethen PB, et al. Methamphetamine and cocaine users: differences in characteristics and treatment retention. *J Psychoactive Drugs* 2000;32:233–238.
81. Rawson RA, Obert JL, McCann MJ, et al. The neurobehavioral treatment manual. Beverly Hills, CA: Matrix, 1989.
82. Rawson RA, Shoptaw SJ, Obert JL, et al. An intensive outpatient approach for cocaine abuse treatment: the Matrix Model. *J Subst Abuse Treatment* 1995;12:117–127.
83. Epstein DE, Hawkins WF, Covi L, et al. Cognitive behavioral therapy plus contingency management for cocaine use: findings during treatment and across 12-month follow-up. *Psychol Addict Behav* 2003;17:73–82.
84. Schmitz JM, Oswald LM, Jacks SM, et al. Relapse prevention treatment for cocaine dependence: group versus individual format. *Addictive Behav* 1997;22:405–418.
85. Marques AC, Formigoni ML. Comparison of individual and group cognitive behavioral therapy for alcohol and/or drug dependent patients. *Addiction* 2001;96:832–837.
86. MTP Research Group. Brief treatments for cannabis dependence: findings from a randomized multi-site trial. *J Consult Clin Psychol* 2004;72: 455–466.
87. Kilmer JR, Cronce JM, Paler RS. Relapse prevention for abuse of club drugs, hallucinogens, inhalants, and steroids. In: Marlatt GA, Donovan D, eds. *Relapse prevention,* 2nd ed. New York: Guilford Press, 2005: 208–247.
88. Maisto SA, McKay JR, O'Farrell TJ. Relapse precipitants and behavioral marital therapy. *Addictive Behav* 1995;20(3):383–393.
89. O'Farrell TJ, Choquette KA, Cutter HSG, et al. Behavioral marital therapy with and without additional couples relapse prevention sessions for alcoholics and their wives. *J Studies Alcohol* 1993;54:652–666.
90. McCrady BS, Epstein EE, Kahler CW. Alcoholics Anonymous and relapse prevention as maintenance strategies after conjoint behavioral alcohol treatment for men: 18-month outcomes. *J Consult Clin Psychol* 2004;72:870–878.
91. McCrady BS, Nathan PE. Impact of treatment factors on outcomes of treatment for substance use disorders. In: Beutler L, Castonguay L, eds. *Empirically supported principles of therapeutic change: integrating common and specific therapeutic factors across major psychological disorders.* New York: Oxford University Press, in press.
92. Maisto SA, Connors GJ, Zwyiak WH. Construct validation analyses on the Marlatt typology of relapse precipitants. *Addiction* 1996;91:89–98.
93. Stout RL, Longabaugh R, Rubin R. Predictive validity of Marlatt's taxonomy versus a more general relapse code. *Addiction* 1996;91:99–110.
94. Marlatt GA. Craving for alcohol, loss of control, and relapse: a cognitive-behavioral analysis. In: Nathan PE, Marlatt GA, Loberg T, eds. *New directions in behavioral research and treatment.* New Brunswick, NJ: Rutgers Center of Alcohol Studies, 1978:271–314.
95. Longabaugh R, Rubin A, Stout RL, et al. The reliability of Marlatt's taxonomy for classifying relapses. *Addiction* 1996;91:73–88.
96. Donovan DM. Marlatt's classification of relapse precipitants: is the emperor still wearing clothes? *Addiction* 1996;91:S131–S137.
97. Kadden R. Is Marlatt's taxonomy reliable or valid? *Addiction* 1996; 91:139–146.
98. Sandahl C. Determinants of relapse among alcoholics: a cross-cultural replication study. *Int J Addict* 1984;19:833–848.

99. Annis H. A relapse prevention model for treatment of alcoholics. In: Miller W, Heather N, eds. *Treating addictive behaviors: processes of change.* New York: Plenum Books, 1986.
100. Miller WR, Westerberg VS, Harris RJ, et al. What predicts relapse? Prospective testing of antecedent models. *Addiction* 1996;91:S155–S171.
101. Hodgins DC, Guebaly N, Armstrong S. Prospective and retrospective reports of mood states before relapse to substance use. *J Consult Clin Psychol* 1995;63:400–407.
102. Carroll KM, Rounsaville BJ, Gawin FH. A comparative trial of psychotherapies for ambulatory cocaine abusers: relapse prevention and interpersonal psychotherapy. *Am J Drug Alcohol Abuse* 1991;17: 229–249.
103. Daley DC, ed. *Relapses: conceptual, research and clinical perspectives.* New York: Haworth Medical Publishing, 1989.
104. Daley DC. *Relapse prevention: treatment alternatives and counseling aids.* Bradenton, FL: Human Services Institute, 1988.
105. Daley DC, Ross JR. *Relapse prevention workbook for sexually compulsive behavior.* Holmes Beach, FL: Learning Publications, 2000.
106. Bandura A. Self-efficacy: toward a unifying theory of behavioral change. *Psychol Rev* 1977;84:191–215.
107. Bandura A. *Self-efficacy: the exercise of control.* New York: Freeman, 1997.
108. Demell R, Rist F. Prediction of treatment outcome in a clinical sample of problem drinkers: self-efficacy and coping style. *Addict Disord Treatment* 2005;4(1):5–10.
109. Maisto SA, Clifford PR, Longabaugh R, et al. The relationship between abstinence for one year following pretreatment assessment and alcohol use and other functioning at 2 years in individuals presenting for alcohol treatment. *J Studies Alcohol* 2002;63(4):397–403.
110. Sklar SM, Annis HM, Turner NE. Development and validation of the Drug-Taking Confidence Questionnaire: a measure of coping self-efficacy. *Addict Behav* 1997;22:655–670.
111. Monti PM, Rohsenow DJ, Swift RM, et al. Naltrexone and cue exposure with coping and communication skills training for alcoholics: treatment process and 1-year outcomes. *Alcohol Clin Exp Res* 2001;25: 1634–1647.
112. Shiffman S, Balabanis M, Paty J, et al. Dynamic effects of self-efficacy on smoking lapse and relapse. *Health Psychol* 2000;19:315–323.
113. Oei TPS, Baldwin AR. Expectancy theory: a two-process model of alcohol use and abuse. *J Stud Alcohol* 1994;55(5):525–534.
114. Smith DE, Seymour RB. The nature of addiction. In: RH Coombs, ed. *Handbook of addictive behaviors: a practical guide to diagnosis and treatment.* New York: Wiley, 2004:3–30.
115. Sale E, Sambrano S, Springer JF, et al. Risk, protection, and substance use in adolescents: a multisite trial. *J Drug Addiction* 2003;33(1):91–105.
116. Jones BT, Corbin W, Fromme K. A review of expectancy theory and alcohol consumption. *Addiction* 2001;96:57–72.
117. Abrams K, Kushner MG. The moderating effects of tension reduction alcohol outcome expectancies on placebo responding in individuals with social phobia. *Addict Behav* 2004;29(6):1221–1224.
118. Demmel R, Nicolai J, Gregorzik S. Alcohol expectancies and current mood state in social drinkers. *Addict Behav* 2006;31(5):859–867.
119. Corbin WR, McNair LD, Carter JA. Evaluation of a treatment appropriate cognitive intervention for challenging alcohol outcome expectancies. *Addict Behav* 2001;26(4):475–488.
120. Rohsenow DJ, Monti PM. Does urge to drink predict relapse after treatment? *Alcohol Res Health* 1999;23:225–232.
121. Tiffany ST, Carter BL, Singleton EG. Challenges in the manipulation, assessment and interpretation of craving relevant variables. *Addiction* 2000;95:177–187.
122. Drummond DC, Litten RZ, Lowman C, et al. Craving research: future directions. *Addiction* 2000;95(Suppl. 2):131–137.
123. Gordon SM, Sterling R, Siatkowski C, et al. Inpatient desire to drink as a predictor of relapse to alcohol use following treatment. *Am J Addict* 2006;15:242–245.
124. Sinha R, Garcia M, Paliwal P, et al. Stress-induced cocaine craving and hypothalamic-pituitary-adrenal responses are predictive of cocaine relapse outcomes. *Arch Gen Psychiatry* 2006;63:324–331.
125. Marlatt GA, Ostafin BD. Being mindful of automaticity in addiction: a clinical perspective. In: Weirs RW, Stacy AW, eds. *Handbook of implicit cognition and addiction.* Thousand Oaks, CA: Sage Publications, Inc., 2006:489–495.
126. Witkiewitz K, Marlatt GA, Walker D. Mindfulness based relapse prevention for alcohol and substance use disorders: the meditative tortoise wins the race. *J Cognit Psychother* 2006;19(3):211–228.
127. Donovan DM, Rosengren DB. Motivation for behavior change and treatment among substance abusers. In: Tucker JA, Donovan DM, Marlatt GA, eds. *Changing addictive behavior: bridging clinical and public health strategies.* New York: Guilford Press, 1999:127–159.
128. Prochaska JO, DiClementa CC. *The transtheoretical approach: crossing the traditional boundaries of therapy.* Malabar: Krieger, 1984.
129. Miller WR, Rollnick S. *Motivational interviewing: preparing people for change,* 2nd ed. New York: Guilford Press, 2002.
130. Rohsenow DJ, Monti PM, Martin RA, et al. Motivational enhancement and coping skills training for cocaine abusers: effects on substance use outcomes. *Addiction* 2004;99(7):862–74.
131. Moos RH, Holahan CJ. Dispositional and contextual perspectives on coping: toward an integrative framework. *J Clin Psychol* 2003;59:1387–1403.
132. Shiffman S. Maintenance and relapse: coping with temptation. In: Nirenberg TD, Maisto SA, eds. Developments in the assessment and treatment of addictive behaviors. Norwood: Ablex, 1987:352–385.
133. Shiffman S. Conceptual issues in the study of relapse. In: Gossop M, ed. *Relapse and addictive behaviour.* London: Tavistock/Routledge, 1989: 149–179.
134. Carels RA, Douglass OM, Cacciapaglia HM, et al. An ecological momentary assessment of relapse crises in dieting. *J Consult Clin Psychol* 2004;72(2):341–348.
135. Maisto SA, Zywiak WH, Connors GJ. Course of functioning one year following admission for treatment of alcohol use disorders. *Addict Behav* 2006;31(1):69–79.
136. Moser AE, Annis HM. The role of coping in relapse crisis outcome: a prospective study of treated alcoholics. *Addiction* 1996;91:1101–1114.
137. Chung T, Langenbucher J, Labouvie E, et al. Changes in alcoholic patients' coping responses predict 12-month treatment outcomes. *J Consult Clin Psychol* 2001;69:92–100.
138. Litt MD, Cooney NL, Morse P. Reactivity to alcohol-related stimuli in the laboratory and in the field: predictors of craving in treated alcoholics. *Addiction* 2000;95:889–900.
139. Litt MD, Kadden RM, Cooney NL, et al. Coping skills and treatment outcomes in cognitive-behavioral and interactional group therapy for alcoholism. *J Consult Clin Psychol* 2003;71:118–128.
140. Marlatt GA. Buddhist philosophy and the treatment of addictive behaviors. *Cognit Behav Pract* 2002;9:44–49.
141. Marlatt GA, Kristellar J. Mindfulness and meditation. In: Miller WR, ed. *Integrating spirituality in treatment: resources for practitioners.* Washington, DC: American Psychological Association Books, 1999:67–84.
142. Marlatt GA, Witkiewitz K, Dillworth T, et al. Vipassana meditation as a treatment for alcohol and drug use disorders. In: Hayes SC, Follette VM, Linehan MM, eds. *Mindfulness and acceptance: expanding the cognitive-behavioral tradition.* New York: Guilford Press, 2004: 261–287.
143. Cooney NL, Litt MD, Morse PA, et al. Alcohol cue reactivity, negative mood reactivity, and relapse in treated alcoholic men. *J Abnorm Psychol* 1997;106:243–250.
144. Shiffman S, Paty JA, Gnys M, et al. First lapses to smoking: within subject analysis of real time reports. *J Consult Clin Psychol* 1996;2:366–379.
145. Baker TB, Piper ME, McCarthy DE, et al. Addiction motivation reformulated: an affective processing model of negative reinforcement. *Psychol Bull* 2004;111:33–51.
146. Stanton M. Relapse prevention needs more emphasis on interpersonal factors. *Am Psychol* 2005;60:340–349.
147. Armeli S, Todd M, Mohr C. A daily process approach to individual differences in stress-related alcohol use. *J Personality* 2005;73(6):1–30.
148. Beattie MC, Longabaugh R. General and alcohol-specific social support following treatment. *Addict Behav* 1999;24:593–606.

149. Dobkin PL, Civita M, Paraherakis A, et al. The role of functional social support in treatment retention and outcomes among outpatient adult substance abusers. *Addiction* 2002;97:347–356.
150. McMahon RC. Personality, stress, and social support in cocaine relapse prediction. *J Subst Abuse Treatment* 2001;21:77–87.
151. Annis H, Davis CS. Self-efficacy and the prevention of alcoholic relapse: initial findings from a treatment trial. In: Baker TB, Cannon DS, eds. *Assessment and treatment of addictive disorders.* New York: Praeger, 1988:88–112.
152. Winters J, Fals-Stewart W, O'Farrell TJ, et al. Behavioral couples therapy for female substance-abusing patients: effects on substance use and relationship adjustment. *J Consult Clin Psychol* 2002;70:344–355.
153. Finney JW, Monahan SC. The cost-effectiveness of treatment for alcoholism: a second approximation. *J Stud Alcohol* 1999;52:517–540.
154. Marlatt GA, Barrett K, Daley DC. Relapse prevention. In: Galanter M, Kleber HD, eds. *Textbook of substance abuse,* 2nd ed. Washington, DC: American Psychiatric Press, 1999.
155. Annis H. A cognitive-social learning approach to relapse: pharmacotherapy and relapse prevention counseling. *Alcohol Alcohol* 1991; 1(Suppl):527–530.
156. National Institute on Drug Abuse (NIDA). *Recovery training and self-help,* 2nd ed. Rockville: NIDA, National Institutes of Health, 1994.
157. Rawson RA, Obert JL, McCann MJ, et al. Relapse prevention models for substance abuse treatment. *Psychotherapy* 1993;30:284–298.
158. Shoptaw S, Reback CJ, Frosch DL, et al. Stimulant abuse treatment as HIV prevention. *J Addict Dis* 1998;17:19–32.
159. Obert JL, McCann MJ, Marinelli-Casey P, et al. The matrix model of outpatient stimulant abuse treatment: history and description. *J Psychoactive Drugs* 2000;32:157–164.
160. Monti PM, Rohsenow DJ, Rubonis AV, et al. Cue exposure with coping skills treatment for male alcoholics: a preliminary investigation. *J Clin Consult Psychol* 1993;61:1011–1019.
161. Gossop M, Stewart D, Browne N, et al. Factors associated with abstinence, lapse or relapse to heroin use after residential treatment: protective effect of coping responses. *Addiction* 2002;97:1259–1267.
162. Boker SM, Graham JS. Dynamical systems analysis of adolescent substance abuse. *Multivar Behav Res* 1998;33(4):479–507.
163. Warran K, Hawkins RC, Sprott JC. Substance abuse as a dynamical disease: evidence and clinical implications of nonlinearity in a time series of daily alcohol consumption. *Addict Behav* 2005;28:369–374.
164. Burgess ES, Brown RA, Kahler CW, et al. Patterns of change in depressive symptoms during smoking cessation: who's at risk for relapse? *J Consult Clin Psychol* 2002;70:356–361.
165. Cinciripini P, Cinciripini L, Wallfisch A, et al. Behavior therapy and transdermal nicotine patch: effects on cessation outcome, affect, and coping. *J Consult Clin Psychol* 1996;64:314–323.
166. Witkiewitz K, Marlatt GA. Modeling the complexity of post-treatment drinking: it is a rocky road to relapse. *Clin Psychol Rev* 2007;27:724–738.
167. Hufford MR, Witkiewitz K, Shields AL, et al. Relapse as a nonlinear dynamic system: application to patients with alcohol use disorders. *J Abnorm Psychol* 2003;112:219–227.
168. Monti P, Adams D, Kadden R, et al. *Treating alcohol dependence.* New York: Guilford Press, 1989.
169. Daley DC. Substance use disorders. In: Daley DC, Salloum IM, eds. *A clinician's guide to mental illness.* New York: McGraw Hill/Hazelden, 2001.
170. Daley DC. Five perspectives on relapse in chemical dependency. *J Chem Depend Treatment* 1989;2:3–26.
171. Daley DC, Marlatt GA. *Therapist's guide for managing your alcohol or drug problem.* San Antonio: Psychological Corporation, 1997.
172. Marlatt GA. Relapse prevention: theoretical rationale and overview of the model. In: Marlatt GA, Gordon JR, eds. *Relapse prevention.* New York: Guilford Press, 1985:108–250.
173. Marlatt GA. Cognitive factors in the relapse process. In: GA Marlatt, J Gordon, eds. *Relapse prevention: a self-control strategy for the maintenance of behavior change.* New York: Guilford, 1985:128–200.
174. McCrady BS. Relapse prevention: a couple's therapy perspective. In: O'Farrell TJ, ed. *Treating alcohol problems: marital and family interventions.* New York: Guilford Press, 1989:165–182.
175. Daley DC, Miller J. *Addiction in your family: helping yourself and your loved ones.* Holmes Beach, FL: Learning Publications, 2001.
176. Zackon F. Relapse and "re-joyment": observations and reflections. *J Chem Depend Treatment* 1989;2(2):67–80.
177. McCusker CG, Brown K. Cue-exposure to alcohol-associated stimuli reduces autonomic reactivity, but not craving and anxiety, independent drinkers. *Alcohol Alcohol* 1995;30(3):319–327.
178. Staiger PK, Greeley JD, Wallace SD. Alcohol exposure therapy: generalization and changes in responsivity. *Drug Alcohol Depend* 1999;57(1): 29–40.
179. O'Connell DF, Alexander CN. *Self recovery treating addictions. Using transcendental meditation and maharishi ayur-veda.* New York: Haworth Press, 1994.
180. Mann K, Lehert P, Morgan MY. The efficacy of acamprosate in the maintenance in alcohol-dependent individuals: results of a meta-analysis. *Alcohol Clin Exp Res* 2004;28:51–63.
181. Kiefer F, Wiedemann K. Combined therapy: what does acamprosate and naltrexone combination tell us? *Alcohol Alcohol* 2004;39:542–547.
182. Bouza C, Magro A, Munoz A, et al. Efficacy and safety of naltrexone and acamprosate in the treatment of alcohol dependence. *Addiction* 2004;99(7):811–828.
183. Rychtarik RG, Connors GJ, Dermen KH, et al. Alcoholics Anonymous and the use of medications to prevent relapse: an anonymous survey of member attitudes. *J Stud Alcohol* 2000;61:134–138.
184. Hughes JR. Combining behavioral therapy and pharmacotherapy for smoking cessation: an update. *NIDA Res Monogr* 1995;150:92–109.
185. Higgins ST, Silverman K, eds. *Motivating behavior change among illicit drug abusers: research on contingency management.* Washington, DC: American Psychological Association, 1999.
186. Daley DC, Zuckoff A. *Improving treatment compliance: counseling and system strategies for substance use and dual disorders.* Center City, MN: Hazelden, 1999.
187. Bradizza CM, Stasiewicz PR, Paas ND. Relapse to alcohol and drug use among individuals diagnosed with co-occurring mental health and substance use disorders: a review. *Clin Psychol Rev* 2006;26:162–178.
188. Kaysen D, Simpson T, Dillworth T, et al. Alcohol problems and post-traumatic stress disorder in female crime victims. *J Traumatic Stress* 2006;19(3):399–403.
189. Ouimette PC, Gima K, Moos RH, et al. A comparative evaluation of substance abuse treatment IV. The effect of comorbid psychiatric diagnoses on amount of treatment, continuing care, and 1-year outcomes. *Alcohol Clin Exp Res* 1999;23(3):552–557.
190. Back SE, Brady KT, Stone SC, et al. Symptom improvement in co-occurring PTSD and alcohol dependence. *J Nerv Ment Dis* 2006;194: 690–696.
191. Simpson TL, Kaysen D, Bowen S, et al. PTSD symptoms, substance use, and Vipassana meditation among incarcerated individuals. *J Traumatic Stress* 2007;20(3):239–249.
192. Najavits LM. Treatment of PTSD and substance abuse: clinical guidelines for implementing seeking safety. *Alcohol Treatment Q* 2004;22:43–62.
193. Cornelius JR, Salloum IM, Ehler JG, et al. Fluoxetine in depressed alcoholics: a double-blind, placebo-controlled trial. *Arch Gen Psychiatry* 1997;54:700–705.
194. Salloum IM, Cornelius JR, Daley DC, et al. Efficacy of valproate maintenance in patients with bipolar disorder and alcoholism. *Arch Gen Psychiatry* 2005;62:37–45.

CHAPTER 66

Richard N. Rosenthal, MD
Richard K. Ries, MD, FAPA, FASAM

Integrating Pharmacological and Behavioral Treatments

Many professionals who prescribe addictions or other medications as part of addictions treatment are faced with the question of what sort of evidence base exists for the "talking part" of what they do, as well as how best to do this. Independent of the impact of pharmacotherapies, several types of brief psychosocial intervention have been established as effective in treatment of drug use disorders, with meta-analyses demonstrating low-moderate to high-moderate effect sizes depending on the specific substance use disorder (SUD) or treatment type (1,2). For busy physicians who treat addicted patients, this may present somewhat of a quandary, especially if that clinician is in a solo practice, is not trained to deliver psychotherapy, or doesn't typically provide those services in the course of daily clinical practice. This chapter provides an overview of the issues regarding the integration of brief psychosocial interventions with medication treatment for addiction and begins with a discussion of a basic psychosocial intervention that clinicians can and should be implementing with all patients. The term *brief* in this context most usually refers to the total number of sessions, but in this chapter may also refer to the relatively brief amount of time that a prescribing clinician has in the context of a 15- to 30-minute medication management session. Such sessions are often of short duration because of limits on insurance or other benefit coverage, or that patients may be getting most of their psychosocial treatment through a structured addictions program, or Twelve Step groups. The rest of the chapter further explicates the evidence base for the various psychotherapeutic interventions for SUD (many of which are found more fully discussed in this volume), and presents principles for integrating brief but more differentiated behavioral interventions into medication management sessions.

CLINICAL SKILLS ANY CLINICIAN SHOULD USE

Engagement Because the outcome of addiction treatment has been related to the time spent in treatment (3,4), techniques that maximize treatment engagement and retention are likely to promote better outcomes. One technique likely to sustain engagement and retention in treatment is to facilitate the therapeutic alliance through psychologic support. Observational studies suggest that psychologic support is among the most prominent and necessary components of management of addicted patients, especially those with more severe dependence (5). As such, clinicians, even very busy ones, should focus special attention supporting the development of a therapeutic alliance with the patient. Alliance building is one of the core tactical techniques of supportive therapy and uses several straightforward approaches accessible to clinicians who may not have had any formal psychotherapy training: expression of interest, expression of empathy, expression of understanding, and repairing a misalliance (6). For example, interest is expressed by the clinician's bringing in his or her knowledge of the patient into the conversation. In assessing primary care quality, more whole-person knowledge (medical history, home/work/school responsibilities, health concerns, and values and beliefs) of the patient by the clinician predicts lower drug and alcohol addiction severity scores on the Addiction Severity Index and lower odds of subsequent substance use in recently detoxified primary care patients (7). It is also important that the clinician is aware that asking too many questions of some patients, especially "why?" questions, can be experienced as intrusive or even an attack, which is off-putting to patients and reduces the likelihood of engagement. Information is best garnered by what, when, where, and how questions, but monitoring patient comfort in this process, because if the patient does not return, such "interrogation" information is not doing them or the clinician much good.

Expression of accurate empathy has a long history as an important psychotherapeutic technique and corresponds to the concept of *reflective listening* used in motivational interviewing (8), as well as the "E" in the BRENDA 1) a biopsychosocial Evaluation; 2) a Report of findings from the evaluation given to the patient; 3) Empathy; 4) addressing patient Needs; 5) providing Direct advice; and 6) Assessing patient reaction to advice and adjusting the treatment plan as needed) therapy for the Penn clinical trials of SUD pharmacotherapies (9). Empathy, which is more than simple care or concern, is expressed by the clinician relating his or her own internal emotional experience to corroborate that of the patient (e.g., "It must've felt terrible to come back after your last binge and find out your drunken behavior was so scary that she'd changed the locks"). The clinician can express his or her understanding by simply stating that he or she "gets" what the patient is communicating, and sometimes paraphrasing what the patient has said. This demonstrates his or her alignment with the patient in a cognitive way, which helps the patient to feel "in sync" with the clinician.

Misalliances occur in all human relationships, and addiction treatment is certainly no exception. However, when patients in substance abuse treatment get frustrated or resentful about the treatment, they frequently drop out of treatment, relapse or both, either of which typically has a negative impact on outcome. Part of the draw of Alcoholics Anonymous (AA) and other mutual help groups is that they can offer a context where an addict can experience not being judged for his or her feelings and actions related to addiction, because there is no cross-talk in the groups, and further it is likely that they will hear others tell similar stories to their own. The willingness of the clinician to entertain a patient's grievances, whether factually based or the result of misconstrual, is a powerful interpersonal reinforcer for patients who may have relatively little experience of a nonjudgmental person willing to listen. Trust (including the experience of the clinician as the patient's agent) is also a factor associated with a lower risk of substance use in detoxified SUD patients in primary care (7). In dealing with the patient's negative sentiments or concerns, it is a useful strategy to first start with practical issues related to the current situation; if the misalliance is not resolved with careful evaluation and response to the actual facts and the patient's experience of them, the clinician can only then tactfully move to discussion of possible problems in the relationship between the patient and the clinician (6). The clinician can clarify the facts or address incorrect assumptions to help support the patient having more accurate perceptions and assumptions.

Example

Clinician: "Hi, how have you been doing since last visit?"

Patient: "Well, it seems that the main thing you want is that I keep taking my meds so it will help the pharmacy budget. Do you get kickbacks or something?"

Clinician: "Wow, it sounds like you are frustrated with something. We've discussed this before; medications are only a part of what addiction treatment and recovery are all about. First, the simple answer to your question is no, I don't get any kickbacks—that would actually be illegal. (Patient frowns) But I get a sense that there's more to this. Can you tell me what this frustration is all about? Did something happen?

Patient: "Um, uh, I threw my naltrexone away 2 weeks ago because my friend told me that it was bad stuff and addicting, and then I relapsed briefly last week. So, I guess you doctors might be right. . . . Anyway, you guys have it so easy."

Clinician: "So you listened to your friend, threw the medications away, and relapsed. Is that accurate?"

Patient: "Yeah."

Clinician: "OK. I wanted to be clear that I understood you. Now, I don't understand what you mean when you say 'you guys have it so easy'?"

Patient: "I don't know, look, I'm just, I don't know . . . (annoyed). . . . I know I screwed up but I guess I'm waiting for the other shoe to drop, and you kick me out of treatment" (looks away).

Clinician: "So to me, it sounds like you're upset with your relapse, and angry at yourself that your stopping medications may have been part of that. Perhaps it's more comfortable for you to be angry at me and the treatment? Did you maybe think I was going to get mad at you and retaliate in some way?

Patient: (shrugs) "Been there, done that."

Clinician: "I hear that you have felt mistreated in the past, in past treatment? Is that right?

Patient: "Right."

Clinician: "But, have I done anything specific in our work together that made you feel this way? I want to address it if I have."

Patient: "Hmmm . . . well, no, not yet."

Clinician: "So, going forward, I need to be mindful of your concern that I'll be unhelpful to you, as others may have done."

Patient: "Huh . . . well, yes." (Turns and gives clinician full eye contact)

Clinician: "What can I do to help get things back on track? I'll help in any reasonable way I can . . . do you want to restart the naltrexone?"

Patient: "You mean I could try it again even though I threw the last bottle away?"

Clinician: "Sure, we can restart it. This stuff can happen as part of recovery. But, can we also take a look at what else happened with your relapse, and how you are dealing with it in your groups and Twelve Step meetings?"

Clinical attention to patient treatment satisfaction is associated with better attendance at outpatient visits for SUD (10).

Motivational Interviewing Motivational interviewing is detailed in Chapter 54 of this text, "Enhancing Motivation to Change," but in short, is a very well researched and evidence-based technique for interacting with patients in such a way as to enhance better communication, engagement, and motivation to change. Compared with a traditional paternalistic and prescriptive approach to the patient's maladaptive choices around substance sue, motivational interviewing encourages internally driven change through a collaborative effort that elicits, through the use of clinical feedback, the patient's own recovery-oriented thoughts and feelings, thus promoting and supporting the patient's sense of autonomy. It is strongly suggested that clinicians read the chapter in this ASAM text and for more detailed information, read the online version of Center for Substance Abuse Treatment Improvement Protocol (TIP 35 *http://www.ncbi.nlm.nih.gov/books/bv.fcgi?rid5hstat5.chapter.61302*). In addition to the standard supportive stance with the patient, the motivational interviewer further explores the patient's feelings and comments, and more specifically "rolls with the resistance." This would be in the service of tipping the patient's "decisional balance" toward higher motivation about treatment engagement and reducing substance use. The clinician would have continued to explore and clarify exactly what the patient was feeling, what the patient wanted to call that feeling, and why they were having it, by restating the patients concerns, supplying statements of empathy and asking for clarification.

Clinician:	"You sound angry—do I have that right?"
Patient:	"No, I don't get angry, but I am frustrated."
Clinician:	"Tell me about this frustration."
Patient:	"Well it just seems that nothing I do works, and I relapsed last week."
Clinician:	"Relapse is usually frustrating, I am sorry that happened."
Patient:	"I thought you would be angry at me."
Clinician:	"No, I am not angry with you, but tell me more about your frustration: what happened? How can I help?"

BEHAVIORAL THERAPIES IN THE CONTEXT OF DETOXIFICATION

It is well-described that the rates of relapse to drug dependence after detoxification are quite high (11). Only about 20% to 50% of patients receive postdetoxification treatment for substance dependence, yet engagement in follow-up treatment increases the time to a second admission for detoxification (12). Systematic review has demonstrated that over and above pharmacologic detoxification for opioid dependence, psychosocial treatments such as contingency management or drug counseling offered in addition demonstrate beneficial effects in terms of completion of treatment (relative risk [RR] 1.68), use of opiate (RR 0.82), follow-up abstinence (RR 2.43), and compliance with clinic visits (RR 0.48) (13). During outpatient opioid detoxification, relapse to opioid use is not uncommon (14,15), but contingency management (CM) improves treatment retention and reduces symptom complaints (16). Thus it appears sensible to provide some form of psychosocial intervention in addition to pharmacotherapy of substance withdrawal, and clearly with opioid dependence. Given that the exposure to treatment during inpatient detoxification is relatively brief and the most important outcome for those in detoxification programs is continued engagement in treatment, motivational interviewing is probably the modality of therapy that best matches the needs of the patient during the interval of treatment (17). This is because detoxification is not a treatment for substance use disorders *per se*, but rather is medical stabilization and an opportunity to engage patients in the work of recovery. With outpatient detoxification, given the generally longer interval of treatment, motivational interviewing with boosters to support continued motivation for treatment engagement, plus some form of CM is a sensible approach to treatment.

MEDICATION ADHERENCE

Medications don't work unless you take them. It is estimated that the overall adherence to medication regimens for general medical disorders such as hypertension, diabetes, and asthma is between 40% and 60%, with factors such as low socioeconomic status, lack of family and social supports, or significant psychiatric comorbidity associated with the lowest percentages (18). It would be surprising if adherence rates for unsupervised addiction medications were higher, and they are not. In a 12-week randomized clinical trial (RCT) of naltrexone versus placebo for alcohol dependence in a clinic setting with 98 subjects, the medication showed only modest effects in reducing alcohol drinking, but the subjects who were highly compliant with taking medication had high naltrexone treatment efficacy on a range of measures (19). Similarly, in the Veterans Affairs Cooperative Study, a randomized placebo-controlled trial of disulfiram for alcohol dependence in 605 subjects showed no difference in the intention-to-treat sample in abstinence rates from placebo, or from an inactive dose of disulfiram. Yet, in a subgroup with high adherence to medication, there were clear improvements in abstinence rates (20).

Thus improved medication adherence could improve the efficacy of pharmacologic interventions for SUD, and it makes sense to propose behavioral interventions that might foster improved medication adherence (21).

Various factors have been identified that adversely affect patients' adherence to a medication regimen. Some of these factors, both intrinsic to patients and external to them are: co-occurring mental disorders, medication side effects, long waiting times, and inadequate understanding of the proposed treatment (22). For short-term pharmacotherapeutic interventions, counseling, written materials and personal phone support may be helpful (23). In general, interventions that are effective in increasing long-term medication adherence, albeit modestly, includes providing information, counseling, reminders, self-monitoring, reinforcement, family therapy, additional supervision or attention, and higher convenience of care (24).

Reid et al. (25) conducted a randomized controlled trial with 40 subjects with alcohol dependence of four to six individual sessions of usual medical care versus a compliance therapy for acamprosate consisting of: exploration of the patient's beliefs and ambivalence about alcohol dependence and the nature of medication and psychosocial treatment; addressing the patient's concerns, symptoms and side effects; supporting patient's evaluation of benefits and consequences of sobriety versus a return to drinking; and support for self-efficacy and continued treatment engagement. Post-hoc analyses of the group that attended at least 50% of the compliance groups demonstrated significantly more days on acamprosate and more days to an extended relapse (3 or more days of more than five drinks) than the usual care group. Therefore psychosocial interventions specifically aimed at supporting medication adherence appear to have clinical impact; however, a common concern in both the acamprosate and the disulfiram studies is that better results may not be caused by better adherence, but rather a common other trait results in both better adherence and better addictions treatment outcome.

Network therapy has as one of its main foci to enlist the aid of the patient's supportive others to assist in optimizing patient adherence with medications. An 18-week randomized controlled trial of network therapy or medication management in opioid-dependent patients receiving daily Suboxone (16 mg) demonstrated higher abstinence rates in the network therapy group (26).

Sometimes strategies designed to promote medication adherence do not demonstrate the magnitude of effects because of patient characteristics or from loss of impact over time. Naltrexone would seem to be a tailor-made medication for opioid dependent patients; however, adherence rates are very poor. Preston et al. (27) conducted a 3-month randomized clinical trial in detoxified patients with opioid dependence ($n = 58$) using CM voucher incentives for adherence to naltrexone, versus random vouchers independent of adherence, versus giving no vouchers. Those getting the contingent vouchers had better treatment retention and a higher number of naltrexone doses taken than either control group. Behavioral naltrexone therapy was a therapy specifically developed to improve retention on oral naltrexone by adding elements of contingency management as above, motivational interviewing and cognitive behavior therapy (CBT), and a significant other for monitoring medication adherence similar to network therapy (28). However, in a 6-month, randomized, controlled trial in heroin-dependent patients, behavioral naltrexone therapy ($n = 36$) improved retention in treatment compared to standard medical management, but overall treatment dropout was very high (>75%) and there was no between-groups difference in the subjects who were very adherent (i.e., >70% of doses) with the medications (29).

MEDICAL MANAGEMENT

Medical Management (MM) is a manualized intervention that is a composite of several different psychosocial interventions focusing on medication compliance and psychosocial treatment engagement and adherence, all of which were integrated for use in the Project Combining Medications and Behavioral Interventions (COMBINE) study (30). The MM intervention is semistructured, and brief in both duration (about nine sessions) and for each session (about 20 minutes after the initial 40-minute session) suitable for delivery in a primary care environment by a medical professional, and with some adaptation, could focus on medications other than that used in COMBINE, and on SUD other than alcohol dependence (31). The manual is available for hard copy order or online *(http://pubs.niaaa.nih.gov/publications/combine/)* and is highly recommended by the authors as probably the most clinically useful, evidence-based practice manual available the addictions clinician who combines medications and psychosocial interventions in typical office visits. The initial intervention has several components, each of which has evidence supporting its use—using targeted feedback of medical information and individualized advice, the intervention motivates the patient toward medication adherence and reduction in harmful substance use, educates the patient about the need for medication, and offers referral to support groups, such as AA. Brief interventions have a substantial evidence base, and brief motivational interviewing type interventions have been demonstrated as more effective than traditional advice giving in the treatment of alcohol and other drug dependence, with small to moderate effect sizes (32–34). Giving the patient self-help materials and supporting involvement in mutual self-help groups each has support in the research literature (35–37). It should be pointed out that in Project COMBINE, the most expensive multisite trial that National Institute on Alcohol Abuse and Alcoholism has performed to date, that evaluated the effect of both psychosocial and medications (acamprosate and naltrexone), that this relatively brief, but well-rounded biopsychosocial therapy alone accounted for the bulk of positive treatment outcome whether the patients took active or placebo medications. Thus MM is a model that the busy clinician can use, whether using medications as part of treatment or not. Further, as mentioned previously, though not yet tested, it is likely that the MM strategy and structure of sessions would also allow apply for better adherence to both psychosocial and psychiatric medication interventions, and thus outcomes, for those with addictions and co-occurring psychiatric disorders.

The intrinsic themes of MM are: educating the patient about the disorder and its specific personal impact; advising the patient about the nature of the treatment, the specific rationale for the medication, and the importance of medication adherence; and recovery support in the form of discussion and advice for implementing medication adherence and alcohol or drug abstinence strategies (38). The initial MM visit takes place after comprehensive clinical evaluation and lasts 40 to 60 minutes. In many cases in clinical practice, this may be shortly after the initial evaluation, but it is optimal to have an interval within which the clinician can compile the relevant medical information necessary for the initial feedback to the patient. In the case of alcohol problems, these data will typically include blood pressure, liver enzymes, other significant labs (e.g., urine or blood), findings on physical exam, recent alcohol intake (days, amount/day), self-reported alcohol problems, and description of specific alcohol dependence or abuse symptoms (30). The MM manual offers a Clinician Report (form A-1) that offers a concise format in which to record the salient data. The clinician reviews the results of the evaluation with the patient, first focusing on the medical data, and then moving to a review of the symptoms of alcohol dependence that the patient endorsed. Any medical concerns of the patient are addressed. The intent is to link the patient's use of alcohol in this case, to each biopsychosocial consequence that has been identified. Having done so, and answering his or her questions, the patient is then given information about alcohol dependence in a clear, nonthreatening, and supportive manner, and advised to stop drinking.

Framing the problem as a routine medical one and offering a friendly "can-do" attitude about treatment and recovery supports the patient in not feeling impugned by the clinician, because patients with SUD are frequently full of shame or hopelessness about their drinking. Communicating a judgmental attitude is likely to engender more resistance to treatment engagement. The clinician advises the patient about the rationale and use of pharmacotherapy as an important medical strategy in assisting recovery. The patient is then instructed about how to take the medicine, and potential side effects are discussed in advance to minimize their contribution to nonadherence (38). The clinician also discusses the rationale of checking the patient's adherence with medication at each subsequent session. The patient's past patterns of medication adherence are evaluated and discussed, so that the patient and clinician together can elaborate a specific plan to assist the patient in remaining adherent with the regimen. The MM manual appendix has a Medication Compliance Plan (form A-13) that can assist the clinician in formalizing the plan with a patient. Finally, the patient is given education and encouragement for attendance at support groups such as AA, and is given brochures and other written materials that have source information on medications, alcohol dependence, and recovery groups. Time is given to the patient to raise questions about the diagnosis or treatment plan (30).

In each of the subsequent visits, which typically range from 15 to 25 minutes, the clinician checks the patient in terms of medical status, appropriate laboratory data, vital signs and weight, and evaluates the blood alcohol concentration. Then the drinking status is asked about, focusing on how the patient coped: with difficulty or ease, the strength of the desire to drink, or in the case of continued drinking, what was the context of use. If the patient is abstinent, other problems, such as an increase in other drug use are evaluated.

Because patients often stop medications when they feel better, it is important that the patient is instructed that even if he or she is doing well in treatment and is abstinent, that is not the time to stop the medication. The patient should be given positive feedback for medication adherence, and the positive health and lifestyle impact of abstinence are reiterated.

If the desire to drink has reduced but the patient is still drinking, that reduction is reinforced as a first step toward change. A nonjudgmental attitude is key in supporting that change may occur slowly, that there may be ups and downs along the way, and that continuing attempts are associated with success. Any positive step, however small, in reduction in use or craving is given positive feedback, and consistent with supportive therapy, the clinician looks for opportunities to provide appropriate, data-based praise (6). If it is earlier in treatment, and the patient is continuing to drink but adherent to the medication, it is important that the patient is told that the medication has not yet had sufficient time to work completely. In addition, the patient is encouraged to attend mutual support groups. In determining the patient's context of use, the patient can be advised to avoid "people, places, and things" associated with use, or to substitute a different healthy pleasure at the time when use usually occurs.

Clinician: "So, how have you been doing over the past week?"

Patient: "I'm taking the naltrexone, but it makes me a little jittery and queasy after I take it."

Clinician: "We discussed that it might do that. Is it severe enough to make you want to stop?"

Patient: "No, It's not too bad. I just distract myself and it gets better as the day goes on. I'm using the plan we talked about!"

Clinician: "Well, it's really good that you are able to continue on it, and usually, those side effects tend to go away over time. Any effects on your desire to drink?"

Patient: "I think so, maybe a little. I hadn't really thought about it. I still get pretty strong urges at times, but I think maybe they're less frequent."

Clinician: "Changes in your desire to drink may be an early sign of a change for you. How well were you able to keep from drinking?"

Patient: "I'm still drinking, but I think it's less—twice this week—Wednesday and yesterday, I started and basically had had enough after two drinks. That's not regular for me. Actually, I didn't even finish the second one yesterday. Funny, I don't know why, I just lost interest!"

Clinician: "Well, you've only been on the medication for a week, and we know it takes time to fully kick in. What's happening with going to AA?"

Patient: "I went to a meeting on the day after I saw you, then I started drinking again and sort of figured 'What the hey?'"

Clinician: "You know, that 'what the hey' attitude frequently comes with the experience of relapse, almost automatically. One of the benefits of going to meetings is that it offers social support for abstinence. Listening to all those stories and folks succeeding in their recovery can really help motivate and support you in your own recovery."

Patient: "I know, I think I need to plan it out in advance, so I know where I'm supposed to go. That way it'll be easier to get to the meetings."

Clinician: "That's an excellent way to anticipate problems in getting support for yourself by planning properly. Can we review? In spite of it giving you some uncomfortable feelings, you are sticking with the medications and coping with unpleasant effects according to your plan, which demonstrates your commitment. And though you briefly relapsed, your alcohol intake has diminished somewhat. All in all, I'd say that was progress. You are making better plans to get to AA meetings; in fact, let's talk about what specific meeting you are going to go to next, where it is, and what you will say when you get there."

The patient who is abstinent but not taking medications as prescribed is given positive feedback for not drinking and the general benefits of abstinence are reinforced. The reasons for the nonadherence (e.g., side effects, forgetting, misinformation) are explored with the patient, and the clinician presents the patient with the information that over time the risks of relapse are reduced on the medication. The compliance plan is amended with strategies addressing the reasons for non-adherence.

The patient, who is nonadherent to medications and is drinking but motivated to stop, is encouraged to engage in treatment more fully. The medical rationale for treatment that was explained in the initial MM visit is repeated. As mentioned, the reasons for nonadherence with medication are explored and the compliance plan is amended with strategies addressing the reasons for nonadherence.

STRATEGIES TO INTEGRATE MEDICATION TREATMENT AND BEHAVIORAL THERAPIES

There is not yet a wealth of empiric data to support the concept, and there clearly has not been a great deal of positive results for attempts at elucidating the beneficial effects of treatment matching (37,39). Nonetheless, because no singular treatment is a "slam dunk," it is still clinically sensible to have an approach to relapse to substance use that places as many barriers as practicable of differing content and strategy in the way of the addict struggling with craving and relapse opportunities. This means that both external and internal structures can be brought to bear in this process, and that combination of different interventions, whether psychosocial or pharmacologic, may have convergent or complementary effects on the inhibition of relapse. In the context of providing an appropriate behavioral therapy platform for use in pharmacotherapy trials, Carroll et al. (40) described the available empirically supported and well-operationalized behavioral therapies as having a range of possible targets such as enhancing medication adherence, reducing attrition, addressing co-occurring problems, promoting abstinence, and targeting specific weaknesses of the pharmacologic agent.

Poldrugo (41) conceptualized the impact of pharmacotherapy for substance use disorders, in this case alcohol dependence, as biologically enhancing mechanisms of either external or internal control. For example, disulfiram, as an aversive agent, would be considered as supporting of external control. Medications that purportedly affected the endogenous reward system, such as neuromodulators like acamprosate, or inhibitors of substance-induced reward like naltrexone, would be considered enhancers of mechanisms of internal control. So, in constructing a combination medication and psychosocial intervention for alcohol dependence, one could consider aligning psychosocial interventions that either augment the control impact of the medication, or offer a complementary control locus. Expanding the concept along similar lines, Mattson and Litten (42) described four strategies for combining medications and behavioral therapies in alcohol dependence, probably the addiction domain best researched for treatment matching and combining behavioral therapy with medication: 1) targeting the same drinking behavior with both the medication and behavioral intervention; 2) medications and therapy each targeting one of two different drinking behaviors; 3) targeting a drinking behavior and a secondary problem that creates a context for drinking or impairs recovery, such as co-occurring mental illness, family problems, or comorbid medical disorders; and 4) adding to a medication regimen a behavioral therapy specifically targeting medication adherence or treatment retention, which was discussed previously. The other strategies will be discussed below, not only in the context of alcohol dependence, but also with other drug dependence.

Using Matching Data to Facilitate Integration In a recent post-hoc analysis of Project MATCH data, alcohol-dependent patients with social networks supportive of drinking had better short-term outcomes if they were assigned to twelve-step facilitation (TSF; 43). This has face validity as a convergent strategy in that TSF attempts to reduce social support for drinking behavior through linkage with the pro-abstinence social support found in AA. Patient characteristics may also interact with the effectiveness of certain types of behavioral intervention. In another Project MATCH data reanalysis using growth mixture modeling, individuals with lower self-efficacy who received CBT drank far less frequently than did those with low self-efficacy who received motivational therapy (44). This also has face validity in that CBT attempts to increase patient's self-efficacy related to abstinence (45). Certain character traits may also have negative impact in the context of specific therapies. For example, across Project MATCH therapies (CBT, MET, and TSF), alcohol-dependent patients ($n = 141$) treated in a more confrontative and directive therapy who had moderate to high trait reactance (the tendency to resist relinquishing control) had worse 1-year alcohol outcomes than those with low trait reactance, but especially so in the MET group (46).

Convergent Strategies Naltrexone has been demonstrated in meta-analyses to be a medication effective in the treatment of alcohol dependence with the greatest effect on reduction in relapse to heavy drinking, modulated either by reductions in cue-induced reward or by reducing the rewarding effects of alcohol, or both (47–50). Recent work by Myrick et al. (51) demonstrates that naltrexone reduces alcohol cue-induced brain activation. Therefore, with naltrexone therapy in alcohol dependence, one could use a complementary behavioral intervention strategy that supported noninitiation of drinking, or a convergent one that increased the likelihood of a slip remaining a slip (a drink or two) rather than becoming a relapse (a binge). Similarly, the craving reduction aspect of naltrexone could be paired as a convergent strategy with the craving attenuating effects of CBT or cue extinction therapy.

In randomized trials of a convergent strategy, Balldin et al. (52) and Heinala et al. (53) found that CBT focused on coping with a slip produced better reductions in relapse to heavy drinking than abstinence-focused supportive therapy when paired with naltrexone. In contrast, O'Malley et al. (54) in a four-cell randomized comparison ($n = 97$) of naltrexone versus placebo, and also CBT versus supportive therapy, demonstrated better cumulative alcohol abstinence rates in the naltrexone-treated patients who were given supportive therapy as compared with CBT. However, taking into consideration that the main effect of naltrexone is reduction in relapse to heavy drinking, the O'Malley et al. (54) study also demonstrated this in the CBT group compared to the group receiving supportive therapy. Anton et al. (55) tested naltrexone against placebo in a 12-week RCT in 131 detoxified alcohol-dependent outpatients who were offered weekly CBT. The group treated with naltrexone had fewer subjects who relapsed, a longer time to relapse to heavy drinking, fewer drinks per drinking day, and higher percentage of days abstinent. Interestingly, the naltrexone-treated group appeared to make better use of CBT—they had more resistance to alcohol-treated thoughts and urges as measured on the Obsessive Compulsive Drinking Scale. More recently, Anton et al. (56) completed a 12-week RCT testing naltrexone versus placebo, combined with either CBT or MET in 120 outpatient alcohol dependent subjects. Again, subjects receiving CBT and naltrexone had significantly fewer relapses to heavy drinking (OR 0.40) than the other groups, and those that did had a longer time to subsequent relapses. It is hypothesized that CBT offers specific skills to deal with craving, high-risk situations, and family conflict that may be a more complete adjunct to the effects of naltrexone than MET provides. Thus, taken together, it is reasonable to provide CBT and naltrexone in combination as a convergent strategy to decrease relapse to heavy drinking in alcohol dependent patients.

Complementary Strategies Stanton and Shadish (57) demonstrated in a meta-analysis of randomized trials that compared to individual and peer group therapy, family and couples therapies have significantly better impact on recovery from substance dependence. As a complementary strategy, behavioral couples therapy (BCT), a well-researched and effective behavioral intervention, can provide elements of increased social support for the patient's efforts to change and contingency for sobriety, whereas disulfiram can assist the maintenance of sobriety through deterrence (58). Meta-analysis of BCT studies demonstrate its superiority over individual interventions for alcohol and drug abuse at treatment follow-up on frequency of use, consequences of use and relationship satisfaction (59). As one part of BCT, the couple enters into a disulfiram contract, an agreement that stipulates that the spouse observes and records on a calendar the patient taking the daily disulfiram dose, the patient and spouse then thank each other for their efforts, and refrain from arguments or discussions about the patient's drinking behavior (60). The structured way of relating around the patient's use of sobriety-supporting medications helps to reduce relationship dysfunction in the couple, which is seen as a major driver of substance use.

In a variant of BCT, Fals-Stewart and O'Farrell (61) used naltrexone contracting with 124 opioid-dependent men and the family members they lived with in a randomized 24-week trial of behavioral family contracting and individual therapy versus individual therapy alone. The behavioral family contracting patients took more doses of naltrexone, were more compliant with scheduled sessions, had longer continuous abstinence, and more opioid and other illicit drug abstinence during and for the year after treatment. They also had fewer drug-related, legal, and family problems at 1-year follow-up. In this example of complementary strategies, behavioral family contracting increased medication adherence and provided social support for continuing opioid abstinence, whereas naltrexone blocked the rewarding effects of opioids. Because the effects of BCT tend to fade over time, as couples tend to regress back toward dysfunctional relating, a study of booster relapse prevention sessions provided to couples after the main treatment had ended supported the maintenance of treatment gains (62).

Other psychosocial interventions may introduce similar convergent factors or complementary factors other than increasing social support or reducing relapse potential, which have equivalent impact as CBT in the context of naltrexone. Latt et al. (63) demonstrated in an RCT ($n = 107$) that naltrexone with adjunctive medical advice in a primary care setting was effective in reducing the relapse to heavy drinking by about 50% irrespective of whether it was accompanied by counseling and supportive therapy. Similarly, in a comparison of CBT and primary care management in 197 alcohol-dependent subjects treated with naltrexone, O'Malley et al. (64) found that the primary care intervention (including referral to and support of AA attendance, medication issues and adherence support, and clinical advice) had similar impact over 10 weeks on reducing relapse to heavy drinking as did CBT. However, the CBT group was better at maintaining days of abstinence over time.

The interaction of bupropion and CM is another complimentary strategy, where the bupropion may affect subjective negative mood and cognitive symptoms post–cocaine withdrawal, and the CM reinforces retention in treatment and rewards abstinence. Poling et al. (65) conducted a 25-week, a double-blind RCT in methadone-maintained, but cocaine-dependent patients ($n = 106$) with four cells: CM that gave vouchers for negative cocaine urine screens and abstinence-related activities and medication placebo, CM and bupropion 300 mg/day, control vouchers for giving urine specimens and placebo medication, or control vouchers and bupropion. Although bupropion had independent effects upon cocaine use over the 12 weeks, results demonstrated that bupropion plus CM significantly improved cocaine outcomes relative to bupropion alone.

Sometimes reasonable complementary strategies don't work synergistically, perhaps because one of the interventions is more robust. Disulfiram is hypothesized to reduce cocaine use through direct impact on neurotransmitter metabolism, reducing the pleasurable effects of cocaine, whereas CBT supports maintenance of abstinence through cognitive restructuring in the form of functional analysis and new skills acquisition (66,67). CBT was tested by Carroll et al. (68) against interpersonal psychotherapy (IPT) in a four cell (disulfiram/CBT; disulfiram/IPT; placebo/CBT; placebo/IPT) 12-week comparison with disulfiram versus placebo in 121 cocaine-dependent patients. Cocaine use was reduced significantly in the disulfiram group, and in the CBT group compared with the IPT group in the context of placebo, but there was no difference between therapies in the context of disulfiram. The effects of the disulfiram on cocaine use were greatest in subjects who were abstinent from alcohol or not alcohol-dependent at baseline suggesting that the effects of disulfiram are not moderated by its effect on alcohol use.

Other Strategies Combination strategies can also target the substance use disorder, and in addition attempt to treat cooccurring mental or medical disorders. It is clear that both disorders need to be targeted independently, although there may be some convergent effects in treating the co-occurring disorder. For example, depression and depressive symptoms have an adverse effect on recovery from SUD. Although it has been reasonable to test a parsimonious treatment such as a selective serotonin reuptake inhibitor to attempt to treat both the depression and the SUD, meta-analysis of this strategy has demonstrated that antidepressant medications are efficacious for the treatment of depression in patients with SUD, but that other interventions are necessary for treating the SUD (69). For example, Stein et al. (70) conducted an RCT of citalopram plus eight sessions of CBT for depression compared with an assessment control condition in 109 active injection drug users with a DSM-IV mood disorder spectrum diagnosis and a Hamilton Rating Scale for Depression (HAM-D) > 13. At follow-up, more than twice the patients receiving the intervention were in remission of the depression, but there was no impact on heroin or cocaine use. In addition to the lack of evidence that treating other co-occurring mental disorders is clinically effective for SUD, some interventions for mental disorders can have adverse impact on SUD. Recent data have suggested that a subset of alcohol dependent patients with Type A alcoholism (later onset) may respond differentially to selective serotonin reuptake inhibitor treatment compared with placebo with reductions in drinking, but that Type B (early onset) alcoholics may actually do worse (71,72).

Patients treated with methadone maintenance often have problems in multiple life dimensions other than substance dependence, and some of these are likely to respond to psychosocial interventions that may also promote abstinence from illicit opioids. Specific gains in psychosocial therapy of methadone-maintained patients tends to be related to the type of therapy (e.g., supportive-expressive, CBT) the patient is exposed to over an in addition to counseling alone, and impacts psychiatric symptoms (73). The improvement in psychologic functioning is correlated with better overall functioning, including SUD, thus it is sensible to provide behavioral therapies to patients on methadone who have psychiatric symptoms (74).

Principles for Care Integration There are no research data to demonstrate whether convergent or complementary strategies have more robust effects. It is likely that there will be individual patient characteristics such as genetics, addiction severity, comorbidity, and drug of choice that will impact what the optimal combination of medications and psychosocial interventions will be. As such, a stagewise approach to recovery may help to guide the clinician as to choosing an appropriate mix of medication and therapy. The clinician can determine what the important tasks are for this stage in treatment. For example, in establishing abstinence, there are several acute issues that typically need to be dealt with: negative mood states and craving, conditioned cues, access to substances, and immersion in contexts supportive of substance use. Thus one could pick treatments based on the impact in those various domains (e.g., reducing social isolation and offering social support for sobriety with mutual self-help groups and TSF, BCT, or network therapy); supporting treatment engagement with motivational interviewing; supporting cognitive and coping skills functioning in early recovery with CBT/relapse prevention or improving baseline cognitive deficits with appropriate medications; reducing alcohol craving with naltrexone, opioid craving with buprenorphine or methadone; supporting self-efficacy and resilience for craving and negative states with CBT; and reducing substance use with CM, and supporting alcohol abstinence with disulfiram or acamprosate. Fortunately, in most cases, appropriately applied interventions are not usually mutually exclusive (e.g., disulfiram and moderation management—if the patient is alcohol dependent, warranting disulfiram, then moderation management is inappropriate because of the patient's loss of control).

CONCLUSION

This chapter has aimed to provide the addiction treatment provider both theoretical and practical information and techniques on the integrated use of medications and psychotherapies for addiction treatment. It is recognized that in today's environment of evidence-based practice that many manualized therapies may be impractical for use in their full form, but that parts of various techniques can be used in an evidence-based manner, and we have supplied rationals for this. Further in this regard, we have strongly advocated that MM (30,38), which is a manualized, evidence-based, and very practical method of such integration be used broadly in the addiction field.

REFERENCES

1. Dutra L, Stathopoulou G, Basden SL, et al. A meta-analytic review of psychosocial interventions for substance use disorders. *Am J Psychiatry* 2008;165:179–187.
2. Miller WR, Wilbourne PL. Mesa Grande: a methodological analysis of clinical trials of treatments for alcohol use disorders. *Addiction* 2002;97:265–77.
3. French MT, Zarkin GA, Hubbard RL, et al. The effects of time in drug abuse treatment and employment on posttreatment drug use and criminal activity. *Am J Drug Alcohol Abuse* 1993;19:19–33.
4. Greenfield L, Fountain D. Influence of time in treatment and follow-up duration on methadone treatment outcomes. *J Psychopathol Behav Assessment* 2000;22:353–364.

5. Nalpas B, Matelak F, Martin S, et al. Clinical management methods for outpatients with alcohol dependence. *Subst Abuse Treat Prev Policy* 2006;1(1):5.
6. Rosenthal RN. Techniques of individual supportive psychotherapy. In: Gabbard GO, ed. *The American psychiatric publishing textbook of psychotherapeutic treatments in psychiatry*, American Psychiatric Publishing, Inc., Washington, DC; 2008:417–445.
7. Kim TW, Samet JH, Cheng DM, et al. Primary care quality and addiction severity: a prospective cohort study. *Health Serv Res* 2007;42(2):755–772.
8. Rogers CR. *Client-centered therapy*. Boston: Houghton-Mifflin, 1951.
9. Pettinati HM, Volpicelli JR, Pierce JD Jr, et al. Improving naltrexone response: an intervention for medical practitioners to enhance medication compliance in alcohol dependent patients. *J Addict Dis* 2000;19: 71–83.
10. Pettinati HM, Monterosso J, Lipkin C, et al. Patient attitudes toward treatment predict attendance in clinical pharmacotherapy trials of alcohol and drug treatment. *Am J Addict* 2003;12(4):324–335.
11. Day E, Ison J, Strang J. Inpatient versus other settings for detoxification for opioid dependence. *Cochrane Database Syst Rev* 2005;2: CD004580.
12. Mark TL, Vandivort-Warren R, Montejano LB. Factors affecting detoxification readmission: analysis of public sector data from three states. *J Subst Abuse Treat* 2006;31(4):439–445. [Epub 2006 Sep 7.]
13. Amato L, Minozzi S, Davoli M, et al. Psychosocial and pharmacological treatments versus pharmacological treatments for opioid detoxification. *Cochrane Database Syst Rev* 2008;(3):CD005031.
14. Iguchi MY, Stitzer ML. Predictors of opiate drug abuse during a 90-day methadone detoxification. *Am J Drug Alcohol Abuse* 1991;17(3):279–294.
15. Sees KL, Delucchi KL, Masson C, et al. Methadone maintenance vs 180-day psychosocially enriched detoxification for treatment of opioid dependence: a randomized controlled trial. *JAMA* 2000;283(10): 1303–1310.
16. McCaul ME, Stitzer ML, Bigelow GE, et al. Contingency management interventions: effects on treatment outcome during methadone detoxification. *J Appl Behav Anal* 1984;17(1):35–43.
17. Soyka M, Horak M. Outpatient alcohol detoxification: implementation efficacy and outcome effectiveness of a model project. *Eur Addict Res* 2004;10(4):180–187.
18. McLellan AT, Lewis DC, O'Brien CP, et al. Drug dependence, a chronic medical illness: implications for treatment, insurance, and outcomes evaluation. *JAMA* 2000;284(13):1689–1695.
19. Volpicelli JR, Rhines KC, Rhines JS, et al. Naltrexone and alcohol dependence. Role of subject compliance. *Arch Gen Psychiatry* 1997;54(8): 737–742.
20. Fuller RK, Branchey L, Brightwell DR, et al. Disulfiram treatment of alcoholism: a Veterans Administration cooperative study. *JAMA* 1986;256:1449–1455.
21. O'Malley SS, Carroll KM. Psychotherapeutic considerations in pharmacological trials. *Alcohol Clin Exp Res* 1996;20(S7):17A–22A.
22. Rohsenow DJ, Colby SM, Monti PM, et al. Predictors of compliance with naltrexone among alcoholics. *Alcohol Clin Exp Res* 2000 Oct;24(10): 1542–1549.
23. Haynes RB, Ackloo E, Sahota N, et al. Interventions for enhancing medication adherence. *Cochrane Database Syst Rev* 2008, Issue 2. Art. No.: CD000011. DOI: 10.1002/14651858.CD000011.pub3.
24. McDonald HP, Garg AX, Haynes RB. Interventions to enhance patient adherence to medication prescriptions: scientific review. *JAMA* 2002;288(22):2868–2879. Review. Erratum in: *JAMA* 2003;289(24): 3242.
25. Reid SC, Teesson M, Sannibale C, et al. The efficacy of compliance therapy in pharmacotherapy for alcohol dependence: a randomized controlled trial. *J Stud Alcohol* 2005;66(6):833–841.
26. Galanter M, Dermatis H, Glickman L, et al. Network therapy: decreased secondary opioid use during buprenorphine maintenance. *J Subst Abuse Treatment* 2004;26:313–318.
27. Preston KL, Silverman K, Umbricht A, et al. Improvement in naltrexone treatment compliance with contingency management. *Drug Alcohol Depend* 1999;54:127–135.
28. Rothenberg JL, Sullivan MA, Church SH, et al. Behavioral naltrexone therapy: an integrated treatment for opiate dependence. *J Subst Abuse Treat* 2002;23(4):351–360.
29. Nunes EV, Rothenberg JL, Sullivan MA, et al. Behavioral therapy to augment oral naltrexone for opioid dependence: a ceiling on effectiveness? *Am J Drug Alcohol Abuse* 2006;32(4):503–517.
30. Pettinati HM, Weiss RD, Dundon W, et al. *COMBINE monograph series, volume 2. Medical management treatment manual: a clinical research guide for medically trained clinicians providing pharmacotherapy as part of the treatment for alcohol dependence.* DHHS Publication No. (NIH) 04-5289. Bethesda, MD: NIAAA, 2004.
31. Fiellin DA, Reid MC, O'Connor PG. New therapies for alcohol problems: application to primary care. *Am J Med* 2000;108(3):227–237.
32. Burke BL, Arkowitz H, Menchola M. The efficacy of motivational interviewing: a meta-analysis of controlled clinical trials. *J Consult Clin Psychol* 2003;71(5):843–681.
33. Rubak S, Sandbæk A, Lauritzen T, et al. Motivational interviewing: a systematic review and meta-analysis. *Br J Gen Pract* 2005;55(513): 305–312.
34. Vasilaki EI, Hosier SG, Cox WM. The efficacy of motivational interviewing as a brief intervention for excessive drinking: a meta-analytic review. *Alcohol Alcohol* 2006;41(3):328–335. Epub 2006 Mar 17. Review.
35. Apodaca TR, Miller WR. A meta-analysis of the effectiveness of bibliotherapy for alcohol problems. *J Clin Psycho*. 2003;59(3):289–304.
36. Nowinski J, Baker S, Carroll K. *Twelve-step facilitation therapy manual: a clinical research guide for therapists treating individuals with alcohol abuse and dependence.* Project MATCH Monograph Series, vol. 1. DHHS Publication No. (ADM)92-1893. Bethesda, MD: National Institute on Alcohol Abuse and Alcoholism, 1992.
37. Project MATCH Research Group. Matching alcoholism treatments to client heterogeneity: treatment main effects and matching effects on drinking during treatment. *J Stud Alcohol* 1998;59:631–639.
38. Pettinati HM, Weiss RD, Dundon W, et al. A structured approach to medical management: a psychosocial intervention to support pharmacotherapy in the treatment of alcohol dependence. *J Stud Alcohol Suppl* 2005;(15):170–178; discussion 168–689.
39. UKATT Research Team. UK Alcohol Treatment Trial: client-treatment matching effects. *Addiction* 2008;103(2):228–238. Epub 2007 Dec 7.
40. Carroll KM, Kosten TR, Rounsaville BJ. Choosing a behavioral therapy platform for pharmacotherapy of substance users. *Drug Alcohol Depend* 2004;75(2):123–134. Review.
41. Poldrugo F. Integration of pharmacotherapies in the existing programs for the treatment of alcoholics: an international perspective. *J Addict Dis* 1997;16(4):65–82.
42. Mattson ME, Litten RZ. Combining treatments for alcoholism: why and how? *J Stud Alcohol Suppl* 2005(15):8–16; discussion 6–7. Review.
43. Wu J, Witkiewitz K. Network support for drinking: an application of multiple groups growth mixture modeling to examine client-treatment matching. *J Stud Alcohol Drugs* 2008;69(1):21–29.
44. Witkiewitz K, van der Maas HL, Hufford MR, et al. Nonnormality and divergence in posttreatment alcohol use: reexamining the Project MATCH data "another way." *J Abnorm Psychol* 2007;116(2):378–394.
45. Kadden R, Carroll KM, Donovan D, et al. Cognitive-behavioral coping skills therapy manual: a clinical research guide for therapists treating individuals with alcohol abuse and dependence. *NIAAA Project MATCH Monograph Series, vol. 3.* DHHS Pub. No. (ADM)92-1895. Rockville, MD: National Institute on Alcohol Abuse and Alcoholism, 1992.
46. Karno MP, Longabaugh R. Less directiveness by therapists improves drinking outcomes of reactant clients in alcoholism treatment. *J Consult Clin Psychol* 2005;73(2):262–267.
47. Bouza C, Angeles M, Muñoz A, et al. Efficacy and safety of naltrexone and acamprosate in the treatment of alcohol dependence: a systematic review. *Addiction* 2004;99:811–828.
48. Rosenthal RN. Current and future drug therapies for alcohol dependence. *J Clin Psychopharmacology* 2006;26[suppl 1]:S20–S29.

49. Rösner S, Leucht S, Lehert P, et al. Acamprosate supports abstinence, naltrexone prevents excessive drinking: evidence from a meta-analysis with unreported outcomes. *J Psychopharmacol* 2008;22(1):11–23.
50. Srisurapanont M, Jarusuraisin N. Naltrexone for the treatment of alcoholism: a meta-analysis of randomized controlled trials. *Int J Neuropsychopharmacol* 2005;8(2):267–280.
51. Myrick H, Anton RF, Li X, et al. Effect of naltrexone and ondansetron on alcohol cue-induced activation of the ventral striatum in alcohol-dependent people. *Arch Gen Psychiatry* 2008;65(4):466–475.
52. Balldin J, Berglund M, Borg S, et al. A 6-month controlled naltrexone study: combined effect with cognitive behavioral therapy in outpatient treatment of alcohol dependence. *Alcohol Clin Exp Res* 2003;27(7):1142–1149.
53. Heinälä P, Alho H, Kiianmaa K, et al. Targeted use of naltrexone without prior detoxification in the treatment of alcohol dependence: a factorial double-blind, placebo-controlled trial. *J Clin Psychopharmacol* 2001;21(3):287–292.
54. O'Malley SS, Jaffe AJ, Chang G, et al. Naltrexone and coping skills therapy for alcohol dependence. A controlled study. *Arch Gen Psychiatry* 1992;49(11):881–887.
55. Anton RF, Moak DH, Waid LR, et al. Naltrexone and cognitive behavioral therapy for the treatment of outpatient alcoholics: results of a placebo-controlled trial. *Am J Psychiatry* 1999;156(11):1758–1764.
56. Anton RF, Moak DH, Latham P, et al. Naltrexone combined with either cognitive behavioral or motivational enhancement therapy for alcohol dependence. *J Clin Psychopharmacol* 2005;25(4):349–357.
57. Stanton MD, Shadish WR. Outcome, attrition, and family-couple treatment for drug abuse: a meta-analysis and review of the controlled, comparative studies. *Psychol Bull* 1997;122:170–191.
58. Azrin NH, Sisson RW, Meyers R, et al. Alcoholism treatment by disulfiram and community reinforcement therapy. *J Behav Ther Exp Psychiatry* 1982;13(2):105–112.
59. Powers MB, Vedel E, Emmelkamp PM. Behavioral couples therapy (BCT) for alcohol and drug use disorders: a meta-analysis. *Clin Psychol Rev* 2008;28(6):952–962. Epub 2008 Feb 16.
60. O'Farrell TJ, Bayog RD. Antabuse contracts for married alcoholics and their spouses: a method to maintain Antabuse ingestion and decrease conflict about drinking. *J Subst Abuse Treat* 1986;3(1):1–8.
61. Fals-Stewart W, O'Farrell TJ. Behavioral family counseling and naltrexone compliance for male opioid-dependent patients. *J Consult Clin Psychol* 2003;71(3):432–442.
62. O'Farrell TJ, Choquette KA, Cutter HS, et al. Behavioral marital therapy with and without additional couples relapse prevention sessions for alcoholics and their wives. *J Stud Alcohol* 1993;54(6):652–666.
63. Latt NC, Jurd S, Houseman J, et al. Naltrexone in alcohol dependence: a randomised controlled trial of effectiveness in a standard clinical setting. *Med J Aust* 2002;176(11):530–534.
64. O'Malley SS, Rounsaville BJ, Farren C, et al. Initial and maintenance naltrexone treatment for alcohol dependence using primary care vs. specialty care: a nested sequence of 3 randomized trials. *Arch Intern Med* 2003;163(14):1695–1704.
65. Poling J, Oliveto A, Petry N, et al. Six-month trial of bupropion with contingency management for cocaine dependence in a methadone-maintained population. *Arch Gen Psychiatry* 2006;63(2):219–228.
66. Baker JR, Jatlow P, McCance-Katz EF. Disulfiram effects on responses to intravenous cocaine administration. *Drug Alcohol Depend* 2007;87(2–3):202–209. [Epub 2006 Sep 18.]
67. McCance-Katz EF, Kosten TR, Jatlow P. Chronic disulfiram treatment effects on intranasal cocaine administration: initial results. *Biol Psychiatry* 1998;43(7):540–543.
68. Carroll KM, Fenton LR, Ball SA, et al. Efficacy of disulfiram and cognitive behavior therapy in cocaine-dependent outpatients: a randomized placebo-controlled trial. *Arch Gen Psychiatry* 2004;61(3):264–272.
69. Nunes EV, Levin FR. Treatment of depression in patients with alcohol or other drug dependence: a meta-analysis. *JAMA* 2004;291(15):1887–1896. Review.
70. Stein MD, Solomon DA, Herman DS, et al. Pharmacotherapy plus psychotherapy for treatment of depression in active injection drug users. *Arch Gen Psychiatry* 2004;61(2):152–159.
71. Kranzler HR, Burleson JA, Brown J, et al. Fluoxetine treatment seems to reduce the beneficial effects of cognitive-behavioral therapy in type B alcoholics. *Alcohol Clin Exp Res* 1996;20(9):1534–1541.
72. Pettinati HM, Volpicelli JR, Kranzler HR, et al. Sertraline treatment for alcohol dependence: interactive effects of medication and alcoholic subtype. *Alcohol Clin Exp Res* 2000;24(7):1041–1049.
73. Woody GE, Luborsky L, McLellan AT, et al. Psychotherapy for opiate addicts. *NIDA Res Monogr* 1983;43:59–70.
74. McLellan AT, Luborsky L, Woody GE, et al. Are the "addiction-related" problems of substance abusers really related? *J Nerv Ment Dis* 1981;169(4):232–239.

SUGGESTED READINGS

Barth J, Critchley J, Bengel J. Psychosocial interventions for smoking cessation in patients with coronary heart disease. *Cochrane Database Syst Rev* 2008 Jan 23;(1):CD006886. Review.

Clark LT. Improving compliance and increasing control of hypertension: needs of special hypertensive populations. *Am Heart J* 1991;121:664–669.

Fals-Stewart W, O'Farrell TJ, Birchler GR. Behavioral couples therapy for substance abuse: rationale, methods, and findings. *Sci Pract Perspect* 2004;2(2):30–41. Review.

Karno MP, Longabaugh R. Does matching matter? Examining matches and mismatches between patient attributes and therapy techniques in alcoholism treatment. *Addiction* 2007;102(4):587–596.

Markowitz JC, Kocsis JH, Christos P, et al. Pilot study of interpersonal psychotherapy versus supportive psychotherapy for dysthymic patients with secondary alcohol abuse or dependence. *J Nerv Ment Dis* 2008;196(6):468–474.

Miller R, Rollnick S. *Motivational interviewing: preparing people to change addictive behavior.* New York: Guilford, 1992.

Prochaska JJ, Delucchi K, Hall SM. A meta-analysis of smoking cessation interventions with individuals in substance abuse treatment or recovery. *J Consult Clin Psychol* 2004;72(6):1144–1156.

Project MATCH Research Group. Matching alcoholism treatments to client heterogeneity: Project MATCH posttreatment drinking outcomes. *J Stud Alcohol* 1997;58:7–29.

Robles E, Stitzer ML, Strain EC, et al. Voucher-based reinforcement of opiate abstinence during methadone detoxification. *Drug Alcohol Depend* 2002;65(2):179–189.

Sees KL, Delucchi KL, Masson C, et al. Methadone maintenance vs 180-day psychosocially enriched detoxification for treatment of opioid dependence: a randomized controlled trial. *JAMA* 2000;283(10):1303–1310.

U.S. DHHS Center for Substance Abuse Treatment Brief Interventions and Brief Therapies for Substance Abuse. *Treatment Improvement Protocol (TIP) Series 34.* DHHS Publication No. (SMA) 99-3353, 1999.

SECTION 9

Mutual Help, Twelve Step, and Other Recovery Programs

SECTION 9

Mutual Help, Twelve Step, and Other Recovery Programs

CHAPTER 67

Jerome E. Schulz, MD, FASAM
Vern Williams, MD
Joseph E. Galligan, MA

Twelve Step Programs in Recovery

Today, millions of people worldwide are living fuller and more complete lives because of their involvement in Twelve Step recovery groups. This discussion of recovery groups will emphasize Alcoholics Anonymous (AA) and its basic philosophy. Other programs—including Al-Anon, Alateen, Narcotics Anonymous, Cocaine Anonymous, and Adult Children of Alcoholics—also will be described.

ALCOHOLICS ANONYMOUS

History AA began in 1935 when a stockbroker (Bill W) met with a physician (Dr. Bob). Bill W was an alcoholic who had a spiritual experience during his fourth detoxification in December 1934, after a visit from a recovering alcoholic friend who was a member of a religious group called the Oxford Movement. A few months later, when a business venture failed during a trip to Akron, Ohio, Bill W's thoughts turned to alcohol as a means to ease the pain. He decided to try to talk to another alcoholic who was also a member of the Oxford Movement. He arranged a meeting with Dr. Bob, an actively drinking alcoholic who was unenthusiastic about meeting with Bill W. A "brief" meeting lasted several hours and marked the beginning of Alcoholics Anonymous. Bill W helped Dr. Bob realize that he suffered from a disease and, in Bill W, Dr. Bob saw someone who had suffered as much as he had from his alcoholism and who was now doing well. Over the following months, Bill W and Dr. Bob began to formulate the basic philosophies of Alcoholics Anonymous, which included reaching out to other alcoholics to help themselves stay sober. The principles that came to guide the organization were published in *Alcoholics Anonymous* (widely known as the "Big Book") in 1939. This publication represented the final break from the Oxford Movement and any apparent connection with a particular religious orientation. It established AA for all alcoholics, including atheists and agnostics.

Overview and Philosophy The preamble of Alcoholics Anonymous, which frequently is read at the beginning of AA meetings, points out many important facts about how AA works:

> *"Alcoholics Anonymous is a fellowship of men and women who share their experience, strength and hope with each other that they may solve their common problem and help others to recover from alcoholism. The only requirement for membership is a desire to stop drinking. There are no dues or fees for AA membership; we are self supporting through our own contributions. AA is not allied with any sect, denomination, politics, organization or institution; does not wish to engage in any controversy; neither endorses nor opposes any causes. Our primary purpose is to stay sober and help other alcoholics to achieve sobriety."*

The Twelve Steps of AA (Table 67.1) describe both the spiritual basis and the necessary actions, which form the backbone of recovery for AA members. AA is a spiritual, not a religious, program. As the AA preamble states, AA is not allied with any sect or denomination. The Twelve Steps have been applied effectively to many other problems in life, such as narcotics, cocaine, gambling, sex, emotions, shopping, and eating disorders.

The Twelve Traditions (Table 67.2), which were formulated in 1945, are the guidelines that help Alcoholics Anonymous

TABLE 67.1 The Twelve Steps of Alcoholics Anonymous

1. We admitted we were powerless over alcohol; that our lives had become unmanageable;
2. Came to believe that a Power greater than ourselves could restore us to sanity;
3. Made a decision to turn our will and our lives over to the care of God as we understood Him;
4. Made a searching and fearless moral inventory of ourselves;
5. Admitted to God, to ourselves, and to another human being the exact nature of our wrongs;
6. Were entirely ready to have God remove all these defects of character;
7. Humbly asked Him to remove our shortcomings;
8. Made a list of all persons we had harmed, and became willing to make amends to them all;
9. Made direct amends to such people wherever possible, except when to do so would injure them or others;
10. Continued to take personal inventory and when we were wrong promptly admitted it;
11. Sought through prayer and meditation to improve our conscious contact with God as we understood Him, praying only for knowledge of His will for us and the power to carry that out; and
12. Having had a spiritual experience (awakening) as the result of these steps, we tried to carry this message to alcoholics, and to practice these principles in all our affairs.

TABLE 67.2 The Twelve Traditions of Alcoholics Anonymous

1. Our common welfare should come first; personal recovery depends on AA unity.
2. For our group purpose there is but one ultimate authority—a loving God as He may express Himself in our group conscience. Our leaders are but trusted servants; they do not govern.
3. The only requirement for AA membership is a desire to stop drinking.
4. Each group should be autonomous except in matters affecting other groups or AA as a whole.
5. Each group has but one primary purpose—to carry its message to the alcoholic who still suffers.
6. An AA group ought never endorse, finance, or lend the AA name to any related facility or outside enterprise, lest problems of money, property, and prestige divert us from our primary purpose.
7. Every AA group ought to be fully self-supporting, declining outside contributions.
8. Alcoholics Anonymous should remain forever nonprofessional, but our service centers may employ special workers.
9. AA, as such, ought never be organized; but we may create service boards or committees directly responsible to those they serve.
10. Alcoholics Anonymous has no opinion on outside issues; hence the AA name ought never be drawn into public controversy.
11. Our public relations policy is based on attraction rather than promotion; we need always maintain personal anonymity at the level of press, radio, and films.
12. Anonymity is the spiritual foundation of all our traditions, ever reminding us to place principles before personalities.

groups survive and function smoothly. The traditions grew out of conflicts that threatened AA's early existence.

Membership and Structure More than 105,000 AA groups with more than 2.0 million members exist in 182 countries worldwide (1). All are guided by the Twelve Traditions, yet no individual or group is "in charge." The General Service Office in New York City serves as a clearinghouse for AA information and publications, under the direction of the General Service Board, which is composed of both alcoholics and nonalcoholics. Neither the Office nor the Board has any authority over AA members or groups. Both are responsible to the AA groups and report annually at the General Service Conference attended by members selected by groups in the United States and Canada. This large, loosely structured, leaderless, democratic system works because AA closely follows the Twelve Traditions. AA has a Web site for further information (*www.aa.org*).

Each AA group is autonomous (as defined in the fourth tradition). This tradition allows AA groups to vary widely in how they apply the Twelve Steps and Twelve Traditions. Membership in AA is simple to obtain: All that is required is to attend a meeting and, according to the third tradition, "have a desire to stop drinking." There is no formal application process or paperwork. Groups may have a phone list so individuals can support and help one another between meetings, but participation is strictly optional. Each member is encouraged to develop his or her personal phone list for use in times of need.

Meetings AA holds both open and closed meetings. Anyone may attend an open meeting, whereas closed meetings are restricted to alcoholics and anyone with a desire to stop drinking. AA meetings usually open with the Serenity Prayer (Table 67.3), after which each participant may introduce himself or herself by saying, "My name is ____, and I'm an alcoholic." There may be several readings, including the Twelve Traditions, "How it Works," the "Promises" (described

TABLE 67.3 The Serenity Prayer of Alcoholics Anonymous

"God grant me the serenity to accept the things I cannot change, the courage to change the things that I can, and the wisdom to know the difference."

Reprinted with permission from Alcoholics Anonymous World Service, Inc.

later), and a daily reflection. At most open meetings, a speaker gives the classic AA talk about "how it was, what happened, and how it is now." Speakers usually talk for an hour or less. They almost never use notes or scripts, because they believe that such spontaneity helps them "talk from the heart and not the head."

In closed meetings, group members may discuss one of the Twelve Steps, a specific topic (such as resentments, fear, or anger), or a reading from *Alcoholics Anonymous*, which serves as the textbook for AA. The Big Book has sold more than 20 million copies in more than 40 languages. An important part of the Big Book, entitled "How it Works" (Chapter 5), often is read at the beginning of AA meetings. The Twelve Steps are part of "How it Works" and also are discussed in the AA publication *Twelve Steps and Twelve Traditions,* the "12 by 12," which describes the important aspects of each of the steps and traditions. AA meetings usually last an hour, and most meetings close with the Lord's Prayer or the Serenity Prayer (described later in the chapter). Many newcomers initially are uncomfortable with the apparent Christian orientation expressed by the Lord's Prayer; however, in the context of AA, the prayer is viewed as a commonly remembered ritual that reminds group members of their need for something other than self in maintaining sobriety. In fact, each group can use any ritual it wishes to open or close the meeting.

Meetings often are followed by socializing over coffee to give members a chance to continue to talk about the meeting topic or just to interact without alcohol—a new experience for most alcoholics. It also gives the newcomer a chance to get to know the other group members.

Types of Groups As AA has grown, many special groups have developed because of the autonomous nature of each AA group. When patients report that they feel uncomfortable at an AA meeting, referral to a special interest group may be helpful. Most large metropolitan areas have special meetings for women, young people, older adults, gays and lesbians, African Americans, and other racial/ethnic groups. Nonsmoking AA meetings are becoming very common. In many areas, there are special meetings for professionals such as nurses, physicians, attorneys, and clergy.

One special group for physicians, psychologists, dentists, veterinarians, educators, and anyone with a doctoral degree is International Doctors in AA (IDAA). IDAA was founded in upstate New York in 1947 by several physicians (three from Canada) and a psychologist. The program is based on the principles of Alcoholics Anonymous. There are more than 6,000 members internationally, many of whom attend the annual IDAA meeting, which is held in different parts of the country (and Canada).

Sponsorship Sponsorship is a basic AA concept. A sponsor generally is someone of the same gender who has been in AA for at least a year. The sponsor becomes a mentor and role model for the newcomer and is an example of how the AA program works. Newcomers are asked to call their sponsors whenever they are thinking about drinking or are having problems (which is very common for newcomers). It also is common for a newcomer to talk with his or her sponsor by telephone between meetings and to meet with the sponsor regularly to discuss progress. The sponsor helps and guides the newcomer to work the Twelve Steps. Newcomers are urged to find a sponsor as soon as possible, and groups often appoint temporary sponsors. AA will provide temporary contacts through the local treatment facilities committee. These temporary contacts can introduce the newcomer to local meetings and members of the fellowship. Sponsorship frequently is a lifelong relationship. After some time in recovery, the AA member may be asked to sponsor a new member. In one 10-year follow up, 91% of alcoholics who became sponsors were in stable sobriety (2).

Anniversaries Sobriety anniversaries are important milestones in AA. Many groups give a "white chip" (a poker chip) to the newcomer attending his or her first AA meeting or the person who has had a relapse and comes back to AA. The white chip signifies surrender and a willingness to try something new to overcome alcoholism. When the newcomer reaches into his or her pocket for drinking money, the chip is a reminder not to drink. Newcomers are given a new chip (different colors) at 1, 2, 3, 6, 9, and 12 months, signifying their continuing sobriety and commitment to recovery. Some groups give out medallions instead of chips. A medallion may have the Serenity Prayer on one side and something about AA on the other side, along with the number of months or years the member has been sober. Anniversaries are special times in AA and may be celebrated with a cake and party. The "dry date," which is the first drug- or alcohol-free day, is an important date for physicians to acknowledge. This date can be put on the patient's problem list along with the diagnosis of alcoholism. Physicians can show support and interest in their patients' recovery by acknowledging anniversaries.

Alcoholics Anonymous Slogans Because many alcoholics suffer permanent cognitive deficits owing to their chronic alcohol intake, AA has many simple slogans and sayings that are repeated frequently at meetings. When recovering alcoholics are having difficulty, these slogans can redirect their thinking and make them less likely to use alcohol or other mood-altering chemicals to overcome their frustration.

The physician's commitment to the patient's recovery is obvious when the physician knows enough about AA to use the slogans.

"One day at a time" is one of the oldest slogans in AA. This slogan emphasizes a basic AA philosophy—that the alcoholic has to be concerned only with today. A lifetime of sobriety can overwhelm many alcoholics. This slogan helps relieve that pressure. This slogan can be applied to drinking and also other life stresses. Alcoholics have all kinds of fears and irrational concerns about what may happen tomorrow, next week, or in the next 100 years. This simple five-word slogan helps them live in the present and take care of just today's problems.

"Easy does it" is another frequently heard slogan. Alcoholics early in recovery tend to want to get everything resolved immediately. They expect years of problems to be resolved the minute they become sober. They frequently want to go on diets, start exercising, quit smoking, and resolve all their personal conflicts. This behavior usually fails and can result in a relapse. "Easy does it" helps recovering alcoholics realize they need to go slowly.

"Let go and let God" emphasizes the spiritual aspect of AA. For alcoholics, attempts to control their drinking can spill over into trying to exert excessive control over other areas of their lives. They overanalyze situations and can develop resentments, which can be fatal errors for the recovering alcoholic. The slogan helps the alcoholic realize that there is a Higher Power ("God, as we understand Him") to help them if they can just "let go." The Serenity Prayer (Table 67.3) has a similar philosophy.

"Keep it simple" is directed toward the alcoholic's knack for complicating things. In AA, members are told not to drink, to go to meetings, to read the Big Book, to work the steps, and to reach out to other suffering alcoholics (doing Twelfth Step work). In other words, they should stay focused and directed on what is important and let go of the rest.

HOW is an acronym frequently heard at AA meetings. It stands for **H**onesty, **O**penness, and **W**illingness. The steps of AA require members to be honest with themselves, with their Higher Power, and with the people around them. For many, this is the first time in their lives (or at least in many years) that they have been truly honest. For most alcoholics, the process of recovery is gradual and does not result in immediate change. Openness helps alcoholics overcome their narrow-minded attitudes. They need to be encouraged to share what they are feeling and to be open to new ideas. They need to be willing to listen, to share feelings, and to try sometimes uncomfortable, new behaviors.

HALT is an acronym that warns alcoholics not to allow themselves to become too **H**ungry, too **A**ngry, too **L**onely, or too **T**ired, because an excess of any of these can lead to relapse.

Serenity Prayer The Serenity Prayer (Table 67.3) is basic to AA. It offers a simple solution to many frustrations that alcoholics (and, for that matter, everyone) experience in life. Almost all AA meetings either open or close with this prayer. Alcoholics use the Serenity Prayer during the day to help them deal with frustrating and stressful situations.

Alcoholics Anonymous Promises An essential aspect of AA recovery is the "Promises," which AA says will happen if a person works the AA program to the best of his or her ability. The promises are as follows:

> *"If we are painstaking about this phase of our development, we will be amazed before we are halfway through. We are going to know a new freedom and a new happiness. We will not regret the past nor wish to shut the door on it. We will comprehend the word 'serenity' and we will know peace. No matter how far down the scale we have gone, we will see how our experience can benefit others. That feeling of uselessness and self-pity will disappear. We will lose interest in selfish things and gain interest in our fellows. Self-seeking will slip away. Our whole attitude and outlook upon life will change. Fear of people and of economic insecurity will leave us. We will intuitively know how to handle situations which used to baffle us. We will suddenly realize that God is doing for us what we could not do for ourselves. Are these extravagant promises? We think not! They are being fulfilled among us—sometimes quickly, sometimes slowly. They will always materialize if we work for them" (3).*

The promises frequently are read at the beginning or end of AA meetings. They help AA members realize that life without alcohol can be rich and rewarding.

NARCOTICS ANONYMOUS

History "We cannot change the nature of the addict or addiction. We can help to change the old lie 'Once an addict, always an addict' by striving to make recovery more available. God help us to remember this difference" (4).

This is the basic premise of Narcotics Anonymous (NA). The concepts of NA began at the U.S. Public Health Service Hospital in Lexington, Kentucky, in 1947 (5). In 1953, a group of AA members, who also were addicts, started a group in Sun Valley, California, from which NA grew. This group emphasized the need for NA to follow the Twelve Steps and Twelve Traditions of AA. NA was formed because of the discomfort many narcotic and other drug addicts felt when attending AA meetings. At NA meetings, members are able to share problems related to drugs other than alcohol. The Twelve Steps are the same, except for Step 1, which in NA is changed from "alcohol" to "addiction," and the Twelfth Step, which in NA is changed from "alcoholic" to "addict." By refocusing from a specific substance (alcohol) to addiction, NA was able to include all drugs.

NA's philosophy is that drug addiction is a disease that is progressive and lifelong and involves more than the use of drugs. Recovery is based on abstinence from all mood-altering drugs, including alcohol. Through the Twelve Steps, the addict is encouraged to work toward freedom, good will, creative action, and personal growth.

Because the drugs they use are illegal, NA members characteristically are suspicious and manipulative early in recovery.

Other group members can help identify these problems in themselves and provide suggestions as to how to overcome them. The goal of recovery is more than abstinence from mood-altering chemicals—it is to live life so that mood-altering chemicals are no longer needed to experience positive feelings. By associating with other people in recovery, the addict is able to see the benefits of being "straight and clean."

Structure and Meetings The structure of NA is almost identical to that of AA. The basic unit is the "group." A World Service Office is NA's information center. There is a Web site *(www.na.org)*. NA meetings are similar to those of AA and generally can be classified as discussion, step, or speaker meetings. Sponsorship is an integral part of the NA program. All newcomers are urged to find a sponsor. The AA slogans and sayings also are used in NA, which estimates that there are approximately 43,900 weekly meetings worldwide (in more than 127 countries) and "hundreds of thousands" of members (6).

Literature NA has its own "Big Book," entitled *Narcotics Anonymous* (7), which outlines the principles of NA and contains the personal stories of early NA members. *Welcome to Narcotics Anonymous* is an excellent NA pamphlet that explains the principles of NA to the interested newcomer. The pamphlet states: "Our message is simple: We have found a way to live without using drugs and we are happy to share it with anyone for whom drugs are a problem." For people in communities without an NA group, the World Service Office provides an *NA Group Starter Kit* that describes how to start an NA group.

COCAINE ANONYMOUS

Cocaine Anonymous (CA) groups exist in many metropolitan areas of the country. CA was founded in Hollywood, California, in 1982 and has a World Service Office in Los Angeles, which hosts a Web site *(www.ca.org)*. CA is based on the Twelve Steps. Its groups are open to anyone who is suffering from addiction to cocaine. The first step of CA is "We admitted we were powerless over cocaine and *all other mind-altering substances*: that our lives had become unmanageable." Most cocaine addicts also attend either Narcotics Anonymous or Alcoholics Anonymous meetings. At NA and AA, they can find people with longer periods of being chemically free. Most cocaine addicts also are addicted to other drugs and alcohol. In 1994, CA published *Hope, Faith and Courage*, which are their stories of recovery.

FAMILY SUPPORT GROUPS

If there are 20 million alcoholics in the United States and the life of each alcoholic affects four other individuals, then approximately 80 million persons are affected by alcoholism in some way. This estimate is very close to the findings of a Gallup poll, which found that 24% of persons interviewed said that their life had been affected by an alcoholic in some way (8). As the field of alcohol and drug addiction has become more sophisticated, the concept of addiction's being a family disease has emerged. Everyone in the family is affected—not just the identified alcoholic or addict. Based on this understanding, Twelve Step support groups for the family members of alcoholics have grown rapidly. These support groups all emphasize that even if the person who is addicted to drugs or alcohol continues to use, the family members can get help. The emphasis is on helping the family member, not the drug- or alcohol-addicted person.

Al-Anon The oldest family program is Al-Anon, which was started by Lois W (wife of Bill W). Early in the history of AA, wives frequently would accompany their husbands to AA meetings. While the men were having their meeting, the wives would get together to talk and support each other. Many members of these groups tried to follow the Twelve Steps and to apply them to their own lives. They began to see that they also were affected by alcoholism and that they needed help and support in their recovery. In 1951, Lois W and several other spouses started their own Clearinghouse, which later became known as Al-Anon Family Group Headquarters and the World Services Office, and published the first Al-Anon literature—*Purposes and Suggestions for Al-Anon Family Groups*. Focusing on themselves, not the alcoholic, was the major theme of this work. This simple philosophy was revolutionary in its meaning and application to people who previously had spent most of their energy and time concentrating on the alcoholic.

Philosophy Like AA, Al-Anon is a spiritual (not religious) program based on Twelve Steps. The steps are similar to AA's, with the exception of Step Twelve, which states:

"Having had a spiritual awakening as the result of these steps, we tried to carry this message to others, and to practice these principles in all our affairs" (9). Two main ideas are stressed by Al-Anon (10): The first is that alcoholism is a disease. This principle is emphasized in the Al-Anon Preamble (Table 67.4), which is read at the opening of most Al-Anon meetings to help members learn to free themselves of feeling responsible for the alcoholic's disease. The second major Al-Anon principle emphasizes that the program is for the relative or friend, not the alcoholic. This idea is emphasized in the Al-Anon welcome:

> *"We who live or have lived with the problem of alcoholism understand as perhaps few others can. We, too, were lonely and frustrated, but in Al-Anon and Alateen we discover that no situation is really hopeless and that it is possible for us to find contentment and even happiness, whether the alcoholic is still drinking or not.*
>
> *"We urge you to try our program. It has helped many of us find solutions that lead to serenity. So much depends upon our own attitudes, and as we learn to place our problem in its true perspective, we find that it loses its power to dominate our thoughts and our lives.*
>
> *"The family situation is bound to improve as we apply the Al-Anon/Alateen ideas. Without such spiritual help, living with alcoholism is too much for most of us. Our thinking becomes distorted by trying to force solutions, and we become irritable and unreasonable without knowing it.*

TABLE 67.4 The Al-Anon Preamble

The Al-Anon Family Groups are a fellowship of relatives and friends of alcoholics who share their experience, strength, and hope in order to solve their common problems.
We believe alcoholism is a family illness and that changed attitudes can aid recovery.
Al-Anon is not allied with any sect, denomination, political entity, organization or institution; does not engage in any controversy; neither endorses nor opposes any cause.
There are no dues for membership. Al-Anon is self-supporting through its own voluntary contributions.
Al-Anon has but one purpose: to help families of alcoholics. We do this by practicing the Twelve Steps, by welcoming and giving comfort to families of alcoholics, and by giving understanding and encouragement to the alcoholic.

> *The Al-Anon/Alateen program is based on the Twelve Steps (adapted from Alcoholics Anonymous) which we try, little by little, one day at a time, to apply to our lives, along with the Serenity Prayer. The loving interchange of help among members and daily reading of Al-Anon/Alateen literature thus make us ready to receive the priceless gift of serenity.*
>
> *"Anonymity is an important principle of the Al-Anon/Alateen program. Everything that is said in our group meetings and member-to-member, must be held in confidence. Only in this way can we feel free to say what is in our minds and hearts, for this is how we help one another in Al-Anon/Alateen (9).*

The Al-Anon program teaches people to look at what they can do to feel better about themselves and to caringly "let go" of the alcoholics. This concept is called "tough love," which means stopping "enabling behaviors" and making the alcoholic responsible for the consequences of his or her drinking and alcoholism. Al-Anon describes this idea in a pamphlet called Detachment (11). Members are encouraged to "let go of our obsession with another's behavior and begin to lead happier and more manageable lives." Al-Anon helps members learn the following:

- "Not to suffer because of the action or reactions of other people
- Not to allow ourselves to be used or abused in the interest of another's recovery
- Not to do for others what they should do for themselves
- Not to manipulate situations so others will eat, go to bed, get up, pay bills, etc.
- Not to cover up another's mistakes or misdeeds
- Not to create a crisis
- Not to prevent a crisis if it is in the natural course of events"

Newcomers often come into Al-Anon with resentments and anger that they have not previously acknowledged. Al-Anon helps them view the alcoholic as someone with a disease instead of someone who is "trying to get them." Step One points out that they are powerless over alcohol and that they have no control over the alcoholic. Steps Two and Three help the person reach outside herself or himself for help from a "Higher Power." "Letting go" of control and trusting a Higher Power are basic concepts of Al-Anon.

Membership and Meetings The Third Tradition of Al-Anon states: "The only requirement for membership is that there be a problem of alcoholism in a relative or friend" (9). There are more than 24,000 Al-Anon groups in 115 countries (12). Al-Anon meetings usually start with the Serenity Prayer, the preamble, and the welcome and are followed by introductions. There are speaker, discussion, and step meetings. The meetings emphasize sharing, support, and encouragement to work on oneself. Meetings usually last an hour and have a standard closing which states in part:

> *"In closing, I would like to say that the opinions expressed here were strictly those of the persons who gave them. Take what you liked and leave the rest.*
>
> *"A few special words to those of you who haven't been with us long: Whatever your problems, there are those among us who have had them too. If you try to keep an open mind, you will find help. You will come to realize that there is no situation too difficult to be bettered and no unhappiness too great to be lessened.*
>
> *"We aren't perfect. The welcome we give you may not show the warmth we have in our hearts for you. After a while, you'll discover that though you may not like all of us, you'll love us in a very special way—the same way we already love you . . ." (9).*

The leader then emphasizes that everything said in the meeting is considered confidential. Frequently there is a social time after the meeting for further support and sharing.

Literature In 1955, Al-Anon published The *Al-Anon Family Groups* (13), which was their first basic book about the program. This book sets down the basic principles of Al-Anon and tells the stories of the founders. In 1995, Al-Anon published *How Al-Anon Works for Families & Friends of Alcoholics*, which is their most recent basic book. Al-Anon also has a book that discusses the Steps and Traditions from an Al-Anon perspective. *One Day at a Time in Al-Anon* (14) is a daily meditation guide that many members read for inspiration and guidance. Al-Anon also publishes 14 other books and more than 50 pamphlets on special topics, such as men in Al-Anon, denial, alcoholism as a family disease, and adult children of alcoholics. (Pamphlets and books are available from Al-Anon Family

Group Headquarters, Inc., 1600 Corporate Landing Parkway, Virginia Beach, VA 23454-5617, or from a local Al-Anon office.)

Alateen Alateen was started by a California teenager in 1957. Alateen is a part of Al-Anon Family Groups specifically for teenagers and follows the Al-Anon Steps and Traditions. Every Alateen group has an active Al-Anon member who serves as a sponsor for the group. The sponsor provides guidance and stability to the group and helps the group stay focused on the Twelve Steps and Twelve Traditions.

A key to being a good sponsor is to guide without dominating. Alateen meetings frequently are held at the same place as Al-Anon meetings but in different rooms. Many schools host Alateen meetings. A referral to Alateen can be made through the local Al-Anon office. Alateen has its own literature especially directed to teenagers. In *Alateen—Hope for Children of Alcoholics* (15), there is a chapter devoted to explaining alcoholism in terms teenagers can understand. Alcoholics are described as anyone and not necessarily "skid row bums." The sources of the alcoholic's obsession, addiction, and compulsion are defined. The family disease concept is discussed, with an emphasis on denial, anger, and anxiety, as well as adolescents' feelings about being "caught in the middle." The alcoholic is described as sick and unable to control his or her alcohol intake or reactions. The slogans are explained, and one chapter contains personal stories to help teenagers feel that they are not alone. At the end of the book, there is a detailed discussion of how to start an Alateen group. A special page labeled "Remember" encourages group members to focus on the common problem of alcoholism and not to gossip, waste time, be impatient, or talk about what happens in the group outside of the group. As the members become older, they are encouraged to attend Al-Anon meetings, which include more than 721 registered Al-Anon adult children groups.

Adult Children of Alcoholics Adult Children of Alcoholics (ACOA) has developed rapidly over the past 35 years. In the 1970s, researchers began trying to identify common characteristics of adults raised in alcoholic homes. In the late 1970s, a small group of previous Alateen members started an Al-Anon meeting called "Hope for Adult Children of Alcoholics." Several books were published on the topic (16–18) and served as the impetus for other support groups for adult children of alcoholics (by some estimates, as many as 30 to 40 million people). Because the movement grew rapidly, it did not have the advantage of time to develop and mature, as did AA and Al-Anon, and many different groups developed. Al-Anon started having special meetings for adult children of alcoholics. Groups such as the National Association for Children of Alcoholics started. There was a lack of clarity about what the groups should and should not do. Many groups had no one who had any extended time in recovery to help provide guidance and direction. Some groups emphasized therapy over support, with heavy confrontation instead of relying on the Twelve Steps and Twelve Traditions. Though these problems may still exist in some groups, most ACOA groups have matured and now offer excellent support for adult children of alcoholics. The national center is Adult Children of Alcoholics World Service Organization (ACA WSO, P.O. Box 3216, Torrance, CA 90510). The center also hosts a Web site (*http://adultchildren.org*).

The "Problem" is read at the opening of meetings:

> *"Many of us found that we had several characteristics in common as a result of being brought up in alcoholic or other dysfunctional households. We had come to feel isolated and uneasy with other people, especially authority figures. To protect ourselves, we became people pleasers, even though we lost our own identities in the process. All the same we would mistake any personal criticism as a threat. We either became alcoholics ourselves, married them, or both. Failing that, we found other compulsive personalities, such as workaholic, to fulfill our sick need for abandonment. We lived life from the standpoint of victims. Having an overdeveloped sense of responsibility, we preferred to be concerned with others rather than ourselves. We got guilt feelings when we trusted ourselves, giving in to others.*
>
> *"We became reactors rather than actors, letting others take the initiative. We were dependent personalities, terrified of abandonment, willing to do almost anything to hold on to a relationship in order not to be abandoned emotionally. We kept choosing insecure relationships because they matched our childhood relationship with alcoholic or dysfunctional parents. These symptoms of the family disease of alcoholism or other dysfunction made us 'co-victims'—those who take on the characteristics of the disease without necessarily ever taking a drink. We learned to keep our feelings down as children and keep them buried as adults. As a result of this conditioning, we often confused love with pity, tending to love those we could rescue. Even more self-defeating, we became addicted to excitement in all our affairs, preferring constant upset to workable solutions. This is a description, not an indictment" (19).*

This is usually followed by the solution:

> *"As ACA becomes a safe place for you, you will find freedom to express all the hurts and fears that you have kept inside and to free yourself from the shame and blame that are carry-overs from the past. You will become an adult who is imprisoned no longer by childhood reactions. You will recover the child within you, learning to love and accept yourself. The healing begins when we risk moving out of isolation. Feelings and buried memories will return. By gradually releasing the burden of unexpressed grief, we slowly move out of the past. We learn to re-parent ourselves with gentleness, humor, love and respect. This process allows us to see our biological parents as the instruments of our existence. Our actual parent is a Higher Power whom some of us choose to call God. Although we had alcoholic or dysfunctional parents, our Higher Power gave us the Twelve Steps of Recovery. This is the action and work that heals us:*

we use the Steps; we use the meetings; we use the telephone. We share our experience, strength, and hope with each other. We learn to restructure our sick thinking one day at a time. When we release our parents from responsibility for our actions today, we become free to make healthful decisions as actors, not reactors. We progress from hurting, to healing, to helping. We awaken to a sense of wholeness we never knew was possible. By attending these meetings on a regular basis, you will come to see parental alcoholism or family dysfunction for what it is: a disease that infected you as a child and continues to affect you as an adult. You will learn to keep the focus on yourself in the here and now. You will take responsibility for your own life and supply your own parenting. You will not do this alone. Look around you and you will see others who know how you feel. We love and encourage you no matter what. We ask you accept us just as we accept you. This is a spiritual program based on action coming from love. We are sure that as the love grows inside you, you will see beautiful changes in all your relationships, especially with your Higher Power, yourself, and your parents" (19).

If physicians are aware of these common characteristics, they can identify patients who are adult children of alcoholics. Until they are identified, these individuals can be overusers of the medical system and frustrating for physicians to treat. By referring patients to ACOA, physicians can be instrumental in helping them start a program of recovery.

Most ACOA meetings last 60 to 90 minutes. They usually start with the Serenity Prayer and a welcome. The Twelve Steps, the problem, and the solution often are read. At some meetings, the characteristics are read. A member may talk about a step or characteristic and how it affects his or her life. Then each member of the group has the opportunity to share his or her feelings about the topic or talk about any other concerns he or she may have. The meeting usually closes with a prayer. Members are invited to socialize after meetings. Newcomers are encouraged to attend six meetings to help them become comfortable with the group and develop the trust that is essential to recovery. Sponsors are an important part of ACOA, and newcomers are encouraged to get a sponsor. Most groups have phone lists and encourage members to call each other for support. As with AA and Al-Anon, an important part of recovery in ACOA is reaching out to others. ACOA members are willing to take people to meetings and can be a helpful resource for physicians.

THE PHYSICIAN'S ROLE

To be able to help patients with addicton, physicians need to be familiar with recovery support groups, especially the Twelve Step programs. The physician can work as a facilitator to help patients attend meetings. Project MATCH (20) showed that trained professionals who support meeting attendance in a positive noncoercive way could improve their patient's acceptance of Twelve Step programs. There are several advantages to referring patients to Twelve Step programs:

- Meetings are free of cost. (AA's Preamble states "There are no dues or fees for AA membership.")
- Meetings are accessible even in the smallest of towns.
- No records are kept of attendance, and anonymity is assured.
- Participants do not have to be sober to attend a meeting. (The only requirement for membership is a desire to stop drinking.)
- Persons from all racial and ethnic backgrounds and socioeconomic groups are welcome. Being unemployed, African American, and unmarried does *not* predict an unfavorable outcome with Twelve Step meeting attendance (21).
- The newcomer develops a feeling of "self-value" as he or she becomes part of the group. Twelve Step groups work supportively with other therapies. They provide the newcomer with many other new positive experiences (22,23).
- Attending group meetings helps overcome the patient's feelings of "terminal uniqueness" and isolation.
- Groups educate patients about the disease process of addiction and hold out the hope of recovery.
- Group members offer newcomers unconditional support as they struggle with early recovery, which the group characterizes as a positive, joyful experience.
- Groups help members learn basic social skills. Members become less self-obsessed and more aware of the feelings of others.
- Groups provide a "reality base" for addicts in recovery, overcoming the isolation and thinking disorders that prevent addicts from comprehending the potential consequences of their behavior and illuminating errors and dangers in the member's thinking.
- Groups help members with the inevitable setbacks experienced in recovery.
- Groups help members constructively use the time formerly occupied by alcohol and drug use.

Making Referrals to Twelve Step Programs In the 1996 triennial AA member survey, only 8% of newcomers reported coming to meetings through a physician's referral. This finding is unfortunate because AA and other self-help programs can be a valuable resource for physicians in helping their addicted patients. There are several ways to refer patients. AA has a listed phone number in most cities and will provide volunteers to contact the patient and explain AA. After obtaining the patient's permission, the physician should initiate contact with the self-help group in the patient's presence. Giving the patient the telephone number with a recommendation to call usually is not successful. Sisson and Mallams (24) randomly assigned newly diagnosed alcoholics to two types of referral. The first group was told to call AA and go to a meeting. The second group was put in direct contact with an AA member while in the physician's office. None of the first group attended a meeting; the entire second group attended a meeting. Most addiction treatment programs incorporate a strong self-help component and will encourage patients to attend Twelve Step meetings as a regular part of their aftercare program.

Alcoholics Anonymous The physician may find it helpful to keep a list of AA members willing to do "Twelfth Step" work. Some physicians accompany patients to AA meetings (nonalcoholic physicians may be allowed to attend closed meetings if they are with patients, or physicians may select an open AA meeting). Though such attendance is time-consuming for the physician, it demonstrates to the patient the physician's sincere belief in the importance of AA to recovery. Physicians can obtain a current list of nearby AA meetings from the local AA office (frequently listed in directories as "Intergroup" or "Central Office"). Such lists usually include a brief description of the type of meeting, whether it is a special interest group, and whether it is nonsmoking.

Other Twelve Step Groups Referrals to NA and Al-Anon are similar to those for AA. In most cities, Al-Anon has a listed phone number. Al-Anon also has a toll-free meeting line (1-888-4AL-ANON) and a public outreach Web site to help professionals and others learn about Al-Anon/Alateen (*www.al-anon.alateen.org*). Frequently, the local AA office may also have information about Al-Anon. The more physicians know about Al-Anon, the more effectively they can make referrals. An excellent way to learn is to talk with Al-Anon members about their experiences with the program and to attend a meeting. It is also helpful for the physician to have a list of Al-Anon members who are willing to take new members to Al-Anon meetings and to encourage patients to attend at least six meetings.

Because there is considerable variation in ACOA groups, physicians must be familiar with the group to which they refer patients. A group can offer support and caring when the pain of being an adult child of an alcoholic begins to surface. The group should not allow "cross-talk" (confrontation or interruptions), so that the meeting feels "safe" to the new member. The purpose of ACOA groups is "to shelter and support newcomers in confronting denial; to comfort those mourning their early loss of security, trust and love; and to teach the skills for reparenting themselves with gentleness, humor, love, and respect" (25). Because alcoholism is an inherited disease, ACOA patients should be screened carefully and referred if there is any suggestion of an addictive disorder. Though ACOA patients may appear to be emotionally stable, they often are fragile under their carefully constructed external shell. They need to be treated with care, understanding, and gentleness by the physician.

Making the Referral Work A knowledgeable, empathetic physician can "prepare" the patient to help overcome the initial fear and apprehension about attending a Twelve Step meeting. The physician should acknowledge the patient's ambivalence (which is not denial) about stopping drinking (26). The following suggestions will help the referral work:

1. Know the meetings in your area and refer each patient to a meeting that will meet his or her needs. Meetings have different "personalities" (27). If they are unhappy with a meeting, help them find another.
2. Help patients make direct contact with members of the group.
3. Give patients a "prescription" to attend a meeting.
4. Tell them what is going to happen at the meeting and how meetings are structured.
5. Encourage them to socialize by arriving early and staying late after the meeting.
6. Encourage patients to pick a *temporary* sponsor early to increase their chances of staying clean and sober. Tell them to pick someone of the same gender with at least 1 year of sobriety. Tell them it is okay to change sponsors if necessary.
7. Talk about their fears and apprehensions about attending a meeting and dispel any inaccurate myths or beliefs they may have about Twelve Step support groups.
8. Encourage them to attend frequent meetings, but initially do not push or coerce them.
9. Schedule them for a follow-up visit to discuss their experience at meetings. If they have been attending regularly, encourage them to pick a "home" group and become more active. Being actively involved in the program is a better predictor of a successful outcome than the number of meetings attended (28).

Potential Problems with Referrals Patient objections to AA and other mutual help groups typically are expressed in the following ways (29).

"I don't believe in God." AA is a spiritual program that is not allied with any particular religion and does not require the members to believe in anything except a Higher Power ("God, as we understand Him"). There are many atheists and agnostics in AA. *Alcoholics Anonymous* (the Big Book) contains an entire chapter for agnostics (Chapter 4), which the physician may recommend to patients who offer this objection.

"I don't like to talk in a group." There is no requirement to talk at an AA meeting. Members can say they "pass" if they do not wish to talk in front of the group.

"I can't stand all the smoke." Nonsmoking group meetings are available in most geographic areas. In others, large groups divide into smoking and nonsmoking sections.

"I don't have a way to get there." Transportation usually can be arranged for an interested newcomer by calling AA.

"I don't want anyone to know about my drinking." Anonymity is a basic concept of AA. Things said in a meeting stay there; no AA member has the right to break the anonymity of another member.

"I can't stay sober." The third tradition of AA clearly states, "The only requirement for AA membership is a *desire* to stop drinking." Many old-timers spent a long time attending meetings before they were able to stay sober, and they understand the plight of the newcomer.

Group Problems The patient may have difficulty identifying with the members of his or her self-help group. If the patient has attended a meeting several times and still has this feeling, he or she should be referred to a different group. In large metropolitan areas, there are many varieties of self-help groups (involving, for example, young people, senior citizens, gays/lesbians, nonsmokers, women, African Americans, and Hispanic Americans).

Twelve Step "Docs" Though AA as an organization encourages members to cooperate with their physicians; individual AA members may give patients inappropriate advice about stopping essential drugs, such as antidepressants, antipsychotics, naltrexone, disulfiram, or other medications. If patients are using these medications, physicians should caution them about this possibility. Frequently, communication between the physician and the patient's sponsor can overcome this problem. It may be wise to tell patients not to discuss their medication at meetings (30).

Gender Orientation Women sometimes have a problem with AA because of the masculine perspective of most AA literature. However, AA groups now are very receptive to women, who do well in the program. There also are AA meetings exclusively for women.

Support in Recovery The patient who participates in a mutual help group may show certain warning signs of an impending relapse. Early in sobriety, patients often experience excessive euphoria, which can lead to overconfidence and relapse. The first sign of a potential relapse may be a patient's unwillingness to discuss the recovery program with his or her physician, a behavior that may indicate the patient has decreased the frequency of or stopped attending meetings. This behavior can lead to the "dry drunk syndrome," which is characterized by irritability and unwillingness to share feelings. The patient loses his or her reality base and reverts to distorted thinking. New resentments and a multitude of other negative feelings can lead to drinking to relieve the pain. At this point, patients may request mood-altering chemicals to relieve anxiety. Such a request is a "red flag" that a relapse may be imminent.

To assess a patient's recovery status, the physician can ask a few simple questions (31).

- "What are you working on in your recovery program and with your sponsor?"
- "What step are you working on?"
- "What meetings are you attending?"
- "How are you using your phone list?"

Patients in a good recovery program will be very open to answering and discussing any of these questions. The questions stimulate patients' thinking about what working a program of recovery really means. Using the information elicited, physicians often can make suggestions about their patients' recovery and decrease the likelihood of a relapse. Physicians also can show an interest in their patients' recovery by acknowledging anniversaries, using the slogans, and caringly asking at each visit about how a patient is doing in his or her recovery. Alcoholism and drug addiction should be included on patient problem lists to help prevent inadvertent prescribing of medications that may endanger recovery. Physicians also can counsel patients during high-risk times, such as periods of extreme stress. Encouraging patients to attend more meetings and contact their sponsor during such periods can prevent relapse. Patients frequently complain to their physicians about AA. By listening attentively to patients' concerns and then encouraging them to continue attending meetings, physicians can allow patients to vent their frustration while maintaining attendance at meetings.

THE TWELVE STEPS IN TREATMENT PROGRAMS

Twelve Step Facilitation (TSF) in the inpatient treatment setting generally follows the constructs and philosophies of the so-called "Minnesota Model." This model integrates the holistic (mind-body-spirit) clinical approach developed by Dan Anderson, Nelson Bradley, and others in Minnesota in the late 1940s, with the spiritual principles of the Twelve Steps of Alcoholics Anonymous (32). This integration began with the founding of Hazelden in Center City, Minnesota in 1949 and was fully established at Hazelden by the early 1960s (33).

From the very beginning, TSF in the inpatient setting has been part of a continuum of care, not a free-standing, one-time intervention. The fundamental "next step" for any patient being discharged from a TSF program is to become a member of Alcoholics Anonymous, Narcotics Anonymous, or some other Twelve-Step program. This membership is intended to be adjunctive to other after-care interventions ranging from residential extended care to personal psychotherapy to weekly continuing-care groups facilitated by treatment professionals. TSF is the very beginning of a lifelong solution to a lifelong problem.

At discharge from a TSF program, the patient will have had the *physical* issues of his or her disease addressed through detoxification and general medical care; the *menta*l issues of his or her disease addressed through interventions coordinated by mental health professionals, as necessary; and the *spiritual* issues of his or her disease addressed through their initial work on the Twelve Steps and through the frequent, and often intense, interaction with other patients. This interpatient interaction accounts for 40% of positive outcomes in TSF programs (34), probably because chemical dependency is a disease of isolation (spiritual death), and TSF fosters connection to other people (spiritual life). Thus, the treatment milieu itself creates the most effective treatment intervention.

Owing to time restrictions, many programs focus their efforts primarily on working through the first three of the twelve steps (though some programs are also able to introduce Steps Four and Five). Regardless of how many steps are addressed, the goals of treatment are to help the patient arrest the course of his or her disease, to develop a belief that this arrestment can be maintained day to day, and to establish the beginnings of an attitude shift that moves the chemically dependent patient's focus from an isolative, cynical orientation toward self, to a communal, hopeful orientation towards the process of recovery. This process tracks the DeClemente-Prochaska (35) stages of change. Most patients entering a Minnesota Model program are precontemplative, and those making the best progress leave in a preparation stage of change.

The spiritual principle of the First Step is honesty and is best exemplified by this statement in *Alcoholics Anonymous*: "We learned that we had to fully concede to our innermost selves that we were alcoholics. This is the first step in recovery" (36). The patient is asked to honestly look at the breadth and depth of his or her use of substances and to establish a direct correlation between escalating use (kinds, frequencies, methods of delivery, and amounts) and escalating unmanageability (legal, financial, personal, social, and occupational difficulties). The chemically dependent person often confuses cause with effect. The thinking error embodied in the statement, "I drink so much because I am not appreciated at work," for instance, can be corrected in the First Step by helping the patient see that the lack of appreciation is probably caused by the drinking, not the other way around. The other dimension of honesty in this phase of treatment is the patient's acknowledgment of the impact of his or her disease on other people. This acknowledgment is essential in order for the patient to progress far enough in his or her program to make direct amends to these people (in Steps Eight and Nine).

The primary barrier to Step One in the inpatient setting is the need for the patient to see that something about his or her baseline state has been unacceptable to him or her (from simple boredom to the residual effects of trauma), that their drug of choice at one time solved this problem for him or her, and that over time, the drug of choice was not only *not solving* the original problem anymore but creating a host of other problems.

Other barriers to progress in the First Step are rationalization/minimization (especially among highly intelligent patients), euphoric recall, anticipatory euphoria from cravings, and comparing one's own experience with mood-altering substances to someone else's experience ("I never did anything like that"). In the inpatient setting, these obstacles are confronted by both staff and other patients so that the patient struggling with the First Step essentially cannot hide the reality of his or her disease any longer.

The spiritual principle of Step Two is faith or hope. By the time a patient enters an ASAM Level Three inpatient program, he or she will often have an equally difficult time thinking of life *with* their drug of choice as thinking of life *without* their drug of choice. The spiritual conundrum for these patients is that there is/was nothing wrong with their value systems, but their behavior is/was consistently in direct contradiction to those value systems. As *Alcoholics Anonymous* puts it: "If a mere code of morals or a better philosophy of life were sufficient to overcome alcoholism, many of us would have recovered long ago. Our human resources, as marshaled by will, were not sufficient; they failed us utterly. We had to find a power by which we could live, and it had to be a Power greater than ourselves" (37).

The patient at this point in treatment has been exposed to a situation from classical psychodynamic therapy—his or her ego has been exclusively servicing his or her id, and the superego has disappeared. The Higher Power (or sometimes Other Power) of TSF is essentially restoration of superego. The belief in restoration to sanity of Step Two is a manifestation of faith/hope that the patient can bring his or her behavior into line with his or her values. Doing so, of course, is impossible if the patient returns to active addiction.

The Minnesota Model is built on a triad of education, fellowship, and therapy. All are brought to bear on Step Two in treatment. Bibliotherapy brings the patient into contact with his or her own spiritual deficit, fellowship allows him or her to share this deficit and hear how others have overcome it, and therapy allows the professional staff to integrate an emerging faith/hope into a promise of a more manageable life. It is important to note here that the TSF approach almost always incorporates an integrated clinical approach to co-occurring disorders in which the chemical dependency and the co-occurring disorder are presented to the patient as two negatively synergistic states of being that require concurrent management. If one has no faith/hope in long-term management of his or her depression, for instance, it is very difficulty for that patient to hang onto faith/hope for a life without intoxicating chemicals.

Barriers to Step Two in TSF programs include confusion between spirituality and religion, negative connotations of the word *God*, lack of trust in the treatment and recovery process, fear of letting go of self-will despite all its negative consequences, distorted views of reality (and thus sanity), and a failure to be rigorously honest in Step One.

The spiritual principle of Step Three is that of surrender—to the program and the Higher (Other) Power one has come to believe in. It is important for the chemically dependent person to step out of his or her self-will because the disease essentially sits in the mental pathways that turn self-will into negative attitudes and behaviors. *Alcoholics Anonymous* puts it thus: "So our troubles, we think, are basically of our own making. They arise out of ourselves, and the alcoholic is an extreme example of self-will run riot, although he usually doesn't think so" (38). Interventions at this point often revolve around helping the patient to accept after-care recommendations, agree to step away from toxic relationships, agree not to socialize with using friends, and commit to Twelve Step programs by making contact with temporary sponsors while still in treatment.

TSF does not require the patient to take any action on Step Three but rather to decide, drawing on the honesty and faith/hope established in the first two steps, to enter into a spiritual program of action (Steps Four to Nine) with resolve. This decision must come from the patient; it cannot be forced by staff and often is arrived at only after the patient has developed faith that the TSF approach works because he has seen it work in more senior peers who are now far less anxious, fearful, and stuck. Again, the importance of the inpatient milieu cannot be overstated: What a patient sees in his or her peers is the "experience, strength and hope" that members of Twelve-Step programs offer to each other.

Steps Four and Five are sometimes touched on in 28-day, intensive residential treatment and are the primary focus of treatment in extended residential care. The difficulty most patients have with Step Four is being able to see those parts of themselves that are worthy and productive. The backward-looking inventory of what becomes "character defects" in Steps Six and Seven helps the patients see how resentment, self-centered fear, and guilt have impeded them and fueled their addictions. Step Five, in which the patient often unburdens him- or herself of something he or she has never told anyone else, is usually done with a spiritual care staff member, with whom conversations are privileged.

The goal of Steps Four and Five is to help the patient identify those aspects of self that have been impediments so that these impediments can be cleared away in Steps Six to Nine in order to make room for those aspects of self that are positive and useful and foster growth.

CONCLUSIONS

Twelve Step programs have more than 70 years' experience in helping alcoholics, addicts, and family members recover from addiction and its consequences. Almost all patients afflicted with addictive disease will have a more rewarding recovery if they actively participate in a Twelve Step program. Physicians can play an important role by helping their patients understand these programs and encouraging them to participate in meetings. Physicians need to know how to use Twelve Step and other support groups effectively to help alcoholics, addicts, and family members recover from the disease of drug and alcohol addiction. By integrating the 12 Steps into treatment programs, the programs can help bridge the gap between treatment and community 12-Step meetings after the patient is discharged.

REFERENCES

1. Anonymous. *A. A. Fact File*, Web site: www.aa.org, 2001.
2. Cross GM, Morgan CW, Mooney AJ, et al. Alcoholism treatment: a ten year follow up study. *Alcohol Clin Exp Res* 1990;14(2):169–173.
3. Anonymous. *Alcoholics Anonymous*, 4th ed. New York: Alcoholics Anonymous World Service, Inc., 2001:83–84.
4. Anonymous. *The triangle of self-obsession*. Van Nuys, CA: Narcotics Anonymous World Service Office, Inc., 1983.
5. Peyrot M. Narcotics Anonymous: its history, structure and approach. *Int J Addict* 1985;20(10):1509–1522.
6. Anonymous. Web site: www.na.org., Van Nuys, CA: Narcotics Anonymous World Service Office, Inc.
7. Anonymous. *Narcotics Anonymous*. Van Nuys, CA: Narcotics Anonymous World Service Office, Inc., 1983.
8. Robertson N. *Getting better inside Alcoholics Anonymous*. New York: Ballantine Books, 1988.
9. Anonymous. *This is Al-Anon*. Virginia Beach, VA: Al-Anon Family Group Headquarters, Inc, 1967 [revised 1998].
10. Anthony M. Al-Anon. *JAMA* 1977;238(10):1062–1063.
11. Anonymous. *Detachment*. Virginia Beach, VA: Al-Anon Family Group Headquarters, Inc., 1979.
12. Al-Anon. Web site: www.al-anon.alateen.org.
13. Anonymous. *The Al-Anon family groups—classic edition*, Virginia Beach, VA: Al-Anon Family Group Headquarters, Inc., 1966.
14. Anonymous. *One day at a time in Al-Anon*. Virginia Beach, VA: Al-Anon Family Group Headquarters, Inc., 1968.
15. Anonymous. *Alateen—hope for children of alcoholics*. Virginia Beach, VA: Al-Anon Family Group Headquarters, Inc., 1973.
16. Wegscheider S. *Another chance*. Palo Alto, CA: Science and Behavior Books, 1981.
17. Woititz J. *Adult children of alcoholics*. Pompano Beach, FL: Health Communications, Inc., 1981.
18. Black C. *It will never happen to me!* Denver: M.A.C. Printing and Publishing Division, 1982.
19. Adult Children of Alcoholics World Services Organization, Inc. Website: www.adultchildren.org. Torrance, CA.
20. Project MATCH Research Group. Matching alcoholism treatment to client heterogeneity: Project MATCH post treatment drinking outcomes. *J Stud Alcohol* 1997;l58:7–28.
21. Miller NS, Verinis JS. Treatment outcome for impoverished alcoholics in abstinence-based program. *Int J Addict* 1995;30(6):753–763.
22. Bassin A. Psychology in action. *Am Psychol* 1975;30(6):695–696.
23. Canavan D. Impaired physicians program-support groups. *J Med Soc N J* 1983;80(11):953–954.
24. Sisson RW, Mallams JH. The use of systematic encouragement and community access procedures to increase attendance at Alcoholics Anonymous and Al-Anon meetings. *Am J Drug Alcohol Abuse* 1981;8(3): 371–376.
25. Jacobson S. The 12-step program and group therapy for adult children of alcoholics. *J Psychoactive Drugs* 1987;19(3):253–255.
26. Miller WR, Rollnick S. *Motivational interviewing: preparing people to change addictive behavior.* New York: The Guilford Press, 1991.
27. Tonigan S, Ashcroft F, Miller W. AA group dynamics and 12-step activity. *J Stud Addict* 1995;56:616–621.
28. Montgomery HA, Miller WR, Tonigan JS. Does Alcoholics Anonymous involvement predict treatment outcome? *J Subst Abuse Treat* 1995;2(4): 241–246.
29. Anonymous. *AA as a resource for the medical profession*. New York: Alcoholics Anonymous World Service, Inc., 1982.
30. Chappel JN, Dupont RL. Twelve-step and mutual-help programs for addictive disorders. *Psychiatr Clin North Am* 1999;22(2):425–445.
31. Chappel JN. Effective use of AA and NA in treating patients. *Psychiatr Ann* 1992;22:409–418.
32. McElrath D. *The quiet crusaders: the untold story behind the Minnesota Model.* Minnesota: Hazelden Foundation, 2001:81.
33. McElrath D. The Minnesota Model. *J Psychoactive Drugs* 1997:29(2): 141–144.
34. Butler Center for Research. *Research update*. Minnesota: Hazelden Foundation, Oct. 2006.
35. Miller W, Rollnick S. *Motivational interviewing: preparing people for change*, 2nd ed. New York: The Guilford Press, 2002:201–216.
36. Alcoholics Anonymous World Services, Inc. *Alcoholics Anonymous*, 3rd [rev.] ed. New York: Author, 1976:30.
37. Alcoholics Anonymous World Services, Inc. *Alcoholics Anonymous*, 3rd [rev.] ed. New York: Author, 1976:44.
38. Alcoholics Anonymous World Services, Inc *Alcoholics Anonymous*, 3rd [rev.] ed. New York: Author, 1976:62.

CHAPTER 68

Barbara S. McCrady, PhD
J. Scott Tonigan, PhD

Recent Research into Twelve Step Programs

Alcoholics Anonymous (AA) is ubiquitous, both in the United States and around the world. In the United States, there are an estimated 53,665 groups and 1,213,269 members (1). Internationally, AA estimates 58,464 groups and 712,342 members. AA also is commonly found in correctional institutions in the United States and Canada, with an estimated 2432 groups and 63,357 members in these facilities (1). The formal structure of AA is similar across nations, though there is some variability in emphasis on different parts of the AA program, and differences in the demography of membership are apparent, depending on the cultural context in which AA occurs (2). Though most addiction professionals have some familiarity with AA and other self-help groups based on Twelve Step principles, professionals' scientific knowledge about AA often is more limited. The past 15 years have witnessed an explosion of research on AA and on treatments designed to facilitate involvement in AA. Despite earlier skepticism about the possibility of conducting research on AA, researchers have used a range of methodologies, including ethnographic methods, epidemiologic studies, longitudinal studies of treatment-seeking and non-treatment-seeking populations, controlled clinical trials, and meta-analyses to develop a body of new research about AA that has some coherence, confirms some previous findings and beliefs, and challenges others. This chapter provides a selective review of earlier research on AA and a more comprehensive review from 1995 through 2007. It addresses several major topics, including patterns of utilization of AA, the unique experiences and views of AA among specific population groups, the effectiveness of AA and treatments designed to facilitate AA involvement, and mechanisms of change associated with involvement with AA and other Twelve Step programs. The chapter concludes with methodologic comments and directions for future research. Research on other Twelve Step programs for substance use disorders is more limited but will be included where relevant data exist.

UTILIZATION OF AA

AA members enter the program by a number of routes, including self-referral or referral by family or friends, referral from treatment centers, or through coercion from the legal system, employers, or the social welfare system.

Population Studies Population surveys provide information on utilization of AA in the general and alcohol-problemed populations. Hasin and Grant (3) examined data from the National Health Interview Survey of 43,809 adults in the United States. Among the survey population, 5.8% had attended AA at some point in their lives. Room and Greenfield's (4) household survey of 2,058 adults revealed similar results:10% of men and 8% of women had attended AA at some point. Room and Greenfield further distinguished between AA attendance for personal problems with drinking and AA attendance for other reasons and found that 3.1% of respondents had attended AA for their own drinking problems. Dawson et al. (5), using data from the National Epidemiological Survey on Alcohol and Related Conditions (NESARC) reported that AA attendance among respondents with a history of alcohol dependence was higher (20.1%).

Help-Seeking Populations A different perspective on the utilization of AA is provided by studies of patterns of help-seeking among individuals seeking assistance for an alcohol problem. Dawson et al. (5), using NESARC data, also reported that among individuals with alcohol dependence who sought help, 78.5% had used AA and other twelve step programs (11.7% using only AA; 66.8% using AA in combination with formal treatment), compared to 88.7% who used professional services (21.9% using only professional treatment; 66.8% using treatment in combination with AA). Timko et al. (6) examined treatment utilization among individuals who first contacted an information and referral center or who underwent alcohol detoxification. One year later, 75% had sought treatment: 18% had attended only AA or another self-help group (24% of help-seekers), 25% had sought only outpatient treatment (33% of help-seekers), and 32% had sought only inpatient/residential treatment (43% of help-seekers). AA involvement was high among treatment seekers, with 66% of outpatients and 68% of inpatients also attending AA. By the time of an 8-year follow-up (7), 17% still had sought no treatment, and 14% had attended only AA. The majority (53%) participated in both formal treatment and AA. Study participants who attended AA (either AA alone or in conjunction with treatment) showed a pattern of remarkably steady and consistent involvement over time: 66 to 91 meetings in the first year, 68 to 97 meetings per year in the subsequent two years, 63 to 71 meetings per year in years 4 to 8, and 46 to 52 meetings per year in years 9 to 16 (8).

Mandated Populations Though there has been considerable controversy about the current criminal justice practice of mandating individuals to attend AA, little research has examined the actual process of criminal justice referral to AA. Speiglman (9) selected four counties in California that varied in the degree to which they used presentencing screening strategies to deal with repeat offenders through the use of driving under the influence (DUI) statutes. Two of the four counties referred cases to AA, referring 37% to 40% of cases. Offenders who were represented by private attorneys were more likely to be referred to AA than those who had public representation. However, among offenders also mandated to parole or to participation in probation-defined treatment, the vast majority (88% to 97%) were required to attend AA. Frequency of attendance also was specified and typically involved two to three required meetings per week. Mandating attendance at AA requires the cooperation of the groups that the offender attends. Information at the AA Web site indicates that

> *"some groups, with the consent of the prospective member, have the A.A. group secretary sign or initial a slip that has been furnished by the court together with a self-addressed court envelope. The referred person supplies identification and mails the slip back to the court as proof of attendance. Other groups cooperate in different ways. There is no set procedure. The nature and extent of any group's involvement in this process [of verifying attendance] is entirely up to the individual group" (10).*

Patterns of Utilization of AA Both cross-sectional and longitudinal studies provide information about patterns of utilization of AA. Data from the Epidemiologic Catchment Area Study (11) suggest that individuals who attend AA or other self-help groups make about twice as many visits to meetings as to professional treatment. Alcohol-dependent persons who attend AA averaged 44.8 visits/person/year, or just under one meeting per week.

Several innovative methodologies have been used to study patterns of affiliation over time. McCrady et al. (12) examined weekly records of AA attendance among outpatients and reported three distinct patterns of affiliation: (1) positive affiliation, characterized by either immediate, regular attendance, or gradually increasing attendance over the course of treatment; (2) negative affiliation, characterized by initially higher rates of attendance that decreased over the course of treatment; and (3) nonaffiliation, characterized by little or no involvement. Morgenstern et al. (13) identified three distinct patterns of posttreatment involvement with AA that were similar to within-treatment findings by McCrady et al. Optimal responders attended meetings daily and often sought advice from AA members, partial responders attended meetings frequently but rarely sought advice from AA members, and nonresponders did not engage with AA. Caldwell and Cutter (14) also examined characteristics of involvement among three groups of alcoholics 10 weeks after treatment. Those with low levels of attendance (fewer than 20 meetings) were least likely to see themselves as alcohol-dependent, less likely to accept the concept of a Higher Power, and least likely to join an AA group. High AA attenders (at least 70 meetings in 10 weeks) saw their drinking problems as the most serious, accepted the concepts of powerlessness and a Higher Power, took advantage of the informal support and sharing associated with AA, and had worked the first five steps in AA. Humphreys et al. (15), in studying patterns of change over time, noted that subjects who were able to attain stable abstinence over a 3-year period initially were actively involved with AA, attending approximately two meetings per week for the first year. However, AA involvement decreased over the following 2 years so that, though remaining abstinent, subjects attended AA rarely, averaging about one meeting per month. Mäkelä (16) studied anniversary announcements published in a Finnish AA newsletter to track AA membership over time. Over 3 consecutive years, he found that the probability of remaining sober and involved with AA was about 67% for those with 1 year of sobriety, 85% for those with 2 to 5 years of sobriety, and 90% for those with more than 5 years of sobriety. More recently, Kaskutas et al. (17) reported on 5-year longitudinal patterns of AA attendance in a treatment-seeking population.

The *low* attendance group participated in AA during the first year after treatment, whereas the *medium* and *high* attendance groups had more consistent attendance over time. Kaskutas et al. also identified a *declining* attendance group that had very high attendance initially but then had dropped off in attendance by the year 5 follow-up. Abstinence rates in year 5 were highest for the two groups still attending AA fairly regularly, were somewhat lower for the group that had declined in attendance, and were lowest for the group that discontinued attendance after the first year.

Smith (18) conducted semistructured interviews with members of AA who had at least 2 years' sobriety to characterize patterns of social affiliation with AA. She described three patterns of affiliation: those who were affiliative from the beginning of involvement, those who were socially distant at first but later became more involved, and those who remained distant from interactions with other group members despite continued attendance at AA meetings. Those who affiliated gradually seemed to have followed a common pattern: first forming a connection with one person in AA; then focusing on specific content of stories told at meetings and through the literature, working the steps with encouragement from the sponsor without much group affiliation; and finally, performing some service work within the organization despite personal discomfort.

Summary Data derived from a number of different methodologies converge in suggesting clearly different patterns of involvement with AA—those who initially are actively involved but taper off over time, those with a steady level of involvement, and those who with a more variable or less engaged type of involvement. Data also suggest that consistent involvement is associated with better outcomes.

FACTORS ASSOCIATED WITH SUCCESSFUL AFFILIATION WITH AA

Despite the diversity of the membership of AA, research shows that certain factors are associated with more successful affiliation with AA. Research to identify characteristics of those more likely to affiliate with AA does not imply that individuals without those characteristics will not affiliate. A number of individual studies have reported characteristics predictive of affiliation with AA, including male gender (4), more serious alcohol problems (3,6,19–21), greater commitment to abstinence (20), more social support to stop drinking (3), less support from and more stress in marriage/intimate relationships (22), fewer psychologic problems such as depression or poor self-esteem (6), use of a more avoidant style for coping with problems (22), and having a greater desire to find meaning in life (23). Most findings, however, are supported by only one recent study, with the exception of severity of alcohol dependence and commitment to abstinence, which seem to be stable predictors of affiliation across multiple studies. Findings are contradictory for some variables, such as education, where affiliation is predicted by greater education among whites but less education among Hispanic Americans; or marital status, where unmarried status predicts affiliation among Hispanics (19), but being married generally is predictive of affiliation in population surveys.

The personal characteristic of spirituality or religiosity has been examined in a series of recent studies. Professionals and the public alike believe that individuals who are more religious will be more successful in AA because of the intrinsically spiritual nature of the recovery program. A recent survey found that program directors in Department of Veterans Affairs (VA) facilities were less likely to refer a patient to AA if the individual was an atheist (24). Winzelberg and Humphreys (25) looked at the relationships among clinician referral to Twelve Step groups, client religiosity, group attendance, and client outcomes. They too found that professionals were less likely to refer patients to Twelve Step groups if the patients engaged in fewer religious behaviors. However, though more frequent religious behaviors predicted Twelve Step meeting attendance, clinician referral to such groups increased attendance regardless of religiosity. Finally, attendance at Twelve Step groups predicted better outcomes, again regardless of religiousness. Tonigan et al. (26) examined religious beliefs and AA affiliation among patients in Project MATCH. They found that clients assigned to Twelve Step facilitation treatment (TSF) were most likely to report increased belief in God, but clients who described themselves as atheists or agnostics generally were less likely to attend AA, even if assigned to TSF treatment, compared to clients who were spiritual or religious in their beliefs. Similar to Winzelberg and Humphreys, Tonigan et al. found that AA attendance was positively associated with outcomes regardless of religious beliefs.

Psychiatric comorbidity is another patient characteristic that could affect AA affiliation. Tomasson and Vaglum (27) determined that the presence or absence of most comorbid disorders was unrelated to AA attendance in an aftercare sample of alcoholics, though the presence of comorbid disorders was associated with higher rates of professional help seeking. Schizophrenia, however, was the one diagnosis associated with lower rates of attendance. In a study of substance abuse patients, Ouimette et al. (28) found that during treatment, individuals with substance abuse only and those with both substance abuse and personality disorders attended Twelve Step meetings more frequently than did substance abusers with psychotic, anxiety, or depression diagnoses. However, in the continuing care phase, there were no significant differences among the groups in frequency of Twelve Step meeting attendance. In a recent comprehensive review of the literature on comorbidity and AA involvement, Bogenschutz (29) also concluded that patients with comorbid psychiatric disorders attended AA at about the same rate as other patients, though attendance was lower for those with psychotic disorder diagnoses (30). He also noted the added benefit of 12-step programs that are specialized for those with comorbid disorders and that mechanisms of change associated with success in AA, such as enhanced self-efficacy and greater social support, are similar for those with and without comorbid disorders.

In Summary Data generally support the view of AA as a program that attracts a diverse membership. However, those with more severe drinking problems and those with a greater commitment to change are more likely to affiliate with AA. Patient religiosity affects clinicians' referrals to AA, and patients with agnostic and atheist beliefs may attend less meetings, but patients who go to AA increase their religiosity regardless of their initial beliefs. Patients with comorbid psychiatric disorders also affiliate with AA, though those with schizophrenia are somewhat less likely to attend.

AA AND POPULATION SUBGROUPS

Two contrasting views of AA lead to different predictions about AA and different population subgroups. One perspective suggests that AA is a program of recovery for a person with alcohol use disorders and that the common experience of alcoholism should supercede superficial individual differences. Because AA groups are autonomous, individual meetings may take on the character of the predominant population in attendance, allowing for meetings that are comfortable for persons of different backgrounds. In the United States, "special interest" groups for certain subpopulations (such as women, gays and lesbians, young people, and certain racial/ethnic groups) are very common (2). An alternative perspective is that, because AA was developed by educated, middle-aged, white, Christian, heterosexual males, its relevance to less-educated, young, or older persons, persons of color, non-Christians, gays and lesbians, or women is suspect. AA's own triennial surveys have found an increase in the proportion of women in AA from about 22% in 1968, to about 35%, leveling off starting in 1989 (31). The average age of AA members responding to AA's triennial survey has increased to about 48 years of age (31), and the triennial survey data as well as observation of AA meetings reveal a broad diversity among the membership in age, occupational status, and race. Research data about the relevance of AA to various subgroups are limited though increasing.

Women Several controlled and qualitative studies have examined women and AA. Recent studies in the United States (22,32) and Sweden (33) have found similar rates of AA attendance in men and women, and the 2004 AA triennial survey reports that about 35% of members responding to the survey were women, rates comparable to the rates of women with alcohol dependence in the general population. Likewise, no substantive gender difference was found in 12-step treatment compliance and engagement in Project MATCH (34). However, men and women may have different reasons for affiliating with AA. For example, Kaskutas (35) studied women attending Women for Sobriety (WFS) meetings, approximately 25% of whom also attended AA. The women attended AA for reasons somewhat different from those for attending WFS: AA was cited as the program most crucial to their staying sober, though the fellowship, support, sharing, and spirituality in AA all were cited as important as well. The women perceived WFS as most valuable for the nurturing atmosphere, involvement with an all-women's program, and exposure to positive female role models. There also may be aspects of AA that make it less appealing to women. In Kaskutas's research, she found that the women in the sample also reported reasons why they did not attend AA, including a feeling that they did not fit in; a perception that AA is too punitive and focused on shame and guilt; disagreement with program principles related to powerlessness, surrender, and reliance on a Higher Power; and a perception that AA is male-dominated. A recent survey of 55 women attending AA (36) found that half the women had experienced "thirteenth-stepping," in which they felt sexually targeted by men in the program. Such experience was less common among women who attended at least some women-only AA meetings. These negative experiences may at least partly explain findings by Humphreys et al. in comparing individuals who were actively involved in AA with those who had been active but then dropped out, that a greater proportion of women than men dropped out of their self-help groups. Women also may use AA differently than do men. Bodin also found that women were more likely than men to call other AA members for help, to have experienced a spiritual awakening, and to have read AA literature.

Cultural, Racial, and Ethnic Subgroups Research on involvement in AA by cultural, racial, and ethnic subgroups is limited. Data reported by Caetano (19) from a national survey showed that, in general, Hispanics, African Americans, and whites tended to endorse equally the basic tenets of the disease model. All groups held fairly positive views of AA (meaning that they would be more likely to recommend it than any other treatment modality). Some variability was noted in support for AA, with 97% of Hispanics, 94% of whites, 87% of African Americans, and 76% of Asian Americans recommending AA as a resource. Caetano also reported that Hispanics in the sample were more likely to have had contact with AA (12%) than either whites or African Americans (5%). AA attendance seems to follow a pattern similar to attitudes about AA. For example, Tonigan et al. (37) reported that in the outpatient arm of Project MATCH, similar proportions of whites, Hispanics, and African Americans attended AA during any follow-up period considered. However, the results from the aftercare arm of the study showed different results: While Hispanics and African Americans did not differ from whites in AA attendance at the beginning of the follow-up period, the two groups differed significantly from whites in having less AA attendance later in follow-up.

Kaskutas et al. (38) examined previous self-help group participation among African American and white treatment seekers. African Americans more frequently reported prior NA or Cocaine Anonymous exposure, with a trend toward more previous AA exposure. Of those who had been exposed to AA in the past, more African Americans (76%) than whites (55%) said they had gone to AA as a part of prior treatment, whereas more whites had gone to AA through other referrals or on their own. Active participation was equivalent for both groups, as measured by mean AA affiliation scale scores. However, analysis of the individual items from the affiliation scale revealed differential types of participation. African Americans were more likely than whites to identify themselves as AA members (64% vs. 54%), to say they had a spiritual awakening through AA (38% vs. 27%), and to have done service at an AA meeting recently (48% vs. 37%). African Americans were less likely than whites to have a sponsor currently (14% vs. 23%) and less likely to have read AA literature recently (67% vs. 77%). These patterns held true after controlling for prior treatment and exposure to AA during treatment. Humphreys et al. (39) reported that among substance abusers who were followed up 1 year after treatment intake, there were no significant racial differences between those individuals who were actively involved in a Twelve Step program and those who were not. When dropouts from Twelve Step groups were compared with those who remained involved, no significant differences were attributable to race/ethnicity. They also found that African Americans who were involved in self-help groups improved more in the areas of drug, alcohol, and medical problems than did African Americans who were not participating. Thus, those authors concluded that members of racial/ethnic groups, such as African Americans, attend and drop out of self-help groups at the same rates as whites; self-help group participation also was found to improve outcomes for African Americans.

A study comparing Hispanics and non-Hispanic whites examined treatment utilization and outcome differences in a treatment-seeking sample (40). They found at 6-month follow-up that Hispanics engaged in more formal treatment sessions but fewer AA meetings than did the non-Hispanic whites. However, alcohol-related outcomes were similar at follow-up for both groups, implying that ultimate outcomes are similar for Hispanics and non-Hispanic whites, despite the finding that they engage in different treatment paths. One possible explanation for the finding that Hispanics participated less in AA is that the Hispanics were more likely to be living with others at intake and thus may have been better able to turn to those persons for social support rather than looking to a support group such as AA. Another possibility is that Hispanics may not have viewed self-help groups as being as effective as formal approaches. Tonigan et al. (37,41) reported on a subsample of Project MATCH participants from Albuquerque, NM. They found that though Hispanics attended fewer AA meetings, they reported being equally or more committed to AA than whites (as evidenced by working the steps, having or being a sponsor, and celebrating AA birthdays), and higher in "god consciousness." AA involvement predicted better drinking outcomes in both Hispanics and whites.

Age-Specific Groups There is some hesitancy about involving adolescents in AA because of their developmental status (42) and concern that adolescent substance use disorders are, in some cases, age-limited phenomena. However, several studies have suggested a strong association between AA/NA involvement and abstinence in adolescents, similar to that found in adults. (These studies are reviewed in the section "The Effectiveness of AA and Treatments Based on AA.") Research to date has focused on adolescents in inpatient treatment programs, arguably the population with the most severe problems. Hohman and LeCroy (43) examined a sample of adolescents who had completed inpatient treatment and reported that about 44% had participated in AA. Adolescents who had attended AA were more likely to have experienced prior treatment, felt more hopeless, had family who had participated less in their treatment program, and currently were more likely to have friends who did not use alcohol or drugs. Kelly et al. (44) found that adolescents were more likely to attend if the AA groups they attended had more age peers. They also found (45) that the severity of the adolescent's alcohol use disorder was correlated positively with motivation to attend AA. An earlier study (46) found that AA attendance was associated with a modest improvement in outcomes 3 and 6 months after inpatient treatment.

Dually Diagnosed Individuals Research on substance abusers with comorbid psychiatric disorders has been focused primarily on a comparison of the substance use, psychiatric, and other life outcomes of those with multiple diagnoses compared to those with substance use disorders alone. Recent research also supports understanding of those dually diagnosed individuals in AA. Pristach and Smith (47) looked at attitudes and participation in AA in a sample of 60 psychiatric inpatients with comorbid alcohol use disorders. The sample was divided by type of disorder, including affective disorders, personality or adjustment disorders, psychotic disorders, and other substance use disorders. Overall, 37% of the sample reported at least weekly attendance at AA. Pro-AA sentiments were common among those involved, and such attitudes were associated with regular past AA attendance. Those who had attended AA previously were more likely to attend AA after treatment than those who had never attended AA; they also reported feeling comfortable with AA. In contrast to Tomasson and Vaglum's (27) finding that alcohol abusers with comorbid schizophrenia were less likely to attend AA, Pristach and Smith found no difference in past AA attendance for schizophrenic individuals compared with other dually diagnosed patients. Polcin and Zemore (48) looked at specific aspects of involvement with AA, using a continuous measure of psychiatric severity (from the Addiction Severity Index) rather than diagnosis. They found that higher psychiatric severity was associated with lower levels of spirituality and less working the 12 steps or serving as a sponsor.

An important implication of the presence of comorbid disorders is the need for prescription medications. The subject of medication use by AA members is a particularly important one, given that medications play a larger role in mental health treatment today, but there are thoughtful cautions raised in the core AA literature about the use of mind-altering drugs (49). In an anonymous survey, Rychtarik et al. (50) assessed AA members' attitudes toward the use of medication, either to prevent relapse or to treat other disorders. (Medications included antidepressants, pain medications, anxiolytics, lithium, antipsychotics, naltrexone, and disulfiram.) The majority (53%) of the sample thought that use of medications to prevent relapse was either a good idea or might be a good idea, 17% reported that they did not like the idea of medication and believed the individual should not take it, and 12% said they would recommend that another member discontinue medication use. About 29% said they had been encouraged to stop taking any type of medication, and an additional 20% had heard of others who had been encouraged to discontinue use. Of those who were encouraged to stop medication use, 31% actually stopped.

Swift et al. (51) predicted that persons with more prior AA exposure would be less likely to take naltrexone for alcohol abuse. They reported that in a treatment-seeking sample, willingness to take naltrexone was unrelated to frequency of past AA meetings attended and, surprisingly, having an AA sponsor was positively related to willingness to take medications, albeit modestly. Naturalistic studies of AA members' perceptions and practices support the counter-intuitive idea that AA exposure has a negligible effect on the use of medications for an alcohol use disorder. Tonigan and Kelly (52), for example, reported that AA affiliation was unrelated to attitudes about the use of medications for drinking problems and that AA members' perceptions did not differ from problematic drinkers who did not attend AA. It seems, then, that though negative messages may be voiced in AA about the use of medications, AA exposure in itself does not deter medication compliance.

Gays and Lesbians Research on the experience of gays and lesbians in relation to AA is quite limited. One ethnographic study (53) recruited lesbians who had been in recovery for at least 1 year. All respondents were familiar with AA; 74% were actively involved. Hall identified three sources of tension for the lesbians in AA. First, they reported a tension between a sense of assimilation and a sense of differentiation. The women said they felt that AA was a program in which people of very different backgrounds could relate because of their common concerns, but at times they viewed AA as a white, male, heterosexist organization. Second, they said they understood the value of the authority of AA as a prescription for sobriety but at times viewed AA more as a program that provided a set of tools for recovery. The perceived sexist language in the AA literature and the lack of focus on lesbian issues made following the program prescriptively a difficult task. Finally, the women said they experienced tension between the strongly individual focus of AA and their perception of the importance of examining issues in a cultural context.

Summary It appears that individuals from minority groups (e.g., women, gays and lesbians, racial/ethnic minorities) have a mixed experience in AA, seeing particular value in the support for sobriety, but also having a different set of experiences with AA, some of which are somewhat negative.

THE EFFECTIVENESS OF AA AND TREATMENTS BASED ON AA

Answering the apparently simple question "Does AA work?" is a challenge. One approach is to look at the success of AA as an organization: The broad dissemination of the program around the world and the large membership suggest that AA has been enormously successful in attracting persons to AA as a program of recovery. The AA triennial surveys also point to the substantial proportion of abstaining, long-term members, as do Mäkelä's (16) studies of stability of sobriety in AA. More difficult questions, however, have less clear-cut answers: "Is AA *the most effective* approach to alcohol dependence?" "Is AA involvement *necessary* to successful resolution of alcohol problems?" "Does AA *lead to* better outcomes or is it simply a correlate? "What are the most effective strategies to *engage* individuals with AA?" Research to answer these questions has used several different methodologies: (1) randomized clinical trials comparing AA or treatments designed to involve individuals in AA to different forms of alcoholism treatment, (2) naturalistic studies of treatments designed to engage individuals with AA, (3) studies examining the unique contribution of AA to the prediction of outcomes in clinical and nonclinical samples, and (4) studies of effective approaches to engaging patients in AA. Review of these four lines of evidence provides some provocative answers to questions about the relative effectiveness of AA.

Randomized Clinical Trials Randomized clinical trials (RCTs) in which persons are randomly assigned to different treatment conditions are considered the most rigorous experimental tests of therapeutic effectiveness. Only three RCTs comparing AA to different forms of treatment have been reported in the research literature, and no RCT has been reported since 1991 (54). Each of the three RCTs has serious methodologic problems, and all used populations mandated to treatment, so it is difficult to draw specific conclusions about the effectiveness of AA from these studies.

AA and Twelve Step–oriented treatments have close conceptual links in their adherence to the classic disease concept of alcoholism, emphasis on abstinence, the importance of AA involvement, and working the Twelve Steps. Differences between AA and other Twelve Step treatment programs are substantial, however, and the two should not be equated. Several important randomized clinical trials of treatments based on Twelve Step principles have been reported over the past several years. The most prominent and visible randomized clinical trial, Project MATCH (23,55–57), was designed to study the interactions between specific patient characteristics and one of three structured 12-week outpatient individual treatments: Twelve Step Facilitation (TSF), motivational enhancement therapy (MET), or cognitive-behavior therapy (CBT). Participants were 1,726 persons with diagnosed alcohol abuse or dependence (952 outpatients and 774 aftercare patients) who were recruited from among 4,481 patients screened at nine participating clinical research units. Participants were assessed thoroughly and then randomly assigned to one of the three treatments. Clinicians were nested within treatments, received extensive training prior to the study, and were carefully supervised throughout. Treatment was delivered over a 3-month period. Individuals assigned to TSF or CBT could receive up to 12 manual-guided treatment sessions, whereas MET participants received up to four treatment sessions over the same 12-week period. All participants were followed up for 15 months from baseline, with research contacts scheduled every 3 months. Participants in the outpatient arm of the study were contacted again 39 months after the initial baseline evaluation, and their functioning during the preceding 3 months was assessed. Though Project MATCH was not designed specifically to study the main effects of the three study treatments, some treatment main effects did emerge. During treatment (56), patients in the outpatient arm of the study were more likely to maintain abstinence or moderate drinking if they received CBT or TSF rather than MET (41% vs. 28%). One year after treatment, patients in the three treatments had comparable outcomes in the percentage of days that they were abstinent and the mean number of drinks consumed per day (23). Two variables favored the TSF treatment: Patients who had participated in TSF treatment were more likely to have maintained continuous abstinence and were less likely to have relapsed to heavy drinking after treatment. At the 3-year follow-up of the outpatient arm of the study, few significant differences among the three treatment conditions were noted, but, as at the 1-year follow-up, patients who had received the TSF treatment were more likely to have been abstinent during the 3 months prior to the 3-year follow-up. Also, compared to patients who had participated in CBT, TSF subjects had a significantly greater percentage of abstinent days during the preceding 3 months (57). Several significant client-treatment matching effects were found. During treatment, no client-treatment match affected drinking (56). However, during the first year after treatment, patients who had low levels of psychiatric symptoms had more days of abstinence if they had received the TSF rather than the CBT treatment (23). Aftercare patients with higher levels of alcohol dependence also had better outcomes with TSF. In contrast, patients who were low in alcohol dependence had better outcomes with CBT (55). A second important matching finding emerged at 3 years: Outpatients whose social networks were highly supportive of their drinking had better outcomes if they received TSF rather than MET treatment (58). Though the positive findings from Project MATCH are significant, most of the matching hypotheses tested were *not* supported, including primary and secondary matching hypotheses related to gender, sociopathy and antisocial personality disorder, other DSM diagnoses, alcoholic subtypes, cognitive impairment or conceptual level, motivation and readiness to change, self-efficacy, assertion of autonomy, meaning seeking, and other aspects of social functioning.

McCrady et al. used an RCT design to study the impact of adding AA to alcohol-focused behavioral couple therapy (ABCT). Participants assigned to the combined AA/ABCT treatment were significantly more likely to attend AA meetings during treatment (59), but AA involvement did not result in better drinking outcomes at either 6 or 18 months after treatment (59,60).

Naturalistic Studies of Treatments Based on Twelve-Step Principles In contrast to randomized clinical trials, which typically include strict experimental controls to maximize internal validity, naturalistic study designs evaluate existing treatment programs and patient populations. Experimental controls are lacking, but the inclusion of a broader sample and the evaluation of extant treatments provide information complementary to that obtained from RCTs. In the largest comparative study of Twelve Step–based treatments, Moos et al. (61) studied 3,698 male veterans being treated at 1 of 15 VA treatment units. The treatment units were classified as Twelve Step–oriented, cognitive behavioral therapy–oriented, or eclectic. No patient was excluded from the study, and 97% of the patients were followed up successfully 1 year after treatment. Overall, patients showed significant decreases in drinking, symptoms of alcohol dependence, and psychological problems and improved in social functioning. Patients who participated in Twelve Step–oriented treatment were about 1.5 times as likely to be abstinent as patients whose treatment was cognitive behavioral in orientation (62). Patients from both types of programs, however, were more likely to be employed than patients whose treatment was more eclectic in focus. Patient-treatment matching also was examined in the VA study (63), but there was no evidence that specific patient characteristics predicted differential response to either Twelve Step–oriented or cognitive behavioral therapy. In the year after treatment, patients from the Twelve Step–oriented programs attended significantly more self-help groups than patients from the cognitive behavioral programs and had significantly fewer outpatient visits and inpatient treatment days, and subsequent costs of treatment were 64% higher for patients who had not participated in a Twelve Step–oriented treatment unit (64).

Single-group evaluations of treatments based on Twelve Step principles typically have studied inpatient treatment programs. Most studies have focused on private treatment centers, whose populations typically are more socially stable than patients in public treatment programs. The largest study of this type (65) reported that 67% to 75% of participants reported abstinence 6 months after treatment, and 60% to 68% abstinent rates at a 12-month follow-up. However, study attrition was substantial, and the investigators estimated that abstinence rates would have been 56% to 65% at 6 months and 34% to 42% at 12 months if patients lost to follow-up were considered to have relapsed. An evaluation of 1,083 patients treated at the Hazelden treatment program (66) reported that at 6 months after discharge, 59% of patients said they had not used alcohol or drugs since discharge; at the 12-month follow-up, 53% said they had not used alcohol or drugs since discharge. Follow-up rates were better than 70%. If patients lost to follow-up are included as treatment failures, adjusted rates of continuous abstinence were 45% at 6 months and 37% at 12 months—results very comparable to those reported by Hoffmann and Miller (65).

AA Involvement and the Prediction of Treatment Outcomes Many studies have examined the contribution of AA attendance and involvement to the prediction of successful resolution of a drinking problem. One of the most consistent and robust findings is that there is a positive correlation between AA attendance and drinking outcomes. Studies of treatment populations in the 1990s (65,67,68) found that patients who attended AA were significantly more likely to be abstinent 1 year after treatment than were those who did not attend AA. Analyses of Project MATCH data by treatment site also found that AA attendance correlated positively with drinking outcomes for all sites (69). More recent studies have reported longer-term follow-ups, with similar results. For example, a 3-year follow-up of participants in a study of posttreatment telephone case monitoring found that mutual help group involvement in years 1 and 2 of follow-up was associated with more abstinence in years 2 and 3 of the study (70). Similar results have now been reported with drug-dependent patients. In a 5-year follow-up, Gossop et al. (71) found a positive association between AA/NA attendance and abstinence from opiates and alcohol but not from stimulants. Two studies have examined the causal relationship between AA attendance and outcomes. In a series of concurrent and time-lagged analyses McCrady et al. (60) found that AA attendance predicted subsequent abstinence throughout 18 months of posttreatment follow-up but that abstinence did not predict AA attendance, thus suggesting a causal relationship between AA attendance and positive outcomes of treatment. Similarly, McKellar et al. (72) reported that the level of AA affiliation 1 year after treatment predicted lower levels of alcohol-related problems 2 years after treatment but that the converse was not the case.

Studies of non-treatment-seeking populations (73) have found that AA involvement was one of a handful of significant predictors of long-term (greater than 5 years) abstinence. Long-term, 8-year (7,74) and 16-year (8) follow-ups of individuals who had presented to an information and referral center or received detoxification found that AA attendance was significantly though weakly correlated with less alcohol consumption, less intoxication, more abstinence, and fewer symptoms of alcohol dependence or alcohol-related problems. They also found that persons who had been involved with AA were more likely to have positive long-term outcomes than those who had received no treatment. Compared to those who received treatment without AA, those who attended AA alone were more likely to be abstinent up to 3 years after initial contact, but outcomes were equivalent at the 8-year follow-up. Outcomes were comparable for persons who attended treatment alone or who combined treatment with AA. Findings from NESARC (5) are remarkably similar. They found that individuals involved with treatment and Twelve Step programs were almost twice as likely to have successful outcomes as those involved with formal treatment alone.

Engaging Patients with AA A recent study examined methods to engage patients in AA. Kahler et al. (75) randomly assigned patients in detoxification to brief advice or motivational enhancement therapy (ME-12) focused on AA attendance. They found that ME-12 resulted in better outcomes than advice for patients without significant experience with AA but that advice was more effective for those with past AA experience. The results suggest that it may be confusing for patients already positively oriented toward AA to be asked to examine their perceptions of the value of AA.

Summary The research literature suggests that involvement with AA clearly is associated with positive outcomes and that AA involvement leads to positive outcomes, rather than simply being a correlate. Data simply do not exist to determine whether AA itself is more effective than different kinds of treatment, but an accumulating body of literature suggests that treatment programs (inpatient and outpatient) based on 12-step principles may be more successful in effecting total abstinence over time and may be more cost-effective than other treatment models. The literature on methods to engage individuals with AA is still very limited, but early findings suggest that methods for engagement may need to vary depending on the individual's past experience with the program.

MECHANISMS OF CHANGE IN AA

With empirical evidence that AA is beneficial for many problem drinkers investigators are now seeking to understand why AA is beneficial. This line of research necessarily involves three integrated aims, and it is important to keep them definitionally distinct. First, investigators are seeking to identify the active ingredients of AA that mobilize behavior change. Such catalysts may include prescribed behaviors such as sponsorship, reading core AA literature, and AA step work but may also include unintended or more subtle processes, such as frequency and nature of social support offered through AA participation. Second, actual active ingredients must produce changes that enhance the probability of successfully changing behavior; active ingredients in and of themselves are not explanations for behavior change. And, third, mobilized changes in an individual must predict later reductions in drinking.

Of the three aims to study why AA is beneficial, investigators have focused most directly on identifying the active ingredients of AA. Historically, the AA meeting has been considered the "dose," and frequency of AA meeting attendance thus indicated the intensity of the dose (76). This monolithic view of AA has yielded to a multidimensional perspective, one that first distinguished between physical exposure and engagement in prescribed AA behaviors. Montgomery et al. (77), for example, distinguished AA *attendance* from AA *involvement*, which included, in addition to attendance, the degree of involvement with various aspects of AA—such as participation during meetings, having a sponsor, leading meetings, working specific steps, or doing Twelfth Step work. They reported that AA involvement and attendance were moderately correlated (0.45); however, involvement, not attendance, correlated with posttreatment alcohol consumption (r = −0.44) in a sample of patients in an inpatient Twelve Step treatment program.

Using Project MATCH data, Tonigan et al. (78) examined the nature of participants' experience with AA. As in other research, there was a positive correlation between AA-related actions and the degree to which patients were abstinent. Tonigan et al. anticipated that there would be two aspects of experience with AA—a subjective dimension and a behavioral dimension. Statistically, however, experiences with AA seemed to reflect one major dimension rather than two. Greater participation was reflected in a combination of factors: a spiritual awakening, God-consciousness, the perception that attending AA meetings was helpful, actually attending AA meetings, being involved with other AA-related practices, and completing more steps. They also found that participation in AA during treatment and in the first 6 months after treatment predicted better drinking outcomes in the second 6 months after treatment (78). Weiss et al. (79) reported similar findings about the importance of commitment to Twelve Step practices, with the important distinction that they were investigating Twelve Step-related benefit among 487 cocaine-dependent adults. In addition to receiving 24 weeks of behavioral counseling, these patients were encouraged to attend Twelve Step programs. Findings indicated that frequency of Twelve Step attendance did not predict later substance use but that a composite measure reflecting engagement in 12-step programs was significantly and positively associated with increased abstinence.

But what of *specific* AA prescribed behaviors and drinking outcomes? Brown and Peterson (80) surveyed AA members' views of the relative importance of different aspects of the AA program. Working the steps, having a sponsor, telling their story at a meeting, and daily meditations were seen as most important. In a second sample, members of AA and other Twelve Step groups were surveyed. Respondents believed in a Higher Power, that they would recover with the help of their Higher Power, and that they were powerless over alcohol or another problem for which they sought help. Additionally, respondents reported a number of behavioral changes that facilitated recovery, including attending group meetings; avoiding people, places, and things associated with their problem; making amends; working the Fourth and Fifth Steps; praying; telling their story at a meeting; and maintaining a regular pattern of sleep.

Research tends to confirm the importance of several AA-related behaviors for abstinence reported by AA members. Pagano et al. (81), for example, in a reexamination of the Project MATCH data set, reported that being an AA sponsor led to a significant reduction in relapse rate at 1 year (e.g., 60% relapse with sponsor versus 78% relapse without sponsor); however, it was relatively rare in this sample (8%; n = 120), suggesting the desirability of encouraging this behavior more often during the treatment experience. Further, investigating whether type of substance use disorder (i.e., alcohol dependence, drug dependence, or both alcohol and drug dependence) moderated the relative benefits of Twelve Step meeting attendance and prescribed behaviors, Witbrodt and Kaskutas (82) found that of seven specific AA behaviors, only having a sponsor predicted positive outcome across substance abuse categories. Secondary benefits of sponsorship have been reported by Kaskutas et al. (17). Specifically, in a 5-year study of 349 alcohol-dependent adults, they reported that sponsorship and frequency of AA attendance were positively associated such that high and medium AA attendees at 5 years had triple the rates of being sponsors as the individuals who had low or declining rates of AA attendance. Other AA program behaviors also appear to predict later improvements, even after statistically controlling for AA fellowship behaviors such as AA attendance. Tonigan and Miller (83), for example, reported that the specific number of AA steps completed at 3-year follow-up and alcohol consumed at 10-year follow-up was significantly and negatively related. Further, Tonigan and Miller (84) reported that commitment to, and understanding of, the 12 steps were significantly and positively predictive of 1-year abstinence.

Less easily classified, AA fellowship behaviors also have been identified as potential candidates to understand what mobilizes mechanisms of change. Essentially, this body of research has focused on the benefits of social support and network support for abstinence provided through AA participation. Involvement in self-help groups, for example, may influence the *nature* of a substance abuser's social network. Humphreys and Noke (85) followed male inpatient substance abusers after treatment and examined AA, NA, or CA participation and social network outcomes. They found that increased group participation predicted both better quality of general friendship and less support of substance use by friends at follow-up. Individuals involved significantly in Twelve Step groups (involved in at least two of three Twelve Step activities measured) actually increased the size of their friendship networks by an average of 16%; those *not* significantly involved in Twelve Step groups showed no change in the size of their friendship networks. The greater increase in social network size was attributable to the fact that those significantly more involved in Twelve Step groups increased their numbers of friends in Twelve Step programs, not because those less involved with Twelve Step groups lost friends. Finally, Humphreys and Noke (85) found that those who had networks composed almost entirely of Twelve Step members experienced better friendship quality than did others who held social networks composed of almost no Twelve Step members.

Evidence suggests that the benefits of social networks supportive of abstinence in Twelve Step programs may vary temporally. In particular, Witbrodt and Kaskutas (82) reported that, for alcohol-dependent adults, network support for abstinence was significantly predictive of abstinence at 6 months but not at 12-month follow-up. The reverse situation was found for drug-dependent individuals in whom the benefits of social support were unrelated to 6-month abstinence but significantly and positively related to 12-month abstinence rates. The exact reasons for this reversal effect are unclear, but it may be related to unintended stimulus cues encouraging illicit drug use during early efforts to achieve abstinence. Also intriguing is the finding that the magnitude of benefit associated with social support for abstinence is different between Twelve Step member provided support and support from others (86). Specifically, at 30- and 90-day follow-up interviews, abstinence rates were twice as high for AA members who reported AA member social support compared to those of AA members reporting social support for abstinence from non-AA sources. Combined, both temporal and social support characteristics appear to moderate the benefit of social support for abstinence, with early AA member support most beneficial for alcohol-dependent individuals.

Given the importance of social network variables in alcohol-treatment outcome in general and AA in particular, recent studies have focused on the role formal treatment can play in facilitating AA-related social network benefit. Litt et al. (87), for instance, designed a treatment to enhance network support either through AA or other social resources such as families and social activities. The network support therapy significantly increased AA involvement and more general support for abstinence from members of their social network. Similar to other studies, both network support and AA involvement correlated positively with treatment outcomes.

Treatment outcome research suggests that social variables also may function as moderators of the relationship between Twelve Step participation and outcome. Though the Project MATCH studies are reviewed elsewhere in this chapter, one study by Longabaugh et al. (58) is of particular interest here. In examining the effects of matching patient characteristics with specific treatment modalities, Longabaugh et al. found that TSF treatment, which aimed to involve patients in AA, was more effective than MET for individuals who had social networks that were supportive of drinking. Those with low support for drinking had similar outcomes, regardless of treatment type. The investigators also found that AA participation mediated the interaction between treatment type and network support for drinking. In other words, TSF treatment emphasized AA involvement and thus helped to create improved social networks, which in turn predicted better drinking outcomes. This was especially true for those individuals who had networks that supported their drinking behavior.

WHAT DO THE AA ACTIVE INGREDIENTS INFLUENCE?

Spirituality The core AA literature specifically posits that as a result of working the 12 steps one will have a spiritual awakening, with benefits including sobriety and increased sense of well being (88,89). Spiritual development therefore seems an ideal candidate to be a central AA-change mechanism. In cross-sectional and longitudinal studies that have employed dozens of different psychometrically validated measures of spirituality and religiosity (e.g., religious beliefs and behavior [90]; spiritual coping questionnaire [91]; brief measure of religiosity and spirituality [92]; daily spiritual experiences [93]) two findings have been reported consistently: (1) AA program and fellowship behaviors are significantly and positively associated with measures of spirituality and religiosity, and (2) the endorsement of spiritual and religious practices increases in amplitude with longer periods of AA affiliation (78,94–96). Based upon a sample (N = 123) of alcohol-dependent adults, for example, Robinson et al. (94) provided estimates of the magnitude of spiritual/religious before and after gains among AA-exposed adults for the first 6 months after outpatient treatment. Before and after changes were largest for the measures that inventoried spiritual and religious *practices*, e.g., prayer (d = 0.33), while before and after changes for measures of spiritual and religious values, beliefs, and meaning were minimal (e.g., d = 10).

Evidence is mixed about the relative importance of spiritual/religious changes for explaining increased abstinence among AA members. In a 3-year follow-up of adult substance abusers who received private and public treatment, for instance, Kaskutas et al. (86) reported that about equal proportions of abstinent adults reported having or not having a spiritual awakening as a result of AA participation. Robinson et al. (94) provide the most compelling evidence that increased spirituality accounts for AA-related benefit. Here, they reported that the average before and after increase in daily spiritual experiences enhanced the odds of reduced heavy drinking at 6 months by 12% after *controlling* for changes in AA involvement. More often, little support for a direct effect of spirituality on subsequent drinking reductions and increased well-being is reported (23,56,97,98).

In the few cases wherein religious and spiritual measures did "significantly" predict later abstinence, the actual magnitude of these relationships was small and was not clinically meaningful (e.g., $r = 0.08$; $p < 0.05$; for Project MATCH baseline religiosity scores and percentage abstinent days at 6-month follow-up [95]). Spirituality, however, may offer secondary benefit. Specifically, Christo and Franey (99) found that, though neither spiritual beliefs nor believing in addiction as a disease predicted drug use outcomes, both predicted NA attendance, which was related to reduced drug use. Clearly, there is strong evidence that the active ingredients of AA (e.g., working the 12 steps) produce, on average, increased spirituality. Whether such increases account for later improvement, however, is open to question at this time. Important to mention is that evidence indicates that self-reported atheists are less likely to attend Twelve Step programs, but those atheists that do affiliate report similar rates of benefit at 1- and 3-year follow-ups relative to self-described spiritual and religious AA members (41,100).

Cognitive Shifts Snow et al. (101) were one of the first teams to investigate the types of cognitive and behavioral processes used by AA members to facilitate change. Half their sample were current members of AA; another 35% had attended at some point. Current members of AA were more likely to use helping relationships, stimulus control ("people, places, and things"), and behavioral management strategies to maintain sobriety. Those who attended more frequently used more behavioral processes of change. Snow et al. also examined the processes of change used by those with the strongest affiliation to AA. They found that those with the greatest affiliation reported greater importance for helping relationships, stimulus control, behavior management, and consciousness-raising processes (101).

Several studies have investigated "AA-specific" cognitive mechanisms in Twelve Step therapy, arguably replicating the mechanisms of change in community-based AA. Morgenstern et al. (102) for example, reported that some cognitive shifts promoted by Twelve Step therapists did predict later improvement (e.g., powerlessness over alcohol), but others did not. Further, Tonigan (103) reported that therapist emphasis on complete abstinence was stronger in Twelve Step therapy relative to motivational enhancement and cognitive behavioral therapies but that this differential emphasis did not explain higher rates of complete abstinence of TSF clients at 1-year follow-up (23). Likewise, using a composite measure of 12-step beliefs Finney et al. (104,105) found modest increases in AA-related cognitions during Twelve Step treatment, but such changes did not explain later abstinence rates. In general, then, we find that cognitive shifts congruent with AA ideology can be successfully mobilized in Twelve Step therapy but that the relative importance of these shifts is mixed, at best, in accounting for increased abstinence.

In contrast, the study of one "nonspecific" therapeutic mechanism in AA has yielded consistent positive findings. Eleven studies have shown, for example, that frequency of AA meeting attendance is associated with gains in abstinence self-efficacy and, in turn, that these gains partially explain AA benefit (20,46,95,106–109). Meta-analytic work (110) further shows that the actual magnitude of the temporal path from AA attendance to self-efficacy gains is, on average, about $r = 0.21$ ($SD = 0.08$), though there was significant variability in this estimate across studies (range, $r = 0.11$ to 0.31). Likewise, these studies also reported positive ($r = 0.33$) but significantly different estimates of the utility of self-efficacy in explaining AA-related abstinence (range, $r = 0.06$ to 0.45). Whether significant variation in the magnitude of relationships was the result of different sample characteristics or in AA practices is speculative because the measure used across these studies to define AA participation, AA meeting attendance, was unfortunately a composite indicator of both AA program and fellowship behaviors.

Summary AA-related benefit occurs because of a tapestry of social interactions, prescribed behaviors, and mobilized psychological processes. There is strong evidence that social support for abstinence in Twelve Step programs is an important element accounting for Twelve Step-related benefit, but evidence also indicates that the nature and temporal benefit associated with such support are complex and are only beginning to be understood. Likewise, consistent support is found for the benefit of two AA-prescribed behaviors: AA meeting attendance and engagement in the AA program by having, and being, an AA sponsor. Because sponsorship is a vital prerequisite for working the 12 steps, an important outstanding question is whether sponsorship per se predicts positive outcome or, alternatively, whether being guided through the 12 steps by a sponsor accounts for AA-related benefit. Contrary to conventional wisdom, cognitive shifts that appear to account for AA-related benefit are not AA-specific. Though changes in many beliefs and values occur among AA-exposed individuals, such changes do not seem to have a direct, and definitive, effect explaining reduced drinking.

FUTURE DIRECTIONS

Research on AA has become increasingly sophisticated over the past decade, and a body of accrued knowledge provides a richer and more articulated research-based picture of AA than was available previously. However, there are important research and conceptual issues not well addressed in the current body of literature.

AA as a Single Entity The program of AA is relatively invariant, but evidence suggests that there is substantial variation in the practice of the AA program (e.g., the fellowship [77,111,112]). Typically, AA-focused research disregards such variation and treats AA as a monolithic entity. This research practice makes several assumptions, ones that probably are not valid. Specifically, (1) the "dose" of AA is fixed and invariant across meetings regardless of meeting type (e.g., speaker, closed, open discussion), size, and membership characteristics, (2) AA group social dynamics do not influence the generation, transmission, or reception of the "dose" of AA, (3) AA social context itself does not account for drinking outcome, directly or indirectly, (4) AA social context and individual characteristics do not interact in accounting for sustaining AA membership or drinking outcome, and (5) the importance of AA social context in accounting for AA-related benefit is temporally invariant (e.g., "unit benefit" of one AA meeting was the same for AA members regardless of length of membership). Though these assumptions have some utility in facilitating prospective demonstrations of general short and long-term AA-related benefit, they may also shackle the continued development of AA-related research and seriously erode the application of evidence-based findings in clinical settings.

Understanding Utilization of and Affiliation with AA Data from AA's triennial surveys and studies of persons in Twelve Step–oriented treatment indicate that the majority of individuals who try AA do not continue or affiliate. Despite reams of research to try to understand what drives initial and sustained involvement with AA, we still have a very incomplete picture of why some individuals affiliate with AA and thrive while others either avoid AA completely or do not stay with the program or benefit. Given that there are few individual characteristics that are consistent predictors of AA involvement and affiliation, research needs to look elsewhere. One untapped area of research is the possibility of key events or experiences that define affiliation or disaffiliation with AA. It is possible that there are key events and experiences at several stages of AA involvement and that these key experiences may be negative or positive. Qualitative and narrative analysis methodologies could be brought to bear in understanding these processes.

Population Subgroups The population of the United States is racially and ethnically diverse. That racial and ethnic diversity is not well represented in AA, but the membership of AA is diverse in age, socioeconomic status, and gender. The research literature, however, provides little information about the experience, utilization, and barriers to use of AA for different groups. Data are particularly scant for young people, older adults, gays and lesbians, persons of color, and persons mandated to attend AA. Culturally informed research methodologies, such as community-based participatory research, may be needed to access populations with limited involvement with AA.

Effectiveness of AA RCTs of AA as a stand-alone program of recovery (separate from treatment), are simply not being conducted. The barriers to conducting such research are considerable, and it may be appropriate to use methodologies other than RCTs to study the effectiveness of AA. However, as AA is the most recommended program of recovery by both lay persons and professionals, it would be useful to have a stronger empirical base to draw upon in making a decision to refer a patient to AA and/or some form of professional treatment. The extant literature on the effectiveness of AA points to two major conclusions: (1) that there appears to be a temporally causal relationship between AA attendance and positive drinking outcomes and (2) that individuals involved with treatments based on Twelve Step principles are more likely to maintain continuous abstinence. It is possible that the core AA message of the necessity of continuous abstinence accounts for the latter finding, but unknown is the possible negative impact of this message should an individual experience a lapse or relapse. This is an open area for future research.

CONCLUSIONS

This chapter has reviewed a substantial body of research on AA and other Twelve Step groups. AA is used widely in the United States, and 6% to 10% of the population has attended an AA meeting, with that rate doubling or tripling among those with drinking problems. Use is growing most quickly among young men, who also are the most likely to be mandated to treatment. Increasingly, the legal system is referring individuals to AA. When individuals seek help voluntarily, a substantial proportion uses AA either as their sole source of assistance or in conjunction with formal treatment. Typically, individuals become actively involved in AA for several months, attending meetings about twice a week. There is, however, considerable variability in patterns of affiliation, with some individuals becoming increasingly committed over time, while others gradually slip away from the program. Longer-term involvement is less common, but those who stay with AA for more than a year are very likely to continue their involvement for many years.

AA is such a heterogeneous organization that it is difficult to draw generalizations about who is most or least likely to affiliate. There is little evidence of problems with affiliation among specific subpopulations, but concerns about aspects of the AA program have been documented, particularly among women. It may be that the presence of special interest groups within AA and modifications of the program at the local level can effectively address these concerns. Overall, data suggest that individuals who have more-severe problems, more concern about their drinking, a greater commitment to staying abstinent, less support from a spouse, a social network supportive of drinking, a history of turning to others for support, and a greater desire to find meaning in their lives may be most likely to affiliate with AA.

Substantial research on mechanisms of change and outcomes associated with AA involvement has been reported. AA involvement clearly is correlated with positive outcomes in terms of reduced drinking, improved psychologic functioning, and better social support. Research suggests that members actively use the core of the AA program: They attend meetings, work the steps, get a sponsor, become sponsors, and tell their story at meetings. Overall, the more active they are with AA, the better are their outcomes. The positive effect of AA seems at least partially attributable to the clear cognitive and behavioral changes that members make and to improved social supports. Other research has focused on treatment programs based in AA philosophy and procedures. Studies of formal treatments that draw from the core beliefs of AA have yielded mixed results, but evidence generally suggests that these programs yield outcomes comparable to or better than programs based in other treatment philosophies. Finally, there is increased methodologic sophistication and creativity in research on AA. Concepts of AA involvement capture more fully the core of the AA program, while several new measures that have good psychometric properties have been developed. A more varied population of problem drinkers is being examined, including subpopulations that differ in age, race/ethnicity, and the presence of comorbid psychiatric disorders. Diverse and complementary methodologies have contributed to a richer, data-based understanding of AA, which should continue to expand over the next decade.

ACKNOWLEDGMENT: *Preparation of this chapter was supported in part by NIAAA grants R01 AA07070 and K02-AA00326-06.*

REFERENCES

1. Alcoholics Anonymous. *Alcoholics Anonymous: Estimates of AA groups and members.* Accessed February 18, 2008, from http:// www.aa.org/ en_ media_resources.cfm?PageID=74.
2. Mäkelä K, Arminen I, Bloomfield K, et al. *Alcoholics Anonymous as a mutual-help movement.* Madison, WI: University of Wisconsin Press, 1996.
3. Hasin DS, Grant BF. AA and other help seeking for alcohol problems: Former drinkers in the U.S. general population. *J Subst Abuse* 1995; 7:281–292.
4. Room R, Greenfield T. Alcoholics Anonymous, other 12-step movements and psychotherapy in the U.S. population, 1990. *Addiction* 1993; 88:555–562.
5. Dawson DA, Grant BF, Stinson FS, Chou PS. Estimating the effect of help-seeking on achieving recovery from alcohol dependence. *Addiction* 2006;101:824–834.
6. Timko C, Finney JW, Moos RH, et al. The process of treatment selection among previously untreated help-seeking problem drinkers. *J Subst Abuse* 1993;5:203–220.
7. Timko C, Moos RH, Finney JW, et al. Long-term outcomes of alcohol use disorders: comparing untreated individuals with those in Alcoholics Anonymous and formal treatment. *J Stud Alcohol* 2000;61:529–540.
8. Moos RH, Moos BS. Paths of entry into Alcoholics Anonymous: consequences for participation and remission. *Alcohol: Clin Exp Res* 2005;29:1858–1868.
9. Speiglman R. Mandated AA attendance for recidivist drinking drivers: ideology, organization, and California criminal justice practices. *Addiction* 1994;89:859–868.
10. Alcoholics Anonymous. *Information on Alcoholics Anonymous.* Accessed February 18, 2008, from http://www.aa.org/ en_information_ aa. cfm? PageID=11.
11. Narrow WE, Regier DA, Rae DS, et al. Use of services by persons with mental and addictive disorders. *Arch Gen Psychiatry* 1993;50:95–107.
12. McCrady BS, Epstein EE, Hirsch LS. Issues in the implementation of a randomized clinical trial that includes Alcoholics Anonymous: studying AA-related behaviors during treatment. *J Stud Alcohol* 1996;57: 604–612.
13. Morgenstern J, Kahler CW, Frey RM, et al. Modeling therapeutic response to 12-step treatment: Optimal responders, nonresponders, and partial responders. *J Subst Abuse* 1996;8:45–59.
14. Caldwell PE, Cutter HSG. Alcoholics Anonymous affiliation during early recovery. *J Subst Abuse Treat* 1998;15:221–228.
15. Humphreys K, Moos RH, Finney JW. Two pathways out of drinking problems with professional treatment. *Addict Behav* 1995;20:427–441.
16. Mäkelä K. Rates of attrition among the membership of Alcoholics Anonymous in Finland. *J Stud Alcohol* 1994;55:91–95.
17. Kaskutas LA, Ammon L, Delucchi K, et al. Alcoholics Anonymous careers: patterns of AA involvement five years after treatment entry, *Alcohol:Clin Exp Res* 2005;29(11):1983–1990.
18. Smith AR. The social construction of group dependency in Alcoholics Anonymous. *J Drug Issues* 1993;23:689–704.
19. Caetano R. Ethnic minority groups and Alcoholics Anonymous: a review. In: McCrady BS, Miller WR eds. *Research on Alcoholics Anonymous: Opportunities and alternatives.* New Brunswick, NJ: Rutgers Center of Alcohol Studies, 1993:209–232.
20. Morgenstern J, Labouvie E, McCrady BS, et al. Affiliation with Alcoholics Anonymous after treatment: a study of its therapeutic effects and mechanisms of action. *J Consult Clin Psychol* 1997;65:768–777.
21. Tonigan JS, Bogenschutz M, Miller WR. Is alcoholism typology a predictor of both Alcoholics Anonymous affiliation and disaffiliation after treatment? *J Subst Abuse Treat* 2006;30:323–330.
22. Humphreys K, Finney JW, Moos RH. Applying a stress and coping framework to research on mutual help organizations. *J Comm Psychol* 1994;22:312–327.
23. Project MATCH Research Group. Matching alcoholism treatments to client heterogeneity: Project MATCH posttreatment drinking outcomes. *J Stud Alcohol* 1997a;58:7–29.
24. Humphreys K. Clinicians' referral and matching of substance abuse patients to self-help groups after treatment. *Psychiatr Serv* 1997;48: 1445–1449.
25. Winzelberg A, Humphreys K. Should patients' religiosity influence clinicians' referral to 12-Step self-help groups? Evidence from a study of 3,018 male substance abuse patients. *J Consult Clin Psychol* 1999;67: 790–794.
26. Tonigan JS, Miller WR, Schermer C. Atheists, agnostics and Alcoholics Anonymous. *J Stud Alcohol* 2002;63:534–531.
27. Tomasson K, Vaglum P. Psychiatric co-morbidity and aftercare among alcoholics: A prospective study of a nationwide representative sample. *Addiction* 1998;93:423–431.
28. Ouimette PC, Gima K, Moos RH, et al. A comparative evaluation of substance abuse treatment: IV. The effect of comorbid psychiatric diagnoses on amount of treatment, continuing care, and 1-year outcomes. *Alcohol: Clin Exp Res* 1999;23:552–557.
29. Bogenschutz B. 12-step approaches for the dually diagnosed: mechanisms of change. *Alcohol: Clin Exp Res* 2007;31:64S–66S.
30. Jordan LC, Davidson WS, Herman SE, Bootsmiller BJ. Involvement in 12-step programs among persons with dual diagnoses. *Psychiatr Serv* 2002;53: 894–896.
31. Alcoholics Anonymous. AA survey shows key role of health caregivers. 2006. Accessed April 23, 2008, from http://www.aa.org/en_press.cfm? PressID=6&thisyear=2006-01-01.
32. Timko C, Finney JW, Moos RH. The 8-year course of alcohol abuse: gender differences in social context and coping. *Alcohol: Clin Exp Res* 2005;29:612–621.
33. Bodin M. Gender aspects of affiliation with Alcoholics Anonymous after treatment. *Contemp Drug Probl* 2006;33:123–141.
34. DelBoca FK, Mattson ME. The gender matching hypothesis. In: Longabaugh R, Wirtz PW eds. *Project MATCH hypotheses: Results and causal chain analyses.* Project MATCH Monograph Series, vol. 8. Bethesda, MD: National Institute on Alcohol Abuse and Alcoholism, 2002:223–238.
35. Kaskutas LA. What do women get out of self-help? Their reasons for attending Women for Sobriety and Alcoholics Anonymous. *J Subst Abuse Treat* 1994;11:185–195.
36. Bogart CJ, Pearce CE. "13th-stepping": Why Alcoholics Anonymous is not always a safe place for women. *J Addict Nurs* 2003;14:43–47.
37. Tonigan JS, Connors GJ, Miller WR. Special populations in Alcoholics Anonymous. *Alcohol Health Res World* 1998;22:281–285.
38. Kaskutas LA, Weisner C, Lee M, et al. Alcoholics Anonymous affiliation at treatment intake among white and black Americans. *J Stud Alcohol* 1999;60:810–816.
39. Humphreys K, Mavis BE, Stoffelmayer BE. Are twelve step programs appropriate for disenfranchised groups? Evidence from a study of posttreatment mutual help involvement. *Prev Hum Serv* 1994;11:165–179.
40. Arroyo JA, Westerberg VS, Tonigan JS. Comparison of treatment utilization and outcome for Hispanics and non-Hispanic whites. *J Stud Alcohol* 1998;59:286–291.
41. Tonigan JS, Miller WR, Juarez P, Villaneuva M. Utilization of AA by Hispanic and non-Hispanic White clients receiving outpatient alcohol treatment. *J Stud Alcohol* 2002;63:215–218.
42. Kelly J, Myers MG. Adolescents' participation in Alcoholics Anonymous and Narcotics Anonymous: review, implications and future directions. *J Psychoactive Drugs* 2007;39:259–269.
43. Hohman M, LeCroy CW. Predictors of adolescent AA affiliation. *Adolescence* 1996;31:339–352.
44. Kelly, JF, Myers, MG, Brown, SA. The effects of age composition of 12-step groups on adolescent 12-step participation and substance use outcome. *J Child Adolesc Subst Abuse* 2005;15:63–72.
45. Kelly, JF, Myers, MG, Brown, SA. Do adolescents affiliate with 12-step groups?: A multivariate process model of effects. *J Stud Alcohol* 2002; 63:293–304.
46. Kelly J, Myers MG, Brown SA. A multivariate process model of adolescent 12-step attendance and substance use outcome following inpatient treatment. *Psychol Addict Behav* 2000;14:376–389.
47. Pristach CA, Smith CM. Attitudes towards Alcoholics Anonymous by dually diagnosed psychiatric outpatients. *J Addict Dis* 1999;18:69–76.

48. Polcin DL, Zemore S. Psychiatric severity and spirituality, helping, and participation in Alcoholics Anonymous during recovery. *Am J Drug Alcohol Abuse* 2004;30:577–592.
49. AA World Services. *The A.A. member—medications and other drugs*. New York: AA World Services, 2006.
50. Rychtarik RG, Connors GJ, Dermen KH, et al. Alcoholics Anonymous and the use of medications to prevent relapse: an anonymous survey of member attitudes. *J Stud Alcohol* 2000;61:134–138.
51. Swift RM, Duncan D, Nirenberg T, Femino J. Alcoholic patients' experience and attitudes on pharmacotherapy for alcoholism. *J Addict Dis* 1998;17:35–47.
52. Tonigan, JS, Kelly, JF. AA-exposure and attitudes of 12-step proscriptions about medications. *Alcohol: Clin Exp Res* 2003;26(5, Supplement):649A (Abstract).
53. Hall JM. The experiences of lesbians in Alcoholics Anonymous. *West J Nurs Res* 1994;16:556–576.
54. Walsh DC, Hingson RW, Merrigan DM, et al. A randomized trial of treatment options for alcohol-abusing workers. *N Engl J Med* 1991;325: 775–782.
55. Project MATCH Research Group. Project MATCH secondary a priori hypotheses. *Addiction* 1997b;92:1671–1698.
56. Project MATCH Research Group. Matching alcoholism treatments to client heterogeneity: treatment main effects and matching effects on drinking during treatment. *J Stud Alcohol* 1998a;59:631–639.
57. Project MATCH Research Group. Matching alcoholism treatments to client heterogeneity: Project MATCH three-year drinking outcomes. *Alcohol: Clin Exp Res* 1998b;22:1300–1311.
58. Longabaugh R, Wirtz PW, Zweben A, et al. Network support for drinking, Alcoholics Anonymous and long-term matching effects. *Addiction* 1998;93:1313–1333.
59. McCrady BS, Epstein EE, Hirsch LS. Maintaining change after conjoint behavioral alcohol treatment for men: Outcomes at 6 months. *Addiction* 1999;94:1381–1396.
60. McCrady BS, Epstein EE, Kahler CW. Alcoholics Anonymous and relapse prevention as maintenance strategies after cojoint behavioral alcohol treatment for men:18-month outcomes. *J Consult Clin Psychol* 2004;72:870–878.
61. Moos RH, Finney JW, Ouimette PC, et al. A comparative evaluation of substance abuse treatment: I. treatment orientation, amount of care, and 1-year outcomes. *Alcohol: Clin Exp Res* 1999;23:529–536.
62. Ouimette PC, Finney JW, Moos RH. Twelve-Step and Cognitive-Behavioral Treatment for substance abuse: a comparison of treatment effectiveness. *J Consult Clin Psychol* 1997;65:230–240.
63. Ouimette PC, Finney JW, Gima K, et al. A comparative evaluation of substance abuse treatment: III. Examining mechanisms underlying patient-treatment matching hypotheses for 12-Step and cognitive-behavioral treatments for substance abuse. *Alcohol: Clin Exp Res* 1999; 23:545–551.
64. Humphreys K, Moos R. Can encouraging substance abuse patients to participate in self-help groups reduce demand for health care? A quasi-experimental study. *Alcohol: Clin Exp Res* 2001;25:711–716.
65. Hoffmann NG, Miller NS. Treatment outcomes for abstinence based programs. *Psychiatr Ann* 1992;22:402–408.
66. Stinchfield R, Owen P. Hazelden's model of treatment and its outcome. *Addict Behav* 1998;23:669–683.
67. Fortney J, Booth B, Zhang M, et al. Controlling for selection bias in the evaluation of Alcoholics Anonymous as aftercare treatment. *J Stud Alcohol* 1998;59:690–697.
68. Johnson E, Herringer LG. A note on the utilization of common support activities and relapse following substance abuse treatment. *J Psychol* 1993;127:73–78.
69. Tonigan JS. Benefits of Alcoholics Anonymous attendance: Replication of findings between clinical research sites in Project MATCH. *Alcohol Treat Q* 2001;19:67–77.
70. Kelly JF, Stout R, Zywiak W, Schneider R. A 3-year study of addiction mutual-help group participation following intensive outpatient treatment. *Alcohol: Clin Exp Res* 2006;30:1381–1392.
71. Gossop M, Stewart D, Marsden J. Attendance at Narcotics Anonymous and Alcoholics Anonymous meetings, frequency of attendance and substance use outcomes after residential treatment for drug dependence: a 5-year follow-up study. *Addiction* 2007;103:119–125.
72. McKellar J, Stewart E, Humphreys K. Alcoholics Anonymous involvement and positive alcohol-related outcomes: cause, consequence, or just a correlate? A prospective 2-year study of 2,319 alcohol-dependent men. *J Consult Clin Psychol* 2003;71:302–308.
73. Schuckit MA, Tipp JE, Smith TL, et al. Periods of abstinence following the onset of alcohol dependence in 1,853 men and women. *J Stud Alcohol* 1997;58:581–589.
74. Timko C, Moos RH, Finney JW, et al. Long-term treatment careers and outcomes of previously untreated alcoholics. *J Stud Alcohol* 1999;60: 437–447.
75. Kahler CW, Read JP, Stuart GL, et al. Motivational enhancement for 12-step involvement among patients undergoing alcohol detoxification. *J Consult Clin Psychol* 2004;72:736–741.
76. Emrick CD, Tonigan JS, Montgomery HA, Little L. Alcoholics Anonymous: what is currently known? In: McCrady BS, Miller WR (eds.). *Research on Alcoholics Anonymous: Opportunities and alternatives*. New Brunswick, NJ: Rutgers Center on Alcohol Studies,1993:41–76.
77. Montgomery HA, Miller WR, Tonigan JS. Does Alcoholics Anonymous involvement predict treatment outcome? *J Subst Abuse Treat* 1995; 12:241–246.
78. Tonigan JS, Miller WR, Connors GJ. Project MATCH client impressions about Alcoholics Anonymous: measurement issues and relationship treatment outcome. *Alcohol Treat Q* 2000;18:25–41.
79. Weiss RD, Griffin ML, Najavits LM, et al. Self-help activities in cocaine dependent patients entering treatment: results from the NIDA Collaborative Cocaine Treatment Study. *Drug Alcohol Depend* 1996;43: 79–86.
80. Brown HP, Peterson JH. Assessing spirituality in addiction treatment. Development of the Brown-Peterson Recovery Progress Inventory. *Alcohol Treat Q* 1991;8:41–50.
81. Pagano ME, Friend KB, Tonigan JS, Stout R. Sponsoring others in Alcoholics Anonymous and avoiding a drink in the first year following treatment: findings from Project MATCH. *J Stud Alcohol* 2004;65: 766–773.
82. Witbrodt J, Kaskutas LA. Does diagnosis matter? Differential effects of 12-Step participation and social networks on abstinence. *Am J Drug Alcohol Abuse* 2005;31:685–707.
83. Tonigan JS, Miller WR. AA practicing subtypes: Are there multiple AA fellowships? [Abstract]. *Alcohol: Clin Exp Res* 2005;295(Suppl):384.
84. Tonigan JS, Miller WR. The relative importance of pretreatment characteristics in predicting AA participation 10 years after treatment [Abstract]. *Alcohol: Clin Exp Res* 2004;285(Suppl):135.
85. Humphreys K, Noke JM. The influence of posttreatment mutual help group participation on the friendship networks of substance abuse patients. *Am J Comm Psychol* 1997;25:1–16.
86. Kaskutas LA, Bond J, Humphreys K. Social networks as mediators of the effect of Alcoholics Anonymous. *Addiction* 2002;97:891–900.
87. Litt MD, Kadden RM, Kabela-Cormier E, Petry N. Changing network support for drinking: initial findings from the Network Support Project. *J Consult Clin Psychol* 2007;75:542–555.
88. Alcoholics Anonymous World Services. *Alcoholics Anonymous* (4th ed.). New York: Author, 1992.
89. Alcoholics Anonymous World Services. *Twelve steps and twelve traditions*. New York: Author, 1981.
90. Connors GJ, Tonigan JS, Miller WR. Measure of religious background and behavior for use in behavior change research. *Psychol Addict Behav* 1996;10:90–96.
91. Pargament KI, Kendall J, Hathaway W, et al. Religion and the problems solving process: three style of coping. *J Sci Study Religion* 1988;27: 90–104.
92. Fetzer Institute. Multidimensional measurement of religiousness/spirituality for use in health research. Kalamazoo, MI: John E. Fetzer Institute, 1999.

93. Underwood LG, Teresi JA. The daily spiritual experiences scale: Development, theoretical description, reliability, exploratory factor analysis, and preliminary construct validity using health-related data. *Ann Behav Med* 2002;24:22–33.
94. Robinson EAR, Cranford JA, Webb JR, Brower KJ. Six-month changes in spirituality, religiousness, and heavy drinking in a treatment seeking sample. *J Stud Alcohol Drugs* 2006;68:282–290.
95. Connors GJ, Tonigan JS, Miller WR. A longitudinal model of intake symptomatology, AA participation and outcome: Retrospective study of the Project MATCH outpatient and aftercare samples. *J Stud Alcohol* 2001;62:817–824.
96. Tonigan JS, Kelly JF. Beliefs about AA and the use of medications: a comparison of three groups of AA-exposed alcohol dependent persons. *Alcohol Treat Q* 2004;22:67–78.
97. Tonigan, JS. Spirituality and AA practices three and ten years after Project MATCH. *Alcohol: Clin Exp Res* 2003;26(5, Supplement):660A (Abstract).
98. Walker SR, Tonigan JS, Miller WR, et al. Intercessory prayer in the treatment of alcohol abuse and dependence: a pilot investigation. *Altern Ther Health Med* 1997;3:79–86.
99. Christo G, Franey C. Drug users' spiritual beliefs, locus of control and the disease concept in relation to Narcotics Anonymous attendance and six-month outcomes. *Drug Alcohol Depend* 1995;38:51–56.
100. Kaskutas LA, Turk N, Bond J, Weisner C. The role of religion, spirituality and Alcoholics Anonymous in sustained sobriety, *Alcohol Treat Q* 2003;21:1–15.
101. Snow MG, Prochaska JO, Rossi JS. Processes of change in Alcoholics Anonymous: maintenance factors in long-term sobriety. *J Stud Alcohol* 1994;55:362–371.
102. Morgenstern J, Bates ME. Effects of executive function impairment on change processes and substance use outcomes in 12-Step treatment. *J Stud Alcohol* 1999;60:846–855.
103. Tonigan, JS. Examination of the active ingredients of Twelve-step facilitation (TSF) in the Project MATCH outpatient sample, *Alcohol: Clin Exp Res* 2005;29(2):240–241.
104. Finney JW, Noyes CA, Coutts AI. Evaluating substance abuse treatment process models: I. Changes on proximal outcome variables during 12-step and cognitive behavioral treatment. *J Stud Alcohol* 1998;59: 371–380.
105. Finney JW, Moos RH, Humphreys K. A comparative evaluation of substance abuse treatment: II. Linking proximal outcomes of 12-step and cognitive behavioral treatment to substance use outcomes. *Alcohol: Clin Exp Res* 1999;23:537–544.
106. Brown TG, Seraganian P, Tremblay J, Annis H. Process and outcome changes with relapse prevention versus 12-Step aftercare programs for substance abusers. *Addiction* 2002;97:677–689.
107. Demmel R, Rist F. Prediction of treatment outcome in a clinical sample of problem drinkers: Self-efficacy and coping style. *Addict Disord Their Treat* 2005;4:5–10.
108. Magura S, Laudet AB, Mahmood D. Role of self-help processes in achieving abstinence among dually diagnosed persons. *Addict Behav* 2003;28:399–413.
109. Moos RH, Moos BS. Paths of entry into Alcoholics Anonymous: consequences for participation and remission. *Alcohol: Clin Exp Res* 2005; 29:1858–1868.
110. Forcehimes A, Tonigan JS. Self-efficacy to remain abstinent and substance abuse: a meta-analysis. *Alcohol Treat Q*, in press.
111. Horstmann MJ, Tonigan JS. Faith development in Alcoholics Anonymous: a study of two AA groups. *Alcohol Treat Q* 2000;18: 75–84.
112. Tonigan JS, Ashcroft F, Miller WR. A group dynamics and 12-step activity. *J Stud Alcohol* 1995;56:616–621.

SUGGESTED READING

Alcoholics Anonymous World Services. *Alcoholics Anonymous*, 4th ed. New York: Author, 1992.

CHAPTER 69

Marc Galanter, MD, FASAM

Spirituality in the Recovery Process

WHAT IS SPIRITUALITY?

Dictionaries define spirituality with phrases such as concerned with or affecting the soul, not tangible or material, or pertaining to God (1). More broadly, it consists of the nonmaterial issues that give a person meaning and purpose in life; these can be found in a person's religious orientation but can also be seen in their ethnic heritage, altruism, humanism, or naturalism. Spirituality infuses some alternative medical therapies that are not grounded in empirical science but have gained popularity because they address symptoms such as anxiety or depression. Given the prominence of Alcoholics Anonymous and related Twelve-Step groups, it can play an important role in the rehabilitation of substance-dependent people.

The issue of spirituality is prominent within contemporary culture, as evidenced in a probability sampling of American adults, among whom 95% of respondents reply positively when asked whether they believe in God or a universal spirit. Responses to a follow-up question survey suggest that this belief affects the daily lives of the majority (51%) of those sampled, who indicated that they had talked to someone about God or some aspect of their faith or spirituality within the previous 24 hours (2).

UNDERSTANDING THE PHENOMENON

Spirituality can be classified among latent constructs such as personality, culture, and cognition. These are not observed directly but inferred from observations of their component dimensions (3). Such constructs are typically multidimensional: understood from the vantage point of more than one discipline. As such, spirituality should be examined from perspectives as diverse as physiology, psychology, and cross-cultural studies. This approach is attempted in this chapter, but it will require expert interdisciplinary collaboration to pursue it to its fullest.

Some researchers have drawn distinctions between the two concepts. In one study, respondents identifying themselves as more spiritual saw God as more loving and forgiving, while those who assessed themselves as more religious saw Him as more judgmental (4). The fellowship of Alcoholics Anonymous is often described as a spiritual program for living (5) but one in which there is no dogma, theology, or creed to be learned (6). The presence of formal doctrine may be considered associated more with religion than with spirituality.

When considered from the perspective of its role in organized religion, the nature of spirituality in a given society is culture-bound, even among Western postindustrial societies. In Sweden, where religious practice had once been an important aspect of the national culture, only 10% of the population indicates that religion is important to them, and fewer than 5% go to church each week (7). This stands in clear contrast to the United States, where these figures are many times higher (87% and 41%, respectively) (2).

AA AS A SPIRITUAL RECOVERY MOVEMENT

How does spirituality relate to recovery from addiction? There is a parallel between the way in which attitudes are transformed in intensely zealous groups and the way in which the denial of illness and the self-defeating behaviors of alcoholics and drug addicts may be reversed through induction into a Twelve-Step group such as AA.

Members of the lay public may conclude that certain health care issues are inadequately addressed by the medical community, particularly when doctors are not sufficiently attentive to the emotional burden that an illness produces. When mutually supportive groups of laymen coalesce to implement a response to this perceived deficit, they may form a spiritual recovery movement (8), one premised on achieving remission based on beliefs independent of evidence-based medicine. Such movements may ascribe their effectiveness to higher metaphysical or nonmaterial forces and claim to offer relief from illness.

AA can be considered as a highly successful example of a spiritual recovery movement, as such movements have three primary characteristics. They (1) claim to provide relief from disease, (2) operate outside the modalities of established empirical medicine, and (3) ascribe their effectiveness to higher metaphysical powers. The appeal of such movements in the contemporary period is due in part to the fact that physicians tend not to attend to the spiritual or emotional concerns of their patients (9).

Clearly, the attitudes and behavioral norms that AA espouses are much more in conformity with the values of the larger culture than those of zealous religious sects. The expectation of avoiding drunkenness in AA, normative in our culture, illustrates this. People who are highly distressed over the consequences of their addiction are therefore candidates to respond to the strong ideologic orientation of AA toward recovery and are operantly reinforced by the relief produced by affiliation with the group's ideology and behavioral norms, all related to abstinence and a spiritually grounded lifestyle. Significantly, AA generates distress in its members by pressing them to give up their addictive behaviors, but the distress associated with this conflict is relieved if they sustain affiliation and cleave to the group.

SPIRITUALITY AS A PSYCHOLOGICAL CONSTRUCT

Two empirically grounded perspectives have played a material role in framing how we conceptualize recovery. One derived from a model of psychopathology modeled on the work of Emil Kraeplin (10). He framed an approach that now characterizes the contemporary medical model for mental disorders, categorizing disease entities diagnosed on the basis of explicit and discrete symptoms. This approach is evident in the development of criteria for substance use disorders employed in recent editions of the symptom-based Diagnostic and Statistical Manual of Mental Disorders (11). From this perspective, a state of remission, colloquially called *recovery* in rehabilitation circles, can take place with the resolution of the specific symptoms listed as diagnostic criteria. A second perspective on recovery derives from behavioral psychology, whose model of stimulus-response sequences has led to the ordering of experience around discrete phenomena that can be observed by a researcher or clinician. From this perspective, recovery can also be defined in terms of observable, measurable responses to substance use, lending credence to recovery as a process defined in behavioral terms.

Both perspectives are well suited to the study of psychopathology and have lent the addiction field approaches to studying addiction as a disorder, one that is compatible with research approaches employing experimental controls that are used in the physical and biologic sciences. Both have, therefore, had heuristic value in promoting a research field that has yielded many advances in addiction treatment. There is a third perspective, however, that is defined on the basis of addicts' reports of their own subjective experience. These experiences are not directly observable by the clinician but are available only as reported through the prism of the person's own introspection and reflection. This model is more difficult to subject to measurement, but instruments are being developed that can be applied for its study, as are discussed later. This approach is inherent in the spiritually oriented psychology of Carl Jung (12), who had a direct influence on Bill W's framing of the Alcoholics Anonymous ethos (13). William James (14), often described as the father of American psychology, also discussed mental phenomena in terms of subjectively experienced mystical or spiritual experience. (In fact, he wrote that "the drunken consciousness is one bit of the mystic consciousness"; p. 378.) The need for spiritual redemption was vital in the writings of Viktor Frankl, who wrote *Man's Search for Meaning* (15) and has recently been espoused with regard to psychotherapy by William Miller (16).

This third perspective is related to the model of spiritually grounded recovery we will discuss here, insofar as it emphasizes the achievement of meaningful or positive experiences rather than a focus on observable, dysfunctional behaviors. Research on this third approach would typically rely on self-report scales, such as those that can be facilitated by development of instruments, such as the Life Engagement Test (17), the General Well-Being Schedule (18), or our own Spiritual Self-Rating Scale (19). We will consider its role in AA, models for how it takes place, and ways in which it can be measured. In this respect, recovery can be understood as a process whereby an abstinent addicted person is moving toward a positive adaptation in life. This movement can take place with varying degrees of success, depending on the person's own innate capacities and the circumstances in which they find themselves.

SPIRITUALLY GROUNDED RECOVERY IN AA

The AA program of recovery is mentioned in numerous places in the Big Book, *Alcoholics Anonymous* (20), and is associated there with such terms as *spiritual experience* and *spiritual awakening* and with working AA's Twelve Steps. Four of the Steps include the word God, which is qualified "as we understood Him." Some clarity is lent to this latter phrase in the Big Book, where it is pointed out that, "with few exceptions, our members find that they have tapped an unsuspected inner resource that they presently identify with their own conception of a Power greater than themselves" (pp. 569–570). Flexibility on the issue of theistic belief is also made clear in one chapter that addresses any alcohol-dependent person "who feels he is an atheist or agnostic," encouraging their membership as well. The text points out for these members that even "We Agnostics . . . had to face the fact that we must find a spiritual basis for life" (p. 44) in order to achieve recovery, implying therein the fellowship's distinction between spirituality and theistic religion.

This issue of theistic connotation, however, is as yet resolved relative to the judicial system, wherein the application of AA is sometimes constrained because of potential church-state conflicts. It is open to question, however, whether the theistic connotations of AA can be modified without vitiating the program's effectiveness. In this relation, it should be noted that in a 5-year follow-up of recovering cocaine-dependent patients, the strength derived from religion and spirituality significantly distinguished those who had a highly favorable outcome from those who did not (21). Additionally, attendance at religious services distinguished significantly between criminal justice clients referred for substance abuse treatment who had a positive outcome and those who did not (22).

In the clinical context, recovery is based on a person's behavioral and physiologic status, which can be assessed by recourse to criteria employed in the DSM. Some of these criteria are also embodied in the Addiction Severity Index (23), which is employed widely in research to evaluate recovery. These items can be assessed relatively easily, as they are premised on observable behavior or delineated by symptomatology described by patient, family member, or clinician.

A spiritually grounded definition of recovery, however, can be useful as well. Such a concept relates to the importance of nondemographic subject factors, originally proposed as quality-of-life issues (24)—among which spirituality can be considered. In this context, a series of suitable criteria for "diagnosing" addiction (a term more apt than *substance dependence*) could be developed. They could then be used to assess the spiritual aspect of recovery associated with the Twelve-Step experience. Resolution of these issues could be considered as important to the spiritual aspect of recovery from addiction. A series of criteria could include items such as the following:

- Loss of sense of purpose due to excessive substance use
- A feeling of inadequate social support because of one's addiction.
- Continued use of a substance while experiencing moral qualms over its consumption
- Loss of the will to resist temptation when the substance is available

Another aspect of the DSM format can be considered as well. The Manual stipulates "course specifiers" of remission, such as "on agonist therapy" and "in a controlled environment." These are included because they are explanatory to the clinician. To them could be added, "fully engaged in a program of Twelve-Step recovery," which would be equally explanatory to many clinicians.

But are spiritually grounded criteria measurable? In recent years, methodologies that have been developed and validated could be used to assess outcome based on such subjectively experienced criteria. They employ a systematic approach to measurement and can be used to describe spiritually-related states:

A. Affective state
   1. A sense of well-being, measured by the General Well-Being Schedule (18) (which we employed) or the Subjective Happiness Scale (25)
   2. Contentment with one's life circumstances, measured by the Satisfaction with Life Scale (26)
   3. Positive affect, assessed with the Positive and Negative Affect Schedule (27), dealing with both variables as separate dimensions rather than bipolar ends of the same scale
   4. Feelings of support, employing a scale for Perceived Social Support (28)

B. Existential variables: Meaningfulness in one's life; assessed by the Purpose in Life Test (29)

C. Flow (the experience associated with engaging one's highest strengths and talents to meet achievable challenges) (30), as measured by Experience Sampling (31) or the Flow Scale (32)

D. Spirituality: The Spirituality Self-Rating Scale, which we developed and applied to both substance-abusing and non-substance-abusing populations (19), as well as other such scales. By means of our own scale, we were able to distinguish different populations of substance abusers' level of spiritual orientation from the of non-substance populations.

E. Personality Assessment: The Classification of Strengths (33), a series of characteristics based on categories of moral excellence drawn from observations across different cultures.

F. AA Involvement: Measures of the degree of affiliation and commitment to the AA fellowship (34).

A methodology for defining recovery based on measurements such as these may not have the same appeal to biomedically oriented clinicians as does the conventional symptom-based approach, as these measurements are based on self-report of the person's subjective state. Furthermore, the enthusiasm of newfound recovery may yield a Hawthorne effect. The biomedical format currently applied in diagnosis, derives from the school of Kraeplin and subsequent investigators, such as those who developed the Feighner criteria (35) in the 1970s, and then in the ensuing DSM system. Spiritual variables, however, have a lineage as well, from William James, Carl Jung, and Bill W.

AA IN THE PROFESSIONAL CONTEXT

The spiritually oriented Twelve-Step approach has been integrated into professional treatment in some settings wherein it serves as the overriding philosophy of an entire program, or in others, where it is one aspect of a multi-modal eclectic approach. The Minnesota Model for treatment, typically located in an isolated institutional setting, is characterized by an intensive inpatient stay during which a primary goal of treatment is to acculturate patients to acceptance of the philosophy of AA and to continue with AA attendance after discharge (36).

Though a variety of exercises are included during the stay, this approach has been criticized as dogmatic (37) because of its sole reliance on the Twelve-Step approach. The outcome of this model, however, has been shown to yield positive results in a survey of patients discharged from one such setting (Hazelden, in Center City, MN) (38), but random assignment of patients treated in Minnesota Model facilities with those treated by means of an alternative approach is needed.

A more eclectic option is illustrated in the integration of Twelve-Step groups into a general psychiatric facility for the treatment of patients with dual diagnoses of major mental illness and substance misuse. The importance of spirituality in such a highly compromised population was evidenced in our studies (19) in which such patients ranked spiritual issues such as belief in God and inner peace higher than tangible benefits such as social service support and outpatient treatment. One inherent advantage of this format is that it benefits from the introduction of an inspirational approach to patients who, as Goffman has pointed out (39), have become degraded by stigmatization owing to their psychiatric disorders.

In summary, spirituality is a matter of personal meaning that is widely accepted. It is also central to the recovery process from addiction for many AA members. The fellowship of AA, in fact, can be considered a movement developed in relation to people's spiritual needs. Though spirituality is subjectively experienced, it can be assessed systematically in given individuals by employing currently available empirical techniques. By such means, an important aspect of addiction recovery can be defined and studied.

REFERENCES

1. Morris W, ed. *The American Heritage Dictionary of the English Language.* Boston: American Heritage Publishing Co., Inc., and Houghton Mifflin Company, 1970.
2. Gallup GH. *Religion in America 2002.* Princeton NJ: Princeton Religious Research Center, 2002.
3. Miller W, Thoresen C. Spirituality, religion, and health. An emerging research field. *Am Psychol* 2003;58:24–35.
4. McCrady B, Miller WN. *Research on Alcoholics Anonymous.* New Brunswick, NJ: Rutgers Center for Alcohol Studies, 1983.
5. Miller W, Kurtz E. Models of alcoholism used in treatment: contrasting AA and other perspectives with which it is often confused. *J Stud Alcohol* 1994;55:159–166.
6. Chappel J. Long-term recovery from alcoholism. *Psychiatr Clin North Am* 1993;16:177–187.
7. DeMarinis V. *Pastoral care, existential health, and existential epidemiology. A Swedish postmodern case study.* Stockholm: Verbum, 2003.
8. Galanter M. Spiritual recovery movements and contemporary medical care. *Psychiatr: Interperson Biol Proc* 1997;60:236–248.
9. Galanter M. *Spirituality and the healthy mind: science, therapy and the need for personal meaning.* New York: Oxford University Press, 2005.
10. Kraeplin E. *Clinical psychiatry: A textbook for students and physicians.* New York: Macmillan, 1902.
11. American Psychiatric Association. *Diagnostic and statistical manual of mental disorders,* 4th ed. (Text revision). Washington, DC: American Psychiatric Association, 2000.
12. Jung C. Instinct and unconscious. In: Read H, Fordham M, Adler G, McGuire W, eds. *The collected works of C. B. Jung.* Princeton, N.J.: Princeton University Press, 1978.
13. Cheever S. *My name is Bill: Bill Wilson—his life and the creation of Alcoholics Anonymous.* New York: Simon & Schuster, 2004.
14. James W. *The varieties of religious experience.* New York: Modern Library, 1929.
15. Frankl V. *Man's search for meaning,* 3rd ed. New York: Touchstone, Simon & Schuster, 1984.
16. Miller WR. ed. *Integrating spirituality into treatment.* Washington, DC: American Psychological Association, 1999.
17. Scheier MF, Wrosch C, Baum A, et al. The life engagement test: assessing purpose in life. *J Behav Med* 2006;29:291–298.
18. Dupuy H. The psychological section of the current health and nutrition examination survey. In: *Proceedings of the Public Health Conference on Records and Statistics* (1972). DHEW Publication HRA 74-1214. Rockville, MD: National Center for Health Statistics, 1973.
19. Galanter M, Dermatis H, Bunt G, et al. Assessment of spirituality and its relevance to addiction treatment. *J Subst Abuse Treat* 2007;33: 257–264.
20. Alcoholics Anonymous World Services. *Alcoholics Anonymous: the story of how many thousands of men and women have recovered from alcoholism.* New York: Alcoholics Anonymous Publishing Inc., 1955.
21. Flynn PM, Joe GW, Broome KM, et al. Looking back on cocaine dependence: reasons for recovery. *Am J Addict* 2003;12:398–411.
22. Brown BS, O'Grady K, Battjes RJ, et al. Factors associated with treatment outcomes in an aftercare population. *Am J Addict* 2004;13:447–460.
23. McLellan AT, Kushner H, Metzger D, et al. The Fifth Edition of the Addiction Severity Index. *J Subst Abuse Treat* 1992;9:199–213.
24. Campbell A, Converse PE, Rogers WL. *The quality of American life.* New York: Russell Sage Foundation, 1976.
25. Lyubomirsky S, Lepper HS. A measure of subjective happiness: preliminary reliability and construct validation. *Social Indicators Res* 1999; 46:137–155.
26. Diener E, Suh EM, Lucas RE, et al. Subjective well-being: three decades of progress. *Psychol Bull* 1999;125:276–302.
27. Watson D, Clark LA, Tellegen A. Development and validation of brief measures of positive and negative affect: the PANAS scales. *J Personal Soc Psychol* 1988;54:1063–1070.
28. Cohen S, Mermelstein R, Kamarck T, et al. Measuring the functional components of social support. In: Sarason IG, Sarason BR eds. *Social support: theory, research and application.* The Hague, Holland: Martinus Nijhoff, 1985:73–94.
29. Crumbaugh JD, Maholick LT. *Manual of instructions for the purpose in life test.* Munster, IN: Psychometric Affiliates, 1969.
30. Csikszentmihalyi M, Larson R. Validity and reliability of the Experience Sampling Method. *J Nerv Ment Dis* 1987;175:526–536.
31. Duckworth AL, Steen TA, Seligman MEP. Positive psychology in clinical practice. *Ann Rev Clin Psychol* 2005;1:629–651.
32. Mayers P. Flow in adolescence and its relation to school experience [Ph.D. thesis]. University of Chicago, 1978, unpublished.
33. Peterson C, Seligman MEP. *Character strengths and virtues: a classification and handbook.* Washington, DC: American Psychological Association, 2004.
34. Humphreys K, Kaskutas LA, Weisner C. The Alcoholics Anonymous Affiliation Scale: development, reliability, and norms for diverse treated and untreated populations. *Alcohol: Clin Exp Res* 1998;22:974–978.
35. Feighner JP, Robins E, Guze SB, et al. Diagnostic criteria for use in psychiatric research. *Arch Gen Psychiatry* 1972;26:57–63.
36. Cook CCH. The Minnesota Model in the management of drug and alcohol dependency: miracle, method or myth? Part I: The philosophy and the programme. *Br J Addict* 1988;83:625–634.
37. Cook CCH. The Minnesota Model in the management of drug and alcohol dependency: miracle, method or myth? Part II: Evidence and conclusions. *Br J Addict* 1988;83:735–748.
38. Stinchfield R, Owen P. Hazelden's model of treatment and its outcome. *Addict Behav* 1998;23:669–683.
39. Goffman E. *Stigma.* New York: Simon & Schuster, 1963.

SECTION 10

Medical Disorders and Complications of Addiction

CHAPTER 70

Richard Saitz, MD, MPH, FACP, FASAM

Medical and Surgical Complications of Addiction

Persons with addictive disorders often do not receive regular health care (1). As a result, their medical care for acute and chronic conditions can be fragmented and inefficient. Furthermore, they miss opportunities to receive preventive health care (2). In addition to the direct effects of intoxication, overdose, and withdrawal, abused substances can affect every body system. Substance abuse and dependence are associated with behaviors that place individuals at risk of health consequences that are not directly related to use of the substance. Regular health care can lead to improved health for persons with addictive disorders (2–5). Such care could be accessed at general medical or specialty addiction treatment delivery sites. This section addresses the wide range of health consequences of alcohol and other drug use, focusing on the most common and most serious illnesses, mainly by organ system. This introductory chapter reviews preventive care, addiction care during medical hospitalization, the medical consequences of substance abuse and dependence, the management of common medical problems in persons with addictive disorders, and consequences in older adults. Preventive care for healthy adults, as well as issues specific to persons with addictive disorders, are presented herein because any health care contact is an opportunity for persons with addictive disorders or dependence to obtain such care. Subsequent chapters address the epidemiology, diagnosis, and management of consequences of substance use in detail, focusing on human immunodeficiency virus and acquired immunodeficiency syndrome (HIV/AIDS); tuberculosis and other infectious diseases; renal and metabolic disorders; endocrine and reproductive consequences; hepatitis, cirrhosis, and other liver diseases; gastrointestinal consequences; neurologic complications; cardiac consequences; respiratory and sleep disorders; pregnancy; injury; and management of addicted surgical patients.

ROUTINE AND PREVENTIVE CARE

In the early 20th century, preventive health care meant a thorough and detailed evaluation focused on examination and testing. The "executive physical," a "one-size-fits-all" approach in which more tests were better, evolved from this approach. Over the past several decades, however, preventive care expert panels have recommended targeted evaluations based on age and other risk factors (6). The rationale for these targeted evaluations is based on the notion that time and resources are limited and, perhaps more important, the recognition that preventive care can result not only in benefit but in harm (such as a perforated colon from a colonoscopy performed as a result of an occult blood test that turns out to be a false-positive test for colorectal cancer). In addition, some preventive testing predicted to offer health benefit has been shown to offer no benefit in terms of length and quality of life when evaluated in controlled clinical trials (e.g., screening chest radiographs in smokers). The approach presented here follows a targeted strategy based on the known effectiveness of interventions. Though disagreements exist among professional and other organizations (and their guidelines) regarding some details, most recommendations are in agreement when it comes to which diseases should be identified during their preclinical stages. Ongoing updates of recommendations by the U.S. Preventive Services Task Force can be accessed at *http://www.ahrq.gov/clinic/uspstfix.htm* (accessed February 3, 2008).

Medical History The medical history in a person with addiction should include the categories of assessment employed for all patients, such as any *current complaints* and the history of that *present illness*, *allergies*, *systems review* (including any symptoms of conditions that could be related to substance use), medications (including over-the-counter and alternative products), and then the *past medical and surgical history*. Questions regarding past history should address hospitalizations and any medical conditions (e.g. cardiovascular, pulmonary, hepatic, renal or neurological diseases and specific illnesses such as cellulitis, pneumonia, hepatitis) that might be related to substance use and might not be volunteered by the patient without direct questions asked by the physician. The *social and family history* is of particular importance. Queries should be made to understand the current living situation, support system, travel history, and immigration status. In an asymptomatic person with an addictive disorder (in addition to a thorough alcohol and drug use history), historical items relevant to preventive care become more of the focus. These assessments should include an assessment of sexual practices and behaviors, including condom use; dental care, including use of floss and brushing with fluoride toothpaste; diet (fat, cholesterol, fruit, grain, vegetable, and overall caloric intake); physical activity; calcium intake; use of lap and shoulder belts when in vehicles; use of helmets when riding a bicycle or motorcycle; presence of a firearm and smoke detector in the household; and cardiopulmonary resuscitation knowledge in the household. These assessments are recommended because they can lead to counseling interventions, depending on the answers. For persons with addictive disorders, screening for depression and anxiety, assessment of sexual practices, intention to conceive a child, and behavior that might lead to injury (including being alert for signs of interpersonal violence) are particularly important. Such patients should be asked specifically about substance use before operating a motor vehicle, riding with intoxicated drivers, heterosexual sex without contraception, and sex while intoxicated. In addition, a thorough history must include past immunizations or courses of chemoprophylaxis (as for tuberculosis or to prevent folate deficiency). People with alcohol use disorders are at higher risk of folate deficiency, and this is of particular importance for women of childbearing age, whose fetuses are at risk of neural tube defects. Additional history is needed to determine if the patient belongs to a high-risk group that would indicate additional preventive interventions. For example, patients should be asked about chronic medical illnesses, whether they live in an institutional setting, contact with active cases of tuberculosis, recency of immigration, cardiovascular risk factors (smoking, cholesterol elevation, family history of heart disease, and diabetes), history or family history of cancer, travel patterns, receipt of blood products, drug injection, and occupation.

Physical Examination The physical examination may be complete and should certainly address body systems related to any reported symptoms.

Vital Signs and Measurements In asymptomatic persons, height, weight, and blood pressure assessments should be performed. The height and weight should be used to determine the body mass index and assess nutritional status.

Skin Skin examination can reveal signs of injection drug use, the wrinkles associated with tobacco use, or the palmar erythema of alcohol dependence.

Head, Eyes, Ears, Nose, and Throat Examination Examination should focus on the oral cavity: Smokers and alcohol users should have a thorough examination of the oral cavity to look for premalignant and malignant lesions to which they are particularly susceptible, synergistically. Tobacco-stained teeth can serve as a focus for discussion. The oral examination may also find the extreme tooth decay associated with methamphetamine use due to xerostomia, tooth grinding, and poor hygiene.

Chest/Cardiovascular Examination Particular attention should be paid to auscultation for cardiac murmurs that may be evidence of past valvular damage from injection drug use.

Abdominal Examination Examination of the liver is advisable, if only to draw attention to the many possible complications of drug and alcohol use. Even asymptomatic persons can have the small hard liver of cirrhosis or the enlarged liver of chronic viral or alcohol-related hepatitis.

Breast Examination Most preventive recommendations include the breast physical examination for adult women when done with mammography for screening, although the evidence for benefit is absent until age 40, when there is less risk from misidentification of benign lesions (6–10). Most masses detected in young women will be benign but may require investigation once detected to rule out malignancy.

Male Genital Examination Testicular examination for young men as well as rectal and prostate examinations (all to screen for cancers) are recommended by some specialty organizations (American Cancer Society and American Urological Association) but not by generalist organizations (American College of Physicians and U.S. Preventive Services Task Force) because of the absence of evidence for benefit (11). The risk of breast cancer is, and prostate and colorectal cancer may be, increased by even moderate alcohol consumption (12–14).

Female Genital Examination Though a pelvic examination without testing (e.g., for cervical cancer) is not routinely indicated, addicted persons are at risk of sexually transmitted diseases, and genital warts, abnormal vaginal discharge, or herpetic lesions can be seen.

Lymph Node Examination Persons with alcohol, tobacco, and other drug abuse should have the cervical, axillary, supraclavicular, and inguinal lymph node regions examined for lymphadenopathy. Tuberculosis, chancroid, syphilis, and HIV are more common in persons with addictive disorders who present with lymphadenopathy. Supraclavicular nodes can be the presenting sign of lung cancer in tobacco users.

Tests Because people with addictions are at risk for many medical illnesses, by various mechanisms, across organ systems and because some tests are widely available and relatively inexpensive, it is reasonable for all such patients to have a complete blood count, a blood sugar, serum creatinine, liver enzymes, and urinalysis at least once. Injection drug users and those with HIV risk factors in particular should have a urinalysis and serum creatinine to assess the presence of silent renal disease.

Routine preventive care for all includes tests for *cardiovascular risk*. All adults should be screened for hypercholesterolemia with a fasting lipid profile (serum low-density lipoprotein, high-density lipoprotein, and total cholesterol and triglycerides) or a random (nonfasting) serum total cholesterol and high-density lipoprotein (15,16). Hypertriglyceridemia is associated with heavy drinking and can be a cause of pancreatitis. Primary prevention—identifying patients with hyperlipidemia who have no clinically evident coronary artery disease—can decrease the risk of heart disease and death. Hematologic testing for preventive purposes includes a serum hemoglobin, mean corpuscular volume (MCV), or a hemoglobin electrophoresis, which should be checked in men and women who might be contemplating parenting. The purpose of the screen is to detect the common thalassemia traits and to provide genetic counseling. An unsuspected anemia or pancytopenia can be found in persons with alcohol use disorders or HIV.

Sexually Transmitted Diseases Adolescent and young adult women and others at high risk should have (urine) chlamydia testing performed. Persons with addictive disorders who have been sexually active or who use injection drugs should be screened routinely for sexually transmitted diseases with a serologic test for syphilis, HIV, and chlamydia (using the ligase chain reaction in a urine or cervical specimen). Recently, the Centers for Disease Control recommended that, in health care settings, all patients be screened for HIV, that HIV testing be done in high-risk patients yearly unless they opt out, and that separate written informed consent not be required. Some state laws do not allow the latter (17). Because of the implications and the potential to trigger relapse, the timing of HIV testing must be individualized, with input from the patient, preferably to a time when recovery is stable. The serologic test for syphilis (rapid plasma reagin or Venereal Disease Research Laboratory) frequently is falsely positive in injection drug users (as is the serum rheumatoid factor and the partial thromboplastin time), reflecting a generalized activation of the immune system. As a result, the screening test should not be used as evidence of syphilis—instead, the result should be confirmed by a treponemal test such as the microhemagglutination test for *Treponema pallidum* or the fluorescent treponemal antibody tests.

Other Infectious Diseases Among other risk factors, persons with alcohol and other drug use disorders without past known tuberculosis should be screened for asymptomatic infection with *Mycobacterium tuberculosis*, using a 5 tuberculin unit intradermal injection read at 48 hours (provided a previous test result is not known to have been positive). A positive test result in such persons is 10 mm of induration (5 mm if immune deficiency is present); in such cases, a chest radiograph should be performed (18). Provided the radiograph is not consistent with active tuberculosis, prophylactic pharmacotherapy should be considered regardless of age (19). Users of injection drugs, those with alcohol abuse, and persons with multiple sexual partners or high-risk sexual activity should have the international normalized ratio (INR), the serum bilirubin, transaminases (aspartate aminotransferase [AST] and alanine aminotransferase [ALT]), and the serum albumin and alkaline phosphatase checked as screening tests for chronic hepatitis and cirrhosis (and the serum albumin for nutritional status as well). The serum pre-albumin will give a more stable view of long-term nutritional status, as it fluctuates less than the serum albumin. Abnormal liver enzymes, INR, or serum bilirubin tests should be followed by hepatitis B (surface antigen and core antibody) and C antibody testing. Previously vaccinated individuals should have the antisurface hepatitis B antibody determined to assess current immunoprotection. Injection drug users and those who practice anal intercourse and who are not from endemic areas should be tested for immunity to hepatitis A.

Cancer Screening Smokers are at higher risk of cervical cancer. All women who have had sexual intercourse should have a cervical cytology (Papanicolaou smears) performed every 1 to 3 years to detect the premalignant lesions of cervical cancer. Human papilloma virus (HPV) testing has become part of cervical cancer routine testing protocols. Yearly mammography should be offered to women, beginning at age 40 or 50. Randomized trials show minimal benefit below the age of 50, and almost half of the women screened will suffer a false-positive and the consequences of further testing to clarify the diagnosis (20). Breast self-examination is of no proven benefit (21) and increases the risk of a benign breast biopsy. Mortality from breast cancer can be decreased by regular physical examination and screening mammography. A family history of breast cancer can indicate the need for earlier testing or referral to a specialist for genetic testing. Prostate cancer screening remains controversial. The serum prostate specific antigen (PSA) test is recommended by some specialty organizations, but many other groups (including all generalist physician organizations) do not. The U.S. Preventive Services Task Force finds insufficient evidence to recommend for or against PSA screening and recommends against screening older (75 years on more) men. They recommend that before any PSA testing, patients be informed about the potential benefits as well as the possible harms of false-positives and unnecessary treatments and their side effects (22). The controversy is due to the current state of the science: Prostate cancer usually has a very long preclinical phase, it is not yet possible to predict accurately which cases will progress, the testing is neither sensitive nor specific, the evaluation for a positive test is invasive, and the treatment results in significant complications (including erectile dysfunction and incontinence). Only one study (of radical prostatectomy) has shown a decrease in cancer-related mortality (23). In that study, only a small fraction of the tumors were PSA-detected. The PIVOT study should help to resolve the controversy (24). Patients who choose to be screened might do so because of the belief they will benefit (a belief shared by some physicians and scientists), but this benefit is by no means certain. Those who are at higher risk of prostate cancer, including African Americans and those with a family history of the disease, may use that information to help make decisions about screening, beginning at age 40. Colorectal cancer screening, however, is not controversial. Colorectal cancer mortality can be decreased in adults aged 50 years and older (younger for those with risk factors or familial disease) by a variety of approaches. Screening is not recommended after age 85 and is of uncertain benefit between 76 and 85 years of age. Currently recommended approaches include yearly fecal occult blood testing, flexible sigmoidoscopy every 5 years, and both procedures or colonoscopy every 10 years (25,26). Positive occult blood testing or sigmoidoscopy should be followed by an examination of the complete colon.

Testing for Other Conditions Older adults (aged 65 or older) should have thyroid function testing (serum thyroid-stimulating hormone) because abnormalities are common, difficult to recognize clinically, and easily treatable. Vision and hearing testing should be performed routinely in older adults. Bone mineral density (BMD) testing should be done for older menopausal women and younger menopausal women with risk factors if an intervention to prevent osteoporosis would be instituted as a result (27). This testing is of particular importance for persons with inadequate calcium intake, excessive alcohol use, physical inactivity, smoking, and a family history of osteoporosis. Persons with addictive disorders can have poor diets, little sun exposure, and minimal intake of milk products; screening for vitamin D deficiency with a 25-hydroxyvitamin D should be considered.

Preventive Counseling All patients should be counseled about healthy dietary habits (limiting saturated fat and favoring fruits, vegetables, legumes, fiber, and grains) and physical activity (at least 20 minutes of aerobic exercise three times a week). All alcohol and other drug abusers should be counseled about safer sexual practices (abstinence and condom use), and injection drug users should be educated about sterile injection practices. Women of childbearing age and their partners should be counseled about contraceptive options. All persons should be counseled that, in addition to their addiction specialty care, they should engage in regular primary and preventive health care with a primary care physician. Linkage of patients to primary medical care has many potential benefits, including improved prevention, management of chronic conditions, coordination of the many health care services needed by patients with addictive disorders, and support in relapse prevention efforts (2,3,28). In addition, because psychiatric illness is so common in addicted patients, linkage to mental health care should be offered when appropriate. This linkage can be accomplished through a primary care physician. Those persons who store or carry weapons should be reminded of gun safety. All patients should be advised about seat belt and helmet use. Referrals for both regular eye and dental care should be routine. Preventive advice about safe lifting is warranted to prevent low-back injury.

Immunizations Immunizations for adults include tetanus, diphtheria, and acellular pertussis (Tdap) vaccine when a tetanus booster is due (for adults younger than 65, or tetanus toxoid for older adults) every 10 years (presuming an initial series has been given); this is particularly important for injection drug users, who can expose themselves to tetanus (29–31). Detailed updated recommendations are published annually (32). Hepatitis B vaccination (a series of three injections) is indicated for injection drug users, health care workers, persons with hepatitis C, sexually active individuals who are not involved in long-term monogamous relationships, and for any adult seeking protection from infection. Hepatitis A vaccination (two injections) is indicated for travelers, those with any chronic liver disease, those who practice anal intercourse, and injection drug users, when negative for immunity (immunoglobulin G to hepatitis A). Pneumococcal vaccination should be administered to all persons aged 65 years and older and those with chronic cardiopulmonary disease (including heart disease, more common in smokers, and reactive airway diseases such as obstructive lung disease and asthma, which are more common in smokers and users of inhaled drugs). Alcoholism is a specific recognized indication for the vaccine, and many practitioners believe other drug addiction also is a reasonable indication. Other indicated vaccines include varicella vaccine for all adults without immunity, zoster vaccine for all older people (age 60 or older), regardless of prior episodes of herpes zoster, and HPV vaccine for all young women (ages 11 to 26).

When childhood vaccinations are unknown, consideration should be given to a primary series for polio; measles, mumps, and rubella; and varicella vaccination. Many adults will have immunity to these diseases but, if unknown, testing is warranted, given that many persons with addictive disorders may be in group living situations, sometimes with children and young adults, in which measles and varicella infections can spread easily. Influenza vaccination should be given yearly to all persons with addictive disorders. It is particularly indicated for those with cardiopulmonary disease and older adults but is cost-effective for general populations, too, and of particular utility for those living in group settings.

Chemoprophylaxis Aspirin is reasonable as primary prevention for myocardial infarction in men, particularly men with risk factors (33). Smoking is a strong risk factor for coronary artery disease. The benefit of aspirin for primary prevention among women is less certain given the results of a randomized trial finding that aspirin lowered the risk of stroke without affecting the risk of myocardial infarction or death from cardiovascular causes (34). However, the benefit of aspirin does not likely outweigh the risks of serious central nervous system or gastrointestinal bleeding in people with alcohol use disorders without symptoms of coronary disease because they are at risk of gastritis, thrombocytopenia, coagulopathy, and trauma. Women of childbearing age should take folate 400 mg daily to prevent neural tube defects (35). Because of the risk of thiamine, vitamin D, pyridoxine, niacin, riboflavin, zinc, and folic acid deficiency in people with alcohol use disorders and those with deficient diets, a daily multivitamin including 400 IU vitamin D, 100 mg thiamine, and 1 mg folic acid can be recommended. If serum 25-hydroxyvitamin D is low, repletion should begin with 50,000 IU vitamin D weekly for 4–8 weeks. Because magnesium deficiency is common in people with alcohol use disorders, replacement by encouraging the use of foods with a high magnesium content (such as peanuts) or a magnesium supplement (magnesium oxide tablets or magnesium hydroxide-containing antacids) is recommended. If the INR is known to be elevated, a trial of vitamin K is warranted, though generally the INR elevation in addicted persons will be due to liver disease and not to vitamin deficiency. Men and women, particularly those with deficient diets, should ensure adequate calcium intake in their diets or should use supplements (1 g elemental calcium daily for all but postmenopausal women, who should receive 1.5 g). Raloxifene, alendronate, ibandronate, and risedronate may be used for the prevention of osteoporosis in postmenopausal women (36–38), though the risks and benefits for addicted persons are difficult to predict. Risks for osteoporosis are higher in people with alcohol use disorders and some other addicted persons, but the interaction between estrogen and alcohol on breast cancer is not clear, and the side effects of the drugs in people who drink heavily and those with liver disease are not well-characterized.

CARE DURING HOSPITALIZATION

Because of the burden of illness carried by persons with addictive disorders, they can require transfer from addiction treatment to a general hospital, or they can be admitted there directly. During a medical hospitalization, three areas deserve particular attention: (1) management of the drug withdrawal, (2) pain management, and (3) common comorbidities (39). Treatment (including brief interventions, which are well suited to medical hospital settings) and withdrawal and pain management are addressed elsewhere in this textbook, but several points are relevant to medical hospitalizations specifically.

Withdrawal When a history of alcohol dependence and recent use is obtained, withdrawal should be anticipated. Symptoms should be treated as they appear. Persons not yet symptomatic with withdrawal but with past alcohol-related seizures or concomitant acute medical or surgical conditions (which increase the risk of withdrawal) should be treated with a benzodiazepine (that is, 10 to 20 mg diazepam or 1 to 2 mg lorazepam to prevent convulsions or delirium) (40). Because the symptoms of withdrawal may not be distinguishable from systemic symptoms of infection, heart disease, or neurologic conditions, treatment for withdrawal should proceed while investigations to identify other treatable medical disorders continue. Though the use of standardized withdrawal scales generally is encouraged, their lack of specificity requires that the information they provide be considered in the context of the coexisting medical illness. Nevertheless, patients hospitalized for withdrawal as well as for other medical conditions have had favorable outcomes when treated with symptom-triggered therapy (41–43). Similarly, opiate and other drug withdrawal should be identified and managed pharmacologically, both for patient comfort as well as to prevent complications of the medical disorder for which the patient was hospitalized. Patients who already are in treatment for opiate or long-acting sedative dependence should have their treating clinician contacted when they are hospitalized, so that any prescribed ongoing treatment can be continued. Similarly, addiction treatment providers should communicate directly with hospital physicians to facilitate appropriate treatment, after obtaining permission from the patient. Doses for patients not on long-acting opiate treatment should be adequate to prevent withdrawal and should be administered to allow treatment of the underlying medical disorder (that is, 10 to 20 mg methadone, repeated in 2 hours, then given daily or in divided doses twice a day). At hospital admission, when deciding on the best treatment for the patient, the patient's disposition at discharge should be anticipated. If the patient plans to abstain from the substance at hospital discharge, the substituted opioid can be tapered if symptoms allow. Alternatively, a dose sufficient to avoid withdrawal can be maintained during the hospitalization for those who intend to continue drug use or to enter a maintenance treatment program. Again, symptoms of withdrawal can mimic medical disorders. In addition to providing comfort and helping to prevent the more serious complications of withdrawal (such as convulsions from alcohol withdrawal), specific treatment of withdrawal controls the autonomic symptoms that can worsen a patient's medical condition (such as tachycardia during a myocardial infarction) and helps the patient cooperate with treatment for the medical condition that prompted hospitalization.

Another consideration for the management of withdrawal in hospitalized patients is the route of administration of the drug. Delirious patients should receive intravenous medications (such as diazepam or lorazepam), whereas others who cannot take medications by mouth should receive medications via a route associated with reliable absorption for the particular drug: lorazepam intramuscularly for alcohol withdrawal or methadone (40% to 50% of the oral dose in three to four divided doses) intramuscularly for opiate dependence.

Pain Pain management often becomes an issue during medical hospitalization of addicted patients. Physicians and nurses may fear providing pain control with opioids when a patient is addicted to them, because of the fear of causing or worsening addiction. This management style generally results in inadequate pain management and frustration for patient and provider alike. Clearly, patients with addictive disorders usually are very tolerant to the substance they use.

In the case of opiate dependence, pain control can be achieved only with substantially higher doses of opioids, with careful reassessment of the dose effect and timing to make appropriate adjustments. Once a dose is determined, pain medications should be given on a regular schedule rather than as needed, to avoid making the patient demand medication to relieve uncontrolled symptoms. Similar principles apply for patients on opioid agonist treatment (44).

Comorbidities Finally, while patients are hospitalized, several comorbidities should be considered. First, because psychiatric comorbidity is common (in particular antisocial personality disorder, anxiety, and depression), attention to behavioral issues is important. Hospital staff members should take extra care to explain hospital procedures, while setting firm limits. Patients should be assured that their medical, psychiatric, and addiction-related symptoms and pain will be attended to. Discussing withdrawal and pain treatment regimens with the patient can help avoid later problems and disagreements and help allay the fears and preconceptions patients may have about providers. Screening for coexisting medical disorders (such as HIV, hepatitis, and tuberculosis) during a medical hospitalization should be considered because the acute care setting may provide the only medical care received by the patient. Nevertheless, when such testing is done, consideration should be given to the patient's readiness to hear and handle the results and to arranging follow-up medical care for the condition. For HIV testing in particular, pretest (reasons for testing, past testing, assessment of risk behaviors, the implications of test results, and the risks and benefits) and posttest counseling must be provided. Most patients in detoxification centers believe HIV testing should be available during detoxification (45). Treatment for coexisting medical and psychiatric conditions should be made available.

MEDICAL CONSEQUENCES OF ALCOHOL, TOBACCO, AND OTHER DRUG USE

Medical consequences of addiction may be due to drug specific effects, methods of administration, contaminants in or vehicles for drugs used, behavioral habits associated with substance use, or common comorbidities (Table 71.1). In this portion of the chapter, the medical consequences of addiction are reviewed and organized by drug and then by organ system or clinical area. More details can be found in the chapters in this section. Though some lifestyle choices and risk behaviors span more than one substance, consequences are discussed once to avoid redundancy.

Alcohol The medical consequences of alcohol use are seen in almost every organ system of the body. Women are more susceptible to many of the effects at lower doses because of less first-pass metabolism of alcohol and lower body weights on average (46). Though moderate drinking can have some beneficial effects for selected individuals, two drinks per day for women and three drinks per day for men increases the risk of death (47,48).

Withdrawal, Seizures, and Delirium Tremens Though the direct medical consequences of alcohol withdrawal (hyperautonomic states, seizures, and delirium) are covered in detail elsewhere in this book, mention is made here because they are common, often are managed in acute care general medical hospitals, and can lead to death. Many patients in withdrawal can be managed as outpatients with or without medication, provided symptoms are minimal and there is little comorbidity that would complicate outpatient management or place patients at higher risk of complications of withdrawal. Alcohol withdrawal symptoms, such as diaphoresis and tremor, begin 6 to 48 hours after the last drink (49). Such withdrawal symptoms may resolve spontaneously or require treatment with benzodiazepines. Benzodiazepines are the only medications proven, compared with placebo, to ameliorate symptoms of withdrawal, to decrease the risk of seizures and delirium and, compared with paraldehyde (50), to speed achievement of a calm but awake state in patients experiencing delirium (40,49). Signs found on physical examination include tremor, moist warm skin, agitation, tachycardia, or hypertension, though these signs may be absent. The tachycardia can complicate underlying medical conditions such as coronary artery disease by precipitating angina or myocardial infarction. Pharmacologic treatment is indicated for asymptomatic patients at higher risk of complications (acute medical, surgical, or psychiatric comorbidity; past seizures; and past delirium) and for those with significant symptoms (on the Clinical Institute Withdrawal Assessment for Alcohol, Revised, a score of more than 8 to 15) to prevent progression to seizures or delirium and for patient comfort (40). Seizures, when they occur, almost always resolve spontaneously. They can recur and generally do so within 6 hours of the first seizure. Benzodiazepines prevent further seizures and progression to *delirium tremens* (DTs). Phenytoin and other anticonvulsants are not indicated unless there is another cause or suspected cause for the seizures in addition to alcohol. DTs (hyperautonomia and disorientation/confusion) should be managed in a setting where frequent and intensive monitoring is possible because of the risk of death from the condition and its treatment. Other medications besides the benzodiazepines can be used as adjunctive therapies, provided the patient receives benzodiazepines. These include beta-blockers for tachycardia determined to be the result of withdrawal, clonidine for hypertension, and haloperidol for psychosis or agitation, when these signs and symptoms fail to respond to benzodiazepines. Other drugs (such as gabapentin and carbamazepine) that can alleviate symptoms, and may even appear to be preferable (for outpatients or to allow earlier participation in counseling) because of less central nervous system depression, should not be used as monotherapy for withdrawal in patients for whom treatment is indicated

TABLE 70.1 Selected Medical Disorders Related to Alcohol and Other Drug Use

Cardiovascular

Alcohol: Cardiomyopathy, atrial fibrillation (holiday heart), hypertension, dysrhythmia, masks angina symptoms, coronary artery spasm, myocardial ischemia, high-output states, coronary artery disease, sudden death

Cocaine: Hypertension, myocardial infarction, angina, chest pain, supraventricular tachycardia, ventricular dysrhythmias, cardiomyopathy, cardiovascular collapse from bodypacking rupture, moyamoya vasculopathy, left ventricular hypertrophy, myocarditis, sudden death, aortic dissection

Tobacco: Atherosclerosis, stroke, myocardial infarction, peripheral vascular disease, cor pulmonale, erectile dysfunction, worse control of hypertension, angina, dysrhythmia

Infection: Endocarditis, septic thrombophlebitis

Cancer

Alcohol: Aerodigestive (lip, oral cavity, tongue, pharynx, larynx, esophagus, stomach, colon), breast, hepatocellular and bile duct cancers

Tobacco: Oral cavity, larynx, lung, cervix, esophagus, pancreas, kidney, stomach, bladder

Injection or high-risk sexual behavior: Hepatocellular carcinoma related to hepatitis C

Endocrine/Reproductive

Alcohol: Hypoglycemia and hyperglycemia, diabetes, ketoacidosis, hypertriglyceridemia, hyperuricemia and gout, testicular atrophy, gynecomastia, hypocalcemia and hypomagnesemia because of reversible hypoparathyroidism, hypercortisolemia, osteopenia, infertility, sexual dysfunction

Opiates: Osteopenia, alteration in gonadotropins, decreased sperm motility, menstrual irregularities

Cocaine: Diabetic ketoacidosis

Tobacco: Graves' disease, azoospermia, erectile dysfunction, osteopenia, osteoporosis, fractures, estrogen alterations, insulin resistance

Any addiction: Amenorrhea

Hepatic

Alcohol: Steatosis (fatty liver), acute and chronic hepatitis (infectious [that is, B or C] or toxic [that is, acetaminophen]), alcoholic hepatitis, cirrhosis, portal hypertension and varices, spontaneous bacterial peritonitis

Opiates: Granulamatosis

Cocaine: Ischemic necrosis, hepatitis

Injection or high-risk sexual behavior: Infectious hepatitis B and C (acute and chronic) and delta

Hematologic

Alcohol: Macrocytic anemia, pancytopenia because of marrow toxicity and/or splenic sequestration, leukopenia, thrombocytopenia, coagulopathy because of liver disease, iron deficiency, folate deficiency, spur cell anemia, burr cell anemia

Tobacco: Hypercoagulability

Injection or high-risk sexual behavior: Hematologic consequences of liver disease, hepatitis C-related cryoglobulinemia and purpura

Infectious

Alcohol: Hepatitis C, pneumonia, tuberculosis (including meningitis), HIV, sexually transmitted diseases, spontaneous bacterial peritonitis, brain abscess, meningitis

Opiates: Aspiration pneumonia

Tobacco: Bronchitis, pneumonia, upper–respiratory tract infections

Injection: Endocarditis, cellulitis, pneumonia, septic thrombophlebitis, septic arthritis (unusual joints, that is, sternoclavicular), osteomyelitis (including vertebral), epidural and brain abscess, mycotic aneurysm, abscesses and soft tissue infections, mediastinitis, malaria, tetanus

Injection or high-risk sexual behavior: Hepatitis B, C, and delta; HIV; sexually transmitted diseases

Neurologic

Alcohol: Peripheral and autonomic neuropathy, seizure, hepatic encephalopathy, Korsakoff's dementia, Wernicke's syndrome, cerebellar dysfunction, Marchiafava-Bignami syndrome, central pontine myelinolysis, myopathy, amblyopia, stroke, withdrawal delirium, hallucinations, toxic leukoencephalopathy, subdural hematoma, intracranial hemorrhage

Opiates: Seizure (overdose and hypoxia), compression neuropathy

Cocaine: Stroke, seizure, status epilepticus, headache, delirium, depression, hypersomnia, cognitive deficits

Tobacco: Stroke, small-vessel ischemia and cognitive deficits

Any addiction: Compression neuropathy.

Nutritional

Alcohol: Vitamin and mineral deficiencies (B_1, B_6, riboflavin, niacin, vitamin D, magnesium, calcium, folate, phosphate, zinc)

Any addiction: Protein malnutrition

(continued)

TABLE 70.1 Selected Medical Disorders Related to Alcohol and Other Drug Use *(continued)*

Other Gastrointestinal
Alcohol: Gastritis, esophagitis, pancreatitis, diarrhea, malabsorption (because of pancreatic exocrine insufficiency, or folate or lactase deficiency), parotid enlargement, malignancy, colitis, Barrett esophagus, gastroesophageal reflux, Mallory-Weiss syndrome, gastrointestinal bleeding
Opiates: Constipation, ileus, intestinal pseudo-obstruction
Cocaine: Ischemic bowel and colitis
Tobacco: Peptic ulcers, gastroesophageal reflex, malignancy (pancreas, stomach)
Any addiction: Overdose from bodypacking

Prenatal and perinatal
Alcohol: Fetal alcohol effects and syndrome
Opiates: Neonatal abstinence syndrome, including seizures
Cocaine: Placental abruption, teratogenesis, neonatal irritability
Tobacco: Teratogenesis, low birth weight, spontaneous abortion, abruptio placentae, placenta previa, perinatal mortality, sudden infant death syndrome, neurodevelopmental impairment

Perioperative
Alcohol: Withdrawal, perioperative complications (delirium, infection, bleeding, pneumonia, delayed wound healing, dysrhythmia), hepatic decompensation, hepatorenal syndrome, death
Opiates: Withdrawal, inadequate analgesia
Cocaine: Hypersomnia and depression in withdrawal, mimicking of postoperative neurologic complications, complications from underlying drug-induced cardiopulmonary disease
Tobacco: Pulmonary infection, difficulty weaning, respiratory failure, reactive airways exacerbations

Pulmonary
Alcohol: Aspiration, sleep apnea, respiratory depression, apnea, chemical or infectious pneumonitis
Opiates: Respiratory depression/failure, emphysema, bronchospasm, exacerbation of sleep apnea, pulmonary edema
Cocaine: Nasal septum perforation, gingival ulceration, perennial rhinitis, sinusitis, hemoptysis, upper airway obstruction, fibrosis, hypersensitivity pneumonitis, epiglottitis, pulmonary hemorrhage, pulmonary hypertension, pulmonary edema, emphysema, interstitial fibrosis, hypersensitivity pneumonia
Tobacco: Lung cancer, chronic obstructive pulmonary disease, reactive airways, pneumonia, bronchitis, pulmonary hypertension, interstitial lung disease, pneumothorax
Injection: Pulmonary hypertension, talc granulomatosis, septic pulmonary embolism, pneumothorax, emphysema, needle embolization
Inhalation: Pulmonary edema, bronchospasm, bronchitis, granulomatosis, airway burns

Renal
Alcohol: Hepatorenal syndrome, rhabdomyolysis and acute renal failure, volume depletion and prerenal failure, acidosis, hypokalemia, hypophosphatemia
Opiates: Rhabdomyolysis, acute renal failure, factitious hematuria
Cocaine: Rhabdomyolysis and acute renal failure, vasculitis, necrotizing angiitis, accelerated hypertension, nephrosclerosis, ischemia
Tobacco: Renal failure, hypertension
Injection or high-risk sexual behavior: focal glomerular sclerosis (HIV, heroin), glomerulonephritis from hepatitis or endocarditis, chronic renal failure, amyloidosis, nephrotic syndrome (hepatitis C)

Sleep
Alcohol: Apnea, periodic limb movements of sleep, insomnia, disrupted sleep, daytime fatigue
Opiates: Insomnia
Cocaine: Hypersomnia in withdrawal
Tobacco: Insomnia, increased sleep latency

Trauma
Alcohol: Motor vehicle crash, fatal and nonfatal injury, physical and sexual abuse
Cocaine: Death during "Russian Roulette"
Opiates: Motor vehicle crash, other violent injury
Tobacco: Burns, smoke inhalation
Any addiction: Sexual and physical abuse

Musculoskeletal
Alcohol: Rhabdomyolysis, compartment syndromes, gout, saturnine gout, fracture, osteopenia, osteonecrosis
Opiates: Osteopenia
Cocaine: Rhabdomyolysis
Any addiction: Compartment syndromes, fractures

to prevent complications. Barbiturates are reasonable alternatives to the benzodiazepines but have a lower margin of safety and no placebo-controlled evidence for efficacy.

Neurologic Consequences Neurologic complications are perhaps some of the most well known. Alcohol intoxication can lead to head trauma. The signs and symptoms of intracranial hemorrhage—particularly subdural hematoma—can be confused with intoxication. Imaging of the brain is indicated when there are signs of significant head trauma and abnormal mental status, focal neurologic deficits are present, or when neurologic symptoms do not resolve with declining alcohol levels. People with alcohol dependence are at higher risk of tuberculosis, which can manifest as tuberculous meningitis (51). DTs are the diagnosis of exclusion (by lumbar puncture) when fever and delirium are present in a person with alcohol dependence. In addition to withdrawal seizures, alcohol can lower the seizure threshold in epileptics, and seizures may be the presenting sign of an intracranial hemorrhage. Moderate drinking may decrease the risk for ischemic stroke (52), but heavy drinking (even at one to two or more drinks a day) (53) increases the risk for ischemic and hemorrhagic stroke, related to an interplay with smoking, trauma, hypertension, folic acid deficiency and hyperhomocystinemia, and cardiomyopathy (54). The overall risk of stroke in women is increased in those who consume just more than one standard drink per day (46).

Cognitive impairment may be caused acutely by Wernicke-Korsakoff disease because of thiamine deficiency, presenting with confusion, ataxia, or nystagmus. Parenteral thiamine, 100 mg administered before glucose, is the initial treatment. Chronically, Wernicke-Korsakoff disease can develop into Korsakoff's syndrome, a memory impairment classically characterized by confabulation. More commonly, chronic alcohol dependence is associated with a nonspecific dementia and volume loss on head computed tomography. Toxic leukoencephalopathy, or damage of cerebral white matter, can contribute to the dementia seen with alcohol dependence (55). Marchiafava-Bignami disease, caused by lesions in the corpus callosum, is rare. Also rare is central pontine myelinolysis, which is seen in conjunction with alcohol dependence and too rapid correction of hyponatremia. Alcoholic cerebellar dysfunction is not so rare; it results in ataxia and incoordination and often is irreversible. People with alcohol dependence can suffer from peripheral neuropathy, usually from vitamin deficiency, pressure on a nerve, or ethanol toxicity. The classic presentation of alcoholic polyneuropathy is of sensory disturbance, including burning, pain, and numbness in a stocking-glove distribution.

Gastrointestinal Consequences Gastrointestinal problems are very common in the patient with alcohol dependence. Alcohol is directly toxic to the gastric mucosa and can lead to gastritis. Gastritis can be asymptomatic or can present as epigastric burning, nausea, vomiting, anemia, or hematemesis (coffee grounds emesis). Vomiting can lead to a Mallory-Weiss tear and hematemesis. Alcohol can lead to stomatitis, esophagitis, duodenitis, esophageal cancer, and gastric cancer. Endoscopy is warranted for persistent reflux symptoms or epigastric pain, particularly if weight loss is present or if patients are aged 40 years and older. Liver and pancreatic consequences of alcohol use are among the most well known. Hepatitis ranges in severity from an asymptomatic elevation of the hepatic transaminases to critical illness with hepatic failure. In alcoholic hepatitis, AST usually is higher than ALT. A higher ALT concentration suggests another or a concomitant etiology, such as hepatitis C, for which alcohol abuse is a risk factor. Heavy alcohol use accelerates the progression to cirrhosis in hepatitis C and interferes with the success of treatment (56,57). Hepatic steatosis can cause elevations in serum transaminases. Though steatohepatitis is best diagnosed by liver biopsy, clinically it often is diagnosed when serology for hepatitis B and C are negative, the abnormality persists with abstinence, and an ultrasound examination is consistent with the diagnosis.

Classic alcoholic hepatitis presents with fever, leukocytosis, right upper-quadrant pain and tenderness, and elevations of the AST concentration out of proportion to ALT elevations. Management consists of abstinence from alcohol as well as supportive care, with attention to fluid and electrolyte balance, vitamin K for coagulopathy, clotting factor replacement when there is active bleeding and coagulopathy, and attention to volume and mental status. Patients with coagulopathy, hyperbilirubinemia, and hepatic encephalopathy are at high risk of death. Corticosteroids have been shown to decrease mortality in selected severe cases of alcoholic hepatitis (hepatic encephalopathy or when 4.6 times the prothrombin time above control in seconds plus the bilirubin is greater than 32 (58). In general, before giving steroids (prednisolone 40 mg a day for 4 weeks followed by a taper), active infection should be excluded. In addition, efficacy is not known for patients with concomitant pancreatitis, gastrointestinal bleeding, or renal failure. Propylthiouracil, colchicine, oxandrolone, and pentoxifylline have shown promising results in some studies (even for mortality in the case of the latter two), though because of limited and conflicting data to date, they are not yet standard treatments (59–65). Cirrhosis can develop in chronic alcohol users either as a consequence of hepatitis C, recurrent alcoholic hepatitis or, simply, chronic heavy use. An increase in the incidence of cirrhosis can be detected in populations drinking two to three standard drinks per day compared with nondrinkers (48,66,67), though heavier amounts are more commonly associated with the condition (that is, 40 to 60 g/day of ethanol for men and less [20 g] for women) (68–71). Cirrhosis leads to hypoalbuminemia, coagulopathy, and hyperbilirubinemia. Hepatocellular carcinoma can occur, particularly when hepatitis C is present (72). It can be cured surgically if detected early enough. Complications of cirrhosis portend a poor prognosis. These complications include hepatic encephalopathy, esophageal or gastric variceal bleeding, ascites and spontaneous bacterial peritonitis, volume overload and edema, and hepatorenal syndrome. When cirrhosis and alcoholic hepatitis coexist, the prognosis is poor (35% to 50% for 4- to 5-year survival), particularly when drinking continues (73,74). End-stage liver disease of many etiologies can be addressed with liver transplantation. Patients transplanted because of alcoholic liver disease have similar survival to those transplanted for other causes of liver failure (75). Many liver transplantation programs have required defined periods of abstinence—often 3 to12 months—(76) before patients will be evaluated for this extensive surgery and scarce resource, though assessing relapse risk without requiring an arbitrary period of abstinence is an alternative approach (77). Furthermore, most transplant recipients do not return to drinking (22% in the first year), and few return to heavy drinking (5% to frequent heavy use in one year, 20% at 5 years) (78). There are few predictors of relapse (other drug use, having needed alcohol rehabilitation, depression, length of pre-transplant sobriety, and having a family history of alcohol dependence) (78,79). Chronic alcohol use increases the risk of acetaminophen toxicity, even at doses of 4 g daily, particularly when the patient has been fasting; cases of fulminant hepatic failure have been reported (80). Pancreatitis often presents as epigastric pain, sometimes radiating to the back, in chronic heavy alcohol users. The other common cause in the United States is gallstones. The serum amylase often is elevated unless there has been chronic pancreatic damage. The amylase is neither sensitive nor specific for pancreatitis (81). In people with alcohol dependence, amylase often is elevated because of chronic parotitis. Abdominal computed tomography is the most sensitive and specific test, but it is not indicated unless the presentation is atypical, fever is present, or the patient does not improve as expected. Severity can range from mild epigastric pain after eating, with some nausea, to a mortal condition complicated by acidosis, adult respiratory distress syndrome, and hypovolemia. Predictors of death include hyperglycemia, anemia, hypoxemia, acidosis, older age, leukocytosis, elevated blood urea nitrogen, lactate dehydrogenase or AST, hypocalcemia, or hypovolemia (82). The only treatment proven to decrease mortality is volume repletion, best accomplished with intravenous normal saline (83). Standard therapy includes nothing by mouth, volume repletion, and pain control by using opiates parenterally. Antibiotics should be considered in the presence of unexplained fever. Surgical consultation should be obtained when other diagnoses are being considered and when consideration is given to necrotizing pancreatitis. When acute episodes resolve, a return to drinking can lead to recurrent episodes and ultimately to constant pain and chronic pancreatitis, loss of pancreatic exocrine function with greasy stools and malabsorption, and even loss of pancreatic endocrine function manifested by hyperglycemia and diabetes (84). The prognosis is markedly worse with any ongoing alcohol consumption (85). Oral pancreatic enzyme supplementation with meals then is indicated, although pain management is difficult and often requires opiates. Serum amylase and lipase often are normal, although calcifications may be seen on abdominal radiographs.

Hematologic Consequences In addition to the iron deficiency anemia that can result from gastrointestinal hemorrhage or chronic blood loss (from variceal bleeding, gastritis, Mallory-Weiss tears, coexisting ulcers, esophagitis, or gastrointestinal cancers), people with alcohol use disorders can develop a pancytopenia (leukopenia, thrombocytopenia, and anemia) from alcohol's direct toxic effects on the bone marrow (86,87). The leukopenia can increase the risk of infections. Splenic sequestration as a result of the splenomegaly associated with cirrhosis and portal hypertension can cause a pancytopenia. People with alcohol dependence often have not only leukopenia but an impaired quantitative and qualitative white blood cell response to infection (87). The thrombocytopenia can lead to serious bleeding (as a result of trauma or varices, for example), when the platelet count is below 50,000. The anemia can be severe. People with alcohol dependence can be folate-deficient, with a megaloblastic anemia. Thus, the MCV, often used to assist in the differential diagnosis of anemia, can be misleadingly normal, with iron deficiency lowering the MCV and hemolytic anemias related to liver disease with reticulocytosis or megaloblastic processes simultaneously increasing it. In these cases, the red cell distribution width should be elevated. The treatment for bone marrow suppression is abstinence, for iron deficiency it is identification of the cause and iron replacement, and for folate deficiency it is folate (after testing for concomitant vitamin B_{12} deficiency and giving treatment, as needed). A reticulocytosis should be seen within 1 to 2 weeks of instituting appropriate treatment. A significant thrombocytosis often develops within days of abstinence. Coagulopathy (manifested as easy bleeding and ecchymoses), confirmed by elevation of the INR and prolongation of the partial thromboplastin time, usually is a result of chronic liver disease, though a trial of vitamin K replacement is warranted at least once. Anemias can be the result of abnormal red blood cell membranes in patients with cirrhosis (that is, spur and burr cell anemia).

Cardiovascular Consequences In addition to the transient hypertension seen during withdrawal, heavy drinking (about two or more standard drinks per day) is associated with chronic hypertension, which can lead to end-organ cardiac, retinal, renal, and vascular damage (88–90). Hypertension can be the result of even low levels of regular consumption. Though persons who in retrospect prove to be safe drinkers of moderate amounts appear to have a lower incidence of coronary heart disease events, chronic heavy drinking can lead to alcoholic cardiomyopathy and congestive heart failure (91). Echocardiogram reveals diffuse hypokinesis and often four-chamber dilation. If left ventricular thrombosis is seen, patients are at higher risk of embolic stroke. Treatment consists of alcohol abstinence (which can, in some cases, lead to an increase in the left ventricular ejection fraction), and standard treatments for congestive heart failure (which include angiotensin-converting-enzyme inhibitors or antagonists, furosemide or other loop diuretics, nitrates, and sometimes digoxin). Evaluation for sustained ventricular dysrhythmias in symptomatic patients is warranted and may lead to antiarrhythmic therapy (with amiodarone) or implantation of an automatic implantable cardioverter defibrillator to decrease the risk of sudden death (92). Anticoagulation with warfarin may be indicated when there is a ventricular clot, but the risk-benefit balance often is unclear, particularly when the patient is not abstinent. Atrial fibrillation ("holiday heart") can occur as a consequence of alcohol use or withdrawal, is not restricted to holidays, and usually resolves spontaneously (93–96). If the dysrhythmia persists after treatment for withdrawal (with benzodiazepines and, in this case, beta-blockers) and abstinence, other etiologies (for example, hyperthyroidism, hypertension, ischemic heart disease, and cardiomyopathy) should be evaluated, and additional treatment (electrical or chemical cardioversion and anticoagulation) should be considered. Moderate drinking (fewer than two standard drinks per day) has been associated with fewer cardiovascular events and decreased mortality in men (but not in average-risk women) (67), although no randomized trials studying important clinical outcomes (e.g., myocardial infarction, mortality) have been done of this pharmacologic agent with known side effects. Furthermore, heavy episodic drinking amounts have adverse cardiovascular consequences (97). The epidemiologic findings of benefit for moderate drinking can be confounded by alternative explanations, such as differences in social characteristics that remain unaccounted for (98–101). Studies have suggested that, if there is a benefit, it may be most pronounced in patients who have the same alcohol dehydrogenase genotype that may predispose them to alcohol dependence (102). Clearly, nondrinkers should not begin to drink for cardiovascular benefit.

Renal and Metabolic Consequences Renal and metabolic consequences of alcohol use often are seen in acute care settings. Hepatitis C can lead to nephrotic syndrome and glomerulonephritis with or without cryoglobulinemia and purpura (103). Cirrhosis can be complicated by the almost always fatal renal ischemic disorder, hepatorenal syndrome. Chronic renal insufficiency may be seen in persons who ingest home-distilled alcohol made with lead equipment (104). Acute renal failure from rhabdomyolysis can occur after alcohol intoxication. Fluid and electrolyte abnormalities are very common and often are minimized and overlooked in people with heavy alcohol use who present for medical care. Many patients with heavy alcohol use who present for medical treatment will be volume-depleted from vomiting, diarrhea, and diuresis. Volume repletion is best accomplished orally, when possible, and with intravenous normal saline, at least until the patient no longer manifests postural changes in blood pressure and heart rate and excess losses are not continuing. Acidosis can be a medical emergency. The first step is to distinguish between a non-anion gap and an anion gap acidosis. If an anion gap is not present, diarrhea is the most common cause in people with heavy alcohol use. If an anion gap is present, the differential diagnosis is broad but, in the people with heavy alcohol use, lactic acidosis (from sepsis, injury, severe pancreatitis, or after convulsion), ketoacidosis, and ingestion should be considered first. To rule out ingestion, in addition to the history (which may be unreliable), the measured serum osmolality should be compared with the calculated osmolality (accounting for the serum ethanol in the calculation). If no osmolar gap is present, ethylene glycol and methanol ingestions are unlikely. If a gap is present, testing for these ingestions should be done though levels are usually not available in time to assist with acute management. These ingestions require prompt treatment with fomepizole, hemodialysis, or both to prevent blindness or death (105). Alcoholic ketoacidosis is common (106,107). The glucose concentration can be high, normal, or low, and the urine ketones can be negative (although serum ketones should be positive). The treatment is volume expansion, and the substrate is given as 5% dextrose in normal saline (preceded by thiamine). In the absence of ketones or an osmolar gap, lactic acidosis is the next most serious diagnosis to consider, mainly because it can be the only clue to an unrecognized etiology (such as myocardial infarction or recent convulsion). Alkalemia is not uncommon in people with heavy alcohol use, either from respiratory alkalosis related to liver disease and hyperventilation or metabolic alkalosis from vomiting. Treatment for withdrawal (holding diuretics if the patient is on them, control of vomiting with antiemetics, and abstinence from alcohol, combined with volume repletion) can help speed the resolution of the alkalemia, which is important because alkalemia can be associated with hypokalemia and hypomagnesemia from secondary hyperaldosteronism. When dextrose is given to malnourished people with heavy alcohol use, severe hypophosphatemia can be unmasked and require treatment (108). Hypomagnesemia is common in people with heavy alcohol use, as a result of diuretic use, hypokalemia, and reversible hypoparathyroidism resulting from impaired parathyroid hormone release when the magnesium cofactor is deficient (109). The latter condition also leads to hypocalcemia, which does not respond to calcium replacement; rather, it responds to magnesium repletion. The hypokalemia often seen in people with heavy alcohol use with hyperaldosteronism from volume depletion and diuretic use will not correct until magnesium is replaced. Serum levels do not reflect total body magnesium stores, so empiric replacement is the best approach. Oral replacement of magnesium and phosphate is possible with magnesium containing antacids and milk, but this approach often is limited by an inability to take food by mouth or by diarrhea (which worsens the deficiencies). Intravenous replacement, with cardiac monitoring in the case of severe hypophosphatemia, may be necessary. Hyperglycemia or hypoglycemia can be seen in people with alcohol use disorders as a result of pancreatic insufficiency or, in the case of end-stage cirrhosis, as a result of depleted glycogen stores, which is a very poor prognostic sign.

Trauma Injury is a common consequence of both alcohol and drug intoxication but may be more likely in people with alcohol problems (110). Trauma, including physical and sexual abuse, can lead to poorer addiction treatment outcomes (111). Alcohol can interfere with balance and coordination, thus predisposing to injury. It also interferes with judgment, and some heavy drinkers already have a predisposition to risk taking. Heavy episodic (sometimes called *binge*) drinking (i.e., exceeding four standard drinks on an occasion for men, three for women) poses a particular risk of injury and accidents (112). Patients who present to emergency departments and trauma centers with serious injuries are far more likely than others to have used alcohol recently (113). The high frequency of injury in persons with heavy alcohol use suggests that facilities where such persons are seen for health care (that is, emergency departments and trauma centers) should routinely screen for alcohol problems and refer patients with alcohol-related disorders for treatment in order to prevent additional injury. Such strategies have proved successful in randomized trials (114). Moreover, addiction specialists should be attuned to the high rates of injury (both past trauma and the risk of future injury) when counseling people with people with alcohol use disorders. Injury can be a motivating factor for discontinuing alcohol use, or a focus of counseling to prevent future injuries.

Infectious Diseases Alcohol can lead to infectious consequences by various mechanisms. People with alcohol dependence can have impaired defenses because of undernutrition, splenic dysfunction, leukopenia, and impaired granulocyte function as well as suppression of the gag reflex during intoxication and overdose. Because of these risks, fever in people with alcohol use disorders must not be attributed to a minor viral syndrome or withdrawal unless other causes have been reasonably excluded. For example, though fever and confusion might be attributable to a postictal state or DTs, cerebrospinal fluid examination is warranted to exclude the possibility of meningitis. Though the treatment is the same as for nonaddicted persons, pneumonia is more common in people with alcohol use disorders, alcoholism increases the risk of mortality, and hospital treatment is more costly because it takes longer (115). Concomitant smoking increases the risk by impairing the mucociliary elevator. Causes include aspiration (commonly of anaerobic organisms), *S. pneumoniae*, atypical organisms, viruses, *Haemophilus influenzae*, and *Klebsiella pneumoniae*.

Tuberculosis is a consideration, particularly when the symptoms are more chronic, weight loss is present, and upper-lobe infiltrates appear on the chest x-ray in people with alcohol use disorders who are homeless, have immigrated from a country where the disease is endemic, are known to have a previous positive tuberculin skin test, or have had contact with an active case. Because HIV is more common in people with alcohol use disorders than in the general population, *Pneumocystis carinii* pneumonia and other opportunistic infections must be considered when pneumonia is diagnosed. Treatment for all of these conditions involves hospitalization in severe cases and antimicrobial therapy directed at the known or likely etiologies, along with observation and treatment for withdrawal symptoms. Other infectious diseases seen in people with alcohol use disorders include sexually transmitted diseases, spontaneous bacterial peritonitis, brain abscess, and meningitis. Meningitis in people with alcohol use disorders has a broader differential diagnosis than in the general population. It can be due to *S. pneumoniae, Listeria monocytogenes*, gram-negative bacilli and, in younger persons, *Neisseria meningitidis*. Brain abscess can result from poor dentition, leading to transient bacteremia and local infection, for example, in a preexisting subdural hematoma. Spontaneous bacterial peritonitis occurs in patients with cirrhosis and ascites. Symptoms can include only fever or abdominal discomfort or encephalopathy, with any one of these symptoms absent. Abdominal tenderness may be minimal or absent. Diagnosis is made by paracentesis, which should be done when there is any clinical suspicion. Spontaneous bacterial empyema can occur when pleural effusion is present (116). Sexually transmitted diseases, including HIV, are more common in people who drink heavily, in part because of sexual risk-taking behavior (117). Treatment for all of these conditions is guided by local epidemiology, frequently updated resources (e.g., *The Medical Letter* or handbooks of antimicrobial therapy), and national treatment guidelines for targeted and empiric antimicrobial therapy (118,119).

Musculoskeletal Consequences Musculoskeletal consequences can occur from the chronic heavy use of alcohol. Intoxication to the point of overdose may result in the individual's remaining in one position for prolonged periods of time. In addition to compression nerve palsies, rhabdomyolysis (with hyperphosphatemia, hyperkalemia, hypocalcemia, and acute renal failure) can develop and cause a compartment syndrome—a surgical emergency that requires release of the pressure by incision of the skin and fascia along with débridement of necrotic tissue. Diagnosis is made when there is a tense edematous limb, often with evidence of trauma, initially with severe pain and later with anesthesia. Because physical signs and symptoms are variable and unreliable, the diagnosis often is pursued with intracompartmental pressures; a newer method, near infrared spectroscopy, shows promise in avoiding delays in treatment (120). Surgical consultation is required. Hyperuricemia and gout are more common in alcohol use disorders. Gout classically presents as podagra, an edematous, exquisitely painful, erythematous great toe. Treatment is with colchicine, using caution in renal or hepatic insufficiency, or indomethacin, using caution in the presence of gastritis or renal insufficiency. The cyclooxygenase-2-specific nonsteroidal anti-inflammatory agents can be effective in gout and have the advantage that they are safer in patients who are at risk of gastrointestinal bleeding, though they have deleterious renal effects. A brief course of corticosteroids or a single injection of adrenocorticotropic hormone may be safer choices for the person with an alcohol use disorder. Chronic treatment in the setting of renal disease, tophaceous gout, or polyarticular gout should be with allopurinol or probenecid. Saturnine gout is diagnosed when the hyperuricemia is associated with past "moonshine" use (121,122). Hyperuricemia can lead to renal insufficiency. Excessive alcohol use (more than one drink a day for women, two for men, and heavy episodic drinking) increases the risk of skeletal fracture. What component of this increased risk is due to a higher risk of trauma and what is attributable to alcohol-related osteopenia is unclear. Though moderate alcohol use can be associated with an increase in BMD (either because of alcohol's effect on estrogens or other hormones or because of a lifestyle factor associated with increased BMD), excessive consumption leads to osteopenia. Heavy alcohol use can lead to osteonecrosis of bone, such as that at the femoral head.

Oncologic Risks Alcohol is a risk factor for a number of cancers. These include malignancies of the lip, oral cavity, pharynx, larynx, esophagus, stomach, breast, liver, intrahepatic bile ducts, prostate, and colon (14). Though most of these cancers are associated with heavy alcohol use, often in association with smoking, the increased risk of the cancers often is detectable in large populations at more moderate levels (48,66,67). For example, breast cancer risk increases with consumption of one to two standard drinks per day on average (12,13).

Pulmonary Consequences Alcohol intoxication can lead to respiratory depression and aspiration, leading to a chemical or infectious pneumonia. Tachypnea can be the result of pulmonary infection, respiratory alkalosis of liver disease, alcohol withdrawal, or compensation for a metabolic acidosis.

Endocrinologic Consequences Alcohol causes sexual dysfunction and hypogonadism in men, both through direct effects on the testes and through secondary effects in chronic liver disease, in which gynecomastia may be seen. Alcohol delays menopause and is associated with menstrual disorders such as dysmenorrhea and metrorrhagia. Amounts as little as one drink per week have been associated with decreased fertility in women (123). Alcohol increases the high-density lipoprotein fraction of cholesterol which, in part, explains observed decreases in coronary artery disease in moderate drinkers; however, it also increases serum triglycerides, which can lead to heart disease, hepatic steatosis, and pancreatitis. Moderate drinking can decrease the incidence of diabetes mellitus but more than three drinks a day increase the risk (124).

Consequences in the Perioperative Patient Heavy alcohol consumption is a risk factor for postoperative complications (125). In the perioperative period, attention must be given to identifying a risk of withdrawal, managing the withdrawal, and managing the pain. Elective surgery can be an opportune time to try to achieve abstinence, both as treatment for alcohol dependence and to prevent perioperative morbidity. This approach can reduce morbidity, as has been demonstrated in at least one randomized trial (126).

Vitamin Deficiencies People with alcohol use disorders are prone to vitamin deficiency because of malabsorption and poor dietary intake (127–131). Alcohol has been associated with deficiencies of fat-soluble vitamins when there is malabsorption because of pancreatic disease and also with deficiencies of thiamine, pyridoxine, niacin, riboflavin, vitamin D, and zinc. Symptoms commonly seen in people with alcohol use disorders may not be due to intoxication or withdrawal. For example, thiamine deficiency can cause confusion and ataxia, whereas diarrhea, abdominal discomfort, amnesia, anxiety, insomnia, nausea, seizure, and ataxia may be the result of pellagra. A clue to this diagnosis is the coexistence of glossitis and rash in sun-exposed areas, but these more specific features may be absent (132). Vitamin replacement is safe and should be done empirically.

Sleep Though alcohol can help people fall asleep, it also can be stimulating and lead to disrupted sleep and daytime fatigue. In people with alcohol use disorders, a drink may be required to sleep, but sleep is quite disrupted (133). This situation also is true of the person with alcohol dependence in recovery, who may relapse because of intolerable insomnia (134). Alcohol increases the risk of obstructive sleep apnea and worsens the disease because of its depressant effects on respiration and relaxation of the upper airway. Alcohol can increase the risk of periodic limb movements of sleep. Treatment of insomnia in the person with an alcohol use disorder involves attention to sleep hygiene as well as pharmacotherapy with drugs with a low or no risk of dependence, such as trazodone.

Fetal, Neonatal, and Infant Consequences Use of alcohol during pregnancy, even in amounts considered to be moderate in nonpregnant adults, can lead to mental retardation and neurobehavioral deficits in children. The fetal alcohol syndrome involves craniofacial abnormalities, neurologic abnormalities, and growth retardation (135). Affected individuals may have some or all of the manifestations of the syndrome. The neurologic disabilities persist into adulthood. Because no safe amount of alcohol during pregnancy has been identified and there is no treatment for the effects of alcohol on the fetus, abstinence is recommended during pregnancy.

Tobacco Tobacco use increases the risk of death. In addition, it causes cosmetic effects such as stained teeth, stained fingers, wrinkles, and many medical illnesses.

Withdrawal Though nicotine withdrawal is not life-threatening, the craving can complicate treatment for other medical illnesses. Nicotine replacement should be provided for medically ill patients who are hospitalized. Bupropion and varenicline are alternatives. Nicotine replacement can precipitate myocardial ischemia, but the alternative, smoking a cigarette, also can do so. Therefore, in general, even smokers with coronary artery disease can use nicotine replacement, unless they are experiencing unstable angina or myocardial infarction.

Neurologic Consequences Tobacco use is associated with atherosclerosis, peripheral vascular disease and, therefore, cerebrovascular disease and ischemic and hemorrhagic stroke. Atherosclerotic disease can involve small vessels and result in cognitive deficits.

Gastrointestinal Consequences Smoking is a cause of gastric and duodenal ulcers. Smoking can cause and exacerbate gastroesophageal reflux disease. Smoking interferes with ulcer healing. These diseases can require pharmacotherapy in addition to smoking cessation, as with histamine type 2 receptor antagonists, proton pump inhibitors, or antibiotics for *Helicobacter pylori*.

Hematologic Consequences Though data are conflicting, smoking is known to have hypercoagulable effects, and it can be a risk factor for deep vein thrombosis (136).

Cardiovascular Consequences Smoking can lead to poorer control of hypertension (137) and causes atherosclerosis. Smokers thus are at higher risk of myocardial infarction and sudden death. Moreover, smoking appears to potentiate the risks of heart attack conferred by hyperlipidemia and diabetes. Smoking can precipitate angina by causing vasospasm and hypercoagulability, and it can precipitate dysrhythmia. Smokers are at higher risk of cerebrovascular disease and stroke and peripheral vascular disease, which leads to intermittent claudication, pain, and loss of limb. Smoking lowers the beneficial serum highdensity lipoprotein subfraction of cholesterol. The risk of heart disease (138) and peripheral vascular disease and stroke morbidity and mortality decreases soon after smoking cessation.

Renal Consequences The renal consequences of tobacco dependence are limited primarily to the effects of atherosclerosis of the renal arteries, which can lead to ischemic renal failure and hypertension from renal artery stenosis.

Injury Though smoking does not increase the level of risk associated with risk-taking behavior, tobacco dependence can lead to house fires, smoke inhalation, and death, as well as other accidental death (139). Anecdotally, smoking in medically ill patients using oxygen has resulted in facial and airway burns and fires.

Infectious Consequences Because of its pulmonary effects, smoking increases the risk of acute and chronic bronchitis and pneumonia. Smokers have more frequent upper respiratory infections. These risks decrease with cessation.

Oncologic Risks Smoking has been associated with the following cancers: oral cavity, larynx, lung, esophagus, bladder, kidney, pancreas, stomach, and cervix. In addition, smokers with one smoking-related cancer are at higher risk for a second one. These risks decrease with cessation.

Pulmonary Consequences Smoking leads to chronic bronchitis and emphysema, collectively referred to as "chronic obstructive pulmonary disease" (COPD). Smoking is the leading cause of both COPD and bronchogenic carcinoma. The risks of both of these mortal diagnoses can be lowered with smoking cessation. Smoking cessation can slow the steady decline in pulmonary function seen in COPD (140). Smoking leads to pulmonary hypertension, interstitial lung disease, and pneumothorax. Though some lung cancers can be treated surgically if detected early, chemotherapeutic approaches have been disappointing. Treatment for COPD is somewhat disappointing, particularly when the patient continues to smoke. Effective treatments include bronchodilators, oxygen for hypoxemia and, less commonly, corticosteroids.

Endocrinologic Consequences Cigarette use is known to increase the risk of Graves' disease (hyperthyroidism) and hypothyroidism (141). Smoking and nicotine itself can increase insulin resistance (including detrimental effects on lipids and glucose) and risk of diabetes. Estrogen is decreased in male and female smokers, as is sperm number and function in men (142,143). Smoking is one of the leading causes of erectile dysfunction, mainly because of atherosclerosis. Cigarette use is associated with decreased BMD, osteoporosis, and fractures.

Consequences in the Perioperative Patient Smoking increases the risk of postoperative pulmonary complications, including pneumonia, atelectasis, reactive airways exacerbations, and respiratory failure. Smoking cessation before elective surgery is advisable, though it should be done at least 2 months before surgery (144–146). Current smokers should pay particular attention to pulmonary toilet perioperatively. Incentive spirometry should be used, along with use of bronchodilators.

Sleep Nicotine increases the time it takes to fall asleep (sleep latency). Abstinence in tobacco-dependent individuals (that is, withdrawal) increases daytime sleepiness.

Fetal, Neonatal, and Infant Consequences Tobacco use during pregnancy causes low birth weight, spontaneous abortion, and perinatal mortality, among other consequences. The risks of sudden infant death syndrome and neurodevelopmental impairment are increased, though studies have had difficulty separating the effects of tobacco, alcohol, nutrition, and social situations.

Opiates, Cocaine, and Other Drugs

The complications of other drugs often are related to route of administration. Injection and inhalation of drugs have particular consequences. In addition to route of administration, drugs have unique organ systems complications.

Injection Drug Use Injection of drugs leads to a break in the skin barrier that protects against infection. As a result, skin and soft-tissue infections are common in injection drug users (147). Most commonly, cellulitis is caused by staphylococci and streptococci. Treatment for minor infections should be with a semisynthetic penicillin or first- or second-generation cephalosporin, a macrolide or clindamycin (148). Vancomycin, linezolid, or daptomycin should be used for infections that worsen on treatment and more severe infections because of the increasing prevalence of methicillin resistance. Abscess usually is caused by *Staphylococcus aureus* and requires surgical drainage in addition to antibiotic treatment. However, one must be aware of local epidemiology and practices because there have been reports of unusual pathogens (for example, *Pseudomonas aeruginosa* and *Serratia* species) and polymicrobial infections from use of saliva to prepare the injection (149,150). Furthermore, injection drug users sometimes use antibiotics obtained without prescription, which places them at risk of infection with resistant organisms. Soft-tissue infections can progress to become serious and life-threatening if fasciitis develops or if there is significant local ischemia, as with cocaine injection (151). Intravenous injection can result in septic thrombophlebitis, as well as arterial injection with embolus and digital ischemia and infection. Injection can lead to venous valvular damage in the extremities, marked by leg ulcers, edema, and a propensity to develop deep vein thrombosis. Though rare, tetanus can develop as a result of nonsterile injection (31,149). Injection drug use spreads blood-borne pathogens when needles or other equipment are shared or when the drug user engages in risky behaviors. Regarding sexually transmitted infections, false-positive screening tests for syphilis often are found in injection drug users. Treponemal specific tests are needed to determine the diagnosis (fluorescent treponemal antibody, or microhemagglutination test for *T. pallidum*). Blood-borne pathogens spread by injection or risky behaviors, including HIV, hepatitis B, hepatitis C, and malaria. Hepatitis B can develop into a chronic infection, and HIV and hepatitis C almost invariably are chronic illnesses that require long-term management strategies by clinicians familiar with the complexities of their care. Hepatitis can lead to cirrhosis and its sequelae, including death, and HIV to opportunistic infections and death. Antiviral drugs for these infections exist (their use is beyond the scope of this introductory chapter). Altered mentation can result from HIV infection and liver disease.

Similarly, opportunistic infections in AIDS can lead to stroke. One of the most serious infectious consequences of injection drug use is bacterial endocarditis. In an injection drug user, as in an alcohol user, fever cannot be taken lightly. If there is an identifiable cause (such as pneumonia or cellulitis), it should be treated. Pneumonia is common in injection drug users, either because of aspiration, septic embolization, or exposure to pathogens such as *M. tuberculosis*. Injection drug users can have septic arthritis in unusual locations (sternoclavicular or sacroiliac joints), spinal epidural or vertebral infections, osteomyelitis, or meningitis. However, a significant proportion of patients with fever and no identifiable cause will have an unrecognized serious illness, most often endocarditis (152). Missing this diagnosis can be fatal. A cardiac murmur may not be present. The classic "textbook" signs of subacute bacterial endocarditis, most of which are immunologic phenomena, often are not present in drug users with acute bacterial, often right-sided (for example, tricuspid valve) endocarditis (153). Therefore, blood cultures should be taken, and close observation (often in the hospital) instituted; many authorities recommend empiric antibiotic treatment while awaiting culture results. If endocarditis is diagnosed, treatment is with bactericidal antibiotics for 4 to 6 weeks. Mycotic aneurysms; endophthalmitis; congestive heart failure; brain, spleen, or myocardial abscesses and emboli; renal failure from interstitial nephritis; pulmonary septic emboli with effusions; stroke; and heart block can complicate the course. Selected uncomplicated cases can be treated with shorter courses (154). Patients who have multiple emboli or hemodynamic decompensation may require surgical intervention and valve replacement.

In addition to infectious complications, injection of drugs can lead to pulmonary talc granulomatosis from injected crushed tablets containing talc, pulmonary hypertension from granulomatous disease or drug-related vasoconstriction, needle embolization, pneumothorax or hemothorax from injection into large central veins gone awry, and pulmonary emphysema related or unrelated to talc granulomatosis. Granulomatosis can occur in the liver from injection of talc. Nephropathy related to injection drug use, primarily because of HIV infection, is a common renal complication. Amyloidosis and nephrotic syndrome can occur because of chronic skin infections. Hepatitis C infection can lead to glomerulonephritis. The coagulopathy that results from liver and kidney disease in injection drug users can lead to neurologic complications—namely, hemorrhagic stroke. Cerebral infarction has resulted from injection of crushed tablets and even of a melted suppository (intravenously and via inadvertent intra-arterial injection) (155).

Inhalation of Drugs Consequences of inhalation that are not related to the specific substance inhaled are primarily pulmonary. Inhalation of drugs has effects related to the size of the particles: larger particles affect the airways, whereas smaller ones reach the alveoli. Complications include granulomatous responses to fibrogenic substances such as talc, chronic bronchitis from inhaled smoke (regardless of whether the drug involved is marijuana, nicotine, cocaine, or others), bronchospasm (as from inhaled cocaine), barotrauma with resultant pneumothorax or pneumomediastinum from prolonged breath holding or stimulant use, hemoptysis from airway irritation, and emphysema from inhaled tobacco, marijuana, or opiates (156,157). Freebasing (inhalation of burned precipitate of cocaine that has been dissolved in a warmed solvent and then dried) can lead to upper airway and facial burns.

Withdrawal Withdrawal from opiates often is seen in patients with medical illnesses who require hospitalization. Though the withdrawal is not fatal in an otherwise healthy person, it should be treated for symptomatic relief to prevent hyperadrenergic states that complicate treatment of the acute medical problems (e.g., coronary syndromes) and to allow the patient to be sufficiently comfortable so that he or she can complete medical treatment and link to addiction treatment.

Neurologic Consequences As with alcohol users, drug users may suffer from incoordination and exposure to risky situations that can lead to injury, including head injury or (in the case of involvement with illegal drugs or difficult social situations) injury from stabbings and gunshots. Seizures can occur as a result of sedative withdrawal (barbiturates and benzodiazepines), stimulant use (methamphetamines and cocaine), or proconvulsant metabolites (meperidine). Similarly, hemorrhagic stroke can occur with use of methamphetamines, phenylpropanolamine, lysergic acid diethylamide, and phencyclidine from hypertension, vasculitis, or other vascular mechanisms. Cocaine use can lead to both hemorrhagic and ischemic strokes (158,159). Anabolic steroids can cause stroke by promoting hypercoagulability. Though classic syndromes of dementia have not been described for users of drugs other than alcohol, chronic cognitive deficits can be seen in users of cocaine, sedatives (barbiturate), and toluene. Neuropathy (including plexopathies and Guillain-Barré syndrome) may be caused by heroin use, compression neuropathy in any drug user, quadriplegia in glue sniffers, and combined systems degeneration from vitamin B_{12} deficiency induced by nitrous oxide use. Parkinsonism can develop from the use of a meperidine analogue, MPTP.

Gastrointestinal Consequences In addition to viral hepatitis, which is almost universal in injection drug users, cocaine itself can cause hepatic necrosis, probably because of ischemia. Ecstasy and phencyclidine use has been reported to cause liver failure (160,161). Androgenic steroids can cause hepatic toxicity. Chronic diarrhea can be a result of laxative abuse, whereas anticholinergic and opiate abuse will cause constipation. "Bodypacking" (transporting cocaine, heroin, or other drugs in bags that are swallowed) can lead to mechanical obstruction of the intestines. Rupture can lead to overdose and death from respiratory arrest or cardiovascular collapse.

Hematologic Consequences Amyl nitrate, isobutyl nitrate, and other "poppers" can cause methemoglobinemia. The arterial partial pressure of oxygen is normal, the saturation is low, and cyanosis is present. Methemoglobin can be measured. The treatment is with methylene blue (162).

Cardiovascular Consequences In addition to the infectious complications of drug abuse that are related to route of administration (endocarditis and myocardial abscess), drugs of abuse can directly affect the heart and blood vessels. Cocaine can cause severe hypertension, cardiac dysrhythmias, angina, myocardial infarction, sudden death, and stroke. As with treatment for hypertension in cocaine users, nitrates and benzodiazepines are first-line agents. For these acute coronary syndromes, oxygen and aspirin are first line as well, and calcium channel blockers (verapamil) and phentolamine are second-line treatments (163). Angioplasty (with anticoagulants as indicated) should be done if infarction is evolving despite medical therapy, and thrombolysis should be given in this situation only if angioplasty is not available. Sedation with a benzodiazepine can be helpful. Labetalol is, in theory, an alternative because of its alpha- and nonselective beta-blocking effects but, because its effects are predominantly beta-blocking, it should be used only if needed after other treatments are tried. Chest pain often occurs during or after cocaine use, but most persons evaluated in emergency departments with chest pain and cocaine use do not have myocardial infarction (164). Nonetheless, heart attacks do occur and are thought to be related to coronary vasospasm, in situ thrombosis, or the accelerated development of atherosclerosis because of cocaine (or underlying atherosclerotic coronary artery disease, from smoking, for example). As with treatment for hypertension in cocaine users, calcium channel blockers, nitrates, and benzodiazepines are preferred. Cardiomyopathy can occur as a consequence of cocaine use (165). Other stimulants (for example, phenylpropanolamine and amphetamines) can produce cardiac complications. Anabolic steroids can lead to coronary artery disease as well as cardiomyopathy.

Drugs with anticholinergic effects (muscle relaxants, antihistamines, and antidepressants) cause tachycardia and can cause dysrhythmias in intoxication or overdose. Inhalants (volatile fluorocarbons) can cause dysrhythmias, as can anesthetic gases.

Renal and Metabolic Consequences Aside from the previously discussed infectious and injection-related renal complications of other drugs of abuse, any drug that leads to sedation with intoxication or overdose (such as, heroin and barbiturates) can lead to muscle compression and rhabdomyolysis and to acute renal failure. Rhabdomyolysis can be seen with amphetamine, cocaine, and phencyclidine use. Persons who abuse prescription drugs (opiates) can present with factitious hematuria (red blood cells in the urine and flank pain, feigning nephrolithiasis) to obtain opiate prescriptions because no radiologic test or procedure is 100% sensitive for kidney stones and because nephrolithiasis is invariably (and appropriately) treated with opiates. Cocaine can lead to accelerated hypertension and renal failure, hypertensive nephrosclerosis, thrombotic microangiopathy, and renal infarction. Amphetamines can result in a drug-related polyarteritis nodosa. Ecstasy use can lead to hyponatremia when users drink excess water to prevent the hypovolemia associated with its use. Toluene inhalation can lead to metabolic acidosis.

Injury Though much of the literature focuses on alcohol as a risk factor for injury, cocaine and other drugs also have been associated with an increased risk of motor vehicle crash and other violent injuries, including fatal shootings (166). Persons in a detoxification program for opiates or cocaine have a very high risk of injury (20% in each of five consecutive 6-month periods) (110).

Infectious Consequences of Drug Use Most of the infectious complications of drug use are related to injection or risky sexual practices, as discussed previously. As with alcohol users, users of other drugs engage in high-risk sexual behaviors that place them at risk of sexually transmitted diseases, including HIV. Diagnosis and treatment are the same as in nondrug users. Similarly, drug users are at risk of pneumonia from aspiration related to overdose and tuberculosis.

Oncologic Risks Though the magnitude of risk remains unclear, marijuana, when smoked, can lead to squamous cell carcinoma of the oral cavity and to lung cancer (167).

Pulmonary Consequences In addition to injection complications, the lungs are affected by many illicit drugs. Drugs that produce sedation with use or overdose can lead to respiratory depression and death. Naloxone and flumazenil can reverse the effects in opiate and benzodiazepine users, respectively. Atelectasis can develop, as can aspiration and chemical pneumonitis; these do not require antibiotic treatment but are managed with airway management, incentive spirometry, chest physiotherapy, and oxygen. More specifically, marijuana use can lead to obstructive lung disease (156) and fungal infection from contamination. Cocaine use can lead to nasal septal perforation, sinusitis, epiglottitis, upper airway obstruction, and hemoptysis, primarily from irritant and vasoconstrictive effects. Cocaine use can lead to pulmonary hemorrhage, edema, hypertension, emphysema, interstitial fibrosis, and hypersensitivity pneumonitis. The treatment for most of these diseases is withdrawal of the cocaine and supportive care, though corticosteroids and bronchodilators are warranted in some cases. Pulmonary hypertension and edema can result from use of stimulants (specifically amphetamines). Opiate use can lead to bronchospasm, as a result of their stimulation of histamine release, and pulmonary edema in the setting of overdose. The pulmonary consequences of sedatives are limited primarily to respiratory depression and arrest from overdose, worsening of sleep-disordered breathing, as well as tachypnea, hyperventilation, and respiratory alkalosis from withdrawal syndromes. Inhalants can lead to methemoglobinemia (treated with methylene blue), tracheobronchitis, asphyxiation, and hypersensitivity pneumonitis. Nitrous oxide can cause respiratory depression and hypoxemia. Anabolic steroids can induce prothrombotic states and lead to pulmonary embolism.

Endocrinologic Consequences Most drugs of abuse can affect hormone levels, particularly thyroid hormones, gonadotropins, antidiuretic hormone, sex steroids, and the hypothalamic-pituitary-adrenal axis, but the clinical implications often are unclear. Opiates can impair gonadotropin release. Clinically, men may have impaired sperm motility, and women may have menstrual and ovulatory irregularities. This mechanism may explain the reduced BMD seen in heroin addicts (168), though etiology is likely multifactorial (169). Cocaine is a risk factor for the more frequent occurrence of diabetic ketoacidosis, in part because of adrenergic effects (170). Barbiturate use can lead to osteomalacia from vitamin D deficiency. The deficiency results from stimulation of the cytochrome hepatic metabolism of substances, including thyroid hormone and hydrocortisone, which are of note when treating patients with these drugs. Clinical metabolic consequences have been clearly linked to use of anabolic steroids. Women develop androgenization, and lipids are adversely affected.

Consequences in the Perioperative Patient Several issues arise in the perioperative period with users of other drugs. First, it is essential to assess (through the history and toxicologic screens) what drugs have been used. Second, attention to and treatment of withdrawal symptoms can avert development of tachycardia and hypertension, which may complicate interpretation of assessments and operative and anesthetic treatments. Third, the anesthesiologist must be informed of any recent drug use because of potential interactions between beta-blockers and cocaine and because of the potentiation of sedative and anesthetic drugs. Finally, anesthesia and pain management generally require much higher doses than usual in the opiate-dependent patient. Nutritional issues often require attention in addicted persons undergoing surgery, as wound healing may be impaired.

Vitamin Deficiencies Nitrous oxide abuse is a well-known cause of vitamin B_{12} deficiency.

Sleep Clearly, stimulants, including caffeine, can suppress sleep, which often is an intended effect. Opioids and nicotine tend to reduce sleep. Benzodiazepines, often used to help with sleep, do reduce the time it takes to fall asleep. Many persons with addictive disorders also experience sleep disturbances, because of the drug used, lifestyles, or comorbid psychiatric conditions. Sleep problems can contribute to the desire to use drugs for self-medication. In fact, opioids are effective for the management of restless legs syndrome and periodic movements of sleep, a treatment an opioid-dependent person may have discovered in the course of illicit use. The management of sleep disorders, particularly insomnia, therefore, is difficult but important in addicted persons. Attention to sleep hygiene (that is, a quiet location, using the bed only for sleep and sex, and elimination of napping) and judicious use of drugs less likely to lead to misuse, such as trazodone, are the best approaches.

Fetal, Neonatal, and Infant Consequences No clear teratogenic effects of opiates are known. Though many studies of the issue have been conducted, studies that did find effects often did not control for the effects of important confounders such as nutrition, alcohol, and tobacco use. However, opiate exposure in utero can lead to the neonatal abstinence syndrome, including seizures. Detoxification, when agreeable to the patient, is best done during the second trimester to prevent this complication. Benzodiazepines have been associated with cleft lip and palate, but the studies of benzodiazepines, like other studies of teratogenesis in drug users, may have been confounded by alcohol use. Toluene use appears to cause an embryopathy, and other inhalants have caused various nonspecific effects, including preterm labor and intrauterine growth retardation. The effects of caffeine in pregnancy are controversial. It probably is relatively safe, although some reports of increased fetal loss suggest minimizing its use during pregnancy. Dextroamphetamine does appear to be associated with teratogenesis. Cocaine can induce teratogenic effects and neonatal irritability and also may cause behavioral and learning disorders. But again, many of these reports are difficult to interpret because other maternal factors (including other drug use, inadequate health care, and malnutrition) might account for the findings (171).

COMMON MEDICAL PROBLEMS IN PERSONS WITH ADDICTIVE DISORDERS

Persons with addictive disorders suffer from the same medical conditions as nonaddicted persons, but addiction can interfere with the disease or its management. A general medical textbook should be consulted about the diagnosis and management of these disorders; however, several points specific to addiction and common medical problems are discussed here.

Treatment adherence is a problem with addicted and nonaddicted persons alike, but it takes on particular importance with the management of chronic medical illnesses. Cardiovascular diseases are the most common cause of death in the United States. Coronary artery disease is particularly common in persons with alcohol and other drug abuse because of concomitant tobacco dependence. The person with addiction and anginal chest pain (which lasts at least 5 minutes, is pressure-like, and often is accompanied by dyspnea, nausea, diaphoresis, and radiation to the jaw or arm) must be taken seriously, with consideration given to a cardiac etiology by examination of the electrocardiogram, cardiac enzymes, and exercise tolerance testing, when appropriate. Angina can be complicated by alcohol, opiate, and sedative withdrawal, as well as cocaine and other stimulant use when the hyperadrenergic states precipitate anginal attacks. Beta blockers are drugs of choice for managing angina (and for preventing death in persons with coronary artery disease) and are helpful in decreasing sympathetic outflow associated with drug withdrawal. They should be administered to persons withdrawing from alcohol, opiates, and sedatives when underlying coronary artery disease is suspected or present, as well as during acute myocardial infarction or unstable angina. However, simultaneous use of beta-blockers and cocaine should be avoided because of the unopposed vasoconstriction that can result. Aspirin is a standard treatment to decrease mortality after myocardial infarction and during unstable angina. Aspirin and other treatments for acute coronary events (heparin, tissue plasminogen activator, and similar anticoagulants) can be problematic in persons who have a potential site for internal bleeding, such as people with alcohol dependence with gastritis or liver disease, or intracranial bleeding that is unrecognized.

Nitrates and calcium channel blockers often are used in the management of coronary heart disease, and there are no particular considerations applicable to addicted patients with these drugs. The diagnosis of hypertension can be problematic in persons with addictive disorders. A single elevated blood pressure should not be equated with the diagnosis of hypertension (172). Blood pressure elevation can be a product of pain, withdrawal, or intoxication, depending on the substance used. Alcohol (and other drugs, such as cocaine) elevates blood pressure. Ideally, hypertension should be diagnosed after at least three blood pressure measurements (140/90 or higher) during prolonged abstinence. Nevertheless, though a diagnosis of hypertension should not be made during detoxification or in an emergency setting (unless end-organ damage is evident), persistent hypertension in a patient who drinks regularly should be managed as hypertension to prevent complications. Treatment of hypertension is the same as in persons without addictive disorders, in that attention to medication adherence for an asymptomatic condition is important, lifestyle modification can help, and many medications are available. Though diuretics are inexpensive, effective, and associated with mortality benefits, they can be somewhat riskier in people with alcohol dependence because of the adverse effects on potassium balance. Beta-blockers are excellent alternatives; however, cocaine users should avoid beta-blockers.

Diabetes is more difficult to manage in persons with addictive disorders, not only because of difficulty with adherence and more erratic eating habits but because of the effects of alcohol on glucose metabolism. Heavy alcohol users are more prone to prolonged and more severe hypoglycemia from the sulfonylurea agents often used to treat type 2 diabetes. Though the thiazolidinediones are relatively contraindicated because of the possibility that they may cause hepatic damage, the evidence is limited that either they or the sulfonylureas will cause adverse events in people who drink alcohol (124). Metformin should not be given to patients with hepatic impairment or those at risk for lactic acidosis. Choices for the management of diabetes in alcohol dependence are difficult; insulin injections are preferred, though use of sulfonylureas with careful monitoring is reasonable. In addition to having etiologic roles in cancers, addiction can lead to difficulties in cancer management. First, any renal, hepatic, or cardiac consequences of addiction can limit the choice of chemotherapeutic agents. Pulmonary consequences of tobacco use may limit surgical options. Finally, pain management can be complicated by ongoing or past addiction.

CONSEQUENCES IN OLDER ADULTS

Alcohol and other drug use can lead to additional consequences in older adults (173). In older adults, lower amounts of alcohol often are associated with adverse consequences because of lower lean body mass and body water, less alcohol dehydrogenase, and impaired ability to develop tolerance. For example, elderly women who drink more than two drinks per day are more likely than nondrinkers to have difficulty with activities of daily living. Similarly, elderly men who drink more than one drink per day are more likely to suffer loss of mobility. Hip fracture, a leading cause of death in older adults, can result from an increased propensity to fall related to alcohol use and to osteopenia. Older adults are more susceptible to injury from motor vehicle crashes and even more so when alcohol is used. Medications (such as antidepressants, interferon for hepatitis C, warfarin, phenytoin, aspirin, and acetaminophen) are less effective or can be harmful when taken with alcohol. Older adults are more susceptible than younger individuals to alcohol's chronic brain-damaging effects, including cognitive deficits, and are less likely to recover completely from those effects. Amounts of alcohol that risk health consequences in the elderly are lower than they are in younger adults. Older adults should drink no more that three standard drinks on an occasion and no more than seven drinks per week on average.

In addition to greater susceptibility, alcohol can cause many consequences in older adults that may be misdiagnosed as other common medical problems. The confusion of alcohol withdrawal delirium may be diagnosed as delirium because of infection. The tremor of withdrawal may be diagnosed as Parkinson's disease or an essential tremor. Dementia, malnutrition, self-neglect, functional decline, sleep problems, and anxiety or depression all may be attributed to "normal" aging when the true cause is alcohol. Similarly, cardiovascular disease and congestive heart failure are common in older adults; alcohol as the cause of cardiomyopathy or exacerbations of congestive heart failure frequently are overlooked. Because many conditions in older adults are multifactorial in origin, perhaps it is best to view alcohol as a contributor to illness. Fractures, seizures, and cerebellar degeneration may be misattributed to other "medical" causes when alcohol is a key contributor. Alcohol can contribute to the occurrence of falls, worsening of chronic illness (such as hypertension), interference with medication adherence and side effects, incontinence, fatigue, neuropathy, sexual dysfunction, and pneumonia. Other drug abuse can lead to similar consequences in the elderly—confusion, falls, and interference with activities of daily living. The effects of smoking are of great significance in older adults because smoking-related diseases often appear with aging and can be exacerbated by continued smoking. Examples include angina, coronary artery disease, and COPD. Prescription drug abuse can lead to physical, functional, and psychosocial impairments.

CONCLUSIONS

Persons with addictive disorders often do not receive adequate medical care. A medical, psychiatric, or addiction health care visit is an opportunity to provide symptom-oriented as well as preventive care or to link such individuals to preventive health care services. Routine health care of the addicted person differs in that the patient almost certainly is at higher risk of disease than are those without addiction. This warrants a targeted approach to the conditions for which the patient is at risk and the risks of which can be ameliorated. During hospitalization for medical reasons, special attention must be directed toward management of withdrawal and adequate pain control. Persons with addictive disorders are at risk of a large number of specific acute and chronic medical illnesses in almost every organ system. Further, the management of unrelated but common medical illnesses is complicated by addiction, its effect on medication adherence, and the direct consequences of the abused substances. Older adults often suffer from a number of chronic disorders including addiction. Beyond worsening the common chronic diseases of aging, addictive disorders can worsen functional status. The subsequent chapters in this section delve into the medical consequences of addiction in greater detail.

ACKNOWLEDGMENT: *The writing of this chapter was supported in part by the National Institute on Alcohol Abuse and Alcoholism (R25 AA 13822, R01 AA 13304, P60 AA 013759, R01 AA 10870) and the National Institute on Drug Abuse (R25 DA 13582, R01 DA 10019).*

REFERENCES

1. Saitz R, Mulvey KP, Samet JH. The substance abusing patient and primary care: linkage via the addiction treatment system. *Subst Abuse* 1997;18:187–195.
2. Samet JH, Friedmann P, Saitz R. Benefits of linking primary medical care and substance abuse services: patient, provider, and societal perspectives. *Arch Intern Med* 2001;161(1):85–91.
3. Laine C, Hauck WW, Gourevitch MN, et al. Regular outpatient medical and drug abuse care and subsequent hospitalization of persons who use illicit drugs. *JAMA* 2001;285(18):2355–2362.
4. Samet JH, Saitz R, Larson MJ. A case for enhanced linkage for substance abusers to primary medical care. *Subst Abuse* 1996;17(4):181–192.
5. Saitz R, Horton NJ, Larson MJ, et al. Primary medical care and reductions in addiction severity: a prospective cohort study. *Addiction* 2005;100:70–78.
6. Agency for Healthcare Research and Quality. *Guide to clinical preventive services.* AHRQ Publication No. 07-05100, September 2007. Rockville, MD: Author, 2007. Retrieved February 3, 2008, from http://www.ahrq.gov/clinic/pocketgd.htm.
7. Kerlikowske K. Efficacy of screening mammography among women aged 40 to 49 years and 50 to 69 years: comparison of relative and absolute benefit. *J Natl Cancer Inst* 1997;22:79–86.
8. Kerlikowske K, Ernster VL. Women should be fully informed of the potential benefits and harms before screening mammography. *West J Med* 2000;173(5):313–314.
9. Kerlikowske K, Grady D, Ernster V. Benefit of mammography screening in women ages 40-49 years: current evidence from randomized controlled trials. *Cancer* 1995;76(9):1679–1681.
10. Sox HC. Benefit and harm associated with screening for breast cancer. *N Engl J Med* 1998;338(16):1145–1146.
11. U.S. Preventive Services Task Force. *Guide to Clinical Preventive Services.* Alexandria: International Medical Publishing, 1996.
12. Fuchs CS, Stampfer MJ, Colditz GA, et al. Alcohol consumption and mortality among women. *N Engl J Med* 1995;332(19):1245–1250.
13. Smith-Warner SA, Spiegelman D, Yaun SS, et al. Alcohol and breast cancer in women: a pooled analysis of cohort studies. *JAMA* 1998;279(7):535–540.
14. Bagnardi V, Blangiardo M. Alcohol consumption and the risk of cancer: a meta-analysis. *Alcohol ResHealth* 2001;25(1):263–270.

15. National Cholesterol Education Program. *Executive summary of the third report of The National Cholesterol Education Program Expert Panel on detection, evaluation, and treatment of high blood cholesterol in adults* (Adult Treatment Panel III). *JAMA* 2001;285(19):2486–2497.
16. Grundy SM, Cleeman JI, Merz CNB, et al. Implications of recent clinical trials for the National Cholesterol Education Program Adult Treatment Panel III Guidelines. *Circulation* 2004;110:227–239.
17. Branson BM, Handsfeld HH. Revised recommendations for HIV testing of adults, adolescents, and pregnant women in healthcare settings. *MMWR* 2006;55(RR14):1–17.
18. American Thoracic Society and the Centers for Disease Control and Prevention. Diagnostic standards and classification of tuberculosis in adults and children. *Am J Respir Crit Care Med* 2000;161(4):1376–1395.
19. American Thoracic Society and the Centers for Disease Control and Prevention. Targeted tuberculin testing and treatment of latent tuberculosis infection. *Am J Respir Crit Care Med* 2000;161(4):221S–2247.
20. Elmore JG, Barton MB. Ten-year risk of false positive screening mammograms and clinical breast examinations. *N Engl J Med* 1998;338(16): 1089–1096.
21. Thomas DB, Gao DL, Ray RM, et al. Randomized trial of breast self-examination in Shanghai: final results. *J Natl Cancer Inst* 2002;94(19): 1445–1457.
22. U.S. Preventive Services Task Force. *Screening for prostate cancer: recommendations and rationale.* Rockville, MD: Agency for Healthcare Research and Quality, 2002. Retrieved February 13, 2008, from http://www.ahrq.gov/clinic/3rduspstf/prostatescr/prostaterr.htm.
23. Holmberg L, Bill-Axelson A, Helgesen F, et al. A randomized trial comparing radical prostatectomy with watchful waiting in early prostate cancer. *N Engl J Med* 2002;347(11):781–789.
24. Wilt TJ, Brawer MK. The prostate cancer intervention versus observation trial. *Oncology* 1997;11:1133–1139.
25. Rex DK, Johnson DA, Lieberman DA. Colorectal cancer prevention 2000: screening recommendations of the American College of Gastroenterology. *Am J Gastroenterol* 2000;95(4):868–877.
26. U.S. Preventive Services Task Force. *Screening for colorectal cancer: recommendations and rationale.* Rockville, MD: Agency for Healthcare Research and Quality, July 2002. Retrieved February 13, 2008, from http://www.ahrq.gov/clinic/3rduspstf/colorectal/colorr.htm.
27. U.S. Preventive Services Task Force. Screening for osteoporosis in postmenopausal women: recommendations and rationale. *Ann Intern Med* 2002;137(6):526–528.
28. Friedmann PD, Saitz R, Samet JH. Management of adults recovering from alcohol or other drug problems: relapse prevention in primary care. *JAMA* 1998;279(15):1227–1231.
29. Gardner P, Peter G. Recommended schedules for routine immunization of children and adults. *Infect Dis Clin North Am* 2001;15(1):1–8.
30. Gardner P, Schaffner W. Immunization of adults. *N Engl J Med* 1993; 328(17):1252–1258.
31. Talan DA, Moran GJ. Update on emerging infections: news from the Centers for Disease Control and Prevention. Tetanus among injecting-drug users—California, 1997. *Ann Emerg Med* 1998;32(3 Pt 1): 385–386.
32. Advisory Committee on Immunization Practices. Recommended adult immunization schedule: United States, October 2007–September 2008. *Ann Intern Med* 2007;147:725–729.
33. Gaziano JM, Skerrett PJ, Buring JE. Aspirin in the treatment and prevention of cardiovascular disease. *Haemostasis* 2000;30(Suppl 3):1–13.
34. Ridker PM, Cook NR, Lee I-M, et al. A randomized trial of low-dose aspirin in the primary prevention of cardiovascular disease in women. *N Engl J Med* 2005;352:1293–1304.
35. Centers for Disease Control and Prevention. Recommendations for the use of folic acid to reduce the number of cases of spina bifida and other neural tube defects. *MMWR* 1992;41(RR-14):1–7.
36. Delmas PD, Bjarnason NH, Mitlak BH, et al. Effects of raloxifene on bone mineral density, serum cholesterol concentrations, and uterine endometrium in postmenopausal women. *N Engl J Med* 1997;337(23): 1641–1647.
37. Hosking D, Chilvers CE, Christiansen C, et al. Prevention of bone loss with alendronate in postmenopausal women under 60 years of age. Early Postmenopausal Intervention Cohort Study Group. *N Engl J Med* 1998;338(8):485–492.
38. McClung MR, Geusens P, Miller PD, et al. Effect of risedronate on the risk of hip fracture in elderly women. Hip Intervention Program Study Group. *N Engl J Med* 2001;344(5):333–340.
39. O'Connor PG, Samet JH, Stein MD. Management of hospitalized intravenous drug users: role of the internist. *Am J Med* 1994;96(6): 551–558.
40. Mayo-Smith MF, American Society of Addiction Medicine Working Group on Pharmacological Management of Alcohol Withdrawal. Pharmacological management of alcohol withdrawal. A meta-analysis and evidence-based practice guideline. *JAMA* 1997;278(2):144–151.
41. Jaeger TM, Lohr RH, Pankratz VS. Symptom-triggered therapy for alcohol withdrawal syndrome in medical inpatients. *Mayo Clin Proc* 2001;76(7):695–701.
42. Saitz R, Mayo-Smith MF, Roberts MS, et al. Individualized treatment for alcohol withdrawal. A randomized double-blind controlled trial. *JAMA* 1994;272(7):519–523.
43. Daeppen JB, Gache P, Landry U, et al. Symptom-triggered vs. fixed schedule doses of benzodiazepine for alcohol withdrawal. *Arch Intern Med* 2002;162(10):1117–1121.
44. Alford DP, Compton P, Samet JH. Acute pain management for patients receiving maintenance methadone or buprenorphine therapy. *Ann Intern Med* 2006;144:127–134.
45. Pugatch D, Levesque B, Greene S, et al. HIV testing in the setting of inpatient acute substance abuse treatment. *Am J Drug Alcohol Abuse* 2001;27(3):491–499.
46. Bradley KA, Badrinath S, Bush K, et al. Medical risks for women who drink alcohol. *J Gen Intern Med* 1998;13(9):627–639.
47. Doll R, Peto R, Hall E, et al. Mortality in relation to consumption of alcohol: 13 years' observations on male British doctors. *Br Med J* 1994; 309(6959):911–918.
48. Holman CD, English DR, Milne E, et al. Meta-analysis of alcohol and all-cause mortality: a validation of NHMRC recommendations. *Med J Aust* 1996;164(3):141–145.
49. Saitz R, O'Malley SS. Pharmacotherapies for alcohol abuse. Withdrawal and treatment. *Med Clin North Am* 1997;81(4):881–907.
50. Thompson WL, Johnson AD, Maddrey WL. Diazepam and paraldehyde for treatment of severe delirium tremens. A controlled trial. *Ann Intern Med* 1975;82(2):175–180.
51. Ogawa SK, Smith MA, Brennessel DJ, et al. Tuberculous meningitis in an urban medical center. *Medicine (Baltimore)* 1987;66(4):317–326.
52. Elkind MSV, Sciacca R, Boden-Albala B, et al. Moderate alcohol consumption reduces risk of ischemic stroke: the Northern Manhattan Study. *Stroke* 2006;37(1):13–19.
53. Mukamal KJ, Ascherio A, Mittleman MA, et al. Alcohol and risk for ischemic stroke in men: the role of drinking patterns and usual beverage. *Ann Intern Med* 2005;142(1):11–19.
54. Renaud SC. Diet and stroke. *J Nutr Health Aging* 2001;5(3): 167–172.
55. Filley CM, Kleinschmidt-DeMasters BK. Toxic leukoencephalopathy. *N Engl J Med* 2001;345(6):425–432.
56. Ohnishi K, Matsuo S, Matsutani K, et al. Interferon therapy for chronic hepatitis C in habitual drinkers: comparison with chronic hepatitis C in infrequent drinkers. *Am J Gastroenterol* 1996;91(7): 1374–1379.
57. Wiley TE, McCarthy M, Breidi L, et al. Impact of alcohol on the histological and clinical progression of hepatitis C infection. *Hepatology* 1998;28(3):805–809.
58. McCullough AJ, O'Connor JF. Alcoholic liver disease: proposed recommendations for the American College of Gastroenterology. *Am J Gastroenterol* 1998;93(11):2022–2036.
59. Akriviadis E, Botla R, Briggs W, et al. Pentoxifylline improves short-term survival in severe acute alcoholic hepatitis: a double-blind, placebo-controlled trial. *Gastroenterology* 2000;119(6):1637–1648.

60. Akriviadis EA, Steindel H, Pinto PC, et al. Failure of colchicine to improve short-term survival in patients with alcoholic hepatitis. *Gastroenterology* 1990;99(3):811–818.
61. Christensen E, Gluud C. Glucocorticoids are ineffective in alcoholic hepatitis: a meta-analysis adjusting for confounding variables. *Gut* 1995; 37(1):113–118.
62. Imperiale TF, McCullough AJ. Do corticosteroids reduce mortality from alcoholic hepatitis? A meta-analysis of the randomized trials. *Ann Intern Med* 1990;113(4):299–307.
63. Orrego H, Blake JE, Blendis LM, et al. Long-term treatment of alcoholic liver disease with propylthiouracil. *N Engl J Med* 1987;317(23):1421–1427.
64. Trinchet JC, Beaugrand M, Callard P, et al. Treatment of alcoholic hepatitis with colchicine. Results of a randomized double blind trial. *Gastroenterol Clin Biol* 1989;13(6-7):551–555.
65. Mendenhall CL, Moritz TE, Roselle GA, et al. A study of oral nutritional support with oxandrolone in malnourished patients with alcoholic hepatitis: results of a Department of Veterans Affairs cooperative study. *Hepatology* 1993;17(4):564–576.
66. Anderson P. Alcohol and risk of physical harm. In: Holder HD, Edwards G, eds. *Alcohol and public policy: evidence and issues*. Oxford: Oxford University Press, 1995:82–113.
67. Thun MJ, Peto R, Lopez AD, et al. Alcohol consumption and mortality among middle-aged and elderly U.S. adults. *N Engl J Med* 1997;337 (24):1705–1714.
68. Batey RG, Burns T, Benson RJ, et al. Alcohol consumption and the risk of cirrhosis. *Med J Aust* 1992;156(6):413–416.
69. Lieber CS. Medical disorders of alcoholism. *N Engl J Med* 1995;333 (16):1058–1065.
70. Norton R, Batey R, Dwyer T, et al. Alcohol consumption and the risk of alcohol related cirrhosis in women. *Br Med J* [Clinical Research Edition] 1987;295(6590):80–82.
71. Parrish KM, Dufour MC, Stinson FS, et al. Average daily alcohol consumption during adult life among decedents with and without cirrhosis: the 1986 National Mortality Followback Survey. *J Stud Alcohol* 1993; 54(4):450–456.
72. Yamauchi M, Nakahara M, Maezawa Y, et al. Prevalence of hepatocellular carcinoma in patients with alcoholic cirrhosis and prior exposure to hepatitis C. *Am J Gastroenterol* 1993;88(1):39–43.
73. Chedid A, Mendenhall CL, Gartside P, et al. Prognostic factors in alcoholic liver disease. VA Cooperative Study Group. *Am J Gastroenterol* 1991;86(2):210–216.
74. Powell WJ Jr, Klatskin G. Duration of survival in patients with Laennec's cirrhosis. Influence of alcohol withdrawal, and possible effects of recent changes in general management of the disease. *Am J Med* 1968;44(3): 406–420.
75. Jain A, Reyes J, Kashyap R, et al. Long-term survival after liver transplantation in 4,000 consecutive patients at a single center. *Ann Surg* 2000;232(4):490–500.
76. Murray KF, Carithers RL Jr. AASLD practice guidelines: evaluation of the patient for liver transplantation. *Hepatology* 2005;41(6):1407–1432.
77. Gish RG, Lee AH, Keeffe EB, et al. Liver transplantation for patients with alcoholism and end-stage liver disease. *Am J Gastroenterol* 1993; 88(9):1337–1342.
78. DiMartini A, Day N, Dew MA, et al. Alcohol consumption patterns and predictors of use following liver transplantation for alcoholic liver disease. *Liver Transpl* 2001,2006;12(5):813–820.
79. DiMartini A, Day N, Dew MA, et al. Alcohol use following liver transplantation. *Psychosomatics* 2001;42:55–62.
80. Schiodt FV, Rochling FA, Casey DL, et al. Acetaminophen toxicity in an urban county hospital. *N Engl J Med* 1997;337(16):1112–1117.
81. Salt WB 2nd, Schenker S. Amylase—its clinical significance: a review of the literature. *Medicine (Baltimore)* 1976;55(4):269–289.
82. Ranson JH, Rifkind KM, Turner JW. Prognostic signs and nonoperative peritoneal lavage in acute pancreatitis. *Surg Gynecol Obstet* 1976;143(2): 209–219.
83. Marshall JB. Acute pancreatitis. A review with an emphasis on new developments. *Arch Intern Med* 1993;153(10):1185–1198.
84. Steer ML, Waxman I, Freedman S. Chronic pancreatitis. *N Engl J Med* 1995;332(22):1482–1490.
85. Lankisch MR, Imoto M, Layer P, et al. The effect of small amounts of alcohol on the clinical course of chronic pancreatitis. *Mayo Clin Proc* 2001;76(3):242–251.
86. Colman N, Herbert V. Hematologic complications of alcoholism: overview. *Semin Hematol* 1980;17(3):164–176.
87. Larkin EC, Watson-Williams EJ. Alcohol and the blood. *Med Clin North Am* 1984;68(1):105–120.
88. Criqui MH. Alcohol and hypertension: new insights from population studies. *Eur Heart J* 1987;8(Suppl B):19–26.
89. Gitlow SE, Dziedzic LB, Dziedzic SW. Alcohol and hypertension: implications from research for clinical practice. *J Subst Abuse Treat* 1986;3(2):121–129.
90. Corrao G, Bagnardi V, Zambon A, et al. A meta-analysis of alcohol consumption and the risk of 15 diseases. *Prev Med* 2004;38(5):613–619.
91. Urbano-Marquez A, Estruch R, Navarro-Lopez F, et al. The effects of alcoholism on skeletal and cardiac muscle. *N Engl J Med* 1989;320(7): 409–415.
92. Hohnloser SH. Implantable devices versus antiarrhythmic drug therapy in recurrent ventricular tachycardia and ventricular fibrillation. *Am J Cardiol* 1999;84(9A):56R–62R.
93. Ettinger PO, Wu CF, De La Cruz C Jr, et al. Arrhythmias and the "holiday heart": alcohol-associated cardiac rhythm disorders. *Am Heart J* 1978;95(5):555–562.
94. Klatsky AL. Alcohol and cardiovascular diseases: a historical overview. *Novartis Found Symp* 1998;216:2–12.
95. Kupari M, Koskinen P. Time of onset of supraventricular tachyarrhythmia in relation to alcohol consumption. *Am J Cardiol* 1991;67(8):718–722.
96. Rich EC, Siebold C, Campion B. Alcohol-related acute atrial fibrillation. A case-control study and review of 40 patients. *Arch Intern Med* 1985;145(5): 830–833.
97. Poikolainen K. It can be bad for the heart, too—drinking patterns and coronary heart disease. *Addiction* 1998;93(12):1757–1759.
98. Camacho TC, Kaplan GA, Cohen RD. Alcohol consumption and mortality in Alameda County. *J Chronic Dis* 1987;40(3):229–236.
99. Kromhout D, Bloemberg BP, Feskens EJ, et al. Alcohol, fish, fibre, and antioxidant vitamins intake do not explain population differences in coronary heart disease mortality. *Int J Epidemiol* 1996;25(4):753–759.
100. Muntwyler J, Hennekens CH, Buring JE, et al. Mortality and light to moderate alcohol consumption after myocardial infarction. *Lancet* 1998;352(9144):1882–1885.
101. Fillmore KM, Kerr WC, Stockwell T, et al. Moderate alcohol use and reduced mortality risk: systematic error in prospective studies. *Addict Res Theory* 2006;14:101–32.
102. Hines LM, Stampfer MJ, Ma J. Genetic variation in alcohol dehydrogenase and the beneficial effect of moderate alcohol consumption on myocardial infarction. *N Engl J Med* 2001;344(8):549–555.
103. Johnson RJ, Gretch DR, Yamabe H, et al. Membranoproliferative glomerulonephritis associated with hepatitis C virus infection. *N Engl J Med* 1993;328(7):465–470.
104. Nolan CV, Shaikh ZA. Lead nephrotoxicity and associated disorders. Biochemical mechanisms. *Toxicology* 1992;73(2):127–146.
105. Brent J. Current management of ethylene glycol poisoning. *Drugs* 2001;61(7):979–988.
106. Fulop M. Alcoholic ketoacidosis. *Endocrinol Metab Clin North Am* 1993;22(2):209–219.
107. Wrenn KD, Slovis CM, Minion GE, et al. The syndrome of alcoholic ketoacidosis. *Am J Med* 1991;91(2):119–128.
108. Knochel JP. Hypophosphatemia in the alcoholic. *Arch Intern Med* 1980;140(5):613–615.
109. Laitinen K, Lamberg-Allardt C, Tunninen R, et al. Transient hypoparathyroidism during acute alcohol intoxication. *N Engl J Med* 1991;324(11):721–727.
110. Rees VW, Horton NJ, Hingson RW, et al. Injury among detoxification patients: alcohol users' greater risk. *Alcohol Clin Exp Res* 2002;26(2): 212–217.

111. Liebschutz J, Savetsky JB, Saitz R, et al. Relationship between sexual and physical abuse and substance abuse consequences. *J Subst Abuse Treat* 2002; 22(3):121–128.
112. Anda RF, Williamson DF, Remington PL. Alcohol and fatal injuries among U.S. adults. Findings from the NHANES I Epidemiologic Follow-up Study. *JAMA* 1988;260(17):2529–2532.
113. Cherpitel CJ. Alcohol and injuries: a review of international emergency room studies. *Addiction* 1993;88(7):923–937.
114. Gentilello LM, Rivara FP, Donovan DM, et al. Alcohol interventions in a trauma center as a means of reducing the risk of injury recurrence. *Ann Surg* 1999;230(4):473–483.
115. Saitz R, Ghali WA, Moskowitz MA. The impact of alcohol-related diagnoses on pneumonia outcomes. *Arch Intern Med* 1997;157(13): 1446–1452.
116. Kirchmair R, Allerberger F, Bangerl I, et al. Spontaneous bacterial pleural empyema in liver cirrhosis. *DigDis Sci* 1998;43(5):1129–1132.
117. Centers for Disease Control and Prevention. Alcohol policy and sexually transmitted disease rates—United States, 1981–1995. *MMWR* 2000; 49(16):346–349.
118. Niederman MS, Mandell LA, Anzueto A, et al. Guidelines for the management of adults with community-acquired pneumonia. Diagnosis, assessment of severity, antimicrobial therapy, and prevention. *Am J Respir Crit Care Med* 2001;163(7):1730–1754.
119. Workowski KA. The 1998 CDC sexually transmitted diseases treatment guidelines. *Curr Infect Dis Rep* 2000;2(1):44–50.
120. Giannotti G, Cohn SM, Brown M, et al. Utility of near-infrared spectroscopy in the diagnosis of lower extremity compartment syndrome. *J Trauma* 2000;48(3):396–401.
121. Ehrlich GE, Chokatos J. Saturnine gout. *Arch Intern Med* 1966;118(6): 572–574.
122. Klinenberg JR. Saturnine gout—a moonshine malady. *N Engl J Med* 1969;280(22):1238–1239.
123. Jensen TK, Hjollund NH, Henriksen TB, et al. Does moderate alcohol consumption affect fertility? Follow up study among couples planning first pregnancy. *Br Med J* 1998;317(7157):505–510.
124. Howard AA, Arnsten JH, Gourevitch MN. Effect of alcohol consumption on diabetes mellitus: a systematic review. *Ann Intern Med* 2004;140: 211–219.
125. Tonnesen H, Kehlet H. Preoperative alcoholism and postoperative morbidity. *Br J Surg* 1999;86(7):869–874.
126. Tonnesen H, Rosenberg J, Nielsen HJ, et al. Effect of preoperative abstinence on poor postoperative outcome in alcohol misusers: randomised controlled trial. *Br Med J* 1999;318(7194):1311–1316.
127. Green PH. Alcohol, nutrition and malabsorption. *Clin Gastroenterol* 1983;12(2):563–574.
128. Hoyumpa AM. Mechanisms of vitamin deficiencies in alcoholism. *Alcohol Clin Exp Res* 1986;10(6):573–581.
129. Lieber CS. Alcohol-nutrition interaction: 1984 update. *Alcohol* 1984; 1(2):151–157.
130. Russell RM. Vitamin A and zinc metabolism in alcoholism. *Am J Clin Nutr* 1980;33(12):2741–2749.
131. Ryle PR, Thomson AD. Nutrition and vitamins in alcoholism. *Contemp Issues Clin Biochem* 1984;1:188–224.
132. Kertesz SG. Pellagra in 2 homeless men. *Mayo Clin Proc* 2001;76(3): 315–318.
133. Stein MD, Friedmann PD. Disturbed sleep and its relationship to alcohol use. *Subst Abuse* 2006;26:1–13.
134. Brower KJ, Aldrich MS, Robinson EA, et al. Insomnia, self-medication, and relapse to alcoholism. *Am J Psychiatry* 2001;158(3):399–404.
135. Anonymous. Prenatal exposure to alcohol. *Alcohol Res Health* 2000; 24(1):32–41.
136. Goldhaber SZ, Grodstein F, Stampfer MJ, et al. A prospective study of risk factors for pulmonary embolism in women. *JAMA* 1997;277(8): 642–645.
137. Buhler FR, Vesanen K, Watters JT, et al. Impact of smoking on heart attacks, strokes, blood pressure control, drug dose, and quality of life aspects in the International Prospective Primary Prevention Study in Hypertension. *Am Heart J* 1988;115(2):282–288.
138. Kawachi I, Colditz GA, Stampfer MJ, et al. Smoking cessation and time course of decreased risks of coronary heart disease in middle aged women. *Arch Intern Med* 1994;154(2):169–175.
139. Leistikow BN, Martin DC, Jacobs J, et al. Smoking as a risk factor for accident death: a meta-analysis of cohort studies. *Accid Anal Prev* 2000;32(3):397–405.
140. Scanlon PD, Connett JE, Waller LA, et al. Smoking cessation and lung function in mild-to-moderate chronic obstructive pulmonary disease. The Lung Health Study. *Am J Respir Crit Care Med* 2000;161(1): 381–390.
141. Winsa B, Mandahl A, Karlsson FA. Graves' disease, endocrine ophthalmopathy and smoking. *Acta Endocrinol (Copenhagen)* 1993;128(2): 156–160.
142. Michnovicz JJ, Hershcopf RJ, Haley NJ, et al. Cigarette smoking alters hepatic estrogen metabolism in men: implications for atherosclerosis. *Metabolism* 1989;38(6):537–541.
143. Vine MF, Margolin BH, Morrison HI, et al. Cigarette smoking and sperm density: a meta-analysis. *Fertil Steril* 1994;61(1):35–43.
144. Bluman LG, Mosca L, Newman N, et al. Preoperative smoking habits and postoperative pulmonary complications. *Chest* 1998;113(4): 883–889.
145. Tisi GM. Preoperative identification and evaluation of the patient with lung disease. *Med Clin North Am* 1987;71(3):399–412.
146. Warner MA, Offord KP, Warner ME, et al. Role of preoperative cessation of smoking and other factors in postoperative pulmonary complications: a blinded prospective study of coronary artery bypass patients. *Mayo Clin Proc* 1989;64(6):609–616.
147. Stein MD. Medical complications of intravenous drug use. *J Gen Intern Med* 1990;5(3):249–257.
148. Stevens DL, Bisno AL, Chambers HF, et al. Practice guidelines for the diagnosis and management of skin and soft-tissue infections. *Clin Infect Dis* 2005;41(10):1373–1406.
149. Cherubin CE, Sapira JD. The medical complications of drug addiction and the medical assessment of the intravenous drug user: 25 years later. *Ann Intern Med* 1993;119(10):1017–1028.
150. Levin MH, Weinstein RA, Nathan C, et al. Association of infection caused by Pseudomonas aeruginosa serotype 011 with intravenous abuse of pentazocine mixed with tripelennamine. *J Clin Microbiol* 1984;20(4):758–762.
151. Murphy EL, DeVita D, Liu H, et al. Risk factors for skin and soft tissue abscesses among injection drug users: a case-control study. *Clin Infect Dis* 2001;33(1):35–40.
152. Samet JH, Shevitz A, Fowle J, et al. Hospitalization decision in febrile intravenous drug users. *Am J Med* 1990;89(1):53–57.
153. Roberts R, Slovis CM. Endocarditis in intravenous drug abusers. *Emerg Med Clin North Am* 1990;8(3):665–681.
154. Di Nubile MJ. Short-course antibiotic therapy for right-sided endocarditis caused by Staphylococcus aureus in injection drug users. *Ann Intern Med* 1994;121(11):873–876.
155. Bitar S, Gomez CR. Stroke following injection of a melted suppository. *Stroke* 1993;24(5):741–743.
156. Johnson MK, Smith RP, Morrison D, et al. Large lung bullae in marijuana smokers. *Thorax* 2000;55(4):340–342.
157. Pare JP, Cote G, Fraser RS. Long-term follow-up of drug abusers with intravenous talcosis. *Am Rev Respir Dis* 1989;139(1):233–241.
158. Johnson BA, Devous MD Sr, Ruiz P, et al. Treatment advances for cocaine-induced ischemic stroke: focus on dihydropyridine class calcium channel antagonists. *Am J Psychiatry* 2001;158(8):1191–1198.
159. McEvoy AW, Kitchen ND, Thomas DG. Intracerebral haemorrhage and drug abuse in young adults. *Br J Neurosurg* 2000;14(5):449–454.
160. Andreu V, Mas A, Bruguera M, et al. Ecstasy: a common cause of severe acute hepatotoxicity. *J Hepatol* 1998;29(3):394–397.
161. Armen R, Kanel G, Reynolds T. Phencyclidine-induced malignant hyperthermia causing submassive liver necrosis. *Am J Med* 1984;77(1): 167–172.
162. Wartenberg AA. Clinical toxicology and substance abuse. In: Kochar MS, Kutty K, eds. *Concise textbook of medicine,* 2nd ed. New York: Elsevier Publishing, 1990:135–160.

163. Lange RA, Hillis LD. Cardiovascular complications of cocaine use. *N Engl J Med* 2001;345(5):351–358.
164. Feldman JA, Fish SS, Beshansky JR, et al. Acute cardiac ischemia in patients with cocaine-associated complaints: results of a multicenter trial. *Ann Emerg Med* 2000;36(5):469–476.
165. Nademanee K. Cardiovascular effects and toxicities of cocaine. *J Addict Dis* 1992;11(4):71–82.
166. Marzuk PM, Tardiff K, Smyth D, et al. Cocaine use, risk taking, and fatal Russian roulette. *JAMA* 1992;267(19):2635–2637.
167. Tashkin DP. Airway effects of marijuana, cocaine, and other inhaled illicit agents. *Curr Opin Pulmon Med* 2001;7(2):43–61.
168. Pedrazzoni M, Vescovi PP, Maninetti L, et al. Effects of chronic heroin abuse on bone and mineral metabolism. *Acta Endocrinol (Copenhagen)* 1993;129(1):42–45.
169. Kim TW, Alford DP, Malabanan A, et al. Low bone density in patients receiving methadone maintenance treatment. *Drug Alcohol Depend* 2006;85(3):258–262.
170. Warner EA, Greene GS, Buchsbaum MS, et al. Diabetic ketoacidosis associated with cocaine use. *Arch Intern Med* 1998;158(16): 1799–1802.
171. Frank DA, Augustyn M, Knight WG, et al. Growth, development, and behavior in early childhood following prenatal cocaine exposure: a systematic review. *JAMA* 2001;285(12):1613–1625.
172. Joint National Committee VI. The sixth report of the Joint National Committee on prevention, detection, evaluation, and treatment of high blood pressure. *Arch Intern Med* 1997;157(21):2413–2446.
173. Blow FC, ed. *Substance abuse among older adults* (Treatment Improvement Protocol 26). Rockville, MD: Substance Abuse and Mental Health Services Administration, 1998.

SUGGESTED READINGS

Barry MJ. Prostate-specific-antigen testing for early diagnosis of prostate cancer. *N Engl J Med* 2001;344(18):1373–1377.

Miller AB, To T, Baines CJ, et al. The Canadian National Breast Screening Study-1: breast cancer mortality after 11 to 16 years of follow-up. A randomized screening trial of mammography in women age 40 to 49 years. *Ann Intern Med* 2002;137(5):305–312.

CHAPTER 71

Howard S. Friedman, MD

Cardiovascular Consequences of Alcohol and Other Drug Use

Alcohol
Nicotine
Cannabis
Opioids
Cocaine
Amphetamines and Related Compounds
Anabolic Steroids

As noted 35 years ago by Samuel Vaisrub (1), though the primary target of addictive psychoactive substances is the brain, the heart does not always remain unmolested. In fact, the use of these substances may have serious cardiovascular consequences. Depending on the drug, the dosage used, and the mode of administration, the cardiovascular effects may range from inconsequential to catastrophic. Because coronary artery disease and stroke are the leading causes of death and disability in most of the world, the effects of these drugs on vasomotion, coagulation, and blood lipids may have serious implications. Often multiple drugs are abused concomitantly; therefore, an understanding of the consequences of their interactions is important. Drug abuse may also be the vehicle by which various contaminating cardiotoxins and microorganisms injure or infect the heart. In this chapter, the cardiovascular consequences of the use of substances that often result in addiction are reviewed.

ALCOHOL

Hemodynamic Effects Though moderate use of alcohol (note that the terms *alcohol* and *ethanol* are used interchangeably in this chapter), defined as no more than two drinks per day in men and no more than one drink in women, may have some cardiovascular benefits (2), even such small amounts of alcohol could have adverse effects in individuals with heart disease, and the consumption of larger amounts can result in serious cardiovascular consequences (3). At plasma concentrations as low as 50 mg/dl (4), ethanol has consistently been shown to depress myocardial contractility (4–6). Because ethanol and its metabolites, acetaldehyde and acetate, also have adrenergic (7) and vasodilatory (8) effects, the direct myocardial depressant actions of ethanol may be obscured when cardiac "pump" function is assessed after ethanol administration. Cardiac output usually increases after alcohol ingestion in healthy subjects, reflecting the changes in heart rate and peripheral resistance that ensue (9,10); by contrast, a more sensitive index of cardiac function, such as left ventricular ejection fraction, generally worsens (7,11).

The explanation for the cardiac muscle depressant actions of alcohol has still not been determined, although various abnormalities have been identified. The heart lacks alcohol dehydrogenase (12), therefore, unlike the liver, it cannot oxidize ethanol (13). However, nonoxidative metabolism with the formation of abnormal esters has been demonstrated (14,15). These fatty acid ethyl esters and their metabolites are potent uncouplers of oxidative phosphorylation (16). Though ethanol can acutely depress mitochondrial respiration (17), the concentrations of phosphocreatine and adenosine triphosphate do not change appreciably even with pharmacologic amounts of alcohol (18); this would suggest that these fatty acid ethyl esters do not have much influence on myocardial energetics. Ethanol has also been shown to affect acutely myocardial metabolism of free fatty acids (19), the major fuel of the heart in a fasted state, and protein metabolism (20) but not glucose metabolism (13). Though these findings are of interest, the changes in myocardial metabolism and energetics are not sufficient to explain the acute myocardial depressant effects of alcohol (18).

Alcohol appears to depress myocardial contractility by direct effects on the contractile process. Ethanol has been shown to reduce the amplitude, duration, and the rate of rise of the myocardial transmembrane action potential, an effect that relates directly to the reduction in contractile force (21). Such changes on myocardial contractility may be related in part to an intracellular acidosis resulting from an ethanol concentration-related inhibition of the acid extruder, Na^+/H^+ exchange (22). The total calcium available to the contractile proteins, measured as light-indicator calcium transients, is also reduced by ethanol (23,24). These changes do not, however, appear to be related to a reduction in calcium entry (25), nor can they be explained by various other abnormalities of cellular calcium kinetics that have been produced by ethanol in experiments that often lack functional or dosage relevancy (26). Even at concentrations lower than those required to affect calcium transients, ethanol depresses contractility, suggesting that ethanol has effects at the level of the myofilament (27). Thus, though alcohol's myocardial depressant actions have been associated with metabolic changes and abnormalities in the contractile process, the factor (or factors) producing these actions appears so far to have eluded investigators.

Ethanol has regional circulatory effects. Alcohol increases skin (28) and splanchnic blood flow (29) but reduces forearm flow (30). Alcohol also decreases pancreatic blood flow (31,32); this change is associated with a reduction in pancreatic oxygenation (33), suggesting that alcohol may produce pancreatitis by an ischemic mechanism.

The effects of alcohol on brain blood flow, however, are not as clear. In experimental studies alcohol has been shown to decrease (34,35), increase (36–38), or produce no change in brain flow (39). The differences may be reconciled by studies that suggest opposite effects of ethanol, which is a cerebrovascular constrictor (34), and its metabolite, acetate, which is a cerebrovascular dilator (8), on the brain circulation. Studies have shown that cerebral blood flow is related inversely to blood alcohol concentrations but directly to blood acetate concentrations (36). Accordingly, with rapid IV administration of alcohol, before the effects of ethanol's metabolites can be seen, cerebral blood flow decreases (35), whereas with *ingestion* of a moderate amount of alcohol, cerebral blood flow increases (36–38). Older patients (older than 62 years) seem to be especially sensitive to the cerebral vasoconstrictor actions of alcohol (36), which may pose an added risk of cerebral circulatory injury in elderly individuals who drink excessively.

In most studies (40,41), but not all (42), ethanol has been found to increase coronary blood flow. In part, this is related to the increased myocardial oxygen requirements that ensue from the increases in heart rate, blood pressure, and cardiac dimensions that generally occur after administration of ethanol (3). Ethanol (43) and its metabolites (8) are coronary vasodilators. Despite these changes, alcohol exerts an unfavorable effect on myocardial ischemia: because the vasculature of the ischemic myocardium is near-maximally dilated, the coronary vasodilatory effects of ethanol occur primarily in arterioles supplying the non-ischemic myocardium, in effect, producing a "coronary steal" (44). Clinical studies have demonstrated findings consistent with this phenomenon (45–47). Individuals with coronary artery disease are more inclined to demonstrate evidence of myocardial ischemia after ingesting alcohol (45–47); moreover, alcohol may mask angina pectoris (47), thereby making the occurrences of myocardial ischemia silent and potentially more dangerous. Also, alcohol may precipitate coronary spasms (48); these spasms often occur several hours after imbibing alcohol, suggesting a "rebound" phenomenon to the vasodilating actions of alcohol and its metabolites.

Alcoholic Heart Disease Excessive alcohol use can result in an array of cardiac abnormalities. From a functional perspective, this ranges from a heart that is hypocontractile, has a reduced output, and is associated with an increased systemic vascular resistance, the findings of alcoholic cardiomyopathy (49), to one that is hyperdynamic, has an increased output, and is associated with a reduced systemic vascular resistance, the findings of decompensated cirrhosis (50,51). Even before such striking abnormalities are evident, subclinical cardiac dysfunction can be detected by noninvasive methods (52–54) and can be demonstrated by tests that measure cardiac reserve (55). Alcohol-related myocardial disease may be present when no obvious heart disease is evident or even when hyperdynamic cardiac function is apparent (56).

Excessive alcohol use leads to myocardial hypertrophy, sometimes with massive increases in heart weight (greater than a kilogram), four-chamber dilation, myocardial necrosis, and interstitial and perivascular fibrosis (57). On electron microscopy, loss of myofibrils, dilation of the sarcoplasmic reticulum, separation of the intercalated disk, and abnormalities of mitochondria may be observed (58,59). When these findings are pronounced, the clinical features of alcoholic cardiomyopathy may become manifest. Cirrhosis does not preclude cardiomyopathy, and when the two conditions are examined for the presence of the other, evidence for their coexistence is not uncommon (60). However, because decompensated cirrhosis is associated with neurohumoral changes that produce a hyperdynamic circulation, the presence of myocardial disease may not be evident by standard clinical measures, such as left ventricular ejection fraction.

The salient cardiovascular feature of decompensated cirrhosis is a reduction of systemic vascular resistance which results in a high cardiac output state (50,51). The diminished systemic vascular resistance is largely a consequence of a generalized vasodilatory response rather than to the presence of arteriovenous shunting (61). The changes in systemic resistance in cirrhosis correlate with changes in hepatic function and are also related to reduced urinary sodium elimination (51). Reduced systemic vascular resistance may be evident even before ascites can be detected by abdominal ultrasound; however, tense ascites, by impeding venous return, can elicit counter-regulatory responses that antagonize the vasodilatory effects of cirrhosis (51).

Some (62–64), but not all (65), experimental models of cirrhosis suggest that nitric oxide might be the mediator of this effect. Studies in humans using nitric oxide synthase inhibitors also support an important role of nitric oxide in the development of increased peripheral blood flow in decompensated cirrhosis (66).

Alcohol-related heart muscle disease (alcoholic cardiomyopathy) is a distinct clinical disorder in people who drink excessive amounts of alcohol who do not have any apparent nutritional deficiencies (67). The relationship between prolonged heavy alcohol use and the occurrence of a dilated, hypocontractile heart is sufficiently strong to suggest that alcohol, acetaldehyde, or some compound formed from these substances, is toxic to the heart (68,69). Despite numerous attempts to replicate this disorder experimentally, however, so far none has adequately reproduced the clinical entity (3).

The development of alcoholic cardiomyopathy appears to require prolonged excessive use of alcohol. People with alcoholism who develop this disorder tend on the average to be 10 years older, have had alcoholism 10 years longer, and drink considerably more than people with alcoholism who maintain normal cardiac dimensions and function (70). However, some people may have a predisposition to getting this condition (71). Though alcoholic cardiomyopathy is seen wherever use of large amounts of alcohol is culturally acceptable, in the United States, 85% to 90% of those with the disease are African American (72).

The inability to reproduce alcoholic cardiomyopathy experimentally and its comparative rarity (in the context of the prevalence of alcohol dependence) suggest that other conditions besides alcoholism may be necessary to produce this disorder. Quebec's beer drinkers' cardiomyopathy may be the prototype of this phenomenon (73). When trace amounts of cobalt, which would ordinarily be nontoxic, were placed in beer to stabilize the foam, a fulminant cardiomyopathy ensued in heavy beer drinkers (73). In experimental studies, alcohol administration exaggerates the myocardial damage produced by trypanosomal (74) and Cocksackie B-3 (75) infections; prolonged alcohol administration also worsens the myocardial injury caused by catecholamines (75).

Hypertension, which is associated with excessive alcohol use (76), may be important in this context. Though the blood pressure elevations in people drinking heavily are often transitory and may abate over several days of abstinence (76), people with alcoholism with transitory hypertension may continue to manifest exaggerated blood pressure responses to stressors after several weeks of abstinence (77). Even when blood pressure is normal, left ventricular wall stress may be elevated (54); moreover, during periods of inebriation, these abnormalities will become exaggerated. The increased left ventricular wall stress and higher heart rates will increase myocardial oxygen consumption. Heart failure might, therefore, ensue as a consequence of the combination of increased myocardial oxygen requirements and the abnormalities of myocardial metabolism and energetics caused by alcohol persisting over many years. Moreover, the occurrence of atrial fibrillation, which is observed more commonly in people who drink heavily (78) or may be seen as a complication of alcoholic cardiomyopathy (72), might produce or worsen myocardial dysfunction (alcohol-related heart muscle disease seen as a manifestation of tachycardia-related cardiomyopathy). The recognition of alcoholism as a cause of congestive heart failure is especially important, because abstinence, especially in the early phases of alcoholic cardiomyopathy, may reverse the abnormalities (72,79,80), whereas continuance of alcohol use will lead inexorably to an unfavorable outcome (72).

Holiday Heart Excessive alcohol use is associated with cardiac arrhythmias. "Holiday Heart" is the term that has been coined to denote the relationship between alcohol use and arrhythmia in the absence of any electrolyte abnormality or evidence of clinical heart disease (81). Often the arrhythmia occurs after binge drinking (78), as implied by the phrase. Though various atrial and ventricular arrhythmias may be seen, people with alcoholism appear to be particularly at risk for atrial fibrillation (78,82). The explanation for this phenomenon is not clear. Though ethanol has been shown to reduce the duration, amplitude and rate of rise of the myocardial transmembrane action potential experimentally (6,21), conditions that would favor the development of atrial fibrillation, such changes have not been observed in the human atrium *in vivo* after administration of alcohol (83,84). However, in individuals who have alcohol-related arrhythmias, the abnormality can often be elicited by programmed electrical stimulation after administration of alcohol (83–85). In some instances, an arrhythmia may be the first manifestation of subclinical alcoholic cardiomyopathy (86). Heavy alcohol use must, therefore, always be considered in individuals with unexplained arrhythmias, especially those having paroxysmal atrial fibrillation.

Experimentally, at least, alcohol has also been shown to have antiarrhythmic actions (87–91). In these studies, ethanol has been shown to increase ventricular fibrillation threshold (89,90), suppress ventricular tachycardia (88), and even shorten the duration of atrial fibrillation (88,91). Whether these findings are just experimental curiosities or have, in fact, clinical significance will require further investigation.

Epidemiologic studies have disclosed an increased incidence of sudden and unexpected deaths in people with alcoholism (92–94). These deaths have been observed in the third through fifth decade of life, in those who have fatty livers at autopsy, and are often found with low blood ethanol concentrations (93,94). The presumption is that these deaths are arrhythmic, perhaps related to hypokalemia, hypomagnesemia, or even alcohol itself. The low blood ethanol concentrations, however, suggest reactions to alcohol withdrawal rather than to alcohol per se as the cause; possible mechanisms might include an arrhythmia from an intense sympathoadrenal reaction (95), post-vasodilatory coronary artery spasm (48) (analogous to weekend angina pectoris in nitrate workers), and small coronary artery thromboses due to rebound hypercoaguability (96). In addition, people with alcoholism develop autonomic neuropathy (97), a condition that might produce arrhythmia by creating cardiac electrical instability. Heavy alcohol use has also been associated with sudden death in individuals with coronary artery disease (94,98), a population already at increased risk for such events. By contrast, in a healthy cohort free of apparent cardiovascular disease, a reduced risk of sudden cardiac death was related to having two to six drinks per week but not with greater or lesser use (99).

Hypertension Alcohol use elevates blood pressure, and heavy alcohol use produces systemic hypertension, an effect that may be intensified during periods of withdrawal. Alcohol and its metabolites, acetaldehyde and acetate, have both direct vasodilatory effects (8) and indirect sympathetic vasoconstrictive actions (100). When alcohol is imbibed (101) or administered intravenously (100), muscle sympathetic nerve traffic (of the peroneal nerve) increases. Initially, blood pressure does not increase, but as blood levels of ethanol decrease (and the vasodilator actions abate) and as sympathetic nerve traffic increases, blood pressure elevates (100). The α-adrenergic blocker phentolamine blocks this vasopressor response, and both the sympathetic neural response and the blood pressure increase are blocked by dexamethasone. The acute hypertensive effects of alcohol are, therefore, mediated centrally, with participation of corticotrophin-releasing hormone, and act directly through α-adrenergic mechanisms (100). Alcohol ingestion also impairs the baroreceptor reflex (102). When alcohol is administered to normotensive subjects, slowing of heart rate to a sudden elevation in blood pressure is attenuated, and the reflex is reset to a higher blood pressure; this effect is directly related to blood ethanol concentrations (102).

Studies have demonstrated clear causal links between alcohol use and blood pressure changes. In individuals with hypertension who use alcohol moderately, within 72 hours of cessation of drinking, blood pressure drops sharply, whereas on resumption, within 48 hours the elevation in blood pressure recurs (103). Even curtailment of alcohol use will lower blood pressure in both normotensive (104) and hypertensive (105) subjects. The effects of alcohol on blood pressure have been found to be related to baseline blood pressure and to the quantity customarily used: Five to six drinks per day for five days had little effect on normotensive, *light* drinkers; elevated only standing blood pressures in hypertensive, *light* drinkers; but increased both supine and standing blood pressure in hypertensive, *moderate* drinkers (106). Experimental studies in animals have also shown that prolonged administration of alcohol elevates blood pressure and changes vascular responsiveness (8,107).

Epidemiologic surveys have demonstrated that the relationship between blood pressure and alcohol is present in diverse populations and that hypertension is more prevalent in individuals who use alcohol excessively (108). The relationship, however, appears to be stronger in men and whites (109). A U- or J-shaped relation between alcohol use and blood pressure had been described in early investigations (108). When adjustments are made for weight and age, the dip tends to disappear (110). Moreover, the association between alcohol use and a *decrease* in blood pressure has been reported mainly in women using alcohol occasionally; it is unlikely that such a small amount of alcohol would exert a persistent biologic effect, suggesting the presence of a hidden confounder. An increase in blood pressure is evident with one or two drinks per day in men, whereas this effect requires three drinks per day in women (109). With menopause, the hypertensive effect of alcohol intensifies (111).

Hypertension is observed frequently in people with alcoholism (76,12). More than half undergoing detoxification have a blood pressure greater than 140/90 mm Hg (112), and a third have a value greater than 160/90 mm Hg (76). Moreover, even when such individuals remain abstinent and their blood pressure returns to normal values, they continue to demonstrate an exaggerated blood pressure response to stressors (76,77), an effect that may last at least for several weeks (77). Alcoholism-associated hypertension appears also to be catecholamine-mediated (76). Almost 90% of people with both alcoholism hypertension undergoing detoxification have elevated plasma epinephrine and when abstinent and their blood pressure normalizes, they still show an exaggerated increment of plasma catecholamines in response to stress (76).

Thus, alcohol has a dual effect on blood pressure. Ethanol and its metabolites, by their vasodilatory actions on the systemic circulation, lower blood pressure; however, alcohol also stimulates the sympathetic nervous system (and probably also the adrenal cortex and medulla) and attenuates the baroreceptor reflex, actions that would elevate blood pressure. Though the elevations of blood pressure associated with habitual use of alcohol disappear after several days of abstinence, people with alcoholism have a proclivity for an exaggerated response of their blood pressure to stressors that may persist for at least several weeks after withdrawal.

Coronary Heart Disease and Stroke Heavy alcohol use is associated with an increased risk of coronary artery disease (113) and stroke (114,115). When used in moderation, however, particularly when there are no heavy drinking episodes (116), alcohol use is favorably related to these conditions (117). The relationships between alcohol consumption and coronary (118) and cerebrovascular diseases (114) can, therefore, be described as U- or J-shaped, initially favorable, with benefit augmenting as use increases, and then unfavorable, with detriment augmenting as use increases (An L-shaped relation has been described for stroke, but this study did not stratify for those with heavy drinking episodes [119].) The adverse effects of alcohol on atherothrombotic diseases can be related to the blood pressure elevations (113,115,120)—and perhaps also to the blood homocysteine elevations (121,122)—caused by alcohol use, whereas the favorable effects appear to be related mostly to the changes alcohol produces on the blood lipid profile (123). Alcohol's effects on hemostasis, its overall antithrombotic actions, would also impact favorably on atherothrombotic events, doing so at a cost of an increased chance of hemorrhagic stroke, a finding in some (124), but not all (119), studies. The effects of alcohol on coronary heart disease and stroke are observed in both men and women, with the U-curve in women located to the left of that in men (a lower dose for both benefit and detriment) (109). Consistent with Bayesian probability, the benefits of moderate ethanol use are evident in those with an increased risk for coronary disease: middle-aged individuals (109) and those with elevated low density lipoprotein cholesterol (125). About 50% of the benefit derived from alcohol consumption on coronary disease mortality can be attributed to an increase in high density lipoprotein cholesterol (126). The effects of alcohol use on hemostasis provide additional benefit. Alcohol use reduces plasma fibrinogen (127), a risk factor for coronary artery disease (128). Alcohol use also reduces platelet aggregability (96); this effect is directly related to the amount of alcohol customarily used, and is exaggerated by a diet high in saturated fats (96). After alcohol is ingested, there is a transient reduction of platelet aggregation, but this is followed by a more prolonged "rebound" enhancement (96). The rebound phenomenon can be antagonized by tannins, which are antioxidants present in red wine (129). Ethanol enhances the antiplatelet actions of aspirin (130). Alcohol use is also positively related to plasma tissue-type plasminogen activator (t-PA), suggesting an alcohol-induced enhancement of fibrinolysis (131).

Alcohol may also exert a protective action on the myocyte subjected to an ischemic/reperfusion injury (132,133). Experimental studies in animals have demonstrated effects of ethanol that are similar to those of ischemic preconditioning (a protective state ensuing from one or more brief periods of ischemia preceding a prolonged ischemic insult that results in reduced myocardial ischemic injury). Such protective action may be triggered by a brief exposure to alcohol (132) or by chronic administration of small amounts of alcohol given over several months (133). Both acute and chronic ethanol preconditioning use signal transduction pathways similar to those of ischemic preconditioning: adenosine receptors, protein kinase C (the epsilon isoform), protein tyrosine kinase, and the mitochondrial potassium channel, K_{ATP} may be activated in both types of myocyte preconditioning (132,133). Paradoxically, the myocardial presence of alcohol at the time of the ischemic insult may actually inhibit the protective processes of ethanol (134) and ischemic preconditioning (135), illustrating the complexity of these relationships.

Given the conflicting experimental findings related to alcohol's myocardial protective actions, it should not be surprising that clinical studies have also produced contradictory results. Though in two case-control studies (136,137) fatal and nonfatal myocardial infarction were less likely to occur in those who used ethanol in the 24 hours preceding the event, in a cohort of patients with acute myocardial infarction (138), no differences were found in the electrocardiographic changes, in the peak creatine kinase levels (as a measure of extent of injury), or in the cardiac complications related to such use of alcohol.

The relation of habitual use of alcohol after an acute myocardial infarction to outcomes is also unclear. Mild to moderate use of alcohol after myocardial infarction, in general (139), and wine in particular (140), has been related to improved survival and fewer complications. However, use of alcohol diminishes after myocardial infarction, particularly when complications ensue (141). When adjustments are made for the propensity not to use alcohol with greater cardiac disability, the reduced incidence of congestive heart failure after myocardial infarction with mild to moderate use of alcohol dissipates (141).

Though the reduced risk of coronary heart disease associated with moderate alcohol use is not related to any specific alcoholic beverage (142), there may be some selective differences. For instance, the tannins in red wine and the vitamin B-6, which is an antagonist of the homocysteine-elevating effects of alcohol (122), in beer, may provide some additional protective advantages for these beverages. However, the beneficial effects of alcohol use can be related to ethanol per se. This is supported by the observation that individuals who have a genetic variation of alcohol dehydrogenase that results in slow metabolism of ethanol have the most protection against myocardial infarction with moderate alcohol use (143). Though the evidence for some benefit of moderate alcohol use is persuasive, which includes numerous confirmatory studies and significant dose-relationships between use and outcomes, the actual value may be less than has been suggested. For instance, a reported 21% decrease in the 12-year incidence of stroke attributable to alcohol use is actually a benefit of only 5.6 per 10,000 per year (119). From an epidemiologic perspective, this may be significant but, in a given individual, the likelihood of benefit is small. Moreover, because the evidence of benefit is based on cohort data, not randomized controlled studies, there are always concerns about a hidden confounder. Individuals who have *one* drink per week have fewer strokes than teetotalers (119). Can such a small amount of alcohol confer this protection, or is there a concealed variable? Similarly, a statistical adjustment for a predictor variable may obscure a detrimental effect of alcohol: If alcohol's adverse effects are the result of raising blood pressure or are a consequence of an interaction with aspirin (for instance, to promote intracerebral hemorrhage), a statistical adjustment for these variables would tend to make the outcomes appear more favorable. In addition, even moderate alcohol use may increase heart rate and blood pressure and depress left ventricular function (3), or produce a "coronary steal" (44), changes that might aggravate congestive heart failure or worsen myocardial ischemia. Thus, encouraging the use of alcohol as a cardiac medicinal would seem to be unwarranted, especially for people with heart disease.

NICOTINE

Cigarette smoking is a leading risk factor for developing cardiovascular diseases (144). The addictive constituent and the agent responsible for most of the adverse cardiovascular effects of smoking tobacco is nicotine. Within a few minutes of smoking a cigarette, heart rate and blood pressure increase (145–147). Though the values begin to decline on cessation of smoking, heart rate and blood pressure remain above baseline for at least 30 minutes (145). These findings can be replicated by administration of nicotine to achieve plasma concentrations observed when smoking a cigarette (148,149). The changes, which can be prevented by adrenergic blockade, are generally accompanied by increases of plasma epinephrine and norepinephrine (145,147). Nicotine exerts its adrenergic actions mainly by release of norepinephrine from nerve terminals (148) and by release of epinephrine from the adrenal medulla (149). A central nervous system stimulatory effect by nicotine is disputed by the observation that muscle sympathetic nerve traffic (of the peroneal nerve) assessed by microneurography decreases as blood pressure increases (146,147). The complex adrenergic response to smoking may account for the lack of elevation of plasma norepinephrine in some studies (146,149). Smoking also attenuates baroreceptor responses to blood pressure elevations (146,147) and the heart rate fluctuations that occur with normal respiration (146).

By its adrenergic actions, smoking exerts a vasoconstrictive effect on most regional circulations. Skin blood flow, reflected by decreases of skin temperature after smoking a cigarette, diminishes (148). Despite an increase in calf muscle vascular resistance, in normal subjects calf blood flow may not change (147). In individuals with symptomatic obstructive peripheral arterial disease, however, smoking would be expected to diminish blood flow and reduce walking distance before calf pain.

The effects of smoking on coronary blood reflect the competing influences of its hemodynamic actions, elevations of heart rate and blood pressure, which evoke an increase in flow, and its direct vasoconstrictive actions, which diminish flow (150–153). The vasospastic coronary actions, which are attenuated by α-adrenergic blockers (151), L-type calcium channel blockers (152), and nitroglycerin (152), but enhanced by β-adrenergic blockers (151), are especially detrimental in the presence of obstructive coronary disease. Smoking worsens coronary artery narrowings (153) and may adversely affect "downstream" collaterals and compensatory arteriolar dilatation (150). Endothelium-dependent coronary blood flow (measured by substance-P stimulation) may also be impaired by smoking, a finding that is exaggerated by the concomitant presence of other coronary risk factors (154). Moreover, the increases in carboxyhemoglobin that occur during smoking impede the delivery of oxygen to tissues (155). Thus, by increasing myocardial oxygen requirements, causing vasospasms, diminishing coronary flow reserve, and interfering with myocardial oxygen delivery, smoking a cigarette causes myocardial ischemia to occur at lower levels of exertion and even at rest in individuals with coronary artery disease (156–158).

Smoking may also cause an acute coronary thrombosis. Smoking even a single cigarette promotes adenosine diphosphate-induced platelet aggregation (159). Several days of smoking has been shown to increase platelet factor 4 and β-thromboglobulin, indicators of platelet activation (160), and to increase the urinary concentrations of the metabolites of thromboxane A_2, the potent platelet aggregatory prostaglandin (160). Increased urinary concentrations of the metabolites of thromboxane A_2 are also observed in chronic smokers (161). In addition, smoking cigarettes may promote coagulation by increasing plasma fibrinogen (160), and it may inhibit fibrinolysis by reducing tissue plasminogen activator (t-PA) activity (154). The elevations of plasma fibrinogen concentration and leukocyte count that occur in smokers would tend to increase blood viscosity (160), thereby contributing to thrombogenesis by slowing blood flow. The associations between smoking cigarettes and thrombogenesis may be of particular concern in women, especially for those using oral contraceptives or receiving hormonal replacement therapy; the risks of thrombotic events in women smokers using oral contraceptives increases sharply after age 35 (144,162). Though the changes in thrombogenesis are not seen with sham smoking or smoking of tobacco-free cigarettes (159), a clear relation between the hemostatic changes that occur with smoking cigarettes and concentrations of nicotine (or cotinine) and catecholamines has not been established (159–161).

Despite the strong relation between cigarette smoking and increases in mortality and morbidity from coronary heart disease (144), people who smoke seem to have better outcomes after an acute myocardial infarction, a relationship that may even be correlated with the number of cigarettes smoked (163). This seemingly paradoxical finding appears to be explained, at least in part, by the younger age at which they have myocardial infarctions and by the lack of association of smoking with other risk factors, but not by the extent of underlying coronary disease (154,163,164). The paramount importance of thrombosis in the pathophysiology of acute myocardial infarction in people who smoke may also explain their enhanced benefit from thrombolytic therapy (163,164). Despite these statistical curiosities, the resumption of smoking after myocardial infarction has an adverse effect on outcomes (144) and must be discouraged.

Smoking promotes atherogenesis (144). Smokers have more extensive atherosclerosis in the coronary arteries, aorta, and peripheral arteries than nonsmokers. Because progression of coronary disease often involves mechanisms related to coagulation, particularly the development of severe narrowings, through a process of plaque disruption, *thrombosis*, and healing (165), by promoting hemostasis, smoking also contributes to atherosclerotic plaque growth. In addition, smoking produces an unfavorable lipid profile, by reducing high-density lipoprotein (HDL)-cholesterol (166), and it adversely affects endothelial function (154).

Nicotine replacement treatment (patches and gum) is used to treat nicotine dependence. Though there have been a few reports of cardiovascular events (acute myocardial infarction, atrial fibrillation, and stroke) associated with their use (167), especially in individuals who continue to smoke, controlled studies have failed to demonstrate a significant risk (167,168). The absence of a detectable risk, when contrasted with the risk in these individuals who continue to smoke cigarettes, has been explained by the sharp reduction in cigarette use even in those who do both and by the elimination of the adverse effects of smoking that are not ascribable to nicotine

(167,168). In brief, given the hazards of smoking, whatever small risks may be related to continued nicotine exposure are offset by the benefits of cessation: a 50% decrease in risk of having a coronary event after 1 to 2 years of abstinence and a continued decline thereafter so that, after 20 years, ex-smokers have a risk comparable to that of nonsmokers (144).

CANNABIS

Cannabis (marijuana) has excitatory effects on the heart (170–176). The cardiac physiologic changes have been related to the major active compound present in the drug, delta-9-tetrahydrocannabinol (Δ-9-THC) (174). Whether cannabis is smoked (170), ingested (Δ-9-THC) (172), or administered intravenously (Δ-9-THC) (173), heart rate increases. The occurrence of isolated premature ventricular impulses has also been observed after smoking cannabis (177,178). Even a single cannabis cigarette may increase heart rate by 50% (176). The increases in heart rate parallel blood concentrations of Δ-9-THC (177) but then tend to level off despite increasing levels (173).

When cannabis is ingested, peak effects occur 3 hours afterward (172), whereas when smoked (175) or when Δ-9-THC is administered intravenously (173), they are evident almost immediately. The increased heart rate that follows smoking cannabis may last for 2 to 3 hours (179). Some tolerance develops over time (175,179), so that the most pronounced heart rate changes would be expected with first-time use. However, even after several weeks of regular use, cannabis will still increase heart rate significantly (175,179). Moreover, after 48 hours of abstinence, tolerance is no longer evident. The heart rate changes occur concomitantly with increased concentrations of urinary epinephrine (171), but not norepinephrine (171), and can be sharply reduced with adrenergic blockade, using either the β-blocker propranolol (170,172), though not in all studies (174,176), or the α_2-agonist clonidine (180). Cannabis' effects on blood pressure are more variable. It may increase (171,181), have no change (173,174), or even decrease systemic blood pressure (182). Though the explanation for this variability is not clear, cannabis use appears to have a vasodilatory action (170,171). When blood pressure increases, this suggests that an increase in cardiac output has offset the decrease in systemic vascular resistance. Decreases of blood pressure are most evident in an upright position (171,172), a finding consistent with the observation that the expected peripheral vasoconstriction after cold exposure or mental stress is attenuated after cannabis use (170). The orthostatic decreases of blood pressure become more evident after several days of drug use, especially when Δ-9-THC is ingested (182,172); hypotension, and even bradycardia, consistent with a vasovagal reaction, may ensue when some individuals assume an upright position after have been given Δ-9-THC (172).

Cardiac output generally increases after the administration of cannabis (173,175,176). The change reflects increases in heart rate and a reduction of total peripheral resistance (vasodilation) (170,171), rather than an improvement in cardiac performance. Stroke volume does not increase, and other, more sensitive measures of myocardial function, such as ejection fraction, do not change (176) or may even decrease (181). The overall cardiovascular changes suggest an adrenomedullary effect. The findings, however, do not fully replicate those of epinephrine, implying the presence of other mechanisms as well.

The hemodynamic changes after cannabis use would not be expected to have any adverse effects in healthy subjects. For persons with heart disease, however, the changes in cardiac dynamics might indeed be detrimental. The increased heart rate, and perhaps also an increase of blood pressure, that occurs with cannabis use will augment myocardial oxygen requirements. When cannabis is smoked, moreover, carboxyhemoglobin increases (183,184). This lowers blood oxygen content and results in more tightly bound oxyhemoglobin, thereby reducing myocardial oxygen delivery (155). As a consequence of such changes, patients with angina pectoris have myocardial ischemia at reduced levels of exertion and a lower heart rate-blood pressure product when they smoke cannabis (183). Worsening of the indices of cardiac performance occurs concomitantly with these changes (181); therefore, individuals with heart failure might experience deterioration of their condition after cannabis use. Moreover, in a study of patients with an acute myocardial infarction, users of cannabis had almost five times the incidence of the event during the 1 hour after their use of cannabis than at other times, suggesting that smoking cannabis might also be a "trigger" of myocardial infarction (185). Thus, even though the explanations for their cardiovascular effects have not yet been clearly elucidated, at least for individuals with heart disease, use of cannabis is harmful.

OPIOIDS

Unlike the other addictive substances reviewed in this chapter, which have little or no cardiac medicinal value, opiates (morphine, in most of the studies cited) are important therapeutic agents: Their use for pain relief in acute myocardial infarction and for treatment of cardiogenic pulmonary edema is well established. When administered intravenously at therapeutic dosages, these drugs have a modest effect on lowering blood pressure (186–190) and reducing heart rate (187,188,190), effects that are independent of the drugs' sedative and respiratory depressive actions (187). Under *experimental* conditions in amounts that exceed therapeutic dosages or amounts used by addicts, opiates (morphine) can evoke intense sympathomimetic effects, manifested by an increased heart rate and blood pressure and an improvement in cardiac performance (191). Though opiates may depress cardiac muscle contractility in isolated preparations (192), a decrease in cardiac output is generally not evident in most (189,190), but not all (193), clinical studies.

Opiates have mild venodilating (194) and more pronounced splanchnic arteriolar vasodilating (195) effects. Such actions may be related, at least in part, to an opioid-induced release of nitric oxide from endothelium (196,197), but not to an apparent direct effect on vascular smooth muscle (198).

Opiates may also have favorable effects on myocardial ischemia. In patients with coronary artery disease, opiates improve myocardial energetics (189) and coronary blood flow (199). Moreover, opiates have a direct protective effect against myocardial ischemia at the cellular level (200,201). Administration of morphine before a prolonged coronary occlusion will reduce myocardial injury analogous to the phenomenon of "ischemic preconditioning." (Brief periods of myocardial ischemia prior to a prolonged episode lessens the injury caused by the prolonged episode.) (200,201). In addition, by actions on the central nervous system (202), by direct effects on the myocyte (203), or by vagally mediated mechanisms (204), or as a combination of such effects, opiates may exert antiarrhythmic effects on catecholamine-mediated (202) and ischemia-related (203) arrhythmias and may increase the threshold for ventricular fibrillation (204). Thus, the overall favorable actions of opioids on the heart may explain why abnormalities of cardiac dimensions and function are generally not found in heroin addicts (205).

Despite the benefits of opiates in the treatment of pulmonary edema, paradoxically, heroin overdose may produce a pulmonary condition resembling cardiogenic pulmonary edema (206). However, heroin-related pulmonary edema, which has also been reported with other opioids (207), generally occurs in the presence of normal cardiac function. The pulmonary edema that characterizes heroin overdose is highly proteinaceous, resembling plasma, consistent with a defect in capillary permeability rather than an elevation of pulmonary capillary pressure (208). This disorder is probably caused by an unusually high opioid-induced release of histamine from pulmonary mast cells (209). The treatment requires maintaining normal blood oxygenation, usually by supplemental oxygen or, if necessary, by noninvasive or mechanical ventilation, until the condition resolves. The major cardiac hazard of injection drug use (IDU), apart from an accidental overdose, is infective endocarditis. Endocarditis in IDUs, however, differs from that seen in the nonaddict by the frequent occurrence on normal valves, the high incidence of virulent microorganisms, such as *Staphylococcus aureus*, *Pseudomonas* species, and fungus, and the increased involvement of right-sided valves, especially the tricuspid (210). Because of the seriousness of this disorder, there must be a high suspicion in any IDU presenting with fever, especially when associated with repeated rigors. Treatment with broad-spectrum antibiotic coverage, that includes an antibiotic against methicillin-resistant *Staphylococcus aureus*, should be initiated whenever this disorder is suspected; a delay while waiting for a positive blood culture or a confirmation of valvular vegetations by echocardiography may result in serious valvular damage. Moreover, the high recidivism of opioid addiction requires that the indications for valve replacement be more rigorous in addicts, because the risk of an infection is higher and the consequences of endocarditis more dire with a prosthetic than with a native valve.

COCAINE

Cocaine is a local anesthetic with potent sympathomimetic actions. The adrenergic effects are the result of blocking presynaptic norepinephrine and dopamine reuptake, thereby making more catecholamines available at postsynaptic receptors (211–213), stimulating the sympathetic nervous system (214), and enhancing the effects of endogenous catecholamines (215,216). As a local anesthetic, cocaine inhibits transmembrane sodium flux during electrical excitation, producing a delay in the upstroke and amplitude of the myocardial action potential; this action diminishes intracellular calcium indirectly (making less sodium available for sodium-calcium exchange) (211). Cocaine may also directly block (L-type channel) calcium entry into the myocyte (217,218), inhibit the release of calcium from the sarcoplasmic reticulum (219), and make the contractile proteins less responsive to available calcium (219). Thus, depending on the dosage and the clinical or experimental conditions, cocaine may produce seemingly contradictory effects, reflecting whether the sympathomimetic or the local anesthetic actions are predominant (219).

Following cocaine use, blood pressure increases, heart rate is generally faster, and in most vascular distributions, arteries constrict (220,221). Depending on the dosage and the susceptibility of the individual to the drug, even a single use of cocaine can result in sudden cardiac death (222), an effect that is related in part to cocaine's arrhythmogenic actions. Cocaine use may cause angina pectoris and acute myocardial infarction; aortic dissection and rupture; ischemic and hemorrhagic stroke; and left ventricular dilation and hypertrophy (212). These cardiovascular disorders are related to the acute and chronic hemodynamic and biochemical effects of the drug. Moreover, people who inject cocaine are at a particularly high risk for bacterial endocarditis (223).

Hemodynamic Effects When cocaine is used or administered systemically, it is a potent vasoconstrictor, elevating systemic vascular resistance and blood pressure in a dose-related fashion (220). Heart rate also elevates as the dosage of the drug increases, though under some experimental conditions slowing may ensue (220). As a consequence of its direct local anesthetic actions, cocaine depresses myocardial function (221,224,225) and attenuates vasoconstriction (224,226); under certain conditions, it might even cause vasodilatation (224). The myocardial depressant actions of cocaine would be most evident when its systemic adrenergic effects are diminished (224) or when baseline myocardial function is depressed (224,227) but may also be observed with high coronary artery concentrations of cocaine (228). Generally, when cocaine is used, increases in heart rate, elevation of blood pressure, myocardial depression, and vasoconstriction ensue.

Because of the autoregulatory properties of the coronary circulation, an increase in coronary blood flow would be expected in response to the augmented oxygen demand caused by cocaine's increase in heart rate and systemic blood pressure. However, measurements of coronary blood flow in humans after the administration of cocaine (approximately half the local anesthetic dosage and between a tenth and a fourth of the amount taken when used illicitly?) demonstrate a reduction (229–232). The decrease in blood flow is also observed in anesthetized dogs even when cocaine does not affect the determinants of myocardial oxygen demand (221). Direct measurements of coronary artery dimensions after this dose of cocaine also show a constriction of coronary epicardial arteries (227,229–231).

The coronary vasoconstrictive actions of cocaine are attenuated by the α-adrenergic blocker phentolamine (229), are enhanced by the β-adrenergic blocker propranolol (230), and are not changed by a drug with both α-adrenergic and β-adrenergic blocker effects, labetalol (233). However, studies demonstrating enhanced vasoconstriction after cocaine by β-adrenergic blockade have all been done with non-cardioselective β-adrenergic blockers; accordingly, whether β_1-adrenergic blockers, which are the preferred drugs in acute myocardial infarction, might still have vasoconstrictive actions, has not been determined. The hemodynamic responses of cocaine follow a bimodal time course: The maximal effects are observed at peak plasma cocaine concentration, and a later secondary effect ensues when the plasma cocaine concentration is at its nadir but the concentrations of its metabolites benzoylecgonine and ethyl methylecgonine are still high (232). Because the vasodilatory modulating actions of the endothelium may be diminished by atherosclerosis, the coronary vasoconstrictive action of cocaine might be even more intense in the presence of coronary artery disease (153).

Some people who use cocaine drink alcoholic beverages, smoke cigarettes, smoke cannabis, or do some combination of these drugs when they use cocaine. Table 71.1 summarizes the hemodynamic effects of these activities. As shown in Table 71.2, though alcohol, smoking cigarettes, smoking cannabis, and cocaine may by themselves increase myocardial oxygen requirements, by increasing systemic blood pressure, heart rate or both, when cocaine use is combined with these other activities, this effect is exaggerated (153,232). Smoking cigarettes also intensifies the ischemic consequences of cocaine by its vasoconstrictive effects on the coronary circulation, including such actions on diseased segments (153); by contrast, alcohol worsens myocardial ischemia by creating a coronary steal, producing arteriolar vasodilation in normal arteries but not in arteries supplying ischemic myocardium, thereby redistributing myocardial blood flow away from the ischemic myocardium (44). Moreover, alcohol intensifies the myocardial depressant actions of cocaine (234). The effect appears to be due mainly to the combined depressant actions of these substances. A metabolite of their interaction, cocaethylene, also has myocardial depressant actions (234) and may continue to exert detrimental effects after cocaine has been metabolized and cocaine's other metabolites are still present. When cocaine is used with cannabis, heart rate is greater than that seen with the same amount of cocaine taken alone, whereas blood pressure changes are comparable to those observed with only cocaine (235,236). When a task is performed together with taking both cocaine and cannabis, the maximal effects of the combination of these drugs on heart rate and blood pressure are intensified (236). Myocardial oxygen requirements are, therefore, greater with a combination of cocaine and cannabis than with the same amount of either drug used alone. Thus, cocaine use, alone or in combination with these other addictive substances, creates an imbalance between myocardial oxygen requirements, which it increases, and myocardial oxygen delivery, which it decreases by coronary arterial and arteriolar constrictive actions (129,153,230). Cocaine is, therefore, a potent agent for producing myocardial ischemia.

Acute Coronary Syndromes In the 1980s, there appeared a number of reports of relatively young people having had an acute myocardial infarction after the use of cocaine (237–240). The average age of these individuals was 31 years, with reports of this condition occurring even in adolescents (240). Though the presence of coronary risk factors, especially heavy cigarette smoking, was observed in most of the patients, some had no known predisposition (240). Both habitual cocaine users and occasional users were at risk for these coronary events (240). The hour after cocaine use appears to be the time of greatest hazard (241).

An acute coronary thrombosis has been found in these individuals on coronary angiography performed within a few hours of the onset symptoms or at autopsy (238–240,242). Angiography after therapeutic or presumed spontaneous thrombolysis generally disclosed patent coronary arteries; multivessel coronary artery stenoses were limited to those individuals at high risk for coronary disease (238–240). By contrast, an autopsy study in cocaine abusers showed coronary occlusive platelet-rich thrombi superimposed on severe luminal narrowing atherosclerosis; plaque rupture, associated with coronary thrombosis in cocaine nonusers, however, was not evident (242). The coronary vasoconstrictive actions of cocaine, especially when intensified by smoking, appears to be a pivotal condition (243).

Cocaine use also appears to promote thrombosis (244–246). Though *in vitro* studies in animals (244) and humans (247) suggest that cocaine may not have a consistent direct action on platelet aggregation or on the formation of vascular and platelet prostaglandins, and may even inhibit platelet function at high concentrations (244), cocaine taken intranasally causes platelet activation, platelet microaggregation, and increased plasma concentrations of platelet factor 4 and β thromboglobulin (246). In addition, when cocaine is taken in this way, inhibition of fibrinolysis may occur as a result of increased plasminogen activator inhibitor (PAI-1) activity (245). Habitual cocaine users have also been found to have an increased percentage of activated platelets (247). Thus, even though the pathophysiology of the acute coronary syndromes related to cocaine use has not yet been fully elucidated, cocaine's demonstrated actions of increasing myocardial oxygen demand, elevating coronary arteriolar resistance, constricting

TABLE 71.1 Salient Cardiovascular Effects of Alcohol and other Drugs

Alcohol
Hemodynamics: Myocardial depression
Increased cardiac output (heart rate increases and/or peripheral resistance decreases)
Increased skin and splanchnic blood flow
Decreased brain and pancreatic blood flow
Increased coronary flow in normal vasculature but decreased flow to ischemic myocardium
Disorders
Dilated cardiomyopathy (sometimes with marked increase of left ventricular wall thickness)
Arrhythmias, especially atrial fibrillation
Systemic, Hypertension
May attenuate (light to moderate use) or promote atherogenesis (heavy use)
Sudden death

Nicotine
Hemodynamics:
Increased heart rate and blood pressure
Vasoconstriction
Promotes myocardial ischemia by increasing myocardial demand and decreasing O_2 delivery
Promotes thrombosis
Disorders
Worsens angina pectoris
Promotes acute coronary syndromes
Promotes atherogenesis

Cannabis
Hemodynamics:
Increases heart rate
Variable effect on blood pressure
Vasodilation
Increases cardiac output (heart rate increases and/or peripheral resistance decreases)
Promotes myocardial ischemia by increasing myocardial demand and decreasing O_2 delivery (increases carboxyhemoglobin)
Disorders
Worsens angina pectoris and promotes acute coronary syndromes

Opioids
Hemodynamics:
Lower heart rate
Lowers blood pressure
Vasodilation
Promotes "ischemic preconditioning"
Disorders
Heroin-related pulmonary edema

Cocaine
Hemodynamics:
Increases heart rate
Increases blood pressure
Myocardial depressant
Vasoconstrictor
Promotes thrombosis
Promotes atherogenesis
Disorders
Atypical chest pain syndrome
Worsens angina pectoris
Promotes acute myocardial infarction
Aortic rupture and dissection
Left ventricular hypertrophy and dilatation (myocarditis/cardiomyopathy)
Arrhythmias
Hypertension, systemic
Stroke
Sudden death

Amphetamines
Hemodynamics:
Increases blood pressure
Increases heart rate (with sharp increases of blood pressure may have reflex slowing)
Promotes thrombosis
Disorders
Promotes acute myocardial infarction
Aortic dissection
Left ventricular hypertrophy and dilation (myocarditis/cardiomyopathy)
Arrhythmias
Pulmonary, Hypertension
Stroke
Sudden death

coronary epicardial arteries, and promoting thrombosis clearly create the milieu for such events.

The diagnosis and treatment of acute myocardial infarction related to cocaine use differs from that of patients who have not used this drug because of the additional detrimental effects of coronary spasms and the concurrence of central nervous system and systemic toxicity (248). The diminished predictive accuracy of the electrocardiogram (248) and the confounding effects of rhabdomyolysis increasing creatine kinase contribute to the difficulty of diagnosing acute myocardial infarction after cocaine use. When compared to other cardiac injury markers, troponin I is the most accurate for the diagnosis of acute myocardial infarction (249). Unless hypotension is present, sublingual nitroglycerin should be administered and IV nitroglycerin infused to counteract the vasoconstrictive effects of cocaine (250); this may be necessary for at least 12 to 24

TABLE 71.2 Drug Effects on Myocardial Oxygen Demand and Coronary Blood Flow

Drug	Rate	SBP	RateXSBP	CBF	CAD-N	CAD-AB
Ethanol	↑	↑/NC/↓	↑	↑	↑	↓[a]
Cocaine	↑	↑	↑	↓	↓	↓
Nicotine	↑	↑	↑	↑/NC/↓	↑/NC/↓	↓
Cannabis	↑↑	↑/NC/↓	↑	↑	↑	UK
Ethanol-Cocaine	↑↑	↑↑	↑↑	↑	↑	↓[b]
Nicotine-cocaine	↑↑	↑↑	↑↑	↓	↓	↓↓
Cannabis-cocaine	↑↑	↑	↑↑	↓	↓	↓

SBP, systolic blood pressure; CBF, coronary blood flow; CAD, coronary artery dimensions; N, normal arteries; AB, stenosed arteries; NC, no change; UK, unknown.

[a]Diminishes blood flow by a "coronary steal."

[b]"Coronary steal" expected.

hours, taking into account the 4 to 6 hours that it may take for the drug to be absorbed from the nasal mucosa (251) and the 24 to 36 hours in which its metabolites may still be found in urine (213). Because cocaine's cardiovascular effects may be in part central nervous system–mediated (248) and pretreatment of experimental animals with diazepam reduces seizures and the mortality of cocaine toxicity (252), benzodiazepine use has been recommended in the management of cocaine-related acute coronary syndromes (248). However, in the only randomized controlled trial comparing diazepam alone or with nitroglycerin to nitroglycerin alone, no hemodynamic or symptomatic benefits were found (253). Despite limited evidence, but with the expectation that benzodiazepines will at least attenuate the excitatory actions of cocaine and its congeners and not produce harm, an American Heart Association consensus statement recommends benzodiazepines in the management of cocaine-related chest pain syndromes (254). In an ST-segment elevation myocardial infarction that has not responded to nitroglycerin and in which symptoms have persisted for not more than 12 hours, coronary angiography should be performed with a view toward coronary angioplasty and stenting; if not available, then an intravenous (IV) thrombolytic drug should be administered, unless there are contraindications to these drugs, such as severe hypertension (255,256). In addition to its analgesic action, morphine attenuates cocaine-induced vasospasm (257) and, therefore, may be considered for unremitting chest pains, though with perhaps some reservations about giving the drug to an abuser. The administration of β-blockers should be deferred at least until after the effects of cocaine and its congeners have dissipated or coronary patency has been established (230). Though IV calcium-channel-blockers have also been shown to alleviate cocaine-induced vasoconstriction (258), then use in this setting should probably be avoided because of their concomitant sympathomimetic actions (259). Reservations about the use of calcium-channel-blockers in this setting have also been expressed in consensus recommendations (254). Antiplatelet drugs and anticoagulants, according to standard practices, should be administered. In treating in-hospital acute myocardial infarction in people who used cocaine, the caveat of "first do no harm" especially applies, because serious complications are the exception and mortality rate is low (260).

Chest pains must be perceived as a symptom for acute myocardial infarction in all suspected users of the drug, though most who have used cocaine who are observed for chest pains do not go on to have a myocardial infarction (261). Monitoring patients in a chest pain observation unit for 9 to 12 hours is generally sufficient to identify those at risk for an acute coronary event (262). The predilection for myocardial ischemia, and for even an acute myocardial infarction (243), may persist for days, and possibly for weeks, after cocaine withdrawal (263), though in most instances this is related to continued cocaine use (262). Counseling people who use cocaine who experience chest pains and those who have had an acute coronary event, who remain at jeopardy for additional heart attacks and even for sudden death, is therefore especially important (240).

Chronic Cardiovascular Effects Cocaine use has also been associated with acceleration of atherosclerosis, myocardial injury and thickening, and vascular complications related to hypertension. Autopsy studies have demonstrated that heavy users of cocaine have worse coronary atherosclerosis than that found in persons 20 years older (264). These findings are consistent with experimental studies showing acceleration of atherosclerosis by cocaine administration in hypercholesterolemic animals (212,265). Cocaine may increase vascular endothelium permeability, allowing more atherogenic lipoproteins to diffuse into the intima, though coronary vasospasm, catecholamine toxicity, and activation of inflammatory cells may also contribute to these findings (265). Chronic and/or acute administration of cocaine have been shown to produce vascular injury and myocardial infarction in hypercholesterolemic and normal cholesterolemic animals; these myocardial infarctions, however, were not associated with coronary thromboses (266).

Myocardial abnormalities have also been observed in cocaine abusers (222,267–269). Focal myocarditis has been reported in 20% of autopsies of cocaine users, whether the deaths were or were not directly attributable to the drug (268). The findings included lymphocytic (and sometimes also eosinophilic) infiltration and myocyte necrosis (268). Such abnormalities, focal necrosis with inflammatory cells, are found in clinical and experimental conditions associated with catecholamine excess (270–272). Myocyte contraction band necrosis (hypereosinophilic-staining bands traversing the cytoplasm), which is a manifestation of clumped sarcomeres and is believed also to be related to catecholamine excess, was a frequent finding in one study of cocaine-associated deaths (267) but not in another (268). Left ventricular hypertrophy has also been found both in autopsies (268) and in clinical echocardiographic studies of chronic cocaine abusers (273). Though cases of acute pulmonary edema (274) and dilated cardiomyopathy (275–277) have been reported in cocaine abusers, it not clear whether any of these occurrences are related to the abnormalities that have been reported at autopsy. Moreover, a role of concomitant heavy alcohol use, an established cause of heart muscle disease, might have been contributory to the findings in some patients (275).

Cocaine use may also exert injurious effects by causing repeated elevations of blood pressure. Regular use of cocaine, moreover, is associated with systemic hypertension (278); therefore, conditions for which hypertension is a risk factor should be more prevalent in habitual users. The finding of increased left ventricular wall thickness and increased heart weight in habitual users of cocaine may be in part related to this association (268,273). The most ominous consequence of hypertension—stroke—has been related to cocaine use in some studies (279) but not in others (278,280). This disparity of findings has been attributed to patterns of drug use. It has been suggested that crack, the smoked cocaine alkaloid that has become a common mode of self-administration, may have insufficient potency to produce marked blood pressure elevations (278,280), thereby obscuring the overall relationship between cocaine abuse and stroke as determined from cohort data. Finally, aortic dissection and rupture, also complications of hypertension, have also been reported in people who use cocaine (281,282). In a *hospital* series (282), 31% of acute aortic dissection were related to the use of crack cocaine within 24 hours of onset of symptoms (average, 12 hours). Patients with cocaine-related aortic dissection were younger and more likely to be black; hypertension, particularly when untreated, was associated with acute aortic dissection, whether it was or was not related to cocaine use (282). Continued use of cocaine after an aortic dissection may result in recurrences (283). By contrast, in a series of *autopsy* cases of aortic dissection in which drug measurements had been made, only 1 of 35 had evidence of previous cocaine use (presence of benzoylecgonine) and then only in association with methamphetamine (284). This discrepancy between hospital admissions and autopsy findings suggests that unlike methamphetamine-associated aortic dissection, crack cocaine-related acute aortic dissection may be less likely to result in an immediate death (282).

Arrhythmogenesis Cocaine may also cause sudden unexpected cardiac death in individuals not having apparent coronary or myocardial abnormalities (222). Such occurrences may be related to the direct and indirect arrhythmogenic effects of the drug. In addition to its sympathomimetic effects, which are due to its central stimulatory effects (214), its peripheral adrenergic reuptake inhibitory actions (211–213), and its enhancing the effects of endogenous catecholamines (215,216), cocaine also has vagolytic actions (285). These neurohumoral properties may explain not only cocaine's effect on heart rate but various atrial and ventricular tachyarrhythmias that might result from enhancing the activity of normal and abnormal pacemaker cells (215).

Cocaine has pronounced direct effects on the myocardial transmembrane action potential as a blocker of several cation channels. Cocaine delays and reduces the amplitude of the upstroke (286), depresses the plateau phase (218), and prolongs the duration of the action potential (218); these changes are related respectively to cocaine's blocking of the sodium channel (286), L-type calcium channel (217,218), and to the delayed rectifier (218) and acetylcholine-activated (285) potassium channels. These findings have been demonstrated at concentrations comparable to those found at autopsy in cocaine-associated deaths (222). Moreover, the electrophysiologic changes have been related to stimulus-induced repetitive responses (286) and to the development of early afterdepolarizations and repetitive triggered responses (218) in the experimental laboratory. The delay in myocardial electrical conduction would also promote reentrant arrhythmias that might develop around scar tissue or occur as the result of acute myocardial ischemia. Electrocardiogram patterns, which may be precursors of ventricular tachycardia, such as a prolongation of the Q-T interval (287) and Brugada's syndrome (right bundle block pattern with characteristic ST segment elevations in leads V-1 through V-3) (288) have also been reported. Wide QRS complex tachycardias, a manifestation of sodium-channel toxicity, have been observed with cocaine overdose (289), especially in the presence of acidemia (290); this arrhythmia may be responsive to sodium bicarbonate and alkalinization (289,290). Thus, cocaine has remarkable electrophysiologic effects that can produce serious cardiac arrhythmias and even sudden death.

AMPHETAMINES AND RELATED COMPOUNDS

Amphetamines (d,l-amphetamine, methamphetamine, methylphenidate, and 3,4-methylenedioxidemethamphetamine [MDMA] are sympathomimetic drugs *without* local anesthetic actions. In addition, PCP and LSD are discussed in this section.) Amphetamines have a common β-phenylethylamine chemical structure, which they share with catecholamines; the differences in their chemical composition determine their modes of action, relative potency and sympathomimetic properties (291). Though these substances differ in their central nervous system and peripheral effects, as a group, they act by stimulating the sympathetic nervous system, by displacing catecholamines or interfering with reuptake from their storage sites, by blocking the actions of monoamine oxidase inhibition, and/or by direct adrenergic actions (291).

Amphetamines produce a dose-dependent elevation of blood pressure and an increase of heart rate (292,293). The magnitude of the changes reflects their relative α_1-adrenergic (elevate blood pressure with reflex slowing of heart rate) and β_1-adrenergic (enhance cardiac contractility and increase heart rate) effects. When amphetamines are taken parenterally, the peak vasopressor effects are evident within a half hour (292), whereas when taken by mouth, the peak changes are observed within 1 to 2 hours (293). Under experimental conditions, amphetamines have been shown to increase systolic and diastolic blood pressure in healthy subjects by 30 and 20 mm Hg, respectively (292,293). The blood pressure elevations dissipate over 3 to 4 hours (292,293). Though for MDMA and methylphenidate an increase in heart rate (20 beats/minute) parallels their blood pressure changes, for amphetamine and methamphetamine only modest heart rate changes are initially observed (the magnitude of the heart rate changes actually having an inverse relation to the blood pressure changes) (292,293). Three to four hours after the administration of amphetamine, methamphetamine, or methylphenidate, as the blood pressure elevations dissipate and the reflex baroreceptor response is attenuated, further heart rate increases ensue (a total change of as many as 20 to 30 beats/minute) that may persist above baseline for 10 hours (292,293). These changes (and accompanying body temperature elevations) may be exaggerated by intense, repetitive activities and crowded conditions (292), which may account for the adverse effects observed when these drugs have been used at discos and "raves" (294,295).

Phencyclidine (PCP) and lysergic acid diethylamide (LSD) also generally increase heart rate and blood pressure (296). In addition to its sympathomimetic effects, in experimental studies, at least, PCP has also been shown to directly enhance myocardial contractility (297), an action that is blocked by calcium channel blockade (298). Such studies using isolated heart muscle preparations have demonstrated that in high dosages, PCP can *slow* heart rate by mechanisms that have not yet been elucidated (298). The mechanisms of actions of LSD, however, are sufficiently different from amphetamines that cross-tolerance does not develop (299). All of these drugs, by their sympathomimetic actions, would also be expected to enhance thrombosis, at least by promoting platelet activation and aggregation, and to produce vasospasms.

In the context of such pharmacologic actions, amphetamines would, therefore, be expected to produce medical complications similar to those of cocaine. Ischemic (300) and hemorrhagic (301) stroke, acute myocardial infarction (302–304), aortic dissection (284), and sudden cardiac death (294,295) have all been related to amphetamine use. Methamphetamine, in particular, has been related to acute aortic dissection (284). In a series of autopsy cases of acute aortic dissection screened for drugs, 20% were related to methamphetamine (284). Ventricular tachycardia and fibrillation have also been observed after IV administration of amphetamines (305). Focal myocyte and contraction band necrosis, features of catecholamine excess, have been reported at autopsy in amphetamine abusers (295), and such findings of myocardial injury may be related to the occurrence of dilated cardiomyopathy in IV amphetamine abusers (306,307). In addition, necrotizing angiitis, indistinguishable from periarteritis nodosa, characterized by fibrinoid necrosis of the intima and media, inflammatory cellular infiltration, and aneurysmal dilatation of small and medium-sized arteries, has been reported in those who used illicit drugs who all used methamphetamine (308), and pulmonary hypertension has been found in users of propylhexedrine (309).

ANABOLIC STEROIDS

Anabolic steroids testosterone and its congeners, are abused largely by athletes intent on improving their performance. Because competitive sports produce changes in cardiac dimensions and variations in the electrocardiogram, often referred to as the "athlete's heart," it should, therefore, come as no surprise that the use of these drugs (which are sometimes used in amounts of 100 to 1,000 times their therapeutic dosages) has been related to abnormalities in the cardiovascular system. Reports of marked cardiac hypertrophy, acute myocardial infarction (sometimes with patent coronary arteries), stroke, and unexpected sudden cardiac death in young athletes using anabolic steroids, and experimental human and animal data demonstrating that these drugs can elevate blood pressure and may have unfavorable effects on blood coagulation and lipids are the basis for this concern (310).

Studies in athletes have demonstrated that anabolic steroids cause fluid retention (311), which in some (312), but not all (311), investigations is associated with an increase in systolic blood pressure. Because left ventricular hypertrophy is a feature of the athlete's heart, the contribution of anabolic steroids to this finding is often controversial (310). The presence of unusually severe hypertrophy on autopsy and evidence of abnormal left ventricular filling disclosed by Doppler echocardiography, so-called diastolic dysfunction, are abnormalities attributed to anabolic steroids (310,313). However, when left ventricular mass is adjusted for body surface area, there are no differences between body builders who use anabolic steroids and those who do not (314). This suggests that cardiomegaly in those who take anabolic steroids is a nonspecific finding related to the generalized organ-enlarging effect of these substances.

Though there are many case reports of various thrombotic complications in young athletes using anabolic steroids (310) and experimental data in rats and guinea pigs demonstrating anabolic steroid-induced increased platelet aggregability, which can be related to the androgenicity of the drug (315), studies in humans have not demonstrated that androgens promote a hypercoagulable state (316). In fact, the evidence suggests that athletes using anabolic steroids have increased plasma protein C and protein S, substances that have anticoagulant actions, and shortened euglobulin lysis times, an indication of enhanced fibrinolysis (316). However, anabolic steroids, especially when taken orally, have adverse effects on blood lipids (314,317). Administration of androgens decreases high-density lipoprotein cholesterol and increases low-density lipoprotein cholesterol (317), producing a lipid profile that favors the development of atherosclerosis. Moreover, the occurrence of an acute myocardial infarction in a young athlete with patent coronary arteries who used anabolic steroids (318) suggests vasospasm may play a role in anabolic-steroid-related cardiovascular toxicity. Thus, though anabolic steroids may be injurious to the heart, the findings are also related to the vigorous exercise and other life-style factors generally seen in users of these drugs.

DEFINITIONS: *Light use of alcohol in men: less than seven drinks each week, not binged*
Moderate use of alcohol in men: 7 to 14 drinks each week, not binged
Heavy use of alcohol in men: more than 14 drinks each week
In women, half the amount for men

REFERENCES

1. Vaisrub S. Cannabis and the cardiovascular system. *J Am Med Assoc* 1973;225:58.
2. U.S. Department of Agriculture, U.S. Department of and Human Health Services. *Nutrition and your health: dietary guide for Americans*, 4th ed. Washington, DC: Author, 1995:40–41.
3. Friedman HS. Cardiovascular effects of ethanol. In: Lieber CS, ed. *Medical and nutritional complications of alcoholism: mechanisms and management.* New York: Plenum Medical Book Company, 1992:359–401.
4. Nakano J, Moore SE. Effect of different alcohols on the contractile force of the isolated guinea pig myocardium. *Eur J Pharmacol* 1972;20: 266–270.
5. Gomes AL, Gimeno MF, Webb JL. Effects of ethanol on cellular membrane potentials and contractility of isolated rat atrium. *Am J Physiol* 1962;203:194–196.
6. Richards IS, Kulkarni A, Brooks SM, et al. A moderate concentration of ethanol alters cellular membrane potentials and decreases contractile force of human fetal heart. *Dev Pharmacol Ther* 1989;13:51–56.
7. Kelbaek H, Gjorup T, Hartling OJ, et al. Left ventricular function during alcohol intoxication and autonomic blockade. *Am J Cardiol* 1987; 59:685–688.
8. Altura BM, Altura B. Microvascular and vascular smooth muscle actions of ethanol, acetaldehyde and acetate. *Fed Proc* 1982;41:2447–2451.
9. Riff DP, Jain AC, Doyle JT. Acute hemodynamic effects of ethanol on normal human volunteers. *Am Heart J* 1969;78:592–597.
10. Blomquist G, Saltin B, Mitchell JH. Acute effects of ethanol ingestion on the response to submaximal and maximal exercise in man. *Circulation* 1970;42:463–470.
11. Delgado CE, Fortuin NJ, Ross RS. Acute effects of low doses of alcohol on left ventricular function by echocardiography. *Circulation* 1975;31: 535–540.
12. Cherrick GR, Leevy GM. The effect of ethanol metabolism on levels of oxidized and reduced nicotinamide-adenine dinucleotide in liver, kidney and heart. *Biochim Biophys Acta* 1965;107:29–37.
13. Lochner A, Cowley R, Brink AJ. Effect of ethanol on metabolism and function of perfused rat heart. *Am Heart J* 1969;78:770–780.
14. Laposata EA, Lange LG. Presence of nonoxidative ethanol metabolism in human organs commonly damaged by ethanol abuse. *Science* 1986; 231:497–499.
15. Lange LG. Nonoxidative ethanol metabolism: formation of fatty acid ethyl esters by cholesterol esterase. *Proc Natl Acad Sci* 1982;79:3954–3957.
16. Lange LG, Sobel BE. Mitochondrial dysfunction induced by fatty acid ethyl esters, myocardial metabolites or ethanol. *J Clin Invest* 1983;72: 724–731.
17. Segel LB. Mitochondrial respiration after cardiac perfusion with ethanol or acetaldehyde. *Alcohol Clin Exp Res* 1984;8:560–563.
18. Aufferman W, Wu S, Parmley WE, et al. Reversibility of acute alcohol cardiac depression: ^{31}P NMR in hamsters. *Fed Am Soc Exp Biol* 1988;2: 256–263.
19. Regan TJ, Koroxenidis G, Moschos CB, et al. The acute metabolic and hemodynamic responses of the left ventricle to ethanol. *J Clin Invest* 1966;45:270–278.
20. Preedy VR, Peters TJ. The acute and chronic effects of ethanol on cardiac protein synthesis in the rat. *Alcohol* 1989;7:97–102.
21. Williams ES, Mirro MJ, Bailey JC. Electrophysiological effects of ethanol, acetaldehyde, and acetate on cardiac tissues from dog and guinea pig. *Circ Res* 1980;47:473–478.
22. Tsai C-S, Loh S-H, Jin J-S, et al. Effects of alcohol on intracellular pH regulators and electro-mechanical parameters in human myocardium. *Res Soc Alcohol* 2005;29:1787–1795.
23. Thomas AP, Sass EJ, Tun-Kirchmann TT, Rubin E. Ethanol inhibits electrically-induced calcium transients in isolated rat cardiac myocytes. *J Mol Cell Cardiol* 1989;21:555–565.
24. Danziger RS, Sakai M, Capogrossi MC, et al. Ethanol acutely and reversibly suppresses excitation-contraction coupling in cardiac myocytes. *Circ Res* 1991;68:1660–1668.
25. Mongo KG, Vassort G. Inhibition by alcohols, halothane and chloroform of the Ca current in single frog ventricular cells. *J Mol Cell Cardiol* 1990;22:939–953.
26. Friedman HS. Cardiovascular effects of alcohol. In: M Galanter, ed. *Recent developments in alcoholism*, vol. XIV. New York: Plenum Publishing Corp., 1998:135–166.
27. Guarnieri T, Lakatta EG. Mechanism of myocardial contractile depression by clinical concentrations of ethanol. *J Clin Invest* 1990;85:1462–1467.
28. Huges JM, Henry RE, Daly MJ. Influence of ethanol and ambient temperature on skin blood flow. *Ann Emerg Med* 1984;13:597–600.
29. Shaw S, Heller EA, Friedman HS, et al. Increased hepatic oxygenation following ethanol administration in the baboon. *Proc Soc Exp Biol Med* 1977;156:509–513.
30. Fewings JD, Hanna JD, Walch JA, Whelan RF. The effects of ethyl alcohol on blood vessels of the hand and forearm in man. *Br J Pharmacol Chemother* 1966;27:93–106.
31. Friedman HS, Lowery R, Shaughnessy Scorza J. The effects of ethanol on pancreatic blood flow in awake and anesthetized dogs. *Proc Soc Exp Biol Med* 1983;174:377–382.
32. Dib JA, Cooper-Vastika SA. Acute effects of ethanol and ethanol plus furosemide on pancreatic capillary blood flow in rats. *Am J Surg* 1993; 166:18–23.
33. Foitzik T, Castillo CF, Rattner DW, et al. Alcohol selectively impairs oxygenation of the pancreas. *Arch Surg* 1985;130:357–361.
34. Altura BM, Altura B, Carella A. Ethanol produces coronary vasospasm: evidence for direct action of ethanol on vascular muscle. *Br J Pharmacol.* 1984;78:260–262.
35. Friedman HS, Lowery R, Archer M, et al. The effects of ethanol on brain blood flow in awake dogs. *J Cardiovasc Pharmacol* 1984;6:344–348.
36. Schwartz JA, Speed NM, Gross M, et al. Acute effects of alcohol administration on regional cerebral blood flow: the role of acetate. *Alcohol Clin Exp Res* 1993;17:1119–1123.

37. Sano M, Wendt PE, Wirsen A, et al. Acute effects of alcohol on regional cerebral blood flow in man. *J Stud Alcohol* 1993;54:369–376.
38. Tiihonen J, Kuikka J. Acute ethanol-induced changes in cerebral blood flow. *Am J Psychiatry* 1994;151:1505–1508.
39. Mayhan WG, Didion SP. Acute effects of ethanol on responses of cerebral arterioles. *Stroke* 1995;26:2097–2102.
40. Mendoza LC, Hellberg K, Rickart A, et al. The effect of intravenous ethyl alcohol on the coronary circulation and myocardal contractility of the human and canine heart. *J Clin Pharmacol New Drugs* 1971;11: 165–176.
41. Friedman HS, Matsuzaki S, Choe SS, et al. Demonstration of dissimilar acute hemodynamic effects of ethanol and acetaldehyde. *Cardiovasc Res* 1979;13:477–487.
42. Hayes SN, Bove A. Ethanol causes epicardial coronary artery vasoconstriction on the dog. *Circulation* 1988;78:169–170.
43. Abel FL. Direct effects of ethanol on myocardial performance and coronary resistance. *J Pharmacol Exp Ther* 1980;212:28–33.
44. Friedman HS. Acute effects of ethanol on myocardial blood flow in the nonischemic and ischemic heart. *Am J Cardiol* 1981;47:61–67.
45. Orlando J, Aronow WS, Cassidy J, Prakash R. Effect of ethanol on angina pectoris. *Ann Intern Med* 1976;84:652–655.
46. Ahlawat S, Siwach SB, Jadish S. Indirect assessment of acute effects of ethyl alcohol on coronary circulation in patients with chronic stable angina. *Int J Cardiol* 1991;33:385–392.
47. Rossinen J, Partanen J, Koskinen P, et al. Acute heavy alcohol intake increases silent myocardial ischemia in patients with stable angina pectoris. *Heart* 1996;75:563–567.
48. Takizawa A, Yasue H, Omote S. Variant angina induced by alcohol ingestion. *Am Heart J* 1984;107:25–27.
49. Brigden W, Robinson J. Alcoholic heart disease. *Br Med J* 1964;2: 1283–1289.
50. Friedman HS, Fernando H. Ascites as a marker for the hyperdynamic heart of Laennec's cirrhosis. *Alcohol Clin Exp Res* 1992;16:968–970.
51. Friedman HS, Cirillo N, Schiano F, et al. Vasodilatory state of decompensated cirrhosis: relation to hepatic dysfunction, ascites and vasoconstrictive substances. *Alcohol Clin Exp Res* 1995;19:123–129.
52. Spodick DH, Pigott VM, Chirife R. Preclinical cardiac malfunction on chronic alcoholism. *N Engl J Med* 1972;287:677–680.
53. Mathews E, Gardin JM, Henry W, et al. Echocardiographic abnormalities in chronic alcoholics with and without overt congestive heart failure. *Am J Cardiol* 1981;47:570–576.
54. Friedman HS, Vasavada BC, Malec AM, et al. Cardiac function in alcohol-associated hypertension. *Am J Cardiol* 1986;57:227–231.
55. Regan TJ, Levinson GE, Oldewurtel HA, et al. Ventricular function in noncardiacs with alcoholic fatty liver: role of ethanol in the production of cardiomyopathy. *J Clin Invest* 1969;48:397–406.
56. Wendt VE, Wu C, Balcon R, et al. Hemodynamic and metabolic effect of chronic alcoholism in man. *Am J Cardiol* 1965;15: 178–184.
57. Alexander CS. Idiopathic heart disease. *Am J Med* 1966;41:213–228.
58. Alexander CS. Electron microscopic observations in alcoholic heart disease. *Br Heart J* 1967;29:200–206.
59. Tsiplenkova VG, Vihert AA, Cherpachenko NM. Ultrastructure and histochemical observations in human and experimental alcoholic cardiomyopathy. *J Am Coll Cardiol* 1986;8:22A–32A.
60. Estruch R, Fernandez-Sola J, Sacanella E, et al. Relationship between cardiomyopathy and liver disease in chronic alcoholism. *Hepatology* 1995;22:532–538.
61. Vorobioff J, Bredfeldt JE, Groszmann RJ. Hyperdynamic circulation in protal-hypertensive rat model: a primary factor for maintenance of chronic portal hypertension. *Am J Physiol* 1983;244:G52–G57.
62. Lee FY, Albillos A, Colombato LA, Groszmann J. The role of nitric oxide in the vascular hyporesponsiveness to methoxamine in portal hypertensive rats. *Hepatology* 1992;16:1043–1048.
63. Seiber CC, Groszmann RJ. Nitric oxide mediates hyporeactivity to vasopressors in mesenteric vessels of protal hypertensive rats. *Gastroenterology* 1992;103:235–239.
64. Pizcueta P, Pique JM. Modulation of the hyperdynamic circulation of cirrhotic rats by nitric oxide inhibition. *Gastroenterology* 1992;103:1909–1915.
65. Sogni P, Moreau R. Evidence for normal nitric oxide-mediated vasodilator tone in conscious rats with cirrhosis. *Hepatology* 1992;16:980–983.
66. Campillo B, Chabrier PE. Inhibition of nitric oxide synthesis in the forearm arterial bed of patients with advanced cirrhosis. *Hepatology* 1995;22:1423–1429.
67. Eliaser M Giansiracusa FJ. The heart and alcohol. *Calif Med* 1956; 84:234–236.
68. Kino M, Imamitchi H, Morigutehi M, et al. Cardiovascular status in asymptomatic alcoholics, with reference to the level of ethanol consumption. *Br Heart J* 1981;46:545–551.
69. Urbano-Marquez A, Estruch R, Navarro-Lopez R, et al. The effects of alcoholism on skeletal and cardiac muscle. *N Engl J Med* 1989;320: 409–415.
70. Fernandez-Sola J, Estruch R, Grau JM, et al. The relation of alcoholic myopathy to cardiomyopathy. *Ann Intern Med* 1994;120:529–536.
71. Fernandez-Sola J, Nicolas JM. Angiotensin-converting gene polymorphism is associated with vulnerability to alcoholic cardiomyopathy. *Ann Intern Med* 2002;137:321–326.
72. Demakis JG, Proskey A, Rahimtoola SH. et al. The natural course of alcoholic cardiomyopathy. *Ann Intern Med* 1974;80:293–297.
73. Morin YL, Foley AR, Martineau G, Roussel J. Quebec beer-drinkers' cardiomyopathy: forty-eight cases. *Can Med Assoc J* 1967;97:881–904.
74. Miller H, Abelmann WH. Effects of dietary ethanol upon experimental trypanosomal (T. cruzi) myocarditis. *Proc Soc Exp Biol* 1967;126: 193–198.
75. Morin Y, Roy PE, Mohiuddin SM, Tasker PK. The influences of alcohol on viral and isoproterenol cardiomyopathy. *Cardiovasc Res* 1969;3:363–368.
76. Clark LT, Friedman HS. Hypertension associated with alcohol withdrawal: assessment of mechanisms and complications. *Alcohol Clin Exp Res* 1985;9:125–130.
77. King AC, Errico AL, Parsons OA, Lovallo WR. Blood pressure dysregulation associated with alcohol withdrawal. *Alcohol Clin Exp Res* 1991;12:478–482.
78. Thorton JR. Atrial fibrillation in healthy non-alcoholic people after an alcoholic binge. *Lancet* 1984;ii:1013–1017.
79. Schwartz L, Sample B, Wigle D. Severe alcoholic cardiomyopathy reversed with abstention from alcohol. *Am J Cardiol* 1975;36:963–966.
80. Molgaar H, Kristensen BO, Basndrup U. Importance of abstention from alcohol in alcoholic heart disease. *Int J Cardiol* 1990;27:372–375.
81. Ettinger PO, Wu CF, De La Cruz C, et al. Arrhythmias and the "holiday heart": alcohol associated cardiac rhythm disorders. *Am Heart J* 1978;95:555–562.
82. Rich EC, Siebold C, Campion B. Alcohol-related acute atrial fibrillation: a case-control study and review of 40 patients. *Arch Intern Med* 1985;145:830–833.
83. Engel TR, Luck JC. Effect of whiskey on atrial vulnerability and "holiday heart." *J Am Coll Cardiol* 1983;1:816–818.
84. Greenspon AJ, Schaal SG. The "holiday heart": electrophysiologic studies of alcohol effects in alcoholics. *Ann Intern Med* 1983;98:135–139.
85. Greenspon AJ, Stang JM, Lewis RP, Schaal SF. Provocation of ventricular tachycardia after consumption of alcohol. *N Engl J Med* 1979;301: 1049–1050.
86. Luca C. Electrophysiological properties of right heart and atrioventricular conducting system in patients with alcoholic cardiomyopathy. *Br Heart J* 1979;42:274–281.
87. Paradise RR, Stoelting V. Conversion of acetyl strophanthidin-induced ventricular tachycardia to sinus rhythm by ethyl alcohol. *Arch Int Pharmacodyn Ther* 1965;157:312–321.
88. Madan BR, Gupta RS. Effect of ethanol in experimental auricular and ventricular arrhythmias. *Jpn J Pharmacol* 1967;17:683–684.
89. Kostis JB, Horstmann E, Mavrogeogis E, et al. Effects of alcohol on the electrocardiogram. *Circulation* 1971;44:558–564.
90. Gilmour RF, Ruffy R, Lovelace DE, et al. Effect of ethanol on electrogram changes and regional myocardial blood flow during acute myocardial ischaemia. *Cardiovasc Res* 1981;15:47–58.

91. Nguyen TN, Friedman HS, Mokraoui AM. Effects of alcohol on experimental atrial fibrillation. *Alcohol Clin Exp Res* 1987;11:474–476.
92. Kramer K, Kuller L, Fisher R. The increasing mortality attributed to cirrhosis and fatty liver in Baltimore (1957–1966). *Ann Intern Med* 1968;69:273–282.
93. Randall B. Sudden death and hepatic fatty metamorphosis. *J Am Med Assoc* 1980;243:1723–1725.
94. Lithell G, Aberg H, Selinus I, Hedstrand H. Alcohol intemperance and sudden death. *Br Med J* 1987;294:1456–1458.
95. Orgata M, Mendelson JH, Mello NK, Majechrowicz W. Adrenal function and alcoholism. *Psychosom Med* 1971;33:159–180.
96. Renaud SC, Ruf JC. Effects of alcohol on platelet functions. *Clin Chim Acta* 1996;246:77–89.
97. Novak DJ, Victor M. The vagus and sympathetic nerves in alcoholic polymyopathy. *Arch Neurol* 1974;30:273–294.
98. Fraser GE, Upsdell M. Alcohol and other discriminants between cases of sudden death and myocardial infarction. *Am J Edpidemiol* 1981;114: 462–476.
99. Albert CM, Manson JE, Cook NR. Moderate alcohol consumption and the risk of sudden cardiac death among male physicians. *Circulation* 1999;100:944–950.
100. Randin D, Vollenweider P, Tappy L, et al. Suppression of alcohol-induced hypertension by dexamethasone. *N Engl J Med* 1995;332: 1733–1737.
101. Grassi GM, Somers VK, Renk WS, et al. Effects of alcohol intake on blood pressure and sympathetic nerve activity in normotensive humans: a preliminary report. *J Hypertens* 1989;7(Suppl 6):S20–S21.
102. Abdel-Rahman ARA, Merrill RH, Wolles WR. Effect of acute ethanol administration on the baroreceptor reflex control of heart rate in normotensive human volunteers. *Clin Sci* 1987;72:113–122.
103. Potter JE, Beevers DG. Pressor effect of alcohol in hypertension. *Lancet* 1984;i:119–122.
104. Puddey JE, Beilin IJ, Vandongen R, et al. Evidence for a direct effect of alcohol on blood pressure in normotensive men. *Hypertension* 1985;7:707–713.
105. Puddey JE, Beilin IJ, Vandongen R. Regular alcohol use raises blood pressure in treated hypertensive subjects. *Lancet* 1987;1:647–662.
106. Malhotra H, Mathur D, Mehta SR, Khandelwal PD. Pressor effects of alcohol in normotensive and hypertensive subjects. *Lancet* 1985;2: 584–586.
107. Chan TCK, Sutter MC. Ethanol consumption and blood pressure. *Life Sci* 1983;33:1965–1973.
108. Friedman HS. Alcohol and hypertension. In: EB Feldman, ed. *Nutrition and heart disease.* New York: Churchill Livingstone, 1990:35–50.
109. Klatsky AL, Armstrong MA, Friedman GD. Alcohol and mortality. *Ann Intern Med* 1992;117:646–654.
110. Cooke KM, Frost GW, Thornell IR, Stokes GS. Alcohol consumption and blood pressure. *Med J Aust* 1982;1:65–69.
111. Fortman SP, Haskell WL, Vranizan K, et al. The association of blood pressure and dietary alcohol: differences by age, sex and estrogen use. *Am J Edpidemiol* 1983;118:496–507.
112. Beevers DB, Bannan LT, Saunders JB, et al. Alcohol and hypertension. *Contrib Nephrol* 1982;30:92–97.
113. Dyer AR, Stamler J. Alcohol consumption and 17-year mortality in the Chicago Western Electric Company Study. *Prev Med* 1980;9: 78–90.
114. Gill JS, Zezulka AV, Shipley MJ, et al. Stroke and alcohol consumption. *N Engl J Med* 1986;315:1041–1046.
115. Wannamethee SG, Shaper AG. Patterns of alcohol intake and risk of stroke in middle-aged British men. *Stroke* 1996;27:1033–1039.
116. Mukamal KJ, Maclure M, Muller JE, Mittleman MA. Binge drinking and mortality after acute myocardial infarction. *Circulation* 2005;112: 3839–3848.
117. Fuchs CS, Stampfer MJ, Colditz GA, et al. Alcohol consumption and mortality among women. *N Engl J Med* 1995;332:1245–1250.
118. Rimm EB. Prospective study of alcohol consumption and risk of coronary disease in men. *Lancet* 1991;338:464–468.
119. Berger K, Ajani UA. Light-to-moderate alcohol consumption and the risk of stroke among U.S. male physicians. *N Engl J Med* 1999;341: 1557–1564.
120. Kozararevic DJ, Vojvodic N, Dawber T. et al. Frequency of alcohol consumption and morbidity and mortality: the Yugoslavia Cardiovascular Disease Study. *Lancet* 1980;1:613–617.
121. Stickel F, Choi S-W, Kim Y-I. Effect of chronic alcohol consumption on total homocysteine level in rats. *Alcohol Clin Exp Res* 2000;24:259–264.
122. Van Der Gaag MS, Ubbink JB, Sillanaukee P, et al. Effect of consumption of red wine, spirits, beer on serum homocysteine. *Lancet* 2000;355:1522.
123. Gaziano JM, Buring JE. Moderate alcohol intake, increase of high-density lipoprotein and its subfractions and decreased risk of myocardial infarction. *N Engl J Med* 1993;329:1829–1834.
124. Donahue RP, Abbott RD, Reed DM, Yano K. Alcohol and hemorrhagic stroke. *J Am Med Assoc* 1986;255:2311–2314.
125. Hein OH, Suadicani P. Alcohol consumption, serum low density lipoprotein cholesterol concentration, and risk of ischemic heart disease: six year follow up in the Copenhagen male study. *Br Med J* 1996;312: 736–741.
126. Suh I, Shaten J, Cutler JA, Kuller LH. Alcohol use and mortality from coronary heart disease: the role of high-density lipoprotein cholesterol. *Ann Intern Med* 1992;116:881–887.
127. Mead TW, Imeson J, Stirling Y. Effects of changes in smoking and other characteristics on clotting factors and the risk of ischemic disease. *Lancet* 1987;2:986–988.
128. Heinrich J, Balleisen L, Schulte H, et al. Fibrinogen and factor VII in the prediction of coronary risk. *Arterioscleros Thrombos* 1994;14: 54–59.
129. Ruf JC, Berger JL, Renaud S. Platelet rebound effect of alcohol withdrawal and wine drinking in rats. Relation to tannins and lipid peroxidation. *Arteriocleros Thrombos Vasc Biol* 1995;15:140–144.
130. Deykin D, Janson P, McMahon L. Ethanol potentiation of aspirin-induced prolongation of the bleeding-time. *N Engl J Med* 1982;306: 852–854.
131. Ridker PM, Vaughan DE, Stampfer MJ, et al. Association of moderate alcohol consumption and plasma concentration of endogenous tissue-type plasminogen activator. *J Am Med Assoc* 1994;272:929–933.
132. Krenz M, Cohen MV, Downey JM. Protective and anti-protective effects of acute ethanol exposure in myocardial ischemia/reperfusion. *Pathophysiology* 2004;10:113–119.
133. Pagel PS, Kersten JR. Mechanisms of myocardial protection produced by chronic ethanol consumption. *Pathophysiology* 2004;10:121–129.
134. Krenz M, Baines CP, Heusch G. Acute ethanol exposure fails to elicit preconditioning-like protection in in situ rabbit hearts because of its continued presence during ischemia. *J Am Coll Cardiol* 2001;37: 601–607.
135. Niccoli G, Altamura L. Ethanol abolishes ischemic preconditioning in humans. *J Am Coll Cardiol* 2008;51:271–275.
136. Jackson R, Scragg R, Beaglehole R. Does recent alcohol consumption reduce the risk of acute myocardial infarction and coronary death in regular drinkers. *Am J Edpidemiol* 1992;136:819–824.
137. McElduff P, Dobson AJ. How much alcohol and how often? Population based case-control study of alcohol consumption and risk of a major coronary event. *Br Med J* 1997;314:1159–1164.
138. Mukamal KJ, Muller JE, Maclure M. Lack of effect of recent alcohol consumption on the course of acute myocardial infarction. *Am Heart J* 1999;138:926–933.
139. Muntwyler J, Hennekens CH, Buring JE. Mortality and light to moderate alcohol consumption after myocardial infarction. *Lancet* 1998;352(9144):1882–1885.
140. De Lorgeril, M Salen P. Wine drinking and risks of cardiovascular complications after recent acute myocardial infarction. *Circulation* 2002; 106:1465–1469.
141. Aguilar D, Skali H Moye LA. Alcohol consumption and prognosis in patients with left ventricular dysfunction after myocardial infarction. *J Am Coll Cardiol* 2004;43:2015–2021.

142. Rimm EB, Klatsky A, Grobbee D, Stampfer MJ. Review of moderate alcohol consumption and reduced risk of coronary heart disease: is the effect due to beer, wine, or spirits. *BMJ* 1996;312:731–736.
143. Hines LM, Stampfer MJ. Genetic variation in alcohol dehydrogenase and the beneficial effect of moderate alcohol consumption on myocardial infarction. *N Engl J Med* 2001;344:549–555.
144. Kannel WB. Update on the role of cigarette smoking in coronary artery disease. *Am Heart J* 1981;101:319–328.
145. Cryer PE, Haymond MW, Santiago JV, Shah SD. Norepinephrine and epinephrine release and adrenergic mediation of smoking-associated hemodynamic and metabolic events. *N Engl J Med* 1976;295:573–577.
146. Niedermaier ON, Smith ML, Beightol LA, et al. Influence of cigarette smoking on human autonomic function. *Circulation* 1993;88: 562–571.
147. Grassi G, Seravalle G. Mechanisms responsible for sympathetic activation by cigarette smoking in humans. *Circulation* 1994;90:248–253.
148. Benowitz NL, Jacob P, Jones RT, Rosenberg J. Interindividual variability in the metabolism and cardiovascular effects of nicotine in man. *J Pharmacol Exp Ther* 1982;221:368–272.
149. Benowitz NL, Gourlay SG. Cardiovascular toxicity of nicotine: implications for nicotine replacement therapy. *J Am Coll Cardiol* 1997;29: 1422–1431.
150. Klein LW, Ambrose J. Acute coronary hemodynamic response to cigarette smoking in patients with coronary artery disease. *J Am Coll Cardiol* 1984;3:879–886.
151. Winnford MD, Wheelan KR. Smoking-induced coronary vasoconstriction in patients with atherosclerotic artery disease: evidence for adrenergically mediated alterations in coronary artery tone. *Circulation* 1986;72:662–667.
152. Winnford MD, Jansen DE, Reynolds GA, et al. Cigarette smoking-induced coronary vasoconstriction in atherosclerotic coronary artery disease and prevention by calcium antagonists and nitroglycerin. *Am J Cardiol* 1987;59:203–207.
153. Moliterno DJ, Willard JE, Lange RA, et al. Coronary-artery vasoconstriction induced by cocaine, cigarette smoking, or both. *N Engl J Med* 1994;330:454–459.
154. Newby DE, McLeod AL, Uren NG. Impaired coronary tissue plasminogen activator release is associated with coronary atherosclerosis and cigarette smoking. *Circulation* 2001;103:1936–1941.
155. Aronow WS, Cassidy J, Vangrow JS, et al. Effect of cigarette smoking and breathing carbon dioxide on cardiovascular dynamics in anginal patients. *Circulation* 1974a;50:340–347.
156. Aronow WS, Kaplan MA, Desiderio J. Tobacco: a precipitating factor in angina pectoris. *Ann Intern Med* 1968;69:529–536.
157. Aronow WS, Swanson AJ. The effect of low-nicotine cigarettes on angina pectoris. *Ann Intern Med* 1969;71:599–601.
158. Barry J, Mead K. Effect of smoking on activity of ischemic heart disease. *J Am Med Assoc* 1989;261:398–402.
159. Levine PH. An acute effect of cigarette smoking on platelet function. A possible link between smoking and thrombosis. *Circulation* 1973;48: 619–623.
160. Benowitz NL, Fitzgerald GA, Wilson, MS Zhang Q. Nicotine effects on eicosanoid formation and hemostatic function: comparison of transdermal nicotine and cigarette smoking. *J Am Coll Cardiol* 1993;22: 1159–1167.
161. Wennmalm Å, Benthin G, Granström EF, et al. Relation between tobacco use and urinary excretion of thromboxane A_2 and prostacyclin metabolites in young men. *Circulation* 1991;83:1698–1704.
162. Castelli WP. Cardiovascular disease: pathogenesis, epidemiology, and risk among users of oral contraceptives who smoke. *Am J Obstet Gynecol* 1999;180:S349–356.
163. Barbash GK, White HD. Significance of smoking in patients receiving thrombolytic therapy for acute myocardial infarction. *Circulation* 1993;87:53–58.
164. de Chillou C, Riff P. Influence of cigarette smoking on rate of reopening of the infarct-related coronary artery after myocardial infarction. *J Am Coll Cardiol* 1996;27:1662–1668.
165. Mann J, Davies MJ. Mechanisms of progression in native coronary artery disease: role of healed plaque disruption. *Heart* 1999;82:265–268.
166. Criqui MH, Wallace RG, Heiss G, et al. Cigarette smoking and plasma high-density lipoprotein cholesterol. *Circulation.* 1980;62(Suppl IV): 70–76.
167. Benowitz NL, Gourlay MB. Cardiovascular toxicity of nicotine replacement therapy. *J Am Coll Cardiol* 1997;29:1422–1431.
168. Kimmel SE, Berlin JA, Miles C, et al. Risk of acute myocardial infarction and use of nicotine patches in a general population. *J Am Coll Cardiol* 2001;37:1297–1302.
169. Kimmel SE, Berlin JA, Miles C, et al. Risk of acute myocardial infarction and use of nicotine patches in a general population. *J Am Coll Cardiol* 2001;37:1297–1302.
170. Beaconsfield P, Ginsburg J, Rainsbury R. Marihuana smoking. *N Engl J Med* 1972;287:209–212.
171. Weiss JL, Watanabe AM, Lemberger L, et al. Cardiovascular effects of delta-9-tetrahydrocannabinol in man. *Clin Pharmacol Ther* 1972;13:671–684.
172. Perez-Reyes M, Lipton MA, Timmons MC, et al. Pharmacology of orally administered Δ-9-tetrahydrocannabinol. *Clin Pharmacol Ther* 1973;14:48–55.
173. Malit LA, Johnstone RE, Bourke DI, et al. Intravenous Δ-9-tetrahydrocannabinol: effects on ventilatory control and cardiovascular dynamics. *Anesthesiology* 1975;42:666–673.
174. Kanakis C, Pouget JM, Rosen KM. The effects of delta-9-tetrahydrocannabinol (cannabis) on cardiac performance with and without beta-blockade. *Circulaton* 1996;53:703–707.
175. Tashkin DP, Levisman JA, Abbasi AS, et al. Short-term effects of smoked marihuana on left ventricular function in man. *Chest* 1977;72:20–26.
176. Shapiro BJ. Cardiovascular effects of cannabis. In: Tashkin DP (moderator). *Cannabis, 1997. Ann Intern Med* 1978;89:539–549.
177. Johnson S, Domino EF. Some cardiovascular effects of marihuana smoking in normal volunteers. *Clin Pharmacol Ther* 1971;12:762–768.
178. Kochar M, Hosko MJ. Electrocardiographic effects of marihuana. *J Am Med Assoc* 1973;225:25–27.
179. Perez-Reyes M, White WR, McDonald SA, et al. The pharmacologic effects of daily marijuanc smoking in humans. *Pharmacol Biochem Behav* 1991;40:691–694.
180. Cone EJ, Welch P. Clonidine partially blocks the physiologic effects but not the subjective effects produced by smoking marihuana in male human subjects. *Pharmacol Biochem Behav* 1988;29:649–642.
181. Prakash R, Aronow WS, Warren M, et al. Effects of marihuana and placebo marihuana on hemodynamics in coronary disease. *Clin Pharmacol Ther* 1975;18:90–95.
182. Benowitz NL, Jones RT. Cardiovascular effects of prolonged delta-9-tetrahydrocannabinol ingestion. *Clin Pharmacol Ther* 1977;18:287–297.
183. Aronow WS, Cassidy J. Effect of marihuana and placebo-marihuana on angina pectoris. *N Engl J Med* 1974;291:65–67.
184. Tashkin DP, Gliedereer F, Rose J, et al. Effects of varying marijuana smoking profile on deposition of tar and absorption of CO and delta-9-THC. *Pharmacol Biochem Behav* 1991;40:651–656.
185. Mittleman MA, Lewis RA, Maclure M, et al. Triggering of myocardial infarction by marijuana. *Circulation* 2001;103:2805–2809.
186. Eckenhoff JE, Oech SR. The effects of narcotics and antagonists upon respiration and circulation in man. A review. *Clin Pharmacol Ther* 1960; 1:483–524.
187. Samuel IO, Clarke SJ, Dundee JW. Some circulatory and respiratory effects of morphine in patients without pre-existing cardiac disease. *Br J Anesthesiol* 1977;49:927–932.
188. Tress KH, El-Sorbky AA. Cardiovascular, respiratory and temperature responses to intravenous heroin (diamorphine) in dependent and non-dependent humans. *Br J Clin Pharmacol* 1980;10:477–485.
189. Sethna D, Moffitt EA, Gray RJ, et al. Cardiovascular effects of morphine in patients with coronary arterial disease. *Anesth Analg* 1982;1982: 109–114.
190. Roth A, Keren G, Gluck A, et al. Comparison of nalbuphine hydrochloride versus morphine sulfate for acute myocardial infarction with elevated pulmonary artery wedge pressure. *Am J Cardiol* 1988;62:551–555.

191. Vatner SF, Marsh JD, Swain JA. Effects of morphine on coronary and left ventricular dynamics in conscious dogs. *J Clin Invest* 1975;55: 207–217.
192. Strauer BE. Contractile responses to morphine, piretanide, meperidine and fentanyl: a comparative study of effects on the isolated ventricular myocardium. *Anesthesiology* 1972;37:304–310.
193. Gould L, Reddy CVR, Oh DC, et al. Hemodynamic effects of morphine in cardiac disease. *J Clin Pharmacol* 1978;18:448–456.
194. Vismara LA, Leaman DM, Zelis R. The effects of morphine on venous tone in patients with acute pulmonary edema. *Circulation* 1976;54: 335–337.
195. Leaman DM, Levenson L, Zelis R. et al. Effect of morphine on splanchnic blood flow. *Br Heart J* 1978a;40:569–571.
196. Stefano GB, Hartman A, Bilfinger TV, et al. Presence of μ^3 opiate receptor in endothelial cells. Coupling to nitric oxide production and vasodilation. *J Biol Chem* 1995;270:30290–30293.
197. Stefano GB, Salzet M, Hughes TK, Bilfinger TV. Δ^2 opioid receptor subtype on human vascular endothelium uncouples morphine stimulated nitric oxide release. *Int J Cardiol* 1998;1:S43–S51.
198. Flaim SR, Vismara LA, Zelis R. The effects of morphine on isolated cutaneous canine vascular smooth muscle. *Res Commun Chem Pathol Pharmacol* 1977;16:191–194.
199. Leaman DM, Levenson L, Zelis R, et al. Effects of morphine sulfate on human coronary blood flow. *Am J Cardiol* 1978b;41:324–326.
200. Schultz JJ, Hsu AK, Gross GJ. Ischemic preconditioning and morphine-induced cardioprotection involve the delta-opioid receptor in the intact rat heart. *J Mol Cell Cardiol* 1997;29:2187–2195.
201. Lliang BT, Gross GJ. Direct preconditioning of cardiac myocytes via opioid receptors and KATP channels. *Circ Res* 1999;84:1396–1400.
202. Rabkin SW. Morphine and morphiceptin increase the threshold for epinephrine-induced cardiac arrhythmas in the rat brain mu opioid receptors. *Clin Exp Pharmacol Physiolo* 1993;20:95–102.
203. Sarne Y, Flitsen A, Oppenheimer E. Anti-arrhythmic activities of opioid agonists and antagonists and their stereoisomers. *Br J Pharmacol* 1991; 102:696–698.
204. Edsilva RA, Verrier RL, Lown B. Protective effects of the vagotonic action of morphine sulphate on ventricular fibrillation. *Cardiovasc Res* 1978;12:167–172.
205. Pons-Lladó G, Carreras F, Borrás X, et al. Findings on Doppler echocardiography in asymptomatic intravenous heroin users. *Am J Cardiol* 1992;69:238–241.
206. Stein AD, Karliner JS. The clinical spectrum of heroin pulmonary edema. *Arch Intern Med* 1968;122:122–127.
207. Bogartz LJ, Miller WC. Pulmonary edema associated with propoxyphene intoxication. *J Am Med Assoc* 1971;215:259–262.
208. Katz S, Aberman A, Frand UI, et al. Heroin pulmonary edema: evidence for increased pulmonary capillary permeability. *Am Rev Respir Dis* 1972;106:472–474.
209. Brashear RE, Kelly MT, White AC. Elevated plasma histamine after heroin and morphine. *J Lab Clin Med* 1974;83:451–457.
210. Andy JJ, Sheikh Ali N, et al. Echocardiographic observations in opiate addicts with active endocarditis. *Am J Cardiol* 1977;40:17–23.
211. Richie JM, Green NM. Local anesthetics. In: Gilman AG, Rall TW, Nies AS, et al., eds. *The pharmacologic basis of therapeutics.* New York: Pergamon Press, 1990:311–331.
212. Kloner RA, Hale SH, Alker K, Rezkalla S. The effects of acute and chronic cocaine use on the heart. *Circulation* 1992;85:407–419.
213. Pitts WR, Lange RA, Cigarroa Hillis LD. Cocaine-induced myocardial ischemia and infarction: pathophysiology, recognition, and management. *Prog Cardivasc Dis* 1997;40:65–76.
214. Shannon RP, Mathier MA, Shen Y-T. Role of cardiac nerves in the cardiovascular response to cocaine in conscious dogs. *Circulation* 2001;103: 1674–1680.
215. Trendelenburg U. The effects of cocaine on the pacemaker of isolated guinea-pig atria. *J Pharmacol Exp Ther* 1968;161:222–231.
216. Greenberg R, Innes IR. The role of bound calcium in supersensitivity induced by cocaine. *Br J Pharmacol* 1976;57:329–334.
217. Josephson I, Sperelakis N. Local anesthetic blockade of Ca^{2+}-mediated action potentials in cardiac muscle. *Eur J Pharmacol* 1976;40:201–208.
218. Kimura S, Bassett AL, Myerburg RJ. Early afterdepolarizations and triggered activity induced by cocaine. A possible mechanism of cocaine arrhythmogenesis. *Circulation* 1992;85:2226–2235.
219. Egashira K, Morgan KG, Morgan JP. Effects of cocaine on excitation-contraction coupling of aortic smooth muscle from the ferret. *J Clin Invest* 1991;87:1322–1328.
220. Wilkerson RD. Cardiovascular effects of cocaine in conscious dogs: importance of fully functional autonomic nervous systems. *J Pharmacol Exp Ther* 1988;246:466–471.
221. Fraker TD, Temesy-Armos PN, Brewster PS, Wilkerson RD. Mechanisms of cocaine-induced myocardial depression. *Circulation* 1990;81: 1012–1016.
222. Shen W-K, Edwards WD, Hammill SC, et al. Sudden unexpected non-traumatic death in 54 young adults: a 30-year population based study. *Am J Cardiol* 1995;76:148–152.
223. Chambers HF, Morris DL, Tauber MG, Modin G. Cocaine use and the risk of endocarditis in intravenous drug users. *Ann Intern Med* 1987; 106:833–836.
224. Perreault CL, Hague NL, Morgan KG, Allen PD Morgan JP. Negative inotropic and relaxant effects of cocaine on myopathic human ventricular myocardium and epicardial coronary arteries *in vitro*. *Cardiovasc Res* 1993;27:262–268.
225. Morcos NC, Fairhurst A, Henry WL. Direct myocardial effects of cocaine. *Cardiovasc Res* 1993;27:269–273.
226. Daniel WC, Lange RA, Landau C, et al. Effects of the intracoronary infusion of cocaine and coronary arterial dimensions and blood flow in humans. *Am J Cardiol* 1996;78:288–291.
227. Hale SL, Alker KJ, Rezkalla S, et al. Adverse effects of cocaine on cardiovascular dynamics, myocardial blood flow, and coronary artery diameter in an experimental model. *Am Heart J* 1989;118:927–933.
228. Pitts WR, Vongpatanasin W, Cigarro JE, et al. Effects of intracoronary infusion of cocaine on left ventricular systolic and diastolic function in humans. *Circulation* 1998;97:1270–1273.
229. Lange RA, Cigarroa RG, Yancy CW, et al. Cocaine-induced coronary-artery vasoconstriction. *N Engl J Med* 1989;321:1557–1562.
230. Lange RA, Cigarroa RG, Flores ED, et al. Potentiation of cocaine-induced coronary vasoconstriction by beta-adrenergic blockade. *Ann Intern Med* 1990;112:897–903.
231. Kuhn FR, Gillis RA, Virmani R, et al. Cocaine produces coronary artery vasoconstriction independent of an intact endothelium. *Chest* 1992;102: 581–585.
232. Pirwitz MJ, Willard JE, Landau C, et al. Influence of cocaine, ethanol, or their combination on epicardial coronary dimensions in humans. *Arch Intern Med* 1995;155:1186–1191.
233. Boehrer J, Moliterno DJ, Willard JE, et al. Influence of labetalol on cocaine-induced coronary vasoconstriction in humans. *Am J Med* 1993; 94:608–610.
234. Henning RJ, Wilson LD. Cocaethylene is as cardiotoxic as cocaine but is less toxic than cocaine plus ethanol. *Life Sci* 1996;59:615–627.
235. Foltin RW, Fischman MW, Pedroso JJ, Pearlson GD. Marijuana and cocaine interactions in humans: Cardiovascular consequences. *Pharmacol Biochem Behav* 1987;28:459–464.
236. Foltin RW, Fischman MW. The effects of combinations of intranasal cocaine, smoked marijuana, and task performance on heart rate and blood pressure. *Pharmacol Biochem Behav* 1990;36:311–315.
237. Coleman DW, Ross TF, Naughton JL. Myocardial ischemia and infarction related to recreational cocaine use. *West J Med* 1982;136: 444–446.
238. Pasternack PF, Colvin SB, Baumann FG. Cocaine-induced angina pectoris and acute myocardial infarction in patients younger than 40 years. *Am J Cardiol* 1985;55:847.
239. Isner JM, Estes M, Thompson PD, et al. Acute cardiac events temporally related to cocaine abuse. *N Engl J Med* 1986;315:1438–1443.
240. Smith HWB, Liberman HA, Brody SL, et al. Acute myocardial infarction temporally related to cocaine use. *Ann Intern Med* 1987;107:13–18.

241. Mittleman MA, Mintzer D, Maclure M, et al. Triggering of myocardial infarction by cocaine. *Circulation* 1999;99:2737–2741.
242. Kolodgie FD, Virmani R, Cornhill JF, et al. Increase in atherosclerosis and adventitial mast cells in cocaine abusers: an alternative mechanism of cocaine-associated coronary vasospasm and thrombosis. *J Am Coll Cardiol* 1991;17:1553–1560.
243. Zimmerman FH, Gustafson GM, Kemp HG. Recurrent myocardial infarction associated with cocaine abuse in a young man with normal coronary arteries: evidence for coronary artery spasm culminating in thrombosis. *J Am Coll Cardiol* 1987;9:964–968.
244. Togna G, Tempesta E, Togna AR, et al. Platelet responsiveness and biosynthesis of thromboxane and prostacycline in response to *in vitro* cocaine treatment. *Haemostasis* 1985;15:100–107.
245. Moliterno DJ, Lange RA, Gerard RD, et al. Influence of intranasal cocaine on plasma constituents associated with endogenous thrombosis and thrombolysis. *Am J Med* 1994;96:492–496.
246. Heesch CM, Wilhelm CR, Ristich J, et al. Cocaine activates platelets and increases the formation of circulating platelets containing microaggregates in humans. *Heart* 2000;83:688–695.
247. Rinder HM, Ault KA, Jatlow PL, et al. Platelet alpha-granule release in cocaine users. *Circulation* 1994;90:1162–1167.
248. Hollander JE. The management of cocaine-associated myocardial ischemia. *N Engl J Med* 1995;333:1267–1272.
249. Hollander JE, Levitt MA, Young GP, et al. Effect of recent cocaine use on the specificity of cardiac markers for diagnosis of acute myocardial infarction. *Am Heart J* 1998;135:245–252.
250. Brogan WC, Lange RA, Kim AS, et al. Alleviation of cocaine-induced coronary vasoconstriction by nitroglycerin. *J Am Coll Cardiol* 1991;18: 581–586.
251. Van Dyke C, Barash PG, Jatlow P, Byck R. Cocaine:plasma concentrations after intranasal application in man. *Science* 1976;191:859–861.
252. Derlet RW, Albertson TE. Diazepam in the prevention of seizures and death in cocaine-intoxicated rats. *Ann Emerg Med* 1989;18:542–546.
253. Baumann BM, Perrone J, Hornig SE, et al. Randomized, double-blind, placebo-controlled trial of diazepam, nitroglycerin, or both for treatment of patients with potential cocaine-associated acute coronary syndromes. *Acad Emerg Med* 2000;7:878–885.
254. McCord J, Jneid H, Hollander JE, et al. Management of cocaine-associated chest pain and myocardial infarction. A scientific statement of the American Heart Association Acute Cardiac Care Committee of the Council on Clinical Cardiology. *Circulation* 2008;117:1897–1907.
255. Hollander JE, Burstein JL, Hoffman RS, et al. Cocaine-associated myocardial infarction: clinical safety of thrombolytic therapy. *Chest* 1995;107:1237–1241.
256. Hoffman RS, Hollander JE. Thrombolytic therapy and cocaine-induced myocardial infarction (editorial. *Am J Emerg Med* 1996;14: 693–694.
257. Saland KE, Hillis LD, Lange RA, Ciagarroa JE. Influence of morphine sulfate on cocaine-induced coronary vasoconstriction. *Am J Cardiol* 2002; 90:810–811.
258. Negus BH, Willard JE, Hillis LD, et al. Alleviation of cocaine-induced coronary vasoconstriction with intravenous verapamil. *Am J Cardiol* 1994;73:510–513.
259. Friedman HS, Rodney E, Sinha B, et al. Verapamil enhances atrial fibrillation by evoking an intense sympathetic neurohumeral effect. *J Invest Med* 1999;47:293–305.
260. Hollander JE, Hoffman RS, Burstein JL, et al. Cocaine-associated myocardial infarction: mortality and complications. *Arch Intern Med* 1995;155:1081–1086.
261. Gitter MJ, Goldsmith SR, Dunbar DN, Sharkey SW. Cocaine and chest pains: clinical features and outcome of patients hospitalized to rule out myocardial infarction. *Ann Intern Med* 1991;115:277–282.
262. Weber JE, Shofer FS, Larkin GL, et al. Validation of a brief period for patients with cocaine-associated chest pain. *N Engl J Med* 2003;348: 510–517.
263. Nademanee K, Gorelick DA, Josephson MA, et al. Myocardial ischemia during cocaine withdrawal. *Ann Intern Med* 1989;111:876–880.
264. Dressler FA, Malekzadeh S, Roberts W. Quantitative analysis of amounts of coronary arterial narrowing in cocaine addicts. *Am J Cardiol* 1990;65: 303–308.
265. Kolodgie FD, Farb A, Virmani R. Pathobiological determinants of cocaine-associated cardiovascular syndromes. *Hum Pathol* 1995;26: 583–586.
266. Núñez BD, Miao L, Klein MA, et al. Acute and chronic cocaine exposure can produce myocardial ischemia and infarction in Yucatan swine. *J Cardiovasc Pharmacol* 1997;29:145–155.
267. Tazelaar HD, Karch SB, Stephens BG, Billingham ME. Cocaine and the heart. *Hum Pathol* 1987;18:195–199.
268. Virmani R, Robinowitz M, Smialek JE, Smyth DF. Cardiovascular effects of cocaine: an autopsy study of 40 patients. *Am Heart J* 1988;15: 1068–1076.
269. Turnicky RP, Goodin J, Smialik JE, et al. Incidental myocarditis with intravenous drug abuse. *Hum Pathol* 1992;23:138–143.
270. Szakács JE, Cannon A. L-norepinephrine myocarditis. *Am J Pathol* 1958;30:425–434.
271. Chappel CI, Rona G, Balazs T, Gaudry R. Comparison of cardiotoxic actions of certain sympathomimetic amines. *Can J Biochem Physiol* 1959;37:35–42.
272. Van Vliet PD, Burchell HB, Titus JL. Focal myocarditis associated with pheochromocytoma. *N Engl J Med* 1966;274:1102–1108.
273. Brickner ME, Willard JE, Eichhorn EJ. Left ventricular hypertrophy associated with chronic cocaine abuse. *Circulation* 1991;84: 1130–1135.
274. Hoffman CK, Goodman PC. Pulmonary edema in cocaine smokers. *Radiology* 1989;172:463–465.
275. Wiener RS, Lockhart JT, Schwartz RG. Dilated cardiomyopathy and cocaine use. *Am J Med* 1986;81:699–701.
276. Chokshi SK, Moore R, Pandian NG, Isner JM. Reversible cardiomyopathy associated with cocaine intoxication. *Ann Intern Med* 1989;111: 1039–1040.
277. Missouris CG, Swift PA. Cocaine use and acute left ventricular dysfunction. *Lancet* 2001;357:1586.
278. Qureshi AI, Suri F, Guterman LR, Hopkins LN. Cocaine use and the likelihood of nonfatal myocardial infarction and stroke. *Circulation* 2001;103:502–506.
279. Kaku DA, Lowenstein DH. Emergence of recreational drug abuse as a major risk factor for stroke in young adults. *Ann Intern Med* 1990;113: 821–827.
280. Qureshi AI, Akbar MS, Czander E, et al. Crack cocaine use and stroke in young patients. *Neurology* 1997;48:341–345.
281. Barth CW, Bray M, Roberts WC. Rupture of the ascending aorta during cocaine intoxication. *Am J Cardiol* 1986;57:496.
282. Hsue PY, Salinas CL, Bolger AF, et al. Acute aortic dissection related to crack cocaine. *Circulation* 2002;105:592–1595.
283. Chang RA, Rossi NF. Intermittent cocaine use associated with recurrent dissection of the thoracic and abdominal aorta. *Chest* 1995;108: 1758–1762.
284. Swalwell CI Davis GG. Methamphetamine as a risk factor for acute aortic dissection. *J Forens Sci* 1999;44:23–26.
285. Xiao Y-F, Morgan JP. Cocaine blockade of acetylcholine-activated muscurinic K^+ channel in ferret cardiac myocytes. *J Pharmacol Exp Ther* 1998;284:10–18.
286. Starmer CF, Lancaster AR, Lastra AA, Grant AO. Cardiac instability amplified by use-dependent Na channel blockade. *Am J Physiol* 1992;262:H1305–H1310.
287. Perera R, Kraebber A, Schwartz M. Prolonged Q-T interval and cocaine use. *J Electrocardiol* 2005;30:337–339.
288. Daga B, Minano A, de la Puerta I, et al. Electrocardiographic findings typical of Brugada syndrome unmasked by cocaine consumption. *Rev Espan Cardiol* 2005;58:1355–1357.
289. Kerns W, Garvey L, Owens J. Cocaine-induced wide complex dysrhythmia. *J Emerg Med* 1997;15:321–329.
290. Wang RY. pH-dependent cocaine-induced cardiotoxicity. *Am J Emerg Med* 1999;17:364–369.

291. Hoffman BB, Lefkowitz RJ. Catecholamines and sympathomimetic drugs. In: Gillman AG, Rall TW, Nies AS, Taylor P, eds. *The pharmacological basis of therapeutics*, 8th ed. New York: Pergamon Press, 1990:187–220.
292. Martin WR, Sloan JW, Sapira JD, Jasinski DR. Physiologic, subjective, and behavioral effects of amphetamine, methamphetamine, ephedrine, phenmetrazine, and methyphenydate in man. *Clin Pharmacol Ther* 1971;12:245–257.
293. Mas M, Farré M, De La Torre R, et al. Cardiovascular and neuroendocrine effects and pharmacokinetics of 3,4-methylenedioxidemethamphetamine in humans. *J Pharmacol Exp Ther* 1999;290:136–145.
294. Kalant H, Kalant OJ. Death in amphetamine users: causes and rates. *Can Med Assoc J* 1975;112:299–304.
295. Milroy CM, Clark JC, Forrest ARW. Pathology of deaths associated with "ectasy" and "eve" misuse. *J Clin Pathol* 1996;49:149–153.
296. Jaffe JH. Drug addiction and drug abuse. In Gillman AG, Rall TW, Nies AS, Taylor P, eds. *The pharmacological basis of therapeutics*, 8th ed. New York: Pergamon Press, 1990:522–573.
297. Temma K, Akera T, Brody TM, Rech RH. Negative chronotropic and positive inotropic actions of phencyclidine on isolated atrial muscle in guinea pigs and rats. *J Pharmacol Exp Ther* 1983;226:885–892.
298. Temma K, Akera T, Ng Y-C. Cardiac actions of phencyclidine in isolated guinea pig and rat heart: possible involvement of slow channels. *J Cardiovasc Pharmacol* 1985;7:297–306.
299. Vaupel DB, Nozaki M, Martin WR, Bright LD. Single dose and cross tolerance studies of β-phenethylamine, d-amphetamine, and LSD in the chronic spinal dog. *Eur J Pharmacol* 1978;48:431–437.
300. Rothrock JF, Rubenstein R, Lyden PD. Ischemic stroke associated with methamphetamine inhalation. *Neurology* 1988;38:589–592.
301. Goodman SJ, Becker DP. Intracranial hemorhage associated with amphetamine abuse. *J Am Med Assoc* 1970;212:480.
302. Ragland AS, Ismail Y, Arsura EL. Myocardial infarction after amphetamine use. *Am Heart J.* 1993;125:247–249.
303. Bashour TT. Acute myocardial infarction resulting from amphetamine abuse: a spasm-thrombus interplay. *Am Heart J* 1994;128:1237–1239.
304. Waksman J, Taylor RN, Bodor GS, et al. Acute myocardial infarction associated with amphetamine use. *Mayo Clin Proc* 2001;76:323–326.
305. Bennett IL, Walker WF. Cardiac arrhythmias following the use of large doses of central nervous system stimulants. *Am Heart J* 1952;44:428–431.
306. Call TD, Hartneck J, Dickenson WA, et al. Acute cardiomyopathy secondary to intravenous amphetamine abuse. *Ann Intern Med* 1982;97:559–560.
307. Croft CH, Firth BG, Hillis LD. Propylhexedrine-induced left ventricular dysfunction. *Ann Intern Med* 1982;97:560–561.
308. Citron BP, Halpern M, McCarron M. et al. Necrotizing angiitis associated with drug abuse. *N Engl J Med* 1970;283:1003–1011.
309. Anderson RJ, Garza HR, Garriott JC, Dimaio V. Intravenous propylhexedrine (Benzedrex) abuse and sudden death. *Am J Med* 1979;67:15–20.
310. Sullivan ML, Martinez CM, Gennis P, Gallagher EJ. The cardiac toxicity of anabolic steroids. *Prog Cardivasc Dis* 1998;41:1–15.
311. Holma P. Effect of an anabolic steroid (metandienone) on central and peripheral blood flow in well-trained athletes. *Ann Clin Res* 1977;9:215–221.
312. Freed DLJ, Banks AJ, Longson D, Burley DM. Anabolic steroids in athletics: crossover double-blind trial on weightlifters. *Br Med J* 1975;2:471–473.
313. De Piccoli B, Giada F, Benettin A, et al. Anabolic steroid use in body builders: an echocardiographic study of the left ventricle. *Int J Sports Med* 1991;12:408–412.
314. Sader MA, Griffiths KA, McCredie RJ, et al. Androgenic anabolic steroids and arterial structure and function in male bodybuilders. *J Am Coll Cardiol* 2001;37:224–230.
315. Johnson M, Ramey E, Ramwell PW. Androgen-mediated sensitivity in platelet aggregation. *Am J Physiol* 1977;232:H381–H385.
316. Ansell JE, Tiarks C, Fairchild VK. Coagulation abnormalities associated with the use of anabolic steroid. *Am Heart J* 1993;125:367–371.
317. Thompson PD, Cullinane EM, Sady SP, et al. Contrasting effects of testosterone and stanozolol on serum lipoprotein levels. *J Am Med Assoc* 1989;261:1165–1168.
318. McNutt RA, Ferenchick GS, Kirlin PC, Hamlin NJ. Acute myocardial infarction in a 22-year-old world class weight lifter using anabolic steroids. *Am J Cardiol* 1988;62:164.

CHAPTER 72

Paul S. Haber, MD, FRACP, FAChAM
Robert Gordon Batey, MD, FRACP, FRCP(UK), FAChAM

Liver Disorders Related to Alcohol and Other Drug Use

Alcoholic Liver Disease
Viral Hepatitis
Toxicity from Co-Injected Materials
Androgenic/Anabolic Steroids

The liver is a major target for the toxicity of alcohol and other drugs of abuse. This chapter describes the more common liver diseases associated with use of alcohol and other drugs (Table 72.1). The emphasis is on clinical manifestations, diagnosis and management.

ALCOHOLIC LIVER DISEASE

Alcoholic liver disease (ALD) is a major cause of morbidity and mortality globally, yet it attracts little concern from the public and health professions in general. Recent research has increased the understanding of the complexity of the pathogenesis of ALD and has improved the capacity of clinicians to detect earlier forms of these liver disorders. Additionally, a greater awareness of treatments for alcohol dependence has decreased the nihilism that has marked many clinicians' attitudes to alcohol-related disorders in general. Early detection of dependence and organ damage followed by specific management strategies improves patient outcomes.

Epidemiology Cirrhosis of the liver (mostly in association with alcohol abuse) is the 12th most common cause of death in America and the fifth most common cause among middle-aged American men. It accounted for 28,085 deaths in 2003, of which 44% were alcohol-related (1). ALD is the second most common indication for liver transplantation in the United States. When it is recognized that many hepatitis C patients requiring transplantation also drink heavily, the full impact of alcohol-related liver disease on health care services can be seen to be massive (2,3).

The population risk of alcohol-related cirrhosis is related to the population level of alcohol consumption. This phenomenon has been demonstrated by comparing rising or falling levels of alcohol consumption in several populations across time and by comparing different populations (4). Well-documented reductions in population alcohol consumption in France and Australia can therefore be expected to lead to reduced prevalence of this disease. By contrast, the prevalence of alcoholic cirrhosis has doubled in the last decade in the United Kingdom in parallel with increased population alcohol use (5).

Risk Factors for Alcoholic Liver Disease Risk factors for alcoholic liver disease include the amount of alcohol consumed, gender, genetic factors, obesity, chronic viral hepatitis, ingestion of hepatotoxins, and nutrition.

Amount of Alcohol Consumed A standard drink contains 14 grams of alcohol. Fatty liver may be observed after a single heavy drinking episode, but more advanced liver disease is typically seen after more than 10 years' consumption at average levels greater than 100 g/day. Population studies demonstrate an increasing risk of cirrhosis above 40 g/day for men and 20 g/day for women, but the majority of those with cirrhosis have drunk more than 100 g/day (6,7). Among very heavy drinkers, the risk rises to approximately 50% but does not reach 100% even at the highest levels of alcohol consumption.

Gender Women appear to be at greater risk of alcoholic liver disease, with that risk rising at lower average levels of alcohol consumption than in men (20 g/day vs. 40g/day in men) (6,8–11). Many factors have been proposed to account for the difference in apparent susceptibility between men and women, but none fully explains this finding. Differences in body composition, average weight, gastric alcohol dehydrogenase activity (accounting, in part, for first pass, gastric alcohol metabolism), hepatic alcohol metabolic rate and liver mass per kilogram of body weight

TABLE 72.1 Associations between Drugs of Abuse and Liver Disease

Hepatic drug toxicity	• Alcohol • MDMA • Cocaine • Heroin • Phencyclidine • Androgenic steroids
Toxic interactions with other drugs of abuse	• Alcohol plus MDMA • Alcohol plus cocaine • Alcohol plus acetaminophen
Systemic effect of drugs leading to liver injury	• Hyper–and hypo–thermia • Shock • Rhabdomyolysis
Infectious complications	• Viral hepatitis: A to D, particularly B and C • Bacteria: SBE, septicemia
Co–injected material	• Talc (hepatic granulomas) • Lead (by–product of metampheta-mine synthesis)
Unrelated to abused drugs	• Fatty liver • Focal Liver Diseases

MDMA-3,4-methylenedioxymethamphetamine

between men and women result in a higher relative alcohol dose in women compared to men drinking the same amount. This is reflected in a higher blood alcohol level for a given amount of alcohol. (12,13). Data suggesting that women have a higher alcohol metabolism rate than men may reflect both a testosterone mediated down-regulation of hepatic alcohol dehydrogenase (14) and a higher liver mass per kilogram of body weight in women (15). There was no gender difference when alcohol elimination was expressed per kilogram of liver. An alternative explanation for a greater female susceptibility to alcohol mediated liver damage may relate to gender differences in endotoxin-induced Kupffer cell activation in alcoholic liver injury (16,17).

Genetic Factors A classic twin study showed that the concordance rate for alcoholic liver disease (ALD) is threefold higher in monozygotic twins compared to dizygotic twins (18) suggesting that genetic factors contribute to the risk of liver disease among those that abuse alcohol. An increasing number of studies report genetic links to both susceptibility to dependence and to tissue injury from alcohol ingestion (19,20). These studies have examined classic genetic markers (such as blood groups and HLA antigens) and genes relevant to the disease process (such as neurotransmitter metabolism, enzymes involved in alcohol metabolism, collagen metabolism and, more recently, the wide variety of proteins involved in the inflammatory process).

Studies of histocompatibility leukocyte antigen (HLA) antigens and collagen gene restriction fragment length polymorphisms (RFLPs) have not revealed consistent associations (21). Alcohol dehydrogenase (ADH) genotypes coding for highly active isoenzyme and aldehyde dehydrogenase (ALDH) coding for a less active isoenzyme have been associated with ALD. These polymorphisms may lead to accumulation of acetaldehyde after alcohol consumption. The findings have not been reproduced in other centers, and their significance remains unclear. The c2 promoter polymorphism of CYP2E1 has been linked to ALD with an odds ratio of 2.4. This allele is uncommon in white persons and can only explain a minority of cases (22). Mutations of the HFE (hemochromatosis) gene are not associated with ALD. Polymorphisms in tumor necrosis factor alpha (TNFα) and interleukin-10 (IL-10) have been recently linked to ALD, but these findings have not been readily replicated, suggesting the mechanisms underlying tissue injury are complex (23,214). The technology to perform genome wide associations is now available and is likely to yield important new information in this field.

Obesity The prevalence of obesity is continuing to rise, and the disorder now affects almost 20% of adult Americans (24). Liver disease is one of its manifestations, and non-alcoholic fatty liver disease (NAFLD) is now recognized as a common and potentially progressive liver disease. NAFLD resembles alcoholic liver disease with respect to the pathological appearance of liver tissue and certain mechanisms of injury (25). There is both experimental and clinical evidence of an alcohol-obesity interaction in the liver. Alcohol-fed rats develop more severe liver disease if given a high fat diet (26). Alcoholics with a high body mass index for at least 10 years are at increased risk of liver disease (27). The effect of weight reduction on alcoholic liver disease has not been documented, but continuing fatty liver disease may explain failure to normalize liver tests in patients who attain abstinence from alcohol.

Chronic Viral Hepatitis Heavy alcohol use is widely recognized as a factor that is associated with advanced liver fibrosis in patients with chronic viral hepatitis, particularly hepatitis C (discussed further in the section "Hepatitis C"). The odds ratio for fibrosis exceeds 200 for heavy (more than 60 gm/day) alcohol use (28). Hepatitis C has been reported to be more common in alcoholics than the general community in a number of studies (2,29) an observation attributed to but not entirely explained by the increased prevalence of injection drug use.

A similar but less marked interaction between the hepatitis B virus and the effect of alcohol on the liver has been ascribed to chronic hepatitis B infection in alcoholics (30), but this interaction is not supported by all studies (31). One possible explanation for this controversy is that the older hepatitis B studies antedated recognition of hepatitis C virus. The studies may have been confounded by unrecognized co-infection with hepatitis C (32).

Ingestion of Hepatotoxins Chronic alcohol consumption is associated with a range of drug interactions that may alter drug effects or increase the risk of liver injury (Figure 72.1). Chronic ethanol consumption increases the hepatotoxicity of a number of compounds including acetaminophen, industrial solvents, anesthetic gases, isoniazid, phenylbutazone and illicit drugs (e.g., cocaine). The induction of cytochrome P450 2E1 (CYP2E1) explains the increased vulnerability of the person who drinks heavily to these substances. CYP2E1 oxidizes

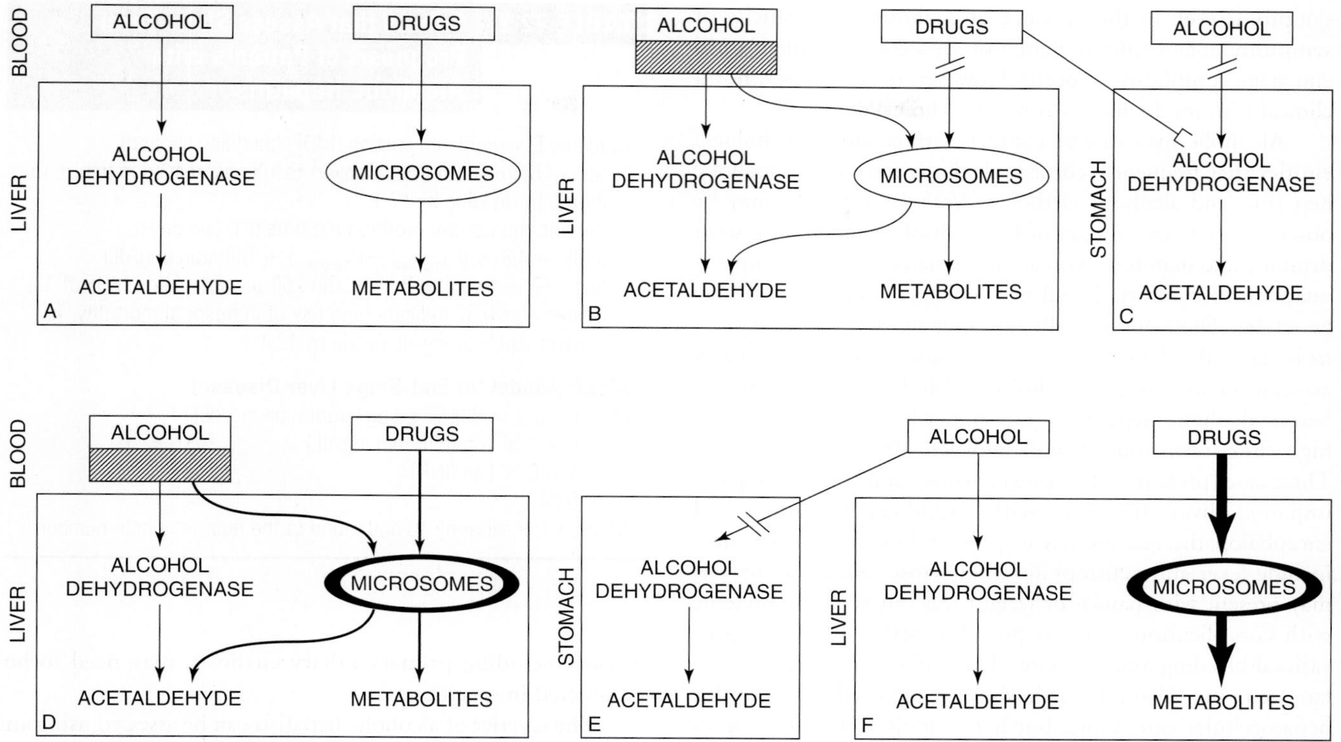

FIGURE 72.1. Schematic representation of ethanol-drug interactions. (Redrawn from Lieber CS. Alcohol and the liver: 1994 update. *Gastroenterology* 1994;106(4):1085–1105. Review.)

ethanol and is induced by chronic alcohol consumption. CYP2E1 also has an extraordinary capacity to activate many xenobiotics (environmental chemicals not normally handled by the liver, such as pesticides) to highly toxic metabolites.

Among patients with alcoholism, hepatic injury associated with acetaminophen has been described after repetitive intake for headaches (including those associated with withdrawal symptoms), dental pain, or the pain of pancreatitis. Amounts well within the accepted rate for the general community (2.5 to 4 g) have been incriminated as the cause of hepatic injury in patients with alcoholism (33,34). It is likely that the enhanced hepatotoxicity of acetaminophen after chronic ethanol consumption is caused, at least in part, by an increased microsomal production of reactive metabolite(s) of acetaminophen. Consistent with this view is the observation that, in animals fed ethanol chronically, the potentiation of acetaminophen hepatotoxicity occurs after ethanol withdrawal (35), at which time production of the toxic metabolite may be at its peak, since at that time competition by ethanol for a common microsomal pathway has been withdrawn. Thus, maximal vulnerability to the toxicity of acetaminophen occurs immediately after cessation of drinking, when there is also the greatest need for analgesia, because of the headaches and other symptoms associated with withdrawal. This also explains the synergistic effect between acetaminophen, ethanol, and fasting (36,37), as these factors all deplete reduced glutathione (GSH). GSH provides a fundamental cellular mechanism for the scavenging of toxic free radicals. Furthermore, CYP2E1 promotes the generation of active oxygen species that are toxic in their own right and may overwhelm the antioxidant system of the liver and other tissues with striking consequences. A similar effect may also be produced by the free hydroxy-ethyl radical generated from ethanol by CYP2E1.

Nutrition For many years, alcohol per se was not thought to be hepatotoxic, and ALD was thought to be fully explained by poor nutrition. Nutritional impairment is universally present in patients with ALD and correlates with the severity of the disease. However, Lieber and DeCarli (38,39) have clearly shown in the baboon model that experimental alcohol administration can lead to progressive liver injury, including cirrhosis, in the presence of an otherwise nutritionally adequate diet. The interaction between alcohol intake and dietary factors is complex as evidenced by studies demonstrating severe injury in animals exposed to high-dose alcohol and either high- or low-fat diets and the impact of dietary modulation on disease outcome (26,40,41).

Nutritional disorders may accelerate progression of ALD. Protein deficiency is a recognized cause for fatty liver owing to impaired apoprotein synthesis required to export lipid from hepatocytes. Choline deficiency is associated with hepatic fibrosis. Vitamin A excess also leads to hepatic fibrosis. Heavy alcohol use is associated with low serum levels of vitamin A and if supplements are inappropriately given, vitamin A toxicity may result, even with normal serum levels (4).

Clinical Features Symptoms and signs are not reliable indicators of the presence or severity of ALD. There may be no symptoms even in the presence of cirrhosis. This paucity of symptoms may facilitate denial of an alcohol problem until end-stage complications occur. However, in some cases, florid clinical features do allow a confident clinical diagnosis.

Alcoholic liver disease comprises three clinicopathologic entities that frequently coexist: alcoholic fatty liver, alcoholic hepatitis, and alcoholic cirrhosis. *Alcoholic fatty liver* may be observed after several days of heavy drinking or in long-term drinking and manifests with anorexia, nausea, and right upper-quadrant discomfort. The liver is enlarged and firm and may be tender. There are typically no other signs. *Alcoholic hepatitis* is classically defined by symptoms and signs of hepatitis in association with heavy alcohol use. Mild cases are common. Severe alcoholic hepatitis is rare but, when present, carries a high short-term mortality of between 30% and 65% (42). These cases present with anorexia, nausea and abdominal pain, impaired liver function with jaundice, bruising, and encephalopathy. Ascites may be present. Systemic disturbances include fever and neutrophilic leukocytosis. *Alcoholic cirrhosis* may present with nausea or weight loss but typically presents with complications such as portal hypertension leading to variceal bleeding and/or ascites, liver failure, and hepatocellular carcinoma. Alcoholic cirrhosis is a recognized risk factor for hepatocellular carcinoma, but it is not clear that there is an association between alcohol abuse and hepatocellular carcinoma in the absence of cirrhosis (43).

TABLE 72.2 Scores that Assess Short-Term Prognosis of Patients with Alcoholic Hepatitis

Maddrey Discriminant Function (MDF) (modified version)
1. Serum Bilirubin (mg/dL). Convert results expressed in (mol/L to mg/dL by dividing by 17.1
2. Patient and Control prothrombin time (PT) (seconds)
   $MDF = 4.6 \times (PT_{patient} - PT_{control}) + \text{Bilirubin (mg/dL)}$
   (e.g., PT 16s, control PT 12s, Bili 250 μmol/L yields MDF of 33)
   Scores above 32 indicate high risk of in-hospital mortality. To convert mol/L to mg/dL divide by 17.1.

MELD (Model for End-Stage Liver Disease)

MELD Score = 0.957 × Log (creatinine mg/dL)
+ 0.378 × Log (bilirubin mg/dL)
+ 1.120 × Log (INR)
+ 0.643
Multiply the score by 10 and round to the nearest whole number.

Diagnosis of Alcoholic Liver Disease

Many cases of ALD are detected only by results of liver tests. The liver tests are a sensitive marker for ALD, but similar findings may be observed in nonalcoholic steatohepatitis and in patients treated with medications such as anticonvulsants. The γ-glutamyl transpeptidase (γGT) level is almost always raised (44) and often exceeds 1,000 U/L. The transaminases are only moderately elevated. Levels above 500 U/L suggest an additional disorder such as acetaminophen ingestion, viral hepatitis, or liver ischemia. The aspartate aminotransferase (AST) exceeds the alanine aminotransferase (ALT) level in most cases, and a ratio of 2:1 AST:ALT is commonly quoted as highly suggestive of ALD. Possible explanations for this observation are that AST is a mitochondrial enzyme and alcoholic injury selectively injures mitochondria. In addition, AST is also found in other tissues subject to alcohol injury including skeletal muscle and heart. If the ALT exceeds the AST, chronic hepatitis C, acetaminophen ingestion, or other causes for hepatocellular injury should be considered. Neutrophilia is found in severe cases but may reflect concomitant sepsis.

The diagnosis of ALD rests on the history of prolonged heavy alcohol ingestion with a compatible clinical and laboratory picture. Other contributing factors that should be routinely considered are ingestion of hepatoxic drugs including herbal preparations and acetaminophen, diabetes mellitus, hepatitis B and C infection, and iron overload. Additional investigations are restricted to atypical cases or those that fail to resolve with abstinence from alcohol. Other explanations for liver disease, including autoimmune hepatitis, Wilson's Disease, alpha-1-antitrypsin deficiency, and cholestatic liver disease including primary biliary cirrhosis, may need to be considered in specific cases.

The severity of alcoholic hepatitis can be assessed using an objective rating scale such as the Maddrey Discriminant Function (MDF) or the Model for End-Stage Liver Disease score (45). These correlate closely with each other and both give an indication of prognosis and may direct the use of specific treatments (Table 72.2).

Role of Liver Biopsy

Liver biopsy has been used for decades to provide invaluable information in a variety of liver disorders. Nevertheless the practice of biopsying the majority of patients with any form of significant liver injury has changed in the past 5 years owing to improvements in noninvasive imaging and diagnostic testing and as patients have become more resistant to the procedure knowing its complications and short falls. Several recent papers have identified the problem of sampling error with biopsies, and the use of the procedure is commonly now restricted to those patients with complex or incompletely understood disease and in those being considered for liver transplantation (46,47). The morbidity of liver biopsy is 0.5%, and the mortality is 0.01% (48), and these risks generally outweigh the benefit of obtaining tissue pathology. Where clinical uncertainty persists, biopsy should always be considered. In life-threatening cases where urgent liver transplantation is being considered, vitamin K or fresh-frozen plasma may be required, to reverse coagulopathy to accomplish biopsies. Transjugular biopsy is validated as a safe procedure in coagulopathic patients (49) but is not widely available and sometimes yields insufficient tissue for diagnosis.

It has been argued that demonstration of the severity of liver damage by biopsy might motivate ambivalent alcohol-dependent patients to adhere more closely to management protocols. However, this has never been validated by clinical studies, and routine use of biopsy could not be justified on this basis.

Pathogenesis The pathogenesis of alcoholic hepatitis is complex and still incompletely understood. New research underscores the multiple factors involved in this disorder (50–52). Damage to the liver in heavy drinking patients is neither predictable nor absolutely preventable. The presence of liver disease reflects the end result of interactions between the host, the toxin (alcohol), metabolic, immunologic, necroinflammatory, and regenerative processes. Ethanol metabolism within the liver leads to the generation of hepatotoxic metabolites. Recent studies demonstrate clearly that alcohol abuse leads to liver injury via oxidative stress (53). This, in association with endotoxin mediated activation of cytokine production by several cell populations within and beyond the liver (50,54,55) leads to progressive fibrogenesis. These broadly described processes interact with each other. Ethanol is metabolized to acetaldehyde and to acetate mainly via ADH and ALDH enzymes, respectively. Acetaldehyde has been shown to affect many aspects of normal cellular functioning, including DNA repair, microtubule assembly, mitochondrial respiration, fatty acid oxidation, and activation of fibrogenesis. High levels of acetaldehyde have been measured in patients with ALD, in part owing to impaired mitochondrial ALDH function (56). High levels of acetaldehyde lead to the production of acetaldehyde/protein adducts, which impact on liver function and disease processes in a variety of ways (57).

A second pathway for alcohol metabolism involves cytochrome P450 2E1, a part of the microsomal ethanol-oxidizing system, that is induced by chronic ethanol consumption (58). A third system involving catalase is generally thought to play a minor role under most circumstances (58).

Oxidative Stress in Alcoholic Liver Disease The induction of cytochrome P450 2E1 (CYP2E1) generates reactive oxygen species (ROS) during oxidation of alcohol (59). Chronic alcohol administration induces selective depletion of mitochondrial glutathione, thus diminishing cellular defense against oxidative stress (60). TNFα release from Kupffer cells and T lymphocytes acts on hepatocytes to generate ROS in hepatic mitochondria (61). Acetaldehyde is highly reactive and binds covalently to normally occurring materials in blood to form compounds known as adducts (such as acetaldehyde-protein adducts and malondialdehyde-acetaldehyde [MAA] adducts) (57,62). Adducts have been shown to cause liver injury in alcohol-fed experimental animals (63), and blood levels of adducts correlate with liver injury in alcoholic humans (64). Acetaldehyde adducts add to ROS in evolving ALD.

Endotoxin is a toxic lipopolysaccharide (LPS) present in the cell wall of all gram-negative bacteria (65). Endotoxin is present in gut flora and may enter the circulation where it binds to a serum protein (lipopolysaccharide-binding protein [LBP]). This complex binds to CD14, a receptor on the surface of Kupffer cells. CD14 lacks an intracellular domain, but interacts with membrane spanning proteins called Toll-like receptors (TLRs) that releases NFκB leading to upregulation of pro-inflammatory cytokines (notably TNFα) (66). This endotoxin pathway has been implicated in human ALD by several findings. Circulating levels of gut-derived endotoxin in alcoholics are increased (67). CD14 is up-regulated in Kupffer cells of alcohol-fed rats (68). Experimental alcoholic liver injury is increased by co-administration of endotoxin (69). However, one study has shown that rats chronically fed alcohol develop tolerance to these effects of endotoxin (70), casting some doubt on the role of endotoxin in this disease. Nonetheless, the intermittent drinker who becomes acutely ill intermittently may still experience bouts of LPS-mediated acute liver injury.

Ethanol itself also contributes to liver injury. Ethanol has been shown to affect intracellular signaling pathways (71,72) by its effects on lipid membranes and its interaction with several cellular proteins, including phospholipases and adenylate cyclase.

Pro-inflammatory cytokines promote tissue damage in experimental alcoholic hepatitis (73). In human ALD, increased plasma levels of IL-1, IL-6, IL-8, and IL-12 have been reported. Interferon-γ and TNFα have also been implicated in human ALD. Anti-inflammatory cytokines such as IL-10 are reduced. Most recently, increased IL-18 (interferon-γ-inducing factor) levels have been reported in the blood (74). Inflammatory factors, including IL-6, might be of fundamental importance for liver regeneration (75). Platelet-derived growth factor (PDGF) has been shown to play an important role in the repair process after acute tissue injury. PDGF is thought to promote effective necrotic tissue removal and the reconstruction of an adequate extracellular matrix network. Long-term ethanol consumption is known to inhibit the regenerative capacity of the liver, possibly via an altered transmission of growth signals through the insulin/insulin receptor substrate-1 (IRS-1)-mediated signal transduction cascade (76).

Progressive liver fibrosis underlies advanced ALD. The major source of hepatic collagen is now known to be the hepatic stellate cell (HSC, or lipocyte, Ito cell or fat-storing cell [77,78]). Similar cells have been isolated in the pancreas (79), the kidneys, and other tissues (80). In early alcoholic hepatic injury, fibrosis is largely pericentral (77) and characterized by accumulation of collagen types 1 and 3, proteoglycans, fibrinonectin, and hyaluronic acid. HSC are activated to become myofibroblast-like, cells that secrete collagen as well as proliferate (77). TGF-β1 is released primarily by macrophages involved in inflammation and is the most potent pro-fibrogenic liver cytokine. HSCs also contribute to matrix degradation during resolution of liver injury. Increasingly, liver fibrosis is seen as a potentially reversible lesion (81).

Treatment of Alcoholic Liver Disease The treatment of ALD rests upon avoidance of further alcohol consumption. Other interventions are reserved for those with particularly severe disease or who are unable to maintain abstinence. There is considerable evidence that survival is increased by maintaining abstinence (82). The improvement with abstinence is so consistent that the γGT falls with an apparent half-life of 26 days (83). Failure to do so suggests continuing alcohol consumption or occasionally another coexisting liver disease such as obesity-related liver disease or drug toxicity. Advanced cirrhosis does not resolve with abstinence, indicating that it is an irreversible lesion, but the activity is reduced, and many very ill patients make striking improvements, often returning to compensated cirrhosis. In practice, it is never too late to stop drinking.

The first issue is to define what level of alcohol consumption to recommend for the patient with liver disease. Those with alcohol dependence or severe liver disease should be given clear advice to remain abstinent long term. However, many patients have only minor abnormalities in liver function tests without clinical evidence of cirrhosis. A typical recommendation is a 6-week period of abstinence followed by repeat liver tests. If these normalize and the patient wishes to resume drinking, consumption within recommended levels may be guided by the results of further liver tests in those who can control their alcohol use. Continuing follow-up in a primary care setting is important, as the major causes of death in mild ALD are extra-hepatic problems such as suicide. Another problem for the generalist physician providing longitudinal and continuous health care is that many patients with alcohol-induced disorders decline referral to a specialist treatment service. Internists and other primary care physicians can readily develop the brief counseling skills to perform motivational interviewing and provide feedback concerning medical progress.

Pharmacotherapies to address alcohol dependence must be used with particular caution in the presence of serious liver disease. A recent study of the use of baclofen in the treatment of alcohol dependence has provided evidence of very positive benefit (84). Further studies are required to replicate the findings but the particular potential benefit is the lack of liver toxicity of baclofen. Disulfiram is contraindicated in advanced liver disease owing to recognized hepatotoxicity. Another issue is the safety of acamprosate and naltrexone in patients with significant liver disease. Acamprosate does not accumulate even in severe liver disease, as the drug is excreted unchanged in the urine and is not metabolized. According to the manufacturers, acamprosate is contraindicated in severe decompensated (Childs C) liver disease, but even in that setting, the risks of treatment should be balanced against the risks of continuing alcohol consumption, and there are no published reports of an adverse effect on liver function. Naltrexone is associated with dose-dependent hepatotoxicity (typically at doses of 300 mg/day), but reactions are most unusual at the standard dose of 50 mg/day. In two studies, liver function tests improved in alcoholics, with no cases of clinically evident hepatotoxicity, indicating the therapeutic effect to reduce alcohol consumption exceeded the potential hepatotoxic effect (85,86). Nonetheless, because of the above concerns, there is little experience with naltrexone in patients with advanced ALD. Nalmefene is a second-generation orally active opiate receptor antagonist that has been reported to have similar efficacy to naltrexone in the treatment of alcohol dependence (87) without reported hepatotoxicity.

In cases where the disease is particularly severe or does not resolve with abstinence, several therapeutic options may be available. None has yet found a definite place in therapy. Propylthiouracil (88,89), colchicine (90), and oxandrolone (91) have been evaluated for the treatment of ALD, but subsequent studies failed to reproduce beneficial effects of these agents. Some agents that can be viewed as "supernutrients" have been found to be effective in nonhuman primates. These include S-adenosylmethionine for the treatment of early aspects of alcohol-induced liver injury (92) and polyunsaturated lecithin for the prevention of fibrosis (93,94). There are some data that both agents are effective in humans. S-adenosylmethionine treatment led to a significantly lower mortality in patients with Childs class B cirrhosis (95). Polyenylphosphatidylcholine is derived from soybeans and comprises a mixture of polyunsaturated phosphatidylcholines, about half of which is dilinoleoylphosphatidylcholine. A large Veterans' Affairs Cooperative Study evaluated this treatment but did not identify any delay in the progression to cirrhosis over the 2 years of the study, though in parallel, the participants substantially reduced their alcohol intake (96).

Selected cases of alcoholic hepatitis may respond to corticosteroids, but this remains controversial despite a number of controlled trials. Prednisolone (40 mg/day for 28 days) has been shown to improve survival of patients with spontaneous hepatic encephalopathy or a high MDF >32; Table 72.2) (42). Widespread use of corticosteroids has been limited by the knowledge that they may exacerbate sepsis, a common complication of severe liver disease. Pentoxifylline (400 mg thrice daily) has also been reported to reduce the mortality of alcoholic hepatitis (97). Pentoxifylline acts by inhibition of TNFα and possibly by improving hepatic perfusion. Replication of this finding by other centers is awaited, but the medication is widely used because it is safe, readily available, and inexpensive. Interleukin 10 (IL-10) is an anti-inflammatory cytokine. There is preliminary evidence that IL-10 may be effective in severe alcoholic hepatitis (MDF >32), but the drug is not available for general use (98).

The management of the complications of cirrhosis, such as ascites and bleeding, lie outside the scope of this chapter. Patients who present with signs of hepatocellular insufficiency or portal hypertension should be evaluated by a gastroenterologist or hepatologist. Advice should be provided to minimize the development of complications. Salt restriction helps reduce fluid retention with edema and ascites whereas prophylactic management of portal hypertension with beta blockers, such as propranalol or esophageal variceal banding, alters prognosis significantly. Once established, ascites is treated by salt restriction with spironolactone and, if necessary, furosemide and bed rest. Paracentesis is effective for diuretic resistant cases. Severe cases may respond to transjugular intrahepatic porta-systemic shunting or surgical shunts. Variceal hemorrhage is treated by transfusion, correction of coagulopathy, nitrate or octreotide infusions, and endoscopic banding. After controlling bleeding, secondary prophylaxis with variceal banding and/or beta blockers reduces the risk of rebleeding. Spontaneous peritonitis is treated by intravenous antibiotics and prophylactic norfloxacin until ascites has resolved. Hepatic encephalopathy may be alleviated by correction of precipitating factors and by decreasing colonic production and absorption of NH_3 with lactulose, a nonabsorbable disaccharide that acidifies the colon content through fermentation. Dietary protein should be adjusted to avoid both deficiency and excess. It was suggested many years ago that *Helicobacter pylori* infection might contribute to hepatic encephalopathy because of its high urease activity, which promotes the conversion of urea to ammonia, one of the precipitating factors of hepatic precoma and coma (99,100). However, there has not been clear benefit from eradication therapy (101).

Liver transplantation is now an accepted treatment option for individuals with advanced liver disease who have stopped drinking (102), but only 5% of patients with end-stage ALD receive transplants. The procedure has been controversial because of ethical concerns about allocation of precious donor livers to individuals with a (mis)perceived self-induced disease, concerns about the chance of a successful outcome in this cohort after transplantation, and concerns about resumption of drinking after a successful transplant. It is unreasonably simplistic to regard ALD as a "self-induced disorder." External factors such as family, peers, and society as a whole encourage the availability and use of alcohol. Genetic factors also contribute to the risk of alcohol dependence, which is considered a chronic relapsing brain disease (103). The 5-year survival after transplantation for ALD is comparable to that of nonalcoholics in series from the United States, Europe, and Australia (104,105). Whereas alcoholics may be at higher risk of some post-transplant problems, there is evidence that the rate of rejection may be lower than for non-ALD (106). Resumption of alcohol consumption remains the major concern and occurs in approximately one-third of survivors (107). Of those one-third that return to drinking, another one-third of them develop life-threatening alcohol-related morbidity such as pancreatitis, recurrent ALD, and noncompliance with immunosuppression resulting in graft rejection (108). These outcomes are comparable to the post-transplantation recurrence rate of other liver diseases. This low rate of recurrent alcohol consumption is better than that observed after other treatments for alcohol dependence. This may be owing to careful case selection for transplantation or the intensity of treatment by the transplant team. Vaillant (109) showed that the prognostic factors that generally predict a favorable outcome for alcoholism treatment are provided by the liver transplant process.

The ideal candidate for transplantation accepts the etiologic role of alcohol in his or her liver disease and has ceased drinking, has strong family supports with a stable home, employment, and enthusiasm to resume interests. Psychosocial evaluation seeks to stratify patients by their risk of relapse for alcoholism. An objective assessment method is highly desirable but has not been devised. The Michigan Alcoholism Prognosis Scale (110) did not predict postoperative drinking (111), possibly as only those with high scores are transplanted. Other prognostic scales have insufficient predictive value to justify rejection of an otherwise suitable candidate (112,113). A simple and objective approach requires 6 months of abstinence before transplantation, and this 6-month rule has been adopted by most transplant centers in the Unites States (114). A recent literature review confirmed that 6 months of pretransplantation abstinence (when patients are very ill) does not predict post-transplantation relapse, and ethical concerns about this practice have been raised (115). Lucey et al. (111) recommend careful individualized assessment.

VIRAL HEPATITIS

Hepatitis A Hepatitis A is an RNA virus that is transmitted by fecal-oral contamination. In underdeveloped countries, almost all children develop IgG antibodies by the age of 10, and acute infection leads to a mild or even clinically inapparent hepatitis. With improving hygiene, the seroprevalence has fallen so that adults in the developed world are now generally susceptible to hepatitis A. The disease becomes increasingly severe with advancing age so that hepatitis A is now less common but often more severe than in the past. The illness does not persist as a chronic infection. Parenteral transmission of hepatitis A is rare owing to the short period of viremia but has been described (116).

The prevalence of hepatitis A IgG antibodies is high among injection drug users (IDUs) and prison inmates in California (117) and Australia (118). Hepatitis A correlated more closely with institutionalization than sharing of injecting equipment, and vaccination of seronegative prison entrants is undertaken in some jurisdictions.

Prevention measures include hygiene precautions to prevent fecal-oral contamination, passive immunoglobulin to household contacts of cases, and active immunization to those at risk. Hepatitis vaccine is given as two injections by intramuscular injection and is safe and effective. Accepted indications for vaccination include occupational risk, travelers, men who have sex with men, and those with chronic liver disease. Vaccination has also been recommended for IDUs (119), but while agreeing that this group is at increased risk of hepatitis A, difficulties of accessing IDUs and the high cost of vaccine limit the usefulness of this strategy (120). Nonetheless, those seronegative IDUs receiving preventive care services should be vaccinated.

Hepatitis B Hepatitis B virus is the most prevalent chronic viral infection of humans. It is readily transmitted among IDUs. Serologic evidence of past hepatitis B infection increases in prevalence with the duration of injecting drug use, which is now the commonest association of hepatitis B infection acquired in adults (121). Other risk groups include people who have more than one sexual partner (heterosexual and sexual contact between men), people from certain ethnic groups (e.g., Asia, Southern European, Mediterranean countries), indigenous people, children of infected parents, and health care workers. The incubation period is 6 weeks to 6 months.

Acute hepatitis B may be preceded by a transient serum-sickness prodrome, with polyarthralgia, fever, malaise, urticaria, and proteinuria (122). The acute illness is characterized by anorexia, nausea, and sometimes vomiting with malaise, jaundice, pale stools, and dark urine. The infection is frequently subclinical. Hepatitis B persists as chronic hepatitis B infection in about 5% of adults, much less often than does hepatitis C (see following section). Acute and chronic hepatitis B are diagnosed by serologic tests, and hepatitis B virus (HBV) DNA testing is now used to define the state of infectivity, risk of HCC and suitability for treatment (Table 72.3). People who remain HBsAg-positive for 6 months have chronic hepatitis B, and the severity of inflammation may vary significantly depending on immune status, viral load

TABLE 72.3 Interpretation of Serological Markers for Viral Hepatitis

	Interpretation	Comments
Hepatitis A		
IgG	Past infection	Persists for life
IgM	Recent infection	Generally indicates acute hepatitis, but may persist after recovery for 18 months
Hepatitis B		
Hepatitis B surface antigen (HBsAg)	Current infection	Positive in both acute and chronic hepatitis B Marker of infectivity
Antibody to hepatitis B surface antigen (HbsAb; anti–HBs)	Immunity (either after infection or vaccination)	Antibody titres >10 IU/L correlate with protection
Hepatitis B core antigen	Not found in peripheral blood	Present in liver tissue
Antibody to hepatitis B core (HbcAb; anti–HBc)	IgG: past exposure to HBV	Anti–HBc + anti–HBs = past infection with recovery; anti–HBc + Hbs Ag = chronic HBV infection
	IgM: (high titre)–acute Hepatitis B (low titre)–active chronic hepatitis B	Distinguishes acute from chronic HBV In chronic HBV, low level titre correlates with ALT level and immune response (some laboratories report all low titre antibodies as negative)
Hepatitis B e antigen (HBeAg)	Acute hepatitis B Chronic active hepatitis B	Marker of infectivity in variety of settings Correlates with HBV–DNA
Hepatitis B viral DNA (HBV–DNA)	Infectivity; active viral replication	Detection by PCR is most sensitive marker of HBV infection HBV–DNA without HbeAg indicates infection with mutant HBV Levels useful to monitor antiviral therapy
Antibody to hepatitis B e antigen (HbeAb; anti–HBe)	Convalescence after acute HBV Marker of lower infectivity	May be associated with active disease, usually with a lower viral load. Less responsive to anti–viral therapy
Hepatitis C Hepatitis C antibody	Positive: indicates exposure to HCV Negative: does not exclude infection if transmission within 3 months; in rare cases HCV infections occur without antibody response	Positive result in subject without any risk factor for HCV is more likely to be a false positive test (confirm this by negative PCR or Recombinant immunoblot assay (RIBA)) Positive HCV antibody does not distinguish past infection from current infection Transplacental passage of HCV antibody makes antibody test unreliable marker of infantile infection for 18 months.
Hepatitis C virus RNA	Positive: confirms antibody result indicating HCV infection	
Hepatitis C viral load	High: $>2 \times 10^6$ copies per ml	High viral load associated with poorer response to therapy
Hepatitis C genotype	I–VI	Type I associated with poorer response to therapy
Hepatitis D (Delta)	Defective virus that requires HBsAg to be viable	
HDV–IgG	Indicates past and/or present infection	
HDV–IgM	Indicates recent or chronic infection	
HDV–RNA	Indicates current viremia	

HAV, hepatitis A virus; HBV, hepatitis B virus; HCV, hepatitis C virus; PCR, polymerase chain reaction (sensitive molecular diagnostic procedure that can detect minute amounts of specific DNA or RNA).

and genotype, co-infection with other hepatitis viruses or HIV, and other external factors such as male sex, ethnic origin, alcohol ingestion or other illicit drug use, and duration of infection. Chronic active hepatitis B is associated with chronic hepatitis, cirrhosis, and hepatocellular carcinoma in a significant minority.

Liver injury results from cell-mediated response to infected hepatocytes. In chronic disease, a series of hepatitis flares may precede viral clearance and recovery. These flares vary in severity from subclinical through to life-threatening. Patients with chronic HBV should be initially assessed with regard to the replication status of the virus and the presence of active liver disease. Patients with persistently abnormal ALT levels or clinical evidence of liver disease should be referred for consideration of antiviral therapy. Patients with chronic HBV may be offered regular screening for HCC, particularly if they have cirrhosis.

Treatment of active chronic hepatitis B is of value in those patients with active liver inflammation (ALT more than twice normal), but it offers no benefit in those with no active liver inflammation at this stage. Treatment with standard and now pegylated interferon-α (IFNα) leads to seroconversion from eAg to eAb status in 30% to 40% compared to spontaneous seroconversion of 15%. The eAg to eAb seroconversion is associated with suppression of viral replication and decreasing hepatic inflammation (123). There is a minimal success rate in clearing the virus with loss of HBsAg (3% to 5%). Treatment can be demonstrated to be cost-effective (124). Loss of HBeAg has been associated with improvements in liver histology and clinical outcome but patients remain infected and infectious. Side effects related to pegylated IFNα are common (see "Hepatitis C" section). The best response to IFNα is seen in white patients who have had the disease for a short time and who have biochemical hepatitis and a low viral load (low HBV-DNA titres). Pegylated IFN-α should be used with extreme caution in patients with HBV-related cirrhosis, as it may induce a flare of hepatitis and lead to hepatic decompensation. Such patients should be assessed for liver transplantation. Immunosuppressive drugs such as cancer chemotherapies are associated with increased HCV viral load and flares of hepatitis such that prophylactic treatment is recommended.

There are now a number of oral antiviral agents available for use in the treatment of HBV-infected patients. These include lamivudine, adefovir, entecavir, and tenofovir. Lamivudine and adefovir were used extensively in the past, but drug resistance is a major problem, with viral and hepatitis breakthrough complicating the management of patients. Currently entecavir is the optimal agent for commencing antiviral therapy as resistance rates at 2 and 3 years remain <3%. Lamivudine resistance affects entecavir efficacy, and resistance rates in those previously treated with lamivudine rise more rapidly. The management of patients with chronic active HBV hepatitis is constantly evolving, and clinicians need to be aware of the latest drug availability and recommendations on usage of these agents. Combination therapy with two or more antiviral agents may prove more effective than serial monotherapy but optimal combinations are yet to be defined. In patients who develop lamivudine resistance, the addition of adefovir to the lamivudine leads to a better outcome than switching from one drug to the other. Most experts now recommend the combination when lamivudine resistance becomes apparent. Other studies have failed to show a benefit from combining interferon alpha with lamivudine in the treatment of HBV.

Hepatitis C Hepatitis C virus (HCV) infection is a major public health problem worldwide (125). It is the most frequently reported notifiable infection in adults, and approximately 3.9 million people are infected in the United States (126). HCV is already the leading indication for liver transplantation, and it is projected that the number of people with advanced liver disease and associated hepatocellular carcinoma (HCC) will double by 2010. HCV is transmitted by blood to blood contact. The most common risk factor is injecting drug use.

Virology HCV, identified in 1989, is an RNA virus from the flavivirus family. It has a single open-reading frame that generates a large viral polyprotein. Viral polymerases ligate this polyprotein into the viral proteins. HCV has recently been cultured *in vitro*, and this has increased understanding of the infectivity and pathobiology of the virus. HCV antibodies in the blood reliably indicate exposure to the virus, but the protective significance of these antibodies remains to be fully defined. Recent studies in active IDUs suggest they are at reduced risk of reinfection when HCV antibodies are present (127).

There are six genotypes of the virus. Genotypes are further divided into subtypes (e.g., a, b, c). The most common genotypes in the United States are types 1 and 3. Reinfection after clearance and co-infection with more than one genotype can occur. Patients with genotypes 2 or 3 respond better to current antiviral therapies than those with other genotypes. The virus alters its genetic structure over time by mutation, leading to the presence of multiple species of virus with similar genetic sequence (quasi-species). This process is thought to allow HCV to evade immune clearance, leading to chronic infection. The continual alteration in genetic structure makes the development of a preventative vaccine difficult.

Transmission

Injecting Drug Use In the United States, Europe, and Australia, the most common risk factor for transmission of hepatitis C infection is IDU (Table 72.4), which accounts for the bulk of incident cases and 91% in Australia (128). HCV prevalence is strongly associated with duration of injecting with an incidence of approximately 20% for each year of IDU (129). Most regular IDUs are infected with HCV, and the incidence is 100% in some populations. Measures to limit the spread of this infection appear to be making only a modest impact, and a recent study demonstrated an incidence of 45 per 100 life years in new injecting users in NSW Australia (130,131). The continuing high incidence appears to be related to the continuing high prevalence of sharing some component of injecting equipment including mixing spoons, filters, swabs, or tourniquets or even on the hands. The continuing epidemic of hepatitis C among IDUs has given rise to calls for wider implementation of infection control procedures such as needle-syringe programs. Distribution of needles is associated with falling HCV transmission in some settings (130,132) but not in all (133).

Sexual transmission rates are generally thought to be very low. An Italian study of the male partners of women infected with contaminated anti-D immunoglobulin showed no evidence of transmission over a combined follow-up period of 862 years (134). Similar findings were found in two other studies (135,136). By contrast, analysis by Alter et al. (137) of the third National Health and Nutrition Examination Survey (NHANES III) database showed that high-risk sexual behavior

TABLE 72.4 Risk Factors for Hepatitis C

High risk
- Sharing contaminated drug injecting equipment: 90% are infected after 10 years.
- Regular or large volume transfusions of blood products prior to 1990: 85%–90% of haemophiliacs are hepatitis C antibody–positive.
- Incarceration: due to the high prevalence of injecting drug use among prisoners and possibly other high-risk events in prisons

Moderate risk
- Body piercing and tattooing: using contaminated equipment
- Mother to baby at birth: occurs in about 10% if mother is RNA-positive

Low risk
- Small-volume blood transfusion prior to 1990
- Sharing toothbrushes, razors, etc.
- Health care worker, needlestick, or sharps injury
- Birth or medical procedure in a country of high HCV prevalence

Very low risk
- Sexual activity: few well–documented cases. The presence of genital ulcerative STDs and/or traumatic sexual practices may increase the risk. Recent outbreaks in HIV-positive men who have sex with men
- Drug use via snorting straws
- Blood transfusion/blood products after 1990

No evidence of increased risk
- Household and casual contacts of people with hepatitis C

was a significant risk factor for hepatitis C in the United States. This conclusion has been challenged (138) because IDU, the major risk factor for hepatitis C infection, was not included in NHANES III so that the effect of other factors such as sexual behavior could have been confounded by IDU (139). Murphy et al. (140) subsequently confirmed that the increased risk of hepatitis C associated with high-risk sexual practices disappeared after adjusting for IDU. Outbreaks of HCV transmission have recently been described in Europe, the United Kingdom, the United States, and Australia among highly promiscuous HIV-positive men who have sex with men (215).

The vertical transmission rate from mother to baby is approximately 5%. The risk is increased if the mother is also HIV-positive, unless she is taking highly active antiretroviral therapy (HAART) (141). The transmission rate was 9.5% from mothers with viremia, but no transmission if the mother was hepatitis C-RNA-negative at the time of delivery (142,143). Hepatitis C RNA has been found in breast milk, but there is no evidence for transmission. Antibody testing of infants should be deferred for 18 months until placenta-transmitted antibody has disappeared. HCV RNA testing at 3 months provides an earlier indication of transmission, but occasionally babies show a transient HCV viremia which is cleared without a persisting HCV infection.

Blood Products The risk of hepatitis C infection in recipients of blood and blood products before 1990 was related to the volume of blood products transfused. The majority of severe hemophiliacs became infected. After screening of blood products for hepatitis C antibody was introduced, the number of people with posttransfusional HCV has reduced markedly. The risk of hepatitis C infection after blood transfusion in Australia was estimated at 1 in 250,000 units transfused (144). Transmission from contaminated anti-rhesus D immunoglobulin was recognized in Ireland and other European countries, many years after its administration (145).

Occupational and Nosocomial Transmission Health care and laboratory staff handling blood and blood products are at risk of contracting hepatitis C. Estimates for the risk of transmission from a needlestick injury range from 0 to 10% (142,146). Transmission of hepatitis C via a needlestick has not been reported where the source was hepatitis C-RNA-negative. Nosocomial transmission of hepatitis C has been reported in a variety of hospital settings, for example in plasmapheresis units (147), in a hematology ward (148), in hemodialysis units (149,150), after colonoscopy (151), and after cardiothoracic surgery (152).

Tattooing Several studies have demonstrated an association between tattooing and hepatitis C infection. In an Australian study of blood donors, the independent relative risk associated with a history of tattooing was 27 (128). Though infection control guidelines for tattooists have been introduced in recent years, the possibility of hepatitis C transmission continues where these guidelines are not followed.

Hepatitis C in Special Populations

Prisoners The prevalence of hepatitis C in prisoners is high, largely owing to the high proportion of IDUs. In Australia, almost 40% of prison entrants are HCV antibody–positive and 65% among prisoners reporting a history of IDU (153,154). Imprisonment has been reported to be associated with hepatitis C even after adjusting for IDU (129,140). It has been suggested that other modes of transmission may occur in prisons owing to high background prevalence with poor hygiene and frequent physical violence (155).

The incidence of HCV among uninfected prisoners is also high (Cameron et al.). Measures that may limit the spread of HCV in the community are frequently not available to prison inmates, including methadone maintenance and needle-syringe programs. Tattooing using unsterilized equipment may also play a role (156).

People Born in Countries of High Hepatitis C Prevalence In Mediterranean, Eastern European, Asian, South American, and African countries, the prevalence of hepatitis C is much higher than in the United States. The prevalence in Egypt for adults is 20%, making this a major community epidemic. The Egyptian hepatitis C epidemic has recently been related to mass inoculations of antischistosomal therapy (157).

Primary Infection Primary infection with HCV is typically subclinical, but mild hepatitis may occur. Fulminant hepatitis is rare. Peak viremia occurs in the preacute or early in the acute phase (weeks 2 to 3), and antibodies appear as early as 4 weeks (average 6 to 8 weeks) using third-generation testing. Clinically evident hepatitis reflects a significant immune response to the virus and may be associated with a higher rate of viral clearance than subclinical infection (up to 40%). A small number of exposed seronegative individuals have evidence of T-cell immunity to HCV, indicating that the virus can be eliminated without detectable antibodies (158). The incidence of this phenomenon is presently unknown. While some studies have reported a high clearance rate of HCV in patients treated with interferon or combination therapy for acute hepatitis C, this approach to treatment cannot be routinely recommended for acute hepatitis C at this time as the illness is generally mild with a significant recovery rate, and current antiviral treatment is costly and carries significant morbidity.

Chronic Infection Between 60% and 75% of patients infected with hepatitis C will develop persistent chronic infection (Figure 72.2). Liver injury predominantly results from immune damage to infected liver cells. After an average of 20 years, approximately 8% of people will develop cirrhosis rising to 20% after 40 years. Progression to cirrhosis is associated with duration of disease, age older than 40 at the time of infection, average alcohol consumption of more than 50 g/day, co-infection with HBV and/or HIV, and male gender. The route of transmission or viral factors such as genotype or viral titre do not appear to play a role (159). The majority of HCV-infected individuals will not die of their HCV disease.

Symptoms of chronic hepatitis C without cirrhosis do not correlate well with disease activity or severity and tend to be nonspecific, mild, and intermittent. The most common is fatigue, with nausea, muscle aches, right upper-quadrant pain, and weight loss. These symptoms are rarely incapacitating, but they can have a detrimental effect on quality of life.

Diagnosis The third-generation enzyme immunoassay for antibodies to hepatitis C is the most practical screening test for hepatitis C infection (Table 72.4). This assay suffers from a high rate of false-positives when used in populations with a low prevalence of hepatitis C, so screening of the general population is not recommended. The antibody tests do not differentiate between current and resolved infection, as the antibody typically takes more than 10 years to disappear after viral clearance.

A positive hepatitis C RNA test indicates the presence of active infection, while a negative test in people with risk factors and positive antibody indicates probable clearance of HCV infection. HCV RNA analysis is particularly useful to assess the status of HCV antibody–positive patients with *normal* liver function tests. Approximately 50% of these patients are HCV-RNA-negative. The test should be repeated 3 to 6 months later and, if again negative, the patient can be reassured the virus has been cleared. Almost all hepatitis C antibody–positive patients with *abnormal* liver function tests have detectable levels of hepatitis C RNA in their blood.

Hepatitis C genotyping and viral load determination should be carried out on all patients considering antiviral therapy for HCV infection. Both of these measures provide information about the likely outcome of therapy and thus assist patient and doctor in determining whether to proceed with treatment. Genotyping may also be used to analyze cases of hepatitis C transmission by identifying the same genotype in the source patient and the recipient.

Management Issues

Access to Health Care and Hepatitis C Information for Injection Drug Users with Hepatitis C

IDUs infected with hepatitis C may be marginalized, indigent, homeless, and frequently experience discrimination. As a consequence, they may lack access to health care (160). It is important to provide culturally appropriate written material that matches the educational level of the patient, as many cannot discuss their illness with others. Specialized outreach clinics held in needle-syringe services, opioid treatment programs, and in prisons have been established. These provide diagnostic evaluation and build a therapeutic relationship to facilitate referral for full

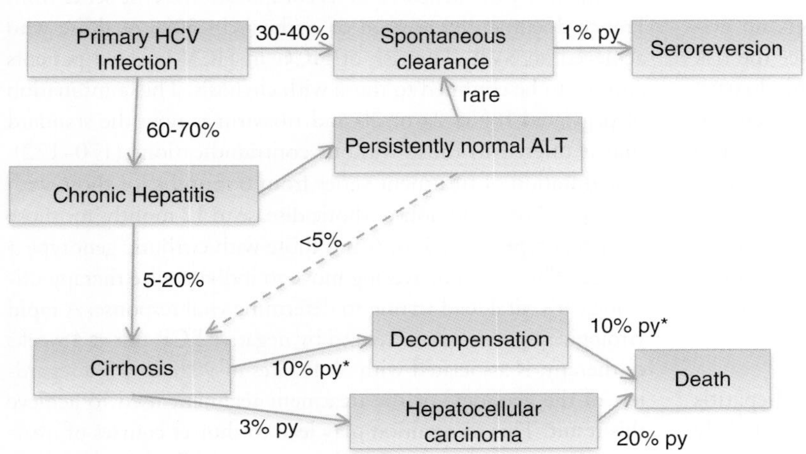

FIGURE 72.2. The natural history of HCV infection. (Adapted from Di Bisceglie AM. Natural history of hepatitis C: its impact on clinical management. *Hepatology* 2000;31:1014–1018.)

evaluation for antiviral therapy along with other substance abuse treatment. Primary care physicians or other health care workers can also engage HCV-infected patients, and clinical guidelines can assist them to provide appropriate management.

Pre- and Post-Test Counseling Issues A diagnosis of hepatitis C often engenders a high level of anxiety that can be exacerbated by misinformation. Adequate time and privacy should be set aside for pre-test counseling. The results of hepatitis C testing should be given in person. Post-test counseling issues include the natural history of the disease, the symptomatology, and privacy issues. Accurate, nonjudgmental language combined with a sincere concern for the patient's welfare helps to build the patient's trust. Clarify the meaning of any colloquial, subcultural terms associated with marginalized groups. Patients are fearful of transmitting hepatitis C to their partners, household contacts, and their children. They can be reassured that the risks are minimal, but contact testing should be offered. Full explanations about the advantages, and limitations of antiviral therapy allow the patient to make an informed choice about treatment options.

Assessing the Severity of the Disease Symptoms, including lethargy, do not correlate with the severity of liver disease. Spider nevi are commonly seen, but the physical signs are nonspecific unless advanced cirrhosis is present. Plasma ALT is the best laboratory indicator of active viral hepatitis, but the level commonly fluctuates and does not correlate well with the stage of liver disease. A normal ALT level does not exclude cirrhosis. Patients with normal ALT levels and those who decline treatment may be monitored in primary care settings by ALT levels two to three times per year and referred if the ALT levels rise. Liver biopsy is no longer considered essential before commencing treatment for HCV infection but, in certain clinical situations, it remains the best investigation for assessing the extent of fibrosis and the likelihood of serious long-term consequences. Newer approaches to defining the extent of hepatic fibrosis using blood tests or devices such as the Fibroscan are reducing the need for biopsy.

Hepatitis A and B Vaccination When there is no evidence of immunity, vaccination is indicated to reduce the risk of further liver injury. Chronic co-infection with other hepatitis viruses is associated with accelerated progression to cirrhosis (161). Hepatitis B vaccination should be offered, and patients with hepatitis C respond well, albeit with lower titres, compared to uninfected controls. An early report of high mortality from hepatitis A in patients with chronic HCV has not been replicated, and vaccination for hepatitis A is appropriate if available. Cost-effectiveness in countries with a low HAV prevalence cannot be demonstrated.

Alcohol Alcohol interacts adversely with chronic hepatitis C in several ways (162). There is now a consensus that daily consumption of alcohol above 40 g has an additive effect on liver inflammation and accelerates the progression of hepatic fibrosis (163). Heavy alcohol use is also associated with increased viral load (164), reduced adherence to therapy, increased risk of progression to HCC, and exacerbation of the skin lesions of porphyria cutanea tarda.

There is no clear evidence concerning adverse effects of moderate levels of alcohol consumption on people with chronic hepatitis C. The National Institutes of Health (NIH) consensus conference in 1997 recommended a maximum of 10 g/day for all people with chronic hepatitis C and abstinence for those with significant disease and those contemplating antiviral therapy (165).

Dietary Guidelines There is no published evidence to support any specific diet in unselected people with hepatitis C. Hepatic steatosis is a feature of hepatitis C, and obesity and type 2 diabetes mellitus are associated with hepatitis C and accelerated progression of fibrosis (166,167). The potential for dietary interventions in selected subjects to control the activity of hepatitis is under investigation.

Management of Risk Factors The presence of HCV infection may increase motivation to participate in alcohol and/or drug dependence treatment, particularly if the patient is seeking antiviral therapy. Avoidance of injecting drug use is the preferred option but it may not be the choice of the patient. Evidence-based harm minimization and abstinence-based treatments should be offered, as described elsewhere in this volume.

Antiviral Treatment The main indication for treatment is active hepatitis with elevated ALT levels and, if performed, biopsy evidence of fibrosis (167a,167b). The main goal of antiviral therapy is sustained virologic response (SVR), defined by a continued normal ALT level and negative hepatitis C polymerase chain reaction (PCR) on more than one occasion at least 6 months after completion of treatment. Individuals with SVR generally remain PCR-negative long term. Several studies have found significant improvements in general health and specific hepatitis C–related symptoms in patients who achieve a sustained response to antiviral therapy (168,169). Those who achieve a sustained response and have no cirrhosis should expect to remain free of cirrhosis and its complications. One series from France documented reversal of cirrhosis in 30% of those who achieved an SVR. The risk of HCC in HCV-infected patients appears to be confined to those with cirrhosis. The combination of pegylated IFNα 2a or 2b and ribavirin is now the standard that is offered to those without contraindications (170–172). The duration of treatment varies from 6 months for those with genotype 2 or 3 and non-cirrhotic disease to 12 months for those with genotypes 1, 4, 5, or 6 and those with cirrhotic genotype 3 disease. There is an increasing move to individualize therapy utilizing early viral load testing to determine viral response. A rapid virologic response, characterized by negative PCR test at 4 weeks of therapy, is associated with SVR rates of 90% to 95% regardless of the genotype or the treatment regiment used to achieve this result. This recognition may lead to shorter courses of treatment for some genotype 2 and 3 patients while detecting those with genotype 1 and 4 disease who are nonresponders at week 12. This allows an appropriate early cessation of treatment, avoiding unnecessary side effects. SVR rates of 75% to 80% are achieved in genotype 2, 3, and possibly 6 infections and 45% to 50% in genotypes 1, 4, and 5 infections. Newer forms of interferon including consensus interferon and albuferon have been shown in studies to be effective, but their use has not replaced standard pegylated interferon at this stage.

Treatment of Special Groups

Human Immunodeficiency Virus Co-Infection The progression of chronic hepatitis C is accelerated in HIV co-infected patients. Treatment of hepatitis C may be indicated in patients with early HIV infection and those stable on HAART, but the response rates reported to date have been lower than in mono-infected groups. Consideration must be given to possible drug interactions and to additive blood abnormalities when treating these co-infected patients.

Patients with Compensated Cirrhosis Patients with compensated cirrhosis may be treated (173). There is some evidence that treatment reduces the risk of hepatocellular carcinoma and decompensation, but these are subject to ongoing trials.

Persistently Normal Aminotransferases Patients who are hepatitis C-RNA-positive and have persistently normal aminotransferase levels generally have mild disease (174). Response rates to treatment have been variable, but a patient requesting treatment to clear the virus and reduce risk of transmission should not be denied access to therapy (175). Most patients can be encouraged not to undergo treatment at this stage, but they should be followed up every 4 to 6 months and treated if the ALT becomes abnormal or if signs of progressive liver disease appear.

Patients with Ongoing Substance Abuse The NIH consensus meeting recommended against treating patients with ongoing substance abuse until substance abuse stabilized (125) and clinicians in hepatology and addiction medicine practice continue to support these recommendations. A number of papers have now demonstrated that patients who continue to use drugs in a controlled fashion and those on methadone or buprenorphine programs can be successfully treated (176,177). There is no clinical evidence that methadone maintenance therapy impairs treatment response, and methadone is encouraged, when indicated, if hepatitis C treatment is contemplated (178). Most IDUs provided all the information about HCV treatment choose to defer treatment until they have stabilized their drug use and social situations.

Side Effects of Therapy

Interferon Flu-like symptoms occur within 4 to 6 hours of the injections, tend to subside within the first month of treatment, and respond to acetaminophen. More persistent side effects are fatigue, alteration in mood, sleep disturbance, moderate suppression of white cell count and platelet count, skin rash, reduction in appetite and weight, dryness of the mucous membranes, and hair loss. Dose reduction or cessation of treatment may be required. Major side effects include severe depression, retinopathy, interstitial fibrosis of the lung, and thyroid disease.

Ribavirin The most common side effect is hemolytic anemia. Other side effects are pruritus, cough, and myalgia. Dose reduction is commonly required, but erythropoietin may improve hemoglobin levels and facilitate full-dose ribavirin therapy. Significant teratogenic effects have been associated with ribavirin. Both women of child-bearing potential and men on treatment must use two forms of effective contraception during treatment and for 6 months thereafter (15 half-lives for clearance of ribavirin).

Contraindications for Treatment Decompensated cirrhosis, pregnancy, lactation, active psychiatric illness, and those who drink more than seven standard drinks a week are at higher risk of side-effects and lower chance of response and are generally not treated. Depression may worsen during therapy, and suicide has been reported. Careful psychiatric assessment and ongoing care may be required (179). Contraindications to ribavirin include end-stage renal failure due to drug accumulation, chronic anemias, a history of cardiovascular dysfunction, and inadequate contraception.

Other Treatments A variety of drugs including amantadine, ursodeoxycholic acid, nonsteroidal anti-inflammatory drugs and venesection to remove iron stores (300 ml on a regular basis till iron stores are normal) have been investigated alone or in combination with alpha interferons. Virologic response rates have been unsatisfactory when these agents are used as monotherapies. None of these agents has contributed to improved SVRs when used in combination with interferon and ribavirin. Alternative medications have been used by a high percentage of HCV-infected patients, but no study has shown an antiviral effect in this disease. Symptomatic improvement and modest ALT reductions have been reported in studies using silymarin or combination Chinese herbal medicine (180,181).

Newer Anti–Hepatitis C Virus Agents A number of new agents designed to impair viral replication have been developed, and some are now being studied in phase 3 clinical trials. Early data show that agents such as Telaprevir (VX 950) can lead to a more rapid viral clearance, but long-term efficacy and safety are still to be proven for these agents. This is a rapidly evolving area with new drugs entering clinical evaluation every year.

Advanced Hepatitis C HCV cirrhosis progresses to HCC at an annual rate of 3% to 5%, and hepatitis C is among the commonest underlying associations of HCC. Once hepatic decompensation occurs, the 5-year survival falls to 50%, and transplantation should be considered rather than antiviral treatment.

Hepatocellular Carcinoma Small primary liver cancers can be resected or treated by local therapies. Cirrhotic patients with HCC are considered for transplantation if there are fewer than three tumeur nodules smaller than 3 cm or a single nodule <5 cm with no extrahepatic spread or vascular invasion. It is currently recommended that such patients undergo 6 monthly screenings with upper abdominal ultrasound and serum alpha-fetoprotein. If abnormalities are found, more extensive evaluation should be undertaken in a specialist liver center.

Liver Transplantation Hepatitis C is now the leading indication for liver transplantation, and the numbers are expected to rise further during the next decade. Patients with cirrhosis should be considered for transplantation if they develop major complications of their cirrhosis indicating a life expectancy of 1 to 2 years without transplantation. The 3-year post-transplantation survival is 84%, equivalent to survival in patients transplanted with other forms of liver disease (182). Before transplantation, patients should be informed of the high risk of hepatitis C recurrence and its potential consequences, including a 10% risk of recurrent cirrhosis at 5 years. Methadone maintenance is no longer considered an absolute contraindication for transplantation (183–185), but careful individualized assessment is required.

Hepatitis D The delta agent is a defective viral RNA particle that cannot replicate without co-infection with hepatitis B. It requires the s Ag of HBV to allow entry to the hepatocyte. Outbreaks of delta virus co-infection with hepatitis B have occurred among IDUs and were associated with high mortality (182). Control of hepatitis B by vaccination will limit the spread of HDV. The diagnosis is by rising titres of IgG antibody or IgM antibody (Table 72.3). Delta infection should be considered in any HBV-positive patient with relapse. Delta hepatitis responds poorly to interferon unless high doses are given for long periods.

Hepatic Bacterial and Fungal Infections Associated with Injecting Drug Use A wide array of infections may occur in the IDU, and these may involve the liver (Chapter 77).

Cocaine Hepatitis Cocaine hepatic injury appears to be uncommon in humans (186) and contributes about 1% to fulminant hepatic failure in several series. Most cases occur in association with systemic heat-shock-like features of cocaine toxicity such as hyperthermia, rhabdomyolysis, hypoxia, and hypotension (187). In some other cases, other drugs, particularly alcohol, have been involved. In experimental animals, cocaine hepatotoxicity is readily demonstrated and is both time- and dose-dependent (188).

The clinical presentation is characterized by a marked increase in serum aminotransferase activities beginning within a few hours of drug ingestion associated with the systemic features of cocaine toxicity listed earlier. Rhabdomyolysis may account for some of the increase in transaminases, as AST and ALT are both present in muscle. The liver biopsy shows coagulative hepatic necrosis typically in a centrilobular distribution, extending to pan-lobular necrosis in extreme cases. Micro- and macrovesicular steatosis may be present, consistent with involvement of mitochondria in hepatic injury.

The mechanism of hepatic injury is thought to involve *hepatic ischemia* and/or *toxic oxidative metabolites*. Hepatic ischemia is a likely mechanism as cocaine is a powerful vasoconstrictor and this action accounts for many of the toxic effects of the drug characterized by impaired systemic perfusion. Hepatotoxicity typically occurs in association with these effects as described. Evidence supporting a role for toxic oxidative metabolites comes from experimental animal models in which hepatotoxicity has been demonstrated to result from the production of metabolites by hepatic metabolism. Usually, more than 90% of cocaine is hydrolyzed by plasma pseudocholinesterase (189). The remainder is metabolized by cytochrome P-450 isoenzymes, including CYP3A1. The hepatotoxic metabolite of cocaine has not been identified with certainty but the oxidative metabolites of N-hydroxynorcocaine may generate reactive alkylating species. The severity of liver toxicity is correlated to the extent of cocaine oxidation by hepatic cytochrome P-450, which is increased by inducers of the cytochrome P-450 system such as phenobarbital and ethanol and reduced by P-450 inhibitors such as cimetidine. In the mouse, chronic cocaine administration induces P-450 3A and may increase the risk of hepatotoxicity (190). Inhibition or deficiency of pseudocholinesterase increases hepatotoxicity by diverting drug toward the P-450 pathway, and induction of pseudocholinesterase may lessen toxicity.

Cocaine is commonly taken with alcohol, and hepatic carboxylesterase generates ethylcocaine (cocaethylene) (191). The same hepatic enzyme also contributes to the non-oxidative metabolism of ethanol to fatty acid ethyl esters (192). Ethylcocaine has similar pharmacologic effects to cocaine but a longer half-life. It may accumulate to higher levels in tissues than cocaine and may be more toxic than cocaine as evidenced by a lower LD50 (193). Nonetheless, a large clinical series found no increase in liver disease among alcoholics using cocaine to those not using cocaine (194).

Pretreatment of experimental animals with cimetidine or cysteine protects against cocaine toxicity and provides additional evidence in support of the metabolic theory of toxicity, but pretreatment is not a clinically feasible approach to therapy in humans. No specific therapy has been shown to be effective, but N-acetylcysteine may be considered.

Ecstasy An increasing number of cases of severe liver failure are being reported (186) leading to fatalities and liver transplantation (195). Two clinical syndromes are emerging (188). One syndrome is similar to cocaine hepatitis and presents shortly after ingestion with systemic toxicity accompanied by severe liver injury. The other presents days to weeks after ingestion with jaundice and pruritus and may proceed to fulminant liver failure. The diagnosis of delayed presentations may be difficult unless specific enquiry about 3,4-methylenedioxymethamphetamine (MDMA) use is made. Biochemically, marked hyperbilirubinemia is noted with a disproportionate increase in AST as compared to ALT. The severity of hepatic dysfunction does not appear to be dose-related (196).

Severe liver injury is a rare event, whereas MDMA use is extremely common, suggesting that other factors may contribute to liver injury. The drug is often taken at "rave" parties where participants dance for hours, predisposing to hyperthermia and volume depletion. Those who suffer from hepatic dysfunction with rhabdomyolysis and hyperpraxia may have an abnormality of muscle metabolism similar to that seen in malignant hyperthermia syndrome. Other individuals may be susceptible on the basis of delayed drug elimination (197). The cytochrome P450 isoenzyme CYP2D6 metabolizes MDMA, and approximately 5% of the population have low activity mutations of this isoenzyme with reduced hydroxylation of MDMA *in vitro* (197). Increased susceptibility to MDMA toxicity *in vivo* has been demonstrated in CYP2D6 deficient mice (198). An immunologic mode of liver injury has been proposed on the basis that rechallenge with ecstasy has produced greater liver damage in the absence of hyperthermia, and liver biopsy features on one patient suggested an autoimmune hepatitis-like injury that resolved spontaneously on withdrawal of the drug (199). There is currently insufficient clinical evidence to evaluate the relative importance of these proposed mechanisms in susceptibility to human disease.

The differential diagnosis of a patient with grossly elevated transaminases includes acute viral hepatitis, toxin ingestion and ischemia. Unexplained liver test abnormalities particularly in young adults with hepatomegaly should prompt inquiry into illicit drug use and a urinary drug screen. A negative drug screen suggests non-drug causes for liver disease but may also result from delayed presentation or consumption of ecstasy tablets not containing MDMA as approximately one in three ecstasy tablets does not contain MDMA (200). Meticulous supportive care should be employed, with rigorous rehydration and active cooling measures (199). The benefit/risk ratio of orthotopic liver transplantation for fulminant hepatic failure remains in question, but there have been survivors of transplantation, and early discussion of cases in liver failure with a liver transplant unit is advised.

TOXICITY FROM CO-INJECTED MATERIALS

It is often suspected that other materials may contribute substantially to toxicity after injecting of illicit drugs, but this problem appears to be most uncommon.

Injection of drugs intended for oral ingestion may lead to accumulation of talc in a dose-dependent fashion at several sites, particularly the lung and liver (186). There is a striking difference between the toxicity of talc in the lung compared to other tissues that may be simply a dose effect (201). Talc is strongly fibrogenic in the lung leading to pulmonary granulomatous disease with a progressive or fatal outcome (202). Talc liver is inconsequential clinically (203). A series of 70 liver biopsies from IDUs with chronic hepatitis was examined under polarizing microscopy, revealing talc particles in two-thirds with no granulomas (204). Another series reviewed the liver biopsy appearances in chronic hepatitis C with and without known IDU. Talc was found in 9 of 109 biopsies, of which only 2 had reported IDU before biopsy. Of the five patients in whom follow-up interview was possible, three admitted to prior IDU after being confronted with the liver biopsy evidence. Thus, the presence of intrahepatic talc was a useful marker of previous IDU but is not sensitive for those with a minimal IDU history.

Lead poisoning has been reported in several patients after amphetamine injecting (186). Lead acetate used in the synthesis of methamphetamine may contaminate the final product. The effects of acute lead poisoning include hepatitis, encephalopathy, and renal impairment. A recent survey of blood lead levels in 92 amphetamine users presenting to the emergency department found no cases of lead toxicity, indicating that this problem is sporadic (205).

Phencyclidine A few cases of liver failure associated with malignant hyperthermia have been reported after phencyclidine use (206). In experimental animals, liver toxicity has been demonstrated without hyperthermia.

Cannabis There is growing concern that regular cannabis use may lead to liver injury either directly or by predisposing the liver to react more damagingly to other insults. The cannabinoid receptor CB1 is linked to profibrogenic activity, and is up-regulated in regular users who may therefore be more at risk of fibrotic complications of diseases such as HCV and ALD. (207,208). Cannabis use is associated with more severe steatosis in HCV-infected individuals (209). Paradoxically, some recent studies have suggested cannabis users with HCV infection do better on antiviral therapy than do non-users (210,211). Currently, it is appropriate to counsel those with liver disease to reduce cannabis use.

Opioids Currently, there are no studies that demonstrate hepatotoxicity from pure preparations of opioid agonists. Antagonists such as naltrexone can cause a minor elevation of liver enzymes in a small percentage of patients, but severe liver disease is not described. Patients commencing naltrexone should have liver tests monitored and the dose suspended if enzymes continue to rise after 2 to 3 weeks. Opioid receptor blockade can protect against certain forms of experimental liver injury by modulating Fas-mediated apoptosis pathways.

Benzodiazepines Regular prescribed benzodiazepine use is not associated with liver damage.

ANDROGENIC/ANABOLIC STEROIDS

Androgenic steroids are increasingly used by athletes and others seeking to build muscle mass. Products may be taken in dietary supplements or by injection. Products purchased via the Internet may contain a range of contaminants that complicate the picture of organ and specifically liver damage. A recent case (not reported) of fulminant liver failure occurring in a young male injecting anabolic steroids was shown to be the result of arsenic toxicity contaminating "black market" pharmaceuticals.

Steroids can produce cholestasis, toxic hepatitis, and hepatic adenomas and carcinomas. Most reports are of small numbers of cases, but the growing number of reports makes it imperative that users are warned of potentially fatal consequences from using these drugs (212–216).

ACKNOWLEDGMENTS: *The authors are grateful to Sarah Hutchinson, Janice Pritchard-Jones, and Gary Nind for assistance in preparation of this chapter. Professor Charles Lieber kindly allowed portions of a similar chapter from the second edition of this text to be reproduced.*

REFERENCES

1. Zakhari S, Li T-K. Determinants of alcohol use and abuse: impact of quantity and frequency patterns on liver disease. *Hepatology* 2007;46: 2032–2039.
2. Rosman AS, Paronetto F, et al. Hepatitis C virus antibody in alcoholic patients. Association with the presence of portal and/or lobular hepatitis. *Arch Intern Med* 1993;153:965–969.
3. Lagging LM, Westin J, et al. Progression of fibrosis in untreated patients with hepatitis C infection. *Liver* 2002;22:136–144.
4. Lieber CS, Leo MA. Alcohol and the liver. In: Lieber CS, ed. *Medical and nutritional complications of alcoholism*. New York: Plenum; 1992: 185–239.
5. Thomson SJ. Chronic liver disease-an increasing problem: a study of hospital admission and mortality rates in England, 1979–2005, with particular reference to ALD. *Alcohol Alcohol* 2008. Advance on-line publication.
6. Pequignot G, Tuyns AJ, et al. Ascitic cirrhosis in relation to alcohol consumption. *Int J Epidemiol* 1978;7:113–120.
7. Batey RG, Burns T, et al. Alcohol consumption and the risk of cirrhosis. *Med J Aust* 1992;156:413–416.
8. Norton R, Batey R, et al. Alcohol consumption and the risk of alcohol-related cirrhosis in women. *Br Med J (Clin Res Ed)* 1987;295: 80–82.
9. Saunders JB, Davis M, et al. Do women develop ALD more readily than men? *Br Med J (Clin Res Ed)* 1981;282:1140–1143.
10. Morgan MY, Sherlock S. Sex-related differences among 100 patients with ALD. *Br Med J* 1977;1:939–941.
11. Parrish KM, Dufour MC, et al. Average daily alcohol consumption during adult life among decedents with and without cirrhosis: the 1986 National Mortality Followback Survey. *J Stud Alcohol* 1993;54: 450–456.
12. Frezza M, di Padova C, et al. High blood alcohol levels in women. The role of decreased gastric alcohol dehydrogenase activity and first-pass metabolism. *N Engl J Med* 1990;322:95–99.
13. Crabb DW. First pass metabolism of ethanol; gastric or hepatic, mountain or molehill. *Hepatology* 1997;25:1292–1294.
14. Teschke R, Wiese B. Sex-dependency of hepatic alcohol metabolizing enzymes. *J Endocrinol Invest* 1982;5:243–250.
15. Kwo PY, Ramchandani VA, et al. Gender differences in alcohol metabolism: relationship to liver volume and effect of adjusting for body mass. *Gastroenterology* 1998;115:1552–1557.
16. Kono H, Wheeler MD, et al. Gender differences in early alcohol-induced liver injury: role of CD14, NF-kappaB, and TNF-alpha. *Am J Physiol Gastrointest Liver Physiol* 2000;278:G652–G661.
17. Iimuro Y, Frankenberg MV, et al. Female rats exhibit greater susceptibility to early alcohol-induced liver injury than males. *Am J Physiol* 1997;272:G1186–1194.
18. Hrubec Z, Omenn GS. Evidence of genetic predisposition to alcoholic cirrhosis and psychosis: twin concordances for alcoholism and its biological end points by zygosity among male veterans. *Alcohol Clin Exp Res* 1981;5:207–215.
19. Marshall SJ, Chambers GK. Genetic aspects of alcohol metabolism: an overview. In: Preedy VR, Watson RR, eds. *Comprehensive handbook of alcohol-related pathology*. London: Elsevier, 2005:31–48.
20. Day CP, Bashir R, et al. Investigation of the role of polymorphisms at the alcohol and aldehyde dehydrogenase loci in genetic predisposition to alcohol-related end-organ damage. *Hepatology* 1991;14:798–801.
21. Lumeng L, Crabb DW. Genetic aspects and risk factors in alcoholism and ALD. *Gastroenterology* 1994;107:572–578.
22. Day CP. Who gets ALD: nature or nurture? *J R Coll Physicians Lond* 2000;34:557–562.
23. Stickel F Osterreicher CH. The role of genetic polymorphisms in ALD. *Alcohol Alcohol* 2006;41:209–224.
24. Mokdad AH, Serdula MK, et al. The continuing epidemic of obesity in the United States. *JAMA* 2000;284:1650–1651.
25. Tilg H, Diehl AM. Mechanisms of disease: cytokines in alcoholic and nonalcoholic steatohepatitis. *N Engl J Med* 2000;343:1467–1476.
26. Tsukamoto H, Towner SJ, et al. Ethanol-induced liver fibrosis in rats fed high fat diet. *Hepatology* 1986;6:814–822.
27. Naveau S, Giraud V, et al. Excess weight risk factor for ALD. *Hepatology* 1997;25:108–111.
28. Alter HJ, Seeff LB. Recovery, persistence, and sequelae in hepatitis C virus infection: a perspective on long-term outcome [in process citation]. *Semin Liver Dis*. 2000;20:17–35.
29. Sata M, Fukuizumi K, et al. Hepatitis C virus infection in patients with clinically diagnosed ALDs. *J Viral Hepatol* 1996;3:143–148.
30. Sherlock S, James D. *Diseases of the liver and biliary system*. Oxford: Blackwell Publishing, 1997.
31. Fong TL, Govindarajan S, et al. Status of hepatitis B virus DNA in ALD: a study of a large urban population in the United States. *Hepatology* 1988;8:1602–1604.
32. Younossi ZM. Epidemiology of alcohol-induced liver disease. *Clin Liver Dis* 1998;2:661–671.
33. Black M. Acetaminophen hepatotoxicity. *Annu Rev Med*. 1984;35: 577–593.
34. Seeff LB, Cuccherini BA, et al. Acetaminophen hepatotoxicity in alcoholics. A therapeutic misadventure. *Ann Intern Med* 1986;104: 399–404.
35. Sato C Matsuda Y, et al. Increased hepatotoxicity of acetaminophen after chronic ethanol consumption in the rat. *Gastroenterology* 1981;80:140–148.
36. Israel Y, Speisky H, et al. Metabolism of hepatic glutathione and its relevance in alcohol-induced liver damage. *Cell Mol Aspects Cirrhosis* 1992;216:25–37.
37. Whitcomb DC, Block GD. Association of acetaminophen hepatotoxicity with fasting and ethanol use [see comments]. *JAMA* 1994;272: 1845–1850.
38. Lieber CS, DeCarli LM. An experimental model of alcohol feeding and liver injury in the baboon. *J Med Primatol* 1974;3:153–163.
39. Lieber CS, DeCarli LM, et al. Sequential production of fatty liver, hepatitis, and cirrhosis in sub-human primates fed ethanol with adequate diets. *Proc Natl Acad Sci U S A* 1975;72:437–441.
40. Nanji AA, Griniuviene B, et al. Effect of dietary fat and ethanol on antioxidant mRNA indiction in rat liver. *J Lipid Res* 1995a;36:736–744.
41. Nanji AA, Sadrzadeh SMH. Dietary saturated fatty acids: a novel treatment for ALD. *Gastroenterology* 1995;109:547–554.
42. Carithers RL, Herlong HF, et al. Methylprednisolone therapy in patients with severe alcoholic hepatitis. A randomized multicenter trial [see comments]. *Ann Intern Med* 1989;110:685–690.
43. Bassendine MF. Alcohol—a major risk factor for hepatocellular carcinoma? *J Hepatol* 1986;2:513–19.
44. Moussavian SN, Becker RC, et al. Serum gamma-glutamyl transpeptidase and chronic alcoholism. Influence of alcohol ingestion and liver disease. *Dig Dis Sci* 1985;30:211–214.
45. Day CP. Treatment of ALD. *Liver transpl* 2007;13:S69–S75.
46. Poynard T, Ratziu V, et al. Appropriateness of liver biopsy. *Can J Gastroenterol* 2000;14:543–548.
47. Ratziu V, Charlotte F, et al. Sampling variability of liver biopsy in nonalcoholic fatty liver disease. *Gastroenterology* 2005;128:1898–1906.

48. Spinzi G, Terruzzi V, et al. Liver biopsy. *N Engl J Med* 2001;344:2030.
49. McAfee JH, Keeffe EB, et al. Transjugular liver biopsy. *Hepatology* 1992;15:726–732.
50. Hill DB, Deaciuc IV, et al. Mechanisms of hepatic injury in ALD. *Clin Liver Dis* 1998;3:703–721.
51. Song Z, Zhou Z, et al. Inhibition of adiponectin production by homocysteine: a potential mechanism for ALD. *Hepatology* 2008;47:867–879.
52. Schuppan D, Afdhal NH. Liver cirrhosis. *Lancet* 2008;371:838–851.
53. Fernandez-Checa JC, Kaplowitz N, et al. Mitochondrial glutathione: importance and transport. *Semin Liver Dis* 1998;18:389–401.
54. Thurman RG II. Alcoholic liver injury involves activation of Kupffer cells by endotoxin. *Am J Physiol* 1998;275:G605–G611.
55. Cao Q, Batey RG. The role of T lymphocytes in the pathogenesis of ALD. In: Preedy VR, Watson RR, eds. *Comprehensive handbook of alcohol-related pathology*. London: Elsevier, 2005:763–773.
56. Korsten MA, Matsuzaki S, et al. High blood acetaldehyde levels after ethanol administration. Difference between alcoholic and nonalcoholic subjects. *N Engl J Med.* 1975;292:386–389.
57. Worrall S, Thiele GM. Modification of proteins by reactive ethanol metabolites: adduct structure, functional and pathological consequences. In: Preedy VR, Watson RR, eds. *Comprehensive handbook of alcohol-related pathology*. London: Elsevier, 2005:1209–1222.
58. Lieber CS, Leo MA. Metabolism of ethanol and some associated adverse effects on the liver and the stomach. *Recent Dev Alcohol* 1998;14:7–40.
59. Lieber CS. Cytochrome P-4502E1: its physiological and pathological role. *Physiol Rev* 1997;77:517–544.
60. Colell A, Garcia-Ruiz C, et al. Selective glutathione depletion of mitochondria by ethanol sensitizes hepatocytes to tumor necrosis factor. *Gastroenterology* 1998;115:1541–1551.
61. Fernandez-Checa JC, Kaplowitz N, et al. GSH transport in mitochondria: defense against TNF-induced oxidative stress and alcohol-induced defect. *Am J Physiol* 1997;273:G7–G17.
62. Xu D, Thiele GM, et al. Detection of circulating antibodies to malondialdehyde-acetaldehyde adducts in ethanol-fed rats. *Gastroenterology* 1998;115:686–692.
63. Yokoyama H, Ishii H, et al. Experimental hepatitis induced by ethanol after immunization with acetaldehyde adducts. *Hepatology* 1993;17: 14–19.
64. Rolla R, Vay D, et al. Detection of circulating antibodies against malondialdehyde-acetaldehyde adducts in patients with alcohol-induced liver disease. *Hepatology* 2000;31:878–884.
65. Schletter J, Heine H, et al. Molecular mechanisms of endotoxin activity. *Arch Microbiol* 1995;164:383–389.
66. Kopp EB, Medzhitov R. The Toll-receptor family and control of innate immunity. *Curr Opin Immunol* 1999;11:13–18.
67. Bode C, Kugler V, et al. Endotoxemia in patients with alcoholic and non-alcoholic cirrhosis and in subjects with no evidence of chronic liver disease following acute alcohol excess. *J Hepatol* 1987;4:8–14.
68. Enomoto N, Ikejima K, et al. Alcohol causes both tolerance and sensitization of rat Kupffer cells via mechanisms dependent on endotoxin. *Gastroenterology* 1998;115:443–451.
69. Bhagwandeen BS, Apte M, et al. Endotoxin induced hepatic necrosis in rats on an alcohol diet. *J Pathol* 1987;152:47–53.
70. Jarvelainen HA, Fang C, et al. Effect of chronic coadministration of endotoxin and ethanol on rat liver pathology and proinflammatory and anti-inflammatory cytokines [see comments]. *Hepatology* 1999;29: 1503–1510.
71. Hoek JB, Thomas AP, et al. Ethanol and signal transduction in the liver. *Faseb J* 1992;6:2386–2396.
72. Hoek JB, Kholodenko BN. The intracellular signaling network as a target for ethanol. *Alcohol Clin Exp Res* 1998;22:224S–230S.
73. McClain C Hill D, et al. Cytokines and ALD. *Semin Liver Dis* 1993;13: 170–182.
74. Hanck C, Singer MV, et al. Systemic enhancement of the mRNA expression of IL–18 in unstimulated PBMC of patients with ALD: correlation with endotoxinemia and sCD14 [Abstract]. *Alcohol Alcoho.* 1999;34: 460.
75. Streetz KL, Luedde T, et al. Interleukin 6 and liver regeneration. *Gut* 2000;47:309–312.
76. Mohr L, Tanaka S, et al. Ethanol inhibits hepatocyte proliferation in insulin receptor substrate 1 transgenic mice. *Gastroenterology* 1998; 115:1558–1565.
77. Friedman SL. Seminars in medicine of the Beth Israel Hospital, Boston. The cellular basis of hepatic fibrosis. Mechanisms and treatment strategies. *N Engl J Med* 1993;328:1828–1835.
78. Wang J, Batey RG. Role of ethanol in the regulation of stellate cell function. *World J Gastroenterol* 2006;12:6926–6932.
79. Apte MV, Haber PS, et al. Periacinar stellate shaped cells in rat pancreas: identification, isolation and culture. *Gut* 1998;43:128–133.
80. Campbell GR, Campbell JH. Smooth muscle diversity: implications for the question; What is a smooth muscle cell? *Biomed Res* 1997;8:81–125.
81. Bonis PA, Friedman SL, et al. Is liver fibrosis reversible? *N Engl J Med* 2001;344:452–454.
82. Alexander JF, Lischner MW, et al. Natural history of alcoholic hepatitis: II. The long-term prognosis. *Am J Gastroenterol* 1971;56:515–525.
83. Orrego H, Blake JE, et al. Relationship between gamma-glutamyl transpeptidase and mean urinary alcohol levels in alcoholics while drinking and after alcohol withdrawal. *Alcohol Clin Exp Res* 1985;9: 10–13.
84. Addolorato G, Leggio L, Ferrulli A, et al. Effectiveness and safety of baclofen for maintenance of alcohol abstinence in alcohol-dependent patients with liver cirrhosis: randomised, double-blind controlled study. *Lancet* 2007;370:1915–1922.
85. Brahen LS, Capone TJ, et al. Naltrexone: lack of effect on hepatic enzymes. *J Clin Pharmacol.* 1988;28:64–70.
86. Croop RS, Faulkner EB, et al. The Naltrexone Usage Study Group. The safety profile of naltrexone in the treatment of alcoholism. Results from a multicenter usage study. *Arch Gen Psychiatry* 1997;54: 1130–1135.
87. Mason BJ, Ritvo EC, et al. A double-blind, placebo-controlled pilot study to evaluate the efficacy and safety of oral nalmefene HCl for alcohol dependence. *Alcohol Clin Exp Res* 1994;18:1162–1167.
88. Orrego H, Kalant H, et al. Effect of short–term therapy with propylthiouracil in patients with ALD. *Gastroenterology* 1979;76:105–115.
89. Orrego H, Blake JE, et al. Long–term treatment of ALD with propylthiouracil. *N Engl J Med.* 1987;317:1421–1427.
90. Morgan TR, Weiss DG. Colchicine treatment of alcoholic cirrhosis: a randomized, placebo controlled clinical trial of patient survival. *Gastroenterology* 2005;128:882–890.
91. Mendenhall CL, Anderson S, et al. Short–term and long–term survival in patients with alcoholic hepatitis treated with oxandrolone and prednisolone. *N Engl J Med* 1984;311:1464–1470.
92. Lieber CS, Casini A, et al. S–adenosyl-L-methionine attenuates alcohol-induced liver injury in the baboon. *Hepatology* 1990;11:165–172.
93. Lieber CS, DeCarli LM, et al. Attenuation of alcohol-induced hepatic fibrosis by polyunsaturated lecithin. *Hepatology* 1990;12:1390–1398.
94. Lieber CS, Robins SJ, et al. Phosphatidylcholine protects against fibrosis and cirrhosis in the baboon [see comments]. *Gastroenterology* 1994;106:152–159.
95. Mato JM, Camara J, et al. S-adenosylmethionine in alcoholic liver cirrhosis: a randomized, placebo-controlled, double-blind, multicenter clinical trial. *J Hepatol* 1999;30:1081–1089.
96. Lieber CS, Weiss DG II. Veterans Affairs Cooperative Study of polyenylphosphatidylcholine in ALD. *Alcohol Clin Exp Res* 2003;27: 1765–1772.
97. Akriviadis E, Botla R, et al. Pentoxifylline improves short–term survival in severe acute alcoholic hepatitis: a double-blind, placebo-controlled trial. *Gastroenterology* 2000;119:1637–1648.
98. Taieb J, Chollet–Martin S, et al. The role of interleukin-10 in acute alcoholic hepatitis. *Alcohol Clin Exp Res* 2000;24:191A.
99. Lieber CS, Lefevre A. Effect of oxytetracycline on acidity, ammonia and urea in gastric juice in normal and uremic subjects. *C R Soc Biology (Paris)* 1957;151:1038–1042.
100. Lieber CS, Lefevre A. Ammonia as source of gastric hypoacidity in patients with uremia. *J Clin Invest* 1959;38:1271–1277.

101. Zullo A, Hassan C, Morini S. Hepatic encephalopathy and *Helicobacter pylori:* a critical reappraisal. *J Clin Gastroenterol* 2003;37:164–168.
102. Kumar S, Stauber RE, et al. Orthotopic liver transplantation for ALD. *Hepatology* 1990;11:159–164.
103. Leshner AI. Addiction is a brain disease, and it matters. *Science* 1997; 278:45–47.
104. Wiesner RH, Lombardero M, et al. Liver transplantation for end-stage ALD: an assessment of outcomes. *Liver Transpl Surg* 1997;3:231–239.
105. Haber PS, Koorey DJ, et al. Clinical outcomes of liver transplantation for ALD. *J Gastroenterol Hepatol* 1999.
106. Van Thiel DH, Bonet H, Gaveler J, et al. Effect of alcohol use on allograft rejection rates after liver transplantation for ALD. *Alcohol Clin Exp Res* 1995;19:1151–1155.
107. DiMartini A, Day N, Dew MA, et al. Alcohol consumption patterns and predictors of use following liver transplantation for ALD. *Liver Transpl* 2006;12:813–820.
108. Neuberger J, Tang H. Relapse after transplantation: European studies. *Liver Transpl Surg.*1997;3:275–279.
109. Vaillant GE. The natural history of alcoholism and its relationship to liver transplantation. *Liver Transpl Surg* 1997;3:304–310.
110. Lucey MR, Merion RM, et al. Selection for and outcome of liver transplantation in ALD. *Gastroenterology* 1992;102:1736–1741.
111. Lucey MR, Carr K, et al. Alcohol use after liver transplantation in alcoholics: a clinical cohort follow–up study. *Hepatology* 1997;25: 1223–1227.
112. Kelly M, Chick J. Predictors of relapse to harmful alcohol after orthotopic liver transplantation. *Alcohol Alcohol* 2006;41:278–283.
113. De Gottardi A. A simple score for predicting alcohol relapse after liver transplantation: results from 387 patients over 15 years. *Arch Intern Med* 2007;167:1183–1188.
114. Everhart JE, Beresford TP. Liver transplantation for ALD: a survey of transplantation programs in the United States. *Liver Transpl Surg* 1997;3:220–226.
115. Weinrieb RM, Van Horn DH, et al. Interpreting the significance of drinking by alcohol–dependent liver transplant patients: fostering candor is the key to recovery. *Liver Transpl* 2000;6:769–776.
116. Hollinger FB, Khan NC, et al. Posttransfusion hepatitis type A. *JAMA* 1983;250:2313–2317.
117. Tennant F, Moll D. Seroprevalence of hepatitis A, B, C, and D markers and liver function abnormalities in intravenous heroin addicts. *J Addict Dis* 1995;14:35–49.
118. Crofts N, Cooper G, et al. Exposure to hepatitis A virus among blood donors, injecting drug users and prison entrants in Victoria. *J Viral Hepat* 1997;4:333–338.
119. Iwarson S. New target groups for vaccination against hepatitis A: homosexual men, injecting drug users and patients with chronic hepatitis. *Scand J Infect Dis* 1998;30:316–318.
120. Shapiro CN, Coleman PJ, et al. Epidemiology of hepatitis A: seroepidemiology and risk groups in the USA. *Vaccine* 1992;10(Suppl 1): S59–S62.
121. Lamagni TL, Davison KL, et al. Poor hepatitis B vaccine coverage in injecting drug users: England, 1995 and 1996. *Commun Dis Public Health* 1999;2:174–177.
122. Sherlock SJ, Dooley J. Virus hepatitis. *Diseases of the liver and biliary system.* Oxford: Blackwell, 1997.
123. Korenman J, Baker B, et al. Long–term remission of chronic hepatitis B after alpha–interferon therapy. *Ann Intern Med* 1991;114:629–634.
124. Dusheiko GM, Roberts JA. Treatment of chronic type B and C hepatitis with interferon alfa: an economic appraisal [see comments]. *Hepatology* 1995;22:1863–1873.
125. National Institutes of Health Consensus Development Conference Panel statement: management of hepatitis C. *Hepatology* 1997;26:2S–10S.
126. Alter MJ. Epidemiology of hepatitis C. *Hepatology* 1997;26:62S–65S.
127. Grebely J, Conway B, Raffa JD, et al. Hepatitis C virus reinfection in injection drug users. *Hepatology* 2006;44:1139–1145.
128. Kaldor JM, Archer GT, et al. Risk factors for hepatitis C virus infection in blood donors: a case–control study. *Med J Aust* 1992;157: 227–230.
129. van Beek I. Infection with HIV and hepatitis C virus among injecting drug users in a prevention setting: retrospective cohort study [see comments]. *BMJ* 1998;317:433–437.
130. MacDonald MA, Wodak AD, Dolan KA, et al. Hepatitis C virus antibody prevalence among injecting drug users at selected needle and syringe programs in Australia, 1995–1997. Collaboration of Australian NSPs [see comments]. *Med J Aust* 2000;172:57–61.
131. Maher L, Li J, et al. High hepatitis C incidence in new injecting drug users: a policy failure? *Aust N Z J Public Health* 2007;31:30–35.
132. Goldberg D, Burns S, et al. Trends in HCV prevalence among injecting drug users in Glasgow and Edinburgh during the era of needle/syringe exchange. *Scand J Infect Dis* 2001;33:457–461.
133. Hagan H, McGough JP, et al. Syringe exchange and risk of infection with hepatitis B and C viruses. *Am J Epidemiol* 1999;149:203–213.
134. Sachithanandan S, Fielding JF. Low rate of HCV transmission from women infected with contaminated anti–D immunoglobulin to their family contacts. *Ital J Gastroenterol Hepatol* 1997;29:47–50.
135. Meisel H, Reip A, et al. Transmission of hepatitis C virus to children and husbands by women infected with contaminated anti–D immunoglobulin. *Lancet* 1995;345:1209–1211.
136. Bresters D, Mauser–Bunschoten EP, et al. Sexual transmission of hepatitis C virus. *Lancet* 1993;342:210–211.
137. Alter MJ, Kruszon–Moran D, et al. The prevalence of hepatitis C virus infection in the United States, 1988 through 1994. *N Engl J Med* 1999;341:556–562.
138. Murphy EL, Bryzman S, et al. Prevalence of hepatitis C virus infection in the United States. *N Engl J Med* 1999;341:2093.
139. Dore GJ, Law MG, et al. Prevalence of hepatitis C virus infection in the United States. *N Engl J Med* 1999;341:2094–2095.
140. Murphy EL, Bryzman SM, et al. NHLBI Retrovirus Epidemiology Donor Study (REDS). Risk factors for hepatitis C virus infection in United States blood donors. *Hepatology.* 2000;31:756–762.
141. Conte D. Prevalence and clinical course of chronic hepatitis C virus (HCV) infection and rate of HCV vertical transmission in a cohort of 15,250 pregnant women. *Hepatology* 2000;31:751–755.
142. Dore GJ, Kaldor JM, et al. Systematic review of role of polymerase chain reaction in defining infectiousness among people infected with hepatitis C virus. *BMJ* 1997;315:333–337.
143. Spencer JD, Latt N, et al. Transmission of hepatitis C virus to infants of human immunodeficiency virus-negative intravenous drug-using mothers: rate of infection and assessment of risk factors for transmission. *J Viral Hepatol* 1997;4:395–409.
144. Whyte GS, Savoia HF. The risk of transmitting HCV, HBV, or HIV by blood transfusion in Victoria. *Med J Aust.*1997;166:584–586.
145. Power JP, Lawlor E, et al. Molecular epidemiology of an outbreak of infection with hepatitis C virus in recipients of anti–D immunoglobulin. *Lancet* 1995;345:1211–1213.
146. NHMRC. A strategy for the detection and management of hepatitis C in Australia. Australian Government Publishing Service, 1997: Publication number 2033.
147. Padron GJ, Rodriguez Z, et al. [Hepatitis C virus in plasmapheresis donors]. *Sangre (Barc)* 1995;40:187–190.
148. Allander T, Gruber A, et al. Frequent patient-to-patient transmission of hepatitis C virus in a haematology ward. *Lancet* 1995;345: 603–607.
149. Dussol B, Berthezene P, et al. Hepatitis C virus infection among chronic dialysis patients in the south of France: a collaborative study. *Am J Kidney Dis* 1995;25:399–404.
150. Okuda K, Hayashi H, et al. Mode of hepatitis C infection not associated with blood transfusion among chronic hemodialysis patients. *J Hepatol* 1995;23:28–31.
151. Bronowicki JP, Venard V, et al. Patient–to–patient transmission of hepatitis C virus during colonoscopy. *N Engl J Med* 1997;337:237–240.
152. Hepatitis C transmission from health care worker to patient, PHLS Communicable Diseases Surveillance Centre: *Commun Dis Rep CDR Wkly* 1995;5:135–139.
153. Crofts N, Stewart T, et al. Spread of bloodborne viruses among Australian prison entrants. *BMJ* 1995;310:285–288.

154. Butler TG, Dolan KA, et al. Hepatitis B and C in New South Wales prisons: prevalence and risk factors. *Med J Aust* 1997;166:127–130.
155. Haber PS, Parsons SJ, et al. Transmission of hepatitis C within Australian prisons [see comments]. *Med J Aust* 1999;171:31–33.
156. Post JJ, Dolan KA, et al. Acute hepatitis C virus infection in an Australian prison inmate: tattooing as a possible transmission route. *Med J Aust* 2001;174:183–184.
157. Frank C, Mohamed MK, et al. The role of parenteral antischistosomal therapy in the spread of hepatitis C virus in Egypt. *Lancet* 2000;355: 887–891.
158. Koziel MJ, Wong DK, et al. Hepatitis C virus–specific cytolytic T lymphocyte and T helper cell responses in seronegative persons. *J Infect Dis* 1997;176:859–866.
159. Poynard T, Ratziu V, et al. Rates and risk factors of liver fibrosis progression in patients with chronic hepatitis C. *J Hepatol* 2001;34: 730–739.
160. Stephenson J. Former addicts face barriers to treatment for HCV. *JAMA* 2001;285:1003–1005.
161. Weltman MD, Brotodihardjo A, et al. Coinfection with hepatitis B and C or B, C and delta viruses results in severe chronic liver disease and responds poorly to interferon–alpha treatment. *J Viral Hepat*ol 1995;2:39–45.
162. Degos F. Hepatitis C and alcohol. *J Hepatol* 1999;31(Suppl 1): 113–118.
163. Ostapowicz G, Watson KJ, Locarnini SA, et al. Role of alcohol in the progression of liver disease caused by hepatitis C virus infection. *Hepatology* 1998;27:1730–1735.
164. Cromie SL, Jenkins PJ, et al. Chronic hepatitis C: effect of alcohol on hepatitic activity and viral titre. *J Hepatol* 1996;25:821–826.
165. Schiff ER. Hepatitis C and alcohol. *Hepatology* 1997;26:39S–42S.
166. Adinolfi LE, Gambardella M, et al. Steatosis accelerates the progression of liver damage of chronic hepatitis C patients and correlates with specific HCV genotype and visceral obesity. *Hepatology* 2001;33:1358–1364.
167. Clouston AD, Jonsson JR, et al. Steatosis and chronic hepatitis C: analysis of fibrosis and stellate cell activation. *J Hepatol* 2001;34: 314–320.
167a. National Institutes of Health Consensus Development Conference Panel Statement: management of hepatitis C. *Hepatol* 1997;26: 25–105.
167b. International Consensus Conference on Hepatitis C. *J Hepatol* 1999; 31 (Suppl 1):1–268.
168. Neary MP, Cort S, et al. Sustained virologic response is associated with improved health–related quality of life in relapsed chronic hepatitis C patients. *Semin Liver Dis* 1999;19:77–85.
169. Ware JE, Bayliss MS, et al. The Interventional Therapy Group. Health-related quality of life in chronic hepatitis C: impact of disease and treatment response. *Hepatology* 1999;30:550–555.
170. Pawlotsky JM. Therapy of hepatitis C: from empiricism to eradication. *Hepatology* 2006;43:S207–S220.
171. McHutchison JG, Gordon SC, et al. Hepatitis Interventional Therapy Group. Interferon alfa-2b alone or in combination with ribavirin as initial treatment for chronic hepatitis C. *N Engl J Med* 1998;339: 1485–1492.
172. Poynard T, Marcellin P, et al. Randomised trial of interferon α2b plus ribavirin for 48 weeks or for 24 weeks versus interferon α2b plus placebo for 48 weeks for treatment of chronic infection with hepatitis C virus. International Hepatitis Interventional Therapy Group (IHIT). *Lancet* 1998;352:1426–1432.
173. Heathcote EJ, Shiffman ML, et al. Peginterferon Alfa-2a in patients with chronic hepatitis C and cirrhosis. *N Engl J Med* 2000;343: 1673–1680.
174. Persico M, Persico E, et al. Natural history of hepatitis C virus carriers with persistently normal aminotransferase levels. *Gastroenterology* 2000;118:760–764.
175. Sangiovanni A, Morales R, et al. Interferon alfa treatment of HCV RNA carriers with persistently normal transaminase levels: a pilot randomized controlled study. *Hepatology* 1998;27:853–856.
176. Davis GL, Rodrigue JR. Treatment of chronic hepatitis C in active drug users. *N Engl J Med* 2001;345:215–217.
177. Edlin BR, Seal KH, et al. Is it justifiable to withhold treatment for hepatitis C from illicit-drug users? *N Engl J Med* 2001;345:211–215.
178. Novick DM. The impact of hepatitis C virus infection on methadone maintenance treatment. *Mt Sinai J Me*d 2000;67:437–443.
179. Dieperink E, Willenbring M, et al. Neuropsychiatric symptoms associated with hepatitis C and interferon alpha: a review. *Am J Psychiatry* 2000;157:867–876.
180. Batey RG, Salmond SJ, et al. Complementary and Alternative medicines in the treatment of chronic liver disease. *Curr Gastroenterol Rev* 2005; 7:63–70.
181. Batey RG, Bensoussan A, et al. Preliminary report of a randomized, double-blind placebo-controlled trial of a Chinese herbal medicine preparation CH-100 in the treatment of chronic hepatitis C. *J Gastroenterol Hepatol* 1998;13:244–247.
182. Levy MT, Chen JJ, et al. Liver transplantation for hepatitis C-associated cirrhosis in a single Australian centre: referral patterns and transplant outcomes. *J Gastroenterol Hepatol* 1997;12:453–459.
183. Lau N, Schiano TD, et al. Survival and recidivism risk in methadone-dependent patients undergoing liver transplantation. *Hepatology* 2000; 32:245A.
184. Rothstein KD, Kanchana TP, et al. Is liver transplantation appropriate in patients on methadone maintenance? *Hepatology* 2000;32:245A.
185. Koch M, Banys P. Liver transplantation and opioid dependence. *JAMA* 2001;285:1056–1058.
186. Riordan SM, Skouteris GG, et al. Metabolic activity and clinical efficacy of animal and human hepatocytes in bioartificial support systems for acute liver failure [editorial]. *Int J Artif Organs* 1998;21: 312–318.
187. Silva MO, Roth D, et al. Hepatic dysfunction accompanying acute cocaine intoxication. *J Hepatol* 1991;12:312–315.
188. Selim K, Kaplowitz N. Hepatotoxicity of psychotropic drugs. *Hepatology* 1999;29:1347–1351.
189. Mallat A, Dhumeaux D. Cocaine and the liver. *J Hepatol* 1991;12: 275–278.
190. Henry JA, Jeffreys KJ, et al. Toxicity and deaths from 3,4-methylenedioxymethamphetamine ("ecstasy"). *Lancet* 1992;340: 384–387.
191. Hearn WL, Flynn DD, et al. Cocaethylene: a unique cocaine metabolite displays high affinity for the dopamine transporter. *J Neurochem* 1991;56:698–701.
192. Heith AM, Morse CR, et al. Fatty acid ethyl ester synthase catalyzes the esterification of ethanol to cocaine. *Biochem Biophys Res Commun* 1995;208:549–554.
193. Andrews P. Cocaethylene toxicity. *J Addict Dis* 1997;16:75–84.
194. Worner TM. Hepatotoxicity is not increased in alcoholics with positive urinary cocaine metabolites. *Drug Alcohol Depend* 1994;35: 191–5.
195. Brauer RB, Heidecke CD, et al. Liver transplantation for the treatment of fulminant hepatic failure induced by the ingestion of ecstasy. *Transpl Int* 1997;10:229–233.
196. Ellis AJ, Wendon JA, et al. Acute liver damage and ecstasy ingestion. *Gut* 1996;38:454–458.
197. Tucker GT, Lennard MS, et al. The demethylenation of methylenedioxymethamphetamine ("ecstasy") by debrisoquine hydroxylase (CYP2D6). *Biochem Pharmacol* 1994;47:1151–1156.
198. Colado MI, Williams JL, et al. The hyperthermic and neurotoxic effects of 'Ecstasy" (MDMA) and 3,4 methylenedioxyamphetamine (MDA) in the Dark Agouti (DA) rat, a model of the CYP2D6 poor metabolizer phenotype. *Br J Pharmacol* 1995;115:1281–1289.
199. Jones AL, Simpson KJ. Review article: mechanisms and management of hepatotoxicity in ecstasy (MDMA) and amphetamine intoxications. *Aliment Pharmacol Ther* 1999;13:129–133.
200. Baggott M, Heifets B, et al. Chemical analysis of ecstasy pills [in process citation]. *JAMA* 2000;284:2190.
201. Kringsholm B, Christoffersen P. The nature and the occurrence of birefringent material in different organs in fatal drug addiction. *Forensic Sci Int* 1987;34:53–62.
202. Pare JP, Cote G, et al. Long-term follow-up of drug abusers with intravenous talcosis. *Am Rev Respir Dis* 1989;139:233–241.

203. Molos MA, Litton N, et al. Talc liver. *J Clin Gastroenterol* 1987;9: 198–203.
204. Allaire GS, Goodman ZD, et al. Talc in liver tissue of intravenous drug abusers with chronic hepatitis. A comparative study. *Am J Clin Pathol* 1989;92:583–588.
205. Norton RL, Burton BT, et al. Blood lead of intravenous drug users. *J Toxicol Clin Toxicol* 1996;34:425–430.
206. Armen R, Kanel G, et al. Phencyclidine–induced malignant hyperthermia causing submassive liver necrosis. *Am J Med* 1984;77: 167–172.
207. Teixeira–Clerc F, Julien B, et al. The endocannabinoid system as a novel target for the treatment of liver fibrosis. *Pathol Biol (Paris)* 2008; 56:36–38.
208. Ishida JH, Peters MG, et al. Influence of cannabis use on severity of hepatitis C disease. *Clin Gastroenterol Hepatol* 2008;6:69–75.
209. Hezode C, Zafrani ES, et al. Daily cannabis use: a novel risk factor of steatosis severity in patients with chronic hepatitis C. *Gastroenterology* 2008;134:432–439.
210. Sylvestre DL, Clements BJ. Cannabis use improves retention and virological outcomes in patients treated for hepatitis C. *Eur J Gastroenterol Hepatol* 2006;18:1057–1063.
211. Fischer B, Reimer J, et al. Treatment for hepatitis C virus and cannabis use in illicit drug user patients: implications and questions. *Eur J Gastroenterol Hepatol* 2006;18:1057–1063.
212. Sanchez–Osorio M, Duarte-Rojo A, et al. Anabolic-androgenic steroids and liver injury. *Liver Int* 2008;28:278–282.
213. The European Association for the Study of Liver Disease. *International Consensus Conference on Hepatitis C.* Paris: Author, 1999.
214. Auguet T, Vidal F, et al. A study on the TNF-alpha system in Caucasian Spanish patients with ALD. *Drug Alcohol Depend* 2008;92:91–99.
215. Danta M, Brown D, Bhagani S, et al. Recent epidemic of acute hepatitis C virus in HIV–positive men who have sex with men linked to high-risk sexual behaviours. *AIDS* 2007;21:983–991.
216. Kafrouni M, Anders RA, Verma S. Hepatotoxicity associated with dietary supplements containing anabolic steroids. *Clin Gastroenterol Hepatol* 2007;51:809–812.

CHAPTER 73

Jose Carlos T. DaSilva, MD, MPH
Derya Bora Hazar, MD

Renal and Metabolic Disorders Related to Alcohol and Other Drug Use

The perception that drug abuse and renal disease are closely intertwined is easily confirmed by a simple survey of the population undergoing chronic dialysis in urban, inner-city hospitals, and clinics. It is likely that the prevalence of present or previous drug addiction in this cohort of individuals surpasses the prevalence in the general population.

The causal links are apparent in some cases (1,2), such as HIV nephropathy, hepatitis C–associated glomerular disease, or subcutaneous injection drug-related amyloidosis.

However, with other diseases, such as accelerated hypertension or subtypes of focal and segmental focal glomerulosclerosis, the relationship, even if strongly suspected, has not been proven definitively.

Most harmful effects of illicit drug use are related to infectious agents inoculated during drug use or acquired owing to high-risk behavior exposures or direct pharmacologic effects of drugs, for example repeated bouts of intense vasoconstriction with cocaine use.

A list of the renal problems thought to be associated with common drugs of abuse is found in Table 73.1. However, the multiplicity of behavioral risk factors and the variety of possible etiologic agents makes it difficult to define a clear-cut relationship between a given drug of abuse and a renal disease. Perhaps a more useful classification for the practitioner features the renal syndromes of presentation that can be related to one or more exposures connected to drug addiction (Table 73.2).

MEASUREMENT OF RENAL FUNCTION

For the physician responsible for any patient with current or past drug abuse or dependence, obtaining a measurement of renal function, serum electrolytes, urinalysis, and urine protein excretion on a regular and frequent basis is mandatory. If proteinuria is present, 24-hour urine quantification is very useful. Using the same 24-hour specimen, a total urine creatinine excretion with a concurrent plasma creatinine will provide a useful estimate of glomerular filtration rate (GFR = urinary creatinine concentration × urinary volume/plasma creatinine concentration/1.73 m^2). The latter is particularly important because many people with drug abuse or dependence have reduced muscle mass or are cachectic. If the compliance with a 24-hour urine collection is a problem, GFR-estimating equations can be used (3), with the caveat that in cases of renal function not at steady-state or elevation of serum creatinine related to increased generation (e.g., rhabdomyolysys), the equations will not apply. Patients with cachexia and cirrhosis often have a serum creatinine values within the "normal range," yet their GFR is markedly diminished. Recent research studies have shown the utility of cystatin C as a marker of renal function in this patient population (4).

Knowledge of GFR is important, not only in assessing renal function but in determining medication dose adjustments. If it is not possible to obtain a 24-hour collection, proteinuria can be estimated by using a spot urine protein-to-creatinine ratio. The ratio represents the approximate protein excretion; for example, a ratio of 3 means an approximate daily excretion of 3 g protein. It should be recognized that, in patients with reduced muscle mass, this ratio will overestimate actual protein excretion. However, it still is very useful in following changes in protein excretion in the same patient over time (5).

TABLE 73.1 Common Drugs of Abuse Associated with Renal Problems

Opiates
- HIV nephropathy
- Hepatitis C–associated glomerulopathies
- Hepatitis B–associated polyarteritis nodosa
- Bacterial endocarditis and acute glomerulonephritis
- Subcutaneous injection ("skin-popping") amyloidosis
- Nontraumatic rhabdomyolysis (muscle compression) and acute renal failure
- Heroin nephropathy.

Cocaine
- Rhabdomyolysis and acute renal failure
- Accelerated hypertension and renal failure
- HIV nephropathy
- Hypertensive nephrosclerosis
- Renal infarction
- Thrombotic microangiopathy and renal failure.

Alcohol
- Hepatorenal syndrome
- Rhabdomyolysis and acute renal failure
- Increased incidence and severity of postinfectious glomerulonephritis
- Electrolyte disorders.

TABLE 73.2 Renal Syndromes Commonly Associated with Drug and Excessive Alcohol Use

Use

Nephrotic syndrome
- Hepatitis B– or hepatitis C–related membranous nephropathy
- HIV nephropathy (IDU)
- Amyloidosis (subcutaneous injection drug use (IDU) ["skin popping"])
- Focal and segmental glomerulosclerosis (IDU).

Nephritic-nephrotic syndrome
- Hepatitis C–related membranoproliferative glomerulonephritis (IDU)
- Hepatitis C–related cryoglobulinemia (IDU).

Nephritic syndrome
- Bacterial endocarditis and acute glomerulonephritis (IDU)
- Postinfectious glomerulonephritis (IDU).

Acute renal failure
- Rhabdomyolysis (alcohol, cocaine, MDMA [ecstasy], opiates)
- Crystal-induced renal failure (indinavir, acyclovir, sulfonamides)
- Thrombotic microangiopathy (cocaine).

Hypertension
- Hepatitis B– or amphetamine-associated polyarteritis nodosa (IDU, amphetamine)
- Accelerated hypertension (cocaine).

NEPHROTIC SYNDROME

Nephrotic syndrome is narrowly defined as heavy proteinuria (>3.5 g/day), hypoalbuminemia, hyperlipidemia, lipiduria, and edema. However, separate components of the syndrome may be absent and, from a diagnostic point of view, heavy proteinuria is sufficient to consider the patient nephrotic.

HIV-Associated Nephropathy In spite of improved survival and decreased incidence of opportunistic infections in HIV-infected individuals taking appropriate antiretroviral therapy, the development of proteinuria and impaired renal function are a harbinger of poor prognosis (6). The most common histologic finding is a form of focal and segmental glomerular sclerosis with collapse of the glomerular tufts, also named *collapsing nephropathy* (7). African American race, low CD4 counts, and positive family history of renal disease are risk factors for the development of HIV-associated nephropathy (HIVAN).

During the years of 1995 and 1999, the incidence of end-stage renal disease (ESRD) due to HIVAN decreased from 8.5% to 6.8%, and the survival on dialysis improved from 52% to 69%, likely the consequence of use of highly active antiretroviral therapy (HAART) (8).

The apparent resistance of white patients with AIDS to developing HIVAN, as compared with African Americans, suggests a genetic predisposition. In fact, more than 90% of patients who develop HIVAN are of African descent (9), and the prevalence of ESRD in relatives of AIDS patients who develop HIVAN is higher than in their counterparts without renal disease (10).

HIVAN can occur at any stage of HIV disease, with presentation in patients who already have an AIDS-defining condition or as the presenting manifestation of AIDS in patients who otherwise are asymptomatic. Most HIVAN patients have CD4 counts of <250 cells/mm^3 (11) and therefore are candidates for aggressive antiretroviral therapy.

The pathogenesis of HIVAN is incompletely understood. It is known that transgenic mice that express HIV proviral constructs in renal tissue develop disease that is identical to HIVAN in humans (12). Moreover, when kidneys from those transgenic mice are transplanted into normal recipients, they develop the typical histologic changes of HIVAN. However, when normal kidneys are transplanted into transgenic mice, renal tissue is unaffected (13). These data suggest a direct role of viral infection rather than the indirect effects of modulation of different cytokines and associated infective agents, which often are encountered in the later stages of AIDS.

Though the typical patient with HIVAN presents with nephrotic-range proteinuria, this massive proteinuria is not usually accompanied by edema or serosal effusions. The urinary sediment contains oval fat bodies and fatty casts and, often, unusually broad waxy casts that, presumably, reflect the dilated tubules of their origin. Ultrasonic evaluation reveals normal-sized or enlarged kidneys that are hyperechoic. The absence of hypertension, even with advanced renal insufficiency, in this largely African American patient population, is intriguing.

Histologic findings with light microscopy in HIVAN include focal and segmental glomerulosclerosis, often with features of collapsing glomerular disease. Interstitial inflammation with microcystic tubular dilatation is regularly noted (14). Immunofluorescence usually is negative. In some cases, electron microscopy reveals tubuloreticular structures that are thought to be associated with ribonucleoproteins and elevated levels of alpha interferon. These structures are typical, but not diagnostic, of HIVAN because they can be found in other diseases, particularly systemic lupus erythematosus.

Renal insufficiency appears very early in the disease and is rapidly progressive, leading to ESRD in a matter of weeks or months. More recently, however, with the use of HAART at earlier stages of HIV infection, a more benign and protracted course can be seen (7,15). In addition, use of angiotensin-converting enzyme inhibitors appears to decrease the magnitude of proteinuria and postpone progression, as drugs of this class do in other glomerular diseases (16,17).

In the past, patients with HIVAN were denied dialysis because of their short life expectancy. Today, dialysis is provided to these patients, and centers are offering stable HIV patients on dialysis the opportunity for renal transplantation. This opportunity reflects the longer survival of HIV patients on renal replacement therapy and the better outlook for patients who respond and are adherent to HAART.

Hepatitis Virus–Associated Nephrotic Syndrome

Hepatitis B- and C-associated nephropathies are, as expected of blood-borne diseases, frequently found among injection drug users (IDUs). All patients presenting with nephritic syndrome of unknown etiology should be tested for hepatitis. The association between hepatitis B and membranous nephropathy is well established, with morphologic studies demonstrating deposition of hepatitis B e antigen in glomerular capillaries (18). It is important to diagnose this cause of membranous nephropathy, because immunosuppressive treatment—often used in the idiopathic form of nephrotic syndrome—actually may enhance ongoing hepatitis B viral replication. Moreover, antiviral therapy may prove beneficial (19–21).

The most common presentation of renal disease in patients with hepatitis C is a combination of nephritic and nephrotic syndromes (i.e., a urine that contains large amounts of protein, red blood cells, and red blood casts; see the following section, "Nephritic-Nephrotic Syndrome"). Less often, membranous nephropathy has been described in association with hepatitis C in IDUs (22,23). The detection of hepatitis C virus protein in the glomeruli of patients with membranous nephropathy (22) strengthens this association.

Heroin Nephropathy Heroin nephropathy has been considered a secondary cause of focal and segmental glomerulosclerosis, often associated with hypertension and slow progression to ESRD. Since HIVAN first was recognized, the diagnosis of heroin nephropathy rarely has been encountered. This rarity may reflect more purified forms of heroin and/or the removal of contaminants that were, in fact, responsible for "heroin nephropathy" or the earlier development of HIVAN in this susceptible group. Patients with focal and segmental glomerulosclerosis, a history of IDU, and infection with hepatitis C may present with a clinical picture similar to that of heroin nephropathy (23).

Subcutaneous Drug Use-Associated Amyloidosis

Chronic suppurative skin infections related to subcutaneous illicit drug injection are known to be associated with secondary amyloidosis with renal involvement (24–26). Clinically, these patients may be very difficult to distinguish from those with HIVAN or hepatitis-related renal disease because they present with nephritic range proteinuria, renal insufficiency, and normal-sized or enlarged kidneys. The evidence of subcutaneous drug injection ("skin popping," or multiple skin scars or draining abscesses) should alert the physician to the possibility of this diagnosis. If alternative diagnoses are possible, a renal biopsy is appropriate to confirm the presence of amyloidosis. In addition to proteinuria and renal insufficiency, tubular dysfunction, including nephrogenic diabetes insipidus and proximal or distal renal tubular acidosis, may be present. New avenues to treat secondary forms of systemic amyloidosis were recently reported (27).

NEPHRITIC-NEPHROTIC SYNDROME

In addition to significant proteinuria, the presence of hematuria, hypertension, and variable degrees of renal insufficiency in the setting of past or present IDU should raise the suspicion of hepatitis C–related glomerular disease. The most common pattern of injury in patients with hepatitis C infection is membranoproliferative glomerulonephritis with or without cryoglobulinemia (28–30). Less commonly, membranous nephropathy (see foregoing) or fibrillary glomerulonephritis and immunotactoid glomerulopathy may be encountered. In the latter two instances, the clinical presentation and light microscopy findings can be indistinguishable from membranoproliferative glomerulonephritis, but organized deposits of fibrils of different sizes are detected on electron microscopy (31).

Though liver function test results often are abnormal, there are many cases in which they are only minimally elevated or within normal limits, and there are no findings in the history or physical examination that point to liver dysfunction (32,33). In cases with associated essential mixed cryoglobulinemia, serum cryoglobulins are detected. In addition, palpable purpura, arthralgias, peripheral neuropathy, and nonspecific systemic complaints may be present. A pattern of serum complement with decreased C4 and normal C3 levels is characteristic of mixed cryoglobulinemia (34). A positive rheumatoid factor is seen inconsistently. Typical renal biopsy features of mixed cryoglobulinemia include intraluminal thrombi in glomerular capillaries and a substructure of curvilinear fibrils in the subendothelial space, which resemble "fingerprints" on electron microscopy.

The use of combination therapy with interferon and ribavirin (Virazole) is accepted even in the absence of specific indications to treat the liver disease. The use of ribavirin is contraindicated when the creatinine clearance is <50 mL/minute because of increased side effects, including severe hemolytic anemia (35).

Coinfection with hepatitis C is found in up to 78% of HIV-infected IDUs (36). The course of nephropathy associated with this dual infection has been reported as aggressive, with rapid progression to ESRD.

NEPHRITIC SYNDROME

The presence of a nephritic urinary sediment (proteinuria, hematuria, and often red blood cell casts), variable degrees of hypertension, and renal insufficiency in the setting of IDU should raise the suspicion of immune complex–mediated glomerulonephritis. In this circumstance, bacterial sepsis and acute bacterial endocarditis are not rare. The most frequent pathogen is *Staphylococcus aureus* (37–42). Less often *Streptococcus viridans*, gram-negative rods, or *Candida* species are isolated. Actual septic embolization of the kidneys is much less common. The latter complication would be recognized by persistent fevers, gross or microscopic hematuria (occasionally accompanied by flank pain), and signs of embolization to other organs. If large renal vessels are occluded, filling defects can be documented by an isotopic renal perfusion scan.

Hypertension and low complement levels (C3) are present less consistently than in poststreptococcal glomerulonephritis, and nephrotic syndrome occurs in a minority of cases (37). Although renal failure may be irreversible in some cases, recovery of renal function usually occurs with treatment of the underlying infection (43).

In patients with postinfectious glomerulonephritis as a manifestation of acute endocarditis or abscesses, histologic features similar to those found with poststreptococcal glomerulonephritis are seen. The pattern is one of acute proliferative glomerulonephritis with neutrophil infiltration and immune complex deposition in the mesangium and capillary walls. A higher incidence and more severe course of postinfectious glomerulonephritis in people with alcohol dependence has been reported, but the specific reasons for this condition are unclear (44–46).

Patients with bacterial endocarditis who develop renal failure days to weeks after the onset of antibiotic therapy should raise the suspicion of acute interstitial nephritis. Suggestive of this diagnosis is the finding, in the urine sediment, of renal tubular and/or white blood cells, often in casts. Eosinophiluria, if found, corroborates the diagnosis, but it has a low specificity and sensitivity for interstitial nephritis.

ISOLATED HEMATURIA

The presence of hematuria should not be assumed to be glomerular in origin, especially in the absence of proteinuria. Obviously, people with addiction can manifest urologic disease unrelated to their drug. Therefore, urologic evaluation may be in order before ascribing isolated hematuria to a parenchymal renal process.

Hematuria may be the only manifestation of immunoglobulin A (IgA) nephropathy, and there appears to be an association between IgA nephropathy and alcoholic cirrhosis. It has been suggested that this association can be related to a decreased clearance of IgA molecules because of arteriovenous shunting away from the reticuloendothelial system. However, IgA deposition is not usually associated with progressive deterioration of renal function and should not preclude liver transplantation in otherwise suitable patients.

IgA nephropathy can occur in patients with HIV infection in whom microscopic or macroscopic hematuria may be the only presenting sign (47,48). Renal biopsy is the only definitive diagnostic tool in these patients. In patients undergoing treatment with antiretroviral medications, particularly indinavir (Crixivan), acyclovir (Zovirax), or large doses of sulfonamides, crystalluria is another possible explanation for hematuria (see the section "Acute Renal Failure"). Such hematuria sometimes is associated with impaired renal function, which usually is reversible after volume expansion and discontinuation of the offending agent.

HYPERTENSION AND RENAL DISEASE

The development of acute hypertension in connection with cocaine use is well recognized and seems to be associated with the release of endothelin 1 and activation of the renin angiotensin system (49,50). The clinical presentations of cocaine intoxication can mimic preeclampsia or scleroderma renal crisis (51,52), and the development of accelerated hypertension and renal failure has been documented by some (53,54) but not other observers (55). This inconsistency may reflect confounding factors, including the intensity and length of exposure, genetic predisposition, and duration of follow-up. The amphetamine-like drug MDMA (3,4-methylenedioxymethamphetamine), also known as "Ecstasy," has been reported to produce accelerated hypertension and acute renal failure (56).

Polyarteritis nodosa has been associated with hepatitis B and drugs of abuse, especially amphetamines. Patients may present with accelerated hypertension and systemic symptoms, including malaise, arthralgias, weight loss, and asymmetric peripheral neuropathy. They may have a necrotizing vasculitis, which can affect medium-sized arteries, including renal, mesenteric, coronary, and (rarely) cerebral circulation. The test result for antinuclear cytoplasmic antibodies usually is negative (57,58). Angiography is the diagnostic procedure of choice. The finding of diffuse microaneurysms with areas of thrombosis and ischemia in multiple organs, including the kidneys, is diagnostic.

Treatment usually is with steroids and cytotoxic agents. Antivirals such as lamivudine or telbivudine may prove to be effective, without the risk of enhanced viral replication with immunosuppression.

Hypertension and progressive renal failure are associated with the ingestion of homemade whiskey (so-called "moonshine"). The nephrotoxic exposure is thought to be the chronic ingestion of lead, which is found in the car radiators used to distill the whiskey. These patients often have hyperuricemia and gout and thus have been labeled with the diagnosis of "saturnine gout" (59).

ACUTE RENAL FAILURE

Rhabdomyolysis The presentation in the emergency department of a young adult with a history of alcohol or illicit drug use (especially cocaine or MDMA), who is agitated, confused, combative, and hyperthermic and who has a urinalysis highly suggestive of this disease (that is, brownish-red urine positive for blood but without red blood cells on microscopy) is a common scenario. Tonic–clonic seizures may have occurred prior to admission. In addition, blood testing usually reveals a markedly elevated serum creatine kinase level.

Drugs associated with rhabdomyolysis include phencyclidine, methamphetamines, MDMA, cocaine, heroin, and alcohol (49,60–63). The presence of volume depletion, hypotension (64), acidosis, and hypoxemia increase the likelihood of acute tubular necrosis.

The mechanism of tubular injury is multifactorial. Precipitating events may include volume depletion, often from fluid sequestered in damaged muscles (potentially several liters); decreased vasodilatory effect of nitric oxide, which is inactivated by myoglobin (65); toxicity of free chelatable iron released from myoglobin (66); and tubular obstruction by pigmented casts (67).

Patients with total-body potassium depletion (e.g., malnourished people with alcohol dependence) may be predisposed to ischemic muscular injury because potassium release at the level of the microcirculation is an important mechanism for vasodilatation that sustains muscle perfusion during physical activity (68). Total-body phosphate depletion is also a predisposing factor, and the hypophosphatemia can be masked at the time of presentation because of phosphate release from injured muscle cells (even producing hyperphosphatemia). In addition to hyperactivity, compression of muscle (crush injury) because of drug induced stupor or coma and immobilization for prolonged periods of time can result in rhabdomyolysis. In the early phase, hypocalcemia can be secondary to deposition of calcium in necrotic muscle cells or precipitation with phosphate released from destroyed muscle cells. Hyperkalemia and hyperuricemia also may be present.

Treatment depends on the phase of the disease at the time of presentation. If severe renal failure is not present, an attempt at volume expansion with isotonic saline is appropriate. In the absence of hypocalcemia, the use of sodium bicarbonate to alkalinize the urine can decrease the toxicity of myoglobin. The role of mannitol (Osmitrol) in this setting is less clear (69). Though in some early series (70) up to 50% of patients required acute dialysis, currently most patients do recover renal function, without the need for renal replacement therapy, perhaps reflecting more aggressive initial volume resuscitation and goal oriented early intensive care interventions.

Crystal-Induced Tubular Injury Acute renal failure has been described with the use of antiviral agents, including acyclovir (71), indinavir (72,73), ritonavir (Norvir) (74), and sulfonamide, usually when they are used in large doses in patients who also are volume-depleted.

The urinary sediment helps to confirm the diagnosis when crystals typical of the ingested drug are present. Recovery of renal function is the rule when the patient is given adequate hydration and is withdrawn from the offending agent or the dose is reduced. Indinavir has been associated with the formation of urinary stones.

Hepatorenal Syndrome Chronic alcohol ingestion can lead to hepatorenal syndrome if liver damage occurs. The pathogenesis and pathophysiology of this syndrome is complex and beyond the scope of this chapter. The interested reader is referred to more complete reviews (75,76).

Briefly, this syndrome is thought to reflect a state of profound renal vasoconstriction and splanchnic vasodilatation associated with severely impaired liver function, often with portal hypertension and ascites. A slow rise in serum creatinine and oliguria, accompanied by low urinary sodium concentration—usually <10 mEq/L—are characteristic of presentation. In this instance, the urinary sediment may not be helpful because it is well known that bilirubin pigmented casts, which are indistinguishable from the "muddy-brown" casts seen in acute tubular necrosis, can be found in patients with jaundice even when they have apparently normal renal function. In addition, because malnutrition and decreased muscle mass are the rule in these patients, the serum creatinine may be within normal limits or minimally elevated, and the blood urea nitrogen may be normal or low, whereas the filtration rate is markedly reduced. This almost uniformly fatal complication can follow episodes of gastrointestinal bleeding, diuresis, or spontaneous bacterial peritonitis; however, many patients, perhaps the majority, have no specific inciting event. The idea that hepatorenal syndrome occurs only in the hospital is not accurate. In fact, the disease often begins days to weeks before hospitalization (77).

Hepatorenal syndrome is a diagnosis of exclusion. If, after cautious trials of volume replacement (salt-poor albumin, not saline) and the removal of any potentially nephrotoxic agent, oliguric acute renal failure does not improve, a diagnosis of hepatorenal syndrome is probable.

The prognosis almost always involves the demise of the patient unless he or she is rescued by successful liver transplantation. A recent study, albeit with few patients, showed improvement in renal function and longer survival through the use of a combination of an oral sympathomimetic agent (midodrine [ProAmatine]) and a somatostatin analogue (octreotide [Sandostatin]) to inhibit endogenous vasodilators (78). This drug combination may help to bridge the gap until liver transplantation is available in suitable candidates.

Hemolytic Uremic Syndrome-Thrombotic Microangiopathy Acute renal insufficiency associated with thrombocytopenic microangiopathic hemolytic anemia has been described in connection with cocaine use (79–81) and possibly also with HIV infection (82). This syndrome can have catastrophic consequences with renal cortical necrosis and permanent loss of renal function, central nervous system involvement with seizures, and the permanent sequelae of ischemic or hemorrhagic strokes.

The pathogenesis of this syndrome is not known but may involve both immunologic and nonimmunologic mechanisms. An auto-antibody directed against the von Willebrand factor cleaving protease has been described in some cases (83). Direct endothelial injury, vasoconstriction, and procoagulant effects of cocaine, which are thought to be involved in cases of renal infarction associated with cocaine abuse (84), may play a part in the development of thrombotic microangiopathic nephropathy.

In such patients, renal biopsy reveals fibrin thrombi in the lumen of glomerular capillaries and occluded interlobular arterioles, with swollen endothelial cells and vessel wall damage. Fibrin and red blood cells are seen in the arteriolar media in the acute phase and with "onion skin" hypertrophy of muscular arteries in the healing phase. These lesions are similar to findings associated with malignant hypertension, systemic sclerosis, and the antiphospholipid antibody syndrome. Early recognition is important because prompt treatment with plasmapheresis and infusion of fresh-frozen plasma can prevent serious complications (85).

TOBACCO USE AND RENAL DISEASE

Tobacco use appears to have a deleterious effect on renal function. Cigarette smoking is related to proteinuria (86), accelerated atherosclerotic vascular disease and, presumably, ischemic nephropathy. In addition, increased risk of progression to renal insufficiency related to tobacco smoking has been documented in patients with diabetes mellitus (87) and severe essential hypertension (88). Moreover, increased risk of sustained proteinuria (86) and poorer prognosis of renal disease have been ascribed to tobacco smoking (89,90).

Accelerated atherosclerotic vascular disease related to cigarette smoking is well known to contribute to the development and progression of ischemic nephropathy. This common cause of renal failure is defined as impaired perfusion to the total renal mass and usually is associated with ischemic manifestations in other organs (brain, myocardium, and lower extremities) (91).

OTHER CAUSES OF RENAL INJURY

Many possible associations between drugs of abuse and renal injury have been suggested, but clear-cut confirmation of these associations is not definitive. Associations suggested from case reports include renal cell carcinoma and anabolic steroids (92), renal infarction and marijuana (93), renal failure and "magic mushrooms" (94), antiglomerular basement membrane disease and cocaine abuse (95,96), cocaine-induced pseudovasculitis (97), acute renal failure and toluene (glue sniffing) (98), granulomatous interstitial nephritis and oxycodone (Oxycontin) use (99), and urinary retention (100) and vasculitis with use of MDMA (101), among others.

Opiates certainly can cause urinary retention, especially in older men who have underlying prostatic hyperplasia. Urinary retention is most commonly seen as an iatrogenic complication of opiate analgesia in the postoperative period (102). Factitious nephrolithiasis has been described (103) and can be a reason for multiple visits to different health care on the part of individuals who seek prescriptions for narcotic drugs. The absence of gross or microscopic hematuria should argue against this diagnosis, stone chemical analysis, if available, may be helpful.

Fluid and Electrolyte Abnormalities among Patients with Drug Abuse Patients who use illicit drugs may present with myriad fluid and electrolyte abnormalities, but few are specifically associated with a particular drug. People with chronic alcohol dependence are the most frequently seen among this group. Patients with chronic alcoholism and recent binge drinking or intercurrent illness that requires abstinence often are admitted with gastrointestinal losses and underlying malnutrition—a scenario for complex and dynamic electrolyte and acid-base problems.

Alcohol-dependent patients, especially if they have been binge drinking and acutely stop, may present with severe anion gap acidosis. Ethanol usually is no longer detectable in the serum on presentation. This condition is a ketoacidosis induced by poor dietary intake, especially carbohydrates, and the inhibition of gluconeogenesis and acceleration of lipolysis by alcohol. The urine test results can be weakly positive or negative for ketones because, in many patients, beta-hydroxybutyrate comprises most of the ketonuria. Standard tablets or dipsticks use the nitroprusside reaction that is positive when acetone or acetoacetate is present but are negative with betahydroxybutyrate.

Other acid-base disturbances seen in alcoholics usually are not life-threatening. They include non–anion gap acidosis secondary to diarrhea, a common finding in this group of patients and, occasionally, renal tubular acidosis. The finding of a reduced serum bicarbonate can represent compensation for respiratory alkalosis. Alcohol misusers may present with this respiratory disturbance that, in part, may be secondary to impaired hepatic metabolism of progesterone, a respiratory stimulant. As with all acid-base disturbances, arterial blood gases, with determination of pH values, are necessary to determine the precise abnormality.

Decreased serum potassium levels often are seen in connection with gastrointestinal losses and secondary hyperaldosteronism. Such loss may be accelerated by the use of diuretics without a potassium-sparing agent. Correction of this electrolyte abnormality is important because hypokalemia can accelerate or worsen hepatic encephalopathy, in part through the enhancement of ammoniagenesis. In addition, hypokalemia (along with hypophosphatemia) increases the risk for rhabdomyolysis. The correction of hypomagnesemia is critical to allow repair of any renal potassium wasting.

One of the most frequent electrolyte abnormalities among people with alcohol dependence is hypomagnesemia (104).

The etiology probably is a combination of poor nutrition and gastrointestinal losses, coupled with direct renal tubular alcohol toxicity (105), which decreases renal magnesium absorption in spite of depleted body stores. Hypomagnesemia often is associated with hypocalcemia because of decreased parathyroid hormone release and bone resistance to parathyroid hormone (106,107). In addition, if chronic pancreatitis and fat malabsorption are present, saponification (complexing) of calcium and magnesium will impair intestinal absorption of these divalent cations. Hypokalemia is worsened by concomitant hypomagnesemia, which promotes kaliuresis (108) and, like hypocalcemia, is refractory to correction unless the magnesium deficit is replaced (109) Severe hypomagnesemia should be treated with slow intravenous infusion, whereas oral replacement can be used for therapy of milder forms of hypomagnesemia.

Hypophosphatemia often is seen in alcoholism and may contribute to rhabdomyolysis and encephalopathy (110,111).

Again, dietary deficiency, increased gastrointestinal losses, and increased renal excretion (46,104) contribute to this deficit.

Toxic Alcohols The ingestion of a toxic alcohol—methanol, ethylene glycol, or isopropyl alcohol—is occasionally seen in an alcohol-dependent patient who has ingested the toxic alcohol as a substitute for ethanol. Methanol is found in solutions used for de-icing and in some paint products, such as varnish or shellac. Ethylene glycol is found in antifreeze. The metabolic products of these alcohols (facilitated by alcohol dehydrogenase) are severely toxic and produce organ damage and anion gap acidosis from the nonvolatile organic acids produced.

Anion gap acidosis usually is the first clue to a toxic alcohol ingestion, but it should be remembered that alcoholic and starvation ketoacidosis are far more common. The presence of an osmolal gap (that is, a difference between the calculated and measured serum osmolality >15) should raise suspicion of a toxic alcohol ingestion when no other reason for this gap is apparent, such as ethanol or mannitol. In cases of ethylene glycol ingestion, the presence of calcium oxalate crystals in the urine is suggestive but not diagnostic.

Treatment used to be directed primarily at inhibition of the production of the organic acids that are the metabolic products of these alcohols, through the use of intravenous ethanol. Ethanol slows the metabolism of the toxic alcohols by competing for alcohol dehydrogenase and thus reduces the production of the toxic organic acid metabolites. Currently, fomepizole, an intravenous medication that competitively inhibits alcohol dehydrogenase more than ethanol, is very effective and safer than an ethanol infusion (112). As long as kidney function is maintained, the alcohol will be removed by renal excretion. With severe intoxication, hemodialysis is used to remove the alcohol and the toxic products efficiently and is useful in the treatment of the concurrent acidosis. Failure to recognize and promptly treat these alcohol intoxications can lead to multiple organ damage (to the brain, liver, and kidney) and, for methanol, to blindness.

Isopropyl alcohol is found in rubbing alcohol and other solvents. It is metabolized to acetone and excreted by the kidneys and the lung. Here, the alcohol itself rather than the products of alcohol metabolism is the toxic agent. Organic acids are not produced, so there is no anion gap acidosis unless there is hypotension to initiate the production of lactic acidosis. Patients usually appear inebriated but without an odor of ethanol on the breath. They often have gastritis, ketonuria, and an osmolal gap.

Inhalants An unusual cause of metabolic acidosis and hypokalemia, encountered more often in teenagers, involves toluene intoxication from glue sniffing. Diagnosis can be very difficult because patients may be reticent to report abuse of this substance. Patients may recover rapidly on admission to the hospital, but recurrent episodes are not uncommon (113). Distal renal tubular acidosis has been described in this setting (114). However, the principal mechanism producing the acidosis seems to involve increased manufacture of hippuric acid derived from toluene metabolism (115).

The hippuric acid is rapidly excreted, leading to a normal anion gap metabolic acidosis. In the distal nephron, acting as a non-reabsorbable anion, hippurate increases the excretion of sodium and potassium. If hippurate is present in sufficient amounts, severe hypokalemia may occur.

MDMA ("Ecstasy") The amphetamine-type drug 3,4-methylenedioxymethamphetamine (MDMA) is also known as *Ecstasy*. Often, users are in a venue (such as a dance club) in which the ambient temperature is high and vigorous physical activity occurs. In such a situation, use of MDMA can lead to agitation, high fever, hyperventilation, and impaired sensorium. This condition leads to increased insensible fluid losses and sets the stage for dehydration (hypernatremia) and volume depletion. The results, unless treated promptly, can include hypotension, shock, brain damage, and rhabdomyolysis with renal failure. The hypernatremia and volume depletion should be treated promptly. If hypotension is present, therapy should be started initially with normal saline to restore organ perfusion. This treatment should be followed by hypotonic fluids to restore isotonicity and to continue to reestablish intravascular volume. Some users have become aware of these problems and try to prevent them through the intake of large amounts of water. The result has been severe hyponatremia with central nervous system symptoms (116).

SUMMARY

In summary, the relationships between drug use and renal diseases range from causality associated with known harmful exposures believed to lead to nephropathies to the peculiar challenges of managing patients with drug-related problems and need for renal replacement therapy, which demands perfect adherence to a therapeutic program and insight in disease process coupled with interest in health promotion and self-care.

The need for vascular access to provide hemodialysis is an avenue leading to infectious complications, related to misuse of dialysis access to self-inject illicit drugs.

If initiation of renal disease is thought in many cases to be traceable to infectious and/or chemical hazards in this patient population, the progression of established nephropathy is certainly accelerated by adherence problems, missed office visits, and sporadic intake of prescribed essential medications.

The family and loved ones involved with an individual with drug addiction problems also develop psychologic and behavior stressors of their own, which will demand attention and sensitivity from the clinician.

Renal and metabolic consequences of illicit substance use are common, may be quite serious, and sometimes are difficult to diagnose and manage. Of course, the best approach for these consequences is primary prevention.

REFERENCES

1. Crowe AV, Howse M, Bell GM, et al. Substance abuse and the kidney. *Q J Med* 2000; 93:147–157.
2. Perneger TV, Klag MJ, Whelton PK. Recreational drug use: a neglected risk factor for end-stage renal disease. *Am J Kidney Dis* 2001;38:49–56.
3. Stevens LA, Coresh,J, Greene T, et al. Assessing kidney function: measured and estimated glomerular filtration rate. *N Engl J Med* 2006;354:2473–2488.

4. Odden MC, Scherzer R, Bacchetti P, et al. Cystatin C levels as a marker of kidney function in human immunodeficiency viruse infection. *Arch Intern Med* 2007;167:2213–2219.
5. Ginsberg JM, Chang BS, Matarese RA et al. Use of single voided urine samples to estimate quantitative proteinuria. *N Engl J Med* 1983309: 1543–1546.
6. Szczech LA, Hoover DR, Feldman JG, et al. Association between renal diseases and outcomes among HIV-infected women receiving antiretroviral therapy or not. *Clin Infect Dis* 2004;39:1199.
7. Izzedine H, Deray G. The nephrologist in the HAART era. *AIDS* 2007;21:409.
8. Gupta SK, Eustace JA, Winston JA, et al. Guidelines for the management of chronic kidney disease in HIV-infected patients: recommendations of the HIV medicine association of the Infectious disease society of America. *Clin Infect Dis* 2005;40:1559–1585.
9. Cantor ES, Kimmel PL, Bosch JP. Effects of race on expression of acquired immunodeficiency syndrome-associated nephropathy. *Arch Intern Med* 1991;151:125–128.
10. Freedman BI, Soucie JM, Stone SM, et al. Familial clustering of end-stage renal disease in blacks with HIV-associated nephropathy. *Am J Kidney Dis* 1999;34:254–258.
11. Winston J, Klotman ME, Klotman PE. HIV-associated nephropathy is a late, not early, manifestation of HIV-1 infection. *Kidney Int* 1999; 55:1036–1040.
12. Klotman PE. HIV-associated nephropathy. *Kidney Int* 1999;56:1161–1176.
13. Bruggeman LA, Dikman S, Meng C, et al. Nephropathy in human immunodeficiency virus-1 transgenic mice is due to renal transgene expression. *J Clin Invest* 1997;100:84–92.
14. D'Agati V, Appel GB. Renal pathology of human immunodeficiency virus infection. *Semin Nephrol* 1998;18:406–421.
15. Szcech LA, van der Horst C, Bartlett JA, et al. Protease inhibitors are associated with a slowed progression HIV-associated nephropathy [abstract]. *J Am Soc Nephrol* 1999;10:116A.
16. Burns GC, Paul SK, Toth IR, et al. Effects of angiotensin converting-enzyme inhibition in HIV-associated nephropathy. *J Am Soc Nephrol* 1997;8:1140–1146.
17. Burns GC, Visitainer P, Mohammed NB. Effect of angiotensinconverting enzyme inhibition on progression of renal disease and mortality in HIV-associated nephropathy [abstract]. *J Am Soc Nephrol* 1999;10:155A.
18. Lai KN, Li PK, Lui SF, et al. Membranous nephropathy related to hepatitis B in adults. *N Engl J Med* 1991;324:1457–1463.
19. Dienstag JL, Eckstein M. Case records of the Massachusetts General Hospital (case 36-1985). *N Engl J Med* 1985;313:622–631.
20. Benhamou Y, Katlama C, Lunel F, et al. Effects of lamivudine on replication of Hepatitis B virus in HIV-infected men. *Ann Intern Med* 1996; 125:705–712.
21. Lai CL, Gane E, Liaw, YF et al. *N Engl J Med* 2007;357:2576–2588.
22. Okada K, Takishita Y, Shimomura H, et al. Detection of hepatitis C virus core protein in the glomeruli of patients with membranous glomerulonephritis. *Clin Nephrol* 1996;45:71–76.
23. Stehman-Breen C, Alpres CE, Fleet WP, et al. Focal segmental glomerulosclerosis among patients infected with hepatitis C virus. *Nephron* 1999;81:37–40.
24. Neugarten J, Galo G, Buxbaum J, et al. Amyloidosis in subcutaneous heroin abusers ("skin poppers' amyloidosis"). *Am J Med* 1986;81:635–640.
25. Tan AU Jr, Cohen AH, Levine BS. Renal amyloidosis in a drug abuser. *J Am Soc Nephrol* 1995;5:1653–1658.
26. Formica R, Perazella MA. Leg pain and swelling in an HIV-infected drug abuser [Office edition]. *Hosp Pract* 1998;33:195–197.
27. Dember LM, Hawkins PN, Hazenberg BPC, et al. *N Engl J Med* 2007; 356:2349–2360.
28. Agnello V, Chung RT, Kaplan LM. A role for hepatitis C virus in type II cryoglobulinemia. *N Engl J Med* 1992;327:1490–1495.
29. Misiani R, Bellavita P, Fenili D, et al. Hepatitis C virus infection in patients with essential mixed cryoglobulinemia. *AnnIntern Med* 1992; 117:573–577.
30. Johnson RJ, Gretch DR, Yamabe H, et al. Membranoproliferative glomerulonephritis associated with hepatitis C virus infection. *N Engl J Med* 19993;328:465–470.
31. Markowitz GS, Cheng JT, Colvin RB, et al. Hepatitis C viral infection is associated with fibrillary glomerulonephritis and immunotactoid glomerulopathy. *J Am Soc Nephrol* 1998;9:2244–2252.
32. Stokes MB, Chawla H, Brody RI, et al. Immune complex glomerulonephritis in patients coinfected with human immunodeficiency virus and hepatitis C virus. *Am J Kidney Dis* 1997;29:514–525.
33. Cheng JT, Anderson HL, Markowitz GS, et al. Hepatitis C virus associated glomerular disease in patients with human immunodeficiency virus coinfection. *J Am Soc Nephrol* 1999;10:1566–1574.
34. Haydey RP, de Rojas MP, Gigli I. A newly described control mechanism of complement activation in patients with mixed cryoglobulinemia (cryoglobulins and complement). *J Invest Dermatol* 1980;74:328–332.
35. Jefferson JA, Johnson RJ. Treatment of hepatitis C-associated glomerular disease. *Semin Nephrol* 2000;20:286–292.
36. Quan CM, Kradjen M, Grigoriew GA, et al. Hepatitis C virus in patients infected with human immunodeficiency virus infection. *Clin Infect Dis* 1993;17:117–119.
37. Neugarten J, Baldwin DS. Glomerulonephritis in bacterial endocarditis. *Am J Med* 1984;77:297–304.
38. Stachura I. Renal lesions in drug addicts. *Pathol Ann* 1985;20(2):83–99.
39. di Belgiojoso GB, Genderine A, Scorza D, et al. Renal damage in drug abusers. *Contrib Nephrol* 1990;77:142–156.
40. Bakir AA, Dunea G. Drugs of abuse and renal disease. *Curr Opin Nephrol Hypertens* 1996;5:122–126.
41. Klevens RM, Morrison MA, Naddle J, et al. Invasive methicillin-resistant *Staphiloccocus aureus* infections in the United States. *JAMA* 2007;298:1763–1771.
42. Hill EE, Vanderschueren S, Verhargen J, et al. Risk factors for infective endocarditis and outcome of patients with staphylococcus aureus bacteremia. *Mayo Clin Proc* 2007;82:1165–1169.
43. Conlon PJ, Jeffries F, Krigman HR, et al. Predictors of prognosis and risk of acute renal failure in bacterial endocarditis. *Clin Nephrol* 1998;49:96–101.
44. Keller CK, Andrassy K, Waldherr R, et al. Postinfectious glomerulonephritis—is there a link to alcoholism? *Q J Med* 1994;87:97–102.
45. Montseny JJ, Meyrier A, Kleinknecht D, et al. Infectious glomerulonephritis (IGN) is unusually frequent and severe in alcoholics [abstract]. *J Am Soc Nephrol* 1994;5:356A.
46. Vamvakas S, Teschner M, Bahner U, et al. Alcohol abuse: Potential role in electrolyte disturbances and kidney diseases. *Clin Nephrol* 1998;49:205–213.
47. Katz A, Bragman JM, Miller DC, et al. IgA nephritis in HIV positive patients: a new HIV associated nephropathy? *Clin Nephrol* 1992;38:61–68.
48. Kimmel PL, Phillips TM, Ferreira AC et al. Idiotypic IgA nephropathy in patients with human immunodeficiency virus infection. *N Engl J Med* 1992;327:702–706.
49. Nzerue CM, Hewan-Lowe K, Riley LJ. Cocaine and the kidney: a synthesis of pathophysiologic and clinical perspectives. *Am J Kidney Dis* 2000;35:783–795.
50. Fine DM, Garg N, Haas M, et al. Cocaine use and hypertensive renal changes in HIV-infected individuals. *Clin J Am Soc Nephrol* 1007;2: 1125–1130.
51. Goodlin RC. Preeclampsia as the great impostor. *J Obstet Gynecol* 1991;164:1577–1581.
52. Lam M, Ballou SP. Reversible scleroderma crisis after cocaine use [letter]. *N Engl J Med* 1992;326:1435.
53. Thakur V, Godley C, Weed S, et al. Case reports: Cocaine-associated accelerated hypertension and renal failure. *Am J Med Sci* 1996;312:295–298.
54. Norris KC, Thornhill-Joynes M, Robinson C, et al. Cocaine use, hypertension, and end-stage renal disease. *Am J Kidney Dis* 2001;38:523–528.
55. Brecklin CS, Gopaniuk-Folga A, Kravetz T, et al. Prevalence of hypertension in chronic cocaine users. *Am J Hypertens* 1998;11:1279–1283.
56. Bingham C, Beaman M, Nicholls AJ, et al. Necrotizing renal vasculopathy resulting in chronic renal failure after ingestion of methamphetamine and 3,4-methylenedioxymethamphetamine ("Ecstasy"). *Nephrol Dial Transplant* 1998;13:2654–2655.
57. Dienstag JL, Eckstein M. Case Records of the Massachusetts General Hospital (case 36-1985). *N Engl J Med* 1985;313:622–631.
58. Samuels N, Shemesh O, Yinnon AM, et al. Polyarteritis nodosa and drug abuse: is there a connection? *Postgrad Med J* 1996;72:684–685.
59. Bennett W. Lead nephropathy. *Kidney Int* 1985;28:212–220.

60. van der Woude FK. Cocaine use and kidney damage. *Nephrol Dial Transplant* 2000;15:299–301.
61. Vanholder R, Sever MS, Erek E, et al. Rhabdomyolysis. *J Am Soc Nephrol* 2000;11:1553–1561.
62. Richards JR, Johnson EB, Stark RW, et al. Methamphetamine abuse and rhabdomyolysis in the ED: a 5-year study. *Am J Emerg Med* 1999;17: 681–685.
63. Murthy BVS, Roberts NB, Wilkes RG. Biochemical implications of ecstasy toxicity. *Ann Clin Biochem* 1997;34:442–445.
64. Fine DM, Gelber AC, Melamed ML, et al. Risk factors for renal failure among 72 consecutive patients with rhabdomyolysis related to illicit drug use. *Am J Med* 2004;117:607–610.
65. Luscher TF, Bock HA, Yang Z, et al. Endothelium-derived relaxing and contracting factors. *Kidney Int* 1991;39:575–590.
66. Zager RA, Burkhart KM, Conrad DS, et al. Iron, heme-oxygenase and glutathione. Effects on myoglobinuric proximal renal injury. *Kidney Int* 1995;48:1624–1634.
67. Heyman SN, Rosen S, Fuchs S, et al. Myoglobinuric acute renal failure in the rat: a role for medullary hypoperfusion, hypoxia, and tubular obstruction. *J Am Soc Nephrol* 1996;7:1066–1074.
68. Knochel JP, Schlein EM. On the mechanisms of rhabdomyolysis in potassium depletion. *J Clin Invest* 1972;51:1750.
69. Zager RA. Combined mannitol and deferoxamine therapy for myoglobinuric renal injury and oxidant tubular stress. Mechanistic and therapeutic implications. *J Clin Invest* 1992;90:711–719.
70. Eneas JF, Schoenfeld PY, Humphreys MH. The effect of infusion of mannitol-sodium bicarbonate on the clinical course of myoglobinuria. *Arch Intern Med* 1979;139:801–805.
71. Sawyer MH, Webb DE, Balow JE, et al. Acyclovir-induced renal failure. Clinical course and histology. *Am J Med* 1988;84:1067–1071.
72. Kopp JB, Miller KD, Mican JA, et al. Crystalluria and urinary tract abnormalities associated with indinavir. *Ann Intern Med* 1997;127:119–126.
73. Tashima KT, Horowitz JD, Rosen S. Indinavir nephropathy [letter]. *N Engl J Med* 1997;336:138–140.
74. Chugh S, Bird R, Alexander EA. Ritonavir and renal failure [letter]. *N Engl J Med* 1997;336:138.
75. Punukollu RC, Gopalswamy N. The hepatorenal syndrome. *Med Clin North Am* 1990;74:933–943.
76. Gines P, Arroyo P. Hepatorenal syndrome. *J Am Soc Nephrol* 1999;8: 1833–1839.
77. Papadakis MK, Arieff AI . Unpredictability of clinical evaluation of renal function in cirrhosis. *Am J Med* 1981;82:945–952.
78. Angeli P, Volpin R, Gerunda G, et al. Reversal of type 1 hepatorenal syndrome with the administration of midodrine and ocreotide. *Hepatology* 1999;29:1690–1697.
79. Kokko JP. Metabolic and social consequences of cocaine abuse. *Am J Med Sci* 1990;299:361–365.
80. Tumlin JA, Sands JM, Someren A. Hemolytic-uremic syndrome following "crack" cocaine inhalation. *Am J Med Sci* 1990;299:366–371.
81. Volcy J, Nzerue CM, Oderinde A, et al. Cocaine-induced acute renal failure, hemolysis, and thrombocytopenia mimicking thrombotic thrombocytopenic purpura. *Am J Kidney Dis* 2000;35:E3–E7.
82. Leaf AN, Laubenstein LJ, Raphael B, et al. Thrombotic thrombocytopenic purpura associated with human immunodeficiency virus 1 (HIV-1) infection. *Ann Intern Med* 1988;109:194–197.
83. Furlan M, Robles R, Galbusera M, et al. von Willebrand factor cleaving protease in thrombotic thrombocytopenic purpura and the hemolytic-uremic syndrome. *N Engl J Med* 1998;339:1578–1584.
84. Sharff JA. Renal infarction associated with intravenous cocaine use. *Ann Emerg Med* 1984;13:1145–1147.
85. Kaplan BS, Meyers KE, Schulman SL. The pathogenesis and treatment of hemolytic uremic syndrome. *J Am Soc Nephrol* 1998;9: 1126–1133.
86. Halimi J-M, Giraudeau B, Vol S, et al. Effects of current smoking and smoking discontinuation on renal function and proteinuria in the general population. *Kidney Int* 2000;58:1285–1292.
87. Stegmayr BG. A study of patients with diabetes mellitus (type 1) and end-stage renal failure: tobacco usage may increase risk of nephropathy and death. *J Intern Med* 1990;28:121–124.
88. Regalado M, Yang S, Wesson DE. Cigarette smoking is associated with augmented progression of renal insufficiency in severe essential hypertension. *Am J Kidney Dis* 2000;35:687–694.
89. Orth S, Ritz E, Schrier RW. The renal risks of smoking. *Kidney Int* 1997;51:1669–1677.
90. Orth SR, Stockmann A, Conradt C, et al. Smoking as a risk factor for end-stage renal failure in men with primary renal disease. *Kidney Int* 1998;54:926–931.
91. Greco RA, Breyer JA. Ischemic nephropathy. *Am J Kidney Dis* 1997;29:167–187.
92. Martorana G, Concetti S, Manferrari F, et al. Anabolic steroid abuse and renal cell carcinoma. *Journal of Urology* 1999;162:2089.
93. Lambrecht GLY, Malbrain MLNG, Coremans P, et al. Acute renal infarction and heavy marijuana smoking. *Nephron* 1995;70:494-496.
94. Raff E, Halloran PF, Kjellstrand CM. Renal failure after eating "magic" mushrooms. *Can Med Assoc J* 1992;147:1339.
95. Peces R, Navascues RA, Br J, et al. Antiglomerular basement membrane antibody-mediated glomerulonephritis after intranasal cocaine use. *Nephron* 1999;81:434–438.
96. Sirvent AE, Enriquez R, Andrada E, et al. Goodpasture's syndrome in a patient using cocaine. *Clin Nephrol* 2007;68:182–185.
97. Friedman DR, Wolfsthal S. Cocaine-induced pseudovasculitis. *Mayo Clin Proc* 2005;80:671–673.
98. Will AM. Reversible renal damage due to glue sniffing. *Br Med J* 1981;283:525–526.
99. Segal A, Dowling JP, Ireton HJC, et al. Granulomatous glomerulonephritis in intravenous drug users: a report of three cases in oxycodone addicts. *Hum Pathol* 1998;29:1246–1249.
100. Bryden AA, Rothwell PJN, O'Reilly PH. Urinary retention with misuse of "Ecstasy" [letter]. *Br Med J* 1995;310:504.
101. Woodrow G, Turney JH. Ecstasy-induced vasculitis [letter]. *Nephrol Dial Transplant* 1999;14:798.
102. Tammela T. Postoperative urinary retention—why the patient cannot void. *Scand J Urol Nephrol* 1995;29(Suppl 175):75–77.
103. Gault HM, Campbell NRC, Aksu AE. Spurious stones. *Nephron* 1988; 48:274–279.
104. Elisaf M, Merkouropoulos M, Tsianos EV, et al. Acid-base and electrolyte abnormalities in alcoholic patients. *Mineral Electrol Metab* 1994;20:274–281.
105. De Marchi S, Cecchin E, Basile A, et al. Renal tubular dysfunction in chronic alcohol abuse—Effects of abstinence. *N Engl J Med* 1993;104 (329):1927–1934.
106. Laitinen K, Lamberg-Allardt C, Tunninen R, et al. Transient hypoparathyroidism during acute alcohol intoxication. *N Engl J Med* 1991;324:721–727.
107. Shis ME. Magnesium, calcium and parathyroid interactions. *Ann N Y Acad Sci* 1980;355:165–178.
108. Kobrin SM, Goldfarb S. Magnesium deficiency. *Semin Nephrol* 1990; 10:525–535.
109. Elisaf M, Milionis H, Siamopoulos KC. Hypomagnesemic hypokalemia and hypocalcemia: clinical and laboratory characteristics. *Mineral Electrol Metab* 1997;23:105–112.
110. Funabiki Y, Tatsukawa H, Ashida K, et al. Disturbances of consciousness associated with hypophosphatemia in a chronically alcoholic patient. *Intern Med* 1998;37:958–961.
111. Nagata N. Hypophosphatemia and encephalopathy in alcoholics. *Intern Med* 1998;37:911–912.
112. Brent J, McMartin K, Phillips S, et al. Fomepizole for the treatment of ethylene glycol poisoning. *N Engl J Med* 1999;340:832–838.
113. Streicher HZ, Gabow PA, Moss AH, et al. Syndromes of toluene sniffing in adults. *Ann Intern Med* 1981;94:758–762.
114. King MD. Reversible renal damage due to glue sniffing [letter]. *Br Med J* 1981;283:919.
115. Carlisle EJ, Donnelly SM, Vasuvattakul S, et al. Glue-sniffing and distal renal acidosis: Sticking to the facts. *J Am Soc Nephrol* 1991;8: 1019–1027.
116. Maxwell DL, Polkey MI, Henry JA. Hyponatremia and catatonic stupor after taking "Ecstasy" [letter]. *Br Med J* 1993;307:1399.

CHAPTER 74

Paul S Haber, MD, FRACP, FAChAM

Gastrointestinal Disorders Related to Alcohol and Other Drug Use

This chapter describes gastrointestinal effects of alcohol and drugs. Excessive alcohol use is associated with injury to all parts of the gastrointestinal tract. Several detailed reviews have been published (1–3). The gastric mucosa is a target for alcohol-related toxicity but also contributes to the oxidation of alcohol. Within the gastrointestinal tract, pancreatitis is an important cause of morbidity and mortality related to excessive alcohol use. Symptoms of intestinal dysfunction are common among people with alcohol dependence and include diarrhea and malabsorption.

Tobacco use is associated with gastroesophageal reflux, peptic ulceration, and gastrointestinal malignancy but appears to protect against ulcerative colitis. Opiates have important effects on gastrointestinal secretion and motility. Other drugs of abuse such as cannabis and cocaine uncommonly affect the gastrointestinal tract. The body-packing syndrome is rare but challenging when encountered.

GASTROINTESTINAL PROBLEMS RELATED TO ALCOHOL

The relative risk of alcohol-related GI toxicity is not well defined and appears to differ between affected tissues and between benign and neoplastic disorders. Similarly, the pattern and type of beverage has not been consistently been shown to predispose to any specific GI effects of alcohol.

Parotids Painless symmetrical enlargement of the parotid glands (termed *sialosis* or *sialadenosis*) is common in patients with alcoholic liver injury (4). It is characterized by the triad of acinar cell hypertrophy, myoepithelial degeneration, and neural degeneration. Salivary secretion is reduced in experimental animals given alcohol. These effects may contribute to progressive dental caries and poor oral mucosal health. The effect of alcohol abuse on salivary function in humans is controversial, with reports of both increased, unaltered (5) and decreased salivary flow (4).

Esophagus Both acute and chronic alcohol consumption are associated with symptomatic gastroesophageal reflux disease (GERD). Reflux episodes were increased by 60 g of ethanol given with a meal to healthy subjects without alcohol dependence (6). These episodes were measured by measurement of esophageal pH for 3 hours after a standard meal, and most were asymptomatic. A number of mechanisms that have been identified may contribute to these effects of alcohol (7). Direct application of 30% ethanol, but not lower concentrations, causes injury to the esophageal mucosa. An acute dose of alcohol reduces lower esophageal sphincter pressure (LESP) (8) and reduced maximal LESP stimulated by a meal (9). Chronic excessive alcohol use is also associated with manometric abnormalities relevant to GERD that recover with a month of abstinence (5,10). These abnormalities were found regardless of the presence or absence of peripheral neuropathy. These studies provide evidence to support the time-honored advice to reduce alcohol consumption in the presence of symptomatic GERD.

Excessive alcohol use was found in most cases of Barrett's esophagus in an early series (11). In a more recent series, excessive alcohol use was not often found in asymptomatic Barrett's (12), but was strongly associated with carcinoma (13).

Alcoholic Gastritis Exposure of the gastric mucosa to 20% alcohol induces gastric mucosal injury. Lower concentrations are not toxic, whereas higher concentrations lead to extensive hemorrhagic injury (14). These lesions are characterized by subepithelial hemorrhages and epithelial erosions. Inflammatory cell infiltration is not a consistent feature. Upper gastrointestinal bleeding is very common among people with alcoholism and may be due to a wide range of pathology, most commonly hemorrhagic gastritis.

The clinical syndrome of alcoholic gastritis has been surprisingly controversial despite considerable study (14,15). There is conflicting evidence concerning the role of alcohol owing to issues with the methodology of many early studies. In addition, most studies were performed before the importance of *Helicobacter pylori* and nonsteroidal anti-inflammatory drugs in the pathogenesis of gastritis was recognized. Brown et al. (16) found that gastritis was not more common in patients with cirrhosis than in healthy controls. Direct application of alcohol to gastric mucosa caused hemorrhagic lesions but these lesions persisted for 24 hours only when the alcohol concentration was greater than 10% (17). Uppal et al. (18) showed that gastritis in people with alcohol dependence was strongly associated with *H. pylori* infection, with histologic and symptomatic relief after eradication of the organism but no improvement with abstinence from alcohol (18). The finding has been confirmed by another group (19). *H. pylori* infection was equally common among a group with heavy alcohol use compared to non-drinking controls (19). The presence of alcohol dehydrogenase (ADH) activity in *H. pylori* organisms may tend to protect the alcohol-drinking host from infection as exposure to alcohol leads to generation of acetaldehyde that may be bactericidal. Healing of established ulcers is not retarded by moderate alcohol consumption (20). Heavier drinking is associated with reduced medication compliance and delayed healing (21).

The clinical term *alcoholic gastritis* is nonspecific and is often used to refer to a broad range of upper-gastrointestinal symptoms experienced by people who drink alcohol excessively. The term *alcoholic gastritis* should be reserved for patients with evidence of gastric mucosal injury in the presence of excessive alcohol intake. It has also been proposed that alcohol may directly induce vomiting by central stimulation of the chemoreceptor trigger zone in the area postrema of the floor of the fourth ventricle in the absence of peripheral disease (22). In addition, bacterial overgrowth has been reported to be more common in people who drink alcohol excessively and may also contribute to upper-abdominal symptoms and diarrhea (23). Given the uncertainty surrounding the etiologic role of excessive alcohol use in gastritis and the broad range of potential explanations for these symptoms, it is appropriate to evaluate patients on an individual basis for specific causes.

Alcoholic Pancreatitis Alcoholic pancreatitis remains a major cause of morbidity among people with alcohol dependence. The incidence appears to have risen in the United States and internationally through the twentieth century (24). UK data confirm this trend and reveal a correlation between rising total community alcohol consumption and the number of hospital admissions for chronic pancreatitis (25). In the past decade, total community alcohol consumption has risen in several countries, particularly the United Kingdom, and there is some evidence that the incidence of alcoholic pancreatitis is rising in parallel (26).

Definitions The term *acute pancreatitis* refers to an acute inflammatory process of the pancreas, with variable involvement of other regional tissues or remote organ systems (27). *Chronic pancreatitis* is characterized by chronic inflammation, glandular atrophy, and fibrosis. Clinically, it manifests pain with exocrine or endocrine insufficiency. Several older ambiguous terms are no longer used: *phlegmon*, *infected pseudocyst*, and *hemorrhagic pancreatitis*. Terms that are retained include *acute fluid collections* (a collection lacking a defined wall, which is common early in the course of the disease and tends to regress spontaneously), *pseudocyst* (a collection of pancreatic juice enclosed by a connective tissue wall arising from disruption of pancreatic ducts and frequently communicating with the duct system), *pancreatic necrosis* (diffuse or focal areas of nonviable pancreatic parenchyma typically associated with peripancreatic fat necrosis and which may be *sterile* or *infected*) and *pancreatic abscess* (a circumscribed collection of pus in or near the pancreas following pancreatitis or pancreatic trauma).

Predisposing Factors Only a minority (fewer than 5%) of people who drink heavily develop clinically evident pancreatic disease, though a postmortem study has shown that pathologic changes in the pancreas are common among those with alcoholism (28). Numerous investigators have attempted to account for this individual susceptibility by studying associations between alcoholic pancreatitis and potential risk factors. These studies have been previously been reviewed (29) and have focused on the amount, type and pattern of alcohol consumption, genetic markers, diet (30), hypertriglyceridemia (31), tobacco consumption (32) and pancreatic ischemia. The genetic markers that have been studied include blood groups, HLA phenotypes (33), α_1-antitrypsin phenotypes (34), cystic fibrosis genotypes (35), cytochrome P450 2E1 (CYP2E1) genotypes, and ADH isoenzyme genotypes. A number of these studies are difficult to interpret owing to small sample sizes, inappropriate controls, and inconsistent findings between studies so there remains insufficient evidence to consider any of the foregoing factors well established. Most recently, a mutation of the gene coding for pancreatic secretory trypsin inhibitor (*SPINK1*) has been described in 5.8% of a cohort with alcoholic pancreatitis compared with 1% in controls with alcoholism, and this important observation has been replicated in an independent study (36). This supports the concept that genetic factors influence susceptibility to pancreatitis, but given that 94% of subjects did not carry this mutation, individual susceptibility to this disease remains largely unexplained.

Etiology The most common associations of acute pancreatitis in Western societies are gallstones and heavy alcohol use, which together account for approximately 75% of cases. Alcohol is the most common cause of pancreatitis in communities with high levels of alcohol consumption (37). Pancreatitis typically occurs in subjects who have consumed more than 100 g alcohol (5–6 drinks) per day for at least 5 to 10 years and rarely if ever follows an isolated episode of heavy drinking. Once the disease is established, episodic heavy drinking often precipitates relapses. Relapses have been described after only 1 day of recurrent drinking. The causative link between alcohol use and pancreatitis for an individual patient is made on clinical grounds by a compatible history and exclusion of other etiologic factors. Pancreatitis is common among people with HIV, particularly in association with heavy alcohol use (38,39).

Other than *gallstones*, relatively common causes for pancreatitis that should be considered include *hypercalcaemia* of any cause and severe *hypertriglyceridemia*. Hypertriglyceridemia (>10 mmol/L [approximately 1,000 mg/dL] with lipaemic serum) of any cause is associated with recurrent attacks of pancreatitis (40). Though alcohol abuse is a known cause of hypertriglyceridaemia, the majority of cases of alcoholic pancreatitis are not associated with marked hyperlipidaemia (31).

Pathogenesis Two important factors leading to tissue injury in pancreatitis are *autodigestion* and *oxidant stress*. Several lines of evidence indicate that activated digestive enzymes play an important role in pancreatitis (41): (1) mutations of the cationic trypsinogen gene that increase pancreatic content of trypsin underlie hereditary pancreatitis (42); (2) activated digestive enzymes are found in both clinical and experimental pancreatitis and can produce cellular necrosis when instilled into pancreatic tissue; and (3) protease inhibitors reduce the incidence of post-ERCP and experimental pancreatitis. Oxidant stress is characterized by the production of reactive oxygen species that are atoms or molecules containing oxygen with an unpaired electron in the outer shell (free radicals). Free radicals are highly reactive and bind to lipids, proteins, and nucleic acids leading to cellular injury (43). Free radicals are generated during experimental pancreatitis (44) from infiltrating leukocytes (45) or possibly within acinar cells (46).

The initiation of alcoholic pancreatitis appears to involve both autodigestion and oxidant stress (Fig. 74.1). Alcohol administration has been reported to increase the tone of the sphincter of Oddi (47) and inhibit pancreatic secretion (48). In experimental animals, alcohol intake impairs the stability of zymogen granules and lysosomes, thereby increasing the possibility of co-localization of digestive enzymes and lysosomal enzymes (36,49). Lysosomal enzymes (particularly cathepsin B) are capable of activating trypsinogen, which in turn can activate other digestive enzyme precursors, resulting in a cascade of autodigestion. Ethanol consumption increases the pancreatic content of the major alcohol-metabolizing isoform of cytochrome P450 (CYP2E1) and increases tissue markers of oxidant stress (50). The progression of the disease involves local inflammation and, when severe, systemic inflammation. A range of cytokines are involved, and these may be detected in blood and pancreatic tissue. These mediators of inflammation include chemokines that act at CCR1, platelet-activating factor (PAF), and substance P (51). Inhibition of these mediators of inflammation has the potential to limit the progression of pancreatitis and prevent serious complications or death but cannot prevent the initial attack.

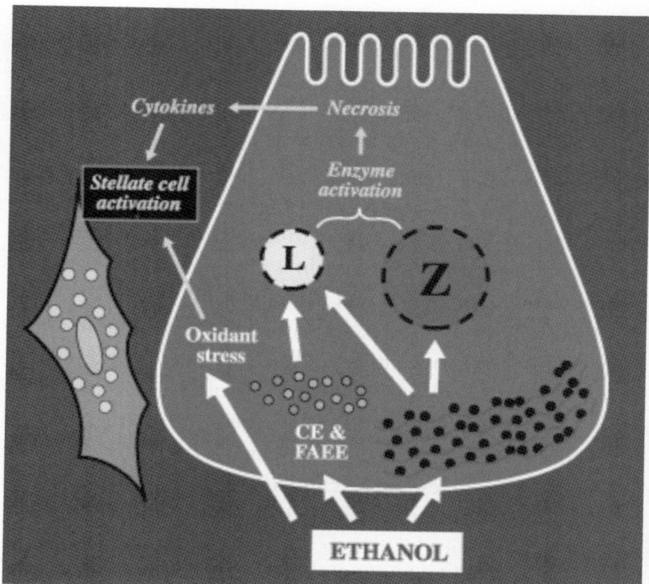

FIGURE 74.1. Overview of the pathogenesis of alcoholic pancreatitis. Ethanol increases pancreatic protein synthesis (•), pancreatic lipids (○) including cholesteryl esters (CE) and fatty acid ethyl esters (FAEE) and generates oxidant stress. These processes increase the protein content of lysosomes (L) and zymogen granules (z) and destabilize their membranes (dotted lines). As a consequence, intracellular activation of digestive enzymes is facilitated, leading to autodigestion. Cellular injury occurs by necrosis and stimulates release of cytokines which promote inflammation, activation of stellate cells and in turn pancreatic fibrosis.

Diagnosis A confident diagnosis of pancreatitis can often be made on the basis of an attack of severe abdominal pain and tenderness with elevation of the serum amylase more than three times the upper limit of normal and with imaging studies suggestive of inflammation in and around the pancreas.

The diagnosis of alcoholic pancreatitis is occasionally difficult. The amylase level does not rise significantly in approximately 10% of cases of acute pancreatitis, including many with alcoholic pancreatitis (52) or in those with delayed presentation. Determination of serum lipase, which remains elevated longer than the serum amylase, may be helpful. A previous report that an increased lipase-amylase ratio was specific for alcohol-induced pancreatitis (53) has not been confirmed (54,55). Amylase levels in the range found in acute pancreatitis may occur in other gastrointestinal disorders, including perforated peptic ulcer and ischemic bowel and in nongastrointestinal disorders, such as bulimia and gynecologic conditions (tubo-ovarian abscess/rupture) and others. Estimation of serum lipase levels does not help distinguish these disorders from pancreatitis because the source of the amylase (intestinal fluid) also contains lipase. In renal failure, serum amylase levels may occasionally be strikingly elevated (56). Salivary gland disease with hyperamylasemia occurs in people with alcohol problems and may be differentiated by fractionation of serum amylase and investigation of the salivary glands. Macroamylasemia is a condition in which amylase forms large complexes with an abnormal serum protein. The disorder is usually found coincidentally in a patient with very high amylase levels but without abdominal pain and is differentiated from pancreatitis by a normal serum lipase and the absence of amylase in the urine. Minor elevations of the serum amylase (less than threefold) may be due to many disorders including administration of morphine with secondary spasm of the sphincter of Oddi. Painless pancreatitis can occur, usually in the setting of a comatose or postoperative patient in whom pain is not appreciated. The diagnosis rests on other clinical and laboratory features.

Gallstones should be excluded by ultrasound examination. In cases with a negative ultrasound, serum alkaline phosphatase or transaminase levels raised at least twofold suggest associated gallstones that may be detected by repeat ultrasonography or endoscopic retrograde cholangiopancreatography (ERCP) (57,58). Magnetic resonance cholangiography (59) and endoscopic ultrasound are increasingly supplanting ERCP for diagnosis of gallstones in this setting. Dilated common bile duct has been recently described in patients on methadone and with opioid dependence in the absence of gallstones (60).

Assessment of Severity Severe pancreatitis carries a risk of mortality and is characterized by presence of organ failure (renal, respiratory, circulatory, gastrointestinal bleeding), local complications (necrosis, abscess or pseudocyst) or systemic alterations (falling hematocrit, rising urea, hypocalcaemia, acidosis, significant fluid sequestration). A number of clinical and laboratory criteria have been developed to identify patients at risk of complications so that they may be treated more intensively at an earlier stage. These objective criteria add little to careful clinical assessment (61), are cumbersome, and not often used clinically. Enzyme levels do not correlate well with disease severity.

The contrast-enhanced CT scan is now widely performed to detect pancreatic necrosis and complications of severe pancreatitis such as fluid collections, pseudocysts and abscesses (62). Some concern has been raised about possible adverse effects of contrast-enhanced CT scanning (63). Studies of intravenous contrast in experimental animals have yielded conflicting findings (64–66). Caution in the unrestricted use of contrast-enhanced CT scans appears warranted. CT scanning without contrast can detect most diagnostic features of pancreatitis and is often performed.

Treatment Severe cases, particularly those associated with respiratory or renal failure, require treatment in an intensive care unit. Initially, patients are treated with bed rest, analgesics, intravenous fluids, and fasting. Opioid analgesia is required, but there is no overall advantage of one opioid over another. Morphine has been reported to have a greater tendency to contract the sphincter of Oddi as compared to meperidine (pethidine) (67). Morphine is a more effective analgesic, is less susceptible to abuse than meperidine, and is usually the drug of choice. Intravenous fluids are given aggressively to restore vascular volume and renal perfusion and hour-by-hour monitoring is required. Patients are initially fasted, partly for symptomatic reasons but also because early refeeding seems to cause clinical relapse. Nutritional support is required if oral intake is not likely to be restored within several days. Total parenteral nutrition (TPN) and enteral feeding (nasogastric or nasojejunal) have been evaluated. Enteral feeding is safer and less expensive, and there is some evidence it may be more effective than TPN (68).

Treatments to reduce pancreatic secretion aim to reduce pressure in the pancreatic duct and consequently reduce the block in exocytosis from pancreatic acinar cells. However, the inflamed pancreas already secretes very little (69), and no beneficial effect has been found from nasogastric suction (70), cimetidine, anticholinergics, glucagon, calcitonin (71), or the somatostatin analog octreotide (72). Protease inhibitors may limit the damage done by activated digestive enzymes. In clinical practice, it is not possible to commence treatment early enough in the attack of pancreatitis for protease inhibitors to be effective, except for post-ERCP pancreatitis, wherein some benefit has been reported. Peritoneal lavage might improve the outcome by removing toxic inflammatory products from the peritoneum but the results of controlled studies have been conflicting (73,74). New approaches that may prove more effective include extended lavage (75) and retroperitoneal lavage using operatively placed cannulae (76). Antibiotics have not been shown to be beneficial for unselected cases of acute pancreatitis for which the prognosis is already excellent (77). In severe pancreatitis, several controlled trials of prophylactic antibiotic therapy have been undertaken, with inconsistent findings (68). In one small controlled study of antioxidant therapy (allopurinol or dimethyl sulfoxide given by enema), there was significant relief of pain in patients with an acute attack of alcoholic pancreatitis (78). More recently, a combination of intravenous antioxidants were ineffective for patients with severe acute pancreatitis (79). These small studies require confirmation before antioxidant therapy can be recommended for routine use in acute pancreatitis.

ERCP with endoscopic sphincterotomy has been shown to reduce the morbidity of patients with unremitting severe gallstone pancreatitis in two randomized controlled studies (80,81). Surgery is uncommonly required, the main indication being necrotising pancreatitis (82). Infected necrosis carries a high morbidity and mortality (83) and requires surgical debridement followed by postoperative lavage (75,83). By contrast, sterile necrosis often improves with conservative therapy alone (84). Pancreatic abscess carries a very high mortality and is an absolute indication for drainage by open surgery or percutaneous techniques. In fulminant cases, multiple procedures may be required. Small pseudocysts may resolve spontaneously, but large or symptomatic ones usually require drainage via endoscopic, percutaneous or operative techniques (85).

Chronic Pancreatitis Recurrent episodes of acute pancreatitis, clinical or subclinical, may lead to chronic pancreatitis. Chronic excessive consumption of alcohol is the most common cause and accounts for approximately 75% of cases.

Clinical Features The main problem is usually pain, and this may be very challenging. Like that of acute pancreatitis, the pain of chronic pancreatitis is typically diffusely located in the upper abdomen and may radiate to the back when severe. Pain tends to increase with meals and decreases appetite and food consumption and often results in weight loss. A minority present without pain for obscure reasons. The other manifestations are diabetes mellitus and steatorrhea. Weight loss is common. Vitamin deficiency is generally subclinical. Investigations reveal malabsorption of fat soluble vitamins and osteopenia.

Treatment Complete abstinence from alcohol is essential to minimize progression of the disease, and this may help to control pain. Reassurance that the disorder is benign with a tendency to slowly remit is helpful. Non-narcotic analgesia may suffice, but opioids are often required and should not be unreasonably withheld. Analgesic dependence or possible misuse should be carefully assessed according to principles described elsewhere in this volume (86). Antidepressants should be tried. Coeliac plexus injection helps about 60% of patients, but pain may recur. The procedure is not often performed owing to limited efficacy, frequent recurrence, and significant complications. Pancreatic enzyme supplements have been evaluated for the treatment of pain, but the evidence is mixed. A trial of 1 month is sufficient to determine whether this works in practice. Octreotide is not effective. There is now evidence from a small placebo-controlled trial that antioxidant therapy may reduce pain and improve quality of life in chronic pancreatitis (49). This study used a combination preparation that contained selenium, beta-carotene, vitamin C, vitamin E, and L-methionine. The relationship between pancreatic duct obstruction and pain is not clear, but relief of obstruction is clinically associated with relief of pain. Endoscopic approaches to dilate pancreatic duct strictures and remove calculi have been developed, and surgery is typically employed for refractory cases. The Whipple procedure or modified Whipple procedures are the most commonly performed procedure. The Puestow procedure (lateral pancreatico-jejunostomy) involves decompression of a dilated pancreatic duct and side-to-side anastomosis onto a roux-en-Y loop of jejunum. Two small randomized trials comparing endoscopic and surgical drainage of dilated pancreatic duct in chronic pancreatitis showed that surgery was associated with better long-term analgesia and quality of life (87,88).

Exocrine failure is treated by dietary modification and pancreatic enzyme replacement. Reduction of dietary fat intake reduces steatorrhea. Pancreatic enzymes are required with each meal and snack. The newer enteric coated microsphere preparations are more potent and are preferred as they release enzymes only in the duodenum, reducing irreversible inactivation of lipase by gastric acid. Histamine-2 receptor antagonists or proton pump inhibitors also limit lipase inactivation due also to failure of pancreatic bicarbonate secretion. Normalization of fecal fat levels does not typically occur. Diabetes mellitus is treated with dietary modification, treatment of malabsorption, and specific therapy. Some patients respond to oral hypoglycemic agents, but most require insulin. The diabetes is "brittle" in that the patient is susceptible to hypoglycemia due to loss of both insulin and glucagon secretion. Long-term surviving patients with this form of diabetes are prone to diabetic complications and should be monitored accordingly.

Small Intestine Diarrhea is common among those who drink alcohol excessively, both acutely and chronically. Multiple factors contribute to this problem, including altered motility, permeability, and nutritional disorders. Small-intestinal mucosal injury can occur after acute or chronic administration of alcohol. Perfusion of the hamster jejunum with 4.8% ethanol caused separation of the tip of the villus epithelium forming blebs (89). These blebs may rupture, leading to denudement of the epithelium. The villus core contracts and loses height within 1 minute of ethanol exposure. This effect is independent of any action on the microcirculation (90) and may be mediated by leukocytes (91) via release of histamine from mast cells and by oxidant stress (90).

Mucosal blood flow is acutely increased with increased endothelial permeability (89). Acute administration of alcohol leads to increased gut permeability, resulting both in abnormal absorption of luminal content (such as endotoxin, which contributes to the pathogenesis of alcoholic liver disease; see Chapter 72) and abnormal leakage of mucosal contents (such as albumin). Ethanol also inhibits absorption of actively transported sugars, dipeptides, and amino acids. Many defects in absorption have been reported in people with alcohol problems, including water (92,93) carbohydrate, lipid, vitamins (notably thiamine, folate), and minerals (calcium, iron, zinc, and selenium) (89). Folate deficiency, common among people with alcohol problems, causes intestinal injury, leading to malabsorption and diarrhea and further loss of folate. Ethanol may exacerbate lactase deficiency, especially in non-whites (94).

Colon Portal hypertension may manifest uncommonly with hemorrhoids and rarely with colonic varices. Colonic varices appear as filling defects on barium enema and may occur in any part of the colon, most commonly in the rectum (15). Alcohol has also been reported to cause nonulcerative inflammatory changes in human colonic epithelium (95). These changes resolved during a 2-week period of abstinence. They were not explained by folate deficiency, as folate levels were normal in 10 of the 11 cases. This form of colitis has the potential to contribute to diarrhea but is not usually recognized clinically, as pathology elsewhere in the gut tends to dominate the clinical picture.

Inappropriate alcohol enema has been reported to cause a chemical colitis (96), and this may result from a toxic effect similar to the direct toxicity of alcohol on the gastric mucosa. Alcohol use has a recognized association with colorectal cancer as indicated below. Finally, alcohol consumption may have at least one beneficial effect on the colon in that it has been linked to a reduced incidence of ulcerative colitis in one study (97).

Alcohol and Gastrointestinal Cancer Alcohol use is a recognized risk factor for several gastrointestinal neoplasms, including tumors of the tongue, mouth, pharynx, larynx, oesophagus, stomach, pancreas, colon, and liver (98–100). Alcohol use has been repeatedly associated with an increased incidence of esophageal (and oropharyngeal) cancer, especially in those who also smoke. Blot reported a 5.8-fold increased risk among those who drink alcohol, a 7.4-fold increased risk among smokers, and a 38-fold increased risk among those who both drank and smoked (101). The effect of alcohol on cancer risk appears to be dose-related. A recent comprehensive Australian overview of the literature reports that relatively modest average daily consumption, 25 g per day, within the guidelines for men in many countries, including the United States, is associated with increased risk of gastrointestinal cancer. For example, consumption of 25 g per day was associated with a relative risk of 1.76 for oropharyngeal cancer and 1.52 for oesophageal cancer, approximately 1.05 for the colon and rectum, and 1.17 for the liver (102). These risks were all statistically significantly greater than 1.0, were adjusted for the confounding effects of smoking, and rose progressively with higher levels of consumption.

In general, the experimental studies have not shown that alcohol is itself a complete carcinogen. Rather, ethanol is a cocarcinogen that increases the cancer risk after exposure to another compound. The effect of ethanol may occur at the initiation, induction, or progression stages of tumor development. For example, alcohol-fed rats given N-nitrosomethylbenzylamine developed more esophageal tumors than did control rats (103). Several mechanisms may contribute to this cocarcinogenic effect of ethanol (104). Ethanol-induced induction of CYP2E1 increases carcinogen activation, potentiation of oxidant stress, diminished DNA repair, suppression of immune responses, and nutritional depletion such as folate deficiency.

With respect to hepatocellular carcinoma (HCC), alcohol abuse has been long recognized as a predisposing factor. Alcohol might contribute to carcinogenesis via mechanisms considered for other tissues and listed earlier, but there is insufficient experimental evidence to conclude that alcohol is a complete hepatic carcinogen (105,106). Most patients have cirrhosis, a condition known to predispose to HCC. Many patients also have other risk factors for HCC, such as chronic hepatitis B, hepatitis C, or exposure to chemical carcinogens such as aflatoxins (105). There have remained a small number of cases of HCC associated with excessive alcohol use without cirrhosis or other contributing factors (107), but it is not clear that this number is greater than would be expected by chance (108).

GASTROINTESTINAL SYMPTOMS ASSOCIATED WITH ABUSE OF PRESCRIPTION DRUGS

Opioids Opioids act on gut function in a complex fashion via all three receptor classes in the brain, spinal cord, and enteric nervous systems. Low doses act at enteric nervous system sites, and higher doses also act within the CNS. Opioids alter both motility and electrolyte absorption, leading to constipation that may be severe, particularly in the elderly. Opioids increase absorption of chloride by both increasing chloride transport and reducing chloride secretion in response to various secretogogues (109,110). These effects in turn increase passive water absorption and reduce colonic volume, exacerbating the tendency to constipation. The motility effects are more prominent for the clinically available opioids. Opioids decrease the frequency of contractions in, and propulsion along, the small bowel and colon (111). Classically, chronic opioid use was thought not to induce tolerance to gut motility, but tolerance and withdrawal have recently been demonstrated in an experimental animal model (111). Tolerance to the gastrointestinal motility effects took longer to develop than

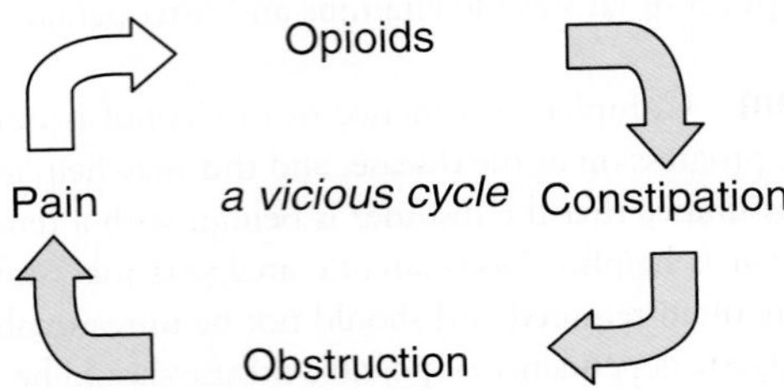

FIGURE 74.2. Opioids increase constipation and in turn obstruction and pain leading to further increase in opioid medication.

to the nociceptive effects and tolerance to the inhibitory effects developed more slowly than that to the excitatory effects. The mechanism(s) by which tissues become tolerant to the effects of opioids have been extensively studied within the CNS (112), but much less is known about the gut effects that are determined by both central and peripheral opioid actions. Among methadone maintenance patients, constipation is common and tends to be worse early in treatment (113,114). The high prevalence of persisting constipation suggests that tolerance to the gut effects of opioids occurs to only a limited extent. In one study, 58% of subjects in methadone maintenance experienced some degree of constipation, and 10% had severe problems (115). Fecal impaction, and even stercoral perforation, have been described (116) and usually respond to increased fluid intake and fiber supplementation to correct for poor dietary intake. Laxatives are not often required, but osmotic agents such as lactulose are the laxatives of choice. The narcotic bowel syndrome is characterized by a picture similar to intestinal pseudo-obstruction (117). The syndrome is characterized by chronic or frequently recurring abdominal pain that worsens with continued or escalating dosages of narcotics (Fig. 74.2). It is attributed to the effects of opioid drugs: on bowel function and opioid-induced hyperalgesia (118). This syndrome responds to withdrawal of opioids and administration of the α_2-agonist clonidine (119). Methylnaltrexone and alvimopan are peripheral opioid receptor antagonists that have recently been reported to relieve constipation without precipitating opioid withdrawal, likely to find greatest application in postoperative and palliative care settings rather than for patients in opioid maintenance programs (120). These latter drugs are not yet available for general use in the United States.

Laxative Misuse Surreptitious laxative misuse is among the more common causes for unexplained chronic diarrhea. It represents an intriguing form of substance misuse but is rare and is typically observed in people without other substance misuse issues. These patients present to family physicians and gastroenterologists. Some are associated with bulimia. Others tend to be older women, and the disorder can be viewed as a form of Munchausen's syndrome. The diagnosis rests on identification of laxatives by stool alkalinization, osmolality studies, or a bag search in the hospital (121).

Misuse of Anticholinergics In high doses, anticholinergic drugs alter mood and are occasionally misused, particularly when prescribed to relieve extrapyramidal symptoms in the mentally ill (122) and among those with limited access to other drugs of abuse. Clonidine and/or buscopan prescribed for opioid withdrawal may also be misused. Patients develop marked constipation and abdominal pain as well as dry mouth and blurred vision. In the author's experience, patients have had previous drug dependence problems and have welcomed an explanation of their symptoms and participated in structured withdrawal.

EFFECTS OF TOBACCO ON GASTROINTESTINAL FUNCTION

Gastroesophageal Reflux Smoking has been linked to exacerbations of reflux symptoms, and cessation of smoking is one of the lifestyle changes traditionally recommended in the treatment of reflux (123). At a practical level, smoking cessation is difficult to achieve and has not been shown to induce remission of reflux or healing of esophagitis. Nicotine has been shown to reduce lower esophageal sphincter pressure and promote gastroesophageal reflux in response to straining during coughing and deep breathing (124). People who smoke cigarettes have also been shown to have delayed acid clearance from the esophagus (125). Not all studies have yielded consistent findings. One recent study found that smoking did not influence basal lower esophageal sphincter pressure or esophageal motility (126). From the foregoing, it is clear that smoking cessation cannot be recommended as sole treatment for reflux, but there is sound evidence that smoking contributes to reflux. It is reasonable to advise patients with GERD to quit smoking based upon the association with reflux, the expectation that GERD might respond favourably to quitting, and to prevent the myriad other adverse effects of smoking.

Peptic Ulceration There is considerable evidence that smoking is involved with peptic ulcer. Smoking increases risk of ulcer according to the number of cigarettes smoked. Heavy smoking is associated with delayed ulcer healing, and the risk of recurrence is increased (127,128). Smoking increases the risk of complications from peptic ulcer (129). Finally, overall ulcer-related mortality is increased in those who smoke as compared to those who do not (130,131). The mechanism by which smoking exacerbates peptic ulcer disease remains unclear.

Pancreatic Disease Evidence from a number of countries provides a clear link between smoking and pancreatic cancer. Several studies have consistently found a moderately increased risk (about threefold) of pancreatic cancer among smokers (132,133).

There have been inconsistent findings concerning the relationship between smoking and pancreatitis (132). In general, most people with alcohol dependence smoke, so it is difficult to separate the effects of tobacco from those of alcohol, which is the major cause for pancreatitis. A case-control study compared tobacco use in a group with alcoholic pancreatitis and a control group who drank at least as much alcohol, did not develop pancreatitis, and were clinically well. The only study using this methodology found no association with smoking (132). Other studies that have found positive associations used less stringent methods (133,134).

Inflammatory Bowel Disease A curious relationship exists between smoking and inflammatory bowel disease. Smoking has been consistently shown to increase the risk of Crohn's disease and to *decrease* the risk of ulcerative colitis (135,136). Somewhat provocatively, smoking may also reduce the severity of established ulcerative colitis, suggesting nicotine has therapeutic potential for this disease. Nicotine influences immune cellular function, increases mucin production, relaxes colonic smooth muscle, increases endogenous glucocorticoids, and influences rectal blood flow and intestinal permeability (137). Less toxic approaches to this form of therapy have been sought and include topical colonic administration of nicotine. These approaches remain experimental at this time (138).

Gastrointestinal Malignancy Smoking has been strongly linked to cancers of the upper aerodigestive tract and pancreas, as discussed earlier. The link between smoking and stomach cancer is weaker but is present in most studies (139).

BODY PACKING

Persons smuggling illicit drugs may ingest large amounts of cocaine, heroin, or other drugs aiming to retrieve the packages after reaching their destination (140). This is referred to as *body packing, cocaine packing,* or *body stuffing syndrome* (141). Multiple packages made from latex condoms, wax, or plastic bags are used and may also be placed retrogradely into the rectum or vagina. The incidence of this practice is unknown. Most cases present in police custody, raising ethical and funding challenges of managing an involuntary patient. Some people may be coerced to smuggle drugs. Cases involving children and pregnant women have been described (140). Hospitals close to international airports may encounter these cases and should consider developing a management policy for this challenging problem. An early report describes 10 cases diagnosed only after death in which as many as 147 packages were found (142). Lethal drug absorption through rubber condoms may occur without rupture. The body packer may present with life-threatening symptoms of intoxication, including seizures and cardiorespiratory collapse, and mechanical obstruction from the ingested drug packets. The largest series comprises 61 cases from Milan, Italy, of which only 2 cases required laparotomy, one each for obstruction and nonfatal drug toxicity (143).

Clinical monitoring constitutes frequent clinical and neurologic assessment and abdominal examination daily to detect complications of acute drug intoxication, bowel obstruction, or perforation. The patient should be kept in hospital until all drug packages have cleared owing to the risk of life-threatening overdose if any rupture. Traub et al. (140) present a detailed review and clinical approach to management. A light solid diet with free liquids may be given. Oily or polyethylene glycol laxatives can be given repeatedly to accelerate passage of packages (144). Plain abdominal x-rays are helpful and can be repeated daily until the gut is cleared, typically 3 to 6 days (145). Dilute contrast has been reported to assist identification of the packages (146). In some cases, CT is required, with potential concerns if repeated examinations are needed. Symptomatic cases may require early surgery (147). Endoscopic removal of packages is not recommended owing to the risk of rupture during manipulation (148). The complication rate was 25% in an early U.S. series (149), but in the recent Italian series, asymptomatic body packers were safely managed conservatively in 59 of 61 cases (143), perhaps related to improved manufacture of drug packages. A variation of this syndrome is referred to as *mini-packing* wherein individual drug users ingest a single packet of drugs in haste to evade police detection (150). Despite ingestion of a lower dose of drug, the risk of life-threatening toxicity remains. In addition, the ingested powder may contain other dangerous drugs (151).

Psychostimulants (Cocaine and Amphetamines)

Cocaine may lead to ischemic injury to the gut leading to intestinal perforation, infarction, or ischemic colitis (152). Young people subjected to prolonged hypotension or hypoxia after opioid overdose may develop ischemic infarction to the gut. These uncommon injuries typically present with abdominal pain and peritonitis but may be occult in a critically ill and unconscious person.

Cannabis Cannabinoid receptors are widely expressed throughout both the upper and lower GI tract and are also expressed on hepatic stellate cells. Consequently, cannabinoids may influence a range of GI functions in health and disease (153). Nausea and vomiting are side effects of many chemotherapeutics and reduce the quality of life of patients with diabetes, cancer, and acquired immune deficiency syndrome. Cannabis (marijuana) and other cannabinoids appear to be effective anti-emetics confirmed by a recent meta analysis (154). The antiemetic effect has been demonstrated in an animal model and is related to the expression of CB1 receptors in the dorsal vagal nucleus (155). Cannabinoids are also involved in inhibition of gastric emptying and gastric acid secretion.

Cannabis has also been linked to a series of cases with hyperemesis (156). These cases presented with a history of several years of cannabis abuse, predating the onset of the vomiting illness. The hyperemesis followed a cyclical pattern every few weeks or months, often for many years, against a background of regular cannabis abuse. Cessation of cannabis, as confirmed by a negative urine drug screen for cannabinoids, led to cessation of the cyclical vomiting illness, and a return to regular cannabis use heralded a return of the hyperemesis weeks to months later. The mechanism was not understood. A further similar case was described in the United Kingdom (157) but the existence of this syndrome remains controversial (158).

REFERENCES

1. Bujanda L. The effects of alcohol consumption upon the gastrointestinal tract. *Am J Gastroenterol* 2000;95;33:74–82.
2. Lieber CS. Interaction of ethanol with other drugs. In: Lieber CS, ed. *Medical and nutritional complications of alcoholism*. New York: Plenum, 1992a:165–183.
3. Preedy VR, Watson RR, eds. *Alcohol and the gastrontestinal tract*. Boca Raton, FL: CRC Press, 1996.
4. Proctor GB, Shori DK. The effects of ethanol on salivary glands. In: Preedy VR, Watson RR, eds. *Alcohol and the gastrontestinal tract* (p. 347). Boca Raton, FL: CRC Press, 1996.
5. Silver LS, Worner TM, Korsten MA. Esophageal function in chronic alcoholics. *Am J Gastroenterol* 1986;81:423–427.
6. Kaufman SE, Kaye MD. Induction of gastro-oesophageal reflux by alcohol. *Gut* 1978;19:336–338.
7. Lieber CS, ed. *Medical and nutritional complications of alcoholism*. New York: Plenum, 1992b.
8. Hogan WJ, Viegas de Andrade SR, Winship DH. Ethanol-induced acute esophageal motor dysfunction. *J Appl Physiol* 1972;32:755–760.
9. Mayer EM, Grabowski CJ, Fisher RS. Effects of graded doses of alcohol upon esophageal motor function. *Gastroenterology* 1978;75: 1133–1136.
10. Keshavarzian A, Iber FL, Ferguson Y. Esophageal manometry and radionuclide emptying in chronic alcoholics. *Gastroenterology* 1987;92: 651–657.
11. Messian RA, Hermos JA, Robbins AH, et al. Barrett's esophagus. Clinical review of 26 cases. *Am J Gastroenterol* 1978;69:458–466.
12. Robertson CS, Mayberry JF, Nicholson DA, et al. Value of endoscopic surveillance in the detection of neoplastic change in Barrett's oesophagus. *Br J Surg* 1988;75:760–763.
13. Gray MR, Donnelly RJ, Kingsnorth AN. The role of smoking and alcohol in metaplasia and cancer risk in Barrett's columnar lined oesophagus. *Gut* 1993;34:727–731.
14. Konturek SJ, Stachura J, Konturek JW. Gastric cytoprotection and adaptation to ethanol. In: Preedy VR, Watson RR, eds. *Alcohol and the gastrontestinal tract*. Boca Raton, FL: CRC Press, 1996:123–141.
15. Feinman L, Korsten MA, Lieber CS. Alcohol and the digestive tract. In: Lieber CS, ed. *Medical and nutritional complications of alcoholism*. New York: Plenum, 1992:307–340.
16. Brown RC, Hardy GJ, Temperley JM, et al. Gastritis and cirrhosis—no association. *J Clin Pathol* 1981;34:744–748.
17. Knoll MR, Kolbel CB, Teyssen S, Singer MV. Action of pure ethanol and some alcoholic beverages on the gastric mucosa in healthy humans: a descriptive endoscopic study. *Endoscopy* 1998;30:293–301.
18. Uppal R, Rosman A, Hernandez R, et al. Effects of liver disease on red blood cell acetaldehyde in alcoholics and non-alcoholics. *Alcohol Alcohol Suppl* 1991;1:323–326.
19. Hauge T, Persson J, Kjerstadius T. *Helicobacter pylori*, active chronic antral gastritis, and gastrointestinal symptoms in alcoholics. *Alcohol Clin Exp Res* 1994;18:886–888.
20. Battaglia B, Di Mario F, Dotto P, Naccarato R. Alcohol intake and acute duodenal ulcer healing. *Am J Gastroenterol* 1990;85:1198–1199.
21. Reynolds JC. Famotidine therapy for active duodenal ulcers. A multivariate analysis of factors affecting early healing. *Ann Intern Med* 1989; 111:7–14.
22. Shen WW. Potential link between hallucination and nausea/vomiting induced by alcohol? An empirical clinical finding. *Psychopathology* 1985;18:212–217.
23. Hauge T, Persson J, Danielsson D. Mucosal bacterial growth in the upper gastrointestinal tract in alcoholics (heavy drinkers). *Digestion* 1997;58:591–595.
24. Go VLW, Everhart JE. Pancreatitis. In: Everhart JE, ed. *Digestive diseases in the United States: epidemiology and impact*. Washington, DC: National Institutes of Health, 1994:615–646.
25. Johnson CD, Hosking S. National statistics for diet, alcohol consumption, and chronic pancreatitis in England and Wales, 1960–1988. *Gut* 1991;32:1401–1405.

26. Yadav D, Lowenfels AB. Trends in the epidemiology of the first attack of acute pancreatitis: a systematic review. *Pancreas* 2006;33:323–330.
27. Bradley EL 3rd. A clinically based classification system for acute pancreatitis. Summary of the International Symposium on Acute Pancreatitis, Atlanta, GA, September 11–13, 1992. *Arch Surg* 1993;128:586–590.
28. Pitchumoni CS, Glasser M, Saran RM, et al. Pancreatic fibrosis in chronic alcoholics and nonalcoholics without clinical pancreatitis. *Am J Gastroenterol* 1984;79:382–388.
29. Haber PS, Wilson JS, Apte MV, et al. Individual susceptibility to alcoholic pancreatitis: still an enigma. *J Lab Clin Med* 1995;125:305–312.
30. Wilson JS, Bernstein L, McDonald C, et al. Diet and drinking habits in relation to the development of alcoholic pancreatitis. *Gut* 1985;26:882–887.
31. Haber PS, Wilson JS, Apte MV, et al. Lipid intolerance does not account for susceptibility to alcoholic and gallstone pancreatitis. *Gastroenterology* 1994;106:742–748.
32. Haber PS, Wilson JS, Pirola RC. Smoking and alcoholic pancreatitis. *Pancreas* 1993;8:568–572.
33. Wilson JS, Gossat D, Tait A, et al. Evidence for an inherited predisposition to alcoholic pancreatitis. A controlled HLA typing study. *Dig Dis Sci* 1984;29:727–730.
34. Haber PS, Wilson JS, McGarity BH, et al. Alpha 1 antitrypsin phenotypes and alcoholic pancreatitis. *Gut* 1991;32:945–948.
35. Norton ID, Apte MV, Dixson H, et al. Cystic fibrosis genotypes and alcoholic pancreatitis: chronic ethanol administration causes oxidative stress in the rat pancreas: cytochrome P4502E1 is present in rat pancreas and is induced by chronic ethanol administration. *J Gastroenterol Hepatol* 1998;13:496–499.
36. Witt H, Apte MV, Keim V, Wilson JS. Chronic pancreatitis: challenges and advances in pathogenesis, genetics, diagnosis, and therapy. *Gastroenterology* 2007;132:1557–1573.
37. Wilson JS, Korsten MA, Pirola RC. Alcohol-induced pancreatic injury (Part I). Unexplained features and ductular theories of pathogenesis. *Int J Pancreatol* 1989;4:109–125.
38. Dutta SK, Ting CD, Lai LL. Study of prevalence, severity, and etiological factors associated with acute pancreatitis in patients infected with human immunodeficiency virus. *Am J Gastroenterol* 1997;92: 2044–2048.
39. Whitfield RM, Bechtel LM, Starich GH. The impact of ethanol and Marinol/marijuana usage on HIV+/AIDS patients undergoing azidothymidine, azidothymidine/dideoxycytidine, or dideoxyinosine therapy. *Alcohol Clin Exp Res* 1997;21:122–127.
40. Greenberger N, Hatch FT, Drummey GD, Isselbacker KJ. Pancreatitis and hyperlipemia: A study of serum lipid alterations in 25 patients with acute pancreatitis. *Medicine* 1966;45:161–174.
41. Haber PS, Pirola RC, Wilson JS. Clinical update: management of acute pancreatitis. *J Gastroenterol Hepatol* 1997;12:189–197.
42. Whitcomb DC, Gorry MC, Preston RA, et al. Hereditary pancreatitis is caused by a mutation in the cationic trypsinogen gene: a gene for hereditary pancreatitis maps to chromosome 7q35. *Nat Genet* 1996;14: 141–145.
43. Freeman BA, Crapo JD. Biology of disease: free radicals and tissue injury. *Lab Invest* 1982;47:412–426.
44. Nonaka A, Manabe T, Asano N, et al. Direct ESR measurement of free radicals in mouse pancreatic lesions. *Int J Pancreatol* 1989;5:203–211.
45. Slater TF. Free-radical mechanisms in tissue injury. *Biochem J* 1984; 222:1–15.
46. Braganza JM, Scott P, Bilton D, et al. Evidence for early oxidative stress in acute pancreatitis. Clues for correction. *Int J Pancreatol* 1995;17: 69–81.
47. Pirola RC. Effects of ethyl alcohol on sphincteric resistance at the choledochoduodenal junction in man. *Gut* 1966;9:557–560.
48. Hajnal F, Flores MC, Radley S, Valenzuela JE. Effect of alcohol and alcoholic beverages on meal-stimulated pancreatic secretion in humans. *Gastroenterology* 1990;98:191–196.
49. Kirk GR, White JS, McKie L, et al. Combined antioxidant therapy reduces pain and improves quality of life in chronic pancreatitis. *J Gastrointest Surg* 2006;10:499–503.
50. Norton I, Apte MV, Haber PS, et al. Cytochrome P-450 2E1 is present in rat pancreas and induced by chronic ethanol administration. *Gastroenterology* 1996;110:A1280.
51. Saluja AK, Steer MLP. Pathophysiology of pancreatitis. Role of cytokines and other mediators of inflammation. *Digestion* 1999;60(Suppl 1): 27–33.
52. Spechler SJ, Dalton JW, Robbins AH, et al. Prevalence of normal serum amylase levels in patients with acute alcoholic pancreatitis. *Dig Dis Sci* 1983;28:865–869.
53. Gumaste VV, Dave PB, Weissman D, Messer J. Lipase/amylase ratio. A new index that distinguishes acute episodes of alcoholic from nonalcoholic acute pancreatitis. *Gastroenterology* 1991;101:1361–1366.
54. Pezzilli R, Billi P, Miglioli M, Gullo L. Serum amylase and lipase concentrations and lipase/amylase ratio in assessment of etiology and severity of acute pancreatitis. *Dig Dis Sci* 1993;38:1265–1269.
55. King LG, Seelig CB, Ranney JE. The lipase to amylase ratio in acute pancreatitis. *Am J Gastroenterol* 1995;90:67–69.
56. Tsianos EV, Dardamanis MA, Elisaf M, et al. The value of alpha-amylase and isoamylase determination in chronic renal failure patients. *Int J Pancreatol* 1994;15:105–111.
57. Goodman AJ, Neoptolemos JP, Carr-Locke DL, et al. Detection of gall stones after acute pancreatitis. *Gut* 1985;26:125–132.
58. Venu RP, Geenen JE, Toouli J, et al. Endoscopic retrograde cholangiopancreatography. Diagnosis of cholelithiasis in patients with normal gallbladder x-ray and ultrasound studies. *JAMA* 1983;249:758–761.
59. Soto JA, Barish MA, Yucel EK, et al. Magnetic resonance cholangiography: comparison with endoscopic retrograde cholangiopancreatography. *Gastroenterology* 1996;110:589–597.
60. Sharma SS. Sphincter of Oddi dysfunction in patients addicted to opium: an unrecognized entity. *Gastrointest Endosc* 2002;55:427–430.
61. Steinberg WM. Predictors of severity of acute pancreatitis. *Gastroenterol Clin North Am* 1990;19:849–861.
62. Kivisaari L, Somer K, Standertskjold-Nordenstam CG, et al. Early detection of acute fulminant pancreatitis by contrast-enhanced computed tomography. *Scand J Gastroenterol* 1983;18:39–41.
63. McMenamin DA, Gates LK Jr. A retrospective analysis of the effect of contrast-enhanced CT on the outcome of acute pancreatitis. *Am J Gastroenterol* 1996;91:1384–1387.
64. Foitzik T, Bassi DG, Schmidt J, et al. Intravenous contrast medium accentuates the severity of acute necrotizing pancreatitis in the rat. *Gastroenterology* 1994;106:207–114.
65. Kaiser AM, Grady T, Gerdes D, et al. Intravenous contrast medium does not increase the severity of acute necrotizing pancreatitis in the opossum. *Dig Dis Sci* 1995;40:1547–1553.
66. Schmidt J, Hotz HG, Foitzik T, et al. Intravenous contrast medium aggravates the impairment of pancreatic microcirculation in necrotizing pancreatitis in the rat. *Ann Surg* 1995;221:257–264.
67. Thune A, Baker RA, Saccone GT, et al. Differing effects of pethidine and morphine on human sphincter of Oddi motility. *Br J Surg* 1990;77:992–995.
68. Pandol SJ, Saluja AK, Imrie CW, Banks PA. Acute pancreatitis: bench to the bedside. *Gastroenterology* 12007;32:1127–1151.
69. Mitchell CJ, Playforth MJ, Kelleher J, McMahon MJ. Functional recovery of the exocrine pancreas after acute pancreatitis. *Scand J Gastroenterol* 1983;18:5–8.
70. Sarr MG, Sanfey H, Cameron JL. Prospective, randomized trial of nasogastric suction in patients with acute pancreatitis. *Surgery* 1986;100: 500–504.
71. Leach S, Gorelick FS, Modlin IM. New perspectives on acute pancreatitis. *Scand J Gastroenterol* 1992;27:29–38.
72. McKay CJ, Imrie CW, Baxter JN. Somatostatin and somatostatin analogues—are they indicated in the management of acute pancreatitis? *Gut* 1993;34:1622–1626.
73. Mayer AD, McMahon MJ, Corfield AP, et al. Controlled clinical trial of peritoneal lavage for the treatment of severe acute pancreatitis. *N Engl J Med* 1985;312:399–404.
74. Stone HH, Fabian TC. Peritoneal dialysis in the treatment of acute alcoholic pancreatitis. *Surg Gynecol Obstet* 1980;150:878–882.
75. Ranson JH, Berman RS. Long peritoneal lavage decreases pancreatic sepsis in acute pancreatitis. *Ann Surg* 1990;211:708–716; discussion, 716–718.

76. Pederzoli P, Bassi C, Vesentini S, et al. Retroperitoneal and peritoneal drainage and lavage in the treatment of severe necrotizing pancreatitis. *Surg Gynecol Obstet* 1990;170:197–203.
77. Bradley EL 3rd. Antibiotics in acute pancreatitis. Current status and future directions. *Am J Surg* 1989;158:472–477; discussion, 477–478.
78. Salim AS. Role of oxygen-derived free radical scavengers in the treatment of recurrent pain produced by chronic pancreatitis. A new approach. *Arch Surg* 1991;126:1109–1114.
79. Siriwardena AK, Mason JM, Balachandra S, et al: Randomized, double blind, placebo controlled trial of intravenous antioxidant (n-acetylcysteine, selenium, vitamin C) therapy in severe acute pancreatitis. *Gut* 2007;56; 1439–1444.
80. Fan ST, Lai EC, Mok FP, et al. Early treatment of acute biliary pancreatitis by endoscopic papillotomy. *N Engl J Med* 1993;328:228–232.
81. Neoptolemos JP, Carr-Locke DL, London NJ, et al. Controlled trial of urgent endoscopic retrograde cholangiopancreatography and endoscopic sphincterotomy versus conservative treatment for acute pancreatitis due to gallstones. *Lancet* 1988;2:979–983.
82. McFadden DW, Reber HA. Indications for surgery in severe acute pancreatitis. *Int J Pancreatol* 1994;15:83–90.
83. Beger HG, Buchler M, Bittner R, et al. Necrosectomy and postoperative local lavage in necrotizing pancreatitis. *Br J Surg* 1988;75:207–212.
84. Bradley EL 3rd, Allen K. A prospective longitudinal study of observation versus surgical intervention in the management of necrotizing pancreatitis. *Am J Surg* 1991;161:19–24; discussion, 24–25.
85. Maule W, Reber HA. 1993 Diagnosis and management of pancreatic pseudocysts, pancreatic ascites, and pancreatic fistulas. *The pancreas: biology, pathobiology, and disease,* 2nd ed. 741–751.
86. Hung CI, Liu CY, Chen CY, et al. Meperidine addiction or treatment frustration? *Gen Hosp Psychiatry* 2001;23:31–35.
87. Cahen DL, Gouma DJ, Nio Y, et al. Endoscopic versus surgical drainage of the pancreatic duct in chronic pancreatitis. *N Engl J Med* 2007;356: 676–384.
88. Dite P, Ruzicka M, Zboril V, Novotny I. A prospective, randomized trial comparing endoscopic and surgical therapy for chronic pancreatitis. *Endoscopy* 2003;35:553–558.
89. Beck IT. Small bowel injury by ethanol. In: Preedy VR, Watson RR, eds. *Alcohol and the gastrointestinal tract.* Boca Raton, FL: CRC Press, 1996:163–202.
90. Dinda PK, Buell MG, Morris O, Beck IT. Studies on ethanol-induced subepithelial fluid accumulation and jejunal villus bleb formation. An *in vitro* video microscopic approach. *Can J Physiol Pharmacol* 1994;72: 1186–1192.
91. Dinda PK, Kossev P, Beck IT, Buell MG. Role of xanthine oxidase-derived oxidants and leukocytes in ethanol-induced jejunal mucosal injury. *Dig Dis Sci* 1996;41:2461–2470.
92. Krasner N, Cochran KM, Russell RI, Carmichael HA,Thompson GG. Alcohol and absorption from the small intestine: 1. Impairment of absorption from the small intestine in alcoholies. *Gut* 1976;17:245–248.
93. Krasner N, Carmichael HA, Russell RI, Thompson GG, Cochran KM. Alcohol and absorption from the small intestine: 2. Effect of ethanol on ATP and ATPase activities in guinea-pig jejunum. *Gut* 1976;17:249–251.
94. Perlow, Baraon, E, Lieber CS. Symptomatic intestinal disaccharidase deficiency in alcoholics. *Gastroenterology* 1977;72:680–684.
95. Brozinsky S, Fani K, Grosberg SJ, Wapnick S. Alcohol ingestion-induced changes in the human rectal mucosa: light and electron microscopic studies. *Dis Colon Rectum* 1978;21:329–335.
96. Herrerias JM, Muniain MA, Sanchez S, Garrido M. Alcohol-induced colitis. *Endoscopy* 1983;15:121–122.
97. Boyko EJ, Perera DR, Koepsell TD, et al. Coffee and alcohol use and the risk of ulcerative colitis. *Am J Gastroenterol* 1989;84:530–534.
98. Franceschi S. Alcohol and cancer. *Adv Exp Med Biol* 1999;472:43–49.
99. Longnecker MP. Alcohol consumption and risk of cancer in humans: an overview. *Alcohol* 1995;12:87–96.
100. Ringborg U. Alcohol and risk of cancer. *Alcohol Clin Exp Res* 1998;22: 323S–328S.
101. Blot WJ, McLaughlin JK, Winn DM, et al. Smoking and drinking in relation to oral and pharyngeal cancer. *Cancer Res* 1988;48:3282–3287.
102. Lewis S, Campbell S, Proudfoot E, et al. *Alcohol as a cause of cancer*. Sydney: Cancer Institute NSW, 2008.
103. Mufti SI, Becker G, Sipes IG. Effect of chronic dietary ethanol consumption on the initiation and promotion of chemically-induced esophageal carcinogenesis in experimental rats. *Carcinogenesis* 1989;10: 303–309.
104. Mufti SI. Alcohol's promotion of gastrointestinal carcinogenesis. In: Preedy VR, Watson RR, eds. *Alcohol and the gastrontestinal tract.* Boca Raton, FL: CRC Press, 1996:311–320.
105. Farber E. Alcohol and other chemicals in the development of hepatocellular carcinoma. *Clin Lab Med* 1996;16:377–394.
106. Misslebeck NG, Campbell TC. The role of ethanol in the etiology of primary liver cancer. *Adv Nutr Res* 1985;7:129–153.
107. Lieber CS, Seitz HK, Garro AJ, Worner TM. Alcohol-related diseases and carcinogenesis. *Cancer Res* 1979;39:2863–2886.
108. Bassendine MF. Alcohol—a major risk factor for hepatocellular carcinoma? *J Hepatol* 1986;2:513–519.
109. McKay JS, Linaker BD, Turnberg LA. Influence of opiates on ion transport across rabbit ileal mucosa. *Gastroenterology* 1981;80:279–284.
110. McKay J S, Linaker BD, Higgs NB, Turnberg LA. Studies of the antisecretory activity of morphine in rabbit ileum *in vitro. Gastroenterology* 1982;82:243–247.
111. Williams CL, Bihm CC, Rosenfeld GC, Burks TF. Morphine tolerance and dependence in the rat intestine *in vivo. J Pharmacol Exp Ther* 1997;280:656–663.
112. Williams JT, Christie MJ, Manzoni O. Cellular and synaptic adaptations mediating opioid dependence. *Physiol Rev* 2001;81:299–343.
113. Langrod J, Lowinson J, Ruiz P. Methadone treatment and physical complaints: a clinical analysis. *Int J Addict* 1981;16:947–952.
114. Yaffe GJ, Strelinger RW, Parwatikar S. Physical symptom complaints of patients on methadone maintenance. *Proc Natl Conf Methadone Treat* 1973;1:507–514.
115. Yuan CS, Foss JF, O'Connor M, et al. Gut motility and transit changes in patients receiving long-term methadone maintenance. *J Clin Pharmacol* 1998;38:931–935.
116. Haley TD, Long C, Mann BD. Stercoral perforation of the colon. A complication of methadone maintenance. *J Subst Abuse Treat* 1998;15: 443–444.
117. Rogers M, Cerda JJ. The narcotic bowel syndrome. *J Clin Gastroenterol* 1989;11:132–135.
118. Grunkemeier DM, Cassara JE, Dalton CB, Drossman DA. The narcotic bowel syndrome: clinical features, pathophysiology, and management. *Clin Gastroenterol Hepatol* 2007;5:1126–1139; quiz, 1121–1122.
119. Sandgren JE, McPhee MS, Greenberger NJ. Narcotic bowel syndrome treated with clonidine. Resolution of abdominal pain and intestinal pseudo-obstruction. *Ann Intern Med* 1984;101:331–334.
120. Yuan CS, Foss JF, O'Connor M, et al. Methylnaltrexone for reversal of constipation due to chronic methadone use: a randomized controlled trial. *JAMA* 2000;283:367–372.
121. Fine KD. Diarrhea. In: Feldman M, Sleisenger MH, Scharschmidt BF, eds. *Sleisenger & Fordtran's gastrointestinal and liver disease*, vol. 1. Philadelphia: Saunders, 1998:128–152.
122. Caplan JP, Epstein LA, Quinn DK, et al. Neuropsychiatric effects of prescription drug abuse. *Neuropsychol Rev* 2007;17:363–380.
123. Pandolfino JE, Kahrilas PJ. Smoking and gastro-oesophageal reflux disease. *Eur J Gastroenterol Hepatol* 2000;12:837–842.
124. Kahrilas PJ, Gupta RR. Mechanisms of acid reflux associated with cigarette smoking. *Gut* 1990;31:4–10.
125. Kahrilas PJ, Gupta RR. The effect of cigarette smoking on salivation and esophageal acid clearance. *J Lab Clin Med* 1989;114:431–438.
126. Bhandarkar PV, Shah SK, Meshram M, et al. Effect of acute and long-term oral tobacco use on oesophageal motility. *J Gastroenterol Hepatol* 2000;15:1018–1021.
127. Sonnenberg A, Muller-Lissner SA, Vogel E, et al. Predictors of duodenal ulcer healing and relapse. *Gastroenterology* 1981;81:1061–1067.
128. Korman MG, Hansky J, Eaves ER, Schmidt GT. Influence of cigarette smoking on healing and relapse in duodenal ulcer disease. *Gastroenterology* 1983;85:871–874.

129. Piper DW, McIntosh JH, Hudson HM. Factors relevant to the prognosis of chronic duodenal ulcer. *Digestion* 1985;31:9–16.
130. Ross AH, Smith MA, Anderson JR, Small WP. Late mortality after surgery for peptic ulcer. *N Engl J Med* 1982;307:519–522.
131. Kurata JH, Elashoff JD, Nogawa AN, Haile BM. Sex and smoking differences in duodenal ulcer mortality. *Am J Public Health* 1986;76:700–702.
132. Chowdhury P, Rayford PL. Smoking and pancreatic disorders. *Eur J Gastroenterol Hepatol* 2000;12:869–877.
133. Talamini G, Bassi C, Falconi M, et al. Alcohol and smoking as risk factors in chronic pancreatitis and pancreatic cancer. *Dig Dis Sci* 1999;44: 1303–1311.
134. Cavallini G, Talamini G, Vaona B, Bovo P, Filippini M, Rigo L et al. Effect of alcohol and smoking on pancreatic lithogenesis in the course of chronic pancreatitis. *Pancreas* 1994;9:42–46.
135. Yen S, Hsieh CC, MacMahon B. Consumption of alcohol and tobacco and other risk factors for pancreatitis. *Am J Epidemiol* 1982;116:407–414.
136. Rubin DT, Hanauer SB. Smoking and inflammatory bowel disease. *Eur J Gastroenterol Hepatol* 2000;12:855–862.
137. Thomas GA, Rhodes J, Ingram JR. Mechanisms of disease: nicotine—a review of its actions in the context of gastrointestinal disease. *Nat Clin Pract Gastroenterol Hepatol* 2005;2:536–544.
138. Sandborn WJ. Nicotine therapy for ulcerative colitis: a review of rationale, mechanisms, pharmacology, and clinical results. *Am J Gastroenterol* 1999;94:1161–1171.
139. Neugut AI, Hayek M, Howe G. Epidemiology of gastric cancer. *Semin Oncol* 1996;23:281–291.
140. Traub SJ, Hoffman RS, Nelson LS. Body packing—the internal concealment of illicit drugs. *N Engl J Med* 2003;349:2519–2526.
141. Malbrain ML, Neels H, Vissers K, et al. A massive, near-fatal cocaine intoxication in a body-stuffer. Case report and review of the literature. *Acta Clin Belg* 1994;49:12–18.
142. Wetli CV, Mittlemann RE. The "body packer syndrome"—toxicity following ingestion of illicit drugs packaged for transportation. *J Forensic Sci* 1981;26:492–500.
143. Aldrighetti L, Paganelli M, Giacomelli M, et al. Conservative management of cocaine-packet ingestion: experience in Milan, the main Italian smuggling center of South American cocaine. *Panminerva Med* 1996;38: 111–116.
144. Hoffman RS, Smilkstein MJ, Goldfrank LR. Whole bowel irrigation and the cocaine body-packer: a new approach to a common problem. *Am J Emerg Med* 1990;8:523–527.
145. Beerman R, Nunez D Jr, Wetli CV. Radiographic evaluation of the cocaine smuggler. *Gastrointest Radiol* 1986;11:351–354.
146. Gherardi R, Marc B, Alberti X, et al. A cocaine body packer with normal abdominal plain radiograms. Value of drug detection in urine and contrast study of the bowel. *Am J Forensic Med Pathol* 1990;11:154–157.
147. Silverberg D, Menes T, Kim U. Surgery for "body packers"—a 15-year experience. *World J. Surgery* 2006;30:541–546.
148. Sleisenger MH, Fordtran JS, Feldman M, Scharschmidt B. *Sleisenger & Fordtran's gastrointestinal and liver disease: pathophysiology, diagnosis, management.* Philadelphia: Saunders, 1998.
149. McCarron MM, Wood JD. The cocaine 'body packer' syndrome. Diagnosis and treatment. *JAMA* 1983;250:1417–1420.
150. Introna F Jr, Smialek JE. The "mini-packer" syndrome. Fatal ingestion of drug containers in Baltimore, Maryland. *Am J Forensic Med Pathol* 1989;10:21–24.
151. Nichols GR, Davis GJ. Body packing with a twist. Death of a salesman [see comments]. *Am J Forensic Med Pathol* 1992;13:142–145.
152. Glauser J, Queen JR. An overview of non-cardiac cocaine toxicity. *J Emerg Med* 2007;32:181–186.
153. Pertwee RG. Cannabinoids and the gastrointestinal tract. *Gut* 2001; 48:859–867.
154. Machado Rocha FC, Stefano SC, De Cassia Haiek R, Rosa Oliveira LM, Da Silveira DX. Therapeutic use of cannabis sativa on chemotherapy-induced nausea and vomiting among cancer patients: systematic review and meta-analysis. *Eur J Cancer Care* (Engl) 2008;17:431–443.
155. Van Sickle MD, Oland LD, Ho W, et al. Cannabinoids inhibit emesis through CB1 receptors in the brainstem of the ferret. *Gastroenterology* 2001;121:767–774.
156. Allen JH, de Moore GM, Heddle R, Twartz JC. Cannabinoid hyperemesis: cyclical hyperemesis in association with chronic cannabis abuse. *Gut* 2004;53:1566–1570.
157. Roche E, Foster PN. Cannabinoid hyperemesis: not just a problem in Adelaide Hills. *Gut* 2005;54:731.
158. Byrne A, Hallinan R, Wodak A. "Cannabis hyperemesis" causation questioned. *Gut* 2006;55:132.

CHAPTER 75

Kevin C. Wilson, MD
Elizabeth Mirabile Levins, MD
Jussi J. Saukkonen, MD

Respiratory Tract Disorders Related to Alcohol and Other Drug Use

The respiratory tract is a unique interface between the body and the environment. The airways of the lung are subject to constant noxious, particulate, and antigenic challenges, which come into close proximity to the vast vascular bed of the lung. The lungs are highly adapted in attenuating such external provocations and in mediating between events at the epithelial and endothelial surfaces. However, a broad variety of addictive drugs present acute or chronic insults to the respiratory system and can overwhelm local capacity for recovery (Table 75.1).

Inhalation, injection, or ingestion of addictive drugs may have adverse effects within the airways, lung parenchyma, and vascular bed. Respiratory complications also may arise from indirect effects of drugs on the central nervous and immune systems.

RESPIRATORY FUNCTION

Addictive drugs can derange the interrelated critical functions of the lungs. The principal function of gas exchange dictates the structure of the respiratory tract. Other functions of the lung are derived from this primary structure–function relationship, including gas exchange, containment and exclusion of foreign materials, immune sampling of antigens, and detoxification and metabolism of proteins, drugs, and other potentially injurious substances.

Inhaled gases and particulate matter travel through the specialized structures of the upper airway into progressively ramifying airways, which terminate in gas-exchanging alveoli. The large surface area of the alveolar spaces and their associated capillary beds provide enormous absorptive capacity for inhaled drugs. Both the cough reflex and the mucociliary escalator are important in ridding the lower respiratory tract of foreign matter. Resident alveolar macrophages ingest particles and pathogens, then process, digest, and transport them to lymph nodes for antigen presentation. Local immune responses recruit other leukocytes, which may further contain or help remove any offending matter through granuloma formation or phagocytosis (1,2).

The pulmonary vasculature provides important defensive functions for the lungs. The circulation carries antioxidants, antiproteolytic agents, and antibodies to the lung to meet ongoing challenges. Significant metabolic functions are performed within the pulmonary vasculature, including removal of drugs (3), vasoactive amines, kinins, and eicosanoids. The pulmonary vascular bed autoregulates flow in response to oxygenation and local concentrations of vasoactive substances. Large numbers of marginated leukocytes and platelets are present within the pulmonary vasculature, but may be mobilized by pulmonary epithelial or endothelial insults, causing exudation, inflammation, and compromise of gas exchange (1,2).

Respiration is under extensive neural control and, consequently, is susceptible to the effects of central nervous system (CNS) depressants and stimulants. Inherent respiratory

TABLE 75.1 Drugs Associated with Pulmonary Complications

Central nervous system stimulants
- Nicotine/tobacco
- Cocaine and crack
- Amphetamines
- 3,4-methylenedioxy methamphetamine (MDMA)
- Methylphenidate
- Caffeine

Central nervous system depressants
- Alcohol/ethanol
- Barbiturates
- Benzodiazepines
- Gamma-hydroxybutyrate (GHB)
- Opioids

Hallucinogens

Marijuana

Volatile substances
- Aromatic hydrocarbons
- Nitrous oxide
- Nitrites
- Refrigerants

automaticity is provided by the medulla oblongata within the brainstem, but this is modulated by the reticular activating system, cerebral cortex, and peripheral sensors. Hypoxic drive comes from the carotid body, which, when stimulated, causes hypotension and bradycardia. Hypoxic drive is blunted by age, obesity, chronic bronchitis, and CNS depressants. C-fiber receptors (including J receptors in lung parenchyma), when stimulated by interstitial edema, microembolism, and chemical products of anaphylaxis, result in tachypnea and dyspnea. Irritant receptors in the epithelium of the larynx and large airways respond to a variety of chemical irritants and mechanical stimuli, resulting in cough, bronchoconstriction, sneezing, laryngospasm, and mucus secretion (1,2). Receptors within the lung and in the brain are responsive to a number of addictive substances.

Addictive drugs may perturb the active processes within the lung, resulting in local inflammation, infections, airway reactivity, impairment of pulmonary vascular integrity, acute lung injury, structural injury, or derangements of gas exchange. Use of numerous substances at the same time often is associated with a variety of injuries, making it difficult to ascribe a particular respiratory complication to a single agent. Coexisting pulmonary pathology may worsen the acute physiologic effects of an addictive drug on the lungs.

COMMON PULMONARY COMPLICATIONS

Several families of drugs cause common respiratory complications, including adverse effects related to respiratory depression, infections, route of consumption, and contaminants.

Respiratory Depression Nearly all of the drugs discussed here may directly inhibit respiration or induce seizures. Patients with respiratory depression usually are somnolent or postictal. Respirations are rapid and shallow, and are accompanied by limited ability to cough. Atelectasis, hypoxemia, hypoventilation, inability to clear secretions, and aspiration may occur. With overdose, lethargy may progress rapidly to stupor, severe respiratory depression, coma, and respiratory arrest. With intravenous drug use, death may occur so rapidly that the needle is still in the vein when the corpse is found.

The diagnosis usually is obvious from the clinical presentation, coupled with a history or signs of drug abuse and a positive toxicology screen. A complete chemistry panel, toxicology screen, electrocardiogram, blood gas, and chest radiograph should be performed. Airway protection is paramount, and patients with known or suspected overdose should be admitted to an intensive care unit for monitoring of their respiratory, neurologic, and hemodynamic status (4,5).

Management generally consists of administration of thiamine, glucose, and naloxone (although the half-life of naloxone is relatively short, temporary improvement may be helpful diagnostically).

Atelectasis In patients with respiratory depression, shallow respirations may not exceed the critical closing volume and may result in airway collapse. Ineffective cough and aspirated oral and gastric secretions, with loss of surfactant, lead to atelectasis. Consequently, unventilated areas are perfused (shunting), which, with lobar or whole-lung atelectasis, may cause significant hypoxemia (2). Incentive spirometry, chest physiotherapy, respiratory suctioning, and supplemental oxygen generally are indicated. Bronchoscopy may be needed for refractory atelectasis in the face of severe hypoxemia or to rule out an endobronchial lesion or aspirated foreign body (6).

Aspiration Pneumonitis Respiratory depression or seizures may cause aspiration of oral secretions or gastric contents. Often the event is only chemical pneumonitis, but this condition may lead to noncardiogenic pulmonary edema and respiratory failure, with or without bacterial super infection. Infiltrates resulting from aspiration may develop within several hours to a few days. Preventive care should be directed toward airway control, maintenance of at least a 45-degree angle, avoidance of oral intake while lethargic, pulmonary toilet, supplemental oxygen, and antibiotics as indicated. Empiric antibiotic coverage for aspiration in the absence of infiltrates and clinical and laboratory indicators of infection may be counterproductive, merely leading to the selection of nosocomial pathogens (7).

Respiratory Infections Chronic users of addictive drugs are susceptible to a variety of respiratory infections. Many drugs have adverse effects on leukocyte function, contribute to malnutrition with resultant immune dysfunction, are injected under septic conditions, or may be contaminated with pathogens. Infectious complications also may be related to coexisting HIV infection, cirrhosis, aspiration, smoking, or lifestyle-related structural lung disease, or inhibition of the mucociliary escalator (8,9). Smoking-related obstructive lung disease may require chronic corticosteroid therapy, which is an immunosuppressant and thus may contribute to infections.

The spectrum of respiratory infections includes sinusitis, acute bronchitis, community-acquired and aspiration pneumonias, septic emboli, tuberculosis, and fungal infection. Patients most often present with acute symptoms of fever, productive cough, dyspnea, and, often, pleuritic chest pain, but general ill health and polymicrobial infections make atypical or subacute presentations common. The chest radiograph may reveal lobar pneumonia, bibasilar or superior segment lower-lobe infiltrates suggestive of aspiration, or nodular infiltrates in the lower lung fields consistent with aspiration. Sputum gram stain can be helpful to confirm lower respiratory infection and indicate whether the specimen is of sufficient quality to make the accompanying sputum culture reliable. Blood cultures are warranted in many patients, especially those who are toxic, ill-appearing, immunocompromised, or otherwise high-risk (e.g., alcohol abuse, intravenous drug abuse). Antibiotics tailored to the suspected pathogen are the therapy of choice.

Respiratory Complications of Contaminants Illicit drugs vary greatly in purity, as they often are adulterated to increase profits. Widely used adulterants include mannitol, cellulose, talc, various sugars, as well as other drugs such as phenobarbital, methaqualone, caffeine, procaine, and noscapine (10). The lungs act as filters, trapping inhaled or injected foreign substances, which may incite local inflammatory or fibrotic responses. Contaminating microorganisms also may lead to pulmonary infection, particularly in immunocompromised hosts, or to hypersensitivity responses (11–15).

The role of herbicides, such as paraquat, in contaminating inhaled drugs and causing pulmonary complications is controversial. Although epidemiologic evidence of paraquat-induced lung injury is lacking, the herbicide has been documented to cause occupational lung disease and acute lung injury in instances of toxic exposure (16,17).

Occupational Lung Disease Agricultural workers may develop pulmonary complications related to the cultivation of certain plants for the drug industry. Such health problems may be obscured because the industry is illicit or barely tolerated and is not subject to occupational safety regulations or to exposure mitigation regimes. Socioeconomic and political factors generally do not allow workers to voice their health concerns. Pneumoconiosis, herbicide-related interstitial fibrosis, and antigen-induced hypersensitivity pneumonitis constitute occupational pulmonary hazards for such agricultural workers (20,21).

Respiratory Complications of Injected Drugs

Opiates, stimulants, and combinations thereof are commonly injected into the veins. The resulting pulmonary complications may be acute or chronic. Acute problems are likely to be severe, including respiratory failure and acute pulmonary edema (4,5). Chronic pulmonary problems include the development of interstitial and bullous lung disease (22,23), endovascular and respiratory infections (22), and tuberculosis (24). Potential pulmonary complications associated with either the drug or its contaminants, or the route of administration, include the following conditions.

Talc Granulomatosis Talc (magnesium silicate) is widely used as a filler in oral medications, which may be crushed and injected, and it is used to adulterate inhaled and injected drugs. A syndrome similar to sarcoidosis may result, with insidious onset of granulomatous interstitial fibrosis (25–29). Dyspnea, particularly with exertion, and cough are the most common symptoms. The retina should be examined in all patients in whom the diagnosis is being considered because talc retinopathy occurs in more than half of patients (25,28).

The chest radiograph is normal in up to half of patients. A diffuse micronodular interstitial opacity may be evident, particularly in the mid-lung zones. These nodules can coalesce to opacify entire lobes as the disease progresses (26). High-resolution computed tomography may reveal diffuse ground glass opacity and confluent perihilar masses, the latter containing areas of high attenuation consistent with talc (27). Pulmonary function tests typically reveal a low-diffusion capacity before any other abnormality (28a). Bronchoalveolar lavage may demonstrate local lymphocytosis and birefringent intracellular or free talc (25,27). Lung biopsy may be required to establish the diagnosis, based on histologic changes of granulomas, mononuclear inflammatory cells, lymphocytes, and fibrosis (27). In advanced stages or if there is associated granulomatous pulmonary arterial occlusion (30,31), pulmonary hypertension and right ventricular failure can occur.

Patients with progressive symptoms and worsening chest radiograph or pulmonary function tests should be given a trial of systemic steroids, although results are highly variable and unpredictable (25).

Pulmonary Hypertension Intravenous drug users may develop chronic pulmonary hypertension from multiple mechanisms, including chronic hypoxemia related to interstitial lung disease and vasoconstriction, or pulmonary arterial thrombosis at sites of foreign body granulomatosis, with subsequent occlusion (angiothrombotic pulmonary hypertension) (30–33). Primary pulmonary hypertension also may occur as a result of HIV-1 infection (34). Patients typically present with interstitial and vascular reactions to talc. Common presentations involve dyspnea on exertion. Physical examination and electrocardiogram may be normal or may show evidence of right ventricular enlargement and failure. Acute, reversible pulmonary hypertension may be associated with injection of sympathomimetics, although it also may due to an effect on cardiac output (35–37). Treatment options include supplemental oxygen for patients who are hypoxemic, anticoagulation for patients at increased risk for venous thromboembolism, and diuretics for patients with pulmonary or peripheral edema. Patients should be referred to a pulmonary hypertension center for hemodynamic evaluation and consideration of advanced therapy (38).

Septic Thromboemboli Septic pulmonary embolism is the most common pulmonary complication among intravenous heroin users (22) and may result from tricuspid endocarditis or from infected injection-site thrombophlebitis (22,25,39). The organism most frequently isolated from sputum or blood cultures is *Staphylococcus aureus* (22).

The patient typically presents in an acute toxic state, with fever, dyspnea, chest pain, and leukocytosis. Radiographic examination of the chest may reveal bilateral necrotizing infiltrates or single or multiple pulmonary lesions, which frequently cavitate. The lesions may coalesce to form large cavities that communicate with a bronchus. Alternatively, infection may be complicated by bronchopleural fistulas, empyema, or pneumothorax.

Antibiotic therapy usually is prolonged. Cases can clear completely, although residual pleural thickening and fibrosis is common (22,25,39).

Needle Embolization Occasionally, needles, especially those used multiple times, may be broken off inadvertently during or after injection. This situation is more likely to occur when less accessible sites are being used. Chest radiograph may demonstrate needle fragments within chest soft tissue or lodged within pulmonary vasculature. No specific therapy or removal is necessary for needle emboli to the lung (40).

Pneumothorax Pneumothorax—unilateral or bilateral—may develop from inadvertent puncture of the lung during attempted needle injection into a jugular or subclavian vessel (41,42). This condition also may result from cavitating septic thromboemboli (43). Large pneumothoraces, those associated with hypoxemia, or those with concomitant empyema, require tube thoracostomy and antibiotics (41–43).

Empyema Cavitating infections from septic emboli, pneumonia, or unclean needles may contaminate the pleural space and lead to empyema (42,43).

Mycotic Aneurysms Septic emboli may lead to the development of mycotic aneurysms of the pulmonary vasculature. Patients may present with evidence of endovascular infection, with or without hemoptysis. Contrast-enhanced computed tomography demonstrates nodular lesions associated with vasculature. This condition may be fatal if there is massive hemoptysis, despite surgical intervention. Patients without hemoptysis may experience resolution of this condition with antibiotic therapy (44,45).

Hemothorax Rupture of a subclavian aneurysm created by multiple injections has been reported to cause a massive hemothorax (46).

Pulmonary Emphysema Bullous emphysema may develop in intravenous drug injectors, either in association with talc granulomatosis or in its absence (23,47–49). The mechanism is unknown.

Respiratory Complications of Inhaled Drugs

Inhalation has become a preferred route for the consumption of many addictive drugs. Delivery of a drug through the lung affords ease of administration, rapid onset of action, dose minimization, avoidance of intravenous injection, and avoidance of the hepatic first pass effect. Drugs may be inhaled nasally ("snorting"), rolled as cigarettes, sprinkled into smoked tobacco, smoked through pipes, or inhaled orally. The route of ingestion may affect the dose delivered and the onset of action. Deep inhalation or smoking may result in an onset of action within seconds, whereas nasal inhalation affords a slightly delayed onset, measured in seconds to minutes (50). Various delivery devices and techniques have been developed to control dose and effects; to provide convenience; and to incorporate cultural, behavioral, and esthetic elements. For example, water pipes, used for smoking a variety of drugs throughout the world (especially Asia), are associated with a café culture and have an esthetic design element. Some water pipes filter smoke and may attenuate a few, but not many, of the detrimental effects of smoked tobacco (51,52).

Inhaled drugs include fine powders, smoked plant material, gases, other volatiles, and combinations of these drugs. Inhaled powders are heterodisperse, varying considerably in size, with a geometric standard deviation >2. The momentum of inhaled particles >6 μm causes them to impact proximally against convoluted upper airway walls and bifurcating large airways of the lung, where they may be absorbed. Smaller particles (1 to 5 μm) are carried by the airstream to the distal airways, where they are deposited chiefly by sedimentation, settling as a result of gravitational forces (1).

Inhalation of talc or other fibrogenic substances may lead to the development of granulomatous inflammation or fibrosis, as discussed earlier. Smoke consists of gas and particulate phases, including carbon monoxide, potentially injurious oxidants, aldehydes, alcohols, nitrosamines, benzene derivatives, and other inorganic and organic substances (53), any of which may cause mucosal injury and inflammation.

Chronic Bronchitis This condition is commonly associated with smoking tobacco, marijuana, cocaine, and other drugs. Cough, dyspnea, and mucus hypersecretion are found in individuals with chronic bronchitis, particularly if they smoke daily. A propensity to airway reactivity and acute bacterial bronchitis may be seen (54,55).

Bronchospasm Airway reactivity often is seen with inhaled heroin, cocaine, tobacco, and marijuana (56–61). Patients typically present with dyspnea, tachypnea, and wheezing, beginning within minutes to hours after inhalation. Sinus tachycardia usually is present. Early blood gases, if drawn, may demonstrate respiratory alkalosis, which may progress to hypercapnia and respiratory acidosis. The chest radiograph typically is clear. Patients are treated with supplemental oxygen, bronchodilators, steroids, and, if severe, mechanical ventilation. Patients with new onset asthma should be assessed for use of inhaled drugs (62).

Barotrauma Inhalation of cocaine, heroin, 3,4-methylenedioxymethamphetamine, marijuana, tobacco, and volatile substances is associated with barotrauma, including pneumothorax and pneumomediastinum. Extreme breath-holding against a closed glottis (a prolonged Valsalva maneuver) in an attempt to increase the drug's effect results in high negative intrathoracic pressure, hyperinflation, alveolar bleb rupture, and dissection of air along peribronchial paths into the mediastinum, pleural cavities, skin, and retropharyngeal space. Some users exhale smoke forcefully into another user's mouth, causing markedly elevated positive airway pressure and, potentially, barotrauma, as well as transmission of respiratory pathogens (63).

Individuals who have developed bullous emphysema from chronic smoking may have spontaneous rupture of a bleb, with resultant pneumothorax. Patients may present with acute chest or back pain and dyspnea, with or without hypoxemia (39, 64,65).

Hemoptysis Hemoptysis may result from mucosal irritation or ulceration anywhere within the respiratory tract (as in epistaxis, sinusitis, or bronchitis), from pulmonary infarct, or from diffuse alveolar hemorrhage (60,65,66).

Pulmonary Emphysema Destruction of lung parenchyma, with resultant pulmonary emphysema, may occur with inhaled tobacco, marijuana, and chronic opium use (67–70).

TOBACCO AND NICOTINE

Within the lung, smoking has profound effects, altering the immunologic and structural milieu. Cigarette tar is associated with a high rate of lung cancer, emphysema, bronchitis, and airway reactivity. Several factors determine the effects of tar and other pyrolysis products on the lung: individual susceptibility to the various adverse effects of smoking varies considerably, and heterozygosity for the gene that causes alpha-1-antitrypsin deficiency may play a role (71,72). The quantity of cigarettes smoked, the years spent smoking, and the manner in which they were smoked (for example, the depth of inhalation) also play a role.

Tobacco smoke induces the elaboration of chemotactic agents for neutrophils and monocytes, as well as mediators that cause epithelial injury and permeability changes (73,74). Pulmonary leukocytes are activated by the local elaboration of cytokines (including interleukin [IL]-8, tumor necrosis factor alpha, and IL-1) and by epithelial cells, fibroblasts, and leukocytes. Neutrophils and macrophages release serine proteases, reactive oxygen species, matrix metalloproteinases, and other potentially injurious cell products (73–79). Imbalance of proteases and antiproteases is thought to play a role in the development of local injury. Elastin and collagen degradation ensues, resulting in a loss of pulmonary architecture and, eventually, of functional gas exchanging units (80,81). T cells and submucosal eosinophils also play a pathogenic role after long-standing injury (74,81–83).

Smoking induces a variety of coexisting pathologies in the lung. Smokers display a more rapid decline in forced expiratory volume in one second (FEV1) than do nonsmokers, which may lead to symptoms such as dyspnea and fatigue. Chronic airflow obstruction is common and, when associated with persistent hypoxemia, may lead to cor pulmonale and pulmonary hypertension. Smoking also increases the risk of lung cancer and lower respiratory tract infections. Smoking cessation may slow the rate of decline of lung function, attenuate symptoms, lower the risk of developing lung cancer, and decrease the incidence of lower respiratory infections (84).

Environmental tobacco smoke has become a major public health issue (85). In children, environmental tobacco smoke contributes to lower respiratory illnesses, chronic respiratory symptoms, middle ear disease, reduced lung function, asthma among children of school age, and wheezing in early childhood. In adults, environmental tobacco smoke appears to increase the risk of lung cancer, cardiovascular diseases, and acute respiratory symptoms and illnesses (86).

Clinical syndromes associated with the use of tobacco include the following.

Chronic Bronchitis In many smokers, a chronic productive cough is present on a daily basis—a common clinical operational definition of chronic bronchitis. More formally, chronic bronchitis is defined as sputum production for at least 3 months in 2 successive years in the absence of other causes of chronic cough. Airway changes in chronic bronchitis are nonspecific, but consist largely of mucous gland hypertrophy of intermediate-sized airways. Overproduction of mucus may overwhelm the mucociliary escalator, which is compromised by tobacco smoke (8). Often, there is associated airway reactivity (54).

Airway Reactivity Smoking tobacco promotes bronchial hyperreactivity, as measured by methacholine bronchoprovocation studies, even in patients without obstructive lung disease (87). Animal studies suggest that early smoke-induced bronchoconstriction is caused by nicotine and is mediated by cholinergic pathways and by tachykinin release from bronchopulmonary C fibers. A delayed and more sustained bronchoconstrictive response is induced by non-nicotinic components of tobacco smoke, which elicit the release of the eicosanoids thromboxane A2, prostaglandin D2, and prostaglandin F2 alpha, acting on airway smooth muscles (88–92). Smokers also have increased numbers of activated leukocytes, which may contribute to asthmatic symptoms (81,82). In some individuals with severe airflow obstruction, there are correlations between total immunoglobulin E (IgE) levels and FEV1, although this correlation is not likely to be related to specific aeroallergens (93).

Patients typically complain of dyspnea, especially with exertion, chest tightness, and cough. Pulmonary function testing may show an obstructive pattern. Tobacco smoke also may exacerbate preexisting asthma. Bronchodilator therapy and inhaled corticosteroids are mainstays of therapy (54,68).

Pulmonary Emphysema Smokers who develop irreversible enlargement of the airspaces distal to the terminal bronchiole, with destruction of the alveolar wall, have pulmonary emphysema. Interstitial fibrosis may occur but is not a major pathologic finding. Centrilobular emphysema in the upper portions of the lungs, as well as paraseptal emphysema in the periphery of the lungs, is commonly found. The latter is associated with the development of large bullae. Hyperinflation and flattening of the diaphragm lead to a mechanical disadvantage for the contractility of the major respiratory muscle (93). There is decreased ability to oxygenate blood, as alveolar septae are destroyed, with loss of the pulmonary capillary bed. These changes, as well as suboptimal ventilation–perfusion relationships, also lead to carbon dioxide retention. There may be associated chronic bronchitis or airway reactivity, or both (69). Pneumothorax may develop from rupture of a subpleural emphysematous bleb.

Pulmonary function testing reveals obstructive lung disease, often with hyperinflation and air trapping. Chest radiography reveals hyperlucent lungs and loss of interstitial marking. Mainstays of treatment include smoking cessation, bronchodilator therapy, trials of inhaled or systemic steroids, judicious use of oxygen, and pulmonary rehabilitation (69).

Interstitial Lung Disease Smoking is associated with an increased risk of developing desquamative interstitial pneumonia, a form of idiopathic interstitial pneumonia (94,95). Patients present with insidiously developing dyspnea, interstitial infiltrates, and restrictive physiology, which may be confounded by concomitant obstructive lung disease, on pulmonary function tests (95). Respiratory bronchiolitis-associated interstitial lung disease, which has radiologic and histopathologic overlap with desquamative interstitial pneumonia (96,97), also may result from smoking.

Open lung biopsy is needed to reliably diagnose and to distinguish among interstitial lung diseases (98). Patients with desquamative interstitial pneumonia or respiratory bronchiolitis-associated interstitial lung disease usually are treated with a trial of systemic corticosteroids (95,97).

Smoking also is a prominent risk factor for the development of pulmonary histiocytosis X (eosinophilic granuloma), because more than 90% of patients with the disease are smokers (99,100). Smoking may precipitate exacerbations of Goodpasture disease, with marked hemoptysis (99).

Pulmonary Hypertension and Cor Pulmonale Chronic hypoxic vasoconstriction of the pulmonary vasculature leads to pulmonary arterial hypertension and right heart strain. Patients may have tachycardia, prominent neck veins, tricuspid insufficiency murmur, right ventricular third heart sound, hepatojugular reflex, and peripheral edema.

Primary therapy consists of optimizing treatment of the cause of the hypoxemia (54,68). As examples, inhaled bronchodilators are indicated if obstructive lung disease is the source of the hypoxemia and immunosuppressive therapy may be indicated if interstitial lung disease is the cause of the hypoxemia. Supplemental oxygen for at least 18 hours per day prolongs survival and improves symptoms. Additional options for primary therapy include anticoagulation for patients at increased risk for venous thromboembolism and diuretics for patients with pulmonary or peripheral edema. After primary therapy is initiated, patients should be referred to a pulmonary hypertension center for hemodynamic evaluation and consideration of advanced therapy.

Pneumothorax Spontaneous pneumothorax may occur as a result of bullous emphysema, with rupture of a subpleural bleb. Occasionally, associated cavitating infections or bronchogenic carcinomas also may cause pneumothorax, usually in association with a pleural effusion (68,101).

Hemoptysis Most often, hemoptysis results from acute bacterial bronchitis, but it may betray the presence of other airway pathology, including bronchogenic carcinoma (68).

Bronchogenic Carcinoma Inhalation of tobacco-specific N-nitrosamines and other carcinogens causes bronchogenic carcinoma in many individuals (102,103). Smokeless tobacco has been linked to the development of malignancies of the aerodigestive tract (104). Tobacco smoke induces widespread epithelial changes, which may predispose to the development of premalignant lesions in association with generalized genetic mutations ("field cancerization") (105). Oncogene mutations, particularly of the *p53* gene, are associated with the development of lung cancer (106). The cumulative risk of lung cancer among heavy smokers may be as high as 30%, compared to only 1% in lifetime nonsmokers (107).

Environmental tobacco smoke also constitutes a risk factor for the development of bronchogenic carcinoma in nonsmokers (108). Other environmental exposures potentially increasing the risk for bronchogenic carcinoma include asbestos and drugs such as crack cocaine and marijuana (105,109).

Smoking cessation reduces the risk of lung cancer, with the extent of risk reduction depending on the duration of abstinence (110). For patients who are unable to quit, smoking reduction also appears to decrease the likelihood of lung cancer, albeit to a lesser extent (111).

Patients may present with asymptomatic, incidentally noted pulmonary nodules or with weight loss, cough, chest or bone pain, fatigue, hoarseness, superior vena cava syndrome, or hemoptysis. Diagnosis may be made by sputum, needle, or bronchoscopic cytologic specimens, endobronchial biopsy, mediastinoscopy, or at the time of surgical resection. Treatment may be definitive, in the case of a completely resected, margin-free solitary pulmonary nodule, or it may entail radiation or chemotherapy, depending on cell type and stage (112).

Hypersensitivity Pneumonitis (Extrinsic Allergic Alveolitis) A variety of molds may be present on tobacco plants, which then are inhaled by workers harvesting the crop or, theoretically, by smokers. In some individuals, these molds, including *Aspergillus* and thermophilic actinomycetes, may induce hypersensitivity reactions on exposure. Workers typically experience amelioration of symptoms when away from work. Clinical features include cough, fever, and obstructive and restrictive findings on pulmonary function testing (20,21). If exposure is long-standing, pulmonary fibrosis may develop (21). Although smoking can lead to serologic evidence of exposure, it is unclear whether hypersensitivity pneumonitis develops in smokers (12).

Lipoid Pneumonia The rare complication of lipoid pneumonia has been reported among chewers and smokers of blackfat tobacco in Guyana, where petroleum jelly is applied to tobacco leaves to moisturize them and enhance their flavor (11). Patients may present with cough and a localized infiltrate, which may suggest chronic pneumonia or bronchogenic carcinoma. The density of the lesion on computed tomography scan usually suggests the diagnosis.

Snuff-Related Pneumonitis In patients with renal failure, snuff has been reported to cause pulmonary infiltrates. The pathogenesis is unclear, but biopsy shows the presence of vegetable fibers and parenchymal necrosis. The syndrome disappears with abstinence (113).

MARIJUANA

Marijuana or hashish may be ingested or smoked as cigarettes or through water pipes of various designs. The pyrolysis products of cannabis are similar to those of cigarettes and exert the same effects on the airway epithelium. The smoke, similar to that of cigarettes, contains tetrahydrocannabinol and other cannabinoids but not nicotine (114,115). Marijuana smoke has deleterious effects on respiration, depositing three times more tar than cigarette smoke and causing a fivefold higher carboxyhemoglobin level in the blood than cigarettes (115). Alveolar macrophages from marijuana smokers do not phagocytose properly, have decreased ability to kill bacteria and tumor cells, and produce decreased amounts of nitric oxide and cytokines, including tumor necrosis factor alpha, granulocyte-macrophage colony-stimulating factor, and IL-6 (116).

Marijuana smoke increases oxidative stress within the lung, causing glutathione stores to be depleted within alveolar macrophages (117). Field cancerization has been shown to occur within the lung, increasing the possibility of lung cancer (105). Cases of squamous cell carcinoma of the oropharynx in heavy marijuana smokers also have been reported in the literature (118).

Obstructive Lung Disease Marijuana smokers may suffer some of the same complications as those who smoke tobacco, including chronic bronchitis and bullous emphysema (69,119). Marijuana smokers' lungs receive more tar because the marijuana cigarettes are not filtered and because inhalation tends to be significantly deeper and is associated with prolonged breath-holding (115). However, chronic obstructive lung disease does not develop consistently, and tobacco smoking, which causes more cellular injury to the bronchial mucosa, may confound causality or even provide an additive effect (55). Moreover, heavy regular marijuana smoking is not associated with accelerated decline in FEV1, as is tobacco smoking (55).

Pathogen-Associated Complications *Aspergillus* and thermophilic actinomycetes have been reported to contaminate marijuana that is smoked (12). These organisms could cause respiratory tract infection or hypersensitivity reactions (12,15). Pulmonary aspergillosis associated with smoking marijuana is reported among immunocompromised patients (13,14). This association may become more important as increasing numbers of immunocompromised patients turn to medicinal uses of marijuana.

Lipoid Pneumonia Respiratory failure because of lipoid pneumonia with pulmonary alveolar proteinosis in a patient with a cadaveric renal transplant has been linked to smoking weed oil prepared from marijuana (120).

Paraquat Lung Paraquat is widely used throughout the world as an herbicide. Massive accidental or intentional exposure to paraquat has resulted in severe multisystem, including respiratory, organ failure (16,17). Workers with chronic occupational exposure and survivors of paraquat poisoning may develop pulmonary fibrosis (19). However, there is no epidemiologic evidence to demonstrate a link between smoking paraquat-sprayed marijuana and pulmonary fibrosis.

Hemp Worker's Lung Nonsmoking workers in the hemp industry display evidence of chronic cough and byssinosis, as manifested by accelerated decline in FEV1. Much of the cultivation of hemp is an industry separate from that of marijuana production, with differing processing techniques. It is not clear whether workers cultivating the same plant, albeit the female of the species, develop a byssinosis-like syndrome.

COCAINE

Cocaine blocks norepinephrine and serotonin reuptake and causes release of norepinephrine, serotonin, and dopamine. Cocaine also has local anesthetic effects, blocking sodium and potassium channel flux, thereby reducing action potentials and inhibiting conduction of nerve impulses. Cocaine crosses the blood–brain barrier and stimulates the CNS where, in addition to the well-known effects on the limbic system, it can increase respiratory rate (121).

Cocaine is inhaled nasally, smoked, injected, and ingested. Approximately 20% to 30% of the inhaled dose actually reaches the lung (122). Cocaine often is combined with nicotine, which has similar effects; with marijuana; and with various depressants, including heroin or morphine ("speedballing") to attenuate the sudden decrease in the sense of euphoria (123). This particular combination has led to a number of high-profile overdose deaths. "Freebasing" is the practice of using volatile solvents to convert cocaine from a salt to a base and to remove adulterants. This potentially incendiary chemical process can lead to extensive cutaneous and inhalational burns. The final freebase product is highly potent and has a rapid onset of action, and thus is likely to induce pulmonary, cardiac, neurologic, and other complications (124).

Cocaine causes fewer tracheobronchial mucosal abnormalities than either smoked tobacco or marijuana, but it may augment the injury induced by those smoked drugs (105). It contributes to field cancerization, increasing the risk of malignancy (105), but epidemiologic studies have not clearly demonstrated a link to cocaine alone (125). However, cocaine is a highly potent bronchoconstrictor when inhaled (126).

Cocaine smoking has prominent effects on vasculature, causing vasoconstriction and permeability changes (126, 127). Reduction in diffusion capacity and increased clearance of inhaled technetium-99 compared with nonsmokers are seen in crack cocaine smokers, reflecting damage to the alveolar–capillary membrane, similar to the abnormality associated with smoking tobacco (128). Cocaine also causes alveolar hemorrhage and noncardiogenic pulmonary edema (128–131). Cocaine thus may induce injury through vasoconstriction and by impairing the integrity of the pulmonary capillary bed.

Cocaine has effects on the immune system, which may contribute to infections or to local inflammatory reactions. It impairs the function of natural killer cells, B and T lymphocytes (132,133). Alveolar macrophages from cocaine users have marked defects in their ability to kill bacteria and tumor cells because of a defect in nitric oxide production (116). After *in vivo* inhalation or injection of cocaine, neutrophils are activated and have enhanced production of IL-8, which has been implicated in a number of inflammatory lung disorders, including acute lung injury (134).

Cocaine may cause a wide range of acute and chronic pulmonary complications, the true incidence of which is not known. Such respiratory complications often cause individuals to seek medical care. Complications may also result from seizure or stroke, including atelectasis, aspiration, and noncardiogenic pulmonary edema (131). Symptoms commonly associated with cocaine use, particularly use of crack cocaine, include cough productive of carbonaceous sputum, pleuritic chest pain, wheezing, dyspnea, and hemoptysis (131).

Barotrauma Barotrauma is common with crack cocaine inhalation and is associated with prolonged and forceful deep inhalation, Valsalva maneuver, or "shotgunning" (forceful exhalation of crack smoke into another individual's respiratory tract) (131).

Upper Airway Complications A variety of upper airway complications are associated with inhaled cocaine, primarily burns and mucosal irritation or inflammation. The latter may result from the vasoconstrictive properties of cocaine and can cause nasal septal perforation, sinusitis epiglottitis, and upper airway obstruction (131,135,136). Aspiration of the nasal septum may occur (137). A vasculitis resembling Wegener granulomatosis in the upper airway has been reported in association with nasal inhalation of cocaine (138).

Bronchitis Both acute and chronic bronchitis may develop from mucosal irritation, as described earlier. Often, there is concomitant tobacco use, which contributes in large measure to airway obstruction (55,131).

Airway Burns Thermal injury, typically associated with freebasing, more commonly involves the upper airway and may cause airway obstruction. Anesthetic properties of cocaine make the oropharynx and tracheobronchial tree susceptible to thermal inhalational injuries (135,136). Lower airway burns may lead to airway or tracheal stenosis, if extensive or circumferential (131).

Bronchospasm Cocaine inhalation, but not injection, causes measurable and clinically significant bronchoconstriction in both asthmatic and nonasthmatic, nonatopic individuals (60). Cocaine-induced bronchoconstriction is thought to be mediated by airway irritant receptors (61). Cocaine inhalation may precipitate life-threatening exacerbations of asthma (131,139).

Bronchospasm tends to be more severe among cocaine users, and cocaine use is associated with inhaled corticosteroid noncompliance and recrudescence of symptoms (59,60,62).

Hemoptysis Hemoptysis may result from mucosal irritation or ulceration anywhere within the respiratory tract (as in rhinitis, sinusitis, and bronchitis), from pulmonary infarct, or from diffuse alveolar hemorrhage (131).

Diffuse Pulmonary Hemorrhage Autopsy studies show high rates of acute and chronic pulmonary hemorrhage (40% to 58%), as well as congestion and pulmonary edema (up to 88%). Diffuse alveolar hemorrhage may be a life-threatening complication (129,131). Cocaine inhalation may incite alveolar hemorrhage in patients with Goodpasture syndrome (132,140).

Pulmonary Edema Cocaine may induce both noncardiogenic and cardiogenic pulmonary edema. The pathogenesis of the latter may involve one or several mechanisms, including high negative intrathoracic pressures associated with inhalation; direct damage to the pulmonary vasculature, causing increased permeability (128,131); or a neurogenic mechanism in which efferent sympathetic stimulation leads to increased pulmonary venous constriction and increased intravascular hydrostatic force, with or without increased pulmonary capillary permeability (141).

Intravenous cocaine, administered to humans in a controlled setting, has a chronotropic effect on the heart but does not cause an increase in pulmonary capillary wedge pressure (37). Cardiogenic edema does occur, related to arrhythmia, coronary vasospasm-induced myocardial ischemia or infarction, or from acute heart failure related to abruptly increased afterload (131). Cocaine given intravenously to dogs proved to have a negative inotropic effect (142), which may result in pulmonary edema.

Pulmonary Vascular Disease and Infarction

Although intravenous cocaine given in a controlled setting was reported not to increase pulmonary vascular resistance, there are case reports of cocaine-induced massive pulmonary artery vasoconstriction and, rarely, pulmonary infarction (143,144). Vasoconstriction, platelet aggregation, and vascular damage and induction of endothelin-1 release may contribute (127, 143–145). Patients may present with symptoms suggestive of pulmonary embolism, with pleuritic chest pain, dyspnea, and hypoxemia, and usually with hemoptysis. Technetium–xenon scintigraphy demonstrates ventilation-perfusion–mismatched defect within the lung. Pulmonary hypertension may develop over time as a result of interstitial lung disease caused by debris deposited in the lung (131). One autopsy series of cocaine-related deaths reported pulmonary artery medial hypertrophy in the absence of talc or other debris in 20% of cases (146).

Eosinophilic Hypersensitivity Pneumonitis ("Crack Lung") A mild Loeffler syndrome has been reported, with transient migratory pulmonary infiltrates and eosinophilia, which may not require treatment (147). A more severe reaction may occur 1 to 48 hours after heavy cocaine smoking; this consists of chest pain, cough with hemoptysis, dyspnea, bronchospasm, pruritus, fever, diffuse alveolar infiltrates without effusions, and pulmonary and systemic eosinophilia (148,149). Elevated circulating IgE may be found; histopathologically, the picture is most consistent with acute eosinophilic pneumonia with extensive IgE deposition. This syndrome may represent an IgE-dependent hypersensitivity response with mast cell degranulation, eosinophil recruitment, and tissue damage. Recurrent episodes may occur with continued cocaine inhalation. It is unclear whether this syndrome is specific to cocaine or to impurities present in the inhaled drug. There is one report of cocaine-related Churg-Strauss vasculitis affecting the lung (150).

Bronchiolitis Obliterans-Organizing Pneumonia

A rare complication of cocaine inhalation (151), bronchiolitis obliterans-organizing pneumonia presents with subacute manifestations, including dyspnea, cough, constitutional symptoms, and patchy—usually peripheral—infiltrates. A variety of inhalational and other insults to the lung are capable of eliciting this type of inflammatory response, but its pathogenesis is obscure. It is diagnosed reliably by open lung biopsy and treated with steroids.

Panlobular Emphysema The mechanism for the development of emphysema is not known. Bullous pulmonary emphysema may develop with chronic cocaine use (49) and may be potentiated by tobacco inhalation.

Interstitial Pulmonary Fibrosis Pulmonary fibrosis may occur as a result of intensive or chronic use of cocaine, either inhaled or injected; silica or talc usually are found histopathologically (152). This complication probably is underrecognized, as it may be subclinical. One autopsy series reported that 38% of patients had evidence of interstitial fibrosis in the lungs (129). Occasionally, the degree of fibrosis is extensive and leads to pulmonary hypertension.

AMPHETAMINES AND OTHER STIMULANTS

Amphetamines—whether ingested, inhaled, or injected intravenously—increase sympathetic stimulation by causing release of biogenic amines and by inhibiting their reuptake. Effects of amphetamines are predominantly cardiovascular and neurologic (153).

Amphetamines were used in the early part of the last century to treat respiratory illness. They have sympathomimetic effects and can induce some bronchodilation and vasoconstriction; consequently, amphetamine inhalers were manufactured for the treatment of asthma. For rhinitis, the Benzedrine nasal inhaler introduced in 1932 contained a large dose of synthetic racemic amphetamine (131). Amphetamines are specifically retained by the lung from the circulation, a property that is exploited for nuclear medicine imaging of the lung (154).

Amphetamines have adverse effects on the immune system, including a decrease in CD4 T-helper cells, an increase in immunosuppressive cytokines (transforming growth factor-beta and IL-10), and a switch from Th1-type cytokines (IL-2 and interferon-alpha) to Th2-type cytokines (IL-4 and IL-10) (155). Such changes may adversely affect the delayed hypersensitivity response to microbial pathogens. Chlorphentermine, an amphiphilic drug, has been reported to cause phospholipidosis in a variety of murine tissues, including the lung, which is associated with impaired phagocytosis (156).

Metabolic Acidosis and Respiratory Alkalosis

Extreme agitation and hyperthermia may result in rhabdomyolysis and severe metabolic acidosis, with an associated increased respiratory drive. A direct central effect also may increase respiratory drive (131).

Barotrauma Pneumomediastinum, subcutaneous, and retropharyngeal emphysema have been reported with the use of inhaled 3,4-methylenedioxymethamphetamine (MDMA or "Ecstasy") (131,157,158).

Respiratory Depression CNS and respiratory depression may be seen, particularly in overdose. Patients are at increased risk of aspiration from a depressed mental status or from seizures (131).

Pulmonary Edema Amphetamines may cause both cardiogenic and noncardiogenic pulmonary edema (131,159,160), as well as myocardial infarction or acute cardiomyopathy. Users also can develop pulmonary edema through a neurogenic mechanism or because of aspiration.

Pulmonary Hypertension Appetite suppressants, such as fenfluramine and its derivatives, may be causal or may hasten the development of pulmonary hypertension. One case-control study reported that the risk of pulmonary hypertension was increased 23 times in patients who used these drugs for more than 3 months (160). The first reported association between pulmonary hypertension and amphetamine use was in Europe in the 1960s, after an increase in cases related to aminorex fumarate. Between 1967 and 1973, 77% of patients with pulmonary hypertension reported use of aminorex fumarate before the onset of symptoms. A 5-year retrospective study of patients referred for evaluation of pulmonary hypertension found that 15 (20%) had used fenfluramine and that 10 (67%) showed a temporal relationship between use of the drug and onset of symptoms (161).

Intravenous injection of methylphenidate has been reported to cause fatal pulmonary hypertension (35). Chronic inhalation of methamphetamine also has been reported to cause pulmonary hypertension (162).

Patients generally complain of exertional dyspnea, have a prominent second heart sound, have jugular venous distension, and have enlarged hila on chest radiograph. Echocardiographic or right-sided catheterization may be performed to obtain pulmonary pressures. Pathology reveals changes similar to primary pulmonary hypertension, with advanced plexogenic pulmonary arteriopathy. Vasodilator therapy with calcium channel blockers, epoprostenol, or an alternative advanced agent may be used in selected individuals, after hemodynamic monitoring ascertains a response to one of these agents. A lack of vasodilator response suggests that pulmonary hypertension is not reversible (38).

One possible explanation for the development of pulmonary hypertension related to fenfluramine use is that the drug increases circulating levels of serotonin and results in vasoconstriction of the pulmonary vasculature. Studies report that plasma serotonin levels are increased in patients with primary pulmonary hypertension. This excess serotonin may lead to pulmonary vasoconstriction and proliferation of pulmonary vascular smooth muscle. Other proposed mechanisms include toxic endothelial injury, hypoxia, vasospasm, vasculitis, and altered balance of mediators of vascular tone, such as eicosanoids (161,163).

Bullous Emphysema Bibasilar bullous pulmonary emphysema, resembling that seen in alpha-1-antitrypsin deficiency, has been reported with injection of methylphenidate (164), but it has not been reported with amphetamines. The pathogenesis of this complication is not known.

CAFFEINE

Caffeine is widely available in food and drinks and in tablet form without a physician's prescription. Caffeine is a phosphodiesterase inhibitor that raises intracellular cyclic adenosine monophosphate, with effects similar to theophylline, including smooth muscle relaxation. Thus caffeine has mild bronchodilator properties. Caffeine actually may falsely elevate the serum theophylline level (165).

Pulmonary complications are rare and usually are associated with a large overdose or unintentional ingestion by children. Respiratory alkalosis, chest pain, seizures, aspiration, respiratory failure, and pulmonary edema associated with cardiac arrhythmias may occur (166).

OPIOIDS

Opioids can have prominent effects on the respiratory and other organ systems because of widespread distribution of opioid receptors throughout the body. Opioids bind to specific receptors, with distribution to the CNS, cardiovascular, immune, and respiratory systems. Opioid receptors in the respiratory tract are found mostly within the alveolar walls, but also are associated with tracheal and bronchial smooth muscle. "Nonconventional" receptors also have been postulated to be active in the lung (167,168).

Opioids have their most dramatic effects on the respiratory system by acting on the CNS. Opioid binding to mu_2 receptors causes a reduction in responsiveness to carbon dioxide and depresses the pontine and medullary centers that regulate respiratory automaticity and cough. Cerebral cortical input also may be inhibited. Consequently, breathing becomes irregular and apnea may develop. Respiratory depression increases progressively as the dose is increased. Maximal respiratory depression occurs within 5 to 10 minutes after an intravenous dose or within 30 to 90 minutes after a subcutaneous or intramuscular dose, with the effects on respiration lasting 4 to 5 hours (169,170).

Opioids may induce respiratory complications through effects on airways, pulmonary vasculature, the immune system, and (indirectly) through the CNS. They can induce histamine release from mast cells (171), which may lead to pulmonary vein constriction, increased pulmonary capillary permeability and pulmonary edema, and bronchoconstriction. Opioids have significant effects on the immune system, which may account for the reported association with infections. Specifically, they may cause defects in T cell and natural killer cell function, macrophage and neutrophil phagocytosis, inhibition of cytosine production by leukocytes, attenuation of antibody responses, inhibition of delayed type hypersensitivity responses, depression of CD4/CD8 ratio, and inhibition of leukocyte chemotaxis (172,173). Opioids can desensitize chemokine receptors in leukocytes, decreasing their chemotactic ability (174). They also can induce programmed cell death of leukocytes (175).

Although morphine often is used for the relief of dyspnea, opioids also can exert adverse effects on the lung, acutely and with chronic abuse. Pulmonary complications account for approximately 20% of opiate-related complications (26,39). Acutely, particularly with inhalational use, opioids may induce bronchospasm, bronchitis, and hypersensitivity pneumonitis. Respiratory depression and failure, pulmonary edema, respiratory infections, chronic bronchitis, septic pulmonary emboli, pulmonary hypertension, and talc-related complications are associated with chronic (particularly intravenous) opioid abuse. Pulmonary edema probably is the most common complication of overdose, while respiratory arrest is the most serious.

Bronchospasm It long has been recognized that asthma exacerbations may be precipitated by heroin use in some people with asthma. Opioids, which cause histamine release potentially through mu receptors or through IgE mediation (171), can induce bronchospasm in histamine-sensitive asthmatics (176), but it is unclear whether histamine-insensitive asthmatics also may be prone to opioid-induced bronchoconstriction. Occupational asthma among workers in a pharmaceutical factory producing morphine was found to be associated with an IgE-mediated mechanism of histamine release (177). Asthma exacerbations also may be precipitated by opioid use (58).

Pulmonary Edema Opioid overdose, particularly with heroin, is a common cause of pulmonary edema in patients younger than 40 years, and it accounts for many drug-related deaths (22,178). As many as 50% of overdose patients present with pulmonary edema. Twenty percent of this group will die (22). The occurrence of pulmonary edema is not limited to intravenously administered drugs (179). Opioid-induced pulmonary edema can occur with the first use of the drug (181), but it is believed to be dose-related rather than an idiosyncratic reaction (180).

Several mechanisms of opioid-induced noncardiogenic pulmonary edema have been offered. One hypothesis suggests that opioids have a direct toxic effect on the alveolar capillary membrane, increasing permeability and allowing fluid extravasation into the alveolar spaces (179). Alternatively, opioids' effect on the CNS may induce a vast neurogenic efferent response that leads to alveolar capillary permeability or pulmonary venous constriction (141,181). Other possibilities include a hypersensitivity reaction or acute hypoxic effect, causing increased alveolar capillary membrane permeability (179). Clinically, this complication manifests as dyspnea and somnolence, usually within minutes, depending on the route of administration.

Rales may be heard bilaterally on physical examination. Progressively, affected individuals become obtunded and cyanotic and develop hypoxemia and hypercapnia (179). The chest radiograph typically reveals interstitial and/or alveolar bilateral infiltrates, often in a perihilar pattern, without cardiomegaly or pleural effusions. The pulmonary capillary wedge pressure usually is within the normal range. The electrocardiogram may be normal or may show arrhythmias and conduction defects.

Treatment is supportive and may include noninvasive or invasive mechanical ventilation, positive end-expiratory pressure, oxygen, and judicious use of diuretics. The clinical and radiographic abnormality generally clears within 24 hours. If there is not improvement within 48 hours, alternative diagnoses should be considered, including aspiration and superimposed pneumonia. It is estimated that as many as 50% to 75% of patients with pulmonary edema develop a superimposed pneumonia (39).

Hypersensitivity Pneumonitis Although uncommon, intranasal heroin has been reported to cause hypersensitivity pneumonitis (182). Patients usually manifest with dyspnea and cough hours to days after inhalation, which may lead to significant hypoxemia. Chest radiograph may show bilateral infiltrates, which may be reticulonodular or coalescent. Treatment includes supplemental oxygen and steroids if compromise is evident and if spontaneous regression does not occur.

ALCOHOL

Alcohol ingestion may cause acute intoxication accompanied by respiratory depression and such common complications as atelectasis, hypoxemia, respiratory acidosis, aspiration, adult respiratory distress syndrome, and respiratory failure (183). Aspiration pneumonia may be associated with loss of airway control or seizures. Alcohol ingestion also may cause worsening of underlying respiratory conditions such as sleep apnea (184). Alcohol depresses respiration by acting directly on the respiratory centers within the brain. Chronic heavy use may lead to cirrhosis, with the development of specific hepatopulmonary syndromes and increased susceptibility to infections. Pneumonia related to *Klebsiella*, *Streptococcus pneumoniae*, tuberculosis, and other pathogens is common among individuals who abuse alcohol chronically (185,186). This condition may stem from malnutrition, concomitant tobacco abuse, immune suppression, and decreased function of the reticuloendothelial system (183,185,186).

Acute Metabolic Acidosis and Respiratory Alkalosis Alcohol may cause metabolic acidosis from alcoholic ketoacidosis, with resultant compensatory respiratory alkalosis (187). Ingestion of other alcohols (such as methanol) may cause wide anion gap acidosis and lead to compensatory respiratory alkalosis (188).

Chronic Respiratory Alkalosis Among patients with cirrhosis, chronic respiratory alkalosis is common, even in the absence of metabolic acidosis. This condition may be due to the respiratory stimulant effect of poorly cleared progesterone and estradiol on the CNS, which has an impaired blood–brain barrier (189).

Asthma Patients with preexisting asthma, particularly those who are histamine sensitive, may experience worsening of asthma symptoms after consumption of alcohol (190–192). However, some individuals actually experience a degree of symptom relief or bronchodilatation (190,193). In a small number of individuals, this relief may be due to the presence of sulfites in wine or other beverages, but it can lead to severe bronchospasm and death (194). A third of asthmatic patients report worsening of symptoms after alcohol consumption, suggesting other operative mechanisms (190,191). In some patients, acetaldehyde, generated from ethanol metabolism, appears to lead to mast cell or basophil degranulation (195). The ensuing release of histamine and other mediators of inflammation induces asthma, as suggested by the ability of chlorpheniramine largely to inhibit ethanol-induced bronchospasm (196). Both heterozygotic and homozygotic mutations in acetaldehyde dehydrogenase genes have been found to correlate with alcohol-induced airway reactivity (198). However, elevated IgE has not been associated with this syndrome (198).

Pulmonary Restriction from Ascites Massive ascites, with or without hydrothorax, may impede diaphragmatic and pulmonary excursion, leading to rapid shallow breathing, dyspnea, atelectasis, and even hypoxemia (199,200).

Hepatic Hydrothorax Cirrhosis with ascites may lead to the formation of pleural effusion. Negative intrapleural pressure generated during inspiration, rather than as a result of decreased plasma oncotic pressure, leads to transdiaphragmatic movement of ascitic fluid into the pleural space. Such fluid often occupies the entire hemithorax, usually on the right side. If refractory to diuretics and other medical therapy, pleurodesis or transjugular intrahepatic portosystemic shunts may be performed, with variable success (201).

Hepatopulmonary Syndrome This syndrome, found in 8% to 15% of patients with cirrhosis, consists of a triad of liver dysfunction, intrapulmonary or other vascular dilatations, and arterial hypoxemia. Arteriovenous shunts are thought to arise from circulating estrogen-like substances, as well as from elevated nitric oxide production in the lung, leading to dyspnea, platypnea, clubbing, and orthodeoxia. Diagnostic elements include evidence of cirrhosis and hypoxemia and the demonstration of a right-to-left shunt by technetium 99-macroaggregated albumin perfusion scan or by bubble echocardiography. Hemodynamic studies often reveal a hyperdynamic cardiac output with low pulmonary vascular resistance, which may be seen in cirrhosis. In general, transjugular intrahepatic portosystemic shunts has been reported to improve the physiologic compromise of hepatopulmonary syndrome (202–205).

Portal Pulmonary Hypertension Approximately 2% of patients with cirrhosis develop pulmonary arterial hypertension. The pathogenesis of this complication is not clear, but it probably is mediated by both mechanical and humoral factors. Vasoactive substances, which ordinarily are cleared or produced by the liver, may induce vasoconstriction or endothelial damage. Pathologically, the lesion is similar to that seen with primary pulmonary hypertension: plexogenic pulmonary arteriopathy, medial hypertrophy, intimal cellular proliferation, and eventual arteriolar dilatation (206,207). Patients usually have exertional dyspnea, but some have incidentally discovered pulmonary hypertension. The physical signs of right-sided heart failure from pulmonary hypertension may be missed in cirrhotic patients, who already may have peripheral edema. Vasodilator therapy may be used judiciously after hemodynamic trials (208).

Liver transplantation has been reported to alleviate portal pulmonary hypertension, but fixed pulmonary hypertension may constitute a relative contraindication because of a poor prognosis (209). Pulmonary hypertension also may develop as a consequence of transjugular intrahepatic portosystemic shunts, which should not be performed in an attempt to treat portal pulmonary hypertension (210).

Adult Respiratory Distress Syndrome Individuals who chronically abuse alcohol are twice as likely as nonusers to develop adult respiratory distress syndrome in response to usual triggers such as aspiration and infection. Epithelial lining fluid from the lung of heavy alcohol users is depleted of glutathione, which is important in mitigating the oxidative stress that plays a role in the pathogenesis of adult respiratory distress syndrome (211). Chronic heavy alcohol is an independent risk factor for adult respiratory distress syndrome and also increases the severity of dysfunction of organs other than the lung in patients with septic shock (212).

SEDATIVE-HYPNOTICS

Sedative-hypnotic drugs may exert significant respiratory depressant effects when abused or when mixed with alcohol and opiates. Benzodiazepines, barbiturates, and gamma-hydroxybutyrate (GHB) bind gamma-aminobutyric acid (GABA) receptors, which normally function as targets for inhibitory neurotransmitters and promote sedation, hypnosis, anxiolysis, anterograde amnesia, and anticonvulsant activity (5,169,213).

GHB is a naturally occurring metabolite of GABA in the CNS. Unlike benzodiazepines and barbiturates, which bind GABA-A receptors, GHB interacts with GABA-B receptors. Other GHB effects include elevation of CNS dopamine, elevation of CNS endorphins, and stimulation of growth hormone release. GHB is abused by bodybuilders and by those seeking its hypnotic and euphoric effects (214). Adverse respiratory effects are mainly related to overdose.

Overdose Barbiturates were the cornerstone of sedative-hypnotic therapy until the 1970s, when they were replaced by the less toxic benzodiazepines. In 1975, sedative-hypnotic drug overdose accounted for approximately 1% of admissions to the medical service and approximately 10% of cases of respiratory failure. One percent to 10% of patients did not survive. Of the patients who died, 40% died of respiratory complications (5). Today, the incidence of sedative drug overdose is substantially lower. In reviews of 1,239 overdose cases from a medical examiner's office, only two deaths were related solely to benzodiazepine overdose (213,215). Benzodiazepine overdose most commonly occurs as part of a polysubstance overdose.

Although barbiturates also may be involved in a polypharmacy overdose, the most common toxic scenario with barbiturates is an accidental or intentional oral ingestion by a seizure patient or member of his or her family (213).

Clinically, sedation may progress to coma, with progressive alveolar hypoventilation and respiratory acidosis. Hypotension, which probably is related to direct myocardial depression and vasodilatation, may follow, with accompanying respiratory arrest (more typically in barbiturate overdose) (213).

Treatment of sedative-hypnotic overdose is supportive and usually entails decontamination with lavage and charcoal adsorption. Supplemental oxygen, airway protection, and mechanical ventilation may be necessary. Most deaths occur as a result of adult respiratory distress syndrome secondary to either a chemical aspiration pneumonitis or bacterial pneumonia (169). The former typically occurs when there is witnessed aspiration during a difficult intubation (5).

In benzodiazepine overdose, the competitive antagonist flumazenil can be administered with caution, but it is short-acting and its ability to reverse the respiratory depressant effects is controversial. Side effects include anxiety, agitation, crying, nausea, and seizures (213).

In barbiturate overdose, elimination can be enhanced with an alkaline diuresis. Dialysis rarely is necessary; however, hemodynamic instability refractory to fluid management is an indication for dialysis. Serum drug levels often rebound after dialysis because of redistribution, necessitating further dialysis (213).

The use of CNS stimulants may increase mortality and is contraindicated (169). In GHB overdose, recovery is rapid, with full return to baseline within several hours (213). Recovery from benzodiazepine and barbiturate overdose is longer in duration. Generally, the prognosis is excellent with supportive care alone.

Withdrawal Syndromes Abrupt cessation of chronically used sedative-hypnotics may lead to withdrawal symptoms. Tachypnea is the most common respiratory manifestation of withdrawal from benzodiazepines, which causes a hyperadrenergic state that increases carbon dioxide production. To eliminate excess carbon dioxide and as a result of anxiety, the individual experiencing withdrawal hyperventilates. Tachypnea always is accompanied by other manifestations of benzodiazepine withdrawal, including anxiety, tremor, headache, diaphoresis, difficulty concentrating, insomnia, hallucinations, or fatigue. It generally occurs 2 to 5 days after the last dose of the drug (213).

Barbiturate withdrawal occurs after two to seven days' abstinence. Agitation, hyperreflexia, anxiety, and tremor are most common, followed by confusion and hallucinations. Up to 75% of patients experience seizures, often refractory to phenytoin. Effective treatment requires reinstitution of a barbiturate or a cross-tolerant medication such as a benzodiazepine. Because seizures are so common in barbiturate withdrawal, airway protection, and management is the primary respiratory issue (213).

Sleep Benzodiazepines can worsen sleep disorders by decreasing the tone of the upper airway muscles and reducing the ventilatory response to carbon dioxide, leading to worse nocturnal hypoxia and pulmonary hypertension (169). Although benzodiazepines can be beneficial in treating sleep disorders by increasing total sleep time and the sense of refreshing sleep, their effect on sleep disorders is difficult to predict.

VOLATILE SUBSTANCES

Abuse of inhalants is highly prevalent throughout the world, particularly among young teenagers. Volatile substances are aromatic and short-chain hydrocarbons, such as toluene, gasoline, butane, butyl and amyl nitrites, and Freon, which are found in adhesives, paints, paint thinner, dry cleaning fluids, refrigerants, and propellants. They are volatile at room temperature. When sniffed or, more commonly, vigorously inhaled within a hermetic container ("huffed"), they are readily absorbed in the lungs. Intoxicating and dysphoric effects follow within seconds (216). Primary acute effects involve the CNS and include lethargy, stupor agitation, hallucinations, dizziness, and seizures (217). Pulmonary complications include severe respiratory depression, barotrauma (pneumomediastinum), persistent cough, and suffocation (217–219).

Methemoglobinemia Butyl and isobutyl nitrites may cause methemoglobinemia, which manifests as cyanosis with normal partial pressure of oxygen. However, oxygen saturation of hemoglobin is low and cooximetry will specifically measure methemoglobin (219,220). Intravenous methylene blue may be administered for treatment (221).

Metabolic Acidosis and Respiratory Alkalosis Metabolic acidosis may occur, with compensatory respiratory alkalosis, resulting from distal renal tubular acidosis or from wide anion gap acidosis. The latter may result from oxidation of toluenes to benzoic acid and conjugation with glycine to form hippuric acid (222).

Asthma Occupational exposure to toluene diisocyanate and other isocyanates may be associated with asthma (223). However, no cases of asthma associated with toluene abuse have been reported. In some cases, an IgE-mediated mechanism may be operative, but in others, multiple mechanisms are at work (224). A hypersensitivity pneumonitis also has been reported with isocyanate inhalation (225).

Tracheobronchitis Nitrates and other inhalants may be directly irritating to airway mucosa and cause chronic cough (226).

Asphyxiation Users of inhalants may develop asphyxiation from plastic bag suffocation or from respiratory depression (227,228).

NITROUS OXIDE

Nitrous oxide is a readily available, often abused substance with euphoric effects. It is a widely used inhalational anesthetic-analgesic agent, which also is used in a variety of commercial products (such as a propellant for whipped cream chargers) (229). Nitrous oxide may bind to the opioid receptors (230).

Pulmonary complications include pneumomediastinum, respiratory depression, and hypoxemia because of displacement of oxygen, leading to asphyxia (229,231,232). Treatment is supportive, including supplemental oxygen and respiratory support (229).

ANABOLIC STEROIDS

Anabolic steroids induce a pro-thrombotic state and may cause pulmonary embolism, strokes, and other forms of thromboses (233,234). Respiratory complications are less common but may occur after stroke, and include atelectasis, pneumonia, and aspiration.

REFERENCES

1. Brugman S, Irvin C. Lung structure and function. In: RS Mitchell, T Petty, M Schwartz, eds. *Synopsis of clinical pulmonary disease*, 4th ed. St. Louis, MO: C.V. Mosby, 1998:1–17.
2. Crofton J, Douglas A. The structure and function of the respiratory tract. In *Respiratory diseases,* 3rd ed. Boston, MA: Blackwell Scientific Publications, 1981:1–79.
3. Foth H. Role of the lung in accumulation and metabolism of xenobiotic compounds—implications for chemically induced toxicity. *Crit Rev Toxicol* 1995;25(2):165–205.
4. Parsons PE. Respiratory failure as a result of drugs, overdoses, and poisonings. *Clin Chest Med* 1994;15(1):93–102.
5. Jay SJ, Johanson WG, Pierce AK. Respiratory complications of overdose with sedative drugs. *Am Rev Resp Dis* 1975;112:591–598.
6. Marini JJ, Pierson D, Hudson L. Acute lobar atelectasis: a prospective comparison of fiberoptic bronchoscopy and respiratory therapy. *Am Rev Resp Dis* 1979;119:971–978.
7. Marik PE . Primary care: aspiration pneumonitis and aspiration pneumonia. *N Engl J Med* 2001;344(9):665–671.
8. Verra F, Escudier E, Lebargy F, et al. Ciliary abnormalities in bronchial epithelium of smokers, ex-smokers, and nonsmokers. *Am J Resp Crit Care Med* 1995;151(3 pt 1):630–634.
9. Sisson JH, Papi A, Beckmann JD, et al. Smoke and viral infection cause cilia loss detectable by bronchoalveolar lavage cytology and dynein ELISA. *Am J Resp Crit Care Med* 1994;149(1):205–213.
10. Kaa E. Impurities, adulterants and diluents of illicit heroin. Changes during a 12-year period. *Forensic Sci Int* 1994;64(2–3):17.
11. Miller GJ, Ashcroft MT, Beadnell HM, et al. The lipoid pneumonia of blackfat tobacco smokers in Guyana. *Q J Med* 1971;40(160): 457–470.
12. Kurup VP, Resnick A, Kagen SL, et al. Allergenic fungi and actinomycetes in smoking materials and their health implications. *Mycopathologia* 1983;82(1):61–64.
13. Hamadeh R, Ardehali A, Locksley RM, et al. Fatal aspergillosis associated with smoking contaminated marijuana, in a marrow transplant recipient. *Chest* 1998;94(2):432–433.
14. Sutton S, Lum BL, Torti FM. Possible risk of invasive aspergillosis with marijuana use during chemotherapy for small cell lung cancer. *Drug Intell Clin Pharm* 1986;20:289–290.
15. Kagen SL, Kurup VP, Sohnle PG, et al. Marijuana smoking and fungal sensitization. *J Allerg Clin Immunol* 1983;71(4):389–393.
16. Lheureux P, Leduc D, Vanbinst R, et al. Survival in a case of massive paraquat ingestion. *Chest* 1995;107(1):285–289.
17. Daisley H, Hutchinson G. Paraquat poisoning. *Lancet* 1998;24;352 (9137):1393–1394.
18. Zuskin E, Mustajbegovic J, Schachter EN. Follow-up study of respiratory function in hemp workers. *Am J Indust Med* 1994;26(1): 103–115.
19. Dalvie MA, White N, Raine R, et al. Long-term respiratory health effects of the herbicide, paraquat, among workers in the Western Cape. *Occup Environ Med Am J Indust Med* 1999;56(6):391–396.
20. Lander F, Jepsen JR, Gravesen S. Allergic alveolitis and late asthmatic reaction due to molds in the tobacco industry. *Allergy* 1998;43(1): 74–76.
21. Huuskonen MS, Husman K, Jarvisalo J, et al. Extrinsic allergic alveolitis in the tobacco industry. *Br J Indust Med* 1984;41(1):77–83.
22. O'Donnell AE, Pappas LS. Pulmonary complications of intravenous drug abuse. *Chest* 1998;94(2):251–253.
23. Pare JP, Cote G, Fraser RS. Long-term follow-up of drug abusers with intravenous talcosis. *Am Rev Resp Dis* 1989;139(1):233–241.
24. American Thoracic Society. Targeted tuberculin testing and treatment of latent tuberculosis infection. *MMWR Morbid Mortal Wkly Rep* 2000; 49(RR-6):1–51.
25. Louria DB, Hensle T, Rose J. The major medical complications of heroin addiction. *Ann Intern Med* 1967;67:1–22.
26. Feigin DS. Talc: understanding its manifestations in the chest. *AJR Am J Roentgenol* 1986;146(2):295–301.
27. Ward S, Heyneman LE, Reittner P, et al. Talcosis associated with IV abuse of oral medications: CT findings. *AJR Am J Roentgenol* 2000;174:789.
28. Waller BF, Brownlee WJ, Roberts WC. Self-induced pulmonary granulomatosis. A consequence of intravenous injection of drugs intended for oral use. *Chest* 1980;78(1):90–94.
28a. Overland ES, Nolan AJ, Hopewell PC. Alteration of pulmonary function in intravenous drug abusers. Prevalence, severity, and characterization of gas exchange abnormalities. *Am J Med* 1980;68(2):231–237.
29. Sharma OP, Kalkat GV. Drug induced clinical syndromes mimicking sarcoidosis. *Sarcoidosis* 1991;8(1):3–5.
30. Genereux GP, Emson HE. Talc granulomatosis and angiothrombotic pulmonary hypertension in drug addicts. *J Can Assoc Radiol* 1974;25(2): 87–93.
31. Hopkins GB. Pulmonary angiothrombotic granulomatosis in drug offenders. *JAMA* 1972;221(8):909–911.
32. Robertson CH Jr., Reynolds RC, Wilson JE 3rd. Pulmonary hypertension and foreign body granulomas in intravenous drug abusers. Documentation by cardiac catheterization and lung biopsy. *Am J Med* 1976; 61(5):657–664.
33. Yakel DL Jr, Eisenberg MJ. Pulmonary artery hypertension in chronic intravenous cocaine users. *Am Heart J* 1995;130(2):398–399.
34. Mehta NJ, Khan IA, Mehta RN, et al. HIV-related pulmonary hypertension: analytic review of 131 cases. *Chest* 2000;118(4):1133–1141.
35. Lewman LV. Fatal pulmonary hypertension from intravenous injection of methylphenidate (Ritalin) tablets. *Hum Pathol* 1972;3(1):67–70.
36. Collazos J, Martinez E, Fernandez A, et al. Acute, reversible pulmonary hypertension associated with cocaine use. *Resp Med* 1996;90(3):171–174.
37. Kleerup EC, Wong M, Marques-Magallanes JA, et al. Acute effects of intravenous cocaine on pulmonary artery pressure and cardiac index in habitual crack smokers. *Chest* 1997;111(1):30–35.
38. Klings ES, Farber HW. Current management of primary pulmonary hypertension. *Drugs* 2001;61(13):1945–1956.
39. Rosenow EC. The spectrum of drug-induced pulmonary disease. *Ann Intern Med* 1972;77:977–991.
40. Kulaylat MN, Barakat N, Stephan RN, et al. Embolization of illicit needle fragments. *J Emerg Med* 1993;11(4):403–408.
41. Lewis JW Jr, Groux N, Elliott JP Jr, et al. Complications of attempted central venous injections performed by drug abusers. *Chest* 1980;78(4): 613–617.
42. Zorc TG, O'Donnell AE, Holt RW, et al. Bilateral pyopneumothorax secondary to intravenous drug abuse. *Chest* 1998;93(3):645–647.
43. Aguado JM, Arjona R, Ugarte P. Septic pulmonary emboli. A rare cause of bilateral pneumothorax in drug abusers. *Chest* 1990;98(5):1302–1304.
44. McLean L, Sharma S, Maycher B. Mycotic pulmonary artery aneurysms in intravenous drug abusers. *Can Resp J* 1998;5(4):307–311.
45. Joseph WL, Geelhoed GW. Surgical sequelae of intravenous drug abuse. *Maryland State Med J* 1974;23(1):70–73.
46. Wayne NG, Spitz WU. Rupture of a subclavian artery aneurysm in a heroin addict. Report of a case. *Rechtsmedizin Zurich* 1978;81(2):147–149.

47. Grellner W, Madea B, Sticht G. Pulmonary histopathology and survival period in morphine-involved deaths. *J Forensic Sci* 1996;41(3):433–437.
48. Smeenk FW, Serlie J, van der Jagt EJ, et al. Bullous degeneration of the left lower lobe in a heroin addict. *Eur Resp J* 1990;3(10):1224–1226.
49. Fullana Monllor J, Garcia Bermejo PA, Pellicer Ciscar C. Bullous emphysema in a cocaine smoker [in Spanish]. *Arch Bronconeumol* 1998; 34(10):514.
50. Cone EJ. Recent discoveries in pharmacokinetics of drugs of abuse. *Toxicol Lett* 1998;102-103:97–101.
51. Kiter G, Ucan ES, Ceylan E, et al. Water-pipe smoking and pulmonary functions. *Resp Med* 2000;94(9):891–894.
52. Lubin JH, Li JY, Xuan XZ, et al. Risk of lung cancer among cigarette and pipe smokers in southern China. *Int J Cancer* 1992;51(3): 390–395.
53. Smith CJ, Hansch C. The relative toxicity of compounds in mainstream cigarette smoke condensate. *Food Chem Toxicol* 2000;38(7):637–646.
54. Wu D, Center D. Chronic bronchitis and bronchiectasis. In: R Goldstein, J O'Connell, J Karlinksy, eds. *A practical approach to pulmonary medicine*. Philadelphia, PA: Lippincott-Raven, 1997:240–252.
55. Fligiel SE, Roth MD, Kleerup EC, et al. Tracheobronchial histopathology in habitual smokers of cocaine, marijuana, and/or tobacco. *Chest* 1997;112(2):319–326.
56. Hughes S, Calverly PMA. Heroin inhalation and asthma. *Br Med J* 1998;297:1511–1512.
57. Aguis R. Opiate inhalation and occupational asthma. *Br Med J* 21989;98:323.
58. Ghodse AH, Myles JS. Asthma in opiate addicts. *J Psychosom Res* 1987;31:41–44.
59. Rome LA, Lippmann ML, Dalsey WC, et al. Prevalence of cocaine use and its impact on asthma exacerbation in an urban population. *Chest* 2000;117(5):1324–1329.
60. Tashkin DP, Kleerup EC, Royal SN, et al. Acute effects of inhaled and IV cocaine on airway dynamics. *Chest* 1996;110(4):904–910.
61. Tashkin DP. Airway effects of marijuana, cocaine, and other inhaled illicit agents. *Curr Opin Pulmon Med* 2001;7(2):43–61.
62. Osborn HH, Tang M, Bradley K, et al. New-onset bronchospasm or recrudescence of asthma associated with cocaine abuse. *Acad Emerg Med* 1997;4(7):689–692.
63. Perlman DC, Perkins MP, Paone D, et al. "Shotgunning" as an illicit drug smoking practice. *J Substance Abuse Treatment* 1997;14(1):3–9.
64. Seaman ME. Barotrauma related to inhalational drug abuse. *J Emerg Med* 1990;8(2):141–149.
65. McCarroll KA, Roszler MH. Lung disorders due to drug abuse. *J Thoracic Imaging* 1991;6(1):30–35.
66. Tashkin DP. Pulmonary complications of smoked substance abuse. *West J Med* 1990;152(5):525–530.
67. Godwin JE, Harley RA, Miller KS, et al. Cocaine, pulmonary hemorrhage, and hemoptysis. *Ann Intern Med* 1989;110(10):843.
68. Karlinsky J. Emphysema. In R Goldstein, J O'Connell, J Karlinksy, eds. *A practical approach to pulmonary medicine*. Philadelphia, PA: Lippincott-Raven, 1997:224–239.
69. Johnson MK, Smith RP, Morrison D, et al. Large lung bullae in marijuana smokers. *Thorax* 2000;55(4):340–342.
70. Da Costa JL, Tock EP, Boey HK. Lung disease with chronic obstruction in opium smokers in Singapore. Clinical, electrocardiographic, radiological, functional and pathological features. *Thorax* 1971;26(5): 555–571.
71. Sandford AJ, Chagani T, Weir TD, et al. Susceptibility genes for rapid decline of lung function in the lung health study. *Am J Resp Crit Care Med* 2001;163(2):469–473.
72. Ishii T, Matsuse T, Teramoto S, et al. Association between alpha-1-antichymotrypsin polymorphism and susceptibility to chronic obstructive pulmonary disease. *Eur J Clin Invest* 2000;30(6):543–548.
73. Sato E, Koyama S, Takamizawa A, et al. Smoke extract stimulates lung fibroblasts to release neutrophil and monocyte chemotactic activities. *Am J Physiol* 1999;277(6 pt 1):L1149–1157.
74. McCusker K. Mechanisms of respiratory tissue injury from cigarette smoking. *Am J Med* 1992;93(1A):18S–21S.
75. Lim S, Roche N, Oliver BG, et al. Balance of matrix metalloprotease-9 and tissue inhibitor of metalloprotease-1 from alveolar macrophages in cigarette smokers. Regulation by interleukin-10. *Am J Resp Crit Care Med* 2000;162(4 pt 1):1355–1360.
76. Shapiro SD. The macrophage in chronic obstructive pulmonary disease. *Am J Resp Crit Care Med* 1999;160(5 pt 2):S29–32.
77. Ofulue AF, Ko M. Effects of depletion of neutrophils or macrophages on development of cigarette smoke-induced emphysema. *J Physiol* 1999;277(1 pt 1):L97–L105.
78. Gadek JE. Adverse effects of neutrophils on the lung. *Am J Med* 1992;92(6A):27S–31S.
79. MacNee W. Oxidants/antioxidants and COPD. *Chest* 2000;117(5 Suppl 1):303S–317S.
80. Snider GL. The pathogenesis of emphysema—twenty years of progress. *Am Rev Resp Dis* 1981;124(3):321–324.
81. Turato G, Zuin R, Saetta M. Pathogenesis and pathology of COPD. *Respiration* 2001;68(2):117–128.
82. Finkelstein R, Fraser RS, Ghezzo H et al. Alveolar inflammation and its relation to emphysema in smokers. *Am J Resp Crit Care Med* 1995;152(5 pt 1):1666–1672.
83. Saetta M, Finkelstein R, Cosio MG. Morphological and cellular basis for airflow limitation in smokers. *Eur Resp J* 1994;7(8):1505–1515.
84. Balfour D, Benowitz N, Fagerström K, et al. Diagnosis and treatment of nicotine dependence with emphasis on nicotine replacement therapy. A status report. *Eur Heart J* 2000;21(6):438–445.
85. Jinot J, Bayard S. Respiratory health effects of exposure to environmental tobacco smoke. *Rev Environ Health* 1996;11(3):89–100.
86. U.S. Department of Health and Human Services (USDHHS). The health effect of involuntary exposure to tobacco smoke. Centers for Disease Control and Prevention, Rockville, MD, 2006.
87. Casale TB, Rhodes BJ, Donnelly AL, et al. Airway responses to methacholine in asymptomatic nonatopic cigarette smokers. *J Appl Physiol* 1987;62(5):1888–1892.
88. Hahn HL, Lang M, Bleicher S, et al. Nicotine-induced airway smooth muscle contraction: neural mechanisms involving the airway epithelium. Functional and histologic studies *in vitro*. *Clin Invest* 1992;70 (3-4):252–262.
89. Hong JL, Lee LY. Cigarette smoke-induced bronchoconstriction: causative agents and role of thromboxane receptors. *J Appl Physiol* 1996; 81(5):2053–2059.
90. Hansson L, Choudry NB, Karlsson JA, et al. Inhaled nicotine in humans: effect on the respiratory and cardiovascular systems. *J Appl Physiol* 1994; 76(6):2420–2427.
91. Lee LY, Lou YP, Hong JL, et al. Cigarette smoke-induced bronchoconstriction and release of tachykinins in guinea pig lungs. *Resp Physiol* 1995;99(1):173–181.
92. Hong JL, Rodger IW, Lee LY. Cigarette smoke-induced bronchoconstriction: cholinergic mechanisms, tachykinins, and cyclooxygenase products. *J Appl Physiol* 1995;78(6):2260–2266.
93. Polkey MI, Hamnegard CH, Hughes PD, et al. Influence of acute lung volume change on contractile properties of human diaphragm. *J Appl Physiol* 1998;85(4):1322–1328.
94. Baumgartner KB, Samet JM, Stidley CA, et al. Cigarette smoking: a risk factor for idiopathic pulmonary fibrosis. *Am J Resp Crit Care Med* 1997; 155(1):242–248.
95. Nagai S, Hoshino Y, Hayashi M, et al. Smoking-related interstitial lung diseases. *Curr Opin Pulmon Med* 2000;6(5):415–419.
96. Heyneman LE, Ward S, Lynch DA, et al. Respiratory bronchiolitis, respiratory bronchiolitis-associated interstitial lung disease, and desquamative interstitial pneumonia: different entities or part of the spectrum of the same disease process? *AJR Am J Roentgenol* 1999;173(6):1617–1622.
97. Yousem SA, Colby TV, Gaensler EA. Respiratory bronchiolitis-associated interstitial lung disease and its relationship to desquamative interstitial pneumonia. *Mayo Clin Proc* 1989;64(11):1373–1380.
98. Aubry MC, Wright JL, Myers JL. The pathology of smoking-related lung diseases. *Clin Chest Med* 2000;21(1):11–35.
99. Murin S, Bilello KS, Matthay R. Other smoking-affected pulmonary diseases. *Clin Chest Med* 2000;21(1):121–137.

100. Hance AJ, Basset F, Saumon G, et al. Smoking and interstitial lung disease. The effect of cigarette smoking on the incidence of histiocytosis X and sarcoidosis. *Ann N Y Acad Sci* 1986;465:643–656.
101. Berk J. Pneumothorax. In: Goldstein R, O'Connell J, Karlinksy J, eds. *A practical approach to pulmonary medicine*. Philadelphia, PA: Lippincott-Raven, 1997:206–233.
102. Schuller HM, Orloff M. Tobacco-specific carcinogenic nitrosamines. Ligands for nicotinic acetylcholine receptors in human lung cancer cells. *Biochem Pharmacol* 1998;55(9):1377–1384.
103. Trump BF, McDowell EM, Harris CC. Chemical carcinogenesis in the tracheobronchial epithelium. *Environ Health Perspect* 1984;55:77–84.
104. Cullen JW, Blot W, Henningfield J, et al. Health consequences of using smokeless tobacco: summary of the Advisory Committee's report to the Surgeon General. *Public Health Rep* 1986;101(4):355–373.
105. Barsky SH, Roth MD, Kleerup EC, et al. Histopathologic and molecular alterations in bronchial epithelium in habitual smokers of marijuana, cocaine, and/or tobacco. *J Natl Cancer Inst* 1998;90(16):1198–1205.
106. Rom WN, Hay JG, Lee TC, et al. Molecular and genetic aspects of lung cancer. *Am J Resp Crit Care Med* 2000;161(4 pt 1):1355–1367.
107. Samet JM, Wiggins CL, Humble CG, et al. Cigarette smoking and lung cancer in New Mexico. *Am Rev Respir Dis* 1998;137(5):1110–1113.
108. Copas JB, Shi JQ. Reanalysis of epidemiological evidence on lung cancer and passive smoking. *Br Med J* 2000;320(7232):417–418.
109. Lee PN. Relation between exposure to asbestos and smoking jointly and the risk of lung cancer. *Occup Environ Med* 2001;58(3):145–153.
110. The health benefits of smoking cessation: a report of the surgeon general. Washington, DC: U.S. Department of Health and Human Services, 1990.
111. Godtfredsen NS, Prescott E, Osler M. Effect of smoking reduction on lung cancer risk. *JAMA* 2005;294(12):1505–1510.
112. Reardon C, Theodore A. Lung cancer. In: Goldstein R, O'Connell J, Karlinksy J, eds. *A practical approach to pulmonary medicine*. Philadelphia, PA: Lippincott-Raven, 1997:129–146.
113. Hoppichler F, Lechleitner M, Konig P, et al. Snuff and recurring pulmonary infiltrations in chronic renal failure. *Lancet* 1992;339(8791):500–501.
114. Van Hoozen BE, Cross CE. Marijuana. Respiratory tract effects. *Clin Rev Allergy Immunol* 1997;15(3):243–269.
115. Wu TC, Tashkin DP, Djahed B, et al. Pulmonary hazards of smoking marijuana as compared with tobacco. *N Engl J Med* 1998;318(6):347–351.
116. Baldwin GC, Tashkin DP, Buckley DM, et al. Marijuana and cocaine impair alveolar macrophage function and cytokine production. *Am J Resp Crit Care Med* 1997;156(5):1606–1613.
117. Sarafian TA, Magallanes JA, Shau H, et al. Oxidative stress produced by marijuana smoke. An adverse effect enhanced by cannabinoids. *Am J Resp Cell Mol Biol* 1999;20(6):1286–1293.
118. Fung M, Gallagher C, Machtay M. Lung and aero-digestive cancers in young marijuana smokers. *Tumori* 1999;85(2):140–142.
119. Fligiel SE, Beals TF, Tashkin DP, et al. Marijuana exposure and pulmonary alterations in primates. *Pharmacol Biochem Behav* 1991;40(3):637–642.
120. Vethanayagam D, Pugsley S, Dunn EJ, et al. Exogenous lipid pneumonia related to smoking weed oil following cadaveric renal transplantation. *Can Resp J* 2000;7(4):338–342.
121. Kreek MJ. Cocaine, dopamine and the endogenous opioid system. *J Addictive Diseases* 1996;15(4):73–96.
122. Fattinger K, Benowitz NL, Jones RT, et al. Nasal mucosal versus gastrointestinal absorption of nasally administered cocaine. *Eu J Clin Pharmacol* 2000;56(4):305–310.
123. McBride DC, Inciardi JA, Chitwood DD, et al. Crack use and correlates of use in a national population of street heroin users. *J Psychoactive Drugs* 1992;24(4):411–416.
124. Hatsukami DK, Fischman MW. Crack cocaine and cocaine hydrochloride. Are the differences myth or reality? *JAMA* 1996;276(19):1580–1588.
125. Mao L, Oh Y. Does marijuana or crack cocaine cause cancer? *J Natl Cancer Inst* 1998;90(16):1182–1184.
126. Tashkin DP, Kleerup EC, Hoh CK, et al. Effects of "crack" cocaine on pulmonary alveolar permeability. *Chest* 1997;112(2):327–335.
127. Om A. Cardiovascular complications of cocaine. *Am J Med Sci* 1992;303(5):333–339.
128. Tashkin DP, Gorelick D, Khalsa ME, et al. Respiratory effects of cocaine freebasing among habitual cocaine users. *J Addict Dis* 1992;11(4):59–70.
129. Bailey ME, Fraire AE, Greenberg SD, et al. Pulmonary histopathology in cocaine abusers. *Hum Pathol* 1994;25(2):203–207.
130. Murray RJ, Albin RJ, Mergner W, et al. Diffuse alveolar hemorrhage temporally related to cocaine smoking. *Chest* 1998;93(2):427–429.
131. Albertson TE, Walby WF, Derlet RW. Stimulant-induced pulmonary toxicity. *Chest* 1995;108(4):1140–1149.
132. Baldwin GC, Roth MD, Tashkin DP. Acute and chronic effects of cocaine on the immune system and the possible link to AIDS. *J Neuroimmunol* 1998;83(1-2):133–138.
133. Xu W, Flick T, Mitchel J, et al. Cocaine effects on immunocompetent cells: an observation of *in vitro* cocaine exposure. *Int J Immunopharmacol* 1999;21(7):463–472.
134. Baldwin GC, Buckley DM, Roth MD, et al. Acute activation of circulating polymorphonuclear neutrophils following *in vivo* administration of cocaine. A potential etiology for pulmonary injury. *Chest* 1997;111(3):698–705.
135. Meleca RJ, Burgio DL, Carr RM, et al. Mucosal injuries of the upper aerodigestive tract after smoking crack or freebase cocaine. *Laryngoscope* 1997;107(5):620–625.
136. Reino AJ, Lawson W. Upper airway distress in crack-cocaine users. *Otolaryngol Head Neck Surg* 1993;109(5):937–940.
137. Libby DM, Klein L, Altorki NK. Aspiration of the nasal septum: a new complication of cocaine abuse. *Ann Intern Med* 1992;116(7):567–568.
138. Armstrong M Jr, Shikani AH. Nasal septal necrosis mimicking Wegener's granulomatosis in a cocaine abuser. *Ear Nose Throat J* 1996;75(9):623–626.
139. Ettinger NA, Albin RJ. A review of the respiratory effects of smoking cocaine. *Am J Med* 1989;87(6):664–668.
140. Garcia-Rostan y Perez GM, Garcia Bragado F, Puras Gil AM. Pulmonary hemorrhage and antiglomerular basement membrane antibody-mediated glomerulonephritis after exposure to smoked cocaine (crack): a case report and review of the literature. *Pathol Int* 1997;47(10):692–697.
141. Smith WS, Matthay MA. Evidence for a hydrostatic mechanism in human neurogenic pulmonary edema. *Chest* 1997;111(5):1326–1333.
142. Lang SA, Maron MB. Hemodynamic basis for cocaine-induced pulmonary edema in dogs. *J Appl Physiol* 1991;71(3):1166–1170.
143. Smith GT, McClaughry PL, Purkey J, et al. Crack cocaine mimicking pulmonary embolism on pulmonary ventilation/perfusion lung scan. A case report. *Clin Nucl Med* 1995;20(1):65–68.
144. Delaney K, Hoffman RS. Pulmonary infarction associated with crack cocaine use in a previously healthy 23-year-old woman. *Am J Med* 1991;91(1):92–94.
145. Hendricks-Munoz KD, Gerrets RP, Higgins RD, et al. Cocaine-stimulated endothelin-1 release is decreased by angiotensin-converting enzyme inhibitors in cultured endothelial cells. *Cardiovasc Res* 1996;31(1):117–123.
146. Murray RJ, Smialek JE, Golle M, et al. Pulmonary artery medial hypertrophy in cocaine users without foreign particle microembolization. *Chest* 1989;96(5):1050–1053.
147. Nadeem S, Nasir N, Israel RH. Loeffler's syndrome secondary to crack. *Chest* 1994;105(5):1599–1600.
148. Kissner DG, Lawrence WD, Selis JE, et al. Crack lung: pulmonary disease caused by cocaine abuse. *Am Rev Resp Dis* 1987;136(5):1250–1252.
149. Forrester JM, Steele AW, Waldron JA, et al. Crack lung: an acute pulmonary syndrome with a spectrum of clinical and histopathologic findings. *Am Rev Resp Dis* 1990;142(2):462–467.
150. Orriols R, Munoz X, Ferrer J, et al. Cocaine-induced Churg-Strauss vasculitis. *Eur Resp J* 1996;9(1):175–177.
151. Patel RC, Dutta D, Schonfeld SA. Free-base cocaine use associated with bronchiolitis obliterans organizing pneumonia. *Ann Intern Med* 1987;107(2):186–187.

152. O'Donnell AE, Mappin FG, Sebo TJ, et al. Interstitial pneumonitis associated with "crack" cocaine abuse. *Chest* 1991;100(4):1155–1157.
153. Albertson TE, Derlet RW, Van Hoozen BE. Methamphetamine and the expanding complications of amphetamines. *West J Med* 1999;170(4): 214–219.
154. Touya JJ, Rahimian J, Corbus HF, et al. The lung as a metabolic organ. *Semin Nucl Med* 1986;16(4):296–305.
155. Pacifici R, Zuccaro P, Lopez CH, et al. Acute effects of 3,4-methylene-dioxymethamphetamine alone and in combination with ethanol on the immune system in humans. *J Pharmacol Exp Therapeutics* 2001;296 (1):207–215.
156. Lehnert BE, Ferin J. Particle binding, phagocytosis, and plastic substrate adherence characteristics of alveolar macrophages from rats acutely treated with chlorphentermine. *J Reticuloendothel Soc* 1983;33(4): 293–303.
157. Quin GI, McCarthy GM, Harries DK. Spontaneous pneumomediastinum and ecstasy abuse. *J Accid Emerg Med* 1999;16(5):382.
158. Onwudike M . Ecstasy induced retropharyngeal emphysema. *J Accid Emerg Med* 1996;13(5):359–361.
159. Call TD, Hartneck J, Dickinson WA, et al. Acute cardiomyopathy secondary to intravenous amphetamine abuse. *Ann Intern Med* 1982;97 (4):559–560.
160. Abenhain L, Moride Y, Brenot F, et al. Appetite-suppressant drugs and the risk of pulmonary hypertension. *N Engl J Med* 1996;335:609–616.
161. Fishman AP. Aminorex to fen/phen: an epidemic foretold. *Circulation* 1999;99(1):156–161.
162. Schaiberger PH, Kennedy TC, Miller FC, et al. Pulmonary hypertension associated with long-term inhalation of "crank" methamphetamine. *Chest* 1993;104:614–616.
163. Herve P, Launay JM, Scrobohaci ML, et al. Increased plasma serotonin in primary pulmonary hypertension. *Am J Med* 1995;99:249–253.
164. Schmidt RA, Glenny RW, Godwin JD, et al. Panlobular emphysema in young intravenous Ritalin abusers. *Am Rev Resp Dis* 1991;143(3): 649–656.
165. Fligner CL, Opheim KE. Caffeine and its dimethylxanthine metabolites in two cases of caffeine overdose: a cause of falsely elevated theophylline concentrations in serum. *J Anal Toxicol* 1998;12(6):339–343
166. Leson CL, McGuigan MA, Bryson SM. Caffeine overdose in an adolescent male. *J Toxicol Clin Toxicol* 1998;6(5-6):407–415.
167. Zebraski SE, Kochenash SM, Raffa RB. Lung opioid receptors: pharmacology and possible target for nebulized morphine in dyspnea. *Life Sciences* 2000;66(23):2221–2231.
168. Fimiani C, Arcuri E, Santoni A, et al. Mu_3 opiate receptor expression in lung and lung carcinoma: ligand binding and coupling to nitric oxide release. *Cancer Lett* 1999;146(1):45–51.
169. Jaffe J, Martin WR. Opioid analgesics and antagonists. In: Gilman AG, Rall TW, Nies AS, et al., eds. *Goodman and Gilman's the pharmacological basis of therapeutics,* 8th ed. Oxford, UK: Pergamon Press, 1990:362–396, 490–494.
170. Sporer KA. Acute heroin overdose. *Ann Intern Med* 1999;130(7): 584–590.
171. Barke KE, Hough LB. Opiates, mast cells, and histamine release. *Life Sci* 1993;53(18):1391–1399.
172. Eisenstein TK, Hilburger ME. Opioid modulation of immune responses: effects on phagocyte and lymphoid cell populations. *J Neuroimmunol* 1998;83(1-2):36–44.
173. Peterson PK, Molitor TW, Chao CC. The opioid-cytokine connection. *J Neuroimmunol* 1998;83(1-2):63–69.
174. Grimm MC, Ben-Baruch A, Taub DD, et al. Opiates transreactivate chemokine receptors: Delta and mu opiate receptor-mediated heterologous desensitization. *J Exp Med* 1998;188(2):317–325.
175. Yin D, Mufson RA, Wang R, et al. Fas-mediated cell death promoted by opioids. *Nature* 1999;397(6716):218.
176. Popa V. Codeine-induced bronchoconstriction and putative bronchial opiate receptors in asthmatic subjects. *Pulmon Pharmacol* 1994;7(5):333–341.
177. Moneo I, Alday E, Ramos C, et al. Occupational asthma caused by Papaver somniferum. *Allergol Immunopathol (Madr)* 1993;21(4): 145–148.
178. Napoli LD, Cigtay OS, Twigg HL, et al. The lungs and drug abuse. *Am Family Phys* 1974;9(3):90–98.
179. Cooper AD, White DA, Matthay RA. Drug-induced pulmonary disease. Part 2: noncytotoxic drugs. *Am Rev Resp Dis* 1986;133:488–505.
180. Rosenow EC 3rd. Drug-induced pulmonary disease. *Dis Mon* 1994;40(5): 253–310.
181. Hakim TS, Grunstein MM, Michel RP. Opiate action in the pulmonary circulation. *Pulmon Pharmacol* 1992;5(3):159–165.
182. Karne S, D'Ambrosio C, Einarsson O, et al. Hypersensitivity pneumonitis induced by intranasal heroin use. *Am J Med* 1999;107(4):392–395.
183. Heinemann HO. Alcohol and the lung. A brief review. *Am J Med* 1977;63(1):81–85.
184. Scanlan MF, Roebuck T, Little PJ, et al. Effect of moderate alcohol upon obstructive sleep apnoea. *Eur Resp J* 2000;16(5):909–913.
185. Cook RT. Alcohol abuse, alcoholism, and damage to the immune system—a review. *Alcohol Clin Exp Res* 1998;22(9):1927–1942.
186. Adams HG, Jordan C. Infections in the alcoholic. *Med Clin N Am* 1984;68(1):179–200.
187. Duffens K, Marx JA. Alcoholic ketoacidosis—a review. *J Emerg Med* 1987;5(5):399–406.
188. Hojer J. Severe metabolic acidosis in the alcoholic: differential diagnosis and management. *Hum Exp Toxicol* 1996;15(6):482–488.
189. Lustik SJ, Chibber AK, Kolano JW, et al. The hyperventilation of cirrhosis: progesterone and estradiol effects. *Hepatology* 1997;25(1):55–58.
190. Vally H, de Klerk N, Thompson PJ. Alcoholic drinks: important triggers for asthma. *J Allerg Clin Immunol* 2000;105(3):462–467.
191. Ayres JG, Clark TJ. Alcoholic drinks and asthma: a survey. *Br J Dis Chest* 1983;77(4):370–375.
192. Zimatkin SM, Anichtchik OV. Alcohol-histamine interactions. *Alcohol Alcohol* 1999;34(2):141–147.
193. Ayres JG, Ancic P, Clark TJ. Airway responses to oral ethanol in normal subjects and in patients with asthma. *J Roy Soc Med* 1982;75(9):699–704.
194. Vally H, Carr A, El-Saleh J, et al. Wine-induced asthma: a placebo-controlled assessment of its pathogenesis. *J Allerg Clin Immunol* 1999; 103(1 pt 1):41–46.
195. Fujimura M, Myou S, Kamio Y, et al. Increased airway responsiveness to acetaldehyde in asthmatic subjects with alcohol-induced bronchoconstriction. *Eur Resp J* 1999;14(1):19–22.
196. Gong H Jr, Tashkin DP, Calvarese BM. Alcohol-induced bronchospasm in an asthmatic patient: pharmacologic evaluation of the mechanism. *Chest* 1981;80(2):167–173.
197. Takao A, Shimoda T, Kohno S, et al. Correlation between alcohol-induced asthma and acetaldehyde dehydrogenase-2 genotype. *J Allerg Clin Immunol* 1998;101(5):576–580.
198. Shimoda T, Kohno S, Takao A, et al. Investigation of the mechanism of alcohol-induced bronchial asthma. *J Allerg Clin Immunol* 1996;97(1 pt 1):74–84.
199. Yao EH, Kong BC, Hsue GL, et al. Pulmonary function changes in cirrhosis of the liver. *Am J Gastroenterol* 1987;82(4):352–354.
200. King PD, Rumbaut R, Sanchez C. Pulmonary manifestations of chronic liver disease. *Digest Dis* 1996;14(2):73–82.
201. Lazaridis KN, Frank JW, Krowka MJ, et al. Hepatic hydrothorax: pathogenesis, diagnosis, and management. *Am J Med* 1999;107(3):262–267.
202. Fallon MB, Abrams GA. Hepatopulmonary syndrome. *Curr Gastroenterol Rep* 2000;2(1):40–45.
203. Fallon MB, Abrams GA. Pulmonary dysfunction in chronic liver disease. *Hepatology* 2000;32(4 pt 1):859–865.
204. Schraufnagel DE, Kay JM. Structural and pathologic changes in the lung vasculature in chronic liver disease. *Clin Chest Med* 1996;17(1):1–15.
205. Abrams GA, Jaffe CC, Hoffer PB, et al. Diagnostic utility of contrast echocardiography and lung perfusion scan in patients with hepatopulmonary syndrome. *Gastroenterology* 1995;109(4):1283–1288.
206. Herve P, Lebrec D, Brenot F, et al. Pulmonary vascular disorders in portal hypertension. *Eur Resp J* 1998;11(5):1153–1166.
207. Robalino BD, Moodie DS. Association between primary pulmonary hypertension and portal hypertension: analysis of its pathophysiology and clinical, laboratory and hemodynamic manifestations. *J Am Coll Cardiol* 1991;17(2):492–498.

208. Kahler CM, Graziadei I, Wiedermann CJ, et al. Successful use of continuous intravenous prostacyclin in a patient with severe portopulmonary hypertension. *Wienr Klin Wochenschr* 2000;112(14):637–640.
209. Kuo PC, Plotkin JS, Gaine S, et al. Portopulmonary hypertension and the liver transplant candidate. *Transplantation* 1999;67(8):1087–1093.
210. Van der Linden P, Le Moine O, Ghysels M, et al. Pulmonary hypertension after transjugular intrahepatic portosystemic shunt: effects on right ventricular function. *Hepatology* 1996;23(5):982–987.
211. Moss M, Guidot DM, Wong-Lambertina M, et al. The effects of chronic alcohol abuse on pulmonary glutathione homeostasis. *Am J Resp Crit Care Med* 2000;161(2 pt 1):414–419.
212. Moss M, Parsons PE, Steinberg KP, Hudson LD, et al. Chronic alcohol abuse is associated with an increased incidence of acute respiratory distress syndrome and severity of multiple organ dysfunction in patients with septic shock. *Crit Care Med* 2003;31(3):869–877.
213. Graudins A, Aaron CK. Sedative-hypnotic poisoning. In: Irwin RS, Cerra FB, Rippe JM, eds. *Intensive care medicine*. Boston, MA: Little, Brown, Company, 1999:1782–1792.
214. Chin RL, Dyer JE, Sporer KA. Gamma-hydroxybutyrate intoxication and overdose. *Ann Emerg Med* 1999;33(4):476.
215. Finkle BS, McCloskey KL, Goodman LS, et al. Diazepam and drug-associated deaths: a survey in the United States and Canada. *JAMA* 1979;242:429–434.
216. Wyse DG. Deliberate inhalation of volatile hydrocarbons: a review. *Can Med Assoc J* 1973;108:71–74.
217. Flanagan RJ, Ives RJ. Volatile substance abuse. *Bull Narc* 1994;46(2):49–78.
218. Cohen S. Glue sniffing. *JAMA* 1975;231(6):653–654.
219. Linden CH. Volatile substances of abuse. *Emerg Med Clin N Am* 1990;8(3):559–578.
220. Curry S. Methemoglobinemia. *Ann Emerg Med* 1982;11:214–221.
221. Wright RO, Lewander WJ, Woolf AD. Methemoglobinemia: etiology, pharmacology, and clinical management. *An Emerg Med* 1999;34(5):646–656.
222. Fischman CM, Oster JR. Toxic effects of toluene; a new cause of high anion gap acidosis. *JAMA* 1979;241(16):1713–1715.
223. Ott MG, Klees JE, Poche SL. Respiratory health surveillance in a toluene di-isocyanate production unit, 1967–1997: clinical observations and lung function analyses. *Occup Environ Med* 2000;57(1):43–52.
224. Raulf-Heimsoth M, Baur X. Pathomechanisms and pathophysiology of isocyanate-induced diseases—summary of present knowledge. *Am J Indust Med* 1998;34(2):137–143.
225. Baur X. Hypersensitivity pneumonitis (extrinsic allergic alveolitis) induced by isocyanates. *J Allerg Clin Immunol* 1995;95(5 pt 1):1004–1010.
226. Covalla JR, Strimlan CV, Lech JG. Severe tracheobronchitis from inhalation of an isobutyl nitrite preparation. *Drug Intell Clin Pharm* 1981;15(1):51–52.
227. Paterson SC, Sarvesvaran R. Plastic bag death—a toluene fatality. *Med Sci Law* 1983;23(1):64–66.
228. Ikeda N, Takahashi H, Umetsu K, et al. The course of respiration and circulation in "toluene-sniffing." *Forensic Sci Int* 1990;44(2–3):151–158.
229. Brouette T, Anton R. Clinical review of inhalants. *Am J Addict* 2001;10(1):79–94.
230. Gillman MA. Nitrous oxide, an opioid addictive agent. Review of the evidence. *Am J Med* 1986;81(1):97–102.
231. LiPuma JP, Wellman J, Stern HP. Nitrous oxide abuse: a new cause of pneumomediastinum. *Radiology* 1982;145(3):602.
232. Wagner SA, Clark MA, Wesche DL, et al. Asphyxial deaths from the recreational use of nitrous oxide. *J Forensic Sci* 1992;37(4):1008–1015.
233. Gaede JT, Montine TJ. Massive pulmonary embolus and anabolic steroid abuse. *JAMA* 1992;267(17):2328–2329.
234. Akhter J, Hyder S, Ahmed M. Cerebrovascular accident associated with anabolic steroid use in a young man. *Neurology* 1994;44(12):2405–2406.

SUGGESTED READINGS

Burrows B, Lebowitz MD, Barbee RA, et al. Interactions of smoking and immunologic factors in relation to airways obstruction. *Chest* 1983;84(6):657–661.

U.S. Public Health Service (USPHS). *Surgeon General's report: the health consequences of smoking: nicotine addiction.* Washington, DC: Government Printing Office, 1998.

U.S. Public Health Service (USPHS). *Targeting tobacco use: the nation's leading cause of death.* Washington, DC: Centers for Disease Control and Prevention, 1998.

CHAPTER 76

John C.M. Brust, MD

Neurologic Disorders Related to Alcohol and Other Drug Use

This chapter addresses neurologic complications of alcohol, tobacco, and other drugs (Table 76.1). The neurologic symptoms and signs of acute toxicity and withdrawal differ widely from agent to agent (see Section 5, "Special Issues in Addiction Medicine"). Opioid overdose causes potentially lethal coma, respiratory depression, and miosis, whereas opioid withdrawal causes flulike symptoms that are hardly ever life-threatening. Cocaine overdose causes delirium, often accompanied by seizures, malignant hyperthermia, or fatal cardiac arrhythmia; cocaine withdrawal causes fatigue and depression. With ethanol (alcohol) and barbiturates, either overdose (coma or apnea) or withdrawal (seizures or delirium) can be fatal. Such symptoms—including the possibility that an individual is using more than one agent or even is intoxicated by one agent while simultaneously withdrawing from another—can confound the interpretation of neurologic symptoms and signs in patients who use and abuse alcohol and other drugs (1,2).

TRAUMA

Trauma frequently affects the nervous system, both peripherally and centrally, and its effects can be masked by coexisting intoxication or other neurologic disturbance. People with alcohol dependence are at particular risk of misdiagnosis. They often have thrombocytopenia and abnormalities of clotting factors, and alcohol acutely enhances blood–brain barrier leakage around areas of cerebral trauma (3). Intracranial hemorrhage always must be considered in a patient who drinks alcohol and who has an altered sensorium; spinal cord injury must be considered in one who is unable to walk.

INFECTION

Parenteral users of any drug are subject to an array of local and systemic infections, including abscesses, cellulitis, pneumonia, sepsis, endophthalmitis, osteomyelitis, and pyogenic arthritis (4). The central and peripheral nervous systems often are affected. Endocarditis, bacterial or fungal, leads to meningitis, cerebral infarction, diffuse vasculitis, abscess (intraparenchymal, subdural, or epidural, including the spinal cord), or subarachnoid hemorrhage from rupture of a septic ("mycotic") aneurysm (5,6). Infectious hepatitis can cause encephalopathy or, because of deranged clotting, hemorrhagic stroke. Vertebral osteomyelitis can cause radiculopathy or spinal cord compression. Tetanus, usually severe, is more common after subcutaneous injection of heroin (7). Botulism occurs at injection sites and, among those who snort cocaine, in the nasal sinuses (8). Malaria has affected users of heroin in endemic areas (9).

Even before the AIDS epidemic, it was recognized that individuals who use alcohol to excess and other drugs often are immunosuppressed. Those with alcohol dependence are prone to develop bacterial or tuberculous meningitis, which always must be considered in someone who drinks excessively with seizures or altered mentation, even when the clinical picture suggests intoxication, withdrawal, thiamine deficiency, hepatic encephalopathy, or hypoglycemia (any of which could coexist). Clinicians should have a low threshold for performing a lumbar puncture in someone with alcohol dependence and altered mentation, even in the absence of fever or stiff neck. HIV-seronegative heroin-addicted patients are also at risk for central nervous system (CNS) infection, including agents such as *Candida* or *Mucor*. Parenteral drug

TABLE 76.1 Drugs Associated with Neurologic Complications

Alcohol
Anticholinergics
Hallucinogens
Inhalants
Cannabis (marijuana)
Opiates
Phencyclidine
Psychostimulants
Sedatives-hypnotics
Tobacco

users with AIDS develop the same neurologic complications as do those with other risk factors for AIDS (10). They are at risk for infection with T-cell lymphotrophic retrovirus type I or type II, with consequent myelopathy (11).

SEIZURES

Seizures can be a feature of either drug toxicity (as with psychostimulants) or withdrawal (as with sedatives or ethanol) (12,13). Seizures associated with amphetamine-like psychostimulants, including smokable methamphetamine ("ice"), usually are accompanied by other signs of overdose (e.g., agitation, psychosis, fever, hypertension, cardiac arrhythmia), whereas cocaine-induced seizures often occur without other symptoms and signs (14). The difference may be related to cocaine's local anesthetic properties; procaine and similar agents are epileptogenic. In animals, cocaine produces a "kindling" effect (repeated fixed doses of the drug progressively lower seizure threshold) (15). Seizures usually occur either immediately or within a few hours of cocaine administration. Seizures occurring many hours after use might be related to the proconvulsant properties of the cocaine metabolite, benzoylecgonine (16). Single grand mal seizures are most common; focal seizures suggest underlying cerebral trauma, stroke, or infection. Status epilepticus tends to be refractory to treatment.

Any route of administration can precipitate a seizure, but new-onset seizures most often follow intravenous administration of cocaine hydrochloride or smoking of alkaloidal "crack"; the reason probably is the higher dose and more rapid delivery to the brain these practices permit. A survey of adolescent cocaine users found that seizures occurred in none of the intranasal users, in 1% of occasional crack smokers, and in 9% of heavy crack smokers (17).

Seizures have occurred in infants being breastfed by cocaine-using mothers (18) and in infants and small children who passively inhaled crack smoke (19).

In animals, opiates are either proconvulsant or anticonvulsant, depending on receptor specificity and seizure model (20). Except possibly in newborns exposed *in utero*, seizures are not a feature of opiate withdrawal. Opiate agonists lower the seizure threshold in humans, but seizures are a sufficiently rare feature of heroin overdose that an alternative cause always should be sought (e.g., concomitant cocaine toxicity, ethanol withdrawal, cerebral trauma, or infection). A case-control study found that heroin use, both past and current, was a risk factor for new-onset seizures independent of overdose, head injury, infection, stroke, or use of alcohol or other illicit drugs (20).

Unlike heroin or morphine, meperidine (Demerol) readily causes myoclonus and seizures through the proconvulsant properties of its metabolite, normeperidine (21). Seizures often follow parenteral use of the mixed agonist-antagonist opiate pentazocine (Talwin) when it is combined with the antihistamine tripelennamine ("Ts and blues"); both drugs are epileptogenic (22).

Phencyclidine blocks N-methyl-D-aspartate receptors and thus would be expected to have anticonvulsant properties; however, at high doses (i.e., 1 mg/kg or more), seizures and myoclonus often are encountered (23,24). Such patients are likely to have other signs of severe overdose, including coma with extensor posturing yet open staring eyes, marked hyperthermia, myoglobinuria, respiratory depression, and hypertension progressing to hypotension. In such patients, anticonvulsant medications are but one aspect of overall management.

Seizures are not an expected toxic feature of hallucinogens (e.g., LSD, mescaline, or psilocin/psilocybin), but they can occur following very high doses (25). Seizures can complicate acute intoxication with inhalants (such as glues, solvents, or aerosols); in fact, toxic seizures and hallucinations are features that distinguish intoxication with inhalants from intoxication with alcohol (26). Seizures accompany severe anticholinergic poisoning (27).

In patients with alcohol dependence seizures can be the result of alcohol-related disorders such as head injury, CNS infection, or stroke. Alcohol also can trigger seizures in subjects with preexisting epilepsy. In such cases, seizures tend to occur after a day or a weekend of heavy drinking; whether small amounts of alcohol significantly lower seizure threshold in epileptics—in other words, whether epileptics should avoid alcohol altogether—is controversial.

The term "alcohol-related seizures" (colloquially, "rum fits") refers to seizures in the absence of epilepsy or other predisposing factors (28). Such seizures most often are a withdrawal phenomenon, occurring within 48 hours of the last drink in persons who have used excessive amounts of alcohol chronically or in binges for months or years. The minimal duration of drinking is uncertain, but the risk is dose-related, beginning at only 50 g absolute ethanol daily (29). Such seizures usually are single or occur in a brief cluster; status epilepticus is infrequent. They usually are grand mal without focality, although focal seizures do occur, and an underlying structural lesion (e.g., an old cerebral contusion) is not always identified. Other symptoms of early withdrawal (tremor or hallucinosis) may or may not be present, and a patient with alcohol withdrawal seizures may go on to develop *delirium tremens* (DTs), but seizures rarely are observed after DTs is present.

Alcohol may cause seizures independently of withdrawal or structural brain lesions. In some alcohol-addicted patients, seizures occur during active drinking or more than a week after the last drink, and a case control study of new onset seizures failed to show a clear temporal correlation between seizures and recent abstinence (29). Animal studies indicate that seizures that occur during alcohol withdrawal are of more than one type, with different time courses, phenomenology, and presumed neuronal mechanisms (30). Alcohol blocks glutamate neurotransmission, and upregulation of N-methyl-D-aspartate receptors theoretically could contribute not only to withdrawal symptoms, including seizures, but also could set the stage for excitotoxicity and permanent neuronal damage (31). Consistent with such a view is evidence that the risk of seizures increases with repeated ethanol detoxification (32).

The diagnosis of alcohol-related seizures requires exclusion of other lesions. Brain computed tomography or magnetic resonance imaging is indicated if seizures are of new onset, and lumbar puncture should be performed if meningitis or subarachnoid hemorrhage is suspected. In patients with alcohol-related seizures, the electroencephalogram usually is normal; claims of a high incidence of photomyoclonic or photoconvulsive response during early withdrawal have not been supported by subsequent studies (33).

Because most alcohol-related seizures occur singly or in brief clusters, by the time a patient is seen it is often too late for effective anticonvulsant pharmacotherapy (although such might be indicated if the diagnosis is in doubt). In animals and humans, phenytoin failed to prevent alcohol seizures (34). Given early enough, intravenous lorazepam does decrease the likelihood of recurrent alcohol seizures over the next several hours (35). Treatment of status epilepticus during alcohol withdrawal is conventional; benzodiazepines and phenobarbital have the advantage (compared with phenytoin) of cross-tolerance with ethanol and, thus, efficacy in treating other withdrawal symptoms, including progression to DTs.

Long-term anticonvulsant medication generally is not indicated in patients with alcohol seizures. Abstainers do not need it, and people who drink excessively do not take it.

As with alcohol, seizures in people with barbiturate dependence occur most often as a withdrawal phenomenon. In a study with volunteers, abrupt withdrawal from oral pentobarbital (Nembutal) or secobarbital (Seconal) that had been taken in a daily dose for several months produced paroxysmal electroencephalographic changes without symptoms in one third of the subjects. Withdrawal from 600 mg/day caused minor symptoms in one half the subjects and a seizure in 10%. Withdrawal from 900 mg or more per day caused seizures in 75% and delirium in 65% (36).

Symptoms after benzodiazepine withdrawal can be difficult to differentiate from those for which the drug was being taken in the first place, but seizures have been reported (37). Also described are paradoxical toxic reactions featuring agitation, hallucinations and, in some cases, seizures (38). Seizures as a toxic effect are described with methaqualone (which sometimes is combined with an antihistamine) and with glutethimide (which has anticholinergic properties) (39). Notorious as a "date-rape drug" is the sedative gamma-hydroxybutyric acid; so are the gamma-hydroxybutyric acid precursors gamma-butyryl-lactone and 1,4-butanediol. An alcohol-like withdrawal syndrome can include seizures, that, however, are also described during overdose (40).

A case-control study found that marijuana was protective against the development of new onset seizures. In animals, the nonpsychoactive cannabinoid compound cannabidiol is anticonvulsant, and limited studies suggest that it can reduce seizure frequency in humans with epilepsy (20).

STROKE

The evidence that alcohol and tobacco are risk factors for stroke is epidemiologic. The evidence that illicit drugs are risk factors for stroke is mostly anecdotal (1).

Systemic complications of parenteral drug abuse, such as hepatitis, endocarditis, or AIDS, predispose to stroke. Heroin nephropathy causes uremia, hypertension, bleeding, and hemorrhagic stroke. Taken parenterally or, in a few cases, sniffed, heroin has caused ischemic stroke in the absence of intermediary conditions or other evident risk factors (41,42). In some reported cases, angiographic changes were consistent with cerebral vasculitis, and laboratory abnormalities (such as blood eosinophilia, hypergammaglobulinemia, and positive Coombs test) suggested hypersensitivity. Other possible mechanisms are systemic hypotension after overdose and embolization of injected foreign material. Intracerebral hemorrhage occurred in a young adult within minutes of intravenous heroin use (43).

During the 1980s, pentazocine (Talwin) combined with tripelennamine (Pyribenzamine) was widely abused in midwestern cities in the United States. Crushed oral tablets were injected intravenously, and cerebral infarcts and hemorrhages were a frequent complication. It is likely that the particulate foreign material passed through secondary pulmonary arteriovenous shunts (22).

Heroin myelopathy may be vascular in origin (44). Acute paraparesis, sensory loss, and urinary retention most often occur shortly after injection and sometimes after a period of abstinence. In some cases, preserved proprioception suggests infarction in the territory of the anterior spinal artery; occasionally symptoms are present in the patient awakening from coma, suggesting "border-zone" infarction secondary to hypotension. In one case, cord biopsy revealed vasculitis (45).

Users of amphetamine-like drugs (especially methamphetamine) are subject to intracerebral hemorrhage, often associated with acute hypertension and fever; routes of administration have been oral, intravenous, or nasal. Hemorrhagic stroke has occurred both in chronic users and after first exposure (1). In some cases, cerebral angiography was consistent with vasculitis, which, in a few instances, was verified at autopsy.

Amphetamine-induced vasculitis, which causes ischemic stroke, appears to be of more than one type. In one report, systemic and CNS necrotizing vasculitis resembled polyarteritis nodosa (46). In other reports, ischemic stroke appeared to be secondary to small-vessel hypersensitivity angiitis. Although some of these cases were based on nonspecific angiographic "beading," cerebral vasculitis was demonstrated in animals receiving repeated doses of methamphetamine over weeks or months (47).

After a case-control study that demonstrated increased risk for hemorrhagic stroke in women using diet preparations containing phenylpropanolamine, the U.S. Food and Drug Administration banned products containing this amphetamine-like psychostimulant (48). Similar association led to a ban on "dietary supplements" containing ephedra ("ma huang") (49).

Intravenous and inadvertent carotid artery injection of crushed methylphenidate (Ritalin) tablets has resulted in ischemic stroke, and foreign body emboli have been found in the brain (50). Angiographic changes suggestive of arteritis were seen in a child who had an ischemic stroke while taking methylphenidate orally for attention deficit/hyperactivity disorder (51).

The designer drug methylenedioxymethamphetamine (MDMA, "Ecstasy") is often used in the setting of "rave" parties, at which frenetic dancing continues for hours at a time. Hypertensive crisis, severe hyperthermia, and both ischemic and hemorrhagic stroke have been reported (52).

Stroke in cocaine users may be secondary to drug-induced cardiac arrhythmia, myocardial infarction, or cardiomyopathy. In many cases, however, cardiac disease, infection, or other risk factors are not evident (53). More than 700 cases of cocaine-related stroke have been reported, about half ischemic and half hemorrhagic. Strokes have followed nasal or parenteral administration of cocaine hydrochloride or smoking of alkaloidal "crack" (54). Ischemic strokes include transient ischemic attacks and infarction of the cerebrum, thalamus, brain stem, spinal cord, and retina. Of patients with hemorrhagic stroke who underwent cerebral angiography, about half harbored saccular aneurysms or vascular malformations. A plausible mechanism for hemorrhagic stroke is surges of systemic hypertension. Alternatively, some ischemic strokes may be the result of direct cerebral vasoconstriction induced by the drug. A study using magnetic resonance angiography in volunteers demonstrated such vasoconstriction during cocaine administration (55). Most autopsies have not shown vasculitis; when present, it consisted of round cell infiltration without vessel wall necrosis. A contributing factor may be cocaine's effects on platelets and clotting factors and the ability of cocaine to accelerate atherosclerosis (1).

LSD, an ergot drug, directly constricts systemic and cerebral arteries, and ischemic stroke has followed ingestion (56).

Phencyclidine causes acute systemic hypertension, which, like the drug's mental effects, can last hours or days. Cerebral infarction, intracerebral and subarachnoid hemorrhage, and hypertensive encephalopathy have followed use of phencyclidine (1,57).

The role of ethanol in stroke is complex. As with coronary artery disease, epidemiologic studies suggest that low-to-moderate doses of ethanol decrease stroke risk, whereas higher amounts increase it. Not surprisingly, reports have been inconsistent. A case control study in New York City found that two drinks per day were protective against ischemic stroke, with a protective trend continuing up to five drinks, but that doses in excess of five drinks per day increased risk. These relationships held for young and old subjects; for whites, African Americans, and Hispanics; and for wine, beer, and spirits (58). In 2003, a meta-analysis of 19 cohort studies and 16 case-control studies found a "J-shaped" association between ethanol consumption and the relative risk of ischemic stroke: consumption of <12 to 24 g/day of ethanol reduced the risk of ischemic stroke (relative risk: 0.72), whereas consumption of more than 60 g/day increased the risk of both ischemic stroke (relative risk: 1.69) and hemorrhagic stroke (relative risk: 2.18). Light-to-moderate ethanol intake did not reduce the risk of hemorrhagic stroke (59).

Possible contributors to the increased risk of occlusive stroke in heavy drinkers include alcohol-related cardiac disease, alcohol-induced hypertension, increased platelet aggregation, acceleration of the clotting cascade, decreased fibrinolysis, direct cerebral vasoconstriction, hemoconcentration, and hyperhomocystinemia secondary to folate deficiency. Protection against ischemic stroke may be related to decreased low-density lipoproteins and increased high-density lipoproteins, increased prostacyclin, decreased platelet aggregation, and decreased fibrinogen levels (1,58).

Tobacco is a major risk factor for both coronary artery and peripheral vascular disease, and case control and cohort studies show that it is a risk factor for ischemic and hemorrhagic stroke as well (1,60–62). Among women smokers, the risk of both ischemic and hemorrhagic stroke is greater in those who take oral contraceptives (63). Risk of stroke decreases, but does not disappear with cessation of smoking.

Possible mechanisms of tobacco's role in stroke include acceleration of atherosclerosis, reductions in oxygen-carrying capacity because of carbon monoxide in tobacco smoke, nicotine-induced endothelial damage, acute elevations of blood pressure and acceleration of chronic hypertension, elevated blood fibrinogen levels, elevated hemoglobin, increased platelet reactivity, and inhibition of prostacyclin formation (1,64).

Anabolic steroids potentiate platelet aggregation, alter fibrinogen, stimulate erythropoietin, and increase systolic blood pressure; strokes have been reported in young athletes using them (65).

ALTERED MENTATION

Excessive alcohol users are at high risk of lasting cognitive impairment through multiple mechanisms that can coexist in the same patient. Head trauma, CNS infection, and hypoglycemia can leave dementia in their wake, while alcoholic liver disease can cause encephalopathy. Nutritional deficiency can result in Wernicke-Korsakoff disease and pellagra.

Wernicke-Korsakoff disease is caused by thiamine deficiency, which, because body stores are limited, can occur after only a few weeks of inadequate intake. In the acute syndrome, mental symptoms evolve over days or weeks to a "global confusional state," with varying degrees of lethargy, inattentiveness, abulia, and impaired memory (66). Usually, but not invariably, present are abnormal eye movements (nystagmus and abduction or horizontal gaze paresis progressing to complete ophthalmoplegia) and ataxic gait (both cerebellar and vestibular in origin), progressing to inability to stand unaided. Without treatment, there is a progression to coma and death and, pathologically, there are histologically distinct lesions in the medial thalamus and hypothalamus, the periaqueductal gray matter of the midbrain, and the periventricular areas of the pons and medulla. With early treatment (intravenous thiamine and multivitamins), recovery begins within hours or days and can be complete, but if treatment is delayed, the mental symptoms evolve into Korsakoff syndrome, an irreversible disorder in which the predominant abnormality is impaired memory, with inability to store or retrieve recent information, varying degrees of retrograde amnesia, and, especially acutely, a tendency to confabulate. Residual nystagmus and gait ataxia also may be present.

Pellagra, caused by nicotinic acid deficiency, consists of skin rash, gastrointestinal lesions (stomatitis and enteritis, with nausea, vomiting, and diarrhea), and mental symptoms, including irritability, insomnia, impaired memory, delusions, hallucinations, dementia, or delirium (67). Untreated pellagra is fatal. With prompt nicotinic acid replacement, recovery can occur over hours or days.

Marchiafava-Bignami disease consists of demyelinating lesions in the corpus callosum and progressive neurologic symptoms, often ending fatally within a few months. Specifically associated with alcoholism, Marchiafava-Bignami disease is rare, and its pathophysiology is unclear. Mental symptoms predominate, with depression, mania, paranoia, and dementia. Seizures are common, and hemiparesis, aphasia, dyskinesia, and ataxia are variably present. The callosal lesions do not explain the devastating neurologic deterioration.

"Alcoholic dementia" refers to progressive mental decline in people with alcohol dependence without apparent cause, nutritional or otherwise (68). Many with alcohol dependence have mental impairment more gradual in onset and more "global" than would be expected with Korsakoff syndrome. Prior episodes of Wernicke syndrome are not identified, and more than memory is affected. Enlarged cerebral ventricles and sulci often are seen on computed tomography or magnetic resonance imaging in people with alcohol dependence, in some reports correlating with cognitive decline and improving with abstinence. Animal studies using pair-fed controls have shown both behavioral and morphologic abnormalities in nutritionally maintained rodents who received chronic ethanol. Changes include loss of dendritic spines and neurons in the hippocampus.

Neuropathologic studies of humans with alcohol dependence without evidence of nutritional deficiency describe neuronal loss in selective regions of brain, especially the superior frontal association cortex (i.e., a pattern unlike that of Wernicke-Korsakoff disease). A study using magnetic resonance spectroscopy and N-acetyl-aspartate confirmed the vulnerability of this region (69). Investigators have correlated frontal lobe damage with particular cognitive or behavioral abnormalities (e.g., difficulty planning, problem solving, and abstracting, as well as disinhibition and lack of insight) (70).

The detrimental effects of alcohol on cognition are dose-related; a review of 19 studies found that 5 or 6 "standard U.S. drinks" daily resulted in "cognitive inefficiencies," whereas 10 or more drinks daily caused serious cognitive impairment (71). On the other hand, numerous epidemiologic studies have shown that mild-to-moderate alcohol intake, compared with abstinence, *reduces* the risk of developing dementia (72). Alcohol's effects on cognition thus follow a J-shaped curve similar to its effects on ischemic cerebrovascular disease, but reducing the likelihood of ischemic stroke does not fully explain the cognitive benefits, which might be related to antioxidant properties of alcoholic beverages (73).

People who use illicit drugs are at risk for altered mentation by indirect mechanisms, including head trauma, infection (especially AIDS), malnutrition, and concomitant alcohol abuse. It is less clear that the drugs themselves cause lasting cognitive or behavioral change. Predrug mental status usually is uncertain, and many people who use drugs are self-medicating preexisting psychiatric conditions (as by using cocaine for depression). People with heroin dependence and tolerance tend to be depressed, irritable, and socially withdrawn, but experience with methadone maintenance treatment shows that the great majority of such patients have normal mental function.

Acute and chronic paranoia are features of psychostimulant abuse; withdrawal depression with stimulants can last for months. However, claims of permanent depression in psychostimulant users (resulting from damage to the dopaminergic mesolimbic "reward circuit") are unproven. Dextroamphetamine damages dopaminergic nerve terminals, MDMA (Ecstasy) damages serotonergic nerve terminals, and methamphetamine damages both dopaminergic and serotonergic nerve terminals. The reversibility of such damage is controversial, as is its correlation with cognitive dysfunction, which is well-documented in users of these psychostimulants (1,74,75). Although lasting cognitive impairment is also described in heavy cocaine users, that drug does not directly damage nerve terminals. Widespread microvascular lesions might contribute to the cognitive dysfunction (76).

Early reports of an "antimotivational syndrome" in cannabis users were not confirmed by later studies. Rigorous neurologic assessment, however, has revealed persistent, if subtle, cognitive impairment in heavy users (77,78). Marijuana use during childhood or adolescence has been implicated as a risk factor for schizophrenia (79).

Sedatives, especially barbiturates, can produce mental clouding or paradoxical hyperactivity in older adults (80). In small children, barbiturates have deleterious effects on IQ; whether these resolve over time is uncertain.

Hallucinogens can produce prolonged adverse reactions, and some users experience flashbacks (the recurrence, days or weeks later, of the drug's original psychic effects in the absence of further drug use). However, it is doubtful that hallucinogens cause permanent cognitive alteration.

Among inhalants, the substance most clearly associated with CNS damage is toluene, which is found in many solvents, paints, and glues. White matter lesions can result in dementia, often accompanied by pyramidal, cerebellar, and oculomotor signs (81). Sniffers of gasoline containing tetraethyl lead have developed lead encephalopathy (82).

Acutely, phencyclidine produces schizophrenia-like symptoms, both positive (agitation, paranoia, delusions, or hallucinations) and negative (autism, loss of ego boundaries, avolition, or catatonia). Permanent neuropsychiatric change has been claimed (83).

MUSCLE, NERVE, AND SPINAL CORD

Acute rhabdomyolysis with myoglobinuria and renal failure has followed use of heroin, methamphetamine, cocaine, or phencyclidine either as a feature of overdose or without other evidence of toxicity (84). In people with alcohol dependence myopathy may consist of asymptomatic elevation of serum creatine kinase, progressive proximal weakness resembling polymyositis, or acute rhabdomyolysis with myoglobinuria. The cause is toxic, not nutritional. Cardiomyopathy may be present (85).

Sensorimotor polyneuropathy is common in people with alcohol dependence. Paresthesias usually begin in the feet and, with progression, may be accompanied by sensory loss and weakness affecting the four limbs, with severe burning pain in the feet. Autonomic symptoms and signs sometimes appear. The cause is both nutritional deficiency and alcohol neurotoxicity. Thiamine deficiency in people who do not drink alcohol produces motor-dominant, rapidly progressive neuropathy affecting predominantly large fibers. Alcoholism without thiamine deficiency produces sensory-dominant, painful, slowly progressive neuropathy affecting predominantly small fibers (86). Most people with alcoholism who have polyneuropathy have a combination of both types. The primary damage is axonal, and so electrodiagnostic studies usually show only mildly reduced nerve conduction velocities, a nonspecific finding. Abstinence and nutritional replenishment are likely to be followed by clinical improvement, although mild distal sensory loss (especially vibratory sensation) can be persistent.

People with alcoholism are subject to pressure palsies from sleeping soundly in unusual positions. Radial nerve palsy with wrist drop and peroneal nerve palsy with foot drop are most common.

Guillain-Barré polyneuropathy and brachial and lumbosacral plexopathy, probably immune-mediated, are described in heroin users (87). Brachial plexopathy has resulted from compression by septic ("mycotic") aneurysm of the subclavian artery. Peripheral nerve injuries follow direct injection of any drug.

"Glue-sniffers' neuropathy" is a severe sensorimotor polyneuropathy that affects users of products containing n-hexane. Quadriplegia can evolve over a few weeks, with incomplete improvement after abstinence (88). Pathologically, axons are distended by masses of neurofilaments, and secondary demyelination occurs.

Nitrous oxide oxidizes cobalamin, and sniffers of nitrous oxide develop a myeloneuropathy that is clinically indistinguishable from combined systems disease. The earliest symptoms usually are paresthesias in the feet and unsteady gait secondary to impaired proprioception. Anemia usually is absent, and serum cobalamin levels generally are normal (89).

OTHER COMPLICATIONS

Severe irreversible parkinsonism developed in a group of drug users in California who were exposed to a meperidine analogue contaminated with 1-methyl-4-phenyl-1,2,3,6-tetrahydropyridine, a metabolite of which is toxic to neurons in the substantial nigra. Levodopa relieved the symptoms, which in some cases were of life-threatening severity, but treatment had to be continued indefinitely, and levodopa-induced dyskinesias were common (90). Positron emission tomography (using 18-F-dopa) of exposed but asymptomatic subjects showed decreased numbers of dopamine-containing neurons, and delayed parkinsonism has developed in previously asymptomatic subjects who used small doses of the drug (91).

Inhaling the vapor of heroin heated on metal foil ("chasing the dragon") resulted in cerebral and cerebellar spongiform leukoencephalopathy in European and North American users. Dementia, ataxia, quadriparesis, and blindness frequently progressed to death, and survivors were left with neurologic residua. The nature of the toxicity is unknown; elevated lactate in the damaged white matter suggests mitochondrial dysfunction (92).

Impaired vision with optic atrophy is common in individuals with alcohol dependence. The optic nerve lesions are mainly the result of nutritional deficiency, but the particular deficiency is uncertain, as are the possible toxicities of alcohol itself and of cyanide in tobacco smoke (93).

Cerebellar degeneration can occur in nutritionally deficient people with alcoholism in the absence of Wernicke-Korsakoff syndrome. The superior cerebellar vermis is preferentially affected, resulting in gait and sometimes leg ataxia, usually without ataxia of the arms or dysarthria (94). As with other central and peripheral nerve complications of alcoholism, both nutritional deficiency and alcohol toxicity are probably contributory. With abstinence and nutritional replenishment improvement is likely, albeit usually incomplete.

Central pontine myelinolysis after overvigorous correction of hyponatremia occurs in both people with alcohol dependence and nondrinkers. Most severely affecting the pontine base, central pontine myelinolysis can cause quadriparesis progressing to locked-in syndrome. Most extensive demyelination can impair consciousness. Extra-pontine myelinolysis can cause ataxia, abnormal behavior, or movement disorders. Lesions can be identified by magnetic resonance imaging, including diffusion-weighted imaging (95).

A man who took large doses of a heroin mixture containing quinine developed blindness. Vision improved when he resumed using heroin without quinine (96).

Chronic cocaine users can develop dystonia or chorea that outlasts drug use by days or weeks, and cocaine can precipitate symptoms in patients with Tourette syndrome (97).

REFERENCES

1. Brust JCM. *Neurological aspects of substance abuse*, 2nd ed. Boston, MA: Butterworth-Heinemann, 2004.
2. Goldfrank LR, Flomenbaum NE, Lewin NA, et al., eds. *Goldfrank's toxicologic emergencies*, 6th ed. Stamford, CT: Appleton, Lange, 1998.
3. Halt PS, Swanson RA, Faden AI.1992; Alcohol exacerbates behavioral and neurochemical effects of rat spinal cord trauma. *Arch Neurol* 49:1178–1184.
4. Richter RW. Infections other than AIDS. *Neurol Clin* 1993;11:591–603.
5. Brust JCM, Dickinson PCT, Hughes JEO, et al. The diagnosis and treatment of cerebral mycotic aneurysms. *Ann Neurol* 1990;27:238–246.

6. Marantz PR, Linzer M, Feiner CJ. Inability to predict diagnosis in febrile intravenous drug abusers. *Ann Intern Med* 1987;106:823–828.
7. Brust JCM, Richter RW. Tetanus in the inner city. *N Y State J Med* 1974;74:1735–1742.
8. Kudrow DB, Henry DA, Haake DA, et al. Botulism associated with Clostridium botulinum sinusitis after intranasal cocaine use. *Ann Intern Med* 1988;109:984–985.
9. Gonzalez-Garcia JJ, Arnalich F, Pena JM, et al. An outbreak of Plasmodium vivax malaria among heroin users in Spain. *Trans Roy Soc Trop Med Hygiene* 1986;80:549–552.
10. Malouf R, Jacquette G, Dobkin J, et al. Neurologic disease in human immunodeficiency virus-infected drug abusers. *Arch Neurol* 1990;47: 1002–1007.
11. Jacobson S, Lehky T, Nishimura M, et al. Isolation of HTLV-II from a patient with chronic, progressive neurological disease clinically indistinguishable from HTLV-I associated myelopathy/tropical spastic paraparesis. *Ann Neurol* 1993;33:392–396.
12. Earnest MP. Seizures. *Neurol Clin* 1993;11:563–575.
13. Alldredge BK, Lowenstein DH, Simon RP. Seizures associated with recreational drug abuse. *Neurology* 1989;30:1037–1039.
14. Pascual-Leone A, Dhuna A, Altafullah I, et al. Cocaine-induced seizures. *Neurology* 1990;40:404–407.
15. Karler R, Petty C, Calder L, et al. Proconvulsant and anticonvulsant effects in mice of acute and chronic treatment with cocaine. *Neuropharmacology* 1989;28:709–714.
16. Konkol RJ, Erickson BA, Doerr JK, et al. Seizures induced by the cocaine metabolite benzoylecgonine in rats. *Epilepsia* 1992;33:420–427.
17. Schwartz RH, Luxenberg MG, Hoffman NG. Crack use by American middle-class adolescent polydrug abusers. *J Pediatrics* 1991;118:150–155.
18. Chaney NE, Franke J, Wadlington WB. Cocaine convulsions in a breast-feeding baby. *J Pediatr* 1988;112:134–135.
19. Bateman DA, Heagarty MC. Passive freebase cocaine ("crack") inhalation by infants and toddlers. *Am J Dis Child* 1989;143:25–27.
20. Ng SKC, Brust JCM, Hauser WA, et al. Illicit drug use and the risk of new onset seizures. *Am J Epidemiol* 1990;132:47–57.
21. Hershey LA. Meperidine and central neurotoxicity. *Ann Intern Med* 1983;98:548–549.
22. Caplan LR, Thomas C, Banks G. Central nervous system complications of addiction to "T's and blues." *Neurology* 1982;32:623–628.
23. McCarron MM, Schultze BW, Thompson GA, et al. Acute phencyclidine intoxication: incidence of clinical findings in 1,000 cases. *Ann Emerg Med* 1981;10:237–242.
24. McCarron MM, Schultze BW, Thompson GA. Acute phencyclidine intoxication: clinical patterns, complications, and treatment. *Ann Emerg Med* 1981;10:290–297.
25. Fisher D, Ungerleider J. Grand mal seizures following ingestion of LSD. *Calif Med* 1967;106:210–211.
26. Morton HG. Occurrence and treatment of solvent abuse in children and adolescents. *Pharmacol Therap* 1987;33:449–469.
27. Mikolich JR, Paulson GW, Cross CJ. Acute anticholinergic syndrome due to jimson seed ingestion. *Ann Intern Med* 1975;83:321–325.
28. Hauser WA, Ng SKC, Brust JCM. Alcohol, seizures, and epilepsy. *Epilepsia* 1988;29(Suppl 2):S66–S78.
29. Ng SKC, Hauser WA, Brust JCM, et al. Alcohol consumption and withdrawal in new-onset seizures. *N Engl J Med* 1988;319:666–673.
30. Gonzalez LP, Czachura JF, Brewer KW. Spontaneous versus elicited seizures following ethanol withdrawal: differential time course. *Alcohol* 1989;6:481–487.
31. Tsai G, Gastfriend DR, Coyle JT. The glutamatergic basis of human alcoholism. *Am J Psychiatry* 1995;152:332–340.
32. Lechtenberg R, Worner TM. Seizure risk with recurrent alcohol detoxification. *Arch Neurol* 1990;47:535–538.
33. Fisch BJ, Hauser WA, Brust JCM, et al. The EEG response to diffuse and patterned photic stimulation during acute untreated alcohol withdrawal. *Neurology* 1989;39:434–436.
34. Alldredge BK, Lowenstein DH, Simon RP. A placebo-controlled trial of intravenous diphenylhydantoin for the short-term treatment of alcohol withdrawal seizures. *Am J Med* 1989;87:645–648.
35. D'Onofrio G, Rathlev NK, Ulrich AS, et al. Lorazepam for the prevention of recurrent alcohol withdrawal seizures. *Ann Emerg Med* 1994; 23:513–518.
36. Fraser HF, Wikler A, Essig CG, et al. Degree of physical dependence induced by secobarbital or pentobarbital. *JAMA* 1958;166:126–129.
37. Fialip J, Aumaitre O, Eschalier A, et al. Benzodiazepine withdrawal seizures. Analysis of 48 case reports. *Clin Neuropharmacol* 1987;10:538–544.
38. Fouilladieu J-L, D'Engert J, Conseiller C. Benzodiazepines. *N Engl J Med* 1984;310:464.
39. Hoaken PCS. Adverse effects of methaqualone. *Can Med Assoc J* 1975;112:685.
40. Snead OC, Gibson KM. Gamma-hydroxybutyric acid. *N Engl J Med* 2005;352:2721–2732.
41. Brust JCM, Richter RW. Stroke associated with addiction to heroin. *J Neurol Neurosurg Psychiatry* 1976;39:194–199.
42. Bartolomei F, Nicoli F, Swaider L, et al. Accident vasculaire cerebral ischemique après prise nasale d'heroine. Une nouvelle observation. *Presse Med* 1992;21:983–986.
43. Knoblauch AL, Buchholz M, Koller MG, et al. Hemiplegie nach injektion von heroin. *Schw Med Wochenschr* 1983;113:402–406.
44. Goodhart LC, Loizou LA, Anderson M. Heroin myelopathy. *J Neurol Neurosurg Psychiatry* 1982;45:562–563.
45. Judice DJ, LeBlanc HJ, McGarry PA. Spinal cord vasculitis presenting as spinal cord tumor in a heroin addict. *J Neurosurg* 1978;48:131–134.
46. Citron BO, Halpern M, McCarron M, et al. Necrotizing angiitis associated with drug abuse. *N Engl J Med* 1970;283:1003–1011.
47. Brust JCM. Vasculitis owing to substance abuse. *Neurol Clin* 1997; 15:945–957.
48. Kernan WN, Viscoli CM, Brass LM, et al. Phenylpropanolamine and the risk of hemorrhagic stroke. *N Engl J Med* 2000;343:1826–1832.
49. Morgenstern LB, Viscoli CM, et al. Use of Ephedra-containing products and risk for hemorrhagic stroke. *Neurology* 2003;60:132–135.
50. Mizutami T, Lewis R, Gonatas N. Medial medullary syndrome in a drug abuser. *Arch Neurol* 1980;37:425–428.
51. Trugman JM. Cerebral arteritis and oral methylphenidate. *Lancet* 1988;1:584–585.
52. Schifano F, Oyefeso A, Webb L, et al. Review of deaths related to taking ecstasy, England and Wales, 1997–2000. *BMJ* 2003;326:80–81.
53. Sloan MA, Kittner SJ, Feeser BR, et al. Illicit drug-associated ischemic stroke in the Baltimore-Washington Stroke Study. *Neurology* 1998;50:1688–1698.
54. Levine SR, Brust JCM, Futrell N, et al. Cerebrovascular complications of the use of the "crack" form of alkaloidal cocaine. *N Engl J Med* 31990;23:699–704.
55. Kaufman MJ, Levin JM, Ross MH, et al. Cocaine-induced vasoconstriction detected in humans with magnetic resonance angiography. *JAMA* 1998;279:375–381.
56. Lieberman AN, Bloom W, Kishore PS, et al. Carotid artery occlusion following ingestion of LSD. *Stroke* 1974;5:213–215.
57. Eastman JW, Cohen SN. Hypertensive crisis and death associated with phencyclidine poisoning. *JAMA* 1975;231:1270–1271.
58. Sacco RL, Elkind M, Boden-Albala B, et al. The protective effect of moderate alcohol consumption on ischemic stroke. *JAMA* 1999;281:53–60.
59. Reynolds K, Lewis LB, Nolen JDL, et al. Alcohol consumption and the risk of stroke. A meta-analysis. *JAMA* 2003;289:579–588.
60. Kurth T, Kase CS, Berger K, et al. Smoking and the risk of hemorrhagic stroke in men. *Stroke* 2003;34:1151–1155.
61. Kurth T, Kase CS, Berger K, et al. Smoking and risk of hemorrhagic stroke in women. *Stroke* 2003;34:2792–2795.
62. Anderson CS, Feigin V, Bennett D, et al. Active and passive smoking and the risk of subarachnoid hemorrhage. An international population-based case-control study. *Stroke* 2004;35:633–637.
63. Goldbaum GM, Kendrick JS, Hogelin GC, et al. The relative impact of smoking and oral contraceptive use on women in the United States. *JAMA* 1987;258:1339–1342.
64. Brust JCM. Stroke and substance abuse. In: Mohr JP, Choi DW, Grotta JC, et al., eds. *Stroke: pathophysiology, diagnosis, and management,* 3rd ed. New York: Churchill-Livingstone, 2004:725–746.

65. Frenchick BS. Are androgenic steroids thrombogenic? *N Engl J Med* 1990;322:476.
66. Victor M, Adams RD, Collins GH. *The Wernicke-Korsakoff syndrome,* 2nd ed. Philadelphia, PA: F. A. Davis, 1989.
67. Serdau M, Hausser-Hauw C, Laplane D. The clinical spectrum of alcoholic pellagra encephalopathy. *Brain* 1988;111:829–842.
68. Brust JCM. Ethanol. In: Spencer PS, Schaumburg HH, eds. *Experimental and clinical neurotoxicology,* 2nd ed. Baltimore, MD: Williams, Wilkins, 2000:541–557.
69. Schweinsburg BC, Taylor MJ, Alhassoon OM, et al. Clinical pathology in brain white matter of recently detoxified alcoholics: a 1-H magnetic spectroscopy investigation of alcohol associated frontal lobe injury. *Alcohol Clin Exp Res* 2001;25:924–934.
70. Brun A, Anderson J. Frontal dysfunction and frontal cortical synapse loss in alcoholism—the main cause of alcohol dementia. *Dementia Ger Cog Disord* 2001;12:289–294.
71. Parsons OA, Nixon SJ. Cognitive functioning in sober social drinkers: a review of research since 1986. *J Stud Alcohol* 1998;59:180–190.
72. Mukamal KJ, Kuller LH, Fitzpatrick AI, et al. Prospective study of alcohol consumption and risk of dementia in older adults. *JAMA* 2003;289: 1405–1413.
73. Brust JCM. Wine, flavanoids, and the "water of life." *Neurology* 2002;59: 1300–1301.
74. Barr AM, Panenka WJ, MacEwan W. The need for speed: an update on methamphetamine addiction. *J Psychiatr Neurosci* 2006;31:301–313.
75. Schilt T, deWin MML, Koeter M, et al. Cognition in novice ecstasy users with minimal exposure to other drugs: a prospective cohort study. *Arch Gen Psychiatry* 2007;64:728–736.
76. Lim KO, Choi SJ, Pomara N, et al. Reduced frontal white matter integrity in cocaine dependence: a controlled diffusion tensor imaging study. *Biol Psychiatry* 2002;51:890–895.
77. Fried PA, Watkinson B, James D, et al. Current and former marijuana use: preliminary findings in a longitudinal study of effects on IQ in young adults. *Can Med Assoc J* 2002;166:887–891.
78. Bolla KI, Brown K, Eldreth D, et al. Dose-related neurocognitive effects of marijuana use. *Neurology* 2002;59:1337–1343.
79. Linszen D, van Amelsvoort. Cannabis and psychosis: an update on course and biological plausible mechanisms. *Curr Opin Psychiatry* 2007;20:116–120.
80. Maytal J, Shinnar S. Barbiturates. In: Spencer PA, Schaumburg HH, eds. *Experimental and clinical neurotoxicology,* 2nd ed. New York: Oxford University Press, 2000:219–225.
81. Filley CM, Heaton RK, Rosenberg NV. White matter dementia in chronic toluene abuse. *Neurology* 1990;40:532–534.
82. Valpey R, Sumi S, Copass MK, et al. Acute and chronic progressive encephalopathy due to gasoline sniffing. *Neurology* 1978;28: 507–510.
83. Fauman B, Aldinger G, Fauman M. Psychiatric sequelae of phencyclidine abuse. *Clin Toxicol* 1976;9:529–538.
84. Richards JR. Rhabdomyolysis and drugs of abuse. *J Emerg Med* 2000; 19:51–56.
85. Fernandez-Sola J, Grav Junyent JM, Urbana-Marquez A. Alcoholic myopathies. *Curr Opin Neurol* 1996;9:400.
86. Koike H, Iijima M, Sugiura M, et al. Alcoholic neuropathy is clinicopathologically distinct from thiamine-deficiency neuropathy. *Ann Neurol* 2003;54:19–29.
87. Dabby R, Djaldetti R, Gilad R, et al. Acute heroin-related neuropathy. *J Periph Nerv Syst* 2006;11:304–309.
88. Pastore C, Izura V, Marheunda D, et al. Partial conduction blocks in N-hexane neuropathy. *Muscle Nerve* 2002;26:132–135.
89. Heyer EJ, Simpson DM, Bodis-Wollner I, et al. Nitrous oxide: clinical and electrophysiological investigation of neurologic complications. *Neurology* 1986;36:1618–1622.
90. Langston JW. MPTP and Parkinson's disease. *Trends Neurosci* 1985;8: 79–83.
91. Calne DB, Langston JW, Stoessl AJ, et al. Positron emission tomography after MPTP. Observations relating to the cause of Parkinson's disease. *Nature* 1986;317:246–248.
92. Kriegstein AR, Shungu DC, Millar WS, et al. Leukoencephalopathy and raised brain lactate from heroin vapor inhalation ("chasing the dragon"). *Neurology* 1999;53:1765–1773.
93. Carroll FD. The etiology and treatment of tobacco-alcohol amblyopia. *Am J Ophthalmol* 1944;27:713–725.
94. Victor M, Adams RD, Mancall EL. A restricted form of cerebellar cortical degeneration occurring in alcoholic patients. *Arch Neurol* 1959;1: 579–688.
95. Uchino A, Yuzuriha T, Murakami M, et al. Magnetic resonance imaging of sequelae of central pontine myelinolysis in chronic alcohol abusers. *Neuroradiology* 2003;45:877–880.
96. Brust JCM, Richter RW. Quinine amblyopia related to heroin addiction. *Ann Intern Med* 1974;74:84–86.
97. Factor SA, Sanchez-Ramos JR, Wiener WJ. Cocaine and Tourette's syndrome. *Ann Neurol* 1988;23:423–424.

CHAPTER 77

Carol A. Sulis, MD

HIV, TB, and Other Infectious Diseases Related to Alcohol and Other Drug Use

Infectious diseases are common complications of alcohol and other drug abuse (1–4). Infections can occur because of a breach in host defenses while a patient is intoxicated, by direct inoculation of bloodborne or environmental pathogens during injection drug use, or as the result of unsafe behaviors. Acute infection accounts for 60% of hospital admissions among injection drug users (referred to as IDUs in this chapter) in the United States each year and complicates a substantial proportion of hospital admissions among others who use drugs (5–8). Cellulitis, cutaneous abscesses, endocarditis, hepatitis, pneumonia, and tuberculosis have been common problems for people who use drugs for decades; malaria, wound botulism, and tetanus have become exceedingly rare; and the acquired immunodeficiency syndrome (AIDS) and infection with type II human T-cell lymphotropic virus (HTLV-II) are relative newcomers.

The two greatest challenges for the clinician are (1) to differentiate the occult or incipient infection from symptoms of intoxication or withdrawal and (2) to recognize an atypical presentation of an infection modified by defective host defenses (splenectomy or AIDS) or the patient's self-medication with antibiotics or analgesics.

This chapter focuses on common infectious consequences of alcohol or other drug abuse. Standard texts and review articles should be consulted for detailed descriptions of the epidemiology, pathophysiology, clinical presentation, and management of infectious disorders.

HOST DEFENSES

Among IDUs, breach of local skin and mucosal barriers by the repeated injection of nonsterile materials and colonization with resistant organisms appears to be more important than deficiencies in phagocytic function or antibody response. Such repeated, nonspecific stimulation of the immune system leads to polyclonal elevation of immunoglobulin, which, in turn, can cause diagnostic confusion in caring for the patient who develops autoantibodies such as rheumatoid factor or who has a biologic false-positive test for syphilis or hepatitis C. Opioids appear to directly modulate immune response, though the magnitude of the effect and the clinical consequences remain uncertain (9–14).

Smokers have defective mucociliary function and are predisposed to the development of sinopulmonary infections caused by encapsulated organisms such as *Streptococcus pneumonia* or *Klebsiella pneumonia* (15). Malnutrition and splenic dysfunction are common among people with alcoholism with cirrhosis, but the magnitude of their contribution to immune dysfunction is difficult to quantify. In contrast, the cell-mediated deficiencies that result from effects on T-lymphocyte function caused by infection with human immunodeficiency virus (HIV), tuberculosis, and other intracellular pathogens are well described (16).

SKIN AND SOFT-TISSUE INFECTIONS

Skin and soft-tissue infections are common among IDUs and often are the reason for hospital admission. The type of infection (cellulitis, abscess, or ulcer), its location and severity, and causative organisms usually are related to the duration and site of injection and local epidemiology (17–20). Clusters of infection caused by unusual pathogens have been reported from California (wound botulism and clostridial myonecrosis), Chicago (*Pseudomonas aeruginosa*), Detroit (*Serratia marcescens*), and Great Britain (*Clostridium novyi* and *Clostridium perfringens*). However, *Staphylococcus aureus* and groups A, C, F, and G beta-hemolytic streptococci are the organisms most often seen (1–3,21–32).

Beginning in 1999, there has been a dramatic increase in the incidence of methicillin-resistant *S. aureus* (MRSA) infection, increasing from 5% to 82% of cases in one study (33). Similar rates of resistance have been described in both community onset and health care–associated invasive MRSA infection (34). Many of the community-onset isolates have discrete genetic and epidemiologic characteristics such as pulsed field gel electrophoresis (PFGE) pattern USA 300 or 400, staphylococcal chromosome cassette methicillin resistance gene type IVa (SCCmec IVa), Panton-Valentine leukocidin production, and sensitivity to trimethoprim-sulfamethoxazole, clindamycin, and vancomycin. Up to 80% of these isolates have been associated with skin and soft-tissue infections. Risk factors for acquisition include use of alcohol, methamphetamine, and injection drugs. The mainstay of therapy is incision and drainage of the wound, judicious use of appropriate antibiotics, and meticulous hygiene (35–40).

IDUs who mix their drugs with saliva or who lick their needles before injecting are particularly prone to the development of polymicrobial infections with viridans streptococci, *Haemophilus* spp., *Eikenella corrodens*, and oral anaerobes. Infection with these organisms also occurs in bite wounds and closed-fist injuries.

Repeated injection of nonsterile, potentially vasoactive opiates can cause ischemic necrosis at the injection site, rendering the damaged areas susceptible to superinfection. Similarly, both inhalation and injection of cocaine cause vasospasm with resulting areas of tissue necrosis serving as a nidus for infection. Streptococcal infection in areas of cocaine-induced tissue ischemia can cause large necrotic ulcers with extensive loss of tissue; such skin ulcers are extremely common among IDUs. Ulcers become colonized with a mixture of environmental pathogens, so surface cultures are not useful in guiding antibiotic selection.

The diagnosis of cellulitis is straightforward: most patients have local signs of pain, redness, and swelling or induration of the skin. However, patients who delay seeking medical care while they attempt to self-medicate with antibiotics or lotions can develop extensive cellulitis, necrotizing fasciitis, or overwhelming sepsis.

Diagnosis of an abscess can be more challenging. Patients may complain of pain or tenderness at the site of a superficial cutaneous abscess and may have erythema, induration, or fluctuance of the overlying skin. A deeper abscess may surround blood vessels (especially in the neck and groin), causing local bland or suppurative thrombophlebitis, or be hidden deep in the mediastinum or epidural space. Deep neck abscess can cause internal jugular vein thrombosis, vocal cord paralysis, airway obstruction, or massive hemorrhage after eroding into the carotid artery. The presentation of deeper abscesses can be quite subtle, and diagnosis often requires radiologic imaging.

In IDUs, necrotizing fasciitis, an infection of the deep fascial structures, can be caused by *Streptococcus pyogenes* (group A beta-hemolytic streptococci) or a mixture of aerobic and anaerobic pathogens and most commonly originates at a soft-tissue injection site. The most important diagnostic clue is the presence of pain or hemodynamic instability out of proportion to the physical findings, which may be quite trivial. Diagnosis can be delayed if the clinician discounts these complaints as evidence of drug-seeking behavior. Classic findings of high fever, crepitus, and progressive edema occur late in the course. Prompt surgical and radiologic evaluations for evidence of fasciitis are crucial for diagnosis. However, imaging studies such as plain films, computerized tomography, or magnetic resonance imaging may show only soft-tissue edema and may be insufficiently sensitive to document extent of soft-tissue involvement, even when gas is present. In patients with necrotizing fasciitis, treatment with antibiotics and urgent surgical exploration with débridement are required to minimize morbidity and maximize the patient's chance for survival.

In all other cases of skin and soft-tissue infection, empiric antibiotic therapy should be directed at the most likely pathogen, then modified when results of cultures of blood or aspirated pus become available. Early surgical evaluation and drainage can minimize morbidity and continued tissue destruction. However, the clinician should carefully evaluate lesions located in the vicinity of blood vessels (especially in the groin), because a mycotic aneurysm can masquerade as an abscess and should not be blindly incised due to the potential for massive hemorrhage.

Management of skin ulcers requires antibiotics and aggressive wound care to minimize loss of function, especially when lesions are located on the hand.

An increasing incidence of infection in large skeletal muscles has been recognized, especially among patients with AIDS (41–45). The clinical presentation resembles that of tropical pyomyositis. Such infections usually are caused by *S. aureus*. Pyomyositis is characterized by the presence of a suppurative collection without myonecrosis, often without prior trauma or local drug injection at the site. Patients may have fever, pain, and swelling in the involved muscle, but often there is little evidence of local inflammation. Diagnosis is made by needle aspiration of pus, with subsequent antibiotic therapy directed by culture results.

Vibrio vulnificus is an unusual cause of cellulitis, soft-tissue infection, and bacteremia in cirrhotic patients who have been exposed to saltwater or shellfish (46–48). Patients complain of nausea, vomiting, fever, hypotension, shock, and hemorrhagic skin bullae. Prognosis is poor, even with aggressive antibiotic and surgical management.

Complications related to infections with the *Clostridium* sp. that cause botulism and tetanus are discussed later, as are epidural and splenic abscess and mycotic aneurysm.

GINGIVITIS

Acute necrotizing ulcerative gingivitis (ANUG, trench mouth, Vincent's angina) is characterized by severe pain, gingival necrosis, and bleeding. Patients often have fever, malaise, and fetid breath. Though associated with a variety of oral flora, the pathogenesis remains uncertain. Development of ANUG appears to be associated with smoking, stress, immunosuppression, and poor oral hygiene. Treatment may include use of antiseptic (chlorhexidine) mouth wash, systemic antibiotics such as penicillin or clindamycin, or débridement.

Extensive tooth decay ("meth mouth") is common among people who chronically use methamphetamine and is thought to be due to a combination of bruxism, decreased saliva production, and poor dental hygiene (49,50). Because aggressive intervention may be required to prevent disease progression, oral health should be evaluated at each visit to facilitate recognition and expedite early referral to a dentist.

ENDOCARDITIS

(Cardiovascular complications also are addressed in Chapter 71.)

Epidemiology and Pathogenesis Infective endocarditis (IE) is the most common cardiac complication of injection drug use (1–3,51–57). IE usually begins during an episode of transient bacteremia. In most cases, microorganisms enter the bloodstream and lodge in a thrombus overlying previously damaged or denuded endothelium. Preexisting cardiac lesions are identified in about three-fourths of patients with IE; they include mitral valve prolapse, prosthetic cardiac valves, or congenital, degenerative, or rheumatic heart disease. In contrast, endocarditis that occurs in structurally normal valves is more likely to be nosocomial in origin, caused by more virulent organisms such as *S. aureus* or occur in an IDU. The resulting lesion, called a *vegetation*, is composed of layers of platelets and fibrin covering clumps of relatively sequestered microorganisms. Though most vegetations are located on heart valves, they can occur on any endothelial surface.

The incidence of endocarditis in the general population is about 5 per 100,000 person years, with regional variations that reflect the prevalence of risk factors in the population. Immunodeficiency (including HIV infection) does not appear to increase the incidence of endocarditis; however, morbidity and mortality from endocarditis increase with increasing immunosuppression (58).

In the non-IDU, IE most often is caused by viridans streptococci (50%) and enterococci (10%). In contrast, in the IDU, IE most often is caused by *S. aureus* (more than 50%), of which variable proportions are methicillin-resistant (34,59). Streptococci (13%), enterococci (7%), and fungi, particularly non-albicans *Candida* species (5%), are much less commonly involved.

Both IDUs and people with alcoholism have a higher proportion of IE because of gram-negative bacilli such as *P. aeruginosa*, *Pseudomonas cepacia*, and *S. marcescens*, although their relative prevalence has significant regional variation (22, 55–57,60–75). A cluster of *P. aeruginosa* endocarditis occurred in Chicago among patients who abused pentazocine and tripelennamine ("Ts and blues") (70,71). This cluster was found to be associated with selective survival of the patients' own bacterial isolates when grown in the presence of these drugs. Outbreaks of *S. marcescens* infection have been reported in Detroit and California, but the reason for the increased prevalence in these locations remains obscure. In one California cluster of *S. marcescens* endocarditis reported in the 1970s, cases were characterized by the development of enormous vegetations that caused almost complete occlusion of the valve orifice in the absence of concurrent valve destruction. Mortality in this outbreak was 70% (73,74). Underlying alcoholism is identified as a risk factor in 40% of episodes of pneumococcal endocarditis, and concurrent meningitis is present in 70% of this subgroup of patients (76–79).

Endocarditis caused by *Bartonella henselae* has been described in homeless people with alcoholism, IDUs, and patients with HIV (80–84). Endocarditis caused by a vast array of additional pathogens has been described in case reports (85–88).

The sustained bacteremia that characterizes IE occurs when microorganisms are released as the vegetation fragments, and the size of the vegetation is related to the type of pathogen. Organisms such as *S. marcescens* and *C. albicans* tend to produce large friable vegetations and bulky emboli.

Clinical Presentation Clinical features usually include fever, accompanied by a panoply of cardiac abnormalities (murmur, conduction delay, congestive heart failure, and valvular dysfunction), complications from emboli or from metastatic seeding of other structures during the bacteremia (causing meningitis, brain abscess, osteomyelitis, or splenic abscess), and a wide spectrum of immune complex mediated phenomena (arthritis, glomerulonephritis, aseptic meningitis, Osler nodes, Roth spots, splinter hemorrhages, and other manifestations of vasculitis) (89–93). Patients may complain of fever, night sweats, anorexia, arthralgias, and myalgias (especially in the low back and upper thighs), and weight loss. However, the presence of IE cannot be predicted in a febrile IDU on the basis of signs and symptoms alone (94,95). Unexplained fever should prompt evaluation for endocarditis.

The most reliable clues are the presence of embolic phenomenon and visualization of vegetations on echocardiography. IDUs have a high incidence of acute IE involving a previously normal tricuspid valve (96,97). As a result, patients have pulmonary symptoms, including cough and pleuritic chest pain from septic pulmonary emboli. Pulmonary infiltrate or effusion occur in 75% to 85%, and evidence of septic pulmonary embolization eventually is present on 90% of chest x-rays. These emboli appear as rounded infiltrates ("cannon balls") early in the course, often in showers, and may undergo central cavitation or be complicated by empyema. Murmurs and congestive heart failure usually are absent in these patients. In contrast, IDUs with left-sided endocarditis have murmur, congestive heart failure, and stigmata of systemic embolization.

Mycotic aneurysms complicate IE in 15% of patients. Most are asymptomatic and resolve with treatment.

Diagnosis After performing a careful history and physical examination, patients should have two or three blood cultures drawn. Hospitalization and treatment with empiric antibiotics often is recommended when adequate outpatient follow-up is uncertain.

Definitive diagnosis requires microbiologic or pathologic proof of infection by histology or by culture of a sample of the vegetation or embolus obtained at surgery or autopsy (98–101). A possible diagnosis is established by demonstrating a characteristic vegetation, valve ring abscess, or dehiscence of a prosthetic valve with echocardiography in a patient with multiple positive blood cultures obtained over an extended period (101–104). However, even a negative transesophageal echocardiogram does not exclude the diagnosis. The probability that endocarditis is present is estimated by using major and minor criteria, as shown in Table 77.1 (101).

Treatment Effective antimicrobial therapy requires identification of the specific pathogen and assessment of its susceptibility to various antimicrobial agents. Empiric therapy should be targeted to the most likely pathogens in the clinical setting (104). Initial therapy with an antistaphylococcal antibiotic is appropriate for most IDUs. Use of vancomycin should be considered in areas with a high prevalence of methicillin-resistant *S. aureus* or penicillin-resistant pneumococcus.

TABLE 77.1 Criteria for the Diagnosis of Infective Endocarditis (Modified Duke University Criteria)

Definite Diagnosis
- Pathologic criteria: Histopathology/microbiology of vegetation, embolized vegetation, or intracardiac abscess grow organisms or show active endocarditis; or
- Clinical criteria:
  a. Two major criteria; or
  b. One major plus three minor criteria; or
  c. 5 minor criteria

Possible diagnosis: One major plus one minor criteria or three minor criteria

No endocarditis: No pathology at surgery or autopsy, clinical resolution with ≤4 days antibiotic therapy, firm alternative diagnosis.

Major criteria
- Blood culture
  a. 2 separate blood cultures positive for either: viridans streptococcus, *Streptococcus bovis*, HACEK (Haemophilus, Actinobacillus, Cardiobacterium, Eikenella, and Kingella) or *Staphylococcus aureus*, or community acquired enterococcus in the absence of a primary focus
  b. Positive blood cultures >12 hours apart
  c. Positive blood cultures 3/3 or majority of ≥4 that are ≥1 hour apart
  d. Positive blood culture for *Coxiella burnetti* or antibody >1:800
- Endocardial involvement
- Echocardiogram positive for endocarditis: oscillating intracardiac mass on a valve or supporting structure, in the path of a regurgitant jet stream, or on implanted material in the absence of alternative anatomic explanation, valve ring abscess, or new dehiscence of prosthetic valve. (TEE recommended in patients with prosthetic valve, or paravalvular abscess.)
- New valvular regurgitant murmur

Minor criteria
- Predisposing heart condition or intravenous drug user
- Fever ≥38°C
- Systemic or pulmonary emboli, mycotic aneurysm, intracranial hemorrhage, conjunctival hemorrhage, Janeway lesions
- Immunologic phenomena: glomerulonephritis, Roth's spot, Osler's node, Rheumatoid factor
- Microbiologic/serologic findings consistent with but not definitive for endocarditis

Adapted from Li JS, Sexton DJ, Mick N, et al. Proposed modifications to the Duke Criteria for the diagnosis of infective endocarditis. *Clin Infect Dis* 2000;30:633–638.

Addition of antibiotics directed against gram-negative pathogens should be considered in geographic regions where an increased prevalence of gram negative endocarditis has been identified by local epidemiology (105).

The chosen antibiotic should be bactericidal and must achieve sufficient levels to permit passive diffusion deep into the vegetation, where microcolonies of the pathogen are located. Ultimately, antibiotic selection should be based on final culture and sensitivity results. The duration of therapy should follow standard guidelines. Most patients require a minimum of 4 weeks of intravenous antibiotics, though shorter courses can be effective in IDUs with uncomplicated tricuspid valve endocarditis. An active IDU should not be discharged with an intravascular access device. Encouraging the patient to remain in a monitored setting for the duration of therapy is one of the most challenging aspects of achieving a successful outcome.

Once effective antimicrobial therapy has been initiated, symptoms of fever and fatigue improve coincident with clearance of bacteremia. Blood cultures for streptococci and enterococci should become sterile after 1 to 2 days. Blood cultures for staphylococci should become sterile after 3 to 5 days, but can take 10 to 14 days to become sterile in patients treated with vancomycin. As a result, short-course therapy cannot be used in regimens containing vancomycin. Blood cultures should be obtained daily, until sterile. If initial blood cultures remain negative, the possibility of culture-negative endocarditis, an undrained focus of infection such as splenic abscess, or an alternative diagnosis should be explored. Diagnostic possibilities are quite extensive and are best assessed with the assistance of an infectious diseases specialist.

When sequelae of endocarditis progress despite appropriate antibiotic management, surgical evaluation is warranted. Surgical intervention should be considered for patients who demonstrate congestive heart failure because of valvular dysfunction that is refractory to medical therapy, multiple clinically relevant emboli despite antibiotic therapy for more than 2 weeks, infection caused by certain pathogens such as fungi or resistant organisms (which rarely respond to medical therapy alone), extension of myocardial abscess, inability to sterilize blood cultures, or infection or dehiscence of a prosthetic valve (106,107). Patients with valve ring abscess should be monitored for the development of conduction abnormalities. These patients may require placement of a temporary pacemaker because of the risk of developing high-grade heart block.

Outcome and Prevention The outcome of an episode of IE is based on many factors, including age of the patient, virulence of the organism, site of the infection, presence of complications (such as congestive heart failure, renal failure, rupture of a mycotic aneurysm, cardiac arrhythmia, conduction abnormalities, or cerebral embolization), and the presence of comorbid conditions such as HIV infection. Left-sided endocarditis is associated with a worse prognosis, as is infection with gram-negative bacilli or fungi. Heart failure remains the leading cause of death.

After cure, patients remain at a substantially increased risk of reinfection, and injection drug use is the most common risk factor for recurrent native valve endocarditis. As a result, patients should follow American Heart Association Guidelines and be given prophylactic antibiotics when undergoing certain invasive procedures (108). Current guidelines recommend prophylaxis only for patients with specific high-risk cardiac conditions who undergo dental procedures that involve manipulation of gingival tissue or the periapical region of teeth or perforation of the oral mucosa. High-risk cardiac conditions include prior endocarditis, prosthetic valve, prosthetic material used to repair valve, congenital heart disease (unrepaired, repaired within 6 months, or repaired with residual defect), or valvulopathy after cardiac transplant. Administration of antibiotics solely to prevent endocarditis is no longer recommended for patients who undergo a genitourinary or gastrointestinal tract procedure. In addition, patients should be counseled about the importance of adopting strategies to reduce the likelihood of transient bacteremia. Other preventative measures include aggressive treatment of skin infections, emphasis on maintaining good dental hygiene, and discussion of the overall benefits of discontinuing illicit drug use.

NONCARDIAC VASCULAR INFECTIONS

Epidemiology and Pathogenesis Both direct injury to blood vessels during injection drug use and vasospasm from cocaine use are associated with endothelial injury and thrombus formation. Bacterial seeding of the thrombus can result in septic thrombophlebitis. Alternatively, a hematoma adjacent to the traumatized or ischemic blood vessel may serve as a nidus for superinfection. An arteriovenous fistula can occur either as a result of a direct injury or from extension of local infection.

A mycotic aneurysm results when emboli to the vasa vasorum cause a mushroom-shaped swelling, especially at arterial bifurcations. Mycotic aneurysm formation classically occurs during episodes of bacterial endocarditis. The damaged arterial wall is seeded during a concurrent or subsequent bacteremia. Mycotic aneurysms complicate 15% of cases of IE. They usually are silent but may become symptomatic in 3% to 5% of patients months or years after completion of appropriate therapy (109–111).

For most noncardiac endovascular lesions, the predominant pathogen is *S. aureus*; however, gram-negative bacilli (especially *P. aeruginosa*) are reported with increased frequency in IDUs.

Clinical Presentation When peripheral blood vessels are involved, clinical findings include fever with local pain, swelling, warmth, and induration. A bruit may be present. Infections of the peripheral vasculature can masquerade as cellulitis or subcutaneous abscess, and blind surgical incision should be avoided (112,113). Thrombosis of larger vessels can be associated with either pulmonary embolization or distal ischemia and may be confused with IE.

A patient with a mycotic aneurysm in the neck or groin may describe a painful, tender, enlarging, pulsatile mass with overlying bruit or thrill, accompanied by various constitutional symptoms. Ischemia of a distal extremity or signs of nerve compression may be present. Two important complications include extension of infection into surrounding soft tissue with abscess formation and massive hemorrhage from aneurysmal rupture. Mycotic aneurysms in the brain complicate 2% to 4% of cases of left-sided endocarditis. Patients complain of unremitting headache, visual disturbances, or cranial nerve palsy.

Patients with endovascular infection may have sustained bacteremia and signs of clinical sepsis. Management of septic thrombophlebitis is controversial but generally includes treatment with both intravenous antibiotics and short-term anticoagulation.

Diagnosis Successful management of a mycotic aneurysm requires early diagnosis before rupture occurs. Misdiagnosis is common, and a high index of suspicion is essential. Arteriographic confirmation remains the standard diagnostic test, though newer radiologic tools such as computed tomographic angiography with contrast enhancement and magnetic resonance angiography are being used with increased frequency.

Treatment Empiric antibiotics can be given after blood cultures have been obtained. Antibiotic choice should reflect local epidemiology and should include an antistaphylococcal agent with additional gram-negative coverage in geographic regions where an increased prevalence of gram-negative endovascular infection has been identified by local epidemiology. The antibiotic regimen should be modified on the basis of culture and sensitivity results and usually is continued for 4 to 6 weeks.

Surgical excision of an enlarging mycotic aneurysm and surrounding infected tissue may be necessary to avoid the catastrophic sequelae of a rupture. Intrathoracic, intraabdominal, and peripheral mycotic aneurysms often require surgical excision. Cerebral mycotic aneurysms usually heal with medical therapy alone but may require neurosurgical intervention if enlarging or bleeding (114).

RESPIRATORY INFECTIONS

(Respiratory problems also are discussed in Chapter 75.)

Epidemiology and Pathogenesis Many factors interfere with host defenses and predispose the patient to infection (7,8,15,115–125). Two important examples include cigarette smoke, which disrupts mucociliary function and macrophage activation, and alteration in the level of consciousness accompanied by depressed gag reflex, which compromises airway protection and permits aspiration of oropharyngeal flora. In addition, alcoholism is associated with oropharyngeal colonization with enteric gram-negative bacilli and abnormal phagocyte function. Injection drug use is associated with a large number of insults, including drug-induced bronchospasm, pulmonary edema, and the development of various types of foreign-body granuloma (cotton, starch, or talc) from contaminants in injected materials. Such nonspecific abnormalities on chest radiograph contribute to diagnostic confusion in a febrile patient with cough. An increased risk of exposure to certain pathogens because of lifestyle (e.g., homelessness or incarceration) and the increased prevalence of HIV infection in this group contributes to the increased risk of infection.

Pneumonia Pneumonia is present in up to one-third of IDUs evaluated for fever and complicates a variable percentage of admissions for treatment of alcohol withdrawal or cocaine intoxication (126,127). Septic pulmonary emboli associated with right-sided endocarditis or septic thrombophlebitis and tuberculosis infection are common. Most pulmonary infections are community-acquired episodes of pneumonia, caused by common respiratory pathogens such as *S. pneumonia*, atypical bacteria (such as *Legionella* or *Chlamydia*), oral anaerobes, or viruses (128,129). IDUs have an increased incidence of pneumonia caused by *Haemophilus influenzae*, *S. aureus*, and *P. aeruginosa*, especially those co-infected with HIV (121–125, 130–135).

Patients with HIV are at higher risk of developing pneumonia. Though *Pneumocystis (carinii) jiroveci* is the major pulmonary pathogen in patients with AIDS, pneumonia caused by *Mycobacterium tuberculosis*, *Mycobacterium avium intracellulare*, cytomegalovirus, and common bacterial and viral pathogens occurs with increased frequency in this group. Lung abscesses can complicate aspiration pneumonia, necrotizing bacterial pneumonia, or septic emboli. Left-sided pulmonic effusion may be a clue to an underlying splenic abscess or bacterial or tuberculous pleuritis.

Evaluation of a febrile person who uses drugs with respiratory symptoms should follow standard guidelines, with empiric management directed at likely pathogens (128,136).

Tuberculosis Tuberculosis is a leading cause of infectious morbidity and mortality worldwide, and one-third of the world population is latently infected. In the United States, only 4% to 6% of the population has latent infections (137). Rates of active disease fell steadily until the mid-1980s, when there was a brief resurgence coincident with immigration patterns and the spread of HIV. HIV infection has contributed to the rising case rates because of the higher likelihood of reactivation as immune function decreases and because of the risk of unusually rapid progression to active disease following new (primary) infection. In addition, patients with HIV have a higher prevalence of extrapulmonary and drug resistant disease (138–151). People who use drugs, especially people with alcoholism and IDUs, have an increased incidence of reactivation tuberculosis for reasons that are unknown (152–154). Injection drug use has been implicated in a large outbreak of multiresistant tuberculosis in New York City, where most transmission occurred in hospitals and jails (155–159). Difficulties in controlling this outbreak were compounded by homelessness and noncompliance with medical therapy.

Infection is spread by the aerosolization of acid-fast bacilli in respiratory secretions. Patients with cavitary disease are particularly infectious because of the high concentration of bacilli in their sputum. Cough-inducing procedures such as bronchoscopy, administration of aerosolized medications (including bronchodilators), and smoking (cigarettes, crack cocaine, and marijuana) can increase transmission.

The classic symptoms of pulmonary tuberculosis include cough with purulent, blood-tinged sputum and increasing malaise, with the development of night sweats and weight loss as the disease progresses. High fever, especially in the evening, is seen with decreasing frequency as the level of immunosuppression increases. Diagnosis is made by culturing *M. tuberculosis* from expectorated sputum. Nucleic acid amplification tests are promising but lack standardization. Tuberculin skin tests generally turn positive 4 to 6 weeks after primary infection but can be negative in up to 25% of patients at the time of diagnosis. Interpretation of the tuberculin test is stratified to reflect a combination of risk factors, including severity of underlying immunosuppression, and should follow standard algorithms (160–167). To avoid nosocomial transmission, patients with a suspicious presentation should be isolated until the diagnosis is excluded.

Extrapulmonary tuberculosis occurs in one-sixth of normal adults and up to 60% to 80% of patients with HIV. Diagnosis is challenging because of the paucity of bacilli in the extrapulmonary sites. Histopathology classically shows giant-cell granulomas with central caseating necrosis. Extrapulmonary seeding commonly causes empyema, meningitis, and vertebral osteomyelitis, and diagnosis generally requires biopsy.

Because of the long delay to obtain culture and sensitivity results, treatment usually is initiated before a definitive diagnosis has been established. Treatment should follow American Thoracic Society Guidelines (161–167). Many patients are started on a four-drug regimen that includes isoniazid, rifampin, pyrazinamide, and ethambutol. Patients should be closely monitored for evidence of disease progression and for the development of treatment-related side effects, such as hepatitis or rash (168–173). The initial regimen is adjusted once sensitivities are known. Duration of therapy is based on the severity of immunosuppression and extent of disease. IDUs are at increased risk of multidrug-resistant tuberculosis (resistant to both isoniazid and rifampin). For these patients, results of sensitivity testing are crucial in planning an effective treatment regimen, which should include at least two active agents.

Medication selection can be particularly troublesome in treating patients with HIV. Drugs may be poorly absorbed because of underlying enteropathy or may have significant interactions with other medications. For example, rifampin should not be used with protease inhibitors or many other medications because of its effect on hepatic catabolism. Directly observed therapy is strongly encouraged when nonadherence is anticipated and often is preferred for patients with risk factors, such as homelessness or addictive disorders.

Most people who use drugs are at increased risk of tuberculosis infection and should have routine tuberculin skin testing. Interpretation of the skin test result and selection of a treatment regimen should follow standard guidelines (160–167). For example, IDUs with more than 10 mm induration on skin testing might be given 6 to 12 months of chemoprophylaxis with isoniazid after active disease is excluded. IDUs with HIV might be given 12 months of isoniazid when there is more than a 5-mm induration on skin testing or after close contact with a case of infectious tuberculosis, regardless of skin test results. Many drug combinations and dosing schedules are available. Rifampin can reduce methadone levels, and patients often require adjustment of their maintenance dose. IDUs with underlying hepatitis or who use hepatotoxins such as alcohol have an increased risk of developing hepatitis when using isoniazid, rifampin, or pyrazinamide. These patients should be monitored for the development of anorexia, abdominal pain, nausea, vomiting, change in color of urine or stool, or jaundice.

Most patients with underlying lung disease are at risk of increased morbidity from influenza and should be offered annual immunization (129). The efficacy of pneumococcal vaccine to prevent invasive disease varies with the population studied. Because there is a clear benefit for most patients with HIV infection and for many patients age 50 or older, administration of the pneumococcal vaccine should be considered as well, particularly in the patient with alcoholism.

HEPATIC AND GASTROINTESTINAL INFECTIONS

(Hepatic and gastrointestinal disorders also are addressed in Chapters 72 and 74.)

Viral hepatitis is common among people who use injection drugs, noninjection drugs, and alcohol and has been extensively reviewed (174–181).

Hepatic cirrhosis results from an irreversible chronic injury to the hepatic parenchyma, which is most often caused by alcoholism or viral hepatitis. Infection is the leading cause of death in patients with cirrhosis (4). Gram-negative enteric bacilli such as *Escherichia coli*, *K. pneumoniae*, and encapsulated respiratory pathogens such as *S. pneumonia* are the most frequent cause of infection in these patients; however, severe infections with many other organisms, including *V. vulnificus*, *Pasteurella multocida*, *Aeromonas hydrophilia*, *Listeria monocytogenes*, *Campylobacter* spp., and tuberculosis, also have been described.

Spontaneous bacterial peritonitis (SBP) is a common and potentially fatal infectious complication in patients with cirrhosis and ascites. Pathogenesis involves translocation of bacteria from the gut to mesenteric lymph nodes and is associated with deficiencies in humoral response and phagocytic function (182,183).

Diagnostic paracentesis should be performed in patients with ascites who have fever. Analysis of ascitic fluid should include gram stain and culture for bacteria, mycobacteria, and fungi; measurement of albumin; absolute and differential white blood cell count; and cytopathology. Empiric antibiotic therapy is directed against suspected pathogens and should be refined once culture results become available. Because gram-negative enteric bacilli and *S. pneumonia* are the most common cause of infection in these patients, a second-generation cephalosporin or a combination of fluoroquinolone plus clindamycin or metronidazole are common starting regimens. Patients who have a low ascitic fluid protein or more advanced liver disease are at increased risk of developing SBP. Some authorities recommend the use of prophylactic antibiotics to prevent SBP in this subset of patients as well as those with a prior episode of SBP.

Tuberculous peritonitis, which is uncommon, usually is diagnosed by peritoneal biopsy and culture.

BONE AND JOINT INFECTIONS

Osteomyelitis Most microorganisms can infect bone. Frequent pathogens include *S. aureus* (60%), *Staphylococcus epidermidis* (30%), streptococci, gram-negative bacilli, anaerobes, mycobacteria, and fungi (10%), and prevalence is related to mode of acquisition. Infection can occur by hematogenous seeding, by introduction after surgery or trauma, or spread from a contiguous focus (184–189). In adults, hematogenous spread of bacteria frequently involves the spine because of the vascularity of the vertebrae. Vertebral osteomyelitis in IDUs usually involves the lumbosacral and cervical spine. Common pathogens include *S. aureus*, gram-negative bacilli (including *P. aeruginosa*), and fungi. Though the original source of these infections may be unknown, most are seeded hematogenously during an episode of bacterial endocarditis or locally from a contiguous soft tissue focus.

Adults may develop osteomyelitis of the hand caused by mouth flora (including *Staphylococcus* spp., *Eikenella corrodens, Pasteurella multocida*, and oral anaerobes) associated with local trauma after bite wounds or closed-fist injury.

Patients with osteomyelitis complain of focal pain and tenderness. Fever is present in two-thirds of patients; erythema, warmth, and swelling are variably present. Lack of signs and symptoms frequently results in a delay in diagnosis.

In vertebral osteomyelitis, associated symptoms result when inflammation extends beyond the spine to cause retropharyngeal abscess, mediastinitis, subdiaphragmatic or iliopsoas abscess, meningitis, or epidural abscess with evidence of spinal cord compression (190). Spinal tuberculosis (Potts disease) is relatively indolent, and patients may have late sequelae and extensive vertebral destruction.

Diagnosis of osteomyelitis is made by biopsy and culture of bone. Computed tomography scan and magnetic resonance imaging are helpful in determining the extent of involvement but are not specific. Blood cultures often are negative, especially when the osteomyelitis resulted from hematogenous seeding during a remote bacteremic infection (such as endocarditis). Antibiotics alone may be sufficient therapy to cure acute osteomyelitis and should be chosen on the basis of isolated pathogens. Use of empiric therapy is suboptimal because of the wide range of potential pathogens. Surgical débridement generally is required for cure when the infection has been present for longer than 6 weeks (chronic osteomyelitis).

As noted earlier, establishing a regimen that is mutually acceptable to the patient and clinician is challenging because of the requirement for prolonged intravenous therapy. This challenge is compounded by the tendency for many physicians to undertreat associated bone pain symptoms; therefore, consultation with a pain management specialist may be beneficial.

Septic Arthritis Septic arthritis occurs when bacteria seed joints previously damaged by trauma, instrumentation, osteoarthritis, or chronic inflammatory conditions. Infection with *S. aureus* is most common, though infection with many other organisms has been reported. Arthrocentesis with culture and microscopic examination of joint fluid are required for diagnosis. Differential diagnosis includes gonorrhea, crystal arthropathy, and a variety of noninfectious etiologies.

Two particular syndromes are more common among IDUs than in the normal population and involve fibrocartilaginous joints, which are most susceptible to hematogenous seeding.

Septic arthritis of the sternoclavicular joint caused by *P. aeruginosa* has been reported primarily in IDUs. Most cases occur without identification of an antecedent infection. Symptoms may be present for several months before the patient seeks evaluation. Complaints include fever, tenderness and swelling over the joint, and decreased range of motion of the ipsilateral shoulder (191). Another unusual presentation is of septic arthritis of the sacroiliac joint or symphysis pubis. Symptoms include fever and various combinations of hip, groin, thigh, or lower abdominal pain that is exacerbated by walking (192–194). In such cases, infection may spread from the joint to contiguous soft tissues and bone. Treatment may require exploratory arthrotomy, with surgical débridement of infected material followed by prolonged antibiotic therapy directed at isolated organisms.

NERVOUS SYSTEM INFECTIONS

People who use drugs are prone to a variety of central nervous system manifestations that may have an infectious origin. Such manifestations are easily missed if symptoms are mistakenly attributed to intoxication or withdrawal. Delirium, acute confusional states, encephalopathy, or coma may accompany overdose, intoxication, infection, or a large number of noninfectious etiologies. Central nervous system mass lesions, seizures, hemorrhage, stroke syndromes, transverse myelitis, and peripheral neuropathies have a similarly broad differential. Clinical features should guide diagnostic strategies, with management based on results of lumbar puncture and neuroradiologic imaging (195).

Endocarditis is the most common cause of central nervous system symptoms in IDUs and can cause meningitis (aseptic or purulent), brain abscess from septic emboli, or hemorrhage from rupture of a mycotic aneurysm. Bacteremia during IE can cause vertebral osteomyelitis, which, in turn, can be complicated by epidural abscess, with evidence of cord compression (196).

Brain abscess and subdural empyema in the absence of endocarditis usually are caused by a varied group of pyogenic bacteria; however, infection with many other organisms, including *Nocardia*, *Aspergillus* spp., *Cryptococcus*, mucormycosis, tuberculosis, and *Toxoplasma gondii*, has been reported, especially in patients coinfected with HIV. Etiology often involves extension from a contiguous focus in the mastoid, ear, or paranasal sinuses; seeding of a preexisting subdural hematoma during an episode of transient bacteremia; or direct inoculation of the subdural space after a traumatic wound. A patient with brain abscess may have nonspecific symptoms such as headache or personality change; and an abscess can attain enormous size before diagnosis. Management includes antibiotics and drainage, if indicated.

In most cases, patients with HIV who have ring-enhancing mass lesions in the brain and appropriate clinical presentation are treated empirically for toxoplasmosis. Symptoms that worsen or fail to improve after 2 weeks should prompt more aggressive evaluation, including consideration of brain biopsy.

Meningovascular syphilis has been reported in a number of patients with HIV, despite presumably effective therapy for primary syphilis infection, and it should be considered in young people who present with a new stroke (197,198).

Contamination of skin ulcers with spores of *Clostridium* spp. can cause neurologic symptoms from elaboration of neurotoxins.

Wound botulism is caused by contamination of injection sites or skin ulcers with *Clostridium botulinum* that release botulinum toxin (199–202). Toxin is absorbed, disseminated, and ultimately binds to specific receptors, where it blocks acetylcholine release, resulting in a descending, symmetric, flaccid paralysis. Fewer than 100 cases were reported between 1951 and 1993. However, over the past 15 years, there has been a dramatic increase in reported cases among IDUs who injected black tar heroin, the dark, gummy substance derived from crude preparations of opium that may be contaminated by spore-containing adulterants such as dirt.

Diagnosis is established by recovering *C. botulinum* from the wound or by detecting toxin in serum, but negative findings do not exclude the diagnosis. Treatment with trivalent or type-specific antitoxin can limit disease progression. Involvement of motor neurons causes respiratory failure, and patients may require respiratory support for several months until synapses are regenerated. Botulism has been reported in a patient with colonization of the paranasal sinuses after intranasal cocaine use (203).

Tetanus is caused by the release of a potent neurotoxin by *Clostridium tetani* at the site of a wound in a person who lacks protective antibody (204–206). Wounds contaminated by dirt, feces, or saliva provide an appropriate anaerobic milieu for these vegetative bacteria. Until the mid-1990s, approximately 100 cases of tetanus per year were reported in the United States. However, since 1995, fewer than 50 cases of tetanus per year have been reported. Most have been associated with acute injury (70%) or chronic wounds (26%). Fifteen to eighteen percent of the reported cases were in IDUs who lacked a history of an acute injury but did inject black tar heroin and presented with infected subcutaneous injection sites. Toxin travels up the axon to spinal neurons, where it blocks the release of glycine and other neurotransmitters used to inhibit afferent motor neurons. Binding results in unrestrained nerve firing with sustained muscle contractions and rigidity. Binding is irreversible, and recovery requires generation of new axon terminals. Symptoms begin 7 to 21 days after injury. Early symptoms of trismus (lockjaw) progress to dysphagia, hydrophobia, and drooling, followed by opisthotonos, with painful flexion of the arms and extension of the legs. The patient remains conscious. Very rarely, localized tetanus can cause weakness limited to a single extremity, but this weakness usually progresses to generalized tetany. Management should include antibiotics, aggressive wound débridement, tetanus immune globulin, and supportive care. Prevention requires protective antibody levels. All patients should be immunized with tetanus toxoid every 10 years after a primary series (or immediately after a high-risk wound if more than 5 years has elapsed since the last booster).

EYE INFECTIONS

IDUs have an increased incidence of bacterial and fungal endophthalmitis as a complication of IE. Many investigators have reported *C. albicans* endophthalmitis as part of a syndrome of disseminated candidiasis in IDUs who injected "brown heroin," presumably related to fungal contamination of the lemon juice used to dissolve the drug (207). The most commonly reported bacterial causes include *S. aureus* and *Bacillus cereus*.

Symptoms of endophthalmitis include acute onset of blurred vision, eye pain, and decreased visual acuity, similar to the symptoms in people who do not use drugs. Diagnosis requires a high index of suspicion; aggressive evaluation and management are required to salvage vision (208).

Cytomegalovirus retinitis is the most common serious intraocular complication of AIDS and generally occurs after reactivation of latent infection in patients with CD4 cell counts of <50, especially those not receiving antiretroviral therapy. Disease is characterized by retinal necrosis and edema that begins peripherally in the eye and may remain asymptomatic until there has been significant retinal destruction or detachment. Symptoms of blurring or loss of vision, floaters, or flashing lights in one or both eyes should always be evaluated with dilated ophthalmoscopy. Characteristic retinal changes include yellow-white, fluffy exudates with associated hemorrhage. Therapy with oral, intravenous, or intraocular antiviral agents can reduce the risk of vision loss. However, patients may develop significant intraocular inflammation associated with immune recovery (immune recovery uveitis) and require aggressive management to prevent permanent loss of vision.

HUMAN IMMUNODEFICIENCY VIRUS AND ACQUIRED IMMUNODEFICIENCY SYNDROME

Tremendous advances have been made in our understanding of the pathophysiology, diagnosis, and management of HIV infection and AIDS since the original description, in 1981, of a cluster of homosexual men with *P. carinii* pneumonia (PCP) and Kaposi sarcoma (209–211). Highlights include the identification of a new cytopathic retrovirus in 1983, the development of a serologic diagnostic test in 1985, and the introduction of antiretroviral therapy in 1987. Comprehensive discussions of the AIDS pandemic, including details of transmission, seroconversion, immunosuppression related to disease stage, use of antiretroviral therapy, and prophylaxis and treatment for opportunistic infections are available (211–218).

Epidemiology and Pathogenesis HIV infection usually is acquired through sexual intercourse, exposure to contaminated blood, or perinatal transmission; the relative frequency of each varies by country. As of December 2007, an estimated 33.2 million persons worldwide were living with HIV/AIDS, 90% in developing countries (214). As of December 2005, AIDS had been reported in 956,019 people in the United States, with 421,873 still alive. Among U.S. adults with known risk factors who were diagnosed between 2001 and 2005, 33% reported injection drug use and another 17% reported sex with an IDU (213). Among children diagnosed with HIV infection between 2001 and 2005, more than 90% of the cases involved transmission from an infected mother. Risk factors for these mothers included injection drug use in 38% and unprotected sex with an IDU in 16% (213). For both men and women, the estimated number of new cases of HIV related to injection drug use has fallen slightly each year for the past several years, perhaps because of emphasis on prevention strategies.

In contrast, evidence from around the world suggests that certain behavioral and social factors are increasing the number of cases associated with unsafe sexual practices. Examples of these factors include little or no condom use, a high prevalence of multiple partners, and women's economic dependence on marriage or prostitution. In these groups, transmission is further enhanced by a high rate of concurrent sexually transmitted infections, especially those causing genital ulcers, and a high level of viremia (viral load) when the patient first is infected (before diagnosis) and again in the late stages of illness (219).

In the past, identification of populations with high risk of exposure to HIV was based on the demographic and geographic distribution of reported AIDS cases. However, as states have implemented laboratory-initiated reporting of positive HIV viral load tests, more and more patients are being identified with a new diagnosis of HIV or AIDS without an obvious behavioral risk or exposure. This incidence reflects the increasing proportion of patients infected by a partner with unrecognized or unreported behavioral risks (220). In response, the Centers for Disease Control and Prevention (CDC) has recommended routine voluntary HIV testing for all patients aged 13 to 64 years (213,221); however, many barriers to testing remain (222,223). Testing can be postponed during acute mental health and addiction exacerbations but should be done, with appropriate communication of results, implications, and treatment options, as soon as patients are prepared to hear the results of testing even if other health problems (including addictions) are not entirely resolved.

In the United States, decreases in AIDS incidence and death began in 1996, in association with the use of potent combinations of drugs known as highly active antiretroviral therapy (HAART). However, to achieve further decreases in AIDS incidence and death, persons infected with HIV must seek testing earlier, agree to take and adhere to therapy, and actively follow risk-reduction strategies to prevent further transmission (221).

Classification Stages of HIV infection range from asymptomatic (latent) through early symptomatic infection (B symptoms) to AIDS. Classification follows CDC criteria and stratifies disease according to the CD4 cell count and the presence of various other criteria (224,225).

Primary HIV infection causes symptoms in 50% to 90% of cases, which occur 2 to 4 weeks after exposure. Symptoms of fever, adenopathy, pharyngitis, rash, and myalgias are reported by more than 50% of patients and last 1 to 4 weeks. Other nonspecific symptoms that have been reported include arthralgias, diarrhea, headache, nausea and vomiting, hepatosplenomegaly, thrush, mucocutaneous ulcers, meningoencephalitis, peripheral neuropathy, cranial nerve palsy, Guillain-Barré syndrome, radiculopathy, cognitive impairment, and psychosis (226–230).

Diagnosis Primary HIV infection should be considered in any patient with a history of potential exposure and compatible symptoms. After performing a careful history and physical examination, the diagnosis is best established by demonstrating the presence of p24 antigen, quantitative HIV RNA, or qualitative HIV RNA in association with negative or indeterminate HIV serology. High-level viremia during the acute illness permits dissemination of virus to the central nervous system and lymphatic tissue. During this period, the patient may have no physical findings except for persistent generalized lymphadenopathy. The lymphatics are a major reservoir of HIV infection, and replication continues during the clinically latent disease stage (231,232). Plasma levels of HIV decline dramatically during the resolution of the symptomatic phase of primary HIV, presumably because of the development of humoral and cellular immune responses, and reach a nadir at 120 days (233). Seroconversion generally occurs at 6 to 12 weeks.

By 6 months after transmission, 95% of patients have developed positive HIV serology and stabilization of viral load, with levels correlating with prognosis (234–236). As the disease progresses, lymph node architecture is disrupted, releasing more HIV, with an accompanying slow but progressive decline in CD4 counts in most patients. The average life expectancy in the absence of treatment is approximately 10 years, and rates of progression appear similar by gender, race, and risk category when adjusted for quality of medical care (237–248).

However, investigators have identified a subset of asymptomatic patients ("long-term nonprogressors") with sustained high levels of CD4 (more than 500 cells/mm^3) for 7 to 10 years in the absence of antiretroviral therapy (249). Correlates of delayed progression include low viral load, preservation of lymph node architecture, increased CD8 cytolytic activity, and a vigorous HIV specific CD4+ T-cell response (250,251). One explanation for delayed disease progression involves the surface chemokine receptor CCR5, which facilitates entry of HIV into macrophages (16,252). Patients with polymorphisms in this receptor appear to progress to AIDS more slowly (10.4 vs. 6.6 years), though transmission of the virus is not affected. Homozygotes are relatively resistant to infection (253,254). Studies with agents that block viral binding to the chemokine receptors are in progress and show promise for future use as antiviral agents.

Most patients are diagnosed months or years after HIV infection. Verification of infection requires that a repeatedly positive enzyme immunoassay screening assay be confirmed by a Western blot that demonstrates at least two characteristic antigens (p24, gp41, or gp120/160).

Once the diagnosis of HIV has been established, all patients should have routine screening tests such as a rapid plasma reagin test for syphilis, tuberculin skin test, cytomegalovirus and toxoplasma immunoglobulin G serology, liver function tests, hepatitis serology, and Papanicolaou tests, in addition to tests such as chest radiograph or ophthalmologic examination as clinically indicated (255).

Treatment The availability of an increasing number of antiretroviral agents and the rapid evolution of new information has introduced extraordinary complexity into the treatment of HIV. Algorithms outline appropriate laboratory monitoring, including measurement of plasma HIV RNA, CD4 cell counts, and HIV drug resistance testing. Guidelines describe when to begin antiretroviral therapy (based on CD4 count and viral load), what drugs to initiate, when and how to change therapy, and special recommendations for pregnant women (216). All pregnant women should be offered counseling and testing for HIV and other sexually transmitted diseases, and women infected with HIV should be treated to maximize their health status and minimize risk to the fetus. Management of patients with HIV/HCV coinfection is particularly challenging (256). When simultaneously initiating HAART and treatment for an opportunistic infection such as tuberculosis or hepatitis, patients with advanced disease must be monitored for the development of the immune reconstitution inflammatory syndrome (215,257,258).

Additional guidelines provide disease-specific recommendations for the use of primary or secondary prophylactic antibiotics for the prevention of the most common, serious opportunistic infections, including PCP, toxoplasmic encephalitis, disseminated *Mycobacterium avium* intracellulare complex, and tuberculosis (217). Immunizations for hepatitis A and B, influenza, and pneumococcus should be administered as needed (259). Therapeutic decisions require a discussion about the benefits and risks of treatment. Antiretroviral regimens are complex, have major side effects, and carry serious potential consequences from the development of viral resistance associated with nonadherence to the drug regimen or suboptimal levels of antiretroviral agents.

Patient education and involvement in therapeutic decisions are especially critical for effective HIV treatment. Past and current high-risk behaviors and exposures that may have resulted in HIV infection should be reviewed and mitigation plans designed to prevent further transmission. Behaviors such as high-risk sexual activity or injection drug use not only increase the risk of HIV transmission to others but can expose the HIV-infected patient to opportunistic pathogens such as herpes simplex virus, cytomegalovirus, *Cryptosporidium*, human papillomavirus (HPV), human herpesvirus type 8, and hepatitis viruses. Ongoing high-risk sexual behavior should prompt discussions about risk reduction and be reviewed at each encounter. Continuing addictive behavior should prompt the offer of referral to addiction treatment services; a history of addictive disorder warrants review of relapse-prevention efforts. Intensive follow-up may be required to assess adherence to treatment and to continue patient counseling to prevent transmission of HIV through unprotected sexual behavior and continued injection of drugs (260). In addition, the patient should receive education and counseling on how to reduce the risk of exposure to opportunistic pathogens associated with food, pets, water, travel, or the environment. It is strongly recommended that care be co-managed with an expert in HIV treatment.

The optimal chance for a prolonged response occurs when an adherent patient initiates combination antiretroviral therapy. Once the decision has been made to initiate treatment, the goals should be maximal and durable suppression of viral load, restoration or preservation of immunologic function, improvement in the quality of life, and reduction of HIV-related morbidity and mortality. Efficacy of therapy is evaluated by monitoring viral load, which should decrease 10-fold by the eighth week and become undetectable (<50 copies per mL) by 6 months after initiation of treatment.

Evidence is promising for at least the short-term efficacy of aggressive therapy on viral load and CD4+ T-cell counts in patients treated at the time of acute HIV seroconversion; however, clinical trials completed to date have been limited by small sample sizes, short duration of follow-up, and the use of suboptimal treatment regimens. Ongoing clinical trials are addressing the question of the long-term clinical benefit of more potent treatment regimens for this group of patients.

The proportion of patients with each of the various AIDS-defining conditions, the rate of disease progression, the rate of AIDS deaths, and the average life expectancy have changed dramatically coincident with the widespread use of HAART and prophylaxis against opportunistic infections (261,262). In the past, patients with advanced HIV disease (defined as CD4 cell count less than 50 cells/mm^3) had a median survival of 12 to 18 months. However, many of these patients had received no antiretroviral therapy or received nucleoside analogues only. Treatment strategies now known to prolong survival include use of HAART, use of primary and secondary prophylaxis for PCP and *Mycobacterium avium intracellulare* complex, and care by a physician knowledgeable about both HIV and primary care (255,263–265). The effect of HAART became apparent in 1996, as the need for inpatient hospitalizations declined and the incidence of AIDS-defining illnesses decreased. Nevertheless, CD4 counts and viral load remain the most important determinants of the rate of progression (266). One important new challenge is to recognize atypical presentations of opportunistic infections during HAART (261,262).

Failure of therapy at 4 to 6 months can be ascribed to nonadherence (including inability to comply with complex dosing schedules), suboptimal levels of antiretroviral agents, viral resistance, and other factors that are poorly understood. Drug-drug or drug-food interactions can profoundly affect the absorption and efficacy of certain medications. For example, methadone levels can be significantly decreased when given with certain protease inhibitors (ritonavir, nelfinavir, or lopinavir) and non-nucleoside reverse transcriptase inhibitors (nevirapine or efavirenz) and often require an increase in methadone maintenance dosage. Conversely, use of maintenance methadone can significantly decrease the level of some nucleoside reverse transcriptase inhibitors (stavudine or didanosine), requiring an increase in antiretroviral dosage. In contrast, limited data suggest that buprenorphine needs no dosage adjustment and is less likely to be associated with adverse events when given with HAART regimens that include efavirenz (267). As noted previously, antiretroviral drug selection often is complicated by the development of side effects. Patients with HIV appear to have a higher incidence of drug-associated toxicity than the general population, especially when renal or hepatic dysfunction is present.

Interactions between the protease inhibitor class and other drugs and foods are extensive and often require dose modification or drug substitution. For example, concurrent therapy with rifampin can decrease the concentration of protease inhibitor by as much as 80%, so its use should be avoided to prevent development of antiretroviral resistance and treatment failure. The combination of a protease inhibitor with terfenadine, astemizole, or cisapride can result in serious cardiotoxicity. The development and severity of these adverse effects often is unpredictable; thus, assessment of toxicity should be performed frequently as part of routine follow-up care. To avoid toxic combinations, a careful review of all medications should be performed by the pharmacist whenever a new agent is added to the patient's regimen. In addition, when side effects occur and acute intervention is required, all drugs should be discontinued simultaneously to minimize development of resistance. Patients whose therapy fails despite apparent adherence should have their regimen changed; this change should be guided by a careful review of past and current medication use and the results of drug resistance testing.

As the epidemiology of AIDS changed, investigators have studied the risks, benefits, and costs of discontinuing chemoprophylaxis against opportunistic infections (268–274). Primary prophylaxis for PCP, MAI, and toxoplasmosis can be discontinued once the CD4 lymphocyte count has increased to at least 200 cells/μL for more than 6 months in response to treatment with HAART (218). Secondary prophylaxis for PCP, MAI, cryptococcosis, and toxoplasmosis can be discontinued once the CD4 lymphocyte count has increased to at least 200 cells/μL for more than 6 months in response to treatment with HAART as long as the patient has completed appropriate therapy and has no symptoms or signs attributable to these pathogens (218). Though patients who respond to aggressive antiretroviral therapy may have prolonged suppression of plasma viremia to below detectable levels, persistent viral reservoirs have been identified in peripheral blood mononuclear cells, particularly CD4 cells (275–282). This reservoir of latent virus must be considered when decisions are made about possible termination of antiretroviral therapy, as viral rebound occurs within 1 to 3 weeks in nearly all patients, is associated with an increased risk of opportunistic infection and death (283), and is generally not recommended. In addition, development of drug resistance, with possible cross-resistance to other drugs, is possible if a sustained reduction in viral load is not maintained.

Prevention A great deal of emphasis has been placed on identification of impediments to successful adherence to chemoprophylaxis. Patients with depression, poor social support, and active addictive disorder are less likely to adhere to clinical regimens (284). Recommendations to improve adherence are discussed elsewhere (285,286). Similarly, patients with HIV who engage in sexual or substance use risk behaviors not only place others at risk of HIV infection but may place themselves at risk of acquisition of opportunistic pathogens. As noted earlier, there should be a formal, ongoing review of risk behaviors. Prevention messages should encourage sexual abstinence or the practice of the correct and consistent use of latex condoms (287–291). Patients should be encouraged to avoid sexual practices that might result in oral exposure to feces (e.g., oral-anal contact) to reduce the risk of intestinal infections (e.g., cryptosporidiosis, shigellosis, campylobacteriosis, amebiasis, giardiasis, and hepatitis A and B). Patients who inject drugs should be encouraged to stop using injection drugs and to enter and complete addiction treatment. If the patient continues to inject drugs, the importance of using a sterile syringe for every injection and the avoidance of sharing any injection-related drug paraphernalia with another person should be emphasized. Such patients should be encouraged to use a needle-exchange program or to safely discard syringes after one use. In areas where needle exchange is illegal, IDUs should be taught to clean their injection equipment with household bleach before use. Patients who are exposed to bloodborne pathogens may be eligible for postexposure prophylaxis (292). Similarly, health care workers who have an unprotected exposure to the blood of these patients should follow CDC guidelines for postexposure prophylaxis, including pretest and posttest counseling (293).

SEXUALLY TRANSMITTED DISEASES

The epidemiology, clinical features, diagnosis, and treatment of sexually transmitted diseases other than HIV/AIDS have been reviewed extensively (294). Though the prevalence is higher in people who use drugs, the presentation, diagnosis, and management of most sexually transmitted diseases are not profoundly influenced by drug use. One exception is that the diagnosis and treatment of syphilis in IDUs may be confounded by an increased prevalence of biologic false-positive nontreponemal screening tests such as venereal disease research laboratory or rapid plasma reagin tests for syphilis.

Recent studies suggest that an increasing number of persons, especially men who have sex with men, are participating in high-risk sexual behaviors (often while intoxicated) that place them at risk of acquiring syphilis, gonorrhea, herpes, chlamydia, HIV, and other sexually transmitted diseases (294–297). Related studies have shown that patients who report heavy drug or alcohol use are most likely to report high-risk sexual behavior and to have HIV infection or syphilis (298–304). The most common high-risk behaviors include multiple recent sexual partners and inconsistent use of condoms (305).

As noted earlier, the clinician and patient should conduct a formal, ongoing review of risk behavior. Prevention messages should encourage safe sex, including the correct and consistent use of latex condoms. In selected patients, use of postexposure prophylaxis may be warranted (292). There are a number of potential complications from sexually transmitted diseases and other infectious diseases that can affect the pregnant woman or her fetus. Pregnant women who use drugs should be screened according to standard protocols and aggressively treated to minimize disastrous maternal or fetal outcomes (306).

Because of the synergistic effect of cigarette smoke in the development of HPV-associated cancers, patients with diagnosed HPV should be strongly encouraged to consider smoking cessation.

Type-one human T-cell lymphotropic virus (HTLV-I) infection is present in widely scattered populations throughout the world and is the etiologic agent in adult T-cell leukemia/lymphoma and HTLV-associated myelopathy. HTLV-II has been reported in IDUs and their sexual contacts, appears to be endemic in IDUs in the United States, and has not been definitively linked to a specific disorder. Patients with HTLV-II infection may be at increased risk of a variety of infections, suggesting an underlying immunologic impairment. Both retroviruses appear to be transmitted by sexual intercourse, administration of blood products, and mother-to-child transmission. No effective therapy exists, and prevention of exposure is the only known method of limiting spread (307).

CONCLUSIONS

Infectious complications in people who use drugs are more frequent, more difficult to diagnose, and more challenging to treat than similar infections in people who do not use drugs. Effective management requires attention to both medical and social issues. An improved outcome can be achieved by emphasizing risk reduction strategies in the context of a strong, ongoing therapeutic alliance.

REFERENCES

1. Cherubin CE, Sapira JD. The medical complications of drug addiction and the medical assessment of the intravenous drug user: 25 years later. *Ann Intern Med* 1993;119:1017–1028.
2. Levine D, Brown P, eds. Infections of intravenous drug abusers. *Infect Dis Clin North Am* 2002;16:535–792.
3. Levine DP, Brown PD. Infections in injection drug users. In Mandell GL, Bennett JE, Dolin R, eds. *Mandell, Douglas, and Bennett's principles and practice of infectious diseases*, 6th ed. Philadelphia: Churchill Livingstone, 2005:3462–3476.
4. Cooper B, Maderazo EG. Alchohol abuse and impaired immunity. *Infect Surg* 1989;3:94–101.
5. Palepu A, Tyndall MW, Leon H, et al. Hospital utilization and costs in a cohort of injection drug users. *CMAJ* 2001;165:415–420.
6. Lucas CE. The impact of street drugs on trauma care. *J Trauma* 2005;59(Suppl 3):S57–60.
7. Moss M, Parsons PE, Steinberg KP, et al. Chronic alcohol abuse is associated with an increased incidence of acute respiratory distress syndrome and severity of multiple organ dysfunction in patients with septic shock. *Crit Care Med* 2003;31:869–877.
8. O'Brien JM, Lu B, Ali NA, et al. Alcohol dependence is independently associated with sepsis, septic shock, and hospital mortality among adult intensive care unit patients. *Crit Care Med* 2007;35:345–50.
9. Alonzo NC, Bayer BB. Opioids, immunology, and host defenses of intravenous drug abusers. *Infect Dis Clin North Am* 2002;16:553–569.
10. Ocasio FM, Jiang Y, House SD, et al. Chronic morphine accelerates the progression of lipopolysaccharide-induced sepsis to septic shock. *J Neuroimmunol* 2004;149:90–100.
11. Vallejo R, de Leon-Casasola O, Benyamin R. Opioid therapy and immunosuppression: a review. *Am J Ther* 2004;11:354–365.
12. Sacerdote P. Opioids and the immune system. *Palliat Med* 2006;20 (Suppl 1):S9–S15.
13. Li Y, Ye L, Peng JS, et al. Morphine inhibits intrahepatic interferon-alpha expression and enhances complete hepatitis C virus replication. *J Infect Dis* 2007;196:719–730.
14. Graham CS, Wells A, Edwards EM, et al. Effect of exposure to injection drugs or alcohol on antigen-specific immune responses in HIV and hepatitis C virus coinfection. *J Infect Dis* 2007;195:847–856.
15. Arcavi L, Benowitz NL. Cigarette smoking and infection. *Arch Intern Med* 2004;164:2206–2216.
16. Dybul M, Connors M, Fauci AS. The immunology of human immunodeficiency virus infection. In Mandell GL, Bennett JE, Dolin R, eds. *Mandell, Douglas, and Bennett's principles and practice of infectious diseases*, 6th ed. Philadelphia: Churchill Livingstone, 2005:1527–1546.
17. Binswanger IA, Kral AH, Bluthenthal RN, et al. High prevalence of abscesses and cellulitis among community-recruited injection drug users in San Francisco. *Clin Infect Dis* 2000;30:579–581.
18. Murphy EL, DeVita D, Liu H, et al. Risk factors for skin and soft-tissue abscesses among injection drug users: a case-control study. *Clin Infect Dis* 2001;33:35–40.
19. DelGiudice P. Cutaneous complications of intravenous drug abuse. *Br J Dermatol* 2004;150:1–10.
20. Gordon RJ, Lowy FD. Bacterial infections in drug users. *N Engl J Med* 2005;353:1945–1954.
21. Brook I, Frazier EH. Aerobic and anaerobic bacteriology of wounds and cutaneous abscesses. *Arch Surg* 1990;125:1445–1451.
22. Levine DP, Crane LR, Zervos MJ. Bacteremia in narcotic addicts at the Detroit Medical Center: II. Infectious endocarditis: a prospective comparative study. *Rev Infect Dis* 1986;8:374–396.
23. Summanen PH, Talan DA, Strong C, et al. Bacteriology of skin and soft-tissue infections: comparison of infections in intravenous drug users and individuals with no history of intravenous drug use. *Clin Infect Dis* 1995;20(Suppl 2):S279–S282.
24. Barg NL, Kish MA, Kauffman CA, et al. Group A streptococcal bacteremia in intravenous drug abusers. *Am J Med* 1985;78:569–574.
25. Lentneck AL, Giger O, O'Rourke E. Group A beta-hemolytic streptococcal bacteremia and intravenous substance abuse. A growing clinical problem? *Arch Intern Med* 1990;150:89–93.
26. Braunstein H. Characteristics of group A streptococcal bacteremia in patients at the San Bernardino County Medical Center. *Rev Infect Dis* 1991;13:8–11.
27. Bernaldo de Quiros JC, Moreno S, Cercenado E, et al. Group A streptococcal bacteremia. A 10-year prospective study. *Medicine* 1997;76: 238–248.

28. Craven DE, Rixinger AI, Bisno AL, et al. Bacteremia caused by group G streptococci in parenteral drug abusers: epidemiological and clinical aspects. *J Infect Dis* 1986;153:988–992.
29. Craven DE, Rixinger AI, Goularte TA, et al. Methicillin-resistant *Staphylococcus aureus* bacteremia linked to intravenous drug abusers using a "shooting gallery." *Am J Med* 1986;80:770–776.
30. Centers for Disease Control and Prevention (CDC). Update: Clostridium novyi and unexplained illness among injecting-drug users—Scotland, Ireland, and England, April–June, 2000. *MMWR* 2000;49:543–545.
31. Centers for Disease Control and Prevention (CDC). Unexplained illness and death among injecting-drug users—Glasgow, Scotland; Dublin, Ireland; and England, April–June, 2000. *MMWR* 2000;49:489–492.
32. Bangsberg DR, Rosen JI, Aragón T, et al. Clostridial myonecrosis cluster among injection drug users: a molecular epidemiology investigation. *Arch Intern Med* 2002;162:517–522.
33. Allison DC, Miller T, Holtom P, et al. Microbiology of upper extremity soft tissue abscesses in injecting drug abusers. *Clin Orthop Relat Res* 2007;461:9–13.
34. Klevens RM, Morrison MA, Nadle J, et al. Invasive methicillin-resistant *Staphylococcus aureus* infections in the United States. *JAMA* 2007;298: 1763–1771.
35. Gilbert M, MacDonald J, Gregson D, et al. Outbreak in Alberta of community-acquired (USA300) methicillin-resistant *Staphylococcus aureus* in people with a history of drug use, homelessness, or incarceration. *CMAJ* 2006;175:149–154.
36. Moran GJ, Krishnadasan A, Gorwitz RJ, et al. Methicillin-resistant *S. aureus* infections among patients in the emergency department. *N Engl J Med* 2006;355:666–674.
37. Paydar KZ, Hansen SL, Charlebois ED, et al. Inappropriate antibiotic use in soft tissue infections. *Arch Surg* 2006;141:850–854.
38. Awad SS, Elhabash SI, Lee L, et al. Increasing incidence of methicillin-resistant *Staphylococcus aureus* skin and soft-tissue infections: reconsideration of empiric antimicrobial therapy. *Am J Surg* 2007;194:606–610.
39. Ruhe JJ, Smith N, Bradsher RW, et al. Community-onset methicillin-resistant *Staphylococcus aureus* skin and soft-tissue infections: impact of antimicrobial therapy on outcome. *Clin Infect Dis* 2007;44: 777–784.
40. Cohen AL, Shuler C, McAllister S, et al. Methamphetamine use and methicillin-resistant *Staphylococcus aureus* skin infections. *Emerg Infect Dis* 2007;13:1707–1713.
41. Blumberg HM, Stephens DS. Pyomyositis and human immunodeficiency virus infection. *South Med J* 1990;83:1092–1095.
42. Schwartzman WA, Lambertus MW, Kennedy CA, et al. Staphylococcal pyomyositis in patients infected by the human immunodeficiency virus. *Am J Med* 1991;90:595–600.
43. Widrow CA, Kellie SM, Saltzman BR, et al. Pyomyositis in patients with the human immunodeficiency virus: an unusual form of disseminated bacterial infection. *Am J Med* 1991;91:129–136.
44. Christin L, Sarosi GA. Pyomyositis in North America: case reports and review. *Clin Infect Dis* 1992;15:668–677.
45. Hsueh PR, Hsiue TR, Hsieh WC. Pyomyositis in intravenous drug abusers: report of a unique case and review of the literature. *Clin Infect Dis* 1996;22:858–860.
46. Wongpaitoon V, Sathapatayavongs B, Prachaktam R, et al. Spontaneous *Vibrio vulnificus* peritonitis and primary sepsis in two patients with alchoholic cirrhosis. *Am J Gastroenterol* 1985;80:706–708.
47. Arnold M, Woo ML, French GL. *Vibrio vulnificus* septicaemia presenting as spontaneous necrotising cellulitis in a woman with hepatic cirrhosis. *Scand J Infect Dis* 1989;21:727–731.
48. Harlow KD, Harner RC, Fontenelle LJ. Primary skin infections secondary to *Vibrio vulnificus*: the role of operative intervention. *J Am Coll Surg* 1996;183:329–334.
49. Saini T, Edwards PC, Kimmes NS, et al. Etiology of xerostomia and dental caries among methamphetamine abusers. *Oral Health Prev Dent* 2005;3:189–195.
50. Shaner JW, Kimmes N, Saini T, et al. "Meth mouth": rampant caries in methamphetamine abusers. *AIDS Patient Care STDS* 2006;20: 146–150.
51. Pelletier LL, Petersdorf RG. Infective endocarditis: a review of 125 cases from the University of Washington Hospitals, 1963–1972. *Medicine* 1977;56:287–313.
52. Bayer AS, Bolger AF, Taubert KA, et al. Diagnosis and management of infective endocarditis and its complications. *Circulation* 1998;98: 2936–2948.
53. Mylonakis E, Calderwood SB. Infective endocarditis in adults. *N Engl J Med* 2001;345:1318–1330.
54. Wilson LE, Thomas DL, Astemborski J, et al. Prospective study of infective endocarditis among injection drug users. *J Infect Dis* 2002;185: 1761–1766.
55. Brown, PD, Levine DP. Infective endocarditis in the injection drug user. *Infect Dis Clin North Am* 2002;16:645–665.
56. Fowler VG, Scheld WM, Bayer AS. Endocarditis and intravascular infections. In Mandell GL, Bennett JE, Dolin R, eds. *Mandell, Douglas, and Bennett's principles and practice of infectious diseases*, 6th ed. Philadelphia: Churchill Livingstone, 2005:975–1022.
57. Beynon RP, Bahl VK, Prendergast BD. Infective endocarditis. *BMJ* 2006;333:334–339.
58. Miró JM, delRio A, Mestres CA. Infective endocarditis and cardiac surgery in intravenous drug abusers and HIV-1 infected patients. *Cardiol Clin* 2003;21:167–184.
59. Tsigrelis C, Armstrong MD, Vlahakis NE, et al. Infective endocarditis due to community-associated methicillin-resistant *Staphylococcus aureus* in injection drug users may be associated with Panton-Valentine leukocidin-negative strains. *Scand J Infect Dis* 2007;39:299–302.
60. Chambers HF, Morris DL, Tauber MG, et al. Cocaine use and the risk for endocarditis in intravenous drug users. *Ann Intern Med* 1987;106: 833–836.
61. Graves MK, Soto L. Left-sided endocarditis in parenteral drug abusers: recent experience at a large community hospital. *South Med J* 1992;85: 378–380.
62. Hecht SR, Berger M. Right-sided endocarditis in intravenous drug users. Prognostic features in 102 episodes. *Ann Intern Med* 1992;117: 560–566.
63. Berlin JA, Abrutyn E, Strom BL, et al. Incidence of infective endocarditis in the Delaware Valley, 1988–1990. *Am J Cardiol* 1995;76: 933–936.
64. Nahass RG, Weinstein MP, Bartels J, et al. Infective endocarditis in intravenous drug users: a comparison of human immunodeficiency virus type 1-negative and -positive patients. *J Infect Dis* 1990;162: 967–970.
65. Chambers HF, Korzeniowski OM, Sande MA. *Staphylococcus aureus* endocarditis: clinical manifestations in addicts and nonaddicts. *Medicine* 1983;62:170–177.
66. Gallagher PG, Watanakunakorn C. Group B streptococcal endocarditis: report of seven cases and review of the literature, 1962–1985. *Rev Infect Dis* 1986;8:175–88.
67. Rapeport KB, Giron JA, Rosner F. *Streptococcus mitis* endocarditis. Report of 17 cases. *Arch Intern Med* 1986;146:2361–2363.
68. Venezio FR, Gullberg RM, Westenfelder GO, et al. Group G streptococcal endocarditis and bacteremia. *Am J Med* 1986;81:29–34.
69. Snyder N, Atterbury CE, Pinto Correia J, et al. Increased concurrence of cirrhosis and bacterial endocarditis. A clinical and postmortem study. *Gastroenterology* 1977;73:1107–1013.
70. Shekar R, Rice TW, Zierdt CH, et al. Outbreak of endocarditis caused by *Pseudomonas aeruginosa* serotype O11 among pentazocine and tripelennamine abusers in Chicago. *J Infect Dis* 1985;151:203–208.
71. Botsford KB, Weinstein RA, Nathan CR, et al. Selective survival in pentazocine and tripelennamine of *Pseudomonas aeruginosa* serotype O11 from drug addicts. *J Infect Dis* 1985;151:209–216.
72. Wieland M, Lederman MM, Kline-King C, et al. Left-sided endocarditis due to *Pseudomonas aeruginosa*. A report of 10 cases and review of the literature. *Medicine* 1986;65:180–189.
73. Mills J, Drew D. *Serratia marcescens* endocarditis: a regional illness associated with intravenous drug abuse. *Ann Intern Med* 1976;84:29–35.
74. Cooper R, Mills J. Serratia endocarditis. A follow-up report. *Arch Intern Med* 1980;140:199–202.

75. Komshian SV, Tablan OC, Palutke W, et al. Characteristics of left-sided endocarditis due to *Pseudomonas aeruginosa* in the Detroit Medical Center. *Rev Infect Dis* 1990;12:693–702.
76. Burman LA, Norrby R, Trollfors B. Invasive pneumococcal infections: incidence, predisposing factors, and prognosis. *Rev Infect Dis* 1985;7: 133–142.
77. Ugolini V, Pacifico A, Smitherman TC, et al. Pneumococcal endocarditis update: analysis of 10 cases diagnosed between 1974 and 1984. *Am Heart J* 1986;112:813–819.
78. Gelfand MS, Threlkeld MG. Subacute bacterial endocarditis secondary to *Streptococcus pneumoniae*. *Am J Med* 1992;93:91–93.
79. Musher DM. Infections caused by *Streptococcus pneumoniae*: clinical spectrum, pathogenesis, immunity, and treatment. *Clin Infect Dis* 1992; 14:801–807.
80. Spach DH, Callis KP, Paauw DS, et al. Endocarditis caused by *Rochalimaea quintana* in a patient infected with human immunodeficiency virus. *J Clin Microbiol* 1993;31:692–694.
81. Spach DH, Kanter AS, Daniels NA, et al. Bartonella (Rochalimaea) species as a cause of apparent "culture-negative" endocarditis. *Clin Infect Dis* 1995;20:1044–1047.
82. Comer JA, Flynn C, Regnery RL, et al. Antibodies to Bartonella species in inner-city intravenous drug users in Baltimore, Md. *Arch Intern Med* 1996;156:2491–2495.
83. Holmes AH, Greenough TC, Balady GJ, et al. *Bartonella henselae* endocarditis in an immunocompetent adult. *Clin Infect Dis* 1995;21:1004–1007.
84. Raoult D, Fournier PE, Drancourt M, et al. Diagnosis of 22 new cases of Bartonella endocarditis. *Ann Intern Med* 1996;125:646–652.
85. Riancho JA, Echevarria S, Napal J, et al. Endocarditis due to *Listeria monocytogenes* and human immunodeficiency virus infection. *Am J Med* 1988;85:737.
86. Bestetti RB, Figueiredo JF, Da Costa JC. Salmonella tricuspid endocarditis in an intravenous drug abuser with human immunodeficiency virus infection. *Int J Cardiol* 1991;30:361–362.
87. Steen MK, Bruno-Murtha LA, Chaux G, et al. *Bacillus cereus* endocarditis: report of a case and review. *Clin Infect Dis* 1992;14:945–946.
88. Ascher DP, Zbick C, White C, et al. Infections due to *Stomatococcus mucilaginosus*: 10 cases and review. *Rev Infect Dis* 1991;13:1048–1052.
89. Weinstein L. Life-threatening complications of infective endocarditis and their management. *Arch Intern Med* 1986;146:953–957.
90. Mansur AJ, Grinberg M, da Luz PL, et al. The complications of infective endocarditis. A reappraisal in the 1980s. *Arch Intern Med* 1992;152: 2428–2432.
91. Omari B, Shapiro S, Ginzton L, et al. Predictive risk factors for periannular extension of native valve endocarditis. Clinical and echocardiographic analyses. *Chest* 1989;96:1273–1279.
92. Robinson SL, Saxe JM, Lucas CE, et al. Splenic abscess associated with endocarditis. *Surgery* 1992;112:781–786.
93. Speechly-Dick ME, Swanton RH. Osteomyelitis and infective endocarditis. *Postgrad Med J* 1994;70:885–890.
94. Marantz PR, Linzer M, Feiner CJ, et al. Inability to predict diagnosis in febrile intravenous drug abusers. *Ann Intern Med* 1987;106:823–828.
95. Weisse AB, Heller DR, Schimenti RJ, et al. The febrile parenteral drug user: a prospective study in 121 patients. *Am J Med* 1993;94:274–280.
96. Frontera JA, Gradon JD. Right-side endocarditis in injection drug users: review of proposed mechanisms of pathogenesis. *Clin Infect Dis* 2000;30:374–379.
97. Moss R, Munt B. Injection drug use and right sided endocarditis. *Heart* 2003;89:577–581.
98. Von Reyn CF, Levy BS, Arbeit RD, et al. Infective endocarditis: an analysis based on strict case definitions. *Ann Intern Med* 1981;94:505–518.
99. Durack DT, Lukes AS, Bright DK. New criteria for diagnosis of infective endocarditis: Utilization of specific echocardiographic findings. Duke Endocarditis Service. *Am J Med* 1994;96:200–209.
100. Bayer AS, Ward JI, Ginzton LE, et al. Evaluation of new clinical criteria for the diagnosis of infective endocarditis. *Am J Med* 1994;96:211–219.
101. Li JS, Sexton DJ, Mick N, et al., Proposed modifications to the Duke Criteria for the diagnosis of infective endocarditis. *Clin Infect Dis* 2000;30:633–638.
102. Lindner JR, Case RA, Dent JM, et al. Diagnostic value of echocardiography in suspected endocarditis. An evaluation based on the pretest probability of disease. *Circulation* 1996;93:730–736.
103. Roe MT, Abramson MA, Li J, et al. Clinical information determines the impact of transesophageal echocardiography on the diagnosis of infective endocarditis by the Duke Criteria. *Am Heart J* 2000;139:945–951.
104. Bonow RO, Carabello BA, Chatterjee K, et al. ACC/AHA 2006 guidelines for the management of patients with valvular heart disease: a report of the American College of Cardiology/American Heart Association task force on practice guidelines. *Circulation* 2006;114:e84–231.
105. Wilson WR, Karchmer AW, Dajani AS, et al. Antibiotic treatment of adults with infective endocarditis due to streptococci, enterococci, staphylococci, and HACEK microorganisms. American Heart Association. *JAMA* 1995;274:1706–1713.
106. Carrel T, Schaffner A, Vogt P, et al. Endocarditis in intravenous drug addicts and HIV infected patients: possibilities and limitations of surgical treatment. *J Heart Valve Dis* 1993;2:140–147.
107. Kaiser SP, Melby SJ, Zierer A, et al. Long-term outcomes in valve replacement surgery for infective endocarditis. *Ann Thorac Surg* 2007;83:30–35.
108. Wilson W, Taubert KA, Gewitz M, et al. Prevention of infective endocarditis: guidelines from the American Heart Association. *Circulation* 2007;116:1736–1754.
109. Tsao JW, Garlin AB, Marder SR, et al. Mycotic aneurysm presenting as Pancoast's syndrome in an injection drug user. *Ann Emerg Med* 1999;34: 546–549.
110. Shaikholeslami R, Tomlinson CW, Teoh KH, et al. Mycotic aneurysm complicating staphylococcal endocarditis. *Can J Cardiol* 1999;15: 217–222.
111. Lee TY, Lee TY, Cheng YF. Subclavian mycotic aneurysm presenting as mediastinal abscess. *Am J Emerg Med* 1998;16:714–716.
112. Tsao JW, Marder SR, Goldstone J, et al. Presentation, diagnosis, and management of arterial mycotic pseudoaneurysms in injection drug users. *Ann Vasc Surg* 2002;16;652–662.
113. Chan YC, Burnand KG. Management of septic groin complications and infected femoral false aneurysms in intravenous drug abusers. *Br J Surg* 2006;93:781–782.
114. Frizzell RT, Vitek JJ, Hill DL, et al. Treatment of a bacterial (mycotic) intracranial aneurysm using an endovascular approach. *Neurosurgery* 1993;32:852–854.
115. Caiaffa WT, Vlahov D, Graham NM, et al. Drug smoking, *Pneumocystis carinii* pneumonia, and immunosuppression increase risk of bacterial pneumonia in human immunodeficiency virus-seropositive injection drug users. *Am J Respir Crit Care Med* 1994;150:1493–1498.
116. Wewers MD, Diaz PT, Wewers ME, et al. Cigarette smoking in HIV infection induces a suppressive inflammatory environment in the lung. *Am J Respir Crit Care Med* 1998;158:1543–1549.
117. Lipsky BA, Boyko EJ, Inui TS, et al. Risk factors for acquiring pneumococcal infections. *Arch Intern Med* 1986;146:2179–85.
118. Bartlett JG, Gorbach SL, Finegold SM. The bacteriology of aspiration pneumonia. *Am J Med* 1974;56:202–207.
119. O'Donnell AE, Pappas LS. Pulmonary complications of intravenous drug abuse. Experience at an inner-city hospital. *Chest* 1988;94: 251–253.
120. Bailey ME, Fraire AE, Greenberg SD, et al. Pulmonary histopathology in cocaine abusers. *Hum Pathol* 1994;25:203–207.
121. Polsky B, Gold JW, Whimbey E, et al. Bacterial pneumonia in patients with the acquired immunodeficiency syndrome. *Ann Intern Med* 1986; 104:38–41.
122. Witt DJ, Craven DE, McCabe WR. Bacterial infections in adult patients with the acquired immune deficiency syndrome (AIDS) and AIDS-related complex. *Am J Med* 1987;82:900–906.
123. Hirschtick RE, Glassroth J, Jordan MC, et al. Bacterial pneumonia in persons infected with the human immunodeficiency virus. Pulmonary Complications of HIV Infection Study Group. *N Engl J Med* 1995;333: 845–851.
124. Caiaffa WT, Graham NM, Vlahov D. Bacterial pneumonia in adult populations with human immunodeficiency virus (HIV) infection. *Am J Epidemiol* 1993;138:909–922.

125. Sullivan JH, Moore RD, Keruly JC, et al. Effect of antiretroviral therapy on the incidence of bacterial pneumonia in patients with advanced HIV infection. *Am J Respir Crit Care Med* 2000;162:64–67.
126. Goss CH, Rubenfeld GD, Park DR, et al. Cost and incidence of social comorbidities in low-risk patients with community-acquired pneumonia admitted to a public hospital. *Chest* 2003;124:2148–2155.
127. de Roux A, Cavalcanti M, Marcos MA, et al. Impact of alcohol abuse in the etiology and severity of community-acquired pneumonia. *Chest* 2006;129:1219–1225.
128. Mandell LA, Wunderink RG, Anzueto A, et al. Infectious Diseases Society of America/American Thoracic Society consensus guidelines on the management of community-acquired pneumonia in adults. *Clin Infect Dis* 2007;44(Suppl 2):S27–S72.
129. Centers for Disease Control and Prevention (CDC). Prevention and control of influenza. *MMWR* 2007;56(RR06):1–54.
130. Janoff EN, Breiman RF, Daley CL, et al. Pneumococcal disease during HIV infection. Epidemiologic, clinical, and immunologic perspectives. *Ann Intern Med* 1992;117:314–324.
131. Rodriguez Barradas MC, Musher DM, Hamill RJ, et al. Unusual manifestations of pneumococcal infection in human immunodeficiency virus-infected individuals: the past revisited. *Clin Infect Dis* 1992; 14:192–199.
132. Steinhart R, Reingold AL, Taylor F, et al. Invasive *Haemophilus influenzae* infections in men with HIV infection. *JAMA* 1992;268:3350–3352.
133. Kielhofner M, Atmar RL, Hamill RJ, et al. Life-threatening *Pseudomonas aeruginosa* infections in patients with human immunodeficiency virus infection. *Clin Infect Dis* 1992;14:403–411.
134. Fichtenbaum CJ, Woeltje KF, Powderly WG. Serious *Pseudomonas aeruginosa* infections in patients infected with human immunodeficiency virus: a case-control study. *Clin Infect Dis* 1994;19:417–422.
135. Centers for Disease Control and Prevention (CDC). Severe methicillin-resistant *Staphylococcus aureus* community-acquired pneumonia associated with influenza—Louisiana and Georgia, December 2006–January 2007. *MMWR* 2007;56:325–329.
136. O'Grady NP, Barie PS, Bartlett JG, et al., Practice guidelines for evaluating new fever in critically ill adult patients. *Clin Infect Dis* 1998;26: 1042–1059.
137. Cantwell MF, Snider DE, Cauthen GM, et al. Epidemiology of tuberculosis in the United States, 1985 through 1992. *JAMA* 1994;272:535–539.
138. Jones BE, Young SM, Antoniskis D, et al. Relationship of the manifestations of tuberculosis to CD4 cell counts in patients with human immunodeficiency virus infection. *Am Rev Respir Dis* 1993;148: 1292–1297.
139. Greenberg SD, Frager D, Suster B, et al. Active pulmonary tuberculosis in patients with AIDS: spectrum of radiographic findings (including a normal appearance). *Radiology* 1994;193:115–119.
140. Castro KG. Tuberculosis as an opportunistic disease in persons infected with human immunodeficiency virus. *Clin Infect Dis* 1995;21(Suppl 1):S66–S71.
141. Havlir DV, Barnes PF. Tuberculosis in patients with human immunodeficiency virus infection. *N Engl J Med* 1999;340:367–373.
142. Markowitz N, Hansen NI, Hopewell PC, et al. Incidence of tuberculosis in the United States among HIV-infected persons. The Pulmonary Complications of HIV Infection Study Group. *Ann Intern Med* 1997;126:123–132.
143. Pablos-Mendez A, Raviglione MC, Laszlo A, et al. Global surveillance for antituberculosis-drug resistance, 1994–1997. World health Organization-International Union against Tuberculosis and Lung Disease Working Group on Anti-Tuberculosis Drug Resistance Surveillance. *N Engl J Med* 1998;338:1641–1649.
144. Shafer RW, Kim DS, Weiss JP, et al. Extrapulmonary tuberculosis in patients with human immunodeficiency virus infection. *Medicine* 1991;70:384–397.
145. Relkin F, Aranda CP, Garay SM, et al. Pleural tuberculosis and HIV infection. *Chest* 1994;105:1338–1341.
146. Frye MD, Pozsik CJ, Sahn SA. Tuberculous pleurisy is more common in AIDS than in non-AIDS patients with tuberculosis. *Chest* 1997;112: 393–397.
147. Diagnostic Standards and Classification of Tuberculosis in Adults and Children. *Am J Respir Crit Care Med* 2000;161:1376–1395.
148. Raviglione MC, Smith IM. XDR tuberculosis—implications for global public health. *N Engl J Med* 2007;356:656–659.
149. Wells CD, Cegielski JP, Nelson LJ, et al. HIV infection and multidrug-resistant tuberculosis: the perfect storm. *J Infect Dis*. 2007;196(Suppl 1):S86–S107.
150. Shah NS, Wright A, Bai GH, et al. Worldwide emergence of extensively drug-resistant tuberculosis. *Emerg Infect Dis* 2007;13:380–387.
151. Centers for Disease Control and Prevention (CDC). *Reported tuberculosis in the United States, 2006*. Atlanta: U.S. Department of Health and Human Services, CDC, September 2007.
152. Reichman LB, Felton CP, Edsall JR. Drug dependence, a possible new risk factor for tuberculosis disease. *Arch Intern Med* 1979;139:337–339.
153. Perlman DC, Salomon N, Perkins MP, et al. Tuberculosis in drug users. *Clin Infect Dis* 1995;1253–1264.
154. Centers for Disease Control and Prevention (CDC). Cluster of tuberculosis cases among exotic dancers and their close contacts: Kansas, 1994–2000. *MMWR* 2001;50:291–293.
155. Frieden TR, Sterling T, Pablo-Mendez A, et al. The emergence of drug-resistant tuberculosis in New York City. *N Engl J Med* 1993;328:521–526.
156. Bloch AB, Cauthen BM, Onorato IM, et al. Nationwide survey of drug-resistant tuberculosis in the United States. *JAMA* 1994;271:665–671.
157. Alland D, Kalkut GE, Moss AR, et al. Transmission of tuberculosis in New York City. An analysis by DNA fingerprinting and conventional epidemiologic methods. *N Engl J Med* 1994;330:1710–1716.
158. Gordin FM, Nelson ET, Matts JP, et al. The impact of human immunodeficiency virus infection on drug-resistant tuberculosis. *Am J Respir Crit Care Med* 1996;154:1478–1483.
159. Centers for Disease Control and Prevention (CDC). Missed opportunities for prevention of tuberculosis among persons with HIV infection—selected locations, United States, 1996–1997. *MMWR* 2000;49: 685–687.
160. Centers for Disease Control and Prevention (CDC). Screening for tuberculosis and tuberculosis infection in high-risk populations. Recommendations of the Advisory Council for the Elimination of Tuberculosis. *MMWR* 1995;44(RR-11):19–34.
161. Centers for Disease Control and Prevention (CDC). Targeted tuberculin testing and treatment of latent tuberculosis infection. *MMWR* 2000;49(RR-6):1–51.
162. Centers for Disease Control and Prevention (CDC). Anergy skin testing and tuberculosis preventive therapy for HIV-infected persons: revised recommendations. *MMWR* 1997;46(RR-15):1–10.
163. Bass JB, Farer LS, Hopewell PC, et al. Treatment of Tuberculosis and tuberculosis infection in adults and children. American Thoracic Society and the Centers for Disease Control and Prevention. *Am J Respir Crit Care Med* 1994;149:1359–1374.
164. Centers for Disease Control and Prevention (CDC). Prevention and treatment of tuberculosis among patients infected with human immunodeficiency virus: principles of therapy and revised recommendations. *MMWR* 1998;47(RR-20):1–58.
165. Horsburgh CR, Feldman S, Ridzon R. Practice guidelines for the treatment of tuberculosis. *Clin Infect Dis* 2000;31:633–639.
166. Centers for Disease Control and Prevention (CDC). Treatment of Tuberculosis. *MMWR* 2003;52(RR11):1–77.
167. Centers for Disease Control and Prevention (CDC). Controlling tuberculosis in the United States. Recommendations from the American Thoracic Society, CDC, and the Infectious Diseases Society of America. *MMWR* 2005;54(RR12):1–81.
168. Halsey NA, Coberly JS, Desormeaux J, et al. Randomised trial of isoniazid versus rifampicin and pyrazinamide for prevention of tuberculosis in HIV-1 infection. *Lancet* 1998;351:786–792.
169. Gordin F, Chaisson RE, Matts JP, et al. Rifampin and pyrazinamide vs. isoniazid for prevention of tuberculosis in HIV-infected persons: an international randomized trial. *JAMA* 2000;283:1445–1450.
170. Centers for Disease Control and Prevention (CDC). Clinical update: impact of HIV protease inhibitors on the treatment of HIV-infected tuberculosis patients with rifampin. *MMWR* 1996;45:921–925.

171. Polesky A, Farber HW, Gottlieb DJ, et al. Rifampin preventive therapy for tuberculosis in Boston's homeless. *Am J Respir Crit Care Med* 1996; 154:1473–1477.
172. Centers for Disease Control and Prevention (CDC). Notice to readers: Updated guidelines for the use of rifabutin or rifampin for the treatment and prevention of tuberculosis among HIV-infected patients taking protease inhibitors or nonnucleoside reverse transcriptase inhibitors. *MMWR* 2000;49:185–189.
173. Centers for Disease Control and Prevention (CDC). Fatal and severe hepatitis associated with rifampin and pyrazinamide for the treatment of latent tuberculosis infection: New York and Georgia, 2000. *MMWR* 2001;50:289–291.
174. Kellerman SE, Hanson DL, McNaghten AD, et al. Prevalence of chronic hepatitis B and incidence of acute hepatitis B infection in human immunodeficiency virus-infected subjects. *J Infect Dis* 2003;188:571–577.
175. Palepu A, Cheng DM, Kim T, et al. Substance abuse treatment and receipt of liver specialty care among persons coinfected with HIV/HCV who have alcohol problems. *J Subst Abuse Treat* 2006;31:411–417.
176. Koziel MJ, Peters MG. Viral hepatitis in HIV infection. *N Engl J Med* 2007;356:1445–1154.
177. Armstrong GL, Wasley A, Simard EP, et al. The prevalence of hepatitis C virus infection in the United States, 1999 through 2002. *Ann Intern Med* 2006;144:705–714.
178. Page-Shafer K, Hahn JA, Lum PJ. Preventing hepatitis C virus infection in injection drug users: risk reduction is not enough. *AIDS* 2007;21: 1967–1969.
179. Neaigus A, Gyarmathy VA, Zhao M, et al. Sexual and other noninjection risks for HBV and HCV seroconversions among noninjecting heroin users. *J Infect Dis* 2007;195:1052–1061.
180. Scheinmann R, Hagan H, Lelutiu-Weinberger C, et al. Non-injection drug use and Hepatitis C Virus: a systematic review. *Drug Alcohol Depend* 2007;89:1–12.
181. Edlin BR, Kresina TF, Raymond DB, et al. Overcoming barriers to prevention, care and treatment of hepatitis C in illicit drug users. *Clin Infect Dis* 2005;40(Suppl 5):S276–S285.
182. Such J, Runyon BA. Spontaneous bacterial peritonitis. *Clin Infect Dis* 1998;27:669–674.
183. Runyon BA, Montano AA, Akriviadis EA, et al. The serum-ascites albumin gradient is superior to the exudate-transudate concept in the differential diagnosis of ascites. *Ann Intern Med* 1992;117: 215–220.
184. Lew DP, Waldvogel FA. Osteomyelitis. *N Engl J Med* 1997;336: 999–1007.
185. Holzman RS, Bishko F. Osteomyelitis in heroin addicts. *Ann Intern Med* 1971;75:693–696.
186. Sapico FL, Montgomerie JZ. Pyogenic vertebral osteomyelitis: report of nine cases and review of the literature. *Rev Infect Dis* 1979;1: 754–776.
187. Sapico FL, Montgomerie JZ. Vertebral osteomyelitis in intravenous drug abusers: report of three cases and review of the literature. *Rev Infect Dis* 1980;2:196–206.
188. Lew DP, Waldvogel FA. Osteomyelitis. *Lancet* 2004;364:369–379.
189. Ziran BH. Osteomyelitis. *J Trauma* 2007;62(Suppl 6):S59–S60.
190. Bass SN, Ailani RK, Shekar R, et al. Pyogenic vertebral osteomyelitis presenting as exudative pleural effusion: a series of five cases. *Chest* 1998;114:642–647.
191. Ross JJ, Shamsuddin H. Sternoclavicular septic arthritis: review of 180 cases. *Medicine (Baltimore)* 2004;83:139–148.
192. Chandrasekar PH, Narula AP. Bone and joint infections in intravenous drug abusers. *Rev Infect Dis* 1986;8:904–911.
193. del Busto R, Quinn EL, Fisher EJ, et al. Osteomyelitis of the pubis. Report of seven cases. *JAMA* 1982;248:1498–1500.
194. Ross JJ, Hu LT. Septic arthritis of the pubic symphysis: review of 100 cases. *Medicine (Baltimore)* 2003;82:340–345.
195. Tunkel AR, Pradhan SK. Central nervous system infections in injection drug users. *Infect Dis Clin North Am* 2002;16:589–605.
196. Darouiche RO. Spinal epidural abscess. *N Engl J Med* 2006;355: 2012–2020.
197. Musher DM, Hamill RJ, Baughn RE. Effect of human immunodeficiency virus (HIV) infection on the course of syphilis and on the response to treatment. *Ann Intern Med* 1990;113:872–881.
198. Centers for Disease Control and Prevention (CDC). Symptomatic early neurosyphilis among HIV-positive men who have sex with men—four cities, United States, January 2002–June 2004. *MMWR* 2007;56:625–628.
199. Bleck TP. *Clostridium botulinum* (botulism). In Mandell GL, Bennett JE, Dolin R, eds. *Mandell, Douglas, and Bennett's principles and practice of infectious diseases*, 6th ed. Philadelphia: Churchill Livingstone, 2005:2822–2828.
200. Passaro DJ, Werner SB, McGee J, et al. Wound botulism associated with black tar heroin among injecting drug users. *JAMA* 1998;279:859–863.
201. Centers for Disease Control and Prevention (CDC). Wound botulism among black tar heroin users—Washington, 2003. *MMWR* 2003;52: 885–886.
202. Werner SB, Passaro D, McGee J, et al. Wound botulism in California, 1951–1998: recent epidemic in heroin injectors. *Clin Infect Dis* 2000; 31:1018–1024.
203. Kudrow DB, Henry DA, Haake DA, et al. Botulism associated with *Clostridium botulinum* sinusitis after intranasal cocaine abuse. *Ann Intern Med* 1988;109:984–985.
204. Bleck TP. *Clostridium tetani* (tetanus). In Mandell GL, Bennett JE, Dolin R, eds. *Mandell, Douglas, and Bennett's principles and practice of infectious diseases*, 6th ed. Philadelphia: Churchill Livingstone, 2005: 2817–2822.
205. Cherubin CE. Clinical severity of tetanus in narcotic addicts in New York City. *Arch Intern Med* 1968;121:156–158.
206. Centers for Disease Control and Prevention (CDC). Tetanus surveillance—United States, 1998–2000. *MMWR* 2003;52(SS03):1–8.
207. Bisbe J, Miro JM, Latorre X, et al. Disseminated candidiasis in addicts who use brown heroin: report of 83 cases and review. *Clin Infect Dis* 1992;15:910–923.
208. Kim RW, Juzych MS, Eliott D. Ocular manifestations of injection drug use. *Infect Dis Clin North Am* 2002;16:607–622.
209. Centers for Disease Control and Prevention (CDC). Pneumocystis pneumonia—Los Angeles. *MMWR* 1981;30:250.
210. Centers for Disease Control and Prevention (CDC). Kaposi's sarcoma and *Pneumocystis* pneumonia among homosexual men—New York City and California. *MMWR* 1981;30:305.
211. Acquired immunodeficiency syndrome. In Mandell GL, Bennett JE, Dolin R, eds. *Mandell, Douglas, and Bennett's principles and practice of infectious diseases*, 6th ed. Philadelphia: Churchill Livingstone, 2005:1465–1719.
212. Mayer KH, eds. HIV/AIDS. *Infect Dis Clin North Am*. 2007;21:1–257.
213. CDC. HIV/AIDS surveillance report, 2005, vol. 17 [revised]. Atlanta: U.S. Department of Health and Human Services, CDC, 2007:1–53.
214. Joint United Nations Programme on HIV/AIDS. UNAIDS. AIDS epidemic update. December, 2007.
215. Panel on Antiretroviral Guidelines for Adult and Adolescents. *Guidelines for the use of antiretroviral agents in HIV-infected adults and adolescents*. Washington, DC: Department of Health and Human Services, October 10, 2006:1–113. Retrieved Nvember 28, 2007, from http://www.aidsinfo.nih.gov/ContentFiles/AdultandAdolescentGL.pdf.
216. Perinatal HIV Guidelines Working Group. *Public Health Service Task Force recommendations for use of antiretroviral drugs in pregnant HIV-infected women for maternal health and interventions to reduce perinatal HIV transmission in the United States*. November 2, 2007:1–96. Retrieved November 28, 2007, from http://aidsinfo.nih.gov/ContentFiles/PerinatalGL.pdf.
217. Kaplan JE, Masur H, Holmes KK, et al. *Guidelines for the prevention of opportunistic infections among HIV-infected persons—2002*. Recommendations of the U.S. Public Health Service and the Infectious Diseases Society of America. *MMWR* 2002;51(RR08):1–46.
218. Benson CA, Kaplan JE, Masur H, et al. Recommendations from CDC, the National Institutes of Health, and the HIV Medicine Association/Infectious Diseases Society of America. *Treating opportunistic infections among HIV-infected adults and adolescents*. Washington, DC: December 17, 2004:1–135. Retrieved November 28, 2007, from http://www.aidsinfo.nih.gov.

219. Beyrer C. HIV epidemiology update and transmission factors: risks and risk contexts-16th International AIDS Conference Epidemiology Plenary. *Clin Infect Dis* 2007;44:981–987.
220. Centers for Disease Control and Prevention (CDC). HIV prevalence, unrecognized infection, and HIV testing among men who have sex with men—five U.S. cities, June 2004–April 2005. *MMWR* 2005;54:597–601.
221. Branson BM, Handsfield HH, Lampe MA, et al. Revised recommendations for HIV testing of adults, adolescents, and pregnant women in health-care settings. *MMWR* 2006;55(RR 14):1–17.
222. Burke RC, Sepkowitz KA, Bernstein KT, et al. Why don't physicians test for HIV? A review of the U.S. literature. *AIDS* 2007;21:1617–1624.
223. Fenton KA. Changing epidemiology of HIV/AIDS in the United States: implications for enhancing and promoting HIV testing strategies. *Clin Infect Dis* 2007;45:S213–S220.
224. Centers for Disease Control and Prevention (CDC). Revision of the CDC surveillance case definition for acquired immunodeficiency syndrome. *MMWR* 1987;36:1–15S.
225. Centers for Disease Control and Prevention (CDC). 1993 Revised classification system for HIV infection and expanded surveillance case definition for AIDS among adolescents and adults. *MMWR* 1992;41(RR–17).
226. Schacker T, Collier AC, Hughes J, et al. Clinical and epidemiologic features of primary HIV infection. *Ann Intern Med* 1996;125:257–264.
227. Niu MT, Stein DS, Schnittman SM. Primary human immunodeficiency virus type 1 infection: review of pathogenesis and early treatment intervention in humans and animal retrovirus infections. *J Infect Dis* 1993;168:1490–1501.
228. Kinloch-de Loes S, de Saussure P, Saurat JH, et al. Symptomatic primary infection due to human immunodeficiency virus type 1: review of 31 cases. *Clin Infect Dis* 1993;17:59–65.
229. Kahn JO, Walker BD. Acute human immunodeficiency virus type 1 infection. *N Engl J Med* 1998;339:33–39.
230. Kelley CF, Barbour JD, Hecht FM. The relation between symptoms, viral load, and viral load set point in primary HIV infection. *J Acquir Immune Def Syndr* 2007;45:445–448.
231. Pantaleo G, Graziosi C, Demarest JF, et al. HIV infection is active and progressive in lymphoid tissue during the clinically latent stage of disease. *Nature* 1993;362:355–358.
232. Schacker TW, Hughes JP, Shea T, et al. Biological and virologic characteristics of primary HIV infection. *Ann Intern Med* 1998;128:613–620.
233. Musey L, Hughes J, Schacker T, et al. Cytotoxic-T-cell responses, viral load, and disease progression in early human immunodeficiency virus type 1 infection. *N Engl J Med* 1997;337:1267–1274.
234. Pantaleo G, Demarest JF, Schacker T, et al. The qualitative nature of the primary immune response to HIV infection is a prognosticator of disease progression independent of the initial level of plasma viremia. *Proc Natl Acad Sci U S A* 1997;94:254–258.
235. Mellors JW, Rinaldo CR, Gupta P, et al. Prognosis in HIV-1 infection predicted by the quantity of virus in plasma. *Science* 1996;272: 1167–1170.
236. Mellors JW, Munoz A, Giorgi JV, et al. Plasma viral load and CD4+ lymphocytes as prognostic markers of HIV-1 infection. *Ann Intern Med* 1997;126:946–954.
237. Maggiolo F, Migliorino M, Pirali A, et al. Duration of viral suppression in patients on stable therapy for HIV-1 infection is predicted by plasma HIV RNA level after 1 month of treatment. *J Acquir Immune Defic Syndr* 2000;25:36–43.
238. Raboud JM, Rae S, Montaner JS. Predicting HIV RNA virologic outcome at 52-weeks follow-up in antiretroviral clinical trials. *J Acquir Immune Defic Syndr* 2000;24:433–439.
239. Grabar S, Le Moing V, Goujard C, et al. Clinical outcome of patients with HIV-1 infection according to immunologic and virologic response after 6 months of highly active antiretroviral therapy. *Ann Intern Med* 2000;133:401–410.
240. Malhotra U, Berrey MM, Huang Y, et al. Effect of combination antiretroviral therapy on T-cell immunity in acute human immunodeficiency virus type 1 infection. *J Infect Dis* 2000;181:121.
241. Mariotto AB, Mariotti S, Pezzotti P, et al. Estimation of the acquired immunodeficiency syndrome incubation period in intravenous drug users: a comparison with male homosexuals. *Am J Epidemiol* 1992;135: 428–437.
242. Margolick JB, Munoz A, Vlahov D, et al. Changes in T-lymphocyte subsets in intravenous drug users with HIV-1 infection. *JAMA* 1992;267: 1631–1636.
243. Margolick JB, Munoz A, Vlahov D, et al. Direct comparison of the relationship between clinical outcome and change in CD4+ lymphocytes in human immunodeficiency virus-positive homosexual men and injecting drug users. *Arch Intern Med* 1994;154:869–875.
244. Galai N, Vlahov D, Margolick JB, et al. Changes in markers of disease progression in HIV-1 seroconverters: a comparison between cohorts of injecting drug users and homosexual men. *J Acquir Immune Defic Syndr Hum Retrovirol* 1995;8:66–74.
245. Vella S, Giuliano M, Floridia M, et al. Effect of sex, age and transmission category on the progression to AIDS and survival of zidovudine-treated symptomatic patients. *AIDS* 1995;9:51–56.
246. Chaisson RE, Keruly JC, Moore RD. Race, sex, drug use, and progression of human immunodeficiency virus disease. *N Engl J Med* 1995;333:751–756.
247. Vlahov D, Graham N, Hoover D, et al. Prognostic indicators for AIDS and infectious disease death in HIV-infected injection drug users. Plasma viral load and CD4+ cell count. *JAMA* 1998;279: 35–40.
248. Sackoff JE, Hanna DB, Pfeiffer MR, et al. Causes of death among persons with AIDS in the era of highly active antiretroviral therapy: New York City. *Ann Intern Med* 2006;145:397–406.
249. Pantaleo G, Menzo S, Vaccarezza M, et al. Studies in subjects with long-term nonprogressive human immunodeficiency virus infection. *N Engl J Med* 1995;332:209–216.
250. Rosenberg ES, Billingsley JM, Caliendo AM, et al. Vigorous HIV-1 specific CD4(+) T-cell responses associated with control of viremia. *Science* 1997;278:1447–1450.
251. McDermott DH, Zimmerman PA, Guignard F, et al. CCR5 promoter polymorphism and HIV-1 disease progression. Multicenter AIDS Cohort Study (MACS). *Lancet* 1998;352:866–870.
252. Magierowska M, Theodorou I, Debre P, et al. Combined genotypes of CCR5, CCR2, SDF1, and HLA genes can predict the long-term non-progressor status in human immunodeficiency virus-1-infected individuals. *Blood* 1999;93:936–941.
253. Telenti A, Ioannidis JPA. Susceptibility to HIV infection—disentangling host genetics and host behavior. *J Infect Dis* 2006;193:4–6.
254. Shrestha S, Strathdee SA, Galai N, et al. Behavioral risk exposure and host genetics of susceptibility to HIV-1 infection. *J Infect Dis* 2006;193: 16–26.
255. Cohen DE, Mayer KH. Primary care issues for HIV-infected patients. *Infect Dis Clin North Am* 2007;21:49–70.
256. Khalsa JH, Kresina T, Sherman K, et al. Medical management of HIV-hepatitis C virus coinfection in injection drug users. *Clin Infect Dis* 2005;41(Suppl 1):S1–S6.
257. Schiffer JT, Sterling TR. Timing of antiretroviral therapy initiation in tuberculosis patients with AIDS: a decision analysis. *J Acquir Immune Defic Syndr* 2007;44:229–234.
258. McIlleron H, Meintjes G, Burman WJ, et al. Complications of antiretroviral therapy in patients with tuberculosis: drug interactions, toxicity, and immune reconstitution inflammatory syndrome. *J Infect Dis* 2007;196(Suppl 1):S63–S75.
259. Centers for Disease Control and Prevention. Recommended Adult Immunization Schedule—United States, October 2007–September 2008. *MMWR* 2007;56:Q1–Q4.
260. Centers for Disease Control and Prevention. Incorporating HIV prevention into the medical care of persons living with HIV: recommendations of CDC, the Health Resources and Services Administration, the National Institutes of Health, and the HIV Medicine Association of the Infectious Diseases Society of America. *MMWR* 2003;52(No. RR-12):1–24.
261. Sepkowitz KA. Effect of prophylaxis on the clinical manifestations of AIDS-related opportunistic infections. *Clin Infect Dis* 1998;26: 806–810.

262. Kaplan JE, Hanson D, Dworkin MS, et al. Epidemiology of human immunodeficiency virus-associated opportunistic infections in the United States in the era of highly active antiretroviral therapy. *Clin Infect Dis* 2000;30(Suppl 1):S4–S14.
263. Palella FJ, Delaney KM, Moorman AC, et al. Declining morbidity and mortality among patients with advanced human immunodeficiency virus infection. HIV Outpatient Study Investigators. *N Engl J Med* 1998;338:853–860.
264. Kitahata MM, Koepsell TD, Deyo RA, et al. Physicians' experience with the acquired immunodeficiency syndrome as a factor in patients' survival. *N Engl J Med* 1996;334:701–706.
265. Aberg JA, Gallant JE, Anderson J, et al. Primary care guidelines for the management of persons infected with human immunodeficiency virus: recommendations of the HIV Medicine Association of the Infectious Diseases Society of America. *Clin Infect Dis* 2004;39:609–629.
266. Giorgi JV, Lyles RH, Matud JL, et al. Predictive value of immunologic and virologic markers after long or short duration of HIV-1 infection. *J Acquir Immune Def Syndr* 2002;29:346–355.
267. McCance-Katz EF. Treatment of opioid dependence and coinfection with HIV and hepatitis C virus in opioid-dependent patients: the importance of drug interactions between opioids and antiretroviral agents. *Clin Infect Dis* 2005;41(Suppl 1):S89–S95.
268. Currier JS. Discontinuing prophylaxis for opportunistic infection: guiding principles. *Clin Infect Dis* 2000;30(Suppl 1):S66–S71.
269. Gulick RM, Mellors JW, Havlir D, et al. 3-year suppression of HIV viremia with indinavir, zidovudine, and lamivudine. *Ann Intern Med* 2000;133:35–39.
270. Furrer H, Egger M, Opravil M, et al. Discontinuation of primary prophylaxis against Pneumocystis carinii pneumonia in HIV-1-infected adults treated with combination antiretroviral therapy. Swiss HIV Cohort Study. *N Engl J Med* 1999;340:1301–1306.
271. Weverling GJ, Mocroft A, Ledergerber B, et al. Discontinuation of Pneumocystis carinii pneumonia prophylaxis after start of highly active antiretroviral therapy in HIV-1 infection. EuroSIDA Study Group. *Lancet* 1999;353:1293–1298.
272. Currier JS, Williams PL, Koletar SL, et al. Discontinuation of Mycobacterium avium complex prophylaxis in patients with antiretroviral therapy-induced increases in CD4+ cell count. A randomized, double-blind, placebo-controlled trial. AIDS Clinical Trials Group 362 Study Team. *Ann Intern Med* 2000;133:493–503.
273. El-Sadr WM, Burman WJ, Grant LB, et al. Discontinuation of prophylaxis for Mycobacterium avium complex disease in HIV-infected patients who have a response to antiretroviral therapy. Terry Beirn Community Programs for Clinical Research on AIDS. *N Engl J Med* 2000;342:1085–1092.
274. Freedberg KA, Scharfstein JA, Seage GR, et al. The cost-effectiveness of preventing AIDS-related opportunistic infections. *JAMA* 1998;279: 130–136.
275. Finzi D, Hermankova M, Pierson T, et al. Identification of a reservoir for HIV-1 in patients on highly active antiretroviral therapy. *Science* 1997;278:1295–1300.
276. Wong JK, Hezareh M, Gunthard HF, et al. Recovery of replication-competent HIV despite prolonged suppression of plasma viremia. *Science* 1997;278:1291–1295.
277. Zhang L, Chung C, Hu BS, et al. Genetic characterization of rebounding HIV-1 after cessation of highly active antiretroviral therapy. *J Clin Invest* 2000;106:839–845.
278. Chun TW, Davey RT, Ostrowski M, et al. Relationship between pre-existing viral reservoirs and the re-emergence of plasma viremia after discontinuation of highly active anti-retroviral therapy. *Nat Med* 2000;6:757–761.
279. Garcia F, Plana M, Vidal C, et al. Dynamics of viral load rebound and immunological changes after stopping effective antiretroviral therapy. *AIDS* 1999;13:F79–F86.
280. Dornadula G, Zhang H, VanUitert B, et al. Residual HIV-1 RNA in blood plasma of patients taking suppressive highly active antiretroviral therapy. *JAMA* 1999;282:1627–1632.
281. Zhang L, Ramratnam B, Tenner-Racz K, et al. Quantifying residual HIV-1 replication in patients receiving combination antiretroviral therapy. *N Engl J Med* 1999;340:1605–1613.
282. Furtado MR, Callaway DS, Phair JP, et al. Persistence of HIV-1 transcription in peripheral-blood mononuclear cells in patients receiving potent antiretroviral therapy. *N Engl J Med* 1999;340: 1614–1622.
283. Strategies for Management of Antiretroviral Therapy (SMART) Study Group. CD4+ count-guided interruption of antiretroviral treatment. *N Engl J Med* 2006;355:2283–2296.
284. Palepu A, Tyndall MW, Joy R, et al. Antiretroviral adherence and HIV treatment outcomes among HIV/HCV co-infected injection drug users: the role of methadone maintenance therapy. *Drug Alcohol Depend* 2006;84:188–194.
285. Mocroft A, Katlama C, Johnson AM, et al. AIDS across Europe, 1994–1998: the EuroSIDA study. *Lancet* 2000;356:291–296.
286. Celentano DD, Lucas G. Optimizing treatment outcomes in HIV-infected patients with substance abuse issues. *Clin Infect Dis* 2007;45 (Suppl 4):S318–S323.
287. Pequegnat W, Fishbein M, Celetano D, et al. NIMH/APPC workgroup on behavioral and biological outcomes in HIV/STD prevention studies: a position statement. *Sex Transm Dis* 2000;27:127–132.
288. Kamb ML, Fishbein M, Douglas JM, et al. Efficacy of risk reduction counseling to prevent human immunodeficiency virus and sexually transmitted diseases: a randomized controlled trial. Project RESPECT Study Group. *JAMA* 1998;280:1161–1167.
289. Sikkema KJ, Kelly JA, Winett RA, et al. Outcomes of a randomized community-level HIV prevention intervention for women living in 18 low-income housing developments. *Am J Public Health* 2000;90: 57–63.
290. The NIMH Multisite HIV Prevention Trial Group. The NIMH multisite HIV prevention trial: reducing HIV sexual risk behavior. *Science* 1998;280:1889–1894.
291. Latka MH, Metsch LR, Mizuno Y, et al. Unprotected sex among HIV-positive injection drug-using women and their serodiscordant male partners: role of personal and partnership influences. *J Acquir Immune Defic Syndr* 2006;42:222–228.
292. Centers for Disease Control and Prevention. Antiretroviral postexposure prophylaxis after sexual, injection-drug use, or other nonoccupational exposure to HIV in the United States: recommendations from the U.S. Department of Health and Human Services. *MMWR* 2005;54(No. RR-2):1–20.
293. Centers for Disease Control and Prevention. Updated U.S. Public Health Service guidelines for the management of occupational exposures to HIV and recommendations for Postexposure Prophylaxis. *MMWR* 2005;54(No. RR-9):1–17.
294. Centers for Disease Control and Prevention (CDC). Sexually transmitted diseases treatment guidelines, 2006. *MMWR* 2006;55(RR11):1–94.
295. Centers for Disease Control and Prevention (CDC). Resurgent bacterial sexually transmitted disease among men who have sex with men: King County, Washington, 1997–1999. *MMWR* 1999;48: 773–777.
296. Centers for Disease Control and Prevention (CDC). Increases in unsafe sex and rectal gonorrhea among men who have sex with men: San Francisco, California, 1994–1997. *MMWR* 1999;48:45–48.
297. Centers for Disease Control and Prevention (CDC). Outbreak of syphilis among men who have sex with men: Southern California, 2000. *MMWR* 2001;50:117–120.
298. Klausner JD, Kent CK, Wong W, et al. The public health response to epidemic syphilis, San Francisco, 1999–2004. *Sex Transm Dis* 2005;32 (Suppl 10):S11–S18.
299. Centers for Disease Control and Prevention (CDC). Primary and secondary syphilis—United States, 2003–2004. *MMWR* 2006;55:269–273.
300. Centers for Disease Control and Prevention (CDC). Methamphetamine use and HIV risk behaviors among heterosexual men—preliminary results from five Northern California counties, December 2001–November 2003. *MMWR* 2006;55:273–277.
301. Adrian M. Addiction and sexually transmitted disease (STD), human immunodeficiency virus, (HIV), and acquired immune deficiency syndrome (AIDS): their mutual interactions. *Subst Use Misuse* 2006;41: 1337–1348.

302. Jeal N, Salisbury C. Health needs and service use of parlour-based prostitutes compared with street-based prostitutes: a cross-sectional survey. *BJOG* 2007;114:875–881.
303. Malow RM, Devieux JG, Rosenberg R, et al. Integrated HIV care: HIV risk outcomes of pregnant substance abusers. *Subst Use Misuse* 2006;41:1745–1767.
304. Raj A, Saitz R, Cheng DM, et al. Associations between alcohol, heroin, and cocaine use and high risk sexual behaviors among detoxification patients. *Am J Drug Alcohol Abuse* 2007;33:169–178.
305. Centers for Disease Control and Prevention (CDC). HIV prevention through early detection and treatment of sexually transmitted diseases—United States. *MMWR* 1998;47(RR-12):1–31.
306. Sulis C. Infectious disease in pregnancy. In Carr PL, Freund KM, Somani S, eds. *The medical care of women.* Philadelphia: WB Saunders Company, 1995:405–422.
307. Blattner W, Charurat M. Human T-cell lymphotropic virus types I and II. In Mandell GL, Bennett JE, Dolin R, eds. *Mandell, Douglas, and Bennett's principles and practice of infectious diseases*, 6th ed. Philadelphia: Churchill Livingstone, 2005:2098–2118.

CHAPTER 78

Sanford Auerbach, MD

Sleep Disorders Related to Alcohol and Other Drug Use

Sleep is a complex physiologic state that is essential for normal function throughout the day. In spite of its critical role, sleep appears to be quite fragile. About 35% of all adults report insomnia at some point during the preceding 6 months and half describe it as serious (1). Given the influence of alcohol and other drugs on sleep, sleep problems are likely to be more prevalent in persons with addictive disorders.

The coexistence of a sleep disorder with an addictive disorder is a complex problem. For example, alcohol consumption can affect "normal sleep" in people without alcohol problems, whereas the patient with alcohol dependence has disrupted sleep while using alcohol and withdrawing from alcohol. Alcohol also has an effect on other sleep-related disorders, particularly obstructive sleep apnea.

This chapter reviews the essential elements of clinical sleep physiology, sleep, the effects of alcohol on both nonalcohol-dependent and alcohol-dependent individuals, and alcohol withdrawal. Finally, the effects of other drugs and alcohol on other specific sleep disorders are considered.

OVERVIEW OF SLEEP

Sleep is essential for normal human function. Wakefulness (lack of sleepiness), vigilance, and performance on monotonous tasks deteriorate after a single sleepless night. Further sleep deprivation leads to more inattentiveness and performance failure. Lack of rapid eye movement sleep is associated with anxiety and excitability, as well as difficulty with concentration and memory. Those deprived of slow wave sleep generally report chronic fatigue, aches, stiffness, uneasiness, and withdrawal.

"Sleep need" is difficult to define, but usually is accepted as the amount of sleep required for optimal function during wakeful periods. Sleep need varies from one individual to the next in a range from 3 to 10 hours of sleep over a 24-hour period (2). These principles apply to sleep that is not interrupted by specific sleep pathology, such as sleep apnea or periodic limb movements.

The relationship of subjective to objective measures of sleep deserves further comment. In the general population, self-reports of sleep time often are subject to both overestimates and underestimates. Overestimates can be attributed, in part, to the fact that an arousal must be at least 5 to 6 minutes in duration if it is to be recalled subsequently as a sustained arousal or period of wakefulness. As a result, sleep punctuated by recurrent, yet brief, periods of arousal may be described as "sound sleep." Similarly, overestimates of sleep duration are not uncommon. This overestimation can be further compounded because healthy older adults may simply accept a decrease in sleep efficiency as a part of normal aging. However, aging also is associated with reduced ability to tolerate sleep deprivation.

Given these influences, it is clear that objective measures of sleep and sleepiness are critical to the study of sleep and the effects of alcohol on sleep. The nocturnal polysomnogram (PSG) is the standard method of determining the presence and stage of sleep by measuring electroencephalographic (EEG), electromyographic, and electro-oculographic activity (3). Similarly, the multiple sleep latency test is a standard and accepted measure of daytime sleepiness; it employs polysomnography while a patient is allowed to take naps on five separate occasions throughout a day (4). The assessment of average sleep latency with such a standardized tool allows a quantification of "sleepiness."

Sleep need often is translated into the concept of "sleep drive." Thus relative sleep deprivation leads to increased sleep drive, whereas napping lends itself to a relative decrease in sleep drive. The change in sleep need with increasing age has been the subject of considerable study, but such studies often are confounded by changes in lifestyle, diet, medication use, napping patterns, and the like. These studies suggest that total sleep over a 24-hour period shows little change as an individual transitions from young adulthood into old age.

Sleep Architecture Understanding normal sleep is an essential prerequisite to understanding sleep disorders. Sleep is a dynamic process, featuring fluctuations in brain wave activity, muscle tone, eye movement, and autonomic activity. It consists of two discrete states: rapid eye movement (REM) and non-rapid eye movement (NREM) sleep. Each can be defined in physiologic terms by using the elements of the PSG: EEG, electro-oculogram, and electromyogram. Formal criteria have been elaborated in a widely accepted manual (3).

NREM NREM sleep has been subdivided into four stages, which are numbered 1 through 4. Stages 3 and 4 usually are consolidated and referred to as *slow wave sleep* (SWS) or *delta sleep*. In brief, each stage is characterized by progressively slower EEG background, lower muscle tone, and decreasing eye movements.

Stage 1 marks the transition from wakefulness to drowsiness. Rhythmic activity is replaced by mixed voltage, 3.0 to 7.0 Hz theta activity, and a decrease in muscle tone. Roving eye movements may be present.

Stage 2 features a similar but slower background EEG, with superimposed "spindles" (low-amplitude, high-frequency, centrally predominant bursts) and K-complexes (high-amplitude, negative or upgoing potential, immediately followed by lower amplitude, positive or downgoing potential, with some faster, low-amplitude activity). Muscle tone may decrease further, whereas eye movements may disappear entirely. Stages 1 and 2 often are referred to as the "light" stages of NREM sleep because of the relatively low arousal threshold.

Stages 3 and 4 (SWS) are characterized by high-amplitude ($\geq$75 microV), slow-wave (0.5 to 2.0 Hz) activity. When the slow wave activity accounts for 20% or more of an epoch, it is considered to be stage 3 sleep. When it accounts for 50% or more, it is considered stage 4. K-complexes and spindles are absent and eye movements are not seen. Muscle tone may be further diminished.

REM REM sleep does not fit into the same staging system as NREM sleep and thus sometimes is referred to as *paradoxical sleep*. Although EEG activity is relatively active, the muscle tone achieves its lowest state over a 24-hour period (relative muscle atonia). REM sleep is characterized by rapid eye movements scattered through the duration of each REM cycle. REM sleep can be further subdivided into tonic (background EEG, relative muscle atonia, hippocampal theta activity) and phasic (rapid eye movements, brief muscle twitches, "saw tooth" waves on the EEG, and pontogeniculo-occipital spikes, as recorded in animals) components. REM sleep is associated with the well-formed dream. Individuals aroused from REM sleep will recall dreams about 80% of the time. NREM arousals may be associated with recall of isolated images or thought fragments, but not the well-formed images of REM sleep.

Nightmares are a reflection of the elements of REM sleep. As the individual initially awakens from a frightening dream and begins to scream, no sound emerges, because he or she still is paralyzed with the muscle atonia of REM. It is noteworthy that these components of REM sleep are not rigidly synchronized. Another example of this loose synchronization can be seen in some normal individuals with sleep paralysis as a benign condition, in which the individual is transiently "paralyzed" as he or she awakens from sleep.

Sleep Rhythms The components of sleep do not occur randomly throughout the course of the night. In fact, a clear pattern emerges from the ultradian or short rhythms of sleep. The "light" stages of NREM are seen first. They are followed by a transition to SWS, followed by lighter stages of NREM again, and then REM sleep. Typically, there are three to four NREM-REM cycles, each lasting 90 to 120 minutes. As the night progresses, the relative amount of time spent in REM increases and the amount of time in SWS decreases. Thus REM usually is skewed toward the end of the sleep period and SWS toward the beginning.

More importantly, sleep-wake rhythms follow a circadian or approximately 24-hour biologic pattern. Sleep-wake is considered a circadian rhythm that is tightly synchronized with circadian variations in core body temperature. The suprachiasmatic nucleus of the hypothalamus in animals, and an analogous structure in humans, with inputs from the retinohypothalamic pathways, has been identified as the endogenous pacemaker. Although individuals may have different periodicities in their clocks ("larks" and "owls"), there are many factors that maintain or influence these rhythms. Although activity levels, social cues, mealtimes, and other external scheduling factors play some role, the most powerful *zeitgeiber* (light-giver) has proved to be exogenous light. Presumably, light exerts its influence through retinohypothalamic input to the suprachiasmatic nucleus (5).

From a clinical perspective, it is helpful to view the usual pattern of sleep-wake in terms of the shifting pattern of core body temperature. The usual evening sleep onset occurs as the core body temperature falls during the "primary sleep permissive" zone. Sleep continues as the core body temperature continues to fall and enters the "sleep maintenance zone." The duration of sleep and REM sleep follows this circadian cycle, with most of REM sleep occurring close to the nadir of the temperature cycle. The temperature then begins to rise, reaching its peak at midday. A secondary dip usually occurs in midafternoon, correlating with a secondary sleep permissive zone or the so-called "siesta" zone. This nap zone usually is followed by a relative plateau that has been related to the "second wind." Similarly, a secondary rise occurs in the early morning hours, usually at about 3 AM, when a secondary arousal time occurs and the individual is susceptible to wakening from any physical or emotional factor (e.g., anxiety, pain, the need to urinate).

UNDERSTANDING SLEEP DISORDERS

For a comprehensive listing of specific disorders and their descriptions, the reader is referred to *The International Classification of Sleep Disorders, revised (ICSD-2*, 2005). This chapter focuses first on problems related to sleep need, sleep rhythms, intrinsic sleep disorders, extrinsic factors, and medical-psychiatric factors. This will then permit a brief discussion of evolving concepts of insomnia, including the concept of primary insomnia.

DRIVE/SLEEP NEED

As noted previously, sleep drive is based on sleep need, which, in turn, assumes sleep need is based on otherwise efficient sleep. Sleep need probably does not change with age after young adulthood (2). It is not uncommon to see an accumulation of "sleep debt" over the course of a week, with the weekend set aside for recovery. These patterns often are related to social and lifestyle decisions.

Identification of an individual's sleep need is the first step in understanding sleep complaints. Careful questioning of the patient is required to account for total sleep time, including both nocturnal sleep and daytime naps.

Timing The sleep-wake circadian rhythm often advances with age toward an early bedtime and early rise time (the lark). A common experience is the transient dysfunction associated with jet lag. This is simply a situation in which the biologic clock suddenly becomes desynchronized from the social environment. Because most people find it easier to "delay" their clocks, it becomes easier for most to fly from the East Coast to the West Coast (which requires an advancement of the rhythm) than from west to east. Typically, it can take a day and a half to recover a 60-minute advancement. Similarly, it takes about a day to recover from a 60-minute delay (one time zone change).

For a variety of social and biologic reasons, there is a tendency for the adolescent to become delayed and the older adult to become advanced. The resulting complaints typically involve insomnia and difficulty in staying awake at other times. Recognition of these disorders leads to the formulation of a treatment plan.

In addition, the circadian rhythm of the older adult appears to be more fragile and susceptible to disruption, as might be seen in shift workers or patients plagued by the nocturnal arousal of chronic pain. It is unclear how much of this change is due to biologic changes in the endogenous oscillator that governs the rhythms, and how much is the result of changes in exogenous factors such as light exposure, lifestyle changes, and physical activity. The rhythm can be manipulated by well-timed bright light exposure. The full range of circadian rhythm disorders, as described in the *ICSD-2*, includes problems related to delays, advancements, and shifting rhythms. The pathophysiology of these disorders may vary, but some can be attributed to jet travel or shift work.

Aging results in a greater sensitivity to time zone or shift work changes. In such situations, there is a significant desynchronization between social and environmental cues and biologic rhythms. The individual attempts to sleep or to stay awake at times that are not closely synchronized to biologic rhythms. Older adults appear to be less tolerant of such desynchronization, as well as dealing with the clinical effects of an advancing rhythm. This implies earlier wake-up times (the lark), which persist despite later sleep onset times. The net result is the need to nap because a sleep debt is acquired.

Intrinsic Sleep Disorders Although there are many intrinsic sleep disorders, the three most common are periodic limb movements of sleep (PLMS), restless legs syndrome (RLS), and obstructive sleep apnea (OSA).

PLMS Periodic limb movements of sleep are characterized by episodes of repetitive, stereotyped limb movements during sleep. Other terms for the condition include *periodic leg movement, nocturnal myoclonus, periodic movements of sleep*, or *leg jerks*. The movements usually involve the legs (unilateral, alternating, or bilateral), although the arms also may be involved. Movements consist of extension of the big toe, in combination with partial flexing of the ankle, knee, and (sometimes) hip. The movements often are associated with partial arousal or overturning, usually too briefly for potential awareness (*ICSD-2*, 2005). There can be marked night-to-night variability in the number of movements (6–8). In some cases, periodic arousals may predominate, with minimal, if any, evidence of limb movements. In such cases, some investigators have referred to the so-called *periodic K-alpha syndrome*.

Clinically, the patient may complain of nonrestorative sleep. Even when the patient reports sound sleep, he or she may thrash about, while the bed partner reports kicking or even bicycling movements.

Typically, an anterior tibialis electromyogram shows contractions with durations of 0.5 to 5.0 seconds (average, 1.5 to 2.5 seconds). Movements generally occur every 5 to 90 seconds (most typically, every 20 to 40 seconds). Although PLMS can occur in any stage of NREM, they are most common in stage 2 and usually disappear in REM (*ICSD-2*, 2005).

The pathophysiology of PLMS remains somewhat obscure. They may be associated with OSA or with the use of antidepressants. Similarly, withdrawal from certain drugs (including anticonvulsants, benzodiazepines, barbiturates, and other hypnotics) may contribute to the development of PLMS. They can be seen in otherwise young, healthy individuals (9).

RLS It has been estimated that RLS is present in 5% to 15% of the general population. It affects both sexes and has been described in both children and adults. The usual presentation is with an urge to move, usually accompanied by uncomfortable sensations. These paresthesias are usually bilateral, often more prominent in the legs than in the arms. The sensations typically are described as burning, tingling, stabbing, aching, or simple pain. Some patients complain of sensations of ants crawling or worms burrowing. Symptoms usually are subjective and vary over the course of the day. They tend to be worse when the individual is relaxing, and especially when preparing for sleep. Patients may have particular difficulties in enclosed areas such as airplanes, cars, or trains. Symptoms are variable and may fluctuate over time, with exacerbations and remissions (10). Some patients develop myoclonus or sudden jerking movements. It is not uncommon to find an overlap with PLMS. PLMS, however, occur during sleep and most commonly in stage 2 NREM sleep. RLS, on the other hand, occurs during wakefulness and interferes with sleep at the transition between wakefulness and sleep.

The pathophysiology of RLS is unknown. Disorders of iron metabolism within the central nervous system and dopaminergic function have been considered. Many medical problems have been found to aggravate the symptoms. Uremia, anemia, and neuropathies have been implicated in many so-called secondary cases. Of particular note in addiction medicine is the observation that RLS may be aggravated or triggered by the use of several medications, including antidepressants, lithium carbonate, neuroleptics, and caffeine (11).

The treatment of RLS usually requires medication. The most commonly used are the dopaminergic drugs such as carbidopa/levodopa or dopaminergic agonists such as ropinirole and pramipexole. Success has also been demonstrated with benzodiazepines (usually clonazepam), anticonvulsants (usually gabapentin), and the opioids. The latter group is of particular interest. Some patients report that they began to use opioids on a regular basis when they received them for an unrelated disorder and realized that they were able to sleep for the first time in years.

OSA OSA is a common syndrome. It is a treatable disorder that accounts for many of the cases of excessive somnolence and insomnia encountered in most sleep centers. It is one of the few diagnoses that make polysomnograms reimbursable by third-party payers.

OSA is characterized by repetitive episodes of sleep-related upper airway obstructions, which usually are associated with oxygen desaturation. OSA can be conceptualized as a disorder emerging from an interaction between anatomy and muscle relaxation as it occurs in sleep. As muscles relax, airflow can generate vibrations in the soft tissues of the upper airway, including the soft palate. Such vibration produces the noise or the snoring. The role of upper airway muscle relaxation in the pathophysiology also means that certain medications, such as benzodiazepines or alcohol, may aggravate the severity of the OSA, presumably, by the enhanced degree of muscle relaxation. In some patients, the snoring appears in isolation; in such cases, the term *primary snoring* is applied.

Further upper airway restriction can result in difficulties along two other dimensions. Muscle relaxation, especially in the upper airway dilator muscles of the oropharynx (often combined with mild anatomic abnormalities) provides the setting for increased airway restriction, which is further enhanced by the negative pressures generated by normal respiration (12).

The sleep disruption may or may not be apparent to the patient because, as noted earlier, brief physiologic arousals may not be recalled. Daytime somnolence often is the prime complaint, although—as in other chronic, progressive disorders—the patient may adapt to and minimize these symptoms. The same patient who denies daytime sleepiness or napping may acknowledge an irresistible urge to doze if allowed to sit in a comfortable chair or when confronted with the monotony of highway driving. Similarly, presenting complaints may be related to difficulties in memory or concentration that reflect suppression of REM sleep (REM sleep is especially vulnerable because of the relative muscle atonia). SWS also can be suppressed and may be associated with complaints similar to those associated with fibrositis or fibromyalgia.

In addition to sleep disruption, there are several cardiopulmonary consequences. Feedback reflexes may be insufficient to cause arousal (arousal produces return of muscle tone on cessation of the respiratory events). Indeed, one might see significant oxygen desaturation with arrhythmia, systemic and pulmonary arterial hypertension, and polycythemia. These changes can become chronic, and recent epidemiologic studies have suggested that OSA plays a role in the development of often-unrecognized hypertension in the general public (13,14).

The severity of OSA thus can be measured in three dimensions: snoring, sleep disruption, and cardiopulmonary consequences. It is not unusual to see some linkage, but the factors may exist independently as well. Manipulation of anatomy or the degree of muscle relaxation can aggravate OSA. Weight gain or supine sleep heightens the anatomic risk factors, whereas use of alcohol, benzodiazepines, and other sedatives enhance muscle relaxation and thus the severity of OSA.

Determination of the severity of OSA is complicated by the arbitrary scoring criteria used in most laboratories, as well as the recent recognition of the upper airway resistance syndrome, where symptoms may be attributed to events that do not meet the formal criteria for the definition of apneas or hypopneas. Fortunately, the establishment of a new scoring system for these events may minimize problems in the future (15). Traditionally, apneas are defined as episodes of 10 seconds' duration in which airflow falls to $<10\%$ of baseline. Obstructive events imply that there is continued respiratory effort (16), although there is some controversy as to how sensitive the effort markers need to be to determine absence of effort of the type seen in central apneas. Hypopneas usually are defined as events of 10 seconds' duration in which airflow drops to 50% of baseline or less, with an associated drop in oxygen saturation or a brief arousal. In upper airway resistance syndrome, "unscoreable" events may be associated with sleep disruption or frequent EEG alpha arousals.

Epidemiologic studies have suggested that snoring occurs in 9% to 24% of middle-age men and in 4% to 14% of middle-age women (17,18), although there is a tendency to underreport snoring (19). The prevalence of OSA in the general male population has been estimated to be 0.4% to 5.9% (19–22), with the incidence in men clearly outnumbering that in women.

Common risk factors include obesity (19,23–25), smoking (21,22,24,26), alcohol consumption (25,27), stroke (28), and age.

Central Sleep Apnea Central sleep apnea (CSA) is a disorder characterized by recurrent episodes of apnea during sleep resulting from temporary loss of ventilatory effort. CSA may be associated with desaturations and arousals, as encountered in OSA. Although CSA is much less frequently encountered when compared with OSA, it does pose a particular potential problem in addiction medicine. There are actually different forms of CSA, including the common form of Cheyne-Stokes respirations that may be associated with congestive heart failure or other central nervous system pathology. A pattern of sleep-related irregular respirations has been referred to as ataxic breathing or Biot's respirations and has been associated with chronic opioid therapy and the risk seems to be related to the morphine dose equivalents (29).

Extrinsic Factors Several extrinsic factors affect sleep, including exercise, the sleep environment, medications, and drug effects.

Exercise long has been recognized as a factor promoting sound sleep (30). Regular exercise, especially in the late afternoon or early evening, is conducive to sleep initiation, either through release of certain endogenous substances or subsequent cooling 5 to 6 hours later, which reinforces circadian factors (31). Inactivity can be a factor in sleep disruption in the young as well as the old, but daytime bed rest is a greater issue in the sleep of older adults (32,33).

Environmental stimuli, such as room temperature and light, often are factors in the initiation and maintenance of sleep. Although arousal thresholds vary from one individual to the next, aging has been associated with increased susceptibility to external arousal (34,35). Often, this increasing susceptibility is not recognized by the patient.

The effect of evening meals is somewhat controversial. The conventional wisdom has been that a light bedtime snack—perhaps with a glass of milk—promotes sleep. This effect has been attributed to tryptophan or to the release of digestive hormones, which can be sedating (36). On the other hand, there are reports that heavy bedtime snacks can be disruptive to sleep. Clinical experience suggests that these effects are variable and need to be assessed in each individual.

Increases in medication and changes in metabolism can contribute to sleep disruption in older adults, as they do in any age group; however, older adults appear to be more susceptible.

Medical and Psychiatric Factors The interaction between sleep and other medical conditions can be quite complex. Certain medical conditions contribute directly to specific sleep disorders such as OSA or RLS. However, other disorders simply lead to problems with the wake-sleep transition at sleep onset or at other times through the night, including the most vulnerable time in the circadian cycle (i.e., 3:00 to 5:00 AM). Sleep disorders have been attributed to nocturia, headache, gastrointestinal illnesses, cardiopulmonary disease, menopause, and chronic pain (37–40).

The role of psychiatric disorders always should be considered in the assessment of sleep disorders. Two specific sleep-related psychiatric disorders have been formally defined. The *ICSD-2* describes an "alcohol-dependent insomnia" in nonalcoholics who use alcohol as a hypnotic for sleep onset for more than 30 days and who may not otherwise meet criteria for alcohol dependence. The DSM-IV describes criteria for a "substance-induced sleep disorder," with subtypes based on the substance used.

Sleep disruption is not uncommon in any person with a comorbid psychiatric syndrome, but most of the attention has been directed toward the relationship between affective disorders and sleep. Insomnia is the prominent feature, although hypersomnia may be seen in depression, especially when the depression is a component of a bipolar disorder (41). Similarly, during manic episodes, one may see periods of sleeplessness, with an apparent reduction in sleep need.

Several PSG features have been associated with depression (42). Sleep disruption with prolonged sleep latency, sleep fragmentation, early morning arousals, decreased sleep efficiency, and daytime fatigue and somnolence have been well documented. Another finding has been an apparent decrease in the amount of SWS, although this observation has been somewhat variable. The most robust feature, however, is a reduction in REM latency. Related features are increased duration of the first REM period and an increase in REM density.

Insomnia In brief, insomnia refers to a pattern of disrupted sleep (e.g., delayed sleep-onset, frequent arousals, early awakening), in an individual given sufficient opportunity to sleep, that is associated with a pattern of daytime distress and symptoms. The requirement of daytime symptoms distinguishes the insomniac from the individual with an insufficient sleep disorder. Insomnia may be transient or chronic, primary, or secondary. Primary insomnia is considered to be independent of other sleep disturbances or the other factors cited previously (*ICSD-2*). The concept of primary insomnia is interesting because most sleep specialists acknowledge that it is fairly uncommon, yet it is the target of all clinical trials of pharmacologic agents seeking a U.S. Food and Drug Administration indication for the treatment of insomnia.

In recent years, there seems to have been a paradigm shift in the approach to insomnia. In a recent consensus statement from a National Institutes of Health summit meeting (June 13–15, 2005), it was concluded that insomnia should be considered a comorbid disorder. This represented a shift from the thinking that insomnia is a symptom and that the emphasis in management should be directed toward the underlying disorder. As an example, one might consider the relationship between pain and insomnia. Although pain may be a causative factor in the development of insomnia, it must also be considered that sleep deprivation may influence pain thresholds and the treatment of insomnia may facilitate the management of pain. Ultimately, it may be reasonable to consider the predisposing, precipitating, and perpetuating factors involved in the individual case (46).

ALCOHOL AND SLEEP

Effect of Alcohol on Sleep in the Individual without Alcohol Dependence The hypnotic properties of alcohol are summarized in Table 78.1. Alcohol probably is the sleep-promoting agent that is most widely used by the general public. In a population survey, 13% of survey respondents ages 18 to 45 years old reported that, in the preceding year, they had used alcohol to assist in sleep onset. Another 2% said they had used alcohol continuously for at least a month for this purpose, whereas 5% said they had used alcohol in combination with another hypnotic agent (44). Despite this wide use, it must be remembered that alcohol can be mildly stimulating (45). The source of the variability in its hypnotic properties is not clear, although animal studies suggest a possible role of age. In at least one study, it was demonstrated that adolescent animals developed a much more rapid tolerance to the hypnotic effects of alcohol than did older animals (46,47), although older males had a tendency to sleep longer (47).

TABLE 78.1 Summary of Effects of Alcohol on Sleep Architecture

Individual without alcohol dependence
Initial half of sleep period
Shortened sleep latency
Decreased REM sleep
Decreased SWS
Second half of sleep period
Shallow disrupted sleep
Increased REM sleep with increased dream (nightmare recall
Sympathetic arousal
Individual with alcohol dependence
Increased sleep latency
Decreased sleep efficiency
Decreased total sleep time
Decreased REM sleep
Decreased SWS
Alcohol withdrawal
Severe insomnia
Severe sleep fragmentation
Rebound of REM sleep
Persistent decreased SWS
Alcohol recovery
Early (initial weeks)
Increased sleep latency
Increased fragmentation
Decreased total sleep time
Increased REM density (exaggerated in depression)
Persistence of decreased SWS
Chronic
Persistence of sleep fragmentation
Persistence of decreased SWS
Recovery relapse
Increased total sleep time
Decreased sleep fragmentation
Increased SWS

REM, rapid eye movement; SWS, slow wave sleep.

The effects of alcohol on the sleep architecture of the individual without alcohol dependence should be considered in terms of both direct effects and immediate withdrawal. Because alcohol is rapidly metabolized, the direct effect of evening alcohol consumption usually is during the sleep cycle. As predicted by the hypnotic effect, sleep latency is shortened and there is an increase in the amount of NREM sleep that occurs at the expense of REM sleep, which is suppressed during the acute phase (48,49). As the effects of the alcohol dissipate, there is a rebound effect, in which sleep becomes lighter and more easily disrupted. REM increases, with an associated increase in dreams and nightmares. There is an increase in sympathetic arousals, with tachycardia and sweating.

As alcohol consumption continues, the hypnotic effects may diminish, but the late sleep disruption persists (50). Ultimately, the net effect is a feeling of fatigue during the individual's waking hours.

Alcohol's hypnotic effects can be seen in infants fed on the breast milk of mothers who consume even small amounts of alcohol. Indeed, it appears that such babies fall asleep more easily, but they seem to sleep less deeply (51). This finding would be predicted from our knowledge of alcohol's effects in older patients. It also has been shown that a woman's daily consumption of small amounts of alcohol in the first trimester of pregnancy is associated with subsequent sleep disruption in infants, when measured by brain electrical activity (52).

It would seem that the hypnotic effects of alcohol should be related to direct effects of alcohol on the central nervous system. Unfortunately, this explanation does not account for the observation that sleepiness can be observed after the alcohol no longer is detectable. Although it is customary to advise patients with sleep difficulties to avoid late evening alcohol, there is evidence that even early evening alcohol consumption may disrupt sleep in the last half of the night (53). This would apply to alcohol consumed even 6 hours before sleep onset (54). Similarly, alcohol administered early in the day has been shown to have a negative effect on multiple sleep latency tests and tests of divided attention, even when given later in the day when alcohol levels are undetectable (54).

Finally, some data suggest that there is a synergistic interaction between alcohol exposure and prior sleepiness. The hypnotic effects seem to be enhanced in the previously sleep-deprived individual (55). In particular, low-dose alcohol administered after a night of reduced sleep is associated with reduced performance on a driving simulator (50,54,56,57). The implication is that, in individuals functioning on reduced sleep, alcohol has an enhanced sedating effect even at low doses, which in turn has an effect on performance in activities such as driving.

It is important to note that many of the conclusions of the studies of the impact of alcohol on the sleep of persons without alcohol dependence have been based on studies of men. A recent study of seven nonalcoholic women (aged 22 to 25) suggested that the impact of alcohol on the sleep of women may be less intense than the impact on the sleep of men (58).

Effect of Alcohol on Sleep in the Individual with Alcohol Dependence It is not uncommon for persons with alcohol dependence to report some combination of insomnia, hypersomnia, circadian rhythm disorders, or parasomnias (abnormal sleep-related behaviors). Such reports usually are reflected in other, more objective measures. Various studies of patients with alcohol dependence have demonstrated increased sleep latencies (time to fall asleep), decreased sleep efficiencies, and decreased total sleep, with reductions in both REM and SWS (59–61). As the dependence continues, patients often report that they no longer are able to initiate sleep without a drink. After a time, the usual rhythms of sleep become quite disrupted.

Dream Content in Alcoholism Although dreams usually are correlated with REM sleep, studies of dream content in people with alcoholism often are conducted without the use of polysomnographic techniques. In general, these studies find that individuals with alcohol dependence suffer from nightly nightmares more often than controls (62,63). In a more general study of patients with substance abuse disorders in a detoxification program, dreaming about drinking was a poor prognostic sign for relapse (64). Others have reported that among people with alcoholism in recovery, dreams about drinking were viewed with concern and were considered a potential trigger for relapse (65).

The use of alcohol to suppress nightmares needs to be considered in the management of other disorders associated with nightmares, such as posttraumatic stress disorder (66). In fact, some patients may have initiated their substance abuse out of a desire to suppress nightmares.

Alcohol, Sleep, and Other Cardiopulmonary Functions In addition to the effect of alcohol on OSA, it is important to be aware of the interaction between chronic obstructive pulmonary disease and alcohol during sleep. For example, alcohol consumption before sleep by patients with chronic obstructive pulmonary disease can worsen nocturnal hypoxemia during sleep (67) and increase ventricular ectopic activity (68).

Sleep in Alcohol Withdrawal The alcohol withdrawal syndrome frequently is marked by severe insomnia and sleep fragmentation. The reduction of SWS during this period has been related to a loss of restful sleep and feelings of daytime fatigue. The rebound of REM sleep has been regarded as a component of the pathophysiology of hallucinations encountered in the withdrawal syndrome. In fact, sleep during withdrawal may consist simply of fragments of REM sleep. It is of some interest that the rebound of SWS does not appear to occur (60).

Nightmares and vivid dreams are not uncommon features of alcohol withdrawal and probably reflect the observed REM "pressure." In fact, it has been speculated that the rebound of REM encountered in acute withdrawal states such as *delirium tremens* may account for much of the associated clinical symptomatology (69,70). It has been speculated that it is the early and abundant REM, with its associated dream content or hallucinations, and the accompanying sympathetic discharge that may account for much of the clinical picture of the *delirium tremens* (71). These views are consistent with attempts to record the sleep of patients with *delirium tremens*, which have found mostly stage 1 NREM and REM, with some evidence of increased muscle tone, even though these findings are clinically inconsistent (72). The increase in muscle activity also has suggested a possible relationship with REM behavior disorder, in which patients lose the muscle atonia of sleep and actually begin to act out their dreams (73).

Sleep During Alcohol Recovery In the alcohol dependent patient, sleep is not immediately recovered with abstinence; in fact, it may require months or even years. In the first 2 to 3 weeks of recovery, increased sleep latency may be seen, accompanied by increased sleep fragmentation and reduced total sleep time. There may be a decrease in SWS and an increase in REM density (74); such an increased density of rapid eye movements suggests an apparent rebound effect. The effects on REM may be exaggerated in patients with secondary depression, who also may exhibit a shortened REM latency (duration of onset of REM after sleep onset) and a greater percentage of sleep time spent in REM sleep (75).

These changes may persist for months or years, with sleep time reduced and fragmented and an elevated percentage of total sleep time spent in REM sleep (74–76). Long-term follow-up of alcohol dependent patients in recovery has demonstrated persistent subjective and objective sleep difficulties. The most prominent feature appears to be a persistent reduction in the amount of SWS as a percentage of total sleep (75,77,78).

Sleep disruption during recovery also has been examined from the perspective of its effect on the patient's efforts to remain sober. For example, it has been demonstrated that the presence of subjective sleep disruption increases the likelihood that the recovering individual will relapse to alcohol use (79). Longitudinal studies have suggested that the persistence of objective and subjective sleep difficulties at about 1 month of sobriety predicts relapse by 5 months (77,79).

A recovering person with alcoholism who begins to drink again will experience an increase in SWS, with an increase in total sleep time and reduction in fragmentation. This response, which involves a perceived immediate improvement in sleep, is thought to contribute to relapse, even though continued alcohol use inevitably leads to further sleep disruption.

Several investigators have attempted to identify the sleep measures that are the most important in predicting relapse. Some studies suggest that the degree of SWS reduction could be correlated with a poorer prognosis for continued recovery 2 months after discharge from an inpatient treatment program (80,81). Subsequent studies, however, suggested that measures of REM sleep were critical in predicting outcome. These studies suggested that measures of REM pressure, as defined by a shortened REM latency, increased REM density, and increased amount of time in REM sleep as a percentage of total sleep, when measured within 2 weeks of initiation of abstinence, were markers of a better prognosis for continued recovery at

3 months after discharge (82–84). In fact, the emergence of these markers of REM pressure is among the most robust predictors of continued recovery at the 3-month mark.

It should be noted that the prognostic value of these sleep measures changes as abstinence progresses. For example, at the 5-month mark, prolonged sleep latency and poor sleep efficiency are predictors of relapse by 1 year, but measures of REM pressure no longer are helpful (78). Prolonged sleep latency (time to sleep onset) has an advantage over other measures because of the relative ease with which it is ascertained.

SPECIFIC SLEEP DISORDERS ASSOCIATED WITH ALCOHOLISM

Alcohol and Sleep-Related Breathing Disorders

Patients with alcohol dependence appear to be at increased risk of developing OSA, especially if they snore (85). A large retrospective analysis suggested that these findings might, in part, be related to an association with smoking in this population and that smoking was the primary agent (25). Nevertheless, alcohol has been found to induce obstructive apnea in healthy asymptomatic men (86), as well as chronic snorers (27,87,88). Alcohol has been shown to increase the frequency and duration of obstructive events in patients with established OSA (27,89).

Two of the essential elements in the pathophysiology of OSA are the anatomy of the upper airway and the degree of relative muscle atonia associated with sleep. The decrease in muscle tone of the upper airway leads to an increase in snoring (27) and inspiratory resistance, with an accompanying reduction in airflow (90,91). Alcohol contributes to a reduction in muscle tone, with a selective reduction in genioglossal activity, thus aggravating any tendency to develop snoring or OSA (90). As a consequence, there is an increase in snoring, as well as interruption in normal nocturnal respiration. The associated sleep disruption then contributes to an increase in daytime fatigue and somnolence. These changes in airflow resistance are sufficient to cause OSA in those who consume moderate to high doses of alcohol in the evening, even if they do not otherwise have OSA (88,90).

Alcohol administration to asymptomatic men has been associated with increased episodes of desaturation, as well as an increase in frequency and duration of hypopneas and apneas (86). Moreover, the depressant effects of alcohol can decrease the likelihood of arousal from an obstructive event, thus prolonging the duration of each respiratory event (77,86,92). In fact, abstinence from alcohol before bedtime is considered an important step in treating OSA (27).

Although alcohol use can induce apneas, and obstructions can worsen established OSA, the relationship of alcohol to the development of OSA varies across populations. Older patients, for example, are more vulnerable to this effect (86). Similarly, the effect is not particularly prominent in normal women (93,94). In some studies of normal male subjects and young nonobese snorers, alcohol exerted minimal effects on the development of OSA (89). Thus it appears that other factors, such as age, the presence of snoring, and perhaps gender, play a role in the development of OSA.

OSA has been related to impaired performance on driving simulators and increased motor vehicle crashes even in the absence of alcohol (54). Alcohol further decreases the performance of the patient with OSA. One small study suggested that a higher-than-expected number of sleep-related respiratory events in detoxified patients might contribute to impaired driving performance (86). In patients with established severe OSA, it has been noted that consumption of two or more alcoholic drinks per day is associated with a fivefold increase in fatigue-related motor vehicle crashes when compared with those who consumed little or no alcohol.

Alcohol and PLMS In at least one survey of a large sleep clinic sample, the risk of PLMS was increased almost threefold by alcohol consumption (95). This increase, however, was not seen in another study in which abstinent patients with a history of alcohol dependence were evaluated and compared with the nonalcohol-dependent group (96). Nevertheless, the potential increase in fatigue and daytime somnolence associated with PLMS can play a role in the management of these patients.

OTHER DRUGS AND SLEEP

Stimulants It is widely accepted that a primary effect of stimulants is to suppress sleep. Studies have demonstrated that stimulants such as amphetamine, methylphenidate, pemoline, or cocaine prolong sleep latency and reduce total sleep time. Stimulants have a specific inhibitory effect on REM sleep, so that there is a prolonged REM latency with a reduction in total REM throughout the sleep period (97). Presumably, this effect is attributable to the dopaminergic stimulation of the arousal system, although serotonergic systems also may be involved (98). When used episodically, these agents contribute to periods of sleeplessness that can last for days, but they usually are followed by a rebound hypersomnia. Tolerance to this effect can develop with continued use, even in those who take these agents for medical disorders such as narcolepsy or attention deficit/hyperactivity disorder (99).

After a period of persistent, chronic use, withdrawal of stimulants often leads to initial insomnia, which may persist (100). The sleep abnormalities encountered in stimulant withdrawal include a rebound effect. In particular, they include a decrease in sleep efficiency, with increased periods of nocturnal wakefulness, increased amounts of REM sleep with a shortened REM latency, and increased stage 1 NREM sleep (101). This effect is similar to the rebound effect encountered in the second half of the night after evening alcohol consumption.

The first 2 weeks of stimulant withdrawal usually are marked by some improvement in measurements of total sleep time, stage 1 NREM sleep, and REM density, even though changes persist.

Opioids The primary effect on sleep of acute administration of opioids to normal subjects or abstinent users is to shorten sleep latency and reduce total sleep time, sleep efficiency, REM sleep, and SWS (102). Chronic use, however, usually leads to tolerance to some of these effects. The REM-suppressing effects of morphine, for example, usually disappear within a week, even though sleep fragmentation may persist (103). Even the longer-acting opioids, such as methadone, contribute to insomnia, with disruption of sleep architecture and increased arousals accompanying chronic administration (104). This also may occur in patients undergoing opioid substitution therapy. The pathophysiology of this effect is not clear, but evidence suggests that the REM-inhibiting properties can be attributed to inhibition of acetylcholine receptors in the pontine reticular formation (105) or to direct agonist effects at specific mu receptors (106).

Opioids play a role in the treatment and management of specific sleep disorders. In particular, they have been found to be quite useful in the management of RLS (107,108) and PLMS (109), although the mechanism of this benefit is not well understood. In fact, anecdotal evidence shows that some patients with RLS or PLMS who are treated with opioids for unrelated disorders become dependent on opioids when they experience the sleep benefits. For example, a patient may suddenly realize that postoperative narcotics allow for marked improvement in sleep that had been interrupted by previously undiagnosed RLS. Opioids play an obvious role in the management of sleep disorders secondary to pain syndromes.

Little has been written about the characteristics of sleep during withdrawal from opioids, but clinical experience suggests that insomnia often is cited as a troublesome feature of withdrawal and requires specific attention.

Nicotine The effects of nicotine on sleep have not been well studied, but the available data suggest that, compared with nonsmokers, smokers experience an increase in sleep latency and an increase in arousals, with resulting poorer sleep maintenance (110). A possible biphasic response is that low doses promote sleep and higher doses disrupt sleep (110,111). Unlike most of the other agents discussed in this chapter, nicotine can increase rather then decrease REM (112).

Withdrawal from nicotine is associated with sleep disruption and increased daytime sleepiness, marked by multiple sleep latency tests (113). The effect of nicotine patches on sleep disruption remains unclear (114). The variability of responses may be due to the anxiety and irritability encountered in nicotine withdrawal.

Some researchers speculate that, in addition to the direct effect of nicotine on sleep mechanisms and architecture, tobacco and the irritation it causes to the upper airway may contribute to OSA (115).

Caffeine The effects of caffeine overlap those of the stimulants. Caffeine has a long history of use to combat fatigue and sleepiness in normal individuals (116), and can trigger insomnia in experimental conditions as well (117). Unlike many other stimulants, caffeine appears to exert its effect by blocking adenosine receptors (118).

Unfortunately, in the clinical setting, patients and clinicians often overlook the effects of caffeine. The half-life of caffeine ranges from 3 to 7 hours, with effects persisting for as long as 8 to 14 hours. Thus the effects of late-morning caffeine intake may continue into the evening. As with other drugs, there is considerable variability in individual responses to caffeine. Thus some individuals may become overstimulated with even 250 mg of caffeine, which is equivalent to about one to two cups of coffee, whereas others develop tolerance and are able to sleep soundly despite heavy consumption.

Caffeine often is used in combination with alcohol and together they can lead to even further aggravation of insomnia. Although alcohol has hypnotic properties, its half-life is much shorter than that of caffeine and its major effects disappear within a few hours. At that point, the rebound effect of alcohol withdrawal and the persistent stimulatory effect of caffeine jointly contribute to further sleep disruption (117).

It is easy to underestimate the effect of abrupt withdrawal of caffeine. Although few formal studies of caffeine withdrawal and its effects on sleep have been conducted, it has been noted that within 18 to 24 hours, some patients develop headache, fatigue, irritability, sleepiness, and flulike symptoms (119).

Benzodiazepines Benzodiazepines represent an interesting group of medications because they often are used in the management of sleep disorders, in addition to being potential drugs of abuse. The primary effect is to reduce sleep latency, increase total sleep time, and reduce nocturnal arousals (120). Unlike the stimulants and caffeine, benzodiazepines have only a minimal effect on REM sleep. With acute and chronic use, there can be an increase in spindle activity and there is a decrease in the amount of SWS (120). The related agents, zolpidem and zaleplon, have similar effects, although it is thought that they have less effect on SWS. The traditional view has been that the sleep-promoting effects are lost within 2 to 3 weeks of use. Recent reviews, however, suggest that the development of tolerance to the hypnotic effects of benzodiazepines is quite variable and that drug effects may persist for extended periods of time. It is likely that this variability is at least partially related to the underlying etiology of the sleep disorder.

Marijuana It has been long been accepted that marijuana and other cannabis-based extracts may contribute to improved quality of sleep either by direct hypnotic activity or by an impact on pain, anxiety, and other chronic difficulties (121,122). Some of the hypnotic effect has been attributed to the ability of cannabinoids to modulate spontaneous neuronal activity and evoke inhibition of the locus coeruleus neuradrenergic neurons (123). The hypnotic properties may be of particular concern in addiction medicine. In a study of chronic marijuana users, abstinence from THC increased ratings of anxiety/depression/irritability and decreased the reported quantity and quality of sleep. It was suggested that these abstinence symptoms may contribute to continued use (124).

The hypnotic effect of marijuana may be a bit oversimplified. Although THC has been usually implicated and its hypnotic properties described, it appears that another major constituent of marijuana, cannabidiol, may actually induce alertness (125). It appears that this alerting system may be modulated by the cannabidiol impact on dopaminergic release and activation of neurons in the hypothalamus and dorsal raphe nucleus.

In addition, there have been a few studies that have looked specifically at the impact of marijuana on sleep architecture. It seems that the acute administration leads to a decrease in REM sleep and an increase in SWS (126,127). Abstinence seems to lead to a rebound effect with a decrease in REM latency and an increase in the relative amount of REM sleep and SWS (128). The long-term administration (more than 7 days) some tolerance probably develops to the SWS effects, but not to the REM sleep effects.

CLINICAL APPROACHES TO SLEEP DISORDERS

The clinical approach to patients with co-occurring sleep addictive disorders poses certain problems. In addition to dealing with specific sleep disorders, it is necessary to address the effect of the substance of abuse on sleep, the effect of withdrawal, and any comorbid psychiatric problems such as depression. In some cases, a drug of abuse may have been masking or inadvertently treating an underlying sleep disorder, as in the case of the therapeutic effects of opioids on RLS. The clinical picture may be further complicated because some of the medications used in the treatment of specific sleep disorders have a potential for abuse. Therefore, a systematic approach is critical.

1. The first step is to obtain a careful history of the amount of sleep actually obtained in a 24-hour period. A diary can be used, but a careful history often elicits the necessary information.
2. The next step is to address the issue of timing and to determine the patient's probable circadian rhythm. This can be complicated by shifting work schedules and other activities. Again, the history is the most powerful tool. A sleep diary can be helpful.
3. Consider the potential for medical or psychiatric issues that can interfere with sleep. These are detected through a careful medical and psychiatric review, including an inventory of medications, exercise, nicotine, alcohol, and other drug use. Give careful attention to symptoms of anxiety, depression, nightmares, and posttraumatic stress.
4. Inquire about possible features of intrinsic sleep disorders. Is there evidence of OSA: snoring, sleep disruption, obesity, hypertension, and morning headache? Is there a reason to suspect PLMS or RLS? Is there a history of sleep-disturbing paresthesias or a history of sleep-related movement disorder?
5. Inquire about the sleep environment. Is the sleep area conducive to the relaxation required to allow the wake-to-sleep transition? This is a relative concept; for example, a television can be hypnotic for some but stimulating for others.

Occasionally, additional diagnostic studies are required. Some of these studies are part of the medical evaluation. Expanded use of a diary can be of value. A PSG should be considered if OSA or narcolepsy is suspected. A PSG also is helpful in evaluating parasomnia (abnormal sleep-related behavior). Finally, a multiple sleep latency test can be helpful in documenting hypersomnia or the presence of early onset REM.

After the evaluation is complete, the clinician can initiate a strategy to address the sleep problem. This approach needs to take the addictive disorder into consideration, because problems underlying the addiction must be addressed and treated. Care must be taken in the selection of medications. Whenever possible, associated medical or psychiatric conditions should be treated. Only then can "intrinsic" sleep disorders be treated.

For example, RLS and PLMS can be treated with medications that are not subject to abuse. OSA usually is treated with continuous positive airway pressure devices. Special attention then can be directed to issues of sleep hygiene, including the following.

- The sleep environment should be modified to allow for the relaxation required for the wake-to-sleep transition. It should be separated from work and play areas. Noise and lighting should be modified to allow for optimal relaxation.
- The times at which caffeine, nicotine, alcohol, and other medications are used should be assessed and adjusted as necessary.
- Regular exercise has been found to improve sleep and should be recommended.
- Adoption of a regular sleep-wake schedule should be encouraged. Napping is permissible, but will reduce the need to sleep at night.
- Finally, the patient needs to be able to separate sleep time from other stressors, allowing for a period of relaxation. The patient should be instructed to leave the bedroom whenever he or she is unable to sleep, to avoid the development of further anxiety.

If the patient still has difficulties with sleep, an underlying cause should be sought. Often, the cause is some form of anxiety disorder that requires direct attention. Relaxation techniques are helpful to some patients, as are medications. The usual sedating or hypnotic agents can be used for transient problems. However, in working with a patient for whom addiction is an issue, it is wise to consider the sedating antidepressants or the more active agents used to treat other anxiety-related disorders, such as the selective serotonin reuptake inhibitors (129–135).

REFERENCES

1. Mellinger GD, Balter MB, Uhlenhuth EH. Insomnia and its treatment: prevalence. *Arch Gen Psychiatry* 1985;42:225–232.
2. Williams RL, Karacan I, Hursch CJ. *Electroencephalography of human sleep: clinical applications.* New York: John Wiley, Sons, 1970.
3. Rechtschaffen A, Kales A. *A method of standardized terminology, techniques and scoring system for sleep stages of human subjects.* Los Angeles, CA: Brain Information Series/Brain Research Institute, 1968.
4. American Sleep Disorders Association (ASDA). The clinical use of the Multiple Sleep Latency Test. *Sleep* 1992;15:265–278.

5. Czeisler C, Richardson G Martin JB. Disorders of sleep and circadian rhythm. In: Wilson JD, Braumwald E, Fauci A, et al., eds. *Principles and practice of internal medicine*. New York: McGraw-Hill, 1991.
6. Mosso S, Dickel MJ, Ashurst J. Night to night variability in sleep apnea and sleep related periodic leg movements in the elderly. *Sleep* 1988;11: 340–348.
7. Billiwise DL, Clarkson MA. Nightly variation of periodic leg movements in sleep in middle aged and elderly individuals. *Arch Gerontol Geriatr* 1988;7:273–279.
8. Edinger JD, McCall WV, Marsh GR, et al. Periodic limb movement variability in older patients across consecutive nights of home monitoring. *Sleep* 1992;15:156–161.
9. Moore P, Jacobsen L. Periodic limb movements in sleep: outcome in supranormal young population. *Sleep* 1991;20:300–306.
10. Allen R, Picchietti D, Hening WA. Restless legs syndrome: diagnostic criteria, special considerations, and epidemiology. A report from the restless legs syndrome diagnosis and epidemiology workshop at the National Institutes of Health. *Sleep Med* 2003;4:101–119.
11. Yang C, White DP, Winkelman JW. Antidepressants and periodic leg movements of sleep. *Biol Psychiatry* 2005;58:510–514.
12. Guilleminault MD, Stohs R. Upper airway resistance syndrome. *Sleep Res* 1991;20:250–257.
13. Morrill MJ, Finn L, Kim H, et al. Sleep fragmentation, awake blood pressure and sleep disordered breathing in a population-based study. *Am J Resp Crit Care Med* 2000;162:2091–2096.
14. Nieto FJ, Young TB, Lind KB, et al. Association of sleep disordered breathing, sleep apnea and hypertension in a large community based study. *JAMA* 2000;283:1829–1836.
15. Iber C, Ancoli-Israel S, Chisson AL Quan, for the American Academy of Sleep Medicine. *The AASM manual for the scoring of sleep and related events*. Westchester, IL: American Academy of Sleep Medicine, 2007.
16. Gislason TH, Aberg H, Taube A. Snoring and systemic hypertension: an epidemiological study. *Acta Med Scand* 1987;232:415–421.
17. Koskenvu M, Kapiro J, Partinen M. Snoring as a risk factor for hypertension and angina pectoris. *Lancet* 1985;1:893–895.
18. Lugaresi E, Partinen M. Prevalence of snoring in sleep and breathing. In: Saunders N, Sullivan CE, eds. *Sleep and breathing*. New York: Marcel Dekker, 1994.
19. Telakivi T, Partinen M, Koskenvuo M, et al. Periodic breathing and hypoxia in snorers and controls: validation of snoring history and association with blood pressure and obesity. *Acta Neurol Scand* 1987;76: 69–75.
20. Cingnotta F, D'Alessandro R, Partinen M, et al. Prevalence of every night snoring and obstructive sleep apnea among 30 to 69 year old men in Bologna, Italy. *Acta Neurol Scand* 1989;79:366–372.
21. Lavie P, Ben-Yosef R, Rubin AE. Prevalence of sleep apnea among patients with essential hypertension. *Am Heart J* 1984;108:373–376.
22. Gislasen T, Almqvist M, Erickssen G, et al. Prevalence of sleep apnea among Swedish men. *J Clin Epidemiol* 1988;41:571–576.
23. Gislason TH, Aberg H, Taube A. Snoring and systemic hypertension: an epidemiological study. *Acta Med Scand* 1987;232:415–421.
24. Schmidt-Norwara WW, Coulas DB, Wiggins C, et al. Snoring in an Hispanic-American population: risk factors and association with systemic hypertension and other morbidity. *Arch Intern Med* 1980;150:87–601.
25. Bloom JW, Kaltenborn WT, Quan F. Risk factors for a general population for snoring: importance of smoking and obesity. *Chest* 1988;93: 678–683.
26. Norton PG, Dunn EV. Snoring as a risk factor for disease: an epidemiological survey. *Br Med J* 1985;291:630–632.
27. Issa FG, Sullivan CE. Alcohol, snoring and sleep apnea. *J Neurol Neurosurg Psychiatry* 1982;45:353–358.
28. Polamaki H, Partinen M, Erkinjuntti T, et al. Snoring, stroke and the sleep apnea syndrome. *Neurology* 1992;42(Suppl 7):75–82.
29. Walker JM, Farney RJ, Rhondeau SM, et al. Chronic opioid use is a risk factor for the development of central sleep apnea and ataxic breathing. *J Clin Sleep Med* 2007;3(5):455–461.
30. Shapiro CM, Warren PM, Trinder J, et al. Fitness facilitates sleep. *Eur J Appl Physiol* 1987;53:1–4.
31. Edinger JD, Morey MC, Sullivan RJ, et al. Aerobic fitness, acute exercise and fitness in older men. *Sleep* 1993;16(4):351–359.
32. Spielman AJ, Sakin P, Thorpy MJ. Treatment of chronic insomnia by restriction of time in bed. *Sleep* 1987;10:145–156.
33. Rubenstein ML, Rothenberg SA, Maherwarren S, et al. Modified sleep restriction therapy in middle aged and elderly insomniacs. *Sleep Res* 1990;19:276.
34. Zepelon H, McDonald CS, Zammit GK. Effect of age on auditory threshold. *J Gerontol* 1984;39:284–300.
35. Harsh J, Purvis B, Badia P, et al. Behavioral responses in older adults. *Biol Psychol* 1990;30:51–60.
36. Southwell PR, Evans CR, Hunt JN. The effects of a hot milk drink on movements during sleep. *Br Med J* 1992;2:429–433.
37. Baker JC, Mitteness LS. Nocturia in the elderly. *Gerontologist* 1989;28: 99–194.
38. Cook NR, Evans DA, Funklestein H, et al. Correlates of headache in a population based cohort study of the elderly. *Arch Neurol* 1989;46:338–344.
39. Hyppa MT, Kronholm E. Quantity of sleep and chronic illness. *J Clin Epidemiol* 1989;42:633–638.
40. Brugge KL, Kripke DF, Ancoli-Israel S, et al. The association of menopause status and age with sleep disorders. *Sleep Res* 1989;18:208.
41. Detre DP, Himmelhoch JM, Swartzburg M, et al. Hypersomnia and manic-depressive illness. *Am J Psychiatry* 1972;128:1303–1305.
42. Benca RM. Mood disorders. In: Kryger MH, Roth T, Dement WC, eds. *Principles and practice of sleep medicine*. New York: WB Saunders, 2000.
43. Spielman AJ, Caruso LS, Glovinsky PB. A behavioral perspective on insomnia treatment. *Psychiatr Clin North Am* 1987;10:541–553.
44. Johnson EA, Roehrs T, Roth T, et al. Epidemiology of alcohol and medications as aids to sleep in early adulthood. *Sleep* 1988;21:178–186.
45. Papineau KL, Roehrs TA, Petricelli N, et al. Electrophysiological assessment (the multiple sleep latency test) of the biphasic effects of ethanol in humans. *Alcohol Clin Exp Res* 1988;22:231–235.
46. Silveri NM, Spear LP. Ontogeny of rapid tolerance to the hypnotic effects of ethanol. *Alcohol Clin Exp Res* 1999;23(7):1180–1184.
47. Silveri NM, Spear LP. Decreased sensitivity to the hypnotic effects of ethanol early in ontogeny. *Alcohol Clin Exp Res* 1998;22(3):670–676.
48. Yules RB, Lippman ME, Freedman DX. Alcohol administration prior to sleep: the effect on EEG sleep stages. *Arch Gen Psychiatry* 1967;16:94–97.
49. Lobo LL, Tuffik S. Effect of alcohol on sleep parameters of sleep deprived healthy volunteers. *Sleep* 1997;20:52–59.
50. Vitello MV. Sleep, alcohol and alcohol abuse. *Addiction Biology* 1997;2:151–158.
51. Mennella JA, Gerish CJ. Effects of exposure to alcohol in mothers' milk on infant sleep. *Pediatrics* 1998;101(5):E2.
52. Scher GS, Richardson GA, Coble PA, et al. The effects of parental alcohol and marijuana exposure: disturbances in neonatal sleep cycling and arousal. *Pediatr Res* 1998;24:101–105.
53. Landolt HP, Roth C, Dijk DJ. Late afternoon ethanol intake affects nocturnal sleep and the sleep EEG in middle-aged man. *J Clin Psychopharmacol* 1996;16:428–436.
54. Roehrs T, Beare D, Zorick F. Sleepiness and ethanol effects on simulated driving. *Alcohol Clin Exp Res* 1994;18:154–158.
55. Zwyghuizen-Doorenbos A, Roehrs T, Timms V. Individual differences in the sedating effects of alcohol. *Alcohol Clin Exp Res* 1990;14:400–404.
56. Zwyghuizen-Doorenbos A, Roehrs T, Lamphere J. Increased daytime sleepiness enhances ethanol's sedative effects. *Neuropsychopharmacology* 1998;1:279–286.
57. Lunley M, Roehrs T, Asker D, et al. Ethanol and caffeine effects on daytime sleepiness/alertness. *Sleep* 1987;10:306–312.
58. Van Reen E, Jenni OG, Carskadon MA. Effects of alcohol on sleep and the sleep electroencephalogram in healthy young women. *Alcohol Clin Exp Res* 2006;30:974–981.
59. Mello MK, Mendelson JH. Behavioral studies of sleep patterns in alcoholics during intoxication and withdrawal. *J Pharmacol Exp Therap* 1970;175:94–112.
60. Allen RP, Wagman A, Fallace LA. Electroencephalic (EEG) sleep recovery following prolonged alcohol intoxication in alcoholics. *J Nerv Mental Dis* 1971;153:424–433.

61. Adamson J, Berdick JA. Sleep of day alcoholics. *Arch Gen Psychiatry* 1973;28:146–149.
62. Cernovsky Z. MMPI, nightmares in male alcoholics. *Percept Motor Skills* 1985;61:841–842.
63. Cernovsky Z. MMPI and nightmare reports in women addicted to alcohol and other drugs. *Percept Motor Skills* 1986;62:717–719.
64. Christo G, Franey C. Addicts' drug related dreams: their frequency and relationship to six-month outcomes. *Substance Use Misuse* 1996;31:1–15.
65. Denizen N. Alcoholic dreams. *Alcohol Treatment Q* 1988;5:133–139.
66. Stewart SH. Alcohol abuse in individuals exposed to trauma—a critical review. *Psychol Bull* 1996;120:83–112.
67. Easton PA, West PA, Weatherall RC, et al. The effect of excessive ethanol ingestion on sleep in severe chronic obstructive pulmonary disease. *Sleep* 1987;10:224–233.
68. Dolly FR, Block AJ. Increased ventricular ectopy and sleep apnea following ethanol ingestion in COPD patients. *Chest* 1983;83:469–472.
69. Rowland RH. Sleep onset rapid eye movement periods in neuropsychiatric disorders: implications for the pathophysiology of psychoses. *J Nerv Ment Disord* 1997;185:730–738.
70. Johnson LC, Burdick JA, Smith J. Sleep during alcohol intake and withdrawal in the chronic alcoholic. *Arch Gen Psychiatry* 1970;22:406–418.
71. Feinberg I. Hallucinations, dreaming and REM sleep. In: Kemp W, ed. *Origin and mechanisms of hallucinations.* New York: Plenum Publishing, 1970:125–132.
72. Wolin SJ, Mello JK. The effects of alcohol on dreams and hallucinations in alcohol addicts. *Ann N Y Acad Sci* 1973;215:266–302.
73. Mahowald MW, Shenck CH. REM sleep parasomnias. In: Kryger MH, Roth T, Dement WC, eds. *Principles and practice of sleep medicine,* 3rd ed. New York: WB Saunders, 2000.
74. Gillin JC, Smith TL, Irwin M. Short REM latency in primary alcoholics with secondary depression. *Am J Psychiatry* 1990;147:106–109.
75. Williams HL, Rundell OH Altered sleep physiology in chronic alcoholics: reversal with abstinence. *Alcohol Clin Exp Res* 1981;2:318–325.
76. Ehlers CL, Phillips E, Parry BL. Electrophysiological findings during the menstrual cycle in women with and without late luteal phase dysphoric disorder: relationship to risk for alcoholism. *Biol Psychiatry* 1996;39: 720–732.
77. Brower KJ, Aldrich MS, Hall JM. Polysomnographic and subjective sleep predictors in alcoholic relapse. *Alcohol Clin Exp Res* 1998;22: 1864–1877.
78. Drummond SPA, Gillin JC, Smith TL. The sleep of abstinent pure primary alcoholic patients: natural course and relationship to relapse. *Alcohol Clin Exp Res* 1998;22:1796–1782.
79. Brower KJ, Aldrich MS, Robinson EA, et al. Insomnia, self-medication and relapse to alcoholism. *Am J Psychiatry* 2001;158:399–404.
80. Allen RP, Wagman AM, Funderburk FR, et al. Slow wave sleep: a predictor of individual responses to drinking. *Biol Psychiatry* 1980;15: 345–348.
81. Wagman AM, Allen RP, Funderbunk FR, et al. EEG measures of functional tolerance to alcohol. *Biol Psychiatry* 1978;13:719–728.
82. Clark CP, Gillin JC, Golshan S, et al. Increased REM density at admission predicts relapse by three months in primary alcoholics with a lifetime history of secondary depression. *Biol Psychiatry* 1998;43:601–607.
83. Clark CP, Gillin JC, Golshan S, et al. Polysomnography and depressive symptoms in primary alcoholism with and without a lifetime history of secondary depression and inpatients with primary major depression. *J Affective Disord* 1999;52:177–185.
84. Gillin JC, Smith TL, Irwin M. Increased pressure for rapid eye movement sleep at time of hospital admission predicts relapse in nondepressed patients with primary alcoholism at three month follow-up. *Arch Gen Psychiatry* 1994;51:189–197.
85. Aldrich MS. Sleep disordered breathing in alcoholics: association with age. *Alcohol Clin Exp Res* 1993;17(6):1179–1183.
86. Tassan V, Block A, Boysen P. Alcohol increases sleep apnea and oxygen desaturation in asymptomatic men. *Am J Med* 1981;71:240–245.
87. Robinson R, White D, Zwilich C. Moderate alcohol ingestion increases upper airway resistance in normal subjects. *Annu Rev Resp Dis* 1985;132: 1238–1241.
88. Miller M, Dawson A, Henricksen S. Bedtime alcohol increases resistance of upper airways and produces sleep apnea in asymptomatic snorers. *Alcoholism* 1988;12:801–805.
89. Scrina L, Broudy M, Nay KN, et al. Increased severity of obstructive sleep apnea after bedtime alcohol ingestion: diagnostic potential and proposed mechanism of action. *Sleep* 1982;5:318–328.
90. Krol RC, Knuth SL, Bartlett D. Selective reduction of genioglossal muscle activity by alcohol in normal human subjects. *Am Rev Resp Disord* 1984;129:247–250.
91. Dawson A, Bigby BG, Poceta JS, et al. Effect of bedtime alcohol on inspiratory resistance and respiratory drive in snoring and nonsnoring men. *Alcohol Clin Exp Res* 1997;21:183–190.
92. Berry RB, Bonnet M, Light RW. Effect of ethanol on the arousal response to airway obstruction during sleep in normal subjects. *Am Rev Resp Disord* 1992;145:445–452.
93. Block AJ, Hellard DW, Slayton PC. Minimal effect of alcohol ingestion on breathing during the sleep of postmenopausal women. *Chest* 1985; 88:181–184.
94. Block AJ, Hellard DW, Slayton PC. Effect of alcohol ingestion on breathing and oxygenation during sleep: analysis of the effects of age and sex. *Am J Med* 1986;80:595–560.
95. Aldrich MS, Shipley JE. Alcohol use and periodic limb movements of sleep. *Alcohol Clin Exp Res* 1993;17:192–196.
96. Le Bon O, Verbanck P. Sleep in detoxified alcoholics: impairment of most standard sleep parameters and increased risk for sleep apnea, but not for myoclonus: A controlled study. *J Stud Alcohol* 1997;58:30–36.
97. Post RM, Gillin JC, Goodwin FK. The effect of orally administered cocaine on sleep of depressed patients. *Psychopharmacology* 1970;37: 59–66.
98. Gillin JC, Pulverenti L, Withers N, et al. The effects of lisuride on mood and sleep during acute withdrawal in stimulant abusers: a preliminary report. *Biol Psychiatry* 1994;35:843–849.
99. Feinberg I, Hibi S, Caveness C, et al. Sleep amphetamine effects in MBDS and normal subjects. *Arch Gen Psychiatry* 1974;31:723–731.
100. Washington WW, Brown BS, Haertzen CA. Changes in mood, craving and sleep during short term abstinence reported by male cocaine addicts. *Arch Gen Psychiatry* 1990;47:861–868.
101. Thompson PM, Gillin JC, Golshan S. Polygraphic sleep measures differentiate alcoholics and stimulant abusers during short-term abstinence. *Biol Psychiatry* 1995;38:831–836.
102. Kay D, Pickworth W, Neider G. Morphine-like insomnia in nondependent human addicts. *Br J Clin Pharmacol* 1981;11:159–169.
103. Staedt J, Wassmuth F, Stoppe G, et al. Effects of chronic treatment with methadone and naltrexone on sleep in addicts. *Eur Arch Psychiatry Clin Neurosci* 1996;246:305–309.
104. Kay D. Human sleep and EEG through a cycle of methadone dependence. *Electroencephal Clin Neurophysiol* 1975;38:35–43.
105. Lydic R, Keifer JC, Baghdoyen HA, et al. Microanalysis of the pontine reticular formation reveals inhibition of acetylcholine release by morphine. *Anesthesiology* 1993;79:1003–1012.
106. Cronin A, Keifer JC, Baghdoyan HA. Opioid inhibition of rapid eye movement sleep by a specific mu receptor agonist. *Br J Anaesthesiol* 1995;74:188–192.
107. Trzepecz PT, Violette EJ, Sateia MJ. Response to opioids in three patients with restless legs syndrome. *Am J Psychiatry* 1984;141:993–995.
108. Walters AS, Wagner ML, Henning WA. Successful treatment of the idiopathic restless legs syndrome in a randomized double-blind trial of oxycodone versus placebo. *Sleep* 1993;16:327–332.
109. Javey N, Walters AS, Henning W, et al. Opioid treatment of periodic leg movements in patients without restless legs syndrome. *Neuropeptides* 1988;11:181–184.
110. Davila DG, Hunt RD, Offord KP, et al. Acute effects of transdermal nicotine on sleep architecture, snoring and sleep disordered breathing in non-smokers. *Am J Resp Crit Care Med* 1994;150:469–474.
111. Gillin JC, Landon M, Ruiz C, et al. Dose-dependent effects of transdermal nicotine on early morning awakening and rapid eye movement sleep time in normal nonsmoking volunteers. *Clin Psychopharmacol* 1994;14: 264–267.

112. Salin-Pascual RJ, Drucker-Colin R. A novel effect of nicotine on mood and sleep in major depression. *Neuroreport* 1998;9:57–60.
113. Prosise GL, Bonnet MH, Berry RB. Effect of abstinence from smoking on sleep and daytime sleepiness. *Chest* 1994;105:1136–1141.
114. Hughes JR, Higgins ST, Bickel WK. Nicotine withdrawal versus other drug withdrawal syndromes: similarities and dissimilarities. *Addiction* 1994;89:461–470.
115. Wetter DW, Young TB, Bidwell TR, et al. Smoking as a risk factor for sleep-disordered breathing. *Arch Intern Med* 1994;154:2219–2224.
116. Kelly TL, Miller NM, Bonnet MH. Sleep latency measures of caffeine effects during sleep deprivation. *Electroencephal Clin Neurophysiol* 1997;102:397–400.
117. Stradling JR. Recreational drugs and sleep. *Br Med J* 1993;305:573–575.
118. Portas CM, Thakkar M, Rainie DG, et al. Role of adenosine in behavioral state modulation: a microdialysis study in the freely moving cat. *Neuroscience* 1997;79:225–235.
119. Hughes JR, Higgins ST, Bickel WK. Caffeine self-administration, withdrawal and adverse effects among coffee drinkers. *Arch Gen Psychiatry* 1994;48:611–617.
120. Mendelson WB. *Human sleep: research and clinical care*. New York: Plenum Press, 1987.
121. Haney M, Gunderson EW, Rabkin J, et al. Dronabinol and marijuana in HIV-positive marijuana smokers caloric intake, mood, and sleep. *J Acquir Immune Defic Syndr* 2007;45:545–554.
122. Paton WD, Pertwee RG. The actions of cannabis in man. In: Mechoulam R, ed. *Marijuana: chemistry, pharmacology, metabolism and clinical effects*. New York: Academic Press, 1973:288–334.
123. Perra Gessa GL. Cannabinoids modulate spontaneous neuronal activity and evoked inhibition of locus coeruleus noradrenergic neurons. *Eur J Neurosci* 2006;23:2385–2394.
124. Haney M, Ward AS, Comer SD, et al. Abstinence symptoms following oral THC administration to humans. *Psychopharmacology* 1999;141:385–394.
125. Murillo-Rodríguez E, Millán-Aldaco D, Palomero-Rivero M, et al. Cannabidiol, a constituent of Cannabis Sativa, modulates sleep in rats. *FEBS Letters* 580. 2006:4337–4345.
126. Feinberg I, Jones R, Walker J, et al. Effects of marijuana extract and tetrahydrocannabinol on electroencephalographic sleep patterns. *Clin Pharmacol Ther* 1976;19:782–794.
127. Feinberg I, Jones R, Walker JM, et al. Effects of high dose delta-9-tetrahydrocannabinol on sleep patterns in man. *Clin Pharmacol Ther* 1975;17:458–466.
128. Liguori A, Brown TW, McCall W. Sleep architecture changes during marijuana withdrawal. *Sleep* 2004;27:54–55.
129. American Psychiatric Association (APA). *Diagnostic and statistical manual of mental disorders, 4th ed* (DSM-IV). Washington, DC: American Psychiatric Press, 1994.
130. National Institutes of Health State-of-the-Science Statement. Manifestations of chronic insomnia in adults, June 13–15, 2005.
131. NIH Consensus and State-of-the-Science Statement, 1983. Available at: http://consensus.nih.gov/1983/1983InsomniaDrugs039html.htm. Accessed November 6, 2008.
132. NIH Consensus and State-of-the-Science Statement, 2005. Available at: http://consensus.nih.gov/2005/2005InsomniaSOS026PDF.pdf. Accessed November 6, 2008.
133. Skoloda TE, Alterman AI, Gottheil E. Sleep quality reported by drinking and non-drinking alcoholics. In: Gottheil EL, ed. *Addiction research and treatment: converging trends*. New York: Pergamon Press, 1979: 102–112.
134. The Diagnostic Classification Steering Committee. *The International Classification of Sleep Disorders Diagnostic and Coding Manual, revised.* Rochester, MN: American Academy of Sleep Medicine, 2005.
135. Van Reen E, Jenni OG, Carskadon MA. Effects of alcohol on sleep and the sleep electroencephalogram in healthy young women. *Alcohol Clin Exp Res* 2006;30:974–981.

CHAPTER 79

Linda C. Degutis, DrPH, MSN
David A. Fiellin, MD
Gail D'Onofrio, MD, MS

Traumatic Injuries Related to Alcohol and Other Drug Use

Alcohol and other drug (AOD) use contributes to a substantial proportion of injury events, including falls, motor vehicle crashes, assaults, drownings, homicides, and suicides. Research evidence suggests that injured patients who also have alcohol and drug problems suffer more frequent and severe complications than other injured patients. These events, in turn, lead to significant morbidity and mortality, with far-reaching implications for the individual, the family, the workplace, and society. This chapter discusses the role of alcohol and other drugs in traumatic injury. It also provides data on the effectiveness of screening instruments for injured patients in emergency department and inpatient settings. The clinician's role in identifying AOD problems in injured patients is discussed, as are the components of brief intervention and referral to treatment.

The objective of the chapter is to provide clinicians with the tools required to incorporate screening and brief intervention into practice for this high-risk group of patients and the motivation to do so. The ultimate goal is to reduce both the risk of injury and the adverse consequences associated with AOD use. Though most of the research done to date relates to alcohol, there is a growing body of literature related to other drugs in the emergency medicine literature that will be referenced throughout the chapter.

EPIDEMIOLOGY OF ALCOHOL- AND OTHER DRUG-RELATED INJURY

Overall Risks There are risks of alcohol-related injuries across the entire spectrum of drinking behavior, from moderate social drinking to alcohol dependence. Nearly 50% of major trauma cases (1) and 22% of minor trauma cases (2) have been found to be alcohol-related. The proportion of positive blood alcohol concentrations (BAC) among injured patients presenting at emergency departments ranges from 6% to 34% (3). Alcohol is a major risk factor for virtually all categories of unintentional and intentional injuries (3–12). Of the 140,000 to 150,000 deaths that occur in the United States each year as a result of traumatic injuries, a significant proportion are related to use of alcohol or other drugs. Data from the 1989 National Health and Nutrition Epidemiologic Survey show that persons who consumed five or more drinks per occasion were twice as likely to die of injuries as nondrinkers and that consuming nine or more drinks on one occasion increased the risk of injury-related death more than threefold (13). Other data support the relationship between alcohol and fatal injuries. Injury is the leading cause of death in the United States for persons aged 1 to 44 years (14), whereas motor vehicle crashes are the leading cause of death for persons ages 5 to 34 years.

Alcohol and Motor Vehicle Fatalities According to the National Highway Traffic Safety Administration, 41% (17,602 people) of motor vehicle fatalities were alcohol-related in 2006, and 11% of people who were injured were in an alcohol-related crash (15). The annual cost of these alcohol-related motor vehicle crashes (MVCs) is approximately $51 billion. More than 50% of those who are arrested for driving under the influence (DUI) have alcohol problems, and many require medical care for injuries related to MVCs. In fact, an arrest for DUI is an independent indicator of risk of death in a future MVC (12). This indicator has been demonstrated to be valid for all age groups, and the association becomes stronger with increased age at the time of DUI arrest.

Almost 40 years ago, Haddon and Bradess (16) documented that alcohol was a factor in about half of single vehicle crashes. The statistic remains true today, as nearly half of the approximately 35,000 fatal MVCs in the United States each year are related to alcohol use (13). Further, alcohol has been implicated as a factor in 40% of crashes involving serious injury, 30% of crashes involving minor injury, and 10% to 15% of minor crashes.

Alcohol and Non-Motor Vehicle–Related Injuries

Alcohol is involved in 42% of pedestrian fatalities, 60% of fatal burns (often related to cigarette smoking), and an unknown percentage of work-related injuries and drownings (17,18). Studies of boating fatalities show that 60% of the victims tested positive for alcohol, and 30% had BACs >100 mg% (19). Alcohol and violence are closely linked. Cherpitel (3) found that persons older than 30 years who sustained violence-related injuries were more likely to have a positive alcohol breath test (for example, Breathalyzer) reading, to report drinking before the event, and to report a significant history of alcohol-related problems as compared with persons who experienced other types of injuries. In a study of adult patients who came to an emergency department for treatment of minor injuries, 6% had positive saliva alcohol tests (SATs) or blood alcohol tests, 9% were positive on at least one question of the CAGE screening questionnaire, and 6% were positive on both the saliva test and the CAGE (2).

Mannenbach et al. (20) examined the scope of alcohol use in a population of 243 injured adolescents. Using urine tests, they found results positive for alcohol use in 33% of adolescent patients injured in MVCs (including 38% of drivers), 37% of patients who attempted suicide, and 44% of assault victims. In another study of adolescents age 12 to 20 years, positive SAT results were found in up to 4% of injured patients who arrived at the emergency department within 6 hours of injury (21). A study comparing drinking problems in injured versus noninjured emergency patients documented that injured patients were more likely to test positive for use of alcohol, to report heavy drinking, to report prior alcohol-related injuries, and to report a history of treatment for alcohol problems than were patients who sought treatment for other disorders (22). This finding was true of patients who were treated in county or community hospital emergency departments, as well as patients who were treated in hospitals affiliated with health maintenance organizations (22). In another study, daily drinking, binge drinking, and heavy drinking each were associated with increased likelihood of injury as the underlying cause of death (14).

Relationship Between Alcohol, Other Drugs, and Injury Elucidating the specific relationship between alcohol, other drugs, and injuries is difficult for several reasons: (1) Few studies have been conducted at the time of injury, (2) there are few standards for reporting data about alcohol and other drug use, (3) alcohol and drug use is underreported on death certificates and hospital discharge data, (4) there is bias in the reporting of alcohol-related deaths, and (5) there is insufficient information on exposure to alcohol and other drugs in control populations (10). In a review of 32 studies of the association between alcohol use and injuries or fatalities from fire and burns, Howland and Hingson (10) found that nearly half of those who died in fires had BACs above 0.10 and that alcohol was an important risk factor for fire and burn injuries associated with cigarette smoking. In addition, studies conducted to determine the role of alcohol in injuries related to boating and swimming have implicated alcohol as a major risk factor for boating fatalities (23).

Work-related injuries, including injuries requiring hospitalization, were found to be more likely in persons who had an average daily intake of five drinks, compared to abstainers, and in those who used psychoactive drugs (11). Finally, onset of alcohol use at ages younger than 21 years was associated with experiencing an alcohol-related injury (24). Studies that have compared alcohol consumption in the general population with that of injured patients in the emergency department demonstrate a clear association between alcohol consumption and injury (3,25–27). One study found that injured patients presenting at the emergency department were five times more likely to report a higher quantity and frequency of alcohol consumption than were control subjects. In that study, positive screening results and recent alcohol consumption (that is, <6 hours before hospital admission) were associated with an increased risk of injury resulting in an emergency department visit (25).

Data derived from studies that have used probability sampling and that compare the prevalence of alcohol problems in patients with and without violence-related injuries indicate, in 10 of 11 studies, that patients with violence-related injuries were more likely to have positive blood or breath alcohol concentrations than those with nonviolent injuries (27). However, the prevalence of a positive BAC in injured patients varied considerably across the studies, because of both the method of measurement and decisions about a cutoff value for a positive test result (27).

Alcohol, Other Drugs, and Trauma Patients Admitted to the Hospital Studies of trauma patients examined those patients with more serious injuries and generally excluded patients who had been discharged from the emergency department to home or patients who were admitted to the hospital for treatment of single-system injuries, such as isolated extremity fractures. Many of the studies were conducted as retrospective reviews of blood alcohol testing and were based on clinical algorithms or subjective decisions by physicians to test, which could lead to selection bias in the samples. In one of the few studies that examined substance use disorders in trauma patients, Soderstrom et al. (28) found that 54% of 1,118 adult trauma patients had a lifetime history of a substance use disorder. In addition, 24% had a current diagnosis of alcohol dependence, and 18% had a current diagnosis of dependence on other drugs. Medical examiners' reports provide insight into the role of alcohol in deaths resulting from traumatic injuries. A meta-analysis of 331 medical examiner studies found that, in 39% of unintentional deaths resulting from injuries, there was evidence of alcohol intoxication (BAC of at least 100 mg/dL) (29). A separate analysis of studies published between 1985 and 1991 implicated alcohol in 35% to 63% of fatal falls and in 13% to 37% of nonfatal falls. In addition, alcohol was identified in 21% to 47% of cases involving drowning fatalities and in 12% to 61% of fatalities from burns (30). In a study of the role of alcohol in bicycle injuries, persons who died were more likely to have had positive BACs (30% vs. 16%) than were those who were injured but did not die (18).

Cocaine Use and Injuries The role of cocaine use in injuries or fatalities has been studied less frequently than that of alcohol. One study that employed medical examiners' records found that as many as 25% of those killed in MVCs had used cocaine within the 24 hours preceding the crash and that 10% had used cocaine and alcohol in combination (31). A separate study found that 31% of homicide victims had used cocaine but failed to find an association between having used cocaine and being killed by a firearm (32). The association between cocaine use and risk-taking behavior leading to fatal injury was evaluated in a unique examination of deaths in participants playing Russian roulette. Illicit drugs or alcohol were detected in 79% of cases of death resulting from Russian roulette and in 61% of control subjects who committed suicide with a handgun (33). An evaluation of 14,842 fatal injuries found evidence of cocaine in 27%. Of these deaths, approximately one-third were the result of drug intoxication, and two-thirds involved traumatic injuries resulting from homicides, suicides, MVCs, and falls (34). Despite these findings, concerns exist that there has been an underestimation of the role of cocaine in injury or fatality based on evidence of underreporting in the federal Drug Abuse Warning Network, which collects data on emergency department visits and drug-related deaths (35).

Drugs and Motor Vehicle Injury Based on the National Survey on Drug Use and Health, an estimated 9.5 million people aged 12 or older, or 4.2% of the population in this age group, reported driving under the influence of illicit drugs. The rate for 2006 was highest among young adults aged 18 to 25 (13%). Other drug use has been identified as a major hazard to road traffic safety. Marijuana is the most prevalent illegal drug used, and studies of trauma patients injured in MVCs have documented the use of benzodiazepines, cocaine, opiates and amphetamines (36). An earlier study of drug use with and without concomitant alcohol use among injured drivers found that 14 (6.6%) of 211 injured drivers tested positive for drugs (amphetamines, barbiturates, benzodiazepines, cocaine, cannabis, and opiates) alone, while 12 (5.7%) of 211 tested positive for alcohol and drugs in combination (37).

EFFECTIVE SCREENING IN INJURED PATIENTS

Principles of Screening Screening involves the identification of disorders in patients without known disease. It is distinct from case-finding, in which patients for whom there is a high clinical index of suspicion of a disease undergo assessment to confirm the diagnosis. Screening is indicated in disorders that meet the following criteria: (1) the disorder has significant prevalence and consequences in the population, (2) there are effective and acceptable treatments for the disorder, (3) early treatment is preferable to later treatment, (4) screening instruments with good operating characteristics are available, and (5) screening instruments are easily administered. Screening for substance use disorders in patients with traumatic injuries meets all of these criteria.

As the foregoing criteria indicate, screening instruments should have specific characteristics to allow for their use in clinical situations. First among these characteristics is good accuracy in identifying patients with the disorder among all those who are screened. Screening tests that are applied to large groups of patients, many of whom do not have the disease, perform best when they have high sensitivity (a low rate of false-negatives) and adequate specificity (a low rate of false-positives). Other desirable features include brevity, utility in diverse demographic and clinical populations, and low cost.

Screening for Alcohol Problems in the Emergency Department Alcohol problems occur across a clinical spectrum in the emergency department (ED). Screening and intervention when needed may take place at almost any time during the ED visit. The important consideration is that there be a protocol or routine for screening and intervention that is based on the resources of the ED. The screening can be part of the history taken by the nurse, physician, or other ED staff member who has been trained in screening. Interventions are dependent upon the specific type of intervention that is needed, whether a brief intervention or a referral to specialized treatment. Patients being admitted to the hospital from the ED may have their screening and interventions when their condition permits, which may mean that the screening and intervention will take place after admission.

At-risk drinking generally is defined as a threshold amount of alcohol consumption per day or week; typically, it is described as "problem," "heavy," or "excessive" drinking (38). This level of alcohol consumption puts patients at risk for future alcohol-related consequences because of the amount they drink or the effect of alcohol on any comorbid medical conditions. However, at-risk drinking may not be associated with ongoing adverse consequences. In contrast, patients with alcohol abuse or dependence experience significant and repeated negative physical and social effects from their alcohol use, often including the cardinal signs of tolerance and withdrawal (39). These diagnostic classifications are useful to clinicians because they allow patients to be stratified according to disease severity and are useful in making treatment recommendations. In addition, the classifications affect the choice of a screening tool for use in identifying patients with alcohol problems in the clinical setting. Studies of screening instruments for alcohol problems in emergency department and trauma settings have focused primarily on the recognition of the most harmful spectrum of alcohol consumption, including alcohol abuse and dependence, and so provide little empirical evidence to guide screening for at-risk drinking. Evidence supports the use of brief, formal screening questionnaires such as the CAGE, TWEAK, or AUDIT (included in the Appendix 2 of this text) in preference to clinical recognition or laboratory analyses such as the BAC or SAT (40–44). Among the screening questionnaires that have been evaluated in emergency departments, the CAGE, TWEAK, and AUDIT are the best studied (45,46). For patients who met the criteria for alcohol dependence:

- Two positive responses on the CAGE had a sensitivity of 76% to 87% and a specificity of 84% to 90%;
- A score of 3 on the TWEAK had a sensitivity of 84% to 89% and a specificity of 81% to 86%;
- A score of 6 on the MAST had a sensitivity of 30% to 71% and a specificity of 92% to 99%; and
- A score of 8 on the AUDIT had a sensitivity of 83% to 91% and a specificity of 81% to 90%.

The first three questions of the AUDIT (which cover quantity, frequency, and intensity of drinking) were shown to have a sensitivity of 97% and a specificity of 65% for harmful or hazardous drinking (47). In contrast, breath alcohol analysis has been shown to have only limited utility in screening, with a sensitivity of 20% to 28% and a specificity of 94% to 97% (41,46). Blood alcohol analysis was similarly disappointing: One study found that the presence of alcohol dependence and other psychoactive substance use disorders was similar in trauma center patients with positive BACs (76%) and negative BACs (62%) (29). The proportion of positive BACs was low even among patients arriving after motor vehicle accidents (48).

In an effort to create a useful and portable screening instrument for alcohol problems in emergency settings, one researcher has combined five questions from the CAGE, TWEAK, and AUDIT to create the Rapid Alcohol Problems Screen (RAPS) (42). One positive response on the RAPS has a sensitivity of 90% to 93% and a specificity of 76% to 78% (44,48) for alcohol dependence and abuse. A reduction of the RAPS instrument to four questions created an instrument with a sensitivity of 93% and a specificity of 87% in one report (42). Though the RAPS instrument appears promising, the wealth of information on the use of the CAGE plus quantity and frequency questions from the AUDIT make these the preferred screening methods at this time.

The operating characteristics of screening instruments for alcohol problems in emergency settings have been shown to vary with ethnicity, gender, and nature of the alcohol problem.

In one study, for example, the CAGE had a sensitivity of 86% in injured African American men and 71% in injured white men. Similar gender and ethnic variations have been seen in the operating characteristics of the AUDIT, TWEAK, MAST, and RAPS (49–51), though the clinical significance of these variations is not clear. Therefore, clinicians who implement screening programs may need to take racial and gender considerations into account in selecting a screening tool. According to Canagasaby and Vinson (52), a single alcohol screening question can be used to detect hazardous or harmful drinking. They suggest the following question: "When was the last time you had more than X drinks in one day?" where X = four for women and five for men, with any time in the past 3 months considered a positive screen (1 drink = 14 g ethanol).

Finally, one study found similar rates of compliance with screening when a straightforward screening questionnaire was used, rather than a questionnaire with alcohol questions embedded among questions on diet, smoking status, and exercise (53). This suggests that straightforward questioning about alcohol use may be appropriate for some populations. There are no comparable screening instruments for drug abuse and dependence other than alcohol. One attempt to identify problems is to add an additional question to the CAGE to ask about specific drugs. Most experts believe that the more specific the question, the better the history obtained, and thus recommend asking about specific classes of drugs (54).

INTERVENTIONS WITH INJURED PATIENTS

Alcohol or other drug-related injury provides a unique opportunity for brief intervention (1,55). The negative consequences of the injury can create what has been described as a "teachable moment"—a unique opportunity to motivate patients to change their behavior or to encourage them to seek further treatment. Empirical evidence supports the hypothesis that the aversive nature of the injury and perception of the degree of alcohol involvement in an injury event are predictive of patients' readiness to change. In a study in an emergency department of patients who were injured in MVCs and who had been drinking alcohol, Cherpitel (56) found that more than one-third connected their alcohol use to the injury event. In addition, the emergency department presents rich opportunities for such interventions, as research shows that a higher proportion of patients in emergency settings than in other settings have alcohol-related problems. One study compared patients from the same metropolitan area who went to an emergency department with those who went to primary care settings and found that the emergency department patients were one-and-a-half to three times more likely to report heavy drinking, negative consequences of drinking, alcohol dependence, or prior treatment for alcohol-related problems than patients in a primary care clinic (22).

Brief interventions can reduce not only alcohol use but the incidence of alcohol-related injuries. A systematic review of the effectiveness of such interventions in preventing injuries evaluated 19 randomized controlled trials and found that treatment for problem drinking was associated with a reduction in suicide attempts, domestic violence, falls, drinking-related injuries, hospitalizations, and deaths (57). In seven trials that compared interventions with a control group, nearly all showed a decrease in injury-related outcomes. The effect size of these decreases ranged from a 27% reduction in drinking-related injuries to a 65% reduction in accidental and violent deaths. Of note, interventions among convicted drunk drivers reduced the number of MVCs and related injuries. It is not clear from this literature, however, whether the mechanism of action of the interventions was reduced alcohol consumption or decreased risk-taking (57).

Brief interventions involve counseling sessions that require 5 to 45 minutes. Such interventions often incorporate the six elements proposed by Miller and Sanchez (58), which are summarized by the mnemonic FRAMES: **F**eedback, **R**esponsibility, **A**dvice, **M**enu of strategies, **E**mpathy, and **S**elf-efficacy. Other elements that have been shown to support the efficacy of brief interventions include goal setting, follow-up, and timing (59).

Multiple studies have demonstrated the efficacy of brief interventions for alcohol problems in a variety of settings (60), including general populations (61–63), and patients in primary care settings (64,65). Results from studies including emergency department patients (66–74) and inpatient trauma centers (75,76) have been mixed. Cohort studies without control groups have demonstrated a significant benefit of brief intervention. Wright et al. (67) reported the results of a study of patients who misused alcohol and who received brief interventions from a health worker in a London emergency department. Of 202 patients enrolled, 71 patients completed the 6-month follow-up. Of these, 46 (65%) reported significant reductions in their alcohol consumption.

In Project ASSERT, Bernstein et al. (66) enlisted health promotion advocates to screen and provide counseling and referral for injured and noninjured emergency department patients, most of whom were alcohol- or drug-dependent. Of 7,118 adult patients screened, 2,931 had evidence of alcohol or drug problems; of those, 1,096 were enrolled in the project. Among the 245 patients assessed at 90-day follow-up, there was a significant reduction in self-reported drug and alcohol use. The results demonstrated a 45% decrease in drug abuse severity score, a 67% reduction in the proportion of subjects reporting use of cocaine or crack, a 62% reduction in the proportion of subjects reporting use of marijuana, a 56% reduction in alcohol use, and a 4% reduction in binge drinking. In addition, more than half the subjects reported that they had acted on a treatment referral. Blow et al. (77) studied four interventions with and without tailored messages and advice for reducing alcohol consumption and consequences in 575 injured patients. Each group significantly decreased alcohol consumption from baseline to 12-month follow-up, with those in the first group significantly decreasing their weekly alcohol consumption by 48.5% ($p < .0001$). In this study, there was no control group for comparison.

The Academic ED SBIRT (screening, brief intervention referral and treatment) Research Collaborative (73) group studied patients who drink over the NIAAA low-risk limits in 14 sites nationwide. A quasi-experimental comparison group was used in which control and intervention patients were recruited sequentially at each site. At 3-month follow-up, the brief intervention group reported consuming 3.25 fewer drinks per week than the controls (B = −3.25 95% CI [−5.75, −0.75]). At-risk drinkers appeared to benefit more from the BI than did dependent drinkers.

In a randomized controlled studies results have been varied. Neumann (71) used a computer-generated brief intervention for at-risk drinkers who presented with minor injury to a German ED. The intervention group had a significant decrease in alcohol intake at 6 months compared with a control group (35.7% decrease compared with 20.5% decrease in controls; $p = 0.006$). This significant decrease persisted at 12-months. Longabaugh et al (69) studied injured adolescent and adult ED patients, and reported a significant decrease in alcohol consumption in both the intervention and the control conditions. Monti et al. (68) divided 74 patients 18 and 19 years of age in a randomized manner to receive either brief intervention or standard care. At 6-month follow-up, the brief intervention group had a significantly lower incidence of drinking and driving, traffic violations, alcohol-related injuries, and alcohol-related problems, including trouble with parents, school, friends, dates, or the police. Over the same time period, patients in both groups significantly reduced their alcohol consumption from baseline. Longabaugh (69) found similar results in the group that received an intervention and booster 1 month later. Daeppen, (72) from Switzerland, studied the efficacy of brief intervention in reducing alcohol use among hazardous drinkers treated in the ED after an injury. He found that there was a similar percentage of participants who reported low-risk drinking at 12 months in all groups; intervention versus those in the control groups with and without assessments (35.6%, vs. 34.0% and 37.0%). D'Onofrio et al. (74) studied all ED patients who screened positive for hazardous and harmful drinking and found that both the intervention group and the control group significantly reduced their alcohol consumption at 12 months. The results were similar whether the patient was injured or not. Whether these mixed results are due to methodologic challenges such as extensive assessments, or enrollment of patients with lower levels of drinking remains to be answered. It is clear that further study is necessary.

In terms of admitted trauma patients, there are also disparate results. Gentilello et al. (75) performed a study in patients who met one of the following eligibility criteria: a positive blood alcohol concentration, an elevated gamma-glutamyl transpeptidase level, or a positive screen on the Short Michigan Alcoholism Screening Test (SMAST). A total of 366 hospitalized, injured patients were randomly assigned to receive a 30-minute intervention or standard care. The intervention was performed by a psychologist and was followed up in 1 month by a letter that summarized the intervention. When followed up at 12 months (54% follow-up rate), the intervention group was found to have decreased alcohol consumption by an average of 21.8 drinks per week, compared with a decrease in the control group of 6.7 drinks per week ($p = 0.03$). The magnitude of the reduction in drinks per week was limited to patients with moderate alcohol problems. At 3 years, follow-up found a 47% reduction ($p = 0.07$) in injuries that required either emergency department or trauma center admission and a 48% reduction in injuries that required hospital admission (also not statistically significant: 95% confidence interval 0.21–1.29).

Sommers et al. (76) studied two types of brief intervention on patients with alcohol-related vehicular injury who were admitted to a trauma center. Patients were randomly assigned into a control group that received simple advice and brief counseling condition. All participants had a significant decrease in alcohol consumption and traffic citations at 12 months as compared with baseline, but there was no difference by condition.

In January 2006 the American College of Surgeons Committee on Trauma passed a resolution mandating that screening and brief intervention services be included as an essential component of Level I Trauma Center verification (77). Though the evidence in the ED/trauma patient is indeed mixed, there is no question that alcohol is associated with injury and that emergency physicians (6) and trauma surgeons (1) are unlikely to incorporate screening and brief intervention into their practices. Barriers cited include lack of education, time, resources, and reimbursement. Moreover, recent reports underscore that education in the use of formal alcohol and drug screening questionnaires is lacking in emergency medicine residency programs (78). Conversely, evidence shows that residents who are exposed to a structured skills-based educational program do improve their knowledge and performance in screening and brief intervention with patients who have alcohol problems (79).

INCORPORATING SCREENING AND BRIEF INTERVENTION INTO PRACTICE

As discussed earlier, screening instruments vary in terms of their effectiveness, availability, ease of administration, and test characteristics (80). In most settings where injured patients are treated, such as emergency departments and trauma centers, time is short, and competing priorities make screening and brief intervention a challenge. Therefore, screens that are short and simple and that can be administered by a variety of providers—nurses, physicians, social workers, and health promotion advocates—have a greater chance of being used.

Screening for alcohol problems in injured patients should detect the entire spectrum of use, including at-risk and harmful drinkers and dependent drinkers. Such detection is important because nondependent drinkers may benefit most from brief intervention and referral to a primary care provider. One screen for alcohol problems that can be adapted to the emergency department and trauma center setting and which has been recommended by the National Institute of Alcohol Abuse and Alcoholism (NIAAA) includes three quantity and frequency questions (to elicit information as to whether the patient exceeds the guidelines for moderate drinking), as well as the CAGE questionnaire (which is better at identifying alcohol dependence (81). Because the CAGE originally was designed for lifetime prevalence, it is helpful, though less well validated, to modify it by specifying "in the past 12 months" (Table 79.1). Asking quantity and frequency questions first, then adding the CAGE questions if the consumption exceeds moderate levels, is one way to use the screens. Another approach is to jump to the CAGE questions for patients who are intoxicated, have high BACs, or in whom dependence is suspected. This approach eliminates the negative connotations and resistance that can occur when attempting to quantify a patient's drinking. More recently (in 2007), the NIAAA has recommended a single question to screen for heavy drinking (see Chapter 18).

TABLE 79.1 Screening for Alcohol Problems in Injured Patients

Ask the NIAAA quantity and frequency questions:

1. On average, how many days per week do you drink alcohol?
2. On a typical day when you drink, how many drinks do you have?
3. What is the maximum number of drinks you had on any given occasion during the past month?

Use the CAGE (In the past 12 months . . .):

C: Have you ever felt you should *C*ut down on your drinking?
A: Have people *A*nnoyed you by criticizing your drinking?
G: Have you ever felt bad or *G*uilty about your drinking?
E: Have you ever had a drink first thing in the morning to "steady your nerves" or get rid of a hangover ("*E*ye opener")?

The screen is positive if:

A positive response on one or more questions from the CAGE and/or at-risk consumption is identified.

At-risk consumption
Men: >14 drinks/wk or >4 drinks per occasion
Women: >7 drinks/wk or >3 drinks per occasion
Both genders older than 65 years:
>7 drinks/week or >3 drinks per occasion

Then assess for:

- Medical problems: blackouts, depression, hypertension, injury, abdominal pain, liver dysfunction, sleep disorders
- Laboratory tests: Liver function tests, macrocytic anemia
- Behavioral problems
- Alcohol dependence

Intervene
If the patient is an "at-risk drinker":

- Advise the patient of his or her risk.
- Set drinking goals.
- Provide referral to primary care.

If the patient is an alcohol-dependent drinker:

- Assess the acute risk of intoxication or withdrawal.

Negotiate a referral for detoxification, to Alcoholics Anonymous, and to primary care.

Reprinted from *The physician's guide to helping patients with alcohol problems* (NIH Publication No. 95-3769). Rockville, MD: National Institute on Alcohol Abuse and Alcoholism, 1995.

Brief interventions may include advice only or incorporate some motivational enhancement techniques. For the at-risk drinker or the patient who has sustained an alcohol-related injury but is not alcohol-dependent, setting goals within safe limits, coupled with a referral to the patient's primary care physician, may be all that is needed. For the patient with nondependent drug use, negotiating abstinence or harm reduction, such as no use while driving, with a referral to primary care may be sufficient. For the patient who is dependent on drugs or alcohol or the clinician who is uncertain as to where a patient fits on the continuum of alcohol and drug problems, the brief intervention becomes a negotiation process to seek further assessment or referral to a specialized treatment program (82).

TABLE 79.2 Brief Intervention for Injured Patients

Raise the subject: "I would like to take a few minutes to talk to you about your alcohol use."
Give feedback: "I am concerned about your drinking. Our screen indicates that you are above what we consider the safe limits of drinking. This level places you at risk for alcohol-related illness, injury, and death."
Compare to norms: Compare with National Institute of Alcohol Abuse and Alcoholism guidelines for moderate alcohol consumption.
Make a connection: "Do you see a connection between your visit and your alcohol use?"
Assess readiness: "On a scale of 1 to 10 (1 being not ready to change: and 10 being very ready), how ready are you to change your drinking pattern?"
Develop discrepancy: So, you enjoy drinking, but you also want to avoid getting hurt.
Elicit a response: "How does all this sound to you?"
Negotiate a goal: "What would you like to do?"
Give advice: "If you stay within the recommended limits (NIAAA guidelines), you will be less likely to experience further illness or injury related to alcohol use. You should never drink and drive."
Summarize, provide agreement form (a plan for change), and primary care follow-up: "This is what I heard you say. . . . Thank you for your time."

The contents of such a brief intervention are outlined in Table 79.2. Using this information, the authors recommend that each institution develop a program and resource list tailored to the needs of its own community.

REFERENCES

1. Gentilello LM, Donovan DM, Dunn CW et al. Alcohol interventions in trauma centers. Current practice and future directions. *JAMA* 1995;74(13):1043–1048.
2. Degutis LC. Screening for alcohol problems in emergency department patients with minor injury: results and recommendations for practice and policy. *Vontemp Drug Probl* 1998;25(3):463–475.
3. Cherpitel CJ. Alcohol and injuries: a review of international emergency room studies. *Addiction* 1993;88(7):923–937.
4. Freedland ES, McMicken DB, D'Onofrio G. Alcohol and trauma. *Emerg Med Clin North Am* 1993;3:225–339.
5. Peppiatt R, Evans R, Jordan P. Blood alcohol concentrations of patients attending an accident and emergency department. *Resuscitation* 1978;6(1):37–43.
6. Lowenstein S, Weissberg M, Terry D. Alcohol intoxication, injuries and dangerous behaviors—and the revolving emergency department door. *J Trauma* 1990;30:1252–1257.
7. Teplin LA, Abram KM, Michaels SK. Blood alcohol level among emergency room patients: a multivariate analysis. *J Stud Alcohol* 1989;50(5):441–447.
8. Wechsler H, Kasey EH, Thum D, et al. Alcohol level and home accidents. *Public Health Rep* 1969;84(12):1043–1050.
9. Antti-Poika I, Karaharju E. Heavy drinking and accidents—a prospective study among men of working age. *Injury* 1988;19(3):198–200.
10. Howland RW, Hingson R. Alcohol as a risk factor for injuries of death due to fires and burns: review of the literature. *Public Health Rep* 1987;102:475–483.
11. Hingson RW, Lederman RI, Walsh DC. Employee drinking patterns and accidental injury: a study of four New England states. *J Stud Alcohol* 1985;46(4):298–303.
12. Brewer RD, Morris PD, Cole TB, et al. The risk of dying in alcohol-related automobile crashes among habitual drunk drivers. *N Engl J Med* 1994;331(1):513–517.
13. Li G, Smith GS, Baker SP. Drinking behavior in relation to cause of death among U.S. adults. *Am J Public Health* 1994;84(9):1402–1406.
14. Centers for Disease Control and Prevention. WISQARS: leading causes of death charts. Retrieved December 5, 2007, from http://www.cdc.gov/ncipc/wisqars/.
15. National Highway Traffic Safety Administration. Traffic Safety Facts 2006—early edition. Washington, DC: Author. DOT HS 810 808, 2007.
16. Haddon W, Bradess VA. Alcohol in the single vehicle fatal accident. *JAMA* 1959;169:1587–1593.
17. Wintemute GJ, Teret SP, Kraus JF, et al. Alcohol and drowning: an analysis of contributing factors and a discussion of criteria for case selection. *Accid Prev* 1990;22(3):291–296.
18. Li G, Baker S, Sterling S, et al. A comparative analysis of alcohol in fatal and nonfatal bicycling injuries. *Alcohol Clin Exp Res* 1996;20(9):1553–1559.
19. Mengert P, Sussman ED, DiSario R. A study between the risk of fatality and blood alcohol concentration of recreational boat operators (Report CG-D-09-92). Washington, DC: U.S. Coast Guard, 1992.
20. Mannenbach MS, Hargarten SW, Phelan MB. Alcohol use among injured patients aged 12 to 18 years. *Acad Emerg Med* 1997;4(1):40–44.
21. Maio RF, Shope JT, Blow FC, et al. Adolescent injury in the emergency department: opportunity for alcohol interventions? *Ann Emerg Med* 2000;35(3):252–257.
22. Cherpitel CJ. Drinking patterns and problems: a comparison of two black primary care samples in two regions. *Alcohol Clin Exp Res* 1999;23(3):523–527.
23. Howland J, Smith GS, Mangione T, et al. Missing the boat on drinking and boating. *JAMA* 1993;270(1):91–92.
24. Hingson RW, Heeren T, Jamanka A, et al. Age of drinking onset and unintentional injury involvement after drinking. *JAMA* 2000;284(12):1527–1533.
25. Borges G, Cherpitel CG, Medina-Mora M, et al. Alcohol consumption in emergency room patients and the general population: a population-based study. *Alcohol Clin Exp Res* 1998;22(9):1986–1991.
26. Cherpitel CJ. Alcohol and casualties: a comparison of emergency room and coroner data. *Alcohol Alcohol* 1994;29(2):211–218.
27. Cherpitel CJ. Alcohol and injuries resulting from violence: a review of emergency room studies. *Addiction* 1994;89(2):157–165.
28. Soderstrom CA, Dischinger PC, Smith GS, et al. Psychoactive substance dependence among trauma center patients. *JAMA* 1992;267(20):2756–2759.
29. Smith GS, Branas CC, Miller TR. Fatal nontraffic injuries involving alcohol: a metaanalysis. *Ann Emerg Med* 1999;33(6):659–668.
30. Hingson R, Howland J. Alcohol and non-traffic unintended injuries. *Addiction* 1993;88(7):877–883.
31. Marzuk PM, Tardiff K, Leon A, et al. Prevalence of recent cocaine use among motor vehicle fatalities in New York City. *JAMA* 1990;263(2):250–256.
32. Tardiff K, Marzuk PM, Leon A, et al. Homicide in New York City. Cocaine use and firearms. *JAMA* 1994;272(1):43–46.
33. Marzuk PM, Tardiff K, Smyth K, et al. Cocaine use, risk taking, and fatal Russian roulette. *JAMA* 1992;267(19):2635–2637.
34. Marzuk PM, Tardiff K, Leon A, et al. Fatal injuries after cocaine use as a leading cause of death among young adults in New York City. *N Engl J Med* 1995;332(26):1753–1757.
35. Brookoff D, Campbell EA, Shaw L. The underreporting of cocaine-related trauma: drug abuse warning network reports vs. hospital toxicology tests. *Am J Public Health* 1993;83(3):369–371.
36. Martins SS, Copersino ML, Soderstrom CA, et al. Risk of psychoactive substance dependence among substance used in a trauma inpatient population. *J Addict Dis* 2007;26(1):71–77.
37. Schepens PJ, Pauwels A, Van Damme V, et al. Drugs of abuse and alcohol in weekend drivers involved in car crashes in Belgium. *Ann Emerg Med* 1998;31(5):633–637.

38. Fiellin DA, Reid MC, O'Connor P. Screening for alcohol problems in primary care: a systematic review. *Arch Intern Med* 2000;160(13): 1977–1989.
39. Fiellin DA, Reid MC, O'Connor PG. Outpatient management of patients with alcohol problems. *Ann Intern Med* 2000;133(10): 815–827.
40. Becker B, Woolard R, Nirenberg T. Alcohol use among subcritically injured emergency department patients. *Acad Emerg Med* 1995;2(9): 784–790.
41. Cherpitel CJ. Screening for alcohol problems in the emergency department. *Ann Emerg Med* 1995;26:158–166.
42. Cherpitel CJ. Screening for alcohol problems in the emergency room: a rapid alcohol problems screen. *Drug Alcohol Depend* 1995;40(2):133–137.
43. Gentilello LM, Villaveces A, Ries R, et al. Detection of acute alcohol intoxication and chronic alcohol dependence by trauma center staff. *J Trauma Injury Infect Crit Care* 1999;47(6):1131–1139.
44. Clifford PR, Sparadeo F, Minugh A, et al. Identification of hazardous/harmful drinking among subcritically injured patients. *Acad Emerg Med* 1996;3(3):239–245.
45. Cherpitel CJ. Analysis of cut points for screening instruments for alcohol problems in the emergency room. *J Stud Alcohol* 1995;56(6):695–700.
46. Cherpitel CJ. Differences in performance of screening instruments for problem drinking among blacks, whites and Hispanics in an emergency room population. *J Stud Alcohol* 1998;59(4):420–426.
47. Minaugh PA, Nirenberg TD, Clifford P, et al. Analysis of alcohol use clusters among subcritically injured emergency department patients. *Acad Emerg Med* 1997;4(11):1059–1067.
48. Chang G, Astrachan BM. The emergency department surveillance of alcohol intoxication after motor vehicle accidents. *JAMA* 1988;260(17): 2533–2536.
49. Cherpitel C, Clark W. Ethnic differences in performance of screening instruments for identifying harmful drinking and alcohol dependence in the emergency room. *Alcohol Clin Exp Res* 1995;22(9):1986–1991.
50. Cherpitel CJ. Comparison of screening instruments for alcohol problems between black and white emergency room patients from two regions of the country. *Alcohol Clin Exp Res* 1997;21(8):1391–1397.
51. Cherpitel CJ. A brief screening instrument for problem drinking in the emergency room: The RAPS4 Rapid Alcohol Problems Screen. *J Stud Alcohol* 1999;61(3):447–449.
52. Canagasaby A and Vinson DC. Screening for hazardous or harmful drinking using one or two quantity-frequency questions. *Alcohol Alcohol* 2005;40:208–213.
53. Adams PJ, Stevens V. Are emergency department patients more likely to answer alcohol questions in a masked health questionnaire? *Alcohol Alcohol* 1994;29(2):193–197.
54. Senay ED. Diagnostic interview and mental status examination. In Lowinson JH, Ruiz P, Millman RB, et al., eds. *Substance abuse: a comprehensive textbook*. Baltimore: Williams, Wilkins, 1997:364–377.
55. D'Onofrio G, Bernstein E, Bernstein J, et al. Patients with alcohol problems in the emergency department: Part 1. Improving detection. SAEM Substance Abuse Task Force. Society for Academic Emergency Medicine. *Acad Emerg Med* 1998;5(12):1200–1209.
56. Cherpitel CJ. Drinking patterns and problems and drinking in the event: an analysis of injury by cause among casualty patients. *Alcohol Clin Exp Res* 1996;20(6):1130–1137.
57. Dinh-Zarr T, Diguiseppi C, Heitman E, et al. Preventing injuries through interventions for problem drinking: a systematic review of randomized controlled trials. *Alcohol Alcohol* 1999;34(4):609–621.
58. Miller WR, Sanchez VC. Motivating young adults for treatment and lifestyle change. In Howard G, ed. *Issues in alcohol use and misuse in young adults*. Notre Dame, IN: University of Notre Dame Press, 1993.
59. Graham AW, Fleming MS. Brief interventions. In Graham AW, Schultz TK, Wilford BB, eds. *Principles of addiction medicine*, 2nd ed. Chevy Chase, MD: American Society of Addiction Medicine, 1998:615–630.
60. Wilk AI, Jensen NM, Havighurst TC. Meta-analysis of randomized control trials addressing brief interventions in heavy alcohol drinkers. *J Gen Intern Med* 1997;12(5):274–283.
61. Heather N, Champion PD, Neville RG, et al. Evaluation of a controlled drinking minimal intervention for problem drinkers in general practice (the DRAMS scheme). *J R Coll Gen Pract* 1987;37(301):358–363.
62. Cox KL, Puddey IB, Morton AR, et al. The combined effects of aerobic exercise and alcohol restriction on blood pressure and serum lipids: a two-way factorial study in sedentary men. *J Hypertens* 1993;11(1):191–201.
63. Nilssen O. The Trömso Study: identification of and a controlled intervention on a population of early-stage risk drinkers. *Prev Med* 1991;20(1): 518–528.
64. Fleming MF, Barry KL, Manwell LB, et al. Brief physician advice for problem alcohol drinkers. A randomized controlled trial in community-based primary care practices. *JAMA* 1997;277(13):1039–1045.
65. Wallace P, Cutler S, Haines A. Randomized controlled trial of general practitioner intervention in patients with excessive alcohol consumption. *Br Med J* 1988;297(9):663–668.
66. Bernstein E, Bernstein J, Levenson S. Project ASSERT: an ED-based intervention to increase access to primary care, preventive services, and the substance abuse treatment system. *Ann Emerg Med* 1997;30(2):181–189.
67. Wright S, Moran L, Meyrick M, et al. Intervention by an alcohol health worker in an accident and emergency department. *Alcohol Alcohol* 1998;33(6):651–656.
68. Monti PM, Spirito A, Myers M, et al. Brief intervention for harm reduction with alcohol-positive older adolescents in a hospital emergency department. *J Consult Clin Psychol* 1999;67(6):989–994.
69. Longabaugh RH, Woolard RF, Nirenberg TD, et al. Evaluating the effects of a brief motivational intervention for injured drinkers in the emergency department. *J Stud Alcohol* 2001;62:806–816.
70. Blow FC, Barry KL, Walton MA, et al. The efficacy of two brief intervention strategies among injured at-risk drinkers in the ED: impact of tailored messaging and brief advice. *Jf Stud Alcohol* 2006;67:568–578.
71. Neumann T, Neuner B, Weiss-Gerlach E, et al. The effect of computerized tailored brief advice on at-risk drinking in subcritically injured trauma patients. *J Trauma Injury Infect Crit Care* 2006;61:805–814.
72. Daeppen JB, Gaume J, Bady P, et al. Brief alcohol intervention and alcohol assessment do not influence alcohol use in injured patients treated in the emergency department: a randomized controlled clinical trial. *Addiction*. 2007;102:1224–1233.
73. The Academic ED SBIRT Research Collaborative. An evidence based alcohol screening, brief intervention and referral to treatment (SBIRT) curriculum for emergency department (ED) providers improves skills and utilization. *Subst Abuse* 2007;28(4):79–92.
74. D'Onofrio G, Pantalon MV, Degutis LC, et al. Brief intervention for hazardous and harmful drinkers in the emergency department. *Ann Emerg Med* 2008 (in press).
75. Gentilello LM, Rivara FP, Donovan DM, et al. Alcohol interventions in a trauma center as a means of reducing the risk of injury recurrence. *Ann of Surg* 1999;230:473–484.
76. Sommers MS, Dyehouse JM, Howe SR, et al. Effectiveness of brief interventions after alcohol-related vehicular injury: a randomized controlled trial. *J Trauma Injury Infect Crit Care* 2006;61(3):523–531.
77. American College of Surgeons Committee on Trauma. Trauma Center Verification Program. Retrieved December 10, 2007, from http://www.facs.org/trauma/verificationhosp.html.
78. Krishel S, Richards CF. Alcohol and substance abuse training for emergency medicine residents: a survey of U.S. programs. *Acad Emerg Med* 1999;6(9):964–966.
79. D'Onofrio G, Nadel ES, Degutis LC, et al. Improving emergency medicine residents' approach to patients with alcohol problems: a controlled educational trial. *Ann Emerg Med* 2002;40:50–62.
80. Schorling JB, Buchsbaum DG. Screening for alcohol and drug abuse. *Med Clin North Am* 1997;81:845–865.
81. Ewing JA. Detecting alcoholism: the CAGE questionnaire. *JAMA* 1984;252:1905–1907.
82. D'Onofrio G. Bernstein E, Bernstein J, et al. Patients with alcohol problems in the emergency department: Part 2.: Intervention and referral. SAEM Substance Abuse Task Force. Society for Academic Emergency Medicine. *Acad Emerg Med* 1998;5(12):1210–1217.

CHAPTER 80

Alan Ona Malabanan, MD, FACE

Endocrine and Reproductive Disorders Related to Alcohol and Other Drug Use

The endocrine effects of alcohol and other drugs are complex. These substances can alter the secretion of hormone-releasing factors and hormones at the level of the hypothalamus and pituitary; alter the synthesis or release of hormones at the level of the thyroid, adrenal, or pancreas; alter hormone action on target organs; and alter hormone economy by affecting their metabolism or binding proteins. Multiple hormone systems can be affected, many of whose actions may conflict, leading to a lack of net clinical effect. When one adds to this inherent complexity the effects on the endocrine system of gender, mental status, and mental illness, the heterogeneity of illicit drugs, the prevalence of polydrug use, the effects of drug withdrawal, and differences between the effects of acute and chronic substance use, it becomes clear that the study of the endocrine effects of alcohol and other drugs is very difficult. Generalizing many of these effects to clinical practice is even more difficult. Therefore, the most clearly recognized and clinically relevant effects are summarized in this chapter (Table 80.1).

DISORDERS RELATED TO ALCOHOL

Hypoglycemia One of the most serious consequences of alcohol abuse is hypoglycemia, which can lead to neurologic damage, coma, seizures, or death. Alcohol causes hypoglycemia by producing malnutrition, reducing the body's production of glucose, and impairing the body's response to hypoglycemia (Fig. 80.1). Though hypoglycemia is an uncommon complication of alcoholism, alcohol use is a common cause of spontaneous hypoglycemia (1).

Unlike other drugs, ethyl alcohol is a significant source of energy, with 7.1 kcal per gram (2). Malnutrition can result from alcohol abuse, as nutrients are replaced by the "empty" calories of alcohol (i.e., alcohol provides energy but no other nutrients such as protein or vitamins). In addition, the normal metabolism of alcohol to acetaldehyde by alcohol dehydrogenase leads to the conversion of nicotinamide adenine dinucleotide (NAD) to its reduced form (NADH), resulting in a decrease in gluconeogenesis. NAD is a cofactor necessary for many of the reactions involved in glucose synthesis. Alcohol does not affect glucose release from glycogen stores, which in a well-fed subject can provide glucose for 12 hours or more. In a prolonged fasting state or in a state of depleted glycogen stores, as seen in malnourished alcoholics, the inability to compensate for hepatic glycogen depletion can lead to hypoglycemia after acute alcohol ingestion.

Alcohol also can impair the body's hormonal responses to hypoglycemia. Several investigators have shown that alcohol impairs the release of cortisol, growth hormone, glucagon, and vasopressin in response to hypoglycemia (3–7). Kolaczynski et al. (8) also found similar alcohol-induced reductions in cortisol, glucagon, and growth hormone levels in response to hypoglycemia but found faster glucose recovery with alcohol use, suggesting alcohol-related peripheral insulin resistance. Kerr et al. (9) found a similar suppression of growth hormone, an insignificant suppression of cortisol, and increased insulin resistance in mildly intoxicated hypoglycemic type 1 diabetics.

There are five classes of alcohol-induced hypoglycemia: simple alcohol-induced fasting hypoglycemia, alcoholic ketoacidosis with hypoglycemia, alcoholic exacerbation of insulin-induced hypoglycemia, alcoholic exacerbation of sulfonylurea-induced hypoglycemia, and alcohol-induced reactive hypoglycemia (1). In simple alcohol-induced fasting hypoglycemia, patients typically present with coma and a blood glucose level of <40 mg/dL. Blood alcohol levels may be

TABLE 80.1 Endocrine Syndromes Associated with Alcohol and Other Drug Use

Alcohol
- Diabetes insipidus
- Gynecomastia
- Hyperadrenalism
- Hyperglycemia
- Hypoglycemia
- Hyperlipidemia
- Hyperprolactinemia (possibly)
- Hypogonadism/infertility
- Hypertension
- Osteoporosis

Amphetamines
- Hyperadrenalism
- Hypertension
- Weight loss

Anabolic steroids
- Gynecomastia
- Hyperlipidemia
- Hypogonadism/Infertility
- Hypertension
- Hyperthyroidism (possibly)
- Virilization

Barbiturates
- Hypoadrenalism (possibly)
- Hypothyroidism (possibly)
- Osteoporosis

Benzodiazepines
- Hypoadrenalism (possibly)
- Hypoglycemia (possibly)
- Syndrome of inappropriate antidiuretic hormone (SIADH) (possibly)

Caffeine
- Hyperglycemia
- Hyperlipidemia (possibly)
- Hypertension
- Osteoporosis (possibly)

Cocaine
- Hyperglycemia
- Hyperprolactinemia
- Hypertension
- Weight loss

Inhalants
- Hypogonadism/infertility
- Hypothyroidism (possibly)
- Osteoporosis (possibly)

Lysergic acid
- None known

Marijuana
- Gynecomastia (possibly)
- Hypoadrenalism
- Hypoglycemia (possibly)
- Hypogonadism/infertility (possibly)

Opioids
- Hyperprolactinemia
- Hypogonadism/infertility
- Osteoporosis

Phencyclidine
- None known

Tobacco/cigarette smoking
- Hyperlipidemia
- Hypogonadism/infertility
- Hypertension
- Hyperthyroidism
- Hypothyroidism (possibly)
- Osteoporosis
- Syndrome of inappropriate antidiuretic hormone

detectable. Because of the mechanism underlying this type of hypoglycemia, patients respond promptly to intravenous dextrose but may not respond to glucagon administration.

Alcoholic ketoacidosis is common. Depletion of NAD resulting from alcohol metabolism leads to the increased production of beta-hydroxybutyrate, acetoacetate, and acetone. Beta-hydroxybutyrate, which is not detectable by routine urine or serum ketone testing, predominates, so the beta-hydroxybutyrate to acetoacetate ratio can be as high as 7:1 to 10:1, as compared to 3:1 in diabetic ketoacidosis. Insulin secretion, which ordinarily prevents development of ketoacidosis, is suppressed by decreased serum glucose levels and high catecholamine levels. The patient usually has a history of chronic heavy alcohol use and may be experiencing nausea, vomiting, abdominal pain, and metabolic acidosis. Blood alcohol levels usually are not detectable. Glucose levels may range from low to mildly elevated but typically are <250 mg/dL. Treatment includes dextrose and volume repletion. Marked hyperglycemia should raise suspicion of concomitant diabetes or diabetic ketoacidosis (10).

Patients with diabetes treated with insulin or sulfonylurea are at risk for severe hypoglycemia with alcohol use (11–13). Cognitive impairment and nonrecognition of hypoglycemia with alcohol use can lead to nontreatment of hypoglycemia in diabetic patients (14,15). Patients with diabetes must be counseled about alcohol use and its hypoglycemic consequences.

Insulin and sulfonylureas should be used with great caution in patients with alcoholism and diabetes, though they often are the only reasonable options for achieving some measure of glucose control in patients who continue to drink heavily. In addition, sulfonylureas and insulin are metabolized in the liver and are more likely to cause severe hypoglycemia in patients with alcoholic cirrhosis than in those without cirrhosis. Agents such as metformin (Glucophage), rosiglitazone (Avandia), and pioglitazone (Actos), which lower glucose but do not produce hypoglycemia, may not be used because of the increased risk of lactic acidosis (metformin) and liver toxicity (rosiglitazone and pioglitazone). Short-acting insulin secretagogues of the meglitinide class, such as repaglinide and nateglinide, have been touted as having less hypoglycemia and might be considered as having a role in patients with alcoholism. However, a recent review by Bolens et al. (16) have reported that hypoglycemia with repaglinide was comparable to that seen with sulfonylureas. Comparison of nateglinide with repaglinide has suggested a lower, albeit statistically insignificant, incidence of hypoglycemia (17). Cases of severe hypoglycemia have been described with repaglinide (18) and nateglinide (19). Alcohol abstinence is recommended, as is consumption of food with alcohol, if alcohol use persists, to minimize the risk of hypoglycemia. Diabetes care in those with alcohol-related liver disease and ongoing heavy alcohol use is difficult, and less stringent glycemic goals as well as early consultation with a diabetologist are reasonable.

Reactive or postprandial hypoglycemia with alcohol use can occur, depending on the carbohydrate composition of the meal consumed. O'Keefe and Marks (20) first described this phenomenon as profound hypoglycemia (mean blood glucose nadir, 48.6 mg/dL) that occurs 3 to 4 hours after the ingestion of alcohol combined with 60 g sucrose (as in gin and tonic). This phenomenon can develop in up to 10% to 20% of healthy subjects and does not appear to occur with saccharin or fructose and alcohol (21). The quinine content of regular tonic, which increases insulin levels, was postulated as the cause of the hypoglycemia, but work by Flanagan et al. (22) suggests that the hypoglycemia develops because of suppression of growth hormone release.

Hyperglycemia Alcoholic pancreatitis can lead to pancreatic exocrine and endocrine insufficiency. When diabetes

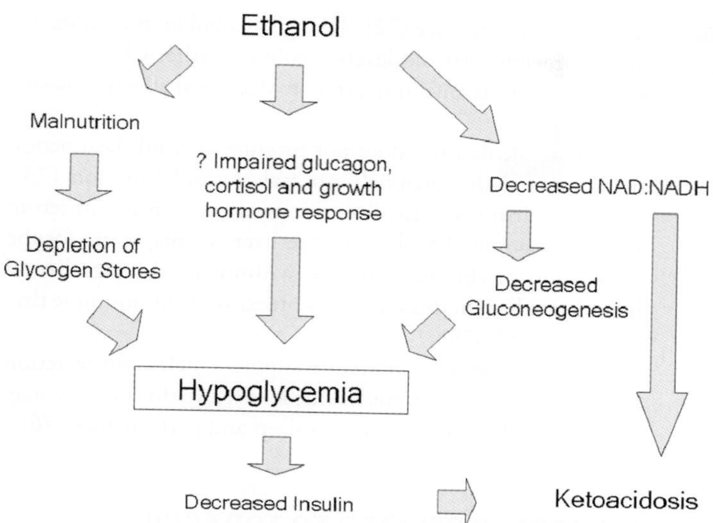

FIGURE 80.1. Alcohol effects leading to hypoglycemia and ketoacidosis.

mellitus results from pancreatic insufficiency, it is an indication that more than 90% of the pancreatic beta cells, which produce insulin, and the alpha cells, which produce glucagon, are destroyed. The secondary diabetes mellitus that results typically is an extremely labile insulin-dependent diabetes, in that patients are absolutely insulin-deficient and have normal or increased insulin sensitivity. Diabetic ketoacidosis results not simply from a lack of insulin but from an increase in the glucagon-insulin ratio. This explains why type 2 diabetics may develop ketoacidosis in the setting of severe infection and the presence of high insulin levels. In patients with pancreatitis-induced diabetes, the lack of glucagon makes the patient somewhat resistant to developing diabetic ketoacidosis but also quite prone to developing hypoglycemia.

Acute ethanol consumption has been shown to increase peripheral insulin resistance, and this topic has been recently extensively reviewed (23). This insulin resistance is localized to skeletal muscle and may be related to ethanol-induced changes in lactate, triglyceride, norepinephrine, hepatic insulin–sensitizing substance, hepatic glutathione and insulin binding. Despite this insulin resistance, postprandial glucose levels may be lower after preprandial consumption of 20 g of alcohol in lean, young healthy adults (24) and 15 g of alcohol after low carbohydrate, high fat meals, in postmenopausal women (25).

Though chronic heavy alcohol use can lead to chronic pancreatitis, pancreatic insufficiency, and subsequent diabetes mellitus, some studies have found an association between moderate alcohol use and improved insulin sensitivity (26–28) and a decreased risk of diabetes mellitus in men (29). Yet others found no effect (30,31). There may be a threshold dose and duration effect as Davies et al. (32) found 30 g daily for 8 weeks was necessary to show decreases in insulin resistance. Daily doses of alcohol greater than 48 g may lead to a loss of this insulin sensitivity (33) resulting in a U-shaped relationship. Increases in adiponectin have been suggested as a cause for this decrease in insulin resistance (34). Ting and Lautt (23) have suggested increases in hepatic glutathione and hepatic insulin–sensitizing substance as a possible etiology for chronic alcohol's effects on insulin resistance.

Reproductive Consequences The reproductive effects of alcohol use are gender-specific. Alcohol use long has been known to cause sexual dysfunction and hypogonadism in men, particularly in those with alcoholic cirrhosis (35). Even in men without liver disease, alcohol use leads to a decrease in testosterone (36), which may be the result of a combination of direct effects on the testicular synthesis of testosterone and hypothalamic-pituitary function (37) or on increases in sex hormone binding globulin, which can lead to a decrease in bioavailable testosterone (38). The incidence of gynecomastia is increased in alcoholic cirrhosis, primarily because of increased levels of androstenedione, a precursor for estrogen synthesis (39). Increased prolactin levels have been found in patients with alcoholic cirrhosis (40), though it may not be present in alcoholics who do not have severe liver disease (41).

In women, the effects of alcohol use depend on menopausal status and hormone therapy use. In premenopausal women and postmenopausal women on estrogen, acute alcohol consumption leads to an increase in estradiol levels through reduced metabolism of estradiol (42). This increase in estrogen level may explain why alcohol use is associated with an increased risk of breast cancer (43) and why alcohol can be associated with a delay in menopause. Women with high or frequent alcohol intake were found to have higher rates of menstrual disorders, including amenorrhea, dysmenorrhea, and irregular menstrual periods. Pregnant women with a high alcohol intake have a higher incidence of miscarriages, placental abruption, preterm deliveries, and stillbirths than do controls (44). An increased risk of infertility was associated with as few as one to five alcoholic drinks a week in a Danish study (45) and with as little as 12 g of alcohol a week (about one drink) in an American study (46). Recent work has found an increase in prolactin levels and decrease in oxytocin levels in lactating women (47) and premenopausal women (48). Despite the increase in prolactin levels, lactating women may have a slight decrease in milk production (49).

Bone Health Consequences Chronic alcoholism is associated with decreased bone mass and an increased risk of skeletal fractures (50–53). African American men may be less susceptible to this bone loss (54). Postmenopausal women who engage in moderate alcohol use may have an increased bone mineral density and a decreased risk of fractures (44).

In addition to alterations in sex hormones and the type of fat malabsorption and vitamin D deficiency associated with liver disease, alcohol use can reversibly impair bone formation by osteoblasts (55–57). Malnutrition and low body mass and decreases in IGF-I a bone growth factor may play a significant role in the decreased bone mass (58,59). In animal studies, parathyroid hormone may help reverse some of the bone loss though continued alcohol use impairs the response (60).

Heavy alcohol use is associated with osteonecrosis of bone (61). Alcohol-associated osteonecrosis of the femoral head may be due in part to lipid or cortisol changes (62) and, in fact, alcohol may be responsible for up to one-third of cases of femoral head osteonecrosis (63).

Other Endocrinologic Consequences Alcohol use increases triglyceride synthesis, leading to hypertriglyceridemia and hepatic steatosis. The increased NADH-NAD ratio leads to increases in alpha-glycerophosphate, which favors hepatic triglyceride accumulation by trapping fatty acids. The excess NADH enhances fatty acid synthesis (2). Alcohol increases the high-density lipoprotein (HDL) fraction of cholesterol, which may be associated with reduced cardiovascular morbidity and mortality (64).

Though glucocorticoid response to hypoglycemia can be impaired by alcohol use, patients with chronic heavy alcohol use have elevated adrenocorticotropic hormone (ACTH) and cortisol production. Rarely, these patients may develop the clinical stigmata of glucocorticoid excess, such as central obesity, moon facies, "buffalo hump," and biochemical evidence of nonsuppressible glucocorticoid excess that is difficult to distinguish from Cushing syndrome. This condition, which has been termed *pseudo-Cushing's syndrome*, reverses with abstinence from alcohol (65).

Alcohol may influence hormones regulating feeding behavior. Leptin levels are decreased acutely after moderate alcohol use (66) and in malnourished alcoholics (67). Ghrelin secretion is similarly reduced, without effects on peptide YY, soon after moderate alcohol intake (68,69). This is somewhat paradoxic given these hormones suppress appetite and alcohol is believed to stimulate appetite.

Alcohol use has effects on body volume and blood pressure status. It transiently decreases vasopressin release, leading to water diuresis (70). This condition can be problematic in patients with partial diabetes insipidus. Acute alcohol use also increases blood pressure, possibly through an increase in norepinephrine (71). Moderate alcohol consumption appears to increase plasma renin activity, though such increases are believed to result from a secondary response to changes in fluid and electrolyte balance (72). Though alcohol by itself does not affect mineralocorticoid levels, alcoholic cirrhosis leads to elevations of aldosterone in response to decreased effective plasma volume.

Acute alcohol use does not produce thyroid dysfunction in patients with previously normal thyroid function (73). Alcoholic cirrhosis of the liver can produce decreases in serum triiodothyronine (T3), because the liver is a major site for the conversion of thyroxine to T3, without producing clinical hypothyroidism in those without preexisting autoimmune thyroid disease (74,75).

Alcohol use was reported to suppress melatonin secretion through increased norepinephrine levels, and this increase may be implicated in disturbances in sleep and performance (76).

DISORDERS RELATED TO TOBACCO

The adverse effects of tobacco on the cardiopulmonary systems are well known. Tobacco smoke contains myriad chemical compounds, most notably nicotine, tar, thiocyanate, 2,3-hydroxypyridine and carbon monoxide, which may have multiple endocrine effects. Many of these effects have been recently reviewed in detail (77).

Thyroid Disease Cigarette smoking increases the risk of Graves' disease, Graves' ophthalmopathy and can lower thyroid-stimulating hormone levels (78–83). Smoking cessation seems to be associated with reduction in the risk for Graves' disease (84). Passive smoke exposure may increase resting metabolic rate and thyroid hormone secretion (85). The increased risk of ophthalmopathy with cigarette smoking may be related to increased fibroblast adipogenesis associated with increased interleukin-1 levels (86).

Smoking may also be associated with decreased levels of serum thyroid autoantibodies (82,87–89) and consequently appear to protect smokers from hypothyroidism (82,89). However, older studies have associated smoking with goiter and hypothyroidism (90,91). This may be a consequence of the thiocyanate present in cigarette smoke, which is a goitrogen that inhibits iodide uptake, hormone synthesis and increases iodine exit from the thyroid (92,93). Smoking may cause hypothyroidism only in those with preexisting thyroid dysfunction and there may be impaired peripheral action of thyroid hormone (94).

Insulin Resistance and Dyslipidemia Cigarette smoking (95), as well as nicotine gum use (96), is associated with an increase in insulin resistance and an increased risk of developing diabetes mellitus (29). Mild decreases in HDL cholesterol and mild elevations in triglycerides, consistent with this insulin resistance, are associated with cigarette smoking (95), though these changes may be due to components of cigarette smoke other than nicotine (97). Both passive smoke exposure and active smoking have been associated with the metabolic syndrome in adolescents (98). Insulin resistance and dyslipidemia may be responsible, in part, for the elevated rates of cardiovascular and atherosclerotic disease associated with cigarette use.

Reproductive Function In women, cigarette smoking is associated with decreases in estrogen levels (99) and, in fact, can enhance estrogen degradation (100). It also is associated with early menopause (101,102) and increased ovarian age and follicular-stimulating hormone levels (103,104). Smoking status does not appear to have an effect on *in vitro* fertilization success (105). In men, cigarette smoking is associated with quantitative and qualitative decrements in sperm (106–108) and with increases in serum estrogen (109).

Bone Health Cigarette smoking is associated with decreased bone mineral density and increased bone loss in postmenopausal women and elderly men (110) and is an independent risk factor for osteoporotic fracture. This risk appears, in part, due to a decrease in intestinal calcium absorption (111,112), resulting in a negative calcium balance. Brot et al. (113) found an association between smoking and decreased serum 25-hydroxyvitamin D,1,25-dihydroxyvitamin, D parathyroid hormone, and osteocalcin levels, suggesting a more complex effect of smoking on calcium and bone metabolism. Cigarette smoking can negate the protective effect of estrogen therapy on the risk of hip fracture in postmenopausal women (114). It also is associated with femoral head osteonecrosis (61), possibly through impairment of vascular function or changes in blood lipids.

Other Endocrinologic Effects Cigarette smoke stimulates antidiuretic hormone release from the pituitary through an airway-mediated mechanism that does not depend on circulating nicotine (115,116). This antidiuretic effect may cause or exacerbate hyponatremia in susceptible patients (117,118). The nicotine found in cigarette smoke can increase the release of catecholamines from the adrenal medulla, which may precipitate a hypertensive crisis for those with pheochromocytoma. In addition, smoking is associated with hypertension and poorly controlled hypertension, apparently through stimulation of the noradrenergic nervous system (119); such hypertension is not angiotensin II–dependent (120).

DISORDERS RELATED TO OTHER DRUGS

Marijuana The major psychoactive component of marijuana is delta-9-tetrahydrocannabinol (THC), though marijuana can contain more than 400 chemicals. Factors including concomitant use of other drugs, variability in smoking technique, and variable potencies of marijuana cigarettes, and development of tolerance to marijuana's effects can make it difficult to generalize from study findings to clinical practice.

Though some investigators have reported that heavy marijuana smoking is associated with low plasma levels of testosterone (121), others report that chronic marijuana use has no effects on plasma testosterone or luteinizing hormone in men (122). Further confusion arises from reports suggesting that smoking marijuana cigarettes acutely suppresses luteinizing hormone in men (123) and premenopausal women in the luteal phase of their menstrual cycle but not in postmenopausal women (124). One study of pregnant marijuana users found no changes in female sex hormones as compared with controls (125). The many conflicting studies make it unlikely that chronic marijuana use affects the reproductive system with any significant clinical relevance. Marijuana has not been found to be teratogenic and has not been found to have consistent effects on pregnancy outcomes.

With regard to other endocrinologic effects, prolonged oral administration of 210 mg THC a day (the equivalent of smoking six marijuana cigarettes) for 14 days significantly suppressed the cortisol and growth hormone response to insulin-induced hypoglycemia, though the THC use did not suppress the cortisol and growth hormone response to values consistent with cortisol or growth hormone deficiency (126). Continued marijuana use has not been found to affect the normalization of the hypothalamic-pituitary-adrenal axis in heroin addicts initiating methadone treatment (127). Adolescents with reported early onset (9–12 years of age) of marijuana use were found to have lower salivary cortisol levels on awakening (128). It is unclear whether the lower salivary cortisol resulted from the early marijuana use or vice versa. Heavy marijuana use may likely cause significant hypoadrenalism or impaired recovery from insulin-induced hypoglycemia only in those with preexisting adrenal disease.

Opiates The endocrine effects of acute administration of opiates occur primarily in the hypothalamus and pituitary. Gonadotropins (follicle-stimulating hormone [FSH] and luteinizing hormone [LH]) are suppressed by inhibition of gonadotropin-releasing hormone secretion. Prolactin secretion is stimulated, while ACTH and cortisol secretion are suppressed (129). Chronic administration of opiates can produce partial tolerance to many of the endocrine effects.

Male gonadal function in methadone and heroin addicts has been found to be variable. In men, methadone use has been associated with a decline in serum testosterone levels and diminished sperm motility (130). Another study looking at methadone, methadone/heroin, and heroin use found normal levels of testosterone, FSH, LH, and prolactin in all but the heroin users, who had elevated prolactin levels (131). All the heroin-addicted, the heroin/methadone users, and 45% of the methadone takers in that study had diminished sperm motility. A third study looked at short-term methadone use in 30 men and found no abnormalities of estrogen, progesterone, or LH, whereas FSH showed lower values than normal and androstenedione, dehydroepiandrosterone, and prolactin noticeably increased in many subjects. Modest variations were noted for testosterone and dihydrotestosterone (132). Other investigators found a decrease in basal FSH and LH levels, with a decrease in pituitary response to gonadotropin-releasing hormone, suggesting a hypothalamic cause for hypogonadism in heroin addicts (133).

The variability in findings may be due in part to the presence of other components, as well as variable doses of opiates, in street preparations of heroin, continued use of heroin in methadone-treated addicts, and the possible effect of malnutrition on the reproductive system. A study of the endocrine effects of long-term intrathecal opioid administration for pain relief found diminished testosterone and LH levels in men but normal FSH and prolactin levels in comparison to control patients with a comparable pain syndrome but who were not treated with opioid (134), suggesting that these are the "pure" opiate effects on the male reproductive system.

In women, more than half of a group of 76 former heroin addicts on methadone maintenance had menstrual irregularities (135). Endocrinologic studies on seven of the women showed alterations in hypothalamic and pituitary function leading to oligo-ovulation. A study of 21 premenopausal women who received chronic intrathecal opioids found 14 to have amenorrhea and 7 to have menstrual irregularity, with decrements in serum LH, FSH, estradiol, and progesterone concentrations (134). In the same study, 18 postmenopausal women had serum LH and FSH levels significantly lower than did postmenopausal control subjects, further indicating impairment of gonadotropin release. Recently, opiates have been found to be competitive inhibitors of human placental aromatase, the enzyme that converts androgens to estrogens (136–138). The clinical implications of this effect and generalizability to other tissues are unclear.

Hypogonadism is a risk factor for osteoporosis. There is evidence showing a decrease in bone density with opiate use (139–143) in both men and women. There is also evidence for increased fracture risk (144,145). The effects on bone may be reversed with cessation of the opiate (139).

Cocaine Cocaine acts primarily by blocking the reuptake of norepinephrine, dopamine, and serotonin at the synaptic junctions, resulting in increased neurotransmitter concentrations. In animal studies, cocaine can stimulate the adrenal medulla to release epinephrine and norepinephrine. By increasing catecholamines, counterregulatory hormones that antagonize insulin, stimulate glucose production, and inhibit glucose clearance, hyperglycemia can result as can diabetic ketoacidosis or hyperosmolar nonketotic hyperglycemia without any other identified precipitants (146,147). Diabetic ketoacidosis appears to occur more frequently in cocaine users, resulting from a combination of omission of insulin therapy and cocaine effects on glucose metabolism (147).

Dopamine is an important physiologic regulator of prolactin and thyroid-stimulating hormone secretion. Acute cocaine use suppresses prolactin secretion with increases in dopamine levels, but with chronic use, dopamine levels become depleted and hyperprolactinemia results (148–150). This hyperprolactinemia persists even after cocaine withdrawal (151). Though acute cocaine use produces rises in ACTH, FSH, and LH (148,152,153), abnormalities of testosterone, cortisol, LH (149) or thyroid function tests (154) have not been found in chronic cocaine users.

Amphetamines Amphetamines, such as dextroamphetamine and methylamphetamine, have not been well studied with regard to the endocrinologic effects of chronic use. They act primarily by stimulating the release of norepinephrine and dopamine. Well-described acute endocrine effects of amphetamine administration include increased corticosteroid release and increased growth hormone release (155–157), each of which can be influenced by the presence of depression (158–162) or other psychoactive medications (163). Though increased salivary cortisol response to D-amphetamine has been associated with personality traits of aggression and thrill seeking (164), the clinical implications of these findings remain unclear. Preexisting hyperthyroidism may increase the risk of death due to Ecstasy (3, 4-methylenedioxymethamphetamine) (165).

Both cocaine and amphetamine have well-known effects on appetite suppression. In 1995, Douglass et al. (166) first described the up-regulation of a peptide in response to the acute administration of cocaine and amphetamine. This peptide is now known as cocaine- and amphetamine-regulated transcript and has been shown to have a role in feeding behavior, interacting with neuropeptide Y (NPY), leptin and cannabinoid (CB1) receptors. Interested readers are referred to a recent review (167).

Caffeine Caffeine is one of the world's most widely used drugs. The many forms in which it is delivered and prepared, including tea, coffee, and caffeinated soft drinks, may contain other bioactive substances such as flavonoids (168) and diterpene (169). This variability has confounded its study.

Caffeine is a neuroendocrine stimulant with action mediated by central adenosine receptor antagonism (170). Ingestion of 250 mg (approximately three cups of coffee) produces a rapid release of epinephrine from the adrenal medulla, which can increase blood pressure (171). Though immediate ingestion of 250 to 500 mg caffeine (equivalent of three to six cups of coffee) has little effect on circulating cortisol, thyroid-stimulating hormone, growth hormone, prolactin, T3 (172), or norepinephrine levels; the ingestion of 250 mg caffeine produces an increased epinephrine and norepinephrine response to tilt-table-testing (171) and increased epinephrine, norepinephrine, cortisol, and growth hormone response to hypoglycemia or low normal glucose levels in normal healthy adults (173) and in insulin-dependent diabetics (174). Tolerance to caffeine can develop with chronic use, so that these neuroendocrine changes do not become clinically relevant except after a period of abstinence, though it has been suggested that caffeine can be a useful treatment for diabetic patients without autonomic neuropathy who have hypoglycemic unawareness (174).

Caffeine may have acute effects on glucose metabolism. Four hundred milligrams of caffeine daily for 1 week decreased insulin sensitivity in caffeine-tolerant young adults (175). Five hundred milligrams of caffeine daily increased average glucose and exaggerated postprandial glucose increases in caffeine-tolerant type 2 diabetics (176). Chronic coffee consumption, however, is associated with a decreased risk of type 2 diabetes mellitus, and this subject was recently reviewed (177).

Caffeine is associated with increased urinary calcium excretion (178) and with decrements in serum-free estradiol (179,180) and serum insulin-like growth factor I levels (181), both of which are important in maintaining bone mass. As such, it is not surprising that caffeine use is associated with an increased risk of fracture (182,183) and an increased risk of reduced bone mass (184,185). However, other studies do not support this increased risk (186,187). Add to this mixture the studies that show that tea can protect against hip fractures (188) and is associated with increased bone density (168), and the overall situation becomes more confusing. If there is an effect of caffeine intake on bone health, it is not likely to be clinically significant.

Benzodiazepines Benzodiazepines act by stimulating gamma-aminobutyric-acid ergic (GABA-ergic) neurons, which usually are inhibitory in function. Many researchers have found that benzodiazepines, such as diazepam (Valium), alprazolam (Xanax), and temazepam (Restoril), suppress basal serum levels of cortisol (189–192) and also suppress the body's cortisol and ACTH response to metyrapone (193), insulin-induced hypoglycemia, corticotrophin-releasing hormone (194), metabolic stress (195), and exercise (196). Such changes potentially could lead to a hypoadrenal crisis or prolonged hypoglycemia in users with preexisting adrenal disease.

Suppression of cortisol response persists despite chronic benzodiazepine use (197); however, this finding may not apply to all benzodiazepines. Ambrosi et al. (198) found that triazolam (Halcion) and flurazepam (Dalmane) did not influence cortisol release in women with insulin-induced hypoglycemia. Chronic diazepam use may decrease basal cortisol levels greater in elderly patients than in young (199).

Benzodiazepines may variably stimulate the release of growth hormone (200), though not all investigators have confirmed this finding (201). This growth hormone response is blunted with long-term benzodiazepine administration (202) and hyperglycemia (203), suggesting that significant clinical effects are unlikely. One case report described a syndrome involving inappropriate antidiuretic hormone secretion associated with use of lorazepam (Ativan) (204).

Barbiturates Barbiturates are known to induce the cytochrome P450 enzyme system, leading to enhanced metabolism of many substances. Among these substances are thyroid hormone, hydrocortisone, and vitamin D. Barbiturate use or abuse can lead to increasing thyroid hormone requirements (205), hydrocortisone requirements, or osteomalacia. Overt hypothyroidism or hypoadrenalism is not likely in the absence of underlying thyroid or adrenal disease.

Inhalants The inhalation of volatile solvents, such as toluene, is known to cause multiple medical complications, such as heart, liver, lung, nerve, and kidney damage (206,207). No specific endocrine consequences have yet been described. However, these solvents can cause renal tubular dysfunction, leading to hypophosphatemia and acidosis, which can affect calcium and bone metabolism. Though recurrent nephrolithiasis was described (208,209), no case of toluene-induced osteomalacia has been described as yet.

Occupational exposure to inhalants is associated with infertility, increased risk of spontaneous abortion, and multiple birth defects. In addition, case reports of children born to those who abuse inhalants have led to the term *fetal solvent syndrome*, reflecting its similarity to fetal alcohol syndrome. Interested readers are referred to the review by Jones and Balster (210).

Anabolic Steroids The anabolic steroids, which are testosterone derivatives, include nandrolone, oxandrolone, oxymetholone, and stanozolol. Male and female athletes often use these substances in efforts to improve athletic performance. The adverse endocrine consequences are a direct result of androgenic effects and suppression of the hypothalamic-pituitary-gonadal axis. These effects include testicular atrophy; decreases in testosterone, LH, and FSH; increases in estrone; and suppression of spermatogenesis in men (211,212). Gynecomastia can result from aromatization of the androgens to estrogen in endogenous androgen suppression. In women, there can be menstrual disturbances, deepening of voice, and development of acne and male-pattern body hair (213).

Anabolic steroids can affect other hormones by decreasing hepatic synthesis of proteins, such as thyroid-binding globulin, sex hormone–binding globulin, vitamin D–binding protein, and HDL cholesterol (212,214). There can be mild thyroidal impairment, as measured by thyroid-stimulating hormone and T3 response to thyrotropin-releasing hormone (215). Clinically relevant sequelae are not present without underlying hyperthyroidism. Other lipid changes include increases in low-density lipoprotein cholesterol and decreases in Lp(a) (216). There are conflicting reports regarding insulin resistance and anabolic steroid use (217,218). Those with preexisting coronary artery disease may be at increased risk because of decreased HDL and increased low-density lipoprotein cholesterol. Hypertension, ventricular remodeling, myocardial ischemia, and sudden cardiac death each have been temporally and causally associated with anabolic steroid use (219). Recent contradicting reports, however, have suggested that androgens may have anti-atherogenic and anti-anginal effects (220–223) in both supraphysiologic and physiologic doses.

No significant changes in adult bone metabolism (parathyroid hormone or vitamin D metabolites) have been reported in patients treated with nandrolone (224). Anabolic steroid use in children, however, may prematurely close epiphyseal growth plates, leading to growth stunting. Growth hormone levels can rise with anabolic steroid use; resolution of the hypothalamic-pituitary-gonadal suppression can take several months (225).

Other Drugs No endocrinologic consequence has been described with phencyclidine or LSD use; further research is required.

REFERENCES

1. Marks V, Teale JD. Drug-induced hypoglycemia. *Endocrinol Metab Clin North Am* 1999;28:555–577.
2. Lieber CS. Ethanol metabolism, cirrhosis and alcoholism. *Clin Chim Acta* 1997;257:59–84.

3. Berman JD, Cook DM, Buchman M, et al. Diminished adrenocorticotropin response to insulin-induced hypoglycemia in nondepressed, actively drinking male alcoholics. *J Clin Endocrinol Metab* 1990;72:712–717.
4. Wand GS, Dobs AS. Alterations in the hypothalamic-pituitary adrenal axis in actively drinking alcoholics. *J Clin Endocrinol Metab* 1991;72:1290–1295.
5. Joffe BI, Seftel HC, Van As M. Hormonal responses in ethanol-induced hypoglycemia. *J Stud Alcohol* 1975;36:550–554.
6. Chiodera P, Coiro V. Inhibitory effect of ethanol on the arginine vasopressin response to insulin-induced hypoglycemia and the role of endogenous opioids. *Neuroendocrinology* 1990;51:501–504.
7. Wilson NM, Brown PM, Juul SM, et al. Glucose turnover and metabolic and hormonal changes in ethanol-induced hypoglycaemia. *Br Med J* 1981;282:849–853.
8. Kolaczynski JW, Ylikahri R, Härkonen M, et al. The acute effect of ethanol on counterregulatory response and recovery from insulin-induced hypoglycemia. *J Clin Endocrinol Metab* 1988;67:384–388.
9. Kerr D, Cheyne E, Thomas P, Sherwin R. Influence of acute alcohol ingestion on the hormonal responses to modest hypoglycaemia in patients with type 1 diabetes. *Diabet Med: J Br Diabet Assoc* 2007;24:312–316.
10. Kitabchi AE, Umpierrez GE, Murphy MB, et al. Management of hyperglycemic crises in patients with diabetes. *Diabetes Care* 2001;24:131–153.
11. Arky RA, Veverbrants E, Abramson EA. Irreversible hypoglycemia: a complication of alcohol and insulin. *JAMA* 1968;206:575–578.
12. Melander A, Lebovitz HE, Faber OK. Sulfonylureas: why, which, and how? *Diabetes Care* 1990;13(Suppl 3):18–25.
13. Richardson T, Weiss M, Thomas P, Kerr D. Day after the night before: influence of evening alcohol on risk of hypoglycemia in patients with type 1 diabetes. *Diabetes Care* 2005;28:1801–1802.
14. Cheyne EH, Sherwin RS, Lunt MJ, et al. Influence of alcohol on cognitive performance during mild hypoglycaemia: implications for type 1 diabetes. *Diabet Med: J Br Diabet Assoc* 2004;21:230–237.
15. Kerr D, Macdonald IA, Heller SR, Tattersall RB. Alcohol causes hypoglycaemic unawareness in healthy volunteers and patients with type 1 (insulin-dependent) diabetes. *Diabetologia* 1990;33:216–221.
16. Bolen S, Feldman L, Vassy J, et al. Systematic review: comparative effectiveness and safety of oral medications for type 2 diabetes mellitus. *Ann Intern Med* 2007;147:386–399.
17. Rosenstock J, Hassman DR, Madder RD, et al., Repaglinide Versus Nateglinide Comparison Study Group. Repaglinide versus nateglinide monotherapy: a randomized, multicenter study. *Diabetes Care* 2004;27:1265–1270.
18. Flood TM. Serious hypoglycemia associated with misuse of repaglinide. *Endocr Pract* 1999;5:137–138.
19. Nagai T, Imamura M, Iizuka K, Mori M. Hypoglycemia due to nateglinide administration in diabetic patient with chronic renal failure. *Diabetes Res Clin Pract* 2003;59:191–194.
20. O'Keefe SJD, Marks V. Lunchtime gin and tonic a cause of reactive hypoglycaemia. *Lancet* 1977;1:1286–1288.
21. Marks V, Wright J. Alcohol-provoked reactive hypoglycaemia. In: Andreani D, Lefebvre PJ, Marks V, eds. *Current views on hypoglycemia and glucagon*. London: Academic Press, 1980:283–295.
22. Flanagan D, Wood P, Sherwin R, et al. Gin and tonic and reactive hypoglycemia: what is important—the gin, the tonic or both? *J Clin Endocrinol Metab* 1998;83:796–800.
23. Ting JW, Lautt WW. The effect of acute, chronic, and prenatal ethanol exposure on insulin sensitivity. *Pharmacol Ther* 2006;111:346–373.
24. Brand-Miller JC, Fatima K, Middlemiss C, et al. Effect of alcoholic beverages on postprandial glycemia and insulinemia in lean, young, healthy adults. *Am J Clin Nutr* 2007;85:1545–1551.
25. Greenfield JR, Samaras K, Hayward CS, et al. Beneficial postprandial effect of a small amount of alcohol on diabetes and cardiovascular risk factors: modification by insulin resistance. *J Clin Endocrinol Metab* 2005;90:661–672.
26. Kiechl S, Willeit J, Poewe W, et al. Insulin sensitivity and regular alcohol consumption: large, prospective, cross sectional population study (Bruneck study). *Br Med J* 1996;313:1040–1044.
27. Razay G, Heaton KW. Moderate alcohol consumption has been shown previously to improve insulin sensitivity in men. *Br Med J* 1997;314:443.
28. Fueki Y, Miida T, Wardaningsih E, et al. Regular alcohol consumption improves insulin resistance in healthy Japanese men independent of obesity. *Clin Chim Acta* 2007;382:71–76.
29. Rimm EB, Chan J, Stampfer MJ, et al. Prospective study of cigarette smoking, alcohol use, and the risk of diabetes in men. *Br Med J* 1995;310:555–559.
30. Cordain L, Melby CL, Hamamoto AE, et al. Influence of moderate chronic wine consumption on insulin sensitivity and other correlates of syndrome X in moderately obese women. *Metabolism* 2000;49:1473–1478.
31. Flanagan DE, Pratt E, Murphy J, et al. Alcohol consumption alters insulin secretion and cardiac autonomic activity. *Eur J Clin Invest* 2002;32:187–192.
32. Davies MJ, Baer DJ, Judd JT, et al. Effects of moderate alcohol intake on fasting insulin and glucose concentrations and insulin sensitivity in postmenopausal women: a randomized controlled trial. *JAMA* 2002;287:2559–2562.
33. Koppes LL, Dekker JM, Hendriks HF, et al. Moderate alcohol consumption lowers the risk of type 2 diabetes: a meta-analysis of prospective observational studies. *Diabetes Care* 2005;28:719–725.
34. Sierksma A, Patel H, Ouchi N, et al. Effect of moderate alcohol consumption on adiponectin, tumor necrosis factor-alpha, and insulin sensitivity. *Diabetes Care* 2004;27:184–189.
35. Lloyd CW, Williams RH. Endocrine changes associated with Laennec's cirrhosis of the liver. *Am J Med* 1948;4:315–330.
36. Gordon GG, Altman K, Southern AL, et al. Effect of alcohol (ethanol) administration on sex-hormone metabolism in normal men. *N Engl J Med* 1976;295:793–797.
37. Van Thiel DH, Lester R, Vaitukaitis J. Evidence for a defect in pituitary secretion of luteinizing hormone in chronic alcoholic men. *J Clin Endocrinol Metab* 1978;47:499–507.
38. Iturriaga H, Lioi X, Valladares L. Sex hormone-binding globulin in non-cirrhotic alcoholic patients during early withdrawal and after longer abstinence. *Alcohol Alcohol* 1999;34:903–909.
39. Kley HK, Niederau C, Stremmel W, et al. Conversion of androgens to estrogens in idiopathic hemochromatosis: comparison with alcoholic liver cirrhosis. *J Clin Endocrinol Metab* 1985;61:1–6.
40. Van Thiel DH, McClain CJ, Elseon MK, et al. Hyperprolactinemia and thyrotropin-releasing factor (TRH) responses in men with alcoholic liver disease. *Alcohol Clin Exp Res* 1978;2:344–348.
41. Agner T, Hagen C, Andersen BN, et al. Pituitary-thyroid function and thyrotropin, prolactin and growth hormone responses to TRH in patients with chronic alcoholism. *Acta Med Scand* 1986;220:57–62.
42. Gill J. The effects of moderate alcohol consumption on female hormone levels and reproductive function. *Alcohol Alcohol* 2000;35:417–423.
43. Zumoff B. The critical role of alcohol consumption in determining the risk of breast cancer with postmenopausal estrogen administration. *J Clin Endocrinol Metab* 1997;82:1656–1657.
44. Bradley KA, Badrinath S, Bush K, et al. Medical risks for women who drink alcohol. *J Gen Intern Med* 1998;13:627–639.
45. Jensen TK, Hjollund NHI, Henriksen TB, et al. Does moderate alcohol consumption affect fertility? Follow up study among couples planning first pregnancy. *Br Med J* 1998;317:505–510.
46. Hakim RB, Gray RH, Zacur H. Alcohol and caffeine consumption and decreased fertility. *Fertil Steril* 1998;70:632–637.
47. Mennella JA, Pepino MY, Teff KL. Acute alcohol consumption disrupts the hormonal milieu of lactating women. *J Clin Endocrinol Metab* 2005;90:1979–1985.
48. Mennella JA, Pepino MY. Short-term effects of alcohol consumption on the hormonal milieu and mood states in nulliparous women. *Alcohol* 2006;38:29–36.
49. Mennella JA. Short-term effects of maternal alcohol consumption on lactational performance. *Alcohol Clin Exp Res* 1998;22:1389–1392.
50. Saville PD. Changes in bone mass with age and alcoholism. *J Bone Joint Surg* 1965;47:492–499.

51. de Vernejoul MC, Bielakoff J, Herve M, et al. Evidence for defective osteoblastic function. A role for alcohol and tobacco consumption in osteoporosis in middle-aged men. *Clin Orthop* 1983;179:107–115.
52. Bikle DD, Genant HK, Cann CE, et al. Bone disease in alcohol abuse. *Ann Intern Med* 1985;103:42–48.
53. Lalor BC, France MW, Powell D, et al. Bone and mineral metabolism and chronic alcohol abuse. *Q J Med* 1986;59:497–511.
54. Odvina CV, Safi I, Wojtowicz CH, et al. Effect of heavy alcohol intake in the absence of liver disease on bone mass in black and white men. *J Clin Endocrinol Metab* 1995;80:2499–2503.
55. Lindholm J, Steiniche T, Rasmussen E, et al. Bone disorder in men with chronic alcoholism: a reversible disease? *J Clin Endocrinol Metab* 1991;73:118–124.
56. Pepersack T, Fuss M, Otero J, et al. Longitudinal study of bone metabolism after ethanol withdrawal in alcoholic patients. *J Bone Miner Res* 1992;7:383–387.
57. Peris P, Parés A, Guañabens N, et al. Bone mass improves in alcoholics after 2 years of abstinence. *J Bone Miner Res* 1994;9:1607–1612.
58. Santolaria F, Gonzalez-Gonzalez G, Gonzalez-Reimers E, et al. Effects of alcohol and liver cirrhosis on the GH-IGF-I axis. *Alcohol Alcohol* 1995;30:703–708.
59. Santolaria F, Gonzalez-Reimers E, Perez-Manzano JL, et al. Osteopenia assessed by body composition analysis is related to malnutrition in alcoholic patients. *Alcohol* 2000;22:147–157.
60. Sibonga JD, Iwaniec UT, Shogren KL, et al. Effects of parathyroid hormone (1-34) on tibia in an adult rat model for chronic alcohol abuse. *Bone* 2007;40:1013–1020.
61. Matsuo K, Hirohata T, Sugioka Y, et al. Influence of alcohol intake, cigarette smoking, and occupational status on idiopathic osteonecrosis of the femoral head. *Clin Orthop* 1988;234:115–123.
62. Chang CC, Greenspan A, Gershwin ME. Osteonecrosis: Current perspectives on pathogenesis and treatment. *Semin Arthritis Rheum* 1993;23:47–69.
63. Antti-Poika I, Karaharju E, Vankka E, et al. Alcohol-associated femoral head necrosis. *Ann Chirurg Gynaecol* 1987;76:318–322.
64. Gaziano JM, Buring JE, Breslow JL, et al. Moderate alcohol intake, increased levels of high-density lipoprotein and its subfractions, and decreased risk of myocardial infarction. *N Engl J Med* 1993;329:1829–1834.
65. Kirkman S, Nelson DH. Alcohol-induced pseudo-Cushing's syndrome: a study of prevalence with review of the literature. *Metabolism* 1988;37:390–394.
66. Rojdmark S, Calissendorff J, Brismar K. Alcohol ingestion decreases both diurnal and nocturnal secretion of leptin in healthy individuals. *Clin Endocrinol* 2001;55:639–647.
67. Santolaria F, Perez-Cejas A, Aleman MR, et al. Low serum leptin levels and malnutrition in chronic alcohol misusers hospitalized by somatic complications. *Alcohol Alcohol* 2003;38:60–66.
68. Calissendorff J, Danielsson O, Brismar K, Rojdmark S. Inhibitory effect of alcohol on ghrelin secretion in normal man. *Eur J Endocrinol* 2005;152:743–747.
69. Calissendorff J, Danielsson O, Brismar K, Rojdmark S. Alcohol ingestion does not affect serum levels of peptide YY but decreases both total and octanoylated ghrelin levels in healthy subjects. *Metab Clin Exp* 2006;55:1625–1629.
70. Oiso Y, Robertson GL. Effect of ethanol on vasopressin secretion and the role of endogenous opioids. In: Schrier RW, ed. *Vasopressin*. New York: Raven Press, 1985:265–269.
71. Howes LG, Reid JL. The effects of alcohol on local neural and humoral cardiovascular regulation. *Clin Sci* 1986;71:9–15.
72. Puddey IB, Vandongen R, Beilin LJ, et al. Alcohol stimulation of renin release in man: its relation to the hemodynamic, electrolyte, and sympatho-adrenal responses to drinking. *J Clin Endocrinol Metab* 1985;61:37–42.
73. Ylikahri RH, Huttunen MO, Härkönen M, et al. Acute effects of alcohol on anterior pituitary secretion of the tropic hormones. *J Clin Endocrinol Metab* 1978;46:715–720.
74. Chopra IJ, Solomon DH, Chopra U, et al. Alterations in circulating thyroid hormones and thyrotropin in hepatic cirrhosis: evidence for euthyroidism despite subnormal serum triiodothyronine. *J Clin Endocrinol Metab* 1974;39:501–511.
75. Hegedüs L, Decreased thyroid gland volume in alcoholic cirrhosis of the liver. *J Clin Endocrinol Metab* 1984;58:930–933.
76. Ekman A, Leppäluoto J, Huttunen P, et al. Ethanol inhibits melatonin secretion in healthy volunteers in a dose-dependent randomized double blind cross-over study. *J Clin Endocrinol Metab* 1993;77:780–783.
77. Kapoor D, Jones TH. Smoking and hormones in health and endocrine disorders. *Eur J Endocrinol* 2005;152:491–499.
78. Bartalena L, Martino E, Marcocci C, et al. More on smoking habits and Graves' ophthalmopathy. *J Endoctinol Invest* 1989;12:733.
79. Hägg E, Asplund K. Is endocrine ophthalmopathy related to smoking? *Br Med J* 1987;295:634.
80. Shine B, Fells P, Edwards OM, et al. Association between Graves' ophthalmopathy and smoking. *Lancet* 1990;335:1261.
81. Prummel MF, Wiersinga WM. Smoking and risk of Graves' disease. *JAMA* 1993;269:518.
82. Belin RM, Astor BC, Powe NR, Ladenson PW. Smoke exposure is associated with a lower prevalence of serum thyroid autoantibodies and thyrotropin concentration elevation and a higher prevalence of mild thyrotropin concentration suppression in the third National Health and Nutrition Examination Survey (NHANES III). *J Clin Endocrinol Metab* 2004;89:6077–6086.
83. Asvold BO, Bjoro T, Nilsen TI, Vatten LJ. Tobacco smoking and thyroid function: a population-based study. *Arch Intern Med* 2007;167:1428–1432.
84. Vestergaard P. Smoking and thyroid disorders—a meta-analysis. *Eur J Endocrinol* 2002;146:153–161.
85. Metsios GS, Flouris AD, Jamurtas AZ, et al. A brief exposure to moderate passive smoke increases metabolism and thyroid hormone secretion. *J Clin Endocrinol Metab* 2007;92:208–211.
86. Cawood T J, Moriarty P, O'Farrelly C, O'Shea D. Smoking and thyroid-associated ophthalmopathy: a novel explanation of the biological link. *J Clin Endocrinol Metab* 2007;92:59–64.
87. Goh SY, Ho SC, Seah LL, et al. Thyroid autoantibody profiles in ophthalmic dominant and thyroid dominant Graves' disease differ and suggest ophthalmopathy is a multiantigenic disease. *Clin Endocrinol* 2004;60:600–607.
88. Strieder TG, Prummel MF, Tijssen JG, et al. Risk factors for and prevalence of thyroid disorders in a cross-sectional study among healthy female relatives of patients with autoimmune thyroid disease. *Clin Endocrinol* 2003;59:396–401.
89. Krassas GE, Wiersinga W. Smoking and autoimmune thyroid disease: the plot thickens. *Eur J Endocrinol* 2006;154:777–780.
90. Hegedüs L, Karstrup S, Veiergang D, et al. High frequency of goiter in cigarette smokers. *Clin Endocrinol* 1985;22:287.
91. Christensen SB, Ericsson UB, Janson L, et al. Influence of cigarette smoking on goiter formation, thyroglobulin, and thyroid hormone levels in women. *J Clin Endocrinol Metab* 1984;58:615–618.
92. Fukayama H, Nasu M, Murakami S, et al. Examination of antithyroid effects of smoking products in cultured thyroid follicles: only thiocyanate is a potent antithyroid agent. *Acta Endocrinol* 1992;127:520.
93. Utiger RD. Cigarette smoking and the thyroid. *N Engl J Med* 1995;333:1001–1002.
94. Muller B, Zulewski H, Huber P, et al. Impaired action of thyroid hormone associated with smoking in women with hypothyroidism. *N Engl J Med* 1995;333:964–969.
95. Targher G, Alberiche M, Zenere MB, et al. Cigarette smoking and insulin resistance in patients with noninsulin-dependent diabetes mellitus. *J Clin Endocrinol Metab* 1997;82:3619–3624.
96. Eliasson B, Taskinen M, Smith U. Long-term use of nicotine gum is associated with hyperinsulinemia and insulin resistance. *Circulation* 1996;94:878–881.
97. Jensen EX, Fusch C, Jaeger P, et al. Impact of chronic cigarette smoking on body composition and fuel metabolism. *J Clin Endocrinol Metab* 1995;80:2181–2185.

98. Weitzman M, Cook S, Auinger P, et al. Tobacco smoke exposure is associated with the metabolic syndrome in adolescents. *Circulation* 2005;112:862–869.
99. MacMahon B, Trichopoulos D, Cole P, et al. Cigarette smoking and urinary estrogens. *N Engl J Med* 1982;307:1062–1065.
100. Jensen J, Christiansen C, Rodbro P. Cigarette smoking, serum estrogens, and bone loss during hormone-replacement therapy early after menopause. *N Engl J Med* 1985;313:973–975.
101. Jick H, Porter J, Morrison AS. Relation between smoking and age of natural menopause. *Lancet* 1972;1:1354–1355.
102. McKinlay SM, Bifano NL, McKinlay JB. Smoking and age at menopause in women. *Ann Intern Med* 1985;103:350–356.
103. Windham GC, Mitchell P, Anderson M, Lasley BL. Cigarette smoking and effects on hormone function in premenopausal women. *Environ Health Perspect* 2005;113:1285–1290.
104. Kinney A, Kline J, Kelly A, et al. Smoking, alcohol and caffeine in relation to ovarian age during the reproductive years. *Hum Reprod (Oxford)* 2007;22:1175–1185.
105. Wright,KP, Trimarchi JR, Allsworth J, Keefe D. The effect of female tobacco smoking on IVF outcomes. *Hum Reprod (Oxford)* 2006;21: 2930–2934.
106. Evans HJ, Fletcher J, Torrance M, et al. Sperm abnormalities and cigarette smoking. *Lancet* 1981;1(8221):627–629.
107. Shaarawy M, Mahmoud KZ. Endocrine profile and semen characteristics in male smokers. *Fertil Steril* 1982;38:255–257.
108. Vine MF, Margolin BH, Morrison HI, et al. Cigarette smoking and sperm density: a meta-analysis. *Fertil Steril* 1994;61:35–43.
109. Barrett-Connor E, Khaw KT. Cigarette smoking and increased endogenous estrogen levels in men. *Am J Epidemiol* 1987;126:187–192.
110. Vogel JM, Davis JW, Nomura A, et al. The effects of smoking on bone mass and the rates of bone loss among elderly Japanese-American men. *J Bone Miner Res* 1997;12:1495–1501.
111. Krall EA, Dawson-Hughes B. Smoking and bone loss among postmenopausal women. *J Bone Miner Res* 1991;6:331–338.
112. Krall EA, Dawson-Hughes B. Smoking increases bone loss and decreases intestinal calcium absorption. *J Bone Miner Res* 1999;14:215–220.
113. Brot C, Jorgensen NR, Sorensen OH. The influence of smoking on vitamin D status and calcium metabolism. *Eur J Clin Nutr* 1999;53: 920–926.
114. Kiel DP, Baron JA, Anderson JJ, et al. Smoking eliminates the protective effect of oral estrogens on the risk of hip fracture among women. *Ann Intern Med* 1992;116:716–721.
115. Husain MK, Grantz AG, Ciarochi F, et al. Nicotine stimulated release of neurophysin and vasopressin in humans. *J Clin Endocrinol Metab* 1975; 41:1113–1117.
116. Rowe JW, Kilgore A, Robertson GL. Evidence in man that cigarette smoking induces vasopressin release via an airway-specific mechanism. *J Clin Endocrinol Metab* 1980;51:170–172.
117. Allen M, Allen HM, Deck LV, et al. Role of cigarette use in hyponatremia in schizophrenic patients. *Am J Psychiatry* 1990;147:1075–1077.
118. Ellinas PA, Rosner F, Jaume JC. Symptomatic hyponatremia associated with psychosis, medications, and smoking. *J Natl Med Assoc* 1993;85:135–141.
119. Cryer PE, Haymond MW, Santiago JV, et al. Norepinephrine and epinephrine release and adrenergic mediation of smoking-associated hemodynamic and metabolic events. *N Engl J Med* 1976;295: 573–577.
120. Ottesen MM, Worck R, Ibsen H. Captopril does not blunt the sympathoadrenal response to cigarette smoking in normotensive humans. *Blood Press* 1997;6:29–34.
121. Kolodny RC, Masters WH, Kolodner RM, et al. Depression of plasma testosterone levels after chronic intensive marihuana use. *N Engl J Med* 1974;290:872–874.
122. Mendelson JH, Kuehnle J, Ellingboe J, et al. Plasma testosterone levels before, during and after chronic marihuana smoking. *N Engl J Med* 1974;291:1051–1055.
123. Cone EJ, Johnson RE, Moore JD, et al. Acute effects of smoking marijuana on hormones, subjective effects and performance in male human subjects. *Pharmacol Biochem Behav* 1986;24:1749–1754.
124. Mendelson JH, Cristofaro P, Ellingboe J, et al. Acute effects of marihuana on luteinizing hormone in menopausal women. *Pharmacol Biochem Behav* 1985;23:765–768.
125. Braunstein GD, Buster JE, Soares JR, et al. Pregnancy hormone concentrations in marijuana users. *Life Sci* 1983;33:195–199.
126. Benowitz NL, Jones RT, Lerner CB. Depression of growth hormone and cortisol response to insulin-induced hypoglycemia after prolonged oral delta-9-tetrahydrocannabinol administration in man. *J Clin Endocrinol Metab* 1976;42:938–941.
127. Nava F, Manzato E, Lucchini A. Chronic cannabis use does not affect the normalization of hypothalamic-pituitary-adrenal (HPA) axis induced by methadone in heroin addicts. *Prog Neuropsychopharmacol Biol Psychiatry* 2007;31:1089–1094.
128. Huizink AC, Ferdinand RF, Ormel J, Verhulst FC. Hypothalamic-pituitary-adrenal axis activity and early onset of cannabis use. *Addiction (Abingdon)* 2006;101:1581–1588.
129. Carlson HE. Drugs and pituitary function. In: Melmed S, ed. *The pituitary.* Cambridge, MA: Blackwell Science, 1995:645–660.
130. Cicero TJ, Bell RD, Wiest WG, et al. Function of the male sex organs in heroin and methadone users. *N Engl J Med* 1975;292:882–887.
131. Ragni G, De Laurentis L, Bestetti O, et al. Gonadal function in male heroin and methadone addicts. *Int J Androl* 1988;11:93–100.
132. Lafisca S, Bolelli G, Franceschetti F, et al. Hormone levels in methadone-treated drug addicts. *Drug Alcohol Depend* 1981;8:229–234.
133. Brambilla F, Resele L, De Maio D, et al. Gonadotropin response to synthetic gonadotropin hormone-releasing hormone (GnRH) in heroin addicts. *Am J Psychiatry* 1979;136:314–317.
134. Abs R, Verhelst J, Maeyaert J, et al. Endocrine consequences of long-term intrathecal administration of opioids. *J Clin Endocrinol Metab* 2000;85:2215–2222.
135. Santen RJ, Sofsky J, Bilic N, et al. Mechanism of action of narcotics in the production of menstrual dysfunction in women. *Fertil Steril* 1975;26:538–548.
136. Zharikova OL, Deshmukh SV, Kumar M, et al. The effect of opiates on the activity of human placental aromatase/CYP19. *Biochem Pharmacol* 2007;73:279–286.
137. Zharikova OL, Deshmukh SV, Nanovskaya TN, et al. The effect of methadone and buprenorphine on human placental aromatase. *Biochem Pharmacol* 2006;71:1255–1264.
138. Zharikova OL, Deshmukh SV, Nanovskaya TN, et al. The effect of methadone and buprenorphine on human placental aromatase. *Biochem Pharmacol* 2006;71:1255–1264.
139. Pedrazzoni M, Vescovi PP, Maninetti L, et al. Effects of chronic heroin abuse on bone and mineral metabolism. *Acta Endocrinol* 1993; 129:42–45.
140. Wilczek H, Stepan J. Bone metabolism in individuals dependent on heroin and after methadone administration. *Casopis lekaru ceskych* 2003;142:606–608.
141. Kinjo M, Setoguchi S, Schneeweiss S, Solomon DH. Bone mineral density in subjects using central nervous system-active medications. *Am J Med* 2005;118:1414.
142. Arnsten JH, Freeman R, Howard AA, et al. HIV infection and bone mineral density in middle-aged women. *Clin Infect Dis* 2006;42: 1014–1020.
143. Kim TW, Alford DP, Malabanan A, et al. Low bone density in patients receiving methadone maintenance treatment. *Drug Alcohol Depend* 2006;85:258–262.
144. Ensrud KE, Blackwell T, Mangione CM, et al., and Study of Osteoporotic Fractures Research Group. Central nervous system active medications and risk for fractures in older women. *Arch Intern Med* 2003;163:949–957.
145. Vestergaard P, Rejnmark L, Mosekilde L. Fracture risk associated with the use of morphine and opiates. *J Intern Med* 2006;260:76–87.
146. Abraham MR, Khardori R. Hyperglycemic hyperosmolar nonketotic syndrome as initial presentation of type 2 diabetes in a young cocaine abuser. *Diabetes Care* 1999;22:1380–1381.
147. Warner EA, Greene GS, Buchsbaum MS, et al. Diabetic ketoacidosis associated with cocaine use. *Arch Intern Med* 1998;158:1799–1802.

148. Heesch CM, Negus BH, Bost JE, et al. Effects of cocaine on anterior pituitary and gonadal hormones. *J Pharmacol Exp Ther* 1996;278:1195–1200.
149. Mendelson JH, Mello NK, Teoh SK, et al. Cocaine effects on pulsatile secretion of anterior pituitary, gonadal, and adrenal hormones. *J Clin Endocrinol Metab* 1989;69:1256–1260.
150. Lee MA, Bowers MM, Nash JF, et al. Neuroendocrine measures of dopaminergic function in chronic cocaine users. *Psychiatry Res* 1990; 33:151–159.
151. Mendelson JH, Teoh SK, Lange U, et al. Anterior pituitary, adrenal, and gonadal hormones during cocaine withdrawal. *Am J Psychiatry* 1988; 145:1094–1098.
152. Mendelson JH, Teoh SK, Mello NK, et al. Acute effects of cocaine on plasma adrenocorticotropic hormone, luteinizing hormone and prolactin levels in cocaine-dependent men. *J Pharmacol Exp Ther* 1992;263:505–509.
153. Teoh SK, Sarnyai Z, Mendelson JH, et al. Cocaine effects on pulsatile secretion of ACTH in men. *J Pharmacol Exp Ther* 1994;270:1134–1138.
154. Dhopesh VP, Burke WM, Maany I, et al. Effect of cocaine on thyroid functions. *Am J Drug Alcohol Abuse* 1991;17:423–427.
155. Besser GM, Butler PWP, Landon J, et al. Influence of amphetamines on plasma corticosteroid and growth hormone levels in man. *Br Med J* 1969;4:528–530.
156. Rees L, Butler PWP, Gosling C, et al. Adrenergic blockade and the corticosteroid and growth hormone responses to methylamphetamine. *Nature* 1970;228:565–566.
157. Dommisse CS, Schulz SC, Narasimhachari N, et al. The neuroendocrine and behavioral response to dextroamphetamine in normal individuals. *Biol Psychiatry* 1984;19:1305–1315.
158. Langer G, Heinze G, Reim B, et al. Reduced growth hormone responses to amphetamine in "endogenous" depressive patients. *Arch Gen Psychiatry* 1976;33:1471–1475.
159. Checkley SA, Crammer JL. Hormone responses to methylamphetamine in depression: a new approach to the noradrenaline depletion hypothesis. *Br J Psychiatry* 1977;131:582–586.
160. Checkley SA. Corticosteroid and growth hormone responses to methylamphetamine in depressive illness. *Psychol Med* 1979;9:107–115.
161. Sachar EJ, Asnis G, Nathan RS, et al. Dextroamphetamine and cortisol in depression: morning plasma cortisol levels suppressed. *Arch Gen Psychiatry* 1980;37:755–757.
162. Halbreich U, Sachar EJ, Asnis GM, et al. Growth hormone response to dextroamphetamine in depressed patients and normal subjects. *Arch Gen Psychiatry* 1982;39:189–192.
163. Nurnberger JI Jr, Simmons-Alling S, Kessler L, et al. Separate mechanisms for behavioral, cardiovascular, and hormonal responses to dextroamphetamine in man. *Psychopharmacology* 1984;84:200–204.
164. White TL, Grover VK, de Wit H. Cortisol effects of D-amphetamine relate to traits of fearlessness and aggression but not anxiety in healthy humans. *Pharmacol Biochem Behav* 2006;85:123–131.
165. Martin TL, Chiasson DA, Kish SJ. Does hyperthyroidism increase risk of death due to the ingestion of ecstasy? *J Forensic Sci* 2007;52:951–953.
166. Douglass J, McKinzie AA, Courceyro P. PCR differential display identifies a rat brain mRNA that is transcriptionally regulated by cocaine and amphetamine. *J Neurosci* 1995;15:2471–2481.
167. Vicentic A, Jones DC. The CART (cocaine- and amphetamine-regulated transcript) system in appetite and drug addiction. *J Pharmacol Exp Ther* 2007;320:499–506.
168. Hegarty VM, May HM, Khaw KT. Tea drinking and bone mineral density in older women. *Am J Clin Nutr* 2000;71:1003–1007.
169. Mensink RP, Lebbink WJ, Lobbezoo IE, et al. Diterpene composition of oils from Arabica and Robusta coffee beans and their effects on serum lipids in man. *J Intern Med* 1995;237:543–550.
170. Snyder SH, Katims JJ, Annau Z, et al. Adenosine receptors and behavioral actions of methylxanthines. *Proc Natl Acad Sci* 1981;78:3260–3264.
171. Debrah K, Haigh R, Sherwin R, et al. Effect of acute and chronic caffeine use on the cerebrovascular, cardiovascular and hormonal responses to orthostasis in healthy volunteers. *Clin Sci* 1995;89:475–480.
172. Spindel ER, Wurtman RJ, McCall A, et al. Neuroendocrine effects of caffeine in normal subjects. *Clin Pharmacol Ther* 1984;36:402–407.
173. Kerr D, Sherwin RS, Pavlakis F, et al. Effect of caffeine on the recognition of and responses to hypoglycemia in humans. *Ann Intern Med* 1993;119:799–804.
174. Debrah K, Sherwin RS, Murphy J, et al. Effect of caffeine on recognition of and physiological responses to hypoglycaemia in insulin-dependent diabetes. *Lancet* 1996;347:19–24.
175. Mackenzie T, Comi R, Sluss P, et al. Metabolic and hormonal effects of caffeine: randomized, double-blind, placebo-controlled crossover trial. *Metab Clin Exp* 2007;56:1694–1698.
176. Lane JD, Feinglos MN, Surwit RS. Caffeine increases ambulatory glucose and postprandial responses in coffee drinkers with type 2 diabetes. *Diabetes Care* 2008;31:221–222.
177. Campos H, Baylin A. Coffee consumption and risk of type 2 diabetes and heart disease. *Nutr Rev* 2007;65:173–179.
178. Massey LK, Opryszek AA. No effects of adaptation to dietary caffeine on calcium excretion in young women. *Nutr Res* 1990;10:741–747.
179. London S, Willett W, Longcope C, et al. Alcohol and other dietary factors in relation to serum hormone concentrations in women at climacteric. *Am J Clin Nutr* 1991;53:166–171.
180. Nagata C, Kabuto M, Shimizu H. Association of coffee, green tea, and caffeine intakes with serum concentrations of estradiol and sex hormone-binding globulin in premenopausal Japanese women. *Nutr Cancer* 1998;30:21–24.
181. Landin-Wilhelmsen K, Wilhelmsen L, Lappas G, et al. Serum insulin-like growth factor I in a random population sample of men and women: relation to age, sex, smoking habits, coffee consumption and physical activity, blood pressure and concentrations of plasma lipids, fibrinogen, parathyroid hormone and osteocalcin. *Clin Endocrinol* 1994;41:351–357.
182. Kiel DP, Felson DT, Hannan MT, et al. Caffeine and the risk of fracture: The Framingham Study. *Am J Epidemiol* 1990;132:675–684.
183. Hernández-Avila M, Colditz GA, Stampfer MJ, et al. Caffeine, moderate alcohol intake and the risk of fractures of the hip and forearm among middle-aged women. *Am J Clin Nutr* 1991;54:157–163.
184. Hernández-Avila M, Stampfer MJ, Ravnikar VA, et al. Caffeine and other predictors of bone density among pre- and perimenopausal women. *Epidemiology* 1993;4:128–134.
185. Yano K, Heilbrun LK, Wasnich RD, et al. The relationship between diet and bone mineral content of multiple skeletal sites in elderly Japanese-American men and women living in Hawaii. *Am J Clin Nutr* 1985;42:877–888.
186. Tavani A, Negri E, La Vecchia C. Coffee intake and risk of hip fracture in women in northern Italy. *Prev Med* 1995;24:396–400.
187. Lloyd T, Rollings N, Eggli DF, et al. Dietary caffeine intake and bone status of postmenopausal women. *Am J Clin Nutr* 1997;65:1826–1830.
188. Kanis J, Johnell O, Gullberg B, et al. Risk factors for hip fracture in men from southern Europe: The MEDOS Study. *Osteopor Int* 1999; 9:45–54.
189. Schuckit MA, Hauger RL, Moneiro MG, et al. Response of three hormones to diazepam challenge in sons of alcoholics and controls. *Alcohol Clin Exp Res* 1991;15:537–542.
190. Zemishlany Z, McQueeney R, Gabriel SM, et al. Neuroendocrine and monoaminergic responses to acute administration of alprazolam in normal subjects. *Neuropsychobiology* 1990;23:124–128.
191. Risby ED, Hsiao JK, Golden RN, et al. Intravenous alprazolam challenge in normal subjects. *Psychopharmacology* 1989;99:508–514.
192. Roy-Byrne PP, Cowley DS, Hommer D, et al. Neuroendocrine effects of diazepam in panic and generalized anxiety disorders. *Biol Psychiatry* 1991;30:73–80.
193. Arvat E, Maccagno B, Ramunni J, et al. The inhibitory effect of alprazolam, a benzodiazepine, overrides the stimulatory effect of metyrapone-induced lack of negative cortisol feedback on corticotrophic secretion in humans. *J Clin Endocrinol Metab* 1999;84:2611–2615.
194. Korbonits M, Trainer PJ, Edwards R, et al. Benzodiazepines attenuate the pituitary-adrenal responses to corticotrophin-releasing hormone in healthy volunteers, but not in patients with Cushing's syndrome. *Clin Endocrinol* 1995;43:29–35.
195. Breier A, Davis O, Buchanan R, et al. Effects of alprazolam on pituitary-adrenal and catecholaminergic responses to metabolic stress in humans. *BiolPsychiatry* 1992;32:880–890.

196. Deuster PA, Faraday MM, Chrousos GP, Poth MA. Effects of dehydroepiandrosterone and alprazolam on hypothalamic-pituitary responses to exercise. *J Clin Endocrinol Metab* 2005;90:4777–4783.
197. Cowley DS, Roy-Byrne PP, Radant A, et al. Benzodiazepine sensitivity in panic disorder: effects of chronic alprazolam treatment. *Neuropsychopharmacology* 1995;12:147–157.
198. Ambrosi F, Quartesan R, Moretti P, et al. Effects of acute benzodiazepine administration on growth hormone, prolactin and cortisol release after moderate insulin-induced hypoglycemia in normal women. *Psychopharmacology* 1986;88:187–189.
199. Pomara N, Willoughby LM, Sidtis JJ, et al. Cortisol response to diazepam: its relationship to age, dose, duration of treatment, and presence of generalized anxiety disorder. *Psychopharmacology* 2005;178:1–8.
200. Monteiro MG, Schuckit MA, Hauger R, et al. Growth hormone response to intravenous diazepam and placebo in 82 healthy men. *Biol Psychiatry* 1990;27:702–710.
201. Levin ER, Sharp B, Carlson HE. Failure to confirm consistent stimulation of growth hormone by diazepam. *Horm Res* 1984;19:86–90.
202. Shur E, Petersson H, Checkley S, et al. Long-term benzodiazepine administration blunts growth hormone response to diazepam. *Arch Gen Psychiatry* 1983;40:1105–1108.
203. Ajlouni K, el-Khateeb M Effect of glucose on growth hormone, prolactin and thyroid-stimulating hormone response to diazepam in normal subjects. *Horm Res* 1980;13:160–164.
204. Engel WR, Grau A. Inappropriate secretion of antidiuretic hormone associated with lorazepam. *Br Med J* 1988;297:858.
205. Hoffbrand BI. Barbiturate/thyroid-hormone interaction. *Lancet* 1979;(October 27):903–904.
206. Streicher HZ, Gabow PA, Moss AH, et al. Syndromes of toluene sniffing in adults. *Ann Intern Med* 1981;94:758–762.
207. Meadows R, Verghese A Medical complications of glue sniffing. *South Med J* 1996;89:455–462.
208. Kaneko T, Koizumi T, Takezaki T, et al. Urinary calculi associated with solvent abuse. *J Urol* 1992;147:1365–1366.
209. Kroeger RM, Moore RJ, Lehman TH, et al. Recurrent urinary calculi associated with toluene sniffing. *J Urol* 1980;123:89–91.
210. Jones HE, Balster RL. Inhalant abuse in pregnancy. *Obstet Gynecol Clin North Am* 1998;25:153–167.
211. Bijlsma JWJ, Duursma SA, Thijssen JHH, et al. Influence of nandrolondecanoate on the pituitary-gonadal axis in males. *Acta Endocrinol* 1982b;101:108–112.
212. Small M, Beastall GH, Semple CG, et al. Alteration of hormone levels in normal males given the anabolic steroid stanozolol. *Clin Endocrinol* 1984;21:49–55.
213. Strauss R, Liggett M, Lanese R Anabolic steroid use and perceived effects in ten weight-trained women athletes. *JAMA* 1985;253:2871–2873.
214. Malarkey WB, Strauss RH, Leizman DJ, et al. Endocrine effects in female weight lifters who self-administer testosterone and anabolic steroids. *Am J Obstet Gynecol* 1991;165:1385–1390.
215. Deyssig R, Weissel M. Ingestion of androgenic-anabolic steroids induces mild thyroidal impairment in male body builders. *J Clin Endocrinol Metab* 1993;76:1069–1071.
216. Hartgens F, Rietjens G, Keizer HA, et al. Effects of androgenic-anabolic steroids on apolipoproteins and lipoprotein (a). *Br J Sports Med* 2004;38: 253–259.
217. Polderman KH, Gooren LJ, Asscheman H, et al. Induction of insulin resistance by androgens and estrogens. *J Clin Endocrinol Metab* 1994;79: 265–271.
218. Hobbs CJ, Jones RE, Plymate SR. Nandrolone, a 19-nortestosterone, enhances insulin-independent glucose uptake in normal men. *J Clin Endocrinol Metab* 1996;81:1582–1585.
219. Sullivan ML, Martinez CM, Gennis P, et al. The cardiac toxicity of anabolic steroids. *Prog Cardiovasc Dis* 1998;41:1–15.
220. English KM, Mandour O, Steeds RP, et al. Men with coronary artery disease have lower levels of androgens than men with normal coronary angiograms. *Eur Heart J* 2000;21:890–894.
221. English KM, Steeds RP, Jones TH, et al. Low-dose transdermal testosterone therapy improves angina threshold in men with chronic stable angina: a randomized, double-blind, placebo-controlled study. *Circulation* 2000;102:1906–1911.
222. Webb CM, Adamson DL, de Zeigler D, et al. Effect of acute testosterone on myocardial ischemia in men with coronary artery disease. *Am J Cardiol* 1999;83:437–439.
223. Webb CM, McNeill JG, Hayward CS, et al. Effects of testosterone on coronary vasomotor regulation in men with coronary heart disease. *Circulation* 1999;100:1690–1696.
224. Bijlsma JWJ, Duursma SA, Bosch R, et al. Lack of influence of the anabolic steroid nandrolondecanoate on bone metabolism. *Acta Endocrinol* 1982a;101:140–143.
225. Alèn M, Rahkila P, Reinilä M, et al. Androgenic-anabolic steroid effects on serum thyroid, pituitary and steroid hormones in athletes. *Am J Sports Med* 1987;15:357–361.

CHAPTER 81

Martha J Wunsch, MD, FAAP, FASAM
Michael F. Weaver, MD, FASAM

Alcohol and Other Drug Use During Pregnancy: Management of the Mother and Child

The prevalence of substance use during pregnancy is substantial. Women addicted to alcohol or drugs may have irregular menstrual cycles, yet still have the ability to conceive, so several months may lapse before an addicted woman realizes that she is pregnant (1). Some women are able to stop using when they learn they are pregnant, but others may have difficulty stopping due to the severity of addiction or withdrawal. Ten percent of pregnant women drink alcohol (2), with 4% reporting heavy episodic drinking (3). The prevalence of illicit drug use varies by drug type during pregnancy, with 8.5% to 15% reporting marijuana use and around 2% using opioids (2), and 1.1% to 9.5% using cocaine (4,5). Perinatal substance use and addiction affects women of all races and socioeconomic levels.

Substance use during pregnancy has significant effects on the developing child as well as the mother. For these reasons, all health care providers should be able to recognize perinatal substance use and addiction and begin to address it to reduce potential complications for the mother and her child.

APPROACH TO THE PREGNANT WOMAN

Pregnancy motivates some women to quit using alcohol and/or illicit drugs. Despite warnings about fetal consequences of smoking and drinking, a significant proportion of pregnant women continue to do so (4). The clinician's role is to begin to motivate substance-using pregnant women (SUPW) to stop using substances and assist with referral for addiction treatment. Whether or not she continues to use, every addicted pregnant woman should be encouraged to continue to engage in prenatal care.

Pregnant women who abuse alcohol or illicit drugs are much more stigmatized than nonpregnant women, so they may deny their drug use, its harmful effects, and the need to seek help (6). Those who provide health care to SUPW should be sensitive to the cultural background and feelings of these patients and provide care in a supportive and nonjudgmental environment. Clinicians should be sensitive to the need for confidentiality regarding substance use diagnoses, because of stigma and potential legal ramifications. In many cases, a woman may have abused alcohol or drugs during a previous pregnancy, experiencing negative consequences such as stigmatization and loss of custody of other children. As the addicted pregnant woman may be wary of health care providers owing to previous experiences, prevention services, diagnosis, and referral to treatment should be available within a prenatal clinic setting. Such a strategy helps to decrease the stigma attached to specialized addiction treatment services.

Encouragement and consistency in approach, expectations, and the message conveyed are as important as the delivery of excellent medical care in the successful engagement and retention in treatment of SUPW (7). Optimal prenatal care should be a collaborative process between an obstetric service, pediatric service, and the addiction treatment program in order to provide the best treatment for the medical disease of addiction and close monitoring of the progress of the pregnancy and, after delivery, her child. Good communication is important among obstetricians, addictionists, primary care physicians, nurses, anesthesiologists, social workers, and legal agencies.

Screening Women with substance use and addiction in pregnancy may not fit the usual stereotype of the person with addiction, which makes early identification and treatment difficult. Though a number of questionnaires have been validated to detect alcohol use, few instruments have been validated for detection of illicit drug use during pregnancy (see Chapter 18, "Sidebar: Screening and Brief Intervention for Pregnant Women") However, certain factors in a patient's history may alert a clinician to the possible presence of substance use during pregnancy such as a family history of substance abuse. Children of alcoholics have a three- to fourfold increase in risk of developing alcoholism themselves (8). The patient who has had frequent encounters with law enforcement agencies needs to be considered at high risk for addiction (9). Women are often introduced to and supplied with drugs by a male partner; therefore, substance use, abuse, or addiction by the current significant other is a concerning history. If any of these risk factors are present, there is increased likelihood of perinatal abuse and/or addiction, and the expectant mother should be asked about drug use.

Asking directly about current substance use can identify the risk of abuse and addiction and guide advice given to women planning conception or currently pregnant. Screening women in a prenatal clinic with specific questions about alcohol and drug holds the promise of reducing substance use during pregnancy (10) (See Chapter 18, "Sidebar: Screening and Brief Intervention for Pregnant Women"). The combination of screening questions and urine toxicology has been shown to be more effective for detection of perinatal addiction than use of either one alone (11).

Common Substances Information from a thorough history (including medical problems and social stressors) and a physical examination can provide clues to use of specific substances during pregnancy. Being alert for these clues and discussing them with SUPW can help enhance honest communication about substance use during pregnancy. Once identified, options for treatment of acute withdrawal syndromes or other pharmacotherapy can be offered to SUPW, if applicable.

Tobacco Forty percent of women who smoke and become pregnant quit during pregnancy (12). All pregnant women should be asked directly about smoking and any attempts to quit. The American College of Obstetricians & Gynecologists recommends clinicians strongly advise all pregnant tobacco users to quit (13). Nicotine replacement helps reduce the amount smoked during pregnancy, which improves birth outcomes (14), and nicotine replacement therapy does not produce fetal complications (15,16).

Alcohol and Sedative-Hypnotics More than 60% of women who use alcohol and become pregnant quit during pregnancy (12). The U.S. Surgeon General's office advises that women who are pregnant or considering pregnancy should not drink alcoholic beverages (2). The majority of women who abuse sedative-hypnotics take one or more benzodiazepines and alcohol, along with barbiturates and other sleeping pills. The smell of alcohol on the breath indicates recent ingestion but not necessarily acute intoxication. Palpation of the abdomen may reveal an enlarged or shrunken liver due to alcoholic hepatitis. Even a minimal neurologic evaluation can reveal altered mental status due to intoxication or acute alcohol withdrawal. Hyperreflexia and tremulousness also prompt consideration of acute alcohol withdrawal.

Progression to severe withdrawal from alcohol or sedative-hypnotics carries a significant mortality risk, so early recognition and treatment are essential. However, the normal physiologic changes that accompany pregnancy can make it difficult to recognize early withdrawal. Table 81.1 displays similarities and differences between sedative-hypnotic withdrawal syndrome and pregnancy. Treatment for acute withdrawal from sedative-hypnotics (including alcohol) in SUPW should be accomplished in an inpatient setting, which allows for medical supervision in collaboration with an obstetrician. Uncontrolled withdrawal symptoms may be life-threatening to both mother and fetus. Benzodiazepines and barbiturates can adversely affect the fetus when given during pregnancy, so this should be taken into account when beginning treatment for acute withdrawal symptoms. However, the risk to both mother and fetus from untreated sedative-hypnotic withdrawal is usually greater than the potential risk to the fetus from exposure to these medications in a controlled setting.

Stimulants Previous pregnancy complications such as preterm labor, premature rupture of membranes, placental abruption, or intrauterine growth restriction may indicate prior complications of stimulant use, especially cocaine or methamphetamine. Respiratory problems in the mother may be a current consequence of intranasal insufflation (snorting) or smoking drugs (17). Atrophy of the nasal mucosa or perforation of the nasal septum (17) indicates snorting of drugs, most often cocaine or methamphetamine. A cough productive of black sputum indicates crack smoking (18).

TABLE 81.1 Pregnancy and Sedative-Hypnotic Withdrawal

Signs and symptoms common to both sedative-hypnotic withdrawal and pregnancy	Signs and symptoms of sedative-hypnotic withdrawal not common to pregnancy
Restlessness	Impaired memory
Insomnia	Distractibility
Nausea and vomiting	Agitation
Hypertension	Tremor
Tachycardia	Fever
Tachypnea	Diaphoresis
Seizures	Hallucinations

The withdrawal syndrome from stimulants is subtle and complex and consists primarily of depression and craving. As abrupt discontinuation of stimulants does not cause gross physiologic sequelae, they are not tapered off or replaced with a cross-tolerant drug during medically supervised withdrawal treatment (19). Pregnant women withdrawing from stimulants should not receive medication except in cases of extreme agitation. Low doses of a benzodiazepine may be used if necessary.

Opioids Use of heroin or abuse of prescription analgesics may continue into pregnancy because attempts to quit lead to obvious withdrawal symptoms, but SUPW may be reluctant to disclose this information. Constipation from opioid abuse may be apparent on abdominal examination. Opioids may be used by injection, especially heroin, so clues on screening that indicate injection drug use are useful. Nearly half of parenteral drug users have a history of acute hepatitis (20). Infections such as endocarditis, recurrent cellulitis, or thrombophlebitis should raise suspicion for injection drug use. Some SUPW hide needle marks by injecting under the tongue, in the axillae, under the breasts, into the legs, between fingers or toes, and under the nails. Track marks are wormlike scars from repeated injection that follow the courses of veins. Look for healed abscess scars from subcutaneous injection.

Opioid withdrawal syndrome during pregnancy can lead to fetal distress and premature labor owing to increased oxygen consumption by both mother and fetus (21). Even minimal symptoms in the mother may indicate fetal distress, as the fetus may be more susceptible to withdrawal symptoms than the mother. Methadone is frequently used to treat acute withdrawal symptoms from illicit opioids. Methadone may be used by a physician for temporary maintenance or detoxification when an addicted patient is admitted to a hospital for an illness other than opioid addiction. This includes admission for evaluation for preterm labor, which may be induced by acute withdrawal. Naloxone should not be given to a pregnant woman except as a last resort in life-threatening opioid overdose, as withdrawal precipitated by an opioid antagonist can result in spontaneous abortion, premature labor, or stillbirth.

Office Care of the Substance-Using Pregnant Woman During prenatal care visits for women in addiction treatment, obstetric clinicians should obtain results of urine drug testing from the addiction treatment program to assess potential fetal effects and encourage abstinence. Addiction in pregnancy involves not only SUPW but also the family and the community. Supportive involvement of the patient's significant others in her treatment should be encouraged.

Routine office visits for prenatal care are opportunities to screen for depression and other mental health issues, as dual diagnosis (coexisting substance use disorder and other psychiatric diagnosis) is not uncommon. Appropriate obstetric care also includes evaluation for sexually transmitted diseases with treatment of the woman and ideally treatment of her partner. Office visits also allow ongoing evaluation of the psychosocial support system for SUPW and may include referral to appropriate community services, if not available in the prenatal clinic setting.

Up to 8% of pregnant women are victims of physical abuse (22), but 34% of SUPW report physical abuse (23). This rate is similar to rates of victimization among nonpregnant substance users, so pregnancy is not a protective factor against domestic violence (24). Physical, sexual, and verbal abuse by a partner are more common among alcoholic women (20), so eliciting a thorough social history adds information about consequences of addiction. These high rates of domestic violence among SUPW should prompt clinicians to ask all pregnant women about the possibility of physical or sexual abuse, especially when substance use is also identified.

Education of pregnant women about childbirth during routine office visits for prenatal care helps prevent problems at the time of delivery, including relapse. Other appropriate care at prenatal office visits includes discussion of a birth plan, education about the potential need for treatment of a substance exposed newborn, appropriate contraceptive methods postpartum, and involvement of the patient's significant other.

Treatment Programs Simple admonitions to stop using are sometimes helpful if the diagnosis of substance use or addiction is made early, but in most cases of addiction are insufficient (25). Therapy for SUPW may begin with detoxification, but this is merely a first step in overall treatment. Addiction treatment is more likely to be effective when begun during pregnancy than afterward (26). Different SUPW are likely to benefit from different types of treatment programs, depending on the drug of choice and severity of addiction, as well as past experience in treatment. However, not all types of treatment have been specifically studied in SUPW, and neither supportive psychotherapy nor relapse prevention has been evaluated in this population (6). In addition to specific formal treatment, Twelve-Step self-help groups can be an important support system for SUPW. The ability of SUPW to follow through with treatment may be compromised by guilt, lack of supportive significant others (including family), and uncertainty about the success of treatment. However, the possibility of having her children reunited with her is often an incentive for a mother to enter treatment. This reduces the burden on the foster care system by assuring the safety of the child in a therapeutic environment.

When planning for addiction treatment in a pregnant woman, factors unique to this population must be taken into account. Access to treatment for SUPW may be limited by factors beyond the control of the woman, such as lack of treatment program openings, transportation problems, lack of childcare, or poverty (27). Comprehensive treatment programs for SUPW are successful (28). Addiction treatment programs must provide childcare to be effective (29,30), but few do so (31). Specialty residential treatment programs for SUPW and/or those caring for an infant are economically justified (32).

Labor and Delivery Women may relapse as they near the end of pregnancy. They may confuse early signs of labor with signs of acute withdrawal, so may use illicit prescription opioids and/or heroin during the early hours of labor and may arrive at the hospital in labor with high concentrations of drugs in the blood from recent use. This increases the chances of fetal stress and distress. Some SUPW may use heroin or illicit prescription opioids immediately before presenting for delivery in anticipation of the pain and stress of labor. Women should be educated about labor and effects of drugs on the fetus, including neonatal withdrawal syndromes. Education of SUPW can prevent frustration that may lead to relapse. The delivery method should be selected based solely on obstetric considerations. The staff on a labor and delivery unit should be aware that women who abuse stimulants may display bizarre and potentially abusive behavior (7).

Delivery is a clinical situation with nearly universal acute pain and a reasonably defined onset and resolution (33). Patients addicted to drugs are subject to pain in the same manner as any other patient, so can benefit from appropriate treatment for pain (34). Addicted pregnant women should be assessed for appropriate analgesia, and anesthesia options and adequate pain management should be provided at the time of delivery. Regional anesthesia may be the procedure of choice during delivery and for postpartum pain. Placement of an epidural catheter with infusion of a local anesthetic such as bupivacaine can reduce or eliminate the need for opioid analgesics. Pain medication should not be withheld based on a history of addiction. Adjust the medication dose based on the patient's reported pain level using a pain scale. One study showed that women on methadone maintenance during pregnancy had similar analgesic requirements and response during labor but required more opioid analgesic after cesarean delivery when compared to women not on methadone maintenance (33). Women who are abusing heroin or prescription opioids or are prescribed chronic opioids (including methadone maintenance) should not receive opioid agonist/antagonist pain medications (such as pentazocine or butorphanol) for acute pain because these medications may cause an acute opioid withdrawal syndrome (35,36). The newborn should not be given naloxone at delivery, as this may precipitate severe withdrawal symptoms (7).

One of the most common complications of addiction and substance use during pregnancy is preterm labor (7) with occurrence varying according to the substance. Rates from opioid use may be as high as 29% to 41% (37,38). Rates for other illicit drugs are generally lower, with around 6% attributable to cocaine (39).

MATERNAL ADDICTION TREATMENT

Different types of addiction treatment programs can be beneficial for SUPW, including Twelve-Step self-help group attendance and/or formal treatment programs. Whether inpatient, residential, or outpatient, these treatments must take into account the challenges facing SUPW to be optimally effective. Pharmacotherapy may be an option for some SUPW, though some medications are contraindicated in pregnancy.

Opioid Maintenance Treatment Medical withdrawal of the pregnant opioid-dependent woman is not recommended because of high rates of relapse to illicit prescription opioid and heroin use and the increased risk to the fetus of intrauterine death. Methadone maintenance is the treatment of choice (40). Being on a stable methadone dose decreases fluctuations in maternal opioid level, which reduces stress on the fetus. Fluctuations between intoxication and withdrawal result in adverse fetal effects, such as premature labor and spontaneous abortion. Illicitly bought heroin is adulterated with other compounds that may be harmful to the fetus, and access to illicit prescription opioids may be unpredictable, so elimination of any opioid use with adequate doses of methadone prevents harm to the fetus from exposure to these other compounds. Improved maternal health and nutrition reduces obstetric complications and improves the health of the infant at delivery. Other advantages of methadone maintenance over illicit opioid use are reduction of criminal activity and decreased disruption of the maternal-child dyad (41). Methadone maintenance enhances the ability of SUPW to participate in prenatal care and addiction treatment, thus giving the woman and her family the opportunity to adequately prepare for the arrival of the infant.

Opioid-dependent pregnant women should be referred to a local methadone maintenance program, if available. Most programs assign high priority to pregnant women, so the patient may be able to enter treatment sooner than if she were not pregnant. Opioid-dependent pregnant women on methadone maintenance are monitored regularly throughout the pregnancy, and the dose is adjusted as necessary. Maternal methadone dose does not correlate with neonatal abstinence symptoms, so maternal benefits of methadone are not offset by harm to the newborn (42). A daily methadone dose over 60 mg is most effective (43). It is not unusual for the methadone dose requirement to increase during the third trimester of pregnancy. This is due to larger plasma volume, decreased plasma protein binding, increased tissue binding, increased methadone metabolism, and increased methadone clearance in the mother. As a result, the half-life of methadone is shortened late in pregnancy, and the woman may experience mild withdrawal symptoms unless adjustments are made to her methadone dose. Splitting the total daily methadone requirement into two doses, given in the morning and evening, is preferred (44,45) if possible. This provides a more even blood concentration throughout each day. Methadone maintenance as part of comprehensive care for pregnant heroin users and illicit prescription opioid users improves maternal psychosocial function and birth outcomes (46).

Sublingual buprenorphine, a partial agonist prescribed for the treatment of opioid addiction, is not yet approved for use in pregnancy but has been used successfully for opioid maintenance in pregnant women (47,48). This medication has been well tolerated by mothers, and the newborns have had a similar incidence of neonatal abstinence syndrome compared to mothers on methadone (49). It is encouraging that early reports of clinical trials and the pregnancies and birth outcomes of pregnant patients prescribed buprenorphine indicate that withdrawal is well tolerated by the newborn (49–52).

Other Pharmacotherapy Some forms of long-term dependence pharmacotherapy are not appropriate for SUPW. Women taking medication for alcohol dependence should stop the medication if they are planning to become pregnant in the near future and immediately upon becoming pregnant. Disulfiram (Antabuse) is contraindicated during pregnancy because of the association with specific birth defects (53), and the effects of acamprosate (Campral) and naltrexone (Revia) have not been studied in pregnancy.

EVALUATION OF THE SUBSTANCE-EXPOSED NEWBORN

Physical examination, social and legal history, maternal history of addiction or of previous treatment, or substance-related obstetrical or medical problems may lead the clinician to request laboratory screening for substances in mother and child. When indicated, infant urine, meconium, and cord blood as well as maternal urine may be tested for legal and illegal drugs of abuse. As with any medical diagnostic evaluation, laboratory evaluation should be accompanied by a review of maternal records, maternal medical and psychiatric history, as well as a complete evaluation of the mother for substance use, abuse, and addiction during the pregnancy (7). A request for infant body fluid testing must be accompanied by informed consent, because testing without this violates the constitutional rights of the mother and child (54). In addition to helping in a diagnostic evaluation, negative results are helpful in validating a mother's history of engagement in treatment, recovery, and abstinence.

Screening of urine, blood, and meconium initially consists of immunologic assays followed by final confirmation of results. As laboratories vary in which substances are tested, the clinician should rely on his or her knowledge of medications and drugs commonly abused in the community and relevant maternal addiction history to direct the specific substances for which to test. For example, if only heroin, morphine, and codeine are requested for analysis and the drugs of abuse in a community are prescription opioids, results may be falsely negative for synthetic and semi-synthetic opioids.

The advantage of testing urine is ease of collection; however, utility is limited, as this provides results only about use and fetal exposure shortly before delivery. Meconium, a dark-green odorless substance produced by the fetal gastrointestinal tract beginning at 13 to 14 weeks of gestation, may also be tested for drugs of abuse as well as alcohol. This is passed by the newborn in bowel movements most often shortly after birth. The advantage of testing meconium is that it provides information about a long window of prenatal exposure, beginning in the second trimester (55). Unfortunately, meconium collection can be more difficult when it is passed in utero before the birth or may take days to collect, and results are not available as quickly as those for urine. Results of meconium and urine for 423 mother-infant pairs for detection of cannabinoids, codeine, morphine, or methadone found that meconium results provided no advantage over analysis of maternal urine and first infant voided urine. Meconium was slightly more effective in testing for cocaine (56). Testing of cord blood is also feasible, providing data about exposure around the time of birth. However, it is less often available and is probably not superior to meconium and urine. In one small study, infant cord blood results for drugs of abuse were concordant with meconium more than 90% of the time for amphetamines, opiates, cocaine, and cannabinoids (57). Finally, the fetus exposed to illicit drugs is more likely to be exposed to alcohol in utero. Recently, significant elevation of four fatty acid ethyl esters in meconium and hair has been investigated as a marker for in-utero alcohol exposure (58,59).

In a newborn, a positive toxicology screen warrants a social work evaluation of the home environment for the health and well-being of the child after discharge from the hospital. Health care practitioners (physicians, nurses, social workers) must be familiar with legislation in their community dictating legal duty to report positive results to Child Protective Services (CPS). CPS workers are responsible for further investigation of the risk to the child, thus optimizing the postpartum environment.

Confirmed or suspected history of addiction in the mother should lead to infant screening for hepatitis B or C, human immunodeficiency virus (HIV), or other sexually transmitted diseases. Infants born to SUPW are at higher risk for these infections because of the association of drug use with high-risk sexual behaviors and intranasal and intravenous routes of administration. Laboratory screening of the child allows for early treatment and may help prevent further transmission or other complications of infection.

NEONATAL INTOXICATION AND ABSTINENCE SYNDROMES

In SUPW using psychoactive substances, polysubstance abuse is the norm rather than the exception. Because of this, determination of specific perinatal effects of individual drugs may be difficult. The signs of intoxication as well as withdrawal from illicit and legal drugs in the neonate are all characterized by autonomic instability, central nervous system (CNS) irritability, and feeding difficulties. The substance-exposed newborn may have poor weight gain, instability in heart rate, respiratory rate, and temperature as well as hyperactivity, irritability, hypertonia or hypotonia, difficulty sucking or excessive sucking, sleep disturbance, and high-pitched cries (60). An abstinence syndrome for intrauterine cocaine exposure has not been clearly defined (61), though effects of cocaine intoxication on neurobehavioral status have been identified. Intoxicated newborns may be irritable, difficult to quiet, and have feeding difficulties (62). Because nicotine is a stimulant, infants born to women who smoke or chew tobacco may also be irritable and difficult to calm. When assessed with the Neonatal Intensive Care Unit Network Neurobehavioral Scale (NNNS), infants exposed to tobacco were more excitable and hypertonic with indications of disturbance in the CNS, gastrointestinal system, and visual response (63). Some investigators have proposed development of a scoring system to describe a nicotine withdrawal syndrome (64).

The duration of intoxication and the onset of withdrawal syndrome will depend upon the time of the last drug exposure, the combination of substances, and the metabolism and excretion of the drug. For example, an infant exposed to cocaine will be irritable, have sleep/wake cycle disruption, and feed poorly, but if the infant has been alcohol-exposed, symptoms may be more severe, as alcohol and cocaine form cocaethylene, a potent stimulant (65). Timing of withdrawal also varies. In the case of the infant exposed to heroin, withdrawal signs will generally emerge in the first 24 hours of life for the newborn if use occurred shortly before birth. In contrast, if methadone is prescribed or abused signs of withdrawal usually present later than with heroin, after 48 hours of life (66). Similarly, though sedative-hypnotic withdrawal is less common than opioid withdrawal syndrome, the newborn exposed to a long-acting benzodiazepine such as diazepam will display withdrawal signs much later than one exposed to short-acting sedative-hypnotics like alprazolam or alcohol. Exposure to benzodiazepines and/or barbiturates in addition to opioids may cause even later onset of opioid withdrawal signs (67). Stimulant exposure may worsen the appearance of opioid withdrawal syndrome because of increased irritability in the newborn with stimulant intoxication.

Neonates with intrauterine drug exposure should be followed up in the hospital for at least 72 to 96 hours after birth to monitor for signs of a neonatal intoxication or withdrawal syndrome. If an infant is discharged prior to this time, the mother and her support network should be educated about signs of neonatal abstinence syndrome (NAS). She will need clear instructions about how to reach a physician to assess the newborn should signs emerge. If more than 7 days has elapsed between the last maternal use and delivery, the incidence of NAS is low (68).

Initial Treatment When the diagnosis of substance use, abuse, or maternal addiction is under consideration; there is known abuse of tobacco; or a urine drug screen has been positive for substances, newborns should have regular assessment for withdrawal or intoxication beginning at birth or as soon as possible. Additionally, an infant born to a mother currently prescribed opioid medication for treatment of her addiction should be monitored closely. Initial treatment of the neonate experiencing NAS should be primarily supportive, as pharmacotherapy may prolong hospitalization and subject the neonate to exposure to medications that may not be indicated (61).

The substance-exposed neonate is easily overstimulated, so ambient light exposure and noise should be minimized. Quieting the infant with swaddling, frequent small feedings, and intravenous replacement of fluids and electrolytes may be required. Indications for pharmacotherapy include seizures; poor feeding, diarrhea or vomiting resulting in dehydration or excessive weight loss; inability to sleep; or significant autonomic instability with bradycardia or tachycardia, apnea or tachypnea, or temperature instability not due to infection. Pharmacotherapy should be considered if the infant is too ill to assess possible withdrawal signs, comorbid medical problems dictate that the infant will not tolerate NAS, or if the infant is not eating well and not thriving as expected. Vomiting and/or diarrhea associated with dehydration and poor weight gain, in the absence of other diagnoses, are relative indications for treatment, even without high total withdrawal scores (61).

Clinical signs and symptoms should not be attributed solely to drug withdrawal or intoxication without appropriate assessment and diagnostic tests to rule out other causes. The differential diagnosis for NAS includes sepsis, hypoglycemia, perinatal anoxia, intracranial bleed, and hyperthyroidism (69). Consultation with a neonatologist may be indicated in cases where presentation is not straightforward, the course is difficult, or the infant is not responding to pharmacotherapy and supportive measures.

Opioids Neonatal opioid withdrawal syndrome occurs in 60% to 80% of infants with intrauterine exposure to heroin or prescription opioids, including methadone and buprenorphine (50,70). The incidence of the syndrome is best described in those cases where SUPW are prescribed an opioid while in treatment. In these cases, historical and laboratory information for most of the pregnancy is available and may assist in treatment of the newborn (71).

Assessment and pharmacologic management of opioid-exposed infants varies across nurseries (72), but the most commonly used and comprehensive assessment is the scoring system developed by Finnegan and Kaltenbach (60) (Fig. 81.1). This scale assesses 21 symptoms with weighted scores, which are evaluated at 2 hours after birth and then every 4 hours. In scoring an infant, considerations of other factors, such as comorbid exposure to tobacco or other stimulants, a noisy environment and overstimulation, or whether the infant is hungry may impact upon results. Pharmacotherapy is usually initiated when the total score is more than 8 for 3 consecutive evaluations; however, some nurseries will utilize a lower score in an infant with comorbid medical problems or a higher score if the infant is feeding well and thriving. After initiation of treatment, the clinician should evaluate and score the infant every 2 hours until the severity score decreases; then scoring resumes every 4 hours.

Another scoring tool, the Lipsitz Withdrawal Score, is used in some nurseries with treatment initiated at a score of more than 4 (73). This assessment has fewer items and may be easier to administer. The NNNS is also used to assess stress and responsiveness in the newborn. The NNNS is sometimes administered in the substance-exposed newborn but is not used alone to guide pharmacologic treatment of opioid withdrawal (74).

Recommendations regarding specific treatments of NAS are hampered by the paucity of controlled trial data supporting

FINNEGAN NEONATAL ABSTINENCE SCORE

Date: ____________ Weight: ____________

System	Signs & Symptoms	Score	Time AM						PM						Comments
Central Nervous System Disturbances	Excessive High Pitched Cry	2													
	Continuous High Pitched Cry	3													
	Sleeps <1 Hour After Feeding	3													
	Sleeps <2 Hours After Feeding	2													
	Sleeps <3 Hours After Feeding	1													
	Hyperactive Moro Reflex	2													
	Markedly Hyperactive Moro Reflex	3													
	Mild Tremors Disturbed	1													
	Moderate – Severe Tremors Disturbed	2													
	Mild Tremors Undisturbed	3													
	Moderate – Severe Tremors Undisturbed	4													
	Increased Muscle Tone	2													
	Excoriation (Specific Area)	1													
	Myoclonic Jerks	3													
	Generalized Convulsions	5													
Metabolic/Vasomotor/Respiratory Disturbances	Sweating	1													
	Fever <101 (37.2-38.2C)	1													
	Fever > (38.4 C and Higher)	2													
	Frequent Yawning (>3-4 Times/Interval)	1													
	Mottling	1													
	Nasal Stuffiness	1													
	Sneezing (>3-4 Times/Interval)	1													
	Nasal Flaring	2													
	Respiratory Rate – 60/min	1													
	Respiratory Rate – 60/min with Retractions	2													
Gastrointestinal Disturbances	Excessive Sucking	1													
	Poor Feeding	2													
	Regurgitation	2													
	Projectile Vomiting	3													
	Loose Stools	2													
	Watery Stools	3													
	TOTAL SCORE														
	Initials of Scorer														

Finnegan, LP, Kron, Re, Connaughton, JF, & Emich, JP, A scoring system for evaluation and treatment of the neonatal abstinence syndrome: A new clinical and research tool. In *Basic and Therapeutic Aspects of Perinatal Pharmacology*, Ed., Moriselli, PL, Garattini, S. & Sereni, F, New York: Raven Press, 139–155, 1975.

The FINNEGAN NEONATAL ABSTINENCE SCORE is for the assessment of infants exposed in utero to psychoactive drugs, particularly opioids/opiates. Evaluator should check signs or symptoms observed at various time intervals and add the scores to obtain a total score. Observation of the scores over the time intervals provides the progression or diminution of symptoms.

FIGURE 81.1. Finnegan neonatal abstinence score.

the efficacy of any one preparation or treatment regimen over another (75). Abuse of other nonopioid drugs such as alcohol and other sedative-hypnotic drugs is a confounder of studies. The Cochrane Database review of NAS concluded that treatment with a substitute opioid, such as morphine, tincture of opium, or methadone, reduces time to regain birth weight and may shorten hospital length of stay (76,77). In these two meta-analyses, phenobarbital and diazepam were found to be less effective in the treatment of seizures, but administration of a CNS depressant did not clearly lead to poorer treatment outcomes. Some investigators report the addition of phenobarbital to an opioid leads to better outcomes (78), whereas others find the CNS depressants fare poorly when compared to treatment with opioids (79,80). In a chart review comparing paregoric to methadone for treatment of neonatal opioid withdrawal, side effect profiles were similar between the two medications. Additionally, there were no differences in time to resolution of symptoms, rate of decrease of symptom severity or length of hospital stay between the two medication groups (81). In the case of SUPW prescribed methadone or buprenorphine for opioid addiction, with no indication of other drug exposure, substitution treatment with an opioid is appropriate when pharmacologic intervention is indicated (Table 81.2).

Other Drugs Symptoms of neonatal sedative-hypnotic withdrawal syndrome, including alcohol, are similar to opioid withdrawal syndrome. In most cases, exposure to alcohol occurs in tandem with other substances, with tobacco the most commonly co-occurring substance. The development of a sedative-hypnotic scoring scale has been difficult because of the predominance of polysubstance exposures and, therefore, there is no specific sedative-hypnotic scoring scale. Seizures are more frequent with alcohol withdrawal than opioid withdrawal syndrome, though given the short half-life of alcohol, even in the newborn, the need for the treatment of alcohol withdrawal is rare (82). Additionally, neonatal benzodiazepine withdrawal syndrome usually resolves spontaneously and does not require specific treatment, though phenobarbital is the agent of choice for severe sedative-hypnotic withdrawal syndrome. Clinical trials comparing dosage, dosing intervals, and the need for serum levels of phenobarbital have not been done. Phenobarbital can be administered orally or intramuscularly at a dose of 2 to 4 mg/kg of body weight every 8 hours (80). After stabilization with reduction of neonatal withdrawal signs, the dose can be tapered by 10% to 20% per day over 5 to 10 days (61).

FETAL EFFECTS OF PSYCHOACTIVE SUBSTANCE USE IN PREGNANCY

A teratogen is a substance that may produce a congenital malformation when used during human or animal gestation. The time of exposure and amount of chemical will affect whether congenital malformations or neurobehavioral problems that persist into later lifetime will occur. In many cases, a "subthreshold exposure" will not lead to malformations, whereas in others a small dose during critical embryogenesis can lead to significant teratogenicity (83). In the human, it is difficult to attribute causation to exposure when there are confounding variables such as malnutrition and concurrent use of other substances. Alcohol and tobacco, alone and in combination with other substances, are known to have the most potential to cause teratogenicity in the human, but psychoactive substance use in pregnancy, whether illicit or medicinal, always involves some degree of risk of teratogenicity to the developing embryo or fetus.

TABLE 81.2 Pharmacotherapy for Neonatal Opioid Withdrawal Syndrome

	Dosing			
Medication	**Induction**	**Titration**	**Stabilization**	**Tapering**
Tincture of opium (diluted solution of 0.4 mg/ml morphine equivalent)	0.1 ml/kg (2 drops/kg) every 4 h with feedings	Increase by 0.1 ml/kg (2 drops/kg) every 4 h as needed to control withdrawal signs	Every 4 h with feedings for 3–5 days	Taper gradually by reducing dose without changing frequency of administration
Paregoric (0.4 mg/ml)	0.1 ml/kg (2 drops/kg) q4h with feedings	Increase by 0.1 ml/kg (2 drops/kg) every 4 h as needed to control withdrawal signs	Every 4h with feedings for 3–5 days	Taper gradually by reducing dose without changing frequency of administration
Methadone	0.05–0.1 mg/kg q6h	Increase by 0.05 mg/kg every 6 h as needed to control withdrawal signs	When stable, give total daily dose once daily, or divided into every-12-h doses	Taper gradually to 0.05 mg/kg, then discontinue (will self-taper as metabolized due to long half-life)

Adapted from American Academy of Pediatrics, Committee on Drugs. Neonatal drug withdrawal. *Pediatrics* 1998;101:1079–1088.

During pregnancy, diagnostic criteria for abuse or addiction need not be met for disruption of fetal growth and development to occur. Exposure in the first trimester can result in significant problems, including pregnancy loss. The majority of development and organogenesis occurs in the first 12 weeks of pregnancy; however, exposure can cause problems during any trimester of pregnancy. Even when maternal history of substance used, amount and mode of use (injection vs. oral), and the timing of use is known, there are multiple factors that affect determination of fetal substance exposure. Substances are often used in combination, confounding the effects of exposure (84). Additionally, recall bias may impact the validity of a retrospective maternal history. Finally, SUPW may feel guilty, ashamed, and overwhelmed when faced with problems in the newborn that are secondary to their addiction and may either under- or overreport their use of substances.

Alcohol In the pregnant woman, when alcohol is consumed it is absorbed into the maternal bloodstream, quickly crosses the placenta, and enters fetal circulation. Alcohol is found in significant levels in the amniotic fluid even after a single moderate dose. As fetal hepatic circulation does not metabolize alcohol as efficiently as in the adult, alcohol is not eliminated from the amniotic fluid as rapidly as it is from maternal circulation (83).

Over the last 40 years multiple diagnostic criteria and schemata have been proposed to describe the spectrum of structural anomalies and neurocognitive disabilities associated with alcohol exposure in pregnancy. Though diagnostic criteria and categorization are under discussion, fetal alcohol syndrome (FAS) is still the currently accepted diagnosis that describes affected individuals. The diagnostic use of fetal alcohol effects has fallen out of favor because of the inherent ambiguity of this diagnostic classification (85). Fetal alcohol spectrum disorders (FASD) is an umbrella term that describes the range of effects that may manifest in an individual whose mother drank alcohol during pregnancy. These effects may include physical, mental, behavioral, and/or learning disabilities with possible lifelong implications (85–89). The term FASD is not intended for use as a clinical diagnosis.

Fetal Alcohol Syndrome When SUPW enter addiction treatment, the addictionist has an opportunity to intervene and prevent further alcohol-affected pregnancies through education. He or she may uncover a significant history of alcohol use in the current or past pregnancies or be the first clinician to become aware of a mother's concern about her child's development. An addictionist can discuss the possibility of a diagnostic evaluation and may conduct the initial screening evaluation for FAS using specific criteria for evaluation (90). The classic phenotype and diagnosis of FAS includes the following:

1. *Evidence of growth retardation (prenatal and/or postnatal)*: Height and or weight equal to or less than the 10th percentile, corrected for racial norms.
2. *Evidence of deficient brain growth and/or abnormal morphogenesis*, including one or more of the following: structural brain anomalies or head circumference equal to or less than the 10th percentile (microcephaly).
3. *Evidence of a characteristic pattern of minor facial anomalies*, including two or more of the following: short palpebral fissures (equal to or less than the 10th percentile), thin vermillion border of the upper lip, smooth philtrum.

Of note, diagnostic criteria for FAS have been clarified by publication of a nomogram for determining palpebral fissure length centiles. Additionally, the 5-point pictorial score for assessing philtrum smoothness and thickness along the vermillion border provides further diagnostic guidance (87,89).

Fetal Alcohol Spectrum Disorders The umbrella term *fetal alcohol spectrum disorder* expands the classification of prenatally alcohol-exposed individuals to include the following:

1. FAS with and without confirmed maternal alcohol exposure.
2. Partial FAS: This diagnostic classification allows for a known or unknown maternal alcohol exposure history. It includes evidence of the characteristic pattern of minor facial anomalies and either evidence of prenatal and/or postnatal growth retardation or structural brain abnormalities or microcephaly.
3. Alcohol-related birth defects (ARBD): Alcohol exposure in pregnancy can cause significant structural defects in multiple organ systems known as ARBD. This includes anomalies in multiple organ systems such as cardiac (atrial septal defect, ventricular septal defect, conotruncal anomalies), skeletal (radioulnar synostosis and vertebral defects), renal (aplastic/hypoplastic/dysplastic kidneys), eyes (strabismus, ptosis, vascular and nerve anomalies), and ears (conductive and sensorineural hearing defects) and may include minor anomalies of the hands, ears, and chest wall with pectus carinatum/excavatum (87).
4. Alcohol-Related Neurodevelopmental Disorder (ARND): In addition to microcephaly and structural abnormalities of the CNS, alcohol exposure may lead to ARND. When the diagnosis of ARND is made, there is evidence of a complex pattern of behavior or cognitive abnormalities inconsistent with developmental level. Additionally, the deficits cannot be explained by genetic predisposition, family background, or environment alone in the exposed child. The child or adult with ARND has marked impairment of complex developmental tasks, higher-level receptive and expressive language deficits, and disordered behavior (91).

For further clarification of the diagnosis and referral of alcohol-exposed individuals, current guidelines are available from the Centers for Disease Control and Prevention (91). The reader is also referred to the comprehensive review by Hoyme et al. (87).

The prevalence of FASD and FAS varies across populations, but affected adults and children are found in all races and ethnic groups. Poverty often leads to higher rates of alcohol abuse, fetal exposure, and FAS as well as FASD (92). In the United States, it is estimated that between 0.5 and 2 per 1,000 live births will meet diagnostic criteria for FAS (92). FASD is more common, encompassing a wider spectrum of effects of exposure, and up to 1% of live births may be affected (93).

After identification of a potential case, the addictionist should refer the family for a multidisciplinary evaluation of the patient, as the differential diagnosis for the clinical features of FAS and FASD includes other genetic syndromes and fetal exposures to other teratogenic substances. Such an evaluation should include a physician skilled in the diagnosis of developmental disabilities, a psychologist with the ability to perform neuropsychologic evaluation, educational specialists, and physical, occupational, and speech and language professionals (87). Addiction clinicians may refer families seeking information about FAS and FASD to the National Organization of Fetal Alcohol Syndrome (NOFAS; *www.nofas.org*).

Sedative-Hypnotic Medications

Barbiturates Barbiturates such as phenobarbital have been evaluated as part of a syndrome of anticonvulsant embryopathy described in infants exposed to anticonvulsant drugs in utero (94). Features include increased major malformations, growth retardation, and hypoplasia of the midface and fingers. The Antiepileptic Drug Pregnancy Registry (AEDPR) enrolled 77 pregnancies to determine the risk of embryopathy with exposure, including phenobarbital as well as mood stabilizers. The AEDPR found the relative risk of major congenital malformations in anticonvulsant-exposed offspring was 4.2, and there was no difference in exposure to phenobarbital when compared to the other medications (95). The maternal use of barbiturates near term, particularly at chronic, high doses, can result in respiratory depression in the neonate and a barbiturate withdrawal syndrome (96).

Benzodiazepines The use of benzodiazepines during pregnancy has been associated with various degrees of teratogenic effects, particularly cleft lip and palate. However, data are conflicting, and heavy benzodiazepine use often is associated with exposure to alcohol and other substances (97,98). Overall, the use of benzodiazepines during pregnancy appears to have a low teratogenic risk (83,96,99). Maternal abuse of benzodiazepines near term has resulted in poor muscle tone and respiratory depression in the neonate (100).

Opioids A review of the animal and human literature provides no evidence that prescribed and illicit use of opioids are in themselves teratogenic (101,102). Other than transmission of infection secondary to injection and intranasal insufflation, the most common ill effect of opioid abuse and addiction in pregnancy is intrauterine growth restriction (IUGR). Growth restriction is a result of poor maternal nutrition and the fluctuations of intoxication and withdrawal from the opioids inherent to the lifestyle and disease of opioid addiction (86,96,103). The offspring of women prescribed opioids for the treatment of pain, with steady-state levels of opioid medications, have no increase in pregnancy complications and deliver infants of normal weight and length (104). The most common complication in these infants is emergence of neonatal opioid withdrawal syndrome. Finally, newborns exposed to opioids chronically through gestation develop physiologic tolerance and rarely have CNS or respiratory depression at birth. In this population, the administration of the opioid antagonist naloxone will result in rapid onset of withdrawal signs.

Stimulants

Cocaine When cocaine is abused by SUPW, the active drug and its metabolites readily cross the placenta. As fetal pH normally is lower than maternal pH and the fetal liver does not metabolize cocaine efficiently, drug is concentrated at higher levels in amniotic fluid. The effects of cocaine are thought to be through direct neurotoxicity by disrupting monoaminergic pathways and causing vascular damage (105,106). Multiple studies over the last decade have identified neurologic, developmental and behavioral deficiencies in the infant, toddler and young child exposed prenatally to cocaine (5,107). Cognitive differences, motor delays, language delays, and fine-motor problems have been identified across multiple studies, and there may be a dose-response effect of cocaine on newborn head circumference (108). However, many confounders of these effects have been identified, not the least of which is the abuse of alcohol by women using cocaine (109). Additionally the teratogenic effect of cocaine on the CNS, heart and genitourinary system are debated as results of large, controlled population studies provide contradictory findings (110).

Methamphetamine The National Toxicology Program Center for Evaluation of Risks to Human Reproduction evaluated the potential for reproductive problems with the therapeutic and nontherapeutic use of amphetamines (111). One of the major concerns of this group was the effect of other factors, including concurrent exposure to other drugs. The report concludes there is some concern about neurobehavioral alterations occurring with prenatal exposure to amphetamines. Additionally the group expressed some concern about growth, and an effect of methamphetamine on growth was found in the multicenter, longitudinal infant development, environment and lifestyle study, with these exposed infants showing higher rates of IUGR (112).

Tobacco Cigarette use exposes the fetus to carbon monoxide, nicotine, and tar, which contains multiple chemicals including cyanide and lead. Disruption of growth has been demonstrated in the animal model and is due to intrauterine hypoxia, a result of carbon monoxide and other metabolites causing reduced uterine blood flow (113). Nicotine is quickly absorbed, crosses the placenta, and is active in the developing CNS, causing developmental neurologic problems (114). An inverse relationship exists between birth weight and the number of cigarettes smoked per day. Neonates born to mothers who smoked during pregnancy weigh an average of 200 grams (range, 100 to 400 grams) less and have lower birth lengths than neonates born to mothers who did not smoke during pregnancy (115). Fortunately, a period of accelerated growth occurs during the first year of life, and generally no differences in body weight or length are observed among these infants at 1 year of age. Finally, neurobehavioral abnormalities have been identified in the newborn period in these infants (63). Multiple studies have examined the causal link between sudden infant death syndrome (SIDS) and smoking. Given the confounding effect of postnatal exposure to cigarette smoking, an analysis of more than 60 studies concluded that nearly one-third of SIDS deaths may be prevented with cessation of smoking in pregnancy (116).

Cannabis Delta-9-tetrahydrocannabinol, the active ingredient in cannabis, easily crosses the placenta, and the fetus is exposed to the active chemical as well as carbon monoxide. Studies of effects on neurodevelopment and growth have produced conflicting results. Additionally, the concurrent use of alcohol and tobacco in pregnancy confounds understanding of the teratogenicity of cannabis.

BREASTFEEDING

Women actively engaged in recovery, including those in addiction treatment, should be encouraged to breastfeed as long as urine drug screens are negative and the mother is negative for HIV (117,118). Breastfeeding builds a strong mother-infant bond while providing optimal nutrition and passive immunization for the child. Women with addiction may struggle with the responsibilities and role of parenthood, sometimes having lost custody of infants and children or having been exposed to addiction in their own families as children. Therefore, successful establishment of breastfeeding by a recovering woman is particularly empowering.

Women can breastfeed while on methadone maintenance (117,118). The American Academy of Pediatrics lists methadone as a medication compatible with breastfeeding (119). Nonetheless, women in methadone maintenance programs are sometimes discouraged from breastfeeding or are told that their "dose is too high." This is in spite of evidence that negligible amounts of methadone are excreted in human milk across the dose range; thus, there is no contraindication to nursing while prescribed methadone (118–122). Though little methadone is transferred in breast milk, small amounts may ease the neonatal withdrawal from opioids. In a study of 190 infant-mother pairs where the majority of the mothers were prescribed methadone, those infants who were breastfed had less severe NAS (123). Buprenorphine is appropriate to be continued for a woman who becomes pregnant while on maintenance treatment, and infants have been breastfed in these cases. Small amounts of buprenorphine are excreted in breast milk, so breastfeeding should also be encouraged in mothers prescribed buprenorphine (124).

An infant may be exposed to psychoactive drugs through breast milk if the mother relapses or is not yet in recovery from drug addiction. The substance-exposed nursing infant will display signs not dissimilar from those seen in the adult abusing a substance. Exposure to nicotine may cause irritability and poor feeding and disrupt sleep in the infant. Similarly, infants can become intoxicated and irritable with exposure to other stimulants such as cocaine and amphetamine. The infant may feed and sleep poorly, have gastrointestinal disturbance with vomiting or diarrhea, and may present with a seizure. Infants exposed to opioids may display intoxication with sedation and poor feeding or may exhibit withdrawal signs and become tremulous, restless, and feed and sleep poorly. Finally, the infant exposed to alcohol may feed and grow poorly, become diaphoretic, and have poor muscle tone. A mother ingesting more than 1g/kg of alcohol each day may have decreased milk letdown, belying the conventional wisdom that alcohol consumption increases letdown and milk production (119).

LEGAL ISSUES

Many states require hospitals to report pregnant women suspected of heavy alcohol or other drug use to local public health authorities or the criminal justice system when they present for delivery, whether she has or has not sought treatment. This reporting may cause SUPW to be even more wary of acknowledging that they have a problem. For this reason, it is very important for a physician who recognizes perinatal addiction to address this with the patient in a compassionate, nonjudgmental manner, thus advocating for both mother and child. Mandatory reporting of positive maternal drug screens or aggressive prosecution of SUPW may cause women to avoid disclosure of addiction during pregnancy. Some SUPW avoid prenatal care and hospital delivery, particularly if they have other children in the custody of Child Protective Services (CPS) or living with relatives, because they fear the loss of their children. However, mandatory reporting legislation may provide an incentive for SUPW to enter treatment prior to delivery in order to avoid potential prosecution. Continued custody of the child may be contingent upon adherence to a treatment plan determined by the CPS. Use of the criminal justice system for coercion to initiate addiction treatment is supported by improved outcomes when SUPW are allowed to retain custody of their infant (26). Every effort should be made to coordinate appropriate placement of the infant (with the mother, another family member, or in foster care) with addiction treatment so the mother can continue to build her bond with the infant. This provides positive motivation for the mother to attend treatment and enter recovery.

Across the nation, in many cases legislators and the courts have ruled that addiction in pregnancy is not a criminal matter (54). Education and support of SUPW about applicable state legislation can help enhance motivation to enter addiction treatment prior to delivery. Laws vary greatly, and criminal prosecution of SUPW should not be supported, as there is no evidence that punitive approaches work (6,125), and laws are often unclear regarding charges of child abuse for SUPW (125).

POSTPARTUM CARE

The link between parental addiction and child maltreatment has been known for many years (126) and has been recently affirmed in the Adverse Childhood Events Study (127). Effectively treating a parent is the most important intervention for the child exposed to substances, both prenatally and during their childhood (128). Particularly in the case of SUPW, the additional stresses of meeting the developmental needs of a newborn and older children, lack of family and social support, depression and other psychiatric problems, inadequate housing or homelessness, exposure to violence, and financial difficulties may pose as much risk to successful child rearing as the diagnosis of addiction (126,129). Comprehensive ongoing maternal addiction treatment, tailored to help the SUPW address other stressors besides addiction, reduces the chance of an adverse outcome for the child. Otherwise these factors can hamper the recovering woman's effectiveness as a parent, thus contributing to the risk of relapse to addiction (130).

If a mother is successful in treatment, she may be able to regain or retain custody of her children. For the woman whose children have been removed from her home, a goal of treatment and recovery should be reunification of her family. Prolonged hospitalization of newborns or foster care for children born to SUPW is an economic burden on society (19). Effective treatment and intervention is cost-effective in the short and long term and becomes the first and most effective prevention intervention for children. For SUPW without addiction, the goal of brief counseling is to prevent a return to hazardous substance use, particularly during a subsequent pregnancy.

After the birth, maternal treatment plans should be expanded to address newborn medical problems such as infection and developmental problems due to substance exposure. Bonding with the infant may be more difficult, so the mother may need to be taught specific skills to calm and feed her infant. Older children may need to be evaluated for developmental problems if the mother is concerned or gives a history of substance use in earlier pregnancies. Communication links developed during the pregnancy should be expanded to include physicians, social workers, and allied health professionals caring for the infant and older children. Such interventions can have a positive impact on development of every child in the family (126,131).

REFERENCES

1. Mitchell JL, Brown G. Physiological effects of cocaine, heroin, and methadone. In: Engs RC, ed. *Women: alcohol and other drugs*. Dubuque, IA: Kendall/Hunt Publishing Co., 1990:53–60.
2. Crome IB, Kumar MT. Epidemiology of drug and alcohol use in young women. *Semin Fetal Neonat Med* 2007;12:98–105.
3. Substance Abuse and Mental Health Services Administration. *Results from the 2003 National Survey on drug use and health: national findings*. Rockville, MD: Author, 2004.
4. National Institute on Drug Abuse. *National pregnancy health survey*. Rockville MD: Author, 1996.
5. Lester BM, El Sohly M, Wright LL, et al. The maternal lifestyle study: drug use by meconium toxicology and maternal self-report. *Pediatrics* 2001;107:309–317.
6. Bolnick JM, Rayburn WF. Substance use disorders in women: special considerations during pregnancy. *Obstet Gynecol Clin North Am* 2003;30:545–558.
7. Wright A, Walker J. Management of women who use drugs during pregnancy. *Semin Fetal Neonat Med* 2007;12:114–118.
8. Zuckerman B, Parker S, Hingson R, et al. Maternal psychoactive substance use and its effect on the neonate. In: Milunsky A, Friedman EA, Gluck L, eds. *Advances in perinatal medicine*. New York: Plenum Press, 1986:125–179.
9. Daley M, Argeriou M, McCarty D, et al. The costs of crime and the benefits of substance abuse treatment for pregnant women. *J Subst Abuse Treat* 2000;19:445–458.
10. Chang G, Wilkins-Haug L, Berman S, Goetz MA. Brief intervention for alcohol use in pregnancy: a randomized trial. *Addiction* 1999;94: 1499–1508.
11. Christmas JT, Knisely JS, Dawson KS, et al. Comparison of questionnaire screening and urine toxicology for detection of pregnancy complicated by substance use. *Obstet Gynecol* 1992;80:750–754.
12. Durham J, Owen P, Bender B, et al. Alcohol consumption among pregnant and childbearing-aged women: United States, 1991 and 1995. *MMWR* 1997;46:3–10.
13. Chapin J, Root W. Improving obstetrician-gynecologist implementation of smoking cessation guidelines for pregnant women: an interim report of the American College of Obstetricians and Gynecologists. *Nicotine Tobacco Res* 2004;6(Suppl 2):S253–S257.
14. Li CQ, Windsor RA, Perkins L, et al. The impact on infant birth weight and gestational age on cotinine-validated smoking reduction during pregnancy. *JAMA* 1993;269:1519–1524.
15. Benowitz NL, Dempsey DA. Pharmacotherapy for smoking cessation during pregnancy. *Nicotine Tobacco Res* 2004;6(Suppl 2):S189–S202.
16. Schroeder DR, Ogburn PL, Hurt RD, et al. Nicotine patch use in pregnancy smokers: smoking abstinence and delivery outcomes. *J Matern Fetal Neonat Med* 2002;11:100–107.
17. Glassroth J, Adam GD, Schnoll SH. The impact of substance abuse on the respiratory system. *Chest* 1987;91:596–602.
18. Warner EA. Is your patient using cocaine? Clinical signs that should raise suspicion. *Postgrad Med* 1995;Aug 98(2):173–176,180.
19. Weaver MF, Schnoll SH. Stimulants: amphetamines, cocaine. In: McCrady BS, Epstein EE, eds. *Addictions: a comprehensive guidebook*. New York: Oxford University Press, 1999:105–120.
20. Abel EL, Sokol RJ. Consequences of alcohol abuse. In: N Gleiche, ed. *Principles and practice of medical therapy in pregnancy*. New Haven, CT: Appleton & Lange, 1992:79–85.
21. Cooper JR, Altman F, Brown BS, et al. Research on the treatment of narcotic addiction: state of the art. In: *NIDA Treatment Research Monograph Series*. Rockville, MD: U.S. Department of Health and Human Services, 1983.
22. Coker AL, Smith PH, McKeown RE, et al. Frequency and correlates of intimate partner violence by type: physical, sexual, and psychological battering. *Am J Public Health* 2000;90:553–559.
23. Haller DL, Miles DR. Victimization and perpetration among perinatal substance abusers. *J Interpers Violence* 2003;18:760–780.
24. Martin SL, Kilgallen B, Dee DL, et al. Women in a prenatal care/substance abuse treatment program: links between domestic violence and mental health. *Matern Child Health J* 1998;2:85–94.
25. Weaver MF, Jarvis MAE, Schnoll SH. Role of the primary care physician in problems of substance abuse. *Arch Intern Med* 1999;159:913–924.
26. Nace EP, Birkmayer F, Sullivan MA, et al. Socially sanctioned coercion mechanisms for addiction treatment. *Am J Addict* 2007;16:15–23.
27. Roberts LW, Dunn LB. Ethical considerations in caring for women with substance use disorders. *Obstet Gynecol Clin North Am* 2003;30: 559–582.
28. Mondanaro J, Reed B. Current issues in the treatment of chemically dependent women. In: *NIDA Research Monograph Series*. Rockville, MD: U.S. Department of Health and Human Services, 1987.
29. Smith IE, Dent DZ, Coles CD, et al. A comparison study of treated and untreated pregnant and postpartum cocaine-abusing women. *J Subst Abuse Treat* 1992;9:343–348.
30. Waterson J, Ettorre B. Providing services for women with difficulties with alcohol or other drugs: the current U.K. situation as seen by women practitioners, researchers and policy makers in the field. *Drug Alcohol Depend* 1989;24:119–125.
31. Howell EM, Heiser N, Harrington M. A review of recent findings on substance abuse treatment for pregnant women. *J Subst Abuse Treat* 1999;16:195–219.

32. French MT, McCollister KE, Cacciola J, et al. Benefit of cost analysis of addiction treatment in Arkansas: specialty and standard residential programs for pregnant and parenting women. *Subst Abuse* 2002;23: 31–51.
33. Meyer M, Wagner K, Benvenuto A, et al. Intrapartum and postpartum analgesia for women maintained on methadone during pregnancy. *Obstet Gynecol* 2007;110:261–266.
34. Weaver MF, Schnoll SH. Abuse liability in opioid therapy for pain treatment in patients with an addiction history. *Clin J Pain* 2002;18: 561–569.
35. Preston KL, Bigelow GE, Liebson IA. Butorphanol-precipitated withdrawal in opioid-dependent human volunteers. *J Pharmacol Exp Ther* 1988;246:441–448.
36. Strain EC, Preston KL, Liebson IA, et al. Precipitated withdrawal by pentazocine in methadone-maintained volunteers. *J Pharmacol Exp Ther* 1993;267:624–634.
37. Fajemirokun-Odudeyi O, Sinha C, Tutty S, et al. Pregnancy outcome in women who use opiates. *Eur J Obstet Gynecol Reprod Biol* 2006;126: 170–175.
38. Lam SK, To WK, Duthie SJ, et al. Narcotic addiction in pregnancy with adverse maternal and perinatal outcome. *Aust N Z J Obstet Gynaecol* 1992;32:216–221.
39. Bada HS, Das A, Bauer CR, et al. Low birthweight and preterm births: etiologic fraction attributable to prenatal drug exposure. *J Perinatol* 2005;25:631–637.
40. Center for Substance Abuse Treatment. *Treatment Improvement Protocol 2: pregnant, substance-abusing women.* Rockville, MD: Author, 1993.
41. Wilson G. Clinical studies of infants and children exposed prenatally to heroin. *Ann N Y Acad Sci* 1989;562:183–194.
42. Berghella V, Lim PJ, Cherpes J, et al. Maternal methadone dose and neonatal withdrawal. *Am J Obstet Gynaecol* 2003;189:312–317.
43. Pond SM, Kreek MJ, Tong TG, et al. Altered methadone pharmacokinetics in methadone-maintained pregnant women. *J Pharmacol Exp Ther* 1985;233:1–6.
44. Wittmann BK, Segal S. A comparison of the effects of single- and split-dose methadone administration on the fetus: ultrasound evaluation. *Int J Addict* 1991:26:213–218.
45. Jarvis MAE, Wu-Pong S, Knisely JS, et al. Alterations in methadone metabolism during late pregnancy. *J Addict Dis* 1999;18:51–61.
46. Batey RG, Weissel K. A 40 month follow-up of pregnant drug using women treated at Westmead Hospital. *Drug Alcohol Rev* 1993;12: 265–270.
47. Fischer G, Etzersdorfer P, Eder H, et al. Buprenorphine maintenance in pregnant opiate addicts. *Eur Addict Res* 1998;4(Suppl 1):32–36.
48. Fischer G, Johnson RE, Eder H, et al. Treatment of opioid-dependent pregnant women with buprenorphine. *Addiction* 2000;95:239–244.
49. Jones HE, Johnson RE, Jasinski DR, et al. Randomized controlled study transitioning opioid-dependent pregnant women from short-acting morphine to buprenorphine or methadone. *Drug Alcohol Depend* 2005; 79:1–10.
50. Ebner N, Rohrmeister K, Winklbaur B, et al. Management of neonatal abstinence syndrome in neonates born to opioid maintained women. *Drug Alcohol Depend* 2007;87:131–138.
51. Fischer G, Ortner R, Rohrmeister K, et al. Methadone versus buprenorphine in pregnant addicts: a double-blind, double-dummy comparison study. *Addiction* 2006;101:275–281.
52. Schindler SD, Eder H, Ortner R, et al. Neonatal outcome following buprenorphine maintenance during conception and throughout pregnancy. *Addiction* 2003;98:103–110.
53. Jessup M, Green JR. Treatment of the pregnant alcohol-dependent woman. *J Psychoactive Drugs* 1987;19:193–203.
54. Harris LH, Paltrow L. The status of pregnant women and fetuses in us criminal law. *JAMA* 2003;289:1697–1699.
55. Gareri G, Klein G, Koren J. Drugs of abuse testing in meconium. *Clin Chim Acta* 2006;366:101–111.
56. Wingert WE, Feldman MS, Kim MH, et al. A comparison of meconium, maternal urine and neonatal urine for detection of maternal drug use during pregnancy. *J Forens Sci* 1994;39:150–158.
57. Montgomery D, Plate C, Alder SC, et al. Testing for fetal exposure to illicit drugs using umbilical cord tissue vs. meconium. *J Perinatol* 2006; 26:11–14.
58. Chan D, Klein J, Koraskov T, et al. Fetal exposure to alcohol as evidenced by fatty acid ethyl esters in meconium in the absence of maternal history for drinking in pregnancy. *Ther Drug Monitor* 2004;26: 474–481.
59. Caprara D, Klein J, Koren G. Baseline measures of fatty acid ethyl esters in hair of neonates born to abstaining or mild social drinking mothers. *Ther Drug Monitor* 2005;27:811–815.
60. Finnegan LP, Kaltenbach K. Neonatal abstinence syndrome. In: Hoekelman RA, Friedman SB, Nelson NM, Seidel HM, eds. *Primary pediatric care,* 2nd ed. St. Louis: Mosby, 1992:1367–1378.
61. American Academy of Pediatrics, Committee on Drugs. Neonatal drug withdrawal. *Pediatrics* 1998;101:1079–1088.
62. Karmel BZ, Gardner JM. Prenatal cocaine exposure effects on arousal-modulated attention during the neonatal period. *Dev Psychobiol* 1996; 29:463–480.
63. Law KL, Stroud LR, LaGasse LL, et al. Smoking during pregnancy and newborn neurobehavior. *Pediatrics* 2003;111:1318–1323.
64. Pichini S, Garcia-Algar O. In utero exposure to smoking and newborn neurobehavior: how to assess neonatal withdrawal syndrome? *Ther Drug Monit* 2006;28:288–290.
65. Chiriboga CA, Kuhn L, Wasserman GA. Prenatal cocaine exposures and dose-related cocaine effects on infant tone and behavior. *Neurotoxicol Teratol* 2007;29:323–330.
66. Fischer G, Jagsch R, Eder H, et al. Comparison of methadone and slow-release morphine maintenance in pregnant addicts. *Addiction* 1999; 94:231–239.
67. Desmond MM, Schwanecke RP, Wilson GS, et al. Maternal barbiturate utilization and neonatal withdrawal symptomatology. *J Pediatr* 1972; 80:190–197.
68. Steg N. Narcotic withdrawal reactions in the newborn. *Am J Dis Child* 1957;94:286–288.
69. Desmond MM, Wilson GS. Neonatal abstinence syndrome: recognition and diagnosis. *Addict Dis Int J* 1975;2:113–121.
70. Fischer G. Treatment of opioid dependence in pregnant women. *Addiction* 2000;95:1141–1144.
71. Lejeune C, Simmat-Durand L, Gourarier L, et al. Prospective multicenter observational study of 260 infants born to 259 opiate-dependent mothers on methadone or high-dose buprenorphine substitution. *Drug Alcohol Depend* 2006;82:250–257.
72. Sarkar S, Donn SM. Management of neonatal abstinence syndrome in neonatal intensive care units: a national survey. *J Perinatol* 2006;26: 15–17.
73. Lipsitz PJ. A proposed narcotic withdrawal score for use with newborn infants: a pragmatic evaluation of its efficacy. *Clin Pediatr* 1975;14: 592–594.
74. Boukydis CFZ, Bigsby R, Lester BM. Clinical use of the Neonatal Intensive Care Unit Network Behavioural Scale. *Pediatrics* 2004;113:679–689.
75. Theis JG, Selby P, Ikizler Y, et al. Current management of the neonatal abstinence syndrome: a critical analysis of the evidence. *Biol Neonate* 1997;71:345–356.
76. Osborn DA, Jeffery HE, Cole M. Opiate treatment for opiate withdrawal in newborn infants. *Cochrane Database Syst Rev* 2005;3: CD002059.
77. Osborn DA, Jeffery HE, Cole MJ. Sedatives for opiate withdrawal in newborn infants. *Cochrane Database Syst Rev* 2005;3:CD002053.
78. Coyle MG, Ferguson A, Lagasse L, et al. Neurobehavioral effects of treatment for opiate withdrawal. *Arch Dis Child Fetal Neonat Ed* 2005; 90:73–74.
79. Kandall SR, Doberczak TM, Mauer KR, et al. Opiate vs. CNS depressant therapy in neonatal drug abstinence syndrome. *Am J Dis Child* 1983;137:378–382.
80. Jackson L, Ting A, McKay S, et al. A randomised controlled trial of morphine versus phenobarbitone for neonatal abstinence syndrome. *Arch Dis Child Fetal Neonat Ed* 2004;89:300–304.
81. Wunsch MJ. A chart review comparing paregoric to methadone in the treatment of neonatal opioid withdrawal. *J Addict Dis* 2006;25:27–33.

82. Robe LB, Gromisch DS, Iosub S. Symptoms of neonatal ethanol withdrawal. *Curr Alcohol* 1981;8:485–493.
83. Pagliaro LA, Pagliaro AM. Drugs as human teratogens and fetotoxins. In: Pagliaro LA, Pagliaro AM, eds. *Problems in pediatric drug therapy,* 4th ed. Washington, DC: American, 2002.
84. Shankaran S, Das A, Bauer CR, et al. Association between patterns of maternal substance use and infant birth weight, length, and head circumference. *Pediatrics* 2004;114;226–234.
85. Aase JM, Jones KL, Clarren SK. Do we need the term "FAE"? *Pediatrics* 1995;95:428–430.
86. Stratton KR, Howe CJ, Battaglia FC. *Fetal alcohol syndrome: diagnosis, epidemiology, prevention, and treatment.* Washington, DC: National Academy Press, 1996.
87. Hoyme HE, May PA, Kalberg WO, et al. A practical clinical approach to diagnosis of fetal alcohol spectrum disorders: clarification of the 1996 Institute of Medicine criteria. *Pediatrics* 2005;115:39–47.
88. Sokol RJ, Delaney-Black V, Nordstrom B. Fetal alcohol spectrum disorder. *JAMA* 2003;290:2996–2999.
89. Astley SJ, Clarren SK. *Diagnostic guide for fetal alcohol syndrome and related conditions: the 4-digit diagnostic code,* 2nd ed. Seattle: University Publication Services, 1999.
90. Jones KL, Smith DW. Recognition of the fetal alcohol syndrome in early infancy. *Lancet* 1973;2:999–1001.
91. Bertrand J, Floyd LL, Weber MK. Guidelines for identifying and referring persons with fetal alcohol syndrome. *MMWR Recomm Rep* 2005;54(RR-11):1–14.
92. May PA, Gossage JP. Estimating the prevalence of fetal alcohol syndrome: a summary. *Alcohol Res Health* 2001;25:159–167.
93. Sampson PD, Streissguth AP, Bookstein FL, et al. Incidence of fetal alcohol syndrome and prevalence of alcohol-related neurodevelopmental disorder. *Teratology* 1997;56:317–326.
94. Nakane Y, Okuma T, Takahashi R, et al. Multi-institutional study on the teratogenicity and fetal toxicity of antiepileptic drugs: a report of a collaborative study group in Japan. *Epilepsia* 1980;21:663–680.
95. Holmes LB, Wyszinski DF, Lieberman E. The AED Pregnancy Registry: a 6 year experience. *Arch Neurol* 2004;61:673–678.
96. Pagliaro AM, Pagliaro LA. *Substance use among children and adolescents: its nature, extent, and effects from conception to adulthood.* New York: John Wiley & Sons, 1996.
97. Iqual MM, Sobhan T, Ryals T. Effects of commonly used benzodiazepines on the foetus, the neonate and the nursing infant. *Psychiatr Ser* 2002;53:39–49.
98. Bergman U, Rosa FW, Baum C, et al. Effects of exposure to benzodiazepine during fetal life. *Lancet* 1992;19:340:694–696.
99. Wikner BN, Stiller CO, Bergman U, et al. Use of benzodiazepines and benzodiazepine receptor agonists during pregnancy: neonatal outcome and congenital malformations. *Pharmacoepidemiol Drug Safety* 2007;16:1203–1210.
100. Sanchis A, Rosique D, Catala J. Adverse effects of maternal lorazepam on neonates. DICP. *Ann Pharmacother* 1991;25:1137–1138.
101. Mellin GW. Drugs in the first trimester of pregnancy and fetal life of Homo sapiens. *Am J Obstet Gynecol* 1964;90:1169–1180.
102. Cobrinik RW, Hood RT Jr, Chusid E. The effect of maternal narcotic addiction on the newborn infant. *Pediatrics* 1959;24:288–304.
103. Pagliaro AM, Pagliaro LA. *Substance use among women.* Philadelphia: Brunner/Mazel, 2000.
104. Wunsch MJ, Stanard V, Schnoll SH. Treatment of Pain in Pregnancy. *Clin J Pain* 2003;19:148–155.
105. Scanlon JW. The neuroteratology of cocaine: background, theory, and clinical implications. *Reprod Toxicol* 1991;5:89–98.
106. Chiriboga CA. Fetal effects. *Neurol Clin* 1993;11:707–728.
107. Lester BM, Tronick EZ, LaGasse L, et al. The maternal lifestyle study: effects of substance exposure during pregnancy on neurodevelopmental outcome in 1-monthold infants. *Pediatrics* 2002;110:1182–1192.
108. Bateman DA, Chiriboga CA. Dose-response effect of cocaine on newborn head circumference. *Pediatrics* 2000;106:E33.
109. Lumeng JC, Howard J, Cabral HJ, et al. Pre-natal exposures to cocaine and alcohol and physical growth patterns to age 8 years. *Neurotoxicol Teratol* 2007;29:446–457.
110. Vidaeff AC, Mastrobattista JM. In utero cocaine exposure: a thorny mix of science and mythology. *Am J Perinatol* 2003;20:165–172.
111. Golub M, Costa L, Crofton K, et al. NTP-CERHR expert panel report on the reproductive and developmental toxicity of amphetamine and methamphetamine. *Birth Defects Res B Dev Reprod Toxicol* 2005;74:471–584.
112. Smith LM, LaGasse LL, Derauf C, et al. The infant development, environment, and lifestyle study: effects of prenatal methamphetamine exposure, polydrug exposure, and poverty on intrauterine growth. *Pediatrics* 2006;118:1149–1156.
113. Suzuki K, Minei LJ, Johnson EE. Effect of nicotine upon uterine blood flow in the pregnant rhesus monkey. *Am J Obstet Gynecol* 1980;136: 1009–1013.
114. Levin ED, Slotkin TA. Developmental neurotoxicity of nicotine. In: Slikker W, Chang LW, eds. *Handbook of developmental neurotoxicity.* Academic Press, 1998:587–615.
115. Andres RL, Day MC. Perinatal complications associated with maternal tobacco use. *Semin Neonatol* 2000;5:231–241.
116. Mitchell EA, Milerad J. Smoking and the sudden infant death syndrome. *Rev Environ Health* 2006;21:81–103.
117. McCarthy JJ, Posey BL. Methadone levels in human milk. *J Hum Lact* 2000;16:115–120.
118. Geraghty B, Graham EA, Logan B, et al. Methadone levels in breast milk. *J Hum Lact* 1997;13:227–230.
119. American Academy of Pediatrics, Committee on Drugs. The transfer of drugs and other chemicals into human milk. *Pediatrics* 2001;108:776–789.
120. Jansson LM, Velez M, Harrow C. Methadone maintenance and lactation: a review of the literature and current management guidelines. *J Hum Lact* 2004;20:62–71.
121. Wojnar-Horton RE, Kristensen JH, Yapp P, et al. Methadone distribution and excretion into breast milk of clients in a methadone maintenance programme. *Br J Clin Pharmacol* 1997;44:543–547.
122. Kuschel CA, Austerberry L, Cornwell M, et al. Can methadone concentrations predict the severity of withdrawal in infants at risk of neonatal abstinence syndrome? *Arch Dis Child Fetal Neonatal Ed* 2004;89: 390–393.
123. Abdul-Latif ME, Piner J, Clews S, et al. Effects of breast milk on severity and outcome of neonatal abstinence syndrome in infants of drug-dependent mothers. *Pediatrics* 2006;17:1163–1169.
124. Marquet P, Chevrel J, Lavignasse P, et al. Buprenorphine withdrawal syndrome in a newborn. *Clin Pharmacol Ther* 1997;62:569–571.
125. Abel EL, Kruger M. Physician attitudes concerning legal coercion of pregnant alcohol and drug abusers. *Am J Obstet Gynecol* 2002;186: 768–772.
126. Nair P, Schuler ME, Black MM, et al. Cumulative environmental risk in substance abusing women: early intervention, parenting stress, child abuse potential and child development. *Child Abuse Neglect* 2003;27: 997–1017.
127. Dube SR, Felitti VJ, Dong M, et al. Childhood abuse, neglect, and household dysfunction and the risk of illicit drug use: the adverse childhood experiences study. *Pediatrics* 2003;111:564–572.
128. Johnson JL, Leff M. Children of substance abusers: overview of research findings. *Pediatrics* 1999;103:1085–1099.
129. Kettinger LA, Nair P, Schuler ME. Exposure to environmental risk factors and parenting attitudes among substance-abusing women. *Am J Drug Alcohol Abuse* 2000;26:1–11.
130. Ingersoll KS, Lu IL, Haller DL. Predictors of in-treatment relapse in perinatal substance abusers and impact on treatment retention: a prospective study. *J Psychoactive Drugs* 1995;27:375–387.
131. Kumpfer KL, Fowler MA. Parenting skills and family support programs for drug abusing mothers. *Semin Fetal Neonatal Med* 2007;12: 132–142.

SUGGESTED READINGS

Arellano CM. Child maltreatment and substance use: a review of the literature. *Subst Use Misuse* 1996;31:927–935.

CHAPTER 82

Daniel P. Alford, MD, MPH, FACP

Surgical Interventions in the Alcohol- or Drug-Using Patient

Surgery may be required for complications of drug and alcohol use such as the management of traumatic injuries, infections of the skin, soft tissue, bones and joints, infective endocarditis, and certain cancers. Because of the high prevalence of substance use, patients who use substances will be among those who are planning to undergo surgery that is unrelated to drug and alcohol use complications. Active substance use and its associated chronic medical conditions can increase the risk of postoperative complications. In a retrospective study of patients presenting with traumatic mandibular fractures in which two thirds had a history of alcohol or drug abuse, postoperative complications including wound infections and poor healing were up to five times more likely in groups with substance abuse compared with nonusers (1). Hospitalization for surgery may be the first time that an addicted patient does not have access to alcohol or other drugs, putting them at risk for withdrawal. Acute withdrawal syndromes may complicate surgery and the postoperative course by presenting as tachycardia, hypertension, anxiety, delirium, pain, and seizures. Therefore providers of perioperative care must identify addiction disorders and be comfortable with the management of substance withdrawal syndromes. The care of patients with addiction disorders is also complicated by a potential mutual distrust that exists between patients and their medical team, with physician fear of being deceived and patient fear of being mistreated and stigmatized (2). Often, preoperative evaluations can be deceivingly simple in this patient population because they are often without known chronic illnesses. However, careful evaluation may detect clinical signs of chronic diseases secondary to alcohol or drug use that increase surgical risk, such as diseases affecting the heart, lungs, kidney, liver, nervous system, and pancreas. In addition, the physiologic stress associated with surgery may bring out subclinical comorbidities not obvious during routine preoperative evaluation. Treating physicians should not expect to cure the patient's alcohol or drug problem during the hospitalization, but should focus on getting the patient through the perioperative period safely and then offering the patient referral to long-term addiction treatment. This chapter focuses on relevant perioperative issues in the alcohol- or drug-using patient.

PERIOPERATIVE CARE OF THE ALCOHOL-DEPENDENT PATIENT

Unhealthy alcohol use is common especially in patients seeking medical and surgical care (3). The prevalence of alcohol use disorders is as high as 40% in emergency room and various surgical inpatient settings and up to 50% in patients with trauma (4). Many chronic medical conditions that can complicate or necessitate surgery, including dilated cardiomyopathy, cirrhosis, pancreatitis, and oral and esophageal cancers, are attributable to alcohol. Alcohol withdrawal is common in hospitalized patients and is up to five times higher in surgical and trauma patients (5). Chronic alcohol use can increase the risk of postoperative complications through immune suppression, reduced cardiac function, and dysregulated homeostasis including alterations in platelet production, aggregation, and changes in fibrinogen levels (6–8). Therefore preoperative screening for alcohol use disorders and withdrawal risk is important.

Preoperative Evaluation In addition to a complete history and physical examination, the preoperative evaluation should assess for the risk of acute alcohol withdrawal and the presence of diseases associated with chronic alcohol use. Physicians often fail to identify alcohol use disorders in medical patients (9). In one study, only 16% of people with alcoholism were identified in the perioperative setting (10). The amount of alcohol consumed is a risk factor for hospital admission (11) and postoperative complications (7). When screening for alcohol use disorders, it is important to remember that patients with unhealthy alcohol use are often asymptomatic and often minimize consumption. Quantity and frequency questions are essential, but are generally not sensitive or specific, with the exception of specific items that have been validated for this purpose (see Chapter 18, "Screening and Brief Intervention"). Laboratory tests such as blood alcohol levels and liver function tests are not sensitive or specific. Adults undergoing preoperative evaluation should be screened using validated questionnaires such as the CAGE questionnaire (see below) or the Alcohol Use Disorder Identification Test. The CAGE (12) questionnaire is brief; however, it is designed to detect alcohol dependence and focuses on the consequences of drinking and may remain positive in patients who are in recovery. The CAGE mnemonic refers the following questions.

Have you ever felt you should *C*ut down on your drinking?
Have people *A*nnoyed you by criticizing your drinking?
Have you ever felt bad or *G*uilty about drinking?
Have you ever taken a drink first thing in the morning (*E*ye-opener) to steady your nerves or get rid of a hangover?

Two or more positive replies to the CAGE questionnaire has a sensitivity of 74% to 78% and specificity of 76% to 96% and is therefore highly suggestive of alcohol dependence (13,14). The Alcohol Use Disorder Identification Test questionnaire is longer, but detects a fuller spectrum of unhealthy alcohol use (15). Screening is covered in more detail in Chapter 18, "Screening and Brief Intervention." Other historical findings suggestive of unhealthy alcohol use include a history of traumatic injuries, marital, social and legal problems, homelessness, and a history of withdrawal and blackout episodes (16). Screening preoperatively in the surgical setting differs from screening in other settings. In the surgical setting, screening for risk of withdrawal and medical comorbidities are the priorities. Consider including one or more of the following questions regarding alcohol withdrawal in the preoperative evaluation:

1. Have you ever gone through alcohol withdrawal, such as having the shakes?
2. Have you ever had problems or gotten sick when you stopped drinking?
3. Have you ever had a seizure or *delirium tremens*, been confused, after cutting down or stopping drinking?

The spectrum of withdrawal ranges from mild tremor, hallucinosis, to seizures and delirium tremens. In the postoperative period, withdrawal can mimic many postoperative complications including acute pain and sepsis. The incidence of alcohol withdrawal in hospitalized patients is as high as 8% and is two to five times higher in hospitalized trauma and surgical patients (6,17). Risk factors associated with severe and prolonged alcohol withdrawal include amount and duration of alcohol use, prior withdrawal episodes, recurrent detoxifications, older age, and comorbid diseases (18). It also important to note that sedatives (e.g., benzodiazepines) and analgesics (e.g., opioids) given during surgery and the postoperative period may delay, partially treat, or obscure some symptoms of alcohol withdrawal. It is important to assess for other drug use as well, because many patients with alcohol abuse use other substances such as benzodiazepines and cocaine. Physical examination should evaluate for evidence of liver, pancreatic, nervous system, and cardiac disease. The spectrum of alcoholic liver disease ranges from fatty liver with normal or mild elevations in liver function tests to acute hepatitis and cirrhosis. Clinical evidence of cirrhosis including jaundice, palmar erythema, gynecomastia, testicular atrophy, spider telangiectases, as well as findings consistent with portal vein hypertension namely splenomegaly, ascites, hemorrhoids, and caput medusa (dilation of the periumbilical veins on the abdominal wall) should be looked for. Pancreatitis can present as acute and chronic abdominal pain as well as exocrine (i.e., malabsorption) and endocrine dysfunction (i.e., glucose intolerance to diabetes mellitus). Pancreatitic calcifications seen on abdominal imaging studies are another clue to chronic pancreatitis. Alcohol-associated dementia occurs in approximately 9% of alcoholics (19). Korsakoff syndrome, hepatic and Wernicke encephalopathy, myelopathies, and polyneuropathies are other nervous system disorders associated with chronic alcohol abuse. These neurologic conditions can worsen during the perioperative period and may be confused with other postoperative neurologic complications. Therefore preoperative baseline mental status and cognition should be assessed and documented. Preoperative evaluation for congestive heart failure should be considered because up to one third of patients with long-standing alcohol abuse have a decreased cardiac ejection fraction (20). Because of the association between alcohol abuse and nicotine dependence, smoking related comorbidities such as coronary heart disease and chronic obstructive pulmonary disease (COPD) should also be evaluated for. Up to 20% of alcohol-dependent patients were found to suffer from COPD in one series (21). Preoperative laboratory studies should include electrolytes, liver function and synthetic tests, coagulation studies, and a complete blood count. Anemia is common in patients with alcohol dependence as well as decreased platelet count from alcohol-associated bone marrow suppression and splenic sequestration. Preexisting anemia may need to be treated preoperatively because these patients are at increased risk of perioperative bleeding secondary to coagulopathies and thrombocytopenia (22). It is also important to identify patients who are in recovery preoperatively because they may have concerns and questions about perioperative exposure to sedative hypnotics and opioid analgesics.

Management of Alcohol Withdrawal One of the most common complications of hospitalized alcohol-dependent patients is withdrawal, with up to 15% at risk for developing seizures or *delirium tremens* (23). The spectrum of alcohol withdrawal ranges from minor symptoms of autonomic hyperactivity including diaphoresis, tachycardia, systolic hypertension to tremor, insomnia, hallucinations, nausea, vomiting, psychomotor agitation, anxiety, and grand mal seizures to life-threatening delirium tremens. In one study, 20% of the alcohol dependent patients admitted to a surgical service developed *delirium tremens* after admission (24). Withdrawal symptoms may appear within hours of decreased intake; however, during the perioperative period, the administration of anesthetics, sedatives, and analgesics may delay the onset of withdrawal for up to 14 days (25). Recognizing withdrawal risk and treating early withdrawal can often prevent the complications of severe withdrawal. Because alcohol withdrawal is especially dangerous during the postoperative period, asymptomatic but at-risk patients should receive prophylactic treatment to prevent withdrawal. Although many medications have been used to treat alcohol withdrawal, benzodiazepines are the drugs of choice for both the prevention and management of alcohol withdrawal (26,27). Preferably benzodiazepines with a long half-life such as diazepam or chlordiazepoxide should be chosen. However, patients with severe liver disease should receive a short-acting agent such as lorazepam to avoid excessive and prolonged sedation. Treatment of withdrawal should be based on the severity of symptoms and signs. The Clinical Institute Withdrawal Assessment Scale for Alcohol, revised, is a validated tool that can be used to rate the severity for alcohol withdrawal (28). This 10-item scale can be completed rapidly and easily at the bedside. Use of the Clinical Institute Withdrawal Assessment Scale for Alcohol, revised, may be difficult to use in the postoperative period in patients unable to verbally communicate and may be less reliable in patients with acute medical or surgical illnesses. Goals for management of alcohol withdrawal include: treatment of withdrawal symptoms, prevention of initial and recurrent seizures, and prevention and treatment of *delirium tremens* (23).

Alcohol Use and Surgical Risk In addition to alcohol withdrawal, numerous observational studies have demonstrated that heavy alcohol use even in the absence of clinical liver disease and even in the absence of alcohol dependence *per se* is an independent risk factor for postoperative complications. Higher rates of postoperative complications were seen after transurethral prostatectomy, colonic surgery, and hysterectomy (29–31). There is a dose-response effect, with increased alcohol consumption in grams being associated with both increased postoperative complications and prolonged hospital stay. The most dramatic differences were in groups who drank greater than 60 g of alcohol (4–5 drinks) per day (32). The postoperative complications reported were an increased rate of infection, bleeding, and delayed wound healing. In a prospective study of patients having colorectal surgery, Tonnesen et al. found an increase in postoperative arrhythmias (33). Patients with chronic alcohol problems also have longer intensive care unit stays, more postoperative septicemia, and pneumonia requiring mechanical ventilation as well as increased overall mortality (34). Five possible pathologic mechanisms have been identified to account for the increased rate of postoperative complications including immune incompetence, subclinical cardiac insufficiency, hemostatic imbalances, abnormal stress response, and wound healing dysfunction (6,7). Chronic alcohol use suppresses T cell–dependent activity and decreases macrophage, monocyte and neutrophil mobilization, and phagocytosis. This immune dysfunction is reversible after abstinence (32). The decrease cardiac function associated with chronic alcohol use is thought to be secondary to direct alteration in the electromechanical coupling and contractility of cardiac myocytes. This alcohol-associated cardiac dysfunction may be reversible, with 50% of patients showing improvement after 6 months of abstinence (35). The hemostatic dysfunction in alcoholics is due to a modification in coagulation and fibrinolysis pathways as well as a decrease in the number and function of platelets (32). Wound healing problems seems related to poor accumulation of collagen (32). Abstinence before surgery decreases postoperative morbidity. Tonnesen et al. preoperatively randomized adults who drank at least five drinks per day who were scheduled for elective colorectal surgery to abstinence for 1 month before surgery versus a usual-care group (36). They observed fewer complications in the abstinent group compared with the usual-care group; however, there was no difference in length of stay or mortality. This is the first study to demonstrate that preoperative abstinence can lead to improved postoperative outcomes.

Alcoholic Liver Disease The spectrum of liver disease associated with the spectrum of unhealthy alcohol use (i.e., risky use to alcohol dependence) includes asymptomatic fatty liver, to acute hepatitis, and finally chronic cirrhosis. Each form of liver disease carries some degree of surgical risk and requires special preoperative considerations.

Alcoholic Fatty Liver Alcoholic fatty liver (hepatic steatosis) occurs in 90% of heavy drinkers and is often asymptomatic and reversible. It can occur after binge or "social" drinking. Signs and symptoms when present include nausea, vomiting, and right upper quadrant pain and tenderness. Laboratory tests often demonstrate a mild elevation in liver transaminases but with preserved liver function with normal bilirubin, albumin, and coagulation studies. These signs and symptoms usually resolve within two weeks of abstinence (37). Patients with fatty liver seem to tolerate surgery well (38); however, there are no known studies evaluating perioperative risk in these patients. It is prudent to delay elective surgery until resolution of clinical signs and symptoms and if possible, abstinence is achieved.

Alcoholic Hepatitis Alcoholic hepatitis is a serious inflammatory disease of the liver, which occurs in up to 40% of heavy drinkers. The pathologic mechanisms include hepatocyte swelling, liver infiltration with polymorphonuclear cells, and hepatocyte necrosis. These patients often present extremely ill with nausea, vomiting, anorexia, abdominal pain, fever, and jaundice. Elevated transaminases and prolonged coagulation studies are common. Surgical risk is very high in this group, with 100% mortality rates reported in older series (39). Therefore alcoholic hepatitis should be considered a contraindication to elective surgery. It is recommended that elective surgery be delayed until clinical and laboratory parameters normalize, sometimes taking up to 12 weeks.

Alcoholic Cirrhosis Cirrhosis occurs in 15% to 20% of heavy drinkers and refers to the irreversible necrosis, nodular regeneration, and fibrosis of the liver. Cirrhosis is associated with abnormal hepatic circulation, resulting in portal vein hypertension. Clinically, patients may present with ascites, peripheral edema, poor nutritional status, muscle wasting, coagulopathies, gastrointestinal bleeding from esophageal varices, encephalopathy, and renal insufficiency as well as hypoxia secondary to hepatopulmonary syndrome and pulmonary hypertension. The need for surgery is common in patients with cirrhosis, with up to 10% requiring a surgical procedure during the last 2 years of life (40). Depending on the stage of cirrhotic disease, surgery can be extremely risky. The most common causes of perioperative mortality in cirrhotic patients are sepsis, hemorrhage, and hepatorenal syndrome (41). Although currently used anesthetic agents are not hepatotoxic, surgical stress in itself causes hemodynamic changes in the liver resulting in postoperative elevations in liver function tests in patients with no underlying liver disease (42). Patients with underlying liver dysfunction are at increased risk for hepatic decompensation during surgical stress because anesthetic agents decrease hepatic blood flow by as much as 50% and therefore decrease hepatic oxygen uptake (43). Intraoperative traction on abdominal viscera may also decrease hepatic blood flow.

Effect of Cirrhosis on Surgical Risk Surgery in patients with cirrhosis is high risk. A study of patients undergoing total knee arthroplasty found that both local and systemic complications were as high as 44% in patients with cirrhosis versus 6% in a control group (44). The preoperative factors associated with increased surgical morbidity and mortality include: emergent surgery, upper abdominal surgery, poor hepatic synthetic function, anemia, ascites, malnutrition, and encephalopathy (45). These patients are at increased risk for uncontrolled bleeding, infections, and delirium. Coagulopathies and thrombocytopenia result in difficult perioperative hemostasis. Ascites increases the risk of intraabdominal infections, abdominal wound dehiscence, and abdominal wall herniation. Nutritional deficiencies result in poor wound healing and an increased risk of skin breakdown and encephalopathy decreases the patient's ability to effectively participate in postoperative rehabilitation. The action of anesthetic agents may be prolonged and increases the risk of delirium. Cholecystectomy is a particularly risky surgery in patients with cirrhosis and portal hypertension because of intraabdominal collateral circulation. This collateral circulation increases the vascularity of the gallbladder bed and places the patient at greater risk for severe perioperative hemorrhage. In a group of patients with cirrhosis undergoing cholecystectomy, those considered decompensated preoperatively by presence of ascites and prolonged coagulation studies had an 83% morality rate compared with 10% in compensated patients (46). In trying to risk stratify patient preoperatively, it is important to look for clinical signs of cirrhosis and portal hypertension. There are two scoring systems in use to predict whether patients with advance liver disease will survive surgery (47). Using a multivariate clinical assessment, the Child and Turcotte Classification made it possible to risk stratify patients with cirrhosis preoperatively. In 1964, the Child and Turcotte Classification stratified cirrhotic patients into three classes based on "hepatic reserve" and therefore surgical risk before portocaval shunt surgery (48). Class A was the most compensated, whereas Class C was the most decompensated group. Variables included laboratory values of bilirubin, and albumin as well as clinical ascites, encephalopathy and nutritional status. Garrison found good correlation between Child and Turcotte Class and abdominal surgical mortality with Class A, B, and C mortality rates of 10%, 31%, and 76%, respectively (49). Some of the limitations of the Child and Turcotte Classification scheme included the subjective nature and interobserver variation in the assessment of nutritional status, encephalopathy, and ascites. In addition, there was variability in the assigning of patients to classes A, B, and C and no accounting for the nature and urgency of the surgical procedure. In an attempt to decrease the subjective nature of the classification scheme, Pugh et al. modified the Child and Turcotte Classification (Table 82.1) (50). The Pugh modification separates hepatic encephalopathy into five grades depending on various signs and symptoms (Table 82.2). The subjective evaluation of nutritional status is changed to objective measured prolongation in prothrombin time and the assignment of class based on a total point score. Using pooled surgical data, the Pugh Classification scheme has proven to be a good preoperative risk stratifier (Table 82.3).

A second scoring system is the Model for End-Stage Liver Disease (MELD), which was designed to predict survival after transjugular intrahepatic portosystemic shunt treatment of bleeding esophageal varices (51). The MELD score is used to prioritize patients for liver transplantation and, more recently, as a predictor of survival after nontransplant surgery (52). The MELD score can be calculated by using an online MELD score calculator at *http://www.unos.org/resources/meldpeldcalculator.asp*.

Preoperative Considerations in Patients with Cirrhosis
Preoperative abstinence should be the goal before all elective procedures. Because coagulopathies may develop as a result of vitamin K deficiency due to malnutrition or intestinal bile salt deficiency, attempts at correction should start with the administration of vitamin K. If there is no effect in 12 hours, it is most likely secondary to decreased hepatic production of coagulation factors and perioperative use of fresh frozen plasma should be considered. Thrombocytopenia secondary to bone marrow

TABLE 82.1 Pugh Classification (Modified Child and Turcotte Classification)

	Points		
	1	2	3
Encephalopathy (grade)	None	1–2	3–4
Ascites	Absent	Slight	Moderate
Bilirubin (mg/dL)	1–2	2–3	>3
Albumin (g/dL)	>3.5	2.8–3.5	<2.8
Prothrombin time (seconds prolonged)	1–3	4–6	>6
International normalized ratio	<1.7	1.7–2.3	>2.3

Class A 5–6 points
Class B 7–9 points
Class C 10–15 points

Adapted from Pugh RN, Murray-Lyon IM, Dawson JL, et al. Transection of the oesophagus for bleeding oesophageal varices. *Br J Surg* 1973;60:646–649.

suppression, hypersplenism, and splenic sequestration should be treated with prophylactic platelet transfusions when counts fall below 20,000/mm^3 (40). In addition, units of packed red blood cells should be on hold in the blood bank. Ascites secondary to portal hypertension and hypoalbuminemia can impede abdominal wall healing, increase the risk of abdominal wall dehiscence and herniation, and restrict effective mechanical ventilation. Therefore ascites should be optimally managed preoperatively with sodium restriction and appropriate diuretic therapy. In patients with peripheral edema, a more aggressive approach including large volume paracentesis (≥5 L) should be considered. Electrolytes should be monitored closely. Perioperative hemodynamic monitoring is often needed because these patients may have large fluid shifts, especially during abdominal surgeries. Preoperative broad-spectrum antibiotics (e.g., norfloxacin, ciprofloxacin) should be considered as prophylaxis against secondary and spontaneous bacterial peritonitis. Renal function should be monitored closely. Perioperative changes in volume status and hemodynamics may adversely affect renal function. These patients are at risk for renal insufficiency secondary to prerenal azotemia as well as developing hepatorenal syndrome. Any potential nephrotoxic agent (e.g., aminoglycoside antibiotics) should be used with extreme caution. Nonsteroidal antiinflammatory drugs and acetaminophen should be used carefully. Many perioperative conditions can exacerbate hepatic encephalopathy such as gastrointestinal bleeding, constipation, azotemia, hypoxia, and the use of sedatives (45). Aggressive preoperative treatment of hepatic encephalopathy using lactulose and dietary protein restriction is recommended. Patients with known gastroesophageal varices should be monitored closely for gastrointestinal bleeding and should be considered for beta-blocker prophylaxis preoperatively. The nutritional status of these patients is usually poor and they are often deficient in thiamine, folate, vitamin C, and B vitamins. Nutritional status should be optimized with multivitamins, thiamine, folate, and nutritional supplementation preoperatively. From a pulmonary standpoint, decompensated cirrhotics may desaturate because of the development of pulmonary shunts in hepatopulmonary syndrome;

TABLE 82.2 Encephalopathy Grade

Grade 0: normal
Grade I: consists of personality changes with altered sleep patterns (e.g., sleep day-night reversal) and inappropriate behavior, constructional apraxia
Grade II: consists of mental confusion, disorientation to time and place, drowsiness, asterixis and fetor hepaticus
Grade III: consists of severe mental confusion, stuporous but arousable, incoherent, asterixis, fetor hepaticus, rigidity, and hyperreflexia
Grade IV: consists of deep coma, unresponsive to stimuli, not arousable, decerebrate and decorticate posturing, fetor hepaticus, decreased muscle tone and decreased reflexes

Adapted from Trey C, Burns DG, Saunders SJ. Treatment of hepatic coma by exchange blood transfusion. *N Engl J Med* 1966;274:473–481.

TABLE 82.3 Pugh Class, Operative Risk, and Operability

Child A 2% to 10% mortality risk
- No limitation
- Normal response to all operations
- Normal ability of liver to regenerate

Child B 6% to 31% mortality risk
- Some limitation in liver function
- Altered response to all operations, but good tolerance with preparation

Child C 20% to 76% mortality risk
- Severe limitation of liver function
- Poor response to all operations regardless of preparation

Adapted from Stone HH. Preoperative and postoperative care. *Surg Clin North Am* 1977;57:409–419.

therefore, continuous monitoring oxygen saturation should be part of the postoperative care. General class-specific guidelines are shown in Table 82.3. There is increasing evidence that laparoscopic procedures in cirrhotic patients may be safer than open procedures regardless of Child classification (38). Patients with cirrhosis undergoing surgery may benefit from a multidisciplinary approach including a hepatologist (and nephrologist if the patient has renal insufficiency).

PERIOPERATIVE CARE OF THE OPIOID-DEPENDENT PATIENT

The goal during the perioperative period is to get the opioid-dependent patient safely through the surgical period. Patients with addictions will not be "cured" of them during their hospital stay and therefore should be encouraged to enroll in long-term addiction treatment at time of hospital discharge. Opioid-dependent persons are at high risk for medical complications, which often require surgical intervention. Most of these complications are a consequence of both active and past high-risk behaviors (i.e., injection drug use [intravenous, intramuscular, subcutaneous "skin popping"]) and the direct toxic effects of the drug and additives being injected. Infections of the skin, soft tissue, bones, and joints are common and often require surgical drainage and débridement. Infectious endocarditis may require emergent or urgent heart valve replacement and will require antibiotic prophylaxis in the future before certain dental procedures (53). Functional bowel obstruction has also been described in chronic opioid users and may require surgical management. Acute hepatitis B and chronic hepatitis C infections are common in intravenous drug users and are the leading causes of liver transplantation (54). Chronic diseases associated with opioid abuse, such as pulmonary hypertension secondary to talc granulomatosis, renal insufficiency secondary to heroin-associated nephropathy, and congestive heart failure from valvular heart disease secondary to endocarditis, HIV syndrome, and chronic hepatitis B and C can all increase surgical risk. Acute opioid withdrawal can also complicate the perioperative period.

Preoperative Evaluation Patients with a history of active injection drug use should be evaluated for a history of endocarditis and the need for antibiotic prophylaxis. These patients should also be evaluated for HIV/AIDS and active hepatitis B and C. Hospitalized patients with active opioid dependence are at risk for acute opioid withdrawal. The onset and severity of withdrawal will depend on which opioid is being used and on the degree of physical dependence, which is related to the duration and amount used. Daily use for at least 3 weeks is generally required before significant physical dependence (and thus clinically significant withdrawal) occurs (55). Heroin withdrawal typically begins within 4 to 6 hours of the time of last use. Withdrawal from long-acting opioids such as sustained release oxycodone (Oxycontin) and morphine (MS Contin), and methadone may not occur for up to 24 to 36 hours. Active opioid use can be verified using urine toxicology tests, whereas injection drug use can be identified by examining the skin for "track marks." Heroin and other semisynthetic opioids will be detected as morphine or codeine in the urine for up to 72 hours. Synthetic opioids (such as methadone, meperidine, and fentanyl) are not usually included in standard urine toxicology screens, so if synthetic opioid abuse is suspected, the laboratory should be asked to test for the specific synthetic opioid of concern. Depending on the opioid of abuse, acute withdrawal usually peaks at 2 to 3 days and can last for up to 14 days. The Clinical Opiate Withdrawal Scale (56) and the Short Opiate Withdrawal Scale (57) are useful clinical opioid withdrawal assessment instruments. Patients who are addicted to opioids may also be addicted to other drugs, such as cocaine or crack, alcohol, or benzodiazepines; these should be the subject of inquiry and laboratory testing (58).

Management of Opioid Withdrawal It is important for providers of perioperative care to be able to recognize and mange acute opioid withdrawal, which is likely in hospitalized opioid-dependent surgical patients. One approach to treating opioid withdrawal in the hospital setting involves treating the physiologic manifestations of acute withdrawal (including the hyperadrenergic signs and symptoms, insomnia, nausea, vomiting, diarrhea, and muscles aches) with clonidine, benzodiazepines, dicyclomine, and nonsteroidal anti-inflammatory drugs. Depending on the patients blood pressure clonidine 0.1 to 0.2 mg orally every 4 to 6 hours is given for the first 48 to 72 hours, with a gradual taper over the next 48 to 72 hours. A much more effective method employs a long-acting opioid agonist such as methadone. In general, trying to convert the dose of opioid the patient is addicted to with an equivalent dose of methadone is unhelpful due to the inexact nature of estimating the actual amount of illicit opioid being used. A starting dose of 20 to 30 mg of methadone orally lessens the signs and symptoms of withdrawal in most patients. The patient should be reassessed for continued withdrawal in 2 to 3 hours; if withdrawal persists, additional doses of 5 to 10 mg may be given, up to a total dose not to exceed 40 mg in 24 hours. After a stable dose has been achieved, it should be given daily to prevent the reemergence of withdrawal. The patient will likely continue to "crave" opioids, but his or her acute withdrawal signs and symptoms should abate. It is important to openly discuss this treatment plan with the patient and nursing staff to avoid unnecessary anxiety and conflict between the patient and healthcare team. If the patient is without food or drink during the perioperative period, he or she should receive 40% of the dose parenterally every 12 hours (e.g., 40 mg by mouth every day = 16 mg intramuscularly every 12 hours). After acute withdrawal is controlled, discussions regarding daily dose taper versus continued daily dose until the day of discharge (as well as postoperative addiction treatment aftercare and referral) should be discussed.

Management of Patients on Opioid Agonist Treatment Approximately 200,000 patients are maintained on opioid agonist therapy in the United States, using methadone or buprenorphine. Such patients should be maintained on their usual maintenance dose during the perioperative period. The correct maintenance dose should be determined by calling the patient's addiction treatment program (e.g., methadone program) or buprenorphine prescriber. The patient's addiction treatment program or physician prescriber should be notified at time the patient is discharged from the hospital to assure continuity of addiction care. Some methadone maintained patients with complicated postoperative courses who have impaired ability to ambulate postoperatively, may be eligible for "medical" take-home doses of methadone from their addiction treatment provider. However, because each methadone clinic has its own policies and procedures on take-home doses, the discharging provider should discuss this possibility with the addiction treatment program's clinical staff.

Management of Acute Pain in Patients on Opioid Agonist Therapy Acute postoperative pain management in patients maintained on long-acting opioid agonist therapy (OAT) can be challenging however guidelines have been published (Table 82.4) (59). The daily methadone or buprenorphine dose a patient receives is not adequate analgesia for acute pain. The lack of analgesia occurs because of the patient's high tolerance to opioids and the pharmacodynamics of methadone and buprenorphine. All methadone- and buprenorphine-maintained patients have a high tolerance to other opioids (cross-tolerance). Cross-tolerance likely is the reason that methadone- and buprenorphine-maintained patients often require higher and more frequent doses of opioid analgesics to adequately treat acute pain. Both methadone and buprenorphine have long plasma half-lives (15 to 40 hours), with different durations of action for analgesia (4 to 8 hours) and for suppression of opioid withdrawal (24 to 36 hours) (60,61). Because the majority of patients on methadone- or buprenorphine-maintenance for opioid addiction are dosed every 24 hours, the potential for even partial pain relief is small. The appropriate treatment of acute pain in these patients includes uninterrupted OAT to address the patient's baseline opioid requirement for their addiction treatment and aggressive pain management. As with all patients suffering acute pain, nonopioid analgesics should be aggressively implemented. However, moderate to severe acute pain will often require opioid analgesics. Continuing the usual dose of OAT, avoids worsening pain symptoms because of the increased pain sensitivity associated with opioid withdrawal. To decrease anxiety, patients should be reassured that their opioid addiction treatment will continue and their pain will be aggressively treated. Because of cross-tolerance with OAT, adequate pain control will generally necessitate higher opioid doses at shorter intervals. Analgesic dosing should be continuous or scheduled rather than as needed. Allowing pain to reemerge before administering the next analgesic dose causes unnecessary suffering and anxiety and increases tension between patient and treatment team. Empiric data on the use of patient controlled analgesia in patients with addiction disorders are limited. One study reported that, although methadone-maintained women had higher pain scores after cesarean section surgery, there was no statistically significant difference in opioid analgesic usage compared with controls (62). Clinical experience supports consideration of patient controlled analgesia use in patients on OAT; increased patient control over analgesia minimizes patient anxiety over pain management. The pharmacologic properties of opioids must be considered when selecting an opioid analgesic for the patient on OAT. Mixed agonist/antagonist opioid analgesics such as pentazocine (Talwin) and butorphanol (Stadol) must be avoided because they are likely to displace the methadone or buprenorphine from the mu receptor, thus precipitating acute opioid withdrawal in these patients.

PERIOPERATIVE CARE OF THE BENZODIAZEPINE-DEPENDENT PATIENT

Benzodiazepines, which are commonly prescribed to treat anxiety, panic attacks, and insomnia have a high abuse potential. Patients who abuse benzodiazepines often are addicted to multiple drugs (63). Some studies have found up to 15% of heroin users and 41% of alcoholics also abuse benzodiazepines (64,65). Therefore patients with addictive disorders should be asked about benzodiazepine use. Chronic benzodiazepine use results in physical dependence, with an acute withdrawal syndrome that can be life-threatening. The withdrawal syndrome ranges from severe anxiety, insomnia, autonomic hyperactivity (including tachycardia and hypertension), to seizures and delirium. Patients with physical dependence to prescribed benzodiazepines should be maintained on their usual dose during the perioperative period to prevent acute withdrawal and subsequent postoperative complications. Patients dependent on illicit benzodiazepines should be maintained on an equivalent dose of long-acting benzodiazepine (e.g., diazepam, chlordiazepoxide) during the perioperative period with psychiatric consultation for guidance on a safe benzodiazepine taper during the postoperative period.

PERIOPERATIVE CARE OF THE NICOTINE-DEPENDENT PATIENT

Nicotine-dependent patients are at risk for pulmonary and cardiac postoperative complications and impaired healing of bones and surgical wounds (66). Asymptomatic smokers are at risk for pulmonary infections due to abnormalities in their respiratory epithelium leading to retained secretions and abnormal lung immune responses (67). A 20 pack-year history and smoking >20 cigarettes a day seems to be the threshold of this increased risk. In observational studies of patients undergoing cardiothoracic surgery, the increased risk decreases only after 8 weeks of smoking cessation and was unrelated to pulmonary function test results (68). Healing is impaired because of decreased tissue oxygenation and inhibition of normal immune responses. Preoperative evaluation should include assessment of physical dependence

TABLE 82.4 Recommendations for Treating Acute Pain in Patients on Opioid Agonist Therapy (OAT)*

Addiction Treatment Issues

- Reassure patient that addiction history will not prevent adequate pain management.
- Continue the usual dose (or equivalent) of OAT.
- Methadone, or buprenorphine maintenance doses should be verified by the patient's methadone maintenance clinic or prescribing physician.
- Notify the addiction treatment program or prescribing physician regarding the patient's admission and discharge and confirm the time and amount of last maintenance opioid dose.
- Inform the addiction treatment maintenance program or prescribing physician of any medications given to the patient during hospitalization because it may show up on routine urine drug screen, such as opioids and benzodiazepines.

Pain Management Issues

- Relieve patient anxiety by discussing, in a nonjudgmental manner, the plan for pain management.
- Use conventional analgesics including opioids to aggressively treat the painful condition.
- Opioid cross-tolerance and patients' increased pain sensitivity will necessitate higher opioid analgesic doses at shorter intervals.
- Write for continuous scheduled dosing rather than as needed orders.
- Avoid using mixed agonist/antagonist opioids such as they will precipitate an acute withdrawal syndrome.

If on methadone maintenance:

- Continue methadone maintenance dose
- Use short-acting opioid analgesics

If on buprenorphine maintenance:

Option
- Continue buprenorphine maintenance
- Titrate short-acting opioid analgesics

Option
- Divide buprenorphine dose to every 6 to 8 h

Option
- Add additional doses of buprenorphine 2 mg every 4 to 6 h for pain.
- Taper back to preoperative buprenorphine dose when acute pain resolves.

Option
- Discontinue buprenorphine maintenance.
- Use opioid analgesics.
- Convert back to buprenorphine when acute pain no longer requires opioid analgesics.

Option (if hospitalized)
- Discontinue buprenorphine.
- Treat opioid dependence with methadone.
- Use short-acting opioid analgesics to treat pain.
- Narcan at bedside.
- Discontinue methadone and convert back to buprenorphine before discharge.

*These recommendations are applicable only when opioid analgesic treatment is determined to be necessary for the treatment of acute pain.

Data from Alford DP, Compton P, Samet JH. Acute pain management for patients receiving maintenance methadone or buprenorphine therapy. *Ann Intern Med* 2006;144:127–134; Book SW, Myrick H, Malcolm R, et al. Buprenorphine for postoperative pain following general surgery in a buprenorphine-maintained patient. *Am J Psychiatry* 2007;164:979.

on nicotine and risk of withdrawal. In addition, preoperative evaluation should include assessment for evidence of cardiovascular disease and COPD. Patients with COPD have a threefold increased risk of postoperative pulmonary complications, including pneumonia (69). Other possible risk factors for pulmonary complications include increased age, duration, and anatomic location of surgery and preoperative sputum production. It is important to assess for upper respiratory infections and to treat with preoperative antibiotics as indicated. Elective procedures should be delayed until any pulmonary infection is resolved. Providers of preoperative care should encourage smoking cessation. Pharmacotherapy, including nicotine replacement, bupropion, and varenicline, consistently increases abstinence rates and should be considered preoperatively. Aggressive perioperative treatment of airflow obstruction should be achieved with inhaled steroids and beta agonists. Preoperative patient education regarding postoperative incentive spirometry use decreases the incidence of postoperative pulmonary complications (69). Nicotine replacement therapy also should be offered postoperatively to patients at risk for nicotine withdrawal.

PERIOPERATIVE CARE OF THE STIMULANT-DEPENDENT PATIENT

Cocaine and methamphetamine may be ingested, snorted, smoked, or taken intravenously. Intravenous stimulant use may result in all the complications attributable to injection drug use such as endocarditis, pulmonary hypertension, hepatitis B and C, and HIV/AIDS. Stimulant use also increases libido and reduces sexual inhibition that also increases the risk of sexually transmitted disease acquisition. Acute stimulant intoxication can be a life-threatening condition because of excessive adrenergic stimulation resulting in acute psychosis, hypertensive crisis, cardiac arrhythmias, sudden cardiac death, seizures, intracranial hemorrhage, myocardial infarction, and cerebrovascular accident. Stimulant users may require surgical interventions due to the acute and chronic affects of these drugs. Cocaine and methamphetamine use can cause bowel ischemia and gangrene resulting from mesenteric vasoconstriction requiring emergent bowel resection. Methamphetamine users may require acute surgical care for traumatic injuries and chemical burns and skin abscesses from compulsive skin-picking. They may require elective surgery for severe periodontal disease. The period of cocaine intoxication is generally brief (~60 minutes) and should not increase the risk of most surgery. However, methamphetamine's longer half-life of 12 hours could adversely affect emergent surgical procedures. Intoxicated patients should be placed in a calm and quiet environment and managed with sedatives such as benzodiazepines. Smoked stimulants can increase surgical risk by causing pulmonary edema. Long-term stimulant use can result in chronic medical conditions, which increase surgical risk such as cardiac dysfunction from prior myocardial infarction or dilated cardiomyopathy. Up to 7% of asymptomatic chronic cocaine users have left ventricular systolic dysfunction (70), although young methamphetamine users were found to have a 3.7-fold increased odds ratio for cardiomyopathy (71). In addition, long-term stimulant use causes left ventricular hypertrophy, a known risk factor for ventricular arrhythmias (72). Therefore it is critically important to identify stimulant use during preoperative assessment and to evaluate carefully for clinical evidence of cardiac disease. Concurrent use of cocaine and alcohol are common, because alcohol prolongs the effects of cocaine through the metabolite, cocaethylene. Cocaethylene increases the rate of cardiac complications (73). Therefore all patients who use cocaine should be screened for concurrent alcohol abuse. Depression and hypersomnolence are common in stimulant withdrawal and may mimic and be confused with other postoperative neurologic complications.

ORGAN TRANSPLANTATION IN PATIENTS WITH ADDICTIONS

Hepatitis B and C infection from injection drug use and alcoholic liver disease are the most common causes of end stage liver disease requiring liver transplantation in the United States. In the past, patients with a history of addictive disorder have been kept off of transplantation lists because of fears of posttransplant noncompliance, with subsequent loss of graft, but also because of moralistic arguments that the patients had "self-inflicted" diseases. In fact, some studies have demonstrated posttransplant relapse rates as high as 49%, with lower overall survival rates in patients who failed to complete addiction treatment (74). Other studies found no difference in 1-year survival rate between alcoholic patients who maintained sobriety and patients who had no history of alcohol abuse (75). In fact, at least among people with alcohol dependence selected for liver transplant, most (71%) abstain or nearly completely abstain and only 7% return to heavy drinking. Furthermore, outcomes (mortality) after liver transplant may be even better among people with alcoholism than among those with other causes of liver failure because those who abstain have no ongoing cause for recurrence, whereas those with hepatitis C infection, for example, often have recurrence. Patients with alcohol dependence who undergo liver transplant are more likely to eventually die from cancer and recurrent infectious hepatitis than they are from recurrent heavy alcohol use complications (76). A recent study identified preoperative risk factors that were predictive of relapse after transplantation which included shorter length of abstinence before transplantation, greater than one episode of alcohol withdrawal before transplantation, younger age at time of transplantation, and alcohol abuse in first-degree relatives (77). A survey of U.S. liver transplantation programs found that most accept applicants with histories of alcohol or drug abuse, but only 56% will accept patients actively receiving methadone maintenance treatment (78). In fact, some programs had policies requiring discontinuation of methadone maintenance before transplantation, which directly contradicts clinical evidence supporting this form of treatment in opioid-dependent patients. It is clear that patients with a history of addiction disorders need to be assessed for risk of relapse and social support systems before being accepted for transplantation. Because organ transplantation in patients with addiction disorders is unusually complex, some medical centers have added addiction specialists to the transplant team (74).

CONCLUSIONS

Patients with addiction disorders have high rates of hospitalization and surgery. The underlying history of addiction may not be apparent initially, but thorough history taking and the use of effective screening tools can elicit information about past or current drug and alcohol abuse. Because of the high prevalence of polydrug abuse, patients who acknowledge an addiction to one substance should be asked about all other substances of abuse. Careful evaluation also can detect clinical signs of chronic diseases of the heart, lungs, and liver related to drug and alcohol abuse. The importance of identifying addiction disorders preoperatively cannot be overstated. Perioperative morbidity associated with acute abstinence syndromes can be prevented with proper preoperative treatment. If possible, elective surgery should be postponed to allow time for complete detoxification. Sedative-hypnotics and opioid analgesics should be used as indicated perioperatively; however, these drugs have a significant abuse potential in patients with a history of addictive disorders, so they should be prescribed with caution. Management of patients with addiction disorders going for surgery often requires consultation with addiction and pain specialists. All patients with active addiction should be encouraged to engage in addiction treatment postoperatively.

REFERENCES

1. Passeri LA, Ellis E, III, Sinn DP. Relationship of substance abuse to complications with mandibular fractures. *J Oral Maxillofac Surg* 1993;51:22–25.
2. Merrill JO, Rhodes LA, Deyo RA, et al. Mutual mistrust in the medical care of drug users: the keys to the "narc" cabinet. *J Gen Intern Med* 2002;17:327–333.
3. Saitz R. Clinical practice. Unhealthy alcohol use. *N Engl J Med* 2005;352:596–607.
4. D'Onofrio G, Bernstein E, Bernstein J, et al. Patients with alcohol problems in the emergency department, part 1: improving detection. SAEM Substance Abuse Task Force. Society for Academic Emergency Medicine. *Acad Emerg Med* 1998;5:1200–1209.
5. Gordon AJ, Olstein J, Conigliaro J. Identification and treatment of alcohol use disorders in the perioperative period. *Postgrad Med* 2006;119:46–55.
6. Spies C, Tonnesen H, Andreasson S, et al. Perioperative morbidity and mortality in chronic alcoholic patients. *Alcohol Clin Exp Res* 2001;25:164S–170S.
7. Tonnesen H. Influence of alcohol on several physiological functions and its reversibility: a surgical view. *Acta Psychiatry Scand* 1992;86:67–71.
8. Zhang P, Bagby GJ, Happel KI, et al. Alcohol abuse, immunosuppression, and pulmonary infection. *Curr Drug Abuse Rev* 2008;1:56–67.
9. Kitchens JM. Does this patient have an alcohol problem? *JAMA* 1994;272:1782–1787.
10. Spies C, Neumann T, Muller C, et al. Preoperative evaluation of alcohol dependent patients admitted to the intensive care unit following surgery. *Alcohol Clin Exp Res* 1995;19 (Suppl. 2):(55A).
11. Andreasson S, Allebeck P, Romelsjo A. Hospital admissions for somatic care among young men: the role of alcohol. *Br J Addict* 1990;85:935–941.
12. Ewing JA. Detecting alcoholism. The CAGE questionnaire. *JAMA* 1984;252:1905–1907.
13. Mayfield D, McLeod G, Hall P. The CAGE questionnaire: validation of a new alcoholism screening instrument. *Am J Psychiatry* 1974;131:1121–1123.
14. Schorling JB, Buchsbaum D. Screening for alcohol and drug abuse. *Med Clin North Am* 1997;81:845–865.
15. Fiellin DA, Reid MC, O'Connor PG. Screening for alcohol problems in primary care: a systematic review. *Arch Intern Med* 2000;160:1977–1989.
16. Chiang PP. Perioperative management of the alcohol-dependent patient. *Am Fam Physician* 1995;52:2267–2273.
17. Foy A, Kay J. The incidence of alcohol-related problems and the risk of alcohol withdrawal in a general hospital population. *Drug Alcohol Rev* 1995;14:49–54.
18. Saitz R. Recognition and management of occult alcohol withdrawal. *Hosp Pract (Minneap)* 1995;30:49–58.
19. Eklund J. Alcohol abuse and postoperative complications. Do we ask the right questions? *Acta Anaesthesiol Scand* 1996;40:647–648.
20. Regan TJ. Alcohol and the cardiovascular system. *JAMA* 1990;264:377–381.
21. Frost EA, Siedel MR. Preanesthetic assessment of the drug abuse patient. *Anesth Clin N Am* 1990;71:453–476.
22. Lindenbaum J. Alcohol and the hematologic system. In: Leiber CS, ed. *Medical and nutritional complications of alcoholism,* New York: Plenum, 1992:241–281.
23. Saitz R, O'Malley SS. Pharmacotherapies for alcohol abuse. Withdrawal and treatment. *Med Clin North Am* 1997;81:881–907.
24. Glickman L, Herbsman H. Delirium tremens in surgical patients. *Surgery* 1968;64:882–890.
25. Spandorfer J. The patient with substance abuse going to surgery. In: Merli GJ, Weitz HH, eds. *Medical management of the surgical patient,* 2nd ed. Philadelphia: WB Saunders Company, 1998:255–262.
26. Mayo-Smith MF. Pharmacological management of alcohol withdrawal. A meta-analysis and evidence-based practice guideline. American Society of Addiction Medicine Working Group on Pharmacological Management of Alcohol Withdrawal. *JAMA* 1997;278:144–151.
27. Mayo-Smith MF, Beecher LH, Fischer TL, et al. Management of alcohol withdrawal delirium. An evidence-based practice guideline. *Arch Intern Med* 2004;164:1405–1412.
28. Sullivan JT, Sykora K, Schneiderman J, et al. Assessment of alcohol withdrawal: the revised clinical institute withdrawal assessment for alcohol scale (CIWA-Ar). *Br J Addict* 1989;84:1353–1357.
29. Tonnesen H, Schutten BT, Jorgensen BB. Influence of alcohol on morbidity after colonic surgery. *Dis Colon Rectum* 1987;30:549–551.
30. Tonnesen H, Schutten BT, Tollund L, et al. Influence of alcoholism on morbidity after transurethral prostatectomy. *Scand J Urol Nephrol* 1988;22:175–177.
31. Felding C, Jensen LM, Tonnesen H. Influence of alcohol intake on postoperative morbidity after hysterectomy. *Am J Obstet Gynecol* 1992;166:667–670.
32. Tonnesen H, Kehlet H. Preoperative alcoholism and postoperative morbidity. *Br J Surg* 1999;86:869–874.
33. Tonnesen H, Petersen KR, Hojgaard L, et al. Postoperative morbidity among symptom-free alcohol misusers. *Lancet* 1992;340:334–337.
34. Jensen NH, Dragsted L, Christensen JK, et al. Severity of illness and outcome of treatment in alcoholic patients in the intensive care unit. *Intensive Care Med* 1988;15:19–22.
35. La Vecchia LL, Bedogni F, Bozzola L, et al. Prediction of recovery after abstinence in alcoholic cardiomyopathy: role of hemodynamic and morphometric parameters. *Clin Cardiol* 1996;19:45–50.
36. Tonnesen H, Rosenberg J, Nielsen HJ, et al. Effect of preoperative abstinence on poor postoperative outcome in alcohol misusers: randomised controlled trial. *BMJ* 1999;318:1311–1316.
37. Ordorica PI, Nace EP. Alcohol. In: Frances RJ, Miller SI, eds. *Clinical textbook of addictive disorders,* 2nd ed. New York: The Guilford Press, 1998:91–119.
38. Rizvon MK, Chou CL. Surgery in the patient with liver disease. *Med Clin North Am* 2003;87:211–227.
39. Greenwood SM, Leffler CT, Minkowitz S. The increased mortality rate of open liver biopsy in alcoholic hepatitis. *Surg Gynecol Obstet* 1972;134:600–604.
40. Patel T. Surgery in the patient with liver disease. *Mayo Clin Proc* 1999;74:593–599.
41. Wong R, Rappaport W, Witte C, et al. Risk of nonshunt abdominal operation in the patient with cirrhosis. *J Am Coll Surg* 1994;179:412–416.
42. Friedman LS, Maddrey WC. Surgery in the patient with liver disease. *Med Clin N Am* 1987;71:453–476.
43. Cowan RE, Jackson BT, Grainger SL, et al. Effects of anesthetic agents and abdominal surgery on liver blood flow. *Hepatology* 1991;14:1161–1166.
44. Shih LY, Cheng CY, Chang CH, et al. Total knee arthroplasty in patients with liver cirrhosis. *J Bone Joint Surg Am* 2004;86-A:335–A:341.
45. Grimm IS, Almounajed G, Friedman LS. Management of the surgical patient with liver disease. In: Merli GJ, Weitz HH, eds. *Medical management of the surgical patient,* 2nd ed. Philadelphia: WB Saunders Company, 1998:193–213.
46. Aranha GV, Sontag SJ, Greenlee HB. Cholecystectomy in cirrhotic patients: a formidable operation. *Am J Surg* 1982;143:55–60.
47. Suman A, Carey WD. Assessing the risk of surgery in patients with liver disease. *Cleve Clin J Med* 2006;73:398–404.

48. Child CG, Turcotte JG. Surgery and portal hypertension. *Major Probl Clin Surg* 1964;1:1–85.
49. Garrison RN, Cryer HM, Howard DA, et al. Clarification of risk factors for abdominal operations in patients with hepatic cirrhosis. *Ann Surg* 1984;199:648–655.
50. Pugh RN, Murray-Lyon IM, Dawson JL, et al. Transection of the oesophagus for bleeding oesophageal varices. *Br J Surg* 1973;60:646–649.
51. Malinchoc M, Kamath PS, Gordon FD, et al. A model to predict poor survival in patients undergoing transjugular intrahepatic portosystemic shunts. *Hepatology* 2000;31:864–871.
52. Suman A, Barnes DS, Zein NN, et al. Predicting outcome after cardiac surgery in patients with cirrhosis: a comparison of Child-Pugh and MELD scores. *Clin Gastroenterol Hepatol* 2004;2:719–723.
53. Wilson W, Taubert KA, Gewitz M, et al. Prevention of infective endocarditis: guidelines from the American Heart Association: a guideline from the American Heart Association Rheumatic Fever, Endocarditis, and Kawasaki Disease Committee, Council on Cardiovascular Disease in the Young, and the Council on Clinical Cardiology, Council on Cardiovascular Surgery and Anesthesia, and the Quality of Care and Outcomes Research Interdisciplinary Working Group. *Circulation* 2007;116: 1736–1754.
54. Aranda-Michel J, Dickson RC, Bonatti H, et al. Patient selection for liver transplant: 1-year experience with 555 patients at a single center. *Mayo Clin Proc* 2008;83:165–168.
55. Kleber HD. Pharmacologic management of opioid withdrawal. Optimizing the treatment and management of substance abuse and addiction (1999 CME Series). San Antonio, TX: Dannemiller Memorial Education Foundation, 1999.
56. Wesson DR, Ling W. The Clinical Opiate Withdrawal Scale (COWS). *J Psychoactive Drugs* 2003;35:253–259.
57. Gossop M. The development of a Short Opiate Withdrawal Scale (SOWS). *Addict Behav* 1990;15:487–490.
58. Joseph H, Stancliff S, Langrod J. Methadone maintenance treatment (MMT): a review of historical and clinical issues. *Mt Sinai J Med* 2000; 67:347–364.
59. Alford DP, Compton P, Samet JH. Acute pain management for patients receiving maintenance methadone or buprenorphine therapy. *Ann Intern Med* 2006;144:127–134.
60. Reisine T, Pasternak G. Opioid analgesics and antagonists. In: Harmon JG, Goodman Gilman A, Limbird LE, eds. *The pharmacological basis of therapeutics,* 9th ed. New York: The McGraw-Hill Company, 1996.
61. Johnson RE, Fudala PJ, Payne R. Buprenorphine: considerations for pain management. *J Pain Symptom Manage* 2005;29:297–326.
62. Paige D, Proble L, Watrous G, et al. PCA use in cocaine using patients: a pilot study. *Am J Pain Manage* 1994;4:101–105.
63. Gold MS, Miller NS, Stennie K, et al. Epidemiology of benzodiazepine use and dependence. *Psychiatr Ann* 1995;25:146–148.
64. Dumont RL. Abuse of benzodiazepines-the problems and the solutions. A report of a Committee of the Institute for Behavior and Health, Inc. *Am J Drug Alcohol Abuse* 1988;14 (Suppl 1):1–69.
65. Ciraulo DA, Sands BF, Shader RI. Critical review of liability for benzodiazepine abuse among alcoholics. *Am J Psychiatry* 1988;145:1501–1506.
66. Warner DO. Preoperative smoking cessation: the role of the primary care provider. *Mayo Clin Proc* 2005;80:252–258.
67. Chalon J, Tayyab MA, Ramanathan S. Cytology of respiratory epithelium as a predictor of respiratory complications after operation. *Chest* 1975;67:32–35.
68. Warner MA, Offord KP, Warner ME, et al. Role of preoperative cessation of smoking and other factors in postoperative pulmonary complications: a blinded prospective study of coronary artery bypass patients. *Mayo Clin Proc* 1989;64:609–616.
69. Jackson CV. Preoperative pulmonary evaluation. *Arch Intern Med* 1988; 148:2120–2127.
70. Bertolet BD, Freund G, Martin CA, et al. Unrecognized left ventricular dysfunction in an apparently healthy cocaine abuse population. *Clin Cardiol* 1990;13:323–328.
71. Yeo KK, Wijetunga M, Ito H, et al. The association of methamphetamine use and cardiomyopathy in young patients. *Am J Med* 2007;120:165–171.
72. Lange RA, Hillis LD. Cardiovascular complications of cocaine use. *N Engl J Med* 2001;345:351–358.
73. Afonso L, Mohammad T, Thatai D. Crack whips the heart: a review of the cardiovascular toxicity of cocaine. *Am J Cardiol* 2007;100:1040–1043.
74. Stowe J, Kotz M. Addiction medicine in organ transplantation. *Prog Transplant* 2001;11:50–57.
75. Starzl TE, Van TD, Tzakis AG. Orthotopic liver transplant for alcoholic cirrhosis. *JAMA* 1988;260:2542–2544.
76. DiMartini A. Natural history of alcohol use disorders in liver transplant patients. *Liver Transplant* 2007;13(11 Suppl 2):S76–S78.
77. Perney P, Bismuth M, Sigaud H, et al. Are preoperative patterns of alcohol consumption predictive of relapse after liver transplantation for alcoholic liver disease? *Transpl Int* 2005;18:1292–1297.
78. Koch M, Banys P. Liver transplantation and opioid dependence. *JAMA* 2001;285:1056–1058.

SECTION 11

Co-occurring Addiction and Psychiatric Disorders

CHAPTER 83

R. Jeffrey Goldsmith, MD
Richard K. Ries, MD, FAPA, FASAM
Christine Yuodelis-Flores, MD

Substance-Induced Mental Disorders

The focus of this chapter is to help clinicians understand, differentially diagnose, and treat person with substance-induced psychiatric syndromes that mimic traditional psychiatric disorders such as depression, anxiety and psychotic disorders. Because all substances of abuse work by altering the same kinds of neurotransmitters that are thought to be involved in these psychiatric disorders, it should not be surprising that many patients with substance abuse, dependence, or withdrawal may appear to be psychiatrically ill, or at least appear to have significant psychiatric symptoms. The fourth edition of the *Diagnostic and statistical manual of mental disorders* (DSM-IV) of the American Psychiatric Association (1) developed new definitions of the substance-induced mental disorders, which differ slightly from the guidelines offered in the revised third edition (DSM-IIIR) (2). This chapter describes the diagnostic criteria in the DSM-IV, reviews the epidemiologic data, and discusses the clinical strategies needed to manage these disorders. Although nine substance-induced mental disorders are given in the DSM-IV (Table 83.1), this chapter will focus on those which are most confounding in terms of differential *psychiatric* presentation (substance-induced psychotic, mood, and anxiety disorders and hallucinogen persisting perceptual disorder.) These will be referred to as substance-induced *psychiatric* disorders. Three others are referred to generically as "organic brain syndrome": substance-induced delirium, substance-induced persisting dementia, and substance-induced persisting amnestic disorder and are not the focus of this chapter nor are substance-induced sexual dysfunction and substance-induced sleep disorder (though substance related sleep disorders are discussed in many of the chapters in this section and others).

PREVALENCE OF SUBSTANCE-INDUCED PSYCHIATRIC DISORDERS

Prevalence of Substance-Induced Mood and Anxiety Disorders

Prevalence rates of substance-induced psychiatric disorders vary considerably depending on the study subjects (treatment-seeking populations versus epidemiologic surveys) and the research diagnostic criteria used to define the disorders (e.g., how long is a substance-induced syndrome defined to last). Brown and Schuckit (3) reported that 42% of the male alcoholics presenting for treatment displayed depressive symptoms in a range comparable to that seen in individuals hospitalized for affective disorder (more than 19 points, which is in the moderate-to-severe range of the Hamilton Depression Rating Scale). The symptoms abated rapidly over the first 2 weeks of abstinence, with only 12% of the subjects still depressed at the end of the second week. In light of this rapid abatement of depressive symptoms, it is significant that the subjects averaged more than nine days of abstinence before the study began.

In a study of similar alcoholic subjects who had been sober for an average of 8 days, Brown et al. (4) reported that 33% of the primary alcoholics (with or without secondary affective disorder) scored in the moderate to severe range for depression, whereas 81% of the subjects with primary affective disorder did so at the end of week 1. By week 4 of the study, none of the patients with primary alcoholism was in the moderate-to-severe range, whereas 67% of the subjects with primary affective disorders were. This finding suggests that all of the subjects with primary alcoholism had alcohol-induced depressive disorder, a number quite comparable to the 30% reported in the earlier study by the same researchers.

TABLE 83.1 DSM-IV Substance-Induced Mental Disorders

- Substance-induced delirium
- Substance-induced persisting dementia
- Substance-induced persisting amnestic disorder
- Substance-induced psychotic disorder
- Substance-induced mood disorder
- Substance-induced anxiety disorder
- Hallucinogen persisting perceptual disorder
- Substance-induced sexual dysfunction
- Substance-induced sleep disorder.

From American Psychiatric Association (APA). *Diagnostic and statistical manual of mental disorders,* 4th ed. (DSM-IV). Washington, DC: American Psychiatric Press, 1994.

Schuckit et al. (5) studied nearly 3,000 alcoholics to test three hypotheses related to substance-induced depression. They hypothesized that (1) there would be more substance-induced depression than major depressive disorder, (2) those with substance-induced depression would have more severe alcohol and drug histories, and (3) those with independent depression would have more first-degree relatives with affective disorder than would the substance-induced group. All three hypotheses were supported by their findings. Among the study population, 15% of 2,495 subjects had an independent depression (group 1), whereas 26% reported information consistent with a substance-induced depression (group 2). Subjects in group 2 drank more alcohol per occasion and drank on more days per week, sought treatment more often, were more likely to have attended Alcoholics Anonymous meetings, and used more marijuana and stimulants than did subjects in group 1 or group 3 (no depression). Women composed about half of the subjects in group 1 (52%), but less than one third of the subjects in group 2 (29.5%) and group 3 (28%). In addition, subjects in group 2 had more antisocial personality disorder than did those in group 1 (28% vs. 22%) or group 3 (28% vs. 15%). Subjects in group 1 had more major anxiety disorder than did those in group 2 (8.4% vs. 4.8%) and the same percentage of mania (1.6% vs. 1.0%).

More recent studies using DSM-IV criteria and structured clinical interviews show a wider variety of results depending largely on the study population used. Kahler et al. (6) looked at substance-induced and independent major depressive disorder in treatment-seeking alcoholics and found that out of 166 alcohol patients with elevated levels of depression, 122 alcoholic patients met the Structured Clinical Interview for DSM-IV (7) criteria for major depressive disorder. Of this group, 61.6% were found to have "pure" substance-induced mood disorder and 15.2% were found to have independent major depressive disorder. The remaining 23.2% had the diagnosis of substance-induced mood disorder with a history of independent major depressive disorder. In contrast to treatment seeking populations, Grant et al. (8) in a major epidemiologic study found the prevalence of substance-induced mood and anxiety disorders to be extremely low in the general population (1.05% for current substance-induced mood disorders and 0.22% for substance-induced anxiety disorders). However, the prevalence of those with current independent mood disorders who reported having both independent and substance-induced mood disorders in the prior year was 7.35%. Of those with current independent anxiety disorders, 2.95% reported having both substance-induced and independent anxiety disorders in the prior year.

It can be very difficult to differentiate between substance-induced and independent depressive disorders and the diagnosis may change if the patient is followed over time. Ramsey et al. (9) studied alcoholics with substance-induced depressive disorder and found that over a course of a year, 26.4% of those diagnosed with substance-induced depressive disorder were reclassified as having an independent major depressive disorder because of meeting full criteria for the diagnosis of major depression after 1 month of sobriety. In this study, those with a history of past independent major depression were five times more likely to be reclassified from substance-induced depression to independent depression. Patients who had lower severity of alcohol dependence were also more likely to be reclassified as having independent major depression. Nunes et al. (10) studied depressive disorders in patients with alcoholism admitted to an inpatient psychiatric unit using the Psychiatric Research Interview for Substance and Mental Disorders and found that 51% of patients had substance-induced depression; however, after following them for a year, 32% of those with substance-induced depression were reclassified as having independent depression.

As with depressive symptoms, anxiety symptoms show similar changes over the early sobriety phase. Several studies have reported high rates of anxiety symptoms among alcoholics in withdrawal, with 80% of alcohol-dependent male subjects experiencing repeated panic attacks during alcohol withdrawal (11). In the same study, 50% to 67% of the alcohol-dependent subjects had high scores on the state anxiety measures, which resembled generalized anxiety and social phobia (11). Brown et al. (12) reported that 40% of recently detoxified alcohol-dependent men scored above the 75th percentile on the state-anxiety subscale of the State Trait Anxiety Inventory. At discharge after 4 weeks, 12% scored that high, whereas at 3-month follow-up, only 5% remained above the 75th percentile. This finding suggests that 35% had an alcohol-induced anxiety disorder. Moreover, if 80% of alcoholic men report withdrawal panic attacks, is this alcohol withdrawal-induced anxiety disorder or is it an independent panic disorder evoked by alcohol withdrawal? Or is it merely anxiety symptoms caused by alcohol withdrawal?

Regarding cocaine-induced depressive disorders, Rounsaville et al. (13), in a study of patients addicted to cocaine examined the current and lifetime prevalence of Research Diagnostic Criteria disorders. They used both strict and less strict criteria in evaluating the depression diagnostic data from the Schedule for Affective Disorders and Schizophrenia-Lifetime (SADS-L). The less strict criteria allowed a diagnosis if the symptoms *ever* had been present, whereas the strict criteria allowed a diagnosis only if symptoms had persisted for 10 or more days after cessation of cocaine use. Using the less strict criteria, major depression was diagnosed in 59% of the subjects, whereas the more strict criteria yielded a 30% prevalence rate. This finding conservatively suggests a lifetime prevalence of about 30% for cocaine-induced depressive disorder. Further, the current rate of major depression was 4.7%, hypomania was 2%, and minor mood disorder was 38% (mania was 0%) (13). (The current diagnoses of minor mood disorders appeared to use the strict criteria, but this was not clarified in the report.) Rounsaville et al. (13) reported a 16% current rate and a 21% lifetime rate of anxiety disorders, but the investigators did not disclose what criteria were used to diagnose anxiety unrelated to cocaine use.

Methamphetamine users are also reported to have high rates of depressive symptoms and suicidal behavior during active use as well as during withdrawal and early abstinence. A large study of psychiatric symptoms among 1,016 methamphetamine users presenting for treatment revealed that depression was the most common symptom reported and 27% had attempted suicide in the past (14).

Prevalence of Substance-Induced Psychotic Disorders In a study designed to examine substance-induced psychotic disorders, Rosenthal and Miner (15) prospectively examined admissions to an acute psychiatric inpatient unit. Over the first year, they found that 30% of the patients admitted met the DSM-IIIR criteria for organic mood disorder, 8% for organic hallucinosis, and 6% for organic delusional disorder. They also found that 15% of the patients with comorbid schizophrenia and substance use disorder and organic delusional disorder or organic hallucinosis were suicidal. Brady et al. (16) evaluated individuals admitted for treatment of cocaine dependence and found that 53% reported transient cocaine-induced psychosis. Caton et al. (17) evaluated psychotic individuals presenting to a psychiatric emergency department in New York and reported a prevalence of 44% for substance-induced psychotic disorder. An Australian study done by McKetin et al. (18) to examine the prevalence of psychotic symptoms among 309 regular methamphetamine users not presenting for treatment found that 13% had psychotic symptoms and 23% had experienced clinically significant psychotic symptoms in the past year. This study reported that the prevalence of psychosis among current methamphetamine users was 11 times higher than among the general population. Pasic et al. (19) in a case-control study of methamphetamine users referred for psychiatric emergency services and found 80% presenting with psychosis compared with only 30% of the non-methamphetamine using patients. In studies conducted in Japan, chronic intravenous methamphetamine use is associated with increased rates of prolonged psychosis persisting for several months to over 2 years after abstinence that closely resembles paranoid schizophrenia (20,21).

Substance-Associated Suicidal Behavior Substance-induced depression can dissipate rapidly, but it is as dangerous as major depressive disorder in terms of the risk of suicide and self-injurious behavior. When completed suicides are investigated, the rate of comorbidity is high. Murphy and Wetzel (22) reported that alcoholic patients had a 60- to 120-fold greater risk of death by suicide than did the non-psychiatrically ill population. Henriksson et al. (23) reported that nearly half (43%) of a group of suicide victims in Finland had alcohol dependence and that 48% of the alcoholics had comorbid depression, 42% had a personality disorder, and 36% had a significant Axis III medical disorder. Young et al. (24) found that persons who had major depressive disorder coexisting with both alcohol and drug dependence were at the highest risk of suicide, even in the absence of pervasive hopelessness. Driessen et al. (25) reported that neither Axis I nor Axis II comorbidity among alcoholics was predictive of suicidal behavior or ideation at 1-year follow-up; however, two Axis I diagnoses or an Axis I with an Axis II diagnosis were predictive. Pages et al. (26) found that alcohol and drug dependence, as well as current use, were associated with greater severity of suicidal ideation among patients with unipolar major depressive disorder. Salloum et al. (27) studied patients who had been hospitalized psychiatrically and found that more than half of the subjects in all three groups studied (with alcohol dependence, cocaine dependence, or alcohol plus cocaine dependence) had a history of suicide attempts. Zweben et al. (14) also found a high prevalence of prior suicide attempts (27%) in methamphetamine dependent patients presenting for treatment. Elliott et al. (28) found that patients who made medically severe suicide attempts had a statistically higher rate of substance-induced mood disorder than did patients who made less severe suicide attempts. There was no difference between the two groups in the prevalence of alcohol abuse or dependence, or in the prevalence of polysubstance abuse or dependence. Moreover, most of the patients with substance-induced mood disorder did not meet the criteria for substance dependence. This finding is consistent with the findings of Asnis et al. (29) and Murphy and Wetzel (22), who argued that alcohol dysregulates mood independent of use patterns, suggesting that some individuals are at risk of severe depression regardless of the chronicity of their alcohol use. Conner et al. (30) analyzed suicidal behavior in 3,729 alcoholic individuals and concluded that both independent and substance-induced depression are associated with suicidal ideation and planning, whereas alcohol-related aggression is correlated with suicide attempts. Aharonovich et al. (31) studied depressed substance-dependent patients who had attempted suicide and found that patients with substance-induced depression were as likely as those with independent depression to have attempted suicide. Ries et al. (32) studied acutely suicidal psychiatric inpatients with substance-induced psychiatric disorders and found that this subgroup had higher severity of suicidal ideation but improved more quickly than other patients and tended to have shorter lengths of stay.

Among schizophrenics, however, Bartels et al. (33) found that it was the severity of the depression, not the substance abuse, which explained suicidal behavior. In contrast, Seibyl et al. (34) reported that schizophrenics who had used cocaine before admission exhibited increased suicidal ideation.

In summary, although a great deal of effort has gone into characterizing substance-induced psychiatric syndromes in both addictions and psychiatric populations, findings are widely variable. Results of prevalence studies in clinical populations are influenced by differences between the populations studied, the diagnostic criteria employed, and the type of interview used. In addition despite the best methods of classification, a significant number of "substance-induced depression" cases turned out to have independent major depression over the following year. However, it is also clear that substance-induced states are common and it is logical that clinical intervention for an alcohol-induced depression would focus on different issues (e.g., getting sober and into recovery) than typical major psychiatric depression (medications and psychotherapy). But what if a patient has both problems? Or a little of one, but a whole lot of the other? Ries et al. (35) have attempted to straddle the "either/or" problem by showing that clinicians can validly classify substance induced syndromes in acute psychiatric patients admitted to an acute county hospital as having 0 = no substance induced effect, 2 = mild substance effect (about 25% of the syndrome being substance related), 3 = moderate substance effect (about 50 % of the syndrome being substance related), or 4 = major substance induced effect (75% or greater substance related). They have suggested that rather than a separate diagnosis, using this system allows for a better clinical description of presenting patients, because in many cases acute psychiatric patients have both conditions at the same time for example: bipolar disorder with acute cocaine-induced paranoia.

SPECIFIC SUBSTANCES: SUBSTANCE-INDUCED SYMPTOMS

The occurrence of psychiatric symptoms as a result of legal and illegal drug use has been well documented. It is common medical knowledge that hallucinogens cause hallucinations, stimulants cause euphoria, and chronic sedative use can result in depression. It is common medical knowledge that in acute withdrawal, alcohol and sedatives cause anxiety. It is less obvious that a distinct set of symptoms appear when psychoactive substances are used over a long period. Symptoms reported for each of the major substances of abuse are reviewed below to establish a basis on which to understand the syndromes that can arise (also see Section 2 of this book).

Caffeine is the most commonly used addictive substance. It is considered a benign drug by many consumers and professionals and has enjoyed an increase in popularity over the past decade. The effects of caffeine include the induction of anxiety with consumption of "large amounts"; however, the range of caffeine doses that can induce anxiety is considerable. Caffeine can increase the frequency of panic attacks in those individuals who are physiologically predisposed to them.

Nicotine is the deadliest psychoactive drug and the third most popular in the United States, with about 25% of the adult population smoking cigarettes, about 5% using smokeless tobacco, and about 5% smoking pipes and cigars. Although there is no indication that nicotine acutely changes mood, there is evidence that nicotine-dependent patients experience more depression than nonusers and that some use nicotine to regulate mood. Whether there is a causal relationship between nicotine use and the symptoms of depression remains to be seen. At present, it can be said only that some persons who quit smoking do experience severe depression, which is relieved by resumption of nicotine use.

Alcohol use is common among American adolescents and young adults. Although light consumption of alcohol is associated with a slight euphoria or "buzz," moderate to heavy consumption may be associated with depression, suicidal feelings, or violent behavior in some individuals. With prolonged drinking, the incidence of dysphoria and anxiety rises, much to the distress of the drinker. In those who are physiologically dependent, one usually sees a hyperadrenergic state that is characterized by agitation, anxiety, tremor, malaise, hyperreflexia, mild tachycardia, increasing blood pressure, sweating, insomnia, nausea or vomiting, and perceptual distortions. After acute withdrawal from alcohol, some persons suffer from continued mood instability, with moderate lows, fatigability, insomnia, reduced sexual interest, and hostility. A few chronic heavy drinkers experience hallucinations, delusions, and anxiety during acute withdrawal, and some have grand mal seizures. Brain damage of several types is associated with alcohol-induced dementias and deliriums.

With *sedatives*, particularly the benzodiazepines, acute use can produce a "high" similar to that seen with alcohol. The drug effects are perceived as relaxing, producing a social ease, but sedatives also can induce depression, anxiety, and even a psychotic-like state with prolonged use and dependence (36). Withdrawal symptoms include mood instability with anxiety or depression, sleep disturbance, autonomic hyperactivity, tremor, nausea or vomiting, transient hallucinations or illusions, and grand mal seizures. A protracted withdrawal syndrome has been reported to include anxiety, depression, paresthesias, perceptual distortions, muscle pain and twitching, tinnitus, dizziness, headache, derealization and depersonalization, and impaired concentration. These symptoms can last for weeks, and some (such as anxiety, depression, tinnitus, and paresthesias) have been reported for a year or more after withdrawal.

Cocaine and *amphetamine* use often are associated with an intense euphoria or "rush," with hyperactive behavior and speech, anorexia, insomnia, inattention, and labile moods (37). The route of administration and the dose alter the intensity of the experience. After a binge of several days, addicts may feel "wired" or "geeked" and stop their use, or they may use other drugs to moderate the agitation.

Individuals occasionally become paranoid and even delusional after prolonged heavy use of cocaine or amphetamine. Unlike other psychotic states, the patient experiencing a paranoid state induced by cocaine has intact abstract reasoning and linear thinking, whereas the delusions, if analyzed, are poorly developed delusions of a nonbizarre nature (38). If abstinence is maintained for several weeks, many stimulant addicts report a dysphoric state that is prominently marked by anhedonia and/or anxiety, but which does not meet the symptom severity criteria to qualify as a DSM-IV disorder (13). This anhedonic state can persist for weeks. Some stimulant addicts report hallucinatory symptoms that are visual ("coke snow") and tactile ("coke bugs"). Sleep disturbances are prominent in the intoxicated and withdrawn states, as is sexual dysfunction.

Methamphetamine intoxication is characterized by euphoria, increased sexuality, and hyperactive, agitated, or violent behavior as well as rapid speech, anorexia, insomnia, and labile moods. Individuals often present with psychotic behavior consisting of reality-based paranoia and hallucinations that can last as little as a couple of hours but as long as several days. Depressive symptoms and cognitive problems as well as hypersomnia, decreased energy, and increased appetite commonly occur during the withdrawal phase. Studies in Japan report that chronic and heavy methamphetamine users, particularly those who use intravenously are reported to have an increased rate of psychosis and depression lasting several months or more that closely resembles paranoid schizophrenia (20,21).

Methylenedioxymethamphetamine (MDMA), more commonly known as "Ecstasy," intoxication produces stimulant effects similar to cocaine and amphetamine as well as empathogenic effects of empathy, a sense of well-being, and sociability. Withdrawal states are characterized by depression, hypersomnia, poor concentration, and fatigue. Chronic methylenedioxymethamphetamine users may develop more severe longer term problems such as dysphoric states and cognitive impairments in memory, concentration, and executive functioning which are thought to be due to serotonergic neurotoxicity (39).

Opiate use is characterized by a "high" or "rush" when the drug is used intravenously or smoked. Unlike the stimulants, opiate-induced euphoria usually is associated with some sedation and manifests as a mellow, sleepy state. If opiates are used for a long period, moderate to severe depression is common. The addict frequently experiences irritability, accompanied by craving, muscle aches, a flulike syndrome, and gastrointestinal symptoms early in withdrawal from drugs such as heroin and morphine. More drug subdues the craving. In withdrawal, some opiate addicts are acutely anxious and agitated, whereas others report depression and anhedonia. Anxiety, depression, and sleep disturbance, in a milder form, can persist for weeks as a protracted withdrawal syndrome. There are reports of an atypical opiate withdrawal syndrome, consisting of delirium after the abrupt cessation of methadone (40). Such patients do not appear to have the autonomic symptoms typically seen in opiate withdrawal.

Hallucinogens such as marijuana, tetrahydrocannabinol, LSD, mescaline, and dimethyltryptamine produce visual distortions and frank hallucinations. Some users experience a marked sense of time distortion and feelings of depersonalization. *Marijuana* and the cannabinoids can augment appetite and cause sedation with euphoria. All hallucinogens are associated with drug-induced panic reactions that feature panic, paranoia, and even delusional states in addition to the hallucinations. A cannabis withdrawal syndrome is described (41,42) that is generally mild and consists of anxiety, irritability, physical tension, depressed mood, decreased appetite, restlessness, and craving. Recent literature has emerged that early use of cannabis is a risk factor for the development of psychotic symptoms later in life (43,44). A few hallucinogen users experience chronic reactions, involving (1) prolonged psychotic reactions, (2) depression, which can be life-threatening, (3) flashbacks, and (4) exacerbations of preexisting psychiatric illnesses. The flashbacks are symptoms that occur after one or more psychedelic trips and consist of flashes of light and afterimage prolongation in the periphery. The DSM-IV refers to flashbacks as "hallucinogen persisting perception disorder" and requires that they be distressing or impairing to the patient (1, p. 234).

Phencyclidine (PCP), an arylcyclohexylamine and dissociative drug, is a hallucinogen used in certain parts of the United States. Popular in the 1970s (45), PCP is known for its dissociative and delusional properties. It also is associated with violent behavior and amnesia of the intoxication (45). Users who once exhibit an acute psychotic state with PCP are more likely to develop another with repeated use (46).

Differential Diagnosis and Treatment Diagnosing and treating a substance-induced mental disorder is very much dependent on the attitude and training of the clinician. Is he or she attuned to the prevalence of alcohol and drug use? Without this awareness, there is less inclination to search for the problem. Does the clinician think that it is relevant to the current problem to take the time to elicit an alcohol and drug use history? Has the clinician received adequate training to counteract the therapeutic nihilism acquired during medical school and residency training? Is he or she adversely affected by the distortions and denial that are exhibited by many alcoholics and drug addicts? Does the clinician routinely seek corroboration of an alcohol and drug use history from family or friends of the patient? Will the clinician order a drug screen? All of these questions hint at behaviors that can make the diagnosis more apparent or allow it to elude identification. Making the diagnosis of a substance use disorder is the first step in the differential diagnosis and treatment of a substance-related problem. In the second step, the substance-induced symptoms must be differentiated from the symptoms of major psychiatric disorders. Finally, the substance-induced disorders must be differentiated from the dual disorders: substance abuse or dependence combined with a comorbid, nonsubstance Axis I disorder. The DSM-IV contains five criteria for substance-induced mood disorders (1).

1. A prominent and persistent disturbance in mood predominates, characterized by (a) a depressed mood or markedly diminished interest or pleasure in activities, or (b) an elevated, expansive, or irritable mood.
2. There is evidence from the history, physical examination, or laboratory findings that the symptoms developed during or within a month after substance intoxication or withdrawal, or medication use is etiologically related to the mood disturbance.
3. The disturbance is not better explained by a mood disorder.

4. The disturbance did not occur exclusively during a delirium.
5. The symptoms cause clinically significant distress or impairment.

Mood Disorders Mood disorders may be the most common substance-induced disorders that clinicians need to consider in arriving at a differential diagnosis. It is important to consider, and make, the substance use diagnosis whenever it is pertinent. There are some guidelines that can help with these diagnoses. Because of denial, the patient may not understand what is happening in his or her life. If the clinician is aware of the prevalence of addictive disorders and the ways in which such disorders typically present, he or she is more likely to take a careful history and to seek confirmation of the history from collateral informants, especially family and friends, but also other health care professionals. Establishing whether there is a relationship between the use of psychoactive substances and the symptoms prominent at the moment is a crucial step. Chronic use of alcohol, sedatives, and opiates can cause depressed mood, as can withdrawal from stimulants and sedatives. Exploring the mood during periods of sustained abstinence from all depressant drugs is critical.

Anxiety Disorders For the substance-induced anxiety disorders, the criteria are almost identical. However, the first is different: prominent anxiety, panic attacks, obsessions, or compulsions predominate. The remaining four criteria are the same as for mood disorder (1). In making the diagnosis of substance use disorder, it is helpful to order a drug screen. Even if the results come back hours after the clinical decision is made, they can be used to confirm the presence of a substance despite the patient's denial. Such a screen also can clarify the history in some future episode. Sometimes addicts report part of their history, but not all. For example, it may be useful to know that both alcohol and cocaine were used by a depressed patient. Although either substance can induce symptoms of anxiety (or depression), a slightly different treatment plan may be necessary for a patient dependent on both. A drug screen may be equally critical to the diagnosis of a substance-induced psychotic disorder. Again, the criteria in the DSM-IV are similar. Hallucinations or delusions must be prominent and are not counted if the individual has insight into the substance-induced nature of his or her cognitive problems. For this reason, the patient's lack of insight, coupled with a drug screen and collateral history, can be important in establishing the use or absence of a psychotogenic drug. The differences among psychiatric symptoms associated with different psychiatric disorders remains elusive. The DSM-IV requires that the diagnosis of anxiety, affective, and psychotic disorders be made only when several criteria are satisfied. First, the anxiety, mood, or cognitive symptoms must be prominent. Second, there must be evidence that a psychoactive substance was used within the preceding month and that the substance is known to cause the symptoms in question. Third, there should not be another cause that better explains the disorder. Fourth, the disorder cannot occur exclusively during the course of a delirium. And fifth, the disorder must cause clinically significant distress or impairment in normal functioning. Although not a criteria for diagnosis, the DSM-IV explains that the assessment should not be made unless the symptoms are judged to be in excess of those usually associated with intoxication or withdrawal. The latter can be problematic if taken literally, because withdrawal can involve extreme symptoms, such as suicidal feelings and panic attacks. In addiction, intoxication can include paranoia and visual hallucinations, feelings of depersonalization, and time distortion. What would it mean to be in excess of such psychotic symptoms?

Case 1 Mr. B is a 46-year-old divorced white man who works as a house painter. He came to the emergency department because of suicidal ideas, which frightened him. He had become increasingly depressed over the preceding month and was afraid that he was "going crazy." He had experienced episodes of depression over the preceding 7 years (since his divorce), but the episodes had not lasted more than a day or two. He also had experienced fleeting suicidal ideas, but had not hurt himself. In the past year, he occasionally had sat with his gun and considered ending it all. At those times, he felt momentarily hopeless. The suicidal and hopeless thoughts lasted for an evening, but were not continuously present for more than a day. He had never been treated psychiatrically for depression. The clinician gathers information suggestive of a depressive syndrome of some kind and must determine whether there are any organic causes, the most common of which would be substance-induced disorder. Mr. B has been hospitalized once, 4 years ago, to be detoxified from alcohol, but he received no treatment for alcoholism after the detoxification. Recently, his drinking has increased to about a case of beer a day. He reports that the alcohol use is the only way he can cope with his depression. He denies any loss of control, but admits to two arrests for driving under the influence (DUI) over the preceding 10 years. He is experiencing difficulty in getting to work on time since becoming depressed and is in trouble with his supervisor. He denies morning shakes and says that he never has experienced *delirium tremens*. Mr. B admits that his ex-wife complained about his drinking. He has had only one period of abstinence for more than a year, while on probation for his second DUI. He felt well during that time. He developed the depressive symptoms in his late 30s, whereas his heavy drinking began in his early 20s. He denies any ongoing medical problems or thyroid problems. He has had some weight loss in the past month because he has not been eating regularly with his heavy drinking, and he has experienced some nausea in the mornings, which made eating breakfast difficult. He denies any use of sedatives, barbiturates, cocaine, or opiates. On mental status examination, Mr. B is found to be a middle-aged white man, who looks more like 55 than 46 years old. He is thin, looks depressed, and smells of alcohol. He is vague about some details and specific about others. He is oriented to person, place, date, and purpose. He is tearful at some times, anxious at others. He seems bewildered about his predicament. He denies having problems with alcohol. He has suicidal ideas about shooting himself, but does not seem motivated to do so. He denies hallucinations and obsessions. He denies any manic episodes. His blood alcohol concentration is 200 mg%. A drug toxicology screen is negative for benzodiazepines, opiates, barbiturates, and cocaine.

Diagnostic Issues Is there a reason to consider a diagnosis of alcohol dependence or abuse for Mr. B? Is depression a prominent symptom? Is there a reason to connect the depressive symptoms to alcohol or drug use or withdrawal? Is the intensity of depression more severe than is usually found with alcohol intoxication alone? Is the depressive mood better explained by a mood disorder? Did the depressed mood occur during a delirium?

Diagnostic Considerations At this point, the clinician has enough information to diagnose alcohol dependence. Mr. B exhibits tolerance, alcohol withdrawal, use despite adverse consequences, impairment of personal relationships, and possibly impairment of occupational function, all related to his use of alcohol. His mood disturbance is prominent and is more severe than that experienced by social drinkers and most alcoholics. His depressive symptoms seem sufficiently severe to suggest major depression; however, there is no evidence of depression at the times that Mr. B is not drinking heavily, suggesting alcohol-induced depressive disorder. The alcohol dependence seems to be primary; that is, it began before the depressive symptoms. This sequence of symptoms also suggests alcohol-induced depressive disorder. It is possible that Mr. B has two independent disorders, alcohol dependence, and major depression; however, there is no evidence of that at present. Finally, there is no evidence of a delirium.

Treatment Issues Safety issues involve ongoing evaluation of the diagnosis, use of medications, and psychosocial therapy.

Treatment Considerations A trial of abstinence is called for in a safe environment with a lot of support. The clinical challenge is to find a safe environment. The risk of alcohol withdrawal delirium and seizures is minimal, suggesting that Mr. B could be managed as an outpatient. However, there are other considerations in this decision. The *ASAM patient placement criteria for the treatment of substance-related disorders, 2nd edition-revised* (*ASAM PPC-2R*) (47) encourage the physician to evaluate the patient's status in six different dimensions. The first is the potential for withdrawal. The second and third are the presence of medical and psychiatric comorbidities. (The seriousness of Mr. B's suicidality, as well as the degree of his anergy and inability to mobilize because of depression, are relevant in this case. The medical comorbidity is minor [possibly gastritis] and should improve with abstinence.) The fourth dimension is the patient's readiness for change. Mr. B appears to seek treatment; however, he may balk at inpatient or outpatient treatment, making his cooperation a major issue. The final two dimensions—the potential for relapse and the presence or absence of a supportive environment—are very pertinent to this patient. If Mr. B has no supportive friends or family who can watch over him and be sure that he gets to therapy sessions, or to the emergency department if his condition worsens, then outpatient therapy becomes risky, particularly given the patient's suicidal ideas. The patient's potential for relapse, including his motivation for abstinence, craving for alcohol while abstinent, and history of prior attempts to quit, is crucial in determining the viability of outpatient treatment. Alcohol-induced depression should remit over the first 2 to 3 weeks of abstinence. Careful follow-up during this period is very important with outpatient treatment because of the severity of Mr. B's symptoms and the possibility that the correct diagnosis is not alcohol-induced depression. However, if he cannot or will not stay sober as an outpatient, it is likely that he will remain depressed or become even more depressed. At this point, residential treatment is essential to break the cycle of addiction and allow the patient's mood to improve. If his mood does not improve with abstinence, a major depression should be considered, and the patient should be given appropriate antidepressant treatment. Anticraving medications such as naltrexone (acamprosate and injectible naltrexone) can be very helpful when the patient is cooperative, somewhat open to the idea of abstinence from alcohol, and willing to engage in some kind of psychosocial follow-up. The same is true of disulfiram. Patients with a firm commitment to sobriety may not need the assistance of such medications. Patients with a strong connection to Alcoholics Anonymous may not be motivated to take such medications because they believe that medications are not appropriate for sobriety; however, Alcoholics Anonymous produces a pamphlet that is quite supportive of both psychiatric care and the use of psychiatric medications.

Case 2 Mr. M is a 59-year-old African American veteran who is divorced and unemployed. He came to the evaluation area at 9:00 AM because of a longstanding problem sleeping that has worsened over the past 2 months. He has been drinking more alcohol to fall asleep, but has been waking after only a few hours of sleep. He experiences hand tremors in the mornings, which resolve with a few shots of whiskey. He has become jumpy and irritable and tends to isolate himself from his friends.

Option A Mr. M has no history of withdrawal seizures or withdrawal hallucinations. He has no history of panic attacks, chronic anxiety, or traumatic life events. His vital signs include blood pressure 148/90, pulse 96, temperature 98.6°F, and respirations 16. Mr. M was detoxified from alcohol within the past year, but refused to enter outpatient treatment. He complained that he was "not going to let the doctors treat him like a 'guinea pig' on the detoxification unit" and that "they just tried to lock up a Black man these days."

Diagnostic Issues Is there a prominent symptom? If so, is this symptom related to drinking? Is there any evidence of other drug use? Is this explained better by another *DSM* disorder? Did the symptoms occur during a delirium? Has this disorder caused symptoms beyond what normally is experienced during alcohol intoxication or withdrawal?

Clinical Considerations At this point, the information available suggests alcohol withdrawal. There also is information suggesting a sleep disturbance, which may be alcohol-induced or related to alcohol withdrawal. Because of the cultural tensions already reported, an effort should be made to rule out an anxiety disorder, as Mr. M may be reluctant to report anxiety symptoms. Efforts should be made to rule out other organic causes of his anxiety and agitation, such as hyperthyroidism, stimulant intoxication, caffeinism, or medication-induced anxiety. A drug toxicology screen would be helpful to rule out stimulant intoxication, caffeinism, and opiate withdrawal. A phone call to a family member or friend may add confidence to the diagnosis and rule out chronic anxiety and paranoid disorders. The symptoms do not seem excessive for alcohol withdrawal, which is the likely diagnosis, given the available information.

Option B Mr. M has no history of withdrawal seizures or withdrawal hallucinations. He has a history of panic attacks, which began after he returned from military service in Vietnam in 1971. He had been in combat for 6 months and had seen a lot of action, which he does not wish to discuss. He becomes more agitated as he talks about combat, eventually cutting off the conversation. He is angry about the way he was treated when he returned to the United States and reports a difficult transition to civilian life. He demonstrates recent heavy drinking, nightmares about combat, flashbacks, relationship problems, and a significant startle reaction to loud noises. He complains of racist treatment by white soldiers and officers in Vietnam and claims that his white superiors sent him on suicide missions.

Diagnostic Issues Is there a prominent symptom? Is there a causal relationship with the drinking? Is there any drug use that could account for the disorder? Is this better explained by another *DSM* disorder? Did the symptoms occur during a delirium? Are the symptoms excessive for alcohol intoxication or withdrawal?

Diagnostic Considerations The patient certainly evidences anxiety as a prominent symptom. However, it still is important to look for a substance dependence disorder and a substance-induced anxiety disorder. It is necessary to clarify the diagnosis of alcohol withdrawal. This patient seems to have a posttraumatic stress disorder (PTSD), alcohol dependence, alcohol withdrawal and, possibly, substance-induced anxiety disorder. Because the engagement of this patient in treatment may depend on which combination of problems he has, it is important for the clinician to obtain collateral information and a toxicology screen. Because the patient's denial may be convincing, it is not sufficient to dismiss substance dependence or a substance-induced disorder based on his history. If the patient's report is the only information available, the clinician must make a treatment decision, while remaining aware that new information could change the diagnosis and treatment plan. Mr. M's vital signs should be monitored to pick up signs of severe alcohol withdrawal. A toxicology screen should be obtained to check for drugs that can cause agitation or anxiety. A chronic history of anxiety, tension, nightmares, and the like is excessive for alcohol-induced anxiety or alcohol withdrawal alone. With this information, the clinician may consider both PTSD and alcohol withdrawal. It will be difficult to diagnose alcohol-induced anxiety in combination with PTSD unless there is a clear history of anxiety that recently has worsened without a psychosocial trigger for the PTSD. More commonly, the clinician will see an acute improvement with sobriety as a sign that there was an alcohol-induced anxiety component.

Treatment Issues Mr. M needs to be engaged in a detoxification setting (followed by an alcohol rehabilitation setting), and his denial needs management in order to expand his awareness beyond the PTSD symptoms. His claims of racism should be addressed as part of the engagement and assessment processes. Mr. M's anxiety should be managed without using benzodiazepines. His sleep disorder should be managed, and the process of relapse prevention initiated.

Treatment Considerations Treatment must be conceptualized in stages. The first stage is detoxification from alcohol (and any other drugs that may be present). With this patient, detoxification can be managed through a careful outpatient regimen if he is able to remain abstinent. If abstinence seems unlikely, if the patient fails at outpatient detoxification, or if a comorbid problem arises that cannot be monitored safely on an outpatient basis, then residential detoxification must be considered. The next stage is the maintenance of sobriety, a stabilization phase. During this stage, the clinician should monitor Mr. M's abstinence and observe the course of the anxiety symptoms. A relapse can increase his anxiety symptoms, which would interfere with attainment of the treatment goals. Such a relapse would require a treatment strategy that focuses on management of denial, motivation, and relapse prevention. If, during abstinence, the anxiety symptoms increase or stay the same, the PTSD probably is severe and medication will be needed. If the anxiety symptoms diminish or are manageable without medication, then counseling may be sufficient. The use of benzodiazepines in alcoholics after detoxification is achieved is controversial, even in the face of severe anxiety. The anxiolytic properties of benzodiazepines are sustained over time; however, many alcoholics request more of this medication. Moreover, craving for drugs is greatest when the drug, or a similar drug, is being used. Thus there always is a concern that benzodiazepines will stimulate the desire for alcohol. Drinking in addition to benzodiazepine use can lead to an "out of control" binge, as well as intoxicated behaviors, which could exaggerate the PTSD symptoms of anxiety and agitation. Disulfiram is a possible safeguard to prevent alcohol use during outpatient treatment, but the patient must be willing to collaborate (that is, take it regularly) if it is to be effective. The use of antipanic medications such as the selective serotonin reuptake inhibitors and other antidepressants would be a safer strategy. The same problem is encountered with the complaints about insomnia. Avoiding sedatives is important. Use of sedating antidepressants like trazodone and doxepin can be very effective and avoids the abuse potential of other sedative drugs.

Option C Mr. M has no history of withdrawal seizures or withdrawal hallucinations. He has had an episode (the day before coming to the emergency department) in which he became frightened, felt short of breath, felt his heart pounding, and worried that he was having a heart attack. This episode was not the first time he has experienced such an attack; he had one 6 months earlier when he quit drinking. He had gone to the emergency room the first time this happened, 5 years ago. The physician then had checked his heart and told him that he was having a nervous attack, not a heart attack. Although Mr. M feels stressed at times, he does not have these attacks regularly. When he stopped his drinking for a year, he felt well and does not recall having a spell during that time. He denies any major, traumatic life events. He was embarrassed to be worried about these anxiety spells, but also fearful that he might have been having a heart attack.

Diagnostic Issues Is there a prominent symptom? Is this symptom related to drinking? Is the symptom better explained by another DSM diagnosis? Is the symptom in excess of the symptoms normally encountered during intoxication or withdrawal?

Diagnostic Considerations There is a prominent symptom of anxiety in this case, and it appears to occur only with drinking. The clinician must think about alcohol dependence, alcohol withdrawal, and alcohol withdrawal-induced panic disorder. The major anxiety disorders should be ruled out, as should PTSD (although certain events, like sexual abuse, may be denied initially). Some attempt to rule out cardiac disease as a cause of the chest pain would be important. Organic causes of anxiety also should be ruled out. It is possible that the patient has a panic disorder that is in a prodromal phase, but this is not the most likely diagnosis. Although patients frequently experience anxiety during alcohol withdrawal, they usually do not experience panic attacks, nor do they typically go to the emergency department in a panic.

Treatment Issues Mr. M should be engaged in a detoxification program and his level of denial and motivation for treatment evaluated. The denial needs to be evaluated and the problem redefined as alcoholism, not panic or heart disease. The possibility of a comorbid anxiety disorder should be explored. The patient then needs to be engaged in an alcohol rehabilitation program. Medications that will enhance the likelihood of sobriety should be considered. The patient should be evaluated for relapse triggers and referred for relapse prevention as appropriate.

Treatment Considerations Treatment should be designed to detoxify Mr. M safely from alcohol, to explore dependence on other drugs, and to keep him sober long enough to determine whether the anxiety disorder abates with sobriety, as an alcohol withdrawal-induced anxiety disorder would. The patient's denial and motivation are important because he must understand the connection between his drinking and his panic. If his awareness of this connection is minimal, then the treatment may have to occur in a setting in which chest pain or panic is the primary focus. He may not accept the focus on his drinking. If this is the case, then referral to a rehabilitation program, either inpatient or outpatient, may not be possible at this time. Ongoing monitoring and working with his denial would be necessary before such a referral could be made. Benzodiazepines would be appropriate only during detoxification; medications that promote sobriety, such as disulfiram or naltrexone, would be appropriate if Mr. M is motivated and able to cooperate. Antipanic medications like the selective serotonin reuptake inhibitors probably would be used if the panic attacks persist with sobriety.

Case 3 A 20-year-old undergraduate presented with a chief complaint of "seeing the air." The visual disturbance consisted of a perception of white pinpoint specks, too numerous to count, in both the central and peripheral visual fields. These specks were constantly present and accompanied by the perception of trails of moving objects left behind as they pass through the visual field. Attending a hockey game became difficult, as the brightly dressed players left streaks of their own images against the white of the ice for seconds at a time. The patient also described the false perception of movement in stable objects, usually in his peripheral visual field, halos around objects, and positive and negative afterimages. Other symptoms included mild depression, daily bitemporal headache, and a loss of concentration, which emerged within the preceding year. The visual syndrome has emerged gradually over the past 3 months, after the patient experimented with the hallucinogenic drug LSD-25 on three separate occasions. The patient fears that he has sustained some kind of "brain damage" from the drug experience. He denies use of any other agents, including amphetamines, phencyclidine, narcotics, or alcohol to excess. He had smoked marijuana twice per week for a period of 7 months at age 17 (48).

Diagnostic Issues Is there a reexperiencing of a perceptual symptom after the use of a hallucinogen? Is this symptom causing significant distress or impairing function? Is this condition better explained by a delirium or another *DSM* disorder?

Diagnostic Considerations This case appears to be hallucinogen persisting perceptual disorder, or flashbacks. It consists of a perceptual disturbance resembling the drug experience (in this case, LSD) at some time after hallucinogen use; it requires that the patient be distressed by the experience. A drug toxicology screen should be obtained to rule out other drugs, despite the patient's denial. The patient appears to have insight and does not seem delusional, nor does he have negative symptoms of schizophrenia. There is no sign of delirium, but this should be considered. An evaluation of his neurologic status would be an important part of this assessment. If consent is given, confirming the patient's story with his family or a friend would be a good idea, because persons with a chronic psychotic condition can, and do, use LSD.

Treatment Issues This patient is frightened by what is happening and is afraid that he has damaged his brain by using drugs. This fear presents a unique opportunity to engage him in some kind of treatment. The question is, what kind of treatment is most appropriate? Because his use of hallucinogens may have been months earlier, it is important to ascertain whether the current problem is anxiety about the flashbacks or is related to current substance abuse or dependence. Although the patient denies being dependent on LSD and does not meet the criteria for abuse or dependence, he may have been dependent on marijuana when he was 17. A careful neurologic evaluation is advised, because there are visual disturbances, difficulties in concentrating, depression, and headaches, all of which could be associated with neurologic illness. Outpatient therapy—either drug rehabilitation or psychotherapy for the fear—probably is sufficient; however, residential treatment may be required if the patient's panic or flashbacks are severe (i.e., if they interfere markedly with his daily routine). Given the patient's anxiety, he may readily commit to abstinence from drugs. If his fears are sufficiently intense, he could develop a panic attack/PTSD-type syndrome, which could become chronic. Classic approaches to the treatment of anxiety should be used, including those discussed in the chapter on anxiety disorders in this section. Although research is lacking, some clinicians use anticonvulsants for such patients on the theory that flashback phenomena are kindled and involve some sort of focal central nervous system hyperactivity.

Case 4 Ms. A is a 35-year-old, white divorced woman who came to the emergency department because of suicidal feelings. She reported feeling very despondent that day, with suicidal ideation, and thought that she needed to be admitted to the hospital to keep her safe. On questioning, Ms. A admits that she smokes crack cocaine, about $100 worth at a time. She recently came off a 4-day binge of crack use. She takes four to six drinks of vodka per day when she uses crack and also has used marijuana.

Diagnostic Issues Is there a prominent symptom? Is this symptom related to drug use? Is this situation better explained by another DSM diagnosis? Did this situation occur exclusively during a delirium? Is this symptom more severe than usually is encountered with intoxication or withdrawal?

Diagnostic Considerations Ms. A has a prominent mood disturbance, which brought her to the emergency department. It is consistent with chronic cocaine use and temporally related to her recent binge. Although her history is not consistent with a DSM mood disorder, it is important to evaluate the possibility. A careful history of mood swings also would be important. If she has been using crack for years, the clinician can expect that she has experienced transient episodes (never more than a few days) of intense depression, even suicidality, with the cessation of cocaine use. At the same time, the clinician can expect that there have been no episodes of prolonged abstinence. Because of the recent onset of this depression, it is not likely to be the result of metabolic problems; however, addicted individuals are not always aware of subtle changes in their bodies, which may be obscured by intoxication. A screening battery is recommended, because nutritional deficiencies often are found and, not infrequently, viral hepatitis (B or C). Unsafe sexual practices and needle sharing make HIV disease a concern. More relevant, the mood disturbance could be alcohol-induced; however, this situation should not coincide with cocaine cessation. The cocaine-induced depression should last only a day or two, whereas alcohol-induced depression likely would last a few days longer with sobriety. Some alcoholics experience marked depression with suicidality during intoxication, which clears with sobriety. Although it is tempting to dismiss substance-induced depression as less significant than a major depressive disorder because the former resolves so quickly, it is important to remember that these episodes are frightening to the individual, that some people make serious suicide attempts, and that a few actually kill themselves. At this point, it appears that the patient has a cocaine withdrawal-induced mood disorder. It would be wise to obtain a toxicology screen to rule out benzodiazepine- or opiate-induced depression. With the history of depression, the clinician should look for manic episodes. Without a careful history of cocaine use and its relationship to the experience of intense moods, up or down, it would be easy to think of manic-depressive illness. Another diagnostic consideration is the possibility that Ms. A has had a social crisis and is homeless. The report of suicidality could be exaggerated to gain admission to housing or hospital. In such a case, there may be a pattern of similar behavior.

Treatment Issues Patient safety and suicidality are the primary issues here. Ms. A needs to be engaged in drug rehabilitation, her denial managed, and her motivation for abstinence enhanced. She needs to be engaged in a comprehensive assessment, with her relapse triggers assessed and relapse prevention initiated as needed.

Treatment Considerations Safety is the first treatment issue in this case because of the patient's depression (suicidality) and the possibility of alcohol withdrawal (*delirium tremens*). The clinician must assess the severity of the suicidal impulse and the social supports available before deciding whether a residential setting is appropriate. The clinician should assess what type of suicidal thoughts the person is having, whether he or she has formulated a plan to carry out the idea, whether he or she has the means to complete the plan, whether he or she has made prior attempts and, if so, if he or she was serious, whether there are other alternatives, and whether the patient is very agitated. A cocaine-induced depression usually is transient when abstinence ensues. Continued cocaine use sustains the cycle of addiction and depression. Outpatient treatment is viable only if the patient can refrain from using drugs and alcohol, and the ability to do so often depends on the degree of support in the patient's environment. Safety from alcohol withdrawal is a potential issue that should be considered; however, it is unlikely that a dangerous withdrawal will occur unless the patient has had *delirium tremens* or seizures in the past (49). Ongoing monitoring is the best precaution and can be handled on an inpatient, as well as an outpatient basis, if the patient is cooperative. Assessing the patient's reliability (ability to follow through) may be difficult if she is previously unknown to the clinician. A variety of factors enter into this assessment, including motivation, denial, awareness, craving, relapse triggers, and availability of a supportive environment. Such an assessment is part of the safety management for this patient. Engagement in a drug and alcohol treatment program will depend on the patient's denial, motivation, and awareness of the centrality of drugs and alcohol, as well as the pull of other social relationships such as children, significant others, and family members who may be dependent on Ms. A. Attention to these psychosocial issues may be the key to engagement. Focusing on a comprehensive assessment, including relapse triggers, can be the way to engage a difficult, ambivalent patient. Inclusion of the family sometimes facilitates engagement, as does admission to a treatment program if the patient is anxious about further drug use and its sequelae. If an individual has been through rehabilitation programs in the past, has relapsed, and has a commitment to abstinence as well as a capacity to remain abstinent, then a focus on relapse prevention may be the appropriate intervention. Such intervention remains part of the art of medicine and hinges on the physician's style of practice, local resources, and managed care practices. It is a complex challenge each time and must be individualized to each situation.

CONCLUSIONS

The substance-induced mental disorders are common illnesses that often are associated with (but are not limited to) substance dependence. Although they frequently are short-lived, these disorders are by no means clinically insignificant. Serious self-injury is reported with the substance-induced mood disorders, and safety is an important clinical issue. This situation can present a clinical dilemma in determining the proper level of care. Most patients with substance-induced mental disorders can be diverted away from traditional psychiatric inpatient treatment, either to dual diagnosis units or to inpatient or outpatient addiction treatment programs in which adequate assessment and appropriate treatment are available. Clinics and residential units that specialize in substance dependent patients who have a comorbid psychiatric illness play an important role when there is diagnostic confusion or when the patient does not respond (or has not responded in the past) to routine psychiatric treatment. Confusion about the diagnosis can delay interventions; therefore, achieving clarification through a comprehensive evaluation is the first order of business, after safety is addressed. Although abstinence is a critical factor in recovery from a substance-induced mental disorder, it is not always the only factor. Regular psychosocial treatments for substance dependence are relevant so long as the patient is behaviorally manageable and not psychotic or delirious. When the patient's behavior is unsafe or wild, a psychiatric unit may be necessary until the patient's behavior is less risky. If a specialized inpatient unit for dual diagnosis is available and can manage the patient's behavior with seclusion, restraints, psychotropic medications, or a locked unit, it may be the best choice. Such patient-treatment matching should be done on an individual basis, depending on the patient's needs, the resources available, and the skills and preferences of the clinicians involved.

REFERENCES

1. American Psychiatric Association (APA) *Diagnostic and statistical manual of mental disorders,* 4th ed. *(DSM-IV).* Washington, DC: American Psychiatric Press, 1994.
2. American Psychiatric Association (APA). *Diagnostic and statistical manual of mental disorders,* 3rd edition, revised *(DSM-IIIR).* Washington, DC: American Psychiatric Press, 1987.
3. Brown SA, Schuckit MA. Changes in depression among abstinent alcoholics. *J Stud Alcohol* 1988;49:412–417.
4. Brown SA, Inaba RK, Gillin JC, et al. Alcoholism and affective disorder: clinical course of depressive symptoms. *Am J Psychiatry* 1995;152:45–52.
5. Schuckit MA, Tipp JE, Bergman M, et al. Comparison of induced and independent major depressive disorders in 2,945 alcoholics. *Am J Psychiatry* 1997;154:948–957.
6. Kahler CW, Ramsey SE, Read JP, et al. Substance-induced and independent major depressive disorder in treatment-seeking alcoholics: associations with dysfunctional attitudes and coping. *J Stud Alcohol* 2002;63: 363–371.
7. First MB, Spitzer RL, Gibbon M, et al. Structured clinical interview for DSM-IV Axis I disorders, New York: New York State Psychiatric Institute, 1995.
8. Grant BF, Stinson FS, Dawson DA, et al. Prevalence and co-occurrence of substance use disorders and independent mood and anxiety disorders: results from the National Epidemiological Survey on Alcohol and Related Conditions. *Arch Gen Psychiatry* 2004;61:807–816.
9. Ramsey SE, Kahler CW, Read JP, et al. Discriminating between substance-induced and independent depressive episodes in alcohol dependent patients. *J Stud Alcohol* 2004;65:672–676.
10. Nunes EV, Liu X, Samet S, et al. Independent versus substance-induced major depressive disorder in substance-dependent patients: observational study of course during follow-up. *J Clin Psychiatry* 2006;67:1561–1567.
11. Schuckit MA, Hesselbrock V. Alcohol dependence and anxiety disorders: What is the relationship? *Am J Psychiatry* 1994;151:1723–1734.
12. Brown SA, Irwin M, Schuckit MA. Changes in anxiety among abstinent male alcoholics. *J Stud Alcohol* 1991;52:55–61.
13. Rounsaville BJ, Anton SF, Carroll K, et al. Psychiatric diagnoses of treatment-seeking cocaine abusers. *Arch Gen Psychiatry* 1991;48:43–51.
14. Zweben JE, Cohen JB, Christian D, et al. Psychiatric symptoms in methamphetamine users. *Am J Addict* 2004;13:181–190.
15. Rosenthal RN, Miner CR. Differential diagnosis of substance-induced psychosis and schizophrenia in patients with substance use disorders. *Schiz Bull* 1997;23:187–193.
16. Brady KT, Lydiard RB, Malcolm R, et al. Cocaine-induced psychosis. *J Clin Psychiatry* 1991;52:509–512.
17. Caton CL, Drake RE, Hasin DS, et al. Differences between early-phase primary psychotic disorders with concurrent substance use and substance-induced psychosis. *Arch Gen Psychiatry* 2005;62:137–145.
18. McKetin R, McLaren J, Lubman DI, et al. The prevalence of psychotic symptoms among methamphetamine users. *Addiction* 2006;101: 1473–1478.

19. Pasic J, Russo JE, Ries RK, et al. Methamphetamine users in the psychiatric emergency services: a case-control study. *Am J Drug Alcohol Abuse* 2007;33:675–686.
20. Ujike H, Sato M. Clinical features of sensitization to methamphetamine observed in patients with methamphetamine dependence and psychosis. *Ann N Y Acad Sci* 2004;1025:279–287.
21. Akiyama K. Longitudinal clinical course following pharmacological treatment of methamphetamine psychosis which persists after long-term abstinence. *Ann N Y Acad Sci* 2006;1074:125–134.
22. Murphy GE, Wetzel RD. The lifetime risk of suicide in alcoholism. *Arch Gen Psychiatry* 1990;47:383–392.
23. Henriksson MM, Aro HM, Marttunen MJ, et al. Mental disorders and comorbidity in suicide. *Am J Psychiatry* 1993;150:933–940.
24. Young MA, Fogg LF, Scheftner WA, et al. Interactions of risk factors in predicting suicide. *Am J Psychiatry* 1994;151:434–435.
25. Driessen M, Veltrup C, Weber J, et al. Psychiatric co-morbidity, suicidal behaviour and suicidal ideation in alcoholics seeking treatment. *Addiction* 1998;93:889–894.
26. Pages KP, Russo JE, Roy-Byrne PP, et al. Determinants of suicidal ideation: the role of substance use disorders. *J Clin Psychiatry* 1997;58: 510–515.
27. Salloum IM, Daley DC, Cornelius JR, et al. Disproportionate lethality in psychiatric patients with concurrent alcohol and cocaine abuse. *Am J Psychiatry* 1996;153:953–955.
28. Elliott AJ, Pages KP, Russo J, et al. A profile of medically serious suicide attempts. *J Clin Psychiatry* 1996;57:567–571.
29. Asnis GM, Friedmen TA, Sanderson WC, et al. Suicidal behaviors in adult psychiatry outpatients, I: Description and prevalence. *Am J Psychiatry* 1993;150:108–112.
30. Connor KR, Hesselbrock VM, Meldrum SC, et al. Transitions to, and correlates of, suicidal ideation, plans, and unplanned and planned suicide attempts among 3,729 men and women with alcohol dependence. *J Stud Alcohol Drugs* 2007;68:654–662.
31. Aharonovich E, Liu X, Nunes E, et al. Suicide attempts in substance abusers: effects of major depression in relation to substance use disorder. *Am J Psychiatry* 2002;159:1600–1602.
32. Ries RK, Yuodelis-Flores C, Comtois KA, et al. Substance-induced suicidal admissions to an acute psychiatric service: characteristics and outcomes. *J Subst Abuse Treatment* 2008;34:72–79.
33. Bartels SJ, Drake RE, McHugo GJ. Alcohol abuse, depression, and suicidal behavior in schizophrenia. *Am J Psychiatry* 1992;149:394–395.
34. Seibyl JP, Satel SL, Anthony D, et al. Effects of cocaine on hospital course in schizophrenia. *J Nerv Ment Di* 1993;181:31–37.
35. Ries RK, Demirsoy A, Russo JE, et al. Reliability and clinical utility of DSM-IV substance-induced psychiatric disorders in acute psychiatric inpatients. *Am J Addictions* 2001;10:308–318.
36. Ashton H. Protracted withdrawal syndromes from benzodiazepines. In: Miller NS, ed. *Comprehensive handbook of drug and alcohol addiction*. New York: Marcel Dekker, 1991:915–930.
37. Gold MS. *Cocaine.* New York: Plenum Publishing, 1993.
38. Mendoza R, Miller BL. Neuropsychiatric disorders associated with cocaine use. *Hosp Comm Psychiatry* 1992;43:677–679.
39. Thomasius R, Petersen KU, Zapletatova P, et al. Mental disorders in current and former heavy ecstasy (MDMA) users. *Addiction* 2005;100: 1310–1319.
40. Levinson I, Galynker II , Rosenthal RN. Methadone withdrawal psychosis. *J Clin Psychiatry* 1995;56:73–76.
41. Budney AJ, Novy PL, Hughes JR. Marijuana withdrawal among adults seeking treatment for marijuana dependence. *Addiction* 1999;94: 1311–1322.
42. Copersino ML, Boyd SJ, Tashkin DP, et al. Cannabis withdrawal among non-treatment-seeking adult cannabis users. *Am J Addict* 2006;15:8–14.
43. Moore TH, Zammet S, Lingford-Hughes A, et al. Cannabis use and risk of psychotic or affective mental health outcomes: a systematic review. *Lancet* 2007;370(9584):319–328.
44. Semple DM, McIntosh AM, Lawrie SM. Cannabis as a risk factor for psychosis: systematic review. *J Psychopharmacol* 2005;19(2):187–194.
45. Giannini AJ. Phencyclidine. In: NS Miller NS, ed. *Comprehensive handbook of drug and alcohol addiction*. New York: Marcel Dekker, 1991: 383–394.
46. Zukin SR, Zukin RS. Phencyclidine. In: Lowinson JH, Ruiz P, Millman RB, et al. eds. *Substance abuse: a comprehensive textbook*. Baltimore, MD: Williams & Wilkins, 1992:290–302.
47. Mee-Lee D, Shulman G, Fishman M, et al. *ASAM patient placement criteria for the treatment of substance-related disorders,* 2nd edition–revised. Chevy Chase, MD: American Society of Addiction Medicine, 2001.
48. Spitzer RL, Gibbon M, Skodol AE, et al., eds. DSM-IV *casebook: a learning companion to the diagnostic and statistical manual of mental disorders,* 4th ed. Washington, DC: American Psychiatric Press, 1994:216.
49. Whitfield CL, Thompson G, Lamb A, et al. Detoxification of 1,024 alcoholic patients without psychoactive drugs. *JAMA* 1978;239: 1409–1410.

CHAPTER 84

Edward V. Nunes, MD
Roger D. Weiss, MD

Co-occurring Addiction and Affective Disorders

OVERVIEW AND DEFINITION OF DSM-IV CRITERIA

Significance Depressive disorders, major depression, and dysthymia are among the most common psychiatric disorders in the general population. Estimates from community surveys show that more than 10% of the general population has experienced a depressive disorder at some point in their lifetime, and the prevalence of substance use disorders is increased by a factor or 2 or more among individuals with major depression (1). Major depression is the most common co-occurring psychiatric disorder encountered among patients presenting for treatment for substance use disorders, with lifetime prevalence rates ranging from 15% to 50% across samples studied from various treatment settings (2). Among drug- and alcohol-dependent patients, major depression has been associated with worse outcome, including worse substance use outcome, worse psychiatric symptoms, and increased suicide risk. Clinical trials suggest that treatment of depression among substance dependent patients with medication or behavioral therapy can improve outcome. Thus, it is very important for clinicians working with substance-dependent patients to be able to recognize and treat depression or make appropriate referrals for treatment.

Bipolar disorder is more rare in the general population, with estimates of the lifetime prevalence of bipolar I disorder ranging from 1% to 3%, and another 1% for bipolar II disorder, and 2% or more having subthreshold disorders in the bipolar spectrum, each of which are associated with moderate to severe functional impairment (3,4). Bipolar disorder is correspondingly less common than major depression among samples of patients seeking treatment for substance use disorders in routine outpatient settings. However, the strength of association between bipolar disorders and substance use disorders is larger than for depressive disorders, with the presence of a bipolar disorder increasing the likelihood a substance use disorder by a factor of 4 or more. Hence, among patients with bipolar disorder, the prevalence of substance use disorders is 40% or more (5), and patients with both substance and bipolar disorders are especially likely to be encountered on inpatient settings or other clinical programs serving psychiatric or dual diagnosis populations. As with unipolar depression, co-occurring bipolar and substance use disorder is associated with worse prognosis, and though clinical trials are more limited, those that have been conducted suggest that proper treatment of bipolar disorder improves substance use outcome. Further, many patients with bipolar disorder (particularly those who have had bipolar disorder for a long time) will present with a depressive syndrome, but the treatment recommendations for bipolar depression are quite different from unipolar depression. Thus, it is very important for clinicians working with substance-dependent patients to be able to recognize bipolar disorder, distinguish unipolar depression from bipolar disorder, and either treat or make appropriate referrals for treatment.

DSM-IV Criteria for Depressive Disorders and Bipolar Disorders A brief overview of DSM-IV mood disorders (6) is provided in Tables 84.1A and 84.1B. Readers who are less familiar with how to take a history to detect these disorders are encouraged to obtain some experience with one of the semi-structured psychiatric diagnostic interviews such as the Structured Clinical Interview for DSM-IV (SCID) (7) or the Psychiatric Research Interview for Substance and Mood Disorders (PRISM) (8). These interviews guide the clinician in how to

TABLE 84.1A Synopsis of Diagnostic Criteria for DSM-IV Depressive Disorders and Important Issues to Consider in Diagnosing Depressive Disorders in Patients Who Are Using Drugs or Alcohol

Overview of DSM-IV criteria	Notes on making the diagnosis in patients using drugs or alcohol
Depressive Disorders Major depressive disorder consists of one or more episodes of major depression, over the course of the lifetime. May occur as single episode, recurrent episodes, or may run a chronic course. Other subtypes include melancholic, atypical, postpartum, psychotic, and catatonic.	Take a careful history of the course of depressive episodes over the lifetime (e.g., age of first onset, age at subsequent episodes, duration and quality of episodes) Relate lifetime course of depression to the lifetime course of substance use and substance use disorders
Major depressive episode At least 2 weeks of persistent core mood disturbance: Depressed mood, and/or Loss of interest or pleasure in most activities plus associated symptoms: Weight loss or gain Insomnia or hypersomnia Psychomotor agitation or retardation Fatigue or loss of energy Feelings of worthlessness or excessive guilt Poor concentration or indecisiveness Thoughts of death or suicide, or suicidal behavior A total of at least 5 symptoms are needed, including either (1) or (2) Symptoms must be persistent: "most of the day, every day" Not due to drug or alcohol use, or another physiological cause such as a medical illness	Most depressive symptoms occur as part of intoxication or withdrawal syndromes of one or more substances (see also Table 84.2), so care is needed in attributing a symptom to a depressive disorder, as opposed to effects of a substance Look for persistence of depressive symptoms ("most of the day every day") through increases or decreases in substance use, or abstinent periods; symptoms that emerge then resolve in step with substance use are more consistent with intoxication or withdrawal effects (e.g., insomnia that occurs only on nights after episodes of cocaine use)
Dysthymic disorder A low-grade but chronic depression–at least 2 years' duration, feeling depressed "most of the day, more days than not," plus at least two associated symptoms (weight disturbance, sleep disturbance, low energy, low self-esteem, poor concentration or indecisiveness, hopelessness). Again, not due to drug or alcohol use, or another physiological cause such as medical illness	Fewer and milder symptoms may be more difficult to distinguish from substance intoxication or withdrawal effects; but chronicity may be more indicative of a disorder that is independent of substance effects Look for the chronicity, and persistence ("most of the day, more days than not") of symptoms, despite ups and downs in levels of substance use or periods of abstinence
Depressive disorder not otherwise specified A residual category for depressive syndromes that fall short of diagnostic criteria for major depression or dysthymia (e.g., not enough symptoms or not sufficient duration or persistence), but appear clinically significant	Little research on this residual category Given fewer and milder symptoms, more concern about distinguishing from intoxication or withdrawal effects But, depressive disorders lie on a continuum and milder forms may still be clinically significant
Substance-induced depression Depressive syndrome that cannot be established to be independent of drug or alcohol use (e.g., by history it seems to occur only during periods of substance use), but depressive symptoms are "in excess of those usually associated with intoxication or withdrawal," and "sufficiently severe to warrant independent clinical attention"	See Table 84.5 and related text for more discussion Bear in mind that this is not simply intoxication or withdrawal effects (a common misconception, encouraged by the term "substance-induced"), but rather mood symptoms "in excess" of substance effects.

Mood disorders, grouped into depressive disorders and bipolar disorders, consist of combinations of mood episodes (major depressive episode, manic episode, hypomanic episode, mixed episode). For detailed criteria, readers are encouraged to study the full DSM-IV criteria and accompanying discussion. Adapted from American Psychiatric Association. *Diagnostic and Statistical Manual of Mental Disorders*, 4th ed. Washington, DC: Author, 1994.

ask about each of the symptoms and apply the DSM-IV criteria, and practice in using them constitutes an excellent training exercise. Mood disorders are divided into depressive disorders (also referred to as *unipolar*), consisting of single or multiple episodes of major depression or dysthymia, and bipolar disorders, which consist of mixtures across the patient's lifetime of episodes of depression and episodes of mania, hypomania, or mixed mood states. The distinction of depressive disorders from bipolar disorders is important, because the relationship to substance use differs, and the treatment implications differ in important ways.

TABLE 84.1B Synopsis of Diagnostic Criteria for DSM-IV Bipolar Disorders and Important Issues to Consider in Diagnosing Bipolar Disorders in Patients Who Are Using Drugs or Alcohol

Synopsis of DSM-IV criteria	Notes on making the diagnosis in patients using drugs or alcohol
Bipolar disorders Bipolar I disorder: at least one episode of mania, or a mixed episode (both mania and major depression criteria are met simultaneously). Often, series of episodes of mania/mixed, and major depression. Bipolar II disorder: episodes of major depression plus episodes of hypomania. Depression may predominate the history. Lifetime course of bipolar I or II over the lifetime may consist of episodes, or be chronic. A rapid cycling pattern is diagnosed when there are at least four episodes in a year (e.g., switches between mania or hypomania and depression).	Take a careful history of the course of depressive episodes over the lifetime (e.g., age of first onset, age at subsequent episodes, duration and quality of episodes) Relate lifetime course of depression to the lifetime course of substance use and substance use disorders Rapid cycling has been associated with substance abuse, though care must be taken not to mistake shifts in mood from euphoric to depressed caused by alternating periods of intoxication and withdrawal
Manic episode At least 1 week of persistently elevated mood (mood may be euphoric, or irritable), accompanied by at least three of the following: Grandiosity, inflated self-esteem (e.g., patient believes they have special powers or insights, e.g., on a mission from God) Decreased need for sleep (sleeps less, yet feels well rested) More talkative, pressured speech, hard to interrupt Flight of ideas—patient may report feeling of racing thoughts, or clinician may observe rapid expression of ideas. Distractibility—attention easily drawn to outside stimuli Increase in activity level—may be goal directed (such as increased activity at school or work, socially, or sexually), or may present as agitation. Excessive involvement in pleasurable activities with high potential for bad consequences (displaying seemingly poor judgment)—e.g., buying sprees (buying large quantities of things the patient may have had little interest in previously), sexual adventures, foolish business ventures. Not due to drug or alcohol use, or other physiological cause	Mania resembles stimulant intoxication (cocaine, amphetamines), including development of psychosis. Other intoxication syndromes, including alcohol, PCP, hallucinogens might also resemble features of mania. Manic-like symptoms that are part of intoxication should resolve quickly as intoxication wears off. Duration (persistence) and severity of symptoms of mania usually make it easy to distinguish mania from intoxication effects.
Hypomanic episode Essentially same criteria as manic episode, but may be of shorter duration (4 days), and not severe enough to meet criteria for mania (no psychosis, no hospitalization, no marked impairment in functioning). There must be a change in functioning, which may cause impairment, but may sometimes enhance functioning (e.g., patient becomes more productive or creative and work)	Milder symptoms may be more difficult to distinguish from substance intoxication, but, again, intoxication symptoms should resolve quickly as intoxication wears off Look for persistence of symptoms, despite ups and downs in levels of substance use or periods of abstinence
Mixed episode Criteria for both major depression and mania are met simultaneously	
Cyclothymic disorder Chronic course (at least two years) with periods of hypomanic symptoms and periods of depressive symptoms (not reaching criteria for major depression)	Fewer and milder symptoms more difficult to distinguish from binge-crash pattern of cocaine/stimulant intoxication and withdrawal. Again, look for persistence of symptoms, despite ups and downs in levels of substance use or periods of abstinence
Bipolar not otherwise specified Residual category for syndromes that fall short of criteria for bipolar I, II, or cyclothymia.	Same caveats re: fewer/mild symptoms as for Cyclothymic Disorder
Substance-induced mood disorder Bipolar syndrome that cannot be established to be independent of drug or alcohol use (seems to occur only during periods of substance use), but symptoms are "in excess of those usually associated with intoxication or withdrawal," and "sufficiently severe to warrant independent clinical attention"	Not simply intoxication or withdrawal effects (e.g., cocaine intoxication symptoms that resolve rapidly after a binge), but rather mood symptoms "in excess" of expected substance effects. There has been little research on substance-induced bipolar disorder, *per se*. Often possible to recognize independent bipolar disorder through a careful history, without needing to invoke the substance-induced category.

Bipolar disorders, consist of combinations of mood episodes (major depressive episode, manic episode, hypomanic episode, mixed episode). For detailed criteria, readers are encouraged to study the full DSM-IV criteria and accompanying discussion. Adapted from American Psychiatric Association. *Diagnostic and Statistical Manual of Mental Disorders*, 4th ed. Washington, DC: Author, 1994.

Depressive Disorders DSM-IV defines a major depressive episode as a period of persistent, relatively severe depression, with multiple associated depressive symptoms (disturbances in weight, appetite, sleep, energy, cognition, self-esteem, suicidal ideation, etc.) lasting at least 2 weeks and interfering with functioning. Dysthymia is a period of milder but chronic depression lasting at least 2 years. Major depressive disorder is diagnosed when there have been one or more major depressive episodes. When interviewing a patient with current depressive symptoms, it is always important to review the lifetime history for past episodes of major depression. Major depression may occur as a single isolated episode or may run a chronic episodic course with multiple recurrences or may be chronic and unremitting. Major depressive episodes may also be superimposed on a chronic dysthymic pattern. At its most severe, there can be psychosis, often involving delusions of paranoia or guilt (e.g., patients begin to believe they have committed a terrible crime and will be punished). The major risk factors for depressive disorders include a genetic component. This is evidenced by heritability estimates from twin and family studies; no "disease genes," per se, have yet clearly identified, and it seems likely that there are multiple genetic factors each with a modest contribution to risk for depression, rather than single major disease genes. Stress (e.g., losses) and trauma are also important risk factors. Thus, in taking a history, it is always important to ask about family history and about stressors and traumatic experiences. DSM-IV also requires that the clinician establish that the depressive disorder is not caused by substance use (abuse, or a medication) or a medical condition (e.g., hypothyroidism, or other systemic illnesses, among others). Thus, a medical history and workup is an important component of the diagnostic evaluation. Finally, when evaluating a patient presenting with a major depressive episode or a syndrome of dysthymia, it is very important to review the history for past episodes of mania, hypomania, or mixed mood episodes. The presence of one of these indicates that the patient has a bipolar disorder.

Bipolar Disorders Bipolar disorders consist of episodes of major depression or dysthymia, alternating with episodes of mania, or hypomania, at some time during the lifetime course. Mania is a severe disturbance consisting of euphoric, expansive, or irritable mood, high energy, less need for sleep (e.g., only a few hours per night), grandiose thinking (e.g., believing one has special powers, religious revelations), and increased speech and activity level. Functioning is severely impaired with disorganized, inappropriate behavior, and patients often become psychotic with hallucinations and delusions that may be grandiose ("I am the messiah") or paranoid ("the CIA is after me"). Mixed states also occur, in which the patient meets criteria for both mania and major depression during the same episode. Hypomania is a milder form of mania, without psychosis and with less functional impairment. In some cases, functioning improves during hypomania with high levels of productivity and creativity. In most cases of bipolar disorder, depressive episodes are predominant with less frequent mania or hypomania. Thus, patients with bipolar disorder often present with major depression, or dysthymia, and a careful lifetime history is needed to determine whether there have been past episodes of mania or hypomania. It is also useful to interview family members about this, as patients themselves often have little insight during mania or hypomania and may not experience these states as abnormal. As with depressive disorders, genetics, stress, and trauma are risk factors, so that family history and history of stress and trauma exposure are again important. Again, DSM-IV requires the clinician to rule out drugs (particularly stimulants), medications, or medical illnesses that might mimic bipolar disorder symptoms.

Distinguishing Substance-Related Mood Symptoms from Mood Disorders The problem of distinguishing mood symptoms caused by substance intoxication or withdrawal or chronic exposure to substances from bona fide mood disorders is one of the pivotal challenges for clinicians working with substance-abusing patients. Hence it is a central focus of this chapter. Mood symptoms (e.g., sadness, apathy, irritability, pessimism, hopelessness, fatigue, anxiety, insomnia, euphoria, hyperactivity) are extremely common among patients with drug or alcohol use problems. Often such symptoms are components of substance intoxication or withdrawal and will resolve with abstinence; in that case, the indicated treatment is aggressive treatment of the substance problem. At other times, the mood symptoms are components of an independent mood disorder that needs to be treated in addition to treating the substance problems.

Table 84.2 provides a summary of the overlap between symptoms of substance intoxication and withdrawal as listed in DSM-IV and DSM-IV symptoms of unipolar and bipolar mood disorders (6). Cannabis withdrawal, although not included in DSM-IV, has been added, as it is now well characterized (9) and likely to be included in DSM-V. As can be seen, there is considerable overlap. It is a worthwhile exercise to review the descriptions in DSM-IV (and the criteria) of the various substance intoxication and withdrawal syndromes. Further, it is clear that chronic substance exposure, perhaps in combination with the high level of stress frequently characterizing the addict lifestyle, often results in considerable depressive symptoms beyond what is listed among DSM-IV intoxication and withdrawal symptoms. This is part of what prompted the creation of the syndrome of Substance-Induced Depression in DSM-IV (6).

Abstinence or Initiation of Substance Abuse Treatment Improves Depression This point cannot be overemphasized. Studies among alcohol- (10-12), opioid- (13), and cocaine-dependent patients (14,15) have documented elevated scores on depression symptom scales that improve substantially after initiation of abstinence upon treatment entry, such as hospitalization for detoxification or initiation of methadone maintenance. Thus, initiation of treatment for the substance use problem and efforts to achieve abstinence should always be a first step in the treatment of patients with co-occurring mood and substance use disorders.

TABLE 84.2 Similarities and Differences between DSM-IV Intoxication or Withdrawal Symptoms and Symptoms of DSM-IV Mood Disorders

	Intoxication or withdrawal symptoms that resemble major depression or dysthymia	Intoxication or withdrawal symptoms that resemble mania or hypomania	Intoxication or withdrawal symptoms that are distinct from symptoms of mood disorder
Alcohol or sedatives	Intoxication: mood lability Withdrawal: anxiety, insomnia	Intoxication: inappropriate sexual or aggressive behavior, mood lability, impaired judgment, impaired functioning, impaired attention Withdrawal: insomnia, agitation, auditory hallucinations	Intoxication: slurred speech, incoordination, unsteady gait, nystagmus, impaired memory, stupor, coma Withdrawal: autonomic hyperactivity (e.g., sweating, increased pulse, blood pressure, temperature), tremor, nausea/vomiting, visual or tactile hallucinations, seizures, delirium
Cocaine or amphetamines	Intoxication: anxiety, anger, psychomotor agitation or retardation, weight loss Withdrawal: dysphoria, fatigue, insomnia or hypersomnia, increased appetite, psychomotor agitation or retardation	Intoxication: euphoria, increased sociability, hypervigilance, anger, impaired judgment, impaired functioning, agitation, auditory hallucinations, paranoia Withdrawal: insomnia, agitation	Intoxication: stereotyped behaviors, vital sign abnormalities, pupillary dilation, sweating or chills, nausea or vomiting, respiratory depression, cardiac symptoms (chest pain, arrhythmias), confusion, coma, dyskinesia, dystonia, seizures, visual or tactile hallucinations or illusions Withdrawal: vivid unpleasant dreams
Cannabis	Intoxication: social withdrawal, anxiety, increased appetite Withdrawal: depressed mood, irritability, anxiety, insomnia, decreased appetite, restlessness	Intoxication: euphoria, impaired judgment Withdrawal: irritability, anger, increased aggression, insomnia	Intoxication: impaired coordination, conjunctival injection, tachycardia Withdrawal: strange dreams, headache, shakiness, sweating, stomach upset, nausea
Opioids	Intoxication: apathy, dysphoria, psychomotor retardation Withdrawal: dysphoria (irritability, anxiety), insomnia, fatigue	Intoxication: euphoria, agitation, impaired judgment or social functioning Withdrawal: irritability, insomnia	Intoxication: pupillary constriction, slurred speech, drowsiness, respiratory depression, stupor, coma (pupillary dilation and other signs of anoxia) Withdrawal: nausea, vomiting, muscle aches, lacrimation, rhinorrhea, pupillary dilation, piloerection, sweating, diarrhea, yawning, fever
Hallucinogens	Intoxication: anxiety, depression, paranoia	Intoxication: euphoria, paranoia, impaired judgment or functioning	Intoxication: ideas of reference, fear of losing one's mind, perceptual changes (depersonalization, derealization, hallucinations, synesthesia), pupillary dilation, tachycardia, sweating, palpitations, tremors, blurred vision, incoordination
PCP	Intoxication:	Intoxication: belligerence, impulsiveness, agitation, impaired judgment or functioning	Intoxication: nystagmus, tachycardia, hypertension, decreased responsiveness to pain, unsteady gait, slurred speech, muscular rigidity, seizures, coma, hyperacusis
Nicotine	Withdrawal: dysphoria, insomnia, irritability, anxiety, difficulty concentrating, restlessness, increased appetite, weight gain	Withdrawal: irritability, impaired concentration, restlessness, insomnia	Withdrawal: bradycardia

Note: The table lists DSM-IV symptoms for intoxication or withdrawal from each of the main substance classes, and shows where there is overlap with similar symptoms of DSM-IV depressive syndromes major depression, dysthymia) in column 2, or bipolar syndromes (mania, hypomania) in column 3. Column 4 lists intoxication and withdrawal symptoms that are not consistent with mood disorder symptoms and would be helpful to distinguish substance effects from mood disorders.

Some Cases of Depression Will Persist Despite Abstinence or Substance Abuse Treatment This point deserves equal emphasis. Despite abstinence or reductions in substance use, some cases of depression will persist. Evidence suggests that a careful clinical history can distinguish mood disorders that are independent of substance use and will persist in abstinence from those that will resolve with abstinence. For example, in a now classic series of studies, Brown and Schuckit (11) divided alcohol-dependent patients entering a 4-week inpatient stay into those with no history of mood disorder, those with a secondary mood disorder onset after the onset of alcohol dependence, and those with a primary mood disorder mood disorder onset prior to the onset of alcohol dependence. All three groups had substantially elevated Hamilton Depression Scale (HDS) scores at the outset. After 1 to 2 weeks of abstinence, the groups with no mood disorder or a secondary mood disorder experienced reductions of more than 50% in their HDS scores with scores dropping into the normal or mildly depressed range, no specific treatment for depression needed. However, in the group with primary mood disorder, there was no change in the depression scores over 3 weeks of abstinence, and two-thirds of those patients had HDS scores greater than 20 after 3 weeks of abstinence, consistent with severe depression. For these patients, aggressive treatment of the alcohol dependence did not take care of the depression, and most clinicians and researchers would now agree that these patients with primary depression, identified with a careful lifetime psychiatric history, need to receive treatment for their depressive disorder in addition to continued treatment for the alcohol dependence.

Importance of the Clinical History Controversy over how to make these distinctions between mood symptoms caused by substances versus mood symptoms that are part of a true mood disorder has characterized the field since the inception of modern psychiatric diagnosis. This will be discussed at greater length in the section on Differential Diagnosis requiring specific treatment. The field has expanded from a narrower view of a "primary" disorder as having prior onset, as in the study of alcohol-dependent patients cited earlier (16), to a broader view articulated in the DSM-IV of independent mood disorders having prior onset or persistence despite a period of abstinence sufficient to rule out substance effect (6). For example, we recently showed that a past history of an independent mood disorder, in the sense of the DSM-IV as operationalized with the PRISM interview (8), distinguished cases of major depression that would persist during abstinence over a 1-year follow-up in a sample of treatment-seeking substance-dependent patients (17). The point to emphasize here is that, in addition to efforts to initiate substance abuse treatment and help the patient attain abstinence, a careful clinical history can help select those patients with independent mood disorders. The history should examine the course of mood symptoms in relation to substance use over the patient's lifetime, looking particularly for onset of a mood disorder syndrome prior to the onset of substance problems, as in the study of alcohol dependence described earlier (16) or the persistence or emergence of a mood disorder during abstinent periods over the lifetime, consistent with the DSM-IV construct of an independent (as opposed to a substance-induced) mood disorder.

Overview of the Chapter The balance of this chapter covers in more detail the epidemiology, differential diagnosis, and treatment of co-occurring mood and substance use disorders. The section on epidemiology examines the prevalence and prognostic significance of co-occurring mood and substance use disorders in community samples and clinical samples typically encountered by practitioners. The next section presents an approach to differential diagnosis of mood disorders in the setting of substance abuse, based on DSM-IV and the latest evidence on diagnostic approaches. The final sections present evidence on treatment for depressive and bipolar disorders co-occurring with substance use disorders. It is hoped that this chapter will provide a useful clinical guideline for physicians and other practitioners working with substance-abusing patients as well as an introduction to the evidence base in the research literature and the gaps in research that need to be filled to further advance the field.

PREVALENCE AND PROGNOSTIC EFFECTS OF CO-OCCURRING MOOD AND SUBSTANCE USE DISORDERS

Since interest in the co-occurrence of mood and substance use disorders began to increase in the 1960s and 1970s, many studies have been published examining the prevalence of mood disorders among substance-dependent samples. The initial generation of studies examined patients being admitted to treatment services for substance use disorders (e.g., inpatient detoxification or rehabilitation units, methadone maintenance clinics). These are particularly useful in establishing the scope of the clinical problem and (when follow-up data were gathered) the prognostic effects. However, in regard to etiology, studies of clinical samples would tend to overestimate the magnitude of association between mood and substance use disorders because of Berkson's bias, namely that high rates of comorbidity can be an artifact of treatment seeking rather than a reflection of a direct relationship between the disorders (18). For example, depression might drive substance-dependent patients to seek treatment, accounting for its high prevalence among treatment seekers without any direct etiologic relationship between the disorders. Studies of comorbidity in community samples drawn from the general population represented a substantial advance in part because they circumvent Berkson's bias. These prevalence studies are also important because they show the evolution of diagnostic methods for addressing the problem of distinguishing mood symptoms from mood disorders, introduced earlier, and the development of the DSM-IV approach to co-occurring disorders, presented later in the section on Differential Diagnosis.

General Population Four major studies of the prevalence of psychiatric disorders among community samples

TABLE 84.3 Odds Ratios[a] Reflecting the Strength of Association, or Co-occurrence, between Alcohol or Drug Dependence Disorders and Affective and Other Selected Disorders

	ECA		NCS				NESARC	
			Alcohol dependence		Other drug dependence			
	Alcohol dependence	Other drug dependence	Men	Women	Men	Women	Alcohol dependence	Other drug dependence
Mood disorders								
Major depressive disorder	1.6	3.7	3.0	4.1	2.0[b]	2.0[b]	3.7	9.0
Dysthymia	2.3	3.6	3.8	3.6	1.3[b]	1.3[b]	2.8	11.3
Bipolar disorder	4.6	8.3	12.0[c]	5.3[c]	—	—	5.7[c]	13.9[c]
Other disorders								
Panic disorder	3.3	4.4	2.3	3.0	—	—	3.6[d]	10.5[d]
Social phobia	1.6	2.2	2.4	2.6	2.6[b]	2.6[b]	2.5	5.4
Posttraumatic stress disorder		—	3.2	3.6	3.0	4.5	—	—
Attention deficit disorder	—	—	2.8[b]	2.8[b]	7.9[b]	7.9[b]	—	—
Antisocial personality	14.7	15.6	8.3	17.0			7.1	18.5

[a]ECA and NCS report odds ratios on lifetime prevalences of co-occurring disorders; NESARC reports odds rations on 12-month prevalences of co-occurring disorders.

[b]For these co-occurring disorders in NCS, odds ratios are reported for men and women combined.

[c]For NCS and NESARC, odds ratios are for bipolar I disorder with a history of full mania.

[d]For NESARC, odds ratios shown are for panic disorder with agoraphobia; odds ratios for panic disorder without agoraphobia were similar.

Note: Data taken from three community surveys: the Epidemiological Catchment Area study (ECA), the National Comorbidity Study (NCS), and the National Epidemiological Survey of Alcoholism and Related Conditions (NESARC). The odds ratio can be interpreted, roughly, as the multiple by which the prevalence of a disorder across the rows (major depression, dysthymia, etc.) is increased when alcohol or drug dependence is present, compared to individuals without alcohol or drug dependence.

drawn from the general population have been conducted in the United States over the recent decades, namely the Epidemiologic Catchment Area Study (ECA) (19), the National Comorbidity Survey (NCS) (20,21), the National Longitudinal Alcohol Epidemiologic Survey (22,23), and the National Epidemiological Study of Alcoholism and Related Conditions (NESARC) (1,3). Table 84.3 summarizes data from ECA, NCS, and NESARC on co-occurrence of mood disorders with alcohol and drug dependence. NLAES data, not shown in Table 84.3, had similar findings for the co-occurrence of major depression and alcohol and drug use disorders but did not include other disorders (bipolar, anxiety, etc.). The data are expressed as odds ratios, which reflect the multiple by which one disorder increases the prevalence rate of the other, hence the strength of association between disorders. For example, an odds ratio of 1.0 indicates that among individuals with a substance-dependence disorder, the prevalence of a mood disorder is the same as in individuals without a substance-dependence disorder; an odds ratio of 2.0 indicates that among individuals with a substance-dependence disorder, the prevalence of a mood disorder is twice that observed among those without substance dependence.

As can be seen in Table 84.3, odds ratios are at least 2.0 for most combinations of disorders, showing that the presence of alcohol or drug dependence at least doubles the odds of a mood disorder, or other disorder, being present. It is notable that the odds ratios for major depression and dysthymia are similar. Thus, though dysthymia is often thought of as a mild version of depression, it should not be discounted in the clinical evaluation; the hallmark of dysthymia is its chronicity, and the presence of chronic depressive symptoms across the course of a substance use disorder, even if the depressive symptoms are milder, should be taken seriously.

For bipolar disorder, the odds ratios are substantially larger than for major depression or dysthymia. Again, when depressive symptoms are present, it is very important to search the history carefully for past episodes of mania or hypomania, as bipolar illness has a particularly strong association with substance use disorders, and it has specific treatment implications that differ from those for unipolar depression. When evaluating a patient with bipolar illness, it is especially important to inquire about substance use problems, as they are likely to be present and to complicate the clinical course.

Common anxiety disorders (social phobia, panic disorder with or without agoraphobia, and post traumatic stress disorders) are also shown in Table 84.3 to illustrate that these too have substantial associations with substance use disorders of at least the same magnitude as major depression or dysthymia. These particular disorders frequently co-occur with major depression or dysthymia and respond to the same antidepressant medications. Further, their cardinal symptoms (fear of social interactions, spontaneous panic attacks and fear of public places, and re-experiencing symptoms triggered by reminders of traumatic events) are distinctive and not attributable to substance toxicity or withdrawal. Thus, when a substance-dependent patient presents with depression, the history should include a detailed inquiry for each of these anxiety disorders. Their presence can be very useful in ruling out substance intoxication or withdrawal as the sole source of mood symptoms. In a patient with chronic substance abuse, it is often difficult to establish in the history whether depressive symptoms are independent of substance use, as so many of those symptoms may be toxic or withdrawal effects of substances. However, the presence of one of these anxiety disorders strongly suggests the presence of an independent disorder, warranting specific treatment.

Attention deficit hyperactivity disorder (ADHD), also shown in Table 84.3, has strong associations with alcohol and drug dependence as well, with odds ratios of 2.8 and 7.9, respectively (24). It is also strongly associated with major depression (odds ratio = 2.7), dysthymia (odds ratio = 7.5), and bipolar disorder (odds ratio = 7.4) (24). The symptoms of inattention and hyperactivity begin in early childhood and can often be recognized in the history as problems with school performance in elementary school, well before the onset of drug or alcohol use. A simple question to ask during the clinical history is, "Tell me what elementary school was like for you," and then follow-up with questions about whether the patient remembers feeling uncomfortable sitting quietly in class, having trouble paying attention to the teacher, daydreaming, trouble staying organized, or getting in trouble for being too active and disrupting the class. The symptoms, particularly poor attention and poor organization skills, often persist into adulthood and are responsible for substantial functional impairment and poor role performance during adulthood (e.g., poor job performance, high divorce rate). This in turn lends itself to the development of depression. Detailed reviews of the comorbidity, diagnosis, and treatment of ADHD among substance-dependent patients can be found elsewhere (2). Briefly, the treatment of ADHD differs from the routine treatment of depression and involves stimulant medications various formulations of methylphenidate or Dexedrine, antidepressant medications with stimulant-like effects on dopamine or norepinephrine systems (e.g., bupropion, tricyclic antidepressants, or the norepinephrine reuptake inhibitor atomoxetine). Thus, in any patient with a substance use disorder and a mood disorder, a careful history for ADHD should be taken and direct treatment of ADHD considered if detected alongside treatment of the mood and substance use problems. A note of caution is that the differential diagnosis between early-onset bipolar disorder and ADHD is difficult and a matter of controversy owing to the substantial similarities between the clinical presentations of these disorders in childhood.

Antisocial personality is included in Table 84.3 to illustrate its strong association with substance use disorders. Substance-dependent patients will often have antisocial features, but it is important to bear in mind that the presence of antisocial features, or disorder, does not rule out the presence of a mood or anxiety disorder, and in fact they often co-occur.

Substance Use Disorder Treatment Populations

Numerous studies have been published examining the prevalence of mood disorders among patients admitted to alcohol or drug treatment programs, mainly inpatient detoxification or rehabilitation units, outpatient programs, or opioid maintenance programs. Reviews of this literature (2) show lifetime prevalence rates of major depression ranging from 20% to 50%, with rates of current major depression in the 10% to 20% range, substantially exceeding rates found in the general population. Bipolar disorder is relatively uncommon in these samples, consistent with its low prevalence rate in the general population. Thus, clinicians seeing patients in these typical addiction treatment settings should expect to see high rates on co-occurring depression and should remain alert for cases of bipolar disorder.

A number of these studies have included a longitudinal follow-up, examining prognostic effects of co-occurring major depression on substance use outcome. A recent review of this literature (2) shows that studies examining a lifetime diagnosis of major depression (i.e., major depression at any point during the lifetime) found little prognostic effect. In contrast, a current diagnosis of major depression has been consistently associated with worse outcome of substance use problems over follow-up periods ranging from 6 months to 5 years. This adverse prognostic effect holds for major depression diagnosed at an initial evaluation (25–28), and for major depression diagnosed during the follow-up period (29,30), among both alcoholics (27–31), methadone maintained opioid addicts (25,26), and cocaine dependent patients (32).

Another important pattern in the results from longitudinal studies is that current depressive symptoms, as measured by an elevated score on a standard scale such as the Beck Depression Inventory (BDI) or Hamilton Depression Scale (HDS), have inconsistent prognostic effects (2). For example, in a study of alcohol dependent inpatients, Greenfield et al. (27) showed that an elevated HDS score at baseline was not associated with outcome across a 1 year follow-up, whereas a diagnosis of major depression at baseline predicted relapse to heavy drinking during follow-up; the latter effect was reduced among patients who were treated with antidepressant medication during the follow-up. Dysthymia (i.e., low-grade chronic depression) has received little study in terms of its prognostic effects on substance use outcome. However, there is some evidence that depressive symptoms have adverse prognostic effects when they persist during or after treatment of a substance use disorder (33,34). This suggests that persistent depression, even if not meeting criteria for major depression, should be taken seriously among substance-dependent patients.

Taken together, these data have clear clinical implications. Depression symptom scales such as the Beck or Hamilton can be useful as screening tools, but these need to be followed up with a careful clinical history, establishing presence or absence of depressive disorder. A past history of a depressive disorder is important information, as it indicates increased risk for depression in the future, but it is current major depression that is most clearly associated with worse outcome among substance-dependent patients and should be attended to in the treatment plan. Chronic low-grade depression, and depression that persists after initiation of treatment for the substance problem also warrant clinical attention.

Psychiatric and Primary Care Populations Among patients presenting in psychiatric and primary care treatment settings for treatment of depression, the prevalence of substance use disorders depends upon the setting and associated severity of the mood disorder. In the STAR*D study, which evaluated and treated more than 4,000 outpatients with major depression in community-based psychiatric and primary care clinics, the prevalence of concurrent alcohol use disorders was 13% and drug use disorders 8%, and a current substance use disorder was associated with a positive family history of substance use disorder (35). Such rates are modest but exceed what would be expected from general population surveys. Among psychiatric inpatients, a more severely ill group, substance use disorders are common among both patients with major depression and bipolar disorder (36). Among patients in treatment for bipolar disorder, substance use disorders are common, with rates of current substance use disorders of 30% or more can (5,36). The co-occurrence of mood and substance use disorders may be especially common among patients with serious co-occurring medical disorders such as HIV (37,38).

It is increasingly clear that the majority of individuals with substance use disorders, depression, and other common mental disorders do not present at specialty treatment settings such as substance abuse treatment programs or even psychiatric clinics. Instead, they often present at the offices of primary care physicians, where substance abuse and depression are likely to go undetected and may be associated with over- or under-utilization of services and poor outcome (39). Patients may be unaware of these problems or may avoid discussing them with health care providers because of the considerable stigma attached to the idea of having such a problem or of seeking treatment at an addiction program or a psychiatrist's office. This presents an important challenge to addiction specialists, suggesting that the need to reach out to these other settings with programs of screening and brief intervention (40).

DIFFERENTIAL DIAGNOSIS

Etiological Relationships between Mood and Substance Use Disorders Beneath the problem of how to diagnose and treat mood symptoms among substance-dependent patients lies the issue that there are multiple different potential etiologic relationships between mood symptoms or syndromes and substance use disorders. A summary of these is presented in Table 84.4, along with possible underlying mechanisms and implications for diagnostic assessment and treatment. A complete review is beyond the scope of this chapter, but each of these relationships and mechanisms has some evidence to support it. In the diagnostic evaluation of a patient with co-occurring disorders, it is useful to think about which of the options in Table 84.4 may be operating. The table also serves to illustrate the complexity involved in co-occurring disorders, particularly when one considers that several of these causal pathways or mechanisms might operate at once.

There are two important clinical implications here. The first is to appreciate the potential complexity and to avoid viewing patients in simplistic terms. All mood symptoms are not caused by toxic and withdrawal effects of substances, nor is all substance abuse caused by underlying psychopathology (as in "self-medication"). The second point is to be cautious in formulating causal mechanisms between co-occurring disorders. For any given patient, it may difficult to prove which of several causal mechanisms may be operating. For example, when depression resolves with treatment of the substance use disorder and reduction in substance use, this is consistent with the inference that depression was a toxic effect of substance abuse. However, it is also possible that there was an independent mood disorder that responded to supportive elements of the behavioral therapy used to treat the substance use disorder, only to re-emerge at some future point.

Pre-DSM-IV Approaches to Co-occurring Mood and Substance Use Disorders The DSM-IV approach to evaluation of comorbidity grew out of previous diagnostic systems and approaches. A review of these is helpful to understanding the current DSM-IV nosology. Each of these systems may be useful in taking a history and formulating the differential for a given patient. A detailed review of the development of diagnostic approaches to psychiatric-substance abuse comorbidity can be found elsewhere. Briefly, the Feighner and Research Diagnostic Criteria, forerunners of DSM-III, formalized the concept of primary and secondary disorders, based on age at onset. When two disorders occur together, the one with earlier age at onset is considered "primary" and the other "secondary." This stands in contrast to the loose use of "primary" and "secondary" to indicate a causal relationship between disorders. The order of onset can be determined reliably (41) and has demonstrated predictive validity, with primary (prior onset) depression distinguishing male alcoholics whose depressive symptoms persist after 3 weeks of abstinence on an inpatient unit (16). However, it also has limitations, being likely to miss cases of independent mood disorders, particularly given the typically early (adolescent) onset of substance use disorders. Further, a true mood disorder may emerge only after the onset of a substance use disorder. Considering the range of possible etiologic relationships between mood and substance use disorders (see Table 84.4), the chronological primary category probably excludes many cases of mood disorder that are clinically significant and warrant clinical attention and treatment.

DSM-III required that a mood disorder not be attributable to the effects of substances or medications, and introduced the category of organic mood disorder, but more specific criteria were not provided. Several research groups subsequently advanced criteria based on expanded notions of the relationship between mood and substance use disorders over time. One system, developed for opioid-dependent populations characterized by chronic use, considered a mood disorder as primary or independent if it emerged during periods of stable substance use and secondary if it emerged during increases or decreases in substance use (26,42). Another considered a mood disorder as primary if either (a) onset of depressive disorder precedes onset of first regular substance use during the lifetime

TABLE 84.4 Summary of Possible Etiological Relationships between Co-occurring Affective Symptoms/Syndromes and Substance Use Disorders

Relationship	Mechanism	Clinical presentation and implications
Substance abuse causes affective symptoms	Substance intoxication, withdrawal, or biologic effects of chronic substance use	Substance use disorder is chronologically primary; mood symptoms resolve with abstinence or reduced substance use; treatment focuses on substance abuse
Substance abuse causes affective syndrome, which then takes on a life of its own	Stress and loss (e.g., relationships, jobs) engendered by substance abuse promote depression; biologic effects of chronic substance exposure trigger a vulnerability to affective disorder	Affective syndrome is chronologically secondary, but persists after abstinence; treat both affective and substance use disorders
Affective syndrome causes substance abuse	Self-medication (taking substances to relieve symptoms of affective disorder—e.g., low mood, low energy, poor sleep in depression; lack of sleep, excessive energy in mania or hypomania)	Affective syndrome is chronologically primary, or emerges during abstinence, preceding relapse; pure self-medication—where self-medication is the only mechanism operating, and treatment can focus exclusively on the affective disorder—is relatively rare
Substance abuse is part of a pattern of increased activity and impulsivity in mania or hypomania	Impulsivity, seeking out new experiences	Substance abuse is chronologically secondary, beginning during episodes of mania or hypomania, and resolves with return to euthymia or depression; treatment can focus on bipolar disorder, but as with pure self-medication, this may be relatively rare
Affective syndrome causes substance abuse, which then takes on a life of its own	Exposure to substances during an episode of affective disorder triggers a vulnerability to substance dependence	Substance abuse is chronologically secondary, but persists after mood disorder is treated; treat both disorders
Independent disorders	Both affective and substance use disorders are common in the general population and will co-occur by chance	Any chronological pattern; each disorder persists during remissions of the other; treat both disorders
Affective and substance use disorders stem from common underlying risk factors	Common genetic factors, stress, trauma	Any chronological pattern; both disorders need to be treated; reduction of stress may help both
Affective symptoms and substance use become related over time	Moods become a conditioned cue triggering substance abuse	Substance use disorder may be chronologically primary, but moods (e.g., sadness, anger) trigger episodes of substance use, or cravings; management of unpleasant moods becomes important part of therapy
Co-occurrence worsens prognosis	Presence of multiple disorders interferes with coping or treatment seeking	Any chronologic pattern; each disorder needs specific treatment
Affective symptoms/syndrome may prompt treatment seeking for substance problems	Affective symptoms (sad mood, trouble sleeping, functional impairment) engender motivation	Any chronological pattern; focus on treatment of substance use, but affective disorder may need to be treated if it persists

(consistent with RDC primary), (b) depressive disorder emerged or persisted during a past episode of prolonged abstinence (abstinence period at least 6 months' duration), or (c) depressive disorder is relatively chronic (e.g., of at least 3 to 6 months' duration in the current episode) (41). Both these systems showed evidence of predictive validity in regard to naturalistic course or response to antidepressant medication treatment (31,43–45).

DSM-IV Independent and Substance-Induced Mood Disorders The DSM-IV committee on substance use disorders forged a substantial advance for the field by synthesizing pre-DSM-IV approaches to define primary or independent mood disorders and creating a new category of Substance-Induced Mood Disorder within the larger section on Mood Disorders. Thus, co-occurring mood disorders in the setting of substance abuse can be categorized as "independent" of substance use or "substance-induced." Because Substance-Induced Mood Disorder is defined as representing mood symptoms that are in excess of the usual effects of substance intoxication or withdrawal, we also recommend construing a third category of "usual effects of substances." The DSM-IV criteria, and our interpretation of them, are summarized in Table 84.5. Because the DSM-IV criteria, as stated, leave some details vague, a suggested operationalization is also included in the table, based on the SCID-SAC (41) and PRISM interviews (8,30).

Independent Mood Disorder Also referred to in the literature as "primary," DSM-IV defines an independent mood disorder as one that precedes the onset of substance abuse or persists during significant periods of abstinence (1 month or more is suggested as the minimum). This is consistent with the prior concepts of RDC primary or subsequent expansions of that concept for longitudinal studies and clinical trials, as reviewed earlier. We have found that the historical data needed to establish these criteria (ages at onset, presence of periods of abstinence, and mood syndromes occurring during abstinent periods) can be determined with good reliability from a clinical history (41), and have established good reliability for the categorical diagnosis with both a modified SCID interview (41) and the PRISM (8).

Substance-Induced Mood Disorder The category of Substance-Induced Mood Disorder was established to recognize the phenomenon of co-occurring mood syndromes that cannot be established as chronologically independent of substance use, yet the mood symptoms seem to exceed what would be expected from mere intoxication or withdrawal effects from the substance(s) the patient is taking. A typical example would be a patient with a long-standing, chronic history of substance abuse with a syndrome consistent with major depression that has occurred only during substance use, yet the syndrome seems substantial enough to warrant specific antidepressant treatment.

Usual Effects of Substances When evaluating patients with co-occurring substance use and mood symptoms, we recommend this third-category "usual effects of substances" be explicitly considered in the differential diagnosis. DSM-IV clearly specifies that the symptoms of either an Independent or a Substance-Induced Mood Disorder must exceed the expected effects of intoxication or withdrawal from the substances the patient is taking (see Tables 84.1A and 84.1B). The term "Substance-Induced" is somewhat confusing in that it implies cause and effect (substances causing mood symptoms). Thus, clinicians may commonly use "substance-induced" to describe intoxication or withdrawal effects, when DSM-IV excludes these from a diagnosis of Substance-Induced Mood Disorder. Thus, we have recommended a more neutral term such as "Substance-Associated" or "Substance-Non-Independent" might be considered for DSM-V (46).

It is true that a DSM-IV Substance-Induced Mood Disorder should, by definition, resolve if abstinence is achieved. On the other hand, it has been shown that if specific criteria are set for making the diagnosis (e.g., the mood disorder has historically never occurred independent of substance use, but full criteria for major depression are met), a substantial proportion of such cases will persist during future abstinent periods and thus, in essence, convert to an independent depression (17,47). Thus, DSM-IV substance induced depression, depending on how it is operationalized, may represent cases in which the status (independent vs. not independent of substance use) is uncertain.

Diagnostic Methods and Predictive Validity of DSM-IV Approach One of the problems with the DSM-IV approach is that the criteria are left vague in some respects, particularly in regard to Substance-Induced Mood Disorder. Table 84.5 highlights those symptoms that are left vague and suggested operationalized criteria in the second column of the table. The Structured Clinical Interview for DSM-IV (7) includes a module for Substance-Induced Mood Disorder, but it essentially asks the interviewer to make a clinical judgment based on the criteria. The PRISM (8,30) is a semi-structured interview that was designed specifically to evaluate mood and other co-occurring psychiatric disorders in the setting of substance use disorders. PRISM provides more specific criteria for Substance-Induced Mood Disorder and its distinction from an independent mood disorder on the one hand or usual effects of substances on the other; and these criteria are reflected in the suggested operationalizations in Table 84.5. To make a diagnosis of Substance-Induced Mood Disorder, PRISM requires full criteria for a mood disorder (e.g., major depression, or dysthymia) to be met, and that each symptom contributing to the diagnosis (e.g., insomnia, loss of appetite, low energy) exceed the expected effects of the substances that the patients is taking, and the interviewer is referred to the DSM-IV criteria sets for intoxication and withdrawal syndromes for the various substances (see Tables 84.1A and 84.1B for symptoms likely to overlap between mood and substance intoxication/withdrawal).

Thus, PRISM establishes criteria for Substance-Induced Mood Disorder that are more specific and stringent than those required by the letter of DSM-IV. Evidence for the predictive validity of the PRISM operationalizations comes from a longitudinal study of substance-dependent patients interviewed with the PRISM at an index hospitalization on a dual diagnosis inpatient unit and then followed for one year (17,30). About half of this sample had a current major depression. About half of the major depressions were diagnosed as Independent and half as Substance-Induced in the current episode. Thus, as experienced clinicians might expect, the prevalence of Substance-Induced Depression in this population was high. A PRISM diagnosis of Substance-Induced Major Depression was associated with failure of the substance use disorder to remit, whereas a diagnosis of Independent Mood Disorder during a period of abstinence in the follow-up was associated with a greater risk of relapse to substance abuse (30). Both disorders were associated with suicidal behavior or ideation (48). Further, of those cases diagnosed with a current Substance Induced Major Depression, more than half converted into an Independent Major Depression over the 1-year follow-up by being shown to persist during at least a 1-month period of abstinence (17). Another study, using similar diagnostic

TABLE 84.5 Summary of DSM-IV Scheme for Classifying Co-occurring Mood and Substance Use Disorders

DSM-IV criteria	Suggested operationalization based on the PRISM or SCID-SAC interviews
Independent Mood Disorder[b] Mood symptoms "precede the onset of substance use" Mood symptoms "persist for a substantial period of time (e.g., about a month) after the cessation of acute withdrawal or severe intoxication" Mood symptoms "substantially in excess of what would be expected given the type or amount of the substance used or the duration of use" "Other evidence" of an independent mood disorder (e.g., a history of recurrent episodes of major depression)	Full criteria for DSM-IV mood disorder are met, and at least one of the following: Age at onset of mood disorder precedes the onset of regular substance use Past episodes of mood disorder occurred during past periods of abstinence (Note: SCID-SAC asks for past abstinence periods of 6 months or more; although this may be unnecessarily long) Mood disorder persists after induction of abstinence in the current episode (Note: DSM-IV recommends persistence of mood disorder during at least one month of abstinence; arguments can be made for shorter or longer durations, although we lean toward shorter—e.g., 2 weeks) Mood disorder is chronic (Note: the symptoms "substantially in excess" (of usual effects of substances) criterion seems difficult to operationalize, as it is a gradation based mainly on clinical judgment; long duration of mood disorder (e.g., 3 to 6 months or more) is more objective)
Substance-induced mood disorder: "Prominent and persistent disturbance in mood" (depressed mood, or loss of interest/pleasure, or elevated/expansive or irritable) Mood symptoms develop during substance intoxication or withdrawal "Mood symptoms are in excess of those usually associated with the intoxication or withdrawal syndrome" "Sufficiently severe to warrant independent clinical attention" Not better accounted for by an independent mood disorder Note: We view the terminology "Substance-Induced" as a likely point of confusion, since it implies the substance causes the symptoms, and clinicians are probably often thinking of intoxication or withdrawal when assigning this diagnosis. But DSM-IV seems clearly to be distinguishing Substance-Induced Mood Disorder as a disorder "in excess" of usual substance effects, warranting "independent clinical attention"	–Full criteria for a DSM-IV mood disorder are met—e.g., "Substance-Induced Major Depression", or "Substance-Induced Dysthymia" (Note: DSM-IV only specifies that the core mood symptoms be present) –PRISM asks the interviewer to judge that each symptom contributing to the diagnosis exceed the usual effects of intoxication or withdrawal of the substances concurrently being taken (e.g., insomnia not better explained by nightly cocaine use), and refers the interviewer to DSM-IV criteria lists for alcohol and drug intoxication and withdrawal syndromes (See Tables 84-1A and 84-1B for overlap of mood and intoxication and withdrawal symptoms) Mood disorder is chronic (Note: symptoms "in excess" of usual effects of substances seems difficult to operationalize as a criterion, since it is a gradation based mainly on clinical judgement; long duration of mood disorder (e.g., 3 to 6 months or more) is more objective, and may be a proxy.
Usual effects of substances: –DSM-IV refers to mood symptoms that "would be expected given the type or amount of substance used or the duration of use", or "those usually associated with the intoxication or withdrawal syndrome" (of the substances being taken). In our view, this implies a third category of Usual Effects of Substances, distinct from Substance-Induced Mood Disorder (see Note above).	PRISM asks the interviewer to judge that each symptom contributing to the diagnosis exceed the usual effects of intoxication or withdrawal of the substances concurrently being taken, and refers the interviewer to DSM-IV criteria lists for alcohol and drug intoxication and withdrawal syndromes

[a]For a complete statement of the criteria see American Psychiatric Assocation (1994, 2000), section on Substance-Induced Mood Disorder. (48a)
[b]DSM-IV terms this "Mood Disorder that is not substance-induced", but in the literature it is commonly referred to as either "Independent" or "Primary".
[c]Structured Clinical Interview for DSM-IV, Substance Abuse Comorbidity Version (41);Psychiatric Research Interview for Substance and Mood Disorders (PRISM) (Hasin et al. …)

Independent Mood Disorder[b], Substance-Induced Mood Disorder, and Usual Effects of substances; and suggestions for operationalization of the criteria based on the SCID-SAC or PRISM interviews[c].

methods, found a similar high rate of conversion to Independent depression over a longitudinal follow-up (47). When predictors of the likelihood of depression occurring over the course of the 1-year follow-up were examined, a past history of independent major depression, and the presence of concurrent anxiety disorders were both associated with increased likelihood of depression (17).

In summary, the data from this longitudinal study (17,30,48) suggest that the PRISM operationalizes a version of Substance-Induced Major Depression that predicts both worse substance use outcome and worse depression outcome and in fact often ends up converting to Independent Major Depression during a follow-up period. The data also highlight the importance of examining the history for the presence of anxiety disorders, which also increased the likelihood of depression during the follow-up. Though more research is needed to examine other potential ways to operationalize it, the PRISM method appears to identify a form of Substance-Induced Depression that is consistent with the spirit of the DSM-IV, namely that it is a clinical syndrome that warrants independent clinical attention.

Ries et al. (2001) tested a much simplified method of operationalizing the DSM-IV approach to co-occurring mood disorders. Specifically, they created a Likert-type scale that asks the evaluating clinician, after completing the clinical history, to rate the degree to which a mood disorder is Independent or Substance-Induced. This is reminiscent of the SCID approach, asking the clinician to make a global judgment of Independent versus Substance-Induced. Mood disorders rated toward the substance-induced end of the spectrum were more likely to remit but were also associated with suicidal ideation and risk (49). This work suggests that the judgment of experienced clinicians can be relied upon to make valid distinctions between substance-induced and independent mood disorders, although experience with psychiatric diagnosis tends to recommend erecting criteria that are as objective as possible in order to maximize reliability and validity.

Diagnosing Bipolar Disorder in the Setting of Substance Abuse Intoxication with cocaine or other stimulants may resemble mania in regard to grandiosity, hyperactivity, talkativeness, impulsivity, insomnia, and paranoia. The impulsivity of alcohol or sedative intoxication may sometimes also resemble that of mania (see Table 84.2). However, full-blown mania (see Table 84.1b) must last for at least a week, during which the symptoms should be persistent, whereas symptoms of intoxication are usually intermittent. For example, in mania, high energy and other symptoms can go on for days despite little or no sleep. In contrast in cocaine intoxication, these symptoms usually last a matter of hours after cocaine use and are followed by a crash with increased sleep and low energy. Further, the marked impairment or psychosis required for mania are usually well in excess of what would be produced by intoxication. For example, cocaine intoxication may produce paranoia that lasts for a few hours and resolves during the crash period, whereas the psychosis characteristic of mania, often either paranoid or grandiose, is persistent. Hence, in establishing a diagnosis of mania, persistence of symptoms over time, and severity of impairment are key markers as well as occurrence of the symptoms during clear periods of abstinence. Frank mania is distinctive, despite ongoing substance use.

Hypomania, which involves the same core symptoms as mania but may be briefer (at least 4 days) and with less impairment in functioning, may be more difficult to distinguish from substance intoxication or withdrawal effects. The same may be true of cyclothymia, which may be difficult to distinguish from alternating periods of intoxication and withdrawal, mimicking hypomanic and depressive symptoms, respectively (see Table 84.1b). Thus, here it is particularly important to try to establish episodes of the mood disturbances during periods of abstinence or pre-dating onset of substance abuse, as recommended, according to the DSM-IV criteria for independent mood disorder.

Rapid cycling bipolar disorder is diagnosed when there have been at least four mood episodes over the past 12 months, punctuated either by periods of remission or by switches in polarity (from mania to depression, or vice versa; American Psychiatric Disorder, 1994). On the order of 20% of cases of bipolar disorder are rapid cycling, and the pattern is associated with greater impairment and poorer response to treatment (50,51). Some evidence suggests that the rapid cycling subtype is associated with increased prevalence of substance use disorders (52). Thus, it is important to look for this pattern in the history. However, as for hypomania or cyclothymia, a pattern or multiple switches in mood states becomes more difficult to distinguish from the ups and downs of substance intoxication and withdrawal. Again, it is important to establish in the history that hypomanic or manic syndromes have persisted over days or weeks before switching to depression as well as seeking to establish occurrence of the symptoms during periods of abstinence.

Substance intoxication is likely to exacerbate the disinhibition and poor judgment associated with mania and is associated with poor medication adherence (53), which promotes relapse. Thus, patients who present to emergency departments or other acute psychiatric settings with worsening mania are likely to also have substance abuse in the clinical picture. However, for most patients with bipolar disorder, particularly those who have had the disorder for an extended period of time, the clinical course predominantly consists of depression, with occasional episodes of mania or hypomania. Thus, in a depressed patient with substance abuse, it is important to carefully review the past history for episodes of mania or hypomania that would indicate that the diagnosis is bipolar disorder. In patients with chronic substance abuse, in whom it is difficult to establish the presence of independent mood symptoms, clear-cut episodes of mania or hypomania, because they are distinctive from the usual effects of substances, are valuable in establishing that an independent mood disorder is indeed present and in need of treatment.

Summary of Recommendations for Diagnosis of Co-occurring Mood Disorders The key challenge for the evaluating clinician is to differentiate mood disorders that are independent of substance use and are likely to require specific antidepressant or mood stabilizing treatment from those syndromes that represent toxic or withdrawal effects of substances and are likely to resolve with treatment of the substance use and achievement of abstinence or reduction of substance use. The accumulated evidence suggests a number of steps that the clinician can take to make this differential (Table 84.6). These include three essential features to establishing a DSM-IV diagnosis of independent mood disorder, embodied in the PRISM interview (8): (a) establishing the presence of a full DSM-IV syndrome (e.g., major depression, dysthymia, hypomania); (b) establishing that each of the component criteria that make up the diagnosis exceeds the symptomatology that might be expected from the substances the patient is taking (e.g., insomnia in a stimulant user); (c) establishing the relative ages of onset and offset of mood disorder episodes in relation to periods of active substance abuse, to determine whether the mood syndrome (including past episodes) precedes the onset of substance abuse or has persisted during abstinent periods; and several associated features that may be helpful in building the case for an independent disorder in difficult differentials; (d) probe for a history of serious suicide attempts (54); (e) probe for a history of co-occurring anxiety disorders (55); (f) probe the developmental history for early onset anxiety disorders or attention deficit hyperactivity disorder; (g) probe the family history for mood, anxiety disorders, or other non-substance axis I disorders (54,56); and (h) document response to past treatment efforts, including psychosocial/behavioral or medication treatments for substance use, and for depression, as this data may guide treatment planning going forward. A thorough clinical history, covering each of these areas, provides a strong basis for determining the presence of an independent mood disorder in substance-dependent patients.

The DSM-IV category of Substance-Induced Mood Disorder is an important advance for the field, allowing clinicians to recognize mood disorder syndromes that cannot be established to be independent, but seem to exceed the usual effects of substances. However, more research is needed on this category to establish more detailed diagnostic criteria. Current evidence suggests that when relatively rigorous criteria are erected (e.g., requiring that a full major depressive syndrome be met, with each symptom exceeding the expected effects of concur-

TABLE 84.6 Summary of Diagnostic and Historical Features Useful in Making the Differential Diagnosis of DSM-IV Independent, as Opposed to Substance-Induced Mood Disorders

Diagnostic/historical feature	Rationale and comment
Essential Diagnostic Features:	
(1) Presence of a full DSM-IV syndrome (e.g., major depression, dysthymia, hypomania)	Essential diagnostic feature
(2) Each component criterion that makes up the diagnosis exceeds what symptomatology might be expected from concurrent substances the patient is taking	Implied in DSM-IV; this feature applies if patient is currently using substances; may also be applied to DSM-IV substance induced mood disorder, as in the PRISM interview (30)
(3) Pattern of relative ages of onset and offset of mood disorder episodes in relation to periods of active substance abuse, such that the mood syndrome (including past episodes) precedes the onset of substance abuse or has persisted during abstinent periods	Essential DSM-IV diagnostic feature. DSM-IV also allows for diagnosis of independent mood disorder if the symptoms substantially exceed what would be expected from effects of substances concurrently taken.
Associated Historical Features:	
(4) History of serious suicide attempts (54)	Serious suicide attempts are associated with depressive and bipolar disorders; suicidality by itself is not a toxic or withdrawal effect of any substance
(5) History of co-occurring anxiety disorders (55) Nunes et al. 2007	Anxiety disorders have symptoms that are distinctive from toxic or withdrawal effects (e.g.,spontaneous panic attacks, agoraphobia, social phobia, re-experiencing symptoms of PTSD) and high co-occurrence with mood disorders
(6) Developmental history for early onset mood, anxiety disorders or attention deficit hyperactivity disorder (ADHD)	Elementary school, if not junior high school, generally precedes onset of substance use, and mood or anxiety disorders sometimes have such early onset; ADHD has early onset, and high co-occurrence with both depressive and bipolar disorder among adults
(7) Family history for mood, anxiety disorders, or other non-substance axis I disorders (54,56)	Mood disorders are heritable, and a positive family history of mood disorder suggests proband may carry similar vulnerability
(8) History of response to prior treatments for substance use disorders and depression	This can be one of the most useful sources of information for treatment planning; treatment approaches (behavioral therapies or medications) that have been successful in the past should be considered to be re-instituted; if treatment approaches have clearly failed despite adequate trials, these might best be avoided.

rent substances, as in the PRISM interview) (8), many of the cases so identified will subsequently persist during an abstinent period and be reclassified as independent (47). Experienced clinicians are able to judge depressions that are substance-induced and likely to resolve with abstinence (49). However, resolution with abstinence does not mean that the Substance-Induced mood syndrome is without prognostic significance, having been associated for example with risk of suicidal behavior (48,49) and failure of substance use disorders to remit after treatment (30). More research is needed on the prognostic and treatment implications of substance-induced mood disorders.

MANAGEMENT OF CO-OCCURRING MOOD AND SUBSTANCE USE DISORDERS

Depressive Disorders

Antidepressant Medication

Effect on Outcome of Depression Antidepressant medication has been the most thoroughly studied treatment modality for co-occurring mood disorders with numerous placebo controlled trials in the literature. Two meta-analyses (57,58) reached similar conclusions that antidepressant medication is more effective than placebo in improving outcome among alcohol-dependent patients with depressive disorders, with the evidence less clear among cocaine- or opioid-dependent patients (the latter may be due to fewer high-quality studies, as some studies found positive results and others not). Nunes and Levin (57) identified 14 placebo-controlled trials of selected patients with depressive disorders (major depression or dysthymia) co-occurring with alcohol, cocaine, or opioid dependence and conducted an in-depth analysis of depression outcome, substance use outcome, and moderators of medication effects. The effect size (Cohen's d; standardized difference between means of Hamilton Depression Scale score at outcome between medication and placebo groups) for the effect of medication on depression outcome was 0.38 (95% confidence interval 0.18 to 0.58), a small to medium-sized effect that is in the same range and that observed in clinical trials of medications for treatment of routine outpatient depression (59). The magnitude of the effect size was strongly related to placebo response—the greater the placebo response, the smaller the effect size.

Effects of Antidepressant Medication on Substance Use Outcome In the Nunes and Levin meta-analysis (57), among studies that showed medium to large effect sizes in favor of antidepressant medication on depression outcome (Cohen's d $>$ 0.5 standard deviations) (44,60–64), an effect size in the medium range was also observed on outcome measures of self-reported quantity of substance use (57), whereas among studies with smaller to zero effects on depression outcome, the effect size for self-reported substance use outcome was near zero (42,43,65–70). However, categorical outcome measures reflecting criteria for remission or substantial improvement in substance use showed smaller differences between medication and placebo and overall modest rates of remission. This suggests the conclusion that treatment of a co-occurring depression with antidepressant medication is helpful in reducing substance abuse when the depression improves, but it is not a stand-alone treatment and cannot be expected to resolve substance problems by itself; concurrent treatment for the substance use disorder (counseling or medication) are also indicated.

Torrens et al. (2005) cast a wider net in their meta-analysis and analyzed placebo-controlled trials of antidepressant medications for substance use disorders, dividing studies into those which did, or did not, require co-occurring depression and focusing on substance use outcomes. They found a significant favorable effect of antidepressant medication among alcohol-dependent patients with depressive disorders, with equivocal findings for cocaine- or opioid-dependent patients with depression, although they conclude that further research in each of these populations is needed.

Results of Recent Trials Results of placebo-controlled trials of antidepressants published since these meta-analyses have produced a similar pattern of results. A placebo-controlled trial of desipramine among cocaine-dependent patients with depressive disorders found a modest effect of medication in improving depression outcome, no direct effect of medication on cocaine outcome, and a moderate placebo response rate (45). Among depressed alcohol-dependent patients, nefazodone (Hernandez-Avila et al., 2005) showed modest beneficial effects of medication on mood outcome and drinking outcome. One large trial of sertraline among alcohol dependent patients showed a high placebo response and no significant effect of medication (71).

Association between Mood Outcome and Substance Use Outcome In addition to the finding that beneficial effects of medication on substance use outcome were observed in trials that demonstrated larger effects of medication on mood outcome (57), some trials also reported the correlation between mood improvement and substance use improvement within the trial dataset. In these analyses, the relationship between improvement in mood and improvement in substance use outcome is consistently strong and positive (44,45,70). One study was able to show clearly that mood improvement mediates the effect of medication on substance use outcome (44), but most such trials lack the power for this type of mediational analysis. Taken together, these data suggests that depression and substance use outcome are causally related, with improvement in mood resulting in improvement in substance use for some patients. However, the direction of causality likely runs in both directions, such that for many other patients it is improvement in substance use that drives improvement in mood.

Moderators of Antidepressant Medication Effect In their meta-analysis, Nunes and Levin (57) also studied moderators of medication effect—that is, features of the trials that predicted greater or lesser effect of medication compared to placebo. These bear detailed discussion, because they are useful in developing guidelines for management of patients with co-occurring depression and substance abuse (Table 84.7).

TABLE 84.7 Factors (Moderators) Associated with Efficacy of Antidepressant Medications in Clinical Trials Among Patients with Co-occurring Depression and Substance Use Disorders, and Implications for Clinical Practice

Moderator	Evidence	Implications for clinical practice
Placebo response	–Low placebo response associated with greater effect of antidepressant medication in both general meta-analysis (57), and another meta-analysis focused on opioid-dependent patients (Nunes, Sullivan, and Levin 2004) –High placebo response associated with lack of effect of antidepressant medication	–Always treat the substance use disorder; in these clinical trials, placebo response represents a response to the background treatment of substance use disorder, which may improve mood without resort to specific antidepressant treatment
Establishment of abstinence before diagnosing depression	–Studies that required abstinence, or enforced abstinence on an inpatient unit prior to diagnosis and treatment of mood disorder, yielded larger medication effects (57)	–Treat the substance use disorder, and try to establish abstinence or reduction in substance use prior to diagnosis and treatment of depression. –Careful clinical history to establish evidence of independent depressive disorder as suggested in DSM-IV (see Tables 84.5 and 84.6 for guidelines on diagnosis)
Class of antidepressant medication	–More consistent evidence for efficacy of tricyclic antidepressants and other noradrenergic or mixed-mechanism antidepressants (57,58) –Less consistent evidence for efficacy of specific serotonin reuptake inhibitors (SRIs), though some studies show robust efficacy of SRIs when depression diagnosed during abstinence (63,64), and many negative studies have high placebo response (57). –SRIs associated with worse drinking outcome among early onset type of alcoholic dependence (not selected for depression, but characterized by early substance onset, antisocial personality features and moderately elevated depression symptoms) (78,79)	–Consider SRIs as first line medication treatment due to good tolerability and safety characteristics in setting of ongoing substance use –Switch to non-SRI antidepressant if SRI trial fails. Tricyclic antidepressants may be considered, but need to weigh risks, including sedation, overdose, seizures. Consider other newer antidepressant medications with noradrenergic or mixed mechanisms of action (e.g., venlafaxine, duloxetine, mirtazapine, nefazodone) –Proceed with caution with SRIs in patients with early onset alcohol or drug dependence and antisocial personality features.
Concurrent manual-guided psychosocial intervention	–Most of the clinical trials of antidepressant medication that were negative implemented a manual-guided psychosocial intervention as the background treatment received by all participating patients (57)	–Initiate treatment of substance use disorder with an evidence based treatment, as elements of that treatment, or resultant improvement in substance use, may improve mood without resort to specific antidepressant treatment
Diagnosis of depressive disorder (vs depressive symptoms)	–Meta-analysis of Torrens and colleagues (2005) found little evidence for efficacy of antidepressants among alcohol or drug dependent patients without depressive disorders, as did meta-analysis of antidepressant medication among opioid-dependent patients (Nunes, Sullivan, and Levin 2004). –Caveats: Noradrenergic antidepressants (bupropion, nortriptline) are effective for nicotine dependence; some limited evidence for efficacy of SRI antidepressants among alcoholics with late-onset alcohol dependence (78,79); some evidence for efficacy of antidepressants among cocaine dependent patients, especially when combined with voucher-incentive therapy (74,75)	–Careful clinical history to establish evidence of independent depressive disorder as suggested in DSM-IV (see Tables 84.5 and 84.6 for guidelines on diagnosis) –More research needed on treatment response to antidepressant medications among patients with DSM-IV Substance-Induced Depression –Bear in mind that antidepressant medications may have beneficial effects for alcohol or drug use that are separate from their antidepressant effects (for example, effect of nortriptyline for nicotine dependence is related not to past history of major depression, but rather to reduction of post-quit dysphoria (117).

Placebo Response Low placebo response rate was the strongest moderator of medication effect, accounting for approximately 70% of the variance in effect sizes across studies (57). Placebo response was quantified as the percent improvement in the Hamilton Depression Scale score between baseline and end-of-study in the placebo group of each respective trial. Studies with low placebo response rates (in the 20% to 30% range) showed large medication versus placebo differences. In contrast, about half the studies had high placebo response rates in the 40% to 60% range, meaning that the Hamilton Depression scale score improved by 40% to 60% in the placebo groups of these studies; for this group of studies, the effect sizes hovered around zero, meaning no benefit of medication over and above placebo. High placebo response is a well-known effect in studies of treatment of depression (59). In the studies of antidepressant treatment of depressed substance abusers, placebo response is particularly meaningful, as it suggests some patients are responding to the background treatment they are receiving, which in most of these trials involved some form of treatment for the substance use disorder. This is part of what underlies our recommendation that treatment of the substance use disorder is a first priority in the management of patients with co-occurring depression and substance abuse. Treatment of the substance use disorder may, in many cases, result in improvement in both substance abuse and depression.

Antidepressant Response in Alcohol-Dependent versus Cocaine- or Opioid-Dependent Samples Consistent with the findings of Torrens et al. (57), they found greater evidence for efficacy of antidepressant medications among depressed alcoholics than among drug dependent patients. In part, this may be owing to the fact that there were more high-quality studies among those dependent upon alcohol, with fewer corresponding high-quality studies of cocaine- or opioid-dependent patients. Also, more of the studies of alcohol-dependent patients had other methodologic features associated with larger medication effects, namely diagnosis of depression during a period of abstinence, treatment with a tricyclic or other noradrenergic medication (as opposed to a specific serotonin re-uptake inhibitory), and absence of a manually guided psychosocial intervention. Each of these moderators, and their implications for clinical guidelines, are discussed in more detail later.

Among studies of the treatment of depression among cocaine- or opioid-dependent patients, there was more heterogeneity of effect across the studies, meaning that there were some studies demonstrating benefits of antidepressants among depressed cocaine (45,61) or opioid-dependent patients (44,72,73) and other studies showing little or no effect (42,67,70). The treatment of depressed cocaine-dependent patients has been studied least. Antidepressant medications have also been studied extensively as a treatment for cocaine dependence without regard to depression, with mainly negative results, although several recent trials suggest antidepressant medications are effective in reducing cocaine use when combined with voucher incentive therapy (74,75).

A meta-analysis of placebo-controlled antidepressant medication treatment studies among depressed opioid addicts (76) cast a wider net than the prior meta-analysis (57), also including studies of antidepressant treatment of patients selected to have elevated scores on depression symptom rating scales without also requiring a formal diagnosis of depression. Most of these trials were conducted among opioid addicts in methadone maintenance treatment. This meta-analysis similarly revealed substantial heterogeneity of effect across trials. Low placebo response was again a strong predictor of benefit of medication over placebo.

Another recent trial recruited from among intravenous opioid addicts not engaged in any treatment and tested a combination of cognitive behavioral therapy (CBT) plus the serotonin re-uptake inhibitor antidepressant citalopram (77). The combined treatment was superior to an assessment-only control condition in terms of proportion achieving remission from depression, and remission was associated with adherence. Most opioid addicts are not engaged in any treatment, and this trial (77) is of particular interest because it suggests the potential of targeting depression as a way of engaging more such patients in treatment. It also suggests the utility of a combined pharmacologic-behavioral treatment approach that may have the potential to benefit more patients than either treatment alone, although a formal trial testing that hypothesis by disentangling effects of therapy and medication has yet to be conducted.

Diagnosis of Depression during a Period of Initial Abstinence Four placebo-controlled trials were conducted among alcohol-dependent patients, who were diagnosed after at least 1 week of abstinence from alcohol (60,60,62). These studies yielded medium to large effects of antidepressant medication on both depression and drinking outcomes. Three of those studies (60,63) worked with hospitalized alcoholics with relatively severe depressive disorders that were shown to persist after detoxification and enforced abstinence on the inpatient unit. In one study, depression was marked by suicidal ideation in many of the patients (63). A fourth study worked with outpatients but required at least 1 week of abstinence prior to making the diagnosis of major depression (62).

In terms of clinical recommendations, this finding seems clearly to suggest that when possible, an effort should be made to help patients initiate abstinence and observe the response of the depression during early abstinence, prior to initiating antidepressant medication. Depression that persists during an initial period of abstinence would be consistent with what DSM-IV would call an independent major depression, and this supports the importance of a careful clinical evaluation and application of DSM-IV criteria for independent major depression. With the advent of managed care and cost containment, hospitalization, particularly of several weeks duration, is less of an option than it was when these studies were conducted; also many patients will resist hospitalization or be unable to set aside work or family responsibilities to go into a hospital. Many of the studies that diagnosed and treated patients entirely on an outpatient basis implemented efforts to obtain a systematic clinical history to establish that depression was independent of substance use on a lifetime basis (see Tables 84.5 and 84.6 and discussion above of differential diagnosis and diagnostic methods). Some of these studies observed significant benefits of medication (44,45,61,62), although others that applied similarly careful historical criteria and methods failed to observe benefits of medication (42,67). A recent large clinical trial among alcohol-dependent patients required both a brief period (1 week) of initial abstinence and a DSM-IV diagnosis of independent major depression using the PRISM interview (see Table 84.5), yet still observed a substantial placebo response rate and no clear advantage of medication (71). One possible explanation is that even independent major depression among alcohol-dependent patients may often respond to the milieu and background psychosocial treatment offered as part of medication trials, resulting in high placebo response and less of a role for medication (see section below on concurrent psychosocial intervention as a moderator of treatment effects in the clinical trials).

Another clinical implication stems from the high level of severity of depression in the inpatient samples and suggests that the greater the severity of the depression, the more consideration should be given to treatment with antidepressant medication from the outset. This is a matter of clinical judgment. For example, a patient with a clear history of independent major depression with suicide attempts, who presents with suicidal ideation, should be considered for initiation of antidepressant medication without delay. As always, this should not distract from initiating and pursuing treatment of the substance dependence.

Class of Antidepressant Medication Interestingly, both meta-analyses (57,58) reached a similar conclusion that the evidence of efficacy for specific serotonin re-uptake inhibitors (SSRIs) is less robust than the evidence for efficacy of tricyclics and other medications with mixed modes of action. Many of the negative studies with SSRIs also had high placebo response rates, which does not suggest an inherent lack of efficacy of the medication. Further, several of the largest effects of medication (vs. placebo) were observed with SSRIs, fluoxetine, or sertraline (64), among hospitalized alcoholics with severe depression.

On the other hand, among placebo-controlled trials with alcoholics not selected specifically for depression, there is evidence that SSRIs may produce worse drinking outcome compared to placebo among patients with type B alcohol dependence (high risk/high severity subtype) (78,79). Type B is characterized by severe alcohol problems, high levels of comorbid psychopathology, and early onset of alcohol problems. In contrast, patients with less severe/late-onset alcohol dependence (type A) may benefit from SSRIs (79). An analogous finding was obtained among patients with posttraumatic stress syndrome (PTSD); sertraline produced worse drinking outcome among patients with severe alcohol problems and later-onset PTSD, whereas sertraline was superior to placebo among patients with early-onset PTSD and less severe alcohol problems (80). The type B subtype of alcohol dependence may have moderate levels of depressive symptomatology (as did the samples in the Kranzler [1996] and Pettinati [2000] studies), but this subtype is more characterized by externalizing psychopathology (e.g., antisocial features, impulsivity). Thus it may be that SSRIs are less effective, perhaps even counterproductive in depressed substance-dependent patients with mixtures of internalizing and externalizing symptoms and markers of high risk for alcohol problems such as early onset, although further research is needed to better evaluate this hypothesis.

In terms of clinical recommendations, SSRIs have the advantage of being generally well tolerated, with less potential for sedation or other adverse effects. In contrast, TCAs generate a number of concerns including risks of sedation, overdose, and seizures. Thus, we would continue to recommend SSRIs as the first-line treatment and move to a non-SSRI antidepressant, such as venlafaxine, duloxetine, mirtazapine, or bupropion, if the SSRI trial fails. The exception might be a patient with early-onset substance use and prominent externalizing symptoms or antisocial personality features, for whom the data suggest caution in the use of SSRIs.

Concurrent Psychosocial Intervention One of the more intriguing findings to emerge from the meta-analysis (57) was that placebo-controlled trials that offered a manually guided psychosocial intervention as the background treatment, received by all participating patients, tended to have high placebo response rates and lesser medication effects (67–69). These were interventions for substance dependence, including various cognitive behavioral interventions or 12-Step facilitation. These interventions generally have components that focus on managing mood symptoms and thus may have inherent antidepressant effects. Also, the focus of the interventions on substance use disorders may result in reduced substance use, which in turn improves mood. The recent multisite sertraline trial, also a negative study with a high placebo response rate, offered all patients a medical management type of intervention, which was manually guided and emphasized abstinence and treatment adherence (71). In terms of clinical recommendations, this finding reinforces the importance of initiating treatment for the substance use disorder as the first step with any patient with co-occurring substance use disorder and depression.

Behavioral Treatments for Depression and Substance Abuse As noted earlier, the findings of the meta-analysis (57) show that manually guided psychosocial interventions were associated with high placebo response rate and lack of difference between medication and placebo. These psychosocial interventions were focused on the substance problems (e.g., cognitive behavioral relapse prevention, 12-Step facilitation) but could also be effective for treating depression in several ways: (a) The psychosocial treatment reduces substance use, which in turn improves mood, or (b) the psychosocial treatment itself exerts antidepressant effects, either through nonspecific supportive aspects of these treatments or owing to specific modules addressing management of moods. Either way, the association with high placebo response suggests that a reasonable first step with a depressed, substance-dependent patient, in whom the presence of an independent mood disorder is less than clear, is to initiate an evidence-based psychosocial treatment for the substance dependence. Effective medications, such as disulfiram, naltrexone (81,82), or buprenorphine should also be considered when appropriate.

There are fewer controlled studies of psychosocial treatments for depression, compared to control treatments, among substance-dependent patients with depression. One small controlled trial found a CBT for depression was superior to control treatment (relaxation therapy) on mood and substance use outcomes (83). Another study found a behavioral treatment combining elements of the community reinforcement approach (CRA) and voucher incentives (84) produced substantial improvements in depression over time, but the relaxation therapy control condition produced equal improvements in outcome (85). Several studies have suggested addition of CBT for depression to smoking cessation treatment improved smoking outcome among patients with histories of major depression or greater severity of depression symptoms (86,87). A small controlled trial found addition of yoga to treatment as usual among alcohol-dependent patients on an inpatient unit produced greater reduction in depressive symptoms, but a large reduction in depression was also observed in controls, and long-term outcome was not reported (88).

A controlled trial among cocaine-dependent patients found that voucher incentives plus the CRA was superior to a control group that received only voucher incentives, not only in terms of improving cocaine use outcome but in reducing depressive symptoms (89). The CRA is designed as a treatment for substance dependence, not depression *per se*. However, CRA places emphasis on developing a behavioral repertoire of pleasant and reinforcing activities (family, friends, recreation, work, etc.) to replace drug taking. Thus, it has much in common with the Behavioral Activation component of CBT for depression (90). Behavioral activation itself has been tested in a small randomized, controlled trial among drug-dependent patients with depressive symptoms and found superior to a treatment-as-usual control on outcome of mood symptoms and satisfaction with treatment (91).

Referral to self-help groups such as Alcoholics Anonymous is one of the most common elements of current practice of substance abuse treatment. One observational study suggests that participation in Alcoholics Anonymous may reduce suicide risk (92).

In summary, these studies, while in some cases small and preliminary, support the effectiveness of behavioral therapies among depressed, substance-dependent patients. Cognitive behavioral approaches focused on depression, and approaches developed for treating substance dependence (such as the CRA) both show promise. In terms of clinical implications, these data further support the conclusion derived from the meta-analysis (57) that in treatment for depressed, substance-dependent patients, consideration should be given to starting with an appropriate behavioral intervention, particularly cognitive behavioral approaches that target depressive symptoms and promote patterns of behavior that may improve depression.

Medication Treatments for Substance Use Disorders

The importance of initiating effective treatment for the substance use disorder among patients with co-occurring depression has already been emphasized, particularly in regard to behavioral/psychosocial treatments. Medication treatments for substance use disorders have received less attention and study in terms of their effects among patients with co-occurring depression, but available evidence is favorable. For example, depressive symptoms decrease substantially during the first 1 to 2 weeks of methadone maintenance treatment for opioid dependence, and about half of major depressive syndromes in patients presenting for methadone maintenance can be expected to resolve during those initial weeks of treatment (44). Naltrexone and disulfiram were both shown to be safe and effective among alcohol-dependent patients with co-occurring psychiatric disorders, including major depression (81,82).

The effect of these treatments is likely attributable to improvement in substance use, which in turn reduces substance-induced depressive symptoms as well as reductions in stress and improvement in functioning that may also occur as effective treatment for a substance problem takes hold. However, it is possible that some of these medications have direct effects on mood as well. For example, buprenorphine has been proposed as a treatment for treatment-resistant depression, based on favorable outcomes in a small case series (93). Conversely, concern has been raised regarding the possibility that naltrexone could worsen depression among opioid-dependent patients (94), although evidence suggests it can be used safely in this population (95). As with any medication treatment, clinicians should remain alert to the possibility that failure to improve or worsening of symptoms might relate to unexpected side effects of the medication.

Adolescents and Treatment of Co-occurring Depression and Substance Abuse Substance use disorders often have their onset in adolescence, as do mood disorders, and the combination is associated with expected risk factors such as abuse (95) and with worse clinical outcome (96). Effective intervention early in the course of these disorders has the potential to improve functioning during adolescence and prevent progression to chronic mood and substance use problems during adulthood. Treatment research on mood and substance use disorders in adolescents lags behind research in adults in part owing to the greater difficulties conducting research in adolescents. Controlled trials of antidepressant medication treatments among depressed adolescents (not selected for substance use disorders) have produced mixed results, often with high placebo response rates. A recent National Institutes of Health–sponsored, multi-site, randomized 2 by 2 trial of fluoxetine and CBT found fluoxetine superior to placebo on depression outcome, with the best outcome overall for the group receiving both fluoxetine and CBT (97,98).

Several open-label trials support the effectiveness of fluoxetine for adolescents with combined depression and substance use disorders (99,100). In the first placebo-controlled trial in this population, adolescents with substance use disorders, major depression, and conduct disorder were randomly assigned to fluoxetine or placebo while all received CBT; fluoxetine was superior to placebo on one of the two main depression outcome measures; the placebo response rate was high with substantial overall improvements in both depressive symptoms, CD symptoms, and self-reported substance use in both fluoxetine and placebo groups; fluoxetine was not superior to placebo on any of the substance use outcome measures, and in fact urine toxicology outcome was slightly better on placebo than on fluoxetine (101). This study supports the effectiveness of combined fluoxetine and CBT for treating adolescents with combined depression and substance abuse. The high placebo response rate here echoes the finding among trials in adults that included a manual-guided intervention as the platform treatment (57) and suggests CBT alone may be effective for many depressed, substance-abusing adolescents. The lack of a favorable fluoxetine effect on substance use outcome, observed here, is reminiscent of concerns, deriving from trials in adults, about poor substance use outcome with serotonin re-uptake inhibitors among type B alcoholics (see discussion earlier). Again, type B is characterized by early onset of alcohol problems and externalizing psychopathology, and this adolescent sample had early onset and carried diagnoses of conduct disorder. The results of the adolescent trial are also consistent with the observation from the meta-analysis (57) that the effect of medication on depression may be more robust than the effect on substance use outcome.

Late Life and Treatment of Co-occurring Depression and Substance Abuse Although often thought of as a disease of youth, substance dependence occurs in the elderly and may be an under-recognized problem in this population. The pattern of substances abused may differ, with more alcohol and prescription drugs problems among the elderly, again, often undiagnosed and untreated (102,103). In addition to depression among the elderly, problems with sleep and painful medical conditions, prompting prescriptions of tranquilizers or narcotic analgesics, no doubt contribute. Sleep problems and pain need to be treated, but clinicians working with the elderly should take a careful history for risk factors (e.g., past history, and family history of substance use problems), proceed cautiously, warn patients of the risks and warning signs of addiction, and monitor patients for the development of warning signs, such as development of tolerance, escalating dose, and substance-related impairment. As treated substance-dependent populations age, as is being observed, for example, among methadone-maintained opioid addicts, the diseases of aging, such as cardiac and pulmonary disease and arthritis, become more prevalent along with depression and other psychiatric disorders, complicating clinical management (104). Importantly, identification and effective treatment of depression (either with pharmacotherapy or behavioral therapy) may improve sleep, pain tolerance, and general functioning, and in that instance could be expected to reduce the need for other prescription medications.

Research on treatment of substance use disorders and co-occurring substance use and depression among the elderly is limited, but results to date are encouraging in suggesting that treatment methods developed for young and middle-aged adults can be cautiously extrapolated to the elderly. Findings include that alcohol intake at treatment outset does not interfere with the treatment of depression (105) and that depression and drinking outcome tend to be correlated (105,106). As these dually diagnosed elderly patients are most likely to present in primary medical or psychiatric care settings, a major challenge is to improve screening and intervention. One large trial showed that an integrated model of care (care for depression and substance abuse within the primary care setting) was superior to a referral-based model in promoting engagement in treatment for depression and alcohol problems (107).

Suicidal Behavior and Co-occurring Depression/Substance Abuse Depression and substance abuse are both important risk factors for suicide, and thus, the potential for suicide needs to be carefully assessed in any patient presenting with this combination of disorders. Recent evidence suggests that both DSM-IV independent and substance-induced depression are associated with increased suicidal thinking and behavior among drug- and alcohol-dependent patients (48,49,54). Other common risk factors for suicide such as family history of suicide, history of trauma, history of irritability or violence, current support systems, and physical illness should also be evaluated (108,109).

In recent years, considerable concern has been aroused by reports of antidepressants being associated with increased risk of suicide, particularly among adolescents and young adults, resulting in the addition of explicit warnings being added to the prescribing information of these medications. Certainly, suicide risk (thinking, intent, and behavior) needs to be followed carefully in any depressed substance-dependent patient during a course of treatment, whether or not it was present at baseline. A general consensus, based on recent data (110,111), is that the benefits of antidepressant treatment (in terms of improved symptoms) outweigh the risks, although exacerbations of suicidal thinking or behavior may occur, and patients should be informed and closely monitored. Among depressed alcoholics admitted to an inpatient unit, most of whom had substantial suicidal thinking at admission, treatment with fluoxetine improved depression and drinking outcome and there were no suicide attempts.

Interventions at the Level of Service Delivery and Primary Care Most patients with depression, substance use problems, or both present not to specialty clinics or practitioners but rather to primary care physicians and settings such as emergency rooms or primary care clinics. Given evidence from randomized controlled trials supporting the effectiveness of treating depression among substance-dependent patients, an important challenge is how to translate this finding into a program of care that is effective and can be implemented in primary health care settings where the majority of such patients with mood depression and/or substance use problems are seen. Watkins et al. (112) conducted a group-level randomized trial in which over 20,000 patients participating in managed care organizations were screened, and those screening positive for depression were randomly assigned to usual care or to one of two quality improvement programs, one focusing on implementation of antidepressant medications and one focused on implementing psychotherapy for depression. The primary care clinics at which these patients were treated were randomly assigned to usual care or to implement one of the two quality improvement programs. For patients with both depression and substance use problems, both quality improvement programs were associated with increased likelihood of prescription of antidepressant medications and improved depression outcome compared to usual care. This study suggests that efforts to increase treatment of combined depression and substance misuse in primary care settings would have favorable effects and should encourage more efforts to develop programs of screening and intervention in primary care settings.

Another important question is whether patients with combinations of psychiatric and substance use disorders benefit when services for both problems are integrated into one treatment program, as opposed to a model in which psychiatric and substance problems are treated at separate programs. One large randomized trial found integrated services for patients with depression or problematic alcohol use resulted in superior outcome compared to a model in which patients were referred out to separate clinics for each problem (107). Whether services are best delivered with an integrated model or through referral out to specialty clinics depends on the availability of integrated services and the severity and complexity of each component problem. Referrals can also be effective, especially when efforts are made to enhance communication between treatment teams and different programs (113).

Depression and the Treatment of Nicotine Dependence The prevalence of nicotine dependence is increased among patients with mood disorders and is very high among patients with substance use disorders. Yet, nicotine dependence is often overlooked during the evaluation and treatment of both mood disorders and substance use disorders—perhaps because it does not cause immediate impairment in the same way as mood or drug and alcohol problems. Nonetheless, nicotine dependence should be a focus of treatment planning, due to its substantial adverse long-term effects on health. Evidence on the co-occurrence of nicotine dependence and depression also serves to illustrate the potential complexity of co-occurring psychiatric and substance use disorders.

Interest in this comorbidity began, in part, with observations that a history of major depression was common among patients seeking treatment to quit cigarette smoking and that a history of depression was an adverse prognostic factor, predicting lower likelihood of successfully quitting smoking (114). Case histories, and a subsequent series, documented the emergence of severe depression after quitting smoking, which resolved only when smoking was resumed, suggesting that nicotine may function like an antidepressant medication for some patients (115). Studies suggest that treatment for nicotine dependence is effective among patients with depression (116). However, few studies have evaluated the treatment of current depression among nicotine-dependent patients, and, in fact, current major depression has been an exclusion criterion from most clinical trials of treatments for nicotine dependence.

Clinical trials of treatments for nicotine dependence have often examined the history of major depression as a moderator, also with surprising findings. These include that noradrenergic antidepressant medications bupropion and the tricyclic nortriptyline are effective agents for promoting smoking cessation, but their effect does not appear to depend upon a history of depression (117,118). For example, in a two-by-two trial, nicotine-dependent patients were randomly assigned to nortriptyline or placebo and to either a cognitive behavioral treatment or a control psychotherapy, and the patients were stratified into those with and without a history of major depression; a history of major depression was not associated with greater effectiveness of nortriptyline, although it was associated with a greater effectiveness of the cognitive therapy; further, analysis of mediators suggested that nortriptyline was having its beneficial effect by reducing the initial dysphoria experienced by patients after they quit smoking (117). Thus, this would appear, perhaps, to be an example of an antidepressant medication having a beneficial effect on substance-induced mood symptoms.

Reminiscent of the questions, raised above, about the effectiveness of SSRI antidepressants among alcohol- or drug-dependent patients, fluoxetine has been found to be ineffective as treatment for nicotine dependence (119) or perhaps even counterproductive (120). An exception is that one trial did find evidence of a beneficial effect of fluoxetine among smokers with more severe depressive symptoms at the outset of treatment (121).

In regard to clinical recommendations, available evidence suggests that patients in treatment for substance use disorders are interested in attempting to quit smoking, and that treatment with nicotine patch and counseling is modestly effective (122). Studies of potentially more powerful medications, including bupropion or varenicline, are needed in substance-dependent populations. Depressed patients, with or without concurrent substance use disorders, should be assessed for smoking, encouraged to make a quit attempt, and assisted in the quit attempt with pharmacotherapy and counseling. Such patients may lack motivation to quit and clinicians should be prepared to address the low motivation. Both depression and other substance use disorders should be concurrently treated as indicated. Patients should be carefully monitored for the emergence of depression, or worsening of depression symptoms, during quit attempts and particularly if the quit attempt is successful.

Summary of Treatment Recommendations for Co-occurring Depression and Substance Use Disorder

(1) Treat the Substance Use Disorder For any patient presenting with drug or alcohol problems, a first priority is always to initiate treatment of the substance use disorder. This is easy to overlook when a clinician is called to consult on a possible depression, or when the patient is most bothered by the depressive symptoms, as the clinical focus may be drawn toward the depression. It is important to recall the substantial evidence, across substances of abuse, that treatment of substance use disorders, especially if abstinence is achieved, is associated with improvement or resolution of depressive symptoms. The substance use disorder may not respond well to the initial treatment regimen, in which case that regimen needs to be adjusted systematically until a good response is achieved. For example, a patient who does not achieve abstinence with initial outpatient treatment should be considered for a brief inpatient stay, addition of a medication (e.g., disulfiram, naltrexone) or adjustment of the dose (e.g., methadone or buprenorphine), or a change in the behavioral therapy regimen. Effective medications for substance use disorders are underutilized in general. Behavioral regimens with a cognitive behavioral emphasis seem particularly promising among patients with co-occurring depression and substance use disorders. A time-honored concern is that depression may become an excuse not to quit substances. In our experience, this is not often the case, as patients with genuine depression along with substance problems are suffering and seek relief from all their problems. But, it is important that the depression and its treatment not distract the clinician or the patient from ongoing aggressive efforts to treat the substance use disorder.

(2) Evaluate the Mood Symptoms All patients presenting for treatment of substance use disorders should receive a brief screening for depression. This can be accomplished during a review of systems in the initial clinical interview or with an instrument such as the Beck Depression Inventory or Hamilton Depression Scale. Patients who screen positive should receive a thorough psychiatric evaluation, according to the DSM-IV, operationalized as suggested earlier (see Table 84.5), to arrive at a DSM-IV diagnostic assessment of either independent depressive disorder, substance-induced depressive disorder, or depressive symptoms as usual effects of substances. The diagnostic evaluation (see Tables 84.5 and 84.6) should also carefully probe for evidence of bipolar disorder (history of mania or hypomania), as the treatment approach for bipolar disorder differs substantially from that of depressive disorders. The diagnostic evaluation should also assess the severity of depression, including suicide risk, as this will influence the urgency with which treatment of depression is initiated. Other disorders that frequency co-occur with depression, including and anxiety disorders and attention deficit hyperactivity disorder (ADHD), should also be assessed, beginning with a thorough developmental history, since these also have distinct treatment implications.

(3) Treat the Depressive Disorder As the evidence reviewed earlier shows fairly clearly, independent major depression or dysthymia among substance-dependent patients should be treated. A guideline such as the Texas Medication Algorithm Project (TMAP) (123,124) can be applied. The evidence (see Table 84.7) suggests two adjustments to the usual approach to treating depression regarding psychotherapy and SRI antidepressants, respectively. The treatment approach outlined in the TMAP emphasizes medication, with psychotherapy as an alternative or adjunct in case initial medication trials fail. Few studies have addressed the efficacy of psychotherapies such as CBT or related approaches (e.g., Behavioral Activation, the CRA) for depressed substance-dependent patients, but those that have suggested favorable results. Also, as reviewed, many of the antidepressant medication trials among substance-dependent patients have shown high placebo response rates, particularly when a manually guided psychosocial intervention was offered to all patients. An advantage of psychotherapy is that it lacks the potential for drug interactions inherent in medication. Thus, it is worth considering as a first-line treatment for depression if personnel trained in the delivery of effective methods are available. To the extent that the depression is more severe, for example with greater symptom levels, impairment, or suicide risk, medication should be preferred as the first-line treatment, perhaps in conjunction with behavioral treatment.

Guidelines such as TMAP (123,124) recommend SSRI antidepressants as the first line of treatment owing to their good tolerability and evidence of efficacy, unless the patient has a history of failure to respond to past adequate trials. However, as reviewed, some evidence suggests SSRIs may be ineffective, or even counterproductive, for some substance-dependent patients, particularly those with early-onset substance use disorders, and externalizing psychopathology (e.g., impulsivity or antisocial traits). SSRIs may still be tried as the first-line antidepressant, presuming there is not a history of prior failed trials, as the good tolerability is an asset. However, practitioners should monitor closely for lack of effect or clinical worsening and be prepared to switch away from an SSRI to an antidepressant with a different mechanism of action. Tricyclic antidepressants have the most convincing evidence of efficacy from clinical trials, although their side effect profile (especially risk of seizures, and cardiac conduction effects) makes them less than ideal for substance-dependent patients. Other medications with noradrenergic or mixed modes of action, such as venlafaxine, duloxetine, mirtazapine, and nefazodone, should be considered, mindful that few clinical trials have tested these agents for treatment of substance abuse plus depression.

Depression among substance-dependent patients may be accompanied by other common psychiatric disorders, which should be identified and treated if present. Anxiety disorders are common among depressed, substance-dependent patients; these also respond to antidepressant medications, although each of the anxiety disorders has specific behavioral interventions with evidence of efficacy (125). More research is needed on the treatment of specific anxiety disorders among substance-dependent patients. ADHD is also common among substance-dependent patients and responds to stimulant medications and noradrenergic antidepressants (e.g., bupropion), although results of clinical trials among substance-dependent patients are mixed so far (126).

Effective treatment of the depression may help to improve the substance use disorder but it is rarely a cure. Hence, ongoing monitoring of substance use and ongoing therapeutic attention to the substance use are needed.

Bipolar Disorder

Pharmacological Treatments

Overview of Medication Treatment for Bipolar Illness

Pharmacologic treatment is the mainstay of the treatment of bipolar disorder. More complete reviews of the pharmacologic management of bipolar disorder can be found elsewhere (127), and the TMAP is a useful guideline (128). Briefly, this can be divided into the management of acute mania or hypomania, the management of bipolar depression, and maintenance medication to prevent relapse once acute episodes have resolved or improved.

Acute mania is typically treated with both a mood stabilizer (lithium or an anticonvulsant) in combination with a neuroleptic. Mood stabilizers that are FDA-approved for treatment of mania include lithium and the anticonvulsant valproate, although carbamazepine and other anticonvulsants have evidence of efficacy as well. The combination is often preferable because mood stabilizers take longer to work, whereas the neuroleptic medications work rapidly and are particularly useful in exerting rapid control over acute manic symptoms such as racing thoughts, agitation, and insomnia, as well as psychosis. Neuroleptic medications of both the first generation (e.g., chlorpromazine, haloperidol, perphenazine) and second generation (so-called atypical neuroleptics such as risperidone, olanzapine, quetiapine) are effective. Frank mania is a medical/psychiatric emergency owing to the potential for psychosis and/or severely impaired judgment, either of which can lead to dangerous and self-destructive behavior. Patients with mania often have little or no insight into their condition and may be uncooperative. Thus, these patients should be brought to an emergency room for acute pharmacologic management and often need hospitalization to fully establish mood stabilization. Substance abuse often accompanies acute mania or hypomania, and brief hospitalization can be invaluable in beginning to bring this under control as well, establishing initial abstinence and evaluating the extent to which manic symptoms are reflective of substance intoxication.

For maintenance treatment after an acute manic episode, mood stabilizers are the mainstay of treatment, with both lithium and valproate having solid evidence of efficacy in preventing relapse. Other anticonvulsants including carbamazepine and lamotrigine have evidence of efficacy as well. Valproate has been favored in recent years, perhaps because lithium has a narrow therapeutic window with serious toxicity and death if the levels become too high, thus requiring careful monitoring and a reliable patient with low risk of overdose. However, lithium is often uniquely effective and should be considered in cooperative patients or in those with a significant other who can be involved to help monitor medication taking. Neuroleptics are less desirable as maintenance treatments because of significant side effects that can develop with chronic use, including tardive dyskinesia, weight gain, and metabolic syndrome. However, a neuroleptic often proves necessary, in conjunction with mood stabilizers, to maintain stable mood. During chronic neuroleptic treatment, clinicians should monitor the motor examination and metabolic parameters, including body mass index, and serum glucose and triglycerides. Three neuroleptics are available as long-acting depot injections: haloperidol (Haldol decanoate), Prolixin (Prolixin decanoate), and risperidone (Risperdal Consta). Though rarely used as the sole treatment, the long-acting injections are especially useful in combination with mood stabilizers or oral neuroleptics for patients who struggle with medication adherence or in whom relapse is regularly preceded by discontinuing medication. The long-acting injection guarantees that at least some mood stabilizing medication is on board, even if the patient stops the other medications, and this can attenuate the severity of the mood relapse and facilitate intervention.

Substance abuse is more likely to occur in manic or hypomanic episodes than in depressive phases of bipolar illness (129), although it can certainly occur in conjunction with depression or during periods of euthymia (normal mood) as well. Hence, clinicians need to be prepared medically to manage acute intoxication or withdrawal. There is little evidence regarding the use of medications for targeted treatment of substance use disorders among patient with bipolar illness. However, as a general principle, if a medication is indicated (e.g., methadone or buprenorphine for opioid dependence, or naltrexone for alcohol dependence) it should be initiated with careful monitoring. Cautions include the fact that disulfiram, arguably the most potent medication for preventing relapse to alcohol dependence (when a significant other can be engaged to monitor the medication), has been associated in rare cases with episodes of psychosis, perhaps owing to its action of inhibiting dopamine beta hydroxylase, which increases brain dopamine levels (130).

In most cases of bipolar disorder, depression is the predominant mood disturbance, with mania or hypomania occurring less frequently. Also, bipolar patients are more likely to present for treatment of depression because depression is painful, whereas mania or hypomania are often experienced as pleasurable. Thus, as noted previously, it is very important to review the history of a depressed patient for evidence of past episodes of mania or hypomania or family history of bipolar illness. The management of bipolar depression differs significantly from the management of unipolar depression, as antidepressant medication, either given alone or in combination with neuroleptics or mood stabilizers, may be less effective than once thought (131) and may be detrimental, inducing mania, mixed mood states, or cycling of mood from mania to depression. Patients with bipolar depression often respond best to a mood stabilizer (lithium or anticonvulsant), and combination of a mood stabilizer with a low to moderate dose of a second-generation atypical neuroleptic: Risperidone (Risperdal), olanzapine (Zyprexa), quetiapine (Seroquel), ziprasidone (Geodon), or aripiprazole (Abilify) can also be effective. Antidepressant medication may be considered if depression persists, and mood stabilizer or neuroleptic treatment is established. Recent evidence has established the efficacy of lamotrigine for bipolar depression (132). Lamotrigine may cause life-threatening skin reaction (Stevens-Johnson syndrome), and thus the medication should be started at low dose (25 mg) and titrated slowly to the target dose range of 100 mg to 300 mg per day, with careful monitoring for dermatologic reactions. However, once a maintenance dose is established without skin problems, lamotrigine is generally well tolerated and often quite effective in treating bipolar depression and preventing relapse. Omega-3 fatty acids, such as contained in fish oil or flax seed or some other vegetable oils, may be useful as adjunctive treatment to exert mood stabilizing effects and prevent relapse in bipolar illness (133). Hence, nutritional supplementation with fish or flax seed oil may be considered as part of long-term management.

Medication Treatments for Co-occurring Bipolar and Substance Use Disorders Compared to unipolar depression, there has been less research focused specifically on pharmacotherapy for co-occurring bipolar disorder and substance abuse, but some studies have been conducted (for a detailed review, see 134). Three double-blind, placebo-controlled trials have been conducted of mood stabilizing anticonvulsant medications. Salloum et al. (139) showed in a double-blind trial among alcohol-dependent individuals with co-occurring bipolar disorder that valproate combined with lithium was superior to lithium plus placebo in reducing the number of heavy drinking days. In another well-designed, placebo-controlled trial among hospitalized adolescents with bipolar and substance use disorders, lithium improved both mood and substance use outcome (135). A third placebo-controlled trial examined carbamazepine among cocaine-dependent patients with or without co-occurring mood disorders (136); the mood disorder group included both major depressive disorder and bipolar disorder, many of those being bipolar II; among the subgroup with mood disorders, carbamazepine improved depression outcome with a trend toward reduced cocaine use as well, whereas the medication had no significant effects in the subgroup without mood disorders. Other open-label trials of anticonvulsant mood stabilizers among substance-abusing bipolar patients have also shown evidence of good tolerability and efficacy, including lamotrigine (137), valproate (138,139), and gabapentin (140). A small, open-label trial showed some promise for lithium among cocaine dependent patient with bipolar spectrum disorders.

Anticonvulsants have been studied as treatments for substance dependence, based on hypotheses of beneficial effects on the pathophysiology of addiction (e.g., augmentation of GABAergic inputs to the brain reward system). For example, one substantial clinical trial suggests the efficacy of topiramate for alcohol dependence (141), and a small trial suggests promise for topiramate (142). The evidence is unclear as to the efficacy of topiramate as a treatment for bipolar disorder, but it does seem to be safe and effective at reducing appetite and body weight among bipolar patients (143). Clinical trials of topiramate among patients with co-occurring bipolar and substance use disorders are needed.

Second-generation neuroleptic medications have also shown promise among patients with co-occurring substance use and bipolar disorders, including small open-label, uncontrolled trials of quetiapine (144), and aripiprazole (145). A recent double-blind, placebo-controlled trial of quetiapine (up to 600 mg per day), added to other mood stabilizers in patients with bipolar disorder (mainly depressed) and substance use disorders (mainly alcohol), showed quetiapine superior to placebo on depression outcome; there was no main effect of quetiapine treatment on substance use outcome, but improvement in drinking outcome measures did correlate with improvement in depression scores (146). Taken together, these results support the efficacy of mood stabilizers both for improving mood and reducing substance use, and one study looked at and found that mood and substance use improvement were correlated.

Taken together, the results of these trials resemble the larger literature on antidepressant medications among unipolar depressed patients (57) in suggesting that appropriate pharmacological treatment of a carefully diagnosed co-occurring DSM-IV independent mood disorder improves outcome of both mood and substance use symptoms. In each of the controlled trials, steps were taken in the diagnostic workup to establish the presence of an independent bipolar disorder (according to DSM-IV criteria), either through establishing persistence of mood symptoms during abstinence on an inpatient unit (135) or through a careful history (136,147). The same caveat applies that such medication treatment is not likely to fully "cure" the substance use disorder, so that specific attention in the treatment plan to behavioral or medication treatment for substance abuse also needs to be considered.

Medications for Substance Dependence Less research has focused on use of medications for treatment of substance use disorders among patients with bipolar disorder. An open-label trial suggests naltrexone, an effective treatment for alcohol dependence, was both safe and associated with both improved mood and improved alcohol use among patients with co-occurring bipolar disorder and alcohol dependence; the majority of patients in that trial were depressed at the outset. A cautionary note, however, was sounded by a report of two cases in which treatment with naltrexone in patients with mania and concurrent alcohol dependence was poorly tolerated, producing marked nausea (148). Similarly, in the open trial of naltrexone, more of the patients who dropped out had mania or hypomania. New onset hypomania has been observed in an opioid-dependent patient after detoxification and induction onto naltrexone (149). This suggests that clinicians should carefully monitor patients with co-occurring bipolar and alcohol use disorders for side effects or clinical worsening when using naltrexone.

Behavioral Treatments

Behavioral Treatment Approaches to Bipolar Disorder Though medications are essential for treating most cases of bipolar disorder, the behavioral approach to the patient is also important to successful management. The goals of behavioral and psychosocial treatment for bipolar disorder include (a) maintaining a treatment alliance and continuity of care; (b) securing adherence to medication treatment, and (c) coping with symptoms and addressing stressors or other circumstances that may lead to symptomatic exacerbations (150,151). Substance abuse may undermine each of these goals, and thus an important related goal is to identify and address substance use problems. Bipolar disorder generally runs a chronic, if waxing and waning, course, and maintaining continuity of care is an essential challenge. Patients may become impulsive or lose insight into their illness, particularly during manic or hypomanic phases, or lose sight of the need for ongoing treatment during periods of remission or relative quiescence of symptoms. Poor adherence to medications is a frequent cause of relapse and poor outcome in bipolar disorder. Patients may be bothered by side effects of medications. Patients may miss certain aspects of their mood fluctuations that are blunted by mood stabilizing medications. Though this is particularly true of manic or hypomanic phases that are often experienced as pleasurable, some patients with bipolar disorder ironically resist the blunting of depressed mood as well, viewing their depression as a reflection of their "true" feelings. Finally, stressful life events such as family conflict, and irregularity of daily routines and the sleep-wake cycle may contribute at a physiologic level to the mood instability of bipolar disorder (150,151).

Several specific behavioral/psychosocial treatments for bipolar disorder have been developed and have shown evidence of efficacy, including psychoeducation (152,153), cognitive behavioral therapy (154,155), interpersonal social rhythm therapy (156–158), and family focused therapy (159,160). Each to varying degrees addresses the common issues outlined earlier, including alliance, understanding the illness and its signs and symptoms, the importance of treatment adherence in general and medication adherence in particular, and the role of stressors and daily routines. Psychoeducation follows a medical model and emphasizes medication adherence, early recognition of symptoms, and social and occupational functioning. In addition to those basic goals, cognitive behavioral therapy seeks to understand and address connections between maladaptive thoughts or behaviors and mood disturbances. Interpersonal social rhythm therapy, derived from interpersonal therapy for depression (156), addresses the impact of relationships on mood fluctuations and also emphasizes the importance of normalizing routines and the sleep-wake cycle and targets disturbances in these areas, particularly disturbances in sleep, as warning signs. Reduced sleep or insomnia are frequently harbingers of mania, and hypersomnia often signals impending depression. Family focused therapy is based on evidence that a stressful family environment has been associated with worse outcome; this treatment approach seeks to reduce tension and improve family functioning and coping strategies. Readers working with bipolar substance abusers are encouraged to become familiar with these approaches. Patients and their families and significant others need to understand bipolar disorder, recognize signs of relapse, and have strategies for how to intervene; each of these approaches affords a range of useful strategies.

Behavioral Treatment Approaches to Co-occurring Bipolar and Substance Use Disorders Integrated group therapy (IGT) (161) is the first group-based behavioral approach developed specifically for patients with both bipolar disorder and substance use disorders and has been shown to be effective in reducing substance use in a randomized, controlled trial (162). IGT is a manually guided group treatment designed to serve as an adjunct to pharmacotherapy for bipolar disorder. It is assumed that the medications are managed during separate individual sessions with each patient's physician. Founded on cognitive behavioral principles and focused on relapse prevention, IGT incorporates aspects of the earlier reviewed behavioral treatments for bipolar disorder while addressing the unique inter-relationships between bipolar disorder and substance abuse.

The core principles of IGT include the idea that similar patterns of thought and behavior promote relapse to both mood episodes and substance abuse, and patients are encouraged to approach their problems as a single disorder—"bipolar substance abuse"—rather than as a pair of disorders. This combats the tendency of patients to view one of the disorders as primary and minimize the other. Each session is focused on a topic, such as "dealing with depression without abusing substances" and "recovery versus relapse thinking." Each session begins with a "check-in" in which group members all report on their week in terms of substance use, mood symptoms, medication adherence, high-risk situations, and coping strategies employed. This is followed by a review of the topic of the previous week, followed by a presentation of the current topic and related coping skills to be learned; patients are given handouts and homework assignments to practice recovery skills during the coming week. The emphasis throughout is on similarities in the relapse and recovery process between the two disorders and the inter-relationships between relapse to substance use and to mood episodes. There is also a strong emphasis on medication adherence, combating pessimism, and on maintaining daily routines and a regular sleep cycle. As IGT is designed as an adjunctive treatment, it can be incorporated into a range of practice settings including either substance abuse treatment programs or psychiatric clinics serving bipolar patients or office-based practice.

An individual cognitive behavioral approach has also been developed for patients with combined substance and mood disorders (163). This approach includes medication monitoring plus 16 individual cognitive behavioral sessions focused on an integrated approach to mood and substance use problems. In a randomized controlled trial among patients with bipolar disorder and substance use disorders, where the control group was medication monitoring alone, patients receiving this CBT had better medication adherence and fewer depressive symptoms compared to controls but no difference in substance use outcome. Interestingly, the opposite pattern was observed in the trial of IGT, in which patients assigned to IGT had superior substance use outcome, but mood symptoms were actually somewhat worse on IGT compared to the Group Drug Counseling control; the latter mood symptoms were in the mild range and could reflect greater awareness and hence greater reporting of mood symptoms on IGT. Nonetheless, taken together, the results of these trials suggest there may be a complementary role for both individual (163) and group (162) CBT approaches to patients with combined bipolar and substance use disorders.

An important line of research has examined the effectiveness of integrated approaches to treatment of patients with severe mental illness and substance use problems, as opposed to the traditional approach of referring patients to different agencies for psychiatric and substance treatment, respectively. In addition to patients with schizophrenia, the severely mentally ill population includes patients with severe cases of bipolar disorder, major depression, or schizoaffective disorder. For example, assertive community treatment (ACT) is carried out by treatment teams that seek to deliver all needed services (e.g., treatment for psychiatric disorder, treatment for substance use disorder, and social services) to patients without resort to outside referrals. ACT and other integrated treatment models have a strong empirical evidence base (164,165), including evidence of efficacy specifically among patients with bipolar and substance use disorders (166). As an alternative to integrated models, efforts to enhance cooperation between separate agencies focusing on diverse combinations of psychiatric and substance problems can also be successful (113).

Summary of Treatment Recommendations for Co-occurring Bipolar Disorder and Substance Use Disorders Again, initiation of effective treatment for the substance use disorder is an important priority. However, the evidence on behavioral or services interventions suggests the importance of approaching the treatment of combined bipolar and substance use disorders simultaneously in an integrated fashion (161,162,165,166). If the diagnostic assessment establishes a clear-cut diagnosis of bipolar I or II disorder, this is almost certainly independent of substance use disorder, and medication treatment for bipolar disorder is generally indicated. Bipolar disorder often runs a severe and disabling course, and medications are usually essential to achieving a good outcome. Several specific behavioral approaches have also been developed, which are useful as adjuncts to medication treatment of bipolar disorder, emphasizing medication adherence, establishing a healthy, well-regulated lifestyle and sleep cycle, and combating cognitions that may promote mood swings or relapses. An acute episode of mania, hypomania, mixed mood episode, or bipolar depression often raises the level of medical emergency, requiring emergency room management and hospitalization. Suicide is a significant risk with bipolar disorder, and patients should be monitored for signs and risk factors. The available evidence on use of mood stabilizers and neuroleptic medications among patients with combined bipolar and substance use disorders suggests these medications are effective in improving both bipolar symptoms and substance use outcome. Guidelines for treatment for medication treatment of bipolar disorder can be followed, bearing in mind that a satisfactory outcome may depend upon combinations of mood stabilizers (e.g., lithium plus an anticonvulsant, combined anticonvulsants), or neuroleptics (e.g., mood stabilizer plus-second generation neuroleptic). For treatment of bipolar depression, lamotrigine or antidepressant medications may be helpful, although the efficacy of the antidepressants is less clear in view of recent controlled trials, and antidepressants may be associated with the emergence of mania or mixed states (the "switch" phenomenon).

When the diagnostic assessment suggests a bipolar spectrum disorder (e.g., cyclothymia or subthreshold bipolar disorder), the differential diagnosis between an independent bipolar disorder and a substance-induced mood disorder may be less clear. This differential is more difficult if the mood swings are less severe, of shorter duration, and consonant with intoxication or withdrawal symptoms of the substances the patient is abusing. In this instance, aggressive treatment of the substance use disorder, combined with careful monitoring of the mood symptoms, may be warranted. Resolution of the mood symptoms with abstinence or improvement in the substance problems would add more credence to the substance-induced diagnosis, although mood swings may occur considerably later. Conversely, persistence of the mood symptoms despite improvement in substance use would suggest that specific treatments for bipolar disorder be considered.

Available evidence suggests that the behavioral management of patients with combined bipolar and substance use disorders is important and should involve approaching both disorders in an integrated fashion, emphasizing common behavior patterns promoting recovery and relapse in both disorders, and the importance of medication adherence and fostering a lifestyle conducive to recovery from both disorders. Manually guided interventions (163) are available, as well as integrated approaches to services for severely ill and disabled patients (165,166).

SUMMARY AND FUTURE DIRECTIONS

This chapter has attempted to serve as a primer on the diagnosis and treatment of mood disorders and presents the evidence on diagnosis and treatment of mood disorders among patients with substance use disorders. Several common themes emerge from the literature on depressive disorders and bipolar disorders co-occurring with substance use disorders. Initiation and maintenance of treatment for the substance use disorder is always a priority that should not be overlooked. Careful diagnostic assessment and a lifetime clinical history are important to making the differential diagnosis between independent mood disorders, requiring specific treatment, and substance-induced mood disorders which may resolve with abstinence or improvement in substance abuse. It is ideal to be able to observe the course of mood symptoms after reduction in substance use or abstinence, although abstinence will not always be achieved among outpatients, and treatment will often need to be initiated without this information. To the extent that they have been tested in clinical trials, independent depressive or bipolar disorders seem to respond to the same medication or behavioral treatments that are effective for mood disorders in the absence of a substance use disorders. Behavioral approaches may be effective as an alternative to antidepressant medication among substance-dependent patients with depression, while among bipolar patients, behavioral techniques have emphasized adherence to mood stabilizing medications and an integrated approach to substance and bipolar problems (166–178).

The conclusions just summarized represent the product of an enormous research effort that has taken place over the last three decades, much of it publicly funded by the NIH and its specific institutes, including NIDA, NIAAA, and NIMH. Progress achieved on the diagnosis and treatment of mood disorders, substance use disorders, and their co-occurrence is gratifying. Still, many questions remain unanswered or only partially answered, and indicate further research. Work is needed on the DSM diagnostic criteria and associated clinical features in order to improve the important differential diagnosis between independent and substance-induced mood disorders and accounting for the unique effects of specific substances. More research is needed on medication and behavioral treatments. There is, to date, only limited research on the prognostic and treatment indications of substance induced mood disorders. Finally, the co-occurrence of mood and substance use disorders invites a range of studies seeking to understand the connection between these domains of disorders at a fundamental biological level. Examples may include studies on the effect of chronic exposure to specific substances (e.g., cannabis, nicotine) on development of mood disorders and vice-versa, using genetics, brain imaging, and other biologic probes. Such research promises to yield insights into the biology of each disorder as well as their combination and should help to place psychiatric diagnosis and treatment on a more pathophysiologic footing, as is the ultimate goal beyond DSM-IV and DSM-V.

ACKNOWLEDGMENTS: *This study was supported by Grants P50 DA09236, U10 DA13035, and K24 DA022412 (Dr. Nunes) and R01 DA15968, U10 DA15831 and K24 DA022288 (Dr. Weiss) from the National Institute on Drug Abuse.*

REFERENCES

1. Hasin DS, Goodwin RD, Stinson FS, et al. Epidemiology of major depressive disorder: results from the National Epidemiologic Survey on Alcoholism and Related Conditions. *Arch Gen Psychiatry* 2005;62(10): 1097–1106.
2. Hasin D., Nunes E., Meydan J. Comorbidity of alcohol, drug and psychiatric disorders: epidemiology. In Kranzler HR, Tinsley JA, eds. *Dual diagnosis and treatment: substance abuse and comorbid disorders*, 2nd ed. New York: Marcel Dekker, 2004:1–34.
3. Grant BF, Stinson FS, Hasin DS, et al. Prevalence, correlates, and comorbidity of bipolar I disorder and axis I and II disorders: results from the National Epidemiologic Survey on Alcohol and Related Conditions. *J Clin Psychiatry* 2005;66(10):1205–1215.
4. Merikangas KR, Akiskal HS, Angst J, et al. Lifetime and 12-month prevalence of bipolar spectrum disorder in the National Comorbidity Survey replication. *Arch Gen Psychiatry* 2007;64(5):543–552.
5. Cerullo MA, Strakowski SM. The prevalence and significance of substance use disorders in bipolar type I and II disorder. *Subst Abuse Treat Prev Policy* 2007;1:2:29.
6. American Psychiatric Association. *Diagnostic and statistical manual of mental disorders*, 4th ed. Washington, DC: Author, 1994.
7. First MB, Spitzer RL, Gibbon M, et al. *Structured clinical interview for DSM-IV-TR Axis I Disorders* (patient edition) (SCID-I/P). New York: Biometrics Research Department, New York State Psychiatric Institute, 2002.
8. Hasin D, Samet S, Nunes E, et al. Diagnosis of comorbid psychiatric disorders in substance users assessed with the Psychiatric Research Interview for Substance and Mental Disorders for DSM-IV. *Am J Psychiatry* 2006;163:689–696.
9. Budney AJ, Hughes JR. The cannabis withdrawal syndrome. *Curr Opin Psychiatry* 2006;19(3):233–238.
10. Schuckit MA. Genetic and clinical implications of alcoholics and affective disorder. *Am J Psychiatry* 1986;143:140–147.
11. Brown SA, Schuckit MA. Changes in depression among abstinent alcoholics. *J Stud Alcohol* 1988;49:412–417.
12. Liappas J, Paparrigopoulos E, Tzavellas G, et al. Impact of alcohol detoxification on anxiety and depressive symptoms. *Drug Alcohol Depend* 2002;68:215–220.
13. Strain EC, Stitzer ML, Bigelow GE. Early treatment time course of depressive symptoms in opiate addicts. *J Nerv Ment Dis* 1991;179(4):215–221.
14. Weddington WW, Brown BS, Haertzen CA, et al. Changes in mood, craving, and sleep during short-term abstinence reported by male cocaine addicts. *Arch Gen Psychiatry* 1990;47:861–868.
15. Satel SL, Price LH, Palumbo JM, et al. Clinical phenomenology and neurobiology of cocaine abstinence: a prospective inpatient study. *Am J Psychiatry* 1991;148:1712–1716.
16. Brown SA, Inaba RK, Gillin JC, et al. Alcoholism and affective disorder: clinical course of depressive symptoms. *Am J Psychiatry* 1995;152(1):45–52.
17. Nunes EV, Liu X, Samet S, et al. Independent versus substance-induced major depressive disorder in substance-dependent patients: observational study of course during follow-up. *J Clin Psychiatry* 2006a;67(10): 1561–1567.
18. Cohen P, Cohen J. The clinician's illusion. *Arch Gen Psychiatry* 1984;41(12):1178–1182.
19. Regier DA, Farmer ME, Rae DS, et al. Comorbidity of mental disorders with alcohol and other drug abuse—results from the Epidemiological Catchment Area (ECA) Study. *JAMA* 1990;263:2511–2518.
20. Kessler R, McGonagle K, Zhao S, et al. Lifetime and 12-month prevalence of DSM-III-R psychiatric disorders in the United States: results from the National Comorbidity Survey. *Arch Gen Psychiatry* 1994;51:8–19.
21. Kessler RC. Epidemiology of psychiatric comorbidity. In Tsuang MT, Tohen M, Zahner GEP, eds. *Textbook in psychiatric epidemiology*. New York: Wiley-Liss, 1995:179–197.
22. Grant B. Comorbidity between DSM-IV drug use disorders and major depression: results of a national survey. *J Subst Abuse* 1995;7:481–497.
23. Grant BF, Harford, TC: Comorbidity between DSM-IV alcohol use disorders and major depression: results of a national survey. *Drug Alcohol Depend* 1995;39:197–206.
24. Kessler RC, Adler L, Barkley R, et al. The prevalence and correlates of adult ADHD in the United States: results from the National Comorbidity Survey Replication. *Am J Psychiatry* 2006;163(4):716–723.
25. Rounsaville BJ, Weissman MM, Crits-Christoph K, et al. Diagnosis and symptoms of depression in opiate addicts: course and relationship to treatment outcome. *Arch Gen Psychiatry* 1982;39:151–156.
26. Rounsaville BJ, Kosten TR, Weissman MM, et al. Prognostic significance of psychopathology in treated opiate addicts; a 2.5 year follow-up study. *Arch Gen Psychiatry* 1986;43:739–745.
27. Greenfield SF, Weiss RD, Muenz LR, et al. The effect of depression on return to drinking: a prospective study. *Arch Gen Psychiatry* 1998; 55(3):259–265.
28. Dixit AR, Crum RM. Prospective study of depression and the risk of heavy alcohol use in women. *Am J Psychiatry* 2000;157(5):751–758.
29. Hasin D, Tsai W, Endicott J, et al. The effects of major depression on alcoholism: five year course. *Am J Addict* 1996;5:144–155.
30. Hasin D, Liu X, Nunes E, et al. Effects of major depression on remission and relapse of substance dependence. *Arch Gen Psychiatry* 2002;59(4):375–380.

31. Rounsaville BJ, Dolinsky ZS, Babor TF, et al. Psychopathology as a predictor of treatment outcome in alcoholics. *Arch Gen Psychiatry* 1987; 44:505–513.
32. Carroll KM, Power ME, Bryant K, et al. One-year follow-up status of treatment-seeking cocaine abusers. Psychopathology and dependence severity as predictors of outcome. *J Nerv Ment Disord* 1993;181:71–79.
33. Brown RA, Monti PM, Myers MG, et al. Depression among cocaine abusers in treatment: relation to cocaine and alcohol use and treatment outcome. *Am J Psychiatry* 1998;155(2):220–225.
34. Curran GM, Flynn HA, Kirchner J, et al. Depression after alcohol treatment as a risk factor for relapse among male veterans. *J Subst Abuse Treat* 2000;19(3):259–265.
35. Davis LL, Frazier EC, Gaynes BN, et al. Are depressed outpatients with and without a family history of substance use disorder different? A baseline analysis of the STAR*D cohort. *J Clin Psychiatry* 2007;68(12): 1931–1938.
36. Brady K, Casto S, Lydiard RB, et al. Substance abuse in an inpatient psychiatric sample. *Am J Drug Alcohol Abuse* 1991;17(4):389–397.
37. Haller DL, Miles DR. Suicidal ideation among psychiatric patients with HIV: psychiatric morbidity and quality of life. *AIDS Behav* 2003;7(2): 101–108.
38. Berger-Greenstein JA, Cuevas CA, Brady SM, et al. Major depression in patients with HIV/AIDS and substance abuse. *AIDS Patient Care STDS* 2007;21(12):942–955.
39. Ford JD, Trestman RL, Tennen H, et al. Relationship of anxiety, depression and alcohol use disorders to persistent high utilization and potentially problematic under-utilization of primary medical care. *Soc Sci Med* 2005;61(7):1618–1625.
40. Babor TF, McRee BG, Kassebaum PA, et al. Screening, brief intervention, and referral to treatment (SBIRT): toward a public health approach to the management of substance abuse. *Subst Abuse* 2007;28(3):7–30.
41. Nunes EV, Goehl L, Seracini A, et al. A modification of the structured clinical interview for DSM-III-R to evaluate methadone patients: test-retest reliability. *Am J Addict* 1996;5(3):241–248.
42. Petrakis I, Carroll KM, Nich C, et al. Fluoxetine treatment of depressive disorders in methadone-maintained opiate addicts. *Drug Alcohol Depend* 1998;50:221–226.
43. McGrath PJ, Nunes EV, Stewart JW, et al. Imipramine treatment of alcoholics with primary depression: a placebo-controlled clinical trial. *Arch Gen Psychiatry* 1996;53:232–240.
44. Nunes EV, Quitkin FM, Donovan SJ, et al. Imipramine treatment of opiate-dependent patients with depressive disorders: a placebo-controlled trial. *Arch Gen Psychiatry* 1998;55:153–160.
45. McDowell D, Nunes EV, Seracini AM, et al. Desipramine treatment of cocaine-dependent patients with depression: a placebo-controlled trial. *Drug Alcohol Depend* 2005;80(2):209–221.
46. Nunes EV, Rounsaville BJ. Comorbidity of substance use with depression and other mental disorders. In *Diagnostic and Statistical Manual of Mental Disorders*, 4th ed. (DSM-IV to DSM-V). *Addiction* 2006;101 (Suppl 1):89–96.
47. Ramsey SE, Kahler CW, Read JP, et al. Discriminating between substance-induced and independent depressive episodes in alcohol dependent patients. *J Stud Alcohol* 2004;65(5):672–676.
48. Aharonovich E, Liu X, Nunes E, et al. Suicide attempts in substance abusers: effects of major depression in relation to substance use disorders. *Am J Psychiatry* 2002;159(9):1600–1602.
48a. American Psychiatric Association. *Diagnostic and Statistical Manual of Mental Disorders*, 4th ed., text revisions. Washington, DC. Author, 2000.
49. Ries RK, Yuodelis-Flores C, Comtois KA, et al. Substance-induced suicidal admissions to an acute psychiatric service: characteristics and outcomes. *J Subst Abuse Treat* 2008;34(1):72–79.
50. Bauer M, Beaulieu S, Dunner DL, et al. Rapid cycling bipolar disorder—diagnostic concepts. *Bipolar Disord* 2008;10(2):153–162.
51. Schneck CD, Miklowitz DJ, Calabrese JR, et al. Phenomenology of rapid-cycling bipolar disorder: data from the first 500 participants in the Systematic Treatment Enhancement Program. *Am J Psychiatry* 2004; 161(10):1902–1908.
52. Kupka RW, Luckenbaugh DA, Post RM, et al. Comparison of rapid-cycling and non-rapid-cycling bipolar disorder based on prospective mood ratings in 539 outpatients. *Am J Psychiatry* 2005;162(7):1273–1280.
53. Manwani SG, Szilagyi KA, Zablotsky B, et al. Adherence to medication in bipolar disorder: a qualitative study exploring the role of patients' beliefs about the condition and its treatment. *Bipolar Disord* 2007; 9(6):656–664.
54. Schuckit MA, Tipp JE, Bergman M, et al. Comparison of induced and independent major depressive disorders in 2,945 alcoholics. *Am J Psychiatry* 1997;154(7):948–957.
55. Preuss UW, Schuckit MA, Smith TL, et al. A comparison of alcohol-induced and independent depression in alcoholics with histories of suicide attempts. *J Stud Alcohol* 2002;63(4):498–502.
56. Schuckit MA, Smith TL, Danko GP, et al. A comparison of factors associated with substance-induced versus independent depressions. *J Stud Alcohol Drugs* 2007;68(6):805–812.
57. Nunes EV, Levin FR. Treatment of depression in patients with alcohol or other drug dependence: a meta-analysis. *JAMA* 2004;291(15):1887–1896.
58. Torrens M, Fonseca F, Mateu G, et al. Efficacy of antidepressants in substance use disorders with and without comorbid depression. A systematic review and meta-analysis. *Drug Alcohol Depend* 2005;78(1):1–22.
59. Walsh BT, Seidman SN, Sysko R, et al. Placebo response in studies of major depression; variable, substantial, and growing. *JAMA* 2002;287: 1840–1847.
60. Altamura AC, Mauri MC, Girardi T, et al. Alcoholism and depression: a placebo-controlled study with viloxazine. *Int J Clin Pharm Res* 1990; (5):293–298.
61. Nunes EV, McGrath PJ, Quitkin FM, et al. Imipramine treatment of cocaine abuse; possible boundaries of efficacy. *Drug Alcohol Depend* 1995;39:185–195.
62. Mason BJ, Kocsis JH, Ritvo EC, et al. A double-blind, placebo-controlled trial of desipramine for primary alcohol dependence stratified on the presence or absence of major depression. *JAMA* 1996;275:761–767.
63. Cornelius JR, Salloum IM, Ehler JG, et al. Fluoxetine in depressed alcoholics: a double-blind, placebo-controlled trial. *Arch Gen Psychiatry* 1997;54:700–705.
64. Roy A. Placebo-controlled study of sertraline in depressed recently abstinent alcoholics. *Biol Psychiatry* 1998;44:633–637.
65. Kleber HD, Weissman MM, Rounsaville BJ, et al. Imipramine as treatment for depression in addicts. *Arch Gen Psychiatry* 1983;40:649–653.
66. Roy-Byrne PP, Pages KP, Russo JE, et al. Nefazodone treatment of major depression in alcohol-dependent patients: a double-blind, placebo-controlled trial. *J Clin Psychopharmacology* 2000;20:129–136.
67. Schmitz JM, Averill P, Stotts AL, et al. Fluoxetine treatment of cocaine-dependent patients with major depressive disorder. *Drug Alcohol Depend* 2001;63:207–214.
68. Pettinati HM, Volpicelli JR, Luck G, et al. Double-blind clinical trial of sertraline treatment for alcohol dependence. *J Clin Psychopharmacol* 2001;21:143–153.
69. Moak DH, Anton RF, Latham PK, et al. Sertraline and cognitive behavioral therapy for depressed alcoholics: results of a placebo-controlled trial. *J Clin Psychopharmacol* 2003;23:553–562.
70. Carpenter KM, Brooks AC, Vosburg SK, et al. The effect of sertraline and environmental context on treating depression and illicit substance use among methadone maintained opiate dependent patients: a controlled clinical trial. *Drug Alcohol Depend* 2004;74(2):123–134.
71. Kranzler HR, Mueller T, Cornelius J, et al. Sertraline treatment of co-occurring alcohol dependence and major depression. *J Clin Psychopharmacol* 2006;26(1):13–20.
72. Woody GE, O'Brien CP, Rickels K. Depression and anxiety in heroin addicts: a placebo-controlled study of doxepin in combination with methadone. *Am J Psychiatry* 1975;132(4):447–450.
73. Titievsky J, Seco G, Barranco M, et al. Doxepin as adjunctive therapy for depressed methadone maintenance patients: a double-blind study. *J Clin Psychiatry* 1982;43(11):454–456.
74. Poling J, Oliveto A, Petry N, et al. Six-month trial of bupropion with contingency management for cocaine dependence in a methadone-maintained population. *Arch Gen Psychiatry* 2006;63(2):219–228.

75. Moeller FG, Schmitz JM, Steinberg JL, et al. Citalopram combined with behavioral therapy reduces cocaine use: a double-blind, placebo-controlled trial. *Am J Drug Alcohol Abuse* 2007;33(3):367–378.
76. Nunes EV, Sullivan MA, Levin FR. Treatment of depression in patients with opiate dependence. *Biol Psychiatry* 2004;56(10):793–802.
77. Stein MD, Solomon DA, Herman DS, et al. Pharmacotherapy plus psychotherapy for treatment of depression in active injection drug users. *Arch Gen Psychiatry* 2004;61(2):152–159.
78. Kranzler HR, Burleson JA, Brown J, et al. Fluoxetine treatment seems to reduce the beneficial effects of cognitive-behavioral therapy in type B alcoholics. *Alcohol Clin Exp Res* 1996;20(9):1534–1541.
79. Pettinati HM, Volpicelli JR, Kranzler HR, et al. Sertraline treatment for alcohol dependence: interactive effects of medication and alcoholic subtype. *Alcohol Clin Exp Res* 2000;24(7):1041–1049.
80. Brady KT, Sonne S, Anton RF, et al. Sertraline in the treatment of co-occurring alcohol dependence and posttraumatic stress disorder. *Alcohol Clin Exp Res* 2005;29(3):395–401.
81. Petrakis IL, Poling J, Levinson C, et al., VA New England VISN I MIRECC Study Group. Naltrexone and disulfiram in patients with alcohol dependence and comorbid psychiatric disorders. *Biol Psychiatry* 2005;57(10):1128–1137.
82. Petrakis I, Ralevski E, Nich C, et al., VA VISN I MIRECC Study Group. Naltrexone and disulfiram in patients with alcohol dependence and current depression. *J Clin Psychopharmacol* 2007;27(2):160–165.
83. Brown RA, Evans DM, Miller IW, et al. Cognitive-behavioral treatment for depression in alcoholism. *J Consult Clin Psychol* 1997;65(5):715–726.
84. Carpenter KM, Aharonovich E, Smith JL, et al. Behavior therapy for depression in drug dependence (BTDD): results of a stage Ia therapy development pilot. *Am J Drug Alcohol Abuse* 2006;32(4):541–548.
85. Carpenter KM, Smith JL, Aharonovich E, et al. Developing therapies for depression in drug dependence: results of a stage 1 therapy study. *Am J Drug Alcohol Abuse* 2008;34(5):642–652.
86. Brown RA, Kahler CW, Niaura R, et al. Cognitive-behavioral treatment for depression in smoking cessation. *J Consult Clin Psychol* 2001;69(3): 471–480.
87. Patten CA, Martin JE, Myers MG, et al. Effectiveness of cognitive-behavioral therapy for smokers with histories of alcohol dependence and depression. *J Stud Alcohol* 1998;59(3):327–335.
88. Vedamurthachar A, Janakiramaiah N, Hegde JM, et al. Antidepressant efficacy and hormonal effects of Sudarshona Kriya Yoga (SKY) in alcohol dependent individuals. *J Affect Disord* 2006;94(1–3):249–253.
89. Higgins ST, Sigmon SC, Wong CJ, et al. Community reinforcement therapy for cocaine-dependent outpatients. *Arch Gen Psychiatry* 2003; 60(10):1043–1052.
90. Hopko DR, Lejuez CW, Ruggiero KJ, et al. Contemporary behavioral activation treatments for depression: procedures, principles, and progress. *Clin Psychol Rev* 2003;23(5):699–717.
91. Daughters SB, Braun AR, Sargeant MN, et al. Effectiveness of a brief behavioral treatment for inner-city illicit drug users with elevated depressive symptoms: the life enhancement treatment for substance use (LETS Act!). *Clin Psychiatry* 2008;69(1):122–129.
92. Mann RE, Zalcman RF, Smart RG, et al. Alcohol consumption, alcoholics anonymous membership, and suicide mortality rates, Ontario, 1968–1991. *J Stud Alcohol* 2006;67(3):445–453.
93. Bodkin JA, Zornberg GL, Lukas SE, et al. Buprenorphine treatment of refractory depression. *J Clin Psychopharmacol* 1995;15(1):49–57.
94. Sullivan MA, Rothenberg JL, Vosburg SK, et al. Predictors of retention in naltrexone maintenance for opioid dependence: analysis of a stage I trial. *Am J Addict* 2006;15(2):150–159.
95. Clark DB, De Bellis MD, Lynch KG, et al. Physical and sexual abuse, depression and alcohol use disorders in adolescents: onsets and outcomes. *Drug Alcohol Depend* 200324;69(1):51–60.
96. Cornelius JR, Maisto SA, Martin CS, et al. Major depression associated with earlier alcohol relapse in treated teens with AUD. *Addict Behav* 2004;29(5):1035–1038.
97. March J, Silva S, Petrycki S, et al., Treatment for Adolescents With Depression Study (TADS) Team. Fluoxetine, cognitive-behavioral therapy, and their combination for adolescents with depression: Treatment for Adolescents With Depression Study (TADS) randomized controlled trial. *JAMA* 2004;292(7):807–820.
98. March JS, Silva S, Petrycki S, et al. The Treatment for Adolescents With Depression Study (TADS): long-term effectiveness and safety outcomes. *Arch Gen Psychiatry* 2007;64(10):1132–1143.
99. Riggs PD, Mikulich SK, Coffman LM, et al. Fluoxetine in drug-dependent delinquents with major depression: an open trial. *J Child Adolesc Psychopharmacol* 1997;7(2):87–95.
100. Cornelius JR, Clark DB, Bukstein OG, et al. Acute phase and five-year follow-up study of fluoxetine in adolescents with major depression and a comorbid substance use disorder: a review. *Addict Behav* 2005;30(9): 1824–1833.
101. Riggs PD, Mikulich-Gilbertson SK, Davies RD, et al. A randomized controlled trial of fluoxetine and cognitive behavioral therapy in adolescents with major depression, behavior problems, and substance use disorders. *Arch Pediatr Adolesc Med* 2007;161(11):1026–1034.
102. Weintraub E, Weintraub D, Dixon L, et al. Geriatric patients on a substance abuse consultation service. *Am J Geriatr Psychiatry* 2002;10(3):337–342.
103. Holroyd S, Duryee JJ. Substance use disorders in a geriatric psychiatry outpatient clinic: prevalence and epidemiologic characteristics. *J Nerv Ment Dis* 1997;185(10):627–632.
104. Lima JE, Reid MS, Smith JL, et al. Medical and mental health status among drug dependent patients participating in a smoking cessation treatment study. *J Drug Issues* (in press).
105. Oslin DW, Katz IR, Edell WS, et al. Effects of alcohol consumption on the treatment of depression among elderly patients. *Am J Geriatr Psychiatry* 2000;8(3):215–220.
106. Oslin DW. Treatment of late-life depression complicated by alcohol dependence. *Am J Geriatr Psychiatry* 2005;13(6):491–500. Ntx vs. placebo controlled trial, all received sertraline;substantial remission/non-relapse rate (42%), relapse correlated with poor response in depression. Late life (age >55)
107. Bartels SJ, Coakley EH, Zubritsky C, et al., PRISM-E Investigators. Improving access to geriatric mental health services: a randomized trial comparing treatment engagement with integrated versus enhanced referral care for depression, anxiety, and at-risk alcohol use. *Am J Psychiatry* 2004;161(8):1455–1462.
108. Roy A. Characteristics of cocaine-dependent patients who attempt suicide. *Am J Psychiatry* 2001;158(8):1215–1219.
109. Phillips J, Carpenter KM, Nunes EV. Suicide risk in depressed methadone-maintained patients: associations with clinical and demographic characteristics. *Am J Addict* 2004;13(4):327–332.
110. Kutcher S, Gardner DM. Use of selective serotonin reuptake inhibitors and youth suicide: making sense from a confusing story. *Curr Opin Psychiatry* 2008;21(1):65–69.
111. Bridge JA, Iyengar S, Salary CB, et al. Clinical response and risk for reported suicidal ideation and suicide attempts in pediatric antidepressant treatment: a meta-analysis of randomized controlled trials. *JAMA* 2007;297(15):1683–1696.
112. Watkins KE, Paddock SM, Zhang L, et al. Improving care for depression in patients with comorbid substance misuse. *Am J Psychiatry* 2006; 163(1):125–132.
113. Rosenheck RA, Resnick SG, Morrissey JP. Closing service system gaps for homeless clients with a dual diagnosis: integrated teams and interagency cooperation. *J Ment Health Policy Econ* 2003;6(2):77–87.
114. Glassman AH. Cigarette smoking: implications for psychiatric illness. *Am J Psychiatry* 1993;150(4):546–553.
115. Glassman AH, Covey LS, Stetner F, et al. Smoking cessation and the course of major depression: a follow-up study. *Lancet* 2001;357(9272):1929–1932.
116. Barnett PG, Wong W, Hall S. The cost-effectiveness of a smoking cessation program for out-patients in treatment for depression. *Addiction* 2008;103(5):834–840.
117. Hall SM, Reus VI, Muñoz RF, et al. Nortriptyline and cognitive-behavioral therapy in the treatment of cigarette smoking. *Arch Gen Psychiatry* 1998;55(8):683–690.
118. Brown RA, Niaura R, Lloyd-Richardson EE, et al. Bupropion and cognitive-behavioral treatment for depression in smoking cessation. *Nicotine Tob Res* 2007;9(7):721–730.

119. Saules KK, Schuh LM, Arfken CL, et al. Double-blind placebo-controlled trial of fluoxetine in smoking cessation treatment including nicotine patch and cognitive-behavioral group therapy. *Am J Addict* 2004;13(5):438–446.
120. Spring B, Doran N, Pagoto S, et al. Fluoxetine, smoking, and history of major depression: a randomized controlled trial. *J Consult Clin Psychol* 2007;75(1):85–94.
121. Blondal T, Gudmundsson LJ, Tomasson K, et al. The effects of fluoxetine combined with nicotine inhalers in smoking cessation—a randomized trial. *Addiction* 1999;94(7):1007–1015.
122. Reid MS, Fallon B, Sonne S, et al. Smoking cessation treatment in community-based substance abuse rehabilitation programs. *J Subst Abuse Treat* 2008;35(1):68–77.
123. Crismon ML, Trivedi M, Pigott TA, et al. The Texas Medication Algorithm Project: report of the Texas Consensus Conference Panel on Medication Treatment of Major Depressive Disorder. *J Clin Psychiatry* 1999; 60(3):142–156.
124. Trivedi MH, Rush AJ, Crismon ML, et al. Clinical results for patients with major depressive disorder in the Texas Medication Algorithm Project. *Arch Gen Psychiatry* 2004;61(7):669–680.
125. Norton PJ, Price EC. A meta-analytic review of adult cognitive-behavioral treatment outcome across the anxiety disorders. *J Nerv Ment Dis* 2007;195(6):521–531.
126. Levin FR. Diagnosing attention-deficit/hyperactivity disorder in patients with substance use disorders. *J Clin Psychiatry* 2007;68(Suppl 11):9–14.
127. Thase ME. STEP-BD and bipolar depression: what have we learned? *Curr Psychiatry Rep* 2007;9(6):497–503.
128. Suppes T, Dennehy EB, Hirschfeld RM, et al. Texas Consensus Conference Panel on Medication Treatment of Bipolar Disorder. The Texas implementation of medication algorithms: update to the algorithms for treatment of bipolar I disorder. *J Clin Psychiatry* 2005;66(7):870–886.
129. Weiss RD, Mirin SM, Griffin ML, et al. Psychopathology in cocaine abusers: changing trends. *J Nerv Ment Dis* 1988;176:719–725.
130. Nunes E, Quitkin F. Disulfiram and bipolar affective disorder. *J Clin Psychopharmacol* 1987;7(4):284.
131. Sachs GS, Nierenberg AA, Calabrese JR, et al. Effectiveness of adjunctive antidepressant treatment for bipolar depression. *N Engl J Med* 2007;356(17):1711–1722.
132. Calabrese JR, Bowden CL, Sachs GS, et al. A double-blind placebo-controlled study of lamotrigine monotherapy in outpatients with bipolar I depression. Lamictal 602 Study Group. *J Clin Psychiatry* 1999;60:79–88.
133. Marangell LB, Suppes T, Ketter TA, et al. Omega-3 fatty acids in bipolar disorder: clinical and research considerations. *Prostaglandins Leukot Essent Fatty Acids* 2006;75(4-5):315–321.
134. Vornick LA, Brown ES. Management of comorbid bipolar disorder and substance abuse. *J Clin Psychiatry* 2006(Suppl 7):24–30.
135. Geller B, Cooper TB, Sun K, et al. Double-blind and placebo-controlled study of lithium for adolescent bipolar disorders with secondary substance dependency. *J Am Acad Child Adolesc Psychiatry* 1998;37:171–178.
136. Brady KT, Sonne SC, Malcolm RJ, et al. Carbamazepine in the treatment of cocaine dependence: subtyping by affective disorder. *Exp Clin Psychopharmacol* 2002;10(3):276–285.
137. Rubio G, Lopez-Munoz F, Alamo C. Effects of lamotrigine in patients with bipolar disorder and alcohol dependence. *Bipolar Disord* 2006;8 (3):289–293.
138. Brady KT, Sonne SC, Anton R, et al. Valproate in the treatment of acute bipolar affective episodes complicated by substance abuse: a pilot study. *J Clin Psychiatry* 1995;56(3):118–121.
139. Salloum IM, Douaihy A, Cornelius JR, et al. Divalproex utility in bipolar disorder with co-occurring cocaine dependence: a pilot study. *Addict Behav* 2007;32(2):410–415.
140. Perugi G, Toni C, Frare F, et al. Effectiveness of adjunctive gabapentin in resistant bipolar disorder: is it due to anxious-alcohol abuse comorbidity? *J Clin Psychopharmacol* 2002;22(6):584–591.
141. Johnson BA, Rosenthal N, Capece JA, et al. Topiramate for Alcoholism Advisory Board, Topiramate for Alcoholism Study Group. Topiramate for treating alcohol dependence: a randomized controlled trial. *JAMA* 2007;298(14):1641–1651.
142. Kampman KM, Pettinati H, Lynch KG, et al. A pilot trial of topiramate for the treatment of cocaine dependence. *Drug Alcohol Depend* 2004;75(3):233–240.
143. Roy Chengappa KN, Schwarzman LK, Hulihan JF, et al. Clinical Affairs Product Support Study-168 Investigators. Adjunctive topiramate therapy in patients receiving a mood stabilizer for bipolar I disorder: a randomized, placebo-controlled trial. *J Clin Psychiatry* 2006;67(11):1698–1706.
144. Brown ES, Nejtek VA, Perantie DC, et al. Quetiapine in bipolar disorder and cocaine dependence. *Bipolar Disord* 2002;4(6):406–411.
145. Brown ES, Jeffress J, Liggin JD, et al. Switching outpatients with bipolar or schizoaffective disorders and substance abuse from their current antipsychotic to aripiprazole. *J Clin Psychiatry* 2005;66(6):756–760.
146. Brown ES, Garza M, Carmody TJ. A randomized, double-blind, placebo-controlled add-on trial of quetiapine in outpatients with bipolar disorder and alcohol use disorders. *J Clin Psychiatry* 2008;69(5):701–705.
147. Salloum IM, Cornelius JR, Daley DC, et al. Efficacy of valproate maintenance in patients with bipolar disorder and alcoholism: a double-blind placebo-controlled study. *Arch Gen Psychiatry* 2005;62:37–45.
148. Sonne SC, Brady KT. Naltrexone for individuals with comorbid bipolar disorder and alcohol dependence. *J Clin Psychopharmacol* 2000;20(1): 114–115.
149. Sullivan MA, Nunes EV. New-onset mania and psychosis following heroin detoxification and naltrexone maintenance. *Am J Addict* 2005; 14(5):486–487.
150. Craighead WE, Miklowitz DJ. Psychosocial interventions for bipolar disorder. *J Clini Psychiatry* 2000;61(Suppl 13):58–64.
151. Scott J, Gutierrez MJ. The current status of psychological treatments in bipolar disorders: a systematic review of relapse prevention. *Bipolar Disord* 2004;6:498–503.
152. Colom F, Vieta E. A perspective on the use of psychoeducation, cognitive-behavioral therapy and interpersonal therapy for bipolar patients. *Bipolar Disord* 2004;6:480–486.
153. Colom F, Vieta E, Martinez-Aran A, et al. A randomized trial on the efficacy of group psychoeducation in the prophylaxis of recurrences in bipolar patients whose disease is in remission. *Arch Gen Psychiatry* 2003;60:402–407.
154. Craighead WE, Miklowitz DJ, Frank E, et al. Psychosocial treatments for bipolar disorder. In Nathan PE, Gorman JM, eds. *A guide to treatments that work*, 2nd ed. New York: Oxford University Press, 2002:263–275.
155. Lam DH, Watkins ER, Hayward P, et al. A randomized controlled study of cognitive therapy for relapse prevention for bipolar affective disorder: outcome of the first year. *Arch Gen Psychiatry* 2003;60:145–152.
156. Frank E, Kupfer DJ, Ehlers LC, et al. Interpersonal and social rhythm therapy for bipolar disorder: Integrating interpersonal and behavioral approaches. *Behav Ther* 1994;17:143–149.
157. Frank E, Swartz HA, Kupfer DJ. Interpersonal and social rhythm therapy: managing the chaos of bipolar disorder. *Biol Psychiatry* 2000;48:593–604.
158. Frank E, Kupfer DJ, Thase ME, et al. Two-year outcomes for interpersonal and social rhythm therapy in individuals with bipolar I disorder. *Arch Gen Psychiatry* 2005;62:996–1004.
159. Miklowitz DJ, Simoneau TL, George EL, et al. Family-focused treatment of bipolar disorder: 1-year effects of a psychoeducational program in conjunction with pharmacotherapy. *Biol Psychiatry* 2000;48:582–592.
160. Miklowitz DJ. Family-focused treatment for bipolar disorder. In Hofmann SG, Tompson MC, eds. *Treating chronic and severe mental disorders: a handbook of empirically supported interventions.* New York: The Guilford Press, 2002:159–174.
161. Weiss RD. Treating patients with bipolar disorder and substance dependence: lessons learned. *J Subst Abuse Treat* 2004;27:307–312.
162. Weiss RD, Griffin ML, Kolodziej ME, et al. A randomized trial of integrated group therapy versus group drug counseling for patients with bipolar disorder and substance dependence. *Am J Psychiatry* 2007;164(1):100–107.
163. Schmitz J, Averill P, Sayre S, et al. Cognitive-behavioral treatment of bipolar disorder and substance abuse: a preliminary randomized study. *Addict Disord Treat* 2002;1:17–24.
164. Grella CE, Stein JA. Impact of program services on treatment outcomes of patients with comorbid mental and substance use disorders. *Psychiatr Serv* 2006;57(7):1007–1015.

165. Drake RE, Mueser KT, Brunette MF. Management of persons with co-occurring severe mental illness and substance use disorder: program implications. *World Psychiatry* 2007;6(3):131–136.
166. Drake R, Xie H, McHugo G, et al. Three-year outcome of long-term patients with co-occuring bipolar and substance use disorders. *Biol Psychiatry* 2004;56:749–756.
167. Brown ES, Beard L, Dobbs L, et al. Naltrexone in patients with bipolar disorder and alcohol dependence. *Depress Anxiety* 2006;23(8):492–495.
168. Brown ES, Perantie DC, Dhanani N, et al. Lamotrigine for bipolar disorder and comorbid cocaine dependence: a replication and extension study. *J Affect Disord* 2006;93(1–3):219–222.
169. Dean AJ, Saunders JB, Jones RT, et al. Does naltrexone treatment lead to depression? Findings from a randomized controlled trial in subjects with opioid dependence. *J Psychiatry Neurosci* 2006;31(1):38–45.
170. Hasin DS, Nunes EV. Comorbidity of alcohol, drug, and psychiatric disorders: epidemiology. In Kranzler HR, Rounsaville BJ, eds. *Dual diagnosis and treatment: substance abuse and psychiatric disorders*. New York: Marcel Decker, Inc., 1988.
171. Hernandez-Avila CA, Modesto-Lowe V, Feinn R, et al. Nefazodone treatment of comorbid alcohol dependence and major depression. *Alcohol Clin Exp Res* 2004;28(3):433–440.
172. Mariani JJ, Levin FR. Treatment strategies for co-occurring ADHD and substance use disorders. *Am J Addict* 2007;16(Suppl 1):45–54.
173. McGovern MP, Xie H, Acquilano S, et al. Addiction treatment services and co-occurring disorders: the ASAM-PPC-2R taxonomy of program dual diagnosis capability. *J Addict Dis* 2007;26(3):27–37.
174. Nunes EV, Quitkin FM, Brady R, et al. Imipramine treatment of methadone maintenance patients with affective disorder and illicit drug use. *Am J Psychiatry* 1991;148(5):667–669.
175. Nunes E, Hasin D, Blanco C. Substance abuse and psychiatric comorbidity: overview of diagnostic methods, diagnostic criteria, structured and semi-structured interviews, and diagnostic markers. In Kranzler HR, Tinsley JA, eds. *Dual diagnosis and treatment: substance abuse and comorbid disorders,* 2nd ed. New York: Marcel Dekker, 2004:61–101.
176. Nunes EV, Rothenberg JL, Sullivan MA, et al. Behavioral therapy to augment oral naltrexone for opioid dependence: a ceiling on effectiveness? *Am J Drug Alcohol Abuse* 2006b;32(4):503–517.
177. Phillips SD, Burns BJ, Edgar ER, et al. Moving assertive community treatment into standard practice. *Psychiatr Serv* 2001;52(6):771–779.
178. Ries RK, Demirsoy A, Russo JE, et al. Reliability and clinical utility of DSM-IV substance-induced psychiatric disorders in acute psychiatric inpatients. *Am J Addict* 2001;10(4):308–318.

CHAPTER 85

Angela E. Waldrop, PhD
Karen J. Hartwell, MD
Kathleen T. Brady, MD, PhD

Co-occurring Addiction and Anxiety Disorders

Numerous studies suggest that anxiety disorders, symptoms of anxiety, and substance use disorders (SUDs) commonly co-occur. The interaction between these disorders and symptoms is not unidirectional, but rather multifaceted and variable. Anxiety disorders may be a risk factor for the development of SUDs. Anxiety disorders modify the presentation and outcome of treatment for SUDs, just as substance use and SUDs modify the presentation and outcome of treatment for anxiety disorders. Anxiety symptoms also emerge during the course of chronic intoxication and withdrawal. Individuals who are defined as having co-occurring anxiety and SUDs should meet criteria for the anxiety disorder independent of periods of acute intoxication and withdrawal. Table 85.1 provides brief descriptions of the major anxiety disorders. In this chapter, the area of co-occurring SUDs and anxiety disorders will be reviewed. Prevalence, diagnostic, and treatment issues will be addressed.

PREVALENCE

General Population A number of epidemiologic studies conducted in the United States over the past 20 years have concluded that anxiety disorders and SUDs co-occur more commonly than would be expected by chance alone (1–3). The National Epidemiological Survey on Alcohol and Related Conditions (NESARC) is the most recent and largest survey study focused on psychiatric and SUDs to date, with a Wave 1 sample of more than 43,000 adults. The study was designed to distinguish between independent (i.e., not attributed to withdrawal or intoxication) and substance-induced mood and anxiety disorders (4). More than 17.7% of respondents with a SUD in the past 12 months also met criteria for an independent anxiety disorder. Approximately 15% of those with any anxiety disorder in the past 12 months had at least one co-occurring SUD (4). The relationship between anxiety disorders and drug use disorders (OR 2.8) was stronger than the relationship between anxiety and alcohol use disorders (OR 1.7). Hasin explored both 12-month and lifetime diagnoses using the NESARC data. For an alcohol use disorder, 12-month prevalence was 8.5% and lifetime prevalence was 30.3%. The odds ratio of alcohol use disorders co-occurring with any anxiety disorder was 1.9 for 12-month diagnoses and 10.4 for lifetime diagnoses (5). Associations between drug use disorders and specific anxiety disorders were virtually all significantly positive ($p < 0.05$). In general, the odds ratios were more positive for abuse compared with dependence and for women compared to men. Marijuana use disorders were the most common drug use disorder among individuals, with anxiety disorders (15.1%) followed by cocaine (5.4%), amphetamine (4.8%), hallucinogen (3.7%), and sedative (2.6%) use disorder (6).

Addiction and Psychiatric Treatment Populations

Because the relationship between anxiety and SUDs is fraught with symptom overlap and diagnostic difficulties, estimates of co-occurring disorders in treatment settings are variable and dependent on diagnostic techniques used and specific disorder being assessed. Specific prevalence estimates will be addressed in more detail in sections focused on individual anxiety disorders. One study of opioid users in a needle exchange program

TABLE 85.1 Brief Description of Major Anxiety Disorders

Panic disorder (PD)	Panic attacks are described as episodes of intense fear and anxiety in the absence of real danger associated with both physical and cognitive symptoms such as rapid heart beat, shortness of breath, shaking, chest pain, nausea, fear of dying or going crazy, derealization, or depersonalization. They can occur in the context of any anxiety disorder, mood disorders, substance-induced disorders, and from some general medical problems. PD is characterized by recurrent unexpected panic attacks followed by persistent worry and concern about additional attacks.
Agoraphobia (AG)	AG is described as anxiety about being in places or situations from which escape may be difficult or help is unavailable, leading to avoidant behavior or marked distress.
Social phobia	Social anxiety disorder (SAD) or social phobia is characterized by a persistent and intense fear of social or performance situations with the fear of embarrassment or humiliation. Anxiety symptoms can be similar to those of a panic attack and may result in a situationally bound panic attack. Feared situations are usually avoided or endured with great distress or anxiety.
Generalized anxiety disorder (GAD)	GAD is characterized by constant and undue worry and anxiety for 6 months or longer, causing significant impairment in functioning or distress.
Obsessive-compulsive disorder (OCD)	OCD is characterized by recurrent excessive obsessions and compulsions that are either time consuming or cause significant impairment or distress.

Descriptions of diagnoses are summarized from the *Diagnostic and statistical manual of mental disorders*, 4th ed. Washington, DC: American Psychiatric Association, 1994.

found that approximately 15% also had a lifetime anxiety disorder diagnosis (12% males and 21% females) (7). In a larger sample of substance use treatment clinics, 80% had at least one co-occurring anxiety disorder and comorbidity had a significant relationship to overall mental distress at initial interview and 6 years later (8).

Primary Care Population Anxiety disorders are common within primary care settings and associated with functional impairment, distress, and high utilization of medical care services (9). Generalized anxiety disorder (GAD) in primary care settings is at least twice the rate reported in general population prevalence estimates (10). Recognition of anxiety is poor with only 23% of anxiety patients recognized within primary care as compared to 56% of depression cases (10). SUDs are also common in primary care settings with estimates that 15% to 20% of men and 5% to 10% of women seen in primary care clinics have problem drinking or an alcohol use disorder (11). The prevalence of primary care practice patients with lifetime use of illicit drugs more than five times was 20%, which is higher than national average (12). Prescription drug misuse and abuse are also common problems in primary care settings. There are very few studies specifically focused on co-occurring disorders in primary care settings. In one large sample of primary care patients, among respondents with panic disorder with or without agoraphobia, 15% also had at least one SUD (13).

SCREENING AND DIFFERENTIAL DIAGNOSIS

One of the most difficult challenges in the area of co-occurring anxiety and SUDs is diagnosis. It is clear that substance use and withdrawal can mimic nearly every psychiatric disorder. Substances of abuse have profound effects on neurotransmitter systems involved in the pathophysiology of anxiety disorders and, with chronic use, may unmask a vulnerability or lead to organic changes that manifest as an anxiety disorder. The best way to differentiate substance-induced, transient symptoms of anxiety from anxiety disorders that warrant treatment is through observation of symptoms during a period of abstinence. Transient substance-related states will improve with time. The duration of abstinence necessary for accurate diagnosis remains controversial and is likely to be based on both the diagnosis being assessed and the substance used. For example, long half-life drugs (e.g., some benzodiazepines, methadone) may require several weeks of abstinence for withdrawal symptoms to subside, but shorter acting substances (e.g., alcohol, cocaine, short half-life benzodiazepines) require shorter periods of abstinence to make valid diagnoses. A family history of anxiety disorder, the onset of anxiety symptoms before the onset of SUD, and sustained anxiety symptoms during lengthy periods of abstinence all suggest an independent anxiety disorder.

Because of the high rate of co-occurrence of anxiety and substance use disorders, screening patients presenting at primary care, substance use, or psychiatric treatment settings is critical. This is especially important considering that early diagnosis and treatment can improve treatment outcomes. A number of screening tools are available and easily integrated into everyday practice. For example, the Mini International Neuropsychiatric Interview has a brief form that contains screening questions for panic disorder, agoraphobia, social phobia, specific phobia, obsessive-compulsive disorder, and posttraumatic disorder (14,15). The screener contains one "yes or no" question for each anxiety disorder and all are based on DSM-IV criteria (Table 85.2). Screening tools such as the

TABLE 85.2 Screening Questions for Anxiety Disorders from the M.I.N.I.

Panic disorder	Have you, on more than one occasion, had spells or attacks when you suddenly felt anxious, frightened, uncomfortable, or uneasy, even in situations where most people would not feel that way? Did the spells surge to a peak, within 10 minutes of starting? CODE YES ONLY IF THE SPELLS PEAK WITHIN 10 MINUTES.
Agoraphobia	Do you feel anxious or uneasy in places or situations where you might have a panic attack or panic-like symptoms, or where help might not be available or escape might be difficult: like being in a crowd, standing in a line (queue), when you are away from home or alone at home, or when crossing a bridge, traveling in a bus, train, or car?
Social phobia	In the past *month*, were you fearful or embarrassed being watched, being the focus of attention, or fearful of being humiliated? This includes things like speaking in public, eating in public or with others, writing while someone watches, or being in social situations.
Generalized anxiety disorder	Have you worried *excessively* or been anxious about several things over the past 6 months?
Obsessions	In the past *month*, have you been bothered by recurrent thoughts, impulses, or images that were unwanted, distasteful, inappropriate, intrusive, or distressing? (e.g., the idea that you were dirty, contaminated *or* had germs, or fear of contaminating others, *or* fear of harming someone even though you didn't want to, *or* fearing you would act on some impulse, *or* fear or superstitions that you would be responsible for things going wrong, *or* obsessions with sexual thoughts, images or impulses, *or* hoarding, collecting, *or* religious obsessions)
Compulsions	In the past *month*, did you do something repeatedly without being able to resist doing it, like washing or cleaning excessively, counting or checking things over and over, or repeating, collecting, or arranging things, or other superstitious rituals?

Adapted from Sheehan DV, Lecrubier Y, *M.I.N.I. Screen*. 5.0.0 ed., 2006.

Mini International Neuropsychiatric Interview can help to identify high-risk individuals, but because of symptom overlap and diagnostic difficulties, a detailed interview is likely to be necessary to fully differentiate substance-induced symptoms from primary mood/anxiety diagnoses.

GENERAL TREATMENT CONSIDERATIONS

In general, treatment efforts addressing psychiatric and substance use disorders have developed in parallel. The integration of services and effective treatments from both fields will be critical to the optimal treatment of individuals with co-occurring disorders. It is important to maximize the use of nonpharmacologic treatments. Learning strategies to self-regulate anxiety symptoms can interrupt the cycle of using external agents to combat intolerable subjective states and help individuals to acquire alternative coping strategies. Among psychosocial treatments, cognitive behavioral therapies are among the most effective for both anxiety disorders and SUDs. Promising pilot work investigating the integration of treatments to develop therapies specifically targeting co-occurring disorders will be discussed in the sections that follow, but much work is left to be done.

Research investigating pharmacotherapeutic treatments for both substance use and anxiety disorders is progressing rapidly. The pharmacotherapeutic treatment of specific anxiety disorders will be discussed in detail later, but some general principles apply. The use of psychotropic medications is sometimes discouraged in SUD treatment settings in a way that can undermine treatment (16–18). Individuals in recovery often have complex and conflicting feelings and attitudes and may see the need for medications as a sign of defectiveness or failure. It is important to address the individual's feelings about taking medications and to emphasize the need for medication adherence in a proactive manner.

In cases where the relationship of psychiatric symptoms and substance use is unclear, the risk/benefit ratio of using medications must be carefully considered. Should the decision to use medication be made, treatment should generally follow routine clinical practice for treatment of the anxiety disorder with some exceptions. It is important to pay attention to potential toxic interactions between the prescription medications and illicit drugs and alcohol in case of relapse. It is also important to use the agent with the least abuse potential.

Despite their effectiveness in immediate relief of panic and other anxiety symptoms, benzodiazepine use is generally avoided in substance-using populations because of their abuse potential. Benzodiazepines may be considered as adjunctive medication during the early treatment phase when activation or latency of onset of the antidepressants is an issue. If a benzodiazepine is prescribed to a patient with a co-occurring substance use disorder, close monitoring for relapse and limited amounts of medication should be given. As a rule, benzodiazepines should be avoided in patients with a current substance use disorder and used with caution in those with a history of substance use. They should be considered for chronic treatment only when other pharmacologic and nonpharmacologic treatment options have been exhausted. If necessary, a benzodiazepine with a low abuse potential such as oxazepam and chlordiazepoxide may be considered.

Finally, the use of agents targeting substance use specifically, such as naltrexone or disulfiram, as add-on treatment for individuals with comorbid SUDs and anxiety disorders is underexplored. In one study of 254 outpatients with alcohol dependence and a variety of comorbid psychiatric disorders, Petrakis et al. (19) investigated the efficacy of disulfiram and naltrexone, or their combination in a 12-week randomized trial. Participants treated with naltrexone or disulfiram, as compared with placebo, had significantly more consecutive weeks of abstinence and fewer drinking days per week. In comparison to naltrexone-treated participants, disulfiram-treated participants reported less craving from pre- to post-treatment. The effects of the medications by specific comorbid psychiatric disorder was not discussed, but active medication was associated with greater symptom improvement (e.g., less anxiety). No clear advantage of combining medications was observed. The use of adjunctive pharmacotherapeutic treatment is likely to become more relevant as pharmacotherapeutic treatment options for SUDs increase.

In the sections that follow, the prevalence rates, differential diagnosis and treatment of GAD, social anxiety disorder (SAD), obsessive compulsive disorder (OCD), and panic disorder will be reviewed. Posttraumatic stress disorder is covered in another chapter and simple phobia will not be covered because most evidence suggests that this disorder has no specific relationship with SUDs.

ALCOHOL AND ANXIETY

The highly comorbid relationship between alcohol and anxiety has received more attention than that of anxiety and other substances of abuse. This is probably because alcohol is legal, readily available, and many individuals with anxiety report using alcohol to relieve anxiety symptoms. However, the relationship between alcohol use and anxiety is complex and probably varies across anxiety disorders. The short-term relief of anxiety from alcohol use in combination with long-term anxiety induction from chronic drinking and withdrawal can initiate a feed-forward cycle of increasing anxiety symptoms and alcohol consumption (20).

GAD In the NESARC study, approximately 90% of individuals with GAD had at least one other co-occurring disorder, and GAD was strongly associated with alcohol use disorders (21). In adolescents, the presence of GAD is associated with a more rapid progression from age of first drink to alcohol dependence (22). GAD follows a chronic course with low rates of remission and frequent relapses/recurrences. Comorbid SUD decreases the likelihood of recovery from GAD and increases the risk of exacerbation (23,24).

Differential Diagnosis GAD symptoms have considerable overlap with acute intoxication from stimulants and withdrawal from alcohol, opiates, sedative, and hypnotic drugs. Because of this, distinguishing substance-induced anxiety symptoms from GAD can be challenging. The DSM-IV diagnostic criteria of GAD require a 6-month duration of symptoms not directly related to the physiologic effects of a substance; however, many substance abusers will have difficulty maintaining abstinence for 6 months, so earlier diagnosis could be important to successful recovery. Careful history taking can establish the timing of GAD relative to the SUD. Both SUDs and GAD can result in significant occupational, social, and health problems, so it can be challenging to discern if the impairments are related to the SUD, GAD, or both. As patients engage in recovery, ongoing assessment of anxiety symptoms will provide valuable information regarding diagnosis and need for continued treatment.

Treatment The most current guidelines for the pharmacotherapeutic treatment of GAD are from the Canadian Psychiatric Association (25). First-line medications include: paroxetine, escitalopram, sertraline, and venlafaxine XR. Second-line agents include: alprazolam, bromazepam (not available in the United States), lorazepam, diazepam, buspirone, imipramine, pregabalin, and bupropion XL. Third-line medications to be considered are mirtazapine, citalopram, trazodone, hydroxyzine, and adjunctive olanzapine or risperidone. Although effective for some individuals, controlled trials do not support the use of beta-blockers. Paroxetine, escitalopram, and venlafaxine have demonstrated long-term efficacy with increasing response rates over 6 months. Because approximately 20% to 40% of patients with GAD relapse within 6 to 12 months after the discontinuation of pharmacotherapy, long-term treatment may be needed (26).

There is little evidence-based research to direct treatment decisions for individuals with GAD and comorbid SUDs. Buspirone has been examined in the treatment of highly anxious alcoholics with mixed results. It has the advantage of minimal interactions with alcohol (27) and low abuse potential (28,29). Although selective serotonin reuptake inhibitors (SSRIs) have not been specifically studied in individuals with co-occurring GAD and SUDs, they are efficacious in the treatment of uncomplicated GAD and relatively safe to use in individuals with SUDs, so would be a reasonable choice in individuals with co-occurring disorders. Bupropion should be avoided or used with caution in individuals at risk for seizures, such as alcoholics with a history of withdrawal seizures (30). Benzodiazepines should be used with caution in this population and never as a first-line agent. Psychosocial treatments are clearly efficacious in the treatment of GAD. Cognitive behavioral therapy (CBT) has been most often used in combination with SUD treatment with goals of managing anxious states without medications (26).

SAD The lifetime prevalence of SAD ranges from 3% to 13% (31,32). In the recent NESARC, the 12-month and lifetime prevalence rates for SAD were 2.8% and 5.0%, respectively (32).

Approximately 20% of individuals with SAD also suffer from an alcohol use disorder (AUD) and the lifetime prevalence of an AUD with SAD (48%) is more than double that of individuals without lifetime SAD (29%) (33). The prevalence of SAD among individuals with AUD is at least 20% (34). Consistent with self-medication, SAD typically precedes AUD onset (35). In one study, SAD was diagnosed in 24.7% of 300 patients hospitalized for AUD and preceded AUD in 90.2% of cases (36).

Differential Diagnosis Symptoms of social anxiety typically precede the onset of SUDs (35). The key symptom, fear of performance or social situations, is specific to SAD and not generally associated with alcohol use or withdrawal making diagnosis easier than it is for other co-occurring anxiety disorders.

Treatment Current treatment recommendations for SAD includes SSRIs or beta-blockers in combination with integrated psychosocial treatment. There are a few studies examining treatment options in comorbid populations. Schade et al. randomized 96 alcohol-dependent patients with comorbid anxiety disorders, including SAD (n = 87) to CBT plus optional fluvoxamine (150 mg/day) versus treatment as usual. There was greater improvement in the combined treatment group in anxiety outcomes. Fluvoxamine was not associated with better outcomes (37).

Two small placebo-controlled studies of paroxetine in co-occurring AUD and SAD have demonstrated significant improvement in social anxiety with paroxetine treatment but no significant group differences in alcohol use in either study (38,39).

In a study of individual CBT for AUD versus concurrent AUD/SUD therapy, those who received concurrent treatment had worse alcohol outcomes (34). The authors hypothesized that exposure to anxiety-provoking social situations in concurrent treatment may have increased drinking to cope (34). Terra et al. followed 300 detoxified alcohol-dependent patients with and without SAD after standard treatment and found no difference in treatment adherence and outcomes; however, individuals with SAD chaired Alcoholics Anonymous meetings less often, were more ashamed of attendance, felt less integrated into the group, and were less likely to feel better after a meeting (40). Individuals with SAD may need treatment targeting their social anxiety before being able to benefit from group interventions. Individual therapy may be better tolerated than group therapy and a period of sobriety and skills training may be important before increasing exposure to social situations.

OCD The association of OCD and AUDs is less robust than for other anxiety disorders. In the National Comorbidity Survey Replication study, OCD was negatively correlated with AUD (41). The Collaborative Study on the Genetics of Alcoholism found no significant increase in rates of OCD in individuals with AUDs (42). Studies in treatment seeking samples also suggest a nonsignificant relationship.

Differential Diagnosis Craving in SUDs has been compared to the intrusive recurrent thoughts that drive behavior in OCD (43), but thoughts and compulsions in individuals with SUDs are restricted to alcohol and drug use and easily distinguished from OCD.

Treatment There are no controlled studies of pharmacologic treatment of co-occurring OCD and SUDs. First-line medications for OCD are clomipramine, fluoxetine, fluvoxamine, paroxetine, and sertraline. In individuals with SUDs, SSRIs are preferable to clomipramine because of more favorable side effect profiles (44). Fals-Stewart and Schafer randomly assigned 60 substance abusers with OCD in a drug-free therapeutic community to combined OCD and SUD treatment, SUD treatment alone, or SUD treatment plus progressive muscle relaxation. At 12 months, the group receiving combined treatment had higher abstinence, longer duration in treatment, and a greater reduction in OCD symptoms (45).

Panic Disorder In the NESARC study, lifetime prevalence of panic disorder (with or without agoraphobia) was 5.1% and was twice as common in women as compared with men (46). Drug dependence was the most strongly associated SUD, although the lifetime risk of alcohol dependence was also elevated (47). In a recent review of the literature, the risk of panic disorder in the presence of AUDs was two to four times higher than in the absence of AUD (48). In the Collaborative Study on the Genetics of Alcoholism, lifetime risk for panic disorder was increased in individuals with AUDs (4.2% vs. 1.0%, respectively) (42).

Differential Diagnosis Alcohol withdrawal can cause panic attacks, which will markedly improve during the first several weeks of abstinence if related to alcohol withdrawal only (42). Alternatively, individuals with panic attacks may use alcohol use to decrease panic symptoms and consequently develop an AUD (48). Panic attacks early in recovery that decrease in frequency may respond to support and reassurance. However, if the panic attacks continue or increase over several weeks of abstinence, the diagnosis of panic disorder should be made. Without treatment, the risk of relapse to alcohol use is increased (49). In one prospective study of alcoholics recruited from acute treatment, panic disorder was the most common diagnosis and was predictive of relapse. After 4 months, approximately 50% of those who had initially met criteria for an anxiety disorder no longer met diagnostic criteria (50). This finding emphasizes the need to carefully track anxiety symptoms early in recovery and to provide normalizing information to patients about common withdrawal symptoms and the typical course of recovery.

Treatment According to current guidelines, four classes of medications—SSRIs, tricyclic antidepressants, benzodiazepines, and monoamine oxidase inhibitors—have approximately comparable efficacy in the treatment of panic disorders (50). As previously discussed, benzodiazepines are generally avoided in individuals with SUDs. The SSRIs fluoxetine, sertraline, paroxetine, and fluvoxamine have each demonstrated effectiveness in clinical trials and are the best choice for individuals with co-occurring panic disorder and SUD (50).

There is an extensive body of literature supporting the efficacy of CBT in the treatment of panic disorder (50). In one controlled trial of standard alcohol treatment versus combined CBT for panic disorder plus AUD (51), improvement of panic symptoms and relapse rates did not differ between the two groups. The authors hypothesized that typical strategies for managing anxiety such as stress management, relaxation training, and relapse prevention present in standard alcohol treatment programs may have made it difficult to detect between-group differences (51).

NICOTINE AND ANXIETY DISORDERS

In the NESARC study, 28% of the participants used tobacco products and 25% were current cigarette smokers (52). The 12-month prevalence rate of nicotine dependence was 13% in the general population and 25% among individuals with anxiety disorders. The risk of anxiety disorder among individuals with nicotine dependence was more than twice that of any other psychiatric disorder. Conversely, the prevalence rates of nicotine dependence were also increased in individuals with anxiety disorders (panic disorder 40%, SAD 27%, and GAD 33%) (52). Despite the strong associations between smoking, nicotine dependence, and anxiety disorders, there has been relatively little investigation of causal connections or treatment. A recent review suggested that smoking, and nicotine in particular, can alleviate anxiety, but other studies indicate that nicotine use and withdrawal can cause anxiety (53). The Development and Assessment of Nicotine Dependence in Youth study followed a cohort of seventh graders for 3.5 years and found a strong association between trait anxiety and all measures of tobacco use and nicotine dependence. A relaxing effect from initial exposure to nicotine, distinct from relief of withdrawal symptoms, was predictive of a sixfold increase in risk for nicotine dependence (54). Smokers with a history of panic attacks have significantly more anxiety-related withdrawal symptoms and shorter quit attempts compared with those without panic attacks (55). Models currently being used to explain the relationship between nicotine dependence and anxiety disorders include conditioning theory, cognitive theory, anxiety sensitivity theory, and stress and coping models (53).

Differential Diagnosis The anxiety and arousal associated with nicotine withdrawal can be distinguished from independent anxiety disorders by the time course. Prospective research suggests that nicotine withdrawal symptoms typically return to baseline within 10 days (56) and anxiety decreases within 4 weeks of quitting among smokers without comorbid psychiatric disorders (57). Anxiety symptoms that persist beyond the withdrawal period warrant further investigation. It is important to note that when individuals enter treatment programs, particularly inpatient treatment, their cigarette smoking is generally significantly curtailed. Anxiety related to nicotine withdrawal should be taken into consideration in any assessment of anxiety in individuals hospitalized for the treatment of either SUDs or psychiatric disorders.

Panic Disorders The relationship between panic disorder and smoking is the best studied of all the anxiety disorders. In the NESARC study, individuals with panic disorder had elevated 12-month prevalence rates of nicotine dependence (52). Daily smoking is associated with an increased risk for the first occurrence of a panic attack or panic disorder and the risk is higher in active smokers than past smokers (58). Early smoking increases the risk for the development of panic disorder (53) and the initiation of smoking may precede the onset of panic disorder by many years (median 12 years) (59). In addition, individuals with panic disorder who smoke regularly report more severe anxiety symptoms and social impairment as compared to nonsmokers (60).

SAD Few studies have investigated the relationship between SAD and smoking. Although some studies have failed to demonstrate a relationship (61), one prospective-longitudinal study of adolescents and young adults found both social fears and SAD were significantly associated with higher rates of nicotine dependence (62). Approximately 50% reported the onset of social anxiety before smoking.

GAD Higher rates of smoking have been observed among individuals with GAD (52,63). In one prospective longitudinal study of adolescents and young adults, heavy smoking (≥20 cigarettes/day) was associated with an increased risk of GAD (21%, OR 5.5) during young adulthood (61). A confounding issue is the high rates of co-occurrence of GAD between other anxiety and depressive disorders.

OCD The prevalence of smoking is the lower in individuals with OCD compared with other anxiety disorders (53). In one prospective longitudinal study of youth, no association between smoking and OCD was found (61). Another study found nicotine-dependent individuals had an increased risk for developing OCD (64). Nicotine administration decreases some forms of compulsive behavior in both human and animal studies and obsessive thoughts can be reduced by transdermal nicotine in humans (53). In one study, nonsmokers with OCD were more symptomatic, worried more, were less self-confident, and less impulsive as compared with smokers with OCD (65). Further research is needed to examine the relationship of nicotine, obsessive compulsive symptoms, and OCD.

Treatment Current guidelines for treating tobacco dependence include a combination of counseling, behavior therapy, and pharmacotherapy. Pharmacotherapy is recommended in all individuals attempting to quit unless there is a contraindication. Medications that reliably increase long-term smoking abstinence include: bupropion SR, all forms of nicotine replacement therapy (nicotine gum, nicotine inhaler, nicotine nasal spray, nicotine lozenge, and nicotine patch) and varenicline (66). Given the high prevalence rates of anxiety disorders among smokers, treatments aimed at the specific needs of this population need to be developed; however, there is little empiric evidence to guide treatment at present. Bupropion treatment can be associated with anxiety and agitation in some individuals, so should be used with caution in anxious patients. Buspirone (up to 60 mg/day) had a beneficial effect on abstinence in highly anxious smokers in one randomized controlled trial in high- and low-anxiety smokers. However, buspirone decreased abstinence in the low-anxiety group and these effects reversed when the drug was withdrawn. No differential effects on abstinence were observed beyond the 3-month follow-up (67). There is little information about the use of nicotine replacement or varenicline for smoking cessation in individuals with anxiety disorders.

In a recent review, Morisette (53) suggested that interoceptive exposure therapy may be helpful in reducing distress and anxiety during withdrawal by teaching individuals to tolerate internal cues such as negative affect, craving, and withdrawal symptoms. Cognitive therapy may also be helpful by addressing maladaptive thoughts associated with both anxiety and tobacco use. Mindfulness and acceptance-based treatments also hold some promise, but much work remains to be done in investigating optimal treatment for nicotine dependence in individuals with anxiety disorders (53).

OPIATES AND ANXIETY DISORDERS

In NESARC, lifetime prevalence of opioid use disorders (OUD) was 1.42% with rates in men double that of women (6). Lifetime prevalence of an OUD was 3.2% in individuals with anxiety disorders. Among individuals with OUDs, lifetime prevalence of any anxiety disorder was 36.3% with a much higher rate in opioid dependence (61%) than opioid abuse (6). In a review of psychiatric comorbidity in OUDs, anxiety disorders were also commonly reported with lifetime rates varying from 8% to 60% (6). In NESARC, lifetime prevalence of SAD was 13% in individuals with OUDs, with a greater association with opioid dependence 21% compared with abuse 10% (6). Across studies, lifetime rates of SAD in individuals with OUDs have been reported between 3% and 39% (68). Approximately one fourth of heroin users in an inner city clinic had evidence of elevated social anxiety. The measures were higher in younger individuals with more ties to nonusing family, friends, and associates who are a source of negative feedback compared to older drug users who were more likely to affiliate with other drug users (69). The lifetime prevalence of panic disorder with agoraphobia, 5%, was lower compared with panic disorder without agoraphobia, 14%, in individuals with OUDs. Panic disorder without agoraphobia rates were higher in opioid dependence 24% than abuse 10% (6). The lifetime prevalence rate of GAD among individuals with OUDs was 11% in the NESARC study with 22% in opioid dependence compared with 7% in opiate abuse (6). In one outcome study, the presence of a comorbid SUD decreased the likelihood of recovery from GAD by nearly fivefold and increased the risk of recurrence threefold (23).

Differential Diagnosis Few studies have investigated diagnostic issues at the interface of OUDs and anxiety disorders. Anxiety is a key feature of opiate withdrawal (70). Stabilization in treatment can significantly reduce withdrawal-related symptoms in as little as 1 week.

Treatment No evidence-based literature exists to guide treatment of co-occurring anxiety and opioid use disorders, however, the general treatment principles discussed above apply. A comprehensive treatment plan is necessary to address the opioid use, anxiety, other comorbid SUDs, and chronic pain if present (68). Initial components should include medical detoxification and consideration of buprenorphine or methadone treatment. Physicians should choose anxiety medications with efficacy for the specific anxiety disorder being treated and with attention to special considerations described in this chapter. Symptoms of chronic pain such as poor sleep, anxiety, and loss of appetite may be misattributed to another psychiatric disorder. Adequate pain treatment may result in resolution of symptoms. Consultation with a pain specialist may be helpful.

MARIJUANA AND ANXIETY DISORDERS

Marijuana is the most frequently used illicit drug in the United States (71). In 2006, 39.8% of Americans age 12 and over had tried marijuana, compared with 29.6% who had tried any non-marijuana illicit drug (71). The relationship between marijuana and anxiety remains unclear. Some studies suggest that marijuana use increases the long-term risk of anxiety (72), others find that marijuana use results in acute anxiety symptoms during intoxication only (73), and anxiety symptoms can develop as part of marijuana withdrawal (72). In a 14-year longitudinal study, individuals who entered the study with a diagnosis of SAD had 6.5 greater odds of developing cannabis dependence after controlling for other relevant factors (74). In another 10-year community longitudinal study that began with adolescents, panic disorder was the anxiety disorder with the strongest association with marijuana use (OR 5.2) and use disorders (OR 5.9). Participants with any anxiety disorder at baseline were more likely to have a lifetime occurrence of cannabis use (OR 1.5) or a use disorder (OR 1.7) with anxiety generally preceding cannabis use. Zvolensky et al. (75) examined marijuana use, abuse, and dependence in a representative sample and found that marijuana dependence, but not use or abuse, was associated with a lifetime risk for panic attacks (OR 2.1).

A recent review attempted to determine order of onset and potential causal relationships between marijuana use and anxiety through the examination of seven longitudinal, population-based studies (76). After controlling for confounding factors, there was little evidence to suggest that marijuana use predicted long-term anxiety or anxiety disorders, but it was associated with transient anxiety reactions (76). Studies suggest that the use of marijuana as a coping strategy may serve to enhance anxiety through an avoidance-anxiety cycle and users who report coping motives for their use also use marijuana more often (77). Anxiety sensitivity is associated with marijuana coping motives (78), suggesting that anxiety may drive marijuana use for some users.

STIMULANTS AND ANXIETY DISORDERS

There is relatively little research on co-occurring anxiety disorders and cocaine, methamphetamine, and amphetamine use. These agents stimulate noradrenergic systems and acute intoxication is often associated with anxiety. Because of these anxiogenic effects, it has been postulated that individuals who are vulnerable to anxiety may be less likely to abuse or become dependent on this class of drugs (79). When anxiety symptoms are reported in individuals with stimulant use disorders, careful attention to the time course of anxiety symptoms relative to stimulant use is critical.

Prevalence In NESARC, the 12-month prevalence of cocaine use disorders was 0.27% and amphetamine use disorders was 0.16%. Thirty-nine percent of individuals with amphetamine use disorders and 31% of those with cocaine use disorders reported lifetime anxiety disorders. Of individuals with anxiety disorders, 4.8% reported lifetime amphetamine use disorder and 5.4% reported lifetime cocaine use disorder (6). Studies of treatment-seeking individuals indicate that anxiety disorders are relatively less common in cocaine-dependent treatment-seeking patients as compared with alcohol and other drug-dependent individuals (80). Myrick and Brady (81) found lifetime prevalence of SAD in a cocaine-dependent population to be 13.9%, with SAD preceding the onset of cocaine dependence in nearly all cases. In one of the few studies examining GAD and drug abuse specifically, Massion et al. (82) found that in a group of subjects with panic disorder or GAD, only 18% had GAD only and 11% had a history of non-alcohol drug abuse or dependence. Crum and Anthony (83) explored the association between cocaine use and OCD and found that the estimated relative risk of OCD among those with cocaine and marijuana and at least one other drug of abuse was 3.2.

In a large sample from the Methamphetamine Treatment Project, participants completed self-report measures of anxiety (84). Women reported higher levels of anxiety than did men. Frequency of methamphetamine use was positively associated with severity of general anxiety and phobic anxiety. In a review of two community surveys, lifetime non-cocaine stimulant use was associated with lifetime diagnoses of nearly every anxiety disorder (85). Onset for SAD preceded use of stimulants and other drugs and onset of GAD tended to occur after stimulant use onset (85). A study of incarcerated women found that the most common form of drug dependence was methamphetamine and about one fourth of the sample had GAD, panic disorder, or posttraumatic stress disorder (86). The results regarding anxiety are difficult to interpret because anxiety and depression were not examined as separate outcomes; however, women with combined anxiety and mood disorders had higher rates of methamphetamine dependence than did those with mood disorder only or those with neither disorder. In a sample of current amphetamine users, one third of respondents reported anxiety symptoms preceding initiation of amphetamine use, two thirds reported experiencing anxiety since initiation of amphetamine use, and at least half reported panic attacks (87).

Diagnosis The compulsive foraging for misplaced cocaine that has been noted in cocaine addicts (88) has commonalities with of OCD. Although this may implicate common neurobiologic processes, these symptoms generally occur only during acute intoxication and withdrawal and do not meet diagnostic criteria for OCD. Cocaine has been reported to precipitate panic attacks in patients without previous panic disorder (89,90). Stimulant withdrawal symptoms may also include low levels of anxiety in the first few days of abstinence (91), so a period of abstinence before diagnosing an anxiety disorder in stimulant abusers is recommended.

Treatment There is a paucity of research focused on the treatment of co-occurring stimulant use and anxiety disorders. In one small case series, patients with cocaine-induced panic disorder had substantial symptom improvement after treatment with carbamazepine or clonazepam (90). Because repeated cocaine administration is associated with neuronal sensitization leading to increased limbic excitability (92), it has been hypothesized that this is the mechanism of cocaine-induced panic. Anticonvulsant agents, such as valproate and carbamazepine, have demonstrated efficacy in the treatment of panic disorder. Panic disorder in patients with comorbid psychostimulant use may be linked to a sensitization mechanism and may respond particularly well to anticonvulsant medications. This hypothesis warrants further investigation.

There are a number of psychosocial treatments with demonstrated efficacy in the treatment of stimulant dependence including contingency management and cognitive-behavioral therapy (93). Clearly, individuals with co-occurring disorders should be engaged in evidence-based psychosocial treatment for their stimulant use. There are no controlled trials of psychosocial treatments designed specifically to address co-occurring stimulant use and anxiety disorders.

CONCLUSIONS

Because of the high co-occurrence of anxiety and substance use disorders and their prevalence in the population, primary care and mental health providers will encounter these conditions frequently in the course of their work. It is essential that providers address substance use patients' anxiety symptoms as a routine part of treatment. This requires careful differential diagnosis, which usually requires at least a brief period of sustained abstinence. It also requires providers to consider the mechanism of action of different medications and to choose those with the lowest risk for abuse. Psychosocial treatments for anxiety and substance use are excellent primary and adjunct treatments for these co-occurring disorders and referrals should be made as necessary.

REFERENCES

1. Regier DA, Farmer ME, Rae DS, et al. Comorbidity of mental disorders with alcohol and other drug abuse. Results from the Epidemiologic Catchment Area (ECA) Study. *JAMA* 1990;264:2511–2518.
2. Kessler RC, Crum RM, Warner LA, et al. Lifetime co-occurrence of DSM-III-R alcohol abuse and dependence with other psychiatric disorders in the National Comorbidity Survey. *Arch Gen Psychiatry* 1997;54:313–321.
3. Kessler RC, McGonagle KA, Zhao S, et al. Lifetime and 12-month prevalence of DSM-III—R psychiatric disorders in the United States: results from the National Comorbidity Study. *Arch Gen Psychiatry* 1994;518–519.
4. Grant BF, Stinson FS, Dawson DA, et al. Prevalence and co-occurrence of substance use disorders and independent mood and anxiety disorders: results from the National Epidemiologic Survey on Alcohol and Related Conditions. *Arch Gen Psychiatry* 2004;61:807–816.
5. Hasin, DS, Stinson, FS, Ogburn, E, et al. Prevalence, correlates, disability, and comorbidity of DSM-IV alcohol abuse and dependence in the United States: Results from the National Epidemiologic Survey on Alcohol and Related Conditions. *Archives of General Psychiatry*, 2007;64:830–842.
6. Conway KP, Compton W, Stinson FS, et al. Lifetime comorbidity of DSM-IV mood and anxiety disorders and specific drug use disorders: results from the National Epidemiologic Survey on Alcohol and Related Conditions. *J Clin Psychiatry* 2006;67:247–257.
7. Kidorf M, Disney ER, King VL, et al. Prevalence of psychiatric and substance use disorders in opioid abusers in a community syringe exchange program. *Drug Alcohol Depend* 2004;74:115–122.
8. Bakken K, Landheim AS, Vaglum, P. Axis I and II disorders as long-term predictors of mental distress: a six-year prospective follow-up of substance-dependent patients. *BMC Psychiatry* 2007;7:29.
9. Gurmankin Levy A, Maselko J, Bauer M, et al. Why do people with an anxiety disorder utilize more nonmental health care than those without? *Health Psychol* 2007;26:545–553.
10. Roy-Byrne PP, Wagner A. Primary care perspectives on generalized anxiety disorder. *J Clin Psychiatry* 2004;65(Suppl 13):20–26.
11. Sullivan E, Fleming MF. *A guide to substance abuse services for primary care clinicians.* Rockville, MD; SAMHSA Center for Substance Abuse Treatment, Public Health Services, United States Department of Health and Human Services, 1997.
12. Manwell LB, Fleming MF, Johnson K, et al. Tobacco, alcohol, and drug use in a primary care sample: 90-day prevalence and associated factors. *J Addict Dis* 1998;17:67–81.
13. Rodriguez BF, Weisberg RB, Pagano ME, et al. Frequency and patterns of psychiatric comorbidity in a sample of primary care patients with anxiety disorders. *Comp Psychiatry* 2004;45:129–137.
14. Sheehan DV, Lecrubier Y. *M.I.N.I. screen.* 5.0.0 ed., 2006.
15. Sheehan DV, Lecrubier Y, Sheehan KH, et al. The Mini-International Neuropsychiatric Interview (M.I.N.I.): the development and validation of a structured diagnostic psychiatric interview for DSM-IV and ICD-10. *J Clin Psychiatry* 1998;59:22–33.
16. Danion JM, Neunreuther C, Krieger-Finance F, et al. Compliance with long-term lithium treatment in major affective disorders. *Pharmacopsychiatry* 1987;20:230–231.
17. Aagaard J, Vestergaard P, Maarbjerg K. Adherence to lithium prophylaxis: II. Multivariate analysis of clinical, social, and psychosocial predictors of nonadherence. *Pharmacopsychiatry* 1988;21:166–170.
18. Keck PE, Jr., McElroy SL, Strakowski SM, et al. Factors associated with pharmacologic noncompliance in patients with mania. *J Clin Psychiatry* 1996;57:292–297.
19. Petrakis IL, Poling J, Levinson C, et al. Naltrexone and disulfiram in patients with alcohol dependence and comorbid psychiatric disorders. *Biol Psychiatry* 2005;57:1128–1137.
20. Kushner MG, Abrams K, Borchardt C. The relationship between anxiety disorders and alcohol use disorders: a review of major perspectives and findings. *Clin Psychol Rev* 2000;20:149–171.
21. Grant BF, Hasin DS, Stinson FS, et al. Prevalence, correlates, co-morbidity, and comparative disability of DSM-IV generalized anxiety disorder in the USA: results from the National Epidemiologic Survey on Alcohol and Related Conditions. *Psychol Med* 2005;35:1747–1759.
22. Sartor CE, Lynskey MT, Heath AC, et al. The role of childhood risk factors in initiation of alcohol use and progression to alcohol dependence. *Addiction* 2007;102:216–225.
23. Bruce SE, Yonkers KA, Otto MW, et al. Influence of psychiatric comorbidity on recovery and recurrence in generalized anxiety disorder, social phobia, and panic disorder: a 12-year prospective study. *Am J Psychiatry* 2005;162:1179–1187.
24. Compton WM, 3rd, Cottler LB, Jacobs JL, et al. The role of psychiatric disorders in predicting drug dependence treatment outcomes. *Am J Psychiatry* 2003;160:890–895.
25. Clinical practice guidelines: management of anxiety disorders. *Can J Psychiatry* 2006;51(8 Suppl 2):9S–91S.
26. McKeehan MB, Martin D. Assessment and treatment of anxiety disorders and co-morbid alcohol/other drug dependency. *Alcohol Treatment Q* 2002;20:45–59.
27. Mattila MJ, Aranko K, Seppala T. Acute effects of buspirone and alcohol on psychomotor skills. *J Clin Psychiatry* 1982;43:56–61.
28. Cole JO, Orzack MH, Beake B, et al. Assessment of the abuse liability of buspirone in recreational sedative users. *J Clin Psychiatry* 1982;43:69–75.
29. Griffith JD, Jasinski DR, Casten GP, et al. Investigation of the abuse liability of buspirone in alcohol-dependent patients. *Am J Med* 1986;80:30–35.
30. Dunner DL, Zisook S, Billow AA, et al. A prospective safety surveillance study for bupropion sustained-release in the treatment of depression. *J Clin Psychiatry* 1998;59:366–373.
31. American Psychiatric Association, *Diagnostic and statistical manual of mental disorders*, 4th ed. Washington, DC: American Psychiatric Association, 1994.
32. American Psychiatric Association. *Diagnostic and statistical manual of mental disorders.* 4th, text revision ed. Washington, DC: American Psychiatric Press, Inc., 2000.
33. Grant BF, Hasin DS, Blanco C, et al. The epidemiology of social anxiety disorder in the United States: results from the National Epidemiologic Survey on Alcohol and Related Conditions. *J Clin Psychiatry* 2005;66:1351–1361.
34. Randall CL, Thomas S, Thevos AK. Concurrent alcoholism and social anxiety disorder: a first step toward developing effective treatments. *Alcohol Clin Exp Res* 2001;25:210–220.
35. Carrigan MH, Randall CL. Self-medication in social phobia: a review of the alcohol literature. *Addict Behav* 2003;28:269–284.
36. Terra MB, Barros HM, Stein AT, et al. Social anxiety disorder in 300 patients hospitalized for alcoholism in Brazil: high prevalence and undertreatment. *Comp Psychiatry* 2006;47:463–467.
37. Schade A, Marquenie LA, van Balkom AJ, et al. The effectiveness of anxiety treatment on alcohol-dependent patients with a comorbid phobic disorder: a randomized controlled trial. *Alcohol Clin Exp Res* 2005;29:794–800.
38. Book SW, Thomas SE, Randall PK, et al. Paroxetine reduces social anxiety in individuals with a co-occurring alcohol use disorder. *J Anxiety Disord* 2008;22:310–318.
39. Randall CL, Johnson MR, Thevos AK, et al. Paroxetine for social anxiety and alcohol use in dual-diagnosed patients. *Depress Anxiety* 2001;14:255–262.
40. Terra MB, Barros HM, Stein AT, et al. Does co-occurring social phobia interfere with alcoholism treatment adherence and relapse? *J Subst Abuse Treatment* 2006;31:403–409.
41. Kessler RC, Chiu WT, Demler O, et al. Prevalence, severity, and comorbidity of 12-month DSM-IV disorders in the National Comorbidity Survey Replication. *Arch Gen Psychiatry* 2005;62:617–627.
42. Schuckit MA, Tipp JE, Bucholz KK, et al. The life-time rates of three major mood disorders and four major anxiety disorders in alcoholics and controls. *Addiction* 1997;92:1289–1304.
43. Modell JG, Glaser FB, Cyr L, et al. Obsessive and compulsive characteristics of craving for alcohol in alcohol abuse and dependence. *Alcohol Clin Exp Res* 1992;16:272–274.
44. Koran LM, Hanna GL, Hollander E, et al. Practice guideline for the treatment of patients with obsessive-compulsive disorder. *Am J Psychiatry* 2007;164:5–53.
45. Chatterjee CR, Ringold AL. A case report of reduction in alcohol craving and protection against alcohol withdrawal by gabapentin. *J Clin Psychiatry* 1999;60:617.

46. Grant BF, Hasin DS, Stinson FS, et al. The epidemiology of DSM-IV panic disorder and agoraphobia in the United States: results from the National Epidemiologic Survey on Alcohol and Related Conditions. *J Clin Psychiatry* 2006;67:363–374.
47. Ormel J, VonKorff M, Ustun TB, et al. Common mental disorders and disability across cultures. Results from the WHO Collaborative Study on Psychological Problems in General Health Care. *JAMA* 1994;272: 1741–1748.
48. Cosci F, Schruers KR, Abrams K, et al. Alcohol use disorders and panic disorder: a review of the evidence of a direct relationship. *J Clin Psychiatry* 2007;68:874–880.
49. Practice guideline for the treatment of patients with panic disorder. Work Group on Panic Disorder. American Psychiatric Association. *Am J Psychiatry* 1998;155:1–34.
50. Kushner MG, Abrams K, Thuras P, et al. Follow-up study of anxiety disorder and alcohol dependence in comorbid alcoholism treatment patients. *Alcohol Clin Exp Res* 2005;29:1432–1443.
51. Bowen RC, D'Arcy C, Keegan D, et al. A controlled trial of cognitive behavioral treatment of panic in alcoholic inpatients with comorbid panic disorder. *Addict Behav* 2000;25:593–597.
52. Grant BF, Hasin DS, Chou SP, et al. Nicotine dependence and psychiatric disorders in the United States: results from the national epidemiologic survey on alcohol and related conditions. *Arch Gen Psychiatry* 2004;61: 1107–1115.
53. Morissette SB, Tull MT, Gulliver SB, et al. Anxiety, anxiety disorders, tobacco use, and nicotine: a critical review of interrelationships. *Psychol Bull* 2007;133:245–272.
54. DiFranza JR, Savageau JA, Rigotti NA, et al. Trait anxiety and nicotine dependence in adolescents: a report from the DANDY study. *Addict Behav* 2004;29:911–919.
55. Zvolensky MJ, Lejuez CW, Kahler CW, et al. Nonclinical panic attack history and smoking cessation: an initial examination. *Addict Behav* 2004;29:825–830.
56. Shiffman S, Patten C, Gwaltney C, et al. Natural history of nicotine withdrawal. *Addiction* 2006;101:1822–1832.
57. West R, Hajek P. What happens to anxiety levels on giving up smoking? *Am J Psychiatry* 1997;154:1589–1592.
58. Breslau N, Klein DF. Smoking and panic attacks: an epidemiologic investigation. *Arch Gen Psychiatry* 1999;56:1141–1147.
59. Amering M, Bankier B, Berger P, et al. Panic disorder and cigarette smoking behavior. *Comp Psychiatry* 1999;40:35–38.
60. Zvolensky MJ, Schmidt NB, McCreary BT. The impact of smoking on panic disorder: an initial investigation of a pathoplastic relationship. *J Anxiety Disord* 2003;17:447–460.
61. Johnson JG, Cohen P, Pine DS, et al. Association between cigarette smoking and anxiety disorders during adolescence and early adulthood. *JAMA* 2000;284:2348–2351.
62. Sonntag H, Wittchen HU, Hofler M, et al. Are social fears and DSM-IV social anxiety disorder associated with smoking and nicotine dependence in adolescents and young adults? *Eur Psychiatry*, 2000;15:67–74.
63. Lasser K, Boyd JW, Woolhandler S, et al. Smoking and mental illness: a population-based prevalence study. *JAMA* 2000;284:2606–2610.
64. Breslau N, Kilbey MM, Andreski P. DSM-III-R nicotine dependence in young adults: prevalence, correlates and associated psychiatric disorders. *Addiction* 1994;89:743–754.
65. Bejerot S, von Knorring L, Ekselius L. Personality traits and smoking in patients with obsessive-compulsive disorder. *Eur Psychiatry* 2000;15: 395–401.
66. Fiore M, Bailey W, Cohen S, et al. *Treating tobacco use and dependence: quick reference guide for clinicians.* Rockville, MD: U.S. Department of Health and Human Services, Public Health Service, 2000.
67. Cinciripini PM, Lapitsky L, Seay S, et al. A placebo-controlled evaluation of the effects of buspirone on smoking cessation: differences between high- and low-anxiety smokers. *J Clin Psychopharmacol* 1995;15:182–191.
68. Strain EC. Assessment and treatment of comorbid psychiatric disorders in opioid-dependent patients. *Clin J Pain* 2002;18:S14–S27.
69. Grenyer BF, Williams G, Swift W, et al. The prevalence of social-evaluative anxiety in opioid users seeking treatment. *Int J Addict* 1992;27: 665–673.
70. Harris AC, Gewirtz JC. Elevated startle during withdrawal from acute morphine: a model of opiate withdrawal and anxiety. *Psychopharmacology (Berl)* 2004;171:140–147.
71. SAMHSA. *Results from the 2006 national survey on drug use and health: national findings.* Rockville, MD: Office of Applied Studies, NSDUH Series H-32, DHHS Publication No. SMA 07-4293, 2007.
72. Raphael B, Wooding S, Stevens G, et al. Comorbidity: cannabis and complexity. *J Psychiatr Pract* 2005;11:161–176.
73. Green B, Kavanagh D, Young R. Being stoned: a review of self-reported cannabis effects. *Drug Alcohol Rev* 2003;22:453–460.
74. Buckner JD, Schmidt NB, Lang AR, et al. Specificity of social anxiety disorder as a risk factor for alcohol and cannabis dependence. *J Psychiatr Res* 2008;42(3):230–239.
75. Zvolensky MJ, Bernstein A, Sachs-Ericsson N, et al. Lifetime associations between cannabis, use, abuse, and dependence and panic attacks in a representative sample. *J Psychiatr Res* 2006;40:477–486.
76. Moore TH, Zammit S, Lingford-Hughes A, et al. Cannabis use and risk of psychotic or affective mental health outcomes: a systematic review. *Lancet* 2007;370:319–328.
77. Bonn-Miller MO, Zvolensky MJ, Bernstein A, et al. Marijuana coping motives interact with marijuana use frequency to predict anxious arousal, panic related catastrophic thinking, and worry among current marijuana users. *Depress Anxiety* 2008;25(10):862–873.
78. Bonn-Miller MO, Zvolensky MJ, Bernstein A. Marijuana use motives: concurrent relations to frequency of past 30-day use and anxiety sensitivity among young adult marijuana smokers. *Addict Behav* 2007;32: 49–62.
79. de Wit H, Uhlenhuth EH, Johanson EC. Individual differences in the reinforcing and subjective effects of amphetamine and diazepam. *Drug Alcohol Depend* 1986;86:1625–1632.
80. Rounsaville BJ, Anton SF, Carroll K, et al. Psychiatric diagnoses of treatment-seeking cocaine abusers. *Arch Gen Psychiatry* 1991;48:43–51.
81. Myrick DH, Brady KT. Social phobia in cocaine-dependent individuals. *Am J Addict* 1996;6:99–104.
82. Massion AO, Warshaw MG, Keller MB. Quality of life and psychiatric morbidity in panic disorder and generalized anxiety disorder. *Am J Psychiatry* 1993;150:600–607.
83. Crum RM, Anthony JC. Cocaine use and other suspected risk factors for obsessive compulsive disorder: a prospective study with data from the Epidemiologic Catchment Area surveys. *Drug Alcohol Depend* 1993;31: 281–295.
84. Zweben JE, Cohen JB, Christian D, et al. Psychiatric symptoms in methamphetamine users. *Am J Addict* 2004;13:181–190.
85. Sareen J, Chartier M, Paulus MP, et al. Illicit drug use and anxiety disorders: findings from two community surveys. *Psychiatry Res* 2006;142: 11–17.
86. Vik PW. Methamphetamine use by incarcerated women: comorbid mood and anxiety problems. *Womens Health Iss* 2007;17:256–263.
87. Vincent N, Schoobridge J, Ask A, et al. Physical and mental health problems in amphetamine users from metropolitan Adelaide, Australia. *Drug Alcohol Rev* 1998;17:187–195.
88. Brady KT, Lydiard RB, Malcolm R, et al. Cocaine-induced psychosis. *J Clin Psychiatry* 1991;52:509–512.
89. Aronson TA, Craig TJ. Cocaine precipitation of panic disorder. *Am J Psychiatry* 1986;143:643–645.
90. Louie AK, Lannon RA, Ketter TA. Treatment of cocaine-induced panic disorder. *Am J Psychiatry* 1989;146:40–44.
91. McGregor C, Srisurapanont M, Jittiwutikarn J, et al. The nature, time course and severity of methamphetamine withdrawal. *Addiction* 2005; 100:1320–1329.
92. Post RM. Cocaine psychoses: a continuum model. *Am J Psychiatry* 1975;132:225–231.
93. Roll JM. Contingency management: an evidence-based component of methamphetamine use disorder treatments. *Addiction* 2007;102(Suppl 1): 114–120.

CHAPTER 86

Douglas Ziedonis, MD, MPH
Aurelia N. Bizamcer, MD
Marc L. Steinberg, PhD
Stephen A. Wyatt, DO
David A. Smelson, PsyD
Adrienne D. Vaiana, BS

Co-occurring Addiction and Psychotic Disorders

The presence of substance use and psychotic symptoms poses special diagnostic and treatment challenges for clinicians in all treatment settings, including mental health, addiction, emergency room, and primary care settings. This chapter focuses on the tasks of assessment, diagnosis, and acute and long-term treatment considerations. The acute management of substance induced psychosis is discussed in addition to the acute and long-term management of individuals with schizophrenia and substance abuse. There is a need for comprehensive assessment and integrated treatment that addresses the multiple diagnoses and problems associated with this co-occurring disorder subtype.

DEFINITION OF PSYCHOSIS

Psychosis is defined as a gross impairment in reality testing that is characterized by severe distortions of perception (as manifested by hallucinations) and severe distortions of thought (as manifested by delusions). It is a nonspecific condition that is associated with a variety of diagnoses and states, including schizophrenia, pervasive developmental disorders, dementias, medical disorders, medications, delirium and toxic states, mood disorders, and substance use disorders. According to the current edition of the *Diagnostic and statistical manual of mental disorders* (DSM-IV) (1), psychotic symptoms include delusions, hallucinations, disorganized speech or behavior, "negative symptoms," and catatonia (Table 86.1). Hallucinations (e.g., auditory, visual, tactile) and delusions (e.g., paranoid, persecutory, grandiose) are labeled *positive symptoms.* Negative symptoms greatly impact interpersonal communication and include flat affect, amotivation, poor attention, anhedonia, indifference, and social withdrawal.

PREVALENCE OF CO-OCCURRING ADDICTION AND PSYCHOSIS

General Population Although addiction is common amongst patients with psychotic disorders in psychiatric treatment settings, schizophrenia has a low prevalence rate of about 1% in the general population. Because of the low frequency of schizophrenia in the general population, large community-based epidemiologic surveys of substance abuse (such as the National Epidemiological Survey on Alcohol and Related Conditions, the National Survey on Drug Use and Health and the National Co-morbidity Survey-Replication) often exclude these disorders from their reports (2). Other epidemiologic analyses of co-occurring disorders didn't report these disorders because of diagnostic uncertainty (3). The Epidemiologic Catchment Area community-based study did report rates of co-occurring addiction and schizophrenia and found that 47% of persons with schizophrenia have a lifetime experience of substance use disorders, including 34% who have an alcohol use disorder and 28% who have a drug use disorder, including 16% abusing cocaine. Of note, about 70% and 90% of patients with schizophrenia are nicotine dependent and that nicotine is not routinely included in reported rates of substance use, making the actual numbers even higher (4,5).

Addiction Treatment Populations Transient substance-induced psychotic symptoms are not uncommon among intoxicated substance abusers; however, addiction

TABLE 86.1 Psychotic Symptoms

- *Catatonia* is a marked and bizarre motor abnormality that is characterized by immobility. It may involve certain types of excessive activity, mutism, resistance to being moved, assumption of unusual body positions, and echoing the sound last heard or action last seen.
- *Delusion* is a firmly held false belief based on in correct inference about reality.
- *Disorganized speech* often presents as looseness of association (get off track) or, in the extreme, can be completely incoherent.
- *Grossly disorganized behaviors* range from childlike silliness to unpredictable agitation. Disorganized behaviors include difficulty in performing activities of daily living, poor hygiene, appearing markedly disheveled, unusual dress, inappropriate sexual behavior, and unpredictable and untriggered agitation.
- *Hallucination* is a sensory perception that has the compelling sense of reality, but occurs without stimulation of the relevant sensory organ.
- *Negative symptoms* are characterized by severe deficits in functioning and include flat affect (clearly diminished range of emotional expressiveness), alogia (poverty of speech), avolition (reduced ability to initiate and complete goals), and anhedonia (loss of interest or pleasure).

treatment programs tend not to include individuals with schizophrenia in longer term rehabilitation treatment programs. In contrast, mental health treatment settings have recognized that their system must address co-occurring disorders for this population, and they have developed "dual diagnosis" or "co-occurring disorders" treatment programs at all levels of care.

Among patients in addiction treatment settings, a range of severity of psychotic symptoms can occur for vulnerable individuals with many substances—including alcohol, cocaine, amphetamine, club drugs, and marijuana. In the addiction treatment setting, the differential diagnosis most often is determined after a period of abstinence, which can vary from hours to months, depending on the drug involved or the duration of use. For example, evidence suggests that chronic amphetamine use can result in long-term neurobiologic changes, which may persist even after prolonged abstinence and present as a protracted psychosis that is phenomenologically similar to schizophrenia (6,7). By contrast, a study of cocaine-induced psychosis by Satel and Lieberman (8) suggested that a psychosis persisting for more than several days is likely to be the product of an underlying psychotic disorder. However, patients who inhale or inject amphetamines at high doses, or who smoke large amounts of marijuana dipped in phencyclidine (PCP) or formaldehyde, may experience psychotic symptoms that can persist for months.

Psychiatric Treatment Populations Mental health treatment settings report rates of current non-nicotine dependence substance use disorders in the population of individuals with schizophrenia in the range from 25% to 75%. However, these epidemiologic data represent a "best guess" as to the true rate of comorbidity, given the challenges of diagnosing substance abuse in the presence of schizophrenia and the problems of diagnosing schizophrenia in the context of a substance use disorder. A Canadian study has shown that of 203 patients with first episode of psychosis, more than half (52%) presented with a comorbid substance use disorder, most often alcohol or cannabis (9). A British survey of 123 patients with first episode of psychosis found that the frequency of substance use is twice that of general population and more common in men, with cannabis being the most frequently used drug (51%), followed by alcohol (43%). Cannabis is increasingly linked to an earlier onset of schizophrenia and increased severity of positive symptoms among schizophrenic patients (9–12). Some data suggest that the use of drugs or alcohol can lead to the earlier onset of schizophrenia in an already vulnerable individual (13). The addition of drugs of abuse often increases and exacerbates psychotic symptoms in psychiatric patients. In this population, ingestion of even relatively small amounts of drug over a short period can result in an exacerbation of psychiatric problems, loss of housing, use of emergency department services, or increased vulnerability to exploitation (sexual, physical, or other) within the social environment. Perhaps because of this sensitivity to psychoactive substances, individuals with schizophrenia appear to progress quickly from substance use to dependence, and some researchers suggest that even small amounts of use are problematic and should be viewed as abuse (14). Medication nonadherence and substance use were found to negatively impact on community survival in a study amongst Australian patients with psychosis (5). Substance use has also been linked to emergence of medication resistance in populations of patients with schizophrenia (15), with involvement with unsafe sexual practices (16) and with poorer prognosis of medical conditions, such as diabetes (17).

Primary Care or Other Health Care Settings Drug-induced exacerbation of psychotic disorders and transient substance-induced psychotic symptoms are not uncommon in the emergency room setting; however, these cases are far less common in general primary care practices. Of the limited research for this category, most has occurred in the emergency room setting (18).

An interesting phenomenon has been reported among inmate populations where some individuals feign psychotic symptoms in order to obtain quetiapine, a sedative atypical antipsychotic drug (19). Another drug reputed to be nonabusable—bupropion (an antidepressant with dual serotoninergic and dopaminergic effects)—has been reported to be abused in the pursuit of an amphetamine-like high (20).

DIFFERENTIAL DIAGNOSIS

A new patient presenting with both psychotic symptoms and active substance abuse can be a diagnostic dilemma and the differential diagnosis must be broad. In evaluating psychotic symptoms, clinicians must consider the possibility that these symptoms are caused by a general medical condition (Table 86.2) or substance intoxication or withdrawal (Table 86.3).

TABLE 86.2 Psychosis Secondary to Medical Conditions

- *Neurologic conditions*: neoplasms, stroke, epilepsy, auditory nerve injury, deafness, migraine, central nervous system infection
- *Endocrine conditions*: hyperthyroid or hypothyroid, parathyroid, or hypoadrenocorticism
- *Metabolic conditions*: hypoxia, hypercarbia, hypoglycemia
- *Fluid or electrolyte imbalances*
- *Hepatic or renal failure*
- *Autoimmune disorders* with central nervous system involvement (systemic lupus erythematosus)
- *Delirium*
- *Dementia*: Alzheimer disease, vascular, HIV-related, Parkinson disease, Huntington disease, head trauma, and the like
- *Neoplasm*: lung.

Psychotic symptoms can occur as the presenting symptom or may be part of a more complex syndrome of cognitive impairment (involving delirium or dementia). Although schizophrenia is the psychotic disorder that is most frequently diagnosed in psychiatric patients, other subtypes of psychotic disorders also must be considered in the differential diagnosis (Table 86.4). Psychotic symptoms can occur in the context of other categories of mental disorders, particularly affective disorders. For example, delusions or hallucinations may be a symptom of major depression or the mania phase of bipolar disorder.

The type and duration of psychotic symptoms are important in making a differential diagnosis. Psychotic symptoms that have a sudden onset and that last no more than 1 month are labeled *brief psychotic disorders*. If the symptoms have been present for less than 6 months, a diagnosis of schizophreniform disorder can be made. If the symptoms last longer than 6 months and include prominent delusions or hallucinations and result in a deteriorating course, with evidence of impaired social and occupational functioning, a diagnosis of schizophrenia or schizoaffective disorder should be considered. (In making a diagnosis of psychotic disorder, the clinician needs to rule out mood disorder, which can present with psychotic symptoms and has a different course, prognosis, and treatment.)

In clinical practice, patients are often seen with a mix of symptoms that may not fit neatly into a diagnostic category such as schizophrenia or manic depression. Schizoaffective disorder is diagnosed when symptoms of a psychotic disorder and a mood disorder (depression, mania, or mixed states) occur during separate time periods. In contrast to major depression with psychotic features, schizoaffective disorder features a period of psychotic symptoms in the absence of mood disorder symptoms. A delusional disorder is diagnosed only when delusional symptoms are present; often, symptoms are well circumscribed and can interfere with functioning to a lesser degree.

Two common scenarios can be problematic for clinicians in establishing a diagnosis of schizophrenia or a substance use disorder. In the first scenario, the clinician is evaluating a new patient who presents with both psychotic symptoms or substance abuse. (In many cases, a definitive diagnosis of a psychotic disorder cannot be established, and treatment of the coexisting psychosis and substance abuse must occur simultaneously.) In the second scenario, the clinician is reevaluating a known psychiatric patient with schizophrenia, who presents with symptoms of an undiagnosed substance use disorder. In some cases, it is very difficult to establish the exact chronology of the onset

TABLE 86.3 Substances That Cause Psychotic Symptoms

During Intoxication

- Sedatives (alcohol, benzodiazepines, barbiturates)
- Stimulants (amphetamine, cocaine)
- Designer drugs ("Ecstasy" and the like)
- Marijuana/THC
- Hallucinogens (LSD, ketamine, psilocybin, and the like)
- Opioids
- Phencyclidines

During Withdrawal

- Sedatives (alcohol, benzodiazepines, barbiturates)
- Anesthetics and analgesics
- Anticholinergic agents
- Anticonvulsants
- Antihistamines
- Antihypertensives
- Antimicrobial medications
- Antiparkinson medications
- Cardiovascular medications
- Chemotherapeutic agents
- Corticosteroids
- Gastrointestinal medications
- Muscle relaxants
- Nonsteroidal anti-inflammatory drugs
- Various over-the-counter medications
- Toxins (anticholinesterase, organophosphate insecticides, nerve gases, carbon monoxide, and volatile substances such as fuel or paint)

TABLE 86.4 DSM-IV Classification of Psychotic Disorders

- Brief psychotic disorder
- Schizophrenia
- Schizophreniform disorder
- Schizoaffective disorder
- Delusional disorder
- Psychotic disorder, Not Otherwise Specified.

From American Psychiatric Association (APA) *Diagnostic and statistical manual of mental disorders*, 4th ed. (DSM-IV). Washington, DC: American Psychiatric Press, 1994.

of the psychotic symptoms and that of substance use. The patient may contribute to a misdiagnosis by downplaying or denying his or her substance-related problems or by pointing to other causes of such problems. One study of patients with schizophrenia who presented at hospital emergency departments found that 33% were recent cocaine users, but half of those persons reported no recent use (21). Thus urine toxicology and alcohol Breathalyzer tests are strongly advised as adjuncts to patients' self-reports. Finally, the clinician should be careful not to dwell exclusively on the amount of substance used, because psychiatric patients suffer more acutely from smaller amounts of a substance than do nonpsychiatric patients.

For many reasons, differentiating schizophrenia from a substance-induced psychotic disorder is not an easy task, especially if the physician does not know whether the patient has a history of serious mental illness. Medication side effects can be mistaken for negative symptoms, and negative symptoms can be mistaken for depression. Substance abusers also may be poorly compliant in taking their medications, so that a presenting psychotic relapse may be the result of noncompliance. In one longitudinal diagnostic study of 165 patients with chronic psychosis and cocaine abuse or dependence, a definitive diagnosis could not be established in 93% of the cases (21). To establish a definitive diagnosis of schizophrenia, the researchers required that a patient meet diagnostic criteria for schizophrenia at some point after 6 weeks of abstinence from psychoactive substances. Patients were interviewed at multiple points over time (using the Structured Clinical Interview and *DSM-IIIR* criteria) (22). Using these strict guidelines, the primary reasons a diagnosis could not be reached were insufficient abstinence (78%), poor memory (24%), or inconsistent reporting (20%) on the part of the patient. A review of hospital records and collateral information addressed the problems of poor memory and inconsistent reporting, leaving insufficient abstinence as the primary barrier to establishing a diagnosis. The researchers' finding that most patients continued to use substances reflects the difficulty of treating persons in this population and underscores the need to make clinical decisions within the context of diagnostic uncertainty.

MANAGEMENT OF CO-OCCURRING PSYCHOSIS AND SUBSTANCE ABUSE

Acute/Subacute The acute management phase includes ongoing assessment and treatment. At the time of the patient's initial presentation for treatment, the clinician should have four primary goals: patient safety, staff safety, elicitation of the patient's history, and formulation of initial impressions that will lead to a set of treatment recommendations. Often, the most appropriate setting for the evaluation of an acutely psychotic patient is a hospital emergency department, although some psychiatric triage settings also are appropriate. Staff members in those settings are trained to treat such patients in an effective and safe manner. An addiction medicine specialist may be asked to participate in the patient evaluation. Patient safety should be addressed by providing a setting in which external stimuli are minimized to ensure the physical safety of the patient and staff members, and to provide a modicum of dignity while the workup is under way. Initial assessment of vital signs should be obtained. Variations in pulse rate, blood pressure, and respiratory function are not uncommon in the presentation of many toxic states.

The patient's mental status should be assessed. Consideration should be given to the need for protection of the airway and possible establishment of intravenous access. Physical restraints are used less frequently in mental health settings, and there is an increased use of a quiet room to reduce a patient's level of anxiety and agitated psychotic symptoms. "Chemical restraints," examples of which include, but are not limited to, benzodiazepines and antipsychotic medications, may be warranted, but should be given only after the primary assessment has taken place, because sedation may be a side effect.

Included in the primary assessment is the gathering of history from anyone with information about the patient before his or her arrival at the hospital. Family, friends, or landlords may be very helpful in reporting the patient's psychiatric, medical, and social history. Emergency personnel or police should be questioned for details of the scene at which they first encountered the patient and their observations of the patient during transport. This information can provide significant insights into the possible involvement of psychoactive substances (as indicated, for example, by a pattern of delirium or a waxing and waning of signs and symptoms).

Initial laboratory information should include a complete blood count, electrolytes, liver enzymes, glucose, blood urea nitrogen, calcium, blood alcohol, and urine analysis with toxicology screen. If the patient lapses into coma, the administration of parenteral thiamine, glucose, magnesium, and naloxone (Narcan) may be appropriate, even before the laboratory results are available. Computed tomography (CT) scanning of the acutely psychotic patient's head always should be considered. Head injury, the severity of which is best confirmed by CT, often results in a confused, bizarre thought pattern that could present as psychosis and that may be associated with substance abuse. However, CT scanning is of little help in differentiating between schizophrenia and drug-induced psychosis (23). If the blood and urine evaluation is not diagnostic and the CT scan is negative, lumbar puncture may be warranted.

The chief challenge in treating this population is to provide integrated treatment while addressing the acute intoxication/detoxification symptoms and the psychotic symptoms. Often the co-occurring disorder treatment also requires a systematic approach to issues that may be of lesser concern in other settings, such as housing, entitlements, rehabilitation, and use of community services. Clinicians who are optimistic, empathic, and hopeful are most helpful to patients in the treatment and recovery processes. Integrated treatment addresses both problems simultaneously, incorporates active outreach and case management efforts, attempts to increase client motivation for abstinence or harm reduction in a realistic manner, integrates mental health and substance abuse approaches, provides broad-based and comprehensive services, and remains flexible in responding to individual needs.

Pharmacological Treatments Clinicians should be aware of the relevant pharmacotherapy for both psychiatric and substance use disorders, including detoxification and maintenance. Medications that best treat schizophrenia include traditional and atypical antipsychotics and, in some cases, long-acting injectable depot antipsychotics. Pharmacotherapy of the acute psychosis induced by substances should be treated symptomatically and managed with short-acting antipsychotic medication, and side effects from these medications should be closely monitored, especially acute dystonias and oversedation. The following discussion focuses on the unique relationship of certain psychoactive substances to the development and acute management of psychotic symptoms.

Management of Drug-Specific Psychotic Symptoms

Alcohol and Psychosis The most obvious psychotic symptoms associated with alcohol use generally occur in the withdrawal stage (24,25). These symptoms are based in the still-undefined interplay of chronic alcohol dependence with the gamma-aminobutyric acid type A, N-methyl-D-aspartic acid (NMDA), and dopamine receptors (26). Symptoms typically are referred to as *alcoholic hallucinosis*; that is, auditory and visual hallucinations that occur in a clear sensorium, often while the patient is alert and well oriented. The auditory hallucinations most often are of the threatening or command type. In this condition, individuals can be in an extremely agitated and paranoid state as a result of the hallucinations and physical discomfort they are experiencing. The onset of this hallucinogenic state has been reported to occur from 12 hours to 7 days after the onset of abstinence from long-term alcohol use. (However, there have been reports of symptom onset having been delayed by as much as 3 weeks.) The most typical time for emergence of symptoms is within 2 days of abstinence (27–29).

Psychotic symptoms, particularly paranoia, may persist for hours to weeks. Some evidence suggests that individuals with symptoms that are prolonged for weeks or months may have a predisposition to a psychotic illness (27). There can be tremendous similarity between this psychotic appearance and schizophrenia.

Paranoia and agitation often are treated with benzodiazepines in the same way one would treat uncomplicated withdrawal. However, in the severely agitated patient with concurrent hallucinations, neuroleptics may be warranted. Withdrawal has been associated with the development of extrapyramidal symptoms, including dystonia, akathisia, choreoathetosis, and parkinsonism (30–32). Particular attention should be paid to the possible development of extrapyramidal symptoms in the patient treated with a neuroleptic drug during acute alcohol withdrawal or in the patient with a primary psychotic illness.

Cannabis and Psychosis In the Epidemiologic Catchment Area study, reported in 1990, the rate of cannabis dependence or abuse in the general population was estimated at a lifetime prevalence of 4.3%, and the comorbid use of cannabis in individuals with schizophrenia was estimated at 6.0% (33). The most frequently reported effects of marijuana at levels of moderate intoxication are euphoria (34–36), an awareness of alteration in thought processes (36), suspiciousness and paranoid ideation (37,38), alteration in the perception of time (39), a sensation of heightened visual perception (40) and, at higher doses, some auditory and visual hallucinations (37,41–43). These effects have been reproduced in the laboratory and appear to be partially dose-dependent. Some evidence suggests that certain users seek the more psychotomimetic effects achieved through chronic high-dose use of marijuana (44). At doses >0.2 mg/kg, the potential for development of psychotic-like symptoms increases dramatically (42). At this level of use, symptoms include suspiciousness, memory impairment, confusion, depersonalization, apprehension, hallucinations, and derealization (35,36,45,46). The symptoms are reported to be transient, although they can recur on repeated administration of the drug (35,47,48).

There is some evidence that chronic use of cannabis is related to the onset of a primary psychotic disorder (35). First-time use, large amounts, and route of ingestion (oral more so than smoked) may be factors in the higher incidence of cannabis-related psychosis (49,50). A study that compared psychotic features in a group of men with psychotic symptoms and high urinary levels of cannabis with such features in psychotic individuals without positive cannabis urine samples showed more hypomania, more agitation, less coherent speech, less flattening of affect, and fewer auditory hallucinations in the cannabis group (49,50). Cannabis use often is associated with a more affective type of psychosis (48).

Typically, the psychosis associated with cannabis is acute and of short duration. However, there are case reports of chronic psychosis attributed to cannabis (51). This is a difficult question to answer for a variety of reasons: Is the patient remaining abstinent? What other drugs might the patient have used? Is there predisposing psychopathology? Frequently, the evaluating clinician must decide whether chronic schizophrenia is secondary to the past use of cannabis. Often this is an issue for both the patient and his or her family. One retrospective study presented evidence showing better premorbid personalities and reduced age of onset in cannabis-using individuals than in the nonusing schizophrenic population (52). Such differences, however, may be secondary to cannabis use, opening the "environmental window" in an already predisposed patient.

Cocaine and Psychosis Transient paranoia is a common feature of chronic cocaine intoxication (8,53), appearing in 33% to 50% of patients. Psychotic symptoms associated with cocaine use are almost exclusively seen in the intoxication phase and rarely extend beyond the "crash" phase in the patient who does not have a primary psychotic illness. There is epidemiologic evidence that men have a greater propensity toward psychosis than women and that Caucasians are affected more frequently than non-whites (54). There are multiple indicators that high-dose use of cocaine over time is strongly associated with the onset of psychotic symptoms (54,55). There also is strong evidence that sensitization occurs with chronic administration of cocaine and amphetamines (56). This sensitization is associated with the type of psychotic symptoms that can occur with repeated use of the stimulants. The psychotic features appear to occur with repeated exposure at lower doses. Onset of psychotic symptoms has been associated with reduction in individual doses and the desire for treatment (54).

The most frequently reported psychotic symptoms related to cocaine use are paranoid delusions and hallucinations. Auditory hallucinations are the most common and often are associated with paranoid delusions. Visual hallucinations are the next most common, followed by tactile hallucinations (54). Visual hallucinations have been associated with chronic mydriatic pupils and the appearance of geometric shapes. Nearly all of the hallucinations are associated with drug use. Evidence suggests that the character of the psychotic symptoms experienced is associated with the setting in which drugs are ingested (57).

Stereotypic behavior also can be associated with psychosis. Such behavior occasionally continues after the intoxication subsides. A study of the phenomenology of hallucinations points to an orderly progression in the development of hallucinations, from early visual hallucinations to tactile forms (58). The study comports with the observation that there is an orderly progression of the effects of cocaine intoxication, from euphoria to dysphoria and finally to psychosis, and that this progression is related to dose, chronicity, and genetic and experiential predisposition (59).

It is very difficult to assess the premorbid evidence of psychotic thinking in individuals who go on to use large repeat doses of cocaine and to forecast the likelihood that they will develop psychotic symptoms. Satel and Edell (60) measured the level of nondrug-psychotic proneness in individuals who had a history of cocaine-induced psychosis, as compared with individuals without such a history. They found strong evidence that there is a greater incidence of low-level psychotic thinking in the abstinent patient who is prone to cocaine-induced psychosis. Whether this is evidence of proneness to the development of psychosis in some individuals as a function of their use of cocaine or an indication of the development of persistent neurobiologic changes concurrent with the onset of cocaine-induced psychosis remains unclear. McLellan et al. (61) examined this question by performing a 6-year follow-up study on drug-dependent individuals who had no initial psychotic symptoms. They found a strong association with psychosis in the amphetamine-dependent population. The nature of the association was unclear, but the investigators speculated that there may be some self-selection of stimulant drugs in this population, or some low-level psychotic thinking that was not identified in the original evaluation.

Amphetamines and Psychosis The first report of psychosis associated with amphetamines was made by Young and Scoville, who in 1938 reported psychotic behavior in a patient who was under treatment for narcolepsy. Since that time, there have been many observations and studies of this association. Rockwell and Ostwald reviewed psychiatric hospital records in 1968 and found that the most common diagnosis of patients admitted with covert amphetamine use was schizophrenia.

Amphetamine psychosis has been described as a three-stage illness. Initially, it is marked by increased curiosity and repetitive examining, searching, and sorting behaviors. In the second stage, these behaviors are followed by increased paranoia. In the final stage, the paranoia leads to ideas of reference, persecutory delusions, and hallucinations, which are marked by a fearful, panic-stricken, agitated, overactive state (56). That the appearance of psychotic-like symptoms in amphetamine users became more prevalent in the late 1960s and 1970s fits what we now know about the pattern of amphetamine use associated with these symptoms. Amphetamine-induced psychosis develops over time in association with large amounts of the drug, delivered by any route of administration. The strongest correlation has been seen in those individuals who use large amounts by intravenous injection.

A common presentation of the psychotic, amphetamine-intoxicated patient involves paranoia, delusional thinking, and (frequently) hypersexuality. The hallucinatory symptoms may include visual, auditory, olfactory, or tactile sensations. However, the patient's orientation and memory usually remain intact. Typically, this altered mental state lasts only during the period of intoxication, although there are reports of it persisting for days to weeks. Treatment should be initiated by providing a safe, secure place for the patient and should reduce external environmental stimuli. Physical restraints should be avoided or used in a time-limited fashion so as not to complicate the presentation with worsening hyperthermia, dehydration rhabdomyolysis, and possible renal failure. One should keep in mind the potential of amphetamines for lowering seizure threshold, inducing hyperpyrexia, and stimulating cardiovascular compromise, particularly in the patient who is using large amounts in a chronic pattern. In such patients, chlorpromazine (Thorazine) should be avoided because of its potential to lower seizure threshold and worsen hyperthermia. Benzodiazepines can be helpful in the treatment of these symptoms. A common initial dose is diazepam (Valium) 10 mg, either intramuscularly or intravenously, then titrated to a level that sufficiently sedates the patient. Patients should be closely monitored for respiratory depression. When using benzodiazepines intramuscularly, the clinician should wait at least 1 hour between doses to avoid inadvertent overdose. It is quite common to see dramatic tolerance to benzodiazepine medications in long-term drug users, so a very high dose may be needed to achieve sedation.

The question of how long the psychosis will last and how likely the patient is to develop a long-term psychotic illness as a result of amphetamine use is not clear. Clinical experience suggests that amphetamine psychosis can last for 3 to 6 months in extreme cases of high-dose use. There is little evidence to suggest that these drugs cause schizophrenia. However, there is a potential for long-term affective instability, a moderate-to-severe anxiety state, and underlying suspiciousness.

Hallucinogens and Psychosis Hallucinogens have a well-documented role, both ceremonial and recreational, in many societies. However, not until the synthesis of lysergic acid diethylamine (LSD) by Hofman in 1943 was a hallucinogen available in large quantities and adopted widely as a recreational drug. A national survey in the United States in 1990 yielded an estimate that 7.6% of the population older than 12 years had ever used a hallucinogen. This number rose to 8.6% in 1993. The percentage of patients admitted to psychiatric hospitals with a diagnosis of "schizophrenia and paranoid disorders" at first admission was 10.9% in 1970, but rose to 24% by 1979 and has remained around 20% since that time. The increase is specific to the population ages 15 to 34 years and correlates with the increased use of hallucinogens in this age group. This finding provides evidence pointing to hallucinogens as a factor in the development of schizophreniform psychosis.

The primary model for hallucinogens is LSD, an indole-type drug with structural similarities to serotonin. Included in this class of drugs are dimethyltryptamine, psilocybin, and psilocin, among others. LSD crosses the blood–brain barrier readily and has a potent affinity for the 5-HT2A receptor. Its half-life is approximately 100 minutes, and the effects wear off in approximately 6 to 12 hours. Initially, there are autonomic changes, which are associated with the early affective instability seen after administration, as manifested in laughter or fearfulness. The associated alterations in perception occur subsequently and feature hallucinations of all kinds. The most common hallucinations are visual; the least common, auditory. The occurrence of synesthesia—the blending of the senses—is uncommon but not unknown. There often is a loss of the concept of time. Paranoia and aggression can be profound, but the more frequent experience is that of euphoria and security. The setting can have an effect on the experience, and much has been written on proper preparation for the "trip."

LSD has a large therapeutic index. Thus the typical emergency visit secondary to use of the drug occurs as a result of anxiety, a concurrent accident, or suicidal behavior. "Talking down" the patient is the most common way to ease his or her anxiety around the psychotic features of LSD and related drugs. The persistently agitated patient may be treated pharmacologically with a benzodiazepine. Neuroleptics have been widely and effectively used to lessen the psychotic-like experience; however, there is a report in the literature of an intensification of the experience following administration of those drugs. If neuroleptics are used, haloperidol (Haldol) 1 to 5 mg, or an equivalent dose of high-potency antipsychotic medication, may be appropriate.

No clear evidence exists that LSD causes a prolonged psychotic-like illness. Attempts at longitudinal studies have yielded insufficient evidence to support this hypothesis. One difficulty in resolving this question is the high rate of adulterants in the formulation of the drugs and the inability to clearly rule out any preexisting psychopathology.

The incidence of the development of schizophrenia after intoxication is not outside parameters one would expect to see in a youthful population. There is evidence that the occurrence of problems after intoxication is greater in those with a preexisting psychiatric illness. The psychiatric diagnosis most commonly associated with post-LSD psychosis is a form of schizoaffective disorder. The appearance of some affective instability—involving a feeling of an altered state of consciousness—and recurrent perceptual disorder, primarily visual, are the most common symptoms seen in patients with associated chronic psychosis. The schizophrenic drug user has been shown to have an earlier age of onset and better premorbid social functioning than the nondrug-using schizophrenic (52,62).

Phencyclidine, Ketamine, and Psychosis The cyclohexylamine anesthetics PCP and ketamine hydrochloride have similar properties. Both result in psychotic-like experiences during intoxication. Evidence suggests that, in the case of PCP, the psychotic-like state can last for prolonged periods beyond the period of intoxication. Soon after PCP was developed in 1957, it was found to be useful in veterinary practice as an anesthetic (10). This finding led to human experimentation and the recognition that administration of the drugs produces a dissociative state. Patients' eyes remain open and scanning during surgery, yet they appear to be "disconnected" from their environments and unable to feel pain (63,64). More alarming are reports of bizarre hallucinations and behaviors during the postoperative period (64). Consequently, PCP never has been released for human use.

Ketamine, at a potency 10 to 50 times lower than PCP, has been shown to produce far fewer of these psychotic-like episodes and was released for use as an anesthetic. Interestingly, children do not appear to develop the associated psychotic-like symptoms.

The history of abuse of these drugs began in the mid-1960s. Street use of PCP increased when prospective users learned that smoking the drug, rather than ingesting it, resulted in fewer unpleasant side effects. It was then that PCP began to be smoked in combination with cannabis (65). The incidence of PCP use increased significantly by 1976, when a survey by the National Institute on Drug Abuse found that 13.9% of 18- to 25-year-olds had experience with the drug (66). At the same time, there was an increase in the number of emergency department visits associated with PCP use. Reports included numerous deaths from toxicity, homicide, suicide, and accidents. A retrospective review of 80 PCP-related deaths showed a strong association with prior affective disorders, aggressive behavior, prior arrests, and a personal crisis in the three months preceding death.

PCP's popularity is attributed to the fact that it can be produced inexpensively and thus frequently is added to the formulation of a variety of drugs sold on the street. A 1975 survey showed that PCP was sold 91% of the time as some other substance—most often, mescaline, LSD, or THC (67). Since that time, the drug seems to have increased in popularity, as suggested by the fact that it more often is sold as PCP, although it still is found as an adulterant in other street drugs.

PCP and ketamine can be smoked, ingested, snorted, or injected intravenously. The drugs are rapidly absorbed and excreted in the urine. The intoxicating effects last for approximately 4 to 6 hours. The recovery period is highly variable. The behavioral effects of these drugs appear to be mediated by their effect on the excitatory amino acid NMDA subtype of glutamate receptor. The high-affinity binding of PCP and ketamine to the NMDA receptor blocks ion exchange, resulting in noncompetitive antagonism of the NMDA receptor (68).

Early observations of patients treated with PCP noted the similarities to dissociative and schizophrenic disorders (69,70). The clinical appearance is that of altered sensory perception, bizarre and impoverished thought and speech, impaired attention, disrupted memory, and disrupted thought processes in healthy individuals. There also may be protracted psychosis (71).

There is considerable symptom variation, depending on dose. At lower doses (20 to 30 ng/mL), one is likely to observe sedation, mood elevation, irritability, impaired attention and memory mutism, hyperactivity, and stereotypy. As serum levels rise to 30 to 100 ng/mL, mood changes, psychosis, analgesia, paresthesia, and ataxia can occur. These levels are associated with profound paranoia, aggression, and violent behavior. Higher levels (>100 ng/mL) can cause stupor, hyperreflexia, hypertension, seizure, coma, and/or death.

Treatment of the acutely disturbing effects of PCP-like drugs can be achieved with benzodiazepines in doses equivalent to diazepam 10 mg and greater, titrated until the patient is satisfactorily sedated. The patient's respiratory status should be continually monitored. There may be a dramatic reduction in aggressive behavior and a significant improvement in the psychotic symptoms. Neuroleptics also can be considered for treatment of the psychotic symptoms. Most typically, a high-potency neuroleptic like haloperidol (1 to 5 mg) is used because of the decreased anticholinergic properties of these drugs. In cases of overdose, the urine may be acidified with ammonium chloride to facilitate urinary excretion. However, metabolic acidosis can result in other problems, including worsening of rhabdomyolysis, and should be considered only in the most extreme cases.

MDMA ("Ecstasy") and Psychosis 3,4-methylenedioxymethamphetamine (MDMA or "Ecstasy") is a representative of a new class of compounds that became popular in the 1980s. A derivative of methamphetamine, MDMA has a mixed spectrum of effects, which are both amphetamine-like and hallucinogenic. MDMA increases the release and inhibits the reuptake of serotonin, dopamine, and norepinephrine from presynaptic neurons, as well as decreasing their degradation by inhibiting monoamine oxidase (72).

Users report enhanced empathy, feelings of closeness to others, euphoria, mood elevation, increased self-esteem, and altered visual perceptions. Hallucinations associated with use generally are mild. Deaths have occurred in cases that presented as a syndrome featuring severe hyperthermia, altered mental status, autonomic dysfunction, and dystonia (73). The mechanism is unclear, but, as with a serotonin syndrome, it may be that MDMA can have a direct effect on the thermoregulatory mechanisms that are potentiated by the context of the drug use. For example, MDMA often is used in the setting of dance parties where there is sustained physical activity, high temperatures, and inadequate fluid intake or dehydration.

Concern about the long-term neurotoxicity of MDMA is growing. Long-term users can suffer serotonin neural injury associated with psychiatric presentation of panic attacks, anxiety, depression, flashbacks, psychosis, and memory disturbances (74). Cases of paranoid psychosis indistinguishable from schizophrenia have been associated with chronic use (75). Although older schizophrenic patients may be less likely to use MDMA, use of it and other designer drugs must be considered and ruled out in patients with new onset of psychotic disorders.

Management of Psychotic Disorder Antipsychotic medications are an important component of the treatment of psychotic disorders. They are instrumental in reducing the long-term positive symptoms of the illness. Despite the advantages of these atypical agents, clinicians should have realistic expectations. Medications should be complemented by psychosocial therapy that engages clients, offers them practical training in interpersonal communication and crisis management, and develops their rehabilitation and recovery skills. The first step in medication management is to consider the best approach to treating the patient's schizophrenia or chronic psychosis. This should be followed by consideration of the potential interactions between the substances abused and the possible medication choices. In general, clinicians should avoid prescribing medications that cause sedation when treating patients who abuse sedating substances. In addition, clinicians generally should avoid prescribing medications with abuse liability.

Patients who present with active substance abuse, psychotic symptoms, and noncompliance can be difficult to manage as outpatients. Improving medication compliance in an outpatient setting can be enhanced by reducing positive and negative symptoms, providing psychoeducation and social skills training in medication management, using motivational enhancement techniques to improve compliance, and switching the route of administration of the medication from oral dosing to a long-acting injected medication, if patients are unable or refuse to take oral medications.

Over the past 12 years, new second-generation antipsychotic medications have been approved by the U.S. Food and Drug Administration for the treatment of schizophrenia. Some of these drugs also have been studied for the treatment of substance use (with and without coexisting schizophrenia) and are the focus of a number of recent review articles (76–78). This class of medication has the added benefit of decreasing extrapyramidal side effects, reducing negative symptoms, and improving cognition when compared with traditional antipsychotics. In addition to acting on the dopamine system, these drugs also bind to the serotonin system, which is thought to play an important role in maintaining cocaine addiction via craving. These findings led researchers to begin examining the mixed dopamine and serotonin antagonist risperidone (Risperdal) in the treatment of cocaine-dependent patients. Results from an open-label, 2-week trial with risperidone in recently withdrawn cocaine-dependent patients (79) suggested that risperidone significantly reduced cue-elicited craving. In a more recent trial, the electroretinogram, a peripheral measure of dopamine, was used to substantiate treatment effects of risperidone in recently withdrawn cocaine-dependent patients. The results suggested that risperidone significantly reduced self-reported craving and that the reduction in craving correlated with electroretinogram amplitude. Similar studies with clozapine (80,81) and olanzapine (82) suggest that these drugs show some efficacy in reducing craving and in preventing relapses to substance abuse among patients with co-occurring cocaine dependence and schizophrenia. Farren et al. (83) recently examined the acute effects of cocaine administration in a sample of eight cocaine addicts who also received clozapine or a placebo. The results suggested that the clozapine had a diminishing effect on the subjective response to cocaine, including the expected high. A study by Brunette et al. (84) indicates that clozapine may also prevent relapses in patients with schizophrenia using alcohol, cannabis, or cocaine. Furthermore, risperidone and clozapine appear to reduce the likelihood of relapse for patients addicted to opioids (85). Risperidone and ziprasidone increased patients' retention into dual diagnosis treatment compared with olanzapine or conventional antipsychotics (86). Some studies, however, show no difference between conventional and atypical antipsychotics used to treat patients with co-occurring disorders (59).

Complications of Substances with Antipsychotic Medications Substances can interact with psychiatric medications used to treat the symptoms of schizophrenia. The interactions are both pharmacokinetic and pharmacodynamic. Most of the substances of abuse interact with psychiatric medications by reducing their effectiveness, but some can alter blood levels of medications and increase side effects. Caffeine in coffee and tea is known to interfere with the absorption and metabolism of psychiatric medications. The metabolism of caffeine occurs through the same liver enzyme affected by cigarette use (cytochrome P450 1A2 isoenzyme). As such, cigarette smoking (the "tar" [polynuclear aromatic hydrocarbons] in cigarettes, not the nicotine) modifies the metabolism of psychiatric medication, including its potential side effects and effectiveness (87). Smoking is known to decrease blood levels of haloperidol, fluphenazine and thiothixene, olanzapine, and clozapine (88–91). Abstinence from smoking increases blood levels of neuroleptic medications. Smokers usually are prescribed approximately double the dose of traditional neuroleptic medications that is given to nonsmokers (92). There is at least one report of clozapine toxicity and seizure in the context of a quit attempt, presumably related to a sudden increase in serum levels of the drug (93). The effect on metabolism is important in making treatment decisions regarding hospitalized patients whose smoking habits are curbed, as well as the patient who is attempting to quit smoking. Substance abuse has been associated with earlier and more severe cases of tardive dyskinesia (94–97). However, other studies concluded that substance abuse had no effect on movement disorders when important covariates were considered (92,98,99).

Additional Medication Decisions After clinicians have chosen a primary medication treatment option that stabilizes the psychotic symptoms, they can consider the use of additional medication, as necessary, to manage comorbid depression, comorbid substance abuse, or another psychiatric problem. For substance use, medications are chosen for specific purposes, including detoxification, relief of protracted abstinence withdrawal, and agonist maintenance. Some adjunctive medications (such as antidepressants) also can address the schizophrenia, helping to reduce and stabilize its negative symptoms. Despite the lack of pharmacotherapy trials among populations with a substance abuse problem and schizophrenia, a growing number of clinicians have reported the benefits of these medications.

Psychosocial Treatment For both acute and longer term treatment, clinical experience and research findings have demonstrated the importance of developing a positive therapeutic alliance as a cornerstone of psychosocial treatment. Patients are more responsive when the therapist consistently acts as a nurturing and nonjudgmental ally (100–106). This is important for both patients with substance induced psychosis as well as schizophrenia and addiction.

Individuals with substance-induced psychosis will benefit from medications as well as a supportive treatment team and environment. This chapter will focus not on this patient population, but rather the individual with co-occurring schizophrenia and addiction. Siris and Docherty (101) maintain that dually diagnosed schizophrenics require such a positive alliance, and that premature termination and psychiatric decline will ensue from a negative alliance, that is, one based on fear, anger, or rejection. This assertion is consistent with the results of focus groups organized by Maisto et al. (107). In those groups, patients with schizophrenia spectrum diagnosis and co-occurring substance use disorders reported that the relationship developed with the therapist was an important part of recovery. Carey (108) has suggested a five-step "collaborative, motivational, harm reduction" approach for working with the dually diagnosed patient. This approach includes (109) establishing and developing a working alliance, (9) helping the patient evaluate the cost-benefit ratio of continued substance use (decisional balance in Motivational Enhancement Therapy (MET), (110) helping the patient develop individual goals, (4) helping the patient build a supportive environment and a lifestyle that is conducive to abstinence, and (5) helping the patient learn to anticipate and cope with crises (108).

Psychosocial treatment requires an awareness of the perceived "self-medication" aspects of why individuals with schizophrenia believe they continue to use substances. Despite the negative consequences associated with substance abuse, some individuals with schizophrenia report that using substances helps them cope with symptoms of their schizophrenia (111,112). They report using substances for pleasure; to alleviate boredom; to relieve feelings of anxiety, sadness, or distress; and to share the excitement of "getting high" with friends who also are using. In one study, the most common reason reported for using substances was "something to do with friends" (113). Some individuals report that substance use reduces their social inhibitions. The self-medication theory suggests that individuals use chemicals to self-medicate the symptoms of schizophrenia; however, the research data supporting this clinical perception are mixed (114). Another self-medication theory suggests that individuals with schizophrenia use substances to help ameliorate the distressing side effects of the medications used to treat their schizophrenia. The term *neuroleptic dysphoria* is used to describe the unpleasant feelings elicited by treatment with conventional antipsychotic medications, including irritability, fatigue, listlessness, and lack of interest or ambition. Although the syndrome often goes unrecognized, rates of neuroleptic dysphoria have been reported as ranging from 5% to 40% (115). One retrospective study reported that patients with a history of neuroleptic dysphoria were four times more likely to develop substance abuse than those without a history of neuroleptic dysphoria (116). Interestingly, many patients hospitalized for psychosis were smoking even before their first hospitalization or initiation of their first antipsychotic medication (61), suggesting a complex relationship between symptoms, medications, and substance use. Some studies suggest that individuals with schizophrenia may smoke to help improve their attention and concentration (117,118). One research group has found that smoking can transiently normalize deficits in auditory physiology (P50 gating) and that this gating abnormality, which is found in individuals with schizophrenia, may be caused by a genetic defect in the nicotinic cholinergic receptors in some individuals (110,117,118). Despite the self-medicating experience of some smokers with schizophrenia, tobacco use is associated with more positive symptoms of schizophrenia (92,99) and more hospitalizations (99,112). Of course, the cross-sectional designs used in these studies do not allow for a causal hypothesis to be tested.

Nonetheless, working with the dually diagnosed patient requires that the therapist be realistic and direct in addressing inconsistencies; however, the manner in which they are approached is crucial. For example, if a patient has recent positive cocaine urine samples, yet denies any use during the preceding month, the clinician must be understanding of the initial stage of recovery, but point out the discrepancy. If there have been overall gains in harm reduction, these should be recognized, and other outcomes should be assessed.

A harm reduction philosophy can be helpful and realistic with the poorly motivated patient who remains uncommitted and ambivalent about the goal of total abstinence (4,108,119). The patient who is in the precontemplation or contemplation stage of change often is unwilling to commit to total abstinence as a short-term goal. Keeping such a patient engaged in treatment often requires finding extrinsic motivators to further the development of the therapeutic alliance (these motivators might include help in obtaining food, clothing, shelter, money management, vocational/training activities, social relationships, and the like). The use of motivational interviewing to develop intrinsic motivation to stop using substances and to maintain compliance with psychiatric treatment also is a useful strategy.

Keeping patients engaged requires efforts to treat their schizophrenia and to provide encouragement and other "rewards" for small steps toward reducing substance use. It is important to evaluate outcomes other than total abstinence; for example, the clinician might assess the patient for reduced quantity or frequency of drug use, participation in treatment or other activities, compliance with medications, progress toward short-term goals, and involvement of family or significant others in treatment.

LONGER TERM MANAGEMENT

Ongoing treatment of psychosis and addiction requires integrated treatment that attempts to reduce the likelihood of relapse to substances, noncompliance with medications, and promotes recovery and wellness. Clinical experience has shown that some psychiatric patients will continue to simultaneously display psychotic symptoms and to actively abuse substances. If the diagnostic assessment was uncertain and the patient is able to achieve prolonged abstinence, the clinician then can consider withdrawing the medication and initiating a medication-free period. Patients who continue to display an affective or psychotic disorder despite a significant period of abstinence may require formal treatment of that disorder. The usual treatment for schizophrenia is long term antipsychotic treatment, psychosocial treatment, and case management as needed. Long-term psychotherapy should consider a dual recovery therapy approach that integrates the best of mental health and addiction psychotherapy. In addition, medications might be helpful in the protracted abstinence phase based on the limited research on this population.

Long-Term Treatment for Alcohol Addiction For the treatment of alcohol use disorders, the U.S. Food and Drug Administration has approved the use of three adjunctive medications: disulfiram, acamprosate, and naltrexone. The clinical record of disulfiram is mixed, and it has yet to be tested in randomized control trials. The possibility of an alcohol-disulfiram reaction requires that it be given only to patients who comprehend the consequences of alcohol consumption when taking disulfiram. According to some clinicians, administration of disulfiram at high doses (1,000 mg) has produced psychotic symptoms in patients not diagnosed with psychotic disorders. Clinical studies of naltrexone in this population are supportive of their use in this population (120). Naltrexone is a relatively safe medication that can be used with patients who are at risk of relapse to alcohol; no alcohol-naltrexone reaction has been reported. Naltrexone's most common side effects include headache and nausea. Naltrexone can precipitate opiate withdrawal, so clinicians should carefully assess patients' use of prescription or illicit opiates and be prepared to manage opiate withdrawal symptoms. Liver function tests should be monitored when using either disulfiram or naltrexone.

For cocaine addiction, clinicians have tried a variety of augmentation medications, including desipramine (Norpramin), selegiline (Eldepryl), mazindol, and amantadine (Symmetrel), all of which aim to produce an increased dopaminergic effect that will reverse or compensate for the neurophysiologic changes stemming from the chronic use of cocaine. There are numerous small studies that suggest some promise for a range of medications; however, there is no strong evidence that any adjunctive medication is more helpful for co-occurring cocaine addiction than excellent integrated psychosocial treatment and that adjusting the primary antipsychotic medication might be the best option (4,100,121).

Psychosocial Treatment Co-occurring disorder treatment programs have used psychosocial interventions in strikingly different ways, but there are core similarities. Some have favored an active outreach case management approach, whereas others have relied more heavily on motivational enhancement therapy in the clinical setting (14,29,100, 102,122–125). Three specific psychosocial treatments that appear fundamental to dual diagnosis treatment include MET (126), relapse prevention (127), and Twelve Step facilitation. However, clinical experience suggests that these three treatment approaches require modification because of the biologic, cognitive, affective, and interpersonal vulnerabilities inherent in schizophrenia. Modifications of conventional substance abuse treatments must take into account the common features of schizophrenia—low motivation and self-efficacy, cognitive deficits, and maladaptive interpersonal skills. These limitations heighten the importance of the treatment alliance (96).

The number and variety of psychosocial interventions for patients with co-occurring addictive and psychotic disorders has expanded, and now ranges from traditional self-help and Twelve Step groups to recent innovations such as community reinforcement (128). The major psychosocial interventions for substance use disorders—MET, relapse prevention, and Twelve Step approaches—require some retooling if they are to address the problems posed by patients with schizophrenia. For such patients, the prognosis for long-term improvement and recovery depends on a treatment design that addresses both patients' addiction and their schizophrenia, that responds to the unique vulnerabilities (cognitive, affective, social, and biologic) of the schizophrenic patient, and that maintains an empathic and collaborative approach. In most cases, treatment of this dual diagnosis subtype is best suited to the mental health setting, provided that mental health staff members receive adequate training in substance abuse and dual diagnosis treatment strategies.

Training programs should be designed to develop basic dual diagnosis assessment and treatment competencies for all staff members. Clinicians should have skills and knowledge in integrating mental health and addiction treatment approaches, with special emphasis on MET, relapse prevention, and Twelve Step facilitation for addiction, as well as social skills training and behavioral therapies for psychiatric disorders. Other helpful strategies include behavioral contracting, community reinforcement approaches, social skills training, money management, peer support/counseling, vocational/educational counseling, and family/network therapies.

The Twelve Step approach has been modified for dually diagnosed individuals, who often have reported some difficulty in engaging in Twelve Step groups, given the perceived stigma toward individuals with serious mental illnesses and the cultural opposition to use of psychiatric medications. Dual Recovery Anonymous meetings can provide a bridge to the Twelve Step movement for patients with dual disorders. Meetings of these groups often are held in mental health settings or social houses. The groups encourage recovery for both problems and emphasize the importance of taking appropriately prescribed medications. Spiritual health also is a focus of the meetings, including connecting with a Higher Power, developing a sense of community, and finding meaning and purpose in life. Clinical experience has shown that individuals with a serious mental illness are eager to talk about spirituality and to develop a stronger sense of hope through the experience of recovery.

Several dual diagnosis treatment approaches with similar behavioral therapy models have been suggested. The Motivation-Based Dual Diagnosis Treatment model employs a stage-matching approach that combines mental health and addiction treatments, based on the patient's motivational level, severity of illness, and dual diagnosis subtype. The Motivation-Based Dual Diagnosis Treatment approach acknowledges the distinctive features of the schizophrenia-addiction subtype (100). The model uses stages of change in assessing the patient and matches treatment strategies and goals (such as abstinence or harm reduction, medication compliance, session attendance, and so forth) to the individual's stage of readiness to change.

MET is a primary psychosocial approach for the patient with poor motivation. However, when the traditional MET approach is used with dually diagnosed patients, clinicians should recognize the need for adjustments, which include:

- The clinician should play a more active role in offering practical, useful solutions to the patient's concerns about everyday survival. The clinician should not assume that dual diagnosis patients have the personal tools or social resources to solve problems effectively while actively engaged in addictive behaviors.
- MET should be formulated as a continuing component of treatment rather than being limited to the four sessions that were envisioned for nonschizophrenic substance users.
- The decision balance intervention, a cornerstone of MET, should be employed so that it fully accounts for the experience of substance use in relation to other and more systemic problems, such as schizophrenia and medication compliance.
- The clinician should acknowledge that dually diagnosed individuals may not consistently accept the diagnosis of schizophrenia, may vary in their willingness to maintain medication for schizophrenia, and may have greater or lesser motivation to stop their substance use.

Attending to the role of motivation is important to the success of the treatment plan. Clinicians must work to strengthen patients' motivation while confronting the effects of schizophrenia and stressing the importance of medications in managing the condition. Prochaska et al. (129) defined motivation in relation to a five-stage scale (precontemplation, contemplation, preparation, action, and maintenance). Individuals enter treatment at various stages and, therefore, interventions need to be tailored accordingly; one author recommends using experiential processes (cognitive and emotional learning) for patients in contemplation or preparation stages, switching to behavioral processes (such as contingency management) for those in action or maintenance phase (130).

Interventions that address individual stages of change have an impact not only on rates of substance use, but also on the severity of psychotic symptoms and on the need for antipsychotics (87). A study that evaluated a group of 295 patients who were diagnosed with both schizophrenia and a substance use disorder concluded that more than half could be described as "low motivated" (i.e., in the precontemplation or contemplation stage), with the degree of motivation related to the substance or number of substances abused (4). Of those patients who abused alcohol, 53% were assessed as having low motivation; the figures for cocaine and marijuana were 65% and 73%, respectively. In another study, a simple five-point Likert scale of current motivation for treatment successfully predicted the dually diagnosed patient's likelihood of achieving abstinence (105). Studies evaluating the impact of MET-based interventions for substance using patients with psychotic disorders show that substance use is decreased, but the major problem with these studies is the high rate of subject loss to observation (40,131). One study shows that MET-based interventions are more effective for patients who use cocaine, whereas the standard psychiatric interview worked better for patients using cannabis.

Certain conditions can work to accelerate a patient's motivation to change through use of external motivators, a realization that led to the development of the community reinforcement approach (132). The community reinforcement approach draws on behavioral therapy principles of contingencies, rewards, and consequences. Because external motivation often is lacking among dually diagnosed patients, the community reinforcement approach searches out a range of possible motivators—disability income, probation, family, and so forth—and uses those motivators to engage, support, and monitor patients in treatment.

Treatment must address not only the effects of low motivation but also potential deficiencies in the cognitive skills known as receiving-processing-sending skills, which allow individuals to act on information in a coherent and productive manner (96). These skills assume basic levels of attention, memory, and reality awareness. In individuals with schizophrenia, such levels often are lower than normal, so that the benefits of traditional relapse prevention treatment, which is built on a cognitive learning model, are sharply reduced (127). Thus the treatment model must be modified and tailored to the dual diagnosis patient, switching the treatment emphasis from cognitive to behavioral approaches as needed.

Traditionally, relapse prevention and Twelve Step facilitation have been used in addiction settings with nonschizophrenic patients, most of whom have a range of social, interpersonal, and problem-solving skills that lead to self-esteem and self-efficacy (133). Self-efficacy, in particular, is directly related to the change processes that influence maintenance and relapse (37,127,134). Relapse prevention and Twelve Step programs can help individuals increase their self-efficacy and self-esteem. However, relapse prevention therapy tends to be administered in a cognitive therapy manner, while clinical experience suggests using a more action-oriented behavioral approach, featuring role playing, modeling, coaching, positive and negative feedback, and homework. Traditional psychiatric approaches of social skills training use this methodology in rehabilitation programs (66,136). The Lieberman modules include psychosis symptom management, medication management, leisure skills, conversation skills, and community reentry. Traditional relapse prevention is easily adapted to work with individuals with schizophrenia with a focus on addressing difficulties in communication and problem solving.

Several exemplary treatment programs for substance abusers with comorbid psychiatric disorders deserve discussion here. The dual diagnosis treatment program at the West Los Angeles Veterans Affairs Medical Center uses an integrated care model, in which treatment teams provide both mental health and substance abuse services. A relapse prevention module was designed in consideration of the cognitive deficits of persons with schizophrenia spectrum diagnoses. Patients are taught and given an opportunity to practice a series of social skills believed to reduce the incidence and severity of relapse. Assertive case management, including housing and advocacy services, also plays an integral part of the treatment program. In addition to medications aimed at relief of psychotic symptoms, patients with comorbid alcohol dependence are offered disulfiram. Finally, patients submit to urine drug screens twice per week. A more detailed description of this treatment program is available from Ho et al. (85).

After the previously mentioned program was developed, enhanced program components were added to meet the needs of substance abuse patients with comorbid psychiatric illnesses. Examples include additional psychiatrist time available to patients, a community reentry module, extra case managers, a specialized relapse prevention module, and a relaxation group. Ho et al. (85) compared patients who attended the program before and after the enhanced services were added. Compared with patients in the original version of the program, patients in the enhanced program showed significantly better abstinence rates at 1 month (60% vs. 30%), 3 months (31% vs. 5%), and 6 months (20% vs. 0%) of treatment. Patients attending the enhanced program also showed superior rates of 30- and 90-day treatment retention compared with patients attending the initial program. The researchers reported that increased use of assertive case management could have played an instrumental role in better engagement in treatment, including improved attendance. This increased exposure to services could have contributed considerably to the improved abstinence rates. Further research could help determine the relative importance of the various therapeutic components.

Bellack and DiClemente (137) described a treatment approach that attempts to compensate for the deficits in motivation, cognition, and social skills commonly seen in patients with schizophrenia. Four treatment modules are used in a rational sequence. Patients first are provided with social skills and problem-solving strategies. Then they are provided with information about the unique difficulties associated with substance abuse in persons with schizophrenia, in addition to information about cravings and triggers for substance use. Motivational interviewing strategies are used, treatment goals are discussed, and behavioral relapse prevention skills are taught.

Patients attend 90-minute sessions twice per week for approximately 6 months. Small groups (six to eight patients) are used to allow for skill rehearsal and individualized attention. Groups are highly structured to compensate for cognitive deficits associated with schizophrenia. Early successes are built into the treatment program to increase client self-efficacy. Treatment focuses on a small number of specific skills so as not to overwhelm the clients cognitively. Additionally, rather than insisting on complete abstinence immediately, the need for flexibility in this population is recognized by focusing on modest treatment goals. Abstinence is reinforced by paying patients a small amount for clean urine test results. Initial data appear promising for this treatment approach. Of the 80 patients examined, none that completed the first 3 weeks of the program subsequently dropped out. Additionally, the overall attrition rate was found to be only 38.5%. Initial substance use outcome data also appear promising (137). A controlled clinical trial of the approach will follow. Dual recovery therapy integrates substance abuse relapse prevention, psychiatric social skills training, MET, and the "recovery language" of Twelve Step programs in linked group and individual treatment sessions (100). MET and recovery language were added to address patients' often low levels of motivation for change and to take advantage of the common lexicon of the Twelve Step programs, with which many patients already were familiar. The resulting treatment is designed to enhance intrinsic motivation for change, bolster the patients' sense of self-efficacy, improve their social skills, and give them tools for coping with high-risk situations. Training is grounded in cognitive-behavioral theory and targets the schizophrenic person's cognitive difficulties (attention span, reading skills, and ability to abstract). The ability to communicate and solve problems is developed through role plays that can be introduced in both group and individual therapy, whereas the understanding and management of their substance use problems are improved through an emphasis on coping strategies (e.g., how to organize one's time). The therapist gives ongoing consideration to both substance abuse and psychiatric problems, monitors their interaction, and adjusts the treatment emphasis accordingly. A patient's motivation to address the symptoms of schizophrenia may not be the same as his or her motivation to address substance use, and treatment is best tailored to the individual's motivation for each problem area.

The first month of dual recovery therapy involves twice-weekly individual sessions. Motivation is assessed and enhanced in these early individual sessions while the therapist works on building a strong therapeutic alliance. A plan for change is discussed, and basic skills that will be necessary for later group sessions are introduced. Subsequent individual sessions focus on reinforcing material discussed in group therapy.

After the first month, once a therapeutic alliance has been established and the client has been prepared for group therapy, the structure shifts from two individual sessions per week to one individual and one group session. These sessions are linked, in that individual sessions are used to reinforce the material discussed during the group sessions. Group sessions follow a standard format, which begins with a relaxation exercise, followed by an update report from each client. Group structure is provided by focusing on a specific topic each week (e.g., relapse prevention, mood management, symptom management, increasing pleasurable activities, communication skills, asking for help, and medication compliance). Because skill-building plays a central role in dual recovery therapy, behavioral rehearsal and role-playing are used regularly.

Recovery Recovery is a journey of healing and transformation enabling a person with a mental health and or substance abuse problem to live a meaningful life in the community of his or her choice while striving to achieve his or her full potential (138). The journey must include transformation of both the mental health and substance abuse. It is often not a linear process and requires the consumer and provider to have patience and respect for the process. In fact, the journey often involves exacerbations and remissions that are all part of the process. Recovery can be reinforced on multiple levels, including the consumer or provider level as well as the systems level. At the consumer or provider level, both parties must first view recovery as a process and have mutual respect for the journey. Both parties must not be frustrated by disruptions or the nonlinearity, as it is the journey that is in fact the recovery. Unfortunately, stigmatization of people with mental health disorders, including substance abuse, has persisted throughout history and can impact recovery. Stigma is manifested by bias, distrust, stereotyping, fear, embarrassment, anger, or avoidance, can be found throughout our society, and can even include people with mental illness and the professionals and health care systems who serve them.

Substance Abuse and Mental Health Services Administration's Center for Mental Health Services Resource Center to Address Discrimination and Stigma provides practical assistance and a wealth of resources for designing and implementing antistigma activities and facilitating the process of recovery. Likewise, consumers and providers should also familiarize themselves with antistigma information contained in such important publications as Substance Abuse and Mental Health Services Administration's *Blueprint for change: ending chronic homelessness for persons with serious mental illnesses and co-occurring substance use disorders* (139) as well as the President's New Freedom Commission's Report on Mental Health *Achieving the promise: transforming mental health care in America* (140). This process of recovery at the provider or systems level can be facilitated via consumers' providers. This can be in the form of direct care and offering the client a roadmap for recovery or at the systems level via resources centers. The New Freedom Commission's findings have helped to pave the way for a broader acceptance of consumer-run services and consumer providers. We are fortunate to be in a time in history when recovery is at the forefront of mental health and substance abuse care and providers, consumers, advocates, and systems are all working together to facilitate these efforts.

Addressing Tobacco Addiction in Recovery Nicotine dependence is very common and a major cause of increased morbidity and mortality in this population. Traditionally, it has received less clinical attention and often has gone untreated, despite the fact that nicotine is the substance most commonly abused by schizophrenics. The development of treatment guidelines can correct this oversight and lead to the inclusion of tobacco dependence as a component in clinical treatment plans (111,141,142). In addition to multicomponent behavioral therapy, treatment for nicotine cessation can include adjunctive medications such as nicotine replacements (transdermal patch, gum, spray, or inhaler), bupropion (Zyban), or varenicline (Chantix). The new atypical antipsychotics can be used to treat negative symptoms and are useful in smoking cessation (also see the discussion in Chapter 52, "Pharmacologic Interventions for Tobacco Dependence").

In patients who were not receiving specific smoking cessation treatment, two studies found significant decreases in nicotine use among patients who were switched from traditional neuroleptics to clozapine (90,117). Although few studies have examined the treatment of tobacco dependence in smokers with schizophrenia, specialized smoking cessation programs appear to benefit this population (4,109,143). In a study evaluating the treatment of tobacco dependence, about 20% of patients with schizophrenia were able to remain abstinent for 6 months with the use of nicotine replacement therapy. This study also showed that intensive psychosocial treatment (weekly individual motivational enhancement therapy combined with weekly relapse prevention group therapy) yielded better outcomes than either individual or group therapy alone (4). In a similar study, Addington et al. (109) found that a significant number of patients with schizophrenia were able to stop smoking by the end of a modified group treatment program sponsored by the American Lung Association.

In the most rigorous study to date, smokers with schizophrenia were randomly assigned to either a specialized smoking cessation group therapy program modified for schizophrenic patients or to a standard American Lung Association group. Smokers in the specially modified group displayed significantly higher rates of continuous smoking abstinence in the last 4 weeks of a 12-week trial than did those in a standard American Lung Association group. Abstinence rates did not differ between groups at the end point, however. When compared with patients prescribed typical antipsychotic medications, patients prescribed atypical antipsychotics showed significantly higher rates of abstinence, lower rates of attrition, and lower levels of expired carbon monoxide (109). An important finding of these studies was that schizophrenic symptoms were not exacerbated in patients who achieved abstinence from cigarettes (109,143,144).

REFERENCES

1. American Psychiatric Association (APA). *Diagnostic and statistical manual of mental disorders,* 4th ed. (DSM-IV). Washington, DC: American Psychiatric Press, 1994.
2. Clark HW, Power AK, Le Fauve CE, et al. Policy and practice implications of epidemiological surveys on co-occurring mental and substance use disorders. *J Subst Abuse Treatment* 2008;34:3–13.
3. Breslau N, Novak SP, Kessler R. Daily smoking and the subsequent onset of psychiatric disorders. *Psychol Med* 2004;34:323–333.
4. Ziedonis DM, Fisher W. Motivation-based assessment and treatment of substance abuse in patients with schizophrenia. *Direct Psychiatry* 1996; 16(11):1–8.
5. Hunt GE, Bergen J, Bashir M. Medication compliance and comorbid substance abuse in schizophrenia: impact on community survival 4 years after a relapse. *Schiz Res* 2002;54:253–264.
6. Schollar E. The long term treatment of the dually diagnosed. In: Solomon J, Zimberg S, Schollar E, eds. *Dual diagnosis: evaluation, treatment, training, and program development.* New York: Plenum Medical Book Co., 1993.
7. Sato M. A lasting vulnerability to psychosis in patients with previous methamphetamine psychosis. *Annals of the New York Academy of Science* 1990;654:160–170.
8. Satel JA, Lieberman JA. Schizophrenia and substance abuse. *Psychiatr Clin N Am* 1991;6(2):401–412.
9. Addington J, Addington D. Patterns, predictors and impact of substance use in early psychosis: a longitudinal study. *Acta Psychiatr Scand* 2006; 115:304–309.
10. Farrelly S, Henry LP, Purcell R, et al. Prevalence and correlates of comorbidity 8 years after a first psychotic episode. *Acta Psychiatrica Scandinavica* 2006;116:62–70.
11. Higgins ST, Budney AJ, Bickel WK, et al. Incentives improve outcome in outpatient behavioral treatment of cocaine dependence. *Arch Gen Psychiatry* 1994;51:568–576.
12. Barnett JH, Werners U, Secher SM, et al. Substance use in a population-based clinic sample of people with first-episode psychosis. *Br J Psychiatry* 2007;190:515–520.
13. Mueser KT, Bellack AS, Blanchard JJ. Comorbidity of schizophrenia and substance abuse: implications for treatment. *J Consult Clin Psychol* 1992;47:1102–1114.
14. Drake RE, Noordsy DL. Case management for people with coexisting severe mental disorder and substance use disorder. *Psychiatr Anns* 1994;24(8):427–431.
15. Kumra S, Thaden E, DeThomas C. Correlates of substance abuse in adolescents with treatment-refractory schizophrenia and schizoaffective disorder. *Schizophr Res* 2005;73:369–371.
16. Meade CS, Sikkema KJ. Psychiatric and psychosocial correlates of sexual risk behavior among adults with severe mental illness. *Comm Ment Health J* 2007;43(2):153–169.
17. Jackson CT, Covell NH, Drake RE, et al. Mortality among persons with co-occurring psychotic and substance use disorders. *Psychiatric Serv* 2007;58(2):270–272.
18. Ziedonis DM, Williams J. When psychosis and substance use coincide in the emergency service. *Psychiatr Issues Emerg Care Settings* 2002; Summer: 3–13.
19. Pierre JM, Shnayder I, Wirshing DA, et al. Intranasal quetiapine abuse. *Am J Psychiatry* 2004;161(9):1718.
20. McCormick J. Recreational bupropion abuse in a teenager. *Br J Clin Pharmacol* 2002;53:214.
21. Shaner A, Roberts LJ, Racenstein JM, et al. Sources of diagnostic uncertainty among chronically psychotic cocaine abusers. Presented at the 149th Annual Meeting of the American Psychiatric Association, New York, May 4–9, 1996.
22. First MB, Spitzer RL, Gibbon M, et al. *Structured clinical interview for axis I DSM-IV disorders-version 2.0.* New York: New York State Psychiatric Institute, Biometrics Research Department, 1995.
23. Wiesbeck GA, Taeschner KL. A cerebral computed tomography study of patients with drug-induced psychoses. *Eur Arch Psychiatry Clin Neurosci* 1991;241:88–90.
24. Isbell H, Fraser HF, Wikler A. An experimental study of the etiology of "rum fits" and delirium tremens. *Q J Stud Alcohol* 1955;16(Suppl): 1–33.
25. Mendelson JH, LaDou L. Experimentally induced chronic intoxication and withdrawal in alcoholics. *Q J Stud Alcohol* 1964;2(Suppl):1–39.
26. Tabakoff B, Hoffman PL. Alcohol addiction: an enigma among us. *Neuron* 1996;16:909–912.
27. Victor M, Hope JM. The phenomenon of auditory hallucinations in chronic alcoholism. *J Nerv Ment Dis* 1958;126:451–448.
28. Scott DF. Alcoholic hallucinosis. *Int J Addict* 1969;4:319–330.

29. Schuckit MA. The history of psychotic symptoms in alcoholics. *J Clin Psychiatry* 1982;43:53–57.
30. Shen WW. Extrapyramidal symptoms associated with alcohol withdrawal. *Biol Psychiatry* 1984;19:1037–1043.
31. Carlen PL, Lee MA, Jacob M, et al. Parkinsonism provoked by alcoholism. *Ann Neurol* 1981;9:84–86.
32. Lang AE. Alcohol and Parkinson's disease. *Ann Neurol* 1982;12: 254–256.
33. Regier DA, Farmer ME, Rae DS, et al. Comorbidity of mental disorders with alcohol and other drug abuse. *JAMA* 1990;264:2511–2518.
34. Hollister LE. Actions of various marijuana derivatives in man. *Pharmacol Rev* 1971;23:349–357.
35. Chopra G, Smith J. Psychotic reactions following cannabis use in East Indians. *Arch Gen Psychiatry* 1974;30:24–27.
36. Ames F. A clinical and metabolic study of acute intoxication with Cannabis sativa and its role in the model psychoses. *J Men Sci* 1958; 104:972–999.
37. Keeler M, Reifler C, Liptzin M. Spontaneous recurrence of marijuana effect. *Am J Psychiatry* 1968;125:384–386.
38. Tart CT. Marijuana intoxication: common experiences. *Nature* 1970; 226:701–704.
39. Renault P. Repeat administration of marijuana smoke to humans. *Arch Gen Psychiatry* 1974;31:95–102.
40. Keeler M, Ewing J, Rouse B. Hallucinogenic effects of marijuana as currently used. *Am J Psychiatry* 1971;128:213–216.
41. Beaubrun MH, Knight F. Psychiatric assessment of 30 chronic users of cannabis and 30 matched controls. *Am J Psychiatry* 1973;130:309–311.
42. Isbell H. Effects of delta-9-trans-tetrahydrocannabinol in man. *Psychopharmacologia* 1967;11:184–188.
43. Waskow IE. Psychological effects of tetrahydrocannabinol. *Arch Gen Psychiatry* 1970;22:97–107.
44. Ghodse H. Cannabis psychosis. *Br J Addict* 1986;81:473–478.
45. Talbott JA, Teague JW. Marijuana psychosis. *JAMA* 1969;210:299–305.
46. Rottanburg D. Cannabis associated psychosis with hypomanic features. *Lancet* 1982;11:1364–1366.
47. Brook MG. Psychosis after cannabis abuse. *Br Med J* 1984;288:1381.
48. Carney P, Lipsedge M. Psychosis after cannabis abuse. *Br Med J* 1984; 288:1381.
49. Tennant FS, Groesbeck CJ. Psychiatric effect of hashish. *Arch Gen Psychiatry* 1972;27:133–136.
50. Chaudry HR. Cannabis psychosis following bhang ingestion. *Brit J Addict* 1991;288:1075–1081.
51. Gersten SP. Long-term adverse effects of brief marijuana usage. *J Clin Psychiatry* 1980;41(2):60–61.
52. Breakey WR, Goodell H, Lorenz PC, et al. Hallucinogenic drugs as precipitants of schizophrenia. *Psychol Med* 1974;4(3):255–261.
53. Manschreck TC, Laughery JA, Weisstein CC, et al. Characteristics of freebase cocaine psychosis. *Yale J Biol Med* 1988;61(2):115–122.
54. Brady KT, Lydiard RB, Malcolm R, et al. Cocaine-induced psychosis. *J Clin Psychiatry* 1991;52(12):509–512.
55. Satel SL, Southwick SM, Gawin FH. Clinical features of cocaine-induced paranoia. *Am J Psychiatry* 1991;148(4):495–498.
56. Ellinwood EH, Sudilovsky A, Nelson LM. Evolving behavior in the clinical and experimental amphetamine (model) psychosis. *Am J Psychiatry* 1973;130(10):1088–1093.
57. Sherer MA. Intravenous cocaine: psychiatric effects, biological mechanisms. *Biol Psychiatry* 1988;24(8):865–885.
58. Siegel RK. Cocaine hallucinations. *Am J Psychiatry* 1978;135:309–314.
59. Post RM. Cocaine psychoses: a continuum model. *Am J Psychiatry* 1975;132(3):225–231.
60. Satel SL, Edell WS. Cocaine-induced paranoia and psychosis proneness. *Am J Psychiatry* 1991;148(12):1708–1711.
61. McLellan TA, Woody GE, O'Brien CP. Development of psychiatric illness in drug abusers. *N Engl J Med* 1979;301(24):1310–1314.
62. Bowers MB. Acute psychosis induced by psychotomimetic drug abuse: clinical findings. *Arch Gen Psychiatry* 1972;27:437–440.
63. Johnstone ME, Evans V, Baigel S. Sernyl (CI-395) in clinical anesthesia. *Br J Anaesth* 1959;31:433–439.
64. Greifenstein FE, DeVault M, Yoshitake J, et al. 1-Arylcyclohexylamine for anesthesia. *Curr Res Anesth Analg* 1958;37:283–294.
65. Liden CB, Lovejoy FH, Costello CF. Phencyclidine: nine cases of poisoning. *JAMA* 1975;234(5):513–516.
66. Levin ED, Conners CK, Silva D, et al. Transdermal nicotine effects on attention. *Psychopharmacology (Berl)* 1998;140(2):135–141.
67. Lundberg GD, Gupta RC, Montgomery SH. Phencyclidine: patterns seen in street drug analysis. *Clin Toxicol* 1976;9:503–511.
68. Cotman CW, Monaghan DT. Chemistry and anatomy of excitatory amino acid systems. In: HY Meltzer, ed. *Pharmacology and toxicology of amphetamine and related designer drugs*. New York: Raven Press, 1987: 197–210.
69. Davies BM, Beech HR. The effect of 1-arylcyclodexylamine (Sernyl) on twelve normal volunteers. *J Ment Sci* 1960;106:912–924.
70. Cohen BD, Rosenbaum G, Luby ED, et al. Comparison of phencyclidine hydrochloride (Sernyl(r)) with other drugs: simulation of schizophrenic performance with phencyclidine hydrochloride (Sernyl), lysergic acid diethylamide (LSD-25), and amobarbital (Amytal) sodium, II: Symbolic and sequential thinking. *Arch Gen Psychiatry* 1962;1:651–656.
71. Fauman B, Aldinger G, Fauman M, et al. Psychiatric sequelae of phencyclidine abuse. *Clin Toxicol* 1976;9:529–538.
72. Battaglia G, DeSouza EB. Pharmacologic profile of amphetamine derivatives at various brain recognition sites: selective effects on serotonergic systems. *NIDA Research Monograph 94*. Rockville, MD: National Institute on Drug Abuse, 1989:240–258.
73. Mueller PD, Korey WS. Death by "ecstasy": The serotonin syndrome? *Ann Emerg Med* 1998;32(3):377–380.
74. Graeme KA. New drugs of abuse. *Emerg Med Clin N Am* 2000;18(4): 625–636.
75. Cash CD. Gammahydroxybutyrate: an overview of the pros and cons for it being a neurotransmitter and/or a helpful therapeutic agent. *Neurosci Biobehav Rev* 1994;18:291–304.
76. Green AI, Brown ES. Comorbid schizophrenia and substance abuse. *J Clin Psychiatry* 2006;67(9):e08.
77. Green AI, Drake RE, Brunette MF, et al. Schizophrenia and co-occurring substance use disorder. *Am J Psychiatry* 2007;164(3):402–408.
78. Smelson D, Dixon L, Craig T, et al. Pharmacological treatment of schizophrenia and co-occurring substance use disorders. *CNS Drugs* 2008; 22(11):903–916.
79. Smelson DA, Losonczy M, Castles-Fonseca K, et al. Preliminary outcomes from a booster case management program for individuals with a co-occurring substance abuse and a persistent psychiatric disorder. *J Dual Diagnosis* 2005;13:47–59.
80. Buckley P. How effective are the second generation antipsychotics? *Int J Psychiatry Clin Pract* 1998;2(Suppl 2):S41–S47.
81. Drake RE, Xie H, McHugo GJ, et al. The effects of clozapine on alcohol and drug use disorders among patients with schizophrenia. *Schiz Bull* 2000;26(2):441–449.
82. Smelson DA, Roy A, Roy M. Risperidone diminishes cue-elicited craving in withdrawn cocaine-dependent patients. *Can J Psychiatry*1997;42(9):984.
83. Farren CK, Hameedi FA, Rosen MA, et al. Significant interaction between clozapine and cocaine in cocaine addicts. *Drug Alcohol Depend* 2000;59(2):153–163.
84. Brunette, MF, Drake, RE, Xie, H, et al. Clozapine use and relapses of substance use among patients with co-occurring schizophrenia and substance use disorders. *Schiz Bull* 2006;32(4):637–643.
85. Ho AP, Tsuan JW, Liberman RP, et al. Achieving effective treatment of patients with chronic psychotic illness and comorbid substance dependence. *Am J Psychiatry* 1999;156(11):1765–1770.
86. Stuyt EB, Sajbel TA, Allen MH. Differing effects of antipsychotic medications on substance abuse treatment patients with co-occuring psychotic and substance abuse disorders. *Am J Addict* 2006;15:166–173.
87. Jarvik ME, Schneider NG. Nicotine. In: Lowinson JH, Ruiz P, Millman RB, eds. *Substance abuse: a comprehensive textbook,* 2nd ed. Baltimore, MD: Williams, Wilkins, 1992.
88. Ereshefsky L, Saklad SR, Watanabe T. Thiothixene pharmacokinetic interactions: a study of hepatic enzyme inducers, clearance inhibitors, and demographic variables. *J Clin Psychopharmacol* 1991;11:296–300.

89. Ereshefsky L. Pharmacokinetics and drug interactions: update for new antipsychotics. *J Clin Psychiatry* 1996;57(Suppl 11):12–25.
90. McEvoy J, Freudenreich O, McGee M, et al. Clozapine decreases smoking in patients with chronic schizophrenia. *Biol Psychiatry* 1995;37(8):550–552.
91. George TP, Sernyak MJ, Ziedonis DM, et al. Effects of clozapine on smoking in chronic schizophrenic outpatients. *J Clin Psychiatry* 1995; 56(8):344–346.
92. Ziedonis DM, Kosten TR, Glazer W. The impact of drug abuse on psychopathology and movement disorders in chronic psychotic outpatients. In: Harris L, ed. *Problems of drug dependence 1994 (NIDA Research Monograph 153)*. Rockville, MD: National Institute on Drug Abuse, 1994.
93. Skogh E, Bengtsson F, Nordin C. Could discontinuing smoking be hazardous for patients administered clozapine medication? A case report. *Therap Drug Monitor* 1999;21(5):580.
94. Dixon L, Haas G, Weiden PJ, et al. Drug abuse in schizophrenic patients: clinical correlates and reasons for use. *Am J Psychiatry* 1991; 148:224–230.
95. Olivera AA, Kiefer MW, Manley NK. Tardive dyskinesia in psychiatric patients with substance use disorders. *Am J Drug Alcohol Abuse* 1990;16(1–2):57–66.
96. Zaretsky A, Rector NA, Seeman MV, et al. Current cannabis use and tardive dyskinesia. *Schiz Res* 1993;11(1):3–8.
97. Binder RL, Kazamatsuri H, Nishimura T, et al. Smoking and tardive dyskinesia. *Biol Psychiatry* 1987;22:1280–1282.
98. Hughes JR, Hatsukami DK, Mitchell JE, et al. Prevalence of smoking among psychiatric outpatients. *Am J Psychiatry* 1986;143:993–997.
99. Goff DC, Henderson DC, Amico BS. Cigarette smoking in schizophrenia: relationship to psychopathology and medication side effects. *Am J Psychiatry* 1992;149:1189–1194.
100. Ziedonis DM, D'Avanzo K. Schizophrenia and substance abuse. In: Kranzler HR, Rounsaville BJ, eds. *Dual diagnosis and treatment: substance abuse and comorbid medical and psychiatric disorders*. New York: Marcel Dekker, 1998:427–465.
101. Siris SG, Docherty JP. Psychosocial management of substance abuse in schizophrenia. In: Herz MI, Docherty JP, Klein SK, eds. *Handbook of schizophrenia, volume 5. Psychosocial therapies,* Amsterdam, the Netherlands: Elsevier Science Publishers, 1990.
102. Docherty JP. The individual psychotherapies: efficacy, syndrome-based treatments, and the therapeutic alliance. In: A Lazare, ed. *Outpatient psychiatry: diagnosis and treatment*. Baltimore, MD: Williams & Wilkins, 1980.
103. Frank AF, Gunderson JG. The role of the therapeutic alliance in the treatment of schizophrenia: relationship to course and outcome. *Gen Psychiatry* 1990;47(3):228–236.
104. Grinspoon L, Ewalt JR, Schader RI. *Schizophrenia: pharmacotherapy and psychotherapy*. Baltimore, MD: Williams & Wilkins, 1972.
105. Rogers CR, Gendlin EG, Kiesler DJ, et al. *The therapeutic relationship and its impact: a study of psychotherapy with schizophrenics*. Madison, WI: University of Wisconsin Press, 1967.
106. Sullivan HS. *Schizophrenia as a human process*. New York: WW Norton, Co., 1962.
107. Maisto SA, Carey KB, Carey MP, et al. Methods of changing patterns of substance use among individuals with co-occurring schizophrenia and substance use disorder. *J Subst Abuse Treatment* 11999;7(3):221–227.
108. Carey KB. Substance use reduction in the context of outpatient psychiatric treatment: a collaborative, motivational, harm reduction approach. *Comm Mental Health J* 1996;32(3):291–306.
109. Addington J, el Guebaly N, Campbell W, et al. Smoking cessation treatment for patients with schizophrenia. *Am J Psychiatry* 1998;155:974–976.
110. Adler LE, Hoffer LD, Wiser A. Normalization of auditory physiology by cigarette smoking in schizophrenic patients. *Am J Psychiatry* 1993;150: 1856–1861.
111. American Psychiatric Association (APA). APA practice guideline for the treatment of patients with nicotine dependence. *Am J Psychiatry* 1996;153(10 Suppl):1–31.
112. Kelly C, McCreadie RG. Smoking habits, current symptoms, and premorbid characteristics of schizophrenic patients in Nithsdale, Scotland. *Am J Psychiatry* 1999;156:751–1757.
113. Test MA, Wallisch LS, Allness DJ. Substance use in young adults with schizophrenic disorders. *Schiz Bull* 1989;15:465–476.
114. Brunette MF, Mueser KT, Xie H, et al. Relationships between symptoms of schizophrenia and substance abuse. *J Nerv Ment Dis* 1997;185:13–20.
115. Weiden PJ, Mann JJ, Dixon L. Is neuroleptic dysphoria a healthy response? *Compr Psychiatry* 1989;30:543–552.
116. Voruganti LN, Heslegrave RJ, Awad AG. Neuroleptic dysphoria may be the missing link between schizophrenia and substance abuse. *J Nerv Ment Dis* 1997;185(7):463–465.
117. Lavin MR, Siris SG, Mason SE. What is the clinical importance of cigarette smoking in schizophrenia? *Am J Addict* 1996;5:189–208.
118. Freedman R, Hall M, Adler LE, et al. Evidence in postmortem brain tissue for decreased numbers of hippocampal nicotinic receptors in schizophrenia. *Biol Psychiatry* 1995;38:22–33.
119. Marlatt GA, Tapert SF. Harm reduction: reducing the risks of addictive behaviors. In JS Baer, GA Marlatt (eds.) *Addictive Behaviors across the life span: prevention, treatment, and policy issues*. Newbury Park, CA: Sage Publications, 1993:243–273.
120. Ziedonis DM, Smelson D, Rosenthal RN, et al. Improving the care of individuals with schizophrenia and substance use disorders: consensus recommendations. *J Psychiatric Pract* 2005;11(5):315–339.
121. McEvoy J, Freudenreich O, Levin ED, et al. Haloperidol increases smoking in patients with schizophrenia. *Psychopharmacology* 1995;119 (1):124–126.
122. Wilkins JN. Pharmacotherapy of schizophrenic patients with comorbid substance abuse. *Schiz Bull* 1997;23:215–228.
123. Drake RE, Osher FC, Noordsy DL, et al. Diagnosis of alcohol use disorders in schizophrenia. *Schiz Bull* 1990;16:57–67.
124. Office on Smoking and Health. *Reducing tobacco use: a report of the Surgeon General.* Atlanta, GA: U.S. Department of Health and Human Services, Centers for Disease Control and Prevention, National Center for Chronic Disease Prevention and Health, 2000.
125. Rosenberg SD, Drake RE, Wolford GL, et al. Dartmouth assessment of lifestyle instrument (DALI): a substance use disorder screen for people with severe mental illness. *Am J Psychiatry* 1998;155(2):232–238.
126. Minkoff K. An integrated treatment model for dual diagnosis of psychosis and addiction. *Hosp Comm Psychiatry* 1989;40(10):1031–1036.
127. Marlatt GA, Gordan JR. *Relapse prevention: maintenance strategies in the treatment of addictive behaviors*. New York: Guilford Press, 1985.
128. Dixon L, Rebori TA. Psychosocial treatment of substance abuse in schizophrenic patients. In: Shiriqui CL, Nasrallah HA, eds. *Contemporary issues in the treatment of schizophrenia*. Washington, DC: American Psychiatric Press, 1995.
129. Prochaska JO, DiClemente CC, Norcross JC. In search of how people change: applications to addictive disorders. *Am Psychol* 1992;47: 1102–1114.
130. Finnell DS. Addictions services—use of the transtheoretical model for individuals with co-occurring disorders. *Comm Ment Health J* 2003; 39(1):3–15.
131. Baker, A, Bucci, S, Lewin, TJ, et al. Cognitive-behavioural therapy for substance use disorders. *Br J Psychiatry* 2006;188:439–448.
132. Hilton T. Pharmacological issues in the management of people with mental illness and problems with alcohol and illicit drug misuse. *Crim Behav Mental Health* 2007;17:215–224.
133. Bandura A. Self-efficacy: toward a unifying theory of behavioral change. *Psychol Rev* 1977;84(2):191–215.
134. Velicer WF, DiClemente CC, Rossi JS, et al. Relapse situations and self-efficacy: an integrative model. *Addict Behav* 1990;15:271–283.
135. Liberman RP, Mueser KT, Wallace CJ, et al. Training skills in the psychiatrically disabled: learning coping and competence. *Schiz Bull* 11986;2:631–647.
136. Foy DW, Wallace CJ, Liberman RP. Advances in social skills training for chronic mental patients. In: KD Craig, MJ McMahon, eds. *Advances in clinical behavior therapy*. New York: Brunner/Mazel, 1983.

137. Bellack AS, DiClemente CC. Treating substance abuse among patients with schizophrenia. *Psychiatr Serv* 1999;50(1):75–80.
138. Substance Abuse and Mental Health Services Administration (SAMHSA), 2006. *National consensus statement on mental health recovery.* Retrieved September 19, 2007: http://mentalhealth.samhsa.gov/publications/allpubs/sma05-4129/.
139. Substance Abuse and Mental Health Services Administration (SAMHSA), 2003. *Co-occurring disorders: integrated dual disorders treatment implementation resource kit user's guide.* Retrieved August 1, 2007: http://download.ncadi.samhsa.gov/ken/pdf/toolkits/cooccurring/IDDTUsersguideAJ1_04.pdf.
140. New Freedom Commission on Mental Health, 2003. *Achieving the promise: transforming mental health care in America. Final report.* DHHS Pub. No. SMA-03-3832. Rockville, MD. Retrieved September 20, 2007: http://www.mentalhealthcommission.gov/reports/FinalReport/FullReport.htm.
141. Fiore MC, Bailey WC, Cohen SJ, et al. *Treating tobacco use and dependence. Quick reference guide for clinicians.* Rockville, MD: U.S. Department of Health and Human Services, Public Health Service, 2000.
142. McEvoy JP, Brown S. Smoking in first-episode patients with schizophrenia. *Am J Psychiatry* 1999;156(7):1120–1121.
143. George TP, Ziedonis DM, Feingold A, et al. Nicotine transdermal patch and atypical antipsychotic medications for smoking cessation in schizophrenia. *Am J Psychiatry* 2000;157:1835–1842.
144. Dalak GW, Becks L, Hill E, et al. Nicotine withdrawal and psychiatric symptoms in cigarette smokers with schizophrenia. *Neuropsychopharmacology* 1999;21:195–202.

CHAPTER 87

Frances R. Levin, MD
John J. Mariani, MD
Maria A. Sullivan, MD, PhD

Co-occurring Addiction and Attention Deficit/Hyperactivity Disorder

This chapter examines two common psychiatric problems, attention deficit/hyperactivity disorder (ADHD), a disorder that manifests itself in childhood, and substance use disorders (SUD), which often occur in adolescence or early adulthood. Although it was thought until recently that most children "grow out" of the problems associated with ADHD (1,2), it has become increasingly clear that most individuals diagnosed with childhood ADHD continue to have impairing symptoms into adulthood (3). Further, the coexistence of a SUD makes it more difficult to treat the ADHD symptoms (4–6). Similarly, untreated ADHD may make it less likely that standard treatments for substance abuse will be as effective (7–11). The overrepresentation of ADHD in substance abusers, the reasons for linkage, the diagnostic issues related to making the diagnosis of ADHD in adult substances abusers, and the implications for treatment will be discussed.

ETIOLOGY OF ADHD

There are numerous etiologies that have been proposed to explain why ADHD occurs. These factors include genetic, environmental, neuroanatomical, neurochemical, and central nervous system insults.

Evidence of a genetic basis for the pathophysiology of ADHD derives from family, twin, and adoption studies as well as molecular genetics research. Twin studies (12,13) have yielded a heritability estimate of 0.8, suggesting that the genetic component is strong, but that environmental factors also play a role. Adoption studies have confirmed that familial clustering of ADHD is due to genetics rather than shared environment (14). Molecular genetics studies support the theory that ADHD is a heterogeneous disorder, dependent on several interacting genes. Prominent among these are the gene for the dopamine transporter and that for the D4 dopamine receptor (DRD4) (13,15,16). Altered DRD4 expression results in reduced receptor effectiveness and increased GABA transmission, thereby decreasing pyramidal cell firing (17,18). Medications that inhibit the dopamine transporter, including methylphenidate and amphetamine, increase synaptic dopamine levels and ameliorate the symptoms of ADHD. Other candidate genes of interest include: (1) SNAP-25, which is associated with neuronal release of dopamine (DA) and shows a statistically significant association with ADHD (13); (2) DBH, which catalyzes the conversion of DA to norepinephrine; the DBH gene mutation 5′ TaqI results in higher DBH enzyme activity, thus lowering DA levels and producing the expression of ADHD symptoms (13); and (3) catechol-O-methyltransferase, in which a single nucleotide substitution (Val/Val) accelerates the degradation of catecholamines, including DA, resulting in decreased attention to relevant stimuli and increased distractibility (19).

Neuroanatomic explanations for ADHD have also been proposed. Neuroimaging studies of ADHD patients have demonstrated reduced volume of the prefrontal cortex (20). The prefrontal cortex is densely populated with DA receptors (especially D1) and norepinephrine receptors, and balanced DA tone in the prefrontal cortex is essential for normal working-memory function and attention regulation (18,21).

Structural imaging studies of ADHD patients have revealed several common findings: smaller volumes in frontal cortex, cerebellum, and subcortical structures (22). Of note, Castellanos et al. (23) found a fixed brain volume abnormality in ADHD: smaller total cerebral brain volumes from childhood through adolescence (23). Another important functional neuroimaging finding has been that the dorsal anterior cingulated cortex shows hypofunction in ADHD on tasks of inhibitory control (24). The hypothesis that dysfunction in frontal-subcortical pathways occurs in ADHD is supported by brain imaging studies implicating the caudate, putamen, and globus pallidus, all of which provide feedback to the cortex for regulation of motor control, inhibition of behavior, and modulation of reward pathways (22,25).

Certain environmental risks have also been associated with ADHD. These include maternal smoking during pregnancy, low birth weight, and low social class. McCormick et al. (26) also demonstrated that in low birth weight children, hyperactivity symptom scores increase as birth weight decreases. Prenatal environmental tobacco smoke is also a strong risk factor for ADHD. In a large nationally representative sample of children ages 4 to 15 years, Braun et al. (27) found that the overall adjusted risk for ADHD was 2.5-fold higher for children exposed prenatally to tobacco smoke. Additional environmental risk factors for the persistence of ADHD symptoms include maternal psychopathology and larger family size (28). Pineda et al. (29) identified several additional environmental factors associated with ADHD, including maternal respiratory viral infection, moderate to severe physical illness in the mother during pregnancy, maternal alcohol exposure, febrile seizures, and moderate brain injury. The finding that traumatic brain injury results in symptoms of ADHD has been documented by a large number of studies (5,30–33).

EPIDEMIOLOGY OF ADHD AND SUDs

ADHD is the most common behavioral disorder of childhood, affecting 8% to 18% of children and adolescents worldwide (34). Given that up to 60% of children with ADHD continue to have symptoms into late adolescence and adulthood (35–37), it was estimated that the rates for adult ADHD in the general population would be from <1% to 5%. This estimate has been in fact substantiated by a recent replication study of the National Comorbidity Survey in which the rate of adult ADHD was found to be 4.4% (38). Clinical experience suggests that many patients do not meet full criteria in adulthood, but do continue to have significant impairment as a result of persistent ADHD symptoms.

Assuming that up to 5% of adults in the general population have impairing symptoms of ADHD, the question arises as to whether ADHD is overrepresented in substance-using populations. There is a strong consensus that the rates of ADHD in substance abuse treatment samples are two to three times the rate found in the general population. Although Weiss et al. (39) obtained low rates of adult ADHD among cocaine (4.7%) and opioid and other depressant drug abusers 0.7%, most prevalence studies have obtained substantially higher rates ranging from 5% to 71%. (40) Interesting, the rates found in opiate-dependent patients have been consistently lower (i.e., 5% to 22%) than rates found in alcohol-dependent samples (33% to 71%). Although the reasons for this difference are somewhat unclear, it may be that persistent opiate use masks the symptoms associated with ADHD. Alternatively, the use of DSM-III or non-DSM criteria, common with the older alcohol studies (41), may have led to somewhat elevated rates. More recent studies that have used structured clinical interviews to assess for symptoms based on DSM-IV criteria have obtained lower rates, with a more constricted range (i.e., 10% to 24%) (42–45). Of note, in four, prevalence rates were not elevated based on any specific drug of abuse. Instead, rates tended to be lower when strict attention was paid to the age-of-onset criterion (i.e., symptoms needed to occur before age of 7) or symptoms that may have been substance-induced were not counted (46). Elevated rates of ADHD among persons with SUD are not confined to treatment samples. Carroll and Rounsaville (7) found that the prevalence of childhood ADHD, although lower among cocaine abusers not seeking treatment than among those seeking treatment (22% vs. 35%) (47), was still higher than that in the general population.

Similarly, SUD appear to be overrepresented in persons with symptoms of ADHD, whether or not they are seeking treatment. Both the ECA Study and the National Comorbidity Survey Replication (NCS) obtained prevalence rates for SUDs within the general population and found that lifetime rates of substance abuse or dependence ranged from 17% to 27% (48,49). In the NCS-replication study, 15.2% of those with ADHD, compared with 5.6% of those without ADHD, had a SUD (38). Biederman et al. (50) found that lifetime prevalence rates for SUD among clinical samples of adults with ADHD was quite high at 52%, compared with 27% in subjects without ADHD. Non–treatment-seeking adults with ADHD were significantly more likely to have alcohol/drug use disorders than were non–treatment-seeking adults without histories of ADHD (51). Taken together, these studies suggest that ADHD and substance use are not independent disorders and that their association is not the result of ascertainment bias.

Individuals with ADHD also have a greater likelihood of nicotine dependence. Adults with ADHD have higher rates of nicotine dependence than the general population (40% vs. 26%). The odds of current smoking in adolescents with clinically significant inattentive ADHD symptoms were 2.8 times greater than for those without inattentive ADHD symptoms (52,53). Analysis of the Longitudinal Study of Adolescent Health, a large perspective epidemiologic survey of adolescents found that for each self-reported inattentive and hyperactive symptom, the risk of lifetime smoking increased. Further, for those reporting ever smoking, increase in symptoms was associated with earlier age of smoking and number of cigarettes smoked (54). In a prospective study, Lambert and Hartsough

(55) noted that individuals with ADHD had early onset of regular smoking and adults with ADHD were more likely to smoke daily than were controls.

THE IMPACT OF HAVING ADHD ALONE AND WITH SUDS

ADHD has substantial morbidity in and of itself. In an individual with ADHD, occupational and social deficits attributed to substance abuse may be due in small or large part to persistent ADHD symptoms. In a recent review, Mannuzza et al. (56) noted that children with ADHD who were followed into adulthood were more likely to have completed less schooling, to hold occupations with less professional or social status, to suffer from poor self-esteem, to have social skill deficits, and to have antisocial personality disorder. Murphy and Barkley (57) found that, as adults, individuals who were diagnosed with ADHD in childhood were more likely to have had their driver's licenses suspended, to have incurred speeding violations, to have quit or been fired from a job, and to have been married multiple times. Persistent ADHD symptoms appear to place these individuals at great risk for antisocial personality disorder and substance abuse (56,58).

Further, adult ADHD exacts an enormous financial cost to society. In a recent economic analysis of administrative health claims, Birnbaum et al. (59) found that adult ADHD conservatively costs the United States more than $31 billion per year in work and health-related costs for patients and their families. In another analysis of the NCS-R (60), adult ADHD was a significant predictor of overall lost work performance (61). Projections based on these data suggest that for the total U.S. civilian labor force approximately 120.8 million lost days of work per year and approximately $19.6 billion salary-equivalent loss per year are associated with ADHD. For the NCS-R respondents who screened positive for current ADHD symptoms, only 16.4% reported that they received treatment for their ADHD symptoms. Another 15.7% reported that they received treatment for an emotional problem without ADHD being the focus of that treatment. This is not surprising given that many individuals with ADHD have additional psychiatric and SUDs (38).

When ADHD symptoms are combined with those of a SUD, the severity of impairment of each disorder is likely to increase. Moreover, the individual's response to addiction treatment is adversely affected by comorbid ADHD. Biederman et al. (28) found that after a period of substance dependence, adults with ADHD were more likely to transition from an alcohol use disorder to a drug use disorder and to continue to abuse substances than were similar patients without ADHD. Likewise, among individuals with a lifetime history of a SUD, those who also had ADHD evinced a longer duration of having a SUD and a slower remission rate (62).

Carroll and Rounsaville (7) compared the clinical course of cocaine use among individuals with and without childhood histories of ADHD. Those with childhood ADHD had an earlier onset of regular cocaine use, more frequent and intense cocaine use, and greater lifetime treatment exposure. Similarly, Levin et al. (63) found that among cocaine-dependent individuals entering a therapeutic community, those with ADHD were less likely to graduate from the program, compared with those with depression (and no ADHD) or those without ADHD or depression. Graduation is an important milestone associated with better long-term outcome. Based on these findings, it is increasingly evident that ADHD may exert a negative effect on the course of a SUD and that treatment needs to be targeted at both the psychiatric and SUDs.

POSSIBLE REASONS FOR LINKAGE OF ADHD AND SUD

Various explanations have been offered for the link between ADHD and SUD, including the presence of a necessary mediating factor, such as conduct disorder, the persistence of ADHD symptoms, low self-esteem, self-medication, genetic factors, and exposure to stimulants in childhood. Prospective studies that have followed children with ADHD into adolescence suggest that a mediating factor—specifically, conduct disorder—substantially increases the likelihood for substance abuse to occur. There is considerable evidence that individuals diagnosed with childhood ADHD who also have conduct disorder as children are more likely to develop problems related to substance use (64–67). Further, in some clinical samples of delinquent adolescents the presence of ADHD is associated with more severe conduct disorder symptoms and greater number of substance dependencies (66). Of note, in a 2-year follow-up study of substance-dependent, conduct-disordered adolescents, severity of initial conduct disorder and age of onset, but not severity of ADHD or treatment duration, predicted worse drug-dependent outcomes (68). Adolescents with ADHD may begin to use drugs even in the absence of conduct disorder. Further, several investigators have found a substantial proportion of individuals with adult ADHD have an ongoing SUD in the absence of ASP (1,50). Thus a critical risk factor for having an ongoing substance abuse in adolescence or adulthood is the persistence of ADHD symptoms. After regular substance use is established, the presence of ADHD symptoms may increase the likelihood of heavy and impairing use.

Impulsivity is another factor than may facilitate the initiation and persistence of drug use among individuals with ADHD. A growing preclinical and clinical literature suggests that impulsivity is associated with increased likelihood of developing or having a substance use problem (69–71). Impulsivity, a common feature of ADHD, is associated with the inability to inhibit responses. More broadly, individuals with ADHD are often thought to have difficulties in executive function including difficulties in impulse control, attention, planning, and goal-directed behavior. Increased impulsivity may facilitate risk-taking behavior, involvement with drug-abusing peers, and poor cognitive skills to weigh the negative consequences of drug experimentation and continued substance use (52,53).

Deregulation and overexpression of the dopamine transporter also have been implicated in the pathophysiology of ADHD (13). The 10-repeat allele of the dopamine transporter gene has been associated with ADHD (72,73) and there are preliminary data to suggest that this transporter variant is associated with a poor methylphenidate response (74,75). In addition, work by Dougherty et al. (76) has showed that dopamine transporter density is significantly higher in adults with ADHD than in healthy controls. Polymorphisms of the D5 dopamine receptor gene (72,77), genes coding for dopamine B-hydroxylase along with other genes involved in serotonin and glutamine transmission have been associated with ADHD (13). However, the "primary candidate genes associated with ADHD are involved in dopamine functioning, lending support to studies implicating catecholamines in the pathophysiology of ADHD" (15,78). Thus it would not be surprising if individuals with ADHD might ameliorate hypodopaminergic function through the use of drugs that increase synaptic dopamine (10).

In a recent review, Kalivas and Volkow (79) note that all abusable substances produce their euphorigenic effects through their direct or indirect release of dopamine in the "reward" system of the brain consisting of the ventral tegmental area of the brain and the nucleus accumbens. With chronic drug use, derangements in the dopaminergic system produce with a relative hypodopaminergic state. Specifically, Kalivas and Volkow adduce evidence from functional imaging studies in addicts revealing that basal prefrontal regulation of behavior is reduced, contributing to the diminished salience of non-drug motivational stimuli and reduced decision-making capacity.

What remains unclear is whether adult substance abusers develop dopaminergic derangements as a result of heavy chronic substance use or had underlying deficits prior to the drug use. If the latter is true, for individuals with hypodopaminergic functioning, in the prefrontal regions of the brain, as documented among individuals with ADHD (80,81) or other psychiatric conditions, such as schizophrenia (82), abusable substances may be more salient and thus more likely to be abused. This concept of a common vulnerability is supported by family genetic studies that have found higher than expected rates of alcohol and substance abuse in non-ADHD–affected relatives of probands who have ADHD but no co-occurring SUD. Further evidence for this link comes from a family-based study evaluating the influence of parental SUD and ADHD on the risk for ADHD in offspring. Wilens et al. (83) determined that the rate of children with ADHD increased among children of parents with neither disorder (3%), children of parents with SUD (13%), children of parents with ADHD (25%), and children of parents with both SUD and ADHD (50%). These results suggest that the offspring of either SUD or ADHD parents are at increased risk for ADHD compared with controls.

A controversial explanation for the observed association between ADHD and substance use is that exposure to stimulants—even that prescribed by treatment providers—increases the likelihood that an individual will develop a problem with stimulants. This heightened risk is thought to occur by the process of behavioral sensitization or patients' belief that, because a stimulant medication has been prescribed, they can use cocaine or other drugs without difficulty. Although Lambert and Hartsough (55) found that adults who had been treated for ADHD with stimulant medications because children were more likely to be daily smokers than were those who had not taken stimulants, other studies suggest that treating ADHD children with stimulants *reduces* the risk of later alcoholism (84) and other SUDs (85). In a meta-analytic review of seven studies that followed ADHD children into adolescence or adulthood, the authors found that those treated with stimulants had a twofold reduction in risk for substance abuse, with the majority of studies (four of seven) finding a reduced risk for SUDs for those treated versus untreated for ADHD (86). The two studies that followed individuals into adolescence, rather than adulthood, obtained more robust findings.

Currently available data do not suggest that treating children with stimulants increases the risk of substance abuse. Further, preclinical and human data suggest that there is a biologically sensitive period, in which active intervention for ADHD may reduce the risk of developing a SUD (87,88). It remains unclear whether stimulant treatment normalizes brain functioning and directly protects adolescents from seeking out agents that increase dopaminergic transmission (89–93). But in a clinical perspective, an untreated child is more likely to function poorly in school, seek out other marginalized peers, and become involved with alcohol or drugs. Clearly, more research is needed to elucidate the relationships among ADHD, its treatment, and the development of SUDs.

DIAGNOSIS OF ADHD

ADHD is characterized by inattention, impulsivity, and hyperactivity. Table 87.1 provides the criteria for childhood ADHD in the fourth edition of the *Diagnostic and statistical manual* (DSM-IV; APA) (94). Importantly, the current criteria require that some symptoms have caused impairment before the age of seven and that impairment must occur in more than one setting. These criteria emphasize both the developmental aspect of the disorder and the fact that childhood behavior problems often are situation-bound. The more settings in which deviant behavior occurs, the more justified one is in saying that the behavior interferes with the child's functioning and therefore warrants a diagnosis. A child who appears distracted and inattentive in only one setting (such as at school), but can listen well and pay attention in other settings may have a learning disability rather than ADHD.

Individuals can meet full criteria for ADHD in three ways: (1) ADHD, inattentive type; (2) ADHD hyperactive/impulsive type, and (3) ADHD, combined type. Individuals who met full criteria in childhood but currently have fewer than six symptoms of inattention or hyperactivity/impulsivity are described as ADHD, in partial remission.

Faraone et al. (95) argue convincingly that the DSM-IV diagnosis of ADHD may be particularly sensitive to developmental changes because the symptoms are performance-based

TABLE 87.1 Criteria for Attention Deficit/Hyperactivity Disorder

A. Either (1) or (2):

1. Six (or more) of the following symptoms of inattention have persisted for at least 6 months to a degree that is maladaptive and inconsistent with developmental level:

Inattention

a. Often fails to give close attention to details or makes careless mistakes in schoolwork, work, or other activities;
b. Often has difficulty sustaining attention in task or play activities;
c. Often does not seem to listen when spoken to directly;
d. Often does not follow through on instructions and fails to finish schoolwork, chores, or duties in the workplace (not due to oppositional behavior or failure to understand instructions);
e. Often has difficulty organizing tasks and activities;
f. Often avoids, dislikes, or is reluctant to engage in tasks that require sustained mental effort (such as schoolwork or homework);
g. Often loses things necessary for tasks or activities (such as toys, school assignments, pencils, books, or tools);
h. Often is easily distracted by extraneous stimuli;
i. Often forgetful in daily activities six (or more) of the following symptoms of hyperactivity-impulsivity have persisted for at least 6 months to a degree that is maladaptive and inconsistent with developmental level.

2. *Hyperactivity*

a. Often fidgets with hands or feet or in seat;
b. Often leaves seat in classroom or in other situations in which remaining in seat is expected;
c. Often runs about or climbs excessively in situations in which it is inappropriate (in adolescents or adults, may be limited to a subjective feeling of restlessness);
d. Often has difficulty playing or engaging in leisure activities quietly;
e. Often is "on the go" or often acts as if "driven by a motor"
f. Often talks excessively.

Impulsivity

a. Often blurts out answers before questions have been completed;
b. Often has difficulty awaiting turn;
c. Often interrupts or intrudes on others (e.g., butts into conversations or games).

B. Some hyperactive-impulsive or inattentive symptoms that caused impairment were present before age 7 years.

C. Some impairment from the symptoms is present in two or more settings (such as at school [or work] and at home).

D. There must be clear evidence of clinically significant impairment in social, academic, or occupational functioning.

E. The symptoms do not occur exclusively during the course of a Pervasive Developmental Disorder, Schizophrenia, or other Psychotic Disorder and are not better accounted for by another mental disorder (such as Mood Disorder, Anxiety Disorder, Dissociative Disorder, or a Personality Disorder).

Code based on type:

- Attention Deficit/Hyperactivity Disorder, Combined Type: if both Criteria A1 and A2 are met for past 6 months.
- Attention Deficit/Hyperactivity Disorder, Predominantly Inattentive Type: if Criterion A1 is met but Criterion A2 is not met for the past 6 months.
- Attention Deficit/Hyperactivity Disorder, Predominantly Hyperactive-Impulsive Type: if Criterion A2 is met but not Criterion A1 is not met for the past 6 months.

Coding note: For individuals (especially adolescents and adults) who have symptoms that no longer meet full criteria, "In Partial Remission" should be specified.

Reprinted with permission from American Psychiatric Association. *Diagnostic and Statistical Manual of Mental Disorders,* 4th ed. (DSM-IV-TR). Washington, DC: American Psychiatric Press, 2000.

rather than experiential. For example, an individual being evaluated for ADHD is asked about his or her behavior (such as how well he or she follows directions or completes tasks), whereas an individual with depression is asked about his or her internal states (such as feelings of sadness or hopelessness) as well as behavioral manifestations (such as changes in sleep pattern or appetite). Often, behaviors that are difficult to perform in childhood become inconsequential in adulthood. Future revisions of the DSM-IV will need to develop new criteria that incorporate symptoms more relevant to the challenges encountered by adults (96).

Validity of the Adult ADHD Diagnosis Until recently, clinicians disagreed as to whether the adult syndrome was a valid disorder. The present diagnostic schema, which requires a constellation of symptoms of either inattentiveness or hyperactivity-impulsivity, represents a revision of the DSM-IIIR designation of "undifferentiated ADHD," in which the disorder was considered to be possible rather than presumable. To be valid, a clinical diagnosis requires: descriptive validity: that is, characteristic signs and symptoms; predictive validity: that is, a specific course of illness and treatment response; and construct validity: that is, data suggesting that an underlying etiology or pathophysiology exist (97). Prevalence and prospective studies (1,50,98), family-genetic studies (50), neuroimaging studies (99), and treatment studies (100,101) all provide data to support the three types of validity described above. Spencer et al. (102) reviewed this evidence and have argued convincingly that adult ADHD is a distinct clinical entity. With greater acceptance of adult ADHD as a valid diagnosis, clinicians have been more likely to assess and diagnose substance-abusing patients with ADHD.

Use of Neuropsychologic Testing to Confirm ADHD Diagnosis There is a widely held acceptance that ADHD is a clinical diagnosis that is best made by carrying out a comprehensive assessment that includes developmental history, learning history, evaluation of other psychiatric comorbidities, and medical evaluation. Although various neuropsychologic tests, electrophysiologic data, and neuroimaging tests have found differences among adults with and without ADHD (103–105), no test has adequate specificity to "diagnose" an individual with ADHD (106,107). However, conclude that continuous-performance tests are the most evidence-based of currently available psychologic tests, demonstrating reasonable sensitivity and specificity and promising positive predictive power (106).

Given the high comorbidity of ADHD with other psychiatric disorders, what is most needed are computer tests that would distinguish ADHD. Computer testing show areas of dysfunction that may or may not be consistent with ADHD. Testing may be useful for treatment or educational planning (106,108,109), because learning disabilities and academic underachievement are common in individuals with ADHD (51,56). Although the utility of these tests in active substance abusing populations has not been established (109), observing how individuals behavior while taking neurocognitive tests can provide useful clinical information. An individual who demonstrates short latency responses, uncritical and careless performance with frequent false starts, off-task behaviors, and concentration problems might indicate the presence of ADHD (110).

Difficulties in Diagnosing Adult ADHD in Substance-Using Populations Although the DSM-IV provides clear-cut criteria for making the diagnosis of adult ADHD, diagnostic ambiguity often arises when one attempts to apply these criteria to individuals who abuse alcohol and other drugs.

Potential Reasons for Underdiagnosis As mentioned earlier, recalling symptoms that began at an early age can be problematic. In assessing a child for ADHD symptoms, child psychiatrists or pediatricians often seek information from a teacher or parent; however, these sources of information may not be available during assessment of the adult patient, particularly a substance-abusing patient. The patient may be estranged from his or her family. Even when an older family member or parent is available, the reliability of the information may be questionable. The older family member may have had an alcohol/drug problem or other dysfunction to a degree that his or her ability to recall the patient's childhood behavior may be limited. Another good way to obtain historical data is to ask the patient to provide elementary school report cards. These can afford an accurate "snapshot" of the patient as a child. Although many parents may not have kept such school records, it is worthwhile to inquire.

If the patient or family cannot recall symptoms before age seven, but does remember substantial impairment related to ADHD symptoms in elementary school it is reasonable to make the late-onset ADHD. NOS diagnosis. However, it is important to inquire specifically about childhood inattention, hyperactivity, and impulsivity, because not all disruptive behavior during the school years can be attributed to ADHD. In some children, learning disabilities, depression, and conduct disorder may better explain such behaviors (either alone or co-occurring with ADHD).

In addition to the lack of good historical information, several other reasons for underdiagnosis of ADHD may be identified. First, many persons with both SUDs and adult ADHD were not diagnosed as children and attribute their impatience, restlessness, or procrastination to character traits of being "hot-headed," "easily bored," or "lazy." Second, many of the consequences of ADHD (such as work failure and poor educational attainment) also are associated with SUD. Persons with undiagnosed ADHD may assume that it is their alcohol or drug use that prevents them from attaining their full potential. Third, patients often develop ways to partially compensate for their ADHD symptoms, so that the symptoms of the disorder may not be obvious to the evaluating clinician. For example, adults who feel restless may learn to get up from the table and serve others as a socially appropriate way to handle their need for increased activity. Fourth, because questions regarding childhood behaviors—particularly behaviors associated with ADHD—may not be part of the "standard" assessment, it is an easy diagnosis to overlook. Unlike depression or psychosis, which cause episodic changes in functioning that may be incapacitating or require hospitalization, the symptoms of ADHD are more chronic and usually do not have such dramatic consequences. The latter are thus less likely to be noticed and attributed to a psychiatric disorder. Finally, the current diagnostic criteria for adult ADHD are problematic and need to be reexamined. As mentioned earlier, some of the symptoms required by the DSM-IV may not be developmentally appropriate and may need to be modified to better characterize the difficulties experienced by adults.

Potential Reasons for Overdiagnosis Screening instruments can be useful in identifying individuals with child and adult ADHD, but overreliance on such instruments can lead to overdiagnosis. The Wender Utah Rating Scale (111) is a self-report instrument that is used to assess individuals for childhood ADHD. Although it has been shown to have some validity among general adult patient populations, its validity among persons with SUDs has not been established. Scored items include affective symptoms, which are not part of the DSM-IV criteria. Therefore this clinical instrument may have utility in the initial screening of substance-abusing patients for childhood ADHD, but it should not replace the clinical interview. Other instruments, such as the ADHD Rating Scale or the Conners ADHD Rating Scale (112), are short screens that help to identify adults who may possibly have ADHD. However, they have not been validated in substance-abusing populations.

Overdiagnosis of adult ADHD also can occur if one ignores the functional impairment criterion. For example, it is common for individuals to procrastinate when faced with difficult projects. The difference is that adults with ADHD have had significant occupational, interpersonal, or psychologic impairment as a result of their impaired ability to start and complete tasks. It is incumbent on the clinician to ensure that a patient's current symptoms of ADHD are not limited to one setting. An individual who is completing difficult projects at home but is unable to finish assigned projects at work may be experiencing job dissatisfaction rather than ADHD. Moreover, the ADHD symptoms need to be impairing, not merely bothersome.

Another way in which the clinician may overdiagnose ADHD is by failing to confirm that a patient shows a continuity of symptoms from childhood into adulthood. Levin et al. (42) have observed that some individuals with cocaine dependence have impairing ADHD-like symptoms that occur only after a period of regular drug use, but they cannot recall having experienced ADHD symptoms in childhood. Therefore, taking a good longitudinal history is key. Further, a good medical evaluation is important because anemia and thyroid problems may mimic some of the symptoms associated with ADHD (107). However, sudden development of "ADHD symptoms" from medical causes should not be confused with ADHD if a good longitudinal history is obtained.

Finally, some individuals may feign symptoms of ADHD to get special consideration with test taking or obtain stimulant medication. Although these possibilities exist, secondary gain is more likely to occur in adolescent, non–drug-dependent groups. In substance-abusing populations, it has been our clinical experience that substance abusers are more likely to be surprised when a clinician suggests that they may have ADHD. Often these patients require psychoeducation to understand why they might have ADHD.

Other Psychiatric Comorbidity Another issue that complicates assessment and often leads to diagnostic confusion is that of additional psychiatric comorbidity. Generally, because ADHD symptoms are present in elementary school and precede the SUD, ADHD can be more readily identified as an independent disorder, compared with disorders that usually are episodic in nature and may occur only after heavy substance use has developed.

The last criterion listed in the DSM-IV for ADHD emphasizes that ADHD should not be diagnosed if the observed symptoms are better accounted for by another mental disorder. Unfortunately, some clinicians may interpret this to mean that if depression or bipolar illness is present, ADHD should not be diagnosed. In reality, these disorders may coexist. For example, common symptoms found in either a depressive disorder or ADHD include inattention, concentration difficulties, and sleep difficulties. In an active substance use, these symptoms can be exacerbated. Similarly, ADHD and hypomania and mania share many symptoms such as distractibility, talkativeness, and increased psychomotor activity.

Kessler, Adler et al. (38) found that 12-month prevalence rates of major depression, bipolar illness, and anxiety disorders were approximately double the rates for non-ADHD adults. The prevalence rate of depression was 18.6% in the ADHD group and 7.8% in the non-ADHD group. Similarly, the prevalence rate of bipolar illness was 19.4% in the ADHD group and 3.1% in the non-ADHD group. The presence of certain symptoms provides helpful clues in discerning whether one or both disorders and present. Individuals with major depression may experience symptoms of inattention, but are less likely to have hyperactivity and talkativeness associated with ADHD. Further, if suicidality is present, this is unlikely to be from ADHD alone.

Bowden (113) found that when treatment-seeking children with bipolar illness were compared with 60 outpatient children with ADHD certain features common to bipolar illness were relatively uncommon in those with ADHD (e.g., elevated mood, grandiosity, flight of ideas). Further, individuals with bipolar illness are more likely to describe discrete periods of increased restlessness, talkativeness, and hyperactivity, and the like, whereas those with adult ADHD will be more likely to describe a life-long constellation of these symptoms to a lesser degree. Importantly, individuals with ADHD typically do not exhibit psychotic symptoms. If these are present, they indicate the likelihood of an additional mood disturbance or a substance-induced psychotic disorder.

Often adults with ADHD have first-degree relatives with ADHD; their presence may suggest that the individual in question has ADHD. However, depression and bipolar illness also are overrepresented in families of individuals diagnosed with ADHD (114,115), complicating the diagnostic picture.

Determining whether an individual has ADHD alone, has multiple psychiatric disorders, or has a psychiatric disorder other than ADHD rests on clinical judgment. Initial treatment is usually focused on the more severe illness present. However, this should not preclude attention to the other disorder when improvement in symptoms of the more severe illness occurs (109). Again, a comprehensive diagnostic assessment that addresses psychiatric comorbidity and pertinent family history is needed before initiating any pharmacotherapy.

TREATMENT OF CO-OCCURRING ADHD AND SUD

Patients with co-occurring ADHD and SUD present a formidable challenge for any clinician treating such individuals. First, as previously described, it is often difficult to accurately diagnose ADHD in patients seeking treatment for SUD, because the symptoms of symptoms of substance use or withdrawal can mimic ADHD. Furthermore, ADHD symptoms are chronic in nature and do not necessarily attract clinical attention on initial presentation for SUD treatment. Finally, because psychostimulants remain the primary treatment modality for ADHD, many clinicians are reluctant to prescribe such medications to patients presenting with SUD. Frequently, consideration of the prospective diagnosis and treatment of ADHD is not part of an initial treatment plan, as the treatment would be deemed "unacceptable" to the SUD program. As the literature regarding the consequences of untreated ADHD grows, the identification and treatment of comorbid ADHD in patients with SUD is an increasing clinical priority.

Compared with other patients with SUDs, individuals with ADHD may have greater difficulties in processing information and in sitting through group meetings—a common format for addiction treatment. Because individuals with ADHD have a tendency to act impulsively, they also may be more likely than those without ADHD to drop out of treatment. Counselors and other patients may find individuals with untreated ADHD to be "frustrating." By recognizing and treating the ADHD, patients' attentional and behavioral problems may be alleviated and as a result their treatment outcomes may be improved.

In this section, we will provide an overview of the pharmacologic and nonpharmacologic therapies available, offer some general guidelines in choosing the most appropriate therapeutic option, and discuss optimal treatment strategies for the treatment of ADHD in a patient with SUD.

PHARMACOTHERAPEUTIC OPTIONS FOR TREATMENT OF ADHD CO-OCCURRING WITH SUD

Amphetamine analogues and methylphenidate have been the most widely studied pharmacotherapies for adult ADHD, although nonstimulant medications, including atomoxetine, tricyclic antidepressants, bupropion, monoamine oxidase inhibitors, alpha-2 agonists, and venlafaxine have been studied as well. Modafinil, a novel stimulant medication with seemingly lower potential for abuse than traditional stimulant medications, has also been studied for the treatment of ADHD. Although there is substantial evidence for the efficacy of these agents in adults with ADHD, there are only a limited number of studies of patients with co-occurring ADHD and SUD.

Stimulant Medications Amphetamine analogues and methylphenidate are the stimulant medications most commonly used to treat ADHD in children and adults in the United States. Methylphenidate is a piperidine derivative that is structurally related to amphetamine, whose mechanism of action is primarily due to dopamine reuptake blockade in the striatum (116). Methylphenidate has been one of the first-line treatments for ADHD in children for decades and has been demonstrated to be safe and effective for the treatment of ADHD in adults (117). Methylphenidate is available in multiple immediate and sustained-release preparations for delayed absorption.

Amphetamine stimulates the cerebral cortex and the reticular activating system primarily by enhancing dopamine release, although it also blocks dopamine reuptake (116). Amphetamine analogs, first-line treatments for childhood ADHD, have also been shown to be effective for the treatment of ADHD in adults (118). Commercially available amphetamine analogs include methamphetamine, dextroamphetamine, and mixed amphetamine salts. Methamphetamine is only available in an immediate-release preparation and is rarely prescribed because of concerns for abuse and diversion. Dextroamphetamine is available in immediate and sustained-release preparations. Mixed amphetamine salts are fixed-combination amphetamine composed of equal amounts of dextroamphetamine saccharate, dextroamphetamine sulfate, racemic amphetamine aspartate monohydrate, and racemic amphetamine sulfate. Mixed amphetamine salts are available in immediate and sustained-release preparations. Side effects most commonly associated with amphetamine and methylphenidate administration include insomnia, emotional lability, nausea/vomiting, nervousness, palpitations, elevated blood pressure, and rapid heart rate. Rare but serious adverse effects include severe hypertension, seizures, psychosis, and myocardial infarction.

Abuse Potential of Psychostimulants Although methylphenidate and amphetamine analogs are widely used in the treatment of ADHD; concern exists with respect to their abuse potential, particularly in patients with SUD. According to the 2003 National Survey on Drug Use and Health, 8.8% of Americans age 12 years or older reported lifetime nonmedical use of prescription stimulant medications (119). Clearly, the risks of using stimulant medications in a population vulnerable to misuse and abuse must be considered carefully.

There is a limited body of evidence available to consider when assessing the risks of using stimulant medications in patients with SUD. In a laboratory double-blind choice procedure, individuals with ADHD significantly chose methylphenidate over placebo (120), whereas other measures of abuse potential were not elevated. In laboratory studies of patients with (121) and without (122) SUD, both methylphenidate and amphetamine analogues demonstrated characteristics associated with abuse potential. Methamphetamine, which is a commonly abused substance (119), has been shown in a laboratory setting to be a positive reinforcer (i.e., individuals exposed to the substance are likely to choose to be exposed again) (123). However, in contrast, a laboratory study of methylphenidate in cocaine-dependent patients receiving treatment showed neither increased neither cocaine craving nor ratings associated with abuse potential (124), suggesting that the therapeutic context may influence subjective effects and abuse potential (125).

The therapeutic use of stimulant medications has been studied in patients with co-occurring adult ADHD and SUD, with mixed reports of efficacy. Methylphenidate has been shown to be effective in uncontrolled trials in reducing ADHD symptoms and cocaine use (46,126). Recently, a three-arm, double-blind, placebo-controlled trial for the treatment of ADHD in cocaine-dependent patients receiving methadone maintenance treatment for opioid dependence was conducted with bupropion and methylphenidate. Neither bupropion nor methylphenidate significantly improved either ADHD symptoms or cocaine use outcomes (4). A double-blind, placebo-controlled trial of methylphenidate in the treatment of co-occurring adult ADHD and cocaine dependence found that methylphenidate improved ADHD symptoms on some measures, but not others, and did not show a reduction in cocaine use (127). In another placebo-controlled, double-blind trial (128), ADHD symptoms were reduced in patients receiving either placebo or sustained-release methylphenidate. For the primary drug use outcome measure there was no superiority of methylphenidate compared to placebo. However, on a secondary outcome measure, proportion in cocaine-positive urine over time, sustained-release methylphenidate showed a greater reduction than placebo. In none of the trials using stimulants was abuse or misuse of prescribed stimulant medication reported.

Further evidence of the feasibility of using stimulant medications for the treatment of co-occurring ADHD and SUD can be found in the literature describing the use of stimulant treatment of cocaine dependence. The results of these studies have been mixed with regard to effects on cocaine use outcomes, with the most consistent positive effects reported for dextroamphetamine (129,130). Dextroamphetamine has also been studied for the substitution treatment of amphetamine dependence (131,132) and this approach has been proven to be successful. Despite concerns that prescription stimulant use may lead to increased craving and cocaine or amphetamine use, this effect has not been reported in the controlled clinical trials conducted to date (4,127,129,130,133,134). In summary, although prescription stimulant medications may be diverted for nonmedical use, clinical data suggest that the use of stimulants in a structured therapeutic context can be accomplished safely.

Use and Misuse of Stimulant Medication One of the greatest concerns that clinicians have when prescribing stimulants is that these medications will be misused by the patient or that the medication will be diverted and misused or abused by others. Misuse is defined as any medication usage that has not been prescribed by the treating physician, including taking medication prescribed to others or taking higher doses than indicated. Misuse should be distinguished from prescription drug abuse or dependence, as underlying motivations for stimulant misuse can vary. McCabe et al. (135) found that among 12th graders, approximately 5% reported using methylphenidate. Further, high school students with poorer grades were more likely to use methylphenidate. For college students, a small overall percentage reported using methylphenidate in the past year (4.1%), with rates being higher in males than females (6.8% vs. 3.5%). Further, McCabe et al. (136) found that the percentage of methylphenidate use was higher in most competitive than least competitive schools (5.9% vs. 1.3%), suggesting that methylphenidate may be used to enhance performance or may be associated with higher socioeconomic status.

Interestingly, the increased risk of illicit use as compared to medicinal use with stimulants is higher than with other medications (137). Individuals who receive medication for ADHD are twice as likely to be asked to divert their medication than those receiving medications for pain, sleep, or anxiety (137). For the 5.4% of undergraduates who had illicitly used prescription stimulants in the past year at one college campus, nearly 60% reported using stimulants to concentrate (138). More than 40% reported using stimulants to increase their awareness with a similar percentage reporting use to get high. Thus the reasons for use are multifactorial and may or may not be associated with abuse or dependence.

Abuse Liability of Short- and Long-Acting Formulations of Prescription Stimulants in the General Population Although many of those who illicitly use stimulants do so for performance enhancement, a substantial number report using to get "high." The studies described here often do not make a distinction between immediate-release preparations and long-acting formulations and there may be substantive differences in the subjective effects and abuse liability of different stimulant preparations. Long-acting preparations of stimulant medications were initially developed to reduce the frequency of dosing and provide consistent therapeutic blood levels throughout the day. However, evidence is accumulating that long-acting preparations may have lower abuse potential and may have particular utility for patients with co-occurring SUD. Because the reinforcing effects of stimulants are associated with rapid changes in serum concentrations (125), sustained-release preparations of methylphenidate or amphetamine, which slow the rate of onset of the drug's effect, are likely to be associated with less positive subjective drug effects.

Kollins et al. (139) found that sustained-release methylphenidate produced fewer subjective effects than immediate-release methylphenidate. In an elegant neuroimaging study conducted by Spencer et al. (140), non–substance-abusing adults without ADHD were administered immediate release methylphenidate or OROS-methylphenidate (Concerta) with similar maximum methylphenidate concentration. Not surprisingly, time to reach maximum concentration and dopamine receptor occupancy was longer in the OROS-methylphenidate group and this was associated with significantly lower ratings of "feeling an effect" or "liking the effect." These data suggest that long-acting stimulants may less likely to be misused for their euphorigenic effects. An additional advantage of delayed-release preparations is greater difficult to using via a nonoral route (e.g., injected, intranasally), which should also reduce the potential for misuse and diversion.

Abuse Liability of Prescription Stimulants in Individuals with ADHD With and Without Active Substance Dependence What is less clear is how common prescription stimulants are abused in ADHD individuals and substance abusers in need of treatment. Whereas MacDonald Fredericks et al. (141) found that non–substance-abusing individuals with ADHD had diminished subjective effects from methylphenidate, under choice procedures, methylphenidate was more likely to be chosen than placebo in nonsubstance-abusing individuals with ADHD (141). Further, in a survey of 300+ college students who received methylphenidate for treatment of ADHD, 22% reported that they had used the medication to get high and nearly 29% reported selling or giving their medication to others (142). In a 10-year longitudinal study of 98 subjects receiving psychotropic medication Wilens et al. found that most ADHD individuals used their medications appropriately. However, those with conduct disorder or SUDs reported more misuse and diversion and there appeared to be more misuse and diversion of immediate-release compared with extended-release stimulants (143). For cocaine-dependent individuals, Collins et al. (144) found that those with ADHD experienced similar subjective effects to cocaine as those without ADHD. However, the subjective effects of cocaine were lessened when cocaine-dependent individuals with ADHD were maintained on higher doses of sustained-released methylphenidate compared with a lower dose of sustained-release methylphenidate or placebo.

Even though misuse and diversion of prescription stimulants, particular long-acting preparations, is not widespread in the general population or substance abusers in treatment, there is reason for concern. In most cases, there is a lack of physician oversight for those individuals who are using stimulants illicitly and therefore, there is no cardiovascular screening or warnings about possible interactions with other stimulants or over-the-counter nonstimulant preparations. It is crucial that patients who are prescribed stimulants for their ADHD, regardless of whether they are current abusers, past substance abusers, or have no history of abuse be warned about the risks associated with prescription stimulant use, understand why it is important not to "share" their medication with others and be given strategies of how to safeguard their medication so that it is not diverted.

Nonstimulant Medications A diverse group of nonstimulant medications has been identified as having some efficacy for the treatment of ADHD, although none has been shown to be therapeutically equivalent to stimulant medications. With the exception of atomoxetine, all nonstimulant medications are "off-label" for ADHD and are generally considered second- or third-line treatments. There are certain instances where nonstimulant medications would be considered first line, such as if a motor tic disorder is present or in the case of cardiovascular disease. It remains controversial whether the presence of even an active SUD represents such a significant risk that the superior efficacy of stimulant medications should be traded off for the lower abuse potential of nonstimulant medications.

Atomoxetine, a centrally acting noradrenergic reuptake inhibitor (145,146), is the only U.S. Food and Drug Administration–approved nonstimulant agent medication for ADHD. The onset of therapeutic effects of atomoxetine are more gradual than that experienced with stimulant medications and takes several weeks to manifest, much akin to antidepressant treatment for depression. Common side effects of atomoxetine include sedation, appetite suppression, nausea, vomiting, and headache. Rare but serious side effects reported in children and adolescents include increased suicidal ideation and hepatotoxicity. Atomoxetine has no known abuse potential, so it is an attractive candidate medication for study in the treatment of ADHD in patients with SUDs, although published data are lacking.

A number of antidepressant agents, typically those with stimulating properties, have been studied for the treatment of ADHD. Tricyclic antidepressants, which block the reuptake of norepinephrine, have some efficacy in reducing ADHD symptoms, but are considered to be less effective than the stimulant medications (147). The dopaminergic antidepressant bupropion has been reported to be effective in the treatment of ADHD (148–150), although when studied in patients with SUD it offered no benefit over placebo (4). Venlafaxine, a norepinephrine-serotonin reuptake inhibitor antidepressant medication, has limited evidence of efficacy in ADHD in uncontrolled clinical trials (151,152). Monoamine oxidase inhibitors have been shown to have efficacy for ADHD, but the potential for hypertensive crises associated with tyramine-containing foods and medications (both illicit and prescribed) limit their utility, and MAOIs should be considered contraindicated in patients with SUD.

Clonidine, a noradrenergic alpha-2 agonist antihypertensive agent, has been shown to be effective for the treatment of ADHD (153). Side effects include sedation, dry mouth, depression, confusion, electrocardiographic changes, and hypertension with abrupt withdrawal. Guanfacine, also a norepinephrine alpha-2 agonist, has limited evidence supporting its efficacy as a treatment for ADHD (154,155). Modafinil, a novel wake-promoting agent that is U.S. Food and Drug Administration–approved for narcolepsy and shift work sleep, has recently been reported to improve ADHD symptoms in children and adolescents (156–158) and limited evidence suggests that it may be effective for adult ADHD as well (159). Further there are some data suggesting that modafinil may have potential as a treatment for cocaine dependence (160) and is deserving of further study in the treatment of co-occurring ADHD and SUD. Although modafinil has some stimulant-like properties (e.g., promoting wakefulness), it has minimal reported abuse potential reported and has not been shown to be as effective as traditional stimulant medications, so for the purposes of discussion it is being grouped with nonstimulant-second line agents.

PHARMACOTHERAPY SELECTION FOR ADHD AND CO-OCCURRING SUD

At present there are no clear-cut guidelines regarding the appropriate use of traditional stimulant medications, methylphenidate and amphetamine analogues, in the treatment of adult ADHD and SUD. Stimulant medications are the gold standard for reducing ADHD symptoms, yet their use carries with it a known risk of misuse and diversion. In choosing between stimulant and nonstimulant agents for co-occurring ADHD and SUD is balancing the risk of untreated ADHD symptoms versus the risk of stimulant misuse and diversion. In developing a treatment plan for co-occurring ADHD and SUD these risks must be considered in light of the individual characteristics of the patient in question. The appropriateness of the medication choice should be regularly reassessed based on the patient's clinical response and overall clinical status. General recommendations for pharmacotherapy management of ADHD and co-occurring SUD follow.

To help organize treatment planning decision making, we propose classifying patients with co-occurring ADHD and SUD into three risk groups: low, moderate, and severe (Table 87.2) The most important clinical variable in considering the use of stimulant medication is whether the SUD is active or in remission. Patients with a remote history of a SUD and a long period of abstinence from substance use likely represent a low-risk group for prescribing stimulant medications. Patients should be counseled that their history of SUD may put them at increased risk and general prescribing precautions should be employed (e.g., use of delayed-release preparations, monitoring prescription renewal times, surveillance for evidence of substance use).

Patients with ongoing substance use, but not consistent with a diagnosis of abuse or dependence, likely represent an increased risk of misuse and diversion of prescription stimulants. For these patients who are elevated risk, additional controls need to be in place to use prescription stimulants safely. More frequent office visits, urine toxicology testing, and monitoring the pattern of substance use are prudent measures. For these patients, nonstimulants may represent desirable alternatives, although with increased likelihood of a less robust response (161).

TABLE 87.2 Suggested Treatment Stratification for Co-occurring ADHD/SUD

- Low-risk group (e.g., 20 years abstinent from alcohol, no current illicit drug use)
  - Brief office intervention
  - Advise of the risk of combining with prescription stimulants with other substances
  - Warn about diversion
  - Ongoing monitoring
  - ADHD response
  - Use/abuse pattern
  - Use delayed absorption formulation when prescribing stimulants
- Moderate-risk group (e.g., some substance use but not current abuse/dependence; misuse of stimulants in past)
  - Include strategies for low-risk group
  - More frequent office visits
  - Very close attention to patterns of alcohol/drug use
  - Urine toxicology testing
  - Use delayed absorption formulation when prescribing stimulants
- High-risk group (e.g., active SUD)
  - Include strategies for moderate risk group
  - May try nonstimulants first
  - If poor response to nonstimulant, switch to long-acting stimulant
  - Require counseling, involvement with self-help group, or referral to appropriate substance abuse treatment
  - If severe SUD may refer for intensive intervention before starting medication
  - May need to avoid stimulants if they have history or current abuser/dependence on prescription stimulants or high risk of diversion of medication (i.e., sold medication in past)

ADHD, attention deficit/hyperactivity disorder; SUD, substance abuse disorder.

Patients with an active SUD represent a high-risk group for prescription stimulant treatment of ADHD. For these patients, given the elevated risk of misuse or diversion, nonstimulant medications are likely to be a first-line choice. However, in cases where response to nonstimulant medications is suboptimal, stimulant medications may be considered in certain circumstances. For example, stimulant treatment of a patient with an active SUD may be indicated in an intensive structured and monitored outpatient treatment program.

Certain precautions are warranted when using stimulants in substance-abusing patients. Keeping careful records of prescriptions written and the number of pills given is crucial. By seeing the patient on a frequent basis, the number of pills per prescription can be reduced, the patient's treatment response can be closely monitored, and any potential interactions between the stimulant and other abused substances can be identified. It should be made clear to patients that urine toxicology screens will be conducted routinely, and that if the patient does not show a clinically significant reduction in alcohol or drug use, other treatment strategies will be implemented. Patients should ingest their medication on a regular schedule, rather than on an as-needed basis, to avoid inadequate and intermittent palliation of symptoms. Our recommendation would be to use long-acting preparations for ADHD in patients with SUD to reduce the potential for misuse although clinical data are lacking to support this approach. Novel delivery systems such as the crush-resistant shell of Concerta (Alza Corporation, Fort Washington, PA) (162) or the recently U.S. Food and Drug Administration–approved methylphenidate skin patch (Daytrana), are more resistant to misuse, and may be desirable alternatives in patients with co-occurring ADHD and SUD.

Finally, persons with co-occurring ADHD and SUD who are treated with stimulants may abuse or divert their medication. Thus these possibilities should be discussed with the patient before a stimulant is prescribed. Similar to the approach in other areas of clinical uncertainty, good clinical judgment becomes crucial when deciding who will benefit from a pharmacologic treatment intervention and which medications should be used. With careful ongoing monitoring and surveillance, emergent problems can be identified early and the treatment plan modified. Possible signs and symptoms of misuse or abuse of prescription stimulant medications include: frequent lost prescriptions or discordant pill counts, demands for immediate-release preparations, continuously escalating doses, psychosis, agitation, and physiologic toxicity (hypertension, tachycardia, or chest pain).

Nonpharmacologic Interventions Compared with the pharmacologic treatment literature, there are even fewer clinical data to suggest which nonpharmacologic approaches work best for persons with substance abuse disorders and adult ADHD. As in the treatment of substance abusers with other psychiatric disorders, concurrently treating the symptoms of both the SUD and the ADHD is more likely to produce a positive treatment outcome than treating one disorder alone. In both the treatment literature for childhood ADHD and for SUDs, positive outcomes are reported with the use of behavioral approaches. Such approaches include contingency management, cognitive-behavioral interventions, and combined pharmacologic and behavioral interventions.

Whereas positive contingencies have been stressed as an appropriate treatment for adults with SUDs (163), there have been no contingency management strategies targeted to persons with both adult ADHD and SUD. Whereas children with ADHD may receive (or lose) a token for following (or breaking) a classroom rule, establishing a token economy system for ADHD behaviors manifested in adulthood would prove more difficult.

Cognitive-behavioral therapy has become an integral part of many addiction treatment programs. The question is whether this approach works equally well for persons with comorbid ADHD and SUD. The use of cognitive interventions for children with ADHD has included "verbal self-instructions, problem-solving strategies, cognitive modeling, self-evaluation, and self-reinforcement." The Multimodal Treatment Study of Children with ADHD (164) demonstrated that combined medication and behavioral treatment did not yield significantly greater benefits than medication management for core ADHD symptoms, but may have provided modest advantages for non-ADHD symptom and positive functioning outcomes (165). Children with ADHD and anxiety responded nearly as well to behavioral treatment as they did to medication management or combined treatment (166). For those ADHD children without a comorbid anxiety disorder, medication or combined treatment was superior to behavioral treatment alone. These data imply that adults with ADHD and comorbid anxiety may do particularly well with behavioral approaches. A randomized trial of cognitive-behavioral therapy plus psychopharmacology versus psychopharmacology alone for adults with ADHD showed a superiority of combined treatment on independently rated ADHD symptoms (167).

Adults, in contrast to children, have a greater potential to understand the effects of ADHD symptoms on their lives and thus may be better able to use cognitive-behavioral approaches. However, such approaches may need to be modified for persons with ADHD and SUD (less emphasis on homework tasks and more emphasis on session work). Weinstein (168) has suggested several attention and memory strategies that may have clinical utility for individuals with ADHD in addiction treatment settings.

Using a manualized relapse prevention approach, Aviram et al. (169) found that the challenge for therapists is to identify the links among the cognitive, behavioral, and physiologic symptoms associated with ADHD and those associated with drug use. Limitations stemming from ADHD, as well as feelings of negative self-worth, may lead to drug use, which is self-reinforcing and further limits the patient's coping abilities. The limitations must be countered in treatment by providing tangible coping skills and techniques, many of which are incorporated into the relapse prevention model.

Two experimental approaches that also might be useful for persons with ADHD and SUD are nodal-link mapping and sensory integration. Nodal-link mapping consists of drawing spatial-verbal displays to represent interrelationships among ideas, feelings, facts, and experiences (170). Although Dansereau et al. (171) did not specifically assess subjects for adult ADHD, they compared the efficacy of nodal-mapping with standard counseling in reducing substance abuse among methadone-maintained patients. Individuals who received standard therapy or had poor attention did less well in methadone treatment. However, mapping-enhanced counseling reduced the negative effects of poor attention.

The other experimental approach, sensory integration, seeks to integrate stimuli in an organized manner. Within an inpatient addiction treatment setting, Stratton and Gailfus (9) found that this technique reduced impulsivity, enhanced anger control and attention span, and improved treatment retention. Although these approaches show promise, there are few controlled trials to guide treatment in the comorbid population.

SUMMARY

Clearly, many questions remain regarding the diagnosis and treatment of persons with co-occurring adult ADHD and SUD. The reliability and validity of screening instruments for both childhood and adult ADHD are yet to be established. Further, the utility of various neuropsychologic tests has not been determined. Although stimulant medications have proved useful in treating adult ADHD, their benefits in active substance abusers is mixed, with some effect in reducing ADHD symptoms and less clear efficacy in reducing drug use. Fewer data exist to support the use of nonstimulants or nonpharmacologic treatment strategies for adults with ADHD and a SUD. Given the substantial subpopulation of persons with SUD and adult ADHD, further research is warranted.

REFERENCES

1. Mannuzza S, Klein RG, Bessler A, et al. Adult outcome of hyperactive boys. Educational achievement, occupational rank, and psychiatric status. *Arch Gen Psychiatry* 1993;50:565–576.
2. Mannuzza S, Klein RG, Bonagura N, et al. Hyperactive boys almost grown up. V. Replication of psychiatric status. *Arch Gen Psychiatry* 1991;48:77–83.
3. Barkley R. *Attention-deficit hyperactivity disorder*, New York: The Guilford Press, 2006.
4. Levin FR, Evans SM, Brooks DJ, et al. Treatment of cocaine dependent treatment seekers with adult ADHD: double-blind comparison of methylphenidate and placebo. *Drug Alcohol Depend* 2007;87(1): 20–29.
5. Levin FR, Bisaga A, Raby W, et al. Effects of major depressive disorder and attention-deficit/hyperactivity disorder on the outcome of treatment for cocaine dependence. *J Subst Abuse Treatment* 2008;34(1):80–89.

6. Carpentier PJ, de Jong CA, Dijkstra BA, et al. A controlled trial of methylphenidate in adults with attention deficit/hyperactivity disorder and substance use disorders. *Addiction* 2005;100:1868–1874.
7. Carroll KM, Rounsaville BJ. History and significance of childhood attention deficit disorder in treatment-seeking cocaine abusers. *Compr Psychiatry* 1993;34:75–82.
8. Levin FR, Evans SM, Vosburg SK, et al. Impact of attention-deficit hyperactivity disorder and other psychopathology on treatment retention among cocaine abusers in a therapeutic community. *Addict Behav* 2004;29:1875–1882.
9. Stratton J, Gailfus D. A new approach to substance abuse treatment. Adolescents and adults with ADHD. *J Subst Abuse Treatment* 1998;15: 89–94.
10. Sullivan M, Levin F. Attention deficit/hyperactivity disorder and substance abuse: diagnostic and therapeutic considerations. In: J Wasserstein, LE Wolf, FF Lefever, eds. *Adult attention deficit disorder: brain mechanisms and life outcomes.* New York: New York Academy of Sciences, 2001, 251–270.
11. White AM, Jordan JD, Schroeder KM, et al. Predictors of relapse during treatment and treatment completion among marijuana-dependent adolescents in an intensive outpatient substance abuse program. *Subst Abuse* 2004;25:53–59.
12. Biederman J. Attention-deficit/hyperactivity disorder: a selective overview. *Biol Psychiatry* 2005;57:1215–1220.
13. Faraone SV, Perlis RH, Doyle AE, et al. Molecular genetics of attention-deficit/hyperactivity disorder. *Biol Psychiatry* 2005;57:1313–1323.
14. Acosta MT, Arcos-Burgos M, Muenke M. Attention deficit/hyperactivity disorder (ADHD): complex phenotype, simple genotype? *Genet Med* 2004;6:1–15.
15. Faraone SV, Biederman J. Neurobiology of attention-deficit hyperactivity disorder. *Biol Psychiatry* 1998;44:951–958.
16. Thapar A, O'Donovan M, Owen MJ. The genetics of attention deficit hyperactivity disorder. *Hum Mol Genet* 2005;14 Spec No. 2:R275–R282.
17. Wang X, Zhong P, Yan Z. Dopamine D4 receptors modulate GABAergic signaling in pyramidal neurons of prefrontal cortex. *J Neurosci* 2002; 22:9185–9193.
18. Staller JA, Faraone SV. Targeting the dopamine system in the treatment of attention-deficit/hyperactivity disorder. *Expert Rev Neurother* 2007;7: 351–362.
19. Drabant EM, Hariri AR, Meyer-Lindenberg A, et al. Catechol O-methyltransferase val158met genotype and neural mechanisms related to affective arousal and regulation. *Arch Gen Psychiatry* 2006;63: 1396–1406.
20. Sowell ER, Thompson PM, Welcome SE, et al. Cortical abnormalities in children and adolescents with attention-deficit hyperactivity disorder. *Lancet* 2003;362:1699–1707.
21. Arnsten AF. Fundamentals of attention-deficit/hyperactivity disorder: circuits and pathways. *J Clin Psychiatry* 2006;67(Suppl 8):7–12.
22. Spencer TJ, Biederman J, Mick E. Attention-deficit/hyperactivity disorder: diagnosis, lifespan, comorbidities, and neurobiology. *Ambul Pediatr* 2007;7:73–81.
23. Castellanos FX, Lee PP, Sharp W, et al. Developmental trajectories of brain volume abnormalities in children and adolescents with attention-deficit/hyperactivity disorder. *JAMA* 2002;288:1740–1748.
24. Bush G, Valera EM, Seidman LJ. Functional neuroimaging of attention-deficit/hyperactivity disorder: a review and suggested future directions. *Biol Psychiatry* 2005;57:1273–1284.
25. Alexander GE, DeLong MR, Strick PL. Parallel organization of functionally segregated circuits linking basal ganglia and cortex. *Annu Rev Neurosci* 1986;9:357–381.
26. McCormick MC, Workman-Daniels K, Brooks-Gunn J. The behavioral and emotional well-being of school-age children with different birth weights. *Pediatrics* 1996;97:18–25.
27. Braun JM, Kahn RS, Froehlich T, et al. Exposures to environmental toxicants and attention deficit hyperactivity disorder in U.S. children. *Environ Health Perspect* 2006;114:1904–1909.
28. Biederman J, Mick E, Faraone SV. Normalized functioning in youths with persistent attention-deficit/hyperactivity disorder. *J Pediatr* 1998;133:544–551.
29. Pineda DA, Palacio LG, Puerta IC, et al. Environmental influences that affect attention deficit/hyperactivity disorder: study of a genetic isolate. *Eur Child Adolesc Psychiatry* 2007;16:337–346.
30. Lewine JD, Davis JT, Bigler ED, et al. Objective documentation of traumatic brain injury subsequent to mild head trauma: multimodal brain imaging with MEG, SPECT, and MRI. *Jo Head Trauma Rehabil* 2007;22:141–155.
31. Anderson V, Anderson D, Anderson P. Comparing attentional skills in children with acquired and developmental central nervous system disorders. *J Int Neuropsychol Soc* 2006;12:519–531.
32. Ziino C, Ponsford J. Selective attention deficits and subjective fatigue following traumatic brain injury. *Neuropsychology* 2006;20:383–390.
33. McAvinue L, O'Keeffe F, McMackin D, et al. Impaired sustained attention and error awareness in traumatic brain injury: implications for insight. *Neuropsychol Rehabil* 2005;15:569–587.
34. Faraone SV, Sergeant J, Gillberg C, et al. The worldwide prevalence of ADHD: is it an American condition? *World Psychiatry* 2003;2: 104–113.
35. Rasmussen P, Gillberg C. Natural outcome of ADHD with developmental coordination disorder at age 22 years: a controlled, longitudinal, community-based study. *J Am Acad Child Adolesc Psychiatry* 2000;39: 1424–1431.
36. Barkley RA, Fischer M, Smallish L, et al. The persistence of attention-deficit/hyperactivity disorder into young adulthood as a function of reporting source and definition of disorder. *J Abnorm Psychol* 2002;111: 279–289.
37. Biederman J, Mick E, Faraone SV. Age-dependent decline of symptoms of attention deficit hyperactivity disorder: impact of remission definition and symptom type. *Am J Psychiatry* 2000;157:816–818.
38. Kessler RC, Adler L, Barkley R, et al. The prevalence and correlates of adult ADHD in the United States: results from the National Comorbidity Survey Replication. *Am J Psychiatry* 2006;163:716–723.
39. Weiss RD, Mirin SM, Griffin ML, et al. Psychopathology in cocaine abusers. Changing trends. *J Nerv Ment Dis* 1988;176:719–725.
40. Wilens TE, Dodson W. A clinical perspective of attention-deficit/ hyperactivity disorder into adulthood. *J Clin Psychiatry* 2004;65: 1301–1313.
41. Wood D, Wender PH, Reimherr FW. The prevalence of attention deficit disorder, residual type, or minimal brain dysfunction, in a population of male alcoholic patients. *Am J Psychiatry* 1983;140:95–98.
42. Levin FR, Evans SM, Kleber HD. Prevalence of adult attention-deficit hyperactivity disorder among cocaine abusers seeking treatment. *Drug Alcohol Depend* 1998;52:15–25.
43. Clure C, Brady KT, Saladin ME, et al. Attention-deficit/hyperactivity disorder and substance use: symptom pattern and drug choice. *Am J Drug Alcohol Abuse* 1999;25:441–448.
44. Schubiner H, Tzelepis A, Milberger S, et al. Prevalence of attention-deficit/hyperactivity disorder and conduct disorder among substance abusers. *J Clin Psychiatry* 2000;61:244–251.
45. King VL, Brooner RK, Kidorf MS, et al. Attention deficit hyperactivity disorder and treatment outcome in opioid abusers entering treatment. *J Nerv Ment Dis* 1999;187:487–495.
46. Levin FR, Evans SM, McDowell DM, et al. Methylphenidate treatment for cocaine abusers with adult attention-deficit/hyperactivity disorder: a pilot study. *J Clin Psychiatry* 1998;59:300–305.
47. Rounsaville B, Carroll K. Psychiatric disorders in treatment-entering cocaine abusers. *NIDA Res Monogr* 1991;110:227–251.
48. Regier DA, Farmer ME, Rae DS, et al. Comorbidity of mental disorders with alcohol and other drug abuse. Results from the Epidemiologic Catchment Area (ECA) Study [see comment]. *JAMA* 1990;264:2511–2518.
49. Kessler RC, McGonagle KA, Zhao S, et al. Lifetime and 12-month prevalence of DSM-III-R psychiatric disorders in the United States. Results from the National Comorbidity Survey. *Arch Gen Psychiatry* 1994;51:8–19.
50. Biederman J, Wilens T, Mick E, et al. Psychoactive substance use disorders in adults with attention deficit hyperactivity disorder (ADHD): effects of ADHD and psychiatric comorbidity. *Am J Psychiatry* 1995;152:1652–1658.

51. Biederman J, Faraone SV, Spencer T, et al. Patterns of psychiatric comorbidity, cognition, and psychosocial functioning in adults with attention deficit hyperactivity disorder. *Am J Psychiatry* 1993;150:1792–1798.
52. Pomerleau OF, Downey KK, Stelson FW, et al. Cigarette smoking in adult patients diagnosed with attention deficit hyperactivity disorder. *J Subst Abuse* 1995;7:373–378.
53. Tercyak KP, Lerman C, Audrain J. Association of attention-deficit/hyperactivity disorder symptoms with levels of cigarette smoking in a community sample of adolescents. *J Am Acad Child Adolesc Psychiatry* 2002;41:799–805.
54. Kollins SH, McClernon FJ, Fuemmeler BF. Association between smoking and attention-deficit/hyperactivity disorder symptoms in a population-based sample of young adults. *Arch Gen Psychiatry* 2005;62:1142–1147.
55. Lambert NM, Hartsough CS. Prospective study of tobacco smoking and substance dependencies among samples of ADHD and non-ADHD participants. *J Learn Disabil* 1998;31:533–544.
56. Mannuzza S, Klein RG. Long-term prognosis in attention-deficit/hyperactivity disorder. *Child Adolesc Psychiatr Clin N Am* 2000;9:711–726.
57. Murphy KR, Barkley RA. Prevalence of DSM-IV symptoms of ADHD in adult licensed drivers: Implications of clinical diagnosis. *J Atten Disord* 1996;1:147–161.
58. Greenfield B, Hechtman L, Weiss G. Two subgroups of hyperactives as adults: correlations of outcome. *Can J Psychiatry Revue Can Psychiatrie* 1988;33:505–508.
59. Birnbaum HG, Kessler RC, Lowe SW, et al. Costs of attention deficit-hyperactivity disorder (ADHD) in the U.S.: excess costs of persons with ADHD and their family members in 2000. *Curr Med Res Opin* 2005; 21:195–206.
60. Kessler RC, Merikangas KR. The National Comorbidity Survey Replication (NCS-R): background and aims. *Int J Methods Psychiatr Res* 2004; 13:60–68.
61. Kessler RC, Adler L, Ames M, et al. The prevalence and effects of adult attention deficit/hyperactivity disorder on work performance in a nationally representative sample of workers. *J Occup Environ Med* 2005; 47:565–572.
62. Wilens TE, Biederman J, Mick E. Does ADHD affect the course of substance abuse? Findings from a sample of adults with and without ADHD. *Am J Addic* 1998;7:156–163.
63. Levin FR, Evans SM, McDowell DM, et al. Bupropion treatment for cocaine abuse and adult attention-deficit/hyperactivity disorder. *J Addict Dis* 2002;21:1–16.
64. Gittelman R, Mannuzza S, Shenker R, et al. Hyperactive boys almost grown up. I. Psychiatric status. *Arch Gen Psychiatry* 1985;42:937–947.
65. Mannuzza S, Klein RG, Addalli KA. Young adult mental status of hyperactive boys and their brothers: a prospective follow-up study. *J Amer Acad Child Adolesc Psychiatry* 1991;30:743–751.
66. Thompson LL, Riggs PD, Mikulich SK, et al. Contribution of ADHD symptoms to substance problems and delinquency in conduct-disordered adolescents. *J Abnorm Child Psychol* 1996;24:325–347.
67. Milberger S, Biederman J, Faraone SV, et al. Associations between ADHD and psychoactive substance use disorders. Findings from a longitudinal study of high-risk siblings of ADHD children. *Am J Addict* 1997;6:318–329.
68. Crowley TJ, Mikulich SK, MacDonald M, et al. Substance-dependent, conduct-disordered adolescent males: severity of diagnosis predicts 2-year outcome. *Drug Alcohol Depend* 1998;49:225–237.
69. Dalley JW, Fryer TD, Brichard L, et al. Nucleus accumbens D2/3 receptors predict trait impulsivity and cocaine reinforcement. *Science* 2007;315:1267–1270.
70. Hoffman WF, Moore M, Templin R, et al. Neuropsychological function and delay discounting in methamphetamine-dependent individuals. *Psychopharmacology* 2006;188:162–170.
71. Kelly TH, Robbins G, Martin CA, et al. Individual differences in drug abuse vulnerability: d-amphetamine and sensation-seeking status. *Psychopharmacology* 2006;189:17–25.
72. Cook EH, Jr., Stein MA, Krasowski MD, et al. Association of attention-deficit disorder and the dopamine transporter gene. *Am J Hum Genet* 1995;56:993–998.
73. Gill M, Daly G, Heron S, et al. Confirmation of association between attention deficit hyperactivity disorder and a dopamine transporter polymorphism. *Mol Psychiatry* 1997;2:311–313.
74. Winsberg BG, Comings DE. Association of the dopamine transporter gene (DAT1) with poor methylphenidate response. *J Am Acad Child Adolesc Psychiatry* 1999;38:1474–1477.
75. Roman T, Rohde LA, Hutz MH. Polymorphisms of the dopamine transporter gene: influence on response to methylphenidate in attention deficit-hyperactivity disorder. *Am J Pharmacogenom* 2004;4:83–92.
76. Dougherty DD, Bonab AA, Spencer TJ, et al. Dopamine transporter density in patients with attention deficit hyperactivity disorder. *Lancet* 1999;354:2132–2133.
77. Giros B, Wang YM, Suter S, et al. Delineation of discrete domains for substrate, cocaine, and tricyclic antidepressant interactions using chimeric dopamine-norepinephrine transporters. *J Biol Chem* 1994;269: 15985–15988.
78. Horst R. The neurobiology of adult ADHD. *Psychiatric Times: Perspective in Psychiatry A Clinical Update*, Vol. Suppl 1(4), 2007.
79. Kalivas PW, Volkow ND. The neural basis of addiction: a pathology of motivation and choice. *Am J Psychiatry* 2005;162:1403–1413.
80. Filipek PA, Semrud-Clikeman M, Steingard RJ, et al. Volumetric MRI analysis comparing subjects having attention-deficit hyperactivity disorder with normal controls. *Neurology* 1997;48:589–601.
81. Valera EM, Faraone SV, Murray KE, et al. Meta-analysis of structural imaging findings in attention-deficit/hyperactivity disorder. *Biol Psychiatry* 2007;61:1361–1369.
82. Jentsch JD, Roth RH, Taylor JR. Role for dopamine in the behavioral functions of the prefrontal corticostriatal system: implications for mental disorders and psychotropic drug action. *Progr Brain Res* 2000;126: 433–453.
83. Wilens TE, Hahesy AL, Biederman J, et al. Influence of parental SUD and ADHD on ADHD in their offspring: preliminary results from a pilot-controlled family study. *Am J Addict* 2005;14:179–187.
84. Paternite CE, Loney J, Salisbury H, et al. Childhood inattention-overactivity, aggression, and stimulant medication history as predictors of young adult outcomes. *J Child Adolesc Psychopharmacol* 1999;9:169–184.
85. Biederman J, Wilens T, Mick E, et al. Pharmacotherapy of attention-deficit/hyperactivity disorder reduces risk for substance use disorder. *Pediatrics* 1999;104:e20.
86. Faraone SV, Wilens T. Does stimulant treatment lead to substance use disorders? *J Clin Psychiatry* 2003;64(Suppl 11):9–13.
87. Wilson JJ. ADHD and substance use disorders: developmental aspects and the impact of stimulant treatment. *Am J Addict* 2007;16(Suppl 1):5–11; quiz 12–13.
88. Carlezon WA, Jr., Mague SD, Andersen SL. Enduring behavioral effects of early exposure to methylphenidate in rats. *Biol Psychiatry* 2003;54: 1330–1337.
89. Hermens DF, Williams LM, Clarke S, et al. Responses to methylphenidate in adolescent AD/HD: evidence from concurrently recorded autonomic (EDA) and central (EEG and ERP) measures. *Int J Psychophysiol* 2005;58:21–33.
90. Lee JS, Kim BN, Kang E, et al. Regional cerebral blood flow in children with attention deficit hyperactivity disorder: comparison before and after methylphenidate treatment. *Hum Brain Map* 2005;24:157–164.
91. Schweitzer JB, Lee DO, Hanford RB, et al. Effect of methylphenidate on executive functioning in adults with attention-deficit/hyperactivity disorder: normalization of behavior but not related brain activity. *Biol Psychiatry* 2004;56:597–606.
92. Pliszka SR, Glahn DC, Semrud-Clikeman M, et al. Neuroimaging of inhibitory control areas in children with attention deficit hyperactivity disorder who were treatment naive or in long-term treatment. *Am J Psychiatry* 2006;163:1052–1060.
93. Shafritz KM, Marchione KE, Gore JC, et al. The effects of methylphenidate on neural systems of attention in attention deficit hyperactivity disorder. *Am J Psychiatry* 2004;161:1990–1997.
94. American Psychiatric Association (APA). *Diagnostic and statistical manual of mental disorders,* 4th ed., text revision. Washington, DC: American Psychiatric Association, 2000.

95. Faraone SV, Biederman J, Friedman D. Validity of DSM-IV subtypes of attention-deficit/hyperactivity disorder: a family study perspective. *J Am Acad Child Adolesc Psychiatry* 2000;39:300–307.
96. Faraone SV, Biederman J, Spencer T, et al. Attention-deficit/hyperactivity disorder in adults: an overview. *Biol Psychiatry* 2000;48:9–20.
97. Spitzer RL, Williams JBW. Classification in psychiatry. In: Kaplan HI, Sadock BJ, eds. *Comprehensive textbook of psychiatry,* 4th ed. Baltimore, MD: Williams & Wilkins, 1985.
98. Weiss RD, Pope HG, Jr., Mirin SM. Treatment of chronic cocaine abuse and attention deficit disorder, residual type, with magnesium pemoline. *Drug Alcohol Depend* 1985;15:69–72.
99. Zametkin AJ, Nordahl TE, Gross M, et al. Cerebral glucose metabolism in adults with hyperactivity of childhood onset. *N Engl J Med* 1990;323: 1361–1366.
100. Spencer T, Wilens T, Biederman J, et al. A double-blind, crossover comparison of methylphenidate and placebo in adults with childhood-onset attention-deficit hyperactivity disorder. *Arch Gen Psychiatry* 1995;52: 434–443.
101. Wilens TE, Biederman J, Prince J, et al. Six-week, double-blind, placebo-controlled study of desipramine for adult attention deficit hyperactivity disorder. *Am J Psychiatry* 1996;153:1147–1153.
102. Spencer T, Biederman J, Wilens T, et al. Is attention-deficit hyperactivity disorder in adults a valid disorder? *Harv Rev Psychiatry* 1994;1:326–335.
103. Mayes SD, Calhoun SL, Crowell EW. Learning disabilities and ADHD: overlapping spectrum disorders. *J Learn Disab* 2000;33:417–424.
104. Johnson DE, Waid LR, Anton RF. Childhood hyperactivity, gender, and Cloninger's personality dimensions in alcoholics. *Addict Behav* 1997; 22:649–653.
105. Johnson DE, Epstein JN, Waid LR, et al. Neuropsychological performance deficits in adults with attention deficit/hyperactivity disorder. *Arch Clin Neuropsychol* 2001;16:587–604.
106. Gordon M, Barkley RA, Lovett BJ. *Tests and observational measures in attention-deficit hyperactivity disorder: handbook for diagnosis and treatment,* 3rd ed. New York: Guilford Press, Inc., 2006.
107. Murphy KR, Gordon M. *Assessment of adults with ADHD in attention-deficit hyperactivity disorder: handbook for diagnosis and treatment,* 3rd ed. New York: Guilford Press, Inc., 2006.
108. Barkley RA, Fischer M, Smallish L, et al. Young adult outcome of hyperactive children: adaptive functioning in major life activities. *J Am Acad Child Adolesc Psychiatry* 2006;45:192–202.
109. Levin FR. Diagnosing ADHD in adults with substance use disorder: DSM-IV criteria and differential diagnosis. *J Clin Psychiatry* 2007; 68:e18.
110. Gascon GG, Johnson R, Burd L. Central auditory processing and attention deficit disorders. *J Child Neurol* 1986;1:27–33.
111. Ward MF, Wender PH, Reimherr FW. The Wender Utah Rating Scale: an aid in the retrospective diagnosis of childhood attention deficit hyperactivity disorder. *Am J Psychiatry* 1993;150:885–890.
112. Conners CK, Erhardt D, Sparrow E. *Conners adult ADHD rating scales.* North Tonawanda, NY: Multi-Health Systems, 2000.
113. Bowden CL. Overcoming the spectrum of obstacles in bipolar disorder. Annual US Psychiatric and Mental Health Congress, New Orleans, 2006.
114. Biederman J, Faraone SV, Keenan K, et al. Family-genetic and psychosocial risk factors in DSM-III attention deficit disorder. *J Am Acad Child Adolesc Psychiatry* 1990;29:526–533.
115. Biederman J, Faraone SV, Keenan K, et al. Further evidence for family-genetic risk factors in attention deficit hyperactivity disorder. Patterns of comorbidity in probands and relatives psychiatrically and pediatrically referred samples. *Arch Gen Psychiatry* 1992;49:728–738.
116. Brunton LL, Lazo JS, Parker KL. *Goodman and Bilman's the pharmacological basis of therapeutics.* New York, McGraw-Hill Book Co., 2006.
117. Faraone SV, Spencer T, Aleardi M, et al. Meta-analysis of the efficacy of methylphenidate for treating adult attention-deficit/hyperactivity disorder. *J Clin Psychopharmacol* 2004;24:24–29.
118. Spencer T, Biederman J, Wilens T, et al. Efficacy of a mixed amphetamine salts compound in adults with attention-deficit/hyperactivity disorder. *Arch Gen Psychiatry* 2001;58:775–782.
119. Results from the 2002 National Survey on Drug Use and Health: National findings. Rockville, MD: Substance Abuse and Mental Health Services Administration, 2003.
120. Fredericks EM, Kollins SH. Assessing methylphenidate preference in ADHD patients using a choice procedure. *Psychopharmacology* 2004; 175:391–398.
121. Stoops WW, Glaser PE, Fillmore MT, et al. Reinforcing, subject-rated, performance and physiological effects of methylphenidate and d-amphetamine in stimulant abusing humans. *J Psychopharmacol* 2004;18: 534–543.
122. Rush CR, Essman WD, Simpson CA, et al. Reinforcing and subject-rated effects of methylphenidate and d-amphetamine in non-drug-abusing humans. *J Clin Psychopharmacol* 2001;21:273–286.
123. Hart CL, Ward AS, Haney M, et al. Methamphetamine self-administration by humans. *Psychopharmacology* 2001;157:75–81.
124. Roache JD, Grabowski J, Schmitz JM, et al. Laboratory measures of methylphenidate effects in cocaine-dependent patients receiving treatment. *J Clin Psychopharmacol* 2000;20:61–68.
125. Volkow ND, Swanson JM. Variables that affect the clinical use and abuse of methylphenidate in the treatment of ADHD. *Am J Psychiatry* 2003;160:1909–1918.
126. Somoza EC, Winhusen TM, Bridge TP, et al. An open-label pilot study of methylphenidate in the treatment of cocaine dependent patients with adult attention deficit/hyperactivity disorder. *J Addict Dis* 2004;23:77–92.
127. Schubiner H, Saules KK, Arfken CL, et al. Double-blind placebo-controlled trial of methylphenidate in the treatment of adult ADHD patients with comorbid cocaine dependence. *Exp Clin Psychopharmacol* 2002;10:286–294.
128. Levin FR, Evans SM, Brooks DJ, et al. Treatment of methadone-maintained patients with adult ADHD: double-blind comparison of methylphenidate, bupropion and placebo. *Drug Alcohol Depend* 2006; 81:137–148.
129. Grabowski J, Rhoades H, Schmitz J, et al. Dextroamphetamine for cocaine-dependence treatment: a double-blind randomized clinical trial. *J Clin Psychopharmacol* 2001;21:522–526.
130. Shearer J, Wodak A, van Beek I, et al. Pilot randomized double blind placebo-controlled study of dexamphetamine for cocaine dependence. *Addiction* 2003;98:1137–1141.
131. Shearer J, Wodak A, Mattick RP, et al. Pilot randomized controlled study of dexamphetamine substitution for amphetamine dependence. *Addiction* 2001;96:1289–1296.
132. White R. Dexamphetamine substitution in the treatment of amphetamine abuse: an initial investigation. *Addiction* 2000;95:229–238.
133. Grabowski J, Rhoades H, Stotts A, et al. Agonist-like or antagonist-like treatment for cocaine dependence with methadone for heroin dependence: two double-blind randomized clinical trials. *Neuropsychopharmacology* 2004;29:969–981.
134. Levin FR, Brooks DJ, Bisaga A, et al. Severity of dependence and motivation for treatment: comparison of marijuana- and cocaine-dependent treatment seekers. *J Addict Dis* 2006;25:33–41.
135. McCabe SE, Teter CJ, Boyd CJ, et al. Prevalence and correlates of illicit methylphenidate use among 8th, 10th, and 12th grade students in the United States, 2001. *J Adolesc Health* 2004;35:501–504.
136. McCabe SE, Knight JR, Teter CJ, et al. Non-medical use of prescription stimulants among U.S. college students: prevalence and correlates from a national survey. *Addiction* 2005;100:96–106.
137. McCabe SE, Teter CJ, Boyd CJ. Medical use, illicit use, and diversion of abusable prescription drugs. *J Am Coll Health* 2006;54:269–278.
138. Teter CJ, McCabe SE, LaGrange K, et al. Illicit use of specific prescription stimulants among college students: prevalence, motives, and routes of administration. *Pharmacotherapy* 2006;26:1501–1510.
139. Kollins SH, Rush CR, Pazzaglia PJ, et al. Comparison of acute behavioral effects of sustained-release and immediate-release methylphenidate. *Exp Clin Psychopharmacol* 1998;6:367–374.
140. Spencer TJ, Biederman J, Ciccone PE, et al. PET study examining pharmacokinetics, detection and likeability, and dopamine transporter receptor occupancy of short- and long-acting oral methylphenidate. *Am J Psychiatry* 2006;163:387–395.

141. MacDonald Fredericks E, Kollins SH. A pilot study of methylphenidate preference assessment in children diagnosed with attention-deficit/hyperactivity disorder. *J Child Adolesc Psychopharmacol* 2005;15:729–741.
142. Upadhyaya HP, Rose K, Wang W, et al. Attention-deficit/hyperactivity disorder, medication treatment, and substance use patterns among adolescents and young adults. *J Child Adolesc Psychopharmacol* 2005;15:799–809.
143. Wilens TE, Gignac M, Swezey A, et al. Characteristics of adolescents and young adults with ADHD who divert or misuse their prescribed medications. *J Am Acad Child Adolesc Psychiatry* 2006;45:408–414.
144. Collins SL, Levin FR, Foltin RW, et al. Response to cocaine, alone and in combination with methylphenidate, in cocaine abusers with ADHD. *Drug Alcohol Depend* 2006;82:158–167.
145. Adler LA, Spencer TJ, Milton DR, et al. Long-term, open-label study of the safety and efficacy of atomoxetine in adults with attention-deficit/hyperactivity disorder: an interim analysis. *J Clin Psychiatry* 2005;66:294–299.
146. Michelson D, Adler L, Spencer T, et al. Atomoxetine in adults with ADHD: two randomized, placebo-controlled studies. *Biol Psychiatry* 2003;53:112–120.
147. Wolraich ML, Wibbelsman CJ, Brown TE, et al. Attention-deficit/hyperactivity disorder among adolescents: a review of the diagnosis, treatment, and clinical implications. *Pediatrics* 2005;115:1734–1746.
148. Conners CK, Casat CD, Gualtieri CT, et al. Bupropion hydrochloride in attention deficit disorder with hyperactivity. *J Am Acad Child Adolesc Psychiatry* 1996;35:1314–1321.
149. Wilens TE, Spencer TJ, Biederman J, et al. A controlled clinical trial of bupropion for attention deficit hyperactivity disorder in adults. *Am J Psychiatry* 2001;158:282–288.
150. Wilens TE, Haight BR, Horrigan JP, et al. Bupropion XL in adults with attention-deficit/hyperactivity disorder: a randomized, placebo-controlled study. *Biol Psychiatry* 2005;57:793–801.
151. Motavalli Mukaddes N, Abali O. Venlafaxine in children and adolescents with attention deficit hyperactivity disorder. *Psychiatr Clin Neurosci* 2004;58:92–95.
152. Olvera RL, Pliszka SR, Luh J, et al. An open trial of venlafaxine in the treatment of attention-deficit/hyperactivity disorder in children and adolescents. *J Child Adolesc Psychopharmacol* 1996;6:241–250.
153. Connor DF, Fletcher KE, Swanson JM. A meta-analysis of clonidine for symptoms of attention-deficit hyperactivity disorder. *J Am Acad Child Adolesc Psychiatry* 1999;38:1551–1559.
154. Scahill L, Chappell PB, Kim YS, et al. A placebo-controlled study of guanfacine in the treatment of children with tic disorders and attention deficit hyperactivity disorder. *Am J Psychiatry* 2001;158:1067–1074.
155. Taylor FB, Russo J. Comparing guanfacine and dextroamphetamine for the treatment of adult attention-deficit/hyperactivity disorder. *J Clin Psychopharmacol* 2001;21:223–228.
156. Biederman J, Swanson JM, Wigal SB, et al. A comparison of once-daily and divided doses of modafinil in children with attention-deficit/hyperactivity disorder: a randomized, double-blind, and placebo-controlled study. *J Clin Psychiatry* 2006;67:727–735.
157. Greenhill LL, Biederman J, Boellner SW, et al. A randomized, double-blind, placebo-controlled study of modafinil film-coated tablets in children and adolescents with attention-deficit/hyperactivity disorder. *J Am Acad Child Adolesc Psychiatry* 2006;45:503–511.
158. Swanson JM, Greenhill LL, Lopez FA, et al. Modafinil film-coated tablets in children and adolescents with attention-deficit/hyperactivity disorder: results of a randomized, double-blind, placebo-controlled, fixed-dose study followed by abrupt discontinuation. *J Clin Psychiatry* 2006;67:137–147.
159. Taylor FB, Russo J. Efficacy of modafinil compared to dextroamphetamine for the treatment of attention deficit hyperactivity disorder in adults. *J Child Adolesc Psychopharmacol* 2000;10:311–320.
160. Dackis CA, Kampman KM, Lynch KG, et al. A double-blind, placebo-controlled trial of modafinil for cocaine dependence. *Neuropsychopharmacology* 2005;30:205–211.
161. Weisler RH, Biederman J, Spencer TJ, et al. Mixed amphetamine salts extended-release in the treatment of adult ADHD: a randomized, controlled trial. *CNS Spectr* 2006;11:625–639.
162. Ciccone PE. Attempted abuse of Concerta. *J Am Acad Child Adolesc Psychiatry* 2002;41:756.
163. Higgins ST, Delaney DD, Budney AJ, et al. A behavioral approach to achieving initial cocaine abstinence. *Am J Psychiatry* 1991;148:1218–1224.
164. A 14-month randomized clinical trial of treatment strategies for attention-deficit/hyperactivity disorder. The MTA Cooperative Group. Multimodal Treatment Study of Children with ADHD. *Arch Gen Psychiatry* 1999;56:1073–1086.
165. Jensen PS, Arnold LE, Swanson JM, et al. 3-year follow-up of the NIMH MTA study. *J Am Acad Child Adolesc Psychiatry* 2007;46:989–1002.
166. March JS, Swanson JM, Arnold LE, et al. Anxiety as a predictor and outcome variable in the multimodal treatment study of children with ADHD (MTA). *J Abnorm Child Psychol* 2000;28:527–541.
167. Safren SA, Otto MW, Sprich S, et al. Cognitive-behavioral therapy for ADHD in medication-treated adults with continued symptoms. *Behav Res Ther* 2005;43:831–842.
168. Weinstein CS. Cognitive remediation strategies: an adjunct to the psychotherapy of adults with attention deficit hyperactivity disorder. *J Psychother Pract Res* 1994;3:44–57.
169. Aviram RB, Rhum M, Levin FR. Psychotherapy of adults with comorbid attention-deficit/hyperactivity disorder and psychoactive substance use disorder. *J Psychother Pract Res* 2001;10:179–186.
170. Dees SM, Dansereau DF, Simpson DD. A visual representation system for drug abuse counselors. *J Substance Abuse Treatment* 1994;11:517–523.
171. Dansereau DF, Joe GW, Simpson DD. Attentional difficulties and the effectiveness of a visual representation strategy for counseling drug-addicted clients. *Int J Addict* 1995;30:371–386.

CHAPTER 88

Linda A. Dimeff, PhD
Katherine Anne Comtois, PhD
Marsha M. Linehan, PhD

Co-occurring Addiction and Borderline Personality Disorder

PREVALENCE OF BORDERLINE PERSONALITY DISORDER TREATMENT AND OUTCOMES FOR BORDERLINE PERSONALITY DISORDER

Borderline personality disorder (BPD) and substance use disorders (SUDs) are both chronic conditions characterized by frequent relapse. BPD, in particular, is considered by many to be difficult, if not impossible, to treat and is often associated with treatment noncompliance, poor treatment outcomes, premature termination of treatment, clinician burnout, and suicide. The combination of BPD and SUD is particularly difficult to treat, as the degree of patient dysfunction and risk exponentially increases. Dialectical behavior therapy (DBT) (1,2) is an efficacious treatment for BPD, including those with SUD (3–5).

This chapter focuses on the prevalence of BPD-SUD comorbidity and the unique clinical challenges encountered in working with patients with BPD. We review the data to date on the treatment for BPD-SUD, including dialectical behavior therapy for substance abusers, an efficacious treatment for multidisordered individuals with BPD and SUD. We then offer a number of suggestions and recommendations to consider in the clinical management of BPD-SUD patients. These include recommendations regarding prescription of potentially lethal drugs to suicidal BPD patients, suggestions for reinforcing functional (vs. dysfunctional) behavior, and validating "valid" behavior. Finally, we review two sets of DBT skills that may be helpful for your BPD patient to learn and practice when in a highly distressing situation.

BORDERLINE PERSONALITY DISORDER DEFINED AND REDEFINED

BPD is a severe Axis II personality disorder characterized by intense and labile negative emotions, including shame, anger, and sadness; significant interpersonal conflict; and extreme behavioral dyscontrol that is characterized by impulsivity and disinhibition. Suicide, suicide attempts, and nonsuicidal self-injury (NSSI; i.e., volitional self-harming behaviors that cause tissue damage such as cutting or burning oneself, swallowing foreign objects, and head banging), and drug abuse (prescription, licit, and illicit) are among the most common impulsive behaviors. DSM-IV diagnostic criteria are summarized in Table 88.1.

Linehan has described BPD as a pervasive disorder of the emotion dysregulation system (1). From this perspective, *all BPD criterion behaviors are understood as functioning to regulate emotions* (e.g., a person uses drugs or cuts as a means of reducing or escaping intense negative emotions) *or are direct consequences of emotion dysregulation* (e.g., verbally attacking someone when angry and destroying the relationship; dissociation; depersonalization; paranoid ideation; catastrophic thinking; and other forms of cognitive dysregulation that occur in a context of intense emotion dysregulation). Indeed, basic biologic research studies (6) have demonstrated that, in comparison to nonclinical/non-BPD individuals, those with BPD have a lower sensitivity to emotional cues (i.e., a small stimulus is all that is required to trigger an emotion in the brain) and high emotion reactivity (i.e., once triggered, the emotions are extreme).

TABLE 88.1 DSM-IV Criteria for Borderline Personality Disorder

Borderline personality disorder (BPD) involves a pervasive pattern of instability of interpersonal relationships, self-image and affects, and marked impulsivity, beginning by early adulthood and present in a variety of contexts, as indicated by five or more of the following:

- Frantic efforts to avoid real or imagined abandonment. (Note: Do not include suicidal or self-mutilating behavior.)
- A pattern of unstable and intense interpersonal relationships, characterized by alternating between extremes of idealization and devaluation identity disturbance, and markedly and persistently unstable self-image or sense of self
- Identity disturbance: markedly and persistently unstable self-image or sense of self
- Impulsivity in at least two areas that are potentially self-damaging such as spending, sex, substance abuse, reckless driving, binge eating. (Note: Do not include suicidal or self-mutilating behavior.)
- Recurrent suicidal behavior, gestures, or threats, or self-mutilating behavior
- Affective instability due to marked reactivity of mood (e.g., intense episodic dysphoria, irritability, or anxiety), usually lasting a few hours and only rarely more than a few days
- Chronic feelings of emptiness
- Inappropriate, intense anger or difficulty in controlling anger such as frequent displays of temper, constant anger, or recurrent physical fights
- Transient, stress-related paranoid ideation or severe dissociative symptoms

Reprinted from American Psychiatric Association 1994 *Diagnostic and statistical manual of mental disorders*, 4th ed. DSM-IV Washington, DC: American Psychiatric Press, 654, with permission.

PREVALENCE OF BORDERLINE PERSONALITY DISORDER AND BORDERLINE PERSONALITY DISORDER–SUBSTANCE USE DISORDER

Between 0.2% and 1.8% of the general population meet criteria for BPD (7). Between 8% to11% of outpatients seeking mental health services (7–9), and between 14% and 20% of inpatients meet criteria for BPD (7,10).

SUDs commonly co-occur with BPD (11) and result in serious and complex behavioral problems. This co-occurrence between BPD and SUDs is second only to mood disorders and antisocial personality disorder in comorbidity prevalence (12). In their extensive review of BPD-SUD comorbidity data gathered from studies published from 1987 to 1997, Trull et al. (11) found that among those seeking substance abuse treatment, rates of BPD ranged from 5.2% (13) to 65.1% (14). Prevalence of current SUDs among patients receiving treatment for BPD range from approximately 25% (15) to 67% (16). Subsequent studies further confirm this significant overlap (17,18). This overlap is not surprising, as impulsiveness is one of the diagnostic criteria for BPD. However, the comorbidity is not entirely due to this overlap in criteria. For example, Dulit et al. (16) found that 67% of current BPD patients met criteria for SUD. When substance abuse was not applied as a criterion of BPD, the incidence dropped to 57%, still a significant portion of the population.

The presence of a personality disorder (PD), such as BPD, among individuals with SUD significantly increases the degree and severity of behavioral dyscontrol and resultant problems. Specifically, individuals with a PD and SUD have higher rates of alcoholism, depression, and more extensive legal and medical problems than patients without personality disorders (19–24) and engage in significantly more high-risk HIV behavior compared to those with SUD only or individuals with a PD but without SUD. Among the personality disorders, BPD was associated with the most severe psychiatric problems (25). When comparing patients with SUD only, BPD only, and BPD with SUD, those with both disorders had more severe psychopathology, engaged in more self-destructive behaviors, and had more suicidal thoughts than those with either SUD or BPD alone (26).

RISK OF SUICIDE AND NONSUICIDAL SELF-INJURY AMONG BORDERLINE PERSONALITY DISORDER

BPD is the only DSM-IV diagnosis for which suicide attempts and/or nonsuicidal self-injuries (SASI) are a criterion, and SASI are thus considered a "hallmark" of BPD. Rates of SASI among individuals diagnosed with BPD range from 69% to 80% (27–31). The suicide rate is 5% to 10% (32,33) and doubles when only those with a previous history of SASI are included (34). Suicidal ideation and behavior among those with BPD endures over time and does not appear to be related to episodic mood disorder, in contrast to suicide attempters of other diagnostic categories (35). Though depressive moods and experiences are related to suicidal behavior in individuals with BPD, Soloff (36) and Mann (37) have both reported an absence of association between suicidal behavior and either comorbid affective disorder or severity of disorder in this population. Functional impairment, however, is extensive and is significantly higher than that associated with non-BPD major depression (38). Patients with BPD and SUD combined may be at higher risk for suicide than BPD patients without SUD or SUD patients without BPD (39). Most leading explanatory models of both suicidal behavior and nonsuicidal self-injury emphasize avoidance or escape from painful emotions, often related to difficult precipitating life events (1,40).

BORDERLINE PERSONALITY DISORDER AND UTILIZATION OF PSYCHIATRIC AND MEDICAL SERVICES

Research over the past two decades indicates that a subset (between 6% and 8%) of the overall population uses a disproportionate amount of inpatient psychiatric services: up to 42% of all admissions (41–46). Research by Hadley et al. (44) indicates that, across sites, 75% to 80% of inpatient treatment dollars are spent on 30% to 35% of patients. Almost three-fourths (72%) of individuals with BPD in a large multisite sample (47) had been admitted for psychiatric hospitalization in their lifetime. Hospitalization was 4.95 times more likely than for comparable individuals with major depression (47). Several studies of high users of inpatient psychiatric hospitalizations found that 9% to 40% of high users are diagnosed with BPD (46,48–51). The 40% figures were reported by Geller (49) and Swigar et al. (48), whose studies focused specifically on the highest users of psychiatric hospitals.

Studies have found that, over their lifetime, 97% of individuals with BPD have received outpatient treatment from an average of 6.1 therapists (52,53). In a large study of treatment-seeking individuals with BPD (47), lifetime rates of most mental health services were high: 95% received individual therapy, 56% group therapy, 42% family or couples psychotherapy, 37% day treatment, and 24% treatment in a halfway house (54). Individuals with BPD were more likely to have received all classes of medications, except hypnotics, than patients with other personality disorders or major depression. Individuals with BPD were twice as likely to have taken antidepressants (47).

Presenting medical concerns frequently include asthma, diabetes, hepatitis, and ulcers, as well as chronic fatigue syndrome, irritable bowel syndrome, and fibromyalgia (55). It is not uncommon for BPD patients to be dismissed as somaticizers because of the large number of somatic complaints they present. Indeed, only a small proportion (4%) of substance-dependent individuals with BPD meet the criteria for somaticization using the SCID I interviews (56). Numerous studies that document a relationship between abuse in childhood and subsequent utilization of primary care and associated high medical costs in adulthood suggest that the high rate of medical problems in individuals with BPD is associated with growing up in a dysfunctional family environment (57–61). Prevalence estimates of childhood abuse in the population with BPD range from 67% to 86% for sexual abuse and 71% for physical abuse, compared with rates of 22% to 34% for sexual abuse and 38% for physical abuse in non-BPD populations (62–66). A recent study compared 200 patients with remitted BPD to 64 patients with active BPD. Patients with remitted BPD were significantly less likely to (1) have chronic fatigue, fibromyalgia, and temporomandibular joint syndrome; (2) be obese or have obesity-related conditions; (3) smoke cigarettes, drink alcohol daily, use pain medications for sustained periods of time, take sleep medication, fail to exercise and (4) have used expensive medical treatment such as emergency rooms and hospitalization (67).

TREATMENT AND OUTCOMES FOR BORDERLINE PERSONALITY DISORDER

Achieving treatment success with BPD patients has been notoriously difficult. Follow-up studies consistently indicate that BPD is a chronic disorder, though the number of individuals who continue to meet diagnostic criteria slowly decreases over the lifespan. Two to three years after index assessment, 60% to 70% of patients diagnosed with BPD continued to meet the criteria (68). Other short-term follow-up studies reported little change in the patients' level of functioning and consistently high rates of psychiatric hospitalization over 2 to 5 years (68–70). Four to seven years after index assessment, 57% to 67% of patients continued to meet the criteria for BPD (71,72). An average of 15 years after index assessment, 25% to 44% continued to meet the criteria (73,74). One study followed up 64 patients with BPD for a mean of 27 years and found most patients showed significant improvement as compared to a previous 15-year follow-up, with only five currently meeting criteria for BPD. The subgroup with dysthymia had significantly poorer outcome on all measures (75).

BPD also has been associated with poorer outcomes in the treatment of Axis I disorders, such as major depression (76), obsessive-compulsive disorder (77), bulimia (78,79), and substance use (25). Analyses of outcomes for individuals with BPD who have received inpatient and outpatient treatment-as-usual (TAU) suggest that traditional treatments are marginally effective at best when outcomes are measured two to three years following treatment (80,81). In pharmacotherapy trials, which often are short-term, dropout rates for individuals with BPD have been very high (82), and compliance has been problematic, with more than 50% of patients reporting misuse of their medications and 87% of therapists reporting medication misuse by their patients.

Despite advances in the treatment of BPD with medications (83–85), it is widely assumed that some form of ancillary behavioral treatment of BPD is necessary (86,87). However, there are few randomized, controlled studies of treatments designed specifically for BPD. In addition to the treatment developed by Linehan et al., several other psychosocial treatments have been evaluated. Marziali and Munroe-Blum (88) found that structured, time-limited group therapy was more effective than individual psychotherapy in retaining patients in treatment, though it did not improve outcome variables. More recently, Bateman and Fonagy (89) demonstrated the efficacy of an 18-month psychoanalytically oriented partial hospitalization program in reducing suicidal behavior; results were maintained at 18-month follow-up during which time the subjects continued the treatment (90).

To date, nine published randomized controlled trials (RCTs) conducted across five research institutions support DBT's efficacy for a number of behavioral problems, including suicide attempts and self-injurious behaviors (91–95), substance abuse (96,97), bulimia (98), binge eating (99), and depression in the elderly (100). These and other studies have also demonstrated the cost-effectiveness of DBT compared to TAU in reducing hospitalization, emergency room visits, medical severity of suicide attempts, and utilization of crisis/respite beds (101–103).

Two of the published RCTs have focused specifically on the application of DBT for individuals with BPD and SUD. Both DBT studies (96,97) were conducted by Linehan et al. at the University of Washington. Comprehensive DBT that included all modes and functions was provided in both trials across a 12-month course of treatment. The assessment phase spanned a total of 16 months, from pretreatment through an assessment 4 months after completion of treatment, and included the collection of urinalyses. The initial RCT compared DBT (n = 12) to community-based TAU (n = 16) among polysubstance–dependent women with BPD (96). In comparison to TAU, DBT subjects were significantly more likely to remain in treatment (64% and 27%, respectively), had significantly reduced their drug use as measured by structured interviews and urinalyses throughout the treatment year, and significantly attended more individual therapy sessions as compared to TAU subjects. Additionally, though subjects in both conditions demonstrated significant improvement in social and global adjustment during the treatment year, only DBT subjects continued to show improvements on these variables at the 16-month follow-up.

The second efficacy trial of DBT (n = 23) utilized a more rigorous control condition (Comprehensive Validation Therapy with Twelve Step; CVT+12 Step) and required that all subjects meet criteria for opiate dependence in addition to BPD. CVT+12 Step is a manualized approach that includes the major acceptance-based strategies used in DBT in combination with participation in a 12-Step program, such as Narcotics Anonymous (NA). CVT therapists focused on validating the client in a warm and supportive atmosphere. Importantly, validation of public and private behaviors only occurred when the behavior was in fact valid; in other words, the behavior was effective in terms of the client's long-term goals, logically consistent with actual data, or an instance of normative behavior. CVT+12-Step subjects were required to attend at least one NA meeting offered weekly at the treatment clinic and facilitated by the CVT therapists, both of whom were members of NA. All subjects were taking levomethadyl acetate, an opiate replacement medication, throughout the initial treatment year followed by continued provision of medication by an external agency after treatment termination. Three major findings emerged from this study. First, results of urinalyses indicated that both treatments were effective in significantly reducing opiate use. However, only DBT subjects maintained these reductions during the last 4 months of treatment. Second, both treatments succeeded in retaining subjects in treatment; however, the CVT+12-Step was exceptionally effective in doing so, as they retained 100% of their subjects (compared to 64% in DBT). Finally, at both posttreatment and at the 16-month follow-up assessment, subjects in both treatment conditions showed statistically significant overall reductions in levels of psychopathology relative to baseline.

DIALECTICAL BEHAVIOR THERAPY IN A NUTSHELL

DBT began as an application of the standard behavior therapy of the 1970s to treat chronically suicidal individuals (104). Its basic premise was that individuals who wanted to be dead did not have the requisite skills to build a life worth living. In developing the treatment, however, it quickly became clear that focusing solely on change would not work. Many suicide attempters were exquisitely sensitive to criticism and prone to emotion dysregulation. An emphasis on change quickly resulted in increased, if not overwhelming, emotional arousal, with clients emotionally "shutting down" and, in some cases, storming out of sessions or attacking the therapist. Dropping the emphasis on change, however, had equally problematic consequences: Clients would view their therapist as ignoring or significantly minimizing their palpable suffering; clients would respond with extreme rage at the therapist for dismissing their problems or would fall into a sea of hopelessness. From either therapeutic stance, (i.e., an exclusive focus on change or on acceptance), clients experienced their therapist as invalidating their needs and experience as a whole. Research by Swann et al. (105) may explain how such perceived invalidation leads to problematic behavior in therapy. Their research revealed that when an individual's basic self-constructs are not verified, the individual's arousal increases, resulting in to cognitive dysregulation and a failure to process new information (106).

To keep the client and therapist in the room and working productively on the client's problems, the therapist had to find a way to simultaneously emphasize both acceptance and change throughout the treatment. This synthesis, when found, engendered additional change and acceptance within the client: The desire to eliminate all painful experiences (including life itself) became balanced with a corresponding effort to accept life's inevitable pain. It was impossible to work on changing one set of problems if the client could not tolerate (at least temporarily) the pain of other problems. Without this tolerance, all problems converged, overwhelming both the client and the therapy. It was as necessary for the client to hold the synthesis of acceptance and change as it was for the therapist. Though treatment of severe disorders requires the synthesis of many dialectical polarities, that of acceptance and change is the most fundamental. It was the necessity of this synthesis that led to considering use of the term *dialectic* as a descriptor of the standard behavior therapy applied in the treatment. This simultaneous embrace of change and acceptance is consistent with the philosophical approach found in Twelve Step programs, captured in the Serenity Prayer (*"God, grant me the serenity to accept the things I cannot change, the courage to change the things I can, and the wisdom to know the difference"*).

From the perspective of the therapeutic dialogue and relationship, dialectics refers to change by persuasion and to making strategic use of oppositions that emerge within therapy and the therapeutic relationship, rather than by formal impersonal logic. By searching for the validity or truth contained with each contradictory position, new meanings within old meanings emerge, thus moving the client and therapist closer to the essence of the subject under consideration. The spirit of a dialectical point of view is never to accept a proposition as a final truth or an undisputable fact. Instead, client and therapist ask, "What is being left out of our understanding?" or "What is the synthesis between these two positions?"

DBT is a comprehensive treatment program composed of five essential functions: improving client motivation to change; enhancing client capabilities; generalizing new behaviors; structuring the environment; and enhancing therapist capability and motivation. The responsibility for fulfilling these functions is spread across four treatment modes: individual therapy, group skills training, telephone consultation, and therapist consultation meetings. More relevant than the treatment mode itself is the extent to which the mode addresses a particular function. For example, ensuring that new capabilities are generalized from the treatment environment to the client's everyday life could be accomplished in various ways based on the treatment setting (e.g., outpatient, inpatient, residential milieu, maximal security prison). Whereas generalization typically occurs via telephone coaching in an outpatient setting, or in a milieu setting, the entire staff might be taught to model, coach, and reinforce use of skills. The individual therapist (who is always the primary treatment provider in DBT)—with the client—is responsible for organizing the treatment so that all functions are met.

The utmost goal of DBT is to aid clients in their efforts to build a life worth living—wherein ultimately they can envision, articulate, pursue, and sustain goals that are independent of their histories of struggle with behavioral dyscontrol, including substance use, and where they grapple with ordinary (vs. extraordinary) problems in living. The emphasis on building a life worth living departs from ordinary expectations of behavioral or "symptom" management and palliative care.

Like other behavioral approaches, DBT includes a hierarchy of behavioral targets, beginning with decreasing imminent life-threatening behaviors (e.g., suicidal and homicidal behaviors), followed by decreasing client and therapist therapy-interfering behaviors (e.g., not attending therapy, dissociating during session, arriving late, attending sessions significantly intoxicated, not attending during the session), decreasing quality-of-life behaviors (e.g., homelessness, probation, Axis I behavioral problems, domestic violence), and increasing behavioral skills. The logic behind the DBT hierarchy of behavioral targets is simple: To address the myriad of problems clients with BPD have that interfere with getting and maintaining a life worth living, the client must first and foremost remain alive, then address problems that interfere with receiving the optimal treatment. When applying DBT to a substance-dependent client with BPD, decreasing drug use and behavioral patterns associated with drug use is typically the highest-order behavioral target within the quality-of-life-interfering behaviors. However, in DBT, quality-of-life targets are chosen by the client to meet his or her ultimate goals. Only when the DBT program is explicitly focused on substance abuse *and* the client commits to this focus is substance abuse required as a top quality of life target.

DIALECTICAL ABSTINENCE IN DIALECTICAL BEHAVIOR THERAPY

A dialectical stance on substance use was developed in recognition that, on the one hand, cognitive-behavioral relapse prevention approaches are effective in reducing the frequency and intensity of relapses after periods of abstinence (107–109) and, on the other hand, "absolute abstinence" approaches are effective in lengthening the interval between periods of use (110,111). "Dialectical abstinence" seeks to balance both approaches by maintaining an unrelenting insistence on total abstinence while the person is off drugs, then shifting to radical acceptance and nonjudgmental problem solving after a slip, followed by a quick return to the absolute abstinence pole the moment the person has stopped using. In DBT, absolute abstinence involves teaching patients specific cognitive self-control strategies that allow them to turn their minds fully and completely to abstinence. Specifically, patients learn how to anticipate and treat willfulness, hopelessness, and waffling on one's commitment to avoiding drugs. Patients learn that the key to absolute abstinence lies in convincing their brains that any use of drugs is completely out of the question. Patients are encouraged to make a commitment to remain abstinent for a specified period of time—a period that is no longer than he or she can commit to with 100% certainty that abstinence will be maintained (and no longer). Like the popular Twelve Step slogan, "Just for Today," the commitment to 100% abstinence may be for only 1 day, for a month, or for 5 minutes, depending on what the individual can commit to with 100% certainty. The commitment then is an act of mental "slamming the door shut" for the specified period of time. At the end of that time, the individual renews his or her commitment to abstinence. In this sense, absolute abstinence is achieved through a series of commitments to slamming the door shut. Hence, abstinence is sought only in the moment and only for a given set of moments.

Other cognitive self-control strategies used during this phase include immediate "adaptive" denial of desires and options to use alcohol or drugs during the specified period of the commitment, practicing radical acceptance of the absence of substance use and the difficulties involved, making an inner resolution that the option to use is left open for the future, and making a promise to one's self that such use will be available when close to death (e.g., learning of a terminal illness). Determining which strategy to use depends on a decision as to which one is most likely to be effective in promoting abstinence and achieving the willingness to maintain it.

The therapist shifts rapidly to the harm-reduction pole of the dialectic once a slip has occurred. Here the emphasis is on practicing "*failing well.*" Like Marlatt's concept of "prolapse" in relapse prevention (RP) (107), lemonade is made from the lemon by mining all there is to learn in the service of preventing future slips. The therapist highlights for the client that all people who attempt new behaviors that are hard and challenging are likely to "fail" before achieving success. Take learning to ride a bike: The new cyclist is likely to fall, potentially several *or more* times, before mastering his or her bike. Key to success lies in learning the relevant factors that seem to result in falling versus staying on the bike. Ideally, when a fall occurs, the cyclist takes stock of the new learning, then gets back on the bike and applies the new insights. In teaching how to fail well, emphasis is placed on "what if" and "just in case" skills. Consistent with a relapse prevention approach (107), the therapist and patient discuss realistic skills the patient can acquire and plans that can be made to address a similar situation in the future. In addition to teaching the patient to learn from past mistakes and encouraging him or her to continue to move forward toward the goal, failing well includes analysis of and reparation for harm done to others. The emphasis on correcting harm is similar to the concept of "making amends" in Twelve Step programs.

APPLYING PRINCIPLES OF DIALECTICAL BEHAVIOR THERAPY IN MANAGEMENT OF BPD PATIENTS

Whether serving as the pharmacotherapist in the context of a DBT treatment team or providing standard, non-DBT medical services to patients with BPD, these DBT-informed principles for clinical management are intended to improve treatment compliance and reduce problems common to patients with BPD.

Principle 1: Do Not Give Lethal Drugs to Lethal People Not all patients with BPD are suicidal or have histories of attempting suicide via overdose. Patients who *do*, however, have a history of attempting suicide by means of drugs should not receive lethal drugs they may use during a crisis as a means of killing themselves. Because the best predictor of future behavior is past behavior, we recommend assessing your patients' history of suicide attempts and the specific means used in those attempts to determine the patient's risk of overdosing on prescribed medications. For those suicidal patients with a history of overdosing on prescription medications, we recommend prescribing nonlethal medications. If it is not possible to prescribe a nonlethal, safe medication, then prescribe a limited non-lethal quantity at a time or have the patient arrange with a friend or family member to hold the bulk of the prescription for him or her.

Principle 2: Combine Pharmacotherapy with a Psychosocial Treatment The rationale for this principle stems from the chronicity and severity of BPD and the absence of data demonstrating that pharmacotherapy is sufficient for BPD patients. (For this reason, pharmacotherapy trials for BPD always include an active psychosocial component [85]). Ideally, the psychosocial treatment is an effective, evidence-based therapy such as DBT (1,2) or mentalization, an 18-month partial hospitalization treatment for BPD (89, 90,112,113). A Clinical Directory of DBT programs who have received DBT Intensive Training through Behavioral Tech, LLC, an organization founded by Marsha M. Linehan, Ph.D., is available through their Web site (*www.behavioraltech.org*). In the absence of a empirically validated treatment for BPD in a patient's region, consider a treatment provider with strong cognitive-behavioral training. The Association for the Advancement of Cognitive and Behavioral Therapy Web site also contains a Clinical Directory of its members (*www.abct.org*).

Principle 3: Do Not Reinforce Dysfunctional, Ineffective Behavior It is not uncommon to inadvertently reinforce (strengthen) dysfunctional behavior, including suicidal behaviors, in the process of attempting to help patients with BPD. In many treatment settings and systems, for example, patients with BPD receive more time, attention, warmth, sympathy, favors, and services (all of which are highly reinforcing for many BPD patients) when their behavior is most extreme, egregious, and dysfunctional. Though this may be temporarily helpful at reducing the immediate problem behavior and perhaps curative for a small percentage of BPD patients, it is seldom effective in the long run. Instead, the problem behavior becomes further strengthened, entrenched as a probable response in similar situations in the future and, ultimately, more difficult to treat. Consider the following examples:

A patient for whom expressions of concern and attention are highly reinforcing is met with extensive and focused attention, expressions of concern, and warmth from three different medical staff at the local emergency room while receiving sutures for a NSSI.

A therapist takes only after-hours telephone calls when her patients are in crisis. Over time, the patient's crises increase, as do the crisis calls. The therapist hypothesizes that the crisis behaviors are in part controlled by an increase in attention during these times. To test the hypothesis, she changes her policy and encourages her client to call to report small daily successes she has had in pursuing her long term goals (e.g., getting a job, enrolling in a vocational program). In a relatively brief period of time, the crises significantly decreased.

A suicidal patient is assigned her most-preferred staff during a one-to-one after a recent suicide attempt made on an inpatient unit.

It is unlikely that anyone intends to strengthen the probability of their patients' dysfunctional behaviors (indeed, most would be aghast at the thought!). Yet, the *proximity* (i.e., occurs after the patient's dysfunctional behavior) and *desirability* (i.e., highly reinforcing or desirable) is likely to nonetheless have this effect. How should a treatment provider respond so as not to inadvertently reinforce dysfunctional behavior? Of course, it all depends on the context, the patient's behavior, and what is in fact reinforcing for him or her. Consider this final scenario: You are meeting with a patient when another patient insists on seeing you right then. He is told that you are unavailable; in response, he begins pounding the wall, escalating in his demand to see you. What do you do? Here are several options:

- Do not make yourself *immediately* available to respond to the request.
- Another staff member on the floor, trained in how to coach emotionally dysregulated patients in skills to tolerate distressing situations without engaging in dysfunctional behavior, is available to encourage and coach the patient to apply adaptive behavioral skill in the moment.
- Wait until the dysfunctional behavior has significantly decreased or ceased and/or an effective, alternative behavior has shown up before seeing him (e.g., the patient makes the request in a way that is interpersonally skillful).
- When you do eventually meet with the patient, validate his feeling of urgency while also communicating your expectation that he makes his requests more skillfully in the future (e.g., uses a gentle, easy manner that demonstrates a willingness to wait until you are available).
- Assess whether your client actually knows how to do the behaviors you are suggesting (e.g., tolerating the distress of having to wait for you when feeling urgent, making the request in a light, easy manner, demonstrating understanding and empathy for your situation and busy schedule). If your patient does not have the necessary skills, teach him one or two and practice their use during your meeting.
- Encourage your patient to practice these skills during moments of mild to moderate distress so he has the skills in his repertoire when he is in greater distress.
- Reinforce your patient, including giving him your time and attention, when he is acting skillfully with you, including imperfect but improved attempts.

Principle 4: Catch the Patient "Being Good" (e.g., Acting Skillfully) Just as it is important *not* to inadvertently reinforce *dysfunctional* behavior, it is equally important to reinforce functional, effective behaviors emitted by the patient. This can be difficult to do for a number of reasons—including the fact that the improvement is barely noticeable and/or it occurs in the midst of other problematic, distressing behaviors. For example, consider a patient who yells loudly and verbally attacks her pharmacotherapist when she does not change the patient's medications or dose. To practice this principle, the pharmacotherapist might initially highlight an instance where the patient is not yelling as loud, or may be yelling loudly but is not simultaneously verbally attacking to reinforce the just noticeable change (e.g., "You know, I wish you weren't yelling as loudly, but I've got to tell you, I'll take the yelling any day over the attacks! It's so much easier for me to hear what you are saying"). The pharamacotherapist would then continue to shape the behavior over time, reinforcing small instances and improvements in the desired direction. Reinforcement can be verbal (e.g., "I *so* appreciate that you made the request the way you just did. I find I work harder to figure out a solution that is going to work for you when you speak to me in a regular voice."), nonverbal (e.g., acting more warm and engaged), and/or functional where he or she actively addresses the patient's requests (e.g., changes the medication or dosage, in this instance).

Two points are noteworthy. First, application of this principle requires paying close attention to the patient's behavior in order to detect "*just noticeable*" improvements to reinforce. Like changing any complex behavior, reinforcement of successive approximations or steps in the direction of the desired behavior is often required. Seldom does a person go from his or her baseline behavior to perfect performance of the behavior with a single reinforcer. Second, what constitutes a reinforcer is highly individualized. For example, though praise or increased attention from an important caregiver can be reinforcing to some patients, others might experience it as aversive. The best way to determine whether something is or is not a reinforcer is to notice the effect the consequence has on the behavior. If the behavior *increases* in response to the consequence, it is likely that the consequence is, in fact, a reinforcer.

Principle 5: Validate Valid Behavior Like most people, patients with BPD often thrive in validating contexts. In our own research, use of validation was associated with treatment retention (97). Treatment providers can always validate how painful or awful something is for the patient, the difficulty of doing something they do not know how to do (particularly in the context of intense emotions, like incredible sadness, shame, or anger), the confusion and/or difficulty they might experience when having to make an important, difficult decision, and the like. However, it is important not to validate maladaptive, ineffective (e.g., invalid) behavior. For example, feeling sad and taking a mini-vacation from grieving after the loss of a loved one by "forgetting" about it for a brief peroid is valid (e.g., it makes sense given the context, is reasonably normative, and is not going to cause the individual or her community harm); shooting up with heroin and cocaine as a means of taking the minivacation is invalid (e.g., it is not normative, does cause harm to the individual and possibly the community, and interferes with developing effective, long-term behavioral skills that are effective).

(To learn more about validation in DBT, read Linehan [114], *Validation in Psychotherapy* and/or contact BTECH [*www.behavioraltech.org*] for information on its online training in the application of validation principles and strategies in DBT.)

Behavioral Skills to Help Your Client Not Use Drugs For most patients with BPD and SUD, drug use and other dysfunctional behaviors function as a means of regulating or escaping negative emotions and tolerating distress (albeit ineffectively). If patients are to succeed in their efforts to get off and stay off drugs, they require a new set of functional behavioral skills to replace their dysfunctional behaviors. Linehan's (2) *Skills Training Manual for Borderline Personality Disorder* includes a plethora of such skills in four modules: **mindfulness** (i.e., skills for being present and "awake" in the moment in ways that move people closer to their "ultimate" or wisest goals and values); **interpersonal effectiveness** (i.e., skills for balancing wants vs. shoulds and priorities with demands, strategies for asking for what you want and say "no" to what you do not want, criteria to determine whether to ask or refuse a request); **emotion regulation** (i.e., strategies for understanding your emotions, stopping unwanted emotions from starting in the first place and skills for intervening once they start); and **distress tolerance (**skills for getting through a crisis without making the situation worse and radical acceptance skills).

Dialectical Behavior Therapy Skills for Newly Abstinent Patients Though most BPD-SUD patients need all skills across all these modules at some time or another in order to successfully maintain their abstinence, distress tolerance skills are particularly important for patients as they get off drugs. DBT Crisis Survival Strategies (2,115), a subcomponent of the DBT distress tolerance skills, are intended to help a person get through an immediate crisis without making matters worse by engaging in dysfunctional behavior, such as using drugs. One set of Crisis Survival Strategies are the Wise Mind "ACCEPTS" skills used to get through a distressing situation through the use of distraction (2,115). Another set involves Self-Soothing the Five Senses. Both sets of crisis survival strategies are intended as *short-term* strategies to get through a crisis (e.g., an intense urge or craving to use drugs, a very upsetting event); they are not intended to feel better or to solve the problem. (Clearly, if solving the problem is possible to do *now*, we would encourage a patient to do that. It is often the case, however, that while the problem can be solved, it cannot be solved this very moment, thus necessitating the use of distress tolerance skills.)

ACCEPTS is an acronym for the following skills: Distract with ***A****ctivities* (e.g., watching a movie, reading a gripping novel, gardening, playing computer games, making music), ***C****ontributing* (e.g., "forgetting" one's own crisis by assisting someone who needs help or doing something thoughtful for someone else such as writing a "thinking of you" card, volunteering, preparing a special meal for someone you care about), ***C****omparisons* (i.e., comparing yourself to those who are less fortunate than you or to times in your own life when things have been even more difficult and painful), *With Opposite* ***E****motions* (i.e., engaging in distracting activities that generate opposite emotions than those prompted by the crisis, such as watching a comedy or scary film, listening to uplifting music if you are feeling sad and having hopeless thoughts), ***P****ushing Away* (i.e., putting the crisis temporarily "on a shelf" so to speak where it can be mentally left, refusing to think about the distressing aspects of the situation, denying the problem for a moment), *With Other* ***T****houghts* (e.g., counting to 10, doing multiplication tables in your head, working crossword puzzles, repeating a word, phrase, or song in order to fill your mind with something other than the immediate crisis situation), and *With Other* ***S****ensations* (e.g., distracting with body sensations such as listening to loud music, getting wet in the rain, squeezing a rubber ball).

Whereas the ACCEPTS skills are intended to distract from the crisis itself, *Self-Soothing the Five Senses* are strategies that can be used when distraction is not possible or preferred. Self-Soothing can take the following forms: with **vision** (e.g., looking at peaceful scenes of nature, lighting a candle and watching the flame, going to an art gallery and looking at beautiful art, sitting in a something that is beautiful hotel lobby); with **smell** (e.g., wearing your favorite perfume, aftershave, or scented lotion; polishing furniture with lemon oil, baking cookies, smelling fragrant flowers, burning a scented candle); with **taste** (e.g., sipping a favorite, soothing, nonalcoholic beverage and/or eating your favorite food, sucking a mint, savoring the tastes fully); with **hearing** (e.g., listen to soothing, calming, beautiful music and/or nature sounds such as birds singing, waves crashing, a stream; hum a favorite tone; pay attention to sounds in your environment); and with **touch** (e.g., wearing clothes that you find compelling to touch, getting a massage, petting a dog or cat, taking a bath with bubbles, applying a cold or hot compress to your face or forehead).

In summary, ACCEPTS skills are intended to help (via distraction) a person get through a crisis situation without throwing fuel on the fire and making it worse. *Self-Soothing the Five Senses* are intended for situations that you cannot or prefer not to distract from. Neither set of crisis survival skills is intended to solve the crisis situation or to make the person feel better. Their function is simply limited to helping the person get through the moment without engaging in dysfunctional behaviors. (Obviously, if the crisis can be easily solved through active problem-solving, this course of action is encouraged as well.)

CONCLUSIONS

BPD and SUDs are both severe, chronic behavioral disorders. In combination, the two disorders pose considerable treatment challenges for both the patient and the clinician. Dialectical behavior therapy, an empirically supported therapy for chronically suicidal patients with BPD, has demonstrated efficacy for substance-dependent persons with BPD. This chapter reviewed the prevalence statistics for BPD with SUD, the risk of suicide and nonsuicidal self-injurious behavior for patients with BPD, and utilization of medical and psychiatric services for BPD patients. We provided a high-level review of DBT, including dialectic abstinence. We presented several principles informed by DBT in managing patients with BPD. Finally, we reviewed several DBT distress tolerance skills that can be of use in assisting patients to get through crises without engaging in dysfunctional behaviors.

REFERENCES

1. Linehan MM. *Cognitive behavioral treatment of borderline personality disorder.* New York: Guilford Press, 1993a.
2. Linehan MM. *Skills training manual for borderline personality disorder.* New York: Guilford, 1993b.
3. Lynch TR, Trost WT, Salsman N, Linehan MM. Dialectical behavior therapy for borderline personality disorder. *Ann Rev Clin Psychol* 2007; 3:181–205.
4. Robins CJ, Chapman AL. Dialectical behavior therapy: current status, recent developments, and future directions. *J Personal Disord* 2004;18 (1):73–89.
5. Salsman NL, Linehan MM. Dialectical-behavioral therapy for borderline personality disorder. *Prim Psychiatry* 2006;13(5):51–58.
6. Lynch TR, Rosenthal MZ, Kosson DS, et al. Heightened sensitivity to facial expressions of emotion in borderline personality disorder. *Emotion* 2006;6(4):647–655.
7. Widiger TA, Frances AJ. Epidemiology, diagnosis, and comorbidity of borderline personality disorder. In: Hales RE, Tasman A, Frances AJ, eds. *Am Psychiatr Press Rev Psychiatry*, vol. 8. Washington DC: American Psychiatric Press, 1989.
8. Kroll JL, Sines LK, Martin K. Borderline personality disorder: construct validity of the concept. *Arch Gen Psychiatry* 1981;39:60–83.
9. Modestin J, Abrecht I, Tschaggelar W, Hoffman H. Diagnosing borderline: a contribution to the question of its conceptual validity. *Arch Psychiatr Nervenkra* 1997;233:359–370.
10. Widiger TA, Weissman MM. Epidemiology of borderline personality disorder. *Hosp Commun Psychiatry* 1991;42:1015–1021.
11. Trull TJ, Sher KJ, Minks-Brown C, Durbin J, Burr R. Borderline personality disorder and substance use disorders: a review and integration. *Clin Psychol Rev* 2000;20:235–253.
12. Widiger TA, Trull TJ. Diagnosis and clinical assessment. *Ann Psychol Rev* 1991;42:109–133.
13. Brooner RK, King VL, Kidorf M, Schmidt CW, Bigelow GE. Psychiatric and substance use comorbidity among treatment-seeking opioid abusers. *Arch Gen Psychiatry* 1997;54:71–80.
14. DeJong CA, van den Brink W, Hartveld FM, van der Wielen, EG. Personality disorders in alcoholics and drug addicts. *Comp Psychol* 1993;34:87–94.
15. Miller NS, Belkin GM, Gibbons R. Clinical diagnosis of substance use disorders in private psychiatric populations. *J Subst Abuse Treat* 1994;11: 387–392.
16. Dulit RA, Fyer MR, Haas GL, Sullivan T, Frances AJ. Substance use in borderline personality disorder. *Am J Psychiatry* 1990;147:1002–1007.
17. Darke S, Williamson A, Ross J, Teesson M, Lynskey M. Borderline personality disorder, antisocial personality disorder and risk-taking among heroin users: fundings from the Australian Treatment Outcome Study (ATOS). *Drug Alcohol Depend* 2003;74:77–83.
18. Swadi H, Bobier C. Substance use disorder comorbidity among inpatient youth with psychiatric disorders. *Aust N Z J Psychiatry* 2003; 37:294–298.
19. Cacciola JS, Alterman AI, Rutherford MJ, Mckay JR, Mulvaney FD. The relationship of psychiatric comorbidity to treatment outcomes in methadone maintained patients. *Drug Alcohol Depend* 2001;61:271–280.
20. McKay JR, Alterman AI, Cacciola JS, Mulvaney FD, O'Brien CP. Prognostic significance of antisocial personality disorder in cocaine-dependent patients entering continuing care. *J Nerv Ment Dis* 2000;188:287–296.
21. Cacciola JS, Alterman AI, Rutherford MJ, Snider EC.. Treatment response of anti-social substance abusers. *J Nerv Ment Dis* 1995;183: 517–523.
22. Ceccero JJ, Ball SA, Tennen H, et al. Concurrent and predictive validity of antisocial personality disorder subtyping among substance abusers. *J Nerv Ment Dis* 1999;187:478–486.
23. Rutherford MJ, Cacciola JS, Alterman AI. Relationships of personality disorders with problem severity in methadone patients. *Drug Alcohol Depend* 1994;35:69–76.
24. Nace EP, Davis CW, Gaspari JP. Axis II comorbidity in substance abusers. *Am J Psychiatry* 1991;148:115–120.
25. Kosten RA, Kosten TR, Rounsaville BJ. Personality disorders in opiate addicts show prognostic specificity. *J Subst Abuse Treat* 1989;6:163–168.
26. Links PS, Heslegrave RJ, Mitton JE, Van Reekum R, Patrick J. Borderline personality disorder and substance abuse: consequences of comorbidity. *Can J Psychiatry* 1995;40:9–14.
27. Stone MH. Long-term outcome in personality disorders. *Br J Psychiatry* 1993;162:299–313.
28. Grove WM, Tellegen A. Problems in the classification of personality disorders. *J Personal Disord* 1991;5:31–41.
29. Gunderson JG. *Borderline personality disorder.* Washington, DC: American Psychiatric Press, 1984.
30. Cowdry RW, Pickar D, Davies R. Symptoms and EEG findings in the borderline syndrome. *Int J Psychiatry Med* 1985;15:201–211.
31. Clarkin JF, Widiger T, Frances A, Hurt SW, Gilmore. Prototypic typology and the borderline personality disorder. *J Abnorm Psychol* 1983;92: 263–275.
32. Frances A, Fyer M, Clarkin J. Personality and suicide. *Ann N Y Acad Sci* 1986;487:281–293.
33. Linehan MM, Rizvi SL, Welch SS, Page B. Psychiatric aspects of suicidal beahviour: personality disorders. In: Hawton K, ed. *International handbook of suicide and attempted suicide.* Sussex, England: John Wiley & Sons, 2000:147–178.
34. Stone MH, Hurt SW, Stone DK. The PI 500: long-term follow-up of borderline inpatients meeting DSM-III criteria: I. Global outcome. *J Personal Disord* 1987;1(4):291–298.
35. Links PS, Heslegrave RJ, Mitton JE, van Reekum R, Patrick J. Borderline personality disorder and substance abuse: consequences of comorbidity. *Can J Psychiatry* 1995;40(1):9–14.
36. Soloff PH. Is there any drug treatment of choice for the borderline patient? *Acta Psychiatr Scand* 1994;379:50–55.
37. Mann JJ. Suicide, aggression, and the depressed patient. In: Siever LJ, Mann JJ, eds. *Aggression and suicide: Neurobiology to treatment.* San Diego, CA: Symposium presented at the meeting of the American Psychological Association, 1997.
38. Skodol AE, Gunderson JG, McGlashan TH, et al. Functional impairment in patients with schizotypal, borderline, avoidant, or obsessive-compulsive personality disorder. *Am J Psychiatry* 2002;159(2):276–283.
39. Links PS, Steiner M, Offord DR, et al. Characteristics of borderline personality disorder: a Canadian study. *Can J Psychiatry* 1998;33:336–340.
40. Williams JM. *Cry of pain: understanding suicide and self-harm.* London: Penguin, 1997.
41. Carpenter MD, Mulligan JC, Bader IA, et al. Multiple admissions to an urban psychiatric center: a comparative study. *Hosp Commun Psychiatry* 1985;36:1305–1308.
42. Geller JL. In again, out again: preliminary evaluation of a state hospital's worst recidivists. *Hosp Commun Psychiatry* 1986;37:386–390.
43. Green JH. Frequent rehospitalization and noncompliance with treatment. *Hosp Commun Psychiatry* 1988;39:963–966.
44. Hadley TR, McGurrin MC, Pulice RT, et al. Using fiscal data to identify heavy service users. *Psychiatr Q* 1990;61:41–48.

45. Surber RW, Winkler EL, Monteleone M, et al. Characteristics of high users of acute inpatient services. *Hosp Commun Psychiatry* 1987;38: 1112–1116.
46. Woogh CM. A cohort through the revolving door. *Can J Psychiatry* 1986;31:214–221.
47. Bender DS, Dolan RT, Skodol AE, et al. Treatment utilization by patients with personality disorders. *Am J Psychiatry* 2001;158(2):295–302.
48. Swigar ME, Astrachan B, Levine MA, et al. Single and repeated admissions to a mental health center: demographic, clinical and use of service characteristics. *Int J Soc Psychiatry* 1991;37(4):259–266.
49. Geller JL. In again, out again: preliminary evaluation of a state hospital's worst recidivists. *Hosp Commun Psychiatry* 1986;4:386–390.
50. Widiger TA, Weissman MM. Epidemiology of borderline personality disorder. *Hosp Commun Psychiatry* 1991;42(10):1015–1021.
51. Surber RW, Winkler EL, Monteleone M, et al. Characteristics of high users of acute psychiatric inpatient services. *Hosp Commun Psychiatry* 1987;38(10):1112–1114.
52. Perry JC, Herman JL, Van der Kolk BA, Hoke LA. Psychotherapy and psychological trauma in borderline personality disorder. *Psychiatr Ann* 1990;20:33–43.
53. Skodol A E, Buckley P, Charles E. Is there a characteristic pattern to the treatment history of clinic outpatients with borderline personality? *J Nerv Ment Dis* 1983;171(7):405–410.
54. Bender DS, Dolan RT, Skodol AE, et al. Treatment utilization by patients with personality disorders. *Am J Psychiatry* 2001;158(2):295–302.
55. Hueston WJ, Mainous AG, Schilling R. Patients with personality disorders: Functional status, health care utilization, and satisfaction with care. *J Fam Pract* 1996;42:54–60.
56. First MB, Spitzer RL, Gibbons M, et al. *User's guide for the Structured Clinical Interview for DSM-IV Axis II Personality Disorders (SCID-II).* New York: Biometrics Research Department, New York State Psychiatric Institute, 1996.
57. Felitti VJ. Long term consequences of incest, rape, and molestation. *South Med J* 1991;84:328–331.
58. Gould DA, Stevens NG, Ward NG, et al. Self-reported childhood abuse in an adult population in a primary care setting. *Arch Fam Med* 1994; 151:252–256.
59. Koss MP, Koss PG, Woodruff W J Deleterious effects of criminal victimization of women's health and medical utilization. *Arch Intern Med* 1991;151:342–347.
60. Lechner ME, Vogel ME, Garcia-Shelton LM, et al. Self-reported medical problems of adult female survivors of childhood sexual abuse. *J Fam Pract* 1993;36:633–638.
61. McCauley JKD, Kolodner K, et al. *JAMA* 1997;277–1362–1368.
62. Bryer JB, Nelson BA, Miller JB, et al. Childhood sexual and physical abuse as factors in adult psychiatric illness. *Am J Psychiatry* 1987;144:1426–1430.
63. Herman JL, Perry JC, van der Kolk BA. Childhood trauma in borderline personality disorder. *Am J Psychiatry* 1989;146:490–495.
64. Ogata SN, Silk KR, Goodrich S, et al. *Childhood sexual and clinical symptoms in borderline patients* [Unpublished manuscript], 1989.
65. Stone MH. Psychiatrically ill relatives of borderline patients: a family study. *Psychiatr Q* 1981;58:71–83.
66. Wagner AW, Linehan MM, Wasson EJ. *Parasuicide: Characteristics and relationship to childhood sexual abuse.* Paper presented at the annual meeting of the Association for Advancement of Behavior Therapy, Washington, DC, 1989.
67. Frankenburg FR, Zanarini MC. Personality disorders and medical comorbidity. *Curr Opin Psychiatry* 2006;19:428–431.
68. Barasch A, Frances AJ, Hurt SW. Stability and distinctness of borderline personality disorder. *Am J Psychiatry* 1985;142:1484–1486.
69. Dahl AA. Prognosis of the borderline disorders. *Psychopathology* 1986; 19:68–79.
70. Richman J, Charles E. Patient dissatisfaction and attempted suicide. *Commun Ment Health J* 1976;123:301–305.
71. Kullgren G. Personality Disorders among psychiatric inpatients. *Nord Psykiastrisktidssr* 1992;46:27–32.
72. Pope HG, Jonas JM, Hudson, JI, et al. The validity of DSM-III borderline personality disorder: a phenomenologic, family history, treatment response, and long term follow up study. *Arch Gen Psychiatry* 1983;40: 23–30.
73. McGlashan TH. The Chestnut Lodge follow-up study: III. Long-term outcome of borderline personality disorder. *Arch Gen Psychiatry* 1986; 43:20–30.
74. Paris J, Brown R, Nowlis D. Long-term follow-up of borderline patients in a general hospital. *Comp Psychiatry* 1987;28:530–535.
75. Paris J, Zweig-Frank H. A 27-year follow-up of patents with borderline personality disorder. *Comp Psychiatry* 2001;42:482–487.
76. Phillips KA, Nierenberg AA. The assessment and treatment of refractory depression. *J Clin Psychiatry* 1994;55:20–26.
77. Baer L, Jenike MA, Black DW, et al. Effect of axis II diagnoses on treatment outcome with clomipramine in 55 patients with obsessive-compulsive disorder. *Arch Gen Psychiatry* 1992;49:862–866.
78. Ames-Frankel J, Devlin MJ, Walsh T, et al. Personality disorder diagnoses in patients wth bulimia nervosa: clinical correlates and changes with treatment. *J Clin Psychiatry* 1992;53:90–96.
79. Coker S, Vize C, Wade T, Cooper PJ. Patients with bulimia nervosa who fail to engage in cognitive behavior therapy. *Int J Eat Disord* 1993;13:35–40.
80. Perry JC, Cooper SH. Psychodynamics, symptoms, and outcome in borderline and antisocial personality disorders an bipolar type II affective disorder. In: McGlashan TH, ed. *The borderline: current empirical research.* Washington, DC: Amercian Psychiatric Press, 1985:21–41.
81. Tucker L, Bauer SF, Wagner S, et al. Long-term hospital treatment of borderline patients: a descriptive outcome study. *Am J Psychiatry* 1987; 144:1443–1448.
82. Kelly T, Soloff PH, Cornelius J, et al. Can we study treat) borderline patients? Attrition from research and open treatment. *J Personal Disord* 1992;6:417–433.
83. Soloff PH. Is there any drug treatment of choice for the borderline patient? *Acta Psychiatr Scand* 1994;379:50–55.
84. Soloff PH. Symptom-oriented psychopharmacology for personality disorders. *J Pract Psychiatry Behavl Health* 1998;4:3–11.
85. Soloff, PH. Psychopharmacology of borderline personality disorder. *Psychiatr Clin North Am* 2000;23:169–192.
86. Skodol AE, Buckley P, Charles E. Is there a characteristic pattern to the treatment history of clinic outpatients with borderline personality? *J Nerv Ment Dis* 1983;171:405–410.
87. Perry JC, Herman JL, Van Der Kolk BA, Hoke LA. Psychotherapy and psychological trauma in borderline personality disorder. *Psychiatr Ann* 1990;20:33–43.
88. Marziali E, Munroe-Blum H. *Interpersonal group psychotherapy for borderline personality disorder.* New York: Basic Books, 1994.
89. Bateman AW, Fonagy P. Effectiveness of partial hospitalization in the treatment of borderline personality disorder: A randomized controlled trial. *Am J Psychiatry* 1999;156:1563–1569.
90. Bateman AW, Fonagy P. Treatment of borderline personality disorder with psychoanalytically oriented partial hospitalization: an 18-month follow-up. *Am J Psychiatry* 2001;158:36–42.
91. Koons CR, Robins CJ, Tweed JL, et al. Efficacy of dialectical behavior therapy in women veterans with borderline personality disorder. *Behav Ther* 2001;32:371–390.
92. Linehan MM, Armstrong HE, Suarez A, et al. Cognitive-behavioral treatment of chronically parasuicidal borderline patients. *Arch Gen Psychiatry* 1991;48:1060–1064.
93. Linehan MM, Heard HL, Armstrong HE. Naturalistic follow-up of a behavioral treatment for chronically parasuicidal borderline patients. *Arch Gen Psychiatry* 1993;50:971–974.
94. Van Den Bosch LMC, Koeter M, Stijnen TV, et al. Sustained efficacy of dialectical behavior therapy for borderline personality disorder. *Behav Res Ther* 2005;439:1231–1241.
95. Verheul R, Van Den Bosch LM, Koeter MW, et al. Dialectical behaviour therapy for women with borderline personality disorder: 12-month randomized clinical trial in The Netherlands. *Br J Psychiatry* 2003;2(182): 135–140.
96. Linehan MM, Schmidt H, Dimeff LA, et al. Dialectical Behavior Therapy for patients with borderline personality disorder and drug dependence. *Am J Addict* 1999;8:279–292.

97. Linehan MM, Dimeff LA, Reynolds SK, et al. Dialectical behavior therapy versus comprehensive validation plus 12-Step for the treatment of opioid dependent women meeting criteria for borderline personality disorder. *Drug Alcohol Depend* 2002;671:13–26.
98. Safer DL, Telch CF, Agras, WS. Dialectical behavior therapy for bulimia nervosa. *Am J Psychiatry* 2001;1584:632–634.
99. Telch CF, Agras WS, Linehan MM. Group dialectical behavior therapy for bing eating disorder: a preliminary uncontrolled trial. *Behav Ther* 2000;31:569–582.
100. Lynch TR, Morse JQ, Mendelson T, Robins CJ. Dialectical Behavior Therapy for depressed older adults: a randomized pilot study. *Am J Geriatr Psychiatry* 2003;11:33–45.
101. American Psychiatric Assocation. Gold award: integrating dialectical behavior therapy into a community mental health program. *Psychiatr Serv* 1998;49:1138–1340.
102. Linehan MM. Development, evaluation, and dissemination of effective psychosocial treatments: stages of disorder, levels of care, and stages of treatment research. In: MD, Hartel Glantz CR, eds. *Drug abuse: origins and interventions.* Washington, DC: American Psychological Association, 1999.
103. Linehan MM, Kanter JW, Comtois KA. Dialectical behavior therapy for borderline personality disorder: efficacy, specificity, and cost-effectiveness. In: Janowsky DS, ed. *Psychotherapy: indications and outcomes* Washington, DC: American Psychiatric Press, 1999:93–118.
104. Linehan MM. Dialectical behavior therapy: a cognitive behavioral approach to parasuicide. *J Personal Disord* 1987;1:328–333.
105. Swann WB, Stein-Seroussi A, Giesler R. Why people self-verify. *J Person Social Psychol* 1992;62:392–401.
106. Linehan MM. Self-verification and drug abusers: implications for treatment. *Psychol Sci* 1997;8:181–183.
107. Marlatt GA, Gordon JR. *Relapse prevention: maintenance strategies in the treatment of addictive behaviors.* New York: Guilford Publications, Inc. 1985.
108. Dimeff LA, Marlatt GA. Preventing relapse and maintaining change in addictive behaviors. *Clin Psychol: Sci Pract* 1998;5:513–525.
109. Carroll KM. Relapse prevention as a psychological treatment: a review of controlled clinical trials. *Exp Clin Psychopharmacol* 1996;4:46–54.
110. Hall SM, Havassy BE, Wasserman DA. Commitment to abstinence and acute stress in relapse to alcohol, opiates, and nicotine. *J Consult Clin Psychol* 1990;58:175–181.
111. Supnick JA, Colletti G. Relapse coping and problem solving training following treatment for smoking. *Addict Behav* 1984;9:401–404.
112. Bateman A, Fonagy P. *Psychotherapy for borderline personality disorder: mentalization based treatment.* Oxford: Oxford University Press, 2004.
113. Bateman AW, Fonagy P. Partial hospitalization for borderline personality disorder: reply. *Am J Psychiatry* 2001;158:1932–1933.
114. Linehan MM. Validation and psychotherapy. In: Bohart A, Greenberg L, eds. *Empathy reconsidered: new direction in psychotherapy.* Washington DC: American Psychological Association, 1997.
115. Linehan MM. *Skills training manual for disordered emotion regulation.* New York: Guilford Publications, Inc., (in press).
116. Jacobson E. *Progressive relaxation.* Chicago: University of Chicago Press, 1938.

SUGGESTED READINGS

McMain S, Sayrs JHR, Dimeff LAD, Linehan MM. Dialectical behavior therapy for individuals with BPD and substance dependence. In: Dimeff LA, Koerner KK, eds. *Dialectical behavior therapy in clinical practice: applications across disorders and settings.* New York: Guilford, 2007:145–173.

Cioffi D, Holloway J. Delayed costs of suppressed pain. *Journal of Personality and Social Psychology* 1993;64:274–282.

Linehan MM. *Cognitive behavioral treatment of borderline personality disorder.* New York: Guilford Press, 1993.

Linehan MM. *Skills training manual for treating borderline personality disorder.* New York: Guilford Press, 1993.

Ling W, Rawson RA, Compton MA. Substitution pharmacotherapies for opioid addiction: from methadone to LAAM and buprenorphine. *J Psychoactuve Drugs* 1994;26:119–128.

Platt S, Bille-Brahe U, Kerkhof A, et al. Parasuicide in Europe: The WHO/EURO multicentre study on parasuicide: I. Introduction and preliminary analysis for 1989. *Acta Psychiatr Scand* 1992;85:97–104.

Smith RG, Monson RA, Ray DC. Psychiatric consultation in somatization disorder: a randomized controlled study. *N Engl J Med* 1986;314(22): 1407–1413.

Tanney BL. Mental disorders, psychiatric patients, and suicide. In: Maris RW, Berman AL, Maltsberger JT, eds. *Assessment and prediction of suicide.* New York: Guilford Press,1992:277–320.

Wegner DM, Gold DB. Fanning old flames: emotional and cognitive effects of suppressing thoughts of a past relationship. *J Person Soc Psychol* 1995;67:782–792.

CHAPTER 89

Joan E. Zweben, PhD
Richard K. Ries, MD, FAPA, FASAM

Integrating Psychosocial Services with Pharmacotherapies in the Treatment of Co-occurring Disorders

The goal of this chapter is to offer assistance to the clinician who is engaged in coordinating addiction and psychosocial treatment services on behalf of patients with co-occurring substance use and psychiatric disorders ("dual disorders"). It focuses on four areas of concern.

First, one of the great strengths of the addiction field is its multidisciplinary teamwork. Though the physician who works in a program with multiple components is an essential part of the health care team, professionals who offer psychosocial interventions also play a major role.

Second, cost constraints now restrict the physician's role far more narrowly than many would prefer. Given these constraints, effective interdisciplinary teamwork often makes the difference between a first-rate program and an average one.

Third, recent developments have expanded opportunities for physicians in office-based practice. Taking advantage of such opportunities requires that physicians become adept at integrating services that are not provided at the office site. The chapter addresses key elements affecting such teamwork and coordination.

Finally, good supervision or collaboration is time-consuming and requires strong facilitation skills at the leadership level. When treatment providers are in conflict, patients suffer. This chapter describes a variety of common situations and dilemmas and offers practical options for handling them.

WORKING WITH COUNSELORS AND PSYCHOTHERAPISTS

Psychosocial interventions typically are provided by practitioners from a variety of disciplines. These range from noncredentialed counselors (usually persons in recovery) to licensed psychologists, social workers, and marriage, family, and child counselors. Such practitioners differ widely in their attitudes, preparation, and skills. They also vary in the degree to which they are accustomed to working with physicians and other medical personnel. Understanding the background and orientation of specific staff can enhance communication and teamwork.

Counselors Noncredentialed counselors have been integrated into treatment teams on inpatient units since the 1950s, when the Minnesota Model was developed at Hazelden and Wilmar (1). Before that time, alcoholism was seen as a psychologic vulnerability to be treated on mental health units; however, this theoretical framework failed to produce effective treatment. Collaboration by the leaders of Hazelden and Wilmar led to an adaptation of the principles of Alcoholics Anonymous (AA) to create a new model within hospital-based treatment. Wilmar and Hazelden eventually blended their approaches to produce the Minnesota Model, which became the prototype of 28-day inpatient programs. Proponents of the model refined their treatment practices and restructured institutional relationships to emphasize collaboration between professional staff and non-credentialed recovering persons. By 1954, counselors without professional degrees shared both responsibility and decision-making authority.

Therapeutic communities (TCs), which developed and expanded in the 1960s, also relied predominantly on noncredentialed staff who were themselves in recovery (2–5). Some of these gifted clinicians and managers subsequently were hired into the private, insurance-funded treatment system, to which they brought their perspective on the importance of developing a culture that supports recovery. Their appreciation of the need to strengthen environmental or microcommunity forces to foster change added an important dimension to the professional model, which typically assumes that professional services are the main—if not the sole—factor in promoting change.

Programs today differ widely in the extent to which they incorporate nonlicensed, recovering personnel. Such personnel are found in short-term, Minnesota Model, chemical dependency inpatient programs, in a growing number of co-occurring disorder programs, and in community-based addiction treatment programs. They also are dominant in therapeutic communities, which have their own conceptual model that integrates Twelve Step elements to varying degrees. Some of these counselors return to school and obtain graduate degrees and licenses, building the cadre of professionals in recovery.

Like licensed staff members, noncredentialed counselors vary widely in talent, experience, and skill. Some have little training, except for occasional in-service training sessions. Others have completed comprehensive credentialing programs and are far more sophisticated than some licensed staff. For example, certificate programs (often attached to universities) may require 200 to 300 hours of course work, plus supervised field placement experience. However, some of these programs teach from an exclusively Twelve Step perspective and do not do justice to alternative approaches or to the empirical literature, while others are more broadly based. The current emphasis on incorporating evidence-based approaches exerts a growing influence on these certificate programs.

Some counselors have superb skills; their "street savvy" and personal experience in recovery produce a highly sophisticated clinician. Others tend toward rigidity ("what worked for me will work for you") and have difficulty tolerating the ambiguities of the complex clinical populations seen today. In short, physicians should draw conclusions about the skill level of the counselors with whom they work from direct observation, not from inferences based on the presence or absence of credentials.

At their best, such counselors also are a powerful role model, a contribution deeply valued by addicted patients, especially those in early recovery.

Licensed Professionals Within addiction treatment settings, one finds licensed professionals, some of whom are recovering, others who are not. Some may be highly knowledgeable, others less so. Though most such professionals have basic clinical skills, their ability and comfort in adapting those skills to the addicted patient population vary greatly. The rigidities of some licensed professionals arise from devotion to theoretical models in which they have extensive training, in addition to their own personality traits. Physicians should be cautious about drawing conclusions from the presence of academic credentials and professional licenses. Unfortunately, graduate schools do not usually integrate thorough training in the assessment and treatment of addiction into their core curricula, even though many of the clinical populations with whom graduates will work are using alcohol and drugs. Typically, such training is provided as an elective (if at all) or in a course mandated by the increasing number of states that require an introductory course for initial licensure or license renewal. Other programs offer extensive training through extension courses or specialized training institutes, and some graduate programs offer addiction treatment as a subspecialty. However, the physician never should assume that a professional is knowledgeable in this area. Professionals may underestimate their own lack of knowledge, preferring to believe that the models they acquired in training can be adapted to treating addiction with little modification, or that specialized knowledge about addictive disorders is unnecessary.

Clinical experience alone may tell little about qualifications. Upon inquiry, a therapist may say, "I've been seeing alcohol and drug users for 20 years." Many therapists have evolved practices with which they have grown comfortable but which bear little relation to those supported by an empirical literature or by the experience of clinicians who are addiction specialists. The comfort level of these therapists is sustained because they do not count, much less study, their dropouts and thus have no objective means of monitoring patient progress in becoming alcohol- and drug-free. (This is of particular concern because many patients report concealing or minimizing their alcohol and drug use during psychotherapy.) In selecting good therapists for referral, physicians should look for evidence of recent systematic training, either through conferences or course work. Such evidence increases the likelihood that the therapist will be familiar with sound treatment practices.

Tensions may be present between recovering and nonrecovering staff and between those with and without professional training and licenses. Passions can run high, and basic concepts can be used to express disapproval or to discredit one's colleagues. The concepts of enabling and codependency in particular lend themselves to disparaging colleagues who take certain positions. They often are used to discourage appropriate forms of helping and to terminate treatment prematurely. Time in treatment is correlated significantly with positive outcomes in a large number of treatment outcome studies (6–9). Thus, the goal is to engage and retain patients in treatment, not to terminate them for manifesting symptoms of their psychiatric or addictive disorder. Physicians also may struggle in dealing with this phenomenon, even though other chronic diseases such as asthma, diabetes, and hypertension have compliance rates comparable to those of addiction treatment (10,11). They may need to be the voice of reason, preventing premature termination of the patient while being mindful of the need to avoid colluding in negative patient behaviors.

Physicians in leadership roles are advised to establish weekly in-service training sessions that address both basic and specialized topics. They can create a multidisciplinary team that has a shared language and is knowledgeable about integrating the treatment of addictive, psychiatric, and medical disorders. Many sources of excellent training materials exist. Some materials are available at no charge (such as the Treatment Improvement Protocols published by the federal Center for Substance Abuse Treatment). These materials can be used to organize on-site training sessions. Securing continuing

TABLE 89.1 Typical Attributes of Addiction Treatment and Psychotherapy, Compared

Typical attributes of addiction treatment	Typical attributes of psychotherapy
1. Structured format	1. Minimal structure
2. Goals less flexible	2. Wider range of goals
3. Alcohol and drug focus	3. Focus on underlying process
4. Monitoring by breath and urine testing	4. No testing; possible negative attitude
5. Varied treatment components	5. One component
6. Active, directive therapists	6. Varied clinical styles

Adapted from Rawson R. Issues in outpatient treatment. Presented at the Medical-Scientific Conference of the American Society of Addiction Medicine, Atlanta, GA, April, 1997, with permission.

education credits for the disciplines represented on staff enhances participation and commitment to a high-quality training sequence.

The National Addiction Technology Transfer Center (*www.nattc.org*) offers a comprehensive list of institutions offering a certificate, associate, bachelor, master, and/or doctoral program in substance use disorders. Also included in this directory are institutions offering a concentration, specialty or minor in the addiction field. It also offers licensing and certification requirements by state and organization.

Collaboration with Psychotherapists in the Community The diversity of psychotherapists in the community can make effective collaboration even more challenging. Table 89.1 describes certain key differences between general psychotherapy and addiction treatment.

Addiction treatment typically is highly structured, with multiple behavioral expectations. Psychotherapy usually has minimal structure other than the scheduled sessions. Psychodynamic therapists in particular may have difficulty incorporating behavioral commitments, whereas eclectic therapists may find this work more comfortable. Most outpatient addiction treatment is abstinence-oriented. Though this goal may be difficult to reach, the goal itself normally does not vary. Abstinence usually is viewed as the foundation that must be in place before meaningful progress can be made on other issues.

Psychotherapy has a wider range of goals and less consistent priorities. Some psychotherapists may not understand or endorse the need for abstinence over some form of controlled use. For example, they may share the view that drinking is "normal." Hence, they see controlled drinking as a reasonable goal, even in patients who have repeatedly demonstrated they cannot moderate their use (12). Addiction treatment makes alcohol and drug use the primary focus, whereas psychodynamic psychotherapy explores the underlying process as a means of bringing about change. If ill-timed, this focus on process can undermine sobriety by elevating anxiety before abstinence is firmly established.

Addiction treatment often includes breath and urine testing if resources permit, whereas psychotherapists rarely arrange such testing, and many consider it invasive and abhorrent. Addiction treatment encompasses a variety of treatment components, whereas psychotherapy usually relies on the therapy sessions themselves as the sole component. Therapists and counselors in addiction treatment are active and directive, whereas psychotherapists in private practice have a variety of styles, which can be more or less compatible with addiction treatment. These differences pose an adaptive challenge to the physician who is arranging for treatment of patients with dual disorders.

USE OF PHARMACOTHERAPIES

Recovering patients who have conditions that require psychotropic or other medications have very special needs. Their specific drug use history makes the use of certain medications highly problematic because of the potential for abuse of the prescribed drug or that use of such a drug will precipitate relapse to the primary drug of abuse. Though this volume offers appropriate prescribing guidelines, patients who present for treatment may be taking medications prescribed by physicians who lack a background in addiction medicine. In settings wherein patients are seen by physicians only when specific problems emerge, counselors need a screening tool that incorporates warning signals (such as prescriptions for benzodiazepines) that indicate a need for physician review.

Recovering patients also have complex feelings and attitudes toward medications that need to be understood and addressed. Many define recovery as living a comfortable and responsible lifestyle without the use of psychoactive drugs. Yet some disorders require the use of psychiatric medications. Family members or Twelve Step program participants may criticize the patient or pressure for discontinuation of medication, generating conflict that undermines treatment. Because physicians often lack adequate time to deal with such issues, these tasks should be delegated specifically to other members of the treatment team. Such providers may need some additional training to handle medication issues.

Achieving Adherence Adherence to treatment recommendations is a key factor in successful treatment outcomes. Hence, physicians should monitor how well the treatment team attends to this issue. Compliance with medication regimens is far from perfect, even in well-educated middle-class patients who do not have a stigmatized illness. Not surprisingly, addicted patients, who often have additional psychiatric and medical disorders, have difficulty in this area. Carefully eliciting patient concerns and objections is worthwhile. Many behavioral strategies yield poor results because no one took the time to identify the real obstacles to compliance. Sympathetic listening, combined with well-timed doses of information, can improve medication adherence significantly.

Physicians can help counselors and psychotherapists to understand and explore these issues in their counseling sessions with patients. Non-physicians vary considerably in their attitudes and education about medication. Time spent on educating therapists usually yields multiple benefits. Certain forms of resistance occur frequently (13). Patients on psychotropic medications often feel ashamed and guilty, believing that they have failed if they cannot master their illness by themselves. Because their illness is not measurable in the same manner as diabetes, it is easier for them to sustain this guilt. For recovering persons, there are added layers of difficulty. Taking a medication to feel better is highly charged, as many link this motive inextricably with their alcohol and drug use. Even in the case of medications such as antidepressants, which produce no feelings of euphoria or "high," such guilt can persist. Some patients report they feel they are "cheating," even though their depression precipitated multiple relapses during the time it was untreated.

Rejecting a recommendation for medication may reflect the "all-or-none" thinking characteristic of the alcohol- or drug-addicted person. The same patient who at one time consumed every available substance becomes horrified at the idea of "putting something foreign in my body" or "relying on drugs." With respect to disulfiram (Antabuse), Banys (14) notes that many patients disdainfully describe it as a "crutch." Even though these are the same patients who used alcohol as a "crutch" for years, they are paradoxically fastidious about this one. Medications such as disulfiram or naltrexone (ReVia) can provide an invaluable (and life-saving) opportunity to alter behavior patterns; however, patients who use these medications may feel unable to take credit for their achievements. Reliance on the medication undermines the sense of mastery that ultimately promotes lasting sobriety; hence, the importance of handling this issue carefully when such treatment adjuncts are used.

Indeed, medication should not be used as a substitute for doing the work of recovery. For example, a patient taking disulfiram can be asked to keep a daily journal describing situations that would have been hazardous if he or she were not on the medication. The patient then can be asked what behaviors need to be strengthened (often assertive behaviors) to create safety even in the absence of medication. The decision to discontinue can be implemented once the patient has developed coping skills for the high-risk situations previously identified.

Adherence with medication regimens can be monitored through refill requests. Patients who are adhering to their regimens initiate contact with their physicians for refills before the existing supplies expire. Prescribing enough doses for a long period deprives the physician of this potential warning signal. Communication with other treatment staff is essential when noncompliance is suspected. Discontinuation of psychotropic medication often is a harbinger of relapse to alcohol and drugs, as distressing psychiatric symptoms begin to reemerge. It also can be an indicator that a relapse to alcohol or other drug use already has occurred.

It is important for counselors to identify medication side effects that influence adherence, discuss them with the patient, and facilitate a plan to coordinate with the physician. For example, Johnson et al. (15) have documented that patients with bipolar disorder are more likely to be consistent about medications that reduce the severity of their depressive episodes and do not cause weight gain or cognitive effects. Supporting the patient in a problem-solving process with the physician is an important role for the counselor.

The physician needs to discuss with the patient and other members of the treatment team the indications for discontinuing medications and the process by which such discontinuation should occur. Many patients with prescriptions for disulfiram report that they have not had discussions with their physicians on this topic. Physicians should clarify that disulfiram is a tool to allow other accomplishments to take place. The patient needs to review his or her progress with program staff, a private therapist, or the prescribing physician before discontinuing medication. Patients who are taking antidepressants may go into denial about their psychiatric disorder once they feel better and thus discontinue use of the medication prematurely. The physician needs to educate both patients and non-physician therapists about the dangers of psychiatric and addiction relapse that attend such a decision.

Control issues are common. Some patients will accept the need for prescribed drugs but will tinker with frequency and dose, much as they did with their illicit substances. Some may operate on the assumption that if one pill is good, three are better, and escalate their dose of medications not usually considered abusable. Drug mixing is another common practice. "Surrendering control of medication use to your physician" is a concept that can prove useful; under such a scenario, any deviation from the prescribed regimen is the subject of inquiry. Patients who are engaged in serious self-examination may spontaneously report such behavior as a residual part of their addictive pattern.

Office-Based Opioid Therapy Recent efforts to reduce barriers to obtaining treatment have created new opportunities and corresponding challenges for physicians who are interested in providing opioid maintenance medications to their patients. Current federal law permits physicians to provide methadone provided they are affiliated with a licensed narcotic treatment program and buprenorphine in an office-based practice.

The U.S. Food and Drug Administration (FDA) has determined that medical maintenance treatment can be provided through program-wide exemptions under the current opioid treatment regulations. Stable, socially rehabilitated patients may receive up to a month's supply of take-home medications, and can reduce the frequency of other clinic visits accordingly. Medication can be provided by the physician's office (if it meets security requirements) or by a pharmacy. This form of office-based opioid therapy (also see Chapter 50, "Special Issues in Office-Based Opioid Treatment") is intended to extend the service continuum to better meet the needs of patients who no longer need the extensive structure of the opioid treatment program or clinic that offers psychosocial services at the clinic site. However, participating physicians should be prepared to recognize relapse warning signs and intervene promptly.

In the event that the patient does not need the more structured interventions available in the clinic, the physician must be prepared to offer relevant alternatives in the community. A psychotherapist with expertise in addiction may be able to provide sufficient assistance if the therapist is clear as to what constitutes an appropriate level of intensity and structure, given the patient's condition. FDA approval of buprenorphine for use by physicians represents a form of office-based treatment with greater complexities. Most patients who are candidates for buprenorphine seek help in the active phase of their addiction, and will need stabilization that includes behavior changes. They differ widely in their level of functioning. To help these patients, it is imperative that treating physicians have arrangements for comprehensive assessment, treatment planning, and referral to appropriate psychosocial services. They also should have a good understanding of the self-help system and how to encourage patients to use it productively. This understanding helps prepare patients to deal with other group members who view their particular medication as incompatible with "true" recovery.

Many patients who seek buprenorphine will have unrealistic expectations as to what the medication can accomplish. They will embrace the view that extensive participation in other treatment and recovery activities is unnecessary. The physician must be prepared to be firm about the commitment required for a serious recovery effort and have a good system of coordination with outside service providers.

RECOVERY-ORIENTED PSYCHOTHERAPY

The many forms of psychotherapy vary considerably in their compatibility with addiction treatment. Therapy funded by insurance has been limited to relatively brief interventions that are limited in scope. They often permit management of the initial crisis that brings the patient to treatment but little beyond that. Patients whose income allows may elect to work with therapists in private practice, many of whom are psychodynamic in orientation. Psychodynamic models assume that a relatively open-ended exploration of emotionally charged issues will increase awareness and lead to change. Such psychotherapy certainly may enhance the quality of recovery, but it has many pitfalls for the patient who needs to establish and consolidate abstinence. Private therapists may refer patients to addiction specialists for collaborative efforts, but potential difficulties exist in the teamwork.

In a recovery-oriented model, the therapist focuses his or her activity according to the tasks faced by the recovering person. These tasks can be conceptualized as recognizing the negative consequences of alcohol and drug use, making a commitment to abstinence, getting clean and sober, and shaping lifestyle transitions to support a comfortable and satisfying sobriety (16).

Engagement For patients who seek psychotherapy without recognizing that their alcohol or drug use is problematic, motivational enhancement strategies have proved beneficial (17–20). The therapist identifies where the patient is on the continuum of readiness to change: *precontemplation*, in which the patient is unaware or barely aware that a problem exists; *contemplation*, in which the patient is weighing the pros and cons of addressing the problem; *preparation*, in which the patient is making some small forays to change behavior (such as cutting down on cigarettes or changing brands); *action*, in which a great deal of time and effort is devoted to making changes; and *maintenance*, or the consolidation of change through relapse prevention strategies and other means (21).

Harm reduction approaches are increasingly available in the community and may be effective as engagement strategies, as damage control, or as sufficient intervention for mild to moderate problems (22). However, many patients with long histories and fairly severe addiction are attracted to harm reduction despite spending decades in fruitless efforts. The abstinence-oriented therapist takes the position that abstinence is the foundation of progress on other issues and makes the alcohol and drug use the primary focus. He or she works to help the patient understand the importance of making abstinence a priority. Patients have many understandable reasons to resist this focus. The therapist must work carefully to examine obstacles that prevent the patient from making a commitment to abstinence, while keeping the patient engaged in treatment. Typically, the obstacles begin with the distress that brought the patient to psychotherapy and include the relationship of that stress to alcohol and drug use.

Addressing the Patient's Self-Medication Hypothesis Patients frequently express strong beliefs that their substance abuse is a form of self-medication and they will be overwhelmed with unmanageable feeling states if they discontinue. They like the rapid change of state that occurs with the use of alcohol and other drugs. It is important for the counselor to explore these beliefs and experiences in detail. It can be important to validate the patient's belief that the substances may appear to help and their effects are generally more rapid than prescribed medication. Patients can be alienated by heavy-handed assertions that "self-medication doesn't work." However, it is usually possible to demonstrate that the overall effect of substance use is to increase the number of crises, hospitalizations, housing instability, poor adherence to medication regimens, and decrease in overall quality of life. Higher-functioning patients may present more subtle challenges. They seek psychotherapy for problems related to self-esteem and well-being. The therapist can help such a patient understand that regular consumption of a central nervous system depressant such as alcohol will inevitably depress mood, even though the initial effect feels like relief. Though the patient believes alcohol is a coping mechanism, he or she needs to be helped to understand that alcohol probably is exacerbating feelings of depressed mood and poor self-worth. In this way, the therapist cultivates in the patient a readiness to commit to at least a brief period of abstinence.

For the counselor or therapist, the key concept to work with is the difference between the initial effects of a drug and the ones that unfold over time. Patients focus on the initial effects and often don't track those that unfold over time. Upon inquiry, most stimulant users concur that over time their depressions become longer and more severe. Patients should be encouraged, through the use of logs and discussion, to monitor longer time frames in an effort to better identify the negative consequences of their drug use. In a study on integrated treatment for bipolar disorder and substance abuse, Weiss et al. (23) noted that patients who believed that their substance abuse had negative impact on their symptoms of bipolar disorder were more likely to stop using substances on their own. In this study, they were able to address this factor in their integrated treatment model, in which the patients were encouraged to think of themselves as having a single disorder—bipolar substance abuse. Successful treatment of this condition involved abstinence from alcohol and other drugs, maintaining good self-care, taking medications as prescribed, and engaging in recovery-related activities. Thus, patients were encouraged to consider both disorders as unitary and primary rather than to succumb to the temptation to minimize one of them.

Integrating Psychosocial Approaches For abstinence to be established, effective interventions tend to be highly structured and focused on developing the behaviors that bring it about. Cognitive-behavioral strategies have been well studied and shown to be effective (24–26). In such therapy, the therapist focuses on how the patient can become and remain abstinent. Insight-oriented exploration is confined to issues relevant to obstacles to abstinence; it is not possible to formulate effective behavioral strategies without clarity as to where problems lie. However, the conventionally trained therapist often tends to widen the exploration too broadly at the beginning of therapy, which may undermine abstinence in its early, fragile stages. The recovery-oriented therapist does not mechanistically focus on behavior but blends approaches while maintaining a clear perspective about the immediate goals to be achieved. Therapists who are not comfortable with a range of intervention strategies do less well with patients at this stage and actually may undermine progress.

Implementation of Evidence-Based Treatments Current emphasis on dissemination and integration of EBT's has brought increasing pressure from funders to use research findings to improve treatment. To facilitate this effort, it is important for physicians in charge of programs to become familiar with some of the complex issues involved in transplanting research-based psychosocial treatments into community programs. This includes the importance of distinguishing between treatment principles and specific interventions (27). When it is desirable to include specific treatments, it is important to appreciate the magnitude of this task. Instructional presentations are only the beginning of a lengthy process that will have to involve demonstrations, the opportunity to role-play with coaching, ongoing clinical supervision, and a supportive organizational culture to be successful. Newly learned behavior takes time to be integrated into the clinician's repertoire, and a supportive atmosphere where forthright feedback is ongoing facilitates adoption of new skills (28).

Collaboration Issues In prescribing medications to address withdrawal phenomena, physicians need to communicate to nonphysician therapists what to expect and what might constitute warning signs of impending problems. For example, the therapist may not be aware that a patient given 3 days' supply of chlordiazepoxide (Librium) for alcohol withdrawal by an addiction specialist also may have obtained a month's supply of diazepam (Valium) from his or her family physician for "back spasm" and thus be in a high-risk situation. Patients who are drinking and using may skip their prescribed medication because they fear their interaction with drugs and alcohol. Physicians should provide guidance to therapists about whether to encourage adherence to medication during these episodes, based on the preferable scenarios. As therapists spend considerable time with their patients, they are in a good position to detect developing problems and initiate communication with the physician or clinician responsible for coordinating care.

Therapists may not understand the importance of urine and breath testing and can weaken cooperation by conveying a sense that it is somehow degrading for the patient to comply with testing requirements. They need to understand that testing often functions as a key element in the support structure for outpatient treatment, permitting lapses to be identified and addressed quickly. Patients should be helped to understand that urine and breath testing serve as a deterrent to impulsive use and make the option of using seem further removed.

Behaviors during the early abstinence period are very similar to those during the active use stage and often include difficulty in structuring time, irritability, sleep disruption, and mood swings. This can threaten the patient's credibility with intimates, to whom he or she may have lied for considerable periods of time while engaged in active drinking or drug use. Drug or Breathalyzer tests relieve anxiety on the part of significant others and protect the patient from the disheartening experience of being mistrusted even as he or she is making progress. Preferably, the patient should be asked to sign appropriate releases for therapists outside the addiction program to be notified of test results.

Ongoing Recovery Issues Late-stage recovery issues require an examination of the lifestyle transitions need to sustain healthy sobriety, so this period resembles conventional psychotherapy in many ways. However, the therapist should have some understanding of relapse precipitants and be able to detect signs of early relapse. Current pressures to shorten the duration of addiction treatment will place more burden on psychotherapists to handle these issues. Structured relapse prevention activities, if undertaken too early in addiction treatment, may not "stick" because it is difficult to deal with late-stage recovery issues while a patient is in early recovery. The conceptual groundwork can be laid early, but the issues are dealt with more effectively at the time they are real. Relapse prevention early in treatment usually is focused on establishing stable abstinence; it is less able to deal with dangers that can manifest after a considerable period of sobriety. Sensitivity to these later relapse issues and a willingness to restore addiction issues to first priority when relapse threatens is a necessary characteristic of the therapist capable of good work with recovering patients.

Addiction treatment providers face a delicate task when collaborating with mental health therapists who are unskilled in dealing with recovering patients. They must inform the patient of appropriate treatment practices without generating distress by criticizing another professional with whom the patient may have a strong relationship. The physician is obligated to educate the patient but must do so with tact and sensitivity to the many complex issues involved in collaboration.

CO-OCCURRING DISORDER PATIENTS IN SELF-HELP GROUPS

Participation in self-help groups is a major element in achieving a positive outcome, so it is important for clinicians to facilitate such participation. Self-help groups are important in two ways: (1) They provide access to a culture that supports the recovery process, from which participants can recreate social networks that are not organized around alcohol and drug use, and (2) they provide a process for personal development that has no financial barriers. Though these goals can be achieved in other ways, for most individuals the self-help system offers the richest resource. Though many different groups exist, Twelve Step programs are the largest self-help system in the world (29).

Many addiction treatment programs systematically promote the use of self-help or mutual-help groups, but physicians in primary care, psychiatry, or other specialties need to consider how best to achieve compliance with a recommendation to participate. Resistance mirrors the patient's conflicts about acknowledging that alcohol or other drugs are a problem and that abstinence is necessary; hence it is not surprising that such feelings are expressed around the issue of meeting attendance. The presence of a coexisting disorder can add additional deterrents to involvement. Though it is understandable that the treating physician or other clinician may be frustrated or even angered by the patient's noncompliance, such a reaction can lead to behaviors that alienate the patient. By contrast, offering an opportunity for the patient to explore these issues is more likely to promote cooperation. Improving willingness is best done by helping the patient to surmount a variety of obstacles, many of which are well known.

Patients with co-occurring addictive and mental disorders may encounter a variety of difficulties in engaging in self-help programs, particularly if they are severely disturbed. For example, they may feel "different" in a way that reduces their sense of belonging. For them, the spirit of fellowship at the meetings may be a source of discomfort or pain. Such feelings may occur not only in patients with psychotic conditions but in those with other problems, such as combat veterans with severe post-traumatic stress disorder, who may feel they rarely hear "their story." Specialized meetings, such as those of Double Trouble groups, may reduce such obstacles, but there are far fewer of these groups than are needed to provide comprehensive coverage throughout the week. Another option is to mainstream such patients into meetings of groups that have a wider tolerance for deviant behavior to achieve a more extensive support system. This requires some process for gathering and sharing feedback on the most hospitable and appropriate meetings in a given community for a particular patient population.

Several common forms of resistance can be anticipated and the patient can be assisted in moving beyond them. Initially, most patients have some form of "stranger anxiety"—an understandable reluctance to enter an unfamiliar group where many or most participants appear to know one another. Encouraging patients to call the central office to find someone to go with them, pairing them with other patients who attend regularly, or encouraging case managers to go with them (at least initially, and perhaps regularly) can reduce some of this awkwardness. Those with social phobias or who describe themselves as isolated may be adamant in their rejection of group activities. Practitioners should not be discouraged by this; many Twelve Step program members readily announce themselves as "loners" but nevertheless maintain active involvement. Because meeting participants generally are friendly and not demanding (or intrusive), many objections diminish once the patient actually has attended.

As part of preparing the patient for Twelve Step participation, the clinician (often a program counselor) can elicit the patient's picture of what occurs in self-help meetings. This affords an opportunity to correct misconceptions and provide a picture of what can be expected (opening rituals, sharing of experiences without direct feedback or "cross-talk"). Patients who object or are ambivalent about calling themselves an addict or alcoholic can be assured that AA is for anyone concerned about drinking and that they can introduce themselves by name only or as a guest. Those who are concerned about "that religious stuff" can be encouraged to attend meetings less dominated by religious overtones, where they can "take what you need and leave the rest."

The concept of powerlessness in the first of the Twelve Steps ("We admitted we were powerless over alcohol—that our lives had become unmanageable") but is problematic for many patients, particularly those who are part of disempowered groups (such as patients with co-occurring mental and substance use disorders, women, or members of ethnic or cultural groups with a painful history of being ineffective and anonymous). Clarification that one gains control over one's life by renouncing struggles to control alcohol or drug use may be reassuring to such individuals but may require some time to be fully understood. The more spiritual aspects of surrendering control often are better appreciated later in recovery. In the early stages, advising patients to "take what you need and leave the rest" may be one of the more effective ways to reduce this obstacle to participation. In some communities, cultural adaptations that stress empowerment may be more attractive. For example, The Reverend Cecil Williams of Glide Memorial Church in San Francisco has adapted Twelve Step elements to the needs of the African American community in a manner that regularly draws crowds from diverse groups (30).

Medications are another issue around which there is much misunderstanding and some genuine hazards. Special preparation is needed for those using psychotropics and some other forms of medication. Despite a well-articulated AA position that medication is quite compatible with recovery (31), it is common to encounter negative attitudes toward medications on the part of AA participants. Patients who already feel vulnerable can be quite shaken by such encounters. It may be helpful to give patients some history about how such negative attitudes were developed (including misuse of medications by addicts and alcoholics and inappropriate prescribing by uninformed physicians). However, AA clearly states that members are not to "play doctor." Patients should be given a copy of the AA pamphlet entitled "The AA Member—Medications and Other Drugs: Report From a Group of Physicians in AA" and provided an opportunity to discuss or role-play potentially difficult situations. It also is possible to find meetings that are more receptive to those on medication. Hospital-based meetings are good candidates in this regard.

For more disturbed patients, additional supports may be useful. For example, the patient can be accompanied to initial meetings by the case manager. As he or she becomes ready to go alone, the case manager can be available by cell phone should the patient encounter problems. Some highly disturbed patients make excellent use of meetings, whereas others incorporate elements such as the higher power into their delusional system. Depending on the state of the patient, some meetings may be overstimulating, leading to disorganization.

The therapist's conceptual orientation also can present obstacles to patient participation in self-help groups. Lack of familiarity with what actually goes on in meetings can lead therapists to accept certain forms of resistance too readily. Brown (12) discusses many ways in which a therapist's belief system can undermine encouraging both abstinence itself and Twelve Step program participation in particular. In the latter case, she notes that, as involvement in AA increases, the patient may cancel or miss therapy appointments and act in other ways that reflect a shift in dependency from the therapist to the AA group. Though addiction specialists may view this as desirable, particularly in early recovery, the therapist may treat it as resistance and fall into a power struggle around loyalties. Some therapists abhor the concept of loss of control, viewing it as a defeat if the patient does not succeed in controlled use. They may dismiss Twelve Step tenets of powerlessness as antithetical to strong self-esteem. Therapists who are more knowledgeable tend to find the Twelve Step philosophy and process quite compatible with psychotherapy and are able to translate concepts back and forth in a manner that reduces confusion and conflict for the patient.

The best preparation for practitioners is first-hand familiarity with self-help programs through a "field trip" to meetings. Interns, residents, and new staff can be asked to attend a specified number of meetings, preferably involving groups recommended by staff or others familiar with community offerings. Those who are not alcoholics or addicts should be advised to select an open meeting and introduce themselves as a student or a guest. Subsequently, they should be provided an opportunity to share their experiences in staff meetings. Those who are in recovery or who have attended some meetings should be encouraged to attend meetings outside of their previous focus. All can be instructed to notice what they felt in anticipation of going (such as resistance or avoidance), what they felt on arriving, what they experienced during and after the meeting, and to share their observations and analyses of the group process, its advantages, and its limitations. Sharing these experiences in a staff meeting or training session can broaden the group's perspective on the variety of experiences possible.

CONCLUSIONS

Interdisciplinary collaboration not only is one of the most challenging aspects of addiction medicine but one that offers the greatest possibility of improving patient outcomes. As with heart disease, the greatest advances in addiction practice are achieved by encouraging patient lifestyle changes, which must be facilitated by all members of the treatment team.

Collaboration is best viewed as a clinical skill as complex as any other—one that is worthy of the time and attention it requires to develop and apply. Members of the treatment team bring to their work diverse attitudes, experiences, and skills that must be understood in order to handle the inevitable conflicts and draw the best from the range of experiences and expertise they represent. Strong physician leadership in fostering teamwork within the program and with other treatment professionals is an essential factor in achieving treatment goals.

REFERENCES

1. McElrath D. The Minnesota Model. *J Psychoactive Drugs* 1997;29(2): 141–144.
2. Deitch DA. The treatment of drug abuse in the therapeutic community: historical influences, current considerations, future outlook. In *Drug abuse in America: problem in perspective*, vol. IV: *Treatment and rehabilitation*. Washington, DC: National Commission on Marijuana and Drug Abuse, 1973:158–175.
3. DeLeon G. The therapeutic community: toward a general theory and model. In: Tims FM, DeLeon G, Jainchill N, eds. *Therapeutic community: advances in research and application*. NIDA Research Monograph 144. Rockville, MD: National Institute on Drug Abuse, 1994.
4. DeLeon G. Residential therapeutic communities in the mainstream: diversity and issues. *J Psychoactive Drugs* 1995;27:13–15.
5. DeLeon G. *The therapeutic community: theory, model, and method*. New York: Springer Publishing Company, 2000.

6. Gerstein DR. Outcome research: drug abuse. In: Galanter M Kleber HD, eds. *Textbook of substance abuse treatment* Washington, DC: American Psychiatric Press, 1994:45–64.
7. Gerstein DR, Harwood HJ. *Treating drug problems*, vol. 1. Washington, DC: National Academy Press, 1990.
8. Hubbard RL, Marsden ME, Rachal JV, et al. *Drug abuse treatment: a national study of effectiveness*. Chapel Hill: University of North Carolina Press, 1989.
9. Simpson DD, Curry SJ, eds. *Drug abuse treatment outcome study*, vol. 11. Washington, DC: Educational Publishing Foundation, 1997.
10. McLellan AT, Lewis DC, O'Brien CP, et al. Drug dependence, a chronic medical illness: implications for treatment, insurance, and outcomes evaluation. *J Am Med Assoc* 2000;284(13):1689–1695.
11. McLellan AT, Metzger DS, Alterman AI, et al. Is addiction treatment "worth it?" Public health expectations, policy-based comparisons. In: Lewis D, ed. *The Macy Conference on Medical Education*. New York: The Josiah Macy Foundation Press, 1995.
12. Brown S. *Treating the alcoholic: a developmental model of recovery*. New York: John Wiley & Sons, 1985.
13. Zweben JE, Smith DE. Considerations in using psychotropic medication with dual diagnosis patients in recovery. *J Psychoactive Drugs* 1989;21(2): 221–229.
14. Banys P. The clinical use of disulfiram (Antabuse): a review. *J Psychoactive Drugs* 1988;20:243–261.
15. Johnson FR, Ozdemir S, Manjunath R, et al. Factors that affect adherence to bipolar disorder treatments: a stated-preference approach. *Med Care* 2007;45(6):545–552.
16. Zweben JE. Recovery oriented psychotherapy: a model for addiction treatment. *Psychotherapy* 1993;30(2):259–268.
17. Miller WR. *Enhancing motivation for change in substance abuse treatment*, vol. 35. Rockville, MD: U.S. Department of Health and Human Services, 1999.
18. Miller WR, Page AC. Warm turkey: other routes to abstinence. *J Subst Abuse Treat* 1991;8:227–232.
19. Miller WR, Rollnick S. *Motivational interviewing: preparing people to change addictive behavior*. New York: Guilford Press, 1991.
20. Miller WR, Zweben A, DiClemente CC, et al. *Motivational enhancement therapy manual*. Rockville, MD: National Institute on Drug Abuse, 1994.
21. Prochaska JO, DiClemente CC, Norcross JC. In search of how people change: applications to addictive behaviors. *Am Psychol* 1992;47: 1102–1114.
22. Washton AM, Zweben JE. *Treating alcohol and drug problems in psychotherapy practice: doing what works*. New York, Guilford Press, 2006.
23. Weiss RD, Kolodziej M, Griffin ML, et al. Substance use and perceived symptom improvement among patients with bipolar disorder and substance dependence. *J Affect Disord* 2004;79(1–3):279–283.
24. Carroll KM. Behavioral and cognitive behavioral treatments. In: McCrady BS, Epstein EE, eds. *Addictions: a comprehensive guidebook*. New York: Oxford University Press, 1999:250–267.
25. Kadden R, Carroll K, Donovan D, et al. *Cognitive-behavioral coping skills therapy manual*. Rockville, MD: National Institute on Drug Abuse, 1995.
26. Matrix Center. *The matrix intensive outpatient program: therapist manual*. Los Angeles: The Matrix Center, 1995.
27. Miller WR, Zweben JE, Johnson W, et al. Evidence-based treatment: why, what, where, when and how? *J Subst Abuse Treat* 2005;29:267–276.
28. Fixsen DL, Naoom SF, et al. Implementation research: a synthesis of the literature. Tampa, FL: University of South Florida, 2005.
29. Alcoholics Anonymous. *Alcoholics Anonymous: 1996 membership survey*. New York: Alcoholics Anonymous World Services, Inc., 1996.
30. Smith DE, Buxton ME, Bilal R, et al. Cultural points of resistance to the 12-step process. *J Psychoactive Drugs* 1993;25(1):97–108.
31. Alcoholics Anonymous. *The AA member—medications and other drugs: report from a group of physicians in AA*. New York: Alcoholics Anonymous World Services, Inc., 1984.

CHAPTER 90

Michael E. Saladin, PhD
Sudie E. Back, PhD
Rebecca A. Payne, MD

Posttraumatic Stress Disorder and Substance Use Disorder Comorbidity

For centuries, the diagnostic condition presently known as posttraumatic stress disorder (PTSD) has been recognized in combat survivors and known by various names, including *soldier's heart, irritable heart, shell shock*, and *combat neurosis*, among others (1). The diagnosis was first formulated and expanded beyond combat-related contexts in the third edition of the *Diagnostic and Statistical Manual of Mental Disorders* (DSM-III), resulting in a growing body of research investigating the etiology, neurobiology, comorbidity, and treatment of the disorder (2). Epidemiologic studies of civilian populations and combat veterans have investigated PTSD and its comorbidities over the past two decades. Results from these studies show that depression, other anxiety disorders, and substance use disorders (SUDs) are common among persons with PTSD. Among civilian populations, the prevalence of lifetime SUDs has been estimated to be between 21.6% and 43.0% in people with PTSD, compared to 8.1% to 24.7% among individuals without PTSD. In one study of Vietnam veterans with PTSD, as many as 75% met criteria for an alcohol use disorder (3). The highly comorbid nature of PTSD and SUDs indicates that persons presenting to treatment for either PTSD or SUD should be screened for both disorders to ensure accurate assessment and appropriate treatment.

In both civilian and combat veteran populations, studies have demonstrated a more complicated clinical course and worse outcomes in persons with comorbid PTSD and SUD. In general, veterans with comorbid PTSD and SUDs have poorer treatment outcomes than those with SUDs alone on various indices of functioning, including more social and legal problems, suicide attempts, and violence (4). They tend to have longer duration of substance use and more symptoms of substance dependence, undergo more episodes of substance abuse treatment, and demonstrate less improvement during treatment than their counterparts with SUDs alone (4). In one study of civilian women (N = 65) with comorbid PTSD and substance dependence, high rates of suicide attempts (21.5%), suicidal ideation, and parasuicidal behaviors were reported (5). Another study examining the health and well-being of civilian men (n = 65) and women (n = 68) with SUDs, with or without comorbid PTSD, found that the presence of comorbid PTSD was associated with significantly more chronic physical, cardiovascular, and neurologic symptoms as well as poorer mental health functional status and well-being (6). These studies are part of a much larger body of literature examining the impact of comorbid PTSD and SUDs on various parameters of functioning and clearly demonstrate the necessity of a thorough understanding and assessment of persons with PTSD-SUD comorbidity. In this chapter, we address the phenomenology, epidemiology, assessment, and treatment of patients with comorbid PTSD and SUDs to assist clinicians in providing informed and effective care.

PHENOMENOLOGY

The current DSM-IV-TR outlines the following criteria necessary to diagnose PTSD: (1) the occurrence of a traumatic event (Criterion A); (2) >1 month of symptoms (Criterion E) within the three symptom clusters of reexperiencing (Criterion B), avoidance (Criterion C), and hypervigilance

(Criterion D); and (3) subsequent impaired functioning or significant distress (Criterion F). The definition of a traumatic event has changed since PTSD was first described in the DSM-III. In the current DSM-IV-TR, it is defined as either an experienced or witnessed event involving "actual or threatened death" or "serious injury or a threat to the physical integrity of self or others" (Criterion A1). To qualify for PTSD, the response must include "intense fear, helplessness, or horror" (Criterion A2) (7). It has been estimated that between 39% and 90% of the population has been exposed to a traumatic event (8). Of those who experience a traumatic event, only 10% to 20% will develop PTSD (9).

There are many ways in which patients with PTSD reexperience (Criterion B) traumatic events. They may report dreams or intrusive memories of the event or behave as if an event were currently happening (i.e., flashbacks). Cues that elicit memories of the trauma(s) may trigger psychologic distress or physiologic reactivity, thus leading to avoidance behaviors (Criterion C). Patients may avoid thoughts, feelings, conversations, activities, places, or people associated with the trauma and demonstrate anhedonia or lack of participation in important life activities. They may be unable to remember portions of the trauma and describe feelings of detachment or a sense of foreshortened future. Affect range may also be restricted. The symptoms of increased arousal (Criterion D) or hypervigilance may involve exaggerated startle response, sleep disturbance, poor concentration, irritability, and/or anger outbursts (7). There are three specifiers that provide information about the duration and onset of symptoms. If symptoms have been present for <3 months, the disorder is considered acute; if symptoms have persisted for more than 3 months, the disorder is described as chronic. If the onset of symptoms is 6 months or more after the traumatic event, the disorder is considered to have a delayed onset.

Exposure to a traumatic event can also lead to a condition known as *acute stress disorder* (ASD). The primary distinction between PTSD and ASD is the duration of symptoms. While PTSD and ASD share many similar symptoms including reexperiencing symptoms, avoidance, increased arousal, and subsequent distress or impairment, ASD can occur for as little as 2 days after exposure to the traumatic event and last up to 1 month afterward. Other symptoms of ASD include dissociative symptoms, such as feelings of derealization, depersonalization, dissociative amnesia, or reduced awareness of the environment.

EPIDEMIOLOGY

The National Comorbidity Survey (NCS), a large-scale epidemiologic survey (N =5877) conducted in the early 1990s, examined psychiatric disorders in the U.S. general population. Using DSM-III-Revised criteria, the NCS found the overall lifetime prevalence rate for PTSD at 7.8% and those with PTSD were two to four times more likely than their counterparts without PTSD to meet criteria for a SUD (10). The National Comorbidity Survey Replication (NSC-R), which took place approximately one decade after the NCS, found a similar overall lifetime PTSD prevalence rate (6.8%) using DSM-IV criteria (11).

The prevalence of comorbid PTSD and SUDs has been examined in various populations, with war veterans being one of the most extensively investigated groups. As mentioned, Vietnam veterans have demonstrated a high prevalence of comorbid PTSD and SUDs. The Vietnam Experience Study found that in veterans with PTSD, 39% met criteria for current alcohol abuse or dependence. Another study of Vietnam veterans found that 98.9% of those with PTSD also met criteria for other disorders, including major depression (28%), antisocial personality disorder (31%), and most commonly, SUD (73%) (12). In Persian Gulf War veterans, the presence of PTSD hyperarousal symptoms at 18 to 24 months after return predicted drug use, but not alcohol use, at 6 years after return (13).

Studies from the civilian population indicate that PTSD and SUDs frequently co-occur. Cottler et al. (14) investigated PTSD and SUDs in the general population and found that individuals with cocaine and opiate use disorders were three times more likely to experience a traumatic event and, subsequently, PTSD rates were significantly higher in this population than in those without an SUD. Careful examination of the civilian data reveals that men and women differ in the prevalence of comorbid psychiatric illnesses and PTSD. The most common comorbid diagnoses in women with PTSD are (in order) depression, other anxiety disorders, and alcohol use disorders. In men (veteran and civilian), the most common comorbidities in those with PTSD are (in order) alcohol use disorders, depression, other anxiety disorders, conduct disorder, and drug use disorders (3).

Finally, distinct populations, including adolescents, young adults, elderly adults, and minorities, have evidenced similar high prevalence rates of comorbid PTSD and SUD (15–18). Collectively, these data indicate a high prevalence of this comorbidity in a variety of clinical populations, suggesting a unique and potent interconnectedness between PTSD and SUDs and raising questions about the chronologic order of onset of these disorders.

ETIOLOGIC RELATIONSHIP BETWEEN PTSD AND SUD

Various theories have been proposed to characterize the development of comorbid PTSD and SUD. One of the most prominent, the self-medication theory (cf. 18–21), postulates that substance use serves to alleviate PTSD symptoms. In one study (22), alcohol dependence was more common in individuals with PTSD and prominent symptoms within the hyperarousal cluster (Criterion D). Likewise, cocaine dependence was more commonly associated with those individuals that demonstrated more avoidance (Criterion C) and flashback symptoms (Criterion B). Therefore, a PTSD and SUD comorbid individual's preference for either a central nervous system depressant or a stimulant may reflect his or her attempt, conscious or otherwise, to alleviate a particular cluster of symptoms. To further complicate matters, withdrawal from substances may closely mimic some symptoms of PTSD (i.e., sleep disturbance, difficulty concentrating, feelings of detachment, irritability) and contribute to a reinforcing cycle of self-medication that fosters the development of a SUD.

The most common competing theory hypothesizes that SUDs precede the development of PTSD. In this model, the probability of developing PTSD is increased via two potential causal pathways. The lifestyle of a substance abuser, which is typically considered to be high risk with dangerous environments and behaviors associated with obtaining or using alcohol or drugs, may increase the likelihood of experiencing a traumatic event and subsequently developing PTSD. Alternatively, the increased anxiety and arousal that accompanies chronic substance use may increase one's biologic vulnerability to develop PTSD after trauma exposure (3).

Last, there is some evidence that other factors may play a role in the development of comorbid PTSD and an SUD. Plausible factors that have been investigated include genetics, common neurophysiologic systems, and conduct disorder. Though the direction of the causal relationship between comorbid PTSD and SUD is likely to vary from one individual to another and further research is indicated, the self-medication hypothesis remains the dominant explanatory model (23,24).

NEUROBIOLOGIC FACTORS IN COMORBID PTSD AND SUD

The model for the human stress response, in which the hypothalamic-pituitary-adrenal (HPA) axis plays an integral role, is also thought to be a key component in the biologic development and maintenance of PTSD. The majority of research to date focuses on the HPA axis and noradrenergic systems, though other systems including dopamine, serotonin, thyroid, and GABA have been investigated and likely play a role (25). Stressor exposure elicits a cascade of neurohormones. The hypothalamus releases corticotropin-releasing hormone (CRH), thereby stimulating the release of adrenocorticotropic hormone from the pituitary gland and finally release of cortisol from the adrenal glands (3).

In patients with PTSD, basal cortisol levels are lower, lymphocyte glucocorticoid receptors are up-regulated, and there is increased suppression of cortisol after dexamethasone administration (3). These findings suggest that glucocorticoid feedback is enhanced in PTSD. Individuals with SUDs commonly report stress as a trigger for relapse, and studies have shown that exposure to stress results in increased craving and salivary cortisol, suggesting HPA axis activation similar to activation in PTSD (3). Furthermore, cerebrospinal fluid CRH levels are elevated in PTSD patients and during acute alcohol withdrawal. Debate continues about the meaning and implications of these findings, and the complex interplay is not yet fully understood.

Noradrenergic dysregulation has also been consistently demonstrated in both PTSD and withdrawal states from chronic alcohol and drug use through laboratory testing (3). Elevated levels of 24-hour plasma norepinephrine and fewer platelet alpha2-adrenergic receptors are some of the findings of both PTSD and withdrawal states of SUDs. This mechanism is the basis for the use of clonidine, an alpha2-adrenergic receptor agonist, in both PTSD and opiate withdrawal (3).

ASSESSMENT OF PTSD IN SUD

Given the high rates of trauma and PTSD among individuals with SUDs, it is important to screen all SUD patients. Numerous interviewer-rated and self-report assessments of PTSD are available (26,27). A recent review found that brief PTSD measures (i.e., 4 to 30 items) appear to perform as well as longer, more complicated measures (28). Accordingly, it cannot be argued that the assessment of PTSD in persons with SUDs is too burdensome from a clinical resource management perspective (i.e., staff/clinician time). In fact, the gains to be achieved in terms of quality of care far exceed any resource expenditures. In this section, we highlight some of the most commonly used and psychometrically sound interview and self-report instruments for assessing PTSD (29).

As a general rule, PTSD assessment should be conducted after a patient has emerged from acute alcohol or drug intoxication and withdrawal (30). In contrast to other anxiety disorders (e.g., generalized anxiety disorder), less abstinence may be required in order to establish a diagnosis of PTSD among SUD patients because of the unique nature of the diagnostic criteria (i.e., requirement of exposure to a criterion A traumatic event). Intrusive PTSD symptoms (e.g., recurrent thoughts or images related to the trauma) are uniquely characteristic of PTSD and are less likely to be mimicked by substance use or withdrawal. Other PTSD symptoms (e.g., irritability or outbursts of anger, sleep impairment) could be exacerbated by the use of, or withdrawal from, alcohol and drugs and should be carefully assessed. The duration of abstinence required before a valid and clinically meaningful assessment of PTSD can be conducted with a patient will vary depending on whether the substance used is short- or long-acting. If there is any diagnostic uncertainty, reassessment of PTSD symptoms as the patient becomes abstinent can provide helpful information (e.g., do PTSD symptoms remit over time with continued abstinence?).

Interviewer-Rated Assessment of Posttraumatic Stress Disorder

Clinician-Administered Posttraumatic Stress Disorder Scale The most widely used interviewer-rated PTSD assessment is the *Clinician Administered PTSD Scale* (CAPS) (31,32). This is a 30-item structured interview that was developed at the

National Center for PTSD and is designed for use by clinicians and trained paraprofessionals. A checklist of potentially traumatic events is included at the beginning of the interview to assess lifetime trauma exposure. Seventeen items assess the frequency and intensity of diagnostic PTSD symptoms (e.g., re-experiencing, avoidance, hyperarousal). In addition, associated features of PTSD (e.g., survivor guilt, homicidality, hopelessness), social and occupational functioning, and global PTSD severity are also rated. Several versions of the CAPS are available, including versions that assess past week, past month, and lifetime symptoms.

Structured Clinical Interview for the Diagnostic and Statistical Manual of Mental Disorders The structured clinical interview (SCID) (33) is a semi-structured interview designed to diagnose most Axis I disorders (e.g., mood, psychotic, anxiety, substance use, and eating disorders). The DSM-III-R SCID (34) was the first comprehensive semi-structured interview for the diagnosis of PTSD. The SCID has been revised to reflect modifications for each version of the DSM. The SCID contains a section that briefly reviews lifetime exposure to traumatic events and the age of occurrence, followed by diagnostic questions to assess PTSD symptoms. If multiple traumas exist, the diagnostic questions are asked in relation to the trauma that has most affected the patient.

Potential Stressful Events Interview and the National Women's Study Posttraumatic Stress Disorder Module The potential stressful events interview (PSEI) and the National Women's Study (NWS) PTSD module instruments were developed by the research group at the National Crime Victims' Research and Treatment Center (Medical University of South Carolina) in Charleston, SC. Though originally developed for use in the NSW, these instruments can be used to assess trauma exposure and PTSD in a variety of populations. The PSEI (35) is a multicomponent instrument for assessing trauma exposure history and PTSD symptomatology (via the NWS PTSD module, which is a component of the PSEI). Using behaviorally specific questions, the PSEI trauma exposure module assesses crime-related (e.g., sexual and physical assault), non-crime-related (e.g., natural disaster, serious accident), and combat-related traumatic events. Age of onset for first and last occurrence of an event is also determined. The NWS PTSD module is a 20-item structured clinical interview that is designed for use by lay interviewers (36). It was derived from the Diagnostic Interview Schedule that was used in the National Vietnam Veterans Readjustment Study. None of the items attempts to link a specific PTSD symptom to a particular traumatic event and so is easily used with individuals with complex trauma histories. Like the CAPS, this instrument has been shown to have strong psychometric properties and can be used to assess PTSD symptomatology in approximately 30 minutes.

PTSD Symptom Scale—Interview (PSS-I) The PSS-I (37,38) is a 17-item semi-structured interview that assesses PTSD symptom frequency and severity over the past 2 weeks. The PSS-I can be administered by trained paraprofessionals.

Structured Interview for PTSD (SIP) The SIP (39) contains 17 items that assess the diagnosis of PTSD and symptom severity. Measures of survivor and behavioral guilt are also included.

MINI International Neuropsychiatric Interview PTSD Module The MINI (40) is a brief structured clinical interview that, like the SCID, assesses most major Axis I psychiatric disorders, including PTSD. The MINI PTSD module assesses diagnostic PTSD symptoms during the past month. Relative to the SCID, this instrument has the advantage of shorter administration time.

Composite International Diagnostic Interview (CIDI) The CIDI (41,42), a standardized interview, assesses most major mental disorders. Unlike the other interviewer-rated measures mentioned in this chapter, the CIDI provides diagnosis according to the International Classification of Diseases, Tenth Edition (ICD-10), which is slightly different from the DSM-IV with regard to PTSD diagnostic criteria. The CIDI is suitable for lay interviewers. Versions are available to assess past 12 months' and lifetime symptoms. In addition, a computerized version of the CIDI is available.

Self-Report Assessment of Posttraumatic Stress Disorder

Impact of Events Scale-Revised The IES-R (43) is a brief and popular 22-item scale for assessing PTSD symptoms in all three of the major categories; re-experiencing, avoidance and arousal. It is a revision of the IES by Horowitz et al. (44), which does not address the arousal category of PTSD symptoms and therefore, the IES-R is more consistent with the DSM-IV (45) diagnostic criteria. Prospective respondents use Likert scales to rate "how distressed or bothered" they were by each specified symptom over the previous week. This instrument has been translated into several different languages (46–49) and has been used with a variety of trauma populations (e.g., earthquake emergency response personnel, earthquake survivors). Though the earlier version of this instrument has been shown to have strong psychometric properties, existing data on the psychometric properties of the IES-R are considered limited, so additional study appears necessary. There are some unpublished data suggesting that the IES-R is a reliable, valid and clinically sensitive measure of PTSD symptomatology when used with traumatized SUD and SUD-PTSD comorbid patients (50).

Posttraumatic Stress Diagnostic Scale The PDS (51) is a user-friendly 49-item Likert-type scale that measures DSM-IV PTSD criteria and symptom severity for all three symptom clusters. This is an updated version of the Foa et al. (52) 17-item self-report PTSD Symptom Scale (PSS-SR) that was based on DSM-III-R (53) criteria. The PDS assesses trauma exposure (12 items) and identifies an individual's most distressing trauma(s). The instrument also assesses trauma features (e.g., physical threat, helplessness) and functional impairment resulting from PTSD symptoms. It has been psychometrically validated on a sample with diverse trauma exposure (51), and it correlates highly with other instruments that measure responses to trauma and has good diagnostic agreement with the SCID. This instrument provides a very efficient means of assessing both type of trauma exposure and PTSD symptomatology. However, like most instruments, it has not been validated on a sample of PTSD and SUD comorbid individuals.

Modified Posttraumatic Stress Disorder Symptom Scale (Self-Report) Like the PDS earlier, the MPSS-SR (54) is based on Foa et al's (52) PTSD Symptom Scale (PSS-SR). It was developed to extend the PSS-SR's symptom frequency assessment to include the assessment of PTSD symptom severity. Not only has this instrument been validated with clinical and nonclinical samples of trauma exposed individuals (55) but it has been shown to have good psychometric properties with respect to the assessment of PTSD symptoms in SUD samples (56,57). Thus, this measure can be used with confidence in screening and assessing PTSD and SUD comorbid individuals.

Mississippi Scale for Combat-Related Posttraumatic Stress Disorder The Mississippi Scale is a widely used 35-item instrument that was developed by Keane et al. (58) to assess combat-related PTSD symptoms. The items for this scale were derived from a sample of 200 items developed by experts. Thirty of the items assess the re-experiencing, avoidance, and arousal symptom categories whereas the remaining five assess guilt and suicidality. Prospective respondents use Likert scales to rate the severity of symptoms since the occurrence of the traumatic event(s). Like the IES-R, the Mississippi Scale has been translated into several languages. Because of its strong psychometric properties (59,60), a civilian version of the instrument has also been developed.

TREATMENT OF PTSD AND PTSD-SUD COMORBIDITY

PTSD has had a relatively brief history as a diagnostic entity and, during that time, a broad range of traditional and specialized therapies have been promoted for its treatment, several of which have received considerable empirical scrutiny. By contrast, there have been very few studies of therapies specifically designed to address PTSD and SUD concurrently. Whether one considers the treatment of PTSD alone or PTSD-SUD comorbidity, treatments tend to fall into two general classes: psychotherapy and pharmacotherapy or, in rare cases, their combination. This section briefly describes, discusses, and evaluates these two general classes of interventions with respect to the treatment of PTSD and PTSD-SUD comorbidity. Though the focus of the following discussion will be on the treatment of PTSD, it should be noted that there is also some evidence that PTSD-SUD comorbid individuals can benefit from interventions that primarily target SUDs (61).

An exhaustive review of the treatment literature is not possible given space limitations; consequently, we have adopted the following focus. First, three types of cognitive behavioral therapies (CBTs) of PTSD will be discussed: (1) exposure-based therapy, (2) cognitive-focused therapy, and (3) anxiety/stress management therapy. CBTs for PTSD are emphasized here because they are widely accepted as the most empirically valid treatments for PTSD (e.g., 62). Additionally, it has been suggested (63) that the treatment of one disorder in dually diagnosed individuals often yields clinical benefits for the untreated comorbidity. This being the case, treatment of PTSD in PTSD-SUD comorbid individuals is important because it can be expected to have positive impact on substance use. Second, we will outline and discuss integrative CBTs for the concurrent treatment of PTSD and SUD. These are relatively recent and comprehensive treatments that make an explicit attempt to concurrently address PTSD and SUD symptomatology. Each treatment will be described in some detail in order to elucidate both unique features and specific commonalities, and important research findings will be briefly outlined. Third, we will examine pharmacotherapies for PTSD and, fourth, we will describe developments in pharmacotherapy for PTSD-SUD comorbidity. These later two sections will be relatively brief, as this type of treatment has not yielded efficacy findings on par with CBT.

On a final note, some investigators have explored the use of psychotherapeutic techniques to prevent the development of PTSD and have found that such single-session critical incident stress debriefing is not only ineffective in preventing the development of PTSD but may be harmful (64). Thus, this chapter will not cover debriefing to prevent PTSD but will instead focus on CBTs designed to treat established PTSD.

Cognitive-Behavioral Therapy for Posttraumatic Stress Disorder

Exposure-Based Therapy There are several forms of exposure-based therapy (65–68) and, as a group, they represent the longest-standing empirically validated psychotherapies for trauma and PTSD. Exposure therapies are based on conditioning (cf. 69–71) or information-processing (72) theories of fear and anxiety, both of which argue that exposure to fear and anxiety-eliciting situations/stimuli (i.e., physical location where a motor vehicle accident occurred) without traumatic outcome (i.e., motor vehicle accident) result in anxiety abatement. Conditioning models assert that fear/anxiety abatement results from behavioral extinction (73), a type of inhibitory learning (cf. 73–75), whereas information-processing theory argues that it occurs via the modification of pathologic elements of a fear-based memory. Procedurally, individuals are either exposed to *in vivo* or imaginal fear-eliciting cues. In the former case, exposure is performed via presentation of physical stimuli associated with traumatic experiences, whereas in the latter case, the fear stimuli are imagined. One of the major advantages of imaginal exposure over in vivo exposure methods is that trauma cues that would otherwise be difficult and/or unethical (i.e., physical conditions present in a combat situation, distant locations where an assault occurred) to use in exposure therapy can easily be integrated into an imagery-based procedure. Both *in vivo* and imaginal procedures aim to reduce/preclude avoidance behavior and promote mastery.

One of the most extensively studied exposure treatments for PTSD is prolonged exposure (PE) therapy. Though this therapy can be practiced in varied forms, its essential features have been detailed in a published manual (76). Briefly, the treatment consists of several primary components, including (1) didactic training about common reactions to traumatic events, (2) relaxation via breathing retraining, (3) prolonged imaginal exposure to the trauma via detailed, therapist guided, recounting of the event(s), and (4) *in vivo* exposure to trauma-related situations that are being avoided because they elicit fear. Though the duration of this therapy can vary, a typical course can be completed in nine sessions, each session lasting about 60 to 90 minutes. In private practice, one of the authors (MES) has achieved substantial therapeutic gains in as few as three sessions of active PE. The authors of the PE treatment manual also suggest a number of PE treatment plan options, two of which contain elements of cognitive therapy and anxiety management as described further. Thus, PE is easily integrated with other forms of therapy.

There is another form of exposure therapy that requires brief consideration. Shapiro (77–79) forwarded an extension of Wolpe's (71) systematic desensitization therapy that she initially named *eye movement desensitization* (EMD) therapy and later added the term *reprocessing* (hence, EMDR therapy) to denote a conceptual shift toward an information-processing interpretation of the therapy's mechanism of action. EMDR is presumed to exert its effects by modifying the neuronal interface between thought, emotion, and memory. Applying EMDR involves a therapist eliciting trauma-related imagery while having the patient develop alternative interpretations of the imagined traumatic event(s). This aspect of EMDR is essentially analogous to exposure with cognitive therapy features. The unique and presumably important feature of EMDR is conducting the imaginal exposure while the patient simultaneously visually tracks the back-and-forth movement of a therapist-manipulated object (e.g., therapist's finger).

Cognition-Focused Therapy There are essentially two therapies that comprise this class, cognitive therapy (CT) and cognitive processing therapy (CPT). CT was originally forwarded as a treatment for depression (80,81) and has subsequently been extended to address anxiety (82,83) and SUDs (84). As applied to PTSD, the therapy is built conceptually around the notion that it is the *meaning* that individuals assign to traumatic events, rather than the traumatic events, which determines duration and intensity of emotion/mood states that ensue. Accordingly, interpretations or meanings that are negatively biased or irrational give rise to negative mood states such as fear and anxiety. The goal of CT, then, is to aid individuals in implementing corrective cognitive procedures to identify and challenge inaccurate, irrational thoughts and beliefs and to replace them with ones that are more evidence-based, rational, and beneficial. Some categories of thinking and belief that would be the focus of CT for individuals with PTSD would be safety/danger, trust and self-concept.

The other therapy in this class, CPT, is similar to CT but has a decidedly more emotional focus. Specifically, Resick and Schnicke (85,86) have developed a specialized or PTSD-specific treatment that combines a cognitive focus with elements of exposure therapy. Though originally developed to address PTSD resulting from sexual assault, it has been extended to victims of other types of trauma (87,88). The therapy has several important elements that are presumed to have therapeutic potency. There is a psycho-education component in which an information-processing model of PTSD is presented. The exposure element consists of a writing-reading task wherein individuals develop a detailed narrative of their traumatic experience(s). The goal of this component is for the individual to maximize emotional processing of the trauma(s) and to identify areas of incomplete processing or conflict concerning the trauma(s). The primary feature of this treatment is the cognitive therapy component that involves identification and challenging of key cognitive distortions. Specific areas of belief that are targeted for challenge relate to themes of safety, trust, power, esteem, and intimacy. The therapy generally concludes with an analysis of beliefs, including changes to dysfunctional thinking, and discussion of future goals. Completion of CPT can be achieved in approximately twelve 60- to 90-minute therapy sessions.

Anxiety Management Therapy Though there are several therapies that could be considered members of this category (e.g., biofeedback and relaxation training) (89), one of the most widely known and studied is stress inoculation training (SIT) (90–92). As applied to PTSD (93,94), the main goal of this therapy is to provide individuals with a sense of mastery over their PTSD symptoms by teaching them a variety of coping skills and then permitting them to practice the skills both inside and outside of treatment sessions. SIT can be used in both individual and group formats and has broad application to a variety of anxiety disorders (e.g., panic disorder). Common elements of SIT are relaxation training, breathing training, thought stopping, self-instruction training, assertiveness training, cognitive restructuring, anger management, and problem-solving training. These skills can be taught and practiced over 8 to 12 sessions and the therapy can be adapted to briefer psycho-educational formats.

Effectiveness of Cognitive-Behavioral Therapy for Posttraumatic Stress Disorder As already noted, the treatments described earlier represent the state of the art with respect to CBT for PTSD. A detailed review of the associated efficacy literature is neither possible, given space limitations, nor necessary as several recent and thorough reviews and meta-analyses of CBT for PTSD have been conducted (62,95–102). An important caveat to the conclusions stated here is that the outcomes from clinical trials involving these therapies may have limited generalizability to PTSD-SUD comorbidity; one recent review (101) noted that 62% of PTSD therapy studies reviewed excluded individuals with a comorbid SUD. With this caveat in mind, there are some general and a few specific conclusions that can be drawn from this literature.

First and foremost, all CBTs produce clinically significant reductions in PTSD symptomatology relative to wait-list or treatment as usual (TAU) comparisons. The treatments also tended to produce appreciable benefits on collateral symptoms of depression and generalized anxiety. The treatments appear to benefit a range of populations including those with civilian and combat-related PTSD. Treatment dropout rates tend to be similar across studies, at approximately 20% to 25%.

Though differences among the treatments are difficult to discern from this vast and complex literature of clinical trials, the reviews do suggest several qualified generalizations can be forwarded. One such generalization is that a combination of *in vivo* and imaginal exposure produces substantial and persistent symptom reduction beyond what can be achieved with anxiety management procedures such as SIT or with cognitive therapy. There is some evidence suggesting that exposure therapy benefits are maximized with the combination of *in vivo* and imaginal exposure and that the addition of other cognitive and anxiety management therapy elements does not appreciably enhance exposure-based therapy outcomes. It also appears that CPT, a cognitive therapy with exposure elements, is as effective as PE in the treatment of rape-related PTSD and that CPT might be more beneficial in addressing trauma-related guilt. This latter observation was echoed in a recent study of industrial accident-related PTSD (103) in which the emotional focus of the PTSD was related to guilt and anger rather than fear and anxiety. The therapy in the study, imagery rescripting and reprocessing therapy (IRRT), combined elements of exposure and cognitive restructuring to transform traumatic imagery into adaptive imagery. IRRT was administered to industrial accident victims who did not benefit from PE. The authors reported an 80% "complete" recovery rate that they tentatively attributed to the therapy's ability to address the predominantly guilt-anger emotional focus of the PTSD. Whether IRRT has benefits beyond those conferred by PE (in general) remains a larger unanswered question, but it appears possible that certain strategic integrations of cognitive and exposure therapy elements may offer benefits that can not be achieved by exposure alone, at least with some subgroups of PTSD afflicted individuals.

Last, EMDR has been the focus of much controversy (104–108) and research, primarily because of the unusual assumption that the rapid saccadic eye movement during imaginal exposure is essential to its efficacy and because EMDR was touted as an especially effective treatment for a variety of disorders, including PTSD. Contrary to these claims, more than a decade of research has shown that the eye movement feature does not appear relevant to treatment outcome (109–115) and that EMDR is no more effective than any other more theoretically grounded exposure therapy (112,114–118). Thus, EMDR is an efficacious treatment for PTSD, but its efficacy is likely attributable to its exposure and cognitive therapy elements.

In sum, the bulk of clinical studies point to exposure therapy (*in vivo* and imaginal combined) as the dominant therapeutic approach for resolving PTSD. Though this assertion may be questionable under some conditions and/or with some subgroups of persons with PTSD, it is consistent with the fact that the Substance Abuse and Mental Health Services Administration has selected PE as its model program for nationwide dissemination.

Integrated Cognitive-Behavioral Therapy for Posttraumatic Stress Disorder–Substance Use Disorder Comorbidity In general, psychotherapy is an important part of treatment for PTSD and SUDs. However, the majority of patients with PTSD and comorbid SUDs receive treatment for the SUD only (119,120). Subsequent to the successful completion of SUD treatment, patients are often, but not always, referred to PTSD treatment. It is unknown how many referred patients actually seek out and complete PTSD treatment. Proponents of this treatment model, known as "sequential" treatment, in which the SUD is first treated and then the PTSD is treated, posit that continued substance use during therapy impedes therapeutic efforts to address PTSD, and that addressing the trauma increases the risk of relapse (121,122). Importantly, there is little empirical data to support these concerns and this general approach to therapy.

"Integrated" treatment models, in which both the SUD and PTSD are simultaneously addressed in therapy, have been developed over the past decade. The findings from studies of integrated treatments show that alcohol and drug use typically decrease significantly and do not increase with the addition of trauma-focused interventions (123–126). Proponents of integrated treatments assert that PTSD symptoms may, at least in part, drive substance use and that untreated PTSD symptoms place SUD patients at risk of relapse. In so far as substance abuse represents self-medication of PTSD symptoms (127), addressing the trauma early in treatment may improve the chances of long-term recovery from addiction (128,129). Furthermore, a substantial proportion of PTSD-SUD comorbid patients express a preference for integrated treatment (119,130,131).

Seeking Safety (SS) is the most widely known and empirically studied integrated CBT (132,133). SS is a 25-session, present-focused, manualized treatment that provides psychoeducation, teaches coping skills and helps clients gain more control over their lives. SS was first developed for adult women in a group modality but has since been expanded to men, adolescents, and individual therapy. The findings from most studies suggest that SS leads to abatement of substance use, PTSD symptoms, and depressive symptoms and improved interpersonal functioning (134,135). In a randomized controlled trial, Hien et al. (136) compared SS to the "gold-standard" substance abuse treatment, Relapse Prevention (RP), and to TAU among 107 women. At the end of treatment, clients who received TAU failed to demonstrate significant improvement, or in the case of PTSD symptoms, worsened over time. In contrast, patients who received either SS or RP demonstrated significant decrease in substance use, PTSD, and psychiatric symptom severity. SS and RP, however, did not differ from one another on treatment outcomes. (See *www.seekingsafety.org* for more detailed information on SS.)

Other integrated CBTs that use exposure-based techniques, the gold-standard psychosocial treatment for PTSD, have also been developed. To date, two small studies have systematically examined an intervention that integrates exposure-based techniques for PTSD with empirically validated treatments for SUDs. Triffleman et al. (126,137) pioneered the effort by developing Substance Dependence Posttraumatic Stress Disorder Therapy (SDPT). SDPT is a 20-week manualized outpatient treatment that utilizes relapse prevention, coping skills, psychoeducation, and in vivo exposure for individuals with PTSD. In a small controlled pilot trial (N = 19) using methadone-maintained primary-cocaine-abusing subjects, SDPT was compared to Twelve-Step Facilitation Therapy. Patients in both groups showed improvements in PTSD and drug use, but no statistically significant differences between treatment conditions were observed. This may have been owing to the small sample size and the short follow-up period of 1 month.

In a larger trial, Brady et al. (123,138) developed a manualized treatment consisting of *imaginal* and in vivo exposure therapy for PTSD combined with cognitive-behavioral relapse prevention for individuals with PTSD and cocaine dependence. The treatment protocol, called Concurrent Treatment of PTSD and cocaine dependence (CTPCD), includes 16 individual sessions. Results from an uncontrolled study (N = 39) showed that patients demonstrated significant pre- to post-treatment reductions in all three clusters of PTSD symptoms, as measured by clinician-rated and self-report measures (123). Significant reductions in cocaine use were also observed. Approximately 10% of urine drug screen tests were positive each week, and this rate did not increase during the course of treatment, as PTSD was more directly addressed with exposure techniques. Symptoms of depression and psychiatric distress showed significant improvement, as well. More controlled trials and larger sample sizes are needed.

One study explored a modified version of CTPCD. In order to use CTPCD among inner-city clients at a community mental health center (CMHC), Coffey et al. (139) created in 2005 the CMHC-CTPCD, which used both individual and group therapy format; consisted of a team-based treatment approach including the individual therapist, the group therapist, case managers, and a psychiatrist; and added a dialectic behavior therapy (DBT) psychosocial skills training group. Preliminary clinical observations indicate that CMHC-CTPCD also leads to reduced trauma-related symptoms, improves SUD outcomes, and is well tolerated (139).

The findings from these and other investigations (140–142) provide evidence that integrated treatments are beneficial to many patients with trauma/PTSD and co-occurring SUDs. They also suggest that imaginal and *in vivo* exposure techniques for PTSD can be used safely and effectively with some SUD patients. Thus, research shows that addressing trauma via present- or past-oriented treatments does not worsen patients' symptoms but rather significantly decreases PTSD, substance use, and general psychiatric distress. More randomized controlled trials are needed, however, to determine whether and for whom integrated PTSD/SUD treatments are superior to SUD-only treatments. More research on the effectiveness of exposure-based techniques among substance-dependent patients is also warranted, as well as studies investigating combined CBT and pharmacotherapy approaches. Related to this latter point, one recent study (143) reported that sertraline treatment of PTSD was significantly augmented by the addition of PE (though the augmentation effect was restricted to persons who were partial responders to sertraline).

Pharmacotherapy of Posttraumatic Stress Disorder

The primary goals of the pharmacologic treatment of PTSD include decreasing PTSD symptoms, improving overall functioning, improving resilience to future stressors, decreasing symptoms of comorbid psychiatric conditions (e.g., depression, SUDs), and reducing risk of PTSD relapse (144). Long-term pharmacologic treatment (e.g., 1 year) is recommended based on evidence that PTSD is likely to return after discontinuation of shorter treatment (64).

Two medications, both selective serotonin reuptake inhibitors (SSRIs), are currently FDA-approved for the treatment of PTSD: sertraline (Zoloft) and paroxetine (Paxil). These are considered the first-line pharmacotherapeutic treatment options for PTSD based on their demonstrated efficacy in treating PTSD and other comorbid conditions and their relative safety in overdose (64,144–149). SSRIs have been shown to diminish all three symptoms clusters of PTSD and improve overall quality of life, particularly among civilian PTSD patients (148).

Though other pharmacologic agents have been investigated for the treatment of PTSD and some have shown promise, none are FDA-approved. As recently reviewed in 2007 by Zhang and Davidson (144), placebo-controlled investigations of dual action serotonergic and noradrenergic medications, such as venlafaxine and mirtazapine, suggest their ability to decrease PTSD symptoms and alleviate sleep disturbances. Though some tricyclic antidepressants (TCAs) and monoamine oxidase inhibitors (MAOIs) have been shown to be effective in improving PTSD and associated symptoms, they are no longer commonly used owing to cardiovascular and anticholinergic side effects, risk of seizures with TCAs, and strict dietary restrictions and risk of hypertensive crisis with MAOIs (150). Findings from other studies examining the use of mood stabilizers and anticonvulsants fail to show clear benefit in the treatment of PTSD (144). Encouraging evidence exists that antipsychotic medications, in particular risperidone, may be beneficial as an augmentation medication to partial responders of SSRIs (144,150). The risk of side effects with the use of antipsychotics, however, needs to be considered when choosing a medication (148). Benzodiazepines, which help alleviate anxiety and sleep impairment, are contraindicated as a monotherapy or preventive strategy based on preliminarily findings that their use was associated with increased risk of PTSD relative to placebo (64,148). Finally, medications that reduce central nervous system activity (e.g., clonidine, prazosin) may be helpful in decreasing nightmares and hyperarousal symptoms, which do not respond particularly well to SSRIs (150). More randomized controlled trials are needed to better assess their spectrum of efficacy.

Research on the pharmacologic prevention of PTSD is limited and methodologically problematic. Consequently there are no medications that effectively prevent/curtail the development of PTSD (144). However, recent translational research has led to findings that would support cautious optimism. Numerous preclinical studies have implicated the noradrenergic system, likely via action in the basolateral amygdala, in both the formation and maintenance of fear-related memories (151–156). A number of studies using fear-conditioning paradigms in animals have suggested a role for the β-adrenoreceptor in memory recall that is prompted by the presentation of cues associated with aversive outcomes (152,157,158). These promising animal studies led to research with human participants suggesting that β-adrenergic antagonists (e.g., propranolol) may selectively interfere with emotional memory (159–161). In one of these studies (161), participants with PTSD and non-PTSD controls treated with propranolol (a β-blocking agent) versus placebo evidenced reduced recall of the emotionally arousing content of a story told to them 1 week earlier. There also are some single-case data and a few preliminary intervention studies of individuals with PTSD suggesting that treatment with propranolol after a traumatic experience can decrease PTSD symptoms (162–164). In addition, there are preliminary data indicating that propranolol administration immediately after trauma cue exposure in individuals with PTSD dampens emotional reactivity during subsequent trauma cue exposure (165). Collectively, these findings suggest that the strategic use of β-blocking agents (e.g., propranolol) may prevent PTSD development or be used in conjunction with exposure-based therapy to dampen PTSD symptoms.

For more information regarding pharmacotherapy algorithms that provide helpful guidance in treating PTSD patients, see the International Psychopharmacology Algorithm Project (*http://www.ipap.org*).

Pharmacotherapy of Posttraumatic Stress Disorder–Substance Use Disorder Comorbidity There is a notable paucity of research on pharmacotherapy for PTSD and comorbid SUDs (166,167). Most studies, however, show promise and suggest that patients with PTSD and comorbid SUDs respond as well to standard PTSD pharmacotherapies as compared to patients without comorbid SUDs.

Several studies have examined the use of SSRIs, the pharmacologic treatment of choice for PTSD, among patients with comorbid SUDs. All of these studies have evaluated sertraline. The first was a small (N = 9) open-label trial among outpatients with alcohol dependence and PTSD (168). Decreases in alcohol use severity (e.g., number of drinking days, number of drinks per day) were shown, and approximately half (4 of 9) were abstinent during the 12-week follow-up period. In addition, significant reductions in all three PTSD symptom clusters were reported.

A second investigation extended the 1995 Brady et al. study (169) and examined the efficacy of 12 weeks of sertraline versus placebo among 94 outpatients with alcohol dependence and PTSD. Both groups showed reduction in alcohol use severity, but no significant between-group differences were revealed. Statistical trends for the sertraline group to demonstrate greater improvement in PTSD symptoms, particularly in intrusion and hyperarousal symptoms, were observed. Follow-up cluster analyses identified that the medication-responsive group tended to have less severe alcohol use and primary PTSD, in which the development of PTSD preceded the onset of alcohol dependence.

A secondary analysis of the Brady et al. (2005) data examined the influence of comorbid depression or other anxiety disorders among patients with alcohol dependence and PTSD who were treated with sertraline or placebo (170). The results indicated that having comorbid depression or a second anxiety disorder did not detract from treatment response to sertraline.

Finally, Zatzick et al. (171) combined case management, motivational enhancement for alcohol use disorders, and pharmacologic treatment for the prevention of PTSD. This intervention, termed *collaborative care*, was compared to TAU among injured surgical inpatients. The preliminary results were encouraging. Though patients in the TAU group evidenced a worsening of PTSD symptoms, patients who received pharmacotherapy did not. Unfortunately, the specific medications used were not reported, so a full understanding of the data is limited. The results for alcohol use severity were also promising but may be attributable to the psychosocial intervention rather than pharmacologic intervention. More research is clearly needed to help advance the pharmacologic treatment of comorbid PTSD and SUDs.

Last, there is developing research indicating a potential for D-cycloserine to enhance exposure-based treatment outcomes with anxiety-disordered individuals (e.g., PTSD) and may also have potential as an innovative treatment for PTSD-SUD comorbidity. The medication, D-cycloserine (DCS), is a partial *N*-methyl-D-aspartate agonist and an FDA-approved antibiotic treatment for tuberculosis. As already noted, exposure-based therapy is founded on the principles of conditioned fear extinction and has demonstrated efficacy in the treatment of several anxiety disorders, including PTSD. Building upon the animal studies demonstrating DCS-facilitated extinction of conditioned fear responses (172–177), a number of recent clinical trials have examined the potential facilitative effects of DCS on extinction of fear-based responses and symptoms associated with anxiety disorders. To date, three published clinical trials have shown that DCS can facilitate extinction of anxiety/fear symptomatology in acrophobia (178), social anxiety disorder (179) and OCD (180). Despite negative findings from one recent study of DCS augmented exposure therapy for subclinical fear of spiders (181), the existing clinical data strongly suggests that DCS might enhance exposure-based treatment outcome for severe anxiety disorders. Accordingly, it seems timely that the effects of DCS augmented exposure therapy should be studied in PTSD-afflicted individuals.

In addition to its potential for advancing exposure therapy for PTSD, the ability of DCS to facilitate extinction might be fruitfully explored with respect to exposure-based treatment of SUDs (cf., 182,183), known as cue exposure therapy (CE). Briefly, CE involves exposing addicted individuals to stimuli that have acquired the ability, via Pavlovian conditioning, to elicit craving and other reactions (e.g., heart rate increases) as a consequence of a long history of contiguous pairings with drug or alcohol administration. These craving and other cue-elicited reactions are assumed to have an important role in the maintenance of, and relapse to, substance use (184–187). The goal of CE is to attenuate or eliminate craving and reactivity via extinction, thereby reducing risk of further substance use (i.e., maintaining abstinence). To date, CE therapy has been associated with modest efficacy (188), but medication developments such as DCS hold promise for bolstering the effects of CE. Furthermore, future clinical studies involving PTSD-SUD comorbid individuals could investigate the possibility of DCS-enhanced outcomes of an integrated exposure-based therapy consisting of PE and CE.

CONCLUDING COMMENTS

As a clinical entity, PTSD is an evolving disorder, and a portion of its evolution relates specifically to our growing understanding of the interface between it and substance use disorders. It is now well-established that SUDs frequently co-occur with PTSD and that this comorbidity is profoundly detrimental to physical and psychologic well-being.

Theory and research about the nature of the causal relationship between the two disorders suggests that even though no single model has received unequivocal empirical support, it appears that PTSD most often precedes SUD onset, threreby lending support to the notion that a SUD may serve to diminish PTSD symptoms (i.e., self-medication hypothesis). Though the contribution of neurobiologic factors to the etiology and maintenance of PTSD-SUD comorbidity are not completely understood, there is considerable evidence of shared causal processes. Chief among these processes is dysregulation of both the HPA axis and noradrenergic systems.

The effective management of PTSD-SUD comorbidity begins with a thorough assessment. Fortunately, thorough does not mean burdensome. There are numerous interview and self-report methods that can be used to efficiently determine the PTSD status of adult civilians and veterans with a comorbid SUD. As always, ensuring that a sufficient period of abstinence has occurred prior to conducting an assessment will enhance the integrity of assessment findings.

Some of the best treatments for PTSD-SUD comorbid individuals are those that concurrently address both disorders. It is unfortunate that such treatments are often unavailable. Nonetheless, there are several highly efficacious cognitive behavioral therapies for PTSD that can be readily employed with comorbid individuals and which often yield collateral benefits for the untreated SUD. Exposure-based interventions (e.g., PE) are considered the gold standard of CBTs, but other cognitive-focused and anxiety-focused therapies have been employed with considerable success. Pharmacotherapy has also been used (with or without CBT) to address PTSD alone or PTSD-SUD comorbidity. Specifically, sertraline and paroxetine are FDA-approved for the treatment of PTSD. Other innovative pharmacotherapies that have the potential to augment exposure-based therapy (i.e., DCS) or disrupt emotional memories (i.e., propranolol) are under investigation. Since treatment of any form can often prove challenging to the recipient, clinicians should employ strategies to enhance retention, such as telephone contact between sessions and continue outpatient care for at least 3 months after treatment completion (189,190).

REFERENCES

1. Sadock B, Sadock VA. *Kaplan & Sadock's synopsis of psychiatry, behavioral sciences/clinical psychiatry*. Philadelphia: Lippincott, Williams & Wilkins, 2003.
2. American Psychiatric Association. *Diagnostic and statistical manual of mental disorders*, 3rd ed. Washington, DC: American Psychiatric Press, Inc., 1980.
3. Jacobsen LK, Southwick SM, Kosten TR. Substance use disorders in patients with posttraumatic stress disorder: a review of the literature. *Am J Psychiatry* 2001;158(8):1184–1190.
4. Young HE, Rosen CS, Finney JW. A survey of PTSD screening and referral practices in VA addiction treatment programs. *J Subst Abuse Treat* 2005;28(4):313–319.
5. Harned MS, Najavits LM, Weiss RD. Self-harm and suicidal behavior in women with comorbid PTSD and substance dependence. *Am J Addict* 2006;15(5):392–395.
6. Ouimette P, Goodwin E, Brown PJ. Health and well being of substance use disorder patients with and without posttraumatic stress disorder. *Addict Behav* 2006;31(8):1415–1423.
7. American Psychiatric Association. *Diagnostic and statistical manual of mental disorders,* 4th ed. [Text revision]. Washington, DC: American Psychiatric Press, Inc., 2000.
8. Hidalgo RB, Davidson JR. Posttraumatic stress disorder: epidemiology and health-related considerations. *J Clin Psychiatry* 2000;61(Suppl 7):5–13.
9. Brunello N, Davidson JR, Deahl M, et al. Posttraumatic stress disorder: diagnosis and epidemiology, comorbidity and social consequences, biology and trea*tment. Neuropsychobiology* 2001;43(3):150–62.
10. Kessler RC, Sonnega A, Bromet E, et al. Posttraumatic stress disorder in the National Comorbidity Survey. *Arch Gen Psychiatry* 1995;52(12):1048–1060.
11. Kessler RC, Berglund P, Demler O, et al. Lifetime prevalence and age-of-onset distributions of DSM-IV disorders in the National Comorbidity Survey Replication. *Arch Gen Psychiatry* 2005;62(6):593–602.
12. Brady KT, Killeen TK, Brewerton T, et al. Comorbidity of psychiatric disorders and posttraumatic stress disorder. *J Clin Psychiatry* 2000;61(Suppl 7):22–32.
13. Shipherd JC, Stafford J, Tanner LR. Predicting alcohol and drug abuse in Persian Gulf War veterans: what role do PTSD symptoms play? *Addict Behav* 2005;30(3):595–599.
14. Cottler LB, Compton WM, Mager D, et al. Posttraumatic stress disorder among substance users from the general population. *Am J Psychiatry* 1992;149(5):664–670.
15. Acierno R, Lawyer SR, Rheingold A, et al. Current psychopathology in previously assaulted older adults. *J Interperson Viol* 2007;22(2):250–258.
16. Kilpatrick DG, Acierno R, Saunders BE, et al. Risk factors for adolescent substance abuse and dependence: data from a national sample. *J Consult Clin Psychol* 2000; 68(1):19–30.
17. Johnson SD, Striley C, Cottler LB. The association of substance use disorders with trauma exposure and PTSD among African American drug users. *Addict Behav* 2006;31(11):2063–2073.
18. Reed PL, Anthony JC, Breslau N. Incidence of drug problems in young adults exposed to trauma and posttraumatic stress disorder: do early life experiences and predispositions matter? *Arch Gen Psychiatry* 2007; 64(12):1435–1442.
19. Khantzian EJ. The self-medication hypothesis of addictive disorders: focus on heroin and cocaine dependence. *Am J Psychiatry* 1985;142(11):1259–1264.

20. Khantzian EJ. Self-regulation and self-medication factors in alcoholism and the addictions. Similarities and differences. *Recent Dev Alcohol* 1990; 8:255–271.
21. Khantzian EJ. The self-medication hypothesis of substance use disorders: a reconsideration and recent applications (see comment). *Harvard Rev Psychiatry* 1997;4(5):231–244.
22. Saladin ME, Brady KT, Dansky BS, et al. Understanding comorbidity between PTSD and substance use disorder: two preliminary investigations. *Addict Behav* 1995;20(5):643–655.
23. Chilcoat HD, Breslau N. Investigations of causal pathways between PTSD and drug use disorders. *Addict Behav* 1998;23(6):827–840.
24. Stewart SH, Conrod PJ. Psychosocial models of functional associations between posttraumatic stress disorder and substance use disorder. In: Ouimette P, Brown PJ, eds. *Trauma and substance abuse: causes, consequences, and treatment of comorbid disorders.* American Psychological Association: Washington, DC, 2003:29–55.
25. Friedman MJ. What might the psychobiology of posttraumatic stress disorder teach us about future approaches to pharmacotherapy? *J Clin Psychiatry* 2000;61(Suppl 7):44–51.
26. Antony MM, Orsillo SM, Roemer L, eds. *Practitioner's guide to empirically based measures of anxiety.* New York: Kluwer Academic/Plenum Publishers, 2001.
27. Wilson J, Keane TM, eds. *Assessing psychological trauma and PTSD.* Guildford Press: New York, 1997.
28. Brewin CR. Systematic review of screening instruments for adults at risk of PTSD. *J Trauma Stress* 2005;18(1):53–62.
29. Elhai JD, Gray MJ, Kashdan TB, et al. Which instruments are most commonly used to assess traumatic event exposure and posttraumatic effects?: a survey of traumatic stress professionals. *J Trauma Stress* 2005;18(5):541–545.
30. Read JP, Bollinger AR, Sharkansky EJ. Assessment of comorbid substance use disorder and posttraumatic stress disorder. In: Ouimette P, Brown PJ, eds. *Trauma and substance abuse: causes, consequences, and treatment of comorbid disorders.* Washington, DC: American Psychological Association, 2003:111–125.
31. Blake DD, Weathers FW, Nagy LM, et al. The development of a clinician-administered PTSD scale. *J Trauma Stress* 1995;8:75–90.
32. Weathers FW, Keane TM, Davidson JRT. Clinician-administered PTSD Scale: a review of the first ten years of research. *Depress Anxiety* 2001; 13(3):132–156.
33. First MB, Spitzer RL, Gibbon M, et al. *Structured clinical interview for DSM-IV-TR Axis I disorders, research version, patient edition (SCID-I/P).* New York: Biometrics Research, New York State Psychiatric Institute, 2002.
34. Spitzer RL, Williams JBW, Gibbon M, et al. The structured clinical interview for DSM-III-R: I. History, rationale and description. *Arch Gen Psychiatry* 1992;49: 624–629.
35. Kilpatrick D, Resnick H, Freedy J. *The potential stressful events interview.* Charleston: Medical University of South Carolina, 1991.
36. Kilpatrick D, Resnick H, Saunders B, et al. *The National Women's Study PTSD module.* Charleston: Medical University of South Carolina, 1989.
37. Foa EB, Tolin DF. Comparison of the PTSD Symptom Scale-Interview Version and the clinician-administered PTSD scale. *J Trauma Stress* 2000;13(2):181–191.
38. Foa E, Riggs DS, Dancu CV, et al. Reliability and validity of a brief instrument for assessing posttraumatic stress disorder. *J Trauma Stress* 1993;6:459–473.
39. Davidson JR, Malik MA, Travers J. Structured interview for PTSD (SIP): psychometric validation for DSM-IV criteria. *Depress Anxiety* 1997;5(3):127–129.
40. Sheehan DV, Lecrubier Y, Sheehan KH, et al. The Mini-International Neuropsychiatric Interview (M.I.N.I.): the development and validation of a structured diagnostic psychiatric interview for DSM-IV and ICD-10. *J Clin Psychiatry* 1998;59(Suppl 20):22–33.
41. Wittchen HU. Reliability and validity studies of the WHO—Composite International Diagnostic Interview (CIDI): a critical review. *J Psychiatr Res* 1994;28(1):57–84.
42. World Health Organization. *Composite International Diagnostic Interview (CIDI).* Geneva, Switzerland: Author, 1993.
43. Weiss S, Marmar CR. The Impact of Event Scale—Revised. In: Wilson J, Keane TM, eds. *Assessing psychological trauma and PTSD.*, New York: Guilford Press, 1997:399–411.
44. Horowitz MJ, Wilner N, Alvarez W. Impact of Event Scale: a measure of subjective stress. *Psychosom Med* 1979;41(3):209–218.
45. American Psychiatric Association. *Diagnostic and statistical manual of mental disorders*, 4th ed. Washington, DC: American Psychiatric Press, Inc., 1994.
46. Kazlauskas E, Gailiene D, Domanskaite-Gota V, et al. Psychometric properties of the Lithuanian version of the Impact of Event Scale-Revised (IES-R). *Psichologija* 2006;33:22–30.
47. Asukai N, Kato H, Kawamura N, et al. Reliability and validity of the Japanese-language version of the Impact of Event Scale-revised (IES-R-J): four studies of different traumatic events. *J Nerv Ment Dis* 2002;190(3):175–182.
48. Baguena MJ, Villarroya E, Belena A, et al. Psychometric properties of the Spanish version of the Impact of Event Scale-Revised (IES-R). *Anal Modif Conduct* 2001; 27(114):581–604.
49. Maercker A, Schutzwohl M. Assessment of post-traumatic stress reactions: the Impact of Event Scale-Revised (IES-R). *Diagnostica* 1998; 44(3):130–141.
50. Rash CJ, Coffey SF, Bashnagela JS, et al. Psychometric properties of the IES-R in traumatized substance dependent individuals with and without PTSD. *Addict Behav* (under review).
51. Foa EB, Cashman L, Jaycox L, et al. The validation of a self-report measure of posttraumatic stress disorder: The Posttraumatic Diagnostic Scale. *Psychol Assess* 1997; 9(4):445–451.
52. Foa EB, Riggs DS, Dancu CV, et al. Reliability and validity of a brief instrument for assessing post-traumatic stress disorder. *J Trauma Stress* 1993;6(4):459–473.
53. American Psychiatric Association. *Diagnostic and statistical manual of mental disorders*, 3rd ed. [Revised edition]. Washington, DC: American Psychiatric Press, Inc., 1987.
54. Falsetti SA, Resnick HS, Resick PA, et al. The Modified PTSD Symptom Scale: a brief self-report measure of posttraumatic stress disorder. *Behav Ther* 1993;16:161–162.
55. Falsetti SA, Resick PA, Resnick HS, et al. *Posttraumatic stress disorder: The assessment of frequency and severity of symptoms in clinical and nonclinical samples.* Boston: Association for the Advancement of Behavior Therapy, 1992.
56. Coffey SF, Dansky BS, Falsetti SA, et al. Screening for PTSD in a substance abuse sample: psychometric properties of a modified version of the PTSD Symptom Scale Self-Report. Posttraumatic stress disorder. *J Trauma Stress* 1998;11(2):393–399.
57. Dansky BS, Saladin ME, Coffey SF, et al. Use of self-report measures of crime-related posttraumatic stress disorder with substance use disordered patients. *J Subst Abuse Treat* 1997;14(5):431–437.
58. Keane TM, Caddell JM, Taylor KL. Mississippi Scale for Combat-Related Posttraumatic Stress Disorder: three studies in reliability and validity. *J Consult Clin Psychol* 1988;56(1):85–90.
59. McFall ME, Smith DE, Mackay PW, et al. Reliability and validity of Mississippi Scale for Combat-Related Posttraumatic Stress Disorder. *Psychol Assess* 1990;2(2): 114–121.
60. McFall ME, Smith DE, Roszell DK, et al. Convergent validity of measures of PTSD in Vietnam combat veterans. *Am J Psychiatry* 1990;147(5): 645–648.
61. Ouimette P, Humphreys K, Moos RH, et al. Self-help group participation among substance use disorder patients with posttraumatic stress disorder. *J Subst Abuse Treat* 2001;20(1):25–32.
62. Nemeroff CB, Bremmer JD, Foa EB, et al. Posttraumatic stress disorder: a state-of-the-science review. *J Psychiatr Res* 2006;40(1):1–21.
63. Tiet QQ, Mausbach, B. Treatments for patients with dual diagnosis: a review. *Alcohol Clin Exp Res* 2007;31(4):513–536.
64. Ballenger JC, Davidson JR, Lecrubier Y, et al. Consensus statement update on posttraumatic stress disorder from the international consensus group on depression and anxiety. *J Clin Psychiatry* 2004;65(Suppl 1):55–62.
65. Brom D, Kleber RJ, Defares PB. Brief psychotherapy for posttraumatic stress disorders. *J Consult Clin Psychol* 1989;57(5):607–612.

66. Foa EB, Danru CV, Hembree EA, et al. A comparison of exposure therapy, stress inoculation training, and their combination for reducing posttraumatic stress disorder in female assault victims. *J Consult Clin Psychol* 1999;67(2):194–200.
67. Hyer L, Woods MG, Bruno R, et al. Treatment outcomes of Vietnam veterans with PTSD and the consistency of the MCMI. *J Clin Psychol* 1989;45(4):547–552.
68. Tarrier N, Pilgrim H, Sommerfield C, et al. A randomized trial of cognitive therapy and imaginal exposure in the treatment of chronic posttraumatic stress disorder. *J Consult Clin Psychol* 1999;67(1):13–18.
69. Mowrer OA. *Learning theory and behavior*. New York: Wiley, 1960.
70. Stampfl TG, Levis DJ. Essentials of implosive therapy: a learning-theory-based psychodynamic behavioral therapy. *J Abnorm Psychol* 1967; 72(6):496–503.
71. Wolpe J. *Psychotherapy by reciprocal inhibition*. Stanford: Stanford University Press, 1958.
72. Foa EB, Kozak MJ. Emotional processing of fear: exposure to corrective information. *Psychol Bull* 1986;99(1):20–35.
73. Pavlov IP. *Conditioned reflexes*. New York: Dover Publications, 1927.
74. Konorski J. *Conditioned reflexes and neuronal organization*. London: Cambridge University Press, 1948.
75. Rescorla RA. Spontaneous recovery. *Learn Memory* 2004;11(5):501–509.
76. Foa E, Rothbaum BO. *Treating the trauma of rape*. New York: The Guilford Press, 1998.
77. Shapiro F, Maxfield L. Eye Movement Desensitization and Reprocessing (EMDR): information processing in the treatment of trauma. *J Clin Psychol* 2002;58(8):933–946.
78. Shapiro F. *Eye movement desensitization and reprocessing: Basic principles, protocols, and procedures*, 2nd ed., New York: Guilford Press, 2001:xxiv, 472.
79. Shapiro F. Efficacy of the Eye Movement Desensitization procedure in the treatment of traumatic memories. *J Trauma Stress* 1989;2(2): 199–223.
80. Beck AT. *Cognitive therapy and the emotional disorders*. New York: International Universities Press, 1976:356.
81. Beck AT. *Cognitive therapy of depression*. New York: Guilford Press, 1979:425.
82. Beck AT, Emery G, Greenberg RL. *Anxiety disorders and phobias: a cognitive perspective* [15th anniversary edition]. Cambridge, MA: Basic Books, 2005:xxxvi, 343.
83. Clark DM. A cognitive approach to panic. *Behav Res Ther* 1986;24(4): 461–470.
84. Beck AT, Wright FD, Newman CF, et al. *Cognitive therapy of substance abuse*. New York: Guilford Press, 1993:xiii, 354.
85. Resick PA, Schnicke MK. Cognitive processing therapy for sexual assault victims. *J Consult Clin Psychol* 1992;60(5):748–756.
86. Resick PA, Schnicke MK. *Cognitive processing therapy for rape victims: a treatment manual.* Interpersonal violence: the practice series, vol 4. Newbury Park, CA: Sage, 1993.
87. Monson CM, Schnorr PP, Resick PA, et al. Cognitive processing therapy for veterans with military-related posttraumatic stress disorder. *J Consult Clin Psychol* 2006; 74(5):898–907.
88. Ahrens J, Rexford L. Cognitive processing therapy for incarcerated adolescents with PTSD. *J Aggress Maltreat Trauma* 2002;6(1):201–216.
89. Silver SM, Brooks A, Obenchain J. Treatment of Vietnam War veterans with PTSD: a comparison of eye movement desensitization and reprocessing, biofeedback, and relaxation training. *J Trauma Stress* 1995; 8(2):337–342.
90. Meichenbaum D. *Stress inoculation training. Psychology practitioner guidebooks*. New York: Pergamon Press, 1985:xi, 115.
91. Meichenbaum D. *Clinical handbook/therapist manual for assessing and treating adults with PTSD.* Waterloo: Institute Press, 1994:600.
92. Meichenbaum D. Self-instructional training. In: Kanfer FH, Goldstein A, eds. *Helping people change*. New York: Pergamon Press, 1975: 357–391.
93. Veronen LJ, Kilpatrick DG. Stress management for rape victims. In: Meichenbaum D, Jaremko ME, eds. *Stress reduction and prevention*. New York: Plenum Press, 1983:341–374.
94. Foa EB, Rothbaum BO, Riggs DS, et al. Treatment of posttraumatic stress disorder in rape victims: a comparison between cognitive-behavioral procedures and counseling. *J Consult Clin Psychol* 1991;59(5): 715–723.
95. Yadin E, Foa E. Cognitive behavioral treatments for posttraumatic stress disorder. In: Kirmayer LJ, Lemelson R, Barad M, eds. *Understanding trauma: integrating biological, clinical, and cultural perspectives*. Cambridge: Cambridge University Press, 2007:178–193.
96. Foa EB, Cahill S. Psychological treatments for PTSD: an overview. In: Neria Y, et al., eds. *9/11: public health in the wake of terrorist attacks*. Cambridge: Cambridge University Press, 2006:457–474.
97. Foa EB. Psychosocial therapy for posttraumatic stress disorder. *J Clin Psychiatry* 2006;67(Suppl 2):40–45.
98. Bisson JI, Ehlers A, Matthews R, et al. Psychological treatments for chronic post-traumatic stress disorder. Systematic review and meta-analysis. *Br J Psychiatry* 2007;190:97–104.
99. Keane TM, Marshall AD, Taft CT. Posttraumatic stress disorder: etiology, epidemiology, and treatment outcome. *Annu Rev Clin Psychol* 2006;2:161–97.
100. Bisson J, Andrew M. Psychological treatment of post-traumatic stress disorder (PTSD). *Cochrane Database System Rev* 2007;3:1–20.
101. Bradley R, Greene J, Russ E, et al. A multidimensional meta-analysis of psychotherapy for PTSD. *Am J Psychiatry* 2005;162(2):214–227.
102. Foa E, Rothbaum BO, Furr JM. Augmenting exposure therapy with other BT procedures. *Psychiatr Ann* 2003;33(1):47–53.
103. Grunert BK, Weis JM, Smucker MR, et al. Imagery rescripting and reprocessing therapy after failed prolonged exposure for posttraumatic stress disorder following industrial injury. *J Behav Ther Exp Psychiatry* 2007;38(4):317–328.
104. Acierno R, Hersen M, van Hasselt VB, et al. Review of the validation and dissemination of eye-movement desensitization and reprocessing: a scientific and ethical dilemma. *Clin Psychol Rev* 1994;14(4):287–299.
105. McNally RJ. EMDR and Mesmerism: a comparative historical analysis. *J Anxiety Disord* 1999;13(1–2):225–236.
106. Herbert JD, Lilienfield SO, Lohr JM, et al. Science and pseudoscience in the development of eye movement desensitization and reprocessing: implications for clinical psychology. *Clin Psychol Rev* 2000;20(8):945–971.
107. Rosen GM, McNally R, Lohr JM, et al. A realistic appraisal of EMDR. *Calif Psychol* 1998;31:25–27.
108. McNally R. Research on eye movement desensitization and reprocessing (EMDR) as a treatment for PTSD. In: Friedman MJ, ed. *PTSD Research Quarterly*. White River Junction, VT: VA Medical and Regional Office Center, 1999:1–8.
109. Lohr JM, Lilienfield SO, Tolin DF, et al. Eye movement desensitization and reprocessing: an analysis of specific versus nonspecific treatment factors. *J Anxiety Disord* 199913(1–2):185–207.
110. Lohr JM, Kleinknecht RA, Tolin, DF, et al. The empirical status of the clinical application of eye movement desensitization and reprocessing. *J Behav Ther Exp Psychiatry* 1995;26(4):285–302.
111. Lohr JM, Kleinknecht RA, Conley AT, et al. A methodological critique of the current status of eye movement desensitization (EMD). *J Behav Ther Exp Psychiatry* 1992; 23(3):159–167.
112. Pitman RK, Orr SP, Altman B, et al. Emotional processing during eye movement desensitization and reprocessing therapy of Vietnam veterans with chronic posttraumatic stress disorder. *Compr Psychiatry* 1996;37(6): 419–429.
113. Lohr JM, Tolin DF, Lilienfeld SO. Efficacy of Eye Movement Desensitization and Reprocessing: Implications for behavior therapy. *Behav Ther* 1998;29(1):123–156.
114. Cahill SP, Carrigan MH, Frueh BC. Does EMDR work? And if so, why?: a critical review of controlled outcome and dismantling research. *J Anxiety Disord* 1999;13(1–2):5–33.
115. Davidson PR, Parker KC. Eye movement desensitization and reprocessing (EMDR): a meta-analysis. *J Consult Clin Psychol* 2001;69(2): 305–316.
116. Rothbaum BO, Astin MC, Marsteller F. Prolonged exposure versus eye movement desensitization and reprocessing (EMDR) for PTSD rape victims. *J Trauma Stress* 2005;18(6):607–616.

117. Macklin ML, Metzger LJ, Lasko NB, et al. Five-year follow-up study of eye movement desensitization and reprocessing therapy for combat-related posttraumatic stress disorder. *Compr Psychiatry* 2000;41(1): 24–27.
118. Renfrey G, Spates CR. Eye movement desensitization: a partial dismantling study. *J Behav Ther Exp Psychiatry* 1994;25(3):231–239.
119. Najavits LM, Sullivan TP, Schmitz M, et al. Treatment utilization by women with PTSD and substance dependence. *Am J Addict* 2004;13(3): 215–224.
120. Young HE, Rosen CS, Finney JW. A survey of PTSD screening and referral practices in VA addiction treatment programs. *J Subst Abuse Treat* 2005;28(4):313–319.
121. Nace EP. Posttraumatic stress disorder and substance abuse. Clinical issues. *Recent Dev Alcohol* 1988;6:9–26.
122. Pitman RK, Altman B, Greenwald E, et al. Psychiatric complications during flooding therapy for posttraumatic stress disorder. *J Clin Psychiatry* 1991;52(1):17–20.
123. Brady KT, Dansky BS, Back SE, et al. Exposure therapy in the treatment of PTSD among cocaine-dependent individuals: preliminary findings. *J Subst Abuse Treat* 2001;21(1):47–54.
124. Foa E, Chrestman K, Riggs DS. *Integrating prolonged exposure therapy and substance abuse treatment.* Hollywood, CA: International Society for Traumatic Stress Studies, 2006.
125. Najavits LM, Schmitz M, Gotthardt S, et al. Seeking Safety plus Exposure Therapy: an outcome study on dual diagnosis men. *J Psychoactive Drugs* 2005;37(4):425–435.
126. Triffleman E. Gender differences in a controlled pilot study of psychosocial treatments in substance dependent patients with post-traumatic stress disorder: design considerations and outcomes. *Alcohol Treat Q* 2000;18(3):113–126.
127. Khantzian E. The self-medication hypothesis of addictive disorders: focus on heroin and cocaine dependence. *Am J Psychiatry* 1985;142(11): 1259–1264.
128. Back SE, Brady KT, Sonne SC, et al. Symptom improvement in co-occurring PTSD and alcohol dependence. *J Nerv Ment Dis* 2006;194(9): 690–696.
129. Ouimette P, Ahrens C, Moos R, et al. Posttraumatic stress disorder in substance abuse patients: relationships to 1 year posttreatment outcomes. *Psychol Addict Behav* 1997;1:34–47.
130. Back SE, Brady KT, Jaaimägi U, et al. Cocaine dependence and PTSD: a pilot study of symptom interplay and treatment preferences. *Addict Behav* 2006;31(2):351–354.
131. Brown PJ, Stout RL, Gannon-Rowley J. Substance use disorder-PTSD comorbidity: patients' perceptions of symptom interplay and treatment issues. *J Subst Abuse Treat* 1998;15(5):445–448.
132. Najavits LM. Seeking Safety: a treatment manual for PTSD and substance abuse. In: Blane HT, Kosten TR, eds. *Guilford Substance Abuse Series.* New York: Guilford Press, 2002.
133. Najavits LM, Weiss RD, Shaw SR, et al. Seeking Safety: outcome of a new cognitive-behavioral psychotherapy for women with posttraumatic stress disorder and substance dependence. *J Trauma Stress* 1998;11(3):437–456.
134. Najavits LM, Ryngala D, Back SE, et al. Treatment for PTSD and comorbid disorders: a review of the literature. In: Foa E, Keane TM, Friedman MJ, eds, *Effective treatments for PTSD.* New York: Guilford Press (in press).
135. Zlotnick C, Najavits LM, Rohsenow DJ, et al. A cognitive-behavioral treatment for incarcerated women with substance abuse disorder and posttraumatic stress disorder: findings from a pilot study. *J Subst Abuse Treat* 2003;25(2):99–105.
136. Hien DA, Cohen LR, Miele GM, et al. Promising treatments for women with comorbid PTSD and substance use disorders. *Am J Psychiatry* 2004;161(8):1426–1432.
137. Triffleman E, Carroll K, Kellogg S. Substance dependence posttraumatic stress disorder therapy. An integrated cognitive-behavioral approach. *J Subst Abuse Treat* 1999;17(1–2):3–14.
138. Back SE, Dansky BS, Carroll KM, et al. Exposure therapy in the treatment of PTSD among cocaine-dependent individuals: description of procedures. *J Subst Abuse Treat* 2001;21(1):35–45.
139. Coffey SF, Schumacher JA, Brimo ML, et al. Exposure therapy for substance abusers with PTSD: translating research to practice. *Behav Modif* 2005;29(1):10–38.
140. Donovan B, Padin-Rivera E, Kowaliw S. Transcend: initial outcomes from a posttraumatic stress disorder/substance abuse treatment program. *J Trauma Stress* 2001;14(4):757–772.
141. Harris M. *Trauma recovery and empowerment: a clinician's guide for working with women in groups.* New York: Free Press, 1998.
142. Toussaint D, van DeMark N, Bornemann A, et al. Modifications to the Trauma Recovery and Empowerment Model (TREM) for substance-abusing women with histories of violence: outcomes and lessons learned at a Colorado substance abuse treatment center. *J Commun Psychol* (in press).
143. Rothbaum BO, Cahill SP, Foa EB, et al. Augmentation of sertraline with prolonged exposure in the treatment of posttraumatic stress disorder. *J Trauma Stress* 2006;19(5):625–638.
144. Zhang W, Davidson JR. Post-traumatic stress disorder: an evaluation of existing pharmacotherapies and new strategies. *Expert Opin Pharmacother* 2007;8(12):1861–1870.
145. Brady K, Pearlstein T, Asnis GM, et al. Efficacy and safety of sertraline treatment of posttraumatic stress disorder: a randomized controlled trial. *JAMA* 2000;283(14):1837–1844.
146. Davidson J, Pearlson T, Londborg P, et al. Efficacy of sertraline in preventing relapse of posttraumatic stress disorder: results of a 28-week double-blind, placebo-controlled study. *Am J Psychiatry* 2001;158(12): 1974–1981.
147. Ipser J, Seedat S, Stein DJ. Pharmacotherapy for post-traumatic stress disorder—a systematic review and meta-analysis. *South Afr Med J* 2006; 96(10):1088–1096.
148. Davidson JR. Pharmacologic treatment of acute and chronic stress following trauma: 2006. *J Clin Psychiatry* 2006;67(Suppl 2):34–39.
149. Marshall RD, Beebe KL, Oldham M, et al. Efficacy and safety of paroxetine treatment for chronic PTSD: a fixed-dose, placebo-controlled study. *Am J Psychiatry* 2001;158(12):1982–1988.
150. Schoenfeld FB, Marmar CR, Neylan TC. Current concepts in pharmacotherapy for posttraumatic stress disorder. *Psychiatr Serv* 2004;55(5): 519–531.
151. Berlau DJ, McGaugh JL. Enhancement of extinction memory consolidation: the role of the noradrenergic and GABAergic systems within the basolateral amygdala. *Neurobiol Learn Mem* 2006;86(2):123–132.
152. Debiec J, Ledoux JE. Disruption of reconsolidation but not consolidation of auditory fear conditioning by noradrenergic blockade in the amygdala. *Neuroscience* 2004;129(2):267–272.
153. Lee JL, DiCiano P, Thomas KL, et al. Disrupting reconsolidation of drug memories reduces cocaine-seeking behavior. *Neuron* 2005;47(6): 795–801.
154. McGaugh JL. Memory—a century of consolidation. *Science* 2000;287 (5451):248–251.
155. Nader K. Memory traces unbound. *Trends Neurosci* 2003;26(2):65–72.
156. Sara SJ. Retrieval and reconsolidation: toward a neurobiology of remembering. *Learn Mem* 2000;7(2):73–84.
157. Cahill L, Pham CA, Setlow B. Impaired memory consolidation in rats produced with beta-adrenergic blockade. *Neurobiol Learn Mem* 2000;74 (3):259–266.
158. Morris RW, Westbrook RF, Killcross AS. Reinstatement of extinguished fear by beta-adrenergic arousal elicited by a conditioned context. *Behav Neurosci* 2005;119(6):1662–1671.
159. Cahill L, Prins B, Weber M, et al. Beta-adrenergic activation and memory for emotional events. *Nature* 1994;371(6499):702–704.
160. O'Carroll RE, Drysdale E, Cahill L, et al. Stimulation of the noradrenergic system enhances and blockade reduces memory for emotional material in man. *Psychol Med* 1999;29(5):1083–1088.
161. Reist C, Duffy JG, Fujimoto K, et al. Beta-Adrenergic blockade and emotional memory in PTSD. *Int J Neuropsychopharmacol* 2001;4(4): 377–383.
162. Pitman RK, Sanders KM, Zusman RM, et al. Pilot study of secondary prevention of posttraumatic stress disorder with propranolol. *Biol Psychiatry* 2002;51(2):189–192.

163. Vaiva G, Ducrocq F, Jezequel K, et al. Immediate treatment with propranolol decreases posttraumatic stress disorder two months after trauma. *Biol Psychiatry* 2003;54(9):947–949.
164. Taylor F, Cahill L. Propranolol for reemergent posttraumatic stress disorder following an event of retraumatization: a case study. *J Trauma Stress* 2002;15(5):433–437.
165. Pitman RK, Brunet A, Orr SP, et al. A novel treatment for posttraumatic stress disorder by reconsolidation blockade with propranolol. *Neuropsychopharmacology* 2006;31(1):S8–S9.
166. Brady KT, Verduin ML. Pharmacotherapy of comorbid mood, anxiety, and substance use disorders. *Subst Use Misuse* 2005;40(13–14):2021–2041, 2043–2048.
167. Lingford-Hughes AR, Welch S, Nutt DJ. Evidence-based guidelines for the pharmacological management of substance misuse, addiction, and comorbidity: recommendations from the British Association for Psychopharmacology. *J Psychopharmacol* 2004;18(3):293–335.
168. Brady KT, Sonne SC, Roberts JM. Sertraline treatment of comorbid posttraumatic stress disorder and alcohol dependence. *J Clin Psychiatry* 1995;56(11):502–505.
169. Brady KT, Sonne S, Anton RF, et al. Sertraline in the treatment of co-occurring alcohol dependence and posttraumatic stress disorder. *Alcohol Clin Exp Res* 2005;29(3):395–401.
170. Labbate LA, Sonne SC, Randal CL, et al. Does comorbid anxiety or depression affect clinical outcomes in patients with post-traumatic stress disorder and alcohol use disorders? *Compr Psychiatry* 2004;45(4):304–310.
171. Zatzick D, Roy-Byrne P, Russo J, et al. A randomized effectiveness trial of stepped collaborative care for acutely injured trauma survivors. *Arch Gen Psychiatry* 2004;61:498–506.
172. Norberg MM, Krystal JH, Tolin DF. *A meta-analysis of D-cycloserine and the facilitation of fear extinction and exposure therapy. Biol Psychiatry* 2008; 63(22):1118–1126.
173. Ledgerwood L, Richardson R, Cranney J. Effects of D-cycloserine on extinction of conditioned freezing. *Behav Neurosci* 2003;117(2):341–349.
174. Ledgerwood L, Richardson R, Cranney J. D-Cycloserine and the facilitation of extinction of conditioned fear: consequences for reinstatement. *Behav Neurosci* 2004;118(3):505–513.
175. Ledgerwood L, Richardson R, Cranney J. D-Cycloserine facilitates extinction of learned fear: effects on reacquisition and generalized extinction. *Biol Psychiatry* 2005;57(8):841–847.
176. Walker DL, Ressler KJ, Lu KT, et al. Facilitation of conditioned fear extinction by systemic administration or intra-amygdala infusions of D-cycloserine as assessed with fear-potentiated startle in rats. *J Neurosci* 2002;22(6):2343–2351.
177. Yang YL, Lu KT. Facilitation of conditioned fear extinction by D-cycloserine is mediated by mitogen-activated protein kinase and phosphatidylinositol 3-kinase cascades and requires de novo protein synthesis in basolateral nucleus of amygdala. *Neuroscience* 2005;134(1):247–260.
178. Ressler KJ, Rothbaum BU, Tannebaum L, et al. Cognitive enhancers as adjuncts to psychotherapy: use of D-cycloserine in phobic individuals to facilitate extinction of fear. *Arch Gen Psychiatry* 2004;61(11): 1136–1144.
179. Hofmann SG, Meuret AE, Smits JA, et al. Augmentation of exposure therapy with D-cycloserine for social anxiety disorder. *Arch Gen Psychiatry* 2006;63(3):298–304.
180. Kushner MG, Kim SW, Donahue C, et al. D-cycloserine augmented exposure therapy for obsessive-compulsive disorder. *Biol Psychiatry* 2007;62(8):835–838.
181. Guastella AJ, Dadds MR; Lovibond PF, et al. A randomized controlled trial of the effect of D-cycloserine on exposure therapy for spider fear. *J Psychiatr Res* 2007;41(6):466–471.
182. Drummond DC, Tiffany ST, Glautier S, et al. Addictive behavior: cue exposure theory and practice. In: Williams JMG, eds. *The Wiley Series in clinical psychology*. Chichester: John Wiley & Sons Ltd., 1995.
183. Drobes DJ, Saladin ME, Tiffany ST. Classical conditioning mechanisms in alcohol dependence. In: Heather N, Peters TJ, Stockwell T, eds. *International handbook of alcohol dependence and problems*. Chichester: John Wiley & Sons, Ltd., 2001:281–297.
184. Childress AR, Ehrman RN, McLellan AT, et al. Conditioned craving and arousal in cocaine addiction: a preliminary report. *NIDA Res Monogr* 1988;81:74–80.
185. O'Brien CP, Childress AR, Ehrman R, et al. Conditioning factors in drug abuse: can they explain compulsion? *J Psychopharmacol* 1998;12(1): 15–22.
186. Sinha R, Fuse T, Aubin LR, et al. Psychological stress, drug-related cues and cocaine craving. *Psychopharmacology (Berl)* 2000;152(2):140–148.
187. Wise RA. The neurobiology of craving: implications for the understanding and treatment of addiction. *J Abnorm Psychol* 1988;97:118–132.
188. Conklin CA, Tiffany ST. Applying extinction research and theory to cue-exposure addiction treatments. *Addiction* 2002;97:155–167.
189. Ouimette P, Brown PJ, eds. *Trauma and substance abuse: causes, consequences, and treatment of comorbid disorders*. Washington, DC: American Psychological Association, 2003.
190. Riggs DS, Rukstalis M, Volpicelli JR, et al. Demographic and social adjustment characteristics of patients with comorbid posttraumatic stress disorder and alcohol dependence: potential pitfalls to PTSD treatment. *Addict Behav* 2003;28(9):1717–1730.

CHAPTER 91

Lisa J. Merlo, PhD
Amanda M. Stone, BS
Mark S. Gold, MD

Co-occurring Addiction and Eating Disorders

This chapter describes issues related to the comorbidity of addiction disorders and disturbances in eating. Anorexia nervosa, bulimia nervosa, binge eating disorder, and obesity are serious clinical conditions with significant medical and emotional consequences. In addition, subclinical presentations of these disorders are common. There are many similarities between obesity, eating disorders, and traditional addiction disorders (i.e., addiction to alcohol and/or drugs), and these disorders are frequently comorbid. Eating disorders can trigger addiction disorder relapses or binges and vice versa. Addiction clinicians must prevent hyperphagia, overeating, and obesity as part of the comprehensive treatment of addictive diseases. Addiction disorders and diseases of eating complicate the assessment, diagnosis, treatment, and long-term recovery processes for both disorders.

DEFINITIONS

Addiction has been summarized as the three Cs: *c*ompulsive use, loss of *c*ontrol, and repetition despite adverse *c*onsequences. Many eating disorders can be similarly described (1), and for this reason have sometimes been included as "behavioral addictions." Clinical and research evidence have demonstrated that pathological attachment to highly hedonic food is similar to a substance use disorder in virtually all spheres (2–4). Whereas addictions can be understood as an individual's biologic sensitivity and pathologic attachment to drugs or alcohol, eating disorders can be described as an unhealthy relationship with food. The eating disorders comprise a category of psychologic illnesses characterized by disturbed eating patterns and dysfunctional attitudes related to food, feeding, and body shape. Currently, the Diagnostic and Statistical Manual of Mental Disorders (DSM-IV) (5) lists three separate eating disorders with specific criteria to differentiate them: anorexia nervosa (AN), bulimia nervosa (BN), and eating disorder not otherwise specified (EDNOS). Symptoms of both AN and BN are rooted in disturbed body image and concerns related to consequences of gaining weight. EDNOS describes either a subclinical presentation of one of the other two disorders or binge eating disorder (BED), which will be described later. More recently, Volkow and O'Brien (6) have proposed adding "obesity" to the Substance Use Disorders section for DSM-V.

AN may be the most widely recognized eating disorder, though it is not well understood by the general public. DSM-IV criteria for the disorder are reviewed in Table 91.1 (5). As described, individuals with AN are characterized by extremely low body weight for their age and height, making their disorder difficult to conceal. Yet, like addiction patients, they are often adamant in their denial of the disorder (7) and may go to great lengths in an attempt to mask their impairment. For example, individuals with AN may attempt to surreptitiously increase their weight for weigh-ins using weights, heavy clothing, or water-loading (8) or hide their symptoms (e.g., by avoiding eating around other people, wearing baggy clothing to hide their emaciated frame, creating/eating elaborate meals when there are witnesses). Just as an individual with alcohol abuse/dependence may boast about high tolerance, individuals with AN rarely have insight into their problem and frequently note significant weight loss as an achievement, despite the medical concerns associated with their condition. Other symptoms include amenorrhea (or delay of menarche) in females, severe disturbance in body image, and a fear of gaining weight. Associated physical symptoms (which may initially provide the

TABLE 91.1 DSM-IV Criteria for Anorexia Nervosa

Individuals display each of the following symptoms:
A. Failure to maintain at least 85% of expected body weight based on gender, age, and height
B. Significant fear of weight gain or being fat, despite underweight status
C. Distorted perceptions of body shape and/or weight, overemphasis of body shape or weight on self-concept, or failure to admit the severity of current underweight status
D. Amenorrhea (i.e., absence of menstruation for at least three cycles in a row) or delayed menarche

Subtypes
A. Restricting type: characterized by restriction of food intake without accompanying binge eating or purging behaviors
B. Binge-eating/purging type: characterized by regular binge eating and/or purging behaviors within the context of a current anorectic episode

Adapted from the *Diagnostic and Statistical Manual of Mental Disorders*, 4th ed. [Text revision]. Washington DC: American Psychiatric Association, 2000:589.

impetus for seeking treatment) include constipation, cold intolerance, lethargy, and in some cases lanugo (fine body hair that develops along the midsection and appendages). AN can result in significant medical complications, including hypothalamic-pituitary-adrenal axis dysfunction, pubertal delay or interruption, growth retardation, bone mass reduction, and osteopenia. Other possible symptoms include bradycardia, hypotension, cardiac arrhythmias, mitral valve prolapse, metabolic alkalosis or acidosis, hypokalemia, hypoglycemia, leucopenia, anemia, carontenemia, acrocyanosis, thrombocytopenia, peripheral neuropathy, hypothermia, dehydration, hair loss, and dry skin (9–11). Similar to addiction populations, the mortality rate for individuals with AN is extremely high. In one longitudinal study, 7% of individuals with AN had died after 8 years (12). Rates of completed suicide in this population range from 0.9% to 6.3% (13).

DSM-IV criteria for BN are outlined in Table 91.2 (5). BN differs from AN in that markedly low body weight is not a required symptom, but presence of binge-eating and compensation for that bingeing are necessary for the diagnosis. Compensatory actions involve purging by self-induced vomiting in approximately 90% of BN cases but can also include misuse of laxatives, diuretics and/or enemas, excessive exercise, or periods of fasting. Because of frequency of vomiting, it is common for dental enamel to show significant erosion (14). Other significant medical complications associated with BN include fluid and electrolyte abnormalities (e.g., hypokalemia, metabolic alkalosis or acidosis), cardiac arrhythmias, parotid enlargement, submandibular adenopathy, menstrual irregularity, constipation, and reproductive problems (11,15).

BED is currently listed in the DSM-IV under the category of Eating Disorder, Not Otherwise Specified. It is being considered for possible inclusion as a separate disorder in the DSM-V. Suggested research criteria are included in Appendix B of the DSM-IV and are outlined in Table 91.3 (5). The

TABLE 91.2 DSM-IV Criteria for Bulimia Nervosa

Individuals display each of the following symptoms:
A. Regular binge eating episodes characterized by:
   (1) eating an abnormally large amount of food within a short time period (e.g., within 2 hours) and
   (2) experiencing a subjective lack of control over one's ability to stop or limit eating during the binge episode.
B. Participation in compensatory behaviors to prevent weight gain (e.g., vomiting; use of laxatives, diuretics, enemas; excessive exercising; fasting)
C. On average, symptoms are present at least two times per week for 3 months.
D. Body shape/weight have excessive impact on one's overall self-evaluation.
E. Symptoms are not present exclusively during an episode of anorexia nervosa.

Subtypes
A. Purging type: characterized by regular purging behaviors (e.g., vomiting or misusing laxatives, diuretics, enemas)
B. Nonpurging type: characterized by participation in only non-purging compensatory behaviors (e.g., fasting or excessive exercise)

Adapted from the *Diagnostic and Statistical Manual of Mental Disorders*, 4th ed. [Text revision]. Washington DC: American Psychiatric Association, 2000:594.

extant literature related to BED is growing rapidly. Though it is similar to BN in that regular binge eating occurs, the key distinction is that individuals with BED do not engage in compensatory behavior for their overeating. Binge eating episodes share many characteristics in common with binge drinking episodes, such as eating rapidly, eating more than intended (e.g., eating until uncomfortably full or bingeing when not hungry), eating alone (often owing to embarrassment or shame regarding the excessive food intake), and feeling disgusted, guilty, or depressed after binge eating. In fact, some have suggested that BED may reflect the consequences of "food addiction" (16,17). Some report feelings of dissociation during episodes of binge eating, and most with BED view their binge eating as unwanted and distressful. Approximately 20% of individuals with BED are overweight, and approximately 70% are obese (18). Additionally, 30% of individuals who are obese are diagnosed with BED (19). The most common medical complications associated with BED result from consequences of morbid obesity, including hypertension, type II diabetes, cardiovascular disease and stroke, osteoarthritis, increased risk for cancer, chronic muscular pain, joint pain, gastrointestinal problems including irritable bowel syndrome, and early menarche (20–22).

Though not currently included in the DSM-IV, obesity represents another serious condition related to a disturbance in eating. Generally, a diagnosis of obesity is made on the basis of an individual's body mass index (BMI) score. BMI is calculated by dividing weight in kilograms by height in meters squared. Standard cut-points are used to determine whether the individual falls within a healthy weight range (i.e., underweight = BMI less than 18.5; normal weight = BMI 18.5

TABLE 91.3 DSM-IV Suggested Research Criteria for Binge Eating Disorder

Individuals display each of the following symptoms:

A. Regular binge eating episodes characterized by:
   (1) eating an abnormally large amount of food within a short time period (e.g., within 2 hours) and
   (2) experiencing a subjective lack of control over one's ability to stop or limit eating during the binge episode.
B. Binge-eating episodes are associated with at least three of the following:
   (1) Abnormally rapid eating
   (2) Continued eating until one feels uncomfortably full
   (3) Eating large amounts of food despite lack of hunger
   (4) Concealing one's eating owing to embarrassment over eating habits
   (5) Experience of self-disgust, depression, or shame after binge episode
C. Individual experiences marked distress as a result of binge eating.
D. On average, binge episodes occur at least twice per week for 6 months or more.
E. Individual does not regularly utilize compensatory behaviors to prevent weight gain, and symptoms are not present exclusively during an episode of anorexia nervosa or bulimia nervosa.

Adapted from the *Diagnostic and Statistical Manual of Mental Disorders,* 4th ed. [Text revision]. Washington DC: American Psychiatric Association, 2000:787.

to <25; overweight = BMI ≥25 to 30, and obese = BMI ≥30). BMI of at least 35 is considered stage 2 obesity. As mentioned previously, obesity is associated with multiple serious health problems.

PREVALENCE

General Population Though eating disorders are most common in Western society, there is evidence of their existence across many cultures (23,24). In general, the prevalence of eating disorders is higher in urban environments (25). Though AN occurs relatively equally among areas of diverse urbanization levels, BN appears to be much more common in cities than in rural areas (26). In addition, upward mobility within the social system is associated with increased risk for eating disorders across various cultures (27–30). As with addiction disorders, heritability appears to be an important factor in the development of eating disorders, with genes accounting for 58% to 71% of the variance for AN (31) and 30% to 83% of the variance for BN (32,33). Unlike addiction disorders, it is commonly accepted that the prevalence of eating disorders is much higher in females, with the incidence of eating disorders in males being approximately one-tenth that of females. However, it is likely that eating disorders have been underdiagnosed among boys and men. Like addiction disorders, eating disorders are often described as diseases of pediatric origin. Symptom onset rarely occurs past the age of 40 years (5), and point prevalence rates are much higher during adolescence and early adulthood. For example, the prevalence of subclinical AN among girls ages 16 to 25 is estimated to be approximately 10% (34). Recent studies have determined the lifetime prevalence of AN in females to be between 0.9% and 1.9% and have found the lifetime prevalence of AN in males to be between 0.29% and 0.3% (35–37). With regard to BN, recent research has demonstrated the lifetime prevalence of BN to be much higher than that of AN, at 1.5% to 2.9% in females and approximately 0.5% in males (35,37). The onset of BN occurs most commonly between the ages of 14 and 22 (35). Finally, recent studies have suggested that BED is the most common eating disorder, with lifetime prevalence rates of 1.9% to 3.5% in females and 0.3% to 2.0% in males (35,37,38). The estimated 12-month and lifetime prevalence of BED greatly exceeds the prevalence of both AN and BN (39,40), reaching up to 1.2% for the previous 12-months, and the prevalence of subclinical binge-eating symptoms is even higher, with rates of 2.1% for the previous 12-months and 4.5% for lifetime occurrence (39). Among the American Latino population, up to 5.61% of individuals demonstrate some binge-eating behavior during their lifetime (41). Given that underreporting is typical in the measurement of disordered eating, the prevalence of BED may be as high as 6 per 100 people (42). BED onset typically occurs later than AN or BN and most frequently in the early to mid-20s, though many patients do not present for treatment until their 40s (43,44). With regard to obesity, the problem extends across all ages, and the number of obese individuals has more than tripled in the last 50 years (45). As of 2004, 31.1% of American adults age 20 or older are obese (i.e., BMI equal to or ≥30) and an additional 2.8% are extremely obese (i.e., BMI equal to or ≥40) (46). Among pediatric populations, the proportion of children ages 6 to 11 years meeting criteria for obesity has more than doubled since 1970 (47). And finally, even half of the poor nations studied in sub-Saharan Africa, Latin America, the Caribbean, East and South Asia, Central Asia, North Africa, and the Middle East currently have rates of overweight/obesity (i.e., BMI equal to or ≥25) that exceed rates of underweight (48).

Much as the prevalence of substance use exceeds the prevalence of substance abuse or dependence, more individuals display subclinical eating disturbances than a full diagnosable eating disorder. These symptoms might include disordered eating patterns and body image concerns. For example, a recent study of middle school and high school students demonstrated that 41.5% of females and 24.9% of males had body shape perception disturbance, 36.4% of females and 23.9% of males had undue influence of weight on self-esteem, and 9.4% of females and 13.5% of males were engaging in compensatory behavior (38). Among college students, 16.3% of females and 9.2 % of males in one study reported binge eating, 18.6% of females and 5.2% of males reported using laxatives, diet pills, or diuretics to promote weight loss, and 17.4% of females and 10.4% of males reported that eating and weight concerns significantly interfered with their academic performance (49). Results of another study suggested that 12% of male college students are dissatisfied with their body shape and 9% engage in disordered eating behaviors (50). Similarly, among pre- and early perimenopausal women without diagnosed eating disorders, approximately 29.2% report dissatisfaction with their eating patterns, 11% report regular binge eating, and 9.2% report a strong fear of gaining weight (51).

Addiction Treatment Populations It is particularly important for addiction clinicians to be familiar with the eating disorders and obesity, as these disorders display relatively high comorbidity with addiction disorders. Drug use, abuse, and dependence can have dramatic and consistent effects on eating. In addition, certain addiction disorders appear to co-occur with specific diseases of eating. Treating one may exacerbate the other, but ignoring one may cause a new life-threatening disease to emerge. Among individuals receiving treatment for an addiction disorder, approximately 0.02% to 3.4% also suffer from an eating disorder (52,53), and it has been estimated that 17% of women with eating disorders have a lifetime history of an addiction disorder (54).

Specifically, results of several studies demonstrate that binge eating is frequently associated with excessive alcohol consumption (55–57). Indeed, up to 57% of men and 28% of women with BED meet criteria for an addiction disorder (58). Thus, any binge eating disorder diagnosis should raise questions regarding alcohol and vice versa. Some research suggests that levels of bulimia are also significantly higher among women abusing alcohol than general population, with greater than two-thirds identifying themselves as "binge-eaters" with or without purging (59). There is anecdotal evidence suggesting that individuals with a history of overeating may develop alcohol or drug abuse after improving their eating habits (e.g., following bariatric surgery). In addition, animal research has demonstrated that abstaining from alcohol may promote bingeing on sugary foods, whereas restricting sugary food intake may promote excessive alcohol consumption (60), and human studies have demonstrated that weight gain frequently occurs after treatment and recovery from addiction disorders (61). However, in the absence of BED, obesity may actually serve a protective function against development of an addiction disorder. Research has demonstrated that, as BMI increases, the percentage of women who have consumed alcohol or smoked marijuana in the previous year decreases significantly (62,63).

Conversely, dieting and purging are frequently associated with the use of cocaine and other stimulants (56,57,64,65). Whereas individuals with food-restricting habits are less likely to abuse stimulants than individuals who binge or purge, they still display increased use of stimulants compared to the general population (56). In fact, results of one study demonstrated that 32% of individuals seeking treatment for cocaine abuse/dependence met criteria for either AN or BN (65). AN patients also frequently abuse prescription and over-the-counter medications and may use drugs to suppress their appetite in order to lose weight. For example, particularly among college students, psychostimulants are misused for weight management as well as cramming for exams and reversing the effects of cannabis smoking on new learning (66). Abuse of caffeine and laxatives are common in all forms of eating disorders (67). In addition, many chronic smokers cite fear of weight gain as a deterrent to their efforts at smoking cessation (68), and presence of an eating disorder may impede treatment efforts in this arena. However, female adolescents with restricting habits are actually less likely to use tobacco, alcohol, and marijuana than is the general population (67).

Psychiatric Treatment Populations Individuals with eating disorders frequently display other psychiatric disorders as well. For example, Blinder et al. (57) recently demonstrated that up to 97% of females treated for anorexia had experienced one or more comorbid psychiatric diagnoses in their lifetime. The rates of psychiatric comorbidity among individuals with AN and BN are not significantly different. The most common axis I psychiatric comorbidity among individuals with AN is a mood disorder, particularly depression, with approximately 94% of AN patients meeting criteria for a depressive disorder (57). Between 56% and 66% of those with an eating disorder experience one or more anxiety disorders (57,69). Obsessive-compulsive disorder is the most common comorbid anxiety disorder, with a prevalence rate between 29.5% and 41% among individuals with AN or BN (69–71). Social phobia is the next most common, with a 20% rate of comorbidity (69,72). Finally, axis II disorders are extremely common among individuals with eating disorders. Research has demonstrated that approximately 68% of patients meet diagnostic criteria for one or more personality disorders (71), though rates vary between 21% and 97% (73). Patients with AN most commonly display cluster C (anxious/avoidant) personality disorders, whereas, those with BN are more likely to display cluster B (dramatic/erratic) personality disorders (73). Finally, individuals with BED are three times more likely to suffer from major depressive disorder than are individuals from the general population (74), and axis II comorbidities are significantly associated with severity of binge eating (58). Obesity is also associated with increased psychiatric conditions, including major depressive disorder and generalized anxiety disorder (75).

Primary Care or Other Health Care Populations Within a family practice setting, the prevalence of AN is estimated to be between 4.2% and 6.3%, and the prevalence of BN is estimated to be between 6.3% and 12.2% (26,76,77). However, rates vary among members of different groups. For example, among female adolescents with type I diabetes, up to one-third of patients exhibit disordered eating behaviors or eating disorders (78). With regard to BED, the prevalence is approximately 5% to 30% among obese individuals (79,80). In fact, there is almost a fivefold increase in risk for BED among individuals whose BMI is at least 40 compared to those whose BMI is within the normal range, and the risk for displaying subclinical binge-eating behavior shows the same trend (81). Heredity may play a role in the development of BED, as 20.2% of individuals who are related to an overweight or obese person with BED also develop BED, compared to only 9.6%

of individuals who are related to an overweight or obese person without BED. Relatives of the BED group are also more likely to have higher current BMI and elevated rates of obesity (81). In addition, among female athletes, rates of subclinical eating disorders range from 15% to 32% (82), and these symptoms also commonly occur among male athletes. Participation in aesthetic sports (e.g., ballet, gymnastics, figure skating) or sports in which "making weight" is required (e.g., wrestling, horse racing) results in increased risk for disordered eating (83).

DIFFERENTIAL DIAGNOSIS

Unfortunately, with the exception of obesity, the detection of eating disorders can be difficult. In fact, research suggests that more than half of individuals with an eating disorder go undiagnosed (84). Even an obesity diagnosis must be made by the physician taking an accurate weight on a reliable scale and measuring the patient's height without shoes. In addition, just as addiction disorder patients are unlikely to self-refer for treatment, eating disorder patients often resist acknowledging their symptoms and impairment or accepting their diagnosis. They may deny or attempt to hide their eating disturbances, even when referred for treatment by a parent or friend. When self-referred, individuals with AN may neglect to mention their disordered eating, instead presenting with nonspecific symptoms such as fatigue/lack of energy or dizziness (85) or associated complaints such as intolerance to cold, throat or abdominal pain, digestive problems, heart palpitations, or changes in drinking or urination (86). In addition, several medical disorders share symptoms with eating disorders, complicating the diagnostic process. For example, hyperthyroidism, diabetes, tumors, gastrointestinal disorders (e.g., inflammatory bowel disease), nutrient malabsorption, immunodeficiency, chronic infections, and Addison's disease may all result in weight changes and associated symptoms (86).

Among addiction disorder patients, detection of eating disorders may be particularly difficult, as substance abuse can lead to symptoms similar to those seen in anorexia nervosa, bulimia nervosa, binge-eating disorder, and even obesity. For example, alcohol-related disorders can include vomiting (as seen in AN and BN) and lethargy (as seen in AN, BN, BED, and obesity). Use of amphetamines, methamphetamine, cocaine, MDMA, and opiates can result in decreased eating and significant weight loss (as in AN), whereas marijuana use may result in binge eating (as in BN, BED, and obesity). In particular, MDMA has attracted some college student users in doses that are markedly lower than doses used as part of the club or party scene (87). As a result, eating disorder symptoms may be written off as secondary to the addiction disorder if a careful assessment is not performed. Regardless of whether an eating disorder is initially suspected, addiction clinicians should specifically inquire about eating disturbances as well as weight-related drug misuse or abuse (e.g., use of "diet pills," laxatives, stimulants). Individuals with eating disorders are unlikely to offer this information spontaneously, but presence of a comorbid eating disorder may affect decisions regarding clinical care.

Ideally, all substance-misusing, -abusing, and -dependent patients should be evaluated for comorbid psychiatric disorders and diseases of eating. All patients would benefit from an analysis of diet, exercise, eating behaviors, and BMI. In particular, patients undergoing treatment for alcohol abuse/dependence should always be evaluated for binge-eating symptoms; those in treatment for stimulant abuse/dependence should always be assessed for purging behaviors and excessive dieting; and patients abusing caffeine or laxatives should always undergo a general eating disorder screening. The addiction clinician should also routinely include an assessment of current and past eating habits when recording a medical history, in order to obtain a comprehensive understanding of the patient and be alert to signs of an underlying or comorbid eating disorder. In addition, as treatment for the addiction disorder progresses, the patient's weight and BMI should be monitored to track significant gain or loss. Many instruments are available to assist with eating disorder screening and assessment. Addiction clinicians may find it helpful to use these questionnaires in their initial evaluation and intermittently throughout treatment. Some example questionnaires are listed below.

Eating Disorders Inventory—Second Edition The Eating Disorders Inventory—Second Edition (EDI-2) (88) has excellent psychometric properties and is the most widely used self-report measure of disordered eating and related symptoms of AN and BN. The 91 items are scored using a forced choice format. The EDI-2 contains eight subscales (e.g., Drive for Thinness, Body Dissatisfaction, Ineffectiveness, Perfectionism, Interpersonal Distrust, Maturity Fears, Bulimia, and Interoceptive Awareness), as well as three provisional subscales (e.g., Asceticism, Impulse Regulation, and Social Insecurity). It is appropriate for individuals 12 and older and can be completed in about 20 minutes.

Eating Disorder Diagnostic Scale The Eating Disorder Diagnostic Scale (EDDS) (89) is a 19-item self-report questionnaire that assesses eating disorder symptoms over the previous 3 months. Most items are scored using a 7-point Likert-type scale. Items assessing overeating and loss of control are structured with an initial yes/no question with follow-up frequency assessment when appropriate. The authors have developed algorithms to determine whether diagnostic criteria are met for AN, BN, and/or BED. The EDDS has demonstrated excellent psychometric properties.

Eating Disorder Examination Questionnaire The Eating Disorder Examination Questionnaire (EDE-Q) (90) is a self-report measure that was based on the EDE interview. It assesses disordered eating behaviors and attitudes over the previous 4 weeks. Like the interview version, the EDE-Q attempts to discriminate between objective and subjective bulimic episodes. The EDE-Q contains 36 items which are scored using a 7-point forced choice scale. It has demonstrated good psychometric properties.

Bulimia Test—Revised The Bulimia Test—Revised (BULIT–R) (91) is a 36-item self-report measure of BN symptoms (e.g., binge eating, compensatory behaviors, and body shape disturbance). Items are scored using a 5-point Likert-type scale. Reliability and validity have been well established, and the BULIT-R has been used with both clinical and nonclinical populations (92). The BULIT-R is recommended for individuals 16 and older.

Binge Eating Scale The Binge Eating Scale (BES) (93) is a 16-item measure used to assess binge-eating symptoms. Eight items measure behavioral symptoms, and eight items measure feelings and cognitions related to binge-eating symptoms. For each item, respondents choose from four statements to determine which statement describes them best. The BES has strong psychometric properties and published cutoffs to determine whether an individual displays clinically significant binge-eating symptoms.

Night Eating Symptom Scale The Night Eating Symptom Scale (NESS) (94) is a self-report instrument that contains 12 items assessing symptoms of night eating syndrome (e.g., percentage of food consumed after supper, frequency of nighttime snacking). Items are rated on a 5-point scale. The NESS has demonstrated treatment sensitivity, but its psychometric properties have not been reported.

Eating Behaviors Questionnaire The Eating Behaviors Questionnaire (EBQ) (95) is a 20-item self-report measure that was developed to assess for symptoms of food addiction. Items were based on modified DSM-IV criteria for substance use disorders and include assessment of tolerance and cravings, as well as distress and impairment related to excessive food consumption. For each item, respondents use a 6-point scale ranging from "never" to "always" to describe their experience of each symptom. Psychometric properties have not yet been studied.

If a patient obtains a positive score on an eating disorder screening questionnaire, the addiction clinician should evaluate further to determine whether immediate eating disorder intervention is necessary. For example, it is important to note that there can be symptom overlap between eating disorders and addiction disorders (weight loss, lethargy, changes in eating habits, etc.), and these symptoms do not necessarily signify a comorbid eating disorder unless the associated symptoms (e.g., body image disturbance, fear of gaining weight, lack of control over eating) are also present.

MANAGEMENT

Like addiction treatment, the treatment of eating disorders can be a long and arduous process marked by alternating periods of relapse and recovery. For serious cases, and particularly for adolescent patients, treatment may commence on a coerced or even involuntary basis through enrollment in an inpatient or residential program. However, as with addiction treatment, the patient is more likely to be successful in treatment if she or he agrees to treatment and is motivated to change his or her behavior. As a result, motivational interviewing interventions may be useful in helping the patient to recognize the need for treatment and to increase his or her willingness to enter and participate in a treatment program (96).

Management of an eating disorder typically involves a multidisciplinary team and includes psychosocial, behavioral, and pharmacologic interventions. Psychotherapy often includes both individual sessions and family sessions. Depending on the severity of symptoms and presence of comorbid addiction or psychiatric disorders, treatment may be administered in outpatient, partial hospitalization, inpatient, or residential settings. Generally, patients who are considered medically or psychiatrically unstable are referred for inpatient care (97). Individuals with comorbid addiction disorders may also be referred for more intensive treatment owing to the increased psychologic strain associated with attempting to simultaneously abstain from two maladaptive coping mechanisms (i.e., substance use and disordered eating) and the increased medical risks associated with these conditions. No matter the treatment milieu or modality, development of a treatment contract specifying goals and expectations related to each disorder may be beneficial.

Biologic Management Whether the patient has a comorbid addiction disorder or not, the medical management of AN begins with a comprehensive medical and neurologic evaluation and treatment of medical comorbidities. While the establishment of weight gain is a goal, it is important to be certain that an electrolyte, cardiac, or other disease does not kill the patient or compromise the patient's ability to be treated or recover. However, in cases of comorbid AN and addiction disorders, once medical issues are resolved, it is generally recommended that addiction treatment take priority unless the patient is at immediate medical risk owing to malnutrition. Once the patient achieves stable sobriety, the treatment for AN may begin. Individuals with AN are generally terrified of gaining weight (much as the addict may be terrified of living without his drug of choice), so weight gain should be implemented gradually (e.g., 0.5 to 1.0 pound per week). The American Dietetic Association recommends nutrition intervention and nutritional counseling by a registered dietician as an integral part of treatment for AN (98). Thus, every addiction counselor should establish contact with a credible a referral source to assist with this component of treatment. Referral to a mental health professional who specializes in eating disorders may also be beneficial for many patients. Among adolescents, weight gain may best be achieved using a family intervention referred to as the *Maudsley method*. This method involves encouraging parents to take an active role in promoting their child's weight regain (99). However neither this method nor other forms of family therapy are generally efficacious for adult patients with AN (100,101). Refeeding treatment for adult patients and some adolescents generally consists of utilizing behavioral reinforcers to reward eating. It has been suggested that parenteral nutrition and nasogastric feeding be avoided, if possible, owing to concerns that the patient may relapse or develop other symptoms (e.g., purging) to compensate for her or his weight gain (102). However, there is some evidence that nocturnal nasogastric feeding may increase weight gain (103). The process of weight regain is often very stressful for patients with anorexia, and the addiction clinician may wish to monitor the patient more closely during this time to assess for signs of addiction relapse.

Thus far, no pharmacologic treatments have proven effective in treatment of the primary symptoms of AN (100,104). However, selective serotonin reuptake inhibitors (SSRIs) may help to decrease associated symptoms such as depression, obsessive-compulsive symptoms, and lack of interoceptive awareness (105,106). Like parenteral feeding, it is recommended that medications to promote weight gain be used judiciously in order to avoid overwhelming the patient. However, use of calcium supplements and a multivitamin are recommended (107). Oral contraceptives or hormone replacement therapy may be prescribed to help regulate the menstrual cycle, mitigate effects of hypoestrogenemia, and minimize bone loss (108,109). Some patients with a comorbid addiction disorder may prefer to avoid prescription medications in order to maintain their focus on sobriety from all mood altering drugs.

As in AN, patients with BN who have a comorbid addiction disorder should be treated first for their addiction. Once in stable sobriety, biologic management of BN generally involves medication with an SSRI. Specifically, fluoxetine has demonstrated efficacy in reducing the core symptoms of BN acutely, and has been shown to lower treatment dropout rates (110,111). The suggested dosage is approximately 60 mg/day. Other medications with demonstrated efficacy include desipramine, up to 300 mg/day (112,113); imipramine, up to 300 mg/day (114,115); and topiramate, titrated from 25 mg/day up to 250 mg/day or 400 mg/day (116,117). With any medication, it is recommended that pharmacotherapy be combined with cognitive-behavioral therapy, as described later (118–121). Individuals with a comorbid addiction disorder who prefer not to take prescription medication should be referred directly for cognitive-behavioral therapy for BN. Among those who are willing to take medications, pharmacotherapy for comorbid psychiatric conditions should also be considered. In addition, given the detrimental effects of digestive juices on tooth enamel and oral health, a dental exam is recommended for those with purging-type BN (119). Similarly, management of other medical complications associated with BN may be necessary. For example, estrogen replacement may be indicated to combat hypothalamic hypogonadism (34). Physicians should monitor patients with BN to assess for fluid and electrolyte abnormalities, cardiac arrhythmias, gastrointestinal symptoms, and reproductive problems. BN patients with comorbid addiction disorders are more likely to have medical complications; a general medical check-up may be indicated for these patients.

Though there is currently no treatment for binge-eating disorder approved by the FDA, experimental treatments of binge eating with various pharmacologic agents have provided positive results. After the BED patient with comorbid addiction achieves sobriety, there are several options for medication management to assist with BED symptoms. For example, several SSRIs (e.g., sertraline, 50 to 200 mg/day; fluvoxamine, 50 to 300 mg/day; fluoxetine, 20 to 80 mg/day; and citalopram, 20 to 60 mg/day) have demonstrated efficacy (122–125). In addition, as with binge drinking, topiramate (50 to 600 mg/day) has shown utility in decreasing the number of binge-eating episodes per week, decreasing BMI, and shortening the time to recovery (126). Sibutramine (15 mg/day) and orlistat (120 mg tid) may also assist patients in their recoveries (127–129). As with AN and BN, pharmacologic treatment of comorbid psychiatric conditions may be warranted if allowable within the patient's sobriety goal. Finally, given that overweight and obesity may be consequences of BED, additional medical management may be necessary to prevent or treat associated conditions (e.g., hypertension, type II diabetes, hypercholesteremia, hyperlipidemia).

Biologic management of obesity is generally considered a three-tiered approach that begins with changes in diet and increased exercise. If additional assistance is needed, medications can be added. For example, sibutramine (which was initially developed as an antidepressant) has demonstrated efficacy in decreasing food consumption and increasing metabolic rate (130). Similarly, Meridia has shown efficacy as an appetite suppressant (131). Another medication, orlistat, has a mechanism similar to that of Antabuse, wherein individuals taking orlistat experience severe gastrointestinal symptoms after eating a high fat meal (130,132). Finally, if treatment using a combination of diet, exercise, and medication does not result in sufficient change, surgical methods may be employed (131). For example Roux-en-Y gastric bypass surgery (133) or lap-band surgery may be considered. Research has demonstrated that these surgeries result in sustained weight loss with decreased prevalence of health conditions (e.g., type II diabetes) related to obesity (134–136). Unfortunately, though these surgeries can be lifesaving for many patients, they are associated with risk of rehospitalization (e.g., owing to ventral hernia repair and gastric revision) (137) and early mortality, particularly in elderly patients (138). In addition, bariatric surgery should not be considered without a full psychiatric evaluation, including an addiction disorder assessment, as psychiatric and substance use comorbidities are common among bariatric surgery candidates (139) and can affect the success of surgery. Clinical evidence suggests that individuals who undergo bariatric surgery may be at increased risk of developing addictions post surgery, and patients with a history of addiction disorders may be particularly at risk.

Psychologic Management As in treatment for addiction disorders, for all eating disorder patients, behavioral intervention strategies can be extremely useful. Many of the same issues arise during therapy for addiction disorders and eating disorders. Thus, participation in addiction treatment may provide a strong foundation from which to work toward management of disordered eating symptoms as well. For example, learning better ways to communicate with family and handle conflict may reduce the need for maladaptive coping through both substance use and disordered eating. Practicing these strategies during addiction treatment may give the patient confidence to implement similar strategies in order to manage the eating disorder symptoms. For example, establishing a daily routine, self-monitoring using a food journal, developing structured meal times, ensuring the availability of nutritional and "safe" foods, and limiting exposure to triggers for bingeing or purging can be effective ways to promote recovery from an eating disorder.

Specifically for AN patients, both family therapy and individual therapy have demonstrated efficacy, though family therapy may be particularly beneficial for younger patients (140,141). Cognitive-behavioral therapy (CBT) has consistently been shown to reduce the risk for relapse and improve outcome (100,142,143) for AN patients. Again, many of the skills developed during CBT for an addiction disorder can be easily transferred to eating disorder treatment (e.g., challenging dysfunctional cognitions, behavioral experiments). As stated previously, management of BN is generally enhanced by combining pharmacotherapy with CBT. CBT is currently recommended as the first-line treatment for BN, given its demonstrated efficacy in multiple trials (144–146). As with AN, treatment for BN should commence once sobriety is attained. CBT can be administered either individually or in a group setting and is generally included as part of both residential and outpatient treatment programs. Among BED patients without comorbid addiction disorders, psychotherapy appears to be most successful when administered as either individual or group CBT (101), though interpersonal psychotherapy has also demonstrated efficacy (147,148). With regard to obesity symptoms, behavioral weight loss strategies have demonstrated positive outcomes in the short term, particularly with regard to weight loss (149); however, CBT appears to be a superior treatment for the symptoms of BED over time (150). Again, when the eating disorder patient has a comorbid addiction disorder, it is important to continue monitoring the patient closely in order to be vigilant for signs of relapse. Therapy should focus on developing new adaptive coping skills to replace the addiction and eating disorder symptoms.

Social Management Eating disorders occur frequently within close-knit groups (e.g., "cliques" of friends, sports teams, sororities), particularly among adolescent females and young adults (151,152). Socially valued behaviors (e.g., food restriction) appear to increase with social proximity, whereas nonvalued behaviors (e.g., binge eating, purging) appear to decrease (153). However, levels of binge eating appear to grow more similar among females as their friendship grows closer (154). As a result, large-scale prevention and intervention programs are important and can be effective in managing the incidence and prevalence of AN, BN, and BED (155,156).

Similarly, social support can be beneficial to individuals as they undergo treatment and recovery. As in addiction treatment, group therapy may be an appropriate and useful component of a comprehensive program. Patients can learn that they are not alone in their struggles with disordered eating, share their challenges and successes, and learn from one another's experiences. However, for individuals admitted to treatment involuntarily (and particularly those with AN), group therapy may be contraindicated. In some cases, this may lead to competition among the patients to be the "thinnest" in the group or sharing of maladaptive strategies to continue losing weight.

Among motivated individuals, and particularly those who have participated successfully in Alcoholics Anonymous (AA) or Narcotics Anonymous (NA), referral to a 12-step program for eating disorders may be beneficial as well. Eating Disorders Anonymous (EDA) follows many of the tenets of AA (e.g., 12 steps and 12 traditions), but—given that food is necessary for survival—it focuses on "balance" rather than "abstinence" as the goal. Eating disorder symptoms (e.g., restricting, bingeing, purging) are viewed as ways of coping with stress, so the program focuses more on developing alternate adaptive coping strategies rather than focusing on eating habits per se. EDA participants are encouraged to work with a sponsor or "buddy" on their path to recovery. Similarly, Overeaters Anonymous (OA) is a 12-step fellowship program following in the tradition of AA. OA meetings focus primarily on the needs of individuals with compulsive eating or binge eating symptoms. It may be particularly useful for individuals who appear to suffer from a food addiction. OA participants view overeating as similar to an alcohol or drug addiction and work toward the goal of abstaining from overeating. Like EDA and other 12-step groups, OA stresses the importance of anonymity within the group, as well as fellowship and spirituality on the road to recovery.

Recovery Issues

Comorbid Addiction Disorders Comorbid addiction disorders may negatively affect treatment prognosis. In fact, eating disorder symptoms may serve as a coping mechanism for some patients with addiction disorders. Thus, as described previously, it is typically recommended that individuals be treated first for their addiction disorder. In addition, when substance abuse is comorbid with AN, it is generally suggested that treatment occur in a residential treatment facility where both issues can be addressed (157). Recovery rates for AN with comorbid substance abuse, especially alcohol abuse, are generally poor; indeed, suffering from these conditions in combination is a strong predictor of fatal outcome (23,158). On the other hand, studies have shown that those receiving treatment for bulimia nervosa as well as an addiction disorder have treatment outcomes similar to those without a history of substance abuse (159,160). Similarly, individuals who suffer from BED with a comorbid addiction disorder show outcomes similar to those without an addiction disorder (58).

General Recovery Rates More generally, research has demonstrated recovery rates for eating disorders to be between approximately 40% and 94%, with recovery rates and outcome for BN being more encouraging than those for AN (161–163). BN generally is not fatal, whereas the mortality rate for those with anorexia nervosa is about 10% (5). In terms of general treatment prognosis, about half of individuals with

AN have good outcomes, approximately 30% display intermediate outcomes, and one in five individuals with AN has a poor outcome. With regard to BN, about 45% of patients display a good outcome, 18% have an intermediate outcome, and 21% have a poor outcome (72). Among BED patients, there is some evidence that the disorder will spontaneously remit over time (164), though other research has suggested a more chronic nature, particularly among patients who are older, more obese, and who meet full diagnostic criteria (165). As is seen among individuals recovering from addiction disorders, the vacillation between dieting (i.e., "abstinence") and overeating (i.e., "active use") is common among individuals struggling with obesity or BED (166).

Disordered Eating after Addiction Treatment After treatment for an addiction disorder, some individuals who are abstaining from drug or alcohol use may compensate for this lack of chemical reinforcement by overeating. Preliminary research has demonstrated significant weight gain among a group of adolescents who completed treatment and maintained abstinence from substances of abuse (61). More research is currently underway to examine this phenomenon among adult patients. In addition, one study has documented the significant rates of past addiction disorders among extremely obese individuals considering bariatric surgery. Kalarchian et al. (167) reported that one-third of these individuals were in recovery from an addiction disorder, whereas fewer than 2% had a current diagnosis. Though information was not available regarding their weight at the time of active substance abuse, clinical experience suggests that it is likely that many of these individuals became obese after treatment for their addiction disorders. In addition, presence of an eating disorder is associated with increased risk for a relapse to substance use. Individuals who are attempting to manage their disordered eating symptoms may turn to drugs or alcohol as an alternate coping strategy. As a result, the addiction clinician should be vigilant to symptoms of overeating or disordered eating among substance use disorder patients and should provide all patients with preventative counseling and referral to a registered dietitian.

Areas for Further Study As mentioned earlier, further research is needed to explore and evaluate the concept of obesity as the consequence of a food addiction. Though various authors have written on this topic (2–4,168), larger controlled and prospective studies are needed to determine the indicators of food addiction and its similarities and dissimilarities with other addictions. In addition, as suggested by Volkow and O'Brien (6), obesity should be considered for inclusion in the DSM-V as an additional mental disorder.

Finally, as research data accumulate demonstrating the similarities among the various eating disorders and addiction disorders, the addiction clinician will likely need to gain further experience with the identification and treatment of these serious diseases. Future work might focus on the development of additional brief screening devices (e.g., a "CAGE"-type questionnaire for eating disorders), as well as alternate treatment strategies built on the principles developed within the field of addiction medicine. For example, eating disorder treatments may capitalize on methods such as contingency management, pharmacotherapies, and long-term residential care for eating disorders and obesity (such as that offered through the Duke Diet & Fitness Center). Addiction clinicians and eating disorder specialists would likely benefit from opportunities to network and share methods and ideas in order to maximize care for these commonly comorbid disorders.

SUMMARY

Eating disorders (e.g., anorexia nervosa, bulimia nervosa, and binge eating disorder) are serious conditions that necessitate timely detection and intervention. These disorders have both psychologic and medical consequences that can be life-threatening. Comorbidity with addiction disorders is common, and it is recommended that all individuals undergoing treatment for an addiction disorder be screened for disordered eating behaviors. When present, serious disordered eating symptoms may complicate treatment for addiction disorders. Individuals should be medically stabilized before beginning addiction treatment. However, once stable, treatment should focus on recovery from the addiction disorder before treatment for the eating disorder commences. Eating disorders and addiction disorders share many similarities with regard to underlying psychopathology and lack of adaptive coping skills. Treatments for both disorders are frequently complementary. Skills learned in the management of an addiction disorder can often be applied to the management of eating disorders, and vice versa.

REFERENCES

1. Volkow ND, Wise RA. How can drug addiction help us understand obesity? *Nat Neurosci* 2005;8:555–560.
2. Wang G, Volkow ND, Thanos PK, et al. Similarity between obesity and drug addiction as assessed by neurofunctional imaging: a concept review. *J Addict Dis* 2004;23:39–53.
3. Gold MS, Frost-Pineda K, Jacobs WS. Overeating, binge eating, and eating disorders as addictions. *Psychiatr Ann* 2003;33:117–122.
4. Stennie KA, Gold MS. Eating disorders and addictions: behavioral and neurobiological similarities. In: Miller NS, ed. *The principles and practice of addictions in psychiatry*. Philidelphia: WB Saunders and Co., 1997.
5. American Psychiatric Association. *Diagnostic and statistical manual of mental disorders*, 4th ed. [Text revision]. Washington, DC, American Psychiatric Association, 2000.
6. Volkow ND, O'Brien CP. Issues for DSM-V: should obesity be included as a brain disorder? *Am J Psychiatry* 2007;164:708–710.
7. Couturier J, Lock J. Denial and minimization in adolescents with anorexia nervosa. *Int J Eat Disord* 2006;39:212–216.
8. Kreipe RE, Birndorf SA. Eating disorders in adolescents and young adults. *Med Clin North Am* 2000;84:1027–1049.
9. Katzman DK. Medical complications in adolescents with anorexia nervosa: a review of the literature. *Int J Eat Disord* 2005;37(Suppl): S52–S59; discussion S87–S89.
10. Miller KK, Grinspoon SK, Ciampa J, et al. Medical findings in outpatients with anorexia nervosa. *Arch Intern Med* 2005;165:561–566.
11. Cartwright MM. Eating disorder emergencies: understanding the medical complexities of the hospitalized eating disordered patient. *Crit Care Nurs Clin North Am* 2004;16:515–530.

12. Eddy KT, Keek PK, Dorer DJ, et al. Longitudinal comparison of anorexia nervosa subtypes. *Int J Eat Disord* 2002;31:191–201.
13. Franko DL, Keel PK. Suicidality in eating disorders: Occurrence, correlates, and clinical implications. *Clin Psychol Rev* 2006;26:769–782.
14. Rytomaa I, Jarvinen V, Kanerva R, et al. Bulimia and tooth erosion. *Acta Odontol Scand* 1998;56:36–40.
15. Mehler PS, Crews C, Weiner K. Bulimia: medical complications. *J Womens Health* 2004;13:668–675.
16. Avena NM, Rada P, Hoebel BG. Evidence for sugar addiction: behavioral and neurochemical effects of intermittent, excessive sugar intake. *Neurosci Biobehav Rev* 2008;32:20–39.
17. Rada P, Avena NM, Hoebel BG. Daily binging on sugar repeatedly releases dopamine in the accumbens shell. *Neuroscience* 2005;134: 737–744.
18. Gruzca RA, Przybeck TR, Cloninger CR. Prevalence and correlates of binge eating disorder in a community sample. *Compr Psychiatry* 2007; 48:124–131.
19. Pagoto S, Bodenlos JS, Kantor L, et al. Association of major depression and binge eating disorder with weight loss in a clinical setting. *Obesity* 2007;15:2557–2559.
20. Bulik CM, Reichborn-Kjennerud T. Medical morbidity in binge eating disorder. *Int J Eat Disord* 2003;34:S39–S46.
21. Raman RP. Obesity and health risks. *J Am Coll Nutr* 2002;21: S134–S139.
22. Pi-Sunyer FX. The medical risks of obesity. *Obes Surg* 2002;12:S6–S11.
23. Keel PK, Klump KL. Are eating disorders culture-bound syndromes? Implications for conceptualizing their etiology. *Psychol Bull* 2003;129: 747–769.
24. Anderson-Fye EP, Becker AE. Cultural aspects of eating disorders across cultures. In: *The handbook of eating disorders and obesity.* London: Wiley, 2003.
25. Hoek HW, Bartelds AI, Bosveld JJ, et al. Impact of urbanization on detection rates of eating disorders. *Am J Psychiatry* 1995;152: 1272–1278.
26. Hoek HW. The incidence and prevalence of anorexia nervosa and bulimia nervosa in primary care. *Psychol Med* 1991;21:455–460.
27. Silber TJ. Anorexia nervosa in blacks and Hispanics. *Int J Eat Disord* 1986;5:121–128.
28. Yates A. Current perspectives on the eating disorders: I. History, psychological and biological aspects. *J Am Acad Child Adolesc Psychiatry* 1989;28:813–828.
29. Soomro GM, Crisp AH, Lynch D, et al. Anorexia nervosa in 'non-white' populations. *Br J Psychiatry* 1995;167:385–389.
30. Becker AE, Burwell R, Gilman S, et al. Disordered eating behaviors and attitudes follow prolonged exposure to television among ethnic Fijian adolescent girls. *Br J Psychiatry* 2002;180:509–514.
31. Klump KL, Miller KB, Keel PK, et al. Genetic and environmental influence on anorexia nervosa syndromes in a population-based twin sample. *Psychol Med* 2001;31:737–740.
32. Kendler KS, Walters EE, Neale MC, et al. The structure of the genetic and environmental risk factors for six major psychiatric disorders in women: phobia, generalized anxiety disorder, panic disorder, bulimia, major depression, and alcoholism. *Arch Gen Psychiatry* 1995;52: 374–383.
33. Bulik CM, Sullivan PF, Kendler KS. Heritability of binge-eating and broadly defined bulimia nervosa. *Biol Psychiatry* 1998;44:1210–1218.
34. Walsh JM, Wheat ME, Freund K. Detection, evaluation, and treatment of eating disorders: the role of the primary care physician. *J Gen Intern Med* 2000;15:577–590.
35. Hudson JI, Hiripi E, Pope HGJ, et al. The prevalence and correlates of eating disorders in the National Comorbidity Survey Replication. *Biol Psychiatry* 2007;61:348–358.
36. Bulik CM, Sullivan PF, Tozzi F, et al. Prevalence, heritability, and prospective risk factors for anorexia nervosa. *Arch Gen Psychiatry* 2006; 63:305–312.
37. Wade TD, Bergin JL, Tiggemann M, et al. Prevalence and long-term course of lifetime eating disorders in an adult Australian twin cohort. *Aust N Z J Psychiatry* 2006;40:121–128.
38. Ackard DM, Fulkerson JA, Neumark-Sztanier D. Prevalence and utility of DSM-IV eating disorder diagnostic criteria among youth. *Int J Eat Disord* 200740:409–417.
39. Hudson J, Hiripi E, Pope HG, Kessler RC. The prevalence and correlates of eating disorders in the National Comorbidity Survey Replication. *Biol Psychiatry* 2007;61:348–358.
40. Hoek H, van Hoeken, D. Review of the prevalence and incidence of eating disorders *Int J Eat Disord.* 2003;34:383–396.
41. Alegria M, Woo M, Cao Z, et al. Prevalence and correlates of eating disorders in Latinos in the United States. *Int J Eat Disord* 2007;40:515–521.
42. Grucza R, Przybeck TR, Cloninger CR. Prevalence and correlates of binge eating disorder in a community sample. *Compr Psychiatry* 2007; 48:124–131.
43. Mussel MP, Mitchell JE, Weller CL, et al. Onset of binge eating, dieting, obesity, and mood disorders among subjects seeking treatment for binge eating disorder. *Int J Eat Disord* 1995;17:395–401.
44. Spurrell EB, Wilfley DE, Tanofsky MB, et al. Age of onset for binge eating: are there different pathways to binge eating? *Int J Eat Disord* 1997; 21:55–65.
45. Parikh N, Pencina MJ, Wang TJ, et al. Increasing trends in incidence of overweight and obesity over 5 decades. *Am J Med* 2007;120:242–250.
46. Ogden C, Carroll MD, Curtin LR, et al. Prevalence of overweight and obesity in the United States, 1999-2004. *JAMA* 2006;295:1549–1555.
47. National Center for Chronic Disease Prevention and Promotion. Defining overweight and obesity, 2004. www.cdc.gov/nccdphp/dpna/obesity/trend/index.htm, accessed December 4, 2008.
48. Mendez M, Monteiro CA, Popkin BM. Overweight exceeds underweight among women in most developing countries. *Am J Clin Nutr* 2005;81:714–721.
49. Hoerr SL, Bokram R, Lugo B, et al. Risk for disordered eating relates to both gender and ethnicity for college students. *J Am Coll Nutr* 2002; 21:307–314.
50. O'Dea JA, Abraham S. Eating and exercise disorders in young college men. *J Am Coll Health* 2002;50:273–278.
51. Marcus MD, Bromberger JT, Wei HL, et al. Prevalence and selected correlates of eating disorder symptoms among a multiethnic community sample of midlife women. *Ann Behav Med* 2007;33:269–277.
52. Hasin D, Sarnet S, Nunes E, et al. Diagnosis of comorbid psychiatric disorders in substance users assessed with the psychiatric research interview for substance and mental disorders for DSM-IV. *Am J Psychiatry* 2006;163:689–696.
53. Castel S, Rush B, Urbanoski K, et al. Overlap of clusters of psychiatric symptoms among clients of a comprehensive addiction treatment service. *Psychol Addict Behav* 2006;20:28–35.
54. Herzog DB, Franko DL, Dorer DJ, et al. Drug abuse in women with eating disorders. *Int J Eat Disord* 2006;39:364–368.
55. Piran N, Robinson SR. Associations between disordered eating behaviors and licit and illicit substance use and abuse in a university sample. *Addict Behav* 2006;31:1761–1775.
56. Conason AH, Sher L. Alcohol use in adolescents with eating disorders. *Int J of Adolesc Med Health* 2006;18:31–36.
57. Blinder BJ, Cumella EJ, Sanathara VA. Psychiatric comorbidities of female inpatients with eating disorders. *Psychosom Med* 2006;68: 454–462.
58. Wilfley DE, Friedman MA, Dounchis JZ, et al. Comorbid psychopathology in binge eating disorder: relation to eating disorder severity at baseline and following treatment. *J Consul Clin Psychol* 2000;68:641–649.
59. Stewart S, Brown, CG, Devoulyte, K., et al. Why do women with alcohol problems binge eat? Exploring connections between binge eating and heavy drinking in women receiving treatment for alcohol problems. *J Health Psychol* 2006;11:409–425.
60. Avena NM, Carrillo CA, Needham L, et al. Sugar-dependent rats show enhanced intake of unsweetened ethanol. *Alcohol* 2004;34:203–209.
61. Hodgkins CC, Jacobs WS, Gold MS. Weight gain after adolescent drug addiction treatment and supervised abstinence. *Psychiatr Ann* 2003;33: 112–116.
62. Kleiner KD, Gold MS, Frost-Pineda K, et al. Body mass index and alcohol use. *J Addict Dis* 2004;23:105–118.

63. Warren M, Frost-Pineda K, Gold MS. Body mass index and marijuana use. *J Addict Dis* 2005;24:95–100.
64. Piran N, Robinson S. The association between disordered eating and substance use and abuse in women: a community-based investigation. *Women Health* 2006;44:1–20.
65. Jonas JM, Gold MS, Sweeney D, et al. Eating disorders and cocaine abuse: a survey of 259 cocaine abusers. *J Clin Psychiatry* 1987;48: 47–50.
66. Teter CJ, McCabe SE, LaGrange K, et al. Illicit use of specific prescription stimulants among college students: prevalence, motives, and routes of administration. *Pharmacotherapy* 2006;26:1501–1510.
67. Stock SL, Goldberg E, Corbett S, et al. Substance use in female adolescents with eating disorders. *J Adolesc Health* 2002;31:176–182.
68. Pomerleau CS, Zucker AN, Stewart AJ. Characterizing concerns about postcessation weight gain: results from a national survey of women smokers. *Nicotine Tob Res* 2001;3:51–60.
69. Kaye WH, Bulik CM, Thornton L, et al. Comorbidity of anxiety disorders with anorexia nervosa and bulimia nervosa. *Am J Psychiatry* 2004;161:2215–2221.
70. Milos G, Spindler A, Ruggiero G, et al. Comorbidity of obsessive-compulsive disorders and duration of eating disorders. *Int J Eat Disord* 2002;31:284–289.
71. Milos G, Spindler A, Schnyder U. Psychiatric comorbidity and Eating Disorder Inventory (EDI) profiles in eating disorder patients. *Can J Psychiatry* 2004;49:179–184.
72. Herzog DB, Nussbaum KM, Marmor AK. Comorbidity and outcome in eating disorders. *Psychiatr Clin North Am* 1996;19:843–859.
73. Westen D, Harnden-Fischer J. Personality profiles in eating disorders: rethinking the distinction between axis I and axis II. *Am J Psychiatry* 2001;158:547–562.
74. Telch CF, Stice E. Psychiatric comorbidity in women with binge eating disorder prevalence rates from a non-treatment seeking sample. *J Consult Clin Psychol* 1998;66:768–776.
75. Kasen S, Cohen P, Chen H, et al. Obesity and psychopathology in women: a three decade prospective study. *Int J Obesity (Lond)* 2007;32:558–566.
76. Currin L, Schmidt U, Treasure J, et al. Time trends in eating disorder incidence. *Br J Psychiatry* 2005;186:132–135.
77. Turnbull S, Ward A, Treasure J, et al. The demand for eating disorder care: an epidemiological study using the general practice research database. *Br J Psychiatry* 1996;169:705–712.
78. Rodin G, Craven J, Littlefield C, et al. Eating disorders and intentional insulin undertreatment in adolescent females with diabetes. *Psychosomatics* 1991;32:171–176.
79. Bruce B, Agras WS. Binge eating in females: a population-based investigation. *Int J Eat Disord* 1992;12:365–373.
80. Bruce B, Wilfley DE. Binge eating among the overweight population: a serious and prevalent problem. *J Am Diet Assoc* 1996;96:58–61.
81. Hudson J, Lalonde, JK, Berry, JM, et al. Binge-eating disorder as a distinct familial phenotype in obese individuals. *Arch Gen Psychol* 2006;63: 313–319.
82. Beals KA, Manore MM. Disorders of the female athlete triad among collegiate athletes. *Int J Sport Nutr Exerc Metab* 2002;12:281–293.
83. Reinking MF, Alexander LE. Prevalence of disordered-eating behaviors in undergraduate female collegiate athletes and nonathletes. *J Athlet Train* 2005;40:47–51.
84. Becker AE, Grinspoon SK, Klibanski A, et al. Eating disorders. *N Engl J Med* 1999;340:1092–1098.
85. Mehler PS. Diagnosis and care of patients with anorexia nervosa in primary care settings. *Ann Intern Med* 2001;134:1048–1059.
86. Pritts SD, Susman J. Diagnosis of eating disorders in primary care. *Am Fam Phys* 2003;67:297–304.
87. Strote J, Lee JE, Wechsler H. Increasing MDMA use among college students: results of a national survey. *J Adolesc Health* 2002;30:64–72.
88. Garner DM. *Eating disorder inventory-2 professional manual.* Odessa, FL. Psychological Assessment Resources, 1990.
89. Stice E, Telch CF, Rizvi SL. Development and validation of the Eating Disorder Diagnostic Scale: a brief self-report measure of anorexia, bulimia, and binge eating disorder. *Psychol Assess* 2000;12:123–131.
90. Fairburn CG, Beglin SJ. Assessment of eating disorders: interview or self-report questionnaire? *Int J Eat Disord* 1994;16:363–370.
91. Thelen MH, Farmer J, Wonderlich S, et al. A revision of the Bulimia Test: the BULIT_R. *Psychol Assess* 1991;3:119–124.
92. Williamson DA, Anderson DA, Jackman LP, et al. Assessment of eating disordered thoughts, feelings, and behaviors. In: Allison DB, ed. *Handbook of assessment methods for eating behaviors and weight-related problems.* Thousand Oaks, CA: Sage, 1995.
93. Gormally J, Black S, Daston S, et al. The assessment of binge eating severity among obese persons. *Addict Behav* 1982;7:47–55.
94. O'Reardon JP, Stunkard AJ, Allison KC, Clinical trial of sertraline in the treatment of night eating syndrome. *Int J Eat Disord* 2004;35:16–26.
95. Merlo LJ. *The Eating Behaviors Questionnaire to assess for food addiction.* University of Florida: Gainesville, FL, 2008.
96. Dunn EC, Neighbors C, Larimer ME. Motivational enhancement therapy and self-help treatment for binge eaters. *Psychol Addict Behav* 2006; 20:44–52.
97. American Psychiatric Association. Practice guidelines for the treatment of patients with eating disorders revisions *Am J Psychiatry* 2000;157:1–39.
98. American Dietetic Association. Position of the American Dietetic Association: nutrition intervention in the treatment of anorexia nervosa, bulimia nervosa, and other eating disorders *J Am Diet Assoc* 2006;106: 2073–2082.
99. LeGrange D. The Maudsley family-based treatment for adolescent anorexia nervosa. *World Psychiatry* 2005;4:142–146.
100. Bulik CM, Berkman ND, Brownley KA, et al. Anorexia nervosa treatment: a systematic review of randomized controlled trials. *Int J Eat Disord* 2007;40:310–320.
101. Wilson GT. Psychological treatment of eating disorders. *Annu Rev Clin Psychol* 2005;1:439–465.
102. Tiller J, Schmidt U, Treasure J. Compulsory treatment for anorexia nervosa: compassion or coercion? *Br J Psychiatry* 1993;162:649–680.
103. Robb AS, Silber TJ, Orrell-Valente JK, et al. Supplemental nocturnal nasogastric refeeding for better short-term outcome in hospitalized adolescent girls with anorexia nervosa. *Am J Psychiatry* 2002;159: 1347–1353.
104. Becker AE. Outpatient management of eating disorders in adults. *Curr Womens Health Rep* 2003;3:221–229.
105. Santonastaso P, Friederici S, Favaro A. Sertraline in the treatment of restricting anorexia nervosa: an open controlled trial. *J Child Adolesc Psychopharmacol* 2001;11:143–150.
106. Fassino S, Leombruni P, Daga G, et al. Efficacy of citalopram in anorexia nervosa: a pilot study. *Eur Neuropsychopharmacol* 2002;12:453–459.
107. Berger MM, Shenkin A. Vitamins and trace elements: practical aspects of supplementation. *Nutrition* 2006;22:952–955.
108. Cumming DC. Exercise-associated amenorrhea, low bone density and estrogen replacement therapy. *Arch Intern Med* 1996;156:2193–2195.
109. Klibanski A, Biller BMK, Schoenfield DA, et al. The effects of estrogen administration on trabecular bone loss in young women with anorexia nervosa. *J Clin Endocrinol Metab* 1995;80:898–904.
110. Berkman ND, Bulik CM, Brownley KA, et al. Management of eating disorders. *Evid Rep Technol Assess* 2006;135:1–166.
111. Goldstein DJ, Wilson MG, Thompson VL, et al. Long term fluoxetine treatment of bulimia nervosa. *Br J Psychiatry* 1995;166:660–666.
112. Walsh BT, Wilson GT, Loeb KL, et al. Medication and psychotherapy in the treatment of bulimia nervosa. *Am J Psychiatry* 1997;154:523–531.
113. Walsh BT, Hadigan CM, Devlin MJ, et al. Long-term outcome of antidepressant treatment for bulimia nervosa. *Am J Psychiatry* 1991;148: 1206–1212.
114. Agras WS, Rossiter EM, Arnow B, et al. Pharmacologic and cognitive behavioral treatment for bulimia nervosa: a controlled comparison. *Am J Psychiatry* 1992;149:82–87.
115. Mitchell JE, Pyle R, Eckert ED, et al. A comparison study of antidepressants and structured group psychotherapy in the treatment of bulimia nervosa. *Arch Gen Psychiatry* 1990;47:149–157.
116. Nickel C, Tritt K, Muehlbacher M, et al. Topiramate treatment in bulimia nervosa patients: a randomized, double-blind, placebo-controlled trial. *Int J Eat Disord* 2005;38:295–300.

117. Hoopes SP, Reimherr FW, Hedges DW, et al. Treatment of bulimia nervosa with topiramate in a randomized, double-blind, placebo-controlled trial. Part 1: improvement in binge and purge measures. *J Clin Psychiatry* 2003;64:1335–1341.
118. Hay PJ, Backaltchuk J. Extracts from "clinical evidence": bulimia nervosa. *BMJ* 2001;323:33–37.
119. Hay PJ. Understanding bulimia. *Aust Fam Physician* 2007;36:708–712.
120. Ramoz N, Versini A, Gorwood P. Eating disorders: an overview of treatment responses and the potential impact of vulnerability genes and endophenotypes. *Expert Opin Pharmacother* 2007;8:2049–2044.
121. Whittal ML, Agras WS, Gould RA. Bulimia nervosa: A meta-analysis of psychosocial and pharmacological treatments. *Behav Ther* 1999; 30:117–135.
122. McElroy SL, Hudson JI, Malhotra S, et al. Citalopram in the treatment of binge-eating disorder: a placebo-controlled trial. *J Clin Psychiatry* 2003;64:807–813.
123. Hudson JI, McElroy SL, Raymond NC, et al. Fluvoxamine in the treatment of binge-eating disorder: a multicenter placebo-controlled, double-blind trial. *Am J Psychiatry* 1998;155:1756–1762.
124. Arnold LM, McElroy SL, Hudson JI, et al. A placebo-controlled, randomized trial of fluoxetine in the treatment of binge-eating disorder. *J Clin Psychiatry* 2002;63:1028–1033.
125. McElroy SL, Casuto LS, Nelson EB, et al. Placebo-controlled trial of sertraline in the treatment of binge eating disorder. *Am J Psychiatry* 2000;157:1004–1006.
126. McElroy SL, Hudson JI, Capece KB, et al. Topiramate for the treatment of binge-eating disorder associated with obesity: a placebo-controlled study. *Biol Psychiatry* 2007;61:1039–1048.
127. Wilfley DE, Crow SJ, Hudson JI, et al. Efficacy of sibutramine for the treatment of binge eating disorder: a randomized multicenter placebo-controlled double-blind study. *Am J Psychiatry* 2008;165:51–58.
128. Appolinario JC, Backaltchuk J, Sichieri R, et al. A randomized, double-blind, placebo-controlled study of sibutramine in the treatment of binge-eating disorder. *Arch Gen Psychiatry* 2003;60:1109–1116.
129. Golay A, Laurent-Jaccard A, Habict F, et al. Effect of orlistat in obese patients with binge eating disorder. *Obes Res* 2005;13:1701–1708.
130. Finer N. Present and future pharmacological approaches. *Br Med Bull* 1997;53:409–432.
131. Salazar S. Assessment and management of the obese adult female: a clinical update for providers. *J Midwifery Womens Health* 2006;51:202–207.
132. Bray GA. Drug treatment of obesity. *Bailliers Best Pract Res Clin Endocrinol Metab* 1999;13:131–148.
133. Virji A, Murr MM. Caring for patients after bariatric surgery. *Am Fam Phys* 2006;73:1403–1408.
134. Dixon JB, O'Brien PE, Playfair J, et al. Adjustable gastric banding and conventional therapy for type 2 diabetes: a randomized controlled trial. *JAMA* 2008;299:316–323.
135. Sjostrom L, Lindroos AK, Peltonen M, et al. Lifestyle, diabetes, and cardiovascular risk factors 10 years after bariatric surgery. *N Engl J Med* 2004;351:2683–2693.
136. Pories WJ, MacDonald KGJ, Morgan EJ, et al. Surgical treatment of obesity and its effect on diabetes: 10-year follow-up. *Am J Clin Nutr* 1992;55:582S–585S.
137. Zingmond DS, McGory ML, Ko CY. Hospitalization before and after gastric bypass surgery. *JAMA* 2005;294:1918–1924.
138. Flum DR, Salem L, Elrod JB, et al. Early mortality among Medicare beneficiaries undergoing bariatric surgical procedures. *JAMA* 2005;15: 1903–1908.
139. Rosenberger PH, Henderson KE, Grilo CM. Psychiatric disorder comorbidity and association with eating disorders in bariatric surgery patients: a cross-sectional study using structured interview-based diagnosis. *J Clin Psychiatry* 2006;67:1080–1085.
140. Robin AR, Siegal PT, Koepke T, et al. Family therapy versus individual therapy for adolescent females with anorexia nervosa. *J Dev Behav Pediatr* 1994;15:111–116.
141. Eisler I, Dare C, Russell GF, et al. Family and individual therapy in anorexia nervosa: a 5-year follow-up. *Arch Gen Psychiatry* 1997;54:1025–1030.
142. McIntosh VV, Jordan J, Carter FA, et al. Three psychotherapies for anorexia nervosa: a randomized, controlled trial. *Am J Psychiatry* 2005;162:741–747.
143. Pike KM, Walsh BT, Vitousek K, et al. Cognitive behavior therapy in the posthospitalization treatment of anorexia nervosa. *Am J Psychiatry* 2003;160:2046–2049.
144. Fairburn CG, Jones R, Peveler RC, et al. Psychotherapy and bulimia nervosa: the longer-term effects of interpersonal psychotherapy, behavior therapy, and cognitive behavior therapy. *Arch Gen Psychiatry* 1993;50:419–428.
145. Goldbloom DS, Olmstead M, Davis R, et al. A randomized controlled trial of fluoxetine and cognitive behavioral therapy for bulimia nervosa: short term outcome. *Behav Res Ther* 1997;35:803–811.
146. Lewandowski LM, Gebing TA, Anthony JL, et al. Meta-analysis of cognitive behavioral treatment studies for bulimia. *Clin Psychol Rev* 1997;17:703–718.
147. Wilfley DE, Agras WS, Telch CF, et al. Group cognitive behavioral therapy and group interpersonal psychotherapy for the nonpurging bulimic individual: a controlled comparison. *J Consul Clin Psychol* 1993;61:296–305.
148. Wilfley DE, Welch RR, Stein RI, et al. A randomized comparison of group cognitive behavioral therapy and group interpersonal psychotherapy for the treatment of overweight individuals with binge eating disorder. *Arch Gen Psychiatry* 2002;59:713–721.
149. Nauta H, Hospers H, Kok G, et al. A comparison between a cognitive and a behavioral treatment for obese binge eaters and obese non-binge eaters *Behav Ther* 2000;31:441–461.
150. Nauta H, Hospers H, Jansen A. One-year follow-up effects of two obesity treatments on psychological well-being and weight. *Br J Health Psychol* 2001;6:271–284.
151. Paxton SJ, Schutz HK, Wertheim EH, et al. Friendship clique and peer influences on body image concerns, dietary restraint, extreme weight-loss behaviors, and binge eating in adolescent girls. *J Abnorm Psychol* 1999;108:255–266.
152. Sundgot-Borgen J. Eating disorders among male and female elite athletes. *B J Sports Med* 1999;33:434.
153. Meyer C, Waller G. Social convergence of disturbed eating attitudes in young adult women. *J Nerv Ment Dis* 2001;189:114–119.
154. Crandall CS. Social contagion of binge eating. *J Pers Soc Psychol* 1988;55:588–598.
155. Becker CB, Smith LM, Ciao AC. Peer-facilitated eating disorder prevention: a randomized effectiveness trial of cognitive dissonance and media advocacy. *J Counsel Psycholo* 2006;53:550–555.
156. Becker CB, Smith LM, Ciao AC. Reducing eating disorder risk factors in sorority members: a randomized trial. *Behav Ther* 2005;36:245–253.
157. Woodside BD, Staab R. Management of psychiatric comorbidity in anorexia nervosa and bulimia nervosa. *CNS Drugs* 2006;20:655–663.
158. Herzog DB, Greenwood DN, Dorer DJ, et al. Mortality in eating disorders: a descriptive study. *Int J Eat Disord* 2000;28:20–26.
159. Mitchell JE, Pyle R, Eckert ED, et al. The influence of prior alcohol and drug abuse problems on bulimia nervosa treatment outcome. *Addict Behav* 1990;15:169–173.
160. Franko DL, Dorer DJ, Keel PK, et al. How do eating disorders and alcohol use disorder influence each other? *Int J Eat Disord* 2005;38:200–207.
161. Couturier J, Lock J. What is recovery in adolescent anorexia nervosa? *Int J Eat Disord* 2006;39:550–555.
162. Katz JL. Eating disorders: a primer for the substance abuse specialist. *J Subst Abuse Treat* 1990;7:143–149.
163. Fichter MM, Quadflieg N. Twelve-year course and outcome of bulimia nervosa. *Psychol Med* 2004;34:1395–1406.
164. Fairburn CG, Brownell K, Cooper Z, et al. The natural course of bulimia nervosa and binge eating disorder in young women. *Arch Gen Psychiatry* 2000;57:659–665.
165. Pope HGJ, Lalonde JK, Pindyck LJ, et al. Binge eating disorder: a stable syndrome. *Am J Psychiatry* 2006;163:2181–2183.
166. Jeffery RW, Drewnowski A, Epstein LH, et al. Long-term maintenance of weight loss: current status. *Health Psychol* 2000;19:5–16.
167. Kalarchian MA, Marcus MD, Levine MD, et al. Psychiatric disorders among bariatric surgery candidates: relationship to obesity and functional health status. *Am J Psychiatry* 2007;164:328–334.
168. Avena NM, Rada P, Hoebel BG. Evidence for sugar addiction: behavioral and neurochemical effects of intermittent, excessive sugar intake. *Neurosci Biobehav Rev* 2008;32:20–39.

SECTION 12

Pain and Addiction

CHAPTER 92

Peggy Compton, RN, PhD, FAAN
Rollin M. Gallagher, MD, MPH
Issam A. Mardini, MD, PhD

The Neurophysiology of Pain and Interfaces With Addiction

INTRODUCTION

The pathophysiology of chronic pain is complex and plastic and brings with it consequences in many life domains. Not unlike addiction, the pathophysiology of chronic pain that is not related to malignancy, which we will term *maldynia* (pathophysiologic pain), in distinction from eudynia (normal pain), does not alone account for the variable expression and psychosocial complexity of this very human condition. Of interest, both scientifically and clinically, is the profound overlap between those neural and opioid systems that regulate pain and those responsible for addiction responses. These observations suggest that the shared physiologic responses in the experience and continuation of both are worthy of examination with the expectation that the clinical coexistence of maldynia and addiction would lead to complex responses: that is, addictive responses altered by the physiologic presence of maldynia and maldynia responses altered by the physiological presence of addiction.

This chapter provides a review of the pathophysiology of maldynia and of the theoretical and clinical evidence for overlap with addiction responses. The mechanisms of pain perception and modulation in maldynia are reviewed, with discussion of those aspects likely to be impacted upon by the presence of addictive disease. In this regard, the role of central sensitization and affective responses (depression, anxiety) to maldynia are discussed, particularly since these co-morbidities also play a role in the phenomenology and treatment of addiction. Finally, ideas about potential sources of interaction between maldynia and addiction are suggested, focusing on how the general state of addiction, inherited characteristics of the individual, and neuroadaptations specific to opioid abuse might affect the co-expression of these phenomena.

CHRONIC PAIN

In contrast to our presently well-established ability to prevent, minimize, and manage acute pain, the management of maldynia often presents a daunting challenge in clinical practice. First, the physiology of pain after initial onset becomes much more complex almost immediately—the longer the pain, the more complex the process. Chronic nociceptive pain, such as from arthritis, involves persistent or episodic *transduction, transmission, modulation* and *perception*, whereas chronic neuropathic pain, from damage to neural tissue such as in neuropathy, is often independent of *transduction, and* involves persistent *transmission, modulation,* and *perception*. These processes will be discussed in more detail.

Although experiments using laboratory-induced nociception in animals can control for much genetic and experiential variability, this is not possible in humans suffering chronic or episodic pain. Every new episode or change in pain intensity, character, or localization activates cognitive processes and emotions that are influenced by current context and meaning that are conditioned by past pain experience. These processes involve interacting neural networks subserved by myriad chemical messengers that communicate among sensory systems and various cognitive-emotional processing and behavioral systems. Because of the uniqueness of each individual's neural system and personal pain experience and the uniqueness of the context of each pain experience, theoretically at least, virtually no two pain experiences are ever the same. Therefore, pain is always an intensely personal experience and clinically always a unique experience. Clinicians caring for patients with maldynia face the challenge of formulating for each patient, to the degree possible in a particular clinical setting, the interaction of biopsychosocial factors and neural processes that activate and perpetuate chronic pain. Then they must devise a feasible treatment plan that has the best chance of remediating the most salient factors to improve outcome (1,2).

Pain Anatomy and Physiology Wall and Melzak's (3) postulation of the gate theory of pain provided the first pathophysiologic model to coherently explain the phenomenology of pain perception and modulation that clinicians observed at the bedside and in clinic.

One author's first memorable clinical experience of the "gating system" occurred when delivering babies for women trained in Lamaze techniques in 1971 to 1973 while in a rural family practice. Women trained with Lamaze breathing and delivering in a secure familiar environment (personalized, informed, longitudinal prenatal care by their doctor in a small hospital in their own community and with a participating family member) would manage childbirth in almost all cases without systemic analgesia and, in many cases, at their preference, without regional blocks, despite the considerable tissue injury and volleys of nociception inherent to the process. Whereas earlier in training, mothers in a culturally foreign and threatening medical setting with no prenatal care (e.g., an urban city hospital) experienced severe pain, high anxiety, and almost always required systemic opioid analgesics and neural blockade.

Like any cogent theory explaining observable phenomena of great clinical salience, the gate theory initiated an explosion of pain science, inspiring a generation of clinical and basic scientists that have dramatically expanded our knowledge about the nature of pain physiology, pathology and experience. A review of the number of pain-relevant articles retrieved in Pub Med using key word indicators, the general term "pain" and the more physiologically specific term "nociception" document the remarkable expansion of available information since the gate theory was published: articles from 1970 to 1979: "pain" 30,138; "nociception" 45; articles from 1980 to 1989: "pain" 60,421, "nociception" 532; articles from 1990 to 1999: "pain" 105,828, "nociception" 1,391; and articles from 2000 to 2007: "pain" 146,654, "nociception" 2,417. This rise constitutes about a 4.9-fold increase for "pain" and a 54-fold increase for the more technical pain term, *nociception*. This new pain science radically changed our understanding of the pathophysiology of different maldynias and has generated a plethora of new treatments targeted at different molecular mechanisms.

Naturally, this new knowledge has led to the common clinical practice of combining treatments, each purportedly targeting different mechanisms in the pathophysiologic matrix of maldynia (1,2,4). Collectively, this additive, integrated approach improves over-all pain control and outcomes in meta-analytic studies (5–8). Although clinical trials comparing a proven single treatment (superior to placebo) to a treatment combining two or more proven treatments are prohibitively expensive, multi-modality treatment to improve functional outcomes, not just pain control, is now standard of care in pain medicine specialty practice. Ultimately, larger clinical databases utilizing standard outcome measures will enable investigators with the analytic power to establish which treatment combinations work best in specific pain conditions (9–11). The establishment of this rapidly growing scientific base, as well as recognition of the prevalence and health care and social costs of maldynia and its inadequate treatment, has created the need for a new specialty, pain medicine, to shepherd this research, to establish and maintain standards of care and specialty training, and to train medical students and non-physician pain specialists (12).

The neurobiological basis of Wall and Melzack's functional gating system, now better understood, provides a conceptual framework for understanding the clinical presentation of pain and helps explain the often complementary effects of these different treatments for pain. Three major "stages" of pain have been proposed involving different neurophysiologic mechanisms depending on the nature and time course of the originating stimulus (3). The three stages are (1) consequences of a brief noxious stimulus, (2) consequences of a prolonged noxious stimulus leading to tissue damage and peripheral inflammation, and (3) the consequences of neurologic damage, including peripheral neuropathies, central pain states, and peripheral and central sensitization. These stages are not mutually exclusive. Their end result is chronic pain perpetuated by one or more of several mechanisms: chronic inflammation; ectopic excitability of pain neurons; structural reorganization of sensory organs in the periphery and central nervous system (CNS) so that touch, movement and temperature changes cause the sensation of pain (discussed in Table 92.1); and loss of descending inhibitory controls. At any given time, one or a combination of these pathophysiologic mechanisms may be contributing to the experience of maldynia.

In stage 1, a sufficiently strong noxious stimuli activates nociceptors leading to depolarization of pain afferents (A delta and C fibers), which transmit the pain message from the peripheral tissue centrally to the dorsal horn of the spinal cord. If the signal is strong enough (many nociceptive neurons firing) and/or repetitive enough, second-order neurons depolarize, sending the message rostrally in the spinal cord to the lateral and medial thalamus. There, lateral projections to the somatosensory cortex convey localization and intensity information, resulting in the conscious perception of pain. Projections from the medial thalamus to the limbic system, specifically the anterior cingulate cortex and insular cortex, activate suffering and the emotional aspect of pain, as in Figure 92.1. Once this entire system is activated, repetitive nociceptor stimulation in the periphery can trigger a hyper-response of the second order neuron, increasing pain despite absence of increased nociceptor input.

The situation changes in stage 2 pain when a noxious stimulus is very intense or prolonged leading to tissue damage and inflammation. Most nociceptors are inactive and unresponsive under normal circumstances; however, cell damage and death from injury or disease and accompanying inflammation can cause an "awakening" of nociceptors, which may spontaneously discharge and become more sensitive to peripheral stimulation (13,14). This state is termed *peripheral sensitization.*

TABLE 92.1 Simple Bedside Examination Findings and their Meaning

Type of allodynia or hyperalgesia	Typical patient complaints	Assessment	Likely mechanism
A. Mechanical allodynia			
Mechanical static	Cannot bear weight of clothing against skin, wear shoes, or carry items	Light manual pressure on skin	Peripheral sensitization (sunburn)
Mechanical dynamic	Brushing of shirt against skin or covers over feet are painful. Avoids being touched.	Stroke skin with very soft brush or cotton	Central sensitization C-fiber input C-fiber loss (*CRPS 1 or 2)
B. Thermal allodynia			
Thermal warm	Pain worsens in sun, cannot cover feet at night	Touch skin with objects at 40°C; pain relieved by contact with cold	Peripheral sensitization (sunburn)
Thermal cold	Using metal knife/ fork is painful; pain is increased in cold room or near freezers in market	Touch skin with objects at 20°C	Central sensitization Central inhibition (CRPS 1 or 2)
C. Hyperalgesia			
Mechanical pinprick	Walking barefoot on beach feels like walking on broken glass	Manual pinprick of skin with pin; von Frey filament	Central sensitization Aδ-fiber input
Thermal cold	Ophthalmic PHN**: cannot tolerate below freezing temperatures	Touch skin with coolants (acetone)	Not known
Thermal heat	Handling hot plates is intolerable	Touch skin with hot object	Peripheral sensitization

*Complex regional pain syndrome: type 1 (reflux sympathetic dystrophy); type 2 (causalgia).

**Post-herpetic neuralgia

The sensitization of nociceptors depends on activation of second-messenger systems by the action of inflammatory mediators released in the damaged tissue, such as bradykinin, prostaglandins, serotonin, and histamine (15). In addition, nociceptor activity is also affected by chemical actions on surface membrane receptors of their axons. Several types of pharmacologic receptors, including opioid, GABA, bradykinin, histamine, serotonin, and, more recently, capsaicin (16), have been identified on the surface membrane of sensory axons.

The consequence of peripheral sensitization is an increase in the depolarization of primary afferent pain fibers after noxious stimulation, leading to an increase in the pain signal to the spinal cord and brain, causing more pain than normal from that stimulus; this is termed *hyperalgesia*. Also in this circumstance, pain can result from what is normally innocuous stimulation, such as light touch that activates sensitized A beta fibers; this is termed *allodynia*. A sunburn provides a good clinical example of a temporary state of peripheral sensitization, whereas arthritis would be a prolonged, chronic state as in Table 92.1.

Along with nociceptor sensitization, changes take place in the central pathways. The central pathways for processing nociceptive information begin at the level of the spinal cord (and medullary) dorsal horn. The interneuronal networks in the dorsal horn transmit nociceptive information not only to neurons that project to the brain but to spinal motor neurons, which leads to enhanced reflex actions in response to a noxious stimulus, including muscle spasm. Other inputs result in inhibition of projection neurons. The balance of these excitatory and inhibitory processes provides an explanatory basis for gate theory of pain transmission (17).

Damage to nerves, such as from disease, amputations, surgery, irradiation, and chemotherapy, can result in spontaneous firing of pain fibers, activated by peripheral stimuli and by sympathetically mediated stress. Continual firing can lead to changes in the spinal cord including alterations of modulatory systems, central sensitization, and neuroplasticity whereby dendritic formation in polymodal afferent fibers promotes pain sensation, causing allodynia. These processes are illustrated in Figure 92.2 (18,19).

In *central sensitization*, persistent noxious input to the CNS sets off a process of enhancement of responsiveness in the dorsal horn neurons that continues independent of primary afferent drive. Central sensitization is thought to be responsible

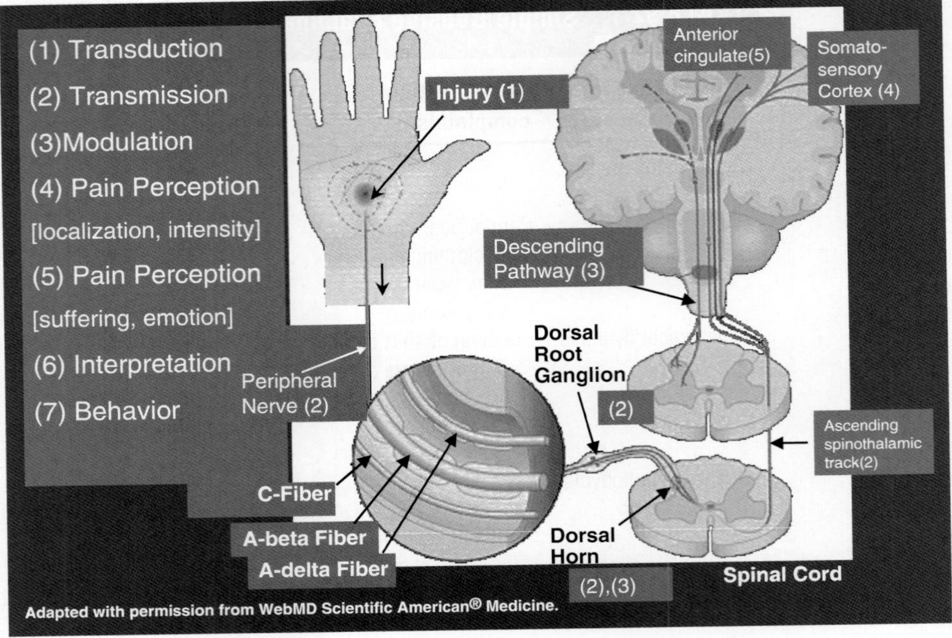

FIGURE 92.1. Anatomy of pain perception.

for the clinical presentation of *secondary hyperalgesia* (hyperalgesia in sites away from the site of initial injury) and *allodynia*. The neurotransmitters contained in the terminals of nociceptive afferents in the dorsal horn include excitatory amino acids, particularly glutamate, and neuropeptides such as substance P, calcitonin gene-related peptides, vasoactive intestinal peptide, somatostatin, and others. The rationale for preemptive analgesia, i.e. when analgesics or neural blocks are given prior to a surgical procedure, is that this is thought to prevent central sensitization (20). Inhibition of nociceptive circuits, mediated by a number of neurotransmitters, including amino acids such as 5-hydroxytryptamine, GABA, and glycine as well as neuropeptides such as enkephalins, form the basis of many pharmacologic interventions.

Stage 3 pain states are abnormal pain states, often termed as *maldynia* (bad pain), which are generally the consequence of chronic inflammation (e.g., arthritis), damage to peripheral nerves (e.g. neuropathy), damage to the CNS (e.g., thalamic stroke, multiple sclerosis) or changes in the CNS itself (e.g., neuroplasticity, central sensitization and alteration in modulatory systems, such as complex regional pain syndrome [RSD]), as in Figure 92.2. *Maldynia* is characterized by a lack of correlation between the intensity of a peripheral stimulus and the intensity of pain (manifest by exaggerated responses to noxious stimuli) and also by pain that is spontaneous or triggered by innocuous physical or psychologic stimuli (21). Descending control from supraspinal centers inhibits ascending nociceptive transmission, and this control is proportional to the afferent nociceptive input by C fibers (19). It has been suggested that loss of a proportion of the normal input after peripheral nerve damage produces a lifting of descending inhibition, which could be responsible for enhanced pain perception, particularly from the phenomenon of hyperpathia, in which there is an exaggerated pain response to a noxious stimulus (14).

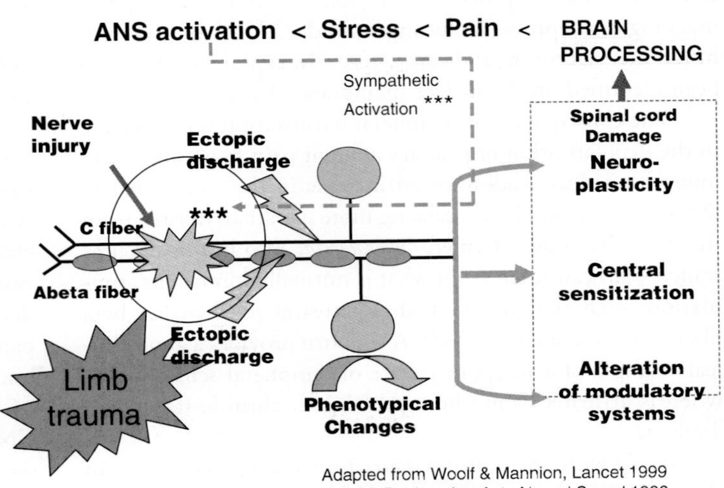

FIGURE 92.2. Maldynia: Neuropathic pain, central sensitization, and stress activation. Key: After injury to first-order nociceptive fibers, they spontaneously and repetitively discharge, activating the biochemical cascade leading to central sensitization and neuroplasticity. Pain activates the stress response, including the sympathetic system, which can also be activated by emotional states such as anxiety or frustration not directly related to pain. Sympathetic terminals on injured nerves and/or nociceptors release norepjnephrine, respectively increasing ectopic discharge of injured nerves and/or lowering nociceptor firing threshold in injured tissue. This pathophysiologic process increases pain such that commonly patients with maldynia are known to "hole up" socially, avoiding interpersonal contact and other situations that might aggravate them and worsen their pain.

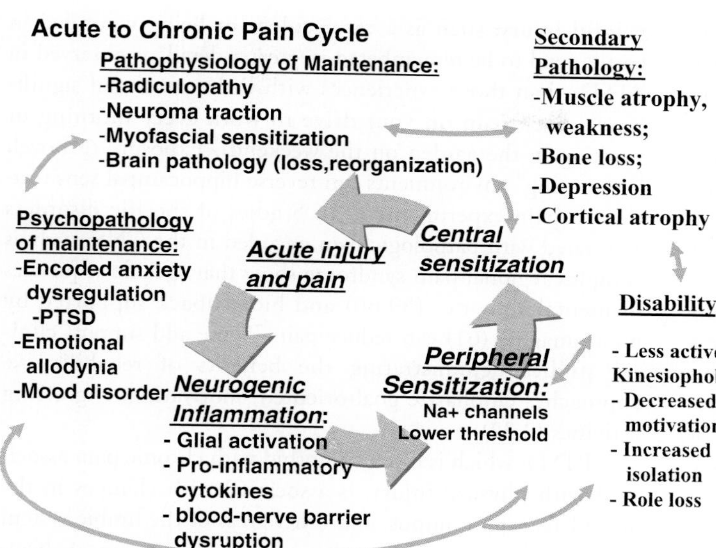

FIGURE 92.3. Acute-to-chronic pain cycle.

However, the development of stage 3 pain may involve genetic, cognitive, and emotional factors that remain to be clarified (17,22). Recent brain imaging studies suggest that more rostral changes in the CNS also mediate sensitization. For example, changes in the hippocampus may sustain potentiation of an initial stimulus for up to a year, which can be reversed by placing laboratory mammals in a challenging novel environment (23). This finding supports a widely held clinical belief in the effectiveness of stimulating, goal-directed activity and exercise in suppressing pain, enabling improvements in functional ability and even reducing the clinical manifestations of central sensitization (e.g., allodynia and hyperpathia). This mechanism is thought to underlie the effectiveness of comprehensive rehabilitation programs for chronic pain. Regions in the cingulate gyrus have now been identified as responsible for modulating behavioral responses to pain, attention to pain, pain-induced fear, and learning and pain (24–26). Figure 92.3 illustrates the phenomenologic sequence of biopsychosocial processes involved in the transition from acute injury to maldynia and related comorbidities and disability. Treatment hence involves a comprehensive approach that identifies the patient's biopsychosocial profile in this pathway and addresses specific pathophysiologic factors that perpetuate pain and pain-related and disease-related impairments and comorbidities.

Pain and Emotions

Emotional states that activate sympathetic arousal, such as anxiety or anger, can increase the level of pain in any episode of acute pain and reactivate or worsen chronic pain. When depression and anxiety disorders, such as posttraumatic stress disorder PTSD and maldynias are comorbid, they complicate each other's treatment, such that treating one condition without treating the other increases the likelihood of treatment failure. Moreover, certain personal traits, such as external locus of control (27,28) and a tendency to catastrophize (29–31), also predict worse outcomes. Finally, comorbid substance abuse may complicate the use of opioid analgesics for pain control. Substance abuse, by interfering with the sustained, goal-oriented behavior needed for functional restoration, leads to poor outcomes of pain treatment generally. The mechanisms for this effect will be discussed in more detail. Thus identifying and managing these comorbidities is critical to effectively treating pain.

Historical Notes on Psychosomatic Concepts

A review of rigorous epidemiologic studies over several decades demonstrate a strong association between depressive and anxiety disorders and chronic pain (32–34). Although chronic pain generally affects psychological health and functional status consistently across cultures (35), the relationship is more complex when considering individual pain diseases. For example, a mechanism for the high association among depression, anxiety disorders, and arthritis is suggested by recent studies linking the presence of depression to an impaired capacity to regulate the inflammatory cascade during stress (36).

The causal direction of the relationships among chronic pain disorders and psychiatric comorbidities and the relative influence of environmental factors and genetic/familial factors—"nature versus nurture"—are also being studied. For example, a series of studies of patients with myofascial facial pain demonstrated that major depression was more common than in community controls (37), that pain and depressed mood seasonally co-varied (38), and, using a family study methodology, that the stress of living with chronic pain increased the risk for depression in persons without a personal or family history of depression (39). This latter study suggests that the stress of living with pain, not familial risk, is the dominant cause of depression comorbidity in chronic facial pain. However, using a similarly rigorous methodology, a series of family studies of community-dwelling adult females with a different pain disease, fibromyalgia, a disorder marked by generalized muscle pain and tenderness with no peripheral pathology, supports the hypothesis that fibromyalgia is a depressive spectrum disorder (40). This and other studies (41) suggest a shared pathogenesis, such as dysfunction in serotonin and norepinephrine systems in fibromyalgia (42–45) and in depression (46,47). Shared genetic risk factors for fibromyalgia (FM) and major depressive disorder (MDD) may also be identified, for example genetic polymorphisms have been demonstrated in serotonin-related genes in fibromyalgia (48–51). Thus, the increase in rates of major depression in families of persons with fibromyalgia, with or without depression, may reflect vulnerability in these neurotransmitter systems that influences both disorders.

The effects of environmental factors on the pathogenesis of pain disorders and depressive disorders may be shared. Stress and trauma, implicated in both facial pain (39) and depression (52–55) are probably specific for different chronic pain disorders. In the only prospective study of a community sample of fibromyalgia and major life trauma (the 9/11 World Trade Center attack), exposure to stress was not associated with an increase in rates of fibromyalgia in controls (community subjects without fibromyalgia), but was associated with increases in pain in community subjects with fibromyalgia already confirmed by research diagnostic criteria (56).

One interpretation of these aforementioned studies is that central states such as fibromyalgia and MDD share a genetic and/or biologically mediated vulnerability to respond to stressful or traumatic events with psychological and pain-related symptoms. This interpretation is consistent with two recent studies, one showing that persons with fibromyalgia symptoms are more likely to develop PTSD in response to a fixed level of exposure to traumatic events (56), another demonstrating that during experimental interpersonal stress, women with fibromyalgia who were primed to experience negative mood prior to stress showed greater subsequent pain elevations than similarly primed women with osteoarthritis (57). Genetic studies suggest that a functional polymorphism in the promoter region of the serotonin transporter gene affects the influence of stressful life events on depression (58), a region that has been implicated in some investigations of fibromyalgia (49,50).

Pain and Anxiety The experimental and epidemiologic evidence points to a strong association between anxiety and pain and anxiety disorders and pain conditions (33), mediated in part by the amygdala, which appears to play a key role in the up- or down-regulation of the emotional response to pain. This "nociceptive amygdala" can be influenced by a wide range of environmental and internal stimuli to modulate the subjective experience of pain.

The hippocampus, a structure with robust connections to the amygdala, is a center for memory formation, storage, and retrieval. It provides information from detailed memories that are processed by the amygdala and given a particular emotional value, which may influence the development of "pain memory" after central sensitization (23). The emotional value the amygdala places on a particular memory is then fed back to the hippocampus, where it integrates this information and either strengthens or weakens the memory. This is why it is believed that events associated with high emotional content, and often painful injury, such as a car accident or being wounded in battle, tend to be remembered in greater detail, as observed in PTSD, than those experiences with little emotional significance (back pain on your drive to work every morning or working in the garden on the weekend). Exposure to novel, "interesting" environments can reverse hippocampal sensitization in pain experiments (23). Studies of specific disorders associated with pathologic pain encoded in the CNS, such as complex regional pain syndrome show that specific sequences of mental activities (59,60) and biofeedback supported by brain imaging (61) can reduce pain. These add support clinical studies demonstrating the benefits of rehabilitative approaches emphasize goal-oriented, motivating, engrossing activities (2,32).

PTSD, which is often comorbid with chronic pain associated with physical injury, is associated with changes in the amygdala, hippocampus, and other areas of the limbic system (the neural circuits of complex emotional experience). Neuroimaging studies have found consistent reductions in either total hippocampal volume or blood flow in men and women with PTSD (62–65).

Other research on structures within this fear circuit has expanded our understanding of how the cortical structures influence the amygdala. Human brain imaging studies have found that the fusiform gyrus, prefrontal gyrus, and anterior cingulate gyrus are preferentially activated in response to fearful stimuli (66,67). The orbitofrontal cortex (OFC), which is involved in the evaluation of risk and reward and social norms, may also have a direct role in regulation of anxiety via its connection to the amygdala (68). The cortex, then, plays an essential role in the categorization, appraisal, and attenuation of our reactions to frightening stimuli, such as pain. These connections are outlined in Figure 92.4. The higher cortical connections to the more primitive fight, flight, and reward circuitry are what allow us to have a degree of conscious recognition and control over these processes. These connections and their conditioning suggest the biologic basis for the effects of behavioral treatments used widely in chronic pain, such as relaxation and biofeedback. They also suggest specific targets for neuromodulation.

More recent functional brain chemistry research has provided neuroanatomic evidence for the overlap between the processing and perception of pain and anxiety. In an experiment comparing patients with chronic low back pain (CLBP) to normal controls, significant differences were found in two regions of the association cortex (OFC and dorsolateral prefrontal cortex [DLPFC]), cingulate gyrus (part of the limbic system) and thalamus (69). The study showed that persons with CLBP have differences in regional brain chemistry in the OFC and DLPFC. Additionally, persons with CLBP and anxiety had changes in brain chemistry suggesting increased interaction between all four brain regions, whereas anxious controls had changes observed only in the OFC. Anxiety and pain, therefore, share common neurochemical pathways and can interact in a way that leads to the reorganization of normal perceptual pathways in the brain.

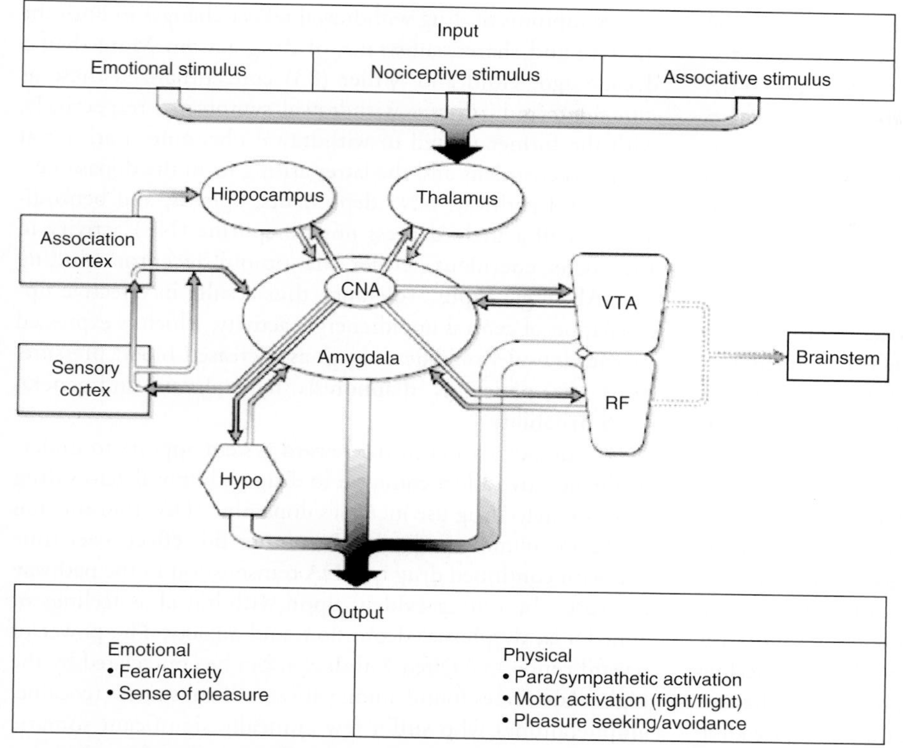

Structures and function:

CNA = Central Nucleus of the Amygdala, [controls output from the amygdala to all other structures in the circuit]

Hypo = Hypothalamus [sympathetic and parasympathetic activation involved in physical fight/flight response]

VTA = Ventral tegmental area. [Dopamine – reward system important for reinforcement of learned behavior. Role in addiction]

RF = Reticular formation [norepinephrine and serotonin output to amygdata. Important role in modulation of amygdala activity]

Thalamus: Principle conduit of information to amygdala from the environment.

Hippocampus: Provides input of stored memory to moderate response to fear.

Cortex: Sends sensory and abstract associative information to amygdala and helps consolidate memory in hippocampus.

FIGURE 92.4. The circuitry of fear. (From Tirado CF, Gallagher RM. The diagnosis and treatment of anxiety and anxiety disorders in chronic spinal pain. In: Slipman C, Wetzel T eds. *Interventional spine: an algorithmic approach.* New York: Elsevier Health Sciences, 2007.)

CLINICAL INTERFACE BETWEEN PAIN AND ADDICTION

Multiple points of interface exist between pain and addiction, and these become significant at the clinical level. Pain and drug reward share common neuroanatomic and neurochemical substrates, and the physiologic sequela of addiction (i.e., tolerance, physical dependence, altered stress response) have clear effects on pain management. Drugs of abuse often have analgesic properties, yet the disease of addiction brings with it physical symptoms, mood states, behaviors, and social losses that serve to worsen the pain experience. The clinical interaction of the pain and addiction is particularly complex in the case of addiction to opioids, as these drugs appear to be imbued with both analgesic and hyperalgesic properties. Further, accumulating genetic data suggest that pain, opioid analgesia, and opioid addiction share similar patterns of gene expression, which become evident in the response of the individual patient.

Physiologic Mechanisms of Addiction Like pain, addiction is an extremely complex human response, with strong behavioral components that cannot be entirely understood by analyzing its physiology. Standard diagnostic criteria for addiction disorders (*Diagnostic and Statistical Manual of Mental Disorders-Revised*) (70) rely only minimally on the more overt physical responses to chronic drug use (such as tolerance and withdrawal), focusing instead on such behavioral consequences as loss of control over drug use and significant disruptions in social role function. By definition, understanding of the molecular and cellular mechanisms underlying addiction disorders is insufficient to convey the actual human experience of addiction. Further, the neural substrate from which both pain and addiction arise cannot be considered static; notable changes to the nervous system are evident with ongoing exposure to pain or addictive drugs.

A full discussion of the physiologic mechanisms underlying addictive disease is provided in Chapter 5, "From Neurobiology to Treatment: Progress against Addiction," and others (Chapters 6–17) describe the different sites and unique mechanisms of action that drugs of abuse have in the CNS, underlying their acute effects and distinctive withdrawal syndromes. All drugs of abuse share an ability to increase dopaminergic activity in the mesolimbic reward pathway—a pathway that, in animal models, has been shown to be responsible for the reinforcing effects of drugs of abuse. In addition, salient and engrained patterns of synaptic strength between the hippocampal memories of drug reward and frontal lobe motivational systems result in the aberrant and dysfunctional behaviors characteristic of the substance use disorders.

Of relevance to issues of pain and pain treatment, the physiology of addiction often is characterized by two incompletely understood yet related allostatic states: *tolerance* and *physical dependence*. This new level of functioning may be manifest both in the systems where drugs of abuse exert discrete actions as well as at shared reward substrate. Importantly, the simple presence of these adaptations in the nervous system does not infer addiction. A pain patient may be tolerant to or physically dependent on an opioid without being addicted to it. Addiction is identified by a cluster of aberrant patterns of behavior that, while partially motivated by these physiologic changes, is evident in much broader domains.

Tolerance Ongoing use of certain psychoactive drugs results in the development of drug tolerance, which is defined as a reduction in response to a given dose of drug after repeated administration (71,72). The neuroadaptations associated with tolerance counter the acute drug effects to maintain system-level homeostasis. A theoretical explanation for the processes underlying tolerance is offered by the opponent process theory of acquired motivation (73). Reflecting homeostatic assumptions, the theory describes how, over the course of repeated exposures to an affectively charged stimulus, a counteracting or opposing emotional response develops, which eventually accounts for habituation to the stimulus to become the predominate feeling state in its absence. Although initially it was rooted in behaviorism, Koob and colleagues (74) advanced the theory by providing evidence for a neurobiologic basis to the opponent processes of tolerance and physical dependence in the case of opioid dependence. Their model predicts that to maintain a "normal" or homeostatic level of reward system activity, "anti-reward" systems are recruited to counteract drug effects, which become stronger with each exposure and extinguish more slowly than the original response (75,76). Upon abrupt drug withdrawal, the tolerance-producing processes are revealed.

Tolerance involves adaptations that occur at both the site of drug action (receptor or ion channel) and in systems distal to the site of drug action (77,78). For example, tolerance to opioids is evident at both the level of the opioid receptor in the locus coeruleus and in the dopaminergic reward pathways afferent to the site of this discrete drug action. Because drugs typically act at selective receptors, tolerance has been conceptualized as a functional "uncoupling" of the receptor from its effector response (opening or closing an ion channel, initiating second-messenger systems); in other words, a certain proportion of receptors are rendered less-than- or nonfunctional, making the drug less effective (and requiring a higher dose to get the same effect that initially was obtained at a lower dose) (78,79). Clinically, the resulting tolerance provides a certain amount of protection for the user, such as with the respiratory depressant effects of opioids or the anesthetic effects of ethanol.

Physical Dependence A related consequence of chronic drug use is physical dependence, which is an altered neurophysiologic state that develops as a result of tolerance. When drug blood level falls below a critical point, the adaptive changes associated with tolerance predominate and become profoundly nonadaptive (80). Suddenly unopposed by drug effects, the sources of tolerance become evident as the characteristic drug-specific withdrawal syndrome (81,82).

Symptoms of drug withdrawal reflect changes in both the discrete and shared substrates of drug action. More than a decade ago, Gold and Miller (83) conceptualized these as *autonomic* and *affective* withdrawal symptoms, respectively, with the former related to withdrawal phenomena arising at the locus coeruleus and the latter arising from the dopaminergic reward pathway. CNS depressants, opioids, and benzodiazepines all acutely depress norepinephrine (NE) activity in the locus coeruleus, either via opioid receptor binding or GABAergic input. Tolerance thus results in effective up-regulation of central noradrenergic activity, which is expressed in withdrawal from these drugs as increased blood pressure, heart rate, peristalsis, diaphoresis, hyperalgesia, and general CNS irritability.

Neuroadaptation in the reward system appears to underlie the negative affect common to drug withdrawal across drug class. Acutely, drug use increases dopamine (DA) transmission in the mesolimbic pathway. To counter this effect, over time and with continued drug use, DA transmission in the pathway decreases, becoming evident upon withdrawal as feelings of anhedonia, dysphoria, depression, and anxiety. The power of reward center–mediated withdrawal can be appreciated by the high relapse rates found among abusers of substances (cocaine, amphetamine) who suffer few clinically significant somatic withdrawal symptoms. Negative affect states such as these are implicated in the development of craving and relapse, both common outcomes of attempting drug abstinence (84).

Role of Stress Of increasing interest to the physiology underlying addiction are the effects of HPA-axis activation, both within the context of addiction and accompanying initial drug use. The potential contributions of abuse and trauma, especially in childhood, to reward responses to addictive drugs is increasingly appreciated (85–87). Both stress and repeated, chronic administration of glucocorticoids to animals have been shown to enhance their behavioral sensitization to addictive drugs, which has prompted the hypothesis that excessive circulating glucocorticoids, as would occur under conditions of chronic stress, function to maintain the sensitized state (88,89). Certainly such trauma, such as a near-fatal automobile crash or physical abuse or rape, is often associated with physiologic pain; thus, the sensitization to drugs of abuse can be intertwined with past experiences with pain.

Analgesic Effects of Drugs of Abuse As points of interface between the physiology of pain and of addiction are considered, it is important to recognize that many classes of abused drugs have demonstrated analgesic properties. The opioids are defined by their direct analgesic effects and, at high doses, alcohol is a potent anesthetic. The sedative hypnotics, particularly benzodiazepines, are used to treat the pain sustained by muscle spasticity secondary to upper motor neuron damage (90,91), and are the standard anxiolytic adjuncts for procedural sedation and analgesia (92,93). CNS stimulants, such as cocaine and caffeine, produce and potentiate analgesia, presumably by increasing neurotransmitter activity in descending inhibitory pain pathways.

Of current interest are the effects of cannabinoids on pain perception. In 1992, Devane and colleagues (94) developed a high-affinity synthetic cannabinoid ligand, confirming the presence of endogenous cannabinoid G-protein-coupled receptors in the human body, with central subtype receptors widely distributed in the cortex, basal ganglia, cerebellum, and hippocampus (95,96). More recently, Mao and colleagues (97) provided good preclinical evidence for an independent THC-responsive antinociceptive pathway that is particularly effective for pain of neuropathic origin. Though clinical trials of cannabinoids in multiple sclerosis have suggested a benefit for neuropathic pain (98,99), human studies of cannabinoid-mediated analgesia have been limited by study size, heterogeneous patient populations, subjective outcome measures, and variable drug pharmacokinetics (100). Interference with glutamate release at the level of the dorsal root ganglia or periaqueductal gray is one hypothesized mechanism by which cannabinoids provide analgesia (101,102).

General Effects of Addiction on Pain Careful examination of the extant literature provides evidence that physiologic states associated with drug addiction can affect or predict nociceptive input, processing and/or modulation in several different ways. Consequences of addictive disease that facilitate the experience of pain are multiple, including associated sympathetic arousal and negative mood states. These changes are related to both the discrete effects of certain classes of drugs and the effects on reward-relevant systems of all drugs of abuse.

For example, important substance-induced disorders or psychological sequelae, including sleep disorders and psychiatric illness, are characteristic of addiction and, as previously noted, can contribute to the experience of chronic pain and decrease the efficacy of analgesic interventions. Addiction commonly co-occurs with anxiety and affective disorders (103,104), which—if unrecognized or untreated—can increase the perception of pain. Depression has been demonstrated to increase the discomfort associated with pain and negatively affect function in studies of chronic pain patients, with symptoms frequently diminishing along with effective antidepressant treatment (105–107).

In addiction, drug use is characterized by frequent and rapid fluctuations in blood levels of the drug. Abused substances tend to be ingested in short-acting formulations and via routes of rapid onset (i.e., inhalation, intravenous) to boost psychoactive effect. These use patterns result in rapidly alternating states of intoxication and subtle (or sometimes full-blown) withdrawal. Both can result in activation of the sympathetic nervous system and thereby contribute to the pain experience. For example, intoxication with cocaine and the CNS stimulants significantly increases central noradrenergic activity, whereas withdrawal from opioids, CNS depressants, and/or sedative-hypnotics do the same related to up-regulated locus coeruleus norepinephrine discharge. Outcomes of noradrenergic overactivity noted during intoxication or withdrawal from these drugs of abuse, including increased muscle tension, anxiety, and irritability, appear to augment, rather than reduce, discomfort in the person/patient with an addiction disorder.

Further, a strong and persistent negative affective state accompanies withdrawal from all drugs of abuse, theorized to be related to overall DA depletion in the reward pathways. When drug-free, the addicted individual suffers from negative symptoms such as anhedonia, prolonged dysphoria, and irritability (84,89) and reports being unable to feel gratification or reward from environmental stimuli. The degree to which affective withdrawal responses contribute to the overall drug-specific withdrawal syndrome varies, with those drugs acting more directly on DA-relevant reward pathways theorized to have a more affectively charged withdrawal. Clearly, the negative feeling states associated with drug withdrawal can augment the subjective discomfort associated with pain.

Finally, and not insignificantly, the interpersonal conflicts, role adjustments, and social support losses that characterize the social context of addiction can worsen the experience of pain, making the individual less able to manage or cope with discomfort. Further, the chaotic and drug-oriented lifestyle of the person/patient with an addiction disorder makes it difficult to comply with prescribed pain management regimes. Empirical support for a worsened pain experience in persons/patients with an addiction disorder has been demonstrated to experimental pain; as compared to matched drug-abstinent ex-addicts and normal controls, persons currently using addictive drugs are significantly less tolerant of cold-pressor (CP) pain, regardless of the particular drug of abuse (108–110).

Unique Effects of Opioid Addiction and Pain The effects of addictive disease on pain become especially pertinent in the case of individuals addicted to opioid drugs, because the class of drug abused also is the primary pharmacologic tool for the treatment of moderate-to-severe clinical pain. Agonist activity at mu-opioid receptors provides a robust and reliable analgesia, making opioids the most powerful and effective treatment for pain known to humans.

Opioid addiction and opioid analgesia are dependent upon opioid agonist activity at the mu-opioid receptor; the reinforcing and analgesic effects of morphine, for example, can be blocked by the administration of mu-receptor antagonists and are absent in mu-opioid receptor gene knock-out mice. Mu-opioid receptors are found throughout body tissues, however, and effects of opioid administration can include activity on immune, respiratory, and gut functions (111). In that the same receptor is central to both addiction and pain systems, it is reasonable to expect that perturbations in the latter might be evident in individuals chronically exposed to opioids (agonists or antagonists) in the context of the former. Although drug reward and analgesia are distinct processes, opioids activate their shared anatomic substrate, the mu opioid receptor, inducing the previously described interrelated CNS changes of tolerance and physical dependence. Opioid addicts may seek psychoactive effects yet are not necessarily immune from the potential effects of these drugs on central and peripheral opioid-relevant pain systems.

That opioid addiction and pain responses might be interrelated is not a new idea. In his early essay describing his clinical observations on patients injecting morphine on a daily basis, physician and author Clifford Albutt (1870) asked,

"Does morphia (sic) tend to encourage the very pain it pretends to relieve?" He continues, "I have much reason to suspect that a reliance upon hypodermic morphia only ended in a curious state of *perpetuated pain*" (112, p. 329). Although poorly explored in the subsequent clinical research, questions about the pain responses of opioid-dependent patients again arose with the institution of methadone maintenance in the 1960s.

Pain and Methadone Maintenance Patients As early as 1965, Martin and Inglis (113) described significantly lower tolerance for cold pressor-induced pain in a sample of incarcerated, known narcotic-abusing females, in comparison to matched non-addict controls. Ho and Dole (114) found that both methadone-maintained (MM) and drug-free opioid persons/patients with an addiction disorder had significantly lower thresholds for CP pain than did matched non-addict sibling controls. Subsequent work supports that, at methadone trough conditions, CP pain *threshold* does not differ between MM and drug-free opioid persons/patients with an addiction disorder but is significantly lower for MM patients in comparison to matched normal controls (109,110,115). Under the same conditions, MM patients' CP pain *tolerance* is less than that in both matched drug-free persons/patients with an addiction disorder (108) and matched controls (109,115). A similar nonsignificant trend for decreased pain tolerance in MM patients was noted for electrical pain stimulation, and a significant analgesic effect for methadone on CP, electrical, and pressure pain 2 to 4 hours after dose was reported (115). With respect to perceived pain severity, Schall and colleagues (116) found no difference between MM and control subjects in their perception of pressure pain (measured on a scale of 1–10) immediately prior to methadone dosing.

These cross-sectional data indicate that MM patients are more sensitive to pain than are matched normal controls. Across electrical and thermal (cold) nociceptive stimuli, methadone patients reliably demonstrate poor tolerance for experimental pain and are, on average, between 42% and 76% less tolerant of CP pain than are normal controls matched on age, gender, and ethnicity (109,110,115,117,118). With appreciable (albeit trough) methadone blood levels, these patients not only receive *no* underlying analgesic effect from daily, high-dose administration of methadone but present a case for the *anti-analgesic* (hyperalgesic) effects of chronic methadone therapy. Pilot data suggest that degree of hyperalgesia varies with the intrinsic activity of the opioid maintenance agent; patients maintained on the partial agonist buprenorphine for the treatment of opioid addiction are less hyperalgesic than those maintained on methadone, a full agonist (110).

Opioid-Induced Hyperalgesia Across this literature, it is of note that the degree of hyperalgesic response to opioid administration (~30% of baseline) is so reliable. Accumulated evidence indicates that opioid administration not only provides analgesia but concurrently sets into motion certain anti-analgesic or hyperalgesic processes, which counteract or oppose the opioid analgesic effects. Ongoing work has culminated in current understanding of what is described as opioid-induced hyperalgesia (OIH), or diminished tolerance for pain following acute and chronic opioid administration (119–126). From this perspective, the pain intolerance of MM patients reflects a latent hyperalgesia secondary to chronic opioid exposure.

Withdrawal Hyperalgesia The observation that chronic opioid administration induces increased pain sensitivity or hyperalgesia is not a new one. The phenomenon of hyperalgesia has long been recognized as a fundamental symptom of the opioid withdrawal syndrome in animal models of physical dependence (127–130), and although not extensively studied, hyperalgesia long has been considered a cardinal symptom of the opioid withdrawal syndrome in humans (71,131). The time course, opioid dose-response relationship, and opioid pretreatment parameters of withdrawal hyperalgesia have been carefully characterized in preclinical models for more than 30 years, such that it arises after single or chronic opioid exposure, can be detected up to 5 days after subcutaneous injection, and increases in intensity with pretreatment opioid dose or intrinsic efficacy (132–135).

Further characterization of the hyperalgesia after opioid administration confirms that although it is present during withdrawal, OIH exists independent of the withdrawal syndrome and can, in fact, be detected in the presence of opioid analgesia (136–138). Demonstrating the key role of the mu-opioid receptor in the development of this hyperalgesia, investigators found diminished OIH development in mouse strains with reduced mu-opioid receptor binding. More recent work has shown that OIH increases in severity with intermittent or naloxone-interrupted opioid dosing (123,139–141). A biphasic response to opioid administration is described such that analgesia is an early response, followed by the longer lasting hyperalgesic state (139,142).

Opioid-Induced Hyperalgesia and Tolerance The presence of hyperalgesia with ongoing opioid use demands reconsideration of the well-described phenomenon of analgesic tolerance. Jasinski (143) suggests that "tolerance occurs not at the (opioid) receptor level but occurs from increased activity of other functional systems to counteract the effects of opioids" (p. 185). The hyperalgesic processes initiated by opioid administration serve to counteract opioid analgesia. As eloquently hypothesized by Colpaert (144,145) and Celerier (139,146–148), that which appears to be opioid analgesic tolerance, and therefore increased opioid need, may in fact be an organismic response to an opioid-induced hypersensitivity to pain. Essentially, opioids lose their analgesic effectiveness in the face of decreased tolerance for pain. That OIH might contribute to the variable and incompletely understood phenomenon of analgesic tolerance in the clinical setting is a paradigm-shifting idea. Analgesic tolerance has long been an untested concern for withholding opioids in the treatment of chronic pain (149,150); re-conceptualizing tolerance as a reflection of OIH in the study of chronic pain management may lead to novel insights into the utility of chronic opioid therapy for this patient population.

Through their preclinical work exploring the molecular mechanisms of hyperalgesic pain states, Mao and colleagues (151–155) demonstrated the similarities between opioid analgesic tolerance and OIH. In an important series of studies, these investigators provide credible evidence that the development of opioid analgesic tolerance via intermittent morphine dosing induces hyperalgesia, whereas animals made hyperalgesic via neuropathic injury concomitantly exhibit opioid analgesic tolerance (results recently were replicated with heroin by Celerier, Laulin, et al., [147]).

Mechanisms of Opioid-Induced Hyperalgesia Various physiologic explanations for the development of OIH have been offered and focus on both spinal and supraspinal systems as the neuroplastic site of action (127,132,156–162). In the work described earlier, Mao and colleagues demonstrated that the common pathway for the development of morphine tolerance/hyperalgesia is activation of ionotropic *N*-methyl-D-aspartate (NMDA) receptors on dorsal horn spinal cord neurons, with subsequent intracellular increases in protein kinase C and nitric oxide. OIH is conceptualized as a variant of central sensitization and, like the hyperalgesia of neuropathic origin (152,163), can be prevented by NMDA-receptor antagonism and calcium channel blockers (139,146,164–167). The latter finding has spurred interest in the potential utility of NMDA-receptor antagonists in pain management as a means to enhance the effectiveness of opioid analgesia (72,168–171) and complements the ongoing work of addiction scientists on the utility of these agents to reverse opioid tolerance and physical dependence (172–176).

Alternatively, Porreca and colleagues (126) have provided good preclinical evidence that OIH may in fact be the result of the activation of descending pain facilitation systems arising from mu-opiate receptor activation (177) in the rostral ventromedial medulla (RVM) (158,178–180). Specifically implicated are opioid-induced increased levels of the pro-nociceptive peptide cholecystokinin (CCK) in the RVM, increases that appear to play a role in the development of opiate analgesic tolerance as well (181). It is suggested that CCK activity in the medulla drives descending pain facilitatory mechanisms, resulting in spinal hyperalgesic responses to nociceptive input (161,178).

Various spinal neuropeptides, distinct from excitatory amino acid systems, have also been implicated in the development of OIH. More than a decade ago, Simonnet's laboratory (182) showed that a single dose of parenteral heroin resulted in significant release of the antiopioid neuropeptide FF from the spinal cord in rats, an effect blocked by the subsequent administration of opioid antagonist naloxone, and inducing a hyperalgesia 30% below baseline. More recent animal work in Porreca's laboratory has demonstrated increased levels of lumbar dynorphin, a kappa opioid agonist with pro-nociceptive activity, after sustained spinal administration of opioid (157,161). Interestingly, the hyperalgesic effects of opioids have been reversed by the administration of an antagonist to the neurokinin-1 receptor, the site of activity for the nociceptive neuropeptide substance P (158). Particularly active in pain of inflammatory origin, substance P involvement suggests a neuro-inflammatory component to the development of OIH (see 180).

Emerging evidence suggests a key role for neuroimmune processes in the development of OIH. (183,184). In this model, exogenously administered opioids are theorized to bind to μ-opioid receptors located on the astrocytes of the blood-brain barrier, activating these and resulting in the subsequent expression and release of pro-inflammatory chemokines and cytokines. Specifically, peripheral immune cells activated in response to opioid administration are hypothesized to bind to glial cells and induce specific classes of central pro-inflammatory (and therefore pro-nociceptive) cytokines, thus resulting in a state of heightened pain sensitivity (183,185).

In support of this hypothesis, Song and Zhao (186), and Johnston and Westbrook (187) have demonstrated that the administration of a glial cell inhibitor (fluorocitrate) reversed the hyperalgesic effect of morphine in acute and chronically treated rats. Further, administration of the cytokine inhibitors interleukin-1β receptor antagonist and interleukin-6 neutralizing antibody have been shown to reverse and/or block morphine-induced hyperalgesia (160,188). As theorized by Watkins and Maier, peripheral inflammation via glial cell activation results in sensitization of spinal neurons pain-processing pathways, both increasing the perception of pain and supporting functional "sickness behaviors" (184,185,189,190). Reviewing the literature, Ossipov and colleagues (138) commented that "opioid-induced abnormal pain may share a molecular signature with pain of inflammatory origin" (p. 320).

Finally, more than 30 years ago, Seigel and colleagues demonstrated a conditioned component to OIH. A robust OIH was observed in animals receiving saline in an environment previously paired with morphine administration (191,192). This work showed that rats receiving acute morphine doses (three to nine doses separated by 48 hours) in a specific environment demonstrate significant hyperalgesia in the same setting as compared to rats receiving morphine unpaired with setting, or saline control rats. Because conditioned responses to medications typically are opposite in direction to unconditional drug effects, the learned responses were ascribed a causal role in the development of drug tolerance.

Clinical Evidence of Opioid-Induced Hyperalgesia As noted, evidence for the existence and characteristics of OIH have been principally established in animal models, making it difficult to extrapolate preclinical findings to the clinical model of the patient with chronic pain. Not only is pain a much more highly modulated experience in humans but it is not entirely clear how pain *tolerance* in humans (point of subjective intolerance of pain, an indicator of hyperalgesia) maps onto putative pain *threshold* or perception (point at which animal withdraws tail, jumps on hotplate) in animals. Further, the development of OIH has been better characterized in animals without pain or with acute pain; thus, its effect and relevance in the setting of clinical chronic pain remain incomplete.

Probably best described is evidence for OIH in postoperative patients who received opioids intraoperatively and perhaps in a dose-dependent manner (193–196). These investigators showed that in patients undergoing various abdominal surgeries, postoperative reports of pain severity and/or opioid consumption were significantly higher in those patients receiving intrathecal or intravenous short-acting opioids (fentanyl and remifentanil) during surgery in comparison to those receiving placebo (194,195) or low-dose opioids (193,196). It is theorized that the increased opioid exposure experienced during surgery-induced hyperalgesic changes, resulting in increased pain perception and opioid need in the postoperative period.

Reports of OIH in patients with chronic pain are much less common and are primarily limited to individuals with malignant pain. Across a number of case studies, the emergence of hyperalgesia and allodynia has been reported in cancer patients on large or rapidly escalating doses of morphine or fentanyl (197–200), in at least one case resolving with discontinuation and switching to a weaker opioid (201). A similar pattern of OIH induced with intrathecal sufentanil and clearing with opioid discontinuation has been described in a single case report of a woman with chronic nonmalignant low back pain (failed back syndrome) (202), suggesting that regardless of the etiology of chronic pain (malignant vs. nonmalignant), OIH becomes evident in certain individuals in the context of high-dose opioid therapy.

Perhaps of most relevance to the clinical situation of chronic pain and ongoing opioid therapy, a single study by Chu and colleagues (203) demonstrated the development of OIH in a small sample of patients with chronic nonmalignant low back pain after 1 month of oral sustained-release morphine treatment (median dose, 75 mg/day). In these six individuals, 30 days of morphine at therapeutic doses not only resulted in analgesic tolerance to challenge doses of remifentanil but also diminished tolerance to CP pain by almost 25% from baseline. Despite appreciating analgesia, the experimental pain responses of these patients suggest the presence of hyperalgesic changes.

Indirect evidence of OIH may be reflected in the large number of chronic pain patients who do not respond to and/or ultimately discontinue chronic opioid treatment; it is unclear the degree to which the development of OIH contributes to poor outcomes in these patients. As noted in several recent meta-analyses of the extant clinical trial data (204–207), the benefits of opioid therapy for chronic nonmalignant pain beyond 6 to 8 weeks of treatment have yet to be demonstrated; thus, potential long-term consequences of opioid therapy, such as OIH, have not been fully evaluated. High rates of dropout (~30%) are reported in these short-term trials (206,208,209), with rates of up to 56% in longer-term open-label follow-up studies (7–24 months) (208). Most commonly attributed to side effects (nausea, constipation, drowsiness, and dizziness), patients also report dropping out owing to a perceived lack of efficacy, perhaps reflecting OIH. Interestingly, and in agreement with Chu and colleagues (203), two groups of investigators (210–212) report findings of pain increasing after opioid titration. Commenting on the large cross-sectional study of Eriksen and colleagues (205), which showed that patients on opioid therapy for the treatment of chronic nonmalignant pain were less likely to achieve key outcomes (pain relief, improved quality of life and functionality) than those not on opioid therapy, Ballentyne (213) warns that "opioids are not a panacea for chronic pain" (p. 4).

Genetic Factors Underlying Pain and Addiction Response Well-recognized individual differences in pain tolerance and opioid response have long been appreciated at the clinical level, and the genetic factors that underlie these differences are increasingly elucidated. For example, heritable differences in hepatic P450 isoenzyme activity affect both the amount of reward and analgesia received from an opioid. Individuals who are extensive "metabolizers" of opioids (i.e., those with high P450 activity) receive less analgesia and reward from a given opioid dose (214–219), theoretically putting them at decreased risk for addiction but increased risk for unrelieved pain (220). Preliminary data suggest that these extensive metabolizers of opioids are less tolerant of CP pain, possibly owing to defects in the endogenous synthesis of opioids (221).

If pain intolerance is, in fact, a genetically determined trait, addicted persons should evidence poor pain tolerance in comparison to controls, regardless of whether they currently are using drugs or are in drug-free recovery. A series of studies by Liebmann and colleagues provide evidence that drug-free opioid persons/patients with an addiction disorder are less sensitive to pain than are controls. These investigators report increased CP pain thresholds in ex-opioid persons/patients with an addiction disorder (in residential treatment) as compared to controls (222–224). Further, Lehofer and colleagues (225) reported that, using guided subjective recall, ex-opioid persons/patients with an addiction disorder rated themselves as less sensitive to pain than did normal controls, both when actively using and when opioid-free. Identified was a distinct subgroup of pain-intolerant ex-opioid persons/patients with an addiction disorder who were almost three times as likely to relapse within 2 years of treatment as pain-tolerant ex-addicts (223). Opioid persons/patients with an addiction disorder with poor pain tolerance may suffer a more severe form of addiction or have difficulty tolerating the discomfort (pain) inherent in detoxification and early abstinence.

Genetics of Pain and Addiction An analysis of the preclinical literature, most notably from the laboratories of Mogil (226,227) and Elmer (228–230), reveals that certain recombinant murine strains differ in both their baseline tolerance for pain as well as the amount of reward or reinforcement they enjoy from opioids. Those strains of animals with poor pain tolerance (i.e., C57, CXBK) find opioids to be highly reinforcing, whereas those with good pain tolerance (i.e., BALB/c, CXBH) receive little reinforcement from opioids (229,231,232). Further, pain-tolerant murine strains receive robust opioid analgesia and demonstrate increased opioid receptor–binding activity as compared to pain-intolerant strains (224,225,233,234).

With the advent of molecular genetics, investigators in both the pain and substance abuse fields have been focusing on polymorphisms in the mu-opioid gene receptor (OPRM) as candidates underlying phenotypes for pain sensitivity (220,235–237), opioid analgesic response (217,238,239), and addiction (240,241). Probably best characterized is the single nucleotide polymorphism A118G of the OPRM, such that normal human subjects with the variant allele have been shown to require almost twice as high a plasma level of morphine to achieve the analgesic response of those with the non-mutated allele (235,242,243). Other genes that have been linked to pain and opioid responses include those that code for the delta opioid receptor (244), the capsaicin-sensing vanillic receptor (244–246), the neurotransmitter enzyme catechol o-methyltransferase (244), and the melanocortin-1 receptor gene (247).

Genetics and Opioid-Induced Hyperalgesia

Genetic differences in response to opioids portend individual variability in the propensity to develop OIH. In a series of studies, Kest and colleagues reported murine strain differences in the development of opioid tolerance (248) and withdrawal severity (249,250), both of which have been ascribed a role in the presentation of OIH. Building upon preliminary evidence for genetic differences in OIH development (123), Liang and colleagues (251) evaluated 16 different strains of inbred mice for the development of thermal hyperalgesia after 4 days of morphine pretreatment and found significant variation amongst strains. Percent reduction in nociceptive thresholds ranged from 4% (LP/J strain) to 36% (AJR/J strain) in these experiments, and interestingly, a strain found to be relatively pain-intolerant (C57BL/6J) in previous work also developed a notable degree of hyperalgesia (24%) after chronic morphine administration.

In a related study, this investigative group evaluated the effects of chronic pain on acute pain and opioid responses across strains of mice (252) and, despite considerable variation, chronic pain induced thermal hyperalgesia and increased sensitivity to morphine analgesia across animals tested. Further, after 4-days of opioid administration, both those with and those without pain demonstrated physical dependence and tolerance, albeit with significant strain variation. Suggesting a shared mechanism for OIH, opioid tolerance and physical dependence, haplotypic genetic analyses revealed that differential expression of a gene coding for the nonspecific P-glycoprotein transporter (*Abcb1b* gene) best accounted for strain-related differences in the development of thermal hyperalgesia after morphine administration (251). Being a transporter for morphine, activity of this glycoprotein appears to play an important role in opioid response across domains.

CONCLUSIONS

Pain is the most modulated of the sensory modalities. How a given, quantifiable stimulus is processed by the nervous system can be modified at the level of the nociceptor, the peripheral nerve, the spinal cord neurons and tracts, the thalamus, or the cortex; modulation typically occurs at one or more of these sites. The unique susceptibility of pain to neuro-modulation portends a significant role for addiction in altering the pain experience. Addiction physiology underlies the processing of stimuli, which by nature provide reward; stimuli that are by nature unrewarding, such as pain, are likely to be preferentially affected by the presence of addiction.

Much of the data providing evidence for overlap between chronic pain and addiction phenomena have been obtained in animal studies, so caution must be exercised in generalizing these to clinical populations. By definition, both pain and addiction are uniquely human conditions; the complexity of each is evident in psychosocial, cognitive, and cultural domains and cannot be replicated in animal models. Hypotheses about how the neurophysiologic overlap between chronic pain and addiction might clinically manifest must take into account how holistic human responses to their combined presence may alter or mask predicted physiologic responses.

Several points of overlap exist between the physiologic bases of pain and addiction. Specific avenues by which the chronic use of addictive drugs might alter the processing of noxious stimuli include the presence of sympathetic stimulation, HPA-axis dysregulation, affective withdrawal, and opioid tolerance. Across this literature, a trend toward decreased pain tolerance in addiction can be discerned; thus, the presence of addictive disease appears to augment the experience of pain.

With respect to opioid addiction specifically, the development or presence of OIH has the potential to complicate the pain management. Less well studied but intriguing is evidence that individuals vary in their propensity to both addiction and pain responses; the link between the two may arise from inborn differences in endogenous opioid system tone. The congruence between the approaches for the treatment of pain and addiction (i.e., cognitive therapy, behavior modification, involvement of family, treatment of concurrent psychiatric disorders, and group support) provides further evidence that these phenomena have similar bases and are not entirely unrelated.

Consideration of the physiologic bases of pain and addiction and how they overlap provides direction for the management of pain in this population. The human phenomena of pain and addiction are not separate but interrelated; knowledgeable management of the former must reflect the extent to which, even at the physiologic level, its expression and response are affected by the latter.

REFERENCES

1. Gallagher RM. Integrating medical and behavioral treatment in chronic pain management. *Med Clin North Am* 1999;83(5):823–849.
2. Gallagher RM. Rational polypharmacy in integrated pain treatment. *Am J Phys Med Rehab (S)* 2005;84(3):S64–S76.
3. Melzack R, Wall PD. Pain mechanisms: a new theory. *Science.* 1965;150 (699):971–979.
4. Gallagher RM. Management of neuropathic pain: translating mechanistic advances and evidence-based research into clinical practice. *Clin J Pain* 2006;22(S1):S2–S8.
5. Cutler RB, Fishbain DA, Rosomoff HL, et al. Does nonsurgical pain center treatment of chronic pain return patients to work? A review and meta-analysis of the literature. *Spine* 1994;19:643–652.
6. Lang E, Liebig K, Kastner S, Neundorfer B, Heuschmann P. Multidisciplinary rehabilitation versus usual care for chronic low back pain in the community: effects on quality of life. *Spine J* 2003;3:270–276.
7. Guzman J, Esmail R, Karjalainen K, et al. Multidisciplinary rehabilitation for chronic low back pain: systematic review. *BMJ* 2001;322: 1511–1516.

8. Guzman J, Esmail R, Karjalainen K, et al. Multidisciplinary bio-psycho-social rehabilitation for chronic low back pain. *Cochrane Database Syst Rev* 2002;(1):CD000963.
9. Rogers WH, Wittink HM, Ashburn MA, et al. Using the "TOPS," an outcomes instrument for multidisciplinary outpatient pain treatment. *Pain Med United States* 2000;1(1):55–67.
10. Rogers WH, Wittink H, Wagner A, et al. Assessing individual outcomes during outpatient multidisciplinary chronic pain treatment by means of an augmented SF-36. *Pain Medicine* 2000;1(1):44–54.
11. Mossey J, Kerr N, Welz M, Gallagher RM. Preliminary evaluation of the Health Background Questionnaire for pain and clinical encounter form for pain. *Pain Med* 2005;6(6):443–451.
12. Fishman S, Gallagher RM, Carr D, Sullivan L. The case for pain medicine as a medical specialty. *Pain Med* 2004;5(3):281–286.
13. Mendell JR, Shehank Z. Clinical practice painful sensory neuropathy. *N Engl J Med* 2003;348(13):1243–1255.
14. Cervero F, Laird JM. Mechanisms of touch-evoked pain (allodynia): a new model. *Pain (Netherlands)* 1996;68(1):13–23.
15. Schaible HG, Schmidt RF. Activation of groups III and IV sensory units in medial articular nerve by local mechanical stimulation of knee joint. *J Neurophysiol* 1983;49(1):35–44.
16. Tal M, Bennett GJ. Extra-territorial pain in rats with a peripheral mononeuropathy: mechano-hyperalgesia and mechano-allodynia in the territory of an uninjured nerve. *Pain (Netherlands)* 1994;57(3):375–382.
17. Willis WD, Westlund KN. Neuroanatomy of the pain system and of the pathways that modulate pain. *J Clin Neurophysiol* 1997;14(1):2–31.
18. O'Connell PJ, Pingle SC, Ahern GP. Dendritic cells do not transduce inflammatory stimuli via the capsaicin receptor TRPV1. *FEBS Lett* 2005;579(23):5135–5139.
19. Fields HL. Pain: an unpleasant topic. *Pain (Netherlands)* 1999;(Suppl 6): S61–S69.
20. Woolf CJ, Mannion RJ. *Lancet* 1999;353:1959–1964.
21. Rome H, Rome J. Limbically augmented pain syndrome (LAPS): kindling, corticolimbic sensitization, and the convergence of affective and sensory symptoms in chronic pain disorders. *Pain Med* 2000;1(1):7–23.
22. Artal N, Bouhassira D. Mechanisms of pain in painful neuropathy. *Acta Neurol Scand* 1999;173:12–24.
23. Abraham WC, Robins A. Memory retention—the synaptic stability versus plasticity dlemma. Trends Neurosci 2005;28(2):73–78.
24. Rainville P, Duncan GH, Price DD, et al. Pain affect encoded in human anterior cingulate but not somatosensory cortex. *Science* 1997;277 (5328):968–971.
25. Rainville P, Duncan GH, Price DD, et al. Pain Affect Encoded in Human Anterior Cingulate But Not Somatosensory Cortex. *Science* 1997;277:968–971.
26. Vogt BA. Pain and emotion interactions in subregions of the cingulated gyrus. *Rev Neurosci* 2005;6:533–544.
27. Iles RA, Davidson M, Taylor NF. Psychosocial predictors of failure to return to work in non-chronic non-specific low back pain: a systematic review. *Occup Environ Med* 2008;65(8):507–517.
28. Gallagher RM, Rauh V, Haugh L, et al. Determinants of return to work in low back pain. *Pain* 1989;39(1):55–68.
29. Vowles KE, McCracken LM, Eccleston C. Patient functioning and catastrophizing in chronic pain: the mediating effects of acceptance. *Health Psychol* 2008;27(Suppl2):S136–S143.
30. Vowles KE, McCracken LM, Eccleston C. Processes of change in treatment for chronic pain: the contributions of pain, acceptance, and catastrophizing. *Eur J Pain* 2007;11(7):779–787. Epub Feb 15, 2007.
31. McWilliams LA, Asmundson GJ. The relationship of adult attachment dimensions to pain-related fear, hypervigilance, and catastrophizing. *Pain* 2007;127(1–2):27–34.
32. Gallagher RM, Verma S. Mood and anxiety disorders in chronic pain. In R. Dworkin and W. Brieghtbart *Psychosocial and Psychiatric Aspects of Pain: A Handbook for Health Care Providers.* Progress in Pain Research and Management, Vol. 27. Seattle: IASP Press, 2004.
33. McWilliams LA, Cox BJ, Enns MW. Mood and anxiety disorders associated with chronic pain: an examination in a nationally representative sample. *Pain* 2003;106(1–2):127–33.
34. McWilliams LA, Clara IP, Murphy PD, et al. Associations between arthritis and a broad range of psychiatric disorders: findings from a nationally representative sample. *J Pain* 2008;9(1):37–44.
35. Gureje O, Von Korff M, Simon GE, et al. Persistent Pain and Well-being: A World Health Organization Study in Primary Care *JAMA* 1998;280:147–151.
36. Miller GE, Rohleder N, Stetler C, et al. Clinical Depression and Regulation of the Inflammatory Response During Acute Stress. *Psychosomatic Medicine* 2005;67:679–687.
37. Gallagher RM, Marbach J, Raphael K, et al. Is there co-morbidity between temporomandibular pain dysfunction syndrome and depression? A pilot study. *Clin J Pain* 1991;7:219–225.
38. Gallagher RM, Marbach J, Raphael K, et al. Seasonal Variation in chronic TMPDS Pain and Mood Intensity. *Pain* 1995;61(1):113–120.
39. Dohrenwend B, Marbach J, Raphael K, Gallagher RM. Why is depression co-morbid with chronic facial pain? A family study test of alternative hypotheses. *Pain* 1999;83:183–192.
40. Raphael K, Janal NM, Nayak S, et al. Familial aggregation of depression in fibromyalgia: a community-based test of alternate hypotheses. *Pain* 2004;110:449–460.
41. Arnold LM, Hudson JI, Hess EV, et al. Family study of fibromyalgia. *Arthritis Rheum* 2004;50(3):944–952.
42. Russell IJ, Michalek JE, Vipraio GA, et al. Platelet 3H-imipramine uptake receptor density and serum serotonin levels in patients with fibromyalgia/fibrositis syndrome. *J Rheumatol* 1992a;19:104–109.
43. Russell IJ, Vaeroy H, Javors M, Nyberg F. Cerebrospinal fluid biogenic amine metabolites in fibromyalgia/fibrositis syndrome and rheumatoid arthritis. *Arthritis Rheum* 1992b;35:550–556.
44. Schwarz MJ, Spath M, Muller-Bardorff H, et al. Relationship of substance P,5-hydroxyindole acetic acid and tryptophan in serum of fibromyalgia patients. *Neurosci Lett* 1999;259:196–198.
45. Yunus MB, Dailey JW, Aldag JC, et al. Plasma and urinary catecholamines in primary fibromyalgia: a controlled study. *J Rheumatol* 1992;19:95–97.
46. Charney DS. Monoamine dysfunction and the pathophysiology and treatment of depression. *J Clin Psychiatry* 1998;59(Suppl 14):11–14.
47. Hirschfeld RM. History and evolution of the monoamine hypothesis of depression. *J Clin Psychiatry* 2000;61:4–6.
48. Bondy B, Spaeth M, Offenbaecher M, et al. The T102C polymorphism of the 5-HT2A-receptor gene in fibromyalgia. *Neurobiol Dis* 1999; 6:433–439.
49. Ebstein RP, Cohen H, Neumann L. An association between FMS and the serotonin transporter promoter region (5-HTTLPR) polymorphism and relationship to anxiety-related personality traits. *Am J Med Genet* 2001;627:105.
50. Gursoy S. Absence of association of the serotonin transporter gene polymorphism with the mentally healthy subset of fibromyalgia patients. *Clin Rheumatol* 2002;21:194–197.
51. Offenbaecher M, Bondy B, de Jonge S, et al. Possible association of fibromyalgia with a polymorphism in the serotonin transporter gene regulatory region. *Arthritis Rheum* 1999;42(11):2482–2488.
52. Kendler KS, Kessler RC, Neale MC, et al. The prediction of major depression in women: toward an integrated etiologic model. *Am J Psychiatry* 1993;150:1139–1148.
53. Riso LP, Miyatake RK, Thase ME. The search for determinants of chronic depression: a review of six factors. *J Affect Disord* 2002;70(2): 103–115.
54. Shrout PE, Link BG, Dohrenwend BP, et al. Characterizing life events as risk factors for depression: the role of fateful loss events. *J Abnorm Psychol* 1989;98(4):460–467.
55. Tennant C. Life events, stress and depression: a review of recent findings. *Aust N Z J Psychiatry* 2002;36:173–182.
56. Raphael KG, Natelson BH, Janal MN, Nayak S. A community-based survey of fibromyalgia-like pain complaints following the World Trade Center terrorist attacks. *Pain* 2002;100(1–2):131–139.
57. Davis MC, Zautra AJ, Reich JW. Vulnerability to stress among women in chronic pain from fibromyalgia and osteoarthritis. *Ann Behav Med* 2001;23:215–226.

58. Caspi A, Sugden K, Moffitt TE, et al. Influence of Life Stress on Depression: Moderation by a Polymorphism in the 5-HTT Gene, *Science* 2003;301(5631):386–389.
59. Moseley GL. Is successful rehabilitation of complex regional pain syndrome due to sustained attention to the affected limb? A randomized clinical trial. *Pain* 2005;114(1–2):54–61.
60. Moseley GI. Graded motor imagery for pathologic pain: a randomized controlled trial. *Neurology* 2006;97:2129–2134.
61. deCharms RC, Maeda F, Glover GH, et al. Control over brain activation and pain learned by using real-time functional MRI (biofeedback) *Proc Natl Acad Sci U S A* 2005;102(51):18626–18631.
62. Bremner JD, et al., MRI and PET study of deficits in hippocampal structure and function in women with childhood sexual abuse and posttraumatic stress disorder. *Am J Psychiatry* 2003;160:924–932.
63. Mohanakrishnan Menon P, Nasrallah H, Lyons J, et al. Single-voxel proton MR spectroscopy of right versus left hippocampi in PTSD. *Psychiatry Research: Neuroimaging* 2003;123:101–108.
64. Lindauer RJL, Vlieger EJ, Jalink M, et al. Smaller hippocampal volume in Dutch police officers with posttraumatic stress disorder. *Biol Psy* 2004;56(5):356–363.
65. Hedges DW, Allen S, Tate D, et al. *Cognitive & Behavioral Neurology* 2003;16(4):219–224.
66. Hadjikhani N, de Gelder B. Seeing fearful body expressions activates the fusiform cortex and amygdala. *Current Biol* 2003;24:2201–2205.
67. Hariri A, Mattay V, Tessitore A, et al. Neocortical modulation of the amygdala response to fearful stimuli. *Biol Psy* 2003;53(6):494–501.
68. Morris JS, Dolan RJ. Dissociable amygdala and orbitofrontal responses during reversal fear conditioning. *Neuro Image* 2004;22:372–380.
69. Hyman S, Nestler E. *The molecular foundations of psychiatry—overview of synaptic neurotransmission*. Washington DC: American Psychiatric Press Inc., 1993:1–239.
70. American Psychiatric Association. *Diagnostic and statistical manual of mental disorders*, 4th ed. Washington, DC: American Psychiatric Press, 1994.
71. O'Brien CP. Drug addiction and drug abuse. In: Brunton LL, Lazo JS, Parker KL eds. *Goodman and Gilman's pharmacological basis of therapeutics*, 11th ed. New York: McGraw-Hill, 2006:607–625.
72. Basbaum AI. Insights into the development of opioid tolerance. *Pain* 1995;61:349–352.
73. Solomon R. The opponent-process theory of acquired motivation: the costs of pleasure and the benefits of pain. *Am Psychol* 1980;35(8):691–712.
74. Koob GF, Stinus L, Le Moal M, et al. Opponent process theory of motivation: neurobiological evidence from studies of opiate dependence. *Neurosci Biobehav Rev* 1989;13:135–140.
75. Koob GF, Le Moal M. Drug addiction, dysregulation of reward, and allostasis. *Neuropsychopharmacology* 2001;24(2):97–129.
76. Koob GF, Le Moal M. Addiction and the brain antireward system. *Annu Rev Psychol* 2008;59:29–53.
77. Christie MJ. Cellular neuroadaptations to chronic opioids: tolerance, withdrawal and addiction. *Br J Pharmacol* 2008;154(2):384–396.
78. Koch T, Höllt V. Role of receptor internalization in opioid tolerance and dependence. *Pharmacol Ther* 2008;117(2):199–206.
79. Chao J, Nestler EJ. Molecular neurobiology of drug addiction. *Annu Rev Med* 2004;55:113–123.
80. Finn AK, Whistler JL. Endocytosis of the mu opioid receptor reduces tolerance and a cellular hallmark of opiate withdrawal. *Neuron* 2001; 32(5):829–839.
81. Bailey CP, Connor M. Opioids: cellular mechanisms of tolerance and physical dependence. *Curr Opin Pharmacol* 2005;5(1):60–68.
82. Redmond DE, Krystal JH. Multiple mechanisms of withdrawal from opioid drugs. *Ann Rev Neurosci* 1984;7:443–478.
83. Gold MS, Miller NS. The neurobiology of drug and alcohol addictions. In: Miller NS, Gold MS eds. *Pharmacological therapies for drug and alcohol addictions*. New York: Marcel Dekker, 1995:31–44.
84. Koob GF, Bloom FE. Cellular and molecular mechanisms of drug dependence. *Science* 1988;242:715–723.
85. Bruijnzeel AW, Repetto M, Gold MS. Neurobiological mechanisms in addictive and psychiatric disorders. *Psychiatr Clin North Am* 2004;27(4): 661–674.
86. Cleck JN, Blendy JA. Making a bad thing worse: adverse effects of stress on drug addiction. *J Clin Invest* 2008;118(2):454–461.
87. Sinha R. The role of stress in addiction relapse. *Curr Psychiatry Rep* 2007; 9(5):388–395.
88. Koob G, Kreek MJ. Stress, dysregulation of drug reward pathways, and the transition to drug dependence. *Am J Psychiatry* 2007;164(8): 1149–1159.
89. Kreek MJ, Koob GF. Drug dependence: stress and dysregulation of brain reward pathways. *Drug Alcohol Depend* 1998;51:23–47.
90. Kita M, Goodkin DE. Drugs used to treat spasticity. *Drugs* 2000;59(3): 487–495.
91. Taricco M, Pagliacci MC, Telaro E, Adone R. Pharmacological interventions for spasticity following spinal cord injury: results of a Cochrane systematic review. *Eur Medicophys* 2006;42(1):5–15.
92. Bahn EL, Holt KR. Procedural sedation and analgesia: a review and new concepts. *Emerg Med Clin North Am* 2005;23(2):503–517.
93. Mazurek MS. Sedation and analgesia for procedures outside the operating room. *Semin Pediatr Surg* 2004;13(3):166–173.
94. Devane WA, Hanus L, Breuer A, et al. Isolation and structure of a brain constituent that binds to the cannabinoid receptor. *Science* 1992;258: 1946–1949.
95. Herkenham M. In: Pertwee RG ed. *Cannabinoid receptors*. New York: Academic Press, 1995:145–166.
96. Matsuda LA, Lolait SJ, Brownstein MJ, et al. Structure of a cannabinoid receptor and functional expression of the cloned cDNA *Nature* 1990; 346:561–564.
97. Mao J, Price DD, Lu J, et al. Two distinctive antinociceptive systems in rats with pathological pain. *Neurosci Lett* 2000;280:13–16.
98. Rog DJ, Nurmikko TJ, Young CA. Oromucosal delta9-tetrahydrocannabinol/cannabidiol for neuropathic pain associated with multiple sclerosis: an uncontrolled, open-label, 2-year extension trial. *Clin Ther* 2007;29(9):2068–2079.
99. Wade DT, Makela P, Robson P, House H, Bateman C. Do cannabis-based medicinal extracts have general or specific effects on symptoms in multiple sclerosis? A double-blind, randomized, placebo-controlled study on 160 patients. *Mult Scler* 2004;10(4):434–441.
100. Hosking RD, Zajicek JP. Therapeutic potential of cannabis in pain medicine. *Br J Anaesth* 2008;101(1):59–68.
101. Palazzo E, Marabese I, de Novellis V, et al. Metabotropic and NMDA glutamate receptors participate in the cannabinoid-induced antinociception. *Neuropharmacology* 2001;40(3):319–326.
102. Palazzos E, de Novellis V, Marabese I, et al. Metabotropic glutamate and cannabinoid receptor crosstalk in periaqueductal grey pain processing. *Curr Neuropharmacol* 2006;4(3):225–231.
103. Nunes EV, Rounsaville BJ. Comorbidity of substance use with depression and other mental disorders. From *Diagnostic and Statistical Manual of Mental Disorders*, 4th ed (DSM-IV) to DSM-V. *Addiction* 2006;101 (Suppl 1):89–96.
104. Schuckit MA. Comorbidity between substance use disorders and psychiatric conditions. *Addiction* 2006;101(Suppl 1):76–88.
105. Begré S, Traber M, Gerber M, von Känel R. Change in pain severity with open label venlafaxine use in patients with a depressive symptomatology: an observational study in primary care. *Eur Psychiatry* 2008;23(3):178–186.
106. Krebs EE, Gaynes BN, Gartlehner G, et al. Treating the physical symptoms of depression with second-generation antidepressants: a systematic review and meta-analysis. *Psychosomatics* 2008;49(3):191–198.
107. Perahia DG, Pritchett YL, Desaiah D, Raskin J. Efficacy of duloxetine in painful symptoms: an analgesic or antidepressant effect? *Int Clin Psychopharmacol* 2006;21(6):311–317.
108. Compton MA. Cold-pressor pain tolerance in opiate and cocaine abusers: correlates of drug type and use status. *J Pain Symptom Manage* 1994;9:462–473.
109. Compton P, Charuvastra C, Kintaudi K, et al. Pain responses in methadone-maintained opioid abusers. *J Pain Symptom Manage* 2000; 20(4):237–245.
110. Compton P, Charuvastra VC, Ling W. Pain intolerance in opioid-maintained former opiate addicts: effect of long-acting maintenance agent. *Drug Alcohol Depend* 2001;63:139–146.

111. Gutstein HB, Akil H. In: Brunton LL, Lazo JS, Parker KL eds. *Goodman and Gilman's pharmacological basis of therapeutics*, 11th ed. New York: McGraw-Hill, 2006:457–590.
112. Albutt C. On the abuse of hypodermic injections of morphia. *Practitioner* 1870;3:327–330.
113. Martin J, Inglis J. Pain tolerance and narcotic addiction. *Br J Sociol Clin Psychol* 1965;4:224–229.
114. Ho A, Dole V. Pain perception in drug-free and in methadone-maintained human ex-addicts. *Proc Soc Exp Biol Med* 1979;162: 392–395.
115. Doverty M, White J, Somogyi A, et al. Hyperalgesic responses in methadone maintained patients. *Pain* 2001;90:91–96.
116. Schall U, Katta T, Pries E, et al. Pain perception of intravenous heroin users on maintenance therapy with levomethadone. *Pharmacopsychiatry* 1996;29:176–179.
117. Athanasos P, Smith CS, White JM, et al. Methadone maintenance patients are cross tolerant to the antinociceptive effects of very high plasma morphine concentrations. *Pain* 2006;120:267–275.
118. Pud D, Cohen D, Lawental E, Eisenberg E. Opioids and abnormal pain perception: new evidence from a study of chronic opioid addicts and healthy subjects. *Drug Alcohol Depend* 2006;82: 218–223.
119. Angst MS, Koppert W, Pahl I, et al. Short-term infusion of the mu-opioid agonist remifentanil in humans causes hyperalgesia during withdrawal. *Pain 2003*;106(1–2):49–57.
120. Angst MS, Clark JD. Opioid-induced hyperalgesia; a qualitative systematic review. *Anesthesiology* 2006;104:570–587.
121. Chu LF, Angst MS, Clark D. Opioid-induced hyperalgesia in humans: molecular mechanisms and clinical considerations. *Clin J Pain* 2008; 24(6):479–496.
122. Koppert W, Angst M, Alsheimer M, et al. Naloxone provokes similar pain facilitation as observed after short-term infusion of remifentanil in humans. *Pain* 2003;106(1–2):91–99.
123. Li X, Angst MS, Clark D. A murine model of opioid-induced hyperalgesia. *Brain Res Mol Brain Res* 2001;86:56–62.
124. Mao J. Opioid-induced abnormal pain sensitivity: implications in clinical opioid therapy. *Pain* 2002;100:213–217.
125. Simonnet G. Opioids: from analgesia to anti-hyperalgesia? *Pain* 2005; 118(1-2):8–9.
126. Vanderah TW, Ossipov MH, Lai J, et al. Mechanisms of opioid–induced pain and antinociceptive tolerance: descending facilitation and spinal dynorphin. *Pain* 2001a;92:5–9.
127. Kaplan H, Fields HL. (). Hyperalgesia during acute opioid abstinence: evidence for a nociceptive facilitating function of the rostral ventromedial medulla. *J Neurosci* 1991;11:1433–1439.
128. Martin WR, Gilbert PE, Jasinski PE, Martin CD. An analysis of naltrexone precipitated abstinence in morphine-dependent chronic spinal dogs. *J Pharmacol Exp Ther* 1987;240:565–570.
129. Sweitzer SR, Allen CP, Zissen MH, Kendig JJ. Mechanical allodynia and thermal hyperalgesia upon acute opioid withdrawal in the neonatal rat. *Pain* 2004;110:269–280.
130. Tilson HA, Rech RH, Stolman S. Hyperalgesia during withdrawal as a means of measuring the degree of dependence in morphine dependent rats. *Psychopharmacologia* 1973;28:287–300.
131. Jasinski DS. Assessment of the abuse liability of the morphine-like drugs (methods used in man). In: Martin WR ed. *Handbook of experimental pharmacology, volume 45: Drug addiction I.* New York: Springer-Verlag, 1977:197–158.
132. Bederson JB, Fields HL, Barbaro NM. Hyperalgesia during naloxone-precipitated withdrawal from morphine is associated with increased on-cell activity in the rostral ventromedial medulla. *Somatosens Mot Res* 1990;7:185–203.
133. Grilly DM, Gowans GC. Acute morphine dependence: effects observed in shock and light discrimination tasks. *Psychopharmacol (Berl)* 1986;88: 500–504.
134. Kim DH, Barbaro NM, Fields HL. Dose response relationship for hyperalgesia following naloxone precipitated withdrawal from morphine. *Soc Neurosci Abstr* 1988;14:174.
135. Kim DH, Fields HL, Barbaro NM. Morphine analgesia and acute physical dependence: rapid onset of two opposing, dose-related processes. *Brain Res* 1990;516(1):37–40.
136. Chu L, Angst M, Clark, D. Opioids in non-cancer pain: measurement of opioid-induced tolerance and hyperalgesia in pain patients on chronic opioid therapy. *J Pain* 2004;5:S73–S86.
137. Holtman JR, Wala EP. Characterization of morphine-induced hyperalgesia in male and female rats. *Pain* 2005;114:62–70.
138. Ossipov MH, Lai J, King T, et al. Underlying mechanisms of pronociceptive consequences of prolonged morphine exposure. *Peptide Sci* 2005;80:319–324.
139. Celerier E, Rivat C, Jun Y, et al. Long-lasting hyperalgesia induced by fentanyl in rats: preventative effect of ketamine. *Anesthesiology* 2000;92: 465–472.
140. Gardell LR, King T, Ossipov MH, et al. Opioid receptor-mediated hyperalgesia and antinociceptive tolerance induced by sustained opiate delivery. *Neurosci Lett* 2005;396:44–49.
141. Ibuki T, Dunbar SA, Yaksh TL. Effect of transient naloxone antagonism in tolerance development in rats receiving continuous spinal morphine infusion. *Pain* 1997;70:125–132.
142. Van Elstraete AC, Sitbon P, Trabold F, et al. A single dose of intrathecal morphine in rats induces long-lasting hyperalgesia: the protective effect of prior administration of ketamine. *Anesth Analg* 2005;101:1750–1756.
143. Jasinski D. Tolerance and dependence to opiates. *Acta Anaesthesiol Scand* 1997;41:184–186.
144. Colpaert FC. System theory of pain and of opiate analgesia: no tolerance to opiates. *Pharmacol Rev* 1996;48:355–402.
145. Colpaert FC. Mechanisms of opioid-induced pain and antinociceptive tolerance: signal transduction. *Pain* 2002;95:287–288.
146. Celerier E, Laulin JP, Larcher A, et al. Evidence for opiate-activated NMDA processes masking opiate analgesia in rats. *Brain Res* 1999;847: 18–25.
147. Celerier E, Laulin JP, Corcuff JB, et al. Progressive enhancement of delayed hyperalgesia induced by repeated heroin administration: a sensitization process. *J Neurosci* 2001;21:4074–4080.
148. Laulin JP, Celerier E, Larcher A, et al. Opiate tolerance to daily heroin administration: an apparent phenomenon associated with enhanced pain sensitivity. *Neuroscience* 1999;89(3):631–636.
149. Finnerup NB, Otto M, McQuay HJ, et al. Algorithm for neuropathic pain treatment: an evidence based proposal. *Pain* 2005;118:289–305.
150. Foley, KM. Opioids and chronic neuropathic pain. *N Engl J Med* 2003; 348:1279–1281.
151. Mao J, Price DD, Mayer DJ. Thermal hyperalgesia in association with the development of morphine tolerance in rats: roles of excitatory amino acids receptors and protein kinase C. *Jof Neurosci* 1994;14: 2301–2312.
152. Mao J, Price DD, Mayer DJ. Experimental mononeuropathy reduces the antinociceptive effects of morphine: implications for the common intracellular mechanisms involved in morphine tolerance and neuropathic pain. *Pain* 1995a;61:353–364.
153. Mao J, Price DD, Mayer DJ. Mechanisms of hyperalgesia and morphine tolerance: a current view of their possible interactions. *Pain* 1995b;62: 259–274.
154. Mayer D, Mao J, Price D. The association of neuropathic pain, morphine tolerance and dependence, and the translocation of protein Kinase C. *NIDA Res Monogr 147.* Rockville, MD: National Institute on Drug Abuse, 1995a:269–298.
155. Mayer D, Mao J, Price D. The development of morphine tolerance and dependence is associated with translocation of protein kinase C. *Pain* 1995b;61:365–374.
156. Dogrul A, Bilsky EJ, Ossipov MH, et al. Spinal L-type calcium channel blockage abolishes opioid-induced sensory hypersensitivity and antinociceptive tolerance. *Anesth Analg* 2005;101:1730–1735.
157. Gardell LR, Wang R, Burgess SE, et al. Sustained morphine exposure induces a spinal dynorphin-dependent enhancement of excitatory transmitter release from primary afferent fibers. *J Neurosci* 2002;2: 6747–6755.

158. King T, Gardell LR, Wang R, et al. Role of NK-1 neurotransmission in opioid-induced hyperalgesia. *Pain* 2005;116:276–288.
159. Lim G, Wang S, Zeng Q, et al. Evidence for a long-term influence on morphine tolerance after previous morphine exposure: role of neuronal glucocorticoid receptors. *Pain* 2005;114:81–92.
160. Raghavendra V, Rutkowski MD, DeLeo JA. The role of spinal neuroimmune activation in morphine tolerance/hyperalgesia in neuropathic and sham-operated rats. *J Neurosci* 2002;22:9980–9989.
161. Vanderah TW, Gardell LR, Burgess SE, et al. Dynorphin promotes abnormal pain and spinal opioid antinociceptive tolerance. *J Neurosci* 2000;20(18):7074–7079.
162. Vanderah TW, Suengaga NM, Ossipov MH, et al. Tonic descending facilitation from the rostral ventromedial medulla mediates opioid-induced abnormal pain and antinociceptive tolerance. *J Neurosci* 2001b; 21:279–286.
163. Mayer DJ, Mao J, Holt J, Price DD. Cellular mechanisms of neuropathic pain, morphine tolerance, and their interactions. *Proc Natl Acad Sci U S A* 1999;96(14):7731–7736.
164. Dunbar SA, Pulai IJ. Repetitive opioid abstinence causes progressive hyperalgesia sensitive to N-methyl-D-aspartate receptor blockade in the rat. *J Pharmacol Exp Ther* 1998;284(2):678–686.
165. Dunbar S, Yaksh TL. Concurrent spinal infusion of MK801 blocks spinal tolerance and dependence induced by chronic intrathecal morphine in the rat. *Anesthesiology* 1996;84(5):1177–1188.
166. Larcher A, Laulin JP, Celerier E, et al. Acute tolerance associated with a single opiate administration: involvement of N-methyl-D-aspartate-dependent pain facilitatory systems. *Neuroscience* 1998;84(2):583–589.
167. Richebe P, Rivat C, Creton C, et al. Nitrous oxide revisited. *Anesthesiology* 2005;105:845–854.
168. Portenoy R, Bennett G, Katz N, et al. Enhancing opioid analgesia with NMDA-receptor antagonists: clarifying the clinical importance. *J Pain Symptom Manage* 2000;19(Suppl 1):S57–S64.
169. Price D, Mayer D, Mao J, et al. NMDA-receptor antagonists and opioid receptor interactions as related to analgesia and tolerance. *J Pain Symptom Manage* 2000;19(Suppl 1):S7–S11.
170. Sang C. NMDA-receptor antagonists in neuropathic pain: experimental methods to clinical trials. *J Pain Symptom Manage* 2000;19(Suppl 1): S21–S25.
171. Weinbroum A, Rudick V, Paret G, et al. The role of dextromethorphan in pain control. *Can J Anaesth* 2000;47(6):585–596.
172. Bisaga A, Popik P. In search of a new pharmacological treatment for drug and alcohol addiction: N-methyl-D-aspartate (NMDA) antagonists. *Drug Alcohol Depend* 2000;59:1–15.
173. Elliott K, Hynansky A, Inturrisi C. Dextromethorphane attenuates and reverses analgesic tolerance to morphine. *Pain* 1994;59(3):361–368.
174. Pasternak G, Kolesnikov Y, Babey AM. Perspectives on the N-methyl-D-aspartate/nitric oxide cascade and opioid tolerance. *Neuropsychopharmacology* 1995;13(4):309–313.
175. Trujillo K. Effects of noncompetitive N-methyl-D-aspartate receptor antagonists on opiate tolerance and physical dependence. *Neuropsychopharmacology* 1995;13(4):301–307.
176. Compton PA, Ling W, Torrington MA. Lack of effect of chronic dextromethorphan on experimental pain tolerance in methadone-maintained patients. *Addict Biol* 2008;13(3–4):393–402.
177. Gardell LR, King T, Ossipov MH, et al. Opioid receptor-mediated hyperalgesia and antinociceptive tolerance induced by sustained opiate delivery. *Neurosci Lett* 2006;396:44–49.
178. Vanderah T, Suenaga N, Ossipov M, et al. Tonic descending facilitation from the rostral ventromedial medulla mediates opioid-induced abnormal pain and antinociceptive tolerance. *J Neurosci* 2001;21(1):279–286.
179. Ossipov MH, Lai J, King T, et al. Antinociceptive and nociceptive actions of opioids. *J Neurobiol* 2004;61:6–148.
180. Ossipov MH, Lai J, King T, et al. Underlying mechanisms of pronociceptive consequences of prolonged morphine exposure. *Biopolymers* 2005;80:319–324.
181. Xie JY, Herman DS, Stiller CO, et al. Cholecystokinin in the rostral ventromedial medulla mediates opioid-induced hyperalgesia and antinociceptive tolerance. *J Neurosci* 2005;25:409–416.
182. Devillers JP, Boisserie F, Laulin JP, et al. Simultaneous activation of spinal antiopioid system (neuropeptide FF) and pain facilitatory circuitry by stimulation of opioid receptors in rats. *Brain Res* 1995;700: 173–181.
183. Leo JA, Tanga FY, Tawfik VL. Neuroimmune activation and neuroinflammation in chronic pain and opioid tolerance/hyperalgesia. *Neuroscientist* 2004;10:40–52.
184. Watkins LR, Maier SF. The pain of being sick: implications of immune-to-brain communication for understanding pain. *Annu Rev Psychol* 2000;51:29–57.
185. Wiesler-Frank J, Maier SF, Watkins LR. Immune-to-brain communication dynamically modulates pain: physiological and pathological consequences. *Brain Behav Immun* 2005;19:104–111.
186. Song P, Zhao ZQ. The involvement of glial cells in the development of morphine tolerance. *Neurosci Res* 2001;39:281–286.
187. Johnston IN, Westbrook RF. Inhibition of morphine analgesia by LPS: role of opioid and NMDA receptors and spinal glia. *Behav Brain Res* 2005;156:75–83.
188. Johnston IN, Milligan ED, Wieseler-Frank J, et al. A role for proinflammatory cytokines and fractalkine in analgesia, tolerance, and subsequent pain facilitation induced by chronic intrathecal morphine. *J Neurosci* 2004;24:7353–7365.
189. Hendrie CA. Naloxone-sensitive hyperalgesia follows analgesia induced by morphine and environmental stimulation. *Pharmacol Biochem Behav* 1989;32:961–966.
190. McNally GP. Pain facilitatory circuits in the mammalian central nervous system: their behavioral significance and role in morphine analgesic tolerance. *Neurosci Biobehav Rev* 1999;23(8):1059–1078.
191. Krank M, Hinson R, Siegel S. Conditional hyperalgesia is elicited by environmental signals of morphine. *Behav Neural Biol* 1981;32: 148–157.
192. Siegel S, Hinson RE, Krank MD. The role of predrug signals in morphine analgesic tolerance: support for a Pavlovian conditioning model of tolerance. *J Exp Psychol* 1978;4:188–196.
193. Chia YY, Liu K, Wang JJ, et al. Intraoperative high dose fentanyl induces postoperative fentanyl tolerance. *Can J Anaesth* 1999;46(9):872–877.
194. Cooper DW, Lindsay SL, Ryall DM, et al. Does intrathecal fentanyl produce acute cross-tolerance to i.v. morphine? *Br J Anaesth* 1997;78(3): 311–313.
195. Hansen EG, Duedahl TH, Rømsing J, et al. Intra-operative remifentanil might influence pain levels in the immediate post-operative period after major abdominal surgery. *Acta Anaesthesiol Scand* 2005;49(10):1464–1470.
196. Guignard B, Bossard AE, Coste C, et al. Acute opioid tolerance: intraoperative remifentanil increases postoperative pain and morphine requirement. *Anesthesiology* 2000;93(2):409–417.
197. Ali NM. Hyperalgesic response in a patient receiving high concentrations of spinal morphine. *Anesthesiology* 1986;65(4):449.
198. Mercadante S, Ferrera P, Villari P, Arcuri E. Hyperalgesia: an emerging iatrogenic syndrome. *J Pain Symptom Manage* 2003;26(2):769–775.
199. Mercadante S, Arcuri E. Hyperalgesia and opioid switching. *Am J Hosp Palliat Care* 2005;22(4):291–294.
200. Sjøgren P, Jonsson T, Jensen NH, et al. Hyperalgesia and myoclonus in terminal cancer patients treated with continuous intravenous morphine. *Pain* 1993;55(1):93–97.
201. Okon TR, George ML. Fentanyl-induced neurotoxicity and paradoxic pain. *J Pain Symptom Manage* 2008;35(3):327–333.
202. Devulder J. Hyperalgesia induced by high-dose intrathecal sufentanil in neuropathic pain. *J Neurosurg Anesthesiol* 1997;9(2):146–148.
203. Chu LF, Clark DJ, Angst MS. Opioid tolerance and hyperalgesia in chronic pain patients after one month of oral morphine therapy: a preliminary prospective study. *J Pain* 2006;7(1):43–48.
204. Chou R, Huffman LH; American Pain Society; American College of Physicians. Medications for acute and chronic low back pain: a review of the evidence for an American Pain Society/American College of Physicians clinical practice guideline. *Ann Intern Med* 2007;147(7):505–514.
205. Eisenberg E, McNicol E, Carr DB. Opioids for neuropathic pain. *Cochrane Database Syst Rev* 2006;3:CD006146.

206. Furlan AD, Sandoval JA, Mailis-Gagnon A, Tunks E. Opioids for chronic noncancer pain: a meta-analysis of effectiveness and side effects. *CMAJ* 2006;174(11):1589–1594.
207. Martell BA, O'Connor PG, Kerns RD, et al. Systematic review: opioid treatment for chronic back pain: prevalence, efficacy, and association with addiction. *Ann Intern Med* 2007;146(2):116–127.
208. Kalso E, Edwards JE, Moore RA, McQuay HJ. Opioids in chronic non-cancer pain: systematic review of efficacy and safety. *Pain* 2004;112(3): 372–380.
209. Fields HL. Should we be reluctant to prescribe opioids for chronic non-malignant pain? *Pain* 2007;129(3):233–234.
210. Caldwell JR, Hale ME, Boyd RE, et al. Treatment of osteoarthritis pain with controlled release oxycodone or fixed combination oxycodone plus acetaminophen added to nonsteroidal antiinflammatory drugs: a double blind, randomized, multicenter, placebo controlled trial. *J Rheumatol* 1999;26(4):862–869.
211. Moulin DE, Iezzi A, Amireh R, et al. Randomized trial of oral morphine for chronic non-cancer pain. *Lancet* 1996;347(8995):143–147.
212. Moulin DE, Palma D, Watling C, Schulz V. Methadone in the management of intractable neuropathic noncancer pain. *Can J Neurol Sci* 2005;32(3):340–343.
213. Ballantyne JC. Opioids for chronic pain: taking stock. *Pain* 2006;125 (1–2):3–4.
214. Bertilsson L, Dahl ML, Dalén P, Al-Shurbaji A. Molecular genetics of CYP2D6: clinical relevance with focus on psychotropic drugs. *Br J Clin Pharmacol* 2002;53(2):111–122.
215. Ingelman-Sundberg M, Johansson I, Persson I, et al. Genetic polymorphism of cytochrome P450. Functional consequences and possible relationship to disease and alcohol toxicity. In: Jansson B, Jornval H, Rydberg U, et al. eds. *Toward a molecular basis of alcohol use and abuse.* Basel, Switzerland: Birkhauser Verlag, 1994:197–207.
216. Gonzalez FJ. Human cytochrome P450: possible roles of drug-metabolizing enzymes and polymorphic drug oxidation in addiction. *NIDA Res Monogr 111*. Rockville, MD: National Institute on Drug Abuse, 1991:202–213.
217. Lötsch J, Skarke C, Liefhold J, Geisslinger G. Genetic predictors of the clinical response to opioid analgesics: clinical utility and future perspectives. *Clin Pharmacokinet* 2004;43(14):983–1013.
218. Maurer PM, Bartkowski RR. Drug interactions of clinical significance with opioid analgesics. *Drug Safety* 1993;8:30–48.
219. Otton SV, Schadel M, Cheung SW, et al. CYP2D6 phenotype determines the metabolic conversion of hydrocodone to hydromorphone. *Clin Pharmacol Ther* 1993;54:463–472.
220. Oertel B, Lötsch J. Genetic mutations that prevent pain: implications for future pain medication. *Pharmacogenomics* 2008;9(2):179–194.
221. Sindrup SH, Poulsen L, Brosen K, et al. (1993). Are poor metabolizers of sparteine/debri Liebmann P, Lehofer M, Schonauer-Cejpek M et al. Pain sensitivity in former opioid addicts. *Lancet* 1994;344:1031– 1032.
222. Liebmann P, Lehofer M, Moser M, et al. Persistent analgesia in former opiate addicts is resistant to blockade of endogenous opioids. *Biol Psychiatry* 1997;42:962–964.
223. Liebmann P, Lehofer M, Moser M, et al. Nervousness and pain sensitivity: II. Changed relation in ex-addicts as a predictor for early relapse. *Psychiatry Res* 1998;79:55–58.
224. Lehofer M, Liebmann P, Moser M, et al. Decreased nociceptive sensitivity: a biological risk marker for opiate dependence? *Addiction* 1997;92 (2):163–166.
225. Sindrup SH, Poulsen L, Brosen K, et al. Are poor metabolizers of sparteine/debrisuquine less pain tolerant than extensive metabolizers? *Pain* 1993;53:335–339.
226. Mogil JS, Przemyslaw M, Flodman P, et al. One or two genetic loci mediate high opiate analgesia in selectively bred mice. *Pain* 1995;60: 125–135.
227. Mogil JS, Wilson SG, Bon K, et al. Heritability of nociception: I. Responses of 11 inbred mouse strains on 12 measures of nociception. *Pain* 1999;80:67–82.
228. Sudakov SK, Goldberg SR, Borisova EV, et al. Differences in morphine reinforcement property in two inbred rat strains: associations with cortical receptors, behavioral activity, analgesia and the cataleptic effects of morphine. *Psychopharmacology (Berl)* 1993;112(2-3):183–188.
229. Elmer GI, Pieper JO, Goldberg SR, George FR. Opioid operant self-administration, analgesia, stimulation, and respiratory depression in mu-deficient mice. *Psychopharmacology (Berl)* 1995;117(1):23–31.
230. Elmer GI, Pieper JO, Negus SS, Woods JH. Genetic variance in nociception and its relationship to the potency of morphine-induced analgesia in thermal and chemical tests. *Pain* 1998;75(1):129–140.
231. Belknap JK, Mogil JS, Helms ML, et al. Localization to chromosome 10 of a locus influencing morphine analgesia in crosses derived from C57BL/6 and DBA strains. *Pharmacol Lett* 1995;57:117–124.
232. Semenova S, Kuzmin A, Zvartau E. Strain differences in the analgesic and reinforcing action of morphine in mice. *Pharmacol Biochem Behav* 1995;50(1):17–21.
233. Berrettini WH, Alexander R, Ferraro TN, et al. A study of oral morphine preference in inbred mouse strains. *Psychiatr Genet* 1994: 81–86.
234. Petruzzi R, Ferraro TN, Kurschner VC, et al. The effects of repeated morphine exposure on mu opioid receptor number and affinity in C57BL/6J and DBA/2J mice. *Life Sci* 1997;61:2057–2064.
235. Edwards RR. Genetic predictors of acute and chronic pain. *Curr Rheumatol Rep* 2006;8(6):411–417.
236. Mogil JS, Yu L, Basbaum AI. Pain genes? Natural variation and transgenic mutants. *Annu Rev Neurosci* 2000;23:777-811.
237. Stamer UM, Stüber F. Genetic factors in pain and its treatment. *Curr Opin Anaesthesiol* 2007a;20(5):478–484.
238. Flores CM, Mogil JS. The pharmacogenetics of analgesia: toward a genetically-based approach to pain management. *Pharmacogenomics* 2001;2(3):177–194.
239. Stamer UM, Stüber F. The pharmacogenetics of analgesia. *Expert Opin Pharmacother* 2007b;8(14):2235–2245.
240. Mayer P, Höllt V. Pharmacogenetics of opioid receptors and addiction. *Pharmacogenet Genom* 2006;16(1):1–7.
241. Ikeda K, Ide S, Han W, et al. How individual sensitivity to opiates can be predicted by genetic analyses. *Trends Pharmacol Sci* 2005;26(6): 311–317.
242. Lötsch J, Geisslinger G. Relevance of frequent mu-opioid receptor polymorphisms for opioid activity in healthy volunteers. *Pharmacogenom J* 2006;6(3):200–210.
243. Mogil JS, Yu L, Basbaum AI. Pain genes? Natural variation and transgenic mutants. *Annu Rev Neurosci* 2000;23:777–811.
244. Kim H, Neubert JK, Miguel AS, et al. Genetic influence on variability in human acute experimental pain sensitivity associated with gender, ethnicity and psychological temperament. *Pain* 2004;109:488–496.
245. Caterina MJ, Leffler A, Malmberg AB, et al. Impaired nociception and pain sensation in mice lacking the capsaicin receptor. *Science* 2000; 288(5464):306–313.
246. McKemy DD, Neuhausser WM, Julius D. Identification of a cold receptor reveals a general role for TRP channels in thermosensation. *Nature* 2002;416(6876):52–58.
247. Mogil JS, Ritchie J, Smith SB, et al. Melanocortin-1 receptor gene variants affect pain and mu-opioid analgesia in mice and humans. *J Med Genet* 2005;42(7):583–587.
248. Kest B, Hopkins E, Palmese CA, et al. Genetic variation in morphine analgesic tolerance: a survey of 11 inbred mouse strains. *Pharmacol Biochem Behav* 2002a;73(4):821–828.
249. Kest B, Palmese CA, Hopkins E, et al. Naloxone-precipitated withdrawal jumping in 11 inbred mouse strains: evidence for common genetic mechanisms in acute and chronic morphine physical dependence. *Neuroscience* 2002b;115(2):463–469.
250. Kest B, Palmese CA, Juni A, et al. Mapping of a quantitative trait locus for morphine withdrawal severity. *Mamm Genome* 2004;15(8):610–617.
251. Liang DY, Liao G, Lighthall GK, et al. Genetic variants of the P-glycoprotein gene Abcb1b modulate opioid-induced hyperalgesia, tolerance and dependence. *Pharmacogenet Genom* 2006b;16(11):825–835.
252. Liang DY, Guo T, Liao G, et al. Chronic pain and genetic background interact and influence opioid analgesia, tolerance, and physical dependence. *Pain* 2006a;121(3):232–240.

SUGGESTED READINGS

Abraham WC, Logan B, Greenwood JM, Dragunow M. Induction and experience-dependent consolidation of stable long-term potentiation lasting months in the hippocampus. *J Neurosci* 2002;22(21): 9626–9634.

Anderberg UM, Marteinsdottir I, Theorell T, von Knorring L. The impact of life events in female patients with fibromyalgia and in female healthy controls. *Eur Psychiatry* 2000;15:295–301.

Centers for Disease Control and Prevention. Minino AM, Anderson RN, Fingerhut LA, Boudreault MA, Warner M. Deaths: Injuries, 2002. National Vital statistics reports; vol 54 no 10. Hyattsville, MD: National Center for Health Statistics, 2006.

Compton WM, Volkow ND. Major increases in opioid analgesic abuse in the United States: concerns and strategies. *Drug Alcohol Depend* 2006;81(2): 103–107.

Fishbain DA, Cutler B, Rosomoff H, Steele-Rosomoff R. Pain facilities: a review of their effectiveness and referral selection criteria. *Curr Rev Pain* 1997;1:107–115.

National Institute on Drug Abuse. *NIDA Infofacts: prescription pain and other medications.* Washington, DC: NIDA, National Institutes of Health, 2005. www.drugabuse.gov/infofacts/PainMed.htlm [accessed March 3, 2006].

Office of National Drug Control Policy, Drug Facts. Prescription Drug Abuse. 2007 http://www.whitehousedrugpolicy.gov/drugfact/prescr_drg_abuse.html [accessed September 8, 2007].

Substance Abuse and Mental Health Services Administration, National Survey on Drug Use and Health: Nonmedical Users of Pain Relievers: Characteristics of Recent Initiates (PDF), 2006. http://www.drugabusestatistics.samhsa.gov/2k6/pain/pain.pdf.

Rome H, Rome J. Limbically augmented pain syndrome (LAPS): kindling, corticolimbic sensitization, and the convergence of affective and sensory symptoms in chronic pain disorders. *Pain Med* 2000;1(1):7–23.

CHAPTER 93

Edward C. Covington, MD
Margaret M. Kotz, DO

Psychological Issues in the Management of Pain

This chapter addresses primarily chronic, nonmalignant pain, as its management differs from that of acute, malignant, and recurrent acute pain. Although the focus is on psychologic interventions, it should be recognized that such interventions are most effective when combined with rehabilitation techniques and with opioid and nonopioid pharmacotherapy.

The last 30 years have seen tremendous advances in understandings of the neurobiology of pain. During this same time there have been numerous new medications and improvements in surgical options and other interventions; yet, despite the progress in acute and postsurgical pain, we have seen no reduction in the prevalence of chronic pain or in its associated disability. In fact, in the case of chronic low back pain, the leading pain-related cause of inability to work, we are devoting far more resources to its diagnosis and treatment, yet have apparently worse functional outcomes now than in the past (1).

This seeming paradox may result in part from our failure to adequately address the psychologic and behavioral components of chronic pain. Numerous studies have compellingly demonstrated that psychosocial variables predict onset, chronicity, and outcomes in back pain more than do somatic variables; however, our health care system is arranged in such a way that the profitability of clinical work is virtually unrelated to the benefit provided to the patient or to society as a whole. Thus treatment may be determined more by incomes than by outcomes, which, under present reimbursement policies, leaves psychosocial approaches underused.

This chapter will review the ways in which psychosocial factors impact patients with chronic pain and strategies for addressing them that have demonstrated benefit. Some strategies are applicable by clinicians for improving outcomes, but others are systemic and societal issues that can be addressed only in the aggregate at policy levels.

Chronic pain has always been with us, and few who live a normal lifespan will fully escape it. It is *disability* related to chronic pain that is more recently of epidemic proportions. Back pain has been called a "20th century health care disaster." It is essentially universal, with a lifetime prevalence of 60% to 80%, and has probably always been so; however, back-related disability has increased exponentially (2). In the United States, about 2% of the work force has compensable back pain at any given time (3). A 2002 survey found that 26% of U.S. adults reported low back pain and 14% reported neck pain in the previous 3 months (4). Worsening impact is indicated by the finding that, in 1997, 20.7% of those with back pain reported limitations in physical function, a figure that rose to 24.7% in 2005 (1). This occurred concomitantly with an increase in medications, techniques for fusion and discectomy, acupuncture, intraspinal adhesiolysis, and intradiscal electrical thermocoagulation, among others, and a liberalization of the availability of opioids for chronic pain.

BIOLOGIC FOUNDATIONS

It may be useful to begin a description of the psychologic components of pain by pointing out what they are not, given our historical tendency to equate unexplained with psychogenic. Thirty years of research into the neurobiology of pain has demonstrated that pain is primarily a creation of the nervous system and, especially in the case of protracted or neuropathic pain, may bear little relation to the degree of peripheral stimulation. The classic picture of pain as a signal transmitted from the receptor to the cortex is a misrepresentation, in that it equates a small part with the whole. Such processes as sensitization (at receptors, dorsal root ganglion, dorsal horn, thalamus, and cortex), descending inhibition and facilitation of pain, and neuroplastic changes (including new sprouting, inhibitory cell death, and phenotypic alterations) account for what were previously considered idiopathic conditions (5,6).

Concepts of "inappropriate" levels of pain for given pathology have also been weakened as large numbers of genetic polymorphisms have been discovered that, in animal models, confer dramatic differences in resistance/vulnerability to various types of pain and in responsiveness to endogenous and exogenous opioids (7).

PSYCHOLOGIC COMPONENTS OF PAIN

The conclusion is inescapable that both the onset of pain and its transition from acute to chronic are determined at least as much by psychologic and environmental factors as by medical ones.

Disease Onset In a 4-year prospective study of 3,020 aircraft workers, job dissatisfaction and poor performance appraisals strongly predicted reports of acute back pain at work (8). Subjects who "hardly ever" enjoyed their jobs were more than twice as likely to report a back injury as those who "almost always" enjoyed their work. Another prospective study of 1,412 pain-free employees confirmed that those dissatisfied with their work were twice as likely to seek care for low back pain during a 12-month period as those who were satisfied, whereas those who felt underpaid were nearly four times as likely, and those in the lowest socioeconomic stratum were almost five times as likely to seek care for low back pain (9). Numerous subsequent investigations have confirmed that first report of a back injury at work is independently predicted by prior low back pain, physical work stress, and psychologic intolerance of the job.

Disease Progression The progression from acute to chronic pain has been studied most thoroughly in low back pain, the leading cause of disability in industrialized nations. Chronicity is highly dependent on demographic, psychosocial, and occupational factors. In a prospective study, progression to chronicity was associated with evidence of nonorganic disease, leg pain, significant self-rated disability at onset, a protracted initial episode, multiple recurrences, and a history of back pain or hospitalization (10). Occupational factors included blue collar jobs, labor requirements beyond the subjects' capabilities, job dissatisfaction, poor performance ratings, and being new at the job. Prior spine-related compensation, sickness payments, and litigation were associated with chronicity. Social and economic predictors included lack of schooling, language problems, low income, and unfavorable family status. In other studies, chronicity was predicted by somatization, depression, catastrophizing, stress, and compensation. Job satisfaction and orthopedic impairment appeared to predict outcome independently.

Even with such objective pathology as acute radicular pain and disc prolapse/protrusion, the only predictive somatic factor was the degree of disc displacement—the less the displacement, the worse the outcome (11). Persistent pain was predicted by depression and coping strategies. Application for retirement at 6 months was best predicted by depression and daily "hassles" at work.

Ironically, much disability may be attributed to the systems designed to help. Workers' compensation systems may be particularly toxic because they often involve delays in diagnosis and treatment, during which time workers must continually prove how sick they are to obtain the care they believe they need. Physicians and attorneys for each side may take polarized and improbable positions (12). The result is that patients who apply for and receive workers' compensation benefits seem to fare worse with virtually all interventions than those not so encumbered.

Litigation is thought to prolong disability, although the issue is controversial. Disability associated with "whiplash" injuries appears much less common in countries with a less developed tort system than the United States, where that complaint accounts for two thirds of all bodily injury claims (13). It may be significant that the rate of compensated whiplash in Saskatchewan, Canada, which had a tort system, was 10 times that of Quebec, which had a no-fault system (14), and that changing the tort system led to apparent reductions in pathology (15). In one study of more than 2,000 low back pain patients, all those who were working at intake returned to work after treatment, except for those in litigation, of whom not one returned to work (12). Vocational failure occurred despite success on other outcome variables. The idea that litigation fosters chronicity of pain and disability is challenged by several authors (16–18); however, litigation does appear to impede performance in domains more amenable to objective measurement than pain (19,20).

Chronic pain syndrome (CPS) is an old term that is still often heard. It must be distinguished from chronic non-malignant pain (CNMP), which, as used here, refers only to pain that is persistent and not associated with progressive tissue destruction. The term *CPS* was used to describe those with inordinate impairment and behavioral abnormalities (21), and was defined as intractable pain of 6 months' or more duration, accompanied by:

- marked alteration of behavior, with depression or anxiety;
- marked restriction in daily activities;
- excessive use of medication and frequent use of medical services;
- no clear relationship to organic disorder; and
- history of multiple, nonproductive tests, treatments, and surgeries.

Thus CPS is predominantly a behavioral syndrome that affects a minority of patients with chronic pain. The term properly directs therapy toward the reversal of regression and away from an exclusive focus on nociception, but does not substitute for a careful diagnosis of the physiologic, psychologic, and conditioning components that compose the syndrome.

Some of the controversy regarding chronic opioid analgesia may be an argument between those who have found opioids useful in treating chronic pain and those who have found them harmful in CPS. Just as tolerance and withdrawal are not synonymous with addiction, so too is chronic pain not synonymous with chronic pain syndrome. However, pain patients who have an active addiction disorder are at risk for chronic pain syndrome as well, because they are prone to inordinate disability, symptom exacerbation, and health care utilization.

Psychologic factors modulate, for better or worse, the intensity with which pain is felt, the associated affective distress, and the extent to which the person is functionally impaired. The psyche enables the majority of people to cope with pain, function despite it, and retain joy in living. It is reasonable to posit a stress-diathesis model in which the degree of disability from a given level of organic pathology varies with the psychologic strengths of the individual, the stresses of the workplace, and the incentives and disincentives for recovery, as well as biologic variance in nociceptive modulation.

Developmental Issues Adverse childhood experiences have been implicated as causes and exacerbating factors in various somatic symptoms (22–26). The factors most often investigated have been deprivation and trauma.

Deprivation, neglect, and abandonment in childhood are thought to leave lasting psychic scars; however, the mechanisms through which they may lead to physical symptoms are unclear. Several studies in the field of attachment theory have suggested that insecure attachment may predispose to increased pain (27). Increased vigilance and anxiety may partially explain this (28). In this regard, it is interesting that Coutinho et al. found that rat pups subjected to separation from their mothers for 3 hours per day during the first 2 weeks of life had symptoms strongly suggestive of human irritable bowel syndrome as adults, in addition to heightened anxiety (29).

Extreme trauma is also associated with multiple unexplained somatic symptoms, including pain, along with affect dysregulation and dissociation (30). Van der Kolk et al. found that there is an apparent spectrum of toxicity, with natural disasters producing fewer symptoms than adult interpersonal trauma, whereas childhood trauma produced the most severe symptoms of all.

Rome and Rome have speculated that psychologic trauma, in a process akin to kindling, can evoke a hypersensitivity not unlike that seen in neurogenic sensitization in pain, and that this hypersensitivity involves cross-sensitization, so that the individuals are hypersensitive to psychic (loss, humiliation) and physical (injury) trauma, both of which elicit both physical and affective symptoms (31). They coined the term *polymodal allodynia*, which seems to well describe the vulnerability experienced by these patients.

Cognitive Factors in Pain The role of cognition in psychiatric conditions has been recognized for more than 15 years (32,33). The underlying premise of cognitive theories is that individuals react not to events *per se*, but to their understanding of them. The terminal cancer patient who is convinced that "the surgeon got it all" will be more content than the healthy hypochondriac who fears occult pathology. Beliefs such as "These exercises must be tearing something loose," "I will resume living after I am well," and "I can't go out if I am in pain" have obvious effects on adaptation. Maladaptive cognitions have the quality of being automatic and habitual, so that they rarely are examined for validity. They are accepted by the patient, even when it is obvious to others that they are illogical.

The Meaning of Pain Cognitive factors affect pain in several ways (34,35). For example, the aversive quality of pain is modified by its interpretation (36,37), so that it is more distressing if thought to presage disaster. One example of maladaptive cognition is catastrophic thinking, a trait associated with poor pain tolerance and coping (38). "Catastrophizing" describes the automatic interpretation of events in catastrophic terms: if a spouse is late returning home, she or he "must have" had an accident. Such catastrophic interpretations as, "The nerves are being crushed," or "I may become paralyzed," increase dysfunction, worsen pain, and hinder coping (39,40). The negative, maladaptive thoughts that reduce pain tolerance include those emphasizing the aversiveness of the situation, the inadequacy of the person to bear it, or the physical harm that could occur (33).

Helplessness Cognitive influences on pain include not only beliefs regarding the pain, but also those regarding the person experiencing it. One's sense of personal power and competence modify coping (41). Seligman's model of learned helplessness in depression suggests that those who feel unable to control events in their lives will respond passively to them, become depressed, and experience increased disability and pain (42). Conversely, belief in self-efficacy is a major determinant of successful coping (43). For example, belief in self-efficacy is associated with better functioning in fibromyalgia and arthritis (44–47).

Locus of Control This refers to the perception that events are determined by one's own behavior ("internal locus of control [LOC]"), as opposed to outside forces, such as family members and physicians ("powerful others"), or chance. In several studies, those with an internal LOC felt and functioned better (48), whereas those with a "chance/external" LOC reported depression and anxiety, felt helpless, and relied on maladaptive coping strategies (49). Internal LOC is associated with successful rehabilitation (50).

Blame Blame attribution can be an important modifying factor in recovery from injury. Chronic pain patients who blame others for their pain report greater mood distress and behavioral disturbance, poorer response to past treatments, and lower expectation of future benefits (51).

Behavioral Contingencies in Pain *Operant conditioning* refers to the process in which behaviors increase in frequency when reinforced. It also addresses effects of punishment. Elimination of reinforcement is followed by "extinction" of the behavior. An essential perspective on operant conditioning is the observation that life could not exist were it not a prominent form of animal learning. An animal must repeat behaviors that led to acquisition of food, water, and a mate, while conserving energy by not repeating behaviors that failed to produce a "reward." Key points regarding operant conditioning include the observations that it often occurs without the knowledge of the trainer or trainee; in most cases, repetition over time is required for the effect to occur, which probably explains why these concepts are more important in chronic conditions than acute ones; and the timing of reinforcement is critical. An immediate small reinforcer may be more powerful than a delayed large one, which is reflected in the human propensity to engage in behaviors that produce immediate small rewards despite substantial delayed adverse consequences.

Because of conditioning, illness behaviors may become less contingent on sensations than on rewards, and may increase or decrease unrelated to nociception. At first glance, the life of a typical pain patient seems to provide remarkably few reinforcers. Poverty, depression, and loss of identity, friendships, and recreational activities are common. Nevertheless, much of the behavior of the pain patient, as with that of the person/patient with alcohol dependence, is maintained by initial consequences that are rewarding. Rest and inactivity initially provide relief; only later does debilitation increase pain.

The idea that "pain behaviors" (e.g., somatically focused conversation, limping, rubbing body parts, remaining bedbound) could be maintained by external reinforcers led to efforts to reduce those behaviors by eliminating reinforcers and reinforcing incompatible behaviors, such as speed-walking. Results were startling, as individuals who had been disabled for years began to exercise, relinquish assistive devices, and engage in conversations about non–pain-related topics (52,53). The operant conditioning-based program developed by Fordyce was soon emulated by hundreds of pain management programs in numerous countries. The rapid response of severely dysfunctional individuals to the environmental contingencies in these programs has lent support to the belief that much functional impairment is maintained by environmental rewards.

It is useful to view disability as a form of pain behavior, because it is strongly influenced by incentives and disincentives for vocational recovery. In the case of chronic pain, positive reinforcers (caretaking, drugs, money) may be less important than "negative reinforcers," such as the avoidance of noxious or hazardous situations. Although disability income is often meager, it is not contingent on one's ability to compete in the work marketplace, or the viability of one's industry in precarious economic times. In the United States, access to health care may be contingent on remaining disabled. On the other hand, when the incentives for wellness are sufficiently powerful, function may be preserved despite serious illness.

There is strong evidence that secondary gain influences pain behavior (54). In a comparison of 3,802 pain patients and 3,849 controls, Rohling et al. found compelling evidence that financial compensation was associated with greater pain and reduced treatment efficacy, whether medical or surgical (55).

Focus on the gain that results from the sick role should not diminish attention to the losses, which include the camaraderie of coworkers, pride in being the breadwinner, identity, and the self-esteem that comes from being a contributor rather than a burden to society and to one's family. Although disability income may provide security, it often does so at the poverty level.

The impact of reinforcement on pain *behavior* begs the question of whether it also modifies pain *perception*. Indeed, Flor studied patients with chronic back pain and found that the presence of a solicitous spouse was associated not only with increased pain reports in response to electrical back stimulation but also with increased activation of pain-sensitive cortical areas, as reflected by electroencephalogram (56). Thus it seems probable that reinforcing pain behavior can actually increase its perception.

Less commonly, gain issues may modify the family's behavior, a phenomenon referred to as *tertiary gain*. For example, a wife whose husband is an unskilled worker in a floundering industry may sense that the family's security is contingent on his disabled status. She therefore may defend his disability and support his helplessness.

Fear and Deconditioning The profound impairment that results from prolonged inactivity often begins with fear of injury. A vicious cycle begins, in which inordinate fear leads to inactivity, which in turn leads to deconditioning and a state of increased fragility, as loss of strength and range of motion increase susceptibility to strains and sprains (57). The fear of injury is compounded by the individual's belief that he is ill or fragile. Kori et al. coined the term *kinesophobia* to denote an irrational fear that movement or activity will lead to reinjury (58). Pain-related fear predicts functional impairment better than does pain severity alone (59,60). It interferes with patients' efforts to focus away from pain onto tasks and other things. (61). Interestingly, this inordinate fear may at times be iatrogenic (62).

Distraction Perceptions, including pain, are amplified when attended to and attenuated by distraction. Patients often respond to chronic pain by retreating into the bedroom, isolating socially, and limiting stimulation in an effort to feel better. These behaviors may so limit competing stimulation that pain becomes all-consuming. ("If life is empty, pain will fill it up.") In contrast, performing a maze task reduced reported pain and activity in the somatosensory association areas and periaqueductal gray/midbrain (as reflected in the positron emission tomography scan) in response to the cold pressor test (63).

Emotional Distress Negative affect that is experimentally induced by reading or by hypnosis reduces experimental pain tolerance (64,65). Chronic pain often is associated with emotional symptoms that do not meet criteria for a psychiatric diagnosis, but nevertheless contribute substantially to overall suffering and require treatment. Depressed mood is extremely common among those with chronic pain and probably reflects a multitude of factors, including pain, loss of gratifying activities, loss of self-esteem/identity, powerlessness, and drug-induced affective changes. Anxiety is also common in chronic pain (66–68) and can both amplify physical symptoms and provide disincentives for recovery; for example, illness may permit escape from feared situations. The cycle of pain-tension-pain reflects the tendency to "brace" to protect an injured part, which can increase musculoskeletal pain. High-anxiety rats have a lowered threshold for pain from innocuous colon distension, suggesting that visceral pains can be modulated by anxiety (69).

More recently, the phenomenon of *anxiety sensitivity*, which essentially refers to an abnormal fear of the normal physical sensations associated with anxiety, has been found to amplify experimental pain and to be associated with muscular, abdominal and head pain, and to impair coping (70,71).

Anger, a major cause of suffering in pain patients, has been somewhat neglected in comparison to other mood states. It seems to increase pain-related suffering and interferes with life activities, while it reduces response to treatment (72,73). Forgiveness, in contrast, seems therapeutic (74).

AXIS I DISORDERS

The four most frequent psychiatric illnesses in pain patients probably are somatoform disorders, anxiety disorders, depression, and substance abuse disorders (67,75). Polatin et al. (76) administered a structured psychiatric interview to 200 chronic low back pain patients entering a functional restoration program. Seventy-seven percent met lifetime criteria and 59% demonstrated current symptoms of at least one psychiatric diagnosis (excluding somatoform pain disorder). The most common diagnoses were major depression, substance abuse, and anxiety disorders. Fifty-one percent met criteria for a personality disorder. Of the patients who had a positive lifetime history of psychiatric syndromes, 94% of those with substance abuse, and 95% of those with anxiety disorders had developed those syndromes before the onset of back pain, whereas depression was equally likely to precede or follow the pain. More recently, the same group reported results of structured diagnostic interviews in 1,300 patients disabled with occupationally related spine pain (77). They found that 65% met criteria for at least one current psychiatric disorder (excluding Pain Disorder, which they described as "nearly universal in this population.)" The most common conditions were major depressive disorder (56%), substance use disorders (14%), anxiety disorders (11%), and personality disorders (70%).

Depression

An extensive literature documents widely varying estimates of the prevalence of depression in CNMP, with figures ranging from 10% to 83% (78). The wide variance reflects differences in settings, methodology, and criteria, as well as the confounding effects introduced by overlap of affective symptoms with those of pain. For example, insomnia from pain and drugs, loss of energy from deconditioning, and guilt from having become a burden all mimic symptoms of mood disorder (33). In a European telephone survey of nearly 19,000 people, Ohayon and Shatzberg found that 75% of those with chronic pain had at lease one core depressive symptom (79). The depression in chronic pain may differ from that usually seen in other settings (80). Although depression is this group is commonly attributed to pain, studies suggest that other factors, such as pain's interference with life activities and its ability to engender a sense of helplessness, are equally important (81). Mood often normalizes in those who acquire a sense of personal empowerment and who resume life involvements. In fact, there seems to be a vicious cycle in which pain behavior, isolation, inactivity, helplessness, depression, loss of reinforcers and distractions, and pain are mutually reinforcing. Improving one element in this series often benefits the others (82). Maruta et al. found that depression in CPS is highly responsive to nonpharmacologic interventions provided in an interdisciplinary pain rehabilitation program, with 98% resolved by discharge, and that recovery persisted at 1-year follow-up.

Dohrenwend et al. interviewed patients with myofascial face pain and their relatives, comparing them with a control group and their relatives (83). Both familial major depression and depressive spectrum disorders were elevated in control probands with major depression, but not in myofascial face pain probands with or without it. This suggests that much of the depression in those with chronic pain is a consequence of the pain, rather than a precursor or coincidental comorbidity.

There is also a well-studied elevated prevalence of pain in those with depression, and Carroll et al found that, in *pain-free* subjects in a population survey, those with high levels of depression were four times more likely to develop problematic spine pain than those without depression (84). Thus it is clear that the arrow of causality in pain-depression comorbidity can point in either direction. In an international study, Gureje et al. found that pain predicts depression and depression predicts pain, and to approximately the same degree (85). In Ohayon's study, if there was at least one core depressive symptom 27.6% had chronic pain, and of those with major depressive disorder, 43.4% had chronic pain (79).

Not only are pain and depression frequently comorbid, but each adversely affects the prognosis of the other, so that unresolved pain impedes depression treatment and vice versa (86,87).

In summary, we can conclude the following:

- Mood disturbance can elicit pain
- Pain can elicit mood disturbance
- Either can exacerbate the other
- Either can make the other treatment-resistant

The greatest fear in depressed patients is, of course, suicide, and in the case of those with CNMP, suicide ideation and behaviors were elevated even after depression was controlled for (88).

Anxiety Disorders

The prevalence of anxiety is elevated in CNMP, with more than 60% of pain clinic admissions suffering significant degrees of anxiety (89) and 28% meeting criteria for generalized anxiety disorder (90). The relationship between panic and pain is likely multifactorial, and involves such disparate elements as hypervigilance, hypothalamic pituitary-adrenal axis (HPA) activation, and the elaboration of alpha receptors on injured nociceptors. That severe trauma promotes somatization is an additional explanation (91). Panic attacks often present with chest or abdominal pain. Because chronic pain often originates with trauma, posttraumatic stress disorder is seen frequently in pain patients. Interestingly, animals that are anxious, whether genetically or from early maternal separation, are vulnerable to induction of visceral hyperalgesia and symptoms suggesting irritable bowel (92,93). Anxiety not only compounds the suffering in CNMP, it also impedes treatment. Baseline anxiety, as well as depression, predicted functional and symptomatic outcome in sciatica (94).

SOMATOFORM DISORDERS AND PSYCHOGENIC PAIN

Psychogenic pain is a concept whose existence is disputed. The term is widely criticized, in part because pain is defined as an *experience,* and to label an experience psychogenic may be tautologous. Additionally, a number of pains thought to be nonphysiologic have subsequently been explained by neurologic plasticity and sensitization. Even granting the validity of the concept, the diagnosis is fraught with difficulty. Nevertheless, pains of various sorts are prominent in somatization disorder, in which there is no evidence of physical disease, and it is certainly worthwhile, if only to avoid costly and potentially harmful studies and treatments, to distinguish complaints based on "hardware dysfunction" from those resulting from "software bugs."

The current term for what was previously called psychogenic pain is *pain disorder associated with psychologic factors* (95). (When medical factors contribute, the diagnosis is "pain disorder associated with medical and psychologic factors.") The criteria require that the pain cause "significant distress or impairment in functioning, that psychological factors be judged to have an important role in the onset, severity, exacerbation, or maintenance of the pain, and that the symptom or deficit not be intentionally produced or feigned." However, the method of determining that psychologic factors are causative is unspecified. Psychogenic pain is analogous to conversion disorders, such as blindness and paralysis, and is similarly typified by nonphysiologic findings on examination and behavioral inconsistencies. Patients may be dramatic, extreme in their denial of nonmedical problems, and cheerful despite a distressing degree of disability. They frequently demonstrate behaviors that are incompatible with the degree of impairment they claim. The diagnosis may encompass several different conditions, given that some individuals appear euthymic and animated and sleep well, whereas others appear to suffer severely, cannot sleep, and even commit suicide. In the authors' experience, a strong indicator of somatization is a patient's inability to discuss nonsomatic issues. If questioned about family, work, or politics, the response rapidly diverges to symptoms, doctors, tests, and treatments. Such behavior is not usually seen even in severe physical illness.

Extreme psychologic trauma leads to multiple somatic symptoms, including unexplained pain. Given the growing evidence that people who report high levels of pain have concordant cortical activation in pain-relevant areas, and that reinforcing pain behavior seems to produce "genuine" increases in pain perception, it is likely that the painful symptoms that follow emotional trauma are physiologically mediated as well.

It is difficult to distinguish conversion symptoms from malingering, because the distinction relies primarily on patient intent and consciousness of the situation, which are not observable. Surveillance may be the only way to diagnose some cases accurately, though grossly discordant findings (e.g., a person who can't tolerate hand touch due to allodynia yet has calluses and grease under the nails), suggest malingering.

Addiction The management of intractable pain can be quite challenging in the presence of comorbid addiction disorder, which tends to magnify complaints, impede diagnosis, and confound interventions. Despite these difficulties, such patients can be treated successfully and they commonly demonstrate the same gratitude for their recovery as do addicted persons in whom pain is not a factor.

The prevalence of addiction disorder in CNMP is disputed. Savage reviewed studies suggesting a prevalence of 3.2% to 18.9% (96). Thus some find a prevalence substantially lower than the population baseline. Such low figures strain credulity for several reasons. Many common causes of CNMP are associated with substance use; for example, low back pain is associated with nicotine and alcohol dependence (97–99). Nicotine may worsen fibromyalgia (100). Chronic pain often follows accidents, which are more common in those who are chemically dependent. Thus the prevalence would be expected to be higher than the population average. A careful study of 414 chronic pain patients in a Swedish rehabilitation hospital found active alcohol or drug misuse or dependence in 23.4%, whereas an additional 9.4% met criteria for remission (101). This figure, which suggests that one in four chronic pain patients has a current substance use disorder and one in three has a lifetime history of such a disorder, is more congruent with the authors' experience.

Addiction disorders are of epidemic proportions in health care settings, have been so for decades, and are largely overlooked. It is instructive that in 1989, among adult inpatients at Johns Hopkins Hospital, positive screens for alcoholism were found in 25% of admissions to medicine, 30% of admissions to psychiatry, 19% to neurology, 12.5% to obstetrics/gynecology, and 23% of those to surgery. Detection rates were <25% in surgery and obstetrics and 25% to 50% in neurology and medicine (102). Thus the likelihood that most substance use disorders is not detected in health care facilities is high. In a Veterans Affairs pain clinic, 27.6% of opioid users met at least abuse criteria (103). Smothers and Yahr found that 14% of U.S. general hospital admissions between the ages of 18 and 44 had chronic illicit substance use (104).

The conclusion seems to be that substance use problems are common in pain patients, but they are also high in health care consumers in general.

The other perspective on the problem of comorbidity is to determine the prevalence of CNMP in those with addiction disorders. Studies of those in methadone maintenance treatment find that 37% to 61% of patients are comorbid for CNMP (105,106). In 531 chemical-dependence inpatients, almost one fourth had CNMP.

Diagnosing addiction disorder in those with CNMP poses special challenges. Two of the major diagnostic criteria of DSM-IV-TR, tolerance and physical dependence, are virtually universal in those on chronic opioid therapy and do not distinguish the person with addiction disorder from those not so afflicted. Continued use despite adverse consequences, which is often an obvious clue to addiction to recreational substances, is less obvious in addiction to prescribed drugs. Falling asleep at inappropriate times can be attributed to pain-induced insomnia, whereas irritability, poor concentration, and regression can be falsely blamed on pain.

Patients with pain have often experienced a major blow to self-esteem as they've become nonproductive and burdensome to loved ones, and they may be especially reluctant to accept a stigmatized diagnosis. They may disavow any similarity between themselves and those who became addicted by recreational substance use.

Diagnosis is also hindered by the lack of consensus as to what constitutes appropriate use of opioids and sedatives. It is now accepted practice to prescribe doses of opioids that were unheard of only a few years ago, and it is often unclear whether opioids are an asset or liability until some time after their elimination. The pain patient who uses analgesics in a nonaddictive fashion is likely to have improved function, whereas addictive use typically impairs function. Perhaps this is because the dose required for psychoactive effects is sufficient to produce intoxication, whereas the analgesic dose usually is not. The addicted pain patient often has the illusion of drug benefit and feels better after ingesting it: "It takes the edge off." This illusion of benefit results if patients are unable to detect the cumulative deleterious effect of a medication when each dose reduces pain. It also represents the fact that peak serum levels are more comfortable than trough levels, which, in the presence of physical dependence, are associated with muscle tension, autonomic arousal, and hyperalgesia. Prescribing physicians may be unaware of the deleterious effects of the drug, and families who witness unwanted drug effects may believe them to be unavoidable and preferable to unrelieved suffering. In the authors' experience, such patients, their families, and their physicians are surprised at the reduction in pain and suffering that occurs after gradual elimination of the drug.

Clues to the presence of addiction in pain patients include frequent intoxication, irritability or other mood changes, inattention to hygiene, inappropriate behaviors, and impaired coordination. Another indicator is provided when, despite apparently generous analgesia, sick role behavior continues to be disproportionate to pathology. Combining other intoxicants with prescription drugs is an obvious clue. Urine toxicology studies facilitate the diagnosis of substance use disorder; however, it must be remembered that typical "dip stick" (immunoassay) technology does not identify synthetics or semisynthetics and that gas chromatography-mass spectrometry (GC/MS) may be needed.

Loss of control may be evidenced by taking handfuls of pills. Patients may be incapable of rationing themselves and use a month's supply in a few days, even in the face of increased pain and withdrawal when their supply is depleted. Patients should be asked about multiple sources of drugs, forged prescriptions, whether their physicians have been concerned about their medication consumption, and whether they found it necessary to change physicians because of this. Generally, a patient who has no history of alcohol or drug abuse, who becomes physically dependent on benzodiazepines or analgesics in the course of pain treatment, who obtains the drugs legitimately, and who has not seemed drug impaired, is not addicted. That is, that chronic high-dose opioids are ineffective does not suggest the presence of an addiction disorder.

Malingering It is somewhat politically incorrect to discuss malingering in the context of CNMP, and indeed it should be. For decades our failure to understand and appreciate the significance of the neurologic processes that generate and amplify pain that is disproportionate to the peripheral stimulus (if any) has led to default diagnoses of psychogenic pain or faking. For this, if no other reason, the burden must be on the clinician to demonstrate the presence of conscious, willful deception before making such a diagnosis. This does not, however, imply that malingering is nonexistent or rare.

Although most authorities hold that willful deception is quite uncommon, supporting data are rarely offered. Fishbain et al. reviewed literature suggesting that malingering is present in 1.25% to 10.4% of chronic pain patients, but found that methodologic flaws precluded conclusions (107). Data from other fields provide hints as to the prevalence of malingering. In patients with unexplained intractable diarrhea, 14% had positive stool examinations for laxatives, although all had denied their use (108). Among 333 persons who claimed compensation for noise-induced hearing loss, the incidence of exaggeration on hearing tests (as determined by cortical evoked response audiometry) was 17.7% (109). Sixty-one percent of litigants for whiplash associated cognitive dysfunction were thought to be malingering, based on a test of feigned cognitive dysfunction (110). Gervais et al. found that fibromyalgia patients who were receiving or seeking disability income were likely to demonstrate faking on tests of exaggerated memory complaints, in contrast to rheumatoid arthritis patients and fibromyalgia patients who were not seeking/receiving disability income (111). Weintraub cites studies showing that 20% to 46% of persons considered purposeful misrepresentation of compensation claims to be acceptable (112).

Such studies do not provide information as to how often such deceptions involve simulated pain. They do suggest keeping an open mind as to the possibility of these phenomena, which probably are more common in individuals seeking compensation or opioids than in those seeking other treatments or diagnoses.

IDENTIFYING PSYCHOGENIC COMPONENTS OF PAIN

A number of findings may support a conclusion that pain and disability are not fully explained by medical pathology.

Pain severity is most easily graded on a 0 to 10 Likert scale. Scores higher than 10 indicate exaggeration (pain greater than "the worst imaginable"), and may reflect a desire to emphasize the severity of suffering present. The McGill Pain Questionnaire contains lists of pain descriptors. Patients who choose predominantly affectively charged terms (e.g., agonizing, torturing, unbearable) are likely to have substantial psychologic components or sequelae of pain.

Pain drawings, in which the person is asked to shade in their area of pain on a human figure, are useful for quickly identifying pains with a particular pattern, such as sciatica, postherpetic neuralgia, or central poststroke pain. The drawing usually depicts pain in discrete, anatomically understandable locations, unless there is a diffuse condition such as fibromyalgia, autoimmune disease, or endocrinopathies. Bizarre locations, multiplicity of pain locations, and pain outside the body may suggest functional components (113).

Functional Impairment Evaluation should always include and assessment of interference with such activities as work, household chores, social and recreational activities, and activities of daily living. It is useful to record "down time"—the hours per day spent reclining, whether a person is housebound, and whether days are spent in night clothes. The concordance between dysfunction and pathology is of major diagnostic import. A rating scale of functional impairment, such as the Pain Disability Index (114) or Sheehan Disability Scale (115), can help to quantify this and also document response to treatment.

Emotional Symptoms Depression, anxiety, and irritability should be noted, along with such symptoms as crying spells and changes in sleep, energy, interest, libido, humor, concentration, appetite, and weight. Suicidality should be assessed. Anxiety and panic attacks should be noted. Posttraumatic stress disorder is suggested by "re-experiencing" symptoms, such as flashbacks, nightmares, and intrusive recollections, anxiety, or hypervigilance with increased startle response, and efforts to avoid situations reminiscent of the original trauma.

Family Response It is most helpful when family and friends accept the person, validate the pain, provide assistance when necessary, and encourage function. Hostility and challenges to the validity of the pain may increase distress and elicit efforts to "prove" the existence of the illness. On the other hand, inappropriate caretaking can promote regression and should be considered a form of "enabling." In such cases it is not unusual for the spouse to speak for the patient and even to "correct" the patient's description of pain.

Stresses Work, family, and entitlement agencies are perhaps the most common stressors mentioned, and the patient may have observed that these issues are related to pain severity. The person who admits to no nonmedical stresses may be in denial (i.e., repressing emotional upset to avoid psychologic discomfort).

Litigation/Disability The presence or absence of disability income may be less relevant than the process of trying to obtain it, which requires continued demonstrations of dysfunction. It is difficult to recover while trying to prove how sick one is.

Collateral Information Poor recollection, drug-induced confusion, and the desire to portray oneself in a favorable light may combine to produce an unreliable history. Relatives and previous physicians may provide critical information regarding substance use, functional impairment, depression, suicide threats, and the like. They also may reveal the converse; for example, corroboration of improved quality of life on opioids, thus confirming treatment efficacy.

Physical Examination It is important to note whether findings are consistent internally and with known pathology, while recognizing that our understanding of pathology is incomplete. Expectations and fear can confound observations, as patients may perform activities in nonfrightening situations that they cannot perform when frightened. Nevertheless, such signs as axial rotation, in which only the hips are rotated, should not affect spine pain (although there is come controversy regarding this). A person who tiptoes should not have breakaway weakness on manual testing of plantar flexion. Limping that is worse with the spouse present, or that changes sides with distraction, suggests nonorganic factors.

Impairment should not exceed pathology. If the complaint is in the lower body, questionnaires should not be completed in the spouse's handwriting. A patient with hand pain should not look to the spouse for help in describing it, and should make his or her own calls for medications.

Important issues include apparent distress, appropriateness of pain behavior, somatic preoccupation, drug effects, and appropriateness of affect to the level of pain and disability. (An animated, euthymic affect is not concordant with pain severity of 10/10.) Inordinate dependence on companions should be noted.

Waddell et al. (116) described nonphysiologic signs in low back pain that are associated with elevations on Minnesota Multiphasic Personality Inventory (MMPI) scales 1 to 3, delayed return to work, and excessive health care utilization (117), and poor surgical outcome.

Mental Status Examination Cognitive function should be assessed for dementia or baseline cognitive limitations that create disincentives to rehabilitation. Locus of control should reflect the patient's acceptance of responsibility for recovery. When everything seems to be contingent on actions of government agencies, the company, the doctors, the lawyer, or the spouse, psychologic issues are likely to impede recovery. When psychologic factors promote illness patients may focus on blame, retribution, and compensation more than on recovery; in treatment, they may show less investment in recovery than does the treatment team. A history of noncompliance with reasonable medical expectations and lack of effort in treatment support this conclusion. Negative reactions to compliments may be noted; that is, the patient may be upset when a peer comments that he or she is showing improvement.

The presence of secondary gain is not a valid indicator of nonorganic symptoms, as patients with clearly organic conditions are equally likely to have gain (118). It does, however, seem that the more patients have to gain by getting well, the more motivated they are to do so.

Testing There are no psychologic tests that can diagnose the cause of a pain disorder. The MMPI has been used for this purpose, but such use has been widely challenged (119). However, it may help to predict treatment outcome (120). Most psychological testing in patients with chronic pain has been for the identification of comorbid psychiatric and substance use disorders. Other tests are designed to quantify pain or functional impairment, or are used primarily as outcome measures.

PSYCHOLOGICAL APPROACHES TO THE TREATMENT OF PAIN

It follows from the above discussion that psychologic interventions should focus on treating psychiatric (including addictive) comorbidity, correcting cognitions, reinforcing healthy behaviors, and reducing such psychophysiologic components as tension and anxiety. Treatment should be prompt and comprehensive in at-risk patients, because the likelihood of return to work decreases rapidly as the duration of sick leave increases (121).

Physical Therapy In the patient with chronic pain, physical therapy is a critical form of psychotherapy. Deconditioning commonly results from fear and causes such psychologic changes as perceived helplessness. A major consequence of deconditioning is that many activities become painful, reinforcing the belief that one is handicapped. Physical therapy thus becomes a form of systematic desensitization for patients who are immobilized and deconditioned because of the fear of reinjury. It is a powerful antidote to "learned helplessness" and directly reduces symptoms such as anxiety and depression (122,123). In addition, reconditioning restores access to previously gratifying and productive activities, thereby indirectly improving mood and self-esteem. Numerous studies confirm the critical role of exercise in chronic back and neck pain in reducing both pain and disability (124–126). In so-called failed back syndrome, exercises plus education produced outcomes that compared favorably with lumbar fusion (127). Although there is evidence supporting the effectiveness of therapeutic massage, passive modalities should be used with caution because of their potential to teach that improvement is achieved by being a passive recipient of others' ministrations, potentially undermining development of self efficacy. It is useful to have the family witness exercises, because they may be more willing to relinquish enabling when they no longer see their loved one as an invalid.

Behavior Modification The management of CNMP has as much to do with behavioral changes as perceptual ones. Pain behaviors may be separated into those that primarily affect nociception (using a heating pad) and those that primarily affect others ("pain talk"). Some behaviors, such as exhibiting a transcutaneous electrical neurostimulation (TENS) device or corset outside clothing, do both. Unwarranted pain behaviors tend to be emitted preferentially in the presence of others, and include moaning, complaining, and holding body parts.

Behavioral change is initiated by changing the environmental consequences of pain behavior. This has been most studied in intensive treatment programs, where social reinforcers can be made contingent on healthy behaviors, whereas pain behaviors are ignored (128). Fifteen randomized controlled trials demonstrated that behavior modification produced reduced pain and analgesic use with improved functional impairment and activity (129). In physical therapy, praise, rest, and other "rewards" should follow goal completion, rather than "trying." Families can learn that unnecessary coddling promotes invalidism. They must learn to distinguish ignoring pain behavior from ignoring the person, and must be encouraged to provide social reinforcers for healthy behavior. This involves a role change from that of caregiver to companion, friend, lover, or playmate.

Although it is apparent how contingency management alters behavior, it is less clear how it changes pain perception and suffering. While some pain reduction may result secondarily from behavioral activation, exercises, etc., Flor's work suggests that avoidance of reinforcement for pain may decrease its perception.

Other behavioral issues in chronic pain are less about contingency management than about education and planning. For example, patients may be extremely sedentary for a time, until they can no longer bear it, then abruptly engage in prolonged vigorous activity—sending them once more to bed, and helping confirm that they should never have tried to function "normally." Educating such patients about pacing their activities, slow gradual escalation of exercise, and planning for activities unlikely to cause pain exacerbations can be quite beneficial in improving quality of life.

Additionally, patients can be assisted in the development of a "wellness plan," that includes strategies for optimizing pain, mood, and function, and for dealing with flares of increased pain.

Education Patients are often bewildered about the significance of their pain, which markedly increases suffering and dysfunction. It is therefore critical to reduce mystery and uncertainty about its cause and import (130). Waddell et al. found that disability from back pain was better accounted for by fear avoidance beliefs than by pain itself (131). These beliefs appear related not to disease severity but to uncertainty of diagnosis. Such an association is a special challenge in caring for patients with chronic low back pain, where a precise anatomic explanation of the pain is unavailable in 80% of cases. Teaching should include the pain pathology, if known, its benign nature, and the difference between hurt and harm, so that patients are not deterred from reconditioning programs that may initially increase pain. In a randomized study of patients who had failed to respond to prior spine surgery, education with exercises was as effective as repeat surgery (127).

Education also should involve families, lest they promote unwarranted regression. Such "enabling" commonly results from misunderstanding the nature of the pain, which activities are harmful, and which are helpful. It is useful to discuss recent neurobiologic discoveries that explain how severe pain can occur with minimal or no peripheral pathology, which accounts for most patient reports that "They can't find the cause of my pain."

Much maladaptive behavior on the part of patients and families can be understood as an inappropriate extension of appropriate *acute* pain management (which is how most *chronic* pain began) into the chronic phase, so that the regression and caretaking that initially protected injured parts and promoted healing come to promote deconditioning, increased pain, and destruction of quality of life. Families should understand that the worst treatment is rest and that activity is beneficial.

Cognitive Behavioral Therapy Cognitive behavioral therapy (CBT) is somewhat of an amalgam of cognitive therapies, relaxation techniques, and behavioral therapy. In this most common psychotherapeutic approach for chronic pain patients are trained to identify, challenge, and alter automatic inappropriate thinking patterns and self-defeating behaviors (132). The goals of CBT are chosen by the patient; however, they typically involve not only improved pain tolerance but also decreased emotional distress and functional restoration. There are various approaches to CBT that share the principle that thoughts largely determine emotional reactions. Therapies are time limited, somewhat didactic in structure, with homework assignments.

As an example, a patient with low back pain may awaken worried about his back and unsure what his pain portends. (Patients' interpretations of physicians' explanations—"Your spine is degenerating."—can lead to considerable fear.) If the patient sits up and has a sudden pain, it may be amplified by his hypervigilance and lead to such conclusions as, "I must be getting up too soon. Perhaps I should spend a few more days at bed rest, or spend the day in the recliner." This decision, based on inaccurate conclusions, promotes further deconditioning, anxiety, loss of pleasurable and productive activities, depressed mood, and a constant focus on somatic themes that drives away those who might otherwise seek out his company, which then leads to feelings of abandonment and betrayal . . . An alternative thought process could be . . . "That really hurts, but most of the pain is probably muscular; after all, everyone's spine is degenerating after the age of 18, and there are 70 year olds running marathons. Perhaps some stretches will help, but in any case the pain always diminishes eventually. In the meantime, perhaps going for coffee with a friend would provide a distraction." It is obvious how inaccurate cognitions can lead to a cascade of emotional and behavioral changes that disable and demoralize the sufferer.

Studies show that CBT leads to improvements in activity, psychologic function, pain, and medication use (133). Meta-analysis of 25 controlled trials confirmed the efficacy of this therapy for pain, mood other than depression, social function, and pain behavior (134). "Learned helplessness" and "external locus of control" can be replaced with the patient's mindset that he is in charge of his life. Thoughts that "these exercises are tearing something loose" can be replaced with "the pain I'm having now probably means that I need to exercise more."

Mindfulness CBT has evolved over the years, and increasingly focuses on such concepts as mindfulness and acceptance. Behavioral therapies initially focused on contingencies for changing patients' behaviors. CBT focused primarily on reducing pain and other (primarily emotional) symptoms. The newer work holds that there can be value in surrender, and that symptom control strategies can be harmful if they fail, dominate the person's life, or lead to loss of important parts of life (135).

Teaching mindfulness meditation has been recently investigated as a technique for improving coping and function in CNMP (136). It has been found that baseline traits of mindfulness are associated with less depression and anxiety and better physical and psychosocial function (137). It was reported to improve pain acceptance and function in elderly patients with low back pain (138), and it was found to improve pain, depression, anxiety, and somatic complaints in women with fibromyalgia (139).

Acceptance As noted by McCracken et al., "Somewhat paradoxically, there may be occasions when helpful change in the quality of a patient's life can only occur when some aspects of the problem are accepted as they are. Change efforts may then be directed away from struggles that keep the person stuck, such as with unwanted thoughts, feelings, or sensations, toward situations that yield overall better results, such as a course of action that is personally meaningful and satisfying." Thus acceptance of pain, which may initially sound like giving up, actually is about changing the things that can be changed and accepting the things that cannot.

In 115 patients being treated for CNMP in the United Kingdom, acceptance of pain and values-based action predicted improvements in pain, pain-related distress, pain-related anxiety and avoidance, depression, depression-related interference with functioning, and physical and psychosocial disability (140). Viane et al. had patients record pain and activities eight times per day and found that pain acceptance was associated with less attention to pain and more engagement, motivation, and efficacy in performing daily activities (141). McCracken and Eccleston assessed various coping strategies, including distraction, ignoring pain, distancing from pain, coping self-statements, and praying along with catastrophizing in 230 CNMP sufferers. These strategies were found to predict pain and distress less robustly than were the variables measuring acceptance (142).

Though these new areas of study have not been fully vetted, they are promising and they are very congruent with clinical observations that the patients who accept the idea that they can't completely eliminate pain and so choose to have a good quality of life despite it are the ones who feel and function best over time.

Stimulus Reinterpretation Pain responses can be reduced through reinterpretation of the stimulus. For example,

"My back is breaking" can be replaced with, "Although it feels as though my back is breaking, it's probably another muscle spasm, and it won't last forever." Catastrophic statements can be identified and reframed. "My back is killing me; I can't stand it anymore," can be changed to, "Although the exercise is painful, ultimately it will help. I've coped with this much pain before and I can again. It always gets better eventually."

Assertiveness Training Those who are uncomfortable directly expressing their desires and declining requests have an intrinsic incentive for remaining "sick." Pain elicits nurture and is an excuse to avoid unpleasant responsibilities or situations. Patients, especially passive ones, may have concerns that assertive training will encourage them to be demanding or unpleasant. It is and should be presented as a strategy for being honest about your own needs and reactions in a way that is respectful of the other person. For example, the assertive alternative to "You're a jerk" might be "I feel really angry when you talk to me in that tone of voice, and I'd prefer that you communicate your point in a friendlier way." A useful slogan for work in this area is, "Say what you mean, and mean what you say, but don't be mean when you say it." As patients set limits on how others treat them, what they're willing to do, and to communicate their needs, the sick role becomes less necessary.

Biofeedback/Relaxation Training Clinical biofeedback/relaxation training (BFT) achieves symptom control by using electronic feedback to teach patients to regulate such functions as skeletal muscle tension, palmar sweating, gastrointestinal motility, and digital blood flow (143). Training in warming the extremities is helpful to patients with Raynaud syndrome (144) and may reduce hypertension (145). It is commonly used to train autonomic responses in complex regional pain syndrome (reflex sympathetic dystrophy) (146). Electromyelogram biofeedback often is used to teach frontalis relaxation and has been used for the treatment of tension headache, fibromyalgia (147), and back pain (148). Both electromyelogram and thermal biofeedback have been used extensively in headache patients (149–151) and masseter feedback may be useful for temporomandibular joint syndrome (152). The indications for BFT are not fully defined and continue to expand into conditions as diverse as rectal pain (153,154), cumulative trauma disorder (155), and vulvodynia (156).

Flor and Birbaumer compared electromyelogram biofeedback training with CBT and conservative medical intervention for chronic musculoskeletal pain. Forty percent of the BFT groups had (2 SD reductions in pain, life interference, and affective distress, versus 17% of the cognitive-behavioral group and 8% of the medical group (157). BFT has been challenged by studies showing that benefit does not correlate with physiologic changes (158), whereas others suggest that it may be no more effective for muscle pain and headache than approaches that do not require electronic equipment, such as autogenic training, progressive muscular relaxation, meditation, or self-hypnosis, all of which facilitate a state of reduced emotional arousal, skeletal muscle relaxation, and reduced autonomic activity (159,160). Many studies of biofeedback have confounded conclusions by combining it with other forms of relaxation training (161). Such studies generally show benefit from the combined approach. There may be a synergistic effect from combining BFT with cognitive therapies (162,163).

Recent studies indicating that pain is associated with a relative increase of electroencephalogram beta-wave activity and a decrease in slower frequencies has led to speculation that electroencephalogram biofeedback ("neurofeedback") may have a general pain-lowering effect. An early (open) study in fibromyalgia supports this (164).

Clinical experience is that patients consistently rate BFT one of the most helpful interventions in a multifaceted, interdisciplinary program. Perhaps this is because, in addition to it specific benefits, biofeedback helps skeptical patients understand the relationship between external and internal events. A patient who witnesses a drop in hand temperature when discussing an employer may be convinced of the importance of stress management in modifying his or her body's responses. Thus BFT may facilitate work in other program components.

Family Therapy It is perplexing that, despite almost universal agreement as to the importance of the family in perpetuating and ameliorating inordinate functional impairment in pain, there is very little literature devoted to the subject of how best to intervene (165–167). There are bidirectional influences—living with a patient who has chronic pain can stress the family financially and often leads to family-wide reductions in recreation and socialization, as well as a sense of obligation to fill the role of caretaker. Role reversal is common, and patients often express remorse for the fact that their small children have begun to parent them. Meanwhile, family responses markedly impact the patient. Overly solicitous responses promote increased pain and decreased function, while rejecting responses promote anger and depression. The optimal response is validation of the person's pain, affection, and acceptance of the person, and the provision of "social reinforcers" for behaviors incompatible with the sick role, while extinguishing sick role behavior.

The distress of family members often warrants specific management. They may find that their lives are controlled by someone else's illness. They feel duty-bound to give, yet receive little. Self-blame and guilt coexist with resentment. They may feel helpless and depressed, and their own lives often become unmanageable. Family discord often becomes a major source of stress for the patient with pain. Individual counseling, group therapy involving family members of pain patients, and conventional family therapy have all been used with success. Restoration of good quality of life to the non–pain sufferers is a valid treatment goal.

Interdisciplinary Pain Rehabilitation Programs

Combined approaches seem more effective than unitary treatments for CNMP. Accordingly, combinations of interventions should be tailored to maximize comfort and function. Interdisciplinary pain rehabilitation programs (IPRPs) combine many elements and, unless they specifically exclude patients with substance use disorders, should have addiction treatment as a major program component. Such programs can dramatically improve the quality of life and functional abilities of disabled pain patients. In a meta-analysis of 65 studies of IPRPs, Flor et al. found improvements in pain, mood, and interference with life activities, including work (168). Health care utilization declined. These benefits were stable over time.

Typical services in multidisciplinary pain rehabilitation programs include:

- education
- reconditioning physical therapy
- medications
- biofeedback/relaxation training
- operant conditioning
- psychotherapy (personal and family)
- detoxification
- addiction treatment
- treatment of psychiatric comorbidity.
- TENS
- interventions such as spinal cord stimulator or nerve blocks may be included

Turk reviewed outcome studies of interdisciplinary programs and found reports of reductions in pain of 14% to 60%, reductions in opioid use of up to 73%, and dramatic increases in levels of activity (169). Forty-three percent more patients were working after treatment than before. One study found a 90% reduction in physician visits. There were 50% to 65% fewer surgeries than in untreated patients and 65% fewer hospitalizations. Thirty-five percent fewer patients were on disability. Turk estimated that IPRPs led to 27 fewer surgeries per 100 patients, for an average of $4,050 saved per patient (at $15,000 per surgery). He estimated overall medical costs at more than $13,000 per year pretreatment and $5,600 in the year after treatment. This suggests a savings of $7,700 per year per patient after treatment. Disability savings were striking, with an estimated $400,000 saved per person removed from permanent disability. [These figures reflect 1995 dollars.]. More recently, Gatchel and Okifuji have reviewed studies of IPRP effectiveness and concluded that such treatment is the most efficacious and cost-effective, evidence-based treatment extant for CNMP (170).

Patients are often apprehensive that increased activity and reduced use of drugs will increase their suffering, and often only the example of patients farther along in the recovery process will encourage them to stay in treatment. Excessive sick role behavior can be conceptualized as similar to addiction-related behavior, in that patients compulsively behave in ways that produce immediate relief, but ultimately increase suffering. They expect to suffer more when they relinquish their customary adaptive strategies, yet in fact they suffer less.

Evidence is compelling that IPRP treatment is the most effective treatment for patients disabled with CNMP, in terms of prolonged symptom reduction, functional restoration, and health care utilization; however, most such programs have ceased operations because of poor reimbursement. Clinically successful programs provided several hours of psychologic intervention daily and several hours of reconditioning (physical therapy/occupational therapy) therapies. It is difficult to bill successfully for such services, and many payers are skeptical of "programs," preferring to pay for single services.

Addressing Pain/Addiction Comorbidity Of the psychologic problems that beset the patient with CNMP, perhaps none is more insidious and difficult to manage than addiction. Addiction (to prescribed substances) is more difficult to diagnose in the presence of CNMP, more difficult to enlist patient efforts to combat, and more difficult to treat. Yet treatment is essential, because addiction recovery seems to be a *sine qua non* for pain recovery—patients may get substantial improvement in pain-related distress and dysfunction even if they continue to have some anxiety, depression, or locus of control issues, but they seem not to recover from chronic pain if they do not establish recovery from addiction.

Diagnosis of Pain/Addiction Comorbidity Impediments to accurate diagnosis previously detailed are further complicated by several issues related to patient willingness to accept the diagnosis. As noted, the person disabled with CNMP is likely to have had problems with low self-esteem and even self-disparagement before pain onset. This is worsened as the person loses the ability to be the breadwinner, to parent, to function sexually, and even to be a desirable dinner guest. In this context, a stigmatized diagnosis may simply be unacceptable.

Second, the person who is addicted to recreational substances, even if in considerable denial, is likely to know that substance use is the reason for job loss, legal consequences, marital discord, and the medical consequences of toxic substances. The person who is addicted to prescribed drugs, on the other hand, is unlikely to experience medical consequences beyond sedation and constipation. Virtually all other consequences, from reduced libido to poverty, can be attributed to pain.

Third, the person/patient with an addiction disorder for whom medications have become a liability is often unable to detect this. Although they report high levels of pain despite high doses of opioids, they find that they feel better after each dose, and have no clue that their pain can drop markedly with opioid elimination.

Finally, the person addicted to medical substances often has the approval of physicians who may perceive the medications as helpful and may lack skills in diagnosing addiction disorders. Family members may believe that the patient could be even worse without the substances. The physician may be unwilling to make a diagnosis that he or she doesn't know how to treat and that feels like adding insult to injury and that he or she feels he or she may have contributed to through prescribing.

Experience suggests that patients often only begin to recognize their addiction late in the process of weaning, because their pain has reduced and their function, cognition, and affect have improved.

Treatment of Pain/Addiction Comorbidity

Contentious Terms

Addicting Drugs and Iatrogenic Addiction Stigmatization of opioids and unwarranted fears of addiction have contributed to a vast amount of avoidable suffering. Thus these terms have been challenged. Experts point out that, although drugs may be rewarding, addiction is a property of the host, not the substance. Additionally they note that no one can "make you a person/patient with an addiction disorder" against your will, and thus the concept of iatrogenic addiction is suspect.

These perhaps anachronistic terms are retained for two reasons. Both reward and addiction are in fact a property of the interaction of a chemical and a person, not of either in isolation, and there is a clear continuum both of addictive potential (crack cocaine >>> tramadol) and of personal vulnerability to addiction. Some, for example, find marijuana aversive, some find it rewarding, some risk their lives to obtain it. Thus the term *addicting* is used in the way that "photosensitizing" is used—it doesn't affect everyone, but suggesting sunscreen is still a good idea.

Iatrogenic addiction may be a scientific oxymoron; however, it is an accepted legal entity. Numerous physicians have been successfully sued for "causing addiction." Clinicians strive to avoid exposing a patient to harm; thus they fear "causing" addiction just as they fear "causing" anaphylaxis. Because the likelihood that addiction will develop in short term treatment is markedly less than that in chronic opioid therapy, many, clinicians who are comfortable providing adequate acute analgesia, may be unwilling to do so chronically.

Conceptually, there are two issues—the treatment of addiction in pain patients, and the treatment of pain in people with addiction disorder. There seem to be no data to determine which treatment should be first, but experience suggests that the pain patient who has an addiction to cocaine, marijuana, or alcohol often responds to traditional addiction care in a setting appropriate to the severity of the disease. In contrast, the person who has become addicted in the course of pain treatment (and perhaps the person who has an "iatrogenic relapse," associated with prescription of opioids after a prolonged period of sobriety) seems to respond better if treatment is initiated in a chronic pain treatment program. It helps when they interact with peers who have also developed addiction without engaging in the behaviors that they stereotypically associate with persons/patients with an addiction disorder. Chronic Pain Anonymous is embryonic, but has applied the Twelve Steps, the principles, and the promises of Alcoholics Anonymous (AA) to chronic pain (171).

The treatment of pain in patients with comorbid addiction raises the question of whether to use opioids, and, if so, how to protect the person's recovery. It is generally considered unethical to withhold opioid analgesia from persons/patients with an addiction disorder (172), yet patients should not be given treatments that fail to help or harm them. Cues associated with prior drug use has considerable potential to trigger relapse, which may explain the clinical impression that opioid therapy with recovering persons/patients with alcohol dependence is often easier and more successful than is the case with recovering opioid-addicted patients. Nevertheless, the concept of cross-addiction suggests that a patient with any prior addiction is at heightened risk for new addiction, even to unrelated substances.

A distinction must be made between acute pain and chronic nonmalignant pain, and between the patient who is actively engaging in substance abuse and the patient in recovery.

Acute Pain Acute injuries and surgery in persons/patients with an addiction disorder, even with sustained recovery, may require more aggressive analgesia than in patients with no addiction history. Although a period of abstinence eliminates apparent drug tolerance, after resumption of use, tolerance is rapidly reestablished in the previously tolerant person or animal. Those on agonist therapy for addiction have special analgesic needs (173).

Patients in recovery may face surgery with trepidation, as they fear having to choose between unrelieved pain and relapse. Some even refuse analgesia in an effort to preserve their sobriety. Experience suggests that this is unnecessary. Patients should be encouraged to inform the surgeon/anesthesiologist in advance of elective procedures that they are in recovery, will likely require higher than usual doses of analgesics, but wish to preserve their sobriety by avoiding their previous drug of choice, transitioning to long-acting oral agents as soon as possible, and making arrangements for safe use of opioids after discharge. The patients should increase their recovery work (e.g., Twelve Step meetings, meetings with addiction counselor) and should notify their addictionologist and sponsor of pending surgery, so that support is in place. It is sometimes helpful to request that a spouse, friend, or sponsor store opioids and bring a supply each day, so that the patient is protected from the temptation of a bottle of opioids within easy reach.

Chronic Pain Appropriate treatment of comorbid pain and addiction remains controversial and there is little data on which to base therapy (174). We must rely on "clinical wisdom" while remembering how often it has proved wrong when data became available.

Opioid Treatment A 1991 survey of state medical board members found that 58% considered it a probable violation of laws and regulations to prescribe opioids for CNMP in a person with a history of opioid abuse (175). A subsequent survey demonstrated a liberalization of this attitude (176); however, many remain reluctant to prescribe opioids to those with substance abuse disorders.

Most studies of chronic opioid therapy in patients with addiction disorder are quite small. In 20 such patients who were treated for >1 year, those who abused medications did so early, and those who did not abuse were more likely to be active in AA, to have stable support systems, and were less likely to be recent polysubstance abusers (177). Those who did not abuse treatment were more likely to benefit from it.

Kennedy and Crowley used methadone and weekly psychotherapy to treat four patients with chronic pain and comorbid substance abuse disorders (178). Three patients remained in treatment (19 to 21 months), stopped needle use or markedly decreased substance abuse, and demonstrated functional improvement.

Currie et al. treated 44 patients with comorbid chronic pain and addiction in cognitive-behavioral groups with emphasis on substance abuse education and relapse prevention (179). Some chose to discontinue opioids because of loss of control. The others were transitioned to longer acting medications (excluding methadone). As-needed opioids were prohibited and, once titrated to the optimal dosage, patients could not obtain additional medication. There were improvements in pain, emotional functioning, and medication requirements. At 12-month follow-up, half the patients were opioid-free, and the remainder had reduced their use from 17 days per month to 12. There was no significant difference in outcomes for opioid and nonopioid users, though those who continued to take opioids appeared to function better. It was suggested that long-acting opioids may provide both analgesia and reduction of cravings.

It is reasonable to conclude that chronic opioid analgesic therapy can help some patients with CNMP if managed meticulously. The issue of ensuring that addiction is being adequately treated is often key to management of the patient with comorbidity.

Miotto et al. have provided recommendations for treating the patient with chronic pain and addiction (180).

- Wean opioids if pain can be managed with nonopioids, although detoxification alone is ineffective treatment for addiction.
- Do not withhold opioids from patients with addiction, but integrate them into a plan to relieve pain and treat addictive disease.
- Address the "false promise" that opioids enable one to avoid pain.
- Provide treatment in a pain center if the primary physician is reluctant to prescribe opioids.
- Require a treatment contract to establish treatment boundaries.
- Educate patients about tolerance, dependence, withdrawal, and interactions between opioids, other medications, and alcohol.
- Optimize adjunctive medications and nonpharmacologic strategies (e.g., physical conditioning, coping skills, daily time management skills, lifestyle modifications).
- Address psychiatric disorders and risk factors—survivors of childhood trauma may require psychotherapy
- Involve families in rehabilitation efforts.
- Consider random urine testing.
- Require drug abuse treatment.
- Slowly titrate opioids to the point of maximum function.
- Monitor analgesic misuse.
- Reevaluate addictive disease if drug seeking persists despite increased dosing in the absence of disease progression.
- Provide multiple dated small prescriptions to those who cannot adhere to instructions.
- Do not replace lost medication.
- Do not expect addiction-controlling doses of methadone to effectively manage pain.
- Expect relapse, especially early in treatment, during stress, or with unrelieved pain. Treat relapse, don't abandon the patient.
- Terminate opioids in the case of selling prescriptions.

Passik and Kirsh echoed several of these suggestions and emphasized the importance of strict contracts and frequent follow-ups with urine toxicology screening (181).

Savage suggested chronic opioid analgesia for patients with addiction whose pain was both distressing and opioid-responsive, and when other therapies failed or were impracticable (182). She noted that stable, relatively high blood levels of opioids could treat both addiction and pain. She advised that risks of treating be balanced against risks of not treating, because unrelieved pain may promote addiction relapse or use of street drugs.

Opioid Selection The goal of opioid selection is to optimize analgesia with minimal risk of relapse. This suggests selection of slow onset, long-acting agents, and avoidance of the fast-in, fast-out products (183).

Mironer et al. compared their patients who successfully continued on opioids with those dismissed because of misuse (184). They found (in retrospective analysis) that some drugs were much more likely to be associated with patient dismissal, and the odds of this (1 being average) were as follows: butorphanol (4.4); propoxyphene (2.5); hydrocodone (1.61); codeine with acetaminophen (1.45); oxycodone immediate release (1.35); oxycodone delayed release (0.73); morphine 12-hour (0.66); transdermal fentanyl (0.23); methadone (0.08).

Several strategies have been proposed to help opioid users remain in control. It is common to request that patients always bring their pill bottles to visits for pill counts. Some clinicians phone patients to bring in the bottle at random times, the idea being that the unpredictable oversight will help the patient to take the drugs as prescribed. Patients may be required to return used transdermal patches to receive a prescription for new patches, thereby demonstrating that they were neither sold, opened, or cut into pieces.

Intrathecal analgesia is somewhat appealing as a strategy for providing opioid therapy to patients who have difficulty controlling their use. Although this route of administration seems resistant to abuse, resourceful persons/patients with an addiction disorder have been able to defeat it (185–187).

Additional Medications Comorbid psychiatric symptoms are the rule in pain and addiction disorder, and their management should also be conducted with an eye to protecting sobriety. There seems little justification for prescribing controlled substances for anxiety, "muscle spasm," and insomnia, because nonaddicting alternatives abound. Most antidepressants have anxiolytic properties and are not subject to abuse (188–191). This is equally true of the antiepileptic drugs commonly used in pain treatment (192). Most so-called muscle relaxants are not habituating, with the exception of carisoprodol, which has no role in the addicted patient. When needed, drugs from both categories (antidepressants and antiepileptic drugs) that have sedative properties can be selected to minimize polypharmacy and unnecessary exposure of vulnerable patients to addicting substances (193).

Nonopioid Treatments It has been compellingly demonstrated over the course of several decades that many patients with chronic pain are more comfortable and functional without opioids (194,195). Lacking accurate predictors, we are limited to therapeutic trials to ascertain which patients will show improved pain, function, and mood and to assess side effects and aberrant behavior.

Our group studied 527 patients treated in a 3- to 4-week pain rehabilitation program, one third of whom had active comorbid addiction (196). Most had failed to rehabilitate with opioid therapy, which was weaned, as were benzodiazepines. Although those with addiction were twice as likely to drop out of treatment (31% vs. 16%) outcome was equally good in those who completed treatment. Treatment included active physical reconditioning, CBTs, and aggressive use of antidepressants and antiepileptic drugs. Mean pain decreased by 40%, mean Beck Depression Inventory decreased from 21 (severely depressed) to 7 (normal), and mean Pain Disability Index decreased from 44.7/70 (markedly impaired) to 20/70 (mild impairment). In all of these variables, patients with addiction disorder did not differ from those without. This suggests a viable option to treating patients with addiction disorder who respond poorly to opioids. In a prior study, we found that patients who fail to respond to moderate-high dose opioids (mean 445 mg oral morphine/day) have pain reduction with opioid elimination as part of a comprehensive treatment approach (197).

Physician Protection The issue of physician self-protection must be raised, because persons/patients with an addiction disorder may seek compensation from physicians who they claim caused their addiction. *De novo* addiction in association with the prescription of opioids, albeit uncommon, does occur and may constitute a compensable injury. A greater risk, however, is that a patient who had a preexisting addiction may falsely believe or claim that the physician caused it. Risk of litigation and sanctions can be minimized by obtaining written informed consent that notes the risk of addiction, meticulously seeking and documenting the presence of prior addiction, careful documentation of unambiguous benefit from opioids (as independently confirmed by family) and weaning when benefit is unclear, and monitoring for development of behaviors suggesting addiction (including urine toxicology), and requiring addiction assessment/treatment as a condition of further opioid prescribing should they appear.

Other Considerations

Self-Help Groups The American Chronic Pain Association is a self-help recovery program for those with chronic nonmalignant pain (198). Its focus is on self-management. Members are encouraged to employ daily relaxation, stretching exercises, and such psychologic tasks as working on goal setting, assertiveness, and avoiding pain behavior. The concept of changing "from a patient to a person" is emphasized. There are fewer than 400 chapters, so it may not be accessible to many. Materials are available to help persons with pain start new groups. The American Chronic Pain Association does not focus on substance use, so participation in AA or Narcotics Anonymous also is essential for pain patients with co-occurring addiction disorders.

Chronic Cancer Pain Although not the focus of this chapter, cancer pain warrants mention for several reasons: First, cancer has become a chronic disease, and thus most of the material in this chapter is relevant to those in prolonged remissions. Additionally, most of the comments of this chapter regarding the importance of treating comorbid depression and anxiety and providing coping skills training can be applied to the cancer patient who is not acutely ill. Physical therapy directed toward maximization of strength and flexibility can reduce discomfort and improve quality of life, while providing distraction. Malignant pain, of course, often is cured and may transition into such chronic non-malignant pains as toxic neuropathy or radiation cystitis, which are forms of CNMP.

Acute Recurrent Pain Special difficulties arise in the treatment of patients with conditions such as inflammatory bowel disease, chronic pancreatitis, sickle cell disease, and other illnesses in which there is recurrent, severe, nociceptive pain and a substantial prevalence of addiction disorders. The literature concerning the long-term treatment of pain in these conditions, with the exception of sickle cell disease, is quite sparse. In the case of sickle cell disease, there is a consensus that proper care of acute pain requires rapid and aggressive titration of opioids, typically those with which the patient reports prior success (199). There is virtually no literature on treating the CNMP that sometimes develops in these patients between episodes (200). Clinical experience with Crohn disease and opioid addiction suggests that the approach described previously for chronic benign pain, combined with primary addiction treatment, is necessary and helpful, but the patients require extensive longitudinal care, which may need to be intense during crises. Treatment frequently requires chronic opioid therapy.

CONCLUSIONS

Physicians confronted with patients who are suffering from intractable pain may experience therapeutic nihilism and hopelessness. This must not be communicated to patients for two reasons. First, the message, "There is nothing more I can do for you," confirms hopelessness and can encourage suicide. Second, it is clear that the most grateful patients are not necessarily those whose pain has remitted in response to clinical interventions. Rather, many patients report that their pain is little changed from admission, but they laugh, walk briskly, take no addicting drugs, and report that their suffering has been largely alleviated. They are optimistic and report that "the pain is on the back burner where I don't much think about it." Thus it is critical to communicate to patients that they can "recover" even when medical interventions have been exhausted. The methods described in this chapter are not sufficient for all patients, even when combined with nonanalgesic medications for pain reduction. Much of the challenge confronting physicians is to identify those in whom psychologic and rehabilitation methods produce satisfactory results, those in whom analgesics are helpful, and those in whom they do harm.

When a patient demonstrates the characteristics of inordinate suffering, medical involvement, disability, or drug use, it is unlikely that solutions will be found external to the patient, whether through pharmacology or technology. Rather, the solution likely will come from the patient's inner resources. It is the physician's task to help that patient find, strengthen, and trust in those resources.

Patient Information Patients often seek information regarding CNMP to better manage their own conditions. The following materials may be useful:

- Learning to Master Your Chronic Pain by Robert N. Jamison
- Managing Pain Before It Manages You by Margaret Caudill
- Mayo Clinic on Chronic Pain by Jeffrey Rome
- Patient To Person: First Steps by American Chronic Pain Association Family Manual (also various tapes, DVDs related to coping with pain); *http://theacpa.org/*

REFERENCES

1. Martin BI, Deyo RA, Mirza SK, et al. Expenditures and health status among adults with back and neck problems. *JAMA* 2008;299:656–664.
2. Waddell G. Low back pain: a twentieth century health care enigma. *Spine* 1996;21:2820–2825.
3. Anderson G. The epidemiology of spinal disorders. In: JW Frymoyer, ed. *The adult spine: principles and practice*. New York: Raven Press, 1991: 107–146.
4. Deyo RA, Mirza SK, Martin BI. Back pain prevalence and visit rates: estimates from U.S. national surveys, 2002. *Spine* 2006;31(23):2724–2727.
5. Giordano J. The neurobiology of nociceptive and anti-nociceptive systems. *Pain Physician* 2005;8(3):277–290.
6. Dubner R. The neurobiology of persistent pain and its clinical implications. *Suppl Clin Neurophysiol* 2004;57:3–7.
7. Lötsch J, Geisslinger G. Current evidence for a modulation of nociception by human genetic polymorphisms. *Pain* 2007;132(1–2): 18–22.
8. Bigos SJ, Battie MC, Spengler DM, et al. A prospective study of work perceptions and psycho-social factors affecting the report of back injury. *Spine* 1991;16(1):1–6.
9. Papageorgiou AC, Macfarlane GJ, Thomas E, et al. Psychosocial factors in the workplace—do they predict new episodes of low back pain? Evidence from the South Manchester Back Pain Study. *Spine* 1997;22 (10):1137–1142.
10. Valat JP, Goupille P, Vedere V. Low back pain: risk factors for chronicity. *Rev Rheumatol (Engl Ed)* 1997;64(3):189–194.
11. Hasenbring M, Marienfeld G, Kuhlendahl D, et al. Risk factors of chronicity in lumbar disc patients. A prospective investigation of biologic, psychologic, and social predictors of therapy outcome. *Spine* 1994; 19(24):2759–2765.
12. Long DM. Effectiveness of therapies currently employed for persistent low back and leg pain. *Pain Forum* 1995;4(2):122–125.
13. Schrader H, Obelieniene D, Bovim G, et al. Natural evolution of late whiplash syndrome outside the medicolegal context. *Lancet* 1996;347: 1207–1211.
14. Spitzer WO, Skovron ML, Salmi LR, et al. Scientific monograph of the Quebec Task Force on whiplash-associated disorders: redefining "whiplash" and its management. *Spine* 1995;20(85):3S–73S.
15. Cassidy JD, Carroll LJ, Cote P, et al. Effect of eliminating compensation for pain and suffering on the outcome of insurance claims for whiplash injury. *N Engl J Med* 2000;342(16):1179–1186.
16. Lord SM, McDonald GJ. Comment. *Pain Med J* 1997;3(1):40–43.
17. Blake C, Garrett M. Impact of litigation on quality of life outcomes in patients with chronic low back pain. *Irish J Med Sci* 1997;166(3): 124–126.
18. Abbott P, Rounsefell B, Fraser R et al. Intractable neck pain. *Clin J Pain* 1990;6:26–31.
19. Larrabee GJ. Exaggerated pain report in litigants with malingered neurocognitive dysfunction. *Clin Neuropsychol* 2003;17(3):395–401.
20. Greve KW, Bianchini KJ, Ameduri CJ. Use of a forced-choice test of tactile discrimination in the evaluation of functional sensory loss: a report of 3 cases. *Arch Phys Med Rehabil* 2003;84(8):1233–1236.
21. U.S. Commission on the Evaluation of Pain. *Report of the commission on the evaluation of pain, appendix C: summary of the National Study of Chronic Pain Syndrome.* Washington, DC: Social Security Administration, Office of Disability, 1987.
22. Payne B, Norfleet MA. Chronic pain and the family: a review. *Pain* 1986;26:1–22.
23. Roy R. Marital and family issues in patients with chronic pain: a review. *Psychother Psychosom* 1982;37:112.
24. Roy R. Pain-prone patient: a revisit. *Psychother Psychosom* 1982;37: 202–213.
25. Bendixen M, Muus KM, Schei B. The impact of child sexual abuse—a study of a random sample of Norwegian students. *Child Abuse Neglect* 1994;18(10):837–847.
26. Walsh CA, Jamieson E, Macmillan H, et al. Child abuse and chronic pain in a community survey of women. *J Interpers Violence* 2007;22(12): 1536–1554.
27. Porter LS, Davis D , Keefe FJ. Attachment and pain: recent findings and future directions. *Pain* 2007;128(3):195–198.
28. McWilliams LA, Asmundson GJG. The relationship of adult attachment dimensions to pain-related fear, hypervigilance, and catastrophizing. *Pain* 2007;127(1–2):27–34.
29. Coutinho SV, Plotsky PM, Sablad M, et al. Neonatal maternal separation alters stress-induced responses to viscerosomatic nociceptive stimuli in rat. *Am J Physiol Gastrointest Liver Physiol* 2002;282:G307–G316.
30. Van der Kolk BA, Pelcovitz D, Roth S, et al. Dissociation, somatization, and affect dysregulation: the complexity of adaptation of trauma. *Am J Psychiatry* 1996;153(7 Suppl):83–93.
31. Rome HP, Rome JD. Limbically augmented pain syndrome (LAPS): kindling, corticolimbic sensitization, and the convergence of affective and sensory symptoms in chronic pain disorders. *Pain Med* 2000;1(1):7–23.
32. Turk DC, Meichenbaum D, Genest M. *Pain and behavioral medicine: a cognitive-behavioral perspective*. New York: Guilford Press, 1983.
33. Turk DC, Rudy TE. Assessment of cognitive factors in chronic pain: a worthwhile enterprise? *J Consult Clin Psychol* 1986;54(6):760–768.
34. Jensen MP, Turner JA, Romano JM, et al. Coping with chronic pain: a critical review of the literature. *Pain* 1991;47:249–283.
35. Affleck G, Urrows S, Tennen H, et al. Daily coping with pain from rheumatoid arthritis: patterns and correlates. *Pain* 1992;51:221–229.
36. Melzack R. Neurophysiology of pain. In: Sternbach RA, ed. *The Psychology of pain*, 2nd ed. New York: Raven Press, 1986.
37. Ahles TA, Blanchard EB, Ruckdeschel JC. The multidimensional nature of cancer-related pain. *Pain* 1983;17:277–288.
38. Weissman-Fogel I, Sprecher E, Pud D. Effects of catastrophizing on pain perception and pain modulation. *Exp Brain Res* 2008;186(1):79–85.
39. Turk DC, Rudy TE. Cognitive factors and persistent pain: a glimpse into Pandora's box. *Cognit Ther Res* 1992;16(2):99–122.
40. Keefe FJ, Brown GK, Wallston KA, et al. Coping with rheumatoid arthritis pain: catastrophizing as a maladaptive strategy. *Pain* 1989;37: 51–56.
41. Ciccone DS, Grzesiak RC. Cognitive dimensions of chronic pain. *Soc Sci Med* 1984;19(12):1339–1345.
42. Seligman ME. Learned helplessness. *Annu Rev Med* 1972;23:407–412.
43. Jensen MP, Turner JA, Romano JM. Self-efficacy and outcome expectancies: relationship to chronic pain coping strategies and adjustment. *Pain* 1991;44:263–269.
44. Maly MR, Costigan PA, Olney SJ. Self-efficacy mediates walking performance in older adults with knee osteoarthritis. *J Gerontol A Biol Sci Med Sci* 2007;62(10):1142–1146.

45. Lefebvre JC, Keefe FJ, Affleck G, et al. The relationship of arthritis self-efficacy to daily pain, daily mood, and daily pain coping in rheumatoid arthritis patients. *Pain* 1999;80:425–435.
46. Buckelew SP, Huyser B, Hewett J, et al. Self-efficacy predicting outcome among fibromyalgia subjects. *Arthrit Care Res* 1996;9(2):97–104.
47. Smarr KL, Parker JC, Wright GE, et al. The importance of enhancing self-efficacy in rheumatoid arthritis. *Arthritis Care Res* 1997;10(1): 18–26.
48. Harkapaa K, Jarvikoski A, Mellin G, et al. Health locus of control beliefs and psychological distress as predictors for treatment outcome in low-back pain patients: results of a 3-month followup of a controlled intervention study. *Pain* 1991;46:35–41.
49. Crisson JE, Keefe FJ. The relationship of locus of control to pain coping strategies and psychological distress in chronic pain patients. *Pain* 1988;35:147–154.
50. Selander J, Marnetoft SU, Asell M. Predictors for successful vocational rehabilitation for clients with back pain problems. *Disabil Rehabil* 2007;29(3):215–220.
51. DeGood DE, Kiernan B. Perception of fault in patients with chronic pain. *Pain* 1996;64(1):153–159.
52. Fordyce WE, Fowler RS, Lehman JF, et al. Operant conditioning in the treatment of chronic pain. *Arch Phys Med Rehab,* 1973;54(9):399–408.
53. Fordyce WE. *Behavioral Methods for chronic pain and illness*. St. Louis, MO: C.V. Mosby, 1976.
54. Fishbain DA, Rosomoff HL, Cutler RB, et al. Secondary gain concept: a review of the scientific evidence. *Clin J Pain* 1995;11:6–21.
55. Rohling ML, Binder LM, Langhinrichsen-Rohling J. Money matters: a meta-analytic review of the association between financial compensation and the experience and treatment of chronic pain. *Health Psychol* 1995;14(6):537–547.
56. Flor H. The functional organization of the brain in chronic pain. In: Bromm SB, Gebhart GF, eds. *Progress in brain research,* vol. 129. Amsterdam: Elsevier Science B.V. 2000:315.
57. Vlaeyen JWS, Linton SJ. Fear-avoidance and its consequences in chronic musculoskeletal pain: a state of the art. *Pain* 2000;85:317–332.
58. Kori SH, Miller RP, Todd DD. Kinisophobia: a new view of chronic pain behavior. *Pain Manage* 1990;3(1):35–43.
59. McCracken LM, Spertus IL, Janeck AS, et al. Behavioral dimensions of adjustment in persons with chronic pain: pain-related anxiety and acceptance. *Pain* 1999;80:283–289.
60. Crombex G, Vlaeyen JWS, Heuts PHTG, et al. Pain-related fear is more disabling than pain itself: evidence on the role of pain-related fear in chronic back pain disability. *Pain* 1999;80:329–339.
61. Crombez G, Van Damme S, Eccleston C. Hypervigilance to pain: an experimental and clinical analysis. *Pain* 2005;116(1–2):4–7.
62. Vlaeyen JW, Linton SJ: Are we "fear-avoidant?" *Pain* 2006;124(3): 240–241.
63. Petrovic P, Petersson KM, Ghatan PH, et al. Pain-related cerebral activation is altered by a distracting cognitive task. *Pain* 2000;85: 19–30.
64. Zelman DC, Howland EW, Nichols SN, et al. The effects of induced mood on laboratory pain. *Pain* 1991;46:105–111.
65. Rainville P, Bao QVH, Chrétien P. Pain-related emotions modulate experimental pain perception and autonomic responses. *Pain* 2005; 118(3):306–318.
66. Poulsen DL, Hansen HJ, Langemark M, et al. Discomfort or disability in patients with chronic pain syndrome. *Psychother Psychosom* 1987;48 (1-4):60–62.
67. Fishbain DA, Goldberg M, Labbe E, et al. Compensation and noncompensation chronic pain patients compared for DSM-III operational diagnoses. *Pain* 1988;32:197–206.
68. Fishbain DA, Goldberg M, Meagher BR, et al. Male and female chronic pain patients categorized by DSM-III psychiatric diagnostic criteria. *Pain* 1986;26(2):181–197.
69. Gunter WD, Shepard JD, Foreman RD, et al. Evidence for visceral hypersensitivity in high-anxiety rats. *Physiol Behav* 2000;69(3):379–382.
70. Keogh E, Cochrane M. Anxiety sensitivity, cognitive biases, and the experience of pain. *J Pain* 2002;3(4):320–329.
71. Thompson T, Keogh E, French CC, et al. Anxiety sensitivity and pain: generalisability across noxious stimuli. *Pain* 2008;134(1–2):187–196.
72. Fernandez E, Turk DC. The scope and significance of anger in the experience of chronic pain. *Pain* 1995;61(2):165–175.
73. Kerns RD, Rosenberg R, Jacob MC. Anger expression and chronic pain. *J Behav Med* 1994;17(1):57–67.
74. Carson JW, Keefe FJ, Goli V, et al. Forgiveness and chronic low back pain: a preliminary study examining the relationship of forgiveness to pain, anger, and psychological distress. *J Pain* 2005;6(2):84–91.
75. Katon W, Egan K, Miller D. Chronic pain: lifetime psychiatric diagnoses and family history. *Am J Psychiatry* 1985;142(10):1156–1160.
76. Polatin PB, Kinney RK, Gatchel RJ, et al. Psychiatric illness and chronic low-back pain. The mind and the spine—which goes first? *Spine* 1993; 18(1):66–71.
77. Dersh J, Gatchel RJ, Mayer T, et al. Prevalence of psychiatric disorders in patients with chronic disabling occupational spinal disorders. *Spine* 2006;31(10):1156–1162.
78. Kramlinger KG, Swanson DW, Maruta T. Are patients with chronic pain depressed? *Am J Psychiatry* 1983;140(6):747–749.
79. Ohayon MM, Schatzberg AF. Using chronic pain to predict depressive morbidity in the general population. *Arch Gen Psychiatry* 2003;60(1): 39–47.
80. Lefebvre M. Cognitive distortion and cognitive errors in depressed psychiatric and low back pain patients. *J Consult Clin Psychol* 1981;49: 517–525.
81. Rudy T, Kerns RD, Turk DC. Chronic pain and depression: toward a cognitive-behavioral mediation model. *Pain* 1988;35:129–140.
82. Maruta T, Vatterott MK, McHardy MJ. Pain management as an antidepressant: long-term resolution of pain-associated depression. *Pain* 1989; 36(3):335–337.
83. Dohrenwend BP, Raphael KG, Marbach JJ, et al. Why is depression comorbid with chronic myofascial face pain? A family study test of alternative hypotheses. *Pain* 1999;83:183–192.
84. Carroll LJ, Cassidy JD; Côté P. Depression as a risk factor for onset of an episode of troublesome neck and low back pain. *Pain* 2004;107 (1–2):134–139.
85. Gureje O, Simon GE, Von Kor M. A cross-national study of the course of persistent pain in primary care. *Pain* 2001;92:195–200.
86. Williams LS, Jones WJ, Shen J, et al. Outcomes of newly referred neurology outpatients with depression and pain. *Neurology* 2004;63(4): 674–677.
87. Kroenke K, Shen J, Oxman TE, et al. Impact of pain on the outcomes of depression treatment: results from the RESPECT trial. *Pain* 2008; 134(1–2):209–215.
88. Ratcliffe GE, Enns MW, Belik SL, et al. Chronic pain conditions and suicidal ideation and suicide attempts: an epidemiologic perspective. *Clin J Pain* 2008;24(3):204–210.
89. Fishbain DA, Goldberg M, Meagher BR, et al. Male and female chronic pain patients categorized by DSM-III psychiatric diagnostic criteria. *Pain* 1986;26(2):181–197.
90. Poulsen DL, Hansen HJ, Langemark M, et al. Discomfort or disability in patients with chronic pain syndrome. *Psychother Psychosom* 1987;48 (1–4):60–62.
91. Van der Kolk BA, Pelcovitz D, Roth S, et al. Dissociation, somatization, and affect dysregulation: the complexity of adaptation to trauma. *Am J Psychiatry* 1996;153:7.
92. Gunter WD, Shepard JD, Foreman RD, et al. Evidence for visceral hypersensitivity in high-anxiety rats. *Physiol Behav* 2000;69(3):379–382.
93. Coutinho SV, Plotsky PM, Sablad M, et al. Neonatal maternal separation alters stress-induced responses to viscerosomatic nociceptive stimuli in rat. *Am J Physiol Gastrointest Liver Physiol* 2002;282(2): G307–G316.
94. Edwards RR, Klick B, Buenaver L, et al. Symptoms of distress as prospective predictors of pain-related sciatica treatment outcomes. *Pain* 2007;130(1–2):47–55.
95. American Psychiatric Association. *Diagnostic and statistical manual of mental disorders*, 4th text revision ed. Washington, DC: American Psychiatric Association, 2000.

96. Savage S. Long-term opioid therapy: assessment of consequences and risks. *J Pain Symptom Manage* 1996;11:274–286.
97. Deyo RA, Bass JE. Lifestyle and low-back pain: the influence of smoking and obesity. *Spine* 1989;14(5):501–506.
98. Kelsey JL, Golden AL, Mundt DJ. Low back pain/prolapsed lumbar intervertebral disc. *Rheum Dis Clin N Am* 1990;16(3):699–716.
99. Atkinson JH, Slater MA, Patterson TL, et al. Prevalence, onset, and risk of psychiatric disorders in men with chronic low back pain: a controlled study. *Pain* 1991;45:111–121.
100. Yunus MB, Arslan S, Aldag JC. Relationship between fibromyalgia features and smoking. *Scand J Rheumatol* 2002;31(5):301–305.
101. Hoffmann NG, Olofsson O, Salen B, et al. Prevalence of abuse and dependency in chronic pain patients. *Int J Addict* 1995;30(8):919–927.
102. Moore RD, Bone LR, Geller G, et al. Prevalence, detection, and treatment of alcoholism in hospitalized patients. *JAMA* 1989;261:403–407.
103. Chabal C, Erjavec MK, Jacobson L, et al. Prescription opiate abuse in chronic pain patients: clinical criteria, incidence, and predictors. *Clin J Pain* 1997;13(2):150–155.
104. Smothers BA, Yahr HT. Alcohol use disorder and illicit drug use in admissions to general hospitals in the United States. *Am J Addict* 2005; 14:256–267.
105. Jamison RN, Kauffman J, Katz NP. Characteristics of methadone maintenance patients with chronic pain. *J Pain Symptom Manage* 2000;1 (1):53–62.
106. Rosenblum A, Joseph H, Fong C, et al. Prevalence and characteristics of chronic pain among chemically dependent patients in methadone maintenance and residential treatment facilities. *JAMA* 2003;289:2370–2378.
107. Fishbain DA, Cutler R, Rosomoff HL, et al. Chronic pain disability exaggeration/malingering and submaximal effort research. *Clin J Pain* 1999;15(4):244–274.
108. Bytzer P, Stokholm M, Andersen I, et al. Prevalence of surreptitious laxative abuse in patients with diarrhea of uncertain origin: a cost benefit analysis of a screening procedure. *Gut* 1989;30(10):1379–1384.
109. Rickards FW, De Vidi S. Exaggerated hearing loss in noise induced hearing loss compensation claims in Victoria. *Med J Aust* 1995;163(7): 360–363.
110. Schmand B, Lindeboom J, Schagen S, et al. Cognitive complaints in patients after whiplash injury: the impact of malingering. *J Neurol Neurosurg Psychiatry* 1998;64(3):339–343.
111. Gervais RO, Russell AS, Green P, et al. Effort testing in patients with fibromyalgia and disability incentives. *J Rheumatol* 2001;28(8):1892–1899.
112. Weintraub MI. Chronic pain in litigation: what is the relationship? *Neurol Clin* 1995;13(2):341–349.
113. Ransford AO, Cairns D, Mooney V. The pain drawing as an aid to the psychologic evaluation of patients with low-back pain. *Spine* 1976;1 (2):127–134.
114. Tait RC, Chibnall JT, Krause S. The Pain Disability Index: psychometric properties. *Pain* 1990;40(2):171–182.
115. Leon AC, Olfson M, Portera L, et al. Assessing psychiatric impairment in primary care with the Sheehan Disability Scale. *Int J Psychiatry Med* 1997;27(2):93–105.
116. Waddell G, McCulloch J, Kummel E, et al. Non-organic physical signs in low-back pain. *Spine* 1980;5:117–125.
117. Gaines WG Jr, Hegmann KT. Effectiveness of Waddell's nonorganic signs in predicting a delayed return to regular work in patients experiencing acute occupational low back pain. *Spine* 1999;24(4):396–400.
118. Raskin M, Talbott JA, Meyerson AT. Diagnosis of conversion reactions. *JAMA* 1966;197:102–106.
119. Main CJ, Evans PJD, Whitehead RC. An investigation of personality structure and other psychological features in patients presenting with low back pain: a critique of the MMPI. In: Bond MR, Charlton JE, Woolf CJ, eds. *Proceedings of the 6th World Congress on Pain*. Amsterdam: Elsevier Science Publishers, 1991:207–217.
120. Turner JA, Calsyn DA, Fordyce WE, et al. Drug utilization patterns in chronic pain patients. *Pain* 1982;12:357–363.
121. Valat JP, Goupille P, Vedere V. Low back pain: risk factors for chronicity. *Rev Rheumatol (Engl Ed)* 1997;64(3):189–194.
122. Dimeo F, Bauer M, Varahram I, et al. Benefits from aerobic exercise in patients with major depression: a pilot study. *Br J Sports Med* 2001;35 (2):114–117.
123. Burleson AM, Covington EC, Scheman J. The benefits of physical conditioning in chronic pain patients. *Am Acad Pain Med* 2008 (poster); available at www.painmed.org/pdf/08scientific_abstracts.pdf.
124. Van Tulder MW, Koes BW, Bouter LM. Conservative treatment of acute and chronic nonspecific low back pain. A systematic review of randomized controlled trials of the most common interventions. *Spine* 1997; 22(18):2128–2156.
125. Van der Velde G, Mierau D. The effect of exercise on percentile rank aerobic capacity, pain, and self-rated disability in patients with chronic low-back pain: a retrospective chart review. *Arch Phys Med Rehabil* 2000;81: 1457–1463.
126. Ljunggren AE, Weber H, Kogstad O, et al. Effect of exercise on sick leave due to low back pain. A randomized, comparative, longterm study. *Spine* 1997;22(14):1610–1616.
127. Brox JI, Reikeras O, Nygaard O, et al. Lumbar instrumented fusion compared with cognitive intervention and exercises in patients with chronic back pain after previous surgery for disc herniation: a prospective randomized controlled study. *Pain* 2006;122(1–2):145–155.
128. Turner JA, Chapman CR. Psychological interventions for chronic pain: a critical review. II. Operant conditioning, hypnosis and cognitive-behavioral therapy. *Pain* 1982;12:23–46.
129. Sanders SH. Operant therapy with pain patients: evidence for its effectiveness. In: Lebovits, AH, ed. *Seminars in pain medicine*. Philadelphia: WB Saunders, 2003:90–98.
130. Williams DA, Thorn BE. An empirical assessment of pain beliefs. *Pain* 1989;36:351–358.
131. Waddell G, Newton M, Henderson I, et al. A fear avoidance beliefs questionnaire (FABQ) and the role of fear avoidance beliefs in chronic low back pain and disability. *Pain* 1993;52:157–168.
132. Fernandez E, Turk DC. The utility of cognitive coping strategies for altering pain perception: a meta-analysis. *Pain* 1989;38:123–135.
133. Compas BE, Haaga DA, Keefe FJ, et al. Sampling of empirically supported psychological treatments from health psychology: smoking, chronic pain, cancer, and bulimia nervosa. *J Consult Clin Psychol* 1998;66(1):89–112.
134. Morley S, Eccleston C, Williams A. Systematic review and meta-analysis of randomized controlled trials of cognitive behavior therapy and behavior therapy for chronic pain in adults, excluding headache. *Pain* 1999;80:1–13.
135. McCracken LM, Carson JW, Eccleston C, et al. Acceptance and change in the context of chronic pain. *Pain* 2004;109(1–2):4–7.
136. Baer, RA: Mindfulness training as a clinical intervention: a conceptual and empirical review. *Clin Psychol* 2003;10(2):125–143.
137. McCracken LM, Gauntlett-Gilbert J, Vowles KE. The role of mindfulness in a contextual cognitive-behavioral analysis of chronic pain-related suffering and disability. *Pain* 2007;131(1–2):63–69.
138. Morone NE, Greco CM, Weiner DK. Mindfulness meditation for the treatment of chronic low back pain in older adults: a randomized controlled pilot study. *Pain* 2008;134(3):310–319.
139. Grossman P, Tiefenthaler-Gilmer U, Raysz A, et al. Mindfulness training as an intervention for fibromyalgia: evidence of postintervention and 3-year follow-up benefits in well-being. *Psychother Psychosom* 2007;76(4):226–233.
140. McCracken LM, Vowles KE. A prospective analysis of acceptance of pain and values-based action in patients with chronic pain. *Health Psychol* 2008;27(2):215–220.
141. Viane I, Crombez G, Eccleston C, et al. Acceptance of the unpleasant reality of chronic pain: effects upon attention to pain and engagement with daily activities. *Pain* 2004;112(3):282–288.
142. McCracken LM, Eccleston C. A comparison of the relative utility of coping and acceptance-based measures in a sample of chronic pain sufferers. *Eur J Pain* 2006;10(1):23–29.
143. National Institutes of Health (NIH), Technology Assessment Panel on Integration of Behavioral and Relaxation Approaches into the Treatment

of Chronic Pain and Insomnia. Integration of behavioral and relaxation approaches into the treatment of chronic pain and insomnia. *JAMA* 1996;276(4):313–338.

144. Karavidas MK, Tsai PS, Yucha C, et al. Thermal biofeedback for primary Raynaud's phenomenon: a review of the literature. *Appl Psychophysiol Biofeedback* 2006;31(3):203–216.
145. Rainforth MV, Schneider RH, Nidich SI, et al. Stress reduction programs in patients with elevated blood pressure: a systematic review and meta-analysis. *Curr Hypertens Rep* 2007;9(6):520–528.
146. Bruehl S, Chung OY. Psychological and behavioral aspects of complex regional pain syndrome management. *Clin J Pain* 2006;22(5): 430–437.
147. Babu AS, Mathew E, Danda D, et al. Management of patients with fibromyalgia using biofeedback: a randomized control trial. *Indian J Med Sci* 2007;61:455–461.
148. Van Tulder MW, Ostelo R, Vlaeyen JW, et al. Behavioral treatment for chronic low back pain: a systematic review within the framework of the Cochrane back review group. *Spine* 2000;25:2688–2699.
149. Sierpina V, Astin J, Giordano J. Mind-body therapies for headache. *Am Fam Physician* 2007;76(10):1518–1522.
150. Astin, JA: Mind-body therapies for the management of pain. *Clin J Pain* 2004;20(1):27–32.
151. Nestoriuc Y, Martin A. Efficacy of biofeedback for migraine: a meta-analysis. *Pain* 2007;128;111–127.
152. Gatchel RJ, Stowell AW, Wildenstein L, et al. Efficacy of an early intervention for patients with acute temporomandibular disorder-related pain: a one-year outcome study. *J Am Dent Assoc* 2006;137(3): 339–347.
153. Gilliland R, Wexner SD, Vickers D, et al. Biofeedback for intractable rectal pain: outcome and predictors of success. *Dis Colon Rectum* 1997; 40(2):190–196.
154. Heah SM, Leong AF, Tan M, et al. Biofeedback is effective treatment for levator ani syndrome. *Dis Colon Rectum* 1997;40(2):187–189.
155. Spence SH, Champion D, Newton-John T, et al. Effect of EMG biofeedback compared to applied relaxation training with chronic, upper extremity cumulative trauma disorders. *Pain* 1995;63(2):199–206.
156. Haefner HK, Collins ME, Davis GD, et al. The vulvodynia guideline. *J Low Genit Tract Dis* 2005;9(1):40–51.
157. Flor H, Birbaumer N. Comparison of the efficacy of electromyographic biofeedback, cognitive-behavioral therapy, and conservative medical interventions in the treatment of chronic musculoskeletal pain. *J Clin Consult Psychol* 1993;61(4):653–658.
158. Rokicki LA, Holroyd KA, France CR, et al. Change mechanisms associated with combined relaxation/EMG biofeedback training for chronic tension headache. *Appl Psychophysiol Biofeedback* 1997;22(1):21–41.
159. Turner JA, Chapman CR. Psychological interventions for chronic pain: a critical review. I. Relaxation training and biofeedback. *Pain* 1982;12:1–21.
160. Linton SJ. Behavioral remediation of chronic pain: a status report. *Pain* 1986;24:125–141.
161. Blanchard EB, Appelbaum KA, Guarnieri P, et al. Five year prospective follow-up on the treatment of chronic headache with biofeedback and/or relaxation. *Headache* 1987;27(10):580–583.
162. Kropp P, Niederberger U, Kopal T, et al. Behavioral treatment in migraine. Cognitive-behavioral therapy and blood-volume-pulse biofeedback: a cross-over study with a two-year follow-up. *Functional Neurol* 1997;12(1):17–24.
163. Turk DC, Greco CM, Zaki HS, et al. Dysfunctional patients with temporomandibular disorders: Evaluating the efficacy of a tailored treatment protocol. *J Consult Clin Psychol* 1996;64(1):139–146.
164. Kayiran S, Dursun E, Ermutlu N, et al. Neurofeedback in fibromyalgia syndrome. *Agri* 2007;19(3):47–53.
165. Lewandowski W, Morris R, Draucker CB, et al. Chronic pain and the family: theory-driven treatment approaches. *Issues Ment Health Nurs* 2007;28(9):1019–1044.
166. Langelier RP, Gallagher RM. Outpatient treatment of chronic pain groups for couples. *Clin J Pain* 1989;5(3):227–231.
167. Flor H, Turk DC, Rudy TE. Pain and families. II. Assessment and treatment. *Pain* 1987;30(1):29–45.
168. Flor H, Fydrich T, Turk DC. Efficacy of multidisciplinary pain treatment centers: a meta-analytic review. *Pain* 1992;49:221–230.
169. Turk DC. Efficacy of multidisciplinary pain centers in the treatment of chronic pain. In: MJM Cohen, NJ Campbell, eds. *Pain treatment centers at a crossroads: a practical and conceptual reappraisal, progress in pain research and management,* Vol. 7. Seattle, WA: IASP Press, 1996:257–273.
170. Gatchel RJ, Okifuji A. Evidence-based scientific data documenting the treatment and cost-effectiveness of comprehensive pain programs for chronic nonmalignant pain. *J Pain* 2006;7(11):779–793.
171. http://www.chronicpainanonymous.org/ Accessed April 20, 2008.
172. American Society for Pain Management Nursing: ASPMN position statement: pain management in patients with addictive disease. *J Vasc Nurs* 2004;22(3):99–101.
173. Mehta V, Langford RM. Acute pain management for opioid dependent patients. *Anaesthesia* 2006;61(3):269–276.
174. Nedeljkovic SS, Wasan A, Jamison RN. Assessment of efficacy of long-term opioid therapy in pain patients with substance abuse potential. *Clin J Pain* 2002;18:539–551.
175. Joranson DE, Cleeland CS, Weissman DE, et al. Opioids for chronic cancer and non-cancer pain: a survey of state medical board members. *Fed Bull J Med Licens Discipline* 1992;79(4):15–49.
176. Gilson AM, Joranson DE. Controlled substances and pain management: changes in knowledge and attitudes of state medical regulators. *J Pain Sympt Manage* 2001;21(3):227–237.
177. Dunbar MB, Katz NP. Chronic opioid therapy for nonmalignant pain in patients with a history of substance abuse: report of 20 cases. *J Pain Symptom Manage* 1996;11(3):163–171.
178. Kennedy JA, Crowley TJ. Chronic pain and substance abuse: a pilot study of opioid maintenance. *J Subst Abuse Treat* 1990;7:233–238.
179. Currie SR, Hodgins DC, Crabtree A, et al. Outcome from integrated pain management treatment for recovering substance abusers. *J Pain* 2003;4(2):91–100.
180. Miotto K, Compton P, Ling W, et al. Diagnosing addictive disease in chronic pain patients. *Psychosomatics* 1996;37:223–235.
181. Passik SD, Kirsh KL. Opioid therapy in patients with a history of substance abuse. *CNS Drugs* 2004;18(1):13–25.
182. Savage SR. Opioid therapy of chronic pain: assessment of consequences. *Acta Anaesthesiol Scand* 1999;43(9):909–917.
183. Busto U, Sellers EM. Pharmacokinetic determinants of drug abuse and dependence: a conceptual perspective. *Clin Pharmacokinet* 1986:11(2): 144–153.
184. Mironer YE, Brown C, Satterthwaite J, et al. Relative misuse potential of different opioids: a large pain clinic experience. American Pain Society, 2000, available at www.ampainsoc.org/db2/abstract/view?poster_id=845#696.
185. Kittelberger KP, Buchheit TE, Rice SF. Self-extraction of intrathecal pump opioid. *Anesthesiology* 2004;101(3):807.
186. Gock S, Wong S, Stormo K, et al. Self-intoxication with morphine obtained from an infusion pump. *J Anal Toxicol* 1999;23(2):130–133.
187. Burton AW, Conroy B, Garcia E, et al. Illicit substance abuse via an implanted intrathecal pump. *Anesthesiology* 1998;89(5):1264–1267.
188. d'Elia G, von Knorring L, Marcusson J, et al. A double blind comparison between doxepin and diazepam in the treatment of states of anxiety. *Acta Psychiatr Scand Suppl* 1974;255:35–46.
189. Bianchi GN, Phillips J. A comparative trial of doxepin and diazepam in anxiety states. *Psychopharmacologia* 1972;25(1):86–95.
190. Rickels K, Downing R, Schweizer E, et al. Antidepressants for the treatment of generalized anxiety disorder. A placebo-controlled comparison of imipramine, trazodone, and diazepam. *Arch Gen Psychiatry* 1993; 50(11):884–895.
191. Kapczinski F, Lima MS, Souza JS, et al. Antidepressants for generalized anxiety disorder. *Cochrane Database Syst Rev* 2003(2):CD003592.
192. Van Ameringen M, Mancini C, Pipe B, et al. Antiepileptic drugs in the treatment of anxiety disorders: role in therapy. *Drugs* 2004;6419:2199–2220.
193. Saletu-Zyhlarz GM, Abu-Bakr MH, Anderer P, et al. Insomnia related to dysthymia: polysomnographic and psychometric comparison with normal controls and acute therapeutic trials with trazodone. *Neuropsychobiology* 2001;44(3):139–149.

194. Finlayson RE, Maruta T, Morse RM, et al. Substance dependence and chronic pain: experience with treatment and follow-up results. *Pain* 1986;26:175–180.
195. Rome JD, Townsend CO, Bruce BK, et al. Chronic noncancer pain rehabilitation with opioid withdrawal: comparison of treatment outcomes based on opioid use status at admission. *Mayo Clin Proc* 2004;79(6):759–768.
196. Scheman J, Van Keuren C, Smith S, et al. Treatment response to chronic pain rehabilitation program among those with an active addiction disorder. The 6th International Conference on Pain and Chemical Dependency, Brooklyn, NY, February 7, 2004.
197. Covington EC, Kotz MM. Pain reduction with opioid elimination. American Academy of Pain Medicine annual meeting: February 13, 2002, San Francisco, CA.
198. http://www.theacpa.org/. Accessed April 20, 2008.
199. Ballas SK. Current issues in sickle cell pain and its management. Current issues in sickle cell pain and its management. *Hematol Am Soc Hematol Educ Program* 2007;2007:97–105.
200. Dunlop RJ, Bennett KC. Pain management for sickle cell disease. *Cochrane Database Syst Rev* 2006(2):CD003350.

CHAPTER 94

James A.D. Otis, MD
Michael Perloff, MD

Nonopioid Treatments in the Management of Pain

Medications can provide effective pain management in most patients. Choosing the appropriate medication requires that the pain state being treated is correctly diagnosed and classified as somatic, visceral, or neuropathic. Nonsteroidal anti-inflammatory drugs and opioids are the principal medications for somatic pain, whereas adjuvant medications such as antidepressants, antiepileptics, anesthetics, and adrenergic agents are useful for neuropathic pain. Severe pain, whether somatic or neuropathic, usually requires opioid therapy. For example, in recent clinical trials, when classic adjuvants (e.g., gabapentin, amitriptyline) failed for moderate to severe neuropathic pain, a good response was demonstrated with tramadol, low-dose methadone, and, of course, morphine (1–3). After the appropriate class of medication has been selected, the choice of a specific drug is determined by its side effects, route of administration, and individual patient characteristics. Balancing the benefits of a drug with the patient's ability to take it is the art of drug therapy. Other treatment modalities include interventional techniques and physical modalities. In the management of chronic pain, these are adjuncts to primary therapy and are not substitutes for pharmacotherapy. This chapter provides an overview of these methods and their indications. (Psychologic approaches, which are integral to a multidisciplinary approach to pain management, are reviewed in Chapter 93. Use of opioid medications is discussed in Chapter 95.)

NONOPIOID PHARMACOLOGIC AGENTS

Many of the medications used to treat pain are not primary analgesics, but have analgesic efficacy under certain conditions. Such medications are classified as adjuvant analgesics. They include antiepileptic drugs, antidepressants, adrenergic agonists, local anesthetics, and muscle relaxants. Other medications are primary analgesics, but are not opioids. Appropriate use of both types of medications can greatly improve analgesia as well as overall pain management.

NONOPIOID ANALGESICS

Nonsteroidal Anti-inflammatory Drugs Nonsteroidal anti-inflammatory drugs (NSAIDs), which are the most widely used analgesics, are indicated for somatic pain of mild to moderate intensity. They are most useful in bone and joint pain, but can be used in conjunction with opioids for all forms of pain. The first NSAID, aspirin, remains the model for all others. Newer compounds have the same presumed mode of action but offer advantages in side effect profiles and ease of use. Although the exact mechanism of NSAID analgesia is unclear, it is thought to be related to the inhibition of cyclooxygenase activity (COX), which in turn inhibits prostaglandin production (4). Prostaglandins sensitize peripheral nerve endings to noxious stimuli and are the key to the inflammatory cascade. There also is evidence that NSAIDs have a role in modulating pain in the central nervous system, particularly at the spinal cord level (5), independent of their anti-inflammatory action (6). It is not clear which mechanism is more important clinically.

All NSAIDs are well absorbed in the gastrointestinal (GI) tract. Most undergo some hepatic conjugation or oxidation and are excreted in urine. For this reason, hepatic and renal impairment can lead to drug accumulation. Generally, NSAIDs that are conjugated require further renal metabolism to be excreted, whereas NSAIDs that predominantly undergo oxidative metabolism in the liver are simply excreted and appear safer in renal failure (tenoxicam and piroxicam) (7). It should be noted that the aforementioned NSAIDs, those requiring hepatic oxidation, are dangerous in patients with liver failure. Overall, most NSAIDs require hepatic and renal clearance; therefore, dose adjustment in these settings is required.

There is a ceiling level to the analgesic effect of NSAIDs, beyond which increasing the dose does not improve analgesia. Unfortunately, this ceiling level varies from patient to patient, requiring individualized titration of dose. Patients have variable responses to the different classes of NSAIDs: some do not respond at all to one class, but have excellent results with a different class.

The toxicity of NSAIDs is well recognized. In elderly persons and patients with renal, hepatic, and hematologic disease, associated side effects are enhanced. For this reason, the usual guidelines regarding dosing need to be adjusted and often cannot be used. Several studies suggest that the rate of significant GI problems is about 10% (8). Nausea and diarrhea are common GI side effects of NSAIDs. Gastric and duodenal ulceration, although less common, are clinically more important. The effects of NSAIDs on the GI tract are thought to be due to prostaglandin inhibition and loss of their protective effect on the gastric mucosa. It does not appear that NSAIDs produce ulceration by a local effect alone, because prostaglandin decrease is seen throughout the entire GI tract. It is difficult to predict which patient will develop GI ulceration. Nausea and abdominal pain are poor warning symptoms of toxicity. Proton pump inhibitors are clinically accepted and suggested by both the American College of Rheumatology and the American Pain Society for patients with GI risk factors when acetaminophen or COX1 alternatives can not be employed (9,10). Prophylaxis with misoprostol can also be useful (9,10), but it is expensive and its long-term effects are unknown. Consequently, it should be reserved for patients who have a known sensitivity to NSAIDs and after proton pump inhibitor (PPI) failure. Renal damage is another major toxic effect of NSAIDs, particularly for patients with compromised renal function (11). NSAIDs should be used very cautiously in these patients. A useful rule of thumb is to avoid the use of NSAIDs in any patient with proteinuria and decreased glomerular filtration rate. Hematologic toxicity, primarily platelet inhibition, can be particularly problematic. Most NSAIDs inhibit platelet aggregation and prolong bleeding time; these effects usually last for about 1 week. Choline magnesium trisalicylate has minimal antiplatelet effect and can be used in patients with platelet dysfunction who would benefit from an NSAID (12).

A variety of other side effects associated with NSAIDs are not well characterized. For example, headache is a common complaint in patients maintained on NSAIDs, as is dizziness, but the mechanism behind these is unclear. The symptoms are often dose-related. Skin reactions can occur as well, usually as an allergic response. Treatment should be discontinued and the patient rechallenged with a different class of NSAID if clinically necessary.

Significant interactions between NSAIDs and other medications are common. The most important of these involve the potentiation of renal and hepatic toxicity of coadministered drugs and the changes NSAIDs can produce in anticonvulsant levels. Dramatic and dangerous increases in serum levels of lithium, widely used in psychiatric therapy, can result from coadministered NSAIDs resulting from decreased renal clearance (13). There is no known interaction between NSAIDs and anti-retroviral medications. Although the major indication for NSAIDs is the treatment of mild to moderate somatic pain (<3 on the visual analog scale), these drugs often are used in conjunction with low-potency opiates for more severe pain. Bone and joint pains are very responsive to NSAIDs, but neuropathic pain usually is not (14). In the author's experience, diffuse myalgias also are generally resistant to these medications, except in the setting of fever. Patients with advanced disease and pain sufficiently severe to interfere with their activities of daily living will require additional medications.

COX-2 Selective NSAIDs In an attempt to decrease the toxicity of traditional NSAIDs, COX-2 selective inhibitors have been developed. Whereas traditional NSAIDs inhibit both COX-1 (which is protective to the gut and important in other constitutive processes) and COX-2 (which is predominantly involved in inflammation and pain), COX-2 selective NSAIDs were thought to affect only the inflammatory pathway. After their introduction, COX-2 inhibitors, celecoxib, valdecoxib, and rofecoxib, were heavily employed because of their therapeutic equality to traditional NSAIDs, but decreased GI side effects. Questions about the importance of COX-2 constitutive expression in vascular endothelium were subsequently raised. Clinical trials and retrospective meta-analysis demonstrated increased myocardial infarctions and strokes in recipients of COX-2 inhibitors compared to traditional NSAIDs (15). Rofecoxib and valdecoxib have been withdrawn from the market. Celecoxib is still available, but with a black box warning for cardiovascular risk. COX-2 inhibitors still have use in specific populations, but considering their cost, absence of analgesic superiority, and the ubiquity of cardiovascular disease, their use over traditional NSAIDs or COX-2 "preferred" NSAIDs (such as meloxicam and nabumetone) should be carefully considered.

Adjuvant Analgesics Medications that have a primary indication other than analgesia, but which have analgesic properties under certain conditions, are termed *adjuvant analgesics*. Most of these medications enhance the body's own pain-modulating mechanisms or the effectiveness of other analgesics. Several different classes of medications are used as adjuvants, including antidepressants, antiepileptics, oral local anesthetics, and adrenergic agonists.

Antidepressants The tricyclic antidepressants (TCAs) have been used for many years for the management of neuropathic pain. Their analgesic effect appears to be independent of their antidepressant actions (16). There is evidence to suggest that their mode of action is to enhance the body's own pain modulating pathways and to enhance opioid effect at the opioid receptors (17). Their onset of action is slow, requiring several weeks for the full drug effect to be achieved. They are most effective for continuous, burning, or dysesthetic pain (18). Although tricyclic antidepressants are a first-line therapy for many forms of neuropathy, they appear to have poor efficacy in HIV neuropathy (19,20). This may be due to the rapid degeneration of nerve fibers in HIV. The greatest analgesic effect is seen with the older, tertiary amine antidepressants, such as amitriptyline, imipramine, and doxepin. Secondary amine tricyclics, such as desipramine and nortriptyline, also are effective and have less sedation and anticholinergic side effects (21). The selective serotonin reuptake inhibitor class does not seem to be as effective for neuropathic pain (22,23). Nevertheless, they can be helpful in managing associated depression and insomnia. Tricyclics are well absorbed from the GI tract and have few interactions with antiretroviral agents. However, they do have a significant number of side effects, the most common of which is sedation. In many cases, this can be avoided by starting at a low dose and instructing the patient to take the medication 10–12 hours before rising, rather than at bedtime. The usual starting dose for amitriptyline is between 10 and 25 mg, and most patients find benefit at ranges between 50 and 150 mg. Some patients do well with doses above and below this range as well. Many of the other side effects seen with tricyclic antidepressants are related to their anticholinergic properties. These include dry mouth, visual blurring, urinary retention, hypotension, and cardiac arrhythmias. Patients often become tolerant to these after some time. Starting at a low dose of 10 mg and escalating at weekly intervals reduces the likelihood of significant discomfort. TCAs are contraindicated in patients with glaucoma, cardiac arrhythmias, and prolonged QTc, and should be used with caution in patients with urinary outlet obstruction.

Some patients are not able to tolerate TCAs and may benefit from some of the newer antidepressants. Paroxetine, in particular, has been found useful in certain forms of painful peripheral neuropathy (24). Similar evidence does not exist for other serotonin norepinephrine reuptake inhibitors. Venlafaxine (mixed neurotransmitter reuptake inhibitor) and duloxetine (SNRI) have shown efficacy in peripheral neuropathy and other pain therapy. In a well designed crossover study venlafaxine (225 mg/day) and imipramine (150 mg/day) similarly improved symptoms of painful polyneuropathy where patients rated pain paroxysms, constant pain, and pressure-evoked pain. The number needed to treat (NNT) was lower in the imipramine group than in those given venlafaxine (2.7 vs. 5.2) (25). Venlafaxine has also been shown to be effective in postmastectomy pain syndrome, without the anticholinergic effects associated with classic TCAs (26). Multiple clinical trials with duloxetine have demonstrated efficacy in restoring functional status and decreasing pain scores in diabetic peripheral neuropathy when given in doses of 60 mg daily or twice daily (27). Duloxetine, at the same dose, has also improved global pain scores in fibromyalgia (with and without comorbid depression) (28). Duloxetine and venlafaxine may be the preferred drugs for the treatment of depression with comorbid pain syndromes, regardless of whether these pain syndromes have classic etiologies (e.g., diabetic peripheral neuropathy, radicular pain) or nonspecific pain associated with depression (29). Advantages over classic TCAs include fewer anticholinergic effects, less alpha blockade (fewer falls), and absence of QTc prolongation.

Anticonvulsants Carbamazepine, phenytoin, gabapentin and several other anticonvulsant/antiepileptic drugs (AEDs) have efficacy in neuropathic pain (30). The exact mode of action varies, but is related to antiepileptic mechanisms and unrelated pathways. It is suspected that AEDs may reduce pain by reducing neuronal excitability and local neuronal discharges. They appear to be helpful in pain syndromes that are characterized by paroxysmal or lancinating pain, as well as burning pain and allodynia (31). Phenytoin has been used for the management of a variety of neuropathic pain syndromes, including trigeminal neuralgia and postherpetic neuralgia (32). That being said carbamazepine remain first-line therapy standard of care (32). The average dose of phenytoin is 300 mg/day. A loading dose of 1 g can be used for acute pain management. Phenytoin has significant drug interactions with a variety of protein-bound medications, including rifampin, methadone, and several antifungal agents. Both phenytoin and carbamazepine induce many cytochrome P450s and glucuronyl transferase enzymes, and can reduce the serum concentration of drugs which are substrates of the same enzymes, including other AEDs, steroids, cyclosporin A, warfarin, cardiovascular, antineoplastic, and psychotropic drugs (33). Dizziness and somnolence are common with phenytoin and usually are dose-related. Serious skin reactions such as Stevens-Johnson syndrome can occur, necessitating discontinuation of the drug. Leukopenia and thrombocytopenia can occur as idiosyncratic reactions. Elevation of liver enzymes is common. Carbamazepine has been well studied and used successfully in a variety of neuropathic pain states (31,34). It appears to be more effective than phenytoin but has several significant side effects, including dizziness, somnolence, and significant leukopenia. Hyponatremia also can occur as an idiosyncratic reaction. Starting at a dose of 100 mg and gradually escalating in 100 mg increments every 3 to 7 days can minimize the dizziness. Close monitoring of the blood count is necessary and limits the utility of this drug in HIV patients. Carbamazepine is known to have significant autoinduction of metabolism and may require escalating doses over time to achieve the same plasma levels and clinical effect. Oxcarbazepine has similar issues clinically. Valproic acid has been used for the management of lancinating pain, with mixed results, and for pain of diabetic neuropathy. There are no large studies demonstrating long-term effectiveness. The large number of drug interactions and significant hepatic dysfunction that can occur with this drug make it a second-line choice.

Several newer AEDs, released in the last 10 to 15 years, have been found to be useful in treating neuropathic pain. Gabapentin is well established and multiple studies have demonstrated efficacy in both lancinating and continuous dysesthetic pain (35–39). It is a remarkably well-tolerated drug with few interactions and a good side effect profile. Treatment usually is started at 100 mg three times per day and then escalated in increments of 100 to 300 mg every 3 to 5 days. Most patients have a response at 300 mg three times per day, but may require dosing up to 3,600 mg/day (39). There is some evidence that doses higher than 3,600 mg to 4,800 mg are not well absorbed, so doses above this range are of questionable utility (40). The most common reported side effect is somnolence, which resolves after the first 2 weeks of therapy. Recent clinical studies have demonstrated that preoperative gabapentin (typically 900 to 1,200 mg/day) reduces the amount of opioid required to achieve adequate postoperative pain control. Accordingly, classic opioid side effects were reduced (vomiting, pruritus, constipation), whereas acute sedation was increased (41). Lamotrigine has showed modest efficacy in treatment of diabetic and HIV neuropathy (42,43); however, because of required slow titration of medication to avoid dermatologic side effects and reduced efficacy compared with gabapentin and pregabalin, lamotrigine appears a poor choice for neuropathic pain therapy. Although topiramate has well established efficacy in migraine prophylaxis, it has little to no efficacy in treatment of acute pain syndromes. Topiramate has not been shown to have efficacy comparable to established agents in the pain syndrome, including lower back pain, radicular pain, diabetic neuropathy, and trigeminal neuralgia.

The newest AED with efficacy in neuropathic pain is pregabalin, which has a very similar profile to gabapentin. Pregabalin binds the alpha2-delta subunit of calcium channels, reducing neurotransmitter release. In multiple large scale trials, 150 to 600 mg/day of pregabalin had good efficacy in controlling neuropathic pain in both postherpetic neuralgia and diabetic peripheral neuropathy (37,44–47). Typically, greater than 50% benefit was quantified with the McGill Pain Questionnaire, average daily pain scores, Patient and Clinical Global Impression of Change, sensory/affective pain scores, and other efficacy measures. These scores were similar to gabapentin trials. Additionally, sleep interference scores improved across multiple studies. Pregabalin is typically initiated at 50 mg three times per day and increased to 100 mg three times per day over a week. Best pain control usually occurs after 1 week of dosing. Dosing of 450 mg/day is typically recommended in fibromyalgia, and various neuropathic pains may require up to 600 mg/day to achieve efficacy. Most common side effects reported were dizziness and somnolence. These were well tolerated and typically resolved with drug habituation. Weight gain is also common. Absolute platelet number can be decreased with pregabalin, thus it should be used with caution in patients prone to thrombocytopenia. Clonazepam is a benzodiazepine with anticonvulsant properties that has been used for lancinating pain. It has utility in the treatment of muscle spasms as well as myoclonus (48,49). Because it produces significant sedation, it is best used in patients who have anxiety or difficulty sleeping. It can produce significant dysphoria and should be used cautiously when depression is present. The usual starting dose is 0.5 mg in the evening, escalating to 2 mg three times per day.

Oral Anesthetics Neuropathic pain has been found to respond transiently to high doses of intravenous local anesthetics, such as lidocaine (50–52). It seems that systemic administration suppresses the activity of dorsal horn cells, which respond to noxious stimulation. Spontaneous firing of damaged cells and axons also is suppressed (53). Tocainide (now off the U.S. market) and mexiletine are oral local anesthetics used for cardiac arrhythmias that have been useful for neuropathic pain. Mexiletine has fewer side effects and has been studied more thoroughly. Evidence of its efficacy is contradictory, but higher dose studies showed benefit. It is useful for continuous dysesthetic pain (54). The starting dose is 150 mg/day, increasing in 150-mg increments every 3 to 5 days, up to a dose of 300 mg three times per day or until side effects occur. The most common side effects are dose-related and include nausea, dizziness, and tremors. Hematologic reactions are idiosyncratic and rare. In this regard, oral local anesthetics may be a good alternative to traditional agents in patients with blood dyscrasias. The efficacy and adverse effects are similar to other drugs used in neuropathic pain (sedation, dizziness), but the acute onset is an advantage to the local anesthetics. A recent meta-analysis by Challapalli et al. reviews oral and intravenous local anesthetics, and validates their efficacy and safety in acute settings (55).

Alpha-Agonists Adrenergic agonists are another type of adjuvant analgesic. There are numerous recent small studies comparing intravenous and oral anesthetics to placebo and drugs that are more classic for neuropathic pain (gabapentin, morphine, carbamazepine). Typically, local anesthetics are used more for acute pain syndromes, inpatient settings, relating to cancer therapy and surgery.

The α2-adrenergic agonists have been studied in a variety of pain syndromes. The mechanisms of action are presumed to be an enhancement of endogenous pain-modulating systems, and, in the case of sympathetically maintained pain, sympatholysis. Clonidine was found to be effective intrathecally in an open study in combination with morphine (57,58). It can be administered epidurally, intrathecally, orally, or transdermally. The major limiting factors in the use of clonidine are hypotension and sedation. Although these are not pronounced in otherwise healthy patients, in the presence of neuropathy, blood pressure fluctuations can be increased. There are few if any other side effects.

Topical Agents Topical agents are useful for several types of continuous pain. In general, they are most effective in pain states that have a predominantly peripheral cause. These include painful neuropathies, herpetic and postherpetic neuralgia, and—occasionally—painful arthropathies. Topical agents alone are usually insufficient to produce total pain relief, but they can be helpful in patients who experience adverse effects from other adjuvant drugs. Capsaicin, a naturally occurring pepper extract, has been found to be useful in reducing neuropathic pain in diabetics (59). The capsaicin preparation is applied to the area of greatest discomfort several times a day. Pain relief does not occur for several days. On initial application, many patients complain of markedly worsened pain and burning. This resolves after several applications and may be due to the local release of Substance P. Unfortunately, the burning can be severe, and patients often are not able to tolerate it. Multiple studies have demonstrated weak to moderate efficacy of capsaicin for neuropathic and musculoskeletal pain (60). It should be reserved for combination therapy or when typical analgesics have failed. In a study of 200 patients with chronic neuropathic pain, pain was significantly reduced by the combination of topical 3.3% doxepin and 0.025% capsaicin. Absolute pain reduction was similar to either agent alone, but with a more rapid onset with the combination (61). A double-blind, randomized, placebo-controlled 3-week study evaluated the efficacy of topical 2% amitriptyline, 1% ketamine, and a combination of both in treating patients with diabetic neuropathy, postherpetic neuralgia, or postsurgical/posttraumatic neuropathic pain. The study used pain assays of change in average daily pain intensity (baseline week vs. final week an 11-point scale) and the McGill Pain Questionnaire, measures of allodynia and hyperalgesia, and patient satisfaction. It was demonstrated that 2% amitriptyline, 1% ketamine, and the combination all produced a good response across all pain scales (62). Additional open-label studies demonstrated greater pain relief with increased concentrations of drug, but no increase in side effects.

Lidocaine patch use has become popular as a treatment for neuropathic pain, and are indicated for pain of postherpetic neuralgia. Off-label, lidocaine patches are often used as palliative agents for patients who have failed other therapies. Typically 5% patches are used: 12 hours on, 12 hours off daily. Side effects are minimal with the exception of local irritation and possible hypersensitivity. In multiple small clinical studies, there was dramatic improvement compared with placebo (63). These studies were small, and there was no comparison to other accepted therapies. Interestingly, a recent randomized open-label comparison of naproxen and lidocaine patch therapy for pain associated with carpal tunnel syndrome showed a clear benefit from both drugs, with patient preference for the lidocaine patch (63).

NSAIDS are the mainstay of musculoskeletal and arthritic pain, and are beneficial adjuncts or primary therapies in many pain syndromes. Diclofenac, as a transdermal patch or gel, is the most commonly prescribed topical NSAID. The diclofenac patch is 1.3% and applied twice daily to affected areas, and the gel is 1% applied four times daily. Side effects are the same as oral diclofenac (GI ulcer, blood dyscrasias, renal and hepatotoxic), but to a markedly lesser extent than systemic. Obviously, dermatologic adverse reactions are possible, including Steven-Johnsons syndrome; thus, naive patients should take caution. Both the diclofenac gel and patch have well studied use in sports injuries and arthritis pain localized to specific joint (64–66). They appear affective when inflammatory pain is limited to a specific target site.

EMLA (eutectic mixture of local anesthetics) is a 1:1 mixture of prilocaine and lidocaine, which can penetrate the skin and produce local anesthesia. It has been helpful in patients with peripheral nerve lesions and in reducing pain associated with venipuncture. EMLA has been particularly helpful in postherpetic neuralgia (67). In the author's experience, the combination of EMLA applied first, followed by capsaicin, has been better tolerated than capsaicin alone, and may be more effective. Compounded ointments of salicylates and NSAIDs also have been used for neuropathic pain, but the data regarding their efficacy are unclear (68). Topical NSAID creams are used for various musculoskeletal pain disorders. Results of pain scales and studies appear to be very much influenced by patient route of administration preference, and are difficult to cross-compare with oral, intravenous, or intramuscular administration of the same NSAID.

Muscle Relaxants Several different classes of medications have muscle relaxant properties. Spasmolytic agents such as baclofen, tizanidine, and benzodiazepines are useful for conditions that produce flexor and extensor spasms because of neural injury, as well as chronic muscle spasm. A group of diverse agents also are classified as muscle relaxants, although their exact mode of action is poorly understood. These include cyclobenzaprine, carisoprodol, methocarbamol, and chlorzoxazone. The latter group has no clear spasmolytic action, but may act through central nervous system depression. Baclofen is a GABAergic drug with affinity for the presynaptic $GABA_B$ receptors. It suppresses excitatory transmitter release and action at the spinal cord level. There is some evidence that it also blocks transmitter release at cutaneous nociceptive nerve endings (69). Patients with spasticity related to multiple sclerosis or upper motor neuron lesion from trauma, cerebrovascular disease, or degenerative disease might benefit from baclofen. There is some anecdotal literature suggesting that it may be useful for facial pain. The major side effects of baclofen are sedation and liver dysfunction. Abrupt discontinuation can result in seizures. Intrathecal administration of baclofen can be useful in patients who develop systemic side effects to the oral form (70). It is also indicated in cerebral palsy, multiple sclerosis, and spastic hemiplegia from trauma or cerebrovascular accident. However, patients may require additional antispasmodic medications. Tizanidine, a newer spasmolytic agent, is a centrally acting $\alpha 2$-adrenergic agonist. Clinical experience suggests that it has antinociceptive properties, particularly in muscle and soft-tissue pain (71). It is as effective as baclofen in decreasing spasticity, but produces less muscle weakness. However, it can be sedating and should not be administered with other adrenergic agonists. Cyclobenzaprine is a tricyclic agent that has been marketed as a muscle relaxant. Its major site of action appears to be in the brainstem, although the exact mechanism of action is unclear. It is indicated for short-term use only. It is quite sedating and should be used cautiously with other serotonin uptake inhibitors. Methocarbamol, carisoprodol, and chlorzoxazone all are older agents whose exact mode of action remains unclear. There are no controlled studies demonstrating clear efficacy for these medications as analgesic agents. Because of their potential for abuse, they should be avoided.

INTERVENTIONAL PROCEDURES

Anesthetic procedures have been a mainstay of pain management. Although there are many effective procedures for acute pain, chronic pain procedures are somewhat more limited. They include infusions and local blocks with anesthetic agents, administration of epidural steroids, implantable drug delivery systems, and implantable neural stimulators.

Anesthetic Infusions Intravenous or oral administration of local anesthetics can produce systemic analgesic effects. It is postulated that the mechanism of action for this phenomenon is the interruption of local reflex arcs, and vasodilation. Additionally, there is evidence that extremely low levels of lidocaine inhibit spontaneaus C fiber activity associated with inflammation (72). This technique has been particularly helpful in the diagnosis and treatment of neuropathic pain syndromes. The usual method is to infuse lidocaine at a rate of 5 mg/kg of body weight over 30 minutes in a monitored setting. The patient usually experiences relief of paresthesias and lancinating pain within 1 hour of the infusion; this relief can persist for several days (73,74). Repeat infusions can be used, although their efficacy may decline. Oral anesthetic agents such as mexiletine also can be used after a loading dose of intravenous lidocaine. Intravenous lidocaine also has been found helpful in certain forms of vascular headache (75).

Trigger Point Injections Local injection of anesthetic into tender areas in muscle, referred to as trigger points, can provide temporary relief in acute and chronic soft-tissue pain. The main indication for these injections is myofascial pain. Considerable controversy exists as to which agents should be injected and how often. In general, a dilute solution of a short-acting local anesthetic (with or without steroid) is injected into the trigger point. Dry needling, or mechanical disruption of the tender area, also can be employed, although it usually is poorly tolerated. The techniques of trigger point injection are described in several texts (76,77). The injections usually are given in conjunction with physical therapy. This maximizes the efficacy of muscle stretching techniques and reduces pain during the recovery phase from an acute injury. For example, in a recent double blind, randomized, crossover trial, patients with myofascial pain syndrome received trigger point injection of either 25 units botulinum toxin A or 0.5% bupivacaine in up to eight facial trigger points and participated in a home exercise program. Patients were crossed over to both study groups and demonstrated good pain control with minimal side effects (78). Patients had similar satisfaction and pain reduction with both agents, but considering botulinum toxin's cost, bupivacaine may be preferred.

Local Neural Blockade Local neural blockade is used principally for the relief of acute pain and for diagnostic purposes. Sequential blocks of individual nerves or spinal levels can help to pinpoint sites of pain generation, but they do not identify the specific disease state that may be producing the pain (79). Neurolytic blocks are reserved for the most intractable cases and for patients with a limited life expectancy (80). The risk of developing a deafferentation pain syndrome is high and increases over time. The local vascular effects and soft tissue damage require that these procedures be performed only by clinicians who have ample clinical expertise in their use. Phenol and absolute alcohol are the most commonly used agents. Both work by destroying peripheral myelin and producing irreversible conduction block. Prolonged administration also is toxic to poorly myelinated axons. Because collateral sprouting can occur, and the peripheral myelin rarely is repaired, ectopic generators can develop in lysed nerves, which may produce a return of the pain locally. Therefore the use of neurolytic blocks should be limited to the most refractory patients and cancer patients (81,82).

Spinal Steroid Injections and Facet Injections

Local steroid injections into either the epidural space or the facet joints have been used in the treatment of mechanical neck and back pain. Although the indications remain controversial, epidural steroids are used in the management of acute or recurrent pain resulting from root irritation with clinical evidence of radicular dysfunction and in nonoperative spinal stenosis (83–85). Double blind comparison of radioguided transforaminal or blindly performed interspinous epidural corticosteroid injections for radicular pain from disc disease with follow up at 6 and 30 days and 6 months favored radioguided transforaminal injections over interspinous epidural on multiple pain scales. Both techniques demonstrated lasting pain relief for months (86). In other studies, transforaminal epidural steroid injections had a success rate of 84%, as compared with 48% for the group receiving saline trigger-point injections for lumbosacral radicular pain secondary to a herniated nucleus pulposus, with an average follow-up period of 1.4 years (87). However, this study was poorly blinded and had operator bias. Epidural injections have also showed benefit in the acute phase of sciatic pain (2 weeks, statistical trend), but failed to help with pain relief and mobility at 6 weeks and 6 months (88).

Facet blocks are useful in patients with neck or back pain with a mechanical component but without radicular signs, presumably arising in the spinal column (68,89–91). The technique of epidural steroid injections is well described in several standard texts (92). Usually, triamcinolone (at a dose of 50 mg) or methylprednisolone (at a dose of 40 to 80 mg) is injected into the epidural space after dilution with either normal saline or a short-acting local anesthetic agent. The injection is performed at the disc level adjacent to the affected nerve roots and sufficient fluid is given to bathe the adjacent nerve roots. Complications are uncommon and usually result from either local irritation or a persistent dural leak. Rare complications include radicular irritation and infection (93). Improvement usually is noted within a week and may persist for several months. A course of three injections generally is given, until pain relief or treatment failure is reached. Efficacy is variable, with most series indicating short-term improvement of acute back pain. Patients who are most likely to benefit have pain of less than 6 months' duration or radicular signs (94–96). Benefits are less convincing in pain related to spinal stenosis (97). Facet blocks are performed with fluoroscopic guidance. Local anesthetic, either 0.5% bupivacaine or 2% lidocaine, is injected at the base of the superior articular process. Relief of pain suggests that the pain generator is within the facet joint (90). Efficacy is quite variable, with prolonged relief usually obtained only after radiofrequency ablation. The routine use of epidural steroids has been questioned, with recent meta-analysis demonstrating modest, short-lived, pain improvement (weeks to months) being agreed on (98,99). There is persisting disagreement regarding the long-term benefit of steroid epidural injections. Some studies see moderate benefit and others find no change in the natural course of the disease with reference to functional impairment, need for surgery, or long-term pain relief (98,99). Lumbar facet injections do appear to give short- and long-term pain benefit (98).

Sympathetic Blockade Sympathetic blockade may reduce pain involving the sympathetic nervous system and the viscera. Sympathetically maintained nociceptive input from the upper extremities, head, and neck can be blocked by infiltrating the stellate ganglion. Thoracic sympathetic paravertebral ganglia receive input from the cardiac and thoracic viscera; their blockade can be helpful in pain originating at those sites. The upper abdominal viscera are innervated by the celiac ganglion, whereas the urogenital viscera are supplied by the superior hypogastric plexus and the ganglion impar. Deep visceral pain can be relieved by blocking the appropriate location. Finally, the lumbar sympathetic ganglia are involved in mediating pain in the lower extremities. Lumbar sympathetic blockade can be very useful in managing ischemic limb pain and neuropathic pain from failed back surgery, as well as chronic regional pain syndromes. The exact mechanisms of involvement of the sympathetic nervous system in peripheral pain are not fully understood (100). In addition, there is poor correlation between the degree of sympathetic dysfunction and response to pain blockade. Therefore, for practical purposes, response to sympathetic blocks is based on the patient's report of pain relief and on changes in skin temperature (101). The indications for stellate ganglion blocks are painful conditions affecting the head, neck, and upper extremities.

Complex regional pain syndromes may be associated with abnormal sympathetic activity; recent small clinical studies have demonstrated that sympathetic ganglionic blockade (stellate ganglia or sympathetic chain blockade with bupivacaine injection) achieved better pain control than selective sympathetic cutaneous modulation (local temperature modulation/thermal suit) (102). In a larger study of 25 complex regional pain syndrome patients, 76% achieved complete or partial relief of pain, with duration of relief being related to the duration of the pain syndrome (those with longer duration having less sustained relief) (103). Both blind and radiographically guided approaches can be used (104), as can repeated blocks. Nevertheless, further studies need to be performed before these techniques are used as standard of care (105). Neurolysis or spinal cord stimulation can be used if significant relief is obtained from temporary blocks. Lumbar sympathetic blockade is used in the diagnosis and therapy of painful and other conditions, presumably associated with a dysfunction of the sympathetic nervous system. These include complex regional pain syndrome types I and II, herpes zoster, amputation stump pain, and inoperable peripheral vascular and vasospastic diseases of the lower extremities. Other indications include selected cases of pelvic pain in which superior hypogastric nerve block cannot be performed (106). Celiac and superior hypogastric blocks, as well as ganglion impar blocks, are used for chronic painful visceral conditions. There are no long-term effectiveness studies of any of these procedures. Radiographic imaging and guidance are mandatory to ensure appropriate anesthetic placement. The major indication for these blocks is chronic cancer-related pain (107,108).

Spinal Cord Stimulation Spinal cord stimulation (SCS) for the management of pain was introduced in 1967. Its actual mechanism is not known, but there are several theories. It is postulated that electrical stimulation produces antidromic blocking of pain transmission at the spinal cord level, spinothalamic tract conductance blocking, and activation of supraspinal pain processing nuclei (109,110). There also is good evidence from cerebrospinal fluid markers of chemical neuromodulatory mechanisms. Studies have shown an increase in serotonin, substance P, and GABA release, as well as a decrease in the presence of excitatory amino acids in response to SCS (111). There are multiple reports of the efficacy of SCS for widely differing chronic pain syndromes (112,113). Generally, it is agreed that SCS is effective in treating pain of neuropathic origin, particularly sympathetically mediated pain and ischemic pain. It appears that SCS has no efficacy in acute pain or pain of nociceptive origin. Because it is known that SCS causes vasodilatation in animal studies, clinicians have used this modality for the treatment of pain resulting from peripheral vascular disease and visceral pain. Peripheral vascular disease remains the leading indication for SCS in Europe today. There are promising results in the use of SCS in pancreatic and pelvic pain, but no large-scale studies of SCS for these indications (114). Recent clinical trials have demonstrated efficacy of SCS in treating select patients with failed back surgery syndrome, refractory angina pectoris, and chronic reflex sympathetic dystrophy that have failed conventional therapy (114–116). SCS implantation is expensive and labor-intensive. Because it usually requires surgical intervention, it should be reserved for patients who have failed more conservative therapies.

PHYSICAL MEDICINE AND REHABILITATIVE THERAPIES

A comprehensive approach to pain management incorporates the use of various physical modalities and rehabilitative therapies. Physical modalities include the therapeutic application of heat, cold, traction, transcutaneous electrical stimulation, acupuncture, and massage. Several excellent texts discuss each of these techniques (117,118). Rehabilitative therapies are aimed at functional restoration and include exercise and conditioning therapies.

Heat Application of heat to muscles or joints can provide analgesia, decrease muscle spasm, and increase flexibility (119,120). It also is very useful in decreasing acute pain in soft-tissue injuries and joint inflammation. Local heat application can be either superficial (as with hot packs, paraffin baths, or hot water) or deep. Deep heat application is accomplished with diathermy and ultrasound, which require training to be performed safely; for this reason, superficial heat application is more widely used. Evidence suggests that pain relief is greater when heat is combined with exercise (121). Deep heat application has been used for many years for deep tissue pain, but several studies suggest that its utility is limited. In a study comparing the relative efficacy of ultrasound, short-wave diathermy, and galvanic current for hip and knee joint pain, the benefits appeared to be similar. There is some evidence that diathermy may worsen postexercise pain (122). Because of the costs associated with deep heat modalities, they should be used in patients only if superficial heat has failed.

Cold The application of cold has a local analgesic effect and reduces inflammatory responses and muscle spasm. Mechanisms that have been postulated for this include altered neural transmission, reduced muscle spasm, altered blood flow to muscle and nerve, and increased endorphin production. Cooling is applied by cold packs, ice massage, hydrotherapy, or vapocoolant sprays, all of which seem to have equal efficacy (123). There is some evidence that cold may produce pain relief faster than heat and may be more effective in acute pain (124).

Transcutaneous Electrical Nerve Stimulation

Transcutaneous electrical nerve stimulation (TENS) has been used for a variety of chronic pain conditions. Initially, it was thought to work by increasing afferent input and turning on inhibitory neurons at the spinal cord level. More recent research indicates that TENS may work by stimulating the sympathetic nervous system and brainstem nuclei and increasing endorphin release (125). It has demonstrated effectiveness in joint pain and acute pain, but little utility in back pain (126). For example, although there is extreme patient variability, TENS has been shown to improve pain and isometric neck strength in chronic neck pain patients over a 6-week period in a trial with greater than 200 patients and placebo comparison (127). Brief trials of TENS should be considered in patients with localized mechanical pain, in conjunction with physical therapy.

Massage Massage is one of the oldest and most widely used techniques for decreasing acute and chronic pain: indeed, descriptions of therapeutic massage can be found in the works of Hippocrates. It is not clear exactly how massage works, although counterirritation and increased blood flow have been proposed as mechanisms. Many different massage techniques are used. The utility of massage seems to be greatest for short-term pain relief after acute injuries (128,129). No studies demonstrate that the benefits of massage in chronic low back or neck pain are any greater than those to be derived from rest and reeducation.

Exercise Pain patients often develop decreased muscle strength, reduced range of motion, and general deconditioning, as well as other functional limitations. Exercise therapy can help overcome those deficits and also reduce pain (130,131). For example, multiple clinical trials show the benefit of exercise therapy in lower back pain. Although results vary, exercise can often help the individual patient and adverse effects are rare (132). Selecting the appropriate exercise therapy is the key to good rehabilitation. In addition to prescribed exercise, simple aerobic exercises such as walking and swimming should be part of chronic pain management. Range of motion exercises (ROM) are designed to reduce stiffness and increase flexibility. Both active and passive ROM can be useful in reducing pain in soft-tissue and joint injuries. It is important to begin with passive ROM and advance to active ROM so as not to overstretch injured tissues, which can decrease tensile strength. ROM therapy can be the first step in rehabilitation and should be used for chronic maintenance therapy as well. Muscle conditioning exercises are useful in increasing strength, endurance, and function. Such exercises are divided into isometric and dynamic forms. Isometric exercise involves muscle contraction without joint movement; it is used to increase muscle tone and strength in preparation for more vigorous exercise. Patients need to be instructed in how to perform isometric exercises so as to avoid excess muscle ischemia and increased intraarticular pressure (130). Dynamic exercise is more vigorous and involves the repetitive contraction and relaxation of muscle groups with joint movement. It is the final step in strengthening muscle groups and involves gradually increasing resistance. Patients usually begin working with elastic bands and move on to progressively greater resistance through use of weights and exercise machines. Determination of an appropriate resistance and training schedule, while monitoring for injury and providing patient education, is essential to a safe and effective dynamic exercise program. Patients need education if exercise is to be an effective part of pain management. Setting specific functional goals rather than focusing on pain reduction is a key part of exercise therapy. In one study of the use of exercise for arthritis pain, patients found that using exercise goals rather than focusing on pain produced better functional outcomes and led to a reduction of pain chronically (131). Patients become discouraged if they focus on pain reduction, because initially exercise may increase pain. Their physician or other caregiver needs to actively reinforce the patient's long-term goals and redirect them to a safe exercise program, despite setbacks.

Acupuncture Acupuncture is a traditional Chinese therapy based on a theory of energy (Qi) flow. Qi is thought to flow along specific channels or meridians which, if blocked, can lead to disease. In classic acupuncture, the practitioner attempts to restore flow by applying treatment at points distributed along the meridians. Needling is the most common method of applying acupuncture, but heat, pressure, and electrical stimulation also have been used (132). Studies have shown that acupuncture produces an increase in endorphin release and modulates the firing of high-threshold, small-diameter nerve fibers (134). The Western approach to acupuncture is based on modulating these elements of pain transmission. Based on the evidence from several controlled studies, acupuncture appears to be effective in controlling the pain of osteoarthritis and fibromyalgia. Study subjects reported significant reduction in pain compared with placebo or pharmacologic treatments (135–137). A recent large (n = 1,162), randomized, multicenter, blinded, parallel-group trial compared verum acupuncture (established points and meridians), sham acupuncture (avoiding points and meridians), and conventional therapy for chronic lower back pain. At 6 months, the response rate (based on pain/ability questionnaire) was approximately 46% in both the verum and sham acupuncture groups, whereas only 27% in conventional therapy (138). It important to recognize that conventional therapy included drugs, physical therapy, and exercise. This study demonstrates the efficacy of acupuncture, but also that patient's expectation in therapy and practitioner encounter may affect outcome (considering sham acupuncture had the same results as verum). There is less evidence to support the effectiveness of acupuncture for neuropathic pain. Nevertheless, there is overwhelming evidence that acupuncture is safe and effective for a variety of somatic pain syndromes, and it should be considered as a treatment option (139).

Botulinum Toxin The use of botulinum toxin (Botox A) for the treatment of focal dystonias has been standard for several years. However, Botox has been found to have multiple effects. By blocking acetylcholine release presynaptically, it not only decreases muscle contraction, but also reduces sympathetic activity and may increase inhibitory interneuron activity at the spinal cord level (140,141). Although some small trials show efficacy, many large scale trials show poor or no efficacy of botulinum toxin for treatment of headache or musculoskeletal pain compared with placebo or conventional therapy (142–144). When pain is directly linked to dystonia or muscle spasm, botulinum toxin has good efficacy (145). The use of botulinum toxin requires knowledge of the muscle groups affected by a particular condition. Electromyographic guidance has been used to identify hyperactive muscles to be targeted in dystonia; the same technique has been used in pain treatment. It is not clear whether this is superior to injection at local areas of spasm or tenderness. Until the long-term effects of chronic botulinum toxin use are known, it would seem reasonable to use the least amount of medication possible by targeting affected muscles by electromyelogram. Usually 40 units of botulinum toxin are injected into large muscles, as in back or neck pain, and 10 units are used for smaller muscle groups in the neck and head. Effects usually are noticeable within 5 to 10 days and may persist for as long as 3 months, at which point the treatment is repeated. Adverse effects usually are associated with local reactions or excessive weakness of affected muscle groups, leading to poor gait or facial drooping.

REFERENCES

1. Raja SN, Haythornthwaite JA, Pappagallo M, et al. Opioids versus antidepressants in postherpetic neuralgia: a randomized, placebo-controlled trial. *Neurology* 2002;59(7):1015–1021.
2. Hollingshead J, Duhmke RM, Cornblath DR. Tramadol for neuropathic pain. *Cochrane Database Syst Rev* 2006;3:CD003726.
3. Morley JS, Bridson J, Nash TP, et al. Low-dose methadone has an analgesic effect in neuropathic pain: a double-blind randomized controlled crossover trial. *Palliat Med* 2003;17(7):576–587.
4. Vane J. Inhibition of prostaglandin synthesis as a mechanism of action for aspirin-like drugs. *Nature* 1971;234:231–238.
5. McCormack K, Brune K. Dissociation between the antinociceptive and anti-inflammatory effects of the nonsteroidal anti-inflammatory drugs. A survey of their analgesic efficacy. *Drugs* 1991;41(4):533–547.
6. Willer JC, De Broucker T, Bussel B, et al. Central analgesic effect of ketoprofen in humans: electrophysiological evidence for a supraspinal mechanism in a double-blind and cross-over study. *Pain* 1989;38(1): 1–7.
7. Davies NM and Skjodt NM. Choosing the right nonsteroidal anti-inflammatory drug for the right patient: a pharmacokinetic approach. *Clin Pharmacokinet* 2000;38(5):377–392.
8. Loeb DS, Ahlquist DA, Talley NJ, Management of gastroduodenopathy associated with use of nonsteroidal anti-inflammatory drugs. *Mayo Clin Proc* 1992;67(4):354–364.
9. Society AP. Guidelines for the management of pain in osteoarthritis, rheumatoid arthritis, and juvenile chronic arthritis. Glenview, IL: American Pain Society, 2002.
10. Recommendations for the medical management of osteoarthritis of the hip and knee: 2000 update. American College of Rheumatology Subcommittee on Osteoarthritis Guidelines. *Arthritis Rheum* 2000;43(9): 1905–1915.
11. Kincaid-Smith P. Effects of non-narcotic analgesics on the kidney. *Drugs* 1986;32(Suppl 4):109–128.
12. Danesh BJ, McLaren M, Russell RI, et al. Comparison of the effect of aspirin and choline magnesium trisalicylate on thromboxane biosynthesis in human platelets: role of the acetyl moiety. *Haemostasis* 1989;19(3): 169–173.
13. Monji A, Maekawa T, Miura T, et al. Interactions between lithium and non-steroidal antiinflammatory drugs. *Clin Neuropharmacol* 2002;25 (5):241–242.
14. Namaka M, Gramlich CR, Ruhlen D, et al. A treatment algorithm for neuropathic pain. *Clin Ther* 2004;26(7):951–979.
15. Caldwell B, Aldington S, Weatherall M, et al. Risk of cardiovascular events and celecoxib: a systematic review and meta-analysis. *J R Soc Med* 2006;99(3):132–140.
16. Chargaff E. A fever of reason the early way. *Annu Rev Biochem* 1975;44: 1–18.
17. Feinmann C. Pain relief by antidepressants: possible modes of action. *Pain* 1985;23(1):1–8.
18. Galer BS. Painful polyneuropathy: diagnosis, pathophysiology, and management. *Semin Neurol* 1994;14(3):237–246.
19. Kieburtz K, Simpson D, Yiannoutsos C, et al. A randomized trial of amitriptyline and mexiletine for painful neuropathy in HIV infection. AIDS Clinical Trial Group 242 Protocol Team. *Neurology* 1998;51(6): 1682–1688.
20. Shlay JC, Chaloner K, Max MB, et al. Acupuncture and amitriptyline for pain due to HIV-related peripheral neuropathy: a randomized controlled trial. Terry Beirn Community Programs for Clinical Research on AIDS. *JAMA* 1998;280(18):1590–1595.
21. Godfrey RG. A guide to the understanding and use of tricyclic antidepressants in the overall management of fibromyalgia and other chronic pain syndromes. *Arch Intern Med* 1996;156(10):1047–1052.
22. Max MB, Lynch SA, Muir J, et al. Effects of desipramine, amitriptyline, and fluoxetine on pain in diabetic neuropathy. *N Engl J Med* 1992; 326(19):1250–1256.
23. Fishbain DA, Cutler R, Rosomoff HL, et al. Evidence-based data from animal and human experimental studies on pain relief with antidepressants: a structured review. *Pain Med* 2000;1(4):310–316.
24. Sindrup SH, Gram LF, Brosen K, et al. The selective serotonin reuptake inhibitor paroxetine is effective in the treatment of diabetic neuropathy symptoms. *Pain* 1990;42(2):135–144.
25. Sindrup SH, Bach FW, Madsen C, et al. Venlafaxine versus imipramine in painful polyneuropathy: a randomized, controlled trial. *Neurology* 2003;60(8):1284–1289.

26. Reuben SS, Makari-Judson G, Lurie SD. Evaluation of efficacy of the perioperative administration of venlafaxine XR in the prevention of postmastectomy pain syndrome. *J Pain Symptom Manage* 2004;27(2):133–139.
27. Armstrong DG, Chappell AS, Le TK, et al. Duloxetine for the management of diabetic peripheral neuropathic pain: evaluation of functional outcomes. *Pain Med* 2007;8(5):410–418.
28. Arnold LM, Pritchett YL, D'Souza DN, et al. Duloxetine for the treatment of fibromyalgia in women: pooled results from two randomized, placebo-controlled clinical trials. *J Womens Health (Larchmt)* 2007; 16(8):1145–1156.
29. Wise TN, Fishbain DA, Holder-Perkins V. Painful physical symptoms in depression: a clinical challenge. *Pain Med* 2007;8(Suppl 2):S75–S82.
30. Johannessen Landmark C. Antiepileptic drugs in non-epilepsy disorders: relations between mechanisms of action and clinical efficacy. *CNS Drugs* 2008;22(1):27–47.
31. Galer BS. Neuropathic pain of peripheral origin: advances in pharmacologic treatment. *Neurology* 1995;45(12 Suppl 9):S17–S25; discussion S35S3–6.
32. McQuay H, Carroll D, Jadad AR, et al. Anticonvulsant drugs for management of pain: a systematic review. *BMJ* 1995;311(7012):1047–1052.
33. Perucca E. Clinically relevant drug interactions with antiepileptic drugs. *Br J Clin Pharmacol* 2006;61(3):246–255.
34. Moosa RS, McFadyen ML, Miller R, et al. Carbamazepine and its metabolites in neuralgias: concentration-effect relations. *Eur J Clin Pharmacol* 1993;45(4):297–301.
35. Houtchens MK, Richert JR, Sami A, et al. Open label gabapentin treatment for pain in multiple sclerosis. *Mult Scler* 1997;3(4):250–253.
36. Chapman V, Suzuki R, Chamarette HL, et al. Effects of systemic carbamazepine and gabapentin on spinal neuronal responses in spinal nerve ligated rats. *Pain* 1998;75(2–3):261–272.
37. Richter RW, Portenoy R, Sharma U, et al. Relief of painful diabetic peripheral neuropathy with pregabalin: a randomized, placebo-controlled trial. *J Pain* 2005;6(4):253–260.
38. Segal AZ and Rordorf G. Gabapentin as a novel treatment for postherpetic neuralgia. *Neurology* 1996;46(4):1175–1176.
39. Rowbotham M, Harden N, Stacey B, et al. Gabapentin for the treatment of postherpetic neuralgia: a randomized controlled trial. *JAMA* 1998;280(21):1837–1842.
40. Elwes RD and Binnie CD. Clinical pharmacokinetics of newer antiepileptic drugs. Lamotrigine, vigabatrin, gabapentin and oxcarbazepine. *Clin Pharmacokinet* 1996;30(6):403–415.
41. Ho KY, Gan TJ, Habib AS. Gabapentin and postoperative pain—a systematic review of randomized controlled trials. *Pain* 2006;126(1–3): 91–101.
42. Simpson DM, Olney R, McArthur JC, et al. A placebo-controlled trial of lamotrigine for painful HIV-associated neuropathy. *Neurology* 2000; 54(11):2115–2119.
43. Eisenberg E, Lurie Y, Braker C, et al. Lamotrigine reduces painful diabetic neuropathy: a randomized, controlled study. *Neurology* 2001; 57(3):505–509.
44. Dworkin RH, Corbin AE, Young JP, Jr., et al. Pregabalin for the treatment of postherpetic neuralgia: a randomized, placebo-controlled trial. *Neurology* 2003;60(8):1274–1283.
45. Sabatowski R, Galvez R, Cherry DA, et al. Pregabalin reduces pain and improves sleep and mood disturbances in patients with post-herpetic neuralgia: results of a randomised, placebo-controlled clinical trial. *Pain* 2004;109(1–2):26–35.
46. Rosenstock J, Tuchman M, LaMoreaux L, et al. Pregabalin for the treatment of painful diabetic peripheral neuropathy: a double-blind, placebo-controlled trial. *Pain* 2004;110(3):628–638.
47. Lesser H, Sharma U, LaMoreaux L, et al. Pregabalin relieves symptoms of painful diabetic neuropathy: a randomized controlled trial. *Neurology* 2004;63(11):2104–2110.
48. Bartusch SL, Sanders BJ, D'Alessio JG, et al. Clonazepam for the treatment of lancinating phantom limb pain. *Clin J Pain* 1996;12(1):59–62.
49. Eisele JH, Jr., Grigsby EJ, Dea G. Clonazepam treatment of myoclonic contractions associated with high-dose opioids: case report. *Pain* 1992; 49(2):231–232.
50. Glazer S, Portenoy RK. Systemic local anesthetics in pain control. *J Pain Symptom Manage* 1991;6(1):30–39.
51. Rowbotham M, Reisner L, HL F. Both IV lidocaine and morphine reduce the pain of post-herpetic neuralgia. *Neurology* 1991;41: 1024–1028.
52. Tremont-Lukats IW, Challapalli V, McNicol ED, et al. Systemic administration of local anesthetics to relieve neuropathic pain: a systematic review and meta-analysis. *Anesth Analg* 2005;101(6):1738–1749.
53. Woolf CJ, Wiesenfeld-Hallin Z. The systemic administration of local anaesthetics produces a selective depression of C-afferent fibre evoked activity in the spinal cord. *Pain* 1985;23(4):361–374.
54. Chabal C, Jacobson L, Mariano A, et al. The use of oral mexiletine for the treatment of pain after peripheral nerve injury. *Anesthesiology* 1992; 76(4):513–517.
55. Challapalli V, Tremont-Lukats IW, McNicol ED, et al. Systemic administration of local anesthetic agents to relieve neuropathic pain. *Cochrane Database Syst Rev* 2005;(4):CD003345.
56. Zeigler D, Lynch SA, Muir J, et al. Transdermal clonidine versus placebo in painful diabetic neuropathy. *Pain* 1992;48(3):403–408.
57. Uhle EI, Becker R, Gatscher S, et al. Continuous intrathecal clonidine administration for the treatment of neuropathic pain. *Stereotact Funct Neurosurg* 2000;75(4):167–175.
58. Rauck RL, Eisenach JC, Jackson K, et al. Intrathecal administration may reduce pain of complex regional pain syndrome: epidural clonidine treatment for refractory reflex sympathetic dystrophy. *Anesthesiology* 1993;79(6):1163–1169.
59. Capsaicin Study Group. Treatment of painful diabetic neuropathy with topical capsaicin. A multicenter, double-blind, vehicle-controlled study. The Capsaicin Study Group. *Arch Intern Med* 1991;151(11): 2225–2229.
60. Mason L, Moore RA, Derry S, et al. Systematic review of topical capsaicin for the treatment of chronic pain. *BMJ* 2004;328(7446):991.
61. McCleane G. Topical application of doxepin hydrochloride, capsaicin and a combination of both produces analgesia in chronic human neuropathic pain: a randomized, double-blind, placebo-controlled study. *Br J Clin Pharmacol* 2000;49(6):574–579.
62. Lynch ME, Clark AJ, Sawynok J, et al. Topical 2% amitriptyline and 1% ketamine in neuropathic pain syndromes: a randomized, double-blind, placebo-controlled trial. *Anesthesiology* 2005;103(1):140–146.
63. Nalamachu S, Crockett RS, Gammaitoni AR, et al. A comparison of the lidocaine patch 5% vs. naproxen 500 mg twice daily for the relief of pain associated with carpal tunnel syndrome: a 6-week, randomized, parallel-group study. *Med Gen Med* 2006;8(3):33.
64. Galer BS, Rowbotham M, Perander J, et al. Topical diclofenac patch relieves minor sports injury pain: results of a multicenter controlled clinical trial. *J Pain Symptom Manage* 2000;19(4):287–294.
65. Bruhlmann P, Michel BA. Topical diclofenac patch in patients with knee osteoarthritis: a randomized, double-blind, controlled clinical trial. *Clin Exp Rheumatol* 2003;21(2):193–198.
66. Mahler P, Mahler F, Duruz H, et al. Double-blind, randomized, controlled study on the efficacy and safety of a novel diclofenac epolamine gel formulated with lecithin for the treatment of sprains, strains and contusions. *Drugs Exp Clin Res* 2003;29(1):45–52.
67. Stow PJ, Glynn CJ, Minor B. EMLA cream in the treatment of post-herpetic neuralgia. Efficacy and pharmacokinetic profile. *Pain* 1989;39(3): 301–305.
68. Rowlingson J. Epidural steroids: do they have a place in pain management? *Am Pain Soc Bull* 1994;3;20–27.
69. Hwang AS, Wilcox GL. Baclofen, gamma-aminobutyric acidB receptors and substance P in the mouse spinal cord. *J Pharmacol Exp Ther* 1989; 248(3):1026–1033.
70. Pirotte B, Heilporn A, Joffroy A, et al. Chronic intrathecal baclofen in severely disabling spasticity: selection, clinical assessment and long-term benefit. *Acta Neurol Belg* 1995;95(4):216–225.
71. Coward DM. Tizanidine: neuropharmacology and mechanism of action. *Neurology* 1994;44(11 Suppl 9):S6–S10; discussion S10–S11.
72. Xiao WH, Bennett GJ. C-fiber discharge evoked by chronic inflammation is suppressed by a long-term infusion of lidocaine yielding nanogram per milliliter plasma levels. *Pain* 2008;137(1):218–228.

73. Boas RA, Covino BG, Shahnarian A. Analgesic responses to i.v. lignocaine. *Br J Anaesth* 1982;54(5):501–505.
74. Kastrup J, Petersen P, Dejgard A, et al. Intravenous lidocaine infusion—a new treatment of chronic painful diabetic neuropathy? *Pain* 1987; 28(1):69–75.
75. Edwards W, Habib F, Burney R, et al. Intravenous lidocaine in the management of various chronic pain states. *Reg Anesthes* 1985;10:1.
76. Maciewicz R, RY C, A S, et al. Relief of vascular headache with intravenous lidocaine. *Cincinnati J Pain* 1988;4:11.
77. Rachlin E. *Myofascial pain and fibromyalgia*. St. Louis, MO: Mosby-Year Book, 1994.
78. Graboski CL, Gray DS, Burnham RS. Botulinum toxin A versus bupivacaine trigger point injections for the treatment of myofascial pain syndrome: a randomised double blind crossover study. *Pain* 2005;118 (1–2):170–175.
79. Travell J. Simon D. *Myofascial pain and dysfunction: the trigger point manual*. Baltimore, MD: Williams & Wilkins, 1983.
80. Winnie A. *Differential neural blockade for the diagnosis of pain mechanisms*. Philadelphia: WB Saunders, 2001.
81. Fields H. Pain modulation and the action of analgesic medications. *Ann Neurol* 1994;35(Suppl):S42–S45.
82. Ramamurthy S, Walsh NE, Schoenfeld LS, et al. Evaluation of neurolytic blocks using phenol and cryogenic block in the management of chronic pain. *J Pain Symptom Manage* 1989;4(2):72–75.
83. Weinstein SM, Herring SA, Derby R, Contemporary concepts in spine care. Epidural steroid injections. *Spine* 1995;20(16):1842–1846.
84. Jain S, Gupta R. *Neurolytic agents in clinical practice*, Philadelphia: WB Saunders, 2001.
85. Abram S. Risk versus benefit of epidural steroids: let's remain objective. *Am Pain Soc Bull* 1994;3:28–29.
86. Thomas E, Cyteval C, Abiad L, et al. Efficacy of transforaminal versus interspinous corticosteroid injection in discal radiculalgia—a prospective, randomised, double-blind study. *Clin Rheumatol* 2003;22(4–5): 299–304.
87. Vad VB, Bhat AL, Lutz GE, et al. Transforaminal epidural steroid injections in lumbosacral radiculopathy: a prospective randomized study. *Spine* 2002;27(1):11–16.
88. Buchner M, Zeifang F, Brocai DR, et al. Epidural corticosteroid injection in the conservative management of sciatica. *Clin Orthop Relat Res* 2000;(375):149–156.
89. Dwyer A, Aprill C, Bogduk N. Cervical zygapophyseal joint pain patterns. I: a study in normal volunteers. *Spine* 1990;15(6):453–457.
90. Bogduk N. International Spinal Injection Society guidelines for the performance of spinal injection procedures. Part 1: zygapophysial joint blocks. *Clin J Pain* 1997;13(4):285–302.
91. Mooney V, Robertson J. The facet syndrome. *Clin Orthop Relat Res* 1976;(115):149–156.
92. Cousins M, Veering B. Epidural neural blockade. In: Cousins MJ, Bridenbaugh P, eds. *Neural Blockade*. Philadelphia: Lippincott-Raven, 1998.
93. Nelson DA. Intraspinal therapy using methylprednisolone acetate. Twenty-three years of clinical controversy. *Spine* 1993;18(2):278–286.
94. Watts RW, Silagy CA. A meta-analysis on the efficacy of epidural corticosteroids in the treatment of sciatica. *Anaesth Intensive Care* 1995; 23(5):564–569.
95. Bowman SJ, Wedderburn L, Whaley A, et al. Outcome assessment after epidural corticosteroid injection for low back pain and sciatica. *Spine* 1993;18(10):1345–1350.
96. Koes BW, Scholten RJ, Mens JM, et al. Efficacy of epidural steroid injections for low-back pain and sciatica: a systematic review of randomized clinical trials. *Pain* 1995;63(3):279–288.
97. Fukusaki M, Kobayashi I, Hara T, et al. Symptoms of spinal stenosis do not improve after epidural steroid injection. *Clin J Pain* 1998;14(2):148–151.
98. Boswell MV, Trescot AM, Datta S, et al. Interventional techniques: evidence-based practice guidelines in the management of chronic spinal pain. *Pain Physician* 2007;10(1):7–111.
99. Armon C, Argoff CE, Samuels J, et al. Assessment: use of epidural steroid injections to treat radicular lumbosacral pain: report of the Therapeutics and Technology Assessment Subcommittee of the American Academy of Neurology. *Neurology* 2007;68(10):723–729.
100. Jaenig W. The sympathetic nervous system in pain. In: Stanton- Hicks M, ed. *Pain and the sympathetic nervous system*. Boston: Kluwer Academic Publishers, 1990.
101. Tahmoush AJ, Malley J, Jennings JR. Skin conductance, temperature, and blood flow in causalgia. *Neurology* 1983;33(11):1483–1486.
102. Schattschneider J, Binder A, Siebrecht D, et al. Complex regional pain syndromes: the influence of cutaneous and deep somatic sympathetic innervation on pain. *Clin J Pain* 2006;22(3):240–244.
103. Ackerman WE, Zhang JM. Efficacy of stellate ganglion blockade for the management of type 1 complex regional pain syndrome. *South Med J* 2006;99(10):1084–1088.
104. Aeschbach A, Mekhail NA. Common nerve blocks in chronic pain management. *Anesthesiol Clin N Am* 2000;18(2):429–459, viii.
105. Cepeda MS, Carr DB, Lau J. Local anesthetic sympathetic blockade for complex regional pain syndrome. *Cochrane Database Syst Rev* 2005;(4):CD004598.
106. Cousins MJ, Reeve TS, Glynn CJ, et al. Neurolytic lumbar sympathetic blockade: duration of denervation and relief of rest pain. *Anaesth Intensive Care* 1979;7(2):121–135.
107. Plancarte R, Amescua C, Patt RB, et al. Superior hypogastric plexus block for pelvic cancer pain. *Anesthesiology* 1990;73(2):236–239.
108. Plancarte R, de Leon-Casasola OA, et al. Neurolytic superior hypogastric plexus block for chronic pelvic pain associated with cancer. *Reg Anesth,* 1997;22(6):562–568.
109. Saade NE, Tabet MS, Soueidan SA, et al. Supraspinal modulation of nociception in awake rats by stimulation of the dorsal column nuclei. *Brain Res* 1986;369(1–2):307–310.
110. Broggi G, Franzini A, Parati E, et al. Neurochemical and structural modifications related to pain control induced by spinal cord stimulation. In: Lazothes Y, Upton A, eds. *Neurostimulation: an overview*. New York: Futura Publishing, 1985.
111. Meyerson BA, Brodin E, Linderoth B. Possible neurohumoral mechanisms in CNS stimulation for pain suppression. *Appl Neurophysiol* 1985;48(1–6):175–180.
112. Spiegelmann R, Friedman WA. Spinal cord stimulation: a contemporary series. *Neurosurgery* 1991;28(1):65–70; discussion 70–71.
113. Kumar K, Nath RK, Toth C. Spinal cord stimulation is effective in the management of reflex sympathetic dystrophy. *Neurosurgery* 1997;40(3): 503–508; discussion 508–509.
114. Kemler MA, Barendse GA, van Kleef M, et al. Spinal cord stimulation in patients with chronic reflex sympathetic dystrophy. *N Engl J Med* 2000;343(9):618–624.
115. Eddicks S, Maier-Hauff K, Schenk M, et al. Thoracic spinal cord stimulation improves functional status and relieves symptoms in patients with refractory angina pectoris: the first placebo-controlled randomised study. *Heart* 2007;93(5):585–590.
116. Kumar K, Taylor RS, Jacques L, et al. Spinal cord stimulation versus conventional medical management for neuropathic pain: a multicentre randomised controlled trial in patients with failed back surgery syndrome. *Pain* 2007;132(1–2):179–188.
117. Tan J. *Practice manual of physical medicine and rehabilitation. Diagnostics, therapeutics and basic problems*. Philadelphia: C.V. Mosby, 1998.
118. Hayes K. *Manual for physical agents*. Upper Saddle River. NJ: Prentice Hall, 2000.
119. Hall J, Skevington SM, Maddison PJ, et al. A randomized and controlled trial of hydrotherapy in rheumatoid arthritis. *Arthritis Care Res* 1996;9(3):206–215.
120. Michlovitz S. Biophysical principles of heating and superficial heat agents. In: Michlovitz S, ed. *Thermal agents in rehabilitation*. Philadelphia: F.A. Davis, 1990.
121. Mayer JM, Ralph L, Look M, et al. Treating acute low back pain with continuous low-level heat wrap therapy and/or exercise: a randomized controlled trial. *Spine J* 2005;5(4):395–403.
122. Svarcova J, Trnavsky K, Zvarova J. The influence of ultrasound, galvanic currents and shortwave diathermy on pain intensity in patients with osteoarthritis. *Scand J Rheumatol Suppl* 1987;67:83–85.

123. Michlovitz S. Cryotherapy: the use of cold as a therapeutic agent. In: Michlovitz S, ed. *Thermal agents in rehabilitation*. Philadelphia: F.A. Davis, 1990.
124. Cote DJ, Prentice WE, Jr, Hooker DN, et al. Comparison of three treatment procedures for minimizing ankle sprain swelling. *Phys Ther* 1988;68(7):1072–1076.
125. Levy A, Dalith M, Abramovici A, et al. Transcutaneous electrical nerve stimulation in experimental acute arthritis. *Arch Phys Med Rehabil* 1987;68(2):75–78.
126. Deyo RA, Walsh NE, Martin DC, et al. A controlled trial of transcutaneous electrical nerve stimulation (TENS) and exercise for chronic low back pain. *N Engl J Med* 1990;322(23):1627–1634.
127. Chiu TT, Hui-Chan CW, Chein G. A randomized clinical trial of TENS and exercise for patients with chronic neck pain. *Clin Rehabil* 2005; 19(8):850–860.
128. Preyde M. Effectiveness of massage therapy for subacute low-back pain: a randomized controlled trial. *CMAJ* 2000;162(13):1815–1820.
129. Triano JJ, McGregor M, Hondras MA, et al. Manipulative therapy versus education programs in chronic low back pain. *Spine* 1995;20(8):948–955.
130. Taubert K. [Massages—necessary or a luxury?] *Z Arztl Fortbild Qualitatssich* 1997;91(2):139–143.
131. James MJ, Cleland LG, Gaffney RD, et al. Effect of exercise on 99mTc-DTPA clearance from knees with effusions. *J Rheumatol* 1994;21(3): 501–504.
132. Hayden JA, van Tulder MW, Malmivaara A, et al. Exercise therapy for treatment of non-specific low back pain. *Cochrane Database Syst Rev* 2005;(3):CD000335.
133. Stux G, Pomeranz B. *Basics of acupuncture*. Berlin: Springer Verlag, 1995.
134. Tsou K. Neurochemical mechanisms of acupuncture. In: Akil H, Lewis J, eds. *Neurotransmitters and pain: control of pain and headache*, vol. 9, Basel, Switzerland: H.G. Karger, 1987:226.
135. Witt C, Brinkhaus B, Jena S, et al. Acupuncture in patients with osteoarthritis of the knee: a randomised trial. *Lancet* 2005;366(9480): 136–143.
136. Martin DP, Sletten CD, Williams BA, et al. Improvement in fibromyalgia symptoms with acupuncture: results of a randomized controlled trial. *Mayo Clin Proc* 2006;81(6):749–757.
137. Witt CM, Jena S, Brinkhaus B, et al. Acupuncture in patients with osteoarthritis of the knee or hip: a randomized, controlled trial with an additional nonrandomized arm. *Arthritis Rheum* 2006;54(11):3485–3493.
138. Haake M, Muller HH, Schade-Brittinger C, et al. German Acupuncture Trials (GERAC) for chronic low back pain: randomized, multicenter, blinded, parallel-group trial with 3 groups. *Arch Intern Med* 2007;167 (17):189–188.
139. NIH consensus statement: acupuncture. Bethesda, MD: National Institutes of Health, 1997:15.
140. Rand MJ, Whaler BC. Impairment of sympathetic transmission by botulinum toxin. *Nature* 1965;206(984):588–591.
141. Hagenah R, Benecke R, Wiegand H. Effects of type A botulinum toxin on the cholinergic transmission at spinal Renshaw cells and on the inhibitory action at Ia inhibitory interneurones. *Naunyn Schmiedebergs Arch Pharmacol* 1977;299(3):267–272.
142. Ojala T, Arokoski JP, Partanen J. The effect of small doses of botulinum toxin A on neck-shoulder myofascial pain syndrome: a double-blind, randomized, and controlled crossover trial. *Clin J Pain* 2006;22(1): 90–96.
143. Aurora SK, Gawel M, Brandes JL, et al. Botulinum toxin type a prophylactic treatment of episodic migraine: a randomized, double-blind, placebo-controlled exploratory study. *Headache* 2007;47(4): 486–499.
144. Silberstein SD, Stark SR, Lucas SM, et al. Botulinum toxin type A for the prophylactic treatment of chronic daily headache: a randomized, double-blind, placebo-controlled trial. *Mayo Clin Proc* 2005;80(9): 1126–1137.
145. Sycha T, Samal D, Chizh B, et al. A lack of antinociceptive or antiinflammatory effect of botulinum toxin A in an inflammatory human pain model. *Anesth Analg* 2006;102(2):509–516.

CHAPTER 95

Seddon R. Savage, MD, MS, FASAM
Ryan Horvath, BA

Opioid Therapy of Pain

Opioids are the most potent analgesic agents clinically available at this time. They have wide efficacy and utility in the treatment of acute and cancer-related pain, and may be helpful as a component of the management of chronic non-cancer-related pain in some patients. With appropriate care, they may be used effectively and safely in persons with addiction disorders. However, opioids may cause euphoria or "reward" in some individuals, which may lead to misuse and, in susceptible individuals, to addiction. This chapter addresses key conceptual, pharmacologic, and clinical issues related to opioids as a basis for weighing the potential benefits and risks of their use in the treatment of pain, and the chapter presents clinical strategies for safe and effective use in persons with, or at risk for, substance use disorders. To provide context, we begin with brief discussions of the historical use of opioids, the prevalence of pain and opioid use and misuse in our society, and contemporary views on the use of opioids in the treatment of pain.

HISTORICAL PERSPECTIVES ON OPIOID USE

Opioids have been used by humans for millennia. One of the first accounts of the use of opioids comes from the Sumerian ideology of hul gil, the "plant of joy," more than 8,000 years ago (1). Theophrastus, the Greek philosopher and popularizer of science, provides the first written account of the use of opium to relieve pain in BC 300. During this time, the Greek physicians Hippocrates and Galen used opium to treat headaches, coughing, asthma, and melancholy. In 1805, morphine was purified from opium, but use did not become widespread until the development of the hypodermic syringe in 1853, which allowed morphine to be introduced directly into the circulatory system.

By the early 1900s, both appropriate therapeutic use of opioids and misuse of opioid were widespread in the United States. Opioids were subjected to regulation, with legal use restricted to "legitimate medical purposes." In 1919, a Federal ruling held that treatment of addiction was "outside the realm of legitimate medical interest," (2) creating a conundrum that allowed physicians to treat pain but not addiction that sometimes occurred in the context of medical use (3). Regulation of opioids continued throughout the 1900s until the 1970 Federal Controlled Substances Act, which further tightened regulation and required registration of providers. With the enhanced regulation, controlled substance designation and the understanding of abuse potential of opioids their use by physicians declined in the latter half of the 20th century. A resurgence in the use of opioids began in the 1990s as treatment of pain became a higher priority and aggressive marketing of newer opioid formulations emerged.

PREVALENCE AND IMPACT OF PAIN

Pain is one of the most common ailments and is the second leading reason for patients to seek medical care (4). More than 80 million Americans report serious pain in any given year, and

86% of these have pain on a chronic basis (5). The most commonly reported pain disorders are headache, lower back pain, arthritis, and other joint pain (6). Pain is also the second leading cause of workplace absenteeism (4) and accounts for an estimated $61.2 billion in lost productivity annually (7). The prevalence of pain among persons with substance use disorders may be significantly higher than that of the general population with, 62% to 80% of patients in methadone maintenance treatment programs and 78% of patients presenting for inpatient substance abuse treatment programs reporting significant chronic pain (8,9). With the enormous social and economic impact of pain on our society, adequate treatment is paramount.

PREVALENCE OF USE AND MISUSE OF PRESCRIPTION OPIOIDS

The therapeutic use of commonly prescribed opioids has increased dramatically recently, with prescriptions for fentanyl and oxycodone rising by 403% and 227%, respectively, between 1997 and 2002. At the same time, prescription opioid misuse has also risen, with increases of 642% and 347%, respectively, for patients presenting to emergency rooms with harm from fentanyl and oxycodone misuse. It should be noted, however, that all opioids save oxycodone were associated with less than 1% of emergency room (ER) visits (10).

While preclinical thefts of opioids (e.g., from pharmacies, manufacturers, and trucks) contribute to diversion of opioids (11) evidence suggests misused opioids are often obtained from clinical sources, either directly from prescribers or through household diversion of prescribed opioids (12). In order to effectively and safely treat pain, while reducing the risk of opioid misuse and diversion, it is critical that prescribing clinicians understand and employ clinical strategies to reduce the risk of diversion of these medications and that patients secure all supplies of opioids.

THE ROLE OF OPIOIDS IN THE TREATMENT OF PAIN

Opioids are essential analgesic agents for the treatment of pain. For the treatment of acute postsurgical or trauma induced pain, opioid therapy is the gold standard of practice. Opioids are also standard in the treatment of cancer pain, occupying steps 2 and 3 of the widely accepted "therapeutic ladder" developed by the World Health Organization (12a). However, there is less consensus regarding the role of opioids in the treatment of chronic non-cancer pain. Chronic pain often has multiple etiologic components that include physiologic, psychosocial, and behavioral factors, and it may similarly impact diverse biopsychosocial domains of experience. Because of this, effective treatment of chronic pain often demands empowerment of the individual through polymodal approaches to pain treatment and to management of residual symptoms. (Such approaches are explored in Chapters 93 and 94). Increasing evidence suggests, however, that opioids may be a helpful component of chronic pain management when, in the judgment of the patient and treating clinician, the potential benefits of use outweigh likely or actual risks of use, compared with those of other treatments. A recent review reporting the results of 26 randomized, controlled clinical trials of relatively short-term study (4 to 32 weeks) opioid therapy for chronic pain found that 25 of 26 documented pain improvement, including improvement of neuropathic pain and, in the studies that assessed function, more than half documented improvement in level of function. The same review found more ambiguous results in available longer-term studies that included case series, surveys, and open-label follow-up studies (13). A recent study published in the *Journal of the American Academy of Family Practice* of 801 primary care patients on opioids for a median duration of 6.5 years, however, found improved quality of life of patients on relatively-low-dose opioid therapy (20 to 40 mg of morphine equivalents per day) compared with patients with chronic pain on no opioid therapy, suggesting long-term treatment efficacy in at least some patients (14). In contrast, an epidemiologic study of 1,906 persons with chronic pain in Denmark, the country with the highest per capita use of opioids in the world, found that those using opioids reported significantly more pain, poorer self-rated health, lower quality of life, lower levels of physical activity and employment, and higher levels of health care utilization than nonusers (15). Clearly more study is needed to understand what subpopulations of patients with chronic pain benefit from opioid therapy and what therapeutic variables are associated with success.

A number of complex issues may affect the long-term prescribing of opioids in some contexts, and many physicians have concerns regarding the use of opioids to treat chronic non-cancer pain that bear careful examination. Primary care physicians, who treat the majority of chronic pain patients, report such concerns as prescription drug abuse, addiction, adverse effects, tolerance, and medical interactions (16). Many of these concerns are addressed later with the goal of empowering physicians to safely and effectively prescribe opioids to patients with chronic pain when appropriate and, more specifically, to provide pain management to patients with a prior history of substance abuse when needed.

SPECIAL ISSUES IN THE USE OF OPIOIDS

Like most medications, opioids have the potential for both intended therapeutic effects as well as unintended side effects. In addition to a range of physical side effects, however, opioids, like other medications that are scheduled as controlled substances under the U.S. Controlled Substances Act (21 USC Sec. 829 01/22/02), deserve special consideration for unintended consequences related to their capacity to provide reward and to produce dependence in some persons. Specific issues include the potential for physical dependence, tolerance, reward, addiction and misuse or diversion for a variety of purposes. These issues may be of less significance in the treatment of acute and cancer pain, given the often time-limited duration of use in these contexts, than in the management of chronic non-cancer-related pain, but a thorough understanding of these issues may enhance decision making in all three contexts. Each issue is considered separately here.

Physical Dependence Physical dependence, as defined by a joint consensus statement of several pain and addictions professional organizations, is a state of adaptation that is manifested by a drug class–specific withdrawal syndrome that can be produced by abrupt cessation, rapid dose reduction, decreasing blood level of the drug, and/or administration of an antagonist (17). Such dependence is an expected occurrence in all patients (with and without addictive disease) after 2 to 10 days of continuous administration of an opioid (18). In an acute pain setting, such dependence generally is not clinically significant, because individuals tend to taper opioids naturally owing to gradual reduction in pain as the acute problem (such as postoperative pain, posttraumatic pain, or medical illness) resolves. However, if pain medications are abruptly stopped or precipitously reduced, a withdrawal syndrome may ensue. The character and intensity of the withdrawal vary, depending on the dose and duration of opioid administration and a variety of host factors, including previous experience with withdrawal, prior long-term administration of opioids, and the patient's expectations regarding withdrawal.

Common symptoms of opioid withdrawal include autonomic signs and symptoms, such as diarrhea, piloerection, sweating, mydriasis, and mild increases in blood pressure and pulse, as well as signs of central nervous system arousal such as irritability, anxiety, and sleeplessness. Craving for the medication is expected in the course of withdrawal, and pain—most often experienced as abdominal cramping, deep bone pain, or diffuse muscle aching—is common (19). Patients with chronic pain may experience an intensified level of their usual pain syndrome during withdrawal. In patients who are physically dependent on opioids, the use of short-acting opioid medications may result in intermittent withdrawal between doses of medication, which may in turn cause an increase in perceived pain (20,21). This may be avoided by using long-acting or continuous medications. Simple physical dependence occurs in any patient when opioids are administered for an extended period of time.

Using the term *addiction* to describe such physical dependence is inaccurate and raises misperceptions about both persons with addiction disorders who become physically dependent on medications despite continuing in a state of recovery and individuals without addiction disorders who become physically dependent on medications without developing the true characteristics of addiction.

Tolerance Tolerance is indicated by the need for increasing doses of a medication to achieve the initial effects of the drug (22). Tolerance may occur both to a drug's analgesic effects and to its unwanted side effects, such as respiratory depression, sedation, or nausea. Many characteristics of opioid tolerance remain poorly understood. Animal studies suggest that tolerance to the analgesic effects of medications occurs in some contexts but not in others (23). Human studies of the management of acute pain document the development of progressive tolerance to the analgesic effects of opioids when they are administered on a continuous basis over a period of several days (24,25). Over a period of weeks to months, however, some studies suggest that the continuing development of progressive tolerance to the analgesic effects of opioids may not routinely occur. Several studies that examined the opioid management of cancer pain suggest that opioid dose requirements increase only during progression of the underlying disease process and that, with stable disease or treatment of painful tissue pathology, the need for medication remains the same or actually decreases (22,26). An 18-month randomized, controlled clinical trial supports the clinical observation that stable opioid doses may provide persistent, if modest, improvement in analgesia over the longer term in some patients with chronic non-cancer pain as well (27).

A number of studies investigated the development of tolerance to specific opioids, with the goal of determining whether opioids of varying efficacy have different profiles with regard to the development of tolerance. Several animal studies have suggested an inverse relationship between analgesic efficacy and tolerance formation; however, no consistent relationship between intrinsic efficacy and tolerance has been demonstrated in human populations (25,28,29).

Most investigators agree that absolute tolerance to the analgesic effects of opioids does not occur (30). That is, opioids may be used over a prolonged period of time in the face of increasing dose requirements yet continue to provide relief of pain. However, in the context of chronic pain not associated with life-threatening illness, such dose escalation may become impractical owing to cost, side effects, or simply unrelenting requirements for dose escalation. In some cases, increasing pain in the absence of progressive pathology may be due not to opioid tolerance but to the related phenomena of opioid-induced hyperalgesia in which opioids actually induce pain (see discussion under "Longterm use side effects"). Based on these issues, there is increasing consensus that very high dose requirements in persons with nonprogressive conditions underlying their chronic pain may signal the evolving failure of opioid therapy. In some cases gradual reduction or elimination of opioids appears to improve pain. Though higher dose requirements appear to be indicated in some patients, it has been suggested on an empirical basis that about 180 mg morphine equivalents per day be considered a point of likely diminishing returns (31). The Dillie study (14) of 801 primary care patients with chronic pain on opioid therapy that is cited earlier found that quality of life was generally best for patients with chronic pain on between 20 and 40 mg of opioid per day compared with those on no opioids or on high-dose therapy. In this study, those on >100 mg morphine equivalents had the lowest quality of life though this may be owing to multiple factors including the underlying pain condition.

Reward Opioids produce reward in many, though not all, individuals. Some persons, in fact, experience dysphoria or no mood changes in association with opioid use. The potential for opioids to produce reward (or euphoria) when used for pain treatment is a critical factor to consider, however, especially when treating persons with co-occurring pain and substance use disorders or risks for substance misuse. A clear understanding of the potential issues that may modulate reward experiences when opioids are used for analgesia may be helpful to optimizing clinical management strategies, particularly in persons at risk for substance misuse.

Mechanisms of Reward Opioids produce reward by binding to GABAergic interneurons that normally inhibit dopamine production in the limbic reward system, preventing them from doing so (32). The resulting increase in dopamine and cascade of secondary effects produces feelings of reward or euphoria. Reward may or may not occur in different individuals along with analgesia when opioids are used for pain and is not itself harmful. In some contexts, particularly terminal illness, euphoria and reward may in fact be valued side effects. However, when euphoria becomes the focus of the use of opioids, particularly in a person with addictive disease, it may undermine pain treatment and become a problem in its own right. Understanding how to limit opioid reward effects therefore may sometimes be helpful.

Most of what is known about the mechanisms that determine reward intensity derives from addiction literature. This knowledge may, however, also apply and provide some guidance in clinical pain treatment settings. Relevant considerations include the rate of increase in brain levels of drug, the blood level of drug relative to individual tolerance, fluctuations in drug blood levels, and the specific receptor profile of the drug with respect to individual receptor variability.

Factors Affecting Reward

Rate of Increase Both animal drug self-administration studies and human drug-liking studies have demonstrated that reward increases when the rate of rise in drug blood levels increases: the faster the onset, the better the rush or high (33). A recent study to determine which properties of prescription opioids make them more attractive for purposes of getting high supported speed of onset as a key value (34). The intravenous route of administration causes a more rapid rise in blood levels and is expected to provide more opioid euphoria than the oral route. Intramuscular and subcutaneous administration provide an intermediate effect. Among opioids given orally, those with an inherently slower time to peak effect (such as methadone or levorphanol) are expected to produce weaker reward effects than opioids with relatively rapid onset, such as immediate-release oxycodone (in Percocet or Tylox), hydrocodone (in Vicodin or Lortabs), or hydromorphone (Dilaudid).

Peak Blood Level Attained The higher the opioid blood level relative to the individual's tolerance for the drug, the greater the reward. An opioid-naive individual with little or no tolerance may experience euphoria with a drug blood level that would cause no significant reward effect in a more tolerant individual. A dose of an opioid given intravenously achieves a higher peak blood level than the same dose administered by the oral route, with subcutaneous and intramuscular again intermediate (Figs. 95.1 and 95.2).

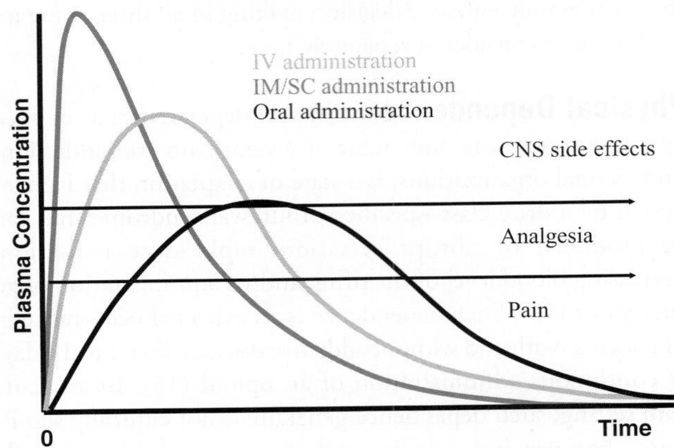

FIGURE 95.1. Routes of administration. (i.v., intravenous; i.m./s.c., intramuscular/subcutaneous; CNS, central nervous system.)

As the rise in blood levels of a drug is associated with onset of euphoria, stable levels generally produce less euphoria than intermittently rising and falling levels. This key principle underlies the effectiveness of methadone maintenance therapy for opioid addiction. And it means that continuous intravenous infusion of an opioid will likely trigger less reward than intermittent boluses and controlled-release opioids (used by the intended route at the intended time interval) or intrinsically long-acting opioids (such as methadone or levorphanol) should be less rewarding than frequently dosed short-acting medications. An exception to this rule is patient-controlled analgesia (PCA), which is not expected to provide significant reward because the incremental doses are very small and spaced at intervals that do not permit a rapid, high rise in blood levels. However, when persons with an active addiction to opioids

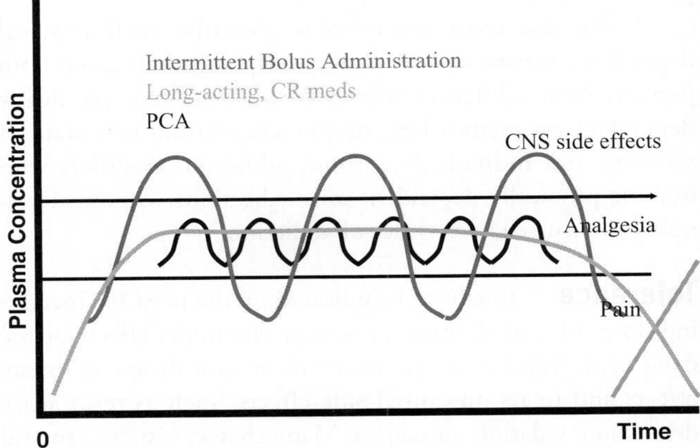

FIGURE 95.2. Schedules of administration. (CR, controlled-release; PCA, patient-controlled analgesia; CNS, central nervous system.)

TABLE 95.1 Limitations of Current DSM-IV Criteria for Identifying Addiction in Pain Patients

DSM-IV substance dependence criteria (Reason not specific for addiction)	Challenges in using criteria to diagnose addiction in opioid analgesia
Tolerance	Expected with prolonged analgesic use
Physical dependence/withdrawal	Expected with prolonged regular analgesic use
Used in greater amounts or longer than intended	Emergence of pain may demand increase dose or prolonged use.
Unsuccessful attempts to cut down or discontinue	Emergence of pain may deter dose taper or cessation.
Much time spent pursuing or recovering from use	Difficulty finding pain treatment may drive time spent pursuing analgesics Time spent recovering from overuse is suggestive of addiction.
Important activities reduced or given up	Valid criteria—activity engagement expected to increase not decline with pain treatment
Continued use despite knowledge of persistent physical or psychologic harm	Valid criteria—no harm anticipated from analgesic opioid use for pain

receive patient-controlled analgesia (PCA) or any intravenous infusion, close supervision is critical to ensure that no tampering with the system occurs.

Receptor Effects As previously discussed, mu opioid agonists are more likely to cause reward than kappa opioid agonists. In light of emerging understanding of mu opioid receptor polymorphism with variable expression of receptors in different individuals—and the differential effects of different opioids on different subreceptor types—different individuals may experience contrasting reward effects as well as unequal analgesic effects from a given opioid. This may explain why patients treated for opioid addiction have different opioids of choice.

Interference of Pain with Reward Some research suggests that people feel less euphoria if they are in pain when given opioids (35). This hypothesis is supported by reports from patients who say that opioids relieve their pain without psychic effects. As well, many patients experience dysphoria or other aversive feelings, rather than euphoria, when given opioids for their pain.

Though concerns regarding drug reward may be relevant for persons at risk for opioid misuse or addiction, they should not deter effective and immediate treatment when opioids are required for relief of significant acute pain. The long-term outcome of addiction is not likely to be strongly affected by use of indicated medications in the short term (13).

Addiction

In the context of pain treatment with opioids, addiction must be defined through the observation of a constellation of maladaptive behaviors rather than by observation of pharmacologic phenomena such as dependence, tolerance, and dose escalation. Addiction in the context of opioid therapy for pain is characterized by the presence of a combination of observations suggesting adverse consequences due to use of the drugs, loss of control over drug use, and preoccupation with obtaining opioids despite the presence of adequate analgesia (17,36). Physical dependence on opioids and the development of tolerance to their effects do not, of themselves, constitute addiction (3,30,36). When the criteria for substance use disorder of the *Diagnostic and Statistical Manual of Mental Disorders*, 4th Edition (37) are used to assess for addiction in the presence of pain, only the criteria that refer to function may be used (36), because other criteria refer only to the expected, nonpathologic sequelae of chronic opioid use (Table 95.1).

Adverse consequences that are suggestive of addiction include persistent over-sedation or euphoria, deteriorating level of function despite relief of pain, or increase in pain-associated distresses such as anxiety, sleep disturbance, or depressive symptoms. Loss of control over use might be reflected in prescriptions used before the expected renewal date, patients who obtain multiple prescriptions, or who obtain opioids from illicit sources. Because of concerns that existing criteria promoted confusion, organizations representing the fields of pain and addiction proposed the definitions outlined in Table 95.2.

Preoccupation with opioid use may be reflected in noncompliance with nonopioid components of pain treatment, inability to recognize non-nociceptive components of pain, and the perception that no interventions other than opioids have any effect on pain (3,36,38). It is important to recognize that such behaviors may occur on an occasional basis for a variety of reasons in the context of successful opioid therapy for pain. By contrast, it is a pattern of persistent occurrences that should prompt concern and further assessment (Table 95.2).

The risk of developing addiction to opioids in the course of opioid therapy for pain is unknown. Early studies led to a perception that the iatrogenic creation of addiction through medical use of opioids was a very frequent occurrence (39,40). In contrast, a number of retrospective surveys of never-addicted medical patients suggested that the development of addiction in the course of long-term opioid therapy for pain was almost negligible (41,42) leading to a likely under-appreciation of the risks. The reality is almost certainly somewhere in between, but the actual rate of occurrence is difficult to assess. Studies of the incidence of addiction in the context of pain treatment have generally examined a wide variety of "aberrant behaviors" rather than specifically assessing for

TABLE 95.2 Definition and Indicators of Addiction in Pain Patients

Addiction

American Society of Addiction Medicine, American Pain Society, American Academy of Pain Medicine

A primary, chronic, neurobiologic disease with genetic, psychosocial and environmental factors influencing its development and manifestations characterized by behaviors that include one or more of the following:

ASAM-APS-AAPM Behavioral criteria	Examples of specific behaviors in opioid therapy for pain
Impaired control over use, compulsive use	Frequent loss/theft reported, calls for early renewals, withdrawal noted at appointments
Continued use despite harm due to use	Declining function, intoxication, persistent over sedation
Preoccupation with use, craving	Nonopioid interventions ignored, opioids only intervention considered, recurrent requests for opioid increase/complaints increasing pain in absence of disease progression despite titration[a]

ASAM, American Society of Addiction Medicine; APS, American Pain Society; AAPM, American Academy of Pain Medicine.

[a]May reflect tolerance or hyperalgesia.

addiction, and they have been variable in methodology, operative definitions, and quality. In addition, many studies that assess opioid use and misuse excluded the highest risk group, those with a prior history of addiction (43).

The prevalence of identified misuse of opioids by patients ranges widely in different studies, between 1% and 38% (44–47). Misuse of opioids, however, can reflect a wide variety of issues as well as addiction. One study of persons presenting for treatment of oxycodone addiction (48) found that 47% (51 of 109) persons had their first exposure to opioids through a prescription for pain and further found that only 31% of this subgroup had prior histories of alcohol or other drug problems, suggesting that a significant number developed de novo addiction to opioids prescribed for pain in the absence of previous addiction disorder. However, the study did not assess for family history of addiction and, therefore, did not shed light on whether such addiction occurred in the context of identifiable biogenetic risk. It also did not provide a denominator that would permit determination of the rate of addiction among those prescribed opioids.

The etiology of addiction in the context of pain treatment likely involves an interplay of biogenetic vulnerability, drug reward effects, and other host and environmental factors including the presence of pain, of stress, and of the psychosocial context of use. The lifetime prevalence of any form of substance dependence (addiction), exclusive of tobacco, is estimated at 3% to 16% of the general population (49). It is reasonable to expect that this portion of the population may be at some level of increased risk for the development of addiction when opioids are used for pain, though the presence of pain may reduce this risk somewhat if it attenuates reward. Nevertheless, it is appropriate to use special care in implementing opioid therapy in patients who have personal or family histories of alcoholism or other addictions. Opioids should not generally be withheld out of fear of addiction when they are indicated for the relief of pain, but the structure of care may be adapted to reduce risks.

When addiction is identified in the course of opioid therapy for pain, it is important to address it aggressively, so that the pain is effectively controlled and to prevent the debilitating sequelae of addiction. Institution of appropriate addiction treatment services, tightening the structure of opioid prescribing in order to help the individual gain control over the medications, and involving the patient's social support system in treatment are important first steps.

Differential Diagnosis of Opioid Misuse Patients misuse opioids for a variety of reasons with a wide range of implications (Table 95.3). It is important to distinguish clinically between different causes of opioid misuse in order to address each case appropriately. The term *opioid abuse* has little clinical utility as it includes a broad spectrum of clinical or behavioral drivers of nonmedical use or misuse and, in its imprecision, fails to provide a basis for resolving the misuse.

The most common cause of misuse, probably, is simply misunderstanding how opioids are supposed to be used; clear written instructions can reduce this type of misuse. Patients may misuse opioids prescribed for pain to obtain relief from depressed feelings, anxiety, insomnia, or discomforting memories; these patients usually will benefit more from more-specific treatments. Patients who have become physically dependent on opioids provided for pain may continue to use the drugs

TABLE 95.3 Differential Diagnosis Misuse of Analgesic Opioids

- Misunderstanding of instructions
- Self-medication of
  - Mood/stress
  - Sleep
  - Disturbing memories
  - Undertreated pain
  - Other
- Elective use for reward or euphoria
- Compulsive use due to addiction

once the pain has resolved in order to avoid withdrawal symptoms; tapering of opioids can usually eliminate dependency without significant withdrawal distress.

Some patients misuse opioids electively in order to experience reward or euphoria as discussed earlier. A subset of patients who have a biogenetic vulnerability and who use opioids electively in a manner that induces euphoria will trigger addiction. This leads to continued compulsive use of opioids in a potentially self-destructive manner that poses significant personal risk.

Finally, some patients exhibit distress and engage in behaviors aimed at obtaining more medication because their pain treatment is inadequate The term *pseudoaddiction* has emerged in the pain literature to describe the inaccurate interpretation of these behaviors in patients who have severe pain that is undermedicated or whose pain otherwise has not been effectively treated (50). Such patients may appear to be preoccupied with obtaining opioids, but their preoccupation reflects a need for pain control rather than an addictive drive. Pseudoaddictive behavior can be distinguished from addiction by the fact that, when adequate analgesia is achieved, the patient who is seeking pain relief demonstrates improved function, uses the medications as prescribed, and does not use drugs in a manner that persistently causes sedation or euphoria. Such behaviors may occur occasionally even in the successful opioid therapy for pain; it is a pattern of persistent occurrences that should prompt concern and further assessment.

CLINICAL MANAGEMENT VARIABLES IN THE USE OF OPIOIDS

Opioids often are the mainstay of treatment of moderate to severe acute pain and cancer-related pain. When used in the long-term treatment of chronic, non-cancer-related pain, they are most often helpful as one component of multidimensional treatment. Goals of pain treatment generally include reduction in pain, enhanced level of function, and improved quality of life.

A number of variables must be considered in planning opioid therapy for pain. In addition to the considerations addressed, important variables include drug selection, dose titration and scheduling, and management of side effects. It also is clinically important to understand how to appropriately change drugs or withdraw medications when indicated. These issues are considered individually.

Drug Selection Opioids produce their pharmacologic effects (both analgesic and side effects) primarily through stimulation of opioid receptors. Stimulation of the mu, kappa, and delta receptors is associated with analgesia and side effects. Most of the commonly used opioid analgesics have predominantly mu receptor activity; however, there are also opioids that have agonist-antagonist and partial mu agonist activity. Each of these opioid classes are considered here.

Mu opioid agonists are the most commonly prescribed class of opioid analgesics and include morphine, oxycodone, hydromorphone, and fentanyl. Pure mu agonists have no ceiling analgesic effect and may be titrated as needed to achieve analgesia. Tolerance to side effects generally occurs more rapidly than tolerance to analgesia, though monitoring for respiratory depression is important, especially in opioid-naive individuals, as doses are increased or specific opioids are changed.

Though most mu agonists are interchangeable if attention is paid to relative dosing potencies and onset and duration of action, emerging evidence suggests that individuals may respond somewhat differently to different opioids. This may be owing to variability in mu opioid receptor expression in different individuals as well as to variable opioid receptor specificity of the different drugs (51). Recently there have been reports of several mu opioid receptor polymorphisms that require higher agonist dosing to achieve maximal analgesic efficacy (52). In addition, some clinically relevant differences between mu agonists long have been apparent (Table 95.4).

Meperidine's usefulness in pain treatment is limited by its short half-life and because, with high dose use, a neurotoxic metabolite—normeperidine—may accumulate, causing irritability, tremors and, potentially, seizures. This is especially relevant in opioid-dependent individuals who may have significant tolerance and correspondingly high dose requirements as well as in patients with renal or hepatic insufficiency.

Propoxyphene, a weak mu agonist, has low analgesic efficacy and some abuse potential and has been associated with seizures. Some clinicians believe it is a reasonable analgesic substitute for nonsteroidal antiinflammatory drugs (NSAIDs) or acetaminophen in some patients who cannot use those drugs. A subset of patients appear to experience more substantial analgesia with propoxyphene than with NSAIDs. However, most experts agree that propoxyphene has limited utility in pain treatment.

Methadone differs from other mu agonists in several ways. It has a long and unpredictable elimination half-life (5 to 130 hours) that necessitates especially careful titration (53). Its dextro-isomer has *N*-methyl-D-aspartate (NMDA) receptor antagonist activity, and it has been suggested that this may result in less tolerance than occurs with other mu opioids and

TABLE 95.4 Opioids Commonly Prescribed for Pain with Key Characteristics

Opioid	Example brands/preparations	Special pain issues	Special misuse issues
Mu Agonists			
Morphine	MSContin (12-h controlled-release [CR]), Kadian, Avinza (24-h CR), Oramorph (intermediate-release [IR])	CR mechanism provides relatively stable blood levels	CR mechanism may be adulterated for misuse
Oxycodone	Percocet (IR and acetaminophen), Percodan (IR and aspirin), OxyContin (12 CR)	CR mechanism provides relatively stable blood level misuse	CR mechanism may be adulterated for misuse
Hydrocodone	Vicodin (IR and acetaminophen), Lortab (IR and acetaminophen)	Most commonly prescribed opioid	Most commonly misused opioid.
Hydromorphone	Dilaudid (IR)		Quick onset, relatively high reward value
Fentanyl	Duragesic (72-h CR patch), Actiq (IR lozenge)	Patch provides very stable blood levels used as prescribed	Less common misuse of patch but dangerous when misused given concentrated dosing
Methadone	Methadose, dolophine	2nd analgesic mechanism: *N*-methyl-D-aspartic acid (NMDA) receptor antagonist. Possibly less tolerance and greater efficacy in neuropathic pain indications	Pharmacologic properties make misuse particularly risky. Recent increased misuse and increased mortality; used to treat opioid addiction
Codeine	Tylenol #3 (IR with acetaminophen)	Prodrug with ceiling effect	
Partial mMu agonists			
Tramadol	Ultram (IR), Ultracet (IR with acetaminophen)	2nd analgesic mechanism (increase serotonin/ norepinephrine); limited dose due to seizures	Relatively low rates of abuse and reward documented, though occur in some persons
Buprenorphine	Subotex (often used off-label for pain)	Partial agonist; ceiling effect; used off-label for pain	Approved for treatment of opioid addiction; some intravenous (i.v.) abuse reported
Kappa opioids		Mu antagonist actions	
Butorphanol	Stadol (intravenous [i.v.] or intranasal)	Rapid onset of intranasal, ceiling analgesic effects	Less reward in some but intranasal route is quick onset
Nalbuphine	Nubain (i.v. only)	Ceiling analgesic effects	Less reward in some than mu medications
Pentazocine	Talwin, Talwin NX (with naltrexone; oral only)	Ceiling analgesic effects	Less reward in some but formulated with naltrexone due to i.v. abuse in 1960s

Savage SR, Passik S, Kirsch K. Challenges in using opioids to treat pain in persons with substance use disorders. National Institutes on Drug Abuse. *NIDA Addiction Science and Clinical Practice* 2008; 4(2) (53a).

in greater efficacy in treating neuropathic pain, though this has not been demonstrated clearly in clinical trials. Further, incomplete cross-tolerance between methadone and other mu opioid agonists requires the use of a much lower than equianalgesic dose of methadone in the patient who is transitioning from other mu agonists (as low as one-tenth the equivalent dose or no more than 30 mg per day is recommended by some) (54). Conversely, however, patients who are changed from methadone to other opioids may experience poor analgesia for reasons that are not fully understood (55). Another mu opioid agonist, levorphanol, is less well studied than methadone but shares a number of its pharmacologic features, including its relatively long half-life and dextro-isomer with NMDA antagonist activity. Methadone is more difficult to use safely than other opioids owing to its variable half-life and multiple drug interactions. Additionally, it causes QTc prolongation and has been associated with torsades de pointes syndrome.

Agonist-antagonist—or kappa agonist—opioids, including pentazocine, nalbuphine, and butorphanol, have predominantly kappa agonist effects while antagonizing the mu receptor. Agonist-antagonist drugs are widely regarded as having less potential for abuse and addiction than the pure opioid agonists, though elective use for reward and the development of addiction to these medications have been observed. Their clinical usefulness as analgesics is limited by a number of factors. The agonist-antagonist drugs exhibit a ceiling effect in terms of analgesia. Their use sometimes is associated with dysphoric reactions. Because of their mu antagonist activity, they may reverse analgesia and precipitate withdrawal in individuals who are physically dependent on mu agonists. Consequently, no clear advantages of agonist-antagonist drugs have been demonstrated in the treatment of pain in persons with addiction disorders, though they may be a reasonable choice in some patients.

Partial mu agonists, including buprenorphine and tramadol, provide analgesia via mu opioid receptors but have relatively low intrinsic efficacy (i.e., they bind mu opioid receptors with high affinity but produce reduced receptor activation compared to full mu agonists). Clinically, they are very different medications. Buprenorphine is available in parenteral, sublingual, and (in Europe) transdermal preparations. It has a long half-life and high receptor affinity and is useful in agonist treatment of opioid addiction. In the United States at this time, buprenorphine's use for analgesia is an off-label use; it is FDA-approved for use in treatment of addiction by clinicians with certification from the Centers for Substance Abuse Treatment to provide this treatment. As an analgesic, it can be used at 6- to 8-hour intervals for moderate to moderately severe pain. It is thought by most observers to have a ceiling effect as an analgesic and, therefore, may not provide continuously increasing analgesia beyond a certain dose titration, though this is currently under study.

Tramadol (Ultram), which generally is used in oral form, has a second mechanism of analgesia through the inhibition of reuptake of serotonin and norepinephrine. Doses are limited by a significant potential for seizures at levels above 400 mg per day, which thus is its effective analgesic ceiling. Tramadol appears to have somewhat less abuse potential than pure mu opioid analgesics, though there are reports of abuse of both medications (56).

Routes of Administration

Opioids may be administered orally, rectally, transmucosally, intravenously, subcutaneously, transdermally, and intraspinally. The oral, enteral, or transdermal routes generally are preferred when feasible because they are less invasive than many other routes and usually provide satisfactory analgesia, even when high doses are required. However, when these routes are not reasonable (as when patients are unable to take medications orally or when rapid titration is necessary), parenteral routes may be preferred. Note that parenteral routes increase both speed of onset and peak blood levels obtained, which may be favorable in terms of analgesia but also may increase reward, a consideration in persons with substance use issues, and may increase sedation and other side effects IV access may be difficult in individuals with a history of injection drug use; for such patients, surgical identification of venous access may be necessary, or continuous subcutaneous infusions may be used. Intramuscular injections also are effective, but this route is increasingly discouraged because of the unnecessary pain involved in repeated injection and variable blood levels with this route of administration. If side effects of systemic use are not acceptable, intraspinal opioids may be indicated. Rectal preparations may be useful for patients who are vomiting or who are unable to take oral medications. Sublingual or transmucosal administration of some preparations is clinically effective as well; these have a rapidity of onset and peak levels generally intermediate to oral and intravenous use.

Dose Titration and Scheduling

Measuring Efficacy The serial use of a pain scale, such as a numerical 0 to 10 rating scale or a visual faces scale indicating variable levels of distress before treatment and at regular intervals during treatment, is helpful in assessing pain and its response to treatment, In treating chronic pain, it is often helpful to inquire about worst pain, best pain, and typical pain experienced in a particular period of time, such as the past week or month, and to document what is an acceptable level of pain that permits satisfactory comfort for the individual as well as function and quality of life. Numerical ratings of satisfactory pain control may be affected by myriad co-occurring issues and experiences so the target numbers viewed as indication of satisfactory treatment must be individualized.

Dose Requirements and Scheduling Considerations

Several factors must be considered in determining the dose and interval of administration that will provide effective analgesia in a given patient for a given problem. The pharmacologic characteristics of each drug in terms of onset, relative potency, and duration of analgesic action must be appreciated and scheduling planned with respect to these. The marked variability among patients in intrinsic responsiveness to opioids must be appreciated and accommodated (22). Finally, the relative tolerance of individuals who have been exposed to opioids on a prolonged basis (whether therapeutically or due to addiction) must be accommodated. Individual who are currently using opioids or have used persistently in the past are likely to be relatively tolerant or may develop rapid tolerance to the analgesic effects of opioids and, therefore, may require relatively high doses at relatively short intervals to achieve analgesia. If the patient used opioids on a daily basis prior to the onset of acute pain, then his or her usual dose of opioids cannot be expected to provide analgesia for acute pain, and additional treatment must be provided.

Long- versus Short-Acting Medications and Scheduled Versus As-Needed In considering medication scheduling, distinctions can be made between short-acting and long-acting medications. Long-acting medications include those that are intrinsically longer-acting, such as methadone or levorphanol, and medications that are long-acting by virtue of being formulated as controlled-release preparations, such as oral controlled-released oxycodone, morphine or oxymorphone, and transdermal fentanyl. Most other opioids are shorter-acting and immediate-release.

When patients have persistent pain on an around-the-clock basis, longer-acting medications may offer several advantages. They provide relatively stable drug blood levels and, therefore, more consistent analgesia than frequent doses of short-acting medications. Fewer peaks and valleys may result in fewer side effects, including less reward. When longer-acting medications are taken on a scheduled basis, patients are less driven to focus on pain and medication use because there is usually less opportunity for pain to break through and less need to watch the clock to note when medication is due.

Despite these theoretical advantages of long-acting or sustained-release opioids, few studies have directly compared analgesia and side effects or reward effects or misuse-related outcomes in persons prescribed different specific opioids or formulations of opioids, for pain. One such study found no significant difference in analgesia or misuse among patients receiving short-acting hydrocodone and others taking longer-acting methadone (57). The theoretical advantages of long-acting opioids, therefore, must be weighed against other clinical indications.

It is important to be aware that most controlled-release opioids can be altered to become immediate-release drugs through chewing, crushing, snorting, or extracting and injecting. Most persons who use prescription opioids to get high do in fact alter them in some way (58). Currently, many pharmaceutical companies are pursuing abuse-resistant formulations, though it is not likely that any system will be entirely abuse-proof. Strategies under development to reduce potential for abuse include embedding the opioid formulation with an opioid antagonist (naltrexone) or aversive medications (such as Ipecac or capsaicin) that are released with tampering and creating a chemical matrix from which the opioid cannot easily be released with chewing, crushing, or chemical extraction.

Shorter-acting medications are more often helpful for intermittent pain or, in association with longer-acting medications, for exacerbation of continuous pain treated with around-the-clock opioids. There are several issues that should be considered, however, regarding the use of short-acting opioids, particularly in prescribing for individuals with, or at risk for, substance misuse. First, pairing the perception of pain with the administration of a rewarding, and therefore potentially reinforcing, drug can theoretically reinforce the perception of pain and lead to increased use of the drug and increasing distress (59,60). Such potential pain reinforcement may be reduced by making opioid use time-contingent or activity-contingent rather than contingent on the experience of pain. In time-contingent dosing, a patient who routinely develops pain in the afternoon and evening, for example, might receive a routine dose of short-acting opioid at noon and 5 PM only. In activity-contingent dosing, someone who has unmanageable pain in association with certain valued activities, such as sitting on hard wooden pews through a church service, might be instructed to take medication 30 minutes before the activity. In addition to reducing reinforcement of pain and medication taking, such strategies may improve pain control by preempting its experience.

In addition, the frequent use of short-acting medications several times a day is thought to result in "on-off effects" as blood levels peak and trough, resulting in alternating analgesia and incipient withdrawal in persons with physical dependency. As the autonomic arousal and muscular tension associated with physiologic withdrawal may facilitate pain, such rebound phenomena may potentially increase pain and associated distress. This can theoretically be avoided by carefully scheduling doses to maintain fairly level blood levels, but stable blood levels are easier to achieve with longer-acting medications.

Scheduling opioid doses in supervised care settings, such as hospitals or nursing homes, also eliminates the need for patients to request medications, which can result in a lag-time in pain treatment and, particularly in patients with substance use disorders, may create a perception that the patient is "constantly seeking opioids." When opioids are scheduled, the patient may decline doses if pain is well controlled.

For constant pain at a moderate level of intensity, when an opioid is indicated, a relatively low dose of a long-acting pure mu agonist (such as methadone or a controlled release preparation of morphine, oxycodone or other opioid) may be appropriate. For severe pain, a pure mu agonist is usually indicated. That should be a drug that does not have a ceiling effect, i.e., it should be a combination product or a mixed agonist-antagonist, and should not have toxic metabolites. If the pain is continuous, patient-controlled analgesia, a continuous parenteral infusion, or long-acting oral or transdermal medications, depending on the context, are appropriate. In the acute or cancer pain context, rescue doses of prn medications are usually provided for breakthrough pain or exacerbations of baseline pain. The frequency of permitted rescue doses must be determined according to the context. When multiple doses are required each day, this generally indicates a need for a higher baseline dose of long-acting medications.

In the chronic non-cancer pain setting, when long-acting opioids are used for continuous baseline pain, some clinicians prefer that patients manage the daily ups and downs of pain with activity pacing and use of nonopioid interventions (heat, ice, stretch, relaxation, etc.) to prevent or address mild exacerbations, rather than using frequent doses of prn medications. Many would provide a few prn doses per month or per week for more major exacerbations of pain to deter unnecessary frequent ER or clinic visits. However, some chronic pain patients have predictable activity-related pain that may require regular prn doses.

PCA can be used successfully for management of acute pain in individuals with addictive disease and sometimes is the preferred method of providing postoperative and posttraumatic pain control. It often is used in the setting of advanced cancer pain as well. PCA allows the patient to self-administer small, incremental doses of opioids intravenously or subcutaneously and thus provides stable analgesic blood levels of opioids. It usually produces more uniform pain relief at a lower total dose of medications than bolus dosing or continuous infusions (24). It avoids peaks (which may cause sedation or intoxication) and valleys (which may result in pain, anxiety, and drug craving). As with scheduled dosing, the use of PCA eliminates the need for the patient to request opioids for pain relief and thus avoids potential conflicts between patients and staff, which can arise when persons with addictive disease request opioids. For persons with significant opioid tolerance, a background infusion may be used with PCA.

Conversely, because PCA requires self-administration, it may create ambivalence in recovering persons and in patients with active addiction who have difficulty limiting their administration of opioids to levels that provide analgesia without intoxication. The latter problem may be managed to some degree through the physician's control of the incremental dose size and frequency and the total dose available over a period of time. In theory, PCA may reinforce pain through the pairing of pain with self-administration of opioids and thus may make cessation of analgesic doses of opioids difficult. In practice, however, these issues rarely arise, probably because the small incremental doses provided by PCA provide relatively little reward.

Enhancing Compliance and Control of Medication Use When scheduled medications are required on an outpatient basis in individuals with addictive disease or other substance use disorders, it is helpful to give specific times for drug administration (for example, "q 8 hours at 7:00 AM, 3:00 PM, and 11:00 PM"), rather than indicating that a drug should be taken three times a day or every 8 hours. This reduces the potential for confusion over dosing and possible resulting misuse.

If an individual has difficulty controlling medication use but needs opioids for pain relief, it may be helpful to have a trusted other, such as a partner or friend, dispense the medications, either by the dose or at time-limited intervals such as every one or two days. Daily or other short-interval dispensing also may be arranged through a visiting nurse, pharmacy, or hospice.

Management of Opioid Side Effects Opioid side effects can be considered in two groups: side effects of acute and long-term opioid use.

Acute Use Side Effects Respiratory depression is a potentially fatal side effect of opioid administration and is a persistent concern throughout treatment when doses are increased or specific opioids changed. Opioid-induced respiratory depression results from depression of brain stem respiratory responses to carbon dioxide (CO_2). Though CO_2 response decreases in a dose-dependent manner with the administration of mu agonists, clinically significant respiratory depression does not usually occur in the course of treating healthy patients with standard analgesic doses of opioids. Respiratory depression may be significant, however, when higher-dose opioids are used for acute pain in opioid-naïve patients, particularly those who are elderly or debilitated. In such patients, respiratory monitoring is important. Pain limits respiratory depression, so care should be taken when a patient using high-dose opioids undergoes a definitive procedure that relieves pain, such as a nerve block or spinal cord ablation. Significant sedation most often is a precursor to respiratory depression and may signal a need to hold medication and adjust the dose. Respiratory depression rarely is a clinical problem in chronic opioid administration because tolerance to the respiratory depressant effects of opioids tends to occur more rapidly than tolerance to their analgesic effects. Patients should be closely observed, however, when doses are abruptly increased or when patients are rotated from one opioid to another. Special care also should be exercised in titrating opioids with long half-lives, such as methadone or levorphanol, because delayed respiratory depression may occur. Reduction of opioid dosage and respiratory support are the first-line treatments for this side effect. An opioid antagonist such as naloxone should be used only in emergency situations owing to the risk of inducing acute abstinence syndrome.

Common physical side effects of opioid use include constipation, nausea and vomiting, urinary retention, pruritus, and myoclonus. Side effects are minimized when opioids are prescribed in a manner that reduces peak blood levels required to sustain analgesia, because higher blood levels may be associated with increased side effects. To achieve stable analgesic blood levels, scheduled doses of long-acting or controlled release opioids may be used when oral preparations are used. Continuous infusions or PCA achieve the same goal when parenteral administration is required. With the exception of constipation, side effects usually are transient and may improve or resolve with continued use of opioids at a stable dose. Side effects sometimes are specific to a particular drug in a particular individual and sometimes can be eliminated by use of an alternative opioid. Persistent physical side effects may be managed through pharmacologic treatments, such as antiemetics for nausea or antihistamines for pruritus.

Constipation is a persistent side effect of opioid use that may not resolve without treatment. The constipating effects of opioids are thought to occur through direct action on opioid receptors in the intestinal wall. This causes a decrease in intestinal motility and results in dehydration of stool. It generally is advisable, therefore, to give both a stool softener and a bowel stimulant to effectively manage constipation. When long-term and/or high dose use of opioids is anticipated, introduction of such treatment on a preemptive basis is recommended.

Hepatic, renal, and other organ toxicity generally are not reported with opioids as they are with many nonopioid analgesics, such as acetaminophen and NSAIDs. However, close observation and dose adjustments may be appropriate in persons who have impaired hepatic or renal function, which may result in reduced drug clearance.

Central nervous system (CNS) side effects of opioids may include sedation, cognitive dysfunction, and affective changes. Sedation and mild cognitive changes are common when opioids are introduced or when the dose is increased, but they usually resolve once a stable therapeutic dose of opioid is achieved and sustained for a period of time (61). Occasionally, however, CNS effects may persist when high doses of opioids are required, particularly when long-acting medications such as methadone are used in elderly or frail patients. Like many other side effects, sedation and cognitive dysfunction may be managed or avoided by changing medications, by continuous administration of the minimum dose necessary to achieve analgesia, or by administration of a treatment medication. When significant persistent opioid-induced sedation occurs in cancer pain patients or patients with other severe intractable pain, stimulants such as methylphenidate and dextroamphetamine may be helpful. The use of stimulant medications, which may be abused by some individuals, requires the same caution in patients with addiction disorder as that required in the use of opioids.

Pain, particularly chronic pain, often is associated with negative mood states such as anxiety or depression. These frequently resolve with effective pain treatment. However, if depression, anxiety, dysphoria, or other distressing affective symptoms occur in the course of analgesic therapy, opioids should be reviewed as a possible contributing factor.

Long-Term Use Side Effects Side effects of long-term opioid use include persisting risk of respiratory depression and constipation (as discussed earlier) as well as the potential for hyperalgesia, hormonal imbalance and immunomodulation.

Increasing evidence suggests that opioids may increase pain in some contexts. Clinical studies and observations suggest that some individuals with pain who use opioids on a long-term basis experience improvement in pain after tapering or simple withdrawal of opioids, without the institution of other major pain interventions (20,62–64). These studies include observations of patients with pain and opioid dependence in both pain treatment and addiction treatment settings. Though increased pain on opioids may have been mediated by on-off (withdrawal-mediated) phenomena associated with use of short-acting opioids in some cases, it is increasingly appreciated that opioids may actually induce hyperalgesia.

One study demonstrated a significantly decreased threshold and tolerance for cold pressor–induced pain in methadone-maintained patients (who had taken their usual dose of methadone), as compared to several control groups of formerly methadone-dependent individuals and persons who had no history of dependence on any drug (65). The presence of hyperalgesia in some patients in the presence of high-dose systemic morphine administration has been well documented (66). The mechanisms of hyperalgesia are not fully defined but appear to involve both glutamate-mediated activation of NMDA receptors and induction of inflammatory cytokines in the CNS (67,68).

The extent to which hyperalgesia occurs in clinical settings and its general clinical relevance for patients who use opioids on a long-term basis is not clear. As more patients with chronic pain of non-cancer origin and normal life expectancy are prescribed opioids for long-term management of pain, controlled studies of the effects of long-term opioids on pain modulation will be important to better understand the circumstances under which hyperalgesia may occur and how best to address the problem.

Hormonal imbalance and immunomodulation are recently recognized sequela of long-term opioid use. Androgen deficiency and osteoporosis have been described in patients receiving long-term methadone and intrathecal opioids (69,70). The current clinical standard of treatment is testosterone replacement for men and estrogen replacement for women when indicated. However, given the current debate concerning the long-term risk of hormone replacement, sex hormone supplementation is controversial.

Numerous studies both in animals and humans have suggested that opioids have immunosuppressive effects (71). More research is needed to elaborate the clinical significance of demonstrated effects and, as pain itself has been demonstrated to have some immunosuppressive effects, the relative balance of effects must be further studies.

Side effects often vary from one opioid to another in different patients. Therefore, rotation from one opioid to another is sometimes helpful in resolving persistent side effects that do not resolve over time or which do not respond to pharmacologic treatment.

Changing Opioids Transition from one opioid or form of opioid to another may be indicated in a number of circumstances (e.g., when unrelenting tolerance occurs to a specific opioid with loss of analgesic efficacy, when a patient on chronic oral opioids becomes NPO, or when significant side effects occur and persist). Opioid rotation often results in improved analgesia when tolerance is present, sometimes on a significantly lower equivalent doses of the new opioid. Rotation back to the original opioid—or an alterative—can occur if tolerance develops to the new opioid over time (72).

When changing from one opioid to another, it is important to understand how to calculate equianalgesic doses of medications and how to modify those doses appropriately in order to maintain analgesia and to avoid serious side effects. There are many ways to calculate opioid equivalency; one method using parenteral morphine as the standard reference is described here.

The first step is to determine the total dose of each opioid used in the previous or usual 24-hour period. Then, using an opioid equivalence table, calculate the equivalent dose of parenteral morphine for each opioid used in the previous 24 hours and add these together; this will yield a number that indicates the total parenteral morphine equivalents of opioid used over the 24-hour period. This subsequently is can be converted to the calculated equivalent 24-hour dose of the new opioid. This 24-hour dose *should be lowered significantly* to accommodate opioid-specific tolerance to the previously used opioid and the potentially greater analgesic efficacy and side effects of the new drug. One-half to two-thirds of the calculated equianalgesic dose often is used as a rule of thumb in switching to many opioids. However, for methadone (and probably levorphanol), which appears to have much less cross tolerance with other opioids and which can accumulate with fatal consequences owing to a long and unpredictable half-life, the percentage should be much lower: one-fifth to one-tenth the calculated dose of methadone but never more than 30 mg oral methadone per day in divided doses as a starting dose has been

TABLE 95.5 Equianalgesic Doses of Opioid Drugs

Drug	Approximate equianalgesic oral dose*	Approximate equianalgesic parenteral dose*
Opioid agonists		
Morphine	30 mg q 3–4 hours	10 mg q 3–4 hours
Codeine	130 mg q 3–4 hours	75 mg q 3–4 hours
Hydromorphone (Dilaudid)	7.5 mg q 3–4 h	1.5 mg q 3–4 h
Levorphanol (Lev-Dromoran)	4 mg q 6–8 h (acute)	2 mg q 6–8 h (acute)
	1 mg q 6–8 h (chronic)	1 mg q 6–8 h (chronic)
Meperidine (Demerol)	300 mg q 2–3 h	75 mg q 2–3 h
Methadone (Dolophine, others)	20 mg q 6–8 h (acute)	10 mg q 6–8 h (acute)
	2–4 mg q 6–8 h (chronic)	2–4 mg q 6–8 h (chronic)
Oxycodone (Percodan, Percocet, Roxicodone, Tylox)	20 mg q 3–4 h	Not available
Opioid agonist/antagonist		
Drugs and partial agonists		
Buprenorphine (Buprenex)	Not available	0.4 mg q 6–8 h
Butorphanol (Stadol)	Not available	2 mg q 3–4 h
Nalbuphine (Nubain)	Not available	10 mg q 3–4 h

***Note:** These should be considered approximate estimates. Equivalencies may vary from individual to individual. Doses are based on single-dose studies and do not necessarily reflect analgesic equivalence with continued dosing. A dose lower than the calculated equianalgesic dose always should be used when switching patients from one opioid to another because of incomplete cross-tolerance between opioids. Special case should be used in changing to methadone or levodromoran because of the pronounced lack of cross-tolerance with other opioids and the potential for delayed respiratory depression due to long half-lives. All patients should be observed carefully for sedation and respiratory depression when opioid doses are initiated or abruptly increased or when a new opioid is used, and doses adapted accordingly.

Caution: Recommended doses do not apply to patients with renal or hepatic insufficiency or other conditions affecting drug metabolism and kinetics.

Caution: Doses are listed for patients with body weight of less than 50 kg; they cannot be used as initial starting doses in infants younger than 6 months of age. Consult the AHCPR Clinical Practice Guideline for Acute Pain Management for recommendations.

suggested as safe dosing when rotating to methadone. The 24-hour dose of the new drug should be given in divided doses at appropriate intervals (Table 95.5).

This method avoids the confusion that arises in trying to convert several medications at different doses and comparing drugs of differing half-lives and potencies. Any calculation, however, should be viewed only as a rough guideline and, when medications are changed, patients should be monitored closely and dosing adapted according to clinical responses. The potential for delayed respiratory depression with opioids that have long half-lives, such as methadone, should be appreciated.

Sometimes the transition from one opioid to another is better tolerated if the patient is gradually "rolled over" from one medication to another. That is, the new medication is increased incrementally over a few days while the old medication is decreased incrementally. This also permits observation of the patient's response to the new drug and adjustment of the dose to avoid side effects and maintain analgesia.

Management of Withdrawal In the acute pain setting, most patients gradually taper their medications without incident as pain gradually improves. However, tapering sometimes is impeded by withdrawal or craving that occurs during troughs in blood levels when physical dependence is present. The goal when tapering an individual who is physically dependent on medications is to provide stable but decreasing blood levels of opioid so as to prevent precipitous troughs. Though stable blood levels usually are only approximated with the use of short-acting medications, most patients do not experience significant withdrawal while gently tapering.

If the patient has been using an intermittently administered medication such as bolus parenteral morphine or oral oxycodone, the interval of administration can be decreased somewhat as the dose is decreased in order to avoid low blood levels of the drug between doses. Alternatively, the patient can be transferred to a continuous parenteral infusion or an equianalgesic dose of a longer acting oral medication (such as methadone, controlled-release morphine, or oxycodone) and the dose gradually reduced. Some patients may benefit from having their medications dispensed daily or dose by dose while tapering in order to assist in controlling use as the dose is decreasing.

If abrupt cessation of opioids is necessary, an acute withdrawal syndrome may be attenuated to some degree through the prescription of alternative medications. Clonidine may be used to attenuate the autonomic signs and symptoms of withdrawal (73); a benzodiazepine or other sedative-hypnotic may be given to reduce irritability, anxiety, and sleeplessness; and a nonopioid analgesic such as an NSAID or acetaminophen may be used to attenuate pain. Antispasmodics are sometimes helpful in reducing abdominal cramping.

CLINICAL PAIN MANAGEMENT

Acute Pain Inadequate treatment of pain increases morbidity after trauma and surgery in the general population (74) whereas optimal pain treatment appears to shorten hospitalizations in similar contexts (75). Pain increases distress and anxiety and, in individuals with substance use disorders, may become a significant risk factor for relapse in those in recovery and for aberrant use in those with active abuse or addiction. Individuals with addictive disease often experience particularly high levels of anxiety in association with the stress of trauma, illness, or surgery, because they fear that their pain will not be adequately managed; this, in turn, can affect how they experience and react to pain. Attention to their concerns may facilitate pain management.

Principles of care that may facilitate safe and effective clinical management of the patient with pain and concurrent substance use disorder include addressing the concurrent addiction disorder directly, identification and treatment of withdrawal when present, provision of effective treatment of pain, accommodation of physiologic dependence on opioids when present, and clear documentation of the treatment plan.

Address the Addiction Disorder An open and nonjudgmental approach to the discussion of substance use concerns may help to facilitate information exchange with patients regarding their use. All too often, health professionals discuss concerns about a patient's substance use among themselves, without bringing the patient into the discussion. When addiction is understood as a medical disorder, it becomes easier to address it in the same manner as any other medical condition, with respectful, but matter-of-fact, concern. Patients with addiction disorders often fear, with some historical basis in reality, that awareness of their problem will negatively affect the manner in which their physicians and other providers approach their care. Therefore, they may not be immediately forthcoming about their addiction disorder or may be anxious about their medical care. In the context of pain treatment, it is helpful to allay such a patient's anxiety by reassuring him or her that the addiction disorder will not be an obstacle to the relief of their pain. For recovering patients, reassurance that effective pain management is not likely to lead to relapse is also helpful.

The patient who is hospitalized for an acute medical problem may be more open to intervention for his or her addiction disorder than he or she would be as an outpatient (76). It is important to capture such windows of opportunity to help bring patients into recovery. Addiction treatment should be offered when addiction is detected in the course of pain treatment. Counseling may be initiated at any time, so long as acute pain is adequately controlled. If the patient does not accept addiction treatment at the time it is offered, it may be helpful to use the acute pain problem to begin to explore the patient's motivation for recovery and to follow-up at future visits. Recovering persons often benefit from increasing their recovery activities during times of stress, such as hospitalization, trauma, and pain.

Many clinicians and individuals in recovery believe that exposure to opioids, sedative-hypnotics or anesthetics—even if not the patient's drugs of choice—may lead to relapse. However, the distress of inadequately treated physical pain may pose an even greater risk of relapse. Effective pain treatment by whatever means, coupled with an active addiction recovery program, probably are the best supports for continued recovery during periods of acute stress, including periods of pain.

Prevent or Treat Withdrawal If a patient is dependent on opioids, it is usually appropriate to continue opioids until the acute pain situation is resolved or effectively managed through use of an alternative approach, such as an epidural catheter. If a nonopioid treatment approach is selected by the patient and physician, opioids can be either tapered gradually to prevent withdrawal or continued at a dose that avoids withdrawal but does not over-sedate the patient. Abrupt cessation of opioids will usually cause acute increase in pain.

It is permissible, under the U.S. Controlled Substances Act, for a treating physician to provide opioids to prevent withdrawal in a patient who is hospitalized for a diagnosis other than addiction. For example, if a patient with heroin addiction is hospitalized with multiple fractures after a motor vehicle crash or with subacute bacterial endocarditis related to heroin use, the treating physician can legally provide opioid medications to prevent withdrawal as well as additional medications for pain. Though opioids for pain treatment can be continued after discharge, opioids can not be provided for treatment of addiction after discharge, except from a licensed addiction treatment program (methadone treatment) or from a certified buprenorphine provider.

An actively drinking patient with alcohol dependence or a patient who is dependent on nonopioid drugs should have withdrawal symptoms treated when they occur in the course of pain treatment. Unrecognized alcohol withdrawal will make pain control difficult to achieve, and physical signs of withdrawal (such as hypertension and tachycardia) may be misinterpreted as reflecting acute pain. Usually, a long-acting benzodiazepine such as oral chlordiazepoxide is an appropriate choice, though other benzodiazepines such as lorazepam or oxazepam may be selected if parental use is required or if hepatic dysfunction is present.

Include the Patient in Clinical Decision Making It is often helpful to include the individual in pain in the decision-making process regarding medication choices, dosing, and scheduling. This provides the patient with a sense of control and allays anxiety as to whether pain will be adequately treated. It also may afford the physician information that is useful in designing an effective treatment regimen. Addicted patients and patients with therapeutic drug dependence often are experienced as to the drug doses they require to meet their basic dependence needs as well as the additional levels required to treat their acute pain. Such consultation may at times lead to a request for a dose beyond that needed for analgesia, so prudence in prescribing is required. If a patient becomes intoxicated or sedated at the prescribed dose, medications can be adjusted to avoid the observed side effects while continuing to provide analgesia.

Provide Effective Pain Relief Pain relief should be provided in an effective and timely manner. Without adequate control of acute pain, it is unlikely that the patient will be able to engage in addiction treatment. Under-treatment of pain also may create craving for pain-relieving medications as well as anxiety, frustration, anger, and other feelings that tend to feed addiction (77). When they are effective, readily available, and safe, non-medication pain treatments—such as cold, transcutaneous electrical neurostimulation (TENS), or regional anesthesia—are preferred by some clinicians and patients over systemic medications for the treatment of acute pain in individuals with addictive disease. When medications are indicated to relieve pain, those that are the least likely to alter mood may be used, if they are effective. Though exposure to dependence or reward-producing drugs may be one component of the development of addiction or relapse to drug use, such exposure alone does not create addiction. When opioids or other such drugs are needed to manage pain, they should be provided at effective doses respecting dosing and scheduling considerations as discussed earlier.

It is important to achieve pain relief with methods that do not confuse, stress, or frustrate the staff or the patient. For example, an epidural infusion of local anesthesia may seem ideal for management of post-thoracotomy pain in a recovering opioid person/patient with an addiction disorder, but if the floor nurses do not know how to manage the required catheters, the patient's overall needs probably will be better met with scheduled or PCA doses of opioids, as potential failure of the epidural may leave the patient in pain and distress and demanding opioids for pain relief. Patients with acute pain should be monitored at regular intervals to assess the effectiveness of analgesia and the presence of side effects with treatment adjusted as indicated. Most patients will naturally taper their medications as the cause of acute pain resolves. Some patients with addiction disorders benefit from the negotiation of a structured tapering of medications on a scheduled basis. Persistent use of opioids despite apparent healing is discussed below.

Accommodate Preexisting Opioid Dependence

Patients Receiving Chronic Methadone for Pain or Addiction Individuals who are physically dependent on opioids that are prescribed for pain or for addiction or who are dependent on street opioids must have their baseline opioid requirements met in addition to receiving additional opioids required for acute pain treatment (38). The average baseline daily dose of opioid should be determined or estimated and either the same drug provided at that dose or an equianalgesic dose of an alternative opioid calculated and provided at a somewhat lower than calculated dose (see method of opioid dosing calculation above).

Most often, a patient receiving methadone treatment of addiction should be continued on his or her baseline methadone dose as an inpatient and provided a different opioid for acute pain, rather than being entirely switched to an alternative opioid or having the methadone increased for pain. This is recommended for several reasons. First, incomplete cross-tolerance of methadone with other mu agonists has been noted and opioid withdrawal from methadone observed in some patients, even in the presence of calculated equianalgesic doses of alternative mu agonists. Second, though an increase in methadone may be effective for pain management, its long half-life makes it relatively difficult to titrate for acute pain. Finally, the use of the same drug for addiction maintenance and for acute pain management may confuse the issues of pain treatment and addiction treatment when the acute pain resolves and it is time to taper the pain medication.

When possible, it is helpful to confirm patients' daily dose of methadone with their methadone treatment program. If the dose cannot be confirmed, it is safest initially to give the dose the patients report in three or four divided doses, particularly if it is a high dose, rather than in a single dose and then to observe the response and adjust according. If a patient cannot take oral medications, methadone can be given parenterally at half the oral dose.

Buprenorphine-Maintained Patients Strategies for managing acute pain in individuals on buprenorphine for treatment of addiction or chronic pain are emerging as experience accumulates. Buprenorphine binds avidly to opioid receptors and thus tends to block the action of other analgesic opioids provided for pain. Thus, it is difficult, though not impossible, to obtain analgesia by adding another opioid. In addition, buprenorphine has kappa opioid receptor antagonist activity that may impact the actions of other opioids (78,79). When acute pain is predicted, such as after elective surgery, in persons on buprenorphine, it is often advisable to discontinue buprenorphine a few days before surgery. Carefully dosed methadone can be added if needed if withdrawal symptoms or craving emerge after stopping buprenorphine while waiting for surgery.

If acute pain occurs unexpectedly, such as after an accident or with an acute illness, in a patient on buprenorphine and opioids are required to relieve pain, mu opioids can usually be aggressively titrated to higher doses to overcome the buprenorphine blockade. Use of an opioid such as intravenous fentanyl, which also binds with high affinity to mu opioid receptors, is often recommended. Opioid titration for acute pain in this setting should be done by an experienced clinician with an intravenous line in place, close monitoring of the patient, and an opioid antagonist such as naloxone available.

Alternatively, if a patient is on a low maintenance dose of buprenorphine (such as 2 to 8 mg per day), sometimes the daily dose of buprenorphine can be increased and given at 6-hour intervals to control pain. However, because of its partial agonist properties and other pharmacologic, buprenorphine may have a ceiling analgesic effect though studies of this are mixed. It is not clear whether continually increasing doses will control more severe pain (80, 80a). Understanding of the analgesic properties of buprenorphine are still in evolution.

Document the Pain Treatment Plan It is important to be clear in communicating the treatment plan to all staff involved in caring for the patient. Stigma and misunderstanding regarding addiction disorders are widespread among health care personnel, and these may lead to inadequate pain management when the primary treating clinician is not available and the plan is not clearly documented. In addition, in the absence of a clear and consistent structure, the patient's disease may result in behaviors that confuse the patient's pain and addiction issues. Written documentation of the plan, displayed in a prominent and accessible location, is usually helpful.

When Pain Persists Beyond Apparent Healing Many factors may lead a patient to complain of pain and to evidence a need for pain medications despite expected and apparent healing from surgery, trauma, illness, or other pain-provoking pathology. Particularly in the patient with an addiction disorder, continuing complaints of pain may lead to concern that the patient is reflecting behaviors of addiction or relapse to addiction. However, it is important to methodically consider other possible explanations before concluding that this is the case.

First, the patient may have an undetected physical problem, related either to the original painful problem or to a separate process. A thorough search for such a cause should be undertaken. The search should include a review of nociceptive causes of pain, such as an abscess or undetected fracture, as well as less common and often overlooked neurogenic causes of pain such as a neuritis, deafferentation pain, central sensitization, or evolving sympathetically maintained pain.

Second, the patient may be physically dependent on analgesic medications and may be experiencing pain related to withdrawal as the medication is discontinued. Withdrawal may mediate pain through a variety of mechanisms, including alterations in sympathetic arousal, changes in muscle tone, and alterations in opiate and other receptor function. Tapering of opioids to avoid withdrawal is described earlier. If increased discomfort occurs during the course of an appropriately crafted medication taper, the patient should be reexamined for an undetected physical origin of the pain. If none is found, the taper can be continued and non-opioid alternatives (such as TENS, NSAIDs, or nerve block therapy) provided to attenuate discomfort during withdrawal. In most cases, the increased discomfort will be transient during and immediately after discontinuation of medications if physical dependence or withdrawal were the cause. If pain persists and no physical cause can be identified, treatment should be as for chronic pain.

A third reason that a patient may continue to seek to continue opioids when the underlying pain condition has resolved is that the medications may be ameliorating non-pain symptoms, such as sleep disturbance, intrusive memories, anxiety, or depression. Opioids have been observed to improve mood in some patients in pain (81), but more-specific treatments usually are indicated and may allow tapering of pain medications in patients whose physiologic pain driver has resolved.

If an undetected physical cause of pain, withdrawal-associated discomfort, or self-medication does not appear to contribute to the patient's need for continued opioids, it is reasonable to reevaluate the patient for addiction to the medication. In a general hospital population, the latter reason is probably less common than the first three possibilities; however, it is relatively more common in the population treated by addiction medicine specialists.

If addiction is suspected, the patient should be observed for behaviors suggestive of addiction, including loss of control, continued use despite harm, and preoccupation with opioid use, with the understanding that any of these may be seen in patients with significant pain that is not effectively treated. The patient's drug and alcohol history, as well as his or her family history of addiction, may be add further useful information.

If the patient has previously been in recovery, reengagement in recovery activities that have been helpful in the past is appropriate. If the patient had an active, untreated addiction disorder at the time of onset of the acute pain or has developed one in the course of treatment, it is appropriate to arrange evaluation and treatment with an addiction specialist if available. If an addiction disorder is diagnosed, the patient's pain medication can be tapered as described earlier and the use of alternative methods for addressing the pain implemented, while treatment for addiction is provided. Unless an underlying physical cause is identified, pain often resolves or improves after discontinuation of medications and treatment of addiction (20,82).

If taper is not possible because of persistent craving or if relapsing use occurs, initiation of opioid agonist therapy for the underlying addiction may be appropriate. If a taper is not possible because of recrudescence of pain despite alternative therapies, continued opioid therapy for pain, coupled with the necessary structure and support (see further), may be selected as a component of chronic pain treatment. If both persistent pain and opioid addiction are present, sometimes combined opioid agonist therapy for addiction and opioid therapy for pain with collaborative care between addiction treatment providers and pain providers is appropriate.

A final consideration in the differential of complaints of persistent pain despite apparent healing is simply that the pain may be factitious. Certainly occasional persons may feign pain in order to divert medications for sale, for personal use, or to share with a family member or friend whose therapeutic needs have not been met. It is appropriate to discontinue opioids if an individual is noted to be diverting medications, as misuse in this manner is both illegal and presents significant risk to the public health.

If the cause of reported persistent pain cannot be identified and there is no evidence that the patient is seeking drugs to sustain an addiction or for purposes of diversion, the clinician has two choices. First, opioids can be continued while the clinician monitors the patient's pain, side effects, and function and continues to screen for a cause of pain. If the patient's quality of life is preserved or advanced without negative consequences, it may be that an undetected basis for the pain is present. The second choice is to gradually taper medications while alternative pain treatment interventions are introduced. Because opioids may induce pain or hyperalgesia in some contexts (83) pain may improve on tapering or discontinuation of the medication. Which choice is appropriate for a particular patient is a decision best made by the clinical care team, with the patient's informed participation.

Cancer-Related Pain Cancer may occur somewhat more frequently in individuals with addiction disorders than in the general population (84), probably because of pathologic effects of many substances of abuse, including tobacco and alcohol. Treatment of cancer-related pain in the patient with addictive disease is similar to that in the person without addictive disease. The comfort of the patient should be the primary goal. Opioids never should be withheld when they are needed for effective pain relief because of concerns regarding the development or perpetuation of addiction. If concerns arise regarding decreased quality of life owing to active addiction, pain control should be continued with appropriate structure to ensure safety (see chronic pain next section) and addiction issues addressed through appropriate interventions. Adjustment of medications may be appropriate to avoid unnecessary side effects or intoxication, but analgesia should be preserved. If the patient has difficulty controlling the use of medications, they should be dispensed in a manner that preserves safety. This may be accomplished by having the medications dispensed by a significant other, by hospice personnel or by a pharmacy.

The "therapeutic ladder" developed by the World Health Organization (WHO) is an accepted model for the treatment of cancer pain (Fig. 95.3) (12). Stage 1 of the ladder is for the management of mild pain and involves the use of nonopioid analgesics such as acetaminophen, aspirin, or an NSAID as well as adjuvant medications such as tricyclics, anticonvulsants, and topical agents for pain-associated symptoms such as sleep, mood problems, or side effects. Stage 2 of the WHO ladder addresses moderate pain. It involves use of a weak opioid preparation that combines opioids with aspirin, acetaminophen, or an NSAID. Adjuvant medications for neuropathic pain and other symptoms should be used as indicated. For patients with continuous moderate pain, it is also reasonable to consider use of a low dose of a long-acting opioid such as methadone or controlled-release oxycodone or morphine. This may avoid the intermittent peak effects of short-acting opioids that some experience as rewarding and which may be disconcerting to some patients in recovery. If these are selected in place of the combination medications, additional acetaminophen or NSAIDs usually should be added for their complementary analgesic effect.

Stage 3 of the WHO ladder, for management of severe pain, involves use of a titratable, potent opioid (such as morphine, oxycodone, fentanyl or hydromorphone) plus nonopioid analgesics and adjuvants as indicated. It is important to note that NSAIDs are particularly effective for bone pain related to metastases, so continuation of these drugs often is important even in the presence of high-dose opioids. Treatment should start as far along the ladder as necessary to achieve pain control. Aggressive titration of opioids is appropriate to control cancer-related pain. Cancer pain usually can be managed with oral or transdermal opioid administration. If oral or transdermal medications are not feasible because of absorption problems, vomiting, or technical problems with transdermal patches, the clinician should consider parenteral treatment, including continuous or PCA intravenous or subcutaneous administration.

When opioids are not sufficient to control pain or have unacceptable side effects, more invasive approaches may be considered. Regional anesthetic techniques such as continuous intraspinal infusions or plexus blocks may provide effective ongoing relief for many types of cancer pain (85). Neuroablative procedures such as celiac plexus block for pancreatic cancer pain, nerve root blocks for pain localized to one or two specific dermatomes (particularly if they serve sensory rather than motor functions, as in single-rib metastases), and others may provide definitive relief in difficult cancer pain situations. Radiotherapy and radiopharmaceuticals may be helpful in selected patients.

Cancer often is accompanied by significant distress arising from fear, grief over impending losses, depression, anger, and spiritual conflict. Because persons with addiction disorders have a tendency to use drugs to relieve such distresses, cancer patients with addictive disease may be at risk to use therapeutically prescribed opioids for symptoms other than pain. Most compassionate physicians would have no issue with the use of opioids to relieve symptoms in the setting of cancer-related

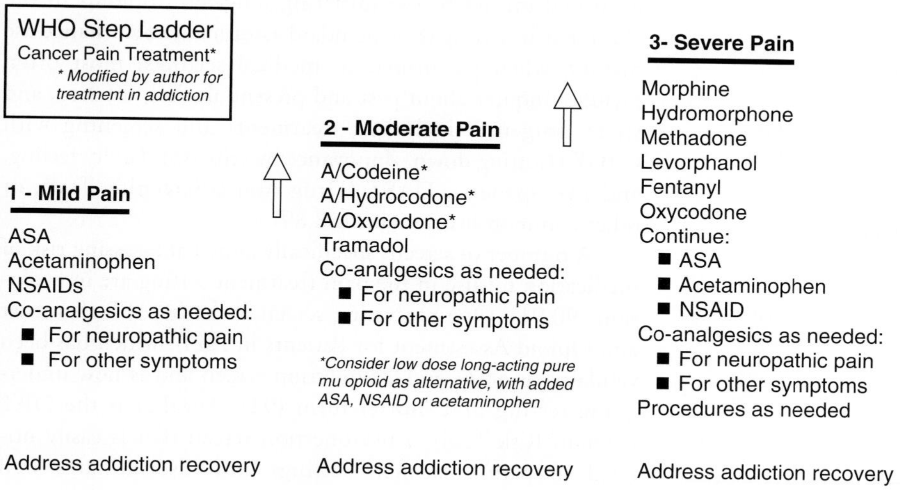

WHO Step Ladder
Cancer Pain Treatment*
** Modified by author for treatment in addiction*

1 - Mild Pain

ASA
Acetaminophen
NSAIDs
Co-analgesics as needed:
- For neuropathic pain
- For other symptoms

Address addiction recovery

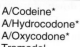

2 - Moderate Pain

A/Codeine*
A/Hydrocodone*
A/Oxycodone*
Tramadol
Co-analgesics as needed:
- For neuropathic pain
- For other symptoms

**Consider low dose long-acting pure mu opioid as alternative, with added ASA, NSAID or acetaminophen*

Address addiction recovery

3- Severe Pain

Morphine
Hydromorphone
Methadone
Levorphanol
Fentanyl
Oxycodone
Continue:
- ASA
- Acetaminophen
- NSAID

Co-analgesics as needed:
- For neuropathic pain
- For other symptoms

Procedures as needed

Address addiction recovery

FIGURE 95.3. WHO step ladder for cancer pain treatment.

pain, if they were effective. However, such use sometimes results in increased distress and greater experience of pain despite massive doses of opioids. Effective non-pharmacologic and pharmacologic means of addressing such stressors are available and should be employed to provide relief. For many individuals in recovery from addiction, the recovery system may provide meaningful support (77). Therefore, it is helpful for the clinician to assess the patient's experience with recovery and to help him or her in sustaining participation in or reengaging with recovery groups, sponsors, and programs if these have been meaningful to the individual in the past.

Chronic non-Cancer-Related Pain Chronic pain may occur for a variety of reasons. Tissue pathology may be ongoing or flare intermittently, stimulating nociceptive (or receptor stimulated) pain, such as in degenerative arthritis, relapsing pancreatitis, or sickle cell disease. Neuropathic pain, such as a neuritis, neuropathy, phantom (or deafferentation) pain, central sensitization (or wind-up) pain, or sympathetically maintained pain may be present after healing from an earlier acute pain problem. Or the experience of pain may have become intractable owing to entrenched psychosocial and behavioral patterns that have emerged over the course of experiencing persistent nociceptive or neuropathic pain. Sometimes all these factors contribute.

Whatever the causes of pain, chronic pain can engender secondary sequela, such as sleep disturbance, mood disturbance, functional disabilities, increased stress, and/or self-medication with alcohol or drugs that that may serve to perpetuate the experience of pain, creating an entrenched and intensified chronic pain syndrome. Active addiction disorders often have similar sequelae to that of chronic pain. Therefore when chronic pain and addiction co-occur, they may reinforce one another (Fig. 95.4), and it is important to address each of these conditions.

It is also important when treating chronic pain to identify and address all secondary problems associated with it. Effective treatment of chronic pain is often multidimensional and requires an active role on the part of the patient in both understanding and managing the pain. Components of effective treatment often include physical approaches, cognitive behavioral techniques, judicious use of interventions, and nonopioid medications. These approaches are discussed in more detail in Chapters 93 and 94. In addition, opioids may be helpful as a component of care in some patients with moderately severe or severe chronic pain. In persons with substance use disorders, the safe and effective long-term use of opioids is challenging and demands a careful balancing of potential risks and benefits, tailored to that individuals. Considerations that may be helpful in achieving this balance are discussed next.

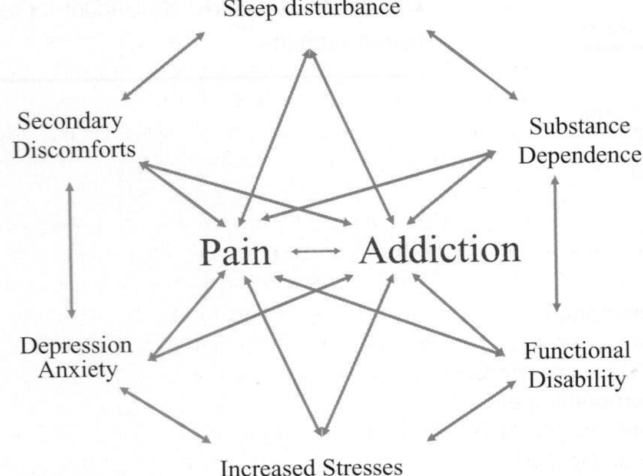

FIGURE 95.4. Synergy of pain and addiction.

Universal Precautions in Opioid Therapy for Chronic Pain Some experts suggest that when opioids are required as a component of chronic pain treatment, a set of universal precautions be used in managing all patients (86). This recommendation is based on the understanding that, similar to the paradigm of universal precautions followed in infectious disease settings, the risk of an individual patient's misusing opioids cannot be reliably predicted and that the misuse of opioids has potentially seriously negative consequences for both the patient and the prescriber. In addition, application of precautions only to selected patients believed to be at higher risk can result in stigmatizing those patients. Therefore, it is argued that, for all patients, care providers should proceed as follows:

- Perform a comprehensive pain assessment.
- Assess psychologic and substance use issues.
- Formulate a differential diagnosis of pain.
- Obtain informed consent for treatment.
- Reach and document a clear treatment agreement.
- Set up a trial treatment period with clear goals.
- Assess and periodically reassess of pain level function and salient other issues.
- Document care thoroughly.

Risk Assessment Though risk cannot always be reliably identified, there is agreement among most clinical experts and regulatory boards that it is important to screen patients for risk of opioid misuse before initiating long-term opioids in the chronic pain setting (87). Standard assessment of substance use history, when performed in medical settings, most often includes inquiry about past and present alcohol, tobacco, and street drug use (including treatment) and screening with CAGE (*C*utting down, *A*nnoyance by criticism, *G*uilty feeling, and *E*ye-openers), DAST (Drug Abuse Screening Test), or other common instruments (88,89).

A number of screens specifically aimed at assessing risk of medication misuse in the pain treatment setting are in evolution (90,91). One promising screen is the SOAPP (Screener and Opioid Assessment for Patients in Pain), which has been validated as a 14- and 20-question screen and is now undergoing testing in a shorter form (92). Another is the ORT (Opioid Risk Tool), a five-question screen that is easily utilized in pain treatment settings and discriminates well

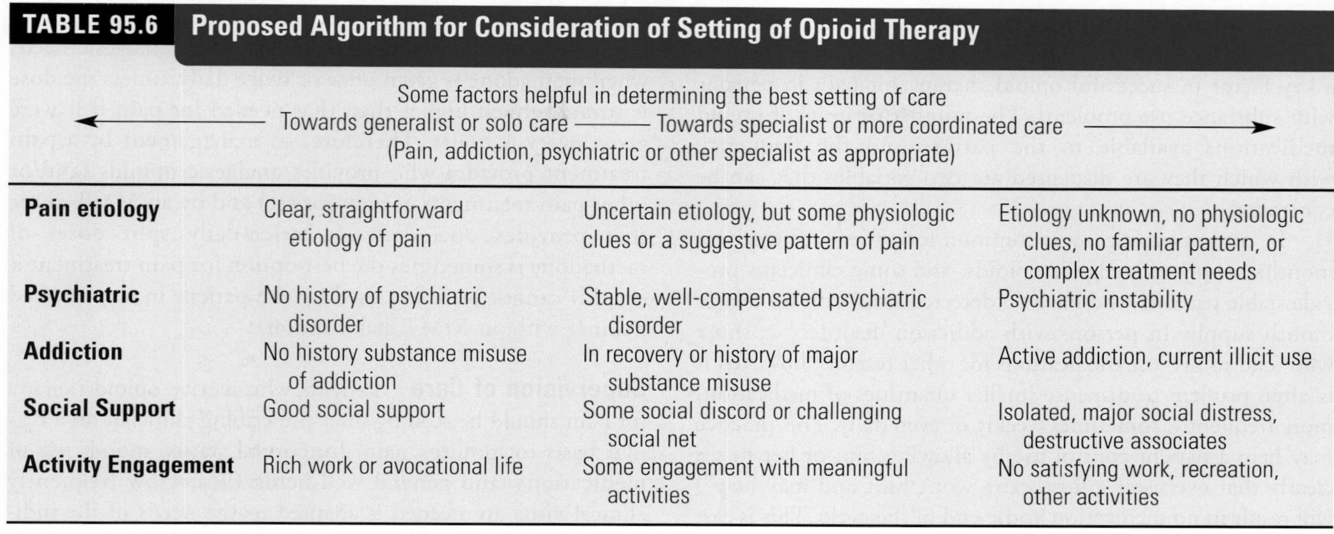

TABLE 95.6 Proposed Algorithm for Consideration of Setting of Opioid Therapy

Some factors helpful in determining the best setting of care
← Towards generalist or solo care —— Towards specialist or more coordinated care →
(Pain, addiction, psychiatric or other specialist as appropriate)

Pain etiology	Clear, straightforward etiology of pain	Uncertain etiology, but some physiologic clues or a suggestive pattern of pain	Etiology unknown, no physiologic clues, no familiar pattern, or complex treatment needs
Psychiatric	No history of psychiatric disorder	Stable, well-compensated psychiatric disorder	Psychiatric instability
Addiction	No history substance misuse of addiction	In recovery or history of major substance misuse	Active addiction, current illicit use
Social Support	Good social support	Some social discord or challenging social net	Isolated, major social distress, destructive associates
Activity Engagement	Rich work or avocational life	Some engagement with meaningful activities	No satisfying work, recreation, other activities

between high- and low-risk patients (93). It is important to be aware that none of these tools has been specifically validated for use in populations with identified substance use disorders. Though not a screen for risk per se, behaviors of concern can be tracked between patient visits in an ongoing fashion with measures, such as the Addiction Behaviors Checklist (94). Another promising tool under development for this purpose is the Current Opioid Misuse Measure (95).

Adapting the Structure of Opioid Therapy to Match Risks

When an increased risk of opioid misuse is perceived, it may be helpful to individualize and tighten the structure of clinical care beyond universal precaution. It is helpful to think in terms of five domains of structure:

- Setting of care (primary care vs. specialty care, clinical care team membership)
- Selection of treatment (risk/benefit assessment of specific medications and treatments)
- Supply of medications (controls on and amounts of medications dispensed)
- Supports for recovery (implementation and documentation of recovery activities) Supervision and monitoring (frequency of visits, toxicology screens, pill counts, other). Though there is some overlap in these areas, attention to each of them should ensure that the clinician has thought through the best options of care for the patient.

Setting of Care

Some patients with pain are best managed in a primary care setting; some in a primary care setting with support from specialists; and some by a specialist with specific skills in an area of need, such as a pain specialist, addiction specialist, or psychiatrist (86). There are advantages and disadvantages to each setting. Primary care providers tend to have broader and more longitudinal knowledge of the patient and are in a better position to integrate care of pain with care of other medical issues. Specialists tend to have more depth of knowledge and expertise in management of a particular aspect of the patient's medical issues and may provide better care when a particular problem is prominent such as addiction or psychiatric instability. Many variables may contribute to determination of the best setting of care for an individual patient. No formula can dictate which professional should manage a particular clinical pain problem, but consideration of a number of variables may be helpful in decision making (Table 95.6). The most appropriate management setting for a patient may change as their presentation changes.

Selection of Treatment

The selection of pain treatments, as with that of most medical treatments, is usually based on determination of which are likely to have the most benefit for the patient with the least risk. The preferences of the patient and the skills and clinical opinions of the care provider are also important factors shaping treatment selection. In a patient with relapsing opioid addiction, cognitive limitations, or certain psychiatric disorders, opioid analgesics may represent a greater risk than for persons without these conditions. This might lead a clinician to select a more invasive or expensive treatment earlier in the course of treatment than with a lower risk patient in whom a trial of opioids would generally be a prerequisite.

For example, usually a trial of pharmacologic therapy including opioid therapy is instituted prior to consideration of spinal cord stimulation (SCS) in a patient with unilateral radiculopathy because of the expense and invasiveness of the procedure. However, in a person with relapsing opioid addiction, an earlier trial of SCS might be justified because the risk/benefit/cost balance is shifted. Similarly, though multiple daily doses of short-acting opioids are often used before initiation of a long-acting (often more expensive) opioid, in a person who experiences reward with each dose of a short-acting opioid (referred to by one recovering patient as "dancing with an old lover"), earlier use of a slow onset, long-acting opioid might be elected if pain is continuous.

Supply of Medications Making opioids available in quantities that relieve pain, while not inviting misuse, may be a key factor in successful opioid therapy for pain in persons with substance use problems. The number of units of opioid medications available to the patient and the frequency with which they are dispensed are two variables that can be controlled.

In current practice, it is common for patients to receive a month's supply of analgesic opioids, and some clinicians provide stable patients who have no detected risks with up to a 3-month supply. In persons with addiction disorders or those who tend to overuse medications for other reasons, however, it is often prudent to dispense smaller quantities of medications more frequently, sometimes weekly or even daily. This practice may help a patient control use by allowing him or her to see clearly that overuse ("a little extra won't hurt and may help") will result in no medication at the end of the cycle. This is easier to see with a week's supply of seven tablets of 24-hour medication than with a month's supply of 120 tablets of every-6-hour medication. Frequent dispensing of small doses can also preserve safety in persons prone to harmful misuse by ensuring that the patient does not have a potentially lethal supply of medications available. A transdermal fentanyl patch, placed in a clinician's office every 72 hours and signed and dated, may be helpful for some patients with recurrent misuse who require opioids for pain. However, note that, except for keeping the total dose dispensed sublethal, no method fully protects a patient who is at risk for major overuse, as all long-acting medications can be altered to cause release of the full dose immediately.

Frequent dispensing can be done by a pharmacy, a clinician's office, or a trusted other such as a family member, though care must be taken that this does not interfere negatively in personal relationships.

Supports for Recovery Many persons with recovering addiction disorders who require opioids for pain treatment benefit from active cultivation of their recovery. What constitutes meaningful recovery activities varies between individuals but may include attendance at self-help meetings, close interaction with a sponsor, work with a counselor, or active participation in a faith community, among others. Addiction professionals may provide an important service to patients and their pain treatment providers by making recommendations on enriching recovery and by supervising the recovery plan while patients are using opioids for pain. In persons with other conditions that may put them at risk for misuse of medications, such as psychiatric disorders or cognitive impairment, engagement of appropriate professionals to assist in management of or accommodation to these disorders is also appropriate.

Persons with relapsing opioid addiction who require opioids for severe chronic pain may sometimes benefit from concurrent methadone maintenance treatment (MMT). Methadone maintenance provides a stable background dose of opioids that blocks craving, blocks the high of other opioids, and provides physiologic homeostasis. However, because the analgesic effects of methadone usually last 6 to 8 hours, MMT alone does not usually meet analgesic needs when methadone is given once or twice daily, unless the dose is titrated much higher than that needed for pain if it were given every 6 hours. Therefore, co-management by a pain treatment provider who provides analgesic opioids (and/or other pain treatments as appropriate) and by an MMT clinic that provides once-daily or twice-daily split doses of methadone is sometimes the best option for pain treatment if opioids cannot be safely used by the patient in a controlled manner without MMT stabilization.

Supervision of Care Patients who receive opioid therapy for pain should be seen by their prescribing clinician on a regular basis to monitor pain, functional status, mood, use of medications, and general well-being (96). How frequently clinical visits are needed is adapted to the needs of the individual patient. Unstable patients or those with more complex problems are seen more often, while stable patients without identified risk factors for misuse and with clearly defined pain problems may be seen less often. Typical intervals for visits vary between once a week and once every 3 months—with monthly intervals most common. In rare cases, daily contact with a clinician is appropriate, or a longer interval beyond 3 months may be acceptable.

Toxicology testing, usually urine drug screens, are increasingly routine as part of supervision of all patients using opioids on a long-term basis in order to document use of the prescribed medication and to identify use of illicit or nonprescribed substances. It is critical, however, that clinicians take care in interpreting the results of the screen and using them to advance the care of patients. Toxicology screen may actually provide a support for recovery in persons with addiction (86). In persons with no appreciated special risks for medication misuse, toxicology testing is often done randomly on an annual basis. For persons at higher risk, testing may be done as often as weekly, especially during periods of high stress.

Another supervision strategy employed by many physicians to promote adherence to the prescribed medication regimen are pill counts. Some clinicians request that patients routinely bring their medications to each appointment and set renewal dates so that there should be residual medications at the visit. Others request patient come in unannounced for pill counts if concerns arise.

A final intervention may be useful if concerns arise that a patient may be diverting part or all of a higher dose of prescribed medications is the "opioid challenge" in which a patient takes a supervised dose of the prescribed medication and stays for observation of its effects through the expected time of peak efficacy. Somnolence or intoxication suggest the dose is not the accustomed dose. An opioid challenge should be done with IV in place and opioid antagonist available for safety.

Recent studies (97–99) have suggested that, with the addition of "structure" and active programs to address substance abuse, pain can be adequately managed in patients with aberrant behaviors and even in some with ongoing substance misuse. In a U.S. Department of Veterans Affairs facility, Wiedemer et al. (99) utilized consultations with clinical pharmacists, signing of second-chance agreements, and simple limit-setting interventions (e.g., more frequent visits, limited supplies of opioids, urine toxicology screening) in patients manifesting aberrant behaviors. Of those referred for this consultation, 45% were able to remain in pain management and had their behavior come under reasonable control, whereas about 38% self-discharged. The Acosta and Haller group (97) demonstrated that a highly intensive psychologic set of interventions, including adherence monitoring, motivational techniques, and cognitive-behavioral techniques, added to a methadone-based pain management program led to a diminution in all nonprescribed opioids and trends toward decreases in nonopioid drug abuse in a group of patients with chronic pain and active drug abuse.

Discontinuation of Opioid Therapy If opioid therapy does not continue to achieve its goals of improved pain, stable or improving function, and enhanced quality of life; if therapy cannot be structured to maintain safety of the patient owing to addictive use; if other concerns such as medications diversion are documented; or if pain resolves, it is sometimes necessary to discontinue opioid treatment. Clarifying the conditions of continued therapy and the conditions under which opioids will be discontinued in the written treatment agreement at the outset of care is enormously helpful when it is necessary to discontinue treatment. Opioids should be tapered (unless a patient has not been using the medication and is therefore not physically dependent) to avoid withdrawal and rebound increase in pain and other interventions used to attenuate pain and any withdrawal symptoms that occur. If addiction is identified, treatment for addiction should be initiated or intensified.

CONCLUSIONS

In the past, medical, legal, public, and regulatory opinions tended to discourage physicians from using opioids for the treatment of pain. With increased scientific and clinical understanding of pain, addiction, and the pharmacology of opioids, this is gradually changing. Numerous initiatives to foster the aggressive treatment of pain have been activated over the past two decades. The American Pain Society, a respected interdisciplinary clinical and research professional association, has produced guidelines on various aspects of pain management among them, one on the principles of analgesic use (100), one an evidence based guideline on the management of cancer pain in adults and children (101) and a soon to be released consensus guideline on the use of opioids in the treatment of chronic non-cancer pain (102). The Federation of State Medical Boards of the United States also has developed guidelines for the use of controlled substances to manage pain. (REFS) These guidelines affirm the right of physicians to use opioids when appropriate to manage all types of pain.

In order to use opioids effectively and safely when they are indicated, physicians must understand pharmacologic and clinical issues related to opioids and carefully structure treatment with respect to the particular benefits and risks for individual patients. Opioids have an important role in relieving human suffering. At the same time, it is important to respect their potential to cause harm in vulnerable individuals. It is to be hoped that, over time, science and clinical experience will provide a fuller understanding of ways to harness the full potential of opioids to relieve suffering while eliminating the potentially negative consequences of their use. In the meantime, the art of medicine should be combined with the science of medicine to give patients the best quality of life possible, given the reality of their clinical diagnoses.

ACKNOWLEDGMENT: *Sections of this chapter have previously appeared in an article by Savage, Passik, and Kirsch published by the National Institutes on Drug Abuse (53a).*

REFERENCES

1. Rasor J, Harris G. Using opioids for patients with moderate to severe pain. *J Am Osteopath Assoc* 2007;107(Suppl 5):ES4–ES10.
2. Webb et al. v. the United States, 1919.
3. Savage SR. Addiction in the treatment of pain: significance, recognition and treatment. *J Pain Symptom Manage* 1993;8(5):265–278.
4. Katz J. Lumbar disc disorders and low-back pain: socioeconomic factors and consequences. *J Bone Joint Surg* 2006;88-A(Suppl 2):21–24.
5. PriCara, Unit of Ortho-McNeil Pharamaceuticals Inc. *Pain in the workplace—a 10-year update of Ortho-McNeil's survey on the impact of pain on the workplace.* Titusville, NJ: Author, 2006.
6. National Center for Health Statistics. *Health, United States, 2006 with Chartbook on trends in the health of Americans.* Hyatsville, MD: Author, 2006.
7. Stewart WF, Riccis JA, Chee E, et al. Lost productive time and cost due to common pain conditions in the U.S. workforce. *JAMA* 2003; 290(18):2443–2454.
8. Jamison RN, Kauffman J, Katz NP. Characteristics of methadone maintenance patients with chronic pain. *J Pain Symptom Manage* 2000;19: 53–62.
9. Rosenblum A, Joseph H, Fong C, et al. Prevalence and characteristics of chronic pain among chemically dependent patients in methadone maintenance and residential treatment facilities. *JAMA* 2003;289: 2370–2378.
10. Joranson DE, Ryan KM, Gilson AM, et al. Trends in medical use and abuse of opioid analgesics. *JAMA* 2000;283:1710–1714.
11. Joranson DE, Gilson AM. Drug crime is a source of abused pain medications in the United States. *J Pain Symptom Manage* 2005;30(4): 299–301.
12. SAMHSA, National Survey on Drug Use and Health, 2005 and 2006.
12a. Agency for Health Care Policy Research. *Cancer pain management: clinical practice guidelines.* Rockville, MD: U.S. Department of Health and Human Services, 1994.
13. Ballantyne JC. Opioid analgesia: perspective on the right use and utility. *Pain Physician* 2007;10(3):479–491.
14. Dillie KS, Fleming MF, Mundt MP, et al. Quality of life associated with daily opioid therapy in a primary care chronic pain sample. *J Am Board Fam Pract* 2008;21(2):108–117.
15. Eriksen J, Bruera E, Ekholm O, Rasmussen NK. Critical issues on opioids in chronic non-cancer pain. An epidemiological study. *Pain* 2006;125:172–179.

16. Bhamb B, Brown D, Hariharan J, et al. Survey of select practice behaviors by primary care physicians on the use of opioids for chronic pain. *Curr Med Res Opin* 2006;22(9):1859–1865.
17. Savage SR, Joranson DE, Covington EC, et al. Definitions related to the medical use of opioids: evolution towards universal agreement. *J Pain Symptom Manage* 2003;26(1):655–667.
18. Portenoy RK. Opioid therapy for chronic nonmalignant pain: a review of the critical issues. *J Pain Symptom Manage Review* 1996;11(4): 203–217.
19. Jaffe J. Opiates: clinical aspects. In Lowinson J, Ruiz P, Millman R, eds. *Substance abuse: a comprehensive textbook.* Baltimore, MD: Williams & Wilkins, 1992:186–194.
20. Brodner RA, Taub A. Chronic pain exacerbated by long-term narcotic use in patients with non-malignant disease: clinical syndrome and treatment. *Mt. Sinai J Med* 1978;45:233–237.
21. Jaffe J, Martin W. Opioid agonists. In: Gilman A, Goodman L, Rall T, et al., eds. *The pharmacologic basis of therapeutics.* New York: Macmillan, 1980:491–531.
22. Foley K. Clinical tolerance to opioids. In: Basbaum A, Besson J, eds. *Towards a new pharmacotherapy of pain.* New York: John Wiley & Sons, 1991:181–203.
23. Collins E, Cesselin F. Neurobiological mechanisms of opioid tolerance and dependence. *Clin Neuropharmacol* 1991;14:465–488.
24. Hill H, Chapman C, Kornell J, et al. Self-administration of morphine in bone marrow transplant patients reduces drug treatment. *Pain* 1990; 40:121–129.
25. Hill H, Coda B, Mackie A, et al. Patient-controlled analgesic infusions: Alfentanil versus morphine. *Pain* 1992;49:301–310.
26. Twycross R. Clinical experience with diamorphine in advanced malignant disease. *Int J Clin Pharmacol Ther Toxicol* 1974;9:184–198.
27. Roth SH, Fleischmann RM, Burch FX, et al. Around-the-clock, controlled-release oxycodone therapy for osteoarthritis-related pain: placebo-controlled trial and long-term evaluation. *Arch Intern Med* 2000;27(160):853–860.
28. Kissin I, Brown P, Bailey E. Magnitude of acute tolerance to opioids is not related to their potency. *Anesthesiology* 1991;75:813–816.
29. Yaksh T. The spinal pharmacology of acutely and chronically administered opioids. *J Pain Symptom Manage* 1992;7:356–361.
30. Portenoy R. Pharmacotherapy of cancer pain. In *Refresher courses on pain management.* Adelaide, Australia: IASP Refresher Courses, 1990:101–112.
31. Jao B. 2000.
32. Hurd YL. Perspectives on current directions in the neurobiology of addiction disorders relevant to genetic risk factors. *CNS Spectr* 2006; 11(11):855–862.
33. Marsch LA, Bickel WK, Badger GJ, et al. Effects of infusion rate of intravenously administered morphine on physiological, psychomotor, and self-reported measures in humans. *J Pharmacol Exp Ther* 2001; 299(3):1056–1065.
34. Butler SF, Benoit C, Budman SH, et al. Development and validation of an Opioid Attractiveness Scale: a novel measure of the attractiveness of opioid products to potential abusers. *Harm Reduct J* 2006; 3:5.
35. Zacny et al. 1996.
36. Sees KL, Clark W. Opioid use in the treatment of chronic pain: assessment of addiction. *J Pain Symptom Manage* 1993;8(5):257–264.
37. American Psychiatric Association. *Diagnostic and Statistical Manual of Mental Disorders,* 4th ed. Washington, DC: American Psychiatric Press, 1994.
38. Wesson D, Ling W, Smith D. Prescription of opioids for treatment of pain in patients with addictive disease. *J Pain Symptom Manage* 1993; 8(5):289–296.
39. Kolb L. Types and characteristics of drug addicts. *Ment Hygiene* 1925; 9:300.
40. Rayport M. Experience in the management of patients medically addicted to narcotics. *JAMA* 1954;165:684–691.
41. Perry S, Heindrich G. Management of pain during debridement: a survey of U.S. burn units. *Pain* 1982;13:12–14.
42. Porter J, Jick H. Addiction rare in patients treated with narcotics. *N Engl J Med* 1980;302:123.
43. Furlan AD, Sandoval JA, Mailis-Gagnon A, et al. Opioids for chronic noncancer pain: a meta-analysis of effectiveness and side effects. *CMAJ* 2006;174(11):1589–1594.
44. Adams NJ, et al. Opioids and the treatment of chronic pain in a primary care sample. *J Pain Symptom Manage* 2001;22(3):791–796.
45. Ives TJ, et al. Predictors of opioid misuse in patients with chronic pain: a prospective cohort study. *BMC Health Serv Res* 2006;6:46.
46. Katz NP, Fanciullo GP. Role of urine toxicology testing in the management of chronic opioid therapy. *Clin J Pain* 2002;18(4 Suppl): S76–S82.
47. Michna E, et al. Urine toxicology screening among chronic pain patients on opioid therapy: frequency and predictability of abnormal findings. *Clin J Pain* 2007;23(2):173–179.
48. Passik SD, et al. Psychiatric and pain characteristics of prescription drug abusers entering drug rehabilitation. *J Pain Palliat Care Pharmacother* 2006;20(2):5–13.
49. Regier D, Meyers JK, Kramer M. The NIMH Epidemiological Catchment Area Study. *Arch Gen Psychiatry* 1984;41:934–958.
50. Weissman DE, Haddox JD. Opioid pseudoaddiction: an iatrogenic syndrome. *Pain* 1989;36:363–366.
51. Somogyi AA, Barratt DT, Collier JK. Pharmacogenetics of opioids. *Clin Pharmacol Ther* 2007;81(3):429–444.
52. Lötsch J, Geisslinger G. Are mu-opioid receptor polymorphisms important for clinical opioid therapy? *Trends Mol Med* 2005;11(2): 82–89.
53. Lugo RA, Satterfield KL, Kern SE. Pharmacokinetics of methadone. *J Pain Palliat Care Pharmacother* 2005;19(4):13–24.
53a. Savage SR, Passik S, Kirsch K. Challenges in using opioids to treat pain in persons with substance use disorders. National Institutes on Drug Abuse. *NIDA Addiction Science and Clinical Practice* 2008;4(2).
54. Wheeler WL, Dickerson ED. Clinical applications of methadone. *Am J Hospice Palliat Care* 2000;17(3):196–203.
55. Moryl N, Santiago-Palma J, Kornick C, et al. Pitfalls of opioid rotation: substituting another opioid for methadone in patients with cancer pain. *Pain* 2002;96:325–328.
56. Cicero TJ, Inciardi JA, Adams EH, et al. Rates of abuse of tramadol remain unchanged with the introduction of new branded and generic products: results of an abuse monitoring system, 1994–2004. *Pharmacoepidemiol Drug Safety* 2005;14(12):851–859.
57. Manchikanti L, Fellows B, Damron KS, et al. Prevalence of illicit drug use among individuals with chronic pain in the Commonwealth of Kentucky: an evaluation of patterns and trends. *J Ky Med Assoc* 2005; 103(2):55–62.
58. Passik SD, et al. Psychiatric and pain characteristics of prescription drug abusers entering drug rehabilitation. *J Pain Palliat Care Pharmacother* 2006;20(2):5–13.
59. Fordyce W. Opioids, pain and behavioral outcomes. *Am Pain Soc J* 1992;1(4):282–284.
60. Højsted J, Sjøgren P. Addiction to opioids in chronic pain patients: a literature review. *Eur J Pain* 2007;11(5):490–518.
61. Zacny J. A review of the effects of opioids on psychomotor and cognitive functioning in humans. *Exp Clin Psychopharmacol* 1995;3: 432–466.
62. Rapaport A. Analgesic rebound headache. *Headache* 1988;28(10): 662–665.
63. Schofferman J. Long-term use of opioid analgesics for the treatment of chronic pain of nonmalignant origin. *J Pain Symptom Manage* 1993; 8(5):279–288.
64. Miller NS, Barkin RL. Effects of opioid prescription medication dependence and detoxification on pain perceptions and self-reports. *Am J Ther* 2006;13(5):436–444.
65. Compton M. Cold pressor pain tolerance in opiate and cocaine abusers: correlates of drug type and use status. *J Pain Symptom Manage* 1994; 9(7):462–473.
66. Sjøgren P, Jensen N, Jensen T. Disappearance of morphine-induced hyperalgesia after discontinuing or substituting morphine with other opioid agonists. *Pain* 1994;59:313–316.

67. Chang G, Chen L, et al. Opioid tolerance and hyperalgesia. *Med Clin North Am* 2007;91(2):199–211.
68. Chu LF, Clark D. Opioid-induced hyperalgesia in humans: molecular mechanisms and clinical considerations. *Clin J Pain* 2008;24(6): 479–496.
69. Paice JA, Penn RD, Ryan WG. Altered sexual function and decreased testosterone in patients receiving intraspinal opioids. *J Pain Symptom Manage* 1994;9(2):126–131.
70. Fortin JD, Bailey GM, Vilensky JA. Does opioid use for pain management warrant routine bone mass density screening in men? *Pain Physician* 2008;11(4):539–541.
71. Sacerdote P. Opioids and the immune system. *Palliat Med* 2006; 20(Suppl 1):9–15.
72. Quigley C. Opioid switching to improve pain relief and drug tolerability. *Cochrane Rev* 2004;3.
73. Jasinski D, Johnson R, Kocher T. Clonidine in morphine withdrawal: differential effects on sign and symptoms. *Arch Gen Psychiatry* 1985; 42:1063–1065.
74. Wattwil M. Postoperative pain relief and gastrointestinal motility. *Acta Chir Scand Suppl* 1989;550:140–145.
75. Jackson D. A study of pain management: patient controlled analgesia versus intramuscular analgesia. *J Intraven Nurs* 1989;12(1):42–51.
76. Graham K, Koren G. Characteristics of pregnant women exposed to cocaine in Toronto between 1985 and 1990. *CMAJ* 1991;144(5): 563–568.
77. McCaffery M, Vourakis C. Assessment and relief of pain in chemically dependent patients. *Orthop Nurs* 1992;11(2):13–26.
78. Robinson SE. Buprenorphine-containing treatments: place in the management of opioid addiction. *CNS Drugs* 2006;20(9):697–712.
79. Vadivelu N, Hines RL. Buprenorphine: a unique opioid with broad clinical applications. *J Opioid Manag* 2007;3(1):49–58.
80. Lutfy K, Cowan A. Buprenorphine: a unique drug with complex pharmacology. *Curr Neuropharmacol* 2004;2(4):395–402.
80a. Yassen A, Romberg R, Sarton E, et al. Buprenorphine induces ceiling in respiratory depression but not in analgesia. *J Anaesth* 2006;96(5): 627–632.
81. Haythornthwaite JA, Menefee LA, Quatrano-Piacentini AL, Pappagallo M. Outcome of chronic opioid therapy for non-cancer pain. *J Pain Symptom Manage* 1998;15:185–194.
82. Finlayson RE, Maruta T, Morse RM, et al. Substance dependence and chronic pain: experience with treatment and follow-up results. *Pain* 1986;26(2):175–180.
83. Mao J, Price D, Mayer D. Mechanisms of hyperalgesia and morphine tolerance: a current view of their possible interactions. *Pain* 1995; 62:259–274.
84. Bruera E, Moyano J, Seifert L, et al. The frequency of alcoholism among patients with pain due to terminal cancer. *J Pain Symptom Manage* 1995;10(8):599–603.
85. Cousins MJ, Bridenbaugh PO. *Neural blockade in clinical anesthesia and management of pain.* Philadelphia: Lippincott Williams & Wilkins,1998.
86. Gourlay DL, Heit HA, Almahrezi A. Universal precautions in pain medicine: a rational approach to the treatment of chronic pain. *Pain Med* 2005;6(2):107–112.
87. American Society of Addiction Medicine. *Public policy statements. Definition related to the use of opioids for the treatment of pain and on the rights and responsibilities of physicians in the use of opioids for the treatment of pain.* Chevy Chase, MD: Author, 1997.
88. Brown RL, Rounds LA. Conjoint screening questionnaires for alcohol and drug abuse. *Wisc Med J* 1995;94:135–140.
89. Gavin DR, Ross HE, Skinner HA. Diagnostic validity of the drug abuse screening test in the assessment of DSM-III drug disorders. *Br J Addict* 1989;84(3):301–307.
90. Akbik H, Butler SF, Budman SH, et al. Validation and clinical application of the screener and opioid assessment for patients with pain (SOAPP). *J Pain Symptom Manage* 2006;32(3):287–293.
91. Dowling LS, Gatchel RJ, Adams LL et al. An evaluation of the predictive validity of the Pain Medication Questionnaire with a heterogeneous group of patients with chronic pain. *J Opioid Manag* 2007;3(5): 257–266.
92. Butler SF, Budman SH, Fernandez K, et al. Validation of a screener and opioid assessment measure for patients with chronic pain. *Pain* 2004; 112(1–2):65–75.
93. Webster LR, Webster RM. Predicting aberrant behaviors in opioid-treated patients: preliminary validation of the Opioid Risk Tool. *Pain Med* 2005;6(6):432–442.
94. Wu SM, et al. The Addiction Behaviors Checklist: Validation of a new clinician-based measure of inappropriate opioid use in chronic pain. *Journal of Pain and Symptom Management* 2006;32(4):342–351.
95. www.painedu.org.
96. Atluri S, Boswell MV, Hansen HC, et al. Guidelines for the use of controlled substances in the management of chronic pain. *Pain Physician* 2003;6(3):233–257.
97. Acosta M, Haller DL. Psychiatric and substance abuse comorbidity influences treatment outcomes in opioid-abusing patients. Paper presented at the College on Problems of Drug Dependency annual meeting, Scottsdale, AZ;2006.
98. Cheatle MD, Gallagher RM. Chronic pain and comorbid mood and substance use disorders: a biopsychosocial treatment approach. *Curr Psychiatry Rep* 2006;8(5):371–376.
99. Wiedemer NL, Harden PS, Arndt IO, et al. The opioid renewal clinic: a primary care, managed approach to opioid therapy in chronic pain patients at risk for substance abuse. *Pain Med* 2007;8(7):573–584.
100. Principles of Analgesic Use, American Pain Society, 6E, 2006. www.ampainsoc.org.
101. Guideline for the management of cancer pain in adults and children. *American Pain Society*, 2005. www.ampainsoc.org.
102. Guideline on the use of opioids for the treatment of chronic non-cancer pain. *American Pain Society*. In press, 2009.

SUGGESTED READINGS

Ives TJ, et al. Predictors of opioid misuse in patients with chronic pain: a prospective cohort study. *BMC Health Serv Res* 2006;6:46.

Katz NP, Fanciullo GJ. Role of urine toxicology testing in the management of chronic opioid therapy. *Clin J Pain* 2002;18(4 Suppl):S76–S82.

Liaison Committee on Pain and Addiction. *Definitions related to the use of opioids for the treatment of pain.* 2001. Available at www.ampainsoc.org. Retrieved (date), from

Savage SR. Long-term opioid therapy: assessment of consequences of risks. *J Pain Symptom Manage* 1996;11:274–286.

Xiangqi Li, Martin S, Angst J, et al. A murine model of opioid-induced hyperalgesia. *Mol Brain Res* 2001;86:56–62.

CHAPTER 96

Aaron M. Gilson, PhD, MS, MSSW
Martha A. Maurer, MSSW, MPH

Legal and Regulatory Considerations in Pain Management

Many pharmacologic and nonpharmacologic treatments are available to relieve pain. Opioid analgesics such as morphine are essential for managing moderate to severe pain from cancer (1–4). Although treating noncancer pain with opioids continues to be controversial (5), currently accepted medical practice standards support practitioners evaluating patients' pain during the initial evaluation and monitoring their pain and functioning during treatment to determine whether opioids are, and remain, an effective therapeutic option (6–8).

Laws and regulations related to the prescribing, dispensing, and administration of controlled substances to patients in pain have changed considerably over the last two decades, often in response to the increased awareness both of the problems of undertreated pain and the risks posed by these substances. Legislatures and regulatory agencies recognize that physicians, pharmacists, and nurses must be able to prescribe, dispense, and administer opioids according to individual patient needs (1,4). However, concerns about opioid side effects, adverse events, and abuse, addiction, and diversion have led to restrictions that have at times marginalized their medical use. This is especially true for patients with pain who also have a substance abuse history or use drugs for nontherapeutic purposes (9–11).

This chapter reviews the laws, regulations, and health care regulatory board policies that govern the use of controlled substances, primarily focusing on opioids, and their possible impact on pain management for patients who abuse, or are in recovery from addiction to, controlled substances.

POLICIES GOVERNING DRUG AVAILABILITY

Before presenting specific examples of relevant policy language, brief definitions are provided of the types of policies that will be discussed. *Law* is a broad term that refers to rules of conduct with binding legal force adopted by legislative or other government bodies at the international, federal, state, or local levels. Laws can be found in treaties, constitutional provisions, court decisions, statutes, and regulations. The most basic laws usually are the statutes enacted by a legislature. A number of laws have been adopted by the states concerning pain management, with Intractable Pain Treatment Acts (IPTAs) the most common form of statutory pain policy.

A *regulation* is an official rule issued by an agency of the executive branch of government. Regulations often are found in an administrative code or code of regulation. Regulations have the force of law and are intended to implement or interpret statutory authority granted to an agency, often to establish what conduct is or is not acceptable for those regulated by the agency (such as physicians, pharmacists, and nurses). Regulations issued by state agencies should not exceed the scope of the agency's statutory authority.

Guideline, as used here, means an official adopted policy statement that is issued by a government agency, such as a state medical board, to express its attitude or position on a particular matter. Although guidelines do not have binding legal force, they may outline parameters or standards of conduct for those who are regulated by an agency. For example, a number of state medical boards have issued guidelines regarding the medical use of opioids that define the conduct the board considers to be within, as well as outside of, the professional practice of medicine. Some pharmacy and nursing boards have issued similar guidelines. Guidelines also include policy statements that may appear in a position paper, report, article, or agency newsletter.

International Policies International treaties, U.S. federal law and regulations, and state laws and regulations govern prescribing and dispensing of controlled substances. Although the control of diversion and the prevention of illicit drug use typically are perceived as the singular purpose of these policies, drug control policy has a second and equally important purpose—to ensure drug availability. According to international treaty, opioids are necessary for pain relief and must be adequately available for medical purposes (12). To achieve a proper balance between availability and control, the United Nations drug control authorities assert that efforts to prevent drug abuse and diversion should not interfere with the availability and medical use of controlled drugs (12,13). Public policies that recognize both control and availability are said to be "balanced" (14–16).

Federal Policies The U.S. Food and Drug Administration (FDA), according to authority granted to that agency by the federal Food, Drug and Cosmetic Act of 1962, ensures that all drugs, including prescription opioid analgesics, are both safe and effective for human use under medical supervision. FDA does not regulate medical practice (17); rather, the states govern health care practice (14). Physicians generally are allowed to prescribe for a medical purpose and in the patient's interest according to their best professional judgment (18); this means that prescribing decisions are medical decisions. Prescription drugs can be prescribed for other than their labeled indications or recommended doses if there is a medical rationale (19).

In addition to FDA regulations, opioids and other controlled substances are subject to federal statutes and regulations because of their abuse liability. The Controlled Substances Act (CSA) (20) is a federal law that establishes the U.S. drug control system, and is intended to achieve both control and availability by paralleling international treaties. The CSA recognizes that controlled substances are necessary for public health and that medication availability must be ensured. The CSA states that "many of the drugs included within this title have a useful and legitimate medical purpose and are necessary to maintain the health and general welfare of the American people" (20, p. 834).

Availability is accomplished through a regulated distribution system that governs import, manufacture, distribution, prescribing, dispensing, and possession. Licensed professionals can prescribe, dispense, and administer controlled drugs for legitimate medical purposes and in the course of professional practice if they have a state license to practice their profession and a valid controlled substances registration from the U.S. Drug Enforcement Administration (DEA). To prevent diversion, the CSA establishes a system of security, record keeping, and monitoring requirements, as well as penalties (both civil and criminal) for violating these requirements. The DEA administers the Code of Federal Regulations (21), which is the regulation that implements the federal CSA.

CSA Drug Schedules The CSA classifies controlled substances into five schedules, according to established medical usefulness and relative abuse liability. Each schedule carries a different penalty for unlawful use. Prescription requirements also vary depending on the schedule of medication prescribed. Schedule I contains the drugs that have no accepted medical use and are available only for scientific research (such as marijuana, methaqualone, and heroin). Schedules II through V contain drugs that are FDA-approved for medical use but have an abuse potential, such as opioids. Opioids considered by the government to have the highest potential for abuse are placed in Schedule II; they include morphine, hydromorphone, oxycodone, oxymorphone, meperidine, and fentanyl. Schedule II also contains such stimulants as amphetamines and methylphenidate, along with some of the older sedatives, including some of the barbiturates. Schedule III contains drugs considered to have less abuse potential than those in Schedule II, and includes opioids such as hydrocodone and codeine combinations, as well as sublingual buprenorphine, indicated for treating addiction. Schedule IV includes opioids with less abuse liability than drugs contained in higher schedules, such as dextropropoxyphene and codeine compounded in smaller doses, benzodiazepines, newer nonbenzodiazepine sedatives, and the stimulant modafinil. Schedule V drugs have the lowest abuse potential, including opioid-containing antitussives and antidiarrheals.

Federal Laws Related to Opioid Prescribing All persons or business entities that manufacture, order, prescribe, or dispense controlled substances must be registered with the DEA. The DEA monitors all transfers of controlled substances within a "closed distribution system." Prescriptions for Schedule II drugs must be in written form and cannot be refilled, whereas five refills are permitted for drugs in Schedules III and IV. A recent addition to federal regulations permits the issuance of multiple prescriptions for Schedule II drugs, written with "do not fill until" instructions, which can be issued sequentially; each of the multiple prescriptions must be dated as of the date they are written (22). Federal law allows oral prescriptions for Schedule II controlled substances in medical emergencies and under specific circumstances (23), but these must be followed with a written prescription within a specified period. For Schedule II prescriptions, federal law also permits partial dispensing (24) for patients in a long-term care facility and faxing (25) for patients in a hospice or a long-term care facility when particular requirements are fulfilled. Federal laws and regulations do not limit, nor have they ever limited, the amount of drug prescribed, the duration for which a drug is prescribed, or the period for which a prescription is valid (although some states do).

The CSA does not permit practitioners to prescribe Schedule II opioids for the purpose of maintenance or detoxification treatment of narcotic addiction. When practitioners have a separate federal registration as an Opioid Treatment Program (OTP) (26), they are allowed to dispense, but not prescribe, narcotic drugs approved for this purpose, such as methadone and buprenorphine, and must comply with federal and state regulations. However, it is important to note that methadone can be prescribed and dispensed to treat pain, just as one would prescribe any other Schedule II opioid analgesic.

The Drug Addiction Treatment Act of 2000 permits physicians to receive a waiver from these rules, so that they can use specifically approved medications for the treatment of opioid addiction. To date, only sublingual buprenorphine (a Schedule III medication) is approved for this purpose. To receive the waiver, the physician must be a certified addictionologist or must complete 8 hours of training and must notify the Center for Substance Abuse Treatment (a component of the Substance Abuse and Mental Health Services Administration) of intent to prescribe this treatment. The notification of intent must document that the physician has the capacity to refer addiction therapy patients for appropriate counseling and other nonpharmacologic therapies.

State Policies Medical practice is regulated at the state, not the federal, level. Therefore numerous state laws, regulations, and guidelines can further limit medical practice using controlled substances. State legislatures have adopted statutes to protect the public (e.g., a Medical Practice Act). The law provides state health care agencies the authority to license and discipline members of their respective professions, by creating oversight boards, such as medical, pharmacy, and nursing boards. Boards may adopt regulations to implement the laws governing health care practice. A board's rule-making procedures are a matter for public input and public record.

Board investigation of a licensee can be initiated by a complaint or by referral from another agency. The procedures used for initial inquiry and investigation into complaints vary greatly among boards. Some boards, according to law, are required to investigate all complaints received, whereas others can exercise discretion. In some states, the mere filing of a complaint against a physician is a matter of public record. Investigations may be prompt, and a case can be dropped because of insufficient evidence or can proceed to disciplinary action. Alternatively, some proceedings can take several years to resolve. If the board finds that violations have occurred, a range of actions may be considered depending on the nature and seriousness of the violations.

Possible disciplinary actions, all of which are reviewable by the state courts, include a warning, education, limiting or revoking prescribing privileges, or license suspension or revocation. Boards also manage programs to identify and treat impaired licensees.

All licensing boards have national organizations: the Federation of State Medical Boards of the United States (FSMB) for medical boards; the National Association of Boards of Pharmacy for pharmacy boards; and the National Council of State Boards of Nursing for nursing boards. These organizations sponsor numerous activities, such as annual meetings, task forces to study specific issues relevant to regulating that profession, and technical assistance, training, policy development, and preparation of model laws and regulations. Health care regulatory boards also disseminate information, including newsletters and statistics about licensees and disciplinary actions.

In addition to professional practice policy, the states have adopted versions of the CSA, as laws to control medications with abuse liability. Typically, these laws are patterned after the National Conference of Commissioners on Uniform State Laws' model Uniform Controlled Substances Act (27,28). Such state laws permit the prescribing, dispensing, and administering of controlled substances for legitimate medical purposes, although most do not specifically recognize the essential medical value of controlled substances, as does the federal CSA. A revised model Uniform Controlled Substances Act was prepared to correct this and other deficiencies (29), but only a few states have adopted the changes, including Colorado, Washington, and Wisconsin. State and local police agencies enforce the criminal provisions of the state controlled substances laws, whereas departments of regulation and licensing, including pharmacy examining boards, manage the administrative aspects (e.g., drug scheduling). Some state agencies have issued regulations that govern controlled substances prescribing and dispensing more strictly than does federal law (examples of which are detailed in the following section) (30,31).

In addition, numerous states have laws that establish prescription monitoring programs (32). At this writing, 36 states have adopted laws that require using an electronic data transfer system to monitor prescriptions for controlled substances. In the past, prescription monitoring programs have been limited to medications in Schedule II, but newer programs monitor drugs in other schedules as well. Generally, these programs enable physicians to quickly determine whether their patients are "multisourcing" (i.e., obtaining controlled substances from multiple providers). Monitoring multiple drug schedules would seem to take the regulatory focus off of Schedule II medications, which research has shown can often motivate practitioners to prescribe lower scheduled medications to avoid being monitored (and has been termed a *substitution effect*) (33). Current prescription monitoring programs typically are administered by state health agencies (such as the Pharmacy Board), rather than law enforcement agencies, and the policies that implement the programs often emphasize that this effort to reduce abuse and diversion should not interfere with appropriate patient care.

In the past, several states required a government-issued serialized prescription form for controlled substances; however, only Texas still requires an official form for Schedule II medications (16).

LEGISLATIVE AND REGULATORY DEFINITIONS OF ADDICTION

The use and definition of addiction-related terminology remains as much a point of confusion for licensing boards and enforcement authorities as for others in the field. Such confusion originates in part from official definitions and expert opinions that historically have characterized addiction in terms of physical dependence, as indicated by the presence of a withdrawal syndrome (11). Almost 50 years ago, the World Health Organization (WHO) replaced the terms *addiction* and *habituation* with *drug dependence*. This represented a major change in philosophy, because dependence was redefined primarily as the use of a drug for its psychic effects. Under the WHO definition, neither physical dependence nor tolerance, alone or together, is sufficient to define drug dependence.

The distinction between physiologic adaptation to a drug (as evidenced by the development of tolerance or a withdrawal syndrome) and compulsive use despite harm currently is reflected in the two primary diagnostic classification systems used by health care professionals: the *International classification of mental and behavioural disorders,* 10th ed., of the World Health Organization (34) and the *Diagnostic and statistical manual*, 4th ed., of the American Psychiatric Association (35). Although a diagnosis of "dependence syndrome" in the *ICD-10* and "substance dependence" in the DSM-IV can include both withdrawal and tolerance, compulsive use that contributes to personal impairment or distress also must be present. As a result, it is unlikely such a diagnosis would apply to patients with pain who are physically dependent because of prolonged opioid therapy, but who are exhibiting no behavioral indications of compulsive use despite harm.

In 1993, the WHO Expert Committee on Drug Dependence further clarified that cancer patients who use opioids should not be considered dependent solely because a withdrawal syndrome would occur if the medication was stopped (36). WHO has continued to reinforce this notion in its statement that ". . . dependence should not be a factor in deciding whether to use opioids to treat the cancer patient with pain" (4, p. 41). To avoid confusion, the term *addiction* is used throughout this article, and is considered synonymous with the current WHO concept of *dependence syndrome* and the APA concept of *substance dependence*.

Accurately using terminology is central to shaping a balanced policy on drug control, especially in the United States where prescribing opioids to maintain addiction is illegal (37). It should be recognized that tolerance and physical dependence denote the body's normal physiological adaptations to the presence of an opioid; thus, a patient being treated with opioid analgesics is likely to become physically dependent. However, when practitioners confuse the development of physical dependence or tolerance with addiction, patients who are prescribed opioids for pain relief can be labeled an "addict," which increases the risk that the patient is denied continued treatment. Weissman and Haddox (38) have coined the term *pseudoaddiction*, which has come to represent the situation in which health care professionals mistake a patient's pattern of pain relief–seeking behaviors, resulting from inadequate pain management, for the type of drug-seeking behavior characteristic of addiction.

Misperceiving patients with pain as drug seekers or persons/patients with an addiction disorder can result in denial of the opioid prescriptions they need for pain management. There is at least one documented case in which a patient with inadequately treated pain illegally called in controlled substances prescriptions to obtain pain relief. Prosecutors viewed the patient as a drug person/patient with an addiction disorder, even though the medical evaluation was positive for pain and negative for an addiction disorder (39).

LEGISLATIVE AND REGULATORY POLICIES THAT INFLUENCE PRESCRIBING

Policies Federal policy has several provisions relevant to pain and addiction.

Defining an "Addict" The CSA defines as an "addict" an individual who "habitually uses any narcotic drug so as to endanger the public morals, health, safety, or who is so far addicted to the use of narcotic drugs as to have lost power of self-control with reference to his addiction" (40). The definition is circular and uses archaic terminology, but nevertheless can be used to determine that a physician prescribed to an "addict." However, the potential to apply this definition to a patient with pain on chronic opioid therapy seems low.

The federal regulation that governed dispensing of methadone for the maintenance or detoxification treatment of opiate addiction historically contributed to confusion between addiction and physical dependence. Admission eligibility for such treatment required that the patient be "narcotic dependent," which was officially defined as "physiologically [in need of] . . . a heroin or morphine-like drug to prevent the onset of signs of withdrawal" (41). Thus numerous patients with chronic pain have been admitted to methadone treatment programs primarily or exclusively to obtain analgesia (42). For example, the director of a California methadone treatment program estimated that, from all patients admitted to the program in the mid-1990s, approximately 200 patients were admitted for the treatment of chronic pain conditions who did not demonstrate behaviors suggesting addiction (43).

The possibility that patients could be admitted to addiction treatment programs only for chronic pain management was minimized when federal regulations governing addiction treatment were modified in 2003 (44). The admission criteria for OTPs now incorporate accepted medical criteria for addiction and characterize "active addiction" as being of at least 1 year's duration. Thus federal regulations no longer contain language that confuses physical dependence with addiction and that provided a loophole allowing admission of patients solely to have their chronic pain treated.

State Policies State policies may vary considerably from international and federal policies. Many state laws do not recognize the value of controlled medications to the public health, as does the federal law (45,46). State laws, regulations, and guidelines/policy statements may unduly limit prescribing and dispensing of controlled substances, and such requirements or restrictions must be considered when making patient care decisions.

Although state laws seek to target illicit drug use without impeding appropriate use, they do neither perfectly. At times policies can interfere with even appropriate care, so practitioners should obtain information concerning the legislative and health care requirements related to the state in which the patient is treated. The full text of pain policies for every state can be found at the University of Wisconsin's Pain and Policy Studies Group website *www.painpolicy.wisc.edu/matrix.htm.*

Studies of state statutes and regulations relevant to pain management began in Wisconsin in the mid-1980s (47–49). Subsequently, national expert groups issued a succession of reports discussing policy content and its possible effect on pain management (27,29,50–53). Many restrictive state policy provisions date back 30 years or more, and appear to have been based on outdated concepts of addiction and the side effects of opioid analgesics.

A series of comprehensive, criteria-based evaluations of the strengths and weaknesses of federal policies, as well as policies in all 50 states and the District of Columbia, has been published since 2000 (16,54–56). Some states restrict the quantity of controlled substances that can be prescribed at one time, or limit the validity of a prescription to a few days. Many states also use imprecise terminology that could legally label patients who are using opioids to treat their pain as persons with an addictive disease (based on the presence of physical dependence). One state requires physicians to report to a government agency those patients to whom they prescribe Schedule II controlled substances for more than several months (16). Other states require that opioid therapy for any patient with chronic pain be provided only after consultation with a specialist with expertise appropriate to the patient's pain (i.e., a patient with chronic pelvic pain would have to see a gynecologist, and a patient with chronic joint pain would need to see a rheumatologist). Finally, several states prohibit chronic opioid therapy to patients with addiction disorder, either completely or unless consultation with an addictionologist is obtained. To address this issue, some states, including California, New York, and Texas, have revised their policies to permit the use of controlled substances to manage chronic pain in patients with an addictive disease (16).

IPTAs Since 1989, a number of state legislatures have adopted IPTAs. Although these policies were designed to reduce physicians' concerns about regulatory scrutiny, they may also unduly restrict physician prescribing and patient access to opioid analgesics (16,30).

Ambiguous language may impede understanding of the laws, especially regarding definitions of intractable pain. The Texas IPTA (57) was the first to be adopted and has served as a model for most other state IPTAs. It defines "intractable pain" as ". . . a pain state in which the cause of the pain cannot be removed or otherwise treated and which, in the generally accepted course of medical practice, no relief or cure of the cause of the pain is possible or none has been found after reasonable efforts" (57, Section 2[3]). Taken in the context of a law governing the use of controlled substances, such a definition implies that physicians' prescribing for chronic pain is outside generally accepted medical practice unless it is done within the parameters of an IPTA. Further, limiting the use of opioids only to patients for whom other efforts have failed seems to relegate them as a treatment of last resort, even when the patient initially presents with severe pain. A balanced approach to drug policy recognizes that physicians should make medical decisions based on individual patients' treatment needs. Also, for some IPTAs, physician immunity from discipline is contingent on obtaining a consultation or evaluation from a specialist in the organ system believed to be causing the pain before prescribing opioids. This requirement does not take into account a physician's expertise or the patient's needs, which in some cases could obviate the need for a consultation.

Because immunity from discipline under some IPTAs is not granted to physicians prescribing to patients who use drugs nontherapeutically, such laws also can unintentionally exclude patients with an addictive disease from pain management (46). These provisions appear to conflict with federal policy, which prohibits physicians from prescribing narcotic drugs only for the *purpose* of maintaining narcotic addiction, but does not prohibit prescribing opioids to *persons* who have both pain and an addictive disease. Such state policies may prohibit treating pain in persons who have addictive disease and a medical problem that causes pain, such as cancer or AIDS. With the recognition that certain IPTA requirements can impede patient care, some states have worked to remove existing ambiguities and restrictions. In 2001, Michigan removed the term *intractable pain* from its statute. More recently, Rhode Island (56) and California (16) repealed many restrictive provisions from their IPTAs and deleted the term and definition of *intractable pain*, which expands the law to govern treating all types of pain.

Perceived Threat of Regulatory Scrutiny IPTAs were created as a mechanism to protect from regulatory discipline health care professionals who prescribe opioids to treat chronic pain. The perception that practitioners need such protection stemmed from a number of articles reporting physicians' reluctance to prescribe opioid analgesics because of concern about being investigated by a regulatory agency (50,58–61). A pilot survey of Wisconsin physicians conducted in 1990 found that more than half reported that they would reduce the dose or quantity, reduce the number of refills, or choose a drug in a lower schedule because of concerns about regulatory scrutiny (62). In addition, 40% of the American Pain Society's physician-members agreed in 1991 that legal concerns influenced their prescribing of opioids for chronic noncancer pain (63).

All state medical board members in the United States were surveyed in 1991 to determine whether medical regulators' knowledge and attitudes about prescribing opioids for chronic cancer and noncancer pain would pose a risk to the physician who provided such treatment (64). Board members were asked their opinions about the legality and medical acceptability of prescribing opioids for more than several months in four patient scenarios involving cancer and noncancer pain, with and without a history of drug abuse of the opioid type. There were five possible responses: such prescribing was (1) lawful and generally acceptable medical practice; (2) lawful, but generally not accepted medical practice and should be discouraged; (3) probably a violation of medical practice laws or regulations and should be investigated; (4) probably a violation of federal or state controlled substances laws and should be investigated; and (5) don't know.

Only 75% of medical board members were confident that prescribing opioids for chronic cancer pain was both legal and acceptable medical practice; 14% felt it was legal, but would discourage it; 5% believed that the practice was illegal and should be investigated. If the patient with chronic cancer pain had a history of opioid abuse, less than half of the respondents (46%) were confident in prescribing opioids and 22% would discourage the practice. Fourteen percent considered the practice to be a violation of medical practice law and 12% viewed it as violating controlled substances laws. When the patient's chronic pain was of noncancer origin, only 12% of respondents were confident that prescribing opioids was both legal and medically acceptable; 47% would discourage it; and nearly one third recommended investigating the practice as a violation of law. Finally, only 1% of respondents viewed the prescribing of opioids for more than several months to a patient with chronic noncancer pain and a history of opioid abuse as legal and acceptable medical practice.

Overall, it appeared that in the early 1990s, many medical board members would discourage or investigate the prescribing of opioid analgesics for chronic pain, particularly if the patient did not have cancer and especially if the patient had a history of drug abuse. It is important to recognize that the presenting problem in each scenario was pain, and not addiction.

Medical board members from all states were resurveyed in 1997 and their responses compared with the 1991 sample (65). Results demonstrated some important improvements in board members' knowledge and attitudes since the early 1990s. Significantly more board members in 1997 considered opioid prescribing to be a lawful and generally acceptable medical treatment for chronic noncancer pain, and for patients with chronic pain and an opioid abuse history. It should be noted, however, that those board members who viewed these prescribing scenarios as lawful still represented only a small percentage of the total sample (only 6%). Nevertheless, the changes in knowledge and attitudes between 1991 and 1997 shows increasing recognition that prescribing opioids for cancer and noncancer pain, with and without a substance abuse history, was an acceptable medical practice.

A third survey was conducted in 2004 to determine whether state board members' views about prolonged opioid prescribing for pain have continued to progress (66). When judging the legality of prescribing opioids for more than several months, respondents in 2004 were significantly more likely to consider this lawful and acceptable medical practice for patients with cancer and noncancer pain, and even when the patient had a history of substance abuse. However, not surprisingly, board members continued to be least confident when considering prolonged opioid prescribing to a patient with chronic noncancer pain who also had a documented drug abuse history, with only 21% considering it lawful and acceptable medical practice. Thus physicians prescribing controlled substances to patients with a prior addiction should be aware that members of their state medical board may subject this practice to heightened scrutiny, and should therefore structure their practice accordingly (e.g., consider appropriate consultation or referral, consider treatment agreements, and thoroughly document rationale for treatment decisions).

Interestingly, a survey of Wisconsin physicians conducted in 2005 showed only 13% of respondents was notably concerned about regulatory investigation for their prescribing practices (67). However, between 35% and 45% of respondents reported at least occasionally changing their opioid prescribing practices in some way because of concern about possible investigation by a regulatory agency. Such changes included prescribing a smaller quantity of medication, limiting the number of refills, and prescribing a lower schedule medication. Another 19% admitted to at least occasionally prescribing a lower dose of medication. This recent evidence suggests that even a perceived low level of concern about disciplinary investigation and sanction can have a notable effect on treatment decisions.

Model Medical Regulatory Policies In 1998, the FSMB adopted a document entitled "Model Guidelines for the Use of Controlled Substances for the Treatment of Pain" (Model Guidelines) to directly address physicians' concern about regulatory scrutiny, and to promote positive state medical board pain policy and greater consistency between the states' policies (51). The Model Guidelines were developed as a cooperative effort between the FSMB and representatives from state medical boards, the American Pain Society, the American Academy of Pain Medicine, the American Society of Law, Medicine and Ethics, and the University of Wisconsin Pain & Policy Studies Group. The FSMB disseminated the Model Guidelines to each state medical board with a request that it be considered and adopted as policy.

The Model Guidelines stated that opioid analgesics may be necessary for the treatment of pain, including pain associated with acute, cancer, and noncancer conditions. If state medical boards adopt this policy, the positive language would communicate to medical professionals that their licensing board recognizes the health benefits of using controlled substances as a part of legitimate medical practice.

The Model Guidelines addressed directly the limitations inherent in medical board policies at that time. Although many board policies did not have an explicit statement of purpose, the Model Guidelines encouraged pain management and clarified that effective pain management was an expected part of good medical practice. In addition, the guidelines recognized that physicians were concerned about regulatory scrutiny, and provided them with information about how the board distinguishes legitimate medical practice from unprofessional conduct. The Model Guidelines made it clear that judgments about the legitimacy of a medical practice were to be based on the patients' treatment outcomes, rather than on the prescription amount or duration.

The Model Guidelines also contained a set of recommended treatment parameters for using controlled substances for pain management, which are based on principles of good medical practice. Seven treatment steps were included: (1) medical history and physical examination, (2) treatment plan with identified objectives, (3) informed consent to treatment, (4) periodic review of treatment, (5) consultation as necessary, (6) accurate and complete medical records, and (7) compliance with both federal and state controlled substances policy. Importantly, the Model Guidelines recognized the need for treatment flexibility, stating that a physician can deviate from the guidelines for good cause shown (51).

Another important advantage of the Model Guidelines was that unambiguous definitions of addiction-related terminology were included. Definitions that conformed to accepted clinical and scientific knowledge were provided for *addiction*, *physical dependence*, *tolerance*, and *pseudoaddiction*. These definitions clarified that physical dependence or tolerance is not sufficient to characterize addiction. Understanding and appropriately using correct terminology decreases the likelihood that health care professionals will diagnose patients using opioid analgesics for pain relief as "addicts" (37,68).

Finally, the Model Guidelines did not exclude patients with addictive disease from being treated for pain with opioids. The FSMB recognized that the decision to prescribe controlled substances to a patient should be based on clinical findings related to the individual patient; however, physicians were urged to "be diligent in preventing the diversion of drugs for illegitimate purposes" (51, p. 1).

In May 2004, the FSMB revised the Model Guidelines, entitled "Model Policy for the Use of Controlled Substances for the Treatment of Pain" (Model Policy) (69). The Model Policy contains substantially the same messages as the 1998 guidelines, but also includes language recognizing that physicians' failure to take action to adequately treat pain is a departure from current practice standards and subject to investigation and discipline. At this writing, 32 states have health care regulatory board policies that are based, either in whole or in part, on the Model Guidelines or Model Policy.

State Medical Board Policies The FSMB's policy templates have contributed to notable improvements in state health care regulatory policy since the late 1990s (70). A recent content evaluation found that there has been a significant increase in the number of state policies that appropriately distinguish "addiction" from physical dependence or tolerance (30); of these policies, health care board policies were more likely than policies created by state legislatures to clarify this correct distinction. However, a few medical board policies also indicate that it would be inappropriate to prescribe controlled substances to a person who not only currently uses drugs nontherapeutically, but "any person previously drug dependent." Such a complete prohibition is in sharp contrast to the FSMB's Model Policy, which establishes no limits for using opioids to treat patients with pain who have an addictive disease or a history of substance abuse, but rather provides the following treatment recommendations.

> . . . *If the patient is at high risk for medication abuse or has a history of substance abuse, the physician should consider the use of a written agreement between physician and patient outlining patient responsibilities. . . . The management of pain in patients with a history of substance abuse or with a co-morbid psychiatric disorder may require extra care, monitoring, documentation and consultation with or referral to an expert in the management of such patients* (69, pp. 6, 7).

Despite this model language, it is evident that a small number of state medical board policies intended to improve access to pain management continue to exclude patients who use (or have used) drugs for other than therapeutic purposes.

Consensus Statement Other national organizations also have attempted to improve and clarify the terms used to describe dependence and addiction. For example, in 2001 the American Academy of Pain Medicine, the American Pain Society, and the American Society of Addiction Medicine jointly published a statement on "Definitions Related to the Use of Opioids for the Treatment of Pain" (71). The statement contains definitions of *addiction*, *physical dependence*, and *tolerance* that reflect the prevailing medical and scientific knowledge about those conditions. The statement was developed through a consensus process to promote a level of consistency that will help optimize both pain management and the treatment of addictive disease, as well as improve communications among health care professionals, regulators, and law enforcement officials (11).

The three organizations created the following definitions and recommended their use:

- *Addiction*: Addiction is a primary, chronic, neurobiologic disease, with genetic, psychosocial, and environmental factors influencing its development and manifestations. It is characterized by behaviors that include one or more of the following: impaired control over drug use, compulsive use, continued use despite harm, and craving.
- *Physical dependence*: Physical dependence is a state of adaptation that is manifested by a drug class specific syndrome that can be produced by abrupt cessation, rapid dose reduction, decreasing blood level of the drug, or administration of an antagonist.
- *Tolerance*: Tolerance is a state of adaptation in which exposure to a drug induces changes that result in a diminution of one or more of the drug's effects over time" (71, p. 2).

These definitions then became the basis for those terms contained in the FSMB's recent Model Policy.

CONCLUSIONS

In recent years, pain management has become a higher priority in the U.S. health care system. This has occurred at the same time that prescription pain medication abuse and diversion has received increased attention, both professionally and in the media (72). The occurrence of these phenomena makes it all the more important to continue emphasizing the critical distinction between pain treatment and addiction. Federal law permits the use of opioids to treat acute and chronic pain, of both cancer and noncancer origins, in patients with drug abuse histories or addictive disease.

However, it is evident that some state policies, and the views of some state medical regulatory board members, can discourage practitioners from prescribing opioid analgesics to the patients who need them for pain relief, but who also have an addictive disease. It is necessary to identify and correct such policies. In addition, health care professionals must be educated about appropriately using controlled substances to manage pain, especially in patients with addictive disease or a substance abuse history, which remains a complex and intensive task.

Trained and experienced practitioners, who are knowledgeable about their state's policies, will be in a much better position to conform to the policy requirements and recommendations while evaluating their patient's medical needs and providing effective treatment.

ACKNOWLEDGMENTS: *The studies described in this article were supported by grants from the Federation of State Medical Boards, Inc., the Robert Wood Johnson Foundation, and the Advocates for Children's Pain Relief. Policy evaluation research conducted in 2006 and 2007 was funded by grants from the American Cancer Society and Susan G. Komen for the Cure, and through a cooperative agreement with the Lance Armstrong Foundation. The authors wish to thank David E. Joranson, MSSW, for his leadership in helping create and guide the U.S. policy research program.*

REFERENCES

1. Miaskowski C, Cleary J, Burney R, et al. *Guideline for the management of cancer pain in adults and children. APS Clinical Practice Guidelines Series, No. 3.* Glenview, IL: American Pain Society, 2005.
2. Portenoy RK, Sibirceva U, Smout R, et al. Opioid use and survival at the end of life: a survey of a hospice population. *J Pain Symptom Manage* 2006;32(6):532–540.
3. Stute P, Soukup J, Menzel M, et al. Analysis and treatment of different types of neuropathic cancer pain. *J Pain Symptom Manage* 2003;26(6): 1123–1131.
4. World Health Organization. *Cancer pain relief: with a guide to opioid availability,* 2nd ed. Geneva, Switzerland: World Health Organization, 1996.
5. Ballantyne JC, Mao J. Opioid therapy for chronic pain. *N Engl J Med* 2003;349(20):1943–1953.
6. Fishman SM. *Responsible opioid prescribing: a physician's guide.* Fine PG, Gallagher RM, Gilson AM, et al., eds. Washington, DC: Waterford Life Sciences, 2007.
7. Nicholson B, Passik S. Management of chronic noncancer pain in the primary care setting. *South Med J* 2007;100(10):1028–1036.
8. Portenoy R, Farrar JT, Backonja M, et al. Long-term use of controlled-release Oxycodone for noncancer pain: results of a 3-year registry study. *Clin J Pain* 2007;23(4):287–299.
9. Katz NP, Adams EH, Benneyan JC, et al. Foundations of opioid risk management. *Clin J Pain* 2007;23(2):103–118.
10. Passik S, Byers K, Kirsh KL. Empathy and failure to treat pain. *Palliat Sup Care* 2007;5:167–172.
11. Savage SR, Joranson DE, Covington EC, et al. Definitions related to the medical use of opioids: Evolution towards universal agreement. *J Pain Symptom Manage* 2003;26(1):655–667.
12. United Nations. *Single convention on narcotic drugs, 1961, as amended by the 1972 protocol amending the single convention on narcotic drugs, 1961.* New York: United Nations, 1977.
13. United Nations. *Convention on psychotropic substances, 1971.* Geneva, Switzerland: United Nations, 1971.
14. Gilson AM, Joranson DE, Maurer MA. Improving state pain policies: recent progress and continuing opportunities. *CA Cancer J Clin* 2007;57(6):341–353.
15. Joranson DE. Why is a balanced policy important, and do we have it now? In: Wilford BB, ed. *Balancing the response to prescription drug abuse, report of a national symposium on medicine and public policy.* Chicago, IL: American Medical Association, Department of Substance Abuse, 1990:1–6.
16. Pain & Policy Studies Group. *Achieving balance in federal and state pain policy: a guide to evaluation,* 4th ed. Madison, WI: University of Wisconsin Paul P. Carbone Comprehensive Cancer Center, 2007.
17. *United States v Evers.* 643 F2d 1043 5th Circuit, 1981.
18. Federal Register. *40 FR 15394.* 1975.
19. Federal Register. *48 FR 26733.* 1983.
20. Controlled Substances Act. Pub L No. 91-513, 84 Stat 1242, 1970.
21. Code of Federal Regulations. *Title 21 CFR Chapter II.*
22. Code of Federal Regulations. *Title 21 CFR § 1306.12(b).*
23. Code of Federal Regulations. *Title 21 CFR §1306.11(d).*
24. Code of Federal Regulations. *Title 21 CFR §1306.13.*
25. Code of Federal Regulations. *Title 21 CFR §1306.11(a).*
26. Code of Federal Regulations. *Title 42 CFR § 8.1 et seq.*
27. National Conference of Commissioners on Uniform State Laws. *Uniform Controlled Substances Act.* Chicago, IL: NCCUSL. Adopted at its annual conference meeting in its Ninety-Ninth Year: Milwaukee, WI, July 13–20, 1990.
28. National Conference of Commissioners on Uniform State Laws. *Uniform Controlled Substances Act.* NCCUSL: St. Louis, MO, 1970.
29. National Conference of Commissioners on Uniform State Laws. *Uniform Controlled Substances Act.* NCCUSL: Chicago, IL. Adopted at its Annual Conference Meeting in its One-Hundred-and-Third-Year: Chicago, IL, July 29–August 5, 1994.
30. Gilson AM, Maurer MA, Joranson DE. State policy affecting pain management: recent improvements and the positive impact of regulatory health policies. *Health Pol* 2005;74(2):192–204.
31. National Association of Boards of Pharmacy. *Survey of pharmacy law, 2000–2001.* Park Ridge, IL: National Association of Boards of Pharmacy, 2000.
32. Joranson DE, Carrow GM, Ryan KM, et al. Pain management and prescription monitoring. *J Pain Symptom Manage* 2002;23(3):231–238.
33. Wastila LJ, Bishop C. The influence of multiple copy prescription programs on analgesic utilization. *J Pharm Care Pain Symptom Control* 1996; 4(3):3–19.
34. World Health Organization. *The ICD-10 classification of mental and behavioral disorders: clinical descriptions and diagnostic guidelines.* Geneva, Switzerland: World Health Organization, 1992.
35. American Psychiatric Association. *Diagnostic and statistical manual of mental disorders,* 4th ed. Washington, DC: American Psychiatric Association, 1994.
36. World Health Organization. *WHO Expert Committee on Drug Dependence: twenty-eighth report.* Geneva, Switzerland: World Health Organization, 1993.
37. Gilson AM, Joranson DE. U.S. policies relevant to the prescribing of opioid analgesics for the treatment of pain in patients with addictive disease. *Clin J Pain* 2002;18(4 suppl):91–98.
38. Weissman DE, Haddox JD. Opioid pseudoaddiction—an iatrogenic syndrome. *Pain* 1989;36:363–366.
39. *State of Wisconsin v. Holly,* Case No. 96 CF 978 1997.
40. Controlled Substances Act. *Title 21 USC §802(1).*
41. Code of Federal Regulations. *Title 21 CFR §291.505(a)(5).*
42. Joranson DE. Is methadone maintenance the last resort for some chronic pain patients? *Am Pain Soc Bull* 1997;7(5):1, 4–5.
43. Tennant FS. *The dilemma of severe incurable, narcotic-dependent pain patients referred to narcotic treatment programs: need for administrative, regulatory, and legislative relief.* West Covina, CA: Research Center for Dependency Disorders and Chronic Pain Community Health Projects Medical Group, 1996.
44. Code of Federal Regulations. *Title 42 CFR §8.12.*
45. Gilson AM. Interpreting changes in state laws and regulations governing the use of controlled substances to treat pain. *Adv Pain Manage* 2007;1(2):60–66.
46. Gilson AM, Joranson DE, Maurer MA, et al. Progress to achieve balanced state policy relevant to pain management and palliative care: 2000–2003. *J Pain Palliat Care Pharmacother* 2005;19(1):7–20.
47. Joranson DE, Dahl JL. Achieving balance in drug policy: the Wisconsin model. In: Hill CS, Jr., Fields WS, eds. *Advances in pain research and therapy,* volume 11. New York: Raven Press, 1989:197–204.

48. Joranson DE, Gilson AM. Improving pain management through policy making and education for medical regulators. *J Law Med Ethics* 1996; 24(4):344–347.
49. Joranson DE, Gilson AM. State intractable pain policy: current status. *Am Pain Soc Bull* 1997;7(2):7–9.
50. Institute of Medicine Committee on Care at the End of Life. *Approaching death: improving care at the end of life*. Washington, DC: National Academy Press, 1997.
51. Federation of State Medical Boards of the United States Inc. *Model guidelines for the use of controlled substances for the treatment of pain*. Euless, TX: Federation of State Medical Boards of the United States Inc., 1998.
52. Jacox A, Carr DB, Payne R, et al. *Management of cancer pain. Clinical practice guideline number 9, AHCPR No. 94-0592*. Rockville, MD: Agency for Health Care Policy and Research, U.S. Department of Health and Human Services, Public Health Service, 1994.
53. Merritt D, Fox-Grage W, Rothouse M, et al. *State initiatives in end-of-life care: policy guide for state legislators*. Washington, DC: National Conference of States Legislatures, 1998.
54. Joranson DE, Gilson AM, Ryan KM, et al. *Achieving balance in federal and state pain policy: a guide to evaluation*. Madison, WI: Pain & Policy Studies Group, University of Wisconsin Comprehensive Cancer Center, 2000.
55. Pain & Policy Studies Group. *Achieving balance in federal and state pain policy: a guide to evaluation*, 2nd ed. Madison, WI: University of Wisconsin Comprehensive Cancer Center, 2003.
56. Pain & Policy Studies Group. *Achieving balance in federal and state pain policy: a guide to evaluations*. Madison, WI: University of Wisconsin Paul P. Carbone Comprehensive Cancer Center, 2006.
57. Texas Intractable Pain Treatment Act. Occupations Code, Title 71. Health-Public, Chapter 6. Medicine, Article 4495c.
58. Hill CS, Jr. The negative influence of licensing and disciplinary boards and drug enforcement agencies on pain treatment with opioid analgesics. *J Pharm Care Pain Symptom Control* 1993;1(1):43–62.
59. Joranson DE, Gilson AM. Controlled substances, medical practice, and the law. In: Schwartz HI, ed. *Psychiatric practice under fire: the influence of government, the media, and special interests on somatic therapies*. Washington DC: American Psychiatric Press, Inc., 1994:173–194.
60. Haddox JD, Aronoff GM. Commentary: the potential for unintended consequences from public policy shifts in the treatment of pain. *J Law Med Ethics* 1998;26(4):350–352.
61. Martino AM. In search of a new ethic for treating patients with chronic pain: what can medical boards do? *J Law Med Ethics* 1998;26(4): 332–349.
62. Weissman DE, Joranson DE, Hopwood MB. Wisconsin physicians' knowledge and attitudes about opioid analgesic regulations. *Wisc Med J* 1991(December):671–675.
63. Turk DC, Brody MC, Akiko Okifuji E. Physicians' attitudes and practices regarding the long-term prescribing of opioids for non-cancer pain. *Pain* 1994;59:201–208.
64. Joranson DE, Cleeland CS, Weissman DE, et al. Opioids for chronic cancer and non-cancer pain: a survey of state medical board members. *Fed Bull J Med Licensure Discipline* 1992;79(4):15–49.
65. Gilson AM, Joranson DE. Controlled substances and pain management: changes in knowledge and attitudes of state medical regulators. *J Pain Symptom Manage* 2001;21(3):227–237.
66. Gilson AM, Maurer MA, Joranson DE. State medical board members' beliefs about pain, addiction, and diversion and abuse: a changing regulatory environment. *J Pain* 2007;8(9):682–691.
67. Zimbal M, Cleary J, Gilson AM, et al. Wisconsin physicians' beliefs and attitudes about the use of opioid analgesics. *J Pain* 2007;7(4 suppl 2):597.
68. Maurer MA, Gilson AM, Joranson DE. Federal and state policies at the interface of pain and addiction. In: Smith H, Passik S, eds. *Pain and chemical dependency*. New York: Oxford University Press, 2008:377–383.
69. Federation of State Medical Boards of the United States Inc. *Model policy for the use of controlled substances for the treatment of pain*. Dallas, TX: Federation of State Medical Boards of the United States Inc., 2004.
70. Gilson AM, Joranson DE, Maurer MA. Improving state medical board policies: influence of a model. *J Law Med Ethics* 2003;31(1):119–129.
71. American Academy of Pain Medicine, American Pain Society, American Society of Addiction Medicine. *Definitions related to the use of opioids for the treatment of pain*. Glenview, IL: AAPM, APS, ASAM, 2001.
72. Gilson AM, Ryan KM, Joranson DE, Dahl JL. A reassessment of trends in the medical use and abuse of opioid analgesics and implications for diversion control: 1997–2002. *J Pain Symptom Manage* 2004;28(2): 176–188.

SECTION 13

Children and Adolescents

CHAPTER 97

Melissa Weddle, MD, MPH
Patricia K. Kokotailo, MD, MPH

Epidemiology of Adolescent Substance Abuse

EPIDEMIOLOGY OF ADOLESCENT SUBSTANCE USE

Epidemiology has historically been defined as "the study of the distribution of a disease or a physiological condition in human populations and of the factors that influence this distribution" (1). Within this framework, epidemiology of adolescent substance use documents the incidence of substance use and correlates of use. Because adolescent substance use may be viewed as a continuum from experimentation to alcohol or drug dependence, it is more helpful to describe use patterns—behaviors that may influence health rather than incidence of disease (i.e., addiction or problem use).

There are several excellent sources of information about prevalence and trends of adolescent substance use including the Monitoring the Future Survey, Youth Risk Behavior Surveillance Survey, and National Survey on Drug Use and Health (Table 97.1). The primary source of information for this chapter is Monitoring the Future, a national survey of drug use that has been administered annually since 1975 and offers a comprehensive view of the factors that influence drug use. In addition to surveying young people about drug use, this survey addresses important factors such as beliefs about the dangers of drugs, and perceived availability.

The 2008 Monitoring the Future surveyed more than 46,000 students from 386 public and private high schools, chosen to offer a nationally representative sample. Between 1975 and 1991, the survey included 12th graders only. Starting in 1991, the survey included 8th and 10th graders. Because this survey is administered within the school setting, groups at high risk of substance use such as truants, dropouts and runaways, are not included, possibly resulting in incidences that are artificially low.

This chapter will review trends of individual substance use including alcohol, tobacco, marijuana, amphetamines, narcotics, cocaine, inhalants, and prescription drugs. Adolescents commonly do use more than one substance, so available information about multiple drug use will be presented. In addition, information about subgroups, examining gender, race/ethnicity, and educational aspirations will be presented. Unless otherwise indicated, all trend and prevalence data is derived from the Monitoring the Future Survey.

PREVALENCE AND TRENDS

Until 1978, use of illicit drugs among 12th graders increased steadily from year to year, then decreased until the early 1990s, again climbing through the decade, and more gradually decreasing in the early years of the 21st century (Fig. 97.1). Since the inclusion of 8th and 10th graders in the 1991 survey, their trends have paralleled those of 12th graders, though at lower levels (2). In 2008, 37% of 12th graders, 27% of 10th graders, and 14% of 8th graders reported use of an illicit drug in the past year (3).

Alcohol As use of other illicit drugs decreased throughout the 1980s, monthly prevalence use of alcohol among 12th graders declined as well, from 72% in 1980 to 51% in 1992 (Fig. 97.2). Daily alcohol use in this group also declined over this period from a peak of 6.9% in 1979 to 3.4% in 1992. The prevalence of drinking five or more drinks in a row within the past 2 weeks (heavy drinking) declined from 41% in 1980 to 23% in 1993. Trends of alcohol use have overall followed the trends of illicit drug, rising and falling in concert (2).

TABLE 97.1 Sources of Adolescent Substance Use Data

Survey	Year initiated	Sample size	Funding agency
Monitoring the Future www.monitoringthefuture.org	1975	45,000	National Institute of Drug Abuse (NIDA)
Youth Risk Behavior Survey www.cdc.gov/HealthyYouth/yrbs	1991	15,000	Centers for Disease Control (CDC)
National Survey on Drug Use and Health www.oas.samhsa.gov/nhsda.htm	1979	25,000 (age 12–17)	Substance Abuse and Mental Health Services Administration (SAMHSA)

In 2008, 39% of 8th graders, 62% of 10th graders, and 72% of 12th graders report having tried alcohol (3). Of greater public health concern is prevalence of episodic heavy drinking, or "binge drinking" (defined as five or more drinks in a row at least once during the past 2 weeks). Heavy drinking was reported in 2007 (the most recent year for which data are available) by 10% of 8th graders, 22% of 10th graders, 26% of 12th graders, and 40% of college students. For secondary school students, binge drinking increased gradually during the 1990s and modestly declined in the early years of the 21st century (2) (Fig. 97.3).

College students show different trends in alcohol use than those for 12th graders or respondents of the same age not attending college. Between 1980 and 1993, college students showed less of a decrease in both monthly prevalence of alcohol use and occasions of drinking. Heavy drinking has changed little among college students with 41% of college students reporting binge drinking in 2007, the same as in 1993. This compares with 34% of age-mates not attending college and 25% of high school seniors (Fig. 97.4). Daily drinking rates of college students have generally been lower than same-age peers not attending college, suggesting a pattern of drinking primarily on weekends, when they tend to drink a lot (4).

For both high school and college students, males report higher rates of binge drinking than females, though the gender differences have narrowed gradually over the duration of the survey (2).

Tobacco Since the survey began in 1975, cigarettes have consistently been the abusable substance most frequently used on a daily basis by high school students. During the 1980s, smoking among adolescents did not decline, even though smoking rates were steadily decreasing among adults. Among 8th and

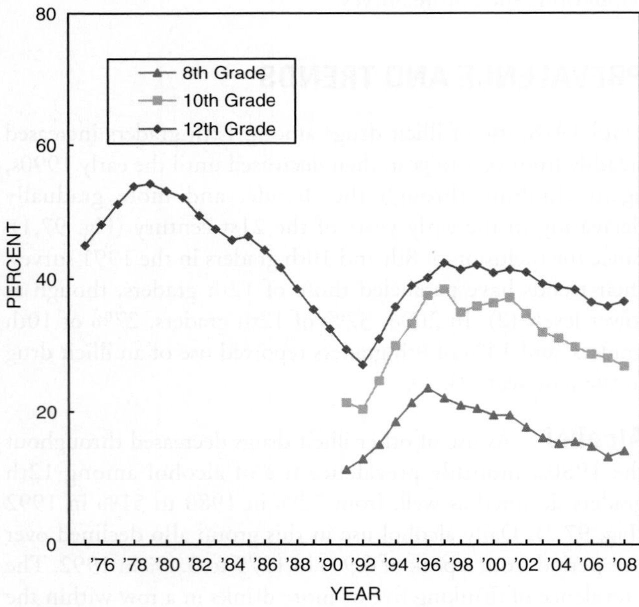

FIGURE 97.1. Illicit drugs. Percentage who have used an illicit drug in the past year. (From The Monitoring the Future study, University of Michigan, http://monitoringthefuture.org/data/08data/fig08_1.pdf.)

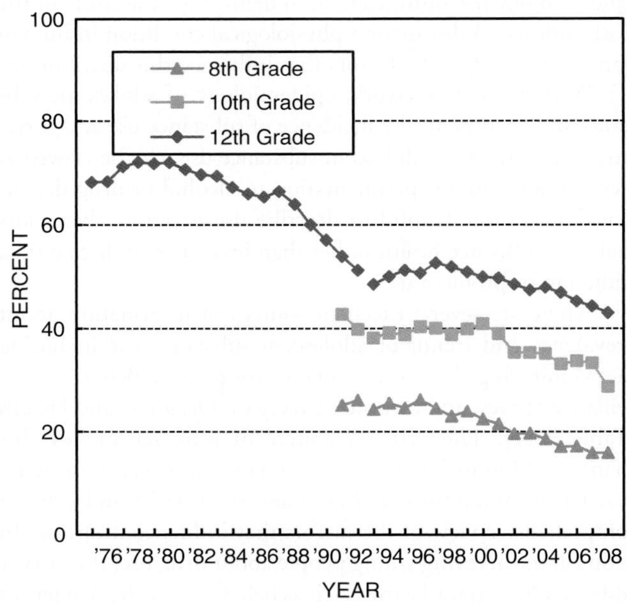

FIGURE 97.2. Alcohol. Percentage who have used in the past 30 days. (From The Monitoring the Future study, University of Michigan, http://monitoringthefuture.org/data/08data/fig08_14.pdf.)

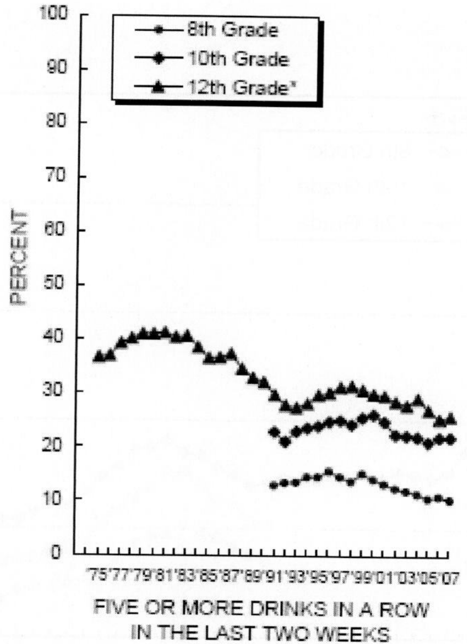

FIGURE 97.3. Alcohol. Percentage who report having five or more drinks in a row in last 2 weeks. (From *Monitoring the Future national survey results on drug use, 1975–2007: Volume 1, Secondary school students,* http://www.monitoringthefuture.org/pubs/monographs/vol1_2007.pdf.)

10th graders, rates of those who report current smoking (defined as having smoked in the past 30 days) increased from 1991 to 1996, reaching a peak of 21.0% and 30.4% respectively and for 12th graders, peaked at 36.5% in 1997 (Fig. 97.5). Since those peaks, rates have steadily decreased for all three groups, with 7.1% of 8th graders, 14.0% of 10th graders, and 20.4% of 12th graders reporting current smoking (2). Between 1975 and 1990, 12th grade boys and girls followed parallel trends of smoking, with a higher percentage of boys reporting daily cigarette use. Since 1991, rates of daily smoking have been similar for boys and girls at all grade levels (5).

Among college students, the peak rate in current smoking (31%) was reached in 1991, then declined moderately until 2006, when a significant decline to 19% was seen, remaining stable at 19.9% in 2007. Daily smoking among college students increased by nearly half from 1994 to 1999, and thereafter decreased, reaching 9.3% in 2007. From 1980 until 1993, college males generally smoked at higher rates than females, but from 1994 through 2007, males and females have smoked at the same rates (4).

Marijuana Of the illicit drugs, marijuana use remains the most prevalent. Before the initiation of the Monitoring the Future study, marijuana use rose sharply during the late 1960s and early 1970s from negligible levels (6). This rise peaked in the late 1970s and then use gradually decreased throughout the 1980s until 1992, when use again rose sharply (Fig. 97.6). During the 1990s, the annual prevalence rates of marijuana rose rapidly peaking at 18.3% in 1996 for 8th graders, 34.8% in 1997 for 10th graders, and 38.5% in 1997 for 12th graders (2). Since 2001, all three grades have showed significant declines in the annual prevalence rates. In 2008, the annual prevalence rates for marijuana were 11%, 24%, and 32% for grades 8, 10, and 12, respectively (3).

Comparison of daily marijuana use between college students, young adults 1 to 4 years past high school, and 12th graders from 1980 on shows highest use has been among the young adults not attending college, and lowest use among 12th graders. Rates between all groups were comparable in the early 1990s, with the rate among young adults increasing more markedly through the late 1990s. In 2007, 3.7% of college students and 5.0% of young adults reported using marijuana on a daily basis (4).

Amphetamines Between 1982 and 1992, annual prevalence rates for nonprescription amphetamine use among 12th graders declined considerably, from 20.3% to 7.1% (Fig. 97.7). Among college students, rates fell even more dramatically over the same interval, from 21.1% to 3.6%.

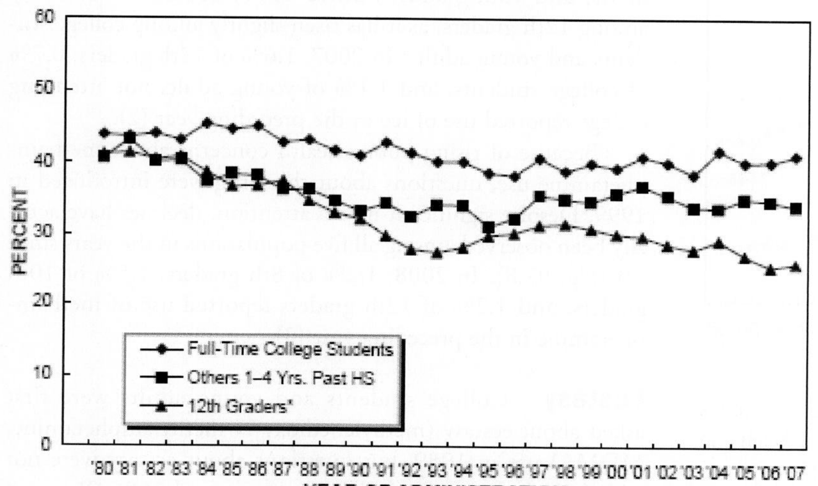

FIGURE 97.4. Alcohol. Percentage who report having five or more drinks in a row in the past 2 weeks: college students, others 1 to 4 years beyond high school, and 12th graders. (*From Monitoring the Future national survey results on drug use, 1975–2007: Volume II, College students and adults ages 19–45,* http://www.monitoringthefuture.org/pubs/monographs/vol2_2007.pdf.)

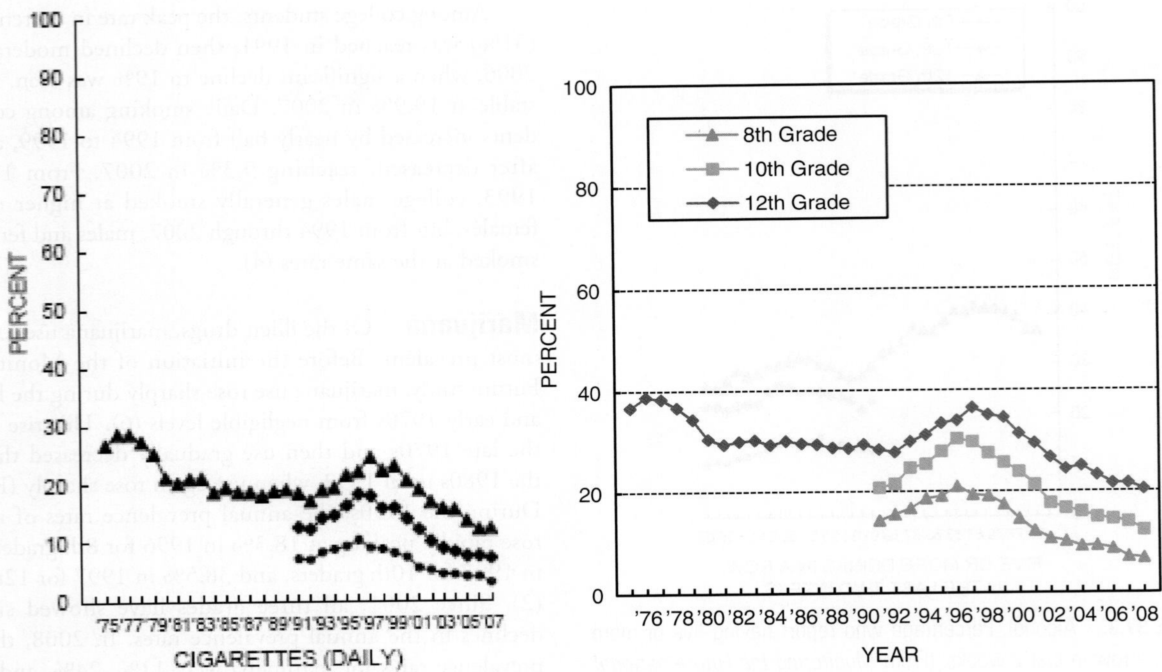

FIGURE 97.5. Cigarettes. Percentage who have used in past 30 days and who have used daily during past 30 days. (From *Monitoring the Future national survey results on drug use, 1975–2007: Volume I, Secondary school students,* http://www.monitoringthefuture.org/pubs/monographs/vol1_2007.pdf (left panel) and http://monitoringthefuture.org/data/08data/fig08_1.pdf (right panel)).

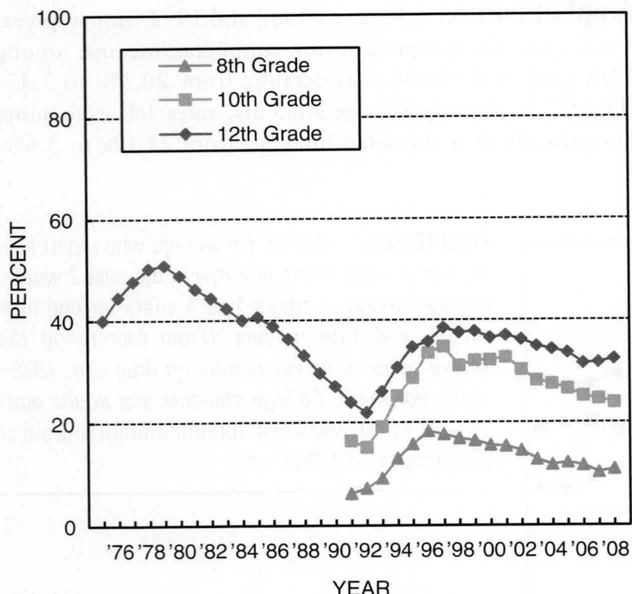

FIGURE 97.6. Marijuana. Percentage who used in past 12 months. (From The Monitoring the Future study, University of Michigan, http://monitoringthefuture.org/data/08data/fig08_11.pdf.)

During the 1990s, annual use increased in all grades, as well as in college students. In 2008, 8th, 10th, and 12th graders reported lifetime prevalence use of 4.5%, 6.4%, and 6.8%, respectively (2).

Methamphetamine Beginning in 1990, Monitoring the Future has included questions about use of "ice" (crystallized methamphetamine, typically smoked). Use of this drug increased during the 1990s among 12th graders, college students, and young adults. Since 1999, use has held steady among 12th graders, as it has risen slightly among college students and young adults. In 2007, 1.6% of 12th graders, 0.7% of college students, and 1.1% of young adults not attending college reported use of ice in the preceding year (2).

Because of rising public health concerns about methamphetamine use, questions about this drug were introduced in 1999. Despite significant media attention, declines have actually been observed among all five populations in the years since (2) (Fig. 97.8). In 2008, 1.2% of 8th graders, 1.5% of 10th graders, and 1.2% of 12th graders reported use of methamphetamine in the preceding year (3).

Ecstasy College students and young adults were first asked about ecstasy (methylenedioxy-N-methylamphetamine, MDMA) use in 1989, but questions about ecstasy were not added to the secondary school surveys until 1996. Between

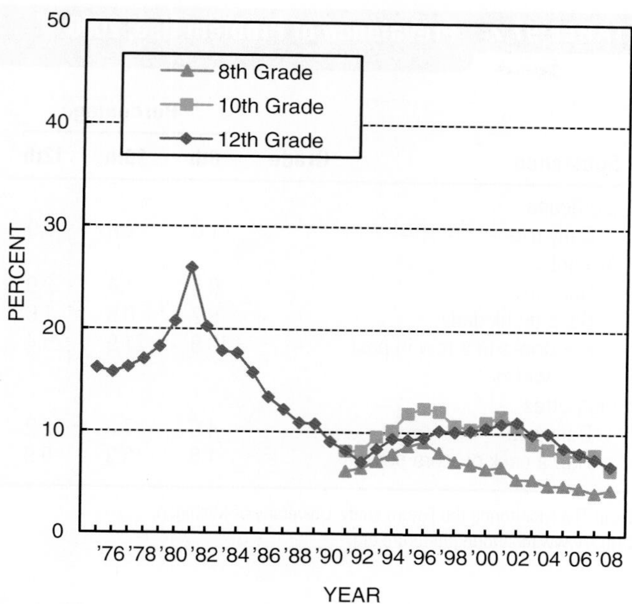

FIGURE 97.7. Amphetamines. Percentage who used in last 12 months. (From The Monitoring the Future study, University of Michigan, http://monitoringthefuture.org/data/08data/fig08_2.pdf.)

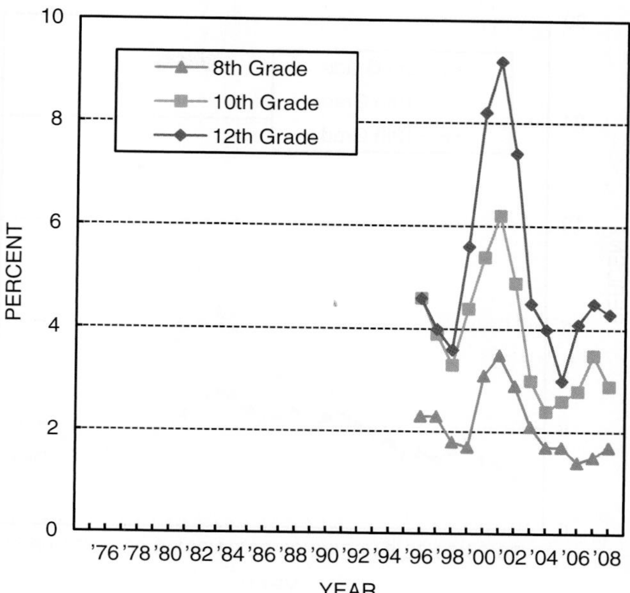

FIGURE 97.9. Ecstasy. Percentage who used in past 12 months. (From The Monitoring the Future study, University of Michigan, http://monitoringthefuture.org/data/08data/fig08_7.pdf.)

1989 and 1994, annual prevalence rates were low for the older age groups, but in 1995, rates increased significantly, from 0.5% to 2.4% in college students. When first surveyed in 1996, 10th and 12th graders had higher rates of annual use (4.6% for both) than the college students (Fig. 97.9). Between 1998 and 2001, use rates increased dramatically in high school students, college students, and young adults. Since 2001, use rates decreased for the next 2 years, and have remained generally stable since 2003 (2). In 2008, 1.7% of 8th graders, 2.9% of 10th graders, and 4.3% of 12th graders reported use of ecstasy in the preceding year (3).

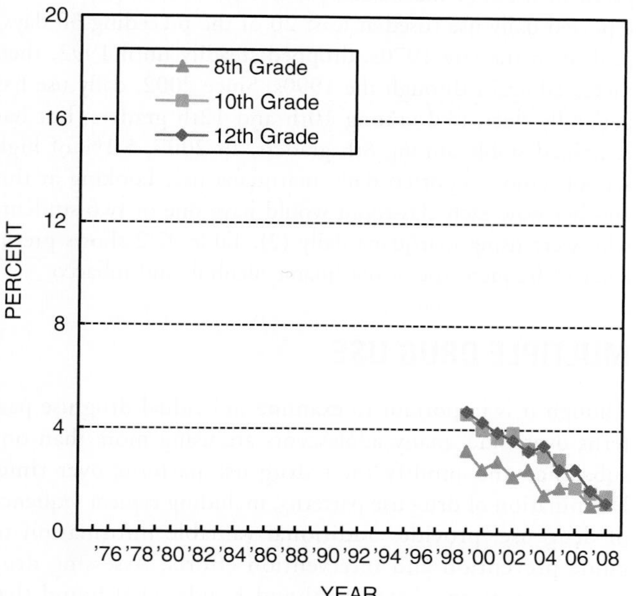

FIGURE 97.8. Methamphetamine. Percentage who used in past month. (From The Monitoring the Future study, University of Michigan, http://monitoringthefuture.org/data/08data/fig08_3.pdf.)

Cocaine Crack cocaine (the rock form of cocaine) use rapidly increased during the early 1980s. Thereafter, annual prevalence dropped sharply, where it has remained quite low, likely because of its perception as a dangerous drug (see sidebar). For powdered cocaine in general, use began to decline a year earlier than for crack. This was likely related to the intense media campaign publicizing the drug's dangers and certainly influenced by the cocaine-related deaths of sports stars Len Bias and Don Rogers (2). In 2008, 1.8% of 8th graders, 3.0% of 10th graders, and 4.4% of 12th graders reported use of cocaine in the preceding year (3).

Inhalants Inhalants include common household substances such as glues, aerosols, and solvents, inhaled to get high. This is the only class of drugs for which use is substantially higher in 8th grade than 10th or 12th grade. Among all high school students, there was a marked increase in inhalant use during the early 1990s, followed by a decrease after 1995 (Fig. 97.10). Since 2002, inhalant use has remained stable (2). In 2008, 8.9% of 8th graders, 5.9% of 10th graders, and 3.8% of 12th graders report inhalant use in the preceding year (3).

Heroin Between 1975 and 1979, the annual prevalence use of heroin among 12th graders fell from 1.0% to 0.5%, then remained stable through 1993. Thereafter, use increased for 8th, 10th, and 12th graders. This upturn was likely related to

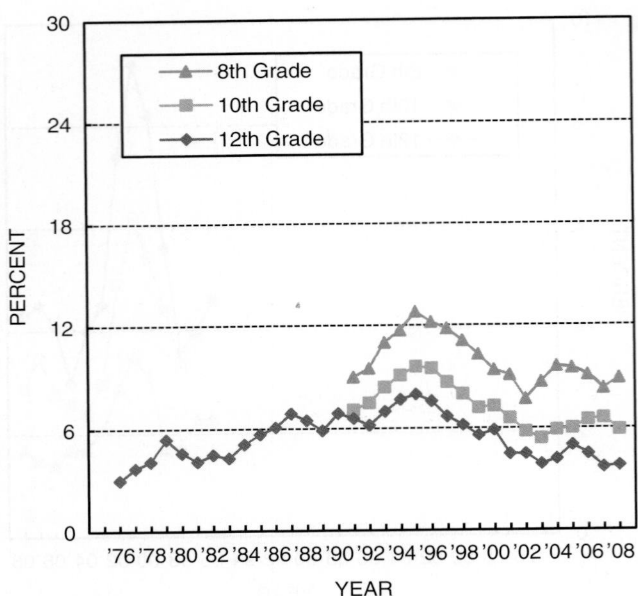

FIGURE 97.10. Inhalants. Percentage who used in past 12 months. (From The Monitoring the Future study, University of Michigan, http://monitoringthefuture.org/data/08data/fig08_12.pdf.)

the decline in perceived risk, as well as the availability of more pure heroin, which allowed use by other means than injection. For 12th graders, college students and young adults, rates doubled or tripled in 1 to 2 years, remaining at the new higher levels for the rest of the decade (2). Between 2000 and 2002, use began to decrease and in 2007, all groups had annual prevalence rates below the recent peaks. In 2008, 0.9% of 8th graders, 0.8% of 10th graders, and 0.7% of 12th graders reported use of heroin in the preceding year (3).

Anabolic Steroids Questions about anabolic steroid use were first included in the 1989 survey. At that time, 1.9% of 12th graders reported annual use, which dropped to 1.1% by 1992, then slowly increased to 1.8% by 1999. Use rose to 2.5% by 2002, where it remained until 2005, when it dropped to 1.5%. Annual prevalence use for 12th graders was 1.4% in 2007. Rates have been substantially lower among girls than boys (2).

Prescription Drugs Overall trends in nonmedical use of opioids, stimulants, and sedative/anxiety medications show increased use since 2000 (2). Young people may perceive prescription drugs as less harmful compared with street drugs, and therefore may be more inclined to use them (7). In a study of Detroit area secondary students in 2005, 20.9% reported lifetime nonmedical use of an opioid, stimulant, sleeping, or sedative/anxiety medication. Lifetime prevalence use was highest for pain medication (17.7%) followed by sleeping (5.9%), sedative/anxiety (3.5%), and stimulant medications (2.4%) (8). Of a sample of 3,939 college students in 2005, 20.2% reported nonmedical use of at least one of these medications. In this group, lifetime prevalence use was highest for pain

TABLE 97.2 Prevalence of Problem Use, 2006

Substance	Grade	Percentage 8th	10th	12th
Marijuana				
Daily use		1.0	2.8	5.0
Alcohol				
Daily use		0.5	1.4	3.0
Been drunk daily		0.2	0.5	1.6
5+ drinks in a row in past 2 weeks		10.9	21.9	25.4
Cigarettes				
Daily use		4.0	7.6	12.2
Half a pack or more per day		1.5	3.3	5.9

From The Monitoring the Future study, University of Michigan, http://www.monitoringthefuture.org.

medication (14.3%), followed by stimulant medication (8.5%), sleeping medication (4.4%), and sedative/anxiety medication (4.4%) (9). Adolescents identify peers and family members as the primary sources for these drugs (10,11).

MORE FREQUENT USE

Much of the previous trend data focuses on annual or lifetime prevalence use of individual drugs. Experimentation is a normal part of adolescent development, and rare or occasional use of a substance may not constitute problem use for most individuals. Frequency of use provides a more accurate measure of problem use. For marijuana, percentage of 12th graders who reported daily use (used at least 20 of the preceding 30 days) peaked in the late 1970s, dropped steadily until 1992, then increased again through the 1990s. Since 2002, daily use has generally decreased among 10th and 12th graders, but has remained stable among 8th graders. In 2007, 5.1% of high school seniors reported daily marijuana use. Looking at this another way, each classroom would have one or two students who were using marijuana daily (2). Table 97.2 shows prevalence of frequent use of marijuana, alcohol, and tobacco.

MULTIPLE DRUG USE

Though it is important to examine individual drug use patterns over time, many adolescents are using more than one substance and modify their drug use patterns over time. Examination of drug use patterns, including typical sequence of drug use, provides additional valuable information to guide prevention and intervention efforts. Assessing drug sequence patterns, Yamaguchi and Kandel (12) found that adolescent drug use typically begins with alcohol or cigarette use, followed by marijuana use, then by other illicit drugs, a finding that has been confirmed by other studies. A more recent study by Golub and Johnson (13) demonstrates a change over time of the probabilities of progression, with those born since the 1960s being substantially less likely to progress from cigarette and alcohol use to marijuana, cocaine, and heroin use.

None of the national surveys cited here includes population information about adolescents who use multiple substances. Drug use patterns of persons admitted to treatment in publicly funded facilities is available through the Drug and Alcohol Services Information System. Of those persons younger than 20 years, 65% reported polydrug use. Of those younger than 20 years, 54% reported polydrug use involving alcohol, and 9% reported alcohol use alone. In this age group, 60% reported polydrug use involving marijuana (or hashish), whereas 22% reported use of marijuana (or hashish) alone (14). Martin et al. found that, among adolescent drinkers, significantly more who have been diagnosed with alcohol dependence or abuse reported recent use of other drugs than drinkers without an alcohol diagnosis (15).

CORRELATES OF SUBSTANCE USE

Among ethnic/racial subgroups, there are varying associations with substance use. When looking at differences among African American, Hispanic, and white students, it is seen that African American 12th graders have consistently lower usage rages than white 12th graders for most drugs. The differences are quite large for many drugs such as inhalants, LSD, powder cocaine, amphetamines, methamphetamine, and tranquilizers. African American students have a lower 30-day prevalence rate of cigarette smoking compared with white students. In the 2007 survey, African American 12th graders were less likely to report heavy drinking (12%) compared with white students (30%) and Hispanic students (23%) (2,5).

Among 12th graders of these three racial/ethnic groups, whites have the highest rates of use of many drugs, including marijuana, hallucinogens, ecstasy, amphetamines, sedatives, tranquilizers, alcohol, getting drunk, cigarettes, and smokeless tobacco. Hispanics have the highest usage rates for some of the more dangerous drugs, such as cocaine, heroin, crack, crystal methamphetamine, and inhalants. In 8th grade, Hispanics have the highest rates for not only these drugs, but for many of the others as well, such as marijuana and binge drinking. This suggests that their considerably higher high school dropout rates may change their relative ranking by 12th grade. For virtually all of the illicit drugs, the three groups have tended to trend in parallel (2).

Comparison of those students who plan to complete 4 years of college with those who do not shows that for all drugs, trends are the same, but those who aspire to complete college use at lower rates. Regarding those who have had five or more drinks in a row in past 2 weeks, the differences between the two groups are narrower among 12th graders than for 8th and 10th graders. For those who smoke cigarettes daily, the differences remain large for all groups, as for the illicit drugs (5).

CONCLUSIONS

Examination of the epidemiology of substance use has played an important role in understanding the etiology of drug use, as well giving valuable insight into the attitudes and norms that influence substance use. Ongoing analysis of use and attitude trends will continue to provide important information for development of public health strategies to combat adolescent substance use. Examination of epidemiologic trends will also aid in the development of research and education priorities to further our knowledge in this area.

REFERENCES

1. Lilienfeld MD. Definitions of epidemiology. *Am J Epidemiol* 1976;107 (2):87–90.
2. Johnston LD, O'Malley PM, Bachman JG, et al. *Monitoring the future national survey results on drug use, 1975–2007: volume I, secondary school students* (NIH Publication No. 08-6418A). Bethesda, MD: National Institute on Drug Abuse, 2008.
3. Johnston LD, O'Malley PM, Bachman JG, et al. (December 11, 2008). *Various stimulant drugs show continuing declines among teens in 2008, most illicit drugs hold steady.* University of Michigan News Services: Ann Arbor, MI [Online]. Available: www.monitoringthefuture.org: accessed 12/16/2008.
4. Johnston LD, O'Malley PM, Bachman JG, et al. *Monitoring the future national survey results on drug use, 1975–2007: volume II, college students and adults ages 19–45* (NIH Publication No. 08-6418B). Bethesda, MD: National Institute on Drug Abuse, 2008.
5. Johnston LD, O'Malley PM, Bachman JG, et al. *Demographic subgroup trends for various licit and illicit drugs. 1975–2006* (Monitoring the Future Occasional Paper No. 67) [Online]. Ann Arbor. Available: www.monitoringthefuture.org; accessed March 10, 2008.
6. Substance Abuse and Mental Health Services Administration. *Results from the 2002 National Survey on Drug Use and Health: national findings* (Office of Applied Studies, NHSDA Series H-22, DHHS Publication No. SMA 03-3836). Rockville, MD, 2003.
7. Hertz JA, Knight JR. Prescription drug misuse: a growing national problem. *Adolesc Med* 2006;17:751–769.
8. McCabe SE, Boyd CJ, Young A. Medical and nonmedical use of prescription drugs among secondary school students. *J Adolesc Health* 2007; 40:76–83.
9. McCabe SE. Screening for drug abuse among medical and nonmedical users of prescription drugs in a probability sample of college students. *Arch Pediatr Adolesc Med* 2008;163(3):225–231.
10. McCabe SE, Boyd CJ. Sources of prescription drugs for illicit use. *Addict Behav* 2005;30:1342–1350.
11. Boyd CJ, McCabe SE, Teter CJ. Medical and nonmedical use of prescription pain medication by youth in a Detroit-area public school district. *Drug Alcohol Depend* 2006;81:37–45.
12. Yamaguchi K, Kandel DB. Patterns of drug use from adolescence to young adulthood. II. Sequences of progression. *Am J Public Health* 1983; 74:668–667.
13. Golub A, Johnson BD. Variation in youthful risks of progression from alcohol and tobacco to marijuana and to hard drugs across generations. *Am J Public Health* 2001;91(2):225–232.
14. The DASIS Report, March 25, 2005. Substance Abuse and Mental Health Services Administration (SAMHSA). *Polydrug admissions: 2002.* Available: www.oas.samhsa.gov; accessed March 10, 2008.
15. Martin CS, Kaczynski NA, Maisto SA, et al. Polydrug use in adolescent drinkers with and without DSM-IV alcohol abuse and dependence. *Alcohol Clin Exp Res* 1996;20(6):1099–1108.

Adolescents' Attitudes Toward Alcohol and Other Drugs

Melissa Weddle, MD, MPH, and Patricia K. Kokotailo, MD, MPH

An adolescent's perception toward alcohol and other drugs influences his or her decision about whether to use those substances. In addition to asking adolescents about history of alcohol and other drug use, Monitoring the Future includes questions about beliefs and attitudes, specifically about perceived harm of individual drugs and the degree to which the adolescent disapproves of the drug. Understanding attitudes about drug use is essential for interpretation of use trends as well as for development of effective interventions.

Overall, the Monitoring the Future data show inverse relationships between the level of drug use and both the perceived risk and disapproval of that drug. Of the illicit drugs, marijuana has the highest level of use and the lowest level of perceived risk and disapproval of use. In contrast, cocaine, perceived as a high-risk drug, has lower levels of use (1).

Over the lifetime of the study, many attitudes and beliefs have changed dramatically. The trends for marijuana use and attitudes strikingly illustrate the relationship between perceived harm and use (Fig.). Between 1975 and 1978, perceived harm of marijuana decreased markedly as use sharply increased. Beginning in 1979, the media gave attention to increasing rates of marijuana use and potential risks of the drug. Subsequently, the attitudes and beliefs among 12th graders shifted during the next decade. In 1992, perceived risk began to drop again, followed by a sharp increase in use beginning in 1993 (2).

Another drug that demonstrates this relationship is ecstasy, first added to the high school survey in 1996 after public health concerns about rising use. Annual prevalence of use peaked in 2001 at 6.2% for 10th graders and 9.2% for 12th graders. In 2002 and 2003, use decreased sharply. Perceived risk of ecstasy changed little until 2001, when it increased sharply, a trend that continued until 2004 (1). Again, amplified media attention to the health consequences of ecstasy have likely contributed to the dramatic decrease in use.

Not surprising, adolescents perceive a drug's harmfulness to be related to the frequency of use. Twelfth graders attribute a lower level of risk to trying most drugs once or twice (experimental use) than they do to regular use of drugs. For marijuana, only 19% of 12th graders associate great risk to experimenting, compared with 55% who see great risk in occasional or regular use (2). Even so, 57% of 12th graders associate great risk with even experimental use

Marijuana: trends in perceived availability, perceived risk of regular use, and prevalence of use in past 30 days for 12th graders. (From *Monitoring the Future national survey results on drug use, 1975–2007: Volume I, Secondary school students:* http://www.monitoringthefuture.org/pubs/monographs/vol1_2007.pdf.)

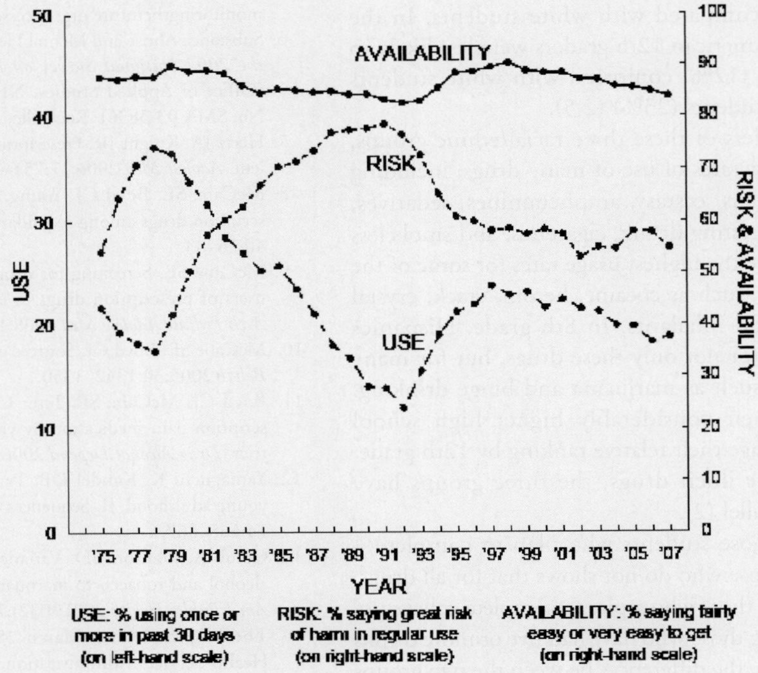

Adolescents' Attitudes Toward Alcohol and Other Drugs *(continued)*

of anabolic steroids, 58% for ecstasy and heroin, and 51% for cocaine (1).

In general, 8th and 10th graders perceive risk similarly to 12th graders, though there are some conspicuous differences. One concerning difference is perceived harm of regular cigarette smoking. Among 12th graders, 77% see great risk in smoking a pack a more per day, but only 61% of 8th graders see great risk. Unfortunately, perceived risk is lowest at ages at which smoking initiation is likely to occur (1). This points to a need for targeted, developmentally appropriate educational interventions for the younger ages.

Another factor in an individual's decision about whether to use a given drug may be the perceived benefits of using that drug. As a new drug becomes available, word may quickly spread about the positive effects, with a delay before information about adverse consequences can be disseminated. Despite the vast amount of available information about the serious health consequences of cigarette smoking, 23% of 12th grade students do *not* believe there is a great risk in smoking a pack or more per day (1). Undeniably, positive associations with cigarettes portrayed in the media, particularly advertising, have contributed to this. For example, after Virginia Slims cigarettes were introduced in the late 1960s, teenaged females sharply increased initiation rates for cigarettes (3). Continued exploration of attitudes about drug use, both the positive and negative, will aid in development of effective prevention programs.

REFERENCES

1. Johnston LD, O'Malley PM, Bachman JG, et al. *Monitoring the future national survey results on drug use, 1975–2007: volume I, secondary school students* (NIH Publication No. 08-6418A). Bethesda, MD: National Institute on Drug Abuse, 2008.
2. Bachman JG, Johnston LD, O'Malley PM. Explaining recent increased in students' marijuana use: impacts of perceived risks and disapproval, 1976 through 1996. *Am J Pub Health* 1998;88(6):887–892.
3. Burns DM, Johnston LD. Overview of recent changes in adolescent smoking behavior, in Changing Adolescent Smoking Prevalence. Monograph 14. U.S. Department of Health and Human Services, 1999.

CHAPTER 98

Kenneth W. Griffin, PhD, MPH
Gilbert J. Botvin, PhD

Preventing Substance Abuse among Children and Adolescents

Substance use and abuse remain important public health problems that contribute significantly to morbidity and mortality in this country and throughout the world. Over the past several decades, significant efforts have been made to understand the epidemiology and etiology of substance use and abuse and to identify effective prevention and treatment approaches. Though at the individual level there is considerable variability in patterns of substance use and abuse, epidemiologic studies show that, from a population perspective, the onset of substance use typically begins during the adolescent years. Many young people initiate substance use by experimenting with alcohol and cigarette smoking with peers during early or mid-adolescence. National datasets show that the prevalence of alcohol, tobacco, and other drug use increases rapidly from early to late adolescence, peaking during the transition to young adulthood. Furthermore, a large body of research has shown that early initiation of substance use is associated with higher levels of use and abuse later in life as well as negative outcomes such as violent and delinquent behavior, poor physical health, and mental health problems (1).

Given the well-established pattern of onset and developmental progression of substance use and abuse, a variety of prevention initiatives for children and adolescents have been developed. Relatively few prevention efforts have focused on adults because the majority of adults with substance abuse problems began use during adolescence. Initiatives to prevent youth substance use include educational and skills training programs for young people in school settings; programs that teach parents ways to effectively communicate with and monitor their children; and community-based programs that combine school and family components with additional educational, mass media, or public policy components (e.g., restricting access to alcohol and tobacco though enforcement of minimum purchasing age requirements). A goal of many prevention initiatives is to prevent early-stage substance use or delay the onset of use. Most aim to prevent alcohol, tobacco, and marijuana use because these are the most widely used substances in our society and pose the greatest risk to the public health. Middle- or junior-high-school-age students are typically targeted because it is during early adolescence that substance use experimentation usually begins to occur. The large body of research examining the efficacy and effectiveness of prevention programs for adolescent substance abuse demonstrates that the most effective approaches target salient risk and protective factors at the individual, family, and/or community levels and are guided by relevant psychosocial theories regarding the etiology of substance use and abuse (2,3).

PREVALENCE RATES AND PROGRESSION OF USE

National survey data demonstrate that the prevalence rates of substance use among adolescents peaked in the late 1970s and early 1980s, fell through much of the remainder of the 1980s, and began to increase again during the 1990s. In recent years, prevalence rates of use for most substances have gradually declined among adolescents but remain problematic. The 2007 Monitoring the Future (MTF) study (4) found that among high school seniors, 37% had used one or more illicit drugs in the last year and 48% had done so during their lifetime. For marijuana use among high school seniors, annual and lifetime prevalence rates were 32% and 42%, respectively; for hallucinogen use, rates were 5% and 9%, respectively; and for amphetamine use, rates were 8% and 12%, respectively. In terms of substances that are legal for adults, the annual prevalence rate for alcohol use among high school seniors was 67%

and the lifetime rate was 73%, and for cigarette smoking the 30-day rate was 22% and the lifetime rate was 47%. Though the rates of use for some substances have decreased in recent years, the MTF study also revealed that nonmedical prescription drug abuse and the misuse of over-the-counter medications such as cough syrup to get high are growing problems among adolescents (4).

Some level of experimentation with substances has become commonplace among young people in contemporary American society. During early adolescence, substance use occurs almost exclusively in a social context. Experimentation typically begins with substances that are readily available, such as alcohol, tobacco, and inhalants. Though many individuals discontinue use after experimentation or fail to progress to the use of other substances, some individuals become regular users and/or progress to marijuana, hallucinogens, and other illicit drugs in a fairly predictable pattern (5). A subset eventually develops patterns of use characterized by both psychologic and physiologic dependence. The likelihood of progressing to more serious levels of substance abuse and disorder is best understood in probabilistic terms. An individual's risk of greater substance use involvement increases at each additional step in the developmental progression. Furthermore, the initial social motivations for substance use eventually yield to those driven increasingly by pharmacologic and psychologic factors (6). Knowledge of the typical patterns and progression of substance use has important implications for the focus and timing of preventive interventions. Prevention programs that effectively target risk factors for alcohol and tobacco use may not only prevent the use of these substances but may reduce or eliminate the risk of using other substances further along the progression.

ETIOLOGY AND IMPLICATIONS FOR PREVENTION

The predictable epidemiologic patterns of substance use onset and progression during adolescence, combined with observations that substance use is frequently linked to important developmental goals and transitions of adolescence, support the notion that substance use and abuse are developmental phenomena. The degree of substance use involvement of any particular teenager is often a function of the negative pro-drug social influences in their environment combined with their individual vulnerabilities to these influences.

Developmental Aspects A developmental perspective on the etiology of substance use is informative in understanding how best to prevent early experimentation with alcohol, tobacco, and other drugs. Adolescence is a key period for experimentation not only with substances but with a wide range of behaviors and lifestyle patterns. Indeed, a great number of changes occur during the years of adolescence, and experimenting with new behavior occurs as part of a natural process of separating from parents, gaining acceptance and popularity with peers, developing a sense of autonomy and independence, establishing a personal identity and self-image, seeking fun and adventure, and/or rebelling against authority. However, many of these same developmental goals can increase an adolescent's risk of smoking, drinking, or using drugs. Indeed, from the point of view of an adolescent, engaging in alcohol, tobacco, and other drug use may be seen as a functional way of achieving independence, maturity, or popularity.

The Importance of Social Influences Research has shown that social influences are the most powerful factors promoting experimentation or initiation of substance use among young people. Modeling of substance use behavior by important others (e.g., parents, older siblings, and especially peers) along with exposure to positive attitudes and expectations regarding substance are the most important types of negative social influence (7). The positive portrayal of substance use and abuse by celebrities in movies, television, and music videos is also a powerful negative influence (8). Advertisements that communicate positive messages about alcohol and tobacco use are likely to promote prosubstance use attitudes, expectancies, and perceived positive consequences of use that can translate into increases in cigarette smoking and alcohol use among young people (9).

Risk and Protective Factors Risk factors that contribute to the initiation, maintenance, and escalation of alcohol, tobacco, and illicit drug use—along with protective factors that offset the effects of risk—occur at the level of the individual, family, school and community.

Individual Level Individual-level factors include cognitive, attitudinal, social, personality, pharmacologic, biologic, and developmental factors (10). Cognitive risk factors for substance use include lack of knowledge about the risks of use and abuse and believing that substance use is "normal" and that most people engage in use. Affect regulation is another important factor in the etiology of substance use, as described in the self-medication hypothesis (11). Psychologic characteristics such as poor self-esteem, low assertiveness, and poor behavioral self-control are associated with substance use. As an individual's substance use increases in frequency and quantity, pharmacologic risk factors become increasingly important. Drugs of abuse such as cocaine, amphetamine, morphine, as well as nicotine and alcohol, have different molecular mechanisms of action but affect the brain in a similar way by increasing strength at excitatory synapses on midbrain dopamine neurons (12). There are likely to be important individual differences in neurochemical reactivity to these drugs that place some individuals at higher risk.

Family Level In addition to the direct modeling of substance use behaviors and positive attitudes regarding use, factors within the family can contribute directly to increased substance use or indirectly by affecting established precursors of substance use such as aggressive behavior and other conduct problems. These family factors include harsh disciplinary practices, poor parental monitoring, low levels of family bonding, and high levels of family conflict. Conversely, parenting practices characterized by firm and consistent limit setting, careful monitoring, and nurturing, open communication patterns with children are protective against substance use and other negative outcomes (13).

School and Community Level Characteristics of schools have been found to be associated with levels of substance use among students (14). When large numbers of students feel disengaged from school—they don't like school, don't feel "part of" their schools, fail academically, feel unsafe at school, or don't have good relationships with teachers—this has been found to be associated with greater substance use prevalence. Similarly, when young people feel disengaged from their communities or feel unsafe in their neighborhoods, this is associated with greater substance use, as is greater levels of community disorganization (15).

TYPES OF PREVENTIVE INTERVENTIONS

The terminology used to describe prevention efforts has evolved over time. Primary prevention interventions are designed to reach individuals in the general population before they have developed a specific disorder or disease. Secondary prevention involves screening and early intervention. Tertiary prevention involves preventing the progression of an established disorder to the point of disability. However, a problem with this terminology is that it is difficult to distinguish the difference between tertiary prevention and treatment because both involve care for persons with an existing disorder. More contemporary terminology for prevention was proposed by the Institute of Medicine (16) as part of a new framework for classifying interventions along a continuum of care that includes prevention, treatment, and maintenance. In this framework, prevention refers only to interventions that occur prior to the onset of a disorder. Prevention is further divided into three types: universal, selective, and indicated interventions. Universal prevention programs focus on the general population and aim to deter or delay the onset of a condition. Selective prevention programs target selected high-risk groups or subsets of the general population believed to be at high risk owing to membership in a particular group (e.g., pregnant women or children of drug users). Indicated prevention programs are designed for those already engaging in the behavior or those showing early danger signs or engaging in related high-risk behaviors. Thus, where recruitment and participation in a selective intervention is based on subgroup membership, recruitment and participation in an indicated intervention are based on early warning signs demonstrated by an individual.

There have been significant advances in the effectiveness of both drug treatment and prevention programs (6). However, treatment remains expensive and labor-intensive and suffers from high rates of recidivism. Prevention is, therefore, a key component in addressing the problem of drug abuse, especially given the increasing availability of effective programs. The first major breakthrough in prevention came at the end of the 1970s in the area of school-based smoking prevention. That work stimulated a great deal of prevention research and led to the development of several promising prevention approaches, including those designed to prevent the use of multiple substances. During the 1980s and up to the present, mounting empirical evidence from a growing number of methodologically sophisticated studies indicates that prevention can be highly effective. In the next several sections of the chapter, we describe contemporary approaches to drug abuse prevention for children and adolescents at the school, family, and community levels.

School-Based Prevention Approaches In the scientific literature on universal prevention programs targeting children and adolescents, schools are the most common implementation site for such programs. School settings are desirable because schools provide access to large numbers of young people, and substance use is seen as inconsistent with the goals of educating our youth. Three types of contemporary approaches to school-based prevention of substance use are (1) social resistance skills training, (2) normative education, and (3) competence enhancement skills training. One or more of these approaches or components may be combined within a single preventive intervention.

Social Resistance Skills These interventions are designed to increase adolescent's awareness of the various social influences to engage in substance use and teach young people specific skills for effectively resisting both peer and media pressures to smoke, drink, or use drugs (17). Resistance skills training programs teach adolescents how to recognize situations in which they are likely to experience peer pressure to smoke, drink, or use drugs along with ways to avoid or otherwise effectively deal with these high-risk situations. Participants are taught ways of handling pressure to engage in substance, including what to say (i.e., the specific content of a refusal message) and how to deliver it in the most effective way possible. Resistance skills programs also typically include content to increase students' awareness of the techniques used by advertisers to promote the sale of tobacco products or alcoholic beverages and teach techniques for formulating counter-arguments to the messages used by advertisers.

Normative Education Because adolescents tend to overestimate the prevalence of smoking, drinking, and the use of certain drugs, normative education approaches include content and activities to correct inaccurate perceptions regarding the high prevalence of substance use (18). This can be done by providing feedback from survey data showing actual prevalence rates collected locally in the classroom, school, or community or by showing the relatively low prevalence rates in national survey data for young teens. Normative education also attempts to undermine popular but inaccurate beliefs that substance drug use is considered acceptable and not particularly dangerous. This can be done by highlighting evidence from national studies showing strong anti-drug social norms and generally high perceived risks of drug use in the population. Material on normative education is often included in social resistance programs.

Competence Enhancement Competence enhancement programs recognize that social learning processes are important in the development of adolescent drug use. However, they also recognize that youth with poor personal and social skills are more susceptible to influences that promote drug use and these youth may be more motivated to use drugs as an alternative to more adaptive coping strategies (19). Competence enhancement approaches typically teach some combination of the following life skills: general problem-solving and decision-making skills; general cognitive skills for resisting interpersonal or media influences; skills for increasing self-control and self-esteem; adaptive coping strategies for relieving stress and anxiety through the use of cognitive coping skills or behavioral relaxation techniques; general social skills; and general assertive skills. In contrast to the more focused drug resistance skills training approaches, competence enhancement programs are designed to teach the kind of generic skills that will have a relatively broad application. The most effective personal and social skills training programs emphasize the application of general skills to situations directly related to substance use and abuse and demonstrate that these same skills can be used for dealing with many of the challenges confronting adolescents in their everyday lives.

Effectiveness of School-Based Prevention There have been a large number of published meta-analyses and systematic reviews of the prevention literature for child and adolescent substance use. In the following sections, we review findings from meta-analyses and systematic reviews of school-based substance use and smoking prevention programs, focusing primarily on those reviews published since 2000.

Meta-Analyses of Substance Use Prevention A recent paper presented a summary of findings from a Cochrane Review on school-based programs for preventing illicit drug use (20). In this meta-analysis, 29 randomized controlled trials (RCTs) evaluating school-based interventions designed to prevent substance use were reviewed. The review focused on illicit drug use and did not include studies that looked at smoking or alcohol use prevention only. The authors classified the interventions as primarily skills-focused, affect-focused, or knowledge-focused. All but 1 of the 29 RCTs were conducted in the United States, and most interventions targeted sixth- and seventh-grade students. Findings from the meta-analysis indicated that, compared to usual curricula, skills-based interventions significantly reduced marijuana use and hard drug use and improved decision-making skills, self-esteem, peer pressure resistance, and drug knowledge. The main conclusion of the meta-analysis was that skills-based programs are effective in deterring drug use, whereas knowledge and affective programs are not effective in changing behavior, a finding consistent with previous meta-analyses of school-based prevention.

Another meta-analysis of the school-based drug prevention literature selected studies in which at least one of the outcomes was tobacco use, those using at least a quasi-experimental design (including a control or comparison group), and those where students were followed up for at least 2 years that included the transition from junior high to high school (21). The primary goal of the review was to summarize the evidence on the long-term effectiveness of prevention programs, defined as effects that last beyond 2 years. Most of the 25 prevention programs included in the meta-analysis reported significant long-term program effects for smoking, alcohol, and/or marijuana use outcomes, with a fairly consistent magnitude of intervention effects across studies. The authors concluded that their analysis demonstrates empirical evidence supporting the long-term effectiveness of social influences programs in preventing or reducing substance use for from 2 to 15 years after the completion of programming. Program effects were less likely to decay over time for interventions that delivered booster sessions as a supplement to the initial program curricula. The authors noted, however, a high level of variability in the methodologic rigor across studies, with most using quasi-experimental rather than true randomized designs.

A third meta-analysis examined 207 universal school-based drug abuse prevention programs that included a control or comparison group in the evaluation design (22). Programs were classified into interactive and noninteractive categories based on a combination of content and teaching methods used. The authors examined a number of program characteristics to identify the attributes of programs that most effectively prevent drug use, including program size, program provider, target substance, intensity or dosage, and grade level, among others. Findings indicated that noninteractive lecture-oriented prevention programs that emphasize drug knowledge or affective development were the least effective. The meta-analysis showed that interactive programs that help students build interpersonal skills were the most effective in preventing substance use behavior. Among these programs, behavioral effects were found to decrease with larger-scale implementations, which may reflect the difficulty in selecting and training the best program providers in large research studies and/or the smaller amount of time each student is given when programs are implemented in larger groups of students.

Meta-Analyses of Smoking Prevention There have been several meta-analyses of school-based smoking prevention programs published since 2000, perhaps because there is a longer history of theory-based preventive interventions implemented for smoking as compared to the use of multiple substances. A recently published Cochrane Review included RCTs of school-based interventions to prevent smoking among children and adolescents (ages 5 to 18) in which study participants were followed up for at least 6 months (23). Included were programs or curricula that focused on information only, social resistance skills, competence enhancement skills, and those programs that included additional intervention components in the community. The main outcome variable was prevalence of nonsmoking at follow-up among those students not smoking at the baseline assessment. The authors included 23 high-quality trials of school-based smoking prevention programs. Most of the intervention studies were social resistance programs, and the authors concluded that half of these interventions produced short-term effects on smoking behavior. The authors concluded that programs focusing primarily on providing information were ineffective. There was, however, evidence supporting the effectiveness of smoking prevention interventions that focused on developing generic social competence among youth as well as for interventions that took a multi-modal approach that included a substantive community component.

A recent meta-analysis of school-based smoking prevention trials was designed specifically to examine long-term effects on smoking, defined as behavioral effects that last until the 12th grade or age 18 (24). The authors included school-based RCTs of smoking prevention with follow-up periods of at least 1 year after intervention and those that had smoking prevalence (defined as at least one cigarette in the past month) as a primary outcome. Of the eight articles included in the meta-analysis, the authors noted that there was significant variability in intervention intensity, presence of booster sessions, length of follow-up, and attrition rates. The authors concluded that that few studies have evaluated the long-term impact of school-based smoking prevention and noted that only one long-term study (25) showed statistically significant decreased smoking prevalence in the intervention group compared to controls. The authors concluded that there was "little to no evidence of long-term effectiveness" of school-based smoking prevention. The article generated a spirited discussion among researchers in a series of letters to the editor and drew criticism from prevention researchers who noted that the findings were inconsistent with several previous meta-analyses and syntheses of the literature (not cited by the authors) that had shown positive short and long-term behavioral effects of school-based smoking prevention.

A third meta-analysis of school-based smoking prevention examined 65 adolescent psychosocial smoking prevention programs among students in grades 6 to 12 published between 1978 and 1997 in the United States (26). Programs were categorized into three prevention approaches (social resistance, social resistance + cognitive skills, and social resistance + cognitive + affective skills) and two delivery settings (school, school + community). Findings from the meta-analysis revealed that program effects on knowledge had the highest effect sizes in the short-term (no more than 1 year) but rapidly decreased over time. Importantly, behavioral effects were observed and persisted over a 3-year period, with the strongest effects on smoking observed with programs that included social resistance combined with cognitive and/or affective skills training activities and/or programs that included both schools and community components in their implementation.

Systematic Reviews of Smoking Prevention Several recent papers have attempted to summarize the evidence regarding school-based smoking prevention research. In one review, the authors concluded that the existing evidence supports findings of decreased prevalence of smoking among students exposed to social influence smoking prevention programs as compared to students in control groups, with the mean difference ranging from 5% to 60%, with duration of 1 to 4 years (27). The authors concluded that the most effective school-based smoking prevention programs are those with sustained application, booster sessions over several years, reinforcement in the community including the involvement of parents and/or the mass media; and those that are part of a comprehensive school health promotion program. In a second review, evidence regarding the effectiveness of tobacco use prevention interventions published since the 1970s was examined (28). In addition to synthesizing the research evidence, the authors supplemented the review by conducting individual interviews and focus groups with practitioners involved in tobacco use prevention programming. They concluded that there is strong evidence that school-based tobacco use prevention programs are effective for most tobacco use outcomes, particularly in the short term. They make several key recommendations for policy, practice, and future research, including that (1) programs should include active learning and skills building activities in order to increase awareness of social and media influences to smoke; (2) school-based programs should be implemented along with other community-wide tobacco control initiatives and maintained until age 18; and (3) programs must be culturally competent and adapted to the needs of various minority communities. A third review of school-based smoking prevention studies published from 1990 to 2002 noted that, with the exception of two programs, "school based curricula alone have been generally ineffective in the long term in preventing adolescents from initiating tobacco use." However, the authors concluded that school-based programs combined with other approaches such as mass media and smoke-free policies can be effective (29).

In summary, several meta-analyses and systematic reviews published since 2000 have examined the effectiveness of school-based substance use and smoking prevention programs. Most of these have found that overall, school-based prevention is effective in reducing smoking and other forms of substance use. There is some debate on the long-term effectiveness of school-based prevention in general, though a handful of programs have shown clear evidence of long-term behavioral effects. Though the methodologic rigor and theoretical bases of prevention programs included in these reviews varied considerably, findings have been useful in identifying characteristics of programs that are most effective. The most effective school-based prevention programs are interactive in nature, focus on building skills in drug resistance and general competence skills, and are implemented over multiple years. School-based programs that have a substantive community component that includes mass media or parental involvement also tend to be more effective than school-only programs. Additional studies have shown, however, that major challenges remain in disseminating evidence-based prevention programs and in adequately preparing prevention providers. Only about 27% of all schools in the United States use 1 of the 10 most effective prevention curricula available (30) and less than one in five providers use effective delivery of prevention program content (31).

Family-Based Prevention Approaches Family-based prevention programs include training in parenting skills, often provided to parents without children present. The specific parenting skills that are taught vary somewhat with the age of the target child or adolescent but may focus on ways to nurture, bond, and communicate with children, how to help children develop prosocial skills and social resistance skills, training on rule-setting and techniques for monitoring activities, and ways to help children reduce aggressive or antisocial behaviors. Prevention programs focusing on family skills often include sessions with the parents and children together (with or without additional parent-only training) that aim to improve family functioning, communication, and practice in developing, discussing, and enforcing family policies on substance abuse (13).

Effectiveness of Family-Based Prevention A recent systematic review evaluated parenting programs to prevent alcohol, tobacco, or drug abuse in children younger than 18 years of age (32). Twenty controlled studies were reviewed, though the rigor of the studies and nature of the interventions varied considerably. Findings indicated statistically significant reductions in alcohol use in 6 of 14 studies, reduction in drug use in five of nine studies, and reduction in tobacco use in 9 of 13 studies. However, three interventions produced increases in alcohol, tobacco, or drug use. The authors concluded that parenting programs can be effective in reducing or preventing substance use and that the most effective programs were those emphasizing both active parental involvement and skills development in the areas of parenting, social competence, and self-regulation skills. The authors point out that little is known about the change processes involved in such interventions and their long-term effectiveness.

In a Cochrane Review of family-based programs for preventing smoking, the authors identified RCTs designed to deter the use of tobacco among children (aged 5 to 12) or adolescents (aged 13 to 18) and other family members (33). The primary outcome was smoking onset among children measured at least 6 months from the start of the intervention. The authors identified nine studies that tested a family intervention against a control group and found that four of these nine had significant positive effects on smoking behavior, though one showed significant negative effects. Five additional RCTs that were identified tested a family intervention against a school intervention. However, none of the parent programs produced significant incremental effects as compared to the school programs alone. The authors concluded that some well-executed RCTs provided evidence that family interventions can prevent adolescent smoking but that RCTs that were less well executed had mostly neutral or negative results. They also concluded that how well the program staff are trained and how well they deliver the program appear to be related to effectiveness, while the number of sessions in the program does not seem to predict effectiveness.

In summary, a variety of parenting skills and family-based drug prevention programs have been studied. Those that focus on both parenting skills and family bonding appear to be the most effective in reducing or preventing substance use. An important limitation of family-based prevention is the difficulty in getting parents to participate; families most at risk for drug use are least likely to participate in prevention programs (34).

Community-Based Prevention Approaches Community-based drug abuse prevention programs typically have multiple components, including some combination of school-based programs, family or parenting components, mass media campaigns, and public policy components such as restricting youth access to alcohol and tobacco, and other types of community organization and activities. The multiple components of a community-based intervention may be managed by a coalition of stakeholders including parents, educators, and key leaders in the community.

Effectiveness of Community-Based Prevention A recent Cochrane Review examined community-based programs to prevent smoking initiation in children and adolescents (35). This qualitative narrative synthesis included RCTs and studies using quasi-experimental designs including a control or comparison group in which the effectiveness of multi-component intervention were compared to no intervention, to a school-only program, or to another single-component intervention. Seventeen studies were included in the review. Among the 13 studies that compared community interventions to no intervention controls, two programs produced lower smoking prevalence in the intervention versus control groups. One of two studies that compared a community intervention to school-only program found behavioral effects on smoking. Two studies found behavioral effects on smoking for multi-component community interventions compared to mass media-only campaigns. The authors concluded that there is some limited support for the effectiveness of coordinated multi-component community prevention programs in reducing smoking among young people and that programs with multiple components prevent smoking behavior more effectively than do programs with a single component.

In summary, multi-component community-based prevention programs can be effective in preventing adolescent substance use, particularly when the different components focus on a coordinated, comprehensive message. A limitation of community-based programs is the expense and high degree of coordination needed to implement and evaluate the type of comprehensive program most likely to be effective.

SUMMARY AND CONCLUSIONS

Substance use and abuse remain important public health problems. The prevalence of alcohol, tobacco, and other drug use increases rapidly from early to late adolescence, peaking during the transition to young adulthood. A variety of prevention initiatives for children and adolescents have been developed for schools, families, and communities. The most effective approaches target salient risk and protective factors and are guided by relevant psychosocial theories regarding the etiology of substance use and abuse. The degree of substance use involvement of any particular teenager is often a function of the negative pro-drug social influences in their environment combined with their individual vulnerabilities to these influences.

Contemporary school-based prevention programs focus on skills building in the areas of drug resistance, life skills, and/or correcting inaccurate beliefs about the high prevalence of substance use. Reviews of the school-based prevention literature have found that overall, theory-based programs can reduce smoking and other forms of substance use. There is some debate on the long-term effectiveness of these programs in general, but a handful of programs have shown clear evidence of long-term behavioral effects. The most effective school-based prevention programs are interactive, focus on building skills in drug resistance and general competence skills, and are implemented over multiple years. School-based programs that include a substantive community component tend to be more effective than are school-only programs. Family-based prevention programs include training in parenting skills and/or group interventions for the entire family that focus on improving family functioning, communication, and family policies on substance abuse. Family interventions that combine parenting skills and family bonding appear to be the most effective. Community-based drug abuse prevention programs typically include some combination of school, family, mass media, public policy, and community organization components. The most effective community programs present a coordinated, comprehensive message across multiple delivery components.

Despite the progress that has been made in the field of drug abuse prevention for children and adolescents, there are several factors that reduce the public health impact of effective school, family, and community prevention programs. Most schools still use non-evidence-based prevention programs, effective family programs often do not reach the families in greatest need, and community programs require substantial financial and human resources. In addition to refining our understanding of the risk and protective factors for substance abuse and translating this knowledge into improved interventions, future research is needed to find ways to effectively disseminate the most promising prevention programs into our schools, families, and communities.

REFERENCES

1. Newcomb MD, Bentler PM. *Consequences of adolescent drug use: impact on the lives of young adults*. New York: Sage, 1988.
2. Hawkins JD, Catalano RF, Miller JY. Risk and protective factors for alcohol and other drug problems in adolescence and early adulthood: implications for substance abuse prevention. *Psychol Bull* 1992;112: 64–105.
3. Petraitis J, Flay BR, Miller TQ. Reviewing theories of adolescent substance use: organizing pieces in the puzzle. *Psychol Bull* 1995;117:67–86.
4. Johnston LD, O'Malley PM, Bachman JG, et al. Monitoring the Future national survey results on drug use, 1975–2006. *Volume I: Secondary school students* (NIH Publication No. 07-6205). Bethesda, MD: National Institute on Drug Abuse, 2007.
5. Kandel D. Stages and pathways of drug involvement: examining the gateway hypothesis. New York: Cambridge University Press, 2002.
6. Hartel CR Glantz MD. *Drug abuse: origins and interventions*. Washington, DC: American Psychological Association, 1997.
7. Welte JW, Barnes GM, Hoffman JH, et al. Trends in adolescent alcohol and other substance use: relationships to trends in peer, parent, and school influences. *Subst Use Misuse* 1999;34:1427–1449.
8. McCool JP, Cameron LD, Petrie KJ. Adolescent perceptions of smoking imagery in film. *Soc Sci Med* 2001;52:1577–1587.
9. Tye J, Warner K, Glantz S. Tobacco advertising and consumption: evidence of a causal relationship. *J Public Health Policy* 1987;8:492–507.
10. Swadi H. Individual risk factors for adolescent substance use. *Drug Alcohol Depend* 1999;55:209–224.
11. Khantzian EJ. The self-medication hypothesis of substance use disorders: a reconsideration and recent applications. *Harvard Rev Psychiatry* 1997;4: 231–244.
12. Saal D, Dong Y, Bonci A, et al. Drugs of abuse and stress trigger a common synaptic adaptation in dopamine neurons. *Neuron* 2003;37:577–582.
13. Lochman JE, van den Steenhoven A. Family-based approaches to substance abuse prevention. *J Prim Prev* 2002;23:49–114.
14. Fletcher A, Bonell C, Hargreaves, J. School effects on young people's drug use: a systematic review of intervention and observational studies. *J Adolesc Health* 2008;42:209–220.
15. Hays SP, Hays CE, Mulhall PF. Community risk and protective factors and adolescent substance use. *J Prim Prev* 2003;24:125–142.
16. Institute of Medicine. Reducing risks for mental disorders: frontiers for preventive intervention research. Washington, DC: National Academy Press, 1994.
17. Hansen WB. School-based substance abuse prevention: a review of the state of the art in curriculum, 1980–1990. *Health Ed Res* 1992;7: 403–430.
18. Hansen WB, Graham JW. Preventing alcohol, marijuana, and cigarette use among adolescents: peer pressure resistance training versus establishing conservative norms. *Prev Med* 1991;20:414–430.
19. Botvin GJ. Preventing drug abuse in schools: social and competence enhancement approaches targeting individual-level etiological factors. *Addict Behav* 2000;25:887–897.
20. Faggiano F, Vigna-Taglianti FD, Versino E, et al. School-based prevention for illicit drugs use: A systematic review. *Prev Med* 2008;46:385–396.
21. Skara S, Sussman S. A review of 25 long-term adolescent tobacco and other drug use prevention program evaluations. *Prev Med* 2003;37:451–474.
22. Tobler NS, Roona M, Ochshorn P, et al. School-based adolescent drug prevention programs: 1998 meta-analysis. *J Prim Prev* 2000;20:275–336.
23. Thomas R, Perera R. School-based programmes for preventing smoking. *Cochrane Database Syst Rev* 2006;3. No. CD001293. DOI: 10.1002/14651858.CD001293.pub2.
24. Wiehe SE, Garrison MM, Christakis DA, et al. A systematic review of school-based smoking prevention trials with long-term follow-up. *J Adolesc Health* 2005;36:162–169.
25. Botvin GJ, Baker E, Dusenbury L, et al. Long-term follow-up results of a randomized drug abuse prevention trial in a white middle-class population. *J Am Med Assoc* 1995;273:1106–1112.
26. Hwang MS, Yeagley KL, Petosa R. A meta-analysis of adolescent psychosocial smoking prevention programs published between 1978 and 1997 in the United States. *Health Ed Behav* 2004;31:702–719.
27. La Torre G, Chiaradia G, Ricciardi G. School-based smoking prevention in children and adolescents: review of the scientific literature. *J Public Health* 2005;13:285–290.
28. Dobbins M, DeCorby K, Manske S, et al. Effective practices for school-based tobacco use prevention. *Prev Med* 2008;46:289–297.
29. Backinger CL, Fagan P, Matthews E, et al. Adolescent and young adult tobacco prevention and cessation: current status and future directions. *Tobacco Control* 2003;12:46–53.
30. Ringwalt CL, Ennett S, Vincus A, et al. The prevalence of effective substance use prevention curricula in U.S. middle schools. *Prev Sci* 2002;3:257–265.

31. Ennett ST, Ringwalt CL, Thorne J, et al. A comparison of current practice in school-based substance use prevention programs with meta-analysis findings. *Prev Sci* 2003;4:1–14.
32. Petrie J, Bunn F, & Byrne G. Parenting programmes for preventing tobacco, alcohol or drugs misuse in children <18: a systematic review. *Health Ed Res* 2007;22:177–191.
33. Thomas RE, Baker P, Lorenzetti D. Family-based programmes for preventing smoking by children and adolescents. *Cochrane Database Syst Rev* 2007;1. No. CD004493. DOI: 10.1002/14651858.CD004493.pub2.
34. Díaz S, Secades-Villa R, Pérez JE, et al. Family predictors of parent participation in an adolescent drug abuse prevention program. *Drug Alcohol Rev* 2006;25:327–331.
35. Sowden A, Stead L. Community interventions for preventing smoking in young people. *Cochrane Database Syst Rev* 2003;1. No. CD001291. DOI: 10.1002/14651858.CD001291.

CHAPTER 99

W. Alex Mason, PhD
J. David Hawkins, PhD

Adolescent Risk and Protective Factors: Psychosocial

The evaluation, management, referral, and long-term care of the adolescent who is seriously involved in substance abuse is marked by the difficulty of such work, the time and expense of treatment, and the frequency with which best efforts nevertheless result in poor outcomes. Our foremost goal should be to prevent the initiation and progression of substance use in young people before the establishment of substance use patterns and outcomes that will be more difficult to alter, including the development of substance use disorders (1).

Advances in cardiovascular disease prevention provide a model for approaching the prevention of substance abuse. Prospective longitudinal studies identified risk factors for heart disease (family history, smoking, high-fat diet, stress, sedentary lifestyle) and protective factors that reduce or buffer heart disease risk (exercise, stress coping skills, healthy eating). Physicians have used this information to determine risk for cardiovascular disease in their patients, assessing family, lifestyle, dietary, and smoking histories; measuring blood pressure; and requesting laboratory studies to measure cholesterol and to determine high-density lipid versus low-density lipid cholesterol. They have used the results of these assessments to advise and prescribe lifestyle changes (exercise, dietary changes, smoking cessation). Through these efforts, the rates of risk factors for cardiovascular disease have decreased dramatically over the past 40 years in the United States (2), with a concomitant decrease in the incidence of cardiovascular disease (3).

Like cardiovascular disease, adolescent substance abuse is a preventable disorder. Current research provides a firm foundation for the physician seeking to reduce risk among young patients before the appearance of substance use, misuse, or abuse. The physician who cares for children and who knows the risk and protective factors can intervene to avert alcohol and drug problems before they arise.

RISK FACTORS

Individual Factors Some children appear to be at greater risk for substance abuse by virtue of their family histories, prenatal and birth experience, temperament, and early and persistent displays of behavioral and emotional problems. A family history of alcoholism increases the risk of alcoholism in children by about four times (4,5), and intergenerational transmission of risk has been observed for other substance use disorders (6,7). Such risk is explained, in part, by genetic influences among both males and females (8,9). However, fewer than 30% of the children of alcoholics develop alcoholism. Physicians should be alert to family history of alcohol or other drug problems when informing their young patients about their own risk for substance abuse and dependence.

Perinatal complications (including preterm delivery, low birthweight, and anoxia) and brain damage (from infectious disease, traumatic head injury, or pre- or postnatal exposure to toxins such as heavy metals, alcohol, tobacco, or cocaine) predispose children to later aggressive behavior, depression and anxiety symptoms, and substance abuse (10–12). In particular, prenatal drug exposure has been shown to increase risk for a host of physical, cognitive, social, and behavioral impairments (13–15), including the development of substance use and misuse (16–20). Physicians who maintain or obtain good birth and trauma histories may see evidence of these risks long before substance use begins. It is important to inform parents and parents-to-be of the risks of alcohol, tobacco, and other drug use during pregnancy and infancy and of the dangers to children of toxins in the home.

Some studies suggest that inherited biologic traits and temperament play a role in substance use behaviors (21,22). High physical activity level (23) and negative emotionality

(24) are temperament dimensions that predict early drug initiation and substance abuse (25). Poor self-control (26) and high sensation seeking (27,28) also increase risk for adolescent substance use and misuse. Attention deficit/hyperactivity disorder, particularly the inattention symptom domain, has been found to predict substance use in late adolescence (29,30), especially when combined with aggressive behaviors or conduct disorder (31). A pattern of persistent conduct problems, including aggressive behavior in childhood, is an early behavioral predictor of risk for later substance abuse (32–34). There is some evidence that serious and persistent depressive symptoms are linked to adolescent substance involvement (35), and the co-occurrence of multiple behavioral and emotional problems can exacerbate risk for substance abuse (36). Primary care physicians can help to reduce risks for later substance abuse by identifying patients who are experiencing behavioral and emotional problems in early childhood and treating or referring them and their parents appropriately. Effective referral would include guiding parents to appropriate parenting resources and training programs for skill development in child management (37).

Various attitudes, perceptions, and beliefs have been shown to predict greater substance use, including alienation and rebelliousness (38,39), positive expectations regarding the effects of alcohol and other drugs (40,41), and beliefs that using substances helps one cope with stress or enhances social interactions (42,43). Prodrug attitudes tend to precede the initiation of drug use in adolescence and continue to develop as drug involvement progresses (44–46). Health professionals should begin to assess substance use attitudes and behaviors when they encounter these signals and be prepared to discuss with their patients who hold attitudes favorable to substance use the harms that can result from the use of substances.

The younger a child is when he or she first initiates the use of alcohol or other drugs, the greater the frequency of substance use (47), the greater the probability of extensive and persistent involvement in the use of illicit drugs (48,49), and the greater the risk of substance misuse and abuse (34,49,50). Each year that the initiation of alcohol or other drug use is delayed can lead to a 4% to 5% reduction in the likelihood of developing later drug use disorders (51,52); therefore, physicians should encourage young people to postpone alcohol use and to avoid the use of tobacco and illegal drugs for their own health and safety. As discussed later, the adoption of strong norms or standards against substance use appears to inhibit substance use initiation.

Family Factors A number of influences within the family context affect the substance use behaviors of children. As mentioned, some family influences are genetic in nature; for example, the link between parent problem drinking and adolescent alcohol involvement is explained in part by genetic factors (53–55). Social factors within the family also play an important role in substance use and misuse. To illustrate, the association between parent and child problem drinking is partly explained by modeling and the transmission of attitudes favorable to alcohol use (56,57). Research shows that risk for substance use increases when parents involve children in their substance-using behaviors, for example, by allowing children to light a cigarette for them (58). Substance use by older siblings increases risk for substance involvement (59–61). In fact, the influence of sibling substance use on adolescents appears to be stronger than that of parental substance use (62). Physicians can help to reduce substance abuse risks by encouraging parents and older siblings to moderate their use of alcohol and other drugs in the presence of children and by not involving children in their own alcohol or drug use behaviors.

Parents who are permissive or who fail to set clear expectations for their children, who are lax in supervision of their children, and who are excessively severe and inconsistent in punishing their children increase their children's risk for substance initiation, use, and abuse (63–67). Parenting difficulties may be evident in office visits or through conversations with parents, but there is no reason to wait for symptoms. Health professionals can reduce drug risks in young patients by encouraging their parents to learn and practice good parenting skills preventatively. Just as participating in childbirth classes helps expectant mothers to prepare for having children, providing or referring parents to developmentally appropriate training opportunities that have been tested and shown to increase family management skills can result in improved parenting, thus reducing the risk of substance abuse (68,69).

Poor family relationship quality increases risk for substance use and abuse. Marital conflict is a stressor that can lead to drug involvement and related externalizing problems among children and adolescents (70,71); indeed, there is evidence that greater risk may come from parental conflict than from parental absence (72). High levels of conflict in the parent-child relationship contribute to risk for higher levels of substance use during childhood and adolescence (73,74). In contrast, positive family relationships appear to discourage the initiation and progression of substance use (63,73,75–77). As noted by Brook et al. (64), such relationships are characterized by parental models of self-control and emotion regulation, high warmth and low conflict in the parent-child relationship, and increased identification of children with their prosocial parents.

Biologic, psychologic, and social factors within the family context interact in contributing to risk for substance use. For example, results from a twin-family study conducted by Dick et al. (78) indicated that low parental monitoring provided opportunities for the expression of genetic predispositions for cigarette smoking among teens, whereas high parental monitoring limited such expression. Chassin et al. (65) found that adolescents' reports of parent-child discussions about smoking were associated with decreased risk for cigarette use among teens with nonsmoking parents but not among teens with smoking parents. Health professionals can ensure that parents know the importance of setting clear expectations for nonuse of alcohol or other drugs during childhood and adolescence; the importance of monitoring their children in developmentally appropriate and nonintrusive ways; the importance of consistent and appropriate punishment for violating family expectations; and the importance of providing recognition to young people for living according to healthy standards. Curricula tested for effectiveness in teaching these skills are available (68,79,80).

School Factors School experiences appear to contribute to substance nonuse, use, and misuse. School engagement, positive scholastic attitudes, and successful school performance have been shown to reduce risk for the initiation and escalation of alcohol, marijuana, and other drug use (81,82). Moreover, positive school experiences can promote resilience by reducing the likelihood of substance use among at-risk youth. For example, though high levels of adolescent substance use are associated with greater risk for substance-related problems, Wills et al. (83) found that the link between substance use and problems was buffered by high levels of academic competence. Conversely, academic problems have been found to predict early initiation of substance use (84,85), levels of use of illegal drugs (86), and substance misuse (87). Adolescents who lose commitment to educational pursuits, as indicated by truancy, little time spent on homework, and a perception that school is unimportant are at greater risk for substance use (88,89). Health professionals can reduce substance abuse risk by inquiring about the academic progress of their young patients, communicating the importance of school success for future health and well-being, and suggesting tutoring or other academically focused interventions for young persons who are not making adequate academic progress.

Peer Factors Having friends who drink, smoke, or use other drugs is among the strongest predictors of adolescent substance use and misuse (64,81,90–93). Associating with substance-using peers can exacerbate the effects of risk factors that originate within the family and other domains (94), synergistically increasing the likelihood of substance initiation, escalation, and abuse. There is evidence that genetic factors contribute to the tendency for certain youth to seek out and form relationships with friends who use alcohol and other drugs (95). Still, research indicates that positive family relationships and school experiences can reduce the likelihood that youth will develop friendships with individuals who use substances (76,96), thereby reducing risk for substance involvement. Though health professionals may have little direct influence over the friendships and peer networks of young patients, helping to promote positive family relationships and school commitments in the ways described earlier can encourage youth to cultivate relationships with friends who avoid substance use.

Interpersonal influences involving the family, school, and peers are particularly important during childhood and adolescence. Whereas parental influences on drug use behaviors tend to be stronger during childhood, peer influences tend to become more important throughout adolescence (97); still, research indicates that parents continue to play an important role in the lives of their children throughout the teen years and even into early adulthood (77). As noted by Newcomb (98), findings such as these illustrate that the salience of predictors can vary depending on an individual's stage of development. This requires that health professionals have an understanding of the changing developmental challenges and competencies of their young patients to identify the predictors that are likely to be most important for a given individual at a particular developmental period.

Contextual Factors Factors in the broader social environment also affect rates of substance use and abuse. Perceived problems with alcohol and drug use in the neighborhood or community predict individual drug use behaviors and drug arrests (99). Rates of use are higher in communities where alcohol or other drugs are inexpensive and readily available (100). Availability and price are influenced by legal restriction or regulation on purchase, by excise taxes, and by market forces. Changes in laws to be more restrictive on alcohol availability (raising the legal drinking age, raising excise taxes on alcohol, limiting alcohol outlets) have been followed by decreases in alcohol consumption and alcohol-related fatalities (101).

Children who grow up in disorganized neighborhoods with high population density, high residential mobility, physical deterioration, and low levels of neighborhood attachment or cohesion face greater risks for drug trafficking as well as drug use and abuse (102–104).

Broad social norms regarding the acceptability and risk of use of alcohol or other drugs also appear to affect the prevalence of substance use and misuse (105–107). One influential way in which such norms are communicated is through the media. Collins et al. (108) found that a high degree of exposure to alcohol advertising (e.g., television ads, in-store displays) among sixth-grade students predicted increased drinking and intentions to drink 1 year later. As further evidence of media effects, depictions of smoking in the movies have been shown to increase risk for smoking initiation (109), and similar findings have been observed for alcohol use (110). Health professionals can reduce substance abuse risks in their communities by urging that policies and laws forbidding the sale of alcohol and tobacco to underage individuals are strictly enforced; by communicating strong normative standards to their patients, their parents, and the public against the use of alcohol, tobacco, or other drugs by children or adolescents; and by participating in groups and coalitions seeking to improve the community.

PROTECTIVE FACTORS

There are factors and processes that protect adolescents against substance abuse, even if they have been exposed to multiple risk factors. In addition to a resilient temperament and high intelligence (111), a general prosocial orientation is a key individual protective characteristic that reduces risk for substance use and abuse (66,112,113). Whereas attitudes and beliefs favorable to substance use increase risk for substance involvement, as noted earlier, a prosocial orientation is characterized by attitudes and beliefs that are inconsistent with substance use and that promote substance nonuse. Indicators of this prosocial orientation that have been shown to have protective effects include bonding to school, religiosity, and an intolerance of deviance (114–118). For example, Wills et al. (83) found that a high value on religion reduced the tendency for life stress to lead to tobacco, alcohol, and marijuana use among adolescents.

The prevalence of adolescents' involvement in different types of substance use has been charted in the United States since the mid 1970s, and fluctuations over the years have been documented (119). These fluctuations reflect, in part, changes in levels of social disapproval and risk perceived to be associated with the use of specific substances by young people (120,121). Changes in perceived harmfulness may be one explanation for the increase in prescription drug misuse among adolescents and young adults that has been documented in recent years (122,123). This highlights the importance of promoting attitudes and beliefs that are incompatible with drug misuse. Physicians are opinion shapers in their communities, especially with respect to matters of health. It is important to advocate abstinence from tobacco use and the use of illegal substances by children and adolescents. With respect to alcohol, the course associated with least health risks is to delay use until adulthood. Health professionals should educate their patients about the harms of substance use and communicate clear norms and standards regarding substances and their use.

Characteristics of the family can provide protection against the initiation of substance use and the development of substance abuse. As mentioned, warm and supportive parental involvement, monitoring, consistent discipline, and clear parental expectations against drug use appear to inhibit substance use and abuse (76,96,124,125). This underscores the importance of good parenting skills throughout development. Health professionals can facilitate good parenting by routinely linking the parents of their patients to developmentally appropriate parenting resources. At a minimum, this means making pamphlets, brochures, books, or videotapes on parenting available in the office and promoting the importance of keeping family bonds strong throughout development. Recently, workshop programs for parents of adolescents have been tested in randomized controlled trials and have been shown to be effective in reducing alcohol and other drug use by their adolescent children (68,79,80). Health care providers should consider offering these effective workshops for parents through their practices to empower parents to prevent substance abuse problems and promote the healthy development of their children.

CONCLUSIONS

The health professional who cares for children and youth can play a critical role in the prevention of substance misuse and abuse and in early intervention with those patients who have begun to use alcohol or other drugs. Knowledge of those factors that place young people at risk and of those factors that can protect against substance abuse is the foundation for assessment, diagnosis, and preventive action. A healthy, open relationship with children and families and an understanding of normal development allow the physician to assess existing and emerging risks for substance abuse across development and across spheres of life. Increasingly, effective approaches for reducing specific risks and enhancing protection have been identified and tested (37,126). The potential to intervene before problems arise is both the opportunity and obligation of those who care for youth.

REFERENCES

1. Sloboda Z, Bukoski WJ. *Handbook of drug abuse prevention: theory, science, and practice*. New York: Kluwer Academic/Plenum Publishers, 2003.
2. Gregg EW, Cheng YJ, Cadwell BL, et al. Secular trends in cardiovascular disease risk factors according to body mass index in U.S. adults. *J Am Med Assoc* 2005;293:1868–1874.
3. Ergin A, Muntner P, Sherwin R, et al. Secular trends in cardiovascular disease mortality, incidence, and case fatality rates in adults in the United States. *Am J Med* 2004;117:219–227.
4. Institute of Medicine. *Pathways of addiction: opportunities in drug abuse research*. Washington, DC: National Academy Press, 1996.
5. Schuckit MA. Biological vulnerability to alcoholism. *J Consult Clin Psychol* 1987;55:301–309.
6. Clark DB, Cornelius JR, Kirisci L, et al. Childhood risk categories for adolescent substance involvement: a general liability typology. *Drug Alcohol Depend* 2005;77:13–21.
7. Tarter R. Are there inherited behavioral traits which predispose to substance abuse? *J Consult Clin Psychol* 1988;56:189–196.
8. Hopfer CJ, Crowley TJ, Hewitt JK. Review of twin and adoption studies of adolescent substance use. *J Am Acad Child Adolesc Psychiatry* 2003;42:710–719.
9. Kendler KF. A population-based twin study of alcoholism in women. *J Am Med Assoc* 1992;268:1877–1882.
10. Allen NB, Lewinsohn PM, Seeley JR. Prenatal and perinatal influences on risk for psychopathology in childhood and adolescence. *Dev Psychopathol* 1998;10:513–529.
11. Bandstra ES, Vogel AL, Morrow CE, et al. Severity of prenatal cocaine exposure and child language functioning through age seven years: a longitudinal latent growth curve analysis. *Subst Use Misuse* 2004;39:25–59.
12. Bendersky M, Bennett D, Lewis M. Aggression at age 5 as a function of prenatal exposure to cocaine, gender, and environmental risk. *J Pediatr Psychol* 2006;31:71–84.
13. Messinger DS, Bauer CR, Das A, et al. The maternal lifestyle study: cognitive, motor, and behavioral outcomes of cocaine-exposed and opiate-exposed infants through three years of age. *Pediatrics* 2004;113: 1677–1685.
14. Singer LT, Minnes S, Short E, et al. Cognitive outcomes of preschool children with prenatal cocaine exposure. *J Am Med Assoc* 2004;291: 2448–2456.
15. Willford JA, Leech SL, Day NL. Moderate prenatal alcohol exposure and cognitive status of children at age 10. *Alcohol Clin Exp Res* 2006;30:1051–1059.
16. Alati R, Al Mamun A, Williams GM, et al. In utero alcohol exposure and prediction of alcohol disorders in early adulthood: a birth cohort study. *Arch Gen Psychiatry* 2006;63:1009–1016.
17. Baer JS, Sampson PD, Barr HM, et al. A 21-year longitudinal analysis of the effects of prenatal alcohol exposure on young adult drinking. *Arch Gen Psychiatry* 2003;60:377–385.
18. Buka SL, Shennasa ED, Niaura R. Elevated risk of tobacco dependence among offspring of mothers who smoked during pregnancy: a 30-year prospective study. *Am J Psychiatry* 2003;160:1978–1984.
19. Day NL, Goldschmidt L, Thomas CA. Prenatal marijuana exposure contributes to the prediction of marijuana use at age 14. *Addiction* 2006;101:1313–1322.
20. Porath AJ, Fried PA. Effects of prenatal cigarette and marijuana exposure on drug use among offspring. *Neurotoxicol Teratol* 2005;27: 267–277.
21. Hinckers AS, Laucht M, Schmidt MH, et al. Low level of response to alcohol as associated with serotonin transporter genotype and high alcohol intake in adolescents. *Biol Psychiatry* 2006;60:282–287.
22. Tarter RE, Kirisci L, Mezzich A, et al. Neurobehavioral disinhibition in childhood predicts early age at onset of substance use disorder. *Am J Psychiatry* 2003;160:1078–1085.
23. Tarter RE, Laird SB, Kabene M, et al. Drug abuse severity in adolescents is associated with magnitude of deviation in temperament traits. *Br J Addict* 1990;85:1501–1504.

24. Measelle JR, Stice E, Springer DW. A prospective test of the negative affect model of substance abuse: moderating effects of social support. *Psychol Addict Behav* 2006;20:225–233.
25. Wills TA, Dishion TJ. Temperament and adolescent substance use: a transactional analysis of emerging self-control. *J Clin Child Adolesc Psychol* 2004;33:69–81.
26. Wills TA, Stoolmiller M. The role of self-control in early escalation of substance use: a time-varying analysis. *J Consult Clin Psychol* 2002; 70:986–997.
27. Cloninger CR, Sigvardsson S, Bohman M. Childhood personality predicts alcohol abuse in young adults. *Alcohol Clin Exp Res* 1988;12: 494–505.
28. Crawford AM, Pentz MA, Chou CP, et al. Parallel developmental trajectories of sensation seeking and regular substance use in adolescents. *Psychol Addict Behav* 2003;17:179–192.
29. Burke JD, Loeber R, White HR, et al. Inattention as a key predictor of tobacco use in adolescence. *J Abnorm Psychol* 2007;116:249–259.
30. Molina BSG, Pelham WE. Childhood predictors of adolescent substance use in a longitudinal study of children with ADHD. *J Abnorm Psychol* 2003;112:497–507.
31. Gittelman RS, Mannuzza RS, Bonagura N. Hyperactive boys almost grown up: I. Psychiatric status. *Arch Gen Psychiatry* 1985;42:937–947.
32. Brook JS, Brook DW, Gordon AS, et al. The psychosocial etiology of adolescent drug use: a family interactional approach. *Genet Soc Gen Psychol Monogr* 1990;116:111–267.
33. Fergusson DM, Horwood LJ, Ridder EM. Conduct and attentional problems in childhood and adolescence and later substance use, abuse and dependence: results of a 25-year longitudinal study. *Drug Alcohol Depend* 2007;88S:S14–S26.
34. Sung M, Erkanli A, Angold A, et al. Effects of age at first substance use and psychiatric comorbidity on the development of substance use disorders. *Drug Alcohol Depend* 2004;75:287–299.
35. Windle M, Windle RC. Depressive symptoms and cigarette smoking among middle adolescents: prospective associations and intrapersonal and interpersonal influences. *J Consult Clin Psychol* 2001;69:215–226.
36. Marmorstein NR, Iacono WG. Major depression and conduct disorder in a twin sample: gender, functioning, and risk for future psychopathology. *J Am Acad Child Adolesc Psychiarty* 2003;42:225–233.
37. Spoth R, Greenberg M, Turrisi R. Preventive interventions addressing underage drinking: state of the evidence and steps toward public health impact. *Pediatrics* 2008;121:S311–S336.
38. Block J, Block JH, Keyes S. Longitudinally foretelling drug usage in adolescence: early childhood personality and environmental precursors. *Child Dev* 1988;59:336–355.
39. Jessor R, Jessor SL. *Problem behavior and psychological development: a longitudinal study of youth.* New York: Academic Press, 1977.
40. Barnow S, Schultz G, Lucht M, et al. Do alcohol expectancies and peer delinquency/substance use mediate the relationship between impulsivity and drinking behaviour in adolescence? *Alcohol Alcohol* 2004;39: 213–219.
41. Goldmann MS, Brown SA, Christiansen BA, et al. Alcoholism and memory: broadening of scope of alcohol-expectancy research. *Psychol Bull* 1991;110:137–146.
42. Cooper ML, Frone MR, Russell M, et al. Drinking to regulate positive and negative emotions: a motivational model of alcohol use. *J Person Soc Psychol* 1995;69:990–1005.
43. Kuntsche E, Knibbe R, Gmel G, et al. Why do young people drink? A review of drinking motives. *Clin Psychol Rev* 2005;25:841–861.
44. Barber P, Lopez-Valcarcel BG, Pinilla J, et al. Attitudes of teenagers towards cigarettes and smoking initiation. *Subst Use Misuse* 2005;40: 625–643.
45. Ellickson PL, Tucker JS, Klein DJ, et al. Antecedents and outcomes of marijuana use initiation during adolescence. *Prev Med* 2004;39: 976–984.
46. Kandel DB. Convergences in prospective longitudinal surveys of drug use in normal populations. In: Kandel DB, ed. *Longitudinal research on drug use: empirical findings and methodological issues.* Washington, DC: Hemisphere Publishing, 1978:3–38.
47. Pitkanen T, Lyyra AL, Pulkinnen L. Age of onset of drinking and the use of alcohol in adulthood: a follow-up study from age 8–42 for females and males. *Addiction* 2005;100:652–661.
48. Kandel DB. Epidemiological and psychosocial perspectives on adolescent drug use. *Am Acad Clin Psychol* 1982;21:328–347.
49. Lynskey MT, Heath AC, Bucholz KK, et al. Escalation of drug use in early-onset cannabis users vs. co-twin controls. *J Am Med Assoc* 2003; 289:427–433.
50. DeWit DJ, Adlaf EM, Offord DR, et al. Age at first alcohol use: a risk factor for the development of alcohol disorders. *Am J Psychiatry* 2000;157:745–750.
51. Grant BF, Dawson DA. Age of onset of drug use and its association with DSM-IV drug abuse and dependence: results from the National Longitudinal Alcohol Epidemiological Survey. *J Subst Abuse* 1998;10: 163–173.
52. Hingson RW, Heeren T, Winter MR. Age at drinking onset and alcohol dependence. *Arch Pediatr Adolesc Med* 2006;160:739–746.
53. Cleveland HH, Wiebe RP. The moderation of genetic and shared-environmental influences on adolescent drinking by levels of parental drinking. *J Stud Alcohol* 2003;64:182–194.
54. Hartman CA, Lessem JM, Hopfer CJ, et al. The family transmission of adolescent alcohol abuse and dependence. *J Stud Alcohol* 2006;67: 657–664.
55. McGue M, Sharma A, Benson P. Parent and sibling influences on adolescent alcohol use and misuse: evidence from a U.S. adoption cohort. *J Stud Alcohol* 1996;57:8–18.
56. Latendresse SJ, Rose RJ, Viken RJ, et al. Parenting mechanisms in links between parents' and adolescents' alcohol use behaviors. *Alcohol Clin Exp Res* 2008;32:322–330.
57. White HR, Johnson V, Buyske S. Parental modeling and parenting behavior effects on offspring alcohol and cigarette use: a growth curve analysis. *J Subst Abuse* 2000;12:287–310.
58. Bush PJ, Iannotti RJ. The development of children's health orientation and behaviors: lessons for substance abuse prevention. In: Jones CL, Battjejs RJ, eds. *Etiology of drug abuse: implications for prevention.* Rockville, MD: National Institute on Drug Abuse, 1985 pp. 45–74.
59. Pomery EA, Gibbons FX, Gerrard M, et al. Families and risk: prospective analysis of family and social influences on adolescent substance use. *J Fam Psychol* 2005;19:560–570.
60. Rende R, Slomkowski C, Lloyd-Richardson E, et al. Sibling effects on substance use in adolescence: social contagion and genetic relatedness. *J Fam Psychol* 2005;19:611–618.
61. Windle M. Parental, sibling, and peer influences on adolescent substance use and alcohol problems. *Appl Dev Sci* 2000;4:98–110.
62. Fagan AA, Najman JM. The relative contributions of parental and sibling substance use to adolescent tobacco, alcohol, and other drug use. *J Drug Issues* 2005;35:869–884.
63. Barnes GM, Reifman AS, Farrell MP, et al. The effects of parenting on the development of adolescent alcohol misuse: a six-wave latent growth model. *J Marriage Fam* 2000;62:175–186.
64. Brook JS, Brook DW, Richter L, et al. Risk and protective factors of adolescent drug use: implications for prevention programs. In: Sloboda Z, Bukoski WJ, eds. *Handbook of drug abuse prevention: theory, science, and practice.* New York: Kluwer, 2003:265–287.
65. Chassin L, Presson C, Rose J, et al. Parenting style and smoking-specific parenting practices as predictors of adolescent smoking onset. *J Pediatr Psychol* 2005;30:333–344.
66. Donovan JE. Adolescent alcohol initiation: a review of psychosocial risk factors. *J Adolesc Health* 2004;35:529.e7–529.e18.
67. Kandel DB, Andrews K. Processes of adolescent socialization by parents and peers. *Int J Addict* 1987;22:319-342.
68. Spoth R, Redmond C, Shin C, et al. Brief family intervention effects on adolescent substance initiation: school-level growth curve analyses 6 years following baseline. *J Consult Clin Psychol* 2004;72:535–542.
69. Velleman RB, Templeton LJ, Copello AG. The role of the family in preventing and intervening with substance use and misuse: a comprehensive review of family interventions, with a focus on young people. *Drug Alcohol Rev* 2005;24:93–109.

70. Harden KP, Turkheimer E, Emery RE, et al. Marital conflict and conduct problems in children of twins. *Child Dev* 2007;78:1–18.
71. Tschann JM, Flores E, Marin BV, et al. Interparental conflict and risk behaviors among Mexican American adolescents: a cognitive-emotional model. *J Abnorm Child Psychol* 2002;30:373–385.
72. Farrington DP. Childhood aggression and adult violence: early precursors and later life outcomes. In: Pepler DJ, Rubin KH, eds. *The development and treatment of childhood aggression*. Hillsdale, NJ: Lawrence Erlbaum, 1991:5–29.
73. Guo J, Hill KG, Hawkins JD, et al. A developmental analysis of sociodemographic, family, and peer effects on adolescent illicit drug initiation. *J Am Acad Child Adolesc Psychiarty* 2002;41:838–845.
74. Wills TA, Sandy JM, Yaeger A, et al. Family risk factors and adolescent substance use: moderation effects for temperament dimensions. *Dev Psychol* 2001;37:283–297.
75. Bronte-Tinkew J, Moore KA, Carrano J. The father-child relationship, parenting styles, and adolescent risk behaviors in intact families. *J Fam Issues* 2006;27:850–881.
76. Simons-Morton B, Chen R. Latent growth curve analyses of parent influences on drinking progression among early adolescents. *J Stud Alcohol* 2005;66:5–13.
77. Wood MD, Read JP, Mitchell RE, et al. Do parents still matter? Parent and peer influences on alcohol involvement among recent high school graduates. *Psychol Addict Behav* 2004;18:19–30.
78. Dick DM, Viken RJ, Purcell S, et al. Parental monitoring moderates the importance of genetic and environmental influences on adolescent smoking. *J Abnorm Psychol* 2007;116:213–218.
79. Haggerty KP, Skinner ML, MacKenzie EP, et al. A randomized trial of Parents Who Care: effects on key outcomes at 24-month follow-up. *Prev Sci* 2007;8:249–260.
80. Mason WA, Kosterman R, Hawkins JD, et al. Reducing adolescents' growth in substance use and delinquency: randomized trial effects of a parent-training preventive intervention. *Prev Sci* 2003;4:203–212.
81. Kandel DB, Kiros G-E, Schaffran C, et al. Racial/ethnic differences in cigarette smoking initiation and progression to daily smoking: a multilevel analysis. *Am J Public Health* 2004;94:128–135.
82. Simons-Morton B. Prospective association of peer influence, school engagement, drinking expectancies, and parent expectations with drinking initiation among sixth graders. *Addict Behav* 2004;29:299–309.
83. Wills TA, Yaeger AM, Sandy JM. Buffering effects of religiosity for adolescent substance use. *Psychol Addict Behav* 2003;17:24–31.
84. van den bree MB, Pickworth WB. Risk factors predicting changes in marijuana involvement in teenagers. *Arch Gen Psychiatry* 2005;62:311–319.
85. van den bree MB, Whitmer MD, Pickworth WB. Predictors of smoking development in a population-based sample of adolescents: a prospective study. *J Adolesc Health* 2004;35:172–181.
86. Bergen HA, Martin G, Roeger L, et al. Perceived academic performance and alcohol, tobacco, and marijuana use: longitudinal relationships in young community adolescents. *Addict Behav* 2005;30:1563–1573.
87. Ellickson PL, Tucker JS, Klein DJ, et al. Prospective risk factors for alcohol misuse in late adolescence. *J Stud Alcohol* 2001;62:773–782.
88. Flory K, Lynam D, Milich R, et al. Early adolescent through young adult alcohol and marijuana use trajectories: early predictors, young adult outcomes, and predictive utility. *Dev Psychopathol* 2004;16:193–213.
89. Henry KL, Huizinga DH. Truancy's effect on the onset of drug use among urban adolescents placed at risk. *J Adolesc Health* 2007;40:358.e9–358.e17.
90. Barnes GM, Hoffman JH, Welte JW, et al. Adolescents' time use: effects on substance use, delinquency, and sexual activity. *J Youth Adolesc* 2007;36:697–710.
91. Mason WA, Hitchings JE, McMahon RJ, et al. A test of three alternative hypotheses regarding the effects of early delinquency on adolescent psychosocial functioning and substance involvement. *J Abnorm Child Psychol* 2007;35:831–843.
92. Newcomb MD, Bentler PM. Substance use and ethnicity: differential impact of peer and adult models. *J Psychol* 1986;120:83–95.
93. Simons-Morton B, Chen RS. Over time relationships between early adolescent and peer substance use. *Addict Behav* 2006;31:1211–1223.
94. Eitle D. The moderating effects of peer substance use on the family structure-adolescent substance use association: quantity versus quality of parenting. *Addict Behav* 2005;30:963–980.
95. Cleveland HH, Wiebe RP, Rowe DC. Sources of exposure to smoking and drinking friends among adolescents: a behavioral-genetic evaluation. *J Genet Psychol* 2005;166:153–169.
96. Mason WA, Windle M. Family, religious, school and peer influences on adolescent alcohol use: a longitudinal study. *J Stud Alcohol* 2001;62:44–53.
97. Huba GJ, Bentler PM. The role of peer and adult models for drug taking at different stages in adolescence. *J Youth Adolesc* 1980;9:449–465.
98. Newcomb MD. Psychosocial predictors and consequences of drug use: a developmental perspective within a prospective study. *J Addict Dis* 1997;16:51–89.
99. Duncan SC, Duncan TE, Strycker LA. A multilevel analysis of neighborhood context and youth alcohol and drug problems. *Prev Sci* 2002;3:125–133.
100. Lambert SF, Brown TL, Phillips CM, et al. The relationship between perceptions of neighborhood characteristics and substance use among urban African American adolescents. *Am J Community Psychol* 2004;34:205–218.
101. Wagenaar AC, Toomey TL. Effects of minimum drinking age laws: review and analysis of the literature from 1960 to 2000. *J Stud Alcohol* 2002;14(Suppl):206–225.
102. Choi Y, Harachi TW, Catalano RF. Neighborhoods, family, and substance use: comparisons of the relations across racial and ethnic groups. *Soc Serv Rev* 2006;80:675–704.
103. Little M, Steinberg L. Psychosocial correlates of adolescent drug dealing in the inner city: potential roles of opportunity, conventional commitments, and maturity. *J Res Crime Delinquency* 2006;43:357–386.
104. Winstanley EL, Steinwachs DM, Ensminger ME, et al. The association of self-reported neighborhood disorganization and social capital with adolescent alcohol and drug use, dependence, and access. *Drug Alcohol Depend* 2008;92:173–182.
105. Beyers JM, Toumbourou JW, Catalano RF, et al. A cross-national comparison of risk and protective factors for adolescent substance use: the United States and Australia. *J Adolesc Health* 2004;35:3–16.
106. Elek E, Miller-Day M, Hecht ML. Influences of personal, injunctive, and descriptive norms on early adolescent substance use. *J Drug Issues* 2006;36:147–171.
107. Verkooijen KT, de Vries NK, Nielsen GA. Youth crowds and substance use: the impact of perceived group norm and multiple group identification. *Psychol Addict Behav* 2007;21:55–61.
108. Collins RL, Ellickson PL, McCaffrey D, et al. Early adolescent exposure to alcohol advertising and its relationship to underage drinking. *J Adolesc Health* 2007;40:527–534.
109. Sargent JD, Beach ML, Adachi-Mejia AM, et al. Exposure to movie smoking: its relation to smoking initiation among U.S. adolescents. *Pediatrics* 2005;116:1183–1191.
110. Sargent JD, Wills TA, Stoolmiller M, et al. Alcohol use in motion pictures and its relation with early-onset teen drinking. *J Stud Alcohol* 2006;67:54–65.
111. Radke-Yarrow M, Sherman T. Children born at medical risk: factors affecting vulnerability and resilience. In: Rolf J, Masten AS, Cicchetti D, eds. *Risk and protective factors in the development of psychopathology*. Cambridge: Cambridge University Press, 1990.
112. Brown TL, Miller JD, Clayton RR. The generalizability of substance use predictors across racial groups. *J Early Adolesc* 2004;24:274–302.
113. Kandel DB, Raveis VH. Cessation of illicit drug use in young adulthood. *Arch Gen Psychiatry* 1989;46:109–116.
114. Ennett ST, Bauman KE, Hussong A, et al. The peer context of adolescent substance use: findings from social network analysis. *J Res Adolesc* 2006;16:159–186.
115. Guo J, Hawkins JD, Hill KG, et al. Childhood and adolescent predictors of alcohol abuse and dependence in young adulthood. *J Stud Alcohol* 2001;62:754–762.
116. Hansen WB, Graham JW. Preventing alcohol, marijuana, and cigarette use among adolescents: peer pressure resistance training versus establishing conservative norms. *Prev Med* 1991;20:414–430.

117. Mason WA, Windle M. A longitudinal study of the effects of religiosity on adolescent alcohol use and alcohol-related problems. *J Adolesc Res* 2002;17:346–363.
118. Walker C, Ainette MG, Wills TA, et al. Religiosity and substance use: test of an indirect-effect model in early and middle adolescence. *Psychol Addict Behav* 2007;21:84–96.
119. Johnston LD, O'Malley PM, Bachman JG. *Monitoring the Future national results on adolescent drug use: overview of key findings, 2006.* NIH Publication No. 07-6202. Washington, DC: National Institute on Drug Abuse, 2007.
120. Bachman JG, Johnston LD, O'Malley PM. Explaining the recent decline in cocaine use among young adults: further evidence that perceived risks and disapproval lead to reduced drug use. *J Health Soc Behav* 1990;31:173–184.
121. Bachman JG, Johnston LD, O'Malley PM. Explaining recent increases in students' marijuana use: impacts of perceived risks and disapproval 1976–1996. *Am J Public Health* 1998;88:887–892.
122. Simoni-Wastila L, Strickler G. Risk factors associated with problem use of prescription drugs. *Am J Public Health* 2004;94:266–268.
123. Substance Abuse and Mental Health Services Administration. *Results from the 2005 National Survey on Drug Use and Health: National findings.* Office of Applied Studies, NSDUH Series H-30, DHHS Publication No. SMA 06-4194. Rockville, MD, 2006.
124. Kosterman R, Hawkins JD, Guo J, et al. The dynamics of alcohol and marijuana initiation: Patterns and predictors of first-use in adolescence. *Am J Public Health* 2000;90:360–366.
125. Zhou Q, King KM, Chassin L. The roles of familial alcoholism and adolescent family harmony in young adults' substance dependence disorders: mediated and moderated relations. *J Abnorm Psychol* 2006;115: 320–331.
126. Hawkins JD, Smith BH, Hill KG, et al. Promoting social development and preventing health and behavior problems during the elementary grades: results from the Seattle Social Development Project. *Victims Offend* 2007;2:161–181.

CHAPTER 100

Deborah R. Simkin, MD

Neurobiology of Addiction from a Developmental Perspective

Addiction, for the purposes of this chapter, will be defined along the DSM-IV-R criteria of substance dependence. The authors will attempt to delineate *genetic*, *biological*, *pharmacological*, and *social* factors that may lead to addiction from a developmental perspective. What factors lead to early experimentation? Is it genes that make youth more susceptible to use, or environment, or both? To answer this, one must understand the role of genes and environment, epigenetics, on the developing brain. In order to illustrate these factors, a case presentation is first discussed; then the author will begin to explore the biopsychosocial components of this case presentation that increased the risk of developing a substance abuse disorder in the case described. As well, the reader is invited to refer to Chapter 1 as background prior to reading this chapter.

Case Presentation

Linda, a 17-year-old female high school student, presents to your office. She is accompanied by her parents, who are worried about drug use. Linda was pulled over by the police after a party for reckless driving. She was found to have an alcohol level of 0.25 and was charged with a DUI. She was ordered by the court to be evaluated and enter a drug treatment program.

Developmental History Mom revealed that, prior to her pregnancy with Linda, she smoked a pack of cigarettes a day and had a glass of wine once a week. She also admitted to using marijuana daily. Upon learning she was pregnant; she stopped smoking both cigarettes and marijuana and stopped drinking. She denied any other drug use. During the delivery, the baby experienced fetal distress owing to a nuchal cord, and the mother had to undergo an emergency C-section. Linda was born blue but did not require intubation. She was described as a colicky child until 4 months of age and experienced slightly below normal weight gain. She had normal developmental milestones but was always hyper and had temper tantrums that would last more than an hour as a toddler. With constant reminders, she responded to praise and rewarding good behavior during her pre-latency years. Linda experienced severe separation anxiety when she went to preschool. When she began kindergarten, mom states that the teacher loved her but she often stated that she was shy at times and also easily distracted and could not seem to finish her work. She struggled with reading in first grade, but her grades did not become a problem until around third grade. At that time, she experienced a re-occurrence of her separation anxiety, accompanied with night terrors. When asked about physical or sexual abuse privately, she revealed she was sexually abused by a neighbor from age 7 to 9 but never told anyone because he threatened to hurt her family. The perpetrator moved away sometime within the past 6 months while she was in 11th grade in high school. As she approached middle school, she continued to struggle with her grades but became an average student. She entered high school and was a good athlete on the soccer team when her parents noted that the students she began to hang around with were skipping school. She quit the soccer team in the beginning of the 10th grade and began skipping school. During this same time period, her parents began to notice extreme mood swings. She would sneak out at night and was found by a neighbor asleep and drunk in their front yard. Her grades were close to failing, and she has been suspended three times for back talking the teachers and carrying cigarettes on campus.

Drug and Alcohol History She reveals that she began experimenting with cigarettes at age 11. She now smokes about four to five cigarettes a day. She began drinking alcohol at the end of seventh grade (age 12). She noticed she was very shy and fearful of not being accepted and began getting drunk during 10th grade (age 15). She now uses to relax and "fit in" when using alcohol. Over the last 6 weeks, she has gotten drunk every weekend. She does not feel she has to use alcohol or marijuana and never uses when she has to study. However, she feels she cannot do well in school because her concentration is poor. She also began experimenting with marijuana during the summer between the 10th and 11th grades. She states that, when she began to drink, she noticed that she could drink more than her friends without getting drunk. She denies any other drug use.

Patient Medical History There is no significant history except for childhood asthma.

Patient Psychiatric History Though told by the school that Linda may need an evaluation for attention deficit hyperactivity disorder (ADHD), her mother did not want to put her daughter on medication and never requested her to be evaluated.

Family Medical History There is a family history for liver problems in a paternal uncle who died of cirrhosis of the liver. He was a person/patient with alcohol dependence. Linda's father has hypertension. Her paternal grandmother died of cancer when she was in the seventh grade. Linda was very close to her because she lived next door and was often at her house when her parents were at work.

Family Psychiatric History Mom was very shy as a child, and, as an adult, suffered from postpartum depression. She was treated with Zoloft, which did relieve her depression. She restarted the medication over the past year owing to the stress she experienced with her daughter's struggles. The uncle who died of cirrhosis of the liver had been diagnosed with posttraumatic stress disorder (PTSD) after serving in the Viet Nam War. He was not treated for the PTSD and continued to drink. Dad's father and mom's father were persons/patients with alcohol dependence, and mom states that dad's drinking has increased recently to 6 to 10 beers every night.

Patient Social History Linda states that she is sexually active but that she is promiscuous only when she is drunk. She does not know whether condoms were always used. Her last period was 2 weeks ago. She sought testing for a sexually transmitted disease and AIDS at a private clinic without her parents' knowledge, and both came back negative. She would like to go to college but is not sure of whether she is smart enough to complete the 4 years required. She began to be attracted to a group of teenagers who were using alcohol. She then started dating a young man who introduced her to this group when she was in 10th grade. She lost interest in soccer and noticed she felt she belonged when "hanging around with them and using marijuana and alcohol" with this group. She has driven when intoxicated but has never used marijuana or alcohol alone. She reveals that, once while drunk, she got in a fight with a friend and hit her. She was never in trouble with the law prior to the present episode but admitted to having stolen beer with a friend from a local store. Linda was very ashamed about both stealing and her sexual activity when drunk. At times, when drunk, she could not remember what she had done. Though Linda feels she is spiraling out of control, repeated efforts by her parents to intervene have failed. Though she is unsure that she can quit drinking, she is willing to try. She wants to get back to sports. She did enjoy her youth group at church but is embarrassed about what she has done in the past and is afraid she would not fit in with this group now.

Family Social History Linda is an only child. Mom finished high school and always had problems with math and reading. Dad was often in trouble for being the "class clown" and finished high school as an average student. There is no history of sexual or physical abuse in either of the parents. Dad has had problems keeping a job as a sales clerk because he is told he is too disorganized. This has put financial stress on the family. Mom works as a bank teller. They have always lived in the same area. There is no cultural diversity in the family. They are Catholic and, though they used to go to church, they have not been able to get their daughter to attend church with them since she got to high school. She was active in the church youth group prior to this. Mom and dad got married when they were just out of high school because mom got pregnant. They have separated on two occasions owing to dad's drinking. This occurred when Linda was 8 years old and again when she was in the seventh grade. From the sixth grade to the present time she has been a child who after school returned home alone until her parents got home from work.

Review of Systems Linda states that it takes her 2 hours to fall asleep. She is wide awake and feels "like I could party all night." She had recurring nightmares when the sexual abuse took place but not anymore. She feels fatigued lately and does not enjoy the things she used to enjoy. Her appetite has decreased, and she has lost 10 pounds. She has a good body image and no signs of an eating disorder. She has no other physical symptoms but notices that she has difficulty getting up in front of the class to speak. She has had flashbacks of the sexual abuse she suffered from age 7 to 9 after she got drunk, and engaged in sex with someone she did not know well. She is hypervigilant in the presence of older men. Overall, she gets much more irritated then she used to be. She cries almost daily and, though she has never had a plan to kill herself, she feels so ashamed that she wishes she would not wake up. Her concentration at school is poor, and she gave up academically in middle school when she could not keep up.

Mental Status Exam Linda's affect is blunted, and she cried several times during the evaluation. She was well-groomed, though wore no makeup. She appeared lethargic. She was underweight. Her judgment in the past was poor, but she seemed motivated to change her behavior. She was oriented, but her concentration was poor. She was unable to remember the three words given to her at the beginning of the mental status exam. She denied any auditory or visual hallucinations and had no delusional thinking. Her speech was slow but not tangential. She was articulate and seemed to appear brighter than the level suggested by her grades. As noted before, she denied suicidal plans but reported some ideation in the past.

BIOPSYCHOSOCIAL ANALYSIS

Constructing a chronologic summary of the biopsychosocial information can help assimilate the important events. This can be done as shown in Figure 100.1.

The impact of each of these events as risk factors for substance abuse is reviewed from a developmental perspective in the next section. When appropriate, the implication of these

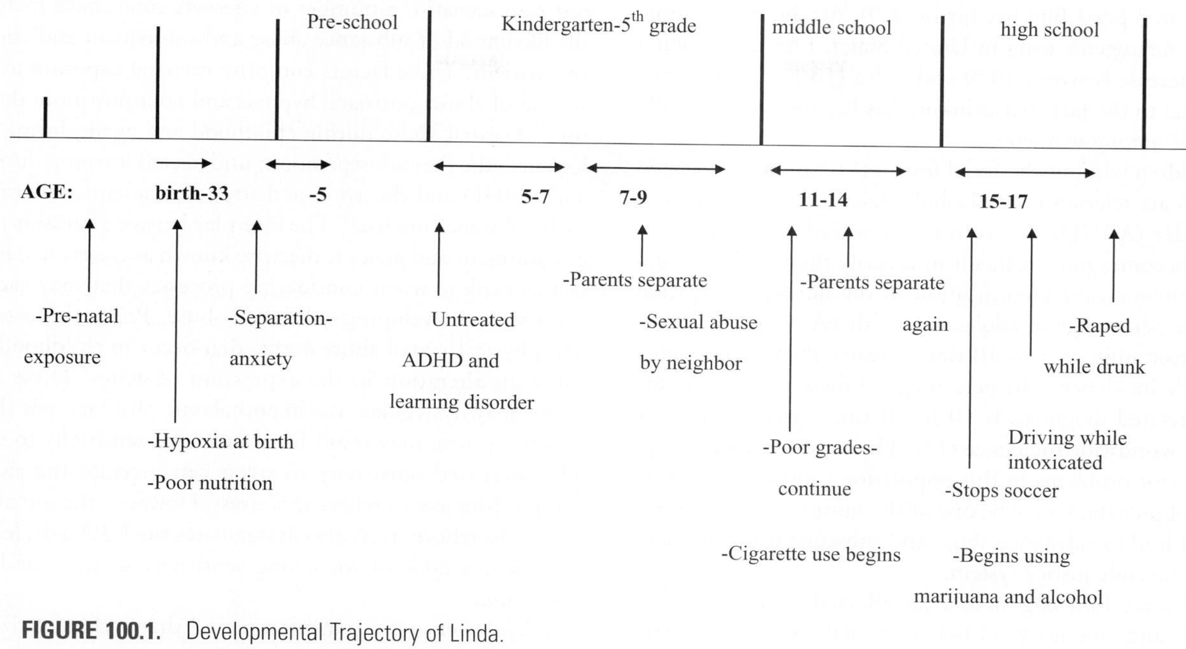

FIGURE 100.1. Developmental Trajectory of Linda.

events on the developing brain from a neurobiologic perspective will be explored in the chapter.

Prenatal Exposure

Though it is unclear whether prenatal exposure to substances of abuse can increase the risk of developing a substance abuse disorder (SUD), studies have shown that prenatal exposure can increase the risk of developing a learning disorder (LD) or comorbid conditions that may increase the risk of abusing drugs and alcohol. In this case study, the fetus was subjected to cigarette and marijuana smoking.

Prenatal Exposure to Nicotine and Marijuana

Prenatal nicotine exposure can increase toddler's negativity, propensity for externalizing disorders, such as ADHD or ADHD symptoms and/or conduct disorders (1,2). Prenatal cigarette exposure has been associated with lower IQ, poorer auditory functioning, and poorer performance on tests requiring fundamental aspects of visual perceptual performance. In contrast, prenatal marijuana exposure did not have a negative impact on IQ, auditory-based behaviors, or basic visual-perceptual skills. Rather, in-utero exposure to marijuana impacted on the application of these skills in problem-solving situations requiring visual integration and analytical skills, as well as sustained attention. A study involving multiple regression analyses (including controls with no exposure) in 18- to 22-year-olds exposed prenatally to marijuana confirmed the effect on visuospatial working memory (3).

Linda's history of early colicky behavior and possible LDs and reading difficulty may have been partly precipitated by early nicotine exposure. However, the fetus was also exposed to marijuana. Consistent patterns of cognitive deficits related to prenatal exposure to marijuana have been found from a longitudinal study (4). The cohort of women included women ranged in age from 18 to 42; half were African American and half white, and most were of lower socioeconomic status. These include IQ deficits and inattention at age 3. At age 6, the history of exposure to heavy marijuana maternal use (one or more cigarettes per day) during the first trimester was associated with lower verbal reasoning scores on the Stanford-Binet Intelligence Scale. Exposure to heavy use during the second trimester predicted deficits in the composite, short-term memory, and quantitative scores on the Stanford-Binet (5). At 6 and 10 years of age, offspring were more impulsive and had more internalizing and externalizing behaviors. At 14 years of age, prenatal marijuana predicted executive function difficulty, attention deficit problems, and an increased risk for substance use. At 16 years of age, externalizing behaviors, psychiatric disorders and substance abuse were associated with prenatal marijuana exposure. All analyses controlled for significant covariates (3). Though Linda's mother stopped using in the first trimester, the use during this time period may have contributed to Linda's reading ability.

Though Linda's mother did not use a substantial amount of alcohol during pregnancy, it is important to mention the potentially severe effects of prenatal exposure to alcohol.

Prenatal Exposure to Alcohol

Though there is little research on the direct effects of substances of abuse on the brain reward circuitry that leads to addiction, research does show a high risk for later alcohol abuse in children exposed to alcohol prenatally (7). Areas affected by early alcohol exposure are discussed further, which lead to increased impulsivity that could promote increased risk for experimentation during adolescence.

Fetal alcohol syndrome (FAS) is the most common non-hereditary cause of mental retardation. The prevalence varies from 0.5 to 3 per 1,000 live births (8,9). Alcohol has become the most teratogenic drug in United States. FAS has shown a sixfold increase between 1979 and 1993 (10,11). This is primarily due to the fact that drinking has become more socially acceptable among women.

Children without the facial features commonly associated with FAS are referred to as alcohol-related neurodevelopmental disorder (ARND). Unfortunately, without the facial features, it becomes more difficult to identify these children, and 60% to 90% escape identification in the normal population (12). The percentage of adolescents with FAS in juvenile justice forensic units is 3 to 10 times greater than the accepted worldwide incidence. The percentage of these youth with any alcohol-related diagnosis is 10 to 40 times greater than the accepted worldwide incidence (13). The cognitive and disruptive behavior problems in this population caused by exposure to alcohol prenatally may be one of the most undiagnosed reasons that lead to substance abuse and subsequent involvement with the juvenile justice system.

There are four cognitive areas affected by FAS/ARND: learning and memory (14–16), visual-spatial processes (15,17), executive function (14–16,18), and attention (19,20).

In another study, auditory processing problems were more impaired in FAS/ARND children than were visual processing problems. The latter information may account for another reason for attention problems with these children (21). Two studies on children with FAS/ARND demonstrated longer reaction times in these individuals. Therefore, children with FAS/ARND may have slower processing speeds that can be confused with attention problems (22,23). These studies stress the importance of evaluating every aspect of attention difficulties in FAS/ARND children.

Prenatal Exposure to Other Substances of Abuse

Though cocaine can cause developmental delays and learning disorders, it is clear that findings once thought to be specific to in-utero cocaine exposure are more likely to be associated with alcohol, tobacco and marijuana and the quality of the child's environment (24). However, a better home environment was found to reduce many of the effects on lower IQ found at age 4 in cocaine-exposed babies (25).

Though the numbers of studies investigating the effect of prenatal caffeine exposure are few, there is little evidence at this time that prenatal caffeine has significant impact on childhood mental and motor development (26).

STRESSORS

Any compromise that would cause fetal distress or hypoxia increases the risk for the development of ADHD or learning disorders, which in turn could lead to an increased risk for substance abuse later in life. However, factors such as trauma, prenatal and postnatal stress, and early-life rearing experiences may alter addiction pathology later in life through changes in gene expression. These changes occur through chromatin remodeling without changes in DNA sequences (27–29). In our case scenario, a number of stressors could have increased the likelihood of substance abuse and subsequent addiction in this patient. These factors comprise prenatal exposure to substances of abuse; postnatal hypoxia and poor nutrition; the history of sexual abuse during childhood and again during adolescence; the parent's separation; undetected learning disorders and ADHD and the associated stress of academic failure; and early substance use itself. The interplay between stressors in the environment and genes (otherwise known as *epigenetics*) is crucial to explore when considering processes that may increase the risk for developing substance abuse. Prenatal, postnatal; and physical/sexual abuse events that occur in childhood may cause an alteration in the expression of genes. These alterations may dysregulate the hypothalamic pituitary axis (HPA) which, in turn, may result in an increased sensitivity to stress. The increased sensitivity to stress can increase the risk for using substances to relieve this stress. However, the use of substances to relieve stress also dysregulates the HPA axis, leading to a vicious cycle of worsening sensitivity to stress and substance use.

Adolescence is a transition period that is characterized by considerable neurobiologic changes and an associated increased propensity for substance use. It is also a time of enhanced sensitivity to stress. Therefore, the vicious circle described earlier may be worsened during adolescence, leading to a steeper spiraling movement toward HPA dysregulation and severity of substance use problems. However, the road to addiction impacted by stress, environment, and developmental factors during adolescence may be modulated by individual genetic background. Studies have suggested an interaction between functional alleles that determine levels of neurotransmitter activity (e.g., dopamine, serotonin), environment (e.g., stress level, family factors), and severity of substance use problems (29). Certain environmental conditions could cause permanent changes in neural circuitry that, in turn, could confer vulnerability for substance abuse and increase the risk of progression from substance abuse to addiction. These factors coupled with the family history of substance abuse may be the reason why Linda moved rapidly from one substance of abuse to another and to addiction.

Stress, Drugs, Reward, and the HPA: Koob's Model-Anti-Reward System The antireward system involves the hypothalamic pituitary axis (HPA) and norepinephrine NE in the brain stress/emotional system and neuropeptide Y (NPY) in the antistress system (29). The role of these systems and the effect on the HPA will be discussed. First, all drugs have positive reinforcing effects. During acute drug use, all drugs of abuse increase dopamine in the shell of the nucleus accumbens (NAc), as well as other areas. Though the HPA can be activated by such things as stress, acute drug use can also activate the hypothalamic pituitary axis (HPA). Both of these processes increase drug reward (30,31). The role of the prefrontal cortex (PFC) in modulating the NAc function will be discussed later. However, the system can still revert to normal or homeostasis if chronic drug use does not occur.

Chronic drug use can induce permanent changes in the motivation to use drugs. One theory that has attempted to explain how this occurs is the opponent-process theory (32). This theory proposes that an affective or hedonic habituation occurs (tolerance) at the same time as a negative affective response develops to abstinence (withdrawal). This would increase the motivation to use drugs to (1) use more drugs to achieve the same effect and (2) ward off the negative effects of withdrawal. However, though all drugs can decrease D2 receptors during chronic drug use, all drugs have the same effect during withdrawal. Another common finding that occurs during withdrawal, though not unique to it, is a hypofunctioning of the orbital frontal cortex (OFC). Other changes that occur during withdrawal include an increase in adrenocorticotropic hormone (ACTH), corticosterone, and corticotrophin-releasing factor (CRF), during overactivation of the HPA axis. Continued use leads to increased CRF and increasing anxiety each time the individual is abstinent.

Furthermore, overactivation of the HPA axis during chronic drug use also increases norepinephrine (NE) in the bed of the stria terminalis of the extended amygdala), which increases sensitivity to stress. Increases in ACTH, corticosterone, CRF, and NE are part of the recruitment of brain stress/emotion systems. In addition, during chronic drug use, NPY decreases in the central and medial nucleus of the extended amygdala. The change in neuropeptide Y (NPY) is referred to as a dysregulation of the brain antistress sytem. All these changes in CRF, NE, and NPY are referred to as the antireward system.

As these events occur, the individual becomes more sensitive to stress each time drugs are used and, therefore, the individual is more likely to seek out drugs to relieve the stress. Each time drugs are used, the continued decrease in reward function in the brain reward system and the increased recruitment of the brain antireward system moves the brain, from a reversible state where homeostasis could have been reinstated, to a more dysregulated state. This dysregulation occurs through a process known as *allostasis*. Allostasis is the attempt of the brain to achieve stability through change. Rather than the allostatic state reaching stability, it instead causes chronic pathologic states and damage. A change in baseline occurs such that environmental events that would normally elicit drug-seeking behavior have more impact; hence, the brain is more sensitive to stress-induced drug seeking (31), and this process involves input into the extended amygdala (29,30). Of course, as noted, if a person has had chronic stressful experiences, like the sexual abuse experienced by Linda in her childhood, and subsequent PTSD symptomatology, this may cause an alteration on the expression of genes that may dysregulate the HPA axis, which would increase the sensitivity to stress and increase the risk for using substances to relieve this stress. Therefore, chronic stressors that occur before drug use occurs may set the stage so that the HPA system is less likely to return to normal once drug use and experimentation begins.

Changes in Brain Reward Circuitry in the Transition to an Addicted State Many teens who abuse substances will not develop an addiction after the maturation of the PFC in the early twenties (33). In those who develop addiction, a conceptualization of addiction neurobiology is helpful toward understanding the role that comorbidity and genes play. Certain comorbid conditions may affect the brain reward circuitry leading to self medication of these comorbid conditions, or genes may be inherited that increase the sensitivity to the reinforcing effects of the drugs on the brain reward circuitry.

First, one must understand how one learns that a stimulus is salient so that the individual will learn to seek out the salient stimuli. When an individual uses cocaine, there is a rapid increase in dopamine in the shell of the NAc. As cocaine is taken intravenously, in this example, dopamine levels increase more rapidly and at higher levels, yielding a more pleasurable high (34). Anticipation of drug reward alone has been associated with dopamine release (34). The evolution of this process is discussed later. In general, the shell of the NAc and dopamine are involved in *acute* drug reinforcement, but the core of the NAc, the basolateral amygdala, and the OFC are involved in *chronic* drug use that leads to addiction. The latter does not involve dopamine but rather the recruitment of glutamatergic efferents from the OFC to the core of the NAc (30,34).

What causes the PFC (anterior cingulate and the orbital frontal cortex) to place less salience on previously salient reinforcers and more salience on drugs of abuse? Chronic drug use causes intracellular changes, leading to circuitry changes, resulting in dysregulation of the reward circuitry involving the PFC, basolateral amygdala, and the core of the NAc. Changes in the intracellular level have been described as three stages: acute, transition, and end/addiction stage (34).

Stage 1: Acute Drug Effects After the acute administration of cocaine, dopamine levels of the nucleus accumbens are elevated with little effect on glutamatergic tone, resulting in increasing locomotor activity and stimulating reward circuits (35,37). Moreover, the D1 dopamine receptor (DRD1) is stimulated, resulting in the following:

- Activation of cAMP-dependent protein kinase (PKA)
- PKA-induced phosphorylation of transcriptional regulator cAMP response element–binding protein CREB
- Induction of early gene products such as cFOS

cFOS causes short-term neuroplastic changes as the molecule cFOS is very unstable. This transcription factor turns on genes that produce dynorphin, which causes dysphoria during early drug withdrawal, and genes that inhibit dopamine and lc opioid receptors, which, in turn, decrease drug reward. cFOS is so unstable that it dissipates in 4 to 12 hours. Therefore, limited exposure to drugs will allow the system to return to normal/homeostasis.

Stage 2: Transition to Addiction Chronic repeated administration of the drug causes stimulation of DRD1 to produce proteins with long half-lives, such as Delta FosB. Delta FosB modulates transcription and synthesis of certain AMPA glutamate receptor subunits and cell-signaling enzymes. A GluR1 glutamate receptor in the ventral tegmental area (VTA) forms after discontinuation of substances such as cocaine. Also, animals with activated Delta FosB have exaggerated sensitivity to the rewarding effects of drugs (35). In addition Delta FosB also increases CdK5, which, in turn, blocks the stimulating effects of cocaine or blocks the anxiolytic effect of alcohol so that, in both instances, more cocaine or alcohol is needed to get the same effect (38). CdK5 may be one of the reasons tolerance occurs in substance abusers. Hence, if the foregoing is true, Delta FosB may increase the rewarding effects of drugs, causing an individual to seek out these rewarding effects more often and, when the individual does, more of the drug must be used to give the same rewarding effect.

Additionally, during chronic drug use and withdrawal periods, there is an increase of G protein binding AGS3. Increased AGS3 levels inhibit D2 receptor signaling and correspondingly increase D1 receptor signaling, which causes increased activity of projections from the PFC (in this case the anterior cingulate and the OFC) to the core of the nucleus accumbens (NAc) which mediates behavior. What do these changes mean? The PFC is involved in salience (see Chapter 1). However, these changes reduce the salience of nondrug motivational stimuli so that normal stimuli such as food are less salient. The PFC becomes hypoactive to previously salient stimuli. However, when drug-associated drug stimuli are available, there is a profound activation of the PFC and glutamatergic drive to the core of NAc, and drug craving occurs. The changes in determining what is now salient (drugs) and the activation of the PFC to the core of the NAc to produce craving moves the brain from a transitional stage to the end-stage of addiction. As previously mentioned, glutamate plays a more important role in drug seeking after chronic drug exposure, versus dopamine playing a role in acute drug use (drug-taking, reinforcement). The NAc core increases release of glutamate in response to stimuli that induce drug seeking and intake. Such stimuli may be a cue previously associated with drug use or a mild stressor.

End-Stage Addiction Changes in protein expression that mediate the transition to addiction may induce changes in protein expression that move from temporary and reversible to permanent.

What effect does glutamate produced by the NAc have on permanent adaptations that lead to continued drug use? Two things occur. First, when presynaptic glutamate is released, the GluR2/3 inhibitory autoreceptor becomes less effective. Less glutamate is released in the NAc after cocaine withdrawal and, therefore, presynaptic inhibitory GluR2/3 tone is decreased, and more glutamate is released in the core of the NAc when a mild stressor occurs or a cue associated with drug use occurs. Increase in glutamate postsynaptically causes an increase in proteins that cause rigid dendritic morphology and signaling. The changes that occur after chronic drug use are more permanent than changes that occur during acute drug use and may be central toward explaining the transition from drug taking, to addiction, and eventually relapse. All relapses can be categorized as due to either (1) drug/behavior re-exposure, (2) cue, or (3) stress.

The amygdala is involved in attaching affective valence to stimuli and has thus been implicated in relapse of all three types mentioned earlier. The basolateral amygdala recognizes motivationally relevant events, triggering the PFC to determine salience, and the PFC then influences the nucleus accumbers, which further mediates behavior (30,34). Hence, this process may reflect a clinical triad that is the phenotype of addiction: (1) loss of control (when the patient continues to use even though there is no enjoyment is using), (2) continued use despite negative consequences, and (3) preoccupation with the drug. The changes that occur after chronic drug use are believed more permanent than changes that occur during acute drug use Adolescent brains not only may be remodeled by this state-dependent process involved in the transition from drug-taking (or perhaps substance abuse) to drug addiction (substance dependence) but may also have trait-dependent, preexisting vulnerabilities in these brain systems. As adolescents may not be able to differentiate between motivationally relevant events (see developmental effects further), when addiction occurs, the PFC may increase the behavior to seek out risky behaviors whether they are relevant or not, or addiction may tune the otherwise more sensitive amygdala found during adolescence into a more sensitive drug state amygdala that now seeks out only drug associated relevant events once drug use begins.

This new allostatic state involved in the transition to addiction involves decreased reward circuitry and increased antireward circuitry. As noted in Figure 100.2, cues would affect the drive to seek out drugs in the VTA and the basolateral amygdala that affect changes in drug circuitry, but changes in the antireward system (that would affect seeking out drugs to relieve stress) would occur in the extended amygdala (29,34).

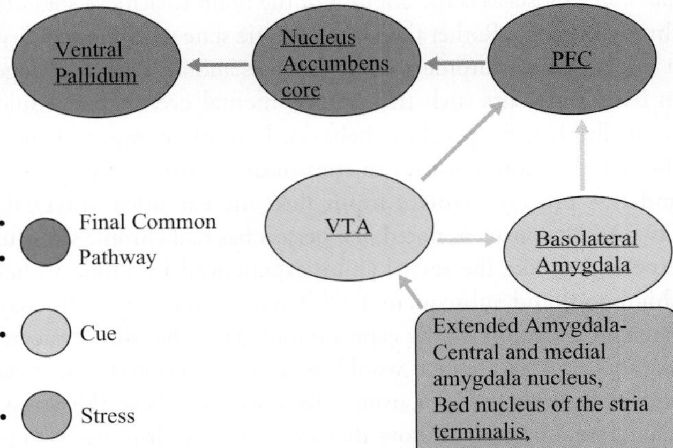

FIGURE 100.2. Role of the reward circuitry and antireward circuitry from a developmental perspective. (Adapted from Koob G, LeMoal M. Addiction and the antireward system. *Ann Rev Psychol* 2008;59: 29–53.)

Role of Genes As noted, stressors can turn on genes that can lead to the dysregulation of the HPA axis. In fact, high alcohol-preferring rats that have increased anxiety-like responses have been shown to have lower NPY activity, which is involved in the antireward system. However, they also have decreased dopaminergic activity. The number of dopamine receptors genetically inherited may play another role in genetic vulnerability. As noted previously, lower D2 receptors may influence PFC so that it no longer recognizes normal reinforcers as salient. The role of D2 receptors may also influence compulsion. When D2 receptors are decreased in the nucleus accumbens, there is a corresponding decrease in metabolism in the orbital frontal gyrus and the cingulate gyrus. The cingulate gyrus initiates the ability to restrain control, and the orbital frontal gyrus shifts attention to what is salient. If the orbital frontal gyrus is destroyed, Volkow believes the drug abuser will continue to use drugs, even if using them is no longer pleasurable. Therefore, if decreased D2 receptors result in decreased metabolism in the cingulate gyrus (so it can no longer inhibit the drive to use drugs) and the orbital frontal gyrus (so that it continues to compulsively use what it sees as salient, drugs, even though it is no longer pleasurable to do so), a person who has inherited decreased D2 receptors would be at more risk for developing SUD (39). In fact, Volkow (40,41) has shown on PET imaging that nonalcoholic family members in alcoholic families had higher than normal D2 receptor levels in the caudate and ventral striatum and metabolism in the anterior cingulate (Brodman area 24/25), orbitofrontal (Brodman area 11), and the prefrontal cortex (Brodman area 9/10). These individuals also had personality scores of positive emotionality on the MMPI. This suggests that higher D2 receptor levels could protect against alcoholism by regulating circuits involved in inhibiting behavioral responses and in controlling emotions. To further illustrate this, Thanos et al. (42,43) increased D2 receptors in mice (by using an adenovirus); alcohol consumption by the mice decreased by 70%. Therefore, people born with an increase in D2 receptors may be at less risk to develop SUD, and those who inherit a decrease in D2 receptors may be more vulnerable. The latter may have been the type of genetic makeup inherited by the young woman discussed in the case scenario.

Couple the decreased D2 receptors with the changes that occur in the motivational circuitry during adolescence (see developmental vulnerability further) and it becomes clear why exposure to substances of abuse during adolescence may increase the risk for developing substance abuse.

Other inherited receptors along with inherited susceptibility to motivational components may increase the risk of SUD. Just as increased D2 receptors may decrease the rewarding effects of drugs during acute drug use and, therefore, increase the risk of addiction, knockout of the mu opioid receptor studied in mice may influence the risk of developing SUD. Mu knockout mice demonstrated not only a decrease in heroin self administration but a decreased rewarding effect of alcohol, nicotine, and cannabinoid (44). These changes cause a negative motivational state during acute abstinence and increase the reaction to stress so that relapse is more probable.

Several representative genes that may be associated with an increased risk for substance use disorders include a lack of a beta 2 subunit on the nicotine receptor, which caused decreases in self-administration (45), and decreased in D1 receptor availability, which caused a decrease in cocaine self-administration in mice (46). Also, a gene encoding the transcription factor FosB/delta Fos B has been found to be associated with high novelty seeking and addiction susceptibility in animals (47).

A gene that has been linked to externalizing disorders has been found for the alpha receptor subunit of the neurotransmitter GABA located on chromosome 4. It is also related to alcohol and drug dependence (48).

Genetic architecture of addiction has also been studied (49). Uhl found 15 small chromosome regions, called "rSA," that contained markers found in multiple studies of addiction to legal and/or illegal substances. Molecular pathways that help maintain the addiction state have been identified that could disrupt or enhance the development of addiction owing to specific genetic variability in these pathways. For instance, a core component of addiction-induced adaptations in glutamatergic transmission has been identified as CAMKII. This component may play a role in the morphologic changes and memory circuits triggered by addictive drugs. Disruption of CAMKII impaired the stabilization of synaptic plasticity and memory consolidation caused by addictive drugs. GnRH, which may play a role in certain emotional behaviors associated with the HPA during stress-induced drug seeking has also been identified (50). Though much more research is needed to further understand the molecular genetics of addiction, additional pharmacotherapies will be discovered.

STUDIES OF INHERITABILITY

This patient's father had a family history for alcoholism. Adoption studies have shown increased risk for alcoholism of adopted-away children of persons/patients with alcohol dependence (51) and increased risk for substance abuse other than alcohol in adopted-away studies (52). However, alcohol use by adoptive parents did not increase risk for alcohol abuse in adoptive children (53).

Adoption studies have shown that genetic susceptibility seemed to be a stronger predictor of risk for substance abuse than exposure to adoptive parents using substances. However, both genetic and environmental influences may be correlated to substance initiation, whereas progression to substance abuse and dependence may be more related to genetic factors alone. In adoption studies conducted by Kendler (54), 485 monozygotic and 335 dizygotic twins demonstrated that cannabis use was influenced by genetic and familial environmental factors, whereas cannabis abuse and dependence were solely related to genetic factors. This was also true for cocaine use versus abuse and dependence (55). Schukit (56) has shown greater tolerance in children of persons/patients with alcohol dependence. In his study, children of persons/patients with alcohol dependence had to use greater proportions of alcohol before the reflex response to a stimulus was delayed to the same degree found in responses of children of nonalcoholics. In children of nonalcoholics, reflex response to a stimulus was delayed to the same degree on lower portions of alcohol. This diminished response to alcohol was also measured by subjective feelings, levels of body sway, electrophysiologic functioning, and change in three hormones.

Personality, Drug History, and Comorbidity Though Koob and LeMoal (29) state that personality, drug history, and comorbidity are more likely to influence drug use later, they all have some root in early childhood and adolescent substance use disorders. Seldom does any patient with a SUD develop substance dependence without some significant precursors in their developmental history, and psychiatric comorbidity may increase the risk or speed of transition from substance abuse to substance dependence.

Drug History Addiction to drugs and alcohol can occur anytime throughout the life of an individual. However, age is a risk factor likely to influence the onset of substance use during childhood and adolescence. In this case scenario, the patient began using cigarettes at age 11, began drinking alcohol at age 12, and began getting drunk at age 15. She began using marijuana at the end of 10th grade. She began getting drunk every weekend as she entered 11th grade. A study of youngsters who began drinking at an early age, 11 to 12 years of age, had a higher probability of meeting the DSM III-R criteria for substance abuse (13.5%) and substance dependence (15.9%) as compared to those who began drinking at age 13 or 14 (13.7% and 9.0%, respectively). Those who drank at age 19 or 20 had rates of 2% and 1%, respectively. Schuckit (57) has noted that the age where a patient with substance abuse was most likely to have started drinking was 13, when first drunk was age 15, had their first problem associated with drinking at age 18, and first dependence was age 25 to 40. Death was most likely to occur by age 60. Important is that rapid progression of SUD occurred often with earlier age of onset and frequency, not duration of use (58,59). Those individuals with earlier onset had a shorter time span from first exposure to addiction than did adult-onset groups (60). Age of onset of heavy drinking also predicted alcohol-related problems (61). Early age of onset also influences higher risks for the use of other substances, as noted in this case scenario. Adolescent-onset adults had higher lifetime rates of cannabis and hallucinogen use disorders, shorter times between the development of their first and second dependence diagnosis, and higher rates of disruptive behaviors and major depression (60). This patient began sneaking out during 10th grade, and her review of systems and mental status indicated that she may have a major depressive disorder.

Screening the patient with the CRAAFT (62) indicates possible substance abuse, possibly substance dependence. Her unidentified and untreated ADHD, PTSD, LDs, and possible major depressive disorder may be factors that are contributing to her persistent use. She does not compulsively use but states she uses now to relax and "fit in" and relieve stress; thus, her substance use may be affecting her HPA axis, making her more sensitive to stress and more likely to use to relieve the stress. As noted before, impulsive use implies possible PFC hypofunctioning whereby the patient may prioritize salience to drug-related stimuli over natural reinforcers. It is difficult to determine whether she is prioritizing drugs as salient because of comorbid conditions, like depression. Anhedonia can diminish pleasure in everyday circumstances, but drug use can also cause anhedonia. It is also difficult to determine whether she is using drugs to ward off the negative effects during withdrawal, such as anxiety, because she has an untreated PTSD and social phobia. Treatment of these conditions, ideally in parallel, may elucidate the salience.

Personality Temperament may explain why some adults continue to demonstrate characteristics of dependence. Both Cloninger (53) and Babor (63) identified personality traits associated with negative prognosis. Cloninger's type 2 and Babor's type B persons/patients with alcohol dependence share common characteristics: early onset of spontaneous alcohol-seeking behavior; diagnosis during adolescence; rapid course of onset; presence of genetic risk factors; deviancy; and greater psychologic vulnerability. Cloninger's type 2 and Babor's type B persons/patients with alcohol dependence may be related to youth who are thought to have conduct disorder. Conduct disorder is thought to be related to genetic vulnerability and negative environmental factors (poverty, parental neglect, marital discord, parental illness and/or parental alcoholism) and is associated with impairment in frontal lobe function, affecting the ability to plan, to avoid harm, and to learn from negative consequences—traits often found in the type 2 or type B persons/patients with alcohol dependence. The same type of personality characteristics were found in kindergartners who had an increased risk for development of SUD in adolescence (64).

More recent research has tried to describe the relationship between personality and risk-taking behaviors in six areas, including smoking, drinking, drugs, sex, driving, and gambling (65). Risk taking across all six areas was related to impulsivity, sensation seeking, aggression, and sociability but not to neuroticism-anxiety and activity.

Though the patient in this case scenario seemed to have many of the characteristics that are found in Cloninger's type 2 and Babor's type B personality types, (early-onset alcohol-seeking behavior, genetic precursors or family history of alcoholism, marital discord, and rapid course of onset of substance abuse), her early personality traits did not suggest an early-onset conduct disorder that would offer a more negative prognosis. In fact, she seems to be very motivated for treatment (66) and did not seem to show any evidence for sensation seeking, aggression (except one time while drunk) or sociability, which would increase her risk taking. Her impulsivity seemed to be related to an untreated ADHD. Her history of separation anxiety and possible social phobia may have led to her using in order to relax and socialize. Her anxiety would have put her at less risk for risk taking. In fact, she was embarrassed by her behavior, especially her history of rape under the influence of alcohol. She is motivated to try to quit abusing substances. Therefore, this patient seemed to be a good candidate for treatment.

Comorbidity Any psychiatric disorders that are not recognized and treated during any developmental stage can increase the risk of substance abuse. The chapters in this text that discuss comorbidity and risk factors will illustrate this. However, there are a few psychiatric disorders that are worth mentioning, which, if untreated, will increase the risk for substance abuse perhaps by making the brain neurobiologically more vulnerable to the development of substance abuse. Therefore, these disorders can be classified as a developmental vulnerability. They are mentioned here briefly. Academic failure and learning disorders are not often given sufficient discussion and, therefore, also are elaborated. Also, as many neuropsychiatric disorders can affect executive function, this may interfere with and undermine treatment. Bolla et al. (67) have shown that abstinent cocaine users show less activation than nondrug users in the left anterior cingulated cortex (ACC) and the right lateral prefrontal cortex (LPFC) and greater activation in the right ACC. All of these findings may impair executive function and further affect decision making once substance use begins, especially if the deficit in executive functioning occurs in undetected and untreated psychiatric disorders.

Mood and Conduct Disorders Though ADHD, major depression, and conduct disorder may be important components of substance dependence, depression may be the primary variable related to substance use disorder in women at any age (68). Though girls are more likely to have internalizing disorders, a study by Couwenbergh et al. (69) has shown that externalizing disorders, especially in boys, were consistently linked to SUDs in treatment-seeking adolescents. Those with conduct disorders had a higher risk of ending up in a juvenile justice system. However, depression in boys may be linked to earlier onset of conduct disorder. In a study of adolescent deviant boys with conduct disorder and comorbid substance abuse reported by Riggs and Whitmore (70), depressed boys were more likely to have ADHD, PTSD, anxiety disorder, and an earlier onset of conduct disorder when compared to nondepressed boys. In this same study, the depressive symptoms did not seem to be relieved after 4 weeks of abstinence.

Hypofunctioning of the OFC and the anterior cingulate has been shown to occur in depressed untreated patients. Hypofucntioning of the PFC in depressed patients may cause disinhibition of the PFC to the amygdala, thereby correspondingly causing a disinhibition of projections to the BNST and hypothalamus. In turn, there would be an increase in CRF. The latter would increase anxiety symptoms and may play a role initially in explaining why people who are depressed "self-medicate." However, during chronic drug use, this may exacerbate the antireward system, which may also increase the use of substances to relieve anxiety (71,72).

Rao (73) identified a unique feature of girls with conduct disorder, SUD, and depression. These girls had more anxiety disorders and elevated cortisol near sleep onset (when the hypothalamic-pituitary system is expected to be more active) than depressed girls without SUD. It is felt that the use of alcohol and/or stress in these girls may be the reason why cortisol levels are much higher than in girls with conduct disorder and depression alone. The role that this may play in treatment, if any, is unclear at this time. However, the role of cortisol (glucocorticsteroids) can influence dopamine transmission in the ventral striatum and the shell part of the NAc and thus may drive the CRF system (29). This may affect the antireward system and increase the likelihood of transition to addiction.

One study has examined the risk of SUD independent of the diagnosis of conduct disorder in late onset bipolar disorder. Wilens (74) has reported that those with adolescent-onset bipolar disorder had an 8.8 times greater risk of developing substance use disorder than those with childhood-onset bipolar disorder, and no other disorder, including conduct disorder, accounted for the risk. This finding may have something to do with the maturation of the nucleus accumbens that seems to occur at a faster rate than the PFC during adolescents (75). This would give greater weight to the intensity of the rewarding effects when using substances during adolescents, especially for youth who have bipolar disorder where they may seek out risky behaviors more often than their adolescent counterparts who do not have bipolar disorder.

Though patients may use substances to self-medicate their manic symptoms, it is clear that the use of multiple substances, such as marijuana and alcohol, may, in reality, make the neurobiologic effect even worse. When patients (aged 18 to 65 years) presented with active marijuana and alcohol use in the manic phase, the marijuana did not decrease the level of the manic state. Thus, though the sensation of feeling calmer may have been experienced by bipolar substance abusers who were manic and using alcohol, the mania symptoms were actually worse in those who presented with bipolar disorder and marijuana and alcohol use than in those with bipolar disorder and alcohol use alone. Use of multiple substances may be a sign of a more progressive addiction, which would likely decrease the ability to inhibit compulsive behavior and the level of mania. Moreover, the type of treatment used may have less effect on those who are actively using marijuana during their presentation with mania and alcohol. In the latter group, those who were treated with lithium and psychosocial therapy (compared with those treated with lithium, valproic acid, or psychosocial treatment alone), had the highest percentage of heavy drinking days as compared to those with bipolar disorder who use alcohol alone (76). The same effect has been studied in adolescents. Geller (77) has shown that bipolar adolescents who also used alcohol had a decrease in manic symptoms and alcohol use when treated with lithium.

Anxiety Disorders Teachers and clinicians will often not recognize children with social phobia because they do not necessarily present with behavioral problems. However, those who are recognized owing to their aggressiveness should also be evaluated for shyness. In one study by Swan (78), the combination of shyness and aggressiveness in boys was a more valid predictor of future cocaine use than a history of aggressiveness alone.

The role of dopamine in the development of social anxiety may help to explain the increased risk of developing substance abuse if social phobia goes untreated. Striatal dopamine reuptake sites were markedly lower in patients with social phobia as compared to controls (79), and there was lower binding of D2 receptors in the striatum of untreated social phobia patients as compared to controls (80). The young woman in the case scenario may have had lower D2 receptors not only owing to her family history for substance abuse but because of her untreated social phobia.

One study of juvenile justice adolescents noted that 11% of juvenile detainees met criteria for PTSD and that more than half had witnessed violence that precipitated their trauma (81). Two direct relationships have been found between childhood trauma and exposure and adult criminal behavior in women. Having been in foster care or adopted was positively related to engaging in sex associated with prostitution. However, early experiences of traumatic events (i.e., death of close relative, serious accidents) were related to engaging violent crime. For African American as well as white women offenders, childhood traumatic events were related to the development of adolescent substance abuse (82). This may help correlate the relationship of stress and its effect on the HPA, which may increase the levels of CRF, ACTH, and cortisol. If a stressor is mild and stimulates the HPA to release CRF and then ACTH, cortisol levels rise in response to ACTH. When cortisol reaches the pituitary gland, it inhibits further release of CRF and ACTH. However, if the stressor is intense; signals in the brain for more CRF outweigh the inhibitory effects of cortisol. In this latter situation, there may be a correspondingly increased risk to use substances of abuse to relieve the anxiety associated with the heightened CRF levels.

The role of the OFC in anxiety disorders correlates to treatment response to cognitive behavioral therapy (CBT) and medications. For example, the higher the magnitude of response of the OFC in fMRI studies prior to treatment inversely correlated with the response to medications but the higher the magnitude of the response of the OFC directly correlated with the response to CBT. If the OFC is hypofunctioning in an individual with an anxiety disorder and a SUD, the patient may not respond to CBT treatment for the anxiety disorder as well as CBT treatment for the substance abuse (83,84).

Attention Deficit Hyperactivity Disorder It is well recognized that ADHD with conduct disorder has a much greater risk for developing substance abuse than ADHD alone. In fact, in a twin study done by Disney et al. (85) of 626 pairs of 17-year-old twins, ADHD did not increase the risk for substance abuse unless it was associated with a co-occurring conduct disorder. Biederman et al. (86) have shown that untreated ADHD has more risk for future substance abuse than ADHD that is treated. If an adolescent has ADHD and is not treated, the risk of developing substance use disorder is two times higher than in those who have ADHD and were treated with stimulants. The role of stimulants in the treatment of ADHD and possible explanations for the decreased risk for substance abuse is discussed further. However, untreated ADHD seems to involve an underactive anterior cingulate and PFC (87,88). The role of the anterior cingulated and PFC in inhibiting impulsivity found with ADHD patients could increase the risk of using substances of abuse and lead to substance abuse and addiction.

Exposure to Stimulants for Treatment of Attention Deficit Hyperactivity Disorder and Attention Deficit Disorder As there is so much controversy over the use of stimulants in the treatment of ADHD and attention deficit disorder (ADD), a common pediatric disease, some point of clarification between the uses of stimulants for medicinal versus recreational drug use should be noted.

First and foremost, one must consider the speed with which substances of abuse move through the blood-brain barrier. Swanson and Volkow (89) have pointed out that the liability of a drug to cause reinforcing acute euphoric feelings in associated with the instant high achieved by using drugs of abuse either by smoking, snorting, or using intravenously. There is a rapid dopamine blockade of dopamine transporters in the ventral striatum (containing the shell of the nucleus accumbens) causing a euphoric high. However, methylphenidate taken orally does not produce this rapid high because it enters the brain barrier more slowly and is less associated with a high that causes a reinforcing effect of the drug. In fact, oral methylphenidate may not induce craving even if it is taken by a subject with cocaine dependence. Volkow et al. (90) have shown that 20 mg of oral methylphenidate will not elicit drug craving unless it is associated with a cocaine cue. Therefore, adolescent substance abusers who have used cocaine or other substances linked to substance abuse should not use stimulants as first-line treatment for ADHD as it is difficult to prevent the drug craving associated with the cues of cocaine use. If the ADHD is severe and no other medication has been helpful in treating the substance-abusing ADHD adolescent, one must be cautious in using stimulants without rigorous relapse prevention, if at all. Care must be used in adolescents using cigarettes who also have ADHD. Upadhyaya, in unpublished research, has shown that nicotine in ADHD patients can reinforce the effects of stimulants, whereas the effects of stimulants are not reinforcing in ADHD patients who did not smoke cigarettes.

Though early use and abuse of alcohol increased the risk of later substance abuse, new studies on the use of stimulants for the treatment of ADHD/ADD may actually decrease the risk of developing substance abuse. Reasons for this may be explained by research done by Castellanos et al. (91). Castellanos reviewed total cerebral volume of treated and untreated adolescents with ADHD. Total white matter in the unmedicated ADHD adolescents was lower than medicated and normals. It is hypothesized that perhaps the trophic effect on myelination, dendritic branching, and length of spines in the treated ADHD youth was somehow protective. How might this occur? Luna (92) has shown that a normal process that occurs during adolescence is an increase in myelination. The effect is an increase in processing speed. Therefore, the lack of myelination may decrease processing speed and these effects may increase the risk for substance abuse related to poor academic success.

Research by Thanos et al. (93) may give further explanation for the role between early use of stimulants for medicinal reasons and decreased risk for development of substance abuse. As noted before, overexpression of D2 receptors reduces alcohol and cocaine self-administration in mice (41,42,94) and decreases drug liking and may be protective against substance abuse in humans (40,43). Thanos found significantly reduced rates of cocaine self-stimulation during adulthood in periadolescent rats treated with 2 mg/kg oral methylphenidate for 8 months as compared to periadolescent rats treated with 1 mg/kg or rats receiving water. The availability of D2 receptors was significantly lower after 2 months of treatment in rats given 1 or 2 mg/kg of methylphenidate compared with control rats, but after 8 months of treatment, it was significantly higher. The rats given 2 mg/kg of methylphenidate at 8 months had greater D2 receptor–binding availability than rats given 1 mg/kg. Therefore, in rodent studies, consistent methylphenidate treatment (started in adolescence) attenuated cocaine self-administration during adulthood. In the case scenario presented here, if this patient had been treated for her ADHD early on, she may not have lost so much potential academically in school, and this may have reduced the risk for the development of substance abuse.

Learning Disorders Academic failure and low commitment to school are other psychobehavioral factors associated with influencing drug use during childhood and adolescence. Beyond early onset of use, poor academic achievement, poor social skills and competence, learning disorders, and poor self-esteem were found to be related to drug abuse (95,96). Hops et al. (97) found that substance abuse at age 14 or 15 could be predicted by academic and social behavior between the ages of 7 and 9. Too often, ADHD is assumed to be the reason for school problems, and a comorbid LD goes undetected. Simkin (98) tested ADHD/ADD children who had responded well to stimulants in elementary school but later began to struggle in middle or high school. Of those tested, 77 children had ADD/ADHD alone or ADD/ADHD with a comorbid anxiety and/or depression, which were well controlled for. Of these children, the average IQ was 122. Ninety-two percent were found to have an auditory processing problem, 70% had a processing speed problem (on the cognitive battery of the Woodcock Johnson-III), and 87% had a disorder of written expression (on the Woodcock Johnson-III). This is extremely important as ADD/ADHD can be confused with processing problems. Tapert et al. (99) found that adolescents with attention difficulties predicted substance abuse and dependency eight years later. This study controlled for substance involvement, education, conduct disorder, family history of substance abuse and learning disorders. The attention difficulties were not necessarily related to ADHD/ADD. Given the foregoing information, the young woman in the case scenario should be evaluated not only for ADHD but also for an LD. This young woman may have had a reading disorder, and proper educational testing should be performed during her evaluation and treatment. Fortunately, this young woman did not end up in a juvenile justice system. However, for youth who do present to a juvenile justice system, these adolescents experience much higher rates of psychiatric disorders thando adolescents in the general population (100). However, what brings them to the attention of the juvenile justice system is an often co-occurring substance abuse disorder. Many of these individuals also have a comorbid LD. In a 2002 report on the California Juvenile Justice system, a pathway was described that denotes how children, beginning in the school system, are identified for risk factors but no appropriate comprehensive evaluation is sufficiently done to prevent entrance into the juvenile justice system (101). First, the child may be identified as having a mental health need at age 5 by a teacher. A referral is made to special education by age 7. Then the child may interact with the mental health and child welfare services by age 9, and inpatient hospitalization may occur by age 12. The pathway ends by entrance into the juvenile justice system by age 14. Windows of opportunities for proper evaluation and intervention are missed along the way. For instance, before a referral to special education occurs, an evaluation for psychiatric disorders should occur or learning difficulties like dyslexia should be identified to reduce the risk of entering the juvenile justice system. In fact, in a study that looked at young offenders and dyslexia, 50% were dyslexic (102).

Early detection of learning disorders is essential to prevent the increased risk for developing substance abuse. However, the timing of the intervention may also be crucial. Wright (103) has suggested that processing problems associated with language impairment, dyslexia, and auditory processing problems is a developmental delay that if not corrected before age 10 may become permanent during adolescence. This does not mean that interventions done after age 9 will not be helpful; however, they may not be as robust since the brain may not be as plastic and responsive to interventions. Therefore, if these disorders are not detected and intervened upon at the appropriate time, a window of opportunity may be lost. Stimulants may help ADD/ADHD but, should learning disorders be detected, accommodations must be made in order to ensure continued success. Early detection of processing problems should occur whenever any child has difficulties with reading in order to prevent the risk of developing substance abuse and involvement with the juvenile justice system.

Schizophrenia In a study by Hambrecht and Hafner (104), a vulnerability hypothesis was constructed to help explain the frequent use of marijuana in patients with schizophrenia. This vulnerability hypothesis was divided into three groups. Frequent use in group 1 may have decreased the threshold for the appearance of schizophrenia as they had used for several years before the onset of the disorder. Group 2 may be made up of a vulnerable group in which the dopaminergic stress factor may precipitate the onset of schizophrenia. This group developed the onset of schizophrenia in the same month they began to use marijuana. Group 3 may use the marijuana to self-medicate, because they developed the onset of marijuana abuse after the onset of the schizophrenia. This vulnerability hypothesis may explain the effects that other substances of abuse may have on the developing brain and how other psychiatric disorders and/or learning disorders may emerge or interplay with drugs of abuse. More research is needed in regard to this hypothesis.

DEVELOPMENT OF THE ADOLESCENT BRAIN

Obviously, if psychiatric disorders and learning disorders are detected early and treated, there is less risk for developing substance abuse. However, adolescence is a time of experimentation. Why do adolescents experiment with risky behaviors? Much of this may be due to the dramatic changes that occur during adolescence. The following is an explanation of these changes.

Though the literature suggests that adolescent cognitive development is progressively increasing during adolescence and that this cognitive control capacity is positively associated with maturation or increased activity within the prefrontal cortex (105–107), adolescence also has shown to be a developmental stage associated with suboptimal choices. Therefore, adolescence seems to demonstrate a nonlinear change in behavior unexpected from what the previous research has illustrated. If cognitive control and an immature prefrontal cortex were the basis for suboptimal choice behavior, then children should look remarkably similar or even worse than adolescents, given their less developed prefrontal cortex and cognitive abilities.Thus, immature prefrontal function alone cannot account for adolescent behavior.

It has been suggested that perhaps researchers should consider adolescence as a period wherein two separate entities are independently working: lack of cognitive control and risk taking. Focusing on these two entities from a neurobiologic level with two different trajectories may give more insight to the reasons behind adolescent behavior (Casey, et al, unpublished). Using recent imaging studies of adolescence (75,108,109), Figure 100.3 depicts this model. On the left (A) is the traditional characterization of adolescence as related almost exclusively to the immaturity of the prefrontal cortex. On the right (B) is our proposed neurobiologic model that illustrates how limbic subcortical and prefrontal top-down control regions must be considered together. The cartoon illustrates different developmental trajectories for these systems, with limbic systems developing earlier than prefrontal control regions. According to this model, the individual is biased more by functionally mature limbic regions during adolescence (i.e., imbalance of limbic relative to prefrontal control) as compared to children, for whom these systems (i.e., limbic and prefrontal) are both still developing; and compared to adults, for whom these systems are fully mature. Further, the model reconciles the contradiction of health statistics of risky behavior during adolescence, with the astute observation by Reyna and Farley (110) that adolescents are able to reason and understand risks of behaviors in which they engage. According to the model in Figure 100.3, in emotionally salient situations, the limbic system will win over control systems given its maturity relative to the prefrontal control system.

DEVELOPMENT OF GOAL-DIRECTED BEHAVIOR

Specifically, a review of the literature suggests that impulsivity diminishes with age across childhood and adolescence (109, 111,112) and is associated with protracted development of the prefrontal cortex (113).

In contrast, to impulse/cognitive control, risk taking appears to increase during adolescence relative to childhood and adulthood and is associated with subcortical systems known to be involved in evaluation of rewards. Human imaging studies that will be reviewed suggest an increase in subcortical activation (e.g., accumbens) when making risky choices (114–116) that is exaggerated in adolescents, relative to children and adults (75,108). These findings suggest different trajectories for reward- or incentive-based behavior, with earlier development of these systems relative to control systems that show a protracted and linear developmental course, in terms of overriding inappropriate choices and actions in favor of goal-directed ones.

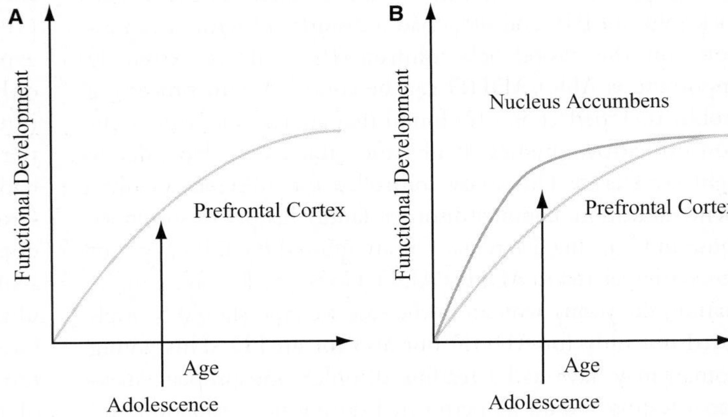

FIGURE 100.3. The traditional explanation of adolescent behavior has been suggested to be due to the protracted development of the prefrontal cortex **(A).** Our model takes into consideration the development of the prefrontal cortex together with subcortical limbic regions (e.g., nucleus accumbens) that have been implicated in risky choices and actions **(B).**

EVIDENCE FROM NEUROIMAGING STUDIES OF HUMAN DEVELOPMENT

Magnetic Resonance Imaging Studies of Human Development Evidence for a developmental model of competition between cortical and subcortical regions is supported by immature structural and functional connectivity as measured by DTI and functional magnetic resonance imaging (fMRI), respectively. Data from recent longitudinal MRI studies indicate that gray-matter volume has an inverted U-shape pattern, with greater regional variation than white matter (117–120). In general, regions subserving primary functions, such as motor and sensory systems, mature earliest; higher-order association areas, which integrate these primary functions, mature later (118,119). For example, studies using MRI-based measures show that cortical gray matter loss occurs earliest in the primary sensorimotor areas and latest in the dorsolateral prefrontal and lateral temporal cortices (118).

In contrast to gray matter, white matter volume increases in a roughly linear pattern, increasing throughout development well into adulthood (118). These changes presumably reflect ongoing myelination of axons by oligodendrocytes enhancing neuronal conduction and communication. Though less attention has been given to subcortical regions when examining structural changes, some of the largest changes in the brain across development are seen in these regions, particular in the basal ganglia (121) (Fig. 100.2) and especially in males (122). A number of studies have related frontal lobe structural maturation and cognitive function using neuropsychological and cognitive measures (120). Specifically, associations have been reported between MRI-based prefrontal cortical and basal ganglia regional volumes and measures of cognitive control (i.e., ability to override an inappropriate response in favor of another or to suppress attention toward irrelevant stimulus attribute in favor of relevant stimulus attribute (123).

Diffuse Tensor Imaging Studies of Human Brain Development The MRI-based morphometry studies reviewed suggest that cortical connections are being fine-tuned with the elimination of an overabundance of synapses and strengthening of relevant connections with development and experience. Relevant to this chapter are the neuroimaging studies that have linked the development of fiber tracts with improvements in cognitive ability. Specifically, associations between measures of prefrontal white matter development and cognitive control in children have been shown via diffuse tensor imaging (DTI). In one study, development of this capacity was positively correlated with prefrontal-parietal fiber tracts (124) consistent with functional neuroimaging studies showing differential recruitment of these regions in children relative to adults.

Using a similar approach, Liston et al. (125) have shown that white-matter tracts between prefrontal-basal ganglia and -posterior fiber tracts continue to develop across childhood into adulthood, but only those tracts between the prefrontal cortex and basal ganglia are correlated with impulse control, as measured by performance on a go/nogo task. The prefrontal fiber tracts were defined by regions of interests identified in a fMRI study using the same task. Across both developmental DTI studies, fiber tract measures were correlated with development, but specificity of particular fiber tracts with cognitive performance were shown by dissociating the particular tract (125) or cognitive ability (124). These findings underscore the importance of examining not only regional but circuitry related changes when making claims about age-dependent changes in neural substrates of cognitive development.

Functional Magnetic Resonance Imaging Studies of Behavioral and Brain Development The ability to measure functional changes in the developing brain with MRI has significant potential for the field of developmental science. Collectively, these studies show that children recruit distinct but often larger, more diffuse prefrontal regions when performing these tasks than do adults. Though neuroimaging studies cannot definitively characterize the mechanism of such developmental changes (e.g. dendritic arborization, synaptic pruning) the findings reflect development within, and refinement of, projections to and from activated brain regions with maturation and suggest that these changes occur over a protracted period of time (107,111,123,126–133).

Studies have begun to focus primarily on the region of the accumbens, a portion of the basal ganglia involved in predicting reward, rather than characterization of the development of this region in conjunction with top-down control regions (prefrontal cortex). However, a recent report of less ventral prefrontal activity in adolescents relative to adults during a monetary decision-making task on risk-taking behavior has been shown (134).

A neurobiologic model proposed by Casey et al. (111) posits that the combination of heightened responsiveness to rewards and immaturity in behavioral control areas may bias adolescents to seek immediate, rather than long-term gains, perhaps explaining their increase in risky decision-making and impulsive behaviors. They hypothesized that relative to children and adults, adolescents would show exaggerated activation of the accumbens, in concert with less mature recruitment of top down prefrontal control regions. Recent work showing delayed functional connectivity between these prefrontal and limbic subcortical regions in adolescence relative to adults provides a mechanism for the lack of top-down control of these regions (Hare et al., in press).

Their findings were consistent with rodent models (2003) and previous imaging studies (135) suggesting enhanced accumbens activity to rewards during adolescence. Indeed, relative to children and adults, adolescents showed an exaggerated accumbens response in anticipation of reward. However, both children and adolescents showed a less mature response in prefrontal control regions than adults. These findings suggest different developmental trajectories for these regions may underlie the enhancement in accumbens activity, relative to children or adults, which may in turn relate to the increased impulsive and risky behaviors observed during this period of development (Fig. 100.4).

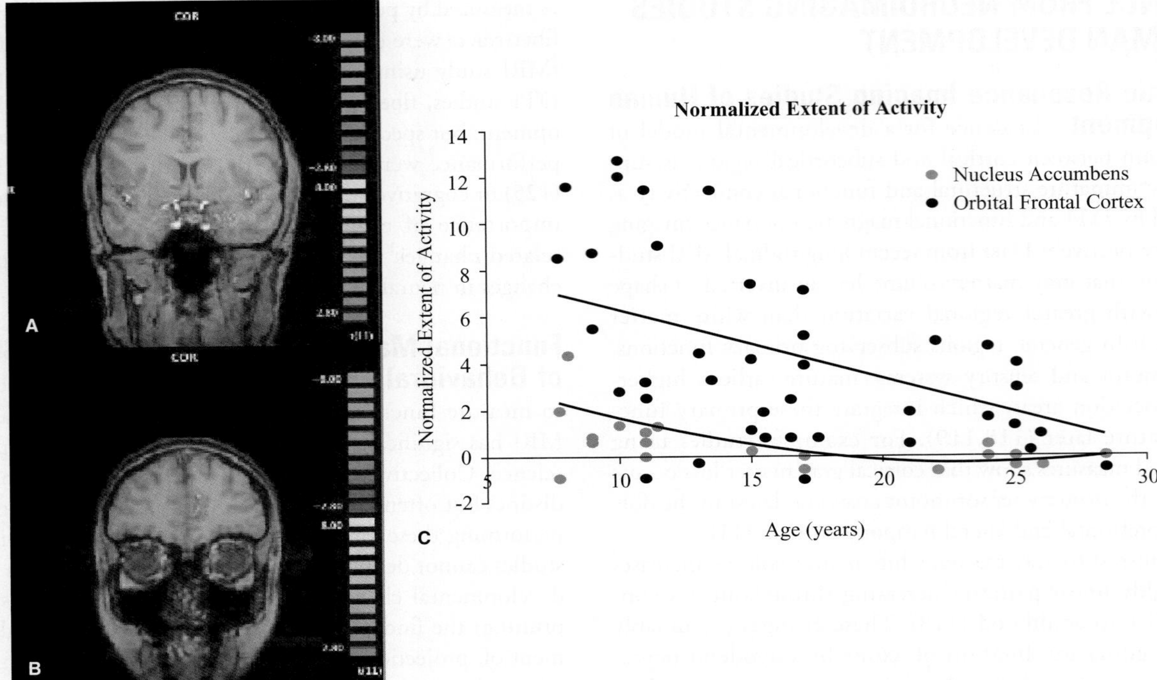

FIGURE 100.4. Localization of activity in anticipation of reward outcome in the nucleus accumbens **(A)** and orbital frontal cortex **(B)**. The extent of activity in these regions is plotted as a function of age, for each individual subject showing protracted development of orbital frontal cortex relative to nucleus accumbens **(C)**. (Adapted from Galvan A, Hare TA, Parra CE, et al. Earlier development of the accumbens relative to orbitofrontal cortex might underlie risk-taking behavior in adolescents. *J Neurosci* 2006;26(25):6885–6892.)

Given evidence of prefrontal regions in guiding appropriate actions in different contexts (136), immature prefrontal activity might hinder appropriate estimation of future outcomes and appraisal of risky choices and might thus be less influential on reward valuation than the accumbens. During adolescence, relative to childhood or adulthood, immature ventral prefrontal cortex may not provide sufficient top-down control of robustly activated reward-processing regions (e.g., accumbens), resulting in less influence of prefrontal systems (orbitofrontal cortex) relative to the accumbens in reward valuation.

Why Would the Brain Be Programmed to Develop this Way? Evolutionarily speaking, adolescence is the period in which independence skills are acquired to increase success upon separation from the protection of the family. Seeking out same-age peers and fighting with parents, which all help get the adolescent away from the home territory for mating, are seen in other species, including rodents, nonhuman primates, and some birds (137). Humans had to engage in high-risk behavior to leave their family and village to find a mate and risk taking at just the same time as hormones drive adolescents to seek out sexual partners. In fact, Luna and Sweeney (92) have suggested that these risk-taking behaviors may be necessary to sculpt the brain in order to reach the adult pattern necessary for efficient processing. Hence, adolescence is a crucial period of plasticity when brain circuitry and behavior are beginning to be established. Risk taking and novelty seeking may provide a mechanism for increasing exposure to the environment necessary for successful sculpting of the brain. However, in today's society when adolescence may extend indefinitely, with children living with parents and having financial dependence and choosing mates later in life, this evolution may be deemed inappropriate. Secondary to the extended adolescence, many high-risk behaviors may be engaged in that may increase chances for harmful circumstances (e.g., injury, depression, anxiety, drug use, and addiction) (138).

BIOLOGIC PREDISPOSITIONS, DEVELOPMENT, AND RISK

Impulsivity plays a major role in risk for developing SUD. Mischel et al. (139) showed that children typically behave in one of two ways: (1) Either they ring the bell almost immediately in order to have the cookie, which means they get only one, or (2) they wait and optimize their gains and receive both cookies. This observation suggests that some individuals are better than others in their ability to control impulses in the face of highly salient incentives and this bias can be detected in early childhood, and they appear to remain throughout adolescence and young adulthood (140). Some theorists have postulated that dopaminergic mesolimbic circuitry, implicated in reward processing, underlies risky behavior (141). Individual differences in this circuitry, such as allelic variants in dopamine-related genes, resulting in too little or too much dopamine in subcortical regions, might relate to the propensity to engage in risky behavior (142). The nucleus accumbens has been shown to increase in activity immediately prior to making risky choices on monetary-risk paradigms (114,115,116) and, as described previously, adolescents show exaggerated accumbens activity to anticipated or rewarding outcomes relative to children or adults (75,108). Collectively, these data suggest that adolescents may be more prone to risky choices as a group (143), but some adolescents will be more prone than others to engage in risky behaviors, putting them at potentially greater risk for negative outcomes. Therefore, it is important to consider individual variability when examining complex brain-behavior relationships related to risk taking and reward processing in developmental populations.

To explore individual differences in risk taking behavior, Galvan et al. (109) recently examined the association between activity in reward-related neural circuitry in anticipation of a large monetary reward with personality trait measures of risk taking and impulsivity in adolescence. Functional MRI and anonymous self-report rating scales of risky behavior, risk perception, and impulsivity were acquired in individuals between the ages of 7 and 29 years. There was a positive association between accumbens activity and the likelihood of engaging in risky behavior across development. This activity varied as a function of individuals' ratings of anticipated positive or negative consequences of such behavior. Those individuals who perceived risky behaviors as leading to dire consequences activated the accumbens less to reward. This association was driven largely by the children, with the adults rating the consequences of such behavior as possible. Impulsivity ratings were not associated with accumbens activity but rather with age. These findings suggest that during adolescence, some individuals may be more prone to engage in risky behaviors owing to developmental changes in concert with variability in a given individual's predisposition to engage in risky behavior rather than to simple changes in impulsivity (Fig. 100.5).

Impulsivity is associated with immature ventral prefrontal development and gradually diminishes from childhood to adulthood (113). The negative correlation between impulsivity ratings and age in the study by Galvan et al. (109) further support this notion. In contrast, risk taking is associated with an increase in accumbens activity (114–116) that is exaggerated in adolescents, relative to children and adults (75,108). Thus, adolescent choices and behavior cannot be explained by impulsivity or protracted development of the prefrontal cortex

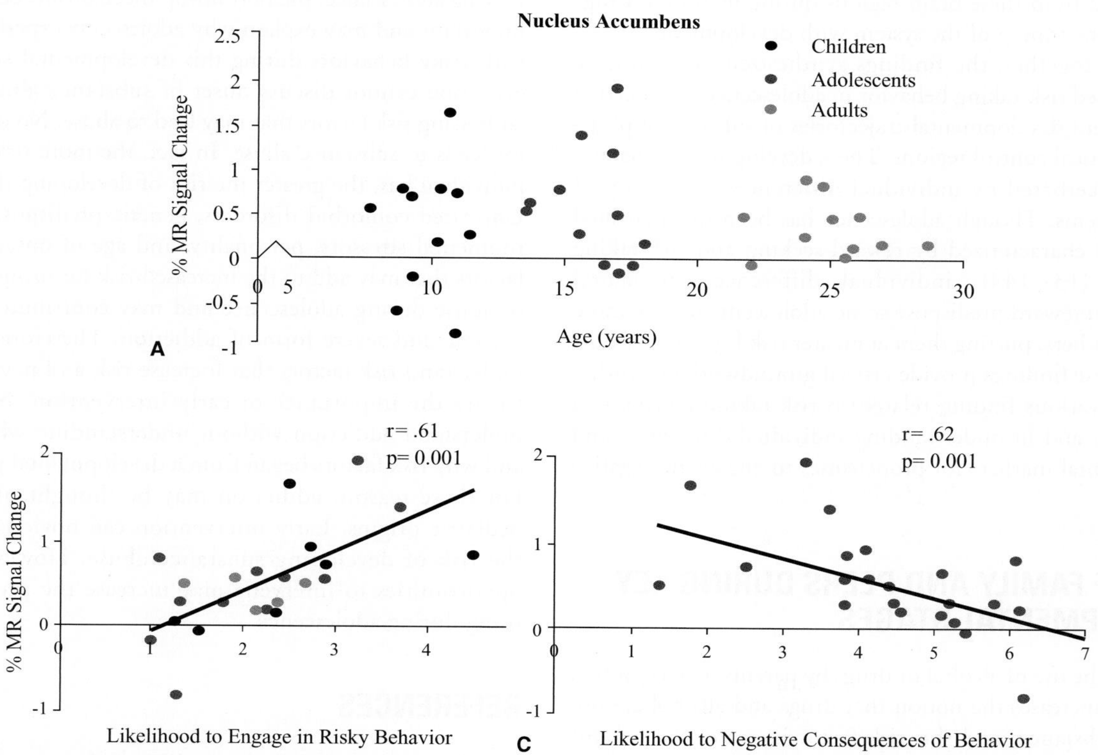

FIGURE 100.5. Adolescents show enhanced activity of the accumbens relative to children and adults **(A)**. Accumbens activity is positively associated with self-ratings of the likelihood of engaging in risky behavior **(B)** and negatively correlated with self ratings of the likelihood of negative consequences of such behavior **(C)**. (Reproduced from Galvan A, Hare T, Voss H, et al. Risk-taking and the adolescent brain: who is at risk? *Dev Sci* 2007;10(2):F8–F14.)

alone, as children would then be predicted to be greater risk takers. The findings provide a neural basis for why some adolescents are at greater risk than others but further provide a basis for how adolescent behavior is different from children and adults in risk taking.

Collectively, these data suggest that though adolescents as a group are considered risk takers (143), some adolescents will be more prone than others to engage in risky behaviors, putting them at potentially greater risk for negative outcomes. These findings underscore the importance of considering individual variability when examining complex brain-behavior relationships related to risk taking and reward processing in developmental populations. Further, these individual and developmental differences may help explain vulnerability in some individuals to risk-taking associated with substance use, and ultimately, addiction.

In conclusion, human imaging studies show structural and functional changes in frontostriatal regions (113,121, 122,144,145) that seem to parallel increases in cognitive control and self-regulation (106,123,129,146). These changes appear to show a shift in activation of prefrontal regions from diffuse to more focal recruitment over time (123,126, 127,130,147) and elevated recruitment of subcortical regions during adolescence (111,129,147). Though neuroimaging studies cannot definitively characterize the mechanism of such developmental changes, these changes in volume and structure may reflect development within, and refinement of, projections to and from these brain regions during maturation suggestive of fine tuning of the system with development.

Taken together, the findings synthesized here indicate that increased risk-taking behavior in adolescence is associated with different developmental trajectories of subcortical pleasure and cortical control regions. These developmental changes can be exacerbated by individual differences in activity of reward systems. Though adolescence has been distinguished as a period characterized by reward-seeking and risk-taking behaviors (137,143), individual differences in neural responses to reward predispose some adolescents to take more risks than others, putting them at greater risk for negative outcomes. These findings provide crucial groundwork by synthesizing the various finding related to risk-taking behavior in adolescence and in understanding individual differences and developmental markers for propensities to engage in negative behavior.

ROLE OF FAMILY AND PEERS DURING KEY DEVELOPMENTAL STAGES

Modeling the use of alcohol or drugs by parents when children are young increases the notion that drugs and alcohol are not harmful substances and this risk factor increases the risk for using as a teen (148). Peers have a stronger influence on adolescents than their parents and not only influence initiation of use but relapse (149,150). Peers have a greater influence during adolescents. Neurobiologic reasons for this can be found in a study by Steinberg et al. (151). Examination of fMRI data indicated that the presence of peers activated certain regions that were not activated when peers were not present during a risky driving game. These regions included increased activity in the medial frontal cortex, left ventral striatum (primarily the accumbens), left superior temporal sulcus, and the left medial temporal structures. This increased activity in the presence of peers was associated with a significant increase in oxytocin, which heightened adolescents' attentiveness to memory for social information. Therefore, after puberty, adolescents are more likely to seek out risky behaviors especially in the presence of their peers. This oxytocin may also explain the role of sex hormones during puberty and the increase in risk-taking behavior. Though sex hormones may not influence the amygdala and the accumbens directly, the influence of sex hormones on oxytocin and the corresponding effect of oxytocin in regulating social bonding and recognition and memory of social stimuli in combination with the reasons for increased risk-taking behavior may more correctly explain the increase in risk taking, especially in the presence of peers.

CONCLUSIONS

As noted by Iacono et al. (152) at the neurobiologic level, behavioral disinhibition can occur via bottom-up mechanisms, whereby stimuli acquire excessive salience or motivational drive is high or via failure of top-down control mechanisms. During adolescence, the bottom-up mechanisms become more important and may explain why adolescents experiment more with risky behaviors during this developmental stage. However, one cannot discuss onset of substance abuse without addressing risk factors that may lead to abuse. No one risk factor leads to substance abuse. In fact, the more risk factors an individual has, the greater the risk of developing the disorder. Untreated comorbid disorders, genetic predisposition, environmental stressors, personality, and age of onset of use are factors that may add to the increased risk for using substances of abuse during adolescence and may contribute to a more chronic and severe form of addiction. Therefore, one must understand risk factors that increase risk and never underestimate the importance of early intervention. No one can understand addiction without understanding when, where, and why risk factors began from a developmental perspective. For these reason, addiction may be thought of as having pediatric origins. Early intervention can obviously decrease the risk of developing substance abuse. However, missed opportunities to intervene may increase the probability of using during adolescence.

REFERENCES

1. Niaura R, Bock B, Lloyd EE, et al. Maternal transmission of nicotine dependence: psychiatric, neurocognitive and prenatal factors. *Am J Addict* 2001;10(1):16–29.
2. Weissmann, MM, Warner, V, Wickramarante, PJ, et al. Maternal smoking during pregnancy and psychopathology in offspring followed to adulthood. *J Am Child Adolesc Psychiatry* 1999;38:892–899.

3. Fried PA, Watkinson B, Gray R. Differential effects on cognitive functioning in 13- to 16-year-olds prenatally exposed to cigarettes and marihuana. *Neurotoxicol Teratol* 2003;25(4):427–436.
4. Day N, Goldschmidt L, Thomas CA. Prenatal marijuana exposure contributes to the prediction of marijuana use at age 14. *Addiction* 2006;101(9):1313–1322.
5. Goldschmidt L, Richardson GA, Willford J, Day NL. Prenatal marijuana exposure and intelligence test performance at age 6. *J Am Acad Child Adolesc Psychiatry* 2008 Mar;47(3):254–263.
6. Smith AM, Fried PA, Hogan MJ, Cameron I. Effects of prenatal marijuana on visuospatial working memory: an fMRI study in young adults. *Neurotoxicol Teratol* 2006;28(2):286–295.
7. Baer JS, Barr HM, Bookstein FL, et al. Prenatal alcohol exposure family history of alcoholism in the etiology of adolescent alcohol problems. *J Stud Alcohol* 1998;59(5):533–543.
8. Streissguth AP, O'Malley KD. Fetal alcohol syndrome/fetal alcohol effects, secondary disabilities and mental health approaches. *Treat Today* 1997;Spring:16–17.
9. National Institutes on Alcohol Abuse and Alcoholism. *Tenth Special Report to the U.S. Congress on Alcohol and Health, Highlights from Current Research.* Washington, DC: U.S. Department of Health and Human Services, 2000:282–338.
10. Centers for Disease Control and Prevention. Updates: Trends in fetal alcohol syndrome-United States, 1979–1993. *MMWR* 1995;44:249–251.
11. Ebrahim SH, Luman E, Floyd RL, et al. Alcohol consumption by pregnant women in the United States 1988–1995. *Obstet Gynecol* 1998;92(2):187–192.
12. Mattson SN, Riley EP, Sowell ER, et al. Neuropsychological comparison of alcohol-exposed children with or without physical features of fetal alcohol syndrome. *Neuropsychology* 1998;12:146–153.
13. Fast DK, Conry J, Loock CA. Identifying fetal alcohol syndrome among youth in the criminal juvenile justice system. *J Dev Behav Pediatr* 1999;20(5):370–372.
14. Mattson SN, Riley EP, Jamigan TL, et al. A decrease in the size of the basal ganglia following prenatal alcohol exposure. A preliminary report. *Neurotoxical Teratol* 1994;16:283–289.
15. Mattson SN, Riley EP, Delis DC, et al. Verbal learning and memory in children with fetal alcohol syndrome. *Alcohol Clin Exp Res* 1996;20(5):810–816.
16. Mattson SN, Goodman AM, Caine C, et al. Executive functioning in children with prenatal alcohol exposure. *Alcohol Clin Exp Res* 1999;23(11):1808–1815.
17. Uecker A, Nadel L. Spatial locations gone awry: object and spatial memory deficits in children with fetal syndrome. *Neuropsychologia* 1996;34(3):209–223.
18. Goldschmidt L, Richardson GA, Day NL. Prenatal alcohol exposure and academic achievement at age six: a nonlinear fit. *Alcohol Clin Exp Res* 1996;20(4):763–770.
19. Coles CD. Critical periods for prenatal alcohol exposure: evidence from animal and human studies. *Alcohol Health Res World* 1994;18:22–29.
20. Mirsky AF, Anthony BJ, Duncan CC, et al. Analysis of the elements of attention: a neuropsychological approach. *Neuropsychol Rev* 1991;2:109–145.
21. Connor PD, Streissguth AP, Sampson PD, et al. Individual differences in auditory and visual attention among fetal alcohol affected adults. *Alcohol Clin Exp Res* 1999;23(8):1395–1402.
22. Streissguth AP, Bar HM, Sampson PD, et al. Attention, distraction, and reaction time at age 7 years and prenatal alcohol exposure. *Neurobehav Toxicol Teratol* 1986;8(16):717–725.
23. Jacobson SW, Jacobson JL, Sokol RJ. Effects of fetal alcohol exposure on infant reaction time. *Alcohol Clin Exp Res* 1994;18(5):1125–1132.
24. Frank DA, Augustyn M, Knight WG, et al. Growth, development, and behavior in early childhood following cocaine exposure. *JAMA* 2000;285(12):1613–1625.
25. Singer MI, Pitchers MK, Hussey D. The relationship between sexual abuse among psychiatrically hospitalized adolescents. *Child Abuse Neglect* 1989;13(3):319–325.
26. Golding J. Reproduction and caffeine consumption—a literature review. *Early Hum Dev* 1995;43:1–14.
27. Stein MB, Schork NJ, Gelernter J. Gene-by-environment (serotonin transporter and childhood maltreatment) interaction for anxiety sensitivity, an intermediate phenotype for anxiety disorders. *Neuropsychopharmacology* 2008;33(2):312–319.
28. Levenson JM, Sweatt JD. Epigenetic mechanisms in memory formation. *Nat Rev Neurosci* 2005;6(2):108–118.
29. Koob G, LeMoal M. Addiction and the antireward system. *Ann Rev Psychol* 2008;59:29–53.
30. Koob G. The neurobiology of addiction: a neuroadaptational view relevant for diagnosis. *Addiction* 2006;101(Suppl 1):23–30.
31. Koob G. Stress dysregulation of drug reward pathways, and the transition to drug dependence. *Am J Psychiatry* 2007;164:1149–1159.
32. Solomon RL, Corbit JD. An opponent-process theory of motivation: I. Temporal dynamics of affect. *Psychol Rev* 1974;81:119–145.
33. Hasin PS, Grant BF, Endicott J. The natural history of alcohol abuse: implications for definition of alcohol use disorders. *Am J Psychiatry* 1990;147:1537–1541.
34. Kalivas PW, Volkow ND. The neural basis of addiction: a pathology of motivation and choice. *Am J Psychiatry* 2005;162:1403–1413.
35. Nestler EJ. Is there a common molecular pathway for addiction? *Nat Neurosci* 2005;8(11):1445–1449.
36. Nestler EJ. Molecular neurobiology of addiction. *Am J Addict* 2001;10:201–217.
37. Nestler , EJ. Delta Fos B: a sustained molecular switch for addiction. *Proc Natl Acad Sci U S A* 2001;98(20):11042–11046.
38. Bibb JA, Jingshan C, Taylor JR, et al. Effects of chronic exposure to cocaine are regulated by the neuronal protein Cdk5. *Nature* 2001;410:376–380.
39. Volkow ND, Wang GJ, Fowler JS, et al. Brain DA D2 receptors predict reinforcing of stimulants in humans: replication study. *Synapse* 2002;46(2):79–82.
40. Volkow ND, Fowler JS, Wang GJ. Role of dopamine in drug reinforcement and addiction in humans: results from imaging studies. *Behav Pharmacol* 2002;13:355–466.
41. Volkow ND, Wang GJ, Begleiter H, et al High levels of dopamine D2 receptors in unaffected members of alcoholic families: possible protective factors. *Arch Gen Psychiatry* 2006;63(9):999–1008.
42. Thanos PK, Volkow ND, Freimuth P, et al. Overexpression of dopamine D2 receptors reduces alcohol self-administration. *Neurochemistry* 2001;78(5):1094–1103.
43. Thanos PK, Rivera SN, Weaver K, et al. Dopamine D2R DNA transfer in dopamine D2 receptor-deficient mice: effects on ethanol drinking, *Life Sci* 2005;77(2):130–139.
44. Gaveriaux-Ruff C, Kieffer BL. Opioid receptor genes inactivated in mice: the highlights. *Neuropeptides* 2002;36:62–71.
45. Walters CL, Brown S, Changeux JP, et al. The beta2 but not alpha7 subunit of the nicotinic acetylcholine receptor is required for nicotine-conditioned place preference in mice. *Psychopharmacol (Berl)* 2006;184(34):339–344.
46. Caine SB, Thomsen M, Gabriel KI, et al. Lack of self-administration of cocaine in dopamine D1 receptor knock-out mice. *J Neurosci* 2007;27(48):13140–13150.
47. Hiroi N, Agatsuma S. Genetic susceptibility to substance dependence *Mol Psychiatry* 2005;10:336–344.
48. Dick DM. Identification of genes influencing a spectrum of externalizing psychopathology. *Curr Dir Psychol Sci* 2007;16:331–335.
49. Uhl GR. Molecular genetics of substance abuse vulnerability: remarkable recent convergence of genome scan results. *Ann N Y Acad Sci* 2004;1025:1–13.
50. Li CY, Mao X, Wei L. Genes and (common) pathways underlying drug addiction *PLoS Comput Biol* 2008;4(1):1–11.
51. Goodwin DW, Schlusinger F., Moller W, et al. Drinking problems in adopted and non-adopted sons of alcoholics. *Arch Gen Psychiatry* 1974;31:164–169.
52. Cadoret RJ, Troughton E, O'Gorman TW, et al. An adoption study of genetic and environmental factors in drug use. *Arch Gen Psychiatry* 1986;43:1131–1136.
53. Cloniger CR, Bohman MC, Sigvardisson S, et al. Psychopathology in adopted out children of alcoholics. The Stockholm Adoption Study. In:

Galanter M, ed. *Recent developments in alcoholism*. New York: Plenum Press, 1985:37–50.

54. Kendler KS, Presscott CA. Genetic and environmental risk factors for cannabis use, abuse, dependence: a study of female twins. *Am J Psychiatry* 1998;155(8):1016–1022.
55. Kendler KS, Presscott CA. Genetic and environmental risk factors for cocaine use, dependence. A study of female twins. *Br J Psychiatry* 1998;173:345–350.
56. Schukit MA. A 10 year study of sons of alcoholics: preliminary results. *Alcohol Alcohol* 1999;(Suppl)1:147–149.
57. Schuckit MA, Daeppen JB, Tipp JE, et al. The clinical course of alcohol-related problems in alcohol dependent and nonalcohol dependent drinking women and men. *J Stud Alcohol* 1998;59(5):581–590.
58. DeWitt DJ, Adlaf EM, Offord DR, et al. Age of first alcohol use: a risk factor for the development of alcohol disorders. *Am J Psychiatry* 2000; 157:745–750.
59. Kandel DB, Yamaguchi K, Chen K. Stages of progression in drug in drug involvement from adolescence to adulthood: further evidence for the gateway theory *J Stud Alcohol* 1992;53(5):447–457.
60. Clark DB, Kirisci L, Tarter, RE. Adolescent versus adult onset and the development of substance use disorders in males. *Drug Alcohol Depend* 1998;49(2):115–121.
61. Lee GP, DeClemente CC. Age of onset versus duration of problem drinking on the alcohol use inventory. *J Stud Alcohol* 1985;46:298–402.
62. Knight JR, Sherritt L, Shier LA, et al. Validity of the CRAFFT substance abuse screening test among adolescent clinic patients. *Arch Pediatr Adolesc Med* 2002;156(6):607–614.
63. Babor TF, Hoffman M, Del Boca FK, et al. Types of alcoholics: I. Evidence for an empirically derived topology based on indicators of vulnerability and solvent. *Arch Gen Psychiatry* 1992;47:599–608.
64. Masse LC, Tremblay RE. Behavior of boys in kindergarten and the onset of substance abuse in adolescence. *Arch Gen Psychiatry* 1997;54:62–68.
65. Zuckerman M, Kuhlman DM. Personality and risk taking: common biological factors. *J Personality* 2000;68(6):999–1029.
66. Prochaska JO, DiClemente C. Transtheoretical theory toward a more integrated model of change. *Psychother Theory Res Pract* 1982;19: 276–288.
67. Bolla K, Ernst M, Kiehl K, Mourotidis M, et al. Prefrontal cortical dysfunction in abstinent cocaine abusers. *J Neuropsychiatry Clin Neurosci.* 2004 Fall;16(4):456–464.
68. Whitmore EA, Milulick SK, Thompson LL, et al. Influences on adolescent substance dependence, conduct disorders, depression, attention deficit hyperactivity disorder, and gender. *Drug Alcohol Depend* 1997; 47(2):87–97.
69. Couwenbergh C, van den Brink W, Zwart K, et al. Comorbid psychopathology in adolescents and young adults treated for substance use disorders: a review. *Eur Child Adolesc Psychatry* 2006;15(6):319–328.
70. Riggs P, Whitmore E. Substance use disorders and disruptive behavior disorders. In: Hendren RL, ed. *Disruptive behavior disorders in children and adolescents. Review of Psychiatry Series,* Washington DC, US American Psychiatric Press 18:133–173.
71. Drevets WC. Orbitofrontal cortex function and structure in depression. *Ann N Y Acad Sci* 2007;121:499–527.
72. Kennedy SH, Evans KR, Krüger S, et al. Changes in regional brain glucose metabolism measured with positron emission tomography after paroxetine treatment of major depression. *Am J Psychiatry* 2001;58(6): 899–905.
73. Rao U, Ryan N, Dahl DE, et al. Factors associated with the development of substance use disorders in depressed adolescents. *J Amer Acad Child Psychiatry* 38(9):1109–1117, Sept., 1999.
74. Wilens TE, Biederman J, Millstein RB, et al. Risk for substance use disorders in youth with child and adolescent onset bipolar disorder. *J Am Acad Child Psychiatry* 1999;38(6):680–685.
75. Ernst M, Nelson EE, Jazbec S, et al. Amygdala and nucleus accumbens in responses to receipt and omission of gains in adults and adolescents. *Neuroimage* 2005;25(4):1279–1291.
76. Saltoum IM, Cornelius JR, Douaihy A, et al. Patient characteristics and treatment implications of marijuana abuse among bipolar alcoholics: results from a double blind, placebo controlled study. *Addict Behav* 2005;30:1702–1708.
77. Geller B, Cooper TB, Sein K, et al. Double blind and placebo controlled study of lithium for adolescent bipolar disorders with secondary substance dependence. *J Am Child Adolesc Psychiatry* 1998;37(2):171–178.
78. Swan N. Early childhood behavior and temperament predict later substance abuse. *National Institute on Drug Abuse Notes* 1995;10:1.
79. Tiihonen J, Kuikka J, Bergstrom K, et al. Dopamine reuptake site densities in patients with social phobia. *Am J Psychiatry* 1997;154:239–242.
80. Schneier FR, Liebowitz MR, Abi-Dargham A, et al. Low Dopamine D2 Receptor Binding Potential in Social Phobia. *Am J Psychiatry* 2000; 157(3):457–459.
81. Abram KM. Posttraumatic stress disorder and trauma in youth in juvenile justice. *Arch Of Gen Psychiatry* 2004;61(4):403–410.
82. Grella C, Stein J, Greenwell L. Association among childhood trauma, adolescent problem behaviors and adverse adult outcomes in substance abusing women offenders. *Psychol Addict Behav* 2005;19(1):43–53.
83. Brody AL, Saxena S, Schwartz JM, et al. FDG-PET predictors of response to behavioral therapy and pharmacotherapy in obsessive compulsive disorder. *Psychiatry Res* 1998;9;84(1):1–6.
84. Rauch SL, Shin LM, Dougherty DD, et al. Predictors of fluvoxamine response in contamination-related obsessive compulsive disorder: a PET symptom provocation study. *Neuropsychopharmacology* 2002;27(5):782–791.
85. Disney ER, Elkins IJ, Mc Gue M, et al. Effects of ADHD, conduct disorder and gender on substance use abuse in adolescents. *Am J Psychobiol* 1997;156(10):1515–1521.
86. Biederman J, Wilens T, Mick E, et al. Pharmacotherapy of ADHD reduces risk for substance use disorder. *Pediatrics* 1999;104(2):20.
87. Mulder MJ, Baeyens D, Davidson MC, et al. Familial vulnerability to ADHD affects activity in the cerebellum in addition to the prefrontal systems. *J Am Acad Child Adolesc Psychiatry* 2008;47(1):68–75.
88. Zhu CZ, Zang YF, Cao QJ, et al. Fisher discriminative analysis of resting-state brain function for attention-deficit/hyperactivity disorder. *Neuroimage* 2008;40(1):110–120.
89. Swanson JM, Volkow ND. Serum and brain concentrations of methylphenidate: implications for use and abuse. *Neurosci Biobehav Rev* 2003;27(7):615–621.
90. Volkow ND, Wang GJ, Telang F, et al. Dopamine increases in striatum do not elicit craving in cocaine abusers unless they are coupled with cocaine cues. *Neuroimage* 2008;39(3):1266–1273.
91. Castellanos FX, Lee PP, Sharp W, et al. Developmental trajectories of brain volume abnormalities in children and adolescents with attention-deficit/hyperactivity disorder. *JAMA* 2002;288(14):1740–1748.
92. Luna B, Sweeney JA. The emergence of collaborative brain function: fMRI studies of the development of response inhibition. *Ann N Y Acad Sci* 2004;1021:296–309.
93. Thanos PK, Michealides M. Benveniste H, et al. Effects of chronic oral methylphenidate on cocaine self-administration and striatal dopamine D2 receptors in rodents. *Pharmacol Biochem Behav* 2007;87(4):426–433.
94. Thanos PK, Taintor NB, Rivera SN, et al. *DRD2* gene transfer into the nucleus accumbens core of the alcohol preferring and nonpreferring rats attenuates alcohol drinking. *Alcohol Clin Exp Res* 2004;28(5):720–728.
95. Scheier LM, Botvin CJ, Drag T, et al. Social skills, competence and drug refusal efficacy as predictors of adolescent alcohol use. *J Drug Ed* 1999;29(3):251–278.
96. Stacy AW, Newcomb MD, Bentler PM. Cognitive motivations and sensation seeking as long term predictors of drinking problems. *J Soc Clin Psychol* 1993;12:1–24.
97. Hops HA, Davis B, Lewin LM. The development of alcohol and other substance use: a gender study of family and peer context. *J Stud Alcohol Suppl* 1999;13:22–31.
98. Simkin D. Adolescent Substance Abuse Textbook of Psychiatry, 8th ed. Sadock B, ed, 2004;2:3470–3490.
99. Tapert SF, Baratta BS, Abrantes BA, Brown SA. Attention dysfunction predicts substance involvement in community youth. *J Am Child Adolesc Psychiatry* 2002;41(6):680–686.
100. Shelton D. Young offenders with emotional disorders. *J Nurs Scholar* 2001;(33)3:259–263.

101. Hartney C, Wordes M., Krisberg B. *Health care for our troubled youth: provision of services in the foster care and juvenile justice systems of California.* National Council on Crime and Delinquency, 2002. available at http://www.nccd-crc.org/nccd/pubs/2002_youth_healthcare.pdf.
102. Kirk J. Reid G. An examination of the relationship between dyslexia and offending in young people and its implications. *Dyslexia* 2001;7(2):77–84.
103. Wright B. Learning Problems, Delayed Development and Puberty. *PNAS* 2004;10(6):9942–9946.
104. Hambrecht M, Hafner H. Cannabis, vulnerability and onset of schizophrenia: an epidemiological perspective. *Aust N Z J Psychiatry* 2000;34:468–475.
105. Yurgelun-Todd D. Emotional and cognitive changes during adolescence. *Curr Opin Neurobiol* 2007;17(2):251–257.
106. Rubia K., Overmeyer S., Taylor E, et al. Functional frontalization with age: mapping neurodevelopmental trajectories with fMRI. *Neurosci Biobehav Rev* 2000;24:13–19.
107. Tamm L, Menon V, Reiss AL. Maturation of brain function associated with response inhibition. *J Am Acad Child Adolesc Psychiatry* 2002;41:1231–1238.
108. Galvan A, Hare TA, Parra CE, et al. Earlier development of the accumbens relative to orbitofrontal cortex might underlie risk-taking behavior in adolescents. *J Neurosci* 2006;26(25):6885–6892.
109. Galvan A, Hare T, Voss H, et al. Risk-taking and the adolescent brain: who is at risk? *Dev Sci* 2007;10(2):F8–F14.
110. Reyna V, Farley F. Risk and rationality in adolescent decision making: implications for theory, practice, and public policy. *Psychol Sci Public Interest* 2006;7(1):1–44.
111. Casey BJ, Thomas KM, Davidson MC, et al. Dissociating striatal and hippocampal function developmentally with a stimulus-response compatibility task. *J Neurosci* 2002;22(19):8647–8652.
112. Casey BJ, Tottenham N, Liston C, Durston S. Imaging the developing brain: what have we learned about cognitive development? *Trends Cogn Sci* 2005;9(3):104–110.
113. Casey BJ, Galvan A, Hare, TA. Changes in cerebral functional organization during cognitive development. *Curr Opin Neurobiol* 2005;15:239–244.
114. Montague PR, Berns GS. Neural economics and the biological substrates of valuation. *Neuron* 2002;36:265–284.
115. Matthews SC, et al. Selective activation of the nucleus accumbens during risk-taking decision making. *Neuroreport* 2004;15:2123–2127.
116. Kuhnen CM, Knutson B. The neural basis of financial risk taking. *Neuron* 2005;47:763–770.
117. Giedd JN. Structural magnetic resonance imaging of the adolescent brain. *Ann N Y Acad Sci* 2004;1021:77–85.
118. Gogtay N, Giedd JN, Lusk L, et al. Dynamic mapping of human cortical development during childhood through early adulthood. *Proc Natl Acad Sci U S A* 2004;101(21):8174–8179.
119. Sowell ER, Thompson PM, Toga AW. Mapping changes in the human cortex throughout the span of life. *Neuroscientist* 2004;10:372–392.
120. Sowell ER, Peterson BS, Thompson PM, et al. W. Mapping cortical change across the human life span. *Nat Neurosci* 2003;6:309–315.
121. Sowell ER, Thompson PM, Holmes CJ, et al. *In vivo* evidence for post-adolescent brain maturation in frontal and striatal regions. *Nat Neurosci* 1999;2(10):859–861.
122. Giedd JN, Blumenthal J, Jeffries NO, et al. Brain development during childhood and adolescence: a longitudinal MRI study. *Nat Neurosci* 1999;2:861–863.
123. Casey BJ, Trainor RJ, Orendi JL, et al. A developmental functional MRI study of prefrontal activation during performance of a go-no-go task. *J Cogn Neurosci* 1997;9:835–847.
124. Nagy Z. Westerberg H, Klingberg T. Maturation of white matter is associated with the development of cognitive functions during childhood. *J Cogn Neurosci* 2004;16:1227–1233.
125. Liston C, Watts R, Tottenham N, et al. Frontostriatal microstructure modulates efficient recruitment of cognitive control. *Cereb Cortex* 2005;16:553–560.
126. Brown TT, Lugar HM, Coalson RS, et al. Developmental changes in human cerebral functional organization for word generation. *Cereb Cortex* 2005;15:275–290.
127. Bunge SA, Dudukovic NM, Thomason ME, et al. Immature frontal lobe contributions to cognitive control in children: evidence from fMRI. *Neuron* 2002;33:301–311.
128. Crone EA, Donohue SE, Honomichl R, et al. Brain regions mediating flexible rule use during development. *J Neurosci* 2006;26(43):11239–11247.
129. Luna B, Thulborn KR, Munoz DP, et al. Maturation of widely distributed brain function subserves cognitive development. *Neuroimage* 2001;13(5):786–793.
130. Moses P, Roe K, Buxton RB, et al. Functional MRI of global and local processing in children. *Neuroimage* 2002;16:415–424.
131. Schlaggar BL, Brown TT, Lugar HM, et al. Functional neuroanatomical differences between adults and school-age children in the processing of single words. *Science* 2002;296:1476–1479.
132. Thomas KM, Hunt RH, Vizueta N, et al. Evidence of developmental differences in implicit sequence learning: an FMRI study of children and adults. *J Cogn Neurosci* 2004;16:1339–1351.
133. Turkeltaub PE, Gareau L, Flowers DL, et al. Development of neural mechanisms for reading. *Nat Neurosci* 2003;6:767–773.
134. Eshel N, Nelson E, Blair RJ, et al. Neural substrates of choice selection in adults and adolescents: development of the ventrolateral prefrontal and anterior cingulate cortices. *Neuropsychologia* 2007;45:1270–1279.
135. Laviola G, Macri S, Morley-Fletcher S, Adriani W. Risk-taking behavior in adolescent mice: psychobiological determinants and early epigenetic influence [abstract]. *Neurosci Biobehav Rev* 2003;27(1-2):19–31.
136. Miller EK, Cohen JD. An integrative theory of prefrontal cortex function. *Ann Rev Neurosci* 2001;24:167–202.
137. Spear LP. The adolescent brain and age-related behavioral manifestations. *Neurosci Biobehav Rev* 2000;24(4):417–463.
138. Kelley AE Schochet T, Landry C. Adolescent brain development: Vulnerabilities and Opportunities: Part 1. Risk taking and novelty seeking. *Ann N Y Acad Sci* 2004;1021:27–32.
139. Mischel W, Shoda Y, Rodriguez MI. Delay of gratification in children. *Science* 1989;244(4907):933–938.
140. Eigsti IM, Zayas V, Mischel W, et al. Predicting cognitive control from preschool to late adolescence and young adulthood. *Psychol Sci* 2006;17(6):478–484.
141. Blum K, Braverman ER, Holder JM, et al. Reward deficiency syndrome: a biogenetic model for the diagnosis and treatment of impulsive, addictive, and compulsive behaviors. *J Psychoactive Drugs* 2000;32(Suppl i–iv):1–112.
142. O'Doherty JP. Reward representations and reward-related learning in the human brain: insights from neuroimaging. *Curr Opin Neurobiol* 2004;14:769–776.
143. Gardener M, Steinberg L. Peer influence on risk taking, risk preference, and risky decision making in adolescence and adulthood: an experimental study. *Dev Psychol* 2005;41:625–635.
144. Jernigan TL, Zisook S, Heaton RK, et al. Magnetic resonance imaging abnormalities in lenticular nuclei and cerebral cortex in schizophrenia. *Arch Gen Psychiatry* 1991;48(10):811–823.
145. Giedd JN, Snell JW, Lange N, et al. Quantitative magnetic resonance imaging of human brain development: ages 4–18. *Cereb Cortex* 1996;(6):551–560.
146. Steinberg L. Risk-taking in adolescence: what changes, and why? *Ann N Y Acad Sci* 2004;1021:51–58.
147. Durston S, Davidson MC, Tottenham N, et al. A shift from diffuse to focal cortical activity with development. *Dev Sci* 2006;(9)1:18–20.
148. Jackson C, et al. A longitudinal study predicting patterns of cigarette smoking in late childhood. *Health Ed Behav* 1998;25(4):436–477.
149. Brook JS, Linkoff IF, Whiteman M. Initiation into adolescent marijuana use. *J Gen Psychiatry* 1980;137:133–142.
150. Brown SA. Recovery patterns in adolescent substance abusers. In: Baer JS, Marlatt GA, McMahon RJ, eds. *Addictive behavior across the life span: prevention, treatment, and policy issues.* Beverly Hills, CA: Sage Publications, Inc., 1993:161–163.
151. Steinberg L. A social neuroscience perspective on adolescent risk taking. *Sci Direct Dev Rev* 2008;28:78–106.
152. Iacono WG, Malone SM, McGue M. Behavioral disinhibition and the development of early-onset addiction: common and specific influences. *Ann Rev Clin Psychol* 2008;4:325–348.

CHAPTER 101

Terri L. Randall, MD
Himanshu P. Upadhyaya, MD, MBBS, MS

Adolescent Cigarette Smoking

Smoking is the leading cause of preventable death in the United States (1). Smoking behaviors begin in childhood (2,3), with even infrequent, experimental smoking by adolescents leading to symptoms of addiction in a matter of weeks (4). Once a teen begins smoking regularly, cessation is difficult (2,5,6). Thus tobacco use among adolescents is an area of considerable public health concern.

Even though the rates of smoking have declined recently, more than 2 million adolescents in the United States are smokers and nearly 4,000 adolescents start to smoke every day (7). Daily smoking, which is probably a good proxy of nicotine dependence, is prevalent in at least 12% of high school seniors and 3% of eighth graders (8). The development of nicotine dependence and success in cessation is inversely related to the age when smoking begins (2,9). Surveys indicate that up to 70% of adolescents try cigarettes and one third of all adolescents are currently smoking (10).

In this chapter, we will review our current understanding of the epidemiology, etiology, comorbidity, assessment, treatment, and prevention of nicotine dependence in adolescents. In this chapter, we will also focus on cigarette use, because the overwhelming majority of the research on nicotine dependence in adolescents is on cigarette smoking. Relatively fewer youth in the United States use smokeless tobacco (chew or snuff), cigars, bidis (a thin South Asian cigarette), kreteks (tobacco and clove cigarette), or water pipes rather than cigarettes (8). These types of tobacco are important areas of discussion especially when considering regional preferences of tobacco use in the United States and in other countries but beyond the scope of this chapter.

EPIDEMIOLOGY

Several surveys collect information on adolescent tobacco and drug use, which is a critical component to understanding and addressing the problem of tobacco in youth. Each year since 1975, Monitoring the Future has surveyed 12th grade (17 to 18 year olds) students in 120 to 146 public and private high schools in the United States. Of note, 15% to 20% of high school students drop out of school before the 12th grade, so these adolescents are not represented in the survey. Since 1991, they have also collected information on eighth and 10th graders, students ages 12 to 13 years old and 15 to 16 years old, respectively (9). Another source of information on substance use in adolescents is the Substance Abuse and Mental Health Services Administrations' National Survey on Drug Use and Health, formerly called the National Household Survey on Drug Abuse. It collects information on the prevalence, patterns, and consequences of drug and alcohol use and abuse in the general population. The respondents of this survey are noninstitutionalized persons ages 12 and older (7). The Global Youth Tobacco Survey is one of the components of the Global Tobacco Surveillance System, a collaboration among the U.S. Centers for Disease Control and Prevention's Office on Smoking and Health, the World Health Organization Tobacco Free Initiative, and other international agencies. It is an anonymous, confidential self-administered questionnaire given to school children ages 13 to 15 years. In 2005, 140 countries participated in the Global Youth Tobacco Survey (11).

According to the Monitoring the Future results for 2006, nearly half of 12th graders have tried cigarettes and more than

20% smoked at least some in the prior month. Among eighth graders, 25% reported having tried cigarettes and 9% smoked in the prior month. Among 8th, 10th, and 12th graders, 4.9%, 7.6%, and 12.2% are daily smokers, respectively. One and one half to 6% of these smokers report smoking a half-pack or more per day. These rates have dropped significantly from 1976 when the past 30-day and daily smoking prevalence was 38% and 29%, respectively. In addition, in 1976, 19% of surveyed youth reported use of a half-pack or more cigarettes per day. The decline in cigarette use may be due to a number of factors, including the increased price of cigarettes, the tobacco industry settlement, prevention activities, restrictions on advertising, and national antismoking campaigns (8).

In 2006, young adults ages 18 to 25 had the highest current use of tobacco products (43.9%) according to the National Survey on Drug Use and Health (7). Among youths age 12 to 17 in 2006, 3.3 million (12.9%) used a tobacco product in the last month and 10.4% used cigarettes (7). They found that the rate of current cigarette use is highest in rural counties. In fact, in rural nonmetropolitan counties, current cigarette use among persons age 12 or older increased from 23% in 2005 to 30% in 2006 (7).

The 2005 results of the Global Youth Tobacco Survey (11) revealed that current tobacco use was highest in the Americas (22.2%) and lowest in the southeast Asia and western Pacific regions (12.9% and 11.4%, respectively). Boys were significantly more likely than girls to use tobacco products (11). Regrettably, nearly one fifth of respondents reported that they were susceptible or likely to begin smoking in the coming year (11).

ETIOLOGY

Like many behaviors, the determinants of adolescent smoking are multifactorial. Several individual and environmental risk and protective factors play a role in determining youths' experimentation, initiation, and maintenance of smoking behaviors.

Psychosocial risk factors for smoking include age, race, socioeconomic status, abuse history, and family structure. Smoking initiation increases with increasing age and grade (12). Youth who begin smoking at younger ages are more likely to become dependent (13) and less likely to stop smoking (5). Native American youths use cigarettes and smokeless tobacco at higher rates than other ethnic groups. In 2004, 72% of Native American 12th graders report ever using cigarettes compared with 53% of non-Native American 12th graders (14). According to the National Survey on Drug Use and Health (which did not include a separate category for Native Americans), the prevalence of current cigarette smoking in young people ages 12 to 17 is highest among Caucasians (12.4%), followed by Latinos (8.2%), and then African Americans (6%) (7). African American adolescents appear to initiate smoking behavior later than Caucasians as rates of smoking among African American adults age 26 and older are about the same as Caucasians (7). A history of verbal, physical, or sexual abuse predicts increased smoking rates in adolescents (15,16). High levels of socioeconomic stress or low socioeconomic status are also risk factors for adolescent smoking (17–19). Being raised in a two-parent family appears to have a protective effect on adolescent smoking (9,20,21). However, a recent study notes that high exposure to deviant peers may nullify the protective effect of being raised in an intact, two-parent family (22).

Several individual risk and protective factors for adolescent smoking behaviors have been identified. Symptoms of depression, anxiety, and attention deficit hyperactivity disorder (ADHD) have all been linked with smoking in youth (23–25). This will be covered more in depth in the Comorbidity section. Novelty seeking (26,27), risk-taking (26,27), and other problem behaviors such as other drug use, early sexual activity, fighting, and poor eating habits are associated with youth smoking (9,28). Individual traits such as low self-esteem and negative self-concept also have been linked with adolescent smoking (9,29,30). Adolescents who have normative views of smoking, such as the belief that the majority of peers smoke, are more likely to be smokers (31). Scholastic achievement (19,32,33), a moderate amount of work (<10 hours per week) (34), and involvement in sports (13) and religious (16,19) activities lessen the risk for youth smoking.

Environmental factors involved in adolescent smoking include parental, peer, and media influences, as well as exposure to secondhand smoke. Increased parental supervision and monitoring is associated with decreased smoking in teens (35–40). This effect may be mediated by limiting exposure to pro-smoking peers (32). Parental smoking is related to higher rates of adolescent smoking possibly by modeling smoking behavior or by teens' perception of parental approval of smoking (37,41).

Compared with parental influences on adolescent smoking, peer factors seem to have a more compelling influence on teen smoking. Youth who have more friends who smoke are more likely to be smokers themselves (39,42). One study reveals that youth reporting peer pressure to smoke are nearly twice as likely to smoke and those with two or more friends who smoke are nine times as likely to smoke (43). Youth with siblings who smoke are also at higher risk for smoking initiation (9).

In 2005, tobacco companies spent more than $13 billion on tobacco advertising and promotion in the United States (44). Greater exposure and receptivity to tobacco marketing is associated with increased smoking susceptibility in youth (45,46). One study estimates that one third of smoking experimentation could be attributed to tobacco promotional activities (47). Surveys estimate that 70% of adolescents try cigarettes (10). Greater exposure to entertainment media influences, such as tobacco use in the movies, has been tied to youths' increased susceptibility to initiate smoking (48) and increased risk of becoming a future smoker (49).

Exposure to environmental smoke may increase the risk of smoking. According to the Global Youth Tobacco Survey, more than half of all students questioned were exposed to secondhand tobacco smoke in public places and more than 40% in their homes (11). Never smokers were significantly less likely than current smokers to be exposed to secondhand smoke at home and in public places in every world region (11). Furthermore, school (50) and home (36) smoking bans are associated with decreased rates of youth smoking perhaps by limiting exposure and perceived approval of cigarette smoking.

Although there is significant literature on the social, individual, and environmental determinants of youth smoking, little is known about the mediators and moderators of the gene and environment interaction that leads to smoking. Researchers have explored the connection of the D2 receptor gene, dopamine transporter gene, and the D4 receptor (DRD4) gene to smoking behaviors (51). Laucht and colleagues (52) found that males with the 7r allele of the dopamine receptor gene (DRD4) had higher rates of lifetime smoking and smoked more cigarettes per day. Their research also confirmed that smokers had higher rates of novelty seeking than those who had never smoked or were nondaily smokers. They found that novelty seeking may serve as mediator between DRD4 status and smoking behaviors.

Also of great interest are the determinants of the transition from nonsmoker to smoker. Dierker and colleagues (53) investigated whether individual risk factor or risk factor constellations predicted transition from nonsmoking to experimental smoking and regular smoking. They found that deviant youth engaging in two to three deviant behaviors such as lying, stealing, running away, skipping school, and unsupervised alcohol use predicted youth who progressed from nonsmoking to experimentation (defined as ever having one puff of a cigarette) over the course of the year assessment period. A relatively low grade point average (lower than a B) predicted the progression from nonsmoker to regular smoker defined as daily smoking of at least one cigarette for 30 days (53).

COMORBIDITIES

Smoking is commonly associated with medical and psychiatric comorbidities in children and adolescents (3,54). Besides the long-term medical consequences of smoking, such as lung cancer and cardiovascular disease, smoking is also associated with more immediate health problems. Children and adolescents who smoke have an increased frequency of respiratory symptoms (i.e., cough and phlegm production), respiratory infections, and a have a decrease in lung function (3,55). Studies indicate that youth smoking also impairs cardiovascular health. Smoking is associated with an increase in atherosclerotic lesions in young people (56). It also is associated with decreases in physical fitness levels in youth (57).

Psychiatric comorbidities associated with smoking in young people include disruptive behavior disorders such as ADHD and conduct disorder, major depression, anxiety disorders, and other substance use disorders (23,24,58,59). Neithammer and Frank (60) conducted a study of 70 consecutive adolescent inpatient admissions to a psychiatric hospital. They found that 96% of the patients had used nicotine and 76% were regular nicotine users (defined as having daily use for 4 weeks or more). According to one longitudinal study, youth with a history of mental illness are 50% more likely to increase their smoking over the course of year than those without a history of mental illness 55 (61).

The incidence of cigarette smoking in adolescents with ADHD ranges from 19% to 46% compared with 10% to 24% in peers (62). Some studies indicate a three times higher rate of smoking daily among adolescents with ADHD compared with those without the disorder (63). Children with ADHD start smoking 1.5 to 2 years earlier than their peers. In addition, they are more likely to become dependent, proceed to daily smoking, and smoke more cigarettes per day (64). Some research indicates that treatment of ADHD may ameliorate the apparent increased risk for smoking (62,65,66). Given the high comorbidity of ADHD and conduct disorder, some researchers believe that the high incidence of nicotine dependence in children and adolescents with ADHD can be explained by the presence of conduct disorder. A diagnosis of conduct disorder at age 11 nearly doubles the odds for nicotine dependence at age 14 and quadruples the odds at age 18, according to one prospective study (67). Elkins and colleagues also found that two or more symptoms of conduct disorder better predicted nicotine dependence compared with inattentive and hyperactive symptoms of ADHD (67).

In addition to the disruptive behavior disorders, investigators have found a link between adolescent cigarette smoking and major depressive disorder (54). Although evidence exists for a bidirectional association between cigarette smoking and major depression, there is more evidence that major depression may be a risk factor for smoking rather than vice versa (68,69). This finding is particularly important because major depression, either past or current, is a poor prognostic indicator in the treatment of nicotine dependence (70,71).

There may be a bidirectional relationship between smoking and anxiety disorders in youth as well. Some evidence indicates that anxious youth start smoking because of peer pressure (72), to facilitate social interactions (25), and to experience the presumed calming effects of nicotine (73). Several studies report that social fears and anxiety disorders are associated with increased rates of nicotine dependence (25,74,75). On the other hand, some evidence indicates that smoking contributes to the development of anxiety disorders (76). Research also indicates that anxiety disorders may play a protective role in youth smoking by delaying the onset of smoking (77).

Tobacco is generally one of the first drugs tried by individuals who use illicit drugs (78,79). Thus cigarette smoking has been conceptualized by some authors as a "gateway" to other substance abuse (80). Youth smoking is associated with increased odds for other substance use disorders (81,82). In one study, male and female smokers had significantly increased odds (OR = 18 and 7.7, respectively) for having a substance use disorder compared with nonsmokers (81). Research also indicates that people who start smoking regularly at an early age are at increased risk for developing substance use disorders compared with later onset smokers or nonsmokers (83). Early-onset smokers are more likely to smoke more heavily, have early onset of drinking alcohol, and have a family history of alcoholism compared with individuals who started smoking at age 17 or older, according to one study's findings (84). Early-onset smoking is also associated with increased odds of cannabis and other drug use (85).

ASSESSMENT

Physicians do not consistently query patients about smoking behavior and frequently do not offer assistance in cessation efforts (86,87). Research shows that brief counseling interventions by physicians are helpful in treating adult substance dependence, however, there are few data regarding physician interventions for youth smoking cessation (86,88). Clinical guidelines recommend that physicians and other health care providers adequately assess children's tobacco use and counsel those who are using tobacco products to quit (88). Assessment of tobacco use should include queries about the types of tobacco used, patterns of use, severity of use, circumstances of use, context of use, benefits and consequences of use, symptoms of withdrawal, and motivation for cessation. The National Cancer Institute has amassed a number of brief questionnaires used as research instruments that clinicians may find helpful in assessing teen smoking (89).

One of the challenging aspects of working with adolescents is facilitating accurate disclosure of behaviors that are generally not socially acceptable for young people, such as sexual relationships and drug use. Assuring adolescents that their responses will be confidential is one way to decrease the likelihood of underreporting or misreporting of sensitive information. Another way is to ask concrete, specific, open-ended questions, "When was the first time you ever had a cigarette, even one puff? Tell me about the first time you tried smoking." The latter question may provide key information about precipitating and perpetuating factors that maintain cigarette use. Depending on the response, the clinician may follow up by asking, "When did you first smoke a whole cigarette?" or "Do you think you will experiment with cigarettes in the future? If one of your best friends offered you a cigarette would you smoke it?" Although cigarettes are the most common tobacco product that youth use, it is important to also ask about cigars, cigarillos, bidis (flavored cigarettes from South Asia), and water pipes (hookahs). In addition, health care providers should inquire about the use of smokeless tobacco, especially because the prevalence of smokeless tobacco has been increasing over the past several years (8).

After assessing if the adolescent has used or is using any tobacco products, the clinician should ask about frequency of use. Clinicians should ask specifically about use during different days of the week as adolescents' use widely varies due to a number of factors including availability, presence of friends who smoke, school attendance, or participation in a sports league. One way to capture this information is the Timeline Follow Back method (90). This method uses a calendar to aid patients in recalling smoking behaviors. Working backward from the day of assessment, weekends, holidays, and special events are used as anchor points to help the youth to mark their cigarette consumption over the past 30 to 90 days.

The clinician may also inquire about the circumstances surrounding smoking episodes such as the child's emotional state and the presence of peers. The Adolescent Smoking Consequences questionnaire (91) has many questions that may help the clinician discuss the triggers and emotions that lead to and maintain cigarette use. Another strategy is to approach the assessment as a behavioral analysis. The provider can ask about the antecedents of smoking as well as the results (feeling more relaxed, feeling more accepted by peers) and any consequences (being punished by parents or parents not discovering use). It is also important for the clinician to ask about children's smoking attitudes and beliefs. Youths' perception of smoking and tobacco harmfulness is inversely proportional to youth smoking prevalence (8). Providing information to correct misinformation (the majority of people do not smoke, smoking does not make one look more attractive to the opposite sex) is helpful in shaping behaviors.

Last, the clinician should also assess whether the child meets criteria for nicotine dependence. Establishing whether the youth is dependent on nicotine is important because those who are dependent on nicotine have more severe symptoms of nicotine withdrawal and have more difficulty with smoking cessation (74). Establishing nicotine dependence in young smokers can be more complicated than in adults because of teen smokers' variable smoking patterns. In our clinical experience, daily smoking of cigarettes for several months can be a marker of dependence for almost all adolescents. However, youth may develop symptoms of nicotine dependence within days of smoking initiation (92). According to the *Diagnostic and Statistical Manual, 4th edition, text revision*, substance dependence is characterized by tolerance, withdrawal, use of the substance for longer periods and in larger amounts; inability to control substance use; use that interferes with important social, occupational, or recreational activities; continued use despite adverse physical or psychologic consequences; and spending an inordinate amount of time obtaining, using, or recovering from the effects of the substance. Not all of these criteria are applicable to smokers in general or in young smokers. For instance, many teens do not believe it is difficult to obtain cigarettes and spend their recreational time with friends smoking (12). Thus the criteria about spending a great deal of time obtaining, using, or recovering from nicotine or that use interferes with social obligations may not apply to teen smokers. The criteria for substance dependence in the International Classification of Disease 10 are similar to *Diagnostic and Statistical Manual, 4th edition, text revision,* but also includes craving, "a strong desire to take the drug."

The diagnosis of nicotine dependence is made using clinical judgment, but there are biochemical markers that can aid in assessment and help track success during cessation efforts. The two most common biomarkers are expired carbon monoxide and cotinine, a metabolite of nicotine. Carbon monoxide monitoring provides information about cigarette smoking over the past several hours, compared with the past several days with cotinine (93). Expired carbon monoxide testing requires specialized equipment (similar to a Breathalyzer). Cotinine can be measured in the saliva or urine by using test strips. Cotinine can also be measured in the serum, but may require shipping to and processing at a specialized laboratory. Of note, cotinine testing may be unreliable in the patient who uses nicotine replacement therapy, because the nicotine in those products will be metabolized to cotinine and lead to positive test results. Biochemical tests may be helpful in monitoring cessation efforts because self-reports are not wholly accurate (94).

TREATMENT

Sixty-six percent of adolescent smokers state that they want to quit and 70% report that they would not have started smoking if they could choose again. However, there is a dearth of quality evidence to guide clinicians in the treatment of youth smoking cessation, especially pharmacotherapy. In fact, recommendations regarding tobacco use in children and adolescents can be conflicting. In 2003, the U.S. Preventative Services Task Force found insufficient evidence to recommend for or against routine assessment, prevention, or treatment for children and adolescent tobacco use (95). Meanwhile, the Public Health Service published its recommendations that clinicians screen adolescents for tobacco use at every visit and counsel users to quit (96). It recommended that clinicians use the behavioral counseling model of the 5As (*ask* about use, advise to quit, *assess* willingness to make a quit attempt, *assist* patient in quitting, and *arrange* follow-up) to guide smoking cessation efforts for all smokers, including adolescents. This intervention, as with most youth smoking cessation programming, is extrapolated from adult treatments. This may be problematic for several reasons. Research indicates that adolescents have different motivations, expectations, beliefs, preparation, and social influences than adults regarding smoking cessation (3). For example, youth overestimate the prevalence of smoking, underestimate the number of peers who have tried to quit, and overestimate the success rate of quitting (97). In addition, youths may have difficulty accessing care given that parental consent may be required for treatment. Internet- and telephone-based quitlines help to fill this void.

There has been relatively little systematic research in the area of smoking cessation in adolescents. Several behavioral and pharmacologic treatments have been tried in adolescents with equivocal results (98). Sussman and colleagues (99) performed a meta-analysis of adolescent smoking cessation interventions published between 1970 and 2003. Of 101 published studies, 48 met their inclusion criteria that the studies had control groups and measured quit rates. The majority of the studies used motivation-enhancement or cognitive-behavioral theory as the basis of their intervention. Overall, the interventions had a small, positive effect on enhancing smoking cessation ($d = 0.29$). The average quit rate was 6.24% and 9.14% for the control and treatment conditions, respectively. Though the effect was small, it remained statistically significant even after 12 months. They also found relatively higher quit rates for programs consisting of at least five sessions and for programming that included cognitive-behavioral, motivation enhancement, or social influence components. Classroom- and school clinic–based programs were relatively more effective settings compared with interventions based at medical clinics, delivered via the computer, or the family.

A Cochrane review published in 2006 found that there is insufficient evidence to test the effectiveness of smoking cessation programs for adolescents. However, they note that interventions based on the transtheoretical model of change and psychosocial interventions show a trend toward effectiveness (100). Recently, emerging evidence suggests that contingency management may be an efficacious psychosocial treatment for smoking cessation in adolescent smokers (101,102).

Colby and colleagues (103) conducted a study of brief motivational interviewing in a medical setting. Eighty-five patients were randomly assigned to one session of motivational interviewing or brief advice to quit smoking. There were no differences between the groups at 1 and 3 months after the intervention. At 6 months, eight patients in the motivational interviewing group compared with one patient in the control group reported 7-day abstinence. However, there was no statistical difference between the groups when cotinine was measured.

A recent study investigated an intervention based on the 5A model of smoking cessation for adolescents (104). Eight pediatric primary care clinics treating 2,700 patients who participated in the study were randomized to either intervention or usual care control condition. The intervention consisted of training clinicians at pediatric primary care clinics in the 5A model of smoking cessation. In addition, former smokers serving as peer-counselors met with patients after their clinic visit and followed-up with four, 10-minute phone calls over the next 5 months. At 6 months, the quit rate was 36.4% for the intervention and 24.6% for the control group (OR: 1.59; CI: 1.06–2.40). However, at 12 months, there was no statistical difference between the intervention and control groups (25.3% and 27.7%, respectively). One limitation of this study is that abstinence was not confirmed by any biochemical markers.

Little is known about which pharmacologic treatments are efficacious for smoking cessation in adolescents. First-line pharmacologic treatments shown to be efficacious in adults and approved by the U.S. Food and Drug Administration include nicotine replacement therapy (e.g., transdermal patch, gum, inhaler, lozenge), bupropion, and varenicline. To date, nicotine replacement therapies such as the transdermal nicotine patch (TNP) and bupropion SR (Zyban) have been the treatments most explored in adolescent smokers. The results of studies examining nicotine replacement therapy have been modest among adolescent smokers. A study of TNP, nicotine gum, and placebo among adolescent smokers found that the TNP group had the highest 3-month abstinence rate (17.6%) compared with 6.5% for the gum and 2.5% for placebo (105).

A small, open-label pilot study with bupropion SR suggested potential efficacy for bupropion SR in adolescents with and without ADHD (106). Muramoto and colleagues (94) conducted one of the first large-scale randomized, placebo-controlled studies of bupropion for adolescent smoking cessation. Three hundred twelve participants were randomized to placebo, 150 mg bupropion, and 300 mg bupropion. The quit rate for the 150 mg bupropion group was not statistically different from the placebo group. However, the average quit rate for the 300 mg bupropion group was 22.6% compared with 11.5% for the placebo group during the 6 weeks of active treatment. Unfortunately, the treatment effects did not carry over after the active treatment ended. They also found that biochemically confirmed quit rates were 14% to 23% lower than self-reported quit rates, highlighting the importance of using biochemical tests to confirm the efficacy of a treatment.

In a study of 211 adolescent smokers randomized to TNP and bupropion (150 mg daily) and TNP and placebo along with counseling, Killen and colleagues found no difference between the groups (107). The percent abstinent was 23% and 28% for bupropion and control group respectively at 10 weeks (OR = 1.05, CI 0.38–2.92). After cessation of the patch and medication, the percent abstinent dropped to 7% and 8% for the bupropion and control group, respectively. The low dose of bupropion used may have played a role in the lack of difference between the groups as well as poor compliance with pharmacotherapy.

Based on the limited data available, behavioral therapy combined with either bupropion SR or transdermal nicotine patch should be used as first line treatment for adolescent smoking cessation. It is common clinical practice in adult smokers to combine nicotine replacement therapy and another medication to increase the chances of success (108). This may be a reasonable strategy among adolescent smokers who have failed a single pharmacologic approach. Given that many smokers require multiple attempts to quit before they can quit completely, clinicians should discuss past quit attempts with adolescents so they are not discouraged by a slip or relapse to smoking. For more in-depth information regarding specific guidelines for use of pharmacotherapy in adolescents, readers are referred to "Youth Tobacco Cessation: A Guide for Making Informed Decisions" (109), which is accessible from the Youth Tobacco Cessation Collaborative website and a review by Upadhyaya and colleagues (110).

PREVENTION

Tobacco use is the leading cause of preventable death in the United States (1). Since the deleterious health consequences of smoking were acknowledged in the 1960s, smoking prevention has been established as a key strategy in controlling smoking in the general population. Prevention interventions that target youth include a variety of different tactics including school-based programs, mass media programming, restrictions on advertising and sales to minors, and environmental programs such as clean-air ordinances mandating nonsmoking schools, businesses, and restaurants.

Thomas and Perera (111) performed a meta-analysis of 23 high-quality randomized controlled trials of school-based smoking prevention programs. The majority (12) of the studies analyzed were social influence interventions. The underlying premise of the social influences approach is that youth lack the skills to deal with social influences that support smoking. The curriculum aims to correct misperceptions that most people smoke, the perceived glamour of smoking, the appeal of cigarette advertising and promotion, and the persuasive effects of peer and sibling smoking. Overall, those studies had a beneficial but not statistically significant effect (effect size = 0.93; CI 0.84–1.03). The authors concluded: "There is little strong evidence that school-based programmes are effective in the long term in preventing uptake of smoking." Their findings agree with those from the Hutchinson Smoking Prevention Project, a large, randomized, high quality, 13-year trial designed to evaluate the impact of a social influences program on smoking prevention that revealed no statistical differences between children who received the intervention and those who did not (112).

In contrast to school-based prevention programs, research suggests that counteradvertising media campaigns may be effective in preventing youth smoking. The "truth" antismoking campaign aims to educate youth about tobacco companies' manipulative marketing and business practices and promote another "brand," the truth. Initial data from Florida's "truth" program reveal that the television campaign lowers smoking prevalence (113) and reduces progression to established smoking among youths (114,115). However, some researchers argue that the decline in prevalence was related to an increase in the cost of cigarettes during the same period (116). Farrelly and colleagues (116) evaluated a national "truth" campaign and a Phillip Morris sponsored campaign, "Think. Don't Smoke," a national campaign, akin to "Just Say No." Youth exposed to the "truth" campaign had decreased susceptibility to smoke in the next year, whereas youth exposed to the "Think. Don't Smoke" expressed an increased intent to smoke in the next year.

Most youth report that obtaining cigarettes is not difficult (8). Research reveals that when laws restricting sales to youth are enforced, it is more difficult for youth to obtain cigarettes (117). However, research does not clearly show whether enforcement of these laws lead to decreased smoking prevalence in youth (118). In addition to laws targeting retailers, there are purchase, use, or possession laws aimed at criminalizing underage use of cigarettes. There is inconclusive evidence about the effectiveness of this legal strategy to limit youth smoking (119). Some critics argue that purchase, use, or possession laws reinforce the idea that smoking is a taboo adult habit and thereby increases its appeal to children interested in assuming adult roles or being rebellious. In addition, critics note that these laws divert attention away from other interventions directed at protecting consumers from the tobacco companies. One legal approach that does decrease youth smoking is higher cigarette prices (50,120).

Clean indoor-air policies are federal, state, local, and institutional policies that reduce exposure to environmental tobacco smoke by prohibiting smoking in public places such as schools, workplaces, restaurants, and bars. These policies have a negative effect on adolescent and young adult smoking

(36,121). Clean indoor air laws may exert their impact by reducing the visibility of role models who smoke, limiting opportunities for youth to smoke alone or in groups, and diminishing the perceived social acceptability of smoking (121). Several studies show that smoking bans in the home, at school, at work, and in the community are associated with less progression to smoking, less consolidation of experimental into regular smoking, and more quitting among adolescents and young adults (36,122). Clean indoor-air policies and media counteradvertising campaigns appear to be some of the most beneficial strategies that have been implemented to prevent and reduce youth smoking.

CONCLUSIONS

Even with the recent decline in cigarette smoking, a significant number of adolescents continue to smoke cigarettes in the United States. In addition, most smokers initiate smoking in adolescence; therefore, prevention and treatment in adolescents should be a high priority. Prevention strategies, such as indoor smoking bans, increased cigarette tax, antismoking advertising campaigns, seem to have made an impact in reducing cigarette smoking among adolescents. There is a good body of literature suggesting that psychosocial treatment for smoking cessation is modestly efficacious in adolescent smokers. Emerging evidence suggests that pharmacotherapies, especially bupropion SR and transdermal nicotine patch, are efficacious in adolescent smokers. More research is needed to examine the efficacy of pharmacotherapies, as well as combination of psychosocial treatments and pharmacotherapies in adolescent smokers.

REFERENCES

1. Center for Disease Control. Annual smoking-attributable mortality, years of potential life lost, and productivity losses—United States, 1997–2001. *MMWR Morb Mortal Wkly Rep* 2005;54(25):625–628.
2. Chassin L, Presson CC, Sherman SJ, et al. The natural history of cigarette smoking: predicting young-adult smoking outcomes from adolescent smoking patterns. *Health Psychol* 1990;9(6):701–716.
3. U.S. Department of Health and Human Services. *Preventing tobacco use among young people: a report of the Surgeon General.* Atlanta, GA: U.S. Department of Health and Human Services, Public Health Service, Centers for Disease Control and Prevention, National Center for Chronic Disease Prevention and Health Promotion, Office on Smoking and Health, 1994.
4. DiFranza JR, Savageau JA, Rigotti NA, et al. Development of symptoms of tobacco dependence in youths: 30 month follow up data from the DANDY study. *Tob Control* 2002;11(3):228–235.
5. Breslau N, Peterson EL. Smoking cessation in young adults: age at initiation of cigarette smoking and other suspected influences. *Am J Public Health* 1996;86(2):214–220.
6. Chassin L, Presson CC, Rose JS, et al. The natural history of cigarette smoking from adolescence to adulthood: demographic predictors of continuity and change. *Health Psychol* 1996;15(6):478–484.
7. Substance Abuse and Mental Health Services Administration. *Results from the 2006 National Survey on Drug Use and Health: national findings.* Rockville, MD: Department of Health and Human Services, 2007.
8. Johnston LD, Bachman JG, Schulenberg JE. *Monitoring the future national survey results on drug use, 1975–2006. Volume I: secondary school students.* Bethesda, MD: National Institute on Drug Abuse, 2007.
9. Tyas SL, Pederson LL. Psychosocial factors related to adolescent smoking: a critical review of the literature. *Tob Control* 1998;7(4):409–420.
10. Massachusetts Medical Society. Trends in smoking initiation among adolescents and young adults: United States 1980-1989. *MMWR Morb Mortal Wkly Rep* 1995;44:521–524.
11. The GTSS Collaborative Group. The global tobacco surveillance system. *Tob Control* 2006;15(Suppl 2):ii1–3.
12. Johnston LD, O'Malley PM, Bachman JG, et al. *Monitoring the future national survey results on drug use, 1975-2006: Volume I, Secondary school students.* Bethesda, MD: National Institute on Drug Abuse, 2007.
13. Escobedo LG, Marcus SE, Holtzman D, et al. Sports participation, age at smoking initiation, and the risk of smoking among U.S. high school students. *JAMA* 1993;269(11):1391–1395.
14. Beauvais F, Thurman PJ, Burnside M, et al. Prevalence of American Indian adolescent tobacco use: 1993–2004. *Subst Use Misuse* 2007; 42(4):591–601.
15. Anda RF, Croft CB, Felitti CJ, et al. Adverse childhood experiences and smoking during adolescence and adulthood. *JAMA* 1999;282(17): 1652–1658.
16. Nichols HB, Harlow BL. Childhood abuse and risk of smoking onset. *J Epidemiol Community Health* 2004;58(5):402–406.
17. Stanton WR, Oei TP, Silva PA. Sociodemographic characteristics of adolescent smokers. *Int J Addict* 1994;29(7):913–925.
18. Milton B, Cook PA, Dugdill L, et al. Why do primary school children smoke? A longitudinal analysis of predictors of smoking uptake during pre-adolescence. *Public Health* 2004;118(4):247–255.
19. Van Den Bree MB, Whitmer MD, Pickworth WB. Predictors of smoking development in a population-based sample of adolescents: a prospective study. *J Adolesc Health* 2004;35(3):172–181.
20. Covey LS, Tam D. Depressive mood, the single-parent home, and adolescent cigarette smoking. *Am J Public Health* 1990;80(11):1330–1333.
21. Isohanni M, Moilanen I, Rantakallio P. Determinants of teenage smoking, with special reference to non-standard family background. *Br J Addict* 1991;86(4):391–398.
22. Eitle D. The moderating effects of peer substance use on the family structure-adolescent substance use association: quantity versus quality of parenting. *Addict Behav* 2005;30(5):963–980.
23. Brown RA, Lewinsohn PM, Seeley JR, et al. Cigarette smoking, major depression, and other psychiatric disorders among adolescents. *J Am Acad Child Adolesc Psychiatry* 1996;35(12):1602–1610.
24. Riggs PD, Mikulich SK, Whitmore EA, et al. Relationship of ADHD, depression, and non-tobacco substance use disorders to nicotine dependence in substance-dependent delinquents. *Drug Alcohol Depend* 1999;54:195–205.
25. Are social fears and DSM-IV social anxiety disorder associated with smoking and nicotine dependence in adolescents and young adults. *Eur Psychiatry* 2000;15:67–74.
26. DiFranza JR, Wittchen HU, Höfler M, et al. Susceptibility to nicotine dependence: the Development and Assessment of Nicotine Dependence in Youth 2 study. *Pediatrics* 2007;120(4):e974–e983.
27. Wills TA, DuHamel K, Vaccaro D. Activity and mood temperament as predictors of adolescent substance use: test of a self-regulation mediational model. *J Pers Soc Psychol* 1995;68(5):901–916.
28. Hawkins Wesley E. Problem behaviors and health-enhancing practices of adolescents: a multivariate analysis. *Health Values* 1992(16):46–54.
29. Bonaguro JA, Bonaguro EW. Self-concept, stress symptomatology, and tobacco use. *J Sch Health* 1987;57(2):56–58.
30. Snow PC, Bruce DD. Cigarette smoking in teenage girls: exploring the role of peer reputations, self-concept and coping. *Health Educ Res* 2003;18(4):439–452.
31. McCool JP, Cameron LD, Petrie KJ. The influence of smoking imagery on the smoking intentions of young people: testing a media interpretation model. *J Adolesc Health* 2005;36(6):475–485.
32. Tucker JS, Martínez JF, Ellickson PL, et al. Temporal associations of cigarette smoking with social influences, academic performance, and

delinquency: a four-wave longitudinal study from ages 13-23. *Psychol Addict Behav.* 2008;22(1):1–11.
33. Bryant AL, Schulenberg J, Bachman JG, et al. Understanding the links among school misbehavior, academic achievement, and cigarette use: a national panel study of adolescents. *Prevention Sci* 2000;1(2):71–87.
34. Ramchand R, Ialongo NS, Chilcoat HD. The effect of working for pay on adolescent tobacco use. *Am J Public Health* 2007;97(11): 2056–2062.
35. Chilcoat HD, Anthony JC. Impact of parent monitoring on initiation of drug use through late childhood. *J Am Acad Child Adolesc Psychiatry* 1996;35(1):91–100.
36. Farkas AJ, Gilpin EA, White MM, et al. Association between household and workplace smoking restrictions and adolescent smoking. *JAMA* 2000;284(6):717–722.
37. Harakeh Z, Scholte RH, Vermulst AA, et al. Parental factors and adolescents' smoking behavior: an extension of The theory of planned behavior. *Prev Med* 2004;39(5):951–961.
38. Simons-Morton B, Crump AD, Haynie DL, et al. Psychosocial, school, and parent factors associated with recent smoking among early-adolescent boys and girls. *Prevent Med* 1999;28(2):138–148.
39. Steinberg L, Fletcher A, Darling N. Parental monitoring and peer influences on adolescent substance use. *Pediatrics* 1994;93(6 Pt 2):1060–1064.
40. Dick DM, Viken R, Purcell S, et al. Parental monitoring moderates the importance of genetic and environmental influences on adolescent smoking. *J Abnorm Psychol* 2007;116(1):213–218.
41. Forrester K, Biglan A, Severson HH, et al. Predictors of smoking onset over two years. *Nicotine Tob Res* 2007;9(12):1259–1267.
42. Ennett S, Faris R, Hipp J, et al. Peer smoking, other peer attributes, and adolescent cigarette smoking: a social network analysis. *Prev Sci* 2008; 9(2):88–98.
43. Simons-Morton B, Haynie DL, Crump AD, et al. Peer and parent influences on smoking and drinking among early adolescents. *Health Educ Behav* 2001;28(1):95–107.
44. U.S. Federal Trade Commission. *Cigarette report for 2004 and 2005,* 2007. Available from: http://www.ftc.gov/reports/tobacco/2007 cigarette2004-2005.pdf. Accessed November 6, 2008.
45. Evans N, Farkas A, Gilpin E, et al. Influence of tobacco marketing and exposure to smokers on adolescent susceptibility to smoking. *J Natl Cancer Inst* 1995;87(20):1538–1545.
46. DiFranza JR, Wellan RJ, Sargent JD, et al. Tobacco promotion and the initiation of tobacco use: assessing the evidence for causality. *Pediatrics* 2006;117(6):e1237–e1248.
47. Pierce JP, Choi WS, Gilpin EA, et al. Tobacco industry promotion of cigarettes and adolescent smoking. *JAMA* 1998;279(7):511–515.
48. Sargent JD, Dalton MA, Beach ML, et al. Viewing tobacco use in movies: does it shape attitudes that mediate adolescent smoking. *Am J Prevent Med* 2002;22(3):137–145.
49. Biener L, Siegel M. Tobacco marketing and adolescent smoking: more support for a causal inference. *Am J Public Health* 2000;90(3):407–411.
50. Powell LM, Tauras JA, Ross H. The importance of peer effects, cigarette prices and tobacco control policies for youth smoking behavior. *J Health Econ* 2005;24(5):950–968.
51. Batra V, Patkar AA, Berrettini WH, et al. The genetic determinants of smoking. *Chest* 2003;123(5):1730–1739.
52. Laucht M, Becker K, El-Faddagh M, et al. Association of the DRD4 exon III polymorphism with smoking in fifteen-year-olds: a mediating role for novelty seeking? *J Am Acad Child Adolesc Psychiatry* 2005;44(5):477–484.
53. Dierker LC, Avenevoli S, Goldberg A, et al. Defining subgroups of adolescents at risk for experimental and regular smoking. *Prev Sci* 2004;5(3):169–183.
54. Upadhyaya HP, Brady KT, Wharton M, et al. Psychiatric disorders and cigarette smoking among child and adolescent psychiatry inpatients. *Am J Addict* 2003;12(2):144–152.
55. Gold DR, Wang X, Wypij D, et al. Effects of cigarette smoking on lung function in adolescent boys and girls. *N Engl J Med* 1996;335(13): 931–937.
56. Zieske AW, McMahan CA, McGill HC Jr, et al. Smoking is associated with advanced coronary atherosclerosis in youth. *Atherosclerosis* 2005;180(1):87–92.
57. Marti B, Abelin T, Minder CE, et al. Smoking, alcohol consumption, and endurance capacity: an analysis of 6,500 19-year-old conscripts and 4,100 joggers. *Prev Med* 1988;17(1):79–92.
58. Kandel DB, Johnson JG, Bird HR, et al. Psychiatric disorders associated with substance use among children and adolescents: findings from the Methods for the Epidemiology of Child and Adolescent Mental Disorders (MECA) study. *J Abnorm Child Psychol* 1997;25(2):121–132.
59. Wu L, Anthony JC. Tobacco smoking and depressed mood in late childhood and early adolescence. *Am J Public Health* 1999;89(12): 1837–1840.
60. Niethammer O, Frank R. Prevalence of use, abuse and dependence on legal and illegal psychotropic substances in an adolescent inpatient psychiatric population. *Eur Child Adolesc Psychiatry* 2007;16(4):254–259.
61. Ismail K, Sloggett A, DeStavola B. Do common mental disorders increase cigarette smoking? Results from five waves of a population-based panel cohort study. *Am J Epidemiol* 2000;152(7):651–657.
62. Lambert NM, Hartsough CS. Prospective study of tobacco smoking and substance dependencies among samples of ADHD and non-ADHD participants. *J Learn Disabilities* 1998;31(6):533–544.
63. Molina BS, Pelham WE. Childhood predictors of adolescent substance use in a longitudinal study of children with ADHD. *J Abnorm Psychol* 2003;112(3):497–507.
64. Kollins S, McClernon F, Fuemmeler B. Association between smoking and attention-deficit/hyperactivity disorder symptoms in a population-based sample of young adults. *Arch Gen Psychiatry* 2005;62: 1142–1147.
65. Upadhyaya H, Rose K, Wang W, et al. Attention-deficit/hyperactivity disorder, medication and treatment, and substance use patterns among adolescents and young adults. *J Child Adolesc Psychopharmacol* 2005; 15(5):799–809.
66. Biederman J, Faraone SV. Attention-deficit hyperactivity disorder. *Lancet* 2005;366:237–248.
67. Elkins IJ, McGue M, Iacono WG. Prospective effects of attention-deficit/hyperactivity disorder, conduct disorder, and sex on adolescent substance use and abuse. *Arch Gen Psychiatry* 2007;64(10):1145–1152.
68. Kandel DB, Davies M. Adult sequelae of adolescent depressive symptoms. *Arch Gen Psychiatry* 1986;43:255–262.
69. Fergusson DM, Goodwin RD, Horwood LJ. Major depression and cigarette smoking: results of a 21-year longitudinal study. *Psychol Med* 2003;33(8):1357–1367.
70. Anda RF, Williamson DF, Escobedo WG, et al. Depression and the dynamics of smoking. A national perspective. *JAMA* 1990;264(12): 1541–1545.
71. Glassman AH, Helzer JE, Covey LS, et al. Smoking, smoking cessation, and major depression. *JAMA* 1990;264:1546–1549.
72. Patton GC, Carlin JB, Coffey C, et al. Depression, anxiety, and smoking initiation: a prospective study over 3 years. *Am J Public Health* 1998;88(10):1518–1522.
73. Kassel JD, Shiffman S. Attentional mediation of cigarette smoking's effect on anxiety. *Health Psychol* 1997;16(4):359–368.
74. DiFranza J, Savageau JA, Fletcher K, et al. Measuring the loss of autonomy over nicotine use in adolescents: the DANDY (Development and Assessment of Nicotine Dependence in Youths) study. *Arch Pediatrc Adolesc Med* 2002;156:397–403.
75. Nelson CB, Wittchen H. Smoking and nicotine dependence. Results from a sample of 14- to 24- year olds in Germany. *Eur Addict Res* 1998;4:42–49.
76. Johnson JG, Cohen P, Pine DS, et al. Association between cigarette smoking and anxiety disorders during adolescence and early adulthood. *JAMA* 2000;284(18):2348–2351.
77. Costello EJ, Erkanli A, Federman E, et al. Development of psychiatric comorbidity with substance abuse in adolescents: effects of timing and sex. *J Clin Child Psychol* 1999;28(3):298–311.
78. Kandel DB, Kessler RC, Maarguiles RZ. Antecedents of adolescent initiation into stages of drug use: a developmental analysis. *J Youth Adolesc* 1978;7(1):13–14.
79. Kandel D, Yamaguchi K. From beer to crack: developmental patterns of drug involvement. *Am J Public Health* 1993;83(6):851–855.

80. Kandel DB, Yamaguchi K, Chen K. Stages of progression in drug involvement from adolescence to adulthood: further evidence for the gateway theory. *J Stud Alcohol* 1992;53:447–457.
81. Chang G, Sherritt L, Knight JR. Adolescent cigarette smoking and mental health symptoms. *J Adolesc Health* 2005;36(6):517–522.
82. Lewinsohn PM, Rohde P, Brown RA. Level of current and past adolescent cigarette smoking as predictors of future substance use disorders in young adulthood. *Addiction* 1999;94(6):913–921.
83. Hanna EZ, Grant BF. Parallels to early onset alcohol use in the relationship of early onset smoking with drug use and DSM-IV drug and depressive disorders: findings from the National Longitudinal Epidemiologic Survey. *Alcohol Clin Exp Res* 1999;23(3):513–522.
84. Grant BF. Age at smoking onset and its association with alcohol consumption and DSM-IV alcohol abuse and dependence: results from the National Longitudinal Alcohol Epidemiologic survey. *J Subst Abuse* 1998;10:59–73.
85. Merrill JC, Kleber HD, Schwarz M, et al. Cigarettes, alcohol, marijuana, other risk behaviors, and American youth. *Drug Alcohol Depend* 1999;56:205–212.
86. McVea KL. Evidence for clinical smoking cessation for adolescents. *Health Psychol* 2006;25(5):558–562.
87. Milne B, Towns S. Do paediatricians provide brief intervention for adolescents who smoke. *J Paediatr Child Health* 2007;43(6):464–468.
88. Fiore M, Bailey W, Cohen S. Treating tobacco use and dependence: clinical practice guideline. Rockville, MD: U.S. Public Health Service, 2000.
89. National Cancer Institute, Tobacco Control Research, and Cancer Control and Population Sciences Home, 2008. Available online from: http://dccps.nci.nih.gov/TCRB/guide_measures.html. Accessed June 20, 2008.
90. Sobell LC, Agrawal S, Sobell MB, et al. Comparison of a quick drinking screen with the timeline followback for individuals with alcohol problems. *J Stud Alcohol* 2003;64(6):858–861.
91. Brandon TH, Baker TB. The smoking consequences questionnaire: the subjective expected utility of smoking in college students. *Psychol Assessment: A Journal of Consulting and Clinical Psychology.* 1991;3(3):484–491.
92. O'Loughlin J, DiFranza J, Tyndale RF, et al. Nicotine-dependence symptoms are associated with smoking frequency in adolescents. *Am J Prevent Med* 2003;25:219–225.
93. SRNT Subcommittee on Biochemical Verification. Biochemical verification of tobacco use and cessation. *Nicotine Tob Res* 2002;4:149–159.
94. Muramoto ML, Leischow SJ, Sherrill D, et al. Randomized, double-blind, placebo-controlled trial of 2 dosages of sustained-release bupropion for adolescent smoking cessation. *Arch Pediatr Adolesc Med* 2007;161(11):1068–1074.
95. U.S. Preventative Services Task Force. *Counseling to prevent tobacco use and tobacco-caused disease.* Rockville, MD: Agency for Healthcare Research and Quality, 2003.
96. Fiore MC, Bailey WC, Cohen SJ. *Treating tobacco use and dependence. Clinical practice guideline.* Rockville, MD: U.S. Department of Health and Human Services. Public Health Service, 2000.
97. Stanton WR, Lowe JB, Gillespie AM. Adolescents' experiences of smoking cessation. *Drug Alcohol Depend* 1996;43(1–2):63–70.
98. Sussman S, Lichtman K, Ritt A, et al. Effects of thirty-four adolescent tobacco use cessation and prevention trials on regular users of tobacco products. *Substance Use Misuse* 1999;34(11):1469–1503.
99. Sussman S, Sun P, Dent CW. A meta-analysis of teen cigarette smoking cessation. *Health Psychol* 2006;25(5):549–557.
100. Grimshaw GM, Stanton A. Tobacco cessation interventions for young people. *Cochrane Database Syst Rev* 2006;(4):CD003289.
101. Krishnan-Sarin S, Duhig AM, McKee SA, et al. Contingency management for smoking cessation in adolescent smokers. *Exp Clin Psychopharmacol* 2006;14(3):306–310.
102. Corby EA, Roll JM, Ledgerwood DM, et al. Contingency management interventions for treating the substance abuse of adolescents: a feasibility study. *Exp Clin Psychopharmacol* 2000;8(3):371–376.
103. Colby SM, Monti PM, O'Leary Tevyaw T, et al. Brief motivational intervention for adolescent smokers in medical settings. *Addict Behav* 2005;30(5):865–874.
104. Pbert L, Flint AJ, Fletcher KE, et al. Effect of a pediatric practice-based smoking prevention and cessation intervention for adolescents: a randomized, controlled trial. *Pediatrics* 2008;121(4):e738–e747.
105. Moolchan ET, Robinson ML, Ernst SM, et al. Safety and efficacy of the nicotine patch and gum for the treatment of adolescent tobacco addiction. *Pediatrics* 2005;115(4):e407–e414.
106. Upadhyaya HP, Brady KT, Wang W. Bupropion SR in adolescents with comorbid ADHD and nicotine dependence: a pilot study. *J Am Acad Child Adolesc Psychiatry* 2004;43:199–205.
107. Killen JD, Robinson TN, Ammerman S, et al. Randomized clinical trial of the efficacy of bupropion combined with nicotine patch in the treatment of adolescent smokers. *J Consult Clin Psychol* 2004;72(4): 729–735.
108. George TP, O'Malley SS. Current pharmacological treatments for nicotine dependence. *Trends Pharmacol Sci* 2004;25(1):42–48.
109. Milton MH, Maule CO, Yee SL, et al.. *Youth tobacco cessation: a guide for making informed decisions.* Atlanta, GA: Centers for Disease Control and Prevention, 2004.
110. Upadhyaya H, Deas D, Brady K. How to help nicotine-dependent adolescents quit smoking. *Cur Psychiatry* 2004;3(9):41–61.
111. Thomas R, Perera R. School-based programmes for preventing smoking. *Cochrane Database Syst Rev* 2006;3:CD001293.
112. Peterson AV Jr, Kealey KA, Mann SL, et al. Hutchinson Smoking Prevention Project: long-term randomized trial in school-based tobacco use prevention—results on smoking. *J Natl Cancer Inst* 2000;92(24): 1979–1991.
113. Sly DF, Heald GR, Ray S. The Florida "truth" anti-tobacco media evaluation: design, first year results, and implications for planning future state media evaluations. *Tob Control* 2001;10(1):9–15.
114. Siegel M, Biener L. The impact of an antismoking media campaign on progression to established smoking: results of a longitudinal youth study. *Am J Public Health* 2000;90(3):380–386.
115. Sly DF, Hopkins RS, Trapido E, et al. Influence of a counteradvertising media campaign on initiation of smoking: the Florida "truth" campaign. *Am J Public Health* 2001;91(2):233–238.
116. Farrelly MC, Healton CG, Davis KC, et al. Getting to the truth: evaluating national tobacco countermarketing campaigns. *Am J Public Health* 2002;92(6):901–907.
117. Gemson DH, Moats HL, Watkins BX, et al. Laying down the law: reducing illegal tobacco sales to minors in central Harlem. *Am J Public Health* 1998;88(6):936–939.
118. Altman DG, Wheelis AY, McFarlane M, et al. The relationship between tobacco access and use among adolescents: a four community study. *Soc Sci Med* 1999;48(6):759–775.
119. Lazovich D, Forster J, Widome R, et al. Tobacco possession, use, and purchase laws and penalties in Minnesota: enforcement, tobacco diversion programs, and youth awareness. *Nicotine Tob Res* 2007;9;Suppl 1:S57–S64.
120. Harris JE, González López-Valcárcel B. Asymmetric peer effects in the analysis of cigarette smoking among young people in the United States, 1992–1999. *J Health Econ* 2008;27(2):249–264.
121. Alesci NL, Forster JL, Blaine T. Smoking visibility, perceived acceptability, and frequency in various locations among youth and adults. *Prev Med* 2003;36(3):272–281.
122. Siegel M. The effectiveness of state-level tobacco control interventions: a review of program implementation and behavioral outcomes. *Annu Rev Public Health* 2002;23(1):45–71.

CHAPTER 102

Sharon Levy, MD, MPH
John R. Knight, MD

Screening and Brief Intervention for Adolescents

Alcohol use is nearly ubiquitous among American adolescents. By senior year of high school, 72.7% of teenagers have consumed alcohol at least once in their lifetime (1). By definition, use of alcohol by adolescents is a developmental norm: That is, we expect that most adolescents will drink alcohol prior to high school graduation, and most of them will not have associated problems or develop substance use disorders. However, all adolescents are at risk of acute consequences such as motor vehicle crashes and other accidents (2), acute overdose, and unwanted sexual activity (3) when they use alcohol. Furthermore, teens that begin drinking at younger ages are more likely to develop chronic alcohol disorders, with significant long-term health consequences, than those who delay the onset of alcohol and drug use until early adulthood (4). We can therefore conclude that all teenage drinking is a health risk behavior, and the level of risk varies from patient to patient.

Use of marijuana by adolescents is also common, with 42.3% of teenagers having tried marijuana at least one time in their lifetime before graduating high school (1). Work by Shedler and Block (5) done in the 1990s found that adolescents who used marijuana were better adjusted than abstainers, who were found to lack social skills. However, more recent studies following up a larger, more demographically diverse group of teenagers over a longer period of time has challenged these results. Work by Tucker et al. (6,7) has demonstrated that teens who abstain from marijuana use through their senior year of high school did better academically and engaged in fewer deviant behaviors than did their peers who used marijuana in social situations, and teens who were solitary users of marijuana faced a wide range of psychosocial and behavioral difficulties that persisted into young adulthood. In addition, marijuana use is associated with multiple health problems, including respiratory burden of carbon monoxide and tar, bronchoconstriction, chronic cough with increased sputum production, suppressed immune function, insulin antagonism, and long-term adverse neurocognitive effects on executive functions such as focus, attention, and ability to filter out irrelevant information. Chronic users are at risk of developing the well-described "amotivational syndrome," leading to a slow, passive withdrawal from school, work, and recreational activities (8). As with data regarding alcohol use, this information suggests that all adolescents who use marijuana are engaging in a health risk behavior and that the level of risk varies based on how the drug is used. Fewer adolescents use drugs other than alcohol or marijuana, and those who do form a particularly high-risk group.

Medical office settings are ideal for early identification of drug and alcohol use by adolescents because they provide a yearly opportunity for a medical professional to interview teenagers in a private and confidential setting. Several professional societies recommend that all adolescents be screened for drug and alcohol use at every primary care visit (9,10). There are several goals to such screening: (1) to determine whether a teen has ever used alcohol or drugs, (2) to determine whether teens that have used alcohol or drugs are at low risk or high risk for developing substance use disorders, (3) to give pertinent health advice to teens who are at risk of acute consequences of alcohol or other drug use, and (4) to refer teens who are at high risk of long-term consequences of substance use to the appropriate level of intervention. This chapter describes screening procedures and tools that can be used in primary care to quickly and accurately determine risk level, brief interventions that can be made with teens of different risk categories, and strategies that encourage teens to follow-up when a referral to more intensive services is required.

OPENING QUESTIONS

Clinicians should begin asking adolescents about substance use and other sensitive questions as soon as the young person is old enough to be interviewed without the parent present. The exact age will vary from patient to patient, falling between 11 and 13 years for most adolescents. After meeting with the parent and patient together, the clinician should ask the parent to leave the room so that she or he can ask the adolescent personal questions. The clinician should review the ground rules of confidentiality while the parent and adolescent are together. Briefly, the clinician should ensure that the details discussed will remain confidential unless the clinician has safety concerns. Determining whether a reported behavior reaches the level of a safety concern is a matter of clinical judgment. Chapter 109, "Liability and Risk Management Issues in Addiction Practice," discusses confidentiality in greater detail.

The Home, Education, Activities/Alcohol, Drugs, Sex, Suicidality (HEADSS) psychosocial interview for adolescents includes questions about alcohol and drug use in the context of a more extensive psychosocial history (11), allowing the interviewer to develop rapport with the adolescent prior to asking more personal questions. When asking about drugs and alcohol (the "D" in HEADSS), the interviewer should ask three straightforward questions: (1) "Have you ever drunk alcohol (more than a few sips)?" (2) "Have you ever smoked marijuana?" (3) "Have you ever used anything else get high, including illicit drugs (like cocaine, heroine or methamphetamine), medications that were not prescribed to you or used in a way other than ordered by a doctor, over the counter medications or inhalant chemicals?"

To maximize the sensitivity of the question, the interviewer should begin the question with "Have you ever . . . ;" however, if the patient is well known to the interviewer or if this is a repeat screening, the interviewer may choose to begin with "Since your last appointment with me . . . ." The interviewer should avoid ambiguous questions, such as "Do you drink/smoke?" as answers to these questions may be interpreted differently by patient and clinician.

Adolescents who report complete abstinence from alcohol and drugs should be given praise and encouragement regarding the good decisions they have made. Any adolescent who reports having used alcohol or drugs should be screened with a developmentally appropriate screening tool.

SCREENING TOOLS

Several tools have been developed to screen patients for high-risk use of alcohol and other drugs. In general, these tools fall into two broad categories: written assessments (such as the AUDIT [12] and POSIT [13]) and oral screens (such as the CRAFFT [14] and CAGE [15]). Written tools have a number of potential advantages-they can be self-administered and completed in a waiting room before the patient is seen by the clinician, and they generally screen for several disorders simultaneously, including mental health, behavioral, and substance use disorders. Both the AUDIT and the POSIT have been well studied and have excellent psychometric properties for screening adolescents. There are also disadvantages to written assessments-patients must have an adequate reading level in order to complete the screen, and screens should be completed in privacy, which is often not possible in a busy waiting room. These assessments also require training and time in order to score and interpret properly.

Oral screens are generally composed of a few questions that an interviewer can ask quickly. The CAGE questions are a popular screen for alcohol disorders and have been shown to have excellent psychometric properties with adults. More recent work, however, has shown that these questions are not developmentally appropriate for adolescents, and their sensitivity is low for identifying high-risk alcohol use among adolescents (16).

The CRAFFT screen is a series of six questions developed to screen adolescents for alcohol and other drug use disorders simultaneously. CRAFFT is a mnemonic acronym: During the past 12 months have you ever (1) Ridden in a **C**ar driven by someone, including yourself, who was high or had been using alcohol or drugs? (2) Used alcohol or drugs to **R**elax, feel better about yourself, or fit in? (3) Used alcohol or drugs while you are by yourself, **A**lone? (4) Forgotten things you did while using alcohol or drugs? (5) Had your **F**amily or **F**riends tell you that you should cut down on your drinking or drug use? (6) Gotten into **T**rouble while you were using alcohol or drugs?

Each "yes" response is scored 1 point. A score of 2 or greater is a positive screen and indicates that the adolescent is at high risk for having an alcohol- or drug-related disorder.

All adolescents who have used alcohol or another drug should be asked the CRAFFT questions or should be screened with an alternative formal screening tool. Recent research has demonstrated that even experienced adolescent medicine specialists significantly underestimate adolescents' risk level when relying on clinical impressions alone (17). Adolescents who report abstinence from alcohol and drugs should be asked whether they have ever ridden in a car with a driver who was high or had used alcohol or drugs. After completing the opening questions regarding alcohol and drug use and the follow-up screen, the clinician can determine the appropriate next step.

SCREEN-SPECIFIC STRATEGIES

No Use: Praise and Encouragement Adolescents that have been abstinent from alcohol and drugs and who have never ridden with an intoxicated driver should receive praise and encouragement from their clinician. Adolescents should be encouraged to discuss drug use or ask questions in the future should the need arise. Statements such as, "It sounds as if you have made smart choices by not using drugs or alcohol.

If that ever changes I hope you will feel comfortable enough to talk to me about it" aim both to praise the young person's abstinence and leave open the opportunity for open communication in the future.

Car +: Contract for life All adolescents who have ridden with an intoxicated driver should receive risk reduction advice. The "contract for life" (18) is a document developed by Students Against Destructive Decisions (SADD) that asks adolescents to commit to never ride with a driver who has been drinking or using other drugs and also asks parents to promise to provide transportation home without any questions if their child is in need. The clinician should explain that the intention of the document is to ensure that the adolescent always has safe transport home and not to avoid conversation between parents and their children. Parents should be encouraged both to praise their children for avoiding riding with an intoxicated driver and to explore the events of such an evening at a later time-when neither adolescent nor parent is intoxicated or angry-with open-ended questions, such as, "How did you end up in this situation?" and "How can you avoid this situation in the future?"

CRAFFT 0-1: Brief Advice Adolescents who report alcohol or other drug use but screen negative (i.e. 0 or 1 on the CRAFFT) are at relatively low risk for meeting criteria for a substance use disorder. These teens should receive brief advice to stop using, such as, "My advice is for you to stop using alcohol or drugs at all, because they pose a serious risk to your health." The clinician should also give specific information related to the health effects of the drug that the teen is using. Any knowledge of the patient's health concerns can be used to target the information. For example, an overweight adolescent who is drinking alcohol might benefit from information regarding the calorie content of beer or mixed drinks. Adolescents who participate in sports will frequently report decreased use of marijuana during the sports season and can be educated about the specific effects of marijuana on the lungs. A sample of brief advice statements is presented in Table 102.1. The clinician should challenge the patient to a time-limited trial of abstinence (e.g., 3 months) and ask him or her to come for a return visit to discuss how it went.

CRAFFT 2 or Above: Brief Assessment Adolescents who screen positive (i.e. CRAFFT score of 2 or more) are at high risk of having a substance use disorder and need further assessment. Clinicians who screen adolescents for substance use should be prepared to perform a limited assessment in order to triage referrals for these patients. The next sections describe office interviewing techniques.

TABLE 102.1 Brief Advice Sample Statements

- As your doctor, I recommend you stop using.
- Smoking marijuana damages your lungs and can affect your sports performance.
- Marijuana directly affects your brain and can hurt your school performance and your future.
- Marijuana use can cause lifelong problems for some people.
- Alcohol can cause high blood pressure, heart problems, and liver problems.
- Alcohol can cause accidents.
- Drug and alcohol use can lead to sexual assault, sexually transmitted diseases, and unintended pregnancies.
- Please don't ever get in a car with someone who has been drinking or using drugs.
- Please don't ever drive a car after using drugs, even if you don't feel high.
- Make arrangements ahead of time for safe transportation.
- Marijuana use can slowly get you into trouble-with your parents, at school, or even with the police.
- Alcohol and marijuana can make you gain weight.
- Marijuana can be laced with other drugs; you never really know what you are getting.

OFFICE INTERVIEWING

Strategies for Interviewing Adolescents For any patient, a nonjudgmental, empathetic interviewing style that accepts the patient's point of view encourages more information sharing than an interrogative style. The interviewer should use open-ended questions to begin the conversation, with an emphasis on the pattern of drug use over time, including whether drug use has increased in quantity or frequency, whether the teen has made attempts at discontinuing drug use, and why and whether attempts have been successful. Information about the pattern of drug use and associated problems is more important in making a diagnosis of a substance-related disorder than the absolute quantity or frequency. At times, cues from the clinician may help the adolescent make connections between drug use and consequences. For example, statements such as, "it seems that your grades started to fall at the same time that you started using more marijuana" may help the adolescent associate the two occurrences. A well-conducted history has therapeutic value as it encourages the adolescent to consider the consequences of drug use that she or he has already experienced.

Substance Use History

Substance of Choice The substance use history should begin with the substance of choice. The clinician should begin with an open-ended question, such as, "Tell me about your history of alcohol use." Cue adolescents to discuss general trends in their substance use (has use been increasing over time?), and get an estimate of the current level of use (about how often do you use now?) For alcohol, ask adolescents how many drinks it takes to get drunk, as a high tolerance for alcohol consumption without feeling drunk may be a signal that the adolescent is genetically susceptible to developing alcohol use disorders, particularly if the family history is positive for alcoholism (19). Also ask whether they have ever had a blackout (i.e. "Have you ever drunk so much alcohol that you could not remember anything, even though you were walking and talking?") as these events indicate significant alcohol intake but may not be considered problematic by some adolescents.

The clinician should ask whether adolescents have had any problems related to their use of substances. Many teens do not connect problems they have experienced with substance use, and cueing by the clinician may be helpful. If the teen denies experiencing problems, the clinician should ask specifically about tension with parents, school problems, decrease in grades or sports performance, suspensions or expulsions from school or sports teams, physical fights, arguments with friends while intoxicated, medical problems, such as overdose or getting sick, unwanted sexual contact, or legal problems/arrests. Stating questions such as, "Some kids say that they feel they could have done better in school if they were not using marijuana. Have you ever felt that way?" may help to draw a connection between substance use and its consequences in a non-threatening manner. The clinician should also ask patients whether they have ever tried to quit, and if so why. Adolescents' reasons for previous quitting attempts provide insight into perceived negative consequences of substance abuse and can be very helpful in personalizing advice.

Review of Other Substances After completing the history for the substance of choice, the clinician should review whether the adolescent has used other substances. If the substance of choice is not alcohol or marijuana, the clinician should ask detailed questions (as earlier) about these substances, as it is unusual for an adolescent to have used other illicit drugs without ever using alcohol or marijuana. However, recently it has become common for teens to misuse prescription (such as narcotics, benzodiazepines, or stimulants) or over-the-counter medications without previous history of alcohol or marijuana use (20).

Substance preferences and slang terms vary by region, and clinicians should be aware of local patterns. Table 102.2 lists common substances of abuse by adolescents. Clinicians should ask adolescents whether they had used any other substances to get high, whether they have been a regular user, and whether they have had problems related to use.

Collateral History At times, substance use by an adolescent will present to a clinician as a report by a parent, from a school, or from another adult. In these cases, the clinician should take a careful collateral history.

If a parent suspects drug use but the child denies using substances, the clinician should have the parent carefully list his or her observations. Substance use often presents with nonspecific complaints, such as staying out late, moodiness, breaking house rules, drop in grades, loss of interest in hobbies, or developing a new group of friends, and these symptoms should always be investigated further, particularly if more than one is present. Lying, stealing, appearing intoxicated, or possessing drugs or paraphernalia are more specific signs of drug use and should raise suspicion whenever present. In some cases, parents will report having caught their child using alcohol or other drugs. In these circumstances, the clinician should ask how the parent approached the child and the child's response. Parent responses to these questions demonstrate the family's attitudes toward drug use and may provide an opportunity for guidance.

As part of a collateral history, the clinician should also ask parents their impression of the frequency of substance use. Adolescents work hard to hide drug use from their parents and, as a result, parents almost always significantly underestimate frequency of their child's drug use (21). Nonetheless, parents' observations and impressions provide a useful piece of clinical information. In addition, the clinician should also ask whether the parents have concerns about other drugs. Occasionally parents will report prescriptions disappearing from the medicine cabinet or finding needles or other paraphernalia in the house. Any such reports should be further explored with the adolescent.

TABLE 102.2 Psychoactive Substances Commonly Used by Adolescents and Common Names

Substance	Common name
Cocaine	Coke or crack
Ecstasy	E
Amphetamines (Ritalin, Adderall, methamphetamine)	Meth, crystal meth
Opioids (Percocet, Vicodin, oxycodone, heroin)	Percs, vics, OC's, oxys
Benzodiazepines (Klonopin, Ativan, Xanax, Valium)	K-pins
Hallucinogens (LSD, PCP, mushrooms)	Dust, acid
Dextromethorphan (cold medications: Robitussin, Coricidin)	DXM, "Triple C"
Inhalants (whipped cream canisters, magic markers, lighter fluid)	Nitrous, whippets
Club drugs (gamma hydroxybutyrate, ketamine, rohypnol)	GHB, K
Other (caffeine pills, diet pills, anti-depressants)	—

TABLE 102.3 Signs of Drug Intoxication, Recovery from Intoxication, and Chronic Use

Drug	Acute intoxication	Recovery from intoxication/withdrawal	Chronic drug use
Alcohol	Fruity smelling breath, disinhibited or silly, clumsiness, vomiting	Headache, nausea, vomiting, dry mouth	Enlarged liver, increased liver enzymes, hypertension
Marijuana	Erythematous conjunctivae, tachycardia, dry mouth, increased talking, euphoria	Anxiety, nervousness	Chronic cough, wheezing
Cocaine	Hyperalert state, increased talking, hyperthermia, nausea, dry mouth, dilated pupils, sweating, cardiac arrhythmias	Depression, anhedonia, insomnia, lethargy, mental slowing	Erosion of dental enamel, gingival ulceration, chronic rhinitis, perforated nasal septum, midline granuloma, cardiac arrhythmias, hypertension, paranoia, psychosis
Amphetamines	Similar to cocaine		Choreoathetoid movement disorders, skin picking and ulcerations
Opioids	Constricted pupils, drowsiness ("nodding"), slowed respirations, bradycardia, slurred speech, slowed comprehension, constipation	Flu-like symptoms, muscle and joint aches, dilated pupils, coryza, lacrimation, sweating, abdominal cramps, nausea, vomiting, diarrhea, hot and cold flashes, piloerection, yawning, tremors, anxiety, irritability	Abscesses, cellulites, phlebitis and scarring (from injection use), chronic constipation, malnutrition
Benzodiazepines	Drowsiness, slowed respirations, slurred speech, slowed comprehension	Seizures (may be life-threatening), anxiety, restlessness	Sleep difficulties, anxiety, personality changes
Hallucinogens	Toxic psychosis, paranoia, anxiety, tachycardia, hypertension, dry mouth, nausea, vomiting	—	Psychosis, depression, personality changes
Inhalants	Euphoria, slurred speech, ataxia, diplopia, lacrimation, rhinorrhea, salivation, irritation of the mucus membranes, nausea, vomiting, arrhythmias	Headaches, sleepiness, depression	Irritation of mucus membranes, changes in neurologic exam
Ecstasy	Euphoria, decreased interpersonal boundaries, tachycardia, hypertension, hyperthermia, sweating, muscle spasms, bruxism, blurred vision, chills, nystagmus	Depression, anxiety, paranoia, dehydration	Cognitive deficits

Physical Exam Adolescents who have a positive screen for high-risk substance use should have a physical exam to look for signs of acute intoxication or chronic drug use. Signs of chronic drug use are rare in teens but should be both discussed with the adolescent and recorded in the chart if present. A list of several signs associated with acute intoxication, withdrawal, and chronic drug use is presented in Table 102.3.

Laboratory Testing Laboratory testing is discussed in detail in (Chapter 19, "Laboratory Diagnosis"). Testing for substances of abuse may be a useful part of an assessment, particularly if a parent or clinician has reasonable concerns and the adolescent denies substance use. If laboratory testing is to be used as part of a medical workup, the clinician should ensure that proper specimen collection, validation, and confirmation techniques are used and that the testing panel will include tests for all suspected substances. Parents and patients should understand that a laboratory test is only one piece of information that must be interpreted in the context of the entire history-a single negative test does not prove that a teenager is not using drugs, and a single positive test does not confirm a substance use disorder. Ethical and confidentiality issues as they relate to drug testing in adolescents are reviewed in the sidebars of Chaper 105, and elsewhere in this text.

SUBSTANCE USE SPECTRUM

The goal of brief assessment is to triage adolescents who screen positive for high-risk substance use to the appropriate level of intervention. Based on the information from the clinical

TABLE 102.4 Stages of Substance Use

Stage	Description
Primary abstinence	No use of alcohol or drugs
Experimentation	The first 1–2 times that a substance is used. At this phase, the adolescent is curious about what it feels like to be intoxicated by a particular substance.
Nonproblematic use	Repeated use in social situations, for recreational purposes only, without associated problems.
Problem use	Use for other than recreational purposes (i.e., to relax or improve mood) or use associated with a single problem (i.e., tension with parents, school suspension)
Abuse	Use that has a negative impact on daily functioning or that is associated with recurrent significant problems (as above) or risks (i.e., driving or babysitting while intoxicated), as defined by DSM-IV-TR[23] criteria below. Patient must meet one or more for a diagnosis of substance abuse: • Failure to fulfill obligations at work, school, or home (e.g., repeated school absences, suspension) • Use in physically hazardous situations (e.g., drinking and driving) • Substance-related legal problems • Continued use despite social or interpersonal problems related to substance
Dependence	Loss of control over a substance, as defined by DSM-IV-TR[23] criteria below. Patient must meet 3 or more criteria for a diagnosis of substance dependence. • Tolerance • Withdrawal • Substance taken in larger amounts or for longer period than intended • Persistent desire or unsuccessful efforts to cut down/control use • Great deal of time spent obtaining, using, or recovering from effects of substance • Important activities given up or reduced because of use • Continued use despite physical/psychologic harm from substance

American Psychiatric Association. Diagnostic and Statistical Manual of Mental Disorders, Fourth Edition. Washington DC: American Psychiatric Association; 2000.

interview, the clinician can conceptualize the adolescents' substance use on a spectrum that varies from primary abstinence to substance dependence. Table 102.4 describes the stages of the spectrum. As with other developmental phenomena, the amount of time spent in any given phase of the spectrum depends on the specific substance and the adolescent's individual characteristics; however, most adolescents will pass through the stages in the identical order.

Nonproblematic use Adolescents whose use is nonproblematic should be advised similarly to other low-risk teens, including brief advice to stop and specific information regarding the health consequences of substance use (see "CRAFFT 0-1: Brief Advice"). The clinician can use information from the brief assessment to direct advice to perceived negative consequences, such as, "You have noticed that marijuana impacts your breathing, leading you to quit during basketball season. Did you know that smoking marijuana is more harmful to your lungs than smoking tobacco?"

Problem Use Adolescents with problem use of any substance should receive a targeted brief intervention, aimed at reducing substance use and related harm. In this chapter, we define "brief intervention" as a small number (i.e., one to three) of individual counseling sessions with an allied mental health provider, such as a psychologist or social worker. This type of intervention could be accommodated in the primary care setting if such staff is available. Motivational enhancement therapy is particularly suited to this type of intervention (23) though other counseling techniques, such as cognitive behavioral therapy and dialectical behavior therapy are also effective. The referring clinician should ensure follow-up after the brief intervention has been completed to discuss the treatment from the patient's perspective and to determine whether the adolescent has made a behavioral change. If the adolescent continues to use substances, a referral to more intensive treatment should be considered. If an adolescent has problem use of a substance but refuses to engage in therapy, the clinician should consider involving parents in the treatment plan.

Abuse Adolescents who meet diagnostic criteria for alcohol or marijuana abuse should be referred for a brief intervention and followed up closely for signs of behavioral change. If substance use continues despite intervention, more intensive treatment may be required.

Adolescents who meet diagnostic criteria for abuse of more than one substance or of a substance other than alcohol and marijuana should be referred to a mental health specialist or a substance abuse specialty program for a detailed assessment and further treatment. In most cases, these adolescents can be treated in the outpatient setting, with group, individual, or family therapy. Parents should generally be included in the treatment plan whenever an adolescent must be referred outside of the primary care setting in order to ensure compliance and maximize therapeutic efficacy. If special circumstances exist that preclude involving parents (such as a history of domestic violence or active parental substance abuse), the clinician should consider involvement from a state agency (such as the department of social services) and/or support from a guardian, such as a grandparent, foster parent, or other relative.

Dependence All adolescents who meet dependence criteria for any substance should be referred to a mental health or substance abuse specialist for treatment. The spectrum of treatment options varies broadly-from outpatient medication programs to intensive outpatient programs, inpatient stabilization units, and residential programs. The range of therapeutic options and services is discussed in detail in Section 4, "Overview of Addiction Treatment."

Any patient who meets dependence criteria for alcohol or benzodiazepines with a history of withdrawal should be referred to the nearest emergency room for medically supervised detoxification, as withdrawal side effects can be life-threatening. Patients who are at risk of withdrawing from opioids, cocaine, or amphetamines can be offered medically supervised detoxification for comfort, though side effects are generally not life-threatening in otherwise healthy adolescents. Adolescents with opioid, cocaine, or amphetamine dependence and underlying medical disorders, such as cystic fibrosis, sickle cell anemia, or heart disease, should be hospitalized for detoxification.

Adolescents referred for specialty care for the treatment of substance dependence should be followed in primary care after the initial phases of treatment. These adolescents can benefit tremendously from the message that they are still accepted at their medical home.

SUMMARY

Substance use is one of the greatest health threats faced by American teenagers. Fortunately, easily implemented substance use screens can quickly and reliably determine which teens are at high risk of having a substance use disorder. Teens who are at low risk, who form the majority of any primary care population, can be effectively advised in a primary care setting. Experienced clinicians can follow-up a positive screen with a brief assessment to determine the appropriate level of care for teens with more serious substance use disorders and make appropriate referrals. Clinicians who routinely screen all adolescent patients for substance use can have a major impact on the health of their patient population.

REFERENCES

1. Johnston L, O'Malley P, Bachman J, Schulenberg J. *Monitoring the Future national results on adolescent drug use. Overview of Key Findings, 2006.* NIH Publication No. 07-6202. Bethesda: National Institute on Drug Abuse, 2007.
2. Eaton DK, Kann L, Kinchen S, et al. Youth risk behavior surveillance—United States, 2007. *MMWR* 2008;57(SS04):1–131.
3. Baskin-Sommers A, Sommers I. The co-occurrence of substance use and high-risk behaviors. *J Adolesc Health* 2006;38:609–611.
4. Li T, Hewitt B, Grant B. Alcohol use disorders and mood disorders: a National Institute on Alcohol Abuse and Alcoholism perspective. *Biol Psychiatry* 2004;56:718–720.
5. Shedler J, Block J. Adolescent drug use and psychological health: a longitudinal inquiry. *Am Psychol* 1990;45:612–630.
6. Tucker J, Ellickson P. Does solitary substance use increase adolescents' risk for poor psychosocial and behavioral outcomes? A 9-year longitudinal study comparing solitary and socail users. *Psychol Addict Behav* 2006; 20(4):363–372.
7. Tucker J, Ellickson P, Collins R, Klein D. Are drug experimenters better adjusted than abstainers and users? A longitudinal study of adolescent marijuana use. *J Adolesc Health* 2006;39:488–494.
8. Schwartz R. Marijuana: an overview. *Pediatr Clin North Am* 1987;34: 305.
9. National Center for Education in Maternal Child Health. *Bright futures: guidelines for health supervision of infants, children and adolescents,* 2nd ed. [rev.]. Washington, DC: Author, 2002.
10. American Medical Association. Guidelines for adolescent preventive services. Chicago: Author, 1997.
11. Goldenring J, Cohen G. Getting into adolescent heads. *Contemp Pediatr* 1988;5(7):75–90.
12. Bohn M, Babor T. The Alcohol Use Disorders Identification Test (AUDIT): validation of a screening instrument for use in medical settings. *J Stud Alcohol* 1995;56:423–432.
13. Rahdert ER, ed. The Adolescent Assessment/Referral System Manual. DHHS Publication No. (ADM) 91–1735 ed: US Dept Health Human Services (PHS) Alcohol, Drug Abuse, and Mental Health Administration; 1991.
14. Knight J, Shrier L, Bravender T, et al. A new brief screen for adolescent substance abuse. *Arch Pediatr Adolesc Med* 1999;153:591–596.
15. Ewing J. Detecting alcoholism: the CAGE questionnaire. *JAMA* 1984; 252:1906–1907.
16. Knight JR, Sherritt L, Harris SK, et al. Validity of brief alcohol screening tests among adolescents: a comparison of the AUDIT, POSIT, CAGE and CRAFFT. *Alcohol Clin Exp Res* 2002;27:67–73.

17. Wilson CR, Sherritt L, Gates E, Knight JR. Are clinical impressions of adolescent substance use accurate? *Pediatrics* 2004;114:e536–540.
18. Students Against Destructive Decisions. *Contract For Life: a foundation for trust and caring.* Marlborough, MA: (on-line). Available at http://www.saddonline.com/contract.htm. Retrieved June 29, 2001.
19. Bierut L, Saccone N, Rice J, et al. Defining alcohol-related phenotypes in humans. *Alcohol Res Health* 2002;26:208–213.
20. Hertz J, Knight J. Prescription drug misuse: a growing national problem. *Adolesc Med Clin* 2006;17:751–769.
21. Fisher S, Bucholz K, Reich W, et al. Teenagers are right-parents do not know much: an analysis of adolescent-parent agreement on reports of adolescent substance use, abuse and dependence. *Alcohol Clin Exp Res* 2006;30:1699–1710.
22. American Psychiatric Association. *Diagnostic and statistical manual of mental disorders,* 4th ed. Washington, DC: Author, 1994.
23. Monti P, Barnett N, O'Leary T. Motivational enhancement for alcohol-involved adolescents. In: Monti P, Colby S, O'Leary T, eds. *Adolescents, alcohol, and substance abuse: reaching teens through brief interventions.* New York: The Guilford Press, 2001:145–182.

CHAPTER 103

Ken C. Winters, PhD
Tamara Fahnhorst, MPH
Andria Botzet, MA
Randy Stinchfield, PhD

Assessing Adolescent Substance Use

ASSESSING ADOLESCENT SUBSTANCE USE

Alcohol and other drug use behaviors by adolescents remains a critical health problem in America, despite regulations against underage use of legal and illicit drugs. From an epidemiologic standpoint, drug use by teenagers is relatively common. According to a recent nationwide survey, Monitoring the Future (1), 51% of 12th graders have used an illicit drug in their lifetime, and nearly one fourth (23.4%) reported use of an illicit drug within the prior month. Also, adolescent-onset of drug use greatly increases the estimated risk for developing a substance use disorder during adolescence and young adulthood (2), and drug use by teenagers can lead to a variety of other negative consequences, including social and health impairments. These impairments include school failure, risky sexual behavior (3,4), delinquency, incarceration, suicidality (5,6), motor vehicle injuries/fatalities (7), possible damage to the brain's memory region (8), and significant medical health care costs (9,10).

Thus precise assessment of adolescent drug use is essential in gaining an accurate understanding of the nature and extent of adolescent drug use, and possible intervention or treatment needs. This chapter will discuss the following issues pertaining to assessment: principles of assessment, self-report, developmental issues, clinical content, assessment process, and instrumentation.

PRINCIPLES OF ASSESSMENT

We distinguish two types of assessment: screening and comprehensive assessment. Screening is the first step in identifying whether a youth may be involved with drugs; comprehensive assessment explores with more depth the extent and nature of the drug involvement, consequential problems, and treatment needs. Thus a screening should not be used to make definitive judgments about whether or not the adolescent has a substance use disorder (i.e., abuse or dependence), nor used as a basis to determine if treatment is needed. Rather, screening results should be used for determining the need for additional assessment. A comprehensive assessment provides a basis for determining if treatment is warranted, and if so, at what level, and for assisting in the development of a comprehensive treatment plan to address the youth's needs. Despite uneven requirements by licensing and accreditation organizations, there is a national trend toward requiring adolescent drug treatment facilities to use at least one adolescent-specific and psychometrically sound assessment instrument as part of intake and treatment planning. Later in this chapter we review nationally recognized screening and assessment tools.

Screening When an adolescent is suspected of using drugs, the assessment process should begin with screening questions about recent drug use quantity and frequency (e.g., How often did you use drugs in the past 6 months?), the presence of adverse consequences of use (e.g., Has your drug use led to problems with your parents?), and situations in which drug use is common (e.g., Do you use drugs before or during school?).

Comprehensive Assessment If the screening suggests a possible drug use problem, the assessor should conduct a more comprehensive assessment in order to determine details of drug use history, consequences of such use, whether the teenager meets criteria for a substance use disorder (SUD), and what other behavioral and mental co-occurring problems may exist. This detailed assessment should include a detailed inquiry into the age of onset and progression of use for specific substances, circumstances, frequency and variability of use, and types of drugs used. The assessor should also inquire about the context of use, which should include the usual times and places of drug use, the attitudes and use patterns of the adolescent's peers, and typical behavioral and social triggers and antecedents that are associated with drug use. The clinician should also ask about direct and indirect consequences of use in the domains of school, social, family, psychologic functioning, and physical/medical problems. Finally, the assessor should evaluate the adolescent's problem recognition and readiness for treatment. These questions may help determine the initial treatment goals.

The determination of a SUD requires that the assessor review the criteria for substance abuse and dependence for specific substances. Abuse criteria focus on negative social and personal consequences as a result of repetitive use; dependence criteria address symptoms associated with the continued use of drugs in the face of negative consequences and loss of control over use (more discussion on these criteria in a subsequent section). The differential diagnosis of adolescent substance use disorders requires consideration that the symptoms of drug use are not due to premorbid or concurrent problems, such as conduct disorder or family issues. Given the frequent comorbidity of SUDs and other psychiatric disorders, it is important that the assessor comprehensively review in timeline fashion the past and present history of psychiatric symptoms. Such a timeline approach can help the assessor sort out the interrelationship between drug use and comorbid psychopathology (11).

DEVELOPMENTAL CONSIDERATIONS

Identifying Clinical Significance It can be difficult to determine when adolescent drug use will have short-term and minimal health effects versus when drug use may escalate to negative long-term repercussions. The high prevalence rate of drug use by teenagers gives some credence to the notion that drug involvement is a normative part of youth. Most often, adolescents use legal drugs (alcohol or tobacco) within a social context (12,13). These so-called *gateway drugs* are readily accessible to minors because of their cultural prominence, legality, and general availability. The majority of youth will not progress beyond the use of these gateway drugs (14), yet some will progress to use illicit drugs and to develop serious problems. For example, based on national data, it is estimated that about 11% of youth (12 to 18 year olds) will use drugs to the point of meeting a current *Diagnostic and statistical manual of mental disorders,* 4th ed. (DSM-IV-TR) criteria (15) for either a substance abuse or substance dependence disorder (16).

Applicability of SUD Criteria The applicability of DSM-IV-TR criteria to adolescent drug use has been met with reservation for several reasons, including: the distinction of abuse and dependence criterion as applied to adolescents are not well-supported by research; some criteria have limited utility among adolescents (e.g., an important criterion for dependence, tolerance, has low diagnostic specificity among adolescents given that this symptom can take extended lengths of time to develop); and the meaning of symptoms for adolescents, who are relatively inexperienced with the effects of drugs, may lead to higher rates of false positive endorsements (e.g., "drinking more than intended" may be endorsed more frequently among teenagers because of poor judgment) (17).

Neurobiology Recent research has indicated that the adolescent brain does not fully develop until early adulthood (18). In some regions of the brain, particularly the prefrontal cortex region that is associated with judgment (resisting impulses and other executive functioning), nearly 50% of the neurons are "pruned" and undergoing transformation during adolescence. Because of this immaturity, there is speculation that the developing adolescent brain may be highly vulnerable to the effects of drug use. Studies with laboratory animals have provided evidence that adolescents differ significantly from adults in their receptivity to the effects of alcohol (19). For example, adolescent rats show decreased sensitivity to the unpleasant effects of alcohol (i.e., vomiting, hangover) and increased sensitivity to the social disinhibitory effects of alcohol as compared with older rats. Adolescent rats also require a larger amount of alcohol to reduce anxiety than older rats (20). If we generalize these findings from animal research, the implication is that adolescents may be less capable of moderating their alcohol intake as compared to adults.

Laboratory animals also provide evidence that exposure to drugs during adolescence influences later neural functioning. After rats were chronically exposed to alcohol during adolescence, they exhibited greater cognitive difficulties than rats that were exposed to the same amount of alcohol in adulthood (21). In regard to human subjects, Tapert and Schweinsburg (8) reported that adolescents with a history of heavy alcohol use had a smaller hippocampus (region of brain responsible for creating memories) compared with a matched control sample (on average, 10% smaller volume in the alcohol use group). The same adolescents revealed an average of 10% less retention compared with the control group on verbal and nonverbal memory tasks. Because prealcohol use brain functioning was not measured, we can not draw any causal conclusions. But these findings emphasize the importance of further study on the possible deleterious effects of alcohol use on the developing brain.

Other Factors Other developmental issues are relevant with respect to assessing adolescent drug use. Clinical studies have revealed both gender differences and similarities with regard to possible psychosocial determinants of drug use. Opland et al. (22) found that girls tend to utilize drug use as a coping mechanism for stress, whereas boys tend to use drugs for the pleasurable effects. Also, delays in social and emotional functioning (23), diminished respect towards authority, and tendencies to be egocentric (24) and to minimize negative consequences (25) may contribute to inaccurate reporting of personal drug use behaviors and to poor motivation to change (26).

SELF-REPORT: VALIDITY AND ALTERNATIVES

The utilization of self-report is a hallmark of a clinical assessment. Convenience, comprehensiveness, low cost, ease of administration, and the perception that the individual is the most knowledgeable reporter have encouraged the use of this method. Self-report approaches or formats include self-administered questionnaire (SAQ), interview, Timeline Follow Back (TLFB) (27), and computer-assisted interview (CAI). SAQs and interviews are the primary approaches used by clinicians. SAQs are completed independently by an individual and traditionally via paper-and-pencil format. An interview (varying in degree of structure) is completed by a trained individual and often yields specific diagnostic data related to SUDs and coexisting psychiatric diagnoses. Lesser used strategies include the TLFB and CAI. The TLFB is a calendar-based tool that compiles a history of drug use over a specified time. TLFB method uses specific dates and events (e.g., birthdays, holidays, vacations) to enhance interviewee recollection to elicit a detailed pattern of recent drug use. The CAI method has been recently used with drug abusing adolescent populations (28). With this method, the respondent completes an interview independently on a computer as the questions are delivered audibly via headphones. This approach may promote a greater sense of privacy while responding to potentially sensitive questions. Research on the concordance of SAQ, interview, TLFB, and CAI formats in clinical and epidemiologic samples is not conclusive, although the data suggest that, for the most part, the various formats yield similar levels of disclosure (29–31).

The overall validity and reliability of the self-report method for assessing adolescent drug use and related problems is still debated in the literature. Stinchfield (32) found that adolescents attending a treatment program for drug dependence generally reported notably more past drug use and consequences compared to disclosures at the start of intervention. In other studies, underreporting occurred more frequently with less socially acceptable drugs, such as cocaine or opiates, compared with marijuana (33,34). Improved urinalysis techniques (immunoassays), and the more recent sophistication of examining hair strands, are being used to corroborate adolescent self-report of drug use (35). Williams and Nowatazki (33) reported that some adolescents disclosed drug use in an interview though the urinalysis conducted immediately after the interview showed a negative finding. Some of this discrepancy was accounted for by limitations in the urinalysis "detection window" for different drugs and because of individuals' varying metabolic rates, but the authors hypothesized that deliberate fabrication, poor memory, and boastfulness may have also been contributing factors (33). These findings are not surprising given the circumstances under which an adolescent assessment may be conducted. Defiance, fear, and apprehension can influence the results of an assessment. In addition, youth may see the assessment as an opportunity to "cry for help" and exaggerate their responses. Despite possible limitations, the validity of self-report for adolescent drug use has been supported by several lines of evidence: only a small percentage of youth endorse improbable questions; adolescent self-reports agree with corroborating sources of information, such as archival records, and for the most part, urinalyses; and the base rate of elevations on "faking-good" and "faking-bad" scales are relatively low (36–39).

Alternatives to Self-Report

Drug Testing Four biologic-based tests (urine, hair, saliva, and sweat) are currently used to detect drugs in the body (35). The main aspect that distinguishes these specimens is the period or window of time for which the drug can be detected. In addition, cost, access, tampering vulnerability, invasiveness, and reliability/validity are other factors that differentiate these biologic sampling procedures. Urinalysis is the most commonly used procedure to detect drug use and validate self-report. The window of detection varies considerably for illicit drugs; the detection period for alcohol is only about 8 hours. Tampering can be minimized by directly monitoring the collection of the urine. Hair analysis has become more commonly used to detect exposure to drugs over a longer period than afforded by urine testing (35), but several variables (e.g., chemical processing, differences in hair structure, growth, porosity, and hygiene, exposure to drugs in the air) (e.g., marijuana smoke) have been shown to affect the concentrations of drugs in the hair (40,41). The testing of saliva and sweat to detect drug exposure is still being refined; their advantages include a noninvasive collection process and the detection of very recent drug use (12 to 24 hours).

Clinical Observation In addition to self-report and biologic tests, direct observation by the assessor for behavioral and psychologic indicators of drug use can be an objective and useful supplement to the assessment process. A simple checklist of items, such as the presence of needle marks, unsteady gate, slurred or incoherent speech, or shaking of hands or twitching of eyelids can indicate problematic use. A 14-item checklist of observable signs that may indicate a drug problem is contained in the Simple Screening Instrument for Alcohol and Other Drug Abuse (42).

Reports from Others Although parent report is relatively valid in the identification of many mental health problems such as attention-deficit hyperactivity disorder (ADHD) and conduct problems, it is unlikely that parents can provide detailed reports about the types, frequency, and quantity of drug use by their son or daughter (38). Collecting information from peers may prove to be a valuable resource especially if the peers are not currently using drugs or are in recovery, although it is very difficult to get peers to participate in the assessment of a friend.

CLINICAL CONTENT

SUD Drug use that goes beyond experimentation and progresses into problematic involvement is formally delineated by various classification systems, with the primary systems including the DSM-IV-TR (15) and the *International Classification of Diseases,* 10th rev. (43).

In the DSM-IV-TR diagnostic system, problem-level drug use is separated into categories of abuse or dependence, as shown in Table 103.1. Abuse symptoms pertain to drug use that increases risk for or results in negative health and social consequences, such as role impairment, physically hazardous use, recurrent substance-related legal problems, and social and interpersonal difficulties resulting from drug use. Abuse symptoms are meant to characterize predependent symptoms; accordingly, an individual must meet at least one of the abuse criteria within the prior 12 months, without obtaining a dependence diagnosis, to receive an abuse diagnosis.

DSM-based dependence, on the other hand, requires the positive endorsement of at least three of seven symptoms, all of which reflect psychologic and physiologic features. Psychologic characteristics refer to continued and compulsive drug use in the face of negative consequences, such as the continuation of drug use despite recognition of drug-induced depression or quitting important social or occupational activities because of drug use. Symptoms indicating physiologic dependence refer to tolerance (i.e., the need for increased amounts to achieve intoxication) and withdrawal (i.e., the development of symptoms such as nausea, anxiety, increased pulse rate, or insomnia

TABLE 103.1 DSM-IV-TR Symptoms of Substance Abuse and Dependence Disorders

Abuse criteria (must endorse at least 1 item in past 12 months and have no dependence diagnosis)

1. **Failure to fulfill role obligations at work, school, or home,** such as:
   - Absences from work/school due to use,
   - Avoiding family activities due to use
2. **Use in physically hazardous situations,** such as:
   - Driving
   - Operating a machine
   - Participating in dangerous activities
3. **Substance-related legal problems,** such as:
   - Possession of an illegal substance
   - Selling or distribution of an illegal substance
   - Minor consumption
4. **Continued use despite social or interpersonal problems,** such as:
   - Physical fights
   - Arguments with loved ones regarding consequences of drug use

Dependence criteria (must endorse at least 3 items in past 12 months)

1. **Tolerance,** defined by:
   - Need for larger amounts of the drug to achieve intoxication
   - Current effect of drug is diminished as compared with previous use of same drug
2. **Withdrawal,** defined by:
   - Two or more symptoms that occur as a result of diminished regular or heavy use, such as increased pulse rate, nausea, anxiety, hand tremors, hallucinations, insomnia
   - Use of same or similar drug to avoid symptoms mentioned above
3. **Using more than intended,** such as:
   - Using for a longer period than intended
   - Using a larger quantity than planned
4. **Desire to cut down or control use,** defined by:
   - Repeated efforts to cut back or quit using substance
   - Efforts to cut back or control use were considered "unsuccessful"
5. **Excessive time spent in obtaining or using the drug,** such as:
   - Driving long distances to obtain drug
   - Spending significant portions of the day using the drug
   - Spending significant portions of the day recovering from use
6. **Activities given up or reduced due to use,** such as:
   - Quitting social or recreational activities
   - Missing appointments or meetings to use the drug or recover from its use
7. **Continued use despite physical or psychological problems,** such as:
   - Continuing to use drugs even though person drug-induced depression
   - Continuing to use drugs even though person suffers from a physical ailment, such as an ulcer, that can be aggravated by drug use

From American Psychiatric Association. *Diagnostic and statistical manual of mental disorders.* 4th ed., text rev. Washington, DC: American Psychiatric Association, Copyright 2000, with permission.

from the cessation of heavy or prolonged drug use). In the DSM-IV-TR, substance abuse and substance dependence criteria are the same for all substances, and the diagnoses of abuse and dependence are hierarchically arranged (i.e., a dependence diagnosis precludes an abuse diagnosis).

One feature of the *DSM*-based definition of SUDs is that none of the criteria directly refer to onset, quantity, and frequency variables. This is not to say that these variables are not important to assess. Indeed, consumption history does produce important information, particularly when data is compared with regularly updated norms of use.

Course of SUDs The clinical course of youth with a SUD indicates the changes and expression of a SUD, as well as the associated functioning over time (44). Understanding the course of adolescent SUDs provides a vital perspective in our understanding of the etiology and prognosis of SUDs. Multiple studies have examined developmental trajectories of adolescent drug use behaviors (26,45), and have found results that support the notion of separate experimental and SUD paths. Developmental trajectories have been characterized as developmentally limited or intermittent, as would be expected in an experimental case, as well as persistent or relatively continuous, suggestive of a SUD. One such trajectory by Lewinsohn et al. (26) found gender differences in alcohol use within a community sample; females had an earlier age of onset for an alcohol use disorder compared to males (14.6 vs. 16.1 years old, respectively), though males developed alcohol-related problems at a faster rate between the ages of 18 and 19 (26). The same sample provided evidence that the average duration of an alcohol use disorder was about 52 weeks for the community sample of adolescents (26).

Some variables have been found to predict the course of SUDs among adolescents in a drug treatment setting. Pretreatment characteristics that are associated with more favorable substance use outcomes include a lower substance use severity level at admission (46), greater readiness to change (47), and fewer conduct problems or other co-occurring psychopathology (48,49). Factors influencing better outcomes during treatment include a longer length of treatment (50) and family involvement in treatment (51). Posttreatment predictors of better outcome include participation in aftercare (52,53), low levels of peer substance use (54), ability to use coping skills (55), and continued commitment to abstain (47). Of all these factors, the posttreatment predictors accounted for more variance in the teenagers' outcomes at 1 year after treatment than did the pretreatment and during-treatment variables. However, it is important to recognize that predictors may change over time, just as the impact of the predictor on the course of SUD may change. For example, Latimer et al. reported that sibling drug use was associated with more frequent drug use during the first 6 months posttreatment, but as time passed, peer drug use became a stronger predictor of SUD course than sibling drug use (56).

Psychosocial Factors Measurement of the various psychosocial dimensions that are related to drug use behaviors provides beneficial information regarding the onset and maintenance factors of the drug use and aids in treatment planning. Dimensions that should be included in the assessment protocol include interpersonal relationships, school and employment, history of criminal justice involvement and delinquency, recreational activities, and sexual behavior. Two additional psychosocial factors merit additional discussion and are addressed in the following paragraphs: peer factors and family environment.

Peer Factors Multiple research studies indicate that peer variables are one of the most prominent factors contributing to the onset and maintenance of drug use. Chilcoat and Breslau (57) found that youth who associate with peers who use drugs were six times as likely to use drugs as those who did not associate with drug-using peers. Similar findings were found by Farrell and Danish (58) and Winters et al. (59). A parallel finding by Guo et al. (60) revealed that adolescents involved with peers exhibiting antisocial behaviors were at a higher risk of initiating illicit drug use. Understanding the intricacies of peer relationships is complex. The nature of this association between drug use and peers could be due to pressure to use drugs from drug-using friends, or to the increased likelihood that drug-using individuals seek out other drug-using peers. Peer influences may also impact the youth's attitudes and expectancies regarding drug use, as well as the youth's access to drugs (61–63).

Family Factors Family influences encompass several variables, including familial genetic risk and parenting practices. Children whose parents suffer from a SUD have been shown to be at increased risk for the development of a SUD (64). Also, other psychopathology in family members, particularly parental antisocial behavior history, is relevant in offspring SUD liability (65–68). Results from twin and family studies provide additional insight into the role of family genetics and home environment on youth drug use. There is converging evidence that the initiation of alcohol use in mid-adolescence is predominantly influenced by factors such as parental monitoring and father's drinking level, rather than genetic factors (69–71). However, after drinking is initiated, it appears the genetic factors increasingly influence the frequency of alcohol and other drug use, as well as the prevalence of SUDs (72). Of course, it is important to keep in mind that even in the face of a presumed SUD heritable liability, a normative developmental outcome is still more common among youth than a disordered course (14).

Parenting factors are strongly associated with adolescent risk for drug involvement, especially factors such as closeness or warmth and control or monitoring. These aspects of parenting reflect characteristics of affection, nurturance, and acceptance of the child by the parent, as well as characteristics of supervising the child's activities and firmness in setting limits (73,74). Several researchers have found increased drug use among adolescents in families that lack closeness or affection, lack effective discipline, lack supervision, have excessive or weak parental control, and have inconsistent parenting (74–79).

Psychological Benefits In spite of the detrimental effects incurred when using drugs, many adolescents use drugs because they serve psychological need states (80). Psychological advantages of adolescent drug use include mood enhancement, stress reduction, and relief from boredom (81). One study found that mood enhancement played a more central role in drug use among youth with a SUD, whereas these psychological benefits were not as important to youth who used drugs infrequently and did not have a SUD (82). Because psychological benefits play such an important role in the attraction and exacerbation of drug use among adolescents, intervention efforts must address these underlying factors.

Co-occurring Mental Health Disorders A very reliable finding in the clinical and epidemiologic literatures is that most adolescents who are involved with drugs have co-occurring psychologic disorders (83–85), and that their presence is a negative sign for recovery (28,86). The most common types of comorbid psychiatric conditions include externalizing disorders (i.e., conduct disorder [CD], oppositional defiant disorder, and ADHD) and internalizing disorders (i.e., depression and anxiety disorders—primarily posttraumatic stress disorder). We will discuss these disorders in more detail.

Coexisting Externalizing Disorders Childhood aggression, rebelliousness, theft, and destructiveness, along with related externalizing disorders such as CD and oppositional defiant disorder, are common among youth with a SUD, as well as among children of parents with a SUD (65,66,68). Prospective research reveals that antisocial behaviors in late childhood, and the initiation of drug use in early adolescence, predict later drug involvement (87,88). The exact relationship between externalizing behavior and SUDs is complex. Three theories have been proposed. One argues that because conduct disorder has been found to predate or contribute to the development of a SUD (89), the resulting poor behavioral inhibition or increased novelty seeking may lead to increased drug use. The second theory is that given that SUDs have been found to precede CD (83) factors that coincide with drug use, such as poor judgment and association with delinquent peers, may act as a catalyst for antisocial behavior and subsequent oppositional defiant disorder or CD. Finally, a third perspective is that CD and drug use may occur concurrently for they may share common environmental and personal risk factors (e.g., socioeconomic status, family, low academic achievement, association with deviant peer group). In this light, these risk factors may act independently or synergistically to impact the severity of the substance use and antisocial behavior (83,90), and both CD and drug use would interact with each other over time to escalate the severity of the other set of symptoms (91).

The relationship between ADHD and SUDs is equally complex, despite the significant amounts of literature that have explored the association. Some studies have found that individuals with a history of ADHD, compared with controls, are more likely to develop substance use and substance-related problems (91–93). Other studies have not found similar relationships (94,95). There is also a large body of research that supports the view that the association of ADHD-drug use problems is mediated by CD (88,94,96,97). But this mediation hypothesis is not a universal finding (98). With regard to tobacco, a commonly cited gateway drug, ADHD has also been linked to its early initiation and increased use (93), and there are indications that this link holds even after controlling for CD (99,100).

Coexisting Internalizing Disorders Internalizing disorders such as anxiety disorders (i.e., posttraumatic stress disorder) and mood disorders (i.e., major depression) may be another pathway associated with SUD (101,102). Children of SUD parents have been found to have increased rates of internalizing disorders and related symptoms (65–67). Among adolescents with a SUD, elevated rates of internalizing disorders and related symptoms have been reported, especially among females as compared with male adolescents with a SUD (103,104). Childhood major depression has been found to be more common with adolescent-onset than with adult-onset SUD (83). These associations do not, however, establish that a causal pathway exists between childhood internalizing disorders and later SUDs. Similar to the "chicken and egg" conundrum that exists with SUDs and externalizing disorders, the specific association between internalizing disorders and SUDs remains indistinct. Researchers have found that symptoms of anxiety and depression may be produced by alcohol or other substances (101,105), whereas others have demonstrated that an alcohol disorder may exacerbate symptoms of posttraumatic stress disorder (106).

Another complicating feature is that data from adolescents with a SUD indicate that both conduct disorders and major depression may coexist in some individuals (107). Prospective longitudinal research that integrates findings for antisocial disorders with findings for internalizing disorders beginning in preadolescence and assesses the sequencing of these characteristics for specific developmental periods (i.e., early adolescence, middle adolescence) is needed to clarify these relationships (88).

Other psychiatric disturbances have also been shown to correlate with adolescent SUD, though at a lower rate. A number of individuals with eating disorders such as bulimia-nervosa have been shown to also abuse substances or have a SUD (108). In addition, adverse life events including childhood maltreatment (i.e., physical abuse, sexual abuse, neglect) have also been found to be associated with the development of a SUD (108).

INSTRUMENTATION

Significant advances have occurred since the mid 1980s in the development and evaluation of adolescent drug abuse assessment instruments (109,110). Most of these measures have been normed on adolescents. Some tools are designed to screen youth at risk for drug problems, whereas other measures provide extensive, diagnostically related information.

Several summaries of adolescent screening and comprehensive assessments exist, including two by the federal government, "Screening Assessment of Adolescents with a Substance Use Disorder" (111) and "Screening and Assessing Youth for Drug Involvement" (110), as part the National Institute on Alcohol Abuse and Alcoholism, 2nd edition, handbook, "Assessing Alcohol Problems: A Guide for Clinicians and Researchers" (112), as well as journal articles (17,109) and book chapters (113). We provide our own syntheses of these various summaries. Inclusion in our overview was the requirement that the instrument was developed specifically for adolescents, its psychometric properties have been reported in a peer-reviewed publication, and user information is available in print (e.g., manual, scoring information), and the instrument's author or publisher is accessible to answer user questions. The synthesis includes both screening and comprehensive instruments.

Screening Instruments Clinicians and researchers working with adolescents have access to a wide range of screening instruments, most commonly self-report questionnaires, to describe the possible or probable presence of a drug problem (see Table 103.2 for a listing). We review four categories of screening tools: alcohol, all drugs (including alcohol), nonalcohol drugs, and multiscreens.

Alcohol Screens There are two contemporary screening tools that focus exclusively on alcohol use. One is the Adolescent Drinking Inventory (ADI) (115). The ADI's 24 items examine adolescent problem drinking by measuring psychologic symptoms, physical symptoms, social symptoms, and loss of control. Written at a 5th-grade reading level, it yields a single score with cutoffs, as well as two research subscale scores (self-medicating drinking and rebellious drinking). The ADI yields high internal consistency reliability (coefficient alpha, 0.93–0.95), and has demonstrated validity in measuring the severity of adolescent drinking problems (e.g., it has revealed a very favorable hit rate of 82% in classification accuracy). The second measure in this group is the 23-item Rutgers Alcohol Problem Index (122). The Rutgers Alcohol Problem Index measures consequences of alcohol use pertaining to family life, social relations, psychological functioning, delinquency, physical problems, and neuropsychologic functioning. Based on a large general population sample, the Rutgers Alcohol Problem Index was found to have high internal consistency (0.92), and, among heavy alcohol

TABLE 103.2 Screening Instruments

Instrument	Purpose	Source	Group used	Norms	Normed groups	Format	Time (min)
Adolescent Alcohol & Drug Involvement Scale (AADIS)	Screen for drug abuse problem severity	114	Adolescents referred for emotional or behavioral disorders	Yes	Substance abusers	14 items, questionnaire	5
Adolescent Drinking Inventory (ADI)	Screen for alcohol use problem severity	115	Adolescents suspected of alcohol use problems	Yes	Normals; substance abusers	24 items, questionnaire	5
CRAFFT	Screen for drug use problem severity	116	Adolescents referred for emotional or behavioral disorders	Yes	Normals; substance abusers	6 items, questionnaire	5
Drug Abuse Screening Test-Adolescents (DAST-A)	Screen for drug use problem severity	117	Adolescents referred for emotional or behavioral disorders	Yes	Substance abusers	27 items, questionnaire	5
Drug Use Screening Inventory-Revised (DUSI-R)	Screen for substance use problem severity and related problems	118	Adolescents referred for emotional or behavioral disorders	Yes	Substance abusers	159 items, questionnaire	20
Personal Experience Screening Questionnaire (PESQ)	Screen for substance use problem severity	119	Adolescents referred for emotional or behavioral disorders	Yes	Normals; substance abusers	40 items, questionnaire	10
Problem Oriented Screening Instrument for Teenagers (POSIT)	Multiscreen for substance use problem severity and related problems	120, 121	Adolescents referred for emotional or behavioral disorders	Yes	Normals; substance abusers	139 items, questionnaire	20–25
Rutgers Alcohol Problem Index (RAPI)	Screen for alcohol use problem severity	122	Adolescents at risk for alcohol use problems	Yes	Normals; substance abusers	23 items, questionnaire	10
Substance Abuse Subtle Screening Inventory-Adolescents (SASSI-A)	Screen for substance use problem severity and related problems	123	Adolescents referred for emotional or behavioral disorders	Yes	Normals; substance abusers	81 items, questionnaire	10–15

users, a strong correlation with *DSM-III-R* criteria for substance use disorders (0.75–0.95) (122).

Screens for All Drugs Another group of screening tools is the relatively short measures that nonspecifically cover all drug categories, including alcohol. Examples of these measures are the Adolescent Alcohol and Drug Abuse Involvement Scale (114), CRAFFT (116,124), Personal Experience Screening Questionnaire (119), and the Substance Abuse Subtle Screening Inventory for adolescents (SASSI) (123). The 14-item Adolescent Alcohol and Drug Abuse Involvement Scale measures drug abuse problem severity scale; a range of reliability and validity evidence for this screen has been reported (114). The CRAFFT is a specialized six-item screen designed to be administered verbally during a primary care interview to address both alcohol and drug use. Its name is a mnemonic device to assist physicians to incorporate six questions during their primary care exams. Based on a study in a large hospital-based adolescent clinic, scores from the CRAFFT were found to be highly correlated with scores from several existing and valid measures, and a cutoff score of 2 has been found to be highly predictive of a drug problem (116,124). The 40-item Personal Experience Screening Questionnaire consists of a problem severity scale (coefficient alpha, 0.91–0.95), drug use history, select psychosocial problems, and response distortion tendencies ("faking good" and "faking bad"). Norms for normal, juvenile offender, and drug abusing populations are available. The Personal Experience Screening Questionnaire is estimated to have an accuracy rate of 87% in predicting the need for further drug abuse assessment (119). The 81-item adolescent version of the SASSI yields scores for several scales, including face-valid alcohol, face-valid other drug, obvious attributes, subtle attributes, and defensiveness. Validity data indicate that SASSI scale scores are highly correlated with MMPI (Minnesota Multiphasic Personality Inventory) scales and that its cut score for "chemical dependency" corresponds highly with intake diagnoses of substance use disorders (125). However, claims that the SASSI can accurately detect *unreported* drug use and related problems have not been empirically justified (126).

Screens for Non-Alcohol Drugs The third category of screening tools pertains to those that screen only non-alcohol drugs. Only one screen falls into this group: the Drug Abuse Screening Test for Adolescents (117), and was adapted from Skinner's (127) adult tool, the Drug Abuse Screening Test. This 27-item questionnaire is associated with favorable reliability data and is highly predictive of DSM-IV-TR drug-related disorder when tested among adolescent psychiatric inpatients.

Multiproblem Screens The final group of screening measures consists of two "multiscreen" instruments that examine several domains in addition to drug involvement. The 139-item Problem Oriented Screening Instrument for Teenagers (121) is part of the Adolescent Assessment and Referral System developed by the National Institute on Drug Abuse. It tests for 10 functional adolescent problem areas: substance use, physical health, mental health, family relations, peer relationships, educational status, vocational status, social skills, leisure and recreation, and aggressive behavior/delinquency. Cut scores for determining the need for further assessment have been rationally established, and some have been confirmed with empirical procedures (120). Convergent and discriminant evidence for the Problem Oriented Screening Instrument for Teenagers has been reported by several investigators (128,129). The Drug Use Screening Inventory-Revised is a 159-item instrument that describes drug use problem severity and related problems. It produces scores on 10 subscales as well as one lie scale. Domain scores were related to *DSM-III-R* substance use disorder criteria in a sample of adolescent substance abusers (130). An additional psychometric report provides norms and evidence of scale sensitivity (118).

Comprehensive Assessment Instruments If an initial screening indicates the need for further assessment, clinicians and researchers can employ various diagnostic interviews, problem-focused interviews and multiscale questionnaires (see Table 103.3 for a listing). These instruments yield information that can more definitively assess the nature and severity of the drug involvement, typically assign a substance use disorder diagnosis, and identify the psychosocial factors that may predispose, perpetuate, and maintain the drug involvement.

Diagnostic Interviews Diagnostic interviews, which focus on *DSM*-based criteria for SUDs, include both general psychiatric interviews that address all psychiatric disorders, and SUD interviews that focus primarily on drug use and related domains of functioning. The majority of the diagnostic interviews are structured; that is, the format directs the interviewer to read verbatim a series of questions in a decision-tree format and the answers to these questions are restricted to a few predefined alternatives. The respondent is assigned the principal responsibility of interpreting the question and deciding on a reply.

There are two well-researched psychiatric diagnostic interviews that address SUDs as well as the full range of child and adolescent psychiatric disorders. The Diagnostic Interview for Children and Adolescents (133) is a structured interview and is used widely among researchers and clinicians. Psychometric evidence specific to substance use disorders has not been published on the Diagnostic Interview for Children and Adolescents, but some of the other sections have been evaluated for reliability and validity (142). An instrument that has undergone several adaptations is the Diagnostic Interview Schedule for Children (DISC) (143,144). Its DSM-IV-TR version is the DISC-Revised (134,145). Separate forms of the interview exist for the child and the parent. As part of a larger study focusing on several diagnoses, Fisher et al. (146) found the DISC-Revised to be highly sensitive in correctly identifying youth who had received a hospital diagnosis of any substance use disorder (n = 8). Both interview forms (parent and child) had a sensitivity of 75%. For the one parent-child disagreement case, the parent indicated that they did not know any details about their child's substance use.

The second subgroup of diagnostic interviews primarily focuses on diagnostic criteria for SUDs. The ADI (131)

TABLE 103.3 Comprehensive Assessment Instruments

Instrument	Purpose	Source	Examples group used	Norms	Normed groups	Format	Time (min)
Diagnostic Interviews							
Adolescent Diagnostic Interview (ADI)	Assess DSM-IV-TR substance use disorders and problems	131	Adolescents suspected of drug use problems	NA	NA	Structured interview	45–60
Customary Drinking and Drug Use Record (CDDR)	Assess DSM-IV-TR substance use disorders and problems	132	Adolescents suspected of drug use problems	NA	NA	Structured interview	10–30
Diagnostic Interview for Children & Adolescents (DICA-R)	Assess DSM-IV-TR child/adolescent disorders	133	Youth suspected mental, behavioral problems	NA	NA	Structured interview	45–60
Diagnostic Interview Schedule for Children (DISC-R)	Assess DSM-IV-TR child/adolescent disorders	134	Youth suspected mental, behavioral problems	NA	NA	Structured interview	45–60
Global Appraisal of Individual Needs (GAIN)	Assess DSM-IV-TR substance use disorders and problems	135	Adolescents suspected of drug use problems	NA	NA	Structured interview	60–90
Problem-Focused Interviews							
Comprehensive Adolescent Severity Inventory (CASI)	Assess drug use and other life problems	136	Adolescents suspected of drug use problems	NA	NA	Semistructured interview	45–55
Teen Severity Index (T-ASI)	Assess drug use and other life problems	137	Adolescents at risk for drug use problems	NA	NA	Semistructured interview	20–45
Multiscale Questionnaires							
Adolescent Self-Assessment Profile (ASAP)	Multiscale measure of drug use and related problems	138	Adolescents suspected of substance use problems	Yes	Normals; substance abusers	225 items, qx	45–60
Hilson Adolescent Profile (HAP)	Multiscale measure of drug use and related problems	139	Adolescents suspected of substance use and related problems	Yes	Normals; substance abusers	310 items, qx	45
Juvenile Automated Substance Abuse Evaluation (JASAE)	Multiscale measure of drug use and related problems	140	Adolescents suspected of substance use problems	Yes	Normals; substance abusers	108 items	20
Personal Experience Inventory (PEI)	Multiscale measure of drug use and related problems	141	Adolescents suspected of substance use problems	Yes	Normals; substance abusers	276 items, qx	45–60

assesses diagnostic symptoms associated with psychoactive SUDs. Other sections provide an assessment of substance use consumption history, psychosocial stressors, and level of functioning. Also, screens for several adolescent psychiatric disorders are provided. The authors have developed a DSM-IV-TR version of the ADI (ADI-R). Evidence that support the interview's psychometric properties have been reported (131, 147,148). A second substance use disorder-focused interview is the Customary Drinking and Drug Use Record (132). The Customary Drinking and Drug Use Record measures alcohol and other drug use consumption, DSM-IV-TR substance dependence symptoms (including a detailed assessment of withdrawal symptoms), and several types of consequences of drug involvement. There are both lifetime and prior 2 years versions of the Customary Drinking and Drug Use Record. Psychometric studies provide supporting evidence for this instrument's reliability and validity (132). The third instrument in this subgroup is the Global Ascertainment of Individual Needs (135). This semistructured interview covers recent and lifetime functioning in several areas, including substance use, legal and school functioning, and psychiatric symptoms. Very favorable reliability and validity data are associated with the Global Ascertainment of Individual Needs, including data for the substance use disorders section when administered to a treatment-seeking adolescent population (149,150).

Problem-Focused Interviews The second major group of comprehensive instruments—problem-focused interviews—measure several problem areas associated with adolescent drug involvement, but do not provide a means to obtain a formal diagnosis of a substance use disorder. The interviews summarized here are adapted from the well-known adult tool, the Addiction Severity Index (151). Thus, these interviews assess drug use history and related consequences, as well as several functioning difficulties often experienced by drug-abusing adolescents.

The Comprehensive Adolescent Severity Inventory (136) measures education, substance use, use of free time, leisure activities, peer relationships, family (including family history and intrafamilial abuse), psychiatric status, and legal history. At the end of several major topics, space is provided for the assessor's comments, severity ratings, and quality ratings of the respondent's answers. An interesting feature of this interview is that it incorporates results from a urine drug screen and observations from the assessor. Psychometric studies on the Comprehensive Adolescent Severity Inventory support the instrument's reliability and validity (136). The other Addiction Severity Index–adapted interview of note is the Teen Severity Index (137). The Teen Severity Index consists of seven content areas: chemical use, school status, employment-support status, family relationships, legal status, peer-social relationships, and psychiatric status. A medical status section was not included because it was deemed to be less relevant to adolescent drug abusers. Adolescent and interviewer severity ratings are elicited on a 5-point scale for each of the content areas. Psychometric data indicate favorable interrater agreement and validity evidence (152). Kaminer has also developed a health service utilization tool that compliments the Teen Severity Index, named the Teen Treatment Services Review (153). This interview examines the type and number of services that the youth received during the treatment episode.

Multiscale Questionnaires The third group of comprehensive instruments consists of the self-administered multiscale questionnaires. These instruments range considerably in terms of length; some can be administered in <20 minutes, whereas others may take a full hour to administer. Yet, as a group, many of them share several characteristics: measures of both drug use problem severity and psychosocial risk factors are provided; strategies are included for detecting response distortion tendencies; the scales are standardized to a clinical sample; and the option of computer administration and scoring are available. Four examples of instruments in this group are briefly summarized. The Adolescent Self-Assessment Profile was developed on the basis of a series of multivariate research studies by Wanberg (138). The 225-item instrument provides an in-depth assessment of drug involvement, including drug use frequency, drug use consequences and benefits, and major risk factors associated with such involvement (e.g., deviance, peer influence). Supplemental scales, which are based on common factors found within the specific psychosocial and problem severity domains, can be scored as well. Extensive reliability and validity data based on several normative groups are provided in the manual. The Hilson Adolescent Profile (139), a 310-item questionnaire (true/false), has 16 scales, 2 of which measure alcohol and drug use. The other content scales correspond to characteristics found in psychiatric diagnostic categories (e.g., antisocial behavior, depression) and psychosocial problems (e.g., home life conflicts). Normative data have been collected from clinical patients, juvenile offenders, and normal adolescents (139). Another true/false questionnaire is the 108-item Juvenile Automated Substance Abuse Evaluation. The Juvenile Automated Substance Abuse Evaluation (140) is a computer-assisted instrument that produces a 5-category score, ranging from no use to drug abuse (including a suggested DSM-IV-TR classification), as well as a summary of drug use history, measure of life stress, and a scale for test-taking attitude. The Juvenile Automated Substance Abuse Evaluation has been shown to discriminate clinical groups from nonclinical groups. The Personal Experience Inventory (154) consists of several scales that measure chemical involvement problem severity, psychosocial risk, and response distortion tendencies. Supplemental problem screens measure eating disorders, suicide potential, physical/sexual abuse, and parental history of drug abuse. The scoring program provides a computerized report that includes narratives and standardized scores for each scale, as well as other various clinical information. Normative and psychometric data are available (141,154).

SUMMARY

Drug use is prevalent among American teenagers. The 2006 Monitoring the Future study found that 66.5% of high school seniors had used alcohol in the past year and 31.5% had used marijuana. Nearly half had tried an illicit drug at least once in their lifetime. Even among 8th graders, 33.6% had already tried alcohol and 20.9% reported illicit drug use in their lifetime (1). Not only do youth have the highest prevalence of drug users within its age group compared with older age groups (13), drug use during adolescence greatly increases the likelihood of developing a later addiction (89). To further complicate the issue, adolescent drug use frequently co-occurs with psychologic disorders (14,155), making the assessment process even more complex. Finally, a large proportion of youth use drugs but do not necessarily meet criteria for a SUD, raising the need for accurate assessment tools. Fortunately, the field consists of multiple psychometrically sound screening and comprehensive measures are available to assess not only level of use, but also patterns of use, accompanying drug use behaviors, SUDs, and comorbidity. The continued development of new and improved biologic assays is a welcomed accompaniment to methods of self-report.

Nonetheless, research is needed to fill important measurement gaps. For many instruments, there are no reports of psychometric data on subpopulations of young people defined by age and ethnicity/race, and most measures have not been formally tested to determine their adequacy as a measure of change (156). A good measure of change should meet the condition that its standard error of measurement is sufficiently minimal to permit its use in detecting small to medium change over time (157). As we have already noted, it is unclear whether the distinction between substance abuse and dependence is diagnostically meaningful when applied to adolescents, and there is a need to improve our measurement of individual abuse and dependence criteria for youth given that some criteria appear to have questionable relevance when applied to young people (17). A related unresolved area is the need for more precise identification of related psychosocial problems that may contribute to the onset and maintenance of drug involvement. Many existing tools assess psychosocial risk factors historically, which is not optimal for more precisely understanding which risk factors recently preceded the drug use or are current consequences of it.

ACKNOWLEDGMENT: *The authors wish to acknowledge the National Institute on Drug Abuse (Dr. Winters, DA017492) and the National Institute on Alcohol Abuse and Alcoholism (Dr. Winters, AA14866).*

REFERENCES

1. Johnston LD, O'Malley PM, Bachman JG, et al. *Monitoring the Future national survey results on drug use, 1975–2004. Volume I: secondary school students* (NIH Publication No. 05-5727). Bethesda, MD: National Institute on Drug Abuse, 2005.
2. Winters KC, Lee S. Likelihood of developing an alcohol and cannabis use disorder during youth: Association with recent use and age. *Drug Alcohol Depend* 2008;92:239–247.
3. Jainchill N, Yagelka J, Hawke J, et al. Adolescent admissions to residential drug treatment: HIV risk behaviors pre- and post-treatment. *Psychol Addict Behav* 1999;13(3):163–173.
4. Mackenzie RG. Influence of drug use on adolescent sexual activity. *Adolesc Med State Art Rev* 1993;4(2):417–422.
5. Kaminer Y. *Adolescent substance abuse.* New York: Plenum Publishing Corporation, 1994.
6. Bolognini M, Plancherel B, Laget J, et al. Adolescent's suicide attempts: populations at risk, vulnerability, and substance use. *Subst Use Misuse* 2003;38(11–13):1651–1669.
7. Kokotailo P. Physical health problems associated with adolescent substance abuse. In: Rahdert E, Czechowicz D, eds. *Adolescent drug abuse: clinical assessment and therapeutic interventions.* NIDA Research Monograph No. 156, NIH Publication No. 95-3908. Rockville, MD: National Institute on Drug Abuse, 1995:112–129.
8. Tapert SF, Schweinsburg AD. The human adolescent brain and alcohol use disorders. In: Galanter M, ed. *Recent developments in alcoholism, vol. 17: alcohol problems in adolescents and young adults: epidemiology, neurobiology, prevention, treatment.* New York: Springer, 2005:177–197.
9. King RD, Gaines LS, Lambert EW, et al. The co-occurrence of psychiatric substance use diagnoses in adolescents in different service systems: frequency, recognition, cost, and outcomes. *J Behav Health Serv Res* 2000;27(4):417–430.
10. DAWN (Drug Abuse Warning Network). *1996 DAWN report.* Washington, DC: Substance Abuse and Mental Health Services Administration, 1996.
11. Riggs PD, Davies R. A clinical approach to treatment of depression in adolescents with substance use disorders and conduct disorder. *J Am Acad Child Adolesc Psychiatry* 2002;41:1253–1255.
12. Kandel DB. Stages in adolescent involvement in drug use. *Science* 1975;0:912–914.
13. Substance Abuse and Mental Health Services Administration (SAMHSA) *Results from the 2004 national survey on drug use and health: national findings* (NDSDUH Series H-28, DHHS Publication No. SMA 05-4062). Rockville, MD: Office of Applied Studies, 2005.
14. Clark D, Winters KC. Measuring risks and outcomes in substance use disorders prevention research. *J Consult Clin Psychol* 2002;70: 1207–1223.
15. American Psychiatric Association. *Diagnostic and statistical manual of mental disorders*, 4th ed. Washington, DC: APA, 1994.
16. Winters KC, Leitten W, Wagner E, et al. Use of brief interventions in a middle and high school setting. *J School Health* 2007;77:196–206.
17. Martin CS, Winters KC. Diagnosis and assessment of alcohol use disorders among adolescents. *Alcohol Health Res World* 1998;22(2):95–105.
18. Giedd J. Structural magnetic resonance imaging of the adolescent brain. In: Dahl RE, Spear LP, eds. *Adolescent brain development: vulnerabilities and opportunities.* New York: New York Academy of Sciences, 2004: 77–85.
19. Spear LP. The adolescent brain and age-related behavioral manifestations. *Neurosci Biobehav Rev* 2000;24:417–463.
20. Varlinskaya EI, Spear LP. Acute effects of ethanol on social behavior and adults rats: role of familiarity of the test situation. *Alcohol Clin Exp Res* 2002;26:1502–1511.
21. Markwiese BJ, Acheson SK, Levin ED, et al. Differential effects of ethanol on memory in adolescent and adults rats. *Alcohol Clin Exp Res* 1998;22:416–421.
22. Opland E, Winters KC, Stinchfield R. Examining gender differences in drug-abusing adolescents. *Psychol Addict Behav* 1995;9:167–175.
23. Noam GG, Houlihan J. Developmental dimensions of DSM-III diagnoses in adolescent psychiatric patients. *Am J Orthopsychiatry* 1990;60: 371–378.
24. Erikson EH. *Identity, youth and crisis.* New York: Norton, 1968.
25. Lewinsohn PM. Rohde P, Seeley JR. Alcohol consumption in high school adolescents: frequency of use and dimensional structure of associated problems. *Addiction* 1996;91:375–390.
26. Cady M, Winters KC, Jordan DA, et al. Measuring treatment readiness for adolescent drug abusers. *J Child Adolesc Subst Abuse* 1996;5:73–91.
27. Sobell LC, Sobell MB. Time-line follow-back: a technique for assessing self-reported alcohol consumption. In: Litten RZ, Allen JP, eds. *Measuring alcohol consumption.* Totowa, NJ: Humana Press, 1992:73–98.
28. Williams RJ, Chang SY. Addiction Centre Adolescent Research Group. A comprehensive and comparative review of adolescent substance abuse treatment outcome. *Clin Psychol Sci Practice* 2000;7:138–166.
29. Dillon F, Turner C, Robbins M, et al. Concordance among biological, interview, and self-report measures of drug use among African American and Hispanic adolescents referred for drug abuse treatment. *Psychol Addict Med* 2005;19(4):404–413.
30. Sarrazin MS, Hall JA, Richards C, et al. The comparison of computer-based versus pencil-and-paper assessment of drug use. *Res Social Work Practice* 2002;12(5):669–683.
31. Stone A, Latimer W. Adolescent substance use assessment: concordance between tools using self-administered and interview formats. *Subst Use Misuse* 2005;40:1865–1874.
32. Stinchfield RD. Reliability of adolescent self-reported pretreatment alcohol and other drug use. *Subst Use Misuse* 1997;32:63–76.
33. Williams R, Nowatzki N. Validity of adolescent self-report of substance use. *Subst Use Misuse* 2005;40:299–311.
34. Harrison LD. The validity of self-reported data on drug use. *J Drug Issues* 1995;25:91–111.
35. Dolan K, Rouen D, Kimber J. An overview of the use of urine, hair, sweat, and saliva to detect drug use. *Drug Alcohol Rev* 2004;23:213–217.
36. Johnston LD, O'Malley PM. The recanting of earlier reported drug use by young adults. *NIDA Res Monogr* 1997;167:59–80.
37. Maisto SA, Connors GJ, Allen JP. Contrasting self-report screens for alcohol problems: a review. *Alcohol Clin Exp Res* 1995;19:1510–1516.
38. Winters KC, Anderson N, Bengston P, et al. Development of a parent questionnaire for the assessment of adolescent drug abuse. *J Psychoactive Drugs* 2000;32:3–13.
39. Winters KC, Stinchfield RD, Henly GA, et al. Validity of adolescent self report of substance involvement. *Int J Addict* 1990–1991;25:1379–1395.
40. Kidwell DA, Blank DL. Environmental exposure: the stumbling block of hair testing. In: Kintz P, ed. *Drug testing in hair.* Boca Raton: CRC Press, 1996:17–68.
41. Rohrich J, Zorntlein S, Pötsch L, et al. Effect of the shampoo Ultra Clean on drug concentrations. *Int J Legal Med* 2000;113:102–106.

42. Substance Abuse and Mental Health Services Administration (SAMHSA). *Simple screening for infectious diseases and drug abuse (Treatment Improvement Protocol Series # 11)*. Rockville, MD: Center for Substance Abuse Treatment, 1994.
43. World Health Organization. *The ICD-10 classification of mental and behavioural disorder: diagnostic criteria for research,* 10th rev. Geneva: World Health Organization, 1992.
44. Brown SA. Drug expectancies and addictive behavior change. *Exp Clin Psychopharmacol* 1993;1:55–67.
45. Schulenberg J, O'Malley PM, Bachman JG, et al. Getting drunk and growing up: trajectories of frequent binge drinking during the transition to young adulthood. *J Stud Alcohol* 1996;57:289–304.
46. Maisto SA, Polloc, NK, Lynch KG, et al. Course of functioning in adolescents 1-year after alcohol and other drug treatment. *Psychol Addict Behav* 2001;15:68–76.
47. Kelly JF, Myers MG, Brown SA. A multivariate process model of adolescent 12-step attendance and substance use outcome following inpatient treatment. *Psychol Addict Behav* 2000;4:376–389.
48. Grella C, Hser Y-I, Joshi V, et al. Drug treatment outcomes for adolescents with comorbid mental and substance use disorders. *J Nervous Mental Dis* 2001;189:384–392.
49. Winters KC, Stinchfield RD, Latimer WW, et al. Long-term outcome of substance dependent youth following 12-step treatment. *J Subst Abuse Treat* 2007;33:61–69.
50. Hser Y-I, Grella CE, Hubbard RL, et al. An evaluation of drug treatments for adolescents in 4 US cities. *Arch Gen Psychiatry* 2001;58(7): 689–695.
51. Liddle HA, Dakof GA. Family-based treatment for adolescent drug use: state of the science. In: Rahdert E, Czechowicz D, eds. *Adolescent drug abuse: clinical assessment and therapeutic interventions.* Rockville, MD: National Institute on Drug Abuse, 1995:218–254.
52. Winters KC, Stinchfield RD, Opland E, et al. The effectiveness of the Minnesota Model for treating adolescent drug abusers. *Addiction* 2000;95:601–612.
53. Winters KC, Stinchfield RD, Latimer WW, et al. Long-term outcome of substance dependent youth following 12-Step treatment. *J Subst Abuse Treatment,* 2007;33:61–69.
54. Winters KC, Lee S, Stinchfield RD, et al. Psychosocial factors associated with long-term outcome of drug-abusing youth following 12-Step treatment. *Substance Abuse.* In press.
55. Myers MG, Brown SA, Mott MA. Coping as a predictor of adolescent substance abuse treatment outcome. *J Substance Abuse* 1993;5:15–29.
56. Latimer WW, Winters KC, Stinchfield RD, et al. Demographic, individual and interpersonal predictors of adolescent alcohol and marijuana use following treatment. Psychol Addict Behav 2000;14:162–173.
57. Chilcoat H, Breslau N. Pathways from ADHD to early drug use. *J Am Acad Child Adolesc Psychiatry* 1999;38(11):1347–1354.
58. Farrell AD, Danish SJ. Peer drug associations and emotional restraint: Causes and consequences of adolescents' drug use? *J Consult Clin Psychol* 1993;61:327–334.
59. Winters KC, Latimer WW, Stinchfield RD, et al. Examining psychosocial correlates of drug involvement among drug clinic-referred youth. *J Child Adolesc Subst Abuse* 1999;9(1):1–17.
60. Guo J, Hill KG, Hawkins JD, et al. A developmental analysis of sociodemographic, family, and peer effects on adolescent illicit drug initiation. *J Am Acad Child Adolesc Psychiatry* 2002;41:838–845.
61. Dishion TJ, Capaldi D, Spracklen KM, et al. Peer ecology and male adolescent drug use. *Development Psychopathol* 1995;7:803–824.
62. Hawkins JD, Catalano RF, Miller JY. Risk and protective factors for alcohol and other drug problems in adolescence and early adulthood: implications for substance abuse prevention. *Psychol Bull* 1992;112: 64–105.
63. Patterson GR, Forgatch MS, Yoerger KL, et al. Variables that initiate and maintain an early-onset trajectory for juvenile offending. *Development Psychopathol* 1998;10:531–548.
64. McGue M. Behavioral genetics models of alcoholism and drinking. In: Leonard KE, Blane HT, eds. *Psychological theories of drinking and alcoholism,* 2nd ed. New York: Guilford, 1999:372–421.
65. Clark DB, Moss H, Kirisci L, et al. Psychopathology in preadolescent sons of substance abusers. *J Am Acad Child Adolesc Psychiatry* 1997;36: 495–502.
66. Earls F, Reich W, Jung KG, et al. Psychopathology in children of alcoholic and antisocial parents. *Alcohol Clin Exp Res* 1988;12:481–487.
67. Hill SY, Muka D. Childhood psychopathology in children from families of alcoholic female probands. *J Am Acad Child Adolesc Psychiatry* 1996; 31:1024–1030.
68. Zucker RA, Fitzgerald HE, Moses HD. Emergence of alcohol problems and the several alcoholisms: a developmental perspective on etiologic theory and life course trajectory. In: Cicchetti, Cohen DJ, eds. *Developmental psychopathology vol. 2: risk, disorder, and adaptation.* New York: Wiley, 1995:677–711.
69. Heath AC, Martin NG. Teenage alcohol use in the Australian twin register: genetic and social determinants of starting to drink. *Alcohol Clin Exp Res* 1988;12:735–741.
70. Iacono WG, Carlson SR, Taylor J, et al. Behavioral disinhibition and the development of substance-use disorders: findings from the Minnesota Twin Family Study. *Development Psychopathol* 1999;11(4): 869–900.
71. Koopmans JR, Boomsma DI. Familial resemblances in alcohol use: genetic or cultural transmission? *J Stud Alcohol* 1996;57:19–28.
72. Rose RJ, Dick DM, Viken RJ, et al. Drinking or abstaining at age 14? A genetic epidemiological study. *Alcohol Clin Exp Res* 2001;25: 1594–1604.
73. Clark DB, Thatcher DL, Maisto SA. Supervisory neglect and adolescent alcohol use disorders: effects on AOD onset and treatment outcome. *Addict Behav* 2005;30(9):1737–1750.
74. Kandel DB. Parenting styles, drug use, and children's adjustment in families of young adults. *J Marr Family* 1990;52(1):183–196.
75. Cleveland MJ, Gibbons FX, Gerrard M, et al. The impact of parenting on risk cognitions and risk behavior: a study of mediation and moderation in a panel of African American adolescents. *Child Develop* 2005; 76(4):900–916.
76. Dishion TJ, Patterson G R, Reid JR. Parent and peer factors associated with drug sampling in early adolescence. In: Rahdert ER, Grabowski J, eds. *Adolescent drug abuse: analyses of treatment research.* Rockville, MD: National Institute on Drug Abuse, 1988.
77. Kosterman R, Hawkins J, Guo J, et al. The dynamics of alcohol and marijuana initiation: patterns and predictors of first use in adolescence. *Am J Public Health* 2000;90:360–366.
78. Patock-Peckham JA, Cheong J, Balhorn ME, et al. A social learning perspective: a model of parenting styles, self-regulation, perceived drinking control, and alcohol use and problems. *Alcohol Clin Exp Res* 2001;25: 1284–1292.
79. Zucker RA, Noll RA. The interaction of child and environment in the early development of drug involvement: a far ranging review and a planned very early intervention. *Drugs Society* 1987;1:57–97.
80. Shaffer HJ. The psychology of change. In: Lowinson J, Ruiz P, Millman RB, et al., eds. *Substance abuse: a comprehensive textbook.* Baltimore, MD: Williams & Wilkins, 1997:100–106.
81. Petraitis J, Flay BR, Miller TQ. Reviewing theories of adolescent substance abuse: organizing pieces in the puzzle. *Psychol Bull* 1995;117: 67–86.
82. Henly GA, Winters KC. Development of problem severity scales for the assessment of adolescent alcohol and drug abuse. *Int J Addict* 1988;23: 65–85.
83. Clark DB, Bukstein OG. Psychopathology in adolescent alcohol abuse and dependence. *Alcohol Health Res World* 1998;22(2):117–121.
84. Kandel DB, Johnson JG, Bird HR, et al. Psychiatric comorbidity among adolescents with substance use disorders: findings from the MECA study. *J Am Acad Child Adolesc Psychiatry* 1999;38(6):693–699.
85. Boys A, Farrell C, Taylor J, et al. Psychiatric morbidity and substance use in young people aged 13–15 years: results from the child and adolescent survey of mental health. *Br J Psychiatry* 2003;182:509–517.
86. Winters KC. Treating adolescents with substance use disorders: an overview of practice issues and treatment outcomes. *Substance Abuse* 1999;20:203–225.

87. Boyle MH, Offord DR, Racine YA, et al. Predicting substance use in late adolescence: results of the Ontario Child Health Study Follow-Up. *Am J Psychiatry* 1992;149:761–767.
88. Clark DB, Parker A, Lynch K. Psychopathology and substance-related problems during early adolescence: a survival analysis. *J Clin Child Psychol* 1999;28:333–341.
89. Clark DB, Kirisci L, Moss HB. Early adolescent gateway drug use in sons of fathers with substance use disorders. *Addict Behav* 1998;23(4):561–566.
90. Donovan JE, Jesso, R. Structure of problem behavior in adolescence and young adulthood. *J Consult Clin Psychol* 1985;53(6):890–904.
91. Barkley RA, Fischer M, Smallish L, et al. Young adult follow-up of hyperactive children: antisocial activities and drug use. *J Child Psychol Psychiatry* 2004;45:195–211.
92. Mannuzza S, Klein RG, Bessler A, et al. Adult outcome of hyperactive boys' educational achievement, occupational rank, and psychiatric status. *Arch Gen Psychiatry* 1993;50:565–576.
93. Milberger S, Biederman J, Faraone SV, et al. ADHD is associated with early initiation of cigarette smoking in children and adolescents. *J Am Acad Child Adolesc Psychiatry* 1997;36:37–44.
94. Biederman J, Wilens T, Mick E, et al. Is ADHD a risk factor for psychoactive substance use disorders? Findings from a four-year prospective follow-up study. *J Am Acad Child Adolesc Psychiatry* 1997;36:21–29.
95. Hechtman L, Weiss G. Controlled prospective fifteen-year follow-up of hyperactives as adults: non-medical drug and alcohol use and anti-social behavior. *Can J Psychiatry* 1986;31:557–567.
96. August GJ, Winters KC, Realmuto GM, et al. Prospective longitudinal study of adolescent drug abuse among community samples of ADHD and non-ADHD participants. *J Am Acad Child Adolesc Psychiatry* 2006; 45:824–832.
97. Lynskey MT, Fergusson DM. Childhood conduct problems, attention deficit behaviors, and adolescent alcohol, tobacco, and illicit drug use. *J Abnorm Child Psychol* 1995;23(3):281–302.
98. Thompson LL, Riggs PD, Mikulich SK, et al. Contribution of ADHD symptoms to substance problems and delinquency in conduct-disordered adolescents. *J Abnorm Child Psychol* 1996;24(3):325–347.
99. Burke JD, Loeber R, Lahey BB. Which aspects of ADHD are associated with tobacco use in early adolescence? *J Child Psychol Psychiatry* 2001;42: 493–502.
100. Molina BSG, Smith BH, Pelham WE. Interactive effects of attention deficit hyperactivity disorder and conduct disorder on early adolescent substance use. *Psychol Addict Behav* 1999;13:348–358.
101. Clark DB, Sayette M. Anxiety and the development of alcoholism: clinical and scientific issues. *Am J Addict* 1993;2:59–76.
102. Clark DB, Miller TW. Stress adaptation in children: theoretical models. In: Miller TW, ed. *Stressful life events: children and trauma.* Madison, CT: International Universities Press, 1998:3–27.
103. Deykin EY, Levy JC, Wells V. Adolescent depression, alcohol and drug abuse. *Am J Public Health* 1987;77:178–182.
104. Martin CS, Lynch KG, Pollock NK, et al. Gender differences and similarities in the personality correlates of adolescent alcohol problems. *Psychol Addict Behav* 2000;14:121–133.
105. Schuckit MA, Hesselbrock V. Alcohol dependence and anxiety disorders: what is the relationship? *Am J Psychiatry* 1994;151:1723–1734.
106. Stewart SH. Alcohol abuse in individuals exposed to trauma: a critical review. *Psychol Bull* 1996;120(1):83–112.
107. Clark DB, Pollock NA, Bromberger JT, et al. Gender and comorbid psychopathology in adolescents with alcohol use disorders. *J Am Acad Child Adolesc Psychiatry* 1997;36(9):1195–1203.
108. Lewinsohn PM, Hops H, Roberts RE, et al. Adolescent psychopathology: 1. Prevalence and incidence of depression and other DSM-III R disorders in high school students. *J Abnormal Psychol* 1993;102: 133–144.
109. Leccese M, Waldron HB. Assessing adolescent substance use: a critique of current measurement instruments. *J Subst Abuse Treatment* 1994;11: 553–563.
110. Winters KC. Adolescent assessment of alcohol and other drug use behaviors. In: Allen JP, Wilson V, eds. *Assessing alcohol problems: a guide for clinicians and researchers,* 2nd ed. Rockville, MD: National Institute on Alcohol Abuse and Alcoholism, 2003.
111. Center for Substance Abuse Treatment. Screening and assessing adolescents for substance use disorders. *Treatment Improvement Protocol (TIP) series #31.* Rockville, MD: Substance Abuse and Mental Health Services Administration, 1999.
112. Allen JP, Colombus M, eds. *Assessing alcohol problems: a guide for clinicians and researchers,* 2nd ed. Rockville, MD: National Institute on Alcohol Abuse and Alcoholism. NIH publication no. 03-3745, 2003. Retrieved February 3, 2006, from http://pubs.niaaa.nih.gov/publications/Assesing%20Alcohol/index.htm.
113. Winters KC, Newcomb M, Fahnhorst T. Substance use disorders In: Hersen, M, ed. *Psychological assessment in clinical practice: a pragmatic guide.* New York: Brunner-Routledge, 2004:393–408.
114. Moberg DP. Screening for alcohol and other drug problems using the Adolescent Alcohol and Drug Involvement Scale (AADIS). Madison, WI: Center for Health Policy and Program Evaluation, University of Wisconsin–Madison, 2003.
115. Harrell A, Wirtz PM. Screening for adolescent problem drinking: validation of a multidimensional instrument for case identification. *Psychol Assessment* 1989;1:61–63.
116. Knight J, Sherritt L, Harris SK, et al. Validity of brief alcohol screening tests among adolescents: a comparison of the AUDIT, POSIT, CAGE, and CRAFFT. *Alcohol Clin Exp Res* 2003;27:67–73.
117. Martino S, Grilo CM, Fehon DC. The development of the drug abuse screening test for adolescents (DAST-A). *Addict Behav* 2000;25: 57–70.
118. Kirisci L, Mezzich A, Tarter R. Norms and sensitivity of the adolescent version of the drug use screening inventory. *Addict Behav* 1995;20: 149–157.
119. Winters KC. Development of an adolescent alcohol and other drug abuse screening scale: personal experience screening questionnaire. *Addict Behav* 1992;17(5):479–490.
120. Latimer WW, Winters KC, Stinchfield RD. Screening for drug abuse among adolescents in clinical and correctional settings using the Problem Oriented Screening Instrument for Teenagers. *Am J Drug Alcohol Abuse* 1997;23:79–98.
121. Rahdert E, ed. *The Adolescent Assessment/Referral System Manual.* Rockville, MD: U.S. Department of Health and Human Services, ADAMHA, National Institute on Drug Abuse, DHHS Pub. No. (ADM) 91-1735, 1991.
122. White HR, Labouvie EW. Towards the assessment of adolescent problem drinking. *J Stud Alcohol* 1989;50:30–37.
123. Miller G. *The Substance Abuse Subtle Screening Inventory—adolescent version.* Bloomington, IN: SASSI Institute, 1985.
124. Knight JR, Sherritt L, Shrier LA, et al. Validity of the CRAFFT substance abuse screening test among adolescent clinic patients. *Arch Adolesc Med* 2002;156:607–614.
125. Risberg RA, Stevens MJ, Graybill DF. Validating the adolescent form of the Substance Abuse Subtle Screening Inventory. *J Child Adolesc Subst Abuse* 1995;4:25–41.
126. Rogers R, Cashel ML, Johansen J, et al. Evaluation of adolescent offenders with substance abuse: validation of the SASSI with conduct-disordered youth. *Crim Justice Behav* 1997;24:114–128.
127. Skinner H. *Development and validation of a lifetime alcohol consumption assessment procedure. Substudy No. 1248.* Toronto: Addiction Research Foundation, 1982.
128. Dembo R, Schmeidler J, Borden P, et al. Use of the POSIT among arrested youths entering a juvenile assessment center: a replication and update. *J Child Adolesc Subst Abuse* 1997;6:19–42.
129. McLaney MA, Del-Boca F, Babor T. A validation study of the Problem Oriented Screening Instrument for Teenagers (POSIT). *J Mental Health U K* 1994;363–376.
130. Tarter RE, Laird SB, Bukstein O, et al. Validation of the adolescent drug use screening inventory: preliminary findings. *Psychol Addict Behav* 1992;6:322–236.
131. Winters KC, Henly GA. *Adolescent diagnostic interview schedule and manual.* Los Angeles: Western Psychological Services, 1993.

132. Brown SA, Myers MG, Lippke L, et al. Psychometric evaluation of the customary drinking and drug use record (CDDR): a measure of adolescent alcohol and drug involvement. *J Stud Alcohol* 1998;59:427–438.
133. Reich W, Shayla JJ, Taibelson C. *The Diagnostic Interview for Children and Adolescents-Revised (DICA-R).* St. Louis, MO: Washington University, 1992.
134. Shaffer D, Fisher P, Dulcan M. The NIMH Diagnostic Interview Schedule for Children (DISC 2.3): description, acceptability, prevalence, and performance in the MECA study. *J Am Acad Child Adolesc Psychiatry* 1996;35:865–877.
135. Dennis ML. *Global Appraisal of Individual Needs (GAIN): administration guide for the GAIN and related measures.* Bloomington, IL: Lighthouse Publications, 1999.
136. Meyers K, McLellan AT, Jaeger JL, et al. The development of the Comprehensive Addiction Severity Index for Adolescents (CASI-A): an interview for assessing multiple problems of adolescents. *J Subst Abuse Treat* 1995;12:181–193.
137. Kaminer Y, Bukstein OG, Tarter TE. The Teen Addiction Severity Index (T-ASI): rationale and reliability. *Int J Addict* 1991;26:219–226.
138. Wanberg K. *Adolescent Self-Assessment Profile (ASAP).* Arvada, CO: Center for Addictions Research and Evaluation, 1992.
139. Inwald RE, Brobst MA, Morissey RF. Identifying and predicting adolescent behavioral problems by using a new profile. *Juvenile Justice Dig* 1986;14:1–9.
140. Ellis BR. *Juvenile Automated Substance Abuse Evaluation (JASAE).* Clarkston, MI: ADE Incorporated, 1987.
141. Winters KC, Stinchfield RD, Henly GA. Convergent and predictive validity of the Personal Experience Inventory. *J Child Adolesc Subst Abuse* 1996;5:37–55.
142. Welner Z, Reich W, Herjanic B, et al. Reliability, validity and parent-child agreement studies of the Diagnostic Interview for Children and Adolescents (DICA). *J Am Acad Child Psychiatry* 1987;26:649–653.
143. Costello EJ, Edelbrock C, Costello AJ. Validity of the NIMH Diagnostic Interview Schedule for Children: a comparison between psychiatric and pediatric referrals. *J Abnorm Child Psychol* 1985;13:570–595.
144. Shaffer D, Schwab-Stone M, Fisher P, et al. Revised version of the Diagnostic Interview Schedule for Children (DISC-R): Preparation, field-testing, and acceptability. *J Am Acad Child Adolesc Psychiatry* 1993; 32:643–650.
145. Shaffer D, Fisher P, Lucas CP, et al. NIMH Diagnostic Interview Schedule for Children Version IV (NIMH DISC-IV): description, differences from previous versions, and reliability of some common diagnoses. *J Am Acad Child Adolesc Psychiatry* 2000;39:28–38.
146. Fisher P, Shaffer D, Piacentini JC, et al. Sensitivity of the Diagnostic Interview Schedule for Children, 2nd edition (DISC-2.1) for specific diagnoses of children and adolescents. *J Am Acad Child Adolesc Psychiatry* 1993;32:666–673.
147. Winters KC, Stinchfield RD, Fulkerson J, et al. Measuring alcohol and cannabis use disorders in an adolescent clinical sample. *Psychol Addict Behav* 1993;7(3):185–196.
148. Winters KC, Latimer W, Stinchfield RD. The DSM-IV criteria for adolescent alcohol and cannabis use disorders. *J Stud Alcohol* 1999;60(3): 337–344.
149. Buchan B, Dennis ML, Tims F, et al. Cannabis use: consistency and validity of self-report, on-site testing & laboratory testing. *Addiction* 2002;97(suppl 1):98–108.
150. Dennis ML, Funk R, Godley SH, et al. Cross-validation of the alcohol and cannabis use measures in the Global Appraisal of Individual Needs (GAIN) and Timeline Followback (TLFB; Form 90) among adolescents in substance abuse treatment. *Addiction* 2004;99(Suppl 2):120–128.
151. McLellan AT, Luborsky L, Woody GE, et al. An improved diagnostic evaluation instrument for substance abuse patients: the Addiction Severity Index. *J Nerv Mental Dis* 1980;186:26–33.
152. Kaminer Y, Wagner E, Plummer B, et al. Validation of the Teen Addiction Severity Index (T-ASI): preliminary findings. *Am J Addiction* 1993;2:221–224.
153. Kaminer Y, Blitz C, Burleson JA, et al. The Teen Treatment Services Review (T-TSR). *J Substance Abuse Treatment* 1998;15:291–300.
154. Winters KC, Henly GA. *Personal experience inventory and manual.* Los Angeles: Western Psychological Services, 1989.
155. Rohde P, Lewinsohn PM, Seely JR. Psychiatric comorbidity with problematic alcohol use in high school students. *J Am Acad Child Adolesc Psychiatry* 1996;35(1):101–109.
156. Stinchfield RD, Winters KC. Measuring change in adolescent drug misuse with the Personal Experience Inventory (PEI). *Subst Use Misuse* 1997;32:63–76.
157. Jacobson N S, Truax P. Clinical significance: a statistical approach to defining meaningful change in psychotherapy research. *J Consult Clin Psychol* 1991;59:12–19.

SUGGESTED READINGS

Donovan DM. Assessment to aid in the treatment planning process. In: Allen J, Colombus M, eds. *Assessing alcohol problems: a guide for clinicians and researchers*, 2nd ed. Rockville, MD: National Institute on Alcohol Abuse and Alcoholism, 2003:125–177.

Grilo CM, Fehon DC, Walker M, et al. A comparison of adolescent inpatients with and without substance abuse using the Millon Adolescent Clinical Inventory. *J Youth Adolesc* 1996;25(3):379–388.

Harrison PA, Fulkerson, JA, Beebe TJ. DSM-IV substance use disorder criteria for adolescents: a critical examination based on a statewide school survey. *Am J Psychiatry* 1998;155:486–492.

Hasin D, Paykin A. Dependence symptoms but no diagnosis: diagnostic orphans in a community sample. *Drug Alcohol Depend* 1998;50:19–26.

Hsieh S, Hollister CD. Examining gender differences in adolescent substance abuse behavior: comparison and implications for treatment. *J Child Adolesc Subst Abuse* 2004;13:53–70.

Kaczynski NA, Martin CS. Diagnostic orphans: adolescents with clinical alcohol symptomology who do not qualify for DSM-IV abuse or dependence diagnosis. Paper presented at the annual meeting of the Research Society on Alcoholism, Steamboat Springs, CO, June 1995.

Kahler C, Read J, Wood M, et al. Social environmental selection as a mediator of gender, ethnic, and personality effects on college student drinking. *Psychol Addict Behav* 2003;17:226–234.

Kaminer Y. Adolescent substance abuse. In: Frances RJ, Miller SI, eds. *The clinical textbook of addictive disorders.* New York: Guilford Press, 1991: 320–346.

Kidwell DA, Lee EH, DeLauder SF. Evidence for bias on hair testing and procedures to correct bias. *Forensic Sci Int* 2000;107:39–61.

Lapham SC, Henley E, Kleyboecker K. Prenatal behavioral risk screening by computer among Native Americans. *Family Med* 199325:197–202.

Martin CS, Kaczynski NA, Maisto SA, et al. Patterns of DSM-IV alcohol abuse and dependence symptoms in adolescent drinkers. *J Studies Alcohol* 1995;56:672–680.

Martin CS, Kaczynski NA, Maisto SA, et al. Polydrug use in adolescent drinkers with and without DSM-IV alcohol abuse and dependence. *Alcohol Clin Exp Res* 1996;20:1099–1108.

Millon T. Classification in psychopathology: rationale, alternatives, and standards. *J Abnorm Psychol* 1991;100(3):245–261.

Moberg DP. Identifying adolescents with alcohol problems: a field test of the Adolescent Alcohol Involvement Scale. *J Stud Alcohol* 1983;44: 701–721.

National Institute on Alcohol Abuse and Alcoholism (NIAAA). *Assessing alcohol problems: a guide for clinicians and researchers.* 2003. NIH publication no. 03-3745. Retrieved February 3, 2006, from http://pubs.niaaa.nih.gov/publications/Assesing%20Alcohol/index.htm.

Newman FL, Ciarlo JA, Carpenter D. Guidelines for selecting psychological instruments for treatment planning and outcome. In: Maruish, ME, ed. *The use of psychological testing and treatment planning for outcomes and assessment,* 2nd ed. Mahwah, NJ: Lawrence Erlbaum Associates, 1999: 153–170.

Pollock NK, Martin CS. Diagnostic orphans: adolescents with alcohol symptoms who do not qualify for DSM-IV abuse or dependence diagnoses. *Am J Psychiatry* 1999;156:897–901.

Pollock NK, Martin CS, Langenbucher JW. Diagnostic concordance of DSM-III, DSM-III-R, DSM-IV, and ICD-10 alcohol diagnoses in adolescents. *J Studies Alcohol* 2000;61(3):439–446.

Reid RW, O'Connor FL, Deakin AG, et al. Cocaine and metabolites in human graying hair: Pigmentary relationship. *J Toxicol Clin Toxicol* 1996;34:685–690.

Sachs H. Theoretical limits of the evaluation of drug concentrations in hair due to irregular hair growth. *Forensic Sci Int* 1995;70:53–61.

Substance Abuse and Mental Health Services Administration (SAMHSA). Youth substance use: state estimates from the 1999 National Household Survey on Drug Abuse. Retrieved December 14, 2005, from www.oas.samhsa.gov/NHSDA/99youthstate/toc.htm.

Tapert SF, Baratta MV, Abrantes AM, et al. Attention dysfunction predicts substance involvement in community youths. *J Am Acad Child Adolesc Psychiatry* 2002;41:680–686.

Tarter RE. Evaluation and treatment of adolescent substance abuse: a decision tree model. *Am J Drug Alcohol Abuse* 1990;16:1–46.

Turner CF, Ku L, Rogers SM, et al. Adolescent sexual behavior, drug use, and violence: increased reporting with computer survey technology. *Science* 1998;280(5365):867–873.

Weinberg NZ, Rahdert E, Collive J, et al. Adolescent substance abuse: a review of the past 10 years. *J Am Acad Child Adolesc Psychiatry* 1998; 37(3):252–261.

Williams JB, Gibbon M, First MB, et al. The Structured Clinical Interview for DSM-III-R (SCID). II. Multisite test-retest reliability. *Arch Gen Psychiatry* 1992;49:630–636.

Willner R. Further validation and development of a screening instrument for the assessment of substance misuse in adolescents. *Addiction* 2000;95: 1691–1698.

CHAPTER 104

Steven L. Jaffe, MD
Ashraf Attalla, MD
Diana I. Simeonova, Dipl-Psych, MA

Adolescent Treatment and Relapse Prevention

Treatment of adolescent substance use disorders involves a number of issues that are quite different from those seen in adults with substance abuse problems. First, the adolescent's biopsychosocial level of development must be considered. For example, it is normal for young adolescents (age 12 to 14 years) to be self-centered, experience mood shifts, and have minimal capacity for introspection. This profile makes therapy with early adolescents very different from the treatment of older adolescents. Second, because adolescents still are developing within a family system, family members must be part of the treatment program. Third, adolescents differ from adults in their patterns of substance use, as adolescents are more apt to use multiple drugs and to use inhalants in early adolescence and club drugs (such as 3,4-methylenedioxymethamphetamine or "Ecstasy," gamma-hydroxybutyrate or GHB, and ketamine) in late adolescence and early adulthood. Fourth, some studies have shown that current comorbidity is more common among adolescents than adults (1), and integrated treatment of the comorbid condition is especially important in adolescents.

After careful evaluation, giving full consideration to the foregoing issues, the physician should make an individualized determination as to the appropriate treatment placement for the substance-involved adolescent. The American Society of Addiction of Medicine has developed placement criteria for adolescent treatment (2) that include the dimensions of treatment readiness, relapse potential, and recovery environment (see Chapter 105, "Placement Criteria and Strategies for Adolescent Treatment Matching").

This chapter describes the treatment approaches most commonly employed in the treatment of adolescents.

TREATMENT MODALITIES

In 1990, Catalano extensively reviewed the literature on adolescent treatment and found that, in residential programs, time in treatment was related to reduced use of alcohol or other drugs. Family participation was associated with better outcome. No treatment modality was significantly better than any other. Catalano could only conclude that some treatment was better than no treatment.

Significant progress has been made in adolescent treatment and relapse prevention in the past two decades. The National Institute on Drug Abuse, the National Institute on Alcohol Abuse and Alcoholism, and the Center for Substance Abuse Treatment have increased their support and direction for controlled studies of adolescent treatment, as well as for the development of clinical researchers to study such treatment. The American Academy of Child and Adolescent Psychiatry has published both a 10-year research review (3) and "Practice Parameters for the Assessment and Treatment of Substance Abuse in Children and Adolescents" (4). Better standardized assessment instruments and adolescent-specific outcome measures have been developed.

A number of treatment approaches have been used alone or in various combinations for the treatment of adolescent substance use, abuse, and dependency disorders. A Treatment Improvement Protocol on adolescent treatment, published by the Center for Substance Abuse Treatment (1999), describes the three most commonly employed treatment approaches as family therapy, Twelve Step–based programs, and therapeutic communities. More recently, a systematic review of the literature on evidence-based psychosocial treatments for adolescent substance abuse (5) concluded that three treatment approaches—multidimensional family therapy, functional family therapy, and group cognitive-behavioral therapy—emerge as well-established models for treatment of this population. The researchers also pointed out that none of the treatment approaches appeared clearly superior and that other therapeutic modalities were efficacious as well. These and other important modalities are reviewed below.

FAMILY THERAPY

Family therapy is the most studied modality in adolescent substance abuse treatment (6). Classic family therapy is based on the hypothesis that there is a connection between family relationships and the development or maintenance of drug abuse. Family therapy targets these specific interpersonal family processes. With structural-strategic family therapy, emphasis is on establishing a coherent family hierarchy, with appropriate rules and authority. Lewis combined a number of different family therapy models to develop a 12-session treatment called the Purdue Model, the goals of which were to decrease family resistance to treatment, to redefine substance use as a family problem, to reestablish parental influence, to interrupt dysfunctional sequences of family behavior, to assess the interpersonal function of the drug abuse, to implement strategies to change family interpersonal functioning, and to provide assertiveness training to the adolescent (7). Families who received this treatment model were found to have significantly decreased adolescent drug abuse compared with families that received parent skill training.

Multidimensional Family Therapy Liddle's multidimensional family therapy (MDFT) has established the most empiric support for efficacy. MDFT is an outpatient family-based treatment that combines substance abuse treatment with multiple system assessments and interventions within the family and the surrounding psychosocial environment. In a randomized clinical trail with 182 marijuana- and alcohol-abusing adolescents, MDFT showed superior improvement among patients compared with a multifamily educational intervention and adolescent group therapy. The treatment improvement was maintained during 6- and 12-month follow-up assessments. At 12 months' follow-up, 45% of MDFT patients reported clinically significant reduction in drug use, compared with 32% and 26% in the adolescent group therapy and the multifamily educational intervention conditions, respectively. Further, at 12 months' follow-up, the MDFT patients demonstrated significantly improved social functioning, as demonstrated by improved academic achievement and family functioning (8).

Brief Strategic Family Therapy This is a manualized family therapy structural-strategic approach developed for Hispanic families with behavior problem youth. A recent randomized trial of 126 youths compared brief strategic family therapy to group therapy (9). Brief strategic family therapy treatment resulted in significant reduction of self-reported marijuana use, and parent-reported conduct problems. Brief strategic family therapy was also more efficacious than group therapy in improving family functioning.

Multisystemic Therapy Henggeler's multisystemic therapy (MST) integrates family therapy with direct interventions in the multiple interacting systems involving the individual, school, peer group, and community. This treatment approach promotes responsible behavior among all family members, and attempts to develop each individual's capacity to manage his or her own problems. Therapists work intensively with each adolescent and family in the home, school, and even neighborhood peer group. MST has demonstrated excellent retention rates and favorable outcomes (10). A randomized clinical trail of 118 juvenile offenders with a diagnosis of substance abuse or dependence, examined MST compared with community service provided through the local office of the state substance abuse commission (11). MST significantly reduced substance use at post-treatment, but the effect was not found at 6- or 12-month follow-up assessments. The total days of out-of-home placement for patients in the MST condition was reduced by 50% at 6-month follow-up compared with patients in the community treatment condition. Henggeler et al. conducted a 4-year follow-up assessment of 80 patients participating in this clinical trail (12). In this study, the findings regarding substance use were mixed, with biologic measures indicating 55% of MST participants to be abstinent compared with 28% of participants in the community treatment condition. However, self-report outcome measures of substance use did not differentiate between treatment conditions. There was a significant decrease of aggressive behavior by the MST. Another study suggested that integrating MST into juvenile drug court improved substance abuse outcomes (13). MST is also integrating Contingency Management to try to improve results.

Functional Family Therapy Functional family therapy integrates behavioral and cognitive interventions with ecological family relationship strategies. A recent study showed functional family therapy and functional family therapy with cognitive-behavioral therapy (CBT0 to be efficacious at 4 months compared with individual CBT or group psychoeducational therapy (14).

Behavioral Family Therapy Azrin combined family therapy with behavior therapy such that parents reinforced drug-incompatible activities, supervised home urge control assignments, and employed written specifications of desired behaviors with contingent reinforcers (15). Abstinence rates at 6 months were 73%, whereas the control group of supportive counseling was only 9%. A more recent study showed equal efficacy to cognitive problem-solving therapy (16).

COGNITIVE-BEHAVIORAL THERAPY

This therapeutic modality combines the learning principles of classical and operant conditioning with approaches to correct cognitive distortions and underlying negative belief systems. Treatment involves teaching the adolescent specific techniques to deal with drugs and alcohol. Specific skills to refuse alcohol and drugs are taught and practiced in role-playing exercises. For example, the adolescent is taught to immediately say "no" in a firm manner, making direct eye contract with the person who offers alcohol or drugs. They are then to suggest an alternative activity or, if that is not successful, to simply tell the person to stop asking.

Cognitive-behavioral coping skills to deal with urges, to manage thoughts of alcohol or drug use, and to handle emergencies and lapses are taught and practiced. Because deficits in coping skills for negative feelings and life stresses contribute to continued substance use, more general coping strategies (such as communication skills, problem-solving strategies, anger and mood management, and relaxation training) also are taught and practiced.

A number of randomized clinical trials provide empirical support for the efficacy of CBT in the treatment of adolescents with substance use disorders. Kaminer et al. compared CBT group therapy with interactional group therapy in adolescents with co-occurring substance use and psychiatric disorders (17). CBT demonstrated a decrease in severity of substance use, but did not produce better results than interactional group therapy at 15-month follow-up. In another study, a randomized clinical trial of 88 predominantly dually diagnosed adolescents compared the treatment efficacy of CBT versus psychoeducational therapy (18). Patients were assigned to one of the two 8-week outpatient group psychotherapy conditions and were assessed at 3 and 9 months' follow-up. Older youth and male participants in the CBT condition showed significantly lower rate of positive urine drug screens than did psychoeducational therapy participants at 3 months' follow-up. Also, self-report decline of substance use was reported from baseline to 3 and to 9 months' follow-up regardless of treatment condition.

Findings from the Cannabis Youth Treatment study provide support for both group and individual CBT interventions for adolescents with substance use disorders (19). Six hundred predominantly white, male cannabis users (average age 16 years) participated in two multisite interrelated randomized clinical trails. The five interventions were: 5 sessions of motivational enhancement therapy plus CBT (MET/CBT5), 12 sessions of MET and CBT (MET/CBT12), family support network), adolescent community reinforcement approach, and MDFT. The main outcome measures were days of abstinence and percent of adolescents in recovery as demonstrated by no use or abuse/dependence problems and living in the community. All Cannabis Youth Treatment interventions across both trials and all four sites produced significant reductions of cannabis use and negative consequences of use from pretreatment to 3 months' follow-up. The treatment gains were sustained through the 12 months' follow-up. Despite the considerable support for family therapy interventions in this population, the MDFT treatment in the second trail did not produce superior outcomes compared with the individual (adolescent community reinforcement approach) and individual/group (MET/CBT5) interventions. The most cost-effective interventions were MET/CBT5 and MET/CBT12 in the first trial and adolescent community reinforcement approach and MET/CBT5 in the second trial. The best predictor of long-term outcome was initial level of change (19).

TWELVE STEP APPROACHES

Although Twelve Step–based treatment is one of the most common treatment models for adolescents, there has been little research into its efficacy.

The Twelve Steps guide changes in actions, thoughts, feelings, and beliefs that an individual slowly undergoes to establish a state of recovery and abstinence from alcohol. Because a person/patient with an addiction disorder cannot use alcohol and drugs in moderation, abstinence is the necessary goal. Working the Twelve Steps is an extremely concrete process that does not require abstract thinking.

The following descriptions present the first five steps, modified to make them meaningful for adolescents (20).

Step 1 "We admitted we were powerless over alcohol—that our lives had become unmanageable." For adolescents, the workbook has the adolescent examine in detail the negative consequences of their alcohol/drug use. Putting their own and others lives in danger, effects on family, school, work, mood, and self-esteem in relationship to alcohol/drug use are explored. The major issue is whether drugs and alcohol are destroying their lives such that they need to stop using to make their lives better. Although many adult programs emphasize the concept of "surrendering" and admitting one is an "addict," these are not useful for adolescents. Rather, enhancing power by doing what one needs to do (such as stop using alcohol and drugs) instead of doing what one wants to do (use alcohol and drugs) is emphasized.

Step 2 "We come to believe that a power greater than ourselves could restore us to sanity." The adolescent workbook approaches this step by recognizing that a child's first Higher Power is the person that raises them. For many drug-abusing/addicted adolescents, their parental figures were neglectful or abusive. Mourning the pain and sadness from the disappointments of their childhood higher powers enables them to begin to develop a sense of something positive in the universe that they can turn to for help. The Higher Power concept is not a religious belief, but a spiritual feeling that one can trust something positive (for example, the group, another person, or nature) to take care of those aspects of one's life that one cannot control. One needs to have trust in the stability of the world and realize one controls one's own behavior, but not what others say or do. For many adolescents, the concrete positive feelings of their relationships to other members become the first Higher Power.

Step 3 "We make a decision to turn our will and our lives over to the care of God as we understand Him." The adolescent workbook interprets this step to involve having the adolescents make a decision to commit themselves to working the Steps and having a positive spiritual power. The teenagers are helped to recognize that they turned over their lives to alcohol and drugs. Now they are being asked to turn their lives over to a positive program.

Step 4 "We made a searching and fearless moral inventory of ourselves." The workbook has the adolescents answer numerous detailed questions covering all aspects of their childhood and present life.

Step 5 "We admitted to God, to ourselves, and to another human being the exact nature of our wrongs." In this step, the adolescent verbalizes an inventory to a counselor or a sponsor.

Twelve Step programs also provide the opportunity to attend free Alcoholics Anonymous or Narcotics Anonymous meetings, which are conducted several times a day in almost every city and town in the United States and most other countries. It is well recognized that adolescents will return to using alcohol and drugs if they return to contact with their alcohol-or drug-using friends. Twelve Step programs provide the opportunity of a recovering peer group. Twelve Step programs also provide mentoring relationships in the form of sponsors. An older member with at least a year of sobriety, the sponsor provides support and guidance on how to work the program to achieve sobriety. Twelve Step programs accept the concept of addiction as a chronic progressive disorder that renders the "addict" unable to control and moderate his or her drinking or drug use. The only viable alternative is complete abstinence (21). For many adolescents, it may be helpful to view themselves as "on the way to becoming an addict," if they do not see themselves as already being one.

Although research on Twelve Step adolescent programs has been sparse, a Comprehensive Assessment and Treatment Outcome Research program (CATOR) residential treatment follow-up study found that teenagers who attended two or more meetings per week were almost six times more likely to report abstinence at 1 year than were those who never attended (22). A study by Winters used improved methodology with a high follow-up contact rate and meaningful comparison groups (23). At 12-month follow-up, those adolescents who completed Twelve Step–based treatment had an abstinence/minor relapse rate of 53%, compared with 27% of those who needed, but did not receive treatment. A recent study of 99 adolescents and Twelve Step attendance following inpatient treatment demonstrated that Alcoholics Anonymous/Narcotics Anonymous attendance was uniquely associated with improved outcome (24). One third were completely abstinent during the first and second 3-month intervals and there was a dramatic reduction in substance involvement with the sample as a whole being abstinent on 82% of the days. The major mechanism identified was that Twelve Step attendance maintained and enhanced motivation for abstinence.

THERAPEUTIC COMMUNITIES

Therapeutic communities (TC) offer long-term treatment (12 to 18 months) to adolescents who have multiple severe problems. In the TC approach, the community itself is part of the treatment process. Residents move through stages of increasing responsibility and privileges. Work, education, group activities, seminars, meals, job functions, and formal and informal interactions with peers and staff form the basis of self-development. The presence of staff members who are themselves in recovery and family involvement are important aspects of TCs.

An outcome study found that 31% of adolescents completed the residential phase of treatment in a TC, whereas 52% dropped out. Treatment completers at 1 year posttreatment had more positive outcomes than those who did not complete treatment, as measured by a reduction in substance use and decreased criminal activity. A recent study examined associations of a multidimensional measure of TC treatment processes (the Dimensions of Change Instrument) with treatment retention and posttreatment outcome in 397 and 207 adolescents in residential treatment, respectively. Although, contrary to the expectation, the researchers did not find an association between Dimensions of Change Instrument and treatment retention, they found that adolescents who stayed in treatment 90 days or more tended to be more involved in self-help activities at the posttreatment follow-up. These adolescents had increased likelihood of attending Twelve Step meetings and having a Twelve Step sponsor after leaving treatment (25).

MOTIVATIONAL TREATMENT

Prochaska and DiClemente have described a series of stages that mark the progress of an individual toward cessation of alcohol or drug use (26). These stages are designated as *precontemplation,* in which the person has no intent to make change regarding substace use, and has little insight into the hazardous nature of his/her substance use; *contemplation,* which is marked by ambivalence in which the person goes back and forth between reasons to change and reasons not to change; *preparation,* in which the person makes a concrete plan for change; *action,* in which the person reduces or ceases use of the substance; and *maintenance,* in which the person develops a lifestyle to avoid relapse. Individuals exhibit different levels of motivation depending on their stage of change. Therapeutic intervention involves helping the patient in an empathetic, nonconfrontational manner to move along the stages. Brief motivational interventions consist of one to four sessions, after an assessment, in which direct feedback and advice is given in a nonconfrontational manner that respects the person's personal responsibility for making a decision.

Monti has studied the use of a single 45-minute emergency department brief motivational interview for adolescents whose injuries are related to alcohol use (27). Follow-up studies found that the adolescents who were exposed to the interventions subsequently had fewer alcohol-related problems. Additional support for the efficacy of motivational treatment is provided by the results of a 4-year follow-up study within a randomized trail of 363 college freshmen who reported drinking heavily in high school (28). This trial indicated that participants receiving an individual preventative intervention had significantly greater reductions in negative consequences compared with high-risk controls. The participants receiving the intervention were also more likely to improve and less likely to worsen regarding negative drinking consequences over a 4-year period.

Intervention Workbook Both motivational interviewing and Twelve Step facilitation therapy develop motivation in the adolescent to stop using alcohol or other drugs through the adolescent's personal recognition of the negative consequences of such use. Jaffe's *Adolescent substance abuse intervention workbook* engages the adolescent in use of this framework to answer concrete, simple questions that explore 12 areas of the adolescent's life that may have been negatively affected by alcohol or other drugs (29). The workbook also compares unhealthy thinking (such as "drugs are fun") with recovery thinking (for example, "but my life is a mess"). Internal motivation is developed by helping the adolescent to conclude that he or she needs to stop using alcohol or other drugs in order to make life better. A recent study of 56 substance-abusing juvenile delinquents in detention who completed the 2-hour workbook intervention demonstrated an increase in recognition of drug harmfulness especially to marijuana, and belief of harmfulness if continues to use as before (30).

Community Reinforcement Approach and Contingency Management Community reinforcement approach (CRA) is a treatment approach originally developed for adults, in which the individual's life is rearranged so that abstinence is more rewarding than drinking. Contingency management involves concrete immediate positive rewards for a closely monitored behavior that usually involves vouchers for negative urines. CRA usually involves contingency management plus behavioral and CBT protocols and functional analyses of drug use. CRA had positive results in the Cannabis Youth Study (19).

The CRA approach closely resembles the "enthusiastic sobriety" adolescent program developed by Meehan (31). This Twelve Step–based program uses young, energetic, enthusiastic, recovering, well-trained counselors. They are role models who demonstrate that one can have fun without drugs or alcohol. The adolescent is asked to try 30 days without alcohol or other drugs. During this time, the adolescent participates in daily groups, meetings, and social functions with recovering peers who make sobriety more fun and rewarding than using drugs and alcohol.

Pharmacotherapy The use of medications in adolescent substance abuse treatment is just beginning to be studied. Nicotine replacement therapy for nicotine dependency, disulfiram aversion therapy for alcohol dependency, naltrexone as a blocker of opiates or to decrease cravings for alcohol, and methadone/buprenorphine as substitution therapy for opioid dependence are some of the strategies being tried (32). Pharmacotherapy of the comorbid disorders (i.e. attention deficit hyperactivity disorder, posttraumatic stress disorder, anxiety, and affective disorders), has been more extensively studied (33). With adolescents, pharmacologic interventions should always be used with psychosocial treatments.

USING MULTIPLE THERAPIES

No single treatment modality has been demonstrated to be clearly superior. All therapies have a significant percentage of failures. Multiple approaches are being integrated in an attempt to improve outcome. For example, family therapies are combined with MET, CBT, contingency management, and Twelve Step treatments in an effort to increase success.

RELAPSE

The most pressing problem in adolescent substance abuse treatment is the enormous relapse rate regardless of the treatment used. Relapse rates are more than 60% at 3 to 12 months after treatment completion. Thus relapse is common and to be expected. With this in mind, it is important not to allow a lapse (return to alcohol or drug use for a few days) to develop into a full relapse (return to use for weeks or months).

When counseling an adolescent during a lapse, the physician should minimize guilt and shame. The emphasis should be on what the adolescent can learn from the lapse: for example, avoiding high-risk situations such as the company of "using" peers, or seeking out a sponsor for help in dealing with intense thoughts and urges to use.

Jaffe describes four pathways that place recovering teens at risk of relapse (34). The most common is involvement with peers who use alcohol or drugs. Even if the adolescent is committed to sobriety, spending time with using peers becomes too tempting and the teen relapses. A second pathway is the presence of comorbid psychiatric disorders. Adolescents with substance abuse disorders have a high incidence (50% to 90%) of other psychiatric disorders, especially mood, behavior, and anxiety disorders. In this pathway, the teen experiences depression, rage, or panic, and relapses in an effort to deal with those symptoms. A third pathway is denial, in which the recovering adolescent decides that he or she is not an "addict" and can use alcohol or other drugs in moderation. The fourth pathway involves subconsciously arranging one's life to be in proximity to alcohol or other drugs.

A recent development is Assertive Continuing Care where continued contact is the responsibility of the therapist. Monitoring by telephone or home visits involves education, support, and reintervention. A study of postresidential adolescents yielded a 52% abstinent rate for marijuana at 3 months for the Assertive Continuing Care group compared with 32% for the usual continuing care (35).

Most adolescents enter treatment because of the external pressure of their family or the law; therefore, internal motivation for abstinence needs to be developed either by MET or a First Step and this usually needs to be repeated many times during the ensuing years.

Recovering adolescents working a Twelve Step program who relapse need to examine the strength of their program and recognize the need for a solid sponsor, a nonusing peer group, and frequent (two or more each week) attendance at Alcoholics Anonymous/Narcotics Anonymous meetings. All relapsing adolescents should be evaluated for comorbid disorders (such as depression or posttraumatic stress disorder), which may require specific treatment.

CONCLUSIONS

Treatment of adolescents cannot be done without considering the developmental stage the youth is going through. The brain may be more susceptible to the influence of drugs and alcohol. The influence of peers may be greater on adolescents than their adult counterparts. Also, the reliance on families which may be very dysfunctional does not allow the adolescent to separate himself or herself from their influence. All of these circumstances may increase the likelihood of relapse and should be considered when treating adolescents.

REFERENCES

1. Kandel D, Johnson J, Bird H, et al. Psychiatric co-morbidity among adolescents with substance use disorders. Findings from the MECA study. *J Am Acad Child Adolesc Psychiatry* 1999;138(6):693–699.
2. Mee-Lee D, Shulman G, Fishman M, et al. *ASAM patient placement criteria for the treatment of substance-related disorders,* 2nd edition-revised (ASAM PPC-2R). Chevy Chase, MD: American Society of Addiction Medicine, 2001.
3. Weinberg NZ, Randert E, Colliver ID, et al. Adolescent substance abuse: a review of the past ten years. *J Am Acad Child Adolesc Psychiatry* 1998;37:252–261.
4. American Academy of Child and Adolescent Psychiatry (AACAP). Practice parameters for the assessment and treatment of children and adolescents with substance use disorders. *J Am Acad Child Adolesc Psychiatry* 2005;44(6):609–621.
5. Waldron HB, Turner CW. Evidence-based psychosocial treatments for adolescent substance use. *J Am Acad Child Adolesc Psychiatry* 2008;37(1): 238–261.
6. Liddle H. Family-based therapies for adolescent alcohol and drug use: research contributions and future research needs. *Addiction* 2004;99 (Suppl 2):76–92.
7. Lewis RA, Piercy FP, Sprenkle DH, et al. Family based interventions for helping drug abusing adolescents. *J Adolesc Res* 1990;5:82–95.
8. Liddle H, Dakof GA, Parker K, et al. Multidimensional family therapy for adolescent substance abuse: results of a randomized clinical trial. *Am J Drug Alcohol Abuse* 2001;27:651–687.
9. Santisteban DA, Coatsworth JD, Perez-Vidal A, et al. Efficacy of brief strategic family therapy in modifying Hispanic adolescent behavior problems and substance use. *J Family Psychol* 2003;17(1):121–133.
10. Henggeler SW, Pickrel SG, Brondino MJ, et al. Eliminating (almost) treatment dropout of substance abusing and dependent delinquents through home-based multisystemic therapy. *Am J Psychiatry* 1999;153: 427–428.
11. Henggeler SW, Pickrel SG, Brondino MJ. Multisystemic treatment of substance-abusing and -dependent delinquents: outcomes, treatment fidelity, and transportability. *Mental Health Serv Res* 1999;1(3): 171–184.
12. Henggeler SW, Clingempeel WG, Brondino MJ, et al. Four-year follow-up of Multisystemic Therapy with substance-abusing and substance-dependent juvenile offenders. *J Am Acad Child Adolesc Psychiatry* 2002; 41(7):868–874.
13. Saldana L, Henggeler SW. Improving outcomes and transporting evidence-based treatments for youth and families with serious clinical problems. *J Child Adolesc Substance Abuse* 2008;17:1–10.
14. Waldron HR, Slesnick N, Brody JL, et al. Treatment outcomes for adolescent substance abuse at 4- and 7-month assessments. *J Consult Clin Psychol* 2001;69:802–813.
15. Azrin NH, Donohue B, Besale VA. Youth drug abuse treatment: a controlled outcome study. *J Child Adolesc Substance Abuse* 1994;3:1–16.
16. Azrin, NH, Donahue B, Teichner GA, et al. A controlled evaluation and description of individual cognitive problem solving and family behavior therapies in dually-diagnosed conduct disordered and substance dependent youth. *J Child Adolesc Substance Abuse* 2001;11:1–43.
17. Kaminer Y, Burleson J. Psychotherapies for adolescent substance abusers: 15 month follow-up of a pilot study. *Am J Addict* 1999;8:114–119.
18. Kaminer Y, Burleson JA, Goldberger R. Cognitive-behavioral coping skills and psychoeducation therapies for adolescent substance abuse. *J Nerv Mental Dis* 2002;190:737–745.
19. Dennis M, Godley SH, Diamond G, et al. The Cannabis Youth Treatment (CYT) Study: main findings from two randomized trials. *J Substance Abuse Treatment* 2004;27:197–213.
20. Jaffe SL. *Step workbook for adolescent chemical dependency recovery: a guide to the first five steps.* Washington, DC: American Psychiatric Press, Inc., 1990.
21. Humphreys K. Professional interventions that facilitate 12 Step self-help group involvement. *Alcohol Res Health* 1999;23:93–98.
22. Harrison PA, Hoffman NC. CATOR report: adolescent treatment completion one year later. St. Paul, MN: Ramsey Clinic, 1989.
23. Winters KC, ed. *Treatment of adolescents with substance abuse disorder* (Treatment Improvement Protocol No. 32). Rockville. MD: Center for Substance Abuse Treatment, Substance Abuse and Mental Health Services Administration, 1999.
24. Kelly JF, Myers MG, Brown, SA. A multivariate process model of adolescent 12-step attendance and substance use outcome following inpatient treatment. *Psychol Addict Behav* 2000;12(4):376–389.
25. Edelen MO, Tucker JS, Wenzel SL, et al. Treatment process in the therapeutic community: associations with retention and outcomes among adolescent residential clients. *J Substance Abuse Treatment* 2007;32: 415–421.
26. Prochaska JO, DiClemente CC. Transtheoretical therapy: toward a more integrated model of change. *Psychother Theory Res Practice* 1982;19: 276–288.
27. Monti PM, Barnett NP, O'Leary IA, et al. Motivational enhancement for school-involved adolescents. In: Monti PM, Colby SM, O'Leary TA, eds. *Adolescents. Alcohol and substance abuse.* New York: Guilford Press, 2001:145–182.
28. Baer JS, Kivlahan DR, Blume AW, et al. Brief intervention for heavy-drinking college students: 4-year follow-up and natural history. *Am J Public Health* 2001;91(8):1310–1316.
29. Jaffe SL. *Adolescent substance abuse intervention workbook: taking a first step.* Washington, DC: American Psychiatric Press, Inc., 2001.

30. Jaffe SL. Pilot study of two hour workbook intervention for juvenile delinquents with substance abuse. Poster presented at the Annual meeting of the American Academy of Psychiatrists in Addiction, San Diego, CA, 2007.
31. Meehan B. *Beyond the yellow brick road–revised.* Denver: Meehan Publishers, 2000.
32. Upadhyaya U, Deas D. Pharmacological interventions for adolescent substance disorders. In: Kaminer Y, Bukstein OG, eds. *Adolescent substance abuse—psychiatric comorbidity and high-risk behaviors.* New York: Taylor, Francis Group, LLC, 2008.
33. Kaminer Y, Bukstein OG, eds. *Adolescent substance abuse—psychiatric comorbidity and high-risk behaviors.* New York: Taylor, Francis Group, LLC, 2008.
34. Jaffe SL. Pathways to relapse in chemically dependent adolescents. *Adolesc Counselor* 1994;55:42–44.
35. Godley MD, Godley SH, Dennis M, et al. Preliminary outcomes from the assertive continuing care experiment for adolescents discharged from residential treatment. *J Substance Abuse Treatment* 2002;23: 21–32.

CHAPTER 105

Marc Fishman, MD

Placement Criteria and Strategies for Adolescent Treatment Matching

Although the fields of adolescent treatment in general, and adolescent treatment outcomes research in particular, are still in their early stages, recent progress has been considerable. Advances have been made in assessment, appreciation of adolescent-specific treatment needs, and development of particular adolescent treatment modalities and techniques. Over the past two decades, much has been learned about the effectiveness and limitations of current adolescent treatment methods and programs.

Compared with the state of the field before 1990—when the effectiveness of adolescent treatment was largely a matter of clinical anecdote, intuition, and deeply held conviction—treatment for adolescent substance use disorders now has clearly and repeatedly been shown to be effective. Reviews of the published literature have shown favorable outcomes out to 1 year after treatment and beyond, across various modalities and levels of care. These results are further enhanced by favorable comparisons of treatment groups to waiting list controls, substance-specific treatments to nonspecific treatment controls, treatment completers to noncompleters, treatment engagers to nonengagers, and carefully organized research-based treatment to loosely organized "treatment as usual" (1–7).

It also is well established that favorable outcomes in treatment of adolescent substance use (including both abstinence and reductions in substance use short of abstinence) are associated with substantial reductions in adolescent morbidity and improvements in psychosocial function. Such improvements in function extend to school, family, criminal behaviors, psychologic adjustment, and other psychosocial domains (5,8).

Although the research to date on adolescent addiction treatment has been very encouraging, there has been very little comparative examination of the broad range of current treatment modalities, levels of care, and program models. Little is known about the differential effectiveness of various treatment strategies, intensities, and treatment program components (9). Perhaps most important, little empiric work has been done to explore hypotheses of adolescent treatment matching and placement. Nevertheless, questions of which patient should receive what treatment have been the subject of extensive expert consideration, with progressive agreement on fundamental principles and approaches. For example, work with adults consistently shows that assessment-based stratification of severity can predict treatment response (10,11). Using insights such as this, consensus-based "best practices" in the area of adolescent treatment matching and placement are steadily improving.

This chapter provides an introduction to the developing area of adolescent treatment matching and placement, with special attention to one particular placement tool, the adolescent patient placement criteria developed by the American Society of Addiction Medicine (ASAM).

DEVELOPMENTAL CONSIDERATIONS IN ADOLESCENT PLACEMENT

One of the most important advances in the field of adolescent treatment is the articulation of approaches that are developmentally specific to the adolescent population. These respond to the principle that adolescents must be approached differently from adults because of differences in their levels of emotional, cognitive, physical, social, and moral development.

Examples of developmental issues that are fundamental to adolescent assessment and treatment include the extremely potent influence of peers and family. Thus it is critical that adolescent assessments include collateral informants, to augment, and clarify (and, often, correct) the history as presented by the adolescent patient. Such key informants may include family, peers, adult friends or surrogate parent figures, school and court officials, court-appointed special advocates, social service workers, and previous treatment providers.

Adolescents' use of substances frequently impairs their emotional and intellectual growth. Substance use can prevent a young person from completing the maturational tasks of adolescence, which involve formation of personal relationships, acquisition of social skills, psychologic development, identity formation, individuation, education, employment, and family role responsibilities. It is one of the special challenges and unique opportunities of adolescent treatment to modify risk factors that are still actively evolving. Adolescent treatment thus often requires habilitative rather than rehabilitative approaches, emphasizing the acquisition of new capacities, rather than the restoration of lost ones.

Younger adolescents have a very narrow view of the world, with little capacity to think of future implications of present actions. Some adolescents may adopt a pseudomature ("streetwise") posture, despite their overall immaturity. Adolescents who live in a chaotic family system may have difficulties with normative expectations of behavioral contingency. Adolescents who have various cognitive difficulties may be delayed or impaired in acquiring abstract thinking. Attempts to reason with an adolescent about the long-term health effects of substance use usually are futile because the adolescent is unable to appreciate such long-term consequences.

These and other developmental issues make adolescents particularly vulnerable. They typically require greater amounts of external assistance and support than adult patients, both to protect them from the sequelae of substance use and to engage them in the recovery process. Most have not yet acquired the skills for independent living and, even without the impairments associated with substance use, must rely heavily on the guidance of adults.

In general, for a given degree of severity or functional impairment, adolescents require greater intensity of treatment than adults. This is reflected in clinical practice by a greater tendency to place adolescents in more intensive levels of care.

THE ASAM PATIENT PLACEMENT CRITERIA

The American Society of Addiction Medicine's *ASAM Patient Placement Criteria for the Treatment of Substance-Related Disorders,* 2nd ed. revised (*ASAM PPC-2R*; 12) is a clinical guide that has been widely adopted to assist in matching patients to appropriate treatment settings. It contains separate sets of criteria for adolescents and adults. The criteria, which have undergone evolutionary change and improvement since publication of the first edition in 1991, rest on the concept of enhancing the use of multidimensional assessments in placement decisions by organizing the assessment of the substance-using adolescent into six dimensions, and specifying appropriate placements according to gradations of problem severity within each dimension.

Assessment-Based Treatment Matching and Clinical Appropriateness The ASAM criteria use decision rules to guide placement in specified levels of care, which exist along a continuum. They also attempt to standardize some of the program specifications for each level of care, including some guidelines for minimum staffing levels and general program components. They do not, however, specify these in detail, nor do they attempt to prescribe program models, approaches, or techniques.

Because the elements of assessment in the *PPC-2R* are not concretely operationalized (as they would be, for example, in standardized instruments of known psychometrics), they certainly allow for and require the use of considerable clinical judgment. They are best used as illustrations of underlying principles of matching, rather than as exact prescriptions or rigid rules.

The ASAM criteria also attempt to avoid assumptions regarding length of service and treatment dose. Rather, they provide guidelines in the form of general decision rules for continued service and discharge/transfer, which are applied to the original admission problems in the six assessment dimensions that led to the initial treatment placement. Under these decision rules, a patient should remain at a given level of care as long as the problems that created the need for admission persist (or new problems requiring that level of care emerge). We may eventually develop knowledge about minimal or optimal doses for various modalities or levels of care, but little work has been done in that area.

The principal goal of the ASAM criteria is to facilitate the process of matching patients in need of treatment for substance use disorders with appropriate treatment services and settings to maximize the accessibility, effectiveness, and efficiency of the treatment experience. The principle of matching on which the criteria are based is that of clinical appropriateness, which emphasizes quality and efficiency over cost. The concept of "clinical appropriateness" contrasts with the more familiar concept of "medical necessity," which has become associated with restrictions on utilization. "Medical necessity" has typically been interpreted in terms of avoiding life-threatening imminent danger, and is related primarily to acute medical or psychiatric concerns (Dimensions 1, 2, and 3). In contrast, "clinical appropriateness" conveys the notion that patients should be treated in the most suitable placements, defined by the extent of their problems and priorities in all six of the ASAM assessment dimensions.

The criteria reflect a tension between an attempt to promote a broader continuum of treatment services on the one hand, and an attempt to reflect the real world of treatment service delivery on the other. As a result, the criteria do not articulate some of the innovative sublevels of intensity and treatment settings that should exist (and in some places already do exist). However, even the "limited" continuum of treatment settings described in the criteria is not yet available in most communities.

The reality of limited availability of services is, of course, a major problem, particularly in the treatment of adolescents. One or more of the levels of care may not exist or be accessible in a given community, in either rural or urban settings. Funding limitations and other resource constraints also are barriers to the availability of a needed treatment setting. Even logistic issues such as waiting lists can render a treatment setting unavailable. And the individual variations in programs within the level of care categories might sometimes mean that specific needed treatment services are unavailable even if an available setting meets the criteria more generally.

When the criteria designate a treatment placement that is not available to a given patient, a strategy must be crafted to provide the patient the needed services in another placement or combination of placements, always erring on the side of safety and effectiveness. This may require increasing the intensity of services, usually through placement at a more intensive level of care.

One of the criticisms of previous editions of the criteria has been that it was too heavily oriented toward private sector and managed care environments. All too frequently, the continuum of services described and the range of benefits implied in the criteria are not available to disadvantaged or public sector populations. However, the *ASAM PPC-2R* outlines a full range of treatment services appropriate to the needs of all drug-involved adolescents, whether they are privately insured, publicly insured, underinsured, or uninsured. Although they may not have access to it, many indigent adolescents may need an even broader continuum of services than those with greater resources. In general, adolescents with fewer supports, less resiliency, and lower levels of baseline functioning may need a higher intensity of services and longer lengths of service at all levels of care than do those with the benefits conferred by economic advantage.

One goal of the current edition has been to broaden the scope of the criteria and more explicitly encompass the circumstances of adolescents in the public sector. For example, there are more specific references to adolescents involved in the juvenile justice system, where many adolescents may have had extended periods of enforced abstinence, but usually have not had active treatment. In this context, the ascertainment of severity and treatment needs should not be made by a narrow standard based on recency of use, but rather by a full multidimensional assessment that emphasizes the adolescent's acquisition of recovery skills and capacity for reintegration into the community. Hopefully, active treatment, including the full continuum of care reflected in the *ASAM PPC-2R*, will increasingly become the rule rather than the exception for adolescents involved in the juvenile justice system.

Treatment at every level of care requires coordination of a broad array of interrelated treatment services to respond to the needs of the individual patient. This is sometimes accomplished by direct provision of multiple treatment services, and sometimes by linkages with other service providers, usually through referral. Examples include psychiatric assessment and treatment, medical assessment and treatment, establishment of a primary care medical "home," psychologic or educational testing for learning disorders, special or alternative education services, family therapies, juvenile justice probation and supervision, foster care support services, public benefit coordination or other social service agency interventions, vocational and prevocational training, child care, transportation, and the like. In general, the greater the adolescent's severity, the greater the need for such broad and diverse, adjunctive services. To deliver this array of services, treatment programs at all levels of care should develop active affiliations with programs and agencies that offer other services or levels of care, and should help patients access treatment fluidly across the continuum. Barriers to treatment integration remain a fundamental and profound problem for the field, which are only recently beginning to be addressed, at least partially in response to adoption of the ASAM criteria by state agencies, third-party payers, and treatment providers.

Placement and Treatment Considerations by Assessment Dimension As discussed earlier, the ASAM criteria organize the assessment of the substance-using adolescent into six dimensions and specify appropriate placements according to gradations of problem severity within each dimension (Table 105.1).

Dimension 1: Intoxication and Withdrawal The *PPC-2R* includes expanded details of the Dimension 1 assessment elements with some breakdown by specific drug classes. This highlights the range of intoxication and withdrawal symptoms, which all too often are overlooked in adolescents, and emphasizes the importance of their treatment. Some clinically prominent examples include memory impairment caused by marijuana intoxication, which can persist for many weeks after abstinence (Substance Induced Persistent Amnestic Disorder); sensory disturbance or "flashbacks" caused by hallucinogens, which can persist for weeks to months after abstinence (Substance Induced Perceptual Distortion); and delirium and other states of cognitive disorganization caused by inhalants, which can persist for weeks or more after abstinence. Another very common example is insomnia as a symptom of extended subacute withdrawal from various substances (including marijuana, opioids, and alcohol), which although not typically thought of as a very severe problem, can be a powerful trigger for relapse.

The approach to detoxification services in the ASAM adolescent criteria is different from that used in the adult criteria, where such services are described in a separate, discrete set of

TABLE 105.1 American Society of Addiction Medicine Patient Placement Criteria Assessment Dimensions

Dimension 1. Intoxication and withdrawal potential
Dimension 2. Biomedical conditions and complications
Dimension 3. Emotional, behavioral, and cognitive conditions and complications
Dimension 4. Readiness to change
Dimension 5. Relapse, continued use potential
Dimension 6. Recovery environment

detoxification criteria. Detoxification is integrated into the adolescent criteria because severe physiologic withdrawal and the need for its management are seen less frequently in adolescents than in adults, given typical patterns of use and duration of exposure. Therefore the provision of detoxification as an "unbundled" or stand-alone service is less common and less needed with adolescents. Nevertheless, withdrawal does occur in adolescents and should not be overlooked. In such cases, the provision of services to manage the withdrawal in a setting separate from other treatment services is clinically undesirable because of the developmental issues involved in the care of adolescents. Moreover, there is no evidence that the kinds of ambulatory detoxification treatments that have become increasingly common for severe withdrawal in adults are effective or desirable in the adolescent population.

Although most adolescents do not develop classic or well-defined physiologic withdrawal symptoms, they may be more susceptible than adults to the development of substance dependence syndromes, including physiologic tolerance. Adolescents have a 1 in 4 chance of developing one of the DSM-IV symptoms of dependence later in life if exposed to alcohol, marijuana, or nicotine before the age of 15, and 4 to 8 times the risk of those not exposed until after age 17 (13). Also, the progression from casual use to dependence can be more accelerated in adolescents than in adults, as well as the progression from dependence on one substance to others (14).

The process of detoxification includes not only the attenuation of the physiologic and psychologic features of intoxication and withdrawal syndromes, but also the process of interrupting the momentum of habitual compulsive use in adolescents. Because of the force of this momentum, and the inherent difficulties in overcoming it even when no clear physiologic withdrawal syndrome is seen, this phase of treatment frequently requires a greater initial intensity to establish treatment engagement and patient role induction. This is critical to the success of treatment because it is so difficult for patients to engage or participate in treatment while caught up in the cycle of frequent intoxication and recovery from intoxication.

Dimension 2: Biomedical Conditions and Complications Although the medical sequelae of addiction generally are not as common or as severe in adolescents as in adults, they certainly need to be considered in treatment placement decisions. Some of the more severe acute and subacute medical complications of substance use include seizures caused by stimulant and inhalant intoxication, traumatic injuries (either accidental or because of victimization) associated with any substance intoxication, respiratory depression caused by opioid overdose (which is increasingly common with cheaper, purer supplies of heroin as well as the increased popularity of diverted prescription opioids, such as sustained-release oxycodone [OxyContin]). Acute alcohol poisoning is a severe medical complication that is more typical of adolescents than adults. The sequelae of injection drug use are well known, including cellulitis, HIV, endocarditis, and hepatitis B and C.

Some of the less severe but more common (and often underrecognized) medical sequelae of substance use include gastritis caused by alcohol use, exacerbation of reactive airway disease caused by smoking marijuana, dental disease caused by poor self-care, and weight loss and malnourishment caused by self-neglect or the appetite suppressing properties of certain drugs. Another notable area of medical complication in adolescents is the exacerbation of chronic illness (such as diabetes, asthma, or sickle cell disease) that results from impaired self-care and poor compliance with indicated medical treatments.

High-risk sexual behaviors are a major problem in adolescents. The associated sexually transmitted diseases commonly seen include chlamydial and gonococcal infections, syphilis, pelvic inflammatory disease, HIV, and hepatitis B virus. Both urethritis in boys and cervicitis in girls are relatively common, but frequently overlooked because they are often asymptomatic. The special needs and medical vulnerabilities of pregnant substance-using teenagers require particular care in selecting treatment services. Overall, the need for contraception and other medical prevention and treatment services related to sexual behaviors in drug-involved adolescents cannot be overemphasized.

Dimension 3: Emotional, Behavioral, and Cognitive Conditions and Complications Drug-involved adolescents typically demonstrate a very high degree of co-occurring psychopathology, which frequently does not remit with abstinence. Many experts estimate that rates of psychiatric comorbidity, or dual diagnosis, are higher in adolescents than in adults (15). Even adolescents who have not been diagnosed with a psychiatric disorder (either because they have not yet had a formal psychiatric evaluation or because subsyndromal symptoms do not meet diagnostic criteria) often have problems in Dimension 3 that need to be considered in making treatment decisions. Examples include hyperactivity or distractibility without a diagnosis of attention deficit hyperactivity disorder, mood lability and explosive temper without a diagnosis of bipolar disorder, or dysphoric mood and loss of interests without a diagnosis of depression. Various nonspecific symptoms—such as problems with anger management or impulse control, suspiciousness, and social withdrawal—also may be substance-induced or substance-exacerbated. And the nonspecific features of immature or impaired executive functioning are very common in drug involved adolescents, including impulsiveness, explosiveness, poor affective self-regulation, poor strategic planning, disinhibition, and the like, even if the descriptive taxonomy of the psychiatric DSM is still primitive in this regard.

The inclusion of cognitive conditions in Dimension 3 emphasizes the importance of cognitive abilities, as well as global or focal cognitive impairments, in an adolescent's functional capacity. Whether cognitive problems are due to preexisting conditions (such as borderline intellectual functioning, fetal alcohol effects, assorted attentional deficits, or learning disorders) (16,17) or are complications of substance use (such as marijuana-induced amnestic disorder), they often contribute to the severity of substance abuse disorders and interfere significantly with treatment and recovery.

To be most effective, physicians and treatment programs must adapt their methods and strategies to respond to adolescents' cognitive vulnerabilities and strengths. It also is critical to consider cognitive function in a developmental perspective, because cognition evolves dynamically over time.

One of the keys to treating adolescents is to use methods that take into account the ways that they learn, responding to issues of normal adolescent development, as well as the delayed development and immaturity that often accompany drug use and co-occurring psychiatric disorders. In general, the delivery of most therapies should be broken down into time-limited components, with frequent breaks, taking into account limitations in youngsters' attention spans. Adolescent engagement and learning are promoted by the use of experiential recovery activities that involve active participation rather than passive reception of information, and that are somewhat energetic, noisy, and fun, while at the same time delivering serious therapeutic content. Engagement also is enhanced by the acknowledgment and even partial endorsement of adolescent culture, including its typical stance of nonconformity with adult and mainstream norms.

Behavior and its management is another prominent developmental feature of adolescent treatment in Dimension 3. Although the expectation of adult, or mature, behavior may be questionable in adult treatment settings, it is certainly absurd in adolescent settings. The acquisition of self-regulation skills is an essential goal of treatment for substance users of all ages, but it also is a work in progress for all adolescents, even without substance use. Adolescent treatment programs must constantly seek a balance between an emphasis on limit-setting and some degree of tolerance for chaos, as part of the necessary recognition that adolescents still are partly children. Moreover, the penchant for mischief among youngsters is not always an indicator of antisocial traits. On the other hand, careful assessment of the broad range of adolescent misbehavior forms the basis of very powerful treatment interventions that target improvements in family monitoring, supervision and behavioral management.

In the *ASAM PPC-2R*, Dimension 3 has been expanded and divided into new subdomains for greater emphasis on psychiatric comorbidity or "dual diagnosis" issues. These subdomains are intended to enrich the detail and guide the assessment of risk and treatment needs for emotional, behavioral, and cognitive problems. The organization of the Dimension 3 severity specifications by subdomains emphasizes that placement decisions emerge out of the assessment of symptomatic functional impairment rather than any specific categorical diagnosis (Table 105.2).

TABLE 105.2 Dimension 3 Subdomains

Dangerousness/lethality
Interference with addiction recovery efforts
Social functioning
Ability for self-care
Course of illness

For example, the subdomain titled "Dangerousness/-Lethality" refers to the extent of risk of imminent harm to self or others. Assessment considerations may include suicidality, assaultiveness, risk of victimization, and exposure to the elements. Treatment decisions in this subdomain focus on safety and protection from dangerous consequences, and may include such interventions as residential containment or high-intensity family monitoring between outpatient sessions.

The subdomain titled "Interference with Addiction Recovery Efforts" refers to the extent to which psychologic and behavioral symptoms are a distraction from treatment participation or engagement. Examples include difficulty attending to treatment sessions because of problems with concentration, difficulty in completing recovery assignments or absorbing treatment materials because of problems with memory or comprehension, inability to attend treatment consistently because of running away, inability to participate in treatment because of disruptive behavior, and distraction caused by preoccupying worries.

The subdomain titled "Social Functioning" refers to the extent to which emotional, behavioral, and cognitive problems cause impairments in meeting responsibilities in major social arenas such as family, school, work, and personal relationships. Examples of assessment considerations in this subdomain include problems managing peer or family conflict, legal and conduct problems, problems with truancy or school performance, ungovernability at home, and narrowing of social repertoire and isolation.

The subdomain titled "Ability for Self-Care" refers to the extent to which the adolescent has problems in managing activities of daily living and personal care. Assessment considerations in this subdomain include behaviors associated with patterns of victimization, high-risk or indiscriminate sexual behaviors, disorganization that interferes with emerging independent living skills, poor self-regulation (or poor cooperation with external regulation) of daily routine, and problems with hygiene or nutrition.

The subdomain titled "Course of Illness" refers to an interpretation of the adolescent's present situation and symptoms in the context of his or her history and response to treatment, with a goal of predicting future course and relative stability. For example, the adolescent's history may suggest that a mood disorder decompensates rapidly with medication noncompliance, suggesting a higher instability and severity than would be the case if the course deteriorates more slowly, and suggesting the need for a more urgent or more intensive treatment response. Other examples include an adolescent who has tended to run away soon after an episode of family conflict, or an adolescent who tends to relapse to substance use after recurrence of depressive symptoms.

Dimension 4: Readiness to Change Assessment of treatment readiness is an essential component of treatment matching for adolescents. In the *ASAM PPC-2R*, Dimension 4 "Readiness to Change," highlights the active, dynamic concept of treatment engagement. Placement decisions based on Dimension 4 will include consideration of whether the adolescent (and related systems, such as the family) is in the "precontemplation," "contemplation," "preparation," or "action" stage of change.

In general, it is likely that effective interventions will be different at various stages of readiness for change. On the whole, adolescents tend to present at earlier stages of readiness to change than do adults because of developmental context. For example, it is external pressures that push them into treatment even more so than adults (18).

It is important to emphasize that engagement and role induction are critical components of treatment. Significant advances have been made in expanding the treatment engagement repertoire from simply and inflexibly attempting to overcome the adolescent's resistance, to appreciating the adolescent's own set of motivations and goals and attempting to enroll those into an evolving treatment agenda. Motivational interviewing and other motivational enhancement techniques have formed the basis of a variety of intervention models at various levels of care, including early intervention (19) and outpatient treatment (20).

Assessments of readiness to change should take into account a variety of change processes, including the processes used by adolescents themselves in effecting self-change (21), the processes used by families in effecting change (22), and the processes used by the external systems that interact with adolescents and their families, such as the coercive influence of the juvenile justice system. It is common to consider readiness for change as a balance of internal experiential contingency motivations (such as social frustrations; symptoms of intoxication or withdrawal; loss of achievements, interests and enjoyment; unpleasant or frightening experiences, including violence, victimization, high-risk motor vehicle use, or unwelcome sexual experiences), and external contingency motivations (such as parental mandates, legal threats, drug testing, peer group affiliations and influences, and loss of status). The question is which of these factors (and others) will have salience, and how and in what setting to make best use of them in enhancing the adolescent's motivation for treatment and change.

Additional factors in treatment engagement include problem identification, help-seeking orientation, self-efficacy, and hopefulness. Cultural factors also are important components in assessing readiness to change, as they influence likelihood of seeking and receiving treatment, likelihood of perceiving treatment as helpful, and consideration of cultural context in devising treatment engagement strategies.

Dimension 5: Relapse, Continued Use, or Continued Problem Potential Dimension 5 entails an estimation of the likelihood of resumption or continuation of substance use. The assessment of relapse potential (or, reciprocally, remission potential) should include a number of key factors. Although not incorporated directly into the criteria, a schema for incorporating four subdomains for more detailed *PPC-2R* Dimension 5 assessments has been proposed (11, p. 345). These subdomains are: (1) historical pattern of use (including amount, frequency, chronicity and treatment response); (2) pharmacologic response to the effects from particular substances (including positive reinforcement such as pleasure with use and cravings, and negative reinforcement such as relief from withdrawal or other negative experiences); (3) response to external stimuli (including reactivity to environmental triggers and acute or chronic stress); and (4) cognitive and behavioral vulnerability and resiliency factors (including traits of impulsivity, passivity, locus of control, and overall coping capacities).

The "historical pattern of use" concept is similar to the "course of illness" subdomain in Dimension 3. That is, history and treatment response are likely to predict future course of illness, including relapse potential. For example, some adolescents are more likely to have a rapid course of full reinstatement of dependence with severe impairment after a single lapse episode, whereas others are likely to have a more indolent course, with only gradual escalation of use. This suggests one means of informing treatment and placement matching decisions on an individualized basis. Response to past treatment also may be a way of using individualized treatment effectiveness as a guide to placement: if a particular dose of treatment or modality or level of care led to a significant period of improvement for an adolescent in the past, then it may suggest the appropriateness of repeating that treatment after a relapse or exacerbation. On the other hand, if a particular dose or placement was not effective in the past, this history may suggest the need for a more intensive intervention.

Dimension 6: Recovery/Living Environment Dimension 6 aims to assess the ability of the adolescent's home environment to support or impede treatment and recovery. For adolescents, the most important features of the recovery environment generally involve family and peers. The need for inclusion of families or other caretakers in assessment and treatment is paramount. In many cases, it is unreasonable to expect that the adolescent will be the initial or most important locus of change. Rather, it often is more effective to help the family improve its approach to monitoring, supervision, and home intervention, with the expectation that the family as the primary locus of change will in turn change the adolescent.

Families, and their needs and involvement, should be considered broadly to encompass a wide range of circumstances, such as extended families, surrogate families, and other caretakers. It also is important to address cultural context and to use cultural competence as a critical tool for engaging families in treatment.

Problems in Dimension 6 that typically affect placement include chaotic home environments in which substance use, illegal behaviors, abuse, neglect or lack of supervision are prominent, or a broader community in which substance use and crime are endemic. Many adolescents have a social network composed primarily or even exclusively of family members or peers who are involved in substance use or criminal behaviors. This social context may portray deviance as normative. There may not be readily apparent role models for the rewards of abstinence. Some adolescents may have had *no* experience of living in an environment that fosters healthy prosocial development and functioning.

TABLE 105.3 American Society of Addiction Medicine Patient Placement Criteria, 2nd Edition, Revised, Adolescent Levels of Care

Level 0.5:	Early intervention
Level I:	Outpatient treatment
Level II:	Intensive outpatient treatment
	II.1 Intensive outpatient
	II.5 Partial hospitalization
Level III:	Residential treatment
	III.1 Clinically managed low-intensity residential
	III.5 Clinically managed medium-intensity residential
	III.7 Medically monitored high-intensity residential/inpatient
Level IV:	Medically managed intensive inpatient (hospital) treatment

Placement and Treatment Considerations by Levels of Care The adolescent levels of care in the *ASAM PPC-2R* are similar to the levels of care described and endorsed in other expert consensus documents (Table 105.3) (23).

Level 0.5

Early Intervention Early intervention services are designed to explore and address the adolescent's problems or risk factors that appear to be related to early stages of substance use. Their goal is to help the adolescent recognize the potentially harmful consequences of substance use, before such use escalates into substance abuse or dependence. Level 0.5 services may be delivered in a variety of settings, including primary care medical clinics, schools (often through organized Student Assistance Programs), social service and juvenile justice agencies, and driving under the influence intervention programs.

Early intervention services are intended to combine prevention and treatment services for youth who are at risk because of their exposure to substances, experimentation, or use. Populations that warrant special attention at Level 0.5 are the children of substance-abusing parents, siblings of substance abusers, and adolescents with other emotional or behavioral problems.

Early intervention is not appropriate for adolescents who qualify for a diagnosis of a substance use disorder. If an adolescent's pattern of substance use has progressed to a point at which it is causing a persistent pattern of impairment, then the applicable treatment services are best provided at a more intensive level of care.

Level I: Outpatient Treatment Outpatient treatment is by far the most frequently used level of care. It may be the initial level of care for an adolescent whose lesser severity of illness warrants this intensity of treatment. Level I also may be employed as a "step-down" program for the adolescent who has made progress at a more intensive level of care.

Outpatient treatment is indicated when safety and progress toward recovery goals can be expected without either the immersion intensity of Level II services or the residential support and protection of Level III services.

One of the advantages of outpatient treatment is the possibility of achieving therapeutic goals in the context of the patient's own home environment, where new behaviors can be practiced and solidified in real life circumstances.

Outpatient services may be useful for the adolescent patient who is in the early stages of readiness to change and who has not yet committed to recovery. Although an adolescent at this stage may require a more intensive level of care (sometimes including coerced treatment) to address dangerousness or high degrees of resistance and denial, such an increase in intensity can be counterproductive in certain situations. An alternative approach is to use a less intensive level of care to engage the resistant adolescent in treatment by enhancing his or her motivation or by modifying the responses of the various systems that affect the adolescent. In such situations, "discovery" may be a more appropriate outpatient treatment goal than "recovery." Such an approach may prepare the adolescent for more intensive treatment services, or even forestall the need for a more intensive level of care.

Outpatient treatment often includes a prolonged continuing care maintenance phase, sometimes referred to as *aftercare*. In this phase, strategies such as relapse prevention and strengthening protective factors are critical components of treatment. This phase focuses on anticipation of difficulties and the guidance of adolescents through the periodic recurrence of stressors without return to or exacerbation of substance use. Even simple ongoing monitoring (such as checking on parental supervision, scrutinizing school performance or peer relationships, and reviewing warning signs and triggers) is a desirable goal of active outpatient treatment. The term *recovery checkups* has sometimes been used to refer to such a monitoring phase in which the intensity/frequency may be low but nevertheless explicitly organized and scheduled rather than triggered only on an ad hoc or as-needed basis.

Level II: Intensive Outpatient Treatment/Partial Hospitalization Intensive outpatient programs (IOPs) generally offer at least 6 hours of structured programming per week. However, the precise number of hours of service delivered is adjusted to meet each patient's needs. Six hours per week will be too few for many adolescents; for example, those who are early in their treatment or who are stepping down from a more intensive level of care may need 9, 12, or even 15 hours a week of IOP services.

Partial hospitalization programs (PHP, also sometimes known as "day programs") generally offer 20 or more hours of clinically intensive programming per week. They feature daily or near-daily contact and thus provide more intensive monitoring and supervision than IOP or Level I outpatient treatment.

Intensive outpatient (Level II.1) programs typically differ from partial hospitalization (Level II.5) programs in the severity of patient disorders that they can manage. Most IOPs have less capacity to effectively treat adolescents who have substantial or unstable emotional or behavioral problems; such patients are better placed in PHPs. Partial hospitalization programs often have direct access to, or close referral relationships with, psychiatric and medical services. They are thus better able than Level II.1 programs to meet needs identified in Dimensions 1, 2, and 3, which may warrant daily monitoring or management, but that can be appropriately addressed in a structured outpatient setting. Some PHPs can provide an intensity of treatment services approaching that of residential care if the patient's home environment can support safety, stability, and treatment progress between PHP sessions.

With both IOPs and PHPs, there are varying approaches to the program schedule and structure. Some programs employ a single fixed schedule of service hours. Others modify their service hours throughout the stages of treatment, tapering the number of hours according to a prescribed schedule. Yet another approach is to match intensity and hours of service flexibly with the severity of the patient's problems.

Adolescent IOPs generally meet after school or work hours, or on weekends. Partial hospitalization may occur during school hours, and many programs, especially if they are longer term, have access to educational services for their adolescent patients. PHP programs that do not provide educational services may coordinate with a school system in order to assess and meet their adolescent patients' educational needs.

Level III: Residential Treatment Although earlier editions of the ASAM criteria treated all adolescent residential treatment as one broad undifferentiated level of care, the *PPC-2R* divides Level III into three sublevels.

- Level III.1: Clinically managed low-intensity residential treatment
- Level III.5: Clinically managed medium-intensity residential treatment
- Level III.7: Medically monitored high-intensity residential/inpatient treatment

Level III.1 (clinically managed low-intensity residential treatment) programs typically are provided in halfway houses and group homes. Such programs offer several hours a week of low-intensity treatment sessions, in addition to their most important feature: a stable living environment, staffed 24 hours per day, which provides sufficient structure and supervision to prevent or minimize relapse or continued use and continued problem potential (Dimension 5). Additional treatment services and intensity may be provided through concurrent involvement in outpatient treatment at Level I or II.

Treatment is directed toward applying recovery skills, preventing relapse, improving social functioning by practicing interpersonal and group living skills, improving ability for self-care by organizing the activities of daily living, promoting personal responsibility through successful concurrent involvement in regular productive activities (such as school or work), developing a social network supportive of recovery, and reintegrating the adolescent into the community and (if appropriate) the family.

Treatment at Level III.1 is most often warranted as a substitute for or supplement to deficits in the adolescent's recovery environment (Dimension 6). Problems in Dimension 6 that might warrant placement in a residential program include home environments that are so abusive, chaotic, or riddled with substance use or antisocial behaviors that extended separation and residential treatment support are required to overcome their toxic influences.

Some adolescents require the structure of a Level III.1 program to achieve engagement in treatment (Dimension 4). Those who are in the early stages of readiness to change may need to be removed from an unsupportive living environment in order to minimize their continued substance use.

The length of stay in a clinically managed Level III.1 program tends to be longer than in the more intensive residential levels of care. In some cases, an extended period in Level III.1 treatment is needed to sustain and consolidate therapeutic gains made at more intensive levels of care because of the adolescent's functional deficits (including developmental immaturity, greater than average susceptibility to peer influence, or lack of impulse control). Longer exposure to monitoring, supervision, and low-intensity treatment interventions is necessary for adolescents to practice basic living skills and to master the application of coping and recovery skills. In some situations, there is no effective substitute for extended residential containment as reliable protection from the toxic influences of substance exposure, problematic or substance-infested environments, or the cultures of substance-involved and antisocial behaviors.

Level III.5 (clinically managed medium-intensity residential treatment) programs include medium-intensity settings such as therapeutic group homes, therapeutic community programs, psychosocial model residential treatment centers, or extended residential rehabilitation programs. As a group, these sometimes are referred to simply as *residential programs.*

Level III.5 programs are designed to provide relatively extended subacute treatments, with the goal of achieving fundamental personal change for the adolescent who has significant social and psychologic problems. The goals and modalities of treatment focus not only on the adolescent's substance use, but also on a holistic view of the adolescent that takes into account his or her behavior, emotions, attitudes, values, learning, family, culture, lifestyle, and overall health. Such programs are characterized by their reliance on the treatment community or milieu as a therapeutic agent of change.

In addition to the stable recovery environment found at Level III.1, these programs use intensive active programming and containment to create a community or milieu that promotes both recovery skills and basic life skills. Critical treatment interventions that require intensity and persistence over extended periods, such as modeling prosocial patterns of behavior and adaptive patterns of emotional responsiveness, have sometimes been likened to "surrogate" or "remedial parenting." Just as important can be the induction into a healthy peer group, with the formation of a group identity that emphasizes recovery and overcoming adversity.

The adolescent who is appropriately placed in a Level III.5 program may have a variety of psychologic or psychiatric problems (Dimension 3). Particularly suitable for Level III.5 treatments are the entrenched patterns of maladaptive behavior, extremes of temperament, and developmental or cognitive abnormalities related to mental health symptoms or disorders. Co-occurring disorders that often require extended treatment at Level III.5 include conduct disorder and oppositional defiant disorder, as well as the persistent patterns of disruptive behavior that may be associated with other disorders, even after they have responded to acute treatment.

Level III.5 programs frequently work with aspects of adolescent temperament—including the impulsive, extroverted, dramatic, antisocial, thrill-seeking, or other personality traits—that may otherwise have the potential to solidify as components of emerging personality disorders. Goals of treatment include overcoming oppositionality through a combination of motivational enhancement, supportive limit setting and judicious confrontation; teaching anger management and acquisition of conflict resolution skills; values clarification and moral habilitation; character molding and education; development of effective behavioral contingency strategies; establishment of a reliable response to external structure; and the internalization of structure through self-regulation skills.

Level III.5 also is appropriate for the adolescent whose problems include severe delinquency and juvenile justice involvement. This level of care often is warranted for adolescents who have severe conduct problems, a progressive history of illegal behaviors, a pattern of emerging criminality, or an incipient antisocial value system. One of the key purposes of Level III.5 treatment for this set of problems is assessment and monitoring of safety, with particular attention to issues of potential safety outside of the contained setting. In this context, treatment must proceed in a contained, safe and structured environment to allow teaching, practicing of prosocial behaviors, and facilitation of healthy reintegration into the community.

Treatment in a Level III.5 program may be used to address problems in treatment engagement and readiness to change (Dimension 4). Many adolescents fail attempts at outpatient treatment out of a lack of engagement, either because of a lack of personal connection to treatment or because the systems surrounding the adolescent (family, school, juvenile justice system, and the like) have not coordinated sufficiently to motivate the adolescent, or both. The immersion experience of a Level III.5 program may be needed to promote treatment role induction and introduce the adolescent into a peer group that is struggling to form a group identity that emphasizes recovery and the need for treatment. An additional goal of treatment at Level III.5 should be to promote coordination of the multiple systems surrounding the adolescent and to help devise and implement motivational strategies for ongoing engagement in treatment.

As with Level III.1, Level III.5 programs may require relatively long stays to allow certain adolescents to acquire basic living skills and mastery of coping and recovery skills. Such patients require the intensity and duration of treatment found in a Level III.5 program to accomplish some of the tasks of habilitation in a temporary "home" (Dimension 6) that can imprint the features of a successful recovery environment.

Level III.7 (medically monitored high-intensity residential/inpatient treatment) programs are appropriate for adolescents whose problems are so severe that they require medically monitored residential treatment, but who do not need the full resources of an acute care hospital or medically managed inpatient treatment program (Level IV). Medically monitored services are provided under the supervision of physicians who are specialists in addiction medicine, and the programs tend to operate under the so-called "medical model."

The adolescent who is appropriately placed in a medically monitored program may have problems in Dimensions 1, 2, or 3 that require direct medical or nursing services. Services typically provided in a Level III.7 program include medical detoxification, titration of a psychopharmacologic regimen, and high-intensity behavior modification. Alternatively, the adolescent may have problems that do not so much require direct medical or nursing services as the overall high intensity of a program and treatment milieu that draws on the staffing pattern and availability of an interdisciplinary professional team.

An adolescent may be admitted directly to a Level III.7 program or transferred from a less intensive level of care if he or she has been refractory to treatment or as bursts of more intensive services become necessary. An adolescent also may be transferred to a Level III.7 program for continuing care from a Level IV program when he or she no longer requires the intensity of services or staffing pattern of a hospital. A fairly common scenario is that of an adolescent who is admitted to a Level IV hospital program on an emergency basis because of a medical or psychiatric crisis situation and then is transferred to a Level III.7 program for further assessment and treatment in a substance-free state to help sort out difficult diagnostic questions regarding subacute intoxication, withdrawal, and co-occurring psychiatric disorders.

Problems in Dimension 3 are probably the most common reason for admission to Level III.7 programs. Such problems include co-occurring psychiatric disorders (such as depressive disorders, bipolar disorders, and attention deficit hyperactivity disorder) or symptoms (such as hypomania, severe disorganization or impulsiveness, and aggressive behaviors).

Treatment at Level III.7 often is necessary simply to orient an adolescent with substance dependence to the structure of daily life using organizing principles other than "getting high" and "being high." Initial forced abstinence through confinement in a Level III.7 program provides many adolescents with a much-needed reintroduction to their own patterns of emotional and cognitive experience without intoxication.

Problems in Dimension 1 that require Level III.7 services include moderate to severe withdrawal or risk of withdrawal; for example, detoxification from heroin or illicit prescription opioids requiring pharmacologic management. Adolescents also may need medically monitored treatment because of acute or subacute intoxication. Lingering drug-induced impairments of cognitive or executive function (for example, by inhalants) or with psychosis (for example, by methamphetamine) may lead to disorganization, poor judgment, aggressiveness, or increased impulsivity. These may require periods of close assessment and high-intensity management.

Level IV: Medically Managed Intensive Inpatient (Hospital) Treatment Level IV medically managed intensive inpatient treatment is delivered in an acute care inpatient setting in which the full resources of a general or psychiatric hospital are available. It is appropriate for adolescents whose acute problems are so severe that they require primary medical and nursing care on a daily basis. Although treatment is specific to substance dependence disorders, the skills of the interdisciplinary team and the availability of support services allow the conjoint treatment of any withdrawal, medical conditions, or psychiatric disorders that need to be addressed. Admissions to Level IV are most commonly provoked by urgent concerns regarding safety or imminent danger.

Level IV treatment tends to be brief, generally consisting of emergency or crisis interventions aimed at stabilization in preparation for transfer to a less intensive level of care for ongoing treatment.

Treatment Dose and Utilization Management The ASAM criteria emphasize the concept of treatment as a dynamic, longitudinal process, rather than a discrete episode of care or particular program enrollment. However, current treatment delivery systems do not generally support the necessary continuum of care. For example, a longitudinal view of treatment might call for the services of a designated care provider to coordinate (or even provide) treatment across discrete placements, but use of such a provider is unusual in most communities and systems of care.

Many difficulties continue to arise over utilization management issues. For example, what is the optimal dose of treatment for adolescents at any level of care? There are no data as yet to answer this and other critical questions. Although the field seems to be moving away from fixed, length of stay-based, program-driven treatment to more flexible, assessment-based, clinically driven treatment, much of the development of adolescent programs has focused on standardized protocols with prescribed content and length of service. There has been little examination of the dose-response relationship for adolescent treatment, and further research into this issue is needed. It may turn out that certain minimum threshold lengths of service are associated with specific therapeutic gains. In particular, the needs of juvenile justice–involved adolescents in public sector programs that use coercive treatment engagement methods (such as a court order or probationary mandate) may be best served by more predictable, though not rigid, lengths of service. Physicians and the courts must collaborate closely to assure that the interests of each adolescent patient are assessed and met.

When a treatment plan is unsuccessful, it calls for reassessment. Reassessment may indicate the need for more treatment, but it also may indicate the need to adopt a different treatment plan with a change in strategy, modality, or scope of treatment. Treatment failure often implies a need for an increase in intensity, but also can suggest a change in approach rather than in level of care. The criteria should be applied within the context of local resources and realistically designed follow-up plans.

Although utilization criteria can be used as an impetus to overcoming treatment barriers through creative systems approaches, they have also been misused as a cynical justification for giving up or limiting payment for care as "fruitless." The ASAM criteria are *not* intended to imply that ongoing problems, even severe treatment-refractory problems (including continued use, lapse, relapse, lack of attendance, lack of participation, and the like) suggest inability to solve treatment problems. Changes in level of care or treatment approach always should be a part of the therapeutic strategy for revision of an overall or longitudinal treatment plan, and never should be motivated by an acceptance of futility or therapeutic nihilism.

Given that substance use disorders often have a chronic, remitting/relapsing course, it is reasonable to expect that treatment must match this chronic course. Treatment may encompass one or several acute episodes, but a treatment plan also must endure over the long term. An older, presumably outdated, approach views discrete time-limited episodes of program enrollment as constituting adequate doses of treatment. In this view, any further continuing care, also typically time-limited, was regarded as "aftercare" rather than ongoing care, as if the active part of treatment were finished.

The more appropriate view of chronic care for a chronic disorder supports a stance of therapeutic optimism and a "never give up" attitude for the treatment-refractory patient. It also reinforces the need for chronic attention and vigilance in response to a chronic vulnerability, even in the improved patient. This view is not incompatible with the common experience that a subset of adolescents, especially those with broader supports and higher levels of premorbid functioning, may respond to more time-limited interventions, or seem to "grow out of" their difficulties with developmental maturation.

A critical feature of successful adolescent treatment across a continuum is ease of transfer across the levels of care. Because payers have not funded more flexible continuums of care and because providers have not developed such systems, it is generally difficult for patients to move back and forth between levels of care at all, much less with coordinated transitions. One reason for prolonged lengths of stay at higher levels of care is the barriers to stepping down to appropriate lower levels. Reciprocally, acute bursts of treatment at higher levels of care often are needed to overcome hurdles at lower levels. Repeated acute episodes of high-intensity care should be an expected modality of treatment for exacerbations, as they would be with any chronic relapsing disorder.

Ongoing treatment at less intensive levels of care to consolidate gains initiated at more intensive levels of care also is a critical feature of successful treatment across a continuum of care. Because enduring treatment effectiveness may be tempered by the attenuation of treatment effect over time, the need for "booster" doses of treatment should be anticipated. Moreover, ongoing active treatment often is required simply to consolidate and sustain therapeutic gains.

Finally, the long-term (sometimes indefinite) maintenance phase of treatment too often is overlooked. Treatment successes, such as a period of abstinence or improvement in functioning, sometimes are misinterpreted as completion of treatment. In fact, long-term maintenance and monitoring of short-term successes are essential goals of active outpatient treatment.

Validation of Placement Criteria The ASAM criteria were developed as a consensus-based guide to "best practices" by committees of experts and diverse stakeholders. As such, their application is not concretely operationalized or based on standardized assessment instruments, and their use clearly relies on the utilization of sound clinical interpretation and judgment.

Encouraging work has been done with the adult ASAM placement criteria to support its validity. Research versions of the criteria, operationalized through standardized assessment instruments to increase reliability, have been shown to have utility and stability as multidimensional severity ratings. Additionally, limited experimental testing of treatment outcomes using earlier versions of the adult criteria has been promising. Work by Gastfriend et al. (11) followed posttreatment outcomes in adults randomized to placements after *ASAM PPC* prescribed matching versus deliberate mismatching. Outcomes were worse when patients received mismatches to the Level of Care of lower intensity instead of the appropriately matched Level of Care prescribed by the *ASAM PPC*.

Unlike the adult placement criteria, there has been very little research on either the reliability or validity of the adolescent criteria. However, preliminary work suggests that clinicians who use the criteria in "real-world" settings are in fact able to discriminate levels of clinical severity. A retrospective analysis of adolescents assigned to placements using the ASAM criteria within a single private provider's system of care found that adolescents referred to inpatient treatment had greater severity than those referred to outpatient treatment (24). Although the two groups were not different demographically, the adolescents placed in inpatient care had significantly greater severity in a variety of substance use indicators, including frequency of use, number of previous treatment episodes, number of diagnoses of dependence as opposed to non-dependent abuse, and prevalence of physiologic dependence (as primarily indicated by the symptom of tolerance). Because adolescent substance abuse is so clearly associated with problems in a wide range of related psychosocial domains, any attempt to stratify severity and treatment needs also must take these into account and not consider substance use alone. This work also demonstrated that patients referred to inpatient treatment based on the ASAM criteria had greater severity on measures of health problems, a variety of mental health symptoms, and conduct problems.

Finally, Dennis' group developed a profile approximating the ASAM assessment dimensions, using calculated subscales from a highly reliable standardized assessment instrument (the Global Assessment of Individual Need). In a retrospective comparison, this standardized research ASAM profile also supported the discrimination of severity and the placement decisions made by clinicians who used their own non-standardized intake assessments and the ASAM criteria (25).

To date, there is no empiric evidence of the effectiveness of adolescent placement or treatment matching criteria based on treatment outcome data. However, there are encouraging preliminary indications that case mix adjustments based on ASAM criteria can help explain a considerable amount of the variance in treatment outcomes for different levels of care (26). These indications suggest that the ASAM criteria, when refined and better operationalized, might in fact lead to predictors of treatment response. There also is work underway to use models of adherence to the ASAM criteria to determine retrospectively whether "appropriate" level of care placements lead to better outcomes.

Further, the Chestnut Health Systems group has refined and expanded its ASAM PPC assessment profile based on the Global Assessment of Individual Need (27) into a computer generated clinical tool, which has proven useful in practice for approximating and highlighting treatment matching needs. Consensus development of computerized algorithmic decision rules based on the Global Assessment of Individual Need is being implemented as an expansion of that tool (28) and will be the subject of future testing and research. The profile of level of care treatment matching is also highlighted by work showing differential patterns of treatment outcomes at different levels of care in community settings (29). Along with a general endorsement of the effectiveness of community treatment, this profile begins to show the effectiveness of level of care sorting with higher severity adolescents appropriately sorted into residential treatment and their outcomes at 12 months showing them improved with severity measures reduced and stabilized at the levels of outpatients.

CONCLUSIONS

At present, the adolescent population is significantly underserved, with fewer than 10% of adolescents who exhibit symptoms of problem drug use in the preceding year ever having received formal treatment (12). It would be a huge advance for these adolescents to receive any treatment at all. It is hoped that the use of organized assessment tools, such as the ASAM criteria, that employ gradations of severity and risk to guide treatment matching and placement decisions will help to create pressure for the creation of the necessary treatment resources.

For the field to take the next steps in understanding treatment effectiveness, and to develop more effective treatments, clinicians must be able to make appropriate and useful treatment matching and placement decisions. To accomplish this, physicians, counselors and other health professionals will need to further operationalize gradations of severity and risk, using more reliable measures, and presumably incorporating standardized instruments. At the same time, it will be important to resist the illusion of technique, and to avoid the error of assuming that the reliability and precision of standardized instruments guarantee validity.

Treatment matching hypotheses and practices must be refined beyond level of care to include specific interventions, services, modalities, and doses. It will be important to discern relevant subtypes that might be expected to be associated with differential treatment response within the heterogeneous population of drug-involved adolescents. (Of course, the validity of such refinements will need to be demonstrated empirically.)

The ASAM adolescent placement criteria continue to evolve in response to ongoing progress in the field of adolescent addiction medicine. The criteria are based predominantly on consensus best practices. As the results of additional adolescent treatment outcome research become available, future revisions of the criteria will be based increasingly on empirically verified principles of treatment matching, placement, and effectiveness. At the same time, the ASAM criteria and other clinical treatment matching guidelines will drive research hypotheses that will lead to improved treatment and treatment access for all adolescents in need.

REFERENCES

1. Williams RJ, Chang SY. Addiction Centre Adolescent Research Group. A comprehensive and comparative review of adolescent substance abuse treatment outcome. *Clin Psychol Sci Pract* 2000;7:138–166.
2. Hser Y, Grella CE, Hubbard RL, et al. An evaluation of drug treatment for adolescents in four U.S. cities. *Arch Gen Psychiatry* 2001;58:689–695.
3. Winters K. Treating adolescents with substance use disorders: an overview of practice issues and treatment outcomes. *Substance Abuse* 1999;20:203–223.
4. Morral A, McCaffrey D, Ridgeway G. Effectiveness of community based treatment for substance abusing adolescents: 12-month outcomes of youths entering Phoenix Academy or alternative probation dispositions. *Psychol Addict Behav* 2004;18:257–268.
5. Dennis M, Godley S, Diamond G, et al. The Cannabis Youth Treatment (CYT) Study: main findings from two randomized trials. *J Subst Abuse Treat* 2004;27:197–213.
6. Muck R, Zempolich K, Titus J, et al. An overview of the effectiveness of adolescent substance abuse treatment models. *Youth Society* 2001;33 (2):143–168.
7. Clemmey P, Payne L, Fishman M. Clinical characteristics and treatment outcomes of adolescent heroin users. *J Psychoactive Drugs* 2004;36(1): 85–94.
8. Brown SA, Myers MG, Vik PW. Correlates of success following treatment for adolescent substance abuse. *Appl Prevent Psychol* 1994;3: 61–73.
9. Dennis M, Dowud-Noursi S, Muck R, et al. The need for developing and evaluating adolescent treatment models. In: Stevens S, Morral A, eds. *Adolescent substance abuse treatment in the United States: exemplary models from a national evaluation study.* Binghamton, NY: Haworth Press, 2002.
10. Gastfriend DR, McLellan AT. Placement matching: theoretic basis and practical implications. *Med Clin N Am* 1997;81:945–966.
11. Gastfriend D, ed. *Addiction treatment matching: research foundations of the American Society of Addiction Medicine (ASAM) patient placement criteria.* Binghamton, NY: Haworth Medical Press, 2003.
12. Mee-Lee D, Shulman GD, Fishman M, et al., eds. *ASAM Patient placement criteria for the treatment of substance-related disorders,* 2nd edition-revised (ASAM PPC-2R). Chevy Chase, MD: American Society of Addiction Medicine, Inc., 2001.
13. Dennis M, McGeary K. Adolescent alcohol and marijuana treatment: kids need it now. *TIE Communique.* Rockville, MD: Substance Abuse and Mental Health Services Administration, Center for Substance Abuse Treatment, 1999.
14. Clark DB, Kirisci L, Tarter RE. Adolescent versus adult onset and the development of substance use disorders in males. *Drug Alcohol Depend* 1998;49(2):115–121.
15. Kandel DB, Johnson JG, Bird HR, et al. Psychiatric disorders associated with substance use among children and adolescents: findings from the Methods for Epidemiology of Child and Adolescent Mental Disorders (MECA) study. *J Abnorm Psychol* 1997;25:121–132.
16. Hops HA, Davis B, Lewin LM. The development of alcohol and other substance use: a gender study of family and peer context. *J Study Alcohol Suppl* 1999;13:22–31.
17. Tapert SF, Baratta BS, Abrantes BA, et al. Attention dysfunction predicts substance involvement in community youth. *J Am Acad Child Adolesc Psychiatry* 2002;41(6):690–696.
18. Deas D, Riggs P, Langenbucher J, et al. Adolescents are not adults: developmental considerations in alcohol users. *Alcohol Clin Exp Res* 2000;24: 232–237.
19. Colby SM, Monti PM, Barnett NP, et al. Brief motivational interviewing in a hospital setting for adolescent smoking: a preliminary study. *J Clin Consult Psychol* 1998;66:574–578.
20. Sampl S, Kadden R. *Motivational enhancement therapy and cognitive behavioral therapy for adolescent cannabis users: 5 sessions, cannabis youth treatment* (CYT) Series, volume 1. Rockville, MD: Center for Substance Abuse Treatment, Substance Abuse and Mental Health Services Administration, 2001.
21. Brown S. Facilitating change for adolescent alcohol problems; a multiple options approach. In: Wagner E, Waldron H, eds. *Innovations in adolescent substance abuse interventions.* Oxford, UK: Pergamon, 2001:169–188.
22. Liddle HA, Hogue A. Multidimensional family therapy for adolescent substance abuse. In: Wagner E, Waldron H, eds. *Innovations in adolescent substance abuse interventions.* Oxford, UK: Pergamon, 2001:229–261.
23. Center for Substance Abuse Treatment Improvement Protocol (TIP) Series 32. Treatment of adolescents with substance use disorders. Washington, DC: SAMHSA, 1999.
24. Godley SH, Godley MD, Dennis ML. Assertive aftercare protocol for adolescent substance abusers. In: Wagner E, Waldron H, eds. *Innovations in adolescent substance abuse interventions.* Oxford, UK: Pergamon, 2001:313–331.
25. Dennis M, Funk R, McDermeit M, et al. Towards better placement and case mix adjustments in adolescent and adult substance abuse treatment systems. Presented at the 8th International Conference on Treatment of Addictive Behavior. Santa Fe, NM, January 1988.
26. Dennis M, Scott C, Godley M, et al. Predicting outcomes in adult and adolescent treatment with case mix vs. level of care: findings from the drug outcome monitoring study. Presentation at the College on Problems of Drug Dependence, San Juan, PR, June 2000.
27. Chestnut Health Systems Lighthouse Institute. The GAIN recommendation and referral summary: a narrative clinical report. www.chestnut.org/L1/gain/index.htm/#GRRS.
28. Stevens L, Dennis M, Fishman M. Using the new GAIN patient placement summary to support individual treatment planning, placement and program evaluation. *Workshop at the joint meeting on adolescent treatment effectiveness,* Baltimore, MD, March 28, 2006. Available online at: www.chestnut.org/LI/Posters.
29. Dasinger L, Shane P, Martinovich Z. Assessing the effectiveness of community-based substance abuse treatment for adolescents. *J Psychoactive Drugs* 2004;36(1):85–94.

Confidentiality in Dealing with Adolescents

Alain Joffe, MD, MPH

Confidentiality is an essential component of health care for adolescents. Without some promise of confidentiality at the beginning of an office visit, the adolescent patient is less likely to disclose information about his or her behaviors, particularly concerning sensitive areas such as sexual activity or substance use. On the other hand, the clinician who promises unconditional confidentiality ("everything you tell me will be kept private") may find himself or herself party to information about very risky behaviors, which he or she has promised not to reveal but that, if allowed to continue, may jeopardize the health of the adolescent. To avoid this clinical conundrum, regardless of the health care setting, health care professionals must understand the key principles underlying confidentiality and its limits.

Physicians demonstrate respect for patients and develop a good working relationship with them by maintaining confidentiality, thereby forming a zone of privacy around the contents of the office visit. This approach maximizes the "patient's willingness to supply information candidly for his or her benefit" (1). A promise of confidentiality is especially important to adolescents, who, from a developmental perspective, are seeking to achieve autonomy from their parents and are learning to make appropriate decisions about a variety of issues, including healthy behaviors and seeking health care. Psychologic research suggests that adolescents demonstrate adult reasoning capacity at approximately age 14 (2). By providing a confidential setting in which adolescents can discuss their concerns, particularly ones they view as sensitive and/or embarrassing or wish to keep private from parents, clinicians help support this critical developmental process.

RESEARCH INTO CONFIDENTIALITY ISSUES

More than two decades of research demonstrate how much value adolescents place on confidentiality. Marks et al. (3) surveyed 649 suburban youth in grades 9 through 12. Only 19% said they would seek care for contraception, 17% for drug use, and 23% for alcohol use if their parents knew of the visit. In contrast, 45% said they would seek care for contraception, 49% for drug use, and 43% for alcohol use under the condition that their parents would not find out.

More recently, Ford (4) used simulated office visits to explore adolescents' views about confidentiality. A total of 562 adolescents from three suburban California high schools were randomized to listen to a standardized audiotape depiction of an office visit. On one tape, the physician promised unconditional confidentiality, on another he or she promised conditional confidentiality, and, on the third, confidentiality was not discussed. Assurances of confidentiality increased the percentage of teenagers who were willing to disclose information about their sexual behaviors, drug use, and mental health concerns from 39% to 46.5%, and increased the percentage willing to seek future health care from 53% to 67%. These studies demonstrate the utilitarian basis for supporting confidentiality for adolescents: many adolescents will not seek health care for sensitive issues unless their expectation of privacy is granted. Furthermore, a recent study demonstrates that it is adolescents with the greatest numbers of risk characteristics—hence, the ones most in need of health care—who are most likely to cite confidentiality concerns as a reason for forgoing needed health care (5). In this study, compared with girls who did not cite confidentiality as a reason, girls who did were more likely to report poor parental communication, endorse higher levels of depressive symptoms, report suicidal ideation and attempts, have unprotected sex, or use alcohol. Boys who cited confidentiality concerns as a reason for forgoing needed health care were more likely to report poor parental communication, endorse higher levels of depressive symptoms, and report suicide attempts in the past year. Studies have also shown that, although many adolescents may forego seeking health care for risky behaviors if parental notification is a prerequisite, they will not stop engaging in the risky behaviors. Hence, failing to afford confidentiality increases the risk of adolescents' delaying seeking or not receiving care until serious consequences arise from undisclosed behaviors (including pregnancy, pelvic inflammatory disease, drug overdose, abuse or dependence, and alcohol-related motor vehicle injuries).

POLICIES ON CONFIDENTIALITY

Physicians' professional organizations long have supported the concept of confidential care for adolescents. In 1967, the American Medical Association adopted a position that the epidemic of sexually transmitted diseases among young people required that minors be able to receive treatment for those infections without parental notification (6). The American Medical Association also opposed regulations that would have required clinicians working in federally funded programs to notify parents when they provided prescription contraceptives to patients under age 18 (7).

In 1988, the American Academy of Pediatrics, the National Medical Association, the American College of

(*continued*)

Confidentiality in Dealing with Adolescents *(continued)*

Obstetricians and Gynecologists, and the American Academy of Family Physicians jointly endorsed recommendations on confidentiality, concluding that "ultimately, the health risks to adolescents are so impelling that legal barriers and deference to parental involvement should not stand in the way of needed care" (8).

The Health Insurance Portability and Accountability Act (1996) and its accompanying Privacy Rule (2001) protects adolescents as much as adults. Adolescents who are legally able to consent to care are generally treated by the Privacy Rule as protected in their own right. The Privacy Rule defers to "state or other applicable law" in terms of parents having access to their children's health information (9). As most states grant adolescents the right to seek confidential care, the Health Insurance Portability and Accountability Act broadly supports confidentiality. However, the specifics of confidentiality protection vary from state to state; hence, clinicians must be knowledgeable about their own state's regulations.

DECIDING WHEN DISCLOSURE IS NECESSARY

How then to handle a situation in which an adolescent discloses information that the clinician believes poses a serious threat to the health of the adolescent? Is it permissible to break confidentiality under these circumstances? Is the clinician required to do so?

Part of the answer lies in what assurance of confidentiality was given to the adolescent. Clearly, some assurance is essential. However, most experts do not recommend a blanket or unconditional assurance, because disclosure is mandated by law in certain circumstances. These include reports of sexual or physical abuse or expression of a clear threat of violence against a readily identifiable individual. Concerns about an adolescent's suicidality also would warrant breaking confidentiality. In such circumstances, the ethical principle of respect for persons, which underlies confidentiality, is overridden by higher ethical principles: "first, do no harm" and obeying the law.

In anticipation of situations such as these, most experts in adolescent health recommend statements that offer conditional confidentiality. Using this approach, the adolescent is assured that most information revealed to the physician will be kept private, but he or she is cautioned that there are some boundaries to the zone of privacy. One sample statement, developed by the American Medical Association's Department of Adolescent Health, is as follows: "I want to assure you that the information we discuss today is between you and me. It's confidential. In other words, I am not going to tell anyone without your permission, unless there is a situation which I believe might threaten your life or another's life or seriously endanger your health" (10). However, recent data suggest that adolescents prefer more specific descriptions of what kinds of discussions will be held confidential (11).

Regardless of the exact assurance the clinician offers, it ultimately rests with his or her judgment as to whether and when a given adolescent's behavior poses a level of risk that warrants a breach of confidentiality. In such cases, the clinician must perform a sufficiently comprehensive assessment to understand how the behavior poses a threat to the adolescent's health.

A belief that a given behavior is wrong in the context of the clinician's own personal, moral, or religious code is not sufficient justification for breaking confidentiality. For example, a personal belief that premarital sex is wrong would not justify disclosing to a parent that an adolescent is sexually active, especially if the adolescent is acting responsibly by taking appropriate steps to protect against sexually transmitted infections or pregnancy. Some clinicians also would argue that, if an adolescent admits to occasionally smoking marijuana but is doing well in school, maintains good relations with his or her parents, and never drives or attends school while "high," then that behavior also does not automatically warrant disclosure.

Even if the clinician concludes that an adolescent's behavior is sufficiently risky to warrant parental involvement, immediate disclosure is not necessarily indicated. The clinician may wish first to discuss his or her concerns with the adolescent and attempt to develop a plan whereby the adolescent can demonstrate a change in the risky behavior. An example would be asking an adolescent who is using marijuana on a regular basis to refrain from smoking for several weeks, with urine testing at the end of that period. In advance, the adolescent would be told that a positive urine test would trigger parental notification.

After a clinician concludes that a breach of confidentiality is warranted, the adolescent should be told in advance and given options about how the disclosure will occur. These might include the adolescent revealing the information to his or her parents in the presence of the clinician, the adolescent telling the parents alone, or the clinician disclosing the information to the parents. In some cases, an adolescent may request that one but not both parents be involved.

SPECIAL CIRCUMSTANCES

The foregoing discussion pertains to typical clinical encounters. In some special circumstances, different rules of confidentiality may apply. For example, the interaction between the adolescent and clinician may be ordered by a

Confidentiality in Dealing with Adolescents *(continued)*

court or required as a condition of return to school. Federal and state regulations also may stipulate conditions of confidentiality for adolescents in drug treatment programs. Under these circumstances, the adolescent, the parents, and the clinician should be clear about the nature of the physician-patient relationship, including the boundaries of confidentiality and who will have access to the adolescent's medical record, including any test results.

REFERENCES

1. National Conference of Commissioners on Uniform State Laws (NCCUSL). *Uniform Health Care Information Act, Uniform Laws Annotated, Part I.* St. Paul, MN: West Publishing Co., 1989: 475–520.
2. Weithorn LA, Campbell S. The competency of children and adolescents to make informed treatment decisions. *Child Development* 1982; 53:1589–1598.
3. Marks A, Malizio J, Hoch J, et al. Assessment of health needs and willingness to utilize health care resources of adolescents in a suburban population. *J Pediatr* 1983;102:456–460.
4. Ford CA, Millstein SG, Halpern-Felsher BL, et al. Influence of physician confidentiality assurances on adolescents' willingness to disclose information and seek future health care. A randomized controlled trial. *JAMA* 1997;278:1029–1034.
5. Lehrer JA, Pantell R, Tebb K, et al. Forgone health care among U.S. adolescents: associations between risk characteristics and confidentiality concern. *J Adolesc Health* 2007;40:218–226.
6. American Medical Association (AMA), Council on Scientific Affairs. Confidential health services for adolescents. *JAMA* 1993;269: 1420–1424.
7. American Medical Association (AMA), Council on Long Range Planning and Development. *AMA Policy Compendium.* Chicago, IL: American Medical Association, 1990:8.
8. American College of Obstetricians and Gynecologists (ACOG). *ACOG Statement of Policy: Confidentiality in Adolescent Health Care.* Washington, DC: The College, 1988.
9. Standards for privacy of individually identifiable health information. Available online at: http://www.hhs.gov/ocr/hipaa/guidelines/guidanceallsections.pdf. Accessed September 1, 2008.
10. Levenberg PB, Elster *AB. Guidelines for Adolescent Preventive Services (GAPS). Implementation and resource manual.* Chicago: American Medical Association, 1995:37–38.
11. Ford CA, Thomsen SL, Compton B. Adolescents' interpretations of conditional confidentiality assurances. *J Adolesc Health* 2001;29: 156–159.

SUGGESTED READING

Hofman AD. A rational policy toward consent and confidentiality in adolescent health care. *J Adolesc Health Care* 1980;1:9–17.

Drug Testing Adolescents in School

Linn Goldberg, MD, FACSM

Laboratory testing for drugs of abuse is found in numerous societal sectors, including the military, business, federal agencies, and organized sports (1–6). Approximately 90% of large companies with more than 5,000 employees have reported a drug testing program (4,7). During the past three decades drug testing has involved Olympic, professional, and U.S. amateur and collegiate athletes (8–10). Drug testing was judged to be a rational approach to reducing drug use among students engaged in middle and high school sports programs in the United States after the U.S. Supreme Court's decision (11), and since that time, more school athletic programs have used drug testing in an attempt to reduce drug use among student-athletes (12–15). A second U.S. Supreme Court case concerning adolescent drug testing during 2003 (16), extended a school's substance use surveillance to include all extracurricular activities.

Although the U.S. Supreme Court has sanctioned drug testing, state courts still can effectively overrule these decisions, based on their state constitution. States have assessed the legality of random student drug testing after the federal courts decisions (17,18). For example, in Oregon, the state Supreme Court agreed with the legality of student-athlete drug testing (17), while the State of Washington Supreme Court overturned its Superior Court and prohibited student drug testing among middle and high school student-athletes as a precondition for participating in school sports (18).

The White House Office of National Drug Control Policy (ONDCP) actively advocates drug testing in schools and published a booklet: *What you need to know about drug testing in schools* (19). The ONDCP has authorized millions of dollars of grants through the U.S. Department of Education, and numerous regional conferences have and are being held throughout the United States (20,21).

TYPES OF DRUG TESTING

Drug testing can be without cause (e.g., no one suspects the persons of using) or there can be "for cause" testing, based on a person's behavior, or after an accident. There is preemployment drug testing, random drug testing in certain businesses such as transportation (e.g., pilots, truck drivers); whereas the military and college, professional, and international sports have random, not for-cause drug testing that may occur at any time (22–25). Also, drug testing is used for rehabilitation from drug addiction and abuse.

Determination of drug use by testing can be done by examination of an individual's urine, blood, hair, sweat, or saliva (22–24). Most programs, including sports, have used urine testing. There are strengths and weaknesses of each test. Although hair analysis may determine drug use that occurred weeks before, it is less likely to determine whether there was very recent substance use. Blood testing, because of its use of needles, is invasive and there is a risk of bleeding, infection and some pain involved.

GOAL OF DRUG TESTING

The goal of a drug testing program can vary, depending on the particular population. From a business perspective, the major aim of preemployment drug screens is more likely to be done to discover drug use, which could indicate whether or not hiring a particular individual will impact the efficiency of their business (e.g., absenteeism, work output) (26). The goal for collegiate, international, Olympic, and professional sports is to ensure competition without the use artificial performance enhancers, which could provide an unfair advantage to the user. Thus, detection, rather than primary prevention of the unhealthy consequences of this level of sports participation, is most important for these policies (27). However, an adolescent drug testing program within the school more than likely has prevention or deterrence as a primary goal, as well as the potential to uncover substance abuse problems, and provide early onset of appropriate treatment.

Thought of in this way, drug testing young student athletes can be reasoned to be a logical extension of the preparticipation physical examination, a procedure designed to detect and protect adolescents from concurrent injury or disease. Central in a physician's report to schools is a medical history, including medication use. Some conditions or prescribed medications may limit certain types of activities. These otherwise "confidential" medical records are reported to schools for the child's safety.

LEGAL ISSUES

As previously mentioned, there have been questions of the legality of drug testing, especially with regard to issues of search and seizure. The U.S. Supreme Court and some federal and state courts have determined that the secondary school environment has a "a special need," wherein suspicionless student drug testing can be used for safety, and discipline and to establish order (11,16,17,28). The issue for the courts was not whether drug testing was an actual deterrent, shown to effectively reduce substance use or abuse, but whether or not it was a legal policy. In 1995, the U.S. Supreme Court sanctioned drug testing in

Drug Testing Adolescents in School *(continued)*

extracurricular school sport activities, wherein there was a balancing between an individual's rights and the need for drug use regulation in schools (16). Justice Clarence Thomas, writing for the majority stated, "it seems self-evident that a drug problem largely fueled by the 'role model' effect of athletes' drug use . . . is effectively addressed by making sure that athletes do not use drugs. By choosing to 'go out for the team' they voluntarily subject themselves to a degree of regulation even higher than that imposed on students generally."

More recently, *Earls v Tecumseh Public School District* (17) upheld expansion of drug testing to other extracurricular activities. Again, Justice Thomas wrote the majority opinion, stating that "individualized suspicion" is not necessary, and that because drug use limits a school's mission and disrupts learning, preemptive measures (e.g., drug testing policies) were deemed to be legal. Despite drug testing being legal in federal courts, state courts can agree with or deny use of student drug testing, based on local laws. For example, in Oregon, the state Supreme Court agreed with the legality of student–athlete drug testing and refused a petition for review (17). In summarizing the Appeals Court decision, Judge Schuman wrote, that with respect to student-athlete drug testing, "They (the plaintiff) neither presented evidence of unreasonableness nor, for that matter, seriously argued that unreasonableness mattered." However, in the state of Washington, the state Supreme Court overturned the decision of its Superior Court and prohibited student drug testing, denying the practice of random testing of middle and high school student–athletes (18). The plurality on the court wrote: "We decline to adopt a doctrine similar to the federal special needs exception in the context of randomly drug testing student athletes." Thus, from state to state, this issue is not final, and schools may have to support their decision to implement drug testing in each individual state.

DRUG TESTING: THE EVIDENCE

Preemployment testing among adults has been shown to have some predictive value. Those testing positive for cannabis/THC appear to be at higher risk for termination, accidents, absenteeism, and disciplinary action (29). A positive cocaine screen has been associated with double the risk of absenteeism and injury (29). In a large study of U.S. postal clerks (30), those testing positive for drug use had 45% higher absenteeism and 40% greater job dismissal rate. To examine the nature and extent of the association between workplace drug testing and worker drug use, Carpenter (31) performed repeated cross-sections from the 2000 to 2001 National Household Surveys on Drug Abuse and the 2002 National Survey on Drug Use and Health. Individuals whose employers perform drug tests were significantly less likely to report past-month marijuana use, even after controlling for a wide array of worker and job characteristics. The overall pattern of results seemed somewhat consistent with workplace drug testing as a deterrent. However, this is not substantiated for adolescents in the school environment.

In general, the support of random drug testing and the positive deterrent effects of drug testing among youth, including those of the White House ONDCP has relied on inference, not well–designed prospective research trials. The ONDCP has stated:

> *Random student drug testing is a powerful public health tool that discourages students from using dangerous, addictive drugs, and confidentially identifies those who may need help or drug treatment. Random testing also promotes a safer, healthier school learning environment.*

There have been a few uncontrolled and nonrandomized reports suggesting that drug testing could have a deterrent effect (32–34), including those among older athletes subject to mandatory testing (35–38). The National Collegiate Athletic Association documented a nearly 50% difference in the use of self–reported anabolic steroid use among Division I football players coincident with initiating drug screening (39). At the same time, Division II football programs, in which there was no threat of testing, reported higher use of anabolic steroids. A study comparing 1,500 athletes from programs with random testing and a group of athletes not subject to testing found less reported use of marijuana, LSD, and barbiturates among athletes who were at risk of urine drug testing (35).

Despite these reports, the statement describing drug testing by Zwerling (40) and workplace drug testing, appears appropriate to describe student drug testing; ". . . a large industry of drug testers has arisen with a financial stake in expanding the market for . . . drug testing." Walsh et al. (41) concluded that drug surveillance is "a public policy instrument that has penetrated far and fast accompanied by almost no credible scientific warrant of effectiveness." Without evidence of deterrent effects among high school student-athletes or those engaged in other extracurricular school activities, the White House ONDCP have not only encouraged schools to implement drug testing programs (42), they have helped establish funds available for schools to implement testing programs (43), despite the fact that drug testing is not considered to be evidence-based, as are many drug prevention education programs (44).

(continued)

Drug Testing Adolescents in School *(continued)*

MORE RECENT RESEARCH

Evidence that considers the deterrent effect of drug testing has begun to emerge. A large epidemiologic investigation of student drug testing was performed by the researchers from the University of Michigan (45). In their study, approximately 18% of the schools contacted reported having a student drug testing program, with a greater number of high schools than middle schools with this policy. Drug use was assessed by self–report questionnaire. Although the study's findings concluded that student drug testing was not associated with (1) students' reported illicit drug use, (2) rates of use among experienced marijuana users, nor (3) was testing associated with illicit drug use among male high school athletes, the study had several design problems that limited the authors' conclusions. First, the study was a cross–sectional design, without a pre and post assessment. Thus it could not be determined whether drug testing was placed in schools with higher initial substance use, which had lowered to reflect other schools' use. Second, despite the large sample size, which should have allowed for very small differences to be detected, the study evaluated schools with different types of testing (e.g., for cause, random, suspicionless). In addition, the authors did not report the level of testing (the percentage or number of tests performed) and quality of the procedures of testing. Most important, the data analysis included students who were not subject to testing, but just attended the schools. For these reasons, the data of this large study cannot be considered to be conclusive.

We performed two prospective drug testing studies (33,46). The pilot investigation of the intervention entitled, SATURN (Student Athlete Testing Using Random Notification) assessed two rural schools in Oregon using identical confidential surveys over a school year (33). One school was to begin a school student–athlete drug testing program, but had not implemented the policy before being in the pilot SATURN study. The other high school was of similar size and selected as a control. The control school had never established a drug testing program before recruitment. Overall, 276 student–athletes took the initial voluntary, confidential survey, and 159 student–athletes in the sample completed the end of the school year questionnaire. Thirty percent of the athletes were tested during the school year. Past 30–day index of illicit drugs and athletic enhancing substances were lower (both $p < .05$) among those athletes in the drug testing school at follow–up, but there were no differences reported in alcohol use. However, some drug use risk factors (all $p < .05$), worsened, including the belief in higher norms of use, belief in lower risk of drugs, and less positive attitudes toward the school, when athletes subject to drug testing were compared with the sports participants at the control school. This suggested potential greater risk of future substance use. Because of the relatively small sample size, the lack of randomization and changes in risk factors, we urged caution before implementing a program without studying its effects.

The larger randomized control SATURN trial, assessed drug testing over 2 years among a single cohort of athletes in five intervention (drug and alcohol testing) schools, compared with six nontesting comparison schools (46). Although drug testing was mandatory, suspicionless, and without previous notification, survey completion was voluntary for all student–athletes. Substance use was serially assessed at the beginning and end of the school year for 2 calendar years. Student–athletes were at risk for random testing during the entire academic year, not only during their sport season, similar to the pilot study. In the analysis, we combined multiple drugs with and without alcohol as a drug index and drug and alcohol index, for both past–month and past–year use. This was done to include students who may switch to substances that were more difficult to detect (e.g., alcohol or club drugs during the testing period).

No differences were found for past-month drug use or for past drug and alcohol use at any of the 4 follow-up over 2 years. However, at two time points (the end of the initial year and after two full school years), student-athletes in the drug testing schools reported less past-year drug use ($p < .01$) when compared with the student athletes in the control schools.

When combining past-year drugs with alcohol use, student-athletes at the drug testing schools reported less use ($p < .05$) at the second and third follow-up, but not at the conclusion of the study. Thus, when combining alcohol with drugs, the deterrent of past–year use vanished at the final testing period. Similar to the pilot investigation, athletes within the drug testing schools reported worsening of some potential risk factors for future drug use. Those included feeling less athletic competence ($p < .001$), having less belief that authorities were opposed to drug use ($p < .01$), and indicating greater risk-taking ($p < .05$). At the final assessment, the athletes in drug testing schools were more likely to believed less in testing benefits ($p < .05$) and less that testing was a reason not to use drugs ($p < .01$).

CONCLUSION

Drug testing is not an established evidence–based policy shown to prevent drug use. Student–athlete and other school–based drug testing have not been evaluated in a

Drug Testing Adolescents in School *(continued)*

randomized control trial more than one time. Its failure to demonstrate reduction in past-month substance use (drug use or drug and alcohol use) suggests that more research with randomized control studies are needed to establish whether there are clear benefits of testing. Because of the potential risk (increasing risk factors for future drug or alcohol use) of testing and the costs of testing (not only the actual test, but the use of school personnel, lost class time, and more expensive tests [e.g., anabolic-androgenic steroids]), it appears prudent that schools wishing to implement prevention programs should do what they do best and educate their students using evidence-based programs. This is especially relevant, because multiple drug education programs have been shown to be effective in preventing substance use both in the short and long term (44).

REFERENCES

1. Fuentes RJ, Rosenberg JM, David A, eds. *Athletic drug reference '95.* Research Triangle Park, NC: Clean Data, Inc., 1995.
2. Programme on Substance Abuse: drug use and sport; current issues and implications for public health. World Health Organization, Jerri Husch, ed. Geneva, Switzerland, 1993.
3. United States Olympic Committee. *National anti-doping program: policies and procedures.* USOC Drug Control Administration Division, Colorado Springs, Colorado, 1996.
4. Peat MA. Financial viability of screening for drugs of abuse. *Clin Chem* 1995;41:805–808.
5. Wadler GI, Hainline B. Drugs and the athlete. Philadelphia, PA: F.A. Davis Company, 1989.
6. Landry GL, Kokotailo PK. Drug screening in the athletic setting. *Curr Problems Pediatr* 1994;344–359.
7. Zwerling C. Drug testing. *JAMA* 1994;272:1467–1468.
8. Mottram DR, ed. *Drugs in sports,* 2nd ed. London: Chapman & Hall, 1995.
9. Fuentes RJ, Rosenberg JM, David A, eds. *Athletic drug reference '95.* Research Triangle Park, NC: Clean Data, Inc., 1995.
10. Ferstle J. Evolution and politics of drug testing. In: Yesalis C, ed. *Anabolic steroids in sport and exercise.* Champaign, IL: Human Kinetics, 1992.
11. *Vernonia School District 47 v Acton.* 15 S Ct 2386 (1995).
12. Hegeman R. Kansas town adopts tough drug testing. Associated Press, September 13, 2006. Available online at: http://www.sfgate.com/cgi-bin/article.cgi?f=/n/a/2006/09/13/national/a11321D03.DTL&hw=drugs&sn=001&sc=1000
13. Florida to begin drug testing of prep athletes. *USA Today,* June 19, 2007. http://www.usatoday.com/sports/preps/2007-06-19-fla-steroids-testing_N.htm.
14. Sterling E. UIL adopts rules for athlete drug testing. *Raymondville Chronicle News,* January 16, 2008. Available online at: http://www.raymondvillechroniclenews.com/news/2008/0116/news/024.html. Accessed September 1, 2008.
15. Temkin B. Teen athletes face drug tests: for 1st time, state requires random testing. Chicago Tribune, January 14, 2008.
16. *Board of Ed. of Independent School Dist. No. 92 of Pottawatomie City. v. Earls* (01-332) 536 U.S. 822 (2002) 242 F.3d 1264, reversed.
17. The Oregon State Supreme Court denied Certiorari in Weber v. Oakridge School District 69 P.3d 1233 (OR 2003). Court of Appeals ruling prevails. Weber v. Oakridge School District 76 Oregon State Supreme Court 16-00-21584; A114141 Appeal from Circuit Court, Lane County.
18. *York v. Wahkiakum Sch. Dist. No. 200.* Supreme Court of the State of Washington, no. 78946-1: March 13, 2008.
19. Office of National Drug Control Policy, Drug Testing in Schools, 2002. Executive Office of the President of the United States, pp. 1–16.
20. Grants for school–based student drug–testing programs CFDA 84.184D. Available online at: http://www.grants.gov/search/ search.do?&mode=VIEW&flag2006=true&oppId=16260. Accessed September 1, 2008.
21. ONDCP takes drug-testing campaign on road. *Join Together* news summary. February 24, 2006. http://www.jointogether.org/news/headlines/inthenews/2006/ondcp-takes-drug-testing.html. Accessed September 1, 2008.
22. SAMHSA proposes updated rules for federal workplace drug testing. The Substance Abuse and Mental Health Services Administration (SAMHSA), Department of Health and Human Services. April 6, 2004. http://www.samhsa.gov/news/newsreleases/040406nr_DWP_guidelines.htm. Accessed September 1, 2008.
23. Pabinger C, Gruber G. World anti–doping regulations for 2005: essential changes for athletes and physicians. *Arch Orthop Trauma Surg* 2006;125(4):286–288.
24. Tokish JM, Kocher MS, Hawkins RJ. Ergogenic aids: a review of basic science, performance, side effects, and status in sports. *Am J Sports Med* 2004;32(6):1543–1553.
25. Bush DM. The U.S. mandatory guidelines for federal workplace drug testing programs: current status and future considerations. *Forensic Sci Int* 2008;174(2–3):111–119.
26. Under the Influence? Drugs and the American work force. Normand J, Lempert RO, O'Brien CP, eds. (Committee on Drug Use in the Workplace, National Research Council/Institute of Medicine.) Washington, DC: National Academy Press, 1994.
27. United States Olympic Committee. National anti doping program: policies and procedures. USOC Drug Control Administration Division, 1996.
28. Estrin I, Sher L. The constitutionality of random drug and alcohol testing of students in secondary schools. *Int J Adolesc Med Health* 2006;18(1):21–25.
29. Zwerling C, Ryan J, Orav EJ. The efficacy of preemployment drug screening for marijuana and cocaine in predicting employment outcome. *JAMA* 1990;264:2639–2643.
30. Normand J, Salyards SD. An empirical evaluation of pre employment drug testing in the United States Postal Service: interim report of findings. In: Gust SW, Walsh JM, eds. *Drugs in the workplace: research and evaluation data.* Rockville, MD: National Institute on Drug Abuse, 1989:111–138.
31. Carpenter CS. Workplace drug testing and worker drug use. *Health Serv Res* 2007;42(2):795–810.
32. Landry GL, Kokotailo PK. Drug screening in the athletic setting. *Curr Probl Pediatr* 1994;24:344–359.
33. Goldberg L, Elliot DL, MacKinnon DP, et al. Drug testing athletes to prevent substance abuse: Background and Pilot study results of the SATURN (Student Athlete Testing Using Random Notification) study. *J Adolesc Health* 2003;32:16–25.
34. Drug Testing in Schools. Case history: testing made the difference: Hunterdon Central regional high school. What you need to know about drug testing in schools. Office of National Drug Control Policy.

(continued)

Drug Testing Adolescents in School *(continued)*

http://www.whitehousedrugpolicy.gov/publications/drug_testing/administering.html#casehx. Accessed September 1, 2008.

35. Coombs RH, Ryan FJ. Drug testing effectiveness in identifying and preventing drug use. *Am J Drug Alcohol Abuse* 1990;16:173–184.
36. Anderson SW, McKeag DB. The substance use and abuse habits of college students athletes. Mission, KS: National College Athletic Association, 1985.
37. Anderson WA, Albrech RR, McKeag DB. A national survey of alcohol and drug use by college athletes. *Phys Sports Med* 1991;19:91–104.
38. National Collegiate Athletic Association. Steroid use drops among student-athletes. September 1, 1993:1.
39. National Collegiate Athletic Association. Only 0.3% ruled ineligible in fall 1993 drug testing. *NCAA News June 4*, 1994:1.
40. Zwerling C. Drug testing. *JAMA* 1994;272:1467–1468.
41. Walsh DC, Elinson E, Gostin L. Worksite drug testing. *Ann Rev Public Health* 1992;13:197–221.
42. Office of National Drug Control Policy, Drug Testing in Schools, 2002. Executive Office of the President of the United States, pp. 1–16.
43. School–based drug testing programs. Office of Safe and Drug Free Schools. http://www.ed.gov/programs/drugtesting/index.html. Accessed September 1, 2008.
44. NREPP: SAMHSA's National Registry of Evidence based Programs and Practices. Available online at: http://www.nrepp.samhsa.gov/. Accessed September 1, 2008.
45. Yamaguchi R, Johnston LD, O'Malley PM. Relationship between student illicit drug use and school drug testing policies. *J School Health* 2003;73(4):159–164.
46. Goldberg L, Elliot EL, MacKinnon DP, et al. Outcomes of a prospective trial of student-athlete drug testing: the Student Athlete Testing Using Random Notification (SATURN) study. *J Adolesc Health* 2007;41(5):421–429.

CHAPTER 106

Marie E. Armentano, MD
Ramon Solhkhah, MD
Deborah R. Simkin, MD

Co-occurring Psychiatric Disorders in Adolescents

Despite recent studies showing that levels of adolescent alcohol and drug use have essentially stabilized, they are sufficiently high to remain a major concern. Given recent increases in the use of "club drugs" such as 3,4-methylenedioxymethamphetamine (MDMA or "Ecstasy"), ketamine, and gamma-hydroxybutyrate (GHB) over the past several years, as well as evidence that the age of first use continues to decline, it is difficult to claim victory in the "War on Drugs."

Adolescents who manifest other psychiatric diagnoses in addition to substance use have elicited increasing concern (1–17).

In fact, adolescents with substance use disorders (SUDs) exhibit a high prevalence of psychiatric disorders compared to the general population (12,18–23). Studies of treatment-seeking SUD adolescents have documented that 50% to 90% also have non-SUD comorbid psychiatric disorders (12,14,24–29). Not only are specific psychiatric disorders associated with alcohol and drug use, but other problems that affect teens—such as suicide, violence, and pregnancy—also are associated with an increased risk of substance use.

In this chapter, the terms *dual diagnosis*, *comorbidity*, and *co-occurring disorders* are used interchangeably to refer to patients who meet the criteria for a substance use disorder and for another psychiatric diagnosis on Axis I or II of the *Diagnostic and Statistical Manual of Mental Disorders,* 4th Edition (DSM-IV-TR) of the American Psychiatric Association (1). The term *substance use disorder* is used to include both abuse and dependence. Adolescents who initially seek treatment for a SUD—the focus of this chapter—may be different from those who seek care for a psychiatric disorder (30,31).

Awareness of the most likely disorders and formulation of an integrated treatment plan is essential. This chapter reviews what is known about comorbidities and offers guidelines for their management and the care of adolescents so affected.

DEFINITIONAL ISSUES

Dual diagnosis issues initially were studied in adults (31–36), leaving the clinician to extrapolate from this research to the adolescent population. More recently, adolescent clinical and community populations have been studied (3,5–8,10,12–14,16,25,37–46).

According to Bukstein and Kaminer (47), however, diagnostic issues related to adolescent substance use continue to be problematic. The criteria that have been developed have not been validated with adolescents, and there may be some discontinuities between adolescent and adult populations (47,48). When diagnostic criteria are based on problem behaviors, it often is not clear whether the behaviors are the result of substance use or of a coexisting or preexisting problem. Though craving and loss of control are included in the criteria, no studies have established whether these actually are present in adolescents (47). Nosology is only the best attempt to make sense of reality; as a result, an imperfect system designed for adults is used to make substance abuse diagnoses in adolescents (47–50).

METHODOLOGIC QUESTIONS

Some of the methodologic questions are identical for adults and adolescents. In both populations, the course and treatment of the same two disorders may vary depending on which one is primary—in other words, which disorder preceded the other (33)—and their relative severity (28,30,34,45,51,52). It is not helpful to assume that all patients with dual diagnoses have the same problems and require the same treatment (45). Though a high prevalence of comorbidity has been reported among adolescent inpatients with SUDs (10,12,13,53–55), it is unclear how many exhibit psychiatric symptoms secondary to the SUDs and how many have a primary or coexisting psychiatric diagnosis.

INCIDENCE AND PREVALENCE

Physicians should know the kinds of comorbidities they are likely to encounter in practice. Until recently, however, large-scale population studies did not focus on adolescents. The National Institute of Mental Health (NIMH) Epidemiologic Catchment Area (ECA) Study (37) attempted to estimate the true prevalence rates of alcohol, other drug abuse disorders, and mental disorders in an adult community and institutional sample of more than 20,000 subjects standardized to the U.S. Bureau of the Census. Of the total, 37% of persons with alcohol use disorders had another mental disorder, with the highest prevalence for affective, anxiety, and antisocial personality disorders. More than half of those with SUDs other than alcohol use had a comorbid mental disorder, including 28% with an anxiety disorders, 26% with an affective disorder, 18% with an antisocial personality disorder, and 7% with schizophrenia. This study verified the widely held impression that comorbidity rates are much higher among clinical and institutional populations than in the general population.

Until very recently, studies involving adolescents were smaller and involved clinical populations. Stowell and Estroff (14) studied 226 adolescents receiving inpatient treatment for a primary substance abuse disorder in private psychiatric hospitals. Psychiatric diagnoses were made 4 weeks into treatment by using a semistructured diagnostic interview. Of the total, 82% of the patients met DSM-IIIR (56) criteria for an Axis I psychiatric disorder, 61% had mood disorders, 54% had conduct disorders, 43% had anxiety disorders, and 16% had substance-induced disorder. Three-fourths of the patients (74%) had two or more psychiatric disorders. Westermeyer et al. (46) found similarly high rates of comorbidity and multiple diagnoses in 100 adolescents 12 to 20 years of age who sought care at two university-based outpatient addiction treatment programs. Of the study group, 22 of 100 had eating disorders, 8 had conduct disorders, 7 had major depressive disorder, 6 had minor depressive disorder, 5 had bipolar disorder, 5 had schizophrenia, and 4 had anxiety disorders. Three had another psychotic disorder, 3 had an organic mental disorder, and 2 had attention deficit/hyperactivity disorder (ADHD).

The distribution of diagnoses as a function of age showed that eating disorder diagnoses and depressive symptoms occurred more frequently in older adolescents (46). Giaconia et al. (39) studied the issue of age in a predominantly white, working-class community sample of 386 individuals 18 years old. They compared adolescents who had met the criteria for one of six psychiatric diagnoses, including SUDs, before and after they were 14 years of age. Adolescents with early onset of any psychiatric disorder were six times as likely to have one, and 12 times as likely to have two, additional disorders by the time they were 18 years of age than were those with later onset of psychiatric disorders (39). This finding suggests that the clinician's index of suspicion for dual diagnosis must be particularly high for younger patients with SUDs.

Burke et al. (37) studied data from the NIMH ECA study to determine hazard rates for the development of disorders and concluded that 15 to 19 years were the peak ages for the onset of depressive disorders in females and for the onset of SUDs and bipolar disorders in both genders.

The National Comorbidity Survey included a large noninstitutional sample of persons aged 15 to 24, though adolescents were not studied separately from young adults (41). Compared with older adults, 15- to 24-year-olds had the highest prevalence of three or more disorders occurring together and of any disorders, including SUDs. In the Methods for the Epidemiology of Child and Adolescent Mental Disorders study rates of co-morbidity were higher in the non-treatment group for conduct disorders (68%) and depression (32%) than those noted in the adolescent treatment sample: 55% and 9%, respectively (56a,40).

DIAGNOSIS AND MANAGEMENT

Controversies aside, psychologists, psychiatrists, and other mental health professionals need to treat the patients they encounter. Some of those patients will have a psychiatric diagnosis. Clinicians will serve such patients well if they (1) conduct a comprehensive evaluation of each patient that includes a mental status examination and an inquiry into other psychiatric symptomatology and obtain information from multiple sources; (2) have a high index of suspicion for comorbidity in adolescents whose conditions do not respond to treatment or who present problems in treatment; (3) individualize treatment to accommodate both the substance use and psychiatric diagnoses; (4) obtain a comprehensive history of alcohol, tobacco, and other drug use; and (5) know when to consult an addiction medicine specialist or mental health professional.

Depressive Disorders Much has been written about the interplay between depression and substance use (3,16,25,28,34–36,38,42,57,58). The emerging concept is that in adolescents (3,12,25,28,47,58) and adults (34–36), two groups exhibit significant depressive symptoms: those individuals who have a substance-induced mood disorder and those who have a primary depressive disorder. The chief symptom of depression consists of a disturbance of mood, which usually is characterized as sadness or feeling "down in the dumps," and a loss of interest or pleasure. Adolescents may report or exhibit irritability instead of sadness. In addition, their depression may be characterized by guilt, hopelessness, sleep disturbances, appetite disturbances, loss of ability to concentrate, diminution of energy, and thoughts of death or suicide.

To meet DSM-IV-TR diagnostic criteria, the patient must exhibit or experience depressed mood most of the day, every day, for 2 weeks (1). Patients with a substance-induced mood disorder may exhibit the same depressive symptoms.

Schuckit (34–36) and Miller (32) stress the importance of distinguishing between primary depressive disorder and substance-induced mood disorder. Studies of adults who abuse substances showed that substance-induced mood disorder dissipates with abstinence, but primary depressive disorders do not and, if left untreated, can interfere with treatment and recovery (32–34,37). Deykin et al. (7,25) interviewed 223 adolescents in residential addiction treatment programs and found that almost 25% met the DSM-IIIR (56) criteria for depression. Of these, 8% met the criteria for primary depression, and the other 16% had a secondary mood disorder. Bukstein et al. (59) studied adolescent inpatients on a dual diagnosis unit and reported that almost 31% had a comorbid major depression, with secondary depressive disorder much more common than primary depressive disorder. Unlike adults, the secondary depression in adolescents did not remit with abstinence (3). This finding, if replicated, would argue for more vigorous treatment of depressive syndromes in adolescents.

During the mental status examination, depressed adolescents may seem taciturn and show poor eye contact and a sad-looking face. They may be poorly groomed or drably dressed and may become tearful during the interview. Often they deny feelings of sadness, though their demeanor states it eloquently. Depression interferes with treatment through lack of concentration, motivation, and hope as well as the tendency toward isolation. Kempton et al. (60) found cognitive distortions, including magnification (all-or-nothing thinking) and personalizing, to be particularly prominent among adolescents with the multiple diagnoses of conduct disorder, depressive disorder, and substance abuse. A depressed adolescent may benefit from a specific cognitive intervention for depression (49,61).

In one study, 126 adolescents with a DSM-IV diagnosis of Major Depression, Conduct Disorders and Substance Use Disorders (SUD) were studied to determine the efficacy of fluoxetine vs placebo. Both groups received cognitive behavior therapy (CBT) for their SUD during the 16 week trial. Rates of depression remission was high in both groups, 75% vs 64% respectively but rates of abstinence were relatively low. Post hoc analysis predicted that remission of depression was a stronger predictor of change in drug use than medication treatment. Therefore, the implication from this study was that depression symptoms may remit in the context of individual outpatient CBT for SUD without pharmacotherapy of abstinence. However, if depression does not remit within the first month of treatment, it appears that starting fluoxetine, with careful monitoring, even if not yet abstinent, is prudent because ongoing depression may prevent abstinence achievement (56a,61a,61b). Serotonin agentsdlike fluoxetine have a safe profile for side effects and may be appropriate considering reports that young substance abusers may have a preexisting serotonin deficit (6,11,62).

If there are doubts about the diagnosis of depression or about how to treat, consultation with a psychiatrist experienced in treating adolescents with SUDs is indicated. If the primary clinician is concerned about possible suicidal behavior, a consultation should be sought without delay (4,38,57).

Bipolar Disorder The diagnosis of bipolar disorder may be among the most difficult to make in children and adolescents and is even more difficult in teens who use alcohol or other drugs. Issues such as changes in sleeping patterns or mood swings can be symptoms of bipolar disorder, substance use, or even normal adolescence. The diagnosis of bipolar disorder certainly should be considered in substance-using youth, particularly those with a binge pattern.

In bipolar disorder, which often begins during late adolescence (5,39,63), the initial symptoms of mania include a persistently elevated, expansive, or irritable mood lasting at least 1 week, accompanied by grandiosity or inflated self-esteem, decreased need for sleep, pressured speech, racing thoughts, increased purposeful activity, and excessive involvement in pleasurable activities, such as spending money, sexual indiscretions, or substance use (1). Wilens et al. (63) have found an increased risk for SUDs in adolescents with bipolar disorder. They reported that those with adolescent-onset bipolar disorder had an 8.8 times greater risk of developing a SUD than those with childhood-onset bipolar disorder, and no other disorder, including conduct disorder, accounted for the risk. Children who were diagnosed and treated appropriately at a younger age had a lower subsequent risk for substance use.

Some patients use substances, particularly alcohol, to calm themselves during a manic phase. Clearly, some of these symptoms also are seen with substance intoxication. If a patient exhibits these symptoms after a period of abstinence, the diagnosis of bipolar disorder should be considered. Valproic acid, carbamazepine, and other anticonvulsants also are used, as are the atypical antipsychotics, such as olanzapine and risperidone (63–65). In a study by Geller (9), when lithium was used, not only were the symptoms of mania decreased but the use of alcohol also decreased. Clinicians should be aware that although the diagnosis of Severe Mood Dysregulation (SMD) is not found in the DSM IV TR, care should be taken in distinguishing SMD from a diagnosis of Bipolar Disorder (65a,65b).

Anxiety Disorders Anxiety disorders are among the psychiatric conditions most often coexisting in adolescents and adults with SUDs. Typically, these conditions include generalized anxiety disorder, panic disorder, social phobia, obsessive-compulsive disorder, and posttraumatic stress disorder. Anxiety disorders often are not detected or treated, especially when present in combination with depression or psychoactive SUDs (5,53). In fact, many adolescents (and adults) believe that drugs and alcohol may contribute to reduction of anxiety and stress, and this belief may lead them to initiate or continue use. Sometimes a closer examination of patients who resist attending self-help meetings may reveal a social phobia or agoraphobia. Social phobia and its importance in terms of early diagnosis cannot be overemphasized. Though many children with social phobia are not recognized early because they are not a behavioral problem in class, children who are referred for evaluation for aggression should be carefully evaluated for social phobia. In a study by Swan (66), the combination of shyness and aggressiveness in boys was a more valid predictor of future cocaine use than a history of aggressiveness alone. Merikangas et al. (67), in the International Consortium of Psychiatric Epidemiology, demonstrated that the onset of anxiety disorders was more likely to precede that of SUDs in all countries. Social phobia was highly comorbid with depressive disorder, somatoform disorder, and SUDs in a study of 1,035 adolescents, ages 13 to 17 (68). To make matters even more confusing, some well-done studies show that teens who *never* use drugs or alcohol may be at higher risk for anxiety disorders later in life.

Panic Disorder Panic attacks are periods of intense discomfort that develop abruptly and reach a peak within 10 minutes. Symptoms include palpitations, sweating, trembling, sensations of shortness of breath or choking, chest discomfort, nausea, dizziness, and fears of losing control or dying. As some of these symptoms also might be seen in substance intoxication or withdrawal, it is important to establish abstinence before making a diagnosis.

Social Phobias Patients with a social phobia may isolate themselves on an inpatient unit or in a group. A careful interview in which anxiety symptoms and family history of anxiety disorders are pursued may be quite revealing.

Behavioral treatment, including relaxation training, often is helpful for anxiety disorders (49). The issue of pharmacotherapy is controversial. Many argue that the use of benzodiazepines is contraindicated in anyone with a history of substance abuse. Buspirone hydrochloride and serotonin reuptake inhibitors have been recommended as nonaddictive antianxiety agents (65). Clinical experience and anecdotal reports suggest that for many, buspirone is ineffective. When treating patients who insist that only benzodiazepines are effective, it often is not clear whether the statement represents drug-seeking behavior or a bona fide observation. If abstinence has been established, adequate trials of behavioral or cognitive therapy (49) and alternative medications have failed, and the patient adheres to the treatment and medication regimen, the judicious use of a long-acting benzodiazepine, such as clonazepam, may be justified.

Posttraumatic Stress Disorder In clinical reports on adolescents, the incidence of severe trauma and symptoms of posttraumatic stress disorder is surprisingly high (7,40,53–55). An adolescent who has been acting out and abusing substances may not have dealt with an earlier trauma, such as physical and sexual abuse or exposure to violence, or with the trauma that may be incurred when abusing substances (54). Symptoms and memories of trauma may manifest themselves only during abstinence.

Trauma and the symptoms associated with trauma should to be considered and inquired about to ensure adequate treatment of adolescents who abuse substances. Care should be taken to acknowledge the trauma without arousing anxiety that will interfere with abstinence and substance abuse treatment. Groups that support self-care and a first-things-first attitude may be the best approach; the patient needs to learn to stay safe, and treatment for substance abuse is a most important aspect of safety. Effective treatments suggests that integrated PTSD- and SUD-focused cognitive-behavioral and family treatment for adolescents with comorbid abuse-related PTSD and SUD may optimize outcomes for this population (68a). In another study comparing treatment as usual (TAU) to a manualized psychotherapy technique called Seeking Safety (SS) on adolescents in an outpatients setting, a variety of domains at posttreatment, including substance use and associated problems, some trauma-related symptoms, cognitions related to SUD and PTSD, and several areas of pathology not targeted in the treatment (e.g., anorexia, somatization) were significantly better in the SS group. Effect sizes were generally in the moderate to high range. Some gains were sustained at follow-up. Therefore, SS appears a promising treatment for this population, but needs further study and perhaps additional clinical modification (68b).

Substance-Induced Mental Disorders In some patients, the use of substances—particularly alcohol, methamphetamine, marijuana, cocaine, ecstasy, hallucinogens, and inhalants—is associated with acute and residual cognitive damage (1,14,60). Acute symptoms may include impaired concentration and receptive and expressive language abilities, as well as irritability. Long-term interference with memory and other executive functions may occur.

The possibility of a substance-induced dementia should be considered in adolescents who have difficulty coping with the cognitive and organizational demands of a structured and supportive program. Some adolescents will be able to use the program if instructions are simplified and if they comprehend information accurately. Improvement in cognitive functioning may be rapid, but the cognitive functioning of some patients continues to improve for as long as a year or more after cessation of the chemical assault to the brain. Some may be left with residual impairments.

Adolescents and their families should be informed of the cognitive consequences of their substance use in a way that does not engender despair but clearly warns against further alcohol or drug use. The presence of cognitive deficits, if they persist, should be considered in rehabilitation, educational, and vocational planning. Such patients need neuropsychologic evaluation and follow-up.

For patients who are exposed to substances of abuse and/or alcohol prenatally, the presence of fetal alcohol syndrome or alcohol- or drug-related neuropsychiatric disorders after birth should be diagnosed with a substance-induced mental disorder secondary to the drug and/or alcohol exposure. Fetal alcohol syndrome is one of the most preventable forms of mental retardation. The distinct facial features make this disorder easier to diagnose than alcohol-related neuropsychiatric disorders, which have no distinct facial features. In fact, 60% to 90% escape identification in the normal population (69). The effect of prenatal cigarette and marijuana smoking, and cocaine use on cognitive ability must also be considered. Prenatal cigarette exposure was associated with lower IQ, poorer auditory functioning, and poorer performance on tests requiring fundamental aspects of visual perceptual performance (70). Marijuana exposure altered neural functioning during visuospatial working memory processing in young adulthood (71). Though cocaine can cause developmental delays and learning disorders, it is clear that findings once thought to be specific to in utero cocaine exposure are more likely associated with alcohol, tobacco, and marijuana and the quality of the child's environment (72).

In fact, a stimulating home environment and high maternal verbal IQ also predicted higher composite IQ scores. Cocaine-exposed boys had lower scores on the Abstract/Visual Reasoning subscale, with trends for lower scores on the Short-Term Memory and Verbal Reasoning subscales, as exposure effects were observed across domains (73).

Learning Disorders Hops et al. (74) found that substance abuse at age 14 or 15 could be predicted by academic and social behavior between the ages of 7 and 9. Therefore, early detection of learning disorders is essential in order to reduce the risk of developing a SUD. Given that some attentional problems are not readily recognized without proper testing, like processing speed deficits and auditory processing problems (75), clinicians should explore other possibilities for attentional problems. In fact, Tapert et al. (76) has shown that attentional difficulties, not necessarily related to attention deficit hyperactivity disorder, predicted substance abuse 8 years later.

Schizophrenia Patients who simultaneously meet the criteria for schizophrenia and a SUD are less likely to receive treatment in an addiction treatment program than in a psychiatric unit (30,52). As the late adolescent years are a time when many schizophrenic disorders begin and the use of substances may precipitate an incipient psychosis, patients with this disorder may seek treatment during the early stages of schizophrenia (13,31,33).

Increasingly, younger schizophrenic patients use substances (31,77,78), some in an attempt to manage or deny their symptoms. Their substance use often interferes with treatment of their psychotic disorder. Such patients are best managed in special dual diagnosis programs for psychotic patients, where the psychosis and the substance use are addressed through integrated mental health and addiction treatment (30,43,52,55,77–80).

Numerous research has indicated that there may be a reward deficiency dysfunction in schizophrenia that underlines the use of substances of abuse to compensate for this reward deficiency (56a,80a) and that clozapine and other atypical agents may be effective in the treatment of co-occurring schizophrenia and SUD (56a,80b). Green, et al. have suggested that clozapine may effective because of its weak blockade of D2 receptors, its potent blockade of norepinephrine alpha 2 receptors and its ability to release norepinephrine in the brain which may allow this medication to ameliorate the brain reward circuit deficit in schizophrenic patients that underlie their substance abuse (56a,80c). Marijuana and alcohol are the two most frequently used substances in these patients and marijuana may trigger psychosis in vulnerable individuals. Marijuana in these individuals may be associated with early onset of schizophrenia and clinicians should be aware of this because marijuana is so widely used by adolescents (56a,80d).

Attention Deficit Hyperactivity Disorder Many professionals involved in the treatment of adolescents with SUDs have noted the large number who also have attention deficit hyperactivity disorder (6,16,17,44,51,81,82). Bukstein et al. (83) postulate that there is no direct connection but that both often coexist with conduct disorder. Crowley and Riggs (6) noted comorbidity with affective, anxiety, and antisocial disorders in the patients and their families.

Treatment should include behavioral and educational interventions. Pharmacotherapy for adolescents has been controversial (83). Riggs et al. (83) have reported some success with the use of bupropion. Wilens et al. (17) suggested that the use of stimulants to treat adolescents for attention deficit hyperactivity disorder may lower the risk of a subsequent SUD. There are few studies on the use of long acting stimulants in the treatment in adolescents with SUD and ADHD. However, in one study, subjects had a significantly greater reduction in ADHD symptoms ($P < 0.001$ for all analyses) during treatment with long acting stimulants compared to placebo. However, there was no significant effect on drug use (83a).

Riggs, et al, have suggested that it is prudent to use non stimulant medications as a first line when treating co morbid ADHD and SUD. However, prior to starting stimulants, the following questions should be asked: 1) Have other non-stimulant medications been tried or are there specific reasons why stimulants make sense as a first line treatment? 2) Is the patient a current substance abuser? 3) If so, has the family been warned about specific potential risks involved in using stimulants? 4) Is the patient reliable and can parents be involved in the distribution of the medication and in the treatment plan? 5) If the patient is a current substance abuser, is he/she motivated and actively involved in treatment? 6) Has the patient had an established period of abstinence? 7) Is there a history of amphetamine or other stimulant abuse? 8) If the individual abused stimulants, what was the reason for the use? To get school work done or get high? (56a).

There is growing evidence of other cognitive interventions that may assist with the improvement of attention, a major component of ADHD. There are no studies that have used these techniques in the treatment of adolescents with SUD and ADHD, but these may prove helpful in the future (83b).

Conduct Disorder and Antisocial Personality Disorder Conduct disorder and antisocial personality disorder are the diagnoses that most often co-occur with substance abuse, particularly in males (6,13,14,16,17,28,34,40,46,51,58). The characteristic symptom of antisocial personality disorder is a pervasive pattern of disregarding and violating the rights of others. The disorder may involve deceitfulness, impulsivity, failure to conform to rules or the law, aggressiveness, and irresponsibility (1). Conduct disorder has similar criteria but includes manifestations that are likely to be seen in younger persons, such as cruelty to animals, running away, truancy, and vandalism.

Many researchers have noted that adolescent SUD usually occurs as part of a constellation of problem behaviors (6,8,40,44,82). Cloninger (84) presented an interesting scheme of hereditary factors on three axes that may account for many psychiatric diagnoses and their interrelationships. The three axes are reward-dependence, harm-avoidance, and novelty seeking. Based on these axes, Cloninger (84) distinguished type 1 and type 2 alcoholic patients. Type 2 alcoholic patients score low on reward dependence and harm-avoidance and high on novelty seeking. Younger alcoholic patients with antisocial personality fit the type 2 classification. The higher prevalence of antisocial personality and conduct disorders among younger alcoholic patients may explain why many clinicians find adolescent substance abusers more difficult to treat.

Horowitz et al. (11) consider many young patients who abuse substances to have a combination of characteristics (such as increased hostility, depression, and suicidal ideation) that suggest an underlying—perhaps neurochemically determined—difficulty with self-regulation and aggression. Adolescents with conduct disorders and antisocial personality disorder need a strong behavioral program with clear limits. If there is a comorbid disorder (such as a mood or attention disorder that can be treated successfully), the adolescent is more likely to do well (6,17,82).

Borderline and Narcissistic Personality Disorders

In addition to psychiatric diagnoses on Axis I, the personality disorders described on Axis II of the DSM-IV are relevant to the treatment of adolescents who abuse substances (1,85,86). Personality disorders are enduring patterns of inner experience and behavior that affect cognition, interpersonal behavior, emotional response, and impulse control. Personality factors often make an adolescent difficult to treat.

Borderline personality disorder is marked by impulsivity and instability of interpersonal relationships, which affect self-image. A marked sensitivity and wish to avoid abandonment, chronic feelings of emptiness, inappropriate and intense anger, and suicidal or self-mutilating behavior are characteristic of borderline personality disorder. In a treatment setting, patients with borderline personality disorder can wreak havoc because of the severe regression often manifested and the divisiveness they often cause among staff.

A pervasive pattern of grandiosity, a need for admiration, and a lack of empathy characterize narcissistic personality disorder. The patient feels unique and entitled to special treatment. A patient with narcissistic personality disorder may have difficulty participating in groups or seeing other people except as need gratifiers.

Both of these personality disorders can present challenges to the clinician and the treatment staff. Powerful negative feelings, conscious and unconscious (28), are easily aroused by patients who are manipulative and full of rage, who feel entitled, and whose behavior saps the emotional strength of the staff (85). If the treatment of a patient requires a great deal of emotional energy, personality issues likely are involved. In such situations, it is essential to be aware of the effect that such patients exert and to take care of the clinical staff as well as the patient.

Eating Disorders The incidence of eating disorders and substance abuse in the adolescent population has increased (15,46,87), so it is not uncommon to find them together. In fact, a fourth of all patients who have an eating disorder either have a history of substance abuse or currently are abusing substances (87).

Anorexia nervosa, which involves weight restriction and increased activity, a distorted body image, and an intense fear of losing control and becoming fat (1), is not as prevalent as bulimia in the general population and among persons who abuse substances. Bulimic patients have been found to have a greater risk for substance abuse than restrictive anorexics (88). However, Bulik et al. (89) have also shown that bulimic women with SUD have higher novelty seeking than bulimic women without SUD. Bulimia involves recurrent episodes of binge eating, sometimes accompanied by compensatory measures (such as vomiting or laxative abuse), and a preoccupation with food and weight. Of all eating disorders, 90% to 95% occur in females (87). Though anorexic patients have a characteristic emaciated appearance, bulimic patients can be any weight. Patients who consistently spend time in the bathroom after meals may be purging.

Persons with an eating disorder may abuse amphetamines to lose weight. Katz (87) postulates that the proneness to substance abuse in bulimic patients may be due to borderline personality features.

CONCLUSIONS

In sum, psychiatric disorders and SUDs often occur together, complicating assessment and treatment. An awareness of the prevalence and manifestations of psychiatric diagnoses is essential to high-quality treatment of adolescents. An ongoing relationship with a psychiatrist who can be available for consultation as needed is helpful. Clinicians also should keep current on psychopharmacologic interventions (65,90). Often, the use of psychiatric medications such as antidepressants, mood stabilizers, psychostimulants, and others is of benefit. However, care must be taken to avoid potential interactions between the illicit drugs and the prescribed medications (91). Also, self-help groups such as Al-Ateen, Alcoholics Anonymous, Narcotics Anonymous, or "Double-Trouble" groups for patients with co-occurring psychiatric and addiction disorders can be a useful adjunct to treatment (92–95).

Careful observation, history taking, and appropriate consultation result in better detection and treatment of comorbid disorders and, ultimately, of the initial substance abuse problem.

REFERENCES

1. American Psychiatric Association. *Diagnostic and statistical manual of mental disorders,* 4th ed [text revision]. Washington, DC: American Psychiatric Press, 2000.

2. Armentano M. Assessment, diagnosis, and treatment of the dually diagnosed adolescent. *Pediatr Clin North Am* 1995;42:479–490.
3. Bukstein O, Glancy LJ, Kaminer Y. Patterns of affective comorbidity in a clinical population of dually diagnosed adolescent substance abusers. *J Am Acad Child Adolesc Psychiatry* 1992;31(6):1041–1045.
4. Bukstein O, Brent DA, Perper JA, et al. Risk factors for completed suicide among adolescents with a lifetime history of substance abuse: a case-control study. *Acta Psychiatr Scand* 1993;88(6):403–408.
5. Burke JD, Burke KC, Rae DS. Increased rates of drug abuse and dependence after onset of mood or anxiety disorders in adolescence. *Hosp Community Psychiatry* 1994;45(5):451–455.
6. Crowley TJ, Riggs PD. Adolescent substance use disorder with conduct disorder and comorbid conditions. In Rahdert E, Czechowicz D, eds. *Adolescent substance abuse* (NIDA Research Monograph 156). Rockville, MD: National Institute on Drug Abuse, 1995:49–111.
7. Deykin EY, Buka SL. Prevalence and risk factors for posttraumatic stress disorder among chemically dependent adolescents. *Am J Psychiatry* 1997;154:752–757.
8. Fergusson DM, Horwood LJ, Lynskey MT. Prevalence and comorbidity of DSM-IIIR diagnoses in a birth cohort of 15 year olds. *J Am Acad Child Adolesc Psychiatry* 1993;2(6):1127–1134.
9. Geller B, Cooper TB, Sun K, et al. Double-blind and placebo-controlled study of lithium for adolescent bipolar disorders with secondary substance dependency. *J Am Acad Child Adolesc Psychiatry* 1998;37:171–178.
10. Grilo CM, Becker DF, Walker ML, et al. Psychiatric comorbidity in adolescent inpatients with substance use disorders. *J Am Acad Child Adolesc Psychiatry* 1995;34(8):1085–1091.
11. Horowitz HA, Overton WF, Rosenstein D, et al. Comorbid adolescent substance abuse: a maladaptive pattern of self-regulation. *Adolesc Psychaitry* 1992;18:465–483.
12. Hovens JG, Cantwell DP, Kiriakos R. Psychiatric comorbidity in hospitalized adolescent substance abusers. *J Am Acad Child Adolesc Psychiatry*1994;33(4):476–483.
13. Kaminer Y, Tarter RE, Bukstein OG, et al. Comparison between treatment completers and noncompleters among dually diagnosed substance-abusing adolescents. *J Am Acad Child Adolesc Psychiatry* 1992;31: 1046–1049.
14. Stowell JA, Estroff TW. Psychiatric disorders in substance abusing adolescent inpatients: a pilot study. *J Am Acad Child Adolesc Psychiatry.* 1992; 31:1036–1040.
15. Westermeyer J, Specker S. Social resources and social function in comorbid eating and substance disorder: a matched-pairs study. *Am J Addict* 1999;8:332–336.
16. Wilcox JA, Yates WR. Gender and psychiatric comorbidity in substance-abusing individuals. *Am J Addict* 1993;2(3):202–206.
17. Wilens TE, Biederman J, Spencer TJ. Attention deficit hyperactivity disorder and psychoactive substance use disorders. *Child Adolesc Psychiatr Clin North Am* 1996;5:73–91.
18. Brook JS, Whiteman M, Cohen P, et al. Longitudinally predicting late adolescent and young adult drug use: childhood and adolescent precursors. *J Am Acad Child Adolesc Psychiatry* 1995;34:1230–1238.
19. Christie KA, Burke JD, et al. Epidemiologic evidence for early onset of mental disorders and higher risk of drug abuse in young adults. *Am J Psychiatry* 1988;145:971–975.
20. DeMilio L. Psychiatric syndromes in adolescent substance abusers. *Am J Psychiatry* 1989;146:1212–1214.
21. Kaminer Y. The magnitude of concurrent psychiatric disorders in hospitalized substance abusing adolescents. *J Abnorm Child Psychol* 1991;25: 122–132.
22. Kandel DB, Johnson JG, Bird H, et al. Psychiatric disorders associated with substance use among children and adolescents: findings from the methods for the epidemiology of child and adolescent mental disorders (MECA) study. *J Abnorm Child Psychol* 1997;25:122–132.
23. Kellam SG, Ensminger ME, Simon MB. Mental health in first grade and teenage drug, alcohol, and cigarette use. *Drug Alcohol Depend* 1980;5: 273–304.
24. Clark DB, Bukstein OG. Psychopathology in adolescent alcohol abuse and dependence. *Alcohol Res Health* 1998;22:117–126.
25. Deykin EY, Buka SL, Zeena TH. Depressive illness among chemically dependent adolescents. *Am J Psychiatry* 1992;149:1341–1347.
26. Kashani JH, Keller MB, Solomon N, et al. Double depression in adolescent substance abusers. *J Affect Disord* 1985;8:153–157.
27. King CA, Naylor MW, Hill EM, et al. Dysthymia characteristic of heavy alcohol use in depressed adolescents. *Biol Psychiatry* 1992;33: 210–212.
28. King C, Ghaziuddin N, McGovern L, et al. Predictors of comorbid alcohol and substance abuse in depressed adolescents. *J Am Acad Child Adolesc Psychiatry* 1996;35:743–751.
29. Milin R, Halikas JA, Meller JE, et al. Psychopathology among substance abusing juvenile offenders. *J Am Acad Child Adolesc Psychiatry* 1991; 30:569–574.
30. Caton CLM, Gralnick A, Bender S, Simon M. Young chronic patients and substance abuse. *Hosp Community Psychiatry* 1989;40:1037–1040.
31. Ries R. The dually diagnosed patient with psychotic symptoms. *J Addict Dis* 1993b;12:103–122.
32. Miller NS. Comorbidity of psychiatric and alcohol/drug disorders: interactions and independent status. *J Addict Dis* 1993;12:5–16.
33. Miller NS, Fine J. Current epidemiology of comorbidity of psychiatric and addictive disorders. *Psychiatr Clin North Am* 1993;16:1–10.
34. Schuckit MA. The clinical implications of primary diagnostic groups among alcoholics. *Arch Gen Psychiatry* 1985;1043–1049.
35. Schuckit MA. Genetic and clinical implications of alcoholism and affective disorder. *Am J Psychiatry* 1986;143(2):140–147.
36. Schuckit MA. Alcohol and depression: A clinical perspective. *Acta Psychiatr Scand* 1994;377(Suppl):28–32.
37. Burke KC, Burke JD, Regier DA, Rae DS. Age at onset of selected mental disorders in five community populations. *Arch Gen Psychiatry* 1990;47: 511–518.
38. Flory M. Psychiatric diagnosis in child and adolescent suicide. *Arch Gen Psychiatry* 1996;53(4):339–348.
39. Giaconia RM, Reinherz HZ, Silverman AB, et al. Ages of onset of psychiatric disorders in a community population of older adolescents. *J Am Acad Child Adolesc Psychiatry* 1994;33(5):706–717.
40. Kandel DB, Johnson JG, Bird HR, et al. Psychiatric comorbidity among adolescents with substance use disorders: Findings from the MECA study. *J Am Acad Child Adolesc Psychiatry* 1999;38:693–699.
41. Kessler RC, Nelson CB, McGonagle KA, et al. The epidemiology of co-occurring addictive and mental disorders: implications for prevention and service utilization. *Am J Orthopsychiatry* 1996;66:17–31.
42. Lewisohn PM, Hops H, Roberts RE, et al. Adolescent psychopathology I: prevalence and incidence of depression and other DSM-IIIR disorders in high school students. *J Abnorm Psychol* 1993;102:133–144.
43. Mason SE, Siris SG. Dual diagnosis: the case for case management. *Am J Addict* 1992;(1):77–82.
44. Morrison MA, Smith DE, Wilford BB, et al. At war in the fields of play: current perspectives on the nature and treatment of adolescent chemical dependency. *J Psychoactive Drugs* 1993;25(41):321–330.
45. Weiss RD, Mirin SM, Frances RJ. The myth of the typical dual diagnosis patient. *Hosp Community Psychiatry* 1992;43:107–108.
46. Westermeyer J, Specker S, Neider J, et al. Substance abuse and associated psychiatric disorder among 100 adolescents. *J Addict Dis* 1994;13(1) 67–89.
47. Bukstein O, Kaminer T. The nosology of adolescent substance abuse. *Am J Addict* 1994;Winter:1–13.
48. Clark DB, Kirisci L, Tarter RE. Adolescent versus adult onset and the development of substance abuse disorders in males. *Drug Alcohol Depend* 1998;49:115–121.
49. Kaminer Y. *Adolescent substance abuse: a comprehensive guide to theory and practice*. New York: Plenum Medical Books, 1994.
50. Weinberg NZ, Rahdert E, Colliver JD, et al. Adolescent substance abuse: a review of the past 10 years. *J Am Acad Child Adolesc Psychiatry* 1998;37:252–261.
51. American Academy of Child and Adolescent Psychiatry. Practice parameters for the assessment and treatment of children and adolescents with substance abuse disorders. *J Am Acad Child Adolesc Psychiatry* 1998;37: 122–126.

52. Ries R, Mullen M, Cox G. Symptom severity and utilization of treatment resources among dually diagnosed inpatients. *Hosp Community Psychiatry* 1994;45:562–568.
53. Clark DB, Bukstein O, Smith MG, et al. Identifying anxiety disorders in adolescents hospitalized for alcohol abuse and dependence. *Psychiatr Serv* 1995;46:618–620.
54. Clark DB, Lesnick L, Hegedus AM. Traumas and other adverse life events in adolescents with alcohol use and dependence. *J Am Acad Child Adolesc Psychiatry* 1997;36:1744–1751.
55. Van Hasselt VB, Ammerman RT, Glancy LJ, Bukstein OG. Maltreatment in psychiatrically hospitalized dually diagnosed adolescent substance abusers. *J Am Acad Child Adolesc Psychiatry* 1992;31(5):868–874.
56. American Psychiatric Association. *Diagnostic and statistical manual of mental disorders,* 3rd ed [Revised] (DSM-IIIR). Washington, DC: American Psychiatric Press, 1987.
56a. Riggs P, Levin F, Green Al, et al. Comorbid psychiatric and substance abuse disorders: recent treatment research. *Subst Abus* 2008;29(3):51–63. Review.
57. Kandel DB, Raveis VH, Davies M. Suicidal ideation in adolescence: depression, substance use, and other risk factors. *J Youth Adolesc* 1991; 20:289–309.
58. Rao U, Ryan ND, Dahl RE, et al. Factors associated with the development of substance use disorder in depressed adolescents. *J Am Acad Child Adolesc Psychiatry* 1999;38:1109–1117.
59. Bukstein O, Brent DA, Kaminer Y. Comorbidity of substance and other psychiatric disorders in adolescents. *Am J Psychiatry* 1989;146(9):1131–1141.
60. Kempton T, Van Hasselt VB, Bukstein OG, et al. Cognitive distortions and psychiatric diagnosis in dually diagnosed adolescents. *J Am Acad Child Adolesc Psychiatry* 1994;33:217–222.
61. Beck AT, Rush AJ, Shaw BF, et al. *Cognitive therapy of depression.* New York: Guilford Press, 1979.
61a. Riggs, PD, Lohman, M, Davies, R, et al. A randomized controlled trial of fluoxetine/placebo and CBT in depressed adolescents with substance use disorders. Abstract, Synposium presented at the 23rd Annual Meeting of the American Academy of Addiction Psychiatry. December 7-11,2005 Scottsdale, Arizona.
61b. Riggs PD, Mikulich-Gilbertson SK, Davies RD, et al. A randomized controlled trial of fluoxetine and cognitive behavioral therapy in adolescents with major depression, behavior problems, and substance use disorders. *Arch Pediatr Adolesc Med* 2007;161(11):1026–1034.
62. Bennett DS, Bendersky M., Lewis M. Children's cognitive ability from 4 to 9 years old as a function of prenatal cocaine exposure, environmental risk, and maternal verbal intelligence. *Dev Psychol* 2008;44(4):919–928.
63. Riggs PD, Mikulich SC, Coffman L, et al. Fluoxetine in drug-dependent delinquents with major depression: an open trial. *J Child Adolesc Psychopharmacol* 1997;7:87–95.
64. Wilens TE, Biederman J, Millstein RB, et al. Risk for substance use disorders in youths with child- and adolescent-onset bipolar disorder. *J Am Acad Child Adolesc Psychiatry* 1999;38:680–685.
65. Kaminer Y. Pharmacotherapy for adolescents with psychoactive substance use disorders. In Rahdert E, Czechowicz D, eds. *Adolescent substance abuse* (NIDA Research Monograph 156). Rockville, MD: National Institute on Drug Abuse, 1995:291–324.
65a. Rich BA, Schmajuk M, Perez-Edgar KE, et al. Different psychophysiological and behavioral responses elicited by frustration in pediatric bipolar disorder and severe mood dysregulation. *Am J Psychiatry* 2007; 164(2):309–317.
65b. Brotman MA, Schmajuk M, Rich BA, et al. Prevalence, clinical correlates, and longitudinal course of severe mood dysregulation in children. *Biol Psychiatry* 2006;60(9):991–997.
66. Wilens T, Spencer T, Frazier J, et al. Psychopharmacology in children and adolescents. In Ollendick T, Hersen M, eds. *Handbook of child psychopathology*. New York: Plenum Publishing, 1998:603–636.
67. Swan N. *Early childhood behavior and temperament predict later substance abuse.* Washington, DC: National Institute on Drug Abuse Notes, 1995;10:1.
68. Merikangas KR, Mehta RL, Molnar BE, et al. Comorbidity of substance use disorders with mood and anxiety disorders: results of International consortium in psychiatric epidemiology. *Addict Behav* 1998;23(6):893–907.
68a. Cohen JA, Mannarino AP, Zhitova AC, et al. Treating child abuse-related posttraumatic stress and comorbid substance abuse in adolescents. *Child Abuse Negl* 2003;27(12):1345–1365.
68b. Najavits LM, Gallop RJ, Weiss RD. Seeking safety therapy for adolescent girls with PTSD and substance use disorder: a randomized controlled trial. *Behav Health Serv Res* 2006;33(4):453–463.
69. Essau CA, Conradt J, Peterman F. Frequency and co-morbidity of social fears in adolescents. *Behav Res Ther* 1999;37(9):831–843.
70. Mattson SN, Riley EP, Gramling L, et al. Neuropsychological comparison of alcohol-exposed children with or without physical features of fetal alcohol syndrome. *Neuropsychology* 1998;12(1):146–153.
71. Fried PA, Watkinson B, Gray R. Differential effects on cognitive functioning in 13- to 16-year-olds prenatally exposed to cigarettes and marihuana. *Neurotoxicol Teratol* 2003;25(4):427–436.
72. Smith AM, Fried PA, Hogan MJ, Cameron I. Effects of prenatal marijuana on visuospatial working memory: an fMRI study in young adults. *Neurotoxicol Teratol* 2006;28(2):286–295.
73. Frank DA, Augustyn M, Knight WG, et al. Growth, development, and behavior in early childhood following cocaine exposure. *JAMA* 2001; 285(12):1613–1625.
74. Bennett Ds, Bendersky M, Lewis M. Children's cognitive ability from 4 to 9 years old as a function of prenatal cocaine exposure, environmental risk, and maternal verbal intelligence. *Dev Psychol* 2008;44(4): 919–928.
75. Hops HA, Davis B, Lewin LM. The development of alcohol and other substance use: a gender study of family and peer context. *J Study Alcohol Suppl* 1999;13:22–31.
76. Simkin DR. Adolescent substance abuse. In Sadock BJ, Sadock VA, eds., *Kaplan and Sadock's Comprehensive Textbook of Psychiatry,* 8th ed. Philadelphia: Lippincott Williams and Wilkins. 2005;2:3470–3490.
77. Tapert SF, Baratta BS, Abrantes BA, Brown SA. Attention dysfunction predicts substance involvement in community youth. *J Am Acad Child Adolesc Psychiatry* 2002;41(6):690–686.
78. Buckley PF. Substance abuse in schizophrenia: a review. *J Clin Psychiatry* 1999;59(Suppl 3):26–30.
79. Minkoff K. An integrated treatment model for dual diagnosis of psychosis and addiction. *Hosp Community Psychiatry* 1989;40:1031–1036.
80. Costello EJ, Costello AJ, Edelbrock C, et al. Psychiatric disorders in pediatric primary care. *Arch Gen Psychiatry* 1988;45:1107–1116.
80a. Juckel G, Schlagenhauf F, Koslowski M, et al. Dysfunction of ventral striatal reward prediction in schizophrenia. *Neuroimage* 2006;29(2): 409–416.
80b. Green Al. Schizophrenia and comorbid substance use disorder: effects of antipsychotics. *J Clin Psychiatry* 2005;66 Suppl 6:21–26. http://www.ncbi.nlm.nih.gov/entrez/utils/fref.fcgi?Prid=3091&itool=Abstract-Plusdef&uid=16107180&db=pubmed&url=http://article.psychiatrist.com/?ContentType=START&ID=10001428
80c. Green Al, Zimmet SV, Strous RD, et al. Clozapine for comorbid substance use disorder and schizophrenia: do patients with schizophrenia have a reward-deficiency syndrome that can be ameliorated by clozapine? *Harv Rev Psychiatry* 1999;6(6):287–296.
80d. Green AL, Drake RE, Brunette MF, et al. Schizophrenia and co-occurring substance use disorder. *Am J Psychiatry* 2007;164(3):402–408.
81. Ries RK. Clinical treatment matching models for dually diagnosed patients. *Psychiatr Clin North Am* 1993;16:167–175.
82. American Academy of Pediatrics, Committee on Substance Abuse. Indications for management and referral of patients involved in substance abuse. *Pediatrics* 2000;106:143–148.
83. Riggs PD. Clinical approach to treatment of ADHD in adolescents with substance use disorders and conduct disorder. *J Am Acad Child Adolesc Psychiatry* 1998;37:331–332.
83a. Szobot CM, Rohde LA, Katz B, et al. A randomized crossover clinical study showing that methylphenidate- SODAS improves attention-deficit/hyperactivity disorder symptoms in adolescents with substance use disorder. *Braz J Med Biol Ries* 2008,41(3):250–257.

83b. Klingberg, T, Forssberg, H, Olesen, P, et al. Computerized training in working memory in children with ADHD-a randomized controlled trial. *J Amer Acad Child and Adol Psychiatry* 2005;44(2):177–186.
84. Riggs PD, Mikulich SC, Pottle LC. An open trial of bupropion for ADHD in adolescents with substance use disorder and conduct disorder. *J Am Acad Child Adolesc Psychiatry* 1998;37:1271–1278.
85. Cloninger CR. Neurogenetic adaptive mechanisms in alcoholism. *Science* 1987;236:410–416.
86. Groves JE. The hateful patient. *N Engl J Med* 1978;298:883–887.
87. Myers WC, Burket RC, Otto TA. Conduct disorders and personality disorders in hospitalized adolescents. *J Clin Psychiatry* 1993;54(1):21–26.
88. Katz JL. Eating disorders: a primer for the substance abuse specialist: I. Clinical features. *J Subst Abuse Treat* 1990;7:143–149.
89. Bulik, C, Sullivan, P, Epstein, L, et al. Drug use in women with anorexia and bulimia nervosa. *Int J Eat Disord* 1992;11:213–225.
90. Bulik CM, Sullivan P, McKee M, et al. Characteristics of bulimic women with and without alcoholism. *Am J Drug Alcohol Abuse* 1994;20(2):273–283.
91. Solhkhah R, Wilens TE. Pharmacotherapy of adolescent alcohol and other drug use. *Alcohol Health Res World* 1998;22:122–125.
92. Wilens TE, Biederman J, Spencer TJ. Case study: adverse effects of smoking marijuana while receiving tricyclic antidepressants. *J Am Acad Child Adolesc Psychiatry* 1997;36:45–48.
93. Brown SA. Recovery patterns in adolescent substance abuse. In Bae JS, Marlatt GA, McMahon RJ, eds. *Addictive behaviors across the life span: prevention, treatment, and policy issues.* Newbury Park, CA: Sage Publications, 1993:161–183.
94. Hohman M, LeCroy CW. Predictors of adolescent AA affiliation. *Adolescence* 1996;31:339–352.
95. Simkin DR. Twelve-step treatment from a developmental perspective. *Child Adolesc Psychiatr Clin North Am* 1996;5:165–175.

SUGGESTED READINGS

American Academy of Pediatrics, Committee on Quality Improvement, Subcommittee on Attention-Deficit/Hyperactivity Disorder. Diagnosis and evaluation of the child with attention-deficit/hyperactivity disorder. *Pediatrics* 1999;105:1158–1170.

Buydens-Branchey L, Branchey MH, Noumair D. Age of alcoholism onset: I. Relationship to psychopathology. *Arch Gen Psychiatry* 1989;46:225–230.

Buydens-Branchey L, Branchey MH, Noumair D, Lieber CS. Age of alcoholism onset: II. Relationship to susceptibility to serotonin precursor availability. *Arch Gen Psychiatry* 1989;46:231–236.

Morrison MA, Smith QT. Psychiatric issues of adolescent chemical dependence. *Pediatr Clin North Am* 1987;34(2):461–479.

Olfson M, Klerman G. The treatment of depression: Prescribing practices of primary care physicians and psychiatrists. *J Family Pract* 1992;35(6): 627–635.

Ross HE, Glaser FB, Germanson T. The prevalence of psychiatric disorders in patients with alcohol and other drug problems. *Arch Gen Psychiatry* 1988;45:1023–1031.

Schuckit MA, Chiles JA. Family history as a diagnostic aid in two samples of adolescents. *J Nerv Ment Dis* 1978;166(3):165–176.

Wolraich MI, Felice ME, Drotar D, eds. *Classification of childhood mental disorders in primary care.* Elk Grove Village, IL: American Academy of Pediatrics, 1996.

SECTION 14

Ethical, Legal, and Liability, Issues in Addiction Practice

CHAPTER 107

H. Westley Clark, MD, JD, MPH, CAS, FASAM
Anton C. Bizzell, MD

Ethical Issues in Addiction Practice

Certain ethical principles are central to medical practice. Foremost among these is the physician's obligation to put the patient's interests first. This is closely followed by respect for the patient's autonomy (which includes the patient's right to make his or her own medical decisions, as well as the right to be left alone) and the patient's privacy or confidentiality. The physician also has a general duty to protect society when the patient's condition poses a threat to others.

Most of the time, these ethical principles are congruent. However, physicians who screen, assess, or treat patients for addictive disorders sometimes find themselves in situations where ethical principles are in conflict (1). For example, a physician who suspects a patient has an addictive disorder may face a conflict between an obligation to put the patient's health first and respect for the patient's autonomy. Should the physician press the patient about his or her substance use and order medical tests out of concern for the patient's health? Or should the physician drop the subject if the patient indicates that he or she does not wish to discuss it out of respect for the patient's autonomy? What should a physician do if the patient's health plan will not pay for the kind of treatment that is needed? Which ethical principles should guide the physician who believes that a patient's addictive disorder poses a danger to the patient's safety: the duty to the patient's health or the duty to protect the patient's privacy? Is coerced treatment ethical (2)?

These questions and others are explored in this chapter. The first section begins with a discussion of the relationship between patient autonomy and the physician's obligation to counsel patients about the health risks of substance use. It then turns to the concept of informed consent and examines the questions raised when a patient is not competent to make his or her own decisions or is not willing to enter treatment voluntarily. The next section concerns privacy of information about a patient's addictive disorders. It begins with a brief discussion of confidentiality of medical information and why it is important. It then turns to an overview of the legal guidelines that govern privacy of medical information. Finally, it examines three situations in which the physician can be called on to resolve an ethical dilemma between the obligation to maintain confidentiality and the duty to protect the patient or society.

PATIENT AUTONOMY

Americans attach extraordinary importance to their right to be left alone. We pride ourselves on having perfected a social and political system that limits how far the government—and others—can intrude on our "space" or control what we do. The principle of autonomy is enshrined in the Constitution, and the courts repeatedly have affirmed the right of citizens to make their own decisions on fundamental issues.

Medicine places a high value on patient autonomy (3). Patients consult physicians on their own initiative when they decide they have reached a level of discomfort with a particular problem. The physician who is consulted by a patient about a condition, such as back pain, is expected to outline the causes and suggest possible preventive measures and available treatments. The physician certainly can make a recommendation, but must recognize that the patient has the right to choose among the recommended treatments or to refuse them altogether. Rarely will a physician consider forcing advice on a patient, even if convinced that the patient is making a wrong choice.

When a patient is in denial about his or her abuse of alcohol or drugs, however, deference to patient autonomy can shift. The principles of autonomy and privacy, so critical to honest communication between physician and patient, can sometimes, in the context of drug and alcohol abuse, seem to work against what the physician sees as the patient's best interests (4).

Dealing with Denial Traditionally, respect for the patient's autonomy has made physicians reluctant to ask questions about areas not directly related to the presenting condition, particularly if those areas are sensitive. Until recent years, patients' annual physicals rarely included questions about alcohol consumption, and physicians were even more reluctant to question patients about drug use. However, a physician who screens or assesses patients for addictive disorders (whether by observing the patient, performing laboratory tests, or administering behavioral questionnaires) is seeking information about lifestyle and personal habits that carry a good deal of stigma. Both patient and physician may view such inquiries as intrusions on the patient's autonomy (as well as his or her privacy).

Nevertheless, when a physician suspects that a patient, who arrives at the office with another presenting complaint, also is abusing drugs or alcohol, he or she must take the initiative if the patient does not raise the issue. In such a case, the physician has an ethical duty to act if there is reason to believe that the patient's use of alcohol or drugs is affecting his or her health.

The difficulty is that raising the issue sometimes is not enough. Denial is an integral part of addictive disorders. Individuals in denial fail to recognize or are reluctant to acknowledge their problem, or they find ways to deny or minimize the extent of their alcohol or drug use because they are ambivalent about giving up such use. What is the proper balance between respect for the principle of autonomy and the physician's responsibility for the patient's health when dealing with a patient in denial? Should the physician raise the issue and then drop it at the slightest hint of resistance on the part of the patient? Or should he or she intervene more forcefully—by talking with the patient, conducting medical tests, or involving the family (5)?

Talking with the Patient To fulfill the ethical responsibility to the patient, the physician should do more than simply raise the issue. He or she should provide relevant information, engage the patient in discussion, and, if the patient shows resistance, follow-up in future visits. How far the physician can intrude on the patient's autonomy will depend a great deal on the strength of the physician-patient relationship.

Unless a firm foundation of trust and understanding has been established, persistent questions or a forceful confrontation can backfire and ultimately strengthen the patient's resistance.

In most cases, it is only the individual with the addictive disorder who can take action to change his or her behavior. Although the physician can supply information and encouragement, it is the patient who must make the decision to change.

Ordering Laboratory Tests Must, or should, a physician obtain the patient's consent before ordering a drug screen? It is most likely that the law does not require the patient's consent. Ordinarily, a physician does not ask a patient to sign a consent form before sending blood or urine for other testing. However, ordering laboratory tests to screen patients for addictive disorders is different. And failing to consult the patient can undermine the physician's efforts to induce the patient to acknowledge the problem.

Screening urine or blood for drugs is not the routine practice in primary care settings. Patients expect to be screened for blood sugar and cholesterol, but they do not expect their physician to screen them for drug use. A patient confronted with the results of a test he or she did not know about and for which he or she did not give consent may feel betrayed by the physician, which is a shorthand way of saying that he or she will be angry that the physician did not show respect for the patient's autonomy (6). The physician runs the risk that such a situation will damage the relationship with the patient. The patient may refuse to participate in any further discussions about alcohol or drug use. Tactically, therefore, the better practice is to obtain the patient's permission for blood or urine tests for alcohol or drugs.

A second reason the physician should obtain the patient's permission before employing laboratory drug screens has to do with the patient's right to privacy. If the physician orders a test, the patient's third-party payer will know about it and perhaps the result as well. The physician's decision to order a drug screen tells the third-party payer a good deal, even if the result is negative. Therefore, it is the patient, not the physician, who should decide whether it is appropriate and necessary for the health insurer to have this information.

A third reason is financial. The patient's third-party payer may not cover drug screens as a matter of course. The advent of managed care has narrowed the range of tests a physician can order on a routine basis. If the patient's insurance carrier or health maintenance organization will not cover the test, the patient should have the opportunity to decide whether he or she is willing to pay for the test out of pocket, a decision that should be made before the test is ordered.

Unfortunately, there is a good chance that if the physician consults the patient and asks permission to perform a drug screen, the patient will refuse to agree to the test. However, this result leaves the door open to further discussion with the patient about possible drug problems. The patient likely will appreciate the physician's concern for his or her autonomy and privacy, and thus may be more open than would be the case if the physician was perceived as acting "behind the patient's back" and therefore could not be trusted. The physician might begin such a discussion by asking, in a neutral way, why the patient does not want to have a drug screen.

The physician is likely to encounter fewer problems if the order is for a test of liver function. Patients are less likely to be surprised that such a test has been ordered, and the test results still provide an opening for a conversation about the health effects of alcohol or drug use.

When the Patient is an Older Adult The physician who suspects an older adult patient is abusing alcohol or drugs must be especially sensitive. As we age, most of us become more sensitive to perceived threats to our autonomy (7). Because of the stigma surrounding addictive disorder, a patient whose physician suggests that he or she may be drinking too much or abusing drugs (legal or illegal) might conclude that the physician is suggesting that whatever brought him or her for a medical visit has an emotional basis or that the patient's functioning or capacity is diminished. If an older adult thinks that his or her autonomy is being threatened, the patient may be more likely to point to the "normal" infirmities of old age as the source of the difficulty, rather than acknowledging a problem with alcohol or other drugs (7).

Most older adults are unaware that the way their bodies metabolize alcohol and drugs (including prescription medications) changes as they age and that the amount of alcohol or drugs they consumed without obvious adverse consequences when they were younger can harm their health and even incapacitate them. Moreover, many older adult patients take multiple prescription drugs to control their cholesterol, blood pressure, diabetes, depression, or anxiety. They may not be aware that their prescription medications can interact with each other and with any alcohol or nonprescription drugs they consume, interfering with the therapeutic effects of their medications. An approach that emphasizes these issues provides a better opportunity to engage an older adult patient in a discussion about addictive disorders without posing a threat to his or her autonomy.

INFORMED CONSENT

Autonomy also is at the root of our belief that a patient has the right to decide what treatment he or she will accept, and even whether he or she will accept treatment at all. When a physician asks a patient to sign an "informed consent" agreement, he or she is affirming that the patient has the right to make decisions about his or her medical care.[1]

"Informed consent" has two components. First, the patient's decision to undergo a course of treatment must be based on knowledge and competency. The physician must give the patient the kind and amount of information the patient needs to make an intelligent ("informed") choice, and the patient must be capable of understanding the information and making a decision. Second, the patient's decision must be voluntary—that is, a product of his or her free will. What happens when one of these conditions cannot be met—when the patient is not fully informed or competent to make a decision for himself or when he is coerced into treatment?

[1]Of course, physicians do not ask patients to sign informed consent forms each time medical decisions are made. When we go for routine blood tests or an electrocardiogram, when we get a flu shot or start an antibiotic for bronchitis, no one asks us to sign a form consenting to treatment. Generally, informed consent forms are used when the patient will undergo an invasive procedure that poses a risk of adverse physical consequences, when the patient chooses a treatment that the physician has warned him may be ineffective, or when the law requires the physician to get informed consent because the test can result in serious adverse *legal* or *psychologic* consequences and asking the patient to sign the form impresses on him the importance of the decision to be made. (For example, in some states, a patient must sign an informed consent form when an HIV test is performed.)

Informed = Knowledge Plus Competency

Information The physician is obligated to give the patient all the information he or she needs to make a decision. This information should include the physician's opinion of the patient's diagnosis, an outline of the available treatment alternatives, a description of what each alternative involves (including its benefits and risks), an explanation of the consequences should the patient decline treatment altogether, and responses to the patient's questions. Often, the physician also helps the patient evaluate the treatment alternatives in accordance with the patient's values, hopes, and fears.

With the growth of managed care, physician and patient no longer have an exclusive relationship. The managed care organization has intruded itself into the relationship. Many managed care contracts shift some financial risk from the managed care company to the physician. In some plans, the contract gives physicians whose patients do not use expensive (or extensive) services a financial bonus. In other plans, the contract limits the services for which the physician will be reimbursed. (Note that such contracts do not limit the services the physician can provide—only those for which he or she will be compensated.) In this way, many managed care plans create incentives that can impinge on medical judgment.

If a physician allows financial incentives or disincentives to influence treatment recommendations, or to discharge a patient who has exhausted benefits under the contract, that physician has placed financial interests before his or her obligation to the patient's health—a clear ethical violation.

Because managed care places (often hidden) limits on certain forms of treatment, ethicists have begun to suggest that the physician should inform the patient about any economic issues that could influence either the physician's recommendation or the patient's decision. Providing "economic informed consent" ensures that the patient knows about any limitations the managed care plan or insurer imposes on treatment before making a decision.

Competence (Decision-Making Capacity) The concept of informed consent is based on the assumption that the patient has "decisional capacity." Decisional capacity means that the patient is able to understand the physician's explanation of the diagnosis, prognosis, treatment alternatives, and likely outcome if treatment is refused, and is able to go through the complex process of assessing that information in accordance with his or her personal system of values. Most patients have decisional capacity. However, the physician may encounter questions about decisional capacity in dealing with two groups: adolescents and older adults.

Issues in Dealing with Adolescents Adolescents do not have the legal same status as full-fledged adults, and there are certain decisions that society does not allow them to make. Below a certain age (which varies from state to state), adolescents must attend school and cannot drive, marry, or sign binding contracts. In some states, the adolescent's right to consent to medical treatment—or to refuse treatment—also differs from an adult's right (6,8).

In more than half the states, adolescents have the right to consent on their own to addictive disorder screening, assessment, or treatment, while in other states, a parent must be notified and/or consent.[2] In states that deem adolescents competent to consent to addictive disorder treatment (and which therefore do not require parental consent), the physician has no ethical dilemma; he or she can provide whatever treatment is appropriate (and to which the adolescent patient consents).

It is in those states that require parental consent or notification that the physician sometimes encounters a complex ethical quandary. The difficulty arises when an adolescent who seeks assessment or treatment refuses to permit communication with a parent. If the physician believes that the adolescent does need treatment, he or she has three choices:

Choice 1: The Physician Can Treat the Adolescent without Consulting a Parent

The Dilemma The physician who treats an adolescent without parental consent or notification is acting in accordance with the ethical principles of putting the patient's health first and respecting the patient's autonomy (and privacy), but may be violating the law (8). Although violation of the parental consent/notification law most likely is not a criminal offense, it could put the physician's professional license at risk or expose him or her to a lawsuit by the adolescent's parents. It is unlikely, however, that a physician treating an adolescent would be faced with either eventuality if the treatment provided is not controversial or intrusive, does not put the adolescent at risk, and is carried out in a responsible, non-negligent manner. In such circumstances, it would be difficult for a parent (or licensing authority) to show that any harm was done. This is particularly true if the physician made a reasoned decision and acted in good faith and out of concern for the adolescent. Contrary to popular belief, most lawyers do not chase after cases that are complex, time-consuming, expensive, and difficult to win. Convincing an attorney to take on such a case would not be easy.

Factors to Consider The physician who is considering whether to offer treatment without parental consent or notification in a state that requires it should consider the following factors.

- The adolescent's age. Society accords adolescents more autonomy as they get older. A physician who might decline to treat a 14-year-old patient without parental consent in a state that requires it might have fewer qualms about treating a 17-year-old patient in similar circumstances.
- The adolescent's maturity. Chronologic age clearly is not the only measure. There are 14 year olds who have maturity beyond their years and emotionally immature 17 year olds with poor social skills and reasoning ability.
- The adolescent's family situation. Adolescents in need of addictive disorder treatment may be estranged from their families. Those who refuse to permit parental notification may have good reason to do so. Forcing them to involve parents who have failed them is neither ethical nor good clinical practice. Reconciliation with the family may be vital to an adolescent's recovery, but circumstances may dictate that it be abandoned or postponed to a later stage of treatment.
- The severity of the adolescent's addictive disorder and the danger it poses to his or her life or health.
- The kind of treatment to be provided. The more intrusive and intensive the proposed treatment, the more risk the physician assumes in treating an adolescent without parental consent. For example, a physician offering an outpatient course of treatment is on firmer ground than one proposing intensive outpatient or residential treatment.
- The physician's possible liability for refusing to treat the patient. State law may impose a duty to treat patients in need.
- The financial consequences. If the physician treats an adolescent without parental consent, he may not be paid.

Choice 2: The Physician Can Refuse to Treat the Adolescent

The Dilemma Refusing to treat the adolescent adheres to the letter of state laws that consider adolescents incompetent to make medical decisions and it shows respect for the patient's privacy, but it may violate the ethical principle that requires the physician to put the patient's health first. In some states, it also violates a law requiring physicians to treat patients in medical need.

Choice 3: The Physician Can Call the Adolescent's Parent to try to Obtain Consent to Treat the Adolescent

The Dilemma Calling the parent and treating the adolescent complies with the letter of state law and is in accordance with the ethical principle that puts the patient's health first. However, it clearly violates the adolescent's right to privacy. Moreover, the federal confidentiality rules complicate this choice. If the physician is subject to the federal confidentiality rules (discussed in a later section), he or she is prohibited from contacting a parent unless the adolescent consents. The sole exception allows a treatment program director to contact a parent when the life or physical wellbeing of an adolescent is threatened.[3]

[2]Presumably, a parent whose child seeks treatment will consent. A parent or guardian who refuses to consent to treatment that a physician believes is necessary to an adolescent's wellbeing could face charges of child neglect.

[3]The federal confidentiality regulations prohibit physicians and others who provide alcohol and drug screening, assessment, and treatment from communicating with anyone, including a parent, unless the adolescent consents. The sole exception allows the director of an addiction treatment program to communicate "facts relevant to reducing a threat to the life or physical wellbeing of the [adolescent seeking services] or any other individual to the minor's parent, guardian, or other person authorized under state law to act in the minor's behalf, when "The program director believes that the adolescent, because of extreme youth or mental or physical condition, lacks the capacity to decide rationally whether to consent to the notification of a parent or guardian," and (2) "The program director believes the disclosure to a parent or guardian is necessary to cope with a substantial threat to the life or physical well-being of the adolesent or someone else" (42 CFR §§2.14(c) and (d)).

Issues in Dealing with Older Adults Most older adults are fully capable of understanding medical information, weighing the treatment alternatives, and making and articulating decisions. A small percentage of older patients clearly are incapable of participating in a decision-making process. In such cases, the older adult may have signed a health care proxy or may have a court-appointed guardian to make such decisions.

The real difficulty arises when a physician is screening or assessing an older adult whose mental capacity lies between those two extremes. The patient may have fluctuating capacity, with "good days" and "bad days," or periods of greater or lesser alertness depending on the time of day. The patient's condition can be transient or deteriorating. Diminished capacity may affect some parts of his or her ability to comprehend information and make complex decisions, but not others.

In caring for an older adult patient whose decisional capacity is less than optimal, how can the physician help the patient to understand the information presented, appreciate the implications of each alternative treatment, and make a "rational" decision, based on the patient's best interests? And what can the physician do if the patient appears to be not competent to make his or her own health care decision? Although there are no easy answers to these questions, there are several possible approaches.

Present Information Carefully The physician can help the patient who appears to have diminished capacity through a gradual information-gathering and decision-making process. Information should be presented in a way that allows the patient to absorb it gradually, clarify and restate information as necessary, and summarize the issues already covered at regular intervals. Each alternative and its consequences should be laid out and examined separately. Finally, the physician can help the patient identify his or her values and link those values to the alternatives. By helping the patient narrow his or her focus and proceeding step by step, the physician may gain assurance that the patient has understood the choices and acted in his or her own best interests (9).

Enlist the Help of a Health or Mental Health Professional If helping the patient through a process of gradual information-gathering and decision-making is not working, the physician can suggest that physician and patient jointly consult a mental health professional or a health professional who is familiar with the patient's history and has a better understanding of the obstacles to decision-making. Or the physician could suggest a specialist who can help determine why the patient is having difficulty and whether he or she has the capacity to give informed consent.

Enlist the Help of Family or Close Friends Another approach is for the physician to suggest that the patient call in a family member or close friend who can help organize the information and sort through the alternatives. Asking the patient who would be helpful could gain endorsement of this approach.

Consult a Family Member or Friend If the patient cannot grasp the information or come to a decision, the physician might ask the patient to allow him to consult a family member or close friend. If the patient consents, the physician should lay out the concerns to the family member or friend. It may be that the patient already has planned for the possibility of incapacity and has signed a durable power of attorney or health care proxy.

Guardianship A guardian is a person appointed by a court to manage some or all aspects of another person's life. Anyone seeking appointment of a guardian must show the court that the individual is disabled in some way by disease, illness, or senility and that the disability prevents that individual from performing the tasks necessary to manage one or more areas of his or her life.

Each state handles guardianship proceedings differently, but some principles apply across the board: Guardianship is not an all-or-nothing state. Courts generally require that the person seeking appointment of a guardian prove the individual's incapacity in a variety of tasks or areas. Courts can apply different standards to different life tasks—managing money, managing a household, making health care decisions, entering contracts. A person can be found incompetent to make contracts and manage money but competent to make his or her own health care decisions (or vice versa), and the guardianship will be limited accordingly.

Guardianship limits the older adult's autonomy and is an expensive process. It should be considered only as a last resort.

VOLUNTARINESS VERSUS COERCION

A growing number of patients in addiction treatment have been forced into such treatment by their families, employers, or the criminal justice system. A spouse may give his or her partner an ultimatum—enter treatment "or else," an employer may require treatment as a condition of retaining a job. A criminal justice agency may require a defendant to enter treatment as a condition of probation, parole, or suspension of charges.

Critics of coerced treatment contend that it is unethical because it violates the principle of autonomy (3–4). Some critics are particularly concerned when it is the criminal justice system that is mandating treatment and holding out the possibility that a criminal defendant will avoid incarceration. Some critics charge that the power imbalance in such circumstances is especially annihilative to autonomy.

Proponents of coerced treatment counter that, although such coercion unquestionably impinges on a patient's autonomy, it does not violate it altogether, even in the criminal context. The patient may not want to enter treatment, but always has a choice and retains the right to refuse. He or she may not like the consequences (losing a spouse, losing a job, or being incarcerated on criminal charges), but still retains the autonomy to make the decision. Proponents also point out that patients who stay in treatment for at least 90 days have better outcomes than those who leave earlier. To the extent that coercion raises retention rates, they argue, it works to improve the odds that the patient will have a positive outcome.

POSSIBLE DEVELOPMENTS

Coming developments in addiction science and treatment will raise additional ethical issues. As pointed out by Ashcroft et al. in a review of ethical issues raised by progress in addiction research, "There is significant potential for great social and individual benefit from developments in this area, but these need to be evaluated alongside some potentially significant risks of harm or limitations on individual freedom that might undermine the value or acceptability of these developments (5)." The authors point out that concerns about the ethical implications of scientific developments is given greater urgency by the stigma and discrimination still attached to addiction and the persons who suffer from this medical disorder.

Areas in which ethical concerns are likely to arise include new approaches to the prevention and treatment of drug addiction, such as vaccinations (10,11); the use of genetic data to predict the effects of drugs on individuals and specific vulnerabilities to addiction (9); the use of neural imaging to identify past, present and potential addiction problems; and the consequences of non-medical use of prescription medications for purposes such as cognitive enhancement (1). In addition, special attention will continue to be given to confidentiality and privacy, because questions continue to be raised about the capacity for informed consent on the part of an addicted patient and thus the true "voluntariness" of their participation in therapeutic interventions (12). Another issue yet to be resolved is the ethical concerns raised by coerced participation in treatment, even when such treatment is judged by professionals to be in the long-term best interests of the individual (13).

ESTABLISHING AN ETHICAL STANCE

The chapter has examined some of the ethical principles at the core of medical practice and considered the ways in which screening, assessing, or treating a patient for addictive disorders can challenge those principles. Physicians can avoid or minimize potential ethical dilemmas if they remain aware of the sources of potential conflict, keep the purposes of the ethical principles in mind, discuss potential conflicts with patients at the beginning of treatment, and take prophylactic steps to reduce conflicts to a few relatively rare situations.

REFERENCES

1. Capron A. Ethical and human rights issues in research on mental disorders that may affect decision-making capacity. *N Engl J Med* 1999;340: 1430–1434.
2. Uhl G. Are over-simplified views of addiction neuroscience providing too simplified ethical considerations? *Addiction* 2003;98:871–874.
3. Morse S. Medicine and morals, craving and compulsion. *Substance Use Misuse* 2004;39:437–460.
4. Husak D. The moral relevance of addiction. *Substance Use Misuse* 2004;39: 399–436.
5. Ashcroft R, Campbell AV, Capps B. *Ethical aspects of developments in neuroscience and drug addiction. Foresight brain science, Addiction and Drugs Project.* London, England: Ministry of Health, 2007.
6. Winters KC, ed. *Screening and assessment for adolescent substance use (Treatment Improvement Protocol 31).* Rockville, MD: Center for Substance Abuse Treatment, 1999.
7. Blow FC. Screening and Assessment for adolescent substance use (Treatment Improvement Protocol 26). Rockville, MD: Center for Substance Abuse Treatment.
8. Winters KC, ed. *Treatment of adolescent substance use (Treatment Improvement Protocol 32).* Rockville, MD: Center for Substance Abuse Treatment, 1999.
9. Wright A, Weinman J, Marteau T. The impact of learning of a genetic predisposition to nicotine dependence: an analogue study. *Tobacco Control* 2003;12:227–230.
10. Murray T. Ethical issues in immunotherapies and depot medications for substance abuse. In: National Research Council and the Institute of Medicine of the National Academies. *New treatments for addiction: behavioral, ethical, legal, and social questions.* Washington, DC: National Academies Press, 2004:188–212.
11. Hall W, Carter L. Ethical issues in using a cocaine vaccine to treat and prevent cocaine abuse and dependence. *J Med Ethics* 2004;30:337–340.
12. Farah M. Emerging ethical issues in neuroscience. *Nat Neurosci* 2002;5: 1123–1129.
13. Ridgely M, Iguchi M, Chiesa J. The use of immunotherapies and sustained-release formulations in the treatment of drug addiction: will current law support coercion? In: National Research Council and the Institute of Medicine of the National Academies. *New treatments for addiction: behavioral, ethical, legal, and social questions.* Washington, DC: National Academies Press, 2004:173–187.

CHAPTER 108

Bonnie B. Wilford, MS

Consent and Confidentiality in Addiction Practice

Consent to Treatment
Confidentiality

CONSENT TO TREATMENT

Americans attach great importance to being left alone. They pride themselves on having perfected a social and political system that limits the degree to which government and others can control what they do. The principle of autonomy is enshrined in the Constitution, and U.S. courts have repeatedly confirmed Americans' right to make decisions for themselves. This tradition is particularly strong in the area of medical decision making: An adult with "decisional capacity" has the unquestioned right to decide which treatment he or she will accept or to refuse treatment altogether, even if that refusal may result in death. (The situation is somewhat different for adolescents because they do not have the legal status of full-fledged adults. There are certain decisions that society will not allow them to make: Below a certain age—which varies by state and by issue—adolescents must attend school, may not marry without parental consent, may not drive, and cannot sign binding contracts. See Section 13 for a discussion of how this affects adolescents' right to consent to treatment.)

Many States require written consent for all types of medical care. This is essential in a climate of increasing patient litigation and questions from insurers. Requests from managed care groups for treatment records that are needed to recertify patients for payment require strict attention to federal confidentiality regulations. Ethical conduct by staff and the program also requires attention and use of specific expectations and standards. Carefully specified grievance procedures are imperative and must be followed in all involuntary termination procedures. The currency of staff credentials may become a legal issue if someone is not properly licensed at the time of an incident or other adverse action.

Adapted by Bonnie B. Wilford, MS, from Treatment Improvement Protocols 32, 40, 43, and 46, produced by the Center for Substance Abuse Treatment of the Substance and Mental Health Services Administration, Rockville, Maryland.

Informed Consent and Agreement for Treatment

The physician should discuss the risks and benefits of treatment with the patient and, with appropriate consent of the patient, the significant other(s), family members, or guardian. In office-based treatment, the patient should receive medications from only one physician and/or one pharmacy when possible.

The physician should employ the use of a written agreement between physician and patient addressing such issues as (1) alternative treatment options; (2) regular toxicologic testing for drugs of abuse and therapeutic drug levels (if available and indicated); (3) number and frequency of all prescription refills; and (4) reasons for which drug therapy may be discontinued (i.e., violation of agreement).

Patients should be seen at reasonable intervals (at least weekly during initial treatment) based upon the individual circumstance of the patient. Periodic assessment is necessary to determine compliance with the dosing regimen and effectiveness of treatment plan and to assess how the patient is handling the prescribed medication. Once a stable dosage is achieved and urine (or other toxicologic) tests are free of illicit drugs, less-frequent office visits may be initiated (monthly may be reasonable for patients on a stable dose of the prescribed medication(s) who are making progress toward treatment objectives). Continuation or modification of opioid therapy should depend on the physician's evaluation of progress toward stated treatment objectives such as (1) absence of toxicity, (2) absence of medical or behavioral adverse effects, (3) responsible handling of medications, (4) compliance with all elements of the treatment plan (including recovery-oriented activities, psychotherapy and/or other psychosocial modalities), and (5) abstinence from illicit drug use. If reasonable treatment goals are not being achieved, the physician should reevaluate the appropriateness of continued treatment.

Consent to the Treatment Plan The written treatment plan should describe the objectives that will be used to determine treatment success, such as freedom from intoxication, improved physical function, psychosocial function, and compliance and should indicate whether any further diagnostic evaluations are planned, as well as counseling, psychiatric management, or other ancillary services. The plan should be reviewed periodically. After treatment begins, the physician should adjust drug therapy to the individual medical needs of each patient. Treatment goals, other treatment modalities, or a rehabilitation program should be evaluated and discussed with the patient. If possible, every attempt should be made to involve significant others or immediate family members in the treatment process, with the patient's consent. The treatment plan should also contain contingencies for treatment failure (i.e., owing to failure to comply with the treatment plan, abuse of other opioids, or evidence that the Schedules III–V medications are not being taken).

CONFIDENTIALITY

Patients expect their caregivers to regard information about them and their treatment as confidential. Medicine historically attaches a high value to patients' privacy because it is critical that patients give their physicians accurate information. By affording privacy protections to medical information, society assures patients that they can discuss sensitive subjects with their physicians without worrying about what use others might make of such information. Nevertheless, the right to privacy is not without limits, and understanding the purpose and implications of those limits frequently poses problems for physicians and other health care professionals.

Basis of Confidentiality Confidentiality is especially important when a patient has an addictive disorder because of the widespread perception that such persons are weak and/or morally impaired. A patient considering treatment might be concerned that, if an insurer or HMO learns that his or her traumatic injuries were related to alcoholism, it will be difficult or impossible to obtain coverage for hospitalization costs or that his or her insurance will be canceled. Similarly, a patient may fear that his or her relationships with a spouse, parents, children, an employer, or friends would suffer if they learned about his or her problems with alcohol or drugs. If a patient has marital problems, information about an addictive disorder could have an effect on divorce or custody proceedings. A patient whose problem becomes known to his employer could lose an expected promotion or his or her job. Adverse consequences such as these can deter patients from admitting to problems with alcohol or drugs and from obtaining treatment for those problems.

Sources of Guidance

Federal Laws In the early 1970s, Congress passed legislation to protect information about patients in addictive disorder treatment and directed the Department of Health and Human Services (DHHS) to issue regulations protecting patients' confidentiality. The law is codified at 42 U.S.C. §290dd-2. The implementing federal regulations, titled "Confidentiality of Alcohol and Drug Abuse Patient Records," are contained in 42 CFR Part 2 (Volume 42 of the Code of Federal Regulations, Part 2).

The federal rules permit disclosures in only nine limited circumstances:

1. When a patient signs a consent form that complies with the regulations' requirements
2. When a disclosure does not identify the patient as a substance abuser
3. When program staff members consult among themselves
4. When the disclosure is to a "qualified service organization" that provides services to the program
5. When there is a medical emergency
6. When the program must report child abuse or neglect
7. When a patient commits a crime at the program or against staff members
8. When the information is for research, audit, or evaluation purposes
9. When a court issues a special order authorizing disclosure

Federal confidentiality rules apply to almost all addictive disorder treatment programs in the United States. They prohibit programs and their counselors from disclosing any information (written or oral) about any applicant, patient, or former patient unless (1) the patient has consented in writing (on the form required by the regulations) or (2) another very limited exception specified in the regulations applies. The rules apply regardless of whether the person seeking information already has the information, has other ways of obtaining it, has official status, is authorized by state law, or has a subpoena or search warrant.

The federal law and regulations restrict communications more tightly in many instances than either the physician-patient or the attorney-client privilege. Violating the regulations is punishable by a fine of up to $500 for a first offense and up to $5,000 for each subsequent offense (42 CFR §2.4).

Physicians who practice primary care probably are not subject to the federal confidentiality law and regulations. However, when a general care practice includes someone whose primary function is to provide addictive disorder assessment or treatment and the practice benefits from "federal assistance," it must comply with the federal rules for handling information about patients who may have alcohol or drug problems.

Though most primary care physicians are not subject to the federal rules, they should handle information about patients' addictive disorders with great care. The best practice for those not subject to the federal confidentiality rules is voluntary compliance.

In 1996, the Congress passed another law, the Health Insurance Portability and Accountability Act, Public Law 104-191 (HIPAA), which mandated the establishment of standards for the privacy of "individually identifiable health information." To carry out that mandate, in December 2000, DHHS issued a set of regulations governing patients' privacy that apply to a wide range of "health care providers." These HIPAA regulations appear in Volume 45 of the Code of Federal Regulations, Parts 160 and 164.

HIPAA regulations are not as restrictive as the federal confidentiality rules. Practitioners who are subject to both sets of rules must follow the more restrictive federal standard.

State Laws State laws also offer some protection to medical information. Most physicians and patients think of these laws as the "physician-patient privilege." Strictly speaking, the physician-patient privilege is a rule of evidence that governs whether a physician can be compelled to testify in a court case about a patient. In many states, however, the laws offer wider protection, and some states have special confidentiality laws that explicitly prohibit practitioners from divulging information about patients without their consent. States often include such prohibitions in professional licensing laws; such laws generally prohibit licensed professionals from divulging information about patients and make unauthorized disclosures grounds for disciplinary action, including license revocation.

Each state has its own set of rules, which means that the scope of protection offered by state law varies widely. Whether a communication (or laboratory test result) is "privileged" or "protected" depends on a number of factors:

- *The type of professional holding the information* and whether he or she is licensed or certified by the state. Most state laws do cover licensed physicians.
- *The context in which the information was communicated.* Some states limit protection to information a patient communicates to a physician in private, in the course of the medical consultation, and do not protect information disclosed to a physician in the presence of a third party, such as a spouse. Other states protect information the patient tells the physician when others are present as well as information the physician gains during examination.
- *The circumstances in which "confidential" information will be or was disclosed.* Some states protect medical information only when that information is sought in a court proceeding. If a physician divulges information about a patient in any other setting, the law does not recognize that there has been a violation of the patient's right to privacy. Other states protect medical information in many different contexts.
- *How the right to privacy is enforced.* State legal protection of medical information is useful only when it is backed by enforcement of the law.

Though enforcement remains relatively rare, states can discipline professionals who violate their patients' privacy, allow patients to sue physicians for damages, or criminalize behavior that violates patients' privacy.

Exceptions Exceptions to any general rule protecting the privacy of information generally include:

- *Consent:* All states permit physicians to disclose information if the patient consents, though states have different requirements about consent. In some states, it must be written; in others, it can be oral. Some states require different consent forms for disclosures about different diseases.
- *Reporting infectious diseases*: All states require physicians to report certain infectious diseases to public health authorities, though states' definitions of reportable diseases vary.
- *Reporting child abuse and neglect*: All states require physicians to report child abuse and neglect to child protective services, though states' definitions of child abuse vary.
- *Duty to warn*: Most states also require physicians to report credible threats a patient makes to harm others.

When Confidentiality Conflicts with Other Principles The laws may differ depending on whether the physician's obligation is to the patient or another individual or class of individuals.

Employer versus Employee To whom does a physician owe loyalty when treating a patient who has been referred by an employer as a condition of retaining a job? Is it to the employer, who is relying on the physician to help the employee recover and remain (or return) to work? Or is it to the patient (the employee)? The employer likely will require reports from the physician on the patient's progress in treatment. What should the physician do if the employee is not attending or complying with treatment? This question appears most starkly when the employee is in a safety-sensitive position and the physician is concerned that his or her behavior poses an immediate risk to other employees or to the public. To which ethical principle should the physician adhere: the obligation to safeguard the patient's privacy or the obligation to protect those who might be harmed by the patient's actions?

The best way to avoid having to grapple with this problem in an emergency (always a difficult and unpleasant experience) is to create agreed-upon ground rules before treatment begins. If an employer requires reports, the physician must have the patient sign a consent form authorizing communications with the employer. Physician and patient must agree on what kinds of information will be reported, and that agreement should be made part of the consent form. (Unfortunately, the patient can revoke his or her consent at any time.) Of course, the employer also must be willing to accept whatever limitations the agreement places on the kinds of information it will receive.

Reports to employers usually include information about attendance and progress in treatment. In most cases, it would be inappropriate for the physician to include detailed clinical information in such reports. However, employers can require more information when safety-sensitive employees are in treatment. Employers may want to hear about positive results from a drug screen test, and the physician may want to be able to report continued drug use by an employee in a safety-sensitive position. The physician can discharge his or her duty to the public at large (and to the employer) without violating the patient's right to privacy if the patient signs a consent form that documents his or her understanding that certain types of behavior would be reported to the employer.

Society versus Patient When a patient presents a danger to others, is the physician's obligation to the patient or to society? Most physicians know that society already has determined that their duty to warn supersedes their duty to protect a patients' privacy. The law requires a warning to the potential victim or someone in a position to protect the potential victim. The duty to warn, however, does not completely nullify the patient's right to privacy. The physician can warn others of potential danger without disclosing extraneous information about the patient, including information about his or her use of drugs and alcohol. Physicians who are subject to federal confidentiality rules are required to issue the warning in a way that minimizes harm to the patient's privacy.

SUGGESTED READINGS

Batki SL, Kauffman JF, Marion I, et al., eds. *Medication-assisted treatment for opioid addiction in opioid treatment programs (Treatment Improvement Protocol 43).* Rockville, MD: Center for Substance Abuse Treatment, 2005. Retrieved http://www.samhsa.gov/centers/csat2002.

Federation of State Medical Boards. *Model policy guidelines for opioid addiction treatment in the medical office.* Dallas: Author, 2002.

Forman RF, Nagy PD, eds. *Substance abuse: administrative issues in outpatient treatment (Treatment Improvement Protocol 46).* Rockville, MD: Center for Substance Abuse Treatment, 2006. Retrieved at http://www. samhsa.gov/centers/csat2002.

Legal Action Center. *Confidentiality and communication: a guide to the federal alcohol & drug confidentiality law and HIPAA, Revised.* New York: Author, 2006.

McNicholas LF, ed. *Clinical guidelines for the use of buprenorphine in the treatment of opioid addiction (Treatment Improvement Protocol 40).* Rockville, MD: Center for Substance Abuse Treatment, 2004. Retrieved http://www.samhsa.gov/centers/csat2002.

Winters KC, ed. *Treatment of adolescent substance use (Treatment Improvement Protocol 32).* Rockville, MD: Center for Substance Abuse Treatment, 1999. Retrieved http://www.samhsa.gov/centers/csat2002.

CHAPTER 109

Theodore V. Parran, Jr., MD, FACP
Robert L. DuPont, MD, FASAM
Bruce D. Lamb, JD, MA

Clinical and Legal Considerations in Prescribing Drugs with Abuse Potential

Most physicians who prescribe controlled substances do so in a legitimate manner that does not warrant scrutiny by federal or state law enforcement agencies. In fact, fewer than 1 in 10,000 physicians have lost their registration to prescribe controlled substances on the basis of a Drug Enforcement Administration (DEA) investigation of improper prescribing (1). Unfortunately, a number of high-profile cases recently brought against physicians for inappropriate prescribing (2) have led some experts to predict that the publicity surrounding such cases can have a "chilling effect" on both physicians and patients (3).

Fear of litigation or censure by regulatory officials need not deter the effective management of patients if physicians approach the diagnostic, treatment, and recordkeeping processes with care. In this regard, the importance of accurate and complete documentation cannot be overemphasized, because accurate and up-to-date medical records become the mechanism that protects both physician and patient (4).

CLINICAL STRATEGIES TO IMPROVE PRESCRIBING

The following strategies are supported by the weight of clinical evidence (5,6).

Patient Assessment Obtaining a history of the patient's past use of medications is an essential first step in appropriate prescribing. Such a history should include very specific questions. For example:

- In the past 6 months, have you taken any medications to help you calm down, keep from getting nervous or upset, raise your spirits, make you feel better, and the like?
- Have you been taking any medications to help you sleep? Have you been using alcohol for this purpose?
- Have you ever taken a medication to help you with a drug or alcohol problem?
- Have you ever taken a medication for a nervous stomach?
- Have you taken a medication to give you more energy or to cut down on your appetite?

The patient history also should include questions about use of alcohol and over-the-counter (OTC) preparations. For example, certain dietary supplements have mood-altering capabilities and often are misused. Many common cold preparations contain alcohol and other central nervous system (CNS) depressant or stimulant ingredients and should not be used in combination with prescribed medications that have CNS depressant effects.

Positive answers to any of these questions warrant further investigation.

Special Precautions for New Patients Many experts recommend that additional precautions be taken when prescribing a controlled drug to a new patient. These might involve the following:

1. *Assessment:* In addition to the patient history and examination, the physician should determine who has been caring for the patient in the past, what drug(s) have been prescribed and for what indications, and what substances (including alcohol, illicit drugs and OTC products) the patient has used. Medical records should be obtained (with the patient's consent).
2. *Emergencies:* In emergency situations, the physician should prescribe no more than 1 day's supply of a drug and arrange for a return visit. At a minimum, the patient's identity should be verified by asking for proper identification.

3. *Limit quantities:* In non-emergency situations, prescribe only enough of a controlled drug to meet the patient's needs until the next appointment. Have the patient *return to the office* for additional prescriptions, as telephone orders do not allow the physician to reassess the patient's continued need for the medication.

Drug Selection Rational drug therapy demands that the efficacy and safety of *all* potentially useful drug classes be reviewed for their relevance to the patient's disease or disorder (7).

When the optimum drug has been selected, the *dose, schedule*, and *formulation* should be determined. These choices often are just as important in optimizing drug therapy as the choice of drug itself. Decisions involve (1) dose (based not only on age, weight, and size of the patient but also on severity of disease, possible loading-dose requirement, and the presence of potentially interacting drugs); (2) timing of administration (such as a bedtime dose to minimize problems associated with sedative effects); (3) route of administration (chosen to improve compliance/adherence as well as to attain peak drug concentrations rapidly); and (4) formulation (e.g., selecting a patch in preference to a tablet or an extended-release rather than an immediate-release formulation).

Most physicians adopt additional safeguards in the use of psychoactive drugs. For example, even when sound medical indications have been established, physicians typically consider three additional factors before deciding to prescribe:

1. The *severity of symptoms*, in terms of the patient's ability to accommodate them. Relief of symptoms is a legitimate goal of medical practice, but using many psychoactive drugs to achieve complete symptomatic relief requires caution.
2. The patient's *reliability in taking medications*, noted through observation and careful history taking. A physician should assess a patient's susceptibility to drug abuse before prescribing any psychoactive drug and weigh the benefits against the risks. The possible development of dependence in patients on long-term therapy should be monitored through periodic checkups.
3. The *dependence-producing potential of the drug*. The physician should consider whether a drug with less potential for abuse, or even a non-drug therapy, would provide equivalent benefits. Patients should be warned about possible adverse effects caused by interactions with other drugs, including alcohol.

At the time a drug is prescribed, patients should be informed that it is illegal to sell, give away, or otherwise share their medication with others, including family members. The patient's obligation extends to keeping the medication in a locked cabinet or otherwise restricting access to it and to safely disposing of any unused supply.

Finally, no treatment program should be left open-ended. Where feasible, planned termination of medication therapy is a reasonable goal because it minimizes drug exposure and contains costs.

Monitoring the Patient's Response to Treatment

Proper prescription practices do not end when the patient receives the prescription from the physician. Plans to monitor for drug efficacy and safety, compliance, and potential development of tolerance must be formulated and clearly communicated to the patient.

Subjective symptoms can be used for monitoring, but some objective clinical signs (e.g., body weight, pulse rate, temperature, blood pressure, drug blood concentration) can serve as early signs of therapeutic failure or unacceptable adverse drug reactions that will require alteration of therapy.

Asking the patient to keep a log of signs and symptoms gives him or her a sense of participation in the treatment program and facilitates the physician's review of therapeutic progress and adverse events.

Simply recognizing the potential for nonadherence, especially during prolonged treatment, is a significant step toward improving medication use. Steps such as simplifying the drug regimen and offering patient education also improve adherence, as do phone calls to patients, home visits by nursing personnel, convenient packaging of medication, and monitoring of serum drug levels.

Finally, the physician should convey to the patient through attitude and manner that any medication, no matter how helpful, is only part of an overall treatment plan.

LEGAL STRATEGIES TO IMPROVE PRESRIBING

Informed Consent Physicians should require informed consent when prescribing controlled drugs. This involves informing the patient of the risks and benefits of the therapy and of the ethical and legal obligations such therapy imposes on both the physician and patient. Such informed consent can serve multiple purposes: (1) providing information about the risks and benefits of drug therapy, (2) fostering adherence to the treatment regimen, (3) limiting the potential for inadvertent drug misuse, and (4) to improve the efficacy of the treatment program.

Informed consent should address the potential for physical dependence and cognitive impairment. Other issues to be addressed including the following:

- Agreement to obtain prescriptions from only one physician and, preferably, from one designated pharmacy
- Agreement to take the medication only as prescribed, with provisions to offer some latitude for the consumption of more or less medication as symptoms dictate
- Acknowledgment that patients are responsible for their written prescriptions, medications, and arranging refills during regular office hours. They also must plan ahead so as not to run out of medication during weekends or vacation periods.
- Terms for informed consent violations, indicating that continued prescribing may be unsafe, and understanding that lack of adherence may result in weaning and gradual or abrupt discontinuation of controlled drug therapy

The informed consent agreement should include a statement instructing the patient to stop taking all other pain medications, unless explicitly told to continue. Such a statement reinforces the need to adhere to a single treatment regimen.

It is helpful to give the patient a copy of the agreement to carry with him or her, to document the source and reason for any controlled drugs in his or her possession. Some physicians provide a laminated card that identifies the individual as a patient of their practice. This is helpful to other physicians who may see the patient and in the event the patient is seen in an emergency department.

Executing the Prescription Order Careful execution of the prescription order form can prevent manipulation by the patient or others intent on obtaining drugs for nonmedical purposes. For example, federal law requires that prescription orders for controlled substances be signed and dated on the day they are issued. Under federal law, every prescription order must include at least the following information:

Name and address of the patient
Name, address and DEA registration number of the physician
Signature of the physician
Name and quantity of the drug prescribed
Directions for use
Refill information

Many states impose additional requirements, which the physician can determine by consulting the state medical licensing board. In addition, there are special federal requirements for drugs in different schedules of the federal Controlled Substances Act (CSA), particularly those in Schedule II.

Drug-seekers are constantly on the lookout for blank forms but also use the names of physicians who recently retired, left the state, or died. Therefore, storing blank prescription order forms in a safe place—as opposed to leaving the pads in examining rooms—is a sound practice. *NOTE: The physician should immediately report the theft or loss of prescription blanks to the nearest field office of the federal DEA and to the state board of medicine or pharmacy.*

When the physician is concerned about a patient's behavior or clinical progress (or the lack thereof), it usually is advisable to seek a consultation with an expert in the disorder for which the patient is being treated *and* an expert in addiction medicine. Physicians place themselves at risk if they continue prescribing controlled drugs in the absence of such consultations.

The Patient Record In the event of a legal or regulatory challenge, detailed medical records documenting what was done and why are the foundations of the physician's defense. Every physician needs to know and understand the federal requirements as well as the laws and regulatory requirements in the state in which he or she practices. This is important because state laws and licensing board rules may differ substantially from the federal requirements and from one state to another. The Board of Medical Licensure or the Board of Pharmacy (or their equivalent) in each state can provide information about the relevant requirements.

At a minimum, patient records should contain the following information:

- *Patient history and physical examination:* The patient record must include a history of all controlled drugs used to treat the patient in the past, any use of illicit substances, and any patient allergies. Regimens tried and failed also should be documented. It is wise to obtain the patient's records directly from physicians who have treated him or her in the past. (Caution should be exercised in accepting records supplied by patients, as these occasionally are fraudulent.) The documentation should include information about the patient's personal and family histories of alcoholism, drug use and addiction, as well any personal history of major depression or other psychiatric disorder.
- *Documentation of the treatment plan:* The treatment plan and goals should be documented in the record so that there is evidence of clear-cut, individualized objectives to guide the choice of therapy. If the patient improves after a brief trial, that should be documented in the record as well, as should regimens tried and failed.
- *Use of consultants:* Whenever the best clinical course is not clear or the patient's response is not as expected, consultation with another physician should be obtained. Generally, the results of the consultation should be discussed with the consulting physician and a written consultation report added to the patient's medical record.
- *Prescription orders:* The patient record must include all prescription orders, whether written or telephoned. Written instructions for the use of all medications should be given to the patient and documented in the record. The prescription order itself should specify both the milligram dose along with the volume of solution to be taken at any given time. Confusion related to ambiguous orders can lead to tragic outcomes, especially early in treatment. The physician should clearly specify the concentration to be used.
- *Informed consent agreement:* As noted earlier, a written informed consent form, signed by the patient, can be helpful in establishing a set of "ground rules" and appropriate expectations (10,11).
- *Monitoring visits:* Medication monitoring visits are billable and can be performed by a nurse. They should be carefully documented in the medical record, in the same manner as a visit with the physician.
- *Treatment results:* The patient's record should clearly reflect the decision-making process that resulted in any given medical outcome. Good records demonstrate that a service was provided to the patient and establish that the service provided was medically necessary. Even if the outcome is less than optimal, thorough records protect both the physician's and the patient's interests.

Inclusion in the patient record of a pharmacy address and telephone number reinforces to the patient the importance of using one only pharmacy to fill all prescriptions.

THE DECISION TO STOP PRESCRIBING

Certain situations may warrant immediate cessation of prescribing. These generally occur when out-of-control behaviors indicate that continued prescribing is unsafe or causing harm to the patient (8). Examples include altering or selling prescriptions, accidental or intentional overdose, multiple episodes of running out early (due to bingeing), egregious doctor shopping, or threatening the physician or staff.

When such events arise, it is important to separate the *person* of the patient from the *behaviors* of the disease by demonstrating a positive regard for the person but no tolerance for the behaviors of the disease.

The essential steps are to (1) stop prescribing, (2) tell the patient that continued prescribing is not clinically supportable (and thus not possible), (3) urge the patient to accept a referral for assessment by an addiction specialist, (4) educate the patient about signs and symptoms of spontaneous withdrawal and urge the patient to go to the emergency department if symptoms occur, and (5) assure the patient that he or she will continue to receive care for the presenting symptoms or condition.

Identification of a patient who is abusing a prescribed controlled drug presents a major therapeutic opportunity. The physician should have a plan for managing such a patient, typically involving work with the patient and the patient's family, referral to an addiction expert for assessment and placement in a formal addiction treatment program, long-term participation in a Twelve Step mutual help program such as Narcotics Anonymous, and follow-up of any associated medical or psychiatric comorbidities (9).

In all cases, patients should be given the benefit of the physician's concern and attention. It is important to remember that even drug-seeking patients often have very real medical problems that demand and deserve the same high-quality medical care offered to any patient.

REFERENCES

1. Kuehn BM. Prescription drug abuse rises globally. *JAMA* 2007;297:1306.
2. McCarthy M. Prescription drug abuse up sharply in the USA. *Lancet* 2007;369:1505.
3. Weaver M, Schnoll S. Addiction issues in prescribing opioids for chronic nonmalignant pain. *J Addict Med* 2007;1(1):2–10.
4. Federation of State Medical Boards of the United States, Inc. *Model guidelines for the use of controlled substances for the treatment of pain.* Dallas: Author, 1998. Retrieved www.fsmb.org.
5. Isaacson JH, Hopper JA, Alford DP, Parran T. Prescription drug use and abuse. Risk factors, red flags, and prevention strategies. *Postgrad Med* 2005;118:19.
6. Compton WM, Volkow ND. Abuse of prescription drugs and the risk of addiction. *Drug Alcohol Depend* 2006;83(Suppl)1:S4.
7. Zacny J, Bigelow G, Compton P, et al. College on Problems of Drug Dependence taskforce on prescription opioid nonmedical use and abuse: position statement. *Drug Alcohol Depend* 2003;69:215.
8. Michna E, Ross EL, Hynes WL, et al. Predicting aberrant drug behavior in patients treated for chronic pain: importance of abuse history. *J Pain Symptom Manage* 2004;28:250.
9. Matzger H, Weisner C. Nonmedical use of prescription drugs among a longitudinal sample of dependent and problem drinkers. *Drug Alcohol Depend* 2007;86:222.
10. Arnold RM, Han PK, Seltzer D. Opioid contracts in chronic nonmalignant pain management. Objectives and uncertainties. *Am J Med* 2006;1119:292.
11. Gourlay DL, Heit HA, Almahrezi A. Universal Precautions in Pain Management. *Pain Med* 2005;6(2):107–112.

CHAPTER 110

Robert L. DuPont, MD, FASAM
Bruce A. Goldberger, PhD, DABFT
Mark S. Gold, MD

Clinical and Legal Considerations in Drug Testing

Drug testing—that is, use of an objective laboratory test for recent use of specific drugs—is useful in deterring and detecting drug use in many settings: physicians' offices, the workplace, schools and athletic programs, and the criminal justice system.

Drug testing identifies recent use of specific drugs, including alcohol and nicotine. It does not identify addiction, or dependence. Though blood and breath (but not urine) alcohol concentrations roughly correlate with level of impairment, tests for drugs and drug metabolites in urine generally do not. Results of drug tests are therefore interpreted as evidence of recent use of specific drugs, rather than as evidence of impairment or dependence. The identification of recent drug use has great value because denial is a cardinal feature of drug abuse and because many drug users do not know which drugs they are taking.

Drug testing has many uses in medicine even though testing has not been included in the curriculum and practical experience of most physicians. Just as with other recently introduced tests in medicine (e.g., functional magnetic resonance imaging or HIV testing), physician education and expert guidelines are needed to make use of the new technologies that greatly enhance medical care. Though drug testing is recognized as important, especially in the evaluation of adolescents, some professional organizations have called on experts, including physicians in the American Society of Addiction Medicine (ASAM), to produce guidelines for their use (1).

This chapter is a practical overview of drug testing for physicians practicing addiction medicine.

EVOLUTION OF DRUG TESTING

Fifty years ago, drug testing was an uncommon, expensive, and laborious component of death investigations, though, drug testing even then was commonly employed in emergency rooms when a drug overdose was suspected. The use of drug testing spread rapidly in the 1970s to substance abuse treatment programs and the criminal justice system. In the 1980s, drug testing became widespread in the workplace following the example of testing in the military, especially in pre-employment testing and in testing of safety- or security-sensitive positions. In addition, in the past decade, drug testing has been used in drug prevention programs including within school systems, in highway law enforcement, and in athletic contests.

Over the past five decades, the technology used for drug testing progressed rapidly, permitting the identification of drugs and their metabolites at far lower concentrations far more economically. At the same time, drug testing expanded to include testing of oral fluid (saliva), hair, and sweat. Because drugs are also present in breath, the future holds the promise of breath testing for drugs of abuse (2). The leading issue in early drug testing—the problem of false-positives—has been virtually eliminated (3).

Drug tests are now available over the counter for home use. When drug testing is conducted by families, it is useful for them to be educated regarding what testing does and does not do and how to handle positive tests most effectively and wisely (4). When drug testing migrated from clinical settings to prevention, because of the controversy over these applications of modern drug testing technology, the use of forensic standards became commonplace for the first time in toxicology. Drug testing is also used in research and evaluation studies to validate self-report on surveys of drug use and to evaluate the effectiveness of treatment programs in reducing drug use by patients (5,6).

SCIENCE OF DRUG TESTING

Though drugs of abuse, including alcohol, are used primarily for their effects on the brain reward centers and are ingested by many routes of administration (oral, intranasal, smoking, and intravenously, among other routes to the brain's reward centers), they are distributed by the blood to all areas of the body. For this reason, drugs and their metabolites can be detected in nearly all body fluids and tissues.

In general, drugs and drug metabolites are detectible in urine for 1 to 3 days after acute administration, though in settings of chronic use they may be detected for longer periods of time, especially marijuana. For marijuana, after a single episode of use, many users have negative urine tests at usual cutoffs within 24 hours and almost all will be negative within 3 to 5 days of last marijuana use. However with chronic use of marijuana, positive urine tests can be obtained for a month or longer.

The immunoassay screening test makes use of the remarkable specificity and sensitivity of the antigen-antibody reaction. Drug test manufacturers previously used bacteria to produce patented antibodies that were highly specific for the tested drugs and drug metabolites. In the early years of drug testing, there was some unwanted cross-reactivity to a few of the antibodies used, but today with improved antibody specificity, there is almost none. The on-site tests described later in this chapter rely on antibodies to detect the low concentrations of drugs and their metabolites in urine and oral fluid.

For standard drug testing, especially when severe consequences from a single positive test may be imposed and when the testing is controversial, an initial immunoassay screening test is followed by a more specific, sensitive, and expensive confirmation test. This two-step process is required for regulated workplace drug testing. In many clinical settings such as the emergency department, drug treatment, and the criminal justice system, only the initial immunoassay test is required, thus reducing the costs of testing and increasing the speed of obtaining results.

When there are controversies or severe consequences to a drug test result, not only is the two-step testing process desirable but the ultimate fail-safe is to retain the positive sample in the original collection container in a frozen state for possible retesting. Such repeat testing is easily done with urine testing. It is the ultimate rebuttal to those who say no drug testing process is completely foolproof. The retained positive urine sample is the standard in regulated workplace drug testing today.

With the advent of bench-top mass spectrometry, the confirmation of drugs and drug metabolites by gas chromatography–mass spectrometry (GC-MS) is now compulsory in many settings, especially when there are serious consequences for a single positive test. The GC-MS identifies the drugs and drug metabolites based primarily on the chemical structure of the compound. It is an accurate method of drug and drug metabolite detection and identification. The current highest standard is the gas chromatography–mass spectrometry–mass spectrometry (GC-MS-MS) or liquid chromatography–mass spectrometry–mass spectrometry (LC-MS-MS), which are breathtakingly expensive and sophisticated technologies.

The question often asked is, "How accurate is the drug test?" When the two-step process (including the immunoassay screen and the MS confirmation) is utilized, the drug identification process is highly accurate. If a specific drug is identified on a drug test of a specimen from a donor, then that drug (or a drug metabolite) was present in the donor's body. An evaluation by a medical review officer (MRO) can validate whether the drug was in the donor's body as a result of a current medical prescription to the donor. While the highest level of science, including the two-step process, the MRO validation and the retained positive specimen are desirable in certain cases, and when there are potential legal challenges, even an immunoassay screen alone is highly reliable for many medical purposes in the identification of specific drugs even though it does not rise to the highest, or forensic, degree of certainty.

ON-SITE VERSUS LABORATORY ANALYSIS

Most drug tests are conducted at clinical laboratories following the collection of the sample at some other site (e.g., at a drug treatment center or a physician's office). The laboratory-testing process usually takes a day or two from the time of collection until the result is available. In recent years, more drug testing is done on-site when the initial immunoassay test is done at the point of collection rather than at a laboratory. In forensic settings, the sample that screens positive on-site is sent to a laboratory for a confirming test before being reported as positive. In many clinical settings, such confirmation is unnecessary, especially when the donor admits recent drug use, as is typically the case.

Having results at the time of collection is enormously useful in many settings. However, on-site tests, especially oral fluid tests, may be less sensitive than laboratory-based analysis. In addition, a confirmation test is not available on-site. On-site tests seldom produce false-positive results—though it does happen. False-negative results may be more common when using on-site test kits, a problem that to some extent mitigates the benefits of immediate results. It is possible to define the extent of the problem of false-negative test results with any on-site device by splitting some samples and sending one sample for laboratory-based testing or, in the case of oral fluid testing, by comparing the oral fluid on-site test results with the results of urine samples taken from the same donors a the same time and then analyzed at a laboratory.

CHOICE OF MATRIX

The choice of a testing matrix relates to the duration after use that drugs and their metabolites are typically detectable, the distribution of the drugs and drug metabolites, the ease of specimen collection, and the resistance to cheating.

Urine is a particularly attractive matrix for drug testing because it is easy to collect (compared to blood), most drugs and drug metabolites can be readily detected in urine without complex extraction processes, and drugs and their metabolites are often detectable for longer periods of time in urine when compared to blood and other fluids such as oral fluid. Nevertheless, there are many settings in which testing for drugs of abuse in oral fluid, hair, and sweat is valuable. For that reason, it is important that physicians using drug tests understand the potential of testing samples other than urine.

Urine Drug testing outside of the medical examiner's office and the emergency department began with urine. There are many reasons to recommend urine as a matrix for drug testing, including that virtually all clinical laboratories perform drug tests on urine samples, creating a highly competitive marketplace that generally works to lower costs and certainly provides abundant alternative drug test suppliers.

When urine drug testing first became widespread in drug abuse treatment and the criminal justice system in the 1970s, the standard was to directly observe the collection—that is, to directly observe the urine leaving the donor and entering the collection cup. However, when drug testing came to the workplace in the 1980s, direct observation was considered objectionably intrusive. To accommodate this objection, unobserved urine collection became common practice. That change opened the door wide for cheating. Donors developed a remarkable range of strategies to cheat on drug tests, which led to one of the more active areas on the Internet and to the publication in 1987 by Abbie Hoffman of a book entitled *Steal This Urine Test* (7). Thus began a cat-and-mouse game that continues to the present time when the Internet provides ready access for drug users to the latest in cheating strategies. Cheating is the Achilles heel for this otherwise attractive matrix. When cheating is suspected, it is useful to use another matrix and/or return to direct observation. There is a robust literature on cheating (8,9).

The determinants of the level of drug and drug metabolites found in urine after a single use of a drug are complex, including the dose of the drug taken and the duration of time between the last drug use and the urine collection of the sample. Also important is how much drug was used over what periods of time in the days prior to the collection of the test sample. A wild card in urine drug concentrations is the amount of fluid recently consumed, because whatever the kidneys excrete of the drug and/or its metabolites is diluted by the fluid excreted by the kidney between the time of the most recent voiding and the time of collection. By special order, creatinine determinations can be used to normalize drug concentrations, thus removing the dilution problem (14,15).

Because urine testing is dominant in the drug-testing marketplace, it is relatively easy and inexpensive to add drugs to the federal government's basic five-drug panel consisting of marijuana, cocaine, PCP, amphetamines, and opiates. This is a major advantage of urine testing as a large proportion of drug abuse is of drugs other than the five on this basic panel (10). This panel is called the SAMHSA-5 because the federal Substance Abuse and Mental Health Services Administration *(www.samhsa.gov)* manages the federal standards for regulated drug testing.

Depending on whether confirming tests and MRO validation are required and on the number of drugs in the panel, urine drug tests cost from about $5 to $30. Both on-site and laboratory-based urine tests are widely available.

Hair Drugs and drug metabolites are incorporated in the hair while it is formed in the hair follicle. Head hair grows approximately one-half an inch a month. The typical hair specimen is 1.5 inches long, thus producing a record of drug use for the prior 90 days. However, as it takes about 1 week for the hair to grow from the base of the follicle to the point where it can be snipped at the level of the scalp, there is no record in hair of drug use for the week prior to sample collection. Alcohol is not incorporated in hair, though alcohol's major metabolites, including ethyl glucuronide (EtG), are detectable in hair samples (11).

Over the course of the 90 days covered by a typical 1.5-inch hair sample, even a few uses of most drugs of abuse are detectable. Marijuana is an exception because levels of THC and metabolites from marijuana are in the body, including in the hair, at significantly lower concentrations than most other drugs of abuse. For this reason, it takes marijuana use of about twice a week for the entire 90 days to produce a positive result at the standard cutoff concentrations. Hair tests are absolutely resistant to cheating because hair collection is always under direct observation.

One problem with urine testing is that recent poppy seed consumption can produce a morphine and/or a codeine positive test result that is difficult to distinguish from heroin use. This makes the urine test virtually useless in identifying heroin use in workplace and other non-clinical settings. Hair samples are not positive for morphine and/or codeine even after repeated consumption of poppy seeds, which makes hair testing an attractive option when urine tests produce positive morphine and/or codeine results in certain settings. Hair testing is an attractive option when cheating is suspected.

Because hair testing gives results that cover the period from 7 to 90 days prior to collection while urine tests provide results that cover the 1 to 3 days prior to collection, these two matrices do not cover the same time periods. When the issue is drug use in the prior 7 days, hair testing has no value. However, in many settings, what is being looked for is prior use of specific drugs of abuse and, in these settings, the question of when the drug use occurred is not particularly relevant. An example of this application is pre-employment testing where cheating on the urine test is a major concern because it is a scheduled test; the sample donors know in advance that they will be tested. This makes cheating on scheduled urine tests all the easier.

Hair testing has been criticized as racially biased because of an early study finding that in a mouse given an antipsychotic drug, there were higher concentrations of the drug found in the black hair on that mouse than in the white hair. It is important to recognize that the claim that hair testing is color-biased is not that black hair or one ethnic or racial group is positive on hair testing without using the drug identified. Rather, the claim is that after drug use, the hair test is more likely to be positive with one hair color than another. In drug testing in general, there is no attempt to normalize the test results for various biologic factors. Instead, the tests are read to a particular concentration in the tested sample. For example, alcohol tests on the highway use the blood alcohol concentration (BAC) of 0.08 as the cut-off for violations for both men and women even though it typically takes less alcohol consumption for a woman to get to this concentration than a man.

With respect to the claim that hair testing is racially biased, there have been several studies using large samples of tested people that have all shown that the proportion testing positive is the same for African Americans and whites based on urine testing, hair testing, and self-report (12–14).

There are no on-site hair tests at this time, though it is possible that on-site hair tests may become available in the future. Thus, only laboratory-based hair tests are available and this from a handful of commercial laboratories. Hair tests typically cost about $40 to $65 per test.

Oral Fluid The liquid content of the oral cavity (e.g., saliva or oral fluid) can be analyzed for drugs of abuse with on-site and laboratory-based techniques. Oral fluid testing is highly resistant to cheating, as the oral fluid sample is collected under direct observation. The big problem with oral fluid testing is that, like hair testing, these tests are relatively insensitive to marijuana use. This means that while the detection of other drugs of abuse is roughly similar for oral fluid testing and urine testing, significantly fewer recent users of marijuana are detected using oral fluid than when using urine for the same people at the same time. The on-site kits for oral fluid testing are particularly prone to miss marijuana use because they are generally less sensitive than the laboratory-based analysis.

In general, oral fluid correlates best with blood testing, with which saliva is in equilibrium, which means that oral fluid testing generally identifies drug use in only the 12 to 24 hours prior to sample collection. Because oral fluid testing is much less common than urine testing, the panel of drugs identified is usually limited to the SAMHSA-5 in on-site kits. Though other drugs and their metabolites are present in oral fluids, as a practical matter today it is impossible to identify use of other drugs of abuse with oral fluid using on-site kits, though laboratory-based oral fluids testing can detect other drugs of abuse.

For many applications, oral fluid testing is widely anticipated to be the test of the future because it does not have the "bathroom problem" that urine does and because it is resistant to cheating. On the other hand, the current sensitivity limits of oral fluid testing leaves much to be desired. The expectation is that in the future, as the technology improves, oral fluid will deliver on its great promise. An oral fluid test typically costs about $15 to $50.

Sweat Because drugs of abuse are contained not only in saliva but in sweat, sweat is an attractive matrix for drug testing. A patch, similar to a nicotine patch worn in smoking cessation, is applied to the tested person. The patch is removed usually after a week or two for analysis at the laboratory. The sweat is collected in an absorbent pad that is protected by a permeable cover that attaches to the skin. The water in sweat evaporates through the covering membrane, leaving the drug and drug metabolites concentrated in the gauze. Sweat testing is prospective from the time the patch is applied, whereas all other drug tests are backward-looking from the time of collection. There is no on-site option for the analysis of drugs and drug metabolites in sweat. Sweat testing is resistant to cheating because the patch puckers when removed and reapplied. A sweat patch test typically costs about $35.

Breath Alcohol is commonly tested in breath and blood, though urine samples can also be tested for recent alcohol use. Drugs of abuse are present in breath at a very low concentration. As the technology of testing improves, it is likely that drugs of abuse will be detected in breath as they now are for alcohol. Breath testing for drugs of abuse is likely to be practical well after oral fluids testing is practical, as both depend on improving technology and the levels in oral fluids, while lower than urine, are far higher than in breath. Nevertheless, the ultimate in drug testing is likely to be with breath testing, which will be resistant to cheating and far easier to collect than urine, oral fluids, or hair.

Testing for Alcohol Since the dose of alcohol needed to produce brain reward is a thousand or more times higher than the dose of the commonly used drugs of abuse, the testing for drugs has been more challenging and more reliant on the evolution of technology.

Alcohol is rapidly metabolized, primarily by the liver, so alcohol levels in the blood fall rapidly—typically to zero within a few hours after the last drink. The acute impairing effects of alcohol are related to the blood alcohol levels as modified by the moderating effects of tolerance and the subject's familiarity with the task being measured. The alcohol level is in equilibrium with the blood at the time the urine leaves the kidneys. The urine in the bladder is a reflection of the blood alcohol levels over the period of time that the urine in the bladder was being produced by the kidneys. For this reason, the urine alcohol level lags the blood level at the time of urination, meaning that the urine alcohol level is lower than the blood alcohol level at the time of urine collection during the ascending slope of the blood level and higher during the descending slope of blood level after drinking stops. The detection window for urine alcohol tests is generally 12 hours or less after drinking has stopped, in contrast to the typical 1 to 3 days for the detection of most drugs of abuse.

The level of alcohol in the urine is of limited value in settings such as highway safety when the BAC standard is typically 0.08. However, in settings in which there is a zero tolerance for alcohol use, such as underage youth, people in drug and alcohol treatment, and people facing legal sanctions for any drinking (as may occur in probation or child custody settings), urine testing for alcohol can be helpful. Urine testing for alcohol is especially practical when drug tests are being done on a urine sample, at which time it is easy to add an alcohol test.

An important recent drug testing option is to test for ethyl glucuronide (EtG) or ethyl sulfate (EtS), both of which are metabolites of alcohol that are found in urine up to 5 to 7 days following the consumption of alcohol. These tests are especially useful in settings where alcohol use is completely prohibited (e.g., people in drug or alcohol treatment and others under supervision that includes a requirement not to use alcohol). A negative EtG test is especially valuable in establishing that the donor of the urine sample has not used alcohol in the prior 5 to 7 days. As most EtG tests are negative, this is valuable information in many settings in which abstinence from drinking is required.

Because the EtG tests may be positive when the donor has used an alcohol hand sanitizer or an alcohol-containing mouthwash, interpreting a positive EtG test result requires clinical judgment, especially if there are severe consequences as a result of a single positive test. When people are subject to EtG testing for alcohol, they need to be warned specifically and in detail in order to avoid alcohol-containing products—which are ubiquitous—or risk getting a positive test result (15).

Comparing Matrices Refer to Table 110.1 for comparison of the clinically available test matrices. There are clinical settings in which each of the four matrices discussed in this chapter is particularly useful. Urine is the default matrix for most drug tests because it is the most familiar and because most clinical laboratories provide these tests. Urine is the matrix that is most practical when special-order tests are required, including tests for drugs that are less commonly used in drug testing. On the other hand, urine has a much shorter detection window than does hair. In addition, urine is the matrix most vulnerable to cheating. Oral fluids are often the most easily obtained matrix, but they can be less sensitive to drug use and have a shorter detection window than urine. Sweat patch testing is prospective—meaning it identifies drug use after the patch is put on—and, like oral fluids and hair testing, sweat patch testing is highly resistant to cheating. Hair testing is particularly helpful in scheduled testing, including pre-employment tests where cheating is common. On the other hand, hair is the most expensive drug test matrix.

Victim and Other Drug Testing Drug use is found in college students who present with accidents, violent arguments, fights, and date rape. Therefore, student health and emergency room personnel routinely perform urine testing on rape and suspected date rape victims (16–19). This is an example of a wide variety of nontraditional settings in which drug testing is increasingly used to identify recent drug use. Another example is the proposal that drug test results be added as a criterion for making the diagnosis of substance use disorders (20).

Smarter Drug Testing Clinicians who use drug tests should be familiar with both laboratory-based and on-site testing techniques and with all four of the commonly used matrices. In many clinical settings, it is desirable to have access to all of these testing options to discourage cheating and to keep track of the relative effectiveness of each type of testing. It is also desirable to test for a wide variety of drugs, at least from time to time, to identify new or unusual drugs that appear among the tested population. The strategy for using wisely the various matrices and for testing for a wide variety of drugs has been described as "smarter drug testing" (21).

INTERPRETATION OF DRUG TEST RESULTS

When interpreting a drug test result, especially when the sample donor denies recent use of an identified drug, it is usually desirable to cast a wide net, seeking the best information available before rending an opinion. Though difficult situations do arise, the vast majority of drug test results are easily interpreted and not disputed by the donors.

When interpreting a disputed or ambiguous drug test result, the physician is wise to consult the laboratory reporting the result, because the laboratories and drug assay manufacturers have highly qualified forensic toxicologists on staff.

In difficult cases, physicians can consult certified MROs, who are physicians certified in the interpretation of drug test results (Table 110.2).

Role of the Medical Review Officer In most clinical settings and in the criminal justice system, it is seldom necessary to have an outside medical expert validate the laboratory results of drug tests because the tests are typically part of an ongoing, often long-term, relationship and because the results of a single positive drug test are unlikely to be severe. In contrast, having professional and independent validation of laboratory positive results is often desirable, and under much regulated drug testing mandatory, in many non-clinical settings where drug testing of particular individuals is much less frequent and where the drug test results may have severe impacts on the tested individual.

An MRO is a physician trained and certified in the interpretation of drug test results (see the Sidebar to this chapter). The MRO receives the laboratory positive result (and in regulated workplace testing, negative results as well) before the results go to the individual or the organization requesting the drug test in order to validate that the proper procedures were maintained, including rigorous chain of custody procedures. In addition, the MRO validates that the laboratory positive drug test result was not the result of a legitimate medical prescription for the tested subject.

Sources of Confusion A confusion that commonly occurs in interpreting drug tests devolves from an assumption that because most drug users use infrequently and almost all drug users minimize (or flatly deny) their drug use and because most drug users use very occasionally, most drug test positives are the result of occasional drug use. Nothing could be further from the truth. Most drug positives are the result

TABLE 110.1 Comparison of Blood, Urine, Hair, Saliva, and Sweat Patch Testing for Drugs of Abuse

Characteristic	Blood	Urine	Hair	Saliva	Sweat patch
Immunoassay screen	Yes	Yes	Yes	Yes	Yes
GC/MS confirmation option (laboratory-based)	Yes	Yes	Yes	Yes	Yes
Chain-of-custody option	Yes	Yes	Yes	Yes	Yes
Medical review officer option	Yes	Yes	Yes	Yes	Yes
Retest of same sample	Yes	Yes	Yes	Yes	Yes
Retain positive samples for retest option	Difficult	Possible	Easy	Difficult	Possible
Common surveillance window	3–12 hr	1–3 d	7–90 d+	3–24 hr	1–21 d
Intrusiveness of collection	Severe	Moderate	None	Slight	Slight
Compatibility of new sample if original test disputed	No	No	Yes	No	No
Number of drugs screened	Unlimited[a]	Unlimited[b]	Large[c]	5+alcohol	5[d]
Cost/sample (SAMHSA-5)	About \$100–\$200	About \$15–\$30	About \$40–\$65	About \$15–\$50	About \$35
Test can distinguish between light, moderate, and heavy drug use	Yes (short term)	No	Yes (long term)	No	Yes (ongoing)
Test resistance to cheating	High	Low	High	High	High
Best application	Post-accident and overdose testing for alcohol and other drugs Blood alcohol concentration level	Reasonable-cause testing Frequent testing of high-risk groups such as those in posttreatment follow-up and the criminal justice system Unannounced, random tests with observed collection	Pre-employment testing Random and periodic testing Testing to determine severity of drug use for referral to treatment Testing of subjects suspected of seeking to evade urine-test detection Opiate addicts claiming poppy seed false-positive	Post-accident and overdose testing for alcohol and other drugs Blood alcohol concentration level Reasonable-cause Testing	Posttreatment testing Maintaining abstinence Opiate addicts claiming poppy seed false-positive Compliance testing in DOT and criminal justice system applications

DOT, U.S. Department of Transportation; GC/MS, gas chromatography/mass spectrometry; NIDA, National Institute on Drug Abuse.

[a]Blood testing for alcohol is routine, costing about \$25/sample, but blood testing for drugs is done by only a few laboratories in the United States. Blood testing for drugs is relatively expensive, costing about \$60 for each drug tested for.

[b]Urine tests for nonroutine drugs are available from most reference laboratories, and costs for broad screens are generally < \$200.

[c]Hair testing is commonly performed for the NIDA 5 (cocaine, opiates, marijuana, amphetamines, and phencyclidine). However, a large number of drugs and metabolites can be detected, and routine broad testing is performed in several toxicology reference laboratories. The cost of non-routine testing of hair is < \$500 in most cases.

[d]Commonly limited to the NIDA 5. Tests can also be performed for alcohol.

of frequent drug use as is easily seen from the fact that most drug tests are conducted in urine that has a window of detection of a few days. That means that unless the drug was used during the days immediately prior to the sample collection, the test will be negative. A study of the probability of a positive test found that 55% of positive tests in random testing are the result of daily or near daily use and that only 7% positive random drug tests are from people who use drugs a few times a year (22).

LIMITATIONS OF DRUG TESTING

Drug tests report the presence or absence of specific drugs and/or their metabolites only when those specific analytes are included in the test panel. In other words, drug tests do not identify recent drug use in general. They identify recent use of the drugs specified on the particular test. This means, for example, that if the test did not specifically include ecstasy (methylenedioxymethamphetamine), the recent use of this

TABLE 110.2 Standard References in Forensic Toxicology

Moffat AC, senior ed. *Clarke's analysis of drugs and poisons,* 3rd ed. London: Pharmaceutical Press, 2004.
Baselt RC. *Disposition of toxic drugs and chemicals in man,* 7th ed. Foster City, CA: Biomedical Publications, 2004.
Karch SB, ed. *Drug abuse handbook.* CRC Press, 2007.
Miller JR, Goldberger BA, eds. *Handbook of workplace drug testing.* Washington, DC: AACC Press, 2008.
Medico-legal aspects of alcohol, 4th ed. , Tucson, AZ: J.C. Garriott, Lawyers & Judges Publishing, 2003.
Jenkins AJ. Goldberger BA, eds. *On-site drug testing.* Washington, DC: AACC Press, 2002.
Levine B. *Principles of forensic toxicology,* 2nd ed. Washington, DC: AACC Press, 2003.
Visit the following Web sites to locate a Medical Review Officer near you.
American Society of Addiction Medicine (ASAM) www.asam.org.
Division of Workplace Programs: Medical Review Officers (Center for Substance Abuse Treatment, Substance Abuse and Mental Health Services Administration, DHHS) http://workplace.samhsa.gov/drugtesting/medicalreviewofficers.

specific drug would not be identified by the test regardless of the clinical significance of its use. A negative drug test does not indicate that the tested individual had not recently used a drug included on the testing panel. A negative drug test result indicates that none of the specific drugs on the test panel was identified at or above the cut-off concentration for that test panel.

Drug testing is valuable in identifying recent use of specific drugs but not in determining impairment, dependence, dose, or recency of drug use. This means drug testing is especially valuable in validating self-report of drug use in surveys and in settings where any use of the identified drug is a violation of the standard for that setting. For example, any use of cocaine or marijuana is strictly prohibited among commercial airline pilots or patients in most substance abuse treatment programs. Though the use of alcohol is legal for adults and generally permitted, there are exceptions (e.g., any identifiable concentration of alcohol is prohibited for a surgeon in an operating room or a physician under the care of a physician health program for dependence or abuse of alcohol (23). For alcohol use by adults in many other settings, the standard for violation relates to the alcohol concentration, so in most states today a BAC of 0.08 or higher is considered evidence of violation of the law.

Drug testing does not permit an estimation of the dose or the recency of drug use. Drug tests are commonly reported as "positive" or "none detected" at specified cut-off concentrations rather than at specific concentrations, unlike blood and breath alcohol tests. For example, a typical urine marijuana positive test is reported as positive at or above a cutoff concentration of 50 ng/mL. In contrast, a typical alcohol test might be reported as 0.05 g/100 mL.

With respect to the use of the drugs that are illegal for everyone, there is a more complex decision to be made about the use of drug tests to identify that use. Parents may be concerned about tobacco or marijuana use and take a hair or demand a urine sample. Drug testing is positively viewed as prevention by many parents (24). Such testing has become controversial, but it is clear that the parents have access to drug testing technology in pharmacies and on the Internet and can choose to pay for testing (25). This new development, without an MRO or plan for confrontation and for how to handle positive test results, needs education for the users of these tests.

Today more than a dozen states have *per se* standards for driving a motor vehicle, making it a violation of the law to have any identifiable concentration of an illegal drug in the driver's body (26). This standard, already applied to commercial drivers, is being more widely adopted throughout the country and in other countries around the world. Similarly, in student drug testing, any drug or metabolite identified in a student is considered a violation of school policy, leading not to arrest or reporting to the police or even suspension from school but to involvement of the student's family in efforts to help the student become drug-free. Here the issue often becomes a question of privacy, a matter subject to litigation, particularly in the public schools where the constitutional protections of the Fourth Amendment apply.

The most common problems today with drug testing relate to potentially misleading negative drug tests. These potential problems include that the donor may have used a drug that was not included in the testing panel, that the donor may have "cheated" on the test, that the drug may have been used outside of the detection window of the test—for example, the amount used was less than required to trigger a positive test result or that the donor may have drunk a sufficiently large amount of water to dilute the sample so the drug or drug metabolite concentration falls below the cut-off concentration required to report it as positive.

In other words, the common problems with drug testing as a practical matter are not the problems of false-positives but that there may well have been recent drug use that was not detected by the drug test. This is not a "false-negative," as the drug or its metabolite typically was not present in the sample at sufficient concentrations to produce a positive test result. For these reasons, a negative result on a drug test should not be overinterpreted. A negative test result means that none of the specific drugs or drugs metabolites on the panel was identified at or above the specified cutoff concentration.

Even with these limitations, drug tests identify far more recent drug use than do self-reports. The simple bottom line is that modern laboratory-based testing for drugs of abuse uses the highest standards of modern analytical technology to produce absolutely accurate findings. Furthermore, the technology of drug testing is continuing to improve rapidly (27,28).

ETHICAL ISSUES

Some pediatricians consider drug testing a breach of the patient-physician relationship, if not a violation of privacy protections unless the adolescent patient specifically consents to the drug testing (29). In this view, involuntary testing is not appropriate in adolescents with decisional capacity—even with parental consent—and should be performed only if "there are strong medical or legal reasons to do so" (30). Such thinking has limited the use of drug tests in a population for whom testing is critical (31). This view does not reflect the compelling need, incessant minimizing, and denial of use by drug users nor does it reflect the legal findings that support drug testing like other essential diagnostic procedures. Still, in some situations—accidents, depression, learning problems, and suicidal ideation, for example—there appears to be a consensus to test adolescents for drugs of abuse, with or without their consent. Even in these settings, however, there is merit to getting the young person to consent to the test. This is especially true when testing is done over time, as one of the primary goals of the testing is prevention. In one recent study, 40% of adolescents who have had an accident tested positive for drugs of abuse in the emergency room (32).

In two landmark Supreme Court cases, the Court has upheld mandatory drug testing in public schools when the testing is linked to participation in athletic or extracurricular activities and for all students when it is voluntary on the part of the student and the students' parents. Private schools have no such legal barrier to mandatory drug testing of all students. Similar legal questions have been answered in workplace drug testing leading also to approval by the Supreme Court of drug testing under specified circumstances. It is the legal battles over drug testing outside of clinical settings that have led to the sometimes elaborate and costly processes that are now routinely applied to drug testing in these settings.

In contrast to drug testing in the workplace and schools, use of testing in the criminal justice system and as part of routine clinical care has not been held to forensic standards, making drug testing more flexible and less costly in these settings. Because in these common clinical settings funding often is severely limited, the major hurdle for drug testing is not legal but financial. The major question in these settings is whether drug testing is thought to be cost-effective. In answering this question, issues to be considered include whether there are consequences to positive and negative drug test results and whether the standard of the program is that the patients be drug-free. When there are consequences and when the standard is that the patients must be drug-free, then drug testing often is vital to the success of the program. Drug testing linked to significant consequences for return to any drug use has been identified as a major reason that the nation's physicians health programs have remarkably high success rates over long periods of time (33).

CONCLUSIONS

Drug testing represents the pinnacle of modern biotechnology. In many non-clinical applications, drug testing now uses forensic standards, the highest laboratory and procedural standards to insure legal defensibility of the result. In both the technology and the process standards, constant changes are taking place that require clinicians using drug testing to keep up with this rapidly evolving area of practice. There are few areas of addiction medicine where drug testing is not central, precisely because drug users are likely to lie about their drug use and because drug users commonly use substances to get high without knowing what is in the substances. A positive drug test confirms recent use of specific drugs whereas a negative drug test helps to establish that abstinence exists as the necessary condition of the patients recovery program (34,35).

It is important for addiction medicine specialists to know how to use drug tests and to know what information drug tests do and do not provide. This chapter summarizes the central features of the rapidly evolving science and practice of drug testing. It provides guidance for additional information, including the latest updates of information about drug testing. Physicians are encouraged to discuss questions about the interpretation of drug test results as well as questions about regulations and legal problems related to drug tests with the laboratories conducting the tests and/or with the manufacturers of test kits as well as with certified MROs.

ACKNOWLEDGMENTS: *The authors express their appreciation to Audrey P. Seymour for her advice and assistance in the preparation of this manuscript.*

REFERENCES

1. Levy S, Harris SK, Sherritt L, et al. Drug testing of adolescents in general medical clinics, in school and at home: physician attitudes and practices. *J Adolesc Health* 2006;38:336–342.
2. Merlo LJ, Goldberger BA, Kolodner D, et al. Fentanyl and propofol exposure in the operating room: sensitization hypotheses and further data. *J Addict Dis* 2008 (in press).
3. Miller NS, Giannini AJ, Gold MS, Philomena JA. Drug testing: medical, legal, and ethical issues. *J Subst Abuse Treat* 1990;7(4):239–244.
4. DuPont RL, Bucher RH. *Guide to responsible family drug and alcohol testing.* Rockville, MD: Institute for Behavior and Health, Inc., 2005.
5. DuPont RL, Newel R, Brethen P. *Drug testing in drug abuse treatment.* Center City, MN: Hazelden, 2005.
6. DuPont RL, Mieczkowski T, Newel R. *Drug testing in the criminal justice system.* Center City, MN: Hazelden, 2005.
7. Hoffman A, Silvers J. *Steal this urine test: fighting drug hysteria in America.* New York, NY: Penguin Books, 1987.
8. Karch SB, ed. *Drug abuse handbook.* Boca Raton, FL: CRC Press, 1998.
9. Liu RH, Goldberger BA, eds. *Handbook of workplace drug testing.* Washington, DC: AACC Press, 1995.
10. Federal Register Notices, Vol. 69, No. 71, Tuesday, April 13, 2004.
11. DuPont RL, Baumgartner WA. Drug testing by urine and hair analysis: complementary features and scientific issues. *Forensic Sci Int* 1995;70:63–76.
12. Mieczkowski T, Newel R. An evaluation of patterns of racial bias in hair assays for cocaine: Black and white arrestees compared. *Forensic Sci Int* 1993;63:85–98.
13. Mieczkowski T, Newel R. An analysis of the racial bias controversy in the use of hair assays. In: Mieczkowski T, ed. *Drug Testing Technology: Assessment of Field Applications.* Boca Raton, FL: CRC Press, 1999.
14. Mieczkowski T, Lerch KM, Kruger M. Police drug testing, hair analysis and the issue of race bias. *Crim Just Rev* 2002;27:124–140.

15. DuPont RL, Skipper GE, White WL. Testing for recent alcohol use. 2008 (in press).
16. Smith K. Drugs used in acquaintance rape. *J Am Pharm Assoc* 1999; 39(3):519–525.
17. Ledray LE. The clinical care and documentation from victims in alleged cases of date sexual assault. *J Emerg Nurs* 2001;27(3):301–305.
18. Mullins ME. Laboratory confirmation of flunitrazepam in alleged cases of date rape. *Acad Emerg Med* 1999;6(9):966–968.
19. El Sohly MA, Salamone SJ. Prevalence of drugs used in cases of alleged sexual assault. *J Anal Toxicol* 1999;23:141–146.
20. DuPont RL, Gold MS. Comorbidity and "self-medication." *J Addict Dis* 2007;26(1):13–23.
21. DuPont RL, Graves H. *Smarter student drug testing*. Rockville, MD: Institute for Behavior and Health, Inc., 2005.
22. DuPont RL, Griffin DW, Siskin BR, et al. Random drug tests at work: The probability of identifying frequent and infrequent users of illicit drugs. *J Addict Dis* 1995;14:1–17.
23. Gold MS, Frost-Pineda K. Random mandatory drug testing: a potential system level solution? *Rapid Response Ann Intern Med* 2006. Retrieved (http://www.annals.org/cgi/eletters/144/2/107#2657).
24. Schwartz R, Silber T, Heyman R, et al. Urine testing for drugs of abuse: A survey of suburban parent-adolescent dyads. *Arch Pediatr Adolesc Med* 2003;157:158–161.
25. Levy S, van Hook S, Knight J. review of Internet-based home drug testing products for parents. *Pediatrics* 2004;A113(4):720–726.
26. State DUID Laws (http://norml.org/index.cfm?Group_ID=6669).
27. DuPont RL, Selavka CM. Laboratory and psychological diagnostic testing. In Galanter M, Kleber HD, eds. *American psychiatric press textbook of substance abuse treatment*, 3rd ed. Washington, DC: American Psychiatric Press, 2003:587–595.
28. DuPont RL, Selavka CS. Testing to identify recent drug use. In Galanter M, Kleber HD, eds. *American psychiatric press textbook of substance abuse treatment*, 4th ed. Washington, DC: American Psychiatric Press, 2007. http://www.appi.org/book.cfm?id=62276.
29. Anonymous. To test or not to test: screening for substance use in adolescents [editorial]. *J Adolesc Health* 2006;38:329–331.
30. American Academy of Pediatrics, Committee on Substance Use. Testing for drugs of abuse in children and adolescents. *Pediatrics* 1996;98:305–307.
31. Casav M. Committee on Substance Abuse and Council on School Health Schools and at home testing for drugs of abuse in children and adolescents: addendum—testing inant. Urine drug screening in adolescents. *Pediatr Clin North Am* 2002;49(2):317–327.
32. Ehrlich PF, Brown JK, Drongowski R. Characterization of the drug-positive adolescent trauma population: should we, do we, and does it make a difference if we test? *J Pediatr Surg* 2006;41:927–930.
33. DuPont RL, McLellan AT, Carr G, et al. How are addicted physicians treated and managed? The structure and function of Physician Health Programs in the United States. *J Subst Abuse Treat* 2007 (in press).
34. The Betty Ford Institute Consensus Panel. What is recovery? A working definition from the Betty Ford Institute. *J Subst Abuse Treat* 2007;33:221–228.
35. Jacobs W, DuPont RL, Gold MS. Drug testing and the DSM-IV. *Psychiatr Ann* 1999;30(9):583–588.

Workplace Drug Testing and the Role of the Medical Review Officer

Robert L. DuPont, MD, FASAM

A medical review officer (MRO) is a physician who verifies chain of custody and interprets drug test results. The MRO receives positive drug test results (and in federally regulated workplace testing, negative results as well) before the results go to the individual or the organization requesting the drug test. At that point, the MROs task is to validate that the proper procedures were maintained, including rigorous chain of custody procedures. In addition, the MRO validates that the positive test results were not the result of a legitimate medical prescription for the tested substance. An example of a common setting in which the MRO overturns a laboratory positive is a workplace positive drug test result for amphetamine in an employee who has a prescription for Adderall to treat attention deficit/hyperactivity disorder (ADHD). In this case, the MRO, after speaking with the employee and verifying that the prescription for the amphetamine is valid for this particular person, downgrades the drug test result and reports it as negative. In such a case, the employer is not informed by the laboratory of the positive test, the fact that the employee has ADHD, or that the employee is using a prescribed medicine for that condition.

REGULATORY FRAMEWORK FOR MEDICAL REVIEW OFFICER PRACTICE

MROs also are experts in the often complex and frequently changing regulations that govern workplace drug testing.

A 1986 Presidential Executive Order directed the U.S. Department of Health and Human Services (DHHS) to develop and publish scientific and technical guidelines for workplace drug testing of federal employees. Those guidelines (1) significantly increased public acceptance of drug testing by establishing rigid certification procedures for laboratories and placing final responsibility for the review of drug tests with a physician—designated, for the first time, as an MRO. The medical review field grew dramatically when, late in 1989, the U.S. Department of Transportation (DOT) mandated testing of transportation workers in safety-sensitive positions (2) and included the requirement for medical review. Further growth occurred as the courts and other government agencies and private employers acknowledged the protection offered by the expertise of a physician and as more employers added MROs to their testing programs, even when not required to do so.

The DOT regulations have been updated several times, including as recently as August 2008 (3). The August 2008 update reflects the latest research data and almost three decades' experience with workplace testing as it focuses especially on the problems of specimen validity to reduce the risk of cheating. Other testing is modeled often after the DOT guidelines because these are the most widely used guidelines and because they have successfully withstood intense legal challenges. In addition to the DOT regulations, which cover testing of commercial drivers, there are separate regulations governing testing of federal workers, employees regulated by the Nuclear Regulatory Commission, the Federal Aviation Administration, and other federal and state organizations. When testing is done under any of these regulations, it is essential that the MRO understand those regulations. This chapter focuses on the DOT regulations because they cover the largest number of workers and because they are considered the gold standard. Most workplace testing is not regulated, but the DOT regulations provide useful guidance even in non-regulated settings.

In the regulations initially promulgated by the DHHS (1), the only qualifications specified for MROs were that such an official must be a "licensed physician with a knowledge of substance abuse disorders." However, it became apparent that additional qualifications would be needed. The 2001 regulations required that MROs not only be licensed but have "clinical experience in controlled substances abuse disorders." They also require attendance at a training course at least once every 3 years and certification by a nationally recognized certifying board (currently, either the Medical Review Officer Coordinating Council or the American Association of Medical Review Officers).

As the laws and regulations governing workplace drug testing change and as drug-using individuals devise ever more challenging ways to "beat" the testing system, the practicing MROs must find ways to keep their knowledge up to date. A list of recommended textbooks and other references as well as suggestions for finding an MRO can be found at the end of this chapter.

CONTRACTUAL ISSUES

Before beginning the process of medical review, the MRO should have a written contract with the employer, spelling out in detail the services to be provided. Medical review is only one of many components of a drug-free workplace program. The successful MRO will either provide the other components or be able to direct the employer to them.

Workplace Drug Testing and the Role of the Medical Review Officer *(continued)*

Organizations called "consortia" or "third-party administrators" (C/TPAs) provide overall program management, policy review, educational materials, training programs, and random sampling of employees and contract out for laboratory, MRO, and collection services. MROs may function as C/TPAs, but they must be careful to follow the regulations that prohibit them from having a financial relationship with laboratories whose tests they review.

INITIATING THE MEDICAL REVIEW PROCESS

The medical review process begins when the MRO receives a drug test result from a laboratory and ends when he or she reports the result. When dealing with urine testing for the so-called SAMHSA 5 drugs (that is, drugs initially specified by the Substance Abuse and Mental Health Services Administration for federally mandated workplace testing programs), it is strongly recommended that MROs work with laboratories that have been certified under the DHHS rules requiring academic credentials, regular inspections, and satisfactory performance on the testing of regularly submitted blind proficiency specimens (4,5). When testing materials other than urine (such as hair, oral fluids, or sweat), laboratory selection involves careful review of quality control procedures and relevant credentials of the laboratory. Consultation with a forensic toxicologist may be desirable.

COLLECTION OF SPECIMENS

Though federal guidelines minimize the MRO's responsibility for collection of laboratory specimens, the MRO is required to check each chain-of-custody form for signatures and collector remarks. In addition to this administrative function, the MRO should confirm that, in cases involving non-negative test results, the chain of custody was not broken. The MRO also should be prepared to evaluate problems of "shy bladder" and issues of dilution, substitution, and adulteration.

Choice of Specimen The choice of specimen (e.g., urine, hair, oral fluid) affects both the detectability of drug use and interpretation of test results. See Chapter 4 for a discussion of the considerations accompanying the various choices.

Negative Results For negative test results, the MROs role is twofold. First, the MRO or his or her assistant reviews the laboratory result to determine whether the specimen is diluted and was within the acceptable temperature range. These conditions need to be reported by the MRO to the employer, and employers need to be advised as to appropriate actions in response. Second, MROs review the Custody and Control Form (CCF) to look for evidence of errors in the collection process. MROs are considered to be the gatekeepers of the drug-testing process and are responsible for verifying that correctable errors are, in fact, corrected if it is possible to do so.

Non-Negative Results Before reporting a result (including positive, adulterated, substituted, and invalid test results) as non-negative, the MRO should be satisfied that (1) the correct specimen was tested (and not somehow mixed up with someone else's, for example); (2) the laboratory accurately performed the necessary analyses; and (3) there was no alternative medical explanation for the non-negative test result. To resolve these questions, the MRO must understand forensic collection and chain-of-custody procedures, know what the toxicology laboratory does, and be familiar with the relevant laws and regulations.

Before a test can be called positive, its designated analyte must test positive both by an approved immunoassay and by confirmation, typically performed with gas chromatography/mass spectrometry (GC/MS) or liquid chromatography/mass spectrometry (LC/MS). The confirmation test is so specific that some have called it a "chemical fingerprint." Screening tests are less specific than LC/MS or GC/MS and may be positive on the basis of compounds that are in some way chemically similar to the sought-after analytes. To discount the possibility of drug tests being read as positive in individuals who may have passively inhaled marijuana or cocaine, the DHHS has established testing cutoff levels, below which an analyte may be present but not reportable. The DHHS certification program primarily addresses the SAMHSA 5 drugs (cocaine, marijuana, phencyclidine [PCP], amphetamines, and opiates). It includes certification only for the testing of controlled substances that are listed in Schedule I or II of the Controlled Substance Act and does not include benzodiazepines or barbiturates, which often are included in non-federally mandated testing panels.

Each employee who has a laboratory-confirmed non-negative test must be offered an opportunity to be interviewed and the relevant paperwork from the laboratory and collection sites reviewed. During this review, the MRO may find it necessary to speak with the designated employer representative (DER), with the individual who collected the urine, with laboratory personnel, and/or with the employee's physician or pharmacy. On occasion, the MRO

(continued)

Workplace Drug Testing and the Role of the Medical Review Officer *(continued)*

may wish to have the worker examined. Additional laboratory testing may be required, possibly including reanalysis of the specimen.

Invalid Test Some specimens cannot be tested because of an interfering substance, because they are too dilute or concentrated, or because their pH is out of range. Some medications interfere with the screening process and, occasionally, adulterating substances have been added. If the laboratory cannot completely identify an adulterant or other interfering substance, the results are reported to the MRO as "invalid." The MRO must review the results, interview the donor, and report the results to the employer as "test cancelled." In most cases, an immediate observed recollection of the urine is ordered. However, if the problem is a legitimate prescription rather than an adulterant, a repeat of the test is not necessary.

Adulterated or Substituted Test If the laboratory can identify an adulterant, the result comes to the MRO as "adulterated." In cases of extreme dilution that is not consistent with human urine, the results are reported to the MRO as "substituted." Adulterated and substituted results also must be reviewed by the MRO and are reported to the employer as "refusal to test," with the reason (e.g., "refusal to test because of adulteration with glutaraldehyde"), unless the donor can demonstrate a valid medical basis for the result.

Recordkeeping When any laboratory report arrives that is not a negative, a chart should be prepared to track all of the relevant paperwork and notes of all MRO interactions with the worker and others. Because the information in such a chart may be subpoenaed, the MRO should treat it with at least as much care as is used in a clinical chart. Under federal testing programs, the MRO is required to keep records of all non-negative tests for 5 years. In practice, this is a good rule for unregulated programs as well. Many MROs retain such records even longer.

THE MEDICAL REVIEW OFFICER INTERVIEW

The MRO obtains the name of the worker from the CCF after the collector transmits it. The MRO then should make at least three attempts to contact the donor at the numbers on the CCF during the 24 hours after the document is received. If the MRO is unable to contact the donor during that time, he or she should ask the DER to contact the donor and inform the donor that he or she should call the MRO within 72 hours. The DER also should warn the donor that if he or she does not contact the MRO, the MRO will report the results to the employer after 72 hours. If contact is made, the MRO should identify the donor by asking him or her to provide the identification number used during the drug test collection (usually the donor's Social Security number). Then the MRO should explain the review process and the role of the MRO in that process. Most important, the MRO must warn the employee that the MRO is required to provide to the employer and/or appropriate government agencies any information disclosed to the MRO during the review process if it might affect the performance of safety-sensitive duties. Some have called this a drug testing "Miranda" warning.

The MRO should tell the individual what drug was detected and ask him or her about medication use that may explain the result. It is not necessary for the MRO to ask about other medicines being taken or about medical treatment except as these may explain the specific drug test result.

REPORTING TEST RESULTS

At the conclusion of the review process, the MRO notifies the donor and employer of the findings, which may be any of the following:

- Negative (including reversals on the basis of legitimate medical explanations) and Negative, dilute;
  - A negative result may include shy bladder with a legitimate medical explanation in an individual who has been examined and found to have no evidence of drug use.
- Positive (including positives confirmed on re-analysis)
- Cancelled, because of
  - Flaws or uncorrected errors,
  - Failure to reconfirm on reanalysis,
  - Invalid specimens with or without medical justification, and
  - Shy bladder in a current employee who has an acceptable medical explanation.
- Refusal to test, because of
  - Specimen adulteration/substitution,
  - Insufficient amount of urine provided without a legitimate explanation,
  - Worker late for test or left the collection site before the test could be completed,
  - Worker refused to permit direct observation of the test as required, or
  - Worker refused to cooperate with the testing process or refused to take a second test when asked to do so.

Workplace Drug Testing and the Role of the Medical Review Officer *(continued)*

THE FUTURE OF MEDICAL REVIEW OFFICER PRACTICE

The contemporary perspective on alcohol and drug abuse in the workplace is rooted in a new understanding of addiction as a biopsychosocial disorder, with a renewed emphasis on brain biology (6,7). As a consequence, MRO practice is challenging and constantly changing, providing physicians who specialize in addiction medicine with an additional arena in which to exercise their expertise and professional interest.

The major challenge for the future of addiction prevention and treatment in the workplace is to develop comprehensive programs that are reasonable as well as tough. Such programs must operate in the public interest in ways that respect not only the interests of all involved but the dignity of workers and their families, including the dignity of persons with addictive disorders. The MRO provides useful oversight of the drug-testing process and the sophisticated interpretation of drug test results to help ensure fairness, accuracy, and the highest level of modern science.

In a free and open society, many hurdles faced by workplace alcohol and drug programs will not be dealt with easily, but they must be addressed if workplace programs are to achieve their full life-saving potential.

FINDING A MEDICAL REVIEW OFFICER

American Association of Medical Review Officers (AAMRO)
www.aamro.com
Division of Workplace Programs (SAMHSA)
http://dwp.samhsa.gov/DrugTesting/
Medical Review Officer Certification Council (MROCC)
www.mrocc.com
U.S. Department of Transportation (DOT)
http://dwp.samhsa.gov/DrugTesting/

SUGGESTED READINGS

American Correctional Association and Institute for Behavior and Health, Inc. *Monograph: Drug testing of juvenile de-tainees*. Washington, DC: U.S. Department of Justice, 1991.

American Psychiatric Association. *Diagnostic and statistical manual of mental disorders*, 4th ed *(DSM-IV)*. Washington, DC: American Psychiatric Press, 1994.

DuPont RL, Newel R, Brethen P. *Drug testing in drug abuse treatment*. Center City, MN: Hazelden, 2005.

DuPont RL, Brady LA. *Drug testing in schools: guidelines for effective use*. Center City, MN: Hazelden, 2005.

DuPont RL, Mieczkowski T, Newel R. *Drug testing in the criminal justice system*. Center City, MN: Hazelden 2005.

DuPont RL, Griffin DW, Siskin BR, et al. Random drug tests at work: the probability of identifying frequent and infrequent users of illicit drugs. *J Addict Dis* 1995;14:1–17.

Gold MS, Frost-Pineda K. Random mandatory drug testing: a potential system level solution? *Rapid Response Ann Intern Med* 2006. Retrieved (http://www.annals.org/cgi/eletters/144/2/107#2657).

Interagency Coordination Group. Action Regarding California Proposition 215 and Arizona Proposition 22. Washington, DC: White House Office of National Drug Control Policy, U.S. Department of Justice, 1997.

Liu RH,Goldberger BA, eds. *Handbook of Workplace Drug Testing*. Washington, DC: AACC Press, 1995.

National Treasury Employees Union v. Von Raab, 489 U.S. 656 (1989).

Schwartz RH. Urine testing in the detection of drugs of abuse. *Arch Intern Med* 1988;148:24-07–2412.

Skinner v. Railway Labor Executives' Association, 489 U.S. 602 (1989).

Swotinsky RB, Smith DS. *Medical review officer manual*, 3rd ed.. Beverly, MA: OEM Press. 2006.

REFERENCES

1. U.S. Department of Health and Human Services. Mandatory guidelines for federal work-place drug testing programs. *Fed Reg* 1998;53:11970.
2. U.S. Department of Transportation. Procedures for transportation workplace drug testing programs. *Fed Reg* 1989;54:11979.
3. U.S. Department of Transportation. 49 CFR Part 40 Procedures for Transportation Workplace Drug and Alcohol Testing Programs. *Fed Reg* 2008;73:123.
4. DuPont RL. Drugs in the American workplace: conflict and opportunity, part II: Controversies in work-place drug use prevention. *Soc Pharmacol* 1989;3:147–164.
5. DuPont RL. Medicines and drug testing in the workplace. *J Psychoactive Drugs* 1990;22:451–459.
6. Nahas GG, Burks TF. *Drug abuse in the decade of the brain*. Amsterdam, The Netherlands: IOS Press, 1997.
7. DuPont RL. *The selfish brain: learning from addiction*. Center City, MN: Hazelden, 2000.

CHAPTER 111

The Hon. Peggy Fulton Hora (Ret.)
The Hon. William G. Schma (Ret.)

Drug Courts and the Treatment of Incarcerated Populations

The number of people who are in jail, prison or under community supervision has skyrocketed in the last decade (1). As of 2005, more than 2.1 million Americans were incarcerated, 4.1 million were on probation and almost a quarter million were on parole (2). With less than 5% of the world's population, the United States has 25% of the world's prisoners (3).

Over the past two decades, it has become abundantly clear that incarceration alone is totally ineffective in addressing alcohol and drug abuse and addiction, let alone recidivism to criminal behavior. Society also has come to realize that prison is a scarce resource best employed to isolate violent offenders from the community. These realizations, coupled with an increased knowledge of the neurobiology of addiction and its treatment, have led to an understanding by the community and the criminal justice system that collaborative projects such as drug treatment courts are the most intelligent way to address this problem.

A drug treatment court (DTC) is a collaborative program of judicially supervised treatment and recovery within the criminal justice system. This specialized system of courts was created to address spiraling numbers of drug-related offenses and offenders, which have swelled court dockets over the past decade. DTCs represent a major retooling of the criminal justice system, as well as a new court role in society as an interdisciplinary, problem-solving community institution with therapeutic implications—in short, a partner in public health (4).

From fewer than a dozen in 1991, the number of DTCs has increased to more than 2,500 today, in communities as diverse as New York City and Las Cruces, NM. DTCs are found in all states, four Federal District, tribal courts (called Healing-to-Wellness Courts) and in 20 countries.

This chapter will examine the theoretical underpinnings of drug treatment courts and explain how they differ from traditional criminal courts. Treatment opportunities in the criminal justice system will be explored, as will the key components of effective DTCs. The chapter will focus on the role of these courts within the treatment community and describe opportunities for collaboration between the court system and the health care community, and particularly addiction specialists (Table 111.1).

DEFINITIONS

A DTC is a judicially supervised, treatment-driven program for nonviolent substance-abusing criminal offenders. It is a collaborative effort that involves judges, prosecutors, defense attorneys, probation officers, treatment providers, and other persons or agencies that interact with addicts whose behavior has brought them into the criminal justice system. Participation by the offender is voluntary.

In this universe, the court serves as a convener and coordinator of related services in a continuum of care for substance-abusing individuals.

DTCs are as varied in form and format as the diverse legal and treatment cultures from which they spring. Some courts divert offenders from the criminal justice system entirely; some accept only misdemeanants, others only felons. There are DTCs solely for alcoholics, or only cocaine or heroin users, whereas others accept anyone whose criminal involvement is related to substance use. There are gender-specific courts and courts that enroll only juveniles. Reentry DTCs recently have emerged to serve adjudicated substance-abusing offenders who are returning to society on parole or probation.

TABLE 111.1 Advice for Assessing Drug Treatment Court Clients

Keep assessments brief. DTCs frequently use the Addiction Severity Index, which can be completed very quickly

Identify clients' expectations. DTCs fully outline the program in participants' handbooks. Treatment providers also explain the DTC to the participant.

Provide clear orientations. The referral to a DTC is made at the time of the defendant's first appearance: arraignment. He or she is referred to the court coordinator before the next court appearance. After viewing the DTC session, the judge reviews the written behavioral contract with each participant. If the defendant wants to proceed, a full orientation with the court coordinator/case manager is scheduled. Each defendant, on request, also is referred to legal counsel to discuss the legal options.

Offer clients options. DTC participation always is voluntary. The participant may opt out at any time and proceed with regular criminal case adjudication.

Keep it simple. The client handbook has clear, understandable information for each participant. Written reminders are given out at every court session. There are written attendance records of meetings and other appointments. Everyone tries to use clear and simple language. Participants who cannot read are helped by other participants who can.

Involve significant others. Family participation is encouraged. Couples counseling and family days are options at the treatment programs. Children and partners always are welcome in court and are identified by name by the judge. "Toxic families" that are detrimental to the participants' recovery are prohibited. Restraining orders may be ordered as part of the program to protect the participant from a spouse, partner, parent, or sibling.

DTC, drug treatment court.

DTCs rely on the principle that the coercive powers of the court system can contribute to recovery from addiction to alcohol and other drugs. Contradicting the popular notion that drug-dependent offenders are best dealt with by adjudication and sanctions, DTCs embrace the scientific premise that alcohol and other drug dependence is a chronic, relapsing medical condition (5). The authoritative and supervisory power of the judge is critical to this approach to treatment. However, the participation of a judge in the rehabilitation process represents a dramatic shift in legal thought and judicial behavior.

A NEW APPROACH TO AN OLD PROBLEM

Through the collaborative efforts of defense attorneys and prosecutors, treatment providers, the court coordinator or case manager, community policing agencies, and probation officials, a criminal defendant in a DTC is given an opportunity to engage in an alternative to the criminal "business as usual" and, in its place, to pursue a program of addiction treatment and recovery.

DTCs employ a series of "carrots and sticks" to induce treatment compliance and lifestyle changes in a criminal defendant. The ultimate payoff for the participant is dismissal of the charges, having a sentence set aside, or imposition of a lesser penalty. By choosing to participate in a DTC, a criminal defendant avoids serving a substantial period of incarceration and gains sobriety and a crime-free lifestyle. "A [DTC] establishes an environment that the participant can understand: a system in which clear choices are presented and individuals are encouraged to take control of their own recovery" (6).

Further, DTCs integrate alcohol and other drug treatment services with justice system case processing. Their operations are defined by 10 key components.

1. Drug courts integrate alcohol and other drug treatment services with justice system case processing.
2. They use a nonadversarial approach; prosecution and defense counsel promote public safety while protecting participants' due process rights.
3. Eligible participants are identified early and promptly placed in the drug court program.
4. DTCs provide access to a continuum of alcohol, drug, and related treatment and rehabilitation services.
5. Abstinence is monitored through frequent alcohol and other drug testing.
6. A coordinated strategy governs DTC responses to participants' compliance.
7. Ongoing judicial interaction with each DTC participant is essential.
8. Monitoring and evaluation measure the achievement of program goals and gauge its effectiveness.
9. Continuing interdisciplinary education promotes effective DTC planning, implementation, and operations.
10. Forging partnerships among DTCs, public agencies, and community-based organizations generates local support and enhances the DTC's effectiveness.

When these components are employed, the courtroom is transformed into an arena in which a judge is the central figure of a team that is focused on the participants' recovery. The prosecutor screens each candidate for eligibility and makes sure each candidate is appropriate for participation in the DTC. The defense counsel verifies that clients know of the voluntary nature of DTC participation, are aware of all their legal options, and make a knowing and intelligent waiver of their rights, including their confidentiality rights. Opposing counsel thus focus on the participant's progress, rather than on the merits of the pending case. A close, interpersonal, and therapeutic relationship develops between the judge and the participant, who is encouraged to develop the tools he or she needs to maintain sobriety and recovery. Participants often enter into written contracts, agreeing to certain behaviors (data show that such contracts are more likely to induce compliance, whether it is taking medication or engaging in addiction treatment) (7). A typical contract includes attending treatment, court dates, self-help meetings, and other appointments on time; complying with all rules; waiving confidentiality; paying fees and fines; taking presumptive urine tests without water-loading, adulteration, or counterfeiting; agreeing to refrain from drinking alcohol or taking other drugs or associating with people who do; abstaining from eating poppy seeds, taking over-the-counter or prescription medications without prior approval, or doing other things that could yield a false result on a urine test; and making a 12- to 18-month commitment to treatment.

Although the judge remains the final arbiter of all issues, he or she receives input from the entire team, including the participant. If a problem arises, such as a use episode, it is not unusual for a participant to arrive in court having already discussed the problem with the treatment provider and a probation officer or court coordinator, who will present a recommendation to the judge (which might involve jail time, increased meetings, or increased urine tests). When participants themselves propose the sanctions, they are more likely to comply with them and not to feel coerced by the "system" or the judge. A person who proposes their own "punishment" is more likely to think it fair (Table 111.2).

TABLE 111.2 Advice on Initiating Treatment with Drug Court Clients

Set clear goals and expectations. Treatment goals for DTCs are sobriety, program retention, and maintenance of a crime-free lifestyle. Goals are explained in the participants' handbook and the written behavioral contract, as well as by the judge, case coordinator, attorneys, and treatment providers.

Establish treatment attendance. Participants must bring written proof of attendance to each court date. Unverifiable meetings are not allowed except in unusual circumstances. For instance, a participant may be going out of town for a business trip and be allowed to attend 12-Step meetings in the area he or she will be visiting. If away for an extended stay, urine testing may be arranged, often with the help of another DTC.

Schedule frequent contacts. Frequent court appearances are a hallmark of DTCs. Daily contact with the case coordinator or treatment provider may be required in volatile relapse situations. At a minimum, weekly contacts are maintained throughout the life of the program in some DTCs.

Use positive incentives to reinforce treatment participation. In the Hayward, CA, DTC, the local Deputy Sheriffs' Association provides the DTC with tickets for Oakland A's games to use as rewards for good performance. There may be a drawing for theater or county fair tickets, a Halloween pumpkin, or a tote bag or tee shirt from the latest conference attended by the judge. To be eligible for the drawing, a participant must have a negative urine test and have attended all meetings. Drawings are held on a random basis and participants who have missed a meeting are quite upset when they are not eligible to participate. One treatment provider awards food vouchers and bus tickets to participants who meet their goals.

Call "no-shows." The court coordinator calls all participants who have failed to appear in court. If there is no response, the bailiff immediately asks the community policing liaison to serve a bench warrant. Through this approach, participants are taught that it is better to appear and test positive than to fail to appear. Program retention and participation lead to negative urine tests; the opposite is not true.

Create a positive environment. Because court appearances are so personalized by the judge, participants develop a positive attitude toward coming to court. Most treatment providers have court meetings so that participants can develop friendships. Participants help each other find jobs and transportation, and even cook Thanksgiving dinner together before marathon holiday meetings. Everyone feels good because of the positive atmosphere in the courtroom.

Enforce "no use" policies for drugs and alcohol. Although there was some initial resistance to uniform "no alcohol" clauses for DTC participants, such requirements now are standard. DTC contracts also include a prohibition on the use of prescription drugs prescribed for others and, of course, prohibit the use of illicit substances.

Establish a daily schedule. Treatment meetings, self-help groups, employment, job training or job seeking, education, volunteer work, and court appointments keep a DTC participant on a tight schedule. Some participants have had to change work shifts and find new employment because working late-night shifts triggered a craving for stimulants to stay awake. Daytime employment and an early bedtime seem to help reduce stimulant craving.

Initiate a schedule for drug testing. Most DTCs require frequent, random, observed urine tests. Night and weekend testing, long-distance testing, and daily testing as a sanction all are employed.

Assess psychiatric comorbidity. Posttraumatic stress disorder and clinical depression are the most commonly observed psychiatric problems among DTC participants. Many DTCs have mutual help groups for cooccurring disorders such a bipolar and schizophrenia. A mental health assessment is ordered for those who are not being program-compliant, rather than assuming that the participant is "treatment resistant." The incidence of comorbidity for this population is very high.

Assess associated compulsive sexual behaviors. Treatment providers who work with stimulant abusers in DTCs have special sex addiction groups. DTCs also offer confidential and anonymous HIV testing and education, as well as testing and education for hepatitis B and C and other sexually transmitted diseases (STDs). Many participants have worked as prostitutes, which raises not only STD issues, but also posttraumatic stress disorder issues that must be addressed in treatment.

Assist with crisis resolution. The court, the case manager, and treatment providers all need to be are aware of the need for suicide and homicide assessment, psychiatric referrals, and necessary medical referrals. Participants may need extra support in times of personal crisis and stepped-up relapse prevention services at these times. The Court may order an emergency psychiatric assessment or additional services.

DTC, drug treatment court.

Confidentiality waivers are mandatory, as are waivers of judicial ethical issues such as the prohibition on *ex parte* communications, simply because the treatment providers, mental health professionals, and physicians must be able to communicate with the court coordinator/case manager and the team. Written waivers that comply with federal statutes are mandatory. Judges must be able to talk to team members individually throughout the week without inhibition. Participants must understand their rights to confidentiality and the judges' prohibition on *ex parte* communication and be willing to provide a written waiver as a condition of entering DTC. This team concept of drug treatment courts uniquely facilitates an individual's treatment progress. It is not unusual for a participant to ask that the arresting officer be present at his or her graduation. Police officers, including the bailiff in the courtroom, become supporters and benefactors rather than enemies. Similarly, supporting actors such a community-based treatment providers, community policing officers, housing authority personnel, mental health professionals, and physicians have a unique new relationship with the courts and a voice not previously heard.

Most DTCs have Three Phases

1. An initiation of abstinence phase, in which the participant comes to court weekly.
2. A treatment phase, in which the participant meets with the judge twice per month.
3. A relapse prevention phase, with monthly court dates.

Frequent contact with and monitoring by the judge is essential to the success of the DTC participant. The court monitors the participant's treatment program, attendance, and drug test results. As the ultimate authority figure in this system, the judge also is important in motivating and encouraging participants. The judge praises, cajoles, kids, threatens, harangues, and does whatever it takes to keep the participant in treatment and recovery. As Dr. John Chappel, Professor of Medicine at the University of Nevada, Reno, sees it, "The role of the judge is to coerce treatment until sobriety becomes tolerable." Treatment may be delivered in a variety of settings: a community-based program, a day treatment model, outpatient, inpatient, residential, or in-custody.

Using graduated sanctions, the court usually begins with the least restrictive model, as indicated by an assessment tool such as the Addiction Severity Index. The participant is moved to more restrictive placements as needed. Placing a participant in a more restrictive environment is not phrased in terms of punishment; rather, participants are encouraged to see the change as necessary to their recovery. At intake, a social needs assessment is completed, along with an alcohol and drug use assessment. Mental health, housing, physical health, employment, education, and other legal entanglements are addressed. Periods of abstinence, confirmed by weekly, random urine tests, are required for each phase—typically at 30, 90, and 180 days.

There is aftercare planning, and participants petition the court to "graduate," typically at about 180 days of sobriety. To receive such approval, the participant must demonstrate a knowledge of addiction and have a plan for relapse prevention. The participant also is invited to become involved in a DTC alumni group. To graduate, the participant must have a clean and sober living environment, as well as full-time employment or full-time student status; all fees and fines must be paid or substantial amounts of volunteer work completed. Graduating participants also must have a drivers' license, insurance, and proof of registration of all vehicles, and be able to show that there are no outstanding tickets or warrants. They must have a high school diploma or GED and either take literacy classes, if they are English-speaking, or enroll in a class for students learning English as a Second Language. The whole person is transformed by the DTC; abstinence alone is not enough.

When a participant submits a positive urine test, misses meetings or appointments, fails to participate, or otherwise breaks program rules, sanctions are imposed immediately. Such sanctions may include payment for the urine test, increased meeting attendance (30 meetings in 30 days, for example), demotion to an earlier phase, requirement to perform volunteer work or short stints of jail time (usually 1 day to no more than 1 week at a time) or, the ultimate sanction, removal from the program and (in a pre-plea model) reentry into the criminal system or (after adjudication) sentencing, including incarceration. Consistent noncompliance may trigger a mental health assessment, as many DTC participants have undiagnosed comorbid mental health problems such as clinical depression, posttraumatic stress disorder, bipolar disorder, or schizophrenia. Program dismissal is reserved for the most serious offenses, such as attempts to falsify or adulterate a urine sample, leaving without permission, or being arrested for a violent offense.

The focus of the DTC team is not on punishment, but on treatment compliance and program retention. Rewards may include an earn-down of program fees, a reduction in the number of court appearances, and awarding of certificates (with much cheering and applause from the audience) to mark the completion of each phase. In a DTC, it is not unusual to hear a public defender recommend jail time, while a prosecutor argues that only increased meetings are required. The adversarial system is put on hold in DTC; defense counsel and the prosecution are equal team members whose interest is in treatment and recovery, not convictions or acquittals. At any point in the process, the participant may opt out of the DTC and into the traditional criminal justice case processing system, with all the attendant rights and remedies.

WHY DRUG TREATMENT COURTS WORK

There is support for DTCs on many fronts and from all factions of the political spectrum (8–11). First, it is clear that coerced treatment works. Research indicates that a person coerced to enter treatment by the criminal justice system is likely to do as well as one who volunteers (12–17). In fact, there is debate about the "voluntariness" of any addiction treatment, because most addicts come to treatment because of legal problems, concerns in their personal lives, problems with job performance, or for health reasons (18). Second, addiction treatment is as successful as treatment for other chronic diseases and saves $7 for every treatment dollar spent (6). Moreover, because of the requirement for interdisciplinary training, DTC judges and other team members are aware of the likelihood of relapse and know how to respond appropriately. DTCs are in a unique position to recognize these temporary setbacks as learning experiences for the participant and the treatment team.

Recent evidence to assess the effectiveness of DTCs (10) examined nine adult drug courts in California. Using a Transactional Institutional Costs Analysis approach, they calculated costs based on every individual's transactions within the drug court or the traditional criminal justice system. This method allowed them to calculate costs and benefits by agency (e.g., public defender's office, court, district attorney). Results in the nine sites showed that the majority of agencies saved money when offenders were processed through a drug court. Overall, for the nine study sites, participation in drug court saved the State more than $9 million in criminal justice and treatment (largely from lower recidivism among drug court participants). Green et al. (19) and Henggeler (13) reported similar results from their study of family drug treatment courts. Werb et al. (20) conducted a similar review of DTCs in Canada, which showed positive near-term outcomes. However, like other investigators, Werb and colleagues point to the need for long-term follow-up studies to reach definitive conclusions about the effectiveness of drug courts.

Courts have come to accept their changing role from neutral, uninvolved arbiter to becoming problem-solvers who look at cases holistically. There also is support for the proposition that judicial job satisfaction is increased if judges work therapeutically (21). The Bureau of Justice Assistance, an arm of the U.S. Department of Justice, recently promulgated trial court performance standards. Standard 4.5 says, "The trial court anticipates new conditions and emergent events and adjusts its operations as necessary" (6). Clearly, DTCs address "new conditions and emergent events."

In 2001, the U.S. Conference of Chief Justices and the Conference of State Court Administrators adopted a joint resolution endorsing DTCs and problem-solving courts based on the drug court model, the first resolution of its kind. The resolution commits all 50 chief justices and state court administrators "to take steps nationally and locally to expand the principles and methods of well functioning drug courts into ongoing court operations." It also pledges to "encourage the broad integration, over the next decade, of the principles and methods employed in problem solving courts into the administration of justice."

Law enforcement support for DTCs is strong because officers see that recovery presents a long-term solution to a community's and an individual's problems with alcohol or other drugs. Formal liaisons between community police and DTCs are encouraged through the Community Policing Mentor Court Network of the National Association of Drug Court Professionals.

THE COURTS AND PHYSICIANS WORKING TOGETHER

"Given what is known about the many social, medical, and legal consequences of drug abuse, effective drug abuse treatment should, at a minimum, be integrated with criminal justice, social, and medical services" (Executive Office of the President, The White House, 2000) (22). DTCs and the criminal justice system can be powerful allies for addiction medicine specialists. Through DTCs, physicians and judges have initiated a whole new dialogue about alcohol and other drug problems. The group Physicians and Lawyers for National Drug Policy, based at Brown University's Center for Alcohol & Addiction Studies, has partnered with the American Judges Association to develop a curriculum for the joint training of judges and physicians. The resulting program was piloted in Fort Worth, TX, in 1999, and replicated in Philadelphia. In each session, 16 local physicians and psychologists met with almost 50 criminal and family law judges for a day of joint training.

The partnership has extended to other venues, as well: judges have participated in Congressional and U.S. mayoral briefings. For the first time, judges presented a panel at the 2000 American Society of Addiction Medicine (ASAM) annual meeting. Addiction medicine specialists teach courses on alcohol and other drug problems at the National Judicial College and in many of the states as well. The time is ripe for local coalitions of judges and other players in the criminal justice system to team up with addiction medicine specialists to educate one another in how to be more effective in working with their mutual clients/patients. Judges in the criminal justice system may have more to say about a patient's treatment that the physician does. Questions relating to involvement with the justice system should be added to patient histories as a case-finding tool for alcohol and other drug problems.

Physicians should acquaint themselves with their local drug treatment courts and, if there isn't one in operation, lead a community coalition to ask that one be established. Most courts have long-range strategic, operational, and action plans developed with community input; DTCs should be part of those plans. Local grand juries, with the help of addiction medicine specialists, should study DTCs and make recommendations for appropriate use of those courts in their own communities. At the very least, state chapters of ASAM should make resource people available to judges who have questions about alcohol and other drug issues. Judges have the power to appoint such physicians as expert advisors to the court. We are at a unique place in our history that will foster these new and exciting collaborations. Let this ASAM chapter, coauthored by two judges, be but a first step (23–41).

REFERENCES

1. Paige M, Harrison & Allen J. Beok, Bureau of Justice statistics, U.S. Dept of Justice, Prison and Jail Inmates at midyear 2005 (2006). Available at (http://www.ojp.us.doj.gov/bjs/pub/pdf/pjim05.pdf).
2. Lauren E. Glaze & Seri Palla, Bureau of Justice statistics, U.S. Dept of Justice, Probation and Parole in the U.S. 2004 (2005). Available at (http://www.ojp.usdoj.gov/bjs/pub/pdf/ppusφ4.pdf).
3. Adam Liptake, *Inmate Count in U.S. Dwarfs Other Nations.* N.Y. Times, 2008; April 23, A1.
4. Hora PF, Schma WG, Rosenthal JTA. Therapeutic jurisprudence and the drug treatment court movement: revolutionizing the criminal justice system's response to drug abuse and crime in America. *Notre Dame Law Rev* 1999;74:439.
5. McLellan AT, Lewis DC, O'Brien CP, et al. Drug dependence, a chronic medical illness: implications for treatment, insurance, and outcomes. *JAMA* 2000;284(13):1689–1695.
6. Bureau of Justice Assistance (BJA). *Trial court performance standards with commentary.* Washington, DC: U.S. Department of Justice, Bureau of Justice Assistance/California Department of Alcohol and Drugs, 1992. CALDATA. Sacramento, CA: The Department, 1997.
7. Winick B. Harnessing the power of the bet: wagering with the government as a mechanism for social and individual change. *Univ Miami Law Rev* 1991;45:737–814.
8. Torgensen K, Buttars DC, Norman SW. How drug courts reduce substance abuse recidivism. *J Law Med Ethics* 2004;32(4 Suppl):69–72.
9. Perry A, Coulton S, Glanville J, et al. Interventions for drug-using offenders in the courts, secure establishments and the community. *Cochrane Database Syst Rev* 2006;3:CD005193.
10. Carey SM, Finigan M, Crumpton D, et al. California drug courts: outcomes, costs and promising practices—an overview of Phase II in a statewide study. *J Psychoactive Drugs* 2006;Suppl 3:345–356.
11. Fulton Hora P, Stalcup T. Drug treatment courts in the twenty-first century: the evolution of the revolution in problem-solving courts. Georgia Law Review 2008;423(3):765.
12. Cooper CS. Drug courts—just the beginning: getting other areas of public policy in sync. *Subst Use Misuse* 2007;42(2–3):243–256.
13. Henggeler SW. Juvenile drug courts: emerging outcomes and key research issues. *Curr Opin Psychiatry* 2007;20(3):242–246.
14. McMurran M. What works in substance misuse treatments for offenders. *Crim Behav Ment Health* 2007;17(4):225–233.
15. Hubbard R, Marsden M, Rachal J, et al. *Drug abuse treatment: a national study of effectiveness.* Chapel Hill, NC: University of North Carolina Press, 1989.
16. Maugh TH II, Anglin MD. Court-ordered drug treatment does work: But some approaches are more successful than others. *Judges' J* 1994; 34(4):10–13.
17. Anglin MD, Hser Y. Legal coercion and drug abuse treatment: research findings and social policy implications. In: Inciardi JA. ed. *Handbook of drug control in the United States.* University of Chicago: Chicago, 1990.
18. Hora PF, Schma WG. Legal intervention. In: White RK, and Wright DG, eds. *Addiction intervention: strategies to motivate treatment-seeking behavior.* New York: Hayworth Press, 1998.
19. Green BL, Furrer C, Worcel S, et al. How effective are family treatment drug courts? Outcomes from a four-site national study. *Child Maltreat* 2007;12(1):43–59.
20. Werb D, Elliott R, Fischer B, et al. Drug treatment courts in Canada: an evidence-based review. *HIV AIDS Policy Law Rev* 2007;12(2–3):12–17.
21. Chase DJ, Hora PF. The implications of therapeutic jurisprudence for judicial satisfaction. *Court Rev* 2000;37:12.
22. National Drug Control Strategy published by The Office of National Drug Control Policy, Executive Office of the President.
23. Barthwell AG. Interventions/Wilmer: a continuum of care for substance abusers in the criminal justice system. *J Psychoactive Drugs* 1995:27–39.
24. Carlson B. Prison-based treatment. *J Psychoactive Drugs* 1995;27(1):39–47.
25. Center for Substance Abuse Treatment. *Treatment improvement protocol series, no. 17.* Rockville, MD: Substance Abuse and Mental Health Services Administration, U.S. Department of Health and Human Services, 1995.
26. Center for Substance Abuse Treatment. *Treatment improvement protocol series, no. 21.* Rockville, MD: Substance Abuse and Mental Health Services Administration, U.S. Department of Health and Human Services, 1995.
27. Center for Substance Abuse Treatment. *Treatment improvement protocol series, no. 23.* Rockville, MD: Substance Abuse and Mental Health Services Administration, U.S. Department of Health and Human Services, 1999.
28. Drug Courts Program Office. *Defining drug courts: the key components.* Washington, DC: Office of Justice Programs, U.S. Department of Justice, 1997.
29. Drug Courts Program Office. *The interrelationship between the use of alcohol and other drugs: summary overview for drug court practitioners.* Washington, DC: Office of Justice Programs, U.S. Department of Justice and the Drug Court Clearinghouse and Technical Assistance Project, American University (NCJ178940), 2000.
30. Drug Strategies Institute. *Keeping score 1996: what are we getting for our federal drug control dollars?* Washington, DC: The Institute, 1996;9–10.
31. Galloway AL, Drapela LA. Are effective drug courts an urban phenomenon? Considering their impact on recidivism among a nonmetropolitan adult sample in Washington State. *Int J Offender Ther Comp Criminol* 2006;50(3):280–293.
32. Inciardi JA. *A corrections-based continuum of effective drug abuse treatment.* Washington, DC: U.S. Department of Justice, National Institute of Justice, 1996.
33. Lipton DS. Prison-based therapeutic communities: their success with drug-abusing offenders. *Natl Inst Justice J* 1996;230:p12.
34. Marlowe DB. Judicial supervision of drug-abusing offenders. *J Psychoactive Drugs* 2006;Suppl 3:323–331.
35. Marlowe DB, Festinger DS, Lee PA, et al. Matching judicial supervision to clients' risk status in drug court. *Crime Delinq* 2006;52(1):52–76.
36. Marlowe DB, Festinger DS, Foltz C, et al. Perceived deterrence and outcomes in drug court. *Behav Sci Law* 2005;23(2):183–198.
37. Office of Justice Programs. *National directory of corrections construction, 1993 supplement.* Washington, DC: National Institute of Justice and Bureau of Justice Assistance, U.S. Department of Justice, 1993.
38. OJP Drug Court Clearinghouse and Technical Assistance Project. *Drug Court Update.* Washington, DC: American University, 2000.
39. Prendergast ML, Hall EA, Roll J, et al. Use of vouchers to reinforce abstinence and positive behaviors among clients in a drug court treatment program. *J Subst Abuse Treat* 2008;35(2):125–136.
40. Roll JM, Prendergast M, Richardson K, et al. Identifying predictors of treatment outcome in a drug court program. *Am J Drug Alcohol Abuse* 2005;31(4):641–656.
41. Warren RK. Re-engineering the court process. Presentation at the Great Lakes Court Summit, Madison, WI, 1998.

Therapeutic Jurisprudence

Bruce J. Winick, JD, and David B. Wexler, JD

Therapeutic jurisprudence is the study of the law's healing potential (1–3). An interdisciplinary approach to legal scholarship that has a reform agenda, therapeutic jurisprudence seeks to assess the therapeutic and counter-therapeutic consequences of the law and how it is applied, as well as to increase the former and diminish the latter. It is an approach to the law that uses the tools of the behavioral sciences to assess the law's therapeutic effects and, when consistent with other important legal values, to reshape law and legal processes in ways that can improve the psychologic functioning and emotional well-being of the individuals affected (4).

PHILOSOPHIC ROOTS OF THERAPEUTIC JURISPRUDENCE

Schma (4) has noted that therapeutic jurisprudence is one of the major vectors of a growing movement in the law "towards a common goal of a more comprehensive, humane, and psychologically optimal way of handling legal matters." In addition to therapeutic jurisprudence, these vectors include (among others) preventive law, restorative justice, facilitative mediation, holistic law, collaborative divorce, and specialized treatment courts. Such specialized courts—"problem-solving courts," as they are becoming known—include drug treatment courts (5), domestic violence courts (6,7), and mental health courts (8,9).

Specialized treatment courts such as drug treatment courts are related to therapeutic jurisprudence (5) but are not synonymous with that concept. Instead, specialized treatment courts often employ the principles of therapeutic jurisprudence to enhance their functioning (10). Such principles include ongoing judicial intervention, close monitoring of and immediate response to behavior, integration of treatment services with judicial case processing, multidisciplinary involvement, and collaboration with community-based and government organizations.

THERAPEUTIC JURISPRUDENCE IN DRUG COURTS

Therapeutic jurisprudence was developed in the late 1980s as an interdisciplinary approach to legal scholarship and law reform. Though drug treatment courts developed independently of therapeutic jurisprudence, they can be seen as taking a complementary approach to the processing of drug cases, inasmuch as their goal is the rehabilitation of the offender. Drug courts use the legal process, and particularly the role of the judge, to accomplish this goal.

Therapeutic jurisprudence already has produced a large body of interdisciplinary scholarship that analyzes principles of psychology and the behavioral sciences and attempts to understand how those principles can be used in the legal system to improve mental health outcomes (1). Recent scholarship has focused on how judges in specialized problem-solving courts can employ the principles of therapeutic jurisprudence in their work (6,7,9). Indeed, a recent symposium issue of *Court Review*, a publication of the American Judges Association, was devoted entirely to therapeutic jurisprudence and its application by the courts (11).

An important insight of therapeutic jurisprudence is that the way in which judges and other legal officers fulfill their roles has inevitable consequences for the mental health and psychologic well-being of the persons with whom they interact. Because drug treatment court judges consciously view themselves as therapeutic agents in dealing with offenders, they can be seen as playing a therapeutic jurisprudence role. In fact, an understanding of the approach of therapeutic jurisprudence and of the psychologic and social work principles it employs can improve the functioning of drug treatment court judges.

Judge-defendant interactions are central to the functioning of drug treatment courts. Judges therefore need to understand how to convey empathy, how to recognize and deal with denial, and how to apply principles of behavioral psychology and motivation theory. They need to understand the psychology of procedural justice, which teaches that persons appearing in court experience greater satisfaction and comply more willingly with court orders when they are given a sense of voice and validation and treated with dignity and respect (Winick, 1999) (11a).

Judges need to know how to structure court practices in ways that maximize their therapeutic potential; for example, even such mundane matters as the ordering of cases in the courtroom can maximize the chance that defendants awaiting their turn before the judge can experience vicarious learning. Offenders who accept diversion to drug treatment court are, in effect, entering into a type of behavioral contract with the court, and judges therefore should understand the psychology of such behavioral contracting and how it can be used to increase motivation, compliance, and effective performance (2,12).

Drug treatment court judges also need to understand how to deal with feelings of coercion on the part of offenders (13). A degree of legal coercion is undeniably present when a drug offender is arrested and must decide whether to face the consequences of trial and potential punishment in the criminal court or instead accept diversion and a course of treatment supervised by the drug treatment court. However, a body of literature on the psychology of choice

(*continued*)

Therapeutic Jurisprudence *(continued)*

suggests that if the defendant experiences this choice as coerced, his or her attitude, motivation, and chances for success in the treatment program may be undermined. On the other hand, experiencing the choice as voluntarily made and non-coerced is more conducive to success. Judges, therefore, should not attempt to pressure offenders to accept diversion to drug treatment court but should remind them that the choice is entirely theirs. A body of psychologic work on what makes individuals feel coerced suggests that judges should strive to treat offenders with dignity and respect, to inspire their trust and confidence that the judge has their best interests at heart, to provide them a full opportunity to participate, and to listen attentively to what they have to say. Judges who treat drug court offenders in this fashion increase the likelihood that the offender will experience treatment as a voluntary choice, will internalize the goals of treatment, and will act in ways that help to achieve those goals.

Though therapeutic jurisprudence can help drug court judges more effectively fulfill their roles in the drug treatment process, it is important to recognize that therapeutic jurisprudence does not necessarily support all actions that may be regarded as protreatment. Nor does therapeutic jurisprudence take a position as to whether increased or decreased criminalization or penalties for possession of drugs are warranted. Indeed, unless there are independent justifications for criminalization, therapeutic jurisprudence would not support continued criminalization solely to provide a stick-and-carrot approach to inducing criminal defendants to accept treatment in a drug court diversion program.

CONCLUSIONS

In summary, therapeutic jurisprudence can contribute much to the functioning of drug treatment courts, and such courts can provide rich laboratories from which to generate and refine approaches to therapeutic jurisprudence. However, the two perspectives are merely vectors moving in a common direction; they are not identical concepts.

Therapeutic jurisprudence and drug treatment courts share a common cause as they strive to understand how legal rules and court practices can be designed to facilitate the rehabilitative process. Each has much to offer the other (14,15).

REFERENCES

1. Wexler DB, Winick BJ. *Law in a therapeutic key: developments in therapeutic jurisprudence.* Durham, NC: Carolina Academic Press, 1996.
2. Wexler DB. Inducing therapeutic compliance through the criminal law. In: Wexler DB, Winick BJ, eds. *Essays in therapeutic jurisprudence.* Durham, NC: Carolina Academic Press, 1991:187–198.
3. Winick BJ. The jurisprudence of therapeutic jurisprudence. *Psychology, Public Policy, and Law* 1997b;3:184–206.
4. Schma W. Therapeutic jurisprudence: using the law to improve the public's health. *J Law Med Ethics* 2005;33(Suppl 4):59–63.
5. Hora PF, Schma WG, Rosenthal JTA. Therapeutic jurisprudence and drug treatment court movement: revolutionizing the criminal justice system's response to drug abuse and crime in America. *Notre Dame Law Review* 1999;74:439–537.
6. Fritzler RB, Simon LMJ. The development of a specialized domestic violence court in Vancouver, Washington utilizing innovative judicial paradigms. *University of Missouri-Kansas City Law Review* 2000;69:139–177.
7. Winick BJ. Applying the law therapeutically in domestic violence cases. *University of Missouri-Kansas City Law Review* 2000;69:33–91.
8. Rottman DB, Casey P. Therapeutic jurisprudence and the emergence of problem-solving courts. *Natl Inst Justice J* 1999:12–19.
9. Casey P, Rottman DB. Therapeutic jurisprudence in the courts. *Behav Sci Law* 2000;18:445–457.
10. Conference of Chief Justices and Conference of State Court Administrators. CCJ Resolution 22 & COSCA Resolution 4. *In support of problem-solving courts.* 2000.
11. Court Review. Special issue on therapeutic jurisprudence. *Court Rev* 2000;37:1–68.

11a. Winick, BJ. Redefining the role of the criminal defense lawyer at plea bargaining and sentencing: A therapeutic jurisprudence/preventive law model, 5. *Psychology, Public Policy, and Low* 1999;1034.

12. Winick BJ. Harnessing the power of the bet: wagering with the government as a mechanism of social and individual change. In: Wexler DB, Winick BJ, eds. *Essays in therapeutic jurisprudence.* Durham, NC: Carolina Academic Press, 1991:219–290.
13. Winick BJ. Coercion and mental health treatment. *Denver University Law Review* 1997;74:1145–1168.
14. Daicoff S. The role of therapeutic jurisprudence within the comprehensive law movement. In: Stolle DP, Wexler DB, Winick BJ, eds. *Practicing therapeutic jurisprudence: law as a helping profession.* Durham, NC: Carolina Academic Press, 2000:465–492.
15. Wexler DB, Winick BJ. *Essays in therapeutic jurisprudence.* Durham, NC: Carolina Academic Press, 1991.

INDEX

Note: Page numbers followed by *f* indicate figures; page numbers followed by *t* indicate tables.

CCS0211